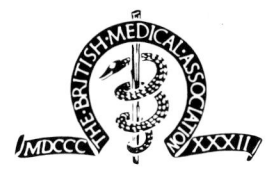

THE BRITISH MEDICAL ASSOCIATION

COMPLETE FAMILY HEALTH ENCYCLOPEDIA

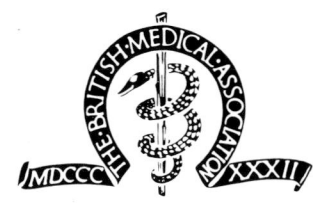

THE BRITISH MEDICAL ASSOCIATION

COMPLETE FAMILY HEALTH ENCYCLOPEDIA

MEDICAL EDITOR

Dr. Tony Smith

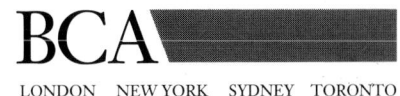

LONDON   NEW YORK   SYDNEY   TORONTO

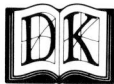

A Dorling Kindersley book

First published in Great Britain in 1990 by Dorling Kindersley
Limited, London
Reprinted twice in 1990
Reprinted twice in 1992
Reprinted 1993
Second edition 1995
Reprinted 1996
Copyright © 1990, 1995 Dorling Kindersley Limited, London
This edition published 1995 by BCA by arrangement with
Dorling Kindersley

The British Medical Association Complete Family Health
Encyclopedia provides information on a wide range of health
and medical topics. The encyclopedia is not a substitute for
medical diagnosis, however, and you are advised always to
consult your doctor for specific information on personal
health matters. The naming of any organization, product, or
alternative therapy in this encyclopedia does not imply BMA
endorsement; the omission of any such names does not indicate
BMA disapproval.

CN 9982

Computerset by Dorchester Typesetting Group Limited, England
Reproduction by Mandarin Offset Limited, Hong Kong
Printed and bound by G. Canale & C., Turin, Italy

PREFACE

Families today put health at the top of their list of concerns. Most people are aware that freedom from disease comes from following a healthy lifestyle, but there is much uncertainty about what is important and what is not. Health programmes on the television and medical articles in magazines may leave people wondering, for example, whether taking vitamins can make up for not taking exercise, or whether an armful of vaccinations is necessary before travelling abroad.

The British Medical Association Complete Family Health Encyclopedia was first published in 1990 and quickly became established as the leading medical reference source for use in the home. In the past five years, medicine has changed a great deal, with rapid advances in our understanding of genetics, new methods of minimally invasive surgery, many new drugs, and wide acceptance of the need for regular health screening. Patients are not prepared to be merely passive recipients of medical care. People now want to be involved with their doctors in decisions that affect their health; they want to know not only what is wrong with them, but also what the choices of treatment are, and what risks are involved.

This new edition of the Complete Family Health Encyclopedia has been expanded and revised to bring it up to date, taking into account the advances made in medicine and the changes in attitudes of patients and their doctors. In contrast to many popular medical books, this encyclopedia does not expound any individual author's theory or market any "breakthrough" treatment or diet. What it does provide is a clear, systematic, illustrated account of current medical knowledge, reviewed and validated by experts selected by the British Medical Association.

Tony Smith.

Dr. Tony Smith
Associate Editor
British Medical Journal

BRITISH MEDICAL ASSOCIATION

Chairman of the Council • Dr. A.W. Macara
Treasurer • Dr. J.A. Riddell
Chairman Journal Committee • Sir Anthony Grabham

MEDICAL REVIEWERS

CONTRIBUTORS

DORLING KINDERSLEY LIMITED

Managing Editor Ruth Midgley
Editors FIRST EDITION Andrea Bagg, Dr. Stephen Carroll, Robert Dinwiddie,
Gail Lawther, Mary Lindsay, Richenda Milton-Thompson, Ricki Ostrov, Martyn Page,
Jillian Somerscales, Tony Whitehorn, Dr. Frances Williams • **Editor** SECOND EDITION Teresa Pritlove
• **Additional editorial assistance from** Maria Adams, Simon Adams, Donald Berwick,
Deirdre Clark, Jean Cooke, Mike Darton, Elizabeth Galfalvi, Ann Kramer, Cathy Meeus, Terence Monaighan,
Theodore Rowland-Entwistle, Ruth Swan, Rena Taylor, Pat White, Kay Wright
Editorial Director Amy Carroll

Managing Art Editors Chez Picthall, Denise Brown
Art Editors Melissa Gray, Caroline Murray
Designers Sandra Archer, Peter Cross, Tina Hill, Gail Jones, Sarah Ponder, Anne Renel,
Tracy Timson, Lydia Umney, Bryn Walls • **Additional design assistance from** Peter Blake, Carol Briggs,
Thomas Keenes, Chris Scollens
Illustrators Karen Cochrane, Paul Cooper, Sandra Doyle, Will Giles, Tony Graham, Brian Hewson,
Chris Jenkins, Kevin Jones, Janos Marffy, Kevin Marks, Coral Muller, Frazer Newman, Nick Oxloby,
Lynda Payne, Sandra Ponder, Patricia Sempron, Mark Surridge, John Temperton, John Woodcock
Picture research Sandra Schneider, Sharon Southren
Production Eunice Paterson, Hilary Stephens

EMERGENCY FIRST-AID TECHNIQUES

Use this quick-reference list to find illustrated first-aid boxes containing step-by-step instructions for performing emergency techniques

Artificial respiration	134	Heatstroke	526
Bleeding, treating	178	Hypothermia	559
Burns, treating	219	Poisoning	813
Cardiopulmonary resuscitation	237	Pressure points	827
Childbirth, emergency	263	Recovery position	863
Choking (adult)	269	Shock	908
Choking (infant and child)	270	Suffocation	958
Electrical injury	392	Unconsciousness	1027
Frostbite	463	Wounds	1085

SYMPTOM CHARTS

Use this quick-reference list to find question-and-answer flow charts that indicate the possible causes and significance of many common symptoms

Abdominal pain	51	Headache	508
Abdominal pain, recurrent	53	Hoarseness or loss of voice	538
Abdominal swelling	56	Intercourse, painful (men)	592
Backache	151	Intercourse, painful (women)	593
Breathing difficulty	210	Menstruation, irregular	678
Chest pain	258	Numbness and tingling	739
Constipation	298	Rash with fever	858
Cough	315	Rash with itching	859
Diarrhoea	354	Tiredness	995
Dizziness	367	Vomiting	1069
Feeling faint and fainting	431	Weight loss	1079
Fever	444		

CONTENTS

HOW TO USE THE ENCYCLOPEDIA ———— 10

HEALTH AND MEDICINE TODAY———— 15

THE A TO Z OF HEALTH AND MEDICINE — 49

DRUG GLOSSARY———————— 1095

INDEX ——————————— 1128

HOW TO USE THE ENCYCLOPEDIA

This highly illustrated encyclopedia is an informative and authoritative guide to all aspects of health and medical care. For swift and easy reference, entries within the main part of the encyclopedia are arranged alphabetically, and longer entries are subdivided into sections, each with a descriptive subheading. Information within entries is presented in clear, concise language, and technical or unfamiliar medical terms are generally explained as they appear.

The main body of the encyclopedia, the **A to Z of Health and Medicine**, contains some 5,000 entries covering a vast range of health, medical,

and medically-related topics. In a one-volume compendium it is obviously impossible to provide separate entries for every single medical term, but many additional terms and topics are discussed within relevant entries.

The encyclopedia also contains a full-colour, introductory section, called **Health and Medicine Today**, which gives useful information on staying healthy and describes the latest advances in diagnosis and treatment. At the back of the book, additional information on generic and brand-name drugs is contained in the **Drug Glossary**. There is also a comprehensive **Index**.

HOW TO FIND THE INFORMATION YOU WANT

All the entries in the **A to Z of Health and Medicine** and in the **Index** are arranged alphabetically using the "letter-by-letter" system. In this system, any spaces or punctuation in the entry titles are ignored. Thus, *Sick building syndrome* is followed by *Sickle cell anaemia* and then by *Sick sinus syndrome*: the fifth letter gives the order.

When the name of a topic consists of more than one word, begin by looking up what seems to be the key word. Thus, for information on general anaesthesia you will find what you want under the heading *Anaesthesia, general*. If the key word is not obvious, you may find it easier to turn first to the **Index**, although many alternative

topic names and common abbreviations are included as short cross-reference entries within the main part of the book. You will also find cross-references within articles. These are indicated by italic type and take several forms. Examples of the different forms are shown and explained in the annotated illustration below.

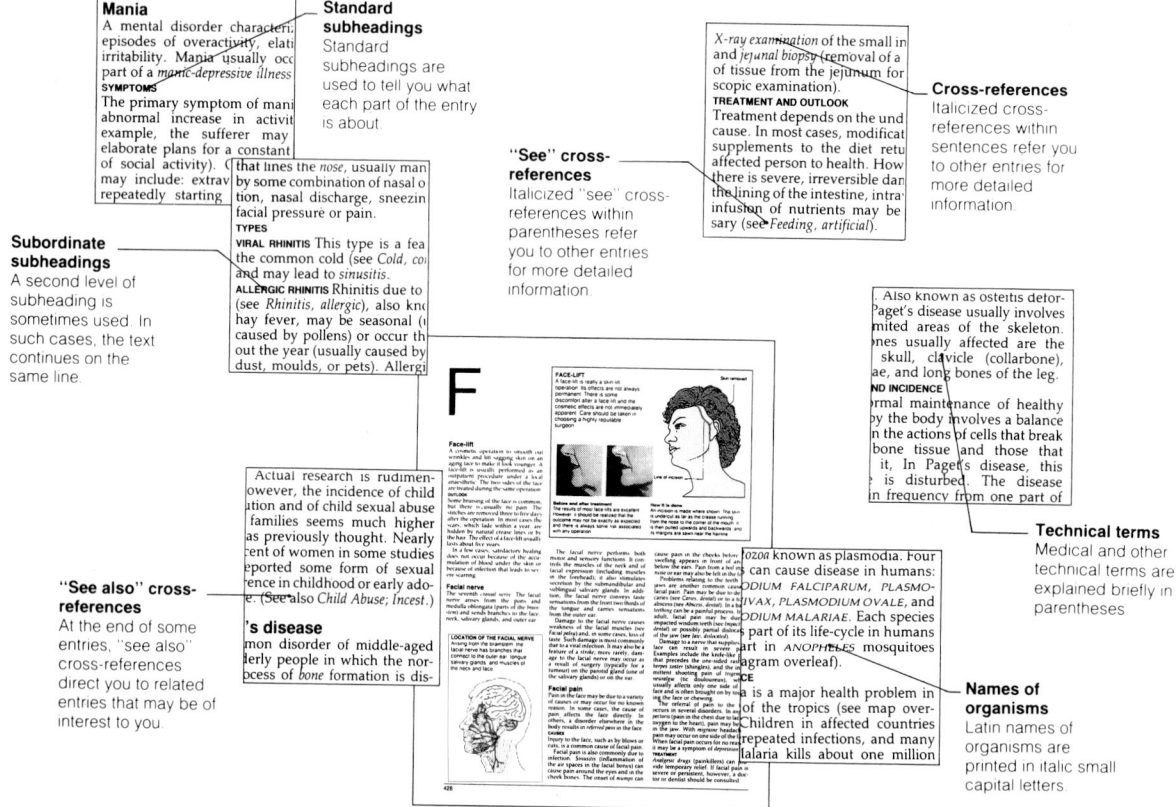

Mania
A mental disorder characteri[zed by] episodes of overactivity, elati[on,] irritability. Mania usually occ[urs as] part of a *manic-depressive illness*
SYMPTOMS
The primary symptom of mani[a is] abnormal increase in activit[y. For] example, the sufferer may [make] elaborate plans for a constant [round] of social activity). C[...] may include: extrav[...] repeatedly starting

Standard subheadings
Standard subheadings are used to tell you what each part of the entry is about.

Subordinate subheadings
A second level of subheading is sometimes used. In such cases, the text continues on the same line.

[...] that lines the *nose*, usually man[...] by some combination of nasal o[bstruc-] tion, nasal discharge, sneezin[g, and] facial pressure or pain.
TYPES
VIRAL RHINITIS This type is a fea[ture of] the common cold (see *Cold, co[mmon]*) and may lead to *sinusitis*.
ALLERGIC RHINITIS Rhinitis due to [allergy] (see *Rhinitis, allergic*), also kn[own as] hay fever, may be seasonal ([if] caused by pollens) or occur th[rough-] out the year (usually caused by [house] dust, moulds, or pets). Allergi[c...]

"See" cross-references
Italicized "see" cross-references within parentheses refer you to other entries for more detailed information.

X-ray examination of the small in[testine] and *jejunal biopsy* (removal of a [sample] of tissue from the jejunum for [micro-] scopic examination).
TREATMENT AND OUTLOOK
Treatment depends on the und[erlying] cause. In most cases, modificat[ion or] supplements to the diet retu[rns the] affected person to health. How[ever, if] there is severe, irreversible dam[age to] the lining of the intestine, intra[venous] infusion of nutrients may be [neces-] sary (see *Feeding, artificial*).

Cross-references
Italicized cross-references within sentences refer you to other entries for more detailed information.

F

Face-lift
A cosmetic operation to smooth out wrinkles and lift sagging skin on an aging face to make it look younger. A face-lift is usually performed as an outpatient procedure under a local anaesthetic. The two sides of the face are treated during the same operation.
PROCEDURE
Some bruising of the face is common, but there is usually no pain. The stitches are removed three to five days after the operation. In most cases the scars, which hide within a year, are hidden by natural crease lines or by the hair. The effect of a face-lift usually lasts about five years.

In a few cases, satisfactory healing does not occur because of the accumulation of blood under the skin or because of infection that leads to severe scarring.

FACE-LIFT
A face-lift is really a skin operation. Its effects are not always permanent. There is some discomfort after a face-lift and the cosmetic effects are not immediately apparent. Care should be taken in choosing a highly reputable surgeon.

[illustration]

How it is done
An incision is made where shown. The skin is undercut as far as the crease running from the nose to the corner of the mouth, is then pulled upwards and backwards, and is margins are sewn near the hairline.

Facial nerve
The seventh cranial nerve. The facial nerve arises from the pons and medulla oblongata (parts of the brain stem) and sends branches to the face, neck, salivary glands, and outer ear.

The facial nerve performs both motor and sensory functions. It controls the muscles of the neck and facial expression (including muscles in the forehead); it also stimulates secretion by the submandibular and sublingual salivary glands. In addition, the facial nerve conveys taste sensations from the front two thirds of the tongue and carries sensations from the outer ear.

Damage to the facial nerve causes weakness of the facial muscles (facial palsy) and, in some cases, loss of taste. Such damage is most commonly due to a viral infection. It may also be a feature of a stroke, more rarely, damage to the facial nerve may occur as a result of surgery (typically for a tumour) on the parotid gland (one of the salivary glands) or on the ear.

LOCATION OF THE FACIAL NERVE
Among them the brainstem the facial nerve has branches that connect to the outer ear, tongue, salivary glands, and muscles of the neck and face.

[illustration]

Facial pain
Pain in the face may be due to a variety of causes or may occur for no known reason. In some cases, the cause of pain affects the face directly; in others, a disorder elsewhere in the body results in referred pain in the face.
CAUSES
Injury to the face, such as by blow or cuts, is a common cause of facial pain. Facial pain is also commonly due to infection. Sinusitis (inflammation of the air spaces in the skull around the nose) can cause pain around the eyes and in the cheek bones. The onset of mumps can

cause pain in the cheeks before swelling appears in front of and below the ears. Pain from a bad tooth nerve or ear may also be felt in the face.

Problems relating to the teeth and jaws are another common cause of facial pain. Pain may be due to an abscess (see Abscess, dental) or to a nerve being disrupted. Jaw disorders, such as temporomandibular joint dysfunction, can also cause facial pain.

Damage to the facial nerve causes weakness of the facial muscles (see part of the face (see *facial palsy*).

Examples include the kinds that precedes the one-sided rash of herpes zoster (shingles) and the painful shooting pains of *trigeminal neuralgia* (tic douloureux), which usually affects only one side of the face and is often brought on by touching the face or chewing.

The referral of pain to the face occurs in several disorders. In some persons pain in the chest due to lack of oxygen to the heart), pain may be felt in the jaw. With migraine headache, pain may occur on one side of the face.

When facial pain occurs for no reason, it may be a symptom of depression.
TREATMENT
Analgesic drugs (painkillers) can provide temporary relief. If facial pain is severe or persistent, however, a doctor or dentist should be consulted.

Actual research is rudimentary [...] owever, the incidence of child [sexual abuse...] ation and of child sexual abuse [in certain] families seems much higher [than] as previously thought. Nearly [per] cent of women in some studies [re-] ported some form of sexual [experi-] ence in childhood or early adole[scen-]ce. (See also *Child Abuse*; *Incest*.)

's disease
[...com]mon disorder of middle-aged [or eld]erly people in which the nor[mal pr]ocess of *bone* formation is dis[rupted].

[...ot]ozoa known as plasmodia. Four [which] can cause disease in humans: [PLASM]ODIUM FALCIPARUM, PLASMO[DIUM V]IVAX, PLASMODIUM OVALE, and [PLASM]ODIUM MALARIAE. Each species [spends] part of its life-cycle in humans [and] part in ANOPHELES mosquitoes [(see di]agram overleaf).

[Malari]a is a major health problem in [many] of the tropics (see map over[leaf).] Children in affected countries [suffer] repeated infections, and many [...] malaria kills about one million [...]

"See also" cross-references
At the end of some entries, "see also" cross-references direct you to related entries that may be of interest to you.

Also known as osteitis deformans, Paget's disease usually involves [li]mited areas of the skeleton. [Bo]nes usually affected are the skull, clavicle (collarbone), [pelvis] and long bones of the leg.
[...] AND INCIDENCE
[No]rmal maintenance of healthy [bone] by the body involves a balance [i]n the actions of cells that break [down] bone tissue and those that [build] it. In Paget's disease, this [balance] is disturbed. The disease [varies] in frequency from one part of [...]

Technical terms
Medical and other technical terms are explained briefly in parentheses.

Names of organisms
Latin names of organisms are printed in italic small capital letters.

HOW TO FIND INFORMATION ON SYMPTOMS

The **A to Z of Health and Medicine** contains individual entries on the whole range of physical and psychological symptoms. In general, you will find the main description of a particular symptom under its common name, if it has one. Thus, for example, *Vomiting* is the main entry and *Emesis*, the medical term for vomiting, is a short cross-reference entry. Alternative names for symptoms also appear in the **Index**.

Symptom charts

The question-and-answer symptom charts will help you understand the significance of common symptoms that have no obvious cause. Each chart singles out possible causes of the symptom, refers you to relevant articles in the encyclopedia, and suggests appropriate action, if any. Start at the top of the chart and answer "yes" or "no" to the series of carefully selected questions until you reach the box that advises you on your particular problem. For the page numbers of all symptom charts, consult page 8.

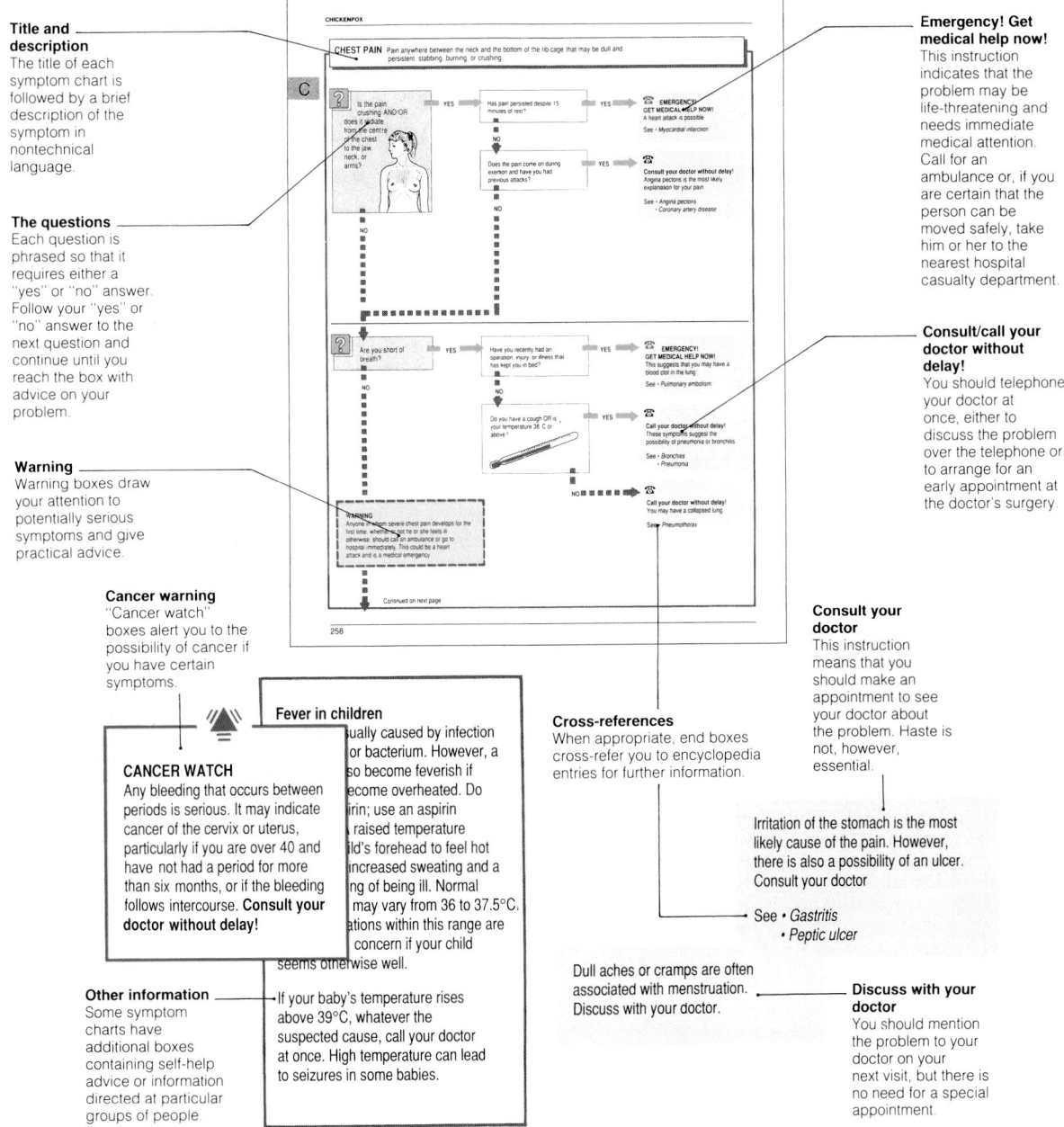

Title and description
The title of each symptom chart is followed by a brief description of the symptom in nontechnical language.

The questions
Each question is phrased so that it requires either a "yes" or "no" answer. Follow your "yes" or "no" answer to the next question and continue until you reach the box with advice on your problem.

Warning
Warning boxes draw your attention to potentially serious symptoms and give practical advice.

Cancer warning
"Cancer watch" boxes alert you to the possibility of cancer if you have certain symptoms.

CANCER WATCH
Any bleeding that occurs between periods is serious. It may indicate cancer of the cervix or uterus, particularly if you are over 40 and have not had a period for more than six months, or if the bleeding follows intercourse. **Consult your doctor without delay!**

Fever in children
...ually caused by infection ...or bacterium. However, a ...so become feverish if ...ecome overheated. Do ...irin; use an aspirin ...raised temperature ...ild's forehead to feel hot ...increased sweating and a ...ng of being ill. Normal ...may vary from 36 to 37.5°C. ...ations within this range are ...concern if your child seems otherwise well.

If your baby's temperature rises above 39°C, whatever the suspected cause, call your doctor at once. High temperature can lead to seizures in some babies.

Other information
Some symptom charts have additional boxes containing self-help advice or information directed at particular groups of people.

Emergency! Get medical help now!
This instruction indicates that the problem may be life-threatening and needs immediate medical attention. Call for an ambulance or, if you are certain that the person can be moved safely, take him or her to the nearest hospital casualty department.

Consult/call your doctor without delay!
You should telephone your doctor at once, either to discuss the problem over the telephone or to arrange for an early appointment at the doctor's surgery.

Consult your doctor
This instruction means that you should make an appointment to see your doctor about the problem. Haste is not, however, essential.

Irritation of the stomach is the most likely cause of the pain. However, there is also a possibility of an ulcer. Consult your doctor

See • *Gastritis*
• *Peptic ulcer*

Cross-references
When appropriate, end boxes cross-refer you to encyclopedia entries for further information.

Dull aches or cramps are often associated with menstruation. Discuss with your doctor.

Discuss with your doctor
You should mention the problem to your doctor on your next visit, but there is no need for a special appointment.

HOW TO FIND INFORMATION ON DISORDERS

The **A to Z of Health and Medicine** has individual entries on all major and many minor disorders. There are also general entries on groups of disorders, such as *Genetic disorders*, or disorders that affect different parts of the body in different ways, such as *Cancer*. These group entries provide an overview and explain the basic disease processes; specific forms, such as *Haemophilia* or *Breast cancer*, are covered in separate entries. Group entries contain cross-references, to more specific entries. If you look up certain group entries in the **Index**, you

will find references to disorders in those groups.

Consult the **Index**, too, if you fail to find an entry on a specific disorder within the **A to Z of Health and Medicine**. You may find that the disorder has an alternative name. For example, if you look up *Decubitus ulcer* in the **Index** you will be directed to the encyclopedia entry on *Bedsores*; decubitus ulcer and bedsore are alternative names for the same condition. In other cases, the **Index** will show you that a specific disorder is covered in a more general entry. For example, con-

ductive deafness is included in the *Deafness* entry.

Disorder boxes

Entries on the main organs and body parts are accompanied by boxed summaries of the various disorders that may affect them. These disorder boxes help you see at a glance the types of problems most often associated with a particular organ or body part. These boxes also cross-refer you to entries on specific disorders and investigation techniques.

Cross-references
Italicized cross-references direct you to entries on specific disorders for more information.

Subheadings
Different disorders are grouped under standard subheadings, allowing you to see at a glance the problems most likely to affect a particular body part.

DISORDERS OF THE BREAST
Problems involving the breasts are usually minor and respond readily to treatment. The most important causes of problems are infection, tumours, and hormonal disturbance.

INFECTION
This is uncommon except during breast-feeding. Nursing mothers may suffer from *mastitis* (inflammation of the breast), usually due to a blocked milk duct. An *abscess* may follow if mastitis is not treated.

TUMOURS
A *breast lump* may be a *cyst* (a fluid-filled sac), a *fibroadenoma* (a thickening of the milk-producing tissue) or other benign tumour, or more rarely, *breast cancer*.

HORMONAL DISORDERS
It is common for women to notice that before *menstruation* their

breasts become bigger and lumpy. Such lumps shrink when menstruation is over. More common are breast pain and tenderness, which often occur just before menstruation or as a result of taking hormones. Hormonal disorders may, rarely, cause *galactorrhoea* (abnormal milk production).
In men, *gynaecomastia* (abnormal breast development) may result from hormonal disturbance or treatment with certain drugs.

INVESTIGATION
Disorders of the breast may be discovered during *breast self-examination* or by your doctor during a physical examination. Special investigations for the breast are *biopsy* and *mammography*.

Abscess
● a collection of pus

Fibroadenoma
● a common benign tumor

Cancer
● a malignant growth

Cyst
● a collection of fluid

Nipple
● discharge

Galactorrhea
● abnormal production of milk

Mastitis
● inflammation of tissue

Illustrations
Some disorder boxes have an annotated illustration showing areas most likely to be affected by different disorders.

Investigation box
A summary of investigation techniques is given here, including italicized cross-references to entries on diagnostic procedures.

HOW TO FIND INFORMATION ON ANATOMY AND PHYSIOLOGY

All body systems (e.g. *Biliary system*) and major organs and body parts (e.g. *Brain* and *Coccyx*) have individual entries in the **A to Z of Health and Medicine**. There are also entries on the senses (e.g. *Vision*) and on other body processes (e.g. *Breathing* and *Blood clotting*). Anatomy and physiology entries explain how the healthy body works and also provide a background for understanding medical disorders.

Most anatomy and physiology entries are accompanied by illustrated boxes. Annotated illustrations show the main structural features of body parts, the location of different body parts in relation to each other, and, for physiology entries, the main stages in important body processes.

Anatomical drawings
Detailed drawings, often with cutaway sections, show the structure of body parts.

Medical images
Pictures obtained by specialized imaging techniques, such as X-rays or scans, are used in many cases.

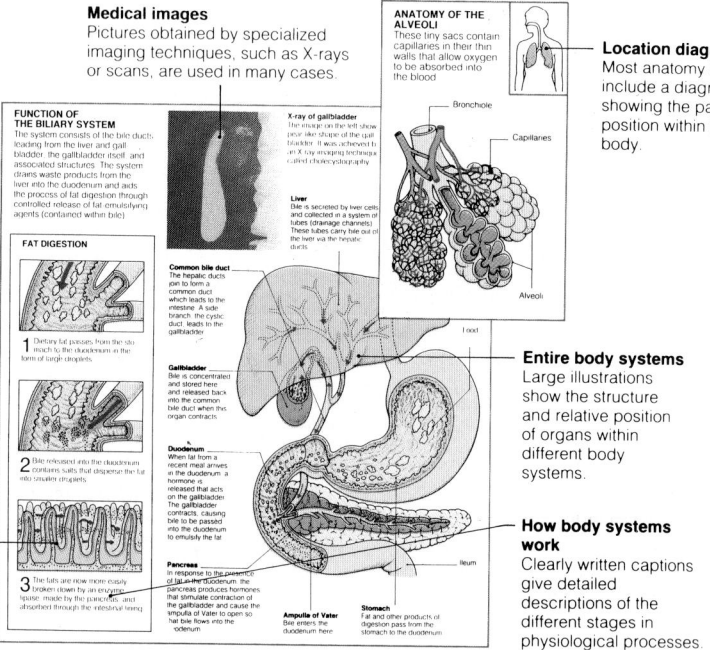

ANATOMY OF THE ALVEOLI
These tiny sacs contain capillaries in their thin walls that allow oxygen to be absorbed into the blood

Location diagrams
Most anatomy boxes include a diagram showing the part's position within the body.

Entire body systems
Large illustrations show the structure and relative position of organs within different body systems.

How body systems work
Clearly written captions give detailed descriptions of the different stages in physiological processes.

HOW TO FIND INFORMATION ON MEDICAL TESTS

Many different tests for diagnosing or monitoring medical conditions have individual entries within the **A to Z of Health and Medicine**. Many of these entries are illustrated by step-by-step diagrams.

More general information on tests is included in the entry headed *Tests, medical*. This entry is accompanied by a table that shows the tests used to investigate different parts of the body and directs you to individual entries within the encyclopedia. You can also find out the various types of tests used to investigate a major body organ by consulting the investigation section of the disorder box for that particular organ.

Entries on specific disorders in the **A to Z of Health and Medicine** cross-refer you to entries on the tests used to diagnose and monitor them.

Illustrations showing techniques
Clear illustrations show a test's most important stages, including, for example, where a needle is inserted in the body or how samples are prepared for testing.

Step-by-step text
Concise captions describe the various stages in each test, including what happens to the patient and how test samples are analyzed in the laboratory.

PROCEDURE FOR CHROMOSOME ANALYSIS

1 Fetal cells are obtained by amniocentesis or by chorionic villus sampling, or white blood cells are obtained from the blood of the baby, child, or adult being tested.

2 These cells are suspended in a medium containing substances that encourage the cells to divide. Chemicals are then added that stop the cells from dividing at a stage where their chromosome content is most easily visible.

3 The cells are then spread on a microscope slide, stained, and a selected few (in which the chromosomes are clearly visible and well separated) have their nuclei photographed or are closely examined through a high-power microscope.

4 The chromosomes are matched up and arranged into the 22 pairs of autosomes together with the sex chromosomes. Study of these reveals any abnormalities.

Test results
Diagrams, photographs, and captions explain the results of the test.

HOW TO FIND INFORMATION ON SURGICAL PROCEDURES

Surgical procedures are described either in individual entries or in the treatment section of disorder entries. In many cases, entries are accompanied by illustrated boxes.

Individual entries on surgical procedures are included under their generally accepted medical names. In many cases, these names are self-explanatory—*Heart-lung transplant* or *Hernia repair*, for example.

If you do not know the name of a particular procedure, look up the encyclopedia entry on the disorder for which it is a treatment, where you will find a description of, or a cross-reference to, the appropriate procedure. Alternatively, consult the **Index**, which lists some popular names. For example, if you look up *Stomach, removal of*, you will be referred to the encyclopedia entry on *Gastrectomy*.

Surgery in progress
True-to-life drawings show surgical procedures in progress and provide an accurate representation of current surgical practice.

Incision sites
A red line superimposed on a photograph of the relevant part of the body shows the position and shape of the surgeon's incision.

HEART-LUNG TRANSPLANT
In this procedure, both the heart and lungs of a patient are removed and replaced with organs taken from a brain-dead donor. The removed heart can sometimes be given to another patient.

HOW IT IS DONE
Heart and lungs must be removed from both donor and patient; the donor organs are then inserted into the patient.

1 The donor heart and lungs must be healthy, and the lungs must match the size of the patient's chest, as measured by chest X-rays.

2 In both donor and patient, the heart and lungs are reached via an incision made in the sternum, and the chest is opened up.

Site of incision

Equipment
Detailed illustrations show the workings of special equipment, such as a heart-lung machine.

3 The patient is connected to a heart-lung machine. It takes over the function of heart and lungs, oxygenating blood taken from the venae cavae and pumping it back to the body via the aorta.

Trachea
Aorta
Right atrium/vena cava

4 In both patient and donor, heart and lungs are removed through cuts in the trachea, aorta, and where the heart connects to the venae cavae. The blood vessels linking donor heart and lungs are left intact.

Tracheal reconnection
Aortic reconnection
Right atrium/vena cava reconnection

WHY IT IS DONE
Subject to availability of a donor, a heart-lung transplant can offer hope to someone who is dying of a terminally chronic lung disease, whether or not he or she is also suffering from heart disease. Diseases treated include emphysema, cystic fibrosis, sarcoidosis, or interstitial pulmonary fibrosis. The heart-lung transplant operation has a better success record than that of lung transplant alone.

5 Insertion of the donor organs into the patient is, in some respects, easier than in the heart transplant, since fewer reconnections have to be made. The main reconnections are between the patient's and donor's tracheas and aortas and between the right atrium of the donor heart and the patient's venae cavae.

These sections were taken from a healthy lung (left) and an emphysematous lung. transplantation of heart and lungs may give an emphysema patient new hope

Step-by-step text and illustrations
Explanatory captions and anatomically correct illustrations take you through the most important stages of surgical procedures. Large numbers show the sequence of events and help you follow the different stages.

Reasons for surgery
Different medical images—such as photographs, X rays, or scans—of diseased tissue show why operations are necessary.

HOW TO FIND INFORMATION ON DRUGS

The **A to Z of Health and Medicine** contains entries on all major drug groups (from *ACE inhibitor drugs* to *Vasodilator drugs*) and on the most important generic drugs (from *Acarbose* to *Zidovudine*). Other information on drugs can be found in general entries, such as *Drug, Drug dependence*, and *Drug poisoning*.

The **Drug Glossary** gives concise information on almost 3,000 generic and brand-name drugs, showing the generic equivalents of brand-name drugs, and identifying the drug groups to which individual drugs belong. Each glossary entry cross-refers you to appropriate entries in the **A to Z of Health and Medicine**.

Drug charts
Selected entries on individual drugs are accompanied by an illustrated chart that summarizes important information about the drug.

Group to which the drug belongs

Forms in which the drug is available

Availability on prescription or over-the-counter

Availability as a generic or under a brand name only

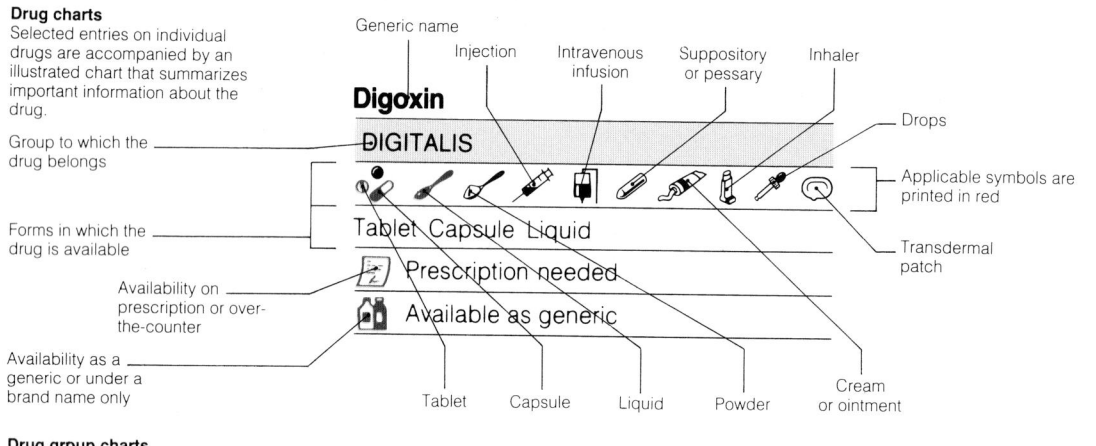

Generic name

Injection

Intravenous infusion

Suppository or pessary

Inhaler

Drops

Applicable symbols are printed in red

Transdermal patch

Digoxin

DIGITALIS

Tablet Capsule Liquid

Prescription needed

Available as generic

Tablet · Capsule · Liquid · Powder · Cream or ointment

Drug group charts
Most drug group entries are accompanied by a chart showing examples of common drugs within the group.

Group name

Division within the main drug group

Generic examples

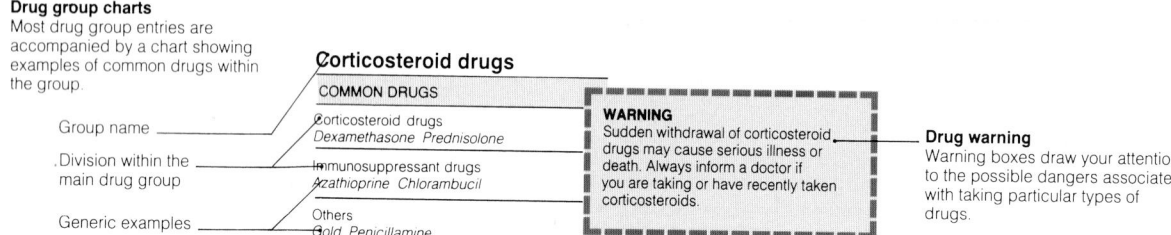

Corticosteroid drugs

COMMON DRUGS

Corticosteroid drugs
Dexamethasone Prednisolone

Immunosuppressant drugs
Azathioprine Chlorambucil

Others
Gold Penicillamine

WARNING
Sudden withdrawal of corticosteroid drugs may cause serious illness or death. Always inform a doctor if you are taking or have recently taken corticosteroids.

Drug warning
Warning boxes draw your attention to the possible dangers associated with taking particular types of drugs.

HOW TO USE THE ENCYCLOPEDIA IN AN EMERGENCY

EMERGENCY FIRST-AID TECHNIQUES

Turn to page 8 for the page numbers of emergency first-aid boxes.

Life-saving and other, less urgent, first-aid techniques are explained in easy-to-follow first-aid boxes. These boxes accompany relevant entries in the **A to Z of Health and Medicine**. All first-aid boxes have a distinctive red border and a special heading. A list of first-aid boxes describing emergency techniques, with their page numbers, is given on page 8.

Distinctive appearance
Bold red borders and special headings make first-aid boxes easy to find.

WARNING
Warning boxes contain essential advice and indicate when professional help should be sought.

WARNING
Frostbite is often accompanied by hypothermia, which must be treated first. Proper medical attention should be sought promptly, but first aid should be given immediately.

DO NOT
- rub the affected parts
- attempt to burst blisters
- warm the affected area with direct heat
- allow the victim to walk on a frostbitten foot

DO NOT
These boxes tell you what not to do when treating an injured person.

Step-by-step
First-aid techniques are clearly described in numbered sequences of text and illustrations.

Close-ups
More detailed illustrations show you exactly what to do.

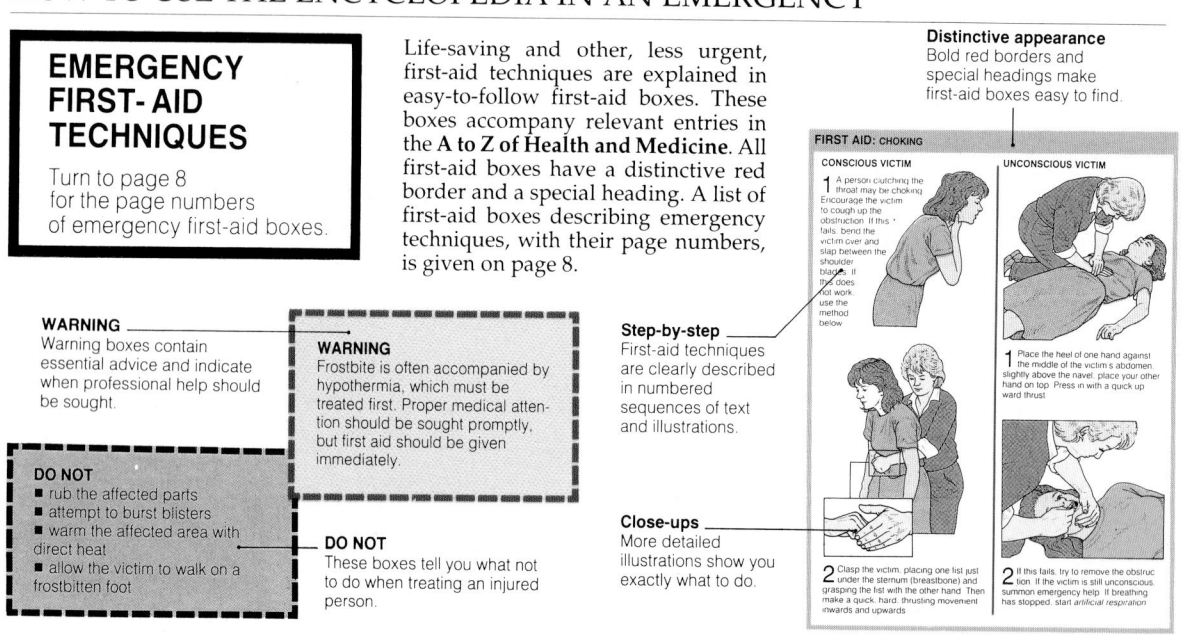

HEALTH AND MEDICINE TODAY

KEEPING HEALTHY

An individual's health is determined partly by inheritance and partly by external factors. Health and longevity tend to run in families, so a person whose grandparents lived beyond the age of 80 is likely to do the same. However, this is not always the case. Even the intrinsically healthiest body can be damaged by neglect or by external factors, especially by the unwise use of drugs, including tobacco and alcohol. With the AIDS epidemic still spreading, it is essential to adhere to safer sex practices and to avoid illicit intravenous drugs.

Good health requires lifelong maintenance of the body. A health-promoting lifestyle in youth not only reduces the chances of premature death from heart disease or cancer but also slows the natural process of aging. Researchers have been able to identify certain factors that speed up the decline of the vital organs—of which the most important are alcohol and tobacco. It has also been possible to identify various factors that slow down the aging process—of which the most important are the taking of regular vigorous exercise and the maintenance of body weight within recommended limits.

A positive approach to health is fundamental to any personal healthcare programme. The fact that you are able to take control of many of the different factors that affect your health means that you can exert a major influence on your own well-being.

Your personal health-care programme does not have to be an unpleasant experience—it is quite simple for you to combine health promotion with enjoyment.

Exercise and your heart
Running is a good way of maintaining cardiovascular fitness and can reduce the risk of heart disease.

SIX WAYS OF KEEPING HEALTHY
By paying attention to each of the following six aspects of personal health care, you can make an important start towards improving or maintaining your individual levels of general health and physical fitness.

Eat sensibly
Eating a balanced diet is a key feature of any personal health-care plan.

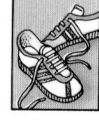
Take exercise
Regular exercise can improve or maintain physical and mental fitness.

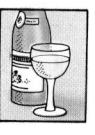
Limit alcohol
Keeping alcohol consumption within safe limits is vital for health.

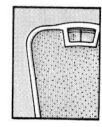
Watch weight
People who are very overweight or underweight tend to die prematurely.

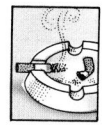
Don't smoke
The link between tobacco-smoking and killer diseases has been proved.

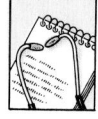
Visit the doctor
Seek medical advice as soon as you suspect a health problem.

Diet and nutrition
Although there are many different views on healthy eating, experts generally agree that diets should be varied and should contain adequate but not excessive amounts of protein, carbohydrates, fats, minerals, and vitamins. You can combine pleasure with health promotion by eating a healthy mix of foods that appeals to your palate.

Alcohol consumption
Excessive alcohol consumption is a major health hazard. Alcohol not only contributes to problems at home and at work, to accidents, and to violent crime, it can also cause irreversible damage to the heart, liver, brain, and nervous system. Limiting alcohol consumption is essential for long-term health.

Tobacco-smoking
Giving up smoking is the single most important measure that any tobacco-smoker can take to improve his or her own health. The life expectancy of nonsmokers is significantly higher than that of smokers. Smoking is a major cause of lung cancer, heart disease, and chronic bronchitis.

Exercise and fitness

Regular exercise benefits every part of your body, enhancing both physical and mental well-being. Different types of exercise vary in the extent to which they improve the three main aspects of health and fitness: heart and lung efficiency, joint suppleness, and muscle power. The best exercises for improving general fitness are aerobic exercises, such as jogging, swimming, and cycling. Most people should be able to select a sport or activity that they find interesting and stimulating as well as beneficial to their health.

Weight control

People who are significantly overweight or underweight tend to die younger than people who are of normal weight. Maintaining a healthy weight involves paying attention to what you eat and drink, and making sure that you take adequate exercise.

Stress control

A certain amount of stress is natural in any demanding or difficult situation, but if feelings of anxiety become persistent, they can become the cause of psychological and physical symptoms. Being able to cope with stress is an important aspect of keeping healthy. You may find that it is helpful to talk problems through with

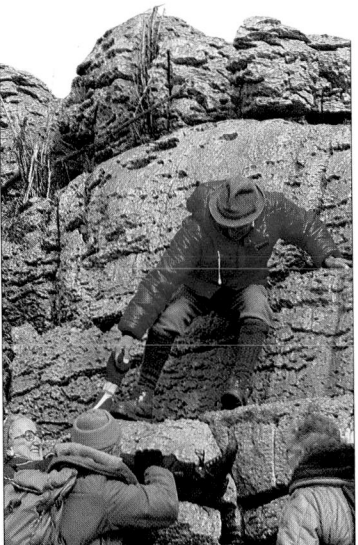

Exercise for life
As you grow older, taking regular exercise will help you maintain the normal functioning of your bones, joints, muscles, tendons, and ligaments. Your joints will stay mobile and your muscle strength, coordination, and confidence will be retained.

family, friends, employers, or professionals. Relaxation techniques can often help relieve tension caused by stress.

Safety measures

Accidents and injury are a major cause of death and disability, especially in young people. Paying attention to basic standards of safety in the home, at work, near water, and particularly on the roads can considerably reduce the risk of accidents. Keeping healthy also depends on keeping safe.

Medical help

People used to believe that medical help was necessary only when they became ill. It is now widely recognized that preventive medicine has an important role to play in maintaining the health of the population at large. Immunization can prevent the outbreak of a range of once common infectious diseases, and screening tests make it possible for certain types of medical problem to be detected at an early stage when they can be treated more easily.

A healthy diet
Healthy food can be appetizing as well as good for you. This attractive display shows some recommended sources of essential nutrients.

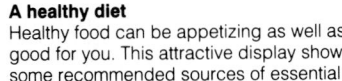

17

EATING WELL

If you eat a balanced diet, you are already well on the way to good health. The function of food is to provide your body with appropriate amounts of the necessary nutrients—fats, protein, carbohydrates, vitamins, minerals, fibre, and water—ideally in as pleasant a form as possible. Many people in the West, however, consume too much fat, salt, sugar, alcohol, and refined food. A diet of this type contributes to numerous health problems, such as diabetes, heart disease, dental decay, liver disease, and some cancers.

THE FOUR FOOD GROUPS

There are four main food groups; a balanced diet should include several servings from each group per day. The "meat" group also contains fish, nuts, and eggs.

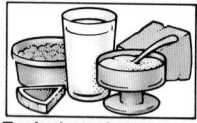

Milk group

Servings required per day: two

Typical servings

Milk	250 ml
Yoghurt, plain	150 g
Hard cheese	35 g
Cottage cheese	100 g

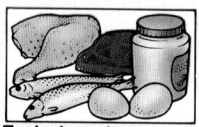

Meat group

Servings required per day: two

Typical servings

Meat, lean	60–90 g
Fish	60–90 g
Eggs	2
Peanut butter	4 tablespoons

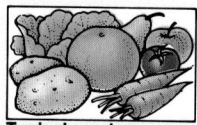

Fruit and vegetable group

Servings required per day: four

Typical servings

Vegetables	100 g
Fruit	100 g
Potato	1 medium
Grapefruit	½ medium

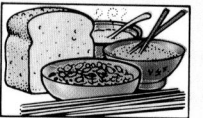

Bread and cereal group

Servings required per day: four

Typical servings

Bread	1 slice
Pasta	150 g (cooked)
Rice	150 g (cooked)
Breakfast cereal	30 g (dry)

Fats

Fats provide energy, and are a structural component of body cells. Fats fall into two main types: saturated and unsaturated.

Saturated fats include most animal fats, such as those found in whole milk, butter, cheese, pork, beef, lamb, and eggs; some vegetable oils are also saturated. Unsaturated fats include most of the fats found in fish and poultry, and in soya, sunflower, and corn oils. A high intake of saturated fats tends to increase the blood levels of cholesterol, which in turn can increase the risk of atherosclerosis and heart disease.

To keep your diet as healthy as possible, reduce your overall intake of fats, and choose unsaturated fats instead of saturated ones whenever possible.

Protein

Protein is needed regularly by the body for growth, and also for the repair and replacement of cells. The main sources of dietary protein are meat, fish, eggs, some dairy products, grains, and pulses.

AN UNHEALTHY MEAL

Although it looks tempting, the meal shown below is high in energy and very high in saturated fats. It contains some protein, but very little fibre and few vitamins.

Eggs
Although they are a good source of protein, eggs are high in cholesterol. Here they have been fried, which has increased their fat and calorie levels substantially.

Potatoes
Potatoes are high in fibre and healthy carbohydrate, but cutting them up small and frying them has drastically boosted their calorie and fat levels.

Parsley
The sprig of parsley used as garnish is the only fresh, uncooked vegetable.

Meat
These fried hamburgers are packed with saturated fats, and may contain unsuspected ingredients— for example, rusk, soya, sugar, monosodium glutamate, salt, water, colourings, preservative, and meat flavourings— as well as meat

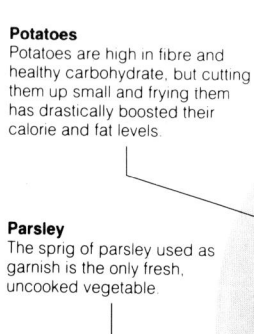

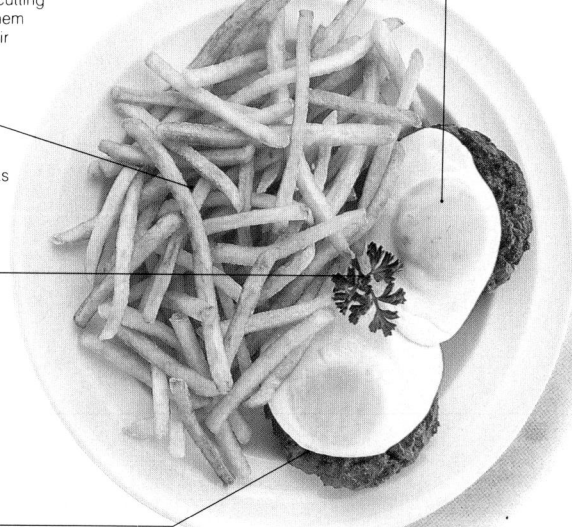

For a healthy diet, choose fish and poultry instead of red meats. Grains and pulses are other good sources of protein.

Carbohydrates

Carbohydrates are the body's main energy source, and are necessary for cell metabolism. There are two main groups: starches, which are found in large amounts in foods such as flour, grains, pasta, bread, and pulses; and sugars, which occur in large amounts in fruits, some vegetables, and foods such as jams, cakes, and sweet drinks.

A high intake of carbohydrates, especially in the form of refined sugar, contributes to obesity and dental decay; obesity in turn can contribute to heart disease, diabetes, and arthritis.

Make your diet healthier by avoiding high-sugar foods. As far as possible, obtain your carbohydrates from relatively low-calorie, high-fibre foods, such as bread, potatoes, and whole-grain cereals.

FOOD HYGIENE

In recent years the incidence of food poisoning—particularly involving bacterial contamination—has risen substantially. You can minimize the risk of infection by following the simple guidelines set out below.

1 Buy the freshest produce you can, and never eat food after its "best before" or "eat by" date. If food smells bad, throw it away, even if it hasn't reached its "best before" date.

2 Store food properly. All food should be covered, wrapped, or put in a clean container; store in the fridge if necessary. Keep raw and cooked foods apart; store raw meats low in the fridge so that they cannot drip on to other foods.

3 Wash your hands thoroughly before handling food, immediately after handling raw meat, and between preparing meat and preparing other foods. Wash fruit and vegetables in clean water before eating or preparing them.

4 Ensure that kitchen surfaces, cutting boards, and cooking utensils are thoroughly clean before use; keep pets away from all food, kitchen surfaces, and utensils.

5 Thaw frozen meats (especially poultry, pork, and seafood) thoroughly before cooking. Don't keep food warm for extended periods; if reheating is necessary, do so quickly but thoroughly on a high heat.

Fibre

Fibre is an indigestible substance found in plants. Although it does not provide the body with any nutrients, fibre is essential for the healthy functioning of the digestive system.

Diets that are low in fibre contribute to constipation, diverticular disease, and some bowel cancers; high-fibre foods provide dietary bulk without excess calories.

Foods that are particularly high in fibre include whole-grain breads and cereals, pulses, nuts, and dried fruits. Fibre is also found in all fruit and vegetables.

Vitamins

Vitamins help to ensure that all the body's cells and organs are functioning well. A balanced diet with plenty of fresh fruit and vegetables provides all the vitamins you need, except during pregnancy. Women planning to become pregnant should take a small supplement of folic acid before conception and for 12 weeks afterwards to minimize the risks of birth defects.

Minerals

Many different minerals, such as calcium, sodium, potassium, iron, zinc, and iodine, are necessary to keep the organs, bones, and muscles functioning properly. A balanced diet usually provides all the necessary minerals.

Water

Water is essential to sustain life. Although most foods contain substantial amounts of water, it is sensible also to drink several glasses of pure water each day.

A HEALTHY MEAL
As this meal shows, healthy eating does not have to be just cottage cheese and carrots. The meal below provides a good variety of taste and texture, but is low in fat and relatively low in calories.

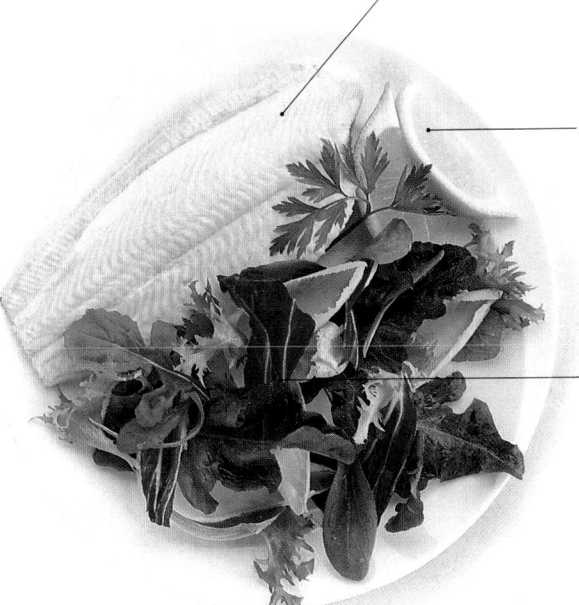

Fish
Grilled, non-oily fish provides a low-calorie nutritious "meat" serving that is also low in fat.

Lemon
Juice from a lemon wedge gives the food extra taste without the fat and sugar of thick, high-calorie dressings.

Vegetables
A mixture of fresh, uncooked salad vegetables provides vitamins, minerals, and fibre without too many calories or any fat content.

EXERCISE AND HEALTH

Regular exercise is an important means of improving health. Exercise keeps the muscles and bones in good health, and also slows down the aging process; it improves fitness levels and increases muscle tone and flexibility, producing a general sense of well-being.

Also, if you exercise regularly and vigorously several times a week you will improve the efficiency of your heart and lungs, and significantly reduce your risk of developing coronary artery disease or of having a myocardial infarction (heart attack).

Types of exercise

There are many different types of exercise, which can be performed to fulfil different functions. For instance, certain exercises may be chosen to improve the efficiency of the heart and lungs, others may be used to improve flexibility, and others to increase muscular strength or physical endurance. A well-balanced exercise programme will contain activities that provide a combination of benefits.

Aerobic exercise is activity that requires the lungs to take in additional oxygen to meet the requirements of the muscles—the kind of exercise that makes you breathless. Activities such as jogging, rowing, cycling, squash, and swimming fall into this category. Aerobic exercise is the best kind of exercise for improving cardiovascular fitness, and also usually improves the strength and flexibility of certain muscle groups at

the same time. For example, jogging improves and strengthens the leg muscles as well as increasing cardiovascular fitness.

Isometric exercise is exercise without movement, in which one group of muscles exerts pressure against an immovable object (a wall, for example) or against an opposing group of muscles. Isometric exercises improve muscle strength, but they do not have any effect on cardiovascular fitness or on flexibility.

Isotonic exercise is a form of exercise in which the body works against its own weight or against an external weight. Weight-lifting and calisthenics (repetitive exercises that have been designed to stretch and strengthen particular muscle groups) are examples of isotonic exercises.

Isokinetic exercise combines elements of isometric and isotonic exercise. This is the kind of exercise usually performed on the sophisticated fitness training equipment found in gymnasiums and sports centres.

Improving health

Exercise improves the blood flow to muscles, providing them with nutrients and removing waste products. Muscles are strengthened and so are the ligaments that attach them to the bones, thus improving the strength and mobility of the joints. The muscle tone is improved and, because the muscles require more energy, fat stored in the body is broken down and utilized, which can lead to a reduction in weight. Specific exercises of the correct

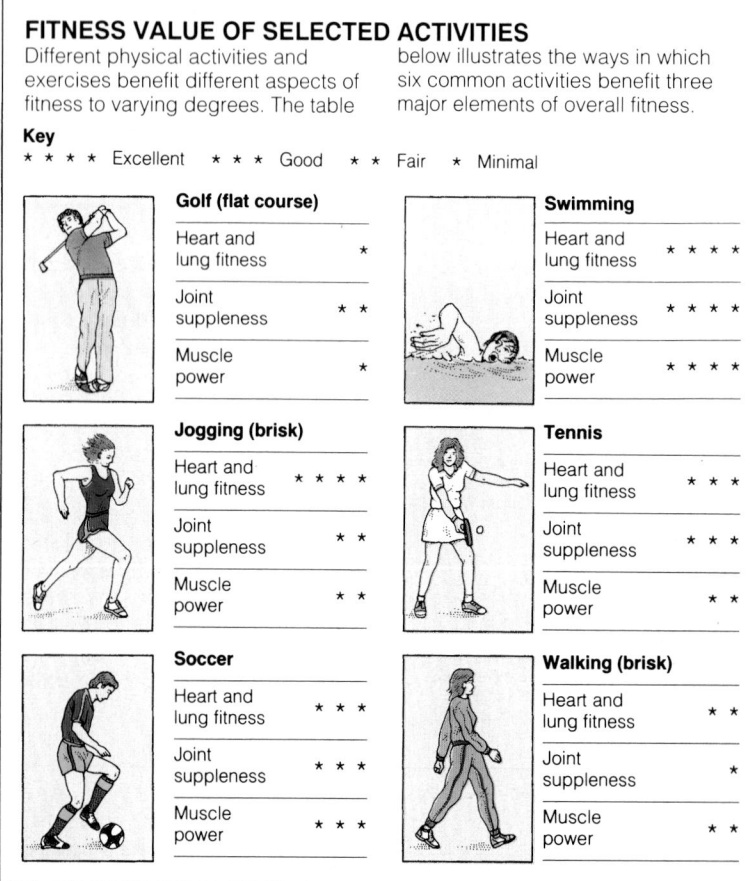

FITNESS VALUE OF SELECTED ACTIVITIES

Different physical activities and exercises benefit different aspects of fitness to varying degrees. The table below illustrates the ways in which six common activities benefit three major elements of overall fitness.

Key

★ ★ ★ ★ Excellent ★ ★ ★ Good ★ ★ Fair ★ Minimal

Golf (flat course)

Heart and lung fitness	★
Joint suppleness	★ ★
Muscle power	★

Swimming

Heart and lung fitness	★ ★ ★ ★
Joint suppleness	★ ★ ★ ★
Muscle power	★ ★ ★ ★

Jogging (brisk)

Heart and lung fitness	★ ★ ★ ★
Joint suppleness	★ ★
Muscle power	★ ★

Tennis

Heart and lung fitness	★ ★ ★
Joint suppleness	★ ★ ★
Muscle power	★ ★

Soccer

Heart and lung fitness	★ ★ ★
Joint suppleness	★ ★ ★
Muscle power	★ ★ ★

Walking (brisk)

Heart and lung fitness	★ ★
Joint suppleness	★
Muscle power	★ ★

ENERGY EXPENDITURE

The table below gives the approximate amount of energy expended during 30 minutes of various activities. The figures are based on levels of exertion likely to be kept up by typical amateurs.

Activity	Energy used
Easy walking	90 kcal
Light gardening	135 kcal
Golf	135 kcal
Housework	135 kcal
Brisk walking	150 kcal
Badminton	170 kcal
Heavy gardening	210 kcal
Gymnastics	210 kcal
Tennis	240 kcal
Hockey	270 kcal
Rugby	270 kcal
Soccer	270 kcal
Squash	300 kcal
Brisk jogging	315 kcal
Cycling	330 kcal
Swimming	360 kcal

THE BODY DURING EXERCISE

During vigorous aerobic activity many of the body's systems are exercised. The illustration shows the effects of strenuous exercise on different parts of the body.

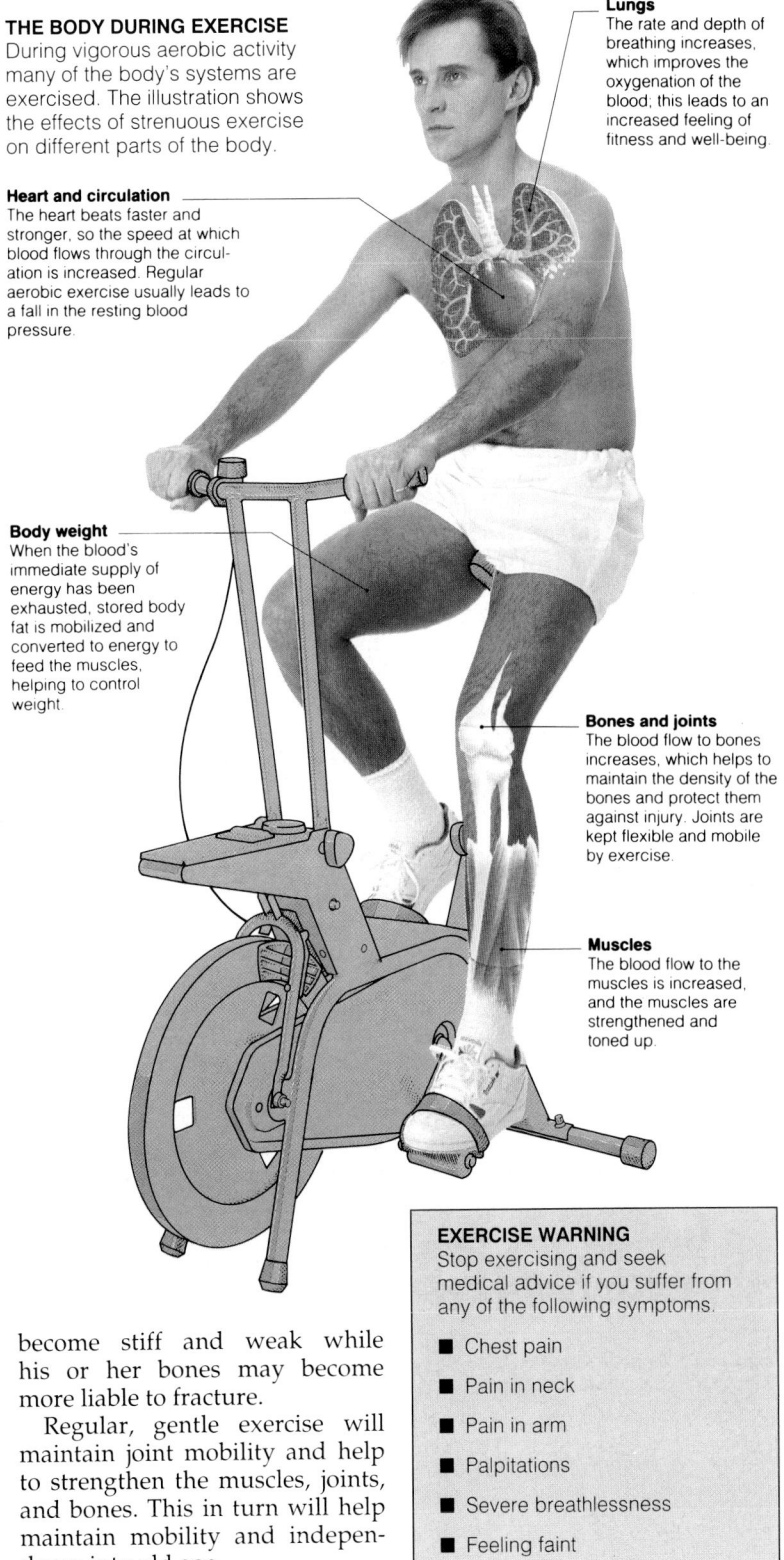

Lungs
The rate and depth of breathing increases, which improves the oxygenation of the blood; this leads to an increased feeling of fitness and well-being.

Heart and circulation
The heart beats faster and stronger, so the speed at which blood flows through the circulation is increased. Regular aerobic exercise usually leads to a fall in the resting blood pressure.

Body weight
When the blood's immediate supply of energy has been exhausted, stored body fat is mobilized and converted to energy to feed the muscles, helping to control weight.

Bones and joints
The blood flow to bones increases, which helps to maintain the density of the bones and protect them against injury. Joints are kept flexible and mobile by exercise.

Muscles
The blood flow to the muscles is increased, and the muscles are strengthened and toned up.

kind can restore mobility to damaged joints and can ease some kinds of back pain.

Avoiding heart disease

Regular aerobic exercise has been shown to reduce the likelihood of coronary artery disease. During aerobic exercise the heart beats more rapidly and more powerfully. This strengthens the heart muscle and improves its efficiency; the blood pressure while at rest is also usually reduced. Aerobic exercise is also thought to help protect the body against the development of atherosclerosis (the accumulation of fatty deposits in the arteries), which can lead to a myocardial infarction.

Exercise in later life

Because mobility—and energy—tend to decrease in later life, an elderly person's joints may become stiff and weak while his or her bones may become more liable to fracture.

Regular, gentle exercise will maintain joint mobility and help to strengthen the muscles, joints, and bones. This in turn will help maintain mobility and independence into old age.

EXERCISE WARNING

Stop exercising and seek medical advice if you suffer from any of the following symptoms.

- Chest pain
- Pain in neck
- Pain in arm
- Palpitations
- Severe breathlessness
- Feeling faint

SMOKING AND DRINKING

Smoking and drinking are two of the greatest enemies of a healthy lifestyle. In recent years, tobacco-smoking and alcohol consumption have both been convincingly implicated in a wide range of health problems. Numerous working days are lost each year through disorders related to smoking or drinking, and both activities increase the risk of cancer and heart disease, and therefore of premature death. Women who smoke or drink during pregnancy risk causing damage to the health of their unborn children.

Both alcohol and nicotine are addictive drugs; people who begin smoking or drinking socially often find themselves, several years later, unable to give up the habit.

The effects of tobacco

The harmful effects of tobacco on the body are mainly due to three constituents of its smoke: nicotine, carbon monoxide, and tar.

Nicotine is a tranquillizer, and is also addictive; it is the absence of nicotine that causes the physical and psychological withdrawal symptoms that may occur when a regular smoker suddenly stops smoking. The presence of carbon monoxide in the blood decreases the amount of oxygen reaching the tissues, and in the long term can lead to atherosclerosis (the accumulation of fatty deposits in the arteries). Tar causes chronic irritation of the respiratory tract, and contains carcinogens (cancer-causing agents).

Smoking and cancer

The link between smoking and lung cancer is well-known; 90 per cent of lung cancer deaths can be attributed to smoking. Lung cancer is, however, only one of the malignant tumours that can be caused by, or aggravated by, tobacco-smoking. Other smoking-related tumours include cancers of the mouth, throat, lip, cervix, and bladder.

Pipe and cigar smokers inhale less smoke than most cigarette smokers and they are therefore somewhat less likely to develop lung cancer; they are, however, more prone to cancers of the mouth and throat.

Other risks of smoking

Many people do not realize that smoking also contributes significantly to numerous other diseases and disorders.

The irritant effect of tobacco smoke causes the respiratory tract to produce excessive sputum (phlegm), leading to the classic "smoker's cough". Tobacco smoke also causes the alveoli (tiny air sacs in the lungs) to lose their elasticity and eventually become fused; this makes them less efficient, and ultimately leads to emphysema. Many heavy smokers die from respiratory failure caused by chronic bronchitis and/or emphysema.

People who smoke also face a great risk of premature death from coronary artery disease. Smokers have been found to suffer more commonly than nonsmokers from angina (chest pain that is caused by inadequate blood supply to heart muscle), and also from the kind of myocardial infarction (heart attack) that does not produce symptoms.

Arterial disease makes smokers more likely than nonsmokers to have a stroke. They are also more likely to develop gastric and duodenal ulcers.

Passive smoking

Passive smoking is the term used to describe the involuntary inhalation of tobacco smoke by people who, themselves, do not smoke. Recent research has shown that nonsmokers who regularly inhale air that is polluted by tobacco smoke suffer measurable ill-effects on their health. The children of smokers have more chest and ear infections than the children of nonsmokers. Adults who work in smoky environments such as bars, or whose workmates or spouses smoke in their company, are at a risk from tobacco-induced cancers that is the equivalent of smoking two to three cigarettes for every day that they are exposed.

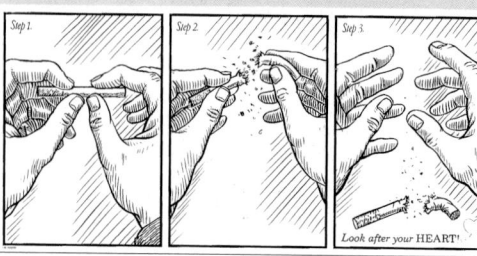

Health education poster Anti-smoking posters, such as the one shown here, have a major part to play in persuading people not to smoke. The link between smoking and heart disease is less well-known than the link between smoking and cancer but is no less serious. For example, the risk of coronary artery disease in a young man who smokes 20 cigarettes a day is about three times that of a nonsmoker.

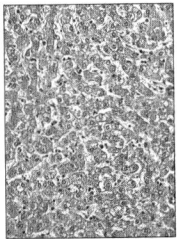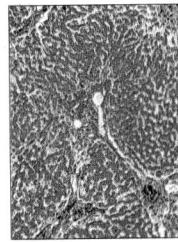

Cirrhosis of the liver
The two photomicrographs above show healthy liver tissue (left), and liver tissue damaged by alcoholic cirrhosis (right). In the healthy liver, the cells are arranged regularly; in the cirrhotic liver, healthy cells have been destroyed by alcohol and replaced by scar tissue (coloured blue). Eventually the cirrhotic liver loses normal function.

Reducing the risk
If you give up smoking, you immediately reduce your chances of developing smoking-related diseases; the more years you subsequently go without smoking, the lower is your risk.

Alcohol and disease
The effects of alcohol on health are more complicated to assess than those of tobacco, the risks of which clearly increase with the amount of tobacco smoked. Research in the UK and the US has shown that people who drink in moderation—an average of two units per day—are at lower risk of

DEATHS FROM CIRRHOSIS
As the population in a given country drinks more, so the death rate from cirrhosis of the liver rises. This graph shows death rates from cirrhosis and other chronic liver disease in four countries in 1990.

As the graph shows, the death rates for England and Wales are slightly lower than for the US. In France and Italy, however, where heavy drinking is more common, the death rate is very much higher.

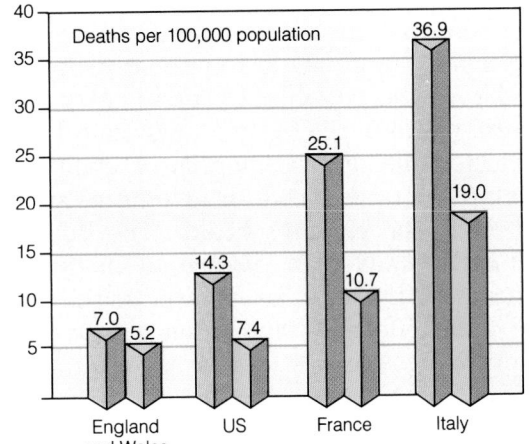

Deaths per 100,000 population

Key: Male / Female

England and Wales — 7.0, 5.2
US — 14.3, 7.4
France — 25.1, 10.7
Italy — 36.9, 19.0

coronary heart disease than those who drink no alcohol at all or those who drink more than three units per day (see box). Alcohol is a danger to health, however, since many people increase their consumption over the years and the risk rises with increased consumption. People who drink substantial amounts on most days may have no social problems from their drinking but may, nevertheless, be damaging their health.

Liver disorders, such as fatty liver, alcoholic hepatitis, and cirrhosis, are common among heavy drinkers. While small amounts of alcohol may protect against heart disease, larger quantities raise the blood pressure and increase the risk of stroke. Heavy drinkers also suffer higher-than-average rates of gastritis, pancreatitis, peptic ulcers, and cancers of the mouth, tongue, pharynx, larynx, oesophagus, and stomach.

Long-term consumption of large amounts of alcohol damages the brain, affecting intellectual abilities. During pregnancy, it is likely to harm the physical and mental development of the unborn child.

Social problems
Alcohol is implicated in a wide range of social problems; it is a significant factor in absenteeism, traffic accidents, drowning, domestic violence, marital breakdown, child abuse, sexual assault, and other violent crimes. Also, there is strong evidence that young people who drink heavily are more likely to experiment with other addictive drugs. For your own sake and for the sake of others, it is sensible to stick to safe drinking limits.

HOW MUCH IS TOO MUCH?
First count how many units of alcohol you drink in a week. Each of the following is one unit:
- half a pint of ordinary beer or lager;
- a glass of wine;
- a single whisky, a vermouth, or a small glass of sherry.

Then check your rating against the table below. Remember that cider and strong beers account for more units of alcohol per half pint than ordinary beers. Remember, too, that home and party measures of drinks are usually larger than pub measures.

Men: 21 units or under per week
Women: 14 units or under per week
Your drinking is within generally safe limits; try not to increase the amount of alcohol you drink. Remember, though, not to drink and drive.

Men: 22-35 units per week
Women: 15-21 units per week
Your drinking level is probably not doing lasting damage if it is spread out evenly through the week, but if it is in two or three binges you could be damaging your health. Try to drink less.

Men: 36-49 units per week
Women: 22-35 units per week
Your drinking is at a level which is likely to do long-term damage to your health. Examine your drinking habits and work out ways in which you can cut down.

Men: 50 units or more per week
Women: 36 units or more per week
Your drinking is almost certainly causing serious damage to your health, and you may well be dependent on alcohol. Cut down your drinking drastically, and seek help if you have trouble doing this.

"If only we'd caught this earlier." All too commonly, it is necessary for a doctor to explain that the disease responsible for a patient's symptoms is too far advanced for a cure to be possible. In many cases, however, modern diagnostic tests could have detected the disease months or even years before the appearance of symptoms or any upset to the patient's health. The detection of early signs of a disease in its hidden, presymptomatic stage allows treatment to be more effective—and often curative; this detection process is known as screening. In recent years, more and more general practices, health centres, and clinics have begun to offer screening programmes for different groups of people.

Some diseases such as muscular dystrophy run in families, while others such as thalassaemia are most common in certain racial groups. Advances in the understanding of genetics have made it possible to screen couples who are planning a family, and who know they are at risk, to check whether they might be carriers of the disease in question, and to give them appropriate advice.

Screening tests

Screening tests may be suitable for the whole population or for subgroups at special risk (such as people over a certain age, people who belong to particular racial groups, people with relatives who have a particular disorder, or people who are employed in hazardous occupations).

Most screening tests need to be performed by doctors or nurses, but it is possible to carry out some types of screening tests yourself—self-examination of the testes or breasts, for example.

Criteria for screening

A good screening test is both sensitive and specific. A test is sensitive if it detects all, or almost all, of the people with the disorder (i.e. there are few false negatives). A test is specific if it does not cause many false alarms (i.e. there are few false positives).

The condition being tested for should be reasonably common (for example, there is not much point screening British people for leprosy). Another criterion for screening is the availability of an effective treatment for the condition at the stage at which it can be detected by the test. Also, there should be good evidence that early diagnosis by screening substantially improves the chance of a cure or of prolonged freedom from symptoms.

These criteria for screening are now fulfilled by a whole range of tests, starting immediately after birth and continuing into old age.

Common screening tests

Newborn infants are examined by a paediatrician, who looks for various conditions, such as heart

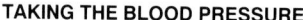

TAKING THE BLOOD PRESSURE
Blood pressure is measured by using a sphygmomanometer (an inflatable cuff attached to a pressure gauge) and a stethoscope to listen for sounds of blood flow. Two pressure readings are recorded: the higher (systolic) pressure and the lower (diastolic) pressure. Blood pressure measurements are conventionally expressed in millimetres of mercury (mm Hg).

During the procedure
With the cuff on one arm, the patient sits with his arm on a firm surface and with the inside of the elbow turned up.

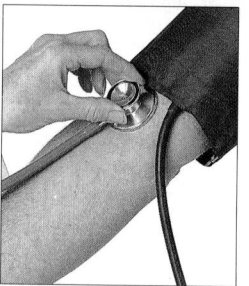

Placing the stethoscope
The doctor positions the end of the stethoscope over the patient's brachial artery at the elbow, just below the sphygmomanometer cuff.

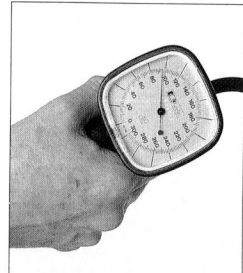

Reading the gauge
The pressure dial of the sphygmomanometer allows the doctor to read the systolic and diastolic blood pressure levels.

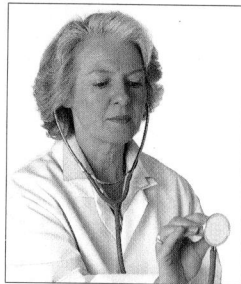

The stethoscope
The stethoscope enables the doctor to hear changes in the flow of blood which are related to blood pressure levels.

defects, and disorders of the brain and nervous system. Blood is taken from newborn infants to test for phenylketonuria (a chemical disorder) and hypothyroidism (a hormonal disorder), which, if undetected, may cause serious illness later in childhood. Infants and children are tested regularly to monitor growth, and to assess mental and physical development (including vision and hearing).

In early adult life, everyone should have their blood pressure measured; this test should then be repeated every three to five years throughout life. Early detection of raised blood pressure is the most useful screening test available, and is both safe and simple. Also important is regular personal measurement of weight.

Screening for cancer

Screening tests for cancer fall into two groups: those appropriate for the whole population, and those for high-risk groups.

All men should learn how to examine their testes regularly for signs of cancer. Cancer of the testis is the most common cancer in men under the age of 40, and is easily curable if detected early.

All women should learn how to examine their breasts, and should begin regular mammographic screening for cancer at the age of 50.

All women who have ever had sexual intercourse should have a cervical smear test every three to five years (more often if they have had a genital viral infection).

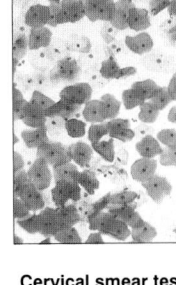 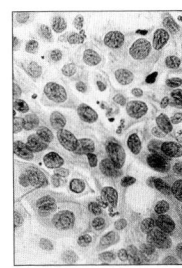

Cervical smear tests
These photomicrographs show the results of a normal smear (above left) and an abnormal smear (above right). The normal smear shows red-stained healthy cells with small nuclei; the abnormal smear shows numerous abnormal blue-stained cells with large, dark nuclei.

Screening tests for several other cancers are still being assessed; a recommendation that the whole population over a certain age should be tested repeatedly has substantial cost implications. Current policy in the UK for cancers of the colon and ovary is to limit screening to the blood relatives of people who have had the cancers.

People aged 50 or more, with relatives who have been treated for cancer of the colon, are recommended to have an annual test for blood in the faeces and, if the test gives a positive result, to have further confirmatory tests followed by a colonoscopy—an endoscopic examination of the interior of the bowel.

Women with relatives who have had a cancer of the ovary may be offered regular ultrasound screening to detect any early evidence of an ovarian tumour. The procedure is painless and carries no risk.

Heel-prick blood test
This blood test is performed eight to 14 days after birth. The baby's heel is pricked and a few drops of blood are collected and sent to the laboratory to be tested for phenylketonuria, an inherited chemical disorder, and for hypothyroidism (thyroid deficiency).

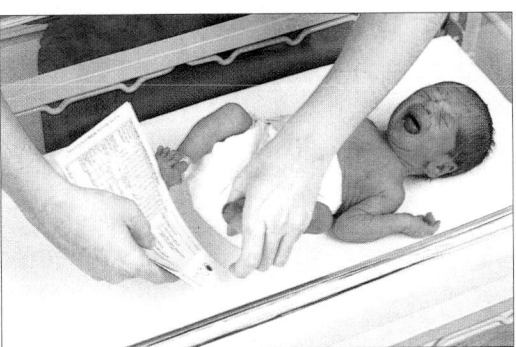

TYPES OF SCREENING TESTS
The table lists tests that can be used to screen people for different conditions.

Antenatal screening tests

Chromosomal abnormalities	•	†
Sickle cell disorders	•	†
Genetic disorders (e.g. muscular dystrophy)	•	†
Haemophilia; thalassaemia	•	†
Anaemia		‡
Blood group (including Rh)		‡
Hepatitis B; HIV infection	•	‡
Rubella; syphilis		‡
Spina bifida (and other malformations)		†

Infant and child screening tests

Hypothyroidism; phenylketonuria	
Sickle cell; thalassaemia	•
Dental caries	
Cataracts; squint; visual defects	
Deafness	
Heart disease, congenital	
Hip dislocation; talipes	
Testes, ectopic or undescended	

Adult screening tests

Hypertension	
Hyperlipidaemia	•
Cervical cancer	
Glaucoma; visual defects	
Breast cancer	
Testicular cancer	
Bladder cancer	•
Intestinal cancer	•

Key
• High-risk groups
† In fetus
‡ In mother

Colour key

- Amniocentesis or chorionic villus sampling
- Blood pressure test
- Blood test
- Cervical smear test
- Dental examination
- Eye test
- Hearing test
- Mammography
- Physical examination
- Ultrasound scanning
- Urine test
- Faeces test

SCREENING 2

Screening for cancer of the prostate is still under evaluation. A blood test for the prostate specific antigen will give a high reading in most men with the cancer, but the level is also raised to some extent in those with a benign enlargement of the gland. Furthermore, almost 90 per cent of men aged 80 or more have small, cancerous growths in their prostate gland, but most are unaffected by these tiny, symptomless tumours. As yet, there is no reliable means of determining which of these early small cancers will cause symptoms later.

After the age of 50, anyone with a family history of intestinal cancer should have an annual test for blood in the faeces. Workers in some industries are more likely to develop some forms of cancer and may benefit from screening; current and past workers in certain chemical industries, for example, should have regular urine tests to check for cancer of the bladder.

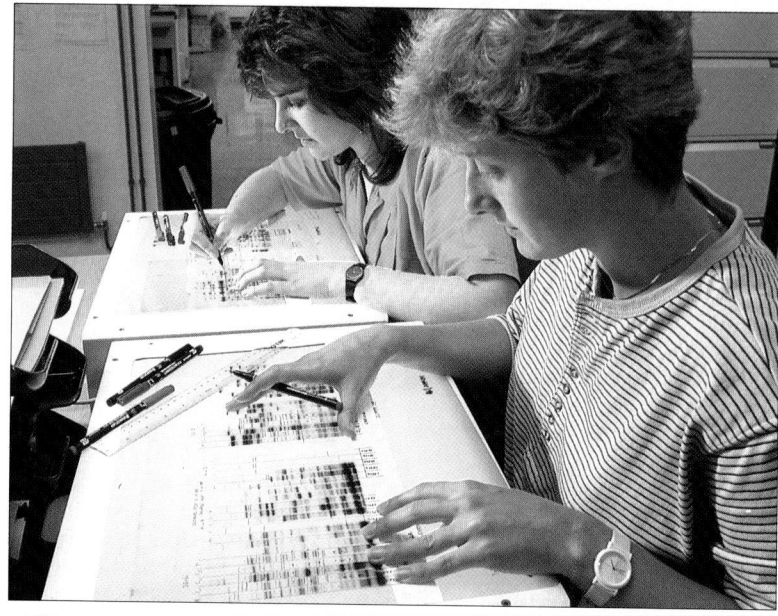

DNA analysis
Advances in laboratory techniques have revolutionized the study of genetic disorders. Suspect regions of DNA can be copied millions of times, providing scientists with large amounts of genetic material for analysis.

Genetic screening

Steady progress has been made in recent years in identifying genetic factors in disease. Many diseases, mostly uncommon, are known to be due to a single gene disorder. People with these conditions inherit a defect in one gene or pair of genes that is the sole cause of the disease. Examples include the brain disorder, Huntington's disease; the eye cancer, retinoblastoma; muscular dystrophy; cystic fibrosis; the haemoglobinopathies, sickle cell disease and thalassaemia; and many biochemical disorders such as Gaucher's disease.

Advances in knowledge have made it possible to treat some of these diseases by providing a regular supply of a missing protein or enzyme, or sometimes by a bone marrow transplant. More often, however, the best that currently can be offered is some form of antenatal screening aimed at reducing the number of sufferers of the disease.

For example, the potentially fatal blood disorder, thalassaemia, occurs only in children who inherit a defective gene from both parents (who are usually entirely healthy). The disorder is especially common in some Mediterranean races such as Greeks, Turks, and Cypriots; genetic testing is now offered to

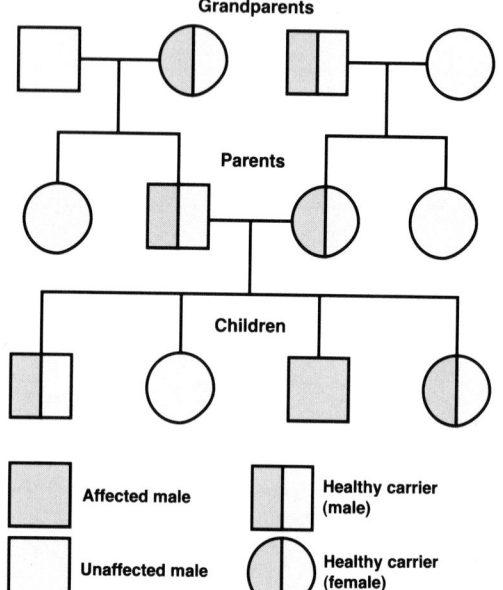

Grandparents

Parents

Children

Affected male

Unaffected male

Healthy carrier (male)

Healthy carrier (female)

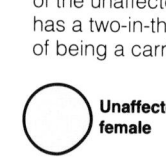

Unaffected female

PATTERN OF INHERITANCE
The diagram shows one of the ways in which an apparently healthy family can have a child with a genetic defect. Two of the four grandparents and both parents are symptomless carriers of the defective gene. When two carriers have children, each child has a one-in-four chance of inheriting the defective gene from both parents and of having the disease. Each of the unaffected children has a two-in-three chance of being a carrier.

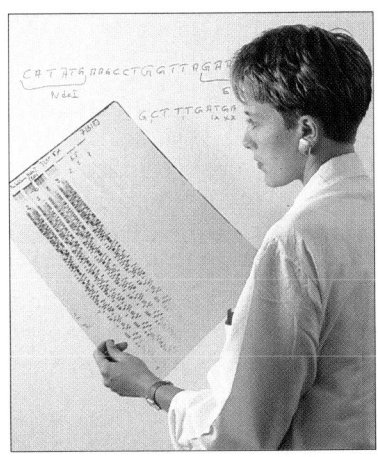

DNA sequencing
This technique is used to compare the chemical structure of the nucleotide chains of defective and normal genes.

all young adults in many communities within these racial groups. If a couple are both found to be carriers of the gene for thalassaemia, there is a one-in-four chance of any children conceived inheriting this gene. Many such couples decide to have a test performed early in the pregnancy, and, if the defective gene is found, they may wish to have the pregnancy terminated.

For less common disorders, such as muscular dystrophy, tests are usually offered only to people from affected families. Sisters of boys with the most common (Duchenne) type of muscular dystrophy have a 50 per cent chance of carrying the defective gene, and most of them welcome the opportunity to find out whether any children they may have run the risk of being affected. As with thalassaemia, couples found to be at risk may choose to have the fetus tested and have the pregnancy terminated if the defective gene has been passed on.

In the coming years even more tests will become available, and couples planning to have a family should ask their relatives whether there have ever been any children in the family who were born with a genetic disorder (such children often die in infancy and relatives may not talk about these past tragedies unless they are specifically asked). Whenever there is a family background that suggests the possibility of genetic disease, couples should consult their doctor before attempting to

have children: advice may be possible on preconceptual nutrition or special precautions as well as on genetic testing.

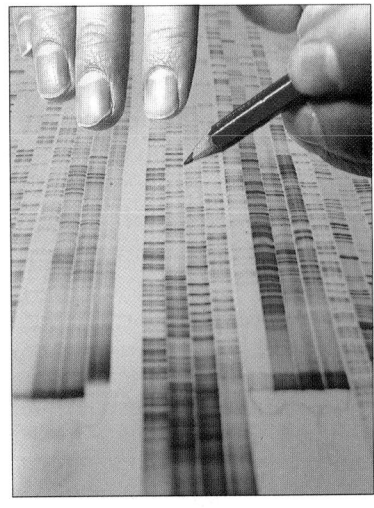

Discovering the gene
The gene responsible for most cases of cystic fibrosis was located in the early 1990s and identified by DNA analysis.

Other screening tests

Regular eye tests are important, particularly after the age of 40. Vision should be checked, and the the interior of the eye examined. Anyone with a family history of glaucoma should have the fluid pressure of the eyes measured at two-yearly intervals from the age of 40 onwards.

Despite the recent publicity concerning cholesterol tests, current medical advice is that they are unnecessary for most people. Doctors recommend blood cholesterol measurement only for relatives of people who have had a heart attack before the age of 50, or for those with other high-risk factors, such as a combination of raised blood pressure and heavy smoking.

The nation's dental health has improved dramatically following many years' use of fluoride toothpaste. Regular dental check-ups are, however, still essential, and are recommended every six months until the age of 21, and every one to two years thereafter.

GENE MUTATIONS

The illustration shows the results of DNA tests on four boys from families known to be affected by the Duchenne type of muscular dystrophy. Genetic probes or markers have been used to pick out the crucial sections of DNA. The column on the far right, which has five bands, comes from a healthy boy; the others are from boys with abnormalities causing the disease.

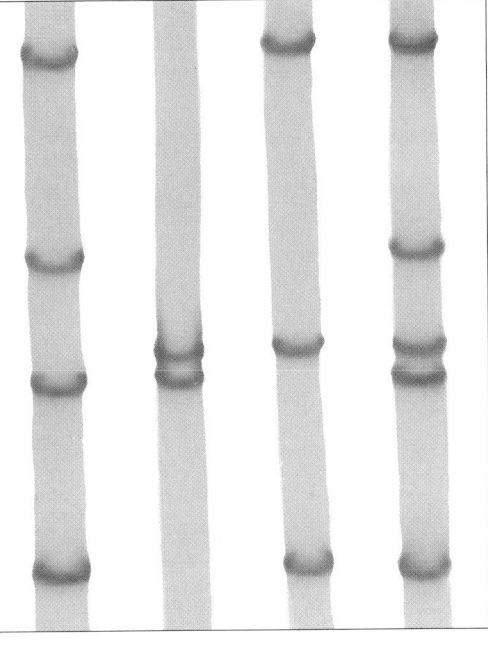

IMMUNIZATION AGAINST DISEASE

A range of dangerous diseases can now be avoided thanks to immunization—the artificial creation of immunity against infection. Smallpox has already been successfully eliminated, and poliomyelitis is no longer seen in the Americas and western Europe. The World Health Organization hopes to eradicate several more diseases in the next decade.

Immunization protects most children completely, but in the rare cases in which an immunized child does catch the disease, the illness is much milder than if the child had not been immunized. No child should be denied immunization without very good reason—not only for the child's sake, but also for that of the community at large.

How immunization works

When an infecting microorganism enters the body, the immune system attacks the invader and produces blood proteins called antibodies, which help to destroy the organism. The immune system is able to "remember" this destruction process, so that if the invader returns, a repeat attack can be mounted faster. This phenomenon is called immunity.

Immunization is the process of creating immunity artificially. It can be done either by passive or by active immunization.

In passive immunization, a person is injected with a preparation of ready-made human antibodies, taken from general blood donors or from people recovering from specific infections. Passive immunization gives immediate protection, but this protection lasts only for a few weeks.

In active immunization, a person is given a vaccine that may contain living, weakened organisms (e.g. measles vaccine), dead organisms (e.g. pertussis vaccine), or weakened forms of bacterial poisons (e.g. diphtheria vaccine). The vaccine stimulates the immune system to produce its own particular antibodies, which provide longer-lasting immunity.

Immunization schedules

For protection against some diseases, only one dose of vaccine is necessary; for other diseases, an initial course followed by booster doses is required.

Your health visitor will probably discuss immunization when your baby is very small, and you will be reminded when the immunizations are due. Premature babies are at greater than average risk from infectious diseases, so every effort should be made to have them vaccinated at the recommended schedule dates. Your child can be immunized by a doctor or nurse at your GP's surgery or your local child health clinic. Most immunizations are given by injection into the upper arm or thigh; polio vaccine is usually given by mouth.

TYPICAL IMMUNIZATION SCHEDULE

Vaccine	2 months	3 months	4 months	13-15 months	4-5 years	10-14 years (girls only)	13 years	15-19 years
Diphtheria	Yes*	Yes*	Yes*		Booster†			
Pertussis (whooping cough)	Yes*	Yes*	Yes*					
Tetanus	Yes*	Yes*	Yes*		Booster†			Booster
Haemophilus influenza b (Hib)	Yes	Yes	Yes					
Poliomyelitis	Yes††	Yes††	Yes††		Booster††			Booster††
Measles				Yes§				
Mumps				Yes§				
Rubella (German measles)				Yes§		Yes		
Tuberculosis							Yes	

Key
* Combined diphtheria, pertussis, and tetanus (DPT) vaccine
† Combined diphtheria and tetanus vaccine
†† Oral vaccine
§ Combined measles, mumps, and rubella (MMR) vaccine

Immunization side-effects

All vaccines are extensively tested for safety and effectiveness. When side-effects do occur, they are usually mild. The risk of harmful side-effects is very small, and for any vaccine this is always less than the risk of serious effects from the disease itself.

Immunization or not?

There are very few genuine reasons why a child should not be immunized; the doctor or nurse will discuss these with you. Vaccination should be postponed if the child is suffering from a feverish illness, but does not need to be put off if he or she simply has a snuffly nose.

If the child has had a severe reaction to a previous dose, or a serious allergic reaction to egg, certain vaccines will not be given. There is no reason why a child with asthma, eczema, or hay fever, or who is older than the scheduled age, should not be immunized.

Live vaccines are generally not given to pregnant women, because of the theoretical risk of harm to the developing fetus; to people suffering from certain forms of cancer or immune system disorders; or to people receiving any treatment that suppresses the immune system.

Travel immunization

Various immunizations are necessary or recommended for people of any age who plan to travel to certain countries where there is a risk of contracting particular infections. You should check your immunization requirements with your doctor, travel agent, or local health centre at least two months before travelling.

TRAVEL PROTECTION

If you travel abroad you may be exposed to potentially serious infections to which you are not immune. Always check the immunizations recommended for your destination, and obtain immunization for the diseases against which you have no current protection.

Disease	Duration of immunity
Cholera	6 months
Hepatitis A	10 years
Meningococcal meningitis	3–5 years
Poliomyelitis	10 years
Rabies	2–3 years
Tetanus	10 years
Tuberculosis	15 years (minimum)
Typhoid fever	3 years
Yellow fever	10 years

PROTECTING YOUR CHILD

For most children, the benefits of immunization far outweigh any slight risks that might be involved. The consequences of catching these avoidable diseases can be very serious, as shown below.

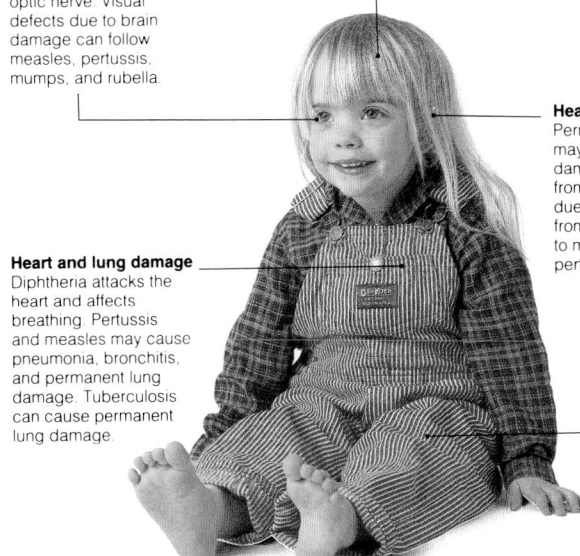

Brain damage
Measles, pertussis, mumps, and rubella can all cause brain inflammation, sometimes leading to permanent brain damage.

Visual defects
Measles can damage the optic nerve. Visual defects due to brain damage can follow measles, pertussis, mumps, and rubella.

Hearing loss
Permanent hearing loss may result from nerve damage due to mumps, from ear infections due to measles, or from brain damage due to mumps, measles, pertussis, or rubella.

Heart and lung damage
Diphtheria attacks the heart and affects breathing. Pertussis and measles may cause pneumonia, bronchitis, and permanent lung damage. Tuberculosis can cause permanent lung damage.

Muscle problems
Poliomyelitis and diphtheria attack the nervous system and may cause muscle paralysis. Tetanus causes painful muscle spasms.

AN ACCEPTABLE RISK

Despite some public fears about the safety of pertussis vaccine, the risks of immunization are much lower than the risks of the disease itself. This graph compares the risk of death or brain damage from pertussis in unvaccinated children with the risk of pertussis vaccination.

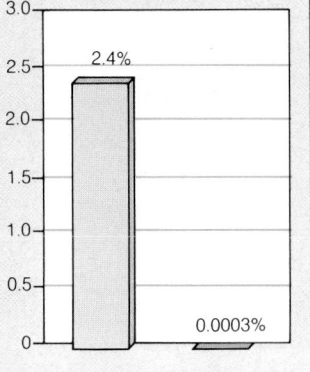

% of children who die or suffer brain damage

2.4%

0.0003%

☐ Not vaccinated against pertussis

▨ Vaccinated against pertussis

DIAGNOSING DISEASE

Diagnosis is the identification by a doctor of a disease process that is causing a person's ill health or other complaint. Without knowing the identity of a disorder, a doctor is able only to relieve symptoms, such as pain or fever. Once the doctor has made a diagnosis, however, it becomes possible to make a prognosis—an estimate of the outcome of a certain disorder—and to begin appropriate treatment.

Diagnosis and prognosis

The concepts of diagnosis and prognosis go back to the fifth century BC, when the Greek physician Hippocrates (c.460-c.377 BC) attempted to identify diseases rather than symptoms, and to describe the sequence of events that occurred in individual diseases. These concepts led to a system of medical training based on pattern recognition that continues to the present day. Doctors are taught to recognize and distinguish diseases by history-taking—during which the doctor asks a series of questions and listens to the patient's own account of the events of the illness—and by performing a physical examination, which may be either general or local depending on the patient's symptoms.

Anatomy and pathology

Diagnosis remained mostly guesswork until the 17th century, when anatomists and pathologists began to make use of dissection to study the structure of the human body, and to investigate the changes that disease causes in body tissues and organs.

The process of diagnosis was also aided by the development in the 17th century of the single-lens microscope, which led to a greater understanding of the structure and function of the body and of the effects of disease.

The 19th century brought another major advance in the history of diagnosis, with the discovery that microorganisms, such as bacteria and fungi, can cause disease. This discovery led to the development of the germ theory of disease by, among others, the French microbiologist and chemist Louis Pasteur (1822-1895) and the German bacteriologist Robert Koch (1843-1910). The germ theory of disease is generally regarded as being one of the most significant achievements in the fields of medical and biological science.

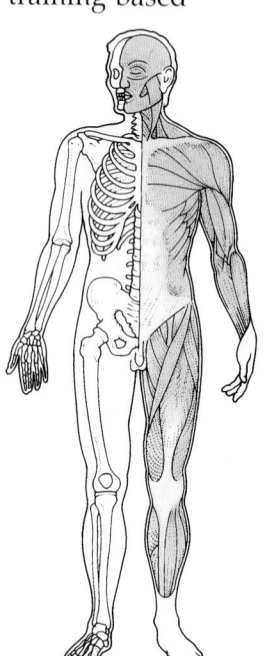

Muscular and skeletal systems
Muscles Muscle biopsy; EMG
Bones Biopsy; imaging techniques (X-ray, CT, MRI, discography, radionuclide scanning); arthroscopy; densitometry; blood tests

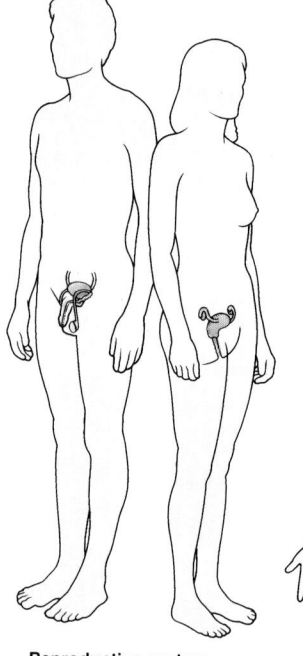

Reproductive system
Men Biochemical analysis of blood and semen; biopsy; culture
Women Endoscopy (laparoscopy, colposcopy, fetoscopy); imaging techniques (mammography, ultrasound, hysterosalpingography); cytology; culture; biopsy; blood tests; amniocentesis; chorionic villus sampling

Respiratory system
Pulmonary function tests; bronchoscopy; culture; biopsy; blood tests; imaging techniques (X-ray, CT, MRI, lung tomography)

Modern diagnostic techniques

Today, doctors still rely heavily on history-taking and physical examination in order to arrive at a diagnosis. However, the speed and accuracy with which diagnoses are made have been greatly increased by the numerous different investigative procedures that can now be performed.

As recently as 50 years ago, the diagnosis of many diseases became certain only after an affected person had died, when his or her body could be fully examined by a pathologist. Nowadays, equal certainty in diagnosis is possible early in the course of a disease, either because it is possible to remove samples of the diseased organs for examination or because diagnostic testing provides a precise, accurate picture of the interior of the body.

The development of these diagnostic methods has led to hospitals being equipped with an enormous range of biochemical, immunological, and microbiological tests on body fluids and tissues. The past 20 years has also seen a revolution in the scale and accuracy of imaging techniques, such as endoscopy, ultrasound, CT scanning, MRI, and PET scanning, which have made it possible to obtain detailed, accurate information about the structure and function of internal organs. Modern diagnostic techniques are able to provide valuable information for doctors, while involving only minimal risk and discomfort to patients.

Some of the most common diagnostic techniques that can be used to investigate disorders affecting the different body systems are listed with the illustrations on these two pages.

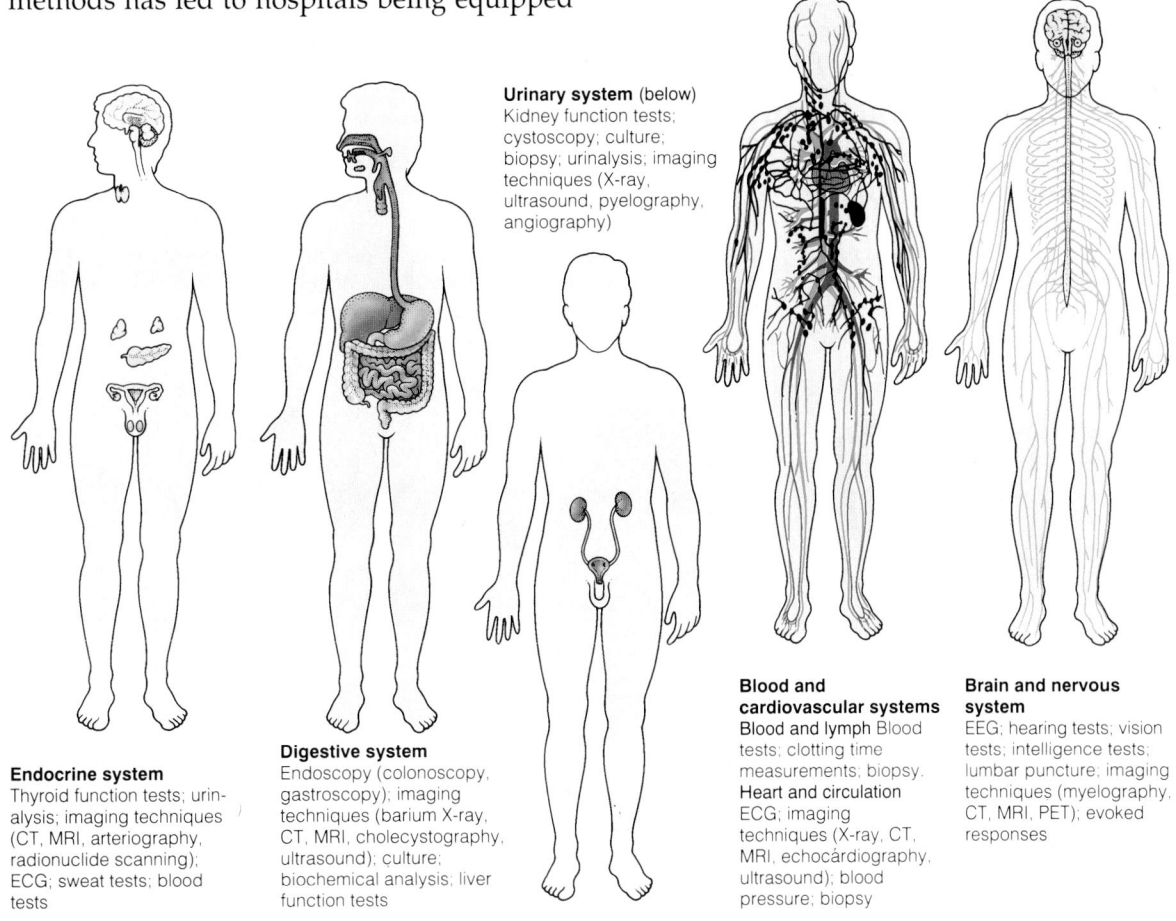

Urinary system (below)
Kidney function tests; cystoscopy; culture; biopsy; urinalysis; imaging techniques (X-ray, ultrasound, pyelography, angiography)

Endocrine system
Thyroid function tests; urinalysis; imaging techniques (CT, MRI, arteriography, radionuclide scanning); ECG; sweat tests; blood tests

Digestive system
Endoscopy (colonoscopy, gastroscopy); imaging techniques (barium X-ray, CT, MRI, cholecystography, ultrasound); culture; biochemical analysis; liver function tests

Blood and cardiovascular systems
Blood and lymph Blood tests; clotting time measurements; biopsy.
Heart and circulation ECG; imaging techniques (X-ray, CT, MRI, echocardiography, ultrasound); blood pressure; biopsy

Brain and nervous system
EEG; hearing tests; vision tests; intelligence tests; lumbar puncture; imaging techniques (myelography, CT, MRI, PET); evoked responses

YOU AND YOUR DOCTOR

Your doctor is trained to diagnose and treat many diseases and disorders. When you consult your doctor about a particular problem, you will find that the consultation typically consists of two main parts. First of these is history-taking, in which the doctor asks you a series of carefully selected questions designed to build up a picture of your problem; second is a physical examination, which confirms or corrects your doctor's first impressions. These two procedures are among the doctor's most important tools.

Before your visit

Before you visit your doctor, check in your own mind just why it is that you want an appointment, and what questions you want to ask. Be totally honest from the outset; for instance, if your specific symptom is that you have an upset stomach, but you also know that you have been feeling run down, tell your doctor about both symptoms—this will enable your doctor to get to the root of the problem more quickly.

If your mind tends to go blank as soon as you get to the surgery, write down your symptoms before you go, and either present the list to the doctor or use it yourself to check that you have not missed anything out. Your doctor is likely to begin by asking you a few questions about your general health—so take a little time before your visit to think over how you have been feeling lately, whether

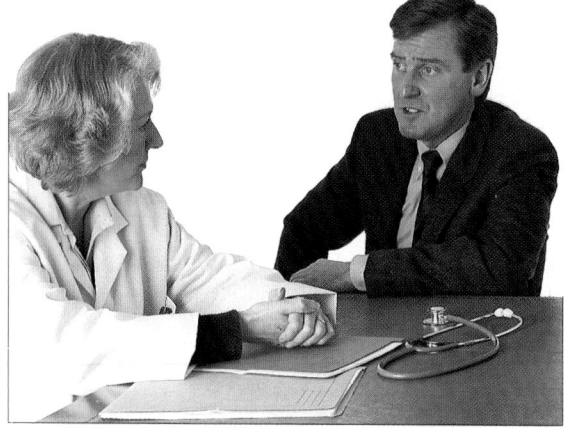

Talking to your doctor
Your doctor will be able to help you most easily if you give him or her a full description of your problem. Always feel free to tell the doctor about anything that is bothering you. He or she will ask you a series of questions designed to help build up a full picture of your problem.

you have noticed any change in your eating habits, bowel habits, or sleeping pattern, and whether you have any particular worries.

Taking the history

The first thing your doctor will want to know is why you have asked for an appointment. Relate your symptoms as simply and clearly as possible, and be as specific as you can. The more clues you can give to the doctor, the easier he or she will find it to diagnose your problem.

While you are relating your symptoms, the doctor will be seeing whether your appearance

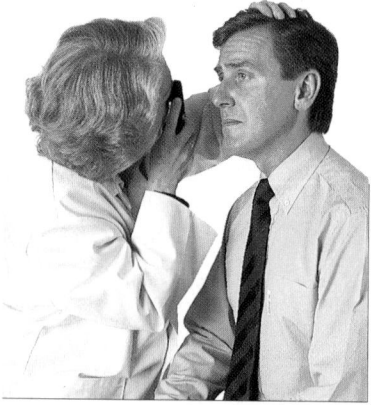

Eye examination
The doctor is using an ophthalmoscope, which uses a deflecting prism to illuminate the inside of the eye.

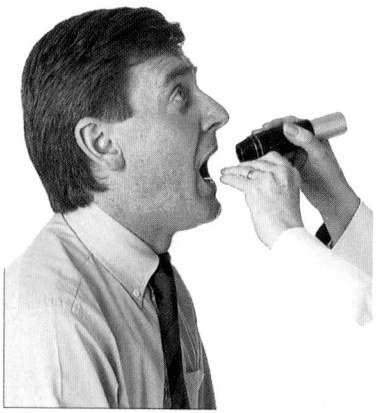

Throat examination
Here the doctor is using a tongue depressor to hold the tongue down, and a torch to illuminate the throat.

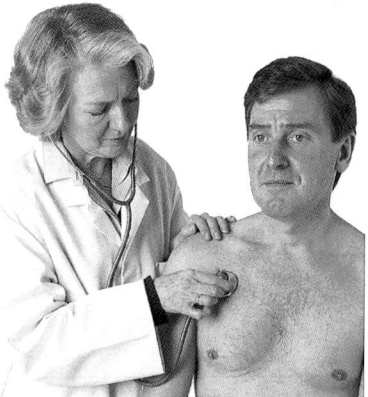

Listening to the chest
A stethoscope is here being used by the doctor to listen for abnormal sounds from the heart or lungs.

gives any clues to your state of health—for example, whether you look generally fit and relaxed, or seem pale, tired, or worried; whether your skin, eyes, hair, and teeth look healthy; and whether you are noticeably overweight or underweight.

Your doctor will make notes on the symptoms you describe, and will then ask you questions to supplement this information: for instance, if you mention that you have a pain in your abdomen, the doctor might ask you about the frequency of your bowel movements. The doctor will also ask you questions about your previous health record and about the medical history of members of your family.

Once your doctor is satisfied that a good picture of your specific symptoms has been built up, he or she might ask you more general questions about your everyday health and lifestyle.

Physical examination

Your doctor may then perform a physical examination. The part or parts of the body that are to be examined will depend on the symptoms that you have described; for instance, if it seems likely that you have a broken arm, the doctor will probably just do a

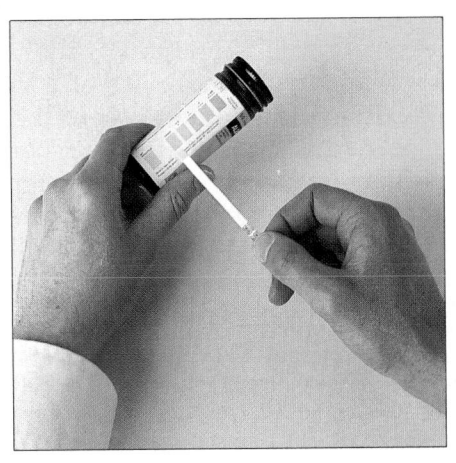

URINE TEST
Urinalysis involves testing a sample of urine to see whether its constituents are abnormal, or present in abnormal quantities. Here, urine is being tested for the presence of protein. A test stick has been dipped in the urine, and has changed colour; the colour is being compared against a chart of possible results.

careful examination of the damaged arm, but if you are feeling under the weather or run down, he or she is likely to do a thorough general examination to see if your main body systems are functioning properly.

Examination techniques that your doctor might use include visual examinations of the ears, eyes, nose, throat, and skin; listening to the chest through a stethoscope; palpating (feeling) body parts such as the abdomen or armpit to detect tenderness or swelling; testing reflexes; and percussion (tapping the chest or abdomen with the fingers to

see from the vibrations whether the different internal organs appear to be normal).

Your doctor may take your temperature to see whether you have a fever, and may also measure your blood pressure, take your pulse, and weigh you. If you are a woman and your symptoms seem to suggest a gynaecological condition, the doctor may perform a pelvic examination, in which the vagina is examined visually and manually to see if the reproductive organs seem to be healthy.

What happens next?

In some cases, your doctor may tell you that further tests are necessary before a diagnosis can be made or confirmed. He or she may ask you to to provide a sample of urine, or may take a blood sample or a throat swab, which will then be sent to a laboratory for various types of analysis. In some cases, your doctor will refer you to a hospital for further examinations and tests.

Once your condition has been diagnosed, an appropriate course of treatment can be recommended. In most cases, treatment will be supervised by your own doctor, but in some cases you will be placed under the care of a hospital doctor.

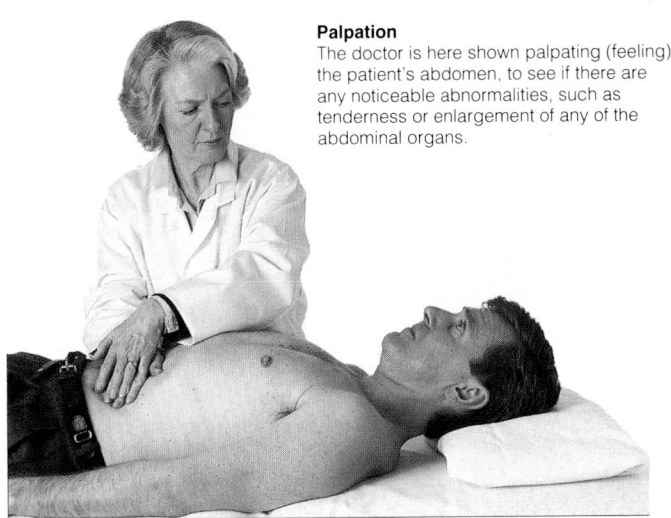

Palpation
The doctor is here shown palpating (feeling) the patient's abdomen, to see if there are any noticeable abnormalities, such as tenderness or enlargement of any of the abdominal organs.

DIAGNOSTIC TECHNIQUES 1

Doctors today can make use of a variety of sophisticated techniques to help them reach an accurate diagnosis. Major advances have been the development of new imaging techniques that provide detailed pictures of internal organs, and fibre-optic endoscopes that enable doctors to look directly into many parts of the body without any need for open surgery. Also of great value in diagnosis are numerous biochemical, immunological, and microbiological tests, as well as techniques of genetic analysis.

X-rays

Following their discovery by Wilhelm Roentgen in 1895, X-rays soon became an important aid to medical diagnosis. Despite the development of newer techniques, X-ray imaging continues to be a widely used and extremely valuable means of seeing inside the body.

X-rays are a form of electromagnetic radiation of extremely short wavelength. They are invisible but blacken photographic film—a property that is used to produce X-ray images. When a beam of X-rays is directed at a part of the body, such as the chest, the rays are absorbed more by dense structures, such as the ribs or heart muscle, than by less dense structures, such as the skin or lungs.

This causes shadows of variable intensity to be cast on to photographic film placed behind the patient. The result is the classic X-ray picture, in which dense tissues appear white, and softer tissues appear as shades of grey.

X-rays cause no sensation when passed through body tissues, but large or frequent radiation doses may damage the skin and internal organs, and may cause cancer in later life. Today, the risk involved in having an X-ray is extremely small, because radiation doses are kept to a minimum.

Contrast X-rays

The development of contrast X-ray imaging techniques has extended the usefulness of X-rays. Fluid-filled or hollow

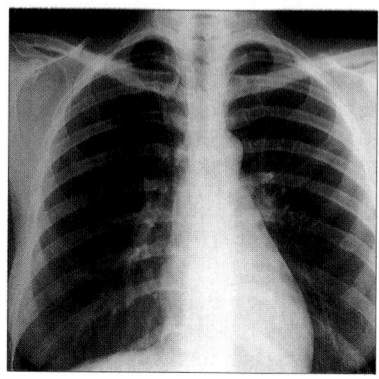

A chest X-ray
The lungs, which are full of air, appear as dark areas on X-ray film; denser structures, such as the heart and skeleton, appear white.

parts of the body that would not show up well on conventional X-rays can be seen clearly on X-rays if they are first filled with a contrast medium (substance opaque to X-rays).

Commonly used examples of contrast X-ray techniques are urography, which is performed to obtain X-ray pictures of the urinary system, and barium X-ray examinations, which are used to investigate the digestive tract. Angiography, in which contrast medium is injected into blood vessels, is used to investigate diseases that alter the appearance of the blood vessels.

Digital subtraction angiography

The technique of digital subtraction angiography uses computers to process images obtained before and after the injection of contrast medium into the patient's bloodstream. The computer subtracts

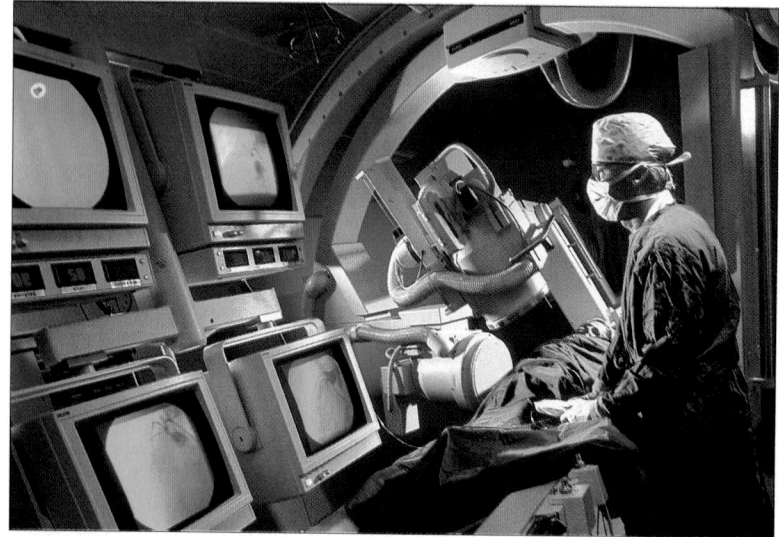

Digital subtraction angiography
This technique is a form of contrast X-ray imaging that uses computers to improve the image. Doctors in this unit watch the screens to monitor the introduction of a contrast medium into the patient's bloodstream and to obtain a clear image of the arteries.

CT SCANNING

CT scanning can be used to obtain images of virtually any part of the body. This technique combines the use of X-rays with computer technology to produce a two- or three-dimensional image of an area. The CT scan included here shows a cross-section through the trunk along the plane shown, at the level of the kidneys. The image has been artificially coloured by computer to make the internal structures (the most important of which have been labelled) more clearly visible.

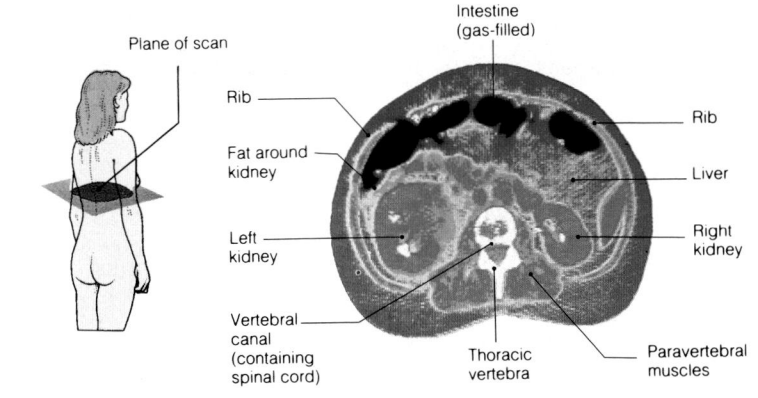

Plane of scan

Intestine (gas-filled)

Rib — — Rib

Fat around kidney — — Liver

Left kidney — — Right kidney

Vertebral canal (containing spinal cord)

Thoracic vertebra

Paravertebral muscles

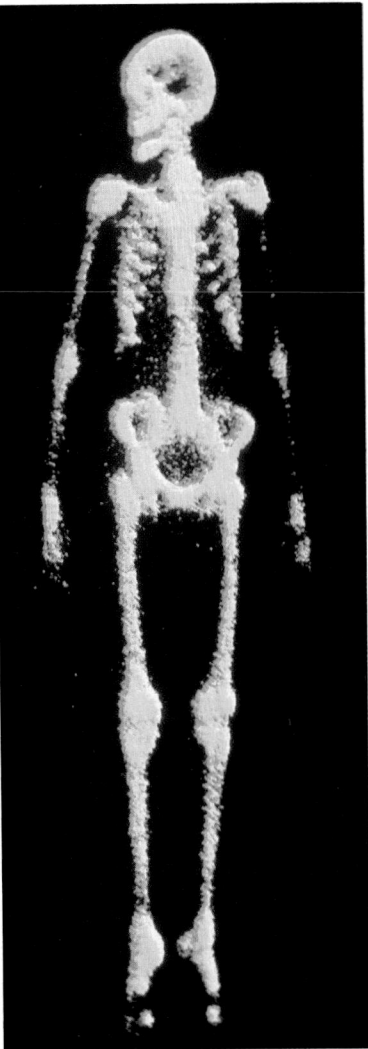

A radionuclide bone scan
This radionuclide bone scan shows a front view of the complete skeleton of a healthy person. Bone scanning is an essential step in assessing treatment for some types of cancer, such as breast cancer, because it can reveal whether or not the cancer has spread beyond its primary site and developed secondary growths in the bones. Cancerous areas appear as bright "hot spots" on radionuclide scans.

(i.e. removes) unwanted background detail, leaving a clear image of the blood vessels.

CT scanning

Conventional X-rays are essentially shadow photographs, but CT (computed tomography) scanning uses X-rays in a completely different way. Multiple beams of X-rays are passed through the body, and their degree of absorption is recorded by sensors. The scanner moves around the patient, emitting and recording X-ray beams from every point. The resulting data are then analysed by a computer, which uses the variations in absorption of the X-rays to construct cross-sectional "slices" through the body.

CT images are more detailed than those produced by conventional X-ray techniques. A further advantage of CT scanning is that images can be manipulated by the computer to obtain a better view of the area under study, or to produce a three-dimensional image. CT scanning was first used, in the early 1970s, for studying the brain. The technique quickly became a first-line test in the investigation not only of brain disorders but also of symptoms affecting virtually every other part of the body.

Radionuclide scanning

Images obtained by conventional X-ray techniques or by CT scanning depend on physical differences (notably in density) among body structures. Imaging by radionuclide scanning utilizes another approach. In this technique, radioactive chemicals are either swallowed by the patient or injected into the bloodstream. These chemicals are taken up by certain organs or tissues, which then give off radiation that can be detected and analysed by a gamma camera.

The amount of radiation emitted by a part of the body depends mainly on the level of metabolic activity of its constituent cells. Thus, cells that are dividing rapidly (such as cancer cells) show up in some cases as "hot spots" on radionuclide scans.

The substances used in radionuclide scanning are usually either radioactive forms of elements that are normally found in the body, such as iodine, or synthetic radioactive elements, such as technetium. The levels of radiation to which the body is exposed in radionuclide scanning are very low, usually considerably lower than in conventional X-rays.

DIAGNOSTIC TECHNIQUES 2

MRI

Unlike X-ray imaging, CT scanning, and radionuclide imaging, MRI (magnetic resonance imaging) does not employ potentially damaging ionizing radiation. Instead, it exploits the natural behaviour of the protons (nuclei) of hydrogen atoms when they are subjected to a very strong magnetic field and radio waves.

For MRI, the patient lies inside a large, hollow, cylindrical magnet in which the body is exposed to a magnetic field many thousands of times more powerful than that of the Earth. Under the influence of the scanner's magnetic field, the protons in the body, which normally point randomly in different directions, line up parallel to each other. A strong pulse of radio waves is then used to knock the protons out of alignment. As the protons realign themselves, they produce detectable radio signals, which are picked up by radio receiver coils in the scanner. A computer then converts these radio signals into a two-

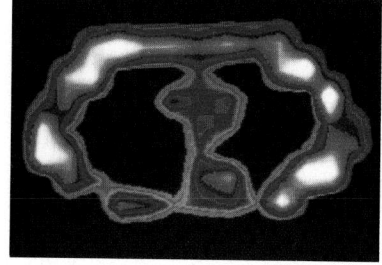 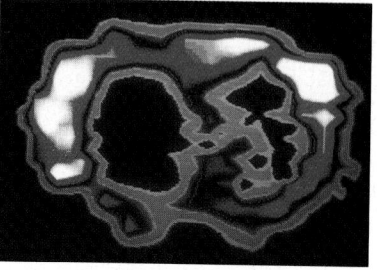

MRI chest scans
These scans show cross-sectional views through a normal chest (above) and through the chest of a patient with a lung tumour (above right). The lungs appear as black areas in the middle and the ribs as yellow-red crescents. The tumour is indicated by the increased blue area and by the affected lung's small size.

dimensional or three-dimensional image based on the strength and location of the signals.

The most abundant sources of protons in the body are the hydrogen atoms in water molecules; an MRI scan thus reflects differences in the water content of tissues.

Superficially, MRI scans look like CT scans. However, MRI scans give a much more detailed picture of the structure of soft tissues because of the differences in water content within these tissues. MRI scans are particularly useful for studying the brain and spinal cord. They are also useful for imaging other soft tissues.

A newer application of MRI, known as magnetic resonance spectroscopy, relies on the detection of other chemical elements, such as phosphorus and calcium. Magnetic resonance spectroscopy can provide useful information on organ function.

Ultrasound scanning

The diagnostic use of ultrasound is based on the principle of naval sonar, in which sound waves are used to locate underwater objects

MRI SCAN OF HEAD
This MRI scan shows a longitudinal section through the middle of the head and upper neck. The image has been artificially coloured to differentiate the internal structures according to differences in water content. MRI scanning is very useful for studying the brain because it allows the detailed structure of the soft brain tissues to be clearly imaged.

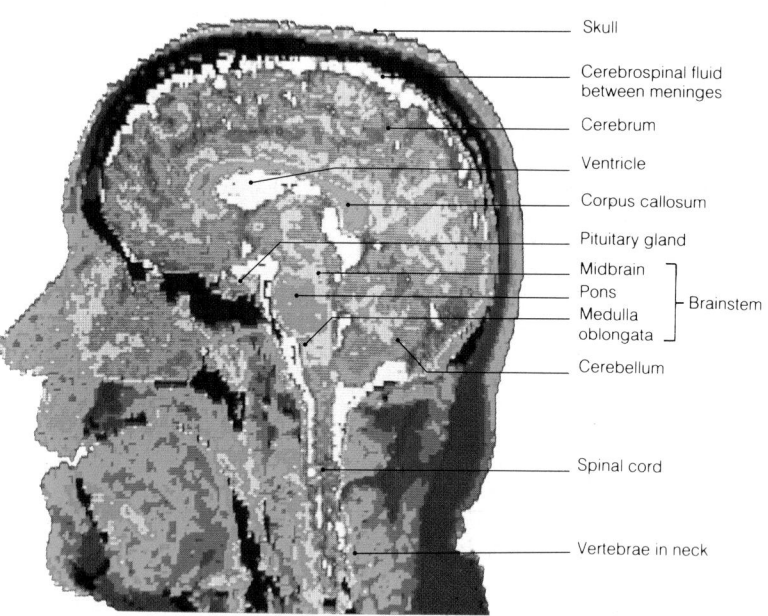

Skull
Cerebrospinal fluid between meninges
Cerebrum
Ventricle
Corpus callosum
Pituitary gland
Midbrain
Pons — Brainstem
Medulla oblongata
Cerebellum
Spinal cord
Vertebrae in neck

by their echoes. Ultrasound scanning causes no discomfort and is thought to be completely safe.

In ultrasound scanning, a device called a transducer is placed on the skin and transmits inaudible high-frequency sound waves into the body, where they are reflected by the internal structures. The transducer detects these echoes, which are converted to numerical data and then displayed directly on a screen or analysed by computer to produce an image of the structures.

The technique is especially useful in obstetrics because it enables the obstetrician to examine the fetus at no known risk to either the pregnant woman or her developing child. Ultrasound waves are converted into an image of the fetus and enable the obstetrician to identify multiple pregnancies, to measure the size of the fetus (so that its age can be assessed), and to detect various defects.

Another ultrasound procedure, known as echocardiography, provides information about the heart, including the structure and flexibility of heart valves, the condition of the heart muscle, and the flow of blood within the heart.

A modification of the basic ultrasound technique makes use of the Doppler effect (the change in pitch that occurs when a sound source is moving relative to the detector) to give information about the rate of blood flow through the heart and blood vessels. This procedure enables the doctor to detect narrowing of blood vessels or turbulence in the flow of blood.

PET scanning

PET (positron emission tomography) scanning is a development of radionuclide scanning. Both techniques use a radioactive substance to produce an image that reflects the level of metabolic activity of cells within the tissues. However, PET scanning, unlike radionuclide scanning, allows a cross-sectional image to be built up.

In PET scanning, a substance that takes part in normal metabolic processes is radioactively labelled (i.e. replaced with a radioactive form of the substance) and then injected into the bloodstream. The radioactive substance is taken up by the most metabolically active areas of tissue, where it emits positrons. The positrons, in turn, release photons, which are then detected by an array of sensors around the patient. The sensors are linked to a computer, which calculates the origins of the photons to construct an image of the distribution of the substance within the tissues.

PET scanning is currently being used for investigating brain tumours, for locating the origin of epileptic activity, and for study-

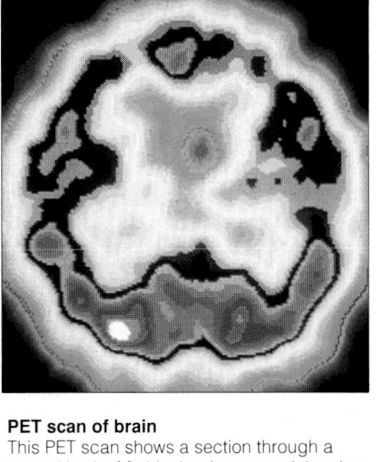

PET scan of brain
This PET scan shows a section through a normal brain. Methionine (an essential amino acid) has been used to show levels of protein synthesis within the brain; different levels of metabolic activity show up as different colours in the scan. Other brain functions can be imaged by using different substances, such as the use of a radioactive form of glucose to show different levels of carbohydrate metabolism.

ing the brain function in various mental illnesses. It is also being used for investigating the heart, and it is expected to be useful for studying other organs.

Biochemical analysis

A doctor may arrange for biochemical tests on samples of blood, urine, and other body fluids such as spinal fluid, saliva, or sweat. These tests may be part of a diagnostic investigation in which the chemical constituents of body fluids are checked primarily to confirm a diagnosis suspected by the doctor. Biochemical tests may also be used to assess the function of a particular organ, such as the liver or kidneys.

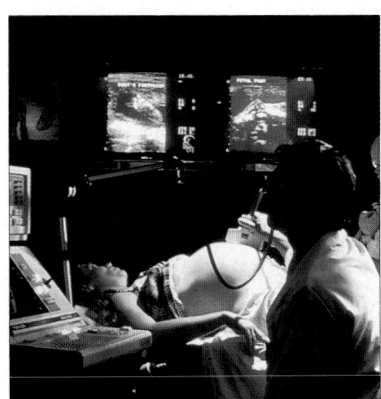

Fetal ultrasound
The photograph (above) shows the ultrasound transducer being passed over the pregnant woman's abdomen, and the ultrasound images being displayed on computer screens. The ultrasound scan (right) shows a 12-week-old fetus, whose body parts are annotated in the accompanying diagram (far right).

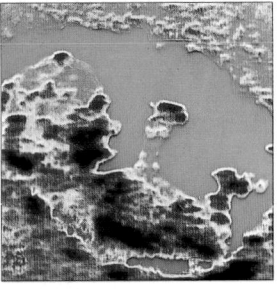

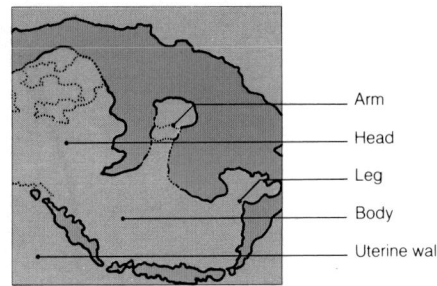

Arm

Head

Leg

Body

Uterine wall

DIAGNOSTIC TECHNIQUES 3

Biopsy

Biopsy is the removal of a sample of tissue or cells from a living patient. Such samples are then examined under a microscope and may be subjected to a variety of biochemical tests. Biopsy thus provides a valuable aid in establishing a precise diagnosis.

Samples of some types of tissue may be removed by passing a hollow needle through the skin and into the target organ or tissue. Other samples may be removed surgically or endoscopically.

Biopsy is useful in the investigation of tumours or cysts in organs such as the breast, ovary, testis, or thyroid. This procedure provides doctors with an important means of determining whether a tumour is benign or malignant, thus allowing appropriate treatment to be carried out. Biopsy can also be used to determine the cause of other disorders, such as unexplained inflammation or degeneration of the liver, kidneys, muscle, or skin.

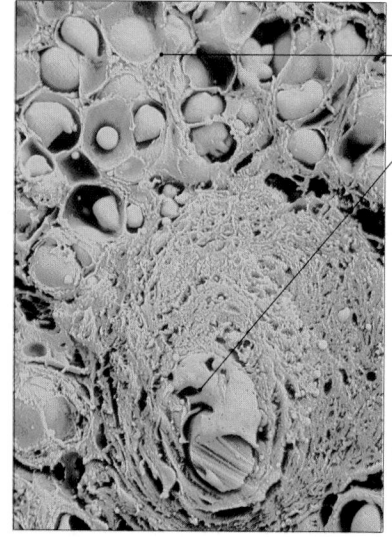

Normal ovarian tissue

Malignant teratoma

Ovarian biopsy sample
The development of biopsy—in which samples of tissue are removed from the body for microscopic analysis—has proved very useful in the diagnosis of a great many disorders. Biopsy samples may be examined in the laboratory under a light microscope or, occasionally, under a scanning electron microscope. This example of a scanning electron micrograph shows a sample of ovarian tissue in which a malignant teratoma (a type of ovarian cancer) can be seen invading the normal ovarian tissue.

Endoscopy

Endoscopy is an investigative procedure that enables a doctor to look directly into a patient's body by means of a viewing instrument known as an endoscope.

Early endoscopes were rigid or partially rigid tubes, sometimes with complex lens systems and interior lighting. The application of fibre-optics in the 1950s gave rise to flexible endoscopes, making the technique more versatile.

Today, many specialized endoscopes, both rigid and flexible, are available, enabling doctors to view virtually any structure in the body, including the digestive tract, nasal sinuses, lungs, bladder, abdominal cavity, and joints. Many endoscopes have attachments for the removal of biopsy samples. Some are fitted with a small video camera, which allows the surgeon to examine the interior of the organ on a screen in the operating theatre. This has led to the development of a new discipline, minimally invasive surgery (see p. 48).

Fetoscopy

Fetoscopy is a procedure for observing a fetus inside the uterus using a fetoscope, a type of endoscope, passed into the uterus via a small incision in the abdomen.

Fetoscopy may be performed if a physical malformation in the fetus, such as spina bifida, is suspected. Attachments on the fetoscope also enable blood or skin samples to be removed to test for certain genetic or other disorders.

ENDOSCOPY OF COLON
The colon can be viewed through a flexible endoscope known as a colonoscope. The technique of colonoscopy is useful in the diagnosis of such disorders as intestinal polyps, inflammatory bowel disorders, and cancer of the large intestine. The inset photograph shows normal intestinal lining as seen through a colonoscope.

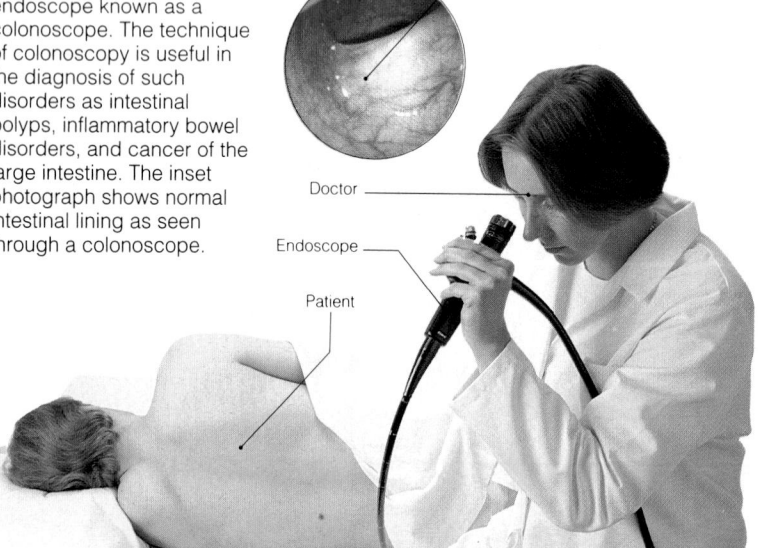

A view through an endoscope showing a healthy colon wall

Doctor

Endoscope

Patient

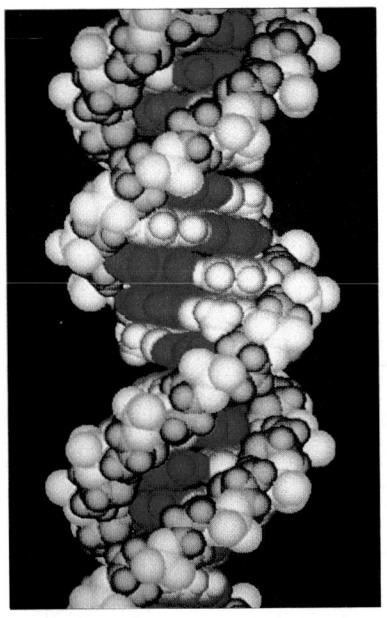

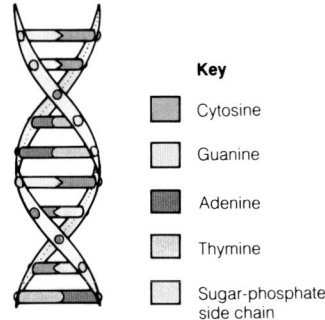

Key

■ Cytosine

□ Guanine

■ Adenine

□ Thymine

□ Sugar-phosphate side chain

Structure of DNA
DNA is a large, double-helix-shaped molecule, as shown in the computer-generated model (left). The DNA molecule consists of two sugar-phosphate side chains linked by the nucleotide bases cytosine, guanine, adenine, and thymine, as shown in the diagram (above). The DNA within each cell carries the 50,000-plus genes that control cellular activities; thus a defective gene may disrupt cellular activity and lead to a genetic disorder, such as cystic fibrosis or haemophilia.

Amniocentesis

Amniocentesis is the removal and testing of a sample of the amniotic fluid that surrounds the fetus in the uterus. Tests on the cells and fluid removed can be used to diagnose certain fetal abnormalities early enough in pregnancy for elective abortion to remain a feasible option. However, because amniocentesis carries a small risk of causing miscarriage, this procedure is recommended only in some cases.

Amniocentesis is technically possible at around the 12th week of pregnancy, but is usually delayed until the 16th to 18th week to reduce to a minimum the risk of causing a miscarriage. Results cannot usually be obtained until the 18th to 20th week of pregnancy.

The sample of amniotic fluid contains fetal cells, which are cultured to provide chromosomes for analysis. Analysis of chromosomes makes it possible to identify chromosomal abnormalities, such as Down's syndrome. Amniocentesis also allows the measurement of various substances in the amniotic fluid. Abnormal levels of such substances may indicate other, non-

chromosomal disorders of the fetus. For example, raised levels of alpha-fetoprotein may indicate spina bifida.

Chorionic villus sampling

Chorionic villus sampling is another method of diagnosing fetal abnormalities. The sample can be taken as early as eight to nine weeks into pregnancy, and testing can usually begin at once. This technique thus gives earlier results than amniocentesis.

Chorionic villus sampling is performed by removing a small sample of tissue from the fetal side of the placenta, and then analysing this sample in the laboratory. The cells in the tissue sample are genetically identical to those of the fetus, and analysis of this sample shows whether the fetus has certain types of chromosomal or genetic disorders.

Genetic analysis

Genetic analysis may be performed in high-risk pregnancies (i.e. when there is a family history of a genetic disorder or when a couple has had a child with such a disorder) to investigate whether a fetus has a disorder of this type,

such as haemophilia or cystic fibrosis. Cell samples for genetic analysis during pregnancy are obtained by amniocentesis or by chorionic villus sampling.

Genetic analysis may also be used to determine whether a person with a family history of a genetic disorder is affected by the disorder, or is a carrier of the disorder and is thus at risk of having affected children.

An important technique in genetic analysis involves the use of genetic probes. A genetic probe is a specific fragment of DNA (the genetic material contained in the chromosomes of all cells) that can be used in laboratory tests to determine whether a particular gene defect is present in an individual's genetic material.

Geneticists are currently building up a complete picture of how human DNA is arranged, showing the position of individual genes in each chromosome. This information is invaluable in the identification of genetic disorders. In many cases, it is not yet possible to detect a defective gene itself. However, for certain gene defects, researchers have identified markers (sections of DNA with a specific base sequence) that very commonly occur on particular chromosomes in association with the defect. The presence of a marker thus provides strong evidence that the associated gene defect is also present.

Sickle cell anaemia
Beta-thalassaemia
Methaemoglobinaemia
Polycythaemia vera

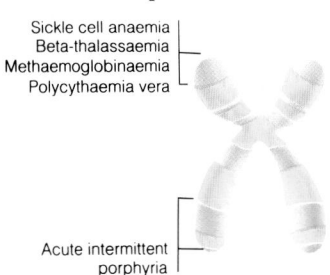

Acute intermittent porphyria

Gene map of chromosome 11
This gene map shows the location of gene defects responsible for various inherited blood disorders, and for the metabolic disorder acute intermittent porphyria. Other gene defects have been located on other chromosomes.

TREATING DISEASE

Most illnesses and injuries are not serious, and most sufferers recover completely within a few days without ever having to see a doctor. In other cases, however, a medical consultation will be necessary, so that a doctor can diagnose the disorder and prescribe suitable treatment. Sometimes a doctor will need to refer patients to a consultant for specialist treatment.

Self-treatment

For treating many disorders, simple self-help measures are all that are needed. Most self-treatments—such as resting in bed, drinking plenty of fluids, or taking over-the-counter medications—are intended to relieve symptoms and to help you feel more comfortable until your illness has run its natural course. Cold remedies, for example, will help relieve the symptoms of nasal congestion, fever, and aches, but will not attack the virus that has caused the cold.

Seeing your doctor

If your symptoms persist, or get worse, you may need to consult a doctor so that your problem can be diagnosed and treated.

If specific treatment is available, the doctor will arrange this. For example, he or she may insert stitches to treat a cut, or may prescribe antihypertensive drugs to treat raised blood pressure. If no specific treatment is available, as in the case of many viral infections, the doctor will provide or advise treatment that will relieve symptoms and help make you feel more comfortable while the disease runs its course.

If your problem requires further medical investigation, or some form of specialist treatment, you will usually be referred by your doctor to a hospital-based consultant. Specialist treatment may involve taking medication, undergoing surgery, or receiving some other form of treatment.

Drug treatment

Until well into this century, doctors had few effective drugs with which to work, and as a result were unable to cure or even to slow down the progress of many diseases. Traditionally, many of the drugs that have proved useful, such as morphine and digitalis, were derived from plants.

The situation changed dramatically in the 1930s, with the introduction of antibacterial drugs, advances in the production of synthetic drugs, and the development of drugs that act on the body's metabolic processes. Since then, progress has been rapid, with the development of an even wider range of effective drugs, and with developments in drug production, such as the application of genetic engineering techniques.

Although immunization began in 1796, when Edward Jenner gave the first smallpox inoculation, it was not until this century that

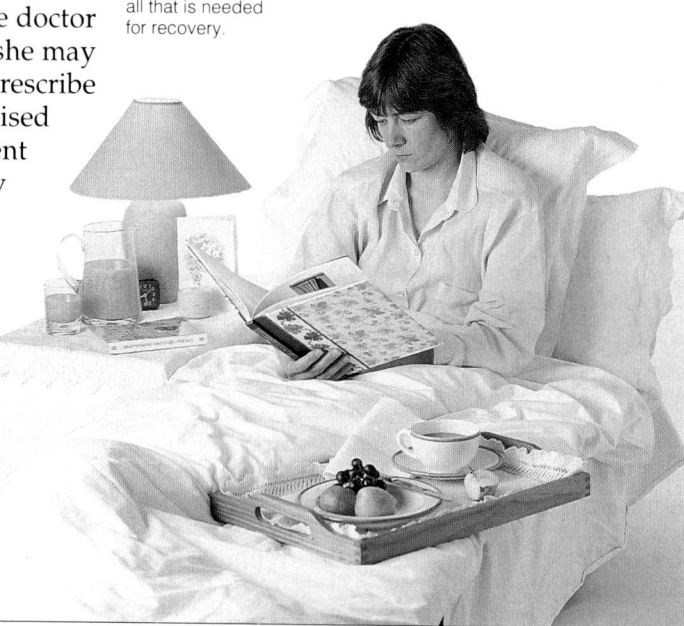

Bed rest
Simply resting in bed may be all that is needed for recovery.

vaccines against other potentially lethal human diseases were developed. Today, vaccines are available against measles, mumps, diphtheria, poliomyelitis, tetanus, pertussis, rubella, tuberculosis, and various other, less common, diseases such as hepatitis, typhoid, rabies, cholera, and yellow fever.

Before any new substance can be marketed as a drug, it must be thoroughly tested for effectiveness and safety, approved by the Committee on Safety of Medicines, and licensed by the Department of Health. The form in which a drug is produced may depend on the nature of the drug itself, the dosage in which it needs to be taken, and the length of time over which it will act.

Surgical treatment

Considerable advances in surgery in the 19th and early 20th centuries—the introduction of general anaesthesia in the 1840s, antiseptic procedures in the 1870s, and blood transfusions in the early 1900s—paved the way for many new surgical techniques.

During the first half of the 20th century, surgery consisted of the cutting out of diseased parts of the body and the repair of injuries.

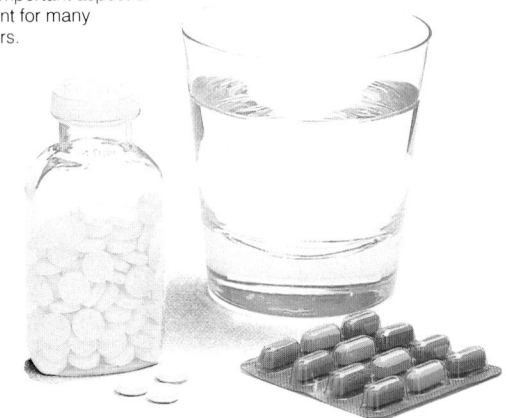

Drug remedies
Over-the-counter drugs or drugs obtained on a doctor's prescription are an important aspect of treatment for many disorders.

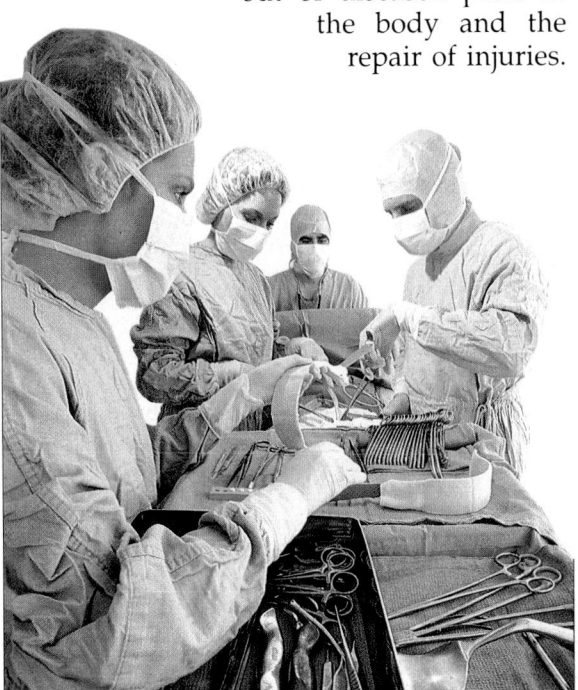

After the Second World War, technological advances enabled surgeons to substitute diseased body parts with man-made joints, valves, and blood vessels, and organs taken from human donors for transplantation. In recent decades, further technological advances have opened up the new disciplines of microsurgery and minimally invasive surgery. Operations are performed—often with the use of lasers—under remote control, using endoscopes and video techniques, which allows greater control and precision.

Other treatments

Drug treatment and surgery are still the primary divisions of medical care, but technological advances have led to the development of other forms of treatment. Radiotherapy plays a central part in the treatment of many forms of cancer, and modern medicine increasingly employs recently developed procedures, such as endoscopy, lithotripsy, and laser treatment, that avoid the need for open surgery. Some new areas of treatment, such as intensive care or neonatology, have become so specialized in recent years that they have developed into separate branches of medicine.

Surgery
Surgical procedures are necessary for the treatment of a wide variety of medical disorders. Surgical operations may be performed under general anaesthesia (as here) or under local anaesthesia.

This century has seen major advances in the treatment of disease. Large numbers of new drugs have been discovered and developed. Many lives are now saved by new intensive-care methods and by techniques such as dialysis and radiotherapy. Surgical advances—including developments in transplant surgery, implant surgery, and microsurgery—have increased the surgeon's range. For some disorders, surgery has been superseded by less invasive techniques, such as lithotripsy, laser treatment, and endoscopy.

Drug treatment

The value of drugs in the treatment of disorders has been known for many thousands of years, and the use of drugs is still an extremely important aspect of medical treatment.

Some drugs, such as aspirin, can be bought over the counter without a doctor's prescription. Other drugs, such as penicillin, can be obtained only on presentation of a prescription to a pharmacist in a shop or hospital pharmacy. Certain drugs, such as the anticancer drug cisplatin, are normally administered only by doctors or nurses in a hospital.

Drugs are available in many different forms, including tablets, capsules, liquids, sprays and inhalers, ointments and creams, suppositories and pessaries, drops, powders, injections, and transdermal patches.

Drug sources

For many centuries, drugs were obtained from diverse natural sources, including many species of plants and animals, and various minerals. More recently, advances in drug production have helped pharmacologists and biochemists to develop an immense range of new drugs. In many cases, these drugs are manufactured synthetically by various chemical processes, or are produced by the newer technique of genetic engineering.

Natural drugs

Drugs that continue to be obtained from natural sources include digoxin, obtained from

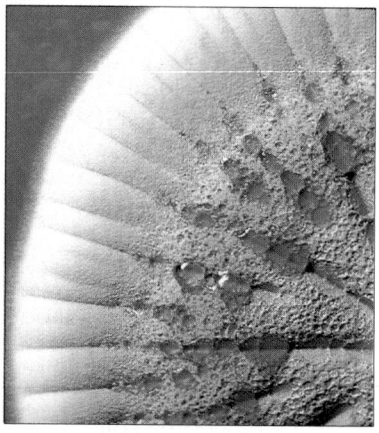

Culture of *PENICILLIUM NOTATUM*
This species of mould was an early source of the antibiotic penicillin. Today, synthetic forms of the drug are usually used.

the foxglove; vinblastine and vincristine, obtained from the periwinkle; and phenoxymethylpenicillin, obtained from a type of penicillin mould.

Other drugs, such as atropine, caffeine, and streptomycin are still sometimes obtained from natural sources but are now more often prepared synthetically.

Drugs from plant sources were originally obtained directly from various parts of the plant. For example, drug preparations could be obtained by grinding a plant's roots or seeds, or by making an infusion of its dried leaves.

Today, most drugs derived from plant sources are obtained in purer form by extracting the active ingredient in the laboratory. For example, morphine and codeine are commercially refined from opium, which is a substance obtained from the unripe seed pods of the opium poppy.

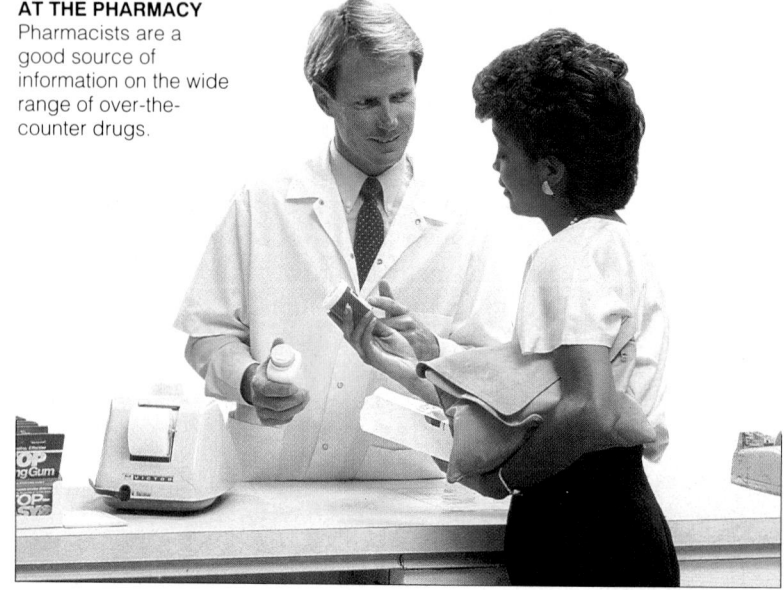

AT THE PHARMACY
Pharmacists are a good source of information on the wide range of over-the-counter drugs.

SOURCES OF DRUGS

Drugs can be placed in one of three categories according to whether they are naturally occurring, synthetically produced, or genetically engineered. At present, most are synthetically produced.

Sources	Drug names	Disorders treated
Natural drugs	Digoxin	Cardiac arrhythmias
	Phenoxymethylpenicillin	Infections
	Vinblastine	Cancers
Synthetic drugs	Cimetidine	Peptic ulcer
	Diazepam	Anxiety
	Paracetamol	Pain
	Propranolol	Hypertension
Genetically engineered drugs	Anistreplase	Coronary thrombosis
	Factor VIII	Haemophilia
	Growth hormone	Growth hormone deficiency
	Human insulin	Diabetes mellitus

Synthetic drugs

The active ingredients of many drugs that were originally derived from natural sources are now produced synthetically from chemicals. Synthetic production ensures that drugs are of consistent potency and that they are available in sufficient quantities when required.

Drugs may also be synthesized to supplement hormones or other body chemicals that are produced in insufficient amounts due to disease. One example is the synthetic drug levodopa, which is given to counteract the deficiency of the natural chemical dopamine that occurs in Parkinson's disease. Drugs developed in this purposeful way to meet particular needs may be further modified chemically to increase their potency and duration of action, or to reduce possible adverse effects.

Genetically engineered drugs

Although technically difficult to achieve, producing a human hormone or other body chemical by genetic engineering is simple in theory. The gene that instructs human cells to produce the hormone is identified, isolated, and inserted into the genetic material of a microorganism such as a bacterium or yeast. The microorganism is then cultured in large vats so that it multiplies and produces large amounts of the hormone for commercial purposes.

Genetic engineering has been applied to the production of human insulin, anistreplase (a tissue-plasminogen activator), factor VIII (used in the treatment of haemophilia), erythropoietin (used to treat some forms of anaemia), human growth hormone, and growth factors to stimulate the bone marrow into producing white blood cells. Diseases such as Gaucher's disease, which is due to lack of the enzyme glucosylceramidase, may now also be treated by replacing the missing enzyme with a genetically engineered substitute.

Gene therapy

The ultimate solution for diseases caused by a faulty or absent gene is to supply the missing gene itself, and in 1990 the first research trials of gene therapy began in the US. Patients with severe combined immunodeficiency were treated by having some of their lymphocytes removed, having the missing gene for adenosine deaminase inserted into these cells, and then having the treated lymphocytes returned to the body. Early results were encouraging, and many other research protocols are now under evaluation.

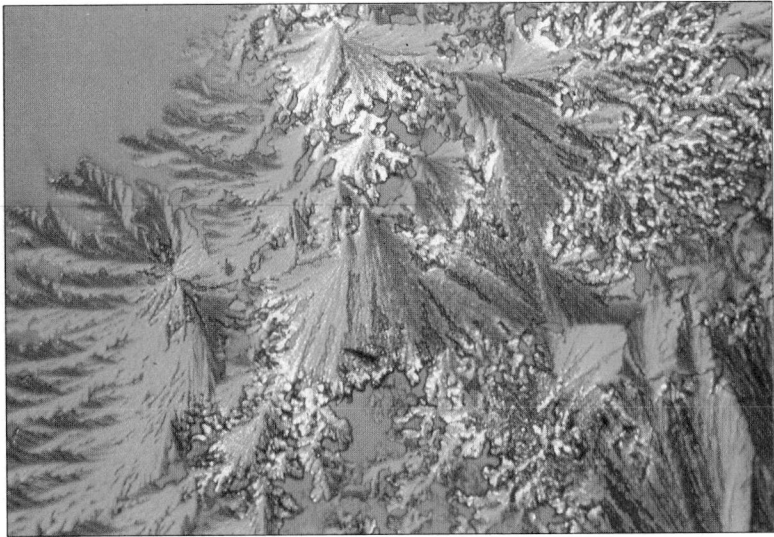

Photomicrograph of adrenaline
Adrenaline (shown here in a polarized light photomicrograph) is an example of the many different drugs that can now be produced synthetically. Naturally occurring adrenaline is a hormone secreted by the adrenal gland. Synthetically produced adrenaline is used to treat cardiac arrest and to control bleeding in surgery.

METHODS OF TREATMENT 2

Intensive care

The intensive care of seriously ill patients is an important aspect of modern medical treatment. The provision of such care has become so specialized in recent years that intensive care is now commonly considered to be a separate branch of medicine. All major hospitals have an intensive-care unit staffed by specially trained medical and nursing staff.

An intensive-care unit contains all the equipment needed to provide continuous monitoring of vital body functions (heart-rate, breathing rate, blood pressure, etc.), and to maintain a stable condition in the patient. Careful monitoring of patients allows any worsening of their condition to be detected and treated at once.

Patients in an intensive-care unit are usually given fluids intravenously through a drip, and nutrients and drugs may also be administered in this way. Many intensive-care patients also need artificial ventilation.

A coronary care unit is a type of intensive-care unit designed to provide care for patients who have had, or are suspected of having had, a myocardial infarction (heart attack).

Neonatal care

Advances in neonatal care have greatly increased the survival rate of newborn babies, especially babies who are born prematurely. The internal organs of premature babies may not be mature enough to cope independently, and many physiological functions, such as those that regulate body temperature, may not be sufficiently well-developed.

Intensive-care equipment in a neonatal unit can support the vital functions of a premature or severely ill baby. For example, an incubator may be used to provide an external environment in which the temperature, humidity, and oxygen levels can be carefully controlled, and in which the baby can be closely monitored.

Many babies in a neonatal unit will also require other support measures, such as the use of a ventilator to maintain breathing, and the use of an intravenous drip or a nasogastric tube for feeding.

Dialysis

A person whose kidneys fail will die within a few days unless the impurities that accumulate in his or her blood can be removed. Removal of impurities from the blood can be achieved artificially by the procedure of dialysis. There are two methods: haemodialysis and peritoneal dialysis.

In haemodialysis, a dialysis machine removes impurities by filtering the patient's blood through a semipermeable membrane immersed in a special dialysis solution. The procedure takes a few hours and is usually necessary several times a week.

In peritoneal dialysis, the patient's abdominal cavity lining is used to filter impurities from the blood into the dialysis solution, which is passed into and out of the abdomen through a tube.

Dialysis may be necessary for only a few days if kidney failure is temporary, but it is also effective as a long-term treatment for permanent kidney failure. In

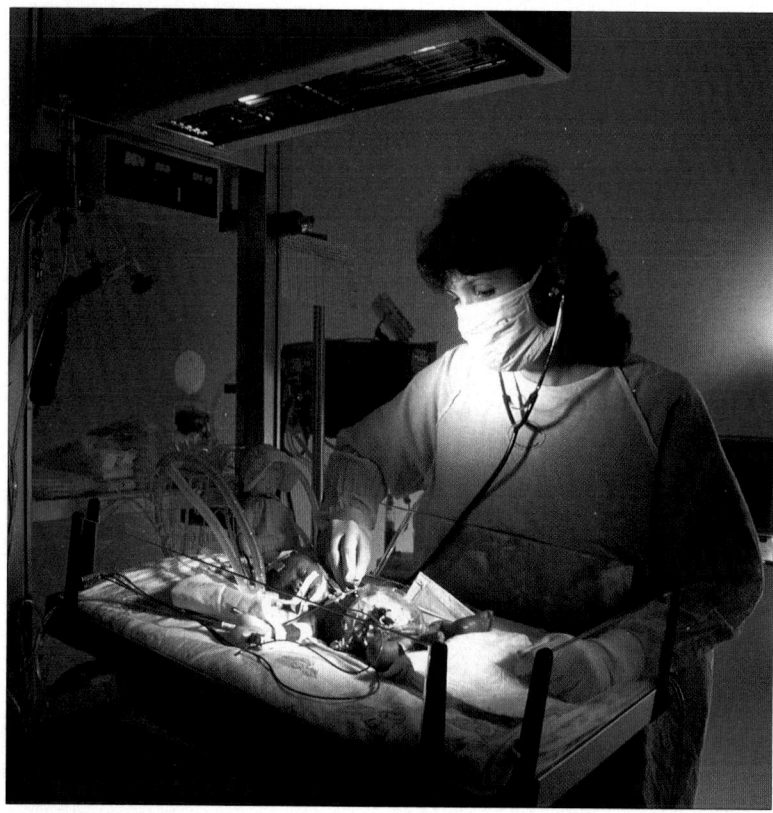

Neonatal intensive care
This photograph, taken in a neonatal intensive-care unit, shows a premature baby being examined after undergoing surgery. The baby is being artificially ventilated to assist breathing and is being given fluids intravenously. The heater above the baby's cot maintains the environment at a controlled temperature.

most cases of permanent kidney failure, however, the best remedy for the patient's condition is a kidney transplant.

Lithotripsy

Extracorporeal lithotripsy is a non-surgical procedure that uses ultrasound to pulverize calculi (stones) in the body. This technique seems likely to replace surgery as the usual treatment for certain types of kidney stones, and is a useful alternative to surgery in the treatment of gallstones.

In lithotripsy, repeated pulses of high-energy ultrasound waves are focused on a stone to break it down into tiny particles; the particles can then be passed out of the body via the urine (in the case of kidney stones) or via the faeces (in the case of gallstones).

Psychiatric treatment

People with mental disorders were formerly incarcerated in remote mental asylums. Today, most sufferers are treated in units within general hospitals or in community settings.

Lithotripsy
This technique involves focusing ultrasound shock waves on a stone until it breaks into tiny fragments that can be passed out of the body. The patient lies on a couch or in a water bath. The doctor uses ultrasound or X-ray imaging to locate the stone, and then positions the patient and the shock-wave emitter for treatment. Shock-wave pulses are then applied until the stone is pulverized.

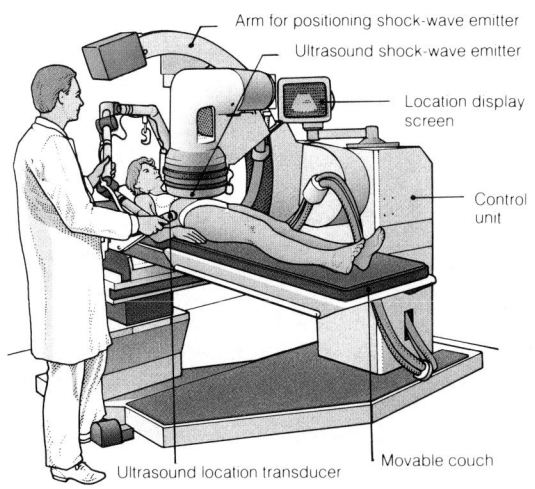

Arm for positioning shock-wave emitter
Ultrasound shock-wave emitter
Location display screen
Control unit
Movable couch
Ultrasound location transducer

The development of antipsychotic drugs and other drugs to treat psychiatric problems has transformed the outlook for many patients with severe mental disorders, such as schizophrenia or manic-depressive illness. Drug therapy enables many people to resume varying degrees of activity within the community.

Psychotherapy may be useful in the treatment of people with neuroses, personality disorders, or forms of abnormal behaviour, such as alcohol dependence or drug addiction. Psychotherapy may take the form of psychoanalysis, group therapy, or counselling.

Radiotherapy

The use of X-rays and implants of radium (a naturally radioactive substance) to treat cancers dates from the turn of this century. Today, X-rays are still used in radiotherapy, but the range of treatment has been greatly expanded to include other forms or sources of radiation (e.g. neutron beams or radioactive varieties of substances such as iodine or yttrium). Damage to surrounding healthy tissue was a significant drawback of early radiation treatment, but with modern technology it is now possible to focus radiation beams more accurately, thereby concentrating them on the tumour and minimizing damage to normal tissue.

Radiotherapy may be used alone to treat some tumours—such as basal cell carcinomas and certain tumours of the pituitary gland—but it is more often used in combination with surgery, chemotherapy, or both of these.

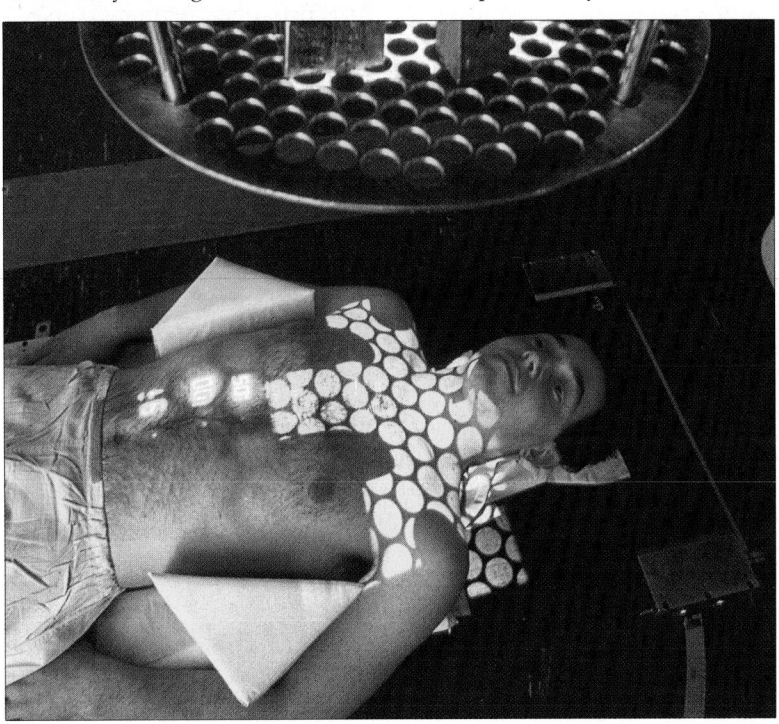

Preparing for radiotherapy
The metal platform between the radiation source and the patient protects against excessive radiation. The illuminated pattern shows the areas to be irradiated.

Surgical treatment

Surgery is the main form of treatment for a great variety of disorders. Common procedures include the removal of diseased tissue or organs, the relief of blockages, the repositioning of displaced structures, the implantation of mechanical or electronic devices, and the transplantation of tissues or organs.

Surgical implants

There are four main problems in replacing a part of the body with an artificial implant. First, the implant must be made of a material that does not provoke the immune system to reject it. Second, it must be tough enough to last for many years, so that the operation does not have to be repeated. Third, a reliable means must be found to secure the implant firmly in position. Fourth, implant surgery requires scrupulous operative techniques

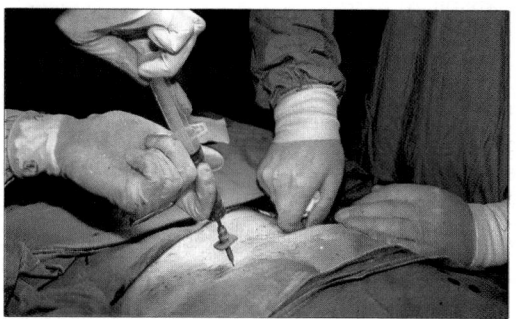

Bone marrow transplant
This photograph shows healthy bone marrow being removed via a syringe from a donor's hip-bone. This marrow will be injected into the recipient's bloodstream after the recipient's own diseased marrow has first been destroyed by radiation. Immuno-suppressant drugs are needed after the operation.

in order to prevent infection of the surrounding tissues.

Today, these problems have largely been solved, and most implants are successful; hip-joint replacements last for 10 years or more in 70 per cent of cases. Furthermore, a wide range of implants is now available: knee and finger joints as well as hip joints; heart valves; artificial lenses for the eyes; sections of blood vessels; and replacements for parts of the skull.

Transplant surgery

In the early days of transplant surgery, the only transplants that were possible without rejection were corneal transplants (which are not subject to rejection because there is no blood supply to the cornea), and those between identical twins; this inevitably limited the number of operations that could be done.

Soon, however, doctors began to treat transplant patients with immunosuppressant drugs to prevent rejection of the new organ. Because drugs that prevent rejection also suppress the immune system, they reduce resistance to infection. Consequently, many early transplant recipients survived the operation but died later as a result of infection.

Gradually, the technical problems were overcome, first with kidney transplants and later with heart and liver transplants.

Improved immunosuppressant drugs were then developed, notably cyclosporin. As a result, the success rates for transplants are now generally high.

The primary problem today is the lack of available donor organs. Many transplants are performed using organs from dead donors, but transplants of kidneys can be

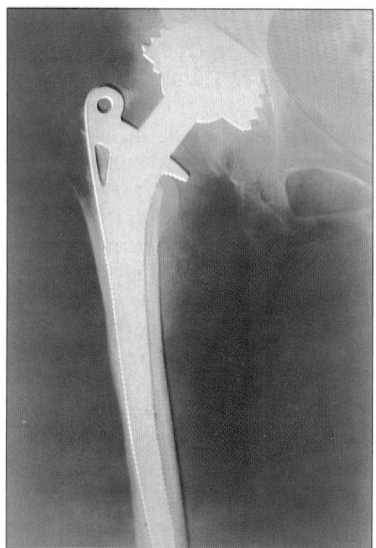

Hip replacement
This coloured X-ray shows a patient's artificial hip joint. The replacement of a damaged hip joint by an artificial substitute is one of the most successful types of implant surgery. Hip-joint replacement is most commonly performed on joints that have been damaged by arthritis.

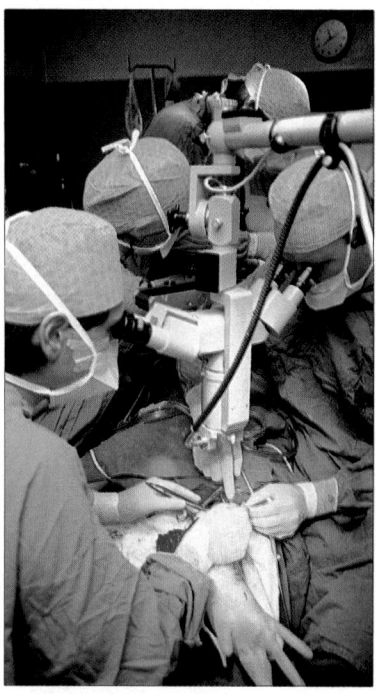

Microsurgical operation
The two surgeons in this photograph are shown performing a delicate microsurgical operation. Each is looking through a binocular eyepiece of an operating microscope, which magnifies the structures being operated on and allows the surgeons to achieve extreme precision.

done from a live donor (usually, but not always, related to the recipient); bone marrow transplants are always done from live donors. Occasionally, tissue from animals is used, for instance the transplantation of heart valves from pigs to humans. The use of fetal tissue and organs for transplantation poses technical and ethical problems that are currently a subject of debate.

Microsurgery

In microsurgery, surgeons use a specially designed microscope, delicate instruments, and fine sutures (stitches) to perform operations on minute structures, such as small nerves or blood vessels. One of the major advantages of microsurgery is that more of the tiny blood vessels and nerves can be preserved, minimizing damage to the tissues being repaired and thus reducing the amount of scar tissue formed.

Microsurgical techniques were pioneered in ear operations for deafness and then developed in eye surgery. Now the techniques are used widely in surgery of the ear, nose, throat, eyes, and nervous system. They have advanced the scope of plastic and reconstructive surgery. Microsurgery has

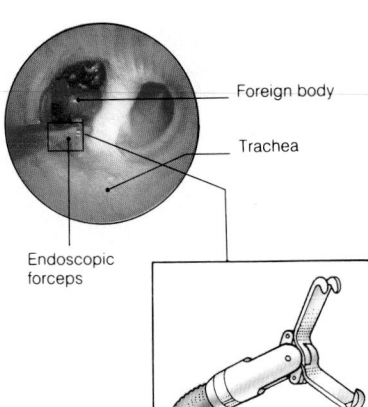

Endoscopic removal of an object
This circular view through an endoscope shows forceps removing an inhaled object from the trachea.

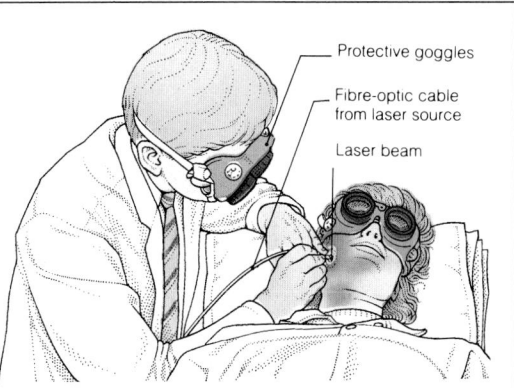

Protective goggles
Fibre-optic cable from laser source
Laser beam

enabled surgeons to reattach severed fingers, toes, and complete limbs. When the vas deferens or fallopian tubes have been divided for contraceptive reasons the cut ends may later be reunited with a good chance of restoring fertility.

Laser surgery

A laser produces a narrow beam of intense energy that surgeons can use as a "light knife" to cut through tissue, usually without causing damage beyond the target area. As it cuts, the laser simultaneously cauterizes blood vessels, thus sealing them and stemming blood flow.

Lasers are widely used in ophthalmology, especially for operations on the retina. Ophthalmic uses include the repair of retinal tears and the destruction of small retinal tumours. Uses in other branches of surgery include the sealing of bleeding arteries in peptic ulcers; the destruction of abnormal cells in various parts of the body, such as the cervix; the treatment of endometriosis; and the removal of some skin blemishes.

Endoscopic surgery

Endoscopes are used not only for diagnosis, but also for performing certain surgical procedures. Special attachments, such as scissors or a wire loop, may be fitted to remove tumours, and sharp-toothed forceps may be used to

grasp and remove foreign bodies. Other operations for which endoscopes are used include the removal of stones from the urinary tract, and the repair of damaged joint cartilage.

Endoscopic surgery is generally safer and easier to perform than conventional surgical techniques. Surgery performed using an endoscope also causes less tissue damage, producing less discomfort and a quicker recovery for the patient.

USES OF ENDOSCOPY
Listed here are some new uses for various types of endoscopy; all these procedures formerly required open surgery.

Endoscope	Possible uses
Arthroscopy	Repair of damaged joint cartilage
Bronchoscopy	Removal of foreign bodies from bronchi
Colonoscopy	Removal of intestinal polyps
Cystoscopy	Removal of bladder calculi (stones)
Fetoscopy	Correction of fetal urinary tract defects
Gastroscopy	Treatment of bleeding peptic ulcers
Laparoscopy	Female sterilization

Foreign body
Trachea
Endoscopic forceps

Minimally invasive surgery

In the late 1980s, the approach to abdominal surgery was transformed by the development of minimally invasive surgery. A laparoscope (a viewing instrument) fitted with a miniature video camera is passed into the abdomen through an opening about 10 mm wide, enabling the surgeon to view the abdominal cavity on a television monitor. Further small openings are made for precision instruments, suction cannulas, and retractors, and the entire operation can be performed without the need for a long surgical incision.

The rapid expansion of minimally invasive surgery has led to the development of new instruments and techniques. Lasers are often used instead of scalpels to cut and shape tissues, and laser-activated tissue glues may be used to join structures together. Basic instruments such as scissors and tissue graspers have been modified to enable them to be passed into the abdomen through an opening only 5–11 mm wide. Long, narrow electrocoagulation instruments have been devised to arrest bleeding quickly—uncontrolled bleeding makes it impossible for the surgeon to see what he is doing. Hydraulic jets are sometimes used (as a substitute for the surgeon's fingers) to separate tissues. Suturing has been largely replaced by the use of miniature stapling devices. Once the operation is completed, the small incisions (usually four) in the abdomen are closed with adhesive strips, leaving little, if any, scarring visible once healing is complete.

The first routine major operation using laparoscopy under video control was gallbladder removal, performed by Dr. P. Mouret, in Lyon, France in 1987. By the early 1990s, surgeons were using minimally invasive techniques to carry out appendicectomies, vagotomies, repair of inguinal hernias, repair of perforated peptic ulcers, many gynaecological procedures, and removal of large sections of colon or a complete, diseased kidney. Large structures of this kind are separated from their attachments, placed in a plastic bag, and reduced to a semi-liquid state before being removed from the body through one of the small openings made in the abdominal wall.

The techniques can also be used for thoracic and head and neck surgery; the greatly enlarged image on the monitor often gives the surgeon a clearer view than that obtained by direct vision.

The advantage of minimally invasive surgery for the patient is that he or she is spared a long surgical incision. The effects of this extend beyond the avoidance of a long scar. Most postoperative pain is caused by the cut through the skin and muscles, the healing of which slows recovery. Conventional surgery for gallbladder removal requires a hospital stay of around 10 days, but after laparoscopic surgery a patient can usually go home after two or three days and regain full mobility within a week.

These substantial savings in length of hospital stay and time off work have to be set against the operation's greater complexity. Operating costs are higher and include the laparoscope and its attachments, disposable items such as trocars and staples, and the fees of the skilled surgeon.

Some laparoscopic procedures, involve a small but important risk of complications such as internal bleeding, which do not occur with open operations. However, since more surgeons have acquired the necessary skills, laparoscopic surgery seems to have become standard for many abdominal and gynaecological operations—with its undoubted advantages of short hospital stay, superior cosmetic result, and rapid recovery.

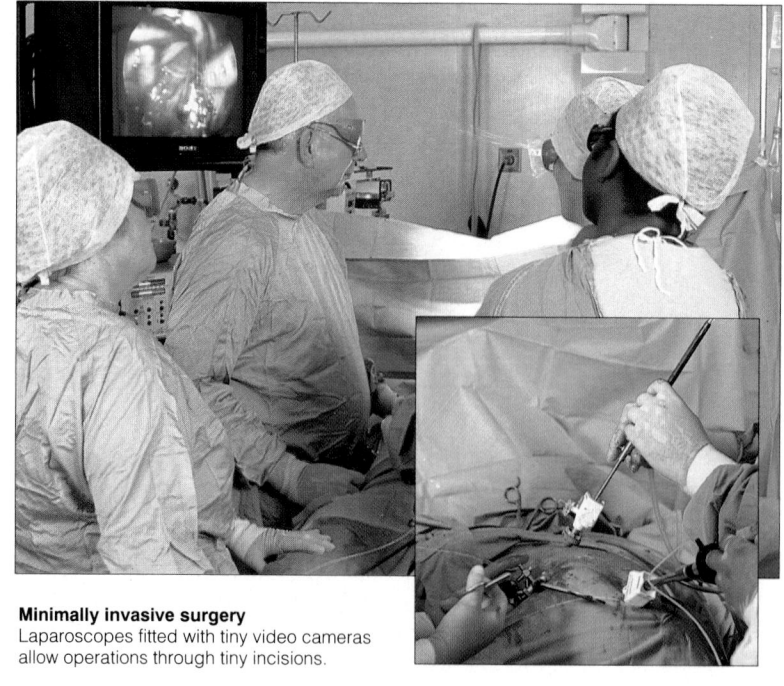

Minimally invasive surgery
Laparoscopes fitted with tiny video cameras allow operations through tiny incisions.

THE A TO Z
OF HEALTH AND
MEDICINE

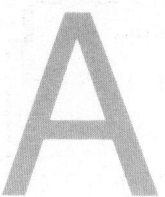

Abdomen

The region of the body between the chest and the hips. The abdominal cavity is bounded by the ribs and the diaphragm above, and by the muscles and bones of the pelvis below, with the spine and the abdominal muscles forming the back, side, and front walls. The abdominal cavity contains the liver, stomach, intestines, spleen, pancreas, and kidneys. In the lower part of the abdomen, enclosed by the pelvis, are the bladder, rectum, and, in women, the uterus and ovaries.

STRUCTURE

The spine, pelvis, and ribs provide attachments for the layers of muscle that make up the abdominal walls. There is a layer of fat between the muscles and the skin; in obese people this layer may be several centimetres thick. The inner surface of the abdominal muscles is covered by a thin membrane, the peritoneum, which

also covers the organs, such as the pancreas and kidneys, that are fixed to the back wall. Folds of peritoneum also cover the mobile organs, such as the stomach and intestines.

Abdomen, acute

The medical term for persistent, severe abdominal pain of sudden onset, usually associated with spasm of the abdominal muscles, vomiting, and fever. These symptoms suggest inflammation of one or more organs in the abdomen and indicate that urgent medical investigation is needed. This usually includes detailed questioning, a physical examination, laboratory tests, and imaging procedures, such as X-rays and ultrasound scanning. A *laparotomy* (surgical exploration of the abdomen) or a *laparoscopy* (internal examination using a viewing instrument) may be necessary in some cases.

CAUSES AND TREATMENT

The most common cause of an acute abdomen is *peritonitis* (inflammation of the membrane that lines the abdomen). Inflammation of any structure in the abdomen may lead to peritonitis—for example, *salpingitis* (inflammation of the fallopian tubes); intestinal disorders, such as *appendicitis*, *Crohn's disease*, or *diverticulitis*; or a perforated *peptic ulcer*. Abdominal injury may also be the cause.

Other possible causes of acute abdomen include urinary tract disorders, such as a stone in the ureter (see *Calculus, urinary tract*), a stone in the duct that drains the gallbladder (see *Gallstones*), or a disorder that stretches the covering of the liver, such as *hepatitis*, or of the kidneys.

In their early stages, these conditions produce similar symptoms, and the doctor will often make observations at regular intervals over several hours before reaching a final diagnosis. Abdominal pain often begins as a vague pain in the centre but then commonly becomes localized to a particular region (such as on the right side in appendicitis). If peritonitis spreads, the abdominal muscles become rigid and the pain generalized.

Treatment depends on the underlying cause, but if the diagnosis is prompt and accurate, the outlook is generally good.

Abdominal pain

Discomfort in the abdominal cavity. Accompanying symptoms may include belching, nausea, vomiting, rumbling and gurgling noises, and flatulence (wind).

CAUSES

Minor degrees of abdominal pain are experienced by everybody at some time, and often the cause is easily recognized—for example, eating unwisely, or an attack of *diarrhoea*.

Many women experience pelvic or lower abdominal pain during part of their menstrual cycle. The pain may occur before or during a period, or around the time of ovulation. Occasionally, the pain is due to a gynaecological disorder, such as *endometriosis* (in which fragments of uterine lining are present in abnormal sites within the abdomen).

A common cause of pain very low in the abdomen is *cystitis* (inflammation of the bladder). Distension of the bladder due to urinary obstruction may also cause pain.

Abdominal colic is the term used for pain that occurs every few minutes as one of the internal organs goes into muscular spasm. Waves of colicky pain may originate in the intestines, bile ducts, ureters, or uterus. Colic is an attempt by the body to overcome an obstruction, partial or total, that may be due to a stone, a tumour, or an area of inflammation. The attacks of colic may become more severe and associated with vomiting—giving the features of an "acute abdomen" (see *Abdomen, acute*).

LOCATION OF THE ABDOMEN

The abdomen is bounded by the lower ribs at the top and the pelvis below. The illustration shows the position of the abdominal organs in an adult woman.

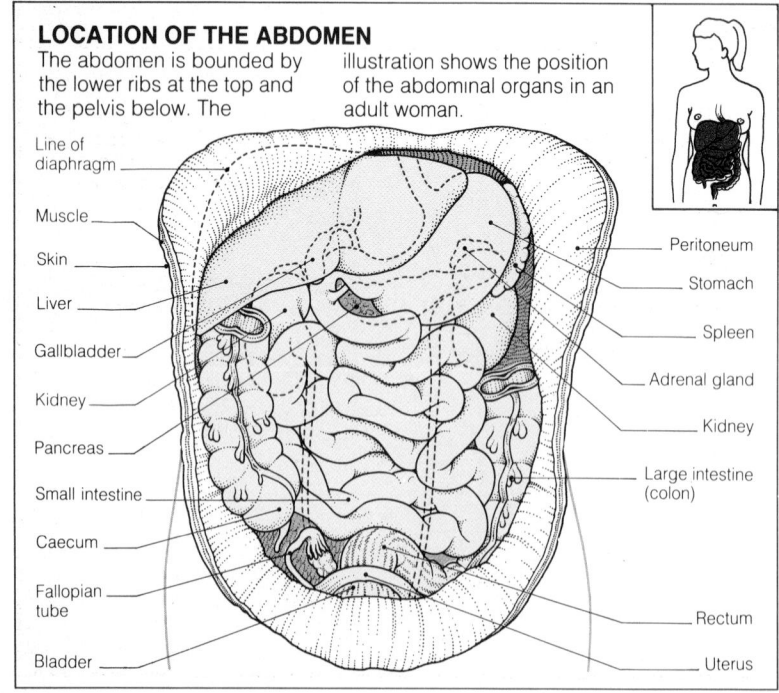

Line of diaphragm
Muscle
Skin
Liver
Gallbladder
Kidney
Pancreas
Small intestine
Caecum
Fallopian tube
Bladder

Peritoneum
Stomach
Spleen
Adrenal gland
Kidney
Large intestine (colon)
Rectum
Uterus

A

ABDOMINAL PAIN General or localized pain between the bottom of the rib cage and the groin that has occurred within the last 24 hours. See also Recurrent abdominal pain chart.

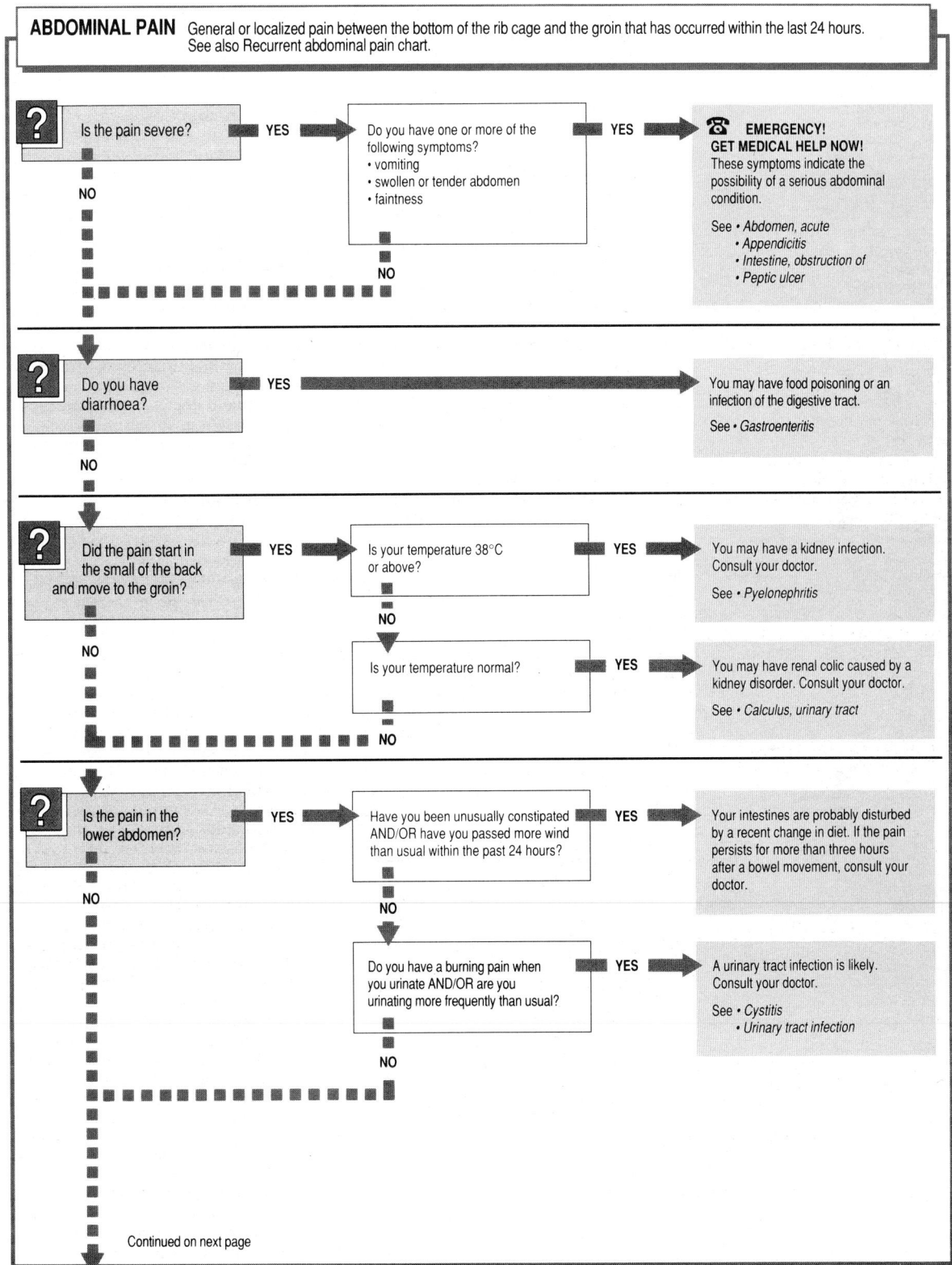

? Is the pain severe?

YES → Do you have one or more of the following symptoms?
- vomiting
- swollen or tender abdomen
- faintness

YES → ☎ **EMERGENCY!**
GET MEDICAL HELP NOW!
These symptoms indicate the possibility of a serious abdominal condition.

See • *Abdomen, acute*
• *Appendicitis*
• *Intestine, obstruction of*
• *Peptic ulcer*

NO

NO

? Do you have diarrhoea?

YES → You may have food poisoning or an infection of the digestive tract.

See • *Gastroenteritis*

NO

? Did the pain start in the small of the back and move to the groin?

YES → Is your temperature 38°C or above?

YES → You may have a kidney infection. Consult your doctor.

See • *Pyelonephritis*

NO

Is your temperature normal?

YES → You may have renal colic caused by a kidney disorder. Consult your doctor.

See • *Calculus, urinary tract*

NO

NO

? Is the pain in the lower abdomen?

YES → Have you been unusually constipated AND/OR have you passed more wind than usual within the past 24 hours?

YES → Your intestines are probably disturbed by a recent change in diet. If the pain persists for more than three hours after a bowel movement, consult your doctor.

NO

Do you have a burning pain when you urinate AND/OR are you urinating more frequently than usual?

YES → A urinary tract infection is likely. Consult your doctor.

See • *Cystitis*
• *Urinary tract infection*

NO

Continued on next page

A

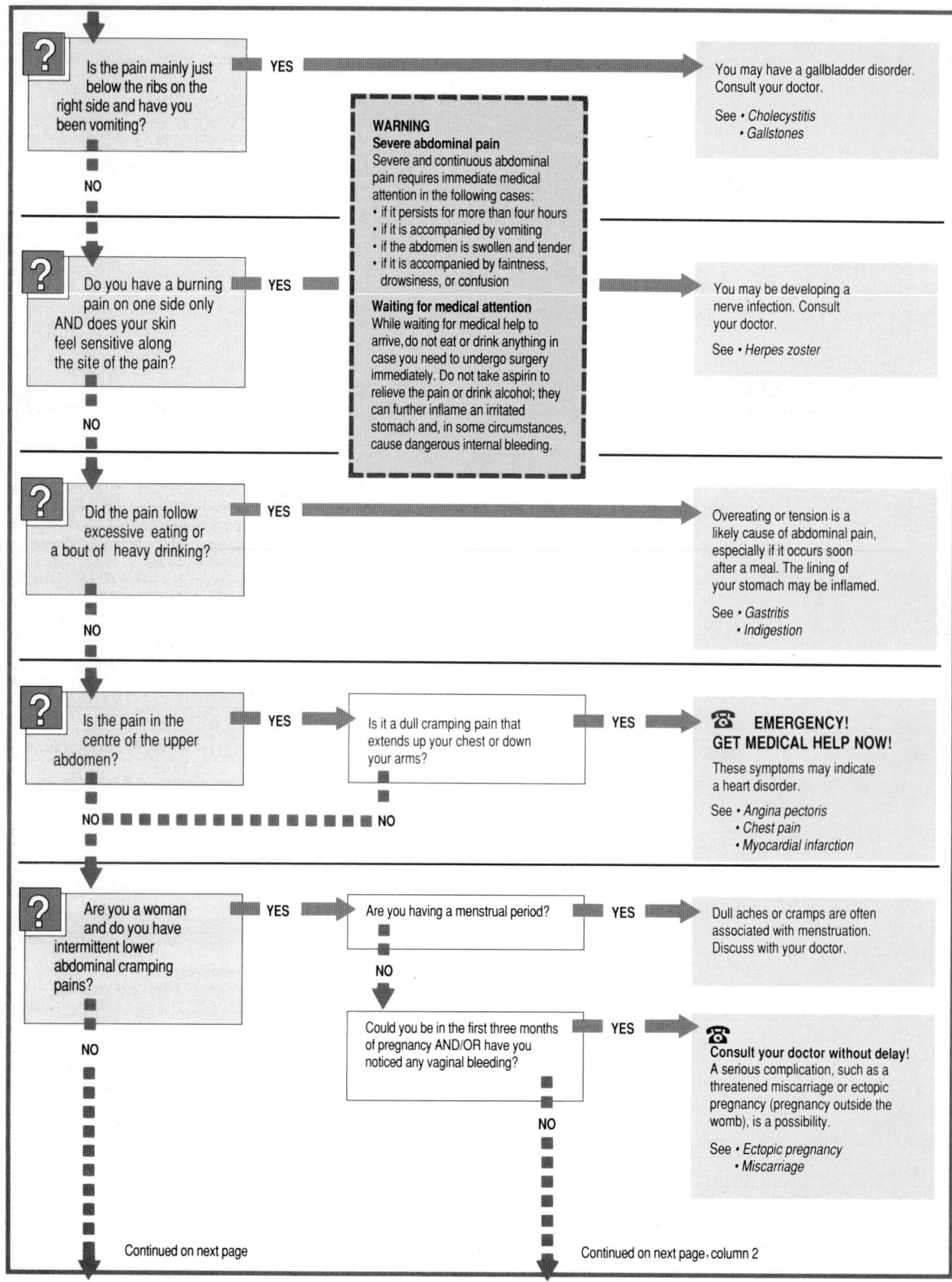

? Is the pain mainly just below the ribs on the right side and have you been vomiting?

YES → You may have a gallbladder disorder. Consult your doctor.

See • *Cholecystitis*
• *Gallstones*

NO ↓

WARNING

Severe abdominal pain
Severe and continuous abdominal pain requires immediate medical attention in the following cases:
• if it persists for more than four hours
• if it is accompanied by vomiting
• if the abdomen is swollen and tender
• if it is accompanied by faintness, drowsiness, or confusion

Waiting for medical attention
While waiting for medical help to arrive, do not eat or drink anything in case you need to undergo surgery immediately. Do not take aspirin to relieve the pain or drink alcohol; they can further inflame an irritated stomach and, in some circumstances, cause dangerous internal bleeding.

? Do you have a burning pain on one side only AND does your skin feel sensitive along the site of the pain?

YES → You may be developing a nerve infection. Consult your doctor.

See • *Herpes zoster*

NO ↓

? Did the pain follow excessive eating or a bout of heavy drinking?

YES → Overeating or tension is a likely cause of abdominal pain, especially if it occurs soon after a meal. The lining of your stomach may be inflamed.

See • *Gastritis*
• *Indigestion*

NO ↓

? Is the pain in the centre of the upper abdomen?

YES → Is it a dull cramping pain that extends up your chest or down your arms?

YES → ☎ **EMERGENCY!**
GET MEDICAL HELP NOW!

These symptoms may indicate a heart disorder.

See • *Angina pectoris*
• *Chest pain*
• *Myocardial infarction*

NO ···· NO ↓

? Are you a woman and do you have intermittent lower abdominal cramping pains?

YES → Are you having a menstrual period?

YES → Dull aches or cramps are often associated with menstruation. Discuss with your doctor.

NO ↓

Could you be in the first three months of pregnancy AND/OR have you noticed any vaginal bleeding?

YES → ☎ **Consult your doctor without delay!**
A serious complication, such as a threatened miscarriage or ectopic pregnancy (pregnancy outside the womb), is a possibility.

See • *Ectopic pregnancy*
• *Miscarriage*

NO ↓

NO ↓

Continued on next page

Continued on next page, column 2

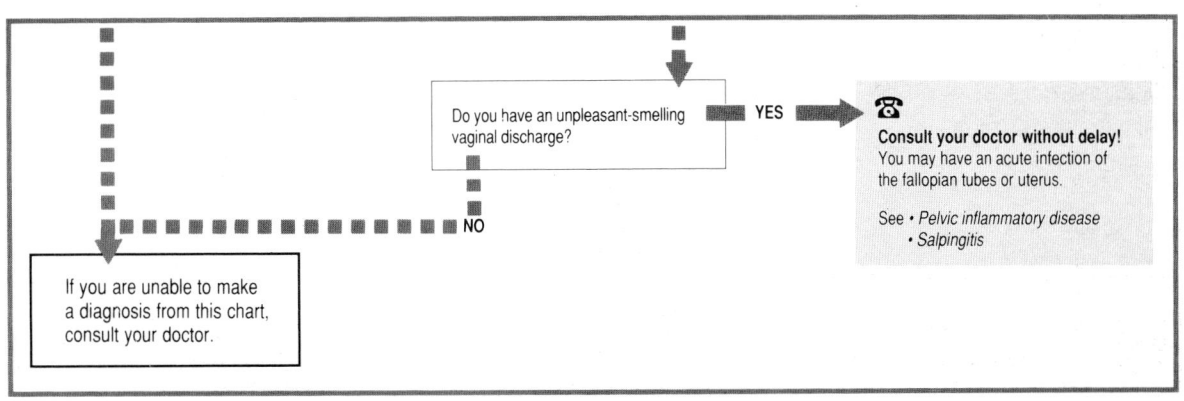

Do you have an unpleasant-smelling vaginal discharge?

YES → ☎ **Consult your doctor without delay!**
You may have an acute infection of the fallopian tubes or uterus.

See • *Pelvic inflammatory disease*
• *Salpingitis*

NO

If you are unable to make a diagnosis from this chart, consult your doctor.

RECURRENT ABDOMINAL PAIN Abdominal pain that has recurred over a week or more.

Pain mainly above the waist

? Do you sometimes get a burning pain in the centre of your chest, especially when you are bending over or lying down?

YES → Leakage of acid into the oesophagus may be causing the pain. This may occur when there is a relaxation of the muscle at the junction of the oesophagus and the stomach, and is most likely if you are overweight.

See • *Heartburn*
• *Hiatus hernia*

NO

? Does the pain come in waves mainly in the upper right side of the abdomen?

YES → Is your temperature 38°C or above?

YES → You may have an inflamed gallbladder. Consult your doctor.

See • *Cholecystitis*

NO

Is the pain temporarily relieved by antacid medicine for indigestion?

YES → Irritation of the stomach is the most likely cause of the pain. However, there is also a possibility of an ulcer. Consult your doctor.

See • *Gastritis*
• *Peptic ulcer*

NO

NO

Does the pain spread from just below the ribs on the right side?

YES → Stones in the tube that connects the gallbladder to the digestive tract may be the cause of this type of pain, especially if you have felt nauseated or have vomited. Consult your doctor.

See • *Gallstones*

NO

Continued on next page

53

A

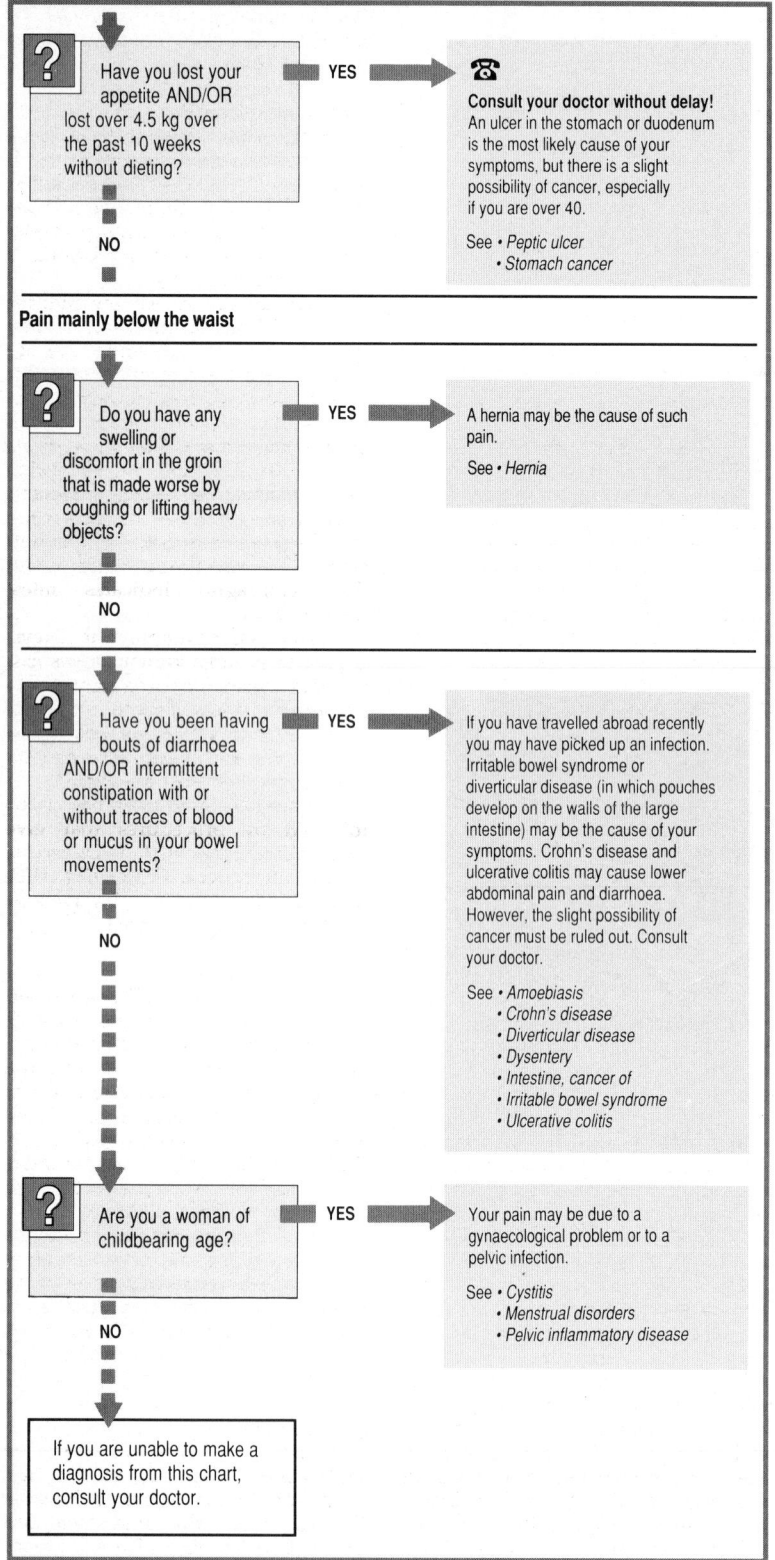

? Have you lost your appetite AND/OR lost over 4.5 kg over the past 10 weeks without dieting?

YES → ☎ **Consult your doctor without delay!**
An ulcer in the stomach or duodenum is the most likely cause of your symptoms, but there is a slight possibility of cancer, especially if you are over 40.

See • *Peptic ulcer*
       • *Stomach cancer*

NO

Pain mainly below the waist

? Do you have any swelling or discomfort in the groin that is made worse by coughing or lifting heavy objects?

YES → A hernia may be the cause of such pain.

See • *Hernia*

NO

? Have you been having bouts of diarrhoea AND/OR intermittent constipation with or without traces of blood or mucus in your bowel movements?

YES → If you have travelled abroad recently you may have picked up an infection. Irritable bowel syndrome or diverticular disease (in which pouches develop on the walls of the large intestine) may be the cause of your symptoms. Crohn's disease and ulcerative colitis may cause lower abdominal pain and diarrhoea. However, the slight possibility of cancer must be ruled out. Consult your doctor.

See • *Amoebiasis*
       • *Crohn's disease*
       • *Diverticular disease*
       • *Dysentery*
       • *Intestine, cancer of*
       • *Irritable bowel syndrome*
       • *Ulcerative colitis*

NO

? Are you a woman of childbearing age?

YES → Your pain may be due to a gynaecological problem or to a pelvic infection.

See • *Cystitis*
       • *Menstrual disorders*
       • *Pelvic inflammatory disease*

NO

If you are unable to make a diagnosis from this chart, consult your doctor.

An increase in the amount of acid formed in the stomach may be associated with the development of a *peptic ulcer*, which produces a recurrent gnawing pain that is temporarily relieved by food, milk, or by taking *antacid drugs*.

Another possible cause of abdominal pain is infection, such as *pyelonephritis* (infection of the kidneys) or *pelvic inflammatory disease* (infection of the female internal reproductive organs). Pain may also be due to *ischaemia* (lack of blood supply), as occurs, for instance, when a *volvulus* (twisting of the intestine) obstructs blood vessels or when a clot forms in one of the intestinal blood vessels.

Tumours affecting any of the abdominal organs can cause pain by stretching the lining of the organ, by pressing on surrounding structures, or by ulcerating or rupturing.

In rare cases, disorders of organs outside the abdomen can cause abdominal pain. For example, pneumonia of the right lower lobe of the lung may produce pain in the upper right part of the abdomen.

Abdominal pain can have a psychological origin. For example, it may result from anxiety, such as that felt by a child starting a new school or an adult changing jobs.

TREATMENT

Many people have recurrent attacks of mild abdominal pain that they learn to recognize as transient. In such circumstances, self-treatment with simple measures is often effective—a milky drink, a hot-water bottle, or simply a night's sleep. Any unusual pain, or pain that is not relieved by vomiting, or that persists for more than six hours, or that is associated with sweating or faintness should be reported to a doctor without delay. Urgent attention is also necessary if the abdominal pain is accompanied by persistent vomiting, by vomiting of blood (which may appear brown), or by the passing of bloodstained or black faeces.

Abdominal pain that is accompanied by weight loss without dieting, or by a change in bowel habits—sudden constipation or attacks of diarrhoea—should also be investigated by a doctor.

INVESTIGATION

The doctor makes a diagnosis based on the patient's detailed description of the pain and its relationship to eating, passing urine, and bowel movements, along with a thorough physical examination.

DIAGNOSING ABDOMINAL PAIN

The doctor conducts a physical examination and listens to the patient's description of the pain. More investigations, such as blood tests or X-rays, may be carried out. If the diagnosis is still in doubt, gastroscopy, colonoscopy or laparoscopy may be performed.

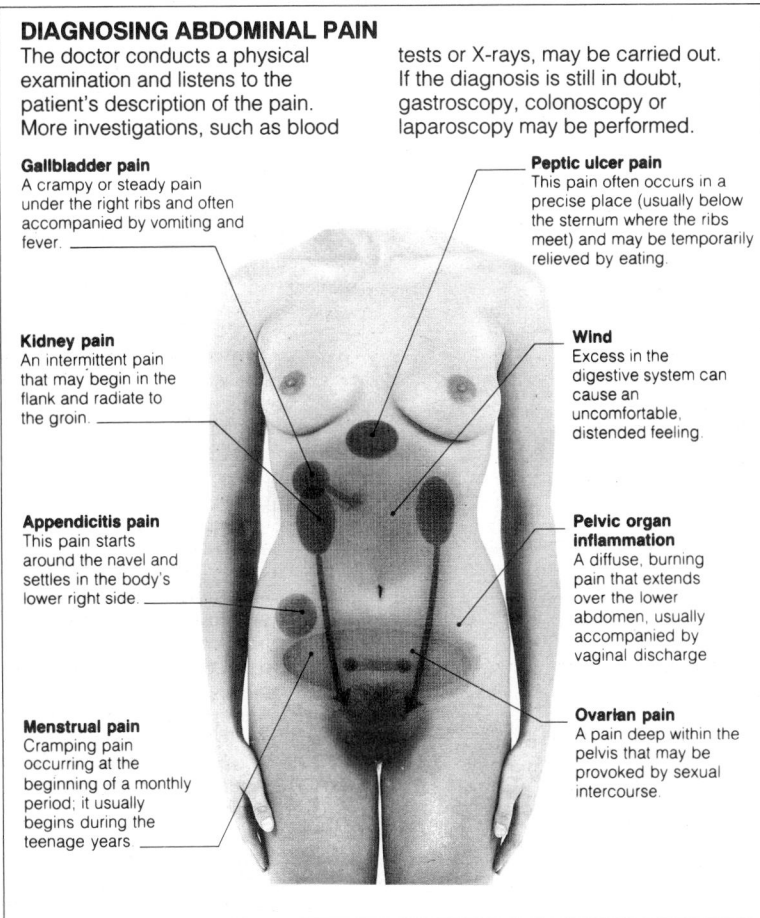

Gallbladder pain
A crampy or steady pain under the right ribs and often accompanied by vomiting and fever.

Kidney pain
An intermittent pain that may begin in the flank and radiate to the groin.

Appendicitis pain
This pain starts around the navel and settles in the body's lower right side.

Menstrual pain
Cramping pain occurring at the beginning of a monthly period; it usually begins during the teenage years

Peptic ulcer pain
This pain often occurs in a precise place (usually below the sternum where the ribs meet) and may be temporarily relieved by eating.

Wind
Excess in the digestive system can cause an uncomfortable, distended feeling.

Pelvic organ inflammation
A diffuse, burning pain that extends over the lower abdomen, usually accompanied by vaginal discharge

Ovarian pain
A pain deep within the pelvis that may be provoked by sexual intercourse.

If there is any doubt about the diagnosis, further investigations may be carried out. The investigations may include a urine test, blood tests, X-rays, and *ultrasound scanning*.

If the cause still cannot be diagnosed after such tests, endoscopic examination (looking into a body cavity with a viewing tube) may be necessary. This may take the form of *gastroscopy* (inspecting the stomach and duodenum), *colonoscopy* (inspecting the large intestine), or *laparoscopy* (inspecting the contents of the abdominal cavity). In some cases, the diagnosis can be confirmed only by an exploratory operation on the abdomen, known as a *laparotomy*.

Abdominal swelling

Distension of the abdomen, which may be due to any of a number of causes. It is the natural result of *obesity* and of enlargement of the uterus during pregnancy, generally noticeable after about 12 weeks.

Some causes of abdominal swelling are harmless. Wind in the stomach or intestine may cause uncomfortable, bloating distension of the whole abdomen. Many women experience lower abdominal distension due to temporary water retention just before a menstrual period.

Other causes may be more serious. For instance, *ascites* (accumulation of fluid in the abdomen) may be a symptom of underlying cancer, heart disease, kidney disease, or liver disease; the swelling may also be caused by *intestinal obstruction* or an *ovarian cyst*.

INVESTIGATION AND TREATMENT
Diagnosis of the underlying cause may involve abdominal X-rays or *ultrasound scanning* to look for abnormalities in the size or shape of the internal organs or for signs of intestinal obstruction. If ascites is present, some of the fluid may be drained for examination. Occasionally, a *laparotomy* (surgical exploration of the abdomen) or *laparoscopy* (internal examination of the abdomen using a flexible viewing tube) may also be necessary. (See also *Abdominal swelling* symptom chart.)

Abdominal X-ray

An X-ray examination of the abdominal contents. An abdominal X-ray is often one of the first steps in the investigation of acute abdominal disease (after the doctor has taken a careful medical history and performed a physical examination).

X-rays do not reveal the internal structure of organs but do show their outlines. Thus a radiologist can see whether any organ is enlarged and is able to spot swallowed foreign bodies within the digestive tract. Useful information is also gained by studying patterns of fluid and gas. Distended loops of bowel containing collections of fluid often indicate an obstruction (see *Intestine, obstruction of*); gas outside the intestine (in most cases under the diaphragm) indicates intestinal *perforation*.

Calcium, which is opaque to X-rays, is present in most kidney stones (see *Calculus, urinary tract*) and a small proportion of *gallstones*; these can sometimes be detected on an abdominal X-ray. Some aortic *aneurysms* contain calcium and therefore are visible.

Abdominal X-rays often need to be followed by procedures that give more information, such as *endoscopy*, *ultrasound scanning*, *CT scanning*, *MRI*, *barium X-ray examinations*, intravenous *pyelography*, or *laparoscopy*.

Abducent nerve

The sixth *cranial nerve*. The abducent nerve supplies only one muscle of each eye, the lateral rectus muscle, which is responsible for moving the eyeball outwards. The abducent nerve originates in the pons (part of the *brainstem*) and passes forwards along the base of the skull, eventually entering the back of the eye socket through a gap between the skull bones.

As a result of its long path inside the skull, the abducent nerve is often damaged in fractures of the base of the skull, or by a disorder, such as a tumour, that distorts the brain. Such damage may give rise to *double vision* or a *squint*.

Abduction

Movement of a limb away from the central line of the body, or of a digit away from the axis of a limb. Muscles that carry out this movement are called abductors. (See also *Adduction*.)

A

ABDOMINAL SWELLING
Generalized swelling over the whole abdomen between the bottom of the rib cage and the groin that is not due to simply being overweight.

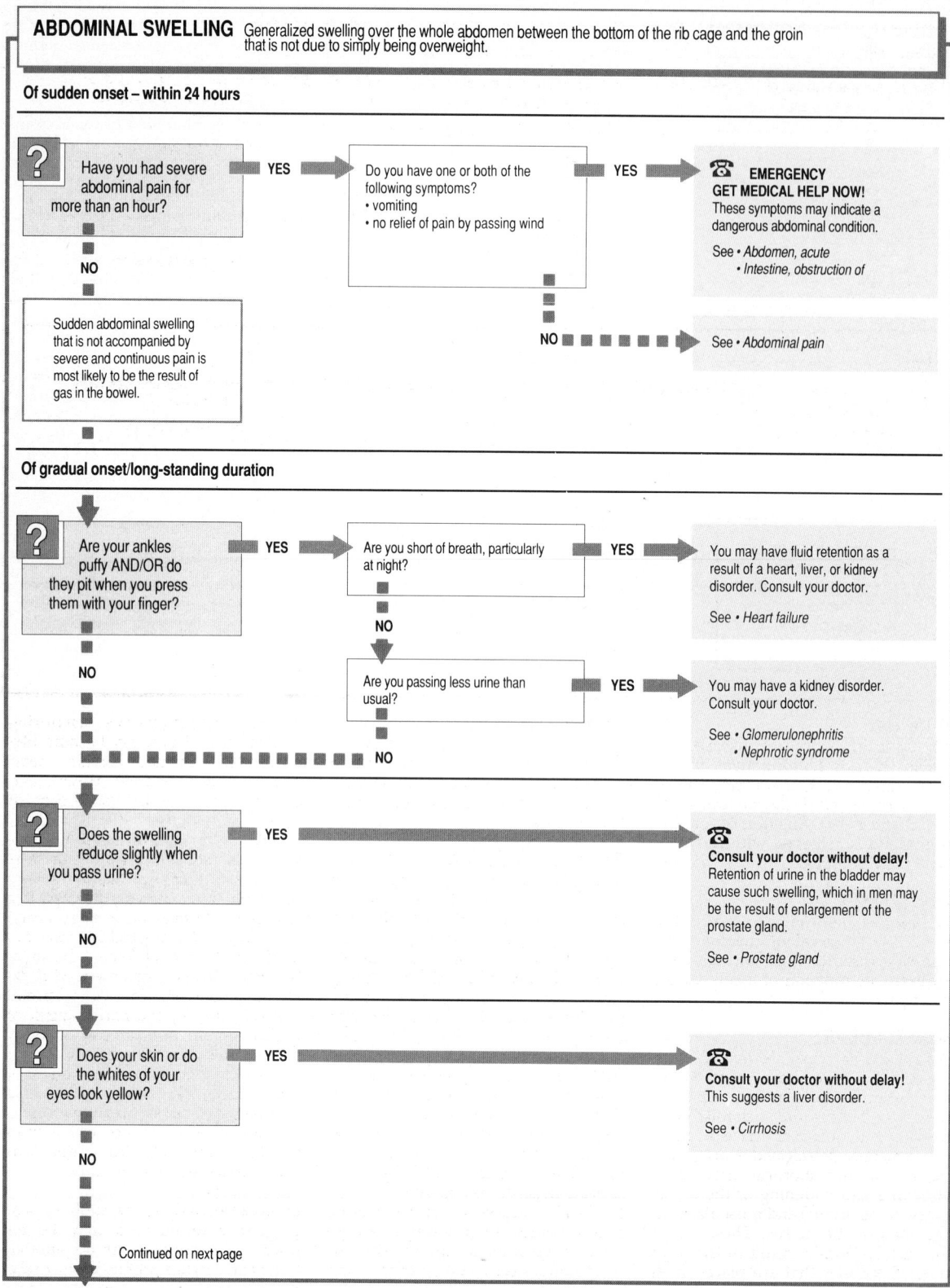

Of sudden onset – within 24 hours

? Have you had severe abdominal pain for more than an hour? — **YES** → Do you have one or both of the following symptoms?
• vomiting
• no relief of pain by passing wind — **YES** → ☎ **EMERGENCY GET MEDICAL HELP NOW!** These symptoms may indicate a dangerous abdominal condition.

See • *Abdomen, acute*
• *Intestine, obstruction of*

NO

Sudden abdominal swelling that is not accompanied by severe and continuous pain is most likely to be the result of gas in the bowel.

NO → See • *Abdominal pain*

Of gradual onset/long-standing duration

? Are your ankles puffy AND/OR do they pit when you press them with your finger? — **YES** → Are you short of breath, particularly at night? — **YES** → You may have fluid retention as a result of a heart, liver, or kidney disorder. Consult your doctor.

See • *Heart failure*

NO

NO

Are you passing less urine than usual? — **YES** → You may have a kidney disorder. Consult your doctor.

See • *Glomerulonephritis*
• *Nephrotic syndrome*

NO

? Does the swelling reduce slightly when you pass urine? — **YES** → ☎

Consult your doctor without delay! Retention of urine in the bladder may cause such swelling, which in men may be the result of enlargement of the prostate gland.

See • *Prostate gland*

NO

? Does your skin or do the whites of your eyes look yellow? — **YES** → ☎

Consult your doctor without delay! This suggests a liver disorder.

See • *Cirrhosis*

NO

Continued on next page

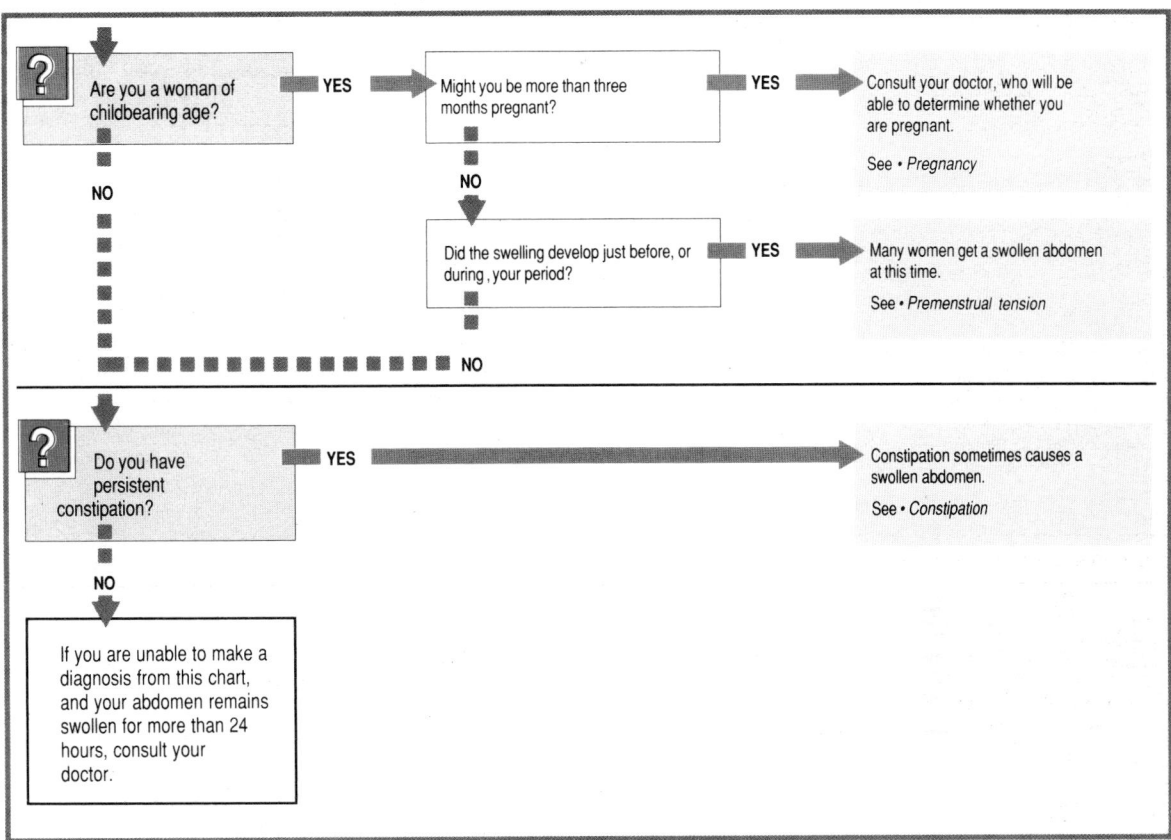

Are you a woman of childbearing age? — **YES** → Might you be more than three months pregnant? — **YES** → Consult your doctor, who will be able to determine whether you are pregnant.

See • *Pregnancy*

NO

NO

Did the swelling develop just before, or during, your period? — **YES** → Many women get a swollen abdomen at this time.

See • *Premenstrual tension*

NO

Do you have persistent constipation? — **YES** → Constipation sometimes causes a swollen abdomen.

See • *Constipation*

NO

If you are unable to make a diagnosis from this chart, and your abdomen remains swollen for more than 24 hours, consult your doctor.

Ablation

The removal of dead or diseased tissue by excision (cutting away with a sharp instrument), *cryosurgery* (freezing), *radiotherapy*, *diathermy* (burning), or *laser treatment*. Ablation of the thyroid gland is achieved with radioactive iodine isotopes.

Abnormality

A physical deformity or malformation, a behavioural or mental problem, or a variation from normal in the structure or function of a cell, tissue, or organ.

Abortifacient

An agent that causes *abortion*. Various substances have been claimed to cause abortion, such as large amounts of castor oil or gin, but such folk remedies are generally ineffective. In medical practice, *prostaglandin drugs* are used to induce abortion; they cause softening and widening of the cervix (neck of the uterus) and muscular contractions of the uterus. These drugs are usually administered in the form of suppositories that are placed high in the vagina.

Abortion

In medical terminology, a word denoting either spontaneous abortion (see *Miscarriage*) or medically induced termination of pregnancy (see *Abortion, induced*).

Abortion, induced

Medically induced termination of pregnancy. In the UK, abortion can legally be performed up to the 28th week of pregnancy but in practice an upper limit of 24 weeks is generally observed. Except in a life-threatening emergency, two doctors must sign a certificate specifying the reasons for the abortion. Under the 1967 Abortion Act, abortion may be performed if continuance of the pregnancy would involve risk to the woman's life, or if there is a risk to the mental or physical health of the woman or her existing children, or if there is a substantial risk of serious handicap to the baby.

MEDICAL REASONS FOR ABORTION
Medically induced abortions may be either therapeutic or elective. A doctor may recommend an abortion for conditions affecting either the woman or the fetus. In the woman, examples of conditions that may worsen during pregnancy and possibly become life-threatening include severe heart disease, chronic kidney disease, and cancer, especially of the breast or cervix.

Fetal conditions, revealed by *ultrasound scanning*, *amniocentesis*, or *chorionic villus sampling*, include severe developmental defects incompatible with normal life (such as *anencephaly*) and serious *chromosomal abnormalities* (such as *Down's syndrome*). Termination may also be recommended if the woman contracts *rubella* (German measles) during the early stages of pregnancy; this virus can severely damage the baby, especially his or her eyes, ears, and heart. Certain other infections in the woman may also damage the fetus. Termination is recommended if the mother has been infected by the *AIDS* virus as this virus can be transmitted to the baby.

HOW IT IS DONE

EARLY ABORTION Up to the ninth week of pregnancy termination may be induced by treatment with a combination of two drugs, mifepristone and a *prostaglandin*. These end the preg-

A

nancy and then induce the uterus to contract and expel the embryo and the placenta; the process usually takes at least 48 hours. If this drug treatment is unsuccessful, a surgical termination will be carried out a week or so later. Up to the 12th week, the pregnancy may be terminated by the surgical technique of vacuum suction curettage, which may be performed under either a general or local anaesthetic. The cervix is dilated with curved metal rods, and a thin plastic tube introduced into the uterus. The tube is connected to a suction apparatus that sucks out the fetal and placental tissues. The gynaecologist then scrapes the lining of the uterus with a curette (a spoon-shaped instrument), to make sure that no placental tissue has been left behind. The tissue may be analysed in a laboratory to confirm that a pregnancy existed and that the tissue appears complete. The reason for such analysis to be carried out is that an *ectopic pregnancy* (development of an embryo outside the uterus) would require more surgery. However, in most cases, the operator knows from his or her examination that there has been a pregnancy and that the uterus has been emptied completely.

Recovery is fast, although strenuous activity should be avoided for several days. There is usually some bleeding, and occasionally mild cramps, for up to a week. A normal period will start four to six weeks after the termination. Sexual intercourse can be resumed after two to three weeks.

LATE ABORTION Between the 12th and 15th week of pregnancy, either the suction procedure used in early abortion or the evacuation procedure described below may be recommended, depending on the facilities available. After the 15th week, it is normally considered safer to perform an abortion by causing the uterus to contract so that the fetus is expelled, as in natural labour. Contractions are induced by introducing a *prostaglandin* hormone into the uterus. This may be done either by injection directly through the woman's abdomen into the amniotic fluid or by infusion, via the cervix, into the gap between the amniotic sac (the membrane that surrounds the fetus) and the uterine wall. Alternatively, a pessary containing prostaglandin may be placed high in the vagina.

It usually takes approximately 12 to 24 hours for the fetus to be expelled, during which time the woman is given analgesic drugs (painkillers). She will remain in hospital for 24 to 48 hours after completion of the termination in order to be monitored for complications.

COMPLICATIONS

If termination is performed in a well-equipped clinic or hospital by a qualified gynaecologist, complications are rare. Infection, resulting in a condition called septic abortion, or serious bleeding occurs in fewer than one per cent of cases. Mortality is less than one woman per 100,000 when abortion is performed before the 13th week, rising to three women per 100,000 after the 13th week. (For comparison, maternal mortality for full-term pregnancy is nine women per 100,000.) Repeated terminations may increase the risk of miscarriage in subsequent pregnancies, although there is little evidence that a single termination affects future fertility.

Illegal abortions, although rare in the UK today, are common worldwide; they carry a high risk of complications, including perforation of the uterus, septic abortion, and severe bleeding. Infertility or death often result.

Abrasion, dental

The wearing away of tooth enamel, often accompanied by the wearing away of dentine (the layer beneath the enamel) and cementum (the bone-like tissue that covers the tooth root), usually through too-vigorous brushing. The areas most commonly affected are the root surface and the front surfaces of the canine and premolar teeth where they emerge from the gum. The depressions produced by abrasion are often sensitive to very cold or hot food or drink, and may require the use of a desensitizing toothpaste and/or protection with a *bonding* agent or *filling*.

Abreaction

The process of becoming consciously aware of repressed thoughts and feelings. In Freudian theory, abreaction ideally occurs via *catharsis*, the open expression of emotions associated with forgotten memories. The term abreaction is sometimes used interchangeably with catharsis but, in its strictest sense, is the result of catharsis. Abreaction is an important part of some forms of *psychotherapy* and is more easily achieved when a recent, specific traumatic event is the source of the patient's symptoms.

Abscess

A collection of pus formed as a result of infection by microorganisms, usually bacteria. The pus is formed from destroyed tissue cells, from leukocytes (white blood cells) that have been carried to the area to fight infection, and from dead and live microorganisms. Usually, a lining (pyogenic membrane) gradually forms around the abscess.

TYPES

Abscesses may develop in any organ and in the soft tissues beneath the skin in any area. Common sites include the breast (see *Breast abscess*) and gums (see *Abscess, dental*). Rarer sites include the liver (see *Liver abscess*) and the brain (see *Brain abscess*).

Common sites for abscesses under the skin include the axilla (armpit) and the groin; these two areas have a large number of lymph glands that are responsible for fighting infection. A collar-stud abscess is one in which a small abscess cavity under the skin connects via a sinus (channel) to a much larger one in deeper tissues.

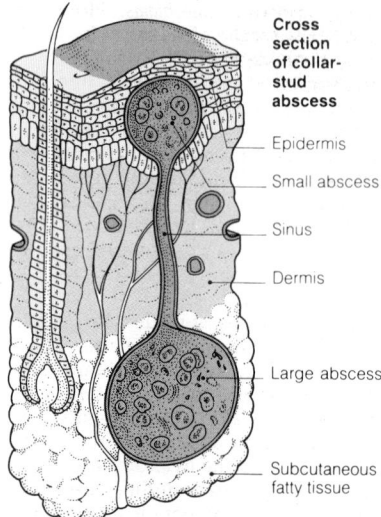

Cross section of collar-stud abscess

Epidermis

Small abscess

Sinus

Dermis

Large abscess

Subcutaneous fatty tissue

CAUSES

Common bacteria, such as staphylococci, are the usual cause, although the bacillus responsible for tuberculosis is an important abscess-forming type. Fungal infections sometimes cause abscesses, while amoebae (single-celled animal parasites) are an important cause of liver abscesses (see *Amoebiasis*). Infectious organisms usually reach internal organs via the bloodstream or penetrate to tissues under the skin by way of an infected wound or bite.

SYMPTOMS AND SIGNS

Symptoms of discomfort or pain depend mainly on the site of the abscess, but most larger abscesses, because they are a source of infection within the body, cause fever (sometimes with chills), sweating, and malaise. Abscesses may produce a sensation of intense pressure and those close to the skin usually cause inflammation with redness, increased skin temperature, and tenderness. Tuberculous abscesses are the exception; hence their description as cold abscesses.

DIAGNOSIS

An abscess within an organ may be apparent from symptoms and signs. Occasionally, the diagnosis is confirmed by imaging techniques, such as *CT scanning*, *MRI*, or *radionuclide scanning* (using radioactively labelled white blood cells or the element gallium, which concentrates in areas where pus has recently formed).

TREATMENT

Antibiotics are usually prescribed to treat bacterial infections, antifungal drugs to treat fungi, and antiamoebic drugs to treat *amoebiasis*. However, the lining of the abscess cavity tends to reduce the amount of drug that can penetrate to the source of infection from the bloodstream. The cavity itself therefore needs to be drained by making a cut in the lining and providing an escape route for the pus, either through a drainage tube (see *Drain, surgical*) or by leaving the cavity open to the skin. Most abscesses require surgical drainage.

OUTLOOK

Many abscesses subside after drainage alone. Others subside after drainage and drug treatment. Some abscesses burst and drain spontaneously through the skin. Occasionally, the presence of an abscess within a vital organ, such as the liver or brain, damages enough surrounding tissue to cause some permanent loss of normal function, or even death.

Abscess, dental

A pus-filled sac in the tissue around the root of a tooth.

CAUSE

An abscess may occur when bacteria invade the pulp (the nerves and blood vessels that fill the central cavity of the tooth), causing the pulp to die. This most commonly happens as a result of dental *caries*, which destroys the tooth's enamel and dentine, allowing bacteria to reach the pulp. Bacteria can also gain access to the pulp when a tooth is injured. Bacteria enter either directly through a fracture or along damaged blood vessels. The infection in the pulp spreads into the surrounding tissue to form an abscess.

Abscesses can also result from *periodontal disease*, in which bacteria accumulate in the deep pockets that form between the teeth and gums.

SYMPTOMS AND SIGNS

The affected tooth aches or throbs, and biting or chewing is usually extremely painful. The gum around the tooth is tender and may be red and swollen. An untreated abscess eventually erodes a sinus (small channel) through the jawbone to the gum surface, where it forms a gumboil (swelling). The gumboil may burst, discharging foul-tasting pus into the mouth, which usually lessens the pain. As the abscess spreads through surrounding tissues and bone, the glands in the neck and the side of the face may become swollen. Eventually, symptoms of infection, such as headache and fever, may develop.

TREATMENT

The dentist will usually try, if possible, to save the tooth by endodontic treatment. To do this, the abscess is drained by drilling through the crown of the tooth and into the pulp cavity to allow the pus to escape. The pulp cavity is then carefully cleaned and disinfected. An antibiotic may be prescribed if the infection has spread beyond the tooth. When the infection has cleared up, the cavity is filled with dental cement (see *Root-canal treatment*), sealed, and crowned.

When an abscess is caused by diseased pulp and the infection cannot be cleared up with endodontic treatment, it is necessary to extract the tooth. *Extraction* removes the source of infection and drains the abscess. Antibiotics are usually prescribed to clear up any residual infection.

An abscess in a periodontal pocket can usually be treated by the dentist passing a probe into the pocket and gently scraping away infected material; sometimes it is necessary to make a small incision in the pocket to reach the abscess. If there is loss of bony support and periodontal ligament attachment due to severe periodontal disease, a dental extraction may need to be performed.

Absence

In medical terminology, a temporary loss or impairment of consciousness that occurs in some forms of *epilepsy*, typically petit mal seizures.

Acanthosis nigricans

A rare, untreatable condition characterized by thickened dark patches of skin in the groin, armpits, neck, and other skin folds. It may occur in young people as a genetic (inherited) disorder, or as the result of an endocrine disorder, such as *Cushing's syndrome*. It also occurs in people with carcinomas (malignant tumours) of the lung and other organs.

Pseudoacanthosis nigricans is a much more common condition, usually seen in dark-complexioned people who are overweight. In this form, the skin in fold areas is both thicker and darker than the surrounding skin, and there is usually excessive sweating in affected areas. The condition may improve with dieting.

Acarbose

A drug used in the treatment of non-insulin-dependent diabetes. It acts on enzymes in the intestines to delay the digestion of starch, which subsequently slows the increase in blood glucose levels after a carbohydrate meal.

Accessory nerve

The 11th *cranial nerve*. The accessory nerve differs from the other cranial nerves in that only a small part of it originates from the brain; most of the nerve comes from the spinal cord.

The part of the nerve originating from the brain supplies many muscles of the palate, pharynx (throat), and larynx (voice-box). Damage to this part of the nerve may give rise to dysphonia (difficulty in speaking) and dysphagia (difficulty in swallowing).

The spinal part of the nerve supplies some large muscles of the neck and back, notably the sternomastoid (which runs from the breastbone to the side of the skull) and the trapezius (a large, triangular muscle of the upper back, shoulder, and neck). Damage to the spinal fibres of the nerve paralyses these muscles.

Accidental death

Deaths due to accidents account for a high proportion of deaths in the age group from five to 34 years, particularly among males. Figures for accidental deaths in the UK are shown in the table (see overleaf).

Nearly half of all male deaths between the ages of 15 and 24 are from road accidents, and alcohol forms the largest added factor. In the 1980s, however, there was a decline in the number of deaths on the road, due in part to compulsory seat-belt legislation.

A

ACCIDENTAL DEATH

Accidents are a very important cause of death in certain age groups, notably those from infancy to the mid-forties. The chart on the right shows the number of deaths from injuries and poisoning (registered in England and Wales in 1990) by age groups for males and females. In all but the oldest age range, many more deaths occur in males than in females.

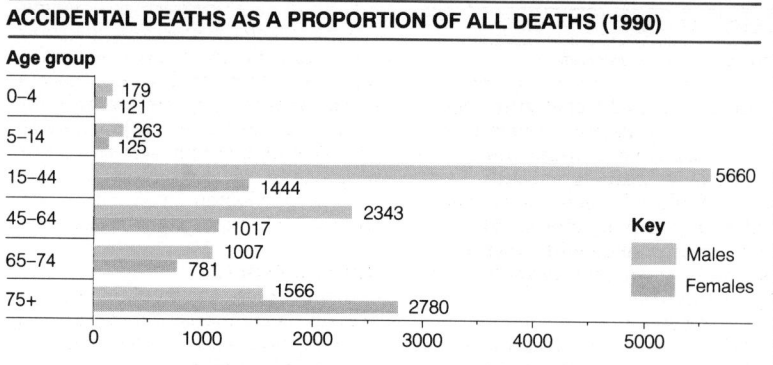

ACCIDENTAL DEATHS AS A PROPORTION OF ALL DEATHS (1990)

Age group

Age group	Males	Females
0–4	179	121
5–14	263	125
15–44	5660	1444
45–64	2343	1017
65–74	1007	781
75+	1566	2780

Key
Males
Females

The home appears to be a very dangerous place, accounting for nearly as many deaths as road accidents. Falls are a leading cause of death overall; in the elderly, they take first place. Most of these falls occur in the home. Young people usually suffer only a bruise when they fall, but, in the elderly, bones are much more brittle, and more than one third of the falls in those over 74 years old result in fracture of the spine, femur (thigh-bone), or wrist. Death often follows as a result of complications associated with the fracture.

Up to the age of one year, an important cause of accidental death is choking on a morsel of food or an object placed in the mouth. Death from smothering by bedclothes, plastic bags, or other material is another major home hazard for infants.

The old are also particularly vulnerable to death from burns or asphyxiation as a result of fires. About half of these victims are over 75.

Every year, about 350 people die in the UK from drowning; three quarters of them are male. Drowning most often occurs when victims are swimming or playing in water. However, drowning can also result from falling into water.

For those aged between 25 and 44, poisoning is almost as common a cause of death as drowning. In many cases, it is due to drug overdose, and suicide may be suspected.

Accidents at work resulting in death have steadily decreased since the beginning of the century; they now account for less than two per cent of all accidental deaths.

Accident proneness

A tendency to have numerous mishaps. Many psychologists doubt that the concept is valid, even though studies have shown that accidents are not distributed evenly among the population according to the laws of chance. A small group of people do seem to have more accidents, but this group changes constantly from study to study and no psychological test has yet identified it.

Accidents may be slightly more common in aggressive and nonconformist men. However, emotional stress is probably the most important factor. Cycles of accidents seem to occur in the months after stressful "life events" regardless of the personality of the person involved.

Accommodation

Adjustment, especially the process by which the eye adjusts itself to focus on near objects. At rest, the eye is focused for distant vision, when its lens is relatively thin and flat. To make it possible to focus on a nearer object, the ciliary muscle of the eye contracts, reducing the pull on the outer rim of the lens, so permitting it to become thicker and more convex.

With age, the lens loses its elasticity and, as a result, accommodation becomes increasingly difficult. This results in a form of longsightedness called *presbyopia*.

Acebutolol

A *beta-blocker drug* commonly used in the treatment of *hypertension* (high blood pressure), *angina pectoris* (chest pain due to impaired blood supply to heart muscle), and certain types of *arrhythmia* (abnormal heart rhythm) in which the heart beats too rapidly.

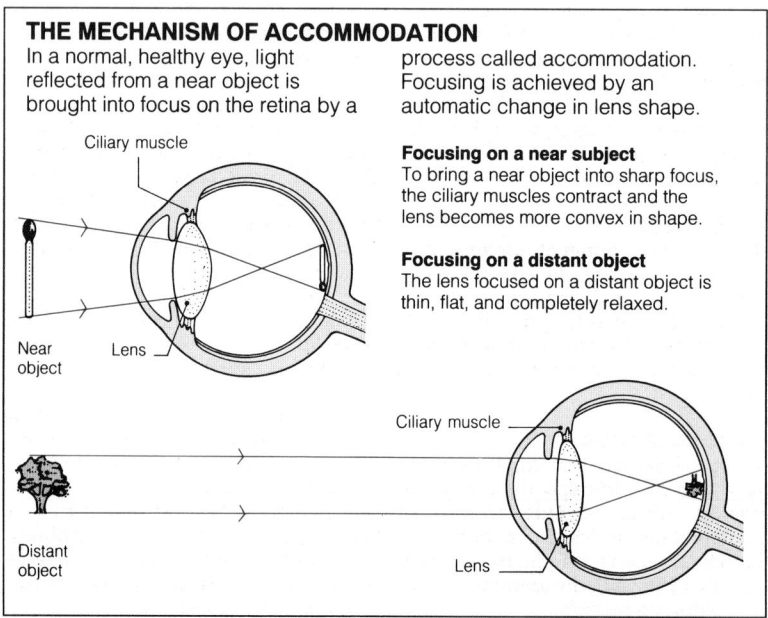

THE MECHANISM OF ACCOMMODATION

In a normal, healthy eye, light reflected from a near object is brought into focus on the retina by a process called accommodation. Focusing is achieved by an automatic change in lens shape.

Focusing on a near subject
To bring a near object into sharp focus, the ciliary muscles contract and the lens becomes more convex in shape.

Focusing on a distant object
The lens focused on a distant object is thin, flat, and completely relaxed.

Ciliary muscle

Near object

Lens

Ciliary muscle

Distant object

Lens

ACE inhibitor drugs

COMMON DRUGS

Captopril Enalapril Lisinopril

A group of *vasodilator drugs* introduced in 1981. ACE inhibitors (*angiotensin*-converting enzyme inhibitors) are used to treat *hypertension* (high blood pressure) and *heart failure* (reduced pumping efficiency). They are often prescribed with other drugs, for example, *diuretic drugs* or *beta-blocker drugs*.

HOW THEY WORK

ACE inhibitor drugs block the action of the enzyme that converts angiotensin (a protein present in the blood) from an inactive form, angiotensin I, to an active form, angiotensin II, which constricts (narrows) blood vessels. By reducing production of angiotensin II, ACE inhibitors reduce constriction of blood vessels, which makes it easier for the blood to flow through them, and thus reduces blood pressure.

POSSIBLE ADVERSE EFFECTS

These include nausea, loss of taste, headache, dizziness, and a dry cough. The first dose may reduce blood pressure so dramatically that the patient collapses; treatment is therefore often started in hospital.

Acetazolamide

A type of drug known as a carbonic anhydrase inhibitor. Acetazolamide is used in the treatment of *glaucoma* (raised pressure in the eyeball) and, occasionally, to prevent or treat symptoms of *mountain sickness* (headache, weakness, or other symptoms occurring at high altitudes).

During treatment with acetazolamide, adverse effects may include lethargy, nausea, diarrhoea, weight loss, and impotence.

Acetic acid

The colourless, pungent, organic acid that gives vinegar its characteristic sour taste. In medicine, acetic acid is an ingredient of antiseptic jellies that are used to restore the normal acidity of the vagina in certain types of vaginal infections.

Acetohexamide

An oral *hypoglycaemic* drug used to treat non-insulin-dependent *diabetes mellitus*. Acetohexamide stimulates the secretion of *insulin*, a hormone that lowers the blood glucose (sugar) level by increasing the amount of glucose absorbed by cells.

Acetylcholine

A type of *neurotransmitter* (a chemical that transmits messages between nerve cells or between nerve and muscle cells). Acetylcholine (sometimes abbreviated to ACh) is the neurotransmitter at all nerve-muscle junctions as well as at many other sites in the nervous system. The actions of acetylcholine are called cholinergic actions and are blocked by *anticholinergic drugs*.

Acetylcysteine

A drug used as an antidote for *paracetamol* overdose. It is also a *mucolytic drug* used in the treatment of chronic *bronchitis*.

HOW IT WORKS

To be effective as an antidote to paracetamol poisoning, acetylcysteine must be given by injection within a few hours of the overdose; it works by reducing the amount of toxic substances produced during the breakdown of paracetamol, thus reducing the risk of liver damage. Taken by mouth, acetylcysteine makes the mucus in sputum less sticky and therefore easier to cough up.

POSSIBLE ADVERSE EFFECTS

In rare cases, vomiting, rash, or breathing difficulty may occur when acetylcysteine is taken in large doses.

Achalasia

A condition in which the muscles at the lower end of the *oesophagus* and the sphincter (valve) between the oesophagus and the stomach fail to relax to let food into the stomach after swallowing.

Food normally stimulates the muscles in the wall of the oesophagus to begin a series of contractions that push food towards the stomach in waves. In achalasia, the sphincter does not relax to allow food to pass from the oesophagus to the stomach, and the lowest part of the oesophagus becomes narrowed, distorted, and blocked with food while the part above widens.

INCIDENCE AND CAUSE

This rare condition can occur at any age, but is unusual before the age of 15. The underlying cause is unknown.

SYMPTOMS AND SIGNS

Symptoms include difficulty and pain with swallowing and pain in the lower chest and upper abdomen. Regurgitated food that may have been swallowed a day or two earlier may cause a foul taste and bad breath. The ability to swallow gradually deteriorates until there is difficulty swallowing liquids as well as solids.

DIAGNOSIS

A barium swallow (a type of *barium X-ray examination*) will show abnormal, ineffective movement of the oesophageal wall and varying degrees of dilatation (widening) of the oesophagus, as well as narrowing at the lowest end of the oesophagus and failure of the sphincter to open after swallowing. *Gastroscopy*, in which a narrow viewing tube is passed down the oesophagus, is used to check the narrowing and to rule out cancer.

In achalasia, the pressure in the area of the lower sphincter is markedly raised; pressure recordings reveal that the sphincter is incompletely relaxed after swallowing.

TREATMENT

Drug treatment is rarely successful. It is possible to widen the oesophagus for prolonged periods by passing a slender rubber bag down it and filling the bag with air or water to stretch the muscles (see *Oesophageal dilatation*). There is also a surgical procedure that cuts some of the muscles at the stomach entrance to widen the passageway for food.

Achilles tendon

The tendon that pulls up the back of the heel. It is formed from the calf muscles (the gastrocnemius, soleus, and plantar muscles) and is attached to the *calcaneus* (heel-bone). The tendon is named after the legendary Greek hero Achilles, who was vulnerable only in the heel.

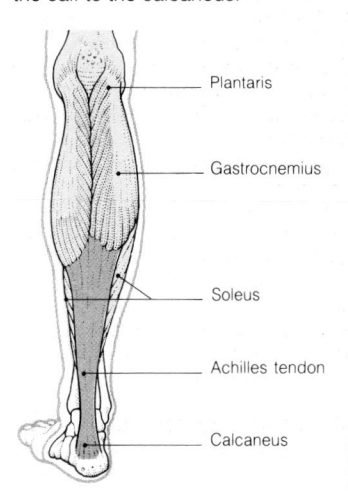

LOCATION OF THE ACHILLES TENDON

The tendon runs from the base of the calf to the calcaneus.

Plantaris

Gastrocnemius

Soleus

Achilles tendon

Calcaneus

A

Minor injuries to the tendon are common. They are usually due to too much exercise, faulty running technique, or wearing incorrect footwear. All of these can cause inflammation of the tendon (*tendinitis*) and tearing of the tendon fibres. In most cases, these conditions clear up with rest and physiotherapy.

Violent stretching of the Achilles tendon can cause it to rupture. In such cases, surgical repair of the tendon may sometimes be necessary, but immobilization of the ankle in a plaster cast may be all that is necessary.

Achlorhydria

Absence of stomach acid secretions. This may be due to chronic atrophic *gastritis* or to an absence or malfunction of acid-producing parietal cells in the lining of the stomach.

About one in every 20 normal people has achlorhydria without symptoms. Achlorhydria in itself is no cause for concern. It is, however, present in some people with stomach cancer, and is also a feature of pernicious anaemia, a blood disorder caused by defective absorption of vitamin B_{12} from the stomach (see *Anaemia, megaloblastic*).

Achondroplasia

A rare disorder of bone growth, present from birth and leading to *short stature* (once called dwarfism). The affected bones are mainly the long bones of the arms and legs. The cartilage that links each bone to its epiphysis (the growing area at its tip) is converted to bone too early, thus preventing further limb growth. Most other bones are able to grow normally.

Affected individuals have short, strong limbs, a well-developed trunk, and a head of normal size except for a somewhat protruding forehead.

INCIDENCE AND CAUSES

In the UK, approximately 2,000 people suffer from achondroplasia. The condition is caused by a gene defect of the dominant variety (see *Genetic disorders*).

The parents of most achondroplastics are of normal stature. In these cases, the abnormality has arisen from a gene *mutation* (new gene defect). However, the children of achondroplastics each have a 50 per cent chance of inheriting the defective gene and of being achondroplastic.

SYMPTOMS AND OUTLOOK

Achondroplasia is usually obvious at birth or during the first year of life, when there is already a noticeable stunting of the limbs relative to the size of the head. Growth of the limb bones slows and stops during childhood, and no treatment is available to alter the outlook. Intelligence and sexual development are not affected, and lifespan is close to normal.

Acid

A substance defined as a donor of hydrogen ions (atoms of hydrogen with positive electrical charges). When mixed with, or dissolved in, water, acid molecules dissociate (split up) to release their constituent ions; all acids release hydrogen as the positive ion (positively-charged ions are called cations, negatively-charged ones are called anions).

A wide variety of substances are acids. Examples of acids within the body include hydrochloric acid, which is a corrosive mineral acid produced by the stomach lining, and many organic acids, such as lactic acid, carbonic acid, ascorbic acid (vitamin C), and pyruvic acid. (See also *Acid-base balance; Alkali*.)

Acid-base balance

A combination of mechanisms that ensures that the body's fluids are neither too *acid* nor too alkaline (*alkalis* are also called bases). The body functions healthily only when its fluids are close to chemical neutrality.

In body metabolism, sugars and fats are broken down and energy is released. This breakdown involves the use of oxygen, and the production of carbon dioxide (which forms carbonic acid when dissolved in water) and organic acids, such as pyruvic acid. Thus, the body's metabolic processes cause fluctuations in the acidity and alkalinity of the blood and other body fluids.

The body has three mechanisms for the maintenance of normal acid-base balance: buffers, breathing, and the activities of the kidneys. Buffers are substances in the blood that tend to neutralize acid or alkaline wastes. Rapid breathing increases the rate at which carbon dioxide is eliminated from the blood, thereby making it less acidic; conversely, slow breathing allows the blood to become more acidic. The kidneys help maintain a constant acidity level in the blood by regulating the amounts of acid or alkaline wastes in the urine.

Disturbances of the body's acid-base balance result in either *acidosis* (excessive blood acidity) or *alkalosis* (excessive blood alkalinity).

Acidosis

A disturbance of the body's *acid-base balance* in which there is an accumulation of acid or loss of alkali (base). There are two types of acidosis: metabolic and respiratory.

CAUSES

In metabolic acidosis, an increased amount of acid is produced by metabolic processes. Ketoacidosis, a form of metabolic acidosis, occurs in uncontrolled *diabetes mellitus* and, to a lesser degree, in starvation. Metabolic acidosis may also be caused by loss of bicarbonate (an alkali) through severe diarrhoea. In kidney failure there is insufficient excretion of acid in the urine. One unusual cause of acidosis is an overdose of aspirin, which may cause an increase in acids produced by cell metabolism.

Respiratory acidosis occurs when breathing fails to remove enough carbon dioxide from the lungs. This causes increased acidity of the blood because the excess carbon dioxide remains in the blood, where it dissolves to form carbonic acid. Impaired breathing leading to respiratory acidosis may be due to conditions such as *bronchitis*, bronchial *asthma*, or *airway obstruction*.

Acid reflux

Regurgitation of acidic fluid from the stomach into the *oesophagus* (the tube connecting the throat to the stomach). Acid reflux is associated with heartburn (a burning pain in the chest) and often leads to *oesophagitis* (inflammation of the oesophagus).

Mild acid reflux is common and of no serious significance. It may occur in pregnancy and often affects people who are overweight.

Acid reflux is attributed to inefficiency of the muscular valve at the lower end of the oesophagus, which permits regurgitation of the acidic fluid. Repeated episodes of discomfort may indicate the presence of a *hiatus hernia* (a weakness in the diaphragm that permits part of the stomach to protrude into the chest).

Acne

A chronic skin disorder caused by inflammation of the hair follicles and the sebaceous glands in the skin.

TYPES

The most common type of acne is acne vulgaris, which mainly affects adolescents. Tropical acne typically affects young white people on unaccustomed exposure to hot, humid environments. Infantile acne, a rare condition affecting male infants, is associated with subsequent severe acne vulgaris in adolescence. Chemical acne is caused by exposure to certain chemicals and oils, and results in acne in unusual sites, such as on the legs. Chloracne is a form of acne caused by exposure to chlorinated hydrocarbon chemicals; many cases occurred following a severe explosion at a chemical factory in Seveso, Italy, in 1976.

INCIDENCE

Acne vulgaris almost always begins during puberty, although it may develop later in life; most adolescent boys and many girls have some acne.

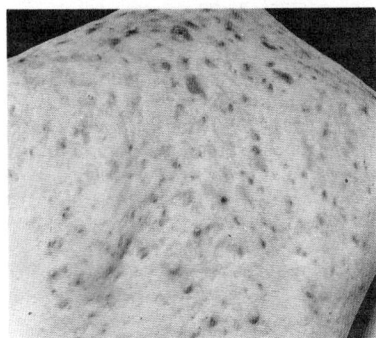

Severe acne
An example of cystic acne, with widespread scarring across the back. Few cases are as extensive as this.

CAUSE

Acne spots are caused by the obstruction of hair follicles by sebum (the oily substance secreted by the sebaceous glands). When a plug of sebum becomes trapped in a follicle, bacteria multiply and the follicle becomes inflamed. The cause of the change in sebum secretion at puberty is uncertain but it seems to be linked with increased levels of *androgen hormones* (male sex hormones). There may also be a genetic factor, since acne can run in families.

Some drugs may bring on or aggravate existing acne (e.g. corticosteroids and androgens, which increase oil production in the skin). Other drugs that can aggravate acne include barbiturates, isoniazid, rifampicin, bromides, and iodides.

Oil and grease may also cause acne. The natural oil from the scalp may cause acne around the hairline. Regular contact with mineral or cooking oils, as may occur in restaurant kitchens, can make the condition worse. Cosmetics with oily bases are also associated with an increased tendency to develop acne.

SYMPTOMS

Acne occurs in areas that have a high concentration of sebaceous glands, mainly the face, centre of the chest, upper back, shoulders, and around the neck. The most common acne spots are comedones (blackheads), milia (whiteheads), pustules, nodules (firm swellings below the skin), and cysts (larger, fluid-filled swellings in the skin). As spots heal, others tend to appear. Healing spots often fade to a pink mark that usually disappears altogether, although some spots, particularly cystic spots, may leave scars. Acne scars often appear as small, depressed pits.

PREVENTION

There are many myths about the prevention of acne, particularly relating to diet. There is no evidence that diet plays any part in causing acne. For example, there is little point in avoiding chocolate. Although washing affected areas does not prevent acne, it may keep it from spreading. The skin should be washed twice daily; more frequent washing is unnecessary, since washing simply removes surface oil.

TREATMENT

There is no instant cure for acne, although many treatments are available to relieve it. Topical (applied to the skin) treatments act by unblocking the pores and removing sebum. They also help to promote healing. Topical applications that are most often used include benzoyl peroxide, retinoic acid, antibiotic lotions, and sulphur-containing creams. Ultraviolet light is often beneficial in treating acne. Exposure to natural sunlight is helpful, and artificial ultraviolet light may be used to treat more severe cases. The spots should not be picked or squeezed; this can worsen the condition and can lead to scarring.

If topical treatment has failed, long-term therapy with oral antibiotics often helps. The antibiotics are prescribed regularly for up to six months at a time. They have an effect not only on the bacteria in the skin but may also have a direct effect on inflammatory cells in acne spots, as well as on sebum production.

The treatment of severe acne has improved with the use of retinoid drugs, which are prescribed only when antibiotics and other measures have not helped. Retinoid drugs reduce oil production and have a drying effect on the skin, but must be taken cautiously because they may cause liver damage and, because they

cause fetal malformations, they must not be given to a woman who might become pregnant.

Acne cysts can often be treated by intralesional therapy (direct injection of a drug into the acne spots), which also helps to reduce scarring. In cases of severe and extensive scarring, *dermabrasion* (removal of the top layer of affected skin) can help to improve appearance.

OUTLOOK

Acne improves slowly over a period of time, often clearing up by the end of the teenage years. With modern treatment, nobody should have severe, scarring acne.

Acoustic nerve

Also called the auditory nerve, the acoustic nerve is the part of the *vestibulocochlear nerve* (the eighth *cranial nerve*) concerned with hearing.

Acoustic neuroma

A rare, benign tumour arising from supporting cells that surround the eighth cranial (auditory or acoustic) nerve, usually within the internal auditory meatus (the canal in the skull through which the nerve passes from the inner ear to the brain).

INCIDENCE AND CAUSES

Acoustic neuromas constitute about five to seven per cent of primary *brain tumours*; there are a few hundred cases each year in the UK. Acoustic neuromas most commonly occur in people between the ages of 40 and 60 and are slightly more common in women than in men.

Usually the cause of acoustic neuromas is unknown. In some cases, however, tumours simultaneously affect the nerves on both sides of the head and may be part of a widespread *neurofibromatosis*, a disease characterized by changes in the nervous system, skin, and bones.

SYMPTOMS AND DIAGNOSIS

Acoustic neuroma can cause *deafness*, *tinnitus* (noises in the ear), loss of balance, and pain in the affected ear. As the tumour enlarges, it may compress the brainstem and cerebellum, causing *ataxia* (loss of coordination). As it expands, the tumour presses on the trigeminal nerve (fifth cranial nerve), causing pain in the face, or on the *abducent nerve* (sixth cranial nerve), causing double vision.

Diagnosis is made by *hearing tests* and tests of balance, such as the *caloric test* or *electronystagmography*, followed by X-rays, *CT scanning*, or *MRI*, to visualize the internal auditory meatus.

TREATMENT

The tumour is treated by surgical removal. Before the operation, CT scanning or MRI is used to show the location of the tumour and its approximate size, so that the surgeon can decide on the best route for removal.

The results of surgery depend on the size of the tumour; in many cases, there is no residual damage to the acoustic nerve and hearing is preserved. Occasionally, however, numbness and weakness of part of the face result from unavoidable damage to neighbouring nerves.

Acrocyanosis

A condition in which the hands and feet turn blue, may become cold, and sweat excessively. Acrocyanosis is caused by spasm of the small blood vessels and is usually aggravated by cold weather.

Acrocyanosis is related to another circulatory disorder, *Raynaud's disease*, in which the skin of the fingers and toes may be damaged by reduced blood flow.

Acrodermatitis enteropathica

A rare, inherited disorder in which areas of the skin (most commonly the fingers, toes, scalp, and the areas around the mouth and anus) are reddened, ulcerated, and covered with pustules (pus-containing spots).

Acrodermatitis enteropathica is caused by an inability to absorb enough zinc from food, and addition of zinc supplements to the diet usually produces a rapid improvement in a person's condition.

Acromegaly

A rare disease characterized externally by abnormal enlargement of the skull, jaw, hands, and feet.

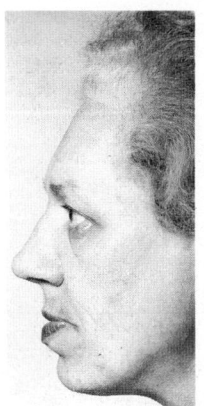

Appearance of acromegaly
The woman in profile at left shows many of the typical features of acromegaly—including lengthening of the face, enlargement of the jaw and nose, and general coarsening of the facial features.

CAUSE AND SYMPTOMS

Acromegaly is caused by excessive secretion of *growth hormone* from the anterior pituitary gland at the base of the brain and is the result of a benign *pituitary tumour*.

If such a tumour develops within the first 10 years of life, the result is *gigantism* (in which growth is accelerated) and not acromegaly. More commonly, the tumour develops after growth in the long bones of the limbs has stopped. This leads to acromegaly, although it may take several years before the symptoms and signs of the condition appear.

Symptoms and signs of acromegaly include enlargement of the hands and feet, coarsening of the facial features, enlargement of the ears and nose, a jutting jaw, and a long face. Sufferers may notice a gradual increase in ring, shoe, glove, and hat size, and deepening or huskiness of the voice. Other possible symptoms are those common to any tumour in the brain, such as headache and visual disturbances.

DIAGNOSIS AND TREATMENT

If a person appears to be developing acromegaly, the level of growth hormone in the blood is measured before and after a quantity of glucose has been administered. Glucose usually suppresses growth hormone secretion; if it has no effect on the blood level of the hormone, this confirms uncontrolled secretion of the hormone by the pituitary gland. *CT scanning* or *MRI* may reveal a tumour or overgrowth of the pituitary gland.

The tumour may be removed surgically or treated by *radiotherapy*. The drug *octreotide* prevents the production of growth hormone, and the drug *bromocriptine* sometimes causes the tumour to become smaller.

Acromioclavicular joint

The joint between the outer end of the clavicle (collarbone) and the acromion (the bony prominence at the top of the shoulderblade).

INJURIES TO THE JOINT

Injuries to the joint are rare. They are usually due to a fall on the shoulder and may result in subluxation (partial dislocation with the bones still in contact) or, rarely, dislocation (complete displacement of the bones).

In subluxation, the synovium (joint lining) and the ligaments around it are stretched and bruised, the joint is swollen, and the bones feel slightly out of alignment. In dislocation, the ligaments are torn, the swelling is greater, and the bone deformity is pronounced. In both subluxation and dislocation, the joint is painful and tender, and movement of the shoulder is restricted.

Subluxation is treated by resting the arm and shoulder in a sling. If the pain and tenderness persist, injection of a corticosteroid and a local anaesthetic into the joint often helps.

Dislocation requires strapping, for about three weeks, around the clavicle and elbow to pull the outer end of the clavicle back into position. Occasionally, an operation may be needed.

Acroparaesthesia

A medical term used to describe tingling in the fingers or toes (see *Pins-and-needles*).

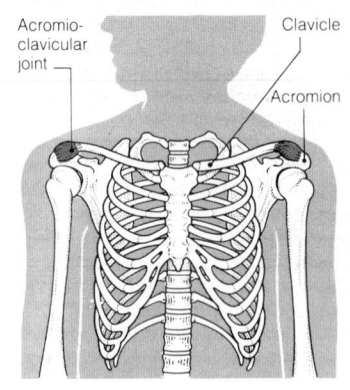

LOCATION OF THE ACROMIOCLAVICULAR JOINT
The joint lies at the junction of the outer end of the clavicle and the acromion.

Acromio-clavicular joint

Clavicle

Acromion

Acrosoxacin

An antibacterial drug of the 4-*quinolone* type used mainly to treat gonorrhoea. The most common side-effects include nausea, vomiting, diarrhoea, headache, and tiredness.

ACTH

The common abbreviation for adreno-corticotrophic hormone (also called corticotrophin). It is produced by the anterior part of the *pituitary gland* and stimulates the adrenal cortex (outer layer of the *adrenal glands*) to release various *corticosteroid hormones*. It is also necessary for the growth and maintenance of the cells of the adrenal cortex.

ACTIONS

ACTH stimulates the adrenal cortex to increase production of *hydrocortisone* (cortisol), *aldosterone*, and *androgen hormones*. Most important is its stimulation of hydrocortisone production.

ACTH production is partly controlled by the *hypothalamus* (an area in the centre of the brain) and partly by the level of hydrocortisone in the blood. When ACTH levels are high, the production of hydrocortisone is increased; this, in turn, suppresses the release of ACTH from the pituitary gland. If ACTH levels are low, hydrocortisone production falls and the hypothalamus releases factors that stimulate the pituitary gland to increase ACTH production.

ACTH levels increase in response to stress, emotion, injury, infection, burns, surgery, and a decrease in blood pressure. The level of ACTH naturally fluctuates in a diurnal (24-hour) pattern.

DISORDERS

A tumour of the pituitary gland can cause excessive ACTH production which, in turn, leads to overproduction of hydrocortisone by the adrenal cortex, resulting in *Cushing's syndrome*. Insufficient ACTH production due, for example, to hypopituitarism (underactivity of the pituitary gland), is rare. When it does occur, it causes *adrenal failure*.

MEDICAL USES

ACTH is used very rarely to treat inflammatory disorders, such as *arthritis*, *ulcerative colitis*, and some types of *hepatitis*. It has also been employed to induce remissions in *multiple sclerosis* but its efficacy in this respect is uncertain. ACTH is also used to diagnose disorders of the adrenal glands.

Acting out

Impulsive actions which may reflect unconscious wishes. The term is most often used by psychotherapists to describe behaviour during analysis when the patient "acts out" rather than reports fantasies, wishes, or beliefs. Acting out can also occur outside psychoanalysis as a reaction to frustrations encountered in everyday life. In this case it usually takes the form of antisocial, aggressive behaviour that may be directed towards oneself (e.g. wrist-cutting) or others.

Actinic

Pertaining to changes caused by the ultraviolet rays in sunlight, as in actinic *dermatitis* (inflammation of the skin) and actinic *keratosis* (roughness and thickening of the skin). Both are caused by overexposure to solar radiation, which is especially likely to occur near the sea in summer and from the snow in winter.

Actinomycosis

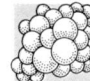 An infection caused by *ACTINOMYCES ISRAELII* or related actinomycete bacteria. These bacteria resemble fungi and cause diseases of the mouth and jaw, pelvis, and chest.

TYPES

The most common form of actinomycosis affects the jaw area. A painful swelling appears, usually under the jaw, and small openings develop in the skin. Pus and characteristic yellow granules discharge through the openings. Poor oral hygiene may contribute to this form of the infection.

Another form of actinomycosis, affecting the pelvis, occurs in women and may cause lower abdominal pain, fever, and bleeding between menstrual periods. This form of actinomycosis has been associated with the use of *IUDs* that do not contain copper. Rare forms of actinomycosis affect the appendix or lung.

DIAGNOSIS AND TREATMENT

A diagnosis of actinomycosis is usually confirmed by finding the typical granules and by identifying the causative bacteria in a culture.

The infection can usually be treated successfully with large doses of a penicillin drug.

Acuity, visual

See *Visual acuity*.

Acupressure

A derivative of *acupuncture* in which pressure instead of a needle is applied.

Acupuncture

A branch of Chinese medicine in which needles are inserted into a patient's skin as therapy for various disorders or to induce anaesthesia.

Traditional Chinese medicine holds that the chi (life-force) flows through the body along meridians (channels); a blockage in one or more of these meridians is believed to cause ill health. Acupuncturists aim to restore health by inserting needles at appropriate sites, known as acupuncture points, on the affected meridians.

A cautious view is taken of acupuncture by orthodox medical practitioners, but some use it to complement other treatments.

HOW IT WORKS

Research suggests that acupuncture causes the release within the central nervous system of *endorphins* (substances resembling morphine), which act as natural analgesics (painkillers).

It has also been suggested that acupuncture may work by inducing a form of hypnosis, or that insertion of the acupuncture needles stimulates the peripheral nerves, acting as a distraction from, or a counter-irritant to, the original pain.

WHY IT IS DONE

Acupuncture has been used successfully as an anaesthetic for dental procedures and surgical operations, and also during labour and delivery (including caesarean sections). Some practitioners use acupuncture to reduce pain after operations and also to relieve chronically painful conditions, such as arthritis, that are not responding to standard treatments.

Acupuncture is claimed to be particularly effective for conditions that affect muscles, bones, joints, eyes, heart, and the digestive, respiratory, and nervous systems; it is also claimed to help in the treatment of addiction, depression, and anxiety.

HOW IT IS DONE

The traditional Chinese doctor recognizes that accurate diagnosis is essential so that the acupuncturist knows which acupuncture points to use. Diagnosis in traditional Chinese medicine is made by examination of the patient's 12 pulses (six in each wrist). Each pulse is believed to give information about the health of a particular body region.

The precise disorder being treated, or the degree of anaesthesia required, determines the temperature of the needle used, the angle of insertion, whether needles are twisted or vibrated while inserted, the speed of insertion and withdrawal, and the length of time the needles remain in position. Some practitioners pass a mild current through the needle to act as a stimulant in unblocking the meridian; others inject homeopathic remedies into the acupuncture point.

RISKS

Currently there are few legal checks on acupuncturists in the UK and no formal qualification is necessary to practise. Infection is a possible risk but good practitioners avoid this by using scrupulous sterilization techniques. It is rare for a blood vessel, body cavity, or organ to be punctured.

Some people find that they experience a temporary exacerbation of their symptoms immediately following acupuncture treatment. Others experience lightheadedness, drowsiness, or exhilaration, although these feelings disappear soon after the treatment session has ended.

Acute

A term often used to describe a disorder or symptom that comes on suddenly. Acute conditions may or may not be severe, and they are usually of short duration. (See also *Chronic*.)

Acyclovir

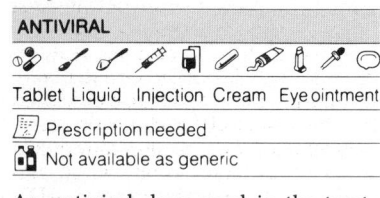

ANTIVIRAL
Tablet Liquid Injection Cream Eye ointment
Prescription needed
Not available as generic

An antiviral drug used in the treatment of *herpes simplex* and *herpes zoster* infections. It has some effect against *Epstein-Barr virus* and *cytomegalovirus* infections. To be effective, acyclovir must be prescribed soon after infection; however, it does not provide a cure, nor does it always prevent attacks from recurring, but it does reduce their severity.

POSSIBLE ADVERSE EFFECTS
Adverse effects are uncommon but wide ranging, and can include nausea and vomiting, disturbances of kidney and liver function, changes in the blood, fatigue, and other neurological symptoms. When the drug is administered by infusion or in the form of an ointment, local reactions are common.

Adam's apple

A projection at the front of the neck, just beneath the skin, that is formed by a prominence on the thyroid cartilage, part of the *larynx* (voice-box). It enlarges in males at puberty.

Addiction

A dependence on, and craving for, a particular drug, such as alcohol, diazepam (a tranquillizer), or heroin. Reducing or stopping intake of the drug may lead to characteristic physiological or psychological symptoms (see *Withdrawal syndrome*), such as tremor or anxiety. (See also *Alcohol dependence; Drug dependence*.)

Addison's disease

A rare disorder in which symptoms are caused by a deficiency of the corticosteroid hormones *hydrocortisone* and *aldosterone*, normally produced by the adrenal cortex (outer part of the adrenal glands). The disease is named after the English physician Thomas Addison (1793-1860). It was invariably fatal before hormone treatment became available in the 1950s.

CAUSES
Addison's disease can be caused by any disease process that destroys the adrenal cortexes. The most common cause is an *autoimmune disorder*, in which a person's immune system produces antibodies that attack the adrenal glands. *Tuberculosis* of the adrenal glands, once the main cause, is now extremely rare.

In addition to the deficient production of aldosterone and hydrocortisone by the adrenal glands, excessive amounts of *ACTH* and other hormones are secreted by the pituitary gland. One of these hormones (called melanocyte-stimulating hormone, or MSH) increases the synthesis of melanin pigment in the skin.

SYMPTOMS AND DIAGNOSIS
Addison's disease generally has a slow onset and chronic course, with symptoms developing gradually over months or years. However, acute episodes, called Addisonian crises, can also occur; they are brought on by infection, injury, or other stresses. The crises occur because the adrenal glands cannot increase their production of aldosterone and hydrocortisone, which normally help the body to cope with stress.

The symptoms of Addisonian crises are mainly due to aldosterone deficiency, which leads to excessive loss of sodium and water in the urine, extreme muscle weakness, dehydration, *hypotension* (low blood pressure),

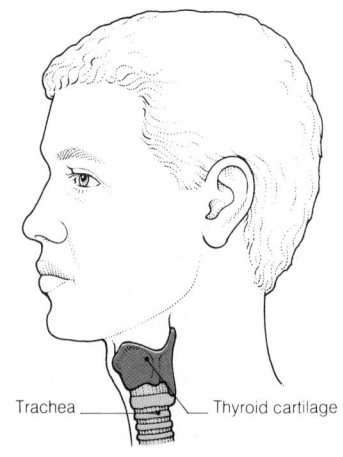

LOCATION OF THE ADAM'S APPLE

This projection at the front of the neck, beneath the skin, is formed by a prominence on the thyroid cartilage.

Trachea   Thyroid cartilage

confusion, and coma. Deficiency of hydrocortisone leads to *hypoglycaemia* (low blood sugar).

Symptoms of the chronic form of Addison's disease include tiredness, weakness, vague abdominal pain, and weight loss. A more specific symptom is darkening of the skin in the creases of the palms and pressure areas of the body, and particularly in the mouth. The darkening is caused by the overproduction of MSH.

Diagnosis is generally made if the patient fails to respond to an injection of ACTH, which normally stimulates the secretion of hydrocortisone.

TREATMENT
Treatment of acute Addisonian crises involves monitoring blood pressure and heart-rate during the rapid infusion of saline and glucose, and supplementary doses of hydrocortisone and fludrocortisone to correct the sodium deficiency and dehydration. Lifelong treatment of the disease requires replacement of the deficient hormones with *corticosteroid drugs*.

Because patients with Addison's disease cannot increase their output of corticosteroid hormones in response to stress, they are at risk during stressful situations, such as infection, surgery, or injury. Their doctors must instruct them in the use of increased doses of corticosteroid drugs at such times so that the body mechanisms that fight infection and promote healing are not impaired.

Adduction

Movement of a limb towards the central line of the body, or of a digit towards the axis of a limb. Muscles that carry out this movement are often called adductors. The opposite movement is called *abduction*.

Adenitis

Inflammation of lymph nodes. Cervical adenitis (swollen, tender lymph nodes in the neck) occurs in certain infections, such as those caused by streptococcal bacteria (especially *tonsillitis*) and infectious *mononucleosis* (glandular fever). In the past, adenitis was often due to scrofula (tuberculous infection of the cervical lymph nodes).

Mesenteric lymphadenitis is inflammation of the lymph nodes in the peritoneum (the membrane that encloses the intestines) caused by a viral infection. Symptoms of mesenteric lymphadenitis—abdominal pain and tenderness—may mimic those of acute appendicitis and may require an operation to confirm a diagnosis.

A

Treatment of adenitis may include analgesic drugs (painkillers), hot compresses or a heating pad, and, if a bacterial infection is suspected, antibiotic drugs. The inflammation usually subsides within a few days.

Adenocarcinoma

The technical name for a *cancer* of a gland or glandular tissue, or for a cancer in which the cells form gland-like structures. An adenocarcinoma arises from epithelium (the layer of cells that lines the inside of organs).

Cancers of the colon (the main part of the large intestine), breast, pancreas, and kidney are usually adenocarcinomas, as are a proportion of cancers of the cervix, oesophagus, salivary glands, and many other organs. (See also *Intestine, cancer of; Kidney cancer; Pancreas, cancer of.*)

Adenoidectomy

Surgical removal of the *adenoids*, usually performed on a child with abnormally large adenoids that are causing recurrent infections of the middle ear or air sinuses. The operation is often performed together with *tonsillectomy.*

Adenoidectomy is generally an operation with minimal after-effects. The patient can usually begin to eat normally the following day.

Adenoids

A midline swelling at the back of the nose, above the tonsils, made up of *lymph nodes* (tissues that contain lymphocytes, which are white cells that help fight infection). These nodes form part of the body's defences against upper respiratory tract infections; they tend to enlarge during early childhood, a time when such infections are common.

DISORDERS
In most children, adenoids shrink after the age of about five years, disappearing altogether by puberty. In some children, however, they become even larger and obstruct the passage from the nose to the throat, causing snoring, breathing through the mouth, and a characteristically nasal voice. They can also block the eustachian tube (which connects the middle ear to the throat), causing infection and deafness.

Obstruction to the flow of secretions behind the nose can result in *rhinitis* (inflammation of the nose), which can spread to the middle ear (see *Otitis media*) and to the air sinuses behind the nose (see *Sinusitis*).

DIAGNOSIS AND TREATMENT To discover whether ear, nose, and throat infections are being caused by abnormally enlarged adenoids, the doctor usually inspects the back of the throat using a mirror with a light attached. Sometimes an X-ray may be taken.

Infections usually respond to antibiotic drugs; however, if infections recur frequently, *adenoidectomy* (surgical removal of the adenoids) may be recommended.

Adenoma

A benign (noncancerous) tumour or cyst that resembles glandular tissue and arises from the epithelium (the layer of cells that lines the inside of organs).

Adenomas of *endocrine glands*, such as the pituitary gland, thyroid gland, adrenal glands, and pancreas, can cause excessive hormone production, leading to disease. Pituitary adenomas, for example, can result in *acromegaly* or *Cushing's syndrome.*

Adenomatosis

An abnormal condition of glands in which they are affected either by *hyperplasia* (overgrowth) or by the development of numerous *adenomas* (benign tumours).

Adenomatosis may simultaneously affect two or more different endocrine glands, such as the adrenal glands, parathyroid glands, pituitary gland, and pancreas.

LOCATION OF THE ADENOIDS
These two glandular swellings are found at the back of the nasal passage above the tonsils. Enlarged adenoids are sometimes implicated in *sleep apnoea*.

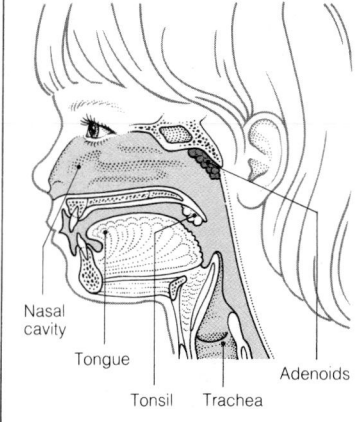

Nasal cavity

Tongue

Tonsil   Trachea

Adenoids

ADH

The abbreviation for antidiuretic hormone (also called vasopressin), which is released from the posterior part of the *pituitary gland* and acts on the kidneys to increase their reabsorption of water into the blood.

ACTIONS
ADH reduces the amount of water lost in the urine and helps control the body's overall water balance. Water is continually being taken into the body in food and drink and is also produced by the chemical reactions in cells. Conversely, water is also continually being lost in urine, sweat, faeces, and in the breath as water vapour. ADH helps maintain the optimum amount of water in the body.

ADH production is controlled by the *hypothalamus* (an area in the centre of the brain), which detects changes in the concentration and volume of the blood. If the blood concentration increases (i.e. the blood contains less water), the hypothalamus stimulates the pituitary to release more ADH. If the blood is too dilute, less ADH is produced; as a result, more water is lost from the body in the urine.

DISORDERS
Various factors can affect ADH production and thus disturb the body's water balance. For example, alcohol reduces ADH production by direct action on the brain, resulting in a temporary increase in the production of urine. Urine production is also increased in *diabetes insipidus*, a disorder in which there is either insufficient production of ADH in the pituitary gland or, rarely, failure of the kidneys to respond to ADH.

The reverse effect, water retention, may result from temporarily increased ADH production after a major operation or serious accident. Water retention may also be caused by the secretion of ADH by some tumours, especially of the lung.

DRUG THERAPY
Synthetic ADH is given via the nose or by injection to treat diabetes insipidus. High intravenous doses cause narrowing of blood vessels and may stop bleeding from *oesophageal varices*. Adverse effects include abdominal cramps, nausea, headache, drowsiness, and confusion.

Adhesion

Joining of normally unconnected body parts by bands of fibrous tissue. Adhesions are sometimes present from birth, but most develop as a result of scarring after inflammation.

Adhesions are most common in the abdomen, where they often form after *peritonitis* (inflammation of the abdominal lining) or after surgery. Sometimes, loops of intestine are bound together by adhesions, resulting in *intestinal obstruction*. In such cases, an operation is usually required to cut the bands of fibrous tissue and free the intestinal loops.

Adipose tissue

A layer of fat just beneath the skin and around various internal organs. After puberty, the distribution of superficial adipose tissue differs in males and females. Adipose tissue makes up a larger proportion of the total body weight of women than of men.

FUNCTIONS AND DISORDERS

Adipose tissue is built up from fat deposited as a result of excess food intake, thus acting as an energy store; excessive amounts of adipose tissue produce *obesity*. The tissue acts as an insulator against loss of body heat, particularly in babies. Adipose tissue helps absorb shock in areas subject to sudden or frequent pressure, such as the buttocks and feet. Adipose tissue also surrounds and cushions the heart, kidneys, and various other internal organs.

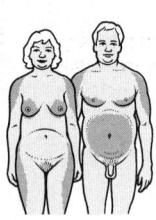

Distribution of adipose tissue
In adult males, adipose tissue accumulates around the shoulders, waist, and abdomen; in women, it accumulates on the breasts, hips, and thighs.

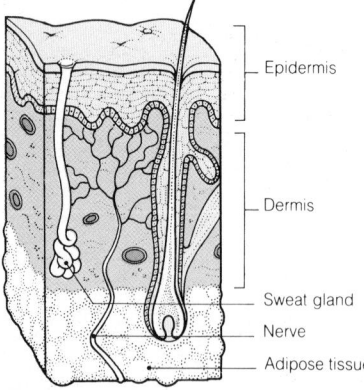

Epidermis

Dermis

Sweat gland

Nerve

Adipose tissue

Adjuvant

A substance that enhances the action of another substance in the body. The term is usually used to describe an ingredient added to a *vaccine* to increase the production of antibodies by the immune system, therefore enhancing the vaccine's efficiency in conferring immunity. Adjuvant chemotherapy is the use of anticancer drugs in addition to surgical removal of a tumour.

Adlerian theory

The psychoanalytical ideas set forth by the Austrian psychiatrist Alfred Adler (1870-1937). Also known as individual psychology, Adler's theories were based on the central idea that everyone is born with natural feelings of inferiority. Life is seen as a constant struggle to overcome these feelings; failure to do so leads to symptoms of neurosis. (See also *Psychoanalytic theory*.)

Adolescence

The period between childhood and adulthood. Broadly speaking, adolescence corresponds to the teenage years. A complex stage of personality development and psychological upheaval, adolescence commences and overlaps with, but is not the same as, *puberty*. Puberty is the period of hormonally regulated development when the secondary sexual characteristics appear, marking the onset of physical and sexual maturity.

FEATURES

Adolescence is a time of much change for the individual and for the adolescent's family. The adolescent must come to terms with the body's physical changes and with the fact that family and society no longer expect or tolerate childish behaviour. During adolescence, the adult's self-identity is formed. This involves achieving reorientation of emotional ties with parents; understanding and developing control and direction of adult sexual and other drives; occupation and career orientation; and eventually developing a mature set of values with responsible self-direction. Adolescence is also a time of forming attitudes and opinions.

Adolescents would like to be independent but many must still rely on adults for emotional and financial support. Family conflicts may arise when adolescents demand increased independence before their parents consider them ready for it.

During the process of achieving an adult identity, the adolescent ceases to define himself or herself only in terms of the adults who are at home and at school. He or she may seek other figures (such as singers or sports personalities) as role models, and may rebel against parental standards and family. Adolescents experiment with views and opinions, with allegiances to peer groups and gangs, and with political movements. They may adopt outrageous fashions of dress, appearance, and behaviour.

Sexual experimentation occurs in fantasy and in reality, alone and with others. Gender identity may be questioned; this may be the time that a person first realizes that he or she is homosexual. Often during adolescence, homosexual behaviour occurs temporarily. Coming to terms with sexual drives may be influenced by the adolescent's perception of his or her parents' relationship.

PROBLEMS

Problems may have physiological, psychological, and/or social origins. Common patterns of adolescent behaviour include moodiness, loss of interest in school, fluctuating school performance, and truancy. Adolescents may worry about their physical appearance, their changing body shape, and whether they are physically attractive. They may feel nervous, may become painfully shy and lacking in confidence. Often they feel very unsure of their personal identity, suffering a so-called "identity crisis". There may be a strong sense of alienation from parents, who may feel they can no longer talk to their children.

Some adolescents are overassertive and strive prematurely for independence. Rebellion against parents is often exaggerated in adolescents who were overdependent on, or overprotected by, their parents during childhood. Childhood deprivation that has resulted in poor *bonding* between child and parents can also lead to rebelliousness. On the other hand, a teenager who remains too dependent may remain stuck in adolescence and not develop sufficiently to make his or her own decisions or to form new relationships outside the family.

Aggressive drives that are not controlled and used constructively can lead to outbursts of temper or other undesirable behaviour. Delinquency is usually a transient phase and may be dealt with by a mixture of firmness and understanding.

Adolescents (and younger children) may become involved in drug or solvent abuse. Youngsters who take drugs to relieve anxiety or depression are more likely to become dependent than others who experiment because of peer-group pressure.

A high proportion of adolescents with serious or prolonged psychological and behavioural problems, particularly delinquency and *drug dependence*, come from disturbed or deprived home environments, where there is poverty, marital disharmony, alcoholism, or psychiatric disturbance in the parents.

Adolescents are often referred for specialist advice because parents or teachers are worried about their behaviour. Only a small percentage of those referred need psychiatric treatment; most have temporary problems that resolve on their own. Family problems or difficulties with relationships may provoke suicide attempts in disturbed adolescents.

Maintaining communication between parents and their offspring is important but not always easy. Parents should give advice on practical problems, such as acne and diet, but should never laugh off or underestimate seemingly minor problems; to do so may undermine the adolescent's confidence. The most valuable support a parent can give an adolescent is to encourage self-confidence and responsibility and thus prepare him or her to cope with adult life.

ADP

Abbreviation for adenosine diphosphate, the chemical that takes up energy released during biochemical reactions to form *ATP* (adenosine triphosphate), the main energy-carrying chemical in the body. When ATP releases its energy, ADP is reconstituted. (See also *Metabolism*.)

Adrenal failure

Insufficient production of hormones by the adrenal cortex (outer part of the *adrenal glands*). It can be acute (of sudden onset) or chronic (of more gradual onset). Adrenal failure may be due to a disorder of the adrenal glands, in which case it is called *Addison's disease*. Alternatively, it may be due to reduced stimulation of the adrenal cortex by *ACTH*, a hormone produced by the pituitary gland (see *Adrenal glands* disorders box).

Adrenal glands

A pair of small, triangular *endocrine glands* (glands that secrete hormones directly into the bloodstream) located above the kidneys. Each adrenal gland can be divided, anatomically and functionally, into two distinct parts: the outer adrenal cortex and the smaller, inner adrenal medulla.

ANATOMY OF THE ADRENAL GLANDS

Also sometimes called the suprarenal glands, the adrenal glands are situated on top of the kidneys. Each one is divided into two regions: the adrenal cortex (which secretes hormones that affect the metabolism) and the adrenal medulla (which is part of the sympathetic nervous system).

Inferior vena cava — Aorta

Adrenal gland

Kidney

Renal vein — Renal artery

Cortex — Medulla

THE ADRENAL CORTEX

This part of the gland secretes a group of hormones called *corticosteroid hormones*, which have a variety of important effects on the body. The adrenal cortex is made up of three zones that can be distinguished under a microscope. The outermost zone secretes the hormone *aldosterone*, which, by inhibiting the amount of sodium excreted in the urine, helps maintain blood volume and blood pressure.

FEEDBACK MECHANISM

The rate at which many glands produce hormones is influenced by other hormones, especially those · secreted by the pituitary gland and the hypothalamus. If the amount of hormone produced is increased, negative feedback mechanisms act on the hypothalamus and pituitary so that they produce less of their stimulating hormones, thus reducing the target gland's activity. If the amount of hormone produced is decreased, the feedback weakens, causing increased production of stimulating hormones.

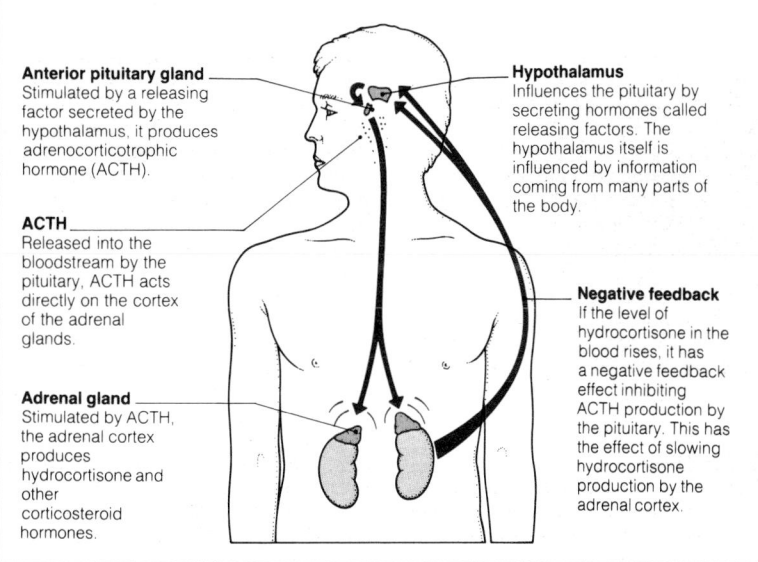

Anterior pituitary gland
Stimulated by a releasing factor secreted by the hypothalamus, it produces adrenocorticotrophic hormone (ACTH).

ACTH
Released into the bloodstream by the pituitary, ACTH acts directly on the cortex of the adrenal glands.

Adrenal gland
Stimulated by ACTH, the adrenal cortex produces hydrocortisone and other corticosteroid hormones.

Hypothalamus
Influences the pituitary by secreting hormones called releasing factors. The hypothalamus itself is influenced by information coming from many parts of the body.

Negative feedback
If the level of hydrocortisone in the blood rises, it has a negative feedback effect inhibiting ACTH production by the pituitary. This has the effect of slowing hydrocortisone production by the adrenal cortex.

A

The inner and middle zones together secrete the hormones *hydrocortisone* (also called cortisol) and corticosterone, as well as small amounts of *androgen hormones* (hormones that stimulate the development of male sex characteristics). Hydrocortisone is the most important human corticosteroid, controlling the body's use of fats, proteins, and carbohydrates. Hydrocortisone and corticosterone also have the effect of suppressing inflammatory reactions in the body and, to a limited extent, the activities of the *immune system*.

Production of hormones by the adrenal cortex is governed by other hormones made in the *hypothalamus* and *pituitary gland*. The rate of hydrocortisone release is controlled by the release of *ACTH* (adrenocorticotrophic hormone) by the pituitary gland, and normally varies during a 24-hour cycle, being minimal at midnight, rising to a peak at around 6 a.m., and then falling slowly during the course of the day. Emotion, stress, and injury are potent stimulators of ACTH and hydrocortisone release; without hydrocortisone, the body is unable to recover properly from stress.

THE ADRENAL MEDULLA

The adrenal medulla is part of the sympathetic division of the *autonomic nervous system*, which is the body's first line of defence against physical and emotional stresses. The adrenal medulla is closely related to nervous tissue and secretes the hormones *adrenaline* and *noradrenaline* in response to stimulation by sympathetic nerves. These nerves are most active during times of stress.

The release of these hormones into the circulation produces effects similar to sympathetic nerve stimulation. The heart-rate and also the force of contraction of the heart muscle increase so that more blood can be pumped around the body, and the airways of the lungs are widened to make breathing easier. The hormones constrict blood vessels in the intestines, kidneys, and liver, and widen blood vessels supplying the skeletal muscles. Consequently, more blood is supplied to the active muscles and less to the internal organs.

Adrenal hyperplasia, congenital

An uncommon disorder, also called adrenogenital syndrome or virilizing adrenal hyperplasia. The condition is present (although not always ap-

parent) from birth. It results from inheritance of a recessive genetic defect (see *Genetic disorders*). The gene defect causes variable *enzyme* defects and blocks the production of the hormones *hydrocortisone* and *aldosterone* by the adrenal glands.

The incidence of congenital adrenal hyperplasia in the UK is about one affected baby per 7,500 live births.

CAUSES AND SYMPTOMS

The enzyme block results in the production of progestogens, which are converted to *androgens* (male hormones) that accumulate in the fetus. In girls, these androgens virilize the genital tract, causing enlargement of the clitoris and some fusion of the labia majora (outer lips of the vulva), resulting in ambiguity of the genitals (see *Sex determination*). About half of the affected males have an enlarged penis, which may be evident at birth or develop later.

Another result of the enzyme defect is that the body is unable to retain salt and water. This may cause dehydration, weight loss, and low blood pressure, and may lead to shock. There may also be hypoglycaemia (low blood sugar).

Normally, hydrocortisone suppresses secretion by the pituitary gland of *ACTH* (adrenocorticotrophic hormone), the hormone that stimulates the adrenal glands. An affected person's adrenal glands produce insufficient hydrocortisone, leading to excessive secretion of ACTH. This causes hyperplasia (enlargement) of the adrenal glands.

The excessive secretion of ACTH and another hormone, called melanocyte-stimulating hormone, causes excessive skin pigmentation, with dark skin creases and dark nipples.

In severe cases, the condition becomes apparent in the first weeks of life. In milder cases, features of the disorder appear later, sometimes producing premature puberty in boys, and delayed menstruation, hirsutism, and potential infertility in girls. These more mildly affected individuals do not usually have problems with salt regulation.

DIAGNOSIS AND TREATMENT

The diagnosis is suggested by the signs and symptoms at birth or later in childhood or adolescence. Congenital adrenal hyperplasia is confirmed by the measurement of corticosteroid hormones in the blood and urine. *Ultrasound scanning* shows the adrenal glands to be enlarged but with no tumour present.

Treatment consists of replacing the missing hormones. If the condition is recognized and treatment started early, normal sexual development and fertility usually follow. Plastic surgery needs to be undertaken in most affected females.

Adrenaline

A naturally occurring hormone, also called epinephrine. Adrenaline has been produced synthetically as a drug since 1900.

Adrenaline is one of two chemicals (the other is *noradrenaline* or norepinephrine) released by the adrenal gland in response to signals from the sympathetic division of the *autonomic nervous system*. These signals are triggered by stress, exercise, or by an emotion such as fear.

Adrenaline increases the speed and force of the heartbeat and thereby the work that can be done by the heart. It widens the airways to improve breathing and narrows blood vessels in the skin and intestine so that an increased flow of blood reaches the muscles, allowing them to cope with the demands of exercise.

USE AS A DRUG

Adrenaline is sometimes given by injection as an emergency treatment for *cardiac arrest* (stopped heartbeat), *anaphylactic shock* (a severe allergic reaction) and acute *asthma* attacks.

During surgery, it is occasionally injected into tissues to reduce bleeding. When combined with a local anaesthetic, adrenaline prolongs the pain-deadening effect by slowing down the rate at which the anaesthetic spreads into surrounding tissues.

Adrenaline eye-drops are used to treat *glaucoma* and they are used during eye surgery because they reduce pressure in the eyeball. Adrenaline can also be used to stop nosebleeds and reduce *nasal congestion*.

POSSIBLE ADVERSE EFFECTS

Regular use of adrenaline as eyedrops may cause a burning pain and, occasionally, blurred vision or pigment deposits on the eye's surface.

In nose-drop form, adrenaline may cause palpitations, restlessness, and anxiety; more recently developed *decongestant drugs* are now usually used to treat nasal congestion.

Adrenal tumours

Rare malignant or benign tumours within the *adrenal glands*, usually causing excess secretion of hormones.

Tumours of the adrenal cortex may secrete aldosterone, causing primary

A

DISORDERS OF THE ADRENAL GLANDS

Excessive or deficient production of hormones by the adrenal glands can occur in a variety of ways. These disorders are uncommon, but may be serious. Disturbed hormone production by the adrenal cortex is more common than disturbance of the adrenal medulla.

CONGENITAL DEFECTS

Congenital *adrenal hyperplasia* affects about one newborn baby in 10,000. The adrenal cortex is unable to synthesize sufficient hydrocortisone and (sometimes) aldosterone, and the baby is ill or fails to thrive. As a side-effect of the reduced hydrocortisone production, the glands are stimulated to produce androgens (male sex hormones) in excess; this can cause masculinization of female babies.

TUMOURS

Growths in the adrenal glands are rare and generally lead to excess hormone production. Excess secretion of aldosterone causes *aldosteronism* (also known as Conn's syndrome), a condition characterized by thirst and high blood pressure. Excess secretion of hydrocortisone causes *Cushing's syndrome*, which has various features including muscle-wasting and obesity of the trunk. Androgens may also be produced to excess, causing masculinization in females.

Tumours of the adrenal medulla include *phaeochromocytoma* and *neuroblastoma*. Excess adrenaline and noradrenaline are secreted.

AUTOIMMUNE DISORDERS

Deficient production of hormones by the adrenal cortex is called *adrenal failure*; if due to disease of the adrenal glands themselves, it is called *Addison's disease*. The most common cause of Addison's disease is an autoimmune process (in which the body's immune system attacks its own tissues). Addison's disease can take a chronic course, characterized by weakness, weight loss, and skin darkening, or an acute form (Addisonian crisis or acute adrenal failure), in which the patient may become confused and comatose.

INFECTION

Destruction of the adrenal glands by *tuberculosis* was once a major cause of Addison's disease but is now uncommon. The onset of an infection or other acute illness in someone with Addison's disease can precipitate acute adrenal failure.

IMPAIRED BLOOD SUPPLY

Loss or obstruction of the blood supply to the adrenals, sometimes as a result of arterial disease, is another possible cause of Addison's disease or acute adrenal failure.

OTHER DISORDERS

In many cases disturbed activity of the adrenals is caused not by disease of the glands themselves, but by an increase or decrease in the blood level of hormones that influence the activity of the glands.

Hydrocortisone production by the adrenal cortex is controlled by the secretion of *ACTH* (adrenocortico-trophic hormone) by the pituitary gland. A tumour or other disorder of the pituitary, or tumours in the lung, breast, and elsewhere, can cause excess ACTH secretion, leading to too much hydrocortisone being produced by the adrenals and, hence, to Cushing's syndrome. Pituitary disease is, in fact, the most common cause of Cushing's syndrome.

Destruction or removal of the pituitary has the opposite effect, stopping ACTH secretion, preventing stimulation of the adrenal cortex, and thus leading to adrenal failure.

INVESTIGATION

Suspected disturbance of adrenal function is investigated by serial measurement of the levels of hormones such as hydrocortisone, aldosterone, adrenaline, and ACTH in the blood and/or urine. Tests may also be carried out to measure the effects of an injected substance that would normally modify the production of a hormone. Such tests can help localize the underlying cause of the disorder—for example, to distinguish Cushing's syndrome due to an adrenal tumour from that due to pituitary disease.

If disease of the adrenal glands themselves is suspected, the glands may be imaged by such techniques as *ultrasound*, *CT scanning*, or *MRI*, which have largely replaced the older methods of *arteriography*, *radionuclide scanning*, and intravenous *pyelography* (to detect distortion of the kidney by an adrenal gland tumour). If a tumour or overgrowth of a gland is present it will usually be detectable by one of these techniques.

---

aldosteronism (also called Conn's syndrome), or hydrocortisone, causing *Cushing's syndrome*.

Tumours of the adrenal medulla may cause excess secretion of adrenaline and noradrenaline. There are two types of tumour affecting the adrenal medulla: *neuroblastoma* and *phaeochromocytoma*. These tumours cause intermittent *hypertension* (high blood pressure) and sweating attacks.

Surgical removal of a tumour, or even a whole adrenal gland, often cures the conditions caused by the excess hormone secretion. (See also *Adrenal glands* disorders box.)

Adrenocorticotrophic hormone
See *ACTH*.

Adrenogenital syndrome
See *Adrenal hyperplasia, congenital*.

Aerobic
Requiring oxygen to live, function, and grow. Humans and many other forms of life are dependent on oxygen for "burning" foods to produce energy (see *Metabolism*). Because of this dependence, they are described as obligate aerobes. In contrast, many bacteria have fundamentally different metabolisms and thrive without oxygen (some of them are even killed by it); such microorganisms are described as *anaerobic*. There are also some bacteria and yeasts (called facultative aerobes) that flourish in oxygen but can also live without it. (See also *Aerobics*.)

Aerobics
Exercises that allow muscles to work at a steady rate with a constant, adequate supply of oxygen-carrying blood. Oxygen is necessary to release energy from the body's stores of fat, glycogen (a starchy material), and sugars.

A

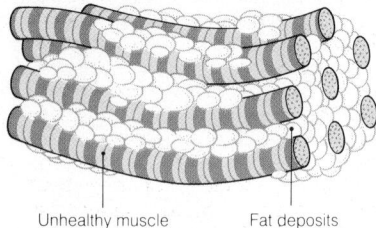

Unexercised muscle

Unhealthy muscle   Fat deposits

Exercised muscle

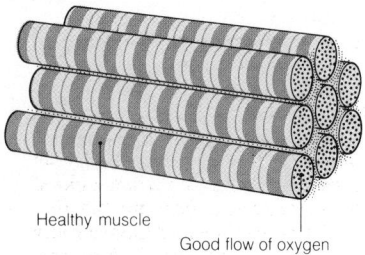

Healthy muscle

Good flow of oxygen

Benefits of aerobic exercise
Regular aerobic exercise improves the condition of the muscles. The supply of blood-carrying oxygen to the muscles is increased and the cells' capacity to use oxygen is consequently enhanced.

During aerobic exercises, such as swimming, jogging, and cycling, the muscles' increased demand for oxygen is met continuously as the rate at which oxygen reaches the muscles keeps pace with the rate at which it is used up. Because of this continual replenishment, the activity can be sustained for long periods.

To fuel aerobic exercise, the muscles use fatty acid rather than glucose, burning it completely to produce energy, carbon dioxide, and water. By contrast, anaerobic exercise relies on a different series of biochemical reactions to obtain energy from the stores of sugar and fat in muscle. The waste products of anaerobic exercise are acidic and, as they accumulate in the muscles, cause muscle fatigue. High-intensity exercises are anaerobic and can be performed for only relatively short periods.

BENEFITS OF AEROBIC EXERCISE
To benefit your health, aerobic exercises should involve the large muscles of the trunk and limbs. In addition, the exercises need to be performed continuously for 20 minutes at least three times a week.

When performed regularly, aerobic exercises improve stamina and endurance. They encourage the growth of capillaries (small blood vessels),

thus improving the supply of blood to the cells. Aerobic exercises also increase the size and number of mitochondria (energy-producing organelles) within muscle cells, thus improving the cells' capacity to use oxygen and increasing the amount of oxygen that the body can use in a given time.

The condition of the heart also improves as the body becomes fitter. The heart-rate becomes slower, both at rest and during exercise; the heart muscle becomes thicker and stronger; and the stroke volume (the amount of blood pumped with each beat) increases. The overall result of these changes is that the heart needs to do less work to achieve the same level of efficiency in pumping blood round the body.

For all-round fitness, which includes strength and suppleness, other types of exercise should be performed as well as aerobics. (See also *Exercise*; *Fitness*.)

Aerodontalgia
Sudden pain in a tooth brought on by a change in surrounding air pressure. Flying at a high altitude in a lowered atmospheric pressure can cause a pocket of air within the dental pulp chamber to expand and irritate the nerve in the root. Common sources of aerodontalgia are improperly fitting fillings, poorly filled root canals, and inflammation of the pulp.

Aerophagy
Excessive swallowing of air. It may occur during rapid eating or drinking or be caused by anxiety. Aerophagy may also be a deliberate action to relieve indigestion by belching. After *laryngectomy* (surgical removal of the larynx), voluntary aerophagy is used to produce oesophageal speech.

Aetiology
The cause of a disease, or the study of the various factors involved in causing a disease.

For some cases of a particular disorder, a specific aetiology can be identified: laboratory studies may show, for example, that an attack of diarrhoea is due to a particular type of bacterium or virus. Other disorders have a multifactorial aetiology: the causative factors of degenerative arthritis, for example, include genetic susceptibility, repeated joint injuries, and being overweight. However, many disorders, such as schizophrenia, are of unknown aetiology.

Affect
A term used to describe a person's mood. The two extremes of affect are elation and depression. A person who experiences extreme moods or changes in moods may have an *affective disorder*. A person whose responses to events seem flat—so that nothing excites, nothing angers—is said to have a shallow, flattened, or reduced affect; this characteristic may be a sign of *schizophrenia* or of an organic *brain syndrome*.

Affective disorders
Mental illnesses characterized predominantly by marked changes in *affect* (mood). Mood may vary over a period of time between *mania* (extreme elation) and severe *depression*. (See also *Manic-depressive illness*.)

Affinity
A term used to describe the attraction between chemicals that causes them to bind together, as, for example, between an antigen and an antibody (see *Immune response*). In microbiology, affinity describes the physical similarity between organisms (for example, viruses). In psychology, the term affinity describes an attraction between two people.

Aflatoxin
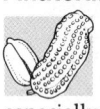 A poisonous substance produced by ASPERGILLUS FLAVUS moulds, which contaminate stored foods, especially grains, peanuts, and cassava. Aflatoxin has been found to cause liver cancer in laboratory animals and is believed to be one of the factors responsible for the high incidence of this cancer in tropical Africa.

Afterbirth
The common name for the tissues that are expelled from the uterus after delivery of a baby. The afterbirth includes the *placenta* and the membranes that surrounded the fetus.

Afterpains
Contractions of the uterus that continue after childbirth. Afterpains are normal and indicate that the uterus is shrinking as it should. They are experienced by many women, especially after a second or subsequent delivery. The pains typically occur during the first few days after delivery and are particularly painful during breast-feeding. Afterpains disappear after a few days but may require analgesic drugs (painkillers).

Agar

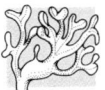 An extract of certain seaweeds with properties similar to those of gelatine. Its full name is agar-agar. It is taken to soften and give bulk to faeces in cases of constipation, and to relieve indigestion and heartburn because of its bland, soothing properties. Another use of agar is as a gelling agent in media for growing bacterial *cultures*.

Age

Of medical significance in diagnosis and in determining treatment, age is usually measured chronologically (in terms of the period of time since birth). However, age can also be measured in terms of physical, mental, or developmental maturity.

PHYSICAL AGE
Physical age can be measured even before birth. The age of a fetus is measured in terms of gestational age. Estimation of gestational age is important in neonatal paediatrics for identifying those babies who are too small for their gestational age and who may have problems because of their low birthweight. Gestational age can be assessed from the date of the woman's last menstrual period and by the size of her pregnant uterus. More accurate determination is made by measuring the size of the fetus by *ultrasound scanning*. The gestational age of a newborn baby can be estimated to within about two weeks by physical examination.

Children vary greatly in the rate at which they develop and grow, but their physical age is a measure of maturity that provides a common scale of development that can be used throughout the period of growth. In adults, physical age is difficult to assess other than through physical appearance. Physical age can be estimated after death by the state of certain organs, particularly by the amount of atheroma (fatty deposits) lining the arteries.

The most useful measure of physical development in children is bone age. Bone age measures how much the bones of a body area have matured, as seen on an X-ray. Measures such as height and weight are less useful as age standards because they vary greatly among individuals of the same chronological age. In contrast, all healthy individuals reach the same adult level of skeletal maturity and each bone passes through the same sequence of changes of shape as it grows.

Assessment of bone age is particularly useful in investigating delayed *puberty* or *short stature* in children. A prediction of the final adult height can be made if the chronological age, bone age, and current height are known.

Dental age is another, though less useful, measure of physical maturity. It can be assessed by counting the number of teeth that have erupted (see *Eruption of teeth*), and by comparing the amount of dental calcification (as seen on X-rays) with standard values in much the same way as bone age is measured.

MENTAL AND DEVELOPMENTAL AGE
Mental age is assessed by comparing scores achieved in intelligence or achievement tests with standard scores for different chronological ages (see *Intelligence tests*).

A young child's age can be expressed in terms of developmental level. Patterns of normal development have been described for children from birth to the age of five years in the fields of speech, vision, hearing, and motor skills (principally walking and delicate hand-eye coordination). Specific tasks in these fields are achieved at certain ages (see *Child development*).

Agenesis

The complete absence at birth of an organ or component of the body, caused by failure of development in the embryo.

Agent

Any substance or force capable of bringing about a biological, chemical, or physical change. An agent can also be a person acting on behalf of someone else. (See also *Reagent*.)

Agent Orange

A herbicide of which the major constituent (50 per cent by volume) is the phenoxy acid herbicide 2,4,5 T. That substance may be contaminated, in manufacture, with the highly toxic poison TCDD, commonly known as dioxin (see *Defoliant poisoning*).

Age spots

Blemishes that appear on the skin with increasing age. Most common are seborrhoeic *keratoses*, which are brown or yellow, slightly raised spots that can occur at any site and sometimes get caught on clothing. Also common in the elderly are freckles, solar keratoses (small blemishes caused by overexposure to the sun), and *De Morgan's spots*, which are red, pinpoint blemishes on the trunk.

Treatment is usually unnecessary for any of these age spots apart from solar keratoses, which may progress to skin cancer. Freezing the keratoses with liquid nitrogen is the usual treatment; they may also be removed surgically under a local anaesthetic.

Most spots are harmless but any unexplained blemish, or one that grows rapidly or bleeds, should be seen by your doctor because of the possibility of skin cancer.

Ageusia

Lack or impairment of the sense of taste (see *Taste, loss of*).

Aggregation, platelet

The clumping together of platelets (small, sticky blood particles). Platelet aggregation takes place when a blood vessel is damaged, forming the first stage of *blood clotting* and thus helping to plug the injured vessel. Aggregation can also have adverse effects. It contributes to the formation of atheroma (the fatty substance that accumulates inside arteries and causes *atherosclerosis*) and thrombi (blood clots), which can cause *thrombosis*.

In the treatment of disorders in which thrombosis plays a part—*coronary artery disease*, for example—drugs such as aspirin, dipyridamole, or sulfinpyrazone may be prescribed to reduce aggregation.

Aggression

A general term for a wide variety of acts of hostility, some of which may be outside the range of normal social behaviour.

CAUSES
Among animals, aggression serves to protect the individual by way of self-defence and in defence of food, territory, and the young. In humans, there seem to be other factors, perhaps based on the needs of prehistoric survival. Some people believe aggression results from frustration, lack of affection, and the attitudes of parents.

EEG studies show changes in brain-wave patterns in people who are continuously aggressive. Aggression centres (for example, the amygdaloid area in the brain) have been described. Brain disease (such as a tumour) or head injury may sometimes result in aggressive behaviour. Even so, such outbursts do seem to be related to events; the person does not start fights for no reason at all, but rather overreacts aggressively to problems.

Androgen hormones, the male sex hormones, seem to promote aggres-

THE PRACTICAL EFFECTS OF AGING

In the body, aging is associated with loss of elasticity in the skin, blood vessels, and tendons. There is also progressive decline in the functioning of organs such as the lungs, kidneys, and liver. Mechanical wear and tear causes cumulative damage to certain organ systems. Brain cells, specialized kidney units, and many other body structures are never replaced after they have reached maturity.

EFFECTS OF AGING

Organ or tissue	Natural effects	Accelerated by
Skin	Loss of elastic tissue causes skin to sag and wrinkle. Weakened blood capillaries cause skin to bruise more easily.	Exposure to sun; smoking.
Brain and nervous system	Loss of nerve cells leads to reduction in ability to memorize or to learn new skills. Reaction time of nerves increases, making responses slower.	Excessive consumption of alcohol and other drugs; repeated head trauma (for example, from boxing).
Senses	Some loss of acuity in all senses, mainly due to loss of nerve cells.	Loud noise (hearing); smoking (smell/taste).
Lungs	Loss of elasticity with age, so that breathing is less efficient.	Air pollution; smoking; lack of exercise.
Heart	Becomes less efficient at pumping, causing reduced tolerance to exercise.	Excessive use of alcohol and cigarettes; a fatty diet.
Circulation	Arteries harden, causing poor blood circulation and higher blood pressure.	Lack of exercise; smoking; poor diet.
Joints	Pressure on intervertebral discs causes height loss; wear on hip and knee joints reduces mobility.	Athletic injuries; being overweight.
Muscles	Loss of muscle bulk and strength.	Lack of exercise; starvation.
Liver	Becomes less efficient in processing toxic substances in the blood.	Damage from alcohol consumption and virus infections.

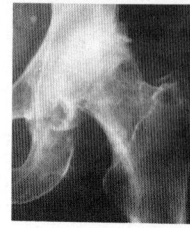

Hip joint in young person
The X-ray shows the rounded head of the thigh-bone (femur) separated by cartilage from the surrounding hip socket.

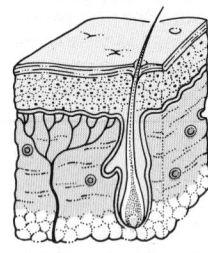

Hip joint in elderly person
This X-ray of an osteoarthritic hip shows almost complete degeneration and disappearance of the cartilage in the joint.

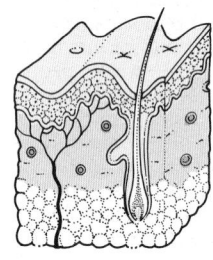

Young skin
The outer skin layer has an appreciable thickness. The deeper layers contain numerous collagen fibres, which give the skin elasticity.

Older skin
The outer layer has become thinned, wrinkled, and prone to injury. There are fewer elastic fibres in the deeper layers.

---

sion, whereas *oestrogen hormones*, the female sex hormones, actively suppress it. Age is another factor, because aggression is more common in adolescence and the early 20s, but becomes increasingly rare the older people get.

Psychiatric conditions associated with aggressive outbursts are *schizophrenia* (especially the catatonic and paranoid types), *antisocial personality disorder*, *mania*, and abuse of amphetamines or alcohol. *Temporal lobe epilepsy*, *hypoglycaemia*, and *confusion* due to physical illnesses are other, less common, medical causes. *Dementia*, whether associated with *Alzheimer's disease* or *alcohol dependence*, may remove control of aggression.

Aging

The physical and mental changes that occur with the passing of time. The aging process is sometimes seen as bringing with it only frailty and increased vulnerability to disease and injury, but many societies value their old people for their wisdom and experience and recognize other virtues that often come with age (e.g. patience and acceptance).

BIOLOGICAL AGING

All animals have a finite lifespan, and the maximum for humans seems to have changed little since biblical times. Very few people live beyond 100 years, and the average lifespan in the absence of disease seems to be about 85 years.

Gerontologists have yet to agree on the biological processes that underlie aging. Among the many theories are the "worn template" concept—that every time cells divide, the copying mechanism is more likely to introduce errors; the accumulated toxins theory, according to which the body is gradually poisoned by the accumulation of chemicals it cannot excrete; and the immune surveillance theory, which postulates that there is a progressive decline in the immune system's ability to detect and destroy microorganisms and developing tumours.

Aging is associated with degenerative changes in various organs and tissues, such as the skin, bones, joints, blood vessels, and nervous tissue (see chart). These changes may be accelerated by factors such as smoking, excessive alcohol consumption, poor diet, insufficient exercise, and excessive exposure of the skin to strong sunlight.

Nevertheless, the evidence of 90-year-olds who have smoked and drunk alcohol all their lives shows that an important factor determining life expectancy is genetic. Just as a person's height is determined by the interaction of diet and environment with the genetic potential inherited from the parents, so lifespan depends to a large extent on heredity.

NORMAL CHANGES
As people age, they discover that their physical performance declines, although not by as much as is often believed. A 60-year-old who has always exercised regularly may retain some 80 per cent of the physical strength and stamina that he or she had at the age of 25. However, the natural decline in lung function limits exertion past the age of about 60. Wound healing and resistance to infection also decline.

Sexual activity past the age of 60 is variable. Prolonged abstinence tends to lead to loss of libido and potency, whereas those who have remained sexually active often find little, if any, decline in their sex life.

As with physical performance, certain of our mental abilities inevitably deteriorate with age. Most people over 60 experience "benign forgetfulness", finding it more difficult, for example, to recall names or telephone numbers. However, *dementia* (a general decline in all areas of mental ability) occurs in fewer than 20 per cent of people older than 80.

AGING AND SOCIETY
In the 20th century there have been dramatic changes in the age structure of developed societies because infant and childhood mortality have declined markedly. Today, few adults under the age of 50 die from natural causes (accidental death is now much more frequent in young adults than death from disease). The result has been a substantial increase in the proportion of people living beyond the age of 65; the proportion living to beyond 75 continues to increase. However, about one third of the people over 75 who are living today have some disability that in some way restricts their everyday activities; improvements in preventive medicine are likely to reduce this proportion in the future.

Agitation
Restless inability to keep still, usually due to underlying anxiety or tension. Agitated people may pace up and down, pluck at clothes or sheets, wring their hands, and start tasks without completing them. Because they cannot relax or concentrate, agitated people constantly repeat such aimless activities.

Agitation is usually caused by worry over a particular situation—a father anxiously awaiting the birth of his child, for example. Persistent agitation is also seen in *anxiety disorders*, especially when there is an underlying physical cause such as alcohol withdrawal. Depressive illness (see *Depression*) in older people is usually accompanied by severe agitation. The restlessness that is sometimes caused by certain drugs, such as the *phenothiazines*, can mimic agitation.

Agnosia
An inability to recognize objects despite adequate sensory information about them reaching the brain via the eyes or ears or through touch. For an object to be recognized, the sensory information about it must be interpreted, which involves recall of memorized information about similar objects. Agnosia is caused by damage to areas of the brain involved in these interpretative and recall functions. The most common causes of such damage are *stroke* and *head injury*.

TYPES AND SYMPTOMS
Agnosia is usually associated with just one of the sensations of vision, hearing, or touch. For example, an object may be recognizable by hearing and sight but not by touch. Some people, after a stroke that damages the right cerebral hemisphere, may seem unaware of any disability in their affected left limbs. This is called anosognosia or sensory inattention.

TACTILE AGNOSIA is an inability to recognize by touch alone objects that are placed in the hands, despite adequate sensation in the fingers.

VISUAL AGNOSIA is an inability to recognize and name objects despite normal vision. Affected people may be able to describe the colour, shape, and size of an object but cannot name what they see or indicate its use.

AUDITORY AGNOSIA is an inability to recognize familiar sounds despite normal hearing.

OUTLOOK
There is no specific treatment for agnosia but some of the lost interpretative ability may return eventually.

Agoraphobia
Fear of going into open spaces and of entering shops, restaurants, or other public places. The condition often overlaps with *claustrophobia* (fear of enclosed spaces), another *phobia*.

The thought of visiting a public place or of mixing with many other people fills sufferers with such dread that they make up any number of excuses to remain at home. If they do venture out, they may have a *panic attack*, which leads to further restriction of activities. Eventually, people with agoraphobia become completely housebound.

People seek psychiatric treatment for agoraphobia more often than for any other phobia. Treatment by *behaviour therapy* is usually successful; *antidepressant drugs* are occasionally needed.

Agraphia
Loss of, or impaired, ability to write, despite normal functioning of the hand and arm muscles, caused by damage to the parts of the cerebrum (the main mass of the brain) that are concerned with writing.

CAUSES
Writing depends on a complex sequence of mental processes, including the selection of words, recall from memory of how these words are spelled, formulation and execution of the hand movements required, and visual checking that written words match their representation in the brain. These processes probably take place in a number of connected regions of the brain. Agraphia may be caused by damage to various parts of these regions (usually within the left cerebral hemisphere) and can be of different types and degrees of severity. The most common reasons for such damage are *head injury*, *stroke*, and *brain tumours*.

Agraphia rarely occurs on its own. It is often accompanied by *alexia* (loss of the ability to read) or may be part of an expressive *aphasia* (general disturbance in the expression of language).

TREATMENT AND OUTLOOK
There is no specific treatment for agraphia. However, some of the lost writing skills may return as time passes after brain injury that is due to a stroke or other event.

Ague
An outdated term for malaria or other diseases causing fever in which the sufferer alternately feels excessively hot and shiveringly cold.

A

AIDS

Acquired immune deficiency syndrome, a deficiency of the *immune system* due to infection with *HIV* (human immunodeficiency virus). Despite vast research efforts, no curative treatment has yet been found, but the progression of the infection and the symptoms and complications may be treated by a variety of *antibiotic drugs, antiviral drugs, anticancer drugs*, and *radiotherapy*. Several vaccines against the HIV viruses have been developed and are undergoing trials.

INCIDENCE

AIDS is not present in all those infected with HIV. The proportion of those infected whose condition progresses to AIDS has varied widely in different countries and different risk groups.

Every year, AIDS develops in one to five per cent of those infected with HIV. The interval between infection and the development of AIDS is highly variable. Around half of those infected develop AIDS within eight to nine years. The proportion who remain well indefinitely has yet to be determined.

Once AIDS has been diagnosed, it is considered fatal. By the end of the 1980s, nearly 100,000 men, women, and children in the US had been diagnosed as having AIDS and about half of them had died. In the UK (by the same date), approximately 2,000 people had been diagnosed as having AIDS, of whom slightly more than half had died.

The main risk groups are homosexual or bisexual men and people who inject themselves with drugs using unsterile needles and syringes. Many people with *haemophilia* also became infected in the early 1980s as a result of receiving infected blood products, but this route of infection has now been closed by better screening of blood. Other risk groups include heterosexual contacts of infected individuals, children born to infected women, and people who have received infected blood transfusions.

HISTORY

In 1981, the Centers for Disease Control (CDC) in Atlanta, Georgia, was alerted to reports of cases of a rare lung infection in previously healthy homosexual men in Los Angeles and then in New York. Infection was found to be with *PNEUMOCYSTIS CARINII*, a protozoan organism that had

---

HOW AIDS HAS BEEN CONTRACTED

Cases (% of people diagnosed as having AIDS in the UK)

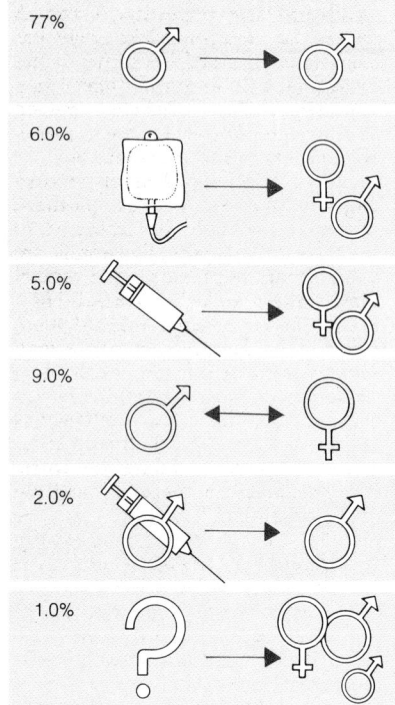

77%
Male homosexual or bisexual activity
This has accounted for most cases to date

6.0%
Receiving infected blood or blood-product transfusions
Most of this group consists of haemophiliacs who were infected before the risk was recognized. Most new cases result from receiving infected blood while abroad

5.0%
Needle-sharing by drug abusers
The number of cases is increasing in this group

9.0%
Heterosexual
In the UK, this has so far accounted for relatively few cases. However, it accounts for a rising percentage of new cases.

2.0%
Multiple risk factors
This group consists of people with more than one risk factor—mainly homosexual males who have also shared needles

1.0%
Other/unknown
This group consists of people who contracted AIDS by another means (e.g. accidental injury with an infected needle), or by unknown means

Up to 1985 only 2 per cent of new HIV infections in the UK had resulted from heterosexual exposure. By the middle of 1992 heterosexual transmission accounted for 30 per cent of new HIV infections in the UK. As with all sexually-transmitted diseases, the risk is greater for people who have multiple sex partners or have sex with prostitutes (or whose partners do). Worldwide, heterosexual sex is now the most common way of becoming infected with HIV.

NO-RISK ACTIVITIES

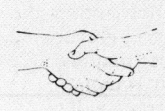
Touching
AIDS virus cannot be transmitted by social contact such as shaking hands.

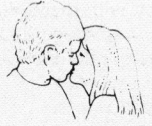
"Dry" kissing
Kissing without exchange of saliva poses no risk of virus transmission.

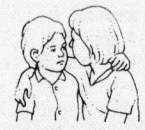
Embracing
There is no risk of transmitting the virus by embracing or cuddling.

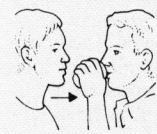
Sharing utensils
The virus cannot be transmitted by sharing a glass or cutlery.

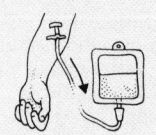
Giving blood
Only sterile needles are used for taking blood from donors

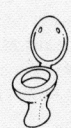
Other contact
The virus cannot be caught from toilet seats or other objects.

previously caused pneumonia only in patients whose immune defences were suppressed.

Later, cases of a rare tumour (*Kaposi's sarcoma*) were reported in young homosexual men; it was recognized as a slow-growing skin tumour previously seen mainly in Africa. In people with AIDS, the tumour behaved much more aggressively and was found in parts of the body other than the skin.

Soon it appeared that there was a rapidly increasing epidemic of conditions associated with depression of the immune system. Several other infections were reported—most of them being *opportunistic infections* (i.e. infections that do not ordinarily affect those with efficient immune defences).

These conditions were observed not only in male homosexuals, but also in intravenous drug users and haemophiliacs, suggesting that transmission was related to blood as well as to sexual activity. An infective cause seemed likely and, in 1984, French and American researchers identified the virus responsible. It was named LAV (lymphadenopathy-associated virus) by the French, and HTLV III (human T-cell lymphotrophic virus, type III) by the Americans. In 1986, the virus was renamed HIV 1; a similar virus, HIV 2, has been found to be the cause of some cases of AIDS in Africa.

THE EFFECTS OF THE VIRUS

The virus infects a type of white blood cell known as the T4, CD4, or T-helper lymphocyte, which is crucial for the regulation of the immune mechanisms. The infected cell may die or the virus may remain dormant in the cell, with the possibility of later reactivation. Many infected individuals have no sign of disease; they are "asymptomatic carriers". Or they have vague complaints, such as weight loss, fevers, sweats, or unexplained diarrhoea. People in this group have been referred to as having AIDS-related complex (ARC).

In its most severe form (i.e. AIDS), HIV infection interferes with the immune system to make the individual susceptible to a variety of infections and cancers, such as Kaposi's sarcoma and *lymphomas*.

METHODS OF TRANSMISSION

HIV has been isolated from blood, semen, saliva, tears, nervous system tissue, breast milk, and female genital tract secretions. However, only semen and blood have been proved to transmit infection.

The major methods of transmission are sexual contact (penis to anus, vagina, or mouth), blood to blood (via transfusions or needle sharing in drug users), and woman to fetus. Other rare methods are through accidental needle injury, artificial insemination by donated semen, and kidney transplants.

"Casual" or household spread does not occur. The infection is not spread by touching or hugging, by breathing the same air, or by sharing cutlery or crockery. Worldwide, heterosexual transmission is the most common way that people become infected with HIV, and it has become increasingly common in the United Kingdom, accounting for around one third of all new infections. In Africa, AIDS affects men and women equally; heterosexual transmission plays a more important role for many reasons, including an increased rate of transmission in people also infected with sexually transmitted diseases such as chancroid.

SYMPTOMS AND SIGNS

Individuals infected with the virus may have no symptoms; others experience a short-lived illness sometimes resembling infectious *mononucleosis*, when they first become infected. Medical examination of those without symptoms may reveal abnormalities, most commonly lymph gland enlargement.

Minor features of HIV infection include skin disorders such as seborrhoeic *dermatitis* (skin inflammation, particularly on the face). More severe features include marked weight loss, diarrhoea, fever, and oral *candidiasis* (thrush).

Other more common or more severe infections in HIV-infected patients include *herpes simplex* infections, *shingles*, *tuberculosis*, salmonellosis, and shigellosis. HIV may also affect the brain, causing a variety of neurological disorders, including *dementia*.

The features of full-blown AIDS include cancers (such as Kaposi's sarcoma and lymphoma of the brain), autoimmune diseases (especially *thrombocytopenia*), and various infections (such as *pneumocystis pneumonia*, severe *cytomegalovirus* infection, *toxoplasmosis*, diarrhoea caused by CRYPTOSPORIDIUM or ISOSPORA, candidiasis, disseminated *strongyloidiasis*, *cryptococcosis*, and chronic or persistent herpes simplex).

DIAGNOSIS

HIV infection may be suspected in someone with lymph gland enlargement or unexplained weight loss if the person is in a high-risk group.

Confirmation of HIV infection involves testing a blood sample for the presence of antibodies to HIV; testing for the virus itself is more difficult. A positive HIV antibody test result indicates exposure to the virus; most antibody-positive individuals are virus carriers. Positive test results are always checked by a confirmatory test. A negative test result may occur in someone who has only very recently come into contact with the virus; for this reason, a negative result should be followed by repeated testing after six months if the individual concerned is in a high-risk group.

Diagnosis of full-blown AIDS is based on positive results to tests for HIV, along with the characteristic infections and tumours.

PREVENTION OF INFECTION

Until a cure or vaccine is found, prevention is the most important measure against AIDS. Risks can be reduced by practising *safer sex*.

Anyone who feels that he or she may have been exposed to the virus may request a blood test, although it is wise to obtain counselling first on the advisability of the test and on the implications of a positive result. A person who knows that he or she has been infected should alter his or her sexual lifestyle to avoid transmitting the virus. An uninfected person should also adopt safer-sex procedures to avoid becoming infected.

Safer-sex techniques involve reducing the number of sex partners; ideally, sex should be restricted to partners whose sexual histories are known. Unprotected anal and vaginal intercourse should be avoided. Hugging, touching, mutual masturbation, and dry kissing are safe. Saliva may contain the virus but is unlikely to be important in transmission; the risk of wet kissing with saliva exchange is unknown. If penile penetration takes place, a condom should be worn. Spermicidal jellies seem to inactivate the virus and should also be used. The risk of oral sex is not fully known, but ejaculation into the mouth should be avoided.

Intravenous drug users should not share needles, so as to prevent the spread of infection; their sexual partners may also be at risk.

In many countries, prostitutes show a high rate of infection. Although rates are very much lower in the UK, prostitutes are a potential means of spread. They should be encouraged to require use of condoms to protect themselves and their clients.

There is a small risk to hospital and other health workers when handling infected blood products or needles. The risk of transmission by needles in

A

CAUSES AND PREVENTION OF AIDS

AIDS is caused by the human immunodeficiency virus (HIV) (right), which consists of some nucleic acid (genetic material) inside two protective shells and an outer envelope. Full-blown AIDS develops in only some people infected with HIV.

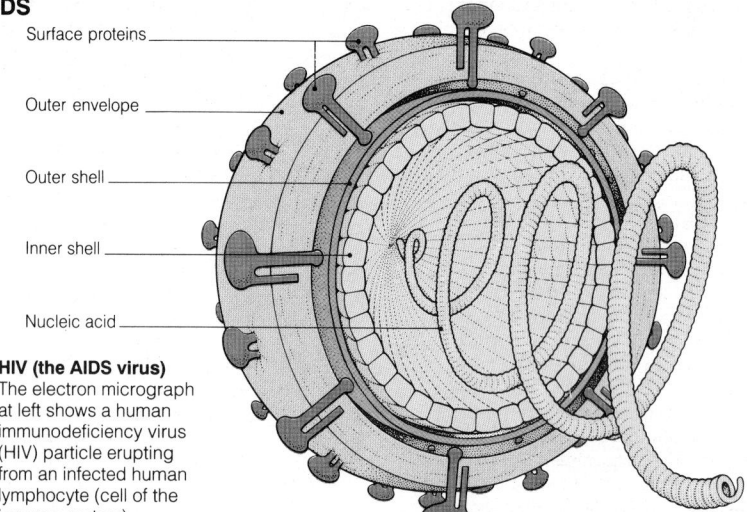

Surface proteins

Outer envelope

Outer shell

Inner shell

Nucleic acid

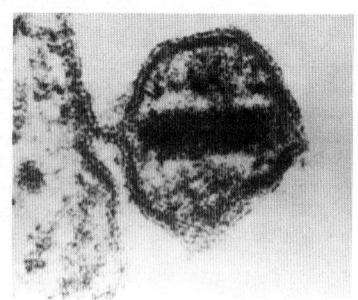

HIV (the AIDS virus)
The electron micrograph at left shows a human immunodeficiency virus (HIV) particle erupting from an infected human lymphocyte (cell of the immune system).

HOW HIV (THE AIDS VIRUS) AFFECTS THE IMMUNE SYSTEM

In a person with a healthy immune system, various types of lymphocytes combat disease organisms.

In a person infected with HIV, the immune system is weakened; in some cases, this may lead to AIDS.

NORMAL IMMUNE SYSTEM

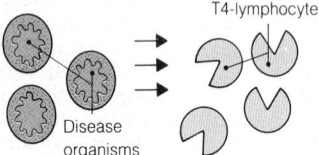

T4-lymphocytes

Disease organisms

1 Disease organisms entering the body alert T4-lymphocytes and other immune system components.

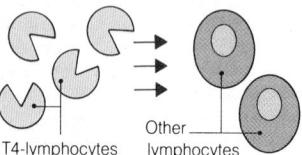

Other lymphocytes

T4-lymphocytes

2 The T4-lymphocytes help regulate the response of other lymphocytes (cells of the immune system).

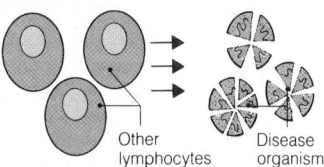

Other lymphocytes

Disease organisms

3 These lymphocytes then counter-attack and destroy the disease organisms by various mechanisms.

IMMUNE SYSTEM IN AIDS VICTIM

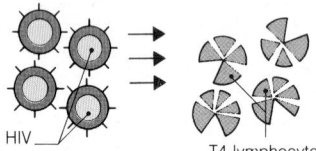

HIV

T4-lymphocytes

1 HIV (the AIDS virus) multiplies within, and ultimately may destroy, the body's T4-lymphocytes.

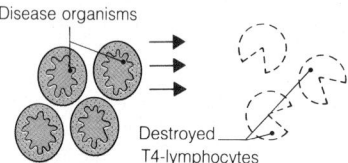

Disease organisms

Destroyed T4-lymphocytes

2 When disease organisms invade, immune responses may fail, due to absence of the vital T4-lymphocytes.

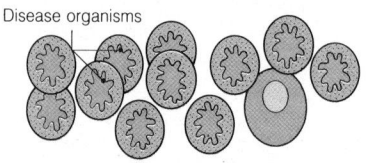

Disease organisms

3 The disease organisms may then overwhelm the immune system and lead to the features of AIDS.

RECOMMENDATIONS FOR PREVENTING THE SPREAD OF AIDS

- Do not have sexual intercourse with persons known or suspected of having AIDS, with many people, or with people who have had many partners.

- Do not use intravenous (IV) drugs. If you use IV drugs, do not share needles or syringes.

- Do not have sex with people who use IV drugs.

- People with AIDS or who have had positive HIV antibody test results may pass the disease on to others and should not donate blood, plasma, body organs, other tissues, or sperm. They should not exchange body fluids during sexual activity.

- There is a risk of infecting (or being infected by) others through sexual intercourse, sharing needles, and, possibly, exposure of others to saliva through oral-genital contact or "wet" kissing. The effectiveness of condoms in preventing infection with HIV is not proved, but their consistent use may reduce transmission, since exchange of body fluids is known to increase risk.

- Toothbrushes, razors, or other implements that could become contaminated with blood should not be shared.

hospitals has, however, been lower than expected; it is minimized if care is taken with all procedures involving sharp instruments.

People in risk groups should not donate blood, semen, or organs. All donated blood, semen, and organs are screened for HIV antibodies; blood products are also heat-treated as a further precaution.

TREATMENT

Those recently infected with HIV will benefit from reassurance and counselling, but will not be offered drug treatment at this stage. On average, people infected with HIV may expect to remain free of symptoms for eight to 12 years, depending on age. However, during that time they may infect others, and should therefore follow safer-sex practices rigorously.

There is no cure for AIDS; supportive treatment is available only for its complications. Repeated measurements of the numbers of T4 white blood cells will indicate the disease's progression. As the white cell count drops, the likelihood of infections increases.

Treatment with antiviral drugs such as zidovudine (AZT), didanosine, and zalcitabine will be started. These drugs, often given in combination, slow the progress of the disease, but have severe side-effects and are not curative. The timing and dosage of drug treatment is continually being assessed in a series of worldwide clinical trials.

Pneumocystis pneumonia is treated with antibiotic drugs (such as pentamidine or co-trimoxazole), but troublesome side-effects often occur and the infection commonly recurs. Treatment of Kaposi's sarcoma by radiotherapy or anticancer drugs is rarely curative.

OUTLOOK

Research is continuing into the development of vaccines and new drugs; and scores of compounds are being tested in the laboratory and in clinical trials. For the foreseeable future, however, prevention will remain the key strategy. Health education and the use of safer-sex techniques have had some impact in slowing the rate of growth of the epidemic, but the numbers infected worldwide in the early 1990s were in excess of 20 million.

AIDS-related complex

A combination of weight loss, fever, and enlarged lymph nodes in a person who has been infected with *HIV* (the *AIDS* virus), but does not actually have AIDS itself. Many people suffering from AIDS-related complex (ARC) will eventually have the features of AIDS.

Air

The colourless, odourless mixture of gases that forms the Earth's atmosphere. Air consists of 78 per cent *nitrogen*, 21 per cent *oxygen*, small quantities of *carbon dioxide* and other gases, and some water vapour.

The balance among the various atmospheric gases is maintained largely by the mutual needs of animals and plants. Animals use oxygen and produce carbon dioxide as a waste product; plants use carbon dioxide and release oxygen in a process called photosynthesis. The level of carbon dioxide in the atmosphere is gradually increasing as a result of extensive deforestation and the large-scale burning of fossil fuels. This disturbance of the atmospheric balance is causing concern among scientists because the raised carbon dioxide levels may lead to significant global warming (the greenhouse effect), which could have potentially disastrous consequences for all life on this planet. (See also *Pollution*.)

Air conditioning

Any system that controls the purity, humidity, and temperature of the air in a building. Air conditioning is important in maintaining comfort and hygienic conditions in hospitals, hotels, offices, and other buildings.

WHY IT IS USED

Air conditioning helps to provide comfortable living and working conditions by acting on air that is already inside rooms and on air that is drawn in from outside. It works by filtering out dust, pollen, smoke, and bad smells, by adding or removing moisture as necessary, and by either cooling or heating the air to keep it at a comfortable temperature. By bringing in outside air that has been filtered and exposed to the antiseptic effect of ultraviolet light, air conditioning may also reduce the risk of airborne infections and allergies.

Hospital sterile units, used for nursing high-risk patients, have air-conditioning units fitted with special bacterial filters that minimize the risk of spreading infection.

DISORDERS

Despite its generally beneficial effects, air conditioning may be responsible for certain disorders. For example, some outbreaks of *legionnaires' disease* (a type of pneumonia) have been linked to contaminated air-conditioning systems; and humidifier fever (a lung disease that causes fever, coughing, and breathing difficulty) is

thought to be caused by the spread of infectious microorganisms (usually fungi) by air conditioning. Air conditioning has also been blamed for some cases of *sick building syndrome*, which is attributed to the physical working environment and produces headache, irritability, and loss of energy.

Air embolism

Blockage of a small artery by an air bubble carried in the blood. Air embolism is rare. In most cases, it is a result of air entering the circulation by way of a vein, either because of an injury or during surgery. Very occasionally, a scuba diver or a person in an aircraft suffers an air embolism as a result of a pressure accident in which lung tissues rupture and air bubbles escape into the bloodstream.

Air pollution

See *Pollution*.

Air swallowing

See *Aerophagy*.

Airway

A collective term for the passages through which air enters and leaves the lungs. The airway is made up of the nasal passages, oral cavity, upper part of the pharynx (throat), larynx (voice-box), trachea (windpipe), bronchi (main air passages in the lungs), and bronchioles (smaller air passages off the bronchi that end with air sacs known as alveoli).

The term airway is also applied to a tube which is inserted into the mouth to hold the tongue forward and allow breathing in an unconscious patient. Preservation of the airway can also be achieved by the insertion of an *endotracheal tube* into the trachea in such a patient, either through the mouth or through an incision in the neck, as in a *tracheostomy* operation. (See also *Respiratory system*.)

Airway obstruction

Narrowing or blockage of the respiratory passages. The obstruction may be due to a foreign body, such as a piece of food, that becomes lodged in part of the upper airway and may result in *choking*. Certain diseases or disorders, such as *diphtheria* and *lung cancer*, affect the airway and can cause obstruction. Additionally, a spasm of the muscular walls of the airway, as occurs in *bronchospasm* (a feature of *asthma* and *bronchitis*), results in *breathing difficulty*. (See also *Artificial respiration*; *Lung* disorders box.)

A

Akathisia

An inability to sit still, occurring occasionally as a side-effect of an *antipsychotic drug* used to treat mental disorders such as schizophrenia and depression. Less commonly, akathisia occurs as a complication of *Parkinson's disease*.

Akinesia

Complete or almost complete loss of movement. It may be due to loss of power in a group of muscles (e.g. as a result of damage to part of the brain by a *stroke*). Akinesia may also occur when muscle power is normal but when the muscles are abnormally rigid (e.g. in *Parkinson's disease*).

Albinism

A *genetic disorder* characterized by a lack of the pigment *melanin* that gives colour to the skin, hair, and eyes. Although rare, albinism occurs in all races. Affected individuals (albinos) suffer visual problems and a tendency to have *skin cancers*.

TYPES

In oculocutaneous albinism (the most common type), the hair, skin, and eyes are all affected. In a severe form of oculocutaneous albinism, the skin and hair are snowy white throughout life (although the tips of the hairs may turn slightly yellow with age). In a less severe form, the skin and hair are white and the irises are almost transparent at birth, but all darken slightly with age and numerous freckles develop on parts of the skin exposed to the sun. In both forms, the eyes are affected by *photophobia* (intolerance to bright light), *nystagmus* (abnormal flickering movements), and, commonly, also by *squint* and *myopia* (shortsightedness).

Other rare types of albinism affect only the skin and hair or the eyes.

CAUSES AND INCIDENCE

The genetic defect results in deficiency of a specific *enzyme*; this deficiency interferes with melanin production in affected tissues. Oculocutaneous albinism shows an autosomal recessive pattern of inheritance, in which there is a one in four chance of a child being affected if both parents have normal skin colouring but carry the gene defect.

The overall prevalence of oculocutaneous albinism is low in Europe and North America—fewer than five people per 100,000 are affected. The prevalence varies in different ethnic groups (e.g. it is higher in the Ibo population in Nigeria).

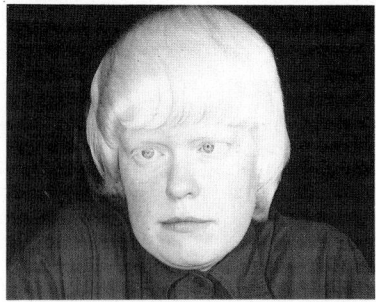

Appearance of albinism
The condition is caused by lack of melanin pigment in the skin, hair, and eyes.

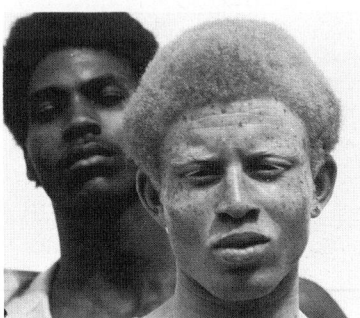

Albinism in an African boy
Albinism is found in people of all races, although it occurs only rarely.

COMPLICATIONS AND TREATMENT

SKIN The most serious complication of oculocutaneous albinism results from the lack of melanin, which normally protects the skin against harmful radiation in sunlight. The skin cannot tan, ages prematurely, and is liable to develop cancers on areas exposed to the sun. Albinos in sunny climates should therefore wear suitable protective clothing.

EYES The visual problems of albinos, such as photophobia and nystagmus, can cause great difficulties, particularly with reading. Expert assessment and treatment should be sought at an early age; in most cases, glasses are needed, preferably tinted to help reduce photophobia.

Albumin

The most abundant protein in the *blood* plasma. Albumin is made in the liver from amino acids that have been absorbed from digested protein.

Albumin has several important functions. It helps retain substances (such as calcium, some hormones, and certain drugs) in the circulation by binding to them and thereby preventing their being filtered out by the kidneys and excreted in the urine.

Albumin is also important in regulating the movement of water between tissues and the bloodstream by *osmosis* (the attraction of water to an area with a higher concentration of salts or proteins). (See also *Albuminuria*.)

Albuminuria

The presence of the protein *albumin* in the urine; a type of *proteinuria*. Normally, the glomeruli (filtering units of the kidneys) do not allow albumin to pass through them and into the urine. Albuminuria therefore usually indicates a failure of the kidneys' filtering mechanisms. Such a failure may be due to a kidney disorder, such as *glomerulonephritis* or *nephrotic syndrome*, or it may be a sign that the kidneys have been damaged by *hypertension*.

Albuminuria can be detected by a simple test on the urine; this test is commonly included in routine medical examinations.

Alcohol

A colourless liquid produced from the fermentation of carbohydrates by yeast. Also known as ethanol or ethyl alcohol, alcohol is the active constituent of alcoholic drinks such as beer, wine, and spirits. In medicine, alcohol is used as an antiseptic and a solvent. *Methanol*, also known as methyl alcohol or wood alcohol, is a related, highly poisonous substance.

Any society where alcohol is freely used is invariably afflicted by the problems of acute *alcohol intoxication* (drunkenness), *alcohol dependence* (habitual, compulsive, long-term heavy drinking), and *alcohol-related disorders* such as liver disorders, heart disease, *hypertension*, *neuropathy*, and *Wernicke-Korsakoff syndrome* (a form of *dementia*). Alcohol is also an important factor in road traffic and industrial accidents, domestic violence, marriage breakdown, child abuse, hooliganism, physical assault, and various other types of crime.

EFFECTS

The effect of alcohol on the *central nervous system* (the brain and spinal cord) is as a depressant, decreasing its activity and thereby reducing anxiety, tension, and inhibitions. Taken in moderate amounts, alcohol gives the drinker a feeling of relaxation and confidence that may enable him or her to socialize more easily. However, any feeling of heightened mental and physical efficiency is illusory. Tests have shown that even a low level of alcohol in the blood slows reactions.

ALCOHOL AND THE BODY

Alcohol is a drug and, even in small amounts, its effects on the body are noticeable. Problems arise when people fail to take into account the effects of alcohol on tasks requiring coordination (such as driving) when they become intoxicated or when they become dependent on the drug. Alcohol dependence can cause early death and is a major factor in crime, marital breakdown, child abuse, accidents, and absenteeism. Prolonged heavy drinking that stops short of dependence still may cause a wide variety of diseases, such as *cirrhosis* of the liver and *cardiomyopathy*.

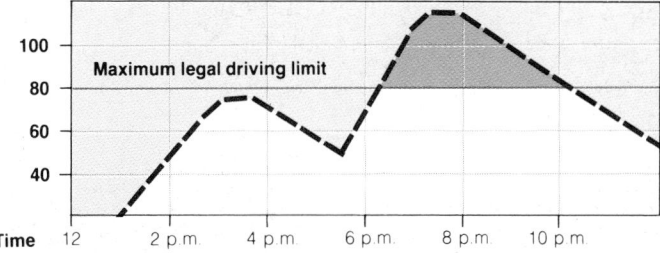

Cumulative effects of alcohol

It takes some time for the body to eliminate even small amounts of alcohol. For instance, if a person has two drinks at lunchtime and then has one or two more drinks early in the evening, his or her cumulative blood alcohol level could be over the legal limit for driving even though several hours have passed.

EFFECTS OF INCREASING BLOOD ALCOHOL LEVELS

Concentration (milligrams per 100 millilitres)	Observable effects
30–50 150–200	Flushed face, euphoria, talkativeness, increased social confidence
50–150 200–350	Disturbed thinking and coordination, irritability, reduced self-control, irresponsible talk and behaviour
150–250 350–500	Marked confusion, unsteady gait, slurred speech, unpredictable shows of emotion and aggression
250–400 500–700	Extreme confusion and disorientation, difficulty remaining upright, drowsiness, delayed or incoherent reaction to questions progressing to coma (a state of deep unconsciousness from which the person cannot be aroused)
400–500 700+	Risk of death due to arrest of breathing (although habitual drinkers may survive even such high levels)

Occasional social drinker

Alcoholic/problem drinker

Alcohol levels in different drinks

Alcoholic drinks come in many forms and contain varying levels of pure alcohol. It can be very difficult to estimate alcohol intake because the strengths of drinks vary. The measures shown here are typical sizes of drinks served in British pubs; they contain approximately equal amounts of pure alcohol.

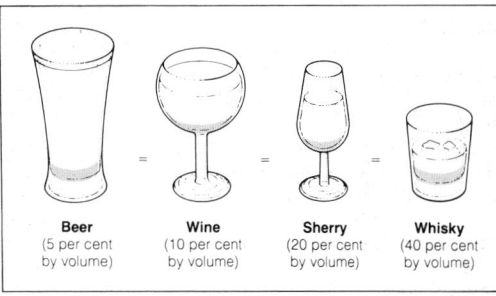

Beer (5 per cent by volume) = **Wine** (10 per cent by volume) = **Sherry** (20 per cent by volume) = **Whisky** (40 per cent by volume)

LONG-TERM EFFECTS ON THE BODY

Persistent heavy drinking eventually damages body tissues; the main effects are shown below.

Liver
The liver is the main organ responsible for metabolizing alcohol from the blood; it manifests many of the long-term effects of heavy drinking. These effects include fatty liver, hepatitis, cirrhosis, and liver cancer.

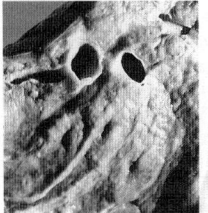

Cirrhotic liver
In this condition, commonly caused by heavy drinking, bands of scar tissue form in the liver, impairing its function.

Brain and nervous system
Alcohol depresses the central nervous system. Prolonged alcohol abuse permanently impairs brain and nerve function.

Skin
Alcohol causes facial flushing, which becomes constant in heavy drinkers.

Heart and circulation
Prolonged heavy drinking can cause coronary heart disease, hypertension, heart failure, and stroke.

Digestive system
Irritation from large amounts of alcohol can cause gastritis and ulcers.

Urinary system
Alcohol acts as a diuretic, increasing urine output. Prolonged heavy drinking can cause renal failure.

Reproductive system
Alcohol increases sexual confidence, but high levels cause impotence.

The more alcohol that is drunk, the greater is the impairment of concentration and judgment. At the same time, the drinker's confidence is increased—a potentially lethal combination while driving. If excessive amounts of alcohol are drunk, poisoning or intoxication results, with effects ranging from euphoria to unconsciousness.

In addition to significantly altering mood and behaviour, alcohol has various physical effects on the body. As a result of peripheral *vasodilation* (widening of the small blood vessels), the face becomes flushed and the drinker feels warm, although in fact a greater amount of body heat is lost. Small amounts of alcohol increase the flow of gastric juices and therefore stimulate the appetite; however, large amounts over a long period can cause erosive *gastritis* (inflammation and superficial ulceration of the stomach lining) and haematemesis (vomiting blood).

The effects of alcohol on sexual behaviour were aptly summarized by William Shakespeare: "It provokes the desire but it takes away the performance."

Regular intake of alcohol adds significantly to the energy content of the diet; pure alcohol provides 700 kcal (2,930 kJ) per 100 g, and habitual drinkers of beer or wine are commonly overweight. People who drink regular, small amounts of alcohol (an average of 2 to 3 drinks a day) have been shown to have lower rates of *coronary heart disease* and possibly of *stroke* than total abstainers. The explanation for these findings is still unclear.

TOLERANCE

Habitual drinkers acquire a tolerance to alcohol. This means that they must drink gradually increasing amounts of alcohol to obtain the same effects. The liver breaks down alcohol at a faster rate, necessitating a greater intake to achieve the same level in the blood. At the same time, nerve cells in the brain become less and less responsive to a given amount of alcohol. Paradoxically, however, after years of drinking, many alcoholics experience a reduced tolerance.

Alcohol dependence

An illness characterized by habitual, compulsive, long-term, heavy consumption of alcohol and the development of withdrawal symptoms when drinking is suddenly stopped. The description "alcohol dependence" is

ALCOHOL AND PREGNANCY

The damage that alcohol can cause a fetus has been recognized only recently. Drinking more than two alcoholic drinks per day (e.g. two measures of spirits, two glasses of wine, or two half-pints of beer) increases the chance of *fetal alcohol syndrome*. This disorder consists of facial abnormalities such as *cleft lip* and *palate*, heart defects, abnormal limb development, and lower-than-average intelligence. This level of drinking also increases the risk of miscarriage. Occasional binge drinking may cause the same effects even if the mother drinks little otherwise. Because a proportion of the alcohol from any drink reaches the baby, there is a risk that drinking even small amounts may disrupt normal development (causing, for example, low birth weight).

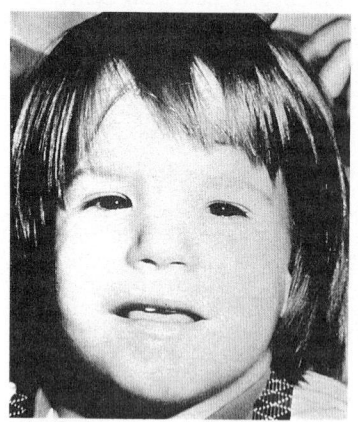

Fetal alcohol syndrome
An affected baby is abnormally short, has small eyes and a small jaw, and may have heart defects or a cleft lip and palate. He or she may suck poorly, sleep badly, and be irritable.

generally preferred medically to "alcoholism", but the terms are often used synonymously.

INCIDENCE

The incidence of alcohol dependence has been rising throughout the world for many years. Statistics on the extent of the problem are difficult to quote with any certainty. Rough estimates indicate that there are approximately one million alcohol-dependent persons in the UK (about one in 60 of the population) and a further million or so who have some trouble controlling their consumption of alcohol.

CAUSES

There is no single cause of alcohol dependence. Three causative factors interact in the development of the illness: personality, environment, and the addictive nature of alcohol. Thus, if all other factors (such as the availability of alcohol) are equal, then inadequate, insecure, or immature personalities are more at risk than more emotionally mature individuals.

Inherited genetic factors probably play a part in causing dependence in some cases, but it is now widely believed that any person, irrespective of environment, genetic background, or personality, can become alcoholic if he or she drinks heavily for a prolonged period.

Environmental factors are important, especially the ready availability, affordability, and widespread social acceptance of alcohol in the individual's national culture and among the

people he or she associates with. Thus alcoholism is much more common in certain countries, occupations, and social groups than others.

Stress is another important factor. Many formerly moderate drinkers begin to drink excessively at times of bereavement. Women may turn to drink when their adolescent children leave home.

Once social and/or psychological factors have induced heavy drinking, the discovery that taking alcohol in the morning relieves the withdrawal symptoms induced by the previous night's drinking tends to accelerate the development of dependence.

DEVELOPMENT OF DEPENDENCE

The development of alcohol dependence can be divided into four main stages, which merge imperceptibly. The time scale of these changes may be from five to 25 years, although the average is about 10 years.

In the first phase, tolerance (being able to drink more alcohol before experiencing its effects) develops in the heavy social drinker. Entering the second phase, the drinker experiences memory lapses relating to events occurring during the drinking episodes. In the third phase, there is loss, or lack, of control over alcohol; the drinker can no longer be certain of discontinuing drinking whenever he or she wants to. The final phase is characterized by prolonged binges of intoxication and by observable mental or physical complications.

Some people halt their consumption, temporarily or permanently, during one of the first three phases.

SYMPTOMS AND EFFECTS

BEHAVIOURAL SYMPTOMS are varied and can include any combination of the following: furtive behaviour (such as hiding bottles); aggressive or grandiose behaviour; personality changes (such as irritability, jealousy, uncontrolled anger, selfishness); frequent changes of job; constant promises to oneself and others to give up drinking; changes in drinking pattern (e.g. switching to early-morning drinking, or changing from beer to spirits); neglect of food intake and personal appearance; and lengthy periods of intoxication.

PHYSICAL SYMPTOMS can also be varied. The drinker may exhibit any of the following: nausea, vomiting, or shaking in the morning; abdominal pain; cramps; numbness or tingling; weakness in the legs and hands; irregular pulse; redness and enlarged capillaries (small blood vessels) in the face; unsteadiness; confusion; lapses of memory; and incontinence. After sudden withdrawal of alcohol, the dependent person may experience *delirium tremens* (severe shakes, hallucinations, and convulsions).

In addition, alcohol-dependent persons are more susceptible than others to a wide variety of specific physical and mental diseases and disorders (see *Alcohol-related disorders*).

Physical and psychological problems may cause difficulties at home and at work. The person's marriage often suffers and there may be financial problems. Suicide threats and attempts may occur.

PREVENTION

Steps for avoiding the development of alcohol dependence include the following: keep to safe limits of alcohol intake as recommended by medical authorities; drink slowly instead of gulping; do not drink on an empty stomach; never drink to relieve anxiety, tension, or depression.

Nobody should ever feel (or be made to feel) embarrassed about refusing an alcoholic drink.

TREATMENT

Many alcoholics require detoxification (medical help in getting over their physical withdrawal symptoms when they stop drinking). Detoxification is followed by long-term treatment. Different methods of treatment—psychological, social and physical—are appropriate for different people, and may be combined.

PSYCHOLOGICAL TREATMENTS involve *psychotherapy* and are commonly carried out in groups. There are various types of *group therapy*.

SOCIAL TREATMENTS include help with problems at work and, in particular, the inclusion of family members in the treatment process.

PHYSICAL TREATMENT is needed only by some alcoholics. It generally includes the use of disulfiram, a drug that sensitizes the drinker to alcohol so that he or she is afraid to drink because of unpleasant side-effects.

Alcoholics are strongly advised to use the self-help fellowship of organizations, such as *Alcoholics Anonymous*, where the alcoholic greatly benefits from meeting fellow sufferers who share their experiences.

Alcoholics Anonymous

A worldwide fellowship of people who readily admit to being alcoholics and who help each other stay sober. Alcoholics Anonymous (AA) was started in 1935 in the US and now consists of an estimated 67,000 local groups and over 1.5 million members in 92 countries. In the UK there are several groups in each large city and at least one group in all but the smallest towns. Contact addresses can be found in telephone directories.

Membership is open to anyone who has a drinking problem and has a desire to become and/or to continue to stay sober. There is no membership fee; the organization relies on voluntary contributions from members. Members are of all races, nationalities, and occupations, and range from people whose health, careers, and relationships were totally destroyed by alcoholism to those who sought help at a much earlier stage of the illness. AA is not affiliated with any sect, political party, institution, or other organization. It has a policy of cooperation with other organizations that fight alcoholism.

Local AA meetings are of two types. At open meetings, which anyone (including members' families) can attend, speakers describe their lives as alcoholics and the effect AA has had in helping them refrain from drinking. At closed meetings, which only members can attend, new members are invited to describe their drinking problems and their difficulties in abstaining. Other members who have had the same experiences suggest methods of staying sober and ways in which other problems can be surmounted. A programme of recovery is

suggested. Many members find that helping other alcoholics is the best way to remain sober themselves.

Members of AA do not reveal the names of other members to people outside AA. The fellowship does not keep membership records, monitor or attempt to control its members, engage or sponsor research on alcoholism, dispense drugs or psychiatric treatment, or provide detoxification, nursing, social services, or vocational counselling.

Alcohol intoxication

The condition, also known as drunkenness, that results from drinking an excessive amount of alcohol, often over a relatively short period (usually about 30 minutes to several hours). Alcohol causes acute poisoning if taken in sufficiently large amounts. It depresses the activity of the central nervous system (the brain and spinal cord), leading to loss of normal mental and physical control.

In extreme cases, a person who drinks a large amount of alcohol over a short period may lose consciousness and even die.

SYMPTOMS

The effects of a large alcohol intake depend on many factors, including physical and mental state, body size, social situation, and acquired tolerance (see *Alcohol*). Thus, a person may become "jocose, lachrymose, bellicose, or comatose" (cheerful, tearful, argumentative, or unconscious). There are wide individual variations. The important factor, however, is the blood alcohol level (see Alcohol and the body chart).

TREATMENT

For intoxication that stops short of coma, no treatment is required. Recovery takes place naturally as the alcohol in the person's body is gradually broken down in the liver.

If a drinker lapses into a coma, medical attention should be sought, particularly if the person is known or suspected to be diabetic or to have been taking another drug, whether prescribed by a doctor (such as a sedative) or illicit (such as cocaine), in addition to alcohol. The person's clothing should be loosened and the mouth and back of the throat checked to make sure there is no obstruction to breathing. No attempt should be made to make the person drink water or to make him or her vomit. If breathing stops, *artificial respiration* should be carried out until breathing restarts or medical help arrives.

A

For a description of the chronic mental, physical, and social effects of long-term heavy drinking, see *Alcohol dependence* and *Alcohol-related disorders*.

Alcoholism
See *Alcohol dependence*.

Alcohol-related disorders
In addition to the many health and social problems that may result from *alcohol dependence*, and the high accident rate associated with *alcohol intoxication*, people who consume large quantities of alcohol are susceptible to a wide variety of physical and mental disorders.

Alcohol consumption can lead to tissue damage and disease by any, or a combination, of three main mechanisms. First, alcohol or its breakdown products from metabolism can have a direct toxic or irritant effect on cells and tissues.

Second, many alcoholics eat little or no nutritious food. Alcohol satisfies their calorie requirements and at the same time reduces appetite through an irritant effect on the stomach. However, alcohol provides no protein, vitamins, or minerals. Consequently, chronic alcoholics are prone to diseases caused by nutritional deficiency, particularly deficiency of thiamine (see *Vitamin B complex*).

Third, a continual high level of alcohol in the blood and tissues can cause wide-ranging disturbances in body chemistry. These disturbances can lead to *hypoglycaemia* (reduced glucose in the blood) and *hyperlipidaemia* (increased fat in the blood), which may contribute to malfunction and disease of such organs as the heart, liver, and blood vessels. Irreversible damage can be done to the heart, liver, and brain, and this may result in premature death.

Aldosterone
A hormone secreted by the adrenal cortex (the outer part of the *adrenal glands*). Aldosterone plays an important role in the control of blood pressure, and in the regulation of sodium and potassium concentrations in the blood and tissues.

Aldosterone acts on the kidneys to decrease the amount of sodium lost in the urine; the sodium is reabsorbed from urine before it leaves the kidneys and is replaced in the urine by potassium. The sodium draws water back into the blood with it, thereby increasing the blood volume and raising the blood pressure.

ALCOHOL-RELATED DISORDERS		
Cancer	High alcohol consumption increases the risk of cancers of the mouth, tongue, pharynx (back of the throat), larynx (voice box), and oesophagus, probably due to irritant action. In each of these cancers, alcohol	consumption along with smoking produces a much higher total risk of cancer than the sum of their separate risks. The risk of *liver cancer*, along with most types of liver disease, is also higher among alcoholics.
Liver damage and disease	Liver diseases caused by a high alcohol consumption include fatty liver, alcoholic *hepatitis*, *cirrhosis*, and liver cancer. They develop in sequence over a period of years. It is thought that a breakdown product of alcohol (acetaldehyde) has a toxic effect on liver cells and is the main cause of these diseases, although nutritional deficiency may also play some part.	The risk of alcoholic hepatitis and cirrhosis developing increases in proportion to the amount of alcohol consumed and the number of years of high consumption; liver cancer develops in about one in five sufferers of cirrhosis. However, about one third of heavy drinkers never get liver disease and in another third, only a fatty liver develops.
Nervous system disorders	Thiamine (vitamin B₁) deficiency, also known as *beriberi* (which disturbs nerve functioning), may develop in alcoholics. The effect of severe deficiency on the brain produces Wernicke's encephalopathy, with symptoms such as confusion, disturbances of speech and gait, and eventual coma. Korsakoff's psychosis may also occur (see	*Wernicke-Korsakoff syndrome*). The effect on the peripheral nervous system (nerve pathways outside the brain and spinal cord) produces polyneuropathy, with symptoms such as pain, cramps, numbness, tingling, and weakness in the legs and hands. Injections of thiamine and resumption of a normal diet can produce a dramatic cure.
Heart and circulatory disorders	Severe thiamine deficiency in alcoholics can cause *heart failure* (reduced pumping efficiency of the heart), usually combined with oedema (fluid collection in the tissues). A high alcohol consumption also	increases the risk of coronary heart disease, of *hypertension* (high blood pressure) and of suffering a *stroke*. Heavy drinkers of certain beers risk *cardiomyopathy*.
Other physical disorders	Other physical diseases and disorders associated with a high alcohol consumption include *gastritis*, *pancreatitis*, and *peptic ulcer*, all probably linked	to an irritant action of alcohol. Heavy drinking during pregnancy carries a risk of the baby being born with *fetal alcohol syndrome*.
Psychiatric illnesses	Alcoholics are more likely than others to suffer from *anxiety* and *depression* (frequently related to financial, work, or family problems) and from paranoia. They are also more likely to	develop *dementia* (irreversible mental deterioration). The incidence of *suicide* attempts and actual suicide is also higher among alcoholics.

The production of aldosterone is stimulated mainly by the action of *angiotensin* II, a chemical produced by a complex series of reactions that involves the enzymes *renin* (released by the kidneys) and converting enzyme. Aldosterone production is also stimulated by the action of *ACTH*, produced by the pituitary gland.

Aldosteronism
A disorder that results from the excessive production of the hormone *aldosterone* from one or both *adrenal glands*. Aldosteronism caused by an *adrenal tumour* is known as Conn's syndrome. Aldosteronism may also be caused by disorders, such as *heart failure* or liver damage, that reduce the

flow of blood through the kidneys. Reduced blood flow through the kidneys leads to overproduction of *renin* and of *angiotensin*, which, in turn, leads to excessive aldosterone production.

SYMPTOMS

Symptoms are directly related to the actions of aldosterone. Too much sodium is retained in the body, leading to a rise in blood pressure; at the same time, excess potassium is lost in the urine. The low potassium level causes tiredness and muscle weakness and impairs kidney function, leading to overproduction of urine, and thirst due to fluid loss.

DIAGNOSIS AND TREATMENT

The diagnosis is suggested by a combination of *hypertension* (high blood pressure), a raised level of sodium in the blood, and a low level of potassium. Further tests may be needed to confirm the diagnosis.

Treatment in all cases includes restriction of salt in the diet and use of the diuretic drug *spironolactone*. This drug blocks the action of aldosterone on the kidneys, leading to increased loss of sodium from the body, lowered blood pressure, and reduced loss of potassium. If the cause of aldosteronism is an adrenal tumour, this may be surgically removed.

Alexander technique

A therapy that aims to improve health by teaching people to stand and move more efficiently.

Developed in the 1920s by F. Matthias Alexander, the technique is based on the belief that bad patterns of body movement interfere with the proper functioning of the body and thus contribute to the development of disease.

The Alexander technique does not claim to take the place of medicine but, by releasing unnecessary muscle tensions, it aims to eliminate or reduce the severity of a wide range of disorders, including back pain, asthma, and stuttering.

Training is carried out in one-to-one sessions with a qualified teacher.

Alexia

Word blindness; the inability to recognize and name written words, thus severely disrupting the reading ability of a person who was previously literate. The disability is caused by damage (e.g. by a *stroke*) to part of the cerebrum (the main mass of the brain) and is a much more severe reading disability than *dyslexia*.

Alienation

Feeling like a stranger, even when among familiar people or places, and being unable to identify with a culture, family, or peer group. Alienation is common in adolescents. It also occurs in people with financial problems or who are isolated by cultural or language differences. In some people, alienation may be an early symptom of *schizophrenia* or part of a *personality disorder*. Feelings of alienation are thought to be a contributing cause of suicide, attempted suicide, and inner-city violence.

Alignment, dental

The movement of teeth by either fixed or removable *orthodontic appliances* (braces) to correct *malocclusion* (incorrect bite).

Alimentary tract

The tube-like structure that extends from the mouth to the anus (see *Digestive system*). It is also known as the alimentary canal.

Alkali

Also known as a base, an alkali is chemically defined as a donor of hydroxyl ions (each of which comprises an atom of hydrogen linked to an atom of oxygen and has an overall negative electrical charge).

Examples of alkalis include *antacid drugs*, such as sodium bicarbonate (bicarbonate of soda) and aluminium hydroxide. Some alkalis, such as caustic soda (sodium hydroxide) are corrosive and cause burns. (See also *Acid; Acid-base balance*.)

Alkaloids

A group of nitrogen-containing substances obtained from plants. *Morphine, codeine, nicotine,* and *strychnine* are examples.

Alkalosis

A disturbance of the body's *acid-base balance* in which there is an accumulation of alkali (base) or a loss of acid.

CAUSES

There are two types of alkalosis: metabolic and respiratory. In metabolic alkalosis, the increase in alkalinity may be caused by taking too much of an *antacid drug* or by losing a large amount of stomach acid as a result of severe vomiting.

Respiratory alkalosis is caused by a reduction in the level of carbonic acid (derived from carbon dioxide) in the blood. This reduction is a consequence of *hyperventilation* (overbreath-

ing), which may occur during a panic attack or at high altitudes due to lack of oxygen. (See also *Acidosis*.)

Alkylating agents

A class of *anticancer drugs*.

Allergy

A collection of conditions caused by inappropiate or exaggerated reactions of the *immune system* to a variety of substances. Many common illnesses, such as *asthma* and allergic *rhinitis* (hay fever), are caused by allergic reactions to substances that in the majority of people cause no symptoms.

In susceptible people, allergies may result from exposure of the skin to a chemical, of the respiratory system to inhaled particles of dust or pollen, or of the stomach and intestines to a particular food. Allergic reactions occur only on second or subsequent exposures to the offending agent, after the first contact has sensitized the body.

TYPES AND CAUSES

The function of the immune system is to recognize *antigens* (foreign proteins) on the surfaces of microorganisms and to form *antibodies* (also called immunoglobulins) and sensitized *lymphocytes* (white blood cells). When the immune system next encounters the same antigens, the antibodies and sensitized lymphocytes interact with them, leading to destruction of the microorganisms.

In allergies, a similar immune response occurs, except that the immune system forms antibodies or sensitized lymphocytes against harmless substances—because these allergens (as they are called) are misidentified as potentially harmful antigens.

The inappropriate or exaggerated reactions seen in allergies are termed *hypersensitivity* reactions and can have any of four different mechanisms (termed Types I to IV hypersensitivity reactions). Most well-known allergies are caused by the Type I variety (also known as anaphylactic or immediate hypersensitivity).

TYPE I HYPERSENSITIVITY REACTIONS Common allergens that can cause Type I reactions include flower, grass, and tree pollens, animal dander (tiny particles of skin and hair), house dust, house-dust mites, yeasts, certain drugs and foods, and constituents of bee and wasp venom. Foods that contain substances that commonly provoke allergic reactions include milk, eggs, shellfish, dried fruits, and nuts.

These allergens cause immediate symptoms by provoking the immune

ALLERGY AND THE BODY

An allergy is an inappropriate response (causing troublesome symptoms) to substances that, in most people, cause no response. The response is mainly to harmless substances that come in contact with the skin, respiratory airways, or the eye's surface. In diagnosing an allergy, the individual's medical history is important. The doctor needs to know whether the symptoms vary according to the time of the day or the season, and whether there are any pets or other likely sources of allergens in the home.

THE MOST COMMON ALLERGENS

Airborne		Foods	
	Grass pollens		Dairy products
	Tree pollens		Eggs
	Spores from moulds		Strawberries
	House-dust mites		Fish and shellfish
	Animal dander		Cereals

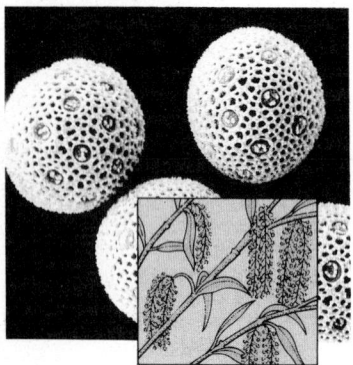

Pollen
Airborne pollen from plants (especially from grasses and trees) may trigger an allergic reaction; symptoms appear during the warmer months. The most common reaction is allergic rhinitis (hay fever), which occurs when pollen is breathed in and irritates the nasal lining.

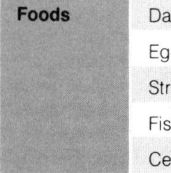

Animal dander
It is often assumed that allergy results from contact with animal hair. In fact, allergy is caused by flakes of dead skin (dander).

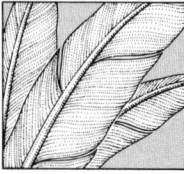

Feathers
Bedding containing feathers may produce an allergic reaction. Instead, use pillows and quilts containing synthetic stuffing.

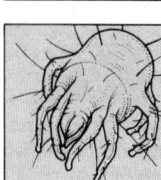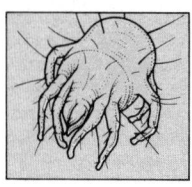

Mites in house dust
Fragments of mites and their faeces in house dust may cause an allergic reaction. Keeping the house dust-free helps.

DIAGNOSING SKIN ALLERGY

Tests are performed to identify specific reactions to allergens. Small amounts of various substances are applied to the skin. A weal indicates sensitivity to a particular allergen

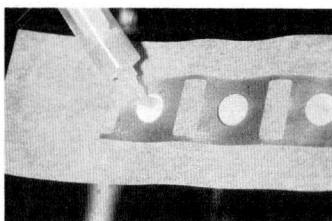

Conducting a patch test
Three different allergens are put on a patch (above left) and taped to the skin.

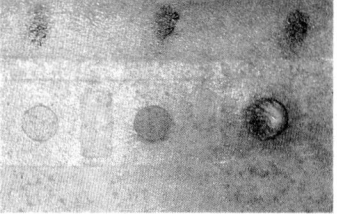

Results are (above right); no reaction; mild inflammation; severe contact dermatitis.

THE ORIGIN OF AN ALLERGY

The immune system is sensitized when it is exposed to an allergen (steps 1 to 3). Symptoms occur when allergens are met again (step 4).

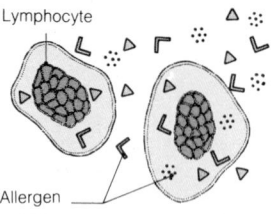

Lymphocyte

Allergen

1 Allergens enter the body and are recognized by lymphocytes (blood cells that form part of the body's immune system).

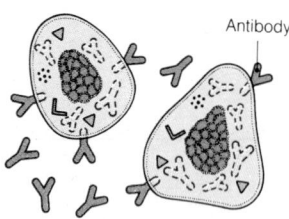

Antibody

2 A few days to weeks later, the lymphocytes produce antibodies specific to the allergens.

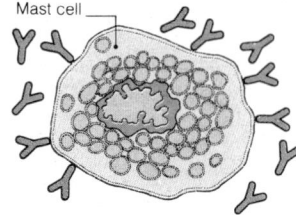

Mast cell

3 The antibodies attach to cells in the tissues called mast cells, which contain packets of histamine.

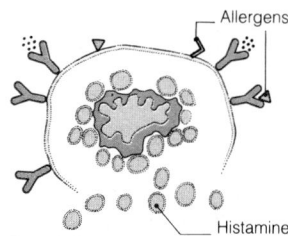

Allergens

Histamine

4 Binding of allergens to antibodies on the surface of mast cells leads to the release of histamine and to the symptoms of allergy.

system to produce specific antibodies, belonging to a type called immunoglobulin E (IgE), which coat cells (called mast cells or basophils) present in the skin and the lining of the stomach, lungs, and upper respiratory airways. When the allergen is encountered for the second time, it binds to the IgE antibodies and causes the granules in mast cells to release various chemicals, which are responsible for the symptoms of the allergy.

Among the chemicals released is histamine, which causes blood vessels to widen, fluids to leak into tissues, and muscles to go into spasm. Symptoms may be restricted to the skin (itchy swelling or rash), upper airways (inflammation or mucus secretion, sneezing in hay fever, and spasm and narrowing of the airways in asthma), eyes (inflammation), or stomach and intestines (vomiting and diarrhoea). Sometimes the symptoms affect several organs, especially when the allergies are to injected drugs, insect venom, or some foods. Particular conditions associated with Type I reactions include asthma, hay fever, *urticaria* (nettle rash), *angioedema*, *anaphylactic shock* (a severe, generalized allergic reaction), possibly atopic *eczema*, and many food allergies.

TYPES II TO IV HYPERSENSITIVITY REACTIONS These reactions have different mechanisms from Type I reactions (see *Hypersensitivity*) and are less often implicated in allergies. However, Type II reactions are responsible for autoimmune haemolytic *anaemia* and *Goodpasture's syndrome*. Type III reactions are responsible for a type of lung disease called allergic *alveolitis* (which includes *farmer's lung*) and for the skin swellings that occur after booster vaccinations. Type IV reactions are responsible for contact *dermatitis*.

It is not known why certain individuals and not others get allergies, although about one person in eight seems to have an inherited predisposition to allergies (see *Atopy*).

TREATMENT
Whenever possible, the most effective treatment for allergy of any kind is avoidance of the relevant allergen. For example, anyone with an allergy to eggs should avoid eating eggs or any dishes containing eggs as an ingredient, and should check the recipes of dishes consumed in restaurants or at parties. If pollen is the allergen, it may be harder to avoid; measures such as keeping car windows closed while driving and closing bedroom windows at night afford some protection.

Drug treatment for allergic reactions includes the use of *antihistamine drugs*, which relieve the symptoms (the itching produced by an insect bite, for example). Most available antihistamine drugs have a sedative effect, which is particularly useful in treating the itching due to eczema because they permit the sufferer to sleep more soundly. Several of the newer antihistamines do not cause drowsiness, making them more suitable for daytime use.

Other drugs, such as *sodium cromoglycate* and *corticosteroid drugs*, can be taken regularly to prevent symptoms from developing. Creams that contain corticosteroids are useful for treating eczema, but prolonged use on the same area can damage the skin. In severe allergic diseases, such as asthma, the use of inhaled or oral corticosteroids may be necessary.

Hyposensitization can be valuable for people who suffer allergic reactions to insect venom, house-dust mites, and some pollens. Gradually increasing doses of the allergen are given to promote the formation of antibodies that will block future adverse reactions. The therapy is effective in about two thirds of cases, but usually requires two to three years of treatment. Hyposensitization can produce mild side-effects, such as itching, swelling, or rashes; occasionally, more serious side-effects occur, such as bronchospasm or anaphylactic shock, and deaths have even occurred in a very few cases. Low-dosage, long-acting methods of desensitization are being researched.

Allopathy

A term that describes conventional medicine as practised by a graduate of a medical school or university granting the degrees of Bachelor of Medicine and Bachelor of Surgery. (See also *Homeopathy*.)

Allopurinol

A treatment for *gout* that works by reducing *hyperuricaemia* (raised levels of uric acid in the blood). Allopurinol does not relieve pain in acute attacks but, taken long term, does reduce the frequency of attacks.

POSSIBLE ADVERSE EFFECTS
These include itching, rashes, and nausea. Occasionally, during the first few weeks of treatment, allopurinol increases the frequency of gout attacks. *Colchicine* or a *nonsteroidal anti-inflammatory drug* may be prescribed to counteract this effect.

Alopecia

Loss or absence of *hair*, which is usually noticeable only on the scalp but which may occur at any hair-bearing site on the body.

TYPES
HEREDITARY ALOPECIA This includes male-pattern baldness, the most common form of alopecia. Normal hair is lost initially from the temples and crown, where it is replaced by fine, downy hair. The affected area gradually widens as the line of normal hair recedes. This pattern of hair loss is inherited; it usually affects men, although young women and women who have passed the menopause are occasionally affected.

Other hereditary forms of hair loss are rare. They may be due to an absence of hair roots or to abnormalities of the hair shaft, causing it to snap under the normal effects of sun, wind, shampooing, and combing.

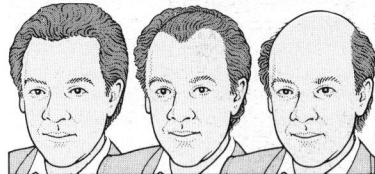

Stages in male pattern baldness
In this common form of alopecia, the man loses hair first from the temples and from the crown; the bald area then gradually widens.

GENERALIZED ALOPECIA In this rare form of alopecia, the hair falls out in large amounts, leaving a nearly invisible covering over the entire scalp. Such hair loss occurs because all the hairs simultaneously enter the resting phase and then fall out about three months later. Regrowth occurs when the underlying cause is corrected.

Causes include various forms of stress, such as surgery, prolonged illness, or childbirth. Many *anticancer drugs* cause temporary alopecia.

LOCALIZED ALOPECIA This may be due to permanent damage to the skin (e.g. by burns or *radiotherapy*). Another common cause of hair loss is trauma to the hair roots. Trauma may be due to excessive pulling of the hair to produce a particular hairstyle or, rarely, to *trichotillomania* (a disorder in which sufferers pull out their hair).

The most common cause is alopecia areata, which produces localized areas of hair loss in which the bald skin looks and feels normal. The cause is unknown. Usually the hair returns to normal within a few months. There is no specific treatment.

Alopecia universalis is a rare, permanent form of alopecia areata that causes all the hair on the scalp and the body to be lost, including the eyelashes and eyebrows.

Ringworm infection of the scalp (see *Tinea*) may cause localized hair loss due to breakage of weakened hair shafts. Other skin diseases, such as *lichen planus, lupus erythematosus,* and *skin tumours,* may also be responsible. The bald skin always looks abnormal in conditions such as these and hair stubble can usually be seen in the affected area.

TREATMENT

Wigs and toupees are often used to disguise alopecia affecting the scalp. *Hair transplants* are sometimes successful as a permanent method of replacing the lost hair. The antihypertensive drug *minoxidil* may cause hair regrowth in some cases.

Alpha-fetoprotein

A protein produced in the liver and gastrointestinal tract of the fetus and by some abnormal tissues in adults.

ALPHA-FETOPROTEIN IN PREGNANCY

Alpha-fetoprotein (AFP) is excreted in the fetal urine into the *amniotic fluid;* the fluid is then swallowed by the fetus, which introduces AFP into the fetal digestive system. Most of the AFP is broken down in the fetal intestine, but some passes from the fetus into the mother's circulation. AFP can be measured in the maternal blood from the latter part of the first trimester of pregnancy, and its concentration rises steadily between the 15th and 20th weeks.

Raised levels of AFP are found in some cases of fetal abnormality and occasionally when the fetus is normal. In *neural tube defects,* such as *spina bifida* or *anencephaly,* excess AFP may leak into the amniotic fluid. AFP levels are also raised in certain kidney abnormalities, and can result from reduced breakdown of AFP in the intestine if the fetus cannot swallow properly due to oesophageal malformation.

AFP levels are also raised in multiple pregnancy (see *Pregnancy, multiple*) and in threatened or actual *miscarriage.* They may be mistakenly thought to be raised if there has been an error in the calculation of gestation dates. AFP levels may be unusually low in pregnancies in which the fetus has *Down's syndrome.*

TESTING AFP LEVELS IN PREGNANCY

Ideally, pregnant women should be offered antenatal screening by measurement of blood AFP and by *ultrasound scanning* at about 16 weeks. Scanning is performed to date the pregnancy, to detect a multiple pregnancy, and to show certain fetal abnormalities. If the blood AFP level is raised, the test is repeated one week later. If the second result is also raised, the woman may be carrying a baby with a neural tube or other defect. An ultrasound scan may strengthen or confirm the suspicion. *Amniocentesis* (removal of a small amount of the fluid surrounding the fetus) may be performed, and further measurements of AFP may be made on the sample. If the level is significantly raised, the chances that the woman is carrying an affected baby are high; a termination of pregnancy (see *Abortion, induced*) may then be considered.

About 10 per cent of cases of neural tube defect are missed during screening because AFP levels are not significantly raised in all such cases. Conversely, in about five cases per 1,000 in which both amniotic fluid and blood levels of AFP are raised, the fetus is normal.

AFP IN ADULTS

In adults, AFP is produced in certain abnormal tissues. Levels are commonly raised in patients with hepatoma (see *Liver cancer*) and in those with malignant *teratoma* of the testes or ovaries. Some patients with cancer of the pancreas, stomach, and lung also have raised levels. Because it is present in abnormal quantities when a person is suffering from certain cancers, AFP is known as a "tumour marker". However, AFP levels are also raised in some noncancerous conditions, including viral and alcoholic *hepatitis* and in *cirrhosis.*

AFP levels can be used to monitor the treatment of hepatomas and teratomas; increasing levels after surgery or chemotherapy are a useful indicator of tumour recurrence.

Alprazolam

A *benzodiazepine drug* used to treat *anxiety, panic attacks,* and *phobias.*

Alternative medicine

Any medical system based on a theory of disease or method of treatment other than the orthodox science of medicine as taught in medical schools.

Every society has its *folk medicine* and traditional healers who use methods and beliefs handed down through the generations. In some cultures, such as in China (see *Chinese medicine*), textbooks of traditional medicine date back several thousands of years. Some systems, such as *acupuncture,* are based on theories of disease that emphasize internal balances. Many cultures have a long tradition of *herbal medicine* and some plant-based remedies have been recognized by orthodox medicine.

The early 19th century brought the development of many new alternative systems, such as *chiropractic, homeopathy,* and *naturopathy.* The popularity of alternative practices declined in the 20th century because of the successes of orthodox medicine—notably vaccines, antibiotics, diuretics, antidepressants, and advances in anaesthesia and surgery. More recently, a small but increasing number of people have questioned the ability of orthodox medicine to provide all the answers. Numerous new and rediscovered disciplines, such as *aromatherapy* and naturopathy, have won a following without conclusive scientific confirmation.

Many alternative practitioners are sympathetic listeners who give sensible advice backed up by treatments that are sometimes successful. The opposition by many practitioners of orthodox medicine to alternative therapies is based on the principle that the essential first step in the treatment of any disorder is accurate diagnosis, which itself requires extensive medical knowledge. Treatment of symptoms without knowing their cause is potentially disastrous if an underlying remediable but progressive condition has not been recognized. Furthermore, some herbal remedies, although based on natural ingredients, may cause adverse reactions in some people and might also be dangerous if taken at the same time as conventional medicines.

Altitude sickness

See *Mountain sickness.*

Aluminium

A light, metallic element which is abundant in bauxite and various other minerals. Aluminium compounds are found in relatively low concentrations in the human body, where they have no known useful function and are almost certainly harmful.

Sources of ingested aluminium in humans include *antacid drugs,* cooking utensils and foil, some baking powders, and food additives such as potassium alum (used to whiten flour) and aluminium calcium silicate (used to keep salt running freely). Most of the aluminium taken into the

A

body is excreted. The remainder is stored in the lungs, brain, liver, and thyroid gland.

Aluminium chloride is a common ingredient in *antiperspirants* and aluminium acetate is used as an *astringent* skin preparation.

ADVERSE EFFECTS
Some industrial processes, such as aluminium processing and explosives manufacturing, may give off minute droplets containing aluminium into the air. Inhalation of such droplets is occasionally associated with various lung diseases, including *fibrosis* of the lungs and *emphysema*.

Prolonged use of antacids containing aluminium hydroxide can cause weakness, tiredness, and loss of appetite. Aluminium chloride in antiperspirants can cause allergic *dermatitis* in susceptible people.

Aluminium-induced *dementia* has developed in some patients undergoing *dialysis* (artificial purification of the blood) due to the aluminium content of the water used; this problem can be prevented by adequate monitoring procedures. There is some evidence suggesting that *Alzheimer's disease* is more common in parts of the UK in which the water supply has high aluminium levels, but most neurologists doubt any causal association between aluminium and the disease.

Alveolectomy
See *Alveoloplasty*.

Alveolitis
Inflammation and thickening of the walls of the alveoli (tiny air sacs) in the lungs. Alveolitis reduces the elasticity of the lungs during breathing and reduces the efficiency of gas transfer between the lungs and the surrounding blood vessels.

CAUSES
Alveolitis is most commonly caused by an allergic reaction to inhaled dust of animal or plant origin, often containing fungal spores. Such allergic alveolitis may be related to occupation, as in cases of *farmer's lung* (caused by spores from mouldy hay), *bagassosis* (caused by spores from mouldy sugar-cane residue), and pigeon fancier's lung (caused by particles from bird droppings).

Fibrosing alveolitis may be an *autoimmune disorder* (a disorder in which the body's defence mechanisms produce antibodies that act against its own tissues). In some cases, fibrosing alveolitis occurs with other autoimmune disorders, such as

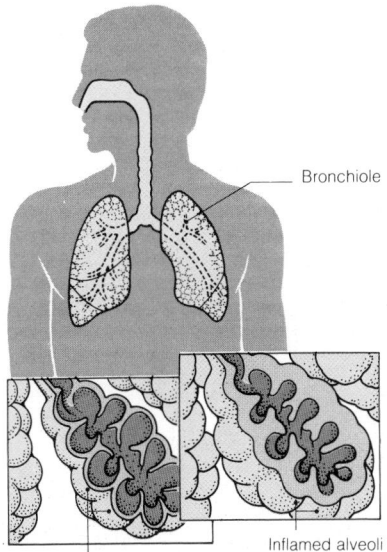

Bronchiole

Normal alveoli

Inflamed alveoli

Signs of alveolitis
The alveoli become inflamed and their walls thicken, causing the lungs to become less elastic and less efficient.

systemic *lupus erythematosus* or *rheumatoid arthritis*.

Radiation alveolitis is inflammation of the alveoli caused by exposure to radiation, usually as a rare complication of *radiotherapy* treatment for lung or breast cancer.

SYMPTOMS AND DIAGNOSIS
Alveolitis usually causes a dry cough and breathing difficulty on exertion.

A chest X-ray usually shows mottled shadowing across the lungs. Blood tests may be performed to look for specific antibodies to an allergen or evidence of an autoimmune disorder. *Pulmonary function tests* show reduced lung capacity without obstruction to air flow through the bronchi. A lung *biopsy* (removal of a sample of tissue for analysis) may be the only way to make a conclusive diagnosis.

TREATMENT AND OUTLOOK
For fibrosing alveolitis, *corticosteroid drugs* may need to be taken indefinitely. For other types of alveolitis, a short course of corticosteroids may relieve symptoms.

If the cause of allergic alveolitis is recognized and avoided before lung damage occurs, there is often no permanent disability. In fibrosing alveolitis, the lung damage progresses despite treatment, causing increasing breathing difficulty and, sometimes, *respiratory failure*. The outlook for radiation alveolitis varies considerably, depending on the severity of the condition.

Alveoloplasty
Dental surgery to remove protuberances and to smooth out other uneven areas from tooth-bearing bone in the jaw. The procedure is performed, before the fitting of dentures, on people whose alveolar ridge underlying the gums would not otherwise be even enough for dentures to be fitted easily or worn comfortably.

Minor alveoloplasty may be performed using a local anaesthetic, but most operations require general anaesthesia (see *Anaesthesia, dental*). An incision is made in the gum, which is then peeled back to expose the uneven bone. The bone is then either reshaped with large bone forceps or filed down to the required shape. Finally, the gum is drawn back over the bone and stitched together again. Some bruising and swelling of the mouth may occur, but the gum usually heals within two weeks.

Alveolus, dental
The bony cavity or socket that supports each tooth in the jaw.

Alveolus, pulmonary
One of a group of tiny, balloon-like sacs at the end of a bronchiole (one of the many small air passages in the lungs) where gases are exchanged during *respiration*. There are approximately 300 million alveoli in each lung, arranged in groups that resemble bunches of grapes.

ANATOMY OF THE ALVEOLI
These tiny sacs contain capillaries in their thin walls that allow oxygen to be absorbed into the blood.

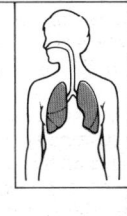

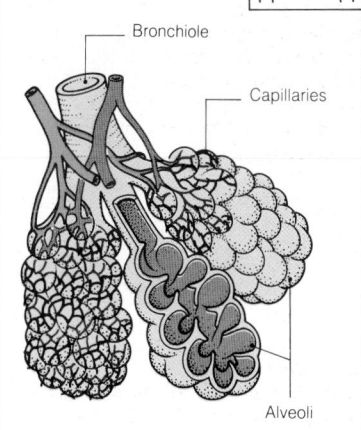

Bronchiole

Capillaries

Alveoli

A

Alzheimer's disease

A progressive condition in which nerve cells in the brain degenerate and the size of the brain substance shrinks. Alzheimer's disease is the single most common cause of *dementia* (a general decline in all areas of mental ability). Although originally classified as a "presenile" dementia, Alzheimer's disease is now known to be responsible for 75 per cent of dementia cases in people over 65 years old. Because of the increasing numbers of elderly people, interest in and research into the causes and treatment of Alzheimer's disease have greatly expanded in recent years. The progress of the disease (which, in most cases, means several years of intellectual and personal decline until death) cannot be arrested.

CAUSES

The cause of Alzheimer's disease has become clearer with recent research. First, there are strong genetic factors. Early onset, or familial Alzheimer's disease, in which symptoms develop before the age of 60, is inherited as a dominant disorder (see *Genetics*). Late onset Alzheimer's disease seems to be associated with one of the three genes for a blood protein, *apolipoprotein* E. Up to 25 per cent of the world's population are thought to have the variant of this protein associated with the disease.

The genes that cause the disease seem to do so by the production within the brain of deposits or plaques of a protein substance known as beta amyloid. There are other chemical abnormalities, too, including a deficiency of the *neurotransmitter* acetylcholine.

INCIDENCE

Onset is rare before the age of 60, but thereafter increases steadily with age. Up to 30 per cent of people over the age of 85 are affected.

SYMPTOMS AND SIGNS

The features of the disease vary among individuals, but there are three broad stages. At first, the patient becomes increasingly forgetful and may try to compensate by writing lists or seeking the help of others. Some deterioration in memory is a feature of normal *aging*, and this alone is not evidence of dementia. Problems with memory due to Alzheimer's disease may cause anxiety and depression.

Forgetfulness gradually shades into a second phase of severe memory loss, particularly for recent events. Victims may remember long-ago events, such as their schooldays, but are unable to recall yesterday's visitors or what they saw on television. They also become disoriented as to time or place, losing their way even in familiar locations. Concentration and numerical ability decline and *dysphasia* (inability to find the right word) is noticeable. Anxiety increases, mood changes are unpredictable, and personality changes soon occur.

In the third stage, patients become severely disoriented and confused. They may also suffer from symptoms of *psychosis*, such as *hallucinations* and paranoid *delusions*. Symptoms are worsened by the patient's disorientation and memory losses and are usually most severe at night. Signs of nervous system disease begin to emerge, such as abnormal *reflexes* (involuntary actions) and incontinence of urine and faeces. Some patients become very demanding, unpleasant, and sometimes violent, and lose all awareness of social norms. Others become docile and helpless. They neglect personal hygiene and may wander purposelessly. Eventually the burden for caring relatives becomes impossible, and full-time hospital care and nursing are often inevitable. Once the patient is bedridden, the complications of *bedsores*, feeding problems, and *pneumonia* reduce life expectancy.

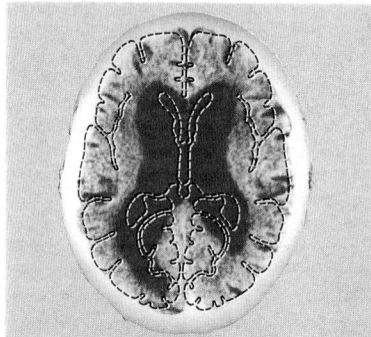

Brain scan in Alzheimer's disease
The volume of the brain substance (grey area) has shrunk markedly. Its normal outline is shown by the dotted line.

DIAGNOSIS

Alzheimer's disease is usually diagnosed from the patient's symptoms and signs. An *EEG* shows slowing of brain waves. *CT scanning* and *MRI* of the brain show evidence of reduced cerebral size. Tests of mental state indicate decreased intellectual ability.

Alzheimer's disease can be definitely diagnosed only by examination of the brain, either by *biopsy* (removal of a sample of tissue for microscopic analysis) or after death. Microscopic examination typically shows loss of nerve cells, specks of brain debris, and tangles of nerves that resemble pieces of unwound string.

Other tests should be performed to exclude other possible causes of symptoms resembling those of Alzheimer's disease. Some 10 per cent of people with such symptoms have a treatable disease (such as *hypothyroidism*, *vitamin B_{12}* deficiency, a *brain tumour*, or a subdural *haematoma*). Other elderly people suffer from depressive pseudodementia, in which they appear to be demented but are actually suffering from the effects of *depression*, which may be treatable.

TREATMENT

The most important aspect of treatment for Alzheimer's disease is the provision of suitable nursing and social care for sufferers and their relatives. A good diet, exercise, and keeping occupied help alleviate anxiety and distress, especially in the earlier stages when the sufferer is still sufficiently aware of his or her condition. *Tranquillizer drugs* can often improve difficult behaviour and help the patient to sleep. Counselling of sufferers' families can help prevent problems and minimize disruption of family life.

People with Alzheimer's disease are often best cared for at home. The provision of suitable day-care and short-stay facilities may reduce the burden on families and enable some people to continue living at home longer than would otherwise be possible. For advanced cases, however, inpatient care may be necessary.

Drugs, such as *tetrahydroaminoacridine* (tacrine), that restore the acetylcholine content of the brain to normal have been evaluated since the mid 1980s, but none has yet been strikingly effective, and side-effects have limited their prolonged use.

Amalgam, dental

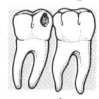

A material used to fill teeth, consisting of an alloy of mercury with one or more other metals. Amalgam is soft enough to be easily workable by the dentist but sets rapidly (within two hours) into a hard, strong solid; it is therefore ideal for use as a filling, especially for back teeth (see *Filling, dental*).

Amantadine

An *antiviral drug* used in the prevention and treatment of *influenza* A. Amantadine has more recently been used to help relieve symptoms of *Parkinson's disease*.

Amaurosis fugax

Brief loss of vision, lasting for periods of seconds to minutes, usually caused by the temporary blockage of small blood vessels in the eye by tiny *emboli* (particles of solid matter such as cholesterol crystals or particles of clotted blood). These emboli are carried in the bloodstream from diseased carotid arteries in the neck or, rarely, from the heart. Sufferers typically experience a loss or dimming of vision, in one eye only, rather like a shade being pulled down or up.

Attacks may be infrequent or may occur many times a day. This symptom should never be ignored since it is a clear warning that the person has an increased risk of *stroke* or *coronary heart disease*. Medical investigation, with special attention to the state of the arteries, is urgently needed.

Ambidexterity

The ability to perform manual skills, such as writing or using cutlery, equally well with either hand because there is no definite *handedness* (preference for using one hand). Ambidexterity is an uncommon and often familial trait.

Amblyopia

A permanent defect of visual acuity in which there is usually no structural abnormality in the eye. In many cases there is a disturbance of the visual pathway between the retina and the brain. The term is also sometimes applied to toxic or nutritional causes of decreased visual acuity, as in tobacco-alcohol amblyopia.

If normal vision is to develop during infancy and childhood, it is essential that clear, corresponding visual images are formed on both retinas so that compatible nerve impulses pass from the eyes to the brain. If no images are received, normal vision cannot develop. If images from the two eyes are very different, one will be suppressed to avoid double vision, and normal vision may not develop in one of the eyes.

CAUSES

The most common cause of amblyopia is *squint* in very young children. In this condition, only one eye points at a selected object and the different image from the other eye is suppressed. Failure to form normal retinal images may also result from congenital *cataract* (opacity of the lens of the eye at birth), and severe, or unequal, focusing errors in a young child, such as when one eye is normal and the other eye has an uncorrected large degree of *astigmatism*, causing a blurred image on the retina. Toxic and nutritional amblyopia may result from damage to the retina and/or optic nerve.

TREATMENT AND OUTLOOK

It is important to treat amblyopia at an early age; after the age of eight, amblyopia usually cannot be remedied. For amblyopia due to squint, patching (covering up the good eye to force the deviating eye to function properly) is the usual treatment. Glasses and/or surgery to place the deviating eye in the correct position may be necessary. Glasses may also be necessary to correct severe focusing errors. Congenital cataracts may be removed surgically.

Ambulance

A vehicle, staffed by trained personnel, for transporting sick, injured, or disabled people. There are two types of ambulance: emergency (front line) ambulances and nonemergency (sitting case) ambulances.

The emergency ambulance crew responds to 999 calls, taking accident victims and severely ill people to hospital. The crew aims to stabilize the patient's condition as much as possible before and during the journey to hospital. The emergency ambulance is staffed by qualified ambulance personnel who undertake a 12-week basic training course and up to one year's supervised practical work.

A nonemergency ambulance is used only to transport people (particularly the disabled or elderly) to hospital outpatient departments and day-care clinics. The ambulance personnel have basic emergency training.

Amelogenesis imperfecta

An inherited condition of the teeth in which the enamel is either abnormally thin or deficient in calcium. Affected teeth may be pitted and discoloured (see *Discoloured teeth*), and, depending on the type of imperfection, may be more susceptible to dental *caries* (tooth decay) and wear.

Amenorrhoea

Absence of menstrual periods. Primary amenorrhoea is defined as failure to start menstruating by the age of 16. Secondary amenorrhoea is the temporary or permanent cessation of periods in a woman who has menstruated regularly in the past.

PRIMARY AMENORRHOEA The main cause of primary amenorrhoea is the delayed onset of *puberty*. The delay is often not due to any disorder but, rarely, it may result from a disorder of the *endocrine system*, such as a *pituitary tumour*, *hypothyroidism* (underactivity of the thyroid gland), an *adrenal tumour*, or *adrenal hyperplasia*. Another rare cause of delayed puberty is *Turner's syndrome*, in which one female sex chromosome is missing.

In some cases, menstruation fails to take place because the vagina or the uterus has been absent from birth, or because there is no perforation in the hymen (the membrane across the opening of the vagina) to allow menstrual blood to escape.

SECONDARY AMENORRHOEA The most common cause of temporary secondary amenorrhoea is *pregnancy*. Periods may also cease temporarily after a woman has stopped taking *oral contraceptives*; periods usually return after six to eight weeks but may not return for a year or longer in some cases. Secondary amenorrhoea may also result from hormonal changes due to emotional stress, *depression*, *anorexia nervosa*, or certain drugs.

Rarely, periods may stop as a result of the same disorders of the endocrine system that can cause primary amenorrhoea. Another possible cause of secondary amenorrhoea is a disorder of the *ovary*, such as polycystic ovary or an ovarian tumour.

Amenorrhoea occurs permanently after the *menopause* or following a *hysterectomy* (a surgical operation to remove the uterus).

INVESTIGATION

Investigation of amenorrhoea usually includes a physical examination and blood tests to measure hormone levels. It may also involve *laparoscopy* to inspect the ovaries, *CT scanning* or *MRI* of the skull to exclude the possibility of a pituitary tumour, and *ultrasound scanning* of the abdomen and pelvis to exclude a tumour of the adrenal glands or ovaries.

TREATMENT

Some women with either primary or secondary amenorrhoea may choose not to have treatment, but in every case the cause should be identified. Ovarian tumours or cysts should be removed surgically. Anorexia nervosa, too, needs treatment because of its long-term threat to health. If a woman with amenorrhoea wants treatment and the cause is an endocrine disorder other than ovarian failure, ovulation can often be induced by treatment with *clomiphene* or *gonadotrophin hormones*.

Amiloride

A potassium-sparing *diuretic drug.* Combined with loop or thiazide diuretic drugs, amiloride is used to treat *hypertension* (high blood pressure) and fluid retention due to *heart failure* or to *cirrhosis* of the liver.

Amino acids

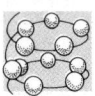 A group of chemical compounds that form the basic structural units of all *proteins.* Each amino acid molecule consists of nitrogenous amino and acidic carboxyl groups of atoms linked to a variable chain or ring of carbon atoms.

Individual amino acid molecules are linked together—by chemical bonds, called *peptide* bonds, between the amino and carboxyl groups—to form short chains of molecules called *polypeptides.* Hundreds of polypeptides are, in turn, linked together—also by peptide bonds—to form a protein molecule. What differentiates one protein from another is the sequence of the amino acids.

There are 20 different amino acids that make up all the proteins in humans. Of these, 12 can be made by the body; they are known as nonessential amino acids, because they do not need to be obtained from the diet. The other eight, known as the essential amino acids, cannot be made by the body and therefore must be obtained from the diet.

The 20 amino acids that make up proteins also occur free within cells and in body fluids. In addition, there are more than 200 other amino acids that are not found in proteins but which play an important part in chemical reactions within cells.

Aminoglutethimide

An *anticancer drug* that is used to treat certain types of breast cancer, prostate cancer, and some endocrine gland tumours.

Aminoglycoside drugs

A group of *antibiotic drugs.* Aminoglycosides are generally reserved for the treatment of serious infections because their use can cause damage to the inner ear or kidneys. Important examples are *gentamicin, neomycin,* and *streptomycin.*

Aminophylline

A drug used to treat chronic *bronchitis, asthma,* and, occasionally, *heart failure.*

HOW IT WORKS
Aminophylline relieves breathing difficulty by widening the bronchi in the lungs. It also dilates (widens) blood vessels, thus improving blood flow from the heart, and increases the production of urine.

POSSIBLE ADVERSE EFFECTS
Nausea, vomiting, headache, dizziness, and palpitations may occur. During long-term treatment, blood tests may be carried out to monitor the level of aminophylline in the body.

Amiodarone

An antiarrhythmic drug used to treat various types of *arrhythmia* (irregular heartbeat). Long-term use of amiodarone may result in inflammation of the liver, thyroid problems, and damage to the eyes and lungs. Because of its possible adverse effects, amiodarone is usually given only when other drugs have not been effective.

Amitriptyline

A tricyclic *antidepressant drug* with a sedative effect. Amitriptyline is useful in the treatment of *depression* accompanied by *anxiety* or *insomnia.* Possible adverse effects include blurred vision, dizziness, and drowsiness.

Amlodipine

A *calcium channel blocker* used to prevent *angina pectoris* and to treat *hypertension* (high blood pressure). Possible adverse effects include oedema (accumulation of fluid in the tissues), flushing, headaches, and dizziness.

Ammonia

A colourless, pungent gas that dissolves in water to form ammonium hydroxide, an alkaline solution (see *Alkali*). Ammonia consists of one nitrogen atom linked to three hydrogen atoms. Ammonia is produced in the body and plays a valuable role in maintaining the *acid-base balance.*

In severe liver damage, the capacity of the liver to convert ammonia to *urea* is diminished. This leads to a high concentration of ammonia in the blood, which is thought to be a cause of the impaired consciousness that occurs in *liver failure.*

Amnesia

Loss of the ability to memorize information and/or to recall information stored in *memory.* Amnesic conditions affect mainly long-term memory (where information is retained indefinitely) rather than short-term memory (where information is retained only for seconds or minutes).

Many people with amnesia have a memory gap that extends back for some time from the onset of the disorder. This condition, known as retrograde amnesia, is principally a deficit of recall. In most cases, the memory gap gradually shrinks over time.

Some people with amnesia are unable to store new information in the period following the onset of illness. The resultant gap in memory, known as anterograde amnesia, extends from the moment of onset of the amnesia to the time when long-term memory resumes (if at all). This memory gap is usually permanent.

CAUSES
Amnesia is caused by damage to, or disease of, brain regions concerned with memory functions. Possible causes of such damage are *head injury,* degenerative disorders (such as *Alzheimer's disease* and other forms of *dementia*), infections such as *encephalitis,* thiamine deficiency in alcoholics leading to *Wernicke-Korsakoff syndrome,* and also *brain tumours, strokes,* and *subarachnoid haemorrhage.* Amnesia can also occur in some forms of psychiatric illness (in which there is no apparent physical damage to the brain). Some deterioration of memory is a common feature of *aging.*

Amniocentesis

A diagnostic procedure in which a small amount of *amniotic fluid* is withdrawn from the *amniotic sac* (the membranous bag that surrounds the fetus in the uterus).

WHY IT IS DONE
The amniotic fluid contains cells and chemicals from the fetus that can be analysed to detect fetal abnormalities, such as *Down's syndrome* and other chromosomal abnormalities. Amniocentesis can also help detect genetic disorders (such as *haemophilia, cystic fibrosis,* and *Tay-Sachs disease*), or developmental disorders (such as *spina bifida*). It is also used to assess fetal disorders, such as *Rhesus incompatibility,* and to check the maturity of the fetal lungs.

HOW IT IS DONE
Amniocentesis is usually performed between the 16th and 18th week of gestation. *Ultrasound scanning* is used to estimate the age and position of the fetus, the placental site, and the amount of amniotic fluid. A needle is then inserted through the abdomen and uterine wall into the amniotic sac, avoiding the fetus and placenta. A syringe is attached to the needle and about 20 to 30 ml of fluid is removed for analysis.

Anaesthesia is not usually required, although occasionally a local anaes-

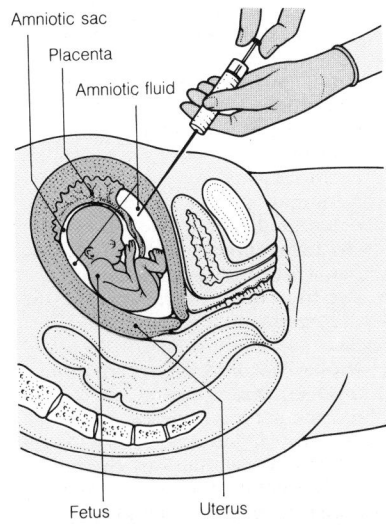

Procedure for amniocentesis
A needle is introduced through the abdomen and uterine wall into the amniotic sac; a sample of amniotic fluid is then withdrawn.

thetic is used. In most cases, the woman can go home soon after the procedure but is advised to rest for about 24 hours.

RESULTS

The amniotic fluid is analysed biochemically and fetal cells are cultured for *chromosomal analysis*. Culturing cells for chromosomal analysis may take up to four weeks and results may therefore not be available until about 20 weeks' gestation.

As well as identifying fetal disorders, chromosome analysis reveals the sex of the fetus. A woman should therefore indicate whether or not she wishes to receive this information. Some laboratories do not report the sex of the fetus.

COMPLICATIONS

Incidence of *miscarriage* or early rupture of the membranes is slightly increased after amniocentesis; recent studies show a risk of about 0.5 per cent. Amniocentesis is therefore usually recommended only when other diagnostic tests such as measurement of the blood concentration of *alphafetoprotein* have revealed a substantial risk of fetal abnormality or there are other compelling medical reasons, such as a family history of a chromosomal abnormality. (See also *Chorionic villus sampling*.)

Amnion

One of the membranes that surrounds the *embryo* and *fetus* in the *uterus*. The outside of the amnion is covered by another membrane called the *chorion*.

Amnioscopy

An obstetric procedure in which an amnioscope (a tapering metal viewing tube) is inserted through the cervix towards the end of pregnancy to allow inspection of the *amniotic fluid* through the intact amniotic membrane. The amnioscope may also be inserted through the cervix during labour to allow a sample of blood to be taken from the fetal scalp, to check the condition of the fetus.

Amniotic fluid

The clear fluid (popularly called the "waters") that surrounds the fetus in the uterus throughout pregnancy. The fluid is contained within the amniotic sac (a thin membrane).

The fetus floats in the amniotic fluid and, in the early months of pregnancy, can move about freely. The amniotic fluid cushions the fetus against pressure from internal organs and protects it from any injury from the mother's movements.

The fluid is produced by the cells that line the amniotic sac and is constantly circulated. It is swallowed by the fetus, absorbed into its bloodstream, and then excreted by the fetal kidneys as urine. Amniotic fluid is 99 per cent water. The remainder consists of dilute concentrations of substances found in *blood* plasma, along with cells and *lipids* (fats) that have flaked off from the fetus.

Amniotic fluid appears during the first week after conception and gradually increases in volume until the 10th week, when the increase becomes very rapid. By 35 weeks' gestation the volume of fluid is about one litre. Thereafter it slowly declines until it is just over half a litre at term, though there is a wide variation between individuals.

In a small number of pregnancies, excessive fluid is formed; this condition is known as *polyhydramnios* or hydramnios. Less frequently, insufficient amniotic fluid is formed; this condition is called *oligohydramnios*.

Amniotic sac

The membranous bag that surrounds the *fetus* and fills with watery *amniotic fluid* as pregnancy advances. The amniotic sac is made up of two membranes, the inner *amnion* and the outer *chorion*.

Amniotomy

Artificial rupture of the amniotic membranes (breaking of the waters) performed for *induction of labour*.

Amoebiasis

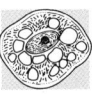

An infection caused by the amoeba *ENTAMOEBA HISTOLYTICA*, a tiny single-celled parasite that lives in the human large intestine. The infection is characterized by recurrent moderate to severe diarrhoea and, occasionally, the development of abscesses in the liver or, more rarely, the brain or lung.

CAUSE AND INCIDENCE

Amoebiasis occurs as a result of drinking water or eating food contaminated by human excreta containing cysts of the amoeba. Once swallowed, the walls of the cysts break down, and the amoebae hatch out to parasitize the large intestine. In the intestine, the amoebae multiply and develop protective capsules, forming new cysts. These cysts are passed out of the body in the faeces, and can survive for long periods before the next person acquires them.

Amoebiasis is prevalent in poor countries where standards of public hygiene and sanitation are low. Although amoebiasis can be acquired worldwide, most sufferers in the UK and other developed countries have contracted the disease in developing countries in the tropics or subtropics. About 500 cases are diagnosed per year in the UK. Deaths from amoebiasis occur occasionally.

PREVENTION

Travellers to countries where sanitary standards are low can reduce their chances of acquiring amoebiasis by drinking only bottled or thoroughly boiled water (chlorine-releasing water-sterilization tablets are not very effective at killing amoebic cysts) and by not eating uncooked vegetables (especially lettuce) or unpeeled fruit.

SYMPTOMS

Some people carry *ENTAMOEBA HISTOLYTICA* in their intestines and excrete cysts but have no symptoms, probably because the strain of amoebae they carry is harmless.

Some strains of amoebae invade and ulcerate the intestinal wall, causing diarrhoea, which may vary in severity from two or more rather loose stools per day, accompanied by rumbling pains in the stomach, to full-blown dysentery, with high fever and the frequent passage of watery diarrhoea accompanied by the passage of blood and mucus. Dysentery often recurs after short intermissions.

Amoebae may spread via the bloodstream to the liver, where they cause abscesses. Symptoms of an amoebic liver abscess include chills, fever, weight loss and painful enlargement

A

of the liver. Liver abscesses sometimes develop in people who are infected with amoebae but who have never had digestive tract symptoms.

TREATMENT

Treatment of all forms of amoebiasis is with drugs such as *metronidazole* or diloxanide, which kill the parasite within a few weeks, leading to full recovery.

Amoebic dysentery

See *Amoebiasis.*

Amoebicides

A group of drugs used to treat *amoebiasis*. Examples include *chloroquine, diloxanide,* and *metronidazole.* They work by killing amoebae in the intestine and in other body tissues.

Amoxapine

An *antidepressant* related to the tricyclic drugs. Possible adverse effects include blurred vision, dizziness, drowsiness, abnormal muscular movements, menstrual irregularities, and breast enlargement.

Amoxycillin

A *penicillin drug* commonly used to treat a wide variety of infections, including *bronchitis, cystitis, gonorrhoea,* and ear and skin infections.

Allergy to amoxycillin causes a blotchy rash and, rarely, fever, swelling of the mouth and tongue, itching, and breathing difficulty.

Amphetamine drugs

COMMON DRUG

Dexamphetamine

A group of *stimulant drugs* with an *appetite suppressant* effect. Their use to treat *obesity* has now been largely abandoned because of dependence problems and abuse. Amphetamines are now used mainly in the treatment of *narcolepsy* (a rare condition characterized by excessive sleepiness).

HOW THEY WORK

Amphetamine drugs stimulate the secretion of *neurotransmitters* (chemicals released by nerve endings), such as *noradrenaline,* which increase nerve activity in the brain and make a person wakeful and alert.

POSSIBLE ADVERSE EFFECTS

Taken in high doses, amphetamines can cause tremor, sweating, palpitations, anxiety, and sleeping difficulties. Delusions, hallucinations, high blood pressure, and, rarely, seizures may also occur. Prolonged use of amphetamines may cause *tolerance*

and physical dependence (see *Drug dependence*).

ABUSE

Amphetamines are abused for their stimulant effects; for this reason, their prescription is controlled by the Misuse of Drugs Act.

Amphotericin B

A drug used to treat fungal infections. Lozenges are used for candidiasis of the mouth. Life-threatening infections, such as *cryptococcosis* and *histoplasmosis,* are treated by injection.

Adverse effects are likely only when amphotericin B is given by injection; these include vomiting, fever, headache, and, rarely, seizures.

Ampicillin

A *penicillin drug* commonly used to treat infections including *cystitis, bronchitis,* and ear infections. Ampicillin is also useful in the treatment of *gonorrhoea, typhoid fever,* and infections of the *biliary system.*

Diarrhoea is a common adverse effect. Some people are allergic to ampicillin and suffer from rash, fever, swelling of the mouth and tongue, itching, and breathing difficulty.

Amputation

Surgical removal of part or all of a limb. Amputation was formerly a common operation, especially in wartime, but is now rarely performed except in the treatment of severe arterial disease and cancer.

WHY IT IS DONE

Until the introduction of *antibiotic drugs* in the early 1940s, amputation was often necessary to prevent the spread of *gangrene* (tissue death) following infection of a wound.

Today, most amputations are performed on patients with *peripheral vascular disease,* in which a combination of *atherosclerosis* and *thrombosis* may completely block the blood supply to a limb, causing gangrene.

Amputation is also sometimes performed to prevent the spread of *bone cancer* or malignant *melanoma* (a type of skin cancer).

HOW IT IS DONE

Before the operation, the surgeon decides where on the limb to operate; the tissue at the amputation site must be healthy if the wound is to heal satisfactorily. Investigative techniques used at this stage include *angiography* (injection into an artery of a solution visible on X-ray) and *thermography* (recordings of body-surface temperatures with a heat-sensitive camera).

During the operation, skin and muscle are cut below the level at which the bone is to be severed to create flaps that will later provide a fleshy stump. Blood vessels are tied off, the bone is sawn through, the area is washed with saline (salt solution), and the flaps of skin and muscle are stitched over the sawn end of bone to form a smooth and rounded stump.

While amputating, the surgeon tries to ensure that nerves are severed well above the stump, reducing the risk of pressure pain when a prosthesis (see *Limb, artificial*) is fitted. However, despite every precaution, a painful *neuroma* (a benign tumour of nerve tissue) sometimes develops in the stump.

In an amputation at the ankle (Syme's amputation), the tough skin of the heel pad is retained to cover the stump. The patient can then place weight on the stump without necessarily having to use a prosthesis.

Amputations below the knee are now more satisfactory than before. Newer techniques for shaping the stump make it easier to fit a prosthesis, and new prostheses, attached by suction rather than straps, are easier to put on and take off.

RECOVERY PERIOD

As the wound heals, bandaging and plaster casts are used to mould the stump to a shape suitable for accepting a prosthesis. The stump is usually swollen for about six weeks after the operation and a permanent prosthesis can be fitted only after it has settled down to a stable size. The patient with a lower limb amputation is usually fitted with a temporary prosthesis during this period to avoid becoming unaccustomed to walking.

For some time after an amputation, some patients have the unpleasant sensation that the amputated limb is still present—a phenomenon known as "phantom limb".

OUTLOOK

The prospect of a person who has had a leg amputation remaining mobile afterwards depends on several factors: age, attitude, general health, the amount of limb lost, and whether the pressure of a prosthesis on the stump causes pain. Some healthy people lead almost as active lives as they did before, but many older people become confined to *wheelchairs.*

Amputation, congenital

The separation of a body part (usually a limb, finger, or toe) from the rest of the body, as a result of the part's blood supply being blocked by a band of *amnion* (fetal membrane) in the uterus. This may result in the affected part being completely separated, or showing the marks of the "amniotic band" after birth. (See *Limb defects*.)

Amputation, traumatic

Loss of a finger, toe, or limb through injury. (See also *Microsurgery*.)

Amyl nitrite

A *nitrate drug* formerly prescribed to relieve *angina pectoris* (chest pain due to impaired blood supply to the heart muscle). Because amyl nitrite frequently causes adverse effects (including headache, hot flushes, palpitations, and restlessness) it has been superseded by other drugs.

Amyl nitrite is sometimes abused for its effect of intensifying pleasure during orgasm.

Amyloidosis

An uncommon disease in which a substance called amyloid, composed of fibrous protein, accumulates in tissues and organs, including the liver, kidneys, tongue, spleen, and heart.

CAUSES

Amyloidosis may occur for no known reason, when it is called primary; more commonly, it is a complication of some other disease, when it is called secondary. Conditions that may lead to amyloidosis include *rheumatoid arthritis*, *multiple myeloma* (a cancer of bone marrow), *tuberculosis*, and some other long-standing infections, such as chronic *osteomyelitis* (bone infection). Exactly why amyloid is deposited in any of these circumstances is not known.

SYMPTOMS AND SIGNS

The symptoms and signs of amyloidosis vary, depending on which part of the body is involved.

Affected organs typically become enlarged. Accumulation of amyloid in the heart may result in *arrhythmias* (disturbances of the heartbeat) and *heart failure* (reduced pumping efficiency). If the stomach and intestines are affected, symptoms such as diarrhoea may develop and the lining of these organs may become ulcerated. In some cases, the joints are affected, causing *arthritis*.

Primary amyloidosis is often characterized by deposits of amyloid in the skin. Slightly raised, waxy spots appear, usually clustered around the armpits, groin, face, and neck.

Some rare forms of amyloidosis are inherited. These forms of the disease tend to involve the nervous system. Symptoms include peripheral *neuropathy*, postural *hypotension*, urinary or faecal *incontinence*, and reduced *sweating*. Death may occur as a result of *renal failure* caused by deposits of amyloid in the kidneys.

DIAGNOSIS AND TREATMENT

Diagnosis depends on microscopic and biochemical examination of a *biopsy* sample of tissue. Affected organs usually have a rubbery consistency and a waxy, pink or grey appearance.

There is no treatment, but secondary amyloidosis may be arrested or even reversed when the underlying disorder is treated.

Amyotrophic lateral sclerosis

See *Motor neuron disease*.

Amyotrophy

Shrinkage or wasting away of a muscle, caused by a reduction in the size of its fibres and leading to weakness. Amyotrophy is usually due to poor nutrition, reduced use of the muscle (as occurs when a limb is immobilized for a long period), or disruption of the blood or nerve supply to the muscle (as can occur in *diabetes mellitus* or *poliomyelitis*).

Anabolic steroids

See *Steroids, anabolic*.

Anaemia

A condition in which the concentration of the oxygen-carrying pigment *haemoglobin* in the blood is below normal. Haemoglobin molecules are carried inside red *blood cells* and transport oxygen from the lungs to the tissues. Under normal circumstances, stable haemoglobin concentrations in the blood are maintained by a strict balance between red cell production in the bone marrow and red cell destruction in the spleen. Anaemia may result if this balance is upset.

By far the most common form of anaemia worldwide is due to a deficiency of iron, an essential component of haemoglobin. However, there are numerous other causes of anaemia, which is not a disease in itself but a feature of many different disorders.

TYPES AND CAUSES

Red blood cells are formed in the bone marrow over a period of about five days from less specialized cells called stem cells. During this time, the cells change their appearance and accumulate haemoglobin. The red cells released from the bone marrow into the blood are called reticulocytes. Over a few days, reticulocytes mature into adult red blood cells. The adult cells circulate in the bloodstream for about 120 days; they age and are eventually trapped in small blood vessels (mainly in the spleen) and destroyed. Some cell components, including iron, are recycled for use in new cells.

The various forms of anaemia can be classified into those caused by decreased or defective production of red cells by the bone marrow (see *Anaemia, aplastic*; *Anaemia, iron-deficiency*; *Anaemia, megaloblastic*) and those caused by decreased survival of the red cells in the blood (see *Anaemia, haemolytic*). The illustrated box shows the main types.

SYMPTOMS

The symptoms common to all forms of anaemia result from the reduced oxygen-carrying capacity of the blood. Their severity depends on how low the haemoglobin concentration in the blood is. Normal blood haemoglobin concentrations are in the range 135 to 180 grams per litre for men and 115 to 160 grams/litre for women. Concentrations below 100 grams/litre can cause headaches, tiredness, and lethargy. Concentrations below 80 grams/litre can cause breathing difficulty on exercise, dizziness due to reduced oxygen reaching the brain, *angina pectoris* due to reduced oxygen supply to the heart muscle, and palpitations as the heart works harder to compensate. General signs include pallor, particularly of the skin creases, the lining of the mouth, and the inside of the eyelids, although this is not a reliable indicator of the severity of the anaemia.

Symptoms also depend upon the speed of development of an anaemia. Slow development of anaemia is tolerated well until it becomes advanced; the sudden development of anaemia causes more immediate symptoms.

Other features may occur with particular forms of anaemia. For example, some degree of *jaundice* occurs in most types of haemolytic anaemia, because the high rate of destruction of red cells leads to an increased level of the yellow pigment bilirubin (produced by the breakdown of the haemoglobin in red cells) in the blood.

DIAGNOSIS

Anaemia is diagnosed from the patient's symptoms and by the measurement of a low level of haemoglobin in the blood. To establish the type and cause of the anaemia, a sample of blood is first examined under the

TYPES AND CAUSES OF ANAEMIA

Anaemia results either from reduced or defective production or from an excessively high rate of destruction of oxygen-carrying red blood cells.

Four of the main types are shown below, but anaemia can have many other causes (such as various forms of leukaemia).

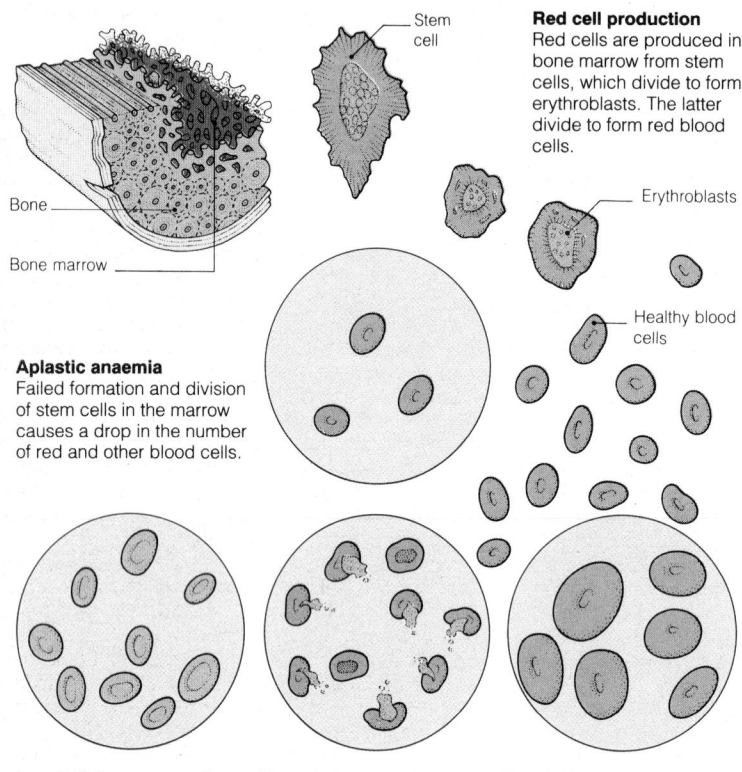

Stem cell

Red cell production
Red cells are produced in bone marrow from stem cells, which divide to form erythroblasts. The latter divide to form red blood cells.

Erythroblasts

Bone

Bone marrow

Healthy blood cells

Aplastic anaemia
Failed formation and division of stem cells in the marrow causes a drop in the number of red and other blood cells.

Iron-deficiency anaemia
Lack of iron prevents the bone marrow from making sufficient haemoglobin for the red cells. The cells produced are small and pale and have a reduced oxygen-carrying capacity.

Haemolytic anaemia
This type includes all anaemias in which the rate of red cell production is normal or high but in which the cells are destroyed at a much faster rate than normal.

Megaloblastic anaemia
A deficient supply of certain vitamins causes the bone marrow to produce red cells that are larger than normal; they also have a reduced oxygen-carrying capacity.

microscope, the numbers of different types of blood cells are counted, and their appearance is noted (see *Blood count*; *Blood film*). A low proportion of reticulocytes suggests that the cause is decreased production of red cells; a high proportion of reticulocytes suggests that cells are being destroyed at a high rate. The size of the red cells—whether small, normal, or large—provides further clues. With some specific forms—for example, *sickle cell anaemia* (a type of haemolytic anaemia)—some of the red cells have an abnormal shape.

Other investigations that may help the diagnosis include examination of cells in the bone marrow by means of a

bone marrow biopsy and measurement of the levels of substances such as folic acid, bilirubin, and vitamin B_{12} in the blood. Sometimes, further investigations must be carried out to establish the exact cause.

Treatment is directed towards correcting, modifying, or diminishing the mechanism or process that is leading to defective red cell production or reduced red cell survival. Anaemia associated with chronic disease or with renal failure responds to long-term treatment with the hormone *erythropoietin*. Anaemias due to genetic disorders such as *thalassaemia* may be treated successfully by bone marrow transplantation.

Anaemia, aplastic

A rare but important type of *anaemia* in which the red cells, white cells, and platelets in the blood are all reduced in number. Aplastic anaemia is caused by a failure of the *bone marrow* to produce stem cells, the initial form of all blood cells.

CAUSES AND INCIDENCE
Treatment of cancer with *radiotherapy* or *anticancer drugs* can interfere with the bone marrow's cell-producing capacity, as can certain viral infections and other drugs. In these cases, the marrow usually recovers and resumes normal production of cells once the cause is removed.

Long-term exposure to the fumes of benzene (a constituent of petrol) or insecticides has been implicated as a cause of more persistent aplastic anaemia, and a moderate to high dose of nuclear radiation (from radioactive fallout or nuclear explosions) is another recognized cause. In about half of all cases an autoimmune process is responsible (see *Autoimmune disorders*). In other people, aplastic anaemia develops for no known reason—a condition that is known as primary or idiopathic aplastic anaemia. This can can occur at any age but is most common around the age of 30.

SYMPTOMS
A low level of red blood cells may result in symptoms common to all types of anaemia, such as fatigue and breathlessness. Deficiency of white cells increases susceptibility to infections, while deficiency of platelets may cause a tendency to bruise easily, bleeding gums, or nosebleeds.

DIAGNOSIS
The disorder is usually suspected from the results of a blood test, particularly a *blood count*, and is confirmed by a *bone marrow biopsy*, in which a small sample of marrow is removed and examined for the presence or absence of blood-forming cells.

TREATMENT
When aplastic anaemia is due to infection or treatment for cancer, transfusions of red cells and platelets are given until the marrow returns to normal. When the anaemia is thought to be due to an autoimmune process, the usual first line of treatment is immunosuppression (therapy to suppress the immune system).

In persistent aplastic anaemia, a *bone marrow transplant* may be carried out if a suitable donor is available. The donor must be someone (usually a brother or sister) whose tissue-type closely matches that of the patient.

A

OUTLOOK

Recovery usually occurs from mild forms of the disease. However, without a bone marrow transplant, severe aplastic anaemia is often fatal.

Anaemia, haemolytic

A form of *anaemia* (a reduced level of the oxygen-carrying pigment *haemoglobin* in the blood) caused by the premature destruction of red cells in the bloodstream—a process known as haemolysis. The bone marrow has the capacity to increase red cell production approximately sixfold over normal rates. Anaemia results only if the shortening of the lifespan of red cells is sufficiently severe to overcome the marrow's reserve capacity.

TYPES AND CAUSES

Haemolytic anaemias can be classified according to whether the cause of the problem is inside the red cells, in which case it is usually an inherited condition, or outside the cells, in which case it is usually acquired later in life.

RED CELL DEFECTS When haemolysis is due to a defect within the red cells, the underlying problem is an abnormal rigidity of the cell membrane (the envelope that surrounds each cell). This causes the cells to become trapped at an early stage of their lifespan in the smaller blood vessels (usually of the spleen) and eventually to be destroyed by macrophages (types of cell which ingest foreign and dead particles).

The abnormal rigidity may result from an inherited defect of the cell membrane (as in hereditary *spherocytosis*), from a defect of the haemoglobin within the cell (as in *sickle cell anaemia*), or from a defect of one of the cell's enzymes. There are only two chemical processes occurring in red cells that are essential to their survival—one that provides energy and one that helps protect the cells from chemical damage. The last process is of great importance; a deficiency of one of the enzymes that catalyses the process, called glucose-6-phosphate dehydrogenase (see *G6PD deficiency*), is a common cause of haemolytic anaemia in some countries but not in the UK. One variety of G6PD deficiency occurs among black people and another variety is most common in Greece (see *Favism*).

DEFECTS OUTSIDE THE RED CELL Haemolytic anaemias resulting from defects outside the red cells fall into three main groups. First are disorders in which red cells are destroyed by mechanical buffeting (e.g. when the lining of the blood vessels is abnormal, when the blood flows past artificial surfaces such as replacement heart valves, or in conditions in which a blood clot has formed inside a blood vessel). In all these conditions, the otherwise normal red cell is physically disrupted by mechanical forces.

In a second group of conditions, the red cells are destroyed by antibodies produced by the *immune system* and directed against the red cells. These immune haemolytic anaemias may occur if foreign blood cells enter the bloodstream, as during an incompatible blood transfusion, or if the immune system becomes defective and fails to recognize the body's own red cells. This is a type of *autoimmune disorder*. Sometimes, the reaction is triggered by a drug such as methyldopa. In *haemolytic disease of the newborn*, the baby's red cells are destroyed by antibodies produced by the mother crossing the placenta. In most cases, however, the cause of immune haemolytic anaemia is unknown.

In a third group of conditions, the red cells are destroyed by microorganisms in the blood. By far the most important cause is *malaria*.

SYMPTOMS AND DIAGNOSIS

People with haemolytic anaemia may have symptoms common to all types of anaemia (such as pallor, headaches, fatigue, and shortness of breath on exertion) or symptoms specifically due to the haemolysis (such as *jaundice*, caused by an excessive concentration in the blood of bile pigments formed from red cell destruction).

The diagnosis of haemolytic anaemia depends on microscopic examination of the blood (see *Blood film*), which often shows a big increase in the number of immature red cells and, with some specific types, red cells that are abnormally shaped. The patient's racial background and medical history may also help establish the diagnosis.

TREATMENT

Some inherited causes of haemolytic anaemia can be controlled by removing the main site of destruction of the red cells—the spleen (see *Splenectomy*). Others, such as G6PD deficiency and favism, are largely preventable by avoiding the drugs or foods that precipitate haemolysis.

Treatment of haemolysis caused by mechanical buffeting of red cells relies on reducing the disruptive forces. Those caused by immune or autoimmune processes can often be controlled by *immunosuppressant drugs*.

More specific treatments may be required in particular cases—for example, the use of antimalarial drugs in haemolysis caused by malaria. Transfusions of red blood cells, or exchange transfusions of whole blood, are sometimes required for emergency treatment of severe life-threatening anaemia.

Anaemia, iron-deficiency

The most common form of *anaemia* (a reduced level of the oxygen-carrying pigment *haemoglobin* in the blood); it is caused by a deficiency of iron, an essential constituent of haemoglobin.

Iron-deficiency anaemia develops if insufficient iron is available to the bone marrow, where haemoglobin is made and packaged into red blood cells. Anaemia occurs when iron loss, along with any extra iron requirements for growth, persistently exceed iron gained from the diet.

Small losses of haemoglobin and iron occur normally from the body through occasional minor bleeding; in women of childbearing age, these losses are much greater due to menstrual blood loss. Small amounts of iron are also shed in skin cells as they peel off from the body surface and in cells from the lining of the bowel which are shed in the faeces. Tiny amounts are lost when red blood cells are destroyed at the end of their lifespan (most of the iron is efficiently repackaged into new red cells).

Because of their menstrual blood losses, women of childbearing age tend to have low, or no, built-up stores of iron and thus tend to become anaemic more quickly if iron losses exceed iron intake. Pregnancy stops the menstrual losses but is replaced by an even greater drain on iron stores (from the baby); hence, pregnant women are at particular risk of iron-deficiency anaemia.

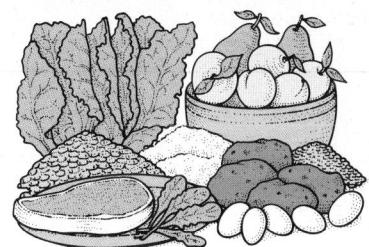

Foods containing iron
Foods such as fruit, wholemeal bread, beans, lean meat, and green vegetables are good sources of iron that help prevent iron-deficiency anaemia.

A

CAUSES

INCREASED LOSSES The main cause of iron-deficiency anaemia is loss of iron at a greater rate than normal as a result of abnormally heavy or persistent bleeding, which may be caused by disease or by particularly heavy periods (see *Menorrhagia*). The diseases most commonly responsible for persistent bleeding are those of the digestive tract, such as erosive *gastritis, peptic ulcer, stomach cancer, inflammatory bowel disease, haemorrhoids*, and bowel tumours, including cancer (see *Intestine, cancer of*). Prolonged treatment with aspirin and aspirin-like *nonsteroidal anti-inflammatory drugs* (NSAIDs) can cause gastrointestinal bleeding. In some countries, *hookworm infestation* of the digestive tract is an important cause of iron-deficiency anaemia.

Blood lost from the lower part of the intestine and from the rectum is bright red and usually noticed when faeces are passed. If the bleeding is in the stomach or upper intestine, it is invisible; when it is excessive, it usually makes the faeces black.

Bleeding may also occur as a result of disorders of the urinary tract (such as *kidney tumours, bladder tumours, cystitis*, or *prostatitis*), in which case it colours the urine.

INSUFFICIENT INTAKE The second most common cause of iron deficiency is poor absorption of iron from the diet, usually as the result of surgical removal of part or all of the stomach (see *Gastrectomy*) but also sometimes due to *coeliac disease*, a disorder that impairs digestion.

The third possible cause of iron deficiency, and the least common, is a diet that does not provide enough iron. Those most affected are old people who live alone and who eat a generally poor diet, children and pregnant women because of their extra needs, and slimmers who reduce their total food intake. Women should be sure to have an iron-rich diet and may be prescribed iron tablets during pregnancy.

SYMPTOMS

The symptoms are those of the underlying cause (e.g. abdominal pain and black faeces in some cases of peptic ulcer), along with brittle nails and a sore mouth or tongue; and those common to all forms of anaemia—fatigue and headaches, and, in severe cases, breathlessness and pain in the centre of the chest.

DIAGNOSIS AND TREATMENT

The diagnosis is made from the measurement of a low level of haemoglo-bin in the blood and from a *blood film* that usually shows the red blood cells to be smaller and paler than normal. When the cause is not clear, investigations such as faecal analysis (for evidence of blood) and *barium X-ray examination* or *endoscopy* (to look for disorders of the digestive tract) may be carried out.

Treatment is for the underlying cause, along with a course of iron tablets or injections (or syrup for children) to build up depleted iron stores and correct the anaemia.

Anaemia, megaloblastic

An important type of *anaemia* (a reduced level of the oxygen-carrying pigment *haemoglobin* in the blood), caused by a deficiency of vitamin B_{12} or another vitamin, folic acid. Either of these deficiencies seriously interferes with the production of red blood cells in the bone marrow. An excess of cells known as megaloblasts appears in the marrow. Megaloblasts give rise to enlarged and deformed red blood cells known as macrocytes.

CAUSES

VITAMIN B_{12} DEFICIENCY Vitamin B_{12} is found only in foods of animal origin, such as meat, fish, and dairy products. It is absorbed from the small intestine after first combining with a chemical called intrinsic factor, produced by the stomach lining. In most diets, there is much more vitamin B_{12} than the body requires; the excess is stored in the liver, where it can last for a few years. If a person on a normal diet acquires a vitamin B_{12} deficiency, it is due not to lack of the vitamin but to an inability to absorb it.

The most common cause of such a deficiency is a failure of the stomach lining to produce intrinsic factor, usually because of an *autoimmune disorder*, in which antibodies are produced that block the production of intrinsic factor. When vitamin B_{12} deficiency anaemia is due to this cause it is known as pernicious anaemia. This disorder has a tendency to run in families, to start in middle age, and to affect women more than men. It is sometimes associated with other disorders, such as *diabetes mellitus* or *myxoedema*. Total gastrectomy (removal of the entire stomach) prevents the production of intrinsic factor by removing its source.

Other causes of defective absorption of the vitamin include removal of part of the small intestine (where vitamin B_{12} is absorbed) and the intestinal disorder *Crohn's disease*.

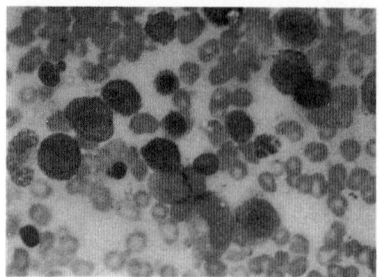

Bone marrow in megaloblastic anaemia
In this microscopic view, some of the large cells are abnormal red cell precursors (megaloblasts).

In a minority of cases, vitamin B_{12} deficiency is the result of a vegan diet, which excludes eggs and dairy products as well as meat and fish.

FOLIC ACID DEFICIENCY Folic acid is present to some extent in many foods, but is found mainly in green vegetables and liver. However, unlike vitamin B_{12}, it is not stored in the body in large amounts; therefore, a constant supply is needed. For this reason, the usual cause of deficiency is a poor diet. The disorder is most common in the poor and in old people living by themselves. It may also occur in people with *alcohol dependence*.

Deficiency can also be caused by anything that interferes with the absorption of folic acid from the small intestine (e.g. disorders such as *Crohn's disease* and *coeliac disease* or removal of part of the small intestine).

Folic acid is required by rapidly dividing cells, as in the fetus, and the requirements during pregnancy are much higher than at other times. For this reason some doctors recommend that women should take folic acid in early pregnancy.

SYMPTOMS

Many people with mild megaloblastic anaemia have no symptoms. In others, symptoms may include any or all of the following: tiredness, headaches, a sore mouth and tongue, weight loss, and *jaundice*. In severe cases there may also be breathlessness, chest pain, and sometimes loss of balance and tingling in the feet due to damage to the nervous system from lack of the vitamins.

DIAGNOSIS

The anaemia is usually first suspected following *blood tests* that show a low level of haemoglobin, a preponderance of large red blood cells, and low levels of either vitamin B_{12} or folic acid or both. The disease is confirmed if a *bone marrow biopsy* (removal of a small sample of marrow for analysis) reveals the presence of large numbers of megaloblasts (abnormal, immature red cells). Tests may also be carried out to discover an underlying cause in cases where this is not clear.

Pernicious anaemia is sometimes diagnosed by a special test, the Schilling test, in which the absorption of vitamin B_{12} into the bloodstream is measured with the vitamin first unbound and then bound to intrinsic factor. If the vitamin is found to be absorbed only when bound to intrinsic factor, it confirms the diagnosis of pernicious anaemia.

TREATMENT
When megaloblastic anaemia is due to poor diet, it can be remedied by adopting a normal diet and taking a short course of vitamin B_{12} injections or folic acid tablets.

If the deficiency is due to inability to absorb vitamin B_{12}, it can sometimes be remedied by treating the underlying cause, but often the power of absorption is lost permanently. A lifelong course of replacement injections of vitamin B_{12} or folic acid tablets is then required.

Anaemia, pernicious
A type of anaemia in which the underlying problem is a disorder of the stomach lining. The lining fails to produce a substance called intrinsic factor, necessary for the absorption of vitamin B_{12} from the intestines into the blood. As a result, a deficiency of vitamin B_{12} develops and without this vitamin, the bone marrow is unable to produce normal red blood cells. (See also *Anaemia, megaloblastic*.)

Anaerobic
Capable of living and growing without oxygen. Many important bacteria are anaerobes and thrive in the intestinal canal or in tissue that has a poor supply of oxygenated blood. These species can cause diseases such as *food poisoning*, *tetanus*, and *gangrene*.

Some human body cells are capable of limited anaerobic activity. For example, when muscular exertion is so strenuous that oxygen is used faster than the blood circulation can supply it, the muscle cells can temporarily work anaerobically. When this happens, lactic acid is produced as waste (instead of the carbon dioxide from *aerobic* activity). The localized acid build-up in the exercising muscle causes fatigue and pain, limiting the time for which anaerobic exercise can be tolerated. Compensation for this

anaerobic activity requires oxygen to convert the lactic acid to glucose or to carbon dioxide, which explains why we need to continue to breathe rapidly after vigorous exertion. The deficit of oxygen that builds up in the muscles during exercise is known as the oxygen debt.

Anaesthesia
Literally, the absence of all sensation; insensibility. Anaesthesia can be induced artificially to abolish pain during surgical procedures and sometimes during childbirth.

Two types of anaesthesia are used for medical purposes: local and general. A patient given a local anaesthetic (see *Anaesthesia, local*) remains conscious and sensation is abolished in only part of the body. This is usually accomplished by injection of drugs that temporarily interrupt the nerve supply from the region to be anaesthetized. Local anaesthetics can also be given in the form of eye-drops, sprays, skin creams, and suppositories. It may be possible to produce local pain relief by using *acupuncture*; this technique is widely used in China and is now being used more widely by Western practitioners.

A patient under general anaesthesia (see *Anaesthesia, general*) is rendered unconscious and maintained in this state with a combination of drugs that are either injected into a vein or inhaled. These drugs affect all parts of the body but have their main sites of action in the brain and spinal cord.

Damage to nerve tissues by injury or disease can produce local anaesthesia. Rarely, anaesthesia may be a result of extreme arousal, as in the case of boxers or soldiers who do not notice painful blows or wounds. Psychological factors may be responsible for numbness, particularly in the hand or foot (see *Conversion disorder*).

Anaesthesia, dental
Loss of sensation induced in a patient to prevent pain during dental treatment. Most dental procedures are carried out using local anaesthesia; general anaesthesia is usually reserved for surgical procedures and special cases.

LOCAL ANAESTHESIA
For minor restorative work, such as fillings, some patients and dentists choose no anaesthesia; otherwise, a local anaesthetic (e.g. lignocaine or bupivacaine) is injected into the gum at the site that is being treated. Sometimes it is not possible to inject directly

into the area to be treated because the gum is painfully inflamed or because there is a risk of spreading an infection in the gum. In these cases, the anaesthetic is injected into or around the nerve a short distance away from the site of operation. This procedure is known as a peripheral *nerve block*. Topical anaesthetics on the surface of the gums are often used in conjunction with injected anaesthetics.

SEDATION
In addition to receiving a local anaesthetic, a patient who is abnormally anxious, agitated, or uncooperative may need to be calmed by sedation. To sedate the patient, an antianxiety agent is given orally or intravenously, or by inhalation. Antianxiety agents include tranquillizer drugs (such as diazepam), nitrous oxide (laughing gas), and barbiturates.

GENERAL ANAESTHESIA
The most common use for general anaesthesia is in surgical procedures such as periodontal (gum) surgery and multiple tooth extractions. General anaesthesia is also used for young children, for people who are allergic to local anaesthetics or who have extremely sensitive teeth, and for those who are unable to cooperate (e.g. because of a mental disorder or physical handicap).

For relatively short dental surgery, general anaesthesia is given by an injection of a barbiturate, such as methohexitone or thiopentone, into a vein. Anaesthesia may then be maintained by the patient breathing a mixture of nitrous oxide, oxygen, and possibly another volatile anaesthetic during surgery.

For longer or more complicated procedures, general anaesthesia is carried out as for other types of surgery (see *Anaesthesia, general*).

Anaesthesia, general
Loss of sensation and consciousness induced to prevent pain and discomfort during surgery. The state of general anaesthesia is produced and maintained by an anaesthetist, who gives combinations of drugs by injection, inhalation, or both. The anaesthetist is also responsible for the pre-anaesthetic assessment and medication of patients, their safety during surgery, and their recovery during the post-anaesthetic period.

HISTORY
Until about the middle of the 19th century, pain relief during surgery relied on natural substances such as alcohol, opium, and cannabis.

A

TECHNIQUES FOR GENERAL ANAESTHESIA

The main phases in the administration of a general anaesthetic are induction (bringing on unconsciousness), maintenance, and emergence (returning the patient to consciousness). Some of the main stages are shown below. Often, to allow surgical manipulation, a muscle relaxant must be given in addition to anaesthetic gases or injections. Because the relaxant temporarily paralyses the breathing muscles, the patient's lungs must be ventilated artificially.

DRUGS USED IN GENERAL ANAESTHESIA

Type	Action	Examples
Drugs given as premedication	Relax patient, abolish pain, reduce saliva and mucus formation	Diazepam, morphine, atropine
Induction agents	Induce unconsciousness	Thiopentone sodium
Anaesthetic gases and volatile agents	Induce and/or maintain unconsciousness	Nitrous oxide, halothane, enflurane, isoflurane
Analgesics	Abolish pain	Morphine, fentanyl
Muscle relaxants	Relax muscles	Pancuronium, vecuronium
Reversal agents	Reverse muscle relaxation	Neostigmine

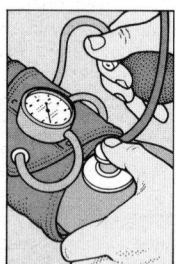

1 Before the operation, the anaesthetist talks to and examines the patient and assesses his or her fitness for anaesthesia and surgery. He or she also answers the patient's questions.

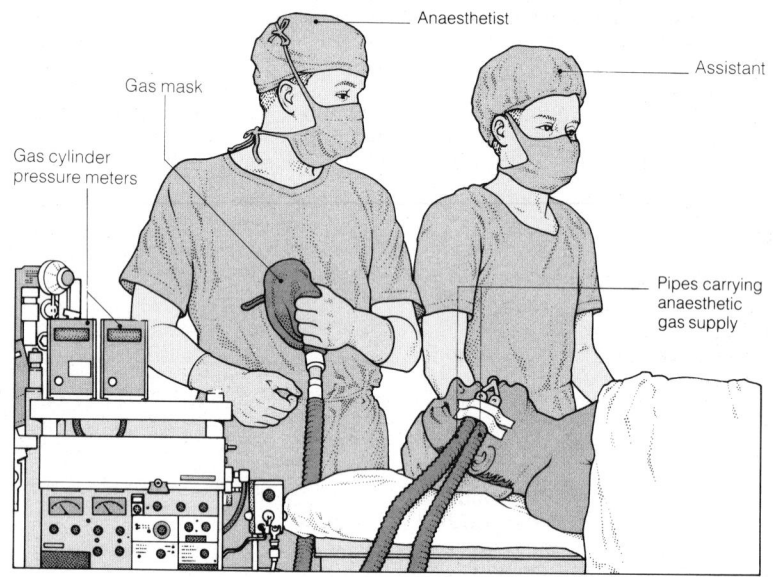

Anaesthetist

Assistant

Gas mask

Gas cylinder pressure meters

Pipes carrying anaesthetic gas supply

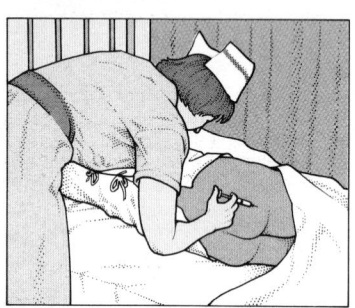

2 Before the operation, premedication may be given. It may include a drug that relieves pain or anxiety and one that prevents excessive salivation.

6 While surgery is in progress, the patient is kept at a level of anaesthesia deep enough to be unaware of the operation. The composition of the gas mixture, and the patient's heart rate, breathing, blood pressure, temperature, blood oxygenation, and exhaled carbon dioxide are monitored. After surgery, anaesthesia is stopped and reversal agents are given if necessary.

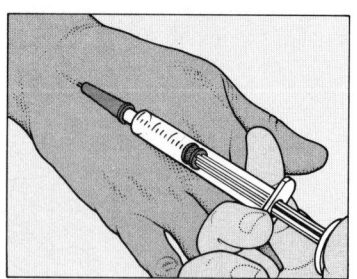

3 The induction agent is usually given via a cannula inserted into a vein. The cannula is left in position so that other drugs can be given rapidly if needed.

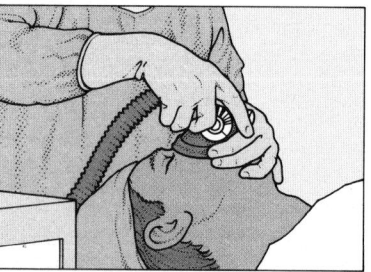

4 Sometimes, anaesthesia is induced or maintained with gases delivered by mask. If no muscle relaxant is used, the patient may be able to continue breathing naturally.

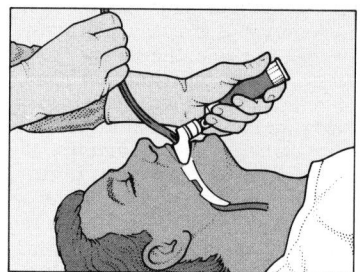

5 In other cases, a breathing tube is inserted for delivery of the anaesthetic gases. If a muscle relaxant is used, artificial ventilation is necessary.

However, the relief obtained was often inadequate and short-lived. It was not until the 1840s that significant progress was made towards solving the problems of inducing unconsciousness in a manner that was safe, easily maintained for long periods, and reversible. *Ether* was first demonstrated successfully in New York in 1842 and Boston in 1846, when a tooth was extracted without pain while the patient was breathing ether. Soon after, the anaesthetic properties of chloroform and nitrous oxide (laughing gas) were discovered, heralding a new era in surgery.

WHY IT IS DONE
The primary objectives of general anaesthesia are to abolish pain, awareness, muscle tone, and cardiovascular reflexes in the patient and so make conditions suitable for surgery or diagnostic procedures.

HOW IT IS DONE
The principal stages in administering, maintaining, and reversing general anaesthesia are shown in the illustrated box.

COMPLICATIONS
The likelihood of any complications depends on the pre-operative condition of the patient, the anaesthetic technique used, and the nature of the operation performed. The longer the operation, the greater the risk of a complication.

General anaesthesia may cause several possible complications. These include nausea, vomiting, *hypotension* (low blood pressure), physical injury (such as chipped teeth and muscle strains), allergic reactions, cardiac *arrhythmia* (irregular heartbeat), respiratory depression (slowed, ineffective breathing), *hypoxia, aspiration* (inhaling vomit into the lungs), and *airway obstruction*.

AWARENESS DURING ANAESTHESIA
It is possible (though rare with modern anaesthetic techniques) for patients to remain aware of events during surgery but, because they have been given muscle-relaxant drugs, to be unable to signal this distressed state to the anaesthetist. The concentrations of anaesthetic agents required to produce adequate anaesthesia in the majority of patients are well documented. In addition, the anaesthetist can detect an inadequate level of anaesthesia by noting physical signs, such as increased sweating and salivation; irregular breathing; changes in muscle tone; spontaneous eye movements; and increases in heart-rate and blood pressure.

Anaesthesia, local
Loss of sensation induced in a limited region of a person's body to prevent pain during examinations, diagnostic or treatment procedures, and surgical operations. Local anaesthesia is produced by the administration of drugs that temporarily interrupt the action of pain-carrying nerve fibres.

HOW IT IS DONE
For minor surgical procedures, such as stitching of small wounds, local anaesthesia is usually produced by direct injection into the area to be treated. When it is necessary to anaesthetize a large area, or when local injection would not penetrate deeply enough into body tissues, a *nerve block* (in which nerves at a point remote from the area to be treated are injected) may be used. Nerves can also be blocked as they branch off from the spinal cord, as in *epidural anaesthesia*, which is widely used during childbirth, and spinal anaesthesia (see *Spinal block*), which is used mainly for surgery of the lower limbs and lower abdomen.

Some parts of the body that are permeable to local anaesthetic drugs can be anaesthetized by applying an anaesthetic drug directly to the area.

The throat, larynx, and respiratory passages can be sprayed before *bronchoscopy*, and the urethra can be numbed with a gel before *catheterization* or *cystoscopy*. An anaesthetic cream can be rubbed on to the skin prior to an injection to make it painless. Other forms of local anaesthetic include anaesthetic lozenges for sore throats, and ointments or rectal suppositories to relieve the discomfort of *haemorrhoids*.

For some procedures, particularly if the patient is anxious, a sedative drug is given in addition to the local anaesthetic.

COMPLICATIONS
Adverse reactions to an anaesthetic drug may occur if the dose is too high or has been absorbed too rapidly. Such reactions include dizziness, loss of consciousness, seizures, and cardiac arrest. In rare cases, people have an allergic reaction to the drug itself. During major (epidural and spinal) blocks, blood pressure may drop, causing reduced blood flow to the brain and heart. Rarely, infections enter the body at the injection site. In a small number of susceptible patients, certain local anaesthetics may rarely cause long-term nerve damage.

LOCAL ANAESTHETICS

Drug	Common uses	How taken
Amethocaine	For surgery on the eye, for relief of pain during dental treatment	Eye-drops, spray, cream
Benzocaine	To treat painful conditions of the mouth and throat, painful anal conditions (e.g. haemorrhoids), skin wounds; used before laryngoscopy	Lozenges, suppositories, spray, cream, ointment
Bupivacaine	As nerve block (e.g. epidural anaesthesia and caudal block)	Injection
Cocaine	For surgery on the nose, throat, and larynx; formerly used in eye operations	Eye-drops, spray, liquid
Lignocaine	For relief of pain during dental treatment; for spinal anaesthesia, nerve blocks (e.g. epidural anaesthesia), eye surgery, and before endoscopic procedures; to treat haemorrhoids	Injection, gel, spray, cream, ointment, liquid, eye-drops, suppositories
Procaine	For relief of pain before surgical and dental treatment	Injection

Anaesthetics

A term for the group of drugs that produce *anaesthesia* and for the medical discipline concerned with their administration.

A specialist who administers anaesthetics is called an anaesthetist. Before a patient goes to the operating theatre, the anaesthetist assesses the condition of the patient's heart, lungs, and circulation. The anaesthetist decides the type and amount of drugs needed to induce and maintain anaesthesia, determines the patient's position on the operating table, watches for signs of trouble, and decides what actions should be taken if an emergency develops. The anaesthetist is also responsible for monitoring the progress of the waking patient, and watching for and treating any complications that might develop.

In many hospitals, the anaesthetist is responsible for the *intensive care* unit, and for emergency resuscitation programmes for inpatients and for casualties in the accident and emergency department.

Anal dilatation

A procedure for enlarging the anus. Anal dilatation is used to treat conditions in which the anus becomes too tight, such as *anal stenosis* and *anal fissure*. It is also used as a treatment for *haemorrhoids*. Anal dilatation can be performed under general anaesthesia by a surgeon, using fingers or an anal dilator. Minor dilatation can be performed by the patient, using a dilator and lubricating jelly.

Reflex anal dilatation, in which the anus dilates abnormally, may occur in certain disorders of the anus, in cases where there has been repeated anal penetration, and, sometimes, without any known cause.

Anal discharge

The loss of mucus, blood, or pus from the anus. *Haemorrhoids*, *anal fissures* (tears in the anal margin), and *proctitis* (inflammation of the rectum) can all cause anal discharge. The production of mucus from the anus tends to irritate the surrounding skin and may cause *itching* of the anus (known medically as pruritus ani).

Analeptic drugs

Drugs that stimulate breathing. Analeptic drugs, which include doxapram and nikethamide, are occasionally used to treat *respiratory failure* in acute flare-ups of chronic bronchitis and after drug overdoses. Analeptic drugs may also be used to hasten recovery from a general anaesthetic, and to treat *apnoea* (absent breathing) in newborn infants.

Analeptics work by stimulating the respiratory centre (a group of nerve endings in the brain stem that control the rate and volume of breathing).

Anal fissure

A fairly common anal disorder caused by an elongated ulcer that extends upwards into the anal canal from the anal sphincter (the ring of muscle that surrounds the anal orifice). The fissure probably originates from a tear in the lining of the anus caused by the passage of hard, dry faeces.

SYMPTOMS

There is usually pain during defaecation and the muscles of the anus may go into spasm. There may be a small amount of bright red blood on faeces or toilet paper.

TREATMENT

The tear often heals naturally in the course of a few days, although spasm of the anal muscles may delay healing. Treatment of recurrent or persistent fissures usually includes *anal dilatation* (a procedure to enlarge the anus) and a high-fibre diet, including wholegrain products, fruits, vegetables, and plenty of fluids, to soften the faeces. Fissures usually heal within a few days after such treatment but surgery to remove the fissure is occasionally necessary.

Anal fistula

An abnormal channel connecting the inside of the anal canal with the skin surrounding the anus.

An anal fistula is occasionally an indication of *Crohn's disease*, colitis, or cancer of the colon or rectum (see *Intestine, cancer of* and *Rectum, cancer of*). In most cases, an anal fistula results from an abscess that develops for unknown reasons in the anal wall. The abscess discharges pus, both into the anus and out on to the surrounding skin.

A fistula is treated surgically by opening the channel, removing the fistulous lining, and then draining the abscess of the pus it contains. The operation is performed under a general anaesthetic.

Analgesia

Loss or reduction of pain sensation. Analgesia differs from *anaesthesia* (loss of all sensation) in that sensitivity to touch is still preserved. (See also *Analgesic drugs*.)

Analgesic drugs

COMMON DRUGS

Nonnarcotic
Aspirin Benorylate Diflunisal Fenoprofen Ibuprofen Nefopam Mefenamic acid Paracetamol Salsalate Sodium salicylate

Narcotic
Buprenorphine Codeine Dextropropoxyphene Diamorphine Dihydrocodeine Morphine Pentazocine Pethidine

> **WARNING**
> Over-the-counter (nonnarcotic) analgesics should only be used for 48 hours before seeking medical advice. If pain persists, becomes more severe, recurs, or differs from pain previously experienced, consult your doctor.

Drugs that relieve pain. The two main types are nonnarcotic and narcotic. Nonnarcotic analgesics include *aspirin; paracetamol;* and *nonsteroidal antiinflammatory drugs* (NSAIDs) such as ibuprofen. Narcotic analgesics include *morphine* and related drugs.

WHY THEY ARE USED

Nonnarcotic analgesics are useful in the treatment of mild or moderate pain (e.g. headache or toothache). For more severe pain, a preparation combining one of the weaker narcotic analgesics (such as *codeine*) with a nonnarcotic analgesic (such as aspirin) is usually prescribed. The most potent narcotic analgesics are used only when other preparations would be ineffective.

HOW THEY WORK

When body tissues are damaged (e.g. by injury, infection, or inflammation), they produce *prostaglandins* (chemicals that trigger the transmission of pain signals to the brain). Nonnarcotic analgesics other than paracetamol work by preventing prostaglandin production. Paracetamol works by blocking the pain impulses in the brain itself, thereby preventing the perception of pain.

Narcotic analgesics act in a similar way to *endorphins* (substances formed within the body that relieve pain). They block pain impulses at specific sites (called opiate receptors) in the brain and spinal cord.

POSSIBLE ADVERSE EFFECTS

Adverse effects are uncommon with paracetamol. Aspirin and NSAIDs may irritate the stomach lining and cause nausea, abdominal pain, and, occasionally, a *peptic ulcer*. Nausea, vomiting, drowsiness, constipation, and breathing difficulties may occur with narcotic analgesics. The stronger narcotic analgesics may also produce a feeling of euphoria.

ABUSE

The euphoric effects produced by some narcotic analgesics have led to their abuse. In most cases, long-term abuse causes *tolerance* and physical dependence (see *Drug dependence*). Both the manufacture and the distribution of strong narcotic analgesics are controlled by law.

Anal stenosis

A tightness of the anus, sometimes referred to as anal stricture. Anal stenosis prevents the normal passage of faeces, causing constipation and pain during defaecation.

The condition may be present from birth, or may be caused by a number of conditions in which scarring has occurred, such as *anal fissure, colitis,* or cancer of the anus. Anal stenosis sometimes occurs after surgery on the anus (e.g. to treat *haemorrhoids*).

Anal stenosis is treated by *anal dilatation* (a procedure to enlarge the anus), which may be performed by the patient.

Anal stricture

See *Anal stenosis*.

Analysis, chemical

Determination of the identity of a substance or of the individual chemical constituents of a mixture. Analysis may be qualitative, as in determining whether or not a particular substance is present, or it may be quantitative, that is, measuring the amount or concentration of one or more constituents. (See also *Assay*.)

Analysis, psychological

See *Psychoanalysis*.

Anaphylactic shock

A rare, severe, frightening, and life-threatening allergic reaction. It is a Type I hypersensitivity reaction (see *Allergy*) that occurs rarely in people in whom an extreme sensitivity to a particular substance (allergen) has developed. The reaction occurs most commonly after an *insect sting* or as a reaction to an injected drug (e.g. penicillin, antitetanus serum, a local anaesthetic, or during *hyposensitization* for an allergy). Less commonly, the reaction occurs after a particular food or drug has been taken by mouth.

HOW ANALGESICS WORK

When tissue is damaged (for example, by injury, inflammation, or infection) the body produces prostaglandins. These substances combine with receptors (specific sites on the surface of cells in the brain and spinal cord). As a result, a signal is passed along a series of nerve cells to the brain, where the signal is interpreted as pain by brain cells. Analgesics (except for paracetamol) work either by preventing the production of prostaglandins or by blocking pain impulses in the brain and spinal cord. Paracetamol works by blocking the pain impulses in the brain itself. This action prevents the perception of pain.

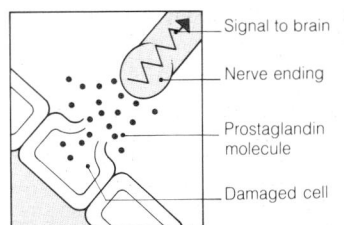

Action of narcotics
When tissue damage occurs, the body produces prostaglandins, chemicals that trigger the transmission of pain signals (above). Normally, the pain signal is transmitted between brain cells, but narcotic drugs (below) combine with opiate receptors to prevent the signals from being transmitted.

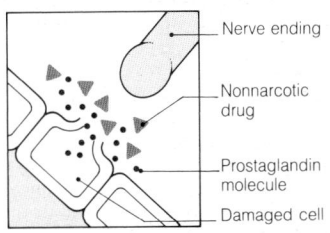

Action of nonnarcotics
Nonnarcotic drugs block the production of prostaglandins (chemicals released in response to tissue damage). This action prevents stimulation of the nerve endings, so that no pain signal passes on to the brain. As a result, these drugs provide pain relief.

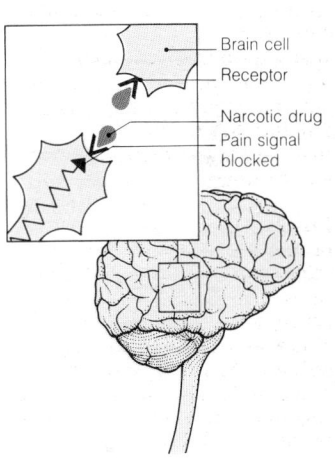

Entry of the allergen into the bloodstream provokes the release of massive amounts of *histamine* and other chemicals that have effects on body tissues. The blood vessels widen, with a sudden severe lowering of blood pressure. Other symptoms include an itchy, raised rash, bronchospasm (constriction of the airways in the lungs), pain in the abdomen, swelling of the tongue or throat, and diarrhoea.

FIRST AID AND TREATMENT

If a person becomes severely ill or collapses soon after an insect sting, injection, or eating a particular food, medical help should be summoned immediately.

The victim should be laid down and the legs raised to improve blood flow to the heart and brain. An injection of *adrenaline* is often life-saving and must be given as soon as possible.

People who have suffered previous severe allergic reactions should carry a preloaded syringe of adrenaline, so that they can inject themselves (if still conscious) or can have the dose administered promptly by someone familiar with the method of injection. Otherwise, medical help should be awaited. If the person's breathing or heartbeat stops, *cardiopulmonary resuscitation* should be performed. In addition to adrenaline (injections of which may need to be repeated until the victim's condition improves), a doctor may also administer *antihistamine drugs* and *corticosteroid drugs*.

Individuals who have suffered anaphylactic reactions to insect venom may respond to a course of desensitizing injections (see *Hyposensitization*, although this treatment itself carries a risk of repetition of the anaphylaxis and therefore should be carried out only by a doctor with a supply of adrenaline and other emergency medications at hand.

Anastomosis

A natural or artificial communication between two tubular cavities or blood vessels that may or may not normally be joined.

A natural anastomosis usually takes the form of two blood vessels joining (see *Arteriovenous fistula*). Surgical anastomosis is used to treat various disorders. For example, if an artery is blocked by *thrombosis* (clot) or *atheroma* (fat deposits), an operation may be performed to remove the blockage and directly connect the two ends of the vessel. Alternatively, an operation to bypass the blockage may be performed by joining a synthetic substitute or a section of a vein from the patient to the artery above and below the obstruction.

Another common use of surgical anastomosis is to treat intestinal obstruction: the obstructed section of intestine may be cut out and the healthy ends joined, or the obstruction may be bypassed by making two openings in a loop of the intestine (one either side of the defective area) and joining together the two openings. (See also *Bypass surgery*.)

Anatomy

The structure of the body of any living thing, and its scientific study. The science of human anatomy dates back to ancient Egyptian times and, together with *physiology* (the study of the functioning of the body), forms the foundation of all medical science. Dissection of human corpses provides the primary source of information for anatomists.

The ancient Greek physician Galen produced many medical treatises containing some anatomical descriptions that are still in use today, but his work is also full of gross errors. It was not until 1543 that the first accurate, comprehensive anatomical text, "De Humani Corporis Fabrica" ("On the structure of the human body"), was produced by the Flemish scientist Andreas Vesalius.

BRANCHES OF ANATOMY

Anatomy as a scientific study today is subdivided into many branches. These include comparative anatomy (the study of the differences between human and animal bodies), surgical anatomy (the practical knowledge required by surgeons, especially recognition of the surface markings of internal organs and the pattern of blood vessels within them), *embryology* (the study of structural changes that occur during the development of the embryo and fetus), systematic anatomy (the study of the structure of particular body systems, such as the urinary system), and *cytology* and *histology* (the microscopic study of, respectively, cells and tissues).

DESCRIPTIVE TERMS

In textbook descriptions of human anatomy, the body is assumed to be standing upright, with the arms hanging down and the palms facing forwards. The body is divided by the median (also called the sagittal) plane into right and left halves, and by the central coronal plane into front (anterior or ventral) and rear (posterior or dorsal) halves.

Every anatomical structure is scientifically named in Latin, but today anatomists prefer to use simpler terms when they exist. For example, the main blood vessel in the thigh is usually called the femoral artery rather than the arteria femoralis.

Ancylostomiasis

See *Hookworm infestation*.

Androgen drugs

Natural or synthetic *androgen hormones* used as drugs; one of the most important of these drugs is *testosterone*.

Androgen drugs are used in the treatment of male *hypogonadism* (underactivity of the testes) to stimulate the development of sexual characteristics, such as growth of facial and pubic hair, enlargement of the genitals, and deepening of the voice. This treatment improves libido and potency but does not increase the production of sperm.

Androgen drugs are also used to stimulate production of new blood cells by the bone marrow in aplastic *anaemia*. They may also occasionally be used in the treatment of certain types of *breast cancer*.

DESCRIPTIVE TERMS IN ANATOMY

The relative positions and movements of body parts are conventionally described with reference to the "anatomical position" (i.e. upright posture with the eyes and palms facing forwards). In this position, the parts of the body can be described in relation to various geometrical planes.

In radiology, body imaging pictures (such as CT and MRI scans) are often taken in a series of transverse planes through part of the body.

Joint movements

Flexion is bending and extension is straightening; abduction is moving away from and adduction moving towards the midline of the body. Other movements are forms of rotation around an axis.

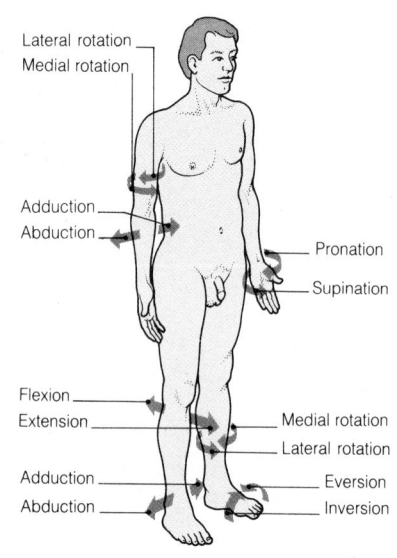

Lateral rotation
Medial rotation
Adduction
Abduction
Pronation
Supination
Flexion
Extension
Medial rotation
Lateral rotation
Adduction
Abduction
Eversion
Inversion

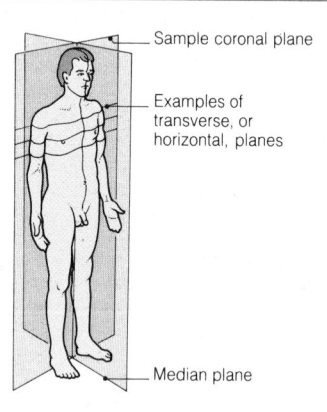

Sample coronal plane
Examples of transverse, or horizontal, planes
Median plane

Planes through the body

The median plane divides the body into right and left halves. Coronal planes are vertical planes at right angles to the median plane; the coronal plane most often referred to divides the body into front and back halves. Transverse planes are horizontal slices through the body.

Androgen drugs have been widely used by athletes and body builders wishing to increase muscle bulk and strength, but this practice has been condemned by doctors as dangerous to health, and has been banned by sports authorities around the world (see *Steroids, anabolic*).

POSSIBLE ADVERSE EFFECTS

Adverse effects include fluid retention, weight gain, increased levels of cholesterol in the blood, and, rarely, liver damage. When taken by women the drugs can cause deepening of the voice and other male characteristics, especially growth of facial hair. Because androgen drugs affect sexual development in babies, they are not prescribed during pregnancy or breast-feeding. They are prescribed with caution during adolescence because they may prematurely halt the growth of the long bones.

Androgen hormones

A group of hormones that cause *virilization* (development of male secondary sexual characteristics, such as the growth of facial hair, deepening of the voice, and increase in muscle bulk).

FORMATION

Androgens are produced by specialized cells in the testes in males and in the adrenal glands in both sexes. The ovaries secrete very small quantities of androgens until the menopause. The most active androgen is *testosterone*, which is produced in the testes. Androgens produced by the adrenal glands are less active than testicular androgens, and have no significant masculinizing effects unless produced to excess.

The production of androgens by the testes is controlled by certain pituitary hormones, called *gonadotrophins*. Adrenal androgens are controlled by *ACTH*, another pituitary hormone.

EFFECTS

Androgens stimulate the appearance of male secondary sexual characteristics at puberty, including enlargement of the penis and growth of facial and body hair. Androgens have what is called an anabolic effect, that is, they raise the rate of protein synthesis and lower the rate at which it is broken down. This increases muscle bulk, especially in the chest and shoulders, and accelerates growth, especially during early puberty. At the end of puberty, androgens cause the long bones to stop growing.

Androgens also promote aggression, a characteristically male trait.

They stimulate sebum secretion, which, if excessive, causes *acne*. In early adult life, androgens promote male-pattern baldness. Absence of androgens protects against male-pattern baldness.

ANDROGEN DEFICIENCY

Adult males may be deficient in androgens if their *testes* are diseased or if the pituitary gland fails to secrete gonadotrophins. Such men are termed "hypogonadal". The effects of androgen deficiency vary according to whether the deficiency develops before or after puberty. Typical effects include decreased body hair and beard growth, smooth skin, a high-pitched voice, reduced sexual drive and performance, underdevelopment of the genitalia, and poor muscle development.

ANDROGEN EXCESS

Overproduction of androgens may be the result of adrenal disorders (see *Adrenal tumours; Adrenal hyperplasia, congenital*), of testicular tumours (see *Testis, cancer of*), or, rarely, of androgen-secreting ovarian tumours (see *Ovary, cancer of*).

In adult males, excess androgens accentuate male physical characteristics. In boys, they cause premature sexual development. Initially they increase bone growth but adult height is reduced because they cause the long bones to stop growing.

In females, excess androgens cause virilization, that is, the development of masculine features such as increase in body hair, deepening of the voice, clitoral enlargement, and *amenorrhoea* (absence of menstruation).

Anencephaly

Absence at birth of the brain and cranial vault (top of the skull). Most affected infants are stillborn or survive only a few hours. Anencephaly is detectable early in pregnancy by measurement of maternal *alpha-fetoprotein*, by *ultrasound scanning*, by *amniocentesis*, or by *fetoscopy*; if anencephaly is detected, termination of the pregnancy may be considered.

Anencephaly is caused by a failure in development of the neural tube (the nerve tissue in the embryo that normally develops into the spinal cord and brain). Maldevelopment of the neural tube may also result in *spina bifida* and *hydrocephalus*. These abnormalities are collectively known as *neural tube defects* and seem likely to have similar causes. Anencephaly occurs in about five in every 1,000 pregnancies, but only in about one third of these does the pregnancy continue to term.

Aneurysm

Abnormal dilation (ballooning) of an artery caused by the pressure of blood flowing through a weakened area. The weakening may be due to disease, injury, or a congenital defect of the arterial wall.

TYPES

Some of the common types, sites, and shapes of aneurysm are shown in the illustrated box overleaf.

A dissecting aneurysm, usually associated with *atherosclerosis*, is a condition in which a longitudinal, blood-filled split forms within the lining of the wall of an artery—usually the aorta—and spreads so that extensive areas of the vessel are weakened. There is usually severe pain and the vessel may rupture. When the aneurysm is located in the aortic arch or the ascending aorta and dissects into the pericardium (membrane surrounding the heart), the pressure of the blood around the heart may be fatal because it prevents the heart from beating.

An aneurysm may sometimes develop in the heart wall due to weakening of the heart muscle as a result of a *myocardial infarction* (heart attack). Such aneurysms seldom rupture but they often interfere with the efficient pumping action of the heart.

A traumatic aneurysm is one caused by mechanical injury that weakens the blood-vessel wall.

CAUSES

An aneurysm may form for several reasons. If the muscular middle layer of an artery is congenitally weak, normal blood pressure causes dilation of the blood-vessel wall at the weak point. *Marfan's syndrome*, a condition in which the middle layer of the wall of the aorta is defective, is often associated with an aneurysm just above the heart. The arterial wall can also be weakened by inflammation, as in *polyarteritis nodosa*.

Most aneurysms of the aorta—usually in the lower part of the vessel—are caused by atherosclerotic weakening of a segment of the wall. Aneurysm of the ascending aorta once commonly resulted from untreated *syphilis* but this is now rare. Aneurysms, known as mycotic aneurysms, may occur in smaller vessels as a result of local infection in *septicaemia*. Aneurysms of arteries in the brain are often termed berry aneurysms because of their size and appearance.

SYMPTOMS AND SIGNS

Symptoms vary according to the type, size, and location of the swelling. Cerebral aneurysms may persist for many years without causing symp-

TYPES OF ANEURYSM

An aneurysm forms when pressure from the blood flow causes a weakened artery wall to distend or forces blood through a fissure.

Aneurysms can form anywhere in the body, although the most common sites are the aorta and the arteries supplying the brain.

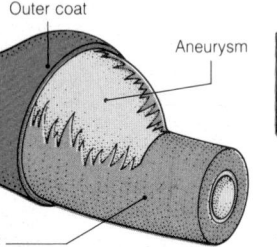

Common aneurysm
This type forms when the tunica media, the artery's middle wall, is weakened; the strong force of the blood flow distends the wall of the artery.

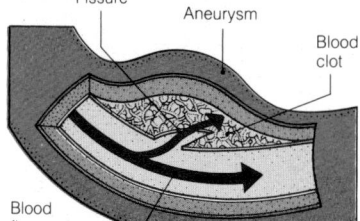

Dissecting aneurysm
This type occurs when there is a fissure in the internal wall of the artery; blood forced through the fissure forms a swelling.

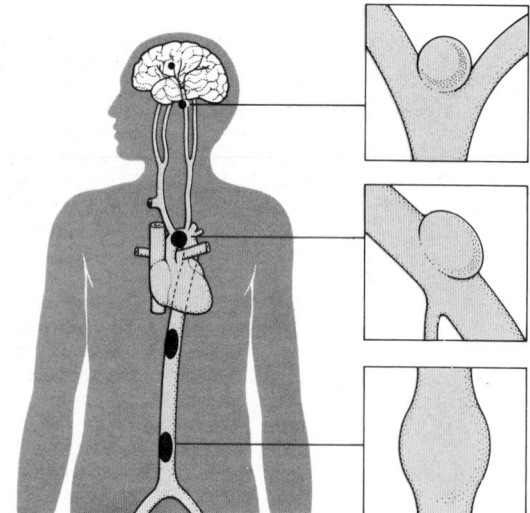

Cerebral (or berry) aneurysm
A swelling where the arteries branch at the brain's base, often caused by congenital weakness.

Saccular aneurysm
A balloon-shaped distension of part of an artery's wall, often seen in aortic aneurysms just above the heart.

Fusiform aneurysm
A distension around an artery's circumference, tapered at both ends, often seen in lower aortic aneurysms.

toms, but the close proximity of the brain makes them very dangerous. Sudden enlargement and bursting of a berry aneurysm produces obvious symptoms and signs, such as paralysis of eye movement, drooping of the lid, dilation of the pupil, rigidity of the neck, severe headache, and unconsciousness (symptoms similar to those of a *stroke*).

Pressure from an aneurysm may damage surrounding structures, especially if the aneurysm is located within the confined space of the skull.

Aneurysms may rupture, sometimes causing fatal blood loss, or, in the case of cerebral aneurysms, may cause severe damage to the brain (see *Subarachnoid haemorrhage*).

Aneurysms of the thoracic (chest) part of the aorta are usually accompanied by hoarseness (due to pressure on a nerve controlling a vocal chord), difficulty swallowing, and chest pain that may be mistaken for myocardial infarction (heart attack). Abdominal aortic aneurysm is sometimes visible as a throbbing swelling and may also cause backache.

DIAGNOSIS
Symptomless aortic aneurysms may be detected by *ultrasound*, and screening is recommended for men over the age of 60 with a family history of the disorder. Cerebral aneurysms may be detected by *CT scanning* or *MRI*. *Angiography* provides more detailed information about all types of aneurysms.

TREATMENT AND OUTLOOK
Treatment varies with the site of the aneurysm and the age and health of the patient. Ruptured or enlarged aneurysms require urgent surgery (see *Arterial reconstructive surgery*). If cerebral aneurysm causes symptoms, surgery is recommended if possible. Nonurgent surgery for aortic aneurysms of the chest offers an 80 to 90 per cent chance of survival. Emergency surgery carries a high risk, and the outlook following a ruptured aneurysm in the chest is poor.

Angel dust

One of the common names for phencyclidine, an illicit drug taken for its hallucinogenic properties. Adverse effects of the drug include slowed breathing rate, agitation, muscle rigidity, vomiting, and convulsions; several deaths have been reported.

Angiitis

See *Vasculitis*.

Angina

A term that describes a strangling or constrictive pain. Angina has become synonymous with the heart disorder *angina pectoris* (chest pain caused by lack of oxygen to the heart muscle, usually a result of poor blood supply). Other types of angina include abdominal angina (abdominal pain after eating caused by poor blood supply to the intestines) and Vincent's angina, pain caused by inflammation of the mouth (see *Vincent's disease*).

Angina pectoris

Pain in the chest due to insufficient oxygen being carried to the heart muscle in the blood. Angina pectoris usually occurs when the demand for oxygen is increased during exercise and at times of stress.

CAUSES
Inadequate blood supply to the heart is usually due to *coronary artery disease*, in which the coronary arteries are narrowed by *atherosclerosis* (fat deposits on the walls of the arteries). Other causes include coronary artery spasm, in which the blood vessels narrow suddenly for a short time but return to normal with no permanent obstruction, *aortic stenosis* (narrowing of the aortic valve in the heart), and *arrhythmias* (abnormal heart rhythms).

Rare causes of angina pectoris include severe *anaemia*, which reduces the oxygen-carrying efficiency of the blood, and *polycythaemia* (increased numbers of red blood cells), which thickens the blood, causing it to slow its flow through the heart muscle. *Thyrotoxicosis* (a disorder caused by excessive production of thyroid hormones) can precipitate angina pectoris by making the heart work much harder and faster than its blood supply will permit.

INCIDENCE
Angina pectoris is a common condition. In men, it usually starts at about the age of 50 but may occur as early as 30; in women, it usually starts later in life.

SYMPTOMS
The chest pain varies from mild to severe and is often described as a sensation of pressure on the chest. It usually starts in the centre of the chest but can spread to the throat, upper jaw, back, and arms (usually the left one) or between the shoulderblades.

The pain usually comes on when the heart is working harder and requires more oxygen—for example, during exercise, when under stress, in extremes of temperature, or during mild exercise soon after a meal. Typically the pain develops at the same stage in daily activities—for example, at the same point on a flight of stairs—and is relieved by a short rest.

Other symptoms may include nausea, sweating, dizziness, and breathing difficulty. These symptoms can, however, be caused by other conditions such as *oesophagitis* (inflammation of the oesophagus), spasm of the oesophagus, arthritis in the upper spine or rib-cage, or a pulled muscle in the chest wall.

A prolonged and usually more severe attack of angina pectoris may be due to *myocardial infarction* (heart attack), in which the heart muscle is permanently damaged.

DIAGNOSIS
Angina pectoris cannot be diagnosed with certainty by a physical examination. Diagnostic tests usually include an *ECG* (measurement of the electrical activity in the heart) while the patient is at rest and a *cardiac stress test* (an ECG performed while the patient is exercising enough to cause chest pain (e.g. while walking on a treadmill). The resting ECG will show no signs of angina (unless an attack is actually in progress), but may show former heart damage.

Blood tests may be performed to look for an underlying cause, such as *anaemia, polycythaemia, thyrotoxicosis,* or *hyperlipidaemia* (abnormally high levels of fat in the blood, which can cause atherosclerosis).

Coronary *angiography* (X-ray examination of the blood vessels) may also be performed.

TREATMENT
Initial treatment attempts to control the symptoms. It is important to stop smoking because nicotine and carbon monoxide contribute to the progressive development of coronary artery disease and make the symptoms worse. Overweight people should lose weight to reduce stress on the heart during exercise.

Attacks of angina pectoris may be prevented and treated by *nitrate drugs,* such as glyceryl trinitrate, which increase the flow of blood through the heart muscle. If nitrates are not effective, or are causing severe headaches due to an increased blood flow through the brain, other drugs may be used, including *beta-blocker drugs* and *calcium channel blockers.*

If *hypertension* (high blood pressure) is found during examination, it is treated with *antihypertensive drugs* to reduce the work load of the heart in pumping blood. Other specific causes can also be treated—for example, arrhythmias with *antiarrhythmic drugs* and hyperlipidaemia with a low-fat diet and/or drugs.

Drug treatment can control the symptoms of angina pectoris for many years, but it cannot cure the disorder. If attacks become more severe, more frequent, or more prolonged, despite drug treatment, and if there is angiographic evidence of advanced narrowing of vessels, then *coronary artery bypass* surgery or *angioplasty* may need to be performed in order to re-establish blood flow to the heart muscle.

OUTLOOK
The effect of angina pectoris on lifestyle depends on the severity of the underlying disease and the effectiveness of drug treatment or surgery. Some people are able to lead a normal life apart from some restriction on strenuous exercise, whereas others are severely disabled.

Angioedema
A type of reaction, also known as angioneurotic oedema, caused by *allergy.* Angioedema is similar to *urticaria* (hives) and characterized by large, well-defined swellings, of sudden onset, in the skin, larynx (voicebox), and other areas. These swellings may last several hours or days if they are left untreated.

INCIDENCE AND CAUSES
Angioedema primarily affects young people (especially those in their 20s) and those with a general tendency towards allergies (see *Atopy*).

The most common cause is a sudden allergic reaction to a food, such as eggs, strawberries, or seafood. Less commonly, it results from allergy to a drug (such as *penicillin*), a reaction to an insect sting or bite, or from infection, emotional stress, or exposure to animals, moulds, pollens, or cold conditions. There is also a hereditary form of the disease.

SYMPTOMS
Angioedema may cause very sudden difficulty in breathing, speaking, and swallowing, accompanied by obvious swelling of the lips, face, and neck.

Angioedema that affects the throat and the larynx is potentially life-threatening because the swelling can block the airway, causing *asphyxia* (suffocation). If the gastrointestinal tract is affected, colic, nausea, and vomiting may occur.

TREATMENT
Severe cases are treated with injections of *adrenaline* and may require intubation (passage of a breathing tube via the mouth into the windpipe) or *tracheostomy* (surgical creation of a breathing hole in the windpipe) to prevent suffocation. *Corticosteroid drugs* may also be prescribed. In less severe cases, *antihistamine drugs* often relieve symptoms.

Angiography
An imaging procedure that enables blood vessels to be seen clearly on X-ray film following the injection of a contrast medium (a substance opaque to X-rays).

WHY IT IS DONE
Angiography is used to detect diseases that alter the appearance of blood vessels. These diseases include *aneurysm* (ballooning of an artery), and narrowing or blockage of blood vessels by *atherosclerosis* (fatty deposits lining artery walls) or by a *thrombus* (abnormal clot) or an *embolus* (fragment carried in the blood). Angiography is also used to detect changes in the pattern of blood vessels that supply organs which have been injured or are affected by a tumour. By noting the abnormal arrangement of blood vessels, the doctor can evaluate the extent of disease and plan treatment accordingly.

Carotid angiography is sometimes performed on patients suffering from *transient ischaemic attacks* (symptoms of *stroke* lasting less than 24 hours) to see whether there is a blockage or substantial narrowing in one of the carotid arteries (in the neck), which supply blood to the brain.

A

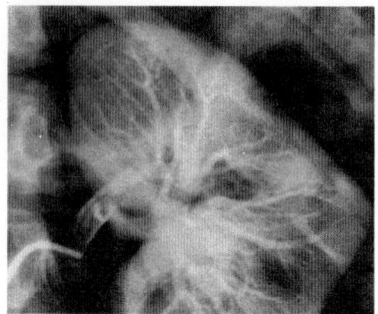

Angiogram of a normal kidney
Contrast medium is passed through the catheter into the kidney's arterial system and a series of X-ray pictures is taken.

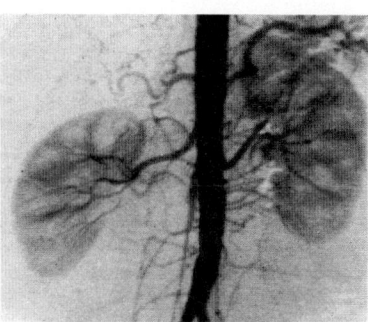

Digital subtraction angiography
Here, the normal kidneys are revealed more clearly because the computer eliminates unwanted information.

Cerebral angiography is used to demonstrate the presence of an aneurysm within the brain or to help pinpoint the position of a brain tumour prior to surgery.

Coronary angiography, which is often combined with cardiac *catheterization*, is carried out to identify the sites of narrowing or blockage in *coronary artery disease*.

HOW IT IS DONE

The contrast medium is usually injected into the blood vessel to be examined through a fine catheter (flexible plastic tube) that is inserted into the femoral artery at the groin, the brachial artery just over the elbow, or a carotid artery.

To insert the catheter, the skin and tissues around the artery are numbed with local anaesthetic and then a hollow needle is inserted through the skin into the artery. A long, thin wire with a soft tip is inserted through the needle, the needle is removed, and the catheter is then threaded over the wire into the blood vessel. Under X-ray control, the tip of the catheter is guided further into the vessel to be examined and contrast medium is injected. A rapid sequence of X-ray pictures (or a continuous recording) is taken so that the blood flow through the vessels can be studied.

Angiography can take from as little as a few minutes to as long as two or three hours.

DIGITAL SUBTRACTION ANGIOGRAPHY

This type of angiography uses computer techniques to process images and subtract (remove) unwanted background information, leaving only an image of the blood vessels to be studied. Digital subtraction angiography requires less contrast medium than conventional angiography and is therefore safer for the patient. In some cases, digital subtraction angiography also makes it possible to avoid injecting the contrast medium directly into affected blood vessels that are not easily accessible by catheter. However, the detail provided by digital subtraction angiography is not always as good as in conventional angiography.

RISKS

Allergy to the contrast medium is a possible adverse effect, but the use of new contrast agents has reduced the risk of a severe reaction to less than one in 80,000 examinations.

Damage to blood vessels can occur at the site of injection or anywhere along the vessel during the passage of the catheter.

OUTLOOK

Angiographic techniques have, in the last few years, been adapted to allow not only diagnosis but also certain types of treatment that, in some cases, eliminate the need for surgery. For example, small balloons can be inflated at the tip of a catheter to expand a narrowed or blocked segment of artery (see *Angioplasty, balloon*), foreign material can be injected to reduce or shut off blood supply to a tumour (see *Embolization*), and medication to control bleeding or to treat tumours can be infused directly into the blood supply to individual organs. (See also *Aortography*.)

Angioma

A benign tumour made up of blood vessels (see *Haemangioma*) or lymph vessels (see *Lymphangioma*).

Angioplasty, balloon

A technique for treating narrowing or blockage of a blood vessel or heart valve by introducing a balloon into the constricted area to widen it.

WHY IT IS DONE

Balloon angioplasty is used in the treatment of *peripheral vascular disease* to increase or restore the flow of blood through a significantly narrowed artery in a limb; it is also used to treat narrowing of the coronary arteries (see *Coronary artery disease*).

COMPLICATIONS

There is a slight risk of damaging the artery or heart valve during this procedure and immediate surgery may be required. In rare cases, a *myocardial infarction* (heart attack) may be caused by prolonged interruption, by the inflated balloon, of blood supply to an area of the heart.

RESULTS

Coronary balloon angioplasty is successful in improving the condition of about two thirds of the patients treated. In three quarters of these cases, the improvement continues after a year; in the remainder, narrowing recurs in the affected vessel, but balloon angioplasty may be repeated successfully.

Angioplasty of peripheral vessels is most successful in treating the iliac and femoral arteries (in the legs), particularly when the affected area is small. After five years, 85 to 90 per cent of iliac arteries treated by angioplasty remain free of obstruction. For femoral arteries, the success rate is 50 to 70 per cent after two years.

New techniques for angioplasty currently under investigation include devices using lasers, cutting drills, and suction to remove the atheromatous deposits blocking the arteries.

Angiotensin

The name of two related proteins involved in regulating blood pressure. The first of these, angiotensin I, is itself inactive and is converted to the second, active form, angiotensin II, by the action of a converting enzyme. Angiotensin II causes narrowing of the small blood vessels in tissues, resulting in an increase in blood pressure. It also stimulates the release from the adrenal cortex (the outer part of each *adrenal gland*) of the hormone *aldosterone*, which also increases blood pressure.

Certain kidney disorders can increase the production of angiotensin II, causing *hypertension* (high blood pressure). Whatever the cause of hypertension, it may be treated with drugs known as *ACE inhibitors* (angiotensin-converting enzyme inhibitors), which work by reducing angiotensin II formation.

PROCEDURE FOR BALLOON ANGIOPLASTY

A blockage or narrowing of a blood vessel may be treated by introducing a balloon catheter into the area and then inflating the balloon to stretch the constricted part. The balloon is then deflated and the catheter withdrawn. The procedure is carried out using a local anaesthetic.

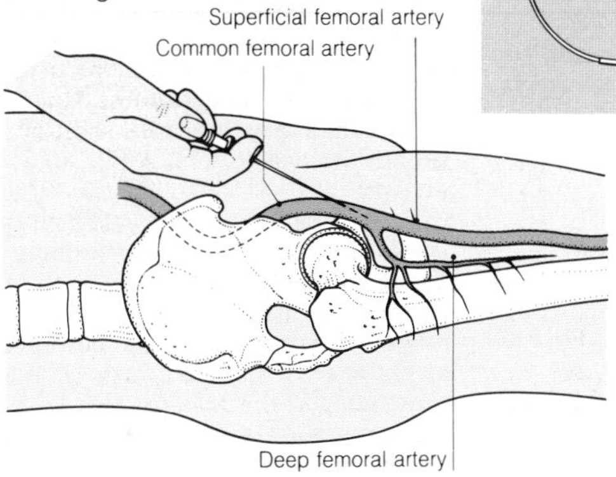

Superficial femoral artery
Common femoral artery
Deep femoral artery

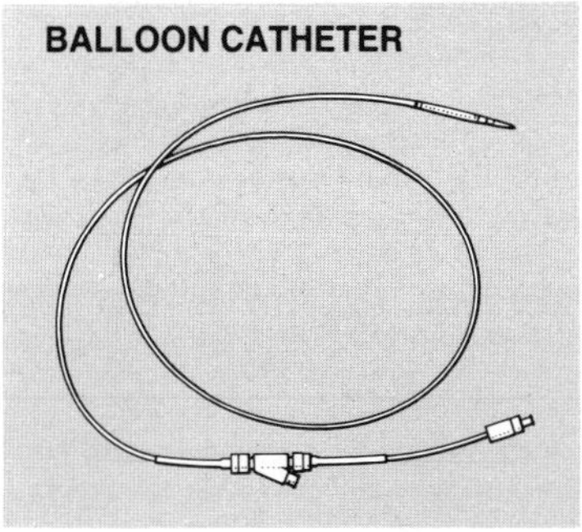

BALLOON CATHETER

How it is done
A hollow needle is inserted into the femoral artery (left). A guide wire is pushed through the needle into the artery, then along it (using X-ray imaging) towards the blood vessel or heart valve to be treated. The steps shown below are then carried out.

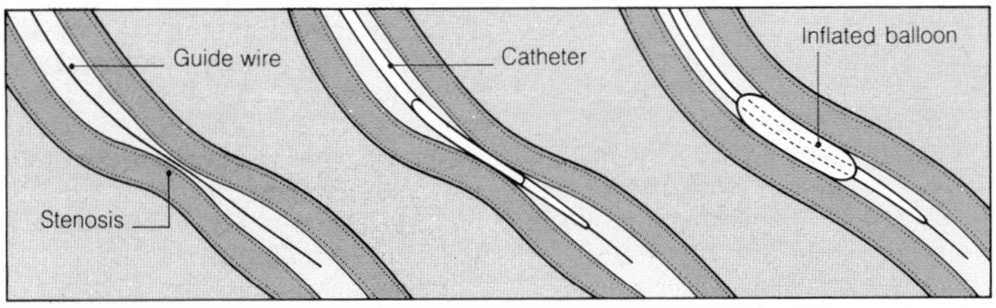

Guide wire — Catheter — Inflated balloon
Stenosis

1 The thin guide wire is manoeuvred through the arteries (using X-ray control) until it is just past the stenosis (narrowing) to be treated.

2 A balloon-tipped catheter (top right) is then threaded over the guide wire and pushed along it until it reaches the narrowed area.

3 A sausage-shaped balloon at the end of the catheter is inflated and deflated a few times to widen the narrowed part, then withdrawn.

Anhidrosis
Complete absence of *sweating*. (See also *hypohydrosis*.)

Animal experimentation
The use of living animals in research and safety testing to provide information about animal biology and about human physiology or behaviour. Animal experimentation is most prolific in developed countries, where medical standards are high and where there is intense concern for public health and safety.

The animals most extensively used in animal experimentation are rats and mice, which are bred for laboratory research. Less than one per cent of experiments involve cats, dogs, farm animals, nonhuman primates, frogs, fish, and birds.

LEGISLATIVE CONTROLS
Animal experimentation is controlled by law in most countries but the controls vary in their stringency. Governments must balance pressures for very tight controls against the weight of scientific opinion, which maintains that animal experiments are indispensable to public health and safety.

TYPES OF EXPERIMENTS
The experiments for which animals are used fall into several groups. One group consists of experiments to test the safety of nonmedical substances, such as pesticides, cleaning chemicals, and cosmetics, before they are released for public use.

Another group includes the many medical experiments in which a condition in an animal corresponds to a human disease. This provides the potential for testing new treatments to discover cures for the disease in the animal and therefore in humans.

Other experiments are performed to discover new drugs and medical procedures or to develop new substances for use in the environment.

ETHICAL OBJECTIONS
Campaigners for animal rights point out that animals suffer in many of these experiments. Sometimes the suffering is an implicit part of the research, as in research to study the mechanism of pain or to create models of painful conditions on which to test analgesic drugs (painkillers). Some of the conditions or effects being studied necessarily cause illness, stress, or pain, such as infecting animals with a disease or studying the irritant or poisonous effects of chemicals.

Two safety tests, often required by law, have received considerable criticism from protest groups and scientists alike. One test is the LD_{50} test, which measures acute toxicity (short-term poisonous effects) by estimating the dose that would kill 50 per cent of the animals in a test group. The other test is the Draize test, which measures irritant damage of chemicals and substances to eyes and skin.

BENEFITS
Experiments on animals have contributed greatly to the advancement of science and have specifically benefited humanity by virtue of new medical and surgical treatments.

In the past 30 years, the incidence of poliomyelitis and other infections has been reduced enormously as a result of vaccines produced after such testing.

Antibiotic drugs developed using animal experiments have also prolonged and saved many lives. Drugs for the treatment of noninfectious disorders, such as arthritis, diabetes mellitus, and hypertension (high blood pressure), are also the result of animal-based research. Surgical treatments may also be developed in animals; the success of transplant operations and microsurgery techniques are notable recent advances.

ALTERNATIVES
Alternatives to animal experiments have been developed and are used whenever possible. Laboratory tests using cultured cells or tissues have replaced many experiments that once involved animals. Other alternatives involve the use of simple organisms, such as bacteria or yeasts, or the computerized or mathematical modelling of an experiment.

A

New techniques have also led in some cases to the replacement of animals as a source of vaccines and hormones. Cell culture techniques have now almost replaced the use of animals in vaccine production, and genetically engineered bacteria and yeasts are increasingly used to produce substances, such as insulin, that were once derived only from animals.

However, even with these newer methods, it is dangerous—and illegal—not to undertake confirmatory studies on animals before releasing a new drug or vaccine.

Animals, diseases from
See *Zoonoses*.

Anisometropia
Unequal focusing power in the two eyes, usually due to a difference in size and/or shape in the eyes. For example, one eye may be normal and the other affected by *myopia* (short-sightedness), *hypermetropia* (long-sightedness), or *astigmatism* (uneven curvature of the cornea).

Significant anisometropia causes visual discomfort because the image formed on one retina differs in size from that formed on the other. Glasses or contact lenses are satisfactory in most cases. In severe cases, however, it is usually better not to sharpen the image in the most affected eye because this would emphasize the difference in image size and increase visual discomfort.

Ankle joint
The hinge joint between the foot and the leg. The talus (uppermost bone in the foot) fits between the two bony protuberances formed by the lower ends of the tibia (shin-bone) and the fibula (outer bone of the lower leg). Strong ligaments on each side of the ankle joint provide support and limit movement. The ankle joint allows up-and-down movements of the foot; other movements of the foot, such as tilting and rotating, occur at joints in the foot itself.

DISORDERS
An ankle *sprain* is one of the most common of all injuries, and is usually caused by twisting the foot over on to its outside edge, which produces overstretching and bruising of the ligaments on the outside of the ankle. Very severe sprains may cause extensive tearing of the ligaments, which requires surgical repair.

Excessive or violent twisting of the ankle can cause a combined fracture

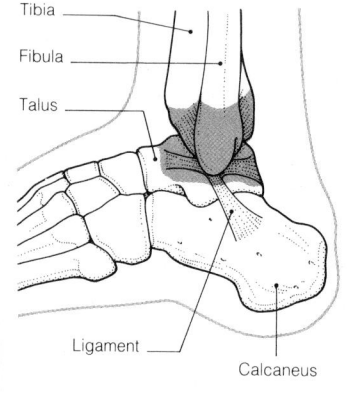

LOCATION OF THE ANKLE JOINT
This hinge joint is formed where the top of the talus fits in between the lower ends of the tibia and fibula.

Tibia

Fibula

Talus

Ligament

Calcaneus

and dislocation (called *Pott's fracture*), in which the fibula breaks above the ankle, and either the tibia breaks or the ligaments tear, resulting in dislocation of the ankle.

Ankylosing spondylitis
An inflammatory disease affecting joints between the vertebrae of the spine and the sacroiliac joints (joints between the spine and the pelvis).

CAUSES AND INCIDENCE
Ankylosing spondylitis is usually of unknown cause. A variant of the disorder is preceded, in some people, either by *colitis* (inflammation of the colon) or *psoriasis* (a skin disease).

Ankylosing spondylitis affects less than one per cent of the population, is more common in men than in women, and has its onset between the ages of 20 and 40 years. The disorder also seems to run in families. A genetically determined *histocompatibility antigen* (HLA-B27) is found much more often in people with ankylosing spondylitis than in the rest of the population.

SYMPTOMS
Ankylosing spondylitis usually starts with pain and stiffness in the lower back and hips, which are worse after resting and especially noticeable in the early morning. Typically, exercise helps reduce the stiffness.

Other, less common, symptoms include pain in the chest (from the joints between the spine and the ribs), loss of appetite, tiredness, and, occasionally, redness and pain in the eyes due to *iritis* (inflammation of the iris). In about one fifth of sufferers, other

joints (e.g. the hips, knees, and ankles) may be swollen and painful. Inflammation of tissues around the heel can cause pain and tenderness.

In time, the inflammation in the spine can lead to *ankylosis* (permanent stiffness and limitation of movement) and *kyphosis* (curvature of the spine). Movement is restricted and expansion of the chest is often limited.

DIAGNOSIS
A diagnosis of ankylosing spondylitis is usually made from the pattern of symptoms, backed up by blood tests and X-rays. Blood tests can be used to assess inflammation and to indicate the presence of the HLA-B27 antigen on white blood cells. At the onset, X-rays of the back may be normal, but later there are signs of increased bone density around the sacroiliac joints. Later still, the spine may show loss of space between joints and bony outgrowths.

TREATMENT
There is no curative treatment but symptoms may be reduced by a programme of heat, massage, and supervised exercise. Regular daily exercise (such as swimming) is advisable to keep the back muscles strong. To prevent curvature of the spine, patients are taught breathing exercises and exercises to improve posture. *Anti-inflammatory drugs* may be prescribed to reduce the pain and stiffness.

OUTLOOK
The inflammatory process tends to become less active with age. With treatment, most people suffer only minor deformity of the spine and are able to lead a normal life.

Ankylosis
Complete loss of movement in a joint caused by fusion of the bony surfaces. Ankylosis may be due to degeneration as a result of injury, infection, or inflammation. Ankylosis may also be produced surgically by an operation to fuse a diseased joint to correct deformity or to alleviate persistent pain (see *Arthrodesis*).

Anodontia
Failure of some or all of the teeth to develop. Anodontia may be due to absence of tooth buds at birth or may be the result of damage to developing tooth buds caused by infection or other widespread disease. Both primary and permanent teeth, or permanent teeth only, may be affected.

If only a few teeth are missing, a *bridge* can fill the gap; if all the teeth are missing, a *denture* is needed.

Anomaly

A deviation from what is accepted as normal, especially a birth defect such as a limb malformation.

Anorexia

The medical term for loss of appetite (see *Appetite, loss of*).

Anorexia nervosa

An eating disorder characterized by severe weight loss, wilful avoidance of food, and intense fear of being fat. *Amenorrhoea* (absence of menstrual periods) is also typical in girls and women. Popularly known as the "slimmer's disease", anorexia nervosa is difficult to treat and is occasionally fatal.

INCIDENCE

Anorexia most often affects teenage girls and young adult women, especially from certain high-risk groups. In the population as a whole, the incidence is one in 100,000; among middle class teenage girls and young women it is one in 100, rising to one in 20 among young female models, ballet dancers, and athletes. Males are affected only very rarely.

FEATURES OF ANOREXIA NERVOSA

Weight loss

Overactivity and obsessive exercising

Tiredness and weakness

Lanugo (baby-like) hair on body, thinning of hair on head

Extreme choosiness over food

Binge eating

Induced vomiting

Use of laxatives to promote weight loss

CAUSES

The causes of anorexia are much debated. Many sufferers seem to be part of close-knit families and to have a special relationship with one of the parents. Some sufferers seem to be particularly anxious to please and tend to be obsessional in their habits.

It is thought that people with anorexia nervosa may see dieting as a way of controlling their lives. It seems as if they do not wish to grow up and are trying to keep their childhood shapes.

Some specialists have suggested that anorexia nervosa is a true *phobia* about putting on weight.

Other specialists believe that anorexia is a symptom rather than a disease, and that the real cause is *depression, personality disorder*, or, rarely, *schizophrenia*. However, it is frequently difficult to identify any such underlying cause.

Hormonal changes related to weight loss and absence of menstruation have led some doctors to regard anorexia nervosa as a physical illness that is caused by a disorder of the *hypothalamus* (part of the brain concerned with hunger, thirst, and sexual development).

SYMPTOMS AND SIGNS

The most obvious sign is emaciation (extreme thinness), with one third or more of the body's weight being lost. In the early stages of the disorder, sufferers are typically overactive, constantly busy, and exercise much of the time. As weight loss continues, they become tired and weak, the skin becomes dry, lanugo hair (fine, downy hair) grows on the body, and normal hair becomes thinner. Starvation causes certain biochemical disorders and disrupts the balance of sex hormones, leading to amenorrhoea in many cases.

Most people with anorexia eat very little and are very choosy about their food. Sometimes they have food binges and then make themselves vomit or take *laxative drugs* or *diuretic drugs* to promote weight loss (see *Bulimia*). Such behaviour occurs because they often feel intensely hungry, even though they may deny this. Food and weight dominate thinking to an extreme degree. Sufferers have a distorted body image and "see" themselves as much fatter than they really are. Drug abuse and alcohol abuse occasionally occur.

TREATMENT

Hospital treatment is often necessary to help the sufferer return to a normal weight. Treatment is usually based on a closely controlled re-feeding programme, combined with individual *psychotherapy* or *family therapy*. Unless a strict watch is kept on feeding, patients tend to hide or throw away food. Occasionally, a system of rewards is used.

Drugs may be needed if there is a depressive or other illness. *Chlorpromazine* is often helpful in the early stages to calm patients and to promote weight gain.

OUTLOOK

Sufferers may need to continue psychotherapy for months or years after they have achieved a more normal weight. Relapses are common whenever there is the slightest stress. About 50 per cent of all patients treated for anorexia nervosa in a hospital continue to have symptoms for many years; five to 10 per cent later die from starvation or suicide.

Anorgasmia

Inability to achieve orgasm (see *Orgasm, lack of*).

Anosmia

Loss of *smell*.

Anoxia

A medical term that means literally a complete absence of oxygen within a body tissue—for example, the brain or a muscle. Anoxia causes a disruption of cell *metabolism* (chemical activity) and cell death unless corrected within a few minutes.

Anoxia is very rare, occurring during cardiopulmonary arrest or asphyxiation, whereas *hypoxia* (the reduction of oxygen supply to a tissue) is a more common problem.

Antacid drugs

COMMON DRUGS

Aluminium hydroxide Magnesium hydroxide Magnesium trisilicate Sodium bicarbonate

---

WARNING
Antacid drugs should not be taken regularly except under medical supervision as they may suppress the symptoms of a more serious disorder or provoke serious complications.

Drugs taken to relieve *indigestion, heartburn, oesophagitis* (inflammation of the oesophagus), *acid reflux* (regurgitation of stomach acids into the oesophagus), and *peptic ulcer*.

TYPES

Antacid drugs usually contain compounds of *magnesium* or *aluminium*, which have a long-lasting effect, or *sodium bicarbonate*, which produces a rapid, short-lived effect. Some antacid drugs also contain alginates, dimethicone, or a local anaesthetic.

HOW THEY WORK

Antacid drugs neutralize stomach acids, an action that helps prevent or relieve inflammation and pain in the upper digestive system.

Antacid drugs also give the stomach lining time to heal when it has been damaged by a peptic ulcer and is therefore sensitive to normal amounts of stomach acid.

ANTENATAL SCREENING PROCEDURES

When performed	Procedure	Reason for procedure
First visit	Blood tests	To check the woman's *blood group* and, sometimes, to check for presence of *hepatitis B* virus which might be transmitted to the baby.
	Cervical smear test (Pap smear)	To test for an early cancer of the cervix (if a test has not been performed recently).
First visit and throughout the pregnancy	Blood tests	To check for *anaemia* in the woman and, in women with Rh-negative blood groups, to look for the presence of Rhesus antibodies.
	Urine test	To check for *proteinuria*, which could indicate a *urinary tract infection* or *pre-eclampsia*.
	Blood and urine test	To check for *diabetes mellitus*.
	Blood pressure check	To screen for *hypertension*, which interferes with blood supply to the placenta and is a sign of pre-eclampsia.
First visit and after any infection	Blood tests	To screen for immunity to rubella which can cause defects in the baby, and for *syphilis* and other possible infections.
First 12 weeks	Chorionic villus sampling	May be performed if there is a risk of certain genetic (inherited) disorders being passed on.
16 to 18 weeks	Ultrasound scanning	Is carried out to date the pregnancy accurately and to detect any abnormalities present in the fetus.
	Amniocentesis	Carried out on older women and those who have children with *spina bifida* or *Down's syndrome* to detect possible abnormalities in the fetus.
	Blood test	In some cases, the amount of *alpha-fetoprotein* in the blood is tested to determine whether the baby has spina bifida.
	Fetoscopy and fetal blood sampling	In some cases, these are carried out if there is doubt about the normality of the baby.
High-risk or overdue pregnancies	Blood and urine tests	May be administered to assess placental function and well-being of the fetus.
	Electronic fetal monitoring	To check on the fetal heart beat.
	Ultrasound scanning	Extra scans may be recommended to assess fetal growth and development, the location of the placenta, and the amount of amniotic fluid.

Alginates included in antacid preparations help to protect the oesophagus against acid reflux. Dimethicone may possibly relieve *flatulence*, and local anaesthetics may numb the pain of oesophagitis.

POSSIBLE ADVERSE EFFECTS

Aluminium may cause constipation and magnesium may cause diarrhoea—these effects may be avoided if a preparation contains both ingredients. Sodium bicarbonate may cause fluid retention and flatulence. Antacid drugs interfere with the absorption of many drugs and a doctor's advice should be sought before taking them with other medication.

Antenatal care

Care of a pregnant woman and her unborn baby throughout pregnancy with the aim of making sure both are healthy at delivery. Such care involves regular tests on the woman and the fetus to detect disease, defects, or potential hazards, and advising the woman on general aspects of pregnancy, such as diet and exercise.

FIRST VISIT

A woman should see her doctor as soon as she believes she is pregnant. She will then usually be referred to an obstetrician, who will take down the medical history of the woman and her family. The obstetrician then examines the woman to confirm that she is actually pregnant and to check her general health. A vaginal examination is usually carried out to check that the reproductive organs and pelvis are normal and to confirm the estimated date of the delivery, which is calculated from the first day of the woman's last period.

The first of a series of screening tests to detect any abnormalities in the woman or baby may be carried out at this visit (see the accompanying antenatal screening procedures chart). Some of these tests, such as *ultrasound scanning* to detect any gross abnormality, usually need to be carried out only once; others, such as *blood tests* or *urinalysis* to detect *anaemia* or *diabetes mellitus* in the woman, may be performed at periodic intervals throughout the pregnancy.

The woman is also given advice about diet and told to avoid smoking (which can stunt the baby's growth) or drinking alcohol (which can result in *fetal alcohol syndrome*).

SUBSEQUENT VISITS

If there are no problems, the woman visits the doctor or midwife every month until the 28th week, then every two weeks until the 36th week, and then weekly until the delivery date, which, on average, is the 40th week from the first day of the mother's last menstrual period. If the pregnancy is a high-risk one—for example, if the woman is over 35 years old or is suffering from *hypertension* or diabetes (see *diabetic pregnancy*)—or if problems develop, visits will be more frequent and, in some cases, the woman may need to be admitted to hospital for closer observation.

At each visit, as well as undergoing the tests detailed in the chart, the woman is weighed, her blood pressure is taken, and the size of the uterus is estimated to confirm that the baby is growing well.

After the 32nd week, the position of the baby in the uterus (whether it is head-down as it should be) is determined, and the degree of engagement (how far the baby's head has descended into the woman's pelvis) is regularly recorded. The woman is also asked about the baby's movements; frequent, pronounced movements usually indicate that the baby is active and healthy.

PREPARATION FOR CHILDBIRTH CLASSES
Childbirth preparation classes are given in hospitals, health centres, community meeting places, or private homes. Such classes aim to provide information on all aspects of pregnancy, labour, and delivery, including advice on exercise, diet, and sexual activity. The woman learns what happens during labour and the different types of pain relief available during it; she may also learn breathing exercises to help her cope better with labour and delivery. (See also *Childbirth, natural*.)

Antenatal screening
Tests carried out during pregnancy to check for abnormalities, disorders or infections in the woman or her unborn baby (see illustrated chart).

Antepartum haemorrhage
Vaginal bleeding after the 28th week of pregnancy.

CAUSES AND INCIDENCE
Antepartum haemorrhage is most commonly due to a problem with the placenta, the organ in the uterus that sustains the developing fetus. The problem may be *placenta praevia*, in which the placenta is positioned abnormally close to the birth canal; placental abruption (detachment of part of the placenta from the wall of the uterus); or bleeding from the edge

of a normally sited placenta. Bleeding can also be caused by *cervical erosion* or other disorders of the cervix or vagina.

Antepartum haemorrhage occurs in approximately three per cent of all pregnancies.

SYMPTOMS
The bleeding is often painless but there may be abdominal pain if the placenta becomes partly separated from the uterus.

INVESTIGATION AND TREATMENT
Admission to hospital is necessary for investigation and treatment. The fetus' heartbeat is monitored to assess the baby's condition. The position of the placenta is located by *ultrasound scanning* (a vaginal examination is not performed as this could damage a low-lying placenta).

In some cases, it is necessary only to keep a careful watch on the conditions of the woman and her baby. If bleeding is severe, the woman is given an *intravenous infusion* and possibly *blood transfusions*. Immediate delivery (possibly by *caesarean section*) may be necessary in some cases to prevent the baby from becoming starved of oxygen.

When delivery is not necessary, the woman usually stays in hospital for at least 48 hours. If the woman is considered to be at risk of further bleeding, which could endanger her or the baby, she may have to stay in hospital until delivery. Otherwise, if the bleeding has stopped and the conditions of woman and baby are considered satisfactory, the woman is allowed to go home—though her condition is carefully monitored for the remaining weeks of the pregnancy.

COMPLICATIONS
Because of good obstetric care, mortality of women and babies today is low. Death of the baby is more likely than maternal death; infant death may be caused by lack of oxygen or by prematurity if bleeding triggers labour.

Anterior
Relating to the front of the body. In human *anatomy*, the term is synonymous with *ventral*.

Anthelmintic drugs

A group of drugs used to treat *worm infestations*. Different types of anthelmintic drugs are used to treat infestation by different types of worms.

Anthelmintic drugs kill or paralyse worms in the intestines, preventing them from gripping the intestinal walls and causing them to pass out of the body in the faeces. To hasten this process, laxative drugs are occasionally prescribed with anthelmintics.

Anthelmintic drugs help kill worms in other tissues by making them more vulnerable to attack by the *immune system*. Once these worms have been killed, they may require surgical removal along with any cysts that the worms have produced.

Possible adverse effects of anthelmintic drugs include nausea, vomiting, abdominal pain, rash, headache, and dizziness.

Anthracosis
An old term for coal worker's *pneumoconiosis*, a lung disease caused by inhalation of large amounts of coal dust over a period of many years.

Anthrax
A serious bacterial infection of livestock that occasionally spreads to humans. The most common form of anthrax in humans is cutaneous anthrax, which affects the skin. Another form, pulmonary anthrax, affects the lungs.

CAUSES AND INCIDENCE
Anthrax is caused by a bacterium, *BACILLUS ANTHRACIS*, which produces spores that can survive dormant for many years in soil and animal products but are capable of reactivation.

Animals become infected by grazing on contaminated land. People may become infected via a scratch or sore if they handle materials from infected animals. Pulmonary anthrax occurs as a result of inhaling large numbers of spores contained in infected animal fibres.

Anthrax is extremely rare in the UK, but serious epidemics have occurred in some developing countries, usually as a result of lapses in control programmes.

SYMPTOMS AND TREATMENT
In cutaneous anthrax, a raised, itchy, area develops at the site of entry of the spores, progressing to a large blister and finally to a black scab, with swelling of the surrounding tissues. Cutaneous anthrax is readily treatable with *penicillin* in its early stages. Without treatment, the infection may spread to lymph nodes and the bloodstream, and may be fatal.

Pulmonary anthrax causes severe breathing difficulty and is fatal in most cases.

A

Antianxiety drugs

A group of drugs used to relieve symptoms of *anxiety*. *Benzodiazepine drugs* and *beta-blocker drugs* are the two main types of antianxiety drugs. Other drugs that may occasionally be used to treat anxiety include *antidepressant drugs*.

WHY THEY ARE USED

Antianxiety drugs are used to provide temporary relief from anxiety when it limits a person's ability to cope with everyday life. In most cases, the underlying disorder is best treated by *counselling, psychotherapy,* or other forms of therapy.

Antianxiety drugs are sometimes used to calm a person before surgical treatment (see *Premedication*) or before a public performance.

HOW THEY WORK

Benzodiazepines promote mental and physical relaxation by reducing nerve activity in the brain; for this reason, they may also be prescribed to treat insomnia. Beta-blockers work by reducing the physical symptoms of anxiety, such as shaking and palpitations.

Antiarrhythmic drugs

A group of drugs used to treat different types of *arrhythmia* (irregular heartbeat). Antiarrhythmic drugs include *amiodarone, beta-blocker drugs, calcium channel blockers, digitalis drugs, disopyramide, lignocaine,* and *procainamide.* The specific drug prescribed by the doctor depends on the type of arrhythmia.

WHY THEY ARE USED

An arrhythmia can reduce the pumping efficiency of the heart, causing breathlessness, dizziness, and chest pain. Antiarrhythmic drugs relieve these symptoms and, in some cases, restore normal heartbeat.

HOW THEY WORK

The heart's pumping action is governed by electrical impulses. Some antiarrhythmic drugs work by altering these impulses within or on their way to the heart. Others affect the response of the heart muscle to the impulses received.

Antibacterial drugs

A group of drugs used to treat infections caused by *bacteria*. Antibacterial drugs share the actions of *antibiotic drugs* but, unlike antibiotics, these drugs have always been produced synthetically.

The largest group of antibacterial drugs are the *sulphonamide drugs*, used mainly for the treatment of *urinary tract infection*.

Antibiotic drugs

COMMON DRUGS

Aminoglycosides
Gentamicin Streptomycin

Cephalosporins
Cefaclor Ceftaxime Cephalexin

Penicillins
Amoxycillin Ampicillin Flucloxacillin Phenoxymethylpenicillin

Tetracyclines
Doxycycline Minocycline Oxytetracycline Tetracycline

Others
Amikacin Erythromycin Neomycin

> **WARNING**
> You must inform your doctor of any previous allergic reaction to an antibiotic drug.

A group of drugs used to treat infections caused by *bacteria*. Originally obtained from moulds and fungi, antibiotic drugs are now produced synthetically.

TYPES

Many antibiotic drugs belong to one of four main types: *aminoglycoside drugs, cephalosporin drugs, penicillin drugs,* and *tetracycline drugs*.

Some antibiotic drugs are effective against only certain types of bacteria. Others, known as broad-spectrum antibiotics, are effective against a wide range of bacteria. The choice of antibiotic drug depends on the type of bacteria and on the site of the infection. This choice is most effectively made by growing a culture of the bacteria and checking its sensitivity to various types of antibiotic.

More than one antibiotic drug may be prescribed to increase the efficiency of treatment and to reduce the risk of antibiotic resistance.

WHY THEY ARE USED

Antibiotic drugs are used to treat bacterial infections. They are also used to prevent infection if a person's *immune system* is impaired or if there is a risk of *endocarditis* (inflammation of the lining of the heart).

ANTIBIOTIC RESISTANCE

Some bacteria develop resistance to a previously effective antibiotic drug. Resistance may occur if a type of bacteria develops a method of growth that is not disrupted by the effects of the drug or if it begins to produce an *enzyme* that breaks down or inactivates the drug.

Resistance is most likely to develop during long-term treatment or if a person fails to take an antibiotic drug as directed by the doctor. Alternative antibiotic drugs are available to treat some bacteria that are resistant to the more commonly prescribed types of antibiotic drugs.

POSSIBLE ADVERSE EFFECTS

Most antibiotic drugs can cause nausea, diarrhoea, or a rash, as well as adverse effects typical of particular types. Antibiotic drugs may disturb the normal balance in the body between certain types of bacteria and

HOW ANTIBIOTICS WORK

Antibiotic drugs are either bactericidal (killing bacteria) or bacteriostatic (halting bacterial growth, allowing the immune system to cope with the infection). Penicillin drugs and cephalosporin drugs are bactericidal; these drugs work by disrupting bacterial cell walls.

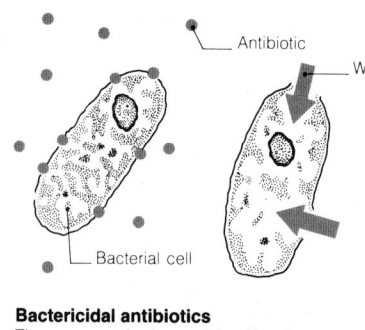
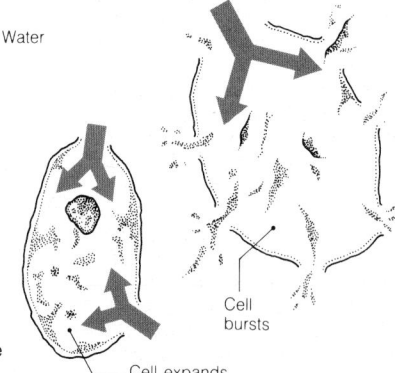

Bactericidal antibiotics
These cause the bacterial cell wall to disintegrate; water is taken into the cell, which expands and then bursts, killing the bacteria.

fungi, leading to proliferation of the fungi that cause oral, intestinal, or vaginal *candidiasis* (thrush). Some people occasionally experience a severe allergic reaction to antibiotic drugs, resulting in facial swelling, itching, or breathing difficulty.

Antibody

A protein that is manufactured by certain lymphocytes (types of white blood cell) to neutralize an *antigen* (foreign protein) in the body. Bacteria, viruses, and other microorganisms commonly contain many antigens; antibodies formed against these antigens help the body neutralize or destroy the invading microorganisms. Antibodies may also be formed in response to *vaccines*, thereby giving immunity against some infections. Antibodies are also known as *immunoglobulins*.

In some cases, inappropriate or excessive formation of antibodies leads to illness. The body's response to certain substances may lead to *allergy*, as in *asthma* or some types of *eczema*. Antibodies against antigens in skin grafts or organ transplants may result in rejection. In some disorders, antibodies are formed against the body's own tissues, resulting in an *autoimmune disorder*; examples of this type of disorder include some forms of arthritis and the *collagen diseases*. (See also *Immune response*.)

Antibody, monoclonal

An artificially produced *antibody* that neutralizes only one specific *antigen* (foreign protein).

Monoclonal antibodies are produced in the laboratory by stimulating the growth of a large clone of antibody-producing cells. (A clone is a group of cells that are genetically identical, or an individual member of such a group.) In effect, this cloning process enables antibodies to be tailor-made so that they will react with a particular antigen.

Monoclonal antibodies are used in the study of human cells, hormones, microorganisms, and in the development of new vaccines. They are also being used experimentally in the diagnosis of some forms of cancer, such as *lymphoma*. In addition, research is being carried out on the use of monoclonal antibodies to treat certain cancers: the antibodies can be directed against specific cancer cells and can, in theory, be used to carry lethal substances, such as radioactive molecules or toxins, to these target cells.

Anticancer drugs

COMMON DRUGS

Cytotoxic
Carboplatin Chlorambucil Cisplatin Cyclophosphamide Doxorubicin Etoposide Fluorouracil Methotrexate Procarbazine Vincristine

Sex-hormone related
Buserelin Ethinyloestradiol Goserelin Medroxyprogesterone Megestrol Stilboestrol Tamoxifen

Drugs used to treat *cancer*. Anticancer drugs are particularly useful in the treatment of *lymphomas*, *leukaemias*, and cancer affecting the ovary or testis. These drugs are sometimes used after surgery or *radiotherapy*.

TYPES
Most anticancer drugs are cytotoxic drugs (drugs that kill or damage cells). Others are synthetic forms of sex hormones and substances related to these hormones (e.g. *androgen drugs*, *oestrogen drugs*, and *progestogen drugs*).

Anticancer drugs are often prescribed in combination to maximize their effects. The choice of drugs depends on the type of cancer, its stage of development, and the general health of the patient.

HOW THEY WORK
All anticancer drugs kill cancer cells by preventing them from growing and dividing. Some cytotoxic drugs work by damaging the cells' *DNA* (genetic material). Others block the chemical processes in the cell that are necessary for growth.

Sex hormones stimulate the growth of certain cancers (e.g. oestrogen stim-

ulates some types of breast cancer). Substances related to these hormones may inhibit growth by blocking their stimulatory effect. The growth of other cancers is sometimes disrupted by a synthetic sex hormone given in high doses. Cancer of the prostate gland, for example, may be treated with the oestrogen drug *stilboestrol* (known as diethylstilbestrol or DES in the US).

POSSIBLE ADVERSE EFFECTS
In the early stages of treatment, nausea, vomiting, and diarrhoea may occur; some cases may be sufficiently serious to make hospitalization necessary.

Anticancer drugs may alter the rate at which noncancerous cells grow and divide. This effect may cause alopecia (hair loss), and reduce the number of blood cells produced by the bone marrow, causing *anaemia*, increased susceptibility to infection, and/or abnormal bleeding. Regular blood tests are usually carried out to monitor blood-cell production.

To minimize adverse effects, anticancer drugs are usually given in short courses with time between each course to enable noncancerous cells to recover from the drugs' effects.

Anticholinergic drugs

COMMON DRUGS

Atropine Belladonna Benzhexol Dicyclomine Hyoscine Ipratropium Mebeverine Orphenadrine Propantheline

A group of drugs that block the effects of *acetylcholine*, a chemical released from nerve endings in the parasym-

---

HOW ANTICHOLINERGICS WORK

Acetylcholine combines with a receptor on the cell's surface. This interaction stimulates activity in that cell (e.g. contraction of a muscle fibre or secretion of a fluid). Anticholinergic drugs block the stimulatory action of acetylcholine by combining with the acetylcholine receptors. This action produces, for example, muscle relaxation (e.g. in the bladder, intestine, and bronchi) and dries up secretions in the mouth and lungs. Anticholinergic drugs are used to treat asthma.

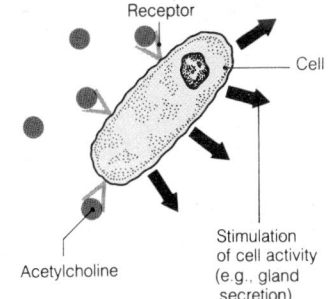

Receptor
Cell
Stimulation of cell activity (e.g., gland secretion)
Acetylcholine

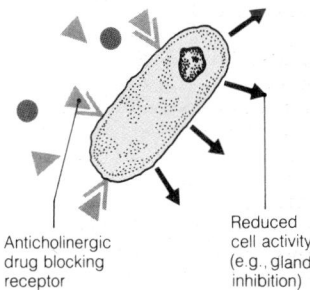

Anticholinergic drug blocking receptor
Reduced cell activity (e.g. gland inhibition)

pathetic division of the *autonomic nervous system*. Acetylcholine triggers activity in a number of cells. For example, it stimulates muscle contraction, increases secretions in the mouth and lungs, and slows the heartbeat.

WHY THEY ARE USED

Anticholinergic drugs are used in the treatment of *irritable bowel syndrome*, urinary *incontinence*, *Parkinson's disease*, *asthma*, and *bradycardia* (abnormally slow heartbeat). They are also used to dilate the pupil before an examination of, or surgical procedure on, the eye. Anticholinergic drugs are also helpful as a *premedication* before general *anaesthesia* and in the treatment of *motion sickness*.

POSSIBLE ADVERSE EFFECTS

Anticholinergic drugs may cause dry mouth, blurred vision, urinary retention, and confusion.

Anticoagulant drugs

COMMON DRUGS

Heparin Warfarin

> **WARNING**
> Many drugs, such as aspirin and alcohol, may increase the risk of an anticoagulant drug causing abnormal bleeding. Always consult your doctor before taking any other drug during anticoagulant treatment.

A group of drugs used to treat and prevent abnormal *blood clotting*. They are used to treat *thrombosis*, and may be used to prevent and treat *stroke* or *transient ischaemic attack* (symptoms of stroke lasting less than 24 hours). Anticoagulant drugs are also prescribed to prevent the development of abnormal blood clotting after major surgery (especially heart valve replacement) or during haemodialysis (see *Dialysis*).

HOW THEY WORK

Heparin increases the activity in the blood of antithrombin III, an enzyme that blocks the activity of other enzymes—known as clotting factors—that are needed for blood to clot. This drug is given by injection and begins to work within a few hours. Most other anticoagulant drugs are taken by mouth and take longer before they become effective. They work by reducing the production of some of the clotting factors.

By disrupting the blood clotting mechanism, anticoagulant drugs prevent an abnormal blood clot from forming. When a blood clot already

exists, anticoagulant drugs stop it from enlarging and reduce the risk of an *embolus* breaking off and blocking another blood vessel. Unlike *thrombolytic drugs*, anticoagulant drugs do not dissolve blood clots that have already formed.

POSSIBLE ADVERSE EFFECTS

Anticoagulant drugs in high doses may cause abnormal bleeding in different parts of the body. As a result, regular *blood-clotting tests* are carried out to monitor treatment.

Anticonvulsant drugs

COMMON DRUGS

Carbamazepine Clonazepam Diazepam Ethosuximide Phenobarbitone Phenytoin Primidone Sodium valproate

> **WARNING**
> Never suddenly stop taking an anticonvulsant drug after long-term treatment; the dose should be reduced gradually or symptoms may return.

A group of drugs used in the treatment of *epilepsy* and other types of *seizure*. Anticonvulsant drugs are taken on a regular basis to reduce the frequency and severity of seizures and as an emergency treatment to stop a prolonged seizure.

Anticonvulsant drugs are also administered to prevent seizures following a serious head injury or some types of brain surgery; they may be given to a child with a high fever who has a history of febrile seizures (see *Convulsion, febrile*).

The choice of drug is largely determined by the type of seizure to be treated. Long-term treatment may require use of more than one type of anticonvulsant drug.

HOW THEY WORK

Seizures are caused by an abnormally high level of electrical activity in the brain. Anticonvulsant drugs have an inhibitory effect that neutralizes this excessive electrical activity and thereby prevents its spread throughout areas of the brain.

POSSIBLE ADVERSE EFFECTS

Anticonvulsant drugs may produce various adverse effects, including reduced concentration, impaired memory, poor coordination, and fatigue. The doctor will try to establish a dose that prevents seizures but minimizes adverse effects. Regular monitoring of blood levels of the drug may be needed to achieve this.

Antidepressant drugs

COMMON DRUGS

Tricyclics
Amitriptyline Clomipramine Doxepin Imipramine Mianserin Nortriptyline

Monoamine oxidase inhibitors (MAOIs)
Isocarboxazid Moclobemide Phenelzine

Others
Fluoxetine Lithium Paroxetine

> **WARNING**
> Food and drink containing tyramine (e.g. cheese and red wine) and certain drugs may produce a dangerous rise in blood pressure if taken during treatment with an MAOI. Always tell your doctor if you are taking an MAOI.

Drugs used in the treatment of *depression*. The two main types are tricyclic antidepressant drugs and monoamine oxidase inhibitors.

HOW THEY WORK

Some antidepressant drugs trigger the release of chemicals in the brain that stimulate nerve activity. Others, notably tricyclic antidepressants and monoamine oxidase inhibitors, prolong the active life of these chemicals after their release. Antidepressant drugs usually take at least 10 days to have any beneficial effect and up to eight weeks to become fully effective.

POSSIBLE ADVERSE EFFECTS

Most antidepressant drugs can cause dry mouth, blurred vision, dizziness, drowsiness, constipation, and difficulty in passing urine; these symptoms often improve as treatment continues. An overdose of an antidepressant drug may cause abnormal heart rhythm, seizures, coma, and, occasionally, death.

Antidiarrhoeal drugs

COMMON DRUGS

Adsorbent agents
Oral rehydration salts

Others
Codeine Diphenoxylate with atropine Loperamide

> **WARNING**
> Do not take antidiarrhoeal drugs regularly except under medical supervision because they may mask a serious underlying disorder.

A group of drugs used to treat *diarrhoea*. Some antidiarrhoeal drugs, including bulking agents, are adsorbent substances; others, including narcotic antidiarrhoeals, reduce the activity of the intestines.

WHY THEY ARE USED

Antidiarrhoeal drugs may be recommended if diarrhoea persists for more than 24 to 48 hours, or if it is causing social problems. The main treatment of severe diarrhoea, however, is replacement of salts and water by oral rehydration therapy (see *ORT*). Antidiarrhoeal drugs are also given to help regulate bowel action in people with a *colostomy* or *ileostomy*.

HOW THEY WORK

Many adsorbent antidiarrhoeal drugs act by taking in the toxic substances that cause diarrhoea, making the faeces more solid. Bulking agents adsorb water from the faeces.

Drugs that reduce the activity of the intestinal wall slow the passage of faeces. As a result, both the fluidity and frequency of bowel movements are reduced. Oral electrolyte solutions are an important part of the treatment of acute diarrhoea since they replace salts lost in the watery motions.

POSSIBLE ADVERSE EFFECTS

Antidiarrhoeal drugs may cause constipation. In cases of diarrhoea caused by an infection, antidiarrhoeal drugs may delay recovery by slowing the elimination of microorganisms.

Bulking agents may cause intestinal obstruction if they are used without drinking sufficient water or if the bowel is narrowed.

Prolonged use of a narcotic antidiarrhoeal drug may cause physical dependence (see *Drug dependence*), producing nausea, abdominal pain, and diarrhoea if the drug is suddenly stopped. *Loperamide* is chemically similar to narcotic antidiarrhoeals, but does not have a narcotic effect.

Antidiuretic hormone
See *ADH*.

Antidote
A substance that neutralizes or counteracts the effects of a poison. The antidote for acid is alkali, and vice versa. A chemical antidote works by combining with a poison to form an innocuous substance, or in some way blocking or diverting the action of the poison. A mechanical antidote prevents the absorption of poison into the blood from the stomach and intestine.

Anti-D(Rh₀) immunoglobulin

Anti-D(Rh_o) immunoglobulin
An *antiserum* that contains antibodies against Rhesus (Rh) D factor (a substance present on the red blood cells of people who have Rh-positive blood). It is given to a woman who has Rh-negative blood after she has given birth to a baby whose blood is Rh positive, which may occur if the baby's father is Rh positive.

Anti-D(Rh_o) immunoglobulin is also given to a pregnant woman with Rh-negative blood after she has had an *amniocentesis*, bleeding episode, *miscarriage*, or *abortion*, or in other instances in which she might have been exposed to fetal blood cells. The injected antibodies destroy any red blood cells from the fetus that have entered the woman's bloodstream. This is important to prevent or reduce the risk that the woman will form her own antibodies against Rh-positive blood, which might adversely affect a subsequent pregnancy. (See also *Haemolytic disease of the newborn*; *Rhesus incompatibility*.)

Antiemetic drugs

COMMON DRUGS

Anticholinergics
Hyoscine

Antihistamines
Cinnarizine Dimenhydrinate Promethazine

Phenothiazines
Chlorpromazine Prochlorperazine Promethazine Thiethylperazine

Others
Metoclopramide Odansetron

> **WARNING**
> An antiemetic drug should not be taken regularly except under medical supervision as it may mask a serious underlying disorder.

A group of drugs used to treat *nausea* and *vomiting* caused by *motion sickness*, *vertigo*, *Ménière's disease*, *radiotherapy*, or certain drugs (especially *anticancer drugs*). Some antiemetic drugs are also used to treat severe vomiting during pregnancy.

Antiemetic drugs are seldom prescribed to treat food poisoning because it is believed that vomiting enables the body to rid itself of harmful substances.

HOW THEY WORK

Some antiemetic drugs reduce nerve activity at the base of the brain and thereby suppress the vomiting reflex. *Antihistamine drugs* and also *anticholinergic drugs* reduce the vomiting associated with vertigo by suppressing nerve activity in the balance centre in the inner ear. Other antiemetic drugs prevent vomiting by relaxing the muscles in the lower part of stomach and so enabling the stomach contents to pass from the stomach into the small intestine.

POSSIBLE ADVERSE EFFECTS

Many antiemetic drugs cause drowsiness. Some antiemetics must not be taken during pregnancy because they may damage the developing fetus.

Antifreeze poisoning
Most antifreeze in the UK contains ethylene glycol, which is poisonous. Antifreeze poisoning is rare. Most cases of poisoning occur as a result of accidental swallowing, although a few people commit suicide by swallowing antifreeze.

SYMPTOMS AND TREATMENT

Drinking antifreeze initially produces the same effects as alcohol intoxication, but vomiting, stupor, seizures, and coma may follow within a few hours; acute *kidney failure* may occur within 24 to 36 hours.

Any person believed to have drunk antifreeze needs immediate medical help. Until such help arrives, small amounts of alcohol (approximately two tots of spirit, such as brandy or whisky) should be given if the person is conscious; alcohol reduces the rate at which antifreeze is metabolized and becomes toxic in the body.

Hospital treatment may include removing the antifreeze from the stomach using a stomach pump (see *Lavage, gastric*), and giving *diuretic drugs*, alcohol, and bicarbonate (by drip into a vein) to correct excess acidity in the body fluids. Haemodialysis (see *Dialysis*) may be required to remove ethylene glycol from the blood and to treat kidney failure.

Antifungal drugs

COMMON DRUGS

Amphotericin B Clotrimazole Econazole Fluconazole Flucytosine Griseofulvin Ketoconazole Miconazole Nystatin Tolnaftate

A group of drugs prescribed to treat infections caused by *fungi*. Antifungal drugs are commonly used to treat different types of *tinea*, including tinea pedis (athlete's foot) and tinea capitis (scalp ringworm). They are also used to treat *candidiasis* (thrush) and rare fungal infections (such as *cryptococcosis*) which affect internal organs.

Antifungal preparations are available in various forms: tablets, lozenges, liquids, creams, injections, and vaginal suppositories.

HOW THEY WORK

Antifungal drugs damage the cell walls of fungi, causing chemicals essential for normal cell function and growth to escape. The fungal cells are unable to survive without these chemicals and die.

POSSIBLE ADVERSE EFFECTS

Preparations applied to the skin, scalp, mouth, or vagina may occasionally increase irritation. Antifungal drugs given by mouth or injection may cause more serious side-effects, including liver or kidney damage.

Antigen

A substance that can trigger an *immune response*, resulting in production of an *antibody* as part of the body's defence against infection and disease. Many antigens are foreign proteins (those not found naturally in the body); they include parts of microorganisms, toxins, and tissues from another person used in organ transplantation. Sometimes, harmless substances (e.g. pollen) are misidentified as potentially harmful antigens by the immune system, resulting in an allergic response (see *Allergy*).

Antihistamine drugs

COMMON DRUGS

Astemizole Azatadine Cetirizine Chlorpheniramine Mebhydrolin Promethazine Terfenadine Trimeprazine Triprolidine

> **WARNING**
> Do not drive or operate potentially dangerous machinery while taking an antihistamine drug until you are certain that the treatment is not causing dizziness or drowsiness or impairing your coordination.

A group of drugs that block the effects of *histamine*, a chemical released during allergic reactions (see *Allergy*).

WHY THEY ARE USED

Antihistamine drugs are used in the treatment of *urticaria* (hives) and other rashes to relieve itching, swelling, and redness. Drugs of this type are also used in the treatment of allergic *rhinitis* (hay fever) to relieve sneezing and a runny nose.

Antihistamine drugs are sometimes included in *cough remedies* and *cold remedies* because they dry up nasal secretions and suppress the nerve centres in the brain that trigger the cough reflex. Antihistamines are also used as *antiemetic drugs* because they suppress the vomiting reflex.

Because many antihistamine drugs have a sedative effect, they are sometimes used to induce sleep, especially when itching keeps the sufferer awake at night. The most recently introduced antihistamines have very little sedative effect.

Antihistamine drugs are usually given by mouth but they may be given by injection in an emergency to aid in treating *anaphylactic shock* (a severe allergic reaction).

HOW THEY WORK

Antihistamine drugs block the effect of histamine on tissues such as the skin, eyes, and nose. Without drug treatment, histamine would dilate (widen) small blood vessels, resulting in redness and swelling of the surrounding tissue due to leakage of fluid from the circulation. Antihistamines also prevent histamine from irritating nerve fibres, which would otherwise cause itching.

POSSIBLE ADVERSE EFFECTS

Many antihistamines cause drowsiness and dizziness. However, the latest generation of antihistamines have virtually no soporific effect. Other possible side-effects of antihistamines include loss of appetite, nausea, dry mouth, blurred vision, and difficulty passing urine.

Antihypertensive drugs

COMMON DRUGS

ACE inhibitors
Captopril Enalapril Lisinopril

Beta-blockers
Atenolol Labetalol Oxprenolol Propranolol

Calcium channel blockers
Diltiazem Felodipine Nifedipine Verapamil

Diuretic drugs
Chlorthalidone Cyclopenthiazide Hydrochlorothiazide

Vasodilator drugs
Hydralazine Minoxidil Prazosin

Others
Clonidine Methyldopa

> **WARNING**
> Never stop taking antihypertensive drugs suddenly as this may cause a dangerous rise in blood pressure.

A group of drugs that are used in the treatment of *hypertension* (high blood pressure) to prevent the development of complications such as *stroke*, *myocardial infarction* (heart attack), *heart failure* (reduced pumping efficiency), and kidney damage.

HOW THEY WORK

Beta-blocker drugs reduce the force of the heartbeat, thereby lowering the pressure of blood flow into the circulation. *Diuretic drugs* increase the amount of salts and water excreted in the urine, although the way in which they lower the blood pressure is not entirely clear.

Other types of antihypertensive drugs cause the blood vessels to dilate (widen), which decreases the resistance to blood flow and thereby lowers the blood pressure.

POSSIBLE ADVERSE EFFECTS

Apart from the side-effects typical of specific groups, all antihypertensive drugs may cause dizziness and fainting as a result of lowering the blood pressure too much.

Anti-inflammatory drugs

Drugs that reduce the symptoms and signs of *inflammation*. (See also *Analgesic drugs*; *Corticosteroid drugs*; *Nonsteroidal anti-inflammatory drugs*.)

Antimalarial drugs

See *Malaria*.

Antiperspirant

COMMON DRUGS

Aluminium chloride

A substance applied to the skin in the form of a lotion, cream, or spray to reduce excessive sweating.

WHY IT IS USED

An antiperspirant is used to prevent the accumulation of sweat, especially in the armpits. When sweat remains on the skin, it creates a moist environment in which bacteria can thrive. The bacteria break down chemicals in the sweat, causing body odour (sweat itself is almost odourless).

High concentrations of antiperspirants are sometimes prescribed to treat *hyperhidrosis* (abnormally profuse sweating). Results of this treatment are variable.

HOW IT WORKS

An antiperspirant reduces the production of sweat by the sweat glands and blocks the ducts that drain sweat on to the surface of the skin.

POSSIBLE ADVERSE EFFECTS

Antiperspirants may cause skin irritation and a burning or stinging sensation. Such effects are more common when high concentrations are used. If the irritation persists when a lower dose is used, treatment should be stopped to prevent *dermatitis*. (See also *Deodorants*.)

Antipsychotic drugs

COMMON DRUGS

Phenothiazines
Chlorpromazine Fluphenazine Perphenazine Thioridazine Trifluoperazine

Others
Haloperidol Lithium

A group of drugs used to treat *psychoses* (mental disorders involving loss of contact with reality), particularly *schizophrenia* and *manic-depressive illness*. Antipsychotic drugs enable many people suffering from mental illness to live relatively normal lives outside mental institutions.

Antipsychotic drugs are also used to calm or sedate people with other mental disorders (such as *dementia*) who have become highly agitated or aggressive.

Antipsychotic drugs include *phenothiazine drugs* and *lithium*, which is used specifically to treat the symptoms of *mania* (abnormal elation and overactivity).

HOW THEY WORK

Most antipsychotic drugs block the action of *dopamine*, a chemical that stimulates nerve activity in the brain. Lithium is thought to reduce the release of *noradrenaline* in the brain.

POSSIBLE ADVERSE EFFECTS

Most antipsychotic drugs can cause drowsiness, lethargy, *dyskinesia* (jerky movements of the mouth, face, and tongue), and *parkinsonism* (symptoms similar to those of Parkinson's disease). Other possible side-effects include dry mouth, blurred vision, and difficulty passing urine. Lithium may cause nausea, diarrhoea, tremor, rash, weight gain, and weakness of the muscles.

Antipyretic drugs

Drugs that reduce fever, such as *aspirin* and *paracetamol*.

Antirheumatic drugs

COMMON DRUGS

Corticosteroid drugs
Dexamethasone Prednisolone

Immunosuppressant drugs
Azathioprine Chlorambucil Methotrexate

Others
Chloroquine Gold Penicillamine Sulphasalazine

A group of drugs used in the treatment of *rheumatoid arthritis* and types of arthritis caused by other *autoimmune disorders* (disorders in which the body's immune system attacks its own tissues)—for example, systemic *lupus erythematosus*. Antirheumatic drugs are prescribed for active disease when *nonsteroidal antiinflammatory drugs* (NSAIDs) fail to relieve pain and stiffness in the joints, or when the disease is causing progressive deformity and disability.

HOW THEY WORK

Antirheumatic drugs limit the damage caused by the immune system by suppressing either the production or activity of white blood cells. Each type of drug works in a different way, but all antirheumatics damp down the inflammation caused by the autoimmune reaction and also slow down the degeneration of the cartilage that lines joints.

The effectiveness of each type of antirheumatic drug varies according to the individual. Beneficial effects do not usually appear for several weeks after starting drug treatment.

POSSIBLE ADVERSE EFFECTS

All antirheumatic drugs may cause serious adverse effects. For example, *gold* and *penicillamine* may cause rashes, blood disorders and kidney damage, *chloroquine* may damage the eyes, and *immunosuppressant drugs* may cause blood disorders. For this reason, regular medical examinations, including blood and urine tests, are carried out during treatment to monitor toxic effects.

Antiseptics

Chemicals applied to the skin to destroy bacteria and other microorganisms and thus prevent *sepsis* (infection). Antisepsis (the use of antiseptics to prevent infection) is not the same as asepsis, which is the creation of a germ-free environment (see *Aseptic technique*). Antiseptics are milder than *disinfectants*, which decontaminate inanimate objects but are too strong to be used on the body.

Antiseptic fluids are generally used for bathing wounds, whereas creams are applied to wounds before they are dressed. Among the more commonly used antiseptics are *iodine*, *hydrogen peroxide*, and *chlorhexidine*.

Antiserum

A preparation containing antibodies that combine with specific *antigens* (foreign proteins), usually components of microorganisms (such as viruses or bacteria). Such antibody-antigen interaction leads to the inactivation or destruction of the microorganisms. Antiserum samples are usually prepared from the blood of animals that have been injected with killed, or live but harmless, strains of particular viruses or bacteria.

Antiserum is usually used, along with *immunization*, as an emergency treatment when someone has been exposed to a dangerous infection such as *rabies* and has not previously been immunized against the infection. The antiserum helps to provide some immediate protection against the infective microorganisms while full immunity is developing. However, such measures are not as effective in preventing disease as earlier (pre-exposure) immunization.

Antisocial personality disorder

Failure to conform to social norms of behaviour. The category of antisocial personality is relatively new and was devised to provide clear guidelines for diagnosing psychiatric disorder. In the past, people displaying antisocial behaviour were classified in a number of ways, for example as "sociopaths" or "psychopaths", but it was argued that these labels described character traits rather than specific illnesses that caused a change in personality or behaviour.

DIAGNOSIS

For a person to be diagnosed as suffering from this type of disorder, the antisocial behaviour must have started before the age of 15 and must not be a result of *mental handicap* or obvious illness. Since there must be evidence of persistent disturbance over a period of time, the term cannot be used to describe anyone under 18 years old. For a positive diagnosis, there must be evidence of disturbances in all of the following areas: performance at work or school; childhood behaviour; personal life; and personal relationships.

In the first area, signs of disturbance include constant job changes; persistent unemployment for no good reason; regular absences from work; and poor school performance. For a positive rate in the second area, at least three of the following must have occurred: truancy; rule-breaking; expulsion from school; lying; stealing; running away from home; excessive drinking; juvenile court appearances; or precocious sexual activity. A positive rating in the third area is given if two or more of the following have occurred: crimes; separation or divorce; fighting; regular drunkenness; money troubles; or periods of homelessness. In the fourth area, a positive rating is given if there is an inability to form or maintain close relationships with family, friends or sexual partners that seems to be due to a basic lack of concern for others.

TREATMENT

The aim of treatment is to alter behaviour; this may include living in *therapeutic communities*, *behaviour therapy*, various forms of *psychotherapy*, and participation in community help programmes. There is a clear overlap with legal punishment, since criminal activity is common, but the debate as to whether people with antisocial personality disorder are "bad" or "mad" remains unresolved.

Antispasmodic drugs

COMMON DRUGS

Dicyclomine Hyoscine Peppermint oil

A group of drugs that relax spasm in smooth (involuntary) muscle in the wall of the intestine or bladder. Antispasmodic drugs are used in the treatment of *irritable bowel syndrome* and *irritable bladder*.

Antispasmodic drugs may have an anticholinergic action (that is, they work by blocking the action of *acetylcholine*, a neurotransmitter chemical released from nerve endings that stimulates muscle contraction).

Possible adverse effects of antispasmodic drugs include dry mouth, blurred vision, and difficulty passing urine. (See also *Anticholinergic drugs*.)

Antitoxin

Any of a variety of commercially prepared substances, each of which contains *antibodies* that can combine and neutralize the effect of a specific toxin released into the bloodstream by bacteria (such as those that cause *tetanus* and *diphtheria*).

Antitoxins are prepared from the blood of animals or humans that have been exposed to particular toxins (either by inoculation or as a result of suffering from the disease) and have therefore produced antibodies against the toxins.

Antitoxins are usually administered by injection into a muscle, under the supervision of a doctor. Occasionally, an antitoxin may cause an allergic reaction; rarely, it causes an *anaphylactic shock* (a severe allergic reaction) requiring emergency treatment.

Antitussive drugs

Drugs that prevent or relieve a *cough*. (See *Cough remedies*.)

Antivenom

 A specific treatment for snake, scorpion, spider, or other venomous animal bites or stings. Antivenom is prepared by inoculating animals, usually horses, with small but increasing amounts of venom from a particular poisonous animal. This provokes the production of *antibodies* that will neutralize the poisons in the venom. A preparation of these antibodies can then be produced from samples of the horse's blood.

In the UK, antivenom treatment is usually needed only for people bitten by exotic snakes in zoos or private collections. Public Health Laboratories and zoos are the usual sources of supply for antivenoms.

Antiviral drugs

COMMON DRUGS

Acyclovir Amantadine Idoxuridine Interferon Zidovudine

A group of drugs used in the treatment of infection by *viruses*. Drugs that kill viruses have proved difficult to develop because viruses live only within body cells and there is a danger that antiviral drugs will damage the host cells as well as the virus. To date, no drugs have been developed that can effectively eradicate viruses and cure the illnesses that they cause.

Immunization is at present more important than drug treatment in fighting serious viral infections. However, some drugs have already proved useful in tackling a few viral infections, particularly those caused by *herpes* viruses. Antiviral drugs reduce the severity of these infections but may not eliminate them completely, so attacks may recur. Other antiviral drugs are currently being developed and used (e.g. to treat *AIDS*).

HOW THEY WORK

Most antiviral drugs destroy viruses by disrupting chemical processes necessary for viruses to grow and multiply within cells. Some antiviral drugs prevent viruses from actually penetrating cells.

POSSIBLE ADVERSE EFFECTS

Antiviral drugs used in treating AIDS carry a high risk of causing anaemia due to bone marrow damage. Most other antiviral drugs rarely cause side-effects. Antiviral creams may irritate the skin. Antiviral drugs given by mouth or injection can cause nausea and dizziness, and, rarely, in long-term treatment, kidney damage.

Antral irrigation

Irrigation of the maxillary antrum (also called the maxillary sinus), one of the nasal sinuses, to diagnose and treat persistent *sinusitis*.

WHY IT IS USED

Antral irrigation is used when sinusitis persists after drug treatment (usually with *antibiotic drugs* and *decongestant drugs*) has failed to provide a cure. Antral irrigation allows a positive diagnosis of infection to be made, and it sometimes also cures the infection.

The normal drainage channel from the antrum into the nose is usually at least partly blocked in chronic sinusitis, causing infected material to build up within the cavity. Antral irrigation creates a temporary opening that allows the contents to be flushed out through the natural opening.

HOW IT IS DONE

A cannula (hollow, flexible tube) is inserted into the antrum, guided by a trocar (sharp, pointed rod). The trocar is inserted into the nostril and pushed through the bony side wall of the nose into the antrum. The trocar is withdrawn, leaving the cannula in place. A syringe is then attached to the cannula and the contents of the sinus are sucked out and sent to the laboratory for bacteriological culture to identify the organism responsible for the infection and to test its sensitivity to various antibiotics.

A large syringe filled with warm saline (salt solution) is attached to the cannula and the antrum is thoroughly washed out by injecting the solution into the cavity and causing it to flow out through the natural sinus opening. Washing out is repeated until the fluid is clear.

RESULTS

Unless sinusitis has been present for so long that permanent damage to the mucosa (lining of the sinus) has occurred, antral irrigation may be curative. However, if the infection fails to disappear after a period of several weeks, and an irrigation confirms that the antrum is still infected, surgery to enlarge the drainage channel may be required.

Anuria

Complete cessation of urine output. Such total failure to pass urine is an indication of a serious problem in the urinary tract because some urine is produced even when a person is severely dehydrated.

Anuria may be caused by a severe malfunction of the kidneys, but a much more common cause is a complete blockage to the flow of urine—due, for example, to enlargement of the prostate gland (see *Prostate, enlarged*), a *bladder tumour*, or a stone (see *Calculus, urinary tract*). Failure of urine production by the kidneys may be due to oxygen depletion as a result of reduced blood flow through the kidneys, as occurs in *shock*, or to severe kidney damage caused by a disease such as *glomerulonephritis*.

Anuria requires urgent investigation to establish the cause and to allow treatment, such as rehydration, or removal of the blockage, to begin. Without treatment, anuria leads to *uraemia* (excess urea and other waste products in the blood) and death.

Anus

The canal at the end of the alimentary tract through which faeces are expelled from the body. About 4 cm long, the anus is an extension of the rectum as it passes backwards and downwards through the pelvic floor. The orifice at the end of the anal canal is open only during defaecation—at other times it is kept closed by the muscles of the anal sphincter. These muscles are arranged in two layers, the internal sphincter, which cannot be controlled voluntarily, and the external sphincter, which can be relaxed at will for defaecation. (See also *Digestive system*.)

Anus, cancer of

A rare cancer of the skin of the anus. Possible early signs of anal cancer are swelling at the outside of the anus

STRUCTURE OF THE ANUS

The anus is a canal at the end of the alimentary tract, with internal and external sphincters to open and close the orifice.

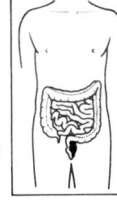

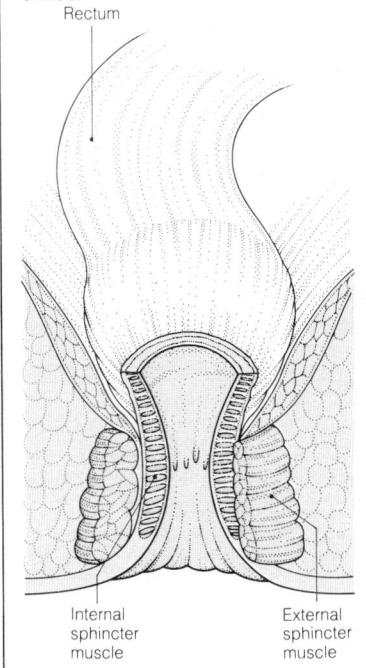

Rectum

Internal sphincter muscle

External sphincter muscle

accompanied by bleeding and discomfort. Surgical removal of the cancer is the usual treatment.

Anus, imperforate

A rare *congenital* abnormality, detected and treated at birth, in which the anal opening appears to be covered over.

TYPES

Classification of the two main types of imperforate anus, high and low, depends on whether or not the bowel ends above or below the pelvic floor. In the high type, the anal canal fails to develop and there is no connection between the rectum and the anus. Many of the normal anal structures, such as the muscles, are missing. The disorder is associated with other abnormalities, especially of the urinary organs. In the low type, there may be only a layer of skin covering the anal opening.

TREATMENT

Treatment for high imperforate anus involves surgery to open up the end of the rectum and join it to the anus. This operation is usually successful and the long-term outlook is good. In some cases, a *colostomy* may be needed.

Treatment for low imperforate anus usually involves surgical removal of the skin over the anus. In addition, *anal dilatation* (a procedure to enlarge the anus) may be needed for several months afterwards.

Anxiety

An unpleasant emotional state ranging from mild unease to intense fear. An anxious person usually feels a sense of impending doom, although there is no obvious threat, and has certain physical and psychological symptoms. A certain amount of

---

DISORDERS OF THE ANUS

Most anal disorders are minor but they may cause considerable discomfort and concern. Many are aggravated by constipation, and may be helped by regular toilet habits, an increased intake of fluids, wholemeal products, fruits, and vegetables to soften the faeces, and the use of glycerine suppositories.

CONGENITAL DEFECTS

Imperforate anus is an uncommon birth defect in which the anus is sealed (see *Anus, imperforate*).

In *anal stenosis*, the anus is too narrow to allow the normal passage of faeces. This is sometimes a congenital abnormality, but it can also result from scarring after surgery for another disorder.

INJURY

Anal fissures originate from small tears in the lining of the anus, usually as a result of straining to pass hard, dry faeces.

TUMOURS

Cancer of the skin around the anus is rare (see *Anus, cancer of*).

OTHER DISORDERS

Haemorrhoids are enlarged blood vessels under the lining of the anus and may cause bleeding during defaecation, itching, and pain.

An *anal fistula* is an abnormal tunnel connecting the inside of the anal canal with the skin surrounding the anus. These fistulas usually result from an abscess in the wall of the anus.

Itching of the anus (pruritus ani) may be a direct result of another disorder, such as an anal fistula, haemorrhoids or *threadworm* infestation.

INVESTIGATION

Investigation of anal disorders is usually by visual inspection, sometimes including *proctoscopy* (use of an internal viewing tube), and digital examination (feeling with a finger). Sometimes a biopsy (specimen of tissue for analysis) or swab may be taken for bacteriological culture.

A

anxiety is normal and serves to improve performance. Anxiety becomes a symptom when it starts to inhibit thought and to disrupt normal everyday activities.

SYMPTOMS AND SIGNS

The most common physical symptoms relate to the chest. They include palpitations (awareness of a more forceful or faster heartbeat), throbbing or stabbing pains, a feeling of tightness and inability to take in enough air, and a tendency to sigh or overbreathe (see *Hyperventilation*).

Muscle tension leads to headaches, spasms in the neck, back pains, grasping too tightly, and an inability to relax. Restlessness, tremor of the hands, and a sense of tiredness are also common. A pins-and-needles sensation or spasm of the arms sometimes follows hyperventilation.

Gastrointestinal symptoms include dryness of the mouth, a feeling of distension, diarrhoea, nausea, changes in appetite, constant belching, and difficulty swallowing. Some sufferers may actually vomit or have severe pain mimicking serious illness.

Other symptoms include sweating, blushing, pallor, dizziness, lightheadedness, yawning, and a frequent need to urinate or defaecate.

People with anxiety usually have a constant feeling that something bad is going to happen. They may fear that they have a chronic or dangerous illness (a fear reinforced by their physical symptoms) or worry about the health or safety of family and friends. Fear of losing control is also common. Anxiety often leads to increasing dependence on others, irritability, a sense of fatigue, and a state of being easily frustrated.

Inability to relax may lead to difficulty getting to sleep and constant waking during the night. Frightening dreams often occur.

Strange but common symptoms are *depersonalization* (the sense of being cut off from oneself) or *derealization* (the sense of being cut off from the world). These symptoms can begin suddenly and last for a long time, leading some people to fear they are becoming insane.

Symptoms of anxiety usually result from an *anxiety disorder*, or are part of another psychological disorder, such as *hypochondriasis*, *depression*, or a type of *psychosexual disorder*.

CAUSES

Three different areas of research have contributed theories for causes of anxiety. Physiological measurements show that anxious individuals have a raised level of *arousal* in the central nervous system, which makes them react more excitedly and adapt more slowly to events. This leads to physical symptoms, such as palpitations, which themselves are unpleasant and reinforce the anxiety.

Psychoanalytical ideas derive from Freud, who coined the term "anxiety neurosis" and believed that anxiety originates from repressed, unresolved childhood experiences. Originally, anxiety was thought to be due to unsatisfied sexual needs, but a better understanding of the importance of *bonding* and of child-parent separations has now led to theories that are based on the fear of losing loved objects. Unconscious conflict can also lead to anxiety.

Behavioural psychologists describe anxiety as a learned response to, for example, pain or mental discomfort. Initially, anxiety drives people to improved performance, but eventually the anxious response becomes a deeply conditioned habit that cannot be controlled and is brought on by the slightest difficulty. Anxiety thus comes to impair performance and thought processes.

TREATMENT

People suffering from anxiety may be helped by reassurance or *counselling*, and, in more severe cases, *psychotherapy* or drug treatment.

Anxiety disorders

A group of mental illnesses in which symptoms of *anxiety* are the main feature. Anxiety disorders include a number of specific syndromes, although there is considerable overlap among them and boundaries are not always clear.

Anxiety disorders are common, affecting roughly four per cent of the population, mainly young adults; the disorders occur equally in men and women and heredity is a contributing factor. Symptoms tend to vary during the course of the illness.

TYPES

Generalized anxiety disorder (the traditional "anxiety neurosis") is diagnosed if the patient has had at least one definite period of anxiety, accompanied by at least one physical or psychological symptom that impairs normal activity. *Panic disorders* are characterized by sudden, intense attacks of panic (extreme, unreasonable fear and anxiety). *Phobias* are dominated by irrational fears that lead to avoidance of certain situations or objects, such as open spaces or spiders. *Post-traumatic stress disorder* is associated with a serious specific event, such as *rape* or a major accident, and symptoms include reliving the event in dreams and a general feeling of numbness and lack of involvement. The principal features of *obsessive-compulsive disorder* are recurrent and persistent thoughts, and ritualized, repetitive behaviour.

TREATMENT

Treatment of anxiety disorders is most effective when there is an identifiable and justified reason for stress. Treatment is more successful in people who have stable underlying personalities. Reassurance, *counselling*, and *psychotherapy* are used, as are *antianxiety drugs* (especially *benzodiazepine drugs*).

Aorta

The main *artery* of the body. The aorta arises directly from the left ventricle (the main pumping chamber of the *heart*) and supplies oxygenated blood to all other arteries except the pulmonary artery (which carries deoxygenated blood from the right side of the heart to the lungs).

DISORDERS

Like other arteries, the aorta can become narrowed as a result of *atherosclerosis* (fat deposits on the walls), which often causes *hypertension* (high blood pressure). There are also specific aortic disorders, notably *coarctation of the aorta* (in which the aorta is abnormally narrow at birth) and *aortitis* (inflammation of the wall of the aorta).

Both aortitis and atherosclerosis can cause an aortic *aneurysm* (ballooning of the vessel wall), which may require surgery to correct impaired blood flow and to remove the risk of rupture and fatal blood loss. (See also *Arteries, disorders of*; *Circulatory system*.)

Aortic incompetence

Leakage of blood through the aortic valve (one of the *heart valves*), resulting in a backflow of blood into the left ventricle (the main pumping chamber of the heart).

CAUSES

Failure of the aortic valve to close correctly may be due to a *congenital* abnormality. Another cause of aortic incompetence is *aortitis* (inflammation of the aorta). Sometimes, the aortic valve leaflets are destroyed by bacterial *endocarditis*, a condition that occurs in intravenous drug users. Aortic incompetence is also found in untreated *syphilis* and is associated with *ankylosing spondylitis* (a disorder

LOCATION AND STRUCTURE OF THE AORTA

From its origin at the left ventricle, the aorta passes upward, curves behind the heart, and runs downward, passing through the thorax (chest) and into the abdomen, where it terminates by dividing into two common iliac arteries. The aorta is thick-walled and large in diameter (about 2.5 cm at its origin) to cope with the high pressure and large volume of blood that passes through it. The thick walls of the aorta have an elastic quality that helps even out the peaks and troughs of pressure that occur with each heart beat.

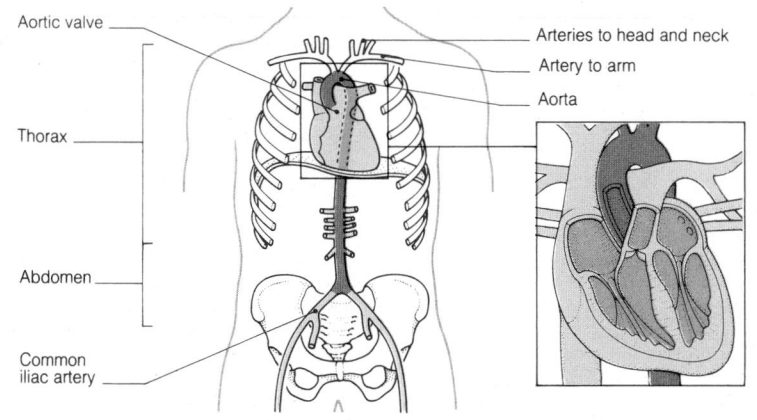

Aortic valve

Thorax

Abdomen

Common iliac artery

Arteries to head and neck

Artery to arm

Aorta

CAUSES

The most common cause is deposition of calcium on the aortic valve, usually associated with *atherosclerosis* (fat deposits). Aortic stenosis may also be due to a *congenital* abnormality. Another cause is *cardiomyopathy* (heart muscle disease) in which thickening of the heart muscle may lead to sub-aortic stenosis (narrowing within the pumping chamber just below the valve). In the past, *rheumatic fever* was a common cause of heart valve damage; today it is rare.

SYMPTOMS AND SIGNS

Aortic stenosis may not cause any symptoms. It is sometimes found during a routine medical examination; the doctor hears a murmur (abnormal heart sound) over the front of the chest wall to the right of the sternum (breastbone) and sometimes up into the neck. Symptoms, when they do occur, include fainting attacks, lack of energy, chest pain on exertion due to *angina pectoris*, and breathing difficulty. Other features include a weak pulse and *cardiomegaly* (enlargement of the heart) at a late stage.

DIAGNOSIS

A *chest X-ray* may show white patches of calcium in the area of the aortic valve. The heart may also appear enlarged on an X-ray.

An *ECG* (measurement of the electrical activity of the heart) may show evidence of thickening of, and strain on, the left ventricle.

Echocardiography (imaging of the heart structures by measuring the pattern of reflection of sound waves from them) usually reveals the diameter of the valve opening and thickness of the valve leaflets, abnormal movement within the aortic valve, and thickening of the walls of the left ventricle. Doppler echocardiography can confirm and measure the reduced flow through the valve.

A cardiac catheter (a flexible tube inserted into the heart through blood vessels) can be fitted with a pressure-measuring device to measure the degree of aortic stenosis; the difference in pressure on either side of the valve reflects the severity of the stenosis (see *Catheterization, cardiac*).

TREATMENT

Before developments in *heart valve surgery*, the outlook for people with aortic stenosis was gloomy; once symptoms developed, the predicted lifespan was only a year or so. Now, provided that valve replacement is performed before irremediable damage to the left ventricle occurs, the outlook is good.

---

affecting the spine), and *Marfan's syndrome* (a congenital disorder of connective tissues). *Rheumatic fever* was once a common cause of aortic incompetence but is now rare. *Atherosclerosis* (fat deposits on the walls of arteries) is associated with aortic incompetence and also with *aortic stenosis* (narrowing of the aortic valve).

SYMPTOMS AND SIGNS

Aortic incompetence may not cause any symptoms. It is sometimes found during a routine medical examination; the doctor hears a murmur (abnormal heart sound) over the front of the chest wall to the left of the sternum (breastbone).

The heart compensates for the backflow of blood into the left ventricle by working harder, until the combination of hypertrophy (muscle thickening) and dilatation (ballooning) of the left ventricle wall eventually leads to *heart failure* (reduced pumping efficiency); this, in turn, results in breathing difficulty and *oedema* (accumulation of fluid).

DIAGNOSIS

A *chest X-ray* may show white patches of calcium in the area of the aortic valve, an enlarged heart, and widening of the aorta.

An *ECG* (measurement of the electrical activity of the heart) may show evidence of thickening of, and strain on, the left ventricle.

Echocardiography (imaging of the heart structures by measuring the pattern of reflection of sound waves from them) will show the diameter of the valve opening and the diameter of the aortic ring, a thickening of the wall of the left ventricle, and reduced movement of the aortic valve. Doppler echocardiography shows the blood flow through the valve.

A cardiac catheter (flexible tube inserted into the heart via blood vessels) is sometimes used to demonstrate the degree of incompetence; a radiopaque substance is injected into the heart through the catheter and X-ray pictures are then taken (see *Catheterization, cardiac*).

TREATMENT

Heart failure resulting from aortic incompetence can be treated with *diuretic drugs* to remove retained fluid from the lungs. *Heart valve surgery* to replace the damaged valve may eventually be necessary, but often not until many years after the condition was first diagnosed.

Aortic stenosis

Narrowing of the opening of the aortic valve (one of the *heart valves*), causing obstruction of blood flow into the circulation. This makes the heart work harder and causes the muscle in the wall of the left ventricle (the main pumping chamber) to thicken.

APGAR CHART

Sign	0	1	2
Colour	Blue, pale	Body pink; extremities blue	Completely pink
Respiratory effort	Absent	Weak cry; irregular breathing	Good strong cry; regular breathing
Muscle tone	Limp	Bending of some limbs	Active motion; limbs well-flexed
Reflex irritability	No response	Grimace (on nasal stimulation)	Cry
Heart rate	Absent	Slow (below 100 beats per minute)	Over 100 beats per minute

Aortitis

Inflammation of the aorta, the large artery that carries blood from the heart to supply all parts of the body except the lungs. Aortitis is a rare condition that occurs in people with *arteritis* (inflammation of the arteries) or untreated *syphilis* and in some people with *ankylosing spondylitis* (a disorder affecting the spine).

Aortitis may cause part of the aorta to widen and its walls to become thinner. This may then lead to the formation of an *aneurysm* (ballooning of the artery), which may burst and cause severe, sometimes fatal, blood loss. Aortitis may also damage the ring surrounding the aortic valve in the heart, leading to *aortic incompetence*, which allows regurgitation of blood back to the heart and may eventually result in *heart failure*.

Aortography

An imaging procedure by which the *aorta* (the main artery leaving the heart) and its branches can be seen on X-ray film after injection of a contrast medium (a substance that is opaque to X-rays).

WHY IT IS DONE
Aortography is used to detect aortic *aneurysm* (ballooning of the aorta) and assess the severity of *peripheral vascular disease* before surgery.

HOW IT IS DONE
Contrast medium is usually injected into the aorta through a fine catheter (flexible plastic tube) inserted either into the femoral artery at the groin, or into the brachial artery on the inside of the elbow. In people with severe arterial disease, the major arteries may be blocked and the contrast medium may have to be injected through a hollow needle directly into the aorta within the lower abdomen.

COMPLICATIONS
There is a small risk of a reaction to the contrast medium. Damage to a vessel during puncture or catheterization can also occur.

Aperient

A mild *laxative drug*.

Apgar score

A system devised by Virginia Apgar, an American anaesthetist, to assess the condition of a newborn baby. Five features are scored at one minute and at five minutes after birth. The features scored are respiratory effort, heart-rate, colour, muscle tone, and reaction to nasal stimulation. Most important are the infant's attempts to breathe and the infant's heart-rate. In general, if these two features are satisfactory, the others will be as well.

Each feature is scored from 0 to 2, making a total of 10 possible points. A low total score of 0 to 3, which will occur if the baby does not breathe or if the heart-rate is too slow, means the baby needs urgent resuscitation. A middle score (4 to 6) indicates that the baby may need medical help. A high score (7 to 10) indicates a well baby.

Parents should not attach undue importance to the Apgar score. It was originally intended to try to quantify the vast changes a newborn goes through in the first minutes of life and to help direct appropriate care.

Aphakia

The absence of the crystalline *lens* from the eye. Aphakia occurs if the lens has been surgically removed, as after *cataract surgery*, or if it has been destroyed by a penetrating injury and subsequently absorbed into the aqueous humour (the fluid within the front part of the eyeball).

Aphakia causes severe loss of focusing in the affected eye or eyes and calls for correction by lens implants, contact lenses, or glasses.

Aphasia

Strictly, a complete absence of previously acquired language skills, caused by a brain disorder that affects the ability to speak and write, and/or the ability to comprehend and read. The term aphasia is also sometimes used interchangeably with the term dysphasia (which more specifically describes disturbance rather than absence of these language skills).

The term aphasia should not be used to describe language difficulties caused by disorders of parts of the body involved in the mechanics of speech (see *Dysarthria*; *Dysphonia*), or by defective hearing or sight.

Related disabilities that may occur, either as a feature of aphasia, or, more rarely, by themselves, are *alexia* (word blindness) and *agraphia* (writing difficulty).

CAUSES
A *stroke* or a *head injury* is the most common cause of brain damage leading to aphasia.

Language function within the brain lies in the dominant cerebral hemisphere (see *Cerebrum*). Two particular areas in the dominant hemisphere, called Broca's and Wernicke's areas (named after their discoverers) and the pathways connecting the two, are known to be important in language skills. Damage to these areas is the most common cause of aphasia.

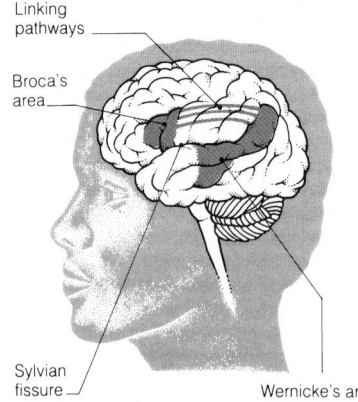

Language function and the brain
Damage to two particular areas (and the pathways between them) in the dominant cerebral hemisphere results in aphasia.

TYPES AND SYMPTOMS

BROCA'S (EXPRESSIVE) APHASIA Damage to Broca's area causes difficulty in the expression of language. Speech is nonfluent, slow, laboured, with loss of normal rhythm. The few words uttered do tend to be meaningful. Writing may also be impaired.

WERNICKE'S (RECEPTIVE) APHASIA Damage to Wernicke's area causes difficulty in comprehension. Speech is fluent but, because of the impaired comprehension, its content is disturbed, with many errors in word selection and grammar, indicating that "internal speech" is impaired. Writing is also impaired and spoken or written commands are not understood.

GLOBAL APHASIA In global aphasia there is a total or near total inability to speak, write, or understand spoken or written words. This is usually caused by widespread damage to the dominant cerebral hemisphere.

NOMINAL APHASIA This is restricted to a difficulty in naming objects or in finding words, although the person may be able to choose the correct name from several offered. Nominal aphasia may be caused by generalized cerebral dysfunction or damage to specific language areas.

TREATMENT AND OUTLOOK

Some recovery from aphasia is usual after a stroke or head injury, although the more severe the aphasia, the less the chances of recovery. *Speech therapy* is the main treatment. (See also *Speech*; *Speech disorders*.)

Apheresis

Also called pheresis, a procedure in which blood is withdrawn from a donor and then reinfused after selected components, such as platelets, white blood cells, or plasma, have been separated and removed.

In therapeutic apheresis, the antibodies causing a disease are selectively removed from the blood. This procedure has proven value in several diseases such as *Guillain-Barré syndrome* and *Goodpasture's syndrome*, but careful assessment in clinical trials has shown that claims for its value in most *autoimmune diseases* were not justified. Research is continuing into an extension of the treatment in which cells are genetically modified before being returned to the body. (See also *Blood donation*.)

Aphonia

Total loss of the voice, usually sudden in onset and caused by emotional stress. A doctor examining the larynx (voice-box) would see that the vocal cords fail to meet as normal when the patient tries to speak, although they come together when the person coughs. Otherwise, there is no detectable abnormality in the larynx.

There is no treatment other than reassurance and *psychotherapy*. The sufferer's voice usually returns as suddenly as it disappeared.

Disease of, or damage to, the larynx usually causes only partial loss of voice production (see *Dysphonia*).

Aphrodisiacs

 Substances thought to stimulate erotic desire and enhance sexual performance. Aphrodisiacs are named after Aphrodite, the ancient Greek goddess of love, beauty, and fertility.

Various substances have been used as "love potions" over the centuries—honey, ginseng, ginger, strychnine, rhinoceros horn, and oysters, among many others. In fact, no substance has a proven aphrodisiac effect, although virtually anything may produce the desired results if the person taking it believes strongly enough that it will work. *Alcohol* can encourage sexual desire by removing inhibitions, but a high blood alcohol level can impair sexual performance.

The male sex hormone *testosterone* is sometimes regarded as a sexual stimulant. In normal men, it has no effect on sexual desire or potency but does reduce sperm production. In men who have a testosterone deficiency, however, the hormone may restore both libido and potency.

Apicectomy

Surgical removal of the tip of a tooth root. Apicectomy may be required as part of *root-canal treatment*.

Aplasia

Incomplete or severely reduced growth and development of any organ or tissue. For example, in bone marrow aplasia, the rate of cell division in the bone marrow is considerably reduced, leading to diminished formation of blood cells of one or all types (see *Anaemia, aplastic*). A number of birth defects—for example, the presence of one or more stunted limbs (see *Phocomelia*)—are a result of incomplete organ formation during prenatal development.

Aplastic anaemia

See *Anaemia, aplastic*.

Apnoea

Cessation of breathing, either temporarily (for a few seconds to a minute or two) or for a prolonged period.

CAUSES

Breathing is an automatic process controlled by the respiratory centre in the brainstem. The respiratory centre sends nerve impulses that regulate contractions of the diaphragm and muscles in the chest wall, thereby controlling the rate and depth of breathing.

Prolonged apnoea can occur if the brainstem is damaged by a *stroke*, by a *transient ischaemic attack* (symptoms of stroke lasting less than 24 hours), or by a *head injury*. Prolonged apnoea can also occur as an effect of certain drugs or as the result of *airway obstruction*, usually by food, drink, vomit, or a small inhaled object.

Deliberate temporary apnoea occurs during *breath-holding attacks* and when swimming underwater. Non-deliberate temporary apnoea can also occur, usually during sleep (see *Sleep apnoea*).

Another type of apnoea occurs in *Cheyne-Stokes respiration*; this is characterized by cycles of deep, rapid breathing alternating with episodes of breathing stoppage.

INVESTIGATION AND TREATMENT

Apnoea requires investigation and treatment of the underlying cause. Treatment may be aimed at relieving any airway obstruction. It may also include the use of respiratory stimulants if the respiratory centre in the brainstem is affected.

Apocrine gland

A gland that discharges cellular material in addition to the fluid it secretes. The term is usually applied to the type of *sweat glands* that appear in hairy areas of the body after puberty.

Apolipoprotein

A protein constituent of *lipoproteins*, the carriers of fat in the bloodstream. Apolipoprotein plays an important part in the growth and repair of nerve tissues. There are three main genetic variants of apolipoprotein E, and one of these seems to determine susceptibility to *Alzheimer's disease*.

Aponeurosis

A wide sheet of tough, fibrous tissue that acts as a tendon (i.e. attaches a muscle to a bone or a joint).

Apoplexy

An outdated term for a *stroke*, resulting in sudden loss of consciousness, paralysis, or loss of sensation.

Apothecary

An obsolete term for a *pharmacist*.

Appendicectomy

Surgical removal of the appendix to treat acute *appendicitis* (inflammation of the appendix).

WHY IT IS DONE

Appendicectomy is carried out to prevent an inflamed appendix bursting and causing *peritonitis* (inflammation of the peritoneum, the abdominal cavity lining) or an abdominal abscess.

Acute appendicitis is often difficult to diagnose and sometimes, because of the dangerous complications that can develop from the condition, a *laparoscopy* is performed (in which a viewing tube, sometimes with a camera attached, is introduced through a small hole made in the abdominal wall). If the appendix appears normal it will be left untouched, since the organ may occasionally prove valuable in the future as a "spare part" tube for reconstructive surgery.

HOW IT IS DONE

If there is time before the operation, the patient is started on a course of antibiotic drugs to prevent the operative wound becoming infected, a serious risk in appendicectomy. The surgeon has two choices of operation: conventional appendicectomy and *minimally invasive surgery*. Until the early 1990s (and still in most parts of the world)

appendicectomy involved making an opening in the abdominal wall large enough for the surgeon to introduce both his instruments and his fingertips (see box). In minimally invasive surgery, three or four small openings are made in the abdominal wall; a laparoscope incorporating a video camera is inserted into one of these, and instruments and suction tubes into the others. In both types of operation, the appendix is identified, clamped, tied off at its base, and removed.

If the appendix has burst, the infected area of the abdominal cavity is washed out with saline (salt solution) and a plastic drainage tube inserted through another small incision to drain off pus. Antibiotics may also be given to prevent peritonitis.

COMPLICATIONS

Possible complications of appendicectomy are infection of the incision wound in the abdominal wall, an abscess at the site from which the appendix was removed, or localized peritonitis.

RECOVERY PERIOD

Following an uncomplicated appendicectomy, the patient is usually able to drink and to eat light food within 24 hours. If a drainage tube has been inserted, it is removed after about 48 hours; the wound seals itself. Normally, the patient can go home after two or three days. Normal physical activ-

ities can usually be resumed after two or three weeks. Recovery may take much longer if there are complications.

Appendicitis

Acute inflammation of the appendix, which is a common cause of abdominal pain and *peritonitis* (inflammation of the lining of the abdominal cavity) in children and young adults.

CAUSES

The cause is usually not known, but appendicitis is sometimes due to obstruction of the appendix by a lump of faeces. The closed end of the appendix beyond the obstruction becomes inflamed, swollen, and infected. This may lead to *gangrene* (tissue death) in the appendix wall, which may perforate (burst).

INCIDENCE

Appendicitis affects about 200 people in 100,000 per year. Although anyone can get appendicitis, it is rare in the very young and very old. It is the most common abdominal surgical emergency in developed countries but is comparatively rare in developing countries.

SYMPTOMS

The first symptom is usually vague discomfort just above and around the navel. Within a few hours this gradually develops into a sharper, more localized pain. This pain is usually most intense in the lower right-hand side of the abdomen.

Symptoms may differ if the appendix is not in the most common position. For example, if the appendix descends behind the caecum, appendicitis may cause little abdominal pain but produce severe pain if the doctor performs a *rectal examination*. If the appendix impinges on the ureter, the urine may become bloodstained.

DIAGNOSIS

Diagnosis can sometimes be difficult because the symptoms of appendicitis are similar to those of many other abdominal disorders. Mesenteric adenitis, which is common in childhood and often follows a viral respiratory infection, has symptoms and signs that resemble those of appendicitis. Disorders of the right *fallopian tube* and *ovary*, *Crohn's disease*, and right-sided *pyelonephritis* (inflammation of the kidney) can also mimic appendicitis. Sometimes a *laparotomy* (surgical investigation of the abdomen) is necessary to confirm or exclude a diagnosis of appendicitis.

COMPLICATIONS

If treatment is delayed, an inflamed appendix may perforate, releasing its contents into the abdomen. At this

---

PERFORMING AN APPENDICECTOMY

The patient is given a general anaesthetic. A small incision is made in the lower right abdomen, above the groin, revealing the caecum (the chamber that links the small and large intestine), to which the appendix is attached.

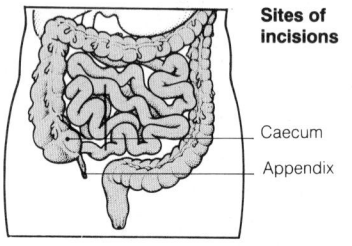

Sites of incisions

Caecum

Appendix

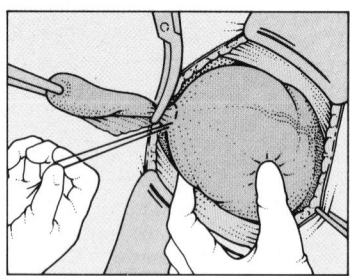

1 The appendix is then carefully and gently brought to the surface of the abdomen, clamped, tied off at the base (where it joins the caecum), and cut off.

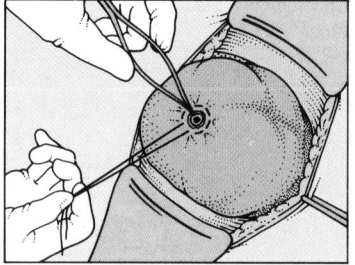

2 The stump is tied with a suture, inverted, and tucked into the caecum with a suture to prevent fluid from leaking into the abdomen.

point, the pain abruptly ceases, but the perforation leads inevitably to peritonitis. In some cases, the omentum (fold of peritoneum covering the intestines) envelops the inflamed appendix; this prevents the spread of infection and results in a localized abscess around the appendix. Peritonitis or an abscess causes a fever (sometimes with chills) as well as increasing pain and tenderness in the abdomen. This pain first appears a few hours to a day or so after the appendix ruptures.

TREATMENT

The usual treatment is *appendicectomy* (surgical removal of the appendix). If an abscess of the appendix is suspected, drainage of the abscess and an appendicectomy may be delayed until the infection has been treated by large doses of antibiotic drugs.

Appendix

A narrow, small, finger-shaped tube that branches off the large intestine. The appendix has no known function. In adults it is usually about 9 cm long, with a thick wall, narrow cavity, and a lining similar to that of the intestine. It contains a large amount of lymphoid tissue, which provides a defence against local infection.

The appendix projects out of the caecum (the first part of the colon) at

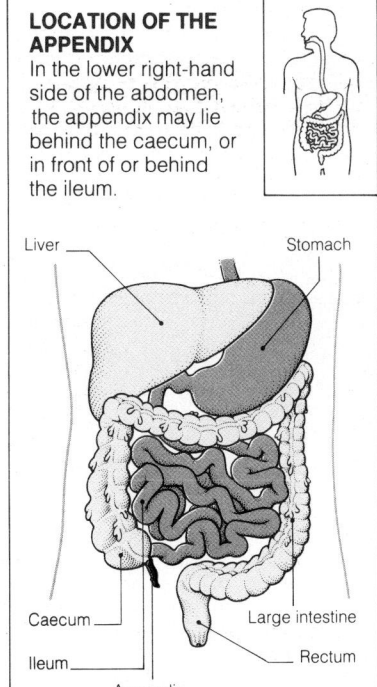

LOCATION OF THE APPENDIX

In the lower right-hand side of the abdomen, the appendix may lie behind the caecum, or in front of or behind the ileum.

Liver

Stomach

Caecum

Large intestine

Ileum

Rectum

Appendix

the lower right-hand side of the abdomen. It may lie behind or below the caecum, or in front of or behind the ileum (part of the small intestine). The position of a person's appendix partly determines the set of symptoms produced by acute *appendicitis* (inflammation of the appendix).

Appetite

A desire for food; a pleasant sensation felt in anticipation of eating, as opposed to *hunger*, a disagreeable feeling caused by the need for food.

Appetite, which is regulated by two parts of the *brain* (the *hypothalamus* and the cerebral cortex), is learned by enjoying a variety of foods that smell, taste, and look good. Ideally, it combines with hunger to ensure that the correct amount of a wide range of foods is eaten to stay healthy to provide proper nutrition for growth in children, and to maintain a proper weight in adults.

Appetite may be lost as a result of various disorders, both physical and psychological (see *Appetite, loss of*).

Appetite, loss of

Known medically as anorexia, loss of appetite is usually temporary and due to an emotional upset or minor feverish illness. Persistent loss of appetite may be a symptom of a more serious underlying physical or psychological disorder and requires investigation by a doctor.

CAUSES

In adolescents and young adults, loss of appetite may be due to *anorexia nervosa* (an eating disorder), or to the abuse of drugs, particularly *amphetamine drugs*. *Depression* or *anxiety* can cause loss of appetite at any age.

Among possible physical causes are a *stroke*, *brain tumour*, or a *head injury* that has damaged the *hypothalamus* or cerebral cortex, the parts of the brain that control appetite. Other physical causes include intestinal disorders, such as *gastritis* (inflammation of the stomach lining, which is common in alcoholics), *stomach cancer*, and *gastric ulcer*, and liver disorders, such as *hepatitis*. Many infectious diseases (*influenza*, for example) can also cause loss of appetite.

Between the ages of about two and four, some children go through a phase of refusing food. If there are no other symptoms, this period of food refusal should be regarded as a normal part of child development.

For a person who is otherwise healthy, a period of two or three days

without food is not harmful, provided that plenty of nonalcoholic fluids are drunk. However, if there are other health problems, particularly *diabetes mellitus*, or if regular medication is being taken, a doctor should always be consulted.

All cases of loss of appetite that last for more than a few days should be investigated by a doctor. Appetite generally returns to normal once any underlying illness has been treated. (See also *Appetite stimulants*.)

Appetite stimulants

There are no known drugs that safely and effectively stimulate the appetite. Lost appetite usually returns when an underlying illness subsides. A variety of drugs (including alcohol, and elixirs containing small quantities of iron, quinine, and strychnine) have been prescribed, but these are rarely effective when there is an underlying physical illness.

Appetite suppressants

COMMON DRUGS
Diethylproprion Fenfluramine Phentermine
These drugs are generally not recommended.

A group of drugs that reduce the desire to eat. Appetite suppressants may be used in the treatment of *obesity*, along with advice on diet and exercise. Some appetite suppressants are nervous system stimulants that are thought to suppress appetite by affecting the *hypothalamus* (part of the brain). Others are bulking agents that, when taken with water before a meal, swell in the stomach to give a feeling of fullness.

POSSIBLE ADVERSE EFFECTS

Adverse effects include dry mouth, dizziness, palpitations, nervousness, restlessness, and difficulty getting to sleep. These symptoms usually disappear after a few days of treatment. Bulking agents may cause flatulence, abdominal pain, and a bloated feeling.

Taking a stimulant appetite suppressant regularly for longer than about six weeks may lead to dependence (see *Drug dependence*). Newer appetite suppressants are less addictive than the *amphetamine drugs* that used to be prescribed.

Apraxia

An inability to carry out purposeful movements despite normal muscle power and coordination. Apraxia is caused by damage to nerve tracts within the cerebrum (the main mass of the brain) that translate the idea for a movement into an actual movement. People with apraxia usually know what they want to do but appear to have lost the ability to recall from memory the sequence of actions necessary to achieve the movement. The damage to the cerebrum may be caused by a direct *head injury*, infection, *stroke*, or *brain tumour*.

TYPES AND SYMPTOMS
Various forms of apraxia are known, each related to damage within different parts of the brain. A person with ideomotor apraxia is unable to carry out a spoken command to make a particular movement—for example, to lick his or her lips—but at other times can be seen making precisely the same movement unconsciously.

Agraphia (difficulty in writing) and expressive *aphasia* (severe difficulty in expressing language) are special forms of apraxia.

TREATMENT AND OUTLOOK
Recovery from events such as a stroke or head injury, and from accompanying syndromes such as apraxia, is highly variable. In most cases, some deficit remains, and it may require considerable effort and patience to relearn lost skills.

APUD cell tumour
A growth, sometimes called an apudoma, composed of cells that produce various hormones. These cells—amine precursor uptake and decarboxylation (APUD) cells—occur in different parts of the body. The cells are similar wherever they are found.

Some tumours of the thyroid gland, pancreas, and lungs are APUD cell tumours, as are a *carcinoid* tumour and *phaeochromocytoma* (a type of adrenal tumour).

Arachnodactyly
Long, thin, spider-like fingers and toes that sometimes occur spontaneously but are characteristic of *Marfan's syndrome*, an inherited connective tissue disease.

Arachnoiditis
An uncommon condition characterized by chronic inflammation and thickening of the arachnoid mater, the middle of the three *meninges* (membranes that cover and protect the brain and spinal cord).

Arachnoiditis may develop up to several years after an episode of *meningitis* (infection of the meninges) or a *subarachnoid haemorrhage* (bleeding beneath the arachnoid). It may be a feature of *syphilis* or of *ankylosing spondylitis* (a disorder affecting the spine). Arachnoiditis may also result from injury or follow procedures, such as *myelography*, in which radiopaque dye is injected into the spinal canal. Usually, however, no cause is found.

The signs and symptoms vary with the extent of the disorder. Arachnoiditis may cause headaches, epileptic seizures, blindness, or slowly progressive spastic paralysis (difficulties with movements due to increased muscle tension) that may affect both legs or all four limbs. There is no effective treatment.

ARC
Abbreviation for *AIDS-related complex*. (See also *AIDS*.)

Arcus senilis
A grey-white ring near the edge of the *cornea* (the transparent front part of the eyeball) that occurs in most elderly people. The ring overlies the outer rim of the iris and is encircled by a narrow zone of unaffected cornea. Arcus senilis is caused by degeneration of fatty material within the cornea.

Arcus senilis develops gradually during adult life, usually starting in the lower part of the cornea, then appearing in the upper part, and eventually affecting the sides to form a complete ring. The ring never spreads to the centre, does not affect eyesight, and is not believed to be related to health.

A similar phenomenon in the young is called arcus juvenilis; this condition may be associated with *hyperlipidaemias* (a group of disorders in which fat levels in the blood are abnormally high).

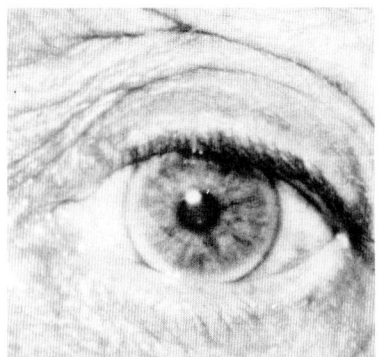

Arcus senilis
The arcus senilis is the lighter ring that overlies the edge of the iris (the coloured part of the eye).

Aromatherapy
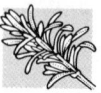
A range of treatments using aromatic oils extracted from plants. Many ancient civilizations, particularly the Chinese, documented the use of essential oils in treating different disorders. Recently, interest in aromatherapy has been rekindled along with other forms of *alternative medicine*. Practitioners claim that aromatherapy can be used to treat a range of disorders, but that it is particularly effective in *psychosomatic* and stress-related conditions.

The patient describes his or her symptoms to the therapist, who chooses the most appropriate oil or oils from a prepared range. The oil is applied in small quantities through massage or is inhaled or incorporated into creams or lotions. Very occasionally the oil is taken internally.

There is no conclusive scientific evidence that the benefits are greater than those that can be achieved by the power of suggestion.

Arousal
The awakening of a person from unconsciousness or semiconsciousness. The term arousal is also used to describe any state of heightened awareness, such as that caused by sexual stimulation or fear. Arousal is regulated by the reticular formation in the *brainstem*.

Arrhenoblastoma
A rare tumour of the ovary, also called andreoblastoma, that occurs in young women. Although the tumour is benign, it secretes *androgen hormones* (male sex hormones) that cause *virilization* (the development of male sex characteristics). Treatment is by surgical removal of the affected ovary.

Arrhythmia, cardiac
An abnormality of the rhythm or rate of the *heartbeat*. Arrhythmia is caused by a disturbance in the electrical impulses within the *heart* (see box opposite). Any isolated irregular beat is called an *ectopic beat* (which does not necessarily indicate the presence of an abnormality).

TYPES
Arrhythmias can be divided into two main groups: the tachycardias, in which the rate is faster than normal (more than 100 beats per minute), and the bradycardias, in which the rate is slower than normal (fewer than 60 beats per minute). The rhythm may be regular, as in the normal heartbeat,

with each beat of the atria (upper chambers) being followed by one beat of the ventricles (lower chambers), or it may be irregular. The beat may originate at the sinoatrial node or in some other area of the heart.

TACHYCARDIAS In *sinus tachycardia*, the rate is raised (100 to 160 beats per minute), the rhythm is regular, and the beat originates in the sinoatrial node. *Supraventricular tachycardia* is faster (with a rate of 120 to 200 beats per minute), the rhythm is regular, and the beat may arise anywhere in the conducting tissue above the ventricles. When rapid, irregular heartbeats (120 to 200 beats per minute) originate in the ventricles, it is called *ventricular tachycardia*.

In *atrial flutter*, the atria beat regularly and very rapidly (200 to 400 beats per minute), but not every impulse reaches the ventricles, which beat at a rate of about 100 to 200 beats per minute. Totally uncoordinated beating of the atria at about 300 to 500 beats per minute is called *atrial fibrillation* and produces completely irregular ventricular beats.

Ventricular fibrillation is a form of cardiac arrest in which the ventricles twitch very rapidly in a completely disorganized manner.

BRADYCARDIAS A slow, regular beat is called *sinus bradycardia*. In *heart block*, the conduction of electrical impulses through the heart muscle is partly or completely blocked, leading to slow, irregular beating. Periods of bradycardia may alternate with periods of tachycardia due to a fault in impulse generation (see *Sick sinus syndrome*).

CAUSES
A common cause of arrhythmia is *coronary artery disease*. In this condition, vessels supplying blood to the heart are narrowed by *atheroma* (fatty deposits) and are unable to supply sufficient blood to the conducting tissue, which becomes damaged as a result. Arrhythmias due to coronary artery disease come on more frequently after a *myocardial infarction* (heart attack).

Sinus tachycardia may be a normal response to exercise or stress; likewise, sinus bradycardia often occurs in healthy athletes.

Caffeine and other drugs can cause tachycardia in some individuals. *Amitriptyline* and some other *antidepressant drugs* can cause serious cardiac arrhythmias if taken in high doses.

SYMPTOMS
Sudden onset of tachycardia can cause palpitations, in which the individual becomes aware of an abnormally fast heartbeat. Any sudden arrhythmia can cause faintness or dizziness due to reduction of blood flow to the brain. If a bradycardia reduces the flow of blood to the lungs, breathing difficulty may occur. If there is underlying heart disease, arrhythmia may lead to *angina pectoris* (chest pain due to reduced blood supply) or *heart failure*.

DIAGNOSIS
The doctor makes a preliminary assessment by feeling the patient's pulse and listening to the heart. The type of arrhythmia is confirmed by an *ECG*, which shows the pattern of electrical activity within heart muscle. In some cases, if the arrhythmia is intermittent, it may be necessary to make continuous ECG recordings for 24 hours using a portable monitor.

TREATMENT
Many different drugs can be used to treat arrhythmias (see *Antiarrhythmic drugs*). When an arrhythmia occurs suddenly after a myocardial infarction, *defibrillation* (application of a short electric shock to the heart) may be necessary to restore the heartbeat to normal.

Artificial *pacemakers* can be used to stimulate heartbeats in cases of heart block. Pacemakers usually consist of a small generating unit implanted under the skin of the chest wall that passes electrical impulses to the heart by means of electrodes.

Arrowroot
A starchy substance obtained from the roots of the West Indian plant *MARANTA ARUNDINACEA*. Traditionally, arrowroot was mixed to a paste with milk or water for use as an easily digestible invalid or baby food.

Arsenic
A metallic element that occurs naturally in its pure form and in various chemical compounds. The term arsenic is also popularly used to refer to the poisonous compound arsenic trioxide.

Arsenic is present in trace amounts in water and many foods and, as a result, most people have minute quantities in their bodies, particularly in their hair and skin.

CARDIAC ARRHYTHMIA

Any disorder that interferes with the generation or transmission of impulses through the heart's electrical conducting system (below) can lead to a disturbance of cardiac rate or rhythm. These ECG recordings show two kinds of arrhythmia: sinus bradycardia and atrial fibrillation.

Sinoatrial node
This is the heart's natural pacemaker from which electrical impulses originate. The impulses spread over the atria, causing them to contract.

Right atrium

Left atrium

Atrioventricular node
Impulses from the sinoatrial node travel to this second node, from which they spread to the ventricles, causing contractions that follow the atrial beats.

Left ventricle

Right ventricle

1 second

1 second

Sinus bradycardia
The heart rate is slow but the rhythm normal, with each atrial beat (small rise) followed by a ventricular beat (spike). Sinus bradycardia is common in athletes, but can also be caused by hypothyroidism.

Atrial fibrillation
The atria beat rapidly and irregularly. Ventricular beats (spikes) do not follow each atrial beat and are irregularly spaced. This arrhythmia is common in the elderly and in people with hyperthyroidism.

A

POISONING

Arsenic has been used intentionally to murder, particularly in fiction, but most poisoning occurs through accidental ingestion, particularly in rural areas, where arsenic is an important constituent of some pesticides. Industrial poisoning from arsenic is nowadays quite rare.

Arsenic poisoning may be acute or chronic. Acute poisoning primarily affects the lining of the intestine and causes the sudden onset of painful symptoms. The victim experiences nausea, vomiting (sometimes with blood in the vomit), diarrhoea, excessive sweating, and burning of the throat, followed by collapse and death if the poisoning is not treated.

Chronic poisoning is usually first noticeable as weakness, tiredness, scaly skin, *keratosis* (thickening of the skin), "raindrop" pigmentation of the skin, and swelling of the lining of the mouth. *Neuropathy* (degeneration of nerves) then sets in, producing tingling and then numbness in the hands and feet. Prolonged absorption of arsenic may cause cancer of the skin and lungs.

INVESTIGATION AND TREATMENT

Arsenic poisoning, once suspected, may be confirmed by analysis of the urine. Treatment of acute poisoning includes washing out the stomach (see *Lavage, gastric*), replacement of lost fluids, treatment for *shock* and pain, and administration of dimercaprol, a drug that helps remove the poison from the body. Chronic poisoning is also treated with dimercaprol.

Arterial reconstructive surgery

An operation to repair arteries that are narrowed, blocked, or weakened.

WHY IT IS DONE

Arterial reconstructive surgery is most often performed to repair arteries narrowed or blocked by *atherosclerosis* (fatty deposits on artery walls). The procedure is also used to repair *aneurysms* (ballooning of blood vessels), which may be *congenital* or due to atherosclerosis. Arterial reconstructive surgery can also be used to repair arteries that have been damaged as a result of injury.

HOW IT IS DONE

A narrowed or blocked section of artery can be bypassed by sewing in a length of vein—usually taken from the patient's leg—above and below the constricted area. This technique is commonly used for coronary arteries (see *Coronary artery bypass*).

For damaged arteries elsewhere in the body, it is more common to cut out the affected section and replace it with an artificial tube or a section of vein taken from another part of the body.

OUTLOOK

Arterial reconstructive surgery is generally successful, depending on the age and health of the patient. Reconstruction of the *aorta* (the main artery carrying blood from the heart) has an operative death rate of up to five per cent, but the risks associated with rupture of an untreated aneurysm are greater. (See also *Angioplasty, balloon*; *Endarterectomy*.)

Arteries, disorders of

Disorders of the arteries may take the form of abnormal narrowing (which reduces blood flow and may cause tissue damage), complete obstruction (which may cause tissue death), or abnormal widening and thinning of an artery wall (which may cause rupture of the blood vessel).

TYPES

ATHEROSCLEROSIS This disorder, in which fat deposits build up on the lining of the artery wall, affects most adults to some extent and is the most common arterial disease. Atherosclerosis can involve arteries throughout the body, including the brain (see *Cerebrovascular disease*), the heart (see *Coronary artery disease*), and the legs (see *Peripheral vascular disease*). Atherosclerosis is the main type of *arteriosclerosis*, a group of disorders that cause thickening and loss of elasticity of artery walls.

HYPERTENSION High blood pressure is another common cause of thickening and narrowing of arteries. Hypertension predisposes people to coronary artery disease and increases the risk of a *stroke* or *kidney failure*.

ARTERITIS This term refers to a group of disorders in which inflammation of artery walls causes narrowing and sometimes blockage.

ANEURYSM This thinning and ballooning of an artery wall may be due to a congenital defect or to atherosclerosis. An aortic aneurysm may result from *aortitis* (inflammation of the aorta wall), which may be part of a generalized arteritis or, rarely today, due to untreated syphilis.

THROMBOSIS A thrombus (blood clot) may form within an artery, causing partial or complete obstruction of the blood flow. Thrombosis occurs most commonly in areas that have already been damaged by atherosclerosis or aneurysm.

EMBOLISM This is the term for obstruction of an artery by an embolus (usually a fragment of thrombus that has broken off from a larger vessel or from the wall of the heart, although it may consist of fat particles from a bone fracture or an air bubble that has formed as a result of a decompression accident in a diver).

RAYNAUD'S DISEASE This is a disorder involving intermittent spasm of small arteries in the hands and feet, usually due to cold. The obstruction to blood flow causes a change in skin colour, numbness, and pins-and-needles. Occasionally, if the obstruction lasts, skin damage and an ischaemic ulcer (see *Ischaemia*) may result.

DIAGNOSIS AND TREATMENT

For the diagnosis and treatment of disorders affecting the arteries, see individual entries on specific disorders.

Arteriography

Another name for *angiography*, a technique for imaging blood vessels.

Arteriole

A blood vessel that branches off an *artery*. Arterioles themselves branch to form *capillaries*. Arterioles are intermediate in size and structure between arteries and capillaries. Arterioles have a high proportion of smooth muscle in their walls, and their nerve supply enables them to be narrowed or widened to meet decreases or increases in the blood-flow needs of the tissues they supply.

Arteriopathy

Any abnormal condition or disorder of an artery. (See *Arteries, disorders of*.)

Arterioplasty

Surgical repair of an artery (see *Arterial reconstructive surgery*).

Arteriosclerosis

A group of disorders that cause thickening and loss of elasticity of artery walls. *Atherosclerosis* is the most common type of arteriosclerosis. Other types include medial arteriosclerosis (in which muscle and elastic fibres from the lining of large and medium-sized arteries are replaced by fibrous tissue) and Monckeberg's arteriosclerosis (in which there are deposits of calcium in the lining of arteries).

Arteriovenous fistula

An abnormal communication or malformation between an artery and a vein. An arteriovenous fistula may be present at birth or may result from injury or infection. A fistula can also be created surgically to provide an easy route of access into the bloodstream. This procedure is useful for people receiving *dialysis*.

If the fistula is close to the skin surface, it may cause a small, pulsating swelling. If several fistulas are present in the lungs, they can impair the uptake of oxygen into the blood, causing *cyanosis* (blue skin colour), breathing difficulty during exertion, and sometimes *coughing up blood*.

If an isolated fistula is causing symptoms, it is usually cut away and the ends of the blood vessels stitched. If there are large numbers of fistulas, surgery is not practicable. Some arteriovenous malformations in inaccessible areas of the brain are treated by *radiotherapy*.

Arteritis

Inflammation of an artery wall, causing narrowing or complete obstruction of the affected artery, reduced blood flow, and, in some cases, *thrombosis* and damage to tissues.

Buerger's disease is an arteritis that affects the limbs, causing pain, numbness, and, in severe cases, *gangrene*.

Polyarteritis nodosa, a serious *autoimmune disorder* (in which the body's defence mechanisms attack its own tissues), can affect arteries in any part of the body, especially the heart and kidneys. It may also cause symptoms such as abdominal and testicular pain, chest pain, breathing difficulty, and tender lumps under the skin.

Temporal arteritis affects arteries in the scalp over the temples, causing headache and scalp tenderness; if the retinal artery is affected, there is a risk of permanent blindness.

A very rare type of arteritis is Takayasu's arteritis, which is thought to be an autoimmune disorder. This disorder usually affects young women and involves the arteries that branch from the first part of the *aorta* into the neck and arms.

Artery

A blood vessel that carries blood away from the *heart*. Systemic arteries carry blood pumped from the left ventricle (lower chamber) of the heart to all parts of the body except the lungs. The largest systemic artery (in fact, the largest artery in the body) is the *aorta*, which emerges directly from the left ventricle; other major systemic arteries branch off from the aorta.

The pulmonary arteries carry blood from the right ventricle of the heart to the lungs. Pulmonary arteries are shorter, thinner-walled, and contain blood under a lower pressure than systemic arteries.

STRUCTURE AND FUNCTION
Arteries are pliable tubes with thick walls that enable them to withstand the high blood pressure to which they are subjected on each heartbeat.

The structure of arteries helps even out the peaks and troughs of blood pressure caused by the heartbeat, so that the blood is flowing at a relatively constant pressure by the time it reaches the smaller blood vessels. These smaller vessels include the *arterioles*, which branch directly off the artery. The arterioles connect to the even smaller *capillaries*. (See also *Arteries, disorders of*.)

STRUCTURE OF AN ARTERY
An artery's walls consist of three layers: a smooth, inner lining, a thick, muscular, elastic, middle layer, and a tough, fibrous outer covering. Veins have thinner walls and most contain valves.

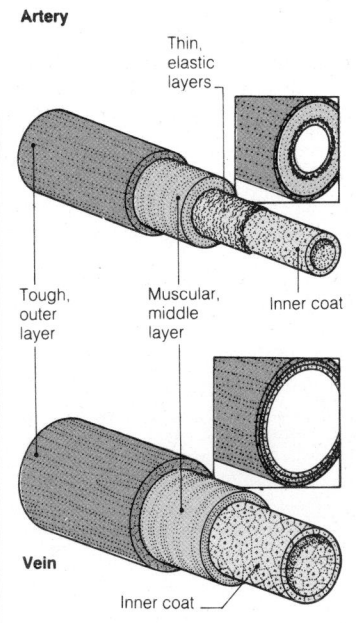

Artery

Thin, elastic layers

Tough, outer layer

Muscular, middle layer

Inner coat

Vein

Inner coat

Arthralgia

A term meaning pain in the joints or in a single joint. (See also *Arthritis*; *Joint*.)

Arthritis

Inflammation of a joint, characterized by pain, swelling, and stiffness. Arthritis is not a single disorder but the name for joint disease from a number of causes. The arthritis may involve one joint or many, and can vary in severity from a mild ache and stiffness to severe pain and, later, joint deformity.

TYPES AND CAUSES
OSTEOARTHRITIS Also known as degenerative arthritis or osteoarthrosis, this is the most common type of arthritis. It results from wear and tear on the joints, although metabolic, genetic and other factors may also contribute. It evolves in middle age, and most commonly troubles older people.

RHEUMATOID ARTHRITIS The most severe type of inflammatory joint disease, rheumatoid arthritis is an *autoimmune disorder* in which the body's *immune system* acts against and damages joints and surrounding soft tissues. Many joints—most commonly those in the hands, wrists, feet, and arms—become extremely painful, stiff, and deformed. Typically, the symptoms occur in people younger than those with osteoarthritis and it is more common in women.

STILL'S DISEASE Also called juvenile rheumatoid arthritis, this disorder is most common in children under the age of four. It usually clears up after a few years, but even then may stunt growth and leave the child with permanent deformities.

SERONEGATIVE ARTHRITIS This is a group of disorders that cause symptoms and signs of arthritis in a number of joints, although blood test results for rheumatoid arthritis are negative. Seronegative arthritis can be associated with skin disorders (such as *psoriasis*), inflammatory intestinal disorders (such as *Crohn's disease*), or autoimmune disorders.

INFECTIVE ARTHRITIS Also known as septic or pyogenic arthritis, this joint disease is caused by the invasion of bacteria into the joint from a nearby infected wound or from *bacteraemia* (infection in the bloodstream). The infected joint usually becomes warm and red as well as painful and swollen. In countries where *tuberculosis* is widespread, infective arthritis may result from invasion of the joint by tubercle bacilli.

Arthritis may also occur as a complication of an infection elsewhere in the body, such as *chickenpox*, *rubella* (German measles), *mumps*, *rheumatic fever*, or *gonorrhoea*; it may also be a complication of *nonspecific urethritis*, in which case the joint inflammation forms part of *Reiter's syndrome*.

ANKYLOSING SPONDYLITIS In this arthritis of the pelvic joints and the spine, the joints linking the vertebrae (spinal bones) become inflamed and the vertebrae fuse. This type of arthritis may also involve other joints, usually the hips and knees.

GOUT This disorder is associated with a form of arthritis in which uric acid (one of the body's waste products) accumulates in joints in the form of crystals, causing inflammation. Gout usually affects one joint at a time.

DIAGNOSIS

The diagnosis is made from the patient's symptoms and signs. To discover the cause, fluid may be withdrawn through a needle from an affected joint. This fluid may then be examined microscopically for the presence of microorganisms, or uric acid or other crystals. Sometimes a *culture* is made from the fluid so that it can be analysed for any infection.

X-rays may be carried out to reveal the type and extent of joint damage. *Blood tests* can reveal the presence of proteins typical of rheumatoid arthritis; a high level of uric acid indicative of gout; or sometimes a high *ESR* (erythrocyte sedimentation rate), indicating inflammation.

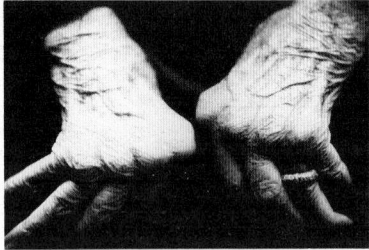

Arthritis in the hands
Severely deformed joints in the hands of an elderly woman who is suffering from rheumatoid arthritis.

TREATMENT

There are specific treatments for the different types of arthritis—for example, *antibiotic drugs* for septic arthritis, *anti-inflammatory drugs* for treating rheumatoid arthritis and osteoarthritis, and *allopurinol* for gout. Many other drugs are used to treat different forms of arthritis, but none seems able to effect a cure.

In a severe attack of arthritis affecting several joints, a few days' bed rest will help settle the inflammation; individual joints can be splinted to reduce the pain, and heat and supervised exercises help keep joint deformity to a minimum. Obese people with arthritis in weight-bearing joints should lose weight.

Diseased joints that have become extremely painful, unstable, or deformed may require *arthroplasty* (replacement of a joint with an artificial substitute) or *arthrodesis* (fusion of the bones in a joint).

OUTLOOK

Arthritis has many forms and varies widely in its effects. Only a few sufferers become severely disabled. Most are able to lead productive lives, although activities may need to be modified to preserve joint function.

Arthrodesis

A surgical procedure in which the two bones in a diseased joint are fused to prevent the joint from moving.

WHY IT IS DONE

If pain and deformity in a diseased joint—caused, for example, by *rheumatoid arthritis*—are so severe that they cannot be relieved by drugs, splinting, and *physiotherapy*, or if a joint has become unstable (usually as the result of an injury), some form of surgery is required. In most cases, the operation of first choice is *arthroplasty* (reconstruction of a diseased joint using artificial replacements), because this procedure retains movement in the joint. However, when arthroplasty is not feasible or fails, arthrodesis may be used.

HOW IT IS DONE

A local anaesthetic may be all that is required for a small joint, such as a finger joint. Otherwise, a general anaesthetic is used. The technique of the operation varies according to the joint being treated, but in most cases cartilage (smooth, shock-absorbing tissue) is removed from the ends of the two bones, along with a surface layer of bone from each. The two ends are then joined so that, when fresh bone cells grow, the ends will fuse. The bones may need to be kept in position with plates, rods, or screws; a *bone graft* may also be carried out in some cases.

In arthrodesis of the knee or ankle, additional immobilization of the joint—by transfixing it with pins inserted through the skin—may be necessary to keep the area stable until healing is complete.

RECOVERY PERIOD

Complete union of the bones can take up to six months but is usually much quicker. In some cases the bones fail to fuse, but often this is irrelevant because fibrous tissue fills the gap between them and is strong enough to provide the same effect and strength as bone fusion.

OUTLOOK

One advantage of arthrodesis over arthroplasty is that, once performed, it needs no regular surveillance or further care; the patient can be reasonably certain that the problem with the joint has been solved permanently.

Arthrography

A diagnostic technique in which the interior of a damaged joint is X-rayed after injection of a radiopaque solution (a solution visible on X-ray) into the joint. The procedure is gradually being replaced by *MRI*, *ultrasound scanning*, and *arthroscopy*.

Arthrogryposis

See *Contracture*.

Arthropathy

A medical term for *joint* disease.

Arthroplasty

Replacement of a joint or part of a joint by metal or plastic components. *Hip replacements* were the first operations of this type to be introduced but replacement of the knee (see *Knee-joint replacement*) has become just as successful and is now performed on similar numbers of patients. Replacement of other joints, including the finger (see *Finger-joint replacement*), shoulder, and elbow, is also routine.

The first attempts to replace part of a damaged hip joint with an artificial substitute were made in the 1930s. In the 1960s, hip replacement operations were revolutionized by developments on three fronts. First, metal and plastic materials were developed that were strong enough to allow a good level of activity while being to some extent self-lubricating; second, cement was used to help fix the artificial joint to the bones; and third, the risk of infection in the joint—a very serious complication—was greatly reduced by the use of *antibiotic drugs*. In many hospitals the surgery is performed in an operating theatre in which the air is filtered and all members of the surgical team wear sterile, all-enveloping clothing.

These principles have now been applied to the full range of replacement joints. Engineers and orthopaedic surgeons are still developing and improving replacement joints of all kinds.

Arthroscopy

Inspection through an *endoscope* (a viewing tube) of the interior of a joint, usually for the purpose of diagnosing a condition affecting that joint. Arthroscopy has rapidly become one of the most frequently performed procedures in orthopaedic surgery, thanks to the development of modern lens systems and brighter lighting by means of fibre-optics.

WHY IT IS DONE

Arthroscopy is most frequently used to inspect the inside of the knee joint. Many conditions affecting the knee do not show up on X-rays and are difficult to diagnose on the basis of symptoms alone. Arthroscopy allows the surgeon to see the surfaces of the bones that come into contact in the joint, the ligaments and cartilages within the joint, and the synovial membrane that lines the internal surface of the joint capsule. Specimens of these structures can be removed for examination and analysis.

Some surgical procedures that used to involve making a large incision to expose the interior of the knee can now be performed arthroscopically. Instruments have been devised that fold down as they are passed through a channel in the arthroscope. Procedures include removal of damaged cartilage, repair of torn cartilage and ligaments, and shaving or drilling the surface of the patella (kneecap). Arthroscopic surgery substantially reduces the time a patient needs to stay in hospital, and the time an athlete is unable to participate in his or her sport.

Artificial insemination

The introduction of semen into the cervix (opening of the uterus) by means of an instrument instead of by sexual intercourse, with the aim of inducing conception and pregnancy.

TYPES

There are two principal types of artificial insemination.

AIH (artificial insemination using the husband's semen) is the use of semen from the woman's permanent sexual partner. It is usually employed for couples who are unable to have intercourse, either because of psychosexual difficulties, such as impotence, or because of physical injury or deformity. Occasionally, AIH may be used when the husband has a low sperm count or a low volume of ejaculate, or if factors such as antibodies in the woman's genital tract create a hostile environment for the sperm. It is also used when semen has been stored from a man who is to undergo treatment (such as chemotherapy) that may make him sterile.

Donor insemination, sometimes called AID (artificial insemination of a donor's semen), is the use of semen from an anonymous donor. It is available to couples if the man is infertile, has a genetic disease, or may be a carrier of such a disease. It may also be used by a woman who wants children but has no male partner.

HOW IT IS DONE

Artificial insemination is carried out at centres that are specially staffed and equipped to obtain and store semen, to carry out the insemination, and to give counselling before and after the procedure.

Fresh semen is usually used for AIH. Donor semen is frozen in liquid nitrogen and then stored; before it is used, the semen is tested to ensure that it does not contain any infection-causing microorganisms. Semen donors must be in good health and are usually screened for as many physical and mental disorders as possible. The viruses causing hepatitis B (see *Hepatitis, viral*) and *AIDS* have been transmitted through donor insemination. To prevent this, all stored semen is placed in quarantine until the donor has been tested for antibodies to these viruses and until test results have been negative on two occasions three months apart. There is no safeguard against the use of sperm from a man who is an unwitting carrier of a genetic disease.

Insemination is carried out by injecting semen into the woman's cervix with a small syringe. Two or three

---

HOW ARTHROSCOPY IS DONE

The procedure is usually performed under general anaesthesia, but sometimes a *nerve block* is used. The joint is distended by injecting air or a saline solution; the instrument is inserted into the joint through a small skin incision. While watching through the endoscope, the surgeon can probe or lift structures to check for damage.

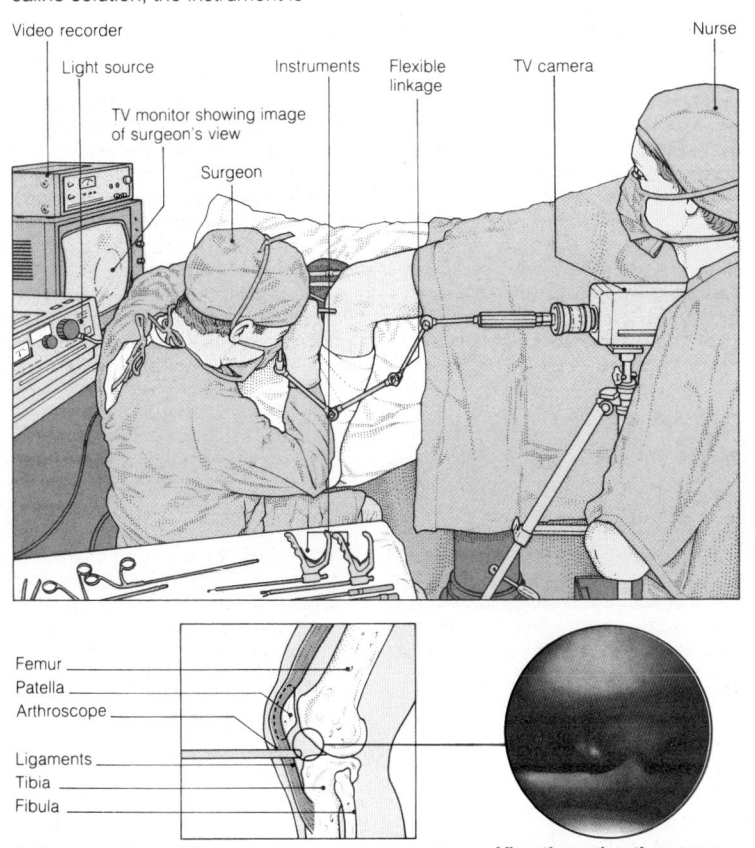

Video recorder
Light source
TV monitor showing image of surgeon's view
Instruments
Flexible linkage
TV camera
Nurse
Surgeon

Femur
Patella
Arthroscope
Ligaments
Tibia
Fibula

Arthroscope in position
An arthroscope is a steel tube containing optical fibres, a lens and a light source.

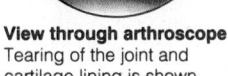

View through arthroscope
Tearing of the joint and cartilage lining is shown.

inseminations are carried out during the two to four optimum days for conception in the woman's menstrual cycle and, unless pregnancy occurs, this procedure is repeated for up to five more cycles.

RESULTS

When fresh semen is used, the success rate of artificial insemination in bringing about pregnancy over a six-month period is 60 to 70 per cent. With semen that has been frozen, the success rate is 55 per cent.

Artificial kidney

The common name for the machine used in *dialysis*.

Artificial respiration

Forced introduction of air into the lungs of someone who has stopped breathing (see *Respiratory arrest*) or of someone whose breathing is inadequate. Artificial respiration may be administered by the mouth-to-mouth or mouth-to-nose method. It may also be given by the use of ventilating equipment administered by anaesthetists (see *Ventilation*).

WHY IT IS DONE

Artificial respiration should be started as soon as possible after someone has stopped breathing; delay in breathing for more than six minutes can cause death. When someone has stopped breathing, there is no rise-and-fall movement of the chest or abdomen, the face becomes blue-grey, and no exhaled breath can be felt. When there is no breathing, it is likely that the heart has stopped beating. If no pulse can be felt in the wrist or neck, cardiac compressions should be carried out in conjunction with artificial respiration (see *Cardiopulmonary resuscitation*).

When breathing is weak or shallow, movements of the chest are minimal and hardly any breath can be felt. If breathing is not restored, the brain is deprived of oxygen; permanent brain damage or death can result.

HOW IT IS DONE

MOUTH-TO-MOUTH RESUSCITATION This is the simplest and most effective method of introducing air into a victim's lungs (see illustrated box). Mouth-to-mouth resuscitation is safe to use on a person whose breathing is weak, shallow, or laboured. Time your exhalations with the victim's inhalations (if any are present).

MOUTH-TO-NOSE RESUSCITATION If the victim has a facial injury, it may be difficult for you to breathe into his or her mouth. In such cases, follow steps 1 and 2 shown in the box. Remove your

hand from the back of the victim's neck and close his or her mouth by lifting the chin. Take a deep breath and seal your mouth around the victim's nose. Blow strongly into the nose. Remove your mouth and hold the victim's mouth open with your hand, so that air can escape. Repeat as for mouth-to-mouth resuscitation every five seconds.

RESUSCITATION OF BABIES AND CHILDREN The method of resuscitating a baby or young child is basically the same as the method of resuscitating an adult, except that you will find it easier to

seal your mouth over both the mouth and nose of the child. Do not tip the child's head back very far, because a child's neck and airway are more fragile than an adult's. Blow gentle breaths of air into the lungs, one breath every two to three seconds (20 to 30 breaths per minute) until the child's chest starts to rise.

Artificial sweeteners

Synthetic substitutes for sugar used by people on slimming diets, by diabetics, and by the food industry. Although saccharin and aspartame

---

FIRST AID: ARTIFICIAL RESPIRATION

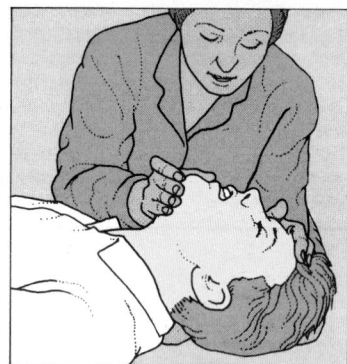

1 If someone stops breathing, send for medical help, but start resuscitation immediately. Lay the victim on his or her back on a rigid surface. If there are no signs of neck injury, gently tilt the victim's head backwards to open the airway. Do this by pressing down on the forehead with one hand while lifting the chin with the fingers of the other hand.

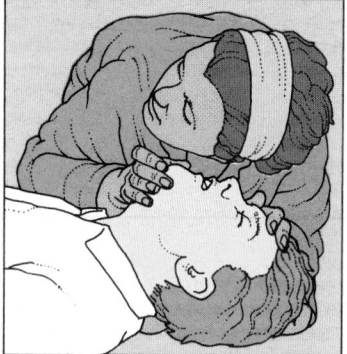

2 Sometimes breathing is restored when the airway is opened by this head tilt, chin lift manoeuvre. Look, listen, and feel for this. See if the chest rises and falls. Place your ear and cheek close to the victim's nose and mouth to hear and feel exhaled air. If none of these signs are present, the victim is not breathing and needs artificial respiration right away.

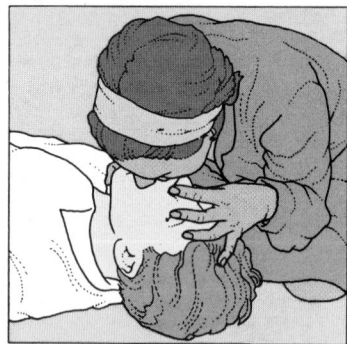

3 Using the hand you have on the victim's forehead, pinch the nose shut with your thumb and index finger. Take a deep breath, seal your mouth around the victim's, and deliver two full breaths, allowing for full deflation of the victim's chest before giving the second. Maintain the head tilt, chin lift throughout, or air may not enter the lungs.

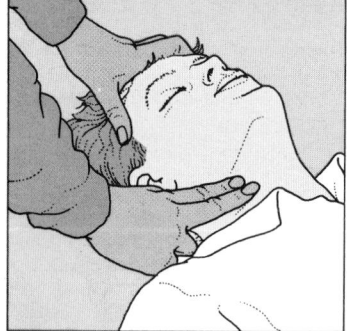

4 Remove your mouth. Check the carotid pulse for seven seconds by placing your index and middle fingers in the hollow between the Adam's apple and the side muscles of the neck. If there is a pulse, but no breathing, continue giving one breath every five seconds until breathing is restored or medical help arrives.

are often recommended for use in slimming diets, they are of questionable value because the appetite compensates for the lack of calories from sugar, and other foods are eaten to maintain the calorie intake.

TYPES
SACCHARIN is 500 to 600 times sweeter than sugar (sucrose), although it has a sour after-taste and provides no calories. It is not suitable for use in baking. Saccharin has been associated with bladder cancer in animal experiments but the risk of associated cancer in humans is negligible.

CYCLAMATE is about 30 times as sweet as sugar, and provides no calories. Unlike saccharin, it can be used in baking without going bitter. Cyclamate was banned in some countries in the late 1960s after it was suspected of causing cancer in animals.

ASPARTAME is about 200 times sweeter than sugar—although its sweetness is destroyed by prolonged heating—and is virtually calorie free in the amounts used. It has no known adverse effects when taken in normal quantities but excessive quantities may cause neurological disorders.

SORBITOL is a sugar substitute that occurs naturally in certain fruits. It is a sugar alcohol which has no effect on the teeth and is used in "sugar-free" sweets and chewing gums. It is used by diabetics but its high calorie value—about 490 kcal (2,050 kJ) per 100 g—makes it unsuitable for use in slimming diets. One problem with using sorbitol is that its slow absorption from the intestine into the bloodstream may cause diarrhoea by drawing fluid into the intestine.

ACESULPHAME is another synthetic sweetener. It is about 130 times as sweet as sugar and is calorie free.

Asbestos-induced diseases
A variety of diseases caused by the inhalation of asbestos fibres. Asbestos is a fibrous mineral formerly used a great deal as a heat- and fire-resistant insulating material. It is also used in brake linings and gaskets. Its use for insulation has declined dramatically over the past 20 years.

TYPES
ASBESTOSIS In this condition, widespread fine scarring occurs in the lungs; this tends to progress even when exposure to asbestos is discontinued. The disease causes breathlessness and a dry cough, eventually leading to severe disability and death.

Asbestosis develops mostly in people who have been heavily exposed to asbestos, such as asbestos miners, workers in asbestos factories, and workers who handle insulation materials. The period from first exposure to development of the disease is seldom less than 10 years and is usually much longer.

Diagnosis is by chest X-ray, which shows widespread shadowing if asbestosis is present. Asbestosis increases the risk of developing *lung cancer* about five-fold in smokers and nonsmokers alike; the combination of cigarette smoking and asbestosis leads to death from lung cancer in about one third of sufferers.

Asbestosis is a *prescribed disease*, which entitles the sufferer to industrial injury benefit. If lung cancer has developed, this is taken into account for the purpose of assessing benefit.

MESOTHELIOMA This is a malignant tumour of the *pleura* (the membrane that surrounds the lungs) or the *peritoneum* (the membrane that lines the abdominal cavity and covers the abdominal organs). In the pleura, mesotheliomas cause pain and breathlessness; tumours in the peritoneum cause enlargement of the abdomen and intestinal obstruction.

There is no treatment for the condition, which usually leads to death within one or two years. The average interval between the first exposure to asbestos and death is between 20 and 30 years. The condition almost exclusively affects those who have worked with blue or brown asbestos; the risk with white asbestos is almost nil.

This is a prescribed disease and about 600 cases a year are reported in the UK.

BILATERAL DIFFUSE PLEURAL THICKENING In this condition, the outer and inner layers of the pleura become thickened, and excess fluid may accumulate in the cavity between them. This combination restricts the ability of the lungs to expand, resulting in shortness of breath. The condition may develop after even short exposure to asbestos and is a prescribed disease. If lung cancer develops, this is considered attributable to the asbestos exposure for the purpose of industrial injury benefit.

PLEURAL PLAQUES These are areas of thickening, called plaques, confined to the outer layer of the pleura. Pleural plaques do not cause symptoms or disability but are detectable on X-rays. The plaques occur commonly in people who have had substantial exposure to asbestos; detection does not usually take place until 20 or more years after first exposure. Sometimes, plaques appear after only a short duration of exposure. Although pleural plaques indicate past exposure to asbestos, they do not indicate a higher than normal risk of developing other asbestos-related diseases. They do not qualify the sufferer for industrial injury benefit.

OUTLOOK
Most of the cases now being diagnosed are the result of working practices that were in effect before 1970. Since then, the use of asbestos has been carefully controlled; fibreglass is used instead of asbestos in insulating materials, and the importation of blue asbestos has been prohibited. Because of the known association with serious disease, asbestos is now handled much more carefully; there are strictly controlled guidelines for the safe removal of old asbestos-containing insulating materials.

Unfortunately, because of the long time lag between first exposure and the development of disease, it is predicted that cases of pleural plaques and mesothelioma will continue to appear into the next century.

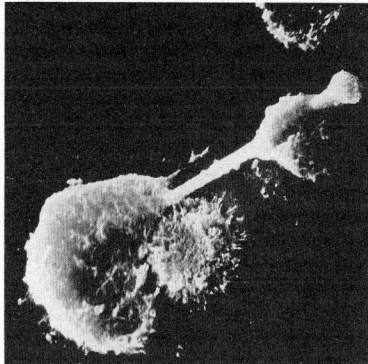

Asbestos fibre in lung
Asbestos is a fibrous mineral that can cause lung disease if inhaled.

Asbestosis
See *Asbestos-induced diseases*.

Ascariasis
Infestation with the worm ASCARIS LUMBRICOIDES. Ascariasis is common worldwide, especially in the tropics. The causative parasite is a pale, cylindrical, tapered roundworm, between 15 and 35 cm in length in adult form, which lives in the small intestine of its human host. One or several worms may be present, but symptoms usually occur only in people with heavy worm infestations.

INCIDENCE AND CAUSES

Ascariasis affects up to 80 to 90 per cent of the population in poorer countries, where children living in rural areas are prone to heavy infestations. In developed countries, such as the UK, less than one per cent of the population have an infestation at any time; these infestations are light and few people are aware of the presence of worms. The disease is spread by ingestion of worm eggs from soil contaminated by human faeces or from uncooked food contaminated with soil containing eggs.

In some dry, windy climates, airborne eggs may be swallowed after being blown into the mouth. The eggs hatch in the intestine, eventually developing into adults, which produce more eggs that are excreted in the faeces. The full cycle of the infestation is shown in the diagram.

SYMPTOMS

Light infestations may cause either no symptoms or occasional nausea, abdominal pain, and irregular bowel movements. A worm may be passed via the rectum or vomited.

A heavy load of worms may compete with the host for food, leading to malnutrition and anaemia, which in children can retard growth.

DIAGNOSIS AND TREATMENT

Ascariasis is diagnosed by finding the worm's eggs during microscopic examination of a person's faeces or, occasionally, finding that an adult worm has been passed in the faeces.

The worm infestation is treated with *anthelmintic drugs*, such as *pyrantel* (which is highly effective in a single dose). The worms are passed via the rectum some days after the drug is taken. The patient usually makes a complete recovery.

Ascites

An excess of fluid in the peritoneal cavity—the space between the two layers of membrane, or peritoneum, that line the inside of the abdominal wall and the outside of the abdominal organs. As much as several litres of fluid may be present, causing abdominal swelling.

CAUSES

Ascites may occur as a feature of any condition that causes generalized *oedema* (excessive accumulation of fluid in the body tissues). The most important of these conditions are congestive *heart failure*, *nephrotic syndrome*, and *cirrhosis* of the liver.

Ascites may occur in *cancer* if metastases (secondary growths) from lung,

LIFE CYCLE OF THE ASCARIS WORM

The person becomes infested by swallowing the eggs. They hatch into larvae in the intestine; the larvae travel in the blood through the wall of the intestine to the lungs, up the windpipe, and are swallowed back into the small intestine. There they become adult worms.

Eggs pass out in faeces to contaminate soil

Food grown in contaminated soil carries eggs to the host

Eggs hatch into larvae in the intestine

Female worms produce large numbers of eggs

Larvae pass in the blood to the lungs

Larvae mature into adult worms in the small intestine

Larvae pass up the wind pipe and are then swallowed

breast, or intestinal tumours are deposited on the surface of the peritoneum. Ascites also occurs when *tuberculosis* affects the abdomen, a condition that is now rare in the UK except among Asian immigrants.

SYMPTOMS

In addition to abdominal swelling and discomfort, ascites may cause breathing difficulty due to pressure on, and immobilization of, the diaphragm, the sheet of muscle that separates the thorax (chest) from the abdomen.

DIAGNOSIS

Ascites is detected during physical examination by a doctor. Diagnosis of the cause involves removing and analysing a sample of ascitic fluid via a sterile needle inserted through the abdominal wall. The fluid is examined under the microscope for malignant cells. Its colour, turbidity (cloudiness), and chemical composition also help identify whether the cause of the ascites is inflammation or a condition such as cirrhosis.

TREATMENT

Treatment depends on the precise cause of the ascites, but in many cases includes bed rest, and fluid and salt (sodium) restriction. Alcohol must not be taken by the patient if liver disease is implicated. *Diuretic drugs*, particularly *spironolactone*, may be prescribed.

If the ascites causes discomfort or breathing difficulty, fluid can be drained from the peritoneal cavity.

Ascorbic acid

The chemical name for *vitamin C*.

Aseptic technique

The creation of a germ-free environment, mainly by the use of *sterilization*, to protect a patient from infection. Aseptic sterilization is distinct from antisepsis, which is the destruction of germs by chemicals (known as *antiseptics*).

WHY IT IS DONE

Aseptic technique is needed for any procedure in which there is a danger of introducing infection into the body. The patient can be contaminated by microorganisms from four main sources: other people, his or her own body, instruments, and the air.

Aseptic technique is used for all surgery in an operating theatre and for other minor surgical procedures, such as inserting a urinary catheter or stitching a wound. Aseptic technique is also needed when caring for patients suffering from diseases, such as *leukaemia*, in which the *immune system* is suppressed and the body's natural defences against infection are reduced as a result.

HOW IT IS DONE

All people who come in contact with the patient must scrub their hands and wear pre-sterilized gowns and disposable gloves and masks. Instruments are sterilized beforehand in an *autoclave* (a chamber containing pressurized steam) and placed ready for use on a trolley that is covered with sterile material.

The area of the patient that is to be operated on is cleaned with antiseptic solutions of *iodine* or *hexachlorophene*, and the surrounding skin is covered with sterile drapes. In addition, before operations on the intestine, the bowel is cleared by giving *laxative drugs* and also sometimes an *enema* to prevent any contamination of the abdominal area by faeces.

When using aseptic technique, care is taken to place used, possibly contaminated, instruments well away from sterile instruments and dressings. In an operating theatre it is important to keep the air and the room scrupulously clean. The windows remain closed and the only air that enters the room is through a special ventilation system that purifies the air and maintains it at a pre-set humidity. (See also *Isolation*.)

Asperger's syndrome

A rare abnormality of development, possibly related to *autism*, that is characterized by subtle abnormalities of social interactions, preoccupation with special interests (such as prehistoric monsters, cars, etc.), and, commonly, by abnormalities of personality (such as a particularly idiosyncratic sense of humour).

The cause is unknown and the disorder is often unrecognized, but it may give rise to major problems of social relationships and oddities of behaviour. Identification of the disorder may help the family to understand the individual's difficulties and allow provision of support and counselling.

Aspergillosis

 An infection caused by aspergillus, a fungus which grows in decaying vegetation; spores of this fungus are usually present in the air all the year round. Aspergillus is harmless to healthy people but causes trouble in certain circumstances. It may grow as a fungus ball in people whose lungs have been damaged by tuberculosis and cause coughing up of blood. In some people with *asthma*, aspergillus grows in the mucus in the bronchi and causes worsening of symptoms and areas of lung collapse. Aspergillus may also cause serious and often fatal infection in people with reduced resistance, such as those with HIV infection, those being treated by *anticancer drugs* for leukaemia or other forms of cancer, or by *immunosuppressant drugs* after *transplant surgery*.

Aspermia

See *Azoospermia*.

Asphyxia

The medical term for suffocation. Asphyxia may be caused by obstruction of a large airway, usually by a foreign body (see *Choking*), by insufficient oxygen in the surrounding air (as occurs when a closed plastic bag is put over the head), or by poisoning with a gas such as carbon monoxide that interferes with the uptake of oxygen into the blood.

The person initially breathes more rapidly and strongly to try to overcome the lack of oxygen in the blood. There is also an increase in heart-rate and blood pressure.

TREATMENT

First-aid treatment consists of *artificial respiration* after first moving the person into the open air and clearing the airway of any obstruction. Untreated asphyxia causes death.

Aspiration

The withdrawal of fluid or tissue from the body by suction. The term also refers to the act of breathing in a foreign body, usually food or drink.

Aspiration *biopsy* is the removal of tissue or fluid for examination by suction through a needle attached to a syringe. The procedure is commonly used to obtain cells from a fluid-filled cavity (such as a breast cyst). It is also used to obtain cells from the bone marrow (see *Bone marrow biopsy*), or from internal organs, when a narrow needle is guided to the site of the biopsy by *CT scanning* or *ultrasound scanning*. The cells obtained are examined under a microscope.

Aspiration pneumonia is inflammation of the lungs due to inhalation of foreign material (e.g. vomit or infected respiratory secretions).

Aspirin

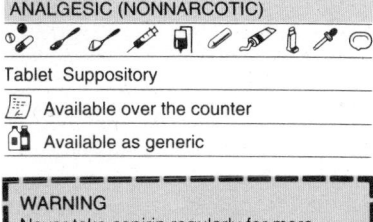

ANALGESIC (NONNARCOTIC)

Tablet Suppository

▤ Available over the counter

▣ Available as generic

> **WARNING**
> Never take aspirin regularly for more than two days except under medical supervision; it may mask the symptoms of a serious disorder.

An *analgesic drug* (painkiller) that has been used for more than 80 years to treat disorders such as headache, menstrual pain, and muscle discom-

fort. Because aspirin has an antiinflammatory action, it is particularly useful in treating joint pain and stiffness caused by types of *arthritis*. Aspirin also reduces fever and is therefore included in some *cold remedies*.

In small doses aspirin reduces the stickiness of platelets (blood particles involved in clotting). This has led to its use in preventing *thrombosis* (abnormal blood clots) in some individuals at risk of having a stroke or *myocardial infarction* (heart attack).

HOW IT WORKS

Aspirin reduces the production of certain *prostaglandins* (hormone-like chemicals) that can be responsible for inflammation, pain, fever, or clumping of platelets.

POSSIBLE ADVERSE EFFECTS

In children there is a slight risk of *Reye's syndrome* (a rare brain and liver disorder). Aspirin should not be given to children except under close medical supervision; in the UK, *paracetamol* is the drug of choice.

Aspirin may cause irritation of the stomach lining, resulting in indigestion or nausea. These side-effects may be reduced by taking the drug with food or by taking a coated tablet that does not release the drug until it reaches the intestine. Prolonged use of aspirin may cause bleeding from the stomach due to *gastric erosion* (disruption of the surface lining of the stomach) or *peptic ulcer* (a deeper penetration of the wall of the stomach or duodenum).

Assay

Analysis or measurement of a substance to determine its presence or effects. A qualitative assay determines only whether a substance is present, whereas a quantitative assay determines the actual amount present.

Biological assays (called bioassays) are concerned mainly with measuring the responses of an animal or specific organ to particular substances. They are used, for example, to assess the effects of a drug or to measure hormone levels. (See also *Immunoassay*; *Radioimmunoassay*.)

Astereognosis

An inability to recognize objects by touch when they are placed in one hand—even though there is no defect of sensation in the fingers or any difficulty holding the object. Testing for astereognosis is part of any detailed examination of the central nervous system. Astereognosis is either leftsided or right-sided; tactile recognition is normal on the other side. If both sides are affected, the condition is called tactile *agnosia*.

Astereognosis and tactile agnosia are caused by damage to parts of the cerebrum (main mass of the brain) concerned with recognition by touch.

Asthenia

An old term meaning loss of strength and energy (see *Weakness*).

Asthenia, neurocirculatory

See *Cardiac neurosis*.

Asthma

Recurrent attacks of breathlessness, characteristically accompanied by wheezing and varying in severity from hour to hour and day to day. The illness often starts in childhood and tends to improve or clear up in early adulthood, but it can develop at any age. Asthma is due to inflammation of the air passages in the lungs; this inflammation commonly becomes chronic and affects the sensitivity of the nerve endings in the airways so that the lungs are easily irritated. In attacks of asthma, the lining of the air passages becomes swollen, causing subsequent narrowing of the airways and reducing the flow of air in and out of the lungs (see *bronchospasm*).

CAUSES

Bronchial asthma can be classified into two main types: extrinsic, in which an allergy (usually to something inhaled) triggers an attack, and intrinsic, in which there is no apparent external cause for the asthma.

The most common *allergens* responsible for extrinsic asthma are pollens, which often also cause allergic *rhinitis* (hay fever), house dust, house-dust mites, animal fur, feathers, and *dander*. Extrinsic asthma may also be triggered by a viral or bacterial respiratory infection, by exercise (especially in cold air), by tobacco smoke or other air pollutants, or by allergy to a particular food or drug.

Intrinsic asthma tends to develop later in life than extrinsic asthma, with the first attack often following a respiratory tract infection. Emotional factors, such as stress or anxiety, may precipitate attacks.

PREVALENCE

About one in 20 of the overall population is asthmatic but about one in 10 among children. It has been estimated that 150,000 school children in the UK suffer from asthma.

Heredity is a major factor in the development of extrinsic asthma. Asthma seems to be becoming more common in developed countries.

SYMPTOMS

Asthmatic attacks vary greatly in their severity, ranging from mild breathlessness to *respiratory failure*. The main symptoms of asthma are breathlessness, wheezing, a dry cough sometimes brought on by exercise, and a feeling of tightness in the chest.

During a severe attack, breathing becomes increasingly difficult, causing sweating, rapid heartbeat, and great distress and anxiety. The sufferer cannot lie down or sleep, may be unable to speak, breathes rapidly, and wheezes loudly.

In a very severe attack, the low amount of oxygen in the blood may cause *cyanosis* (bluish discoloration) of the face, particularly the lips, and the

THE CAUSE OF ASTHMA

Breathlessness and wheezing in asthma is caused by narrowing of the bronchioles (small airways in the lungs). Asthma can be triggered by a wide variety of stimuli, including exercise, infection, pollen, and dust, which would have no effect on non-asthmatic people.

Inflammation of the linings of these bronchioles causes an increased production of sputum (phlegm), which makes the obstruction worse. A dry cough often develops as the sufferer attempts to clear the airways.

TREATMENT OF AN ASTHMA ATTACK

Attacks are treated by inhalation of a bronchodilator drug from an inhaler or from a nebulizer.

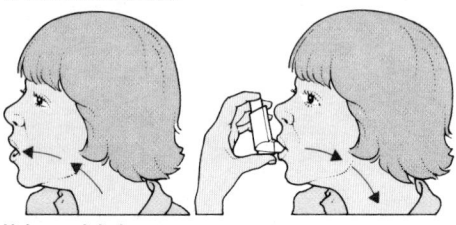

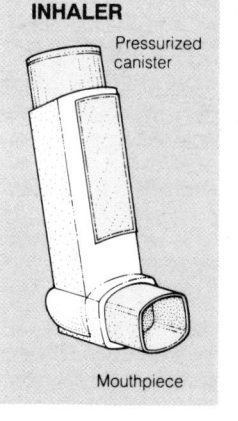

INHALER

Pressurized canister

Mouthpiece

Using an inhaler
To use the inhaler correctly, exhale first; then take in a slow, deep breath while you release the drug by depressing the canister. Two puffs should increase air flow within 15 minutes.

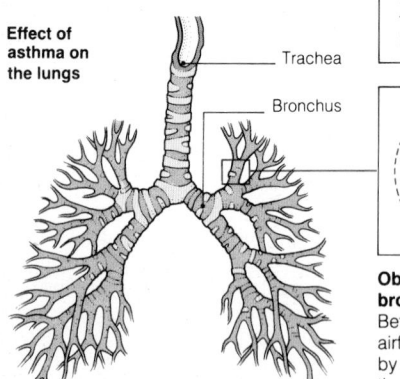

Effect of asthma on the lungs

Trachea

Bronchus

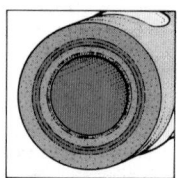

Obstructed bronchiole
Before treatment, airflow is obstructed by a narrowing of the bronchiole.

Healthy bronchiole
Inhalation of the bronchodilator widens the bronchiole and improves airflow.

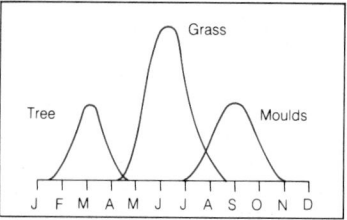

Grass

Tree

Moulds

J F M A M J J A S O N D

Seasonal asthma
When symptoms occur only during a few months, the cause is likely to be allergy to pollen or spores.

skin may become pale and clammy. Such attacks may be fatal.

PREVENTION

Although there is no cure for asthma, attacks can be prevented to a large extent. For sufferers from extrinsic asthma, tests are available to discover whether any of the common allergens is responsible for triggering attacks; if a specific cause is discovered, steps can be taken to avoid it. For example, if the house-dust mite is responsible, mattresses, pillows and quilts (in which the mites flourish) should be enclosed in airtight plastic covers and the home should be kept as free from dust as possible.

Hyposensitization (a course of injections of the allergen) is fashionable in some countries but is little used in the UK because careful trials have shown little or no benefit. Much more successful in preventing attacks are prophylactic (preventive) drugs, such as *sodium cromoglycate* and inhaled *corticosteroid drugs*. To be effective, they must be taken several times daily, usually through an inhaler.

TREATMENT

Every sufferer from asthma should have a treatment plan agreed with his or her doctor to deal with the day-to-day management of the disorder. This usually involves measuring the severity of symptoms and setting out the steps to be taken if the symptoms worsen. The air flow in and out of the lungs may be measured with a *peak-flow meter*; daily or twice daily measurements will give early warning of worsening of the asthma. Once an attack has started, a prophylactic drug has limited effects and a *bronchodilator drug*, such as *salbutamol*, is needed to relax and widen the airways. Bronchodilator drugs are usually inhaled from small pressurized aerosol cans (see illustration). Inhalation technique is very important. For young children and those who have difficulty with aerosols, various devices are advisable to make the procedure easier (e.g. a Nebuhaler) or the drug can be taken in powder form from a Rotahaler. Oral *theophylline* preparations may also be used to prevent or treat attacks. Long-term treatment with oral corticosteroids may be necessary for people with chronic continuing asthma if all other treatments have failed.

EMERGENCY PROCEDURE

Most asthma attacks either pass naturally or can be controlled using a bronchodilator; but sometimes an attack may be so severe that it fails to respond to the recommended drug dosage. In this case, the dose should be repeated. If it has no effect, a doctor should be consulted or the person taken to hospital, where treatment may include the use of oxygen and a powered ventilator.

OUTLOOK

More than half of the children who suffer from asthma grow out of it completely by the age of 21; in a proportion of the remainder, attacks become less severe as they grow older. With modern drug treatment, even people who suffer repeated attacks as adults can expect to live a normal life. In most cases, quality of life need not be impaired (demonstrated by the success of world-class athletes who have had asthma). However, a small minority continue to suffer from disabling asthma despite being on optimum treatment.

Asthma, cardiac

Breathing difficulty caused by accumulation of fluid in the lungs that causes bronchospasm and wheezing. This response is usually due to reduced pumping efficiency of the left side of the heart (see *Heart failure*), causing congestion and increased pressure of blood circulation through the lungs, and the accumulation of fluid in the lungs.

Although cardiac asthma has a different cause from the more familiar bronchial asthma, the two conditions have similar symptoms, including wheezing and breathing difficulty. A chest X-ray may show fluid in the lungs. Treatment is primarily for heart failure but may include use of bronchodilator drugs.

Astigmatism

A condition in which the front surface of the cornea does not conform to the normal "spherical" curve. Although the eye is perfectly healthy, the corneal surface has discrepancies in its curvature, with the result that magnifying power in one direction is greater than in the other.

A minor degree of astigmatism is normal and glasses are not necessary to correct it. More severe astigmatism causes blurring of lines set at a particular angle. A person with astigmatism might see horizontal lines clearly but vertical lines blurred, or the blurring may occur in an oblique meridian.

TREATMENT

Ordinary spherically curved spectacle lenses cannot correct astigmatism. Correction requires lenses with little optical power in the "normal" meridian but greater curvature in other meridians. These "cylindrical" lenses must be framed at a precise angle.

Hard contact lenses can bridge over the anomalous corneal curve and present an even spherical surface for focusing; they give excellent vision in astigmatism. Ordinary soft lenses tend to mould to the astigmatic curve.

Astringent

COMMON DRUGS

Aluminium acetate Potassium permanganate Silver nitrate Zinc sulphate

A substance that causes tissue to dry and shrink by reducing its ability to absorb water. Astringents are widely used in *antiperspirants* and skin tonics. They are also used to promote healing of broken or inflamed skin. Astringent drugs are used to treat *otitis externa* (inflammation of the ear canal) and watering of the eye due to minor irritation. Astringents may cause burning or stinging when applied.

Astrocytoma

A type of malignant *brain tumour*. Astrocytomas are the most common type of *glioma*, a tumour arising from the glial (supporting) cells within the nervous system, and are composed of cells called astrocytes.

Astrocytomas most commonly develop within the cerebrum (the main mass of the brain). Although all types are very serious, they are classified in four grades (I to IV) according to their rate of growth and malignancy. A grade I astrocytoma is a slow-growing tumour that may spread widely throughout the brain but may be present for many years before causing symptoms. A grade IV astrocytoma is a very fast-growing tumour that causes rapid development of disabling symptoms.

Symptoms are similar to those caused by other types of brain tumour. Diagnostic tests include *CT scanning* or *MRI* and, often, *angiography*. Few astrocytomas can be completely surgically removed.

Asylum

An outdated term for an institution that provides care for those who are mentally ill.

Asymptomatic

A medical term that means without *symptoms*—those indications of illness noticed by the patient (as distinct from signs, which are observed by the doctor). Examples of conditions that may be asymptomatic include *hypertension* (high blood pressure), which is usually discovered during a routine blood pressure test, and *diabetes mellitus*, which is often diagnosed from a blood or urine test. Most disorders are asymptomatic in their early stages. In the case of *cancer*, much effort has been made to devise screening tests to detect tumours at their early, asymptomatic stage.

Asystole

A term meaning absence of the heartbeat (see *Cardiac arrest*).

Ataxia

Incoordination and clumsiness, affecting balance and gait, limb or eye movements, and/or speech.

CAUSES

Ataxia may be caused by damage to the *cerebellum* (part of the brain concerned with coordination) or to the nerve pathways that carry information to and from the cerebellum.

Possible causes include injury to the brain or to the spinal cord. In adults, ataxia may be caused by drug or *alcohol intoxication* (the most common cause), by a *stroke* or *brain tumour* affecting the cerebellum or brainstem, by a disease of the balance organ in the ear, or by *multiple sclerosis* or other types of nervous system degeneration. In rare cases, ataxia is a result of untreated *syphilis*. In children, causes of ataxia include acute infection, brain tumours, and the inherited condition *Friedreich's ataxia*.

SYMPTOMS

Symptoms depend on the site of damage within the nervous system, although an awkward gait is common to most forms. The typical ataxic gait is lurching and unsteady, like that of a drunk person, with the feet widely placed. If the damage is to nerves that carry sensory information from joints and muscles to the cerebellum, sensory ataxia results. In such cases, the person's unsteadiness is worse when the eyes are closed. Damage to parts of the brainstem concerned with eye movements often cause controlling *nystagmus* (jerky eye movements).

Damage to the cerebellum itself usually causes slurred speech as well as an unsteady gait. Sometimes, if damage is confined to one side of the cerebellum, incoordination is confined to the limbs on the same side and is often accompanied by a tremor in the limbs during purposeful movements. When walking, the person often has a tendency to veer or fall towards the affected side. Other features may include decomposition of

complex actions into their component parts, producing jerky movements, and "overshoot" when attempts are made to touch or pick up objects.

DIAGNOSIS AND TREATMENT

Discovery of the cause of ataxia may be helped by *CT scanning* or *MRI*. Treatment depends on the cause.

Atelectasis

Collapse of part or all of a lung caused by obstruction of the bronchus (the main air passage through the lung) or the bronchioles (smaller air passages). When this happens, air already in the lung cannot be breathed out and, instead, is absorbed into the blood, leading to the collapse of all or part of the lung. After collapsing, the lung loses its elasticity and cannot take in air; consequently, the blood passing through it can no longer absorb oxygen or dispose of carbon dioxide.

In an adult, atelectasis is usually not life-threatening, because unaffected parts of the lung (or, if the whole lung has collapsed, the other lung) expand to compensate for the loss of function in the collapsed area. However, when a lung collapses in a newborn baby—because mucus has blocked a bronchus—the baby's life is at risk. (For lung collapse caused by a perforation of the outer covering of the lung, see *Pneumothorax*.)

CAUSES AND INCIDENCE

Obstruction of a bronchus is usually due to one of four mechanisms. First, secretions of mucus in the bronchus or bronchioles may accumulate and cause blockage. This can happen after an abdominal or chest operation that has made coughing difficult due to pain; in a baby at birth; in *asthma*; or in certain infections, such as *pertussis* (whooping cough) in children or chronic *bronchitis* in adults.

Second, an accidentally inhaled *foreign body*, such as a peanut, may stick in the bronchus; this is more common in children than in adults. Third, a benign or malignant *tumour* in the lung may block the bronchus. Fourth, enlarged lymph nodes (which occur in *tuberculosis*, other lung infections, or some forms of *cancer*) may exert pressure on the airway.

SYMPTOMS, DIAGNOSIS, AND TREATMENT

The main symptom is breathing difficulty. There may also be a cough and chest pain, depending on the underlying cause.

The condition is diagnosed by physical examination of the chest and *chest X-rays*. Treatment is aimed at the cause of the blockage. If the cause is an

accumulation of mucus, the patient will be given chest *physiotherapy*, including encouragement to clear the chest by coughing or deep breathing and use of *postural drainage*.

Once the obstruction has been removed, the collapsed lung usually reinflates gradually, although some areas of it may be permanently damaged or scarred.

Atenolol

A *beta-blocker drug* commonly used in the treatment of *hypertension* (high blood pressure), *angina pectoris* (chest pain due to impaired blood supply to heart muscle), and certain types of *arrhythmia* (irregular heartbeat).

Atheroma

Fatty deposits on the inner lining of an artery that can cause *atherosclerosis*.

Atherosclerosis

A disease of the arterial wall in which the inner layer thickens, causing narrowing of the channel and thus impairing blood flow.

The narrowing is due to the development of raised patches called plaques in the inner lining of the arteries. These plaques consist of a substance called atheroma, a mixture of low-density lipoproteins (see *Fats and oils*), decaying muscle cells, fibrous tissue, clumps of blood platelets, *cholesterol*, and sometimes calcium; they tend to form in regions of turbulent blood flow and are found most often in people with high concentrations of cholesterol in the bloodstream. The number and thickness of plaques increase with age, causing loss of the smooth lining of the blood vessels and encouraging *thrombus* (abnormal blood clot) formation. Sometimes, a fragment of thrombus breaks off and forms an *embolus*, which travels through the bloodstream and blocks smaller vessels.

INCIDENCE

Atherosclerosis is responsible for more deaths in the UK than any other condition. Atherosclerotic heart disease involving the coronary arteries is the most common single cause of death, accounting for one third of all deaths (see *Coronary artery disease*); atherosclerotic interference with blood supply to the brain (causing *stroke*) is the third most common cause of death after cancer. Atherosclerosis also causes a great deal of serious illness by reducing the blood flow in other major arteries, such as those to the kidneys, legs, and intestines.

CAUSES

Certain risk factors increase the probability that atherosclerosis will develop. These risk factors are cigarette smoking, *hypertension* (high blood pressure), male gender, obesity, physical inactivity, a high level of cholesterol in the blood, poorly controlled *diabetes mellitus*, family history of arterial disease, and, possibly, an anxious or aggressive personality.

The risk of atherosclerosis increases with age, probably in part because of the length of time it takes for the plaques to develop. The influence of gender is illustrated by comparing men with premenopausal women: in the group aged 35 to 44, coronary artery disease kills six times as many men as women.

PREVENTION

Modifications of the risk factors, especially early in adult life, can markedly reduce the probability that atherosclerosis will develop or can at least delay its manifestations. Smoking should be stopped, blood pressure checked regularly, and hypertension treated. Diet should be low in saturated fats and obesity should be avoided. If cholesterol levels remain high despite a low-fat diet, drug therapy to reduce the cholesterol levels may be warranted. Meticulous control of diabetes mellitus is important. Regular exercise is of great value in maintaining the health and efficiency of the heart and circulation.

SYMPTOMS

Unfortunately, atherosclerosis produces no symptoms until the damage to the arteries is severe enough to restrict blood flow. Restriction of blood flow to heart muscle due to atherosclerosis can cause *angina pectoris*. Restriction of blood flow to the muscles of the legs causes intermittent *claudication* (pains in the legs brought on by walking and relieved by rest). Narrowing of the arteries supplying blood to the brain may cause *transient ischaemic attacks* (symptoms and signs of a *stroke* lasting less than 24 hours) and episodes of dizziness.

DIAGNOSIS

A medical history and examination will reveal much about the health of the circulation, but special investigation may be necessary. Blood flow in an artery can be investigated by *angiography* (X-rays after injection of a radiopaque substance), *Doppler* ultrasound scanning, or *plethysmography* (a technique that produces a tracing of the pulse pattern).

TREATMENT

Medication can do little for atherosclerosis that has developed over many years, but prolonged treatment to lower the blood cholesterol and (if necessary) the blood pressure will halt the progress of the disease and may eventually reverse it. *Anticoagulant* and *vasodilator drugs* may be useful in the control of symptoms, but they have no curative value.

Surgical treatment may be recommended for people who are unresponsive to medical treatment or who have a high risk of suffering serious complications. Balloon *angioplasty* may be used to open up narrowed vessels and improve blood supply. The blood supply to the heart muscle can be restored by *coronary artery bypass* surgery. Large atheromatous and calcified arterial obstructions can be removed by *endarterectomy*, and entire segments of diseased peripheral vessels can be replaced by woven plastic tube grafts (see *Arterial reconstructive surgery*).

Athetosis

A nervous system disorder, characterized by slow, writhing, involuntary (uncontrollable) movements, most often seen in the head, face, neck, and limbs. The movements commonly include facial grimacing, with contortions of the mouth and lips. Often, the affected person also has difficulty balancing and walking. In some cases the muscles are abnormally flaccid (floppy), while in others they are spastic (tense).

Very commonly, athetosis is combined with *chorea* (involuntary fidgety movements)—a combination called choreoathetosis. Both conditions arise from damage to the *basal ganglia*, clusters of nerve cells deep within the brain that are concerned with the control of movements. Causes include

ARTERIAL DEGENERATION IN ATHEROSCLEROSIS

Atherosclerosis is narrowing of the arteries caused by plaques on their inner linings. These plaques are composed mainly of fats deposited from the bloodstream. They disrupt the normal flow of blood through the affected artery. Men are affected earlier than women because premenopausal women are protected by natural oestrogen hormones.

RISK FACTORS

Cigarette smoking

Hypertension

Male gender

Obesity

Physical inactivity

Diabetes mellitus

Heredity

Aggressive personality

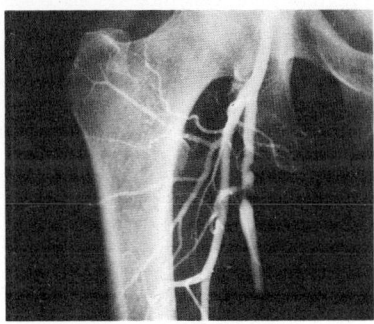

X-ray showing atherosclerosis
The leg arteries shown here appear as bright channels. One is narrowed at a point corresponding to the dark gap.

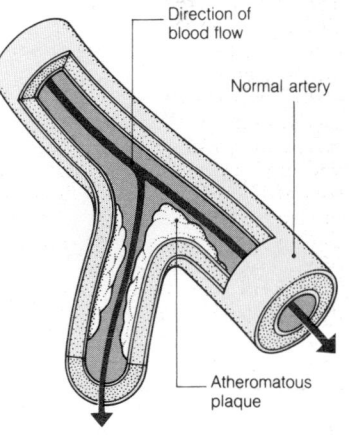

Direction of blood flow

Normal artery

Atheromatous plaque

Atherosclerotic artery
A deposit of atheromatous plaque disrupts normal blood flow through the artery at the point where it branches. This occurs because of the greater level of turbulence in this area.

damage to the brain prior to or around the time of birth (see *Cerebral palsy*), *encephalitis* (brain infection), degenerative disorders such as *Huntington's disease*, or the use of certain drugs such as *phenothiazine drugs* or *levodopa* derivatives. If drug treatment is the cause, the abnormal movements may stop when the drug is withdrawn.

Athlete's foot

A common skin condition in which the skin between the toes becomes itchy and sore, may crack and peel away, and occasionally blisters. The webs between the fourth and fifth toes are most often involved. Athlete's foot is rare in young children and is associated with wearing shoes and sweating; the condition is rare where most people go barefoot.

CAUSES

Athlete's foot is usually caused by a dermatophyte (a type of fungal) infection, known medically as tinea pedis, but may be caused by bacteria. Secondary infection occurring through skin cracks is bacterial.

TREATMENT

Athlete's foot sometimes clears up without medication. Careful drying of the affected area is necessary; wearing dry cotton socks or sandals may help. Disinfecting the floors of showers and locker rooms helps control the spread of infection.

Most fungal infections respond to treatment with *antifungal drugs*, such as tolnaftate, miconazole, or an undecenoate compound.

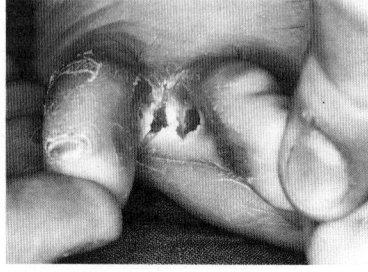

Athlete's foot
The typical appearance shows fissuring in the cleft between the fourth and fifth toes. There is usually an annoying itch.

Atony

Complete loss of tension in a muscle, so that the muscle is completely flaccid (floppy). Atony can occur in some nervous system disorders or after injury to nerves. The arm muscles may become atonic after injury to the *brachial plexus* (nerve roots in the neck passing into the arm).

Atopy

A predisposition to various allergic reactions (see *Allergy*). Atopic individuals have a tendency to suffer from one or more allergic-based disorders, such as *asthma*, *eczema*, *urticaria* (nettle rash), and allergic *rhinitis* (hay fever).

The mechanism that causes the predisposition is not fully understood, although various theories have been proposed.

There is a distinct genetic, or inherited (familial), basis to atopy—the relatives of atopic individuals are much more likely than the average person to be atopic (even after allowance is made for bias caused by similarities of environment).

ATP

The abbreviation for adenosine triphosphate, the chief energy-carrying chemical in the body. (See also *ADP*; *Metabolism*.)

Atresia

The *congenital* absence or closure of a body opening or canal, caused by a failure of development while in the uterus. Examples are *biliary atresia*, in which the bile ducts between the liver and duodenum are absent; *oesophageal atresia*, in which the oesophagus comes to a blind end; pulmonary atresia, in which the pulmonary artery between the right side of the heart and the lungs is closed off; and anal atresia (see *Anus, imperforate*), in which the anal canal is narrowed and shut off. Most forms of atresia require surgical correction early in life.

Atrial fibrillation

A type of irregular heartbeat (see *Arrhythmia, cardiac*) in which the atria (upper chambers of the heart) beat irregularly and very rapidly (300 to 500 beats per minute) Not all these beats pass through the atrioventricular node (the impulse carrier between the atria and the ventricles, the lower chambers of the heart). As a result, the ventricles beat irregularly at a rate of 80 to 160 beats per minute.

CAUSES

Atrial fibrillation can occur in almost any long-standing heart disease in which there is enlargement of the atria. It is common in rheumatic heart disease (see *Rheumatic fever*), *thyrotoxicosis* (overactivity of the thyroid gland), and atherosclerotic heart disease.

SYMPTOMS AND SIGNS

Sudden onset of atrial fibrillation can cause *palpitations* (awareness of fast heartbeat) or *angina pectoris* (chest

pain due to reduced blood supply). The inefficient pumping action of the heart can reduce the output of blood into the circulation by as much as 30 per cent. Blood clots in the atria may enter the bloodstream and become lodged in an artery (see *Embolism*). This is most serious when it affects the main artery to the lungs, causing *pulmonary embolism*, or an artery in the brain, causing *stroke*.

DIAGNOSIS

The pulse is irregular in rate and strength and does not correspond with the heart-rate; many heartbeats audible at the heart fail to reach the wrist because the heart has contracted prematurely when only partly filled with blood. The diagnosis of atrial fibrillation is confirmed by an *ECG*, which shows the electrical activity within the heart.

TREATMENT

The first step usually is to control the heart-rate by giving *digoxin* or, in certain instances, intravenous *verapamil*. If the fibrillation is of recent onset, treatment is directed at remedying the cause—for example, treatment for thyrotoxicosis, or replacement of heart valves damaged by rheumatic heart disease. Atrial fibrillation of recent onset can often be reversed by *defibrillation* (application of a short electric shock to the heart).

If atrial fibrillation is long-standing, or is combined with severe heart disease, the likelihood of reversing it is small. In this case, control of the heart-rate with digoxin is continued and *beta-blocker drugs* are sometimes also used. In most cases *anticoagulant drugs* are given to reduce the risk of embolism.

Atrial flutter

A type of irregular heartbeat (see *Arrhythmia, cardiac*) in which the atria (upper chambers of the heart) beat very rapidly at 200 to 400 beats per minute. At these rates the atrioventricular node, the conducting mechanism between the atria and the ventricles (lower chambers of the heart), is unable to respond to every beat. As a result, the ventricles beat only once to every two, three, or four beats of the atria. The condition generally occurs in people over 40 who have severe heart disease.

Some people with atrial flutter have no symptoms; others may complain of palpitations (an awareness of a fast heartbeat). The condition can lead to *heart failure* (reduced pumping action of the heart) or *angina pectoris* (chest pain due to reduced blood supply).

When treatment is urgent, *defibrillation* (application of a short electric shock to the heart) may be effective. For nonurgent treatment, *digoxin* may be prescribed.

Atrial natriuretic peptide

A substance produced in the muscular wall of the atria (upper chambers of the heart). It is released into the bloodstream in response to an increase in atrial muscle tension caused, for example, by *heart failure* or by some types of *hypertension*.

Atrial natriuretic peptide increases the amount of sodium excreted in the urine; sodium draws water out with it, decreasing the volume of water in the circulation and helping to lower the blood pressure. Atrial natriuretic peptide also lowers the blood pressure by causing blood vessels to dilate (widen) so that blood can flow more easily.

Children with congenital heart disorders causing heart failure (see *Heart disease, congenital*) have high levels of atrial natriuretic peptide. These levels fall after successful surgery to correct the abnormality.

Atrium

Either of the two (right and left) upper chambers of the *heart*.

ANATOMY OF THE ATRIUM

The left atrium receives oxygenated blood from the pulmonary veins; the right atrium receives deoxygenated blood from the venae cavae.

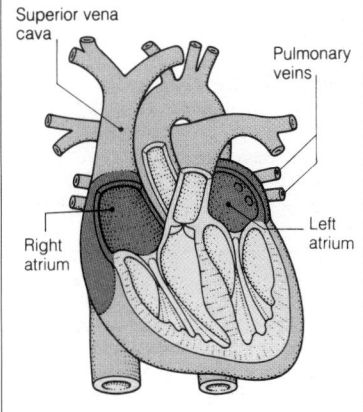

Superior vena cava

Pulmonary veins

Right atrium

Left atrium

Atrophy

Shrinkage or wasting away of a tissue or organ due to a reduction in the size or number of its cells. Atrophy is commonly caused by disuse (such as when a limb has been immobilized in a plaster cast) or by inadequate cell nutrition due to poor blood circulation. Atrophy may also occur during prolonged serious illness, when the body needs to use up the protein reserves in the muscles. Other, less common, causes include nerve damage that partly or completely immobilizes part of the body, and lack of a specific *enzyme* or *hormone* needed to stimulate growth of a cell or an organ.

Atropine

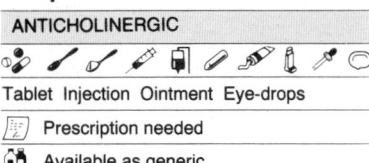

ANTICHOLINERGIC

Tablet Injection Ointment Eye-drops

Prescription needed

Available as generic

A drug derived from *belladonna*. Atropine is used to treat *iritis* (inflammation of the iris) and *corneal ulcer*. It is also used in young children to dilate (widen) the pupil of the eye for the purpose of examination.

Atropine is commonly given as a *premedication* before general *anaesthesia* to reduce secretions from the lungs and is also used as an emergency treatment for *bradycardia* (abnormally slow heartbeat).

Atropine is occasionally prescribed for its antispasmodic effects. It is sometimes combined with an *antidiarrhoeal drug* to relieve abdominal cramps accompanying diarrhoea.

POSSIBLE ADVERSE EFFECTS
Adverse effects include dry mouth, blurred vision, abnormal retention of urine, and, in the elderly, confusion. Atropine eye-drops are rarely given to adults because they cause disturbance of vision lasting two to three weeks and may precipitate acute *glaucoma* in a susceptible person.

Attachment

An affectionate bond between individuals, especially between parent and child (see *Bonding*), or between a person and an object, as in the case of a young child and a security object such as a blanket or a doll. The attachment gives emotional satisfaction.

The term attachment is also used to note the joining of a muscle or tendon to a bone.

Audiogram

A graph produced as a result of certain *hearing tests* that shows the hearing threshold—that is, the minimum audible decibel level (loudness)—for each of a range of sound frequencies.

Audiology

The study of hearing, especially of impaired hearing that cannot be corrected by drugs or surgery.

Audiometry

Measurement of the sense of hearing. The term often refers to specific *hearing tests* in which a machine is used to produce sounds of a defined intensity (loudness) and frequency (pitch) and in which the hearing in each ear is measured over the full range of normally audible sounds.

Auditory nerve

Also called the acoustic nerve, the part of the *vestibulocochlear nerve* (the eighth *cranial nerve*) concerned with the sense of hearing.

Aura

A peculiar "warning" sensation that precedes or marks the onset of a *migraine* attack or of a seizure in a person suffering from *epilepsy*.

A migraine attack may be preceded by a feeling of elation, unusual well-being, excessive energy, or drowsiness. The sufferer comes to recognize these as warning signs of an attack. Thirst or a craving for sweet foods may develop. An attack of migraine may also be heralded by flashing lights seen before the eyes, blurred or tunnel vision, or difficulty in speaking. Weakness, numbness, or tingling of one half of the body may occur. As these symptoms subside, the migraine headache pain begins.

An epileptic aura may be a distorted perception, such as a hallucinatory sound or smell, or a sensation of movement in part of the body. One type of attack (in people with *temporal lobe epilepsy*) is often preceded by a vague feeling of discomfort in the upper abdomen, sometimes accompanied by borborygmi (rumbling, gurgling bowel sounds) and followed by a sensation of fullness in the head.

Auranofin

A *gold* preparation used as an *antirheumatic drug* in the treatment of *rheumatoid arthritis*. Auranofin, unlike other gold preparations, is effective when taken by mouth.

Auricle

Another name for the pinna, the external flap of the *ear*. The term was also once used as a synonym for *atrium* (one of the two upper chambers of the heart). Ear-like appendages of the atria are still called auricles.

Auriscope

An instrument for examining the ear, also called an *otoscope*.

Auscultation

The procedure of listening to sounds within the body to assess the functioning of an organ or to detect the presence of disease. The sounds are heard through a stethoscope.

To listen to the heart, the doctor places the stethoscope at four points on the chest, corresponding to the location of the heart valves. With the patient sitting up, in a semi-reclining position, or lying on his or her left side, the doctor listens for any abnormality in the rate and rhythm of the heartbeat and for heart *murmurs* or other abnormal *heart sounds* that might indicate a heart defect.

When listening to the lungs, the doctor places the stethoscope on many different areas of the front and back of the chest. The patient breathes normally and then takes deep breaths while the doctor compares the sounds of the air movement on the left and right sides. Abnormal breath sounds may indicate *pneumonia, bronchitis,* or *pneumothorax.* Additional sounds (called crepitations) that resemble crackling or bubbling are caused by fluid in the lungs. Wheezing sounds result from spasm of the airways, usually as a result of *asthma*. In *pleurisy*, a scratching sound can be heard, produced by inflamed areas of the lung rubbing together.

The doctor may also test for vocal resonance by asking the patient to whisper something. The sound produced is louder if there is pus in the lung (e.g. as a result of pneumonia) because sound is transmitted better through an affected, pus-containing lung than through normal air-containing lung tissue.

Blood vessels near the skin surface (usually the carotid artery in the neck, the abdominal aorta, and the renal artery) may be listened to for bruits (sounds made by turbulent or abnormally fast blood circulation). Such sounds occur when blood vessels are narrowed (e.g. by fatty deposits in *atherosclerosis*) or widened (e.g. by an *aneurysm*), or when heart valves are narrowed or damaged (e.g. by *endocarditis*).

The abdomen is auscultated for borborygmi (loud rumbling, gurgling sounds made by the movement of air and fluid in the intestine) and for abnormal bowel sounds. The former may have no significance; the latter may indicate *intestinal obstruction.*

Autism

A condition in which a child is unable to relate to people and situations and may show an obsessive resistance to any change.

INCIDENCE

Autism is rare, affecting about two to four children in every 10,000. Nearly three times more boys than girls are affected, and it seems more common

---

PROCEDURE FOR AUSCULTATION

A doctor's examination often includes auscultation — listening to sounds within the body using a stethoscope. Some organs make sounds during normal functioning.

Examples are the movement of fluid through the stomach and intestine, the opening and closing of heart valves, and the flow of air through the lungs and airways. However, the presence of

abnormal sounds usually indicates disease of that tissue. The obstetrician listens to the baby's heartbeat as part of routine examination during pregnancy.

STETHOSCOPE

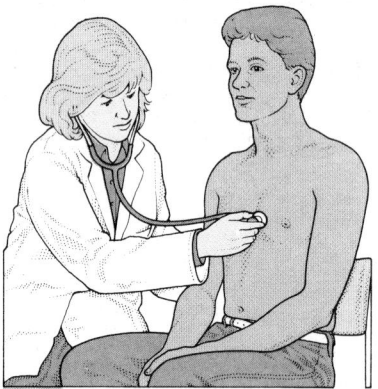

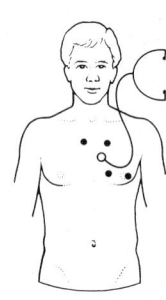

The heart
The stethoscope is usually placed at four places on the chest overlying the sites of the heart valves. The doctor listens for the presence of murmurs, clicks, and extra heart sounds that may indicate disease of a heart valve.

Using a stethoscope
The end is held against the skin. The diaphragm picks up most noises, while the bell detects quiet, deep noises.

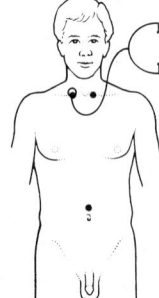

Carotid artery and abdominal aorta
The doctor may listen to the flow of blood through a blood vessel that passes just beneath the skin. The presence of bruits (sounds of turbulence) usually indicate abnormal narrowing or widening of an artery.

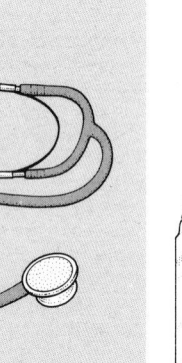

The abdomen
The doctor may listen to the abdomen for the sounds made by movement of fluid through the intestine. A disorder of the intestine may cause these sounds to be absent, abnormal, or very loud.

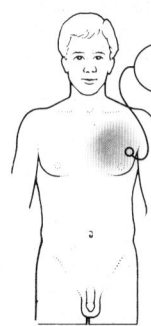

The lungs
The doctor places the stethoscope over several different areas of the chest and back to listen to sounds made during breathing. The presence of crackles and dry or moist wheezes indicates various types of lung disease.

among the higher social classes. Autism is by definition evident before the age of 30 months and is usually apparent within the first year of life.

CAUSES

The precise causes of autism are unknown, but evidence points to a physical basis. Because about one quarter of autistic children have signs of a neurological disorder and because epileptic seizures develop at adolescence in nearly one third of sufferers, it is likely that there is a subtle form of brain damage. The earlier theory that lack of warmth from parents was a cause is now rejected.

SYMPTOMS AND SIGNS

Often, autistic children are normal for the first few months of life before becoming increasingly unresponsive to parents or other stimuli. The first sign may be an inability to fix on the mother's face. Resistance to being cuddled may cause the child to scream to be put down when picked up.

The child remains aloof from parents and other people and fails to form relationships. He or she avoids eye-to-eye contact, has a preference for playing alone, and is often indifferent to the feelings of others and to social conventions.

Extreme resistance to change of any kind is an important feature. The child reacts with severe tantrums to alteration in routine or interference with activities. Rituals develop in play and often the child becomes attached to unusual objects or collections, or obsessed with one particular topic or idea. This wish for sterile "sameness" makes it very difficult to teach the autistic child new skills.

Delay in speaking is very common. The autistic child lacks the ability to understand or copy speech or gestures and responds to sounds inappropriately. Even when speech is acquired, it is immature, unimaginative in content, and has a robot-like sound. The child often makes up words and echoes what has been said.

There may be other behavioural abnormalities, such as walking on tiptoe, flicking or twiddling fingers for hours on end, rocking, self-injury, sudden screaming fits, and *hyperactivity*. Unusual fears and difficulty in learning manual tasks are also common in autistic children.

Despite all these bizarre symptoms, appearance and muscular coordination are normal. Some autistic children have an isolated special skill, such as an outstanding rote memory or musical ability.

TREATMENT

There is no known effective treatment. Special schooling, support and *counselling* for parents and families, and sometimes *behaviour therapy* (e.g. to reduce violent self-injury) can be helpful. Medication is useful only for specific problems, such as *epilepsy* or *hyperactivity*.

OUTLOOK

Outlook depends on intelligence and language ability. Only about one sixth of autistic children can lead any form of independent life; the majority need special, sometimes institutional, care.

Autoclave

An apparatus that produces steam at high pressure within a sealed chamber; the resulting high temperature of the water vapour destroys microorganisms. Autoclaving is used in hospitals as a means of sterilizing surgical equipment (see *Sterilization*).

Autoimmune disorders

Any of numerous disorders, including *rheumatoid arthritis*, insulin-dependent *diabetes mellitus*, and systemic *lupus erythematosus*, caused by a reaction of the individual's *immune system* against the organs or tissues of his or her own body.

The function of the immune system is to respond to invading microorganisms (for example, bacteria or viruses) by producing antibodies or sensitized lymphocytes (types of white blood cell) that will recognize and destroy the invaders. Autoimmune disorders occur when these reactions inexplicably take place against the body's own cells and tissues, producing a variety of disorders.

The disease-producing processes in autoimmunity are termed *hypersensitivity* reactions, of which there are several types. These reactions are similar to the reactions that occur in *allergy* except that in autoimmune disorders the hypersensitivity response is to the body itself rather than to an outside substance.

CAUSES

The immune system normally distinguishes "self" from "nonself". Some lymphocytes are capable of reacting against self, but these lymphocytes are generally suppressed. Autoimmune disorders occur when there is some interruption of the normal control process, allowing lymphocytes to escape from suppression, or when there is an alteration in some body tissue so that it is no longer recognized as "self" and is consequently attacked.

The exact mechanisms causing these changes are not fully understood, but bacteria, viruses, and drugs may play a role in triggering an autoimmune process in someone who already has a genetic (inherited) predisposition. It is speculated that the usual inflammatory response of tissues to these agents somehow provokes an abnormal "sensitization" response to the tissues involved.

TYPES

Autoimmune processes can have various results—for example, slow destruction of a particular type of cell or tissue, stimulation of an organ into excessive growth, or interference in its function. Organs and tissues frequently affected by autoimmune processes include the endocrine glands (such as the thyroid, pancreas, and adrenal glands), components of the blood (such as the red blood cells), and the connective tissues, skin, muscles, and joints.

AUTOIMMUNE DISORDERS

Autoimmune disorders are a group of conditions in which the immune system attacks the body's own tissues as if they were foreign substances. The reasons why these disorders develop are unclear but genetic factors may play a role. Women are more often affected than men. An individual who has one autoimmune disorder may develop others.

An autoimmune disorder may primarily affect a specific organ or cell type, or may affect various organs. The following are examples of conditions that are, or are thought to be, autoimmune.

Specific (organs or cells affected)
Addison's disease (adrenal glands)
Autoimmune haemolytic anaemia (red blood cells)
Autoimmune chronic active hepatitis (liver)
Autoimmune infertility (sperm or ovary)
Diabetes mellitus type 1 (pancreas)
Goodpasture's syndrome (lung and kidney)
Graves' disease (thyroid gland)
Hashimoto's thyroiditis (thyroid gland)
Idiopathic thrombocytopenic purpura (platelets)
Myasthenia gravis (muscle receptors)
Pernicious anaemia (stomach lining)
Vitiligo (melanocytes)

Nonspecific
Behçet's syndrome
Rheumatoid arthritis
Sjögren's syndrome
Systemic lupus erythematosus

Specific autoimmune disorders are frequently classified into organ-specific and non-organ-specific types. In organ-specific disorders, the autoimmune process is directed mainly against one organ. Examples (with the organ affected) include *Hashimoto's thyroiditis* (thyroid gland), pernicious *anaemia* (stomach), *Addison's disease* (adrenal glands), and insulin-dependent *diabetes mellitus* (pancreas).

In non-organ-specific disorders, autoimmune activity is widely spread throughout the body. Examples are systemic *lupus erythematosus* (SLE), *rheumatoid arthritis*, and *dermatomyositis*. Some autoimmune diseases fall between the two types. Sometimes, patients may experience several organ-specific or non-organ-specific diseases simultaneously. However, there is little overlap between the two ends of the spectrum.

TREATMENT

The first principle in treating any autoimmune disorder is to correct any major deficiencies. This may involve replacing hormones, such as thyroxin or insulin, that are not being produced by a gland. Alternatively, it may involve replacing components of the blood by transfusion.

The second principle is to diminish the activity of the immune system; this necessitates a delicate balance, controlling the disorder while maintaining the body's ability to fight disease in general. The drugs most commonly used are *corticosteroid drugs*. More severe cases can be treated with other more powerful *immunosuppressant drugs* such as cyclophosphamide, methotrexate, and azathioprine, but all of these drugs can damage rapidly dividing tissues, such as the bone marrow, and so are used with caution. Drugs that act more specifically on the immune system (for example, by blocking a particular hypersensitivity reaction) are being developed.

Automatism

A state in which behaviour is not controlled by the conscious mind. The individual carries out movements and activities without being aware of doing so, and later has no clear memory of what happened. Episodes of automatism, which is uncommon, start abruptly and usually last a few seconds or minutes at the most.

Automatism may be the main symptom of *temporal lobe epilepsy*; this diagnosis can be confirmed by *EEG*. Other causes include *dissociative disorders*, hysteria, alcohol intoxication, *drug abuse*, and *hypoglycaemia* (low blood sugar level).

Autonomic nervous system

The part of the *nervous system* that controls the involuntary, seemingly automatic, activities of organs, blood vessels, glands, and a variety of other tissues in the body. The autonomic nervous system consists of a network of nerves divided into two parts: the sympathetic nervous system and the parasympathetic nervous system.

In general, the sympathetic nervous system heightens activity in the body—quickening the heartbeat and breathing rate as if it were preparing the body for a *fight-or-flight response*. The parasympathetic system has the opposite effect.

The two systems act in conjunction and normally balance each other. However, during exercise or at times of stress or fear, the activity of the sympathetic system predominates, while during sleep the parasympathetic system exerts more control.

SYMPATHETIC NERVOUS SYSTEM

The sympathetic nervous system consists of two chains of nerves that pass from the spinal cord throughout the body to the organs and other structures they control. Into these tissues the nerve endings release the *neurotransmitter* chemicals *adrenaline* and *noradrenaline*. The system also stimulates the release of adrenaline from the adrenal glands into the bloodstream.

Among the most important effects produced by the neurotransmitters of the sympathetic nervous system are acceleration and strengthening of the heartbeat, widening of the airways, widening of the blood vessels in muscles, and narrowing of the blood vessels in the skin and abdominal organs (to increase blood flow through the muscles). In addition, the neurotransmitters decrease the activity of the digestive system, dilate the pupils of the eyes, and produce the contractions in the male urethra by which semen is ejaculated at orgasm.

PARASYMPATHETIC NERVOUS SYSTEM

The parasympathetic nervous system is composed of one chain of nerves that passes from the brain and another that leaves the lower spinal cord. The nerves are distributed to the same organs and structures that are supplied by the nerves of the sympathetic system. The parasympathetic nerves release the neurotransmitter *acetylcholine*, which has effects opposite to those produced by adrenaline and noradrenaline. The parasympathetic nervous system also helps to produce and maintain erection of the penis.

EFFECT OF DRUGS

Certain disorders can be treated by giving drugs that affect the autonomic nervous system. *Anticholinergic drugs*, for example, block the effect of acetylcholine, which can reduce muscle spasms in the intestine. *Beta-blocker drugs* block the action of adrenaline and noradrenaline on the heart and thus slow the rate and force of its beat.

Autopsy

A postmortem examination of the body, usually to determine the precise cause of death. An autopsy is sometimes required by law.

In instances of unnatural death or death in suspicious circumstances or where a doctor feels unable to issue a certificate of the cause of death, the Coroner (or in Scotland the Procurator Fiscal) may order an autopsy to be performed as part of his or her inquiry.

When the circumstances of death are not suspicious, but when examination of the body and organs after death will be useful in advancing knowledge of the disease causing death, and thus helping in the care of future patients, hospitals and doctors often seek the permission of the next of kin to perform an autopsy. Relatives are free to refuse such consent.

Autosuggestion

Putting oneself into a receptive hypnotic-type state as a means of stimulating the body's ability to help itself. The idea that symptoms could be relieved merely through attitude was put forth by the Frenchman Emile Coué at the end of the nineteenth century. He observed that, if people accepted a doctor's suggestion that a treatment would be effective, it was often enough to make it so. He thought that it might be possible for people to make suggestions to themselves with equally effective results.

As an aid to achieving the necessary relaxed state for successful autosuggestion, Coué advocated repetition of the catchphrase "Every day in every way, I am getting better and better." Although autosuggestion enjoyed only brief popularity, some techniques used today are based on its premise. For example, in one method used to control anxiety symptoms, people are taught muscular relaxation (*biofeedback*) techniques and then learn to summon up calming imagery or pleasant thoughts.

FUNCTIONS OF THE AUTONOMIC NERVOUS SYSTEM

The autonomic nervous system is responsible for controlling the involuntary body functions, such as sweating, digestion, and heart-rate. The system affects smooth muscles, such as those of the airways and the intestine, rather than the striated muscles, which are under the body's voluntary control.

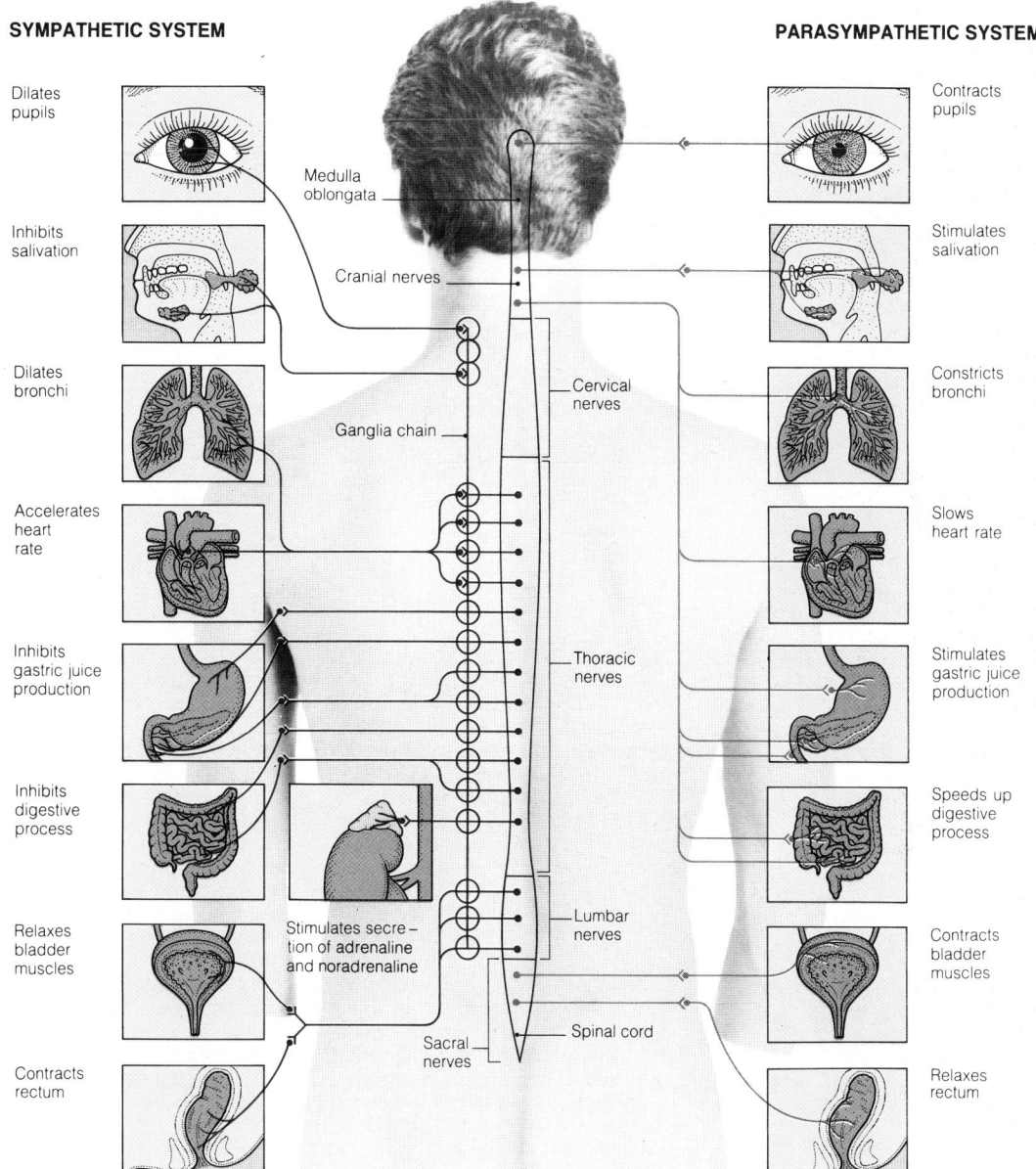

SYMPATHETIC SYSTEM

Dilates pupils

Inhibits salivation

Dilates bronchi

Accelerates heart rate

Inhibits gastric juice production

Inhibits digestive process

Relaxes bladder muscles

Stimulates secretion of adrenaline and noradrenaline

Contracts rectum

Medulla oblongata

Cranial nerves

Ganglia chain

Cervical nerves

Thoracic nerves

Lumbar nerves

Sacral nerves

Spinal cord

PARASYMPATHETIC SYSTEM

Contracts pupils

Stimulates salivation

Constricts bronchi

Slows heart rate

Stimulates gastric juice production

Speeds up digestive process

Contracts bladder muscles

Relaxes rectum

The autonomic nervous system

The autonomic nervous system is divided into two systems: the sympathetic nervous system and the parasympathetic nervous system. The sympathetic system is primarily concerned with preparing the body for action; it predominates at times of stress or excitement. The sympathetic system stimulates functions such as heart-rate and sweating and dilates the blood vessels to the muscles so that more blood is diverted to them. Simultaneously, it subdues the activity of the digestive system. In contrast, the parasympathetic nervous system is concerned mainly with the body's everyday functions such as digestion and the excretion of waste products; this system dominates during sleep. The parasympathetic system slows the heart-rate and stimulates the organs of the digestive tract. Most of the time, activity is balanced between the two systems, with neither dominating. Both of the systems play an important part in sexual arousal and orgasm in both men and women.

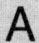

Aversion therapy

An outdated form of *behaviour therapy* in which unpleasant stimuli, such as electric shocks, are applied to suppress unwanted behaviour. It has been used to help treat self-injurious behaviour in people who are mentally handicapped. Other forms of therapy are, in general, now considered to be more appropriate.

Aviation medicine

The medical speciality concerned with the physiological effects of flight and the causes and treatment of medical problems during air travel. Aviation medicine includes assessment of the fitness of aircrew and sometimes of passengers to fly, the management of medical emergencies in the air, the consequences of special types of flight (e.g. in helicopters, high-altitude aircraft and spacecraft), and the investigation of aircraft accidents.

EFFECTS OF REDUCED OXYGEN

Increasing altitude causes a fall in air pressure and with it a fall in the pressure of oxygen. *Hypoxia* (a seriously reduced oxygen concentration in the blood and tissues) is a serious threat to anyone who flies at altitude.

If aircraft cabins were not pressurized, the oxygen saturation of the blood would fall from nearly 100 per cent on the ground to about 80 per cent at 3,000 m. To avoid the development of hypoxia, airliners are kept at a pressure equivalent to an altitude of about 2,500 m during flight, although the cruising altitude may be as high as 12,000 m (even higher in Concorde). This means that the cabin pressure is about 30 per cent less than at ground level but much higher than the outside pressure during flight. Any sudden failure of the aircraft's pressure hull leads to a rapid fall in cabin pressure, with a risk of hypoxia and *decompression sickness*. Rapid decompression in civil aircraft is extremely rare, but passengers and crew are provided with oxygen masks for use in emergencies while the aircraft descends to a safe altitude.

ANXIETY AND HYPERVENTILATION

Hypoxia or, more commonly, anxiety during flight can lead to *hyperventilation* ("overbreathing"), in which increased breathing efforts result in excess loss of carbon dioxide. This alters the acidity of the body and gives rise to symptoms such as tingling around the mouth, muscle spasms, and lightheadedness. The symptoms of hyperventilation are themselves likely to increase anxiety.

Although flying can be an exhilarating experience, many people are anxious at some stage of a flight; others suffer an acute fear of flying and may need mild pre-flight sedation. If symptoms of hyperventilation develop, the treatment is to rebreathe air from a paper bag held over the nose and mouth, which reduces the loss of carbon dioxide.

DECOMPRESSION SICKNESS

Aviator's decompression sickness has the same causes as the condition that affects scuba divers and deep tunnel workers. It is not a risk for passengers on normal flights, except when there is a marked, rapid depressurization in the cabin or when a passenger has recently been exposed to pressure changes (usually through scuba diving, which is best avoided in the 24 hours before a flight).

PRESSURE EFFECTS ON BODY CAVITIES

The changes in altitude or cabin pressure during a flight affect the body's gas-containing cavities, principally the middle ears, facial sinuses, lungs, and intestines. When pressure drops during ascent, the volume of gas in these cavities increases; on descent, the gas volume decreases as pressure outside the body rises.

On ascent, unless there is a catastrophic fall in pressure, air from the lungs is harmlessly released via the trachea (windpipe), air in the large intestine and stomach can also escape freely (although trapped gas in the small intestine can give rise to a feeling of fullness), and air in the middle ears and sinuses can leave via ducts linking them to the back of the nose.

It is during descent that pressure changes in the ears and sinuses may fail to keep up with cabin repressurization. Unless preventive measures are taken, this may lead to pain and, rarely, damage (see *Barotrauma*).

ACCELERATION AND DECELERATION

The accelerative forces experienced by civil aircraft passengers are mild, even during take-off and descent, and no precautions are necessary other than the wearing of a seat-belt. Military aircraft pilots, on the other hand, may experience severe accelerations and must wear special suits and use a reclined seat to prevent pooling of blood in the feet, which would cause immediate loss of consciousness.

OTHER EFFECTS

Motion sickness is usually less of a problem for air than for road or sea travellers. Passengers prone to motion sickness may benefit from taking an anti-motion sickness preparation.

Air travel allows the rapid crossing of several time zones within a short period, which can affect sleep-waking cycles, causing *jet-lag*.

CONDITIONS AFFECTING PASSENGER SUITABILITY FOR AIR TRAVEL

Conditions	Comments
Lung disease (such as chronic bronchitis or emphysema) Severe anaemia Heart condition (such as angina pectoris, heart failure, or recent heart attack)	The lowered cabin pressure (and thus the oxygen level) at higher altitudes aggravates an already impaired ability to oxygenate the blood and/or tissues and may cause severe respiratory distress or collapse. Seek your doctor's advice. Flying may be possible if you are able to walk 50 metres without breathlessness or chest pain.
Recent stroke	Seek your doctor's advice. You may need to wait some weeks before flying.
Recent surgery to inner or middle ear, abdomen, chest, or brain; a recently collapsed lung or a fractured skull	Seek your doctor's advice. You may need to wait before flying to avoid damage to your hearing mechanism from the expansion of gas trapped in the chest, abdomen, or skull.
Pregnancy	No flying after 34 to 36 weeks on most airlines.
Newborn baby	An infant should not fly until at least 48 hours old.
Psychiatric disorder	May need trained escort.
Infectious disease, terminal illness, or vomiting	May be refused entry to aircraft. Check with airline.

Most aircraft passengers are well able to tolerate travel in the comfort of a pressurized cabin. Those with pre-existing disorders, however, are advised to seek medical advice before undertaking a journey by air, especially if the condition is likely to be made worse by even the mild hypoxia induced at normal cabin pressures.

Most large airlines have a medical department staffed by doctors specially trained in aviation medicine, who are responsible for the health care of the airline staff. The doctors also give advice on the transportation of sick passengers, the provision of training and equipment to deal with illness during a flight, and the maintenance of airline hygiene.

Avitaminosis

Any condition that results from an insufficiency of one or more *vitamins*. Avitaminosis (also called hypovitaminosis) may be due to an inadequate dietary intake of vitamins, or a digestive disorder that causes *malabsorption* (impaired absorption of nutrients from the intestine).

Avulsed tooth

A tooth that has become completely dislodged from its socket as the result of an accident. The tooth should be carried to the dentist immediately in a glass of milk or cool water, or in a loosely wrapped, damp cloth. The dentist will reimplant the tooth into the socket as rapidly as possible, and immobilize it with a splint (see *Reimplantation, dental*). If the tooth is reimplanted within 30 minutes of the accident, and the patient is young, it will reattach itself to the socket in 90 per cent of cases.

Avulsion

The tearing away of a body structure from its point of attachment.

Avulsion may be due to an injury—for example, when a severe ankle sprain stretches ligaments on the outside of the ankle, causing a small fragment of bone to be torn away from the fibula (outer lower leg-bone).

Avulsion may also be performed deliberately as part of a surgical procedure. In the surgical treatment of *varicose veins*, for example, the stripping of veins from the leg is described as an avulsion.

Axilla

The medical name for the armpit.

Axon

The thin, elongated part of a *neuron* (nerve cell) that conducts nerve impulses. Many axons in the body are covered with a fatty *myelin* sheath.

Ayurvedism

See *Indian medicine*.

Azathioprine

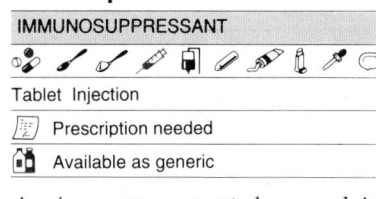

IMMUNOSUPPRESSANT		
Tablet Injection		
Prescription needed		
Available as generic		

An *immunosuppressant drug* used in the treatment of severe *rheumatoid arthritis* and other *autoimmune disorders* (in which the *immune system* attacks the body's own tissues). Azathioprine is prescribed when other treatments (e.g. *corticosteroid drugs* and other *antirheumatic drugs*) fail to slow the progress of the disease or to improve symptoms. Azathioprine is also among the drugs used to prevent organ rejection after *transplant surgery*.

Azathioprine reduces the efficiency of the body's immune system by preventing lymphocytes (types of white blood cells) from multiplying. Lymphocytes destroy foreign proteins (those not normally found in the body) and, in autoimmune disorders, attack body proteins that the immune system considers to be foreign.

Abnormal bleeding and increased susceptibility to infection may occur as a result of reduced blood cell production by the bone marrow; regular blood tests are carried out to monitor these effects.

Azithromycin

An *antibiotic* used to treat infections of the skin, chest, throat, and ears. It is also used to treat genital infections caused by *chlamydia*.

Azoospermia

The absence of sperm from semen; an important cause of *infertility* in males. Azoospermia may be caused by a disorder present at birth or may develop later in life. The condition is thought to affect about one male in 100.

Congenital azoospermia may be the result of a chromosomal abnormality, such as *Klinefelter's syndrome* (the presence of an extra sex chromosome); failure of the testes to descend into the scrotum; absence of the vasa deferentia (the ducts that carry sperm from the testes to the seminal vesicles, the sacs where sperm is stored before ejaculation); or *cystic fibrosis*, a genetic disease affecting the lungs and pancreas that may also cause defects of the vasa deferentia. *Orchitis* caused by mumps may result in azoospermia or oligospermia (fewer than normal numbers of sperm).

In some males, azoospermia is due to puberty failing to take place, usually because the pituitary gland produces insufficient follicle-stimulating hormone (*FSH*), which is necessary for sperm production. In other males, puberty occurs but the testes fail to function properly. This disorder may also cause azoospermia.

The most common cause of azoospermia in later life is *vasectomy*, the sterilization operation in which the vasa deferentia are cut and tied off. Another cause is blockage of the ducts, which may follow a *sexually transmitted disease*, *tuberculosis*, or surgery on the groin (usually performed to repair a *hernia* or to lower undescended testes in a boy).

Azoospermia can also develop because of temporary or permanent failure of the testes to produce sperm. This can follow *radiotherapy*, accidental radiation exposure, treatment with certain drugs (particularly *anticancer drugs* and the antidiarrhoeal drug *sulphasalazine*), and prolonged exposure to heat, insecticides, or industrial chemicals. In some cases, production of sperm ceases permanently for no known reason.

The diagnosis is made by analysing at least two samples of semen, given a month apart, for the presence of sperm. Other tests are carried out to discover or confirm the cause.

Injections of FSH may cause puberty to develop, and surgery can sometimes unblock ducts closed by infection. Most other causes of azoospermia are untreatable and a sufferer who wishes to become a parent must do so by *artificial insemination* of his partner with donor sperm or must adopt a child.

AZT

The abbreviation for azidothymidine, the former name for *zidovudine*.

Aztreonam

An *antibiotic* used to treat some types of meningitis and infections by certain types of bacteria including *PSEUDOMONAS*.

B

Babinski's sign

A reflex movement in which the big toe bends upwards when the outer edge of the sole of the foot is scratched. In adults, Babinski's sign indicates damage or disease of the brain or the spinal cord. In babies, Babinski's sign is a normal reflex.

Baby blues

A common name for a mild form of depression that may occur after childbirth. Such depression almost always disappears without treatment, but can occasionally develop into a more serious depressive illness. (See *Postnatal depression.*)

Bacampicillin

A type of *penicillin drug.*

Bacilli

Rod-shaped *bacteria.* Bacilli are responsible for many diseases, including tuberculosis, pertussis (whooping cough), tetanus, typhoid fever, and diphtheria (see *Infectious disease*).

Back

The area between the shoulders and the buttocks. The back is supported by the spinal column (see *Spine*), which is bound together by ligaments and supported by muscles that also control posture and movement.

DISORDERS

Problems involving the back are numerous. They arise from a number of causes affecting the spine, and can involve disorders of bones, muscles, ligaments, tendons, nerves, and joints in the spine. These disorders can cause *back pain.* (See also *Spine* disorders box.)

Backbone

See *Spine.*

Back pain

Most people suffer from back pain at some time in their lives. In many cases, no exact diagnosis is made because the pain gets better with rest and because *analgesic drugs* (painkill-

ers) are used before any tests, such as *X-rays*, are performed. In such cases, doctors use the term "nonspecific back pain".

CAUSES

Nonspecific back pain is one of the largest single causes of working days lost through illness in the UK. People most likely to suffer from back pain are those whose jobs involve much heavy lifting and carrying, or those who spend long periods sitting in one position or bending awkwardly. Overweight people are also more prone to back pain—their backs carry a heavier load and they tend to have weaker abdominal muscles, which help provide back support.

Nonspecific back pain is thought to be due to a mechanical disorder affecting one or more structures in the back. The disorder may be a ligament strain, a muscle tear, damage to a spinal facet joint, or prolapse of an intervertebral disc.

In addition to pain from a damaged structure, spasm of surrounding muscles will cause additional pain and tenderness over a wider area and can cause temporary *scoliosis* (abnormal sideways curvature of the spine).

Abnormalities of a facet joint and *disc prolapse* (slipped disc) can both cause *sciatica* (pain in the buttock and down the back of the leg into the foot), resulting from pressure on a sciatic nerve root as it leaves the spinal cord. Coughing, sneezing, or straining will increase the pain. Pressure on the sciatic nerve can also cause pins-and-needles in that leg, and weakness in muscles activated by the nerve. Rarely, pain may radiate down the femoral nerve at the front of the thigh.

Osteoarthritis in the joints of the spine can cause persistent back pain. *Ankylosing spondylitis* (an inflammatory disorder in which arthritis affects the spine) causes back pain and stiffness with loss of back mobility. *Coccydynia* (pain and tenderness at the base of the spine) may occur after a fall in which the coccyx has struck the ground, during pregnancy, or spontaneously for unknown reasons.

Fibrositis is an imprecise term sometimes used to describe pain and tenderness in muscles. It may affect the back. Fibrositis is often worse in cold and damp weather and is occasionally associated with feeling unwell. Unlike other causes of back pain, fibrositis is not accompanied by muscle spasm or restriction of back movement. It often improves when treated with *nonsteroidal anti-inflammatory drugs.*

Pyelonephritis can cause back pain with pain and tenderness in the loin, fever, chills, and pain when passing urine. Cancer in the spine can cause persistent back pain that disturbs sleep and is not relieved by rest.

SELF-HELP

Back pain and sciatica may improve by resting on a firm mattress or board. Analgesic drugs and the application of heat to the back can help relieve pain. However, if pain persists, is very severe, or is associated with weakness in a leg or problems with bladder control, a doctor should be consulted without delay.

INVESTIGATION

Examination of the back may show tenderness in specific areas and loss of mobility of the back. Weakness or loss of sensation in the legs implies pressure on a nerve root, which requires prompt investigation.

X-rays of the spine may show narrowing between the intervertebral discs, osteoarthritis, *osteoporosis*, ankylosing spondylitis, compression fracture, stress fracture, *bone cancer*, or *spondylolisthesis* (displacement of vertebrae). X-rays will not reveal ligament, muscle, facet joint, or disc damage. To reveal pressure on a nerve root (due to disc prolapse, for example), *myelography, CT scanning*, or *MRI* is performed.

TREATMENT

If a specific cause is found for back pain, treatment will be for that cause. Acute nonspecific back pain is treated with periods of rest and use of analgesic drugs. Chronic nonspecific back pain is more difficult to treat. Treatment may include *aspirin* and related drugs, *nonsteroidal anti-inflammatory drugs*, or *muscle-relaxant drugs*; *acupuncture* or spinal injection; or exercise, spinal *manipulation*, wearing a surgical *corset*, or spinal surgery.

Baclofen

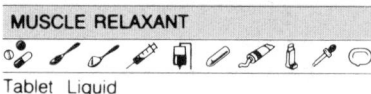

MUSCLE RELAXANT	
Tablet Liquid	
Prescription needed	
Available as generic	

A *muscle-relaxant drug* that blocks nerve activity in the spinal cord. Baclofen relieves muscle spasm and stiffness that have been caused by injury to the brain or spinal cord, by a *stroke*, or by neurological disorders such as *multiple sclerosis*. Baclofen does not cure the underlying disorder but

BACKACHE Pain and/or stiffness in the back that may be continuous or intermittent.

Of recent origin

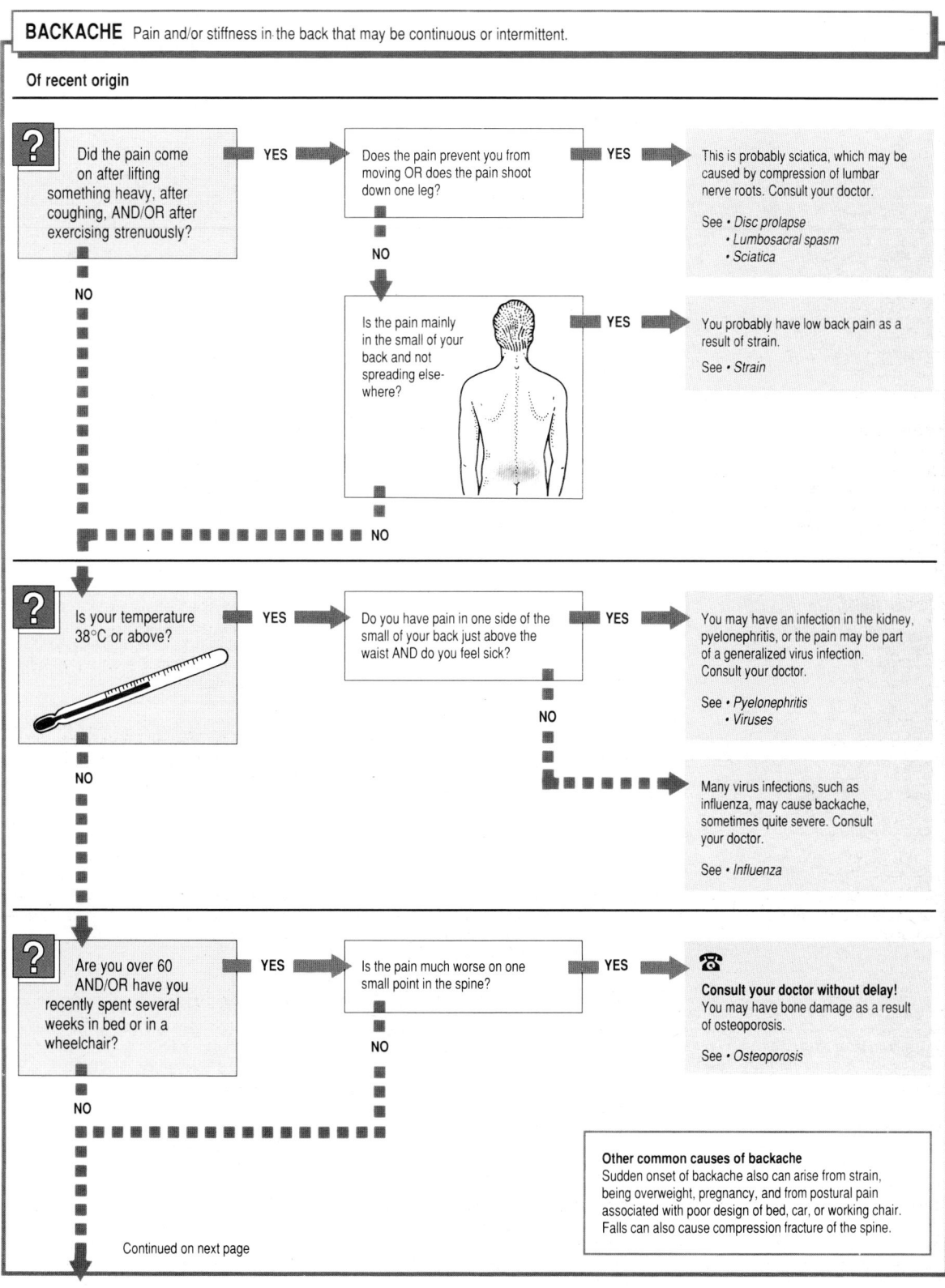

? Did the pain come on after lifting something heavy, after coughing, AND/OR after exercising strenuously?

→ **YES** → Does the pain prevent you from moving OR does the pain shoot down one leg?

→ **YES** → This is probably sciatica, which may be caused by compression of lumbar nerve roots. Consult your doctor.

See • *Disc prolapse*
 • *Lumbosacral spasm*
 • *Sciatica*

NO ↓

Is the pain mainly in the small of your back and not spreading else-where?

→ **YES** → You probably have low back pain as a result of strain.

See • *Strain*

NO →

? Is your temperature 38°C or above?

→ **YES** → Do you have pain in one side of the small of your back just above the waist AND do you feel sick?

→ **YES** → You may have an infection in the kidney, pyelonephritis, or the pain may be part of a generalized virus infection. Consult your doctor.

See • *Pyelonephritis*
 • *Viruses*

NO →

Many virus infections, such as influenza, may cause backache, sometimes quite severe. Consult your doctor.

See • *Influenza*

NO ↓

? Are you over 60 AND/OR have you recently spent several weeks in bed or in a wheelchair?

→ **YES** → Is the pain much worse on one small point in the spine?

→ **YES** → ☎

Consult your doctor without delay!
You may have bone damage as a result of osteoporosis.

See • *Osteoporosis*

NO ↓

NO →

> **Other common causes of backache**
> Sudden onset of backache also can arise from strain, being overweight, pregnancy, and from postural pain associated with poor design of bed, car, or working chair. Falls can also cause compression fracture of the spine.

Continued on next page

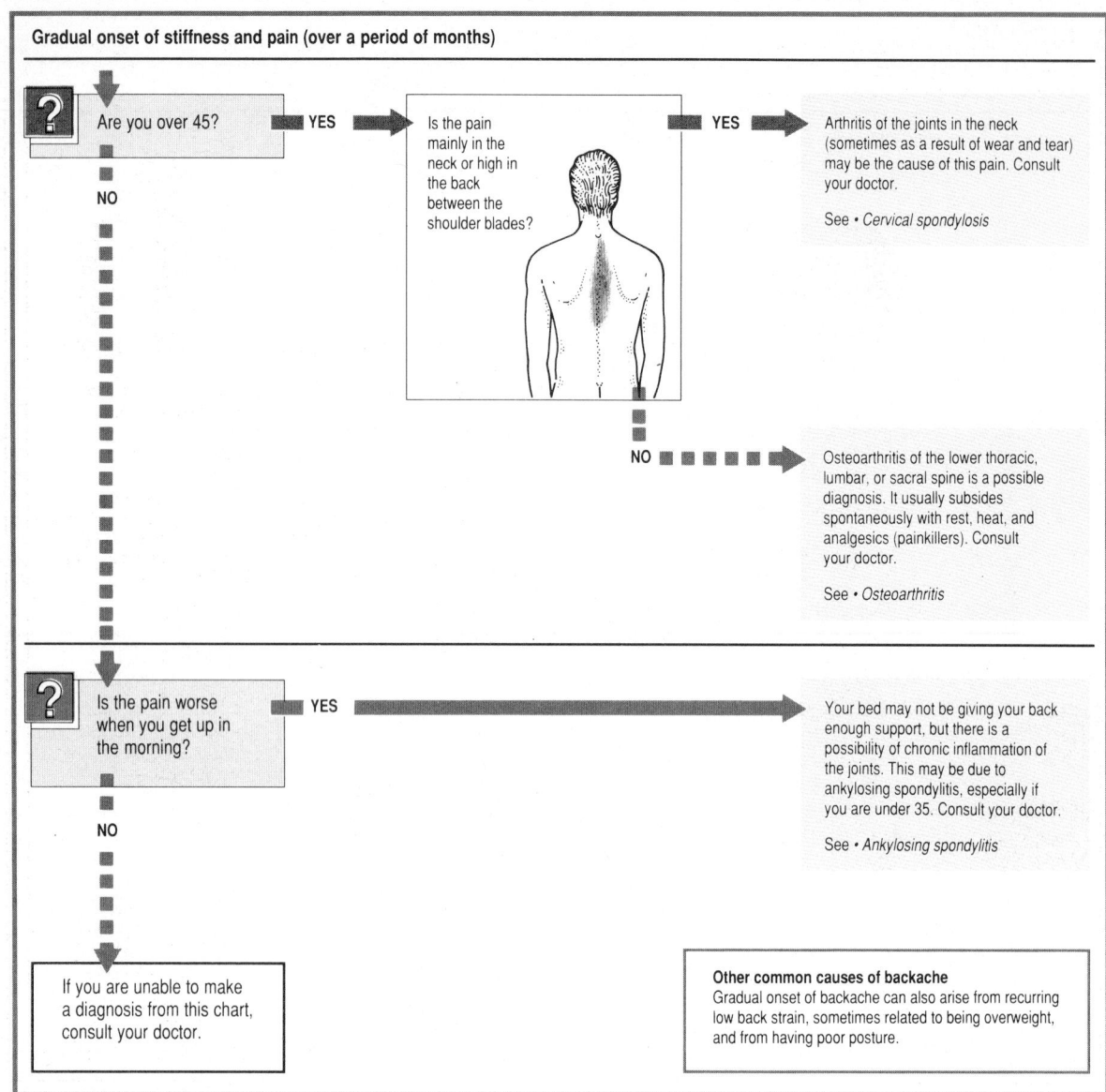

Gradual onset of stiffness and pain (over a period of months)

Are you over 45? — YES →

Is the pain mainly in the neck or high in the back between the shoulder blades? — YES → Arthritis of the joints in the neck (sometimes as a result of wear and tear) may be the cause of this pain. Consult your doctor.

See • *Cervical spondylosis*

NO →

NO → Osteoarthritis of the lower thoracic, lumbar, or sacral spine is a possible diagnosis. It usually subsides spontaneously with rest, heat, and analgesics (painkillers). Consult your doctor.

See • *Osteoarthritis*

Is the pain worse when you get up in the morning? — YES → Your bed may not be giving your back enough support, but there is a possibility of chronic inflammation of the joints. This may be due to ankylosing spondylitis, especially if you are under 35. Consult your doctor.

See • *Ankylosing spondylitis*

NO →

If you are unable to make a diagnosis from this chart, consult your doctor.

Other common causes of backache
Gradual onset of backache can also arise from recurring low back strain, sometimes related to being overweight, and from having poor posture.

often allows *physiotherapy* to be more effective, and makes walking and performing tasks with the hands easier.

To reduce the risk of adverse effects, such as drowsiness and muscle weakness, the dose of the drug is usually increased slowly under medical supervision until the desired effect is achieved.

Bacteraemia

The presence of bacteria in the bloodstream. Bacteraemia occurs for a few hours after many minor surgical operations and may also occur with infections such as tonsillitis.

In people with abnormal heart valves, due to a congenital defect or to scarring from previous rheumatic fever, the bacteria may cause *endocarditis* (inflammation of the heart lining and valves). If bacteraemia affects a person whose *immune system* has been weakened by illness or a major surgical operation, *septicaemia* and *septic shock* may follow.

Bacteria

A group of single-celled *microorganisms*, some of which cause disease. Commonly known as "germs", bacteria have been recognized as a cause of

disease for over a century, but it is still not fully understood why some people become ill while others remain well when exposed to the same sources of infection. Abundant in the air, soil, and water, most bacteria are harmless to humans. Some, indeed, are beneficial, such as those that live in the intestine and help break down food for digestion. Bacteria that cause disease are known as pathogens.

Bacteria were discovered by Antonj van Leewenhoek in the 17th century following development of the microscope, but it was not until the mid-19th century that the French

BACK PAIN

Most people experience back pain some time in their lives, but in most cases it is not serious and the problem corrects itself before investigation takes place. However, some kinds of back pain can be related to a specific disorder. In the diagram below, you will find the most common sites affected by back pain.

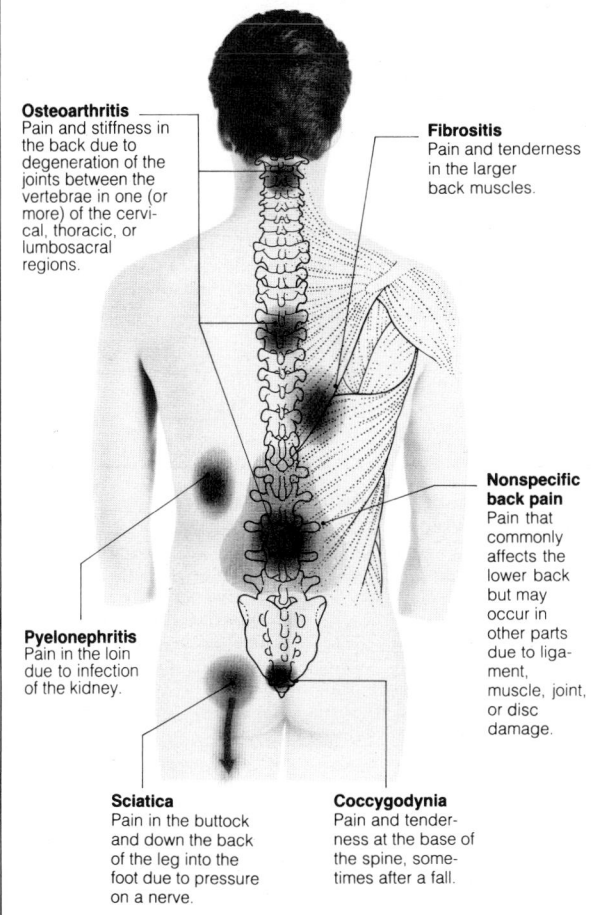

Osteoarthritis
Pain and stiffness in the back due to degeneration of the joints between the vertebrae in one (or more) of the cervical, thoracic, or lumbosacral regions.

Fibrositis
Pain and tenderness in the larger back muscles.

Nonspecific back pain
Pain that commonly affects the lower back but may occur in other parts due to ligament, muscle, joint, or disc damage.

Pyelonephritis
Pain in the loin due to infection of the kidney.

Sciatica
Pain in the buttock and down the back of the leg into the foot due to pressure on a nerve.

Coccygodynia
Pain and tenderness at the base of the spine, sometimes after a fall.

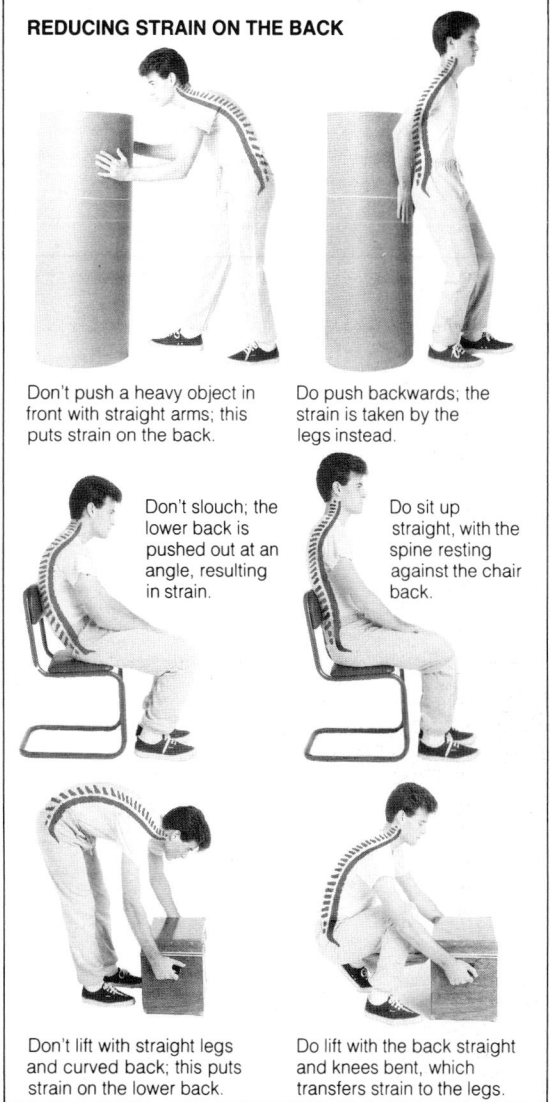

REDUCING STRAIN ON THE BACK

Don't push a heavy object in front with straight arms; this puts strain on the back.

Do push backwards; the strain is taken by the legs instead.

Don't slouch; the lower back is pushed out at an angle, resulting in strain.

Do sit up straight, with the spine resting against the chair back.

Don't lift with straight legs and curved back; this puts strain on the lower back.

Do lift with the back straight and knees bent, which transfers strain to the legs.

scientist Louis Pasteur established beyond doubt that they were the cause of many diseases.

TYPES

Pathogenic (disease-producing) bacteria are classified, on the basis of shape, into three main groups: cocci (spherical); bacilli (rod-shaped); and spirochaetes or spirilla (spiral-shaped).

Among the wide range of diseases caused by cocci are pneumonia, tonsillitis, bacterial endocarditis, meningitis, toxic shock syndrome, and various skin disorders.

Diseases caused by bacilli include tuberculosis, pertussis (whooping cough), tetanus, typhoid fever, diphtheria, salmonellosis, shigellosis (bacillary dysentery), legionnaires' disease, and botulism.

Bacteria from the third, and smallest group, the spirochaetes, are responsible for syphilis, yaws, leptospirosis, and Lyme disease.

GROWTH, MOVEMENT, REPRODUCTION

The bacteria that colonize the human body thrive in warm, moist conditions. Some are aerobic—that is, they require oxygen to grow and multiply—and so they are most commonly found on the skin or in the respiratory system. Anaerobic bacteria thrive where there is no oxygen—deep within tissue or wounds.

Many bacteria are naturally static and, if they move around the body, do so only in currents of air or fluid. Some, however, such as salmonella (responsible for food poisoning and typhoid) are highly motile, moving through fluid by lashing with their flagella (whip-like, filamentous tails).

Bacteria reproduce by dividing into two cells, which in turn divide, and so on. Under ideal conditions (exactly the right temperature and sufficient nourishment for all cells), this division can take place every 20 minutes, an extremely rapid rate of reproduction. After only six hours, a single bacterium can have multiplied to form a colony of more than 250,000 bacteria. This very rarely happens, however, because ideal conditions rarely occur and in a healthy individual the body's *immune system* destroys the invading bacteria.

As well as dividing, some types of bacteria—such as, for example, clostridia (responsible for botulism, tetanus, pseudomembranous colitis, and anthrax)—also multiply, in a much more restricted way, by each producing a spore. A spore is a single new bacterium, protected by a tough membrane, that can survive high temperatures, dry conditions, and lack of nourishment.

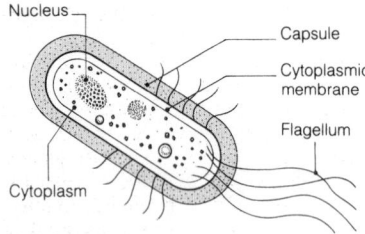

Magnified bacterium
A typical bacterial cell enlarged to approximately 20,000 times its normal size.

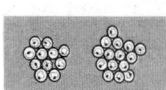

Staphylococcus
(causes boils)

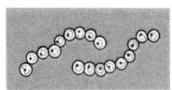

Streptococcus
(causes sore throat)

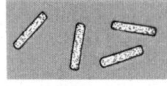

Salmonella typhosa
(causes typhoid fever)

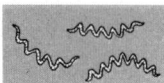

Spirochaeta
(causes syphilis)

Common types of bacteria

HOW BACTERIA ENTER THE BODY
Bacteria can enter through the lungs if droplets breathed, coughed, or sneezed out by an infected person are inhaled. Diseases caught thus include diphtheria, and pertussis.

The digestive tract can become infected if contaminated food is eaten. Bacteria may be present in food at its primary source, or brought to it by flies or by people preparing it with contaminated hands.

Microorganisms that enter the genito-urinary system include those causing sexually transmitted diseases (e.g. syphilis, pelvic inflammatory disease, and gonorrhoea).

Bacteria can penetrate the skin in various ways: through hair follicles (which may cause boils); through superficial wounds, such as cuts or abrasions (which may lead to erysipelas); or through deep wounds (as in the case of tetanus).

HOW BACTERIA CAUSE DISEASE
Bacteria produce poisons that are harmful to human cells. If they are present in sufficient quantity and the affected person is not immune to them, disease results. Some bacteria release poisons known as endotoxins, which can cause fever, haemorrhage, and shock. Others produce exotoxins, which account for the major damage in diseases such as diphtheria, tetanus, and toxic shock syndrome.

RESISTANCE BY THE BODY
The body's first means of preventing invasion by harmful bacteria are the substances hostile to bacteria in the skin, lining of the respiratory tract, digestive tract, and genito-urinary system. The eyes are protected by an enzyme in the tears, and the stomach secretes hydrochloric acid, which kills many of the bacteria found in food and water.

If the bacteria break through these defences, two types of white blood cell attack them: neutrophils engulf and destroy many of the bacteria, and lymphocytes produce antibodies against them. The antibodies attack the bacteria directly. After an infection, antibodies remain in the blood for a considerable time—many years in the case of typhoid and scarlet fever—so that any further attacks of the disease are usually prevented or are mild.

TREATMENT OF BACTERIAL DISEASE
The response of the immune system to bacterial illness is sometimes enough by itself to bring about recovery, but in many cases medical treatment is necessary. The main form of treatment is *antibiotic drugs*, given either by mouth or by injection. Some, such as penicillin, are bactericidal (destroy the invading bacteria); others, such as tetracycline, are bacteriostatic (prevent them from multiplying further), permitting the immune system to overcome the invaders.

Some diseases—among them diphtheria, tetanus, botulism, and gas gangrene—are treated by the injection of an antiserum. This is a fluid taken from the blood of a person or a horse who has been given a series of immunizing injections and whose blood therefore contains antibodies against the disease organisms.

Superficial inflammation and infected wounds may be treated with antiseptic solutions.

PREVENTION
Immunity to certain bacterial diseases (for example, diphtheria, typhoid, pertussis and tetanus) can be acquired by active *immunization* (injection with weakened or killed forms of the bacteria or their poisons).

People with infections should take steps to prevent their spread; those with respiratory infections should keep away from crowded places to prevent the possibility of droplet infection, and should always use a handkerchief when coughing or sneezing. Food handlers should be meticulous about their health and personal hygiene.

Any wound should be washed with an antiseptic solution to destroy bacteria, and then covered with a clean, dry dressing. (See also *Infectious disease*.)

Bactericidal
A term used to describe any substance that kills bacteria. (See *Antibacterial drugs*; *Antibiotic drugs*.)

Bacteriology
The study of *bacteria*, particularly of the types that cause disease. The pioneer of this science was the French scientist Louis Pasteur (1822-1895), who was the first to prove that bacteria are the cause and not the result of illness. He was followed by the German physician Robert Koch (1843-1910), who not only discovered a large number of the bacteria responsible for particular diseases but also laid down the principles for isolating and identifying disease-producing bacteria on which modern bacteriology is based.

METHODS OF IDENTIFYING BACTERIA
To discover which bacterium is causing a disease, it must be isolated. A throat swab or a specimen of urine, faeces, blood, spinal fluid, sputum, or pus is first taken from an infected person. This material is then examined by one of three main methods.

STAINING The application of special stains makes it possible to look at and differentiate bacteria under the microscope. In a sample treated with Gram's stain, for example, staphylococci or streptococci bacteria turn purple, whereas many other types, such as salmonella, turn red.

CULTURE For this method of examination, the sample material is introduced into a nutrient, where the bacteria multiply and can be identified by their appearance and growth re-

CULTURING AND TESTING BACTERIA

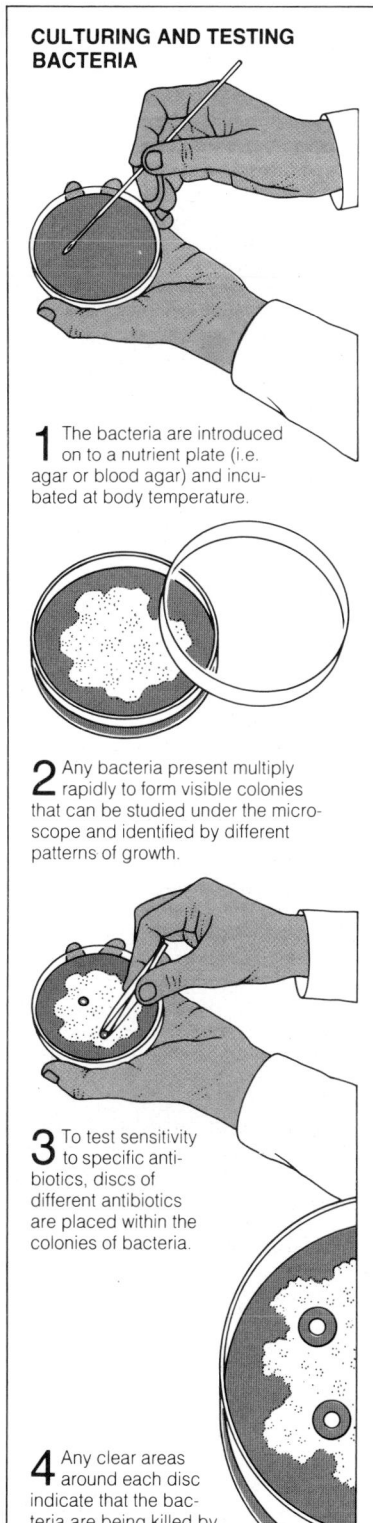

1 The bacteria are introduced on to a nutrient plate (i.e. agar or blood agar) and incubated at body temperature.

2 Any bacteria present multiply rapidly to form visible colonies that can be studied under the microscope and identified by different patterns of growth.

3 To test sensitivity to specific antibiotics, discs of different antibiotics are placed within the colonies of bacteria.

4 Any clear areas around each disc indicate that the bacteria are being killed by a particular antibiotic.

quirements. Different antibiotics are introduced and their effects studied to see which will be effective in treating the infection (see box).

ANTIBODY TESTING This is done by extracting serum from the blood of an infected person and adding it to a sample of the type of bacteria suspected of causing the infection. If the suspicion is correct, antibodies against the bacteria already present in the serum will visibly clump together with the bacteria in the sample.

Bacteriostatic

A term used to describe a substance that stops the growth or multiplication of bacteria. (See *Antibacterial drugs*; *Antibiotic drugs*.)

Bacteriuria

The presence of *bacteria* in the urine. A small, harmless number of bacteria may be found in the urine of many healthy people, so bacteriuria is of significance only if more than 100,000 bacteria are present in each millilitre of urine, or if 100 white blood cells (pus cells) per millilitre are present.

Bad breath

See *Halitosis*.

Bagassosis

An occupational disease affecting the lungs of workers who handle mouldy bagasse (the fibrous residue of sugarcane after the juice has been extracted). Bagassosis is one cause of allergic *alveolitis*, a reaction of the lungs to inhaled dust that contains fungal spores.

Acute attacks usually develop four to five hours after inhalation of dust. The symptoms may include shortness of breath associated with wheezing, fever, headache, and cough; typically they last no more than 24 hours. Repeated exposure to dust may lead to permanent lung damage, chronic sickness, and weight loss. Protective measures taken by industry have now made the disease rare.

Baker's cyst

A firm, walnut-sized, fluid-filled lump behind the knee. A Baker's cyst is caused by increased pressure within the knee joint due to a build-up of fluid in a disorder such as *rheumatoid arthritis*. The cyst is created by a backward "ballooning out" of the synovial membrane covering the knee joint.

Most Baker's cysts are painless. Some disappear spontaneously, perhaps after many months. Occasion-

ally, a cyst may rupture, causing fluid to seep down between the layers of the calf muscles. A ruptured cyst may produce pain and swelling.

Diagnosis may be assisted by *arthrography* (imaging of the joint with X-rays after injection of a radiopaque substance). Treatment may consist simply of a supportive bandage. In some cases, surgical removal of the cyst is required.

Balance

The ability to remain upright and move without falling over. Keeping one's balance is a complex process that relies on a constant flow of information about body position to the brain. Integration of this information and a continual flow of instructions from the brain enable various parts of the body to perform the changes needed to maintain balance.

Information about body position comes from three sources: the eyes, which give visual information about the body's position relative to its surroundings; sensory receptors (called proprioceptors) in the skin, muscles, and joints, which provide information about the position and movement of the different parts of the body; and the three semicircular canals of the labyrinth in the inner ear, which detect the direction and speed of head movements. The part of the brain called the cerebellum collates this information and instructs muscles to contract or relax to maintain balance.

DISORDERS

Various disorders can affect balance, particularly disorders of the inner ear, such as *labyrinthitis* (inflammation of the labyrinth of the ear) and *Ménière's disease* (abnormally high pressure of fluid in the labyrinth). In some cases, *otitis media* (inflammation of the middle ear) may also affect the inner ear and disturb balance. In addition to loss of balance, these disorders often cause *dizziness* or *vertigo*, and impaired hearing.

Damage to nerve tracts in the spinal cord, which carry information from proprioceptors, may occur as a result of spinal tumours, disorders of the circulation, nerve degeneration due to deficiency of vitamin B_{12}, or, rarely, tabes dorsalis (a complication of *syphilis*). These disorders produce a distinctive, wide-based, clumsy gait.

A tumour or stroke that affects the cerebellum may cause not only clumsiness of the arms and legs, but also speech disorders and other features of impaired muscular coordination.

Balanitis

Inflammation of the glans (head) of the penis and foreskin. The main symptom is a painful or itchy penis, and the entire area may be red and moist. Causes include infection with bacteria or fungi, *phimosis* (tight foreskin), or irritation by chemicals in clothing or contraceptive cream. Infection may be the result of poor hygiene, but fungal infections such as *candidiasis* (thrush) are usually contracted from a sexual partner.

Washing the penis (including under the foreskin), applying a soothing cream (your doctor will recommend one), and taking a course of *antibiotic drugs* will relieve the symptoms. If balanitis recurs frequently, or if the cause is phimosis, *circumcision* (removal of the foreskin) may be recommended.

Baldness

See *Alopecia*.

Balloon catheter

A flexible tube with a balloon at its tip, which, when inflated, keeps the tube in place or applies pressure to an organ or vessel.

USES

The oldest and simplest type, the Foley catheter, is used to drain urine from the bladder. This catheter is passed into the bladder and sterile

water is then pumped into one channel to inflate the balloon, which prevents the catheter from dropping out. Urine flows out of the bladder through a second channel.

Balloon catheters are sometimes used when a blood vessel has been blocked by a blood clot. The end of the catheter is passed through the clot, the balloon is inflated, and, when the catheter is withdrawn, the balloon pulls the clot out with it. This procedure is called balloon *embolectomy*.

A catheter with a sausage-shaped balloon is used to expand narrowed arteries. In many cases this technique, known as balloon *angioplasty*, avoids the need for surgery, although narrowing of the vessel may recur.

Another use of the balloon catheter is to treat bleeding *oesophageal varices* (widened veins in the lower part of the oesophagus), a life-threatening complication of some kinds of liver disease. The tube is passed down the oesophagus and into the stomach, where a balloon at the tip keeps the tube in position. Another balloon higher up the tube is inflated to compress the vein walls; this usually stops or controls the bleeding until the patient can be prepared for surgery.

Another type of balloon can be placed by a narrow catheter into a blood vessel, inflated with a quick-setting durable material, detached, and left in permanent position, thereby completely shutting off blood flow in that vessel. These catheters are used to control bleeding or to starve a tumour of its blood supply.

Balm

A soothing or healing medicine applied to the skin.

Bambuterol

A bronchodilator drug that is converted to *terbutaline* in the body and has similar actions.

Bandage

A strip or tube of fabric used to keep *dressings* in position, to apply pressure, to control bleeding, or to support a sprain or strain.

Roller bandages are the traditional type and are still the most widely used. Tubular gauze bandages are quicker and easier to apply than roller bandages, but they require a special applicator. They are mainly used for small cuts, grazes, and burns on areas that are awkward to bandage, such as a finger. Triangular bandages are used to make *slings*. (See also *Wounds*.)

Barbiturate drugs

COMMON DRUGS

Amylobarbitone Butobarbitone Phenobarbitone Quinalbarbitone Thiopentone

> **WARNING**
> Barbiturates may be habit forming; if taken with large amounts of alcohol, they may cause death.

A group of *sedative drugs* that work by depressing activity within the brain. Barbiturates were formerly in wide use as *antianxiety drugs, sleeping drugs,* and *anticonvulsant drugs*. Today, their use is strictly controlled because they are habit-forming and widely abused. An overdose can be fatal, particularly in combination with alcohol.

WHY THEY ARE USED

Phenobarbitone is still often used as an anticonvulsant drug in the treatment of *epilepsy*, and thiopentone remains a drug of choice for inducing anaesthesia (see *Anaesthesia, general*). However, *benzodiazepine drugs* and other nonbarbiturate drugs have now largely replaced barbiturates in the treatment of sleeplessness and anxiety. Barbiturates which are occasionally used today to induce sleep include amylobarbitone, butobarbitone, and quinalbarbitone.

HOW THEY WORK

The sedative action of barbiturate drugs is produced by the drug molecules blocking the conduction of stimulatory chemical signals between nerve cells in the brain and reducing the ability of the cells to respond.

Barbiturates, especially phenobarbitone, also reduce the sensitivity of brain cells to abnormal electrical activity. This action is beneficial in the treatment of epilepsy because it reduces the likelihood of seizures.

POSSIBLE ADVERSE EFFECTS

Adverse effects include excessive drowsiness, staggering gait, and, in some cases among the very young and old, excitability. The depressant effect of barbiturates on the brain (including suppression of the respiratory centre) is dangerously increased by alcohol.

Barbiturates are likely to produce *drug dependence* if used for longer than a few weeks; withdrawal effects (which may include sleeplessness, twitching, nightmares, and convulsions) may occur when regular treatment is suddenly stopped. Tolerance, in which increasingly large doses are needed to produce the same effect, often develops.

TYPES OF BALLOON CATHETER

Irrigation tube for fluid to wash out bladder

Sterile water tube

Tube to drain urine from bladder

Embolectomy catheter

Inflatable balloon

Urinary catheter

FIRST AID: APPLYING BANDAGES

TUBULAR BANDAGE

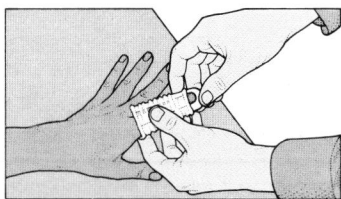

1 Cut a length of tube gauze about two and a half times the length of the finger and put it all on to the applicator. Push the applicator over the finger and hold on to the end of the gauze.

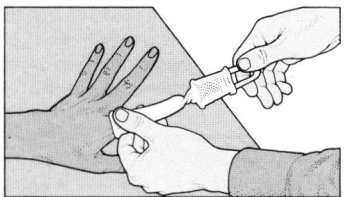

2 Still holding the gauze end on the finger, gently pull back the applicator, leaving the tube of gauze in position. Then twist it once or twice, but not more, or you may impair circulation.

3 Push the applicator back on to the finger; again, hold on to the two gauze ends, then pull it off again leaving two layers in position. Secure the ends of the gauze with tape.

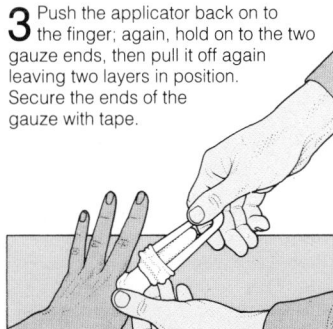

ROLLER BANDAGE

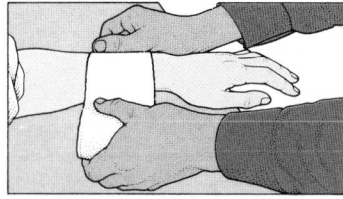

1 Place the end of the bandage on the arm and hold it firmly while you make a straight turn with the rolled end to secure it.

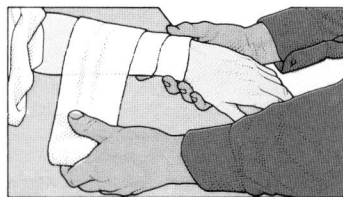

2 Work up the limb, making a series of spiral turns so that each successive turn covers two thirds of the previous one.

3 Complete the bandaging with a straight turn, cut off the spare bandage roll, and secure the end with a safety pin, adhesive tape, or bandage clip.

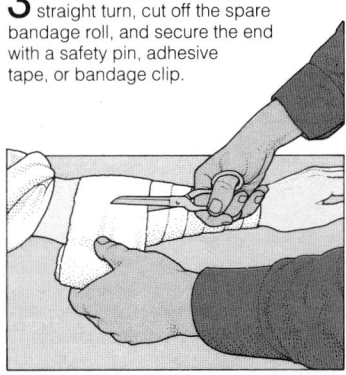

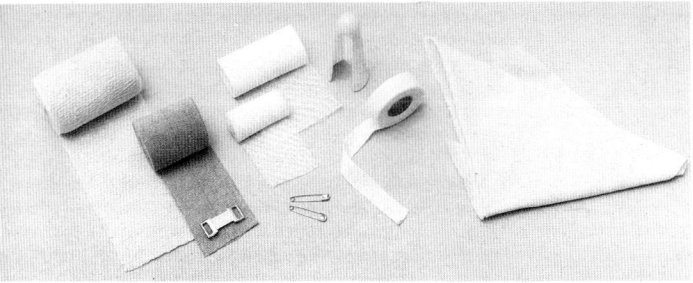

Bandaging equipment
Shown (from left) are crepe roller bandages, a bandage clip, gauze roller bandages, safety pins, a tubular bandage applicator, a roll of tubular bandage, and a triangular bandage.

Barium X-ray examinations

A group of procedures used to detect and follow the progress of some diseases of the gastrointestinal tract. Powdered barium sulphate mixed with water is passed into the part of the tract that needs to be examined and *X-ray* pictures of the area are taken. Because barium, a metallic element, is opaque to X-rays, it provides an image of the tract on the X-ray film.

WHY THEY ARE DONE

Barium X-rays are carried out less often since the development of *endoscopy*, but they provide a useful alternative in the assessment of patients with swallowing difficulty, abdominal pain, bloodstained vomit, bleeding from the rectum, a change in bowel habits, persistent diarrhoea or constipation, and unexplained weight loss.

Disorders that can be detected by barium X-rays include narrowing or inflammation of the oesophagus, disorders of the swallowing mechanism, hiatus hernia, stomach and duodenal ulcers and tumours, inflammatory bowel disease, diverticular disease, Crohn's disease, coeliac disease, and tumours or polyps in the colon.

HOW THEY ARE DONE

Barium X-ray examinations are generally carried out on an outpatient basis. No anaesthetic is required. A fluorescent screen connected to the X-ray machine enables the radiologist to follow the progress of the barium through the gastrointestinal tract, and to see any abnormalities outlined by the barium. Permanent records of the examination are provided by X-ray photographs or video recordings.

Because barium sulphate liquid dries out as its water content is absorbed in the colon, it often causes constipation. Patients may therefore need a fibre-rich diet, plenty to drink, and in some cases laxatives to get rid of the chemical.

TYPES OF EXAMINATION

Different types of barium X-ray examination are used to investigate the gastrointestinal tract.

BARIUM SWALLOW, BARIUM MEAL, BARIUM FOLLOW-THROUGH These are used to investigate disorders of the upper gastrointestinal tract: barium swallow for the oesophagus, barium meal for the lower oesophagus, stomach, and duodenum, and barium follow-through for the small intestine.

In a barium swallow examination, the patient usually takes in enough air with the barium to facilitate double-

B

contrast imaging. If a double-contrast barium meal examination is required, it is necessary to give carbonated barium, usually with gas-producing tablets or granules. Double-contrast imaging is usually not possible for a follow-through examination because it is too difficult to introduce air into the small intestine.

Barium swallow and meal take about 10 minutes to perform; follow-through may last up to five hours.

BARIUM SMALL-BOWEL ENEMA Also called enteroclysis, this single-contrast X-ray technique provides a more detailed examination of the small intestine than the barium follow-through because more barium reaches the

area. Sedation may be necessary because the procedure, which takes 20 to 25 minutes, can cause discomfort.

BARIUM ENEMA This technique is used to investigate disorders of the lower gastrointestinal tract: the large intestine and rectum. For a single-contrast image, the large intestine is filled with diluted barium liquid. For a double-

---

BARIUM X-RAY PROCEDURES

BARIUM SWALLOW, MEAL, AND INTESTINAL FOLLOW-THROUGH

1 No food or drink is permitted for six to nine hours beforehand

2 At the examination, the patient swallows a glass of barium mixed with a flavoured liquid, or is given a piece of bread or a biscuit soaked in barium if a disorder of the swallowing mechanism is being investigated.

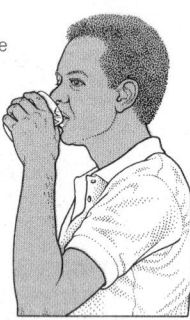

3 The radiographer then takes X-ray pictures. For a barium swallow, the patient stands; for a barium meal, the patient lies on the table in different positions; for a barium follow-through, the patient lies on the right side and X-rays are taken at intervals until the barium has progressed through the small intestine.

BARIUM SMALL-BOWEL ENEMA

1 No food or drink is permitted for nine hours beforehand.

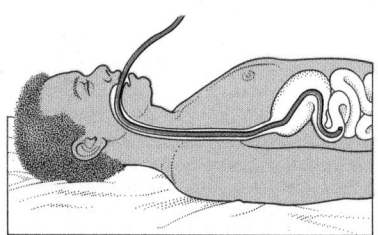

2 At the examination, the patient lies down and the radiographer or the radiologist passes a fine tube through the mouth or nose, down through the stomach and duodenum, and into the small intestine.

3 Barium is then passed down the tube directly into the small intestine.

BARIUM ENEMA

1 For successful examination, the large intestine needs to be as empty and clean as possible, since faeces can obscure or simulate a polyp or tumour. For this reason the patient's intake of food and fluids is sometimes restricted for a few days before the examination, and laxatives are given.

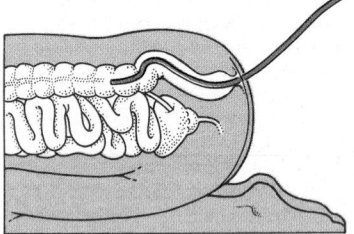

2 The patient lies face-down on the X-ray table.

3 The radiographer or the radiologist introduces barium into the intestine through a tube inserted into the rectum.

X-RAY TECHNIQUES
There are two different techniques.

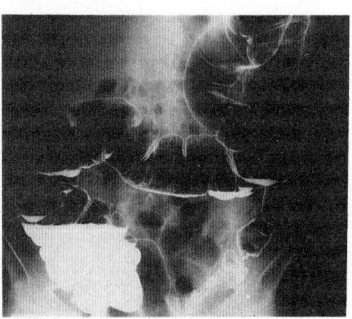

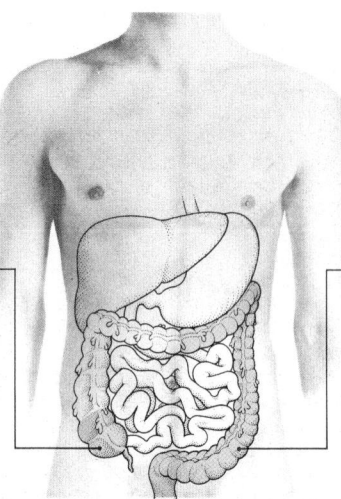

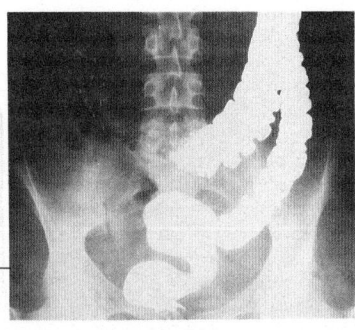

Double-contrast technique
Air, as well as barium liquid, is introduced into the tract. As a result, the barium does not fill the tract but forms only a film on its inner surface. This provides an image of small, surface abnormalities that would not be visible using the single-contrast technique.

Single-contrast technique
The section of intestine is filled with barium liquid, which provides an outline image that shows up prominent abnormalities.

contrast examination, a smaller quantity of more concentrated barium liquid is introduced, followed by air. The whole procedure lasts about 20 minutes, and in most cases causes only mild discomfort.

After the examination, a small amount of barium is expelled from the body immediately, and the rest is excreted later in the faeces.

Barotrauma

Damage or pain, mainly affecting the middle *ear* and facial *sinuses*, caused by the effects of a change in surrounding air pressure. Air travellers are the largest group at risk, but scuba divers face similar problems (see *Scuba-diving medicine*).

CAUSE

When an aircraft ascends to cruising height, cabin pressure is usually reduced by about one third (to a pressure equivalent to an altitude of about 2,500 m). A "popping" sensation may be felt as air, trapped at ground-level pressure in the middle ears and facial sinuses, escapes via the eustachian tubes and sinus ducts (which, respectively, link the middle ears and sinuses to air passages at the back of the throat).

When the aircraft descends, cabin pressure is increased again and becomes greater than the pressure within the ears and sinuses. Some pain may be felt as the eardrum is pushed inwards. To ease this, air needs to be reintroduced into the middle ears and sinuses to equalize the internal and external pressures. This "ear clearing" can be achieved by vigorous swallowing or by forcibly breathing out with the mouth closed and the nose pinched (the Valsalva manoeuvre).

If the sinus ducts or eustachian tubes are blocked with mucus, as commonly occurs during a head cold, equalizing pressure by using the ear-clearing methods described above may be difficult or impossible. Minor damage can occur if pressure equalization is prevented or delayed, or if the Valsalva manoeuvre is carried out over-enthusiastically. The damage usually involves rupture of tiny blood vessels in the walls of the middle ears, or in the membranes lining the inside of the sinuses.

Changes in pressure sufficient to rupture the eardrum are unlikely to occur during ordinary airline flights but rupture may be suffered by scuba divers or high-altitude pilots (see *Eardrum, perforated*).

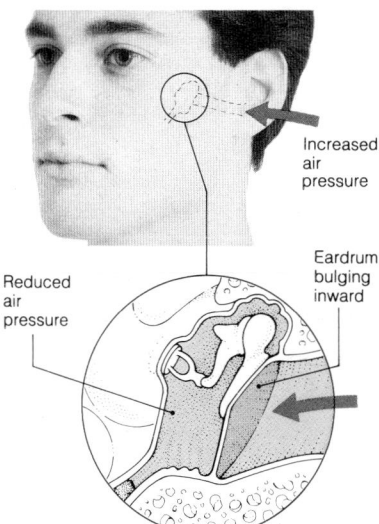

Mechanism of barotrauma
The diagram above shows the location of the middle ear, and pressure changes when the eustachian tube is blocked and there is an increase in surrounding air pressure.

Increased air pressure

Eardrum bulging inward

Reduced air pressure

PREVENTION

Anyone with a severe head cold should avoid flying if possible. If flying is unavoidable, a nasal spray containing a *decongestant drug* should be used shortly before aircraft descent. Air travellers should also know how to perform the Valsalva manoeuvre. Infants should be breast- or bottle-fed during descent; the baby's sucking and swallowing has the same effect as the Valsalva manoeuvre.

SYMPTOMS

Pain in the ears, or over the cheekbones and forehead, during aircraft descent is a warning of pressure differences. Minor pressure damage in the middle ear, called barotraumatic otitis, may cause continued pain, some hearing loss, and *tinnitus* (ringing in the ears) for a few days; pressure damage within the facial sinuses, called barotraumatic sinusitis, may also cause pain, and possibly a discharge of mucus or blood for a couple of days.

TREATMENT

In most cases, no treatment is necessary and symptoms wear off within hours or a couple of days. However, if an infection is present, these symptoms may become worse and persist for several days. If sinus pain persists or a discharge from the nose is noticed, symptoms that suggest infection, medical advice should be sought. Treatment may be required. (See also *Aviation medicine*.)

Barrier cream

A cream used to protect the skin against the effects of irritant substances and of excessive exposure to water. (See also *Sunscreens*.)

Barrier method

A method of preventing pregnancy by blocking the passage of sperm to the uterus, for example, by using a condom or a diaphragm. (See *Contraception, barrier methods of*.)

Barrier nursing

The nursing technique by which a patient with an infectious disease is prevented from infecting others (see *Isolation*).

Bartholin's glands

A pair of oval, pea-sized glands whose ducts open into the vulva (the folds of flesh that surround the opening of the vagina). During sexual arousal these glands secrete a fluid that helps to lubricate the vulval region.

DISORDERS

Infection of Bartholin's glands causes bartholinitis, in which an intensely painful red swelling forms at the opening of the ducts. Treatment is with *antibiotic drugs*, *analgesic drugs* (painkillers), and warm baths.

If infection produces an *abscess*, the affected gland is cut open and drained, usually under general anaesthesia. Should abscesses recur, an operation may be performed, either to convert the duct into an open pouch (see *Marsupialization*), or to remove the gland completely.

If an infection narrows the duct by scarring, the gland may not be capable of emptying, and a Bartholin's cyst, a painless swelling of the duct, may form. The cyst may become repeatedly infected, in which case marsu-

B

BARTHOLIN'S GLANDS
These glands are located on each side of the entrance to the vagina.

Vagina

Vulva

Bartholin's glands

Anus

B

pialization or removal of the gland is needed. Even if both the Bartholin's glands are removed or destroyed by infection, other glands in the vagina are capable of secreting adequate amounts of lubricants.

Basal cell carcinoma

A type of skin cancer that occurs most commonly on the face or neck, also known as a rodent ulcer. The cells of the tumour closely resemble, and are possibly derived from, cells in the basal (innermost) skin layer.

INCIDENCE
Basal cell carcinoma is the most common skin cancer in the UK, with an estimated overall incidence of at least 30,000 cases per year.

Fair-skinned people over 50 are the most commonly affected (dark and black-skinned people are affected only rarely). The incidence is much higher among people living in sunny climates, especially those with outdoor occupations; in parts of the US and Australia, over half the white population has had a basal cell carcinoma by the age of 75.

CAUSE
Direct skin damage from the ultraviolet radiation in sunlight is thought to be the cause in most cases. Dark-skinned people are protected by the larger amount of *melanin* (a pigment that absorbs ultraviolet radiation) in their skin.

SYMPTOMS
More than 90 per cent of basal cell carcinomas occur on the face, often at the side of an eye or on the nose, but the tumour can appear virtually anywhere on the body. It starts as a small, flat nodule and grows slowly, eventually breaking down at the centre to form a shallow ulcer with raised edges. Diagnosis is confirmed by microscopic examination of a sample of cells from the tumour.

Without treatment, the growth gradually invades and bites deeper into surrounding tissues. Fortunately, basal cell carcinomas virtually never spread to other parts of the body.

PREVENTION
Individuals at risk, particularly fair-skinned people, should avoid over-exposure to strong sunlight by wearing protective clothing and sun hats, and using *sunscreen* preparations containing *para-aminobenzoic acid* (PABA).

TREATMENT AND OUTLOOK
The tumour can be destroyed by *cryosurgery* or *radiotherapy* or it may be removed surgically. Treatment usually results in a complete cure, although new tumours may develop in people who do not take adequate preventive measures. (See also *Melanoma, malignant*; *Squamous cell carcinoma*; *Sunlight, adverse effects of*.)

Basal ganglia

Paired nerve cell clusters in the *brain*, deep within the cerebrum (main mass of the brain) and upper part of the brainstem. The basal ganglia play a vital part in producing smooth, continuous muscular actions and in stopping and starting movement.

Disease or degeneration of the basal ganglia and their connections may lead to the appearance of involuntary movements, trembling, and weakness, as occur in *Parkinson's disease*.

Battered baby syndrome

Injuries to a child that suggest repeated physical assault. Such injuries often include bruises, burns, and fractures. Usually the full extent of past injuries is apparent only when the child is examined medically and the complete skeleton is X-rayed. (See *Child abuse*.)

B-cell

See *Lymphocyte*.

BCG vaccination

A vaccine that provides immunity against *tuberculosis*. BCG is prepared from an artificially weakened strain of bovine (cattle) tubercle bacilli, the microorganisms responsible for the disease. The initials BCG stand for "bacille Calmette-Guérin", after the two Frenchmen who developed the vaccine in 1906.

WHY IT IS DONE
In the UK, BCG vaccination is commonly given to children aged 12 to 13 if it is thought they may need protection against tuberculosis in early adult life. Treatment policies are kept under review, taking account of changes in the incidence of disease in Britain and the spread of tuberculosis through bacteria resistant to the common drugs.

BCG vaccination is also given to immigrants, especially those from Africa and the East, and to newborn babies of Asian parents. Household contacts of people with tuberculosis are also vaccinated, as are others at special risk, such as doctors, nurses, laboratory staff, and other hospital staff.

HOW IT IS DONE
Except in newborn babies, a *tuberculin test* is performed first and only those with negative reactions (no immunity) are vaccinated.

The vaccine. is usually injected into the upper arm. About six weeks later a small pustule appears. This normally heals completely, leaving a small scar.

An occasional complication is development of a chronic ulcer because the pustule fails to heal.

Beclomethasone

A *corticosteroid drug* prescribed as a nasal spray to relieve the symptoms of allergic *rhinitis* (hay fever) and as an inhaler to treat *asthma*. Beclomethasone controls nasal symptoms by reducing inflammation and mucus production in the nose. In asthma, it reduces the inflammation of the air passages that underlies the disease and so relieves the main symptoms—wheezing and coughing. If an asthma attack becomes severe, the dose of beclomethasone may be increased. However, the action of the drug is slow, and its full effect takes several days to become apparent.

Beclomethasone is a front-line treatment in the management of asthma and is often combined with *bronchodilator drugs*. Adverse effects may include hoarseness, throat irritation, and, rarely, fungal infections in the mouth. Irritation may be prevented by thoroughly rinsing the mouth and gargling with water after each inhalation.

Beclomethasone is also prescribed as a cream or ointment to treat skin inflammation caused by *eczema*.

Becquerel

A unit of radioactivity (see *Radiation units* box).

Bed bath

A method of washing a person who is confined to bed. To give a bed bath, wash and dry a small area at a time, keeping the rest of the person covered to prevent chilling.

Bedbug

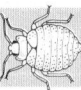
A flat, wingless, brown insect 5 mm long and 3 mm wide. Bedbugs live in furniture, especially beds, and floors during the day and emerge at night to feed on humans by sucking blood. They are not known to transmit any diseases but their bites cause itching sores that may become infected.

Bedpan

A metal, plastic, or fibre container into which a patient confined to bed can defaecate and, if female, urinate. Male patients use a *urinal* for urination. In the past, bedpans and urinals were used routinely, but today unless the patient is immobile, the use of the toilet or a bedside *commode* is considered to be less stressful.

Bed rest

A term used to describe periods spent in bed. It may be an essential part of treatment in certain illnesses, such as rheumatic fever, and for some types of injuries, such as a fractured vertebra or a slipped disc.

Prolonged bed rest may involve various risks for the patient, among them muscle wasting, *bedsores*, weakness, depression, and loss of calcium leading to bone demineralization and urinary tract *calculi* (stones). People recovering from an operation are at special risk of developing deep vein thrombosis (see *Thrombosis, deep vein*) and, especially if elderly, of contracting *pneumonia*. To prevent these problems, patients today are encouraged to be physically active while in bed and to get out of bed sooner than in the past.

Bedridden

A term used to describe a person who is unable to leave bed due to illness or injury. People most likely to be bedridden are the very elderly, the terminally ill, and those paralysed as the result of an accident.

Beds, hospital

Special beds for nursing sick or injured patients may be used in hospitals and sometimes at home.

TYPES

STANDARD HOSPITAL BED This bed is made of metal to allow it to be disinfected, mounted on wheels for ease of movement, jointed to allow tilting in any direction, and adjustable in height. The higher position is used for nursing procedures; the lower position allows the patient to get in and out of bed easily. A firm mattress provides support for the patient while various procedures are being performed.

TURNING FRAMES These beds, including the Stryker frame and the Foster frame, enable patients with extensive burns, multiple injuries, pelvic and spinal fractures, or spinal cord injuries to be turned with a minimum of handling and without disturbing body alignment. The patient lies prone or supine on a canvas-covered frame. When turning is required, a second canvas is placed on top of the patient, both canvases (with the patient sandwiched between) are rotated through 180 degrees, and the top canvas is then removed.

REVOLVING CIRCULAR BED This bed is used for the same purposes as manual turning frames, but allows the patient to be placed in a variety of sitting or standing positions at any angle between vertical and horizontal. It is particularly useful for patients with spinal cord injury who may develop hypotension (lowered blood pressure) when sitting or placed upright after being immobilized in a horizontal position for a prolonged period. Gradual rehabilitation of patients is also facilitated because they can adjust gradually from lying flat to standing upright, while remaining supported.

AIRBEDS AND WATERBEDS Beds with air- or water-filled mattresses can help prevent bedsores by providing uniform support for the patient's whole body. Airbeds are more commonly used than waterbeds because they are lighter and more comfortable for patients. A modern type of airbed, the ripple-bed, has a small motor that alternately fills and empties coils inside the mattress with air, creating a rippling effect. The continuous motion stimulates the patient's circulation, which, it is claimed, helps to keep the skin healthy and less susceptible to bedsores. (See also *Burns*.)

BALKAN FRAME This is used for the attachment of traction apparatus. It incorporates a hanging bar so that the patient can pull himself or herself up.

Bedsores

Also known as decubitus ulcers or pressure sores, these are ulcers that develop on the skin of patients who are bedridden, unconscious, or immobile. They commonly affect victims of stroke or *spinal injuries* that result in a

---

PREVENTING BEDSORES

Once a bedsore has developed it will heal only if pressure on it is minimized, so good nursing care of a bedridden, immobile patient is crucial. The patient's position should be changed at least every two hours and it is important to wash and dry pressure areas carefully, especially if there is incontinence. Barrier creams can be used for additional protection.

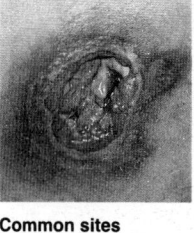

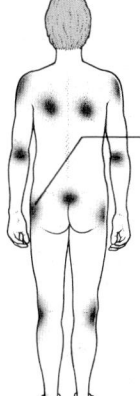

Common sites
These include the shoulders, elbows, lower back, hips and buttocks, knees, ankles, and heels.

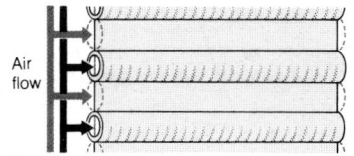

Ripple-bed mattress
A rippling effect is created by pumping air in and out of the mattress, so stimulating the circulation.

Cushions and pillows
These can be used to relieve pressure by placing them between the knees and under the shoulder.

Sheepskins
A sheepskin under the buttocks and bootees under the heels relieve pressure.

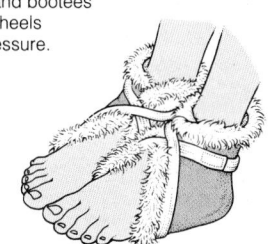

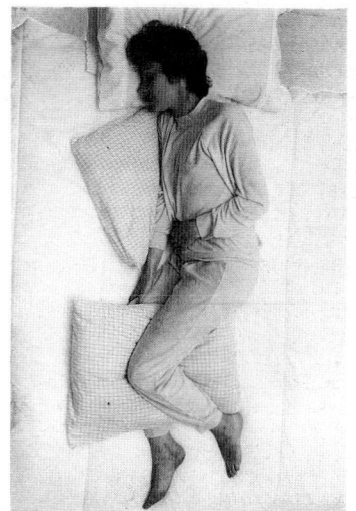

B

loss of sensation. Constantly wet skin, caused by *incontinence*, may also be a contributory factor.

Bedsores start as red, painful areas that become purple before the skin breaks down, developing into open sores. Once the skin is broken, the sores often become infected, enlarged and deeper, and are very slow to heal. Deep, chronic ulcers may require treatment with *antibiotic drugs*, packing with plastic foam, and possibly *plastic surgery*. New medications for preventing and treating bedsores are constantly being evaluated.

Bed-wetting

The common name for poor bladder control at night. (See *Enuresis*.)

Bee stings

See *Insect stings*.

Behavioural problems in children

Behavioural problems occasionally occur in all children; specialist management is called for when they become frequent and disrupt school and/or family life. *Enuresis* (bed-wetting), sleep difficulties, *tantrums*, feeding difficulties, truancy, disobedience, stealing, jealousy, aggressive attitudes towards siblings, *alcohol intoxication*, and *drug abuse* are all common problems. When a particular form of disturbed behaviour continues for a long time or forms part of a larger pattern, it becomes a cause for concern. Almost inevitably, however, stressful external events, such as moving home, changing schools, peer pressure, birth of a sibling, divorce, remarriage, hospitalization, chronic disease in the family or child, unemployment, or death in the family may produce periods of problem behaviour.

MANAGEMENT

BABIES Most problems resolve themselves over a matter of months; your health visitor or doctor will discuss any concerns you may have. (See also *Colic, infantile*; *Crying in infants*; *Feeding, infant*.)

TODDLERS Parents need to be realistic and consistent in their expectations, and should encourage a degree of decision sharing. Consistent and appropriate discipline should be exercised. Toilet-training should be delayed until a child is physically and emotionally ready. Separations from parents and changes in activity should be carefully planned. Parents who exercise adequate self-control provide the best model for a toddler who is having dif-

ficulty controlling explosive feelings. (See also *Breath-holding attacks*; *Head-banging*; *Toilet-training*.)

EARLY CHILDHOOD Parents should take a positive approach and concentrate on rewarding good behaviour rather than punishing bad behaviour, which tends to exaggerate difficulties or create new ones. Close cooperation is needed between home and playgroup/school because children often behave badly in only one place. (See also *Nightmares*; *Thumb-sucking*.)

MIDDLE CHILDHOOD/ADOLESCENCE Firm, but not punitive, parental treatment can help the child at this stage. If the child's difficulties persist and there are stressful family events, it may be useful to seek professional advice. Drug or alcohol abuse (or suspicion that they are taking place) require immediate medical attention.

OUTLOOK

Parents who find a baby difficult to care for may find they can cope better when the child is older. When an older child's behaviour is linked to a deterioration in the family situation, improvements can be expected when the circumstances improve. Whether family problems persist or are resolved, professional advice should be sought if the child's behaviour continues to be difficult. Even when the family situation is satisfactory, worried parents can often benefit from professional advice.

TYPES OF PROBLEM, BY AGE

Babies up to 18 months	Sleeping and feeding difficulties, colic, crying
Toddlers and small children 1-4 years	Head-banging, tantrums, biting, breath-holding attacks, separation anxiety, poor social interaction, difficulty changing from one activity to another, toilet-training problems
Early childhood 4-8 years	Nail-biting, thumb-sucking, aggression, clinginess, anxiety about illness and death, nightmares, enuresis
Middle childhood/ adolescence 9-18 years	Lying, stealing, smoking, truancy, disobedience, aggression, low achievement in school, drug or alcohol use, running away, sexual promiscuity

Behaviourism

An American school of *psychology* founded by John Broadus Watson early in this century. He argued that, because behaviour, rather than experience, was all that could be observed in others, it should constitute the sole basis of psychology.

Behaviour therapy

A collection of techniques, based on psychological theory, for changing abnormal behaviour or treating anxiety. Behaviour therapy can be effective in the treatment of phobic and obsessional disorders and certain kinds of sexual and marital problems.

The concept of behaviour modification originated with animal psychologists, but the techniques have been expanded and refined by clinical psychologists in the last decade. Treatment relies on two basic ideas: that exposure to a feared experience under safe conditions will render it less threatening, and that desirable behaviour can be encouraged by using a system of rewards. Aversion therapy—using punishment to discourage undesirable behaviour—was used in the past, particularly in the treatment of alcoholics and drug addicts, but was found to be ineffective in the long term.

TYPES

EXPOSURE THERAPY Also called desensitization, this consists of exposing the patient in stages to the cause of his or her anxiety. At the same time, the patient is taught to cope with anxiety symptoms by using relaxation techniques. The intensity of the anxiety-provoking stimulus is gradually increased until eventually the patient is able to deal with the full situation.

FLOODING Instead of being introduced to the cause of the phobia in stages, the patient is confronted with the anxiety-provoking stimulus at once, but with the support of the therapist. The patient remains in this situation until his or her feelings of anxiety eventually disappear.

RESPONSE PREVENTION The patient is prevented from carrying out an obsessional task. This technique is used in combination with other methods.

MODELLING The therapist acts as a model for the patient, performing the anxiety-provoking activity first, so that the patient may copy.

HOW IT IS USED

TREATMENT OF PHOBIC DISORDERS This treatment is dependent on exposure therapy, through which the patient is helped to face the feared situation. In agoraphobia (fear of open spaces), for example, the therapist accompanies the sufferer on a short journey, providing emotional support. Relaxation techniques may help prevent anxiety. Gradually, the distance travelled from home is increased, and the therapist withdraws from the treatment as the sufferer gains confidence.

Similar techniques of gradual exposure may also help people with animal phobias, flying phobias, or other phobias in which there is a specific fear.

TREATMENT OF OBSESSIONAL RITUALS This consists of three aspects: prevention, exposure, and modelling. For example, a patient with a hand-washing compulsion would be prevented from carrying out the washing rituals. At the same time, exposure to materials that the patient might consider contaminated is encouraged, with the therapist acting as a model by touching the "contaminated" objects first.

TREATMENT OF MARITAL AND SEXUAL PROBLEMS This is based on *Marriage guidance*; partners reward each other for pleasing behaviour. (See also *Sex therapy*.)

Behçet's syndrome

A rare disorder in which the main symptoms are recurrent mouth ulcers, genital ulceration, and inflammation of the eye. The condition was first described by the Turkish dermatologist Hulusi Behçet (1889-1948).

The cause is unknown, but the condition is strongly associated with a genetically-determined *histocompatability antigen*, HLA-B5. It is uncommon in the UK, but more common in some Middle Eastern countries.

Treatment is difficult and may require *corticosteroid drugs* or *anticancer drugs*. The condition often becomes chronic.

Belching

The noisy return of air from the stomach through the mouth. Swallowing air is usually an unconscious habit which may be a result of eating or drinking too much too quickly. When a person belches, he or she swallows air, which may cause further belching. Sometimes, belching alleviates discomfort caused by indigestion. During pregnancy, belching briefly helps relieve nausea and heartburn, which disappear after delivery of the baby.

Belladonna

An extract of the deadly nightshade plant, containing *alkaloids* including *atropine*, which has been used medicinally since ancient times. Women

used to apply belladonna to their eyes to dilate the pupils (the name in Italian means beautiful lady). In modern medicine, belladonna alkaloids are used as *antispasmodic drugs* to treat gastrointestinal disturbances. (See also *anticholinergic drugs*.)

Bell's palsy

The most common form of *facial palsy*.

Bendrofluazide

A thiazide *diuretic drug* used to treat *hypertension* (high blood pressure) and *heart failure*.

Bends

A popular term for *decompression sickness*, especially for the severe bone and joint pains that are a common symptom in divers who rise to the surface too rapidly.

Benign

The term used to describe a relatively mild form of a disease. For example, a benign tumour will not spread throughout the body, whereas a *malignant* or cancerous tumour may do so if it is not removed at an early stage.

Benorylate

A *nonsteroidal anti-inflammatory drug* containing both *aspirin* and *paracetamol*. Benorylate is mainly used to relieve joint pain and stiffness in *osteoarthritis* and *rheumatoid arthritis*. Benorylate is longer acting than aspirin or paracetamol alone and needs to be taken only twice a day. Side-effects are not usually serious; the aspirin in the drug may cause nausea or indigestion.

Benzodiazepine drugs

COMMON DRUGS
Sleeping drugs *Flunitrazepam Flurazepam Loprazolam* *Lormetazepam Nitrazepam Temazepam*
Sedatives *Alprazolam Bromazepam* *Chlordiazepoxide Clobazam* *Clorazepate Diazepam Lorazepam* *Medazepam Oxazepam*

WARNING
Benzodiazepine drugs may be habit-forming; if taken with large amounts of alcohol they may dangerously increase the alcohol's effect.

Among the best-known and most widely prescribed drugs in the world, benzodiazepines are used mainly as

tranquillizer drugs to control symptoms of *anxiety* or *stress* and as *sleeping drugs* for *insomnia*.

WHY THEY ARE USED
For the treatment of anxiety, benzodiazepines are given for short periods to promote mental and physical relaxation. They reduce feelings of agitation and restlessness, slow mental activity, and relax the muscles.

Most benzodiazepine drugs have a strong sedative effect and help to relieve insomnia. They cause drowsiness and sleep when given in a higher dose than that used to treat anxiety.

Benzodiazepines are also used in the management of alcohol withdrawal and in the control of *epilepsy*.

HOW THEY WORK
Benzodiazepines promote sleep and relieve anxiety by depressing brain function. By interfering with chemical activity in the brain and nervous system, they reduce the communication between nerve cells. This leads to a reduction in brain activity, which is increased in proportion to the amount of drug taken.

POSSIBLE ADVERSE EFFECTS
Minor adverse effects include daytime drowsiness, dizziness, and forgetfulness. Benzodiazepines may also cause unsteadiness and slow reactions, thus impairing the ability to drive or operate machinery.

The main risk of benzodiazepines is that regular users may become psychologically and physically dependent on them. For this reason, they are usually given for courses of two to three weeks or less. When benzodiazepines are stopped suddenly, withdrawal symptoms, such as excessive anxiety, nightmares, and restlessness, may occur. When they are taken for longer than two weeks, they should be withdrawn gradually under medical supervision.

Benzodiazepine drugs have been abused for their sedative effect.

Benzoyl peroxide

An *antiseptic* agent used in the treatment of *acne* and fungal skin infections (see *Fungal infections*), particularly tinea pedis.

Bereavement

The emotional reaction following the death of a loved relative or friend. A bereaved person's feelings will vary in intensity according to his or her level of maturity and the nature of emotional problems or conflict in the bereaved person prior to the loss. Also involved is the nature and quality of the bereaved person's relationship with the deceased and the kind of relationship they shared before the death. The expression of grief is individual to each person, but there are recognized stages of bereavement, each characterized by a particular attitude.

STAGES OF BEREAVEMENT

Numbness, hallucinations, and an unwillingness to recognize the death are defence mechanisms against admitting, and therefore accepting, the loss and associated pain. Numbness is the pervading feeling that enables the bereaved person to get through the funeral arrangements and family gatherings. This stage may last from three days to three months. Often, the reality of the death does not penetrate completely at this time, and many people continue to behave as if the dead person were still alive. Hallucinations, too, are a common experience among the recently bereaved. They may consist of a sense of having seen or heard the dead person, or of having been aware of his or her presence. This can be comforting for some people, but others may find it disturbing.

Depression is a reaction to loss. Once the numbness wears off and the bereaved person can know and feel that a loss has occurred, he or she may be overwhelmed by feelings of anxiety, anger, and despair that can develop into a depressive illness (see *Depression*). Gastrointestinal disturbances and *mental disorders* may occur and there is a risk of attempted suicide. An increase in the intake of alcohol, tranquillizers, and other drugs is common, as are insomnia, malaise, agitation, and tearfulness.

Gradually, but usually within two years, the bereaved person adjusts to the loss and begins to make positive plans for the future. This process can involve periods of pain and despair, alternating with periods of enthusiasm and interest; eventually, positiveness usually triumphs over despair. Research suggests, however, that the death of a spouse may increase the mortality for people in every age group, although there is little consistent information on the length of survival after widowhood. Survival may depend on whether a bereaved person can develop other relationships.

SUPPORT AND COUNSELLING

Family and friends can often provide the support a bereaved person needs, but sometimes other factors can impede the recovery process. Outside help may be required and may be given by a social worker, health visitor, member of the clergy, or self-help group. For some people, however, the care of a psychiatrist is necessary when depression, apathy, and lethargy obstruct any chance of recovery. In these cases, specialized *counselling* and *psychotherapy* should be encouraged by the person's family and friends. (See also *Stillbirth*.)

Beriberi

A metabolic disorder resulting from a lack of thiamine (vitamin B_1) in the diet. In developed countries, the illness is seen only in people who are starving or on an extremely restricted diet (such as alcoholics).

Breast-fed babies can develop beriberi if their mother's milk is seriously deficient in thiamine due to severe dietary restriction.

CAUSES

Thiamine, found in wholemeal cereals, meat, green vegetables, potatoes, and nuts, is essential for the metabolism of carbohydrates. Without it, the brain, nerves, and muscles (including the heart muscle) are unable to function properly.

INCIDENCE

Beriberi occurs among underfed populations in developing countries. The illness was once a major problem in the Far East among people subsisting on rice from which the thiamine rich outer layer had been removed, but improved milling and a better overall diet has led to a dramatic decline in the disorder.

SYMPTOMS AND SIGNS

Two forms of the illness—"dry" and "wet" beriberi—are recognized. In dry beriberi, the thiamine deficiency mainly affects the nerves and skeletal muscles. Symptoms include numbness, a burning sensation in the legs, and wasting of the muscles. In severe cases, the patient becomes emaciated, virtually paralysed, and bedridden.

In wet beriberi, the main problem is *heart failure* (inability of the heart to keep up with its task of pumping blood). This in turn leads to congestion of blood in the veins, and *oedema* (swelling caused by fluid accumulation) in the legs, and sometimes also in the trunk and face. Other symptoms include poor appetite, rapid pulse, and breathlessness. As the heart failure worsens, breathing becomes difficult and, without medical treatment, the patient will die.

DIAGNOSIS AND TREATMENT

The diagnosis is usually obvious from the symptoms and environmental factors; it can be confirmed by a test of the levels in the blood of lactic and pyruvic acids, which accumulate because carbohydrates cannot be completely metabolized.

Treatment consists of thiamine, given orally or by injection, which brings a rapid and complete cure. Since other vitamin deficiencies are also likely, a permanent improvement in diet is also needed.

Berylliosis

An occupational disease caused by the inhalation of dust or fumes containing beryllium, a metallic element which, with its compounds, is used in high-technology industries, such as nuclear energy, electronics, and aerospace.

Short exposure to high concentrations of beryllium may lead to an episode of severe *pneumonitis* (lung inflammation), characterized by coughing and breathlessness. Exposure over many years to smaller concentrations may lead to permanent lung and liver damage. The lung changes may lead eventually to severe breathlessness after the slightest exertion.

Treatment with *corticosteroid drugs* can help alleviate the symptoms of berylliosis but does not alter the course of the illness. The main emphasis is on preventing the disease through adequate protection against the inhalation of beryllium fumes.

Beta-blocker drugs

COMMON DRUGS
Cardioselective
Acebutolol Atenolol Betaxolol Bisoprolol Metoprolol
Noncardioselective
Nadolol Oxprenolol Pindolol Propranolol Labetolol Timolol

> **WARNING**
> Do not suddenly stop taking a beta-blocker; a severe recurrence of your previous symptoms and a significant rise in blood pressure may result.

A group of drugs, also known as beta-adrenergic blocking agents, prescribed principally to treat heart disorders. They have been used since the 1960s and although other, newer drugs have been found to treat many of the conditions for which they are effective, beta-blockers are still prescribed widely today.

WHY THEY ARE USED

Beta-blocker drugs are used in the treatment of *angina pectoris* (chest pain due to insufficient oxygen reaching

HOW BETA-BLOCKERS WORK

Beta-blockers block beta-receptors — specific sites on body tissues where *neurotransmitters* (chemicals released from nerve endings) bind. There are two types of beta-receptor: beta$_1$-receptors found in heart tissue and beta$_2$-receptors found in the lungs, blood vessels, and other tissues. At these receptors, two chemicals, adrenaline and noradrenaline, are released from nerve endings in the *sympathetic nervous system*, the part of the involuntary nervous system that enables the body to deal with stress, anxiety, and exercise. These neurotransmitters bind to beta-receptors to increase the force and speed of the heartbeat, to dilate the airways to increase air flow to the lungs, and to dilate blood vessels.

Cardioselective beta-blockers combine predominantly with beta$_1$-receptors; noncardioselective beta-blockers combine with both types.

Beta-blockers slow heart-rate and reduce the force of contraction of heart muscle. These effects can be used to slow a fast heart-rate and regulate abnormal rhythms.

Beta-blockers prevent angina pectoris attacks by reducing the work performed by the heart muscle and so the heart's oxygen requirement. High blood pressure is reduced because the rate and force at which the heart pumps blood into the circulation is lowered.

The effect of blocking beta-receptors on muscles elsewhere in the body is to reduce the muscle tremor of anxiety and an overactive thyroid gland. Beta-blockers can help to reduce the frequency of migraine attacks by preventing the dilation of blood vessels surrounding the brain, which is responsible for the headache. In glaucoma they lower pressure in the eye by reducing fluid production in the eyeball.

the heart muscle), *hypertension* (high blood pressure), and cardiac *arrhythmia* (irregular heartbeat). Beta-blockers are sometimes given after a *myocardial infarction* (heart attack) to reduce the likelihood of further damage to the heart muscle.

Beta-blockers may also be given to prevent *migraine* attacks and to reduce the physical symptoms of *anxiety* (such as palpitations, tremor, and excessive sweating). They may be given to control symptoms of *thyrotoxicosis* (overactive thyroid gland). A beta-blocker is sometimes given in the form of eye-drops to treat *glaucoma* (raised fluid pressure in the eyeball) by lowering the fluid pressure.

HOW THEY WORK
See explanatory box.

POSSIBLE ADVERSE EFFECTS
By reducing heart-rate and air flow to the lungs, beta-blockers may reduce an individual's capacity for strenuous exercise, although this may not be noticed if physical activity is already limited by heart problems.

Beta-blockers may worsen the symptoms of *asthma*, *bronchitis*, or other forms of lung disease. They may also reduce the flow of blood to the limbs and thus aggravate *peripheral vascular disease*.

If long-term treatment with beta-blockers is abruptly withdrawn, there may be a sudden severe recurrence of the patient's symptoms and a significant rise in blood pressure. These problems can be avoided by gradually decreasing the dose.

Betahistine

A drug used to treat *Ménière's disease* (a disorder of the inner ear). Taken regularly, betahistine reduces the frequency and severity of the attacks of nausea and vertigo that characterize this condition. Betahistine is thought to work by reducing pressure in the inner ear, possibly by improving blood flow in the small blood vessels. Adverse effects are rare but may include headache and nausea.

Betamethasone

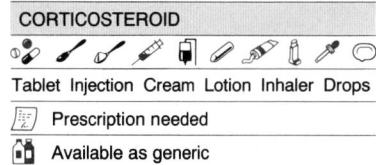

CORTICOSTEROID					
Tablet	Injection	Cream	Lotion	Inhaler	Drops

	Prescription needed
	Available as generic

A *corticosteroid drug* used to treat inflammation. Betamethasone is applied to the skin to treat *eczema* and

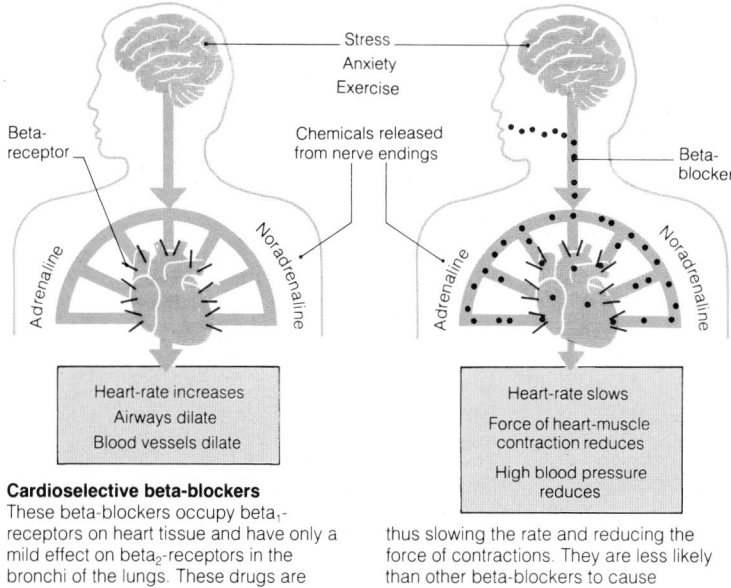

Stress
Anxiety
Exercise

Beta-receptor

Chemicals released from nerve endings

Beta-blocker

Adrenaline — Noradrenaline

Adrenaline — Noradrenaline

| Heart-rate increases |
| Airways dilate |
| Blood vessels dilate |

| Heart-rate slows |
| Force of heart-muscle contraction reduces |
| High blood pressure reduces |

Cardioselective beta-blockers
These beta-blockers occupy beta$_1$-receptors on heart tissue and have only a mild effect on beta$_2$-receptors in the bronchi of the lungs. These drugs are used in the treatment of heart disorders to reduce the workload of the heart,

thus slowing the rate and reducing the force of contractions. They are less likely than other beta-blockers to cause breathing difficulty.

Types of beta-receptors
Beta$_1$-receptors occur mainly in the heart muscle; beta$_2$-receptors are found in the lungs, blood vessels, and certain tissues. Beta-blocker drugs bind to beta-receptors, thereby blocking neurotransmitters.

Key
Beta$_1$-receptor
Beta$_2$-receptor
Neurotransmitter
Beta-blocker
Blocked beta-receptor

contact *dermatitis*, particularly when the skin is infected. Betamethasone is also prescribed to treat allergic *rhinitis* (hay fever).

Betamethasone is taken by mouth to treat severe cases of asthma and *arthritis*. It is also occasionally used to reduce cerebral oedema (swelling of the brain) and in mothers about to deliver prematurely, to lessen the baby's risk of developing *respiratory distress syndrome*.

POSSIBLE ADVERSE EFFECTS

Adverse effects are unlikely to occur when betamethasone is inhaled or used as ear-drops. This is because the dose that reaches the bloodstream is low. A higher dose may be absorbed when the drug is applied to the skin and for this reason betamethasone should be applied only sparingly and for short periods. Even when used with caution, betamethasone can cause thinning of the skin. It may also aggravate a skin infection and is therefore sometimes prescribed with an *antibiotic drug*. Taking betamethasone tablets for a prolonged period or in high doses can cause adverse effects typical of other corticosteroid drugs.

Bethanidine

A drug used to treat severe *hypertension* (high blood pressure) that has not responded to other drugs. Adverse effects may include dizziness, diarrhoea, and impotence.

Bezoar

A ball of food and mucus, vegetable fibre, hair, or other indigestible material, in the stomach. Bezoars are rare in adults except after partial *gastrectomy* (removal of part of the stomach). Trichobezoars (composed of hair) may form in children or emotionally disturbed adults who nibble at, or pull out and swallow, their hair.

Bezoars can cause loss of appetite, constipation, nausea and vomiting, and abdominal pain. If they pass into the intestines, they may cause an obstruction (see *Intestine, obstruction of*). Bezoars are diagnosed by means of a *barium X-ray examination* or *endoscopy* (passing a viewing tube down the digestive tract), and are removed by washing out the stomach (see *Lavage, gastric*), by use of a pincer attachment on the endoscope, by surgery, or by use of drugs that break down the protein portion of the bezoar.

Bi-

The prefix meaning two or twice, as in bilateral (two-sided).

Bicarbonate of soda

See *Sodium bicarbonate*.

Biceps muscle

The name, meaning "two heads", given to a muscle originating at one end as two separate parts, which then fuse. The biceps in the upper arm bends the arm at the elbow and rotates

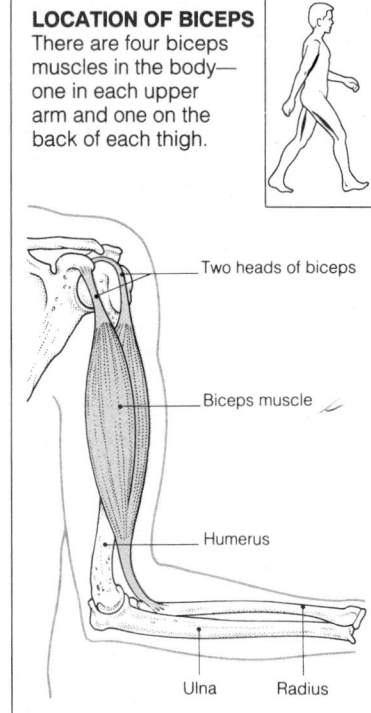

LOCATION OF BICEPS
There are four biceps muscles in the body—one in each upper arm and one on the back of each thigh.

Two heads of biceps

Biceps muscle

Humerus

Ulna   Radius

the forearm; the biceps at the back of the thigh bends the leg at the knee and extends the thigh.

Bicuspid

A term meaning to have two cusps (curved, pointed structures). It is used, for example, as a means of describing certain *heart valves* and as an alternative name for a premolar tooth (see *Teeth*).

Bifocal

A term used to describe a spectacle lens with two different focal lengths. Glasses with bifocal lenses make corrections for both close and distant vision.

Bilateral

A term that means affecting both sides of the body, or affecting both organs if they are paired (for instance, both ears in bilateral deafness).

Bile

A greenish-brown liquid secreted by the *liver*. It carries away waste products formed in the liver and also helps to break down fats in the small intestine so that they can be digested.

The waste products in bile include the pigments *bilirubin* and biliverdin, which give it its greenish-brown colour. The other main constituents are bile salts and *cholesterol*. Bile salts aid in the breakdown and absorption of fats.

Bile passes out of the liver via the bile ducts and is then concentrated and stored in the gallbladder until, after a meal, it is expelled and enters the duodenum via the common bile duct. At the end of the small intestine, most of the bile salts are reabsorbed into the bloodstream to be recycled into bile by the liver. Bile pigments are normally excreted from the body in the faeces, which they colour dark brown. (See also *Biliary system*; *Cholestyramine*.)

Bile duct

Any of the ducts by which *bile* is carried from the liver, first to the gallbladder and then to the duodenum (the first section of the small intestine).

STRUCTURE

The bile duct system starts as tiny tubular canals called canaliculi that surround the liver cells and collect the bile. The canaliculi join together to form a network of bile ducts of increasing size, which emerge from the liver, on the underside, as the two hepatic ducts.

These ducts join within or just outside the liver to form the common hepatic duct. Another duct—the cystic duct, lying just beyond the junction—branches off to the gallbladder, which lies in a hollow on the undersurface of the liver. The continuation of the common hepatic duct past the junction with the cystic duct is known as the common bile duct, and leads directly into the duodenum. (See also *Biliary system*.)

Bile duct cancer

See *Cholangiocarcinoma*.

Bile duct obstruction

A blockage or constriction of any of the ducts that carry bile from the liver to the gallbladder and then to the duodenum (see *Biliary system*).

The obstruction results in *cholestasis* (accumulation of bile in the liver), and the development of *jaundice* due to accumulation of *bilirubin* in the blood. Prolonged bile-duct obstruction over many years can lead to secondary *biliary cirrhosis*, a serious type of advanced liver disease.

CAUSES

The bile ducts can become blocked or narrowed for a variety of reasons. Perhaps the most common cause is *gallstones*, which have usually formed in the gallbladder and escaped into the common bile duct.

A tumour of the pancreas (see *Pancreas, cancer of*) may compress the lower end of the common bile duct. Occasionally, cancers of other organs may spread to the biliary system and cause obstruction. *Cholangiocarcinoma* (cancer of the bile ducts) is a very rare cause of blockage.

Bile duct obstruction is a rare side-effect of certain drugs, such as tranquillizers, antibacterials, and sex hormones. It may also be caused by trauma, such as injury during gallbladder operations, by *cholangitis* (inflammation of the bile ducts), and, very rarely, by the entry of various flukes or worms into the ducts.

SYMPTOMS

All patients develop "obstructive" jaundice, which is characterized by pale-coloured faeces (due to lack of the normal bilirubin content) and dark urine (due to excess bilirubin content) as well as a yellow skin colour. Some patients also complain of itching, caused by the presence of bile salts in the skin.

Other symptoms depend on the cause of the biliary obstruction—for example, abdominal pain with gallstones, or weight loss with many types of cancer.

DIAGNOSIS AND TREATMENT

Liver-function tests may suggest an obstruction, the site of which can be confirmed by *ultrasound scanning* and *cholangiography* or *ERCP*.

If bile duct obstruction is due to a drug, the drug should be discontinued. In other cases, an obstruction can sometimes be removed by surgery or by means of an attachment to an *endoscope* (viewing instrument) passed down the digestive tract and up the common bile duct.

When the obstruction is due to a cancer that is too advanced for surgical removal, the obstruction is usually bypassed to relieve the jaundice. This may be done by joining a loop of intestine either to the gallbladder or to the biliary system above the blockage. Alternatively, a tube may be pushed through the blockage, either from the intestinal side using an endoscope, or with catheters from the liver side of the duct (using X-rays to track the catheters). The tube is left in place for bile to flow through.

Bilharzia

An alternative name for the tropical parasitic disease *schistosomiasis*.

Biliary atresia

A rare disorder, present from birth, in which the bile ducts, either outside or inside the liver, fail to develop or have developed abnormally. As a result, bile cannot flow through the ducts to the duodenum (the first part of the small intestine) and becomes trapped in the liver (see *Cholestasis*). Unless the atresia is treated, secondary *biliary cirrhosis* will develop and may prove fatal.

The main signs of biliary atresia are deepening *jaundice*, usually beginning a week after birth, and the passing of dark urine and pale faeces.

DIAGNOSIS AND TREATMENT

If biliary atresia is suspected, blood tests and a *liver biopsy* (removal and microscopic examination of a small sample of liver tissue) are performed. If these tests show that the baby's jaundice is not due to a different cause, such as *hepatitis*, an operation may be performed to examine the liver and bile ducts directly. If this confirms the diagnosis of biliary atresia, surgery is carried out to bypass the ducts by joining a loop of small intestine directly to the liver. If this fails, or if the jaundice recurs, a *liver transplant* is the only possible treatment.

Biliary cirrhosis

An uncommon form of liver *cirrhosis* that results from disease or defects of the bile ducts. There are two types: primary and secondary biliary cirrhosis. Both types are characterized by *cholestasis* (accumulation of bile in the liver), which impairs liver function.

PRIMARY BILIARY CIRRHOSIS

In this type of biliary cirrhosis, the bile ducts within the liver become inflamed and are destroyed. The cause is unknown, but the disease seems to be associated with a malfunction of the *immune system*. Middle-aged women are the group most commonly affected.

The first symptom is itching, followed later by *jaundice*, an enlarged liver, and sometimes abdominal pain, fatty diarrhoea, and *xanthomatosis* (the appearance of fatty deposits under the skin). *Osteoporosis* may develop. Over a number of years the patient may develop other symptoms of liver cirrhosis and *liver failure*.

The disease is diagnosed by *liver-function tests*, by *liver biopsy*, and by *cholangiography* or *ERCP*. Drug treatment has been aimed mainly at relieving symptoms, such as itching, and minimizing complications. A *liver transplant*, if available, provides the only long-term cure.

SECONDARY BILIARY CIRRHOSIS

This results from prolonged *bile duct obstruction* or *biliary atresia* (absence or abnormality of the bile ducts from birth). The symptoms and signs include abdominal pain and tenderness, liver enlargement, fevers and chills, and sometimes blood abnormalities. Treatment is as for bile duct obstruction or biliary atresia.

Biliary colic

A severe pain in the upper right quadrant of the abdomen usually caused by the gallbladder's attempts to expel *gallstones* or the movement of a stone in the bile ducts. The pain is extremely severe and often lasts for up to an hour. It may mimic the pain of a heart attack and may radiate to the right shoulder or penetrate through to the centre of the back.

Injections of an *analgesic drug* (painkiller) and an *antispasmodic drug* may be given to relieve the colic. Tests such as *cholecystography* or *ultrasound scanning* are usually carried out to determine whether gallstones are definitely present; if they are, *cholecystectomy* (surgical removal of the gallbladder) may be considered.

Biliary system

The organs and ducts by which *bile* is formed, concentrated, and carried from the *liver* to the duodenum (the first part of the small intestine). Bile removes waste products from the liver and carries bile salts, necessary for the breakdown and absorption of fat, to the intestine.

Bile is secreted by the liver cells and collected by a system of tubes that mirrors the blood supply to the organ. This network of bile-drainage channels carries the bile out of the liver by way of the hepatic ducts, which join together to form a common duct that opens into the duodenum at a controlled orifice called the ampulla of Vater. Bile does not pass directly into the duodenum but is first concentrated and then stored until needed in the gallbladder, a pear-shaped reservoir lying in a hollow under the liver, to which it gains access by way of the cystic duct.

When food is eaten, the presence of fat in the duodenum causes the secretion of a hormone, which opens the ampulla of Vater and causes the gallbladder to contract, squeezing stored bile via the cystic and common bile ducts into the duodenum. In the duodenum, bile salts emulsify the fat, breaking it down to a kind of milk of microscopic globules.

DISORDERS

The main disorder of the gallbladder is the formation of *gallstones*, which can have multiple complications affecting the entire biliary system (see *Gallbladder* disorders box). The main disorders of the bile ducts are congenital *biliary atresia* (absence or abnormality of the bile ducts from birth) and *bile duct obstruction*, which may itself be caused by gallstones or by other causes. Bile duct obstruction can have important complications affecting the liver.

Biliousness

A term commonly and erroneously used to describe nausea or vomiting. More accurately, however, biliousness describes a condition in which bitter bile is brought up to the mouth from the stomach.

Bilirubin

The main pigment found in *bile*. Bilirubin is produced by the breakdown of *haemoglobin*, the pigment in red blood cells. Bilirubin is the yellow pigment associated with *jaundice*. Products

---

FUNCTION OF THE BILIARY SYSTEM

The system consists of the bile ducts leading from the liver and gallbladder, the gallbladder itself, and associated structures. The system drains waste products from the liver into the duodenum and aids the process of fat digestion through controlled release of fat-emulsifying agents (contained within bile).

FAT DIGESTION

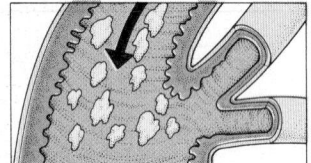

1 Dietary fat passes from the stomach to the duodenum in the form of large droplets.

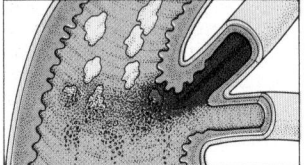

2 Bile released into the duodenum contains salts that disperse the fat into smaller droplets.

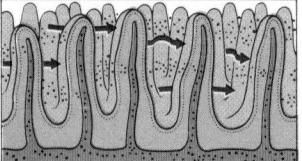

3 The fats are now more easily broken down by an enzyme, lipase, made by the pancreas, and absorbed through the intestinal lining.

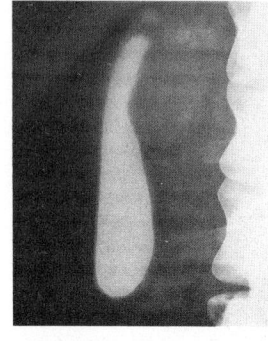

X-ray of gallbladder
The image on the left shows the pear-like shape of the gallbladder. It was achieved by an X-ray imaging technique called cholecystography.

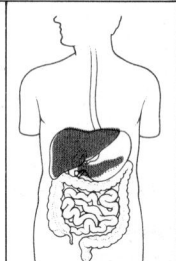

Liver
Bile is secreted by liver cells and collected in a system of tubes (drainage channels). These tubes carry bile out of the liver via the hepatic ducts.

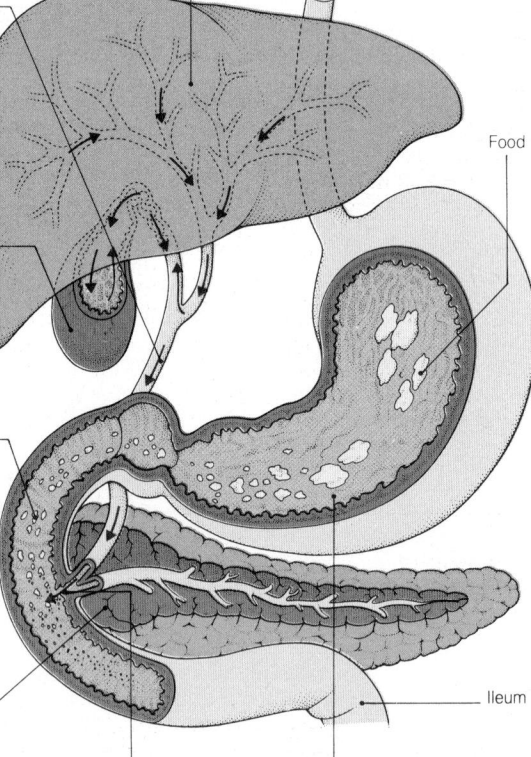

Common bile duct
The hepatic ducts join to form a common duct, which leads to the intestine. A side branch, the cystic duct, leads to the gallbladder.

Gallbladder
Bile is concentrated and stored here and released back into the common bile duct when this organ contracts.

Duodenum
When fat from a recent meal arrives in the duodenum, a hormone is released that acts on the gallbladder. The gallbladder contracts, causing bile to be passed into the duodenum to emulsify the fat.

Pancreas
In response to the presence of fat in the duodenum, the pancreas produces hormones that stimulate contraction of the gallbladder and cause the ampulla of Vater to open so that bile flows into the duodenum.

Ampulla of Vater
Bile enters the duodenum here.

Stomach
Fat and other products of digestion pass from the stomach to the duodenum.

Food

Ileum

formed from the breakdown of bilirubin are responsible for the brown colour of faeces.

Billings' method

A technique (also called the mucus inspection method) in which a woman notes changes in her normal vaginal discharge to predict the time of ovulation for purposes of *contraception* or *family planning*.

Billroth's operation

A type of partial *gastrectomy* in which the lower part of the stomach is removed. Devised by the Viennese surgeon Theodor Billroth, it was the first successful stomach operation and is still one of the standard operations for treating *peptic ulcer* and certain types of stomach tumour.

Binet test

The first *intelligence test* that attempted to measure higher mental functions rather than more primitive abilities, such as reaction times. It was devised by Alfred Binet and Theodor Simon for French schoolchildren in 1905.

Bio-

A prefix that describes a relationship to life, as in biology, the science of life.

Bioavailability

The amount of a drug that enters the bloodstream and thus reaches the tissues and organs throughout the body, usually expressed as a percentage of the dose given. In this way, the effectiveness of various means of administration or types of preparation can be compared. For instance, intravenous administration produces 100 per cent bioavailability since the drug is injected directly into the bloodstream. Drugs given by mouth have a much lower bioavailability, because only a proportion of the drug can be absorbed through the digestive system; some drugs may be broken down in the liver before reaching the general circulation.

Preparations with equal bioavailabilities are described as bioequivalent. (See also *Drug*.)

Biochemistry

A science that studies the chemistry of living organisms, including human beings. The human body is made up of millions of cells that require nutrients and energy, and which grow, multiply, and die. The chemical processes involved in providing cells with energy, eliminating their wastes,

repairing damage, cell growth, and normal and abnormal cell division are all studied by biochemists.

Life is maintained by a huge number of chemical reactions that are carried out inside cells and that link together in a complex way. These reactions together make up the *metabolism* of the body. The reactions which produce energy and break down food and body structures are termed catabolism, and those which build up body structures and store away food are termed anabolism. Overall, large-scale regulation of all these processes is a function of *hormones* (chemicals secreted into the bloodstream by the *endocrine glands*), whereas regulation of individual metabolic reactions is carried out by *enzymes* (biological catalysts).

Some vital chemical processes occur in every cell in the body. Other chemical processes are confined to specialized cells that make up the tissues of particular organs; for example, liver cells store and chemically modify the digestion products of food, and kidney cells help to control the amounts of various substances in the blood (such as certain minerals), as well as regulating the amount of fluid in the body.

There is a constant interchange between fluids, which move in and out of cells, and blood and urine. As a consequence, biochemists can learn about the chemical changes going on inside cells from measurements of the various minerals, gases, enzymes, hormones, and proteins in blood and urine. Such tests are used to make diagnoses, to screen people for disease, and to monitor the progress of a disease and its treatment. The most important biochemical tests are *blood tests* (such as *liver-function tests*), *kidney-function tests*, and *urinalysis*.

Biofeedback training

A technique in which a person uses information about a normally unconscious body function, such as blood pressure, to gain conscious control over that function.

WHY IT IS USED
Biofeedback training may help in the treatment of various stress-related conditions, including certain types of *hypertension* (high blood pressure), *anxiety*, and *migraine*.

HOW IT IS DONE
The doctor connects the patient to a recording instrument that can measure one of the unconscious body activities: blood pressure, pulse rate,

body temperature, muscle tension, the amount of sweat on the skin, brain waves, or stomach acidity. The patient receives information (feedback) on the changing levels of these activities from alterations in the instrument's signals—a flashing light, a fluctuating needle, or a sound changing its tone.

After some experience with the technique, the person starts to become aware of how he or she is feeling whenever there is a change in the recording instrument's signal. *Relaxation techniques* may also be used to bring about a change in the signal; the response of the biofeedback machine may indicate which methods of relaxation are most effective.

With time, the patient learns to change the signals at will, by consciously controlling the body function being tested. Once acquired, this control can be exercised without the instrument.

Biomechanical engineering

A discipline that applies engineering principles and methods to the human body to explain how it functions and to treat disorders. Joint movements, the reaction of bone to stress, and the flow of blood are among the body activities that can be looked at in terms of these principles. Practical applications include the design of artificial joints, plaster casts, kidney dialysis machines, and artificial heart valves.

Biopsy

A diagnostic test in which tissue or cells are removed from the body for examination under the microscope. Most biopsies are minor procedures that require no sedation, but some require local or general anaesthesia. Biopsy is an accurate method of diagnosing many illnesses, including cancer. The term biopsy is also commonly used for the cell or tissue sample itself (although the term biopsy specimen is more correct).

WHY IT IS DONE
Microscopic examination of tissue (*histology*) or of cells (*cytology*) usually gives a correct diagnosis. Biopsy is valuable for discovering whether a tumour is benign or malignant, since a malignant tumour usually has many features that clearly distinguish it from a benign tumour. In the case of a malignant tumour, biopsies of the surrounding tissue and the lymph nodes can be done to determine whether the cancer has spread. Another important use of biopsies is

B

to determine the cause of unexplained infections and inflammations.

HOW IT IS DONE

INCISIONAL BIOPSY This consists of cutting away a small piece of skin or muscle for analysis. Usually only a local anaesthetic is required.

NEEDLE BIOPSY A needle is inserted through the skin and into the organ or tumour to be investigated. The needle may be fitted with a cutting tip to help remove a piece of tissue for examination. Aspiration biopsy is another type of needle biopsy in which the cells that are sucked from a tumour are examined cytologically. Usually, only a local anaesthetic is required.

Until recently, if the target area could not be felt through the skin, or the organ was not accessible by endoscopic biopsy (see below), the doctor would have to work blindly, relying only on experience and a knowledge of anatomy, so that deep-needle biopsy was almost never done. Today, guided biopsy, using *ultrasound scanning* or *CT scanning* to precisely locate the tissue to be biopsied and follow the progress of the needle, makes the procedure far more accurate, safe, and productive. In addition, the recent use of very fine needles for biopsies allows for safe sampling of tumours in organs such as the salivary glands and pancreas, in which sampling with larger needles was considered dangerous.

ENDOSCOPIC BIOPSY An *endoscope* (viewing tube) is passed into the organ to be investigated and an attachment (such as forceps to remove tissue or brushes to remove cells) is used to take a sample.

The procedure, which usually requires sedation, is used to take samples from the lining of accessible hollow organs and structures, such as the lungs, bladder, oesophagus, stomach, and colon.

OPEN BIOPSY This is part of an operation, usually requiring a general anaesthetic, in which the surgeon opens a body cavity, such as the chest or abdomen, to reveal a diseased organ or tumour, and removes a sample of tissue. Open biopsy is carried out when neither guided nor endoscopic biopsy is possible, or when it is likely that the organ or tumour will require removal. Prompt analysis of a tissue sample can enable the surgeon to decide whether to remove the entire diseased area immediately, so making a second operation unnecessary.

EXCISIONAL BIOPSY If a lump is found in the skin or an organ, such as the

BIOPSY PROCEDURES

NEEDLE (ASPIRATION) BIOPSY

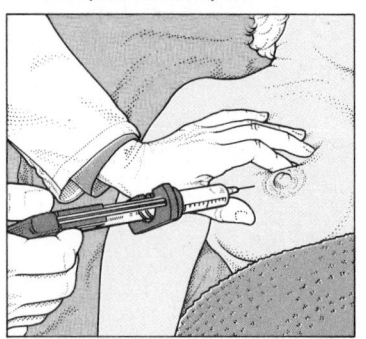

1 The area is usually first numbed with local anaesthetic, although occasionally a general anaesthetic is required. A needle attached to a syringe is then inserted into the cyst or tumour to be investigated and cells are sucked out to be examined cytologically.

2 Before examination, the fluid is sometimes spun at high speed in a centrifuge and a small amount is placed on a slide.

3 The cells are then fixed (preserved) and finally stained for viewing. The cytologist examines individual cells for abnormalities, paying particular attention to the size, shape, and structure of the nucleus.

Cells as seen through microscope

INCISIONAL BIOPSY

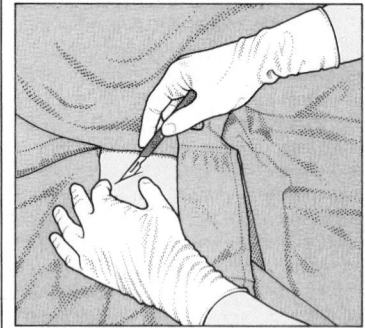

1 The area is first numbed with a local anaesthetic and a section of tissue is cut away. The wound is then stitched.

2 The tissue is then embedded in wax so that it is given a firm consistency suitable for slicing. This process usually takes 24 hours.

3 The tissue is then cut into ultra-thin slices and transferred to a slide. The pathologist conducts an examination, looking for distortion or alteration of tissue structure.

Tissue sample as seen through microscope

ENDOSCOPIC BIOPSY

If an area of abnormal tissue is to be removed for further examination, the forceps attachment, shown here, is passed through an endoscope to remove the piece of tissue.

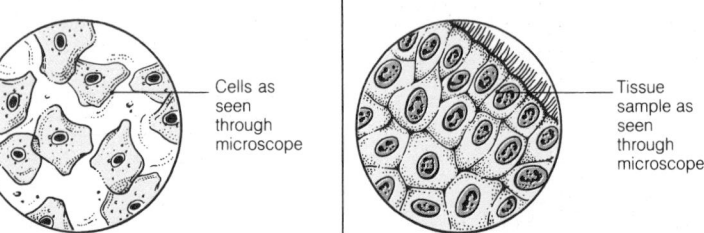

Endoscope

Forceps attachment

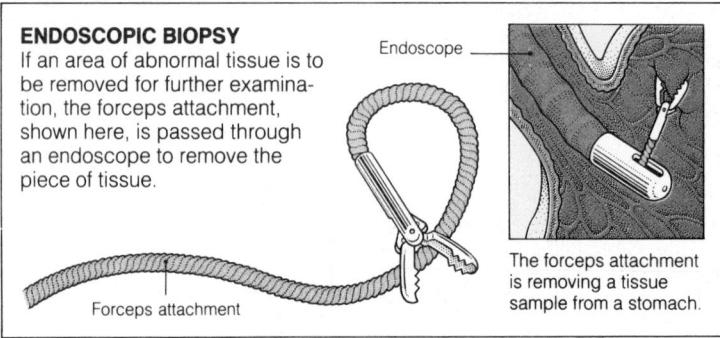

The forceps attachment is removing a tissue sample from a stomach.

breast, the surgeon may remove the lump completely and send the whole specimen for laboratory examination. If an abnormality is detectable only by an imaging technique, such as *mammography*, injected dye or fine wire probes may be used to identify the abnormal area for the surgeon.

OBTAINING A RESULT
Most biopsy samples need careful preparation for detailed examination. For a tissue sample, this usually involves embedding the sample in wax and then *staining* it with dyes to show up structures more clearly or to identify particular constituents, such as *antibodies* or *enzymes*. In special cases, a sample may be examined under an electron *microscope*—for example, to determine the origin of certain tumours.

In the investigation of infections and inflammations, a tissue sample may be tested with specific antibodies. In some cases, a tissue *culture* may be required.

Many of the more specialized techniques for preparing biopsy specimens prolong the time required to make an exact diagnosis but allow for greater accuracy and more precise information about the outlook for patients with certain diseases.

Biorhythms
A term used to describe physiological functions that vary in a rhythmic way (e.g. the menstrual cycle, which repeats itself approximately every 28 days in fertile women).

Most biorhythms are based on a daily or circadian (24-hour) cycle. Our bodies are governed by an internal clock, itself regulated by *hormones* (chemicals secreted into the bloodstream by the *endocrine glands*). Periods of sleepiness and wakefulness may be affected by the level of melatonin secreted by the pineal gland in the brain. Release of melatonin is stimulated by darkness and suppressed by light. When the normal regular division between night and day is distorted by air travel to a distant time zone, the body's internal clock is disrupted and the result is *jet-lag* (the symptoms of which could theoretically be relieved by the administration of melatonin).

Cortisol, secreted by the adrenal glands, also reflects the sleeping and waking states, being low in the evening and high in the morning.

The applications of biorhythms are still being explored. For example, many asthmatics feel worse in the morning due to the cyclic release of

hormones. This finding has implications for the management of their condition, and research groups are studying the optimum time of day for the administration of *bronchodilator drugs* and other drugs that interact with body functions that undergo rhythmic variations.

Biphosphonates
Biphosphonate drugs slow bone metabolism. They are used to treat *Paget's disease* and to reduce the high calcium levels in the blood associated with destruction of bone by secondary cancer growths.

Bipolar disorder
An illness characterized by swings in mood between opposite extremes (see *Manic-depressive illness*).

Birth
See *Childbirth*.

Birth canal
The passage, extending from the cervix (neck of the uterus) to the introitus (vaginal opening), through which the baby passes during *childbirth*.

Birth control
Limitation of the number of children born, either to an individual or within a population. Most people in developed nations now practise birth control; as a result, their population growth rates have decreased. Furthermore, in some countries, political and social pressures are applied to couples in an attempt to reduce population growth. Nevertheless, the total world population is still increasing rapidly (see box).

WORLD POPULATION
The rapid rate of population growth is a major problem. Reduction in infant and child mortality, due to better sanitation and disease control, has increased the number of people reaching their reproductive years. Because the world's population is doubling every 35 years, the task of adequately feeding, educating, and employing people is becoming increasingly difficult.

World population growth
The chart on the right shows growth from 1750 to 1990.

Distribution by continent
The diagram below shows the 1990 population of each continent, given also as percentages of total world population.

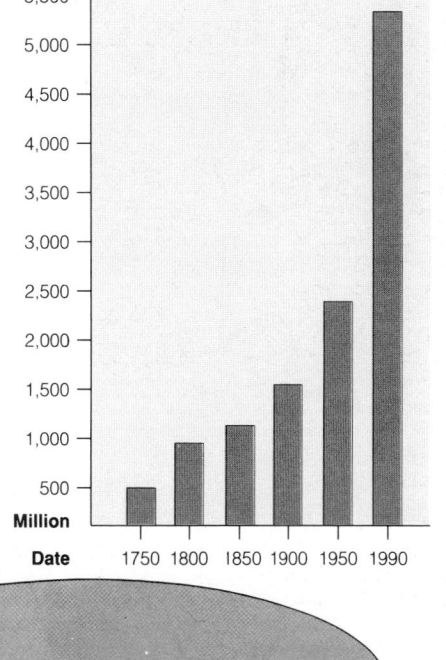

Million

Date 1750 1800 1850 1900 1950 1990

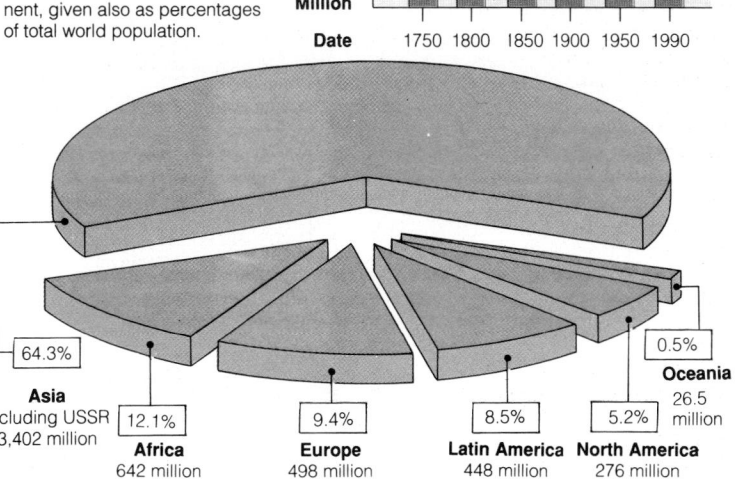

64.3%
Asia
including USSR
3,402 million

12.1%
Africa
642 million

9.4%
Europe
498 million

8.5%
Latin America
448 million

5.2%
North America
276 million

0.5%
Oceania
26.5 million

B

Family planning allows men and women to choose if and when to have children; *contraception* and abortion (see *Abortion, induced*) can prevent unwanted pregnancies.

Birth defects

Abnormalities obvious at birth or detectable early in infancy. Also called congenital defects, they encompass both minor abnormalities, such as *birthmarks*, and serious disorders such as *spina bifida* (a failure of the spinal column to close completely). Approximately 5 per cent of infants in the UK have a major or minor defect at birth; about two thirds of the defects are minor ones.

CAUSES

Birth defects may have a variety of different causes, but unknown factors also play a part. Among the recognized causes of birth defects are the following.

CHROMOSOME DEFECTS Some children are born with more or fewer than the normal 23 pairs of *chromosomes* (thread-like structures in cell nuclei that carry the information necessary for normal development)—or there are extra or missing parts of chromosomes (see *Chromosomal abnormalities*). In *Down's syndrome*, for example, where there is an extra chromosome, there is a higher incidence of congenital heart disease and intestinal defects.

GENETIC OR HEREDITARY DEFECTS These may be inherited from one or both parents (see *Genes; Genetic disorders*).

Examples of genetic defects obvious at birth are *achondroplasia* and *albinism*.

DRUGS AND OTHER HARMFUL AGENTS Certain drugs can damage the fetus if taken by the mother during early pregnancy, the most notorious examples being *thalidomide*, a sedative widely prescribed in the late 1950s and early 1960s but now prescribed only very rarely, and *isotretinoin*, used to treat acne. Both drugs should be given to women only if they are prepared to avoid becoming pregnant during the period of treatment.

Smoking by the mother can harm the fetus; some constituents of tobacco smoke diminish the baby's growth. Alcohol can have a similar effect and may also affect the development of the brain and face (see *Fetal alcohol syndrome*). Drugs and chemicals that can harm the fetus in this way are collectively called *teratogens*.

IRRADIATION Irradiation of the embryo in early pregnancy—for example, if a woman is X-rayed before the pregnancy is recognized or if she receives *radiotherapy* for cancer—can cause abnormalities. However, great care is taken to prevent radiation from reaching the embryo if a woman is known to be (or might be) pregnant.

Radiation damage to the unborn child may also occur from atomic radiation or radioactive fallout (following a nuclear explosion or leak from a nuclear reactor). Heavy doses of radiation, as occurred at Hiroshima in 1945 for example, can cause serious

mental and physical handicaps at birth. Even very small doses of radiation increase the child's risk of developing *leukaemia* later in life (see *Radiation, hazards of*).

MATERNAL INFECTIONS Certain illnesses during pregnancy can cause birth defects. If a woman who has not been immunized against *rubella* (German measles) contracts the disease during the first three months of pregnancy, there is a 50 per cent chance that her child will suffer brain, eye, ear, or heart abnormalities. Other types of infection, such as *toxoplasmosis*, may cause inflammation of the eyes, liver, spleen, and various other organs in the fetus.

PHYSICAL FACTORS IN THE UTERUS If the developing baby has too little fluid around it, its limbs may become distorted. *Talipes* (club-foot) is thought to occur in this way.

Apart from defects of known cause, many others occur, the causes of which are unknown. Among the more common are abnormalities of the brain and spinal cord. In the embryo these structures develop from a simple, fluid-filled tube of nerve tissue. Interference in its development can lead to *spina bifida* with or without *hydrocephalus*.

The heart and blood vessels in a fetus develop from what in the embryo is a central muscular tube. If development of the cardiovascular system is impaired, a congenital heart disorder may result—for example, patent ductus arteriosus, septal defect, coarctation of the aorta, or transposition of the great vessels (see *Heart disease, congenital*).

Other common defects include *cleft lip and palate*, both of which result from a failure of the two halves of the fetal face and palate to join completely.

PREVENTION

Steps can be taken to minimize the risk of an abnormal child being born. For example, before starting a family, *genetic counselling* should be obtained if either parent has relatives who have genetic or hereditary abnormalities. All women should make sure they are immune to rubella.

A woman should not smoke during pregnancy and should drink alcohol in moderation only. Unless prescribed by a doctor, drugs of any kind should be avoided during the first three months of pregnancy.

Various tests may be carried out when there is a possibility that a fetus may have some defect. Tests include *amniocentesis* (taking a sample of amniotic fluid from the uterus), blood

BIRTH DEFECTS (per 10,000 live births in England and Wales in 1991)

Defect	Number	Cause
Talipes (club-foot)	13	Multifactorial
Hypospadiasis and epispadiasis	10.5	Multifactorial
Congenital heart defects	8.2	Multifactorial
Polydactyly	7.9	Multifactorial
Cleft lip	7.5	Multifactorial
Down's syndrome	6.3	Chromosome abnormality
Syndactyly	5.5	Multifactorial
Brain and/or spinal cord malformations	4.6	Multifactorial
Ear malformation	3.9	Multifactorial
Cleft palate	3.7	Multifactorial
Limb defects	3.7	Multifactorial
Exomphalos	2.3	Multifactorial
Rectal and anal atresia and stenosis	1.8	Multifactorial
Hydrocephalus (without spina bifida)	1.5	Multifactorial
Spina bifida	1.5	Multifactorial
Eye defects	1.2	Multifactorial

tests to detect the level of *alpha-fetoprotein* (AFP) in the mother, *chorionic villus sampling* (removing a sample of tissue from the placenta), genetic tests on fetal blood cells separated from the mother's blood, and *ultrasound scanning*.

Birth injury

Damage sustained during birth. All babies suffer at least minor trauma, such as abrasions or minor bruising. Bruising and swelling of the scalp during a vaginal delivery is sometimes marked (see *Cephalhaematoma*).

More serious injury can occur, particularly if the baby is born prematurely or has difficulty passing through the mother's birth canal—for example, in a difficult *breech delivery*. Birth injuries are less common today, however, partly because more babies are delivered by *caesarean section*.

In breech deliveries, nerves in the shoulder region are sometimes injured, causing temporary paralysis in the arm. The face, likewise, may be paralysed temporarily if the facial nerve is traumatized by forceps. Fractures of bones, such as the clavicle (collarbone), humerus (upper-arm bone), and femur (thigh-bone), are another hazard of difficult deliveries. The bones usually heal easily.

Many cases of *cerebral palsy*, *mental handicap*, and *epilepsy* were once attributed to birth injury, but it is now considered that most of these problems are due to prenatal factors. Poor nutrition, smoking, maternal alcohol intake, bleeding during pregnancy, and prematurity are among the factors that can lead to brain damage or abnormal brain development. (See *Birth defects*; *Brain damage*.)

Birthmark

An area of discoloured skin present from birth. The most common birthmarks are *moles* and freckles; these and other types of melanocytic *naevus* (various flat, brown to blue-grey skin patches) are malformations of pigment cells.

Strawberry marks (bright red, usually protuberant areas) and port-wine stains (purple-red, flat, often large areas) are *haemangiomas* (malformations of blood vessels). Strawberry marks often increase in size in the first year but 90 per cent disappear after the age of nine years. Port-wine stains seldom fade.

Unsightly moles can be removed from late childhood onwards by *plastic surgery*. Some port-wine stains can now be caused to fade by *laser treatment*,

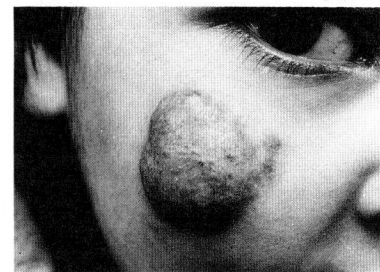

Birthmark
Strawberry marks—a common type of birthmark caused by malformation of blood vessels—are usually bright red, protuberant, and spongy.

which is best undertaken after the age of about 17 years. The most successful results have been in young adults.

Birthpool

A pool of warm water in which a woman in labour may give birth so that her baby emerges under the water. This method of delivery became popular in France, the United States, and Britain during the late 1980s and early 1990s, and was claimed to make labour less painful and distressing. It has not been evaluated in controlled clinical trials, and some unexplained deaths have occurred to infants delivered in this way.

Birthweight

The average full-term infant weighs 3.4 kg at birth. Few babies weigh less than 2.5 kg or more than 4.5 kg.

A baby's birthweight depends on a number of factors, including the size and ethnic origin of the parents. Small parents tend to have small babies. In the UK, Asian infants tend to be smaller than white or black infants. Baby boys weigh, on average, slightly more than baby girls.

Babies who weigh less than 2.5 kg at birth are classified as being of low birthweight. About one half of these babies are small due to *prematurity*—that is, they were born before the 37th week of pregnancy. Others are small because they have been undernourished in the uterus, where the placenta was insufficient, for example, because the mother had *pre-eclampsia* or smoked heavily during pregnancy.

Oversized babies are often born to mothers who have *diabetes mellitus*.

Bisexuality

Sexual interest in members of both sexes that may or may not involve sexual activity. Between what are regarded as the two ends of the human

sexuality spectrum—exclusive heterosexuality and exclusive homosexuality—there exists a continuous spectrum of bisexuality. Sexuality is determined by a person's sexual desires as well as his or her actual sexual behaviour. Thus, the term bisexual includes those who suppress homosexual desires and behave exclusively as heterosexuals.

Sexual preference may vary during a person's lifetime. Alfred Kinsey, who conducted a broad study of human sexual habits in the US during the 1940s, developed a scale that allowed him to rate the relative amounts of heterosexual and homosexual activity and/or responses at different periods in a person's life. He concluded that, at some stage in their adult life, half the population engaged in both heterosexual and homosexual activity, or reacted sexually to persons of both sexes.

Bismuth

A metal, salts of which are used in tablets to treat *peptic ulcer* and in suppositories to treat *haemorrhoids* (piles). Bismuth salts adhere to ulcers of the stomach and duodenum and form a protective coating over them, thus promoting healing.

Bismuth preparations taken by mouth may colour the faeces black, simulating the presence of blood. The tongue may darken and occasional nausea and vomiting may also occur.

Bite

See *Occlusion*.

Bites, animal

Any injury inflicted by the mouthparts of an animal—from the tiny puncture wounds of bloodsucking insects to the massive injuries caused by shark or crocodile attacks. For discussion of special problems caused by bites of venomous snakes, spiders, insects, and other venomous animals, see *Snake bites*; *Spider bites*; *Insect bites*; *Venomous bites and stings*.

INCIDENCE
The greatest number of animal attacks worldwide come from dogs, mainly strays. In England and Wales about 200,000 people annually are bitten badly enough by a dog to seek hospital treatment. A few deaths each year result from dog bites, and occasionally from the bites of other domestic animals, such as horses, cattle, and pigs.

Wild animals that have killed or caused serious injuries to humans include lions, tigers, elephants, rhinoceroses, hippopotamuses, buffaloes, bears, wolves, hyenas, and wild pigs. Small mammals, such as rodents, cause less extensive injury but many have razor-sharp teeth and there is a high risk of infection.

About 100 shark attacks occur worldwide each year, of which half are fatal. In Africa, more than 1,000 people die annually from crocodile attacks. Other aquatic creatures capable of inflicting a serious bite include barracudas, piranhas, and moray and conger eels.

THE MAIN HAZARDS

TISSUE DAMAGE The biological function of the mouth is to obtain food and prepare it for digestion. Teeth, especially those of carnivores, are well-adapted to tearing, crushing, and macerating tissues and bones, and can inflict severe and extensive mechanical injury.

BLOOD LOSS Severe injuries and lacerations to major blood vessels can lead to loss of a large amount of blood and physiological *shock*.

INFECTION An animal's mouth is heavily populated with bacteria and other microorganisms that thrive on food residue and debris. These organisms can produce serious secondary infection, especially in wounds where there is already extensive tissue damage. *Tetanus* is a particular hazard of animal bites.

RABIES In countries where *rabies* is present (including most European countries but not the UK), any mammal may potentially harbour the rabies virus and transmit it by a bite. Worldwide, dog bites are by far the most common source of rabies infection in humans. The UK, because it was separated from the Continent, has remained free from rabies to date. Strict quarantine is enforced at airports to prevent the importation of potentially infected animals.

TREATMENT

Medical advice should be sought for all but minor injuries—or if there is any possibility of rabies. Treatment usually includes wound cleaning and examination (under anaesthesia, if necessary). The wound will usually be left open and dressed, rather than stitched, because closing the wound tends to encourage the multiplication of bacteria that have been transmitted by the bite. Preventive antibiotic treatment, and an antitetanus injection, may also be given.

In the case of bites abroad, the animal that inflicted the bite should if possible be held and checked for rabies. Sometimes, an antirabies vac-

cine or serum may need to be given. (See also *Bites, human*.)

Bites, human

Wounds caused by one person biting another. In general, these wounds are more serious than animal bites due to a higher complication and infection rate. People bite each other more often than might be supposed—commonly in the course of fights, as part of a general pattern of *child abuse*, or during sexual play.

HAZARDS

Human bites rarely cause serious tissue damage or blood loss. However, infection from any microorganisms in the mouth is as likely, or even more likely, than with animal bites, particularly if the bite is deep. There is a risk of *tetanus* infection.

The viruses responsible for hepatitis B (see *Hepatitis, viral*), herpes simplex, *AIDS*, and *rabies* are present in the saliva of those affected. Transmission of hepatitis B and AIDS by a bite is a theoretical hazard. Human cases of rabies are extremely rare, and the risk of being bitten by a human victim would be generally confined to doctors and nurses caring for the patient.

TREATMENT

Treatment for any bite that penetrates the skin is as for *Bites, animal*.

Black death

The medieval name for bubonic *plague*. One feature of the disease is bleeding beneath the skin, causing dark blue or black bruises. This, along with the fact that in medieval times the disease was fatal in over 50 per cent of cases, accounts for the name.

Black eye

The bruised appearance of the skin around the eye, usually following an injury. Any direct blow damages the many small blood vessels beneath the skin, causing blood to leak and collect there.

Because the skin around the eyes is loose and transparent, bruising is darker in this area than on other parts of the body. A cold compress held over the eye will help to relieve the discomfort.

Blackhead

A semi-solid, black-capped plug of greasy material blocking the outlet of a sebaceous (oil-forming) gland in the skin. Blackheads occur most commonly on the face, chest, shoulders, and back, alone or in groups, and are associated with increased sebaceous

gland activity, which is normal in adolescents. Blackheads are a characteristic feature of certain types of *acne*.

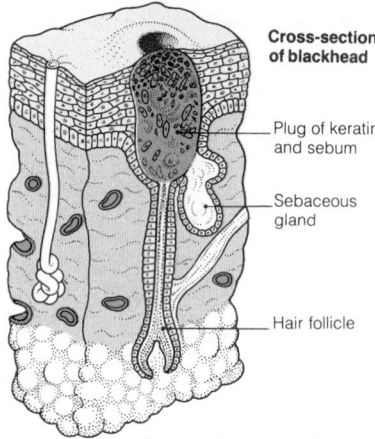

Cross-section of blackhead

Plug of keratin and sebum

Sebaceous gland

Hair follicle

Blackout

A common term for loss of consciousness (see *Fainting*.)

Black teeth

See *Discoloured teeth*.

Blackwater fever

An occasional and life-threatening complication of falciparum *malaria* (the most dangerous form of malaria). The condition is brought on by a sudden increased rate of destruction of red blood cells. The breakdown products of the cells find their way via the kidneys into the urine and cause it to darken, hence "blackwater". Other symptoms include loss of consciousness, fever, chills, and vomiting.

Bladder

The hollow, muscular organ in the lower abdomen that acts as a reservoir for *urine*. The adult bladder can hold half a litre or more of urine. It lies behind the pubic bone, hidden within and protected by the bony pelvis.

The bladder walls consist of muscle and an inner lining called urinary epithelium. At the back are the two ureters, which carry urine to the bladder from the kidneys. At the lowest point of the bladder—the neck—is the opening into the urethra; this is normally kept tightly closed by a ring of muscle (the urethral sphincter).

FUNCTION

The bladder's function is to collect and store urine until it can be expelled from the body at a suitable time.

Full control over bladder function takes several years to develop. In infants, emptying of the bladder is an

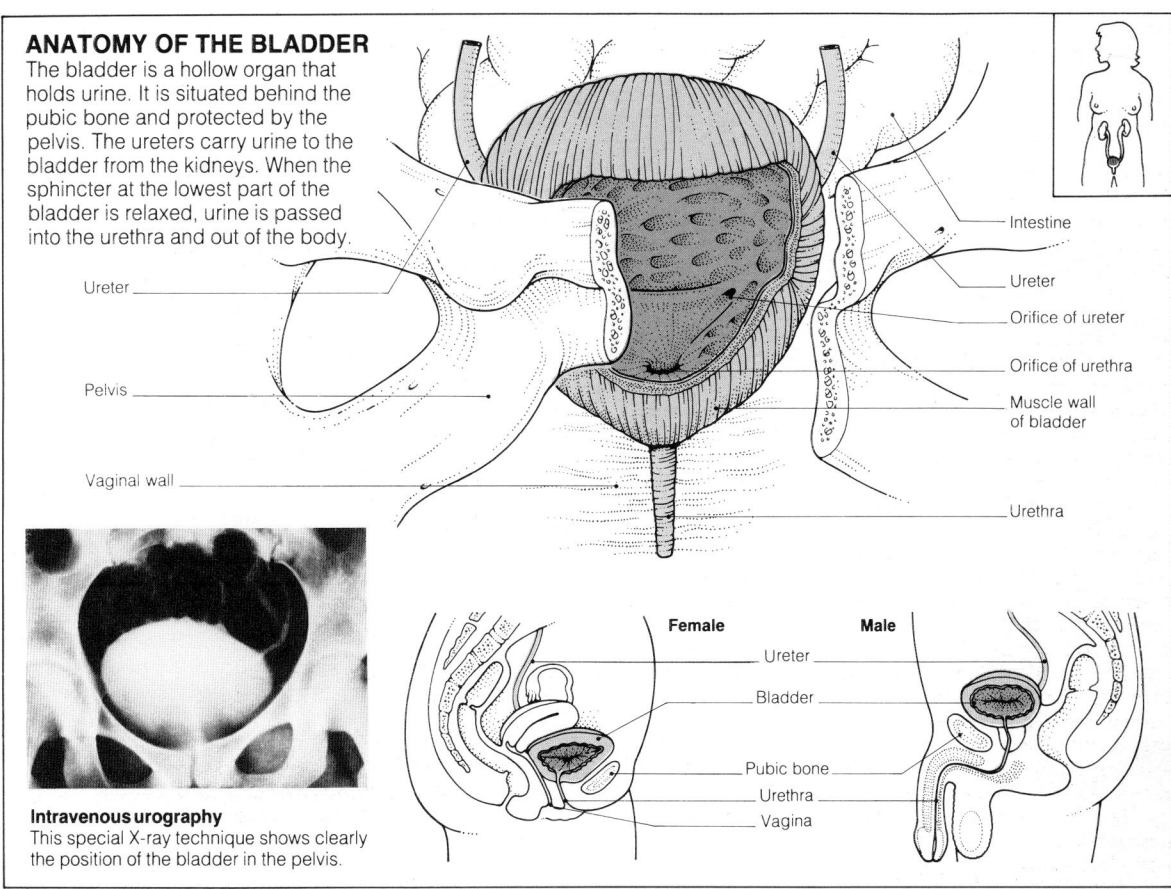

ANATOMY OF THE BLADDER

The bladder is a hollow organ that holds urine. It is situated behind the pubic bone and protected by the pelvis. The ureters carry urine to the bladder from the kidneys. When the sphincter at the lowest part of the bladder is relaxed, urine is passed into the urethra and out of the body.

Ureter

Pelvis

Vaginal wall

Intestine

Ureter

Orifice of ureter

Orifice of urethra

Muscle wall of bladder

Urethra

Intravenous urography
This special X-ray technique shows clearly the position of the bladder in the pelvis.

Female   Male

Ureter

Bladder

Pubic bone

Urethra

Vagina

---

entirely automatic or *reflex* reaction. When the bladder fills and stretches beyond a certain point, signals are sent to the spinal cord. Nerve signals from the spinal cord then cause the urethral sphincter to relax and the main bladder muscle to contract, thus expelling urine via the urethra.

As the child grows, he or she gradually develops the ability to delay emptying. Stretching of the bladder is registered consciously (as discomfort) in brain centres, which, if desired, can then send nerve signals suppressing the emptying reflex. Eventually, however, the bladder becomes so full and stretched that the urge to pass urine is overwhelming.

Children vary in the age at which they achieve perfect bladder control and, in particular, night-time control. Most children are dry at night by the age of five years, but some take longer (see *Enuresis*).

Defective bladder function, leading to problems such as *incontinence* and *urinary retention* can have a variety of causes. (See *Bladder* disorders box.)

Bladder cancer
See *Bladder tumours*.

Bladder tumours
Growths originating in the inner lining of the bladder. Many bladder tumours are *papillomas* (small wart-like growths), which tend to recur, and eventually may become cancerous. Other, more malignant growths tend to spread inwards, into the bladder cavity, but may also spread through the bladder wall to nearby organs, such as the rectum, colon, prostate gland, or uterus, and to the lymph glands and pelvic bones.

INCIDENCE AND CAUSES
Bladder cancers account for about five per cent of all cancers diagnosed in the UK, with about 10,000 new cases (leading to about 5,000 deaths) per year. Almost three times as many men as women are affected, and the average age at diagnosis is 65 years.

Certain groups are at increased risk, notably smokers and workers in the dye and rubber industries. Exposure to carcinogenic substances used in these industries or in tobacco smoke is the presumed cause in these groups. Bladder cancer is also common in areas of the tropics where the parasitic infection *schistosomiasis* is prevalent.

PREVENTION
Avoiding smoking is the principal means of reducing the personal risk. The incidence of occupational bladder cancer has been reduced by protective measures in the industries concerned and by screening of those who have been exposed in the past.

SYMPTOMS
Haematuria (blood in the urine) is the main symptom. Passing urine is usually painless, but a bladder infection may develop, and the passage of urine then becomes painful and frequent. Sometimes, a tumour may obstruct the entry of a ureter into the bladder, causing back pressure and pain in the kidney region, or may obstruct the urethral exit, causing difficulty in passing urine.

DIAGNOSIS AND TREATMENT
Bladder tumours are investigated by *cystoscopy* (passage of a slim viewing

DISORDERS OF THE BLADDER

The most important causes of bladder problems are infection, tumours, *calculi* (stones), or impairment of the bladder's nerve supply.

INFECTION

Infection of the bladder, better known as *cystitis*, is particularly common in women, mainly because of the much shorter female urethra, which provides less of a barrier to bacteria. In men, infection is usually associated with obstruction to the flow of urine from the bladder by, for example, tumours of the bladder or an enlarged prostate gland. In some parts of the tropics, the parasitic worm infection *schistosomiasis* (bilharzia) is a common cause of bladder problems.

TUMOURS

Bladder tumours may be benign or malignant and are more common in men than in women. They are usually painless in the early stages and may cause *haematuria* (blood in the urine) or obstruction to the outflow of urine from the bladder. The latter may also be caused by a tumour or enlargement of the prostate and result in partial or complete *urine retention* and stagnation in the bladder.

Tumours of the spinal cord may affect the nerves controlling the bladder, leading either to retention or *incontinence*.

CALCULI

Calculi (stones) in the bladder, caused by the precipitation from solution of substances present in the urine, are an uncommon problem in the UK. They mainly affect men and usually result from urinary retention and/or a long-standing urinary tract infection. In some other parts of the world, such as Southeast Asia, they are more common and are often associated with a low-protein diet.

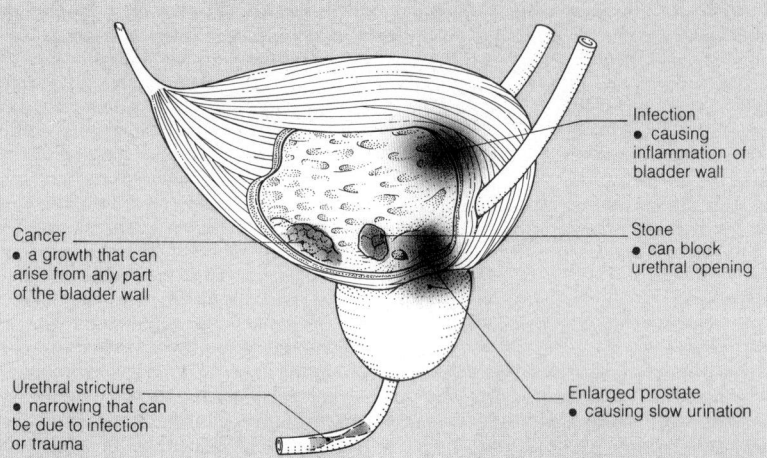

Cancer
● a growth that can arise from any part of the bladder wall

Urethral stricture
● narrowing that can be due to infection or trauma

Infection
● causing inflammation of bladder wall

Stone
● can block urethral opening

Enlarged prostate
● causing slow urination

INJURY

Injury to the bladder is uncommon. It may occur, however, if the pelvis is fractured when the bladder is full. Such injury typically occurs in traffic accidents. The bladder ruptures and urine leaks into the abdominal and pelvic cavities.

Damage to the nerves involved in bladder control may severely disrupt bladder filling and emptying, causing either incontinence or urinary retention, depending on the site of the injury. In the UK, the most common cause of such damage is spinal cord injury due to road traffic accidents. Nerves that control the bladder may also be damaged by a prolapsed intervertebral disc.

OTHER DISORDERS

Disturbance of bladder control can also result from nerve degeneration found in conditions such as *diabetes mellitus*, *multiple sclerosis*, or *dementia*.

An unstable or *irritable bladder* is a common condition in which the urge to empty the bladder occurs frequently. It is not fully understood but is sometimes associated with a *urinary tract infection* or prolapse of the uterus. Many other underlying conditions, most com-

monly tension or anxiety, can cause frequent urination.

Failure to achieve bladder control by the age of three or four is termed *enuresis* (bed-wetting); this may be due to a treatable physical cause, such as urinary tract infection, or to emotional problems but more often results from delayed maturation of the nervous system.

INVESTIGATION

Various methods are used to investigate bladder disorders. Urinary tract infection is diagnosed by culturing a urine sample. The bladder can be viewed directly by *cystoscopy*. X-ray studies include micturating *cystourethrography*, which normally shows only the bladder and urethra, and intravenous *urography*, which shows the whole urinary tract except the urethra. *Cystometry* measures bladder capacity in relation to pressure.

---

tube up the urethra into the bladder) and by *biopsy* (removal of a sample of tissue for microscopic analysis). Early tumours are usually cut out or treated by *diathermy* (heat destruction) via the cystoscope. Tumours recur in at least 60 per cent of cases, so regular follow-up cystoscopy is necessary. Recurrences may be treated surgically or with a solution of *anticancer drugs* introduced into the bladder.

In the case of a more widely spread cancer, treatment is usually by *radiotherapy*, though if this fails, more drastic surgery to remove the bladder (see *Cystectomy*) may be necessary.

OUTLOOK

This varies according to what stage the growth has reached when first diagnosed. If a tumour is diagnosed and treated early, the long-term prospects are excellent. However, if

cancer has spread beyond the bladder wall, the chances of survival for more than five years are poor.

Bleaching, dental

A cosmetic procedure for lightening some types of *discoloured teeth*, including nonvital "dead" teeth. The surface of the affected tooth is painted with chemical oxidizing agents and then exposed to ultraviolet light.

Bleeding

Loss of blood from the *circulatory system* caused by damage to the blood vessels or by a *bleeding disorder*. Bleeding may be visible (external) or concealed (internal). Rapid loss of more than 10 per cent of the blood volume can cause symptoms of *shock*, with faintness, pallor, and sweating.

CAUSES

The most common cause of bleeding is an injury. The speed with which blood flows from a cut depends on the type of blood vessel damaged: blood usually oozes from a capillary, flows from a vein, and spurts from an artery. If an injury does not break open the skin, blood collects around the damaged blood vessels close under the skin to form a *bruise*.

Damage to internal blood vessels may be the result of inflammation, infection, an ulcer, or a tumour. Any lost blood that mixes with other bodily fluids such as sputum (phlegm) or urine will be noticed quite readily; bleeding in the digestive tract may make vomit or faeces appear darker than usual because the blood is partially digested. Sometimes, internal bleeding is not discovered until severe *anaemia* develops.

Bleeding that is not caused by injury usually requires medical investigation. The exceptions are an occasional *nosebleed* and bleeding during *menstruation*. The amount of blood lost during menstruation varies from woman to woman and from month to month. Menstrual blood loss is only a problem if it is very heavy or frequent, when it might lead to iron-deficiency anaemia.

Bleeding disorders

A group of conditions characterized by bleeding in the absence of injury or by abnormally prolonged and excessive bleeding after injury.

Bleeding disorders result from defects in the mechanisms by which bleeding is normally stopped (see *Blood clotting*). These mechanisms are blood coagulation, plugging of damaged blood vessels by platelets, and constriction of blood vessels.

Defects in the coagulation system tend to cause deep bleeding into the gastrointestinal tract, the muscles, and the joint cavities. Defects of the platelets or blood vessels usually produce superficial bleeding into the skin, gums, or lining of the intestine or urinary tract. However, bleeding may occur anywhere in the body with any type of bleeding defect.

COAGULATION DEFECTS

These disorders usually result from deficiencies of the enzymes (called coagulation factors) that take part in blood clotting, or from the enzymes being abnormal. Blood-clot formation is very slow and the clots are weak and do not seal blood vessels securely. Coagulation defects may be congenital (present from birth) or acquired later in life.

CONGENITAL The principal congenital coagulation defects are *haemophilia*, *Christmas disease*, and *von Willebrand's disease*. In each of these, one of the coagulation factors is either absent from the blood or is present in only small amounts.

Haemophilia and Christmas disease are similar disorders, resulting from deficiencies of two different coagulation factors, called factor VIII and factor IX, respectively. The inheritance of these disorders is sex-linked (see *Genetic disorders*), which means that normally only males are affected. In the UK, about 5,000 people have haemophilia and about 1,000 have Christmas disease.

Von Willebrand's disease is also an inherited disorder in which there is a factor VIII defect, but one that affects both sexes roughly equally. About five persons per 100,000 are affected.

Individuals with bleeding disorders may suffer from bruising, internal bleeding, abnormally heavy menstrual periods, and excessive bleeding from wounds. In severe cases, sufferers may bleed recurrently into joints such as the knee.

ACQUIRED Deficiencies of coagulation factors may develop at any age as a result of severe liver disease, digestive system disorders that prevent the absorption from the diet of *vitamin K* (required to make some coagulation factors), or the use of *anticoagulant drugs*, such as warfarin, that prevent normal production of coagulation factors. As with congenital bleeding disorders, a severe bleeding tendency may result.

One particularly complex coagulation disorder is disseminated intravascular coagulation (DIC), which may be triggered by any of a variety of circumstances. In DIC, there is aggregation of platelets and clotting within small blood vessels. Subsequently, coagulation factors are used and broken up in the blood faster than they can be replaced by the liver, and severe bleeding may result. Paradoxically, anticoagulant drugs are sometimes used to interfere with clotting activity

in this condition, but in most cases this very serious condition does not improve until the underlying problem (for example, infection or cancer) is brought under control.

Coagulation defects are investigated by *blood-clotting tests* such as the prothrombin time. Treatment is based on giving the patient transfusions of the missing coagulation factor or factors in fresh blood or fresh frozen plasma. These factors can be made synthetically using genetic engineering, but most are still obtained from human blood provided by volunteer donors. Transmission of some viral infections (e.g. hepatitis B and C (see *Hepatitis, viral*) and *HIV* infection) has occurred in the past, but blood is now checked for harmful viruses and discarded if necessary. Blood products are also heat-treated in an attempt to destroy viruses.

PLATELET DEFECTS

Bleeding may occur if there are too few platelets in the blood—a condition called *thrombocytopenia*. The main feature of this disorder is surface bleeding into the skin and gums, causing multiple small bruises.

Occasionally, the platelets are present in normal numbers but function abnormally, with resultant bleeding. Defects of platelet function may be inherited, may be associated with the use of certain drugs (including *aspirin*), or may be a complication of certain bone marrow disorders such as myeloid *leukaemia*.

Platelet defects are investigated by tests, such as measuring bleeding time and clotting time, and various other tests of platelet aggregation (clumping). Whatever the cause, the main treatment consists of transfusions of platelets from single donors or from "pools" (obtained from several normal blood transfusions). The transfusions need to be given every one to three days until the underlying defect has been corrected and the body is again producing its own healthy platelets.

BLOOD-VESSEL DEFECTS

In rare cases, abnormal bleeding is caused by a blood-vessel defect. In the past, *scurvy* (a disorder caused by vitamin C deficiency) was a common and often fatal disorder of this type, affecting sailors, polar explorers, and anyone with a diet lacking fresh fruit and vegetables. Today, mild scurvy is occasionally seen in elderly people on a poor diet.

Elderly people and patients on long-term courses of *corticosteroid drugs* may suffer mild abnormal bruising due to loss of skin support to the smallest blood vessels. Treatment is rarely required.

Bleeding gums

See *Gingivitis*.

Bleeding, treatment of

Part of the body's response to internal or external loss of blood is to constrict the damaged blood vessels and to cause blood to clot at the site of injury. At the same time, blood flow may be reduced in the skin and muscles to make sure that the brain, kidneys, and other vital organs are adequately supplied. Loss of a large volume of blood quickly causes a dramatic fall in blood pressure, accompanied by weakness, confusion, pallor, and sweating as the body tries to compensate; this state is known as *shock*.

First-aid measures have two objectives: to minimize blood loss and to help the body cope with the loss. In most cases, bleeding can be stopped, or at least slowed, by direct pressure (see box).

PROFESSIONAL TREATMENT

When bleeding is severe, intravenous infusions of saline solution and plasma preparations may be given to help replace fluids lost from the circulation. If a large amount of blood is lost, *blood transfusion* may also be required. Large wounds may need closing with sutures (stitches), which are effective in stopping bleeding from scalp injuries and also reduce the extent of scarring. If bleeding within the abdomen is suspected following an accident, *CT scanning* and/or exploratory surgery may be needed. If bleeding within the skull is compressing the brain, a hole will be drilled in the skull to relieve the pressure.

Severe bleeding may require treatment in the operating theatre. During operations, bleeding from small blood vessels is controlled by clamping them with forceps and then either tying them or sealing them by *diathermy* (the application of a high-frequency electric current).

Blepharitis

Inflammation of the eyelids, with redness, irritation, and scaly skin at the lid margins. The patient may note burning and discomfort in the eyes and flakes or crusts on the lashes. Occasionally, the surface of the eye may also be inflamed and red. In some cases, the roots of the eyelashes become infected, and small ulcers form. Blepharitis is common, tends to

recur, and is sometimes associated with dandruff of the scalp or eczema.

The problem can often be cleared up by removing the scales with cotton-wool moistened with warm water. Blepharitis of the lid margins frequently recurs, especially after periods of stress or illness, or when aggravated by dust or tobacco smoke, and requires further treatment. Ulcerated eyelids need medical attention. Severe cases of blepharitis may lead to *corneal ulcers*. Various eye-drops reduce discomfort even though they cannot prevent recurrences.

Blepharoplasty

A cosmetic operation to remove wrinkled, drooping skin from the upper and/or lower eyelids. The operation is usually done under local anaesthesia and takes about one and a half hours. The patient can usually go home the same day.

FIRST AID: TREATING BLEEDING

SIMPLE CUT

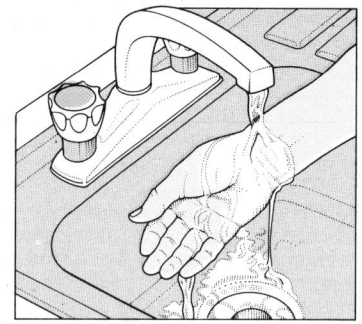

1 Wash your hands before dealing with the cut. Then, if the cut has dirt in it, rinse it lightly under lukewarm running water until it is clean, being careful not to touch the spout.

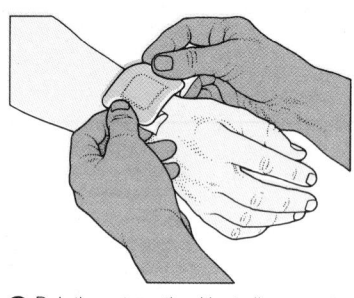

2 Dab the cut gently with sterile gauze to dry it. Then dress the cut with an adhesive dressing.

DEEP CUT

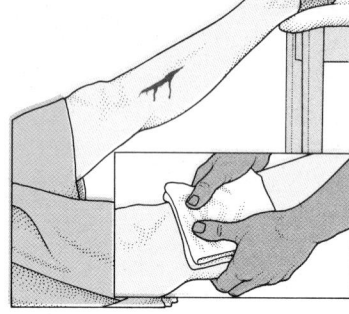

1 Raise the injured part and support it. Put a sterile dressing on the wound and apply firm pressure to control bleeding.

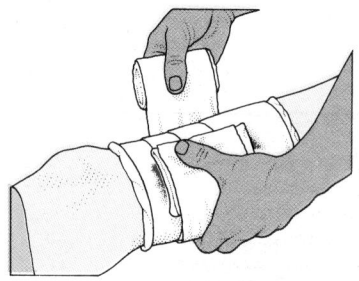

2 If blood seeps through, do not remove the dressing as this may disturb clots and restart bleeding. Put other dressings on top of the first one and bandage all dressings snugly.

WHY IT IS DONE

As a person grows older, the skin loses some of its fat, and much of its elasticity, becoming droopy and creased. This process may be accelerated by worry or sudden weight loss. As a result, the eyelids become baggy. Removing the excess skin can greatly improve appearance.

HOW IT IS DONE

On the upper lids a horizontal fold of skin is removed from the centre of each lid so that the resultant scar runs in a natural crease line. On the lower lids the incision is made just below the eyelashes, so that the scar will be in the shadow of the lashes and extend into a smile wrinkle. The baggy skin is pulled upwards and outwards, the excess is removed, and the wound is then stitched.

RECOVERY PERIOD

After the operation, ice-packs and pads soaked with witch-hazel solution are applied to both eyes, to reduce swelling and bruising. The patient is advised to repeat these applications at home. Swelling usually subsides within three days but bruising may last for two weeks.

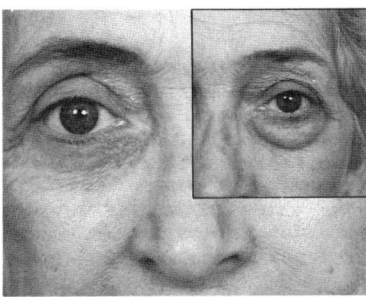

Appearance before (inset) and after
Blepharoplasty involves removal of a crescent-shaped section of skin and underlying fat from each eyelid.

Some of the stitches are removed three to five days after the operation, the rest seven to 10 days after. The scars usually fade to fine, unnoticeable marks after six to 12 months.

Blepharospasm
Involuntary, prolonged contraction of one of the muscles that controls the eyelids, causing the eyes to close. It may be due to *photophobia* (abnormal sensitivity of the eyes to light), *blepharitis* (inflammation of the eyelids), *anxiety*, or *hysteria*. Treatment is aimed at remedying the cause.

Blind loop syndrome
A condition in which abnormal faeces occur due to a redundant area or dead end (blind loop) in the small intestine. Blind loop syndrome is characterized by *steatorrhoea* (pale yellow, foul-smelling, fatty, bulky faeces that are difficult to flush away), together with general sickness, tiredness, and weight loss. The syndrome is usually the result of surgery but may be *congenital* (present at birth).

The blind loop interferes with the normal flow of bowel contents, resulting in stagnation. Bacteria other than the usual dominant inhabitants of the bowel proliferate in the loop and spread into other areas of the intestine, where they interfere with the absorption of nutrients, including fat and vitamin B_{12}.

Antibiotic treatment, usually with a *tetracycline drug*, may be successful. If not, surgery to remove the blind loop usually cures the condition.

Blindness
Inability to see. Generally, the term blindness refers to a severe loss of *vision* that cannot be corrected with ordinary *glasses*. Precise definitions of blindness and of partial sight vary. In the UK, blindness is usually defined as a corrected *visual acuity* of 3/60 or less in the better eye, or a *visual field* of no more than 20 degrees in the better eye. Partial sight is a lesser degree of visual disability, which affects employment or normal living.

INCIDENCE
It is estimated that over 40 million people in the world are partially or totally blind. *Vitamin A* deficiency alone accounts for blindness in millions of children living in developing countries of Africa, Asia, and South America.

In the UK, just over 100,000 people are registered as legally blind, and a further 50,000 as partially sighted.

CAUSES
Blindness may result from injury, disease, or degeneration of the eyeball, of the optic nerve or nerve pathways connecting the eye to the brain, or of the brain itself.

EYEBALL Normal vision depends on the uninterrupted passage of light from the front of the eye to the light-sensitive retina at the back. Anything that prevents light from reaching the retina can cause blindness.

Various disorders may impair the transparency of the cornea at the front of the eye. In *Sjögren's syndrome*, an inability to produce tears leads to *keratoconjunctivitis sicca*, which, if severe, causes the cornea to cloud over. Other causes of a cloudy cornea include vitamin A deficiency, accidental chemical damage, infections, and injury. *Corneal ulcers* can also cause blindness because they leave scars after healing. The most common causes of such ulcers are severe attacks of certain infections, among them *ophthalmia* neonatorum (inflammation of the conjunctiva in

---

AIDS FOR THE BLIND
There are many ways in which life can be made easier for the blind person, and there are now a number of specially designed and adapted devices available. These include braille writers, mathematical apparatus, and home appliances, as well as aids for helping the blind person get around outside the home.

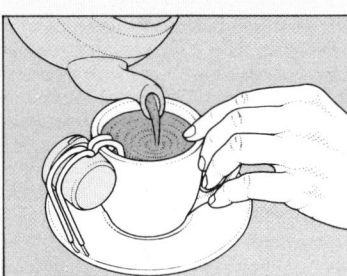

Liquid level indicator
This device measures liquid being poured into a cup or glass. Two sets of prongs are connected to a bleeper. A short set of prongs measures almost to the top, while the long set measures small amounts in the bottom. A bleep sounds when the liquid makes contact with the prongs.

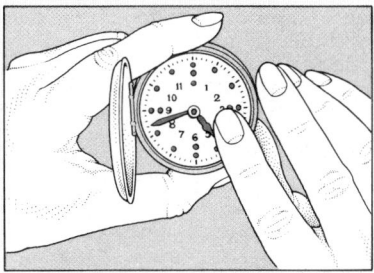

Pocket watch
Strengthened hands and raised dots make it easier for a blind person to "read" numerals: three dots are at 12, two are at 3, 6, and 9, and one is at each of the other hour positions.

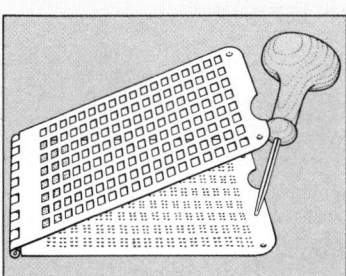

Pocket braille maker
This frame produces braille on one side of the paper. A special pointed stylus is used to make the braille indentations; a stencil keeps the stylus in the right place. The braille can be read without removing the paper from the frame.

B

newborn babies), *trachoma* (most common in hot, overcrowded regions), *herpes simplex*, and bacterial ulcers.

Inflammation of the iris, ciliary body, or choroid—a condition known as *uveitis*—can cause loss of vision. The inflammation may occur in association with *tuberculosis, sarcoidosis, syphilis, toxocariasis,* or *toxoplasmosis,* but often occurs for no known reason.

Cataract (cloudiness of the lens) is a common cause of blindness. It is usually the result of the lens becoming less transparent in old age, but is occasionally present from birth or develops in childhood.

Diabetes mellitus, hypertension, or injury can cause bleeding into the cavity of the eyeball. In *hyphaema,* blood enters the aqueous humour (watery substance in front of the lens). *Vitreous haemorrhage* is bleeding into the jelly-like vitreous humour behind the lens.

Disorders of the retina are a common cause of blindness. They include age-related *macular degeneration* (degeneration of the central area of the retina, which occurs in old age), *retinopathy* due to diabetes or hypertension, *retinal artery occlusion* or *retinal vein occlusion* (blockage of the blood flow to or from the retina), *retinal detachment,* tumours such as *retinoblastoma* and malignant *melanoma* of the eye, and *retinal haemorrhage* (bleeding into the retina), caused by diabetes, hypertension, vascular disease, or injury.

In *glaucoma,* another common cause of blindness, excessive pressure in the eyeball causes degeneration of nerve fibres at the front end of the optic nerve. The most common type of glaucoma can cause loss of side vision, which may not be noticed until the disease is well advanced.

OPTIC NERVE AND NERVE PATHWAYS The light energy received by the retina is transformed into nerve impulses that travel along the optic nerve and nerve pathways into the brain. Conduction of these impulses may be impaired by pressure from a tumour in the orbit (the bony cavity that contains the eyeball) or in the brain; by interference with the blood supply to the optic nerve, caused by diabetes mellitus, hypertension, a tumour, injury, or *temporal arteritis*; by *optic neuritis* (inflammation of the optic nerve that may occur in *multiple sclerosis*); by toxic amblyopia, which is caused by the poisonous effects of certain chemicals; or by nutritional deficiency amblyopia, which is caused by a lack of certain essential nutrients in the diet.

BRAIN Nerve impulses from the retina eventually arrive in a region of the *cerebrum* (main mass of the brain) called the visual cortex. Here, the nerve impulses are analysed and interpreted to provide conscious images. Blindness can be caused if there is pressure on the visual cortex from a *brain tumour* or *brain haemorrhage*, or if a *stroke* reduces the blood supply to the cortex.

Finally, apparent blindness may be related to *hysteria*, a reaction to severe stress in which physical symptoms develop without any physical cause, or to *malingering*.

DIAGNOSIS AND TREATMENT

Anyone who suffers a loss of vision, whether partial or complete, should consult a doctor immediately. Various types of *vision tests* can be done.

Often, the cause can be ascertained by direct examination of the eye, including ophthalmoscopy, slit-lamp examination, tonometry, and perimetry. Electrical activity produced in the brain following visual stimulation can be measured by visual potentiometry (see *Evoked responses*). The age and medical history of the patient, the patient's account of the development of the sight loss, and other signs and symptoms, may provide important clues to the diagnosis. In a few cases, *ultrasound scanning, CT scanning,* or *MRI* may be performed to look for any abnormalities in the eyes, orbits, structures around the optic nerves, or brain. *Fluorescein* angiography (a technique for photographing the vessels of the eye) may be used to study the retina and choroid. Treatment depends on the underlying cause. If the loss of vision cannot be corrected, the patient may then be registered as legally blind or partially sighted. Certain services and benefits may then be available. (See also *Eye*; *Vision, loss of.*)

Blind spot

The small, oval-shaped area on the retina of the eye where the optic nerve joins the eyeball. The area is not sensitive to light because it has no light receptors (nerve endings responsive to light).

To demonstrate the presence of the blind spot, mark an X on a piece of paper and a dot 15 cm to the right. While holding the paper at arm's length, shut your left eye and look at the X with your right eye. Slowly move the paper towards you until the dot disappears. This is the point at which the image of the dot has fallen on your right eye's blind spot.

Blister

A collection of fluid beneath the outer layer of the skin that forms a raised area, usually oval or circular in shape. Large blisters (more than 1 cm in diameter) are sometimes called bullae; small blisters are sometimes called vesicles.

The fluid in a blister is serum that has leaked from blood vessels in underlying skin layers after minor damage. The fluid is usually sterile and the blister provides valuable protection to the damaged tissue.

CAUSES

Common causes of blisters are *burns* (including *sunburn*) and friction—for example, from an ill-fitting shoe.

A number of skin diseases can also cause blisters. These include *eczema, impetigo, erythema multiforme,* and *epidermolysis bullosa,* the bullous disorders *pemphigoid, pemphigus,* and *dermatitis herpetiformis,* and some types of *porphyria.*

Small blisters develop at an early stage in the rashes of the viral infections *chickenpox, herpes zoster* (shingles), and *herpes simplex*; these blisters contain infectious virus particles that may spread the infection.

TREATMENT

A blister is best left to heal on its own. It should not be burst, because the underlying damaged tissue could become infected. In the case of large, troublesome, or unexplained blisters, consult your doctor. Bullous disorders are potentially serious and expert advice is needed.

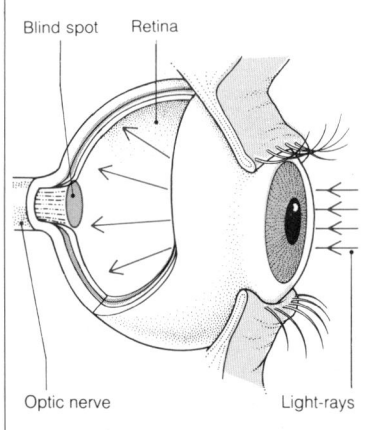

LOCATION OF BLIND SPOT
The blind spot is a minute area on the retina that lacks light receptors and so is not light-sensitive.

Blind spot   Retina

Optic nerve   Light-rays

Blocked nose

See *Nasal congestion; Nasal obstruction.*

Blocking

Inability to express true feelings or thoughts, usually as a result of emotional or mental conflict. In Freudian-based psychotherapies, blocking is regarded as originating from repression of painful emotions in early life. Successful treatment is thought to depend on putting patients in touch with these unconscious feelings.

A very specific form of thought blocking occurs in *schizophrenia*. In this disorder, trains of thought are persistently interrupted involuntarily, to be replaced by new ones that are totally unconnected with the first. (See also *Psychotherapy.*)

Blood

The sticky red fluid that circulates in our veins, arteries and capillaries. Its main function is to act as the body's transport system, but blood also plays an important role in the defence against infection.

The average-sized adult has about five litres of blood. At rest, roughly this same volume of blood is pumped each minute by the heart via the arteries to the lungs and all other tissues, then returned to the heart in veins, in a continuous circuit (see *Circulatory system*). During exercise, the heart may pump blood at a rate of 30 litres or more a minute.

Almost half the volume of blood consists of *blood cells*; these include red blood cells (or erythrocytes), white blood cells (or leukocytes), and platelets (or thrombocytes). The remainder of the blood volume is a watery, straw-coloured fluid called plasma, which contains dissolved proteins, sugars, fats, salts, and minerals.

BLOOD CELLS
The main function of red blood cells is to act as containers for *haemoglobin* (a pigmented protein that contains iron). Haemoglobin carries oxygen from the lungs to the tissues, where the oxygen is exchanged for the waste product carbon dioxide (see *Respiration*). White blood cells play an important part in the defence against infections and cancers, and also contribute to inflammation (see *Immune system*). Platelets are essential to the arrest of bleeding and to the repair of damaged blood vessels. The platelets clump together to block small holes in blood vessels, and the clumps release chemicals that begin the process of *blood clotting*.

PLASMA
Blood plasma is a straw-coloured fluid, consisting mainly of water (95 per cent), with a salt content very similar to that of seawater. Levels of the many other dissolved constituents in plasma vary from time to time. Measurements of these constituents are useful to doctors in the diagnosis of disease (see *Blood tests; Liver-function tests*). Important constituents of plasma include the following.

NUTRIENTS These are transported to the tissues after absorption from the intestinal tract or after release from storage depots such as the liver. Nutrients include sugars (principally glucose), fats, amino acids (required by cells to make proteins), and various vitamins and minerals. Immediately after a meal rich in fats, the blood plasma has a milky appearance as a consequence of its high fat content.

WASTE PRODUCTS The main waste product of tissue metabolism is *urea* (produced by the breakdown of proteins), which is transported in the plasma to the kidneys; abnormally high blood urea levels occur in *kidney failure*. The waste product from the destruction of haemoglobin is a yellow pigment called *bilirubin*. This is normally removed from the plasma by the liver and excreted in the *bile*. Bilirubin levels become abnormally high in liver disease, or in haemolytic *anaemia*, in which there is excessive destruction of red blood cells.

PROTEINS These include substances, such as fibrinogen, that are involved in the processes of blood coagulation, and others that act to inhibit coagulation (see *Blood clotting*). Plasma proteins, such as *immunoglobulins* (also called *antibodies*), and *complement*, are part of the immune system. Another important plasma protein is *albumin*. The large size of the protein molecules prevents them from escaping from the blood into the tissues; this helps to keep water in the blood (by a mechanism called osmotic pressure) and thus maintain blood volume.

HORMONES These are chemical messengers produced by various glands of the *endocrine system* and transported in the blood to their target organs.

Blood cells

Cells present in blood for most or part of their lifespan. These include red blood cells, which make up about 40 per cent by volume of normal blood, and white blood cells and platelets, which make up less than five per cent of the total volume.

All types of blood cells are formed in the bone marrow by a series of divisions from one type of cell called a stem cell.

RED BLOOD CELLS

These are also called RBCs, red blood corpuscles, or erythrocytes. They carry oxygen from the lungs to the tissues, where they exchange the oxygen for the waste product carbon dioxide (see *Respiration*).

FORMATION Red blood cells are formed from stem cells in the bone marrow by a process (called erythropoiesis) that takes about five days. Their formation requires an adequate supply of nutrients, including iron, amino acids, and the vitamins B_{12} and folic acid. The rate at which RBCs are formed is influenced by a hormone called erythropoietin, which is produced by the kidneys.

Immature red blood cells just released into the bloodstream from the marrow are called reticulocytes; over a period of two to four days, these develop into mature red blood cells. Reticulocytes are easily recognized in blood by means of special staining techniques, and a count of their numbers provides doctors with a helpful estimate of the rate at which RBCs are being formed.

STRUCTURE AND FUNCTION In 1 cu. mm of blood there are about five million red blood cells, each of which is disc-shaped, about 0.0075 mm in diameter, and much thicker around the edge than at the centre. This shape gives each cell a relatively large surface area, which helps it absorb and release oxygen molecules, and allows the cell to distort as it squeezes through narrow blood vessels.

Each red blood cell is packed with large quantities of *haemoglobin*, a pigmented protein that contains iron. Haemoglobin is highly efficient at "binding" (combining chemically) with oxygen when the oxygen concentration is high (in the lungs), and at releasing the oxygen when the oxygen concentration is low (in the tissues). Oxyhaemoglobin, formed when oxygen combines with haemoglobin, is responsible for the bright red coloration of oxygenated blood (which flows mainly through arteries). Most venous blood is darker in colour, because it contains the unbound (deoxygenated) form of haemoglobin.

Each red blood cell also contains *enzymes*, minerals, and sugars, which provide energy for the cell's *metabolism* and maintain its shape, structure, and elasticity.

B

The surface structure of red blood cells varies slightly among individuals, and this provides the basis for classifying blood into groups (see *Blood groups*).

AGING AND DESTRUCTION The normal lifespan of red blood cells in the circulation is about 120 days. (Blood in blood banks must be discarded after three to four weeks, by which time the proportion of dead cells has reached significant levels.) As red blood cells age, their internal chemical machinery wears out, they lose elasticity, and they become trapped in small blood vessels in the spleen and other organs; they are then destroyed by a type of white blood cell called a macrophage. Most components of the haemoglobin molecules are reused, but some are broken down to form the waste product *bilirubin*.

DISORDERS Abnormalities can occur in the rate at which RBCs are formed or destroyed, in their numbers in the blood, and in their shape, size, and haemoglobin content, causing various forms of *anaemia* and *polycythaemia* (see *Blood* disorders box).

WHITE BLOOD CELLS

 These are also called WBCs, white blood corpuscles, or leukocytes; their principal role is to protect the body against infection and to fight infection when it occurs. White blood cells are bigger than red blood cells (up to 0.015 mm in diameter) but much less numerous (about 7,500 per cu. mm of blood). They generally spend a much shorter part of their lifespan than red blood cells in the blood itself.

There are three main types of white blood cells, called granulocytes, monocytes, and *lymphocytes*.

GRANULOCYTES White blood cells of this type are also called polymorphonuclear leucocytes. Under the microscope, they are seen to contain granules and have an oddly shaped nucleus. Granulocytes are themselves of three types, called neutrophils, basophils, and eosinophils. Of these, the most important are neutrophils, which are responsible for isolating and destroying invading bacteria (pus consists largely of neutrophils). The

action of neutrophils in "swallowing" bacteria has led to their being called phagocytes (literally "engulfing cells"). Neutrophils remain in the blood for only about six to nine hours before moving through blood-vessel walls into the tissues, where they survive for a few more days. Eosinophils play a part in allergic reactions and increase in numbers in response to certain parasitic infections. Basophils are involved in inflammatory and allergic reactions.

MONOCYTES These cells are also a type of phagocyte; they circulate in the bloodstream for about six to nine days and play an important part in the *immune system*.

LYMPHOCYTES Many of these are formed in the lymph nodes rather than the bone marrow. They play a central role in the immune system, roving around the body between the bloodstream, the lymph nodes, and the channels between the lymph nodes.

T-type lymphocytes are responsible for the delayed hypersensitivity phenomena (see *Allergy*) and produce substances known as lymphokines,

---

CONSTITUENTS OF BLOOD

Blood is pumped around the body in veins and arteries, transporting oxygen from the lungs to the tissues, and carbon dioxide from the tissues to the lungs. Blood also carries nutrients such as sugars, fats, and proteins that have been absorbed from the intestine, and hormones produced by a variety of glands. Waste products that are released from cells are carried in the blood to be broken down in the liver or excreted from the kidneys.

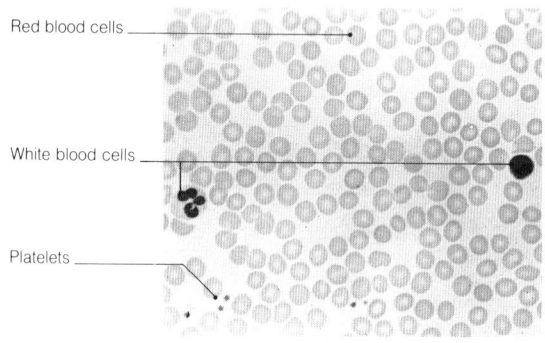

Red blood cells

White blood cells

Platelets

Normal blood smear
This is the appearance of normal blood under a microscope. The dominant feature is the abundance of red blood cells, which make up almost half the blood volume. Two white blood cells (a granulocyte at left and a lymphocyte) can be seen; the platelets are the tiny dark particles.

White blood cells
These cells protect the body against infection and fight it when it occurs. They are bigger than red blood cells but fewer in number. Each of the three main types (granulocytes, monocytes, and lymphocytes) plays a different role in dealing with infection.

Platelets
The smallest type of blood cell produced in the bone marrow; they play an important part in blood clotting.

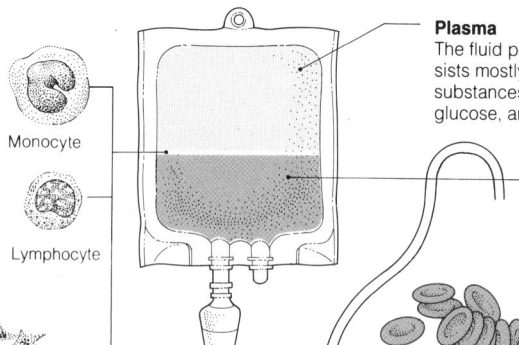

Monocyte

Granulocyte   Lymphocyte

Plasma
The fluid part of the blood that consists mostly of water. It carries substances such as proteins, fats, glucose, and salts.

Red blood cells
These disc-shaped cells are formed in the bone marrow and carry oxygen from the lungs to the rest of the body. They have a large surface area and a flexible shape.

which affect the function of many cells. T-type lymphocytes also moderate the activity of other lymphocytes called B-type cells. These B-type lymphocytes form the *antibodies* that protect us against second attacks of certain diseases (such as measles). Individual lymphocyte cells may survive for anywhere between three months and 10 years.

DISORDERS The *leukaemias* are disorders in which there is a disorganised proliferation of WBCs in the bone marrow. WBCs may also be too few in number (see *Blood disorders*). In *AIDS*, certain T-lymphocytes are infected by *HIV* (the AIDS virus), which results in dysfunction of the immune system, and increased risk of certain types of infection and cancers.

PLATELETS

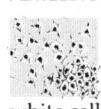
These are the smallest type of blood cell (0.002 mm to 0.003 mm in diameter), more numerous than white cells but less numerous than red cells (about 250,000 per cu. mm of blood). Like other blood cells, they originate from stem cells in the bone marrow. Platelets survive in blood for about nine days.

FUNCTION Platelets circulate in the blood in an inactive state, but under certain circumstances they begin to stick to blood-vessel walls and adhere to each other. These activities play a very important part in the arrest of bleeding and in *blood clotting*. The same processes can also lead to the unwanted formation of thrombi (clots) in intact blood vessels (see *Thrombosis*), and to fatty deposits on blood-vessel walls (see *Atherosclerosis*).

Because of their role in clot formation, platelets are sometimes also called thrombocytes.

DISORDERS Abnormal platelets, or a lack of platelets in the blood, can lead to some types of *bleeding disorder*.

BLOOD CELLS IN DIAGNOSIS
Microscopic examination of blood preparations may reveal not only blood-cell abnormalities characteristic of various diseases, but also healthy variations in the numbers of white blood cells produced in response to infections. For example, the number of neutrophils is raised in response to bacterial infections. The same is also true of lymphocytes in some viral infections.

The numbers, shapes, and appearance of the various types of blood cell are of great value to doctors in the diagnosis of disease (see *Blood count*; *Blood film*).

Blood clotting

Solidification of blood. Blood begins to clot within seconds of the skin being cut. The clot helps seal the damaged blood vessels, which also constrict to keep blood loss to a minimum. Blood clotting is not always helpful, however. Thrombi (clots) formed inside major blood vessels are the cause of many heart attacks, strokes, and other disorders (see *Thrombosis*).

The blood-clotting process has two parts: the activation and clumping of platelets in the blood; and the formation of fibrin filaments (see box overleaf).

To prevent the formation of clots inside healthy blood vessels, the blood also contains mechanisms that act to discourage clotting and to dissolve clots. These balance the proclotting mechanisms; normally, the balance is tipped in favour of clot formation only when a blood vessel is damaged.

PLATELET AGGREGATION
Platelets have to be "activated" before they will clump together. This occurs when they come into contact with damaged blood-vessel walls or with artificial surfaces (such as glass), when blood flow is turbulent, or when platelets are acted on by certain chemicals secreted into the blood.

Once activated, platelets first become sticky, adhering to surfaces. They then change shape from discs into spiny spheres, enmeshing with each other. Finally, they release chemicals that activate other platelets, start the process of fibrin formation, and cause blood vessels to contract.

FIBRIN FORMATION
This process, also called coagulation, is triggered by chemicals released either by activated platelets or by tissues following injury. It results from a complex series of reactions in the blood plasma called the coagulation cascade. With each step in the cascade, a coagulation factor in the plasma is converted from an inactive to an active form. The active form of the factor then activates several molecules of the next factor in the series— and so on until, in the final step, a factor called fibrinogen is converted into fibrin.

Provided all the participating factors are present, the activation of just one molecule of the first factor in the series can lead to the explosive production of up to 30,000 molecules of fibrin at the site of injury.

The factors involved in the coagulation cascade are numbered I,II, and V to XIII. Factor I is fibrinogen and

factor II, its immediate precursor in the cascade, is called prothrombin. Most of the coagulation factors are made in the liver.

An adequate supply in the diet of *vitamin K*, found in green vegetables, is required for the manufacture of certain factors.

ANTICLOTTING MECHANISMS
Separate mechanisms act to prevent unwanted platelet activation and fibrin formation.

Platelet activation is inhibited mainly by a substance called prostacyclin (a type of *prostaglandin*), which is secreted by the walls of healthy blood-vessels.

Fibrin formation is discouraged by various mechanisms. First, a number of inhibitory enzymes (types of protein) circulating in the blood neutralize activated coagulation factors. The most important of these is called antithrombin III. Second, a further series of enzymes is activated at the same time as the coagulation cascade. These enzymes form a substance called plasmin that breaks down fibrin (see *Fibrinolysis*). In addition, blood flow tends to discourage coagulation by washing away active coagulation factors from areas where they are being formed, and the liver deactivates any excess coagulation factors.

DEFECTS AND DISORDERS
Defects can occur for a wide variety of reasons in the clotting (or anticlotting) mechanisms, tipping the balance either in favour of a tendency to bleed or to form clots.

Some people carry a genetic defect that prevents them from making sufficient amounts of one of the coagulation factors. In other cases, abnormally few platelets are produced, insufficient vitamin K (which is required to make certain coagulation factors) is absorbed from the diet, or excessive amounts of the enzymes that inhibit coagulation are produced. Any of these conditions may result in a tendency to bleed excessively (see *Bleeding disorders*).

On the other hand, sometimes the balance is tipped abnormally in favour of coagulation and clotting. Possible causes include an increase in the levels of coagulation factors (as can occur in late pregnancy or when using some oral contraceptives), a decrease in the level of enzymes that inhibit coagulation (as can occur in some forms of liver disease), or a sluggish blood flow through a particular area. The result may be thrombosis (abnormal clot formation).

B

Conditions in which there is a tendency for clot formation are often treated with *anticoagulant drugs* such as heparin or warfarin. Heparin exerts its anticoagulant effect by increasing the activity of antithrombin III, which neutralizes activated coagulation factors; warfarin works by disrupting the production of coagulation factors by inhibiting the action of vitamin K. Because of the delicate balance between the clotting and anticlotting mechanisms in blood, the use of anticoagulant drugs must be monitored frequently to prevent the development of severe bleeding.

Blood-clotting tests

Tests performed to screen for and diagnose *bleeding disorders*. These disorders usually result from deficiencies or abnormalities of platelets or of blood coagulation factors (see *Blood clotting*).

Bleeding disorders caused by low numbers of platelets are detected by a *blood count* in conjunction with a test of the bleeding time.

Bleeding time may be measured by nicking the skin of the ear or the forearm and timing the interval before bleeding stops. The normal range is three to eight minutes.

Reduced platelet activity results in a prolonged bleeding time.

Various tests are used to assess the activity of blood coagulation factors, the most frequently performed being prothrombin time and activated partial thromboplastin time (named after two coagulation factors). The time taken for the patient's blood to clot is measured after addition of calcium and other substances that promote the coagulation process; the results are compared with the time taken for normal blood to clot under the same conditions. Abnormal results may indicate deficiency of a specific coagulation factor, as occurs in *haemophilia*, or of many coagulation factors, as occurs in liver disease.

Anticoagulant drug therapy is designed to prolong the prothrombin time or the clotting time and to reduce the risk of *thrombosis* (abnormal clotting) in susceptible people. Anyone taking anticoagulant drugs should have regular clotting tests to ensure that the dosage is not excessive, which could cause bleeding.

Blood count

Also called full blood count, this test measures haemoglobin concentration, and the numbers of red blood cells, white blood cells, and platelets in 1 cu. mm of blood. The proportion of various white blood cells is measured and the size and shape of red and white cells is noted.

A blood count is the most commonly performed blood test. It is important for diagnosing *anaemia* or conditions in which the number of blood cells is abnormally high (such as white blood cells in *leukaemia*) or abnormally low (such as platelets in *thrombocytopenia*).

About 1 to 2 ml of blood is required for a blood count, which is usually performed by an automatic analyser.

Blood culture
See *Culture*.

Blood donation

The process of giving blood so that it can be used in *blood transfusion*. In most cases, whole blood is taken from the donor and broken down later into components for storage. Recently, a new method called apheresis has been introduced, which involves extracting only a specific blood component from the donor. Whole blood donation takes about 45 minutes, including the medical check, while apheresis takes about two and a half hours.

HOW BLOOD CLOTS

Clotting describes the solidification of blood anywhere in the body. Clotting occurs almost immediately at the site of a cut and helps limit blood loss by sealing damaged blood vessels. However, if abnormal clotting occurs in major blood vessels, heart attacks, strokes, and other disorders may occur. The clotting process has two main parts—platelet activation and the formation of fibrin filaments.

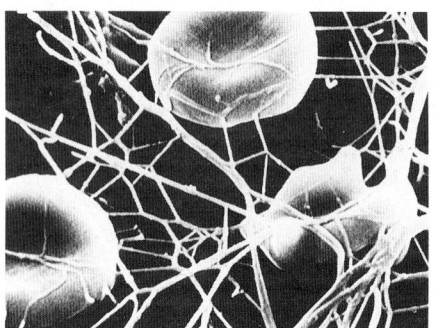

Red blood cells enmeshed in fibrin filaments
Fibrin is formed by a chemical change from a soluble protein, fibrinogen, which is present in the blood. The fibrin molecules aggregate to form long filaments, which enmesh blood cells (see left) to form a solid clot. The conversion of fibrinogen to fibrin is the last step of the "coagulation cascade", a series of reactions in the blood triggered by tissue injury and platelet activation.

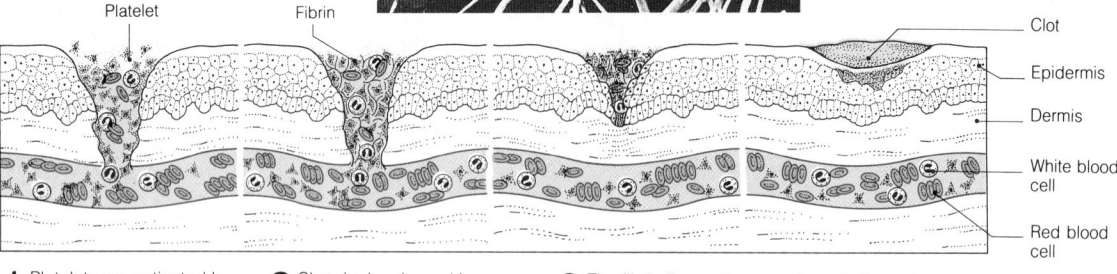

Platelet   Fibrin

Clot
Epidermis
Dermis
White blood cell
Red blood cell

1 Platelets are activated by coming into contact with damaged blood vessel walls, where they become sticky and then clump at the site of injury and adhere to the damaged blood-vessel wall.

2 Chemicals released by platelets and damaged tissues stimulate coagulation factors within the blood to form filaments of fibrin at the site of injury.

3 The fibrin filaments enmesh the platelets along with red and white blood cells.

4 Once the cut blood vessel is plugged by the mass of fibrin, platelets, and red and white blood cells, the fibrin filaments contract to form a solid clot.

DISORDERS OF THE BLOOD

Abnormalities can occur in any of the components of blood — the red blood cells (RBCs), white blood cells (WBCs), platelets, and numerous constituents of plasma.

Anaemia (a deficiency of the red cell pigment *haemoglobin* and a consequent reduction in the blood's oxygen-carrying capacity) is by far the most common blood disorder. It has many different possible causes. In *polycythaemia* there are too many red blood cells. In *leukaemia* excessive numbers of abnormal white blood cells crowd out the normal cells from the bone marrow.

Defects in the platelets and in the clotting mechanisms may lead to any of various *bleeding disorders*. Unwanted clot formation (*thrombosis*) may result from circumstances that overactivate the blood-clotting mechanisms.

Deficiencies of the proteins in blood plasma include hypo-albuminaemia (*albumin* deficiency) and agammaglobulinaemia (gamma-globulin deficiency). Known causes of blood disorders include the following.

GENETIC DISORDERS

In these disorders there is an inherited abnormality in the production of some component of blood. People with *sickle cell anaemia* and *thalassaemia* produce an abnormal type of haemoglobin that makes their red blood cells more fragile; those with *haemophilia* fail to produce enough of one of the factors involved in blood clotting. Disorders of this kind are present from birth and continue throughout life.

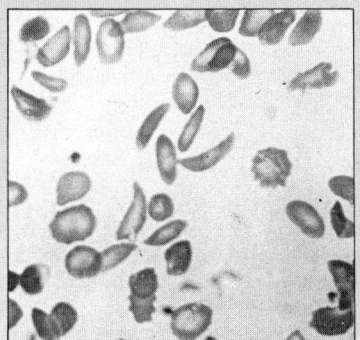

Sickle cell anaemia
In this genetic (inherited) disorder, the red blood cells are abnormally fragile and have a characteristic sickle shape.

NUTRITIONAL DISORDERS

Loss of regular amounts of blood over an extended period may mean that iron (required to make haemoglobin) is lost faster than it can be replaced in the diet (see *Anaemia, iron-deficiency*).

If insufficient amounts of the vitamins B_{12} or folic acid reach the bone marrow, it produces fewer red blood cells, which are abnormally large (see *Anaemia, megaloblastic*). The vitamin deficiency may be due to a poor diet or, more often in developed countries, to a failure to absorb vitamin B_{12} correctly from the intestinal tract.

INFECTION

Multiplication of bacteria in the blood is termed *septicaemia*.

Many other microorganisms (i.e. viruses, fungi, protozoa, and other parasites) may infect the blood at some stage in their life-cycle. Some organisms (notably those responsible for *malaria*) may actually attack and destroy red blood cells and so cause anaemia (see *Anaemia, haemolytic*).

TUMOURS

All types of leukaemia are the result of a type of cancer of the bone marrow, causing overgrowth of abnormal white blood cells and destruction of healthy marrow. In polycythaemia vera, a similar process occurs, except that mainly red cells are produced to excess. Another type of bone marrow cancer called *multiple myeloma* can cause an excess of certain proteins in the blood plasma.

POISONS

Carbon monoxide directly impairs the functioning of red blood cells by displacing oxygen bound to haemoglobin within the cells. Lead poisoning causes defective red blood cell production. Some snake and spider venoms destroy red cells and/or provoke clotting. Septicaemia describes the multiplication of bacteria in the blood; *toxaemia* describes the presence of metabolic poisons in the blood.

DRUGS

Certain drugs can cause blood abnormalities as a side-effect. For example, co-trimoxazole, thiazide diuretics, and carbimazole may depress the production of white blood cells and/or platelets; chloramphenicol and sulphonamides may depress all blood

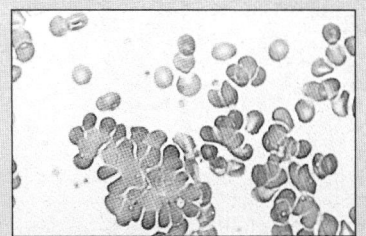

Cold agglutinin disorder
This is a rare blood disorder in which the body develops antibodies to its own red blood cells, causing them to clump together. This effect is especially marked in cold conditions when the clumps of cells reduce blood flow to the limbs.

cell production; methotrexate and phenytoin may interfere with red cell production.

Too high a dose of *anticoagulant drugs* can cause a bleeding tendency through excessive disruption of clotting mechanisms.

RADIATION

High doses of radiation (received at the time of therapy or from nuclear explosions or radioactive leaks from nuclear reactors) can severely damage the bone marrow, causing depression of all blood cell production (see *Anaemia, aplastic*).

OTHER DISORDERS

Albumin — an important protein in the blood plasma — may become deficient either as a result of liver disease (reduced production) or kidney disease (loss of albumin in the urine).

Liver disease may also cause *hyperbilirubinaemia* (excess bilirubin in the blood), anaemia, and deficiencies of some of the clotting factors. Kidney disease causes *uraemia* (excess urea in the blood), sometimes anaemia (possibly due to decreased production of the hormone erythropoietin), and also complex changes in blood chemistry.

INVESTIGATION
Blood disorders are investigated principally by various *blood tests*, such as the *blood count, blood smear,* and *blood-clotting tests,* and by *bone marrow biopsy.*

B

Any healthy adult can potentially be a blood donor. Volunteer donors are first interviewed about their medical history. Anyone who has had *anaemia, cancer,* types of *heart disease, malaria,* or *hepatitis,* or who has been exposed to *HIV* (the *AIDS* virus) may be disqualified. Pregnant women are also disqualified. A blood sample usually taken from a finger or earlobe, is then tested for anaemia; body temperature, pulse, and blood pressure are also checked.

Most regular donors of whole blood give blood twice a year, but those with rare *blood groups* may be asked to give more often. Donors may safely give plasma or platelets by apheresis as often as 15 times per year, provided a whole blood donation is not made between apheresis procedures.

HOW IT IS DONE

WHOLE BLOOD DONATION While the donor lies down and relaxes, a needle attached to a tube is inserted into the forearm. Up to 500 ml of blood (about one tenth of the total volume in the circulation) is slowly withdrawn into a plastic bag containing anticoagulant to prevent the blood from clotting. Most people feel no effects from giving blood. A few may feel faint or sick and should rest or lie down for a few minutes. All donors should avoid strenuous exercise for about five hours afterwards and should drink plenty of water and fruit juices.

The blood is taken to a transfusion centre, where it is tested for hepatitis B virus, syphilis, and antibodies to HIV. The blood will not be used for transfusion if any of these are present. After being classified into blood groups, the blood is stored in a blood bank, either whole or separated into its different components (see *Blood products*).

APHERESIS This technique allows only a blood component, such as plasma, platelets, or white cells, to be withdrawn from the circulation. For example, with one type of machine about 500 ml of the donor's blood is taken from one arm, circulated through a closed, sterile separator system, and then returned to the other arm minus the component being collected. This withdrawal and return is repeated six to eight times, and collects an amount of component that would normally require six to eight donors. Because only a single donor may be required to provide a patient with a sufficient quantity of a particular component, the risk of reaction or hepatitis transmission is reduced.

Blood film

A test that involves smearing a drop of blood on to a glass slide so that it can be examined under a microscope. The blood film is stained with special dyes to make the blood cells show up more clearly.

The shape and appearance of blood cells are inspected for any abnormality, such as sickle-shaped red blood cells in *sickle cell anaemia* or abnormal lymphocytes in infectious *mononucleosis*. The relative proportions of the different types of white blood cells can also be counted. This examination, called a differential white cell count, may be helpful in diagnosing infection or *leukaemia*. Blood films are also used in diagnosing infections, such as *malaria*, in which the parasites can be seen inside the red blood cells.

Blood films are usually done together with a full *blood count*.

Blood gases

A test for determining the acidity-alkalinity (pH) and the concentrations of oxygen, carbon dioxide, and bicarbonate in the blood.

Blood oxygen and carbon dioxide values are useful in diagnosing and monitoring *respiratory failure*. Bicarbonate and acidity reflect the *acid-base balance* of the body. This may be disturbed in conditions such as diabetic ketoacidosis, aspirin poisoning, hyperventilation (overbreathing), or repeated vomiting.

Modern apparatus can quickly measure blood gases using a few drops of blood. Blood for analysis is usually taken from an artery rather than from a vein and possibly from the interior of the heart.

Blood groups

Systems of classifying blood according to the different marker proteins on the surface of red blood cells. These marker proteins—called *antigens*—affect the ability of the red blood cells to provoke an *immune response*. Blood group typing is essential for safe *blood transfusion*.

TYPES

ABO GROUPS Attempts in the 19th century and earlier at transfusing blood from one living person to another were sometimes successful but sometimes caused serious illness and even death. In 1900 the German pathologist Karl Landsteiner began mixing blood taken from different people and found that some mixtures were compatible while others were not. He discovered two types of anti-

gens on the surface of the red blood cells—these he called A and B. According to whether a person's blood contains one or other antigen, both, or neither, it is classified as type A, B, AB, or O. Landsteiner found that the fluid part of some people's blood contained *antibodies*—anti-A and/or anti-B—that reacted with the antigens. People with the A antigen (blood group A) have anti-B antibodies; people with the B antigen (blood group B) have anti-A antibodies; those with both the A and B antigens (blood group AB) have no anti-A or anti-B antibodies; people with no A or B antigens (blood group O) have both anti-A and anti-B antibodies. A person cannot safely be transfused with blood of a group containing antigens to which he or she has antibodies (see table on next page).

In the UK, the most common of the ABO blood groups is A, followed by O, then B, and finally AB. The precise frequency of each group differs between races.

RHESUS FACTORS Another blood-group system, the Rhesus system (Rh factors), was discovered in 1940 by Landsteiner during experiments on Rhesus monkeys. This system involves several antigens, the most important of which is factor D. This factor is found in the blood of 85 per cent of people, who are called Rh positive, while 15 per cent lack the factor and are Rh negative. Individuals are therefore classed as, for example, "O positive" or "AB negative" on the basis of their ABO and Rh blood groups.

The importance of this group relates mainly to pregnancy in Rh-negative women since, if the baby is Rh positive, the mother may form antibodies against the baby's blood (see *Rhesus incompatibility*). An Rh-negative mother is therefore given antibodies directed against factor D after delivery to prevent her developing anti-D antibodies, which might cause *haemolytic disease of the newborn* in subsequent Rh-positive infants.

Transfusion of Rh-positive blood into an Rh-negative patient can cause a serious reaction if the patient has had earlier blood transfusions containing the Rh antigen.

OTHER GROUPS

Since the discovery of the ABO and Rh factors, about 400 other antigens have been identified, but these rarely cause transfusion problems.

USES

TRANSFUSION AND CROSS-MATCHING The ABO and Rh groups are used to categorize blood stored in blood banks. When a blood transfusion is given, the recipient's blood group is determined and blood of the same group is located in the bank. Each unit (about 500 ml) of blood to be given is first tested against a small sample of the patient's blood to exclude the small possibility that the two might be incompatible because of a reaction due to one of the other blood groups. This test is known as cross-matching and takes a short time to perform. In an emergency, the circulation can usually be maintained by transfusion of plasma solutions until blood has been matched. Once commonplace, it is now exceptional for unmatched blood of the appropriate group to be given.

INHERITED DISORDERS Some blood groups are associated with particular disorders. For example, blood group A is more common in people suffering from cancer of the stomach, while blood group O is more common in those with peptic ulcer.

PATERNITY CASES An individual's blood group is determined by the genes inherited from his or her parents. Identification of blood group can be used in a paternity case to establish that a man could not have been the father of a particular child. It cannot be shown positively that a man is the father by blood grouping, but, with genetic analysis, paternity can now be proved with virtual certainty (see *Paternity testing*).

CRIMINAL INVESTIGATION Blood found at the scene of a crime can be grouped according to the various red blood cell antigens present. New techniques of genetic analysis allow identification of the blood of a suspect with virtual certainty (see *Genetic fingerprinting*).

ANTHROPOLOGY The ABO blood groups are found in all people, but the frequency of each group varies with race and geographical distribution. Study of blood groups can therefore aid anthropologists in investigating, for

CHANGES IN BLOOD PRESSURE

Raised or lowered blood pressure can be caused by various factors. During pregnancy it tends to rise but then returns gradually to its previous level after birth. Certain drugs also affect blood pressure as a side-effect. During the day (below) a normal person's blood pressure fluctuates according to activity. Hypertension (abnormally high blood pressure) is treated with weight loss, sodium restriction, drugs, and modification of lifestyle.

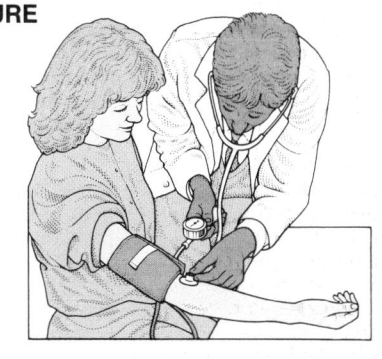

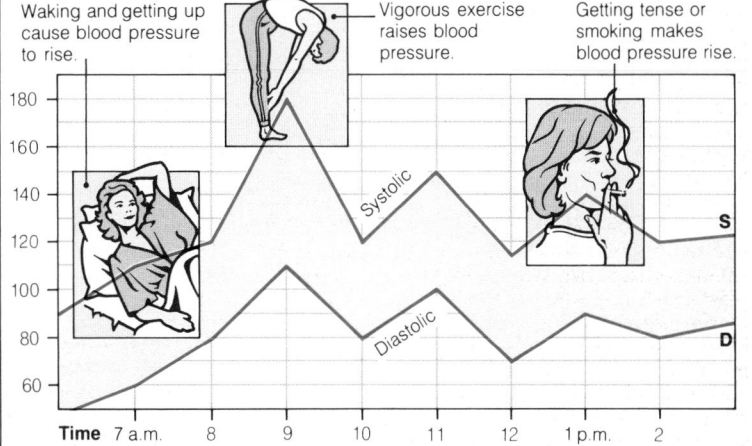

Waking and getting up cause blood pressure to rise.

Vigorous exercise raises blood pressure.

Getting tense or smoking makes blood pressure rise.

Systolic

Diastolic

S

D

Time 7 a.m. 8 9 10 11 12 1 p.m. 2

example, the origins and migrations of various populations.

Blood level

The concentration of a given substance in the blood plasma or serum. Sodium, potassium, and glucose levels are commonly measured in routine *blood tests*. The police may order the measuring of blood alcohol levels in connection with traffic offences. For this purpose, the legal limit in the UK is 80 mg of alcohol per 100 ml of blood.

Blood loss

See *Bleeding, treatment of*.

Blood poisoning

A common name for *septicaemia* with *toxaemia*, an often life-threatening illness caused by multiplication of bacteria and their formation of toxins in the bloodstream. Septicaemia may be a complication of infection (e.g. an infected wound or burn). It was once a feared and fatal complication of childbirth (see *Puerperal fever*). In some infective conditions, *septic shock* may be caused by toxins released by bacteria. The mort-

ality rate of septicaemia, once high, has been greatly reduced by treatment with *antibiotic drugs* and intensive therapy for shock. (See also *Bacteraemia*.)

Blood pressure

The pressure exerted by the flow of blood through the main arteries. Blood pressure rises and falls as the heart responds to the varying demands made by the body during different activities, such as exercise, stress, and sleep. Two types of pressure are measured. Systolic, the highest, is the pressure created by the contraction of the heart muscle and the elastic recoil of the aorta (the main artery leaving the heart) as blood surges through it. Diastolic pressure (the lowest) is recorded during relaxation of the ventricles between beats; it reflects the resistance of all the small arteries in the body and the load against which the heart must work. The pressure wave transmitted along the arteries with each heartbeat is easily felt as the *pulse*.

MEASURING BLOOD PRESSURE

Blood pressure is measured using a *sphygmomanometer*. This instrument

BLOOD GROUP COMPATIBILITY

		Donor blood group			
		A	B	AB	O
Recipient blood group	A	▲	●	●	▲
	B	●	▲	●	▲
	AB	▲	▲	▲	▲
	O	●	●	●	▲
Key	▲ Compatible		● Incompatible		

B

consists of a cuff with an air bladder connected to a tube and bulb (for pumping air into the bladder), and a gauge for indicating the air pressure being exerted. The soft rubber cuff of the sphygmomanometer is inflated around the upper arm until it is tight enough to stop the flow of blood in the main artery in the arm. The cuff is then gradually deflated until, by listening to the artery through a *stethoscope*, the blood can first be heard as a beat forcing its way along the artery. This is recorded as the systolic pressure. The cuff is then deflated further until the beat disappears and the blood flows steadily through the now open artery—giving the diastolic pressure.

In special circumstances, blood pressure may also be measured by miniature devices attached to an artery or by a continuous recording for 24 hours or more while a person leads his or her daily life.

Blood pressure is recorded by giving the systolic pressure and diastolic pressure, expressed as millimetres of mercury (mm Hg). This unit was adopted because the earliest equipment used a glass column filled with mercury to measure the pressure directly. Today, some sphygmomanometers use a spring gauge with a round dial. A healthy young adult has a blood pressure reading of about 110/75 (i.e. 110 mm Hg systolic and 75 mm Hg diastolic). This often rises normally with age, to about 130/90 at age 60. Abnormally high blood pressure is known medically as *hypertension*; abnormally low pressure is termed *hypotension*.

Blood products

After *blood donation*, blood is stored either whole or separated into its various components. Each product has a particular use in *blood transfusion*.

WHOLE BLOOD

This is used to restore blood volume after sudden severe bleeding—for instance, after a traffic accident or during major surgery. Whole blood keeps for only three to four weeks after donation.

PACKED RED CELLS

These are prepared by removing part of the liquid plasma. Concentrated red cells are used to treat patients with some forms of chronic *anaemia* that have not responded to drug treatment. The red cells provide the necessary haemoglobin without overloading the recipient with fluid, which can result in, or aggravate, *heart*

failure. Concentrated red cells can also be used to treat babies with *haemolytic disease of the newborn*.

WASHED RED CELLS

This is blood that has had the white blood cells and/or plasma proteins removed, thus reducing the chances of an allergic reaction occurring in patients, such as those with chronic anaemia, who require transfusions over a long period.

FROZEN RED CELLS

Red cells can be preserved for long periods if stored at very low temperatures. This technique is used to preserve red cells belonging to rare blood groups.

PLATELETS

Platelets play an important part in normal blood clotting. Their low level in some blood disorders causes patients to bruise easily and to suffer from internal bleeding. Patients with such disorders may benefit from transfusions of platelets that have been extracted from whole blood and then concentrated. If necessary, platelets from several donors can be given during one transfusion.

WHITE BLOOD CELLS

Granulocytes, a type of white blood cell, can be separated from normal blood, or from the blood of patients with chronic myeloid (granulocytic) *leukaemia*, who have an excess of these cells. Patients with life-threatening infections accompanied by low levels of granulocytes may be treated with granulocytes if they are not responding to antibiotic drugs.

FROZEN FRESH PLASMA

This is prepared by separating and freezing plasma as soon as possible after blood collection. Rich in clotting factors, fresh plasma is used to correct many types of bleeding disorder.

PLASMA PROTEIN SOLUTIONS

The liquid part of any whole blood not used within three weeks of collection can be converted into a concentrated solution of albumin (the main protein in plasma). The solution can be stored for long periods. Its chief use is in treating *shock*, resulting from severe blood loss, until whole blood compatible with the patient's blood group becomes available. Purified albumin preparations are used to treat *nephrotic syndrome* (a kidney disorder causing albumin loss in the urine) and chronic liver disease (in which production of albumin is deficient).

CLOTTING FACTORS

Concentrates of clotting factors VIII and IX can be prepared for the treatment of *haemophilia* and *Christmas dis-*

ease. Because blood from many donors is required to produce one small batch of clotting factor, it must be heat-treated to reduce the risk of *hepatitis* or *AIDS* virus transmission.

IMMUNOGLOBULINS

Immunoglobulins (also called antibodies) occur in the blood of healthy individuals who have recovered from the common viral diseases. These nonspecific immunoglobulins can be taken from the blood plasma, concentrated, and given by injection (see *Immunoglobin injection*) to protect, by passive *immunization*, people who are unable to produce their own antibodies or who are likely to be exposed to *hepatitis A*. Nonspecific immunoglobulins can also be given intravenously in large doses to treat certain *autoimmune disorders*, such as thrombocytopenic *purpura*.

Specific antibodies (taken from patients who have recovered from a particular infection or who have been specifically immunized against one) are given as passive immunization to protect especially susceptible patients from specific infections. For example, varicella-zoster virus antibodies are given to children with leukaemia who are exposed to chickenpox, and pseudomonas antibodies are given to patients suffering from burns.

Anti-D immunoglobulin, a type of specific antibody, is obtained from the blood of patients sensitized to the Rh blood group factor. If anti-D immunoglobulin is given to an Rh-negative mother within 60 hours of her giving birth to an Rh-positive baby, it will prevent *haemolytic disease of the newborn* in any other babies she might have.

Blood smear

See *Blood film*.

Blood tests

Analysis of a sample of blood to give information on its cells and proteins and any of the chemicals, antigens, antibodies, and gases that it carries. Since blood is the main transport system of the body, such tests can be used to check on the health of major organs, as well as on respiratory function, hormonal balance, the immune system, and metabolism.

TYPES

HAEMATOLOGICAL TESTS These involve looking at the components of the blood itself, including examination of the numbers, shape, size, and appearance of blood cells, and testing the function of clotting factors. The most important haematological tests are *blood count*, *blood film*, *blood clotting tests*, and *blood group* tests.

BIOCHEMICAL TESTS These measure chemicals in the blood, such as glucose, sodium, potassium, uric acid, urea, enzymes, gases, digested foods, and drugs. (See *Acid-base balance*; *Kidney-function tests*; *Liver-function tests*.)

MICROBIOLOGICAL TESTS These look for microorganisms in the blood, such as bacteria, viruses, fungi, and parasites, and the antibodies formed against them. (See *Culture*; *Immunoassay*.)

HOW THEY ARE DONE
The most convenient site for taking a blood sample is a vein at the bend in the elbow. A tourniquet is applied to the upper arm, and the blood is withdrawn through a needle into a syringe. The procedure causes only mild discomfort. Up to 20 ml of blood may be required, but, as the circulation contains 4 to 5 litres, loss of this small proportion has no harmful effect. If only a few drops are needed, they may be obtained by pricking a finger. Rarely, tests may require a sample of arterial blood, which is taken from the elbow, wrist, or groin; this is a more difficult procedure and causes some discomfort.

The sample may be allowed to clot, leaving its clear serum for examination, or an anticoagulant may be added to allow study of the cells and clotting factors. The sample is then sent to the laboratory, where one or more of the hundreds of available tests are carried out. In some laboratories, modern computerized analysers are used to perform many different tests simultaneously on one small sample of blood. The printed results compare each value with the accepted normal range for that test. Each laboratory produces its own normal ranges that depend on the method and the ingredients of the test, and sometimes on the age and sex of the patient. Some tests may be performed at the bedside or in a doctor's consulting room. Some, such as blood glucose, may be performed by patients on themselves.

Blood transfusion
The infusion of large volumes of blood or blood components directly into the bloodstream, performed mainly to remedy severe blood loss or to correct chronic anaemia.

Before the discovery of the major *blood groups* earlier this century, blood transfusion was a hazardous undertaking, often causing severe reactions

and even death. Growing knowledge of the complex properties of blood and its components has now made transfusion a safe procedure, although still not without possible complications.

WHY IT IS DONE
Blood transfusion may be needed by a patient who has bled severely after an accident or who has lost a lot of blood during an operation. It may also be required after internal bleeding—for example, from a bleeding *peptic ulcer*. Chronic *anaemia* that does not respond to medication may require treatment by blood transfusion (for example, in conditions such as *thalassaemia* and *leukaemia*).

In an exchange transfusion, nearly all of the recipient's blood is replaced by donor blood. It is most often needed in *haemolytic disease of the newborn*, when abnormally high levels of bilirubin in the blood might cause brain damage.

HOW IT IS DONE
Before a transfusion is performed, blood must be cross-matched to ensure compatibility. This procedure involves taking a sample of the recipient's blood, identifying the blood groups, and matching it with suitable donor blood. This is done by mixing some of each blood sample and examining it to make sure there are no *antibodies* in the recipient's plasma that would damage the donor blood cells. Blood can usually be cross-matched in one hour or less. If the patient is losing blood very rapidly, it may not be possible to wait. In this case, O Rh-negative (universal donor) blood that has not been cross-matched, plasma protein solution, or a plasma substitute may be given until tested blood becomes available.

The donor blood is transfused into an arm vein. Usually, each unit (about 500 ml) of blood is given over one to four hours; in an emergency 500 ml may be given in a couple of minutes. The amount of blood required depends on how much has been lost or on the severity of anaemia. During transfusion, the patient's pulse, blood pressure, and temperature are measured regularly, and, if there is any sign of an adverse reaction, the transfusion is stopped.

COMPLICATIONS
If blood has not been cross-matched reliably, antibodies in the recipient's blood may cause incompatible donor cells to haemolyse (burst). The most severe reactions can result in *shock* or *kidney failure*. Less severe reactions can produce fever, chills, a rash, or

delayed anaemia. Transfusion reactions can also occur as a result of allergy to transfused white cells, plasma proteins, or platelets.

Infections, such as with *HIV* (the *AIDS* virus), hepatitis B and C (see *Hepatitis, viral*), *syphilis*, and *malaria*, can occur if donor blood has not been adequately screened. All blood for transfusion is now carefully tested and the risk of infection is extremely small.

In elderly or severely anaemic patients, transfusion can overload the circulation, leading to heart failure. *Diuretic drugs*, which cause fluid loss, may need to be given simultaneously to avoid this. In patients with chronic anaemia who require regular transfusion over many years, excess iron may accumulate (a condition called haemosiderosis) and cause damage to various organs, such as the heart, liver, and pancreas. Dangerous build-up of iron can be relieved by giving the drug desferrioxamine.

Blood transfusion, autologous
The use of a person's own blood, donated on an earlier occasion, for *blood transfusion* during or after surgery. Autologous transfusion is used to avoid the risk that blood from another donor might be infected.

Autologous transfusions were first performed on a large scale in the early 1960s for certain major operations, and services continued to develop to some extent during the 1970s. Fear of AIDS during the 1980s created a demand for much greater availability and use of this technique.

WHY IT IS DONE
Autologous transfusion eliminates the slight but serious risk of transmitting *HIV* (the *AIDS* virus) or the hepatitis B and C viruses (see *Hepatitis, viral*) from contaminated blood. It also eliminates the less significant risk of transmitting *cytomegalovirus*, *malaria*, and *syphilis*.

Another advantage of autologous transfusion is that there is no risk of a transfusion reaction occurring as a result of incompatibility between donor and recipient blood.

Autologous transfusion has been used illegally by people associated with professional sports. Carried out just before a sporting event, "blood doping" increases the oxygen-carrying capacity of the circulation and thus improves stamina.

HOW IT IS DONE
Blood can be withdrawn (in the same way as for *blood donation*) in several sessions at least four days apart and

up to three days before surgery is planned. A total of up to about 3.5 litres of blood can be removed and stored. Blood may also be salvaged during an operation, filtered and processed, and returned to the circulation, thereby reducing the need for transfusion of donated blood.

Blood vessels

A general term for arteries, veins, and capillaries. (See *Circulatory system*.)

Blue baby

An infant with a cyanotic (bluish) complexion, especially of the lips and tongue, caused by a relative lack of oxygen in the blood. This is usually due to a structural defect of the heart or the major arteries leaving the heart. The defect allows some of the deoxygenated blood returning to the right side of the heart to be pumped straight back into the circulation instead of first going to the lungs to receive oxygen, or results in too little blood passing into the lungs because of a blocked or narrowed pulmonary artery. Such defects may need to be corrected surgically. (See *Heart disease, congenital*.)

Blue bloater

A term used by doctors to describe the appearance of some patients with lung disease (see *Lung disease, chronic obstructive*).

Blurred vision

A common term used to indicate indistinct, fuzzy, or misty visual images. Blurred vision should not be confused with *double vision* (diplopia). Blurred vision can occur in one or both eyes, for episodes of varying lengths of time, and can develop gradually or suddenly. Sometimes only part of the field of vision is affected. Any change in vision should be brought to the attention of your doctor.

CAUSES
Blurred vision is most commonly due to refractive errors—*myopia* (short-sightedness), *hypermetropia* (long-sightedness), and *astigmatism* (unequal curvature of the front of the eye). These defects can easily be rectified by glasses or contact lenses.

Many people notice gradual changes in near vision from the age of 40 onwards—their vision for close work becomes progressively less sharp, causing problems with small print and the need for reading glasses or bifocals for close-up reading to correct the blur. This is due to *presbyopia* (decreased ability to focus near

objects). If a person has been short-sighted, he or she may simply need to take off the glasses to see close objects after the age of 40.

Vision may be impaired, or blindness caused, by damage, disease, or abnormalities affecting the tear film, cornea, iris, lens, aqueous humour, vitreous humour, retina, or the nerve pathways behind the eye. These nerve pathways may be damaged by a tumour, *head injury*, or *stroke*.

Blushing

Brief reddening of the face and sometimes the neck caused by widening of the blood vessels close to the skin's surface. Blushing is usually an involuntary reaction to embarrassment. In some women, blushing is a feature of the *hot flushes* that occur during the *menopause*. Flushing of the face occurs in association with *carcinoid syndrome*.

Body contour surgery

Operations performed to remove excess fat, skin, or both, from various parts of the body, especially the abdomen, thighs, and buttocks. Diet and exercise are the proper means of reducing the fat content of the body, and surgery is not a substitute. Operations may improve appearance where accumulations of fat or excess skin persist in certain areas after successful weight control.

TYPES
ABDOMINAL WALL REDUCTION In this reshaping operation, often called abdominoplasty, excess skin and fat are removed from the abdomen. The operation may benefit people who retain an excess of skin following weight loss or pregnancy.

Abdominal wall reduction is carried out under general anaesthesia and requires a hospital stay of from two to three days. The surgeon makes a horizontal "bikini" incision in the skin as low down on the abdomen as possible, then cuts upwards between the fat and muscle layers. The flap of skin and fat is pulled down and the excess is removed. Sometimes, when the amount to be removed is particularly large, a vertical incision is required in addition to the horizontal one. In many cases, the umbilicus (navel) must be moved to a higher position because it has been pulled down with the flap. At the end of the operation, the skin is stitched together. Drains are inserted into the wound and left in place for several days to prevent the risk of blood or serum collecting, which can lead to infection.

To minimize the size of the scar or scars, the patient should avoid tension on the wound and walk with the trunk slightly flexed for several weeks. Despite taking care, the final scar is often not as narrow as the patient and surgeon would like.

REDUCTION OF THIGHS AND BUTTOCKS For thigh reduction, excess fat and skin are removed through an incision along the "stocking-seam line". For buttock reduction, the scar is planned to lie in the crease line separating the thighs and buttocks. In both cases, the scars are often wide and unattractive, and the reduction seldom satisfies the patient. There is also a risk of complications. The skin surrounding the wound often dies, leading to infection and delayed healing, which may necessitate skin grafting.

SUCTION LIPECTOMY To overcome the problem of noticeable scars, instruments have been developed to remove fat through "key-hole" incisions. A suction instrument is inserted through a small skin incision and moved back and forth under the skin to break up large areas of fat, which can then be sucked out through the instrument. However, because of the plentiful blood supply within the fat, there may be significant blood and fluid loss, which must be treated by the surgeon to prevent shock or anaemia. In addition, the total amount of fat that can be removed at one time is limited. Suction lipectomy is useful in improving the appearance of people who have localized areas of excess fat, but cannot be used as a substitute for weight control. Minor irregularities and dimpling of the skin commonly occur after surgery.

Body odour

The smell caused by sweat on the skin surface. Sweat itself has no odour, but, if it remains on the skin for a few hours, bacterial decomposition may lead to body odour. The sweat may also smell strongly after garlic, curry, or other spicy foods have been eaten. Bacterial decomposition of sweat occurs most noticeably in the armpits and around the genital area, because the *apocrine glands* in these areas contain proteins and fatty materials favourable to the growth of bacteria. Sweat from other areas of the body is mainly salt water, which does not encourage bacteria to grow. Feet are an exception because they are under warm, airless conditions for many hours—the perfect environment for bacteria and fungi to flourish.

If body odour is a problem, the most effective treatment is to wash all over at least once daily. After washing, the use of a deodorant containing an antiperspirant will prevent sweat from reaching the surface of the skin.

Boil

An inflamed, pus-filled area of skin, usually an infected hair follicle (the tiny pit from which a hair grows). Common sites include the back of the neck and moist areas such as the armpits and groin. A more severe and extensive form of a boil is a *carbuncle*.

The usual cause of boils is infection with the bacterium STAPHYLOCOCCUS AUREUS. Some people carry this organism in their noses or other sites, but often the source of an infection cannot be traced.

SYMPTOMS
A boil starts as a red, painful lump. As it swells it fills with pus and becomes rounded, with a yellowish tip (head). Recurrent boils may occur in people with known or unrecognized *diabetes mellitus* or other conditions in which general body resistance to bacterial infection is impaired.

TREATMENT
Do not burst a boil, as this may spread the infection. A hot compress applied every two hours will relieve discomfort and hasten possible drainage and healing. Showering, instead of bathing, reduces the chance of spreading the infection.

If the boil is large and painful, consult your doctor. He or she may prescribe an antibiotic, or may open the boil with a sterile needle to allow the pus to drain. Large boils occasionally need to be lanced with a surgical knife, usually using local anaesthesia.

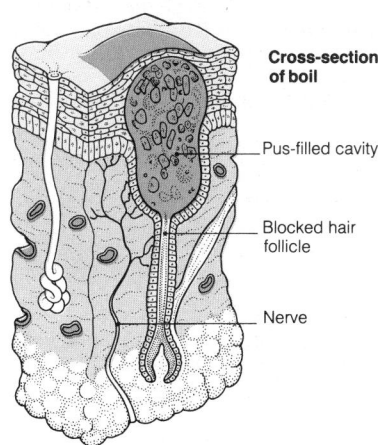

Cross-section of boil

Pus-filled cavity

Blocked hair follicle

Nerve

Bolus

A soft mass of chewed food that is produced by the action of the tongue, teeth, and saliva. In this form, food is easily swallowed and passed through the oesophagus.

The term bolus is also used to describe a drug dose that is rapidly injected into a vein.

Bonding

The process by which a strong psychological and emotional tie is established between a parent and newborn child. Bonding is essential for a baby's healthy emotional development.

Ideas about bonding were developed from studies of geese, monkeys, and other animals. Goslings were observed attaching themselves to and following the first moving object they saw after birth. Monkeys deprived of their mothers failed to develop normal parental instincts. However, most monkeys in the experiment developed normally when they were given an inanimate mother substitute, especially a furry one that could be held and cuddled.

Bonding is a reciprocal process in which baby and parent respond to each other's gestures and expressions. A failure to bond may occur if a baby is ill or premature and has to be separated from his or her parents (by being placed in an incubator directly after birth), but such babies usually bond normally if given special attention at a later stage. Bonding problems may occur if a new parent's own early family experiences failed to provide a good model of parent-infant interaction. However, such people can be taught successful ways to interact with their newborns.

Lack of bonding may increase the risk of neglect or *child abuse* and may lead to delayed emotional development, depression, and inability to develop satisfactory relationships in adulthood.

Most studies indicate that working mothers may bond as successfully as nonworking mothers and that children can fare well with more than one primary care-giver (of either sex) as long as all care-givers are loving and consistent.

Bonding, dental

Dental techniques that use plastic resins and veneers made of acrylic or porcelain to repair, restore, or improve the appearance of damaged or defective *teeth*. Dental bonding is sometimes used as an alternative to

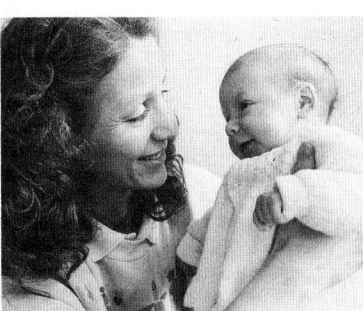

The bonding process
By maintaining eye-to-eye and frequent physical contact, bonding gradually becomes established.

crowning (see *Crown, dental*), and may also be used as a preventive technique to protect the teeth.

WHY IT IS DONE
Bonding techniques are sometimes suitable for treating teeth that are badly stained, chipped, broken, or malformed. Bonding may also be used to fill the gaps between teeth that are too widely spaced, or to rebuild decayed back teeth. In some cases, bonding is performed before the attachment of (*orthodontic appliances*). Bonding can be used as a protective measure when the roots of the teeth are exposed or when teeth are particularly sensitive to changes in temperature. Plastic sealants are sometimes applied as a preventive measure, to prevent the build-up of bacteria in the deep grooves of the back teeth.

HOW IT IS DONE
There is usually no need for anaesthesia during bonding procedures.

The dentist begins by applying a weak acid solution to the tooth—a technique sometimes known as acid-etching. This roughens the surface of the tooth so that it will hold the resin, which is applied to the tooth in liquid form.

If a portion of a tooth needs rebuilding, or is missing completely, the resin can be shaped on the tooth. The resin is then hardened either chemically or by the application of a special light. The bonded surface is then smoothed and polished.

If bonding is carried out on badly stained or highly visible teeth, a porcelain or acrylic veneer may be applied over the resin.

RESULTS
Bonding can improve both the structure and the appearance of teeth. Typically, however, the procedure must be repeated after about five years.

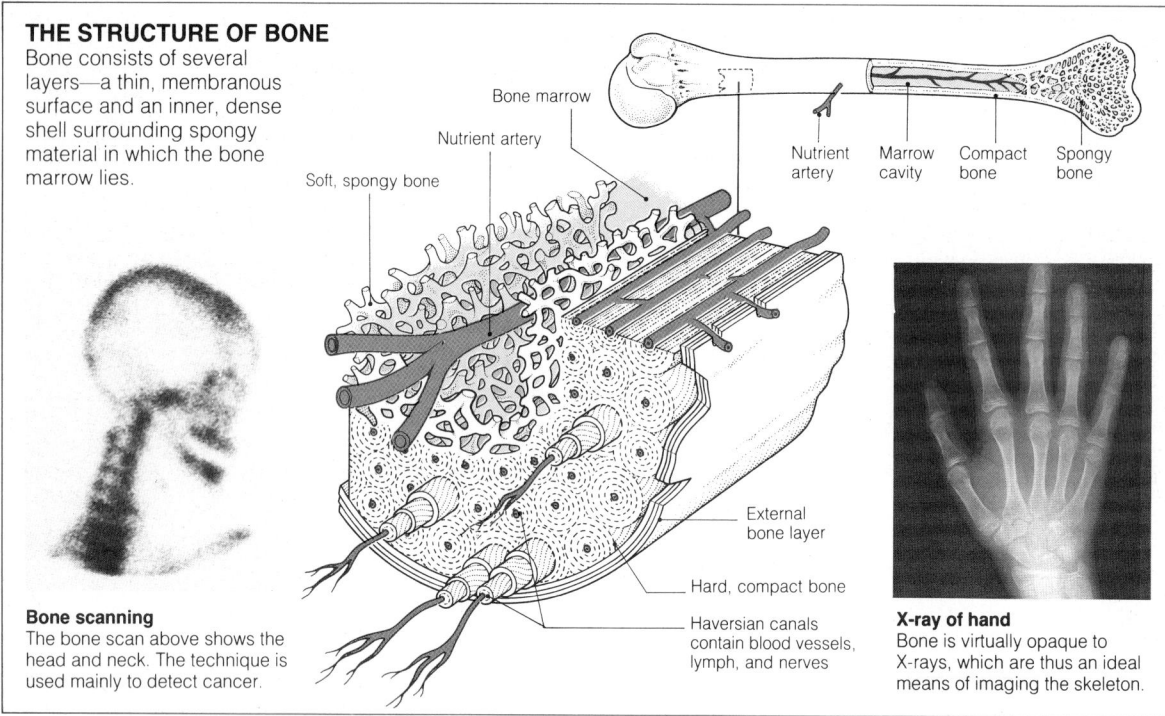

THE STRUCTURE OF BONE

Bone consists of several layers—a thin, membranous surface and an inner, dense shell surrounding spongy material in which the bone marrow lies.

Bone marrow

Nutrient artery

Soft, spongy bone

Nutrient artery

Marrow cavity

Compact bone

Spongy bone

External bone layer

Hard, compact bone

Haversian canals contain blood vessels, lymph, and nerves

Bone scanning
The bone scan above shows the head and neck. The technique is used mainly to detect cancer.

X-ray of hand
Bone is virtually opaque to X-rays, which are thus an ideal means of imaging the skeleton.

Bonding materials are weaker than natural tooth enamel and thus chip more easily. Bonded teeth may also become stained by certain types of food and drink. Because bonding materials are less hard-wearing than the materials used for dental crowns, crowning may sometimes be a more suitable technique for the repair of badly damaged back teeth.

Bone

The structural material of the *skeleton*. Bone contains calcium and phosphorus, which make it hard and rigid; the arrangement of fibres in bone makes it resilient and strong.

STRUCTURE

The surface of bone is covered with periosteum, a thin membrane that contains a network of blood vessels and nerves. Beneath the periosteum is a hard, dense shell that is known as compact, ivory, or cortical bone. Inside this shell the bone has a mesh-like structure and is known as spongy, cancellous, or trabecular bone. The central cavity found in some bones and the spaces in spongy bone contain a fatty tissue, *bone marrow*, in which the red cells, platelets, and most white blood cells are formed.

The hard structural bone underneath the periosteum is formed of columns of bone cells; each column

has a central hollow called a haversian canal. These canals are important for the nutrition, growth, and repair of the bone. The direction of the canals corresponds with the mechanical forces acting on the bone. Bone is insensitive; any sensation comes from the nerves in the periosteum.

FUNCTIONS

The bones of the skeleton provide a rigid framework for the muscles; parts of the skeleton protect the body's organs (the heart and lungs in the bony thoracic cavity, the brain in the skull, and the uterus and bladder in the bony pelvis). Bones, together with the joints and muscles, form the locomotor system.

GROWTH

The growth of bone is a balance between the activity of its two constituent cells, osteoblasts and osteoclasts. Osteoblasts encourage deposition of the mineral calcium phosphate on the protein framework of the bone. Osteoclasts remove mineral from the bone. The actions of these cells are controlled by hormones: growth hormone secreted by the pituitary gland, the sex hormones oestrogen and testosterone, the adrenal hormones, parathyroid hormone, and the thyroid hormone thyrocalcitonin. These hormones also maintain the calcium level in the blood within

close limits; any fall below the normal range affects the nerves and muscles.

Most bones begin to develop in the embryo during the fifth or sixth week of pregnancy, when they take the form of cartilage. This cartilage begins to be replaced by hard bone, in a process known as *ossification*, at around the seventh or eighth week of pregnancy; the process is not complete until early adult life. At birth many bones consist mainly of cartilage, which will ossify later. The *epiphyses* (the growing ends of the long bones) are separated from the bone shaft by the epiphyseal plate. Some bones, such as some skull bones, do not develop from cartilage and are known as membranous bones.

Bone abscess

A localized collection of pus in a bone (see *Osteomyelitis*).

Bone cancer

Malignant growth in bone. Bone cancer may originate in the bone itself (primary bone cancer); more commonly, it occurs as a result of cancer spreading from elsewhere in the body (secondary bone cancer). The cancerous growth replaces bone, causing pain and sometimes swelling. It also makes the bone more likely to fracture without preceding injury. Bone cancer that affects the spine may cause collapse or crushing of vertebrae (spinal bones), damaging the spinal cord, and thus causing weakness or paralysis of one or more limbs.

PRIMARY BONE CANCER

All forms of primary bone cancer are rare. The type that occurs most often is *osteosarcoma*, which most frequently affects the leg bones of children and young adults. Symptoms of osteosarcoma are pain, tenderness, and swelling, typically just above or just below the knee. X-rays, bone scans (see *Bone imaging*), and *biopsy* may be used to confirm the diagnosis.

Other types of primary bone cancer include *chondrosarcoma* (originating from cartilage) and *fibrosarcoma* (from fibrous tissue). Bone cancer can also start in the bone marrow (see *Ewing's sarcoma; Multiple myeloma*).

The treatment of osteosarcoma, chondrosarcoma, and fibrosarcoma depends on the extent to which the disease has spread. If it remains confined to bone, amputation may be recommended. Alternatively, radiotherapy or chemotherapy, or both, may be used to control the tumour. With modern *anticancer drugs*, the outlook has improved.

SECONDARY BONE CANCER

Secondary, or metastatic, bone cancer, is more common than primary bone cancer; it usually occurs later in life. The cancers that spread readily to bone are those of the breast, lung, prostate, thyroid, and kidney. Bone metastases occur commonly in the spine, pelvis, ribs, and skull.

In secondary bone cancer, pain is usually the main symptom and is often worse at night. Affected bones are abnormally fragile and may fracture, even without preceding injury. Such a fracture (a pathological fracture) may be the first indication that a person has cancer.

Imaging studies will confirm the presence of secondary bone cancer. If the original site of the cancer is not obvious, further tests may be needed to identify it.

Secondary bone cancers from the breast and prostate often respond to hormone therapy. Growth of prostate tumours may be inhibited with oestrogen or hypothalamic hormones and in some breast tumours by *hormone antagonists*. Sometimes the most effective treatment is removal of the ovaries, testes, or adrenal glands. Fractures may require orthopaedic surgery, including the use of pins and plates inserted in the bone.

DISORDERS OF THE BONE

Bone is affected by the same types of disorders as other body tissues, but its hard, rigid structure makes for extra complications. If a bone receives a direct blow or suffers from repeated stress it may *fracture*. If it becomes infected (for instance, due to *osteomyelitis* or a *bone abscess*), the resulting inflammation may interfere with the blood supply, leading to death of part of the bone.

GENETIC DISORDERS

Several genetic (inherited) conditions may affect bone growth; these include *achondroplasia* and *osteogenesis imperfecta*. Such disorders often result in *short stature*.

NUTRITIONAL DISORDERS

Lack of calcium and vitamin D in the diet may result in *rickets* in children and *osteomalacia* in adults; in both conditions the bones become soft and lose their shape.

HORMONAL DISORDERS

If the pituitary gland produces excess growth hormone before puberty, there is an overgrowth of bones and other organs leading to *gigantism*. Excess parathyroid hormone causes *bone cysts. Osteoporosis* is also frequently due to other hormonal disturbances.

TUMOURS

Several different types of benign and malignant growth can affect bones (see *Bone tumour; Bone cancer*).

DEGENERATION

Degenerative disorders of bone become more common in old age. In *osteoarthritis* there is wearing of the bone surface in a number of joints.

AUTOIMMUNE DISORDERS

Here the body's *immune system* attacks its own tissues. The main autoimmune disorder that may affect bones is *rheumatoid arthritis*.

OTHER DISORDERS

Paget's disease involves thickening of the outer layer of the bones while the inside becomes spongy.

INVESTIGATION

Bone disorders are investigated by techniques such as *X-rays, CT scanning*, and *radionuclide scanning*, by *biopsy*, and by biochemical *blood tests* to look for any abnormalities in the levels of hormones or nutrients such as calcium and vitamin D.

Bone cyst

An abnormal cavity in a bone, usually filled with fluid. Bone cysts typically develop at one end of a long bone. The presence of a cyst is often discovered by chance after there has been a bone fracture at the site of the cyst. A minor operation that involves scraping the cyst and filling the cavity with bone chips usually cures the condition.

Bone graft

An operation in which a small piece of bone is taken from one part of the body to repair bone damage in another part. The bone graft is attached to the defective bone, and provides a protein that stimulates bone growth. Although the bone graft eventually dies, it acts as a scaffold upon which new bone can grow.

WHY IT IS DONE

A bone graft has four main uses: to encourage a fracture to heal, to restore bone lost through injury, to replace bone removed surgically because of disease, and to provide a peg to join the bones of a diseased or unstable joint. A bone graft may also be used in cosmetic surgery to improve the shape of the face and skull.

HOW IT IS DONE

The bone from which the graft is to be taken is exposed and a portion removed. The most common sources are the iliac crests (upper part of the hip-bones). These bones contain a large amount of the inner, spongy bone, which is especially useful for getting grafts to "take". Other sources are the ribs, which provide curved bone, and the ulna (in the forearm), which provides excellent bone pegs.

The bone that needs treatment is exposed and the graft fixed to it with screws or wires. After the area has been stitched, a plaster cast is applied to keep the graft in place.

RECOVERY PERIOD

Bruising and pain at the site from which the graft was taken clear up within a week or two, and the only large scars left are those where bone has been taken from the iliac crests.

B

X-rays are taken to check the progress of healing, which usually is well under way after about six weeks.

Most bone graft operations succeed in permitting formation of new bone as strong and efficient as the old.

Bone imaging
Techniques for providing pictures that show the structure or function of bones, used for the detection of disease or injury.

TYPES
Because X-rays are more fully absorbed by bone than by other tissues, X-ray images show bone structure clearly. This makes them ideal for diagnosing fractures and injuries and also for revealing tumours and infections that cause changes in bone structure. A more detailed examination of small changes or abnormalities hidden by surrounding structures is provided by tomography (taking X-ray pictures at different depths of the structure being examined) or by CT scanning. MRI shows tumours and infections and the effect of diseased bone on surrounding muscles, ligaments, and fat. Either CT scanning or MRI is useful in looking for disc prolapse (slipped disc) in people with low back pain.

Radionuclide scanning is used to reveal bone function by showing the rate of blood flow to the bone and of cell activity within it. The technique is used mainly to determine whether cancer has spread to bone. It can also give useful information on bone injuries, infections, tumours, arthritis, and metabolic disorders, such as rickets, that affect bone.

Bone marrow
The soft fatty tissue found in bone cavities; it may be red or yellow. Red bone marrow is a blood-producing tissue present in all bones at birth. During the teens, it is gradually replaced in some bones by less active yellow marrow. In adults, red marrow is confined chiefly to the spine, sternum, (breastbone), ribs, clavicles (collarbones), scapulae (shoulderblades), pelvis (hip-bones), and skull bones.

Red bone marrow is the factory for most of the blood cells—all of the red cells and platelets and most of the white cells. Stem cells (cells whose descendants specialize into different cell types) within the red marrow are stimulated to form blood cells by erythropoietin, a hormone originating in the kidney. The blood cells go through various stages of maturation

in the red marrow before they are ready to be released into the circulation. Yellow marrow is composed mainly of connective tissue and fat. If the body needs to increase its rate of blood formation, some of the yellow marrow will be replaced by red.

Sometimes marrow fails to produce sufficient numbers of normal blood cells, as occurs in aplastic anaemia (see Anaemia, aplastic) or when marrow has been displaced by tumour cells. In other cases, marrow may overproduce certain blood cells, as occurs in polycythaemia and leukaemia.

Bone marrow biopsy
A procedure to obtain a sample of cells from the bone marrow (aspiration biopsy) or a small core of bone with marrow inside (trephine biopsy). The sample is usually taken from the sternum (breastbone) or the iliac crests (upper part of the hip-bones).

Microscopic examination of the bone marrow gives information on the development of the various components of blood and on the presence of cells foreign to the marrow. It is useful in the diagnosis of many blood disorders, including anaemia, leukaemia, bone marrow failure, and certain infections. It can also show whether bone marrow has been invaded by lymphoma (a cancer of lymphatic tissue) or cells from other tumours.

Trephine biopsy requires a long, thick needle for removal of the bone core, usually from the iliac crest. Trephine biopsy is used when tumour growth makes aspiration impossible, or when the bone marrow structure needs to be examined. Bone marrow biopsy may be performed repeatedly to monitor the response of a disease to treatment.

Bone marrow transplant
The technique of using normal bone marrow to replace malignant or defective marrow in a patient. In allogeneic bone marrow transplantation (BMT), healthy bone marrow is taken from a donor who has a very similar tissue-type to the recipient's—usually a brother or sister. In autologous BMT the patient's own bone marrow is used. Either type of BMT is performed only in centres that specialize in this procedure.

WHY IT IS DONE
Because the procedure itself carries certain risks, BMT is used only in the treatment of serious, mostly potentially fatal blood and immune system disorders, including severe aplastic

anaemia (see Anaemia, aplastic), thalassaemia, sickle cell anaemia, leukaemia, severe combined immunodeficiency (see Immunodeficiency disorders), and some inborn errors of metabolism (see Metabolism, inborn errors of).

HOW IT IS DONE
ALLOGENEIC BMT Blood samples are taken from the patient and the prospective donor to assess compatibility of tissue-types.

Before transplantation is carried out, all of the recipient's marrow (healthy and diseased) must first be destroyed. This is achieved by treatment in the form of cytotoxic drugs or radiation. Destroying the marrow prevents rejection of the donated cells and also kills any cancer cells present. After this has been done, the patient is nursed in a single room with reverse isolation facilities to minimize the risk of infection. The procedure for removing bone marrow from a donor and transplanting it into the patient is shown in the illustrated box.

AUTOLOGOUS BMT Bone marrow is taken from the patient (usually a person who has a malignant disease) while his or her disease is in remission (not active) and stored by cryopreservation (a tissue-freezing technique). Before being frozen, the marrow is usually treated in an attempt to eliminate any remaining malignant cells. If the disease recurs, the stored bone marrow can then be thawed and reinfused into the patient, after first destroying all his or her bone marrow as in allogeneic BMT.

COMPLICATIONS
Infection can be a major problem during the recovery period, and isolation nursing procedures must continue for about four to six weeks until the new marrow is producing adequate numbers of white blood cells.

In allogeneic BMT, the other dangerous complication is the rejection process known as graft-versus-host disease (GVHD). GVHD occurs when lymphocytes in the donor bone marrow recognize their new host (recipient) environment as foreign. Symptoms include rash, jaundice, and diarrhoea. Immunosuppressant drugs, such as cyclosporin and corticosteroid drugs, prevent and treat rejection. The risk of GVHD may be reduced by removing the T-cells from the bone marrow with monoclonal antibodies (see antibody, monoclonal) before it is reinfused.

Complications may continue to arise for long periods after a bone marrow transplant.

PERFORMING A BONE MARROW TRANSPLANT

Normal bone marrow is used to replace malignant or defective marrow. In the allogeneic procedure, healthy marrow is taken from a donor. In the autologous procedure, the patient's own healthy marrow is used.

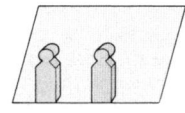

With one sibling there is a 25% chance of finding a compatible donor.

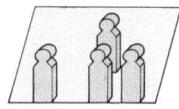

With three siblings there are three opportunities for a 25% chance of finding a donor.

Finding a donor
The more siblings one has, the greater the chance of finding a donor. With three or more siblings, the chances are good.

HOW IT IS DONE

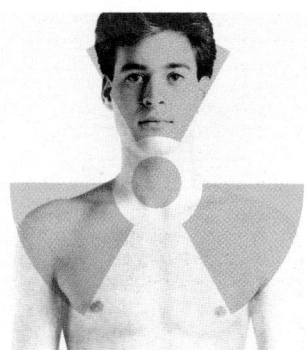

1 Before transplantation, all the recipient's marrow is destroyed by treatment with drugs or radiation. Destroying the marrow kills any cancer cells.

3 After aspiration, the bone marrow is transfused intravenously into the patient. The bone marrow cells find their way through the circulation into the patient's marrow cavities, where they start to grow.

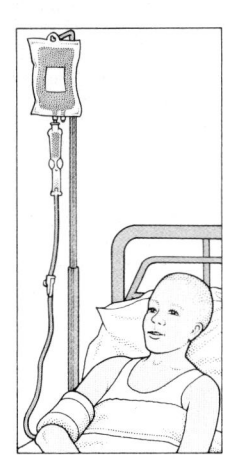

SITES OF BONE MARROW

Red or yellow in colour, bone marrow is a soft, fatty tissue found in the cavities of bones. In newborn babies, red bone marrow is present in all bones; during the teen years, most is replaced by yellow marrow'. The marrow used for transplants is red.

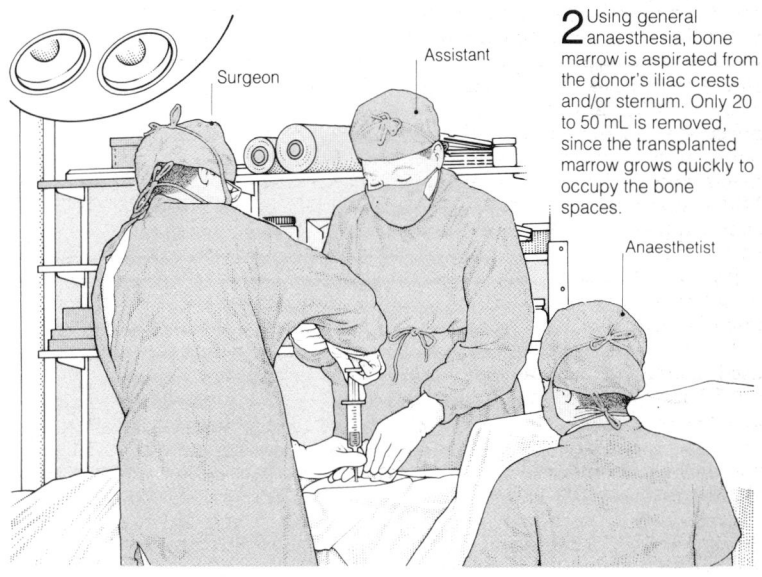

Bone marrow

Soft, spongy bone

Hard, compact bone

Bone marrow seen under the microscope

2 Using general anaesthesia, bone marrow is aspirated from the donor's iliac crests and/or sternum. Only 20 to 50 mL is removed, since the transplanted marrow grows quickly to occupy the bone spaces.

Surgeon

Assistant

Anaesthetist

ASPIRATION BIOPSY

A hollow aspiration needle is introduced into the bone (iliac crests or sternum). A stylet (a thin, sharp lance) is passed through the needle and advanced (using small, twisting movements) through the bone cortex. The stylet is removed. Bone marrow is sucked out from the cortex into a syringe connected to the needle.

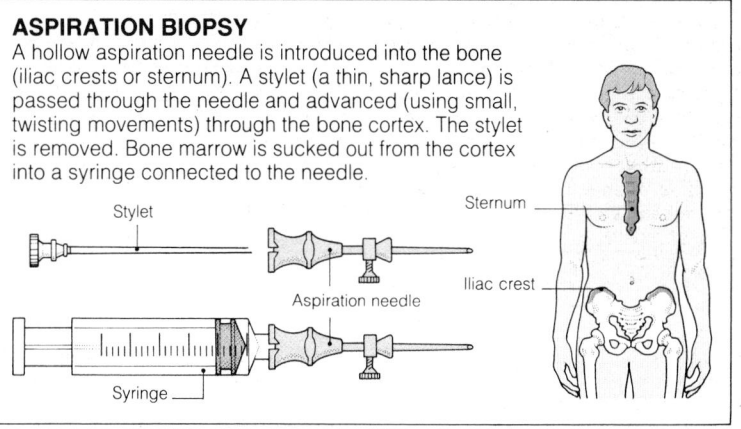

Stylet

Aspiration needle

Syringe

Sternum

Iliac crest

B

Bone tumour

A swelling occurring in a bone. Bone tumours may be malignant (see *Bone cancer*) or benign (noncancerous).

Benign bone tumours are classified into different types. The most common is an *osteochondroma*, a mixed swelling of bone and cartilage that often begins in childhood. Other types are *osteoma*, a smooth, rounded bone swelling, and chondroma, which is made up of cartilage cells and occurs mainly in the hands or feet (see *Chondromatosis*). Osteoma and chondroma are painless and may affect any bone in the body. No treatment is necessary unless the tumour becomes very large or unsightly, or causes symptoms by pressing on other structures (such as arteries or nerves). In such cases, the tumour can be removed surgically.

Another type of benign bone tumour is an osteoclastoma (also called a giant cell tumour). This tumour, which usually occurs in the arm or leg of a young adult, is tender and painful and should be removed.

Booster

A follow-up dose of *vaccine* given to reinforce the effect of a first course.

Borborygmi

A name for the audible bowel sounds that are a normal part of the digestive process. They are caused by movement of air and fluid through the intestine. In some people they may be accentuated during times of anxiety.

Borborygmi may be affected by some disorders of the *intestine*, and doctors listen to the bowel sounds as an aid to diagnosis.

Borderline personality disorder

A form of personality disorder falling between neurotic and psychotic levels. The person with a borderline personality disorder is usually incapable of maintaining stable relationships. Mood changes are often rapid and inappropriate. Frequent, angry outbursts are common, as are impulsive, self-damaging acts such as gambling, shoplifting, or suicide attempts. This term is more commonly used in the US and there is disagreement as to its exact nature.

Bornholm disease

One of many names for epidemic *pleurodynia*, an infectious viral disease that is characterized by severe chest pains and fever.

BOTTLE-FEEDING

The parent's back should be supported firmly with feet flat on the floor. The baby should be cradled snugly with the head supported well above the level of the stomach. Eye contact should be maintained.

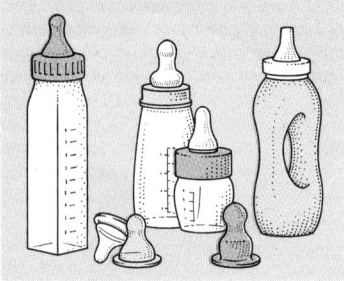

Types of bottle
Bottles, and their teats, come in various shapes and sizes. Some come ready-filled with milk formula.

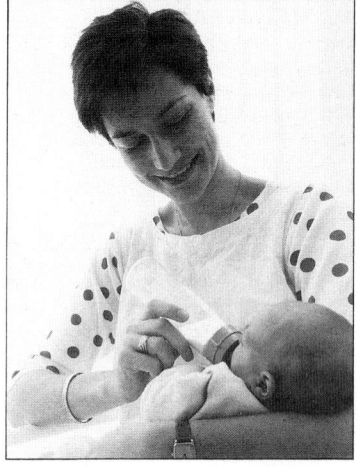

Technique
The bottle must be kept tilted and the flow of milk maintained at a good rate but not so fast as to cause choking.

Bottle-feeding

A method of infant feeding using a milk preparation usually based on modified cow's milk. Although *breast-feeding* is preferable and recommended where possible, parents may choose bottle-feeding. With bottle-feeding, there is no fluctuation in the quality or quantity of the milk, and the baby's intake can be measured and regulated.

PREPARING THE FEED
Milk powder must be measured accurately and mixed with water to the correct strength as indicated on the container. The proportions of protein, fat, lactose (milk sugar), and minerals are similar to those in human milk and vitamins are added. No extra milk powder, sugar, or cereal should be added to the feed.

It is essential that strict rules of hygiene be observed when preparing infant feeds because bacteria thrive in warm milk. All equipment must be cleaned thoroughly and sterilized using one of two methods.

ASEPTIC STERILIZATION This technique involves sterilizing all bottles, teats, and caps before use by immersing them in boiling water and storing them in an antiseptic solution such as sodium hypochlorite. The feed is then prepared using boiled water and can be used immediately after it cools to a lukewarm temperature.

TERMINAL STERILIZATION This method involves sterilizing the prepared milk along with the bottles in a special

steam sterilizing unit or saucepan. Up to six feeds—enough for one day—may be prepared at once and stored in the refrigerator. The feed may be warmed for use by standing the bottle in a pan of hot water, or by placing it in an electric warmer. Do not use a microwave oven; this method of warming may alter the nutritional value of the feed. Any unused milk must be discarded immediately.

PROBLEMS
If feeds are carefully prepared, equipment sterilized, and bottles given with warmth and cuddling, problems should be rare. However, parents should guard against overfeeding; the correct amount for an infant is based on his or her weight and expected weight for age. There is some variation in requirements, however.

A more serious long-term problem for some bottle-fed infants concerns the proteins and peptides found in cow's milk. Early exposure to these (which are not present in breast milk) may sensitize the infant to cow's milk protein and result in allergic reactions in later life. If there is a history of allergy in the family, feeding an infant with a non-milk protein formula may be recommended to prevent an allergic reaction in the child; consult your doctor. (See also *Feeding, infant*.)

Botulism

A rare but serious form of poisoning caused by eating improperly canned or preserved food contaminated with a toxin produced by the bacterium *CLOSTRIDIUM BOTULINUM*. The toxin causes progressive muscular paralysis and other disturbances of the central and peripheral nervous system.

CAUSES AND INCIDENCE
CLOSTRIDIUM BOTULINUM is found in soil and untreated water in most parts of the world and is harmlessly present in the intestinal tracts of many animals, including fish. It produces spores that resist boiling, salting, smoking, and some forms of pickling. These spores, which multiply only in the absence of air, cannot normally infect humans, but thrive in improperly preserved or canned food where they produce the toxin. If such food is eaten, absorption of even minute amounts of toxin can lead to severe poisoning. Botulism is extremely rare in the UK, with no cases reported in most years.

SYMPTOMS AND TREATMENT
Symptoms of botulism usually first appear between eight and 36 hours after eating contaminated food. The symptoms include difficulty swallowing and speaking, nausea, vomiting, and double vision. Prompt treatment with an antitoxin brings the risk of death down to less than 25 per cent. (See also *Food poisoning*.)

Bowel
A common name for the large and/or small *intestines*.

Bowel movements, abnormal
See *Faeces, abnormal*.

Bowel sounds
See *Borborygmi*.

Bowen's disease
A rare skin disorder that sometimes becomes cancerous. The disorder consists of a flat, regular-shaped, patch of red, scaly skin, usually on the face or hands. Treatment consists of removing the diseased patch of skin surgically or destroying it by freezing or *cauterization*. The disorder is unlikely to recur.

Some doctors believe that a person who has had Bowen's disease is at increased risk of developing cancer of the lung, kidney, or large intestine later in life.

Bowleg
An outward curving of bones in the legs. Bowlegs are common in very young children and are a normal part of development. The curve usually straightens as the child grows, but, if

the bowing is severe, is on one side only, or persists beyond the age of six, a doctor should be consulted. An operation may be needed.

Rarely, leg deformity is a result of bone disease, particularly *rickets* (a vitamin D deficiency) in children.

Brace, dental
See *Orthodontic appliances*.

Brace, orthopaedic
An appliance worn to support part of the body or to hold it in a fixed position. An orthopaedic brace may be used to correct or halt the development of a deformity, to aid mobility, or to relieve pain. (See *Caliper splint*; *Corset*; *Splint*.)

Brachialgia
Pain or stiffness in the arm. Brachialgia is often accompanied by pain, tingling, or numbness of the hands or fingers, and weakness of hand grip. It may indicate an underlying disorder such as *frozen shoulder* or nerve compression from *cervical osteoarthritis* (arthritis in the bones of the neck).

Brachial plexus
A collection of large nerve trunks that pass from the lower part of the cervical spine (in the neck) and the upper part of the thoracic spine (in the chest) down the arm. These nerve trunks divide into the musculocutaneous and axillary, median, ulnar, and radial nerves which both control muscles in and receive sensations from the arm and hand.

INJURIES
Injuries to the brachial plexus are an important and fairly common cause of partial or complete loss of movement and sensation in the arm. Damage to the brachial plexus sometimes occurs during birth, with an increased risk in *breech delivery*. In adults, a common cause of brachial plexus injury is a fall from a motorcycle.

Injury is usually a forcible separation of the neck and shoulder, due to a fall pushing the shoulder downwards or to a blow to the side of the neck that stretches or tears upper nerve roots in the plexus. Damage to these roots causes paralysis in muscles of the shoulder and elbow.

Injury to lower nerve roots in the plexus, causing paralysis of muscles in the forearm and hand, can result from a forcible blow that lifts the arm and shoulder upwards.

In severe injuries, both the upper and the lower nerve roots of the brachial plexus are damaged, producing complete paralysis of the arm.

Paralysis may be temporary if the stretching was not severe enough to tear nerve fibres.

TREATMENT Treatment of a brachial plexus injury depends on the extent and severity of nerve damage. Possible investigational procedures include *EMG* (electromyography) to demonstrate which nerves are still intact, and *myelography* (X-ray examination of the spinal cord after injection of a contrast medium).

Nerve roots that have been torn can be repaired by nerve grafting, a *microsurgery* procedure often performed with good results. However, if a nerve root has become separated from the spinal cord, surgical repair will not be successful.

In the event of permanent paralysis of a particular group of muscles in the arm, function can be improved by a muscle or *tendon transfer* operation to provide an alternative structure to perform a particular movement. *Physiotherapy*, with exercises continued at home, helps restore function after a successful nerve graft operation and can also help to reduce *contractures* in paralysed muscles.

OTHER DISORDERS
Apart from injuries, the brachial plexus may be affected by the presence of a *cervical rib* (extra rib), infections, tumours, or *aneurysms*.

Bradycardia
An adult heart-rate of below 60 beats per minute. Most people have a heart-rate of between 60 and 100 beats per minute, the average being 72 to 78. Many athletes and healthy people who exercise regularly and vigorously have perfectly normal bradycardia. In others, however, bradycardia may indicate an underlying disorder such as *hypothyroidism* (underactivity of the thyroid gland) or *heart block*. Bradycardia may also occur as a result of taking *beta-blocker drugs*.

Profound or sudden bradycardia may cause a drop in blood pressure and symptoms such as loss of energy, weakness, and fainting attacks. Bradycardia occurs in a *vasovagal attack*, a condition in which the vagus nerve slows the heart-rate, dilates blood vessels, and causes fainting.

Braille
A system of embossed dots that enables blind people to read and write. It was developed by the Frenchman Louis Braille and is now accepted for all written languages, music, mathematics, and science.

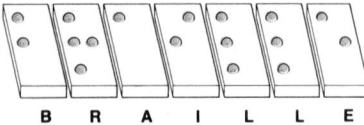

Example of Grade I braille
In this system, each letter is represented by its own pattern of dots.

The braille system is based on six raised dots, which can be arranged in different combinations. There are two types. In Grade I, each symbol represents an individual letter or punctuation mark. In Grade II, symbols represent common letter combinations or words. This second form is more widely used.

Brain

The major organ of the *nervous system*, located in the *cranium* (skull). The brain is the organ of thought, speech, and emotion, but its primary role in humans—just as in animals—is as the body's control centre.

The brain and spinal cord constitute the *central nervous system* (CNS). The CNS controls basic functions such as heart-rate, breathing, and body temperature. The brain receives, sorts, and interprets sensations from the nerves that extend from the CNS to every other part of the body; it initiates and coordinates the motor output involved in activities such as movement and speech.

Three main structures are easily recognized: the *brainstem*, *cerebellum*, and, above the brainstem, the large forebrain, much of which consists of the *cerebrum* (see illustrated box opposite). Extending from the brain are 12 pairs of *cranial nerves*; some of these have a sensory function, some a motor function, and some are both sensory and motor.

BRAINSTEM AND CEREBELLUM

These parts of the brain are the oldest in evolutionary terms, and their structure and function differ little between humans and other mammals. The brainstem is concerned mainly with control of vital functions, such as breathing and blood pressure, and the cerebellum with muscular coordination, balance, and posture.

Both these brain regions operate below the level of consciousness by *reflex* action, a system by which particular stimuli or patterns of stimuli evoke preprogrammed or automatic responses. The brainstem and cerebellum receive sensory information (about temperature, pressure, posi-

tion, or pain) from sensory receptors scattered throughout the body. They then transmit the appropriate response—for example, to muscles in the blood vessels or limbs to change blood pressure and flow or alter posture.

FOREBRAIN

The forebrain consists of a central group of structures and nerve nuclei (nerve-cell groups) above the brainstem and, enclosing these, the relatively huge cerebrum.

CENTRAL STRUCTURES These act mainly as links between parts of the cerebrum above and brainstem below. They include the two egg-shaped *thalami*, which serve as relay stations for sensory information passing towards the cerebrum. Beneath them, the *hypothalamus* is a tiny region involved in the regulation of body temperature, thirst, and appetite; it also influences sexual behaviour, aggression, and sleep. The hypothalamus has close connections with the *pituitary gland*, which produces hormones that affect other glands and in this way controls growth, sexual development, metabolism, fluid balance, and numerous other physiological variables. Encircling the thalami, a further complex of nerve centres, called the *limbic system*, is thought to be involved in the handling of emotions, some memory functions, and the processing of olfactory (smell) sensations.

CEREBRUM The two hemispheres that make up the cerebrum project upwards and outwards from the centre of the forebrain to form an almost continuous egg-shaped mass. The cerebrum constitutes nearly 70 per cent of the weight of the entire nervous system.

The surfaces of the hemispheres are folded into deep clefts so that only one third of the total surface is visible. Certain of the sulci (fissures) separating gyri (folds) are particularly noticeable and divide the surface into distinct lobes—occipital, parietal, temporal, and frontal—named after the main bones of the skull that overlie them. The two halves of the cerebrum are connected by the corpus callosum.

The cerebral cortex (the outer surface of the cerebrum) consists of grey matter, with nerve cells arranged in six layers. This is the region concerned with conscious thought, sensation, and movement. It operates in a similar way to the more primitive parts of the brain, except that incoming sensory information undergoes a far more detailed analysis. Various conscious processes, such as perception,

memory, thought, and decision-making, take place between the reception of sensory information and the output of a motor response. Actions initiated by output from the cortex—speech, movement, writing—can be extremely complex in form.

Beneath the cortex, much of the cerebrum consists of tracts of nerve fibres forming white matter; these tracts connect various areas of the cortex to each other and to nerve centres in the centre of the forebrain and brainstem. Deeper within the hemispheres are groups of cells named the *basal ganglia*; they are connected to the brainstem and cerebellum and are involved in relaying and modifying motor output from the cerebral cortex, signalling and coordinating movements to skeletal muscles.

Though the cerebrum is symmetrical in appearance, some higher activities such as speech and writing are controlled from one cerebral hemisphere, the dominant one. In right-handed people this is the left hemisphere; even in left-handed people the left side is usually dominant. The nondominant side plays an important role in visual/spatial orientation and may also be involved in artistic/creative thought.

PROTECTION AND NOURISHMENT

The whole of the brain and spinal cord is encased in three layers of membranes, called the *meninges*. The *cerebrospinal fluid* circulates between two of these layers and also within the four main brain cavities called *ventricles* (one in each cerebral hemisphere, a third in the centre of the forebrain, and a fourth in the brainstem). This cerebrospinal fluid helps nourish the brain and also helps cushion it from injury when the head is moved quickly or receives a blow.

The brain as a whole also has an extensive blood supply. Blood comes from a circle of arteries fed by the internal *carotid arteries* (which run up each side of the front of the neck to enter the base of the skull) and from two vertebral arteries that run parallel to the spinal cord. The brain receives about 20 per cent of the heart's output of blood. (See also *Brain* disorders box overleaf.)

Brain abscess

A collection of pus, surrounded by inflamed tissues, within the brain or on its surface. Along with *brain tumours* and other space-occupying brain abnormalities, abscesses cause symptoms due to raised pressure within the skull

STRUCTURE OF THE BRAIN

The brain has three main parts—the brainstem (an extension of the spinal cord), the cerebellum, and the forebrain, much of which consists of the two large cerebral hemispheres. Each hemisphere consists of an outer layer, or cortex, which is rich in nerve cells and called grey matter, and inner areas rich in nerve fibres, called white matter. The surface of each hemisphere is thrown into folds called gyri separated by fissures called sulci. The two hemispheres are linked by a thick band of nerve fibres, the corpus callosum. Deep within the forebrain are various central structures, which include the thalamus, hypothalamus, basal ganglia, and pituitary gland.

The brain has a consistency like jelly and, in adults, weighs about 1.4 kg. It is protected by membranous coverings, the meninges, within the skull.

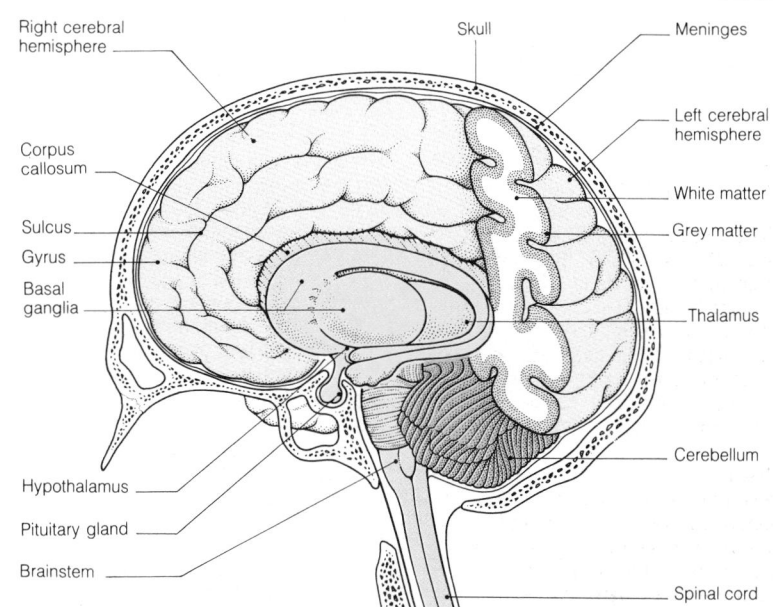

Right cerebral hemisphere — Skull — Meninges — Left cerebral hemisphere — White matter — Grey matter — Corpus callosum — Sulcus — Gyrus — Basal ganglia — Thalamus — Hypothalamus — Pituitary gland — Brainstem — Cerebellum — Spinal cord

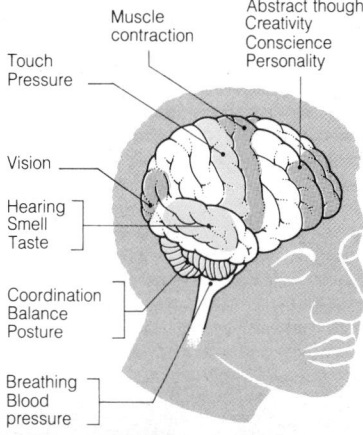

Muscle contraction — Abstract thought Creativity Conscience Personality — Touch Pressure — Vision — Hearing Smell Taste — Coordination Balance Posture — Breathing Blood pressure

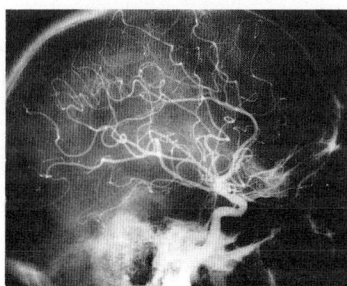

Postcentral gyrus — Precentral gyrus — Parietal lobe — Frontal lobe — Occipital lobe — Cerebellum — Temporal lobe

Lobes
These are broad surface regions of each hemisphere that are named after the overlying bones of the skull. The four main regions are the frontal, parietal, temporal, and occipital lobes.

Special areas
Some brain areas are associated with specific functions—for example, the occipital lobe with vision, and the cerebellum with balance and coordination. Touch and pressure sensation is perceived within the postcentral gyrus. Muscle movements are controlled from the precentral gyrus; speech is controlled from an area in the frontal lobe of the dominant hemisphere.

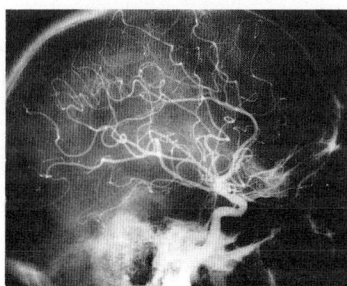

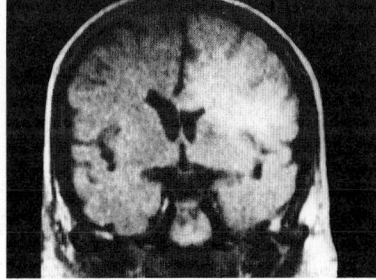

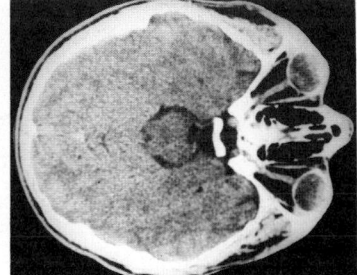

Angiography
This technique makes blood vessels clearly visible. The angiogram above shows the carotid artery and its branches.

Magnetic resonance imaging
This technique is used mainly to reveal abnormalities that are otherwise undetectable. In the MRI scan above, the white mass to the upper right is a tumour.

CT scanning
The CT scan above shows a "slice" through the head. The nose and eyeballs are visible at the right; the small circular area in the centre is the brainstem.

B

DISORDERS OF THE BRAIN

Defects and disorders of the brain have much the same causes as disease in other body organs. One special feature of the brain, however, is that it is packed inside a rigid casing, the skull, so any space-occupying *brain abscess*, *brain tumour*, or *haematoma* (large blood clot) following a *head injury* or *brain haemorrhage* creates raised pressure that impairs the function of the whole brain. Another special feature is that brain cells destroyed through injury or disease cannot be replaced, so the loss in function can be more difficult to reverse.

Some diseases and defects in the brain are localized in a small region and may thus have a specific effect—for example, *aphasia* (speech loss). More often, damage is more diffuse and, because the brain has so many related functions, the symptoms can be varied and numerous.

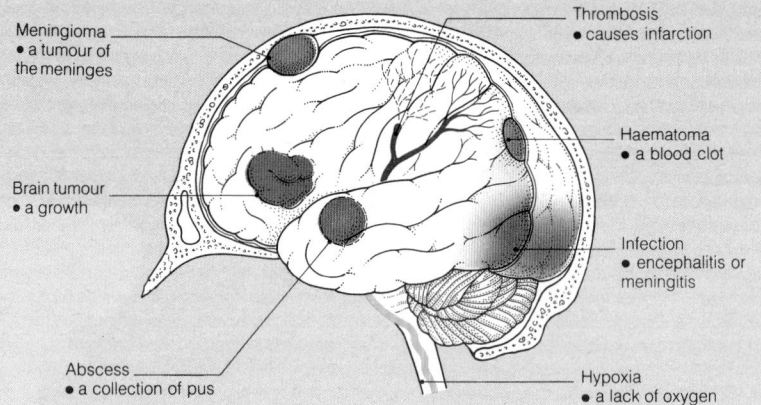

Meningioma
• a tumour of the meninges

Brain tumour
• a growth

Abscess
• a collection of pus

Thrombosis
• causes infarction

Haematoma
• a blood clot

Infection
• encephalitis or meningitis

Hypoxia
• a lack of oxygen

CONGENITAL DEFECTS

Babies may be born with brain defects due to genetic or chromosomal disorders, as in *Down's syndrome*, *Tay-Sachs disease*, or *cri du chat syndrome* (all of which are associated with mental deficiency). Structural defects that arise during fetal development may be fundamental and untreatable, as in *microcephaly* (small head), or fatal, as in *anencephaly* (congenital absence of the brain). Others are potentially correctable, even while the fetus is still in the uterus, as in *hydrocephalus* (water on the brain).

IMPAIRED BLOOD AND OXYGEN SUPPLY

These are two of the most important causes of brain dysfunction because brain cells can survive only a few minutes without oxygen. *Hypoxia* (lack of oxygen) affecting the brain as a result of asphyxiation during the process of birth is one of the causes of *cerebral palsy*. Later in life, cerebral hypoxia can result from an accident such as choking or from arrest of breathing and heartbeat following electrocution or drowning.

From middle age onwards, the most important affliction of the brain is *cerebrovascular disease* impairing blood supply to one or several brain regions. If an artery within the brain becomes blocked or ruptures leading to haemorrhage, the result is a *stroke*.

INJURY

Although protected by the skull, the brain may be damaged by heavy blows to the head or following skull fracture as a result of falls, high-speed impacts, bullet wounds, or other physical violence (see *Head injury*).

INFECTION

Infection within the brain, called *encephalitis*, or of the membranes surrounding the brain, called *meningitis*, is uncommon today. Meningitis is usually caused by a bacterial infection. Encephalitis can be caused by any one of numerous viruses, of which the best known and most dangerous are the *rabies* and *herpes simplex viruses*.

An abscess (localized pocket of infection) in the brain may result from spread of infection from the ear, sinuses, or elsewhere in the body (see *brain abscess*).

TUMOURS

Tumours that affect the brain may be primary (arising from tissues inside the skull) as in *gliomas*, *meningiomas*, *acoustic neuromas*, and *pituitary tumours*, or secondary (arising from cancer cells that have spread through the bloodstream from tumours in the lungs, breasts, or elsewhere). See *Brain tumours*.

DEGENERATION

Multiple sclerosis, a progressive disease of unknown cause in which the nerve sheaths (composed of myelin) are destroyed, starts most commonly in early adulthood.

Degenerative brain diseases, such as *Alzheimer's disease* (a type of dementia) and *Parkinson's disease*, are particularly important causes of disability among the elderly.

OTHER DISORDERS

Disorders characterized by their symptoms rather than any obvious cause include *migraine*, *narcolepsy* (excessive episodic sleepiness), and idiopathic *epilepsy* (epilepsy of unknown cause), though epileptic seizures can also have specific causes, such as a tumour.

Disorders of thought, emotion, or behaviour are generally described as psychiatric or *mental illnesses*. Often, there is no obvious physical brain defect or disorder, although, with many important mental illnesses, such as *depression* and *schizophrenia*, there seems to be an underlying disturbance of brain chemistry. Some psychiatric illnesses, collectively called organic *brain syndromes*, by definition have a physical cause.

INVESTIGATION

Many different procedures may be used to investigate disorders of the brain. A full *physical examination* will include assessment of brain function by means of tests of mental abilities and state, sensation, movement, muscle tone, and reflexes. Electrical activity within the brain may be measured by means of an *EEG*. Physical abnormalities may be looked for using *brain imaging* techniques, such as *angiography*, *CT scanning*, or *MRI*. A *lumbar puncture* may be performed to look for evidence of an infection or a degenerative disorder.

and local damage to nerve tracts. The most common sites of brain abscesses are the frontal and temporal lobes of the *cerebrum* in the forebrain.

CAUSES AND INCIDENCE
Brain abscesses may follow head injury but most cases result from the spread of infection from elsewhere in the body. Approximately 40 per cent of abscesses result from middle ear or sinus infections. Other causes include infection following a penetrating brain injury, and blood-borne infection, most commonly in patients with acute bacterial *endocarditis* or some types of *immunodeficiency disorders*. Abscesses due to blood-borne infection are often multiple.

SYMPTOMS
The commonest symptoms are headache, drowsiness, and vomiting. There may also be visual disturbances, fever, epileptic seizures, and symptoms due to local brain damage—for example, partial paralysis or speech disturbances.

DIAGNOSIS AND TREATMENT
The diagnosis is suggested by *CT scanning* or *MRI* (magnetic resonance imaging) of the brain. Treatment consists of a high dosage of antibiotics and usually surgery. A hole may need to be made in the skull (see *Craniotomy*), and the abscess is then cut open and drained of pus.

OUTLOOK
Brain abscesses prove fatal in about 10 per cent of cases, and the remaining patients often suffer some residual impairment of brain function. *Epilepsy* is common, so *anticonvulsant drugs* are often prescribed after removal or drainage of the abscess.

Brain damage
Degeneration or death of nerve cells and tracts within the brain. Damage may be localized to particular areas of the brain—causing specific defects of brain function, such as loss of coordination or difficulty with speech—or may be more diffuse, causing mental or severe physical handicap.

DIFFUSE DAMAGE
The most important cause of diffuse brain damage is prolonged cerebral *hypoxia* (insufficient oxygen reaching the brain). This may occur during birth; a baby's brain cannot tolerate a lack of oxygen for more than about five minutes. At any age, hypoxia may result from *cardiac arrest* (heart stoppage) or *respiratory arrest* (cessation of breathing), or from causes such as poisoning, drowning, or *status epilepticus* (prolonged convulsions).

Diffuse damage may also occur through the accumulation in the brain of substances poisonous to nerve cells—as in untreated *phenylketonuria* or *galactosaemia*, or as a result of inhaling or ingesting environmental pollutants such as compounds of lead or mercury (see *Minamata disease*).

Other possible causes include infections of the brain, such as *encephalitis* or, very rarely, brain damage following *immunization*.

LOCALIZED DAMAGE
Localized brain damage may occur as a result of *head injury*, especially penetrating injury, at any age. It may occur later in life as a result of a *stroke, brain tumour*, or *brain abscess*.

At birth, local damage to the *basal ganglia* (nerve-cell centres deep within the brain) caused by a raised blood level of *bilirubin* (formed from the destruction of blood cells in *haemolytic disease of the newborn*) leads to a condition called *kernicterus*. This condition is characterized by disorders of movement and sometimes by mental deficiency. The basal ganglia may also be damaged by carbon monoxide.

SYMPTOMS AND TREATMENT
Brain damage that occurs before, during, or after birth may result in *cerebral palsy*, a condition characterized by paralysis and abnormal movements, and often associated with *mental handicap* and sometimes *deafness*.

Victims of head injury, stroke, or other causes of localized or diffuse brain damage may also be left with any of a range of handicaps, including disturbances of movement, speech, or sensation, mental handicap, or epileptic seizures.

Nerve cells and tracts in the brain and spinal cord do not recover their function if they have been destroyed (nerves in the limbs or trunk regenerate slowly after being cut or crushed). Nevertheless, some degree of improvement may be expected after brain damage as the victim learns to use other parts of the brain and other muscle groups in the body. Treatment towards this goal often involves teamwork on the part of doctors and specialists in *physiotherapy, speech therapy*, and *occupational therapy*.

Brain death
The irreversible cessation of all functions of the entire brain, including the *brainstem*. The recognition of brain death, as defined above, has allowed doctors to certify death in situations where the lungs and heart continue to function (with machine assistance) but where death has occurred based on the absence of brain function. (See also *Death*.)

Brain failure
See *Brain syndrome, organic*.

Brain haemorrhage
Bleeding within or around the brain, caused either by injury or by spontaneous rupture of a blood vessel. There are four possible types: *subdural hae-*

SITES OF BRAIN HAEMORRHAGE
Haemorrhages within the skull fall into four main categories—extradural, subdural, subarachnoid, and intracerebral haemorrhages—according to the site of the bleeding in relation to the brain and its protec-tive coverings, the meninges. The causes and effects of the bleeding and the outlook for the patient vary among the categories.

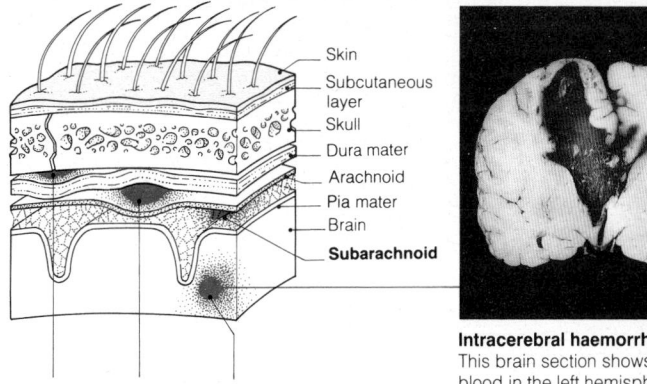

Skin
Subcutaneous layer
Skull
Dura mater
Arachnoid
Pia mater
Brain
Subarachnoid

Extradural Subdural Intracerebral

Intracerebral haemorrhage
This brain section shows a mass of blood in the left hemisphere.

morrhage, *extradural haemorrhage, subarachnoid haemorrhage*, and *intracerebral haemorrhage*.

CAUSES AND SYMPTOMS

Extradural and subdural haemorrhages usually result from a blow to the head (see *Head injury*); symptoms may include headache, drowsiness, confusion, and the development of paralysis on one side of the body. These symptoms may develop within hours in extradural haemorrhage but much more slowly (over weeks or months) in subdural haemorrhage. Hospital investigation and treatment is urgently required.

Subarachnoid and intracerebral haemorrhages usually occur spontaneously (i.e. without any head injury) and are the result of rupture of *aneurysms* or small blood vessels in the brain. Middle-aged and elderly persons with untreated *hypertension* are at highest risk. Subarachnoid haemorrhage is characterized by sudden violent headache and/or loss of consciousness. Intracerebral haemorrhage is one of the three main types of *stroke*; symptoms may include collapse, speech loss, and paralysis of the muscles of the face or an arm or leg. Subarachnoid and intracerebral haemorrhages are medical emergencies.

Brain imaging

Techniques that provide pictures of the brain; they are used to detect injury or disease. The introduction of computerized scanning has brought tremendous growth in this field in the past decade.

TYPES

CONVENTIONAL X-RAY TECHNIQUES The simplest and longest established method of obtaining images of the brain is to take *X-ray* films. X-rays reveal distortion or erosion of the bony skull caused by a fracture, *brain tumour*, *brain abscess*, or *aneurysm*. Unless the brain substance itself is calcified in a localized area due to disease, plain X-rays cannot detect disease of the brain matter.

Angiography involves injecting a contrast medium that shows up on X-rays into one of the arteries supplying the brain, and then taking X-ray pictures. This technique shows up the blood vessels in the brain, and is used to investigate *subarachnoid haemorrhage*, aneurysms, abnormalities of the blood vessels, and other circulatory disorders.

SCANNING TECHNIQUES *CT scanning* was first conceived in 1971 specifically to study the brain. Unlike conventional X-rays, this method gives images of the brain substance; it gives especially clear pictures of the ventricles (fluid-

filled cavities) and can reveal tumours, blood clots, strokes, aneurysms, and abscesses. Contrast medium is often administered to help differentiate normal from abnormal brain tissue.

MRI produces better images of the brain than CT scanning. It is especially helpful in showing tumours of the posterior fossa (back of the skull). MRI does not involve radiation. Nevertheless, CT remains the first choice for patients with acute head injuries who are accompanied by large amounts of medical equipment, and those who cannot remain immobile. MRI cannot be used on patients with pacemakers or mechanical heart valves.

Some special types of scanning give information about both the function and the structure of the brain. PET (positron emission tomography) scanning uses positron emitting radionuclides; SPECT (single photon emission CT) uses gamma emitters, is less expensive, but gives less precise information. These techniques allow measurement of both blood flow within the brain and metabolic activity.

Ultrasound scanning is used only in premature or very young babies because ultrasound waves cannot penetrate the bones of a mature skull. Ultrasound scanning is particularly useful in detecting *hydrocephalus* and ventricular haemorrhage in premature babies and, because no radiation is involved, repeated scans can be performed safely.

Brainstem

A stalk of nerve tissue that forms the lowest part of the brain and links with the spinal cord. The brainstem acts partly as a highway for messages travelling between other parts of the brain and spinal cord, but also connects with 10 of the 12 pairs of *cranial nerves* and controls basic functions, such as breathing, vomiting, and eye reflexes. The activities of the brainstem are below the level of consciousness and operate largely on an automatic basis.

STRUCTURE

From the spinal cord upwards, the brainstem consists of three main parts called the medulla, pons, and midbrain. Attached to the back of the brainstem is a separate part of the brain, the *cerebellum*, which is concerned principally with balance and coordinated movement. Running longitudinally through the middle of the brainstem is a canal, which widens in the pons and medulla to form the fourth *ventricle* (cavity) of the brain,

which contains the circulating *cerebrospinal fluid*.

MEDULLA The medulla resembles a thick extension of the spinal cord. It contains the nuclei (nerve-cell centres) of the ninth to 12th cranial nerves, by which it receives and relays taste sensations from the tongue and relays signals to muscles involved in speech and in tongue and neck movements. It also contains the vital centres—groups of nerve cells involved in the automatic regulation of heart-beat, breathing, blood pressure, and digestion—and sends and receives information regarding these functions via the 10th cranial or *vagus nerve*.

Many of the nerve tracts running through the medulla cross over in its lower portion so that the right side of the body links up with the left side of the brain and vice versa.

PONS The pons is wider than the medulla and contains thick bundles of nerve fibres that connect with the cerebellum, which lies directly behind. It also contains the nuclei for the fifth to eighth cranial nerves and thus relays sensory information from the ear, face, and teeth, as well as the signals that move the jaw, adjust facial expressions, and produce some eye movements.

MIDBRAIN The midbrain is the smallest section of the brainstem, above the pons. It contains the nuclei of the third and fourth cranial nerves, which control eye movements and the size and reactions of the pupil. It also contains cell groups such as the substantia nigra and red nuclei, which are involved in the smooth coordination of limb movements.

RETICULAR FORMATION Throughout the brainstem are numerous nerve-cell groups collectively known as the reticular formation. The reticular formation is believed to act as a watchdog on sensory information entering the brain, alerting the higher brain centres to new or important sensory stimuli that may require a conscious response. Our sleep/wake cycle is controlled by the reticular formation, and many *sleeping drugs* and *stimulant drugs* are believed to exert their actions through their effects on this part of the brain.

DISORDERS

The brainstem is susceptible to the same disorders that afflict the rest of the central nervous system (see *Brain disorders* box). Damage to the medulla's vital centres is rapidly fatal, while damage to the reticular formation may cause *coma*. Damage to specific cranial nerve nuclei can have specific effects—*facial palsy* in the case of the

LOCATION OF THE BRAINSTEM

The brainstem is a 7.5-cm-long stalk of nerve cells and fibres that joins the upper spinal cord to the rest of the brain.

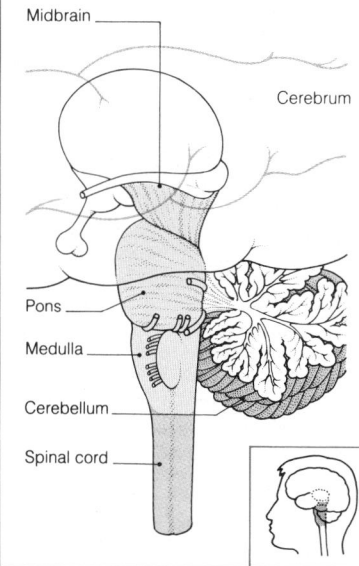

Midbrain

Cerebrum

Pons

Medulla

Cerebellum

Spinal cord

seventh cranial (facial) nerve and tongue-wasting with the 12th cranial (hypoglossal) nerve. Degeneration of the substantia nigra in the midbrain is thought to be a cause of *Parkinson's disease*.

Brain syndrome, organic

Disturbance of consciousness, intellect, or mental functioning of organic (physical) as opposed to psychiatric origin. Possible causes include degenerative diseases such as *Alzheimer's disease*, metabolic imbalances, infections, certain drugs, toxins, vitamin deficiencies, or the effects of injury, *stroke*, or tumour.

SYMPTOMS
In acute organic brain syndrome, symptoms range from slight confusion to stupor or *coma*, and may also include restlessness, disorientation, memory impairment, hallucinations, and delusions (see *Delirium*). The chronic form results in a progressive decline in intellect, memory, and behaviour (see *Dementia*).

TREATMENT
Treatment relies on discovering and, if possible, dealing with the underlying cause. Treatment is more likely to be successful with the acute form. In chronic cases, irreversible *brain damage* may already have occurred. (See also *Psychosis*.)

Brain tumour

An abnormal growth in or on the brain. Although not always malignant, all brain tumours are serious because of the build-up of pressure in the brain and compression of adjoining brain areas that occur as the tumour expands.

TYPES
Brain tumours may be primary growths arising directly from tissues within the skull, or metastases (secondary growths) spread via the bloodstream from tumours elsewhere in the body, mostly the lung or breast.

The cause of primary brain tumours is not known, although possible associations have been found with vitamin deficiency in the mother's pregnancy and with prolonged exposure to electrical power fields. About 60 per cent are *gliomas* (frequently malignant), which arise from the brain substance. Other primary tumours include *meningiomas*, arising from the meningeal membranes covering the brain; *acoustic neuromas*, arising from the acoustic nerve; and *pituitary tumours*, arising from the pituitary gland. All of these tumours are benign.

Certain types of primary brain tumours mainly affect children and are often situated in the back of the brain. These include two types of glioma called *medulloblastoma* and cerebellar *astrocytoma*.

Secondary growths, or metastases, are always malignant and may be found in more than one organ.

INCIDENCE
In the UK, about 3,000 to 3,500 new cases of primary brain tumour, leading to about 2,600 deaths, are diagnosed per year. They occur most commonly around the age of 50 years, although a significant number of children are also affected; each year several hundred children in the UK die from a primary brain tumour.

In addition, about 18,000 persons annually die of cancer that includes metastases in the brain.

SYMPTOMS
Brain tumours cause symptoms by several mechanisms. Compression of brain tissue or nerve tracts near the tumour may cause muscle weakness, loss of vision, or other sensory disturbances, speech difficulties, and, in about 20 per cent of cases, epileptic seizures.

The presence of an expanding tumour can increase pressure within the skull, causing headache, vomiting, visual disturbances, and impairment of mental functioning. If the circulation of cerebrospinal fluid is obstructed by the tumour, *hydrocephalus* may result.

DIAGNOSIS
Many different techniques are used to locate the site of a brain tumour and to establish the extent of its spread. The most important are *CT scanning*, *MRI*, special *X-ray* studies, and *angiography*.

TREATMENT
When possible, tumours are removed by surgery after opening the skull (see *Craniotomy*), but many malignant growths are inaccessible or too extensive for removal. The outlook in these cases is poor; fewer than 20 per cent of patients survive for a year after the initial diagnosis. In cases where a tumour cannot be completely removed, as much as possible of it will be cut away to relieve pressure in the brain. *Radiotherapy* or *anticancer drugs* may also be given.

Corticosteroid drugs are often prescribed to reduce the swelling of tissue around a tumour, thus temporarily relieving symptoms.

Bran

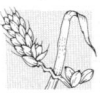

The fibrous outer covering of grain. Eating bran regularly, either in breakfast cereals or added to food, raises the *fibre* content of the diet. This helps prevent *constipation* and thus reduces the risk of intestinal disease.

Branchial disorders

A group of disorders resulting from abnormal development of the branchial arches in the *embryo*. Branchial disorders include branchial cyst and branchial fistula.

A branchial cyst is a soft swelling, about 2 to 5 cm across, that appears on the side of the neck in early adult life. The swelling contains a pus-like or clear fluid that is rich in cholesterol. Diagnosis is made by identifying cholesterol crystals in a few drops of the fluid drawn from the cyst by means of a needle and syringe. Treatment is by surgical removal.

A branchial fistula is an abnormal passage between the back of the throat and the external surface of the neck, where it appears as a small hole usually noted at birth. If the hole in the neck does not extend to the back of the throat, it is termed a branchial cleft sinus; it may be present at birth or may form if a branchial cyst becomes infected and ruptures. A branchial fistula or cleft sinus may discharge mucus or pus, in which case the fistula or sinus may be removed surgically.

Brash, water

See *Waterbrash*.

Braxton Hicks' contractions

Short, relatively painless contractions of the uterus during pregnancy. In early pregnancy, Braxton Hicks' contractions may be felt by a doctor performing an internal examination. In late pregnancy, they may be felt by the woman and seen by looking at the abdomen. Sometimes they are mistaken for labour pains, although they occur as isolated contractions, have no effect on the cervix, and are not as uncomfortable as the contractions of true labour.

Breakbone fever

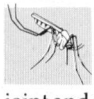 A tropical, mosquito-spread, viral illness also called *dengue*. One symptom of the illness is severe joint and muscle pain, hence the name "breakbone".

Breakthrough bleeding

Vaginal bleeding or staining ("spotting") between menstrual periods when taking an *oral contraceptive*, especially a low-dose preparation. Breakthrough bleeding is most common during the first few months of taking the pill, when the body is adjusting to alterations in hormone levels. Loss of blood during pregnancy, or when an oral contraceptive is not being taken, may be a symptom of a serious underlying disorder (see *Vaginal bleeding*).

Breast

In addition to its primary function of nourishing a baby with milk, the female breast is a secondary *sexual characteristic*, and is regarded by society as a symbol of femininity, beauty, and eroticism. The size, shape, and appearance of breasts vary from one woman to another. The male breast is an immature version of the female breast.

STRUCTURE

The female breast consists mainly of 15 to 20 lobes of milk-secreting glands embedded in fatty tissue. The ducts of these glands have their outlet in the nipple, which is surrounded by the areola, the circular area of pigmented skin. The breast contains no muscle, but bands of fine ligaments that weave between the fat and lobules are attached to the skin and determine the breast's height and shape.

The skin over the breast is somewhat smoother, thinner, and more translucent than over much of the rest of the body. The areola skin is particularly thin, and contains sweat glands, sebaceous glands, and hair follicles.

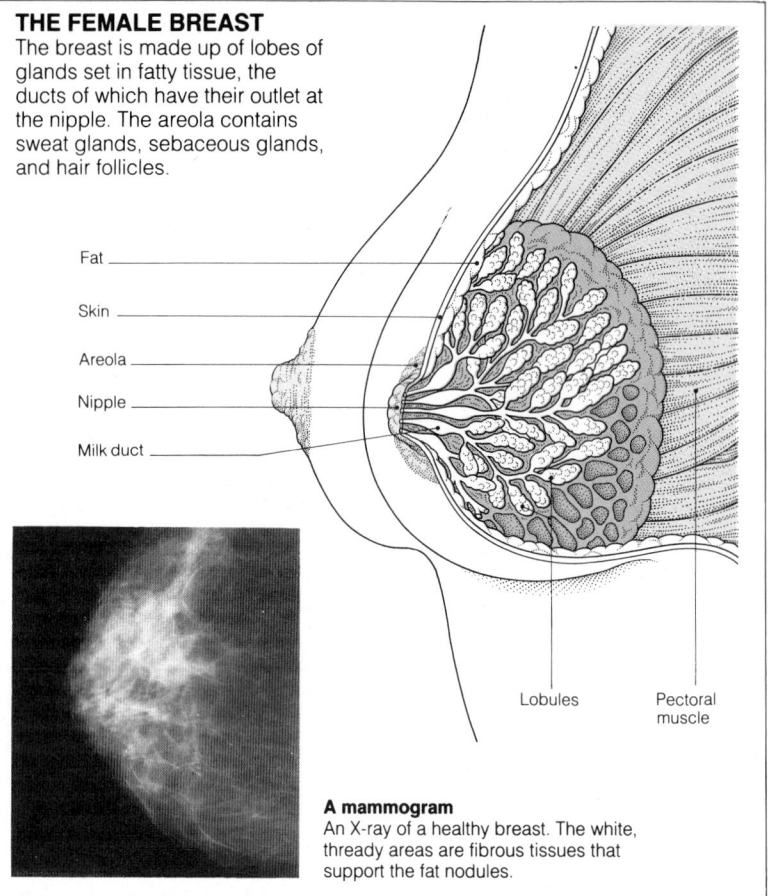

THE FEMALE BREAST

The breast is made up of lobes of glands set in fatty tissue, the ducts of which have their outlet at the nipple. The areola contains sweat glands, sebaceous glands, and hair follicles.

Fat

Skin

Areola

Nipple

Milk duct

Lobules

Pectoral muscle

A mammogram
An X-ray of a healthy breast. The white, thready areas are fibrous tissues that support the fat nodules.

The nipple is very sensitive to touch; contraction of its muscle fibres results in erection, which is a sign of sexual arousal or cold.

The size and shape of the breasts of mature women not only vary between individuals, but also at different times—during the menstrual cycle, during pregnancy and lactation, and after the menopause.

FUNCTION

During pregnancy, oestrogen and progesterone, secreted by the ovary and placenta, cause the milk-producing glands to develop and become active and the nipple to enlarge in preparation for *breast-feeding*. Just before or after childbirth the glands in the breast produce a watery fluid called colostrum, which contains proteins and antibodies to protect the newborn baby against infection. Within about three days the colostrum is replaced with milk, whose production is stimulated by the hormone prolactin, released from the anterior pituitary gland.

BREAST DEVELOPMENT

The breasts start to grow from mammary buds when the fetus is about five months old. At birth there is a nipple with rudimentary milk ducts. At *puberty*, a girl's breasts begin to develop—the areola swells and the nipple enlarges. This is followed by an increase in glandular tissue and fat, which enlarge the breast. Eventually, the breast becomes rounded and the areola flattens.

Breast abscess

A collection of pus in the mammary gland, usually in a woman who is lactating (producing milk). Breast abscesses develop if acute *mastitis* (inflammation of the breast, usually due to infection) is not treated promptly with *antibiotic drugs*. They occur most commonly during the first month after a woman's first delivery.

SYMPTOMS

The initial symptoms are of acute mastitis: the breasts become increasingly tense and tender, and the woman may also develop fever and chills. The abscess develops in one area, which becomes very firm, red, and extremely painful.

TREATMENT AND PREVENTION

Simple *analgesic drugs*, such as paracetamol, provide some pain relief. The abscess is treated by surgical incision and drainage of the pus under general anaesthesia. Breast infections can be prevented by cleaning and drying the breasts carefully after each feed. Breast abscesses are less likely to occur if the breasts are emptied regularly, making engorgement (overfilling) and the development of mastitis less likely.

Breastbone

A common name for the *sternum*.

Breast cancer

The most common cancer in women. One woman in every 14 will develop breast cancer at some time in their lives. More than half of these will die from the disease. Around 14,000 women, most of whom are over 65, die from breast cancer each year in England and Wales.

The incidence of breast cancer has increased slightly but steadily—by around 1 per cent each year—in western countries this century.

Mortality from breast cancer (taking account of age) has hardly changed, but, in the early 1980s, research in Sweden and the Netherlands suggested that deaths could be cut by about one third by mammographic screening of whole populations of women. Other studies indicate the great importance of breast examination by women and their doctors in diagnosing breast cancer in its early stages: most deaths occur because the disease has already spread beyond the breast when first detected.

CAUSES

Current theories of the cause of breast cancer are focused on genetic and hormonal influences. Breast cancer in women under the age of 50 is often linked to genetic factors. Women with two relatives who have developed the disease in their thirties or forties are at increased risk and should consult a genetic specialist, who may advise annual mammographic screening or other tests. The incidence of breast cancer is known to be raised in women whose menstrual periods began at an early age and whose menopause was late; in those who had no children or had their first child in their late 20s or 30s; and in those with mothers or sisters who had breast cancer. Diet also plays a part. The disease is rare in Japan, which has a low-fat diet, but Japanese women living in the US and eating an American diet have the same rate of breast cancer as Americans. Tall, heavy women have more breast cancer than short, thin ones. Breast cancer may also be more common in women who have had certain types of nonmalignant tumours removed.

Several research studies in the late 1980s suggested that prolonged use of oral contraceptives might increase the risk of a woman's developing breast cancer before the age of 35. Such tumours are, however, rare so if there is any increase in breast cancer due to the pill, the overall effect is small. Furthermore the risk is balanced by the pill's effect in lowering the incidence of cancer of the ovary and uterus. The introduction of the pill, 25 years ago, does not seem to have affected the slight but steady rise in breast cancer in Europe and North America this century.

SYMPTOMS

The most common site of a malignant breast tumour is the upper, outer part of the breast. The lump is usually felt rather than seen and in most cases is not painful. Other symptoms include a dark discharge from the nipple, retraction (indentation) of the nipple, and an area of dimpled, creased skin over the lump. In 90 per cent of the cases only one breast is affected.

DIAGNOSIS

Monthly examination of the breasts (see *Breast self-examination*) has not been shown to reduce mortality from breast cancer but it does allow detection of any changes in the breast and nipples at an early stage. Mammography is available through the NHS to women aged 50 to 65 and to younger women with the disease in the family. Private clinics offer mammography on request. Research studies have consistently shown that mammography

---

DISORDERS OF THE BREAST

Problems involving the breasts are usually minor and respond readily to treatment. The most important causes of problems are infection, tumours, and hormonal disturbance.

INFECTION

This is uncommon except during breast-feeding. Nursing mothers may suffer from *mastitis* (inflammation of the breast), usually due to a blocked milk duct. An *abscess* may follow if mastitis is not treated.

TUMOURS

A *breast lump* may be a *cyst* (a fluid-filled sac), a *fibroadenoma* (a thickening of the milk-producing tissue) or other benign tumour, or more rarely, *breast cancer*.

HORMONAL DISORDERS

It is common for women to notice that before *menstruation* their breasts become bigger and lumpy. Such lumps shrink when menstruation is over. More common are breast pain and tenderness, which often occur just before menstruation or as a result of taking hormones. Hormonal disorders may, rarely, cause *galactorrhoea* (abnormal milk production).

In men, *gynaecomastia* (abnormal breast development) may result from hormonal disturbance or treatment with certain drugs.

INVESTIGATION

Disorders of the breast may be discovered during *breast self-examination* or by your doctor during a physical examination. Special investigations for the breast are *biopsy* and *mammography*.

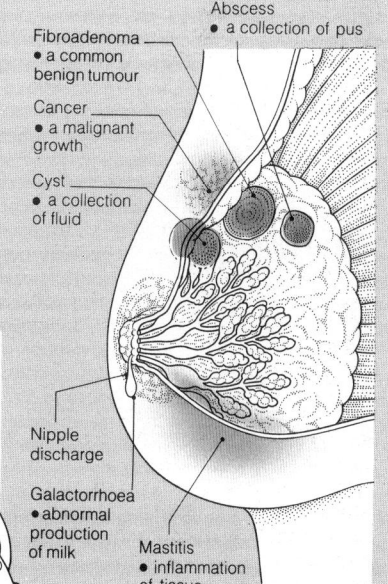

Fibroadenoma
• a common benign tumour

Cancer
• a malignant growth

Cyst
• a collection of fluid

Abscess
• a collection of pus

Nipple discharge

Galactorrhoea
• abnormal production of milk

Mastitis
• inflammation of tissue

reduces mortality from breast cancer in women over 50 but no such benefit has been shown in younger women.

A woman who discovers a lump in her breast should report it to her doctor immediately. A mammogram may be appropriate at this time. If the doctor suspects that the lump is merely a *cyst* (a fluid-filled tissue sac), it can be aspirated (i.e. the fluid can be withdrawn) and may disappear completely. Where there is a possibility that the lump may be a malignant tumour, a *biopsy* will be carried out. This may be an outpatient procedure in which breast tissue is withdrawn with a hollow needle, causing little discomfort, or an operation to remove all or part of the lump; in either case the suspect tissue will be examined under the microscope.

If cancer is discovered, blood tests, X-rays, and scanning will determine whether the disease has spread to other parts of the body, such as the bones or liver.

TREATMENT

Surgical removal of the tumour achieves a cure (as defined by survival for 20 years) in one third of women with breast cancer. Studies have shown survival is not improved by extensive operations (such as radical *mastectomy*); many surgeons recommend lumpectomy (simple removal of the tumour), combined with *radiotherapy* and/or *anticancer drugs*. The treatment given depends on the woman's age, the size of the tumour, whether or not there are signs of spread to the lymph nodes under the arm, and the sensitivity of the tumour cells to hormones as determined in the laboratory by a technique called oestrogen receptor testing.

Secondary tumors in other parts of the body, which may be present at the time of the initial diagnosis or may develop years after apparently successful treatment, are treated with anticancer drugs and hormones. Such treatment usually relieves symptoms and prolongs life.

OUTLOOK

If cancer is treated early, the outlook is optimistic; either a complete cure or years of good health can be expected. Regular check-ups are needed to detect any recurrence or cancer in the other breast. Breast self-examination should be carried out monthly and mammograms should be performed periodically. If the cancer recurs, it can be controlled for years by drugs, radiotherapy, and, in some cases, further surgery.

Breast enlargement
See *Mammoplasty*.

Breast-feeding
The natural method of infant feeding from birth to weaning. Human milk contains the ideal balance of nutrients for the human baby and provides valuable antibodies to protect the child against infections, such as *gastroenteritis*. Breast-feeding also provides the mother and child with a physical closeness that strengthens the bond between them.

HOW TO BREAST-FEED

Ideally, the baby should be put to the breast as soon after delivery as possible. Once sucking has begun, the mother should ensure that the whole of the areola (the dark area around the nipple) is in the baby's mouth. This helps to stimulate the milk flow and can prevent soreness caused by the baby chewing on the nipple. In the first few days after birth, the baby should be encouraged to suck frequently, but for only a few minutes at a time. This provides him or her with valuable colostrum, and also stimulates the breasts so that a consistent and plentiful milk supply is established. During the first few weeks a baby should be fed on demand to make sure that the milk supply is maintained. Babies may want to feed from once every hour or two, to once every three or four hours.

PROBLEMS

Engorged breasts are common in early lactation; they are uncomfortable and can prevent the baby from sucking properly. Expression of milk, either manually or with a *breast pump*, usually solves the problem.

Sore or cracked nipples, often a problem in the early weeks, may be relieved by using a nipple shield. Alternatively, the milk may be expressed and given by bottle.

A possible complication of breast-feeding is infection leading to an abscess, indicated by soreness and inflammation on the surface of the breast. Early treatment with *antibiotic drugs* may mean that breast-feeding can continue.

Sometimes breast-feeding problems have an emotional basis. A few women regard their breasts as having a primarily sexual function and find the whole feeding process distasteful. Others fear feeding may spoil the shape of their breasts and may resent the intensive commitment to the child that breast-feeding requires.

A woman whose baby always seems unsatisfied after feeds may doubt the quality or quantity of her milk. If she is in good health, eating a nutritious diet, and getting enough rest, then her milk supply should be adequate, and she may simply need reassurance and encouragement.

MANAGING BREAST-FEEDING

The mother should wear comfortable, loose, front-opening clothes and a nursing bra that provides good support. She should rest her back, firmly cradling the baby in the crook of her arm, with the baby's head well above stomach level.

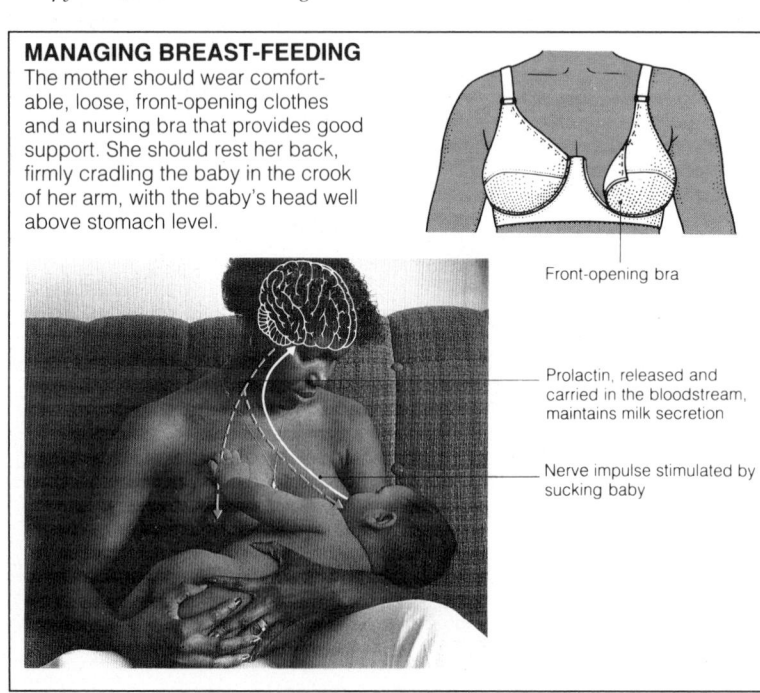

Front-opening bra

Prolactin, released and carried in the bloodstream, maintains milk secretion

Nerve impulse stimulated by sucking baby

Sometimes, despite continuing efforts by the mother, the baby remains hungry or the process of feeding is painful. A change to *bottle-feeding* or supplementing the breast with the bottle is the likely answer, and should not be seen as failure or a reason for guilt. (See also *Feeding, infant.*)

Breast lump

Any mass, cyst, or swelling that can be felt in the breast tissue. At least 80 per cent of lumps are benign; the remainder are malignant (see *Breast cancer*). All breast lumps need to be checked by a doctor.

CAUSES AND TYPES

The most common cause of a breast lump is *fibroadenosis* (also known as chronic mastitis or fibrocystic disease), in which one or more cysts (fluid-filled tissue sacs) develop. Occurring mainly between the ages of 30 and 50, fibrocystic disease usually causes one or both breasts to become lumpy and tender in the week or so before a menstrual period starts.

Another common cause of a breast lump is found most often in young women and usually results in a single lump called a *fibroadenoma*. This benign growth is usually round, firm, and rubbery, causes no pain, and can be moved about beneath the skin using the fingertips.

There are also several less common forms of breast lump: breast cancer, lipoma, intraductal papilloma, and cystosarcoma phylloides.

A lipoma is a benign, painless tumour, made up of fatty tissue, that sometimes changes the size and shape of the breast.

An intraductal papilloma is a wart-like growth within a duct of the milk-producing glands. The most common symptom is a discharge from the nipple; the discharge may be clear, dark or bloody. There may also be a pea-sized lump beneath the nipple. Intraductal papillomas are harmless but may become malignant.

A cystosarcoma phylloides is a rare tumour of connective tissue that can grow to an enormous size very quickly. It is usually benign and only rarely becomes malignant.

SEEKING MEDICAL ADVICE

All women should examine their breasts regularly each month (see *Breast self-examination*) to detect any significant changes. If a new lump or any change in a long-standing lump is detected, or if there is any discharge from a nipple, it should be reported to a doctor.

DIAGNOSIS AND TREATMENT

Since a physical examination cannot reveal whether or not a growth is benign, *mammography* and/or *biopsy* (analysis of a sample of tissue removed either by needle aspiration or by surgery) will be arranged.

Cysts can be drained in a simple outpatient procedure. Other lumps can be removed surgically. (For the treatment of malignant tumours, see *Breast cancer.*)

Breast pump

A simple device, consisting of a rubber bulb and a glass or plastic tube and reservoir, that is used to draw milk from the breasts. The pump is used to relieve overfull breasts during early lactation and to express milk for future use. Most pumps are hand-operated, although an electrically operated version is also available.

Breast reconstruction
See *Mammoplasty.*

Breast reduction
See *Mammoplasty.*

Breast self-examination

A visual and manual examination of the breasts carried out by a woman to detect lumps and other changes that might indicate the presence of early breast cancer. Although *mammography*

EXAMINING YOUR BREASTS

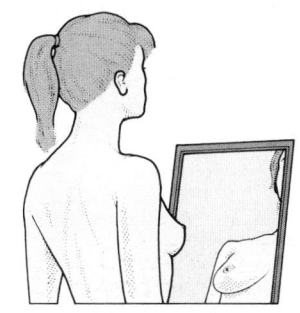

1 Once a month after your period, examine your breasts. With arms by your side, look in a mirror and get to know their general appearance, shape, and size. Be alert to changes.

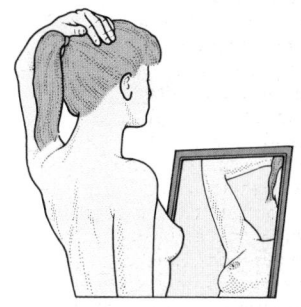

2 Raise each arm in turn above your head, looking for changes in appearance. Turn from side to side, looking at the outline of the breasts for any changes.

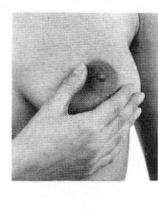

3 Gently squeeze the nipples to see whether there is any discharge.

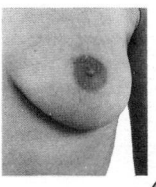

4 Examine the skin surface for peculiarities. Orange-peel texture could indicate the presence of a lump.

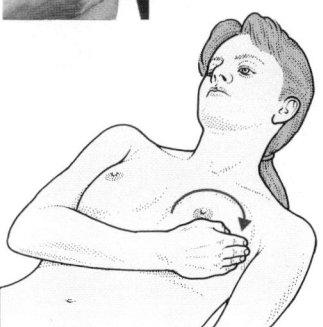

5 Lie on your back with a pillow under your shoulders and head, one arm by your side. Using the flat of your hand, work around the outer parts of the breast in a clockwise direction.

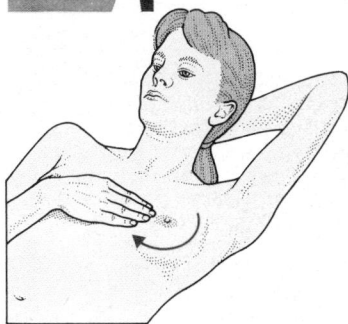

6 Raise your arm above your head and examine the inner parts of the breast. Stretching the tissue makes detection of lumps easier. Feel also along the top of the collarbone and into the armpit.

B

(breast X-ray) has been shown to be more effective in reducing mortality from breast cancer, self-examination allows early detection of all kinds of breast disease and should be carried out at about the same time every month.

WHY IT IS DONE

Breast cancer is the leading cause of death among women aged 35 to 54 years. It is curable, however, if diagnosed at an early stage. Self-examination allows early changes and small lumps (less than 1 cm in diameter) to be detected, and enables treatment to be undertaken when the chances of cure are greatest.

Breast tenderness

Soreness or tenderness of the breasts, often accompanied by a feeling of fullness in one or both breasts. Breast tenderness is relatively common just before menstruation (see *Premenstrual syndrome*), in early pregnancy, or during lactation.

Most cases of breast tenderness are thought to be due to hormonal changes (particularly increased levels of oestrogen or progesterone) affecting the cells of the breast, causing them to retain excess fluid. This explains why *oral contraceptives* cause, or make worse, breast tenderness in some women. Conversely, very low dose oral contraceptives may reduce breast tenderness in some women.

Tenderness during lactation may be due to engorgement with milk or to *mastitis* (inflammation of breast tissue as a result of infection).

At other times, and in the absence of other symptoms (such as a *breast lump*, *nipple discharge*, or hot, inflamed skin over the breast), breast tenderness is unlikely to be due to a serious underlying disorder. *Breast cancer* is usually painless.

Breath-holding attacks

Periods during which an infant or toddler holds his or her breath, usually as an expression of pain, frustration, or anger. It is thought that children may unconsciously bring on these attacks to exert control over their parents.

The child usually begins to cry, expels air from the lungs, and then holds his or her breath, becoming red or even blue in the face after a few seconds. The child may faint temporarily, but breathing quickly resumes as a natural reflex, ending the attack. Breath-holding sometimes results in twitching that resembles a seizure. Although breath-holding attacks may

be alarming to parents, they are usually harmless.

CAUSES AND INCIDENCE

Breath-holding attacks occur in one to two per cent of toddlers. They are most common between the ages of one and two years, particularly in children with determined personalities. Children at this age are just beginning to see themselves as individuals and are trying to determine the extent of their power over the environment. They may quickly learn that breath-holding attacks annoy or frighten parents, and may use them as a means of manipulation.

MANAGEMENT

Breath-holding attacks should be ignored as far as possible. If the child is rewarded by gaining increased attention from parents, then he or she will continue to have the attacks. As soon as the child realizes there is nothing to be gained, the attacks will stop. Firm, patient, and consistent handling will help prevent attacks. Parents who are anxious about their child's breath-holding should consult a doctor for advice, but attacks will usually stop in any case by the time the child is four.

Breathing

The process by which air passes into and out of the lungs to allow the blood to take up oxygen and dispose of carbon dioxide. Breathing is controlled by the respiratory centre in the brainstem; no conscious effort is needed to inhale and exhale air, but the depth and rate of breathing can be altered voluntarily.

During exercise, when the heart and muscles need more oxygen, reflexes lead to a rapid increase in the breathing rate. This can vary in an adult from 13 to 17 breaths per minute at rest up to 80 breaths per minute during vigorous exercise. A newborn baby breathes at a rate of approximately 40 breaths per minute.

HOW AIR ENTERS THE LUNGS

When air is inhaled (inspiration), the diaphragm, which is dome-shaped when relaxed, contracts and flattens. The muscles between the ribs contract and pull the rib-cage upwards and outwards. This movement increases chest volume, causing the lungs to expand and suck in air. When air is exhaled (expiration), the chest mus-

---

BREATHING

Inhalation and exhalation occur between 13 and 17 times a minute at rest, and up to 80 times a minute during vigorous exertion. A normal, resting inhalation takes in about 400 ml of air; a deep breath, up to 4 litres.

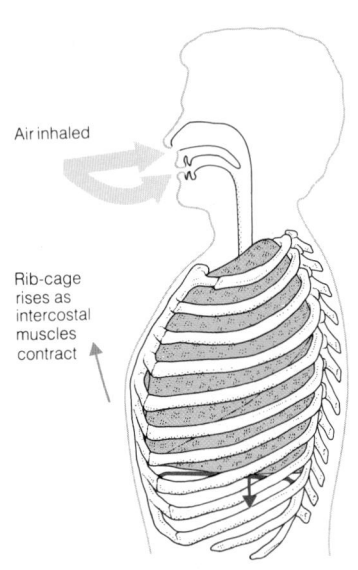

Air inhaled

Rib-cage rises as intercostal muscles contract

Diaphragm contracts

Inhalation
Air is drawn into the lungs as the intercostal muscles (between the ribs) contract, causing the rib-cage to rise, and the diaphragm contracts and flattens.

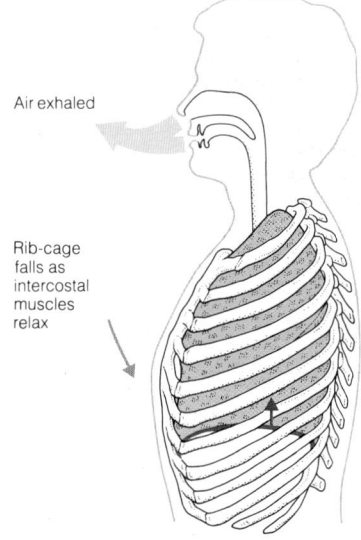

Air exhaled

Rib-cage falls as intercostal muscles relax

Diaphragm relaxes

Exhalation
Air is expelled from the lungs as the intercostal muscles relax, causing the rib-cage to fall, and the diaphragm relaxes and resumes its domed shape.

cles and diaphragm relax, causing the rib-cage to sink and the lungs to contract, squeezing out air.

The lungs do not fill completely during inhalation or empty completely during exhalation. In normal, quiet breathing, only about one tenth of the air in the lungs passes out to be replaced by the same amount of fresh air. This new air (tidal volume), mixes with the stale air (residual volume) already held in the lungs.

A man's lungs hold up to about 6 litres of air, and a woman's lungs about 4.25 litres. At rest, about 400 ml of air is taken into the lungs during normal inspiration; a deep breath can take in as much as 3 to 4 litres of air. (See also *Respiration*.)

Breathing difficulty

Distressed breathing that includes a change in the rate and depth of breathing. Breathing difficulty may occur when the effort required to breathe is increased, or when breathing movements are causing pain. Symptoms that may accompany breathing difficulty include a feeling of tightness in the chest, coughing, wheezing, or chest pain.

CAUSES

Breathing difficulty may be caused by any condition that affects the flow of air into and out of the lungs, the transfer of oxygen from lungs to the blood, the circulation of blood through the lungs, or control of breathing by the brainstem. Breathing difficulty can occur either at rest, or when more oxygen is needed by the body during exercise or illness.

LACK OF FITNESS The heart and lungs of an unfit person cannot respond adequately when there is an increased need for oxygen, so the increased effort needed to breathe causes discomfort. This problem can be overcome by fitness training.

EXCESS WEIGHT Overweight people often experience difficulty in breathing during exertion; this occurs partly because they are unfit and partly because of the increased effort needed to carry their excess weight. In Pickwickian syndrome, the breathing centre in the brainstem of very obese people does not function efficiently, which results in irregular patterns of breathing.

ANXIETY Severe anxiety during times of stress or tension can bring on attacks of *hyperventilation*. These attacks are associated with a feeling that it is impossible to get a good breath, which in turn leads to further overbreathing.

BRAINSTEM DAMAGE Damage to the breathing centre in the brainstem due to a *stroke* or a *head injury* can reduce or increase breathing activity. This may also happen as a side-effect of certain drugs. In certain instances, breathing may need *ventilator* assistance.

ALTITUDE Being at high altitude can cause a person to become breathless because there is less oxygen present in the surrounding air, making it necessary for the lungs to work harder to provide the body with sufficient oxygen. Swelling of the brain and fluid in the lungs are serious features of altitude sickness (see *Mountain sickness*).

ANAEMIA In all types of anaemia, there is insufficient *haemoglobin* to carry oxygen around the body. If anaemia is severe, the lungs need to work harder to supply the body with oxygen, resulting in breathlessness.

CIRCULATION DISORDERS Breathing difficulty intensified upon exertion may be caused by a reduced circulation of blood through the lungs. This may be due to *heart failure* (reduced pumping efficiency of the heart), to *pulmonary embolism* (blockage of blood vessels in the lungs by blood clots), or to *pulmonary hypertension* (increased pressure in the arteries in the lungs).

AIRWAYS BLOCKAGE Breathing difficulty due to air-flow obstruction may be caused by chronic *bronchitis* (in which mucus and thickened walls block the airways), by *asthma* or an allergic reaction (in which there is narrowing of the air passages), or by *lung cancer* (if the tumour blocks a large airway).

LUNG DAMAGE Breathing difficulty may also be due to inefficient transfer of oxygen from the lungs into the bloodstream. Temporary damage to lung tissue may be due to *pneumonia, pneumothorax* (collapsed lung), *pulmonary oedema* (fluid in the lung), or *pleural effusion* (fluid around the lung). Permanent lung damage may be due to *emphysema*, a condition in which the walls of the *alveoli* (small air sacs in the lungs) are destroyed.

PAIN Any pain in the chest that is made worse by chest or lung movement can make normal breathing difficult and painful. A fractured rib, for example, results in pain at the fracture site during breathing or movement of the torso. *Pleurisy* is associated with pain in the lower chest and often in the shoulder tip of the affected side.

SKELETAL DISORDERS Abnormalities of the skeletal structure of the thorax (chest), such as severe *scoliosis* or *kyphosis* (conditions in which there are abnormal curvatures of the spine), may cause breathing difficulty by impairing normal movements of the rib-cage.

Breathing exercises

Techniques for learning to control the rate and depth of breathing. Breathing exercises are used for therapeutic purposes and to aid in *relaxation*.

WHY THEY ARE DONE

PHYSIOTHERAPY Breathing exercises are sometimes recommended for people with chronic chest diseases, such as chronic *bronchitis*. They can also help people with *anxiety disorders* who breathe too deeply and rapidly and as a result disturb the chemical make-up of their blood.

Breathing exercises are important after surgery, because post-operative patients often breathe shallowly and avoid coughing because of pain. In these circumstances, poor air exchange and the build-up of secretions can lead to collapse of segments of the lung or to collapse of a lobe of the lung, particularly in patients who are overweight or who smoke. Deep breathing promotes coughing and keeps the lungs clear.

RELAXATION In *yoga*, deep rhythmic breathing is used to achieve a state of relaxation. During *childbirth*, breathing exercises relax the mother and also help to control contractions and reduce pain.

HOW THEY ARE DONE

Breathing exercises aim to teach people to inhale through the nose, while expanding the chest, and then to exhale fully through the mouth, while contracting the abdominal muscles. (See also *Physiotherapy*.)

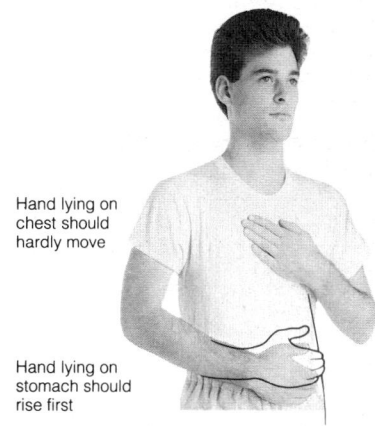

Hand lying on chest should hardly move

Hand lying on stomach should rise first

Practising breathing
This exercise can be done unsupervised. A second person may apply gentle pressure to the chest or abdomen to help you become aware of the muscle groups used.

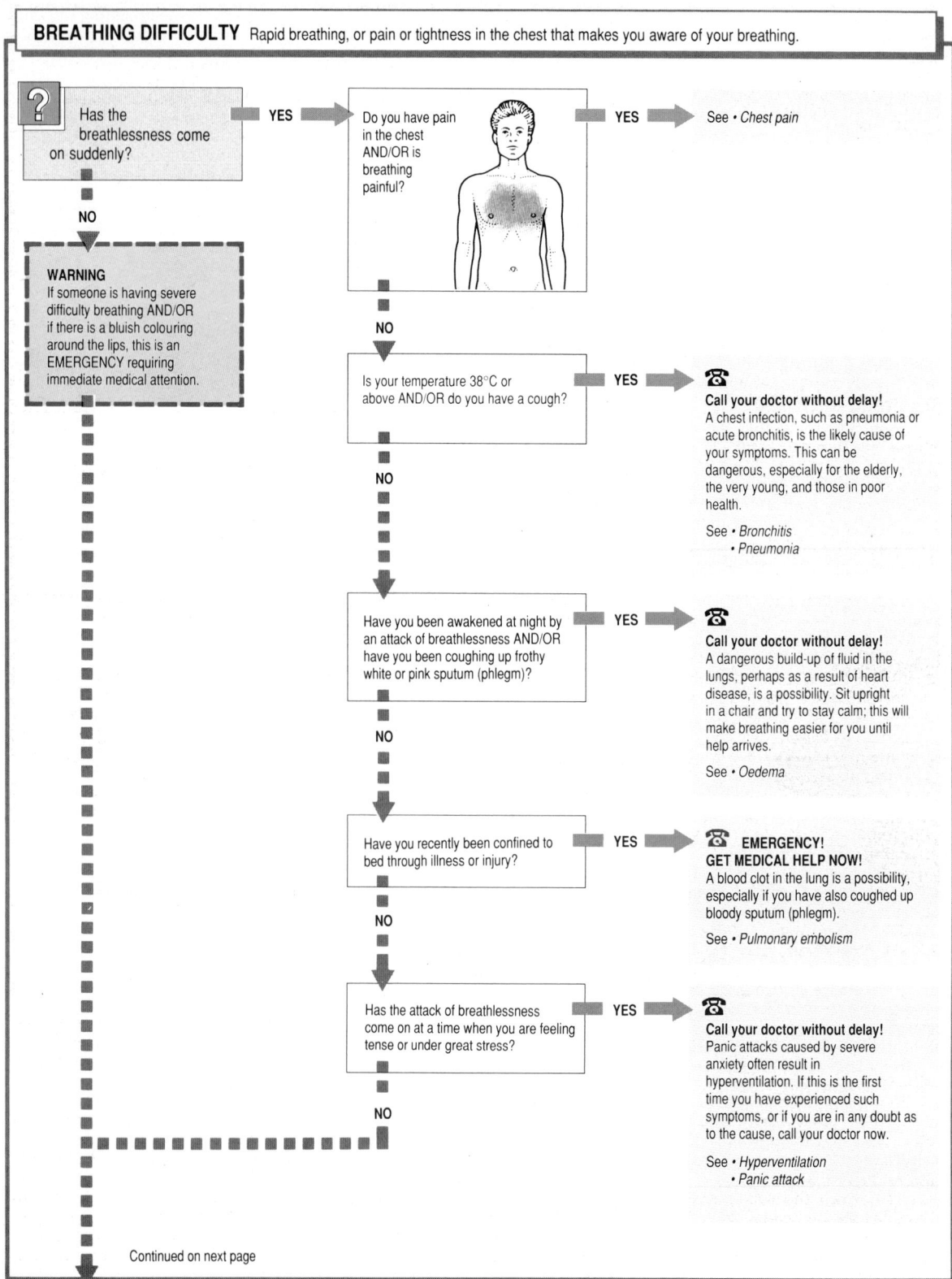

BREATHING DIFFICULTY Rapid breathing, or pain or tightness in the chest that makes you aware of your breathing.

Has the breathlessness come on suddenly?

YES → **Do you have pain in the chest AND/OR is breathing painful?**

YES → See • *Chest pain*

NO ↓

WARNING
If someone is having severe difficulty breathing AND/OR if there is a bluish colouring around the lips, this is an EMERGENCY requiring immediate medical attention.

NO ↓ (from chest pain question)

Is your temperature 38°C or above AND/OR do you have a cough?

YES → ☎ **Call your doctor without delay!**
A chest infection, such as pneumonia or acute bronchitis, is the likely cause of your symptoms. This can be dangerous, especially for the elderly, the very young, and those in poor health.

See • *Bronchitis*
      • *Pneumonia*

NO ↓

Have you been awakened at night by an attack of breathlessness AND/OR have you been coughing up frothy white or pink sputum (phlegm)?

YES → ☎ **Call your doctor without delay!**
A dangerous build-up of fluid in the lungs, perhaps as a result of heart disease, is a possibility. Sit upright in a chair and try to stay calm; this will make breathing easier for you until help arrives.

See • *Oedema*

NO ↓

Have you recently been confined to bed through illness or injury?

YES → ☎ **EMERGENCY!**
GET MEDICAL HELP NOW!
A blood clot in the lung is a possibility, especially if you have also coughed up bloody sputum (phlegm).

See • *Pulmonary embolism*

NO ↓

Has the attack of breathlessness come on at a time when you are feeling tense or under great stress?

YES → ☎ **Call your doctor without delay!**
Panic attacks caused by severe anxiety often result in hyperventilation. If this is the first time you have experienced such symptoms, or if you are in any doubt as to the cause, call your doctor now.

See • *Hyperventilation*
      • *Panic attack*

NO

Continued on next page

B

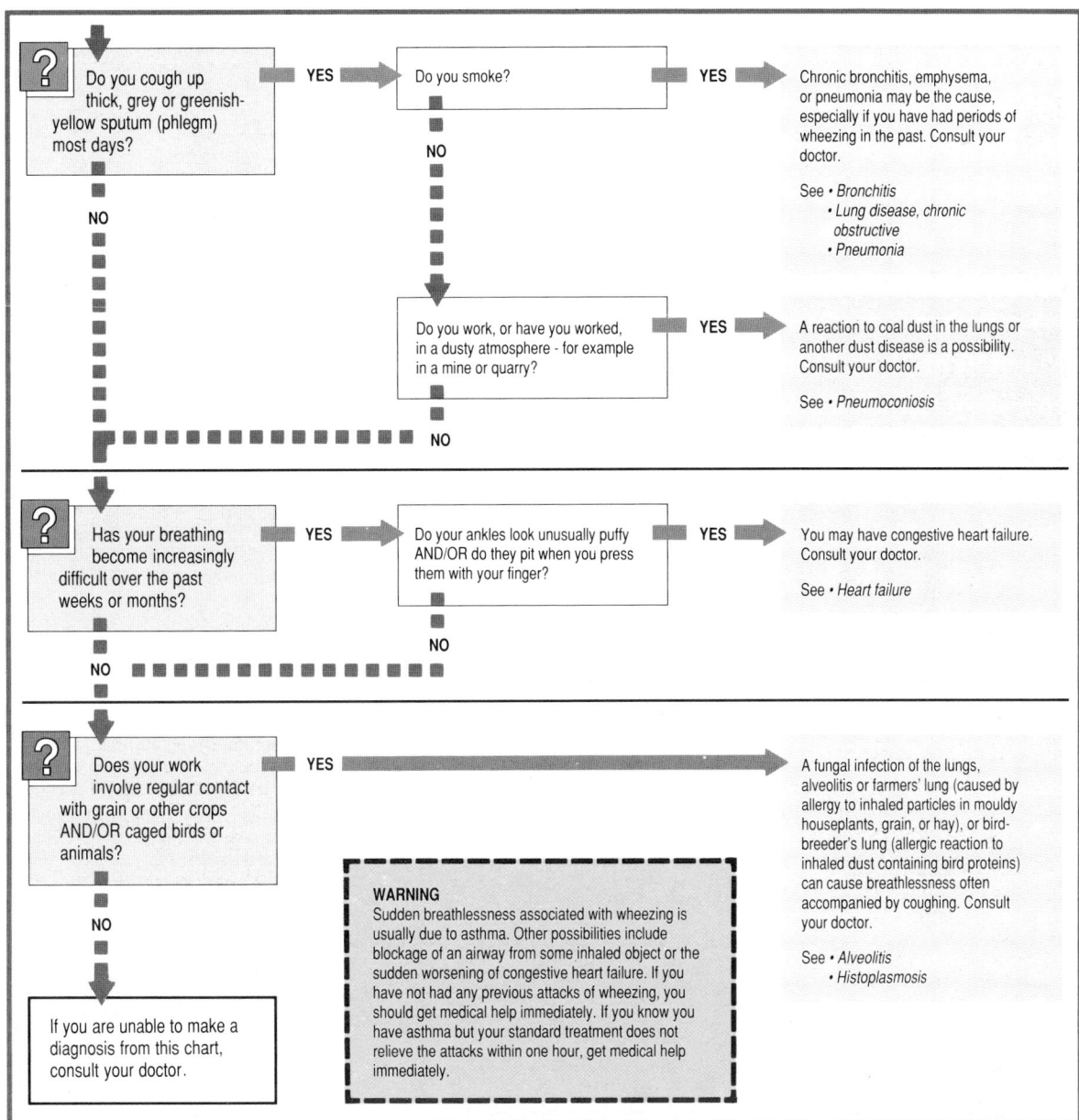

Do you cough up thick, grey or greenish-yellow sputum (phlegm) most days?

YES → Do you smoke?

YES → Chronic bronchitis, emphysema, or pneumonia may be the cause, especially if you have had periods of wheezing in the past. Consult your doctor.

See • *Bronchitis*
• *Lung disease, chronic obstructive*
• *Pneumonia*

NO → Do you work, or have you worked, in a dusty atmosphere - for example in a mine or quarry?

YES → A reaction to coal dust in the lungs or another dust disease is a possibility. Consult your doctor.

See • *Pneumoconiosis*

NO

Has your breathing become increasingly difficult over the past weeks or months?

YES → Do your ankles look unusually puffy AND/OR do they pit when you press them with your finger?

YES → You may have congestive heart failure. Consult your doctor.

See • *Heart failure*

NO

Does your work involve regular contact with grain or other crops AND/OR caged birds or animals?

YES → A fungal infection of the lungs, alveolitis or farmers' lung (caused by allergy to inhaled particles in mouldy houseplants, grain, or hay), or bird-breeder's lung (allergic reaction to inhaled dust containing bird proteins) can cause breathlessness often accompanied by coughing. Consult your doctor.

See • *Alveolitis*
• *Histoplasmosis*

NO

WARNING
Sudden breathlessness associated with wheezing is usually due to asthma. Other possibilities include blockage of an airway from some inhaled object or the sudden worsening of congestive heart failure. If you have not had any previous attacks of wheezing, you should get medical help immediately. If you know you have asthma but your standard treatment does not relieve the attacks within one hour, get medical help immediately.

If you are unable to make a diagnosis from this chart, consult your doctor.

Breathlessness

Rapid, shallow breathing to provide the body with sufficient oxygen. Breathlessness occurs as a normal response to exercise or exertion. It may also occur as a result of some underlying disorder (see *Breathing difficulty*).

Breech delivery

A birth in which the baby's bottom emerges before the head.

By around the 32nd week of pregnancy, most babies have assumed a head-down position in the uterus, but about three to four per cent take up a breech presentation, with the head at the top of the uterus. Often, one of two twins may present as a breech. At 34 weeks, some obstetricians try to turn a baby with a breech presentation into the head-down position.

If this attempt fails, the baby is left in the breech presentation until delivery. A breech delivery adds to the problems of both mother and baby because the baby's bottom does not push its way through the birth canal as efficiently as the head. Usually, an *episiotomy* is performed to ease the baby's passage, and obstetric *forceps* are commonly used to ensure smooth emergence of the head.

If a baby with a breech presentation has a large head or if the mother's pelvic girdle is small, delivery by *caesarean section* may be decided upon before she goes into labour. Some obstetricians recommend caesarean section for most breech babies, particularly if the baby is a footling presentation (feet-first) or if a woman has not had a previous vaginal delivery, as there is an increased risk of *birth injury*. In other instances, the decision regarding caesarean section is based on the results of investigations including *X-rays* and *fetal heart monitoring*.

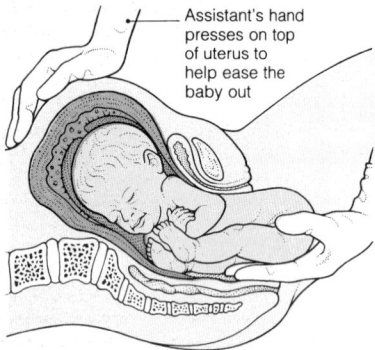

Delivering a breech baby
The buttocks are delivered first and then the legs. An episiotomy may be performed before the head is delivered.

Bridge, dental

False teeth (usually no more than four) attached to natural teeth on either side of a gap left by a missing tooth or teeth. A bridge is fitted to enable the person to bite properly and to speak clearly, and to avoid problems resulting from shifting or drifting of the remaining natural teeth.

Bridges for the front of the mouth are usually made of gold alloy faced with porcelain. Bridges for the back of

the mouth are commonly made of gold or gold alloy without a facing. Unlike a *denture*, a bridge has no baseplate (artificial gum) and cannot be removed by the wearer.

Bright's disease

Another name for *glomerulonephritis*, a kidney disease that was first described by Dr. Richard Bright (1789-1858), a doctor at Guy's Hospital, London.

British Dental Association

The professional association for dentists in the UK, founded in 1880, which acts as the spokesman and negotiator for the dental profession. Membership of the British Dental Association (BDA) is voluntary and is open to any dentist.

The BDA is a registered trade union and its main function is to negotiate with the government, via the Department of Health and appropriate ministers, on terms and conditions of service for dentists.

Through its publications and meetings, the BDA also plays an educational role and keeps its members up-to-date on all matters relating to dentistry. The "British Dental Journal" provides information on clinical and scientific topics. A newspaper, "BDA News", concentrates on political matters (such as fees for check-ups).

The BDA is not the regulating body for dentists. This responsibility

is held by the General Dental Council, which determines whether a dentist can practice and investigates complaints against dentists.

British Medical Association

The professional association for doctors in the UK, founded in 1832, which acts as the spokesman and negotiator for the medical profession. Membership of the British Medical Association (BMA) is voluntary and is open to any practitioner registered with the *General Medical Council* (the regulating body of the medical profession).

The BMA is a registered trade union and much of its work is concerned with negotiation of fees and salaries with the Department of Health and other bodies that employ doctors. It regularly gives evidence on behalf of doctors to committees of inquiry, Parliamentary select committees, etc.

The association also has a long tradition of promoting scientific activities for its members; it publishes each week the "British Medical Journal", one of the leading medical journals in the world, together with around 20 more specialist journals. It has also published many influential reports, such as "The Drinking Driver" and "The Medical Effects of Nuclear War". The BMA organizes regular scientific meetings in Britain and overseas and maintains in London a comprehensive medical library.

Brittle bones

Bones with an increased tendency to fracture. Brittle bones are a feature of the disorder *osteoporosis* (thinning of the bones), which is common in women after the menopause, and may occur in people who are confined to bed, who are taking *corticosteroid drugs*, or who are suffering from certain hormonal disorders. In *osteomalacia* (a disorder caused by deficiency of *vitamin D*), the bones become soft and have an increased tendency both to become deformed and to fracture.

A rare cause of brittle bones and frequent fractures is the inherited connective tissue abnormality *osteogenesis imperfecta* (sometimes called brittle-bone disease).

Broken tooth

See *Fracture, dental*.

Broken veins

See *Telangiectasia*.

Bromides

Substances formerly prescribed as

FITTING THE BRIDGE

The most common type of bridge consists of one or more false teeth attached to a crown on each side of

a gap. The natural teeth are shaped to receive the crowns, which are then cemented into place.

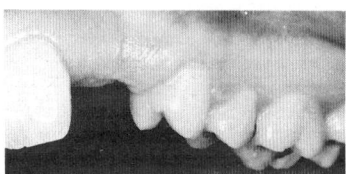

1 Two complete teeth are missing. A bridge of two false teeth and three crowns can be attached.

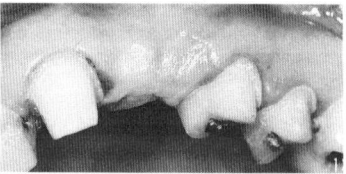

2 The three healthy teeth are shaped so that they can receive the crowns on either side of the gap.

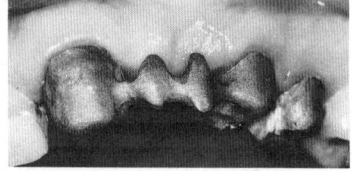

3 A cast-metal subframe made from an impression is tried out in the mouth and any necessary alterations are made.

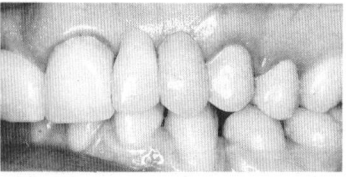

4 The finished bridge is in position, showing the new porcelain teeth cemented to the metal base.

sedative drugs in the treatment of *anxiety* or as *anticonvulsant drugs* in the treatment of *epilepsy*. Bromides are no longer prescribed because of their unpleasant side-effects, which include loss of sex drive, acne, tremor, lack of coordination, and confusion.

Bromocriptine

A drug that inhibits the secretion of the hormone *prolactin* by the anterior pituitary gland.

WHY IT IS USED

Bromocriptine is helpful in treating disorders associated with excessive prolactin production. Such conditions include *galactorrhoea* (abnormal milk production), some types of female and male infertility, severe premenstrual breast discomfort, and benign pituitary tumours, including *prolactinomas* and tumours that cause *acromegaly* (abnormal tissue and bone growth). Bromocriptine can also be used to suppress lactation in women who do not wish to breast-feed.

A few years after its development in the 1960s, bromocriptine was also found to be effective in relieving the symptoms of *Parkinson's disease*. It has almost the identical characteristics of *dopamine*, the chemical that is lacking in the brains of persons with Parkinson's disease. Bromocriptine is used to treat patients in the advanced stages of Parkinson's disease when other drugs have failed or are unsuitable.

ADVERSE EFFECTS

Nausea and vomiting are the most common adverse effects. Low doses are unlikely to cause serious adverse effects but ulceration of the stomach occurs in rare cases. High doses may cause drowsiness and confusion. Women who have prolactinomas treated with bromocriptine may regain their fertility.

Bronchiectasis

A lung disorder in which one or more bronchi (the air passages leading from the trachea) are distorted and stretched, and have damaged linings. Bronchiectasis is most common in childhood and results in chronic infections that may persist into later life.

CAUSES AND INCIDENCE

Bronchiectasis was formerly common and was usually caused by childhood chest infections such as measles, pertussis (whooping cough), tuberculosis, or severe bacterial pneumonias. As these infections have been controlled by *immunization* and by *antibiotic drugs*, so the incidence of bronchiectasis has plummeted. Child-

hood bronchiectasis is now virtually extinct in developed countries. It is still sometimes seen as a complication of cystic fibrosis.

SYMPTOMS

The main symptom of chronic lung infection in bronchiectasis is a cough that produces green or yellow sputum (phlegm) containing pus and occasionally flecks of blood. The sputum sometimes causes bad breath. If the disease is extensive, it causes shortness of breath.

DIAGNOSIS AND TREATMENT

The diagnosis is usually made from the symptoms. The extent of damage to the bronchi can be determined by *chest X-rays* or by *bronchography* (an imaging technique in which X-rays are made after a radiopaque substance has been injected into the bronchi).

Symptoms can usually be controlled by antibiotic drugs and by *postural drainage*; the patient is taught to lie in a position that allows pus and fluid to drain from the affected areas of lung so that they can be coughed up more easily.

If severe symptoms persist despite these measures, surgery may be recommended to remove the damaged lung areas.

Bronchiolitis

An acute viral infection of the lungs, mainly affecting babies and young children, in which the bronchioles (the smaller airways in the lungs that branch off from the bronchi) become inflamed.

CAUSES AND INCIDENCE

The most common cause of bronchiolitis is the respiratory syncytial virus (RSV), but other viruses may also be responsible. Adult bronchiolitis may follow *bronchitis*, brought on by an influenza virus.

Winter epidemics of bronchiolitis tend to occur every two or three years. The viruses responsible can be transmitted from one person to another in airborne droplets, and a virus that may cause only a moderate head or chest infection in an adult can cause severe bronchiolitis in an infant. People who are suffering from a head or chest infection should therefore minimize contacts with babies.

SYMPTOMS

The symptoms of bronchiolitis are a cough, rapid breathing, fever, and, in severe cases, a cyanotic (bluish) complexion due to shortage of oxygen. The doctor will often hear crepitations (bubbling noises) in the child's lungs through a stethoscope.

TREATMENT

If a baby or young child has a cold and a cough that suddenly worsens, leading to rapid and laboured breathing, a doctor should be consulted.

Sometimes no treatment is necessary but, in more severe cases, sufferers may be admitted to hospital, where *oxygen therapy* and *physiotherapy* (to clear the mucus from the bronchioles) can be given. Occasionally, sufferers are put on an artificial *ventilator* until normal breathing is restored. With prompt treatment, sufferers usually recover completely within a few days.

Antibiotic drugs are ineffective against the viral infection, but may be prescribed to prevent any secondary bacterial infection. Adults with bronchiolitis are commonly treated with *corticosteroid drugs*.

Bronchitis

Inflammation of the bronchi, the airways that connect the trachea (windpipe) to the lungs, resulting in a cough that may produce considerable quantities of sputum (phlegm). Two forms of the disease are recognized—acute bronchitis (of sudden onset and short duration) and chronic bronchitis (persistent over a long period and recurring over several years). Both are more common in smokers and in areas with high atmospheric pollution. (See also *Bronchitis, acute*; *Bronchitis, chronic*.)

Bronchitis, acute

A form of *bronchitis* that develops suddenly and usually clears up within a few days except in people with a low resistance to infection.

CAUSES AND INCIDENCE

Acute bronchitis is usually a complication of a viral infection such as a cold or influenza, but may also be caused by the effect of air pollutants. Bacterial infection may cause acute bronchitis or may occur as a further complication of acute bronchitis when this has other causes.

Attacks occur most often in winter. Smokers, babies, the elderly, and people with lung disease are particularly susceptible.

SYMPTOMS

The inflammation of the mucosal lining of the bronchi causes swelling and congestion, and pus is formed. The principal symptoms are wheezing, shortness of breath, and a persistent cough that produces yellow or green sputum. There may also be discomfort behind the sternum (breastbone) and a raised temperature.

TREATMENT

Symptoms may be relieved by humidifying the lungs, either using a humidifier in the home, or by inhaling steam directly (taking care to avoid burns). Drinking plenty of fluids helps loosen the sputum so that it can be coughed up more easily.

Most acute bronchitis clears up without further treatment, causing no further trouble. Complications, such as *pneumonia* and *pleurisy*, develop only in exceptional cases. However, a doctor should be consulted in any of the following circumstances: if there is severe breathlessness, if there is no improvement after three days, if blood is coughed up, if the temperature is above 38.3°C, or if the patient has underlying lung disease.

If the doctor suspects there is a bacterial infection, *antibiotic drugs* will be prescribed, but these are of no use if the infection is caused by a virus.

Bronchitis, chronic

A form of *bronchitis* in which sputum is coughed up on most days during at least three consecutive months in at least two consecutive years. The disease commonly results in widespread narrowing and obstruction of the airways in the lungs. It often coexists with (and may contribute to the development of) another lung disease, *emphysema*, in which the alveoli (air sacs) in the lungs become distended (widened). Chronic bronchitis and emphysema together are sometimes called chronic obstructive lung disease (COLD) or chronic obstructive airways disease (COAD).

CAUSES AND INCIDENCE

Smoking is the main cause of chronic bronchitis. It stimulates the production of mucus in the lining of the bronchi and thickens the bronchi's muscular walls and those of the bronchioles (smaller airways in the lungs), resulting in narrowing of these air passages. The passages then become more susceptible to infections, causing further damage. Atmospheric pollution can have the same effect.

Chronic obstructive lung disease is more common in the UK than anywhere else in the world. It is also the most common cause of loss of work in the UK, accounting for nearly 30 million working days lost per year.

About three million persons in the UK suffer from the disease. Most sufferers are over 40, and male sufferers outnumber female sufferers by two to one. The disease is most prevalent in industrial cities and among smokers, and is more common in manual and unskilled workers than white-collar workers (even after adjusting for differences in smoking habits). There are 30,000 deaths annually in England and Wales from chronic obstructive lung disease.

SYMPTOMS AND COMPLICATIONS

The symptoms vary depending on the extent of the emphysema. When emphysema predominates, breathlessness is the main problem, there is little sputum, and the illness shows little fluctuation with the seasons. When bronchitis predominates, (usually in cigarette smokers) the cough is the main symptom, with large amounts of sputum in winter.

As the disease progresses, often with the development of emphysema, the lungs become more resistant to the flow of blood, resulting in *pulmonary hypertension* (increased pressure in the arteries supplying blood to the lungs) and strain on the right side of the heart, as it must increase its work to pump blood through the lungs. The patient may suffer severe breathlessness. Sometimes, *heart failure* develops, further reducing the oxygen in the blood and causing a cyanotic (bluish) complexion. *Oedema* (swelling caused by fluid collection) then develops in the legs and ankles due to the back pressure in blood vessels as a result of the heart failure.

People with chronic bronchitis usually have two or more episodes of acute viral or bacterial infection of the lungs every winter. Occasionally, blood may be coughed up, requiring medical investigation to exclude the possibility of *lung cancer*.

PREVENTION

A reduction in atmospheric pollution in towns and cities over the last few decades has reduced the incidence of chronic bronchitis, but the most important preventive measure is for people to stop (or never to start) smoking, as this is by far the most important cause of the disease. Waiting until symptoms develop may be too late to halt its course.

DIAGNOSIS AND TREATMENT

Before starting treatment, the doctor may decide to investigate the severity of the patient's condition by *chest X-rays*, *blood tests*, *sputum* analysis, and *lung-function tests*.

HOW BRONCHODILATORS WORK

When bronchioles become narrow following contraction of the muscle layer and swelling of the mucous lining, the passage of air is impeded. Bronchodilator drugs relax the muscles surrounding bronchioles by acting on the nerve signals that govern muscle activity. Sympathomimetic and anticholinergic drugs interfere with nerve signals passed to the muscles through the autonomic nervous system. Sympathomimetics enhance the action of neurotransmitters that encourage muscle relaxation. Anticholinergics block the neurotransmitters that trigger muscle contraction. Xanthine drugs relax muscle in the bronchioles by a direct effect on the muscle fibres, but their precise action is not known.

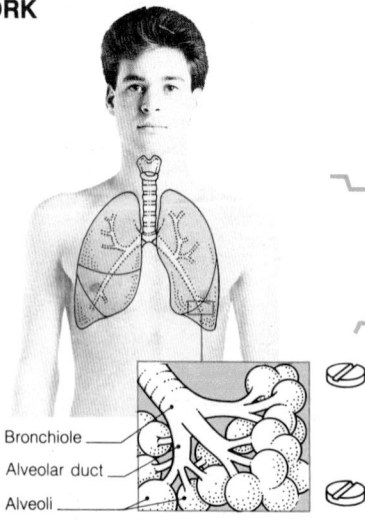

Bronchiole

Alveolar duct

Alveoli

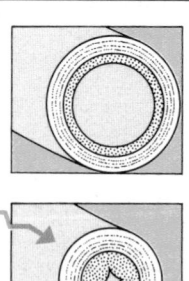

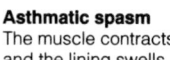

Normal bronchioles
The muscle surrounding the bronchioles is relaxed, leaving the airway open.

Asthmatic spasm
The muscle contracts and the lining swells, narrowing the airway.

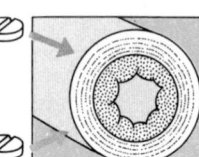

After drug treatment
The muscles relax, opening the airway, but the mucous lining remains swollen.

To relieve breathlessness, the doctor may prescribe an inhaler containing a *bronchodilator drug* (a drug that relaxes and widens the bronchi). Certain patients may benefit from inhaling oxygen from oxygen cylinders or an oxygen concentrator kept at home. Efforts may be made to help the patient cough up sputum. *Antibiotic drugs* may be given to treat or prevent bacterial lung infection.

The disease often shows an inexorable progression, with increasing shortness of breath leading to early retirement; eventually the sufferer may become housebound.

Bronchoconstrictor

A substance that causes constriction (narrowing) of the airways in the lungs. Bronchoconstrictors, such as *histamine* or methyl choline, are sometimes given by inhalation to provoke an attack of *asthma* (in order to confirm the diagnosis), or to test the effectiveness of a *bronchodilator drug*.

Bronchodilator drugs

COMMON DRUGS
Sympathomimetics
Fenoterol Pirbuterol Reproterol
Rimiterol Salbutamol Terbutaline
Anticholinergics
Ipratropium
Xanthines
Aminophylline Theophylline

> **WARNING**
> If your inhaler is not helping your symptoms, call your doctor.

A group of drugs that widen the bronchioles (small airways in the lungs) to increase the flow of air and improve breathing. Narrowing of the airways may be caused by contraction of the bronchiole walls and/ or by congestion with mucus.

TYPES

Three main groups of drugs are used as bronchodilators: sympathomimetic drugs, *anticholinergic drugs*, and xanthine drugs. Sympathomimetic drugs are primarily used for the rapid relief of breathing difficulty. Anticholinergic and xanthine drugs are more often used for the long-term prevention of attacks of breathing difficulty.

Drugs can be given by *inhaler*, in tablet form, or, in severe cases, by *nebulizer* (a type of inhaler that uses air and/or oxygen under pressure to propel a watery suspension of the drug into the lungs) or by injection.

WHY THEY ARE USED

Bronchodilator drugs are used to improve air-flow into the lungs, especially in the treatment of *asthma* and chronic *bronchitis*.

HOW THEY WORK

The action of bronchodilators is described in the box opposite.

POSSIBLE ADVERSE EFFECTS

Sympathomimetic drugs may cause palpitations and trembling. Anticholinergic drugs may cause dry mouth, blurred vision, and difficulty passing urine. Xanthine drugs may cause headaches and palpitations.

Inhaled bronchodilator drugs are not absorbed by the body in large amounts and serious side-effects are therefore uncommon. However, because of the possible effect of sympathomimetic and xanthine drugs on heart-rate, these drugs are prescribed cautiously for people who have heart problems, high blood pressure, or an overactive thyroid gland. Anticholinergic drugs may not be suitable for men who have enlarged prostate glands or for people who have a tendency to glaucoma.

Bronchography

An X-ray procedure for examining the bronchi, the main air passages of the lungs. Bronchography was formerly used to diagnose the *bronchiectasis*, but has now been largely replaced by other imaging techniques, such as *CT scanning* or lung *tomography*, and by the use of *bronchoscopy*.

HOW IT IS DONE

After the patient has been given mild sedation and/or a local anaesthetic, contrast medium (a substance opaque to X-rays) is introduced into the lung through a hollow flexible tube (either a cannula or a bronchoscope). X-ray pictures are then taken of the bronchi to detect any abnormalities. When the procedure is finished, the contrast medium is partly coughed up and partly absorbed into the bloodstream.

Bronchopneumonia

The most common form of *pneumonia*. Bronchopneumonia differs from the other main type of pneumonia (lobar pneumonia) in that the inflammation is spread throughout the lungs in small patches rather than being confined to one lobe. Bronchopneumonia is often the actual cause of death in patients who are chronically ill from other conditions.

Bronchoscopy

Examination or treatment of the bronchi, the main airways of the lungs, by means of a hollow tube or a fibre-optic *endoscope* (viewing tube with a light and lens attached).

PERFORMING BRONCHOSCOPY

There are two kinds of bronchoscope. The rigid type is passed into the bronchi via the mouth and requires anaesthesia. The flexible, fibre-optic bronchoscope (a narrower tube formed from light-transmitting fibres) can be inserted through either the mouth or nose. It is used after giving only a mild sedative and/or local anaesthetic and it reaches farther into the lungs. Both types of bronchoscope can be fitted with forceps, and the instrument also has attachments for performing laser therapy and cryosurgery. (See also *Endoscopy*.)

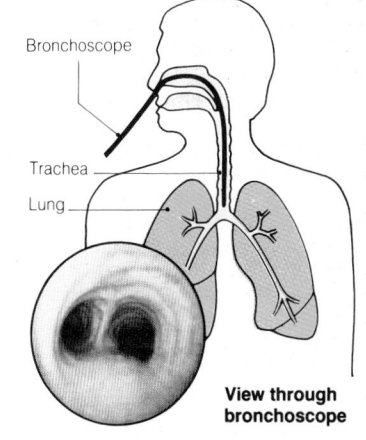

Bronchoscope

Trachea

Lung

View through bronchoscope

THE BRONCHOSCOPE

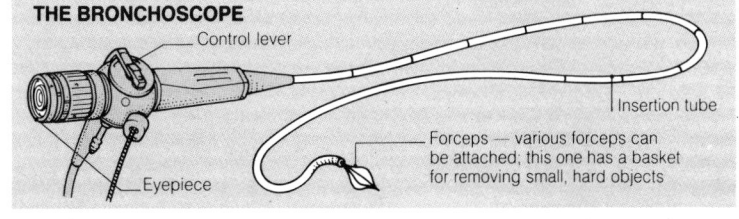

Control lever

Eyepiece

Insertion tube

Forceps — various forceps can be attached; this one has a basket for removing small, hard objects

The two main uses of bronchoscopy are to aid in diagnosing and treating certain lung disorders. Apart from inspecting the bronchi for abnormalities, diagnostic procedures include collecting samples of mucus, obtaining cells from the outermost distant airways of the lungs, and taking biopsy specimens (small samples of tissue), all for analysis or microscopic examination. The bronchoscope is also sometimes used in a type of X-ray investigation called *bronchography*.

Among the various forms of treatment possible are removing thick secretions of mucus or inhaled foreign bodies, destroying growths, and sealing off damaged blood vessels. The last two are carried out by *laser therapy*, *diathermy*, or *cryosurgery* (a tissue-freezing technique) by means of attachments to the bronchoscope.

Bronchospasm

Temporary narrowing of the bronchi (airways into the lungs) caused by contraction of the muscles in the walls of the bronchi, by inflammation of the lining of the bronchi, or by a combination of both.

Contraction and relaxation of the airways is controlled by the autonomic nervous system. Contraction may also be caused by the release of substances during an allergic reaction.

When the airways are narrowed, flow of air out of the lungs causes wheezing or coughing. The most common cause of bronchospasm is *asthma*, though other causes include respiratory infection, chronic lung disease (including *emphysema* and chronic *bronchitis*), *anaphylactic shock*, or an allergic reaction to chemicals.

Bronchus

A large air passage in a lung. Each lung has one main bronchus, originating at the end of the trachea (windpipe). This main bronchus divides into smaller branches known as segmental bronchi, which further divide into bronchioles.

Bronchus, cancer of

See *Lung cancer*.

Brown fat

A special type of fat, found in infants and some animals, but not in healthy adults. It is located between and around the scapulae (shoulderblades) on the back. Brown fat is a source of energy and helps infants to maintain a constant body temperature.

Brucellosis

A rare bacterial infection, caught from farm animals and dairy products, that may cause a feverish illness.

CAUSES AND INCIDENCE

The disease is caused by various species of *BRUCELLA*, which may be transmitted to humans from affected cattle, goats, and pigs. Farm workers, veterinary surgeons, and people who work in slaughterhouses have the highest risk of infection. The bacteria enter the bloodstream through a cut or are breathed in.

In countries where milk pasteurization is not the rule, the disease can be caught by drinking milk or by eating unpasteurized dairy products, including cheese. Brucellosis has been eliminated from farm animals in the UK.

SYMPTOMS

Acute brucellosis consists of a single bout of high fever, shivering, aching, and drenching sweats, which last for a few days. Other symptoms include headache, poor appetite, backache, weakness, and depression. Untreated severe cases may lead rarely to potentially fatal complications, such as *pneumonia* or *meningitis*.

In chronic brucellosis, bouts of the illness recur over months or years.

DIAGNOSIS AND TREATMENT

A definite diagnosis of brucellosis is made from blood tests. The disease is treated by bed rest and *antibiotic drugs*.

Bruise

A discoloured area under the skin, caused by leakage of blood from damaged capillaries (tiny blood vessels). At first, the blood appears blue or black; then the breakdown of *haemoglobin* turns the bruise yellow.

To reduce the pain and swelling of a large bruise, place a cloth soaked in ice-cold water over it for 10 minutes. If a bruise does not fade after about one week, or if bruises appear for no apparent reason or are severe after only minor injury, a doctor should be consulted as these may be indications of a *bleeding disorder*. (See also *Black eye*; *Purpura*.)

Bruits

The sounds made in the heart, arteries, or veins when blood circulation becomes turbulent or flows at an abnormal speed. This happens when blood vessels become narrowed by disease (as in *arteriosclerosis*), when heart valves are narrowed or damaged (as in *endocarditis*), or if blood vessels dilate (as in an *aneurysm*). Bruits are usually heard through a *stethoscope*.

Bruxism

Rhythmic grinding or clenching of the teeth that usually occurs during sleep but may be done unconsciously when a person is awake. Bruxism may develop at any age. The chief underlying causes are emotional stress and minor discomfort or unevenness when the teeth are brought together.

Continued bruxism may cause wearing away and loosening of the teeth, and stiffness in the jaw. If the underlying problems cannot be resolved, a biteplate worn at night will minimize the damage.

BSE

The abbreviation for bovine spongiform *encephalopathy*.

Bubonic plague

The most common form of *plague*, characterized by the development of a bubo (swollen lymph node) in the groin or armpit early in the illness.

Buccal

An anatomical term, from the Latin word for cheek, that means relating to the cheek or mouth.

Buck teeth

Prominent upper incisors (front teeth), which protrude from the mouth and are often splayed out at an angle to each other. Buck teeth are easily damaged and may be susceptible to decay because they are not moistened by saliva.

CAUSES

The malpositioning of the teeth is probably an inherited trait rather than acquired (for example, by faulty eating habits). Often, the person's upper jaw is relatively large compared with the lower jaw, and the lips do not close over and exert a controlling influence on the position of the teeth. Rarely, the malpositioning may be the result of an abnormally large tongue gradually displacing the teeth forwards. Often, there is an overall crowding of teeth within the upper jaw. Buck teeth formerly occurred in conjunction with mouth breathing due to enlarged *adenoids*, but this has become less common.

TREATMENT

Orthodontic treatment involves gradually coaxing the teeth back into position with a removable brace (see *Brace, dental*), or, in more extreme cases, with a fixed *orthodontic appliance*). To create room for the incisors, other crowded teeth may sometimes need to be extracted.

Budd-Chiari syndrome

A rare disorder in which the veins draining blood from the liver become blocked or narrowed. Blood then accumulates in the liver, which swells. The blockage leads to serious *liver failure*, and to *portal hypertension* (back pressure in the blood vessels due to abnormally slow blood flow through the liver).

Treatment is aimed at removing the cause of the vein obstruction—which may be a blood clot, pressure on the veins from a liver tumour, or a congenital abnormality of the veins. In most cases, however, treatment has only a limited effect and, unless a *liver transplant* can be performed, most patients die within two years.

Budesonide

A *corticosteroid drug* given by inhalation in the treatment of bronchial *asthma*. Budesonide has a local anti-inflammatory action on the airways that makes it useful in the prevention of asthma attacks. It is administered as a metered-dose aerosol or in powder form from a turbohaler. Side-effects include hoarseness, throat irritation, and, rarely, fungal infections in the mouth. Irritation may be prevented by gargling and thoroughly rinsing the mouth with water after each inhalation.

Buerger's disease

A rare disorder, also called thromboangiitis obliterans, in which the arteries, nerves, and veins in the legs, and sometimes those in the arms, become severely inflamed. Narrowing of the arteries blocks off blood supply to the toes and fingers, eventually causing *gangrene* (tissue death).

The disease occurs mainly in men under the age of 45 who smoke heavily. Most have a history of *phlebitis* (vein inflammation). The main symptom is pain in the hands and feet. In cold conditions, sufferers' hands turn white, then blue, and then red (see *Raynaud's phenomenon*).

Sufferers must stop smoking to halt the disease's progress. *Vasodilator drugs* may be prescribed to widen blood vessels, but are rarely effective. If gangrene develops, affected limbs, toes, or fingers usually have to be amputated.

Bulimia

An illness characterized by bouts of gross overeating usually followed by self-induced vomiting. These activities are often kept secret, so the exact prevalence of the disorder is not known, but most sufferers are girls or women between the ages of 15 and 30.

CAUSES

Bulimia is often a variant of *anorexia nervosa*. In both disorders, the sufferer has a morbid fear of fatness. After months or years of eating sparsely, sufferers may develop a constant craving for food and begin to binge, but the fear of becoming overweight remains and prompts self-induced vomiting. Sometimes, large doses of *laxative* drugs are used to expel food rapidly.

Occasionally, a person may develop bulimia without a history of anorexia.

SYMPTOMS

People with bulimia may be of normal weight or only slightly underweight, although some are extremely thin. Bingeing and vomiting may occur once or several times a day. In severe cases, repeated vomiting can lead to dehydration and potassium loss, causing weakness and cramps. The gastric acid in vomit may damage the teeth. Sufferers are often highly distressed about their compulsions and may be depressed and sometimes suicidal.

TREATMENT AND OUTLOOK

The sufferer must first be persuaded to accept treatment. Similar to the treatment for anorexia nervosa, it includes supervision and regulation of eating habits, and, sometimes *psychotherapy* and/or *antidepressant drugs.* In many cases there is a risk of relapse weeks or even months after ending treatment.

Bulla

A large air- or fluid-filled bubble, usually in the lungs or skin.

Lung bullae in young adults are usually *congenital* defects. In later life, lung bullae develop in patients with the lung disease *emphysema* as the alveoli burst and join together. Skin bullae are simply large, fluid-filled *blisters*.

Bumetanide

A powerful, short-acting loop *diuretic drug*. Bumetanide is used to treat oedema (fluid retention) resulting from *heart failure, nephrotic syndrome,* or liver *cirrhosis*. It is particularly useful in people with impaired kidney function who do not respond well to thiazide diuretics. Given by injection, it is often used as emergency treatment for pulmonary oedema (fluid in the lungs).

ADVERSE EFFECTS

Adverse effects can include rash and muscle pain. There may also be weakness due to excessive potassium loss in the urine, which may be prevented by taking a supplement or a potassium-sparing diuretic with bumetanide.

Bundle branch block

See *Heart block.*

Bunion

A thickened, fluid-filled *bursa* (pad), overlying the big toe joint. The underlying cause is *hallux valgus*, in which the joint at the base of the big toe projects outwards while the tip turns inwards. Bunions can be very painful.

TREATMENT

Without treatment, any bunion will get worse. To remedy a small bunion, wear properly fitting shoes and a special toe pad to straighten the big toe and keep it in position. Large bunions may require surgery.

HOW BUNIONS FORM

A bunion results from rubbing of a shoe against an abnormal outward projection of the joint at the base of the big toe (a hallux valgus), leading to irritation and inflammation. The joint abnormality is often itself due to the wearing of narrow, pointed shoes with high heels, although it can also result from an inherited weakness in the joint.

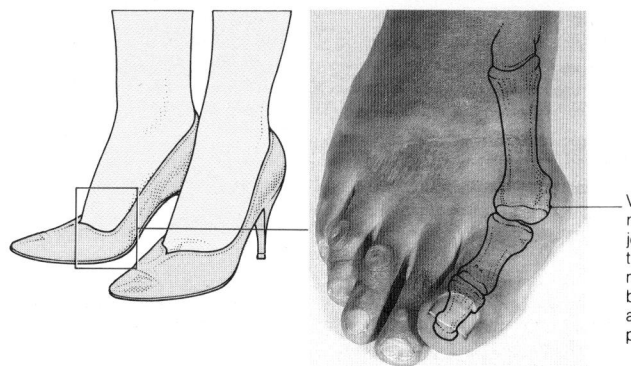

Valgus deformity of the joint between the first metatarsal bone and the adjoining phalanx.

CARE OF BURN PATIENTS

Burn patients need specialized nursing care and equipment. Air-fluidized therapy units encourage tissue repair by providing a clean, dry, temperature-controlled environment. A filtered air-flow activates millions of tiny glass beads in the tank; oxygen, nutrients, and antibiotics are transported to the wound site, while body fluids are drained away.

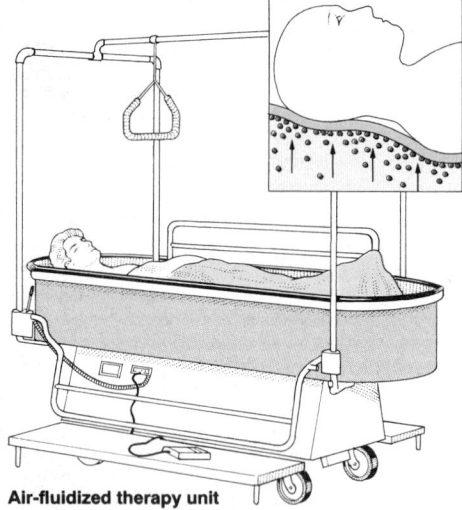

Air-fluidized therapy unit

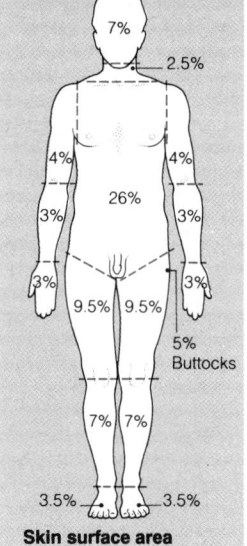

Skin surface area
This is a rough guide to what percentage each area represents of the total skin area (percentages do not total 100 due to rounding).

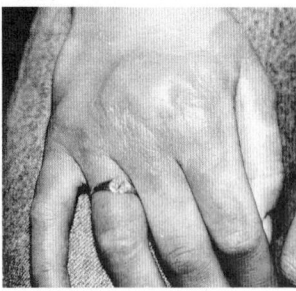

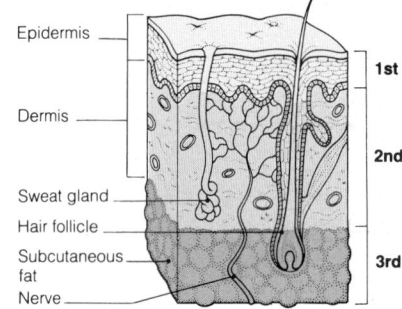

Epidermis

Dermis

Sweat gland

Hair follicle

Subcutaneous fat

Nerve

1st

2nd

3rd

Degrees of burns
Burns are divided into three categories. First-degree burns affect the epidermis and skin may peel; second-degree burns cause blisters; third-degree burns destroy the whole of the skin's thickness and require special treatment.

DEATHS FROM BURNING IN ENGLAND AND WALES IN 1990

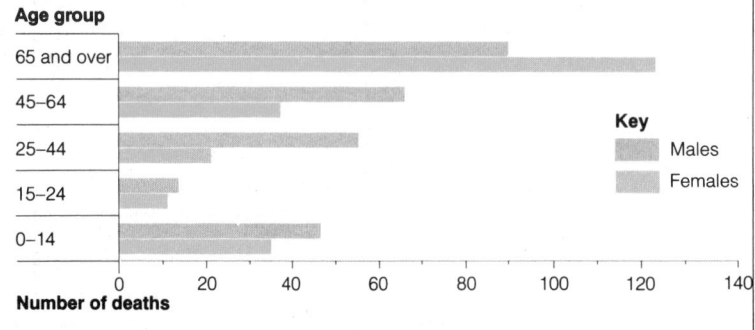

Age group

65 and over

45–64

25–44

15–24

0–14

Key
Males
Females

Number of deaths

Buphthalmos

A large, prominent eyeball in an infant, resulting from increased pressure inside the eyeball due to congenital *glaucoma*. Treatment usually involves surgery to reduce pressure, otherwise the child's sight is progressively damaged.

Burkitt's lymphoma

A cancer of lymph tissues that is characterized by an enlarging tumour or tumours within the jaw or abdomen, or both.

INCIDENCE
Burkitt's lymphoma is confined almost exclusively to children living in low-lying, moist, tropical regions of Africa and New Guinea. A few cases have occurred among a wider age group in North America and Europe.

CAUSE
The growths are believed to be an abnormal response to a common virus, the Epstein-Barr virus. The distribution of the disease in Africa closely follows that of *malaria*; it is thought that malaria in childhood may alter the body's immune response to the Epstein-Barr virus, which triggers growth of the lymphoma.

TREATMENT
Anticancer drugs or *radiotherapy* give complete or partial cure in about 80 per cent of cases. (See also *Lymphoma*.)

Burns

Each year in England and Wales over 1,000 people are burned or scalded badly enough to require admission to hospital, and on any one day they occupy more than 350 hospital beds. Burns are most common in children and older people; many are due to accidents in the home, which are usually preventable.

TYPES
Skin is a living tissue, and even brief heating above 49°C damages its cells.
FIRST-DEGREE BURNS cause reddening of the skin and affect only the epidermis, the top layer of the skin. Such burns heal quickly, but the damaged skin may peel away after a day or two. *Sunburn* is a common example of a first-degree burn.

SECOND-DEGREE BURNS damage the skin more deeply, causing the formation of blisters. However, some of the dermis (deep layer of the skin) is left to recover, and as a result these burns usually heal without scarring, unless they are very extensive.

THIRD-DEGREE BURNS destroy the full skin thickness. The affected area will look white or charred, and, if the burn is very deep, muscles and bones may be exposed. Even if very localized, third-degree burns will need specialist treatment and possibly skin grafts to prevent scarring.

ELECTRICAL BURNS can cause extensive damage with minimal external skin damage. Because the electric current may cause heart damage, electrical burns require evaluation by a doctor.

EFFECTS AND COMPLICATIONS

Extensive first-degree burns (such as sunburn) cause pain, restlessness, headache, and fever, but are not life-threatening.

In second- or third-degree burns affecting more than 10 per cent of the body surface, the victim will be in a state of *shock*, with lowered blood pressure and a rapid pulse. This is caused by the loss of large quantities of fluid (and its constituent proteins) from the burned area. Shock may be fatal if not treated by intravenous fluid replacement.

When the skin is burned, it can no longer protect the body from contamination by airborne bacteria. The infection of extensive burns may cause fatal complications if effective treatment with antibiotic drugs is not available.

Victims who have inhaled smoke may develop swelling and inflammation of the lungs and may need specialist care for burns of the eyes and respiratory passages. People who die in burning buildings usually suffocate long before their bodies are burned.

PROFESSIONAL TREATMENT

The burn is covered with a non-stick dressing to keep the area moist, since drying slows healing. Every effort is made to keep the skin area scrupulously clean by reverse *isolation* nursing. If necessary, analgesic drugs (painkillers) are given, and antibiotic drugs are prescribed if there is any sign of the wound being infected. Shock is treated by intravenous fluids through a drip inserted into a vein, usually in the arm.

For extensive second-degree burns, when there is slow healing, or when there is a fear of infection, a topical antibacterial agent such as silver sulphadiazine is used. *Skin grafts* are used early in treatment to minimize scarring. Third-degree burns always require skin grafting if scarring is to be avoided. Extensive burns may require repeated plastic surgery.

Length of hospital stay can vary from a few days in some cases to many weeks in the case of severe and extensive burns. Patients with extensive burns are usually treated at a specialist burns centre.

FIRST AID: TREATING BURNS

MINOR BURNS

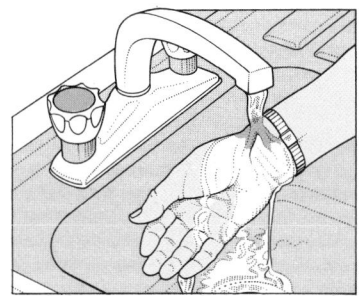

1 Immerse the burned area immediately in cold, running water.

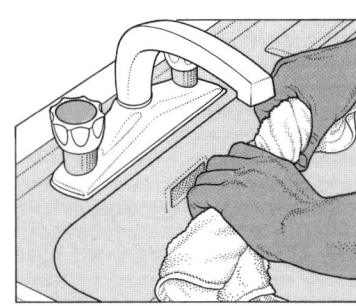

2 Or apply a cold-water compress (a clean towel or handkerchief) until the pain diminishes.

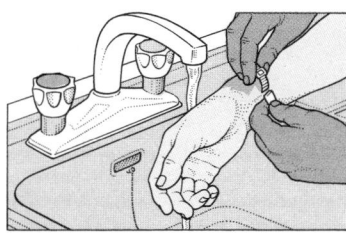

3 Remove any watches, bracelets, rings, belts, or constricting clothing from the area before it begins to swell.

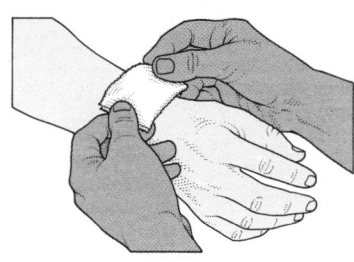

4 Dress the area with a clean (if possible, sterile), nonfluffy material.

MAJOR BURNS

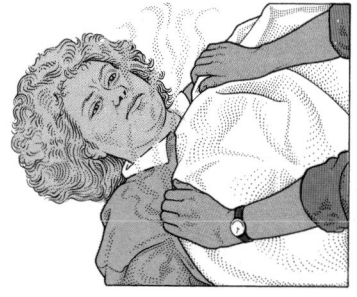

1 If a person's clothing is on fire, douse the victim with water or wrap him or her in a blanket and place on the ground.

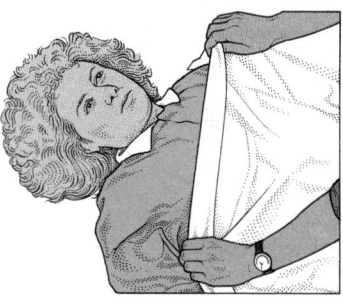

2 Do not remove clothing that is stuck to the wound, but cover any exposed burned areas with a dry, clean, nonfluffy cloth to stop infection; secure with a bandage.

DO NOT
- use adhesive dressings on burns
- apply butter, oil, or grease
- apply lotions or creams
- prick blisters with a pin or otherwise interfere with the injured area
- use fluffy materials on wounds

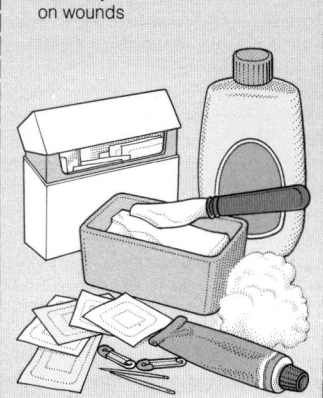

Burping

Another term for *belching*.

Burr hole

A hole made in the skull by a special drill with a rounded tip (burr). The hole is made to relieve pressure on the brain, often resulting from the accumulation of blood between the inside of the skull and the brain after a *head injury*. The burr hole relieves the potentially fatal pressure by allowing the blood to drain.

Several burr holes may be made as part of a *craniotomy*, in which a section of the skull is removed to allow access to the brain and surrounding tissues.

Bursa

A fluid-filled pad that acts as a cushion at a pressure point in the body—often near a joint, where a tendon or muscle crosses bone or other muscles. The important bursae are around the knee, elbow, and shoulder.

A *bunion* is a thickened bursa at the base of the big toe.

Bursitis

Inflammation of a *bursa*, causing pain and swelling due to accumulation of fluid. Bursitis is usually the result of pressure, friction, or slight injury to the membrane surrounding the joint. Less commonly, it may be caused by bacterial infection.

TYPES

Prepatellar bursitis ("housemaid's knee") is caused by prolonged kneeling on a hard surface, tibial tubercle bursitis ("clergyman's knee") from kneeling on a more upright surface, and olecranon bursitis ("student's elbow") from prolonged pressure of the elbow point against a desk or table. Another common form is subdeltoid bursitis (affecting the shoulder), which, if left untreated, may result in *frozen shoulder*.

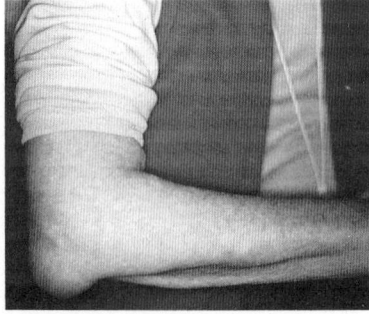

Bursitis of the elbow
This condition produces a fluid-filled swelling around the point of the elbow.

TREATMENT

Rest is the usual treatment. Bursitis usually subsides after a few days as the fluid is reabsorbed into the bloodstream. Application of an ice-pack may help relieve pain. Bacterial bursitis usually requires treatment with *antibiotic drugs*.

If swelling persists, a doctor may drain the bursa using a needle and syringe and apply a pressure bandage for a few days to stop the fluid from reforming. An injection of a *corticosteroid drug* may also be given.

In rare, recurrent cases, bursectomy (a minor operation to remove the bursa) may be performed. Under general anaesthesia, a small incision is made in the skin over the bursa, and the lining of the bursal sac is completely removed to prevent it from regrowing.

Bypass operations

Procedures to bypass the blockage or narrowing of an artery or vein or any part of the digestive system.

TYPES

Arteries can become blocked or narrowed in *atherosclerosis*. Most often affected are the carotid arteries (in the neck), the coronary arteries (in the heart), and the iliofemoral arteries (leading to the legs). Obstructions can be bypassed using sections of artery or vein (taken from the patient) or using synthetic tubing.

Surgeons have attempted to bypass blocked arteries in the brain by joining points above the blockage to an artery in the neck. Known as extracranial-intracranial bypass, this procedure has had little success, and is now rarely used.

Veins are bypassed most often in patients with diseases of the liver that cause portal hypertension (increased pressure in the veins draining the intestinal tract) and bleeding oesophageal varices (enlarged veins in the lower oesophagus). These bypasses are called *shunts*.

Intestinal bypasses are most commonly employed in patients with cancer. If tumour growth is too extensive for surgical removal, symptoms may be relieved by joining the sections of intestine at either side of the blockage. An obstructed bile duct may be diverted into the intestine lower down the digestive tract. Intestinal bypass operations for the treatment of *obesity* have largely been replaced by operations to reduce the capacity of the stomach. (See also *Arterial bypass*; *Coronary artery bypass*.)

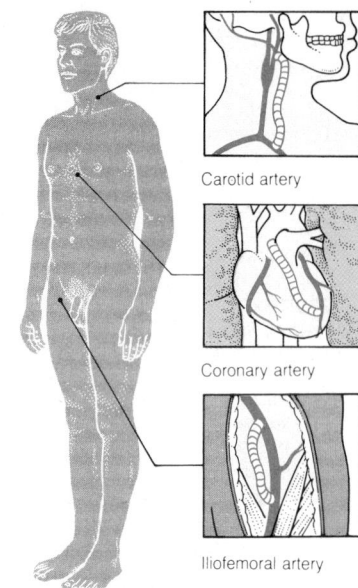

Common bypass locations
The carotid and coronary arteries and the iliofemoral vessels are the most common locations for bypasses.

Byssinosis

A lung disease caused by an unknown agent in the dust produced during the processing of flax, cotton, hemp, or sisal. Byssinosis was once a common problem among cotton mill workers in the UK, but recently it has become less prevalent due to better dust control and the decline of the textile industry. It remains common in India and other developing countries.

SYMPTOMS

Byssinosis produces a feeling of tightness in the chest and shortness of breath that may become chronic. At first, symptoms are most pronounced at the start of the working week, but gradually they become troublesome on every working day. In chronic byssinosis (the risk of which is increased by smoking), the sufferer is short of breath even when away from work. *Respiratory failure* may develop when lung damage has become extensive, but this is quite uncommon.

TREATMENT AND PREVENTION

Bronchodilator drugs and other drugs used to treat *asthma* may relieve symptoms, but the answer to the problem is prevention. This is achieved by treatment of raw textiles before processing, reduction of dust levels, and the wearing of face masks.

Byssinosis is a *prescribed disease* and sufferers are entitled to industrial injury benefit.

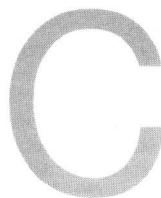

Cachexia

An appearance of profound illness and severe weight loss. Cachexia is usually caused by extreme starvation or by a serious underlying disease such as cancer or tuberculosis.

Cadaver

A dead human body used as a source of transplant organs or preserved for anatomical study and dissection.

Cadmium poisoning

The toxic effects of cadmium, a tin-like metal. Poisoning due to the inhalation of cadmium dust or fumes is an industrial hazard, the effects of which vary according to the duration and severity of exposure. Acute exposure may lead to *pneumonitis* (inflammation of the lungs). Exposure over a long period can lead to urinary tract *calculi* (stones), *kidney failure*, or *emphysema* (a form of permanent lung damage).

Cadmium poisoning may also be caused by eating vegetables grown in cadmium-rich soil or by consuming food or drink that has been stored in cadmium-lined containers. Cadmium is known to accumulate in the body (especially in the kidneys) throughout life. Although cadmium has been implicated in the development of high blood pressure in animals, a causative link has not been proved in humans.

Caecum

The first and widest part of the large intestine. The caecum is joined to the *ileum* (the last part of the small intestine) and to the ascending *colon*. Projecting from the caecum is the short tube known as the *appendix*. (See also *Digestive system*.)

Caesarean section

An operation to deliver a baby from the uterus through a vertical or horizontal incision in the abdomen. Caesarean section is performed when it is impossible or dangerous to deliver the baby vaginally. In the past 15 years the number of caesarean sections per-

formed in the US has increased dramatically to around 25 per cent of all births. In the UK, the increase has been less dramatic, with around 13 per cent of all babies being delivered by caesarean section in the early 1990s.

HOW IT IS DONE

The procedure for performing a caesarian section is shown in the illustrated box (see overleaf).

RECOVERY PERIOD

After the operation, the mother is given *analgesic drugs* (painkillers) as required. She is usually allowed to take fluids after 12 hours and to eat after 24 hours. The recovery period tends to be quicker if *epidural anaesthesia* rather than general anaesthesia (see *Anaesthesia, general*) is used. Provided there are no problems, the usual hospital stay is around a week after the operation.

Café au lait spots

Coffee-coloured patches on the skin. Café au lait spots are usually oval in shape, may measure several centimetres across, and may develop anywhere on the skin. The presence of only a few such spots is usually of no significance. Larger numbers of café au lait spots may be a sign of *neurofibromatosis*, a hereditary disorder of the sheaths that surround nerve fibres. In neurofibromatosis, café au lait spots are commonly accompanied by multiple small nodules in and on the skin.

Caffeine

A *stimulant drug* that occurs naturally in coffee beans, tea leaves, cocoa beans, and cola nuts commonly used in drinks. Caffeine is used in some drug preparations.

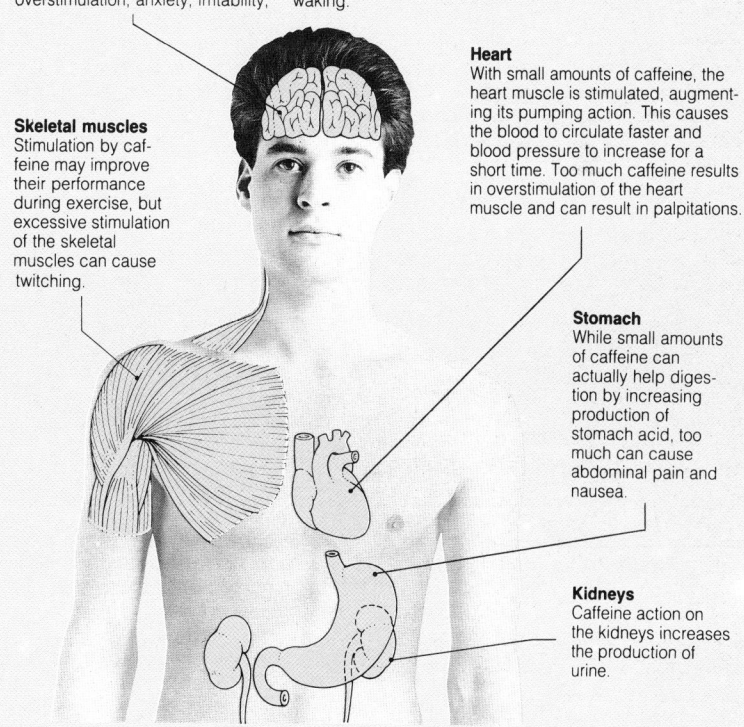

EFFECTS OF CAFFEINE ON THE BODY

Caffeine has a stimulant effect on all organs and tissues. It acts directly on individual cells by affecting their chemical reactions, and indirectly by increasing the release from the adrenal glands of adrenaline and noradrenaline, hormones that stimulate cell activity.

Brain
Small amounts of caffeine stimulate the brain cells, helping to reduce drowsiness and fatigue. Concentration is improved and reactions are speeded up. Large amounts cause overstimulation, anxiety, irritability, and restlessness. This is why consuming caffeine before going to bed can cause insomnia and a hangover in the morning, with excessive fatigue and drowsiness on waking.

Skeletal muscles
Stimulation by caffeine may improve their performance during exercise, but excessive stimulation of the skeletal muscles can cause twitching.

Heart
With small amounts of caffeine, the heart muscle is stimulated, augmenting its pumping action. This causes the blood to circulate faster and blood pressure to increase for a short time. Too much caffeine results in overstimulation of the heart muscle and can result in palpitations.

Stomach
While small amounts of caffeine can actually help digestion by increasing production of stomach acid, too much can cause abdominal pain and nausea.

Kidneys
Caffeine action on the kidneys increases the production of urine.

C

PROCEDURE FOR A CAESAREAN SECTION

A caesarean section allows delivery of a baby through a horizontal or vertical cut in the abdominal and uterine walls. The mother is given epidural anaesthesia, so that she remains conscious during the procedure, or general anaesthesia.

HOW IT IS DONE

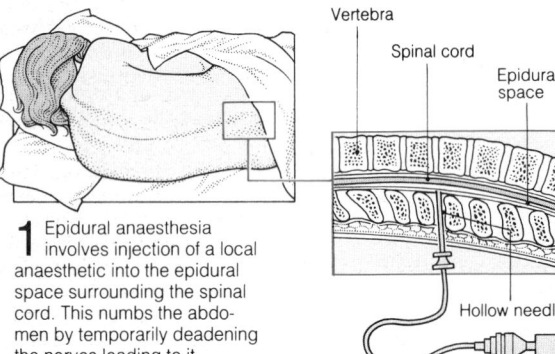

Vertebra
Spinal cord
Epidural space
Hollow needle

1 Epidural anaesthesia involves injection of a local anaesthetic into the epidural space surrounding the spinal cord. This numbs the abdomen by temporarily deadening the nerves leading to it.

WHY IT IS DONE

The operation is necessary if the baby is unable to fit through the mother's pelvis or shows signs of *fetal distress* (lack of oxygen) before the cervix is fully dilated. Other reasons for performing a caesarean section include a placenta (afterbirth) that is lying close to the cervix (placenta praevia), scarring on the uterus from previous surgery, unsuccessful induction of labour, *breech* presentation, and *postmaturity*.

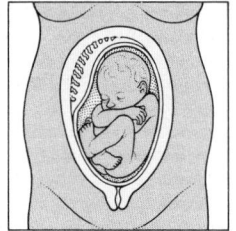

Breech presentation

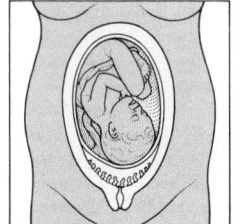

Placenta praevia

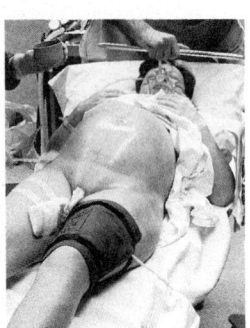

2 A *catheter* is inserted into the bladder to empty it. The abdomen is then opened, usually through a horizontal incision made just above the pubic bone. This type of cut heals most effectively.

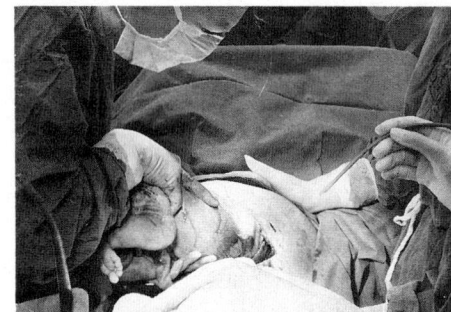

3 The amniotic fluid is drained off by suction. The baby is delivered through an incision in the lower part of the uterus, the umbilical cord is cut, and the afterbirth removed.

4 The incisions in the uterus and abdomen are then sewn up. The mother is given an injection of ergometrine to make the uterus contract and stop any bleeding.

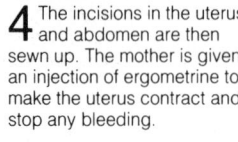

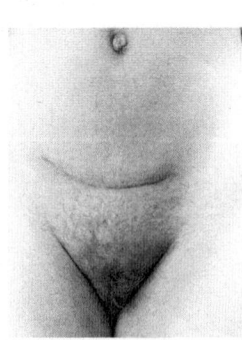

5 The resulting scar is hardly noticeable and comes below the "bikini line".

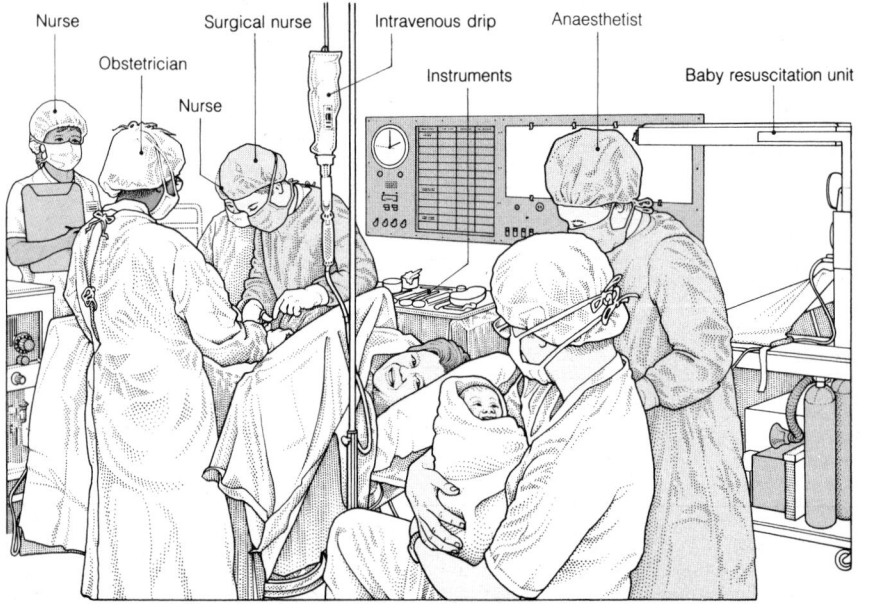

Nurse
Obstetrician
Nurse
Surgical nurse
Intravenous drip
Instruments
Anaesthetist
Baby resuscitation unit

Caffeine in drinks generally produces unpleasant side-effects, such as agitation and tremors, only when consumed in large quantities or by particularly sensitive individuals. People who regularly consume large amounts of caffeine (e.g. more than five cups of coffee per day) often find that their *tolerance* to the substance has increased, making it necessary for them to increase their intake to obtain the equivalent stimulant effect. They may also suffer withdrawal symptoms, such as tiredness, headaches, and irritability, if they go without caffeine for even as little as a few hours (see *Drug dependence*).

Because of its stimulant effect, caffeine can improve short-term athletic performance and its use is therefore banned for sports competitions (see *Sports, drugs and*).

Caffeine is often included in various drug preparations, particularly in combination with certain *analgesic drugs* (painkillers). However, its value is questionable, because it does not enhance the painkilling effect. Caffeine is combined with *ergotamine* in several drugs for the early preventive treatment of migraine.

CAFFEINE LEVELS (mg per cup)	
Tea, weak	50
Tea, strong	80
Coffee, weak	80
Coffee, strong	200
Cocoa	10-17
Cola	43-75

The strength and method of preparation determine exact amounts of caffeine present (in mg per cup).

Calamine

A pink substance consisting of zinc oxide and iron oxide that is applied to the skin in the form of ointments, lotions, or dusting powders. Calamine has a protective, cooling, and drying effect, and is used to relieve skin irritation and itching. It is sometimes combined with a local anaesthetic (see *Anaesthesia, local*), a *corticosteroid drug*, or an *antihistamine drug*. Bandages impregnated with calamine are sometimes used to protect leg ulcers.

Calcaneus

The heel-bone. The calcaneus is one of the tarsal bones and is the largest bone in the *foot*.

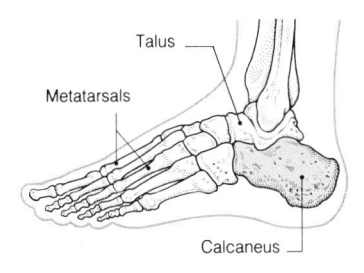

LOCATION OF THE CALCANEUS
This is the largest tarsal bone, projecting backwards beyond the leg bones.

Talus
Metatarsals
Calcaneus

DISORDERS
The calcaneus may be fractured as a result of falling from a height on to the heels. Minor fractures usually do not cause problems and are treated by putting the foot and leg in a cast. A more serious fracture, with compression of the bone, may cause permanent damage to the joints involved in turning the foot in and out, leading to pain and stiffness that are aggravated by walking.

The *Achilles tendon* is fixed to the back of the heel-bone and controls the up and down movement of the foot. The point at which the tendon joins the bone may be strained by excessive or prolonged stress from the pull of the tendon—for example, in some *running injuries*. In children this area of bone is still growing and occasionally becomes inflamed and painful (see *Osteochondrosis*).

Tendons of the sole of the foot are fixed under the heel-bone; the associated muscles are important in supporting the arches of the foot. Inflammation around these tendons (as in plantar *fasciitis*) causes pain and tenderness under the heel when standing or walking. A calcaneal spur (a bony protrusion from this part of the calcaneus) occurs in some people with plantar fasciitis and also sometimes in people with healthy feet.

Calciferol

An obsolete name for vitamin D_2; it is now known as ergocalciferol (see *Vitamin D*).

Calcification

The deposition of calcium salts in body tissues. Calcification is part of the normal process of bone and teeth formation and is necessary for the healing of fractures. Calcification can

occur in an injured muscle and is common in arteries affected by *atherosclerosis*. It may also occur if the blood calcium level is raised as a result of a disorder of the *parathyroid glands*.

Calcification, dental

The deposition of calcium crystals in developing teeth. Calcium and phosphorus salts are carried in the blood supply to the teeth, where the crystals make up 96 per cent of tooth enamel and 70 per cent of dentine. Calcification of primary teeth begins in the fetus at between three and six months gestation; calcification of permanent teeth (other than the wisdom teeth) begins between birth and four years.

Abnormal calcification occurs in amelogenesis imperfecta, an inherited disorder of the enamel (see *Hypoplasia, enamel*). The affected teeth have a thin, grooved covering due to incomplete calcification. Another cause of abnormal calcification is the absorption of high levels of fluoride (see *Fluorosis*).

Calcinosis

A condition in which there is abnormal deposition of *calcium* salts in various tissues, such as the skin, muscles, or *connective tissues*. The abnormal calcium deposits form nodules within the affected tissues. Calcinosis tends to be associated with an underlying connective tissue disorder, such as *scleroderma* or *dermatomyositis*.

The term "calcinosis" is usually combined with another word to signify which part of the body is affected—for example, calcinosis cutis affects the skin. (See also *Calcification*.)

Calcitonin

A hormone produced by the *thyroid gland*. Calcitonin helps to control the level of *calcium* in the blood by slowing the rate at which calcium is lost from the bones.
WHY IT IS USED
A synthetic form of calcitonin is used to treat *Paget's disease*, in which the bones grow abnormally and become deformed, causing pain and an increased risk of fracture. Given by injection, calcitonin halts abnormal bone formation in about a week and can relieve pain within a few months.

Calcitonin is also used to treat *hypercalcaemia* (abnormally high levels of calcium in the blood) caused by overactivity of the *parathyroid glands* or by cancer of the bone. Calcitonin helps relieve the nausea and vomiting that result from hypercalcaemia by quickly reducing the level of calcium in the

C

blood. Calcitonin may be prescribed in conjunction with a *corticosteroid drug* that also decreases the calcium level in the blood.

POSSIBLE ADVERSE EFFECTS
Calcitonin does not usually cause any troublesome adverse effects. Gastrointestinal reactions, such as nausea, vomiting, and diarrhoea, usually diminish with continued use.

Calcium

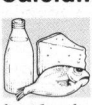
The most abundant mineral in the body, with several important functions. Calcium is essential for the functioning of cells, for muscle contraction, for the transmission of nerve impulses from nerve endings to muscle fibres, and for blood clotting. In the form of calcium phosphate it makes up the hard basic constituent of teeth and bones. An average-sized person carries about 0.9 to 1.1 kg of calcium, mostly in the bones.

The main dietary sources of calcium are dairy products, eggs, fish (when the bones are eaten), and some vegetables (e.g. green, leafy vegetables). Calcium may be added to flour.

CONTROL OF CALCIUM LEVELS
Vitamin D and certain hormones help control the overall amount of calcium in the body by regulating the amount of calcium absorbed from food, and the amount removed from the body by the kidneys (which filter excess calcium from the blood and excrete it in the urine).

Control of calcium levels is achieved by the actions of two hormones: parathyroid hormone (produced by the *parathyroid glands*) and calcitonin (produced by the *thyroid gland*). Normally the blood plasma carries less than 0.1 per cent of the body's total amount of calcium—the optimum amount for the efficient functioning of cells throughout the body. When the level of calcium in the blood falls to a low level, the parathyroid glands release more parathyroid hormone, which raises the blood calcium level by helping to release calcium from the enormous reservoir in the bones. When the blood calcium level rises to a high level, the thyroid gland releases more calcitonin, which counteracts the effects of parathyroid hormone and lowers the calcium level.

DISORDERS OF CALCIUM METABOLISM
Abnormally high or low levels of calcium in the blood may seriously disrupt cell function, particularly in muscles and nerves. Having too much calcium in the blood is called *hypercal-*

caemia and having too little is called *hypocalcaemia*. (See also *Calcium channel blockers*; *Mineral supplements*.)

Calcium channel blockers

COMMON DRUGS

Diltiazem Felodipine Nifedipine Verapamil

A relatively new class of drug used in the treatment of *angina pectoris* (chest pain due to an inadequate blood supply to heart muscle), *hypertension* (high blood pressure), and certain types of cardiac *arrhythmia* (irregular heartbeat).

HOW THEY WORK
In the treatment of angina pectoris and high blood pressure, calcium channel blockers work by interfering with muscle contraction. They prevent the movement of calcium across the membrane that lines muscle cells, which is an essential part of the mechanism of muscle contraction. This action decreases the work of the heart in pumping blood, reduces the pressure of blood flow through the body, and improves the circulation of blood through heart muscle.

Calcium channel blockers also slow the passage of nerve impulses through heart muscle, which helps correct certain types of arrhythmia.

POSSIBLE ADVERSE EFFECTS
Adverse effects of calcium channel blockers are mainly related to their action of increasing blood flow through tissues. These effects include headaches, facial flushing, and dizziness (usually on standing). Such effects, however, generally disappear with continued treatment.

Calculus

A deposit on the teeth (see *Calculus, dental*) or a small, hard, crystalline mass formed from substances occurring in fluid, such as bile, urine, or saliva. The usual sites for such calculi are the gallbladder and bile ducts (see *Gallstones*), the kidneys, ureters, or urinary bladder (see *Calculus, urinary tract*), and the salivary ducts. Stones may be symptomless or may cause severe pain and may then need to be treated (by being dissolved, shattered, or surgically removed).

Calculus, dental

A hard, crust-like deposit found on the crowns and roots of teeth. Also known as tartar, calculus is formed when mineral salts from saliva are deposited in existing *plaque*. These minerals, mainly calcium and phos-

phorus, make up about 70 per cent of the calculus; the rest is organic material and bacteria.

TYPES
Supragingival calculus, which forms above the gum margin on the crowns of teeth, is usually white or yellowish. It commonly occurs on the inside surfaces of the lower incisors and on the outer surfaces of the upper molars—areas close to the duct openings of the salivary glands.

Subgingival calculus, which forms below the gum margin, is more evenly distributed around all the teeth. Possibly because of breakdown products of blood from the gums, subgingival calculus is brown or black, and is visible if the gum is gently parted from the tooth. It may show through the gum as a dark area.

Both types of calculus are hard and are therefore difficult to remove; the subgingival variety may be more difficult to remove because of its location and degree of calcification.

EFFECTS AND TREATMENT
Being porous, calculus is impossible to keep clean and continually becomes covered by plaque. The irritant effect of toxins in plaque and calculus causes progressive inflammation and destruction of the gums and supporting structures of the teeth (see *Periodontitis*). Calculus should be completely removed on a regular basis by professional *scaling*. Careful *oral hygiene*, professional cleaning, and elimination of stagnation areas, such as poorly finished fillings, should diminish or slow its recurrence.

Calculus, urinary tract

A stone in the kidneys, ureters, or bladder, caused by precipitation from solution of the substances in urine.

INCIDENCE
The incidence of stones varies in different parts of the world. Kidney and ureteral stones are more common than bladder stones in developed countries; bladder stones are relatively more common in developing countries.

In the UK, about 40,000 people each year are diagnosed as having a kidney or ureteral stone. Such stones are three times more common in men than in women and the incidence is highest in the summer months, perhaps because the urine is more concentrated because of loss of fluid in sweat. Stones tend to be a recurrent problem; about 60 per cent of patients treated for a stone develop another within seven years.

COMPOSITION AND CAUSES

KIDNEY AND URETERAL STONES There are various types of kidney and ureteral stones. In the majority of cases, there is no identifiable underlying cause, although mild chronic dehydration (for example, due to inadequate water consumption in a hot climate) may play a part, as may a prolonged period of confinement to bed.

About 70 per cent of kidney and ureteral stones consist mainly of calcium oxalate and/or phosphate. Oxalate is an end-product of body *metabolism* and is present naturally in the urine. The salt it forms with calcium dissolves poorly. An abnormally high level of oxalate in the urine predisposes to stone formation and may be related to a diet containing food or drinks with a high oxalic acid content (for example, rhubarb, spinach, leafy vegetables, and coffee). Stones containing calcium are in some cases the first evidence of a disturbance of metabolism associated with *hyperparathyroidism* (overactivity of the parathyroid glands).

About 20 per cent of calculi are termed infective stones and are linked with chronic *urinary tract infection*. These calculi consist of a combination of calcium, magnesium, and ammonium phosphate and are associated with a high ammonium content and alkalinity of the urine produced by the action of bacteria on urea (a substance in urine). In the kidney, an infective stone may fill the entire network of urine-collecting ducts and the top part of the ureter, forming a large, oddly shaped "staghorn" calculus.

Stones consisting mainly of uric acid comprise about 5 per cent of the total and may occur in people with *gout*, people with some cancers, and people with chronic *dehydration*.

Other, uncommon types of stone occasionally occur. Those formed from the amino acid cystine affect people with cystinuria (an inherited *metabolic disorder*).

BLADDER STONES In poorer countries, bladder stones usually develop as a result of a diet that is low in phosphate and protein. In developed countries, they usually result from obstruction to the flow of urine from the bladder and/or a long-standing urinary tract infection. The composition of bladder stones varies according to the acidity or alkalinity of the urine, but in the UK the most common type consists of calcium oxalate.

SYMPTOMS

The most common symptom of a stone in the kidney or ureter is *renal colic* (a severe pain in the loin). The most common symptom of a bladder stone is difficulty in passing urine.

DIAGNOSIS

Investigation of a suspected calculus usually starts with examination of the urine, which may reveal red blood cells and the presence of crystals. The degree of acidity or alkalinity of the urine may reflect the type of stone involved. About 90 per cent of urinary tract calculi are visible on X-rays, which show the site of the stone; this can be confirmed by intravenous or retrograde *urography*. These special X-ray techniques also indicate any obstruction of the urinary tract above the stone, which can be monitored by *ultrasound scanning*. If a metabolic disorder is a suspected cause of the stone, chemical analysis of the blood and urine may be performed to look for high levels of calcium, phosphate, urate, or cystine.

TREATMENT

Renal colic is treated with bed rest, a narcotic analgesic drug (painkiller), and adequate fluid intake to encourage passing of the stone through the ureter, bladder, and urethra. The majority of stones less than 5 mm in diameter are passed in the urine at home with relatively few problems.

In the case of larger stones, or if an infection or obstruction to urinary flow is present, surgical treatment may be needed to prevent damage to the kidney. The traditional method of removing stones from the ureter or the junction between the ureter and kidney is by surgery under general anaesthesia. Stones in the bladder and lower ureter can be crushed and removed by *cystoscopy* (passage of a slim viewing tube and crushing device up the urethra into the bladder) or by ureterorenoscopy (passage of a similar tube into the ureter).

Methods introduced in the 1980s for the removal of kidney, ureteric, and bladder stones substantially changed the approach to their treatment. The first line of treatment is extracorporeal shock wave *lithotripsy*, which disintegrates stones by focusing

---

URINARY TRACT CALCULI

Symptoms vary according to the site of the stone. Small stones in the kidney often cause no symptoms until they start to pass down the ureter, resulting in *renal colic*, a sudden pain in the flank that moves towards the groin. The pain is acute, sharp, and intermittent and may cause nausea and vomiting. There may also be haematuria (blood in the urine). Bladder stones, which affect men far more often than women, can cause difficulty in passing urine, a poor flow rate, and dribbling. Some stones may be associated with recurrent episodes of *urinary tract infection*. Any obstruction to urine flow may result in rapid kidney damage and acute severe infection termed *pyelonephritis*.

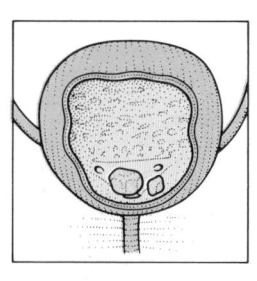
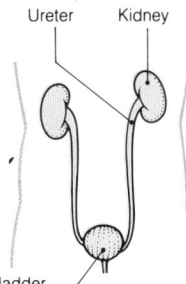
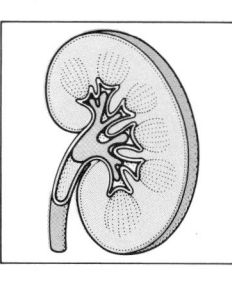

Ureter   Kidney

Bladder

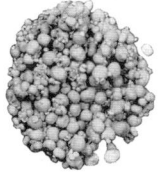
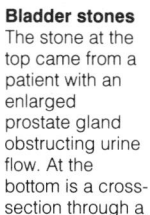

Bladder stones
The stone at the top came from a patient with an enlarged prostate gland obstructing urine flow. At the bottom is a cross-section through a much larger stone.

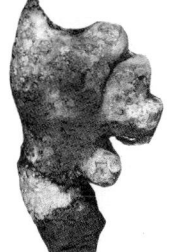

Staghorn calculus
Stones of this type form within and fill the pelvis of the kidney (at the top of the ureter). They are linked with urinary tract infection.

C

shock waves on them from outside the body; and sometimes an ultrasonic probe is inserted into the body in order to break up large stones. Traditional methods are still used in some cases.

If a stone is thought to have developed because of a metabolic disorder, the patient may be prescribed a diet, and possibly drugs, to lower the content in the urine of the substance from which the stone is formed; it may also be necessary to maintain a high fluid intake. These methods may act to dissolve an existing stone and may help prevent recurrences.

Stones associated with hyperparathyroidism are treated by methods appropriate to their location; in most cases a parathyroid gland tumour is responsible for the condition and this is removed.

Calendar method

A method of *contraception*, also called the rhythm method, that entails abstaining from sexual intercourse around the time of ovulation, which is predicted on the basis of the length of previous menstrual cycles.

The calendar method is unreliable because a woman's menstrual cycle may vary, and therefore the time of ovulation can be estimated only approximately. There are now more scientific and effective contraceptive methods of this type. (See *Contraception, natural methods*.)

Calf muscles

The muscles extending from the back of the knee to the heel. The *gastrocnemius muscle* starts behind the knee and forms the bulky part of the calf. Under it is the soleus muscle, which starts lower down from the back of the *tibia* (shin). These muscles join to form the *Achilles tendon*, which connects them to the heel.

Contraction of the calf muscles pulls the heel up to produce a springing movement through the toes. This movement is important in walking, running, jumping, and hopping.

Pain can occur because of *cramp*, *sciatica* (inflammation of the sciatic nerve), or, more rarely, deep vein *thrombosis*. The calf muscles may be affected by *claudication* (a cramp-like pain brought on by walking and quickly relieved by rest).

Caliper splint

An orthopaedic device used to exert control on a deformed leg or to support a leg weakened by a muscular

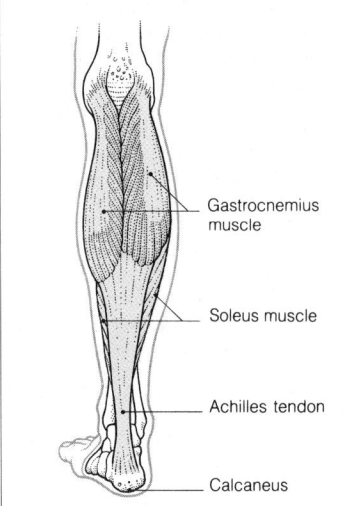

LOCATION OF CALF MUSCLES
The gastrocnemius and soleus join to form the Achilles tendon.

Gastrocnemius muscle

Soleus muscle

Achilles tendon

Calcaneus

disorder, making it possible for the person to stand and walk. For example, a person who has lost the ability to flex the foot upward, and, as a result, drags the toes on the ground with each step, can be fitted with a splint that keeps the foot permanently at right angles to the leg and thus allows walking.

A caliper splint consists of one or two vertical metal rods attached to leather or metal rings worn around the limb. A caliper splint extending only below the knee is sufficient to control the position of the ankle. Longer splints may be jointed to allow knee movement.

Callosity

See *Callus, skin*.

Callus, bony

A diffuse growth of new soft *bone* that forms around a healing *fracture*. The callus is eventually replaced by stronger bone with a more organized structure. A callus can sometimes be felt as a lumpy deformity around a fracture site and is visible on an X-ray. Presence of a callus provides evidence that healing has started. As healing continues, the original shape of the bone is restored.

Callus, skin

An area of thickened skin, caused by regular or prolonged pressure or friction. Manual labourers develop calluses on the palms of their hands, jog-

gers on the soles of their feet, and guitarists on the tips of their fingers.

Calluses may also develop if body weight is borne unevenly—for example, if there is a persistent deformity affecting one foot. A *corn* is a callus on a toe.

TREATMENT
If a callus on the foot becomes troublesome or painful, a chiropodist should be consulted. He or she can pare away layers of thickened skin with a scalpel. Calluses caused by foot deformities almost always recur unless the underlying problem is corrected—either surgically or by using a moulded insole in the shoe.

Caloric test

A method of discovering whether a person with *vertigo* (dizziness) and hearing loss has a diseased labyrinth (part of the inner ear).

The outer-ear canal of one ear is briefly flooded with water at different temperatures above and below normal body temperature. This flooding sets up convection currents in the semicircular canals situated within the inner ear.

If the labyrinth is normal, *nystagmus* (rapid reflex flickering of the eyes) occurs for a predictable period. If the labyrinth is diseased, nystagmus will either not occur or will stop sooner than normal. The presence and duration of the nystagmus may be observed directly or be recorded electrically using the technique of *electronystagmography*.

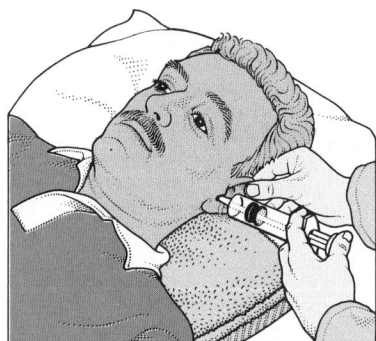

Performing a caloric test
The doctor floods the outer ear with water at different temperatures and watches for reflex flickering of the eyes.

Calorie

A measure of energy. Strictly, one calorie is the amount of energy needed to raise the temperature of 1 g of water by 1°C. In medicine and dietetics, the energy content of foods and the energy used to perform various activities is sometimes measured in units called kilocalories, which are equal to 1,000 calories. These two units are often confused because both are referred to as calories. However, the medical unit is abbreviated as Cal or kcal, whereas the ordinary, "small" calorie is abbreviated as cal.

When the daily calorie intake is the same as the amount of energy expended, a person's weight usually remains constant. If intake exceeds expenditure, weight is usually gained; if expenditure exceeds intake, weight is usually lost. In general, fats contain the most calories per unit weight—9 kcal per g compared with carbohydrates and proteins at 4 kcal per g.

The use of calories as a measure of energy is gradually being replaced by the joule; 1 calorie equals 4.2 joules. (See also *Calorimetry; Diet and disease*.)

Calorie requirements

See *Energy requirements*.

Calorimetry

The measurement of the *calorie* (energy) value of foodstuffs or the energy expenditure of a person.

Direct calorimetry is the usual method of calculating the calorie value of small amounts of a particular foodstuff. This calorie value may then be converted to the number of calories in a typical serving. After being weighed and placed in a special sealed container, called a bomb calorimeter, the food is ignited; the calorimeter is then immersed in a known volume of water. The rise in the temperature of the water when the foodstuff is completely burned up is used to calculate the calorie value.

Energy production in humans is more easily measured indirectly. It has been found that every litre of oxygen taken into the body produces 4.8 kilocalories of energy. Therefore, to calculate energy production, it is only necessary to measure oxygen uptake. This can be done by comparing the percentage of oxygen in inspired and expired air.

Cancer

Any of a group of diseases in which symptoms are due to the unrestrained growth of cells in one of the body organs or tissues. Malignant tumours most commonly develop in major organs, such as the lungs, breasts, intestines, skin, stomach, or pancreas, but they may also develop in the nasal sinuses, the testes or ovar-

CANCER-CAUSING AGENTS

The table gives a rough estimate of the proportion of cancer deaths that can be attributed to various specific agents or behaviours. Smoking is particularly implicated in lung and bladder cancers, and alcohol in cancers of the tongue, pharynx, and oesophagus. Sexual and reproductive behaviour affect the risk of cervical cancer (the more sexual partners a woman has, the higher the risk) and of breast cancer (having children while relatively young protects against this cancer). Note the importance of dietary factors.

CANCER-CAUSING AGENTS	
Agent	% of cancer deaths
Natural constituents of food	35
Tobacco	30
Sexual and reproductive history	7
Occupational hazards	4
Alcohol	3
Food additives	1
Other	20

ies, or the lips or tongue. Cancers may also develop in the blood-cell-forming tissues of the bone marrow (the *leukaemias*) and in the lymphatic system, muscles, or bones.

Cancers are not the only type of abnormal growth, or *neoplasm*, that occur in the body. However, a cancer differs from a *benign tumour*, such as a *wart* or a *lipoma*, in two important ways. As it grows, it spreads and infiltrates the tissues around it and may block passageways, destroy nerves, and erode bone. Cells from the cancer may spread via the blood vessels and lymphatic channels to other parts of the body, where these *metastases* form new, satellite tumours.

INCIDENCE

Cancer is a process that has affected humans since prehistoric times and is just as common in domestic and farm animals, birds, and fish. It affects more than one in four people in the UK at some time in their lives and is the second most common cause of death (after heart disease), accounting for about 150,000 deaths annually or one fifth of the total number of deaths. Altogether about 220,000 cases of cancer are registered every year. Apart from childhood cancers, which may be associated with events during pregnancy, such as exposure to radiation, most adult cancers are a feature of the aging process.

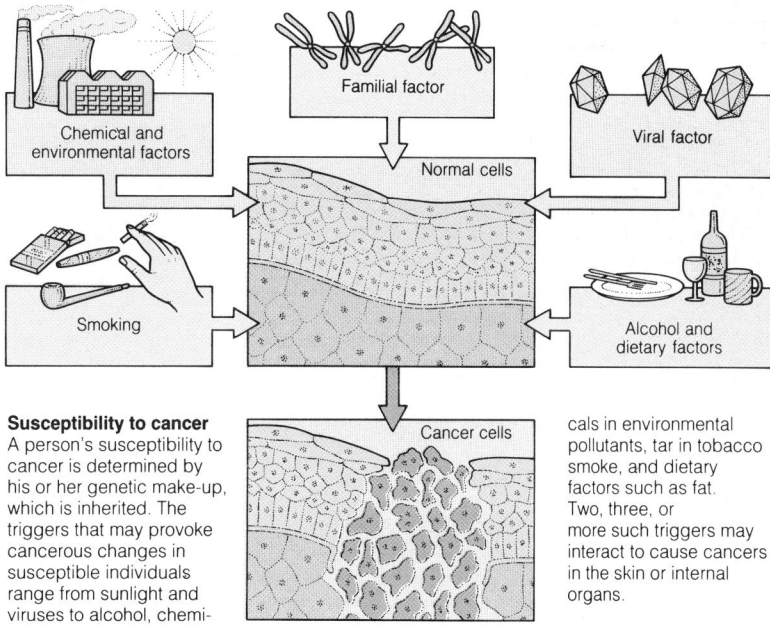

Susceptibility to cancer
A person's susceptibility to cancer is determined by his or her genetic make-up, which is inherited. The triggers that may provoke cancerous changes in susceptible individuals range from sunlight and viruses to alcohol, chemi-cals in environmental pollutants, tar in tobacco smoke, and dietary factors such as fat. Two, three, or more such triggers may interact to cause cancers in the skin or internal organs.

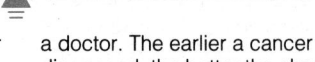

INCIDENCE OF CANCER

The likelihood of cancer developing varies with age. A 20-year-old has a very low likelihood of it developing by the age of 30, but the risk roughly doubles between 30 and 40, and doubles again for each decade thereafter. Whatever the cause of death in someone aged 90, careful examination of the internal organs will often reveal a small cancer that may not have caused any symptoms. Localized cancer of the prostate is an almost universal finding in elderly men. Thus, while cancer seems to be much more common than in the past, this is mostly due to the increasing numbers of old people in the population.

CANCER WARNING SIGNS

Cancer may cause a variety of minor symptoms. Any that persist for several days should be checked by a doctor. The earlier a cancer is diagnosed, the better the chance of there being a cure.

Rapid weight loss without apparent cause
A scab, sore, or ulcer that fails to heal within three weeks
A blemish or mole that enlarges, bleeds, or itches
Severe recurrent headaches
Difficulty swallowing
Persistent hoarseness
Coughing up bloody sputum (phlegm)

Persistent abdominal pain
Change in shape or size of testes
Blood in urine, with no pain on urination
Change in bowel habits
Lump or change in breast shape
Bleeding or discharge from nipple
Vaginal bleeding or spotting between periods or after menopause

Cancer site

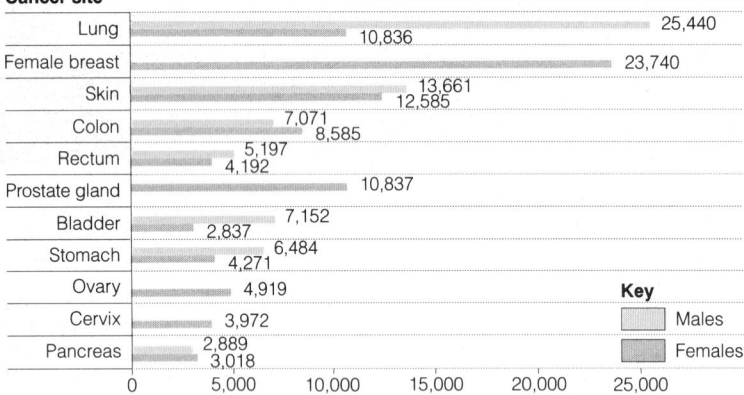

Cancer site	Males	Females
Lung	25,440	10,836
Female breast		23,740
Skin	12,585	13,661
Colon	7,071	8,585
Rectum	5,197	4,192
Prostate gland	10,837	
Bladder	7,152	2,837
Stomach	6,484	4,271
Ovary		4,919
Cervix		3,972
Pancreas	2,889	3,018

Incidence (total new cases men or women)

Key
Males
Females

Incidence of common cancers

The chart (left) shows the total numbers of new cases of the common cancers registered in England and Wales in 1987. (These figures were published in 1993—there is a long delay.) Lung cancer remains the most common cancer in men, and breast cancer the most common in women, and both still have a high mortality rate despite advances in treatment. The high number of skin cancers in both men and women has to be seen in the context that most of these cancers are cured. The greater number of bladder cancers in men is partly explained by the link between these cancers and industrial chemicals.

WORLD INCIDENCE RATES FOR COMMON CANCERS

Site of origin of cancer	% affected in high-incidence area by age 75	Low-incidence area
Skin	20 Queensland, Australia	Bombay, India
Oesophagus	20 Northeast section of Iran	Nigeria
Lung and bronchus	11 England	Nigeria
Stomach	11 Japan	Uganda
Cervix	10 Colombia	Jewish Israel
Prostate	9 US (blacks only)	Japan
Liver	8 Mozambique	England
Breast	7 British Columbia, Canada	Non-Jewish Israel
Colon	3 Connecticut	Nigeria
Uterus	3 California	Japan
Mouth	2 Bombay, India	Denmark
Rectum	2 Denmark	Nigeria
Bladder	2 Connecticut	Japan
Ovary	2 Denmark	Japan
Nasopharynx	2 Chinese Singapore	England
Pancreas	2 Maori New Zealand	Bombay, India
Larynx	2 São Paulo, Brazil	Japan
Pharynx	2 Bombay, India	Denmark
Penis	1 Parts of Uganda	Jewish Israel

Age group

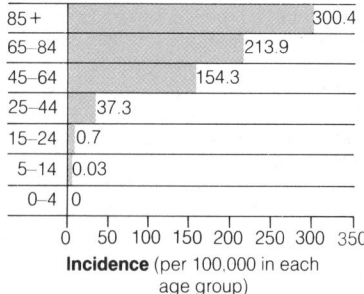

Age group	Incidence
85+	300.4
65–84	213.9
45–64	154.3
25–44	37.3
15–24	0.7
5–14	0.03
0–4	0

Incidence (per 100,000 in each age group)

Incidence of breast cancer with age

Breast cancer is almost nonexistent under the age of 25. Over 25, the incidence rises rapidly, from 37.3 cases per 100,000 women in the 25-44 age group, to more than 300 cases per 100,000 in the over-85s.

CAUSES

The growth of a cancer begins when the *oncogenes* (genes controlling cell growth and multiplication) in a cell or cells are transformed by agents known as *carcinogens*.

Once a cell is transformed into a tumour-forming type (malignant transformation), the change in its oncogenes is passed on to all offspring cells. A small group of abnormal cells is thus established, and they divide more rapidly than the normal surrounding cells. Usually the abnormal cells show a lack of *differentiation*—that is, they no longer perform the specialized task of the cells of their host tissue—and may escape the normal control of hormones and nerves. Thus, they are in effect parasites, contributing nothing to their host tissue but continuing to consume nutrients.

Years may pass before the growth of cells becomes large enough to cause symptoms, although the rate of growth varies according to the tissue of origin. Current estimates suggest that some cancers of the lung and breast may be present for well over five years before they cause symptoms. During this "occult" phase, metastases may be seeded in the liver, lungs, bones, or brain, and, in these circumstances, a purely surgical cure is impossible because the cancer has already spread far beyond the primary site of origin.

SYMPTOMS

The range of symptoms produced by cancers is vast. The symptoms depend on the site of the growth, the tissue of origin, and the extent of the growth. Symptoms may be a direct feature of the growth (e.g. lumps or skin changes) or they may be derived from obstruction or bleeding into passageways, such as the lung airways, gastrointestinal tract, or urinary tract, or from disruption of the function of a vital organ. Tumours pressing on or disturbing nerve tracts can cause nervous system disorders and pain. Some tumours lead to the overproduction of hormones, with complications and effects far distant from the site of the growth. Unexplained weight loss is a feature of many types of cancer.

Some important warning signals that always warrant investigation by a doctor are shown in the accompanying table (see opposite page).

DIAGNOSIS

Both the means of diagnosing cancer at an early stage (when the chances of cure are highest) and the range of

TREATMENT OF CANCER

The treatment of many cancers is still primarily surgical; excision of an early tumour will often give a complete cure. Because there may be small, undetectable metastases at the time of operation, surgery is commonly combined with *radiotherapy* and *anticancer drugs*. The aim of these treatments is to suppress, or arrest, the rate of cell division in any tumour cells left after surgery. Anticancer drugs often have unpleasant side-effects because it is sometimes difficult to target specific drugs effectively, and normal cells and tissues may be disrupted along with the tumour cells.

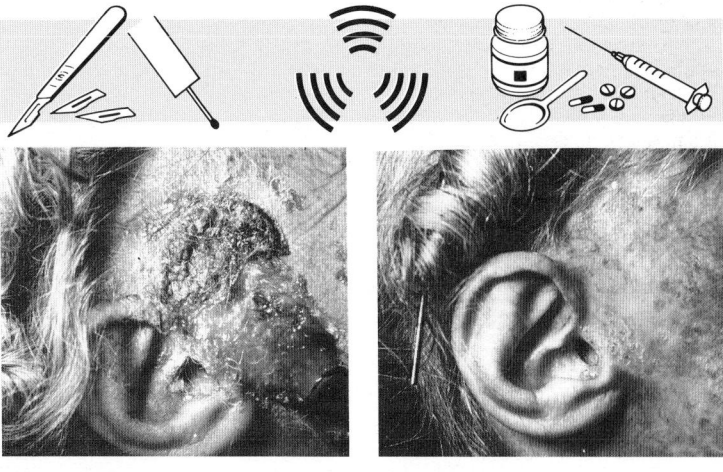

Before radiotherapy
The photograph shows a skin cancer in front of the ear before treatment.

After radiotherapy
This was the appearance a few weeks later, after a course of radiotherapy.

treatments available have improved dramatically in the past decade.

Screening tests (for early breast cancer, cancer of the cervix, and intestinal cancer) have reduced mortality from these tumours. For most tumours, however, diagnosis generally occurs after the appearance of symptoms, is based on the doctor's examination of the patient, and is confirmed by microscopic examination of tissue cells obtained by *biopsy* (cancer cells look different from normal cells). New scanning and imaging techniques give more information while causing less discomfort to the patient.

There are four main types of tests: cytology tests, imaging techniques, chemical tests, and direct inspection (see chart overleaf).

OUTLOOK

Almost half of all cancers are today cured completely, and cure and survival rates for various years after diagnosis continue to improve. For disease of certain organ systems, the diagnosis of a cancer may actually provide a better outlook than some of the alternative diagnoses. Cure and survival rates and the chances of recurrence do, however, differ markedly according to the organ or tissue affected.

For more information on cancers of individual organs—their incidence, causes, symptoms, treatment, and outlook—refer to the organ in question (e.g. *Breast cancer; Lung cancer; Stomach cancer*).

Cancerphobia

An intense fear of developing cancer, out of proportion to the actual risk, so that the sufferer's behaviour and lifestyle are significantly altered. A cancerphobic person becomes convinced that any symptoms (e.g. skin problems, constipation, or difficulty in swallowing) are signs of cancer and seeks medical advice. Instead of paying sensible attention to diet and prevention (such as giving up smoking), he or she adopts extreme behaviour (for example, prolonged washing rituals, avoidance of social contact, bizarre eating habits) typical of *obsessive-compulsive disorder*. *Psychotherapy* or *behaviour therapy* may be of benefit. (See also *Phobia*.)

TYPES OF CANCER TEST

Cytology tests	These tests reveal the shedding of abnormal cells. One example is the *cervical smear test*, an investigation in which cells are scraped from the cervix and examined microscopically to	detect potential or early cancer of the cervix. Another example is the urine cytology test, periodically carried out on those working in manufacturing industries where bladder cancer is a known risk.
Imaging techniques	These can sometimes reveal early cancerous changes in tissue. A notable example is the special low-dose X-ray technique used in *mammography* to detect early cancer of the breast. Research	with *ultrasound scanning*, which produces images of internal organs, suggests that it may provide a means of screening for cancer of the ovary.
Chemical tests	These tests can reveal the presence of substances that are indicative of cancer—for example, microscopic amounts of blood in	the faeces, and high levels of the enzyme acid phosphatase in the blood.
Direct inspection	Inspection of the interior of organs subject to cancer is usually carried out with an *endoscope* (a tube with a viewing lens), which is passed into the organ to be examined. Examples of this technique are	*colonoscopy, gastroscopy, cystoscopy,* and *laparoscopy*. These procedures are usually carried out only when clinical suspicion has been aroused.

Cancer screening

Tests carried out on groups of people to detect early signs of cancer. To warrant their use, screening tests must have a high rate of accuracy, must be safe, and must cause minimal discomfort. Effective treatment must also be available. Screening tests are most effectively carried out among those particularly susceptible to cancer, either because of their occupation or lifestyle, or because of a genetic predisposition.

In theory, regular check-ups, including radiological and laboratory tests, might be expected to detect cancers at an early, treatable stage. In practice, several of the more common cancers—notably lung and pancreas cancers—are rarely detected by screening tests before they cause symptoms.

Nevertheless, tests proven to be effective include those for cancers of the cervix, breast, bladder, and colon, while tests are being evaluated for early diagnosis of ovarian and prostate cancers.

Cancrum oris

A condition, also called *noma*, in which ulcers and tissue destruction occur in and around the mouth. Cancrum oris commonly affects malnourished children in poor tropical countries.

Candidiasis

Infection by the fungus CANDIDA ALBICANS, also known as thrush or moniliasis. It most commonly affects the vagina but also affects other areas of mucous membrane, such as inside the mouth, or moist skin.

CAUSES AND INCIDENCE
The fungus that causes candidiasis is normally present in the vagina and mouth. Its growth is kept under control by the bacteria usually present in these organs. If *antibiotic drugs* destroy too many of the bacteria, or the body's resistance to infection is lowered, the fungus may multiply excessively.

Certain disorders, notably *diabetes mellitus*, and the hormonal changes that occur in pregnancy or when a woman is taking *oral contraceptives*, may also encourage growth of the CANDIDA ALBICANS fungus.

Candidiasis can be contracted by sexual intercourse with an infected partner, and about 60,000 cases are reported annually by sexually transmitted disease clinics in the UK. Candidal infection is much more common in women than in men. Candidal infection of the penis is uncommon but is more likely to occur in men who have not been circumcised.

Candidiasis may spread from the genitals or mouth to other moist areas of the body. It may also affect the gastrointestinal tract, especially in people who have impaired immune systems. In infants, candidiasis sometimes occurs in conjunction with *nappy rash*.

SYMPTOMS
Vaginal candidiasis may cause a thick, white, "cottage cheese" discharge from the vagina and/or vaginal itching and irritation. There may also be discomfort when passing urine. However, some women have no symptoms. In men, infection of the penis usually causes *balanitis* (inflammation of the head of the penis).

Oral candidiasis produces sore, creamy-yellow, raised patches in the mouth. Candidiasis that affects the skin folds or the nappy area takes the form of an itchy red rash with flaky white patches.

DIAGNOSIS AND TREATMENT
Candidiasis is diagnosed by examination of a sample of the white discharge or patches. Treatment is with an *antifungal drug*, such as nystatin, clotrimazole, miconazole, or econazole nitrate. Drugs are usually prescribed in the form of vaginal suppositories or creams to be applied to the affected area. Simultaneous treatment of sexual partners is recommended to prevent reinfection.

Treatment is usually successful but the condition tends to recur. People with a tendency to skin candidiasis should keep the skin as dry as possible, and women who take *oral contraceptives* may be advised to consider changing to another, nonhormonal, method of contraception.

Canine tooth

See *Teeth*.

Cannabis

Psychoactive preparations derived from the hemp plant CANNABIS SATIVA. (See *Marijuana*.)

Cannula

A plastic or metal tube with a smooth, unsharpened tip for inserting into a blood vessel, lymphatic vessel, or body cavity in order to introduce or withdraw fluids.

To insert a cannula, the doctor first punctures the site with a long, thin needle, slides the cannula over it, and then withdraws the needle. Alternatively, he or she may insert a trocar (sharp-pointed rod) inside the cannula and remove it once the vessel has been entered.

Cannulas are frequently used for *blood transfusions* and *intravenous infusions* and for draining *pleural effusions*. In certain circumstances, such as when blood is required for testing over a period of time, the cannula may be left in place for several days.

Cap, contraceptive

A barrier method of contraception in the form of a latex rubber device placed directly over the cervix to prevent sperm from entering. (See *Contraception, barrier methods of.*)

Capgras' syndrome

The *delusion* (false belief) that a relative or close friend has been replaced by an impostor. Also known as the "illusion of doubles", Capgras' syndrome is seen most frequently in paranoid *schizophrenia*, but also occurs in organic disorders (see *Brain syndrome, organic*) and *affective disorders.*

Capillary

Any of the vessels that carry blood between the smallest arteries, or arterioles, and the smallest veins, or venules (see *Circulatory system*). Capillaries form a fine network throughout the body's organs and tissues. It is through the thin capillary walls that blood and cells exchange their constituents (see *Respiration*).

Capillaries have a diameter of approximately 0.008 mm—not much wider than the red blood cells that flow through them. The capillary walls are permeable to substances such as oxygen, glucose, carbon dioxide, and water, which can thus move freely between the blood and the tissue fluid that surrounds all cells.

STRUCTURE OF CAPILLARIES

These minute blood vessels have permeable walls to allow transfer of oxygen, glucose, and water from blood to tissues.

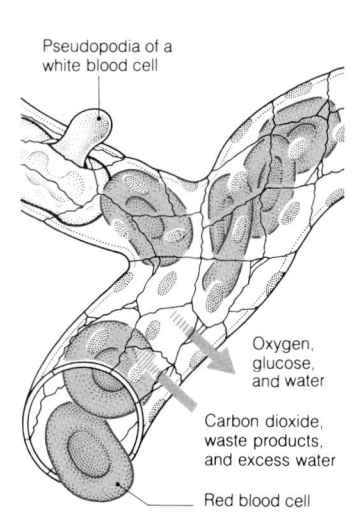

Pseudopodia of a white blood cell

Oxygen, glucose, and water

Carbon dioxide, waste products, and excess water

Red blood cell

The capillaries are not open to blood flow all the time; they open and close according to different organs' requirements for oxygen and nutrients. Thus, when a person is running, most of the capillaries in the leg muscles are open, but at rest many are closed. The opening and closing of skin capillaries plays an important role in *temperature* regulation. Blood flow through each capillary is controlled by a tiny circle of muscle at its entrance.

DISORDERS

A direct blow to the body may rupture the thin capillary walls, resulting in bleeding under the surface of the skin and causing swelling and bruising.

Capillaries become more fragile in the elderly, in people taking high doses of *corticosteroid drugs*, and in sufferers from *scurvy* (vitamin C deficiency). All such people have a tendency to *purpura* (small blue-purple areas of bleeding under the skin).

Capillary *haemangiomas* are benign tumours of the capillary wall that may cause a red patch of variable size and shape on the skin or mucous membranes. Such haemangiomas may be congenital (present at birth) or they may develop later in life.

Capping, dental

See *Crown, dental.*

Capsule

An anatomical structure enclosing an organ or body part; examples include the capsules of the liver, kidneys, joints, and eye lenses.

The term capsule is also used to describe a hard or soft shell, usually made of gelatine, containing a drug. Capsules are taken by mouth and have two main advantages over solid tablets. Firstly, their elongated shape makes them easier to swallow. Secondly, they make it easier for patients to take solid or liquid medications that would otherwise have an unpleasant taste or smell.

Some capsules have a special coating to prevent the release into the stomach of drugs that may have an irritant effect. Others are designed to release their contents into the small intestine at a slow, steady rate so that a drug need be taken less frequently than if it was in the form of a conventional capsule or tablet.

Capsulitis

Inflammation of a capsule around an organ or other body part. Inflammation of the capsule of the shoulder joint is a feature of *frozen shoulder.*

Captopril

The first member of a new class of drugs, the *ACE inhibitors*, used in the treatment of *hypertension* (high blood pressure) and *heart failure.*

Caput

The Latin word for head. The term caput is also used to refer to the face, skull, and all associated organs, to the origin of a muscle, or to any enlarged extremity, such as the caput femoris, the head of the femur (thigh-bone). However, the term most commonly refers to the caput succedaneum, a soft swelling in the scalp of newborn babies. The swelling occurs as a result of pressure on the baby's head during labour and usually disappears after a few days.

Carbamazepine

ANTICONVULSANT

Tablet Liquid

Prescription needed

Available as generic

An *anticonvulsant drug*, introduced in 1960, chemically related to the tricyclic *antidepressant drugs.*

WHY IT IS USED

Carbamazepine reduces the likelihood of seizures caused by abnormal nerve signals in the brain and is mainly used in the long-term treatment of *epilepsy*. It has less of a sedative effect than many other anticonvulsant drugs.

Carbamazepine is also prescribed to relieve *neuralgia* (the intermittent severe pain caused by damage to, or irritation of, a nerve). Carbamazepine is occasionally prescribed to treat certain psychological or behavioural disorders, such as *mania.*

POSSIBLE ADVERSE EFFECTS

There may be some sedative effect, especially if alcohol is consumed.

Carbenoxolone

An *ulcer-healing drug* that is used to treat stomach ulcers. Carbenoxolone is thought to work by stimulating the production of mucus that forms a protective coating over the lining of the stomach. Carbenoxolone is also given in the form of a special capsule for the treatment of duodenal ulcers; the capsule releases the active drug in the duodenum after it passed through the stomach. A gel containing carbenoxolone is also available for the relief of mouth ulcers.

Adverse effects of carbenoxolone are usually caused by a loss of potassium or an increase in sodium levels in the body and include headache and muscle weakness.

Carbimazole

A drug used to treat *hyperthyroidism* (overactivity of the thyroid gland). Carbimazole may take several weeks to take full effect and *beta-blocker drugs* are therefore often used in addition to carbimazole to help control symptoms in the interim.

Long-term treatment with carbimazole may reduce production of blood cells by the bone marrow; regular blood cell counts may be carried out to monitor this effect. Other possible adverse effects include headache, dizziness, joint pain, and nausea.

Carbohydrates

A group of compounds composed of carbon, hydrogen, and oxygen which supply the body with its main source of energy.

TYPES AND SOURCES

There are two groups: available carbohydrates, which are metabolized (chemically changed) in the body, and unavailable carbohydrates, which can not be broken down by human digestive *enzymes*.

Monosaccharides	glucose, galactose, fructose
Disaccharides	sucrose, lactose, maltose
Polysaccharides	starch cellulose

Types of carbohydrates
Monosaccharides are the simplest, consisting of a single saccharide molecule. Disaccharides consist of two saccharide molecules linked together. Polysaccharides consist of a long chain of many saccharide molecules. The most important carbohydrate is starch.

The available carbohydrates include starches (complex carbohydrates) and sugars (simple carbohydrates) and are found in cereals, root crops, and fruits. The unavailable carbohydrates include cellulose and hemicellulose, which pass through the body virtually unchanged and make up the bulk of what is known as dietary fibre (see *Fibre, dietary*).

The term refined carbohydrate usually refers to sucrose refined from cane or beet, with no other nutrients. Cornflour (corn starch) is another refined carbohydrate, consisting of pure starch with no other nutrients.

CARBOHYDRATE METABOLISM

The monosaccharides or simple sugars—glucose (grape sugar), galactose (a milk sugar), and fructose (fruit sugar)—are absorbed into the bloodstream unchanged; the disaccharides (double sugars) such as sucrose and lactose (a milk sugar) have to be broken down to the simple sugars first, and so do the starches.

The monosaccharides (principally glucose) are then absorbed through the intestinal wall and into the bloodstream for distribution throughout the body. Certain cells, such as brain cells and red blood cells, must have a constant supply of glucose to survive. Some of the glucose is used immediately by these cells, which ''burn'' it in a series of biochemical reactions to generate energy (see *Metabolism*). The rest of the glucose is conveyed to the liver, muscles, and fat cells where it is converted into *glycogen* (animal starch) and fat for storage. When more energy is needed, this glycogen is converted back to glucose, which reenters the bloodstream for distribution around the body.

Fat cannot be converted to glucose but can be burned as fuel to conserve glucose. Unlike glucose, galactose and fructose cannot be used directly by the body's cells and so must first be converted by the liver to glucose; thereafter, the fate of this glucose is the same as that of glucose absorbed directly into the bloodstream from the intestine.

When the blood glucose level is high, such as after a meal, carbohydrate metabolism is primarily controlled by *insulin*, a hormone secreted by the *pancreas*. Insulin restores the glucose level to normal by stimulating its uptake by the liver, muscles, and adipose cells for storage as glycogen and fat. In the disorder *diabetes mellitus*, carbohydrate metabolism is disturbed by a deficiency of insulin, and carbohydrates cannot enter most cells for storage.

The action of insulin is balanced by that of *glucagon*, another hormone produced by the pancreas. When the blood sugar level is low—for example, after fasting overnight or after exercise—insulin secretion diminishes and glucagon stimulates the conversion of glycogen to glucose for release into the bloodstream. Adrenaline and corticosteroid hormones produced by the *adrenal glands* at times of stress also act to raise the blood sugar level.

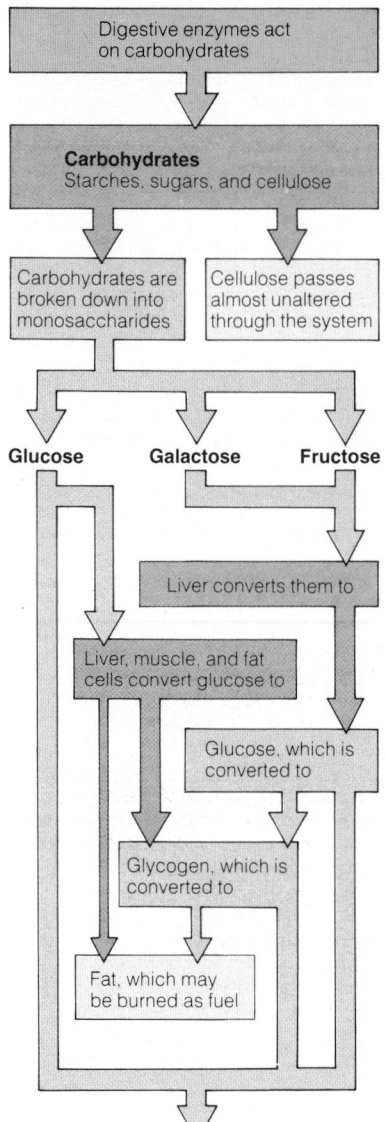

CARBOHYDRATE METABOLISM

Digestive enzymes act on carbohydrates

Carbohydrates
Starches, sugars, and cellulose

Carbohydrates are broken down into monosaccharides

Cellulose passes almost unaltered through the system

Glucose **Galactose** **Fructose**

Liver converts them to

Liver, muscle, and fat cells convert glucose to

Glucose, which is converted to

Glycogen, which is converted to

Fat, which may be burned as fuel

Glucose is absorbed into the bloodstream for distribution throughout the body or is used directly by body cells.

Carbon

A nonmetallic element that is present in all organic molecules (the fundamental molecules of all living organisms), such as *proteins*, *fats*, and *carbohydrates*, and also in some inorganic molecules, such as *carbon dioxide*, *carbon monoxide*, and *sodium bicarbonate*. Pure carbon exists in nature as the major constituent of diamonds, coal, *charcoal*, and graphite (pencil lead).

Carbon dioxide

A colourless, odourless gas. Carbon dioxide is present in small amounts in the air and is an important by-product of normal *metabolism* in the body. Carbon dioxide consists of one carbon atom (symbol C) linked to two oxygen atoms (symbol O) and has the chemical formula CO_2. When cooled and compressed, carbon dioxide forms a white solid, *dry ice*, which is used in *cryosurgery*.

Carbon dioxide is a waste product of metabolic reactions that break down various substances, especially carbohydrates and fats, to generate energy. Waste carbon dioxide is carried by the blood to the lungs, where it is released and breathed out. One of the factors controlling the rate of breathing is the level of carbon dioxide in the bloodstream. When a person exercises, the amount of carbon dioxide produced increases, and the resultant high level in the bloodstream causes the person to breathe more rapidly to eliminate the carbon dioxide and to take in more oxygen.

Carbon monoxide

A colourless, odourless, poisonous gas. Carbon monoxide is present in the exhaust fumes of petrol engines and is also produced by inefficient burning of coal, gas, oil, or bottled gas in domestic heating appliances. It consists of one carbon atom (chemical symbol C) linked to one oxygen atom (symbol O) and has the chemical formula CO.

POISONING

Carbon monoxide is poisonous because it binds with *haemoglobin* (the oxygen-carrying molecule in red blood cells) and prevents it from carrying oxygen. As a result, the tissues are deprived of oxygen and asphyxiation occurs. Continued inhalation of the gas may lead to permanent brain damage or even death.

The initial symptoms of carbon monoxide poisoning—which may sometimes be mistaken for those of food poisoning—are dizziness, headache, nausea, and faintness. The most important step in first-aid treatment is to take the victim into the fresh air; continued exposure to the gas will lead to loss of consciousness. If the victim has stopped breathing, give *artificial respiration* and get emergency medical aid. Even if the victim seems to recover completely when taken into the fresh air, it is advisable for him or her to consult a doctor to make certain that there are no long-term effects.

Carbon tetrachloride

A colourless, poisonous, volatile liquid with a characteristic odour. Carbon tetrachloride is present in some home dry-cleaning fluids and is sometimes used as an industrial solvent. It consists of one carbon atom (symbol C) linked to four chlorine atoms (symbol Cl) and has the chemical formula CCl_4.

Carbon tetrachloride is a dangerous chemical; it can produce dizziness, mental confusion, and liver and kidney damage if it is inhaled or drunk. Symptoms of poisoning include abdominal pain, nausea, headache, and convulsions. Because its use is controlled, poisoning by carbon tetrachloride is now rare in the UK.

Carbuncle

A cluster of interconnected *boils* (painful, pus-filled, inflamed hair roots). Carbuncles are usually caused by the bacterium STAPHYLOCOCCUS AUREUS; they generally begin as single boils, then spread. Common sites are the back of the neck and the buttocks.

Carbuncles are less common than single boils. They mainly affect people who have a lowered resistance to infection, in particular, people with *diabetes mellitus*.

TREATMENT

Anyone with a carbuncle should see a doctor, who will usually prescribe an *antibiotic drug*. The application of hot *compresses* may encourage the pus-filled heads of the boils to burst and thus relieve pain. After the boils have burst, the carbuncle should be covered with a dressing until it has healed completely. Occasionally, incision and drainage (with removal of the core of the carbuncle) are necessary if drainage and healing do not occur on their own.

Carcinogen

Any agent capable of causing *cancer*, such as tobacco smoke, high-energy radiation, or asbestos fibres.

CHEMICAL CARCINOGENS

Chemicals are the the largest group of carcinogens. Among the most important are polycyclic aromatic hydrocarbons (PAHs), which occur in tobacco smoke, pitch, tar fumes, and soot. Exposure to PAHs may lead to cancer of the respiratory system or skin.

Other major chemical carcinogens are certain aromatic amines. These chemicals are used principally in the chemical and rubber industries and may cause bladder cancer after prolonged exposure.

PHYSICAL CARCINOGENS

The best-known physical carcinogen is high-energy *radiation*, including nuclear radiation and *X-rays*. High doses of high-energy radiation destroy individual cells (an effect utilized in *radiotherapy* to destroy tumours), and very high doses may kill people within a few hours. Lower doses may not kill cells but may sometimes cause malignant changes.

Radiation affects most easily those cells which divide quickly—for example, the precursors of white blood cells in the bone marrow, so causing leukaemia.

Exposure over many years to ultraviolet radiation in sunlight can cause skin cancer, particularly in people who are fair-skinned.

Asbestos fibres are another known physical cause of cancer. White asbestos may cause lung cancer, particularly in workers who are exposed to the fibres for long periods, who already have *asbestos-induced diseases* of the lungs, and who smoke. Blue asbestos and, to a lesser extent, brown asbestos can cause *mesothelioma* (a tumour of the membranes that surround certain body cavities and organs).

BIOLOGICAL CARCINOGENS

Very few biological agents cause cancer in humans. SCHISTOSOMA HAEMATOBIUM, one of the blood flukes responsible for the tropical disease *schistosomiasis*, can cause cancer of the bladder, where it lays its eggs. ASPERGILLUS FLAVUS, a fungus that contaminates stored grain and peanuts, produces the poison *aflatoxin*, which is believed to be a cause of liver cancer.

Certain viruses have been associated with cancer. The papilloma virus is believed to play a part in the causation of cancer of the cervix, the hepatitis B virus has been implicated in liver cancer, and the Epstein-Barr virus is considered to be a factor in the causation of *Burkitt's lymphoma*, a malignant tumour of the jaw and abdomen which occurs mainly among children in Africa. *Kaposi's sarcoma* is probably associated with a virus (possibly cytomegalovirus). Although not caused directly by *HIV* (the *AIDS* virus), Kaposi's sarcoma is seen more frequently in individuals who have HIV infection.

SCREENING

Any substance that could possibly be carcinogenic, such as a food additive, cosmetic, or chemical for use in drugs, must be screened before it is allowed to be manufactured. One major preliminary test is to expose a certain strain of bacteria to the substance, and, if *mutation* (genetic change) occurs in the bacteria, the substance is regarded as a suspect carcinogen. It is then tested on laboratory animals, such as rats. If an increased incidence of tumours occurs in the test animals, no licence is usually granted to manufacture the substance for public sale.

AVOIDING CARCINOGENS

In industry, known carcinogens are either banned or allowed only if their use is considered essential, if exposure to them is strictly limited, and if regular medical screening is provided for workers using them, as, for example, in the nuclear fuel industry and hospital X-ray departments.

Outside industry, the individual is exposed to very few known, unavoidable, high-risk carcinogens. However, given the long latent period from exposure to the development of cancer for most carcinogens, it would be prudent to regard handling of any chemical repeatedly as something to be done with the maximum of care. (See also *Carcinogenesis*.)

Carcinogenesis

The development of a *cancer* (a malignant tumour) caused by the action of certain chemicals, viruses, constituents of the diet, radiation, or unknown factors on cells that are primarily normal.

Cancer-causing factors are called *carcinogens*. Carcinogens are believed to alter the *DNA* (genetic material) within cells, particularly the structure of certain genes called *oncogenes* which normally control the growth and division of cells. An altered cell divides abnormally rapidly and passes on the changes in its genetic material to all its offspring cells. Thus, a group of cells becomes established that is not affected by the body's normal restraints on growth.

Carcinoid syndrome

A rare condition characterized by bouts of facial flushing, diarrhoea, and wheezing. Carcinoid syndrome is caused by an intestinal or lung tumour, called a carcinoid, that secretes excess quantities of the hormone serotonin.

Symptoms usually occur only if the tumour has spread to the liver, or arises from the lung.

DIAGNOSIS AND TREATMENT

Carcinoid syndrome is diagnosed by measuring the level of a breakdown product of serotonin in the urine.

The condition is sometimes treated by surgical removal of the tumour from the intestine or lung, and from the liver as well, if possible. In most cases, surgical treatment is unlikely to be helpful, and in these circumstances symptoms may be relieved by drugs that block the action of serotonin.

Carcinoma

Any malignant tumour (*cancer*) arising from cells in the covering surface layer or lining membrane of a body organ. A carcinoma is thus distinguished from a *sarcoma*, which is a cancer arising in bone, muscle, or connective tissue. Carcinomas include all the most common cancers of the lungs, breast, stomach, skin, cervix, colon and rectum (parts of the large intestine). The terms cancer and carcinoma tend to be used interchangeably but are not strictly synonymous.

Carcinomatosis

The presence of malignant tissue in many different sites of the body due to the spread of cancer cells from an original malignant tumour.

SYMPTOMS

The sufferer experiences weight loss, lack of energy, and other symptoms depending on the site of the *metastases* (secondary or offspring tumours). Metastases in the lungs may cause coughing or breathlessness; in the liver they may cause jaundice.

DIAGNOSIS AND TREATMENT

A diagnosis of carcinomatosis may be confirmed by *X-rays* or by *radionuclide scanning* of the bones and lungs, by biochemical tests, or during an operation or postmortem examination. An operation to remove the primary (original) tumour will not help someone with carcinomatosis unless the primary tumour is producing a hormone that is directly stimulating growth of the metastases. *Anticancer drugs* or *radiotherapy* may be given to deal with the metastases, sometimes following removal of a primary carcinoma.

Metastases associated with some cancers (of the testis, prostate, and thyroid glands) may be treated with drugs or hormones, and a prolonged abatement of symptoms, and even cure, is now common. Metastases from lung and intestinal cancers are less responsive to treatment and, in such cases, the outlook is not good.

Cardiac arrest

A halt in the pumping action of the heart due to cessation of its rhythmic, muscular activity.

CAUSES

The most common cause is a *myocardial infarction* (heart attack), but other causes include *respiratory arrest*, *electrical injury*, *hypothermia*, loss of blood, drug overdose, and *anaphylactic shock*.

DIAGNOSIS AND TREATMENT

A person with cardiac arrest collapses suddenly, with loss of consciousness, absence of pulse, and no breathing movements. A person who is breathing cannot have suffered from a cardiac arrest.

An absolutely certain diagnosis can be made only by measuring the electrical activity of the heart by *ECG*, but *cardiopulmonary resuscitation* should be started immediately to minimize the risk of brain damage.

As soon as adequate help arrives—most hospitals have a cardiac arrest team on standby—the diagnosis can be confirmed by ECG. This test distinguishes between *ventricular fibrillation* and *asystole*, which are the two types of heart muscle disturbance that can lead to cardiac arrest.

Ventricular fibrillation is the random, uncoordinated contraction of individual heart muscle fibres. This may be corrected by *defibrillation* (an electric shock to the heart).

Asystole is the complete absence of heart muscle activity and is more difficult to reverse. It may respond to intravenous injection of *adrenaline* and calcium or in extreme cases to direct injection of adrenaline into the heart. An electrical *pacemaker* may also stimulate the heart in asystole.

In all cases of cardiac arrest the balance of the chemical constituents of the blood is disturbed, making the blood more acidic; an intravenous infusion of sodium bicarbonate is usually given to correct this. Other drugs, such as lignocaine, can also be administered intravenously to stabilize the heart muscle.

OUTLOOK

Between one fifth and one third of patients whose heartbeat is restored after cardiac arrest recover sufficiently to leave hospital (however, a substantial number of these die within the following year). In the remainder, the damage to the heart or brain is too extensive for recovery to be possible.

Cardiac massage

See *Cardiopulmonary resuscitation*.

Cardiac neurosis

Excessive anxiety or fear about the condition of the heart. It usually occurs after a *myocardial infarction*

C

(heart attack) or heart surgery but may also occur in people who have had no previous heart trouble.

The sufferer experiences symptoms that mimic those typical of heart disease—chest pain, tightness in the chest, lethargy, palpitations, and breathlessness—and may be reluctant to exercise or to return to work for fear of bringing on these symptoms. Examination and investigation of the heart by a doctor will reveal no physical cause for the symptoms.

Psychotherapy may help the patient overcome fears and anxieties. If it does not, the patient may not be able to return to a normal, active life.

Cardiac output

The volume of blood pumped by the heart in a given time (usually per minute). Cardiac output can be used as a measure of how efficiently the heart is working. At rest, a healthy adult heart pumps between 2.5 and 4.5 litres of blood per minute; during exercise this figure may rise to as much as 30 litres per minute. A low figure during exercise is a sign that the heart muscle is damaged or that major blood loss has occurred.

Cardiac stress test

A type of *fitness test* carried out on people who experience chest pain, breathlessness, or palpitations during exercise. The test is used to determine whether the patient has *angina pectoris* and signs of *coronary artery disease*. A cardiac stress test may also be performed in conjunction with *radionuclide scanning* to identify any damaged areas of heart muscle.

HOW IT IS DONE
The patient is attached to an *ECG* machine, which records the pattern of the heart's electrical activity. He or she then performs an exercise, such as walking on a treadmill. A diagnosis of angina is confirmed if there are specific changes in the wave pattern shown on the *ECG* recording as the intensity of exercise is increased.

The test is performed under close medical supervision, with resuscitation facilities immediately available. If at any time the patient suffers chest pain, becomes breathless, or feels sick, the test is stopped immediately.

Cardiology

The study of the function of the *heart*; the investigation, diagnosis, and medical treatment of disorders of the heart and blood vessels, especially *atherosclerosis* and *hypertension*.

Anatomically and physiologically, the heart occupies a central position in the body. It has a single function—to pump blood first to the lungs and then to the rest of the body—but the sequence of events in each heart contraction is complex.

Reduced pumping efficiency of the heart can have various underlying causes, including *arrhythmias*, *coronary artery disease* (in which the blood supply to the heart muscle is impaired), *cardiomyopathy* (in which the muscle itself is abnormal), and *heart valve disorders*.

Disease of the lungs and blood vessels can also have adverse effects on heart function. Some babies are born with structural defects of the heart and/or major blood vessels that emerge from it (see *Heart disease, congenital*).

Heart disorders are now the leading cause of death in the UK. The study of the heart in health and disease is thus a large part of the training of every doctor; general practitioners are familiar with the treatment of patients with common disorders, such as coronary artery disease and hypertension.

For more expert investigation and treatment, a person with a heart problem may be referred to a cardiologist (heart specialist), who may perform tests such as *echocardiography*, and detailed interpretation of *ECGs* (electrocardiograms) and *chest X-rays*. A cardiologist may, in turn, refer a patient to a cardiovascular surgeon if surgical treatment is necessary.

The past 10 years have seen rapid advances in the understanding of heart disease, its causes, its investigation, and its treatment.

Cardiomegaly

Enlargement of the heart. In some cases, cardiomegaly takes the form of hypertrophy (thickening) of the heart muscle; in others, it takes the form of dilatation (increase in volume) of one or more of the heart chambers.

CAUSES
Hypertrophy of the heart muscle occurs in any condition where the heart has to work harder than normal to pump blood around the body. Such conditions include *hypertension* (increased blood pressure), which causes the wall of the left ventricle (main pumping chamber) to thicken; *pulmonary hypertension* (increased blood pressure in the lungs), in which the wall of the right ventricle thickens; and one type of *cardiomyopathy* (disease of the heart muscle), in which either or both ventricles may thicken.

Dilatation of a heart chamber may be due to heart valve incompetence (failure of a valve to close properly after a contraction). For example, in *aortic insufficiency*, failure of the aortic valve to close completely allows blood to flood back from the aorta into the left ventricle after each contraction, eventually enlarging the chamber. Certain types of cardiomyopathy can also lead to swelling of a chamber.

SYMPTOMS
There are no symptoms until enlargement reaches a point where the heart is no longer capable of coping with additional stress (for example, as a result of exercise or infection). This reduces the efficiency of the heart as a pump and leads to *heart failure*, causing breathlessness and swelling of the legs and hands.

DIAGNOSIS AND TREATMENT
Cardiomegaly is diagnosed by physical examination, *chest X-ray*, and *ECG* (measurement of electrical impulses in the heart). Treatment is directed at the underlying disorder.

Cardiomyopathy

Any disease of the heart muscle that causes a reduction in the force of heart contractions and a resultant decrease in the efficiency of circulation of blood through the lungs and to the rest of the body. The disease may have an infectious, metabolic, nutritional, toxic, autoimmune, or degenerative cause, but in many cases the cause is unknown.

TYPES
Cardiomyopathies fall into the following three main groups: hypertrophic, dilated, and restrictive.

Hypertrophic cardiomyopathy is usually a familial (inherited) disorder of unknown cause in which there is abnormality of the heart muscle fibres.

In dilated cardiomyopathy, muscle cell metabolism (chemical activity) is abnormal, and the walls of the heart tend to dilate (balloon out) under pressure. The cause of the abnormal cell metabolism is unknown.

Restrictive cardiomyopathy is caused by scarring of the endocardium (the inner lining of the heart) or by *amyloidosis* (infiltration of the muscle with a starch-like substance).

Heart muscle disorders may also be due to poisoning (e.g. by excessive consumption of alcohol) or to a vitamin or mineral deficiency (e.g. lack of vitamin B_1).

INCIDENCE
Cardiomyopathies are less common than other types of heart disease. The specific incidence of the different

C

types is unknown because in many cases of cardiomyopathy there are few or no symptoms. Sometimes the damage to the heart muscle is discovered only at an autopsy after the individual has died from an unrelated cause.

SYMPTOMS AND SIGNS

Symptoms usually include fatigue, chest pain, and palpitations due to an increased awareness of the heartbeat or to an abnormal heart rhythm such as *atrial fibrillation* (rapid, uncoordinated contractions of the upper chambers of the heart).

Heart failure (reduced efficiency of the heart's pumping action) can cause breathing difficulty and oedema (swelling due to accumulation of fluid) of the legs and hands.

DIAGNOSIS

A *chest X-ray* usually shows enlargement of the heart outline. *Echocardiography* shows the thickened heart muscle and confirms the absence of valvular disease.

The diagnosis can be confirmed by examining a *biopsy* sample of heart muscle under the microscope to show muscle cell abnormalities.

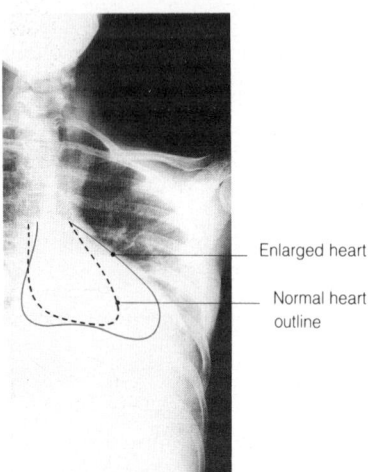

Enlarged heart

Normal heart outline

Chest X-ray showing cardiomyopathy
The heart has become much enlarged, due to the heart muscle abnormality.

TREATMENT

If, as is often the case, the cause remains unknown, there is no specific treatment. Treatment of symptoms may include the use of *diuretic drugs* to control heart failure and *antiarrhythmic drugs* to correct abnormal heart rhythm. For those with alcoholic cardiomyopathy, stopping all intake of alcohol is essential. *Immunosuppressant drugs* are occasionally helpful.

In many cases, heart muscle function steadily deteriorates, and the only option left is a *heart transplant*.

Cardiopulmonary resuscitation

The administration of the life-saving measures of external cardiac compression massage and mouth-to-mouth resuscitation (see *Artificial respiration*) to someone collapsing with *cardiac arrest* (cessation of heartbeat).

It is vital to restore the circulation of oxygen-carrying blood to the brain as quickly as possible because permanent brain damage is likely if the brain is starved of oxygen for more than three to four minutes.

WHEN TO GIVE CARDIOPULMONARY RESUSCITATION

Before starting cardiopulmonary resuscitation it is important to establish that the victim has suffered a cardiac arrest and has not simply fainted. A person who has had a cardiac arrest will be unresponsive and have no (or very slight) breathing motions. Skin colour will be extremely pale, or bluegrey, especially around the lips. The person's heart will not seem to be beating. No pulse will be felt in the wrist or neck, and no heartbeat will be heard when the chest is listened to. (If the person is breathing, no matter how slowly, then the heart will probably still be beating, even if no pulse can be felt.)

HOW TO GIVE CARDIOPULMONARY RESUSCITATION

See illustrated box opposite.

Cardiotocography

See *Fetal heart monitoring*.

Cardiovascular

A term that means pertaining to the heart and blood vessels.

Cardiovascular disorders

Disorders of the heart, blood vessels, and blood circulation. (See *Heart disorders box*; *Arteries, disorders of*; *Veins, disorders of*.)

Cardiovascular surgery

The branch of surgery concerned with the heart and blood vessels. Cardiovascular surgery includes operations to prevent or repair damage caused, for example, by congenital heart disease (see *Heart disease, congenital*), *atherosclerosis* (fat deposits on arterial walls), or a *myocardial infarction* (heart attack). Procedures performed include *heart valve surgery*, *coronary artery bypass*, and *heart transplant*.

Cardioversion

Another name for *defibrillation*.

Carditis

A general term for inflammation of any part of the heart or its linings. Carditis may be one of three kinds: a *myocarditis* (inflammation of the heart muscle), usually caused by a viral infection; an *endocarditis* (inflammation of the internal lining of the heart chambers and heart valves) usually due to a bacterial infection; or a *pericarditis* (inflammation of the outer lining of the heart), possibly with *effusion* (collection of fluid). The latter is usually due to a viral or bacterial infection, but may be associated with a *myocardial infarction* (heart attack) or, occasionally, may be caused by an *autoimmune disorder*, such as systemic *lupus erythematosus* (SLE).

Caries, dental

Tooth decay; the gradual erosion of enamel (the protective covering of the tooth) and dentine (the substance beneath the enamel).

CAUSES

Plaque is the main cause of tooth decay (see illustrated box overleaf). The most common sites of initial decay are areas where plaque easily becomes trapped, such as the grinding surfaces of the back teeth (which have minute grooves in them), the lateral (side) edges of adjacent teeth, and near the gum line.

INCIDENCE

An encouraging sign in industrialized countries over the past 10 to 15 years has been the significant decline (of 35 to 50 per cent) in dental caries among children. The evidence suggests that, of the various factors probably responsible, the most important is water *fluoridation*, which strengthens enamel. The addition of *fluoride* to toothpaste has also played a part.

SYMPTOMS

Early decay does not usually cause any symptoms. The chief symptom of advanced decay is toothache, which may be aggravated by eating very sweet, hot, or cold food. Decay may also cause bad breath.

TREATMENT

Treatment consists of drilling away the area of decay and filling the cavity (see *Filling, dental*) with either dental amalgam (a mercury alloy) or cement (a composite resin that matches the colour of the tooth).

In cases of advanced decay, it may be necessary to remove the infected pulp (the central, living part of a

FIRST AID: CARDIOPULMONARY RESUSCITATION

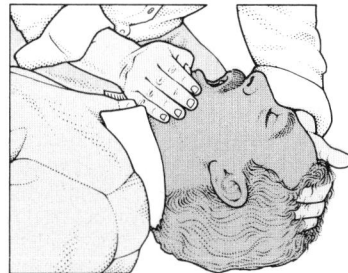

1 First make sure the airway is clear. Then look and listen for signs of breathing. Listen for air escaping and feel for air flow. Feel for the pulse.

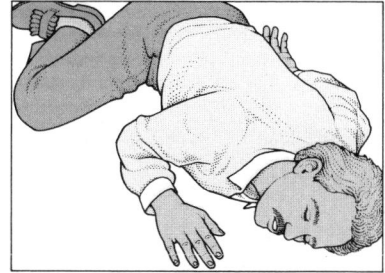

2 If the victim is breathing, place in the *recovery position*—if not, SHOUT FOR HELP then begin mouth-to-mouth resuscitation; prolonged resuscitation requires assistance.

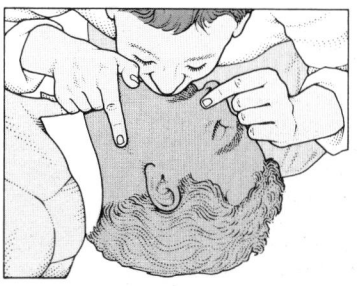

3 Pinch the victim's nose shut, take a breath, seal your lips around the mouth, and blow. Your breath contains enough oxygen for the victim's needs.

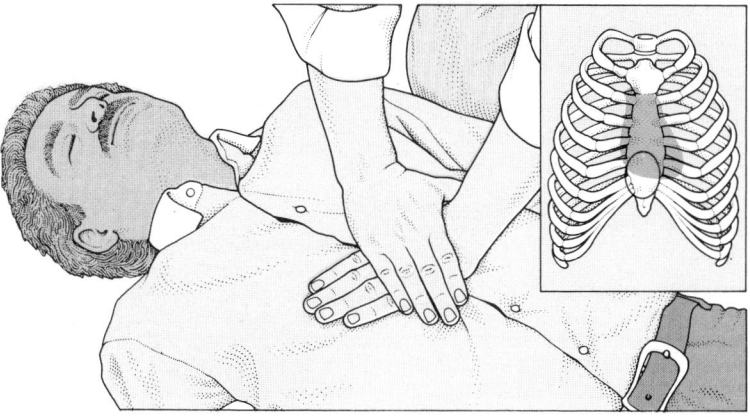

4 If breathing does not restart and you cannot detect a pulse or heartbeat, start cardiac compression. Press with the heel of one hand placed on top of the other.

5 It is vital to apply pressure at the correct point—the lower part of the breastbone. Keep the pressure well clear of the victim's ribs.

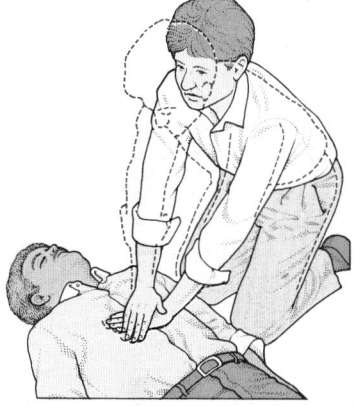

6 If you are on your own, the rate of compression should be 80 per minute, with two breaths given after every 15 compressions.

WARNING

Cardiopulmonary resuscitation is a life-support technique that is used in a medical emergency when the victim is not breathing and when it is possible that his or her heart has stopped beating.
Although restoring the victim's breathing can be performed effectively at the time of the crisis by following the instructions here, restoring the victim's circulation if the heart has stopped beating (cardiac compression) cannot be learned effectively in an emergency. For this reason, cardiac compression, and all phases of cardiopulmonary resuscitation, should be learned through formal instruction. Practising the technique regularly and taking refresher courses are also recommended.

WITH TWO RESCUERS

If two rescuers are available, one should perform cardiac compression and the other mouth-to-mouth resuscitation (one breath to five compressions). Sixty compressions should be given per minute, with 1 to 1.5 seconds pause after every five compressions.

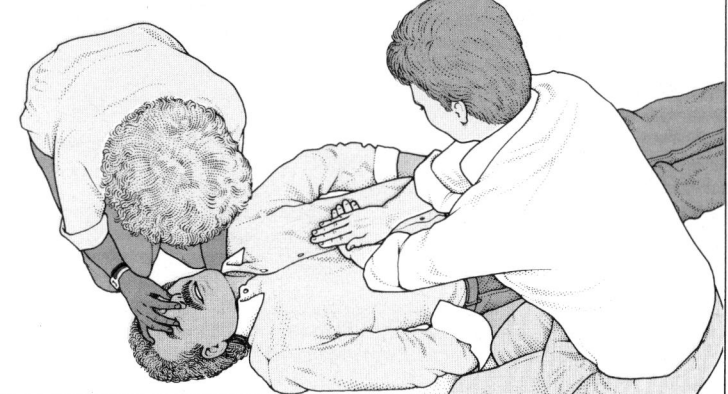

tooth) and replace it with a filling (see *Root-canal treatment*) or to extract the tooth (see *Extraction, dental*).

PREVENTION

Our modern diet makes it unlikely that we can completely avoid dental caries even by taking the most scrupulous preventive measures. However, it is possible to reduce the risk of caries considerably by consuming less sugar and other refined carbohydrates and by practising good oral hygiene, such as regular toothbrushing.

Sweet food should be eaten only at mealtimes; snacks between meals should be limited. From the beginning of a child's life, careful attention to diet is essential to minimize the harmful effects of refined carbohydrates. Babies should not be given a bottle of milk, fruit juice, or other sugar-containing liquid to comfort them or get them to sleep; this habit can cause extensive early tooth decay.

Teeth need brushing thoroughly each day with fluoride toothpaste, and dental floss should be used to clean between the teeth. A dentist should be visited regularly for check-ups. (See also *Oral hygiene*.)

Carotene

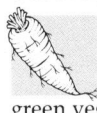

An orange pigment found in carrots, tomatoes, and various other coloured plants, including leafy green vegetables.

Most of the carotene absorbed from food is converted in the walls of the intestine to *vitamin A*, which is essential for normal vision and the health of the skin and other organs.

Excessive intake of carotene-containing foods, especially carrots, results in carotenaemia (abnormally high blood levels of carotene). This condition is harmless, but does cause yellowing of the skin, especially of the palms and soles. It can be differentiated from jaundice because the eyes remain white. The abnormal pigment rapidly disappears if carrots or other such carotene-containing plants are omitted from the diet.

Some recent research indicates that carotene may have some protective effect against certain types of cancer but this is far from proven.

Carotid artery

Any of the four principal arteries of the neck and head. There are two common carotid arteries (left and right), each of which divides into two main branches (internal and external).

The left common carotid artery arises from the *aorta* (main blood vessel leading from the heart) just above the heart, and runs up the neck on the left side of the *trachea* (windpipe). Just above the level of the *larynx* (voicebox) it divides into two, forming the left internal carotid and the left external carotid arteries. The right common carotid artery arises from the subclavian artery, which branches off the aorta, and then follows a similar path to the left common carotid, but on the other side of the neck.

The external carotid arteries have multiple branches, which supply most of the tissues in the face, scalp, mouth, and jaws. The internal carotid arteries enter the skull to supply the brain (via cerebral branches) and eyes (via ophthalmic branches). At the base of the brain, branches of the two internal carotids and the basilar artery join to form a ring of blood vessels called the circle of Willis. Narrowing of these vessels may be associated with *transient ischaemic attack* (TIA), while obstruction causes a *stroke*.

The carotid arteries have two specialized sensory regions in the neck, called the carotid sinus and the carotid body. The former monitors blood pressure; the latter monitors the oxygen content of the blood and helps regulate breathing.

Carpal tunnel syndrome

Numbness, tingling, and pain in the thumb, index, and middle fingers that often worsens at night. The condition may affect one or both hands and is sometimes accompanied by weakness in the thumb.

CAUSES AND INCIDENCE

The condition results from pressure on the median nerve where it passes into the hand via a gap (the "carpal tunnel") under a ligament at the front of the wrist. The median nerve carries sensory messages from the thumb and some fingers and also motor stimuli to the muscles in the hand; damage to the nerve causes sensory disturbances, particularly numbness or tingling, and weakness.

CAUSES OF TOOTH DECAY

The primary cause of tooth decay is dental *plaque*, a sticky substance that forms on the teeth. Plaque consists of food remains, mucus-saliva by-products, and the bacteria that live in the mouth. The bacteria feed mainly on the fermentable carbohydrates (simple sugars and starches) in food, and, in breaking them down, create an acid that gradually destroys enamel, forming a cavity. If the process is not checked, the dentine is eroded next, enlarging the cavity and enabling the bacteria to invade the pulp at the centre of the tooth.

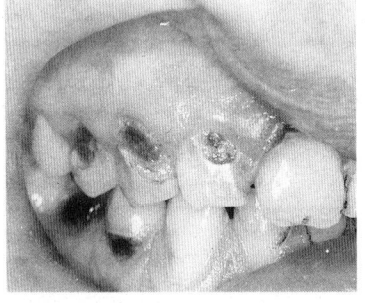

Severe dental caries
Example of caries affecting the necks of several upper and lower teeth.

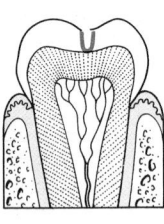

1 Acid produced in the breakdown of food gradually destroys enamel, forming a cavity.

2 Unchecked, decay spreads to the dentine.

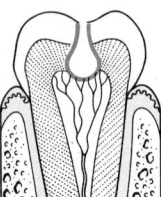

3 The cavity continues to enlarge, enabling the bacteria to invade exposed pulp at the tooth's centre.

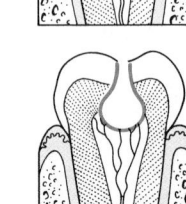

4 If untreated, the infected pulp will die and the tooth will be destroyed.

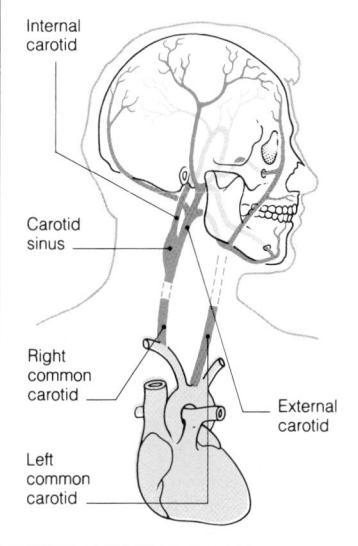

LOCATION OF CAROTID ARTERY
The common carotid on each side divides to form internal and external branches.

Internal carotid

Carotid sinus

Right common carotid

Left common carotid

External carotid

Carpal tunnel syndrome is a common occupational disease of workers using word processor or computer keyboards, and of middle-aged women in whom there is no obvious occupational cause. It is quite frequent in pregnancy, in women who have begun using *oral contraceptives* or who suffer from *premenstrual syndrome*, and in men or women suffering from *rheumatoid arthritis*, *myxoedema*, or *acromegaly*.

DIAGNOSIS AND TREATMENT
The diagnosis may be confirmed by measuring the passage of nerve impulses through the median nerve to the muscles of the hand. The condition often disappears without treatment. Resting the affected hand at night in a splint may alleviate symptoms. If symptoms persist, a small quantity of a *corticosteroid drug* may be injected under the ligament in the wrist. If this fails to help, surgical cutting of the ligament may be performed to relieve the pressure on the nerve.

Carrier

A person who is able to pass on a disease to others without actually suffering from it. Carriers may transmit infectious diseases to others, or pass on inherited diseases to their offspring.

A carrier who harbours potentially harmful bacteria or viruses may unknowingly transmit an infectious disease such as typhoid fever or hepatitis B. The carrier may never have had symptoms of the disease, or may have had an infection in the past with apparently complete recovery.

Inherited disease may be transmitted if a parent who shows no signs of having a particular disease carries a gene for it. For example, a woman who carries the gene for the bleeding disorder haemophilia does not have the disease herself but may pass the gene on to some of her children; if one of her sons receives the gene, he will develop haemophilia.

Car sickness
See *Motion sickness*.

Cartilage

A type of connective tissue (a material that holds body structures together). Cartilage is not as hard as *bone* but nevertheless forms an important structural component of many parts of the skeletal system, such as the *joints*. Much of the fetal skeleton is formed entirely of cartilage, which is then gradually converted to bone by a process known as *ossification*.

Cartilage consists of specialized cells called chondrocytes embedded in a matrix, or ground substance, that comprises varying amounts of *collagen*, a gel-like substance. There are three main types of cartilage: hyaline, fibrocartilage, and elastic, each with a different proportion of collagen and each with different functions.

TYPES
Hyaline cartilage is a tough, smooth tissue that lines the surfaces of joints, such as the knee, providing an almost frictionless layer over the bony parts of the joint. If the lining becomes worn (as occurs in *osteoarthritis*) or damaged, joint movement may be painful or severely restricted.

Fibrocartilage contains a large amount of collagen and is solid and very strong. It makes up the intervertebral discs between the bones of the spine and the shock-absorbing pads of tissue that are found in joints.

Elastic cartilage is soft and rubbery. It is found in various structures, notably the outer ear and the *epiglottis*.

Cast

A rigid casing applied to a limb or other part of the body to hold a broken bone or dislocated joint so that it will heal in the correct position. Most casts are made using bandages impregnated with plaster of Paris. The bandages are applied wet to the injured part and harden as they dry. Modern

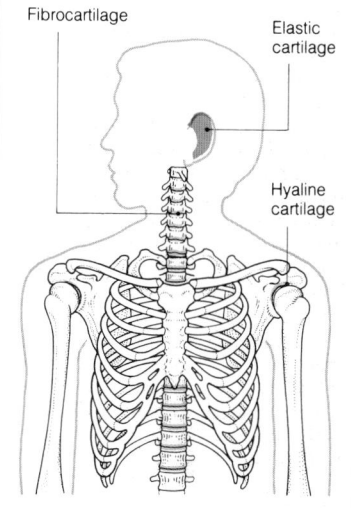

TYPES OF CARTILAGE
The three main types contain different proportions of collagen and differ in their toughness and elasticity.

Fibrocartilage

Elastic cartilage

Hyaline cartilage

fibreglass casts are stronger and lighter than plaster but are more expensive and difficult to apply. Casts are removed using an electric saw that cuts through the cast but does not damage the skin.

A back slab is a type of cast that covers only half the affected limb and is held in place with straps. A back slab is used if swelling at the site of injury is likely, or as a temporary measure pending the insertion of a pin to secure a broken bone.

Castor oil

A colourless or yellow-tinged oil obtained from the leaves of the castor oil plant. When given orally, castor oil irritates the lining of the small intestine and within two to six hours causes a powerful *laxative* action that completely empties the bowel. This effect helps in preparing patients for X-rays of the intestine. Castor oil should not be used as a regular treatment for *constipation* because of its strong, rapid effect.

Zinc and castor oil ointment is a soothing, moistening cream used to treat conditions such as nappy rash.

Castration

The removal of the testes (see *Orchidectomy*) or ovaries (see *Oophorectomy*).

Castration is performed to remove a diseased organ or to reduce the

C

amount of *testosterone* (male hormone produced in the testes) or *oestrogen* (female hormone produced in the ovaries) in the body. The procedure may be used in the treatment of breast and prostate cancers because oestrogen stimulates the growth of some breast cancers and testosterone stimulates the growth of cancer of the prostate. Castration in adulthood has no immediate effect on libido (sexual desire), although libido may be reduced in the long term.

In former times, castration was performed to preserve the high-pitched voices of boy singers and to emasculate male slaves who guarded harems.

Catalepsy

A physical state in which the muscles of the face, body, and limbs are maintained in a semi-rigid position. Catalepsy may last for many hours, during which time neither the expression nor the bodily position will alter, no matter how uncomfortable. Attempts to change the person's position will meet with resistance or the unyielding adoption of a new position. Catalepsy occurs mainly in people with *schizophrenia*, *epilepsy*, or a *conversion disorder*, but may also be caused by brain disease and some drugs.

Cataplexy

A sudden loss of muscle tone, causing the victim to collapse, without any loss of consciousness. Cataplexy usually lasts for a few seconds and is triggered by emotions, particularly laughter. A rare cause of sudden involuntary falls, cataplexy occurs almost exclusively in those suffering from *narcolepsy* and other *sleep disorders*.

Cataract

Loss of transparency of the crystalline *lens* of the *eye*. Cataract is due to changes in the delicate protein fibres within the lens, similar to the changes that occur in cooked egg whites.

Cataract never causes complete blindness, because even a densely opalescent lens will still transmit light. However, with increasing loss of transparency, the clarity and detail of the image is progressively lost. Even at a fairly advanced stage, a cataract may not be apparent to an external observer, and it is only when the front part of the crystalline lens becomes densely opaque that whiteness is visible in the pupil.

Cataract usually occurs in both eyes, but in most cases one eye is more severely affected than the other.

INCIDENCE

Most cataracts occur in elderly people. In fact, almost everyone over 65 has some degree of cataract, but usually the opacification is minor and often confined to the edge of the lens, where it does not interfere with vision. Opacification tends to progress with age, so that most people over 75 have minor visual deterioration from cataract.

CAUSE

Most cataracts in the elderly have no known cause but they are so common that they might be considered a part of the normal aging process. Exposure to ultraviolet radiation increases the risk, and cataract is more common in tropical countries than in Europe and North America. It occurs more often in those who spend most of their lives outdoors.

Congenital cataract (a cataract that is present from birth) may be due to infection of the mother early in pregnancy, especially with the *rubella* (German measles) virus, or to the toxic effects of drugs taken during pregnancy. Congenital cataract may also occur in infants who have *Down's syndrome* or a variety of rare genetic conditions, such as *galactosaemia*.

Cataract may be caused by direct injury to the eye, and is almost inevitable if a foreign particle enters the crystalline lens. Cataract is common in people with *diabetes mellitus* and may develop at an early age if blood sugar levels are very high. Other possible causes of cataract include prolonged intake of *corticosteroid drugs*, poisoning by substances such as naphthalene (found in mothballs) or ergot (formed in stored grain contaminated by a certain type of fungus). In addition to the link with ultraviolet radiation, cataract may also be caused by exposure to other types of radiation including infra red, microwave, and X-rays.

SYMPTOMS

Cataract is entirely painless and causes only visual symptoms. The onset of these symptoms is almost imperceptible, and progress is nearly always very slow.

The main symptom is progressive loss of visual acuity (increased blurring of vision). Increased density in the lens often increases its light-refracting power so that the person becomes shortsighted. This may temporarily permit a person who was previously longsighted to read without using his or her reading glasses.

Colour values are often disturbed, with dulling of blues and accentuation of reds, yellows, and oranges; the full perception of colour is strikingly re-

stored after surgery. Often the lens' opacities cause scattering of light-rays and, even at a fairly early stage, may seriously affect night driving. However, many sufferers are barely aware of these effects and notice only that they cannot see as well as before.

TREATMENT

If normal clear images are to be perceived, the opacified lens must be removed surgically and the refracting power of the eye restored by a spectacle lens, a contact lens, or by a replacement lens implanted during the operation. Provided the eye is otherwise healthy, *cataract surgery* gives excellent results in most cases.

Cataract surgery

Removal of an opacified lens from the eye to restore sight. Cataract extraction is most often performed when the opacification of the lens has developed to a point where the person feels it seriously impairs his or her vision.

Once a cataract has developed, changes to the lens are irreversible and vision can be restored only by removing the opacified lens and replacing it with an artificial lens. In the past, patients were forced to wear very strong, highly magnifying ("pebble") glasses, which were often uncomfortable and caused distortion at the edges of the narrowed field of vision. By replacing the removed lens with a tiny plastic implant, fixed permanently in the eye during the operation, the need to use such thick glasses can now usually be avoided.

HOW IT IS DONE

Each surgeon uses a slightly different technique, but a typical cataract operation is described in the illustrated box (see opposite).

Sometimes the whole lens is removed, in its capsule, by means of a probe that can be made to freeze to the lens (the lens may first be loosened by means of a digestive enzyme injected into the front chamber of the eye). In this case, the lens is replaced by an implant that either clips into the pupil or is fitted in front of the iris. Another technique involves placing the implant within the capsule of the lens, after removing all its contents; the implant is supported by loops or flanges which keep it in a central position. Alternatively, the implant may be placed in front of the pupil.

By taking pre-operative measurements of the curvature of the cornea and (using an ultrasonic method) of the length of the eye, it is often possible to calculate the power of the

PROCEDURE FOR CATARACT SURGERY

In a normal, healthy lens there is no interference with the passage of light-rays. Even with peripheral opacities, vision is not limited until the central zone is affected. Dense nuclear opacities, such as that shown right, result in deteriorating vision and cannot be restored to transparency, hence the need for surgical replacement.

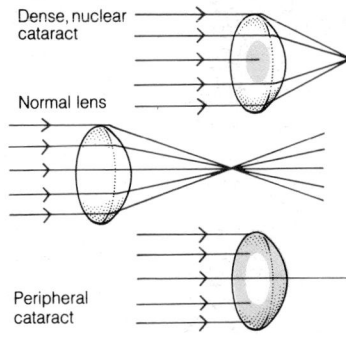

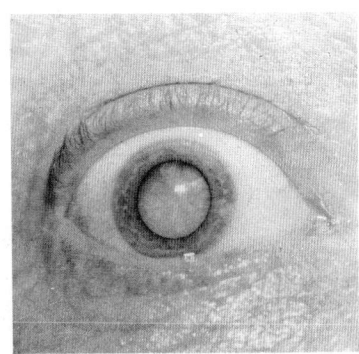

1 In preparation for surgery, measurements are taken of the cornea and of the length of the eye, in order to calculate the power of the lens implant needed to restore vision fully. The operation may be performed using general or local anaesthesia; there is no pain in either case. Instruments of remarkable delicacy and precision are used to carry out the procedure, usually with the help of microscope magnification.

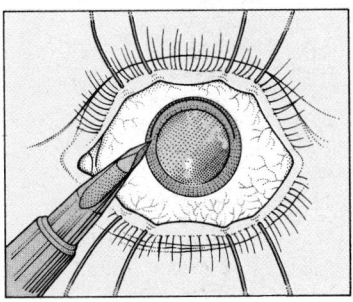

2 Before the operation, drops are used to widen the pupil so that most of the front surface of the lens is exposed. An incision is made around the upper edge of the cornea using an instrument with a diamond tip.

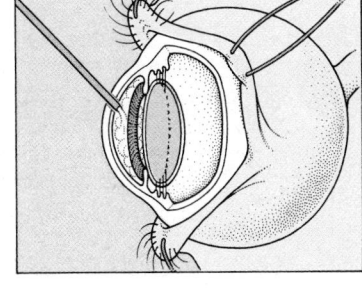

3 A small quantity of a clear gel (sodium hyaluronate) is injected to maintain a space between the back of the cornea and the lens.

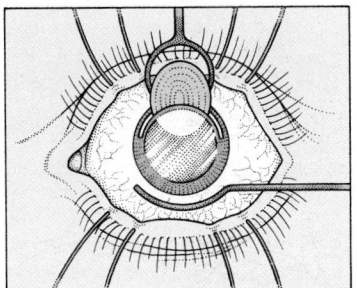

4 A large part of the centre of the front capsule of the lens is then removed and the hard nucleus of the lens carefully removed. The soft remaining parts of the lens are then cleared away, leaving the back of the capsule.

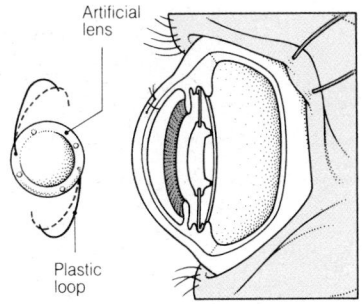

5 The artificial implant is slipped into the natural lens capsule; plastic loops hold it in place. The corneal incision is sewn up with fine nylon thread about half the diameter of a human hair.

implant lens needed to restore normal vision to the patient. Some patients, however, continue to need to wear glasses after the operation, at least for reading.

There are, however, some cataract patients for whom intraocular lens implants are unsuitable. This group consists mainly of people with a history of other eye disease. Some surgeons also advise against intraocular lenses in young people because the lifespan of the implant has not been established. Contact lenses can offer these people excellent vision postoperatively, and many people now wear such lenses.

RECOVERY PERIOD

Most patients can leave hospital within a couple of days of the operation. In some cases, the patient may be discharged on the same day, provided that facilities for specialist supervision during the next few days are available.

The corneal incision takes about a month to heal, but it is usually about two months before the corneal curvature has ceased to alter. Glasses may not be fitted until then.

The results of treatment are usually excellent provided no other cause of visual deterioration is present.

Catarrh

Inflammation of a *mucous membrane* causing an increase in the amount of mucus secreted. Catarrh is usually due to infection or to allergy, and may affect the nose (see *Rhinitis*), the middle ear (see *Glue ear*), or the sinuses (see *Sinusitis*).

Catatonia

A state characterized by abnormalities of movement and posture. An affected person appears to be awake but makes no voluntary movements. He or she may adopt rigid, often bizarre, postures, which may be maintained against resistance. Catatonia is a feature of a rare form of *schizophrenia* and also occurs in some types of brain disease.

Catharsis

A term meaning purification. Catharsis is used to refer to the process of evacuation of the bowels. In *psychoanalytic theory*, it refers to the process of expressing or acting out feelings and memories that were previously repressed. The term was originally used in psychiatry by Sigmund Freud, who believed that the revival of "forgotten" memories and the expression of the emotions associated with them could bring relief from anxiety, tension, and other symptoms.

The patient may be hypnotized or given drugs to bring on a suggestive state that allows the traumatic memory to be recalled and the emotions associated with the memory to be openly expressed. *Psychodrama*, which involves dramatic recreation of events, is another method used to help patients achieve emotional release. This method is claimed to be particularly successful in the treatment of *post-traumatic stress disorder*.

Cathartic

A term that means having the power to purify or cleanse. A cathartic is a drug that stimulates movement of the bowels (see *Laxative drugs*).

Catheter

A tube used to drain or inject fluid, or to apply pressure to a vessel. Catheters are commonly used to drain urine from the bladder (see *Catheterization, urinary*). Other types are used to sample blood from the heart or to inject dye into the blood vessels during X-ray screening (see *Catheterization, cardiac*). Catheters are also used to unblock or widen obstructed blood vessels, or to control bleeding. (See also *Balloon catheter*.)

Catheterization, cardiac

A diagnostic test in which a fine, sterile *catheter* (tube) is introduced into the heart, via a blood vessel, to investigate its condition.

The technique is used to diagnose and assess the extent of congenital heart disease (see *Heart disease, congenital*) and *coronary artery disease*. It is also used to diagnose as well as to treat some disorders of the *heart valves* (see *Valvuloplasty*). Cardiac catheterization enables the pressure within the heart chambers to be measured, blood samples to be taken, and samples of tissue from the heart lining to be removed for analysis.

Cardiac catheterization may cause temporary disturbance of the heart rhythm and is therefore used only to investigate disorders that might become life-threatening.

HOW IT IS DONE

The procedure, which causes little discomfort, is performed under local anaesthesia. A small incision is made in an artery or vein and the catheter introduced. The tube is passed along the blood vessel and into the heart. Catheterization of the left side of the heart is carried out via an artery in the thigh or elbow. Investigation of the right side of the heart is performed via a vein in the groin or elbow.

Once the catheter is in position, it can be used to measure blood pressure within the heart, withdraw blood to measure its oxygen content, or inject a *radiopaque* substance into the heart so that its cavities can be X-rayed.

After the catheter has been removed, the blood vessel through which it was passed is put under firm pressure and kept under observation. No further treatment is usually needed.

Catheterization, urinary

Insertion of a sterile *catheter* (tube) into the bladder to drain urine.

WHY IT IS DONE

Urinary catheterization is most often performed when a person is unable to empty the bladder normally or is suffering from incontinence (see *Incontinence, urinary*). Patients with urinary incontinence associated with neurological disorders may be given permanent catheters or are taught to carry out self-catheterization.

Urinary catheterization may be necessary during certain operations in which a full bladder might obstruct the surgeon's view of surrounding organs. The procedure is also carried out to allow careful monitoring of urine production by patients who are critically ill.

Urinary catheterization is also performed for tests of bladder function, such as *cystometry* and micturating *cystourethrography*.

HOW IT IS DONE

There are two principal techniques: urethral catheterization (described in the illustrated box below) and suprapubic catheterization.

Suprapubic catheterization is used if it is not possible to pass a catheter up the urethra (e.g. if the urethra is abnormally narrow). The skin of the lower part of the abdomen is cleaned with an antiseptic solution and a local anaesthetic is injected under an area of skin overlying the bladder. A small incision is then made with a scalpel blade and a suprapubic catheter is inserted into the bladder through the abdominal wall.

CATHETERIZATION OF THE BLADDER

The catheter is usually passed into the bladder through the urethra. Before this is done, the doctor or nurse cleans the surrounding area with antiseptic solution to avoid introducing infection into the urinary tract. The procedure usually takes about 10 minutes.

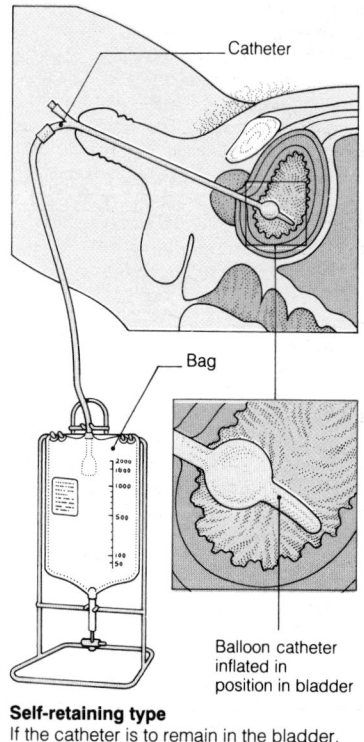

Catheter

Bag

Balloon catheter inflated in position in bladder

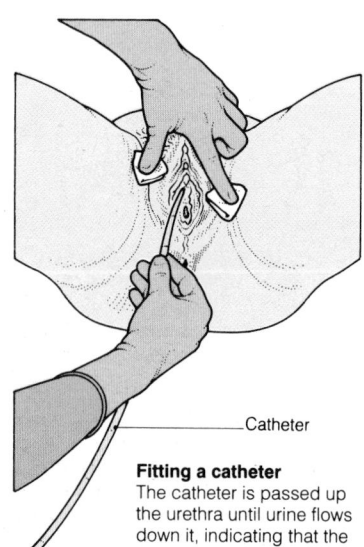

Catheter

Fitting a catheter
The catheter is passed up the urethra until urine flows down it, indicating that the tip is in the bladder.

Self-retaining type
If the catheter is to remain in the bladder, a self-retaining type is used. This catheter has a balloon at its tip that can be inflated and filled with sterile water.

RISKS

There is a risk that urinary catheterization may lead to *urinary tract infection* even though the procedure is performed under sterile conditions.

CAT scanning

An abbreviation for computerized axial tomographic scanning, more commonly known as *CT scanning*.

Cat-scratch fever

An uncommon disease that usually develops after a scratch or bite by a cat and is due to infection with a small bacterium called ROCHALIMAEA HENDELAE, which is transmitted by the cat. The cat itself is not ill. Three quarters of cases occur in children, and the disorder is most common in autumn and winter.

SYMPTOMS

Symptoms usually appear three to 10 days after a bite or scratch. In some cases there is no apparent break in the skin, although contact with a cat is sometimes reported. The main sign of illness is a swollen lymph node near the scratch. The node may become painful and tender and, in rare cases, may produce a discharge. A small, infected blister sometimes develops at the original site of skin injury. A fever, rash, and headache may also occur.

DIAGNOSIS AND TREATMENT

The diagnosis is confirmed by *biopsy* (removal of a small tissue sample for microscopic analysis) of the swollen lymph node and by the results of a skin test. Analgesic drugs (painkillers) may be needed to relieve fever and headache. A severely infected lymph node or blister may have to be surgically drained. In most cases, the illness clears up completely within two months. There is no need to destroy the cat.

Cats, diseases from

Cats carry various parasites and infectious organisms that can be spread to humans. Some are specific to cats, others affect dogs as well. A well-cared for cat poses no serious threat to human health, but cat owners should be aware of possible problems.

SPECIFIC DISEASES

Rabies is the most serious disorder that can be contracted from an infected cat. Although there is no rabies in the UK, anyone who is bitten by a cat (or any other mammal) in a country where rabies is present should see a doctor immediately.

Cat-scratch fever is an uncommon illness that usually follows the scratch or bite of a cat. The cause of the illness is a small bacterium called ROCHALIMAEA HENDELAE that the cat transmits.

Cats commonly carry the protozoan (single-celled parasite) TOXOPLASMA GONDII, which is the cause of *toxoplasmosis*. A form of the parasite is present in the cat's faeces. In most cases, the infection causes few or no symptoms, but, if a woman is infected during pregnancy, the parasites may gain access, via the placenta, to the fetus. Infections in early pregnancy can lead to spontaneous abortion or severe malformation; infections that occur later in pregnancy can cause nervous system disorders and sometimes blindness in early childhood. Pregnant women should not change cat litter boxes.

Cat faeces may also carry eggs of the cat roundworm, a possible cause of *toxocariasis*. In rare cases, a larva from an ingested roundworm egg may migrate to and lodge in an eye, causing deterioration of vision or even blindness. This most commonly occurs in children who have been playing in soil or sand that is contaminated by dog or cat faeces infected with roundworm eggs.

Of the more common problems, a substantial number of *tinea* (ringworm) fungal infections of the skin—particularly scalp ringworm—probably come from cats. Unlike dogs, cats are little affected by the fungus, but its presence can be demonstrated by examining the fur under ultraviolet light, which causes fluorescence of infected skin and hairs.

Bites from cat *fleas* are common; many bites blamed on midges and mosquitoes are actually caused by fleas. The fleas may jump on to humans to feed, particularly in warm weather and if the cat is absent. Flea bites are most common around the ankles and lower leg, and can be intensely irritating.

Some people develop allergic reactions to dander (tiny scales derived from animal skin and fur and present in the air) and consequently may suffer from *asthma* or *urticaria* when a cat is in the house.

PREVENTION

Serious diseases from cats are easily avoided by good hygiene—in particular, thorough washing of the hands if there is any chance they have been contaminated by cat faeces. Young children should be discouraged from playing with cats and other animals, except under supervision, until they have become aware of the risks of poor hygiene. Animals that are obviously ill should be seen by a veterinary surgeon, and routine health care should include regular worming and flea treatment.

Cauda equina

A collection of nerve roots that descends from the lower part of the *spinal cord* and occupies the lower third of

HOW CATS TRANSMIT INFECTION

There are three main routes by which an infection or parasitic disease may be spread.

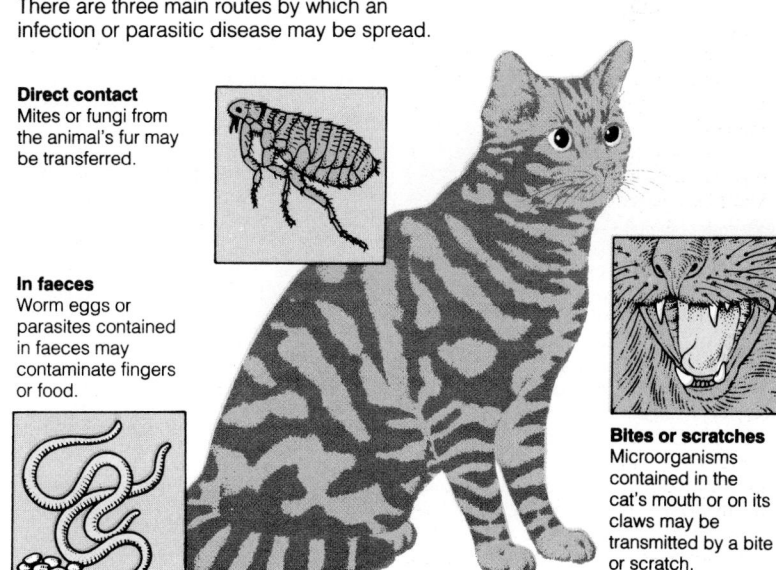

Direct contact
Mites or fungi from the animal's fur may be transferred.

In faeces
Worm eggs or parasites contained in faeces may contaminate fingers or food.

Bites or scratches
Microorganisms contained in the cat's mouth or on its claws may be transmitted by a bite or scratch.

C

the spinal canal (the central space within the spine). This "spray" of nerves resembles a horse's tail.

Caudal

Denoting a position towards the lower end of the spine. Caudal literally means "of the tail".

Caudal block

A type of *nerve block* in which a local anaesthetic is injected into the lower part of the spinal canal (the central space within the spine). Caudal block is sometimes used for obstetric and gynaecological procedures.

Cauliflower ear

A painful, swollen distortion of the pinna (ear flap) resulting from blows or friction that have caused bleeding within the soft cartilage framework. The condition occurs most commonly in rugby football players.

TREATMENT
If the ear swells after injury, an ice-pack should be used to reduce the swelling. In severe cases, a doctor should be consulted. Blood can be drained from the ear using a needle and syringe, and a pressure bandage applied. Despite these measures, repeated injury may lead to a severely distorted ear, and plastic surgery is sometimes needed to improve the appearance.

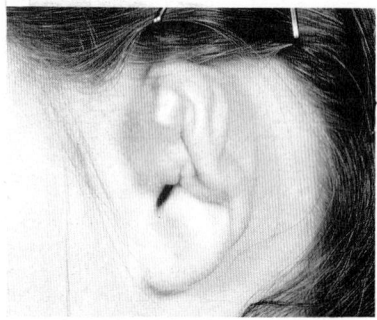

Example of cauliflower ear
Deformity of the shape of the ear, with loss of normal folds of skin.

Causalgia

A persistent, burning pain, usually in an arm or leg. The skin overlying the painful area may be red and tender or may be blue, cold, and clammy.

Causalgia usually occurs as the result of injury to a nerve by a deep cut, limb fracture, or gunshot wound. In some cases, the pain may be aggravated by emotional factors or even by normal sensations, such as touch or a cold breeze.

Treatment is usually unsatisfactory but a few patients benefit from *sympathectomy*, an operation in which nerves are severed.

Caustic

A term applied to any substance that has a burning or corrosive action on body tissues or has a burning taste. An example is caustic soda, the common name for sodium hydroxide.

Caustic substances can destroy body tissues and therefore should not be used without adequate protection, such as rubber gloves. If a caustic chemical is spilled on to the skin or splashed into the eye, wash it off immediately with a gentle stream of running water, taking care not to wash the chemical on to other areas of skin or into the other eye.

Cauterization

The application of a heated instrument or a *caustic* chemical to tissues in order to destroy them, to stop them from bleeding, or to promote healing within them.

In the past, heat was widely used to destroy *haemorrhoids* (piles), to treat *cervical erosion*, and to stop bleeding during operations. Cauterization has now been largely replaced by *electrocoagulation* (the use of high-frequency electric current), which is more efficient and easier to use. Chemicals such as silver nitrate are still used to destroy warts.

Cavernous sinus thrombosis

Blockage by a *thrombus* (abnormal blood clot) of a venous sinus (widened channel for venous blood) deep within the skull behind an eye socket. Cavernous sinus thrombosis usually occurs as a complication of a bacterial infection in an area drained by the veins entering the sinus. At first, only the veins behind one eye are affected but, within two or three days, the thrombosis may spread to the sinus behind the other eye. This serious condition has become rare since the advent of *antibiotic drugs* to treat bacterial infections.

CAUSES
Among the infections that can lead to cavernous sinus thrombosis are *cellulitis* (a severe skin infection) of the face; infections of the mouth, eye, or middle ear; *sinusitis* (infection of the air spaces of the facial skull); and *septicaemia* (infection in the bloodstream). Picking at a small, infected pimple at the angle of the nose may also spread infection to the sinus.

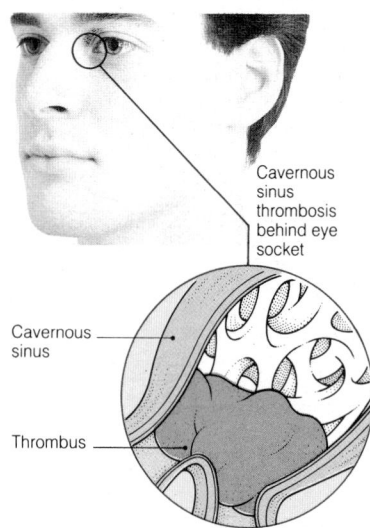

Cavernous sinus thrombosis behind eye socket

Cavernous sinus

Thrombus

Thrombus in cavernous sinus
The cavernous sinus is found behind the eye socket, deep within the skull.

Rarely, the thrombosis is caused by a tumour pressing on the veins or by *polycythaemia* (an excessive concentration of red cells in the blood).

SYMPTOMS
The patient is usually critically ill. The symptoms are severe headache, high fever, pain in and above the affected eye, loss of sensation in the cornea and on the forehead due to pressure on the fifth cranial nerve, and *proptosis* (protrusion of the eyeball) due to swelling around and behind the eye. Vision may become blurred and eye movements paralysed due to pressure on the optic nerve and on other cranial nerves controlling the muscles that move the eyes.

TREATMENT
Treatment is with antibiotic drugs to treat the infection and *anticoagulant drugs* to prevent the blood clot enlarging. Treatment can save vision in the affected eye or eyes; if untreated, blindness will result, and the infection may prove fatal.

Cavity, dental

A hole in a tooth, commonly caused by dental caries (see *Caries, dental*).

Cefaclor

A common cephalosporin-type antibiotic drug. (See *Cephalosporin drugs*.)

Cell

The basic structural unit of the body. Each person consists of billions of cells, structurally and functionally

CELL TYPES

Despite their fundamental similarities, the cells of the body are differentiated to perform specific tasks, such as carrying oxygen (red blood cells), destroying invading microorganisms (white blood cells), manufacturing hormones (secretory cells in glands), and so on. Some cells (nerve cells, for instance) cannot be replaced once destroyed, while other cells (those that form fingernails, for instance) continue to function even after death. Cells can be grouped into four main types according to their underlying similarities.

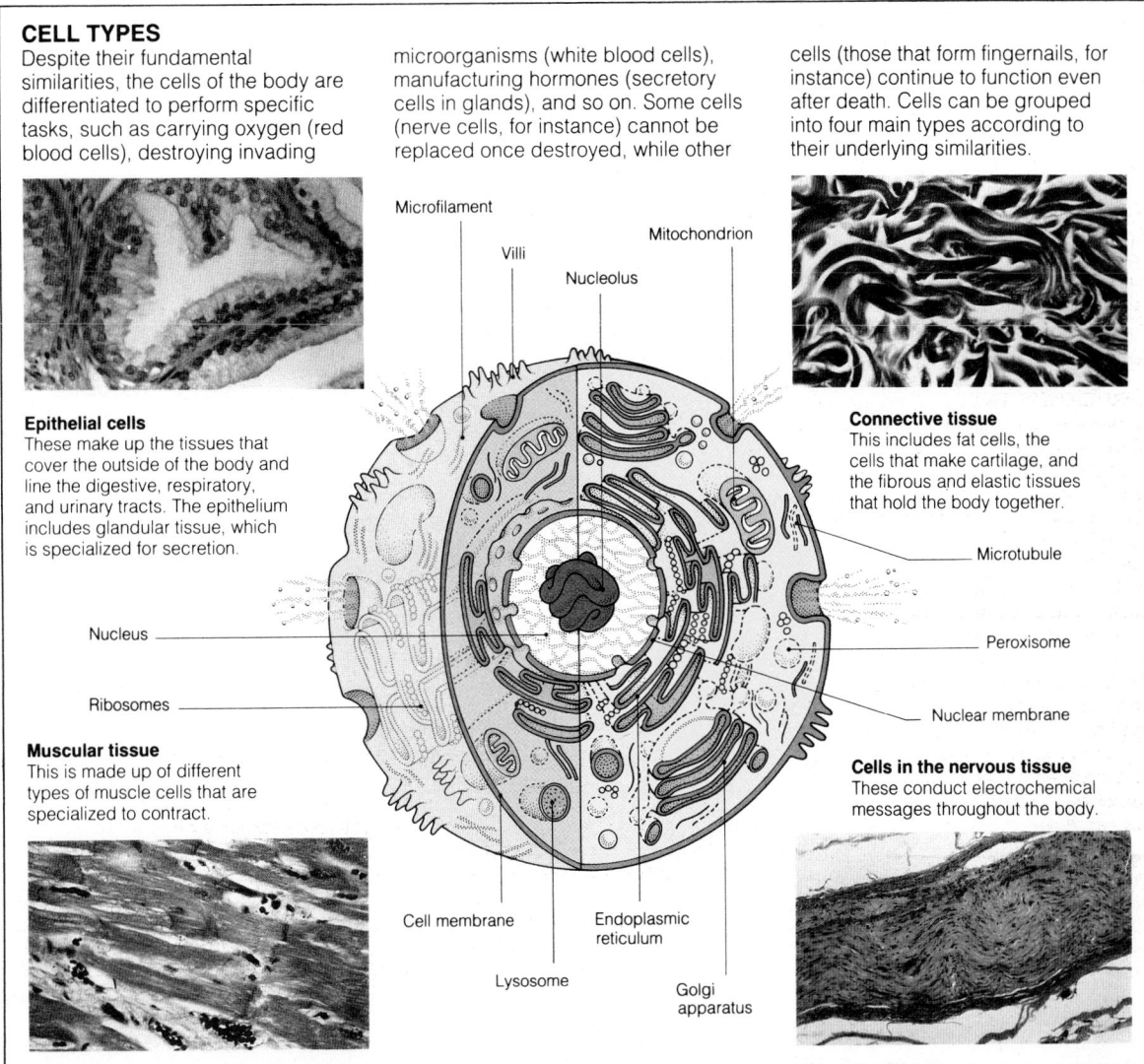

Microfilament

Villi

Nucleolus

Mitochondrion

Epithelial cells
These make up the tissues that cover the outside of the body and line the digestive, respiratory, and urinary tracts. The epithelium includes glandular tissue, which is specialized for secretion.

Nucleus

Ribosomes

Muscular tissue
This is made up of different types of muscle cells that are specialized to contract.

Connective tissue
This includes fat cells, the cells that make cartilage, and the fibrous and elastic tissues that hold the body together.

Microtubule

Peroxisome

Nuclear membrane

Cells in the nervous tissue
These conduct electrochemical messages throughout the body.

Cell membrane

Endoplasmic reticulum

Lysosome

Golgi apparatus

integrated to perform the nearly infinite number of complex tasks necessary for life.

There is enormous variation among cells in the body. For example, mature red blood cells are only about 0.0075 mm in diameter and are so highly specialized for their function of transporting oxygen that they lack some of the internal structures normally found within other cells, such as a nucleus. In contrast, individual nerve cells may be 1 m or more in length and are specialized to perform their function of transmitting electrochemical messages (nerve impulses).

Despite detailed differences, most human cells are basically similar in structure. Each cell is an invisibly small bag containing a fluid material called cytoplasm, surrounded by an outer "skin" called the cell membrane. Within the cytoplasm are the nucleus (except in red blood cells) and various other specialized structures, known collectively as organelles.

CELL MEMBRANE
Formed from a double layer of fatty material and proteins, the cell membrane envelops and holds the cell together. Its other main function is to regulate the passage of materials into and out of the cell, thereby enabling useful substances (such as nutrients and oxygen) to enter the cell, and waste materials (such as carbon dioxide) and substances for use elsewhere in the body (hormones, for example) to leave it. Small molecules can pass freely through the cell membrane, but larger molecules require special molecular transport systems to cross the membrane.

NUCLEUS
The control centre of the cell, the nucleus governs all major activities and functions. The nucleus exerts its influence by regulating the amount and types of *proteins* made in the cell. Proteins have two main functions. Large, structural proteins make up the tough building materials of the body (such as muscle fibres). Smaller proteins called *enzymes* regulate all functions and activities of the cell.

The *chromosomes* (genetic material of the cell), in the form of the *nucleic acid* known as *DNA*, are situated in the nucleus. This DNA contains the instructions for *protein synthesis*. These instructions are conveyed into the cytoplasm by a type of *RNA*, another nucleic acid. Particles called ribosomes in the cytoplasm play a major part in decoding these instructions for the purpose of protein synthesis.

OTHER ORGANELLES

In addition to the nucleus, the cell contains various other organelles, each with a specific role.

The endoplasmic reticulum is a single sheet of membrane twisted into complex folds. The sheet has rough and smooth areas. Rough endoplasmic reticulum is covered with tiny round "beads"—the ribosomes that help produce proteins.

Once completed, the proteins are transferred to another membrane system, the Golgi apparatus, which resembles a series of stacked plates. Here protein structures are modified and packaged into vesicles budded from its surface.

Energy is generated from the breakdown of sugars and fatty acids by organelles called mitochondria. These are shaped like coffee beans and have a complex, folded inner surface. Cells with high energy requirements, such as muscle or liver cells, have a large number of mitochondria.

Many cell processes involve substances that would damage the cell if they came into contact with the cytoplasm, so they are contained within special vesicles called lysosomes and peroxisomes. Lysosomes are the cell's major digestive structures in which enzymes break down large particles, such as bacteria. Peroxisomes neutralize toxic substances.

CYTOPLASM

Modern techniques for studying the structure of cells have shown that the cytoplasm contains a network of fine tubes (microtubules) and filaments (microfilaments) known as the cytoskeleton. This network gives the cell a definite shape and allows it to move. In addition, microfilaments support microvilli (small projections from the surface of the cell), which help to increase the surface area of the cell. Microfilaments also form micromuscles, which can produce contractions and movements of the cell.

Cell division

The processes by which cells multiply. There are two main types of cell division, *mitosis* and *meiosis*. The former gives rise to daughter cells that are identical to the parent cell. The latter gives rise to egg and sperm cells, which differ from their parent cells in that they have only half the normal number of *chromosomes*.

Cellulitis

A bacterial infection of the skin and the tissues beneath it. Cellulitis is most commonly caused by streptococci bacteria, which enter the skin via a wound.

SYMPTOMS

The face, neck, or legs are the usual sites. The affected area is hot, tender, and red, and the patient may be feverish and have chills.

Untreated cellulitis complicating a wound may progress to *bacteraemia* and *septicaemia* or, occasionally, to *gangrene*. Before the advent of *antibiotic drugs*, cellulitis was an occasional cause of death. Facial infections may spread to the eye socket. Very rarely, cellulitis occurs after childbirth and may spread to the pelvic organs.

Any form of cellulitis is likely to be more severe in people with reduced resistance to infections, such as people with *diabetes mellitus* or any type of *immunodeficiency disorder*.

TREATMENT

The usual treatment is a *penicillin* antibiotic (or *erythromycin* in the case of patients who are allergic to penicillin). Drugs may have to be taken for up to two weeks to clear an infection. (See also *Erysipelas*.)

Celsius scale

A temperature scale in which the melting point of ice is zero degrees (0°C) and the boiling point of water is 100 degrees (100°C). On this scale, normal body temperature is 37°C (equivalent to 98.6°F). The scale is named after the Swedish astronomer Anders Celsius (1701-1744). Centigrade is an obsolete name for the same scale.

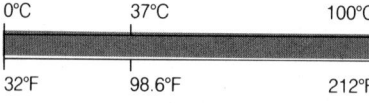

0°C	37°C	100°C
32°F	98.6°F	212°F

To convert a Celsius temperature to Fahrenheit, multiply by 1.8 (or nine fifths), then add 32. To convert Fahrenheit to Celsius, subtract 32 then multiply by 0.56 (or five ninths). (See also *Fahrenheit scale*.)

Cementum

The bone-like tissue that surrounds the root of a tooth (see *Teeth*).

Centigrade scale

The obsolete name for the *Celsius scale*.

Central nervous system

The anatomical term for the brain and spinal cord, often abbreviated as CNS. The central nervous system works in tandem with the *peripheral nervous system* (PNS), which consists of all the nerves that carry signals between the CNS and the rest of the body.

The overall role of the CNS is to receive sensory information from organs, such as the eyes, ears, and receptors within the body, analyse this information, and then initiate an appropriate motor response (for example, contracting a muscle).

The analytical stage may be very short and simple for information that goes no further than the spinal cord or lower areas of the brain (see *Reflex*), but may be complex and prolonged for information that reaches higher, conscious brain centres.

In anatomical terms, the CNS consists of nerve cells or neurons and supporting tissue; the PNS is made up of nerve fibres extending from cells in the CNS. In functional terms, injury or disease affecting the CNS usually causes permanent disability, whereas recovery is sometimes possible after repairing damage to the PNS. (See also *Nervous system*.)

Centrifuge

A machine that separates the different components of a body fluid, such as blood or urine, so that they can be analysed as an aid to diagnosis. The liquid is placed in a container that is spun at high speed around a central axis, and the centrifugal force (force moving away from the centre) separates groups of particles of varying density. Blood, for example, can be separated into red cells, white cells, and its remaining constituents.

Cephalexin

A common cephalosporin-type antibiotic drug. (See *Cephalosporin drugs*.)

Cephalhaematoma

An extensive, soft swelling on the scalp of a newborn infant, caused by bleeding into the space between the cranium (skull) and its overlying fibrous covering (the periosteum or pericranium). The swelling is due to pressure on the baby's head during delivery, causing rupture of small blood vessels.

Although possibly alarming, a cephalhaematoma is not serious and

C

no treatment is necessary. However, the cephalhaematoma should not be handled unnecessarily. The swelling gradually subsides as the blood clot is reabsorbed, although this may take many weeks.

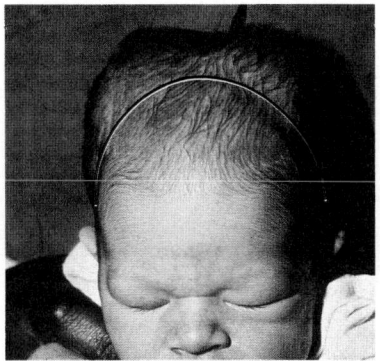

Bilateral cephalhaematoma
This baby was born with a cephalhaematoma on both sides of the scalp at the back of the head. The red line superimposed on the photograph indicates the normal outline of the head.

Cephalic

Relating to the head, as in cephalic presentation, the head-first appearance of a baby in the birth canal.

Cephalosporin drugs

COMMON DRUGS

Cefaclor Cefadroxil Cefotaxime Ceftriaxone Cefuroxime Cephalexin Cephamandole Cephazolin Cephradine

A group of *antibiotic drugs* derived from the fungus CEPHALOSPORIUM ACREMONIUM. Cephalosporin drugs were discovered in Sardinia in 1948. A large number of synthetic cephalosporin drugs have since been produced, which are effective against a wide range of infections.

WHY THEY ARE USED
Cephalosporins are widely used to treat infections of the ear, throat, and respiratory tract. They are also particularly useful in the treatment of *urinary tract infections* (which are often caused by bacteria that are resistant to penicillin-type antibiotics) and are used to treat *gonorrhoea* that is resistant to other antibiotics. Cephalosporins are also sometimes used after surgery to reduce the incidence of wound infections.

The drugs in this group may be used in patients allergic to penicillin-type antibiotics. However, approximately 10 per cent of those people allergic to penicillins are also found to be allergic to cephalosporins.

HOW THEY WORK
Cephalosporins interfere with the development of bacterial cell walls and inhibit the production of protein within the bacterial cells. As a result, the bacteria die. However, some types of bacteria produce an enzyme (a protein that stimulates chemical reactions) called beta-lactamase that can inactivate some of the older varieties of cephalosporin drugs. The newer drugs in the group are not affected by this enzyme.

POSSIBLE ADVERSE EFFECTS
Some people who take cephalosporins develop an allergic reaction causing rash, itching, and fever. In very rare cases, *anaphylactic shock* (a severe allergic reaction that causes collapse) occurs.

Cerebellar ataxia

Jerky, staggering gait and other uncoordinated movements caused by disease or damage to the *cerebellum*. Other features include *dysarthria* (slurred speech); hand tremor and "overshoot" when an attempt is made to touch something; and *nystagmus* (abnormal jerky eye movements).

Possible causes include *stroke, multiple sclerosis, brain tumour*, damage caused by *alcohol dependence*, and degeneration of the cerebellum due to a hereditary disorder.

Cerebellum

A region of the brain concerned primarily with the maintenance of posture and balance and with the coordination of movement.

STRUCTURE
The cerebellum is a rounded structure located behind the *brainstem*, to which it is linked by thick nerve tracts. The cerebellum accounts for about 11 per cent of the whole brain weight and, with its convoluted surface, appears similar to the *cerebrum* (the main mass of the brain).

Outwardly, the cerebellum consists of two hemispheres flanking the vermis, which is a small protrusion from the brainstem. The cortex (outer part) of the hemispheres consists of numerous parallel ridges separated by deep fissures, so that only one sixth of the surface is visible. From the inner side of each hemisphere, three nerve fibre stalks, or peduncles, arise; these link up with different parts of the brainstem. All the signals between the cerebellum and the rest of the brain travel along these nerve tracts.

Microscopically, a cross-section of the cerebellum shows the nerve fibres from these tracts fanning out towards the convoluted cortical surface. The cortex itself consists of grey matter (interconnected nerve cells) arranged in three main layers. Prominent in the middle layer are large cells called Purkinje's cells, each of which may interconnect with up to 100,000 other cells.

FUNCTION
Via its connections to the brainstem, the cerebellum receives information from organs such as muscle tendons and the balance organ in the inner ear. Much of this information concerns the body's posture and the state of contraction or relaxation of its muscles. Using this information, the cerebellum, working in concert with the *basal ganglia* (nerve cell clusters deep within the brain), fine-tunes the orders sent to muscles from the motor cortex in the cerebrum, resulting in smoothly coordinated movements and balance.

DISORDERS
Disease or damage to the cerebellum may result in *cerebellar ataxia*, characterized by jerky, staggering gait, slurred speech, and other uncoordinated movements. *Alcohol intoxication* impairs cerebellar function and thus may produce symptoms similar to those of cerebellar disease.

LOCATION OF CEREBELLUM
The cerebellum is found behind the brainstem and is connected to it by nerve tracts.

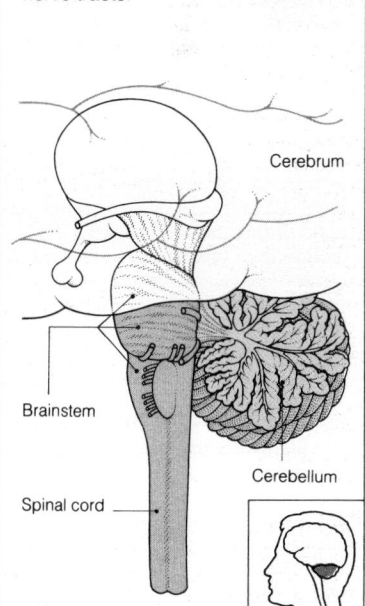

Cerebrum

Brainstem

Cerebellum

Spinal cord

C

Cerebral haemorrhage

Bleeding within the brain caused by rupture of a blood vessel. (See *Intracerebral haemorrhage*.)

Cerebral palsy

A general term for disorders of movement and posture resulting from damage to a child's developing brain in the later months of pregnancy, during birth, in the newborn period, or in early childhood. These disorders are nonprogressive (i.e. the disability does not increase with time).

A child with cerebral palsy may suffer from *spastic paralysis* (abnormal stiffness and contraction of groups of muscles), *athetosis* (involuntary writhing movements), or *ataxia* (loss of coordination and balance). The degree of disability is highly variable, ranging from slight clumsiness of hand movement and gait to complete immobility. Other nervous system disorders, such as hearing defects or epileptic seizures, may be present. Many affected children are also mentally handicapped, although some are of normal or high intelligence.

About two to three children per 1,000 have cerebral palsy, although the incidence varies between countries. There has been only a slight reduction in cases in the past 20 years.

CAUSES

In more than 90 per cent of cases the damage occurs before or at birth. Probably the most common cause is cerebral *hypoxia* (poor oxygen supply to the brain).

A maternal infection spreading to the baby within the uterus is an occasional cause. A rare cause is *kernicterus*, which results from an excess of bilirubin (bile pigment) in babies with *haemolytic disease of the newborn*. The baby is severely jaundiced, and the bile pigment damages the *basal ganglia* (nerve cell clusters in the brain concerned with control of movement).

Following birth, possible causes include *encephalitis* (inflammation of the brain) or *meningitis* (inflammation of the brain's protective coverings), *head injury*, or *intracerebral haemorrhage* (bleeding within the brain).

SYMPTOMS

Cerebral palsy may not be recognized until well into the baby's first year. Sometimes, some of the infant's muscles are initially hypotonic (floppy), and the parents may notice that the baby in some way does not "feel right" when held. There may also be feeding difficulties. Delay in sitting up without support is another early sign.

Once the disability is apparent, most affected children fall into one of two groups—a spastic group, in which the muscles of one or more limbs are permanently contracted and stiff, thus making normal movements very difficult, and a smaller, athetoid group, characterized by involuntary writhing movements.

Children in the spastic group may be affected by diplegia (in which all four limbs are affected, but the legs more severely than the arms), hemiplegia (in which the limbs on just one side of the body are affected, usually the arm worse than the leg), or by quadriplegia (in which all four limbs are severely affected, not necessarily symmetrically). In each case, muscle stiffness begins to appear from the age of about six months onwards. Normal balance is disrupted and the limbs settle in abnormal positions—for example, in diplegia the affected legs cross in scissor-like fashion, and in hemiplegia the affected arm is tucked up at the side of the body, with both the elbow and wrist bent.

The diplegic child has delayed development in many movement skills and has difficulty learning to walk. In hemiplegia the limbs on the affected side grow slowly; there may be some sensory deficiency from the affected side of the body.

In quadriplegia, it may be difficult to know whether the child's arms or legs are the worst affected; mental retardation is usually severe. Often, the child never learns to walk.

Mental handicap, with an IQ below 70, occurs in about three quarters of all children with cerebral palsy, but the exceptions are important and occur particularly among athetoids; many athetoids and some diplegics are highly intelligent.

The features of most types of cerebral palsy change as the child gets older, often for the better with patience and skilled treatment.

DIAGNOSIS

Parents of babies who are "at risk" from cerebral palsy—for example, babies born prematurely or those who have had particularly difficult births—are generally encouraged to take the child more frequently for routine check-ups by a doctor, who will test with particular care for any abnormalities in the baby's muscle tone and reflexes, and for any delay in reaching various developmental milestones (see *Child development*). The diagnosis may rely on a combination of abnormalities being present.

TREATMENT

Although cerebral palsy is incurable, much can be done to help children affected by it. Abilities need to be recognized and developed to the full, as much stimulation as possible should be offered, and loving patience must be shown.

Physiotherapy is required to teach an affected child how to develop muscular control and maintain balance. This therapy is often given initially at a special school or clinic and then continued at home, possibly with the use of special equipment.

Inadequate speech can be helped greatly by *speech therapy*. For children who cannot speak at all, sophisticated techniques and devices have been developed to teach them how to communicate nonverbally.

Every attempt is made to place children with mild cerebral palsy in normal schools, but those who are severely affected need the special help and facilities that are available at schools for the physically and/or mentally handicapped.

OUTLOOK

Children with only moderate disability have a near-normal life expectancy and, with the help of social services, most of those who can move around and communicate effectively grow up to lead a relatively independent and normal life.

Cerebral thrombosis

The formation of a *thrombus* (blood clot) in an artery in the brain. The clot may completely block the artery, cutting off the supply of blood, nutrients and oxygen to a region of the brain, causing a *stroke*.

Cerebrospinal fluid

A clear, watery fluid that circulates between the ventricles (cavities) within the brain, the central canal in the spinal cord, and the space between the brain and spinal cord and their protective coverings, the meninges. Cerebrospinal fluid contains dissolved glucose (sugar), proteins, and salts, and some lymphocytes (white blood cells).

The fluid functions as a shock-absorber, helping to prevent or minimize damage to the brain and spinal cord after a blow to the head or back.

Examination of cerebrospinal fluid, usually obtained by *lumbar puncture*, is important in the diagnosis of many conditions affecting the brain and spinal cord, including *meningitis* and *subarachnoid haemorrhage*.

Accumulation of cerebrospinal fluid within the skull during fetal development or in infancy may cause the skull to become enlarged—a condition known as *hydrocephalus*.

Cerebrovascular accident

Sudden rupture or blockage of a blood vessel within the brain, causing serious bleeding and/or local obstruction to blood circulation, and leading to features of nervous system disturbance commonly called a *stroke*.

Blockage may be due to *thrombosis* (clot formation) or to *embolism* (a fragment or air bubble carried in the blood). Rupture of different blood vessels may cause different patterns of bleeding—such as *intracerebral haemorrhage* (bleeding within the brain) or *subarachnoid haemorrhage* (bleeding around the brain).

Cerebrovascular disease

Any disease affecting an artery within, and supplying blood to, the brain—for example, *atherosclerosis* (narrowing of the arteries) or constitutional defects or weaknesses in arterial walls causing *aneurysm* (a balloon-like swelling in an artery). The disease may eventually lead to a *cerebrovascular accident* (sudden blockage or rupture of a blood vessel), which most commonly leads to the features of *stroke*. Extensive narrowing of blood vessels throughout the brain can be a cause of *dementia*.

Cerebrum

The largest and most developed part of the brain, and the site of most conscious and intelligent activities. The cerebrum consists of two large outgrowths from the upper part of the brainstem (an extension of the spinal cord) called the cerebral hemispheres. Together these outgrowths form an almost continuous mass that envelops much of the rest of the brain.

For size relative to body weight, and also for sophistication, the human cerebrum is unmatched in the animal kingdom, except arguably by that of some marine mammals, such as dolphins. Its complexity dwarfs that of the most advanced man-made machines and, although its structure and function are understood in broad terms, much of its workings remain a complete mystery.

STRUCTURE

Like the rest of the brain, the cerebrum consists of billions of interconnected nerve cells, arranged in layers or in clusters called nuclei, together

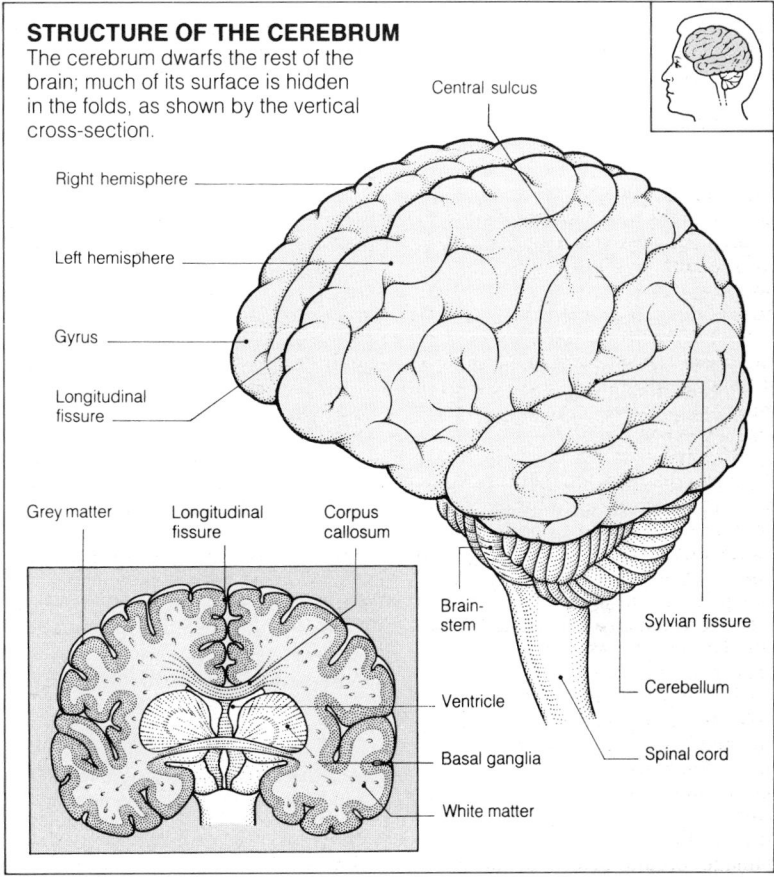

STRUCTURE OF THE CEREBRUM
The cerebrum dwarfs the rest of the brain; much of its surface is hidden in the folds, as shown by the vertical cross-section.

Central sulcus
Right hemisphere
Left hemisphere
Gyrus
Longitudinal fissure
Grey matter
Longitudinal fissure
Corpus callosum
Brainstem
Sylvian fissure
Cerebellum
Ventricle
Spinal cord
Basal ganglia
White matter

with nerve fibres, the long filamentous outgrowths from nerve cells along which electrical messages (nerve impulses) pass to other cells. These fibres are organized into bundles, or nerve tracts, like electrical cables. Both the nerve cells and their fibres lie in a matrix of supporting cells, called glial cells, which provide both physical support and some metabolic requirements (e.g. energy, nutrients, or structural components) for the nerve cells.

Each cerebral hemisphere contains a central cavity, called a ventricle, which is filled with *cerebrospinal fluid*. Much of the rest of each hemisphere falls into three main layers: an inner layer surrounding the ventricle and consisting of clusters of nerve cells called the basal ganglia; a middle layer of "white matter" consisting mainly of tracts of nerve fibres; and an outer surface layer, known as the cerebral cortex or "grey matter", which is about 1 cm deep and consists of several layers of interconnected nerve cells.

The surface of each hemisphere is thrown into a series of folds, called gyri, separated by fissures called sulci; much of the cortex is hidden within the folds. Broad surface regions, or lobes, of each hemisphere are named after overlying bones; the four main regions are the frontal, parietal, temporal, and occipital lobes.

The pattern of cortical folding is not precisely the same for everyone, but some of the gyri and sulci are constant and easily recognized on the surface of any brain. They have been given names by anatomists. The parietal and frontal lobes, for example, are separated by the central sulcus, and the temporal lobe from the frontal by the sylvian fissure. The longitudinal fissure is a deep cleft running front to back over the entire surface of the cerebrum, thus separating the two hemispheres. By reference to such landmarks, the location of any point on the surface of the cortex can be specified with some precision.

The nerve fibres forming much of the white matter in each hemisphere are of three main types: association fibres that link areas of cortex within a single hemisphere; projection fibres that link areas of the cortex to central brain structures and to the brainstem below; and commissural fibres, collected into a thick band called the corpus callosum, that link the two hemispheres. A continuous stream of information, in the form of electrical impulses, flows along these fibres between groups of nerve cells.

FUNCTION

Much of the sensory information from organs such as the eyes and ears and from sensory receptors in the skin has its final destination in the cerebral cortex, where it is sorted, analysed, and generally integrated until finally it is perceived as images, sound, touch sensations, and the like. Different levels of analysis are thought to correspond to the distinct layers of neurons in the cortex, with full conscious sensation probably occurring only in the top few layers.

Certain sensory modalities are specifically located within particular cortical regions—for example, visual perception is located within a part of the occipital lobe called the visual cortex. If this part of the brain is seriously damaged, vision is lost completely. Touch and pressure sensations are consciously perceived along the postcentral gyrus, immediately behind the central sulcus that divides the frontal and parietal lobes. Other cortical regions, mainly in the temporal lobe, are associated with auditory (hearing), olfactory (smell), and gustatory (taste) sensations, although less specifically so. If these areas are destroyed, sensation is dulled considerably, but not lost altogether. It seems that some primitive sensations (e.g. smell and pain) may be perceived below the level of the cortex.

In addition to sensory areas, there are also specific "motor" areas concerned with the initiation of signals for movement by the skeletal muscles. The main motor area of the cortex is in the frontal lobe, along the precentral gyrus, immediately in front of the central sulcus. Again, it seems that not all movements are initiated from the cortex. Some learned, semi-automatic programmes of movement, such as those for walking, are delegated to lower brain regions, leaving the cortex free to deal with newly formulated, skilled movements.

Linked to the more clearly defined sensory and motor areas are association areas of the cortex, which integrate information from various senses. The association areas also perform functions such as comprehension and recognition, memory storage and recall, arithmetical calculation, thought and decision-making, or are involved in the conscious experience of emotions. Whereas many of the sensory and motor areas are on both sides of the cerebrum (serving the opposite side of the body), some of these other cortical functions are localized to one hemisphere. The "dominant" hemisphere (the left in almost all right-handed and many left-handed people) tends to control logical functions such as word comprehension, language, speech, and numeration, whereas the nondominant hemisphere is concerned with spatial relationships and emotional responses such as colour appreciation.

In general, the more complex the function, the less well localized it is. However, the areas responsible for the comprehension of words (heard and read) and for language expression are located within clearly defined areas of the dominant hemisphere. The comprehension region (Wernicke's area) is close to the part of the cortex concerned with sound perception; the region concerned with language expression (Broca's area) is close to the motor region controlling the muscles used in speech.

Of all the regions of the cerebrum, the functions of the frontal lobe are the least understood, and for this reason it is sometimes termed a "silent area". Information on the activity of this and some other areas derives mainly from study of the symptoms of local damage or disease.

DISORDERS

Damage to the cerebrum may be the result of direct physical trauma, (see *Head injury*), *intracerebral haemorrhage* or other forms of *stroke*, *brain tumours*, *encephalitis* (inflammation of the brain), or to some types of poisoning, nutritional deficiency, and degenerative processes.

Damage to particular regions may cause specific syndromes. Examples are mental apathy and self-neglect (or other personality change) resulting from frontal lobe damage, or the loss of sensory discrimination, tactile *agnosia* (loss of the ability to recognize objects by touch), and geographic disorientation (losing one's way even in a familiar area), which may occur with parietal lobe injury. Disease of the temporal lobe may cause *amnesia* (loss of memory), strange hallucinations of smell, sight, and sound, and *aphasia* (loss of the ability to comprehend or express language) if the dominant hemisphere is affected. Specific visual defects result from damage to the occipital lobe.

Often, however, cerebral disease causes nonspecific symptoms such as epileptic convulsions or headaches.

Certification

An outmoded term for the process of completing the necessary legal documents for a person's commitment to a mental institution for compulsory detention and treatment. (See *Mental Health Act*.)

Cerumen

The wax-like yellowish substance commonly found in the external ear canal (see *Earwax*).

Cervical

Relating to the neck or to the cervix (neck of the uterus).

Cervical cancer

See *Cervix, cancer of*.

Cervical erosion

A condition affecting the cervix (neck of the uterus) in which a layer of cells more characteristic of those found in the inner lining of the cervix appear on its outside surface—as though the cervix had been turned inside out. The layer of cells contains many that are column-shaped and of a glandular (mucus-forming) type. The term "erosion" is something of a misnomer as there is no loss of tissue or ulceration of the cervix. The cervix may, however, be more fragile and have a tendency to bleed and secrete more mucus than normal.

CAUSES

Some women are born with cervical erosion and have no symptoms. Other possible causes include injury to the cervix during labour (which may cause glandular tissue to appear on the outer surface of the cervix during healing) and long-term use of *oral contraceptives*.

SYMPTOMS

Most women with cervical erosion have no or few symptoms. Those that do have symptoms usually complain of a vaginal discharge, especially in the week prior to a period, or bleeding between periods or after intercourse. Inspection of the cervix shows a reddened area on the surface that may bleed easily when touched. This appearance needs to be distinguished from cervical cancer by means of a *cervical smear test* and perhaps *colposcopy* (examination of the cervix with a viewing instrument).

TREATMENT
Only women with symptoms need to be treated. Treatment by local destruction of glandular tissue includes *cauterization, cryosurgery* (freezing), *diathermy* (heat destruction), or *laser treatment*. The areas of destroyed glandular tissue are replaced in time by a layer of normal squamous (flat) cells.

Cervical incompetence
Abnormal weakness of the cervix (the neck of the uterus) that can result in recurrent *miscarriages*. Normally, the cervix remains closed until labour begins. However, if the cervix is incompetent, it may gradually widen from about the 12th week of pregnancy onwards because of the weight of the fetus within the uterus, or may suddenly open during the middle third of pregnancy.

CAUSES AND SYMPTOMS
Cervical incompetence may be suspected if a woman has had two or more miscarriages after the 14th week of pregnancy. About one fifth of women who have recurrent miscarriages have cervical incompetence.

The obstetrician may be able to detect the cervical widening by performing an internal pelvic examination. The condition may also be diagnosed by *ultrasound scanning*.

TREATMENT
When a woman with cervical incompetence becomes pregnant, a suture (stitch) is tied, like a purse string, around the cervix. This is performed during the fourth month of pregnancy under an epidural or general anaesthetic. After the operation, the patient stays in the hospital for a few days, and may be advised to rest frequently in bed throughout the remainder of the pregnancy. The suture is left in position until the pregnancy is at or near full term. It is then cut so that the mother can deliver the baby normally.

Cervical mucus method
A form of contraception based on periodic abstinence from intercourse according to the changes in the mucus secreted by a woman's cervix. (See *Contraception, natural methods of.*)

Cervical osteoarthritis
A degenerative disorder, also known as cervical spondylitis, that affects the joints between the cervical vertebrae (bones in the neck).

Because the degenerative changes are associated with aging, the condition mainly affects middle-aged and elderly people. An X-ray of almost everyone over the age of 50 would show some evidence of cervical osteoarthritis, but most people have no or only minor symptoms.

Occasionally, the degeneration may be started by an injury—for example, a whiplash neck injury sustained in a road traffic accident.

SYMPTOMS
The main symptoms are pain and stiffness in the neck. Pressure on nerves passing between the affected vertebrae may cause pain in the arms and shoulders, numbness and tingling in the hands, and a weak grip. Symptoms tend to flare up from time to time, with intervening periods of only mild discomfort.

Other symptoms include dizziness, unsteadiness, double vision and headache brought on by turning the head. These symptoms are caused by pressure on blood vessels running through the vertebrae up to the brain. Rarely, pressure on the spinal cord itself can cause weakness or even paralysis in the legs, and loss of bladder control.

DIAGNOSIS AND TREATMENT
People who have persistent minor symptoms or symptoms that are becoming worse should consult their doctor. X-rays and possibly other tests will be performed.

Treatment of severe neck pain and stiffness may include rest, *heat treatment*, supporting the neck in a collar, *traction* of the neck, and the use of *analgesic drugs* (painkillers). *Physiotherapy*, including *diathermy*, ultrasound, massage, and exercises to improve neck posture and movement, is useful when the pain has eased. People with pressure on the spinal cord may benefit from a surgical procedure to relieve pressure on the cord (see *Decompression, spinal canal*).

Cervical rib
A *congenital* abnormality in which the lowest of the seven cervical vertebrae (neck bones) has overdeveloped to form a *rib*. The cervical rib lies parallel to and above the first normal rib. The abnormality varies from a small bony swelling to a fully developed rib and may occur on one or both sides. The cause is unknown.

SYMPTOMS
Often, there are no symptoms and the cervical rib is discovered only when an X-ray of the chest or neck is taken for some unrelated reason. Symptoms

may develop in early adult life, when the rib begins to press on the lower part of the *brachial plexus* (the group of nerves passing from the spinal cord into the arm), causing pain, numbness, and pins-and-needles in the forearm and hand. These symptoms can often be relieved by changing the position of the arm.

DIAGNOSIS AND TREATMENT
An X-ray will show the presence of a cervical rib, but other possible causes of pain and tingling in the hand or arm (such as *carpal tunnel syndrome* or a *disc prolapse*) still need to be excluded.

Symptoms due to a cervical rib can sometimes be reduced by exercises to strengthen the shoulder muscles and to improve the posture. Severe or persistent symptoms may require surgical removal of the rib.

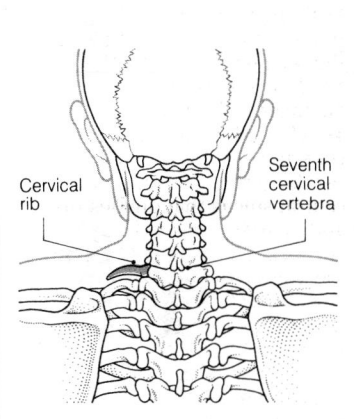

LOCATION OF CERVICAL RIB
The overdeveloped seventh cervical vertebra forms a rib parallel to a normal one.

Cervical rib

Seventh cervical vertebra

Cervical smear test
A test to detect abnormal changes in the cells of the cervix (the neck of the uterus) and thus to prevent the development of cervical cancer (see *Cervix, cancer of*).

WHY IT IS DONE
The test offers a 95 per cent chance of detecting dysplasia (abnormal cell changes) which, if not discovered and treated, could become cancerous.

Cervical smears can also detect viral infections of the cervix, such as *herpes simplex* and wart virus infection (see *Warts, genital*).

WHEN IT IS DONE
A woman should have a cervical smear within six months of first having sexual intercourse. A second

smear should be performed six to 12 months later (because of the small chance of missing an abnormality on one smear) and, if no abnormality is found, subsequently at approximately three-yearly intervals for the rest of her life. More frequent tests may be needed in women who change sex partners often or whose partner changes sex partners frequently.

Cervical smears may be performed by general practitioners or at well woman or family planning clinics.

RESULTS

If the cells in the cervix appear normal, no further treatment is required. However, if the cells appear abnormal, the smear is graded according to the cervical intra-epithelial neoplasia (CIN) classification system: CIN1 (mild dysplasia), CIN2 (moderate dysplasia), or CIN3 (severe dysplasia/early cancer). All abnormal smears are followed either by repeat smears or by *colposcopy* (examination of the cervix with a viewing instrument) and *biopsy* (removal of small samples of tissue for microscopic analysis) of any suspicious areas. There are two types of cervical biopsy: punch and cone (see illustration opposite).

Areas confirmed as abnormal by biopsy are treated by *electrocoagulation* or *laser* (both of which use heat to destroy tissue) or by *cryosurgery* (which uses cold to destroy tissue). Treatment is sometimes carried out at the same time as colposcopy if the abnormal area is small and well-defined. If a woman is pregnant, treatment is usually delayed until after delivery.

If colposcopy is not available, or if the extent of the severe dysplasia cannot be identified, treatment is by *cone biopsy*, an operation to remove a core of cervical tissue.

Cervical spondylosis

An alternative name for *cervical osteoarthritis*.

Cervicitis

Inflammation of the cervix (the neck of the uterus). Cervicitis is usually due to an infection, such as *gonorrhoea*, *chlamydial infection*, or genital *herpes*. Cervical infection may also follow injury to the cervix during childbirth or surgery on the uterus. There are acute and chronic forms of cervicitis.

SYMPTOMS

Acute cervicitis is often symptomless and may not be discovered until the cervix is examined for some other reason. The cervix is inflamed and there may be a discharge from it.

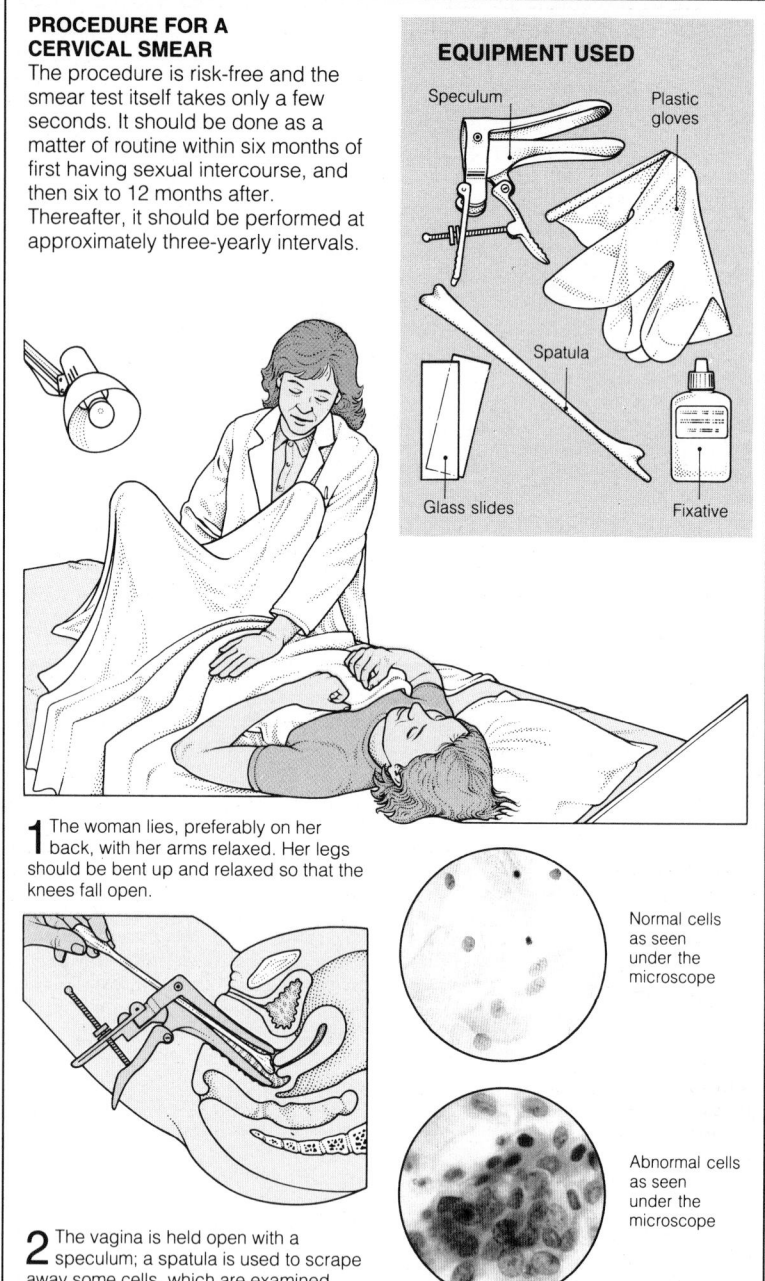

PROCEDURE FOR A CERVICAL SMEAR

The procedure is risk-free and the smear test itself takes only a few seconds. It should be done as a matter of routine within six months of first having sexual intercourse, and then six to 12 months after. Thereafter, it should be performed at approximately three-yearly intervals.

EQUIPMENT USED

Speculum

Plastic gloves

Spatula

Glass slides

Fixative

1 The woman lies, preferably on her back, with her arms relaxed. Her legs should be bent up and relaxed so that the knees fall open.

2 The vagina is held open with a speculum; a spatula is used to scrape away some cells, which are examined under the microscope.

Normal cells as seen under the microscope

Abnormal cells as seen under the microscope

Chronic cervicitis may produce a vaginal discharge, bleeding from the vagina after sexual intercourse or between periods, and pain low in the abdomen, sometimes felt only during sexual intercourse.

COMPLICATIONS

Untreated cervicitis can spread to cause *endometritis* (inflammation of the lining of the uterus), *salpingitis* (inflammation of the fallopian tubes), or *pelvic inflammatory disease*.

If a pregnant woman has cervicitis, her baby may be infected during delivery, resulting in neonatal *ophthalmia* (an eye infection) or, less commonly, in *pneumonia* caused by chlamydial infection.

BIOPSY OF THE CERVIX

If a woman has recurrent abnormal smears, colposcopy and biopsy of suspicious areas will be performed. If the abnormal area cannot be seen completely by colposcopy, a larger sample of tissue is removed by cone biopsy. This procedure is used for treatment as well as diagnosis.

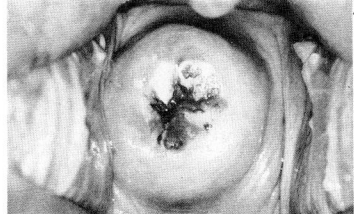

View of cervix
The photograph shows the end-on appearance of the cervix after a biopsy specimen has been taken from its tip.

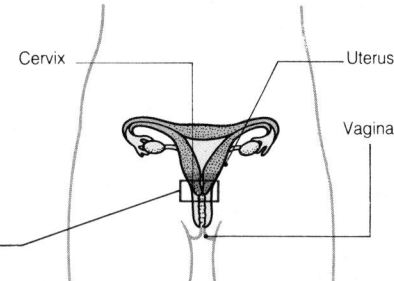

Cervix — Uterus

Vagina

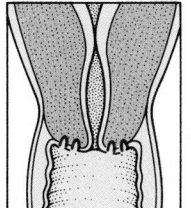

Punch biopsy
If regions of the cervix look abnormal, but not serious enough for full biopsy, minute fragments of the cervix are removed for examination.

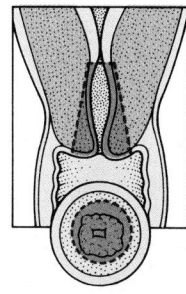

Cone biopsy
Using general anaesthesia, a cone-shaped piece of the cervix (containing an area with abnormal cells) is removed with a scalpel. The resulting crater is repaired by stitching flaps of tissue over the wound. Alternatively, the wound may be left open and diathermy or freezing used to stop any bleeding. Lasers (left) may be used to destroy abnormal tissue.

DIAGNOSIS AND TREATMENT

A woman who has the symptoms described should see her doctor, who will probably examine her cervix and take swabs of any discharge so that the microorganism responsible for the discharge can be identified.

Treatment is with *antibiotic drugs*, especially a *tetracycline* or *penicillin drug*, or with an *antiviral drug*, such as *acyclovir*, depending on the cause of infection. If symptoms persist, the inflamed area of the cervix may be cauterized by *electrocoagulation, cryotherapy,* or *laser treatment* to destroy the infected tissue.

Cervix

A small, cylindrical organ, several centimetres in length and less than 2.5 cm in diameter, comprising the lower part and neck of the uterus. The cervix separates the body and cavity of the uterus from the vagina. Running through the cervix is a canal, through which sperm can pass from the vagina into the uterus and through which blood passes during *menstruation*. The cervical canal forms part of the birth canal during *childbirth*.

The bulk of the cervix consists of fibrous tissue with some smooth muscle. This tissue makes the cervix into a form of sphincter (circular muscle) and allows for the great adaptability in its size and shape required during *pregnancy* and childbirth.

FUNCTION

After puberty, mucus is secreted from glandular cells in the canal. The function of this mucus is to assist the entry of sperm into the upper cervix, which acts as a sperm reservoir. In the middle of the menstrual cycle, this mucus becomes less viscous and more favourable for the passage of sperm. Within the cervix, the sperm are protected and provided with energy by the mucus.

During pregnancy, the internal muscular fibres increase in size, thus lengthening the cervix, which acts as a barrier for retention of the foetus. Towards the end of pregnancy there is a general shortening of the cervix in readiness for labour and delivery. During labour the central canal widens to up to 10 cm in diameter to allow the baby to pass from the uterus. Soon after childbirth the muscles in the cervix contract and the canal returns to its original size.

Cervix, cancer of

Cancer of the cervix (neck of the uterus) is one of the most common cancers affecting women worldwide, and in many areas is becoming more common. Untreated, it may spread to most of the organs in the pelvis. The chances of cure depend very much on what stage the cancer has reached when first detected.

TYPES

Cervical cancer has well-defined precancerous stages. Before any cancer appears, abnormal changes occur in cells on the surface of the cervix, referred to as dysplasia, which can be detected by a *cervical smear test*.

ANATOMY OF THE CERVIX

The cervix contains a central canal for passage of sperm and menstrual blood, and for childbirth. Both the canal and outer surface of the cervix are lined with two types of cells: mucus-secreting glandular cells and protective squamous cells.

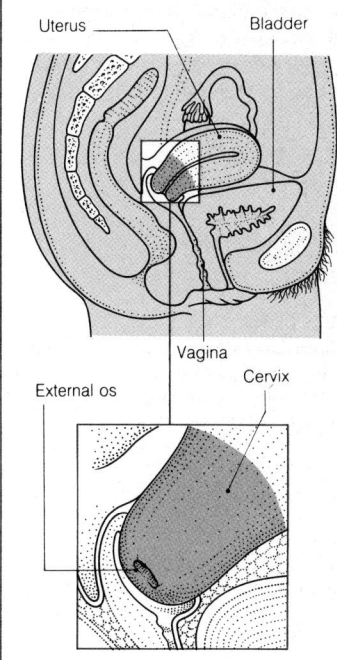

Uterus

Bladder

Vagina

Cervix

External os

C

DISORDERS OF THE CERVIX

The cervix (neck of the uterus), with its central position in the female reproductive tract, is susceptible to injury, infections, and tumours.

INJURY

Minor injury to the cervix is common during childbirth, especially if labour has been prolonged or if forceps have been used to deliver the baby's head. These injuries usually take the form of a laceration (tear) in the side wall. Usually they can be repaired immediately after delivery, but rarely they may extend into the tissues surrounding the uterus and lead to internal bleeding, requiring major surgery.

Injury may also occur if the cervical canal is excessively dilated (widened) in the process of an abortion, especially if the woman has not had children. However, the risk of such injury is extremely small if the abortion is carried out in a well-equipped hospital or clinic by a qualified gynaecologist.

When an injury does occur, there is a danger that the muscle fibres within the cervix will be damaged or weakened, leading to a condition called *cervical incompetence*. The ability of the cervix to retain a fetus in the uterus is impaired, with a risk of miscarriage unless the weakness is repaired.

INFECTION

Cervical infections are common and usually sexually transmitted, but may cause no or few symptoms. *Gonorrhoea* and *chlamydial infections* are the two most frequent and are sexually transmitted. These infections may spread to the lining of the uterus or to the fallopian tubes with a risk of causing infertility (see *Cervicitis; Endometritis; Salpingitis*).

Wart
• a benign growth caused by a virus

Tear
• a rare occurrence caused by childbirth or abortion

Infection
• causing inflammation of the cervix

Polyp
• a form of benign growth on the cervix

Erosion
• cells normally in the cervical canal appearing on the cervix

Cancer
• a malignant growth arising from abnormal cells in the cervix

Trichomoniasis is another common infection affecting the vagina and cervix; it is also sexually transmitted and caused by a protozoan parasite.

Viral infections of the cervix are becoming more common, especially those due to the human papilloma or wart virus and the herpes simplex virus. These infections are sexually transmitted and are associated with warts or herpetic ulcers in other parts of the reproductive tract (see *Warts, genital; Herpes, genital*). Both have been linked to cancerous and precancerous conditions of the cervix.

TUMOURS

Growths may be benign or malignant (cancerous). The former are usually present in the form of a polyp.

Malignant growths are always preceded by changes in the surface layer of cells, called cervical dysplasias. These changes can be detected by a cervical smear test and alert the gynaecologist to the need for possible further investigation and treatment to prevent a cancer from developing (see *Cervix, cancer of*).

OTHER DISORDERS

Mucus-forming cells typical of those usually found in the cervical canal may appear as a layer on the outer surface of the cervix, causing a tendency to bleed. This condition is readily treated (see *Cervical erosion*).

INVESTIGATION

Investigation is by means of an internal examination (see *Pelvic examination*), a *cervical smear test*, and, in cases of suspected cancer or a precancerous condition, a *colposcopy*.

Mild dysplasia may later revert to normal, but any woman who has an abnormal cervical smear should undergo further investigation and possible follow-up smears.

If more severe dysplasia or early cancer is detected, it can be treated and cured completely.

CAUSES

There are two main types of cervical cancer. Both can occur before or after the *menopause*.

SQUAMOUS TYPE This is by far the most common type of cervical cancer and is almost certainly the result of some process that occurs during sexual intercourse, possibly involving an infectious organism acquired from the male partner. Recent evidence suggests that the organism is a strain of the human papillomavirus (wart virus). A woman in a sexual relationship with a man who has genital warts (see *Warts, genital*) has about a one in three risk of developing a precancerous condition of the cervix.

There are over 40 different strains of human papillomavirus, but traces of "high risk" strains, especially HPV16 and HPV18, have been found in 90 per cent of squamous-type cervical cancers and in 50 to 70 per cent of precancerous conditions.

Other factors are also known to predispose a woman to cancer of the cervix. Smokers are at higher risk than nonsmokers, possibly because smoking impairs the *immune system* (natural defences against infection) and thus allows entry and proliferation of a causative virus. An alternative explanation is that the chemical *carcinogen* in cigarettes is absorbed into the bloodstream and excreted into the cervical secretions. Additional evidence in favour of this theory is the observation that the incidence of cervical cancer is affected by the smoking habits of women's male partners.

The sexual behaviour of a woman and her male partner or partners strongly influences her chances of developing the disease. The earlier a woman and/or her partner first started having sex, and the greater the number of sexual partners they have had, the higher the risk that she will develop a precancerous condition.

ADENOCARCINOMA The causes of this much rarer type of cervical cancer are unclear. Both sexually active women and those who have never had intercourse are susceptible.

INCIDENCE

Overall, there are about 4,500 cases of cervical cancer diagnosed in the UK per year, with about 1,600 deaths from this cause. Although the incidence of diagnosed cervical cancer and precancerous conditions has been increasing in the UK for several years, the death rate has been decreasing, and should continue to do so due to more widespread, regular, and efficient cervical smear testing.

SYMPTOMS

The precancerous stages cause no symptoms whatsoever. Symptoms of the malignant stage are also initially few. Eventually, a woman will notice vaginal bleeding or a bloodstained discharge at unexpected times—between periods, after intercourse, or after the menopause.

If left untreated, the cancer spreads from the cervical surface into the deeper parts of the cervix and then out into the pelvic tissues, causing pain. Eventually the cancer spreads to the bladder, rectum, and surrounding pelvic tissue.

DIAGNOSIS

The precancerous stages can be detected only by a cervical smear test or by *colposcopy* (inspection of the cervix with a viewing instrument). All sexually active women are advised to have a cervical smear test soon after their first experience of sexual intercourse, again six to 12 months later, and at intervals of approximately three years thereafter.

Diagnosis of more advanced stages may be made from a cervical smear, colposcopy, *cone biopsy,* or from a doctor seeing areas of ulceration or cauliflower-like growths on the cervix after symptoms are experienced.

TREATMENT

If a persistent area of abnormality or localized early cancer is diagnosed by colposcopy and biopsy and can be seen in its entirety, destruction is by *electrocoagulation, diathermy,* or *laser treatment* (all of which use heat to destroy tissue), or by *cryosurgery* (which uses cold). All methods except diathermy can usually be carried out painlessly under local anaesthesia. Success rates for complete removal after one application of laser or diathermy are about 95 per cent. If a woman is pregnant, treatment of precancerous conditions or early cancer is usually delayed until after delivery.

If an area of abnormality or cancer has spread into the cervical canal, close inspection of a cone biopsy may show that this procedure has removed all the diseased tissue. In all other cases of spreading cancer, treatment will depend on the extent of the spread, the age of the patient, and the doctor's recommendation for surgery or *radiotherapy.*

In more advanced cases, when the tumour has spread to the organs of the pelvis, radiotherapy is given. In certain specialized centres, radical surgical techniques may be employed for selected patients, in which the bladder, vagina, cervix, uterus, and rectum may all be removed.

Survival rates (five or more years after treatment) are about 50 to 80 per cent for early spreading cancer, whether treated by surgery or radiotherapy. For later-stage disease, survival rates drop to 10 to 30 per cent, but improve to about 30 to 50 per cent among those selected patients who undergo radical surgery.

Cestodes

The scientific name for tapeworms—a group of long, flat, multisegmented parasites. (See *Tapeworm infestation.*)

Chagas' disease

An infectious parasitic disease found only in parts of South and Central America and spread by certain insects commonly called "cone-nosed" or "assassin" bugs. The disease is named after the Brazilian physician Carlos Chagas (1879-1934).

The parasites responsible for Chagas' disease are single-celled organisms called trypanosomes, very similar to those that cause *sleeping sickness* in Africa. They live in the bloodstream and can also affect the heart, intestines, and nervous system.

Symptoms include swelling of the lymph nodes and fever. Long-term complications include damage to the heart. Treatment is unsatisfactory. A drug called nifurtimox kills trypanosomes in the blood but has unpleasant side-effects.

Chalazion

A round, painless swelling in the upper or lower eyelid, sometimes known as a meibomian cyst. The swelling is caused by obstruction of one of the meibomian glands that lubricate the edge of the eyelids. If the swelling is large, pressure on the cornea at the front of the eye can cause blurring of vision.

Chalazions can occur at any age and are particularly common in people suffering from the skin conditions *acne, rosacea,* or seborrhoeic *dermatitis.* If the cyst becomes infected, the eyelid becomes more swollen, red, and painful. About one third of chalazions disappear without any treatment, but large cysts usually need to be removed surgically (from behind the eyelid) under local anaesthetic.

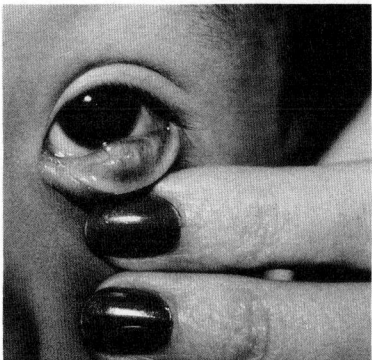

A chalazion on the lower lid
Many small chalazions disappear spontaneously. Larger ones may require surgery.

Chancre, hard

An ulcer, usually on the genitals, that develops during the first, or primary, stage of the sexually transmitted disease *syphilis.*

Chancroid

A sexually transmitted disease found mainly in the tropics; it is characterized by painful ulcers on the genitals and enlarged lymph nodes in the groin. Also known as soft chancre or soft sore, the disorder is caused by the bacterium HAEMOPHILUS DUCREYI.

The infection is relatively rare in Europe; most cases occur in sailors or travellers who have had contact with prostitutes in tropical countries. Generally, fewer than 100 cases are diagnosed in the UK annually.

Prompt treatment with *antibiotic drugs* is usually effective. If the disease is not treated, abscesses can form in the groin and leave deep scars.

Chapped skin

Sore, cracked, rough skin on areas that have been repeatedly wet, inadequately dried, or exposed to the cold. The hands and face (particularly the lips) are the most commonly affected areas.

Chapping occurs when the skin becomes excessively dry due to lack, or removal, of the natural oils that help keep it supple. This tends to happen in cold weather because the oil-secreting glands produce less oil. Repeated washing or wetting removes the oils.

Chapped skin can often be prevented by using protective gloves or *barrier creams* and by drying the skin carefully. Skin that has already become chapped usually responds well to applications of a rich, lanolin-based hand cream or face cream.

Character disorders

See *Personality disorders.*

Charcoal

A form of carbon. Charcoal's principal medical use is as an adsorbent agent in the emergency treatment of some types of poisoning and drug overdose.

Charcot-Marie-Tooth disease

An inherited muscle-wasting disease that mainly affects the legs. (See *Peroneal muscular atrophy.*)

Charcot's joint

A joint damaged by injuries that have gone unnoticed because of loss of sensation affecting the joint. (See *Neuropathic joint.*)

Check-up

See *Examination, physical.*

Cheilitis

Inflammation, cracking, and dryness of the lips. Cheilitis can be caused by ill-fitting dentures, a local infection, allergy to cosmetics, too much sunbathing, or deficiency of riboflavin (vitamin B_2). In riboflavin deficiency, the corners of the mouth are chiefly affected. Until the underlying problem is remedied, a soothing skin cream will relieve the soreness.

Chelating agents

Chemicals used in the treatment of poisoning by metals such as lead, arsenic, and mercury. Chelating agents act by combining with these metals to form less poisonous substances. *Penicillamine* is a commonly used chelating agent.

Chemist

The common term for a pharmacist, the health professional who prepares drugs, makes up prescriptions and supplies them, and who also gives advice on the treatment of common and minor illnesses.

Chemotherapy

The treatment of infection or cancer by the use of drugs that act selectively on the cause of the disorder. Drugs that are used in chemotherapy may also have substantial effects on normal tissue.

Infections are treated by *antibiotic drugs,* which may be either bactericidal (killing bacteria) or bacteriostatic (stopping further bacterial growth and allowing the body's immune system to take over and destroy the bacteria). In the same way, *anticancer drugs* act either by destroying tumour cells or by stopping them from multiplying.

One problem with chemotherapy is that natural selection leads to the emergence of resistant bacteria or cells. This effect is minimized by the discriminatory use of antibiotics, and, in cancer chemotherapy, by giving several different types of anticancer drugs simultaneously.

A further problem with cancer chemotherapy is that the drugs act on all rapidly dividing cells, not just tumour cells. Thus, they may affect the bone marrow, the intestinal lining, the hair follicles, the ovaries and testes, and the mouth, sometimes causing severe side-effects. Antibiotic drugs act selectively on bacterial cells, which have a different structure from human cells. Antibiotic chemotherapy therefore has generally less serious side-effects than cancer chemotherapy.

Chenodeoxycholic acid

A chemical in *bile* that reduces the amount of *cholesterol* released by the *liver* into the bile.

Chenodeoxycholic acid is sometimes prescribed as a treatment for small *gallstones* if they contain mainly cholesterol and no calcium. Treatment takes several months, during which time progress is monitored by *X-rays*

or *ultrasound scanning* of the *gallbladder.* Chenodeoxycholic acid may cause diarrhoea and, rarely, liver damage. It should not be taken during pregnancy because of possible adverse effects on the fetus.

Chest

The upper part of the trunk. Known technically as the *thorax,* the chest extends from the base of the neck down to the *diaphragm.*

Chest pain

Chest pain usually does not have a serious cause, although occasionally it may be a symptom of an underlying disorder that requires medical attention. The pain may occur in the chest wall (in the skin, the underlying muscles, or the ribs) or in an organ within the chest.

CAUSES

The most common causes of pain in the chest wall are a strained muscle (which usually follows exercise) or an injury, such as bruising or a broken rib (due to a blow, fall, or other accident).

Pressure on a nerve root attached to the spinal cord may result in a sharp pain that travels to the front of the chest. This pain may be caused by *osteoarthritis* of, or injury to, the vertebrae, or, more rarely, a *disc prolapse.*

Pain in the side of the chest may be due to *pleurodynia* (inflammation of the muscles between the ribs and the diaphragm associated with a viral infection).

The viral infection *herpes zoster* (shingles) may cause pain in the chest wall. The pain, which is severe, runs along the course of a nerve and is followed by a rash of blisters in the area of skin supplied by the nerve.

In *Tietze's syndrome,* inflammation at the junctions of the rib cartilages causes pain on the front of the chest wall which increases with movements of the chest.

Within the chest, pain may be caused by *pleurisy* (inflammation of the pleurae, the membranes surrounding the lungs and covering the inner surface of the chest wall), which may be brought on by *bronchitis, pneumonia,* or, rarely, by *pulmonary embolism* (a blood clot lodged in an artery in the lungs). The pain of pleurisy is worse when the sufferer breathes in.

Malignant tumours of the lung (see *Lung cancer; Mesothelioma*) may cause pain as they grow and press on the pleura and ribs.

Acid reflux (regurgitation of acid fluid from the stomach into the oesophagus) may lead to heartburn, a burning pain behind the sternum. Heartburn may also be a symptom of *hiatus hernia*.

Various heart disorders can cause chest pain. Most common of these is *angina pectoris*, which is due to the heart muscle receiving too little blood (and therefore oxygen), commonly as a result of *coronary artery disease*. The pain, which resembles that of severe indigestion or of a heavy weight pressing on the chest, is felt in the centre of the chest and may spread outwards to the throat, jaw, or arms (usually the left one). It usually occurs when the work load of the heart muscle is increased by exertion, and is relieved by rest.

Myocardial infarction (damage to the heart muscle due to an inadequate blood supply) produces pain in the same areas as angina but the pain is more severe and persistent.

The pain of acute *pericarditis* (inflammation of the pericardium, the membrane that surrounds the heart) is also felt in the centre of the chest. In some cases the pain is severe enough to resemble the pain of a heart attack. It can often be relieved by leaning forwards. Acute pericarditis is rare and tends to occur in young adults after or with a viral infection.

Mitral valve prolapse has been associated with many symptoms, including chest pain. The chest pain may be sharp and left-sided.

Chest pain may also be a result of anxiety and emotional stress. (See *Hyperventilation; Panic attack.*)

INVESTIGATION AND TREATMENT
Chest pain not associated with a trivial cause (such as bruising from a minor injury) should receive medical attention. Whether or not emergency treatment is necessary depends on the type and location of the pain and on the accompanying symptoms.

The treatment of chest pain depends on the underlying cause. For example, antibiotics may be prescribed for chest pain caused by pneumonia, and surgery may be necessary for the treatment of a malignant lung tumour or for some cases of coronary artery disease. (See also *Chest pain* symptom chart overleaf.)

Chest X-ray
One of the most frequently performed medical tests, usually carried out to examine the heart or lungs. The procedure is simple, quick, and painless, and is normally performed on an outpatient basis. Mobile equipment

DIAGNOSING CHEST PAIN
To make an accurate diagnosis of the underlying cause, it is important for the patient to describe the location, quality (e.g. burning, pressing, or sharp), severity, and duration of the pain, any factors that relieve it or make it worse, and any other symptoms, such as breathing difficulty. In addition, the doctor will perform a physical examination, including listening to chest sounds with a stethoscope and feeling for areas of tenderness in the chest wall. He or she may also arrange for other diagnostic procedures to be carried out.

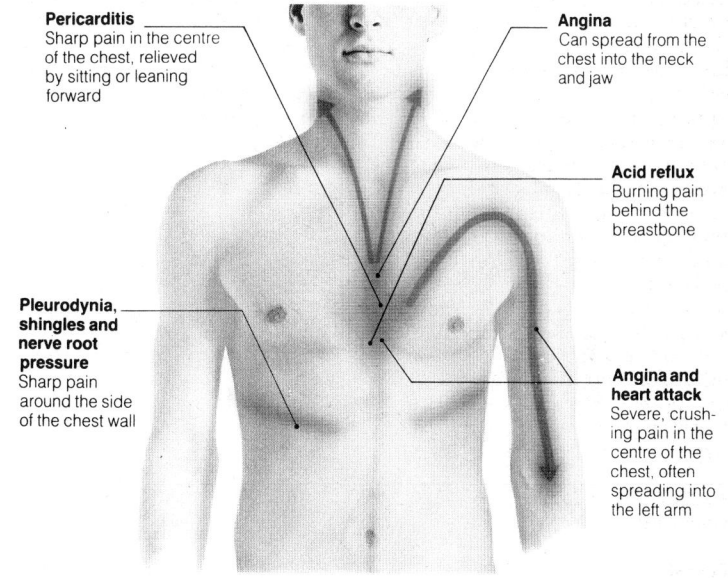

Pericarditis
Sharp pain in the centre of the chest, relieved by sitting or leaning forward

Angina
Can spread from the chest into the neck and jaw

Acid reflux
Burning pain behind the breastbone

Pleurodynia, shingles and nerve root pressure
Sharp pain around the side of the chest wall

Angina and heart attack
Severe, crushing pain in the centre of the chest, often spreading into the left arm

means that it can also be used (although somewhat less accurately) at the bedside of patients in hospital, and in patients' homes.

WHY IT IS DONE
Chest X-rays are usually used to confirm a diagnosis in patients suspected of having a heart disorder, such as enlargement of a heart chamber, or a lung disease, such as tuberculosis or lung cancer.

HOW IT IS DONE
The X-ray stand holds a film in a large, flat cassette positioned at chest level. The patient stands between the film and the X-ray machine, facing the film cassette with the chest touching it and the chin projecting over the top. The hands are placed on the hips and the elbows swung forwards, to move the shoulderblades to the side so that they do not obscure the lungs. A lead apron or screen protects the lower half of the body from radiation.

The patient takes (and holds) a deep breath while the radiographer operates equipment that passes X-rays for a fraction of a second through the upper trunk from the back. The resul-

tant X-ray picture provides an image not only of the heart and lungs but of major blood vessels, bones, and joints. (See also *X-rays*.)

Cheyne-Stokes respiration
An abnormal pattern of breathing in which the rate and depth of respiration varies rhythmically. Deep, rapid breathing gradually becomes slower and shallower until breathing actually stops for some 10 to 20 seconds. Respiration then resumes, with deep, rapid breathing, and the cycle repeats itself. Each cycle lasts a few minutes.

Cheyne-Stokes respiration may be caused by disease or malfunctioning of the part of the brain that controls breathing (as occurs in some cases of *stroke, head injury, metabolic disorder*, or drug overdose). It may also occur as a result of *heart failure* and in some healthy people at high altitudes, especially during sleep.

Chickenpox
A common and mild infectious disease of childhood, characterized by a rash and slight fever. It is sometimes

CHEST PAIN
Pain anywhere between the neck and the bottom of the rib-cage that may be dull and persistent, stabbing, burning, or crushing.

? Is the pain crushing AND/OR does it radiate from the centre of the chest to the jaw, neck, or arms?

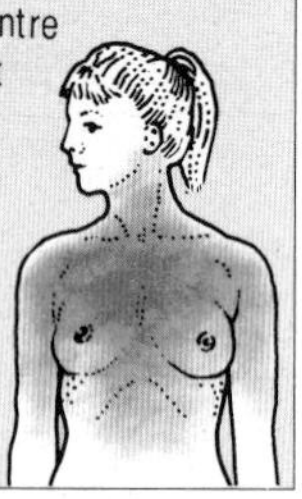

→ YES → Has pain persisted despite 15 minutes of rest?

→ YES → ☎ **EMERGENCY! GET MEDICAL HELP NOW!** A heart attack is possible.

See • *Myocardial infarction*

NO ↓

Does the pain come on during exertion and have you had previous attacks?

→ YES → ☎ **Consult your doctor without delay!** Angina pectoris is the most likely explanation for your pain.

See • *Angina pectoris*
• *Coronary artery disease*

NO ↓

NO ↓

? Are you short of breath?

→ YES → Have you recently had an operation, injury, or illness that has kept you in bed?

→ YES → ☎ **EMERGENCY! GET MEDICAL HELP NOW!** This suggests that you may have a blood clot in the lung.

See • *Pulmonary embolism*

NO ↓

Do you have a cough OR is your temperature 38°C or above?

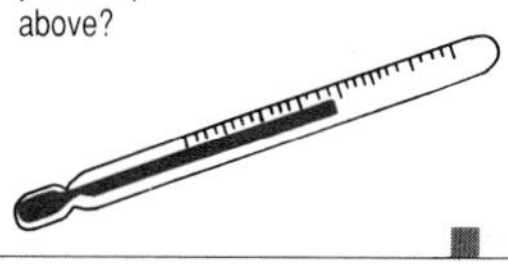

→ YES → ☎ **Call your doctor without delay!** These symptoms suggest the possibility of pneumonia or bronchitis.

See • *Bronchitis*
• *Pneumonia*

NO → ☎ **Call your doctor without delay!** You may have a collapsed lung.

See • *Pneumothorax*

NO ↓

WARNING
Anyone in whom severe chest pain develops for the first time, whether or not he or she feels ill otherwise, should call an ambulance or go to hospital immediately. This could be a heart attack and is a medical emergency.

Continued on next page

C

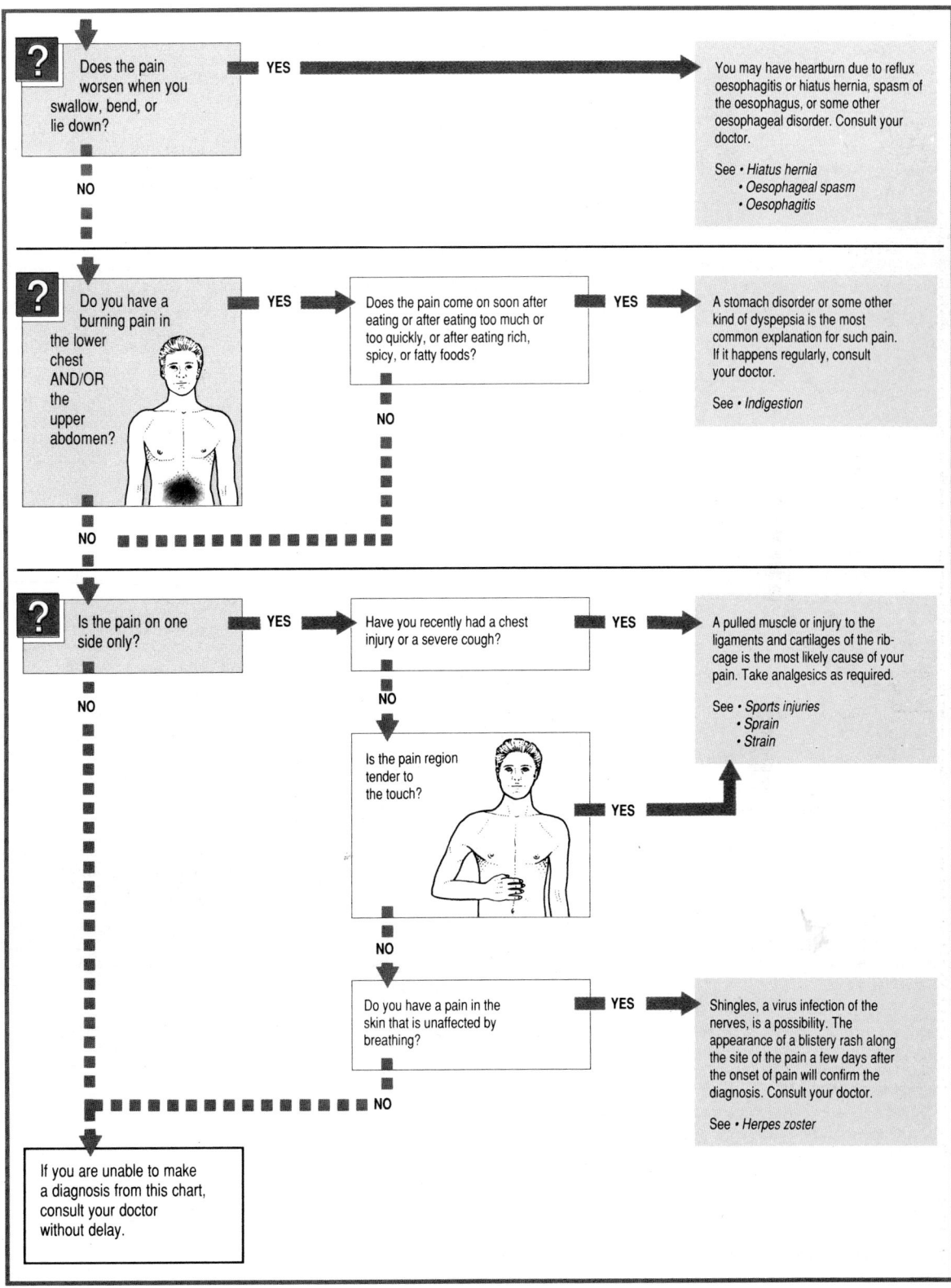

? Does the pain worsen when you swallow, bend, or lie down?

YES → You may have heartburn due to reflux oesophagitis or hiatus hernia, spasm of the oesophagus, or some other oesophageal disorder. Consult your doctor.

See • *Hiatus hernia*
• *Oesophageal spasm*
• *Oesophagitis*

NO

? Do you have a burning pain in the lower chest AND/OR the upper abdomen?

YES → Does the pain come on soon after eating or after eating too much or too quickly, or after eating rich, spicy, or fatty foods?

YES → A stomach disorder or some other kind of dyspepsia is the most common explanation for such pain. If it happens regularly, consult your doctor.

See • *Indigestion*

NO

NO

? Is the pain on one side only?

YES → Have you recently had a chest injury or a severe cough?

YES → A pulled muscle or injury to the ligaments and cartilages of the rib-cage is the most likely cause of your pain. Take analgesics as required.

See • *Sports injuries*
• *Sprain*
• *Strain*

NO

Is the pain region tender to the touch?

YES →

NO

Do you have a pain in the skin that is unaffected by breathing?

YES → Shingles, a virus infection of the nerves, is a possibility. The appearance of a blistery rash along the site of the pain a few days after the onset of pain will confirm the diagnosis. Consult your doctor.

See • *Herpes zoster*

NO

NO

If you are unable to make a diagnosis from this chart, consult your doctor without delay.

C

called varicella. Chickenpox is rare in adults; when it does occur it usually takes a more severe form.

INCIDENCE AND CAUSE

Throughout the world, most people have had chickenpox by the age of 10. The disease is caused by the varicella-zoster virus. Although an attack confers lifelong immunity, the virus remains dormant within nerve tissues after the attack and may reappear later in life to cause *herpes zoster* (shingles).

The virus is spread from person to person in airborne droplets. Patients are highly infectious from about two days before the rash appears until about a week after.

In most children, chickenpox is no more than an inconvenience. However, adults who have never had the disease should avoid it by staying away from children with chickenpox and also from anyone with shingles. Women in the final stage of pregnancy should be particularly careful, since the disease may be serious in pregnancy and the newborn child may develop a severe attack.

SYMPTOMS

Two to three weeks after infection, a rash appears behind the ears, in the armpits, on the trunk, upper arms, and legs, inside the mouth, and sometimes in the trachea (windpipe) and bronchial tubes, causing a dry cough. The rash comes in crops appearing after 12 to 48 hours and consists of clusters of small, red, itchy spots that become fluid-filled blisters, 2 to 3 mm in diameter, within a few hours. After several days the blisters dry out and form scabs. Children usually have only a slightly raised temperature, but an adult may have severe *pneumonia* with breathing difficulties and fever. Those taking *immunosuppressant drugs* are more susceptible to a severe form of the disease. Rarely, *encephalitis* (inflammation of the brain) occurs as a complication.

DIAGNOSIS AND TREATMENT

Diagnosis is usually obvious from a simple examination of the patient. In most cases, rest is all that is needed for a complete recovery, which usually takes place within 10 days in children, but over a longer period in adults.

Paracetamol can be taken to reduce fever, and *calamine* lotion relieves the itchiness of the rash. In severe cases, *acyclovir* (an antiviral drug) may be prescribed, but it must be used early in the course of the disease.

Children should be discouraged from scratching the blisters, which could lead to secondary bacterial infection and so to scarring (keeping the child's nails short is a good idea).

Specific antivaricella-zoster *immunoglobulin* has been used to prevent outbeaks in nurseries. Experimental *vaccines* have been tried but so far their use has been confined to high-risk groups such as children on treatment for leukaemia.

Chigoe

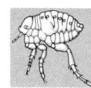 A painful, itchy, pea-sized swelling caused by a sand flea (also called the jigger or burrowing flea). When stepped on, the flea penetrates into the skin of the feet, under the toenails, or between the toes.

The chigoe flea lives in sandy soil only in Africa and tropical America. The burrowing fleas are pregnant females, which lay their eggs under the skin.

Avoidance involves wearing shoes or sandals outdoors in tropical countries (this also protects against *hookworms*). In the event of a suspected chigoe infestation, consult a doctor. Chigoe fleas should be removed with a sterile needle and the wounds treated with an antiseptic.

Chilblain

An itchy, purple-red swelling, usually on a toe or finger, caused by excessive constriction (narrowing) of small blood vessels below the surface of the skin in cold weather.

Chilblains are most common in the young and the elderly, and women are more susceptible than men. Chilblains generally heal without treatment; talcum powder may partially relieve itching. People susceptible to chilblains can help prevent them by keeping their feet and hands warm in cold weather.

Child abuse

Any form of physical or emotional mistreatment or mismanagement of a child, by acts or omissions that cause actual or potential harm to the child's health, well-being or development, or expose the child to unnecessary risk or suffering. Child abuse includes the use of a child for sexual purposes.

Cases of child abuse today are coming to light with increasing frequency, probably not just because such abuse may be more widespread, but also because there is a greater awareness of the problem.

Child abuse occurs at all levels of society. The problem appears to be more common in lower socioeco-nomic groups, possibly because of the greater stress on unsupported families with poor living standards. However, child abuse may be less easily recognized in higher socioeconomic groups.

The person injuring the child is usually a parent, but may be a step-parent, a parental friend or cohabitee, a guardian, or a sibling.

CAUSES

Being deprived or ill-treated when young seems to predispose people to abuse their own children by repeating the pattern of their own experience. This is particularly likely if the abused people have become parents at an early age, when they are too immature and inexperienced to cope with the stress and demands made on them by a young child. *Alcohol dependence, drug dependence*, or emotional disturbances are other causative factors, since they may lessen a parent's self-control.

A child born following an unwanted pregnancy may be at increased risk of abuse, as may a child whose *bonding* relationship with the mother was disturbed at birth.

Children under three years old are at greatest risk of physical abuse or emotional abuse because they are very demanding and are not old enough to be reasoned with.

PHYSICAL ABUSE

Physical injury, also called nonaccidental injury (NAI), is the most readily recognized type of abuse. The term "battered baby" refers to this form of abuse. The incidence is six per cent in Western Europe and the US. One per cent end in the child's death.

Inflicting injury on a child is most often an impulsive act, the result of a sudden loss of temper. Infants and toddlers may be picked up and shaken vigorously, which can damage the eyes and rupture blood vessels in the brain, and eventually cause severe brain damage. Slaps or punches are usually delivered to the head, resulting in black eyes and other facial bruises, cuts on the inner lip, and bone fractures. Injuries of abuse (e.g. scalds or cigarette burns) present different characteristics from injuries that occur accidentally and may reveal to a paediatrician or other examiner that, whatever the reason given for them by the parents, deliberate infliction is the real cause.

Premeditated, repeated physical assault is rare. When it does occur, it is a sign that a parent is severely disturbed and that the risks to the child are grave. These types of assault can

C

lead to multiple fractures, damage to internal organs, and even to death. Such abuse is sometimes accompanied by deliberate neglect, with no attempt made to feed or clothe the child adequately.

Physical abuse may also take the form of giving drugs to a child—for example, to sedate an overactive toddler or sometimes to poison a child deliberately. Addictive drugs are also sometimes given, with obvious risks.

A child with nonaccidental injuries is usually admitted to hospital for full examination and tests. He or she may then be removed from home while members of the health, social, and educational services, often a member of the police and sometimes a legal representative, assess the case and decide on the best course of action at a case conference. The child's interests remain paramount, but the parents, who may be under great stress, should be treated sympathetically.

EMOTIONAL ABUSE OR NEGLECT

Neglect of physical and emotional needs, such as love, stimulation, and guidance, is another form of abuse which courts have recognized only more recently. Such abuse is often unintentional, arising from the parents' lack of understanding of their child's needs. The parents may themselves be emotionally disturbed and require psychiatric help.

Indications that a child is being emotionally abused include failure to thrive, slow development, poor learning ability, and lack of normal emotional responses. Emotionally deprived children are often insecure, have poor self-esteem, and find it difficult to relate to others.

The diagnosis is usually confirmed when the child begins to put on weight and become more responsive after being taken into hospital or into care for observation. Management of the situation is aimed at the family as a whole and is the same as for physical abuse.

SEXUAL ABUSE

Sexual abuse can be defined as the use of a child for the sexual gratification of an adult. Sexual abuse of children has been increasingly recognized in recent years. Most frequently, sexual abuse occurs within the family; usually the victim is a girl, although adolescent boys may also be at risk. Sexual exploitation of both sexes occurs in pornography and prostitution.

Most cases of sexual abuse consist of a father, close relative, or family friend taking advantage of a girl's affection to obtain sexual gratification from her. This form of abuse is usually secretive, because of the man's awareness of the gravity of the offence, and is morally coercive, because of the power he holds over the girl.

Sexual abuse may come to light because of an obvious complaint from the child, a relative, or friend, or the child may display disturbed behaviour or have symptoms of a *sexually transmitted disease*. Police, psychiatrists, and social workers usually cooperate in managing the problem, the main aims being to prevent further sexual abuse and to rehabilitate the child through therapy.

Childbed fever

See *Puerperal fever*.

Childbirth

The process by which an infant moves from the uterus to the outside world. Childbirth normally occurs at between 38 and 42 weeks' gestation (pregnancy), timed from the mother's last normal menstrual period.

For most women in developed countries, who receive proper medical care during pregnancy (see *Antenatal care*) and delivery, childbirth presents no serious problems. In developing countries, however, the number of women who die from childbirth remains high (see *Maternal mortality*).

Specialized equipment and the availability of *blood transfusions* and *antibiotic drugs* have made childbirth much safer for mother and baby. However, increased concern among women that childbirth has become overmechanized in many hospitals has led to the popularity of "natural childbirth", which advocates the avoidance of unnecessary medical intervention. Many hospitals now recognize the right of women to choose the type of birth they would like, provided their wishes are compatible with safety. Women are encouraged to make "birth plans" with their midwives and obstetricians and to discuss matters such as possible methods of pain relief and preferred positions during delivery.

ONSET OF LABOUR

It is often difficult to know when labour has started. During the last three months of pregnancy the uterus starts to contract in preparation for the birth, and these *Braxton Hicks' contractions* may be mistaken for the start of labour. However, when contractions become progressively more painful, regular, and at shorter intervals, then labour has probably started. Two other events may also happen. The mucous plug that has blocked the cervical canal during pregnancy may be expelled as a bloody discharge. This is called a "show" and means that the cervix is beginning to stretch. Rupture of the membranes that surround the amniotic fluid in which the baby floats may occur at any time up to delivery. The leakage of amniotic fluid, called "breaking of the waters", varies

PAIN RELIEF IN LABOUR AND DELIVERY

Method	Why given	Possible effects on baby
Narcotic analgesics	Routine pain relief during labour	Less responsive at birth; respiratory problems, particularly in premature babies
Epidural	Routine pain relief during labour and childbirth, forceps delivery, and caesarean section	Brief drop in fetal heart-rate; fetal monitoring is recommended during and after the procedure
Paracervical block	Pain relief during active labour (after the fetal head is engaged)	Drop in fetal heart-rate; respiratory problems
Pudendal block	Forceps delivery	None
Local anaesthetic into perineum	Forceps delivery, episiotomy, and repair of perineal tear	None
General anaesthesia	Caesarean section	Reduced responsiveness at birth; respiratory problems, particularly in premature babies

C

STAGES OF BIRTH

At the onset of labour, painful and regular contractions begin and the cervix starts to dilate. The mother is usually examined vaginally every two to four hours to assess the extent of dilation. The duration of labour depends on several factors, but primarily on whether it is a first or subsequent baby. *Fetal heart monitoring* is often performed, and the frequency, strength, and duration of the mother's contractions are recorded. During the second stage contractions become stronger and the woman feels the urge to push; however, she is advised to push only during a contraction. Once delivered, the baby is usually placed on the mother's abdomen, but may first be warmed, dried, and checked by a midwife or doctor.

ELECTRONIC FETAL MONITORING

This may be carried out if the fetus is at risk, or as a routine procedure. The detecting device is linked to a monitoring machine.

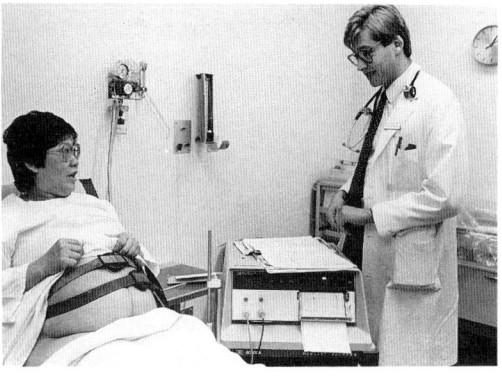

Printout

Fetal heart rate

Uterine contractions

Detecting devices

Here, the baby's heartbeat is picked up by a metal plate strapped to the mother's abdomen (lower belt). A plate beneath the upper belt detects the mother's contractions.

An alternative method is to attach to the baby's head an electrode linked to the monitor by a wire led through the mother's vagina.

THE FIRST STAGE

With the first contractions, the normally thick, tough cervix becomes thinned and softened and is gradually pulled up until it becomes effaced (merged with the walls of the uterus). The cervix then begins to dilate (open) with each contraction. It is fully dilated when the opening is approximately 10 cm in diameter. This stage can take 12 hours or more for first babies, but only a few hours for subsequent babies.

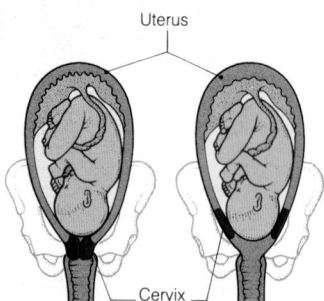

Uterus

Cervix

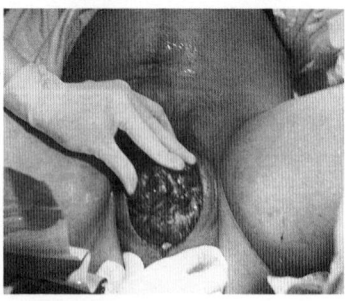

The head emerges
At this point, an episiotomy is sometimes performed to prevent tissues from tearing.

THE SECOND STAGE

As the baby's head descends, it reaches the pelvic floor muscles, which cause the head to rotate until eventually the baby's chin is pointing down to the woman's rectum. As the baby is pushed farther down, the anus and perineum (the area between the genitalia and anus) begin to bulge out, and soon the baby's head can be seen at the opening of the vagina. As the head emerges, the perineal tissues are stretched very thin; sometimes it is necessary to perform an *episiotomy* to prevent the tissues from tearing. As soon as the baby's head emerges, it turns so that it is once more in line with the baby's body; the midwife usually helps this rotation.

With the next few contractions, first one shoulder and then the other is delivered; then the rest of the baby slides out. After delivery, the umbilical cord is clamped and cut.

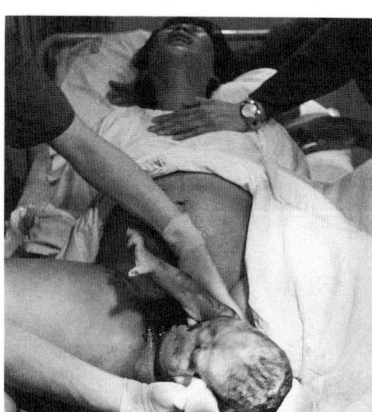

Delivery of the baby
Once both shoulders are out, the rest of the baby emerges easily.

THE THIRD STAGE

Within three to 10 minutes after the baby's birth, the placenta (afterbirth) is usually expelled. Drugs such as ergometrine or oxytocin may be used to aid in its expulsion, or the placenta may have to be manually removed by an obstetrician. Any tears or incisions are cleaned and stitched. This may be done while the mother holds her baby.

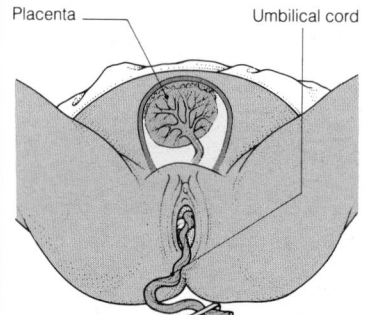

Placenta

Umbilical cord

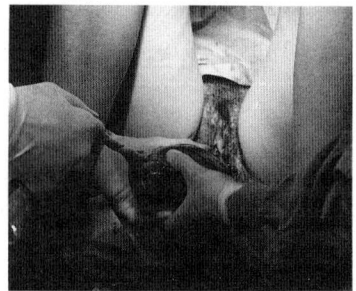

Placenta being delivered
The placenta is usually expelled within a few minutes of the baby's birth.

FIRST AID: EMERGENCY CHILDBIRTH

PREPARING FOR THE BIRTH

1 Summon medical help and reassure the mother. Stay calm—most births are normal and natural.

2 Wash hands and scrub nails under running water. Do not dry them. Wash hands frequently during the birth. Make sure everything you use is clean: bedding, sheets, towels, and cloths.

3 Prepare a flat surface, using a clean sheet or towel, a plastic sheet, or fresh newspaper.

4 Prop the mother up with pillows. Her legs should be bent and apart, and the feet flat.

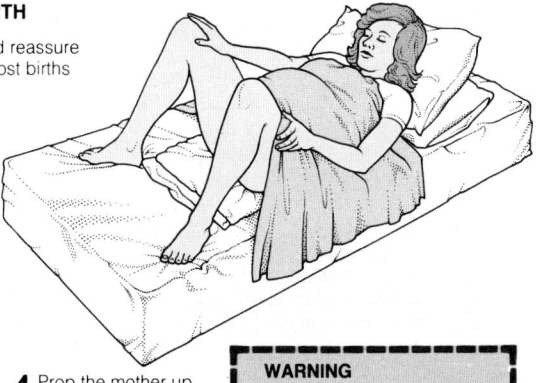

WARNING
DO NOT attempt to delay the birth by crossing the mother's legs or pushing in the baby's head. This is very harmful.

YOU WILL NEED

- Sterilized scissors (boil for 10 minutes and wrap in clean cloth).
- Clean pieces of string, boot laces, or strips of cloth about 22 cm long for tying the cord.
- Container in case the mother vomits.
- Container or plastic bag for the afterbirth (which must be taken to a doctor for examination).
- Sanitary towels or clean cloth to place over the mother's vagina after the birth.
- Cradle (or a box or drawer) and soft blanket for the baby.

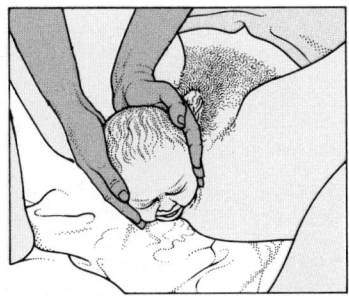

1 As the baby's head emerges, support it with cupped hands. If a membrane covers the face, tear it with your hands and remove quickly. If the cord is looped around the neck, ease it gently over the head. DO NOT touch the baby's head until it is out.

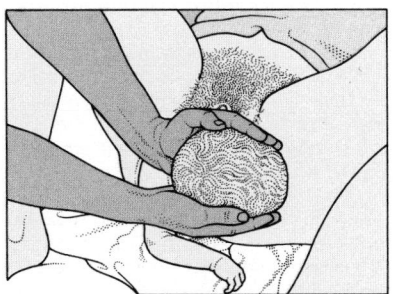

2 Support the shoulders as they emerge. One appears first, the second follows easily if you carefully raise the head. DO NOT pull on the baby's head.

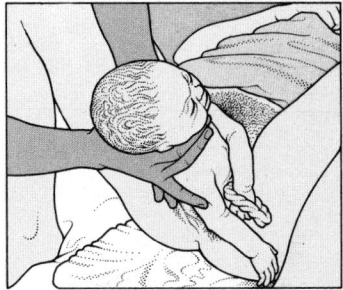

3 Support the body as it comes out. Using a clean cloth, wipe away any mucus or blood from the baby's mouth.

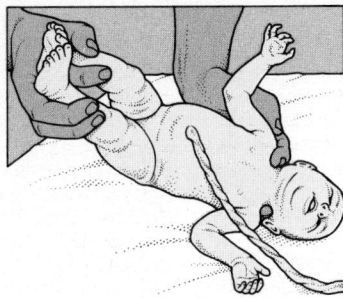

4 If the baby fails to breathe immediately, hold the head lower than the body to drain mucus away. DO NOT slap the baby on the back. Blow hard on the chest or tap the soles of the feet. If these methods fail, start *artificial respiration*.

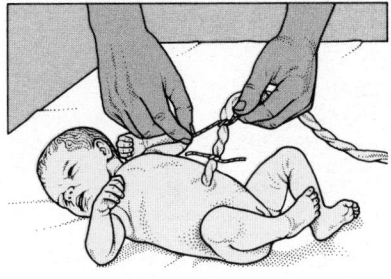

5 When the cord has stopped pulsating, tie it firmly once 15 to 20 cm away from the baby and again 5 to 10 cm away. Cut between the ties with sterilized scissors. Wrap the baby and place him or her on the mother's abdomen.

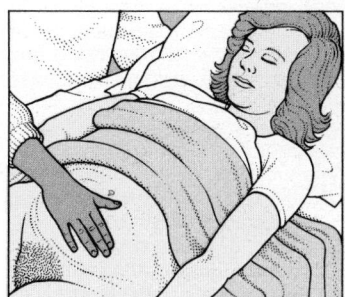

6 The afterbirth is delivered within 10 minutes. To help control blood flow, place a hand on the mother's abdomen and gently massage the uterus every few minutes until it feels firm. DO NOT pull on the cord to deliver the afterbirth.

C

from woman to woman. It may be a slow trickle of fluid from the vagina, or it may be a sudden gush.

STAGES OF LABOUR

Labour is divided into three stages (see illustrated box on p.262 for details). The first stage covers the period from the onset of labour until the woman's cervix is fully dilated. The second stage lasts from full dilatation of the cervix until delivery of the baby. The third stage lasts from delivery of the baby until the placenta (afterbirth) has been expelled.

Childbirth, complications of

Difficulties and complications occurring after the onset of labour. These complications may be associated with the mother or the baby, or both. Some are potentially life-threatening, particularly to the baby, because they may impair its oxygen supply and cause brain damage (see *Fetal distress*).

MATERNAL PROBLEMS

If contractions begin, or if the membranes rupture, before 37 weeks' gestation, premature labour may occur, with the risk of delivery of a small, immature baby who may not be developed adequately to survive (see *Prematurity*). Drugs such as salbutamol or ritodrine can sometimes stop premature labour. However, if the gestation is more than 34 weeks and hospital conditions are suitable, or if other complications are present, it may be safer to allow labour to progress. Premature rupture of the membranes can also lead to infection in the uterus; the baby must be delivered as soon as possible and the infection treated with *antibiotic drugs*.

Slow progress early in a normal labour is most often the result of failure of the cervix to dilate, usually due to inadequate contractions of the uterine muscles. This problem is often treated by giving intravenous infusions of synthetic *oxytocin* to augment the naturally occurring oxytocin that causes the muscles of the uterus to contract during labour.

The mother may tire during a long labour so that she is unable to push strongly enough, or the muscular contractions of the uterus may be ineffective; in these cases, *forceps delivery*, *vacuum extraction*, or even *caesarean section* may be required.

A major hazard in childbirth is blood loss. Bleeding before labour (*antepartum haemorrhage*) or during labour (intrapartum haemorrhage) may be due to premature separation of the placenta from the wall of the

uterus or, less commonly, to a condition called *placenta praevia* in which the placenta lies over the opening of the cervix instead of being attached to the wall of the uterus. Blood loss after the delivery (*postpartum haemorrhage*) is usually due either to failure of the uterus to contract normally after the child has been expelled or to retention of part of the placenta. With blood transfusions, complications from haemorrhage have decreased dramatically in the last 40 years.

In rare instances, women suffer from *eclampsia* (convulsions associated with raised blood pressure) during or just prior to the onset of labour. If eclampsia occurs, it is treated by giving *anticonvulsant drugs* and oxygen, and by inducing labour or performing a caesarean section.

FETAL PROBLEMS

If the baby is in a *malposition* (not lying in the normal head-down position in the uterus), vaginal delivery may be difficult or impossible. A baby in the breech position (bottom downwards) can be delivered vaginally, although delivery by caesarean section may be preferable (see *Breech delivery*). A baby lying horizontally is always delivered by caesarean section because the arm and shoulder usually become jammed in the pelvis.

Multiple pregnancies (see *Pregnancy, multiple*) may be a problem during delivery because it is often difficult to predict the position of the second or subsequent babies. It is also more likely that such babies will be born prematurely.

FETAL-MATERNAL PROBLEMS

Sometimes the mother's pelvis is too small in proportion to the baby's head (a condition known as cephalopelvic disproportion), making vaginal delivery impossible or hazardous. In these cases, delivery by caesarean section is usually necessary.

Childbirth, natural

The avoidance of unnecessary medical intervention during the delivery of a baby, especially the use of relaxation techniques as a means of coping with pain and minimizing the use of drugs during labour.

Natural childbirth techniques are taught by a number of organizations, of which best known in the UK is the National Childbirth Trust (NCT). Natural childbirth classes are taught by midwives or other qualified childbirth educators. Pregnant women and their partners usually attend classes during the last three months of the

pregnancy. Involvement of the partner is an important feature of the natural childbirth method.

The primary purpose of the classes is to teach relaxation techniques, often using breathing exercises, to help women cope with the pain of uterine contractions. Relaxation techniques help a mother to be aware of muscle tension and to relax during labour. Involvement of the woman's partner helps him to provide full encouragement and support during labour.

The classes also supply information about female anatomy, the physiology of pregnancy, fetal development, labour, delivery, and the postnatal period. Other topics (such as nutrition, breast-feeding, and parental skills) are also covered.

Child development

Children acquire physical, mental, and social skills in well-recognized stages called developmental milestones. Although there is wide variation in the rate at which each child progresses, most children develop certain skills by a predictable age (see illustrated box overleaf).

FACTORS AFFECTING DEVELOPMENT

A child becomes capable of developing certain skills only as his or her nervous system matures. The time taken for maturity to develop is determined genetically for each individual and modified by environmental factors in the uterus and after birth. For instance, girls often begin to walk and/or talk at an earlier age than boys. Premature children miss out on some growing time in the uterus; the time they take to progress should be calculated from the full-term pregnancy date, not the actual date of birth.

Sight and hearing are both crucial to a child's general developmental progress; any defect will affect the child's ability to watch, listen, learn, and imitate. Intelligence also affects a child's development, especially in the acquisition of speech and the ability to coordinate muscles for precise movements, such as holding a pencil.

The home environment plays an important part in developing the child's potential for certain skills. Speaking to and playing with children is essential for language development and for practising new physical skills. Introducing children to other children at the age of two or three years provides them with plenty of stimulation.

HOW A CHILD DEVELOPS SKILLS

Reflex actions present at birth (see *Reflex, primitive*) gradually disappear as the child learns to perform voluntary actions and develops sufficient muscle strength and control to perform them. Often, the child's actions progress from seemingly unconnected movements to the ability to control part of his or her body. In most children, development begins with control of the head and progresses down the body until control of the arms, trunk, and legs is attained. Walking is achieved in numerous stages, from lying with the head raised, to sitting unsupported, crawling, standing unsupported, toddling, and, finally, walking unaided.

A baby begins to develop hand-eye coordination from birth. He or she watches objects, learns to focus and judge distances, and develops the connection of seeing and doing by watching his or her hands. Both hand-eye and body-limb coordination can be encouraged in an older child (by practising ball games, for example).

At birth, a child communicates his or her needs by crying. Once vision and hearing are sufficiently developed, a child watches the parent's mouth intently to learn how to smile and listens to the parent speaking before attempting to imitate sounds. A child is able to concentrate on learning only one skill at a time, often forgetting a recently mastered skill that will appear again some time in the future.

DEVELOPMENTAL MILESTONES

When assessing the development of a child, specialists in child development look at abilities in four main areas: locomotion; hearing and speech; vision and fine movement; and social behaviour and play. All children acquire skills in much the same order—for example, a child will not stand before learning to sit. The rate at which these skills are acquired varies enormously; a more detailed professional investigation is necessary only if a child's progress is significantly slower than average or if the parent is concerned for some other reason (see *Developmental delay*).

Child guidance

A multidisciplinary diagnosis and advice team service for a child who is suffering from emotional or *behavioural problems*. These may include poor school performance, disruptive or withdrawn behaviour at school or at home, breaking the law, or *drug abuse*.

SOURCES OF HELP

Trained professionals from a number of disciplines offer help to such children and their families. A doctor will arrange referral to the most appropriate team for assessment and, possibly, therapy.

Psychiatrists are medical doctors with a special interest and training in the field of mental problems. Their techniques may range from *psychotherapy* to treatment with drugs. The latter are rarely used.

Clinical and educational *psychologists* are nonmedical specialists whose main role is diagnosis and assessment by means of intelligence and personality tests. They may also assess a child's progress during treatment. Many clinical psychologists also provide psychotherapy.

Psychiatric social workers are also nonmedical specialists. They are specially trained to deal with family problems and relationships within the family. In some instances they may be given legal responsibility for children who have severe personality or family problems.

These specialists often work closely together, either in hospital paediatric departments, schools, or special child-guidance clinics.

HOW IT IS DONE

Various methods of assessment and therapy may be employed, depending on the age of the child and the particular problem involved. For young children, *play therapy* may be used for diagnosis, by observing the child's behaviour during play, and also for therapy, by providing an environment in which the child can express his or her emotions freely.

For older children, *counselling* or psychotherapy may be tried. For the child who has fallen behind in schoolwork or is thought to have a learning difficulty, examination of intellectual performance may be required.

Group therapy may be used as a means of helping older children. Various interactions develop within a group and under the guidance of a professionally qualified group leader, these interactions can be examined and discussed to help children gain insight into their problems.

Family therapy may be used in cases where there are conflicts and difficulties between the child and one or both parents.

Chill

A shivering attack accompanied by chattering teeth, pale skin, goose pimples, and feeling cold. Chill frequently precedes a *fever*. Repeated or severe shivering suggests serious illness and a doctor should be consulted.

Chinese medicine

Most of the various techniques of traditional Chinese medicine are based on the theory that there is a universal life-force, called chi, which manifests itself in the body as two complementary qualities known as yin and yang. According to traditional beliefs, the vigorous yang and restraining yin must be balanced, and the chi must flow evenly for good health. An imbalance in the yin and yang and disruption of the flow of chi produce illness. Traditional Chinese treatments therefore aim to restore the yin-yang balance and normalize the flow of chi. To achieve this aim various techniques have evolved, notably *acupressure*, *acupuncture*, Chinese *herbalism*, and *t'ai chi*.

In general, these treatments are incompatible with orthodox Western medicine and most doctors do not recommend them. However, some techniques may help when standard treatment has not been effective.

Chinese restaurant syndrome

A short-lived illness that some people develop after eating food containing *monosodium glutamate* (MSG). Only about five per cent of the population is susceptible to it.

Monosodium glutamate is present naturally in some foods, such as soya beans and some types of seaweed, used in Chinese cooking. The substance is also used as a flavour-enhancing *food additive* in many types of "fast foods".

SYMPTOMS AND PREVENTION

The most common symptoms, which usually occur within three hours of a meal, are pain in the neck and chest, palpitations of the heart, feeling hot, and headache. Nausea, dizziness, and other symptoms have also been reported, and some people compare Chinese restaurant syndrome to the effects of migraine.

The symptoms pass and have no long-term effects. Affected people should avoid food containing MSG as an additive.

Chiropody

The examination, diagnosis, treatment, and prevention of diseases and malfunctions of the foot and its related structures. Chiropody is concerned with many different types of foot problems, including walking disorders in children, ankle injuries in adolescents, fractures in athletes and joggers, *bunions* and *hammer toes* in men and women of all ages, and care

CHILD DEVELOPMENT

LOCOMOTION

By 6 months, babies lift up their heads and chests and roll from front to back and from back to front. They can sit up with support, bounce up and down, and bear weight on their legs if supported.

9-month-old children try to crawl, sit without support, pull themselves up to standing or sitting positions, and step purposefully on alternate feet if supported.

1-year-old children crawl on hands and knees, walk around furniture (holding on), and may walk alone or with one hand held.

At 18 months, children can walk well with feet closer together, can stoop to pick up objects, run with care, walk upstairs with one hand held, and crawl backwards downstairs.

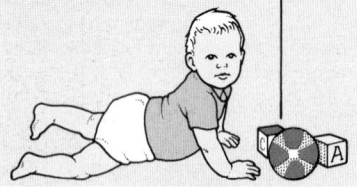

VISION AND FINE MOVEMENT

By 6 months, babies look intently at everything and everybody. They follow moving objects with their eyes and reach out for objects with one or both hands. Objects are transferred from hand to hand and brought to the mouth.

9 month olds are visually very alert. Grasp involves mostly the index and middle fingers. They can manipulate objects with both hands, but have difficulty voluntarily releasing grasped objects.

1-year-old children can grasp small objects well and release grasped objects easily. Both hands are used equally. They can hold a block in each hand and bang the blocks together.

At 18 months, children can build a tower of three blocks (when shown), enjoy turning pages of a book, can grip a crayon, scribble, and make dots. They may use one hand more than the other.

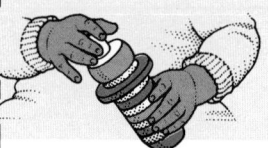

HEARING, UNDERSTANDING, AND SPEECH

By 6 months, babies turn their heads to locate sources of sound and have begun to understand the tone of their mother's voice. They enjoy making vowel sounds and tuneful noises. They laugh, chuckle, and squeal.

9 month olds listen to sounds and understand "no" and other words. They babble in long strings (making sounds such as ba-ba, da-da, ma-ma) and start using sound to attract attention. (Deaf babies' utterances are monotonous and do not develop in complexity.)

1-year-old children turn when they hear their own names. They have some understanding of how other people feel, know what most household objects are used for, may babble meaningfully to themselves, and may say two or three words.

At 18 months, children comprehend short communications spoken directly to them, but do not understand the difference between statements, commands, and questions. Vocabulary may contain six to 20 words.

SOCIAL BEHAVIOUR AND PLAY

6 month olds enjoy looking at their images in mirrors and playing peekaboo games. They can grasp objects and also shake, bang, and otherwise manipulate them. However, they will not look for objects that are shown and then hidden. They are shy with strangers.

9 month olds look for objects that are shown and then hidden, thus showing the beginnings of memory. They imitate hand clapping, wave bye-bye, and show great determination in getting objects. They continue to be shy with strangers.

1-year-old children spend less time putting objects in their mouths and more time releasing objects—throwing them, dropping them, putting them in boxes. They play pat-a-cake and like to be around a familiar adult to whom they demonstrate affection.

At 18 months, children actively explore their homes. They enjoy putting things in and taking things out of boxes and looking at picture books. They use spoons and cups and can take off their shoes and socks. They are also determined, impetuous, selfish, and cannot be reasoned with. They alternate between clinging to a familiar adult and struggling to break free.

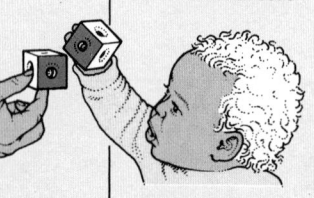

C

LOCOMOTION

2 year olds climb furniture and walk up and down stairs (with two feet to each step).

3 year olds can climb with agility, throw and kick balls, ride tricycles, and run around corners.

4 year olds walk up and down stairs with one foot on each step, and can stand, walk, and run on tiptoe.

5 year olds can stand and hop on one foot, and are skilful in rolling, sliding, and swinging.

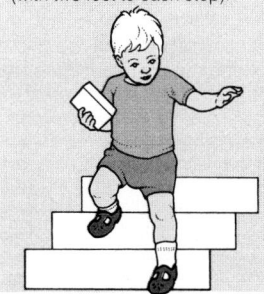

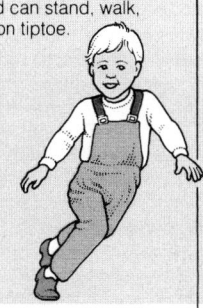

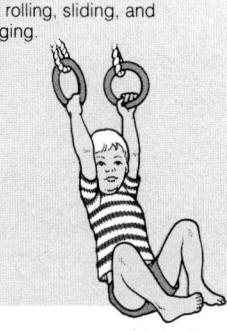

VISION AND FINE MOVEMENT

2 year olds can build towers of six or seven blocks, can unscrew a lid, and show a definite right- or left-handedness.

3 year olds hold crayons with an adult grasp and can undo buttons, but may need help buttoning them up. Their handedness is clearly established.

4 year olds hold a pencil with a mature grasp, can copy simple letters (i.e. O,T,H, or V), and can build a tower of more than 10 blocks.

5 year olds can match 10 or 12 colours, can copy many more letters, and can draw the full body of a person with a recognizable head and facial features.

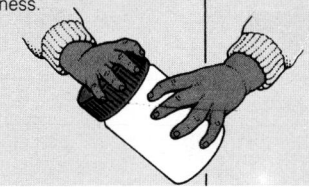

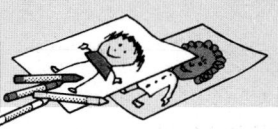

HEARING, UNDERSTANDING, AND SPEECH

2 year olds begin to listen to general conversation. They obey simple instructions and can use 50 or more words meaningfully. They constantly talk to themselves and can put two or more words together to communicate.

3 year olds listen to general conversation and enjoy nursery stories. They understand the difference between statements, commands, and questions. They have large vocabularies and speak clearly in sentences, but there may be some errors.

4 year olds can repeat softly spoken words at a distance of 1 m. They speak fluently and with correct grammar, and can provide their full names, ages, and addresses. They tell long stories, confusing fact and fantasy.

5 year olds enjoy reciting rhymes, telling stories, and having books read to them.

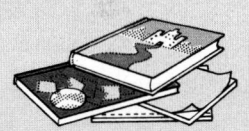

SOCIAL BEHAVIOUR AND PLAY

2 year olds ask the names of everything and enjoy participating in nursery rhymes and songs. They ask for food and drink and indicate toilet needs. They begin to play with toys more imaginatively, though they may not like to share them. They are constantly demanding and will throw tantrums if their desires are thwarted.

3 year olds constantly ask questions. They can dress and undress and eat with a fork and spoon. They are dry and clean during the day and sometimes at night. Three year olds can play with toys imaginatively and will share with others. They can be reasoned with and have fewer tantrums. They are also more affectionate to younger siblings.

4 year olds continue to ask questions constantly. They are more independent and skilful in dressing, undressing, eating, and washing. They need to play with other children and can share with others. They can understand past, present, and future.

5 year olds ask the meaning of abstract words. They like to build complex structures out of bricks or other objects. They continue in imaginative and dramatic play. They enjoy companionship and understand the need for rules and fair play. They have an understanding of time and are generally sensible, restrained, and independent.

C

of foot ulcers, toenails, and infections of the feet in people who have *diabetes mellitus.*

To qualify as a State Registered Chiropodist, students must complete a full-time three-year course at a chiropody school approved by the Society of Chiropodists. They are trained to use pharmaceutical preparations, specialized dressings, and local anaesthetics, and become skilled in the use of mechanical and electrical techniques to treat foot problems and restore normal use of the foot. Some chiropodists take additional postgraduate training in surgery.

Chiropractic

An alternative system of treatment based on the theory that disease is due, at least in part, to abnormal nerve functioning. Instead of relying on drugs and surgery for treatment, chiropractors treat a whole range of disorders by manipulation of the spine. Most doctors who practise orthodox medicine do not believe that chiropractic has a firm scientific basis.

Chlamydial infections

Chlamydiae are a group of microorganisms, intermediate in size between bacteria and viruses, that cause various infectious diseases in humans and animals (particularly birds). Like viruses, chlamydiae can multiply only by first invading the cells of another life-form; otherwise, they behave more like bacteria than viruses and are susceptible to treatment with antibiotic drugs.

Two main species of chlamydiae cause disease in humans. Different strains of CHLAMYDIA TRACHOMATIS cause various types of genital, eye, and lymph node infections. CHLAMYDIA PSITTACI mainly affects birds, but is occasionally spread to humans to cause a lung infection.

CHLAMYDIA TRACHOMATIS INFECTIONS

GENITAL INFECTIONS In the tropics, strains of ACHLAMYDIA TRACHOMATIS cause the sexually transmitted disease *lymphogranuloma venereum.*

In developed countries, by far the most important impact of CHLAMYDIA TRACHOMATIS is as a cause of *nonspecific urethritis* (NSU). This is the most common sexually transmitted disease in the UK; CHLAMYDIA TRACHOMATIS can be isolated from the urethras of at least 50 per cent of men with NSU and is also present in the genital tracts of about 20 per cent of women attending clinics for sexually transmitted diseases.

In men, nonspecific urethritis may cause a discharge from the penis and complications such as swelling of the testes, which, if untreated may lead to infertility. In women, the equivalent condition, nonspecific genital infection (NSGI), is usually symptomless, but may lead to *salpingitis* (inflammation of the fallopian tubes) which may cause infertility.

Treatment is with *antibiotic drugs,* such as *tetracycline* or *erythromycin,* and is usually rapidly successful. Treatment of sexual partners is advisable to prevent reinfection.

EYE INFECTIONS A child born to a woman with a chlamydial infection of the cervix may acquire an acute eye infection called neonatal *ophthalmia.*

In parts of Africa and Asia, usually where hygiene is poor, certain strains of CHLAMYDIA TRACHOMATIS cause *trachoma.* This serious eye disease is the main cause of blindness worldwide.

CHLAMYDIA PSITTACI INFECTION

The only disease that can be caused by CHLAMYDIA PSITTACI in humans is a type of pneumonia called *psittacosis.* It is a rare infection, usually contracted from parrots, parakeets, pigeons, or poultry. The disease can be treated with antibiotic drugs but is sometimes fatal in elderly and debilitated patients.

Chloasma

A condition, also called melasma, in which blotches of pale brown skin pigmentation appear on the forehead, cheeks, and nose.

Chloasma sometimes develops during pregnancy. In some cases, the spots merge, forming the so-called "mask of pregnancy". More rarely, chloasma occurs in women who have been taking oral contraceptives or around the time of menopause.

The pigmentation is aggravated by sunlight. It usually fades gradually, but may be permanent or recur in successive pregnancies. There is no treatment, although avoiding direct sunlight and changing the brand of oral contraceptive (if appropriate) may help.

Chloral hydrate

One of the oldest *sleeping drugs* in use today. Chloral hydrate is mainly used as a short-term treatment for insomnia, especially in the elderly.

Chlorambucil

An *anticancer drug* used to treat some types of cancer, including *Hodgkin's disease* and cancer of the ovary.

Chloramphenicol

An *antibiotic drug* widely prescribed in the form of eye-drops or ointment to treat *conjunctivitis* caused by a bacterial infection.

Chloramphenicol tablets or injections carry a risk of causing aplastic *anaemia* (inability of the bone marrow to produce blood cells) and are therefore used only to treat serious infections that are resistant to safer types of antibiotics.

Chlorate poisoning

Toxic effects caused by chemicals present in some defoliant weedkillers.

Swallowing of chlorates can cause kidney and liver damage, corrosion of the intestine, and methaemoglobinaemia (a chemical change in the blood pigment *haemoglobin*). Symptoms of poisoning include ulceration in the mouth, abdominal pain, and diarrhoea. Even small doses can prove fatal, especially in children, and medical help should be obtained immediately if poisoning is suspected.

Weedkillers that are spilled on the skin or into the eyes should be washed off with plenty of water.

Chlordiazepoxide

A *benzodiazepine* drug used mainly to treat anxiety, but also in the management of alcohol withdrawal.

Chlorhexidine

A type of disinfectant. Chlorhexidine is widely used to cleanse the skin before surgery or before a blood sample is taken. It is also used to wash out the bladder as a treatment for *urinary tract infection* in people who have a permananent urinary *catheter.*

Chlorhexidine occasionally causes skin irritation; bladder irrigation with a concentrated solution may cause haematuria (blood in the urine).

Chlorine

A poisonous, yellowish-green gas with very powerful bleaching and disinfecting properties. If inhaled in even very small amounts, chlorine gas is highly irritating to the lungs; inhalation of large amounts is rapidly fatal.

Chloroform

A colourless liquid producing a vapour that acts as a general anaesthetic when inhaled. Formerly, chloroform was widely used for operative procedures but because it caused a high incidence of liver damage and heart problems it has now been replaced by safer drugs.

Chloroform is still occasionally used in some countries as an emergency anaesthetic for major first aid or field surgery. It is also sometimes used as a flavouring and preservative for other medicines, although research has indicated that it may be carcinogenic.

Chloroquine

A drug used in the prevention and treatment of *malaria* and occasionally as an *antirheumatic drug*.

When taken to prevent malaria, chloroquine is usually prescribed with other drugs because some strains of malaria parasite are now resistant to it. Chloroquine remains the main treatment for acute attacks of malaria.

Chloroquine is also used to treat *rheumatoid arthritis* and *lupus erythematosus* that have not responded to treatment with other drugs.

Possible side-effects include nausea, headache, diarrhoea, rashes, and abdominal pain. Since long-term treatment (as for rheumatoid arthritis) can damage the retina, regular eye tests are usually carried out.

Chlorpheniramine

An *antihistamine drug* used in the treatment of allergies such as allergic *rhinitis* (hay fever), allergic *conjunctivitis*, *urticaria* (hives), and *angioedema* (allergic facial swelling). It is also an ingredient of some over-the-counter *cold remedies*.

Chlorpromazine

ANTIPSYCHOTIC

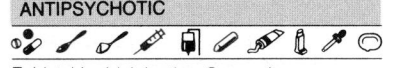

Tablet Liquid Injection Suppository

📋	Prescription needed
🔒	Available as generic

The first *antipsychotic drug* to be marketed. Introduced in the early 1950s, it remains one of the most widely used drugs of this group. It is also sometimes used as an *antiemetic drug*.

WHY IT IS USED
Chlorpromazine is used primarily in the treatment of schizophrenia, mania, and other disorders in which confused or abnormal behaviour may occur. It does not cure the underlying disorder, but does relieve particular symptoms. Chlorpromazine reduces delusional and hallucinatory experiences, which are the major features of psychotic illness. It may also help to reduce the irritability and overactivity that are characteristic of manic illnesses.

Chlorpromazine is also used in the treatment of nausea and vomiting, especially if caused by drug treatment, radiotherapy, or anaesthesia.

POSSIBLE ADVERSE EFFECTS
Chlorpromazine sometimes produces serious side-effects, including *parkinsonism* (a movement disorder), slow reactions, and blurred vision. It may also cause *photosensitivity* (increased sensitivity of the skin to light).

Chlorpropamide

A drug used to treat non-insulin-dependent *diabetes mellitus*. (See *Hypoglycaemics, oral*.)

Choking

Partial or complete inability to breathe due to an obstruction of the airway, usually by food, drink, or an inhaled or swallowed foreign body. If the blockage is only partial, the choking person can usually inhale enough air to cough out the obstruction. If the airway is completely blocked, the person will be unable to breathe and, unless the blockage is cleared, he or she will die of suffocation.

CAUSES
Choking is caused by blockage of any part of the airway—the pharynx (throat), larynx (voice-box), trachea (windpipe), or bronchi (air passages from the trachea into the lungs). Most cases of choking occur when food or drink "goes down the wrong way", that is, when it enters the trachea and bronchi instead of passing from the pharynx into the oesophagus. Although this can be alarming, it is normally corrected by coughing.

FIRST AID: CHOKING

CONSCIOUS VICTIM

1 A person clutching the throat may be choking. Encourage the victim to cough up the obstruction. If this fails, bend the victim over and slap between the shoulder-blades. If this does not work, use the method below.

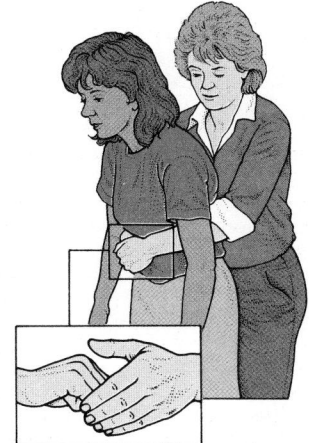

2 Clasp the victim, placing one fist just under the sternum (breastbone) and grasping the fist with the other hand. Then make a quick, hard, thrusting movement inwards and upwards.

UNCONSCIOUS VICTIM

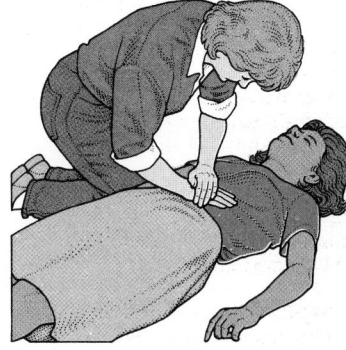

1 Place the heel of one hand against the middle of the victim's abdomen, slightly above the navel; place your other hand on top. Press in with a quick upward thrust.

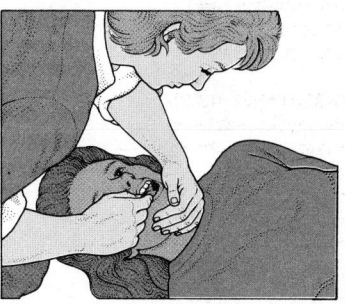

2 If this fails, try to remove the obstruction. If the victim is still unconscious, summon emergency help. If breathing has stopped, start *artificial respiration*.

Obstruction by something that partially blocks the airway is more serious. In adults the cause is usually a fishbone or a piece of meat. In children, who are more vulnerable to this type of choking because their airways are narrower, the obstruction is often a peanut or small plaything, such as a bead. Less commonly, choking may be due to inhaling vomit.

TREATMENT

Emergency medical help should be summoned if the obstruction cannot be cleared. The doctor will probably try to clear the blockage manually; if this fails, an emergency *tracheostomy* (making an incision into the trachea and inserting a tube through it into the lungs) will be performed. When the airway has been restored, the doctor can use a laryngoscope, broncho-scope, or oesophagoscope (viewing tubes through which instruments can be passed) to locate and clear the obstruction (see *Laryngoscopy*; *Bronchoscopy*; *Oesophagoscopy*).

Cholangiocarcinoma

A malignant growth in one of the *bile ducts* that carries bile from the liver and gallbladder to the small intestine. The disease is very rare in the UK, with just a few hundred cases each year, although more common in certain parts of Africa and Asia. The cause of the cancer is unknown. The main symptoms of cholangiocarcinoma are *jaundice* and weight loss.

Cholangiography

A procedure that enables the *bile ducts* to be seen on X-ray film after filling them with a contrast medium (a substance opaque to X-rays).

WHY IT IS DONE

Cholangiography is used when people who have had their gallbladders removed are suspected of having biliary stones. Biliary stones are similar to gallstones, but they form in the bile ducts instead of the gallbladder. Cholangiography is usually employed as a follow-up to *ultrasound scanning* if this has failed to establish the presence of stones. Cholangiography is also performed during a *cholecystectomy* (operation to remove the gallbladder) to ensure that no stones have been left behind in the bile ducts. Cholangiography is also useful for diagnosing narrowing or tumours of the bile ducts.

HOW IT IS DONE

The contrast medium may be injected slowly into a vein, in which case the liver will excrete it several hours later in bile into the ducts. More satisfactory images can be obtained by injecting the contrast medium directly into the ducts. This may be done either through an endoscope (a flexible viewing instrument) passed into the ducts via the mouth, stomach, and duodenum (see *ERCP*), or by means of a long, fine needle inserted through the abdomen into the liver. Once the ducts have filled, X-ray pictures are taken and any stones are apparent.

Cholangitis

Inflammation of the common bile duct (see *Biliary system*). There are two types: acute ascending cholangitis and sclerosing cholangitis.

ACUTE ASCENDING CHOLANGITIS

This type is usually due to bacterial infection of the duct and its content of bile. It generally results from blockage of the duct—by a gallstone, tumour, following surgery, or, in some parts of the world, by entry of a worm or fluke into the duct (see *Bile duct obstruction*). The infection moves up the duct and may affect the liver.

The main symptoms are recurrent bouts of jaundice, abdominal pain, and chills and fever. Attacks may vary from mild episodes to a severe, life-threatening illness with *septicaemia* (spread and multiplication of bacteria in the bloodstream) and *kidney failure* from toxins circulating in the blood.

The infection is usually diagnosed from the patient's symptoms, although investigations such as *liver-function tests* and *ultrasound scanning* may also be carried out.

Mild cases are treated with *antibiotic drugs* and a high intake of fluids. In severe cases, if there is no improvement within 24 hours, the infected material is drained from the bile duct by surgery or endoscopy.

Once the patient has recovered, the cause of the blockage must be determined and appropriate treatment of the cause of the obstruction provided (see *Bile duct obstruction*).

SCLEROSING CHOLANGITIS

In this rare condition, all the bile ducts, within and outside the liver, become narrowed. Sclerosing cholangitis leads to *cholestasis* (stagnation of bile in the liver), chronic jaundice, and itching of the skin due to excess levels of the bile pigment bilirubin in the blood and skin. The liver is progressively damaged.

No treatment is available other than the possibility of a *liver transplant*. The drug *cholestyramine* may be prescribed to relieve itching.

Chole-

A prefix that means relating to the bile or the biliary system, as in cholelithiasis (the formation of stones in the biliary system).

Cholecalciferol

An alternative name for vitamin D_3 (see *Vitamin D*).

Cholecystectomy

Surgery to remove the gallbladder.

WHY IT IS DONE

Cholecystectomy is usually performed to deal with the presence in the gallbladder of troublesome *gallstones*, often because they are causing recurrent attacks of *biliary colic*. Many surgeons advocate cholecystectomy at an early stage to treat acute *cholecystitis*

FIRST AID: CHOKING

INFANT

Straddle the baby over your arm with the head lower than the trunk, supporting the head by holding the baby's jaw. Deliver four back blows between the shoulderblades.

UNCONSCIOUS CHILD

Place the heel of one hand slightly above the navel and well below the rib-cage. Place the other hand on top and press down with a quick, upward thrust.

C

(inflammation of the gallbladder). Emergency cholecystectomy is occasionally required to treat perforation (rupture) of the gallbladder or *empyema* (an accumulation of pus). Many gastroenterologists believe that it is unnecessary to remove a gallbladder that contains stones unless the stones are causing symptoms.

HOW IT IS DONE

Cholecystectomy may be performed using conventional surgery as shown in the illustrated box. More commonly, it is performed laparoscopically using *minimally invasive surgery*. A *laparascope* fitted with a video camera is introduced into the abdominal cavity through a small incision; further instruments are passed through two or three other incisions. While watching the video monitor, the surgeon removes the gallbladder using either diathermy or laser methods. Laparascopic surgery takes longer, but the patient is spared a large surgical incision, and recovery is substantially quicker.

RISKS AND OUTLOOK

The chief risk of cholecystectomy is inadvertent damage to the common bile duct. However, the outcome is generally good—symptoms are relieved completely in 90 per cent of patients. About three weeks should be allowed for recovery from the operation. Loss of the gallbladder has little adverse effect on the digestive system.

Cholecystitis

Inflammation of the gallbladder, causing severe abdominal pain. There are two types: acute and chronic.

CAUSES

Acute cholecystitis is usually caused by a *gallstone* obstructing the outlet (cystic duct) from the gallbladder. The trapped bile becomes concentrated by absorption of its water content and causes chemical irritation of the gallbladder walls; this is followed by bacterial infection of the stagnating bile.

Repeated mild attacks of acute cholecystitis can lead to chronic cholecystitis, in which the gallbladder shrinks, its walls thicken, and it ceases to store bile. Medical opinions differ on whether chronic cholecystitis produces recognizable symptoms that justify surgery.

SYMPTOMS AND COMPLICATIONS

The main symptom of acute cholecystitis is severe constant pain in the right side of the abdomen, just under the ribs, which worsens on movement. The pain is accompanied by fever and, occasionally, *jaundice*.

In some cases complications develop. These may include a form of

PROCEDURE FOR CHOLECYSTECTOMY

Conventional surgery (pictured here) takes about one hour; laparoscopic surgery takes approximately twice as long, although the same steps are followed for both techniques.

With the patient under general anaesthesia, an incision is made under the rib-cage on the right-hand side; the cut may be vertical, horizontal, or oblique, according to the patient's build.

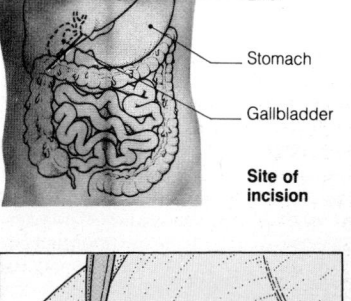

Liver

Stomach

Gallbladder

Site of incision

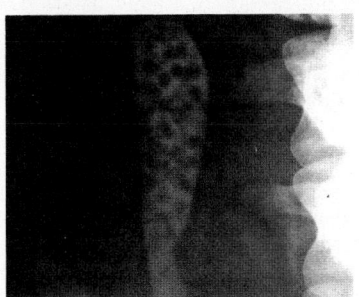

1 Gallstones, as shown by an ultrasound scan or by a cholecystogram (X-ray image of the gallbladder) such as the one above, increase in prevalence with age.

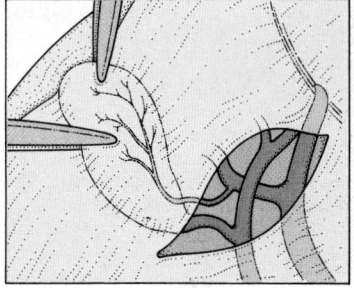

2 After an incision has been made, the liver is pulled up to expose the gallbladder. The thin membrane covering it is incised so that the cystic duct and artery can be identified.

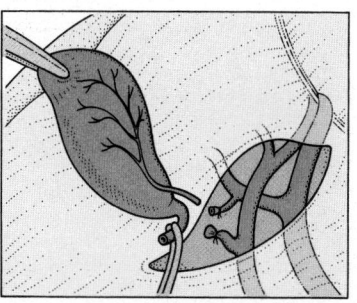

3 The artery to the gallbladder and the cystic duct leading from it are tied and cut, and the gallbladder is removed. If the person has jaundice, X-rays are taken to ensure that there are no stones in the common bile duct. If the X-ray reveals the presence of stones, they are removed.

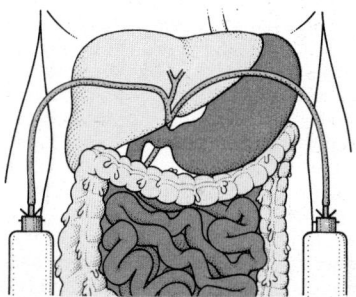

4 Drains are placed under the liver (and in the bile duct if it was opened) and the abdominal incision is closed. The two drains are removed, respectively, 48 hours and eight to 10 days later, after another X-ray shows there are no more stones.

empyema (in which the gallbladder fills with pus) and *peritonitis* (inflammation of the lining of the abdominal cavity) if the gallbladder bursts. In either case, the patient requires urgent surgical treatment.

The ill-defined gastrointestinal symptoms attributed to chronic cholecystitis are indigestion, vague pains in the upper abdomen, nausea, and

belching. These symptoms may be aggravated by eating fatty food.

DIAGNOSIS AND TREATMENT

A doctor makes a provisional diagnosis of acute cholecystitis by listening to a description of the symptoms and by performing a physical examination. The patient is usually admitted to hospital at once and given *analgesic drugs* (painkillers), *antibiotic drugs,* and an

C

intravenous infusion to provide nutrients and fluid. *Ultrasound scanning* or *radionuclide scanning* may be used to make a firm diagnosis and exclude other possible causes of *abdominal pain*, such as a duodenal ulcer or pancreatitis.

Acute cholecystitis usually subsides without urgent surgery but, to prevent recurrences, most patients are advised to have a *cholecystectomy* (surgical removal of the gallbladder). This operation can be performed either during the initial attack or after an interval of several weeks. Cholecystectomy is usually recommended for chronic cholecystitis although the results are less certain.

Cholecystography

An X-ray procedure for examining the gallbladder and common bile duct after they have been filled with a contrast medium (a substance opaque to X-rays). The technique is used mainly to detect gallstones, usually as a follow-up to *ultrasound scanning* if this test has failed to enable a definite diagnosis to be made. Cholecystography is not usually the procedure chosen first to study the gallbladder and it is now performed much less often.

HOW IT IS DONE
The patient swallows tablets containing a contrast medium, which, after about 12 hours, is excreted by the liver into the bile. The opaque bile is stored by the gallbladder, which then shows up when X-ray pictures are taken. Gallstones, which do not absorb the contrast medium, appear on the X-ray film as "holes".

Cholera

An infection of the small intestine caused by the comma-shaped bacterium *VIBRIO CHOLERAE.* Cholera results in profuse watery diarrhoea, which in severe untreated cases can lead to rapid dehydration and death. Infection is always acquired by swallowing contaminated food or water.

HISTORY, CAUSE, AND INCIDENCE
Cholera has been known for centuries in northeast India, where outbreaks of the disease occur regularly. In the 19th century, with the opening up of world trade routes and the increase in Muslim and Hindu pilgrimages, cholera spread throughout the world, causing millions of deaths in epidemics.

During the first half of the 20th century cholera was confined to Asia, but in 1960 the seventh pandemic spread from Indonesia to the rest of Asia, Africa, and the Mediterranean coast. In 1993 a new strain of cholera, 0139,

was identified in Bangladesh as a cause of, potentially, the eighth pandemic. Immunity from earlier strains seemed not to protect against the new one.

A few cases of cholera occur in the UK in most years, mainly among travellers who have returned from visits to Asia or Africa. Occasionally, outbreaks are reported in areas bordering the Mediterranean. Usually the victim has eaten shellfish, which seem to be capable of harbouring the cholera bacterium.

SYMPTOMS
Cholera starts suddenly, between one and five days after infection, with diarrhoea, often accompanied by vomiting. More than 500 ml of fluid may be lost each hour in the diarrhoea and, if not replaced, this loss of fluid may cause death within only a few hours. The fluid loss is brought about by the action of a toxin produced by the cholera bacterium that greatly increases the passage of fluid from the bloodstream into the large and small intestines.

TREATMENT
Cholera is treated by replacing the lost fluid with drinks of water containing the correct proportions of various salts and sugar (see *Oral rehydration therapy*). However, if dehydration develops despite fluid replacement by mouth, the patient may be given extra fluid by means of *intravenous infusion*. *Antibiotic drugs*, especially *tetracycline*, can shorten the period of diarrhoea and infectiousness.

With adequate rehydration, patients usually make a full recovery. However, in major epidemics following natural disasters, there may be insufficient supplies of clean water or so many people may be affected that few are left to nurse the sick.

PREVENTION
Worldwide, cholera is controlled by improving sanitation—in particular by ensuring that sewage is not allowed to contaminate water supplies that will later be used for drinking. Travellers to cholera-infected areas should restrict themselves to water boiled before drinking or to bottled drinks from reliable sources.

A vaccine that provides some protection against the disease is advisable when travelling to Africa and to the Middle and Far East. The protection it gives is short-lived (six months) and precautions still must be taken with drinking water. Usually, no country insists that travellers arriving directly from Europe or the US have a cholera vaccination certificate, but regulations

change from time to time, and a certificate is sometimes required if travel has been via a cholera-infected area. International travellers should therefore check vaccination requirements before departure.

Cholestasis

Stagnation of *bile* in the small *bile ducts* within the liver, which leads to a characteristic type of *jaundice* and to liver disease. The obstruction to the flow of bile may be intrahepatic (within the liver) or extrahepatic (in the bile ducts outside the liver).

CAUSES
Intrahepatic cholestasis may occur as a result of viral *hepatitis* (inflammation of the liver) or as a side-effect of a number of drugs.

The bile ducts outside the liver can become blocked or constricted for various reasons, including gallstones or tumours (see *Bile duct obstruction*); rarely, the ducts are absent from birth (see *Biliary atresia*).

TREATMENT
In the case of viral hepatitis, there is no specific treatment; the flow of bile improves gradually as the liver inflammation resolves. Drug-induced cholestasis usually disappears if use of the causative drug is stopped.

Extrahepatic bile duct obstruction and biliary atresia can often be treated surgically to ensure a free passage of bile from the liver to the duodenum.

Cholesteatoma

A rare but serious condition in which skin cells proliferate and debris collects within the middle ear.

Cholesteatoma usually occurs as a result of a long-standing *otitis media* (middle-ear infection) together with a defect in the eardrum (see *Eardrum, perforated*). In such cases, skin may grow inwards from the ear canal into the middle ear. If the cholesteatoma continues untreated, it may grow and damage the small bones in the middle ear and surrounding bony structures.

Cholesteatoma requires surgical removal either through the eardrum or by *mastoidectomy* (excision of the mastoid bone behind the ear together with the cholesteatoma). If there is residual deafness, reconstructive surgery may be performed; alternatively, a hearing-aid may be required.

Cholesterol

Chemically a *lipid*, cholesterol is an important constituent of body cells. It is also involved in the formation of *hormones* and bile salts and in the transport of fats in the bloodstream to tissues throughout the body. Most cholesterol in the blood is made by the liver from a wide variety of foods, but especially from saturated *fats*. However, a small amount of cholesterol is absorbed directly from cholesterol-rich foods, such as eggs and dairy products.

Both cholesterol and fats (triglycerides) are transported around the body in the form of *lipoproteins*. These are particles with a core, made up of cholesterol and triglycerides in varying proportions, and an outer wrapping of *phospholipids* and apoproteins ("carrier" proteins).

CHOLESTEROL-RELATED DISEASES

The level of cholesterol in the blood—which can be measured by analysis of a blood sample—is influenced by diet, heredity, and metabolic diseases such as *diabetes mellitus*. There is overwhelming evidence that a high blood cholesterol level increases the risk of developing *atherosclerosis* (accumulation of fatty deposits on the inner lining of arteries), and with it the risk of *coronary artery disease* or *stroke*.

Assessment of an individual's risk of developing atherosclerosis depends firstly on a measurement of the total cholesterol concentration in the blood. Those with levels below 5.2 mmol/L need no further investigation, but those with higher levels should have further biochemical tests, since the risk of developing atherosclerosis can be assessed more accurately by measuring the proportions of different types of lipoproteins in the blood. In general, cholesterol in the blood in the form of high-density lipoproteins (HDLs) seems to protect against arterial disease; conversely, cholesterol in the form of low-density lipoproteins (LDLs) or very low-density lipoproteins (VLDLs) is a risk factor.

People with *hyperlipidaemias* (inherited metabolic disorders) are at high risk of atherosclerosis and may need drug treatment and low-fat diets to lower the levels of lipids in their blood. However, most people found to have raised levels of total cholesterol rarely need drug treatment. They can lower the cholesterol concentration to a safe level by eating a sensible low-fat, high-fibre diet, and by keeping their weight within the recommended range.

Cholestyramine

A *lipid-lowering drug* used to treat some types of *hyperlipidaemia* (high levels of fat in the blood). Cholestyramine reduces the amount of *bile* salts reabsorbed

into the blood from the small intestine. By reducing the level of bile salts in the circulation, cholestyramine increases the need for the liver to convert *cholesterol* into bile salts, thereby reducing high levels of cholesterol in the blood.

Cholestyramine is also used to treat diarrhoea caused by abnormal digestion of fats, a feature of disorders such as *Crohn's disease*.

Chondritis

Inflammation of a *cartilage*, usually caused by mechanical pressure, stress, or injury. Costochondritis is a form of chondritis affecting the cartilage between the ribs and the sternum (breastbone). This causes tenderness over the sternum and pain if pressure is exerted on the ribs at the front of the chest. Chondritis affecting the cartilage lining the hip and knee joints may eventually lead to *osteoarthritis*.

Chondro-

A prefix that denotes a relationship to *cartilage*, as in chondroblast, a cell that forms cartilage.

Chondromalacia patellae

A painful disorder of the knee, also known as anterior knee pain. The condition most commonly affects adolescents, in which the cartilage directly behind the patella (kneecap) is damaged. When, rarely, it occurs in adults, the condition is known as retropatellar arthritis.

CAUSE

The cause is uncertain. One theory is that certain knee injuries or activities in which the knee is bent for long periods (e.g. horse-riding) weaken the inner part of the quadriceps (main thigh muscle). As a result of this weakness, the patella is tilted when the knee is straightened; instead of sliding smoothly across the lower end of the femur (thigh-bone) it rubs against it, roughening the smooth cartilage that covers both bones.

SYMPTOMS AND DIAGNOSIS

Pain is felt when the knee is straightened and is particularly bad when using stairs. After examination, the doctor may order *X-rays*, but these do not normally show any specific signs and their main purpose is to exclude other possibilities.

TREATMENT AND OUTLOOK

Analgesic drugs (painkillers) may be given to relieve tenderness in the knee. In many cases, the condition improves without further treatment. If symptoms persist, treatment consists of strengthening the inner part of

the quadriceps by exercises or electrical stimulation, which usually clears up the problem. If pain still persists, arthroscopic surgery may be needed to confirm the diagnosis and to smooth the joint surface. Surgery may sometimes be needed to alter the angle of the patella permanently, thus preventing further friction on the cartilage. In rare severe cases, it is necessary to remove the patella—an operation that hinders mobility surprisingly little.

Chondromatosis

A condition in which multiple benign tumours, called chondromas, arise within bones. The tumours consist of cartilage cells and most commonly develop in the bones of the hand.

Usually the tumours cause no symptoms, but occasionally they lead to thinning of the lining of the bone and a resultant fracture, which may occur without any causative injury.

Chondrosarcoma

A cancerous growth of cartilage that can develop within a bone or on its surface, occurring most commonly within large bones, such as the femur (thigh-bone), tibia (shin), and humerus (upper-arm bone). Chondrosarcoma is one of the more common types of primary *bone cancer;* overall, however, the incidence of bone cancers in the population is low.

Chondrosarcoma usually occurs in middle age and may develop from a benign tumour (see *Chondromatosis; Dyschondroplasia*) or from a previously normal area of bone. It causes pain, swelling, and, occasionally, tenderness. X-rays show an abnormal area of bone. The tumour grows slowly and does not spread until its later stages, so amputation of the bone above the tumour usually results in a permanent cure.

Chordee

Abnormal curvature of the penis, usually downwards. Chordee most often occurs in males with *hypospadias,* a birth defect in which the urethral opening lies on the underside of the penis instead of at the tip. Corrective surgery is usually performed when the child is between one and three years old. Untreated chordee may make sexual intercourse very difficult.

Chorea

A condition characterized by irregular, rapid, jerky movements, usually affecting the face, limbs, and trunk. These movements are involuntary and, unlike *tics*, they are not pre-

C

dictable, but occur at random. Sometimes they resemble fragments of coordinated movements. Chorea disappears in sleep. Chorea is sometimes combined with athetosis (continuous writhing movements), a condition known as *choreoathetosis.*

TYPES AND CAUSES

Chorea arises from disease or disturbance of structures deep within the brain, in particular the paired nerve cell groups called the *basal ganglia.* Chorea is a feature of *Huntington's disease* and *Sydenham's chorea.* It may also occur in pregnancy, when it is called chorea gravidarum. Chorea may be a side-effect of certain drugs, including *oral contraceptives,* drugs used to treat some psychiatric disorders, and drugs used to treat *Parkinson's disease*; the choreic movements usually disappear when the drug is withdrawn.

TREATMENT

If chorea has occurred as a drug side-effect, the drug may be withdrawn and a substitute prescribed. If there is an underlying disease, the doctor may prescribe a drug that inhibits the nervous system pathways concerned with movement.

Choreoathetosis

A condition that is characterized by uncontrollable movements of the limbs, face, and trunk, which combine the jerky, rapid fidgeting movements characteristic of *chorea* and the slower, continuous writhing movements of *athetosis.*

Choreoathetosis may occur in children with *cerebral palsy* or as a side-effect of certain drugs.

Choriocarcinoma

A rare malignant tumour that develops from the *placenta* in the uterus. It is a type of trophoblastic tumour (a tumour derived from cells in the placental attachment of . the fertilized ovum to the wall of the uterus).

INCIDENCE AND CAUSES

Choriocarcinoma occurs in about one in 20,000 pregnancies, usually as a complication of a *hydatidiform mole* (a benign tumour of the trophoblast). Much less frequently, choriocarcinoma follows an abortion; very rarely, it develops after a normal pregnancy. Occasionally, the tumour may not develop until months or even years after the pregnancy.

If untreated, the tumour invades and destroys the walls of the uterus and may spread to the vagina and vulva. Distant spread may occur to the liver, lungs, brain, and bones.

SYMPTOMS

The tumour may become apparent because of persistent bleeding from the vagina after an abortion or for more than eight weeks after childbirth. There may be no early symptoms, the disease being suspected and diagnosed only after the cancer has spread to the lungs, causing symptoms such as breathlessness and coughing up of blood, or to the brain, producing mental changes.

DIAGNOSIS

Successful treatment depends upon diagnosing the disease at an early stage. Diagnostic tests include *ultrasound scanning* and measurement of the blood and urine levels of human chorionic gonadotrophin (HCG), a hormone normally produced by the placenta. Abnormally high levels of HCG are found in patients with trophoblastic diseases.

Women who have had a hydatidiform mole must have regular examinations for at least two years after it has been removed to check that there are no signs of choriocarcinoma. In the UK, such women are registered in a national scheme that ensures that they are regularly asked to submit specimens of urine for HCG testing.

TREATMENT

Treatment of choriocarcinoma is with *anticancer drugs,* especially *methotrexate. Hysterectomy* (surgical removal of the uterus) may be necessary if persistent bleeding occurs despite drug treatment. The use of anticancer drugs has dramatically reduced the mortality from this once highly lethal cancer. Nowadays, if the tumour is detected early, nearly all patients should be cured.

Chorion

One of the two membranes that surround the *embryo.* The chorion lies outside the *amnion,* has small finger-like projections called the chorionic villi, and develops into the *placenta.*

Chorionic villus sampling

A method of diagnosing abnormalities in a fetus in which a small sample of chorionic tissue is taken from the edge of the placenta and analysed in the laboratory. The cells in the villi come from the embryo and therefore have the same chromosome makeup. Laboratory examination of these cells can be used to detect many genetic and chromosomal abnormalities. Chorionic villus sampling (CVS) is usually performed in the first three months of the pregnancy.

It may also be performed in the middle months of pregnancy.

Chorionic villus sampling is a possible alternative to *amniocentesis* in some cases. Chorionic villus sampling can be performed earlier in the pregnancy than amniocentesis. It also has the advantage that the results of *chromosome analysis* are available sooner after the test.

WHY IT IS DONE

The procedure is usually performed to determine whether a pregnant woman who has a family history of—or who is otherwise at increased risk of having a child with—a chromosomal disorder, such as *Down's syndrome,* or a genetic disease, such as *thalassaemia,* is carrying a child affected by the condition. Because the test can also identify the sex of the fetus, it can be performed on a woman who is a known carrier of a sex-linked disease (such as the bleeding disorder *haemophilia*) to predict the child's chance of having the disease.

HOW IT IS DONE

Chorionic villus sampling is an outpatient procedure. In some cases the woman is sedated before the sample is taken. The procedure takes about half an hour.

The most common procedure is to introduce a cannula (hollow tube), with a syringe attached, through the abdominal wall into the uterus. The position of the cannula is checked by ultrasound scanning and when it is in contact with the chorion, a small sample of chorionic villi is sucked into the syringe.

Sometimes the cannula is inserted into the uterus via the vagina, but this technique is used less commonly than transabdominal sampling.

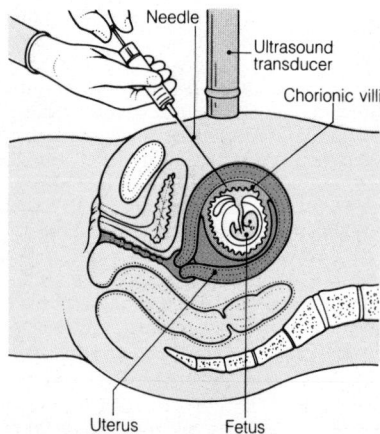

Sampling via the abdomen
A few chorionic villi are sucked through a hollow needle from the placenta.

After removal, the villi are transferred to the laboratory. The cells are grown in an appropriate *culture* medium to allow *chromosome analysis* to be carried out.

RESULTS

If the test reveals genetic abnormalities in the fetus, the parents may choose to terminate the pregnancy (see *Abortion, induced*).

RISKS

Chorionic villus sampling occasionally causes complications, such as perforation of the amniotic sac (the membrane that encloses the fetus), bleeding, and infection. The test itself seems to increase the risk of pregnancy loss by about one per cent above the usual miscarriage rate of three to four per cent in all pregnancies at this stage.

The main advantage of CVS lies in providing the woman with the choice of having an abortion in the first three months of pregnancy rather than facing the increased health risks and emotional strain of a late abortion (as is the case when amniocentesis is employed).

Choroid

A layer of tissue containing many blood vessels that lies at the back of the *eye* behind the retina. Pigment between the blood vessels is visible through an *ophthalmoscope* (see *Eye, examination of*). The choroidal vessels supply nutrients and oxygen to the light-sensitive cells in the retina and to surrounding tissues in the eye.

Choroiditis

Inflammation of the *choroid*. Choroiditis may occur on its own or as part of a generalized inflammation affecting the whole eye. It is commonly caused by infections such as *toxocariasis* or *toxoplasmosis*, more rarely by *sarcoidosis*, *syphilis*, and *histoplasmosis*, or may have no obvious cause.

Treatment may include *corticosteroid drugs* for the inflammation, and *antibiotic drugs* for any causative infection.

Christian Science

A religious movement founded by Mary Baker Eddy. Following a near-fatal accident in 1862, she supposedly was healed after reading one of the New Testament healing miracles. Eddy devoted the rest of her life to spreading the ideas of Christian Science. Strict Christian Scientists reject orthodox medicine and will, for example, refuse to allow themselves or members of their families to receive blood transfusions, opting to die rather than break the faith.

Christmas disease

A rare type of *bleeding disorder* caused by a defect in the blood coagulation mechanism (see *Blood clotting*). Christmas disease has very similar features to another bleeding disorder, *haemophilia*, and is sometimes called haemophilia B. It is named after a man named Christmas, the first patient in whom the disease was shown to be distinct from haemophilia, and was first described in 1952.

Both Christmas disease and haemophilia are *genetic disorders* in which there is deficient production of one of the proteins in blood. In Christmas disease the deficiency is of a protein called factor IX, while in haemophilia the deficiency is of the protein factor VIII.

Chromium

A metallic element, which is essential for life because of its vital role in the activities of several *enzymes* (substances that promote biochemical reactions in the body). Chromium is required only in minute amounts (see *Trace elements*); chromium deficiency is unknown.

In excess, chromium is toxic, although poisoning is rare. Chromium produces inflammation of the skin and, if inhaled, damages the

---

STRUCTURE OF CHOROID

The choroid thickens around the lens to form the ciliary body. Ciliary muscles found between it and the lens contract to control the lens' shape.

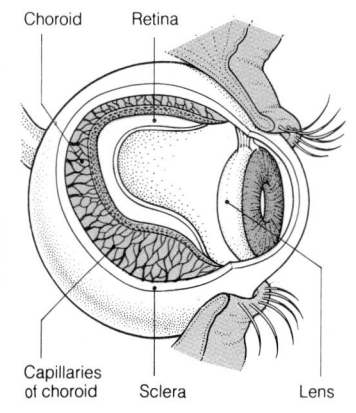

Choroid   Retina

Capillaries of choroid   Sclera   Lens

---

nose. People exposed to certain chromium fumes also have an increased risk of developing *lung cancer*.

Chromosomal abnormalities

Variations from normal in the number or structure of *chromosomes* contained within a person's cells. In most cases, the chromosomal abnormality is present in all the cells; it may have anything from a lethal to virtually no effect, depending on the particular type of abnormality.

INCIDENCE AND CAUSES

About one in every 200 babies born alive has a chromosomal abnormality. Among fetuses that have been spontaneously aborted, about one in two has such an abnormality; this suggests that most chromosomal abnormalities are incompatible with life and that those seen in babies born alive are generally the less serious ones.

The cause in most cases is some fault in the process of chromosome division, either during the formation of the egg or sperm, or during the first few divisions of the fertilized egg. Occasionally, one of the parents has an abnormal arrangement of his or her own chromosomes.

TYPES

A complete extra set of chromosomes per cell is called polyploidy and is lethal. Other chromosomal abnormalities can be classified according to whether they involve the 44 autosomes or the two sex chromosomes. Abnormalities affecting the autosomes are slightly less common than abnormalities of the sex chromosomes, but autosomal abnormalities tend to produce more serious and widespread effects.

AUTOSOMAL ABNORMALITIES

An extra autosome means that one of the 22 pairs of autosomes occurs in triplicate instead of as a pair—a phenomenon called *trisomy*. The most common trisomy, occurring in about one in 650 live births, is *Down's syndrome*; it is due to the presence of three chromosomes labelled number 21. Other trisomies are rare and usually cause multiple physical defects and death soon after birth. All trisomies are more common with advancing maternal age.

Sometimes, a part of a chromosome is missing (for instance, in *cri du chat syndrome*) or an extra bit is present and joined to another chromosome.

All these autosomal abnormalities, as well as causing physical defects of varying severity, tend to cause mental handicap as well.

C

Occasionally, a person has a normal chromosomal complement, but part of one chromosome is not in its proper position; instead, it is joined to another chromosome—a phenomenon called *translocation*. The person is normal, but some of his or her children may suffer from an abnormality through inheriting too much or too little chromosomal material.

SEX CHROMOSOME ABNORMALITIES

About one girl in 2,500 is born with only one X chromosome in her cells instead of two—a condition known as *Turner's syndrome*. The chromosome annotation for this defect is 45 XO (meaning 45 chromosomes, including a single X chromosome), compared with the normal female chromosome annotation of 46 XX (meaning 46 chromosomes, including two X chromosomes). Turner's syndrome causes characteristic physical abnormalities, defective female sexual development, and infertility.

All other sex chromosome abnormalities involve extra chromosomes. A boy born with one or more extra X chromosomes has *Klinefelter's syndrome*. The annotation for this is usually 47 XXY or 48 XXXY. Klinefelter's syndrome occurs in about one in 500 male births, although it is often not diagnosed until puberty. The con-

dition causes defective male sexual development, infertility, and, in some cases, mild mental handicap.

Some women are born with an extra X chromosome (47 XXX) and men with an extra Y chromosome (47 XYY). These people are usually normal physically, but may have an increased risk of mild mental handicap and perhaps psychological problems. The presence of the extra chromosome is recognized only if a special attempt is made to discover it.

DIAGNOSIS AND TREATMENT

Abnormalities are diagnosed by *chromosome analysis*, which is now possible early in pregnancy using *chorionic villus sampling*. Because of the fundamental nature of chromosomal abnormalities—affecting every one of a person's cells—no "cure" is possible. Many disorders caused by autosomal chromosome defects result in early death. Others, including Down's syndrome, are compatible with the survival of a physically and mentally handicapped individual. Children and adults with Down's syndrome, although handicapped, can usually integrate well into the community. Hormonal or surgical treatment, or both, can help correct some of the developmental defects of Klinefelter's and Turner's syndromes.

Anyone with a child or other member of the family with a chromosomal abnormality should obtain *genetic counselling* to establish the risk of his or her future children being affected and also to discuss other considerations of family planning. Fortunately, the risk of an abnormality recurring within a family is usually low.

Chromosome analysis

Study of the chromosomal material in an adult's, child's, or unborn baby's cells to discover whether a *chromosomal abnormality* is present or to establish its nature.

WHY IT IS DONE

Certain fetuses have a higher-than-average chance of being born with a chromosomal abnormality, in particular if the mother is over 35 years old, if she has previously given birth to a child with a chromosomal defect, or if either the mother or father carries a defect or *translocation* (rearrangement) of his or her chromosomes.

In such cases, the parents are usually offered, at around the 16th week of pregnancy, chromosome analysis of cells that can be obtained from the fetus by a technique called *amniocentesis*. Some centres offer an alternative, *chorionic villus sampling*, which may have greater

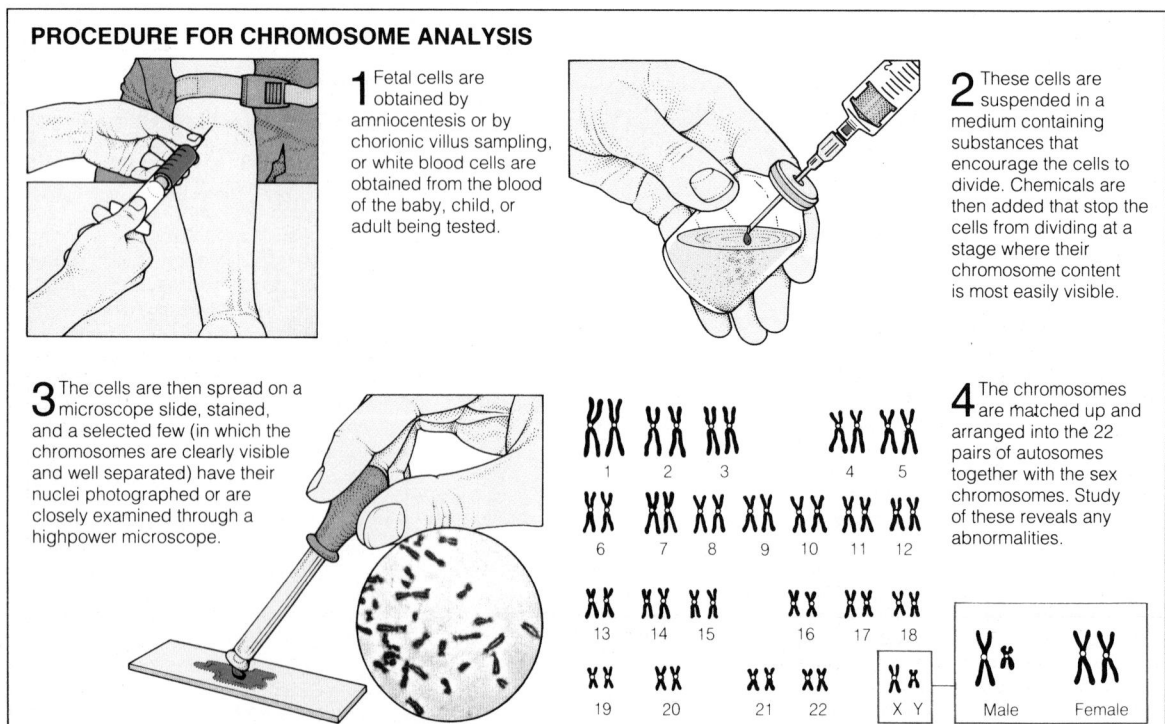

PROCEDURE FOR CHROMOSOME ANALYSIS

1 Fetal cells are obtained by amniocentesis or by chorionic villus sampling, or white blood cells are obtained from the blood of the baby, child, or adult being tested.

2 These cells are suspended in a medium containing substances that encourage the cells to divide. Chemicals are then added that stop the cells from dividing at a stage where their chromosome content is most easily visible.

3 The cells are then spread on a microscope slide, stained, and a selected few (in which the chromosomes are clearly visible and well separated) have their nuclei photographed or are closely examined through a highpower microscope.

4 The chromosomes are matched up and arranged into the 22 pairs of autosomes together with the sex chromosomes. Study of these reveals any abnormalities.

risks (regarding loss of the fetus), but which can be carried out as early as eight weeks into pregnancy. This permits a much earlier and safer abortion, should one be chosen. Neither test will be performed unless the parents would want the pregnancy terminated if the fetus were abnormal.

If no abnormality is found, the test spares the parents anxiety. If a serious abnormality is discovered, such as one that would lead to the infant having *Down's syndrome,* termination of the pregnancy is offered, along with *genetic counselling* to assess the chances of a subsequent pregnancy being affected.

Chromosome analysis is also carried out when a baby is stillborn, or is born with physical abnormalities that suggest a chromosome defect. The analysis clarifies the nature and type of defect, which in turn will affect the genetic and other counselling given to the parents.

Analysis of a person's sex chromosomes may also be carried out for any of the following reasons: establishing the chromosomal sex of a child in cases where the genitals have an ambiguous appearance (see *Genitalia, ambiguous*); confirming or excluding the diagnosis of sex chromosome abnormalities such as *Turner's syndrome* and *Klinefelter's syndrome;* or the investigation of *infertility.*

Chromosomes

Thread-like structures present within the nuclei of cells. Chromosomes carry the inherited, genetic information that directs the activities of cells and, thus, the growth and functioning of the entire body.

All the cells of any one person (with the exception of egg or sperm cells) ordinarily carry precisely the same chromosomal material. This is because everyone develops, by a process of cell division, from a single, fertilized egg cell and, with each cell division, the chromosomal material originally present in the fertilized egg is faithfully copied. A rare exception to this rule is seen in people with *mosaicism,* in which some of a person's cells contain one set of chromosomal material and other cells contain a slightly different set.

Although most chromosomal material is the same for everyone, certain parts differ from one person to another; these differences make each person (with the exception of identical twins) unique. Chromosomes determine physical characteristics, such as

sex, hair texture and colour, skin and eye colour, nose shape, height, and (probably to a lesser extent) mental abilities and personality.

Each chromosome contains up to several thousand *genes* (hereditary units) arranged in single file along its length. A single gene is responsible for just one small aspect of body chemistry (e.g. the synthesis of a particular enzyme).

STRUCTURE AND NUMBERS

Chemically, a chromosome consists of an extremely long chain of the hereditary substance *DNA* (deoxyribonucleic acid) along with a coating of protein. This combination of DNA and protein is called chromatin. The sequence of chemical units, or bases, in the DNA provides the coded instructions for cellular activities. Each cell contains the chemical machinery for decoding these instructions (see *Genetic code; Nucleic acids*).

Although DNA chains are relatively enormous (compared, for example, with a molecule of water), their long,

filamentous shape means that chromosomes cannot normally be seen in cell nuclei, even with the aid of a powerful microscope. But, shortly before any cell divides, its DNA molecules contract (probably by forming into tight coils) and, if cell division is chemically halted and the cell stained with a dye, the chromosomes can be seen with a microscope as dark rods in the nucleus, a few thousandths of a millimetre long.

This technique has shown that human cells (with the exception of egg and sperm cells) normally contain 46 chromosomes consisting of 23 pairs.

AUTOSOMAL AND SEX CHROMOSOMES

Of the 23 pairs of chromosomes, 22 are the same in both sexes and are called autosomal chromosomes. The two members of a pair cannot be told apart under the microscope—being alike in their length, the position of their centromeres (constrictions at a point along their lengths), and in other aspects—but at the molecular level they differ slightly, in particular in the

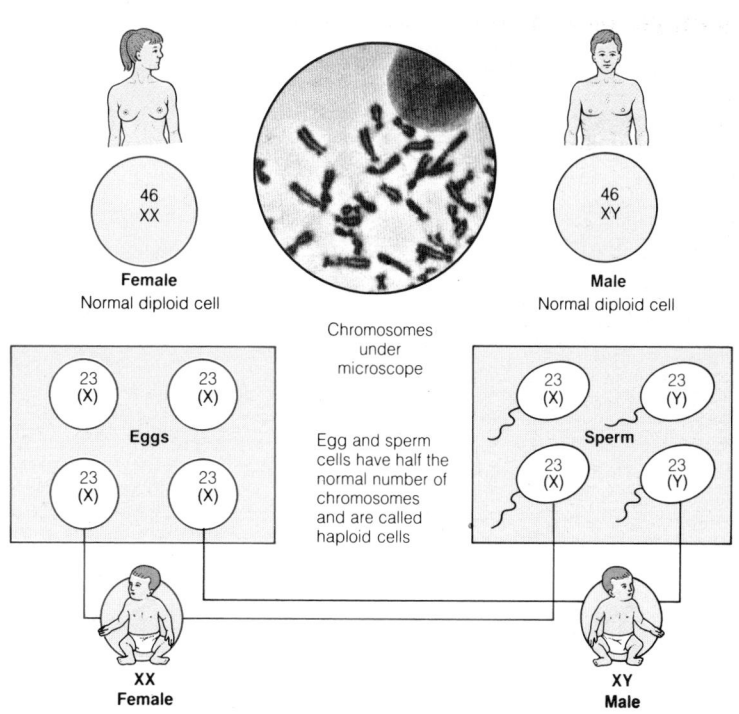

EGG AND SPERM CELLS

These differ from other body cells in that they contain only 23 chromosomes—one from each of the 22 autosome pairs plus an X chromosome (in the case of an egg)

and either an X or a Y (in the case of a sperm). Because they have only half the normal complement, they are said to be haploid, while other cells are called diploid.

Female
Normal diploid cell

46
XX

Male
Normal diploid cell

46
XY

Chromosomes under microscope

23
(X)

23
(X)

Eggs

23
(X)

23
(X)

Egg and sperm cells have half the normal number of chromosomes and are called haploid cells

23
(X)

23
(Y)

Sperm

23
(X)

23
(Y)

XX
Female

XY
Male

C

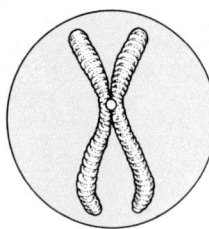

Most chromosomes have a constriction called a centromere that divides them into long and short "arms"

Appearance of chromosomes
This is the appearance just after a chromosome has copied itself. The two copies are joined at the centromere.

sequence of chemical bases in their DNA. One member of each pair is derived originally from a person's mother and the other from the father.

The remaining two chromosomes are called sex chromosomes. In females they form a pair and are called X chromosomes. Again, they look alike but differ slightly at the molecular level. In males, however, the two sex chromosomes are completely different. One is an X chromosome, but the other is a much shorter chromosome called the Y chromosome. The Y chromosome is believed to provide all the information for the development of male sexual characteristics. In its absence, the female pattern of development occurs.

As with the autosomal chromosomes, one of a person's sex chromosomes (an X) has originated from the mother's ovum and the other (an X in girls and a Y in boys) from the father's sperm.

CHROMOSOME DIVISION
When a cell divides, its components are duplicated into the two offspring cells; this applies also to the chromosomes. Shortly before division, the DNA in each chromosome is copied. This means that, when the chromosomes are viewed just before division, they appear not as single but as double rods, conjoined in the region of their centromeres. This gives all 46 chromosomes (not just the sex chromosomes) an X-shaped appearance in the nuclei. As the normal cell division (*mitosis*) proceeds, these duplicated chromosomes are pulled apart, dividing at the centromeres, so that each daughter cell receives a single copy of each of the usual 46 chromosomes.

When egg or sperm cells are formed (a process known as *meiosis*) there are two important departures from the normal process of chromosome division. First, after the DNA has been copied, but before division takes place, some sections of chromosomal material are exchanged between the two members of all the paired chro-

mosomes. This helps ensure that each of a person's eggs or sperm contains a different combination of chromosomal material—and helps explain why all brothers and sisters (except identical twins) have a unique appearance.

The second difference is that, because eggs and sperm receive only 23 chromosomes, their formation requires two consecutive divisions—a first one in which the 46 duplicated chromosomes in the parent cell are split into two groups of 23, followed by a second division in which the 23 duplicated chromosomes in each daughter cell are pulled apart. Thus, the original parent cell gives rise to four separate egg or sperm cells.

DISORDERS
Defective chromosome division during the formation of eggs and sperm—or more rarely during the first few divisions of a fertilized egg—can lead to various *chromosomal abnormalities*. The precise nature of the abnormality can be investigated by detailed *chromosome analysis*.

Chronic
A term describing a disorder or set of symptoms that has persisted for a long time. In some disorders, such as chronic active *hepatitis*, the time is specified as six months or longer.

Chronic disorders are usually contrasted with acute ones (of sudden onset and short in duration). In addition to the difference in duration between the two, the term acute suggests the presence of symptoms such as high fever, severe pain, or breathlessness, with a rapid change in the patient's condition from one day to the next. By contrast, a person with a chronic infection shows little change in symptoms from day to day and may be able, with some difficulty, to carry out his or her daily activities.

A person with a chronic disease may experience an acute exacerbation (flare-up) of symptoms. Also, people who have had an acute illness such as a *stroke*, or who have been injured in an accident, may be left with permanent disabilities, but their condition is not chronic. A chronic disorder implies a continuing disease process with progressive deterioration (sometimes despite treatment).

Chronic fatigue syndrome
See *Myalgic encephalomyelitis*.

Chronic obstructive lung disease
See *Lung disease, chronic obstructive*.

Cimetidine

ULCER HEALING		

Tablet Liquid Injection

📝 Prescription generally needed

🔒 Not available as generic

An H$_2$-*receptor antagonist* used as an *ulcer-healing drug*. Introduced in 1976, cimetidine reduces the secretion of hydrochloric acid in the stomach and, by doing so, promotes healing of gastric and duodenal ulcers (see *Peptic ulcer*) and reduces *oesophagitis* (inflammation of the oesophagus).

Cimetidine usually relieves symptoms within one to two weeks and heals an ulcer in over 75 per cent of cases after one to two months. Once the ulcer has healed, a maintenance dose of cimetidine is often prescribed; without such treatment the chance of an ulcer recurring is high.

There is a slight risk that cimetidine may temporarily relieve the symptoms of *stomach cancer* in its early stages, and thus delay the diagnosis. Cimetidine is therefore usually prescribed for periods of no longer than two months unless investigations, such as *gastroscopy* and *barium X-ray examinations*, have ruled out the possibility of cancer.

POSSIBLE ADVERSE EFFECTS
Dizziness, sleepiness, and fatigue occasionally occur, as do rashes. Other rare side-effects include gynaecomastia (enlargement of the breasts in men) and impotence. Cimetidine may interfere with the breakdown by the liver of certain anticoagulant and anticonvulsant drugs.

Cinnarizine
An *antihistamine drug* used mainly to control nausea and vomiting caused by travel sickness. Cinnarizine is also prescribed to reduce nausea and vertigo resulting from disorders of the inner ear, such as *labyrinthitis* and *Ménière's disease*. In high doses, cinnarizine has a vasodilator effect and is used to improve circulation in some cases of *peripheral vascular disease* and *Raynaud's disease*.

Possible adverse effects include drowsiness, lethargy, dry mouth, and blurred vision.

Circadian rhythms
Any biological pattern based on a cycle approximately 24 hours long, also called a diurnal rhythm. (See also *Biorhythms*.)

Circulation, disorders of

Conditions affecting the flow of blood from the heart around the body. (*See Arteries, disorders of; Veins, disorders of; Capillary.*)

Circulatory system

The *heart* and blood vessels, which together are responsible for maintaining a continuous flow of blood throughout the body. Also called the cardiovascular system, the circulatory system provides all body tissues with a regular supply of oxygen and nutrients, and carries away carbon dioxide and other waste products.

STRUCTURE AND FUNCTION

The circulatory system consists of two main parts: the systemic circulation, which comprises the blood supply to the entire body except the lungs and the pulmonary circulation to the lungs, which is responsible for reoxygenating the blood (see the box overleaf).

The systemic circulation begins at the left side of the heart, where the left atrium receives oxygen-rich blood from the pulmonary circulation. The blood is ejected from the left atrium to the left ventricle, a powerful pump that sends the blood out through the *aorta*, the body's main artery. Other arteries branching off the aorta carry the blood all over the body, into the arterioles (small arteries) that supply the various organs. The arterioles branch further into a network of capillaries. These extremely fine blood vessels have thin walls to allow oxygen and other nutrients to pass easily from the blood into the tissues, and carbon dioxide and other wastes to pass in the opposite direction.

The capillaries deliver the deoxygenated blood into venules (small veins), which join to form veins. These carry the blood into the *venae cavae*, the body's two main veins, which then return the blood to the right atrium of the heart.

From the right atrium, the blood enters the pulmonary circulation. It passes to the right ventricle, which pumps the blood through the pulmonary artery to the lungs. Here, carbon dioxide passes out of the blood, and oxygen enters. The reoxygenated blood then returns through the pulmonary veins to the left atrium of the heart, where it re-enters the systemic circulation.

Within the systemic circulation there is a bypass to the liver called the portal circulation. Capillaries carrying nutrient-rich blood from the stomach, intestine, and other digestive organs join to form venules which, in turn, meet to form veins. These then merge to form the portal vein, which conveys the blood to veins, venules, and capillaries in the liver. Nutrients pass from the capillaries into the liver cells for processing and storage or re-entry into the general circulation, and the blood continues to rejoin the main systemic circulation via the inferior vena cava.

On its journey from the heart to the tissues, blood is forced along the arteries at high pressure. However, on the return journey through the veins and back to the heart, the blood is at low pressure. It is kept moving by the muscles in the arms and legs compressing the walls of the veins, and by valves in the veins preventing the blood from flowing backwards. (See also *Lymphatic system; Respiration.*)

Circumcision

Removal of the foreskin of the penis. Circumcision may be performed on newborn male babies for religious reasons. It may also be carried out on older children or on adults.

WHY IT IS DONE

Circumcision is a religious ritual practised for many centuries by Jews and Muslims. It is performed routinely in some countries for reasons of hygiene, but British paediatricians do not usually recommend the operation in healthy babies, and in Britain fewer than 10 per cent of teenage boys have been circumcised.

Medical reasons for circumcision include a foreskin that is tight (see *phimosis*) causing ballooning on urination, or recurrent attacks of *balanitis* (infection under the foreskin due to retained secretions). The foreskin may also be removed because it is tight and painful during intercourse, or because of attacks of paraphimosis (painful compression of the shaft of the penis by a retracted foreskin).

HOW IT IS DONE

In newborn babies, circumcision can be done using a local anaesthetic; in older children and adults, general anaesthesia is used.

The operation consists of carefully cutting away the inner and outer layers of the foreskin and then stitching the raw edges together. A dressing is not usually required. The patient can usually return home the same day.

Circumcision, female

Removal of all or parts of the clitoris, labia majora, and labia minora, sometimes combined with narrowing of the entrance to the vagina. The operation is common in parts of Africa. In the early 1980s it was estimated that more than 84 million women in 30 countries had been circumcised.

There is absolutely no valid medical purpose for the procedure. Circumcision may cause retention of urine, injuries during sexual intercourse, and may also lead to loss of sexual desire and other psychological problems. Childbirth is likely to be made more hazardous.

There are strong moves to end the practice completely, but so far with little success in some countries.

Cirrhosis

A disease of the *liver* caused by chronic damage to its cells. Bands of *fibrosis* (internal scarring) break up the normal structure of the liver. The surviving cells multiply to form regeneration nodules (islands of living cells separated by scar tissue). Because these nodules are inadequately supplied with blood, liver function is gradually impaired—for example, the liver no longer effectively removes toxic substances from the blood (see *Liver failure*). In addition, the distortion and fibrosis of the liver leads to *portal hypertension* (high blood pressure in the veins from the intestines and spleen to the liver), which can cause serious complications.

INCIDENCE AND CAUSES

In the UK, about 4,000 cases of cirrhosis are reported each year and there are about 2,500 deaths each year as a direct result of chronic liver disease and cirrhosis.

Heavy alcohol consumption is the most common cause of cirrhosis in developed countries. The risk is related to the amount of alcohol consumed rather than the type, and women are more susceptible to the condition than men (see *Alcohol*).

Hepatitis (inflammation of the liver) can lead to cirrhosis. Chronic viral hepatitis (particularly when caused by the hepatitis B and C viruses) is the most common cause of cirrhosis in the Middle and Far East and Africa (see *Hepatitis, viral*). A special pattern of liver inflammation called chronic active hepatitis is usually present before the cirrhosis develops (see *Hepatitis, chronic active*). Autoimmune chronic active hepatitis, with similar liver changes but with no obvious viral infection, occurs in developed countries.

Rarer causes of cirrhosis include diseases and defects of the *bile ducts*, which can cause primary or secondary *biliary cirrhosis; haemochromatosis*, in

C

C

CIRCULATORY SYSTEM

The heart and blood vessels create a continuous flow of blood around the body to provide tissues with oxygen and nutrients. The system also removes waste products. The systemic circulation deals with the supply of blood to all parts except the lungs; the pulmonary system reoxygenates the blood.

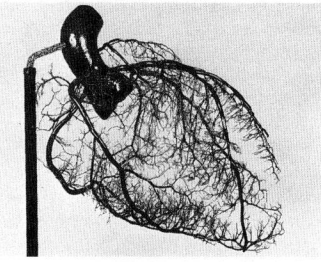

Resin cast of coronary arteries

Shown (left) is a cast of the arrangement of blood vessels that supply the heart muscle. The larger vessels are the coronary arteries; these branch off the root of the aorta, the massive artery that receives oxygenated blood from the heart. The coronary arteries and their branches supply blood and oxygen to all parts of the heart muscle.

SYSTEMATIC CIRCULATION

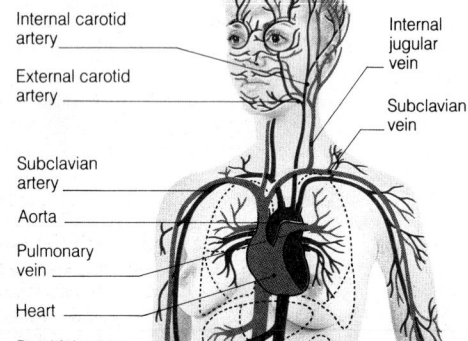

Internal carotid artery
External carotid artery
Subclavian artery
Aorta
Pulmonary vein
Heart
Brachial artery
Superior mesenteric artery
Inferior vena cava
Radial artery
Iliac vein
Femoral artery
Peroneal artery

Internal jugular vein
Subclavian vein
Femoral vein
Great saphenous vein
Small saphenous vein

Key

■ Oxygenated blood

■ Deoxygenated blood

PULMONARY CIRCULATION

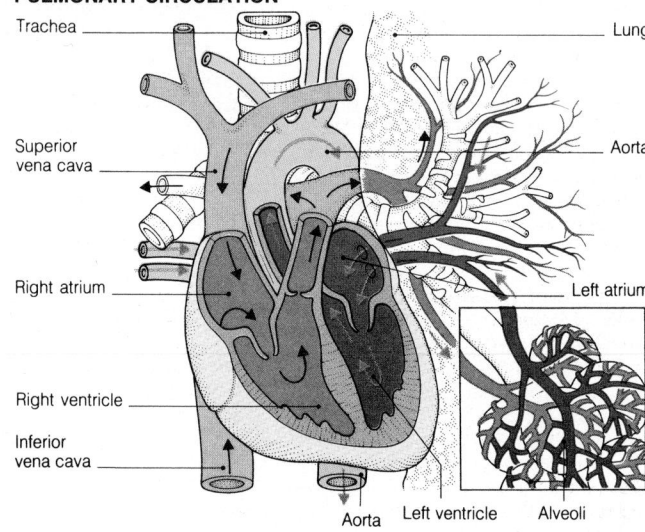

Trachea
Superior vena cava
Right atrium
Right ventricle
Inferior vena cava
Aorta

Lung
Aorta
Left atrium
Left ventricle
Alveoli

Blood is pumped by the left side of the heart, via arteries, to the body, where it gives up oxygen. It then drains, via the venae cavae, to the right side, is pumped to the lungs, receives oxygen from the alveoli, and returns to the left side.

CAPILLARY NETWORK

All tissues contain a network of tiny blood capillaries. Blood enters these from the arterioles and is drained by venules.

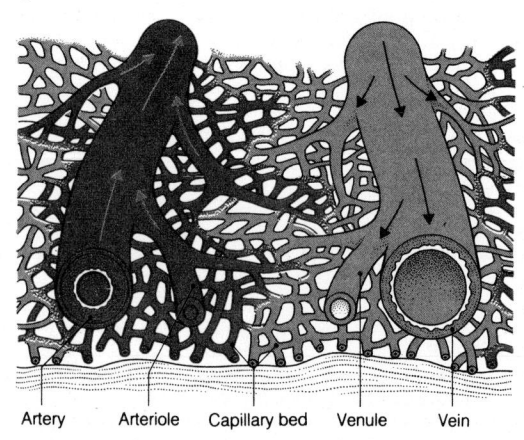

Artery   Arteriole   Capillary bed   Venule   Vein

which increased iron absorption occurs; *Wilson's disease*, in which there is an increase in copper absorption; *cystic fibrosis*, in which the bile ducts become obstructed by sticky mucus; and "cardiac cirrhosis", in which *heart failure* has led to long-standing congestion of blood in the liver.

SYMPTOMS AND SIGNS
There may be no symptoms of cirrhosis; the disease may not be discovered until a routine medical examination or blood test is performed for another reason. The most common symptoms are mild *jaundice, oedema* (fluid collection in the tissues), confusion, and vomiting of blood. Examination may detect enlargement of the liver and spleen.

In men, enlargement of the breasts and loss of body hair are thought to be due to an abnormality in the sex hormone balance caused by liver failure associated with cirrhosis.

COMPLICATIONS
Cirrhosis may lead to various complications, any of which may be the first sign of the condition. *Ascites* (collection of fluid in the abdominal cavity) can occur because of low protein levels in the blood and high blood pressure in the veins leading to the liver. The high pressure in these veins also leads to *oesophageal varices* (enlarged veins in the wall of the oesophagus), which can rupture, causing vomiting of blood. *Confusion* and *coma* can result from the accumulation of toxic materials poisonous to the brain that would normally be processed and detoxified by a healthy liver. *Hepatoma* is a primary cancer of liver cells that may complicate any form of cirrhosis.

DIAGNOSIS
Although the symptoms and signs of cirrhosis, or the results of *liver-function tests*, may suggest cirrhosis, the diagnosis is usually confirmed by *liver biopsy* (removal of a sample of tissue for microscopic analysis), which may also point to the underlying cause. Special blood tests and *cholangiography* (X-rays of the bile ducts) may be performed to exclude the rarer causes.

TREATMENT
The cirrhotic process can be treated by slowing the process causing liver-cell damage. Abstinence from alcohol can lead to substantial improvement. In some cases, specific treatment for the underlying cause may be available.

Ascites may be controlled by giving *diuretic drugs* and sometimes by reducing salt intake. Bleeding oesophageal varices can be obliterated by injecting them with a sclerosant solution (a liquid that blocks off the affected

veins) via a gastroscope (see *Gastroscopy*). The pressure in the veins can be reduced by using a *shunt* operation to divert the blood supply away from the engorged, dilated veins.

Confusion can usually be improved by measures that reduce the level of toxic waste and other poisonous substances circulating in the blood. Such measures may include reducing protein in the diet and giving *antibiotic drugs* to reduce the number of bacteria in the intestines. In most cases, however, a *liver transplant* may offer the best chance of a long-term cure.

Cisapride
A drug used to treat symptoms of gastro-oesophageal reflux, such as *indigestion* and *heartburn*, and delayed stomach emptying associated with *diabetes mellitus* and some other diseases. Adverse effects include abdominal cramps and diarrhoea, and, rarely, headaches, dizziness, and convulsions.

Cisplatin
An *anticancer drug* used especially to treat some cancers of the testis and ovary. Cisplatin can be used on its own or with other anticancer drugs.

Clap
A slang term for the sexually transmitted infection *gonorrhoea*.

Claudication
A cramp-like pain in one or both legs that develops on walking and may eventually cause a limp.

The usual cause of claudication is blockage or narrowing of arteries in the legs due to *atherosclerosis* (see *Peripheral vascular disease*). Patients typically have to stop walking after a particular distance because of pain in the calves. After a short rest, they may be able to resume walking. This is called intermittent claudication.

A rarer cause is spinal stenosis (narrowing of the canal carrying the spinal cord), causing pressure on nerve roots that pass into either leg.

Claustrophobia
Intense fear of being in enclosed spaces, such as lifts or small rooms, or of being in crowded areas. Claustrophobia may originate from a previous bad experience involving an enclosed space. *Behaviour therapy* is the usual form of treatment.

Clavicle
The medical name for the collarbone. These two slightly curved bones, one

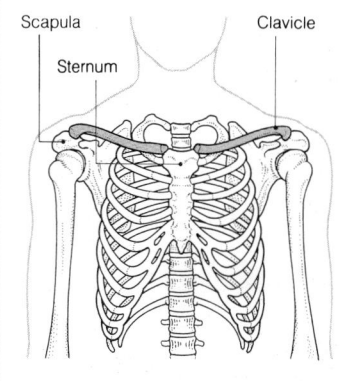

LOCATION OF CLAVICLE
The two slightly curved bones join the top of the sternum to the shoulders and help support the arms.

Scapula

Clavicle

Sternum

on each side, form joints with the top of the sternum (breastbone) and the scapula (shoulderblade). The clavicles support the arms and transmit forces from the arms to the central skeleton.

The ligaments that link each clavicle to the sternum and scapula are very strong, which explains why the clavicle is rarely dislocated but frequently broken. Most fractures occur as a result of a fall on to the shoulder or an outstretched arm. When the clavicle is broken, the arm must be supported by a *sling* and a figure-of-eight bandage used to keep the broken ends of the clavicle together for about three weeks until the fracture has healed.

Claw-foot
A deformity of the foot, also known as pes cavus, in which there is an exaggerated arch and turning under of the tips of the toes. The disorder may be present from birth or may result from disturbance or damage to the nerve or blood supply to the muscles of the foot.

The condition can be helped by using a moulded insole in the shoe to redistribute body weight evenly over the foot. Occasionally, surgical cutting of a tendon on the underside of the foot may be performed in an attempt to flatten the foot.

Claw-hand
A deformity of the hand in which the fingers are permanently curled. It is caused by injury to the ulnar nerve. Treatment includes repair of the damaged nerve, if possible. Other-

C

wise, symptoms may be relieved by using splints to hold the fingers straight or by surgical cutting of a tendon in the wrist to allow the fingers to straighten.

Claw-toe

A deformity of one or more toes. The end of an affected toe bends downwards so that the toe curls under itself. The cause is unknown. A painful corn may develop on the tip of the toe or over the top of the bent joint.

Protective pads can sometimes relieve excessive pressure from footwear. In severe cases, surgical treatment of the toe may be needed.

Cleft lip and palate

Cleft lip is a vertical, usually off-centre split in the upper lip that may be a small notch or may extend up to the nose. In some cases the upper gum is also cleft or notched, and the nose is crooked. Although cleft lip is also sometimes known as hare lip, this term properly refers only to a midline cleft lip, which is extremely rare.

Cleft palate is a gap that most commonly runs along the midline of the palate (the roof of the mouth that separates the mouth from the nasal cavity). The cleft may extend from the back of the palate forward to behind the teeth and allow open communication with the nasal cavity. Many people with cleft palate are partially deaf and may have other *birth defects*. In some cases the lip or palate is cleft on both sides.

Cleft lip and palate are present from birth, occurring either singly or together. About one in 870 babies is born with one or both deformities. Of every nine affected babies, two have only a cleft lip, three have only a cleft palate, and four have both. Inheritance is complicated but one third of those affected have relatives with one or both deformities.

DIAGNOSIS AND TREATMENT
All babies should be routinely examined for cleft lip and cleft palate immediately after birth. Babies with a cleft lip can breast-feed, but those with a cleft palate must be bottle-fed using a special teat.

Surgery, usually at about three months, can repair a cleft lip so that it looks almost normal, and there are rarely any speech defects. A cleft palate is usually repaired when the baby is about one year old; in some cases, further operations, dental management, and speech therapy are also necessary.

Clergyman's knee

Inflammation of the bursa (fluid-filled sac) that acts as a cushion at the pressure point over the tibial tubercle (the bony prominence below the knee). The inflammation is caused by prolonged kneeling. (See *Bursitis*.)

Climacteric

The *menopause*, which indicates the end of menstruation (and thus fertility) in the female. Strictly speaking, the "menopause" refers to the last menstrual period and the "climacteric" refers to the interval of time—months or years—during which symptoms may occur due to falling levels of female sex hormones.

Clindamycin

An *antibiotic drug*. Clindamycin has severe side-effects and is used only to treat serious infections that do not respond to other antibiotic drugs.

Clitoridectomy

An operation to remove the clitoris (see *Circumcision, female*).

Clitoris

Part of the female genitalia. A small, sensitive, erectile organ, the clitoris is located just below the pubic bone and is partly enclosed within the folds of the *labia*. The clitoris is richly supplied with nerves and blood vessels. During sexual stimulation, the clitoris swells and becomes more sensitive.

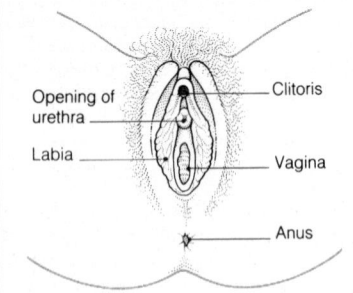

LOCATION OF CLITORIS
The clitoris is a small, sensitive, erectile organ located just below the pubic bone, partly enclosed within the labia.

Opening of urethra — Clitoris

Labia — Vagina

— Anus

Clofibrate

A *lipid-lowering drug* that reduces high levels of *cholesterol* and triglycerides (see *Fats and oils*) in the blood. Clofibrate is sometimes used to treat certain types of *hyperlipidaemia*.

Clomiphene

A drug used to treat female *infertility* caused by failure to ovulate. Multiple births may occur.

HOW IT WORKS
Normal *ovulation* (the release of a ripened egg from one of the ovaries) is stimulated by the action of two *gonadotrophins* (follicle-stimulating hormone and luteinizing hormone) released from the *pituitary gland*. This secretion is stimulated by chemicals released by the *hypothalamus*.

Failure to ovulate, one of the most common causes of infertility, is usually due to an abnormally low production of these gonadotrophins. Clomiphene works by blocking the action of *oestrogen hormones* in the hypothalamus. Oestrogens normally reduce the output of gonadotrophins from the pituitary gland. As a result, the production of gonadotrophins is increased and sometimes ovulation is stimulated. Occasionally, clomiphene must be given with gonadotrophins before ovulation will occur.

POSSIBLE ADVERSE EFFECTS
Minor side-effects include hot flushes, nausea, headache, breast tenderness, and, occasionally, blurred vision. All usually improve when the dose is reduced or if a gonadotrophin is also taken. Between five and 15 per cent of the women who take clomiphene develop *ovarian cysts*. These cysts shrink when the dose is reduced.

Clomipramine

A tricyclic *antidepressant drug* used mainly as a long-term treatment for *depression*. Clomipramine is less sedating than many other antidepressants and is particularly useful when depression is associated with irrational fears and obsessive behaviour.

Possible adverse effects include dry mouth, blurred vision, and constipation. If an overdose is taken, clomipramine may cause dangerously abnormal heart rhythms and coma.

Clonazepam

A *benzodiazepine drug* mainly used as an *anticonvulsant drug* to prevent and treat epileptic fits. Clonazepam is particularly effective in preventing petit mal attacks in children. Possible adverse effects include drowsiness, dizziness, fatigue, and irritability.

Clone

An exact copy. In medicine the term usually refers to one of three main types: clones of cells, clones of genes, and clones of organisms.

Clones of cells are all descended from one original cell. Many types of cancer are thought to be cellular clones derived from one abnormal cell. Monoclonal antibodies (substances obtained from a clone of cells) have been used to identify certain types of cancer and infection (see *Antibody, monoclonal*).

Clones of genes are duplicates of a single gene. Gene cloning is a valuable research tool, because once several copies of a gene have been made the gene can be studied in detail.

Clones of organisms can be produced by removing the nuclei from cells of one individual and transplanting them into the egg cell of another individual. When these eggs mature into living plants or animals, they are all identical as they contain only the genes of the donor nuclei. To date, this process has been successful only with simple organisms.

Clonidine
An *antihypertensive drug* (a drug used to treat high blood pressure). Clonidine works by reducing nerve impulses from the brain to the heart and circulatory system.

When clonidine is given in high doses, sudden stopping of the drug may lead to a dangerous rise in blood pressure. Rarely, an unexpected rise in blood pressure develops when clonidine is given with a *beta-blocker drug*.

Other possible adverse effects, more common in patients on high dosages, include drowsiness, dizziness, dry mouth, and constipation. Such effects often decrease with continued treatment or may require a reduction in dose.

Clonus
An abnormal response of a *muscle* to stretching. Muscles normally respond to being stretched by contracting once and then relaxing. In clonus, stretching sets off a rapid series of muscle contractions.

Clonus is a sign of damage to nerve fibres that carry impulses from the motor cortex within the *cerebrum* of the brain to a particular muscle. One typical example of clonus is called ankle clonus. A doctor may demonstrate this in the course of an examination by forcibly jerking the front of the foot upwards, thus stretching the muscles of the calf, which are then triggered into a series of rhythmical contractions. Clonic muscle contractions are also a feature of seizures in grand mal *epilepsy*.

Clotrimazole
A drug used to treat yeast and fungal infections, especially *candidiasis* (thrush). (See *Antifungal drugs*.)

Clove oil

A colourless or pale-yellow oil distilled from the dried flower-buds of EUGENIA CARYOPHYLLUS. Clove oil is sometimes used to relieve abdominal pain due to *flatulence*, but its main use today is in flavouring pharmaceuticals. Applied externally, clove oil is germicidal and mildly analgesic (painkilling). It is also used as a domestic remedy for toothache, but repeated application may damage the gums.

Cloxacillin
A penicillin-type antibiotic used to treat infections with staphylococcal bacteria. (See *Penicillin drugs*.)

Clubbing
Thickening and broadening of the tips of the fingers and toes, usually with increased curving of the fingernails and toenails.

Clubbing is associated with certain chronic lung diseases, including *bronchiectasis*, *lung cancer*, fibrosing *alveolitis*, and lung *abscess*; and with heart abnormalities that result in *cyanosis* (bluish complexion due to lack of oxygen in the blood). Clubbing is also occasionally associated with the inflammatory bowel diseases *Crohn's disease* or *ulcerative colitis*. Rarely, clubbing may be inherited, in which case it is not a sign of any disease.

Club-foot
A deformity of the foot, present from birth. (See *Talipes*.)

CNS
An abbreviation for *central nervous system* (the brain and spinal cord).

CNS stimulants
Drugs that increase mental alertness. (See *Stimulant drugs*.)

Coagulation, blood
The main mechanism by which blood clots (solidifies). Coagulation involves a complex series of reactions in the blood plasma (the fluid part of blood as distinct from the blood cells). The end result of this process is the formation of an insoluble substance called fibrin, which provides much of the framework for a blood clot. (See also *Blood clotting*.)

Coal tar
A thick, black, sticky substance distilled from coal. Coal tar is a common ingredient of ointments and some medicinal shampoos. These preparations, which often also contain *antiseptics* and *corticosteroid drugs*, are prescribed for skin and scalp conditions such as *psoriasis* and some forms of *dermatitis* and *eczema*.

Coarctation of the aorta
An abnormality, present from birth, in which there is a localized narrowing of the aorta (the large artery that supplies blood from the left side of the heart to the rest of the body).

The narrowing occurs in the part of the aorta that supplies blood to the lower part of the body, including the legs; blood supply to the upper part of the body is not affected. In order to compensate for the reduction in blood supply to the lower part of the body, the heart works harder, causing *hypertension* (abnormally high blood pressure) in the upper part of the body, while the blood pressure in the legs is normal or low.

The cause is unknown. Coarctation of the aorta occurs in about 10 per cent of babies born with heart defects (see *Heart disease, congenital*), or in about one in 5,000 of all babies.

SYMPTOMS AND DIAGNOSIS
The symptoms often first appear in early childhood and depend on the degree of abnormality of the blood pressure. Symptoms may include headache, weakness after exercise, cold legs, and, rarely, breathing difficulty and swelling of the legs due to *heart failure*.

A physical examination of the child usually reveals the following abnormalities associated with the defect: a murmur (abnormal heart sound), weak or absent pulses in the groin, lack of synchronization between groin and wrist pulses, and higher blood pressure in the arms than in the legs. The diagnosis is confirmed by X-rays of the chest that show bulging of the aorta on either side of the narrowed segment, among other abnormalities.

TREATMENT AND OUTLOOK
Surgery is necessary to prevent progressive hypertension, even when there are no symptoms. The narrowed segment of the aorta is removed and the two ends rejoined. The operation is usually performed between the ages of four and eight. Despite successful repair of the aorta, high blood pressure may persist, requiring drug treatment to lower it.

C

C

Cobalamin
A cobalt-containing complex molecule that forms part of *vitamin B₁₂*.

Cobalt
A metallic element and a constituent of *vitamin B₁₂*. Radioactive cobalt is used in *radiotherapy*.

Cocaine
A drug obtained from the leaves of ERYTHROXYLON COCA and similar plant species indigenous to parts of South America.

WHY IT IS USED
Cocaine was once used as a local anaesthetic (see *Anaesthesia, local*), mainly for minor surgical procedures on the eye, ear, nose, or throat. It is sometimes sprayed on to the back of the throat before examination of the lungs or stomach with an *endoscope*. Because of its potential for abuse, cocaine has largely been replaced by other local anaesthetics.

The onset of anaesthesia is rapid and the effects last for about one hour. Cocaine also constricts blood vessels, helping to localize its effect. However, some cocaine is usually absorbed into the bloodstream; this may interfere with the action of chemical *neurotransmitters* in the brain, producing feelings of euphoria and increased energy.

ABUSE
The effects of cocaine on the brain have led to its abuse. Regular inhaling of the drug can damage the lining of the nose. Continued use can lead to psychological dependence (see *Drug dependence*), and *psychosis* may develop if high doses are taken. Overdose

can cause seizures and *cardiac arrest*. "Crack", a purified form of cocaine, produces a more rapid and intense reaction that also wears off very quickly; it has caused deaths due to adverse effects on the heart. (See also *Drug abuse*.)

Cocci
Spherically shaped *bacteria* that cause various infections (see *Staphylococcal infections*; *Streptococcal infections*).

Coccydynia
A pain in the region of the *coccyx*. Coccydynia is usually caused by a fall in which the base of the spine strikes a hard surface. It may also be caused by prolonged pressure on the coccyx due, for example, to habitual slouching in a chair or to use of the *lithotomy position* during childbirth. Occasionally, coccydynia may occur for no obvious reason.

Treatment may include the application of heat, injections of a local anaesthetic, and manipulation, but these measures are not always successful. The pain usually eases in time with or without treatment. In very rare cases of persistent, incapacitating pain, surgical removal of the coccyx may be considered.

Coccyx
A small triangular bone at the base of the *spine*. The coccyx consists of four tiny bones that are fused together; it is all that remains of the tail-bone structure of our evolutionary ancestors.

Together with a much larger bone called the *sacrum*, which lies above it, the coccyx forms the back section of the *pelvis*—a bowl-shaped, bony structure that provides protection to lower abdominal organs such as the uterus and bladder and supports the upper body.

There is very little relative movement between the coccyx and sacrum. Later in life, the coccyx and sacrum commonly fuse together.

Cochlea
The spiral-shaped organ in the inner ear that transforms sound vibrations into nerve impulses for transmission to the brain.

Cochlear implant
A device for treating severe deafness that consists of one or more electrodes surgically implanted inside or outside the *cochlea* in the inner ear. Unlike a *hearing-aid*, which amplifies sounds, the implant receives and passes on electrical signals. It cannot restore

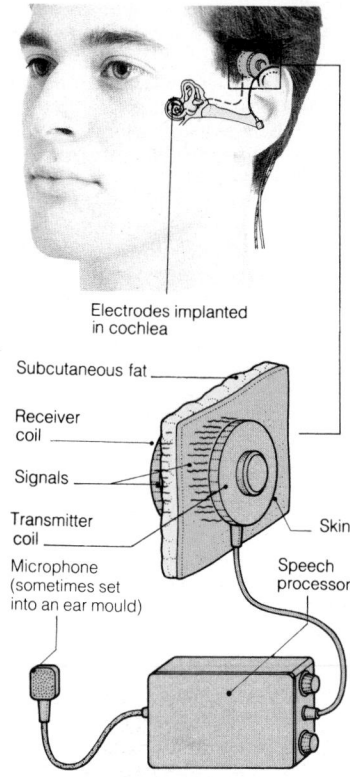

Electrodes implanted
in cochlea

Subcutaneous fat

Receiver
coil

Signals

Transmitter
coil

Microphone
(sometimes set
into an ear mould)

Skin

Speech
processor

How a cochlear implant works
Sounds picked up by the microphone are converted into electronic signals by the processor and relayed to the external transmitter, which sends them through the skin to the receiver. The waves then travel along the wire to the electrodes in the cochlea.

normal hearing but may allow a greater understanding of speech.

WHY IT IS DONE
Some children who are born deaf and some adults who become deaf have such profound deafness that a conventional hearing aid is no help at all. However, if some nerve connections exist, it may be possible to stimulate them, and this is what the implant achieves.

HOW IT IS DONE
An operation is carried out to implant one or more tiny electrodes either inside or outside the cochlea. At the same time, a miniature receiver is implanted under the skin, either behind the ear or in the lower part of the chest. A wire connecting the electrodes to the receiver is also implanted at this time.

Directly over the implanted receiver, the patient wears an external transmitter, which is connected to a sound processor and a microphone.

ANATOMY OF COCCYX
The coccyx consists of four fused bones at the base of the spine. With the sacrum, it forms the back of the pelvis.

Four bones of
coccyx fused
together

OUTLOOK

In general, an implant enables the user to hear the rhythms of speech, and sometimes also the intonation of the voice. Understanding obtained through lip-reading is increased, and the deaf person is able to converse more effectively.

Experience with implants for profoundly deaf children has shown that around half are able to understand speech without lip-reading. Their recognition of words improves with time, and early treatment improves the chances of a good result. In adults the usefulness of an implant for any particular person cannot be predicted. Some patients are greatly helped by the implant and can understand and repeat simple words without needing to lip-read. Others find that their comprehension of lip-reading is increased. However, a final group are not helped at all by the implant, either because the signal is poor, an electrical fault occurs, or an infection develops and the implant has to be removed.

Codeine

ANALGESIC ANTIDIARRHOEAL COUGH REMEDIES
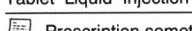
Tablet Liquid Injection
📇 Prescription sometimes needed
📖 Available as generic

A narcotic *analgesic drug* (painkiller), derived from the opium poppy plant. Codeine, used since the early 1900s, is not as strong as some other narcotic analgesics and is often used in combination with other analgesic drugs.

WHY IT IS USED

Codeine is most useful in the relief of mild to moderate pain. It is also used as a *cough remedy*, because it suppresses the part of the brain that triggers coughing, and as an *antidiarrhoeal drug*, because it slows down muscle contractions in the intestinal wall.

POSSIBLE ADVERSE EFFECTS

Codeine may cause dizziness and drowsiness, especially if taken with alcohol. When taken over a long period, codeine may cause constipation and be habit-forming.

Cod-liver oil

A pale-yellow oil obtained from the liver of fresh cod. Cod-liver oil is a valuable source of *vitamin A* and *vitamin D*. Before vitamin drops became common, cod-liver oil was often given to children as a dietary supplement to ensure the healthy development of bones and skin. Excessive use may be dangerous.

Coeliac disease

 An uncommon condition, known also as gluten enteropathy, in which the lining of the small intestine is damaged by gluten, a protein found in wheat, rye, and certain other cereals. The damage causes *malabsorption* (failure to absorb nutrients from the intestine), weight loss, and deficiencies of some vitamins and minerals. This can lead to *anaemia* and skin problems. Faeces are bulky, foul-smelling, and contain large amounts of fat and other nutrients.

CAUSE

Damage to the intestinal lining seems to be due to *hypersensitivity* (an abnormal immunological response). The *immune system* becomes sensitized to gluten, reacting in the same way as it would to an infection or foreign body. The abnormal reaction is limited to the intestinal lining, and the practical result is that the villi (frond-like projections) from the lining become flattened, seriously impairing nutrient absorption.

INCIDENCE

The proportion of people affected by coeliac disease differs greatly among populations. In the UK it affects about 40 per 100,000 people (about 25,000 in all). In the west of Ireland the incidence is 300 per 100,000. In Africa and Asia, coelic disease is very rare.

Coeliac disease tends to run in families—relatives of patients are much more likely than other people to have the disease themselves—and most patients may be shown to have a particular set of *histocompatibility antigens*.

SYMPTOMS AND SIGNS

The severity of the disease varies, and many of those who suffer some damage to the intestinal lining never develop symptoms.

In babies, symptoms usually develop within six months of the introduction of gluten into the diet. The faeces become bulky, greasy, pale, and foul-smelling, and the baby loses weight, becomes listless and irritable, and produces a lot of intestinal gas, which makes the abdomen swell. Defective absorption of iron may lead to anaemia (see *Anaemia, iron-deficiency*). Defective absorption of folic acid (a vitamin) may lead to megaloblastic anaemia (see *Anaemia, megaloblastic*). Vomiting may occur, and sometimes the baby develops acute diarrhoea, becoming dehydrated and seriously ill.

In adults, symptoms usually develop gradually over months or years. Symptoms may include vague tiredness, breathlessness, weight loss, diarrhoea, vomiting, abdominal pain, and swelling of the legs. Some patients develop a chronic, distinctive rash called *dermatitis herpetiformis*.

DIAGNOSIS

A firm diagnosis is made by means of jejunal *biopsy*, in which a small sample of tissue is taken from the lining of the upper small intestine via a tube passed through the stomach under X-ray guidance. Three biopsies may be performed over a period of time—one when the patient is eating a diet that contains gluten, another when he or she is on a gluten-free diet, and a third when gluten is again introduced into the diet. A change in the intestinal lining during the second and third stages indicates that gluten is causing the illness. Tests on the blood, urine, and faeces may be performed to show the level of malabsorption.

TREATMENT AND OUTLOOK

The only treatment required is a life-long gluten-free diet; all foods containing wheat, rye, or barley must be avoided (many sufferers are also advised to avoid oats).

Specially manufactured substitute foods, such as gluten-free bread, flour, and pasta are available. There is no restriction on meat, fish, eggs, dairy products, vegetables, fruit, rice, and corn.

Within a few weeks of the start of a gluten-free diet, symptoms clear up and the sufferer starts to regain lost weight and to enjoy normal health.

Cognitive-behavioural therapy

A method of treating mental disorders based on the idea that the way we perceive the world and ourselves (our cognitions) influences our emotions and behaviour.

A person suffering from *depression* may believe that all undesirable events are due to his or her behaviour and that all desirable events are due to chance. The therapist shows the patient that these interpretations may be false, suggests more positive ways of thinking, and encourages the patient to try out these new ideas during his or her everyday activities.

Because cognitive-behavioural therapy is based on the manner in which each person relates to the environment, it allows treatment to be more specifically tailored to the individual's needs than do more traditional forms of *behaviour therapy*.

Coil

Any of the various types of intraute-rine contraceptive device (see *IUD*).

Coitus

Sexual intercourse (from the Latin word for a going together).

Coitus interruptus

The contraceptive technique in which the male partner withdraws his penis from the vagina before ejaculation occurs. This technique is not reliable as a contraceptive method, because sperm may sometimes be released before orgasm occurs. Coitus interruptus has been blamed for *psychosexual dysfunction* in both men and women. (See also *Contraception*.)

Colchicine

A drug extracted from the autumn crocus flower. Colchicine has been in use since the 19th century as a treatment for *gout*. Although it has now been mainly superseded by newer drugs (because it causes many side-effects), colchicine continues to be used both as a treatment for acute attacks of gout and to reduce the frequency of attacks.

Cold, common

A viral infection that causes inflammation of the mucous membranes lining the nose and throat, resulting in a stuffy, runny nose and sometimes also a sore throat, headache, and other discomfort.

CAUSES

Almost 200 viruses, all broadly similar in their effects, are known to cause colds. The most common belong to one of two groups—the rhinoviruses and the coronaviruses.

Most colds are contracted by breathing in virus-containing droplets that have been sneezed or coughed into the atmosphere or by rubbing the eyes or nose with fingers that have picked up a virus by hand-to-hand contact or by handling contaminated objects, such as hand towels.

INCIDENCE

Almost everyone occasionally gets a cold. The incidence is highest among schoolchildren (who may have as many as 10 colds a year) and declines with increasing age. On average, a young adult has two or three colds per year, an elderly person has one or none at all. The reason for this is that children at school are exposed to a host of different viruses to which they have not yet become immune and which they pass to one another.

Adults gradually build up immunity against a wide variety of viruses responsible for colds.

Colds are most frequent in winter, probably because people tend to spend more time during these months crowded together indoors.

SYMPTOMS

Most colds are what are popularly known as head colds—that is, infections confined to the nose and throat. The first symptoms are often a tickle in the throat, a watery discharge from the nose, and sneezing. In some cases the discharge may thicken and become yellow or green. Other symptoms may develop—watering eyes, a slight fever, a sore throat, a cough, aching muscles and bones, headache, listlessness, and chills.

In some cases, infection spreads and causes *laryngitis, tracheitis* (inflammation of the trachea, or windpipe), acute *bronchitis, sinusitis,* or *otitis media* (inflammation of the middle ear). In these cases, a more serious secondary bacterial infection may follow.

Colds can also aggravate existing respiratory disorders, such as *asthma,* chronic bronchitis, and chronic ear infections. They may also reactivate dormant HERPES SIMPLEX virus, causing *cold sores.*

TREATMENT

Most colds clear up within a week or so. A doctor should be consulted only if this fails to happen, if the infection has spread beyond the nose or throat, or if the cold has aggravated a chronic chest infection or ear disorder. If a secondary bacterial infection is suspected, *antibiotic drugs* may be given.

PREVENTION

Many people believe there are ways of preventing colds—by avoiding cold drafts and dampness, for instance, or by taking large quantities of vitamin C—but there is no scientific evidence that any such measures work.

OUTLOOK

The search to find a cure for the common cold continues. In volunteer experiments, the drug *interferon* has proved effective in preventing and reducing the severity of colds, but has caused local inflammation. Another area of research involves the use of synthetic *antigens* (substances that stimulate the immune system to produce antibodies).

Cold injury

Localized tissue damage caused by chilling—as distinct from *hypothermia,* which refers to generalized chilling; the two may occur together.

The most serious form of cold injury is *frostbite,* a hazard of very cold, dry conditions. The frostbitten area of skin and flesh is frozen, hard, and white; it may be caused by exposure to the cold air sometimes coupled with restriction of the blood supply to the affected area.

Immersion foot is another type of cold injury, occurring when the legs and feet have been cold and damp for many hours or days, and blood supply to the feet has been restricted by tight-fitting footwear.

In established frostbite and immersion foot, the main risk is that blood flow will be slowed so much that the tissues will die, leading to *gangrene* (tissue death). Treatment may take several months.

Less serious forms of cold injury include *chilblains,* caused by rapid rewarming of the skin after being out in cold weather, and *chapped skin* of the lips, nose, and hands from exposure to cold, windy conditions.

Cold remedies

Preparations for the relief of symptoms of the common cold. Many different preparations are available over-the-counter. The main ingredient is usually a mild *analgesic drug* (painkiller), such as *paracetamol* or *aspirin,* which helps to relieve aches and pains. Other common ingredients include *antihistamine drugs* and *decongestant drugs,* which help to reduce nasal congestion, and caffeine, which acts as a mild stimulant. *Vitamin C* is frequently included in cold relief products, but there is no evidence that it speeds recovery.

Cold sore

A small skin blister, usually around the mouth, caused by the HERPES SIMPLEX virus. Usually, several blisters occur together in a cluster.

CAUSE AND INCIDENCE

The strain of the virus usually responsible for cold sores is called HSV1 (HERPES SIMPLEX virus type 1). Most people—perhaps as many as 90 per cent worldwide—are infected by HSV1 at some time in their lives. The first attack may pass unnoticed or may cause an illness resembling influenza and painful ulcers in the mouth and on the lips—a condition called gingivostomatitis.

Subsequently, the virus lies dormant in nerve cells, but in some people it is occasionally reactivated, causing cold sores. Such sores tend to recur when a person with the virus is exposed to hot sunshine or a cold wind, is suffering from a common cold or other infection, or is feeling run down; women seem more likely to develop cold sores around the time of their menstrual periods. Some people are afflicted regularly throughout the year. Prolonged attacks can occur in people with an underlying disease that affects their immunity to infection, or in those taking *immunosuppressant drugs* (transplant or cancer patients, for example.)

SYMPTOMS

An outbreak is often preceded by a telltale tingling in the lips. The blisters are small at first but soon enlarge, sometimes causing itching, irritation, and soreness. Within a few days they burst and become encrusted. Most disappear within a week.

TREATMENT

If cold sores are particularly troublesome, a doctor may prescribe *idoxuridine* paint or the antiviral drug *acyclovir* (in tablet or cream form) to soothe them. Both treatments are most effective if given as early as possible after symptoms develop.

No effective preventive treatment is available, although some people find that applying a lip salve before exposure to the sun does help prevent outbreaks. (See also *Herpes simplex*.)

Colectomy

The surgical removal of part or all of the *colon* (the major part of the large intestine).

WHY IT IS DONE

A partial colectomy may be performed to relieve severe cases of *diverticular disease* or to remove either a malignant tumour in the colon or a narrowed part of the intestine that is obstructing the passage of faeces.

A total colectomy is carried out in cases of *ulcerative colitis* that cannot be controlled with drugs; in cases of long-standing ulcerative colitis in which *colonoscopy* (examination of the colon through a viewing instrument) suggests there may be a hidden malignancy; and in cases of familial *polyposis coli*, a rare condition in which potentially malignant growths stud the lining of the colon.

HOW IT IS DONE

In a partial colectomy, the diseased section of the colon is removed and the two ends of the severed colon are joined together; they fuse in a matter of weeks. A temporary *colostomy* (which allows the discharge of faeces from the large intestine through an artificial opening in the abdominal

wall) may also be required. The temporary colostomy is closed when the rejoined colon has healed.

In a total colectomy the whole of the large intestine is removed; the rectum (last part of the large intestine) may be removed or left in place. If the rectum is removed, an *ileostomy* (similar to a colostomy, but involving the small instead of the large intestine) is performed. If the rectum is left in place, the ileum (the last part of the small intestine) may be joined directly to it.

RECOVERY PERIOD

The patient is usually in hospital for eight to 12 days. After discharge, it may take up to two months or so at home to recover from the operation. A patient with an ileostomy or colostomy should receive training—before leaving hospital and preferably from a specialist nurse—on caring for the opening in the abdomen.

OUTLOOK

The bowel usually functions normally after most partial colectomies. If a large section of the colon has been removed, or if the ileum has been joined directly to the rectum, the greatly reduced ability of the intestines to absorb water from the faeces can cause diarrhoea. *Antidiarrhoeal drugs*, such as *codeine, loperamide*, or *diphenoxylate*, may be required.

Colic

A severe, spasmodic pain that occurs in waves of increasing intensity, reaches a peak, and then abates for a short time before returning. The intermittent increase in pain occurs when the affected part of the body contracts.

Colic in a bile duct (see *Biliary colic*) or in the urinary tract (see *Renal colic*) is often the result of obstruction by a stone. Intestinal colic may be due to obstruction of the intestine (see *Intestine, obstruction of*), to intestinal infections, or simply to intestinal gas. (See also *Colic, infantile*.)

Colic, infantile

Episodes during which an infant, who is otherwise completely well, is irritable, cries or screams excessively, and draws up the legs.

CAUSES AND INCIDENCE

Infantile colic is thought to be due to spasm in the intestines, although there is no proof of this, and the cause of the presumed spasm is unknown. The condition is common, occurring in approximately one in 10 babies. It often first appears around the third or fourth week of life. Usually it clears up without treatment by the age of 12

weeks, hence the popular name "three-month colic". The condition is harmless, although it can be highly distressing to a tired parent.

SYMPTOMS

The baby cries or screams incessantly, draws up the legs towards the stomach in a characteristic position, may become red in the face, and may pass wind. Episodes of colic tend to be worse in the evenings and do not respond to the usual means of comforting the infant, such as feeding, cuddling, or nappy changing.

If the baby seems to be ill between the bouts of colic, is failing to gain weight satisfactorily, or has diarrhoea, constipation, or a fever, a doctor should be consulted because the baby may have a more serious underlying problem.

TREATMENT

No treatment is usually required. *Antispasmodic drugs* have sometimes been given for infantile colic in the past, but these drugs are not now generally recommended for babies under six months old.

Distracting the baby by nappy changing, cuddling, or bathing may help. The baby may be soothed by rhythmic activities such as being taken for a car ride, being rocked, or being placed face-down on a lap while his or her back is stroked. Other possibly helpful measures include using white noise (e.g. static from a radio), applying warmth (e.g. from a warm face-cloth) to the baby's abdomen, carrying the baby in a front sling, or giving the baby a dummy.

Parental anxiety is likely to make the baby even more irritable, and parents should try to avoid becoming overtired.

Colistin

One of the polymyxin group of *antibiotic drugs*. Colistin is used only to treat severe infections that are resistant to other antibiotics, as there is a risk that it may damage the kidneys and nerve tissue. It is also used in eye drops for local eye infections.

Colitis

Inflammation of the *colon* (part of the large intestine) causing diarrhoea, usually with blood and mucus. Other symptoms may include abdominal pain and fever.

CAUSES

Colitis may be due to infection by various different types of microorganism, such as *CAMPYLOBACTER* and *shigella* bacteria, viruses, or amoebae.

C

Antibiotic drugs may sometimes provoke a form of colitis; prolonged use commonly has a direct irritative effect on the colon. In some cases, antibiotics cause colitis by killing some types of bacteria that normally live in the intestine and allowing the proliferation of *CLOSTRIDIUM DIFFICILE* bacteria, which produce a toxin that irritates the colon.

Ischaemia (impairment of blood supply) of the intestinal wall is a very rare cause of colitis in the elderly. Intestinal ischaemia is usually due to *atherosclerosis* (accumulation of fatty deposits on the inner lining of arteries).

Colitis is a feature of *ulcerative colitis* and *Crohn's disease*, which are serious intestinal disorders of unknown origin that most commonly start in young adulthood.

Other disorders that can cause symptoms similar to those of colitis include *proctitis* (inflammation of the rectum), *diverticulitis* (inflammation of pouches in the colon), or cancer of the colon (see *Colon, cancer of*).

DIAGNOSIS

A doctor may suspect colitis if severe diarrhoea, with or without blood or mucus, persists for more than five days despite eating no solid foods and restricting the diet to clear fluids (such as water, tea, or soups). The doctor will then usually send a sample of faeces to a laboratory to be examined for the presence of microorganisms.

If no infection is found, *sigmoidoscopy* (inspection of the rectum and colon with a viewing instrument) or *colonoscopy* (inspection of the colon with a viewing instrument) may be performed to look for any inflammation or ulceration of the lining. A *biopsy* (removal of a sample of tissue for microscopic analysis) of inflamed areas or ulcers may be performed to look for the changes of ulcerative colitis or Crohn's disease. A barium enema (see *Barium X-ray examinations*) may be performed to look for any areas of narrowing or severe inflammation in the colon.

TREATMENT

Colitis caused by an infection usually clears up without treatment. However, *CAMPYLOBACTER* infections are sometimes treated with the antibiotic drug *erythromycin*, amoebic infections with *metronidazole*, and clostridium infections with metronidazole or *vacomycin*.

Colitis caused by ischaemia is treated by surgical excision of the diseased section of colon.

Crohn's disease and ulcerative colitis are treated with *corticosteroid drugs*, with other drugs such as *sulphasala-*

zine, or by a special diet and vitamin supplements. Surgery does not cure these diseases and is reserved for the treatment of complications.

Collagen

A tough, fibrous *protein*. Collagen is the body's major structural protein, forming an important part of *tendons, bones,* and *connective tissues*. Because of its tough, insoluble nature, collagen helps hold together the cells and tissues.

Collagen diseases

Two groups of diseases are referred to as collagen diseases—true collagen diseases and connective tissue diseases. True collagen diseases are uncommon, usually inherited, and due to faulty formation of *collagen* fibres. Features of these diseases include thin, slack skin, and poor wound healing.

Connective tissue diseases are types of *autoimmune disorder* (in which the *immune system* reacts against the body's organs or tissues). These disorders often affect blood vessels and produce secondary connective tissue damage. Diseases of this type are sometimes called collagen vascular diseases. They include *rheumatoid arthritis*, systemic *lupus erythematosus, polyarteritis nodosa, scleroderma*, and *dermatomyositis*.

Collarbone

The common name for the *clavicle*.

Collar, orthopaedic

A device worn to treat neck pain or instability. There are two basic types: soft, usually made of foam, and stiff, usually made of foam reinforced with plastic.

A soft collar can provide pain relief by limiting movement of the neck, by transferring some of the weight of the head from the neck to the chest, and by providing local warmth. Stiff collars may be used to provide support when a fractured neck has almost healed or when the cervical vertebrae (neck bones) have become unstable for some other reason.

College of Health

A self-help organization for patients that provides telephone information on waiting lists and common diseases and symptoms. It also helps health authorities to monitor and improve the service they offer to their patients.

Colles' fracture

A break in the *radius* (one of the lower-arm bones) just above the wrist, usually caused by a fall.

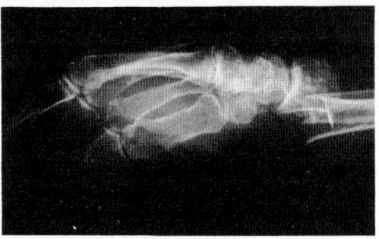

X-ray of Colles' fracture
The wrist has been pushed back over the broken bone. This gives a classic "dinner fork" appearance when viewed from the side.

In a Colles' fracture the wrist and hand are displaced backwards, resulting in restriction of movement and severe pain and swelling. Colles' fracture is the most common type of fracture in people over 40.

CAUSES

Colles' fracture usually occurs when someone stumbles when walking or slips on an icy pavement and puts out a hand to lessen the impact of the fall. Such a fall rarely produces a fracture in a young person, but it may be enough to break a bone weakened by *osteoporosis*, an invariable feature of aging. When a young person suffers a Colles' fracture, it is usually the result of a more violent injury and often extends to the wrist joint itself.

TREATMENT AND OUTLOOK

The two ends of the broken bone are usually manipulated back into position, under a local or a general anaesthetic, and a plaster *cast* is applied. Healing usually takes up to six weeks. When the cast is removed, the wrist may be stiff and exercise may be needed to restore its flexibility.

Minor deformity of the wrist may result from Colles' fracture, but movement of the hand and wrist usually returns to normal. In cases where the injury was extensive, however, there is an increased likelihood that arthritis (see *Osteoarthritis*) will develop.

Colloid

A state of matter similar to a suspension. A typical suspension—milk, for example—consists of insoluble particles of a substance suspended in a liquid. These particles are large and heavy enough to be separable from the liquid by centrifugation (spinning at high speed). A colloid is basically the same, except that its particles are significantly smaller and lighter than those of a suspension; they can be separated from the remaining part of the colloid only by ultracentrifugation (spinning at extremely high speed).

In medicine, colloid preparations containing *plasma proteins* (proteins in the fluid portion of blood) or certain complex carbohydrate molecules may be given to treat *shock*.

The term colloid is also used to refer to the protein-containing material that fills the follicles of the *thyroid gland*.

Colon

The major part of the large intestine. The colon is a segmented tube, about 1.3 m long and 6.5 cm wide, that forms a large loop in the abdomen. Its segments, known as haustrations, give it an irregular outline.

The colon consists of four sections: the ascending, transverse, descending, and sigmoid colon. The ascending colon extends up to a sharp bend just below the liver. The transverse colon loops across the abdomen below the stomach. The descending colon passes down the left side to the brim of the pelvis, adopts an S-shaped course of variable length (the sigmoid colon), and finally connects with the *rectum* on the lower left of the abdomen.

STRUCTURE

The colon is a muscular tube with a lubricated inner lining. Its walls have four layers. The outermost layer,

---

LOCATION OF COLON
A segmented tube within the abdomen, the colon takes the form of a large, roughly M-shaped, loop about 1.3 m long and 6.5 cm wide.

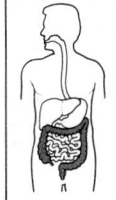

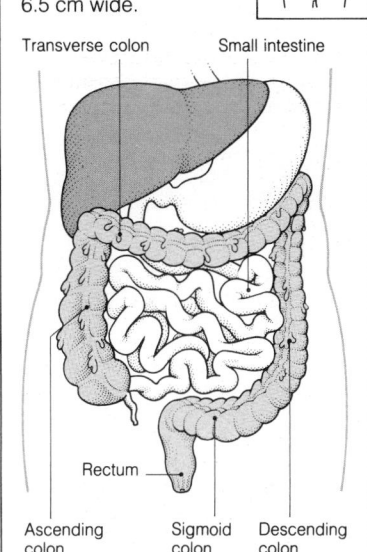

Transverse colon   Small intestine

Rectum

Ascending colon   Sigmoid colon   Descending colon

---

called the serous coat, is a tough, fibrous membrane with a smooth outer surface. This membrane protects the colon from damage when intestinal movements cause it to rub against the abdominal wall.

The next layer consists of three bands of longitudinal muscles and an inner band of circular muscles. Rhythmic contractions and relaxations of these muscles (*peristalsis*) squeeze the intestinal contents through the colon.

Inside the muscular layer is the third layer, the submucous coat. It consists of *connective tissue*, blood vessels, and lymphatic vessels.

The innermost layer is the mucous coat, which contains numerous tubular glands, which produce large amounts of mucus to lubricate the passage of digested material through the colon. Unlike the small intestine, the mucous coat of the colon (and the rest of the large intestine) is not folded into *villi* (finger-like projections).

FUNCTION

The functions of the colon are, principally, to absorb water (and also a small amount of mineral salts) from the digested material passing through the colon and to concentrate indigestible waste for expulsion as *faeces*.

When the intestinal contents enter the colon, digestion has been completed and the material is in the form of a liquid. As this liquid passes through the colon, the water and salts it contains are absorbed into the blood vessels in the submucous coat. By the time the intestinal contents pass out of the colon into the rectum, almost all the water has been absorbed and the contents are in the form of faeces. (See also *Digestive system; Intestine* disorders box.)

Colon, cancer of

A malignant tumour of the *colon* (the major part of the large intestine). The colon is one of the most common of all cancer sites. About 25,000 cases of cancer of the large intestine (colon and rectum) occur in the UK each year, of which about two thirds are cancers of the colon. Cancers of the large intestine account for about 20 per cent of all cancer deaths in the UK.

CAUSES

Approximately 5 per cent of cancers of the colon occur in families with an inherited predisposition to the disease, and several different types have been identified and associated with different genes. Blood relatives of those who have developed cancer of the colon before the age of fifty should undergo

genetic testing for one of the familial cancer genes, and may be advised to undergo regular screening.

In most cases of cancer of the colon, however, the precise cause is not known, but there are a number of possible contributory factors.

The higher incidence of cancer of the colon in Western countries suggests an environmental, probably dietary, factor. It is thought that a high-meat, high-fat, and low-fibre diet encourages the production and concentration of *carcinogens*.

Cancer of the colon frequently occurs in assocation with some other diseases of the colon, such as *ulcerative colitis* and familial *polyposis*.

SYMPTOMS

An inexplicable change in bowel movements (either constipation or diarrhoea) lasting for 10 days or so may be one of the first symptoms of cancer of the colon.

Blood mixed in the faeces (as opposed to the blood from *haemorrhoids*, which usually coats the faeces) is another important warning signal. However, if the cancer is high up in the colon, blood can be detected only by chemical tests.

There may be pain and tenderness in the lower abdomen. Sometimes, however, there are no symptoms until the cancer grows so big that the intestine becomes obstructed (see *Intestine, obstruction of*) or perforates (ruptures).

DIAGNOSIS AND TREATMENT

The chances of cure for cancer of the colon and rectum depend critically on early diagnosis (see *Cancer screening*). The most widely used screening test, the *occult blood* test, is for microscopic traces of blood in the faeces. Research in the UK and the US has shown that people over fifty, who regularly undergo this test, substantially reduce the risk of dying from the disease. If the test is positive, *sigmoidoscopy* (inspection of the colon and rectum with a viewing instrument), and *colonoscopy* (inspection of the colon with a viewing instrument) may be carried out.

Treatment depends on the stage of development of the cancer, but, in most cases, a partial *colectomy* (removal of part of the colon) is performed. The diseased tissue and a small amount of surrounding normal tissue are removed and the cut ends are sewn together to re-establish the channel. If the disease is extensive, surgery may not be possible.

OUTLOOK

The long-term prospects vary according to the stage the disease has reached when it is discovered. More than 50 per cent of patients survive in good health for at least five years after a colectomy. Nonsurgical treatments merely arrest the growth and spread of the cancer and are not curative. The earlier the tumour is detected, the greater the chances of a full recovery after treatment. Anyone over the age of 50 who experiences an inexplicable change in bowel movements should see a doctor without delay. (See also *Rectum, cancer of.*)

Colon, disorders of

See *Intestine* disorders box.

Colon, irritable

See *Irritable bowel syndrome.*

Colonoscopy

Examination of the inside of the *colon* (the major part of the large intestine) by means of a long, flexible, fibre-optic viewing instrument called a colonoscope (see *Endoscopy*).

WHY IT IS DONE

Colonoscopy is used to investigate symptoms (such as bleeding from the bowel) and to look for disorders of the colon, such as colitis, polyps (small, benign, grape-like growths), and cancer. Attachments at the end of the instrument enable the doctor to take biopsy specimens (small samples of tissue or cells for microscopic analysis), or to remove polyps.

HOW IT IS DONE

The patient takes *laxative drugs* for one or two days before the examination to empty the colon of faeces. Because the procedure causes slight discomfort, the patient is lightly sedated beforehand. The colonoscope is passed into the colon through the anus and guided along the length of the colon, which the operator examines through a viewing lens. A complete examination of the entire colon can take from 10 minutes to a couple of hours.

Colon, spastic

See *Irritable bowel syndrome.*

Colostomy

An operation in which part of the *colon* (major part of the large intestine) is brought through an incision in the abdominal wall and formed into an artificial opening to allow the discharge of faeces into a lightweight bag attached to the skin. The colostomy may be temporary or permanent.

WHY IT IS DONE

In a severely ill patient, a temporary colostomy may be carried out as an emergency measure to deal with an obstruction or perforation in the large intestine that is preventing the patient from passing faeces. The colostomy is made above the obstruction and, by allowing the faeces to discharge, enables the patient to become well enough to undergo a partial *colectomy* (an operation to remove part of the large intestine) to remove the obstruction. A temporary colostomy may also be performed at the same time as a colectomy in order to allow the colon to heal without faeces passing through it. Temporary colostomies are closed when the rejoined colon has healed.

A permanent colostomy is needed if all or part of the rectum or anus must be removed (e.g. to treat cancer of the rectum), making normal defaecation impossible.

RECOVERY PERIOD

For two or three days after the operation the patient is fed intravenously. He or she is then given a light diet and begins to pass faeces through the stoma (artificial opening) into a lightweight bag that is attached by adhesive seals to the skin around the stoma. After a bowel movement, the bag is exchanged for a new one.

During this period the patient should receive advice and training from a specialist stoma care nurse on how to look after the stoma and on how to change the colostomy bag.

After leaving hospital, the patient usually needs to convalesce for up to several weeks before returning to normal activities. The stoma care nurse will make visits to check progress.

OUTLOOK

A person with a colostomy may eventually establish an almost normal bowel routine. The bowel usually discharges faeces into the bag once or twice a day; the bag is then changed.

A person with a colostomy can expect to lead a normal life after he or she has fully recovered from the operation. There are usually no complications. Occasional problems, such as prolapse (protrusion) of part of the colon through the abdominal opening, or blockage to the passage of faeces due to narrowing of the stoma, can usually be treated surgically.

PROCEDURE FOR COLOSTOMY

An incision is made in the abdominal wall and either a small loop of the colon or (if the rectum and anus have been removed) the severed end of the colon is pulled through. If a loop of the colon is used, an opening is made in it large enough for the faeces to pass through. The edges of this opening or the edges of the severed end of the colon are stitched to the skin at the edge of the abdominal incision to create a stoma (artificial opening).

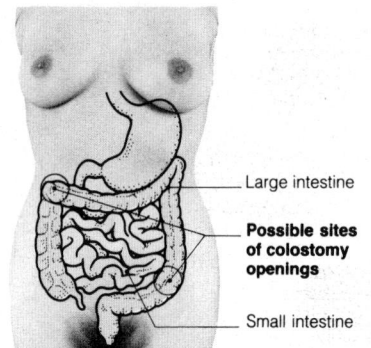

Large intestine

Possible sites of colostomy openings

Small intestine

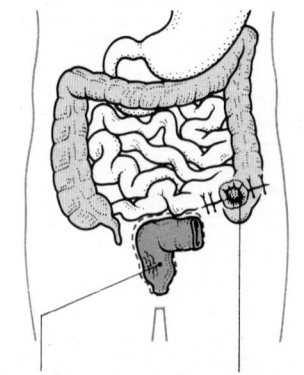

Diseased part of rectum removed

Open end of bowel brought through to skin surface

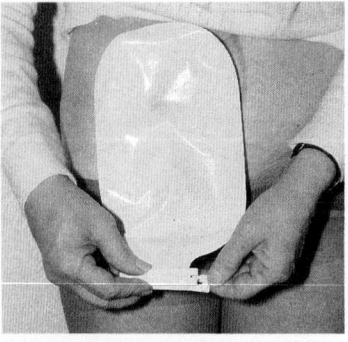

Position of colostomy bag
The bag is attached to the skin around the stoma by adhesive seals. After a bowel movement, a new bag is attached.

Colostrum

The thick, yellowish fluid produced by a mother's breasts during the first few days after childbirth. Colostrum is replaced by mature breast milk about four to five days after birth. Compared with mature breast milk, colostrum contains less fat and sugar, and more minerals and protein. It has a high content of *lymphocytes* (white blood cells) and *immunoglobulins*, which help protect the baby from infection.

Colour blindness

See *Colour vision deficiency*.

Colour vision

The ability to discriminate different parts of the colour spectrum (see illustrated box). Colour vision probably evolved as an aid to finding or catching food.

THE COLOUR SPECTRUM

Light perceived by the human eye consists of electromagnetic radiation (energy waves) with wavelengths between about 400 and 700 nanometres (a nanometre is a millionth of a millimetre).

Going from the short to the long end of this spectrum, different wavelengths produce the sensations of violet, indigo, blue, green, yellow, orange, and red when they impinge upon the retina of the eye and stimulate nerve signals, which are processed in the rear of the brain.

COLOUR VISION

Light, consisting of radiation of various wavelengths, is focused on the retina, where light-sensitive rod and cone cells are stimulated to emit nerve impulses. Some initial processing of this "signalling" occurs in the ganglion cells of the retina, before impulses pass to the brain via the optic nerve.

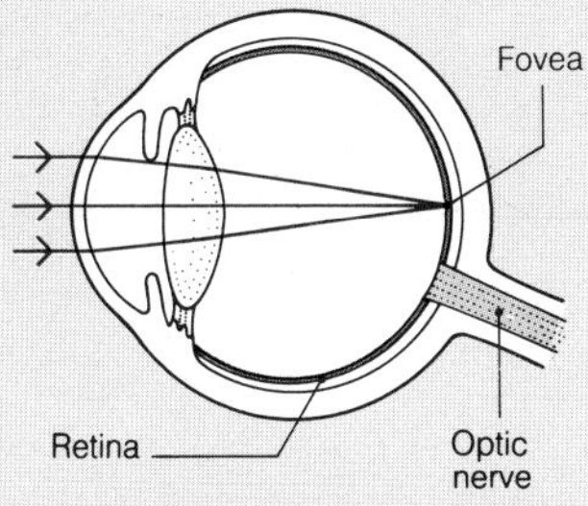

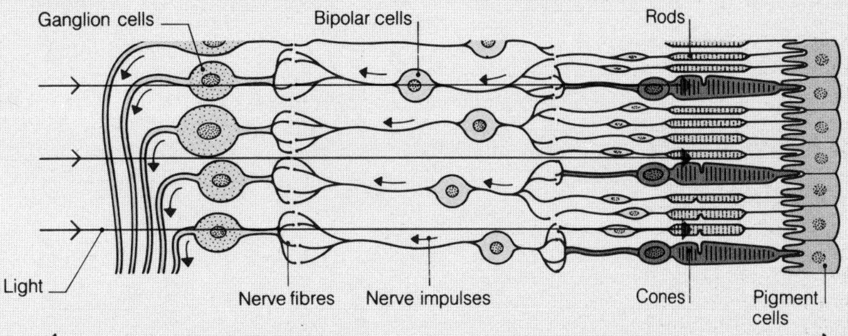

Location of colour-sensitive cells
Light passes through the whole thickness of the retina before striking the rods and cones. Colour vision depends mainly on the cones, concentrated in a region of the retina called the fovea.

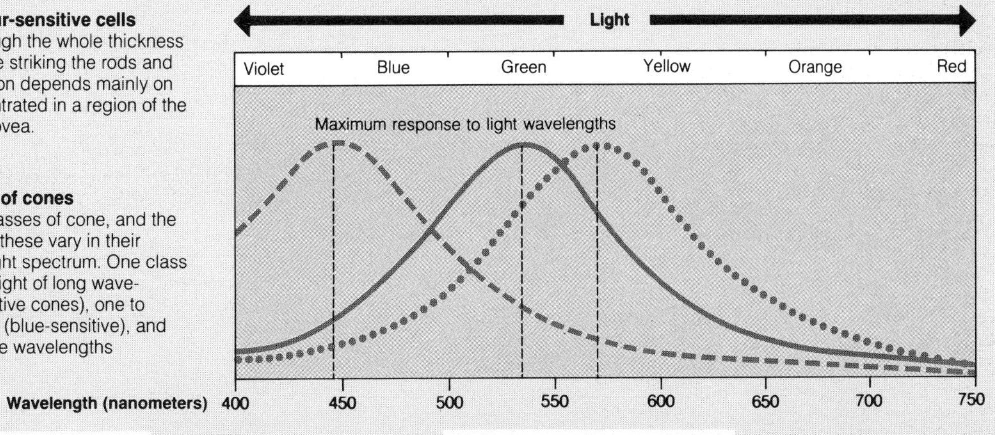

Colour response of cones
There are three classes of cone, and the graph shows how these vary in their response to the light spectrum. One class responds best to light of long wavelengths (red-sensitive cones), one to short wavelengths (blue-sensitive), and one to intermediate wavelengths (green-sensitive).

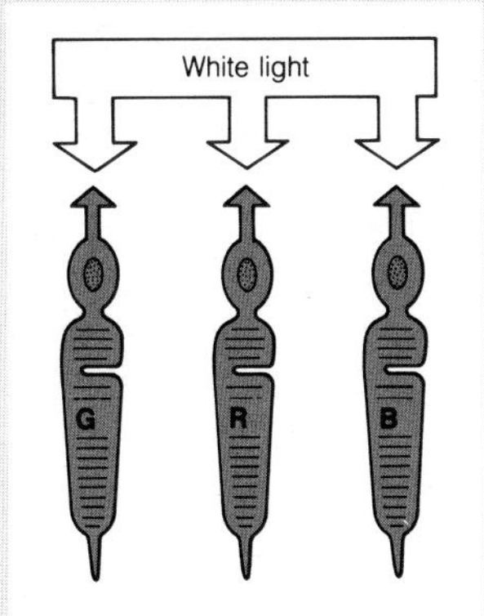

Response to white light
White light consists of a mixture of all wavelengths (colours), so it stimulates all three classes of cone to signal equally. This pattern of response produces the sensation of whiteness in the brain.

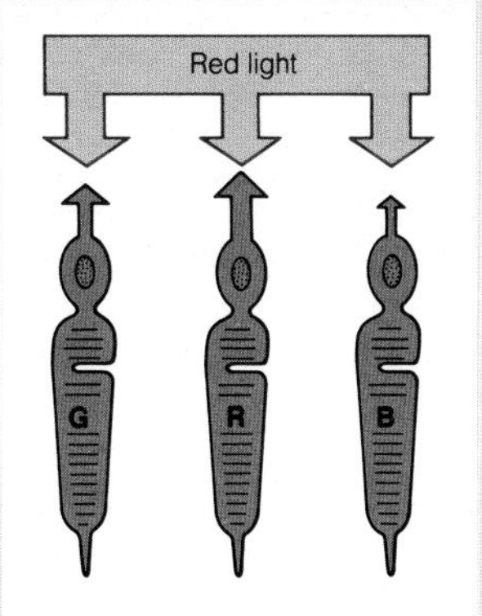

Response to red light
Light with a long wavelength (red light) produces a strong response from red-sensitive cones, a weak response from blue-sensitive cones, and an intermediate response from green-sensitive cones. This pattern of signalling is interpreted as the colour red in the brain.

Key
G Green-sensitive
R Red-sensitive
B Blue-sensitive

C

Light consisting of a single wavelength—pure spectral colour—is rare in nature. The light reflected or emitted by most objects consists of a complex mixture of many different wavelengths, known as a spectral mixture. White light consists of a fairly uniform mixture of all wavelengths of the visible spectrum. The number of possible spectral mixtures is infinite, and a major task of the retina and brain is to sort and interpret the information available in order to produce a usefully large but finite number of perceivable colours (estimated at several million).

CONE FUNCTION

The light-sensitive cells in the retina are of two main types, rods and cones. Of these types, the rods vary little in their response to different light wavelengths, and thus play little, if any, part in colour vision. The cone cells, of which there are roughly four million to seven million per eye, play the major part and are more concentrated within a central area of the retina called the macula lutea; about 25,000 of the cones are in the fovea in the centre of this area. Consequently, colour vision is most accurate for objects viewed directly and is poor at the periphery of vision. Colour perception also requires a minimum level of total available light—below this level, only the rods respond, and everything is seen as shades of grey. When light impinges upon a cone, it causes a structural change in pigment contained within the cone, which in turn causes the cone to emit an electrical impulse. Light of any wavelength and of sufficient intensity, in general, causes all cones to respond to some extent, but any single cone responds better (i.e. produces impulses more frequently) to certain wavelengths than others. Overall, it has been found that there are probably three classes of cone, responding maximally to light wavelengths of 445, 535, and 570 nanometres. Any particular light wavelength produces a unique overall pattern of response from all the cones together, and consequently any two wavelengths produce different patterns of response.

This offers some explanation of how the retina distinguishes light of different wavelengths, but gives few clues as to how information about complex mixtures of wavelengths is sorted, transmitted to the brain, and interpreted. The retina seems to contain other cells that receive, analyse, and compare the signals coming from several classes of cone. Further integration of the signals is accomplished as they are carried to the brain, where additional processing occurs, allowing for the perception of colour. (See also *Colour vision deficiency*; *Eye*; *Perception*; *Vision*.)

Colour vision deficiency

Any abnormality of the *colour vision* system that causes difficulty distinguishing between certain colours. Such deficiencies are of various types and differ markedly in degree. Mild forms of deficiency, which are by far the most common, allow vision that is completely adequate for most purposes.

True "colour blindness" (monochromatism), in which the world is seen only in shades of black, white, and grey, is extremely rare.

CAUSES AND TYPES

Most cases of colour vision deficiency are caused by an inherited defect of the light-sensitive pigment in one or more classes of cone cell in the retina and/or an abnormality or reduced number of the cone cells themselves. Acquired colour vision deficiency may result from certain retinal and optic nerve diseases or from injury.

The two common types of hereditary colour vision deficiency are reduced discrimination of light wavelengths within the middle (green) and long (red) parts of the visible spectrum. In the more severe cases, a person with green deficiency (deuteranopia) has great difficulty distinguishing oranges, greens, brown, and pale reds. For a person with severe red deficiency (protanopia) all reds are markedly dulled. These inherited defects are usually sex-linked (see *Genetic disorders*), i.e. the majority of those affected are male, although women may carry the defect and pass it on to some of their children.

A further very small group have a blue deficiency, called tritanopia, which may be inherited or due to the toxic effects of poisons or drugs on, or degenerative processes of, the retina or optic nerve.

INCIDENCE

Among white people of European origin, about eight per cent of males and less than one per cent of females have either green or red deficiency. The prevalence is generally lower in people of Asian origin and even lower among black people. The prevalence of both blue deficiency and monochromatism may be as low as one affected person per 100,000.

SYMPTOMS

Most people with defective colour vision have no reason to suspect there is anything abnormal about the way they see, because they have no ready access to how other people see the world and because most cases are mild and do not interfere with everyday activities. Most cases come to light only when a person is noticed making mistakes with colour discrimination, such as confusing close shades of colours, or when the person's colour vision is tested.

DIAGNOSIS AND MEASUREMENT

Colour vision is commonly tested, by means of special colour plates under daylight conditions, during childhood or on entry to occupations for which good colour discrimination is needed.

More complicated testing may also be used. The anomaloscope shines a variable mixture of green and red lights, and the person is asked to adjust the mixture until it appears the same as a fixed yellow light. If the adjusted mixture looks far too red or too green to someone with normal vision, the subject of the test is colour defective. The severity of the defect is also measurable in this way.

OUTLOOK

People with the common, inherited, types of colour vision deficiency retain the defect for life. It could be important for them to know about the abnormality, especially if they are considering an occupation that depends on colour discrimination. In particular, a person who is severely colour deficient could be dangerous in certain jobs, such as that of pilot, train driver, or electrician. Mild colour vision deficiencies, however, rarely cause trouble.

Colposcopy

Visual inspection of a woman's *cervix* (neck of the uterus) and *vagina* under illuminated magnification. The procedure is performed with a colposcope, a viewing instrument using a series of lenses to give different degrees of magnification.

WHY IT IS DONE

Colposcopy is performed to recognize or exclude the presence of any areas of precancerous tissue or early cancer in the cervix (see *Cervix, cancer of*). In most cases, the gynaecologist has been alerted by an abnormal *cervical smear test*, by smears that repeatedly show inflammation or infection, or by an abnormal appearance of the cervix during visual inspection at the time of a vaginal examination.

Colposcopy is a painless procedure requiring no anaesthetic. With the woman in the lithotomy position (lying on her back with legs apart and supported), the vagina and cervix are exposed using a speculum (an instrument that widens the opening and separates the walls of the vagina). The exposed tissues are first wiped with a dry sponge; the area is then washed with a solution of either dilute acetic acid or saline. The tissues are visually inspected under magnification to identify any suspicious-looking areas.

The applied solution causes any precancerous areas to show up either white (instead of their natural pink state) or with a characteristic surface pattern due to abnormal blood vessels. Once any such areas are seen, a *biopsy* sample of the tissue can be obtained.

If the biopsy sample shows cells typical of severe dysplasia (abnormal growth) or an early cancer, treatment is required. If the whole of the abnormal area can be seen during colposcopy, the abnormal tissue can be destroyed by *diathermy, cryosurgery,* or *laser treatment*. If any of the abnormal area is within the cervical canal and therefore out of sight of the colposcope, a *cone biopsy* (removal of a conical section of the cervix for inspection) is needed.

Coma
A state of unconsciousness and unresponsiveness distinguishable from *sleep* in that the person does not respond to external stimuli (e.g. shouting or pinching) or to internal stimuli (e.g. a full bladder).

CAUSES
Coma results from disturbance or damage to areas of the brain involved in conscious activity or the maintenance of consciousness—in particular, parts of the *cerebrum* (the main mass of the brain), upper parts of the *brainstem*, and central regions of the brain, especially the *limbic system*.

The damage may be the result of a *head injury*, or of an abnormality such as a *brain tumour, brain abscess,* or *intracerebral haemorrhage*; all are shown by *brain imaging* techniques.

More often, there has been an accumulation of poisonous substances that intoxicate brain tissues (due to a drug overdose, advanced liver or kidney disease, acute alcoholic intoxication, or in uncontrolled *diabetes mellitus*) or there has been impairment of blood flow to some brain areas, leading to cerebral *hypoxia* (lack of oxygen). *Encephalitis* (inflammation of the brain) and *meningitis* (inflammation of the brain's protective coverings) can also cause coma.

SYMPTOMS
Varying depths of coma are recognized. In less severe forms, the person may respond to stimulation by uttering a few words or perhaps moving an arm. In severe cases, the person fails to respond in this way to repeated vigorous stimuli. However, even deeply comatose patients may show some automatic responses—they continue to breathe unaided, may cough, yawn, blink, and show roving eye movements, indicating that the lower brainstem, which controls these responses, is still functioning.

Measurement of variations in the depth of coma is important in assessment and treatment. Variations can be recorded by systems that classify the coma according to the person's verbal behaviour, the movements he or she makes, and the state of the eyes (whether open, shut, or roving).

A person may remain alive for many years in a state of deep coma provided the brainstem is still functioning (and also provided he or she receives appropriate nursing care). If the lower brainstem is damaged or diseased, the vital functions of coughing, swallowing, and breathing are impaired and artificial ventilation and maintenance of the circulation may be needed to maintain life. Complete irreversible loss of brainstem function leads to death (see *Brain death*).

Combination drug
A preparation that contains more than one active, therapeutic substance. A common example of a combination drug is the antibiotic co-trimoxazole, which contains sulphamethoxazole and trimethoprim.

Comedo
Another name for a *blackhead*.

Commensal
A usually harmless bacterium or other organism that normally lives in or on the body. Occasionally, commensals may cause disease, especially in people with impaired immunity.

Commode
A portable chair that contains a removable toilet bowl in its seat. Commodes are useful for patients who are not confined to bed but who are not mobile enough to use the toilet.

Communicable disease
Any disease caused by a microorganism or parasite that can be transmitted (directly or indirectly) from one person or animal to another. (See also *Contagious; Infectious disease*.)

Compartment syndrome
A painful cramp caused by compression of a group of muscles within a confined space. An example is *shin splints* (also known as tibial compartment syndrome), which affects the muscles on the outer side of the shin.

The condition may occur if muscles have become enlarged as a result of intensive training or injury. During exercise, blood flow into muscles increases and they expand slightly. In compartment syndrome, the muscles are compressed, causing cramps due to obstruction of the blood flow through them. Cramps induced by exercise usually disappear when the exercise is stopped. Severe cases may require *fasciotomy* surgery to improve blood flow and prevent development of a permanent *contracture* (deformity caused by shrinkage of tissues).

Compensation neurosis
Psychological reaction to injury affected by the prospect of financial compensation, also called accident or "traumatic" neurosis.

Symptoms in compensation neurosis vary from person to person, but headache, dizzy spells, loss of concentration, anxiety, and mild depression are common, as are neurological symptoms, such as pain and tingling in the legs or numbness in the affected part. Symptoms do not depend necessarily on the severity of the injury.

Some specialists consider the neurosis to be a genuine and persistent psychiatric reaction; others insist it is an attempt, conscious or unconscious, to manipulate the situation for profit. Repeated medical assessments, legal wrangling, and contradictory experts make this one of the most difficult areas of psychiatric diagnosis. Backing the idea of a genuine organic disorder, recent studies have shown that some people's symptoms persisted even after a satisfactory settlement of their insurance claims.

Complement
A group of proteins in *blood* plasma. Complement is an important part of the *immune system*, destroying foreign cells. The complement system is usually activated by reactions between antigens and antibodies.

C

Complex

A term meaning a group or combination of related items. In medicine it is used, for example, to refer to a combination of signs and symptoms forming a syndrome (as in *Eisenmenger complex*) or to a collection of substances that share a similar structure or function (as in *vitamin B complex*).

In psychology, a complex is a group of unconscious ideas, beliefs, and memories that have great emotional importance. The term was first used by Sigmund Freud and Carl Jung to sum up psychological states deriving from experiences and relationships in childhood. The *Oedipus complex* is an important example, affecting all levels of adult behaviour and attitudes.

Compliance

The degree to which patients follow medical advice. Research suggests that the degree of compliance is generally greater among patients who are provided with adequate information. For example, patients are more likely to comply with a drug treatment if they know whether the drug is likely to produce side-effects and under what circumstances the drug should be discontinued.

Complication

A condition that results from a preceding disorder or from the treatment of that disorder. For example, in a case of *appendicitis*, the inflamed appendix may rupture, spreading infection throughout the abdominal cavity and causing a serious complication called *peritonitis*. The childhood condition *mumps* occasionally has complications that may be serious, particularly *encephalitis* (inflammation of the brain) or *orchitis* (inflammation of the testes). Recovery from an operation may be complicated by *wound infection*.

Compos mentis

Latin for "of sound mind".

Compress

A pad of lint or linen applied, under pressure, to an area of skin, and held in place by a bandage. The pad may be soaked in ice-cold water or wrapped around ice to provide a cold compress for reducing pain, swelling, and bleeding under the skin after an injury (see *Ice pack*).

Compresses that have been soaked in hot water increase the circulation and are useful for bringing boils to a head. A dry compress may be used to stop bleeding from a wound (see

Bleeding first-aid box) or may be smeared with medication to help treat an infected area of skin.

Compression syndrome

A collection of symptoms caused by pressure on a nerve that supplies the muscles in a particular area of the body and carries sensations from that area. The symptoms may include numbness, tingling, discomfort, and muscle weakness. The best known is *carpal tunnel syndrome* (which affects the hand), caused by pressure on the median nerve as it passes under a ligament in the wrist.

Compulsive behaviour

See *Obsessive-compulsive disorder*.

Computed tomography

Another name for *CT scanning*.

Computer-aided diagnosis

The doctor makes a diagnosis by considering the patient's symptoms and medical history, examining the patient, and, when necessary, making use of special tests and procedures. The computer has made possible many new investigative procedures, such as *CT scanning* and *MRI* (see *Imaging techniques*). It can also be used to aid diagnosis in the following ways.

PROBABILITY-BASED SYSTEMS
With probability-based systems the computer is used to store vast quantities of information involving cases of many different disorders. For example, it may be programmed with the details of thousands of cases of stomach pain—giving, for each patient, the exact type, location, and duration of the pain, accompanying symptoms, and the relevant medical history, together with the eventual diagnosis. A doctor confronted with a new case of stomach pain can enter the details into the computer, which, in a matter of seconds, will compare them with those already stored in its memory. It will then print out a list of the most likely diagnoses.

Although such computers are currently used in comparatively few hospitals, they are proving valuable in the treatment of people isolated from medical services, such as oil-rig crews or deep-sea divers. If someone becomes ill, the computer may be used to diagnose whether the case is an emergency requiring the person to be transported to a hospital.

PATTERN-RECOGNITION SYSTEMS
Computers can also be programmed to recognize and interpret visual data.

One example is the examination of cells under a microscope. The computer has the ability to recognize abnormal cells. This could be of great future significance in certain types of *blood count* (e.g. a differential white blood cell count) and also in *cervical smear tests*, in which cells taken from the cervix are examined under a microscope for early signs of cancer. At present, each of the millions of smears taken annually needs examination by a laboratory technician, who can check only a comparatively small number per day.

Conception

The *fertilization* of a woman's *ovum* (egg) by a man's *sperm*, followed about five days later by implantation of the resultant blastocyst in the lining of the *uterus*, thus starting a *pregnancy*. (See also *Contraception*.)

Concussion

Brief unconsciousness, usually lasting only a few seconds, that follows a violent blow to the head or neck. The loss of consciousness is due to disturbance of the electrical activity in the brain, and in most cases is not associated with any damage. Nevertheless, concussion should always be reported to a doctor because of the possibility of serious consequences.

Among the more common causes of concussion are traffic accidents, sports injuries, falls, industrial accidents, and blows received in fights.

SYMPTOMS AND TREATMENT
Common symptoms immediately following concussion include confusion, inability to remember events immediately before the injury, dizziness, blurred vision, and vomiting. The more prolonged the period of unconsciousness, the more severe and persistent symptoms tend to be.

Repeated concussion—as happens, for example, to some boxers—can damage the brain and cause the "punch-drunk" syndrome: slow thinking, impaired concentration, and slurred speech.

Anyone who has been knocked out should see a doctor, who will usually advise 24 hours of bed rest, either in hospital or at home, under observation. The person should not drive a car or play any sport during this time. If new symptoms develop, such as drowsiness, difficulty breathing, repeated vomiting, or visual disturbances, they should be reported to the doctor immediately since they could signify damage to part of the brain or an *extradural haemorrhage* (bleeding between the skull and the outside of the brain).

The initial symptoms usually start to clear within a few days. If they fail to do so, medical opinion should be sought again, at which time the doctor may wish to have the condition investigated further. (See also *Head injury*.)

Conditioning

The formation of a specific response or type of behaviour to a specific stimulus in the environment. Theories of conditioning are based largely on the work of the Russian physiologist Ivan Pavlov and the American psychologist B.F. Skinner.

TYPES

CLASSICAL CONDITIONING If a stimulus that consistently produces a particular response is paired repeatedly with a second stimulus (which would not itself produce the response), the second stimulus (the conditioned stimulus) will eventually produce the response even without the presence of the first stimulus (the unconditioned stimulus).

Classical conditioning was described by Pavlov, who demonstrated the phenomenon in dogs. He noted that food (the unconditioned stimulus) caused dogs to salivate (the unconditioned response). He found that if a bell (the conditioned stimulus) was rung immediately before the food was presented to the dog, the dog would eventually produce the conditioned response of salivating when it heard the bell alone, without any food being presented.

Pavlov noted that a conditioned response to a specific conditioned stimulus would also occur in response to a similar conditioned stimulus. Thus, a dog conditioned to salivate when shown a round object would also salivate, although not as much, when shown an elliptical one. He also found that the conditioned response would eventually fade unless reinforced by occasional pairing of the conditioned with the unconditioned stimulus.

OPERANT CONDITIONING The central concept of this type of conditioning is that behaviour can be modified by a system of rewards and/or punishments.

Much of the early work in this field was done by B.F. Skinner, who demonstrated the phenomenon in laboratory animals. Skinner placed a hungry rat in a box. It moved randomly about the cage, but occasionally accidentally pawed a lever, which released a pellet of food. Eventually the rat learned that the action of pressing the lever led to the reward of food. Thus the rat became conditioned to press the lever whenever it wanted food.

EFFECTS

Many behavioural psychologists believe that all behaviour is learned by a process of conditioning. They regard some psychiatric problems as inappropriate behaviour patterns that have been learned through conditioning. Treatment for these disorders can also be based on the principles of conditioning, which can be used to modify inappropriate behaviour patterns (see *Behaviour therapy*).

Condom

A barrier method of contraception in the form of a thin latex rubber or plastic sheath placed over the penis before intercourse. In addition to their contraceptive effect, condoms provide both partners with some degree of protection against the sexual transmission of disease. (See *Contraception, barrier methods of*.)

Condom, female

A barrier method of contraception in the form of a vaginal sheath inserted before intercourse. (See *Contraception, barrier methods of*.)

Conduct disorders

A group of behavioural disturbances, occurring in childhood or adolescence, in which the individual persistently and repetitively violates the rights and privileges of others. These violations may include vandalism, arson, assault, and robbery, as well as less aggressive forms of behaviour such as truancy, substance abuse, and persistent lying. (See also *Behavioural problems in children; Adolescence*.)

Condyloma acuminatum

See *Warts, genital*.

Cone biopsy

A surgical technique in which a conical or cylindrical section of the lower part of the *cervix* (neck of the uterus) is removed.

WHY IT IS DONE

A cone biopsy is performed if a woman has had an abnormal *cervical smear test* or a series of abnormal smears, and if visual inspection of the cervix by *colposcopy* has failed to delineate the exact area of cancer or a precancerous condition (see *Cervix, cancer of*). Sometimes a cone biopsy is performed if a smear test suggests the presence of cancer, but colposcopy has failed to detect any abnormality on the outer surface of the cervix or at the entrance to the canal. In the latter cases there may be a precancerous area or cancer confined to the cervical canal, out of sight of the colposcope.

Cone biopsy can now be accomplished by *laser treatment* or by *cryosurgery*. (See also illustrated box on biopsy of the *Cervix*.)

Confabulation

The use of a fictional story to make up for gaps in memory. Confabulation differs from lying in that it is motivated by the need to make sense of one's past rather than by a desire to deceive a listener. The phenomenon occurs most commonly in chronic alcoholics suffering from *Wernicke-Korsakoff syndrome*. It also occurs in some people with head injuries.

Confidentiality

The ethical principle that a doctor does not disclose to others information given in confidence by a patient. This concept was introduced by the ancient Greek physician Hippocrates and has been adopted by medical associations in all countries.

The doctor's responsibility for maintaining confidential records has become more difficult with modern trends in medical practice. Clinics and health centres may have scores of medical and ancillary staff with access to records. In hospitals with computerized records, thousands of staff members may have such access. To prevent breaches in confidentiality, everyone working in a medical setting is expected to understand and respect the code of confidentiality. Some computer systems make it possible to render the sensitive sections of medical records secure.

The patient's consent to disclosure is required before a doctor may give confidential information to an employer, insurance company, or lawyer. When required by law to disclose confidential information, a doctor (unlike a lawyer) does not have any "privilege" that allows refusal. A doctor who persists in refusal is in contempt of court.

Doctors who treat children are expected to discuss their findings with the parents. As children mature, a point is reached at which their confidences merit the same respect as those of adult patients. In general, doctors believe that they should respect a child's request for confidentiality.

C

Most legal systems require doctors to override confidentiality in certain circumstances. For example, they are required to notify specified infectious diseases; if patients with certain of these diseases refuse treatment, the health authorities may be informed so that treatment or isolation may be imposed by law. Doctors are also generally required to notify the police if they treat gunshot wounds or know of other serious crimes.

Doctors who breach confidentiality without legal justification may be sued in the civil courts and damages may be awarded against them. They may also be brought before the ethical committee of their professional body, which may have the right to suspend or cancel their legal right to practise.

Confusion

A disorganized mental state in which the abilities to remember, think clearly, and reason are impaired.

TYPES AND CAUSES

Confusion can be acute or chronic. Acute confusion can arise as a symptom of *delirium*, in which the activity of the brain is affected by fever, drugs, poisons, or injury. Elderly people are particularly prone to acute confusional states from these causes, and especially from certain drugs (e.g. *antianxiety drugs* or *alcohol*).

Chronic confusion is often associated with *alcohol dependence*, long-term use of antianxiety drugs, and certain organic (physically based) mental disorders. Chronic confusion is a feature of *dementia*, a brain disorder commonly caused by the progressive degeneration and death of brain cells.

SYMPTOMS AND SIGNS

People who are acutely confused are temporarily unable to organize their thoughts. They may also suffer from terrifying hallucinations and may behave in a violent and abusive manner. Few people are able to recollect the period of confusion once it has passed.

Chronic confusion is generally noticeable by features such as absent-mindedness, poor short-term memory, and a tendency for the sufferer to repeat himself or herself. Chronically confused people may also become depressed and frustrated, but they are less likely to become aggressive or violent. Many of the conditions responsible for chronic confusion tend to be slowly progressive.

DIAGNOSIS AND TREATMENT

The cause of a person's confusion can often be diagnosed from a detailed description of the symptoms (often from a relative) and a general physical examination of the patient. In some cases, further tests may be necessary for an accurate diagnosis.

Treatment varies a great deal, depending on the underlying cause, and can often produce a marked improvement. *Sedative drugs* may be of benefit to some people who are acutely confused. Drugs are of little help to elderly chronically confused patients, for whom skilled, supervised care is the most important aspect of treatment.

Congenital

A term that means "present at birth". Thus, a congenital abnormality may have been inherited from the parents, may have occurred as the result of damage or infection in the uterus, or may have occurred at the time of birth. Congenital abnormalities are often also called *birth defects*.

Note that "congenital" does not mean the same as "hereditary". Not all congenital abnormalities are inherited, and many hereditary diseases (such as *Huntington's chorea*) are not apparent at birth.

Diseases and disorders that are neither congenital nor inherited but which are caused by external factors—for example, infection, injury or poisoning—are termed "acquired".

Congestion

A term that usually refers to the accumulation of an excessive amount of blood, *tissue fluid*, or *lymph* in part of the body.

A major cause of congestion is an increase in the flow of blood to a particular area of the body, as occurs in inflammation. Another possible cause of congestion is reduced drainage of blood from the affected area, as can occur in *heart failure*, in venous disorders such as *varicose veins*, and in *lymphatic disorders*.

In *nasal congestion*, inflammation of the nasal lining is accompanied by an increase in mucus production.

Congestive heart failure

See *Heart failure*.

Conjunctiva

The transparent membrane covering the sclera (white of the eye) and lining the inside of the eyelids. Cells in the conjunctiva produce a fluid (similar to tears) that lubricates the lids and the cornea. Blood vessels within the conjunctiva are normally invisible to the naked eye, but become engorged in *conjunctivitis* and other inflammatory conditions.

Conjunctivitis

Inflammation of the conjunctiva, causing redness, discomfort, and a discharge from the affected eye. Conjunctivitis is very common: at least one person in 50 who visits a doctor does so because of this complaint.

CAUSES AND TYPES

The common causes are infections (especially in children) and allergy (more common in adults).

INFECTIVE CONJUNCTIVITIS Most conjunctival infections are caused by bacteria (e.g. staphylococci), which are spread by hand-to-eye contact, or by viruses associated with a cold, sore throat, or illness such as *measles*. Viral conjunctivitis sometimes occurs in epidemics, spreading rapidly through schools and other groups.

Newborn babies occasionally develop conjunctivitis soon after birth, a condition known as neonatal *ophthalmia*. This condition results from the spread of infection from the mother's cervix during birth and may be caused by various microorganisms, including those responsible for *gonorrhoea*, genital *herpes*, or *chlamydial infection*. The infection may spread to the entire eye and can cause blindness.

Keratoconjunctivitis is an inflammation of both the conjunctiva and the cornea; it is often due to a viral infection. *Trachoma* is a serious form of conjunctivitis; it is caused by a type of chlamydial infection that is most common in tropical countries.

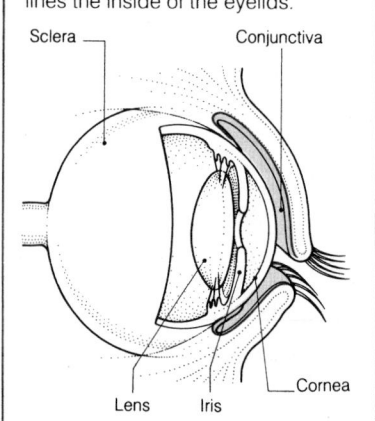

LOCATION OF CONJUNCTIVA
This transparent membrane covers the white of the eye and lines the inside of the eyelids.

Sclera

Conjunctiva

Lens

Iris

Cornea

ALLERGIC CONJUNCTIVITIS An allergic response of the conjunctiva may be provoked by a variety of substances, including cosmetics (such as mascara), contact lens cleaning solutions, and pollen.

SYMPTOMS

All types of conjunctivitis cause redness, irritation, itching, discharge, and occasionally photophobia (abnormal sensitivity to bright light). In infective conjunctivitis the discharge contains pus and may cause the eyelids to be stuck together in the morning. In allergic conjunctivitis the discharge is clear, and the eyelids are often swollen.

DIAGNOSIS

Diagnosis is made from the appearance of the eye. If an infection is suspected, swabs may be taken to find out the causative organism, especially in a newborn baby when an exact diagnosis may be needed.

TREATMENT

Warm water is used to wash away the discharge and remove any crusts on the eyelids.

Suspected infections are treated with eye-drops or ointment containing an *antibiotic drug* (such as *chloramphenicol*). Viral conjunctivitis tends to get better without treatment.

Allergic conjunctivitis may be relieved by the use of eye-drops containing an *antihistamine drug*. Occasionally, eye-drops containing a *corticosteroid drug* may be prescribed provided that there is definitely no accompanying infection (which could be worsened by a corticosteroid).

Connective tissue

The material that holds together the various structures of the body. Some structures are made up of connective tissue, notably *tendons* and *cartilage*. Connective tissue also forms the matrix (ground substance) of *bone* and the nonmuscular structures of *arteries* and *veins*.

Connective tissue diseases

See *Collagen diseases*.

Conn's syndrome

A disorder caused by the secretion of excessive amounts of the hormone aldosterone by a benign tumour of one of the adrenal glands. (See also *Aldosteronism*.)

Consciousness

An awareness of self and surroundings, so that a person knows what he or she is doing and intends to do. The awareness is dependent on sensations (especially visual and auditory), memories, and experiences.

Such awareness requires intact brain function, particularly within the *cerebrum* (the main mass of the brain) and the reticular system in the *brainstem*. The content of consciousness relies heavily on the functions of the cerebrum—for example, on memory and the interpretation of sensations—while wakefulness is linked with the reticular system.

Although a person may be conscious, a great deal that goes on within the brain is still below the level of consciousness. In psychological terms this activity is referred to as *subconscious* activity.

Disturbance of consciousness leads to impaired attention, concentration, and understanding. Thought processes become slowed and memory fails. There appears to be a lack of direction to thoughts and actions. Although patients can be stimulated to respond, their responses are faulty. As the level of arousal deteriorates, the person may eventually pass into a state of *stupor* and then *coma*.

Consent

The legal term describing a patient's agreement to a doctor performing an operation, arranging drug treatment, or carrying out diagnostic tests. Strictly, consent is valid only if the patient has been fully informed about the purpose of the procedure, the likely outcome, and both common and rare complications and side-effects that may arise.

AVAILABILITY OF INFORMATION

Even as recently as the 1960s many doctors believed it necessary to conceal much of the information about an illness and its treatment from the patient and his or her family. At that time few doctors told patients they had cancer, even when the illness was at an advanced stage, and few told such patients that they would die. Similarly, few doctors discussed the small risk of serious complications or death that accompanies any surgical procedure requiring an anaesthetic, or explained the full range of side-effects possible from treatment with a particular drug.

This concealment was justified by the medical profession in the paternalistic belief that the doctor knew best, and that patients were unable to understand technical terms or concepts. The consumer rights movements of the 1960s and 1970s swept away such ideas, and doctors now recognize that patients expect full and frank information about illness and its treatment. Nevertheless, in many countries, including the UK, doctors are still allowed to conceal rare hazards if they believe that such a policy is in the patient's best interests.

The amount of detailed information offered to patients varies from doctor to doctor. Some distribute printed information sheets before asking patients to sign consent forms, while others discuss the issues at length. Many doctors tell patients that they will answer their questions honestly, but will not force unwanted information on them.

When the investigation or treatment is carried out solely for the patient's benefit the explanations may be fairly brief, but more detail must usually be offered when patients are asked to take part in research studies that may be of no direct benefit to them as individuals. Under these circumstances the purpose of the study must be explained along with all its hazards. Consent to a research procedure is invalid if any pressure was placed on the patient (for example, by suggestions that participation in the study would ensure preferential treatment by a surgeon).

WITHHOLDING CONSENT

Consent cannot be given by children or by people with serious mental disorders. Consent may be given (or withheld) on their behalf by parents or relatives. On several occasions in recent years, however, the courts have been asked to intervene and overrule the consent of relatives to withhold treatment from newborn children with severe handicaps. This action by the courts is based on the doctrine that the law forbids euthanasia or assisted suicide, whether or not consent is given by or on behalf of the patient. Consent may not be given on behalf of children or the mentally ill for research procedures that would be of no benefit to them as individuals.

Constipation

The infrequent or difficult passing of hard, dry *faeces*. In most cases constipation is harmless, but occasionally it may be a symptom of an underlying disorder, especially if it is of recent onset in an adult over 40. Many people worry that they do not move their bowels often enough, but, in fact, regularity and comfort of bowel action are more important than fre-

C

CONSTIPATION Infrequent or difficult passing of hard bowel movements.

? Have you always tended to suffer from constipation?

YES → Do you often resist the urge to move your bowels because you are too busy?

YES → This can lead to an eventual loss of normal bowel reflexes. You should try to reestablish a regular habit by always going to the toilet when you feel the urge.

NO ↓

Have you used laxatives regularly for a long time?

YES → Overuse of laxatives can eventually make your bowel inactive. Stop taking the laxatives and try adding bran and extra fruit to your diet instead.

See • *Laxative drugs*

NO ↓

NO ↓ (from first question)

Dietary fibre
This should be an essential part of everyone's diet because it provides bulk to help the large intestine carry away body wastes. Not only does it help prevent constipation and certain diseases of the large intestine but it may also help lower the level of fats in the body.

→ Your constipation is probably due to a lack of fluid, fruits, vegetables, and whole-grain cereals in your diet. Increase your intake. If no improvement results, consult your doctor.

See • *Fibre, dietary*

? Has defaecation become painful?

YES → A tear in the lining of the anus or haemorrhoids may cause such pain. Consult your doctor.

See • *Anal fissure*
• *Haemorrhoids*

NO ↓

? Do you have lower abdominal pain?

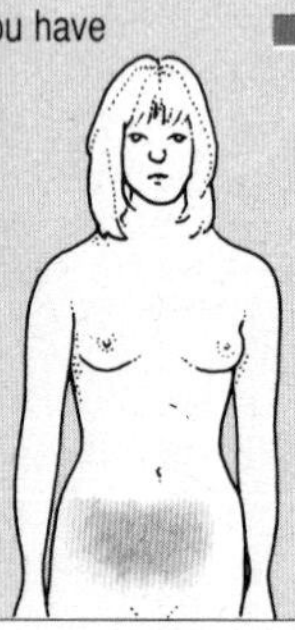

YES → Have you had similar episodes of pain and constipation for many years?

YES → You probably have an irritable bowel. Consult your doctor.

See • *Irritable bowel syndrome*

NO ↓

☎
Consult your doctor without delay!
An irritable bowel or diverticular disease (pouches in the walls of the large intestine) may cause such symptoms. However, the slight possibility of intestinal cancer must also be ruled out.

See • *Diverticular disease*
• *Intestine, cancer of*
• *Irritable bowel syndrome*

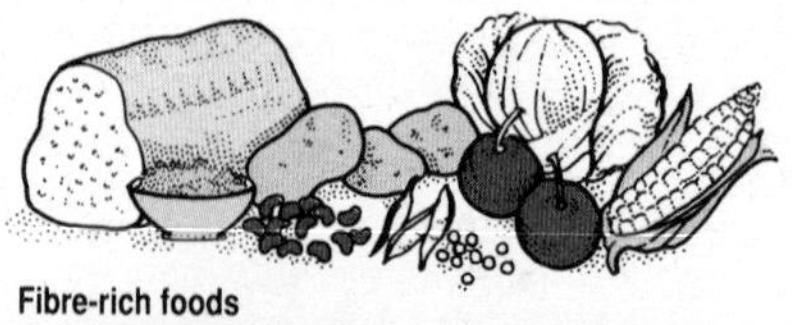

Fibre-rich foods
Fruit, leafy vegetables, potato skins, whole-meal bread and cereals, dried peas and beans, and bran are all examples of high-fibre foods.

NO ↓

Continued on next page

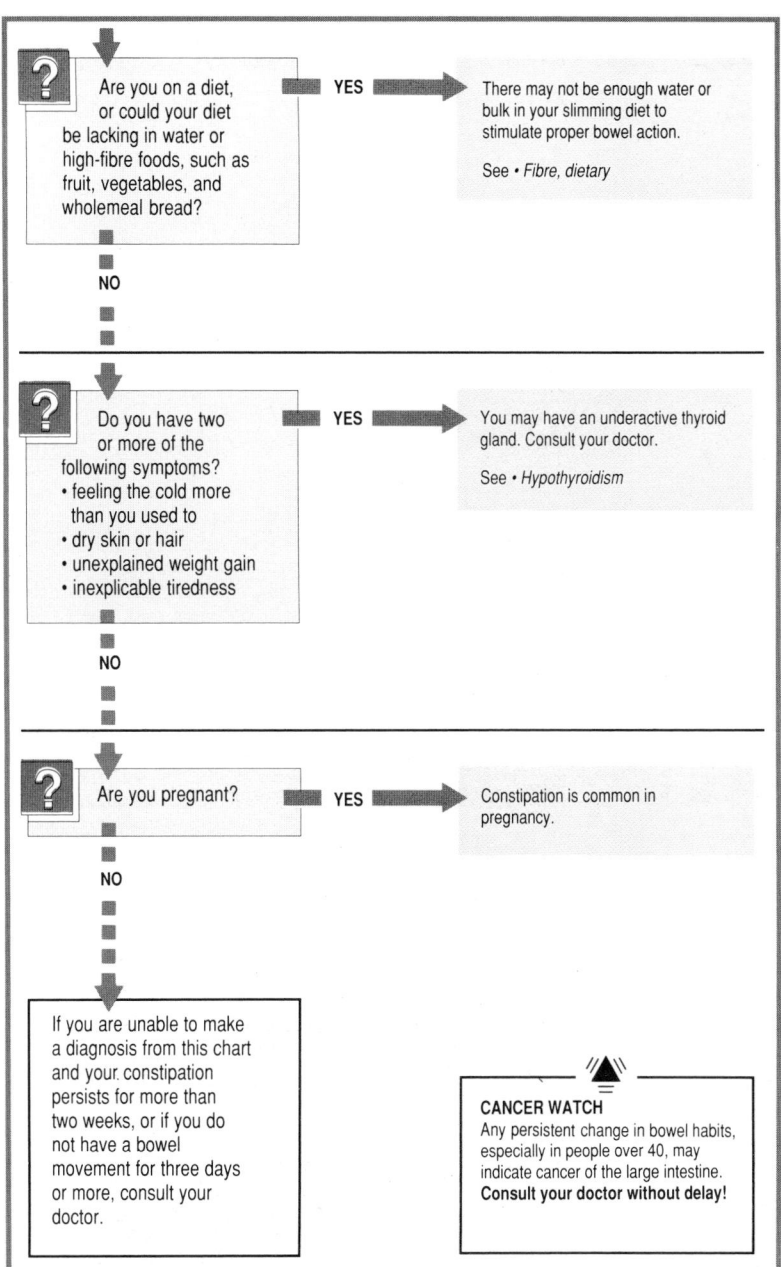

Are you on a diet, or could your diet be lacking in water or high-fibre foods, such as fruit, vegetables, and wholemeal bread?

YES → There may not be enough water or bulk in your slimming diet to stimulate proper bowel action.

See • Fibre, dietary

NO

Do you have two or more of the following symptoms?
• feeling the cold more than you used to
• dry skin or hair
• unexplained weight gain
• inexplicable tiredness

YES → You may have an underactive thyroid gland. Consult your doctor.

See • Hypothyroidism

NO

Are you pregnant?

YES → Constipation is common in pregnancy.

NO

If you are unable to make a diagnosis from this chart and your constipation persists for more than two weeks, or if you do not have a bowel movement for three days or more, consult your doctor.

CANCER WATCH
Any persistent change in bowel habits, especially in people over 40, may indicate cancer of the large intestine. **Consult your doctor without delay!**

quency. However, any persistent change in the pattern of bowel movements should be investigated by a doctor to rule out the possibility of a serious disorder.

CAUSES
The most common cause of constipation in developed countries is insufficient *fibre* in the diet. Fibre, which is found in foods such as wholemeal bread, fresh fruit, and vegetables, provides the bulk that the muscles of

the *colon* (the major part of the large intestine) need to stimulate propulsion of the faeces.

Lack of regular bowel-moving habits is another cause of constipation. This may be the result of poor toilet-training in childhood or of repeatedly ignoring the urge to move the bowels. In the elderly the latter is sometimes due to immobility. Another cause of constipation in some elderly people is weakness of the

muscles of the abdomen and the pelvic floor, which prevents adequate pressure when attempting to move the bowels.

In people suffering from *haemorrhoids* (piles) or an *anal fissure* (a crack in the skin around the anus), the pain experienced on passing faeces can be severe enough to inhibit the initiation of bowel movements.

In *irritable bowel syndrome*, the person may experience intermittent constipation, sometimes alternating with diarrhoea. In *hypothyroidism*, colonic contractions slow down and result in chronic constipation. Narrowing of part of the colon—due to *diverticular disease* or cancer (see *Colon, cancer of*), for example—is another possible cause of constipation.

INVESTIGATION
A doctor usually investigates the condition by obtaining a detailed case history, carrying out a physical examination, and sometimes arranging for special tests.

TREATMENT
Prolonged use of *laxative drugs* can impair the normal functioning of the colon, and their use should generally be avoided except in cases where straining to pass faeces will aggravate another existing condition, such as haemorrhoids.

Constipation can usually be cured by a few self-help measures—establishing a regular routine for using the toilet, acting on any urge to move the bowels, increasing the amount of fibre in the diet, and drinking more fluids. If constipation continues despite these measures, medical advice should be obtained.

A doctor should also be consulted if constipation occurs after years of normal bowel habits, or if it is accompanied by blood in the faeces, pain on moving the bowels, loss of a sense of well-being, or weight loss.

Constriction
A narrowed area, or the process of narrowing, as of the pupil.

Contact lenses
Very thin, shell-like, transparent discs fitted on the *cornea* (the transparent outer coating of the eye) to correct defective *vision*. Contact lenses alter the power of the cornea by replacing the existing outer surface with a plastic surface that is curved to compensate for the visual defect.

Leonardo da Vinci in 1508 was the first to describe the possibility of using contact lenses. The first lens was

C

made by Eugen Frick in 1887; it was made of glass and covered the entire front surface of the eye. The conventional small hard lens made of transparent plastic was first introduced in the 1940s and many millions have been used since.

WHY THEY ARE USED

Contact lenses can correct most of the defects in vision for which glasses are prescribed and can correct some conditions that glasses cannot.

Vanity and convenience account for most contact-lens wear. Unlike glasses, contact lenses are almost undetectable when worn, generally do not fall off, do not get covered with rain, and normally do not mist up.

Contact lenses are useful for some people with particular optical problems or medical conditions. For people who have extreme *myopia* (shortsightedness) or who have had cataracts removed, contact lenses may be preferable to glasses because glasses can produce considerable distortion of vision in these cases. Contact lenses can also be useful for hiding scars on the surface of the cornea. Patients with irregular corneas (such as may follow corneal disease, corneal injury, corneal ulceration, or corneal grafting) may be helped by contact lenses.

TYPES

HARD PLASTIC LENSES These give good optical vision, are long-lasting and durable (possibly five years or more of use), inexpensive, and easy to maintain. However, they are sometimes difficult to tolerate and occasionally fall out; severe pain can result if grit gets into the eye and under the lens. When the lenses are removed after prolonged wear, vision with glasses may be temporarily blurred.

HARD, GAS-PERMEABLE LENSES Introduced in the early 1980s, these have the same visual qualities as hard plastic lenses, but are more comfortable and easier to get used to because they allow oxygen to pass through the lens to the eye. However, they are less durable (possibly giving up to five years of wear) and more expensive.

SOFT LENSES Also called hydrophilic (having a strong affinity for water) lenses, these are the most comfortable because of their high water content, which can range from 38 to 80 per cent. They are usually easy to wear from the beginning, can be worn for long periods, and are ideal for occasional use since the eye generally tolerates them for short periods of time despite infrequent wearing. Soft lenses can correct myopia and *hyper-*

CARE AND INSERTION OF CONTACT LENSES

Hard lenses may require several solutions, one for cleaning, one for wetting, and possibly one for storage. If used, the storage solution is washed off before lens insertion. The wetting solution is used before inserting a lens in the eye.

Care of soft lenses is more complicated. Because the lenses are permeable and absorb any chemicals they come in contact with, the solutions must be weaker. Disinfection with a chemical or heating system is required to prevent contamination and infection. Two or three solutions may be necessary, but intermittent cleaning with a third system, such as an enzyme tablet or an oxidizing agent, is also required to remove mucus and protein.

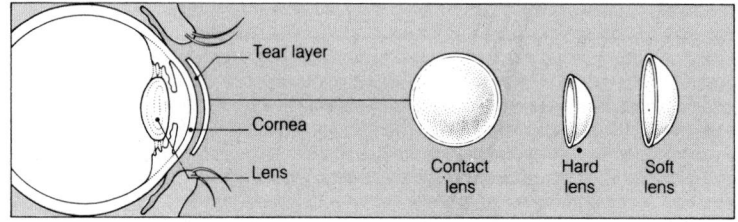

Tear layer
Cornea
Lens
Contact lens
Hard lens
Soft lens

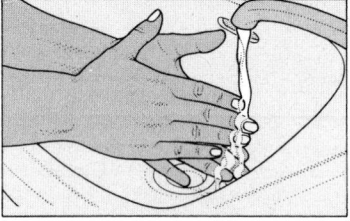

1 Wash your hands thoroughly under running water and carefully rinse off all traces of soap.

Inverted lens

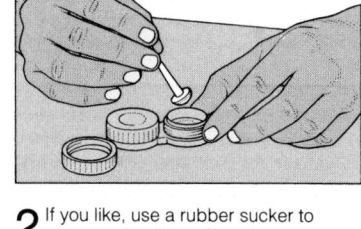

2 If you like, use a rubber sucker to remove a hard lens from its container. Rinse the lens thoroughly.

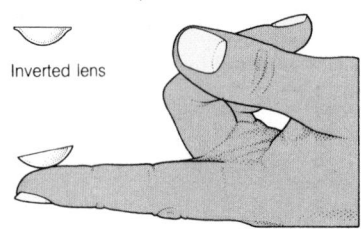

3 Place the lens on your index finger. If it is a soft lens, make sure that it has not turned inside out. If it has, you will see an out-turned rim.

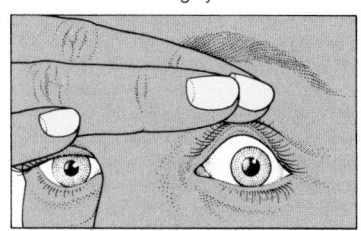

4 Keep both eyes open, hold the upper lid open, and look straight ahead or at the lens as you bring it up to your eye.

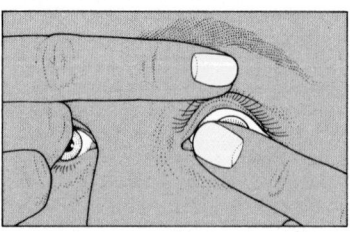

5 Place the lens on your eye. Look downwards and then release the lid. If necessary, the lens may be centred by gently massaging the eyelid (the photograph on the right shows a hard lens correctly positioned).

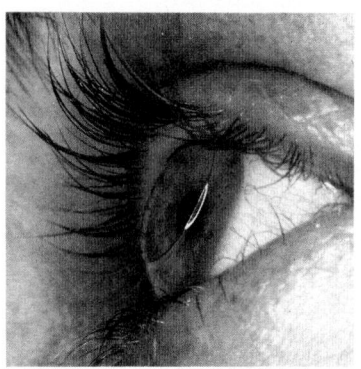

metropia (longsightedness). They cannot correct much *astigmatism* because, being flexible, they mould themselves to the shape of the eye, and thus cannot correct the irregularly shaped cornea that is the cause of this condition. Other drawbacks of soft lenses include fragility, a relatively short life (12 to 18 months), more complicated maintenance, and a higher price than hard lenses.

Extremely thin, specially designed soft lenses with a high water content can be worn for periods of up to one month. These "extended-wear" contact lenses may increase the risks and dangers of infection.

SPECIAL LENSES Rigid, scleral lenses, which cover the whole of the front of the eye, are used to hide eyes disfigured by injury or disease. Hard or soft bifocal contact lenses can be produced, but can be difficult to fit, and vision may not be satisfactory.

Toric contact lenses (lenses of uneven surface curvature) are a type of soft lens used to correct high degrees of astigmatism; such lenses can be made in all materials.

CARE

Basic care procedures are shown in the illustrated box opposite. Periodic follow-up examinations are needed to ensure that the lenses continue to fit correctly and that they are not harming the eyes.

PROBLEMS

A few people are unable to wear contact lenses because they have particularly sensitive eyes, difficult optical requirements, or poor personal hygiene habits.

Lenses can irritate the eye because of dryness due to problems with tear production, which may be inadequate, especially in older people.

Hard plastic contact lenses may cause abrasion of the cornea if they are worn for too long. Symptoms are pain and excessive tear production. Covering the affected eye with a patch and/or applying eye-drops containing *antibiotic drugs* usually clear up symptoms within 24 hours.

Some people who wear soft lenses develop sensitivity of the eyes and lids either to the maintenance solutions or to altered mucus. Symptoms include decreased lens tolerance, stinging, increased lens movement, increased mucus, and redness of the conjunctiva. An affected person must generally stop wearing contact lenses for several months and then start again with new lenses and a different type of maintenance solution.

Other problems that may occur with any type of contact lens are infections, redness of the eye, and unexpected changes in the eye itself. Contact lens wear should be stopped and an eye examination arranged if the eyes become red or infected, if vision is blurred, or if the lenses become uncomfortable.

Contact tracing

A service, provided by clinics treating *sexually transmitted diseases* (STDs), that aims to control their spread.

WHY IT IS DONE

If a person is diagnosed as having an STD, it may be possible to identify from whom it was caught and to whom it may have been passed on. If these contacts are encouraged to have an examination and to receive treatment if necessary, the spread of the disease can be reduced. Contacts may be infected although they may have no obvious symptoms.

Contact tracing is also sometimes undertaken for infections such as tuberculosis, meningitis, and some imported tropical diseases.

HOW IT IS DONE

At clinics involved in the treatment of sexually transmitted infections, trained health workers interview patients after their diagnosis to explain the nature of the disease, its mode of transmission, and the complications that might occur if the disease is left untreated. Patients are also given printed leaflets, which they are recommended to give to their contacts, and which advise the contacts of the need for treatment.

Contagious

A term describing a disease that can be transferred from one person to another by ordinary social contact, such as by sharing a home or workplace. All contagious diseases, such as the common cold, chickenpox, or measles, are infectious, but many *infectious diseases*, such as typhoid, syphilis, or AIDS, are not contagious (being spread by other means of transmission, such as contamination of food or water by infected human excreta, by sexual contact, or by contaminated blood).

Contraception

The control of fertility to prevent *pregnancy*. Contraception can be achieved by various methods, which work by preventing the formation of ova (eggs) by the woman, stopping sperm from meeting an ovum in the fallopian tube

(thus preventing fertilization), or preventing a fertilized ovum from implanting in the lining of the uterus.

METHODS

Contraception may be achieved or attempted in the following ways: by total abstinence from *sexual intercourse*; by methods involving periodic abstinence from intercourse (see *Contraception, natural methods of*); by *coitus interruptus*; by barrier methods, including the use of condoms, diaphragms, cervical caps, spermicides, and contraceptive sponges (see *Contraception, barrier methods of*); by hormonal methods, including the use of *oral contraceptives*, implants, and injections (see *Contraceptives, injectable*); by intrauterine devices (see *IUDs*); by postcoital methods (see *Contraception, postcoital*); or by sterilization of the male (see *Vasectomy*) or female (see *Sterilization, female*).

Breast-feeding was once considered to be a method of contraception because frequent suckling causes changes in the hormone levels in the body that can prevent ovulation. The unreliability of the effect on ovulation is, however, too great for breast-feeding to be considered a contraceptive method today.

MEASURING CONTRACEPTIVE EFFECTIVENESS

Contraceptives are measured not so much by their effectiveness as by their failure rate. The failure rate is the rate of pregnancies per 100 woman-years of use (i.e. the number of pregnancies among 100 women using the method for one year, or 50 using it for two years). The lower the failure rate, the more effective and useful the contraceptive. Failure rates do not take into account the fact that failures are more likely in the first year of use, while the woman is getting used to the method.

There are two ways of defining contraceptive effectiveness: theoretical, or "method", effectiveness; and "use" effectiveness (i.e. the effectiveness in actual use).

THEORETICAL (METHOD) EFFECTIVENESS This is the effectiveness of a particular contraceptive method when used exactly as prescribed by the manufacturers, the doctor, or the clinic. Theoretical failure rates are usually much lower than the failure rates of contraceptives in actual use.

USE EFFECTIVENESS This measures the effectiveness of the method under all circumstances. It takes into account pregnancies resulting from incorrect use (for example, forgetting to take the pill or not putting on a condom correctly). Use effectiveness is almost always markedly lower than theoretical effectiveness in "user-dependent" methods, such as barriers. With "nonuser-dependent" methods, such as IUDs and sterilization, there is less of a difference.

RISKS INVOLVED IN CONTRACEPTIVE METHODS
Risks vary a great deal depending on the method. Perhaps the greatest risk in all cases is failure of the contraceptive method, which can lead to unwanted pregnancy and all that this entails (such as an elective *abortion*, possible danger to the health or life of the mother, or danger to the health of any existing children).

Risks inherent in contraceptives themselves must also be weighed against the benefits. Hormonal contraceptives have been linked with *cardiovascular disease*, particularly in women over the age of 35 who smoke, and there is some evidence of a link with *breast cancer* in women under the age of 35. IUDs may be associated with an increase in *pelvic inflammatory disease*, particularly in women who have more than one sex partner; and sterilization carries the risks of a surgical operation.

CONTRACEPTIVE RESEARCH
New forms continue to be investigated although the constraints of licensing authorities, the great cost, and the paucity of funds have slowed the pace. However, a few of the promising lines of research are as follows.

HORMONAL CONTRACEPTION New forms of hormonal contraception include the use of *luteinizing hormone-releasing hormone* (a hormone that regulates the release of other hormones that control the ovulatory cycle), which may be given as a nasal spray.

MIFEPRISTONE Formerly known as RU-486, mifepristone is a progesterone antagonist that is used for the medical termination of pregnancy (see *Abortion, induced*). Mifepristone is effective as a postcoital contraceptive and it could be used as an oral contraceptive, but neither of these uses had been licensed in Britain in 1994.

STEROIDAL VAGINAL RINGS Made of silicone-rubber containing a progestogen, these are at an advanced stage of development. They are inserted into the vagina where they release the progestogen, which acts directly on the reproductive organs.

PINPOINTING OVULATION Various methods to determine the exact time of ovulation continue to be researched; this would be of considerable help in improving natural methods of contraception.

VACCINES These are being studied, but still present problems. Vaccines are being developed against sperm, against the outer coat of the ovum, and against the hormone that helps maintain a pregnancy.

THE MALE PILL This continues to be researched, but so far without much practical progress. The main problem is that the testes are continually producing millions of sperm, while the ovaries have a definite number of ova present at birth and release only one each month—making suppression of ovulation simpler than suppression of sperm production.

Contraception, barrier methods of

The use of a device and/or chemical to block or otherwise stop sperm from reaching the ovum, thus preventing fertilization and pregnancy. Barrier contraceptives include the condom (placed over the erect penis); and the diaphragm, the cervical cap, the contraceptive sponge, and the female condom, which are all placed within the vagina. Spermicides are recommended in combination with barrier devices for maximum protection.

Barrier methods, especially condoms, are advisable for people with more than one sex partner because they help to prevent the sexual transmission of diseases such as *AIDS* and hepatitis B (see *Hepatitis, viral*).

TYPES

CONDOM A sheath of fine, latex rubber or plastic, about 17 cm long, usually lubricated for ease of application. A condom normally has a teat at its end to hold ejaculated sperm. Condoms are available over-the-counter in various sizes, colours, and textures; also, some types are precoated with spermicide.

A condom should be carefully rolled on to the erect penis before intercourse. The tip of the condom should be squeezed as it is rolled on, so that no air is trapped in the end (trapped air may lead to bursting of the condom when ejaculation occurs). The rim of the condom should be held close to the penis when it is withdrawn from the vagina, which should occur after orgasm but before the erection subsides.

DIAPHRAGM This is a hemispherical dome of thin rubber with a metal spring in the rim. It fits diagonally across the front wall of the vagina, with the top part of the rim up behind the cervix (neck of the uterus) and the opposite edge of the rim resting on the ledge above the pubic bone.

Diaphragms are available in a range of sizes and must be properly fitted by a nurse or a doctor. The size and type of diaphragm required is determined by each individual's anatomy.

A diaphragm must be used with a spermicidal agent and be left in place for six hours after intercourse. Without disturbing the diaphragm, additional spermicide should be used if intercourse is repeated within the six-hour period.

CERVICAL CAP Smaller and more rigid than the diaphragm, this latex rubber device fits tightly over the cervix (rather than covering the vaginal vault), where it is held in place by suction. There are three types: the cervical cap, which is thimble-shaped; the vault cap, which is bowl-shaped; and the vimule cap, which combines features of both the cervical and vault caps. Caps are often used by women who cannot use diaphragms because of anatomical changes, such as prolapse of the uterus or of the front wall of the vagina. As with the diaphragm, a cap must be properly fitted by either a nurse or doctor, and should be used with a spermicide.

CONTRACEPTIVE SPONGE This device is a disposable circular polyurethane foam sponge about 5 cm in diameter and 5 cm thick that is impregnated with spermicide. The sponge incorporates a loop for easy removal. Before being inserted high into the vagina, the sponge should be moistened with water to activate the spermicide. It should be left in position for at least six hours after intercourse.

FEMALE CONDOM This is a new type of barrier contraceptive. Female condoms are similar to male condoms but are larger and have rings to hold them in the vagina during intercourse.

SPERMICIDE A wide range of spermicides is available, including aerosol foams, creams, jellies, pessaries, soluble plastic film, or foaming tablets, which are placed in the vagina as near to the cervix as possible. Some preparations are recommended for use with a condom, diaphragm, or cap. Others are intended to be used alone; they are inserted into the vagina using a syringe-like applicator. Some spermicides should not be used with rubber barrier devices.

Spermicides should be applied shortly before intercourse; a fresh application is needed when intercourse is repeated or prolonged. Spermicides must be used in accordance with the manufacturer's instructions because the length of time for which

METHODS OF CONTRACEPTION

There are various methods of contraception: the natural methods, barrier methods, hormonal methods, and postcoital methods. Sterilization interferes with part of the male or female reproductive system to render the individual infertile.

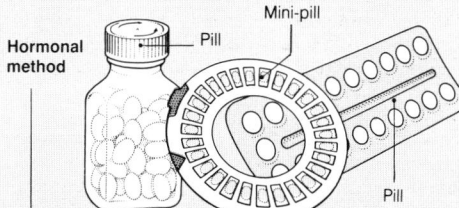

Hormonal method

Pill

Mini-pill

Pill

The pill

Prevents ovulation, changes the cervical mucus to prevent sperm penetration, or alters the uterine lining to prevent implantation.

Barrier method

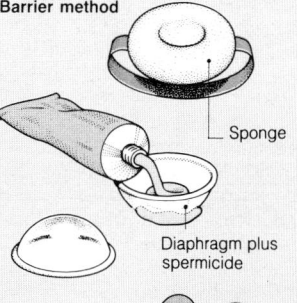

Sponge

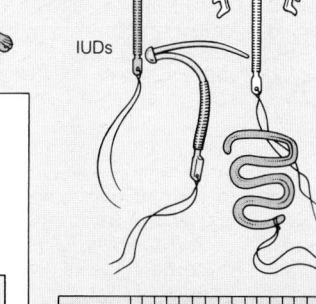

Diaphragm plus spermicide

Caps

IUDs

Hormonal implant

Capsules containing a progestogen are inserted into the arm, where they release progestogen into the blood.

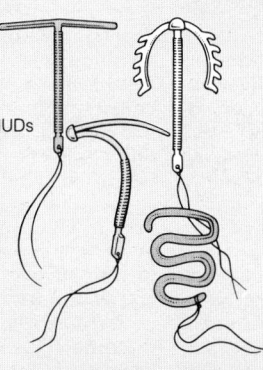

Diaphragm in position

Held in place over the cervix by means of a coiled metal spring in its rim, the diaphragm prevents sperm from reaching the cervix.

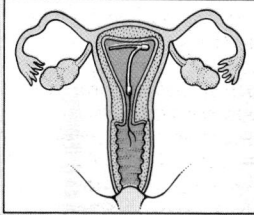

IUD in position

A small piece of moulded plastic with string attached, sometimes with copper or a female hormone added. The IUD is worn in the uterus.

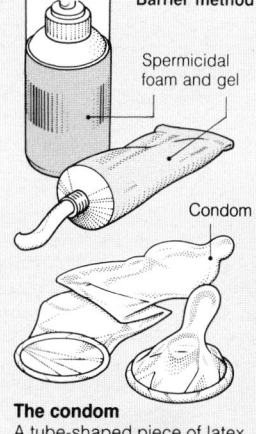

Barrier method

Spermicidal foam and gel

Condom

The condom

A tube-shaped piece of latex rubber that usually has a teat to hold ejaculate. It should be used with spermicide, examined for holes before use, and have all air squeezed out of the tip to prevent bursting. The rim should be held during withdrawal to stop the condom from slipping off.

STERILIZATION

Offers an almost completely safe and reliable form of birth control. It is usually irreversible. It has no effect on the production of sex hormones, so a man produces sperm-free semen and a woman produces normal eggs.

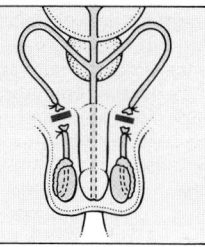

Male sterilization (vasectomy)

The vas deferens on each side is cut so that sperm cannot pass from testes to penis.

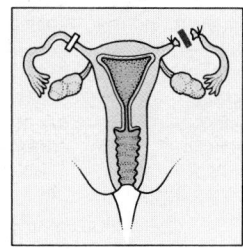

Female sterilization

Two cuts are made below the navel, and a laparoscope is inserted. An attachment to this is used to seal off the tube ends.

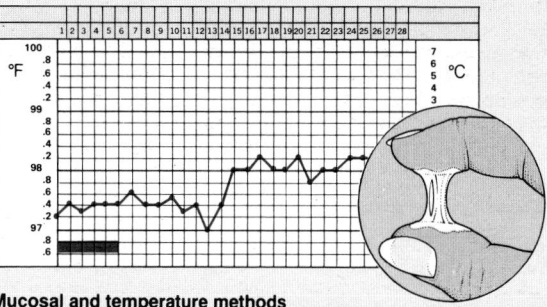

Mucosal and temperature methods

The temperature method involves charting the woman's temperature to ascertain whether ovulation has taken place. The mucosal method involves studying the cervical mucus throughout the woman's menstrual cycle.

C

they remain effective varies. They should not be washed away until six to eight hours after intercourse.

EFFECTIVENESS

If used consistently and correctly, employing both mechanical and chemical means, barrier methods can be highly effective in preventing conception. Failure rates in actual use vary between four and seven pregnancies per 100 woman-years of use for the male condom, diaphragm, or contraceptive cap; nine to 16 pregnancies per 100 woman-years of use for the contraceptive sponge; and 20 to 30 pregnancies per 100 woman-years of use for spermicides used alone. The effectiveness of the female condom is not yet known. (See *Contraception* for the definition of woman-years.)

Contraception, hormonal methods of

The use by women of synthetic progestogens, frequently combined with synthetic oestrogens, to prevent pregnancy. The best-known form of hormonal contraception is the contraceptive pill (see *Oral contraceptives*). Contraceptive hormones can also be administered in the form of *contraceptive implants* or by injection (see *Contraceptives, injectable*).

Hormonal methods of contraception work by suppressing ovulation in most (although not all) menstrual cycles, and by acting on the cervical mucus to make it thick and impenetrable to sperm. They also cause thinning of the endometrium (lining of the uterus).

Contraception, natural methods of

Periodic abstinence from sexual intercourse to avoid conception. All natural methods of contraception attempt to pinpoint the fertile period around the time of ovulation, so that intercourse can be avoided on the days when *fertilization* might occur.

Natural methods of contraception need great motivation on the part of the couple, with a strong commitment to abstain from intercourse when there could be a possibility of pregnancy. They are the only forms of contraception permitted by the Roman Catholic church.

TYPES

CALENDAR METHOD This is the oldest method of natural contraception. The calendar method attempts to predict a woman's fertile period with reference to the length of her menstrual cycle,

EFFECTIVENESS (FAILURE RATES) OF CONTRACEPTIVE METHODS

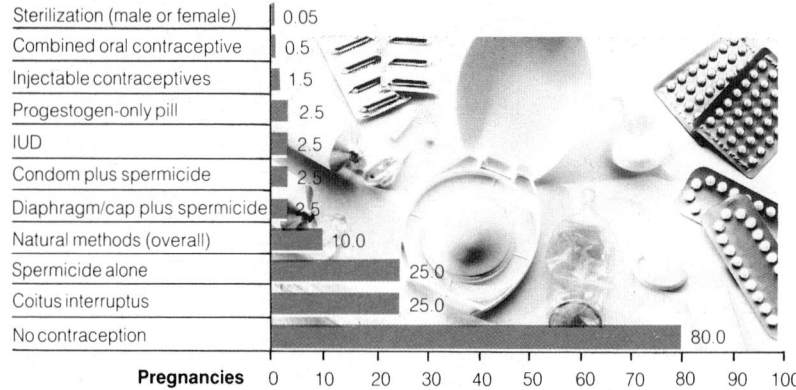

Method	Pregnancies
Sterilization (male or female)	0.05
Combined oral contraceptive	0.5
Injectable contraceptives	1.5
Progestogen-only pill	2.5
IUD	2.5
Condom plus spermicide	2.5
Diaphragm/cap plus spermicide	2.5
Natural methods (overall)	10.0
Spermicide alone	25.0
Coitus interruptus	25.0
No contraception	80.0

Pregnancies 0 10 20 30 40 50 60 70 80 90 100

The chart shows the approximate number of pregnancies that can be expected if 100 couples use a given contraceptive method, or none at all, for one year.

making the assumption that ovulation occurs 14 days before menstruation. Because of its high failure rate, this method has now been largely superseded by other natural methods of contraception.

TEMPERATURE METHOD Also known as the basal body temperature method, this method makes use of the fact that a woman's body temperature is higher in the second half of the menstrual cycle, after ovulation has taken place. The temperature should be taken at the same time each day (normally first thing in the morning), using a special ovulation thermometer marked in fractions of degrees. Intercourse is not considered safe until there has been a sustained temperature rise for at least three days.

CERVICAL MUCUS METHOD This method attempts to pinpoint the fertile period by observing and charting the amount and appearance of the mucus secreted by the cervix (neck of the uterus) during the menstrual cycle. Menstruation is followed by "dry" days when the mucus forms a thick plug that blocks the cervix. The mucus then becomes thick and viscid and appears at the vulva. At about the time of ovulation it turns thin, watery, elastic and slippery, and flows more easily. A few days after ovulation it begins to become thick and viscid again, and this state lasts until the start of the next menstrual period.

Using the cervical mucus method, intercourse should be avoided from the first appearance of mucus after the dry days until four days after the last appearance of the thin, watery mucus that occurs around the time of ovulation.

SYMPTOTHERMAL METHOD This method combines the temperature and the cervical mucus methods. Intercourse is permitted during the dry days after menstruation, but must stop as soon as mucus is felt. Intercourse can be resumed only when both the sustained rise in temperature and the four-day period after the last appearance of thin, watery mucus have taken place.

SIDE-EFFECTS

Once the techniques have been mastered and a woman can observe and chart the necessary changes, there are no provable side-effects. There is, however, a supposition that a higher incidence of miscarriages or birth defects could occur among pregnancies that result from a failure of these methods because of the fertilization of so-called "aged" ova by "aged" sperm. This supposition has been neither completely proved nor disproved.

Contraception, postcoital

An attempt to prevent pregnancy following unprotected sexual intercourse. Postcoital contraception is normally used only in exceptional circumstances and must be provided soon after intercourse. Methods are not 100 per cent effective, and women are advised to have a pregnancy test a month after treatment to ensure that they are not pregnant.

TYPES

There are two main types of postcoital contraception: use of *oral contraceptives* (sometimes known as the "morning after pill") and use of an *IUD* (coil).

ORAL CONTRACEPTIVES This must be started not later than 72 hours after unprotected intercourse. The most common method is to give two high-dose oral contraceptive pills as soon as possible, followed by a further two pills 12 hours later. Treatment sometimes causes nausea and vomiting, and an *antiemetic drug* may be needed at the same time.

IUD For use as a postcoital method of contraception, an IUD must be inserted within five days of unprotected intercourse.

Contraception, withdrawal method of
See *Coitus interruptus*.

Contraceptive
Any agent that diminishes the likelihood of conception. Contraceptives can be hormonal (such as oral contraceptives), chemical (such as spermicides), or mechanical (such as condoms). (See also *Contraception*.)

Contraceptive implant
A hormonal method of contraception in which long-acting contraceptive drugs are inserted under the skin. Contraceptive implants consist of small capsules containing a *progestogen drug*. The implants remain active for several years, steadily releasing progestogen into the bloodstream. Fertility returns soon after the implants are removed.

Contraceptive implants are very effective and may be suitable for women who want long-term protection against pregnancy and who are unable to use *oral contraceptives* or an *IUD*. (See also *Contraception, hormonal methods of*.)

Contraceptives, injectable
A hormonal method of contraception in which long-acting *progestogen drugs* are given by injection. Injectable contraceptives are administered every two or three months.

Injectable contraceptives may be suitable for women who want long-term protection against pregnancy and who are unable, or who do not want, to use *oral contraceptives* or an *IUD*. Injectable contraceptives are extremely effective, with a failure rate of only two per 100 woman-years (see *Contraception* for the definition of woman-years).

Side-effects may be troublesome, especially during the first few months of use. There may be menstrual disturbances, such as heavy or scanty periods, irregular periods, or amenorrhea (absence of periods). Other pos-

sible side-effects include weight gain, headaches, and nausea. Even if side-effects are severe, there is no way of neutralizing the activity of injectable contraceptives once they have been administered. The drug must run its normal two-to-three month course.

The return of fertility may be delayed for some time after injections are discontinued.

Contractions, uterine
The spasms of rhythmic, squeezing muscular activity that affect the walls of the *uterus* during *childbirth*. These true labour contractions differ from *Braxton Hicks' contractions*, which are milder contractions that are often noticeable during the last few weeks of pregnancy. True contractions are characterized by the discomfort they cause, by their regularity, and by the fact that they increase in strength and frequency from the start of the first stage of labour.

Contracture
A deformity caused by shrinkage of tissue in the skin, muscles, or tendons. Contractures may restrict the movement of joints.

Skin contractures commonly occur as a result of scarring following extensive burns. Other types of contracture may be caused by inflammation and shrinkage of *connective tissues* (materials that surround body structures and hold them together).

Examples include *Dupuytren's contracture*, which affects tendons and fibrous tissue in the hand, and *Volkmann's contracture*, in which muscle fibres in the arm are damaged, usually by reduced blood supply following an injury.

Contraindication
Any factor in a patient's condition that makes it unwise to pursue a certain line of treatment—such as drug therapy or surgery.

Controlled trial
A method of testing the value of a treatment—such as a new drug—or comparing the effectiveness of different treatments.

WHY IT IS DONE
The effectiveness of a treatment cannot accurately be assessed simply by administering it to a group of sick people and seeing if their conditions improve. With many illnesses, a significant proportion of patients tend to get better even if the treatment they are given is useless. Reasons for this

phenomenon include the healing properties of time, the psychological reassurance of the doctor, and the fact that both the patient and doctor believe the treatment will work (the so-called *placebo* effect). A controlled trial is a scientific attempt to unravel the true effect of a treatment from the psychological side benefits of "being treated".

HOW IT IS DONE
In a typical controlled drug trial, a sample of patients with the illness that the drug is thought to cure is randomly split into two groups. It is checked that the groups are well-matched in age, sex, social class, etc. One group is given a normal course of the drug—for example, a pill to be taken every day. The other patients—called the control group—are given an identical course of treatment, except that their pills are "dummy", or placebo, tablets, containing none of the drug being tested, but only an inert substance such as starch. Alternatively, the control group may be given a well-established drug treatment but with the drug disguised to appear identical to the test drug.

After a predetermined period, the two groups are assessed medically. If the improvement in the illness has been significantly greater in the patients given the test drug over those given the dummy tablets, this suggests that the drug does have a real curative effect. Any benefits (or side-effects) of treatment separate from the pharmacological effects of the drug have been accounted for (or "controlled") by the use of identical treatment regimens for the two groups.

To be of any use, controlled trials must be conducted "blind"—that is, the patients do not know whether they are receiving the real or the dummy treatment. In a further refinement—the "double-blind" controlled trial—neither the patients nor the doctors who assess them know who is receiving which treatment. The results of trials require detailed and careful statistical analysis before any conclusions can be drawn.

Contusion
Damage to the skin and underlying tissues from a blunt injury such as a fall; the skin may be grazed and the tissues bruised.

Convalescence
The recovery period following an illness or a surgical operation during which the patient regains strength be-

C

fore returning to normal activities. The convalescent period can vary from one or two days (following an infection such as influenza or tonsillitis) to several weeks (following a heart attack or a major operation). Special convalescent homes were formerly popular for patients of all ages, but today such homes are generally reserved for the elderly.

Conversion disorder

A psychological disorder in which it is thought that painful emotions are repressed and unconsciously converted into physical symptoms. The repressed idea is expressed symbolically by the particular bodily symptom. For instance, a paralysed right arm may represent guilt over an injury that the patient, using that arm, inflicted on another person; mutism may represent sexual guilt, the mouth symbolizing the vagina.

This disorder serves mainly to relieve anxiety, but the sufferer may also "benefit" by gaining sympathy and avoiding responsibility. Such symptoms may also be part of other psychiatric or organic disorders.

Treatment requires *psychotherapy* involving exploration of the person's history and childhood experiences.

Convulsion

See *Seizure*.

Convulsion, febrile

Twitching or jerking of the limbs with loss of consciousness occurring in a child after a rapid rise in temperature. Febrile convulsions are common; about one child in 20 has one or more attacks. The seizures tend to run in families, are usually not serious, and occur mainly in children between six months and five years old.

CAUSES AND SYMPTOMS

Febrile convulsions are caused by an immaturity of the temperature-lowering mechanism in the brain, allowing the temperature to rise too rapidly in response to an infection, commonly *measles, roseola infantum, influenza,* or an upper respiratory tract infection, such as *pharyngitis, tonsillitis* or *otitis media* (inflammation of the middle ear). The sudden rise in temperature excites the brain cells, causing them to discharge impulses to the muscles, which then contract. There is no underlying brain defect; seizures triggered by fever are distinct from those triggered by *meningitis* or *encephalitis,* which are infections of the central nervous system.

The child loses consciousness and his or her arms and legs twitch uncontrollably for a few minutes. After regaining consciousness, the child may be drowsy.

TREATMENT

During a seizure, objects that could be harmful should be moved out of the child's way. Biting the tongue is rare and no attempt should be made to prevent this happening by wedging the mouth open (which can cause cuts and broken teeth). Once the seizure is over, the child should be placed in the *recovery position*. Every effort should be made to lower the temperature by sponging the child's face and body with lukewarm water, and by using a fan (if one is available).

If the child has not had a seizure before, a doctor should be consulted; if the seizure lasts for more than five minutes, an ambulance should be called. In some cases, investigative tests, such as a *lumbar puncture,* are performed to determine whether the seizure has a serious cause, such as *meningitis*. Drug treatment with *diazepam* or *paraldehyde* may be given to control the seizure or to avert further episodes. Treatment may also be given for an underlying infection.

PREVENTION

If an infectious illness develops in a susceptible child, parents can often prevent seizures from occurring by reducing the child's temperature. *Paracetamol* should be given at the first signs of fever and repeated every four to six hours as necessary; you should give the full dose for the child's weight as instructed on the package. Most of the child's clothing should be removed, and he or she should be cooled by sponging the face and body with lukewarm water and also by using a fan if possible.

OUTLOOK

Most children who have febrile convulsions are completely normal and suffer no ill effects from the attacks. A second seizure occurs in about 30 to 40 per cent of cases, usually within the following six months. In most children, the risk of developing *epilepsy* (recurrent seizures) is very small. However, recurrences are more likely if a child has a pre-existing abnormality of the brain or nervous system, if the first febrile convulsion was limited to only part of the body (e.g. one side) or was prolonged (longer than 15 minutes), and if there are family members with epilepsy. Children with all of these factors have about a one in 10 chance of developing epilepsy.

Cooley's anaemia

A term formerly used to refer to the inherited blood disorder beta *thalassaemia* major.

Copper

A metallic element that forms an essential part of several *enzymes* (substances that promote biochemical reactions in the body). Copper is needed by the body only in minute amounts (see *Trace elements*); deficiency is very uncommon.

Copper poisoning is rare, occurring mainly in people who drink homemade alcohol distilled using copper tubing. Symptoms of poisoning include nausea, vomiting, and diarrhoea. Copper excess may also result from *Wilson's disease,* a rare inherited disorder of copper metabolism.

Co-proxamol

An *analgesic drug* (painkiller) that contains *paracetamol* and the weak narcotic analgesic dextropropoxyphene. Co-proxamol is widely used for the relief of mild to moderate pain that has not responded to paracetamol or other nonnarcotic analgesics alone.

Possible adverse effects include dizziness, drowsiness, constipation, nausea, and vomiting. Co-proxamol may be habit-forming if taken regularly over a long period. Overdose is dangerous because high doses of paracetamol can damage the liver and dextropropoxyphene may interfere with breathing.

Cordotomy

An operation to divide bundles of nerve fibres within the *spinal cord*.

Cordotomy is performed to relieve persistent pain that has not responded to treatment with strong *analgesic drugs* (painkillers) or *TENS* (transcutaneous electrical nerve stimulation). In theory, cordotomy can treat pain anywhere in the body, depending on the part of the cord that is operated on. In practice, however, it is often difficult to locate precisely the nerves responsible for pain in the upper part of the body, and the operation is most frequently performed for pain in the lower trunk and legs, usually on patients with cancer.

Corn

A small area of thickened skin on a toe, caused by the pressure of a tight-fitting shoe. People with high foot arches are affected most, because the arch increases the pressure on the tips of the toes when walking.

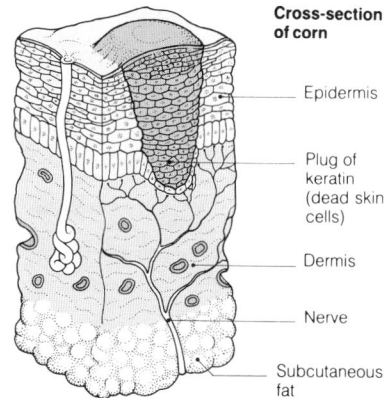

Cross-section
of corn

— Epidermis

— Plug of
keratin
(dead skin
cells)

— Dermis

— Nerve

— Subcutaneous
fat

If a corn is painful, the obvious solution is to change to shoes that fit more comfortably; the corn should then gradually disappear. A spongy ring or corn pad—available at chemist shops in various sizes—can be placed over the corn to ease pressure. If the corn persists, a chiropodist can remedy the problem by paring away the thickened skin with a scalpel.

Cornea

The front part of the tough outer shell of the eyeball. The cornea is transparent and is shaped like a thin-walled cap or dome. It is about 12 mm in diameter, less than 1 mm thick, and has a convex front surface like the front of a camera lens. At its circumference the cornea joins the sclera (white of the eye), which is easily seen. The cornea itself, being transparent, is less obvious. The black pupil and the coloured iris are visible beneath it.

The cornea performs two main functions: it helps focus light-rays on to the retina at the back of the eye and it protects the front of the eye. To warn of possible damage, the cornea's surface is extremely sensitive, and small scratches and foreign bodies are thus very painful.

The cornea must be kept moist (by tears) to remain healthy. This function is performed by the lacrimal gland and the mucus-secreting and fluid-secreting cells in the eyelids and conjunctiva (the thin lining of the rest of the surface of the eye and the inside of the eyelids). The cells that form the inner cell layer of the cornea in adults cannot reproduce themselves. If they are severely damaged, there may be permanent corneal clouding, because one of the functions of the cell is to pump excess water out of the cornea to keep it transparent.

Corneal abrasion

A scratch or defect in the epithelium (outer layer) of the cornea. The abrasion may be caused by a small, sharp particle in the eye (see *Eye, foreign body in*) or by an injury—for example, by a twig or hairbrush.

Corneal abrasions usually heal quickly but may meanwhile cause severe pain and photophobia (abnormal sensitivity to bright light) and increased production of tears.

Pain may be relieved by covering the eye with a patch, by *analgesic drugs* (painkillers), and, if the eye muscles go into spasm, by eye-drops containing cycloplegic drugs (drugs that paralyse the ciliary muscles in the eye). Eye-drops containing *antibiotic drugs* are usually also given to prevent any risk of bacterial infection, which could cause serious corneal ulceration, abscess, or even blindness.

Corneal abrasions usually heal completely within a few days, but (rarely) they may recur, probably because the new epithelium fails to stick properly to the underlying tissue. Patching the eye, application of bland ointments, and even prescription of a soft "bandage" contact lens may be tried.

Corneal graft

The surgical transplantation of corneal tissue. Most corneal grafts are homografts, in which tissue is taken from a human donor and put into the eye of a recipient with a corneal disorder. A much smaller number are autografts, in which a person's cornea is simply repositioned—for example, it may be rotated to a position in which the effect of a scar on the corneal surface is lessened. Donor corneal tissues can now be stored for days for future use. The term "eye bank" is used for the organization that handles the donor corneas.

WHY IT IS DONE

A corneal graft is carried out when a patient has an eye with good visual potential (most of the eye is healthy) but with substantially impaired vision caused by a cornea that is scarred or clouded (see *Cornea* disorders box).

HOW IT IS DONE

The patient is given a general or a local anaesthetic. The diseased area of the cornea is then cut out and replaced with a similarly shaped piece of donor tissue, which is fastened in place with stitches. Most corneal grafts are full-thickness but if the back part of the cornea is healthy, the cornea is sometimes split, with only the front, diseased part removed and replaced.

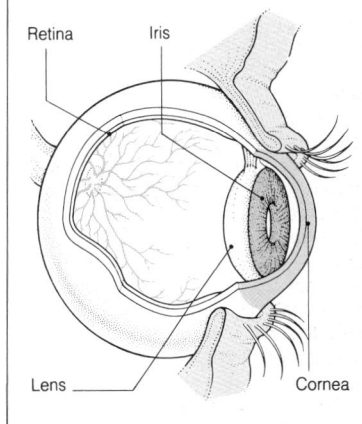

LOCATION OF CORNEA
The cornea is a transparent thin-walled dome forming the front of the eyeball. It consists of five layers of differing thickness.

Retina

Iris

Lens

Cornea

OUTLOOK

The success rate for corneal grafts is high, but depends on the type of corneal disorder (certain corneal problems have lower transplant success rates than others). Generally, however, corneal grafts have a much better chance of success than other types of transplant. This is because the healthy cornea has no blood vessels, so there is less access for the white blood cells, which bring about rejection of donor tissue. Matching certain features of the donor's and recipient's immune systems (see *Histocompatibility antigens*) has also improved the success rate of corneal grafts. Unlike the recipients of other transplants, there is usually no need for the recipient of a corneal graft to receive *immunosuppressant drugs* to lessen the chance of rejection of the graft.

Corneal transplant

See *Corneal graft.*

Corneal ulcer

A break, erosion, or open sore in the outer layer of the *cornea*, sometimes extending into the underlying stroma (middle layer).

CAUSES

The most common cause is a *corneal abrasion* (scratch), but an ulcer may also be produced by chemical damage, or by infection with various bacteria, fungi, or viruses (particularly with the *herpes simplex* virus or the virus that causes *herpes zoster*).

C

Certain eye conditions may make an ulcer more likely—for example, *keratoconjunctivitis sicca* (dry eye), eyelid deformities such as *entropion* or *ectropion,* or diminished sensation in the cornea, which more easily permits injury to occur.

SYMPTOMS, DIAGNOSIS, AND TREATMENT
Corneal ulcers are very painful, though chronic ones may become less so. They are easily recognized by a doctor who introduces some fluorescein dye into the eye and shines a blue light on it; the fluorescein fills the ulcer and reflects back green light.

Superficial, noninfectious ulcers caused by mechanical injury usually heal quickly. If an infection is suspected, swabs will be taken to identify the causative microorganism and the doctor will then prescribe suitable drug treatment. Sometimes, a predisposing eye condition may need to be treated in addition to the ulcer. Noninfectious ulcers that fail to heal quickly sometimes respond to a "bandage" contact lens or to *tarsorrhaphy* (temporary joining of the eyelids).

Coronary
Strictly, a term used to describe any structure that encircles like a crown (from "corona", the Latin word for crown). In practice, the term usually refers to the coronary arteries that encircle and supply the heart. In popular usage, coronary often means a *coronary thrombosis* or a *myocardial infarction* (heart attack).

Coronary artery bypass
An operation to circumvent narrowed or blocked coronary arteries by grafting on additional blood vessels to transmit blood flow.

Coronary artery bypass may be performed when symptoms of *coronary artery disease* have not been relieved by drugs and other measures, such as weight loss, stopping smoking, and the adoption of a sensible diet and lifestyle. Balloon *angioplasty* (in which the narrowed segment of artery is stretched by a small balloon) is often recommended as a simpler alternative for patients with mild to moderate coronary artery disease and good heart function. Bypass surgery may then be postponed until it is clearly needed.

HOW IT IS DONE
A decision to carry out coronary artery bypass surgery is based on identification of the sites of blockage using *angiography* (an X-ray technique). Surgery—performed under general anaesthesia—usually requires two surgeons and lasts up to five hours. The heart is temporarily stopped, and blood circulation and oxygenation is taken over by a *heart-lung machine.* The procedure is described in the illustrated box.

RECOVERY AND OUTLOOK
After a coronary artery bypass, the patient spends two to four days in an

---

DISORDERS OF THE CORNEA
The cornea is a living structure, much like very specialized skin, and is prone to many disorders.

CONGENITAL DEFECTS
These are rare. Microcornea (smaller than normal) or megalocornea (bigger than normal) may occur in one or both eyes. In *buphthalmos,* or "ox-eye", the entire eyeball is distended from *glaucoma* (raised pressure in the eye). This often leads to haziness of the cornea.

INJURY
Trauma to the cornea is common and is usually minor, a frequent occurrence being a *corneal abrasion* (scratch) caused by a particle in the eye or by overuse of contact lenses. An abrasion may become infected and progress to a *corneal ulcer.* Penetrating corneal injuries can cause scarring with loss of transparency, which may lead to severe impairment of vision.

Chemical injuries to the cornea can result from acid or alkali splashes, the latter being the more serious. All contact with corrosive substances is dangerous, and immediate flushing of the eye with large volumes of water is essential if sight is to be saved.

The term *keratopathy* can be applied to any corneal disorder, but is also used more specifically for certain types of corneal damage.

Actinic keratopathy is damage to the outer layer of the cornea by ultraviolet light. Exposure keratopathy is the damage done to a cornea deprived of the normal protection afforded by the tear film and the blink reflex.

INFLAMMATION
Keratitis means inflammation of the cornea. However, because the cornea contains no blood vessels, true inflammatory reactions are uncommon.

INFECTION
The cornea can be infected by viruses, bacteria, and fungi. Some of these cause ulceration, which may lead to penetration. *Herpes simplex* is especially dangerous.

NUTRITIONAL DISORDERS
Keratomalacia is the result of vitamin A deficiency and is common in severely undernourished children. The cornea becomes soft and often perforates. Keratomalacia is a major cause of blindness in some tropical countries.

DEGENERATION
Degenerative conditions occur mainly in the elderly, and are more common in previously damaged eyes. Corneal changes include calcium deposition, thinning, and spontaneous ulceration.

OTHER DISORDERS
Keratoconjunctivitis sicca (dry eye) occurs when the tear film is inadequate. This is a feature of *Sjögren's syndrome,* the *Stevens-Johnson syndrome,* and various rheumatic disorders. Corneal dystrophies are inborn errors of corneal structure or function that may appear at various ages and may lead to opacification. One form of dystrophy is *keratoconus,* in which the cornea thins and bulges forwards into a conical shape. Oedema (fluid accumulation) of the cornea occurs when the endothelium (inner layer) fails to prevent the internal fluid of the eye from entering the cornea, so impairing vision.

INVESTIGATION
Corneal disorders are examined under high magnification, using a slit-lamp microscope. In the majority of cases, the appearance of the various conditions is characteristic and diagnosis is straightforward. Corneal ulcers may require gentle scraping so that samples can be obtained for viral, bacterial, or fungal *culture* in the pathology laboratory.

CORONARY ARTERY BYPASS

This is now the most common and successful major heart operation in the Western world. Each year some 10,000 people in the UK undergo the operation, which can relieve them from dependence on drug treatment for heart disease and restore them to active life.

HOW IT IS DONE

Coronary artery bypass is a major procedure, requiring two surgeons and lasting up to five hours.

1 The first surgeon makes an incision down the centre of the patient's chest. The heart is then exposed by opening the pericardium.

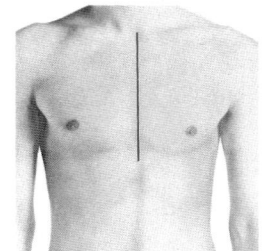

2 Simultaneously, several incisions are made in the leg, and a length of vein removed.

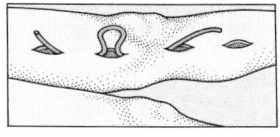

Site of incision

3 Before any incisions are made in the coronary arteries, the patient is connected to a heart-lung machine. This takes over the function of the heart and lungs while the surgeon repairs the heart.

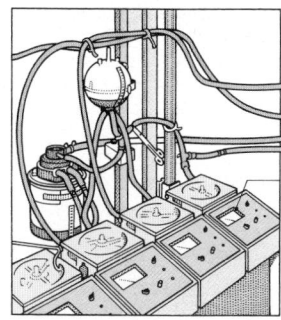

Heart-lung machine

4 A section of the vein taken from the leg is then sewn to the aorta and to a point below the blockage. If several arteries are blocked, they can be bypassed by using other sections from the same leg vein, or an arterial graft may be taken from the chest.

5 The heart-lung machine is disconnected, allowing blood to flow back into the coronary arteries.

WHY IT IS DONE

Narrowed coronary arteries are unable to supply the heart muscle with a sufficient amount of blood; as a result, it becomes starved of oxygen. This may cause angina (chest pain) or heart tissue damage. By attaching lengths of a vein taken from the leg (or in some cases a length of mammary artery) to the aorta and to a point below the blockages, the narrowed or blocked sections can be bypassed.

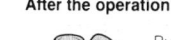

Before the operation

Diseased coronary artery

Affected area

Coronary arteries

After the operation

Bypass

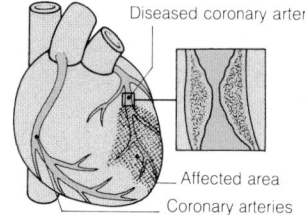
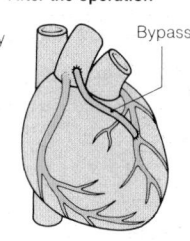

First surgeon prepares heart for bypass

Second surgeon removes vein from leg

Anaesthetist

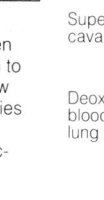

Oxygenated blood from heart-lung machine

Superior vena cava (tied off)

Deoxygenated blood to heart-lung machine

Inferior vena cava (tied off)

Pericardium

Aorta

Bypass

Coronary arteries

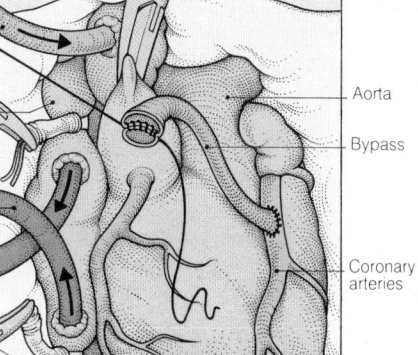

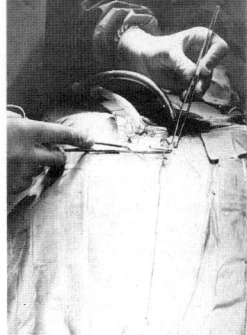

6 Finally, the breastbone is wired together, and pericardium and chest are sewn up.

C

intensive care unit, where his or her heart and other body functions are carefully monitored. The hospital stay is generally about 10 to 12 days, and return to work is usually possible after about six weeks.

Long term, the outlook is good, although the bypass grafts may eventually become blocked by a recurrence of the same disease process that narrowed the coronary arteries in the first place. Follow-up studies have shown that more than half the grafts are still functioning ten years after the operation.

Coronary artery disease

Damage to, or malfunction of, the heart caused by narrowing or blockage of the coronary arteries, which supply blood to the heart muscle. The two most common features of coronary artery disease are *angina pectoris* (chest pain caused by insufficient blood supply to the heart muscle) and acute *myocardial infarction* (heart attack).

INCIDENCE

The rate of coronary artery disease in the UK (especially in Scotland and Northern Ireland) is one of the highest in the world. In the UK, coronary artery disease accounts for one third of all deaths between the ages of 45 and 64. In most developed countries, deaths from the disease have dropped in the past 20 years; in the UK a small decline has occurred since the early 1980s but the rates are still high. Part of this decline is thought to be due to better medical treatment of *hypertension* (raised blood pressure), one of the causes of coronary artery disease, and part is due to improved surgical treatment of narrowed coronary arteries. Also, emergency treatment of heart attacks has improved, and people are adopting a less heart-disease-prone lifestyle by taking more exercise, eating a healthier diet, and smoking less.

CAUSES

The symptoms of coronary artery disease are caused by reduction in the blood flow to the heart muscle. The coronary arteries are first narrowed and may eventually be blocked by plaques (patches) of atheroma (cholesterol-rich fatty deposits) which can cause *atherosclerosis*. Further narrowing or blockage may be caused by thrombi (blood clots) formed on the roughened surface of the plaques.

Atherosclerosis has many interrelated causes, including smoking, lack of exercise, being overweight, and having a raised blood cholesterol level (which itself is linked in part with a diet rich in dairy and animal fats). Other im-

portant factors include a genetic predisposition and diseases such as *diabetes mellitus* and hypertension.

The importance of personality traits, behaviour, and stress as causes of coronary artery disease is still disputed. Some doctors believe that heart attacks are more frequent in people with "type A" personalities. Such individuals are always in a hurry, checking the time, impatient with delays, and interrupting colleagues in mid-sentence—but they are also doers and achievers.

There is some evidence that heart attacks occur more frequently in people who are depressed after the death of a relative, loss of a job, or some other adverse life event. However, the medical consensus is that these psychological and behavioural factors are less important than physical factors—smoking, unhealthy diet, high blood pressure, and lack of exercise.

SYMPTOMS

In its early stages, atherosclerosis of the coronary arteries is symptomless. The first symptom is usually either angina pectoris or a heart attack.

The pain of angina pectoris is typically brought on by exertion and relieved by rest. The pain is a dull ache in the middle of the chest or a feeling of pressure that may spread up to the neck or down the arms (the left arm more commonly than the right). In some cases the pain occurs only in an arm or in the neck. The pain comes on predictably after a certain amount of exertion—after walking halfway up the stairs, for instance—and disappears after resting for a minute or so.

Angina occurs when the heart muscle is working hard and getting too little blood for the amount of effort

being expended. If the blood supply to part of the muscle is cut off completely by a blood clot or spasm in one of the coronary arteries (a coronary thrombosis), the result is an acute myocardial infarction (a heart attack)—death of a portion of the heart muscle. The main symptom is intense chest pain of the same type as angina, but not relieved by rest and not necessarily brought on by effort; the victim may also become cold, sweat profusely, feel weak and nauseated, or lose consciousness as the heart's pumping action is weakened and shock ensues.

Angina and myocardial infarction may lead to disturbances in the electrical conduction system of the heart with resulting *arrhythmias* (heartbeat abnormalities) ranging from *ectopic beats* (misplaced beats) to *tachycardia* (rapid beats) and *ventricular fibrillation* (ineffective fluttering of the heart muscle). The latter causes rapid loss of consciousness and is fatal if not treated within a few minutes.

DIAGNOSIS AND INVESTIGATION

A myocardial infarction may produce such clear-cut symptoms that the diagnosis is in no doubt. Confirmatory tests may include *ECG* (electrocardiography) and measurement of the level of substances called cardiac enzymes released into the blood by damaged muscle. The conditions of patients who have intermittent attacks of angina are usually assessed by ECG both at rest and during exercise (see *Cardiac stress test*).

When the angina is persistent, severe, changing in quality, or of recent onset, the patient's condition is assessed by various *heart imaging* techniques. These imaging procedures

---

DEATH RATES FROM HEART DISEASE (per 100,000 in group 35 to 74)

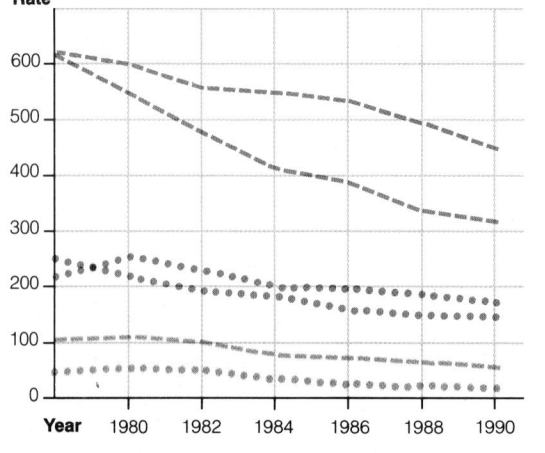

The downward-sloping graphs for the US probably result from a combination of healthier living and better treatment of heart disease. In the UK, death rates have remained more constant, while Japan has always had a low rate. Note the higher death rates in men.

Key

- – – – US Males
- • • • • US Females
- – – – UK Males
- • • • • UK Females
- – – – Japan Males
- • • • • Japan Females

include *echocardiography* and *radionuclide scanning* as well as coronary *angiography* (injection of a radiopaque substance into the arteries, followed by X-ray). Investigation results establish the precise extent of the narrowing of the arteries and the condition of the heart muscle, thereby determining the best choice of treatment.

TREATMENT

Angina may be relieved by a range of drugs that improve blood flow through the coronary arteries and/or reduce the workload on the heart during exercise. These drugs include glyceryl trinitrate and other *nitrate drugs, beta-blockers, calcium channel blockers,* and *vasodilator drugs.* Arrhythmias are commonly treated with beta-blockers, calcium channel blockers, and specific *antiarrhythmic drugs.* If the heart's pumping action is weak, it may sometimes be improved by vasodilators or *digoxin.*

If drug treatment fails to relieve the symptoms, or if investigation shows extensive narrowing of the coronary arteries, blood flow may be improved by *coronary artery bypass* surgery (in which a vein graft is used to circumvent the narrowed segment). If the disease is localized to one or two segments of artery, it may be possible to relieve blockages using balloon *angioplasty* (a technique by which a narrowed segment of artery is stretched by a small balloon).

A heart attack is usually treated initially in a hospital *coronary care unit.* Treatment may be given with *thrombolytic drugs* in an attempt to dissolve the blood clot in the coronary artery, the affected artery may be widened by angioplasty or may be immediately bypassed by surgery, or treatment may simply be aimed at allowing the heart to recover by a natural process of healing.

OUTLOOK AND PREVENTION

Coronary artery disease is a disease of middle to old age, but its foundations are laid in the teens and early adult life. The chances of developing the disease can be considerably reduced by an "anticoronary" lifestyle. The person who has never smoked, exercises regularly, is the correct weight, has normal blood pressure, and eats a prudent diet is unlikely to develop symptoms of coronary artery disease until late in life.

Even when symptoms develop, treatment can do a great deal to halt their progression. Studies of patients treated by coronary bypass surgery for disease affecting all the major coronary arteries have shown that 80 to 90 per cent are still alive five years after the operation. Survival is even better among those with less extensive disease; they can usually be treated with drugs. Survival is substantially improved in patients who give up cigarette smoking.

Coronary care unit

A small ward, specially staffed and equipped for the care of acutely ill patients who are suspected of being in the process of suffering, or who have suffered, a *myocardial infarction* (heart attack). In the unit, patients are kept under close surveillance and given immediate treatment if a complication such as *cardiac arrest* (cessation of heartbeat), *arrhythmia* (irregular or very rapid or slow heartbeat), or *heart failure* occurs.

A coronary care unit usually holds only five to 10 people, and the ratio of specially trained nurses to patients is high: one-to-one or one-to-two. The ward is equipped with monitoring equipment that provides a continuous record of each patient's heart rhythm, respiratory rate, and blood pressure, and contains specialized equipment for providing treatment, such as *defibrillation* to restore normal heart rhythm and *ventilation* to help the patient breathe.

Coronary heart disease

Disease of the arteries that supply blood to the heart muscle, causing damage to, or malfunction of, the heart. (See *Coronary artery disease.*)

Coronary thrombosis

Narrowing or blockage of one of the coronary arteries (which supply blood to the heart muscle) by a thrombus (blood clot). This causes a section of the heart muscle to die because it has been deprived of oxygen.

Coronary thrombosis is one of the main processes involved in *coronary artery disease,* the major cause of death in the UK. Sudden blockage of a coronary artery causes an acute *myocardial infarction* (death of a portion of heart muscle). The terms coronary thrombosis and myocardial infarction thus tend to be used interchangeably, but the latter is the more precise medical term for heart attack.

Coroner

A public officer appointed to inquire into any death of which the cause is unknown, or when it is suspected or known to result from unnatural causes, such as a road accident, poisoning, or an industrial injury. A coroner is most often informed when the deceased was not attended by a doctor during the final illness. If there are any uncertainties about the cause of death, the coroner will order a postmortem examination before issuing a death certificate. If the death is thought to be due to unnatural causes, the coroner will hold an inquest, sometimes before a jury. In Scotland, the duties of the coroner are encompassed by the Procurator Fiscal.

Cor pulmonale

Enlargement and strain of the right side of the heart due to chronic lung disease. Damage to the lungs increases resistance to blood flow from the heart through the branches of the pulmonary artery and causes pulmonary hypertension (increased pressure in the pulmonary artery). The resultant "back pressure" strain on the heart may eventually cause right-sided heart failure with *oedema* (fluid collection in the tissues). (See *Pulmonary hypertension.*)

Corpuscle

Any minute body or cell, particularly red and white *blood cells* or certain types of nerve endings.

Corset

A device worn around the trunk to treat *back pain* and spinal injuries or deformities (see *Spine* disorders box).

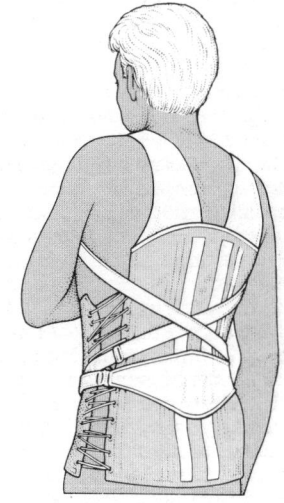

Spinal corset
Most often prescribed for back pain, this type of corset is usually made of cotton stiffened with metal or plastic.

Soft corsets, usually made of cotton fabric stiffened with plastic or metal, have straps enabling them to be tightened. Most commonly prescribed for back pain, corsets work in the same way as the belts worn by weightlifters—by increasing pressure on the abdomen they take the weight of the trunk off the lower spine. They also restrict painful movements and help keep the back warm.

Rigid corsets are made of plaster or lightweight plastic and must be moulded to the body. They are used to immobilize and support a spinal column that has become unstable through injury, or to help correct faulty alignment of the spine.

Cortex

The outer layer of certain organs, such as the brain, kidneys, or adrenal glands. The innermost region of some organs and other body structures is called the *medulla*.

Corticosteroid drugs

COMMON DRUGS

Beclomethasone Betamethasone Cortisone Dexamethasone Fludrocortisone Hydrocortisone Prednisolone Prednisone

---
WARNING
Sudden withdrawal of corticosteroid drugs may cause serious illness or death. Always inform a doctor if you are taking or have recently taken corticosteroids.

A group of drugs similar to the natural corticosteroid hormones produced by the cortex of the *adrenal glands*.

WHY THEY ARE USED

Corticosteroid drugs have a wide variety of uses. They are prescribed as hormone replacement therapy to patients with an inadequate level of natural corticosteroids caused by *Addison's disease*, following surgical removal of the adrenal glands, or when the *pituitary gland* has been destroyed by disease, surgery or irradiation.

Corticosteroid drugs are used in the treatment of inflammatory intestinal disorders, such as *Crohn's disease* and *ulcerative colitis*. *Temporal arteritis* needs urgent treatment with corticosteroids to reduce inflammation in the artery leading to the retina and so prevent blindness.

Other disorders that often improve with corticosteroid treatment include *asthma*, *rheumatoid arthritis*, *eczema*, *iritis* (inflammation of the iris), and

allergic *rhinitis* (hay fever). The injection of corticosteroids around an inflamed tendon or joint may relieve pain in disorders such as *tennis elbow* and *arthritis*.

Corticosteroid drugs are also used to suppress the immune system to prevent rejection of a transplanted organ (see *Transplant surgery*) and in the treatment of some types of cancer, such as a *lymphoma* or *leukaemia*.

POSSIBLE ADVERSE EFFECTS

The incidence and severity of any adverse effects depends on the dosage, the form in which the drug is given, and the duration of treatment.

Adverse effects are uncommon when corticosteroids are given in the form of a cream or by inhaler because only small amounts are absorbed into the bloodstream.

Corticosteroid tablets taken in high doses for long periods may cause *oedema* (accumulation of fluid in tissues), *hypertension* (high blood pressure), *diabetes mellitus*, *peptic ulcer*, *Cushing's syndrome*, *hirsutism* (excessive hairiness), inhibited growth in children, and, in rare cases, *cataract* or *psychosis*.

High doses of corticosteroid drugs also increase susceptibility to infection by impairing the body's *immune system* (natural defences).

Long-term treatment with corticosteroid drugs suppresses production of *ACTH* (adrenocorticotrophic hormone) by the pituitary gland, which in

turn suppresses production of corticosteroid hormones by the adrenal glands. Sudden withdrawal of the drugs may lead to *adrenal failure*, which may result in collapse, coma, and even death.

Corticosteroid hormones

A group of hormones produced by the *adrenal glands* that control the body's use of nutrients and the excretion of salts and water in the urine.

Corticotrophin

An alternative name for *ACTH* (adrenocorticotrophic hormone).

Cortisol

Another name for *hydrocortisone*, an important corticosteroid hormone produced by the *adrenal glands*. The level of cortisol in the blood is used to measure the function of the *pituitary gland* and the adrenal glands.

Cortisone

A synthetic *corticosteroid drug* used to reduce inflammation in severe allergic, rheumatic, and connective tissue diseases. It is also used as a replacement hormone in *Addison's disease*, in which there is a corticosteroid hormone deficiency, and after removal of the *adrenal glands*.

Coryza

A term for the nasal symptoms of the common cold (see *Cold, common*).

HOW CORTICOSTEROIDS WORK

When given as hormone replacement therapy, corticosteroids supplement or replace natural hormones. Large doses have an anti-inflammatory effect as they reduce the production of prostaglandins. They also suppress the immune system by reducing the release and activity of white blood cells.

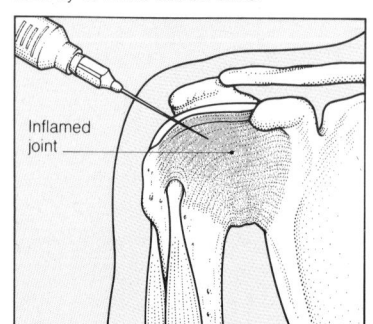

Inflamed joint

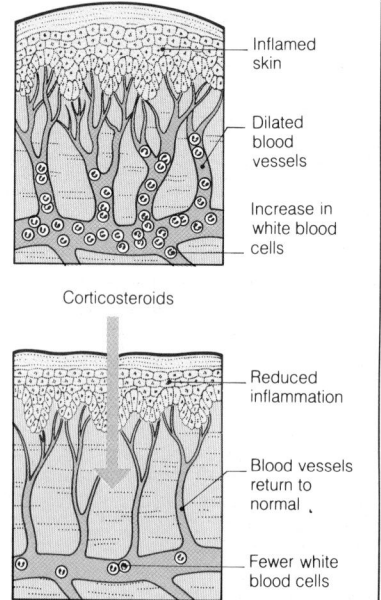

Inflamed skin

Dilated blood vessels

Increase in white blood cells

Corticosteroids

Reduced inflammation

Blood vessels return to normal

Fewer white blood cells

Cosmetic dentistry

Procedures to improve the appearance of the teeth. In many cases, these treatments are also necessary to restore or prevent further damage to the teeth and/or gums.

Teeth that are out of alignment can become decayed because the bite is incorrect (see *Malocclusion*) and because the teeth are hard to keep clean. Such teeth can be moved into proper position by fitting an *orthodontic appliance* (brace). Correction is usually best carried out during childhood, when the teeth and jaws are still growing and developing, but can also be performed in adults.

The main use of a *crown* is to restore normal tooth structure and thus prevent further damage when a tooth is severely decayed or has been broken. However, crowns can also be fitted primarily for cosmetic reasons when a front tooth is damaged or discoloured; in this case a porcelain crown is fitted because of its similarity in colour to the natural teeth.

Bonding is a relatively new technique that has a wide range of cosmetic uses. It can be used to treat chipped or malformed teeth, to close small gaps between front teeth, or to cover stained or discoloured teeth. In some cases it can be used instead of a crown for front teeth.

Teeth that have become discoloured because the pulp is dead or has been removed may be treated by bleaching (see *Bleaching, dental*).

Cosmetic surgery

An operation performed primarily to improve the appearance of an individual rather than to improve function or to cure disease.

WHY IT IS DONE

Cosmetic surgery can improve appearance in a number of ways. Skin blemishes can be removed, and the appearance of an unsightly scar improved. The shape and size of the nose, chin, jaw, or breasts can be altered. Excess skin and fat, and any unsightly creases or marks that come with age or loss of weight, can be removed from the eyelids, face, breasts, or stomach.

An individual's expectations of the benefits of cosmetic surgery are often too great, however. Cosmetic surgery will not produce a dramatic change in personality or cure depression that a person attributes to his or her appearance. Nor can it reproduce an exact replica of someone else's features. Some procedures (such as *face-lifts* and

hair transplants) may need to be repeated over the years; other procedures (such as *body contour surgery*) may result in uneven residual fat and unattractive scarring. Anyone contemplating cosmetic surgery should first discuss the operation in detail with his or her doctor.

Costalgia

Pain around the chest due to damage to a rib or to one of the intercostal nerves (which run beneath the ribs). A broken rib produces pain and tenderness over the affected part of the ribcage. The pain is made worse by deep breathing and often persists for several weeks after the original injury.

Damage to one of the intercostal nerves is most commonly a result of an attack of the viral infection *herpes zoster* (shingles). The pain is difficult to treat successfully and tends to persist for several months or longer.

Cot death

See *Sudden infant death syndrome*.

Co-trimoxazole

An *antibacterial drug* that contains trimethoprim and sulphamethoxazole. Co-trimoxazole is commonly prescribed for the prevention and treatment of urinary tract infections, and the treatment of infections of the respiratory tract, gastrointestinal tract, skin, and ear. It is also used to treat prostatitis, gonorrhoea, and pneumocystis pneumonia.

Possible adverse effects include nausea, vomiting, sore tongue, rash, and, rarely, blood disorders and jaundice.

Cough

A reflex action to try to clear the airways of mucus, sputum (phlegm), a foreign body, or other irritants or blockages. A cough is said to be productive when it brings up mucus or sputum, and unproductive, or dry, when it does not.

CAUSES

Many coughs are due to irritation of the airways by dust, smoke, or gases, or by mucus dripping from the back of the nose because of chronic *sinusitis*. Another common cause of coughs is inflammation of the upper respiratory tract, usually due to a viral infection (see *Cold, common*; *Laryngitis*; *Pharyngitis*; *Tracheitis*).

In a child, inflammation of the upper respiratory tract can cause narrowing of the airways, leading to *croup*

TYPES OF COSMETIC SURGERY

There are various different cosmetic surgery procedures, some of the more commonly performed of which are shown below. The different procedures vary in the permanency of their results and in the likelihood of achieving a satisfactory appearance.

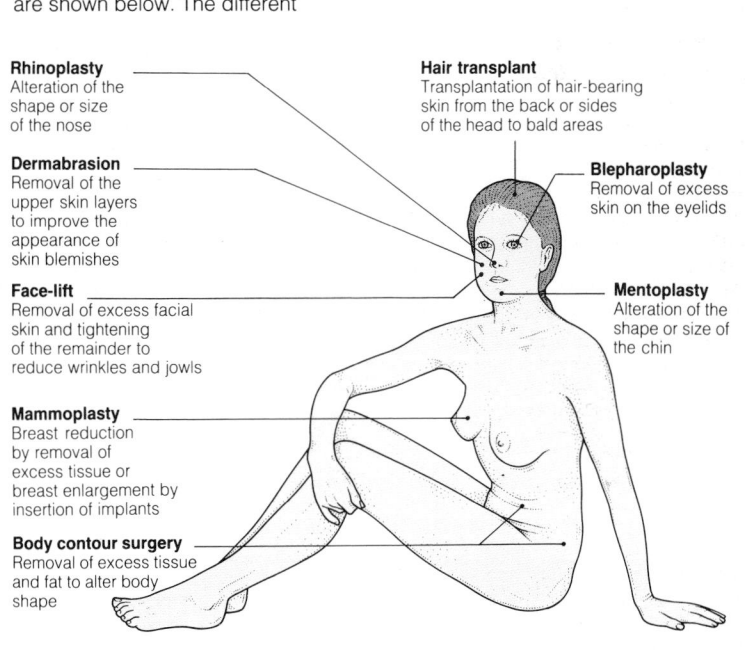

Rhinoplasty
Alteration of the shape or size of the nose

Dermabrasion
Removal of the upper skin layers to improve the appearance of skin blemishes

Face-lift
Removal of excess facial skin and tightening of the remainder to reduce wrinkles and jowls

Mammoplasty
Breast reduction by removal of excess tissue or breast enlargement by insertion of implants

Body contour surgery
Removal of excess tissue and fat to alter body shape

Hair transplant
Transplantation of hair-bearing skin from the back or sides of the head to bald areas

Blepharoplasty
Removal of excess skin on the eyelids

Mentoplasty
Alteration of the shape or size of the chin

C

(a condition that is characterized by hoarseness, noisy breathing, and a barking cough) and breathing difficulty. Infection with the bacterium *BORDETELLA PERTUSSIS* produces the characteristic cough of *pertussis* (whooping cough).

Bronchitis (inflammation of the bronchi, the air passages into the lungs) produces thick mucus and sputum and causes severe coughing. The disorder may be brought on by an infection, but often occurs as a result of smoking (see *Cough, smoker's*). In *bronchiectasis* (distortion or widening of the bronchi), a large amount of infected sputum accumulates in the bronchi, making the sufferer cough persistently.

Bronchospasm (temporary narrowing of the bronchi) causes a dry cough that is usually worse at night. It is a feature of *asthma*, but may also be due to infection or an allergic reaction.

The damage to lung tissues caused by *pneumonia* (inflammation of the lungs) results in a painful productive cough. Damage to the lungs brought about by pulmonary *oedema* (accumulation of fluid in the lungs) produces a cough that is dry at first, but which later may bring up frothy, blood-stained sputum. The cough associated with viral bronchitis and viral pneumonia is often dry and persistent, and may interrupt sleep.

Various chronic lung infections, notably *tuberculosis*, may cause a cough. Many *pneumoconioses* (dust diseases of the lungs) also cause a cough, which is usually accompanied by shortness of breath.

An inhaled foreign object, such as a peanut, that lodges in the larynx causes violent coughing to relieve *choking*. If the object travels further down and blocks a bronchus, inflammation and mucus will be produced at the site of obstruction, leading to a persistent cough.

Lung cancer and, less commonly, other tumours of the air passages usually first cause a mild cough and then a more severe one that may produce bloodstained sputum.

A cough may be a side-effect of *ACE inhibitor drugs*. Sometimes, especially in children, coughing may be a nervous reaction to stress.

SELF-HELP

In some cases, a dry cough may be relieved by sucking throat lozenges or by drinking warm, soothing drinks, such as honey and water. If these are ineffective, narcotic *cough remedies* help to relieve symptoms and may be particularly useful at bedtime to permit sleep.

Productive coughing is the body's way of unblocking airways that are obstructed by mucus or sputum and, in such cases, cough suppressants should be avoided because they can do more harm than good. An expectorant cough medication and/or drinking lots of fluids can help to loosen mucus or sputum if there is difficulty coughing it up.

A doctor should be consulted if any cough persists for more than a week, is severe, or is accompanied by symptoms such as chest pain, green sputum, coughed-up blood, or breathing difficulty.

TREATMENT

Treatment for a cough depends on the underlying disorder. For example, an *antibiotic drug* may be given for a bacterial infection; a *bronchodilator drug* and/or a *corticosteroid drug* for asthma; *breathing exercises* and *postural drainage* (lying in a position that allows mucus to drain from the bronchi) for bronchiectasis and chronic bronchitis; and surgery or *radiotherapy* for cancer.

Coughing up blood

Known medically as haemoptysis, coughing up blood is due to rupture of a blood vessel in the airways, lungs, nose, or throat.

Coughed-up blood may be in the form of bright-red or rusty-brown streaks or clots in or on the sputum (phlegm), a pinkish froth, or, more rarely, pure blood. The form it takes depends as much on the size of the ruptured blood vessel as on the underlying cause. Coughing up blood should not be confused with blood in the mouth, which is usually due to a nosebleed or to bleeding gums.

Because of the possibility of a serious underlying disorder, all cases of coughing up blood require medical assessment.

CAUSES

Any disorder that causes a persistent *cough* can produce haemoptysis by putting strain on the blood vessels in the airways.

The most common cause of coughing up blood is an infection—such as *pneumonia*, *bronchitis*, or *tuberculosis*—in which inflammation of the bronchi (airways into the lungs) and alveoli (air sacs) damages a blood-vessel wall. Similarly, in *bronchiectasis* the bronchi become enlarged and distorted, which can lead to rupture of a blood vessel and coughing up blood.

Another cause of coughing up blood is congestion in, and subsequent rupture of, blood vessels within the lungs. Congestion can be due to *heart failure*, *mitral stenosis* (narrowing of the mitral valve in the heart), or pulmonary embolism (blood clot lodged in an artery in the lungs).

A malignant tumour can lead to coughing up blood by eroding the wall of a blood vessel in the larynx (voice-box), bronchi, or alveoli.

INVESTIGATION AND TREATMENT

A *chest X-ray* may be carried out. Anyone who smokes, who is older than 40, whose chest X-rays are abnormal, or who has coughed up blood more than once may require *bronchoscopy*, a diagnostic procedure in which a flexible viewing instrument is passed into the lungs. In about one third of cases, however, no underlying cause is found.

Treatment depends on the cause, but may include *antibiotic drugs*, *anticoagulant drugs*, and *diuretic drugs*.

Cough remedies

COMMON DRUGS

Expectorants
Ammonium chloride

Cough suppressants
Antihistamines Codeine Dextromethorphan

A bewildering variety of over-the-counter medications is available for treating a *cough*. Most cough remedies consist of a syrupy base to which various active ingredients and flavourings are added.

Two main groups of drugs are used: expectorants, intended for coughs that are producing sputum (phlegm), and cough suppressants, intended for dry coughs. It is important to select the correct type of medication—a cough suppressant taken for a sputum-producing cough may interfere with the coughing up of sputum and delay recovery.

HOW THEY WORK

Expectorants "loosen" a cough by stimulating the production of watery secretions in the lungs. Some expectorants also have a mucolytic action (a direct effect on the sputum that makes it less sticky).

Cough suppressants act on the part of the brain that controls the coughing reflex. Drugs with this effect include some *antihistamine drugs* and the narcotic analgesic drug *codeine*.

POSSIBLE ADVERSE EFFECTS

All cough suppressants have a sedative effect and may cause drowsiness.

C

COUGH A noisy expulsion of air from the lungs that may produce sputum (phlegm) or be "dry."

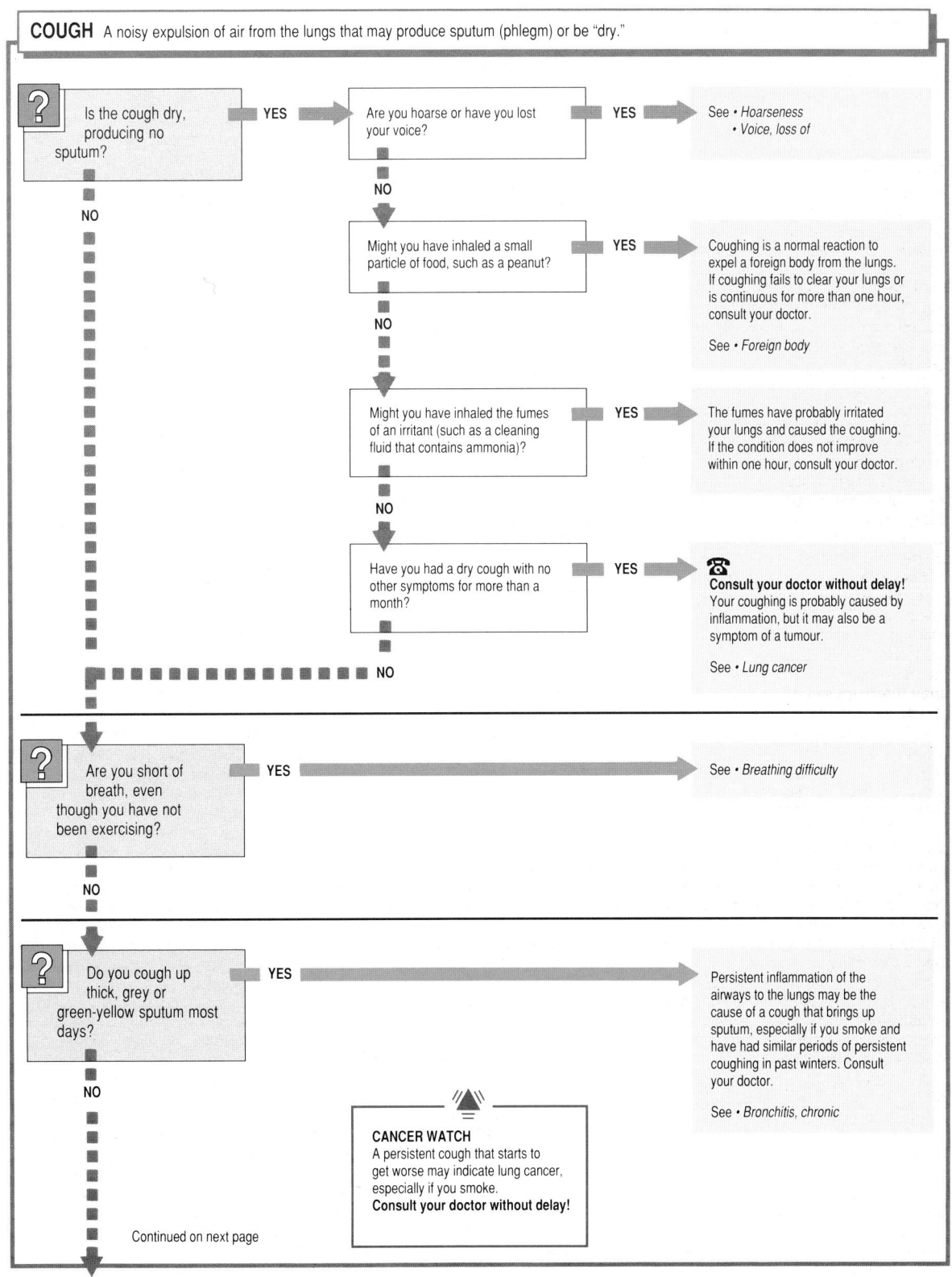

? Is the cough dry, producing no sputum?

YES → Are you hoarse or have you lost your voice?

YES → See • *Hoarseness*
• *Voice, loss of*

NO ↓

Might you have inhaled a small particle of food, such as a peanut?

YES → Coughing is a normal reaction to expel a foreign body from the lungs. If coughing fails to clear your lungs or is continuous for more than one hour, consult your doctor.

See • *Foreign body*

NO ↓

Might you have inhaled the fumes of an irritant (such as a cleaning fluid that contains ammonia)?

YES → The fumes have probably irritated your lungs and caused the coughing. If the condition does not improve within one hour, consult your doctor.

NO ↓

Have you had a dry cough with no other symptoms for more than a month?

YES → ☎ **Consult your doctor without delay!** Your coughing is probably caused by inflammation, but it may also be a symptom of a tumour.

See • *Lung cancer*

NO →

NO (from first question) ↓

? Are you short of breath, even though you have not been exercising?

YES → See • *Breathing difficulty*

NO ↓

? Do you cough up thick, grey or green-yellow sputum most days?

YES → Persistent inflammation of the airways to the lungs may be the cause of a cough that brings up sputum, especially if you smoke and have had similar periods of persistent coughing in past winters. Consult your doctor.

See • *Bronchitis, chronic*

NO ↓

CANCER WATCH
A persistent cough that starts to get worse may indicate lung cancer, especially if you smoke.
Consult your doctor without delay!

Continued on next page

C

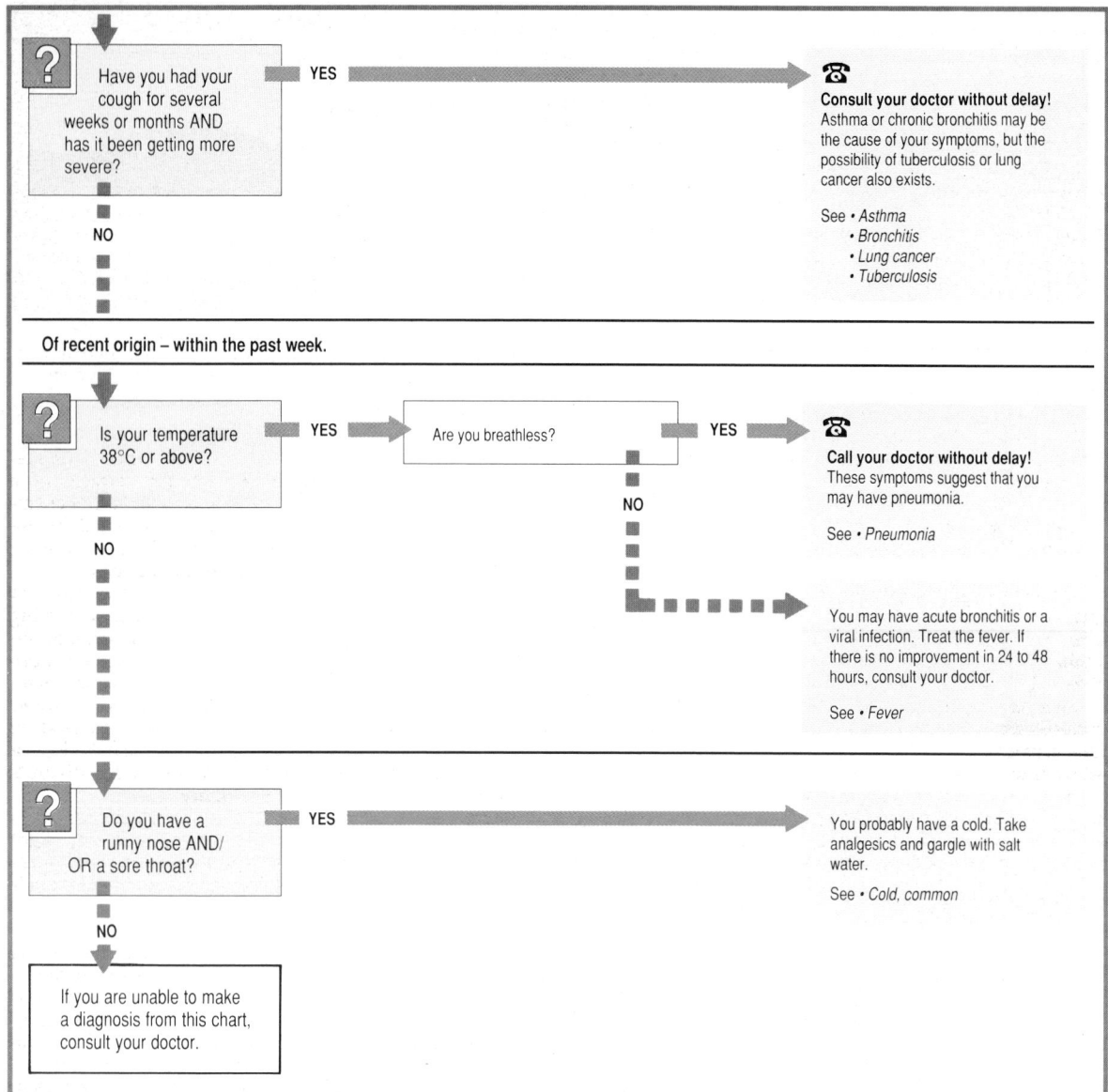

Have you had your cough for several weeks or months AND has it been getting more severe?

YES → ☎ **Consult your doctor without delay!**
Asthma or chronic bronchitis may be the cause of your symptoms, but the possibility of tuberculosis or lung cancer also exists.

See • *Asthma*
    • *Bronchitis*
    • *Lung cancer*
    • *Tuberculosis*

NO

Of recent origin – within the past week.

Is your temperature 38°C or above?

YES → Are you breathless? **YES** → ☎ **Call your doctor without delay!**
These symptoms suggest that you may have pneumonia.

See • *Pneumonia*

NO (from "Are you breathless?") → You may have acute bronchitis or a viral infection. Treat the fever. If there is no improvement in 24 to 48 hours, consult your doctor.

See • *Fever*

NO (from temperature)

Do you have a runny nose AND/OR a sore throat?

YES → You probably have a cold. Take analgesics and gargle with salt water.

See • *Cold, common*

NO

If you are unable to make a diagnosis from this chart, consult your doctor.

Using cough remedies to alleviate the symptoms of a persistent cough may delay diagnosis of a serious disorder.

Cough, smoker's
A recurrent cough that is very common among smokers, particularly heavy smokers and those who have smoked for a long time. In many cases, the sufferer becomes accustomed to his or her cough and regards it as normal.

Usually, coughing is triggered by the accumulation of thick sputum (phlegm) in the airways (a feature of chronic *bronchitis*), which is caused by inflammation of the airways due to smoking. There is no such thing as a "normal" cough.

TREATMENT
Stopping smoking usually stops the persistent cough, although this does not happen immediately. In general, the longer the person has been smoking, the longer the cough will persist after giving up.

Because of the association between smoking and *lung cancer*, it is essential for a smoker to seek medical advice about his or her cough, particularly if there is any change in its frequency or character. (See also *Tobacco-smoking*.)

Counselling
Advice and psychological support given by a health professional and usually aimed at helping a person cope with a particular problem (for example, bereavement or cancer treatment). A more general exploration of a person's feelings and attitudes, not aimed at one particular problem, is sometimes included in the definition.

WHY IT IS DONE
Counselling can help people with problems at school, work, or within the family; provide advice on medical problems, family planning, abortion, and sexual and marital problems; help

people deal with drinking and drug problems; and provide support during various life crises.

Doctors may use a counselling style when interviewing a patient whose medical problem is complicated by personal circumstances, or when the patient's reason for consulting the doctor is not clear.

HOW IT IS DONE

Some counselling, especially for genetic disorders (see *Genetic counselling*) or the treatment of cancer, consists mainly of providing personalized information in a setting in which the patient, or client, is encouraged to ask questions and express any doubts and uncertainties.

Techniques used in psychotherapeutic counselling are essentially similar. The counsellor encourages the individual to make statements about his or her feelings, experiences, and problems. These statements can then be discussed and explored for inconsistencies as a means of helping the individual develop a greater and more realistic understanding of his or her problems.

Usually, counselling is a one-to-one activity. However, in some situations, such as *sex therapy*, representatives of a particular point of view or gender model may take part (for example, one male and one female counsellor). This is termed co-counselling. Counselling may also occur in small groups. (See also *Child guidance*; *Family therapy*; *Marriage guidance*; *Psychotherapy*.)

Cowpox

An infection caused by the *VACCINIA* virus, which usually affects cows.

An attack of cowpox used to confer immunity against *smallpox* (now extinct) because the viruses responsible for the two diseases were very similar. This fact was the basis of smallpox vaccination. Vaccinia virus, which gave its name to "vaccination", continued to be used as smallpox vaccine until smallpox was eradicated in the 1970s.

Coxa vara

A deformity of the hip in which the angle between the neck and head (ball) of the femur (thigh-bone) and the shaft of the femur is reduced, resulting in shortening of the leg and a limp.

CAUSES

The most common cause of coxa vara is injury—either a fracture of the neck of the femur or, during adolescence, injury to the developing part of the

head of the bone. The deformity can also occur if the bone tissue in the neck of the femur is soft instead of firm, so that it bends under the weight of the body. This softening may be congenital (present at birth) or it may be the result of a bone disorder such as *rickets* or *Paget's disease*.

SYMPTOMS, DIAGNOSIS, AND TREATMENT

The symptoms are pain and stiffness in the hip and difficulty in walking. The disorder is diagnosed by *X-rays*, which reveal the deformity.

Treatment depends on the underlying condition. In some cases, an operation may be performed to cut the deformed part of the bone and reposition the two ends at the correct angle (see *Osteotomy*). This usually eases the condition so that the patient can walk with only minor discomfort.

Crab lice

See *Pubic lice*.

Cradle cap

A condition common in babies in which thick, yellow scales occur in patches over the scalp. Cradle cap is harmless if the scalp skin does not become infected. The condition tends to recur.

Cradle cap is a form of seborrhoeic *dermatitis*, which may also occur on the face, neck, behind the ears, and in the nappy area. The skin in these areas may look red and inflamed.

TREATMENT

Cradle cap is best treated by daily use of a simple shampoo, such as cetrimide solution. Alternatively, warm olive oil or arachis oil may be rubbed into the baby's scalp and left on overnight to loosen and soften the scales, which can then be gently washed off the following day. This procedure may need to be repeated for several days until all the scales have been loosened and washed off.

The baby's hair should be brushed daily using a clean soft-bristled brush. This will also help loosen the scales.

If the condition seems to be worsening or if the skin looks inflamed, a doctor should be consulted. A mild ointment containing an *antibiotic drug* and a *corticosteroid drug* may be prescribed for use until the condition improves.

Cramp

Painful spasm in a muscle caused by excessive and prolonged contraction of the muscle fibres. Cramps are a common occurrence and usually last only a few moments.

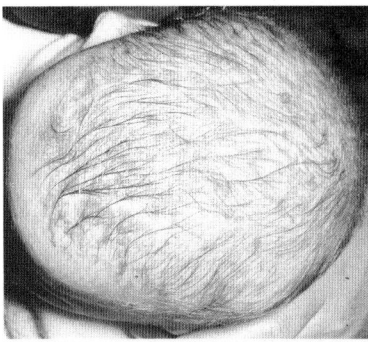

Appearance of cradle cap
Most prevalent between 3 and 9 months of age, it is not clear why cradle cap occurs, but it is not a result of poor hygiene.

CAUSES

Cramps often occur during or immediately after exercise because of a build-up of lactic acid and other chemicals in the muscles (caused by increased muscular activity) and small areas of muscle-fibre damage.

Cramps can also occur during any repetitive movement, such as writing (see *Cramp, writer's*), or through sitting or lying in an awkward position. Anything that causes profuse sweating, such as a fever, very hot weather, or prolonged exercise, can lead to cramps in resting muscles; the loss of sodium salts in the sweat disrupts muscle cell activity.

Cramps at night usually have no known cause. In some cases, night cramps may be due to *peripheral vascular disease* (narrowing of blood vessels in the legs).

TREATMENT

Cramp can be relieved by massaging or stretching the muscles involved. If cramps occur regularly at night, your doctor may prescribe a drug containing calcium or quinine, which can help prevent painful recurrences.

If cramps persist for longer than about an hour, they are likely to be due to a more serious condition and medical attention should be sought immediately.

Cramp, writer's

Painful spasm in the muscles of the hand, which makes writing or typing impossible. In most cases the muscles in the hand are still able to perform other tasks, indicating that the problem may be psychological in origin. However, writer's cramp does not respond to psychotherapy. Drug treatment has also been found to have little effect. Writer's cramp sometimes improves if the hand is rested for

C

a few months, but often the problem is permanent. Occasionally the other hand becomes affected.

Cranial nerves

Twelve pairs of nerves that emerge directly from the brain—as opposed to the *spinal nerves*, which connect with the spinal cord. All but two of the cranial nerve pairs connect with nuclei in the *brainstem* (the lowest section of the brain). The other two (the olfactory and optic nerves) link directly with parts of the *cerebrum*. All the nerves emerge through various openings in the cranium (skull surrounding the brain); many then soon divide into several major branches.

Craniopharyngioma

A tumour of the pituitary gland. Craniopharyngioma is very rare, with a few hundred cases in the UK each year. More than half of those affected are under 20 years old.

Symptoms include headaches, vomiting, defective vision, stunted growth, and failure of sexual development. If untreated, a craniopharyngioma may result in permanent brain damage.

Craniopharyngiomas are identified by *brain imaging* techniques and are usually removed surgically.

Craniosynostosis

The premature closure of one or more of the joints (known as synostoses or *sutures*) between the curved, flattened bones of the *skull* (cranium); also called craniostenosis.

Craniosynostosis is three times more common in boys than in girls. It may occur before birth, and one third of those affected have other *birth defects*. It also may occur in an otherwise healthy baby, or in a baby affected by another disorder such as rickets. The condition occasionally runs in families.

If all of the skull joints are involved, the growing infant's brain may be compressed and the pressure inside the skull may increase. If the abnormality is localized, the head may be deformed.

DIAGNOSIS AND TREATMENT
The diagnosis is made from the outward appearance of the skull and from skull *X-rays* or *CT scanning*. If the brain is compressed, treatment must be undertaken to prevent brain damage. An operation is performed to separate the skull bones by cutting away the fused edges and separating the bony plates.

Craniotomy

Removal of part of the skull to carry out an operation on the brain, such as for the removal of a sample of tissue for analysis, removal of a tumour, or drainage of an abscess or blood clot.

After the operation, the bone is replaced and the membranes, muscle,

FUNCTIONS OF CRANIAL NERVES

Some cranial nerves are principally concerned with delivering sensory information from organs, such as the ears, nose, and eyes, to the brain. Others carry messages that move the tongue, eyes, and facial (and other) muscles, or stimulate glands such as the salivary glands. A few have both sensory and motor functions. One of the nerves—the 10th cranial, or *vagus nerve*—is one of the most important components of the *parasympathetic nervous system*, which is concerned with maintaining the rhythmic automatic function of the internal body machinery. It has branches to all the main digestive organs, the heart, and the lungs.

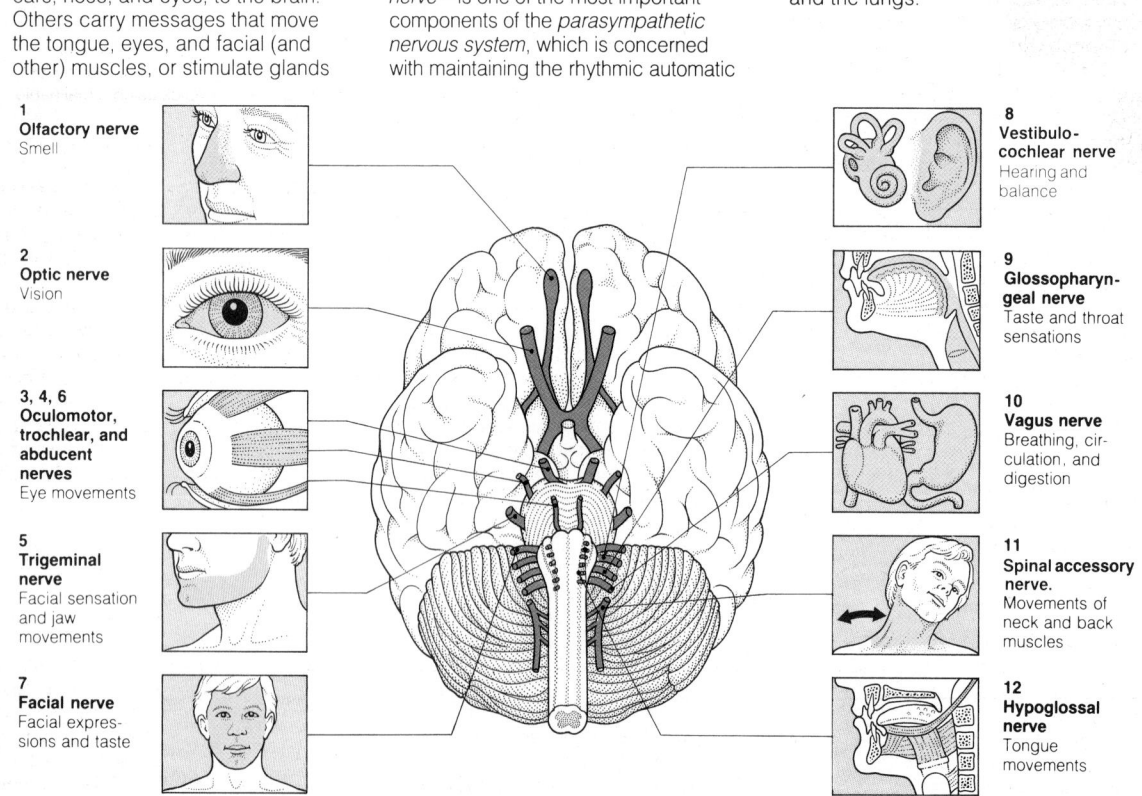

1
Olfactory nerve
Smell

2
Optic nerve
Vision

3, 4, 6
Oculomotor, trochlear, and abducent nerves
Eye movements

5
Trigeminal nerve
Facial sensation and jaw movements

7
Facial nerve
Facial expressions and taste

8
Vestibulo-cochlear nerve
Hearing and balance

9
Glossopharyngeal nerve
Taste and throat sensations

10
Vagus nerve
Breathing, circulation, and digestion

11
Spinal accessory nerve.
Movements of neck and back muscles

12
Hypoglossal nerve
Tongue movements

and skin are sewn back into position. After successful surgery, patients usually leave hospital within a week, and will generally experience mild headaches for a time, but little real pain.

Cranium

The part of the *skull* around the brain.

Cream

A thick, semi-solid preparation used to apply medications to the skin for therapeutic or prophylactic (preventive) purposes. Creams are useful in the treatment of dry skin conditions because their high water content gives them a moisturizing effect.

Creatinine clearance

See *Kidney-function tests*.

Crepitus

The grating sound heard, and the sensation felt, when two rough surfaces rub together. Crepitus may be experienced when the ends of a broken bone rub against each other, or in *osteoarthritis* when the cartilage that covers the bony surfaces of a joint has worn away and the roughened areas of the joint grind against each other. The sound is usually audible to the naked ear. Fainter sounds, audible through a *stethoscope*, are produced in the lung as a result of inflammation—due to pneumonia, for example.

The term crepitus is also used to describe the sounds made when an area of air under the skin (see *Emphysema, surgical*) or *gas gangrene* (gas within infected tissues) is pressed.

Cretinism

A *congenital* condition that is characterized by stunted growth, mental handicap, and coarse facial features in infants. Cretinism results from absent or insufficient thyroxine (a *thyroid hormone*) production by the thyroid gland at birth.

A routine test is performed to screen for the condition in all newborn infants in the UK. A complete cure is possible by means of replacement therapy with thyroxine provided the condition is recognized early. (See also *Hypothyroidism*.)

Creutzfeldt-Jakob disease

A very rare degenerative condition of the brain thought to be due to a slow virus (one that causes no signs of disease until many months or years after the original infection).

In most instances, no source of infection is discovered. However,

PROCEDURE FOR CRANIOTOMY

Before the operation, all or part of the patient's scalp is shaved. After a general anaesthetic has been given, layers of skin, muscle, and membrane are cut away from the skull at the planned operation site and the bone is cut with a saw. The lid of bone is then either lifted back on a hinge of muscle or removed completely. The dura (the outer membrane lining the brain) is then opened to reveal the inner membranes and the brain.

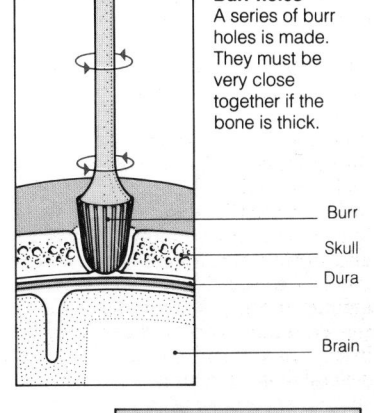

Burr holes
A series of burr holes is made. They must be very close together if the bone is thick.

Burr

Skull

Dura

Brain

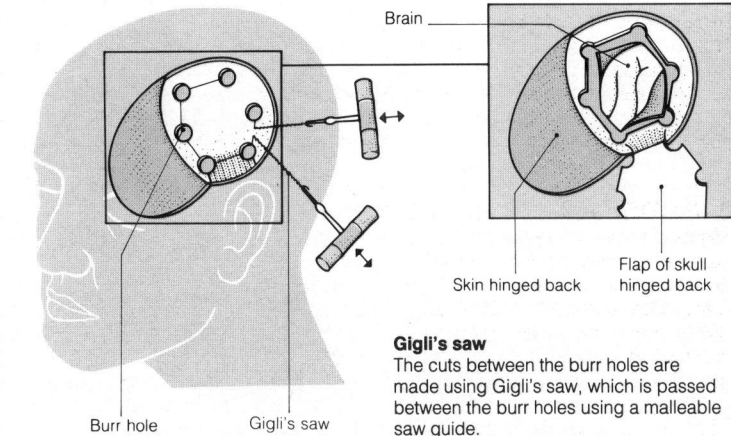

Brain

Flap of skull hinged back

Skin hinged back

Burr hole   Gigli's saw

Gigli's saw
The cuts between the burr holes are made using Gigli's saw, which is passed between the burr holes using a malleable saw guide.

rarely, infection has been linked with brain surgery when instruments contaminated by the virus have been used, and with transplant of an infected cornea. It has also been linked with treatment with human *growth hormone* or *gonadatrophin hormones* extracted from pituitary glands after death. Hormones from this source are no longer used; current preparations are made by genetic engineering, or extracted from urine, and carry no risk.

The condition causes progressive *dementia* and *myoclonus* (sudden muscular contractions). Muscular coordination diminishes, the intellect and personality deteriorate, and blindness may develop. As the disease progresses, the power of speech is lost and the body becomes rigid. There is no treatment and death usually occurs within three to 12 months of onset.

Cri du chat syndrome

A *congenital* condition characterized by a cat-like cry due to a small larynx. Mental handicap, poor brain de-

velopment, a small head, an unusual rounded face with small jaw and wide spacing between the eyes, a low birth weight, and shortness of stature are other typical features.

Cri du chat syndrome is rare and is the result of a *chromosomal abnormality*; a portion of one particular chromosome is missing in each of the affected individual's cells.

No treatment is possible. The child needs special care and schooling if he or she survives infancy. (See also *Genetic counselling*.)

Crisis

A term that describes a turning point in the course of a disease (marking the onset of either recovery or deterioration), an emergency, or a distressing time of emotional difficulty (such as divorce, or a serious illness or death in the family). In medicine, the term was in common use before the advent of antibiotics when patients who had lobar *pneumonia* would be watched for the crisis.

C

Crisis intervention

The provision of immediate advice or help to people with acute personal or sociomedical problems.

Many voluntary organizations have been established to help people in crisis. Help may also be available at walk-in centres or social services departments. In addition to other crisis services, these centres may offer *counselling*, usually with the aim of helping clients cope with crises rather than of providing longer-term help.

Critical

A term used to mean seriously ill, or to describe a crucial state of illness from which it is uncertain whether the patient will recover.

Crohn's disease

A chronic inflammatory disease that can affect any part of the gastrointestinal tract from the mouth to the anus. Crohn's disease may cause pain, fever, diarrhoea, and loss of weight.

The most common site of inflammation is the terminal ileum (the end of the small intestine where it joins the large intestine). The intestinal wall becomes extremely thick due to continued chronic inflammation, and deep, penetrating ulcers may form. The disease tends to be patchy; areas of the intestine that lie between diseased areas may appear to be normal, but are usually mildly affected.

CAUSES AND INCIDENCE
The cause is unknown. It may represent an abnormal allergic reaction or may be an exaggerated response to an infectious agent, such as a bacterium or a virus. There is a slight genetic predisposition (inherited tendency) to develop the disease.

The incidence of Crohn's disease varies between countries. In the UK, about 3,000 to 4,000 new cases are diagnosed each year. The incidence seems to have increased over the last 30 years. A person may be affected at any age, but the peak periods are adolescence and early adulthood and after the age of 60.

SYMPTOMS
In young people, the ileum is usually involved, and the disease causes spasms of pain in the abdomen, diarrhoea, and chronic sickness due to loss of appetite, anaemia, and weight loss. The ability of the small intestine to absorb food is reduced. In the elderly, it is more common for the disease to affect the rectum and cause rectal bleeding. In both groups, the disease may also affect the anus,

resulting in chronic abscesses, deep fissures (cracks), and fistulas (abnormal passageways).

Crohn's disease can also affect the colon (the major part of the large intestine), causing bloody diarrhoea. In rare cases, the disease also affects the mouth, oesophagus, stomach, and duodenum (the upper part of the small intestine).

Complications may affect the intestines or may develop elsewhere in the body. The thickening of the intestinal wall may narrow the inside of the intestine so much that an obstruction occurs.

About 30 per cent of patients with Crohn's disease develop a fistula. Internal fistulas may form between loops of intestine. External fistulas from the intestine to the skin of the abdomen or the skin surrounding the anus may follow a surgical operation (or the rupture of an abscess) and may cause leakage of faeces on to the skin.

Abscesses (pus-filled pockets of infection) form in about 20 per cent of patients. Many of these abscesses occur around the anus, but some occur within the abdomen.

Complications in other parts of the body may include inflammation of various parts of the eye, severe arthritis affecting various joints of the body, *ankylosing spondylitis* (an inflammation of the spine), and skin disorders (including *eczema*).

DIAGNOSIS
If the symptoms suggest Crohn's disease, a physical examination may reveal tender abdominal swellings that indicate thickening of the intestinal walls. *Sigmoidoscopy* (examination of the sigmoid colon and rectum with a viewing instrument) may confirm the disease's presence in the rectum. X-rays using barium meals or barium enemas (see *Barium X-ray examinations*) will show thickened loops of intestine with deep fissures. It may be difficult to differentiate between Crohn's disease that affects the colon and *ulcerative colitis*, an inflammatory bowel disease that is limited to the large intestine, but *colonoscopy* (examination of the colon using a flexible viewing instrument) and *biopsy* (removal of a sample of tissue for microscopic examination) may help in doubtful cases. In addition, blood tests may show evidence of protein deficiency or *anaemia*.

TREATMENT
Sulphasalazine and related drugs may be given by mouth to try to control the inflammatory process and *corticosteroid*

drugs may be given by mouth or as enemas. Patients suffering from severe acute attacks may require admission to hospital for blood transfusion, intravenous feeding, and intravenous administration of corticosteroid drugs. The severity of the disease fluctuates widely, and patients are usually under long-term medical supervision.

Some patients find that particular foods exacerbate their symptoms. Others may benefit from a high-vitamin, low-fibre diet.

A surgical operation to remove damaged portions of the intestine may be needed to treat chronic obstruction or blood loss. If the small intestine is involved, the surgeon will remove as little of the intestine as possible, seeking only to remove the most affected parts since the surgery is not curative.

If the large intestine is involved, surgery may involve removal of narrowed obstructing segments.

Emergency surgery may sometimes be required to deal with an abscess. Simple drainage of an abscess will produce an external fistula, but occasionally the patient is too ill for any further treatment. Surgery may also occasionally be required for obstruction, perforation (rupture), or severe bleeding.

OUTLOOK
The disease is chronic and the symptoms fluctuate over many years, eventually subsiding in some patients. Many patients require surgical treatment at some stage to deal with complications of the disease. The recurrence rate after surgery is high, although recurrences may be delayed for many years.

Some patients in whom the disease is localized remain in normal health indefinitely and seem to be cured. There is no predisposition to intestinal cancer.

Crossbite

A type of *malocclusion* in which some or all of the lower front teeth overlap the upper front teeth. In a normal bite, the reverse is true.

Cross-eye

A type of *strabismus* (squint) in which one or both eyes turns inwards relative to the other.

Cross-matching

A procedure used to determine compatibility between the blood of a person who requires a *blood transfusion* and that of a blood donor.

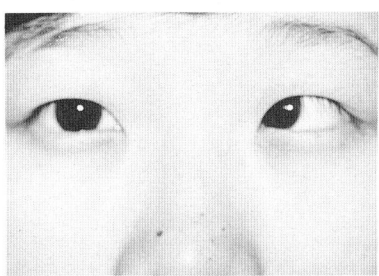

Appearance of cross-eye
Many cases of cross-eye can be corrected to improve appearance and vision.

Red blood cells from the donor are mixed with serum from the recipient, and red blood cells from the recipient are mixed with serum from the donor. After a short time, the mixtures are examined on a glass slide under a microscope. Grouping together of the red cells to form a small clump indicates the presence of antibodies in the serum, showing that the blood is not compatible. If no clumping occurs, the donor's blood may be safely transfused to the recipient.

Croup

A term meaning a harsh sound, applied to a condition due to narrowing and inflammation of the airways in infants and young children. Croup causes hoarseness, stridor (a grunting noise during breathing), and a barking cough. It is very common in children up to the age of about four years.

In older children and adults, the airways are wider and the cartilage in the wall is stiffer, so that the effect of any swelling or inflammation is less marked.

CAUSES

Croup may be caused by a viral or bacterial infection that affects the larynx (voice-box), the epiglottis which covers the larynx (see *epiglottitis*), or the trachea (windpipe). Infectious croup tends to occur in winter. Other causes include *diphtheria*, *allergy*, spasm caused by deficient *calcium* in the blood, and the inhalation of a *foreign body*, such as a peanut.

TREATMENT

Most cases are mild and pass quickly. A parent should remain calm and comfort the child; once soothed, the child will be able to breathe more easily. Providing a warm mist for the child to inhale (e.g. by using a room humidifier or putting wet towels over radiators) may also help.

If a child is distressed and you are concerned, you should call your doctor. If the child is struggling to breathe or turns blue, medical help should be obtained immediately. The child should be taken to hospital where he or she may be given humidified oxygen in a tent. If breathing is seriously obstructed, treatment involves either the passage of a tube down the throat or an operation called a *tracheostomy*, in which a tube is passed into the throat through the neck to bypass the obstruction. In either case, the tube can usually be removed within a few days and complete recovery takes place after a few more days.

Crowding, dental

See *Overcrowding, dental*.

Crown, dental

An artificial replacement for the crown of a tooth (the part above the gum) that has become decayed, discoloured, or broken. A porcelain crown is usually used on front teeth because of its similarity in colour to natural teeth, but back teeth require the greater strength of a crown made from gold or from porcelain fused to metal.

Cruciate ligaments

Two ligaments in the knee that pass over each other to form a cross (hence their name, from the Latin word "crux", meaning cross). The ligaments form connections between the femur (thigh-bone) and tibia (shin) inside the knee joint.

The role of the cruciate ligaments is to prevent overbending and over-straightening at the knee joint. Consequently, if these ligaments are torn, the knee joint becomes unstable and may cause pain.

Crush syndrome

Damage to a large amount of body muscle—most commonly as a result of a serious road traffic accident—causing *kidney failure*. Protein pigments rel-

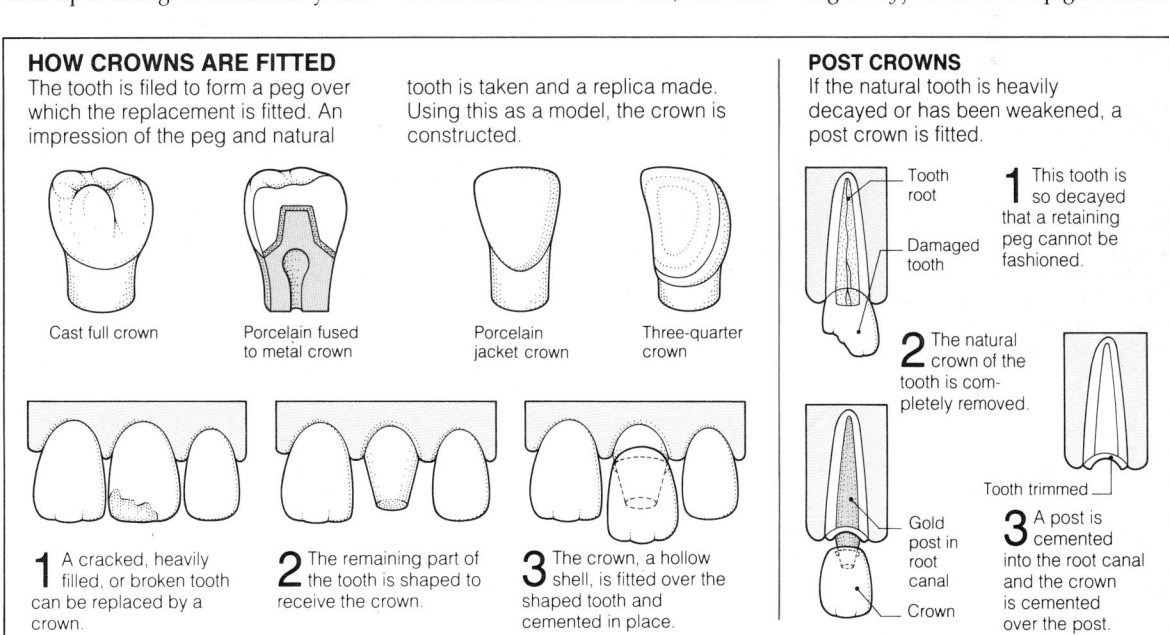

HOW CROWNS ARE FITTED
The tooth is filed to form a peg over which the replacement is fitted. An impression of the peg and natural tooth is taken and a replica made. Using this as a model, the crown is constructed.

Cast full crown

Porcelain fused to metal crown

Porcelain jacket crown

Three-quarter crown

1 A cracked, heavily filled, or broken tooth can be replaced by a crown.

2 The remaining part of the tooth is shaped to receive the crown.

3 The crown, a hollow shell, is fitted over the shaped tooth and cemented in place.

POST CROWNS
If the natural tooth is heavily decayed or has been weakened, a post crown is fitted.

Tooth root

Damaged tooth

1 This tooth is so decayed that a retaining peg cannot be fashioned.

2 The natural crown of the tooth is completely removed.

Tooth trimmed

Gold post in root canal

Crown

3 A post is cemented into the root canal and the crown is cemented over the post.

C

eased into the bloodstream from the damaged muscles temporarily impair the functioning of the kidney. As a result, some substances normally excreted in the urine build up to toxic levels in the blood. Without treatment the kidney failure may be fatal but treatment by *dialysis* gives the kidneys a chance to recover their function.

Crutch palsy

Weakness or paralysis of muscles in the wrist, fingers, and thumb due to pressure under the arm affecting the nerves that supply these muscles. Such pressure may be caused by a crutch pressing tightly under the arm—hence the name.

A crutch will cause crutch palsy only if it is too tall for the individual and is used for prolonged walking. A crutch should fit comfortably under the arm when standing upright, with the hand taking much of the weight.

Crutch palsy can also occur if a person falls asleep with one arm over the back of a chair so that the top of the chair presses into the armpit. In many cases, the person has fallen asleep after a bout of drinking, giving the disorder its common name of Saturday night palsy.

Symptoms usually improve without treatment because nerve damage is only temporary. Rarely, exercises are needed to strengthen the wrist and fingers.

Crying in infants

Occasional crying in a baby is normal. It is the baby's only means of communicating a need. Only when the baby is inconsolable or the crying is unusual in any way should it be regarded as signifying a problem.

CAUSES
Crying in infants is a response to needs or discomforts, such as hunger, thirst, a wet or soiled nappy, tiredness, interrupted sleep, a desire to be comforted, feeling hot or cold, boredom, or separation from parents. Most healthy babies stop crying when their needs are attended to.

Persistent crying, when it is not due to a persistently ignored or unrecognized need, may be a baby's reaction to the overwrought state of a parent. In a minority of cases, it may be due to an unrecognized physical cause such as intolerence of cow's milk, an illness, commonly an ear or throat infection, or a viral fever. Persistent crying may indicate maltreatment (see *Child abuse*).

TREATMENT
A crying baby should always be attended to. The idea that attending to

a crying infant is "giving in" is wrong. Persistent lack of attention is believed to have an adverse effect on emotional development in later life.

If a baby continues to cry after a feed and a change of nappy, parents should make sure that their child is not uncomfortable or too hot or cold, and should try to comfort the baby. A baby sling can be used to provide continuous physical contact. The baby may also prefer being propped up in a chair rather than lying flat, so that he or she can look around.

Parents should try to get as much sleep as possible, and should put aside at least one period during the day for relaxation. If the baby cries at night, parents should take turns attending to him or her.

Medical advice is usually necessary only if a baby cries persistently despite all attempts to soothe him or her, if a normally quiet baby starts to cry a lot, if a baby also has diarrhoea, vomiting, fever, or seems unwell, or if a baby cries only weakly or not at all. Parents should not attribute these more serious symptoms to teething or colic without first consulting their doctor.

Cryo-

A prefix meaning ice cold. It is often used to indicate that a procedure uses freezing or low temperatures.

Cryopreservation

The preservation of living cells by freezing. The technique is used chiefly to store human eggs, sperm, and blood for later use.

WHY IT IS DONE
If a woman is infertile because of blocked fallopian tubes, eggs can be removed from her ovaries and then frozen and stored until they can be used for *in vitro fertilization*.

Treatment of cancer by means of radiotherapy or chemotherapy carries the slight risk of damaging sperm. If the man wants to retain the option of future fatherhood, a sample of his sperm is collected before treatment begins and frozen for possible later use in *artificial insemination*. Sperm from donors can also be frozen and used later to enable a woman whose husband is infertile to bear a child.

Plasma and blood belonging to rare blood groups can be preserved by freezing and stored in a blood bank for long periods until needed.

HOW IT IS DONE
The cells to be preserved are first immersed in a fluid, usually glycerol. Glycerol enters and surrounds the

cells so that they are protected from the normally destructive effect of freezing. The temperature is progressively lowered as the concentration of protecting fluid is increased until the final storage temperature of about -180°C is reached.

OUTLOOK
Apart from widespread cryopreservation of cells, there has also been some success with freezing and reusing small areas of tissue, such as the cornea and portions of skin. This has led to experimental work on the possibility (as yet unfulfilled) of cryopreservation of major organs, such as the heart, liver, and kidneys, taken from people who have recently died, for transplantation. This would enable transplants to be carried out on a normal surgical timescale rather than as a race against time.

Cryosurgery

The use of temperatures below freezing to destroy tissue. The term is also applied to the use of cold during surgery to produce adhesion between an instrument and body tissue. Cryosurgery has been in common use only for the past decade; in many cases it is proving to be a useful alternative to more traditional forms of surgery or radiotherapy.

WHY IT IS DONE
Because cryosurgery causes only minimal scarring, it is particularly valuable for dealing with malignant tumours in the cervix and in major organs, such as the liver or intestines, in which heavy scarring can block vital openings or channels.

Cryosurgery is a good method for operating on tiny structures in the eye, and has proved particularly useful in *cataract surgery* and for treating *retinal detachment*.

Cryosurgery is also a common technique for removing *warts, skin tags*, some birthmarks, and certain types of skin cancer, such as *basal cell carcinoma*. *Haemorrhoids* (piles) and other anal disorders can be treated rapidly and effectively.

HOW IT IS DONE
Treatment of an internal tumour with cryosurgery is a major operation requiring a general anaesthetic. The growth is destroyed in one of two ways—by applying a metal probe cooled to the temperature of liquid nitrogen (about -160°C), or by spraying it with liquid nitrogen.

Cryosurgery on the skin and for haemorrhoids is usually performed on an outpatient basis. The procedure, using a cooled metal probe, is virtually painless because the extreme cold paralyses the nerves in the skin. After treatment, a blister develops, which may weep for a few days before healing. Although there is little scarring, the treated area may show up as a patch of paler skin.

Cryotherapy
The use of cold or freezing in treatment. (See also *Cryosurgery*.)

Cryptococcosis
A rare infection caused by inhaling the fungus CRYPTOCOCCUS NEOFORMANS. This fungus is found throughout the world, especially in soil contaminated with pigeon droppings. Infection with the fungus may cause *meningitis* (inflammation of the coverings of the brain and spinal cord) or granular growths in the lungs, skin, or elsewhere. Most, but not all, cases occur in people whose resistance to infection has been drastically lowered by diseases such as *AIDS* and *Hodgkin's disease* or by treatment with *immunosuppressant drugs*.

SYMPTOMS
Meningitis is the most usual, and serious, form that the illness takes. Symptoms include headache, stiffness in the neck, fever, drowsiness, blurred vision, and a staggering gait. If the infection is not treated, it may end in coma and death. When the disease attacks the lungs it causes chest pain and a cough, sometimes with sputum (phlegm); there may also be a skin rash of ulcerating spots.

DIAGNOSIS AND TREATMENT
Cryptococcal meningitis is diagnosed from a sample of fluid drawn from the spine. An X-ray may be needed to detect any damage to the lungs, and laboratory examination of the sputum, lung *biopsy* (removal of a sample of tissue for microscopic analysis), and *bronchoscopy* (inspection of the bronchi with a viewing instrument) may be needed.

Most cases in which only the lungs have been infected need no treatment. When the meninges have been affected, a combination of *amphotericin B* and another *antifungal drug* flucytosine is usually given for about six weeks. Although these drugs are usually effective, relapses can occur.

Cryptorchidism
A developmental disorder of male infants in which the testes fail to descend normally into the scrotum. (See *Testis, undescended*.)

Cryptosporidiosis
A type of diarrhoeal infection caused by *protozoa*. Cryptosporidiosis may be spread from person to person, or from domestic animals (especially calves) to people. The disease is most common in children but also occurs in male homosexuals.

The main symptom is usually an attack of watery diarrhoea that lasts about a week. There may also be fever, nausea, and abdominal pain. The infection may be much more severe in people whose *immune system* is suppressed, especially those with *AIDS*.

Diagnosis of cryptosporidiosis is confirmed by microscopic examination of a sample of faeces. Treatment, other than *rehydration therapy*, is not usually necessary, except in immunosuppressed patients.

CT scanning
A diagnostic technique in which the combined use of a computer and *X-rays* passed through the body at different angles produces clear cross-sectional images ("slices") of the tissue being examined. CT (computed tomography) scanning—also known as CAT (computed axial tomography) scanning or whole body scanning—provides clearer and more detailed information than X-rays used by themselves. CT scanning also has the advantage of tending to minimize the amount of radiation exposure.

WHY IT IS DONE
The first CT scanner, which came into operation in 1972, was developed to study the brain. Since then, CT brain scanning has revolutionized the diagnosis and treatment of tumours, abscesses, and haemorrhages in the brain, as well as strokes and head injuries. These once required tests, such as *angiography* and ventriculography (an outmoded technique for imaging the ventricles of the brain), that were not only difficult to perform, lengthy, and not always clear-cut in their findings, but also entailed some risk to the patient. CT scanning, on the other hand, is simple, quick, accurate, and involves only modest exposure to radiation (see box overleaf).

As well as being essential for the study of the brain, CT scanning is invaluable in investigating disease of any part of the trunk. It is particularly useful for locating and imaging tumours, and for facilitating needle *biopsy* (removal of a sample of tissue via a needle).

RESULTS
Using the information produced by the scanner, a computer constructs cross-sectional images of the tissue under examination. These images, displayed on a TV screen, reveal soft tissues (including tumours) more clearly than normal X-ray pictures. The images are particularly valuable in brain scans due to their sharp definition of the ventricles (fluid-filled spaces). The images can be manipulated electronically to provide the best view of the area of interest, and adjacent two-dimensional "slices" can be reconstructed to produce three-dimensional representations as well as images in different planes.

Culture
A growth of bacteria or other microorganisms, cells, or tissues cultivated artificially in the laboratory.

WHY IT IS DONE
Microorganisms are collected and cultivated to enable the cause of an infection to be accurately diagnosed. Cultivation produces larger numbers of microorganisms in a form suitable for further tests.

Healthy cells are cultured to diagnose various disorders prenatally and for studying chromosomes. Human tissues, such as skin, may be cultured to produce larger amounts for use in grafting. Other tissues, notably human *amnion* and monkey kidney, are cultivated to provide a medium in which viruses can be grown and identified in the laboratory; viruses will multiply only within living cells.

HOW IT IS DONE
MICROORGANISMS The type of specimen collected from the patient depends on the suspected site of infection. For example, a throat swab is taken if a streptococcal throat infection is suspected, a urine specimen is collected if urinary tract infection is thought likely, a sputum sample if respiratory infection is suspected, or a faeces sample if gastrointestinal infection is suspected. Likewise, a blood sample is cultured if the blood is thought to be infected. Bacteria, fungi, and, occasionally, viruses may be cultured directly from the blood.

The specimen is collected in a sterile container and is incubated at body temperature in a carefully chosen culture medium. Liquid or solid culture media, usually agar gel or meat-based broth, are used for culturing bacteria. These media contain various nutrients chosen for the particular needs of the organism suspected of causing the infection; the media may also contain ingredients to discourage the growth of other organisms.

C

C

PERFORMING A CT SCAN

CT scanning combines the use of a computer and X-rays passed through the body at different angles to produce clear cross-sectional images of areas of body tissue. Before the scan is carried out, a contrast medium may be injected to make blood vessels, organs, or abnormalities show up more clearly; a drink of contrast medium may be given to highlight loops of intestine.

1 The patient lies on a table that can be moved up or down to allow easy transfer and accurate positioning within the machine.

A central sliding cradle in the table moves the patient, at a controllable rate, into the machine

The machine can be tilted in either direction to allow precise areas to be X-rayed

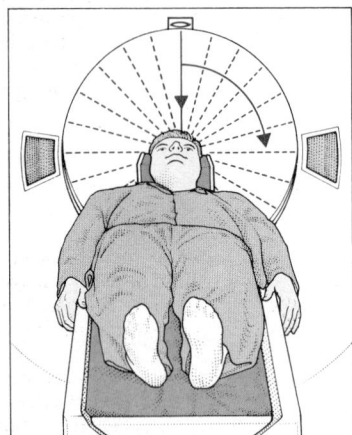

2 A great number of X-ray beams, each of low dosage and lasting only a fraction of a second, are passed through the body at different angles as the scanner rotates around the patient.

Right kidney
Spinal cord
Spine
Rib
Abnormal left kidney
Cysts
Cysts
Gas in stomach   Liver

3 The amount of X-rays absorbed by different tissues is recorded by detectors in the scanner and transformed by a computer into an image, which is interpreted by a radiologist.

Any bacteria present will multiply to form visible colonies. The type of bacteria can be identified by noting the appearance of the colony, by chemical tests, and by examining the bacteria under the microscope. Bacterial cultures can be tested with various antibiotics to determine which antibiotic may be the most effective against a particular infection.

CELLS AND TISSUES For the diagnosis of prenatal abnormalities, cells are collected by *amniocentesis* or by *chorionic villus sampling*. Cells for studying chromosomes (see *Chromosome analysis*) are cultured from white blood cells or cells gathered from the inside of the cheek. Cells and tissues to be used for analysis, for growing viruses, or for grafting are cultured in a small amount of fluid containing nutrients essential for their growth.

Cupping

An ancient form of treatment used to draw blood to the surface of the skin. Although cupping fell out of favour during the development of modern medicine, it is still used in folk healing in some countries, such as China and Turkey. Common conditions treated include bronchitis, asthma, and musculoskeletal pains.

A small vessel—commonly a glass jar, animal horn, ceramic vessel, or a bamboo tube with a closed end—is applied to the skin and heated. When it cools and the air inside contracts, a partial vacuum is created, causing the skin to be sucked into the vessel, producing a rounded area of inflammation. Believers in this form of treatment think that the inflammatory response is therapeutic.

Curare

An extract from the bark and juices of various trees which has been used for centuries by South American Indians as an arrow poison. The principal active ingredient is tubocurarine, a drug that inhibits muscle contractions by interfering with the action of *acetylcholine*, a *neurotransmitter* (chemical released from nerve endings). Curare kills by causing widespread muscle paralysis in the victim.

Cure

To treat successfully; that is, to restore to normal health after an illness. The term usually means the complete disappearance of a disease rather than just a halt in its progress. Any medication or therapy used in the treatment of an illness may also be called a cure.

In general, infections may be cured, as may some tumours. By contrast, chronic conditions, such as *osteoarthritis*, or endocrine deficiency diseases, such as *hypothyroidism* (underactivity of the thyroid gland), are never cured but instead undergo remission or are controlled with long-term hormone treatment.

Curettage

The use of a sharp-edged, spoon-shaped surgical instrument called a curette to scrape abnormal tissue, or tissue for analysis, from the lining of a body cavity or from the skin. Curettage is commonly used to remove infected material from an abscess, to scrape tissue from the lining of the uterus as part of a *D and C* (dilatation and curettage) operation, and to remove small growths from the skin. (See also *Curettage, dental*.)

Curettage, dental

The scraping of the wall of a cavity or other surface with a dental *curette* (a narrow, spoon-shaped, scaling instrument). It is one method used in the treatment of simple periodontal pockets occurring in *periodontitis*. The curette is used to remove the lining of the periodontal pocket as well as diseased tissue from the lateral surfaces of the root. This enables the healthy, underlying tissue to reattach itself to the root surface.

Curette

A spoon-shaped surgical instrument for scraping away material or tissue from an organ, cavity, or surface.

Curling's ulcer

A type of *stress ulcer* (a disruption in the lining of the stomach or duodenum following any severe injury, infection, or shock) that occurs specifically in people who have suffered extensive skin burns. Ulcers develop about 24 hours after the burns and are usually small and multiple. Diagnosis and treatment are as for other types of stress ulcer.

Cushing's syndrome

A hormonal disorder caused by an abnormally high level of corticosteroid hormones in the bloodstream. The excess may be caused by overactivity of the *adrenal glands,* which normally produce corticosteroid hormones, or by prolonged administration of *corticosteroid drugs*. Cushing's syndrome can occur at any age, but is most common in middle age.

CAUSES AND INCIDENCE
Most cases of Cushing's syndrome today are caused by prolonged use of corticosteroid drugs, which are widely used to treat inflammatory conditions such as *rheumatoid arthritis, inflammatory bowel disease*, and *asthma*. Such cases are usually mild; the patient is often described as having cushingoid features rather than Cushing's syndrome.

Cushing's syndrome is sometimes produced directly by an *adrenal tumour* that causes excessive secretion of corticosteroids. The condition may also

be caused indirectly by overactivity of the *pituitary gland,* often due to a *pituitary tumour*. The pituitary gland controls the activity of the adrenal glands by producing a hormone called ACTH (adrenocorticotrophic hormone); this stimulates the cortex (outer part) of the adrenal glands to grow and secrete excess corticosteroids. Cases caused by pituitary overactivity (sometimes called Cushing's disease) are much more common in women.

Some lung cancers and various other tumours may also lead to Cushing's syndrome by secreting ACTH and thus leading to excess secretion of corticosteroids by the adrenal glands. This cause of Cushing's syndrome is more common in men.

SYMPTOMS
People with Cushing's syndrome have a characteristic appearance. The face appears round ("moon-faced") and red, the trunk tends to become obese with a humped upper back, and the limbs become wasted. Acne develops and purple stretch marks may appear on the abdomen, thighs, and breasts. The skin is thin and bruises easily. The bones become weakened by *osteoporosis* and are more likely to fracture. Women may become increasingly hairy. Affected people are more susceptible to infection and may suffer from peptic ulcers.

Mental changes often occur, causing *depression, paranoia,* or sometimes *euphoria. Insomnia* may be a problem. Patients may develop *hypertension* (high blood pressure) and *oedema* (fluid collection in the tissues). About one fifth of patients develop *diabetes mellitus*. In children, Cushing's syndrome may suppress growth.

DIAGNOSIS
Anyone suspected of having Cushing's syndrome should be examined by an endocrinologist. Confirmation of the diagnosis may require measurement of ACTH levels in the blood and of corticosteroid levels in the blood and urine. *CT scanning* or *MRI* of the adrenal and pituitary glands may be performed to look for abnormalities.

TREATMENT
If corticosteroid drugs are the cause, Cushing's syndrome will usually disappear if the dose of drugs is gradually reduced.

If the cause is shown to be a tumour or overgrowth of an adrenal gland, the gland is removed surgically. If the cause is a pituitary tumour, the gland is removed surgically or the tumour is shrunk by irradiation and medication. Patients subsequently need hormone

replacement therapy to compensate for lack of production of adrenal and pituitary hormones.

Cusp, dental

One of the protrusions on the grinding surface of a tooth (see *Teeth*).

Cutaneous

A term meaning relating to the skin.

Cutdown

The creation of a small incision in the skin over a vein in order to gain access to the vein. A doctor may perform a cutdown if a vein cannot be identified through the patient's skin when it is necessary to take blood or to give intravenous fluid.

CVS

See *Chorionic villus sampling*.

Cyanide

Any of a group of substances that contain a carbon atom and a nitrogen atom bound together by a triple chemical bond. Most cyanides are highly poisonous.

The poisonous effects of cyanides are due to their ability to block a specific *enzyme* (cytochrome oxidase) which plays an essential role in the uptake of oxygen by cells. This blocking action deprives cells of the ability to utilize oxygen, which, in turn, produces a rapid progression of symptoms from breathlessness, through paralysis and unconsciousness, to death.

Because of their toxicity, the use of cyanides in industry (such as in electroplating, "case hardening", and polymer manufacture) is carefully controlled. Hydrogen cyanide is used to kill rodents and to fumigate buildings. It has also been used in gas chambers. Certain other cyanides are powerful eye irritants and are used in some tear gases.

Cyanocobalamin

A name for *vitamin B$_{12}$*.

Cyanosis

A bluish coloration of the skin and mucous membranes (such as the lining of the mouth) due to too much deoxygenated *haemoglobin* in the blood. Cyanosis is generally most obvious in the beds of the fingernails and toenails, and on the lips and tongue.

Cyanosis is most commonly due to slow blood flow through the skin in low temperatures (the familiar sign of turning blue with cold). In such cases,

C

C

where no other symptoms are present, cyanosis does not indicate a serious underlying disease.

In other cases, cyanosis requires medical investigation as it may be a sign of a serious disorder. Cyanosis of the fingers and toes even in relatively warm conditions may indicate poor peripheral blood circulation (see *Peripheral vascular disease*). Cyanosis may also be a sign of a heart or lung disorder, such as *heart failure*, a heart disorder present at birth (see *Heart disease, congenital*), lung damage, or *pulmonary oedema* (fluid in the lungs).

Cyclopenthiazide

A thiazide *diuretic drug* used to reduce oedema (fluid retention) in people with *heart failure*, kidney disorders, *cirrhosis* of the liver, and *premenstrual syndrome*. Cyclopenthiazide is also frequently prescribed to treat *hypertension* (high blood pressure).

Possible adverse effects include lethargy, loss of appetite, leg cramps, dizziness, rash, and impotence.

Cyclophosphamide

An *anticancer drug* used mainly in the treatment of *Hodgkin's disease* and *leukaemia*, often in combination with other anticancer drugs. Cyclophosphamide is also useful as an *immunosuppressant drug*, helping prevent rejection of a transplanted organ by modifying the body's natural defences against foreign cells. Cyclophosphamide is also used occasionally to treat certain connective tissue diseases such as severe systemic *lupus erythematosus*.

Possible adverse effects are as for other anticancer drugs; there may also be a severe form of *cystitis*.

Cycloplegia

Paralysis of the ciliary muscle of the *eye*. Cycloplegia impedes *accommodation* (the process by which the shape of the lens adjusts to focus light rays from near objects on to the retina).

Cycloplegia may be induced by drugs, known as cycloplegic drugs, to facilitate examination of the eye.

Cyclosporin

An *immunosuppressant drug* that suppresses the body's natural defences against abnormal cells. Cyclosporin was introduced in 1984.

WHY IT IS USED

Cyclosporin's immunosuppressant action is of particular use following *transplant surgery*, when the body may start to reject the transplanted organ

unless the immune system is damped down. Cyclosporin is now widely used following many different types of transplant surgery, including heart, kidney, bone marrow, liver, and pancreas transplants. Its use has considerably reduced the risk of tissue rejection and also the need for large doses of *corticosteroid drugs*. Cyclosporin may need to be taken in oral form for an indefinite period following transplant surgery.

POSSIBLE ADVERSE EFFECTS

Because cyclosporin reduces the effectiveness of the immune system, people being treated with this drug have an increased susceptibility to infection. Any 'flu-like illness or localized infection requires immediate treatment by a doctor.

Swelling of the gums and increased hair growth are fairly common side-effects. Cyclosporin has also been found to cause kidney damage in some people. Regular monitoring of kidney function is therefore necessary for people being given this drug. If signs of kidney damage, such as proteinuria (protein in the urine), are detected, the dose of cyclosporin may need to be reduced or another drug substituted.

Cyclothymia

A personality characteristic typified by marked changes of mood. Cyclothymic individuals may change, for no apparent reason, from being cheerful, energetic, and sociable to being gloomy, listless, and withdrawn. Mood swings may last for days or months and may follow a regular pattern. Sometimes there are periods of relatively normal behaviour.

Cyclothymia resembles *manic-depressive illness* in some respects but the mood swings of cyclothymia are less severe; in some cases there is a family history of manic-depressive illness. People with cyclothymia who are predominently "high" may have successful careers; others may resort to episodes of heavy drinking or difficult behaviour.

Cyproterone acetate

A synthetic hormone that blocks the action of *androgen hormones* (male sex hormones) and has effects similar to those of *progesterone hormone* (a female sex hormone).

Cyproterone acetate is used in the treatment of cancer of the prostate (see *Prostate, cancer of*). It is also occasionally used to reduce male sex drive. Cyproterone acetate may be

prescribed in combination wih an *oestrogen drug* to treat women with severe acne or excessive hair growth.

Possible adverse effects, which usually diminish as treatment continues, include breast tenderness and weight gain.

Cyst

An abnormal lump or swelling, filled with fluid or semi-solid material, that may occur in any body organ or tissue.

Many different processes cause the development of cysts. Some types, such as *sebaceous cysts* in the skin, result from blockage of the ducts leading from fluid-forming glands. Others, such as *ovarian cysts* or *Baker's cysts*, form as a result of abnormal activity or growth of a fluid-forming tissue when there is no means for the fluid to escape. Cysts may also form around parasites in diseases such as *hydatid disease* or *amoebiasis*. A *dermoid cyst* is a type of skin cyst that may contain particles of hair follicles, sweat glands, nerves, and teeth.

Cysts are usually harmless in themselves but may sometimes disrupt the function of the tissues in which they grow; in some cases this may necessitate surgical removal of the cyst.

Cyst-/cysto-

Prefixes that denote the bladder, as in *cystitis* (inflammation of the bladder) and *cystoscopy* (endoscopic examination of the bladder).

Cystectomy

Surgical removal of the bladder. Cystectomy must be followed by the creation of an alternative passageway for the expulsion of urine, usually via a specially constructed channel emerging in a stoma (mouth-like opening) in the lower abdomen (see *Urinary diversion*). Cystectomy is a means of treating cancer of the bladder (see *Bladder tumours*).

HOW IT IS DONE

Before undergoing surgery, cystectomy patients are advised to discuss the operation and its consequences with their doctors and with a stoma care nurse.

The basic steps in the procedure are shown in the illustrated box opposite. Cystectomy is accompanied by removal of the prostate gland and seminal vesicles in men, and by removal of the uterus, ovaries, and fallopian tubes in women.

OUTLOOK

Patients need to adapt to wearing an external pouch for the collection of urine and to learn about care of the stoma. Many patients are able to return to an active and healthy life.

Removal of the reproductive organs with the bladder results in infertility. Cystectomy also usually causes impotence in men (due to damage to nerve tracts involved in penile erection).

Cysticercosis

An infection characterized by the presence of cysts, in muscles and the brain, formed by the larval stage of the pork *tapeworm*. Cysticercosis is very rare in developed countries.

Cystic fibrosis

An inherited disease, present from birth, characterized by a tendency to chronic lung infections and an inability to absorb fats and other nutrients from food. The disease is also called "mucoviscidosis" because the main feature is secretion of viscid (sticky) mucus which is unable to lubricate and flow freely in the nose, throat, airways, and intestines.

When cystic fibrosis (CF) was first identified in the 1930s, before effective *antibiotic drugs* were available, almost all sufferers died in early childhood. However, since 1975 the outlook has changed dramatically. With more advanced methods of diagnosis and treatment, including the use of a wide range of antibiotics, over two thirds of CF sufferers now survive into adult life, although few of them are in perfect health. But despite the improved outlook CF remains a serious and potentially fatal disorder.

CAUSES AND INCIDENCE

CF is caused by an inherited defect in a *gene* on chromosome 7 (see *Chromo-somes*). The defect is of the recessive type, which means that it must be inherited in a double dose (one gene from each parent) before any outward abnormality is apparent (see *Genetic disorders*). People who inherit the defective gene in a single dose (from one parent only) are called "carriers"; they are usually unaware of the fact and have no symptoms.

Among Western Europeans and white Americans, about one person in 20 to 25 is such a "carrier". The chance that any (random) procreating white couple are both carriers is roughly one in 500 to 600. In this event, each of their children has a one in four chance of inheriting the defective gene from both parents and of being born with CF. The incidence of the disease is thus about one per 2,500 live births. The incidence in Jewish, Asian, and African populations is much lower.

Identification of the defective gene has enabled the protein that it forms (the cystic fibrosis transmembrane conductance regulator) to be studied. The biochemical abnormality in CF is a fault in the movement of ions such as sodium and chloride across cell membranes, which leads to defective mucus formation. The effect is that glands in several organs do not function properly. Most seriously, the glands in the lining of the bronchial tubes produce thick mucus, which predisposes the person to chronic lung infections. A further serious malfunction is poor or absent secretion of pancreatic enzymes, which are involved in the breakdown of fats and their absorption from the intestines; this deficiency causes malnutrition. Sweat glands are also affected and secrete excessive amounts of sodium chloride (common salt).

SYMPTOMS AND SIGNS

The pattern of development of the disease, and the severity of its features, varies considerably. In some cases it is obvious soon after birth, in others it escapes detection for months or years.

In a typical case, the child passes unformed, pale, oily, and foul-smelling faeces, and, in some cases, will fail to thrive. In many cases, growth is stunted and the child suffers from recurrent upper respiratory tract and chest infections, causing constant coughing and breathlessness. Without early diagnosis and treatment, *pneumonia, bronchiectasis,* and *bronchitis* develop, and the lungs become damaged.

Infertility occurs in the majority of male sufferers and some affected females. Some otherwise healthy adult males have been diagnosed as having

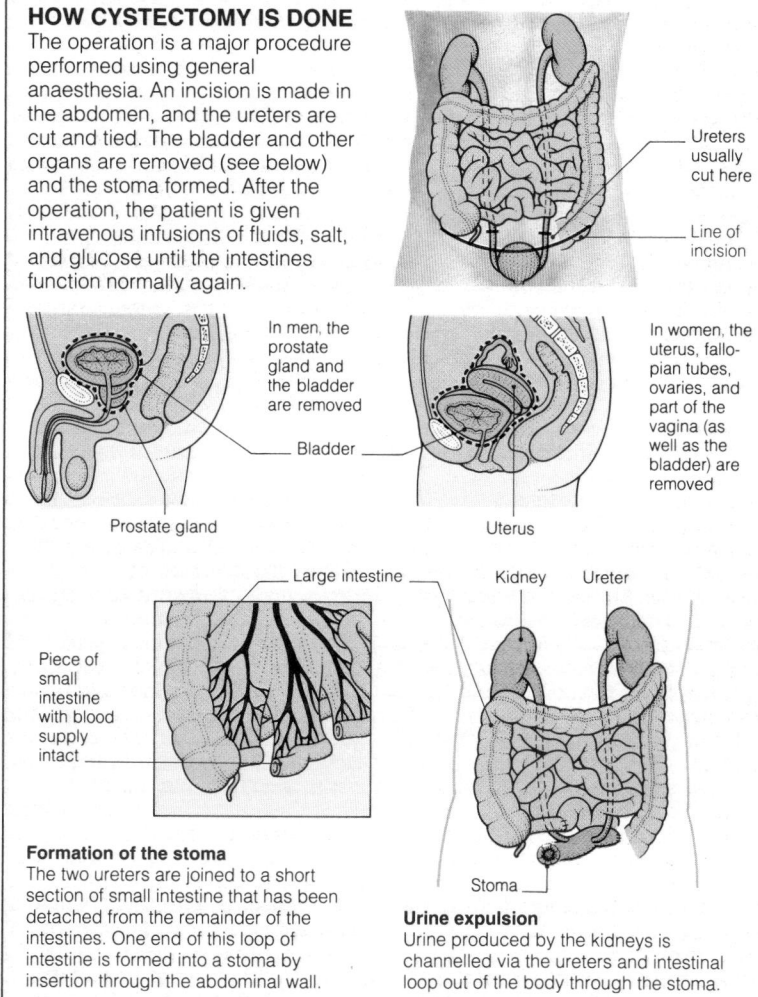

HOW CYSTECTOMY IS DONE

The operation is a major procedure performed using general anaesthesia. An incision is made in the abdomen, and the ureters are cut and tied. The bladder and other organs are removed (see below) and the stoma formed. After the operation, the patient is given intravenous infusions of fluids, salt, and glucose until the intestines function normally again.

Ureters usually cut here

Line of incision

In men, the prostate gland and the bladder are removed

Bladder

Prostate gland

In women, the uterus, fallopian tubes, ovaries, and part of the vagina (as well as the bladder) are removed

Uterus

Large intestine

Piece of small intestine with blood supply intact

Kidney   Ureter

Stoma

Formation of the stoma
The two ureters are joined to a short section of small intestine that has been detached from the remainder of the intestines. One end of this loop of intestine is formed into a stoma by insertion through the abdominal wall.

Urine expulsion
Urine produced by the kidneys is channelled via the ureters and intestinal loop out of the body through the stoma.

C

CF after attending an infertility clinic. *Heatstroke* and collapse may occur in hot climates due to the excessive loss of salt in the sweat.

DIAGNOSIS AND TREATMENT

Suspicious symptoms should be reported to a doctor as soon as they are noticed because the sooner intensive *physiotherapy* and treatment with appropriate antibiotic drugs is started, the less lung damage will be caused by chest infections. Once cystic fibrosis is suspected, the diagnosis is easily confirmed or refuted by simple laboratory tests, including a sweat test.

Confirmation of the diagnosis and supervision of treatment is best carried out from a special centre staffed by paediatricians, nurses, and physiotherapists who have a particular knowledge of the disease.

To enable food to be properly digested, *pancreatin* (a replacement pancreatic enzyme preparation) must be taken with meals. The diet needs to be rich in calories and proteins, and a vitamin supplement is often prescribed. These measures bring about weight gain and more normal faeces.

AFFECTED FAMILIES

The parents of a child with CF must assume that any subsequent child has a one in four chance of being born with the disease. Unaffected siblings of affected people have a two in three chance of being "carriers", creating problems if they are thinking of co-parenting with someone who also has CF in the family. Advice can be obtained through *genetic counselling.*

One particular mutation has been shown to be responsible for around 70 per cent of all cystic fibrosis, but approximately 200 other mutations have been identified; about 20 of these are quite common. Almost all carriers of CF can now be identified with near certainty. It is not yet feasible to test the whole population, but families in which individuals have been found to have CF can now be tested.

If a couple planning a family are both found to be carriers of the same mutation, the chance of the child having the disease is one in four. One possible approach is for them to have several ova fertilized by *in vitro fertilization* and have the embryos tested before implantation in the uterus. Alternatively they may choose to conceive naturally and then have the fetus tested, at around the 8th or 9th week of pregnancy, by *chorionic villus sampling*, or later in pregnancy by *amniocentesis.* The parents may choose to terminate the pregnancy if the fetus is affected.

OUTLOOK

The highly specialized treatment given to CF sufferers today provides them with a much better quality of life. Even so, most suffer permanent lung damage and have a much shorter life expectancy. Some have been treated by a *lung* or *heart-lung transplant* with good results. The hope is that specific *gene therapy* may eventually be introduced, possibly using an aerosol to access the lining of the air passages in the lungs.

Cystitis

Inflammation of the inner lining of the *bladder*, usually caused by a bacterial infection. Anything that obstructs the voiding of urine from the bladder, or leads to incomplete voiding of urine, tends to encourage infection; stagnant urine in the bladder or urethra (the tube leading from the bladder to the exterior) provides a good breeding ground for bacteria.

INCIDENCE AND CAUSES

In women, cystitis is common because the urethra is short, making it easier for infective agents to pass from the urethral opening up into the bladder. The bacteria may come from the vagina or from the intestine via the anus. Most women have cystitis at some time. A *calculus* (stone) in the bladder, a *bladder tumour*, or a *urethral stricture* increases the risk of infection due to obstruction of urine flow.

In men, cystitis is rare (because of the longer urethra) and usually occurs only in the presence of an obstruction, which in most cases is due to an enlarged *prostate gland* compressing the urethra where it leaves the bladder. Less commonly, the obstruction is due to a urethral stricture.

In children, cystitis is often due to a structural abnormality of the ureters (tubes that carry urine from the kidneys to the bladder) at the point at which they enter the bladder, allowing reflux (backward flow) of urine into the ureters when the bladder muscle contracts. This leads to incomplete voiding of urine and to subsequent infection.

Another possible source of infection is the introduction of a catheter (drainage tube) into the bladder—a procedure used to drain urine in a variety of circumstances (see *Catheterization, urinary*), including the treatment of incontinence and urinary retention. Diabetics are particularly susceptible to urinary tract infections.

SYMPTOMS

The main symptom of cystitis in both sexes is a frequent urge to pass urine, with only a small amount of urine passed each time. Passing urine is accompanied by pain, which is usually of a burning or stinging nature. Sometimes, the urine is foul smelling or contains blood. There may be a fever and occasionally chills and continuous discomfort in the lower abdomen. Children may have no urinary symptoms but may develop a fever or cry when passing urine.

DIAGNOSIS

The diagnosis of a urinary infection can be confirmed by examining a sample of urine under the microscope, looking for pus cells, and by growing bacteria in a *culture*. When no infection is found in someone with symptoms of cystitis, the diagnosis may be *urethritis* (inflammation of the urethra), bacterial *prostatitis* (in men only), or *urethral syndrome* (in women only), in which the cause is thought, in some people, to be trauma to the urethra from sexual activity.

TREATMENT

People with symptoms of cystitis should drink large quantities of fluids to help flush out the bladder (which should be emptied completely every time urine is passed) and should keep the urine alkaline by taking a teaspoon of sodium bicarbonate in water every six hours. Women who are prone to cystitis should empty the bladder as soon as possible after intercourse.

If an infection is present, *antibiotic drugs* are prescribed to destroy the bacteria and prevent the infection from spreading to cause *pyelonephritis* (infection of the kidneys).

In many cases, the doctor will start the patient on a course of antibiotics, especially when there are pus cells in the urine, before waiting for the result of the urine culture. The doctor will then check the results of the culture to confirm the presence of an infection and to check the sensitivity of the bacteria to various antibiotics.

Prompt treatment of cystitis with antibiotic drugs usually settles the infection within 24 hours. More tests are performed on any man or child who has cystitis, and on women who suffer from recurrent infection. (See also *Urinary tract infection*.)

Cystocele

A swelling at the front and top of the vagina formed where the bladder pushes against weakened tissues in the vaginal wall. Weakened tissues may be associated with descent of the uterus from its normal position down into the vagina (see *Uterus, prolapse of*).

A cystocele may not cause symptoms, but occasionally the urethra (through which urine drains from the bladder to the exterior) is pulled out of position. This may cause stress *incontinence* (leakage of urine on coughing, lifting, or sneezing) or the bladder may not empty completely when urine is passed. The urine remaining in the bladder may then become infected, causing frequent and painful urination (see *Cystitis*).

Exercises to strengthen the pelvic floor muscles (which support the bladder, uterus, and other pelvic organs) may help relieve the symptoms (see *Pelvic floor exercises*). In many cases, surgery is needed to lift and tighten the tissues at the front of the vagina.

Cystometry

A procedure carried out to provide information about normal bladder function and about abnormalities either of the nerves supplying the bladder or of the bladder muscle itself. Cystometry measures changes in pressure as the bladder fills. It also shows the total bladder capacity and detects any residual urine after the bladder has fully contracted.

WHY IT IS DONE
Cystometry is used to investigate urinary *incontinence* or poor bladder emptying caused by damage to the bladder muscles (following childbirth or pelvic surgery, for example) or to disruption of the nerve control of these muscles (as in *Parkinson's disease* or *diabetes mellitus*).

HOW IT IS DONE
The examination, which takes about 20 minutes, is performed by a urologist or a trained urological technician. It is usually done on an outpatient basis and no anaesthetic is required. A catheter (flexible tube) and a probe for measuring pressure are inserted into the bladder and sometimes the rectum. The bladder is gradually filled with water or carbon dioxide and a series of pressure readings is taken.

Cystoscopy

The examination of the *urethra* and *bladder* cavity using a cystoscope (viewing instrument inserted up the urethra). Modern cystoscopes have a metal sheath with interchangeable lenses, allowing a viewing angle ranging from zero to 120 degrees.

WHY IT IS DONE
Cystoscopes have both diagnostic and therapeutic uses. Diagnostic uses include inspection of the bladder cavity for calculi (stones), *bladder tumours*, and sites of bleeding and infection, as well as the obtaining of individual urine samples from the *ureters* to look for the presence of infection or tumour cells. It is also possible to inject radiopaque dye into the ureters via the cystoscope, allowing the taking of X-rays to investigate the site of any obstruction to the flow of urine. This procedure is known as retrograde pyelography (see *Urography*).

Many diseases of the urethra and bladder lend themselves to treatment via the cystoscope. For example, bladder tumours can be removed, analysed under the microscope, and treated with diathermy or laser; calculi can be crushed or removed with basket forceps from the bladder or ureter; and stents (narrow tubes) can be inserted into a ureter to relieve any obstruction.

Cystostomy

The surgical creation of a hole in the bladder. A cystostomy is usually performed to drain urine when the introduction of a *catheter* (flexible tube) into the bladder via the urethra is inadvisable or impossible.

Cystourethrography, micturating

An X-ray procedure for studying a person's bladder while he or she is passing urine. Micturating cystourethrography is most commonly performed on young children who have had urinary infections. The technique allows detection of reflux of urine (backflow of urine up the *ureters*) as the bladder contracts. In severe cases, reflux leads to repeated infection and possible kidney damage.

-cyte

The suffix that denotes a cell. A *leukocyte* is a white blood cell; an *erythrocyte* is a red blood cell.

Cyto-

The prefix used to describe a relationship to a cell, as in *cytology*, the study of cells.

Cytology

The study of individual cells, as distinct from *histology* (the study of groups of cells forming a tissue). The main application of cytology in medicine is to detect abnormal cells; it is thus used extensively to diagnose cancer. Cytology is becoming more important in *antenatal screening* for certain fetal abnormalities. A cytologist is a specialist in this field.

APPLICATIONS
The best known use of cytology is screening for cancer of the cervix, a procedure known as a *cervical smear test*. A scraping of cells from the cervix and vagina is examined under a microscope; if the cells show precancerous changes, the woman's condition can be observed and she can be treated before cancer develops.

C

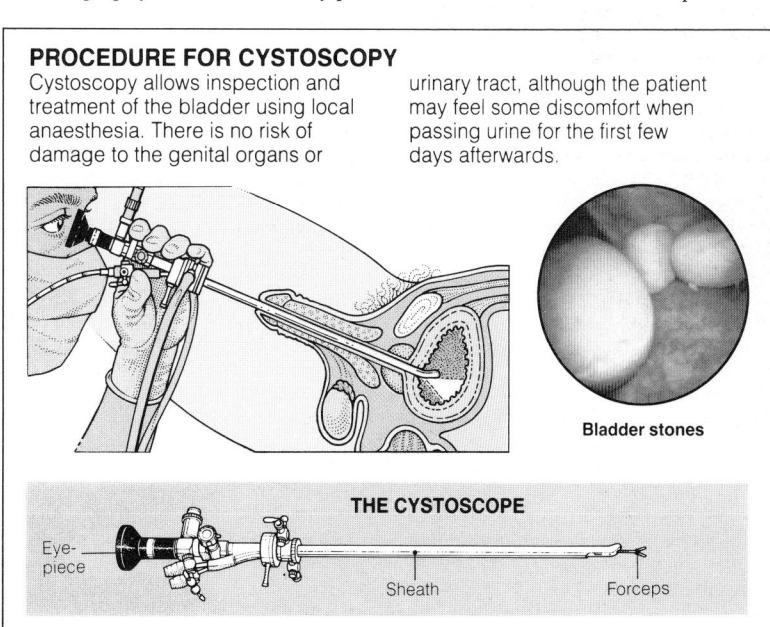

PROCEDURE FOR CYSTOSCOPY
Cystoscopy allows inspection and treatment of the bladder using local anaesthesia. There is no risk of damage to the genital organs or urinary tract, although the patient may feel some discomfort when passing urine for the first few days afterwards.

Bladder stones

THE CYSTOSCOPE

Eye-piece

Sheath

Forceps

C

CYTOLOGY METHODS

Cells for cytological examination are obtained in several ways, depending on the part of the body being investigated. Recent improvements in imaging techniques have made it possible to collect cells from previously inaccessible sites. If the cytologist can make a definite diagnosis from a cell sample removed from a tumour using a very fine needle, the patient may be spared an exploratory operation.

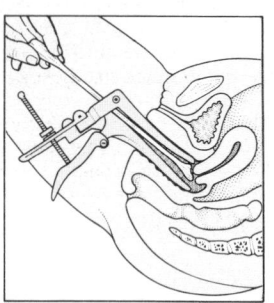

Cells from the cervix
These are scraped away with a spatula.

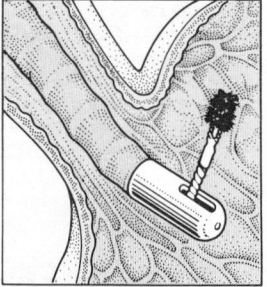

Cells from the respiratory tract or oesophagus
These are usually obtained by using an *endoscope* and small brush or suction tube.

Cells from body fluids
These are obtained either by passing the fluid through a filter or by centrifugation.

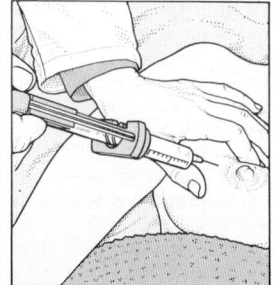

Aspiration biopsy
A very fine needle can be accurately passed into a suspected tumour and a biopsy sample of cells removed.

Cytology is also used to confirm (or exclude) the diagnosis of other cancers. Coughing up of blood may be due to lung cancer, but a cytological examination of cells in a sample of sputum (phlegm) will help determine whether or not cancer is actually the cause. Similarly, cytology is valuable in detecting recurrent tumours in people who have already been treated for cancer. It is used particularly in cases of bladder cancer, in which tumours tend to recur after the original cancer has been successfully treated. Regular urinary cytology can detect any recurrent tumours at an early stage. Cytology may be helpful in determining the cause of conditions such as *pleural effusion* (fluid in the pleural cavity around the lungs) and *ascites* (fluid in the abdominal cavity). Examination of cells in a sample of fluid usually indicates whether the condition is caused by cancer or an infection.

Fine-needle aspiration *biopsy* of internal organs is growing as a method of diagnosis that utilizes cytology. A needle is guided to the organ (often with the help of *ultrasound* or *CT scanning*) and a sample taken for examination. The procedure may eliminate the need for surgical biopsy or a major operation.

The other major application of cytology is in various screening techniques for the early detection of fetal abnormalities such as Down's syndrome. The most widely used of these techniques is *amniocentesis*, in which a sample of the fluid that surrounds the fetus is removed and the cells in the fluid are examined for abnormalities. *Chorionic villus sampling* is a newer technique that can be performed earlier in the pregnancy. Usually, the cells must be cultured before an analysis can be made.

MODERN DEVELOPMENTS

Various cytological techniques are being developed to improve the ability to detect abnormal cells. Cells aspirated from various organs or tissues, as well as cells from cervical smears, can be studied further by the technique of *flow cytometry* (which uses a laser beam to scan cells and produce an image of the cells' DNA contents, thus differentiating between benign and malignant cells).

The use of monoclonal antibodies—highly specific proteins that react with only one particular type of protein on the surface of a cell (see *Antibody, monoclonal*)—makes it easier to detect small numbers of abnormal cells in the midst of many normal ones, thereby improving the sensitivity of cytological tests for cancer. A refinement of this technique involves labelling the monoclonal antibodies with special fluorescent stains, which make the antibodies stand out clearly against a dark background.

Other modern techniques have made it possible to detect abnormalities in *chromosomes* and even in individual *genes*. Such procedures have a potentially wide application for prenatal screening for genetic disorders and chromosomal abnormalities, but many of them are still in the developmental stage and are not yet generally available.

Cytomegalovirus

One of the family of *herpes* viruses. Cytomegalovirus has the unique effect of causing the cells that it infects to take on a characteristic enlarged appearance.

Infection with the cytomegalovirus (CMV) is extremely common. Approximately 80 per cent of adults have *antibodies* to the virus in their blood (an indication of previous infection). CMV infection may cause an illness resembling infectious *mononucleosis* (glandular fever), but in most cases it produces no symptoms.

More serious CMV infections can occur in people who have impaired immunity, such as the elderly and those with *AIDS*. A pregnant woman can transmit the virus to her unborn child; this could cause malformations and brain damage in the child.

Cytopathology

The study of the microscopic appearances of cells in health and disease. (See also *Cytology*.)

Cytotoxic drugs

A group of drugs that kill or damage cells; a type of *anticancer drug*. Cytotoxic drugs primarily affect abnormal cells but they can also damage or kill healthy cells, especially those that are multiplying rapidly.

D

Dacryocystitis

Inflammation of the tear sac, which lies between the inside corner of the eyelids and the nose.

CAUSES

Dacryocystitis usually results from blockage of the duct that carries tears from the tear sac to the nose. Inflammation may be followed by bacterial infection of fluid trapped in the tear sac. In infants, the tear duct may fail to develop normally. In adults, the cause of the duct blockage is usually unknown. Rarely, it follows an injury; more often, it follows inflammation in the nasal region.

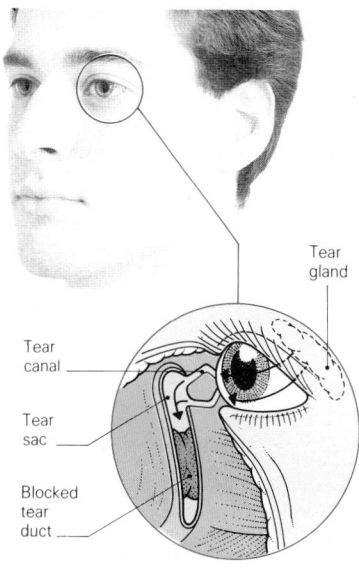

Mechanism of dacryocystitis
Inflammation of the tear sac occurs when the duct that carries tears from the tear sac becomes blocked.

SYMPTOMS

Usually only one eye is affected. There may be pain, redness, and swelling in the area between the inner corner of the eyelids and the nose. Occasionally, pus discharges from the inner corner. Prior to infection in the tear sac, the only symptom may be a watery eye due to obstruction of the duct.

TREATMENT

Irrigation can sometimes clear the obstruction. A *cannula* (fine tube) is introduced into one of the drainage openings into the tear duct and saline flushed through it. Antibiotic eyedrops or ointment are prescribed to treat infection. In infants, massage of the tear sac can empty the sac and sometimes clear a blockage.

If irrigation and antibiotics fail to clear up the symptoms, a dacryocystorhinostomy (surgery to drain the tear sac into the nose) can be performed. In the infirm and elderly, if recurrent infection is a problem, the tear sac may be removed.

Danazol

A drug used in the treatment of *endometriosis* (a condition in which fragments of the tissue that normally lines the uterus occur elsewhere in the pelvic cavity), fibrocystic breast disease (breast tenderness and lumpiness that worsen before menstruation), and *menorrhagia* (heavy periods).

HOW IT WORKS

Danazol suppresses the release of *gonadotrophin hormones* (pituitary hormones that stimulate activity in the ovaries). This reduces the production and release of oestrogen from the ovaries. The change in hormone levels usually prevents ovulation and causes irregularity or absence of periods.

Danazol is usually administered in courses lasting a few months. The disorder may recur after treatment has been discontinued.

POSSIBLE ADVERSE EFFECTS

Adverse effects may include nausea, dizziness, rash, back pain, weight gain, and flushing. Pregnancy should be avoided while taking (and shortly after taking) danazol because the drug can cause masculine characteristics in a female fetus.

D and C

A gynaecological procedure in which the endometrium (lining of the uterus) is scraped away. D and C is an abbreviation for dilatation and curettage. The procedure is commonly used to diagnose the cause of and treat *menorrhagia* (heavy menstrual bleeding) and other disorders of the *uterus*. D and C is also used as a means of terminating a pregnancy (see *Abortion, induced*) and may sometimes be carried out following a *miscarriage*. D and C is increasingly being replaced by an endoscopic technique in which a hysteroscope is used to remove the endometrium (see *Endometrial ablation*).

HOW IT IS DONE

D and C is usually carried out under general anaesthesia. The cervix is dilated (stretched open) so that a *curette* (a spoon-shaped surgical instrument) can be inserted into the uterus to scrape away the endometrium. The scrapings may then be examined under a microscope to assess the condition of the uterus.

RESULTS

Removal of the endometrium causes no side-effects and it may be beneficial if the lining has thickened, causing

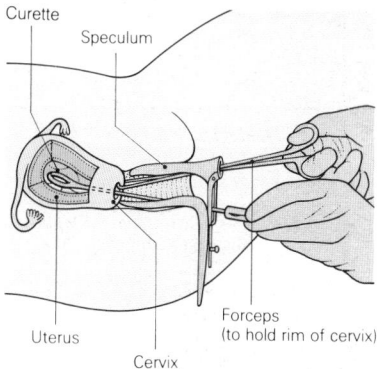

Procedure for D and C
The vagina is dilated with a speculum, the cervix is dilated, and a curette is inserted into the uterus to scrape away the endometrium.

heavy periods. The endometrium soon grows again during the menstrual cycle (see *Menstruation*).

Dander

Minute scales shed from an animal's skin, hair, or feathers. Dander from humans and pets floats in the air or settles on a surface, making up a large proportion of household dust.

Some people are allergic to animal dander and develop symptoms of allergic *rhinitis* (hay fever) or *asthma* if they breathe in the scales.

Dandruff

A common, harmless, but irritating condition in which dead skin is shed from the scalp, often producing unsightly white flakes in the hair and on the collar and shoulders of clothes. The usual cause of the condition is seborrhoeic *dermatitis,* an itchy, scaly rash on the scalp, which may also occur on the face, chest, and back.

TREATMENT

The hair should be shampooed frequently with an antidandruff shampoo. If this fails, a doctor may prescribe a cream or lotion containing a *corticosteroid drug* to be applied to the

D

scalp or a cream containing an *antifungal drug*, which sometimes helps (even though dandruff is not a fungal infection). Whatever the type of treatment, dandruff usually requires constant control.

Dantrolene

A *muscle-relaxant drug* used to relieve muscle spasm caused by *spinal injury*, *stroke*, or neurological disorders such as *cerebral palsy* or *multiple sclerosis*. Dantrolene does not cure the underlying disorder, but often leads to a gradual improvement in mobility.

Dapsone

An *antibacterial drug* used to treat *Hansen's disease* (leprosy) and *dermatitis herpetiformis*, a rare disorder of the skin. Combined with pyrimethamine, it is used to protect against malaria.

Dapsone may cause nausea, vomiting, and, rarely, damage to the liver, red blood cells, and nerves. During long-term treatment, blood tests are carried out regularly to monitor liver function and the number of red cells in the blood.

Daydreaming

Conjuring up pleasant or exciting images or situations in one's mind during waking hours. Everyone daydreams to some extent, but it may be more common during unhappy or stressful periods in a person's life.

Children and teenagers may spend a lot of time daydreaming. In general, this is not a cause for concern unless schoolwork and/or relationships suffer, in which case it may be advisable to seek professional help.

Day surgery

Surgical treatment carried out in a hospital or clinic without an overnight stay. Improvements in *anaesthesia* and the increasing use of *minimally invasive surgery* have made many operations simpler and less stressful for patients; many procedures formerly requiring a stay of several nights in hospital are now carried out on a day-surgery basis. The patient needs to be accompanied by a relative on the journey home, and needs the cooperation of his or her general practitioner. A few patients treated by day surgery develop complications that require them to stay in hospital, but this is usually a precaution and is no cause for alarm.

DDT

The generally used abbreviation for the insecticide dichloro-diphenyl-trichloro-ethane. Developed in Switzerland in the early 1940s, DDT was much more effective than earlier insecticides and it became an important weapon against insect-transmitted diseases, particularly in hot climates. A disadvantage of DDT is that some insects have become resistant to its toxic effects. Moreover, this resistance is genetically determined, so that a DDT-resistant insect may pass the resistance on to its offspring. (See also *Pesticides*.)

Deafness

Complete or partial inability to hear. Total deafness is rare and is usually congenital (present from birth). Partial deafness, ranging from mild to severe, is most commonly the result of an ear disease, injury, or degeneration of the hearing mechanism with age.

All deafness is either conductive or sensorineural. Conductive deafness results from faulty propagation of sound from the outer to the inner ear, usually through damage to the eardrum or the three connected bones in the middle ear—the malleus, incus, and stapes. In sensorineural deafness, sounds that reach the inner ear fail to be transmitted to the brain because of damage to the structures within the inner ear or damage to the acoustic nerve, which connects the inner ear to the brain.

CAUSES

CONDUCTIVE DEAFNESS In an adult, the most common cause of conductive deafness is *earwax* blocking the outer ear canal. Less commonly, *otosclerosis* (in which the stapes loses its normal mobility) may be the cause. In a child, *otitis media* (middle-ear infection) and *glue ear* (collection of sticky fluid in the middle ear) are by far the most common causes of this type of deafness.

Rarely, conductive deafness can be caused by *barotrauma* (damage to the eardrum or middle ear due to sudden pressure changes in an aircraft or under water) or by a perforated eardrum (see *Eardrum, perforated*) following injury, a middle-ear infection, or surgery on the ear.

SENSORINEURAL DEAFNESS Defects of the inner ear are sometimes congenital, due to an inherited fault in a chromosome, to *birth injury*, or to damage to the developing fetus—for example, as the result of the mother having had *rubella* (German measles) during pregnancy. Damage to the inner ear may also occur soon after birth as the result of severe *jaundice*.

Sensorineural deafness that develops in later life can be caused by damage to the cochlea and/or labyrinth due to prolonged exposure to loud noise, to *Ménière's disease*, to certain drugs (such as *streptomycin*), or to some viral infections. The cochlea and labyrinth also degenerate naturally with old age, resulting in *presbyacusis*.

Damage to the acoustic nerve may be the result of an *acoustic neuroma* (a benign tumour on the nerve). As the acoustic neuroma enlarges, it causes increasing deafness.

INCIDENCE

Deafness at birth is sensorineural and incurable. Such deafness is rare, occurring in only about one in 1,000 babies. Deafness that develops in young children is usually conductive and curable. This type of deafness is quite common. As many as one quarter of the five-year-olds starting school have some degree of hearing loss as a result of previous middle-ear infections.

The hearing mechanism gradually degenerates with age, and about one quarter of the population over 65 needs a hearing-aid.

SYMPTOMS, SIGNS, AND DIAGNOSIS

A baby suffering from congenital deafness fails to respond to sounds, and, although crying is often normal, he or she does not babble or make the other baby noises that usually precede speech. These symptoms may be first noticed by a parent.

In a young child, a health visitor or doctor will conduct *hearing tests* during the child's regular check-ups to detect any hearing loss, which is usually due to glue ear.

In an adult who has started to become deaf, sounds heard are not only quieter than before but are also distorted and less clear, high tones are less audible than low ones, the sounds "s", "f", and "z" are not heard, and speech may be difficult to understand if there is background noise. Deafness in one ear may be noticed only when that ear alone is used (for example, when using the telephone).

Deafness may be accompanied by *tinnitus* (noises in the ear) and *vertigo* (dizziness and loss of balance). It sometimes causes confusion, *paranoia*, and auditory *hallucinations*, and can lead to withdrawal and *depression*.

Examination of the ear with an *otoscope* (a viewing instrument with a light attached) can show if the outer-ear canal is obstructed by wax, or if the eardrum is inflamed, perforated, or has fluid behind it.

To determine whether deafness is conductive or sensorineural, hearing tests are carried out.

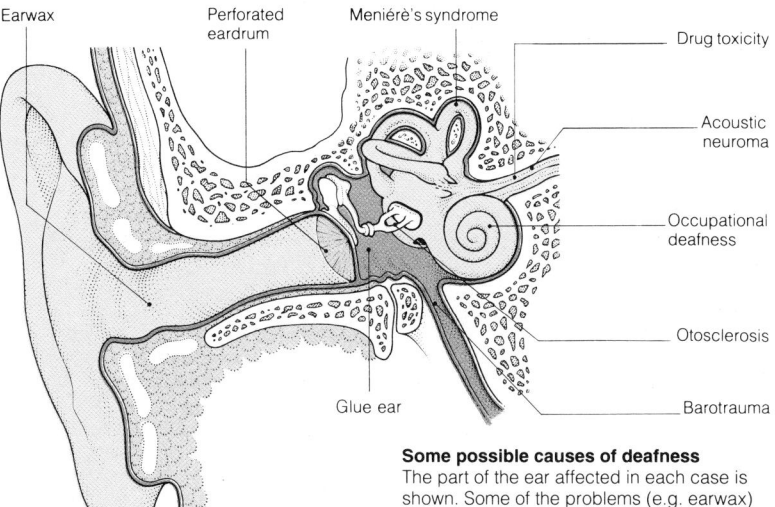

Earwax — Perforated eardrum — Menière's syndrome — Drug toxicity — Acoustic neuroma — Occupational deafness — Glue ear — Otosclerosis — Barotrauma

Some possible causes of deafness
The part of the ear affected in each case is shown. Some of the problems (e.g. earwax) cause conductive deafness; others (e.g. drug toxicity) cause sensorineural deafness.

TREATMENT
Children born deaf need special instruction if they are to learn to speak. The process is a long and difficult one, but eventually many children can communicate effectively, often with sign language.

Conductive deafness in children due to glue ear is treated by an operation to drain the fluid from the middle ear through a hole in the eardrum (see *Myringotomy*). While awaiting surgery, a child should sit at the front of the classroom to hear as much as possible.

When conductive deafness is caused by wax in the ear, a doctor or nurse can remove the wax by syringing the ear with warm water.

A perforated eardrum is usually allowed to heal of its own accord, but, if it has not done so after two or three months, a surgical repair, called *tympanoplasty*, is often carried out.

Conductive deafness due to otosclerosis is usually treated by *stapedectomy*, an operation in which the fixed stapes is replaced with an artificial substitute.

Hearing-aids are sometimes used to lessen deafness caused by otosclerosis, in which case the hearing-aid may take the form of a bone-conducting device that transmits sound to the inner ear through a vibrating pad touching the bone behind the ear. The main use of hearing-aids, however, is in the treatment of sensorineural deafness, which cannot be cured because the structures of the inner ear are too delicate to allow surgery to be performed on them.

The hearing-aids used in these cases increase the volume of sound reaching the inner ear by means of an amplifier and an earphone that fits into the outer ear.

A technological advance in the treatment of sensorineural deafness is the *cochlear implant*, in which electrodes that can receive sound signals are implanted in the inner ear. Implants have proved successful in helping children born profoundly deaf to learn how to speak.

Lip-reading is an invaluable aid for all deaf people, whatever the type and severity of their deafness. People addressing a deaf person should remember to face him or her and not shout, which only distorts sounds.

Various household aids, such as an amplifier for the earpiece of a telephone, are available. (See also *Ear; Hearing*.)

Death

Permanent cessation of all vital functions; the end of life. The classic indicators of death are the permanent cessation of the function of the heart and lungs and in the overwhelming majority of cases these remain the criteria by which a doctor diagnoses and certifies death.

During the 1960s, however, medical technology advanced to the stage where artificial (machine-assisted) maintenance of breathing and heartbeat became possible in cases where the lungs and heart would otherwise have stopped functioning due to gross structural brain damage. This prompted a re-examination of concepts of death and the development of criteria for the diagnosis of *brain death*. This is defined as the irreversible cessation of all functions of the entire brain, including the brainstem.

An individual can thus now be certified legally dead if there is either irreversible cessation of circulatory and respiratory functions or if the criteria for brain death are satisfied.

DIAGNOSIS OF DEATH
The determination of death is considered to be a medical diagnosis. However, doctors are expected to exercise their medical judgment within a defined legal framework.

The diagnosis of death under normal circumstances, when the individual is not on a *ventilator* (breathing machine), is based on absence of spontaneous breathing, absence of heartbeat, and on the pupils being dilated (wide open) and unresponsive to light.

The criteria for diagnosing brain death are based on the determination of the irreversible cessation of brain function. There must be clear evidence of irreversible damage to the brain; persistent deep coma; no attempts at breathing when the patient is taken off the ventilator; and absence of brainstem function (e.g. no response of the pupils to light, no grimacing in response to painful stimuli, and no involuntary blink when the surface of the eye is touched). The guidelines warn that this assessment might not be reliable if the patient is intoxicated, has a very low body temperature, or is in shock. (See also *Death, sudden; Mortality*.)

Death, sudden

Death that occurs unexpectedly in a person who previously seemed to be healthy and who had not complained of any symptoms of illness (deaths due to *accidents* are excluded).

The most common cause of sudden death in adults is *cardiac arrest*. People older than about 35 who die from cardiac arrest are frequently found at *autopsy* (postmortem examination) to have had *coronary artery disease*, and may have died as a result of *myocardial infarction* (heart attack) or cardiac *arrhythmia* (irregularity of heartbeat); younger victims are often found to have had an undiagnosed congenital heart abnormality. *Cardiomyopathy* may cause sudden death at any age, and its presence may have been totally unsuspected.

Sudden death may also occur in people suffering from unsuspected

D

D

myocarditis, stroke, or pneumonia. Other less common causes include anaphylactic shock, asthma, and suicide.

To reduce the risk of sudden death from heart disease, any person about to begin an exercise programme after a period of inactivity should consult a doctor for a check-up, especially if exertion causes chest pain, breathlessness, extreme fatigue, or palpitations, or if he or she is overweight, smokes, or has a family history of coronary artery disease.

In infants (mainly up to one year old), death that occurs without warning is called sudden infant death syndrome (SIDS) or cot death. The causes of SIDS are unknown, although there are several theories.

Cases of sudden death must be reported to the coroner, who decides whether or not an autopsy should be performed.

Debility

Generalized weakness and lack of energy. Debility may be caused by a physical disorder (such as anaemia) or by a psychological disorder (such as depression).

Debridement

Surgical removal of foreign material and/or dead, damaged, or infected tissue from a wound or burn to expose healthy tissue. Such treatment promotes healthy healing of badly damaged skin, muscle, and other tissue.

Decalcification, dental

The dissolving of minerals in a tooth. Dental decalcification is the first stage of tooth decay. It is caused by the bacteria in plaque acting on refined carbohydrates (mainly sugar) in food to produce acid. After prolonged or numerous exposures, the acid causes changes on the surface of the tooth. The decalcified area can be seen as a chalky white patch when the plaque is brushed away. The process is partly reversible at this stage if a mineralizing solution is applied.

If the decalcification penetrates the enamel, it spreads along the junction between the enamel and dentine, and then into the dentine. Lack of professional treatment at this stage will permit bacteria to enter the pulp. Further destruction of dentine will then be caused by bacterial enzymes, and the pulp, once infected, may die. (See also Caries, dental.)

Decay, dental

See Caries, dental.

Decerebrate

The state of being without a functioning cerebrum (the cerebral hemispheres and associated structures), which is the main controlling part of the brain. This situation occurs when the brainstem (the upward extension of the spinal cord) is severed, which effectively isolates the cerebrum.

Deciduous teeth

See Primary teeth.

Decompression sickness

A hazard of divers (both recreational and professional) and of others who work in or breathe compressed air or other gas mixtures. It is also known as the "bends" and was formerly known as caisson disease. Decompression sickness results from the formation of gas bubbles in the diver's tissues during ascent from depth.

CAUSES AND INCIDENCE

The amount of gas that can be held dissolved in a tissue (such as blood or body fat) increases with pressure (i.e. as a diver descends underwater) and decreases when the pressure is released. At depth, divers accumulate large quantities of inert gas in their tissues from the high-pressure gas mixture they breathe (see Scuba-diving medicine); if air is being breathed (as is usual for recreational divers), the main inert gas is nitrogen.

When the diver ascends, pressure falls and the gas can no longer be held within the tissues; if the pressure reduction is rapid, the gas may form bubbles—just as bubbles form in a bottle of beer when the cap is flipped off. The bubbles may block blood vessels, causing various symptoms.

Trained divers and industrial compressed air workers avoid problems by allowing the excess gas that has built up in their tissues to escape slowly via the blood into their lungs during controlled, very slow ascent or release of pressure.

SYMPTOMS

Symptoms may appear any time within 24 hours after a dive. Common symptoms include skin itching and mottling, and severe pains in and around the larger joints, particularly the shoulders and knees. Symptoms of impairment of the nervous system (such as leg weakness, visual disturbances, or problems with balance) are particularly serious, as is a painful, tight feeling across the chest, which may indicate the presence of bubbles in the vessels that supply the heart and in the circulation to the lungs.

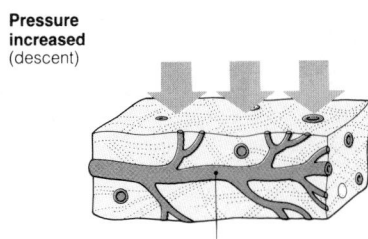

Pressure increased (descent)

Inert gas dissolved in tissue fluids and blood

Pressure reduced (ascent)

Bubbles form in blood vessels and tissues

Bubble blocking blood vessel

How decompression occurs
On ascent, pressure is reduced rapidly and the gas may form bubbles that may, in turn, cause symptoms. Divers avoid this by ascending slowly.

TREATMENT

Any diver with the symptoms described should be transported immediately to, and placed inside, a recompression chamber. Pressure within the chamber is raised by pumping in air; this causes the bubbles within the diver's tissues to redissolve, and the symptoms to disappear. Subsequently, the pressure in the chamber is slowly reduced, allowing the excess gas to escape safely via the blood and lungs.

OUTLOOK

If treated promptly by recompression, most divers with the "bends" make a full recovery. However, in serious, untreated cases, there may be long-term complications such as partial paralysis. Repeated episodes lead to degenerative disorders of the bones and joints.

Decompression, spinal canal

A surgical procedure to relieve pressure on the spinal cord or on a nerve root emerging from the cord.

WHY IT IS DONE

Pressure on the spinal cord may be due to a disc prolapse, to a tumour (in most cases benign) of the membranes surrounding the cord or of the cord itself, to a narrow spinal canal, which may be present from birth or caused by osteoarthritis, or to fracture of the vertebrae after an accident. Any of these conditions can cause weakness or paralysis of the limbs and loss of bladder control.

HOW IT IS DONE

To treat major disc prolapses and tumours, a *laminectomy* (removal of the bony arches of one or more vertebrae) to expose the affected part of the cord or nerve roots must be performed. Severely prolapsed discs are cut away and affected nerve roots are freed from surrounding tissues. Sometimes a surgeon may approach the spinal cord from the front.

When pressure is being caused by a tumour or abscess in a vertebra, the affected section of bone is removed. If a large portion of bone is removed, bone grafting is carried out at the end of the operation.

RECOVERY PERIOD

Confinement to bed in a flat position is necessary initially, with measures taken to prevent *bedsores* and *physiotherapy* given to keep the leg muscles strong. Usually a patient can get up within a few days. Heavy lifting must be avoided for several weeks.

OUTLOOK

Recovery of movement, sensation, and bladder control, and achievement of pain relief after treatment depend on the severity and duration of the pressure before the operation, the success of the surgery in relieving the pressure, and whether damage was sustained by the cord and nerves during the operation.

Decongestant drugs

COMMON DRUGS

Ephedrine Oxymetazoline Phenylephrine Phenylpropanolamine Pseudoephedrine Xylometazoline

WARNING
Symptoms worsen when, after several days of treatment, decongestants are suddenly withdrawn. Use only in low doses for a short time.

Drugs used to relieve *nasal congestion.* Small amounts of these drugs are present in many over-the-counter *cold remedies,* which are available in tablet or nose-drop form. Decongestant drugs are commonly used in the treatment of upper *respiratory tract infections,* especially in patients susceptible to *otitis media* (middle-ear infection) or *sinusitis* (sinus infection).

POSSIBLE ADVERSE EFFECTS

Taken by mouth, decongestant drugs may cause tremor and palpitations;

THE ACTION OF DECONGESTANTS

Decongestants work by narrowing blood vessels in the membranes that line the nose. This action reduces swelling, inflammation, and the mount of mucus produced by the nasal lining.

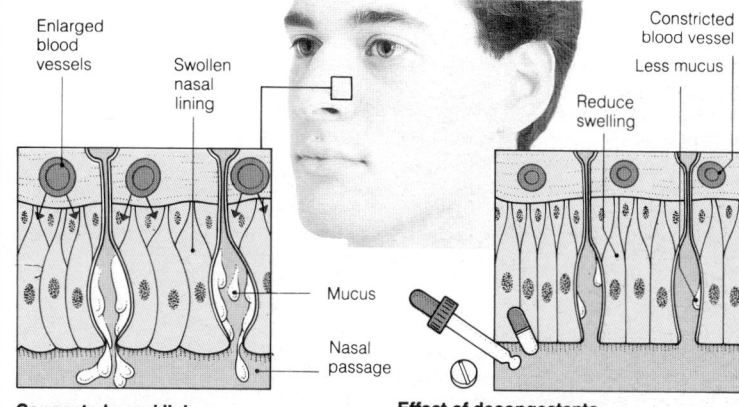

Enlarged blood vessels
Swollen nasal lining
Mucus
Nasal passage
Constricted blood vessel
Less mucus
Reduce swelling

Congested nasal lining.
When blood vessels enlarge in response to infection or irritation, increased amounts of fluid pass into the lining, which swells and produces more mucus.

Effect of decongestants
Chemicals stimulate constriction of the blood vessels in the nasal lining, which reduces swelling, mucus production, and nasal congestion.

they are therefore not usually prescribed if a person has heart disease. In the form of nose-drops, only small amounts are absorbed into the blood and adverse effects are unlikely.

If decongestant nose-drops are taken for several days and then stopped, congestion frequently recurs and may be worse than that for which the drug was taken. For this reason, decongestants should be taken for as short a time as possible.

Decubitus ulcer

See *Bedsores.*

Defaecation

The expulsion of *faeces* from the body via the anus.

Defence mechanisms

Techniques used by the mind in order to cope with unpleasant or unwelcome events, experiences, impulses, or emotions.

For example, death of a relative normally provokes grief and/or anger. One defence against these emotions may be repression—refusing to recognize these feelings and appearing to be unaffected by the event. Another reaction is denial—carrying on as though the relative is still alive.

A person who feels guilty about hating his or her father may transfer this hate to another person or turn the bad feelings towards himself or herself.

Disturbing impulses may take the opposite form in conscious thought. For instance, a person with strong sexual feelings may be excessively prudish or inhibited.

The body's defence mechanisms against infection are described under *immune system.*

Defibrillation

A technique in which a brief electric shock is administered to the heart, usually via two metal plates placed on the wall of the chest. It is also called cardioversion. The technique is performed to treat some types of *arrhythmia* (irregular or rapid heartbeat). The sudden burst of electricity through the heart converts *fibrillation* (rapid, uncoordinated heartbeat) or *tachycardia* (rapid heartbeat) back into a normal, regular heartbeat. Occasionally a drug, such as lignocaine, is injected into a vein before the procedure to try to stabilize the heart rhythm.

Defibrillation can be carried out as an emergency procedure to treat *ventricular fibrillation,* which most commonly starts after a *myocardial infarction* (heart attack). It may also be used to treat an arrhythmia that has lasted several hours or days.

Defoliant poisoning

The toxic effects of chemicals that are applied to plants to kill them by causing their leaves to drop off. Com-

D

D

monly used as weedkillers, defoliants are poisonous if swallowed. They should therefore always be kept in clearly labelled containers and stored out of the reach of children. The most widely used defoliant weedkillers are sodium chlorate, potassium chlorate (see *Chlorate poisoning*), and *paraquat*.

Another well-known group of defoliants are the phenoxy herbicides which may be contaminated with dioxin, a substance that is highly toxic to humans. One such herbicide (known as Agent Orange) was used by US forces in the Vietnam war. Phenoxy herbicides have also occasionally been released into the atmosphere as a result of industrial accidents. Allegations have been made that Agent Orange (due to its dioxin content) caused nerve and other disorders in many Vietnam veterans, Vietnamese civilians and others exposed to it (as well as birth defects in their children), but an Australian Royal Commission that reported in 1985 found no links with disease in servicemen or their children.

Deformity

Any malformation or distortion of part of the body. Deformities may be *congenital* (present from birth) or they may be acquired as a result of injury, disease, disorder, or disuse.

Most congenital deformities are relatively rare. Among the more common are club-foot (*talipes*) and *cleft lip and palate*.

Injuries that can cause deformity include burns, torn muscles, broken bones, and dislocated joints. Among the various diseases and disorders that may cause deformity are infections, such as *tuberculosis* and *Hansen's disease* (leprosy); damage to or disorders of nerves, such as paralysis of the facial nerves; some deficiency diseases, such as *rickets*; and a condition of unknown cause called *Paget's disease* of the bone.

Disuse of a part of the body—as a result of being bedridden or confined to a wheelchair, for example—can lead to deformity through stiffening and *contracture* (shortening) of unused muscles or tendons.

Many deformities can be corrected by *plastic surgery*, various orthopaedic techniques (including surgery), exercise, or by a combination of these methods. For example, cleft lip and palate are now treated by surgery during childhood, with good results in most cases.

It is often possible to prevent the development of a deformity due to disuse by ensuring that the patient gets regular exercise and by teaching him or her exercises that can be performed at home.

Degeneration

Physical and/or chemical changes in cells, tissues, or organs that reduce their efficiency. Degeneration is a feature of aging and may also be due to a disease process. Other known causes include injury, reduced blood supply, poisoning (by alcohol, for example), or a diet deficient in a specific vitamin. (See also *Degenerative disorders*.)

Degenerative disorders

A blanket term covering a wide range of conditions in which there is progressive impairment of both the structure and function of part of the body. This definition excludes diseases caused by infection, inflammation, altered immune responses, chemical or physical damage, or malignant change. Many of the features of aging, such as wrinkling of the skin, are due to degenerative changes in body tissues, but, in degenerative disorders, the changes come on earlier in life, are more rapid, and typically affect some organs and not others.

Microscopic examination of an organ affected by degenerative disease often shows that the number of specialized cells or structures is reduced and that their place has been taken by *connective tissue* or scar tissue.

Some diseases, such as *Creutzfeldt-Jakob disease*, were once thought to be degenerative disorders but later proved to be due to slow viruses. *Parkinsonism* (a disorder that shares the symptoms of *Parkinson's disease*) may be traceable to poisoning—with carbon monoxide or with MPTP, an impurity formed during the illegal manufacture of one of the many *designer drugs*. Future research may identify specific infective or environmental causes for other disorders that are at present thought to be degenerative disorders.

NERVOUS SYSTEM

Among degenerative disorders affecting the nervous system the most common is *Alzheimer's disease*, the main cause of presenile and senile *dementia*. In *Huntington's disease*, dementia is combined with disorders of movement. Here, susceptibility to the degenerative changes in the brain is due to an abnormality in a single gene; the disease is transmitted from one generation to the next in a dominant pattern of inheritance (see *Genetic disorders*). In Parkinson's disease and in degenerative disorders that affect the *cerebellum*, abnormalities of movement are the main features. In *motor neuron diseases*, including *Werdnig-Hoffmann disease*, the prime symptom is muscular weakness.

EYES

Blindness in early adult life can be caused by a condition called Leber's *optic atrophy*, which is due to loss of nerve cells in the retina. *Retinitis pigmentosa*, another retinal degeneration, can cause blindness in childhood, but some vision may be preserved until late middle age. Both disorders have a genetic basis. By contrast, senile *macular degeneration* is not an inherited condition and rarely develops before the age of 60.

JOINTS

The most familiar degenerative disorder is *osteoarthritis*, also sometimes known as degenerative joint disease. Susceptibility to the condition seems to run in families; it also develops in sports enthusiasts and manual workers who have repeatedly damaged their joints. The prime features of osteoarthritis are thinning and destruction of the cartilage covering the surfaces of the joints, and overgrowth and distortion of the bone around affected joints.

ARTERIES

Some hardening of the arteries seems to be a feature of aging. In some individuals, however, the degenerative changes in the muscle coat of these blood vessels are unusually severe and calcium deposits may be seen on X-ray films (as in Monckeberg's sclerosis, a type of *arteriosclerosis*).

MUSCLES

Degeneration of muscles occurs in a group of genetic disorders, known as *muscular dystrophies*, which cause distinctive patterns of muscular weakness and are sometimes associated with increased muscle bulk.

Deglutition

The medical term for *swallowing*.

Dehiscence

The splitting open of a partly healed wound; the term is most commonly used to refer to the splitting open of a surgical incision that has been closed with sutures or clips.

Dehydration

A condition in which a person's water content has fallen to a dangerously low level. Water accounts for about 60 per cent of a man's weight and 50 per cent of a woman's, and the total water content must be kept within fairly narrow limits for healthy functioning of cells and tissues (see *Water*).

The concentration of mineral salts and other substances dissolved in the body's fluids must also be kept within a narrow range. In many cases of dehydration, the body's salt content, in addition to the water content, has been depleted.

CAUSES

Normally, dehydration is prevented by the sensation of thirst, which encourages a person to drink when the body is short of water. This mechanism may fail because water is not available or because of high losses of water from the body.

Even in a temperate climate, a minimum of 1.5 litres of water is lost by an adult every 24 hours through the skin via perspiration, from the lungs into the air, and in the urine to rid the body of waste products. Severe dehydration is likely to develop within a few days if no water is taken. In a hot climate, an extra 2 to 5 litres of water may be lost in sweat every day, or up to 10 litres a day in someone doing hard physical work. Large amounts of water may also be lost in vomit or diarrhoea, particularly if the diarrhoea is profuse and watery (as in *cholera*) or in the urine of anyone with uncontrolled *diabetes mellitus, diabetes insipidus,* and some types of *kidney failure.* In all these cases, the thirst sensation may not encourage sufficient water intake to balance the losses.

Babies tend to become dehydrated more rapidly than adults because their normal water loss per hour makes up a much higher proportion of their water content.

SYMPTOMS AND SIGNS

Symptoms and signs of water depletion include severe thirst, dry lips and tongue, an increase in heart-rate and breathing rate, dizziness, confusion, and eventual coma. The skin looks dry and loses its elasticity. Any urine passed is small in quantity and dark-coloured. If there is also salt depletion (usually as a result of heavy sweating, vomiting, or diarrhoea), additional symptoms may include lethargy, headaches, cramps, and pallor.

PREVENTION

When living in a hot climate, or when suffering from a fever, vomiting, or diarrhoea, the simplest rule is to drink enough water to produce urine that is consistently pale. This often means drinking well beyond the point of thirst (possibly 0.5 litre of water every hour during the heat of the day).

Salt losses from heavy sweating need to be replaced either in the diet or by adding a quarter of a teaspoon of table salt to each 0.5 litre of drinking water. Bottled mineral water can help maintain the intake of salts. For vomiting and diarrhoea, *rehydration therapy* is needed; special salt and glucose rehydration mixtures can be purchased from chemists. Children are particularly susceptible to severe dehydration by diarrhoea and it is worth taking a supply of these mixtures if planning a visit to a warm country with small children.

TREATMENT

Once dehydration has developed, fluid and salt replacement may be required at a far faster rate than that needed simply to prevent dehydration. In severe cases of dehydration, fluids must be given intravenously. The water/salt balance has to be carefully monitored by blood tests and adjusted if necessary.

Déjà vu

French for "already seen". A sense of having already experienced an event that is happening at the moment. Déjà vu is a common phenomenon that has never been properly explained. Some people believe that it is due to an unconscious emotional response caused by similarities between the current event and some past experience. Others believe that a neurological "short circuit" results in the experience registering in the memory before reaching consciousness. Frequent occurrence of déjà vu may sometimes be a symptom of *temporal lobe epilepsy.*

Delhi belly

One of many popular names for *gastroenteritis* and infective diarrhoea caused by eating food contaminated by microorganisms or their toxins.

Delinquency

Behaviour in a juvenile that in an adult would be considered a crime. The term is often extended to include non-criminal behaviour, such as playing truant, running away from home, drinking alcohol, or *drug abuse.*

Juvenile delinquency is probably caused by a combination of factors—social, psychological, and biological—but relatively few offenders suffer from a definite mental disorder or mental handicap.

Child guidance or *family therapy* may be recommended for juvenile delinquents and their families. Persistent

offenders are sometimes sent to special schools and may be taken into care or made wards of court.

Delirium

A state of acute mental confusion, commonly brought on by physical illness. The symptoms are those of disordered brain function, and vary according to personality, environment, and the severity of illness. Failure to understand events or remember what has been happening, increased anxiety, physical restlessness, and sudden swings of mood occur as delirium worsens. At its most severe, the patient may hallucinate, suffer from *illusions* (for example, seeing nurses as threatening monsters), lapse into a terrified panic, and resort to shouting and violence. Usually the symptoms are worse at night, because of sleep disturbance and the fact that darkness and quiet make visual illusions more likely.

CAUSES

While any severe illness may underlie this state, high fever and disturbances of body chemistry are commonly present. Children and older people are most susceptible, particularly after major surgery or when there is a pre-existing brain disturbance such as *dementia.* Drugs, various poisons, and alcohol are common precipitants.

TREATMENT

Treatment is of the underlying physical disorder, with appropriate nursing to reduce anxiety. Suitable lighting, calm and clear communication, appropriate seclusion, and known, trusted attendants are all important. Particular attention must be paid to fluids and nutrition, but *tranquillizer drugs* (such as *haloperidol* or *thioridazine*) are sometimes necessary to reduce the physical restlessness. The control of infection by *antibiotic drugs* has made delirium much rarer than formerly.

Delirium tremens

A state of confusion accompanied by trembling and vivid *hallucinations*. It usually arises in chronic alcoholics after withdrawal or abstinence from alcohol, often following admission to hospital with an injury or for a surgical operation.

SYMPTOMS AND SIGNS

In the early stages, symptoms include restlessness, agitation, trembling, and sleeplessness. Overactivity of the *sympathetic nervous system* causes a rapid heartbeat, fever, dilation (widening) of the pupils, and profuse sweating

D

that may lead to dehydration. Confusion follows, with visual and sometimes auditory hallucinations, and the patient appears terrified. Convulsions may also occur. Symptoms usually subside within three days.

TREATMENT
Treatment consists of rest, rehydration, and sedation in hospital. *Sedative drugs* used include *chlorpromazine, chlordiazepoxide,* or chlormethiazole. Injections of vitamins, particularly of thiamine (see *vitamin B complex*), may be given, because some of the features of delirium tremens seem to be linked with thiamine deficiency (see *Wernicke-Korsakoff syndrome*).

Delivery

Expulsion or extraction of a baby from the mother's uterus. In most cases the baby lies lengthwise in the uterus with its head facing downwards and is delivered head first through the vaginal opening by a combination of uterine contractions and maternal effort at the end of the second stage of labour (see *Childbirth*).

If the baby is lying in an abnormal position (see *Breech delivery; Malpresentation*), if uterine contractions are weak, or if there is disproportion between the size of the baby's head and the mother's pelvis, a *forceps delivery* or *vacuum extraction* may be required; these are called operative deliveries. In some cases, vaginal delivery is impossible or potentially dangerous to the mother or the baby, and *caesarean* section is necessary.

Deltoid

The triangular muscle of the shoulder region that forms the rounded flesh of the outer part of the upper arm, and passes up and over the shoulder joint. The wide end of the muscle is attached to the scapula (shoulderblade) and the clavicle (collarbone). The muscle fibres converge to form the apex of the triangle, which is attached to the humerus (upper-arm bone) about halfway down its length.

The central, strongest part of the muscle raises the arm sideways. The front and back parts of the muscle twist the arm.

Delusion

A fixed, irrational idea not shared by others and not responding to reasoned argument. The central idea in a paranoid delusion involves persecution or jealousy. For instance, a person may believe that he or she is being poisoned or that a partner is persis-

LOCATION OF THE DELTOID
The deltoid muscle of the shoulder region forms the rounded, outer part of the upper arm and is attached to the scapula and clavicle.

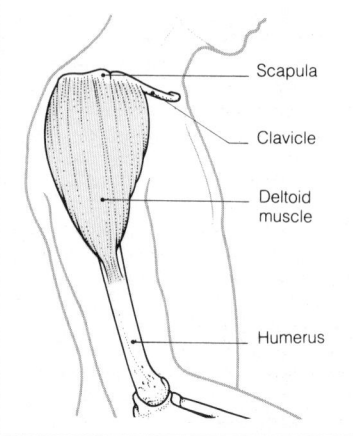

Scapula

Clavicle

Deltoid muscle

Humerus

tently unfaithful (see *Paranoia*). A person who is suffering from delusions of grandeur may believe, for example, that he or she is a member of the royal family.

Persistent delusions are a sign of serious mental illness, notably *schizophrenia* and *manic-depressive illness.* (See also *Hallucination; Illusion.*)

Dementia

A general decline in all areas of mental ability. Dementia is usually due to brain disease and is progressive, the most obvious feature being decreasing intellectual ability.

INCIDENCE
Dementia is the great health problem of modern developed societies, since long life is creating an increasing proportion of elderly citizens. Some 10 per cent of those aged over 65 and 20 per cent of those aged over 75 are affected to some degree by dementia.

CAUSES
Traditionally, dementing illnesses were divided into presenile (under 65 years of age at onset) and senile (over 65 years). This is now regarded as an artificial division, although treatable causes are more common in the younger age group. Such causes include *head injury, brain tumour, encephalitis, myxoedema, syphilis,* pernicious *anaemia,* and *alcohol dependence.* However, only some 10 per cent of cases are due to one of these "reversible" illnesses.

In almost all cases, dementia is due to *cerebrovascular disease,* including

strokes, or to *Alzheimer's disease.* Cerebrovascular disease is often due to narrowed or blocked arteries in the brain and can sometimes be helped by treatment of *hypertension* or heart disease. However, recurrent loss of blood supply to the brain usually results in deterioration that characteristically occurs gradually but in stages. Research into drug treatments such as *tetrahydroaminoacridine* for Alzheimer's disease have given disappointing results; improvement is usually slight, and side-effects are often troublesome.

SYMPTOMS
The person with dementia may not remember recent events, may become easily lost in a familiar neighbourhood, may fail to grasp what is going on, and may become confused over days and dates. These symptoms tend to come on gradually and may not be noticed at first. People also tend to cover up their problems by *confabulation* (making up stories to fill the gaps in their memories). Sudden emotional outbursts or embarrassing behaviour (such as urinating in public) may be the first obvious signs of the condition.

Commonly, the person's failures in judgment result in the magnification of his or her unpleasant personality traits; families may have to endure unreasonable demands, accusations, pilfering, and even physical assault. *Paranoia, depression,* and psychotic *delusions* may occur as the disease worsens. Irritability or anxiety, of which the patient retains some awareness, gives way to a shallow indifference towards all feelings. Personal habits deteriorate, clothes and possessions become soiled and dirty, and speech becomes incoherent. Demented individuals may then need total nursing care for feeding, toilet, and physical activities.

TREATMENT
While appropriate treatment of certain illnesses is effective in arresting decline (such as surgery for a brain tumour or thyroid hormone replacement for myxoedema), management of the most common Alzheimer-type illness is based on the treatment of symptoms. The patient should be kept clean and well-nourished in comfortable surroundings with good nursing care. *Sedative drugs* will be given for obvious restlessness or paranoid beliefs. These measures can help ease the distress for both patient and family. Timing of a transfer to suitable hospital or custodial care must be sensitively organized.

Research into medication to alleviate memory loss and intellectual decline has shown some promise, but no truly effective treatment is yet available. Several experimental drugs that increase the amount of the chemical *acetylcholine* in the brain have produced remissions in some patients in clinical trials but these drugs also have serious side-effects.

Dementia praecox

An outdated term for severe *schizophrenia*, especially that developing in adolescence or early adulthood.

De Morgan's spots

Harmless red or purple raised spots in the skin, about 2 mm across, which usually affect middle-aged or elderly people. De Morgan's spots are also called cherry spots or cherry angiomas and consist of a cluster of minute blood vessels. With increasing age they become more numerous but do not increase in size. The spots are of no significance, although they may bleed if injured.

Demyelination

Breakdown of the fatty sheaths that surround and electrically insulate nerve fibres. The sheaths provide nutrients to the nerve fibres and are vital to the passage of electrical impulses along them. Demyelination "short-circuits" the functioning of the nerve, causing loss of sensation, coordination, and power in specific areas of the body. The affected nerves may be within the central nervous system (CNS), comprising the brain and spinal cord, or may be part of the peripheral nervous system, which links the CNS to the body's sense receptors, muscles, glands, and organs.

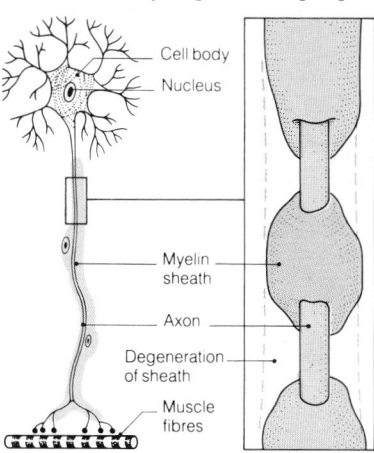

Mechanism of demyelination
The fatty myelin sheaths that surround and insulate nerve fibres break down, causing the affected nerves to "short-circuit".

Patches of demyelination are the prime feature of *multiple sclerosis*, a disease with symptoms that include blurred vision, muscle weakness, and loss of coordination. The cause of the demyelination is not known. In many cases, attacks of demyelination alternate with periods of partial or complete recovery of nerve function.

Encephalomyelitis is a rare disorder in which there is inflammation of nerve cells within the CNS and sometimes areas of demyelination. It may be due to a viral infection or very rarely to an allergic-like reaction following immunization.

Dendritic ulcer

A type of *corneal ulcer* characterized by thread-like extensions that branch out in various directions from the centre. The ulcer is commonly caused by infection of the cornea by the *herpes simplex* virus.

Dengue

 A tropical disease caused by a virus spread by the mosquito AEDESA EGYPTI. It occurs in Southeast Asia, the Pacific region, parts of Africa, South and Central America, and the Caribbean. There have also been occasional outbreaks in Mexico, Puerto Rico, and the US Virgin Islands.

Symptoms and signs appear five to eight days after a bite by an infected mosquito and include fever, headache, rash, and severe joint and muscle pains. These symptoms often subside after about three days, recur a few days later, and then subside again. Serious complications are uncommon. Full recovery may take several weeks. The symptoms of severe muscle and bone pain have led to the alternative name of breakbone fever.

No specific treatment is available for dengue, although *analgesic drugs* (painkillers) may relieve symptoms. No vaccine is available at present; avoidance involves personal protection against mosquito bites in areas where the disease is prevalent (see *Insect bites*).

Densitometry

The measurement of bone density, as determined by the concentration of calcified material.

WHY IT IS DONE
Densitometry is used to confirm the presence of *osteoporosis* (wasting away of bone substance) or to diagnose *rickets* in young children. It is also useful in assessing the response of these conditions to treatment.

HOW IT IS DONE
The most accurate way to measure bone density is by analysing the weight and content of a bone *biopsy* sample. However, this technique is time-consuming and requires an operation to remove the sample. *CT scanning* provides detailed pictures of internal bone structure, which enable changes in bone density to be seen.

A relatively new densitometry technique is single or dual photon absorption, in which the pattern of absorption of a beam (or beams) of radiation as it passes through the bone is analysed on an electronic counter. The dual photon method is used to evaluate the mineral content of the type of bone found in the vertebrae and most other bones where fractures from osteoporosis occur.

Density

The "compactness" of a substance, defined as its mass per unit volume. Because of the close relationship between mass and weight (a mass achieves weight when acted on by gravity) the densities of substances can be compared directly by weighing standard volumes of them under the same gravitational conditions. For instance, a cubic centimetre of lead always weighs much more than a cubic centimetre of wood when weighed at the earth's surface; lead is therefore denser than wood.

In radiology, the term density relates to the amount of radiation absorbed by the structure being X-rayed. Bone, which absorbs radiation well, appears white on X-ray film. By contrast, a lung, which contains mostly air, absorbs very little radiation and appears dark on film. The same holds true in *CT scanning* and *MRI*. (See also *Specific gravity*.)

Dental emergencies

Injuries or disorders of the teeth and gums that require immediate treatment because of severe pain and/or because delay could lead to poor healing or complications.

A tooth that has become avulsed (completely dislodged from its socket) should be gently washed, reimplanted as rapidly as possible (see *Reimplantation, dental*), and then immobilized with a splint. The success rate is about 90 per cent if the tooth is out of its socket for 30 minutes

D

or less and the patient is young. An extruded tooth (one that is partly dislodged from its socket) should be manipulated back into the socket within a few minutes of the injury.

A direct blow to a tooth may cause a fracture (see *Fracture, dental*). Sometimes a blow hard enough to fracture teeth may also fracture the jaw; the fractured parts may need to be wired together to allow them to heal (see *Wiring of the jaw*).

Toothache may be so severe that eating and sleeping are disturbed. Temporary pain relief can be gained by placing a sedative dressing in the tooth until the cause of the pain can be treated. The most severe dental pain is usually caused by an abscess (infection). This is treated either by *antibiotic drugs* to reduce the swelling, or by draining the abscess (see *Abscess, dental*), followed by endodontic treatment. Swelling, pain, and inflammation may also occur around an impacted or erupting wisdom tooth, and the jaw may become stiff and difficult to open. This requires immediate treatment to prevent the infection from spreading (see *Impaction, dental*).

Vincent's disease (see *Gingivitis, acute ulcerative*) comes on suddenly and causes pain, inflammation, ulceration, and bleeding of the gums. It is a destructive condition, and professional treatment should be sought as quickly as possible.

Dental examination

Examination of the mouth, gums, and teeth by a dentist. A dental examination may be performed as a routine check at least once a year or as part of the assessment of the condition of a person complaining of a symptom.

WHY IT IS DONE

Routine examinations enable dental caries (tooth decay) and diseases of the gums and mouth to be detected and treated at an early stage before they cause serious damage. The examinations also allow the efficiency of *oral hygiene* to be checked.

It is particularly important for children to have their teeth examined regularly by a dentist so that the replacement of primary teeth by permanent teeth can be monitored. If any problems occur, such as crowding, the dentist can refer the child for *orthodontic* treatment at the correct stage.

HOW IT IS DONE

Before the examination, the dentist or dental hygienist usually asks about the patient's general health, especially if it is the person's first visit or the first visit for a long time. Understanding the person's general health is important since it can affect the type of treatment that is recommended. A person with a heart-valve disorder, for example, may be under increased risk of contracting bacterial *endocarditis* after extraction of a tooth or any other dental treatment. Particular care is also needed when treating people with *diabetes mellitus* or people who have had *hepatitis*. The dentist should also ask about any drugs the patient is taking; people taking certain drugs can react badly to anaesthesia. The dentist also needs to know whether the patient is allergic to drugs such as *penicillin drugs*.

If a patient is complaining of pain, the dentist will ask him or her questions, such as when the pain was first noticed and whether it is continuous or intermittent.

The dentist begins by noting the general appearance of the patient and by examining the face and neck externally. The face is inspected for puffiness that might indicate a dental *abscess* and the neck for swollen lymph glands, which may be caused by an infection of the mouth or teeth. The dentist may also feel the *temporomandibular joint* (jaw joint) for any abnormal movements.

The dentist next examines the patient's bite and the teeth as a whole, noting any tilted, rotated, overlapping, or missing teeth and observing points of contact between teeth, and the presence of any excessive movement in a tooth when the patient makes chewing movements.

Using a mirror to see the backs of the teeth and into the back of the mouth, the dentist then examines individual teeth, using a metal instrument to probe for cavities or chips. Fillings and crowns are inspected for fit, jagged edges, and signs of erosion or cracks. If teeth are missing, the alveolus (bone that surrounds and supports the teeth) is examined for signs of abnormality, especially if the patient is to be fitted with a prosthodontic appliance, such as a dental

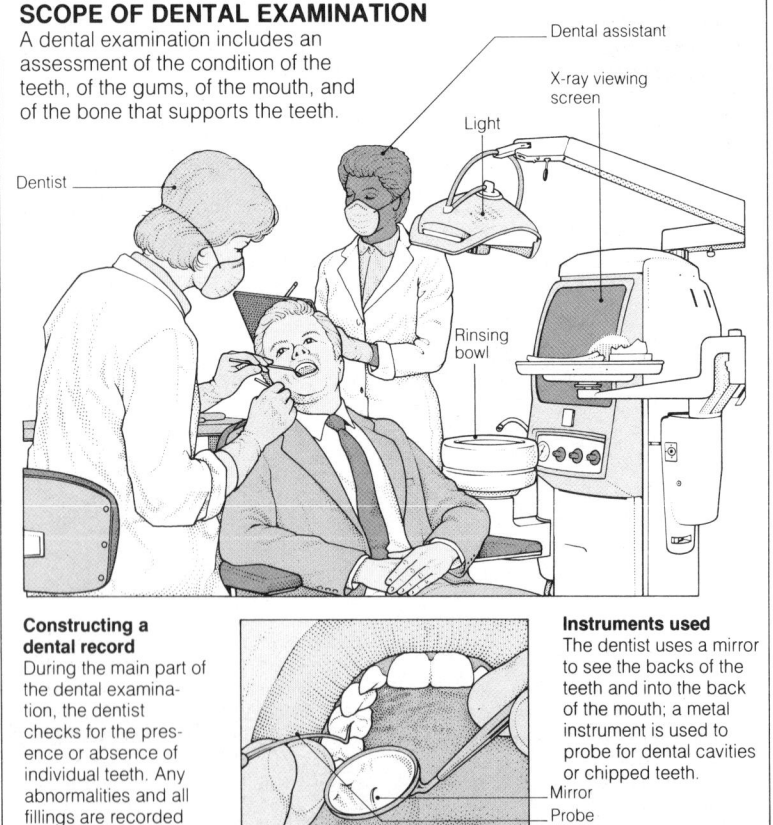

SCOPE OF DENTAL EXAMINATION
A dental examination includes an assessment of the condition of the teeth, of the gums, of the mouth, and of the bone that supports the teeth.

Dentist

Dental assistant

X-ray viewing screen

Light

Rinsing bowl

Constructing a dental record
During the main part of the dental examination, the dentist checks for the presence or absence of individual teeth. Any abnormalities and all fillings are recorded by the assistant.

Instruments used
The dentist uses a mirror to see the backs of the teeth and into the back of the mouth; a metal instrument is used to probe for dental cavities or chipped teeth.

Mirror

Probe

bridge. If the patient wears a *denture*, this is checked to make sure that it still fits properly.

The gums and inside of the mouth are examined for signs of disease. Gums that are red, puffy, or receding or that bleed easily when touched with the probe may indicate *gingivitis* or *periodontitis*. White discoloration of the inside of the mouth may signify *candidiasis* or *leukoplakia*.

Finally, the dentist assesses the accumulation of plaque and calculus on the teeth; this indicates the efficiency of the patient's oral hygiene. *Dental X-rays* are an integral part of the examination in some 95 per cent of new patients.

Dental extraction
See *Tooth extraction*.

Dental X-ray
An image of the teeth and jaws that provides information essential for detecting, diagnosing, and treating conditions that can threaten oral and general health. The part to be imaged is placed between a tube emitting *X-rays* and a photographic film. Because X-rays are unable to pass easily through hard tissue (such as teeth and bone), a shadow of the teeth and bone is seen on the film.

WHY IT IS DONE
X-rays can reveal disorders of the teeth and surrounding tissues that a dentist would not see during a normal visual examination of the mouth. Small caries (areas of decay), abscesses, cysts, tumours, and other disorders can be detected and treated before obvious signs and symptoms have developed, thereby avoiding serious long-term damage. Early identification of dental problems, such as impacted teeth, allows treatment to be carefully planned and carried out at an early stage.

RISKS
The amount of radiation received from dental X-rays is extremely small, and the risk of any harmful effects is negligible. However, a woman who is, or suspects she may be, pregnant should tell her dentist, who may postpone X-rays until after the pregnancy, or will cover her abdomen with a leaded apron (which blocks X-rays) while the X-rays are taken.

Dentifrice
A paste, powder, or gel used with a toothbrush to clean the teeth. Although brushing without a dentifrice removes food debris and some dental *plaque*, a slightly abrasive dentifrice is needed to remove the remaining plaque and the pellicle (a thin film formed from saliva).

A dentifrice contains the following: a mild abrasive—usually an insoluble salt, such as dicalcium phosphate; synthetic detergents; binding and moistening agents; thickening agents; flavourings; and colourings. Most dentifrices also contain *fluoride*, use of which has resulted in a dramatic drop in the incidence of dental *caries*.

Various desensitizing dentifrices are available for use on teeth that are sensitive because of exposed dentine near the gum margin.

Dentine
Hard tissue surrounding the pulp of a tooth (see *Teeth*).

Dentistry
The science or profession concerned with the teeth and their supporting structures. Dentistry involves the prevention, diagnosis, and treatment of disease, injury, or malformation of the teeth, gums, and jaws. The majority of dentists work in general dental practice; others practise in a specialized branch of dentistry.

Dentists in general practice undertake all aspects of dental care, including cleaning teeth, filling cavities, extracting teeth, correcting problems with tooth alignment, and fitting crowns, bridges, and dentures. They also check for cancer of the mouth, perform cosmetic procedures (such as bonding), and give general advice on how to care for the teeth and gums.

Dentists in general practice may refer patients to a consultant in one of the specialized branches of dentistry.

D

TYPES OF DENTAL X-RAY
There are three different types of X-ray. Each is useful for revealing particular problems.

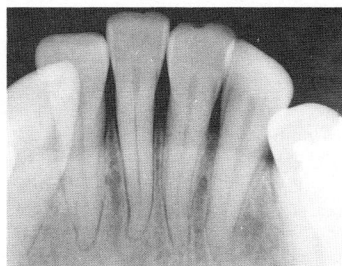
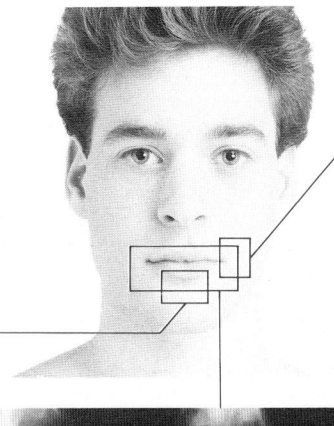
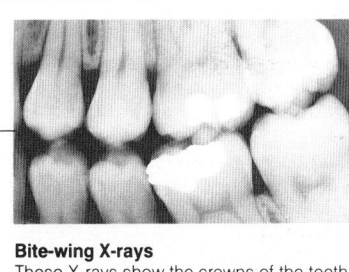
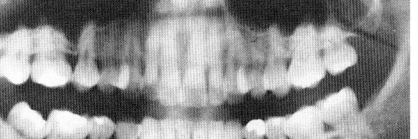

Bite-wing X-rays
These X-rays show the crowns of the teeth. They are useful for detecting areas of decay between teeth and changes in bone caused by periodontal (gum) disease. The film is in a holder with a central tab on to which the patient bites.

Periapical X-rays
These X-rays give detailed pictures of whole teeth and the surrounding gums and bone. They show unerupted or impacted teeth, root fractures, abscesses, cysts, tumours, and the characteristic bone patterns of some skeletal diseases. The film, in a protective casing, is placed in the patient's mouth and is held in position behind the teeth to be X-rayed.

Panoramic X-rays
These X-rays show all the teeth and surrounding structures on one large film. They are invaluable for finding unerupted or impacted teeth, cysts, jaw fractures, or tumours. Pictures are recorded continuously on to film as the camera swings around from one side of the jaw to the other.

D

Orthodontics concerns the moving of improperly aligned teeth to improve function and appearance. *Prosthetics* concerns the provision of bridgework and dentures to replace missing teeth and the provision of substitutes for missing oral tissues. Two branches specialize in the treatment of diseases: *endodontics* involves the treatment of diseases of the pulp, while *periodontics* involves the treatment of disorders that damage the supporting structures of the teeth, such as the gums.

Dental hygienists are qualified to carry out scaling (the removal of calculus from the teeth) and to demonstrate methods of keeping the teeth and gums healthy (see *Oral hygiene*).

Dentition

The characteristics of a person's *teeth*, including the number and arrangement in the jaw. The term is also used to describe the *eruption of teeth*.

Denture

An appliance that replaces missing natural teeth. A denture consists of an acrylic (tough plastic) and/or metal base mounted with acrylic or porcelain teeth. A natural appearance is achieved by choosing artificial teeth of the size, colour, and shape that closely resemble the original teeth and that blend with the contours of the face.

FITTING

The dentist takes impressions of the upper and lower gums. The impressions are removed from the mouth and allowed to harden. Models are then made by pouring plaster of Paris into the hardened impressions. Denture baseplates created from these models will fit the mouth accurately, but, to ensure that the bite will be correct when the artificial teeth are positioned, the dentist must also record the relationship of the upper and lower jaw. This is done by having the patient bite on to wax-rimmed plates (bite blocks) that can be trimmed to indicate the correct relative positions of the jaws.

Using the bite blocks as a guide, a temporary denture with the teeth waxed into position is then produced. The patient tries it on so that the dentist can make adjustments to the position or choice of teeth. When the dentist and patient are satisfied with the bite and appearance, the wax is replaced by acrylic, and the finished, polished dentures are fitted at the patient's next visit. Additional visits may be needed to ease any part of the baseplate that is uncomfortable.

TYPES OF DENTURES

Partial dentures	Partial dentures are used when only some teeth are missing. They fill unsightly gaps, make chewing easier, maintain clear speech, and keep the remaining teeth in position. Teeth on either side of a gap may tip (making cleaning more difficult) or drift (placing unnatural stress on the	tissues of the mouth). Partial dentures are held in place by metal clasps that grip adjacent teeth or by clasps combined with metal rests (extensions of the denture plate that rest on the tooth surface).
Full dentures	Full dentures are needed when there are no teeth left in the mouth. They stay in place by resting on the gum ridges and, in the case of upper dentures, by	suction. Fitting is usually delayed for several months after extraction of teeth to allow the gums to shrink and change shape as they heal.
Immediate dentures	Immediate dentures are fitted immediately after extraction of teeth. They protect the gum and control bleeding from extraction sites. Since a toothless period is avoided, they are particularly useful	for replacing front teeth. However, they can be expensive and require follow-up visits for refitting or relining so that they fit comfortably.

Dentures fitted immediately after tooth extraction usually require extra visits so that adjustments to the fit can be made as the tissues heal. Often a new acrylic lining is fused to the existing baseplate after healing is complete. Sometimes a soft lining (made of impression material) is inserted temporarily to minimize pain.

Deodorant

A substance that removes unpleasant odours, especially body odours. Deodorants may contain *antiseptics* to destroy bacteria, perfume to mask odours, and *antiperspirants* to reduce the production of sweat.

Deodorant preparations are a useful aid against body odour caused by decomposition of sweat by bacteria on the skin.

People who have had a *colostomy* or an *ileostomy* can reduce odour by taking deodorant drugs, such as bismuth, by mouth and by putting deodorant liquids into the stoma bags.

Deoxyribonucleic acid

See *DNA*; *Nucleic acids*.

Dependence

Psychological or physical reliance on persons or drugs. An infant is naturally dependent on parents, but, as he or she grows, dependence normally wanes. Some adults never become fully independent and make excessive demands for love, admiration, and help from others.

Alcohol and drugs (such as opiates, amphetamines, and tranquillizers) may induce a state of physical or emotional dependence in users. A person who is dependent may develop physical symptoms (such as sweating and abdominal pains) or emotional distress if deprived of the drug. The pattern of dependence varies with the drug and with the personality of the individual. (See also *Alcohol dependence*; *Drug dependence*.)

Depersonalization

A state of feeling unreal, in which there is a sense of detachment from self and surroundings. Depersonalization is frequently accompanied by *derealization*, in which the world is experienced as unreal. Depersonalization, which is rarely serious, usually comes on suddenly and may last for moments or for hours.

Depersonalization may sometimes occur in people who are otherwise perfectly healthy, especially if they are tired or worried. More often, depersonalization occurs in people with *anxiety disorders*, especially when *hyperventilation* takes place during a *panic attack*. Other causes of depersonalization include drugs (such as *LSD* or *marijuana*), *migraine*, and *temporal lobe epilepsy*.

Depilatory

A chemical hair remover, such as barium sulphide, in the form of a cream or paste. Depilatories are used to remove hair for cosmetic reasons and also in the treatment of *hirsutism* (excessive hairiness).

HOW THEY WORK

Depilatories dissolve hair at the surface of the skin. They do not affect the hair root and therefore do not permanently remove the hair.

POSSIBLE ADVERSE EFFECTS

Depilatories may cause an irritant reaction, with inflammation and swelling. It is advisable to test them first on a small area of skin (they are not usually recommended for use on the face). Depilatories should not be used after a hot bath or shower. Heat increases blood flow to the skin and opens pores, thus increasing the amount of chemical that is absorbed into the body.

Depot injection

An intramuscular (into a muscle) injection of a drug that is specially formulated to give a slow, steady release of its active chemicals into the bloodstream. Depot injections usually contain a much higher dose than that normally given by injection. Release of the drug is slowed by the inclusion of substances such as oil or wax. The release of the active drug can be made to last for hours, days, or weeks, depending on the formulation.

A depot injection is useful for patients who may not take their medication correctly. It also prevents the necessity of giving a series of injections over a short period. Examples of drugs given by depot injection include hormonal contraceptives (see *Contraception, hormonal methods of*), corticosteroid drugs, and antipsychotic drugs.

Disadvantages of this type of injection include side-effects caused by the uneven release of the drug into the bloodstream and prolonged adverse reactions caused by the long-acting nature of the treatment.

Depression

Feelings of sadness, hopelessness, pessimism, and a general loss of interest in life, combined with a sense of reduced emotional well-being. Most people experience these feelings occasionally, in many cases as a normal response to a particular event. For example, it is natural to feel depressed when a close relative dies. However, if the depression occurs without any apparent cause, deepens, and persists, it may be a symptom of any of a wide range of psychiatric illnesses. When a person's behaviour and physical state are also affected, it then becomes part of a true depressive illness.

SYMPTOMS

Symptoms vary with the severity of the illness. In a person with mild depression, the main symptoms are anxiety and a variable mood. Sometimes he or she has fits of crying that occur for no apparent reason. A person with more serious depression may suffer from loss of appetite, difficulty in sleeping, loss of interest and enjoyment in social activities, feelings of tiredness, and loss of concentration. Movement and thinking may become slowed; in some cases, however, the opposite occurs, and the person becomes extremely anxious and agitated. Severely depressed people may have thoughts of death and/or *suicide,* and feelings of guilt or worthlessness. In extreme cases, they may have *hallucinations* or *delusions* (believing, for example, that someone is poisoning them).

Intensity of symptoms often varies with the time of day. Most depressed people feel slightly better as the day progresses, but in some people the symptoms are worst at night. As a depressive illness progresses, the symptoms become more and more prominent. Finally, the person may become totally withdrawn and spend most of the time huddled in bed.

CAUSES

Usually, a true depressive illness has no single obvious cause. It may be triggered by certain physical illnesses (such as a viral infection), by hormonal disorders (such as *hypothyroidism*), or by hormonal changes after childbirth (see *Postnatal depression*). Some drugs, including *oral contraceptives* and *sleeping drugs,* are contributing factors. If the depression is part of a *manic-depressive illness,* inheritance may play a part, since this illness tends to run in families.

Some people become depressed during the winter months of most years (see *Seasonal affective disorder syndrome*) probably in response to the long hours of darkness.

Aside from these biological causes, social and psychological factors may play a part. Lack of a satisfactory mother-child relationship may lead to depression in later life (see *Bonding*), especially when it is combined with difficult social circumstances. For example, a woman whose mother died early in her life may be particularly vulnerable if she has to cope with bringing up a child on her own. Depression may also be related to the number of disturbing events or changes in a person's life.

INCIDENCE

Depression is the most common serious psychiatric illness. Some 10 to 15 per cent of people suffer from it at some time in their lives, especially the milder forms. The more severe manic-depressive type affects only about one to two per cent of depressed people, but the incidence of all forms of the illness increases with age. This may be due to social isolation, failing mental powers, and physical illness.

Depression appears to be more common in women, with about one in six seeking help for depression at some time in their lives (as opposed to only one in nine men). This may be a true difference or may result from the fact that women are more prepared to visit doctors for their depressive symptoms while men may be more likely to resort to alcohol, violence, or other expressions of discontent.

TREATMENT

There are three main forms of treatment for depression, depending on the type and severity of the illness.

Psychotherapy, whether individual or in a group, is most useful for those whose personality and life experiences are the main causes of their illness. Many types of therapy are available, such as an informal, purely practical approach to problem-solving, or the more structured approaches of *cognitive-behavioural therapy* and *psychoanalysis.*

Drug treatment is used for people with predominantly physical symptoms. *Antidepressant drugs* are usually effective in more than two thirds of these patients, provided the drugs are taken in a sufficient dosage over a long enough period of time.

ECT (electroconvulsive therapy), which is given under a general anaesthetic, is usually reserved for treating severely depressed people, especially if they are suffering from delusions or have failed to respond to other forms of treatment. ECT is effective and safe, and may be life-saving; the only side-effect may be mild, temporary memory impairment. Trials have demonstrated that ECT relieves severe depression faster than drugs.

OUTLOOK

Despite the effectiveness of drug treatment, suicide remains a serious risk for sufferers from depression. Nearly half of all deaths in people suffering from recurrent depression are suicides. The risk can be lowered substantially by maintenance treatment with antidepressant drugs. The newer antidepressants, such as serotonin

D

D

re-uptake inhibitors, have fewer side-effects than the older drugs, and are therefore more suitable for long-term preventive treatment.

Studies of large numbers of patients treated for depression in the 1980s showed that around 40 per cent made a good, sustained recovery and returned to normal life, while around 10 per cent eventually killed themselves. These results should be improved by the more general use of long-term drug treatment.

Derangement

An outdated term for severe mental disorder. It was first used in the 19th century to describe the idea of an orderly mind that had become "disarranged". Today, the term derangement is usually applied to wild, disturbed behaviour rather than to a specific mental state.

The term derangement also applies to disorders of the ligaments in the knee joint (i.e. internal derangement of the knee).

Derealization

Feeling that the world has become unreal. It usually occurs with *depersonalization* and shares the sudden onset, symptoms, and causes of that condition. Sufferers commonly describe the feeling as "looking at the world through a glass screen". Derealization may be caused by excessive tiredness, *hallucinogenic drugs,* or disordered brain function.

Dermabrasion

Removal of the surface layer of the skin by high-speed sanding to improve the appearance of scars, such as those of *acne,* or remove tattoos. The skin is numbed with a local anaesthetic and the surface is removed by a spinning abrasive wheel. Healing takes about two weeks and the full effect of the treatment is apparent after two months.

Dermatitis

Inflammation of the skin, sometimes due to an allergy but in many cases occurring without any known cause. Many types of dermatitis are better known as *eczema* (for example, atopic, discoid, infantile, and hand eczema).

Apart from eczemas, the three main forms of skin inflammation are seborrhoeic dermatitis, contact dermatitis, and photodermatitis.

SEBORRHOEIC DERMATITIS

This is a red, scaly, itchy rash that develops on the face (particularly the nose and eyebrows), scalp, chest, and back. On the scalp it is the most common cause of *dandruff.* The rash often develops during times of stress, but its exact cause is unknown. Generally, the treatment of dermatitis must be tailored to each case. Applying *corticosteroid drugs* and/or drugs to kill microorganisms is often helpful. It is important to avoid scratching affected areas or exposing them to irritating substances such as detergents.

CONTACT DERMATITIS

In this type of dermatitis, the rash is a reaction to some substance that comes in contact with the skin. The reaction may result from a direct toxic effect of the substance or it may be an allergic response.

Among the more common causes of the reaction are detergents (including traces left in washed clothes), nickel (e.g. in watch straps, bracelets, necklaces, and the fastenings of underclothes), chemicals (e.g. in rubber gloves and condoms), certain plants (e.g. ragweed), certain cosmetics, and some medications in the form of creams, lotions, or drops.

The type of rash varies considerably according to the substance causing it, but it is often itchy, and may flake or blister; distribution of the rash corresponds to the skin area that has been in contact with the causative substance. Rashes may be treated with corticosteroid medications.

If the causative substance is not known, it may be possible to identify it by a patch test (see *Skin tests*). Once the offending substance is identified, it may be possible to avoid it.

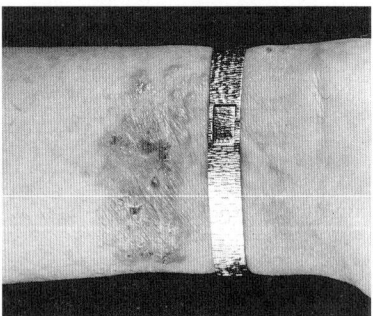

Contact dermatitis
Reaction to the nickel in a watch strap produced the itchy, blistering rash on the inside of the wrist shown above.

PHOTODERMATITIS

This type of dermatitis occurs in people whose skin is abnormally sensitive to light. In the most common form of photodermatitis, a cluster of spots or blisters develops on any part of the body exposed to the sun (see *Photosensitivity*).

Dermatitis artefacta

Any self-induced skin condition. Dermatitis artefacta may range from a mild scratch self-inflicted by someone under stress to severe and extensive mutilation by a psychologically disturbed person.

The skin damage may take any form—ulcers, blisters, or scratches. The damage often has a symmetrical or bizarre pattern and, to the trained eye, does not resemble that seen in any skin disease.

Dermatitis herpetiformis

A chronic skin disease in which clusters of tiny, red, intensely itchy blisters occur in a symmetrical pattern on various parts of the body, most commonly the back, elbows, knees, buttocks, and scalp.

The disease usually develops in adult life and is believed to be related to *coeliac disease,* a condition in which the small intestine is allergic to gluten, a constituent of wheat and certain other cereals. One of the symptoms of coeliac disease is chronic diarrhoea, which also occurs in some people with dermatitis herpetiformis. Both conditions often improve after treatment with a gluten-free diet.

Dermatology

The branch of medicine concerned with the *skin* and the disorders that affect it. Also included in this specialty are the hair and nails, together with their various disorders. Problems include everything from wrinkles, warts, and hair loss to acne, athlete's foot, and skin cancer.

Diagnostic techniques used in dermatology include *skin biopsy* (removal of a sample of tissue for microscopic analysis). Methods of treatment include drug therapy, surgery, and the destruction of unwanted growths by *cryosurgery* (freezing), *electrocautery* (burning), *laser treatment,* and *radiotherapy.*

Dermatopathology is the study of the microscopic appearance of diseased skin tissue.

Dermatome

An area of skin supplied with nerves from one spinal root (see *Nervous system*). The entire surface of the body is an interlocking mosaic of dermatomes, the pattern of which is very similar from one person to another.

Loss of sensation in a dermatome signifies damage to a particular nerve root, the most usual cause of which is a *disc prolapse*. The rash in *herpes zoster* (shingles) is usually confined to one dermatome.

Dermatome, surgical
A surgical instrument for cutting variable thicknesses of skin for use in skin grafting. Types include a drum dermatome, which permits removal of skin pieces of a precise thickness, and an electric dermatome, which makes it possible to remove long strips of skin.

Dermatomyositis
A rare, sometimes fatal, disease in which the muscles and skin become inflamed, causing weakness of the muscles and a skin rash.

CAUSES AND INCIDENCE
The disorder belongs to a group of illnesses called the *autoimmune disorders*, in which, for reasons that are not fully understood, the *immune system* (body's defences against disease) starts attacking the body's own tissues. Dermatomyositis is sometimes associated with underlying cancer of an internal organ. Two thirds of people suffering from dermatomyositis are middle-aged women.

SYMPTOMS
The first sign is often a red rash on the bridge of the nose and cheeks, followed by a purple discoloration on the eyelids and sometimes a red rash on the knees, knuckles, and elbows. Muscles then start to become weak, stiff, and painful, particularly those in the shoulders and pelvis where the limbs join the trunk. The skin over the affected muscles feels thicker than normal. Sometimes the muscle pains precede the rash. The sufferer may also experience bouts of nausea, weight loss, and fever.

DIAGNOSIS AND TREATMENT
The diagnosis is confirmed by blood tests, *EMG* (electromyography) to detect the electrical activity of muscles, and a skin or muscle *biopsy* (removal of a small piece of tissue for microscopic analysis).

Treatment is with *corticosteroid drugs* and/or *immunosuppressant drugs* (to reduce the inflammation) and *physiotherapy* (to prevent muscles from scarring and shrinking as they heal).

OUTLOOK
In about 50 per cent of cases, full recovery occurs after a few years. In about 30 per cent, the disease is persistent, causing muscle weakness. In the remaining 20 per cent, it eventually affects the lungs and other organs and may be fatal.

Dermatophyte infections
A group of common fungal infections affecting the skin, hair, and nails, also known as *tinea* and, popularly, as ringworm.

Dermographism
Greater than normal sensitivity of the skin to mechanical irritation, to the extent that firm stroking leads to the appearance of itchy wheals (raised areas), which are slightly darker than the surrounding skin. The term dermographism literally means "writing on the skin", and in fact it is sometimes possible with a few finger strokes to write visible words on a sufferer's back.

Dermographism (also called dermographia) is a form of *urticaria* (nettle rash) and is most common among fair-skinned people with a tendency to allergic conditions such as *eczema*.

Dermoid cyst
A benign tumour with a cell structure similar to that of skin, and containing hairs, sweat glands, and sebaceous glands. Dermoid cysts may also contain fragments of cartilage, bone, and even teeth. The cysts may occur in various parts of the body.

Dermoid cysts account for about 10 per cent of all ovarian tumours. Ovarian dermoid cysts range in size from a few millimetres to 10 or more centimetres in diameter. They may cause discomfort and abdominal swelling, but only rarely do they become malignant (cancerous).

Dermoid cysts in the skin most commonly occur on the head or neck, causing a small painless swelling. This type of dermoid cyst is usually congenital (present from birth) and contains only skin structures.

Surgical removal of dermoid cysts is recommended in most cases. (See also *Teratoma*).

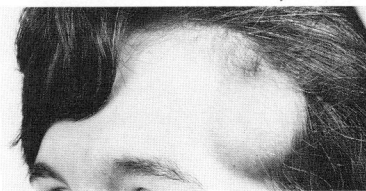

Appearance of dermoid cyst on head
The growth is firm, painless, and has an inner cavity that contains a fatty substance and sometimes hair, teeth, and bony material.

Dermoid tumour
See *Dermoid cyst*.

Desensitization
A technique, used in *behaviour therapy* for treating *phobias*, in which the patient is gradually exposed to the cause of the fear.

Desensitization, allergy
See *Hyposensitization*.

Designer drugs

> **WARNING**
> Designer drugs carry a high risk of *drug dependence*, with severe withdrawal reactions, and of *drug poisoning*, causing effects such as brain damage.

A group of illegally produced chemicals that mimic the effects of specific drugs of abuse. Made in illicit laboratories, these drugs are cheap to produce and thus undercut the street prices of drugs such as *LSD* and *amphetamine drugs*.

Designer drugs are often made in such a way that their structures are subtly different from those of the drugs they imitate. As a result, these drugs may circumvent laws controlling the manufacture and distribution of drugs in some countries.

TYPES
Designer drugs can be divided into three major groups: those derived from narcotic *analgesic drugs* (painkillers) such as meperidine and fentanyl; drugs that mimic amphetamines such as *ecstasy*; and variants of phencyclidine (PCP), a *hallucinogenic drug* originally used in animal anaesthesia.

POSSIBLE ADVERSE EFFECTS
Designer drugs are highly potent. Some derivatives of fentanyl, for example, are between 20 and 2,000 times more powerful than *morphine*; this has led to a high incidence of death due to *drug poisoning*.

Amphetamine derivatives cause brain damage at doses only slightly higher than those required for a stimulant effect. Although they have been abused as aphrodisiacs, amphetamine derivatives commonly impair orgasm in both men and women and may prevent erection.

Many designer drugs contain impurities. For example, a substance known as MPTP, contained within a meperidine derivative, has caused permanent brain damage resulting in *parkinsonism*. Phencyclidine variants often cause seizures and psychosis.

Desmoid tumour

A growth, usually in the abdominal wall. The tumour is hard, with a well-defined edge.

Desmoid tumours occur most frequently in women who have had children. Stretching or bruising of the abdominal muscle fibres during pregnancy may be a factor in their development. Desmoid tumours may also arise at the sites of old surgical incisions in the abdomen or elsewhere in the body, and they are often regarded as overgrowths of scar tissue.

Surgical removal is the usual treatment, although recurrence of the growth at the same site is common.

Detergent poisoning

The toxic effects that occur as a result of swallowing the cleaning agents in shampoos, laundry powders, and cleaning liquids. Detergent poisoning causes vomiting, diarrhoea, and a swollen abdomen. Victims should drink large quantities of fluids to dilute the detergent.

Development

The process of growth and change by which an individual matures physically, mentally, emotionally, and socially. Development takes place in the following major phases: during the first two months of pregnancy (see *Embryo*); to a lesser extent, during the rest of pregnancy (see *Fetus*); during the first five years of life (see *Child development*); and during *puberty* and *adolescence*.

Developmental delay

A term used when a baby or young child has not achieved new abilities within the normal time range and has a pattern of behaviour that is behind what is appropriate for his or her age.

Development is an increase in abilities—physical, mental, emotional, and social—and is a well-orchestrated process, with new abilities and new patterns of behaviour appearing at given ages, while existing patterns of behaviour change and sometimes disappear (see *Child development*).

Delays may be of varying severity and may affect any or all of the major areas of human achievement (i.e. development of the ability to walk upright, of fine hand-eye coordination, of listening, language, and speech, and of social interaction). Developmental delay is not a term used for slow increase in physical size (see *Growth; Short stature*) or for late appearance of sexual characteristics

(see *Puberty; Puberty, delayed*). The term is not usually applied to children over the age of five.

In general, the child who is slow in one or two aspects of development and is of average or perhaps advanced ability in others, needs to be distinguished from the child who is delayed in most aspects. When there is a significant delay in a few aspects, there may be a specific (although often not obvious) disability such as a visual or hearing impairment, which, if adequately treated, may allow the child to catch up. Children who are developmentally delayed in most aspects usually have a more generalized problem—for example, lack of adequate stimulation and teaching at home or a slowness to learn because of limited intellectual abilities.

CAUSES

Some important causes of generalized developmental delay are shown in the accompanying table. It is important to remember that a child born prematurely will reach most developmental milestones later than other children. Parents should take into account how old the baby would be if he or she had been born at the normal time rather than prematurely. Causes of delay in specific areas are as follows.

WALKING AND MOVEMENT SKILLS There is an enormous time range within which most children learn to walk; most begin between the ages of nine and 15 months, but a child who crawls fast and efficiently may delay longer.

In most late walkers, no serious cause is found. Late walking is an inherited feature in some families and is probably due to delayed maturation of the nervous system. Such children learn to walk a few months later than other children, and from then on usually develop new skills at a normal rate. Other children develop slightly unusual patterns of locomotion—for example, creeping on their abdomens or shuffling on their bottoms. These traits also tend to run in families. Such children may miss out on the crawling stage. They eventually stand and walk and from then on follow the normal developmental sequence in all other developmental aspects.

A more specific reason for delayed walking and other skills is weakness of the leg muscles and other muscles. This can occur in boys with *muscular dystrophy* and in children with *spina bifida*. *Cerebral palsy* is a disorder that affects all aspects of motor development; it may cause slowness and difficulty in gaining control of the head,

CAUSES OF GENERALIZED DEVELOPMENTAL DELAY

Unsatisfactory parental interaction (e.g. lack of affection, stimulation, or teaching, or lack of consistent and constant guidelines of acceptable behaviour).

Severe visual impairment. Vision is vitally important for normal development in all areas. Children learn to recognize objects by sight before learning their names, they learn about sounds by seeing which objects make which sounds, and they become motivated to crawl and walk by the desire to explore the surroundings they see. (See *Vision, disorders of; Blindness*.)

Severe hearing impairment. (See *Deafness*.)

Limited intellectual abilities. (See *Mental handicap*.)

Damage to the brain before, during, or after birth, or in infancy. The results of damage depend on which parts of the brain are damaged and on severity. (See *Brain damage; Cerebral palsy*.)

Severe disease of other organs and systems of the body. (See *Nutritional disorders; Heart, Bone, Muscles*, and *Kidney* disorder boxes.)

neck, and back muscles during the first few months of life, as well as delay in sitting and walking.

HAND-EYE COORDINATION Any defect of vision or of the nerves and muscles used to control fine finger movements may be a cause of delayed manipulative skills. However, the most common cause is not a specific abnormality but lack of experience; stimulation and encouragement are extremely important in the acquisition of these skills. If a child has only large toys to play with and is not encouraged to use the small finger muscles, skills involving these muscles will be delayed. Similarly, if a child is left lying down for most of the time instead of in a sitting position, the hands will not be in the correct position to acquire certain skills.

RESPONSE TO SOUND If a child is unresponsive to sound it may be due to *deafness*. However, children who are not talked to may show a lack of interest in the human voice, although they may respond normally to other sounds. Children exposed continually to a great deal of noise may show a general lack of interest in sound.

A rare cause of unresponsiveness to the human voice is *autism*. An affected child can hear normally but shows little interest in human contact of any kind. Although unresponsive to human voices, autistic children often become obsessively interested in particular sound-producing toys.

SPEECH AND LANGUAGE The most important cause of delayed speech is a hearing problem. Another common cause is lack of stimulation (when parents do not talk to the child sufficiently). In other cases (more commonly in boys than girls), delayed speech runs in families. Twins are often late talkers, perhaps because they may receive less individual parental attention. Some twins develop a private language that includes idiosyncratic words and nonverbal communication.

Children exposed to two or more languages may show signs of speech delay and may confuse the languages. However, many children become naturally bilingual or trilingual with no difficulties.

Any generalized difficulty with muscle control can affect speech production; muscle control can be a particular difficulty in children with *cerebral palsy*. Damage to, or structural defects of, the speech muscles, larynx (voice box), or mouth may also cause speech difficulties, as may any disorder affecting the speech area of the brain (see *Aphasia; Dysarthria; Dysphonia; Speech disorders*).

BLADDER AND BOWEL CONTROL Children vary enormously in the age at which control of bowel and bladder function is acquired. Usually bowel function is acquired first. Delay in bladder control is much more common than delayed bowel control. There are many possible causes (see *Encopresis; Enuresis; Soiling*).

ASSESSMENT

In many instances, the parents are the first to notice that their child is not acquiring new skills at the same rate as his or her peers. A doctor should be consulted. Problems are sometimes detected during one of the developmental checks that are carried out routinely in child and well-baby clinics. These checks are performed by family doctors, paediatricians, or other health professionals at varying ages,

but usually at birth, six weeks, six to eight months, 12 to 15 months, two years, three years, and five years.

If developmental delay is discovered, the first step is to establish the cause by undertaking a full assessment. This examination usually includes hearing and vision testing, a full physical examination, and thorough developmental assessment. Further investigation is arranged as necessary. It may include referral to a paediatrician, neurologist, psychologist, speech therapist, occupational therapist, or physiotherapist.

TREATMENT

Once the severity of the delay and the probable cause have been discovered, the appropriate treatment can be arranged. In many cases, the parents can be reassured that there is no serious abnormality and that their child can be expected to develop normally without any specific treatment. Sometimes advice is given regarding suitable toys and other forms of education and stimulation.

Treatment may include a course of *speech therapy* or *family therapy*, or provision of *glasses* or a *hearing-aid*. In some cases it is felt that the child's best interests are served by admission to a special school or unit for children with specific difficulties: for example, a school for physically handicapped children, or a language unit.

Whatever the cause of the developmental delay, children can be helped to achieve their full potential by the provision of appropriate therapy. Parents are often of prime importance in providing this help.

Deviation, sexual

A form of sexual behaviour in which intercourse between adults is not the final aim. Instead, the man (deviation is rare in women) achieves erection and orgasm in other ways, such as by being whipped or wearing women's clothes. Forms of sexual deviation include *exhibitionism, fetishism, frottage, necrophilia, paedophilia, sadomasochism*, and *transvestism*.

Dexamethasone

A *corticosteroid drug* prescribed as a nasal spray to relieve *nasal congestion* caused by allergic *rhinitis* (hay fever) and as eye-drops in the treatment of *iritis* (inflammation of the iris). Dexamethasone is given in tablet form to treat severe cases of *asthma* and to reduce inflammation of the brain due to *head injury, stroke*, or a *brain tumour*.

Occasionally, dexamethasone may be injected into an inflamed joint to relieve pain and stiffness caused, for example, by *osteoarthritis*.

POSSIBLE ADVERSE EFFECTS

Dexamethasone in the form of a nasal spray or eye-drops may cause minor local side-effects, such as nosebleed or eye irritation. When prescribed for a prolonged period or in high doses, dexamethasone tablets may cause the adverse effects common to the corticosteroid group of drugs.

Dexamphetamine

A central nervous system stimulant. (See *Amphetamine drugs; Stimulant drugs*). Dexamphetamine may be used to treat *narcolepsy* (a rare condition characterized by excessive sleepiness). Paradoxically, it is also used to treat children with *hyperactivity*, although the reason it helps this condition is not known.

Dexamphetamine has no place in the management of depression or obesity.

ABUSE

Because of its stimulant properties, dexamphetamine has become a drug of abuse. It is one of a group of drugs commonly referred to as "uppers". If use is prolonged, the stimulant effects lessen and a higher dose must be taken to produce the desired effect. In an overdose, dexamphetamine can cause seizures and hypertension (high blood pressure).

Dextrocardia

A rare condition, present from birth, in which the heart is situated in, and points towards, the right-hand side of the chest instead of the left. The heart may also, but not necessarily, be malformed. Sometimes, the position of the abdominal organs is also reversed, so that the liver is on the left-hand side and the stomach on the right. When all organs are on the opposite side of

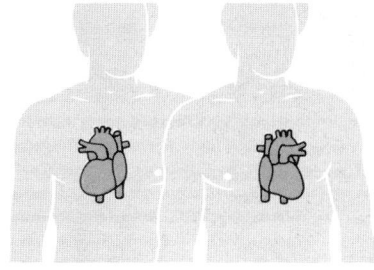

Abnormal position　　Normal position

Heart positions
In dextrocardia, the heart is situated in, and points toward, the right-hand side of the chest instead of the left.

the body from where they are customarily found, the condition is known as *situs inversus*.

The cause of dextrocardia is unknown. No treatment is necessary unless the heart is malformed, in which case surgery may be required.

Dextromethorphan

A cough suppressant available over-the-counter as an ingredient in a number of *cough remedies*.

Dextromoramide

A narcotic *analgesic drug* (painkiller) derived from the unripe seeds of the opium poppy, dextromoramide is used for the relief of severe pain following injury or surgery and during long-term illnesses, such as cancer. It relieves pain quickly but has only a short duration of action. This drug is less likely to cause sedation and constipation than *morphine* but, as with other narcotics, regular use can produce *drug dependence*.

Dextropropoxyphene

A weak narcotic *analgesic drug* that is included in some compound analgesic preparations. It works rapidly and relieves mild to moderate pain for about four hours. Possible adverse effects of dextropropoxyphene are drowsiness, dizziness, nausea, and vomiting. It should not be taken with alcohol; an overdose combined with alcohol can be very dangerous. Regular use can cause *drug dependence*.

Dextrose

Another name for *glucose*, one of the monosaccharide sugars. Dextrose is absorbed from digested *carbohydrates* through the intestinal wall into the bloodstream. It is also available in the form of tablets, as an injection for use in the emergency treatment of *hypoglycaemia* (low blood sugar level), and as a component of infusion fluids used for intravenous feeding (see *Feeding, artificial*).

DH

Abbreviation for the Department of Health, the Government structure that oversees the *National Health Service* in Britain. There are separate departments for England, Scotland, and Northern Ireland; the Welsh Office is responsible for the Health Service in Wales.

The Secretary of State for Health has overall responsibility for the whole department, assisted by one or more ministers of state.

The administration of the NHS is the task of the National Health Service Management Board, which includes the chief medical and nursing officers.

Diabetes, bronze

Another name for *haemochromatosis*, a rare disease in which excessive amounts of iron are deposited in tissues such as the liver, pancreas, and skin. Its name comes from the bronze skin coloration and *diabetes mellitus* that usually develop in sufferers.

Diabetes insipidus

A rare condition that is characterized by polyuria (the passing of large quantities of dilute urine) and polydipsia (excessive thirst) to compensate. These symptoms also occur, in a milder form, early in *diabetes mellitus*, a more common disease that differs in other ways from diabetes insipidus.

CAUSES
Diabetes insipidus usually results from a failure of the *pituitary gland* to secrete *ADH* (antidiuretic hormone). Normally, this hormone reduces the amount of water passed by the *kidneys* into the urine. Diseases of the pituitary gland, including damage from injury or a tumour, can cause failure of ADH secretion. The condition may temporarily follow brain surgery.

Rarely, the disease is due to failure of the kidneys to respond to normal levels of ADH, when it is called nephrogenic diabetes insipidus. This type is usually congenital (present from birth), but may result from kidney disease or from certain drugs.

SYMPTOMS, DIAGNOSIS, AND TREATMENT
A person with diabetes insipidus may pass between five and 20 litres of urine every 24 hours, provided this output is matched by the intake of water. If not, *dehydration* may occur, leading to confusion, stupor, and coma.

Diabetes insipidus is usually treated with synthetic ADH, in the form of a nasal spray. ADH is ineffective for people with nephrogenic diabetes insipidus; in such cases, treatment consists of a combination of a low-sodium diet and, paradoxically, thiazide *diuretic drugs*.

Diabetes mellitus

A disorder caused by insufficient or absent production of the hormone *insulin* by the *pancreas*. Insulin is responsible for the absorption of glucose into cells for their energy needs and into the liver and fat cells for storage. If there is a deficiency, levels of glucose in the blood become abnor-

mally high, causing polyuria (the passing of large quantities of urine) and polydipsia (excessive thirst). The body's inability to store or use glucose causes weight loss, hunger, and fatigue. Diabetes mellitus also results in disordered *lipid* (fat) metabolism and accelerated degeneration of small blood vessels. Apart from the symptoms of thirst and polyuria, the disease has nothing in common with the much rarer disorder *diabetes insipidus*.

There are two main types of diabetes mellitus. Insulin-dependent (type I) diabetes, the more severe form, usually first appears in people under the age of 35 and most commonly between the ages of 10 and 16. It develops rapidly. The insulin-secreting cells in the pancreas are destroyed, probably as a result of an *immune response* after a viral infection, and insulin production ceases almost completely. Without regular injections of insulin, the sufferer lapses into a coma and dies. The other main type, non-insulin-dependent (type II) diabetes, is usually of gradual onset and develops mainly in people over 40. In many cases it is hidden and discovered only during a routine medical examination. Not enough insulin is produced for the body's needs, especially when the person is overweight. Often the body is resistant to the effects of insulin. In most cases, insulin-replacement injections are not needed; instead, a combination of dietary measures, weight reduction, and oral medication controls the condition.

CAUSES AND INCIDENCE
Diabetes mellitus tends to run in families. However, of those who inherit the genes responsible for the insulin-dependent form, only a small proportion eventually develop the disease. In these cases, the disorder is thought to be the delayed result of a viral infection that damaged the pancreas several years earlier. In the case of non-insulin-dependent diabetes, a greater proportion of the people who are predisposed by heredity actually go on to develop the disease.

Although obesity is the main factor leading to the unmasking of latent diabetes, it may be indicated by certain illnesses (among them *pancreatitis* and *thyrotoxicosis*), certain drugs (including some *corticosteroid drugs* and *diuretic drugs*), infections, and pregnancy (see *Diabetic pregnancy*).

In the UK about 1.4 persons per 1,000 develop insulin-dependent diabetes by the age of 16; overall, this form of the disease affects about

D

60,000 people in the UK. Non-insulin-dependent diabetes is more common, affecting about 600,000 people in the UK.

DIAGNOSIS

A doctor who suspects diabetes mellitus in a patient can often obtain confirmation by testing a sample of urine for its glucose level. Further confirmation is obtained when significantly high glucose levels are found in blood samples following an overnight fast or from samples taken two hours after a meal. Glucose-tolerance tests are sometimes required.

TREATMENT

The aims of treatment are to prolong life, to relieve symptoms, and to prevent long-term complications. Suc-

cess depends on keeping the level of blood glucose as near normal as possible through maintenance of normal weight, regular physical activity, careful dietary management, and, if necessary, injections of insulin.

In people with insulin-dependent diabetes, treatment consists of regular self-injections—between one and four times a day—with insulin (either obtained from animals or of a human type synthesized by *genetic engineering*). In addition, the person must follow a diet in which carbohydrate intake is regulated and spread out over the day according to a consistent timetable. By these means, marked fluctuations in the glucose levels in the blood can be avoided.

Disturbances in the careful balance between insulin and glucose intake can result in *hyperglycaemia* (too much glucose in the blood), causing the symptoms of the untreated disease, or *hypoglycaemia* (too little glucose in the blood), which can cause weakness, confusion, dizziness, sweating, and even seizures and unconsciousness. To help prevent this, people with either type of diabetes mellitus are advised to monitor their blood and/or urine glucose levels regularly with do-it-yourself testing kits (see illustrated box below). As a precaution against an attack of hypoglycaemia, insulin-dependent diabetics need to carry some sugar or glucose with them at all times.

LIVING WITH DIABETES MELLITUS

As the level of glucose in the blood rises, the volume of urine required to carry it out of the body is increased, causing not only a frequent need to urinate but also constant thirst. The high levels of sugar in the blood and urine impair the body's ability to fight infection, leading to urinary tract infections (such as *cystitis* and *pyelonephritis*), vaginal yeast infections (*candidiasis*), and recurrent skin infections.

Because the body's cells are starved of glucose, the sufferer feels weak and fatigued. The cells are able to obtain some energy from the breakdown of stored fat, resulting in weight loss. However, the chemical processes involved in this breakdown of fat are defective (especially in insulin-dependent diabetics) leading to the production of acids and substances known as ketones, which can cause coma and sometimes death.

Other possible symptoms of undiagnosed diabetes include blurred vision, boils, increased appetite, and tingling and numbness in the hands and feet.

Symptoms develop in all untreated insulin-dependent diabetics, but symptoms develop in only one third of those who have the non-insulin-dependent type. There are many people suffering from a mild form of the disease who are unaware of it. The disease is often diagnosed only after complications of the diabetes have been detected.

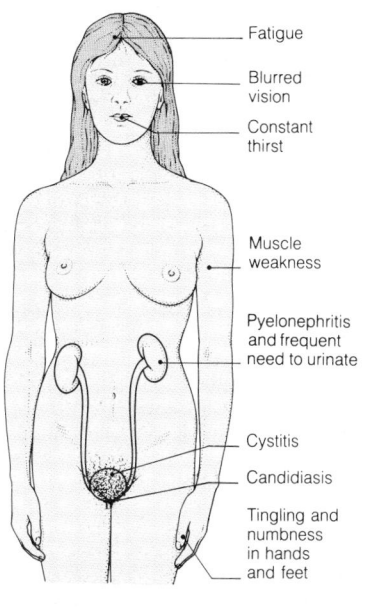

- Fatigue
- Blurred vision
- Constant thirst
- Muscle weakness
- Pyelonephritis and frequent need to urinate
- Cystitis
- Candidiasis
- Tingling and numbness in hands and feet

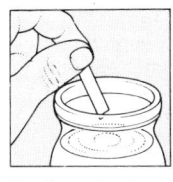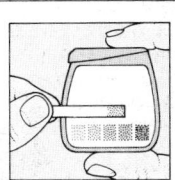

Testing urine for glucose
Urine can be tested for glucose by means of a chemically impregnated strip dipped into a sample of urine. The resulting colour change in the strip is compared with a chart to indicate the glucose level.

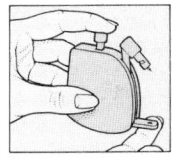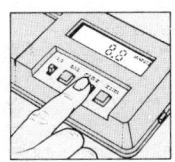

Direct testing of blood glucose
A pricking device is used to obtain blood, which is spread on a chemically coated strip. The strip is inserted into an instrument that reads the blood glucose.

DEVICES FOR INJECTING INSULIN

Insulin can be injected using a disposable syringe and needle or a pen with refill cartridges (below), or it may be infused continuously from a portable pump (right).

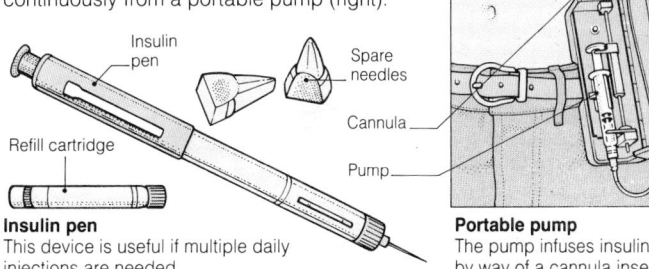

- Insulin pen
- Spare needles
- Cannula
- Pump
- Refill cartridge

Insulin pen
This device is useful if multiple daily injections are needed.

Portable pump
The pump infuses insulin by way of a cannula inserted through the skin.

D

For difficult-to-control diabetes, an insulin pump is an alternative treatment for those who are willing to monitor their blood glucose levels carefully. Insulin is continuously infused from a refillable pump through a needle implanted in the skin. In some people, however, control is no better than that from multiple daily injections.

In non-insulin-dependent diabetes, because the pancreas does produce some insulin, the disorder can often be controlled by dietary means alone (regulating the carbohydrate intake with meals spaced out over the day). This not only lowers the blood glucose level, but also reduces weight. If diet fails to lower the glucose level sufficiently, *hypoglycaemic* tablets (oral antidiabetic drugs that stimulate the pancreas to produce more insulin) may be prescribed, although these are ineffective unless dietary restrictions are observed.

All people with diabetes need regular advice from their doctors so that any complications can be detected and treated at an early stage. Diabetics should wear or carry information identifying them as diabetics in case of an emergency.

COMPLICATIONS
Complications eventually develop in a large number of diabetics; but these are less likely if there has been good control. Complications include *retinopathy* (damage to the retina, the light-sensitive area at the back of the eye, and the blood vessels serving it) which may need laser treatment to prevent blindness, peripheral *neuropathy* (damage to nerve fibres), and *nephropathy* (kidney damage) which occasionally requires dialysis and/or a kidney transplant. Ulcers on the feet, which in severe cases can develop into *gangrene,* are an additional risk, but with good foot care they can usually be prevented.

Diabetics also have a higher-than-average risk of *atherosclerosis* (accumulation of fatty deposits on the inner lining of arteries), *hypertension* (high blood pressure), other *cardiovascular disorders,* and *cataracts* (opacities in the lens of the eye).

There are, however, people who have lived full and active lives with diabetes mellitus for 50 years or more with few complications.

OUTLOOK
With modern treatment and sensible self-monitoring, almost all diabetics can look forward to a normal lifespan. The life expectancy of people who have well-regulated, insulin-dependent diabetes is little different from that of nondiabetics. Those with the non-insulin-dependent illness have a slightly reduced life expectancy because of circulatory and heart disorders; however, these disorders were often already present when the diabetes was diagnosed.

Diabetic pregnancy
Special precautions are necessary for pregnant women with pre-existing *diabetes mellitus,* and also for those women who develop diabetes during pregnancy (a condition known as gestational diabetes).

PRE-EXISTING DIABETES
Nearly all women with established diabetes mellitus can have a normal pregnancy, provided that the diabetes is well-controlled throughout. It is important to plan the pregnancy and to make sure that the blood glucose level is under particularly good control before and at the time of conception; otherwise there is a slightly increased chance of the baby being malformed. (No special precautions are needed by a diabetic man who is planning to become a father.) If control is poor during the pregnancy, there may be an increase in the amount of glucose reaching the baby (which makes the baby grow faster than normal) and this may cause difficulties at birth. Conversely, the growth of infants of diabetic mothers may be stunted; these babies may have complications in the days immediately after birth.

GESTATIONAL DIABETES
Gestational diabetes is most often detected in the second half of pregnancy, when increased glucose appears in the urine or the baby is found to be bigger than expected when a doctor examines the mother's abdomen (although these findings do not always mean the mother is diabetic). It appears that the mother does not produce enough insulin to keep the blood glucose levels normal during the pregnancy. Some obstetricians now screen for diabetes at 26 weeks. True gestational diabetes disappears with the delivery of the baby, but can be a sign of future diabetes in up to three quarters of these mothers.

CARE
Diabetic pregnancies must be supervised at hospital antenatal clinics. Some hospitals offer pre-pregnancy clinics for those with established diabetes to help women achieve good control before conception. At many hospitals, the care of diabetic women in pregnancy is shared between an obstetrician and a physician who is a specialist in diabetes. Stringent control over blood glucose levels, especially towards the end of pregnancy, is the key. If there are complications or the baby is large, early delivery may be considered.

The chances that the baby of a diabetic parent will become diabetic are about one in 100 and, if both parents are diabetic, about one in 20.

Diagnosis
The determination by a doctor of the nature and cause of a person's problem. Usually this entails identifying both the disease process—pneumonia or cirrhosis of the liver, for example—and the agent responsible, such as pneumonia due to legionnaires' disease, or cirrhosis due to alcohol. Diagnosis is part science and part art; an experienced doctor relies not only on his or her scientific knowledge and experience, but also on intuition to recognize the pattern of an illness and establish a diagnosis.

THE MEDICAL HISTORY
The patient's own account of his or her illness is perhaps the most important part of the diagnostic procedure. This history provides vital clues, which can then be augmented by questions from the doctor in an exchange that may last some 20 to 30 minutes in a complex case or if the doctor has not previously seen the patient. What the doctor is looking for is a pattern of symptoms that is strongly suggestive of a single disease. For example, the features of a migraine headache, duodenal ulcer, enlarged prostate gland, or angina pectoris are often unmistakable.

In some circumstances the doctor may not attempt to reach a final diagnosis. If a patient has had a sore throat for only 48 hours, the doctor may be content to treat the condition symptomatically, attempting to relieve the symptoms while he or she is waiting for the results of a throat culture or other tests.

However, when symptoms have been more prolonged, the doctor will want to reach at least a provisional diagnosis before beginning treatment, partly because any treatment is likely to affect the symptoms and thus make diagnosis more difficult.

EXAMINATION AND TESTS
Tests may be ordered after a physical examination and the formation of a provisional diagnosis.

STEPS IN DIAGNOSING A CONDITION

A doctor may go through several steps to ascertain the cause of a person's problem. The medical history, physical examination, and tests may prove vital clues. A doctor usually makes at least a provisional diagnosis before beginning any treatment because treatment can mask symptoms, making the doctor's task of establishing an exact diagnosis more difficult.

Taking the medical history

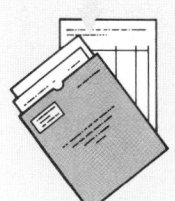

Perhaps the most important part of the diagnostic procedure is the patient's own account of his or her illness — the medical history. "Listen to the patients, they are telling you their diagnosis" is the traditional teaching given to medical students. Many doctors believe that the medical history provides the strongest basis for ascertaining a diagnosis. The added information derived from the physical examination is small, but, at times, critical.

Conducting a physical examination

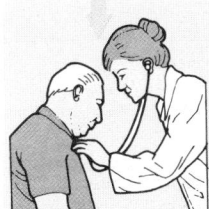

After the medical history has been obtained, the doctor has in mind a short list of probable diagnoses. A physical examination helps shorten the list. The doctor is then left with a differential diagnosis. A differential diagnosis is a group of possible diseases that could account for the patterns of symptoms and signs (i.e., physical findings, such as enlargements of lymph nodes or tenderness in a specific region of the abdomen).

Ordering special tests

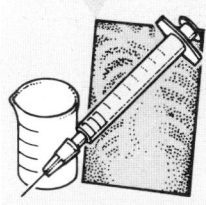

Next, based on his or her working diagnosis, the doctor may order a series of laboratory tests on the blood (and sometimes the urine) and may also arrange for diagnostic imaging of suspect organs by techniques such as *ultrasound scanning, X-rays,* *CT scanning, MRI,* or *radionuclide scanning.* The results of these tests either confirm the doctor's working diagnosis or narrow the possibilities so the doctor may be confident that he or she has found the correct diagnosis.

Using a computer

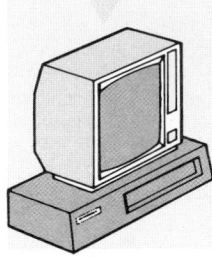

Doctors today also use computer systems and algorithms to help reach a diagnosis. Both approaches rely on analysis of large numbers of patient records to quantify probabilities and to devise an orderly series of questions — a decision tree. The main purpose of computer assistance is to remind the doctor of the full range of possible diagnoses for a particular set of symptoms, thereby making it less likely that any possibility will be overlooked. It remains the task of the doctor to integrate the facts and decide upon a diagnosis.

Confirmation of a diagnosis may be obtained in a variety of ways, including tissue biopsy, culture of microorganisms, or finding the cause by surgery. If specific treatment (either with drugs or by surgery) relieves the symptoms and cures the patient, the diagnosis is likely to have been correct—although it is also possible that the patient may have recovered spontaneously and the treatment may simply have coincided with the time of recovery. Alternatively, if the patient dies, a pathologist can usually, but not always, determine by postmortem examination what the disease process was (see *Autopsy*).

Dialysis

A technique used to remove waste products from the blood and excess fluid from the body as a treatment for *kidney failure.*

WHY IT IS DONE

The main function of the kidneys is the maintenance of *electrolyte* and water balance and the excretion of waste products. One fifth of the blood pumped by the heart goes to the kidneys; the kidneys filter approximately 1,500 litres of blood daily. From this volume of blood, the kidney reabsorbs important elements, such as sodium, potassium, calcium, amino acids, glucose, and water. The kidneys excrete, as urine, the protein breakdown product nitrogen in the form of urea, as well as other excess minerals, toxins, and drugs.

In people whose kidneys have been damaged, this process may fail—either suddenly (in acute kidney failure) or gradually (in the chronic form of the disease). Wastes start to accumulate in the blood, with harmful, sometimes even life-threatening, effects. In severe cases, the function of the kidneys must be taken over by the artificial means of dialysis. In cases of acute kidney failure, dialysis continues until the kidneys recover and start functioning normally again. However, in chronic kidney failure, patients may need to undergo dialysis for the rest of their lives or until they can be given a *kidney transplant.* Dialysis therapy may not always be appropriate if kidney failure is part of an otherwise rapidly fatal disorder.

HOW IT IS DONE

There are two methods of dialysis. Haemodialysis, which filters out wastes by passing blood through an artificial kidney machine, was pioneered early in the 1940s. Peritoneal dialysis, which makes use of a natural filtering membrane within the body's abdomen, (the peritoneum), was developed in the early 1970s.

In most cases, haemodialysis is performed in outpatient dialysis centres by trained staff nurses, but many patients now undergoing dialysis carry it out themselves with a kidney machine installed at home.

Peritoneal dialysis may be performed in a hospital, but an increasing number of patients are now able, once

PROCEDURE FOR DIALYSIS

There are two methods of removing wastes from the blood and excess fluid from the body when the kidneys have failed. The first, haemodialysis, may also be used as emergency treatment in some cases of poisoning or drug overdose. It makes use of an artificial kidney (or "kidney machine") and can be carried out at home. Peritoneal dialysis, also done in the home, requires an abdominal incision (which is performed in the hospital).

HOW HAEMODIALYSIS IS DONE

1 Access to the bloodstream for dialysis is obtained by a shunt or an *arteriovenous fistula* connecting an artery to a vein.

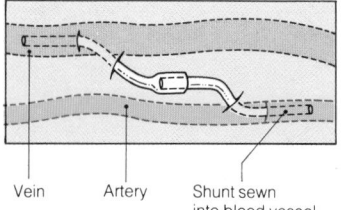

Vein   Artery   Shunt sewn into blood vessel

2 A needle connected to plastic tubing passes blood to the artificial kidney and back to the patient. The artificial kidney consists of many layers of special membrane.

Machine that prepares dialysate

Blood into kidney machine

Dialysate to and from kidney machine

4 The dialysate is discarded and the purified blood is returned to the patient. Each session lasts two to six hours.

Artificial kidney machine

Blood out of kidney machine

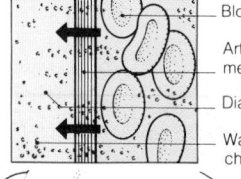

3 The membrane separates the patient's blood from a special fluid called dialysate. Wastes, toxic molecules, and excess fluid pass from the blood into the dialysate.

Blood cell

Artificial membrane

Dialysate

Waste chemicals

Shunt

WHY IT IS DONE

In people with damaged kidneys, the process of maintaining the balance of electrolytes and water, and of excreting waste products, may fail, causing harmful, if not life-threatening, effects. Dialysis can take over the function of the kidneys until they start working normally again. Or dialysis can function for the kidneys for the rest of a seriously affected person's life if a kidney transplant is not performed.

Diseased kidney
The kidney at right was removed from a person with adult polycystic kidney disease—one of many disorders that may damage kidney function to the extent that dialysis is needed.

HOW PERITONEAL DIALYSIS IS DONE

1 A small abdominal incision is made (using a local anaesthetic); a catheter is inserted through it into the peritoneal cavity. Dialysate from a bag attached to the catheter passes into the cavity, where it is left for several hours.

Spinal column

Catheter

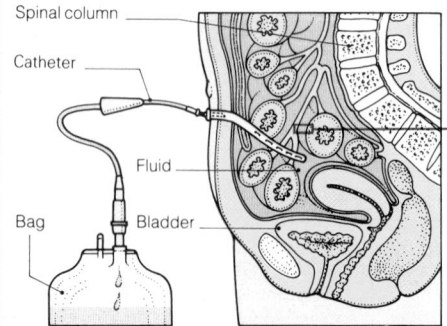

Fluid

Bag   Bladder

Blood cell

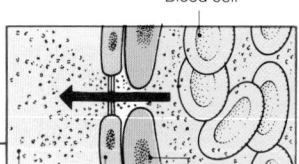

Fluid   Peritoneal membrane   Capillary wall

2 Waste products and excess water from the blood vessels lining the peritoneal cavity seep through the peritoneal membrane into the cavity and mix with the dialysate. The fluid is then allowed to drain out (by the release of a clamp) through the catheter and into the empty dialysate bag.

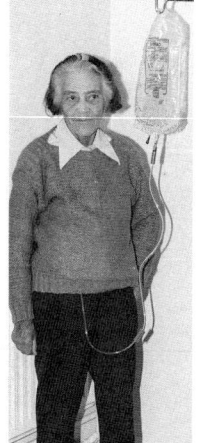

3 The bag is discarded and replaced with a bag containing fresh dialysate. The procedure, which takes about an hour, can be performed during the day or overnight.

the catheter has been inserted into the abdomen, to carry out the dialysis themselves at home, a procedure known as continuous ambulatory peritoneal dialysis (CAPD).

For patients with chronic kidney failure, haemodialysis needs to be carried out several times a week. In the treatment of acute kidney failure, the process is carried out more intensively over a period of days or weeks until the kidneys are working normally again. Complications of haemodialysis may include weakening of the bones (see *Osteomalacia*; *Osteodystrophy*), *anaemia*, infections, and *pericarditis*. Complications of peritoneal dialysis are the same as for haemodialysis, plus *peritonitis*.

OUTLOOK
Long-term dialysis enables people who would once have died from chronic kidney failure to live relatively normal lives. Their diet and fluid intake may need to be restricted somewhat and they may not feel completely well. However, many do return to full or part-time employment. Since the patient's health is invariably affected in the long run, many doctors feel that dialysis should

be replaced with a kidney transplant, which, if successful, can bring about a dramatic restoration of general health.

Diamorphine
A synthetic, narcotic *analgesic drug* (painkiller) which is similar to *morphine*. Diamorphine is an alternative name for heroin.

Diamorphine is used medically to relieve severe pain caused by injury, surgery, myocardial infarction (heart attack), and painful chronic diseases, such as cancer. It is also used to relieve distress in acute heart failure, and is occasionally used as a cough suppressant when other remedies have been ineffective.

Because of the risk of dependence, diamorphine is prescribed with caution. Other adverse effects include nausea, vomiting, and constipation. (See also *Heroin abuse*.)

Diaphragm, contraceptive
The most commonly used female barrier method of contraception, in the form of a hemispherical dome of thin rubber with a metal spring in the rim. The diaphragm is individually fitted. (See *Contraception, barrier methods*.)

Diaphragm muscle
The dome-shaped sheet of muscle that separates the thorax (chest) from the abdomen. The diaphragm is attached to the spine, ribs, and sternum (breastbone).

The diaphragm plays a vital role in breathing. For air to be drawn into the lungs, the muscle fibres of the diaphragm contract, thereby pulling the whole diaphragm downwards. This action enlarges the chest, and air passes into the lungs to fill the increased space. (See also *Breathing*.)

Diarrhoea
Increased fluidity, frequency, or volume of bowel movements, as compared to the usual pattern for a particular person. Diarrhoea itself is not a disorder but is a symptom of an underlying problem.

Acute diarrhoea affects almost everybody from time to time—usually as a result of eating contaminated food or drinking contaminated water. These attacks normally clear up within a day or two with or without treatment. Chronic diarrhoea may be the result of a serious intestinal disorder and requires investigation by a doctor.

Diarrhoea can be very serious in infants because of the risk of severe, potentially fatal, *dehydration*. Elderly people are also at risk of dehydration as a consequence of diarrhoea.

DIARRHOEA IN ADULTS
Normally, the *colon* (the major part of the large intestine) absorbs much of the water from the liquid food residues that pass through it, producing semi-solid *faeces*. However, if the intestinal contents pass through the colon too quickly, or if the small intestine is inflamed and secretes fluid into the faecal material, diarrhoea may result.

CAUSES Acute diarrhoea starts abruptly and usually lasts from a few hours to two or three days. The most common cause is *food poisoning*. Diarrhoea that affects two or more people within six hours of them sharing a meal usually indicates that the food has been contaminated by toxins from STAPHYLOCOCCUS bacteria. Toxins from CLOSTRIDIUM bacteria cause diarrhoea within six to 12 hours after eating. If diarrhoea develops 12 to 48 hours after eating, it may be due to contamination by bacteria such as SALMONELLA or CAMPYLOBACTER, or by a virus such as the rotavirus or Norwalk virus. Infective *gastroenteritis* may also be acquired as a result of droplet infec-

---

ANATOMY OF THE DIAPHRAGM
The diaphragm is attached to the spine, the lower pairs of ribs, and the lower end of the sternum (breastbone). The muscle fibres of the diaphragm converge on the central tendon, a thick, flat plate of dense fibres. There are openings in the diaphragm for the oesophagus, phrenic nerve (which controls diaphragm movements and hence breathing), and the aorta and vena cava blood vessels.

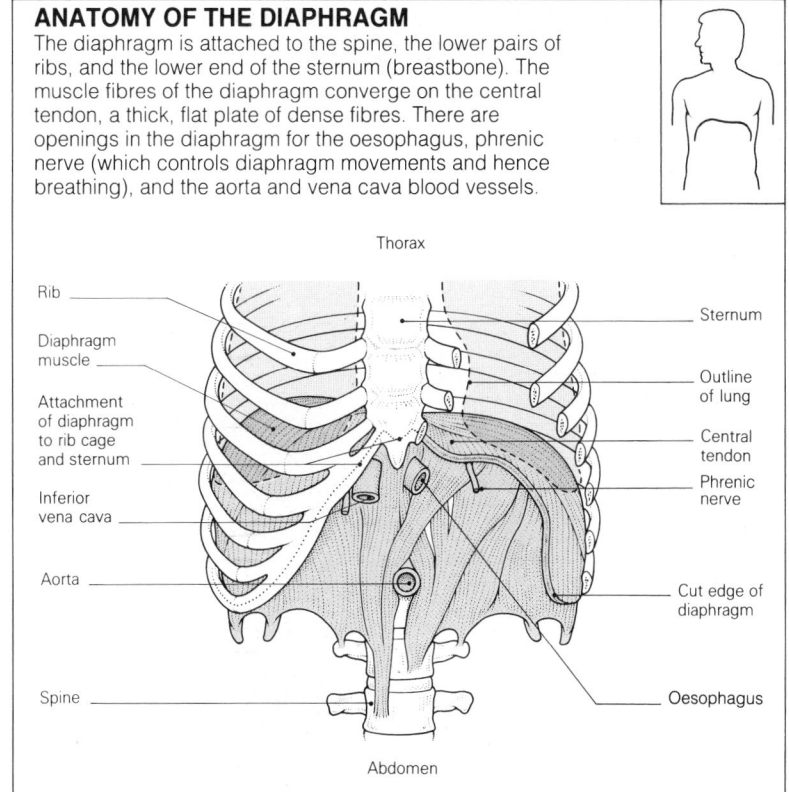

Thorax

Rib

Diaphragm muscle

Attachment of diaphragm to rib cage and sternum

Inferior vena cava

Aorta

Spine

Sternum

Outline of lung

Central tendon

Phrenic nerve

Cut edge of diaphragm

Oesophagus

Abdomen

D

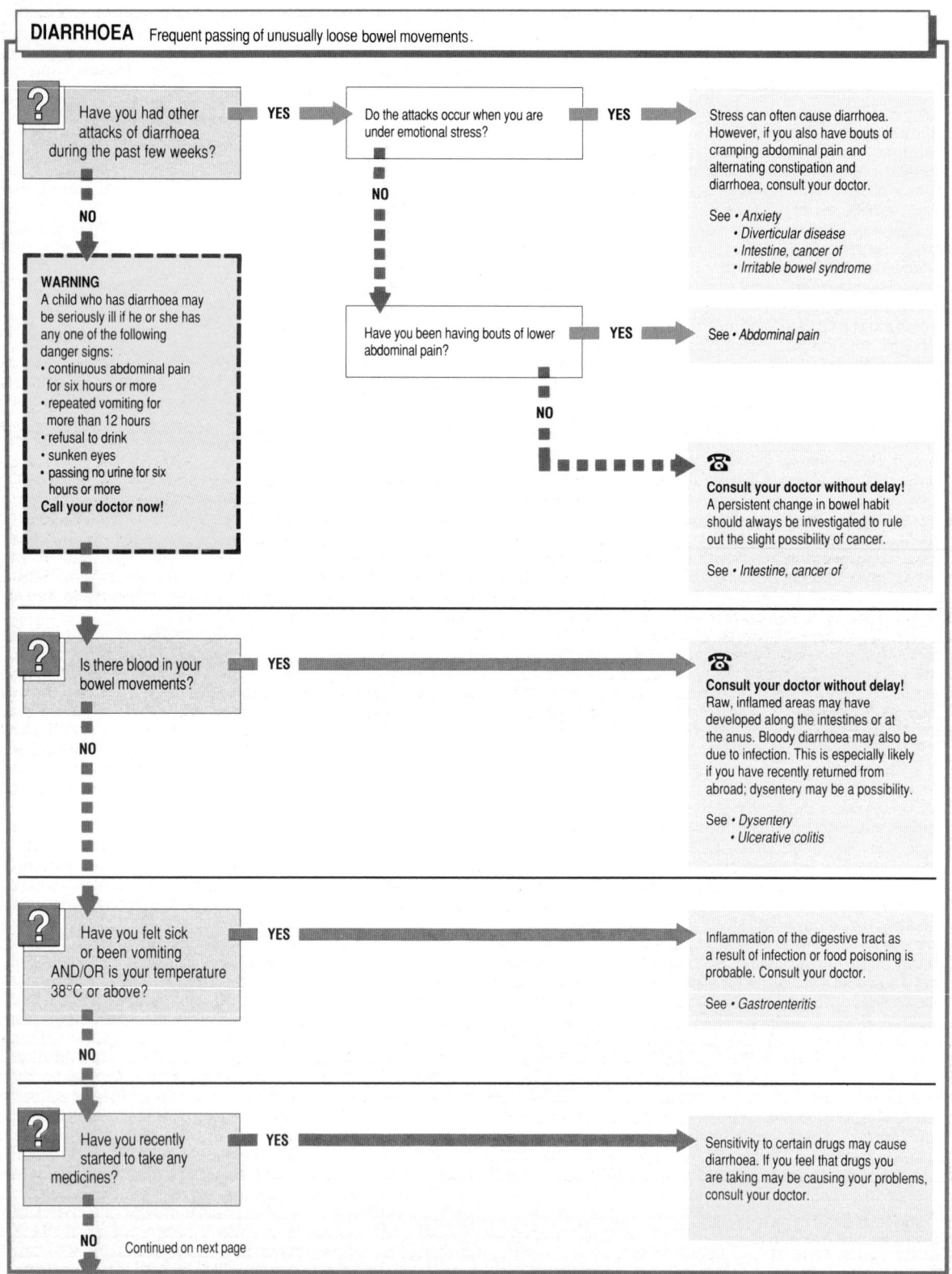

DIARRHOEA Frequent passing of unusually loose bowel movements.

Have you had other attacks of diarrhoea during the past few weeks?

YES → **Do the attacks occur when you are under emotional stress?**

YES → Stress can often cause diarrhoea. However, if you also have bouts of cramping abdominal pain and alternating constipation and diarrhoea, consult your doctor.

See • *Anxiety*
• *Diverticular disease*
• *Intestine, cancer of*
• *Irritable bowel syndrome*

NO ↓

Have you been having bouts of lower abdominal pain?

YES → See • *Abdominal pain*

NO ↓

☎
Consult your doctor without delay!
A persistent change in bowel habit should always be investigated to rule out the slight possibility of cancer.

See • *Intestine, cancer of*

NO ↓

WARNING
A child who has diarrhoea may be seriously ill if he or she has any one of the following danger signs:
• continuous abdominal pain for six hours or more
• repeated vomiting for more than 12 hours
• refusal to drink
• sunken eyes
• passing no urine for six hours or more
Call your doctor now!

↓

Is there blood in your bowel movements?

YES → ☎
Consult your doctor without delay!
Raw, inflamed areas may have developed along the intestines or at the anus. Bloody diarrhoea may also be due to infection. This is especially likely if you have recently returned from abroad; dysentery may be a possibility.

See • *Dysentery*
• *Ulcerative colitis*

NO ↓

Have you felt sick or been vomiting AND/OR is your temperature 38°C or above?

YES → Inflammation of the digestive tract as a result of infection or food poisoning is probable. Consult your doctor.

See • *Gastroenteritis*

NO ↓

Have you recently started to take any medicines?

YES → Sensitivity to certain drugs may cause diarrhoea. If you feel that drugs you are taking may be causing your problems, consult your doctor.

NO ↓ Continued on next page

D

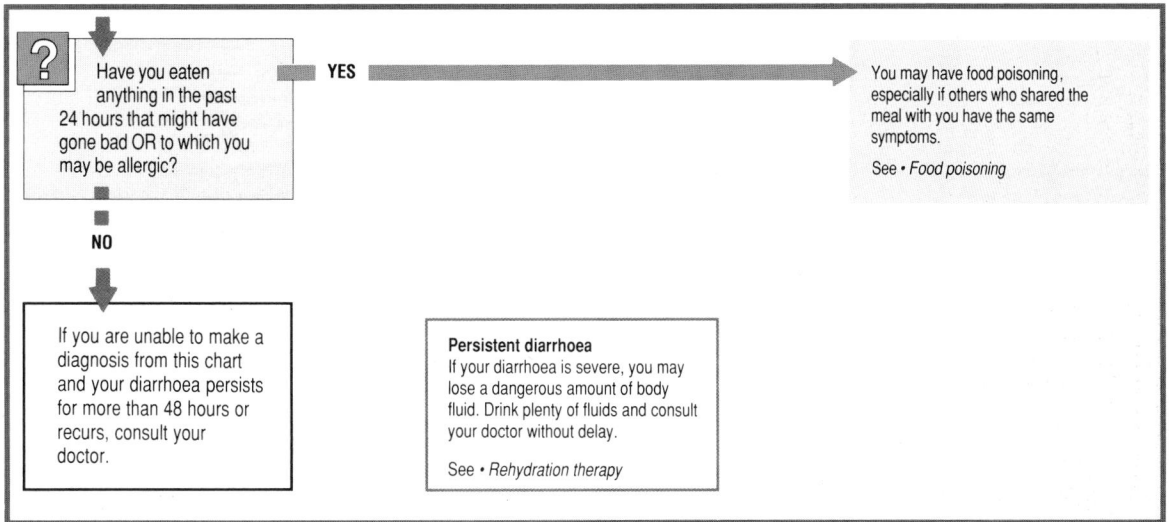

? Have you eaten anything in the past 24 hours that might have gone bad OR to which you may be allergic?

YES → You may have food poisoning, especially if others who shared the meal with you have the same symptoms.

See • *Food poisoning*

NO ↓

If you are unable to make a diagnosis from this chart and your diarrhoea persists for more than 48 hours or recurs, consult your doctor.

Persistent diarrhoea
If your diarrhoea is severe, you may lose a dangerous amount of body fluid. Drink plenty of fluids and consult your doctor without delay.

See • *Rehydration therapy*

---

tion, with adenoviruses or echoviruses, for example. Acute diarrhoea may be caused by interference with the intestinal flora (harmless bacteria in the intestine) as a result of travel to a country where these bacteria are of a different type.

Other causes of acute diarrhoea include anxiety and, less commonly, *shigellosis* (bacillary dysentery), *typhoid fever* and *paratyphoid fever,* drug toxicity, *food allergy,* and *food intolerance.* In the case of shigellosis and amoebic dysentery (see *Amoebiasis*), there may be blood in the faeces.

Chronic diarrhoea generally takes the form of repeated attacks of acute diarrhoea. Causes include *Crohn's disease, ulcerative colitis, diverticular disease,* cancer of the colon (see *Colon, cancer of*), *thyrotoxicosis,* and *irritable bowel syndrome.* In all of these conditions, except thyrotoxicosis and irritable bowel syndrome, the bowel movements may contain blood.

TREATMENT The water and electrolytes (salts) lost during a severe attack of diarrhoea need to be replaced to prevent dehydration. It is possible to buy ready-prepared powders of electrolyte mixtures to be added to a specific amount of water. Half a litre of the oral rehydration liquid should be drunk every hour, and no solid food eaten, until the diarrhoea subsides. Alternatively it is possible to make up an oral rehydration solution: dissolve one teaspoon of salt and eight teaspoons of sugar (which helps the intestine absorb the water and salt) in one litre of water. It is important to be accurate with the quantities as too much salt may cause further dehydration.

Antidiarrhoeal drugs should generally not be taken to treat attacks of diarrhoea resulting from infection since they may prolong the illness. They may be useful, however, if the diarrhoea is disabling or is associated with abdominal pain. Examples are *codeine* phosphate, *diphenoxylate* and *loperamide.*

Diarrhoea that recurs, persists for more than a week, or is accompanied by blood in the bowel movements requires investigation by a doctor to discover the underlying cause. In addition to taking the patient's case history, the doctor will probably arrange for a *culture* of the faeces to determine whether or not infection is the underlying cause. If it is not, other tests may be carried out, such as a barium enema or meal (see *Barium X-ray examinations*), *sigmoidoscopy,* and a *biopsy* of the rectum. These tests enable the doctor to discover the underlying cause of the diarrhoea; treatment will be for that cause.

DIARRHOEA IN INFANTS
Most cases of diarrhoea in infants are acute and carry the risk of rapid dehydration (especially when accompanied by vomiting). Dehydration can be fatal unless countered quickly.

CAUSES In the past 20 years many viruses that may cause diarrhoea in infancy have been identified, including rotavirus, astrovirus, calcivirus, and adenoviruses. By the age of five most children will have been infected with all of these and will have developed immunity. The illnesses caused vary in severity; viral gastroenteritis can damage the lining of the small intestine, thereby impairing its ability to absorb nutrients, and can cause a temporary deficiency of the enzyme lactase. The

latter may lead to lactose intolerance (inability to absorb sugar from milk), which may produce secondary diarrhoea that can last for several weeks.

TREATMENT An infant with diarrhoea should not be fed milk. He or she should be given an electrolyte mixture (obtainable from a chemist) to replace lost water and salts.

If the diarrhoea clears up within 24 hours, milk can be gradually reintroduced over a 24-hour period. The first feed should consist of one part milk to three parts water, the second of equal parts of milk and water, the third of three parts milk to one part water, and the fourth of undiluted milk.

If the diarrhoea persists for more than 48 hours, a doctor should be consulted.

A doctor should be called urgently if the infant shows signs of dehydration at any stage during the illness. Signs of dehydration include drowsiness, unresponsiveness, prolonged crying, loose skin, glazed eyes, a depressed *fontanelle* at the front of the head, and a dry, sticky mouth and tongue. (See also *Rehydration therapy.*)

Diastole
The period in the heartbeat cycle when the heart muscle is at rest; it alternates with the period of muscular contraction (*systole*).

Diathermy
The production of heat in a part of the body using high-frequency electric currents or microwaves. The heat generated can be used to increase blood flow and to reduce deep-seated pain in rheumatic and arthritic conditions.

By using large currents, enough heat can be produced to destroy tumours and diseased parts without causing bleeding. A diathermy knife is an instrument used by surgeons to coagulate bleeding vessels or to separate tissues without causing them to bleed (see *Electrocoagulation*).

Diathesis

A predisposition towards certain disorders. For example, a bleeding diathesis is present when a *bleeding disorder* (such as *haemophilia*) makes a person susceptible to prolonged bleeding after an injury. A diathesis may be inherited or may be acquired as a result of an illness.

Diazepam

BENZODIAZEPINE ANTICONVULSANT MUSCLE RELAXANT

Tablet Injection Suppository

Prescription needed

Available as generic

One of the best known and most widely used *benzodiazepine drugs*. Diazepam is used mainly to treat *anxiety* and *insomnia*. It is also prescribed as a *muscle-relaxant drug* (for example, to treat back-muscle spasm), and as an *anticonvulsant drug* in the emergency treatment of *epilepsy*. It is often used to treat alcohol withdrawal symptoms.

POSSIBLE ADVERSE EFFECTS

Diazepam may cause drowsiness, dizziness, and confusion; driving and hazardous work should therefore be avoided. Alcohol increases the sedative effect of the drug and should be avoided during the use of diazepam.

Like other drugs in this group, diazepam can be habit-forming if taken regularly, and its effect may diminish with prolonged use. Individuals who have taken diazepam regularly for more than two weeks should never stop their treatment suddenly. Instead, they should gradually decrease the dose under medical supervision to avoid withdrawal symptoms (which may include anxiety, sweating, and, rarely, following large doses, fits).

Diclofenac

A *nonsteroidal anti-inflammatory drug* (NSAID) used to relieve pain and stiffness in different types of *arthritis*. It is also prescribed to hasten recovery following injury to muscles or ligaments. Possible adverse effects include nausea, abdominal pain, and peptic ulcer.

Diet

See *Nutrition*.

Diet and disease

Until recently, medical concern about diet in developed countries focused on dietary deficiencies in the poor. Today, deficiency diseases are very rare in developed countries (except in alcoholics, people with malabsorptive intestinal disorders, and people on extremely restricted diets). Instead, many common disorders are due partly to overconsumption of certain foods.

In poorer developing countries, dietary deficiencies remain a major problem. Starvation or malnutrition may result in *marasmus* or *kwashiorkor* in children; specific vitamin deficiencies may cause *rickets* or blindness due to *keratomalacia*. Lack of certain vitamins in adult life may lead to *beriberi*, *pellagra*, or *scurvy*.

FATS

Virtually all people in developed countries have some degree of *atherosclerosis* (narrowing of arteries by deposits of fatty material), which can lead to cardiovascular diseases (such as *coronary artery disease*, *stroke*, and *peripheral vascular disease*). A major cause of atherosclerosis is a high level of *cholesterol* in the blood which most nutritionists believe to be due to a high intake of saturated *fats*, found in meat, eggs, and dairy products. The disease is much less common in countries (such as Japan) in which fat in the diet is minimal and mostly unsaturated.

CALORIES

Obesity places a person at greater risk of disorders such as *diabetes mellitus*, stroke, coronary artery disease, and *osteoarthritis*. The cause is an excess intake of *calories*. About one third of people in developed countries is overweight (10 per cent or more above the accepted weight range for a given height) and a few of them are obese (20 per cent or more above the range).

ALCOHOL

Overconsumption of *alcohol* can lead to *cirrhosis* of the liver, brain damage (see *Wernicke-Korsakoff syndrome*), peripheral *neuritis*, and *cardiomyopathy*, and has been linked with *pancreatitis*, oesophageal cancer (see *Oesophagus, cancer of*), and many other disorders. People with *alcohol dependence* tend to become malnourished.

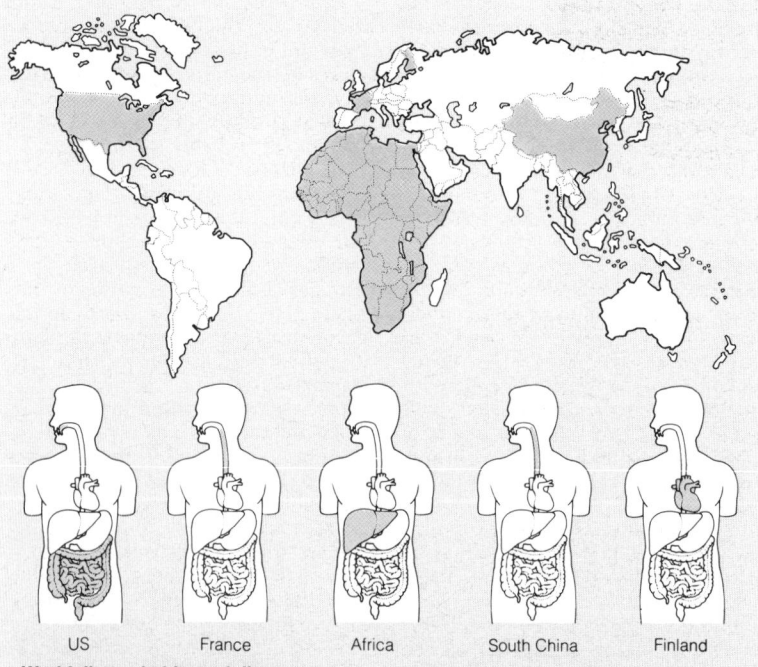

US   France   Africa   South China   Finland

World dietary habits and disease
In the US, bowel cancer may be more common because of high fat, low fibre consumption; dental caries are caused by high sugar intake. Coronary artery disease is common among Finns because of their fatty diets; in France, alcoholic drink is blamed for the frequency of oesophageal cancer; in South China, certain fungi in food cause oesophageal cancer; and in Africa, aflatoxins may cause liver cancer.

FIBRE

The part played by diet in digestive disorders is less clear than its contribution to cardiovascular disease and obesity, but there is evidence suggesting that lack of fibre may be an important factor in some illnesses. Fibre—found in foods such as wholemeal bread and vegetables—provides bulk to enable the large intestine to work effectively and also helps regulate the absorption of nutrients in the small intestine. Lack of dietary fibre has been implicated in intestinal disorders such as *diverticular disease*, chronic *constipation*, and *haemorrhoids*.

SALT

In developed countries, *hypertension* (high blood pressure) is far more prevalent than in developing countries. One theory is that some people are genetically susceptible to develop high blood pressure in middle age if they consume too much salt. For this reason, some nutritionists consider it prudent not to have a high salt intake.

VITAMINS

Classic vitamin deficiency diseases such as rickets are now virtually unknown in developed countries. However, many people's diets still contain too few natural vitamins; supplements of multivitamin preparations are less satisfactory than a diet rich in natural vitamins (see Good Dietary Habits box, above right). Pregnant women need high intakes of B group vitamins to reduce the risk of the embryo having a *neural tube defect*; high intakes of vitamins A and C have been shown to lower the risk of cancer in later life.

DIET AND CANCER

Studies of cancer in different countries suggest that diet may be an important factor. High vitamin intakes are protective, but a high intake of fat has been linked with cancer of the bowel (see *Colon, cancer of*) and *Breast cancer*. Mouldy foods are known to cause cancer of the oesophagus and *liver cancer*, and research groups are examining many other associations.

FOOD ALLERGIES

Although many illnesses are commonly ascribed to food allergy, a definite link can be proved in only a few cases. They include those suffering from *coeliac disease*, as the result of an intolerance to gluten, a protein in cereals; and people who develop a rash after eating shellfish or soft fruit (see *Urticaria*). Some *asthma* attacks and *eczema* may be due to an allergy to eggs and dairy products; and an allergy to food additives, such as colourings, may be a factor in eczema and *irritable bowel*

syndrome. Some doctors believe that allergy to food additives is a major cause of behavioural disorders, such as *hyperactivity* in children, but research suggests that this association is rare.

Treatment for self-diagnosed food allergy should always be supervised by a doctor. It is a time-consuming process in which suspected items in the diet are excluded one at a time.

A PRUDENT DIET

Although the connection between certain types of food and disease has not been proved in all cases, enough evidence exists to indicate that it is wise to make sure your diet is low in fats and sugar and high in fibre. The fats and sugar should be replaced with starchy foods and cereals. (See also *Nutritional disorders*).

Dietetics

The application of nutritional science to the maintenance or restoration of health. Dietetics involves not only a detailed knowledge of the composition of foods, the effects of cooking and processing, and dietary requirements, but also psychological aspects, such as eating habits (see *Nutrition*).

Differentiation

The process by which the cells of the early *embryo*, which are almost identical and have not yet taken on any particular function, gradually diversify to form the distinct tissues and organs of the more developed embryo.

In cancer terminology, the word means the degree to which the microscopic appearance of a tissue resembles normal tissue.

Diffusion

The spread of a substance (by movement of its molecules) in a fluid from an area of high concentration to one of lower concentration, thus producing a uniform concentration throughout.

Diflunisal

A *nonsteroidal anti-inflammatory drug* (NSAID) used to relieve joint pain and stiffness in *osteoarthritis*, *rheumatoid arthritis*, and other types of arthritis. It is also prescribed to treat back pain, sprains, and strains. Occasionally, it is prescribed to ease pain after a minor operation or dental treatment. Diflunisal may cause nausea, indigestion, diarrhoea, and a rash.

Digestive system

The group of organs that breaks down food into simple chemical components that the body can absorb and use for energy and for building and repairing cells and tissues.

The digestive system consists of the digestive tract (also known as the alimentary tract or alimentary canal) and various associated organs. The digestive tract is basically a tube through which food passes; it consists of the *mouth*, *pharynx* (throat), *oesophagus* (gullet), *stomach*, *intestines* (the small intestine, comprising the *duodenum*, *jejunum*, and *ileum* and the large intestine, comprising the *caecum*, *colon*, and *rectum*), and the *anus*. The associated digestive organs—such as the *salivary glands*, *liver*, and *pancreas*—secrete digestive juices that break down food as it passes through the tract.

Food and the products of digestion are moved through the intestine, from the throat to the rectum, by *peristalsis* (waves of muscular contractions of the intestinal wall).

THE DIGESTIVE PROCESS

The human diet is made up of foods consisting of nutrients and energy sources (*vitamins*, *minerals*, *carbohydrates*, *proteins*, and *fats*), residues (mainly vegetable *fibre*), and water. Most vitamins and minerals are absorbed into the bloodstream without change. However, before other nutrients can be absorbed into the bloodstream, they must be broken down by digestive agents into simpler substances with smaller molecules.

Part of food breakdown is physical, performed by the teeth, which cut and

D

THE DIGESTIVE PROCESS

Digestion starts when food enters the mouth. It continues as the food is propelled through the digestive tract by waves of muscular contractions (peristalsis). The digestive process also involves other organs (the salivary glands, liver, gallbladder, and pancreas), which produce enzymes and acids that help break down the food.

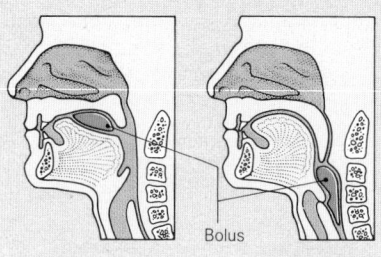

Bolus

Swallowing

In the mouth, food is cut and ground by the teeth and mixed with saliva, which softens food and breaks down certain carbohydrates. After swallowing, the food mass (bolus) enters the oesophagus.

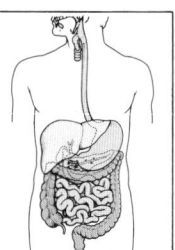

ACTION OF DIGESTIVE AGENTS

Agent or enzyme (where produced)	Digestive action
Amylase (mouth and pancreas)	Converts starch (a form of carbo-hydrate) to maltose
Sucrase, maltase, and lactase (pancreas and small intestine)	Break down vegetable and milk sugars into glucose, fructose, and galactose
Hydrochloric acid (stomach) Pepsin (stomach) Trypsin (pancreas) Peptidase (small intestine)	Assist in the breakdown of proteins into polypeptides, peptides, and amino acids
Lipase (pancreas) Bile salts and acids (liver — stored in the gallbladder)	Break down fats into glycerol and fatty acids

TIME SCALE

The approximate period food spends in each part of the digestive system is shown below.

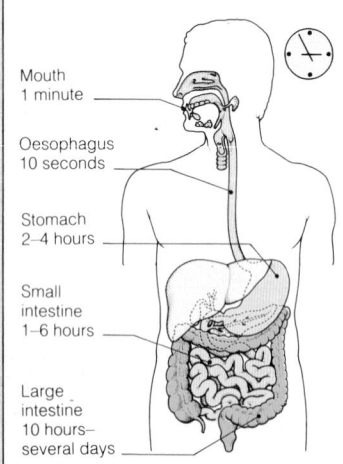

Mouth
1 minute

Oesophagus
10 seconds

Stomach
2–4 hours

Small intestine
1–6 hours

Large intestine
10 hours–several days

Oesophagus

Food is carried down the oesophagus by peristaltic action and enters the stomach.

Stomach

Food is broken down further by churning and by the action of hydrochloric acid and digestive enzymes secreted by the stomach lining. Food remains in the stomach until it is reduced to a semi-liquid consistency (chyme), when it passes into the duodenum.

Duodenum

As food travels along the duodenum, it is broken down further by digestive enzymes from the liver, gallbladder, and pancreas. The duodenum leads directly into the small intestine.

Small intestine

Additional enzymes secreted by glands in the lining of the small intestine complete the digestive process. Nutrients are absorbed through the intestinal lining into the network of blood vessels and lymph vessels supplying the intestine. Undigested matter passes into the large intestine (the colon).

Colon

Water in the undigested matter leaving the small intestine is absorbed through the lining of the colon. The residue passes into the rectum.

Rectum

Undigested matter enters this final part of the large intestine and is expelled.

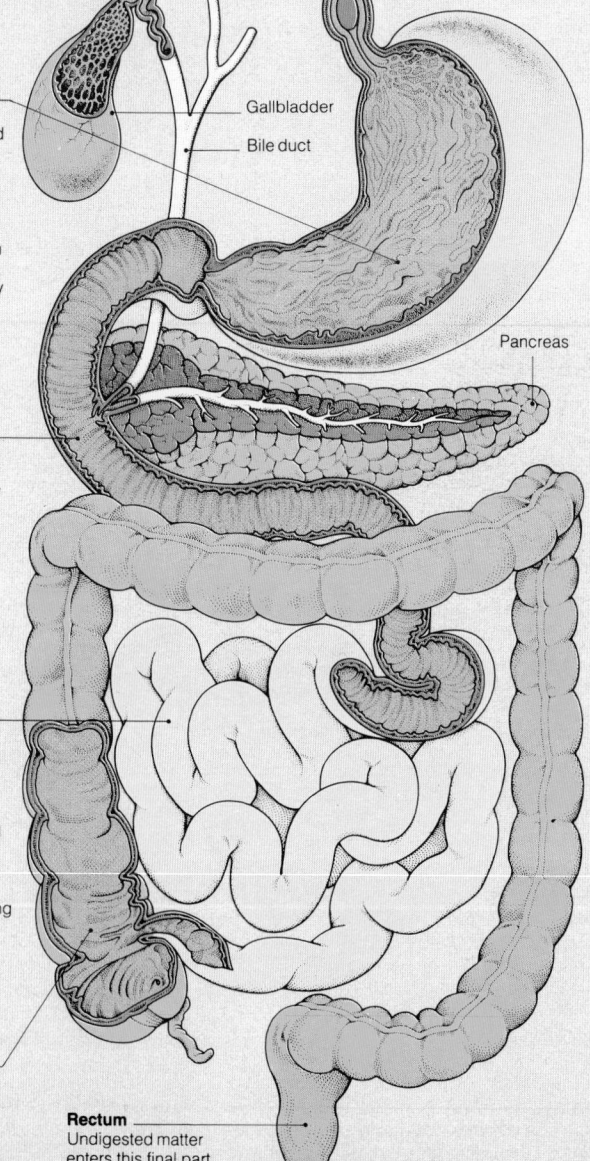

Gallbladder

Bile duct

Pancreas

Anus

chew food, and the stomach, which churns it. The rest of the process is chemical, performed by the action of *enzymes*, acids, and salts.

Carbohydrates, which are provided mainly by starchy and sugary foods, are the body's principal source of energy. The digestive process eventually converts all carbohydrates (except those that make up dietary fibre) to three simple forms of sugar: glucose, fructose, and galactose.

Proteins, which are found in abundance in meat, fish, eggs, cheese, peas, beans, and lentils, are essential for the growth, replacement, and repair of cells. Proteins are broken down into *polypeptides*, *peptides*, and *amino acids*.

Fats (also known as lipids), which are found in meat and dairy products, and also in oily plant foods such as peanuts and avocados, provide energy and some of the materials for cell building and maintenance. They are broken down into *glycerol*, glycerides, and *fatty acids*.

The digestive process begins in the mouth, where the teeth chop food and the salivary glands secrete saliva, which lubricates the food and contains enzymes that begin to break down carbohydrates. The mouth also contains sensory nerves, in the taste buds on the tongue. The tongue manipulates food in the mouth and forms it into small balls (called boli) for easy swallowing.

From the mouth, food passes into the pharynx, which then pushes it into the oesophagus. The oesophagus does not contribute to the breakdown or absorption of food products; its sole function is to squeeze food down into the stomach. In the stomach, food is mixed with hydrochloric acid and pepsin produced in the stomach lining; these help break down proteins. The stomach also breaks down food mechanically by its continual churning action. When the food has been converted to a semi-liquid consistency, it passes into the duodenum.

The liver produces bile salts and acids, which are stored in the gallbladder and then released into the duodenum. These salts and acids help break down fats. The pancreas also releases digestive juices into the duodenum, and these juices contain enzymes that further break down carbohydrates, fats, and proteins. The final breakdown stages are completed in the small intestine, carried out by enzymes produced by glands in the lining of the intestine.

As the products of the breakdown of digestion pass through the small intestine, they are absorbed by its thin lining and then pass either into the bloodstream or into the lymphatic system.

Finally, the food residue passes into the large intestine, where much of the water it contains is absorbed by the lining of the colon. Undigested matter is then expelled, via the rectum and anus, as faeces.

DISORDERS

Some digestive system disorders disrupt the digestive process, either because they obstruct the passage of food, or because they interfere with the breakdown or absorption of nutrients. Other conditions have little effect on the digestion of nutrients but produce gastrointestinal symptoms.

Digestive system disorders result from various causes, including birth defects, inherited biochemical disorders, parasitic infections, and chronic allergic conditions. (See also disorder boxes for *Mouth, Oesophagus, Stomach, Liver, Gallbladder, Pancreas,* and *Intestine*.)

Digitalis drugs

A group of drugs that are extracted from the leaves of plants belonging to the foxglove family. Digitalis drugs are used to treat various heart conditions. The most commonly used drugs in this group are *digoxin* and *digitoxin*.

Digital subtraction angiography

See *Angiography*.

Digitoxin

A *digitalis drug*. Digitoxin is used to treat *heart failure* (reduced pumping efficiency) and certain types of *arrhythmia* (irregular heartbeat).

Digoxin

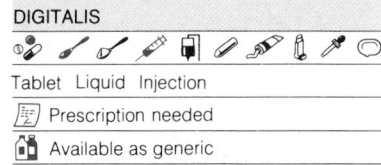

DIGITALIS
Tablet   Liquid   Injection
Prescription needed
Available as generic

The most widely used of the *digitalis drugs*. Digoxin is used in the treatment of *heart failure* (reduced pumping efficiency) and certain types of *arrhythmia* (irregular heartbeat), such as *atrial fibrillation* (a rapid, irregular beating of the heart muscle).

HOW IT WORKS

Digoxin increases the force of heart muscle contractions, making the heart work more efficiently. It also slows down abnormally rapid impulses as they pass between the atria (upper chambers of the heart) to the ventricles (main chambers of the heart), which allows the ventricles time to fill up with blood and empty normally with each contraction.

POSSIBLE ADVERSE EFFECTS

If digoxin is to be effective, the dose must be just below that of a toxic dose. The patient must therefore be given regular blood tests to ascertain the digoxin level. An excessive dose may cause loss of appetite, nausea, vomiting, and headache. Digoxin occasionally disrupts the normal heartbeat, causing *heart block* (an abnormally slow rate of contraction).

Adverse effects are more likely if the potassium level in the body is low. Patients who are also taking *diuretic drugs* (and therefore are more likely to become deficient in potassium) are given regular blood tests to monitor potassium levels.

Because digoxin is removed from the body mainly in the urine, careful attention to dosage is needed in patients with kidney disease; measurement of plasma concentrations of the drug may be needed to avoid the risk of toxicity.

Dilatation

A condition in which a body cavity, tube, or opening is enlarged or stretched due to normal physiological processes or because of disease.

The term dilatation also refers to procedures for achieving such enlargement, as in dilatation and curettage.

Dilatation and curettage

See *D and C*.

Dilation

A term that is sometimes used as an alternative to *dilatation*.

Dilator

An instrument for stretching and enlarging a narrowed body cavity, tube, or opening.

Diltiazem

A *calcium channel blocker* used in the treatment of *hypertension* (high blood pressure) and *angina pectoris* (chest pain due to impaired blood supply to heart muscle). Taken regularly, diltiazem reduces the frequency of angina attacks, but acts too slowly to relieve pain in an acute attack.

D

Diltiazem may cause headache, appetite loss, nausea, constipation, and swelling of the ankles.

Dioxin

The name of a group of chemicals that are among the most highly toxic substances known. They are contaminants of some defoliant weedkillers (see *Defoliant poisoning* and *Agent Orange*). Dioxins have also been detected in minute traces in some bleached paper products.

Diphenhydramine

An *antihistamine drug* that is used to treat various allergic disorders, such as *urticaria* (nettle rash) and allergic *rhinitis* (hay fever).

Diphenhydramine is also prescribed as an *antiemetic drug* to relieve nausea and vomiting in pregnancy and to prevent *motion sickness*. It is used as an ingredient in some *cough remedies* because of its cough-suppressant effect.

POSSIBLE ADVERSE EFFECTS
Diphenhydramine often causes drowsiness and, because of its sedative effect, has occasionally been used to treat *insomnia*. Driving and hazardous work should be avoided if the drug is causing sedation. Other possible side-effects include dry mouth and blurred vision.

Diphenoxylate

An *antidiarrhoeal drug* chemically related to the narcotic *analgesic drugs* (painkillers). Diphenoxylate works by reducing the contractions of the muscles in the walls of the intestine, thus slowing down the frequency of bowel movements.

POSSIBLE ADVERSE EFFECTS
In normal doses, drowsiness and abdominal pain occur in rare instances. When taken in high doses, diphenoxylate produces euphoria due to its narcotic ingredient. Adding *atropine* to the preparation prevents abuse; a dose high enough to produce euphoria causes unpleasant side-effects, such as dry mouth, flushing, blurred vision, and vomiting.

Diphtheria

An acute bacterial illness that causes a sore throat, fever, and, sometimes, more serious or even fatal complications. Diphtheria was one of the most important causes of childhood death worldwide until the 1930s. Since then, mass immunization has made it extremely rare in developed countries. Diphtheria is still a hazard in some developing countries and is a risk for nonimmunized travellers to such countries.

CAUSES AND INCIDENCE
Diphtheria is caused by the bacillus *CORYNEBACTERIUM DIPHTHERIAE*. It may live in the skin or in the nose of a person immune to the disease or, during an infection, may multiply in the throat or skin. Serious complications are caused by a toxin released by the bacterium into the blood.

The few cases that occur in the UK are invariably among immigrants from developing countries. In these countries, the disease is usually caught from a healthy "carrier" of diphtheria bacilli, who harbours the organisms in his or her nose or skin and spreads them through the air or by touch. These carriers have acquired immunity to the illness, having in the past recovered from a relatively mild infection.

SYMPTOMS
When a nonimmune person is infected by the bacterium, it usually multiplies in the throat, giving rise to a membrane that appears over the tonsils and may spread over the palate or downwards to the larynx (voice-box) and trachea (windpipe). This may cause breathing difficulties and a husky voice. Other symptoms include enlarged lymph nodes in the neck, an increased heart-rate, and mild fever. Sometimes, infection is confined to the skin, where it may cause no more than a few yellow spots or sores with an appearance similar to *impetigo*.

Life-threatening symptoms develop only in nonimmune people and are caused by the bacterial toxin. Occasionally, victims collapse and die within a day or so of developing throat symptoms. More often they are recovering from this condition when *heart failure* or paralysis of the throat or limbs develops. These later complications can occur up to seven weeks after onset of infection in the throat. If victims survive the disease they make a complete recovery.

PREVENTION
The *DPT vaccine* (against diphtheria, pertussis, and tetanus) is given routinely in three spaced doses during the first year of life. The practice of immunizing against diphtheria must continue, despite the extreme rarity of the disease in developed countries, because carriers may bring the infection from countries where the disease is more common; if large numbers of children were not immune, there could be an epidemic.

Those travelling to developing countries who are in doubt as to whether or not they were immunized against diphtheria as children should have their immune status checked. People who are not immune should be vaccinated.

Spread of effective immunization programmes to all countries could eventually eradicate diphtheria (as smallpox has been eradicated), although this possibility is not envisaged at present.

TREATMENT
Penicillin drugs kill diphtheria organisms in the throat but are ineffective against the toxin in the blood. If diphtheria is suspected, an *antitoxin* (derived from the blood of immunized horses) must be given as soon as possible in addition to penicillin. If severe breathing difficulties develop in a patient, a *tracheostomy* (surgical introduction of a breathing tube into the windpipe) may be necessary.

Victims are kept in isolation until no diphtheria bacilli can be detected in the nose and throat (by swabs taken on six consecutive days).

Diplopia

The medical term for *double vision*.

Dipsomania

A form of *alcohol dependence* in which periods of excessive drinking and craving for drink alternate with periods of relative sobriety.

Dipyridamole

A drug that reduces the stickiness of platelets in the *blood* and thus helps prevent the formation of abnormal blood clots within arteries.

Dipyridamole is used together with *aspirin* or *warfarin* to prevent the formation of clots following *heart-valve surgery*. It may also be given to people who have recently had a *myocardial infarction* (heart attack) or undergone *coronary artery bypass* surgery. Dipyridamole may also reduce the frequency of *transient ischaemic attacks* (symptoms of stroke lasting less than 24 hours).

Possible adverse effects include headache, flushing, and dizziness.

Disability

A measurable physical or mental loss or impairment, which may be temporary or permanent.

A distinction may be made between disability and *handicap*, defining disability as the physical disorder (e.g. muscle weakness or blindness) and handicap as the extent to which a dis-

PHYSICAL AIDS FOR THE DISABLED

A variety of articles exist that are specially designed or adapted to assist disabled people in performing everyday activities. Aids include prostheses, supports, and mobility aids that enable disabled people to function more efficiently, as well as equipment designed to help them perform specific tasks more easily.

Devices that help vision, hearing, and movement improve the ability of disabled people to cope with all aspects of everyday life. Such devices include walking frames, glasses, hearing-aids, artificial limbs, corsets, and wheelchairs. Ventilators, home dialysis, and artificial feeding devices are life-sustaining aids.

There are various household aids available that can help people cook, feed themselves, wash, dress, use the toilet, and get in and out of beds and chairs. Specially designed furniture and other devices can help disabled parents care for their children. Sexual aids can facilitate an active sex life.

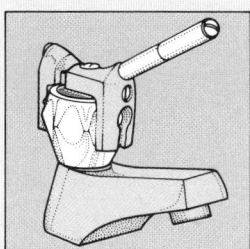

Tap turner
A device that helps grip and turn taps.

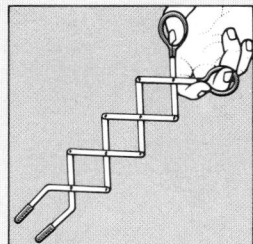

Tongs
Extending tongs to pick up dropped items. Closes up to fit in pocket or handbag.

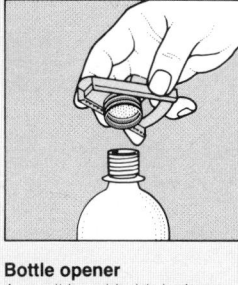

Bottle opener
A small hand-held device designed to grip and open small bottle tops.

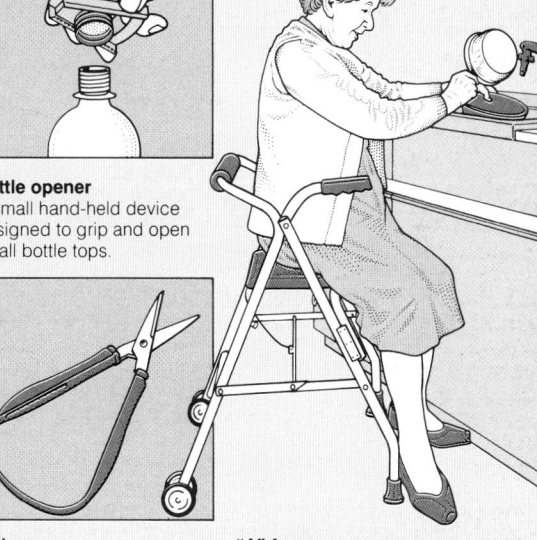

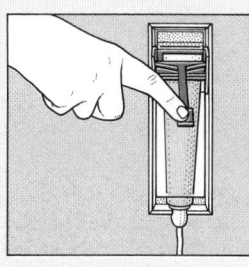

Cutlery
A range of knives, forks, and spoons with thick, moulded handles for easy manipulating.

Toothpaste extruder
A wall-mounted device that dispenses toothpaste with minimal finger pressure.

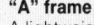

Scissors
Self-opening scissors with easy-grip handles.

"A" frame
A lightweight walking frame that doubles as a seat and can be folded flat.

---

order impairs normal functioning. Thus two people with the same disability may suffer different degrees of handicap because one person manages to cope with everyday living better than the other. In practice, however, the distinction between disability and handicap is vague and the two terms are often used interchangeably. (See also illustrated box showing aids for the disabled; *Rehabilitation*.)

Discharge

A visible emission of fluid from an orifice or a break in the skin (such as a wound or burst boil). Discharge may be a normal occurrence, such as some types of *vaginal discharge*, or may be due to infection or inflammation, such as occurs in *rhinitis* (inflammation of the lining of the nose), *urethritis* (infection of the urethra), and *proctitis* (infection of the rectum).

Disc, intervertebral

A flat, circular, plate-like structure containing *cartilage* which lines the joints between adjacent *vertebrae* (bones) in the *spine*.

Each intervertebral disc is composed of a hard, outer layer and a soft, jelly-like core. The material acts as a shock absorber to cushion the vertebrae during movements of the spine, and to minimize jarring when jumping or running.

With increasing age, intervertebral discs may wear out, becoming less supple and more susceptible to damage from injury. One of the most common forms of damage is a *disc prolapse*, in which part of the disc's soft centre bulges out through a weak area in the hard, outer layer. This may compress a spinal nerve root and produce symptoms, such as muscle weakness and/or pain in the back and leg.

Disclosing agents

Dyes that make the *plaque* deposits on teeth more visible so that they can be seen and removed. When giving

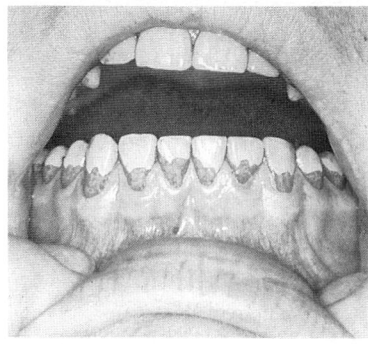

Plaque revealed by disclosing agent
Bacteria, mucus, and food debris build up quickly as plaque if teeth are not brushed and flossed regularly.

D

information about *oral hygiene,* a dentist or dental hygienist may apply a disclosing solution to the teeth to show the presence of harmful dental plaque and pellicle (a film formed from saliva), and to demonstrate an effective method of tooth cleaning.

Discoloured teeth

Teeth tend naturally to darken with age. The red pulp tissue in the centre of the tooth, which makes young teeth look bright, gradually recedes while at the same time more dentine is laid down around it, resulting in the tooth's dull yellow colour.

Both the tooth's surface and its internal structures are liable to be stained by a variety of substances introduced into the mouth or carried by the blood supply. Extrinsic stains, those found on the tooth's surface, are common, but are usually easily removed by polishing and can be prevented by regular tooth cleaning. Intrinsic stains, those within the tooth's substance, are permanent. Many stains, both extrinsic and intrinsic, can be covered or diminished with cosmetic dental procedures, such as *bonding* and *bleaching.*

EXTRINSIC NONMETALLIC STAINS
BROWNISH-BLACK DEPOSIT Smoking tobacco or chewing betel nuts can lead to staining due to accumulation of tars and resins. The discoloration may be worse on the inside surfaces of the teeth.

BLACK STAIN A firmly attached black or brown line, close to and following the contour of the gum, usually on the inside surfaces of the upper back teeth. More common in children, it is thought to be due to pigment-producing bacteria.

GREEN STAIN A heavy, "furry", greyish-green stain, firmly attached close to the gum, usually on the front surfaces of the upper front teeth. It is most commonly found in children and may be due to staining of remnants of developmental membrane by colour-producing bacteria.

DULL YELLOW STAIN This may be due to discoloration of *plaque* by dyes in foodstuffs; it is easily removed.

BROWN SPOTS Dark areas near the gum line may be due to areas of thinned enamel becoming stained by tea or other foods. Brown coloration may also result if the areas become remineralized (i.e. if the enamel is built up again through deposition of calcium and phosphate from saliva).

ORANGE-RED STAIN This may be caused by pigment-producing bacteria; it is easily removed.

STAINED DENTINE With advancing age, the full thickness of enamel may be worn away in parts and the dentine becomes stained by dyes in foods.

EXTRINSIC METALLIC STAINS
Stains of this type may follow the use of medicines containing metallic salts. Iron-containing liquids stain the teeth brown. Inhalation of metallic dust by metal workers (prior to stringent safety measures) caused accumulation of metals in the plaque. Brass, copper, lead, bronze, and other copper alloys caused a bluish-green stain, iron produced brown staining, and mercury led to black staining.

INTRINSIC STAINS
BLACK TEETH Teeth may darken following the death of the pulp or the removal of the pulp during *root-canal treatment.* Darkening is caused by the decomposition of red blood cells that pass from damaged blood vessels in the pulp into the dentine.

TETRACYCLINE STAINING The antibiotic drug *tetracycline* is absorbed by developing teeth and causes discoloration of primary or permanent teeth. Which teeth are affected depends on the stage of tooth development at the time it is absorbed, the amount taken, and the type of tetracycline prescribed. Tetracycline given to a pregnant woman often causes discoloration of her child's teeth. If mildly affected, the teeth will appear yellow but, if severely affected, they will be brown or blue-violet.

After the age of seven years, discoloration is less likely to occur, because all the crowns of the important teeth are already formed.

FLUOROSIS Mottling of the tooth enamel occurs if excessive amounts of fluoride are taken during development of the enamel (see *Fluorosis*).

OTHER CAUSES *Hepatitis* during infancy may cause yellow-brown discoloration of the primary teeth due to the inclusion of bile pigments in the developing teeth. The teeth of children with *congenital* malformation of the *bile ducts* may be similarly affected. Congenital erythropoietic *porphyria* (a rare inherited disorder) causes reddish-brown or purple discoloration.

Disc prolapse

A common, painful disorder of the *spine,* in which an invertebral *disc* ruptures and part of its pulpy core protrudes, causing painful and at times disabling pressure on a nerve.

About 95 per cent of disc prolapses occur in the lower back, but they can affect any part of the back or the neck.

CAUSES AND INCIDENCE
Although a prolapsed disc may sometimes be caused by a sudden strenuous action (such as lifting a heavy weight or twisting violently), it usually develops gradually as a result of degeneration of the discs with age.

People between the ages of 30 and 40 are the most likely to suffer from a disc prolapse. Over the age of 30, discs start to dehydrate and become less resilient but, after 40, extra fibrous tissue forms around them, increasing their stability.

Disc prolapses are slightly more common in men than in women, and their incidence is higher in people who spend long periods sitting without a break.

DIAGNOSIS
Many other disorders may cause back and leg pain or neck and arm pain, and various tests may be needed to arrive at a firm diagnosis. After the doctor has examined the spine and tested movement and reflexes in the affected arm or leg, he or she may arrange for tests, which can include the following: *X-rays, CT scanning, MRI,* and *EMG* (tests of electrical activity in the muscles).

If a certain nerve root is suspected of being compressed, a local anaesthetic may be injected into its lining; if this relieves the pain, the location of the trouble is confirmed.

TREATMENT
In most cases, symptoms are relieved by bed rest and a variety of other measures (see illustrated box). However, if the pain is persistent, if muscle, bladder, or bowel function are impaired, surgical techniques, such as decompression of the spinal canal (see *Decompression, spinal canal*) or *chemonucleolysis* may be necessary.

Disc, slipped

See *Disc prolapse.*

Disinfectants

Substances that kill microorganisms and thus prevent infection. The term is usually applied to strong chemicals that are harmful to human tissue and so are used to decontaminate inanimate objects, such as items of medical equipment. Decontaminants that are safe for human tissue are known as *antiseptics.*

Dislocation, joint

Complete displacement of the two bones in a joint so that they are no longer in contact, usually as a result of injury. (Displacement that leaves the bones in partial contact is called *subluxation*.) Dislocation is usually accompanied by tearing of the joint ligaments and damage to the joint capsule (the membrane that encases the joint); it is the tearing that makes the injury so painful. Injury severe enough to cause dislocation often also causes fracture of one or both of the bones involved.

SYMPTOMS AND COMPLICATIONS

Dislocation restricts or prevents the movement of the joint and is usually accompanied by severe pain. The joint looks misshapen and soon swells. In some cases, dislocation is followed by complications. For example, dislocation of the spinal vertebrae resulting from a severe back injury can damage the spinal cord, sometimes causing paralysis below the point of injury.

SYMPTOMS AND TREATMENT OF DISC PROLAPSE

A prolapsed disc in the lower back causes low back pain and, if the sciatic nerve root is compressed, *sciatica* (pain running down the back of the leg from the buttock to the ankle), sometimes accompanied by numbness and tingling. Low back pain and sciatica are usually aggravated by coughing, sneezing, bending, and sitting for long periods. Prolonged pressure on the sciatic nerve can lead to weakness in the muscles of the leg.

A prolapsed disc in the neck causes neck pain, stiffness, and, if the root of a nerve that is in the arm is compressed, tingling and weakness in that arm and hand.

In rare cases, pressure is exerted on the spinal cord itself, sometimes leading to paralysis of the legs and loss of bladder or bowel control.

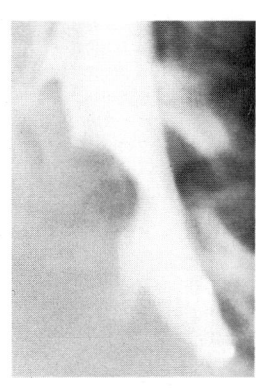

Before treatment
X-ray showing the prolapsed disc protruding into the spinal cord, affecting the nerve from that point downwards.

The sections of the spine

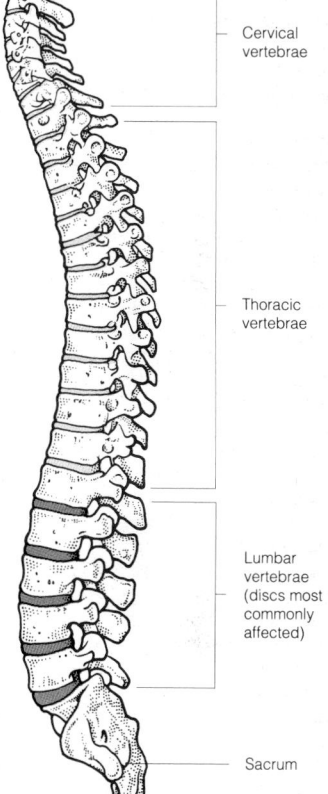

- Cervical vertebrae
- Thoracic vertebrae
- Lumbar vertebrae (discs most commonly affected)
- Sacrum
- Coccyx

Cross-section of a prolapsed disc
The fibrous outer layer is ruptured and some of its pulpy interior protrudes and presses on a spinal nerve root.

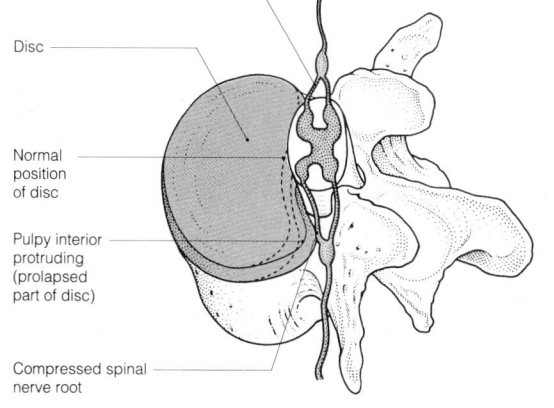

- Normal spinal nerve root
- Disc
- Normal position of disc
- Pulpy interior protruding (prolapsed part of disc)
- Compressed spinal nerve root

TREATMENT

Disc prolapse often responds to bed rest (lying flat on the back on a firm mattress for a few weeks) and analgesics; later, a supportive collar or corset and special exercises are helpful. If these measures fail and the nerve root compression is producing muscle weakness, an operation may relieve the pressure (see *Decompression, spinal canal*).

The head should be supported, and the shoulders, hips, and ankles aligned (as illustrated below) to ease pressure on the spine.

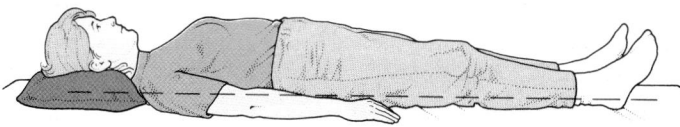

D

Dislocation of the shoulder or hip joint can damage major nerves in the arm or leg, which again sometimes results in paralysis.

Rarely, the tissue around a dislocated joint, usually the shoulder, becomes so weakened that after the joint has mended only minimal pressure causes another dislocation.

TREATMENT

FIRST-AID A person without medical qualifications should not attempt to manipulate the joint back into position because of the risk of seriously damaging nerves around the joint or making an accompanying fracture worse. A *splint* or, in the case of a dislocated shoulder, a *sling* should be applied to prevent movement of the joint. The victim should not take any food or drink because a general anaesthetic will probably be required when the bones are reset.

PROFESSIONAL The joint is usually first X-rayed to see whether a fracture is present. Then the bones are manipulated back into their proper position as quickly as possible, or, when manipulation is not feasible, an operation may be performed to reset them. After either procedure, the joint is usually immobilized by means of a splint or plaster cast to allow it to heal without disturbance. Recurrent dislocation is treated by surgery to shorten and tighten the ligaments of the joint, thus strengthening it.

Disopyramide

An *antiarrhythmic drug* used to treat abnormally rapid heartbeat, such as may occur after a *myocardial infarction* (heart attack). Disopyramide reduces the force of heart muscle contraction and, as a result, may occasionally aggravate pre-existing *heart failure*. Other possible adverse effects of the drug include dry mouth, constipation, and blurred vision.

Disorientation

Confusion as to time, place, or personal identity. The experience is similar to being awakened from a deep sleep. The disoriented person's speech and behaviour tend to be muddled, and he or she is often unable to answer simple questions about time, date, present location, name, or address.

Disorientation is usually caused by *head injury*, *intoxication*, or a chronic brain disorder, such as *dementia*. It may occasionally be due to *somatization disorder* (a psychological illness). (See also *Confusion*; *Delirium*.)

Displacement activity

The transference of feelings from one object or person to another. This is usually a conscious act, performed to obtain emotional relief in a manner that will not cause harm to oneself or to another person. For example, a person who is angry may hit a wall or throw something rather than risk harming someone else.

Displacement is regarded as an unconscious *defence mechanism*, by some psychotherapists. Disturbing or unwelcome feelings are prevented from entering consciousness by being transferred to another person or object. An understanding of this unconscious process is an important part of the interpretation of a patient's dreams during *psychoanalysis*.

Dissociative disorders

A group of psychological illnesses in which a particular mental function becomes cut off from the mind as a whole. Although the process of dissociation is common in everyday life (e.g. not hearing what is said because of concentration on another task), taking disassociation to extremes can lead to serious problems.

A common type of dissociative disorder is hysterical amnesia. The affected person is unable to remember his or her name or personal history, but can still speak, read, and learn new material (see *Hysteria*). Other forms of this disorder are *fugue*, *depersonalization*, and *multiple personality*. (See also *Conversion disorder*.)

Distal

A term describing a part of the body that is further away from another part with respect to a central point of reference, such as the trunk. For example, the fingers are distal to the arm with the trunk as the reference point. The opposite of distal is *proximal*.

Disulfiram

A drug that acts as a deterrent to drinking *alcohol*. Disulfiram is prescribed for people who request help for *alcohol dependence*. Treatment with disulfiram is usually combined with a counselling programme.

HOW IT WORKS

Alcohol is normally converted in the liver to acetaldehyde, which in turn is broken down to form acetic acid. Disulfiram slows down the breakdown of acetaldehyde, resulting in an increased level of this toxic substance which causes flushing, headache, nausea, dizziness, and palpitations.

These unpleasant symptoms usually start within an hour of drinking alcohol and can last for several hours.

POSSIBLE ADVERSE EFFECTS

Drowsiness and a metallic or garlic taste in the mouth frequently occur. These symptoms usually disappear within a few days as the body adapts to the drug. Occasionally, large amounts of alcohol taken during treatment can cause unconsciousness; a person taking disulfiram should carry a warning card indicating that he or she is taking the drug.

Dithranol

```
WARNING
Dithranol should not be applied to raw
or blistered areas of skin
```

A drug used to treat *psoriasis* (a skin disorder caused by excessive skin cell production). Dithranol, which is prescribed as an ointment, paste, or cream, works by slowing the rate at which skin cells multiply. This effect is sometimes boosted by ultraviolet light treatment (see *Phototherapy*). The normal method of use is to apply dithranol daily, leaving it on for between 30 minutes and an hour before washing it off.

POSSIBLE ADVERSE EFFECTS

Dithranol commonly causes skin inflammation, which may be relieved by application of a *corticosteroid drug*. The skin around patches of psoriasis can be protected from inflammation by applying *petroleum jelly*.

Dithranol may cause temporary staining of the skin and hair; it also stains clothing. Gloves and old clothing should therefore be worn when applying the drug.

Diuretic drugs

COMMON DRUGS

Thiazide
Bendrofluazide Chlorothiazide
Chlorthalidone Cyclopenthiazide

Loop
Bumetanide Frusemide

Potassium-sparing
Amiloride Spironolactone Triamterene

A group of drugs that help remove excess water from the body by increasing the amount lost as *urine*.

TYPES

The various types of diuretic drug differ markedly in their speed and mode of action.

THIAZIDE DIURETICS These diuretics cause moderate diuresis (increased urine production) and are suitable for prolonged use.

LOOP DIURETICS So called because they act on the region of the kidneys called Henle's loop, these are fast-acting, powerful drugs, especially when given by injection. Loop diuretics are particularly useful as an emergency treatment for *heart failure.*

POTASSIUM-SPARING DIURETICS These are often used along with thiazide and loop diuretics, both of which may cause potassium deficiency.

CARBONIC ANHYDRASE INHIBITORS Drugs that block the action of carbonic anhydrase (an enzyme that affects the amount of bicarbonate ions in the blood); these diuretic drugs cause moderate diuresis but are effective only for short periods.

OSMOTIC DIURETICS These are powerful diuretics that are used to maintain urine production after serious injury or major surgery.

WHY THEY ARE USED
By increasing the production of urine, diuretic drugs reduce the amount of water in the circulation and thus reduce the *oedema* (fluid retention in

tissues) that causes breathlessness and ankle swelling in *heart failure, nephrotic syndrome* (a kidney disorder), and *cirrhosis* of the liver. Diuretics can also relieve bloating and breast tenderness in *premenstrual syndrome.*

Diuretic drugs lower the blood pressure and are therefore used in the treatment of *hypertension* (high blood pressure). Carbonic anhydrase inhibitors are sometimes used to treat *glaucoma* (abnormally high fluid pressure in the eyeball).

POSSIBLE ADVERSE EFFECTS
Diuretic drugs may cause chemical imbalances in the blood, most commonly hypokalaemia (low levels of potassium in the blood). Symptoms of this condition include weakness, confusion, and palpitations. Treatment usually consists of a course of potassium supplements or a potassium-sparing diuretic drug. A diet rich in potassium (containing plenty of fruits and vegetables) may be helpful.

Some diuretic drugs may raise the level of uric acid in the blood, and thus increase the risk of *gout.* Certain types of diuretics increase the blood sugar level, an effect that can cause or aggravate *diabetes mellitus.*

Diurnal rhythms
A biological pattern based on a daily cycle; also called *circadian rhythms.* (See also *Biorhythms.*)

Diverticula
Small sacs or pouches that protrude externally from the wall of a hollow organ (such as the colon or the oesophagus). Diverticula are thought to be caused by pressure forcing the lining of the organ though areas of weakness in the wall. The presence of diverticula in the walls of the intestines is the characteristic feature of *diverticular disease.*

Diverticular disease
The presence of small externally protruding sacs or pouches known as *diverticula* in the wall of the intestines and any symptoms or complications caused by their presence.

Diverticula may form in any part of the intestine but usually affect the lower part of the *colon* (the major section of the large intestine). The cause is not conclusively established, but diverticula are thought to arise when pressure forces the lining of the colon through areas of weakness in the intestinal wall.

The term *diverticulosis* merely signifies the presence of diverticula in the intestine. *Diverticulitis* is a complication produced by inflammation due to obstruction and, occasionally, perforation (formation of a hole) in one or more diverticula.

Diverticulitis
Inflammation of *diverticula* in the intestine, particularly in the *colon.* It is a form of *diverticular disease* and a complication of *diverticulosis.*

Diverticulitis is associated with perforation (rupture) of diverticula and may lead to the formation of abscesses in the tissue around the colon. In exceptional circumstances, perforation may lead to *peritonitis* (inflammation of the lining of the abdomen). Bleeding of the intestinal wall may occur. Other complications of diverticulitis include the development of a stricture (narrowed section) in the intestine, or of a *fistula,* an abnormal channel that connects the affected part of the intestine to another part of the intestine or to the bladder or vagina.

SYMPTOMS AND SIGNS
Diverticulitis may cause fever, vomiting, abdominal pain, and rigidity of the abdomen over the area of the intestine involved. An abscess may be felt as a tender lump when a

---

HOW DIURETICS WORK
The normal filtration process of the kidneys (which takes place in the tubules) removes water, salts (mainly potassium and sodium), and waste products from the bloodstream. Most of the salts and water are returned to the bloodstream, but certain amounts are expelled from the body along with the waste products in the urine.

Diuretic drugs interfere with this normal kidney action. Osmotic, loop, and thiazide diuretics reduce the amount of sodium and water taken back into the blood, thus increasing urine volume. Other diuretics increase blood flow through the kidneys and thus the amount of water they filter and expel in the urine.

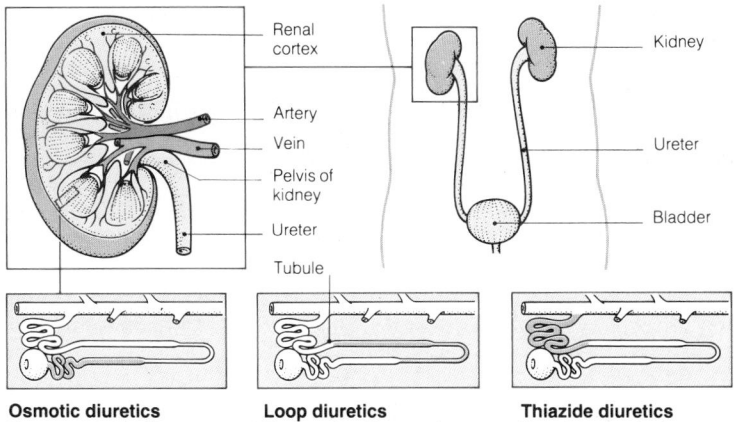

Renal cortex
Artery
Vein
Pelvis of kidney
Ureter
Tubule

Kidney
Ureter
Bladder

Osmotic diuretics
These act on the first part of the tubules to reduce water reabsorption into the bloodstream.

Loop diuretics
These take effect on the middle part of the tubules and block sodium and chloride reabsorption.

Thiazide diuretics
These act on the last part of the tubules to reduce reabsorption of sodium into the bloodstream.

D

doctor examines the abdomen. Intestinal haemorrhage may produce bleeding from the rectum.

TREATMENT
Diverticulitis usually subsides with bed rest and *antibiotic drugs*. In severe cases, a liquid diet or *intravenous infusion* may be required. Surgical treatment may be needed if perforation causes a large abscess or peritonitis, if bleeding cannot be controlled, or if a stricture develops. In most cases requiring surgery, the diseased section of the intestine is removed and the remaining sections are joined together. Some patients are given a temporary *colostomy* (an operation in which part of the colon is brought to the abdominal wall to form an opening for the discharge of faeces).

Diverticulosis

The presence of *diverticula* in the intestine, particularly in the *colon*. Diverticulosis is a form of *diverticular disease*. Complications, which are uncommon, include intestinal haemorrhage and *diverticulitis*.

CAUSES AND INCIDENCE
Lack of adequate dietary fibre (see *Fibre, dietary*) is believed to play an important role in the development of diverticulosis. The incidence of the condition increases with age: it is rare before the age of 20 but is found in more than half of all people aged over 80 in Western Europe and the US. In developing countries, however, diverticulosis is very rare.

SYMPTOMS
Symptoms occur in only 20 per cent of patients with diverticulosis and usually result from spasm or cramp of the intestinal muscle near diverticula.

Many patients have symptoms of *irritable bowel syndrome*, which may coexist with diverticulosis. In such patients, symptoms include a bloated sensation, episodes of pain in the lower abdomen, and changes in bowel habits (constipation, diarrhoea, or alternating attacks of both).

Intestinal haemorrhage may produce bleeding from the rectum.

DIAGNOSIS
Diverticula of the colon are easily diagnosed by *barium X-ray examination* or by *colonoscopy* (inspection of the colon with a flexible viewing instrument). A doctor should also investigate the possibility of cancer of the large intestine (see *Colon, cancer of*; *Rectum, cancer of*) in patients with symptoms of diverticulosis; tumours developing in affected areas may be difficult to diagnose.

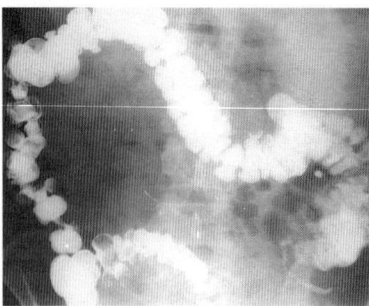

X-ray showing diverticulosis
In this X-ray taken after a barium meal, the bright, winding tube is the patient's colon. The knobs on its outer surface are diverticula.

TREATMENT
In patients with muscle spasms that cause cramps, a high-fibre diet, fibre supplements, and *antispasmodic drugs* may relieve symptoms. A high-fibre diet has also been shown to reduce the incidence of complications. Bleeding from diverticula usually subsides without treatment, but occasionally requires surgical treatment such as that for diverticulitis. Otherwise, surgery is rarely necessary.

Diving medicine

See *Scuba-diving medicine*; *Decompression sickness*.

Dizziness

A sensation of unsteadiness and light-headedness. Dizziness may be a mild, brief symptom that occurs by itself, or it may be part of a more severe, prolonged attack of *vertigo* (characterized by a spinning sensation) accompanied by nausea, vomiting, sweating, or fainting.

CAUSES
Most attacks of dizziness are harmless and are caused by a momentary fall in the pressure of blood to the brain, as can occur, for example, when getting up quickly from a sitting or lying position (a phenomenon called *postural hypotension*). Postural hypotension is more common in the elderly and in people taking *antihypertensive drugs* to treat high blood pressure. Similar symptoms may result from a temporary, partial blockage in the arteries that supply the brain—a *transient ischaemic attack* (symptoms of stroke lasting less than 24 hours).

Other causes of dizziness include tiredness, stress, fever, *anaemia, heart block* (impairment of electrical activity within the heart muscle, causing slow, uncoordinated beating of the

individual heart chambers), *hypoglycaemia* (low blood sugar level), and *subdural haemorrhage* (bleeding between the outer two membranes that cover the brain).

Dizziness as part of vertigo is usually due to a disorder of the inner ear, the *acoustic nerve*, or the *brainstem*.

The principal disorders of the inner ear that can cause dizziness and vertigo are *labyrinthitis* and *Ménière's disease*. In labyrinthitis, the labyrinth (the fluid-filled canals in the inner ear which play a vital role in balance) becomes inflamed, usually as a result of a viral infection. In severe cases, any movement of the head causes vomiting and fainting. In Ménière's disease (a degenerative disease of the inner ear), the dizziness and vertigo are often associated with *deafness* and *tinnitus* (noises in the ear).

Disorders of the acoustic nerve are relatively rare causes of dizziness and vertigo. They include *acoustic neuroma* and cases of *meningitis* in which the acoustic nerve is affected.

Disorders of the brainstem that can cause dizziness and vertigo include *migraine* that involves blood vessels in the brainstem; *brain tumours* that press on the brainstem; and *vertebrobasilar insufficiency* (narrowing of the blood vessels that supply part of the brainstem). Vertebrobasilar insufficiency, which is often due to *cervical osteoarthritis* (arthritis of the neck region of the spine), produces pain and dizziness on turning the head or moving the neck.

DIAGNOSIS AND TREATMENT
Brief episodes of mild dizziness usually clear up after taking a few deep breaths, or, if this fails, after resting for a short time.

Severe, prolonged, or recurrent dizziness should be investigated by a doctor, who will make a diagnosis from a description of the symptoms, from a physical examination, and, in some cases, from the results of further diagnostic tests.

Treatment, when necessary, depends on the underlying cause. For example, certain cases of dizziness and vertigo due to a disorder of the inner ear may be treated with *antiemetic drugs* or with *antihistamine drugs*.

DNA

The commonly used abbreviation for deoxyribonucleic acid, the principal molecule carrying genetic information in almost all organisms; the exceptions are certain viruses that

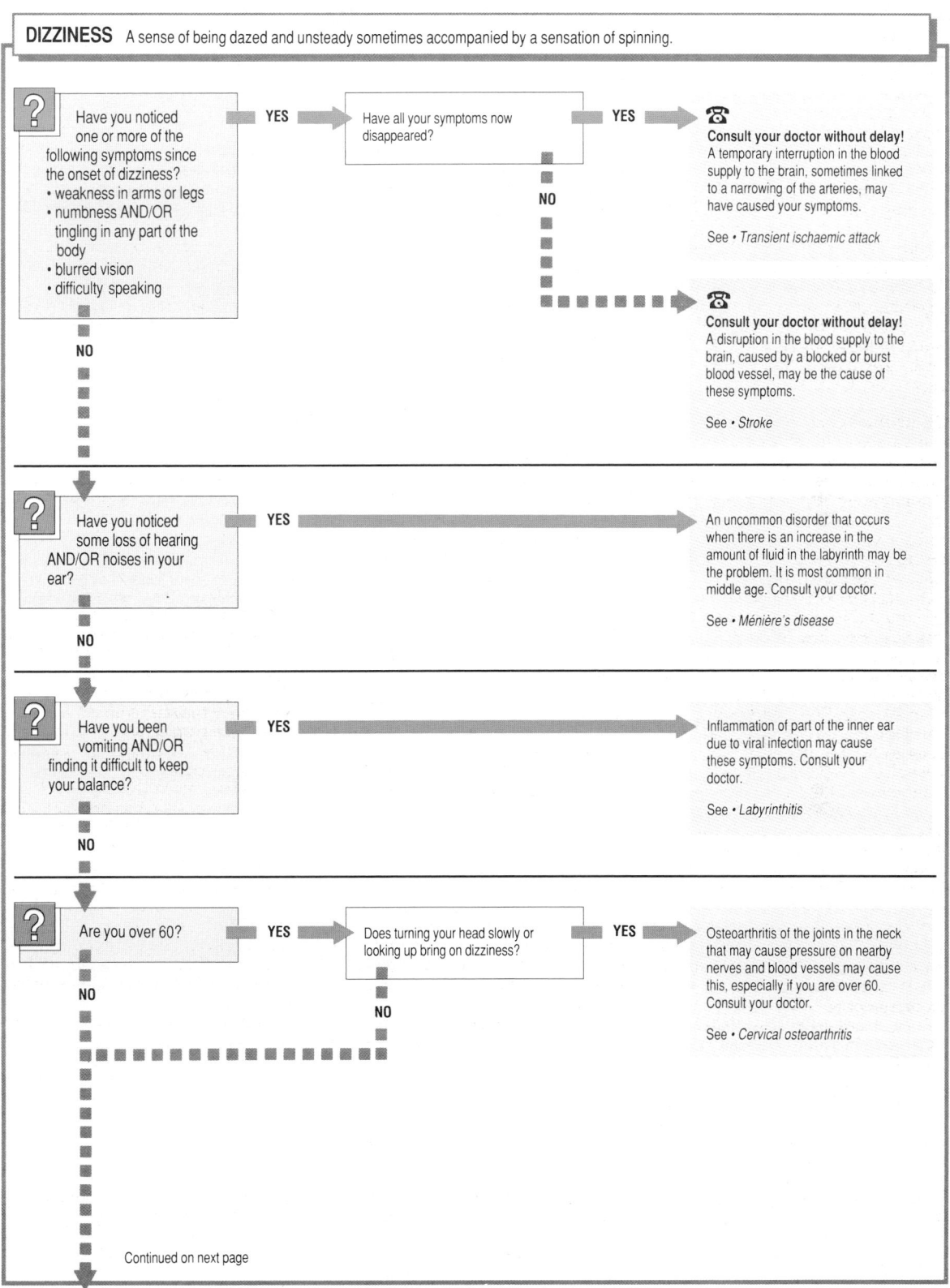

DIZZINESS A sense of being dazed and unsteady sometimes accompanied by a sensation of spinning.

D

? Have you noticed one or more of the following symptoms since the onset of dizziness?
• weakness in arms or legs
• numbness AND/OR tingling in any part of the body
• blurred vision
• difficulty speaking

YES → Have all your symptoms now disappeared?

YES →

☎ **Consult your doctor without delay!** A temporary interruption in the blood supply to the brain, sometimes linked to a narrowing of the arteries, may have caused your symptoms.

See • *Transient ischaemic attack*

NO

☎ **Consult your doctor without delay!** A disruption in the blood supply to the brain, caused by a blocked or burst blood vessel, may be the cause of these symptoms.

See • *Stroke*

NO

? Have you noticed some loss of hearing AND/OR noises in your ear?

YES → An uncommon disorder that occurs when there is an increase in the amount of fluid in the labyrinth may be the problem. It is most common in middle age. Consult your doctor.

See • *Ménière's disease*

NO

? Have you been vomiting AND/OR finding it difficult to keep your balance?

YES → Inflammation of part of the inner ear due to viral infection may cause these symptoms. Consult your doctor.

See • *Labyrinthitis*

NO

? Are you over 60?

YES → Does turning your head slowly or looking up bring on dizziness?

YES → Osteoarthritis of the joints in the neck that may cause pressure on nearby nerves and blood vessels may cause this, especially if you are over 60. Consult your doctor.

See • *Cervical osteoarthritis*

NO

NO

Continued on next page

367

D

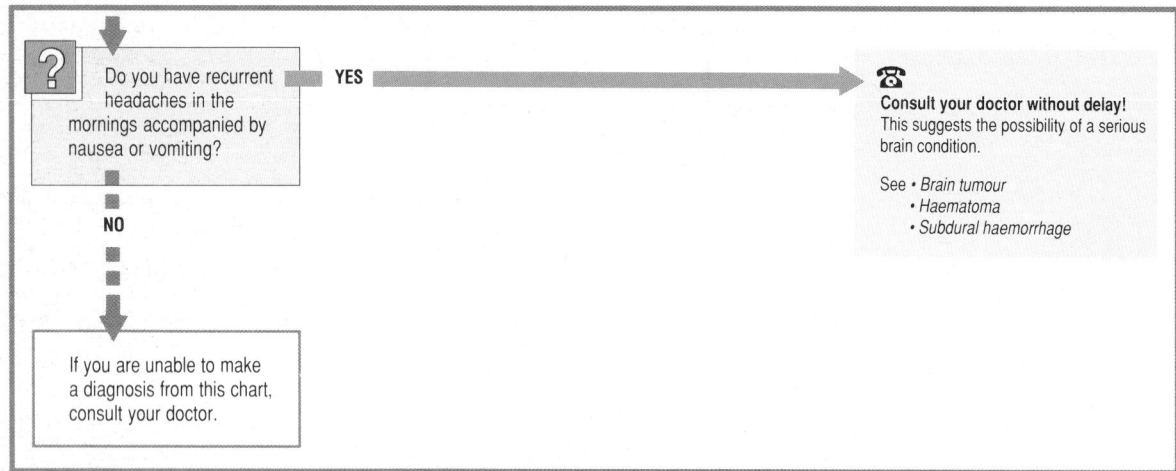

Do you have recurrent headaches in the mornings accompanied by nausea or vomiting?

YES

☎ **Consult your doctor without delay!**
This suggests the possibility of a serious brain condition.

See • *Brain tumour*
• *Haematoma*
• *Subdural haemorrhage*

NO

If you are unable to make a diagnosis from this chart, consult your doctor.

use *RNA* (ribonucleic acid) to carry genetic information. DNA is found in the *chromosomes* of cells; its double-helix structure allows the chromosomes to be copied exactly during the process of cell division. (See also *Nucleic acids.*)

DNA fingerprinting
See *Genetic fingerprinting.*

Dogs, diseases from
A number of infectious or parasitic diseases may be acquired from contact with dogs. Such diseases may be caused by viruses, bacteria, fungi, protozoa, worms, insects, or mites living in or on a dog.

Dogs and humans share various parasites. Many of these parasites show a marked preference for dogs, but may accidentally transfer to humans who stroke a dog's fur or touch contaminated faeces.

Overall, diseases contracted from dogs, especially the more serious ones, are uncommon and must be looked at together with the psychological benefits and pleasure that owners derive from their pets.

SPECIFIC DISEASES
The most serious disease that can be caught from a dog is *rabies*, usually transmitted by a bite. The UK is free of rabies but travellers to countries where rabies exists should treat any dog bite, particularly if the dog is a stray, with suspicion. Dog bites can also cause serious bleeding and shock and may become infected.

Two potentially serious, although rare, diseases caused by the ingestion of worm eggs from dogs are *toxocariasis* and *hydatid disease*. Toxocariasis is mainly an infection of children. The

passage of worm larvae through the body can cause allergic symptoms, such as *asthma*, and, rarely, a larva may lodge in an eye and cause blindness. Hydatid disease can lead to the harmful presence of cysts in the liver, lungs, brain, or elsewhere. Usually, however, sheep, not people, pick up the infection and then reinfect dogs; the disease is most common in sheep-rearing areas.

In the tropics, walking barefoot on sand or soil previously contaminated with dog faeces can lead to infection with dog *hookworms*.

Bites from dog *fleas* are an occasional nuisance. The fleas inhabit places in a house where the dog habitually rests and, if the dog is absent,

Ticks and fleas
Ticks may transfer from a dog's fur; fleas inhabit the pet's resting places and can cause irritating bites.

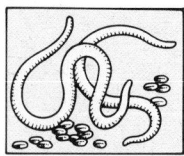

Worms and eggs
Worm eggs in dog faeces are a more serious danger than adult worms.

Transmission of infection
Transmission from faeces occurs when a person (often a child) directly handles a dog's faeces or anus (or contaminates his or her fingers with faecal material from the soil or from the dog's fur) and transfers infective

may jump on to humans for a meal. *Ticks* and *mites* from dogs, including a canine version of the *scabies* mite, are other common problems. The fungi that cause *tinea* (ringworm) infections cause progressive hair loss in dogs and can be caught by humans.

Some people become allergic to animal *dander* (tiny scales derived from fur or skin and present in household dust) and have such symptoms as asthma or *urticaria* (nettle rash) when a dog is in the house. (See also *Cats, diseases from; Zoonoses.*)

Domperidone
An *antiemetic drug* used to relieve the nausea and vomiting that occurs in some gastrointestinal disorders or

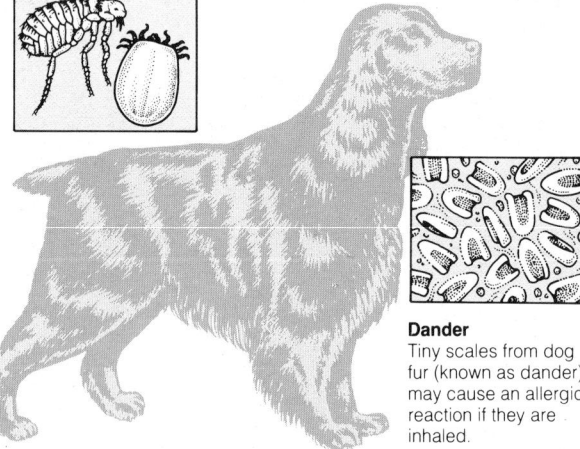

Dander
Tiny scales from dog fur (known as dander) may cause an allergic reaction if they are inhaled.

organisms to his or her mouth. Infection can also occur from eating food that has been contaminated with dog faeces. Other means of transferring infection are through saliva and direct contact with an infected dog.

during treatment with *anticancer drugs* or *radiotherapy*. Adverse effects of the drug, which are rare, may include breast enlargement and secretion of milk from the breast.

Donor

A person who provides blood for transfusion, tissues or organs for transplantation, or semen for artificial insemination.

Many individuals carry donor cards to indicate that they have bequeathed all or parts of their bodies to be used, should they die unexpectedly, for the treatment of others. The bequest may also be made by the next-of-kin at the time of death.

Donors should be free of cancer (other than primary brain cancer), should be free of serious infection (such as hepatitis B), and should not carry HIV (the AIDS virus). Organs are usually taken from people between the ages of three and 65.

In general, organs for transplantation must be removed within a few hours of *brain death*, and before or immediately after the heartbeat has stopped. An organ is used only if it is completely healthy.

In about one third of kidney transplants, the kidney is provided by a living donor. The living volunteer is usually a sibling or parent whose body tissues match well on the basis of *tissue-typing*. Tests are performed to make sure that both kidneys are healthy before one is removed for transplantation. A healthy donor's life is not shortened because the remaining kidney grows to compensate for the kidney that has been removed.

Suitable related donors whose tissue-types match may also provide bone marrow for transplantation and sometimes skin for grafting. (See also *Artificial insemination; Blood donation; Bone marrow transplant; Organ donation; Transplant surgery*.)

Dopamine

A *neurotransmitter* (chemical released from nerve endings) found in the brain and around some blood vessels. Dopamine blocks activity in specific nerves and is important in the control of body movements. A deficiency of dopamine in the *basal ganglia* (groups of nerve cells deep within the brain) causes *Parkinson's disease*.

Synthetic dopamine is injected as an emergency treatment for shock caused by a *myocardial infarction* (heart attack) or *septicaemia* (blood infection) and as a treatment for severe *heart*

COMMONLY DONATED BODY PARTS

The organs that are most frequently donated are kidneys, corneas, heart, lungs, liver, and pancreas.

Blood for transfusion and semen for artificial insemination are also given by donors.

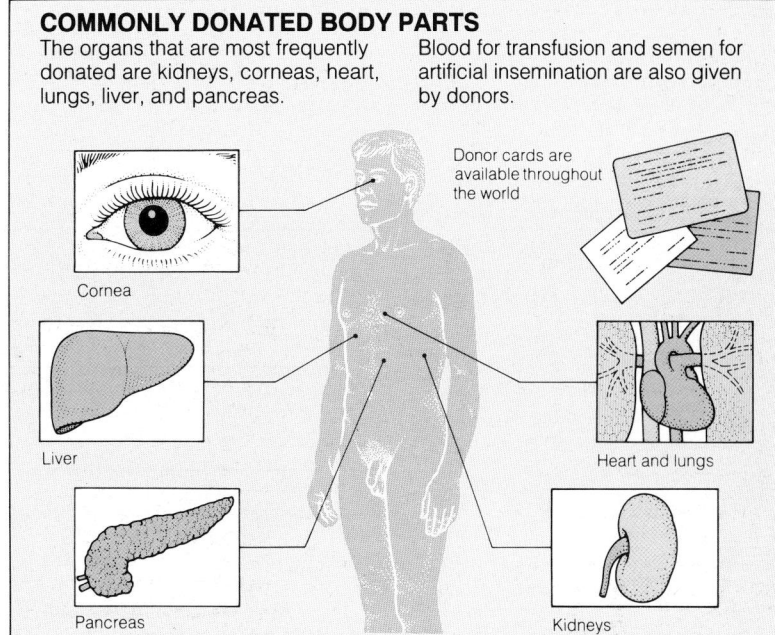

Donor cards are available throughout the world

Cornea

Liver

Pancreas

Heart and lungs

Kidneys

failure that has not responded to other drugs. Dopamine increases the efficiency of the heartbeat and helps return the blood pressure to normal.

Doppler effect

A change in the frequency with which waves from a given source reach an observer when the source is in rapid motion with respect to the observer.

When a fast-moving train blows its whistle as it passes through a station, a person standing on the platform hears an apparent increase in pitch (frequency) as the train approaches and then a lowering of pitch as the train passes and is moving away. In fact, the whistle gives off a constant pitch, but it seems to rise and then fall to the person on the platform because the wavelengths of the sound from the approaching train are progressively foreshortened whereas the wavelengths from the receding train are stretched. This change in the perceived frequency of sound as a result of movement is called the Doppler effect or Doppler shift.

The Doppler effect is utilized in various medical *ultrasound scanning* techniques. In these techniques, an emitter sends out pulses of ultrasound (inaudible high-frequency sound) of a specific frequency. When these pulses bounce off a moving object—blood flowing through a blood vessel or the beating heart of a fetus in the uterus,

for example—the frequency of the echoes is changed from that of the emitted sound (the Doppler effect in action). A special sensor detects the frequency changes and, for the examples above, converts this data into information about how fast the blood is flowing or the rate at which the fetal heart is beating.

Doppler ultrasound techniques are also used to measure blood pressure in superficial blood vessels and to detect air bubbles in *dialysis* and *heart-lung machines*.

Dorsal

Relating to the back, located on or near the back, or describing the uppermost part of a body structure when a person is lying face-down. For example, dorsalgia is pain in the back, and the dorsal part of the hand is the back of the hand. In human anatomy, the term dorsal means the same as posterior. The opposite of dorsal is *ventral* (anterior or front).

Dose

A term used to refer to the amount of a drug taken at a particular time, or to the amount of radiation an individual is exposed to during one session of *radiotherapy*.

DRUG DOSE

The dose of a drug can be expressed in several ways: in terms of the weight of its active substance, usually in milli-

D

grams; in terms of the volume of liquid to be drunk, usually in millilitres; or in terms of its biological activity potential (its effects on body tissues as calculated in a laboratory), a value usually given in units or international units.

It is not possible to compare the effects of two different drugs from the same group on the body simply by comparing the size of the doses. This is because some drugs are "stronger" (more potent) than others, just as various alcoholic drinks differ in their alcohol content.

RADIATION DOSE

The dose of radiation received during a session of radiotherapy is expressed in units called rads or grays (see *Radiation units* box). These units are a measure of the amount of radiation absorbed by body tissues. Different types of body tissue are able to absorb different amounts of energy from the same beam of radiation.

Dothiepin

A tricyclic *antidepressant drug* used in the long-term treatment of depression. As dothiepin has a sedative action, it is particularly useful when *depression* is accompanied by *anxiety* or *insomnia*. Dothiepin takes several weeks to have its full effect. Possible adverse effects include blurred vision, dizziness, flushing, and rash.

Double-blind

A type of *controlled trial*—the aim of which is to test the effectiveness of a treatment or to compare the benefits of different treatments. Double-blind trials differ from other types of controlled trials in that neither the patients taking part nor the doctors who assess the treatments know which patients are receiving which treatment. This eliminates any conscious or unconscious expectations (on the part of the patients and doctors) about which treatment will be most effective, which might affect the results of the trial.

For example, a new drug and an older, standard treatment might be compared by having the two drugs made up (by a person who otherwise takes no part in the trial) in identical capsules and giving them to different groups of patients on a random selection (chance) basis. The patients are later examined by one or more doctors. Only after all assessments have been made is the identity of the drug that was given to each patient revealed—usually by the person who originally prepared the capsules.

Double vision

The seeing of two instead of one visual image of a single object, also known as diplopia.

CAUSES

Double vision is usually a symptom of a squint, although not all types of squint produce double vision. Paralytic squint is a type that commonly causes double vision; in this type, movement of the eye in a particular direction is impaired due to paralysis of one or more of the eye muscles. Tilting or turning the head can sometimes overcome the double vision.

A tumour in the eyelid pressing on the front of the eyeball may cause temporary image separation by distorting the shape of the front of the eye and thus causing a slight displacement in the path of light-rays entering that eye (and thus variation in the points at which they are focused on the retina). A tumour or blood clot behind the eye that prevents the normal movement of the eyeball may also be a cause of double vision.

In endocrine-related *exophthalmos*, protrusion of the eyeballs is the result of an underlying hormonal disorder. In exophthalmos, double vision results from swelling and weakness of the eye muscles, causing abnormal alignment and motion of the eyes.

Rarely, double vision arises because of an abnormality within the eye. For example, *lens dislocation* may cause some light-rays to pass through the lens and others to pass around it, thereby causing separate images to fall on the retina.

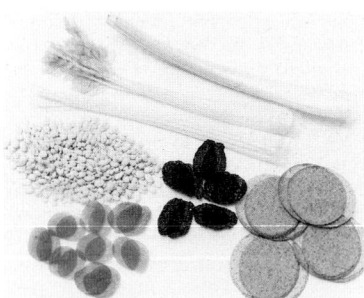

Example of double vision
Two images, rather than a single image, are seen. Prompt investigation by a doctor is required.

DIAGNOSIS AND TREATMENT

A child with a squint that may be causing double vision should be seen by a doctor for diagnosis and treatment. Without treatment in early childhood, squint can lead to the development of *amblyopia* (lazy eye).

The onset of double vision in adult life needs immediate investigation to exclude the possibility of a tumour, aneurysm, and/or nervous system abnormality. The double vision could be a symptom of a serious underlying disorder that requires prompt medical attention. Treatment depends on the cause.

Douche

Introduction of water and/or a cleansing agent into the vagina using equipment consisting of a bag and tubing with a nozzle attached.

In the past, douches were used by some women after sexual intercourse to cleanse the vagina and to try to prevent conception. They were also used by women who were worried about having excessive or offensive vaginal discharge. Douches were sometimes recommended to treat vaginal infections and were also used after vaginal repair operations.

Today, doctors rarely recommend douches for any reason. Douching is unnecessary for purposes of hygiene because the vagina is normally slightly acidic and cleans itself. As a method of *contraception*, douching is completely ineffective. Furthermore, use of a douche can be harmful, because it may introduce infection into the vagina or may spread an existing vaginal infection into the uterus or fallopian tubes.

Down's syndrome

A *chromosomal abnormality* resulting in mental handicap and a characteristic physical appearance. Down's syndrome was originally named "mongolism" because it was thought that the facial features of affected children resembled those of Mongolians. The term "mongolism" is no longer used by the medical profession.

CAUSES

The cause of Down's syndrome remained a mystery until 1959, when researchers discovered that each of the body cells of people with Down's syndrome has one too many chromosomes—47 instead of the normal 46. Because the extra chromosome is number 21 (affected individuals have three, instead of two, number 21 chromosomes), the disorder is also called trisomy 21.

There are several possible reasons for the chromosomal abnormality. In most cases it is the result of a failure of the two chromosomes numbered 21 in a parent cell to go into separate daughter cells during the first stage of sperm or egg cell formation (see *Chromosomes*). Some eggs or sperm are therefore formed with an extra number 21 chromosome and, if one of these takes part in fertilization, the resulting baby will also have the extra chromosome. This type of abnormality is particularly likely if the mother is aged over 35, suggesting that defective egg formation, rather than sperm formation, is usually at fault.

A less common cause is a chromosomal abnormality in either parent, known as a *translocation*, in which part of one of the parent's own number 21 chromosomes has joined with another chromosome. The parent is unaffected except for the high risk of having children with Down's syndrome. The chromosomal translocation may be familial, and relatives who are at risk of having an affected child should be tested by a blood sample for *chromosome analysis*.

INCIDENCE
About one in 650 fetuses has Down's syndrome; the frequency rises steeply with increased maternal age to around one in 40 in women aged over 40. Routine screening tests early in pregnancy, including measurement of the blood concentrations of alphafetoprotein and human chorionic gonadotrophin, indicate those fetuses likely to have the syndrome. In such cases, the mother will be offered chromosome analysis, in which samples of fetal cells are removed by *chorionic villus sampling* or *amniocentesis*. If the fetus is found to have trisomy 21, the parents may consider termination of the pregnancy.

SYMPTOMS
Most people with Down's syndrome have eyes that slope up at the outer corners and folds of skin on either side of the nose that cover the inner corners of the eye. The face and features are small, the tongue is large and tends to protrude, the head has a flattened back, and the hands are typically short and broad. The degree of mental handicap varies. A Down's syndrome child's IQ may be anywhere from 30 to 80. Virtually all affected children are capable of a limited amount of learning, including in some cases the ability to read. Down's syndrome children are usually affectionate, friendly, and cheerful, and they get along well with other members of the family.

About one quarter of Down's syndrome children have a heart defect at birth (see *Heart disease, congenital*). They also have a higher-than-average incidence of intestinal *atresia* (narrowing at some point in the intestines),

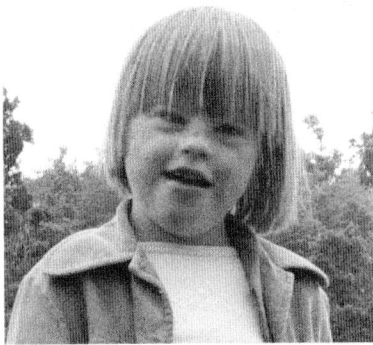

Typical features The eyes slope upwards at the outer corners and the inner corners are covered, the facial features are small, and the tongue is large and tends to stick out. The back of the head is usually flat.

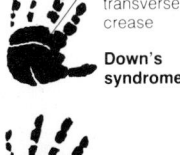

Inward-curving finger
Single transverse crease
Down's syndrome

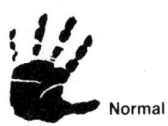

Normal

congenital *deafness*, and acute *leukaemia*. Children with Down's syndrome are especially susceptible to repeated ear infections. They also have an increased frequency of instability of the joints in the neck. In 1983, Special Olympics Inc. advised against people with Down's syndrome taking part in certain sports unless they had been medically certified to be free of risk. More recently these restrictions have been eased. For unknown reasons, *atherosclerosis* (narrowing of arteries by deposits of fatty material), which leads to an increased risk of heart disease, tends to develop early in adults affected by Down's syndrome.

DIAGNOSIS
Because of the distinctive physical features, Down's syndrome is usually recognized soon after birth. The diagnosis is confirmed by a count of the chromosomes in white blood cells taken from a blood sample (see *Chromosome analysis*).

TREATMENT
Although there is no cure for the mental handicap, children with Down's syndrome can make the most of their capabilities if they receive constant educational and environmental stimulation. Institutional care is sometimes necessary, but affected children are generally happiest in a sympathetic home environment. It is possible to alter the facial appearance by plastic surgery.

OUTLOOK
Until recently (less than a generation ago) most Down's syndrome children did not survive beyond their teens because of the high incidence of defects present from birth as well as their susceptibility to infection. Advances in medical and surgical techniques, together with improved long-term care facilities, have extended the life expectancy of sufferers from Down's syndrome, although they still tend not to survive beyond early middle age.

Doxorubicin
An *anticancer drug*, given by injection, often with other anticancer drugs. Doxorubicin is used to treat a variety of cancers, including *leukaemia*, *Hodgkin's disease*, and *lung cancer*.

Doxycycline
A *tetracycline drug*. Doxycycline has been found to be more effective than most other tetracycline antibiotics in the treatment of chronic *prostatitis* (inflammation of the prostate), *pelvic inflammatory disease*, and attacks of chest infection in chronic *bronchitis*. Doxycycline is also used to treat severe attacks of traveller's diarrhoea (see *Gastroenteritis*).

Because its action lasts longer than that of some other tetracyclines, doxycycline needs to be taken only once or twice a day.

Possible adverse effects, such as nausea and indigestion, can be reduced by taking doxycycline with food; absorption of doxycycline, unlike that of many other tetracyclines, is not impaired if the drug is taken with food.

DPT vaccination
An injection that provides immunity against *diphtheria*, *pertussis* (whooping cough), and *tetanus*; also known as triple vaccine.

HOW IT IS DONE
DPT vaccine is given as a course of three injections at around the ages of two, three, and four months. The precise age at which the injections are given is variable. A booster dose of diphtheria and tetanus vaccine is given at nursery or primary school entry age.

WHY IT IS DONE
DPT vaccination causes the body to produce *antibodies* against diphtheria, pertussis, and tetanus infections. The vaccine does not provide complete immunity to diphtheria, but it does reduce the risk of serious illness with the infection. Because DPT was not routinely administered in the UK until the 1940s, any adult exposed to

diphtheria should be checked for immunity. If a blood sample shows that there are no antibodies against the disease, diphtheria vaccine will then be administered.

The pertussis vaccine does not provide absolute protection, but children who have been immunized suffer from only a mild version of the disease and are unlikely to become seriously ill, whereas the disease can be fatal in unimmunized children. The protection gradually wanes, so adults can get the infection. In adults, the disease is mild, but adults can infect unimmunized children.

Protection against tetanus is not permanent; it needs to be "boosted" with another shot every 10 years or at the time of any dirty, penetrating injury if vaccination has not been performed within the last five years.

RISKS

In the cases of diphtheria and tetanus, the life-threatening feature of the infection is a toxin (poison) produced by the bacteria. The vaccine contains toxoids—modified versions of the diphtheria and tetanus toxins—that stimulate the formation of antibodies. Because the toxoids are chemicals not organisms, reactions to them are rare.

Pertussis vaccine consists of killed bacteria, which stimulate the formation of antibodies. It is more likely than the other components of the vaccine to provoke a reaction and commonly causes slight fever and some irritability for a couple of days after the vaccination. More serious reactions include signs of irritation of the brain and nervous system, which may lead to *seizures* (convulsions), and an allergic reaction, which may lead to sudden breathing difficulty and *shock*. Such serious reactions occur in fewer than one in 100,000 vaccinations. Permanent damage from the vaccine is even rarer.

Fears about the safety of the pertussis vaccine led many parents in the UK to refuse pertussis vaccination for their children in the mid-1970s and early 1980s. The result was an epidemic of pertussis. Between 1977 and 1983, several hundred children died as a result of pertussis infection; some cases of permanent brain damage or lung damage occurred as well.

Doctors are now agreed that for most children, the benefits of DPT vaccination outweigh the minimal risk from the vaccine. Vaccination should be postponed if the child has a feverish illness. The pertussis element of the vaccine should not be given to children who have reacted severely to a preceding dose of the vaccine, or to children who have a brain abnormality or who have suffered from seizures. The pertussis element may also not be recommended for children whose parents or siblings have a history of *epilepsy*, or for some children with disorders of the nervous system and with *developmental delay*.

Drain, surgical

An appliance inserted into a body cavity or wound to release air or to permit drainage.

TYPES

The simplest drains are soft rubber tubes that pass from a body cavity into a dressing. More sophisticated drains are wide-bore tubes that connect to a collection bag or bottle. A valve prevents air or fluid from passing back into the body. Another type, corrugated drains, have a series of curved ridges to help collect fluid from a wound. Suction drains consist of a thin tube with many small holes to help collect fluid or air, which is drawn into a vacuum bottle. Suction can also be applied to a drain by means of a vacuum pump. A T-shaped drain is used to remove bile from the biliary system after surgery.

Dream analysis

The interpretation of a person's dreams as part of *psychoanalysis* or *psychotherapy*. First developed by Sigmund Freud, the technique is based on the idea that a person's repressed feelings and thoughts are revealed in dreams, but in a disguised manner. The therapist unravels the significance of the dream by using a knowledge of the patient's character to interpret symbols, and by asking the patient for any associations suggested by the dream.

Dreaming

Mental activity that takes place during *sleep*. Evidence strongly suggests that dreaming occurs only during periods of REM (rapid eye movement) sleep, which last for about 20 minutes and occur four or five times a night.

PHYSIOLOGY

Although arguments about the exact function of dreams persist, the physiological aspects of dreams are well understood. By using an *EEG* to record the electrical activity of the brain, it is possible to describe various phases of sleep in terms of their different electrical patterns. Compared to other phases, the REM phase is

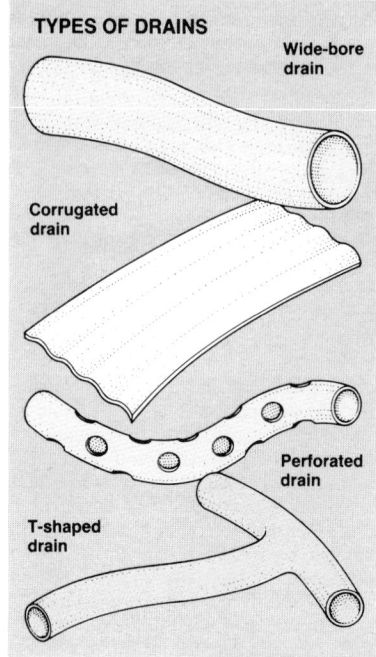

TYPES OF DRAINS

Wide-bore drain

Corrugated drain

Perforated drain

T-shaped drain

active, as if the sleeper were awake but drowsy. Blood flow and brain temperature increase and there are sudden changes in heart-rate and blood pressure. All this may indicate that the brain is restoring itself for further activity.

Dreaming can be seen as a parallel process in which the mental impressions, feelings, and ideas that have been taken in during the day are sorted out. The content of dreams therefore closely represents the day's preoccupations—with the ideas and memories distorted by the lack of a conscious and awake mind.

People roused during periods of REM sleep report especially vivid dreams, but those who wake normally after normal dream activity has ended may not remember dreaming at all.

SIGNIFICANCE

As a proportion of total sleep, REM sleep is much greater in young babies and after head injury. This suggests that REM sleep may have an important role in promoting brain activity. Whether or not dreams have an important psychological role is more controversial. Depriving people of their dreams by constantly waking them during REM phases was once thought to cause severe psychological disorders, but this is now less generally accepted. Some *hypnotic drugs* suppress REM sleep without causing obvious psychological harm.

Dressings

Protective coverings for *wounds*. Dressings are placed directly on to wounds and may be used to control *bleeding*, to absorb secretions, or to prevent contamination by bacteria or foreign material such as dirt.

Dressings should be large enough to cover a wound completely. They should be sterile so that they do not introduce bacteria that could cause infection. A dressing should also be absorbent in order to prevent the accumulation of sweat; otherwise, the skin around the wound becomes moist and soft, thus encouraging infection. Unless a wound needs regular cleaning, dressings should be left undisturbed. Wounds should be covered for as short a time as possible.

APPLYING A DRESSING

The basic procedure for applying a dressing is shown in the illustrated box below.

TYPES

ADHESIVE BANDAGES Available in a range of sizes, these consist of absorbent pads held in place by waterproof adhesive backings. They are commonly used to protect small wounds, such as cuts and abrasions, but may also be used to cover surgical wounds. **GAUZE** Usually applied in layers, gauze is made of cotton or a synthetic material and is used to cover larger wounds. It is held in place by a bandage or a length of adhesive strapping. The gauze is usually applied dry, but ribbon gauze, soaked in a substance that promotes healing, may be used for packing deep wounds. Prepacked, sterile, unmedicated dressings consist of layers of fine gauze and a pad of absorbent cotton attached to a roller bandage.

NONSTICK DRESSINGS These dressings consist of a nonadherent contact layer of perforated polyethylene or viscose with an impregnated gauze pad backing. Such dressings do not adhere to wounds and can be removed without disturbing newly formed tissue.

IMPROVISED DRESSINGS In an emergency, almost any clean, dry, and absorbent material (e.g. a handkerchief or piece of sheeting) may be used to cover a wound if a sterile dressing is not available. Cottonwool or other fibrous materials should not be used because the fibres may become embedded in the wound.

Dressler's syndrome

An uncommon condition, also called postinfarction syndrome, that may occur after a *myocardial infarction* (heart attack) or after heart surgery. The condition is characterized by fever, chest pain, *pericarditis* (inflammation of the membrane surrounding the heart), and *pleurisy* (inflammation of the membrane surrounding the lungs).

Dressler's syndrome is thought to be an *autoimmune disorder*. The body's immune system produces *antibodies* (proteins with a defensive role) which are directed against the damaged areas of heart muscle.

The features of the condition first appear any time between a few days and several weeks after a myocardial infarction or heart surgery. The diagnosis is confirmed by detecting specific antibodies in the blood. Treatment with *aspirin* usually clears the condition, although, in some more severe cases, treatment with *corticosteroid drugs* is needed.

Dribbling

A term commonly used to denote involuntary leakage of urine (see *Incontinence, urinary*) or of saliva from the mouth.

Dribbling of saliva, also known as drooling, is normal behaviour in infants up to the age of about 12 months. Dribbling of saliva in an adult may simply be due to poorly fitting dentures or may be the result of facial paralysis, *dementia*, or another serious disorder of the nervous system, most commonly *Parkinson's disease*. Dribbling of saliva may also be caused by obstruction to swallowing.

Drip

See *Intravenous infusion*.

Drop attack

A brief disturbance affecting the nervous system, causing a person to fall suddenly to the ground without warning. Unlike in *fainting*, the per-

---

FIRST AID: DRESSINGS

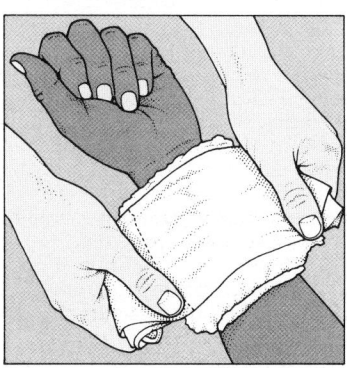

1 Remove outer protective wrapping, being careful not to touch the gauze. If possible, wash your hands before touching the unwrapped dressing. Then hold the dressing, gauze-side down, over the wound.

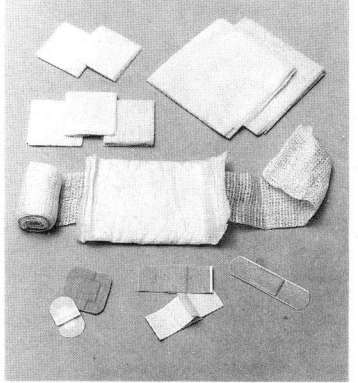

Assorted dressings
In addition to sterile dressings, plain gauze and a variety of sticking plasters can be used.

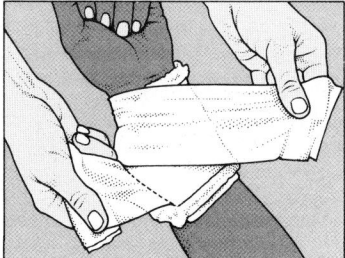

2 Wind the short end of the bandage once around the arm and dressing. Bandage firmly (not tightly) and cover the gauze pad.

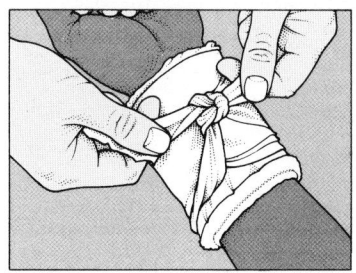

3 Secure the bandage by tying the two ends over the gauze pad using a reef knot (left end over right end, and under; right end over left end, and under).

D

son may not lose consciousness, but injuries can occur to the hands, face, or knees as a result of the fall.

CAUSES AND INCIDENCE
Although drop attacks can affect all age groups, elderly women are the most commonly affected. The causes are not fully understood, although in some cases there may be a fall in blood flow to nerve centres in the *brainstem*.

Occasionally, elderly men may experience a drop attack while passing urine or while standing. Lowered blood pressure or an abrupt alteration in heart rhythm may be involved; it is advisable for a man who has previously had an attack to sit down while urinating.

Another rare cause of drop attacks is a block in the flow of cerebrospinal fluid around the brain, usually in patients with a type of *hydrocephalus*. Also sometimes described as drop attacks are akinetic seizures (a rare form of *epilepsy*), in which the sufferer falls suddenly to the ground and briefly loses consciousness but does not have muscular spasms.

TREATMENT
There is no treatment for drop attacks in the elderly. Akinetic seizures respond to *anticonvulsant drugs*.

Dropsy

An outmoded term for generalized *oedema* (fluid collection in body tissues). In the past, many people were certified dead "due to dropsy", which, however, is not a disease in itself, but merely a sign of malfunction in the body (especially congestive *heart failure* or kidney disease).

Drowning

Death caused by suffocation and *hypoxia* (lack of oxygen) associated with immersion in a fluid.

In about four fifths of drownings the person has inhaled liquid into the lungs; in the other fifth, no liquid has entered the lungs—a condition called dry drowning (see *Drowning, dry*). People who are resuscitated after prolonged immersion are said to be victims of "near drowning".

INCIDENCE AND CAUSES
Drowning accounts for about 350 deaths a year in England and Wales. Many more are victims of near drowning. Worldwide, possibly as many as 200,000 people drown annually.

Many victims are competent swimmers who have failed to take into account factors such as tidal currents (or undertow) and have become tired, and then panicked. A relatively small number of victims are nonswimmers. Other drowning circumstances include floods, sinkings, immersion in very cold water after falling through ice, and infant drownings, which can occur in very shallow water.

Over one third of drowning victims have a significant amount of alcohol in their blood upon postmortem examination. Alcohol intoxication impairs judgment and at the same time reduces physical coordination—an extremely dangerous combination before swimming.

Some methods of minimizing the risks of a drowning accident are shown in the box below.

MECHANISM OF DROWNING
The thrashing movements that a panicking person makes at the surface of the water are incapable of keeping the body afloat, and the person begins taking in small amounts of water. Initially, automatic contraction of a muscle at the entrance to the windpipe—a mechanism called the laryngeal reflex—prevents water from entering the lungs and instead it enters the oesophagus and stomach. However, the laryngeal reflex impairs breathing, which can quickly lead to hypoxia and to loss of consciousness.

If the person is buoyant at this point and floats face-up, his or her chances of survival are reasonable because the laryngeal reflex begins to relax and normal breathing may recommence.

FIRST AID AND TREATMENT
If a person is panicking at the surface of the water, he or she should be thrown any large item that will float. Ideally, the person in difficulties should be approached in a boat and reached out for. If approached by swimming, an attempt should be

---

DROWNING: RESCUE METHODS
Throwing the victim something to hold on to is useful if he or she is still conscious and has not panicked.

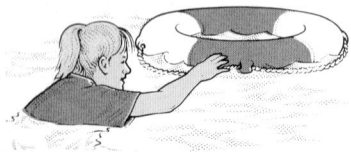

Rescuing from a boat
After grasping the victim's arms, it may be necessary to "bounce" him or her in the water to gain momentum for a lift into the boat. When there are two rescuers, one can enter the water to assist.

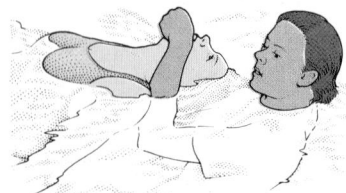

Otherwise, approach the victim in a boat or, if no boat is available, reach him or her by swimming.

Throwing a buoy or line
If no life-buoy is available, use any large object that floats. It should preferably have a rope attached to pull the person to safety (a rope alone may be sufficient).

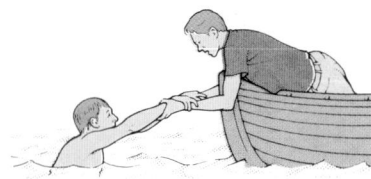

Towing
A panicky victim may need to be calmed before making contact; otherwise, he or she may struggle. During the tow ashore, it is important to keep the victim's face above water.

MEASURES THAT MAY HELP PREVENT DROWNING ACCIDENTS

1 Never jump into deep water without ensuring that there is an easy and obvious method of exit.

2 Wear a life-jacket or buoyancy device for all water sports (such as sailing and windsurfing).

3 Swim only in pools or from public beaches designated as safe and patrolled by lifeguards.

4 Do not drink alcohol before swimming or taking part in water sports of any kind.

5 Children should always be supervised when swimming and when they are taking baths.

6 Children should never walk on an iced-over pond or river unless the ice has first been tested by an adult.

made to calm the person before contact is made, otherwise he or she may struggle, possibly causing the rescuer to drown as well.

The victim should be supported with his or her head above water and towed to the nearest boat or shore. An ambulance should be called and the person's medical condition assessed. If breathing and/or the pulse (felt in the neck) is absent, resuscitative measures should be started (see *Artificial respiration; Cardiopulmonary resuscitation*). These measures should be continued until an ambulance or doctor has arrived.

Because of the operation of a primitive reflex, known as the "diving reflex", which preserves a minimal blood supply to the brain, victims can sometimes be resuscitated despite a long period of immersion in very cold water (which reduces the body's oxygen needs) and the initial appearance of being dead. In all cases of successful resuscitation, the person should be sent to a hospital for investigation and observation. Life-threatening symptoms may develop some hours after rescue, because water may have passed from the lungs into the blood and the lining of the lungs may have been damaged.

Drowning, dry

A form of *drowning* in which no fluid enters the lungs. About one fifth of fatal drowning cases are "dry". Victims of dry drowning have a particularly strong laryngeal reflex, which diverts water into the stomach instead of the lungs, but at the same time impairs breathing.

Drowsiness

A state of consciousness between full wakefulness and *sleep* or *unconsciousness*. Drowsiness is medically significant if it is abnormal, that is, if a person fails to awaken after being shaken, pinched, and shouted at, or wakes but relapses into drowsiness.

Abnormal drowsiness may be the result of a *head injury*, high fever, *meningitis* (inflammation of the membranes that surround the brain and spinal cord), *uraemia* (excess urea in the blood due to *kidney failure*), or *liver failure*. Alcohol or drugs may also produce this effect. In a person with *diabetes mellitus*, drowsiness may be due to *hypoglycaemia* (low blood sugar), usually as a result of taking too much insulin, or to *hyperglycaemia* (high blood sugar) due to inadequate control of the disorder.

Abnormal drowsiness should be treated as a medical emergency and professional help should be called immediately.

Drug

Any chemical substance that alters the function of one or more body organs or changes the process of a disease. Drugs include prescribed medicines, over-the-counter remedies, and substances, such as alcohol, tobacco, and drugs of abuse, that are used for non-medical purposes. Many foods and drinks contain small quantities of substances classed as drugs—tea, coffee, and cola drinks, for example, all contain *caffeine*, which is both a *stimulant drug* and a *diuretic drug*.

Each drug normally has three names: a detailed, descriptive chemical name; a shorter, generic name (see *Generic drug*) that has been officially approved; and a specific brand name chosen by the company that manufactures the drug.

Drugs are either licensed for prescription by a doctor only or are over-the-counter preparations available at a chemist or supermarket.

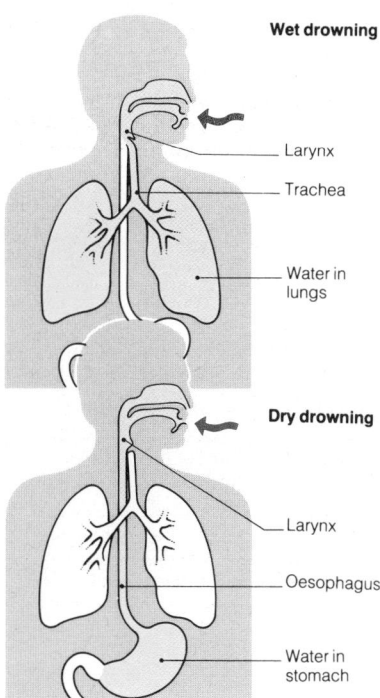

Wet drowning

— Larynx

— Trachea

— Water in lungs

Dry drowning

— Larynx

— Oesophagus

— Water in stomach

Types of drowning
In four fifths of deaths due to drowning, the victim has inhaled liquid into his or her lungs. In the other fifth, no liquid is present in the lungs (dry drowning). In both cases, death is by suffocation.

SOURCES

Formerly, all drugs were naturally occurring substances extracted from animals, plants, and minerals. Today, most drugs are produced artificially in the laboratory, ensuring a purer preparation with a predictable potency (strength) that is safer for medical use. Some drugs, such as *insulin* and *growth hormone*, are now mainly synthesized by means of *genetic engineering* procedures.

New drugs are discovered in a number of ways: by screening a substance for different types of activity against a disease; by making alterations to the structure of an established drug; or, occasionally, by finding a new application for a drug that is being used for another condition.

CLASSIFICATION

A drug is classified in one of the following ways: first, according to its chemical make-up (a *corticosteroid drug*, for example); second, according to the disorder it treats (an *antihypertensive drug*, for example, is used to treat high blood pressure); or, third, according to its specific effect on the body (the effect of a diuretic drug, for example, is to produce diuresis, that is, to increase the volume of urine excreted).

EVALUATION

All new drugs are tested for their efficiency and safety. Tests usually go through three stages: laboratory trials on animals; laboratory trials on human volunteers; and, finally, clinical trials on patients.

The Department of Health (DH) will issue a licence if studies provide evidence of the drug's efficacy and safety according to strictly defined standards. The DH also establishes standards of quality, purity of the preparation, and adequate labelling.

Evaluation continues even after a drug has become widely prescribed. A drug's licence may be withdrawn if toxic effects are reported frequently or if even a few patients develop serious illness attributable to the drug. Doctors report any adverse effects from particular drugs to the Committee on Safety of Medicines (CSM).

WHY DRUGS ARE USED

Drugs can be used in the treatment, prevention, or diagnosis of a disease. They are prescribed to relieve physical or mental symptoms, to replace a deficient natural substance (such as a *hormone*), or to stop the excessive production of a hormone or other body chemical. Some drugs are given to destroy foreign organisms, such as bacteria or viruses. Others, known as *vaccines*, are given to stimulate the body's *immune system* (natural defences) to form *antibodies*.

Antibiotic drugs, diuretic drugs, *analgesic drugs* (painkillers), and *tranquillizer drugs* are among the most commonly prescribed drugs. The most frequently used over-the-counter preparations include analgesics, *cough remedies*, *cold remedies*, *vitamin supplements*, and *tonics*.

HOW DRUGS WORK

Drugs act on cells in the body or the infecting organism by stimulating or blocking chemical reactions. In many cases, this action occurs because the drug mimics a chemical that occurs naturally in the body.

Some drugs act by binding (becoming attached) to a drug receptor (a specific site on the cell's surface that matches up with the chemical structure of the drug). This triggers a change in chemical activity within the cell. Other drugs work by being absorbed into the cell, where they affect the chemical processes directly.

Drugs may also have a *placebo* effect, which occurs as a result of the individual's expectations of the drug's action.

METHODS OF ADMINISTRATION

Drugs are given in different forms and in different ways (see table). These methods depend on many factors, including the severity of the illness, the part of the body being treated, the properties of the drug, and the speed and duration of action required.

ELIMINATION

Drugs taken by mouth that are not absorbed in the intestine are excreted in the faeces. Drugs that have entered the bloodstream are eliminated via the kidneys, in the urine. Some drugs are broken down into inactive forms in the liver by *enzymes* before being eliminated.

COMPLIANCE

If drug treatment is to be beneficial, the full course must be taken as instructed by a doctor. It is estimated that as many as two out of every five people who are prescribed a drug do not take it properly, if at all. Reasons for noncompliance include failure to understand instructions, fear of possible reactions, adverse effects, or simply not bothering to take the drug.

DRUG INTERACTIONS

Taking drugs together or in combination with food or alcohol may produce effects on the body that differ from those occurring when a drug is taken on its own. Such drug interactions

METHODS OF ADMINISTERING DRUGS

How taken		Action
By mouth		Drugs are digested and absorbed from the intestine in the same way as nutrients. How quickly the tablet or liquid works depends on how rapidly it is absorbed. This, in turn, depends on such factors as the drug's composition, how quickly the drug dissolves, and the effect of digestive juices on it.
By injection		Drugs given by injection have a very rapid effect. Injection is also used if digestive juices would destroy a drug.
As a cream, anal or vaginal suppository, pessary, nasal spray, or by inhaler		These drugs have a local effect on the parts of the body that are exposed to them as well as a systemic (generalized) effect if some of the drug is absorbed into the bloodstream from the site of application.

occur if chemicals in the different substances act on the same receptors or if one chemical alters the absorption, breakdown, or elimination of another.

Doctors commonly make use of interactions to increase the effectiveness of a treatment; combinations of drugs are often prescribed to treat infection, cancer, or hypertension (high blood pressure). Many interactions, however, are unplanned; they may reduce the benefit from a drug or increase its level in the blood and cause adverse effects.

Patients undergoing long-term drug treatment may be advised to carry cards that warn of potentially dangerous interactions from treatment that may be given during an emergency. Patients should tell their doctors about any other drugs they are taking to prevent interactions with drugs the doctor may prescribe.

ADVERSE EFFECTS

Most drugs can produce adverse effects—harmful or unpleasant reactions that result from a normal dose of the drug. These adverse effects can be divided into predictable adverse reactions, which result from the chemical structure of the drug, and bizarre (unpredictable) reactions, which are unrelated to the drug's normal chemical effects on body cells.

Predictable adverse reactions are due to the difficulty in targeting a drug on a single organ. For example, *anticholinergic drugs* prescribed to relieve spasm in the intestine also cause blurred vision and dryness of the mouth. Symptoms may wear off as the body adapts to the drug; other-

wise, they usually are relieved by reducing the dose or increasing the interval between doses.

Any change in the absorption, breakdown, or elimination of a drug (caused, for example, by liver or kidney disease) that increases its concentration in the blood will increase the risk of predictable adverse effects.

Bizarre drug reactions may be due to a genetic disorder (for example, lack of a specific enzyme that usually inactivates the drug), an allergic reaction, or the formation of *antibodies* that damage tissue. Common side-effects of this type include a rash, facial swelling, or jaundice. Occasionally, *anaphylactic shock* (a severe allergic reaction), characterized by breathing difficulty or collapse, may occur. Bizarre drug reactions usually make it necessary to withdraw the drug.

Many drugs cross the placenta and some adversely affect growth and development of the fetus. Most drugs pass into the breast milk of a nursing mother and some will have adverse effects on the baby.

A drug is useful only if its overall benefit to the patient outweighs the risk and severity of any adverse effects. Research on new drugs partly aims to discover preparations that act selectively on target organs to avoid unwanted effects on other tissues.

Drug abuse

The use of a drug for a purpose other than that for which it is normally prescribed or recommended. Among the many reasons for drug abuse are the desire to escape from reality or achieve a mystical experience, curiosity about a drug's effects, and the search for self-awareness.

Commonly abused drugs include *stimulant drugs*, such as *amphetamine drugs*; central nervous system depressants, such as *alcohol* and *barbiturate drugs*; *hallucinogenic drugs*, such as *LSD*; and *narcotic drugs*, such as *cocaine* and *heroin*. Certain types of drug are sometimes abused to improve performance in sports (see *Sports, drugs and*; *Steroids, anabolic*).

Problems resulting from drug abuse may arise from the adverse effects of the drug, from accidents during intoxication, and from the habit-forming potential of many drugs, which may lead to *drug dependence*.

Drug addiction

Physical or psychological dependence on a drug. (See *Drug dependence*.)

Drug dependence

The compulsion to continue taking a drug, either to produce the desired effects that result from taking it, or to prevent the ill-effects that occur when it is not taken.

TYPES

Drug dependence takes two forms: psychological and physical. A person is psychologically dependent if he or she experiences craving or emotional distress when the drug is withdrawn. In physical dependence the body has adapted to the presence of the drug, causing the symptoms and signs of *withdrawal syndrome* when the drug is withdrawn. Withdrawal is usually associated with severe physical and mental distress.

CAUSES AND INCIDENCE

Drug dependence develops as a result of regular and/or excessive use of a drug. Large numbers of people are dependent on *nicotine* in tobacco, on the *caffeine* in coffee and tea, and on *alcohol*. A significant proportion of the population is dependent on *tranquillizer drugs*.

Dependence develops most frequently with drugs that alter the individual's mood or behaviour. The speed with which a drug acts on the body is another factor in the development of dependence. Intravenous drug abuse, for example, produces a rapid effect on the body, which reinforces the habit of injecting the drug.

Some people seem to be more susceptible to dependence than others. Factors that usually play a part include pressure from friends and associates, and environmental factors, such as poverty, unemployment, disrupted family life, and the availability of drugs. Hereditary factors may also play a part.

SYMPTOMS AND SIGNS

A mild withdrawal reaction may cause yawning, sneezing, a runny nose, watering eyes, and sweating. More severe reactions include diarrhoea, vomiting, trembling, cramps, confusion, and, rarely, fits and coma. These symptoms are usually relieved if the drug is taken again.

Withdrawal symptoms probably occur because the body has become adapted to the continuous presence of the drug, which reduces the release of certain natural chemicals (e.g. nicotine affects production of *adrenaline* and similar substances). When the drug is no longer taken or is withheld, the chemical deficiency is exposed.

COMPLICATIONS

Drug dependence may cause physical problems, such as lung and heart disease from tobacco-smoking and liver disease from drinking excessive amounts of alcohol. Mental problems, such as anxiety and depression, are common during withdrawal. Dependence may also be associated with drug tolerance, in which an increasingly higher dose of the substance is needed to produce the desired effect.

Complications may occur as an indirect result of dependence. For example, people who inject a *narcotic drug* may become ill and die from *hepatitis* or *AIDS*, contracted as a result of introducing infection into the bloodstream via a dirty needle. In other cases, abusers may suffer from an overdose because of confusion about the dosage or because they take a purer, more potent preparation than they are used to. Social problems often result from the disruption of family life and from criminal acts carried out to pay for drugs.

TREATMENT

Controlled withdrawal programmes are available in special centres and larger hospitals. These programmes usually offer supervised reductions in dose. Alternative, less harmful drugs may be given, as well as treatment for withdrawal symptoms. Social service agencies and support groups may provide follow-up care.

OUTLOOK

Successful treatment requires motivation on the part of the dependent person. Problems frequently recur when people return to the circumstances that originally gave rise to drug abuse and dependence.

Drug overdose

The taking of an excessive amount of a drug, which may cause toxic effects. (See *Drug poisoning*.)

Drug poisoning

The harmful effects on various organs of the body as a result of taking an excessive dose of a drug.

CAUSES AND INCIDENCE

Drug poisoning may be accidental or deliberate. Accidental poisoning is most common in young children under the age of five years who swallow coloured tablets thinking they are sweets. Child-resistant drug containers have helped reduce this risk. In adults, accidental poisoning usually occurs in elderly or confused people who are uncertain about their treatment and dosage requirements. Accidental poisoning may also occur during *drug abuse*.

Deliberate self-poisoning is usually unsuccessful and is done as a cry for help (see *Suicide*; *Suicide, attempted*). The drugs that are most commonly taken in overdose are *benzodiazepine drugs*, *antidepressant drugs*, *paracetamol*, or *aspirin*. Homicide may involve the administration of a drug by another person.

TREATMENT

In dealing with a drug overdose, first-aid measures depend on the condition of the patient. If the patient is unconscious, ensure that the *airway* is clear and that there is normal breathing and a pulse before rolling the patient into the *recovery position* and summoning emergency help. If the person is not breathing, *artificial respiration* should be started.

Any individual who has taken a drug overdose and any child who has swallowed tablets that belong to someone else should be seen by a doctor. It is important to identify the drugs which have been taken. Drug containers and any drugs that are near the victim may provide vital clues; save any you find. Contact a hospital casualty department or your GP for advice. If the victim is fully conscious, you may be advised to induce vomiting by sticking a finger down his or her throat or by giving an *emetic* if one is available.

Some drugs taken in excess may cause *hypothermia*; if this occurs, keep the victim warm with blankets.

Treatment in hospital may involve washing out the stomach using several litres of water passed down a tube through the mouth and oesophagus (see *Lavage, gastric*). However, this procedure is effective only if it is performed within a few hours of taking the overdose.

Charcoal may be given by mouth in some cases to reduce the absorption of the drug from the intestine into the bloodstream. Increased production of urine may be induced by an *intravenous infusion* to speed up the elimination of the drug from the bloodstream; the infusion solution will be either acidic or alkaline depending on the drug taken.

Antidotes are available only for specific drugs. Such antidotes include *naloxone* (given to reverse breathing difficulty caused by *morphine*), methionine (given to reduce the formation of toxic substances from paracetamol in the liver), and *chelating agents* such as desferrioxamine (given to absorb and inactivate iron).

COMPLICATIONS
Drug poisoning may cause drowsiness and breathing difficulty (due to effects on the brain), irregular heartbeat, and, rarely, cardiac arrest, fits, and kidney and liver damage. Monitoring of the heartbeat by *ECG* is usually carried out for the first 24 to 48 hours after poisoning with a drug that is known to have effects on the heart. *Antiarrhythmic drugs* are prescribed to treat any heartbeat irregularity as it develops. Fits are treated with *anticonvulsant drugs*. In some serious cases, the patient requires artificial *ventilation* because of severe drug-induced breathing difficulty.

Blood tests to monitor liver function and careful monitoring of urine output are carried out if the drug is known to have any toxic effect on the liver or kidneys.

Dry eye
See *Keratoconjunctivitis sicca*.

Dry ice
Frozen *carbon dioxide,* also known as carbon dioxide snow. Unlike most substances, carbon dioxide changes directly from a gas to a solid when it is cooled, without first passing through a liquid phase. In practice, dry ice is produced by allowing carbon dioxide gas stored under pressure to escape through a small nozzle. This rapid expansion cools the carbon dioxide to about -70°C, and dry ice is formed as a powder. This powder is then compressed into cakes.

Dry ice is sometimes applied to the skin in *cryosurgery,* a freezing technique used, for example, to destroy *warts* and *naevi*.

Dry socket
Infection at the site of a recent tooth extraction, causing pain, bad breath, and an unpleasant taste. Dry socket is a complication of about four per cent of extractions. It occurs most commonly when a blood clot fails to form in the tooth socket after a difficult extraction, such as removal of an impacted wisdom tooth (see *Impation, dental*). Infection may also develop following a normal extraction if the blood clot becomes dislodged (for instance, because of excessive rinsing of the mouth). In some cases, the clot itself may become infected, or infection may already have been present before extraction. The inflamed socket appears dry, and exposed bone, which may be dead and fragmented, is often visible.

TREATMENT
The socket is gently irrigated to remove debris, and may then be coated with a soothing, anti-inflammatory paste, such as a mixture of zinc oxide and eugenol (oil of cloves). The infection usually begins to clear up within a few days. *Antibiotic drugs* may help prevent dry socket but are not usually effective once the condition is established.

DSM IV
The fourth, and most recent, edition of the "Diagnostic and Statistical Manual of Mental Disorders", published by the American Psychiatric Association in 1994. DSM IV provides criteria for classifying psychiatric illnesses and is widely accepted in other countries.

Dual personality
See *Multiple personality*.

Duct
A tube or a tube-like passage leading from a gland to allow the flow of fluids—for example, tears through the tear ducts.

Dumbness
See *Mutism*.

Dumping syndrome
Symptoms including sweating, faintness, and palpitations resulting from the rapid passage of food from the stomach into the upper intestine. Dumping syndrome mainly affects people who have had a partial or total *gastrectomy* (surgical removal of the stomach).

The symptoms may occur within about 30 minutes of eating (early dumping), or after 90 to 120 minutes

(late dumping, usually due to low blood sugar and potassium levels). Some tense people may have symptoms of dumping even though their stomach is intact.

CAUSES
Gastric surgery interferes with the normal mechanism for emptying food from the stomach (see *Digestion*). If a meal that is rich in carbohydrates is "dumped" too quickly from the stomach, the upper intestine may swell and excessive amounts of certain hormones are released into the bloodstream. These excess hormones, with the intestinal swelling, cause the symptoms of early dumping.

As sugars are absorbed from the intestine, they rapidly increase the blood glucose level, causing an excess amount of *insulin* to be released. The abnormally high insulin level may in turn later lower the blood sugar level below normal, causing the symptoms of late dumping.

A person who has had a gastrectomy can avoid symptoms by eating frequent, small, dry meals that do not contain refined carbohydrates such as white sugar. Symptoms may also be prevented by lying down after a large meal. Drug treatment is not often successful, but adding *guar gum* to food to slow the emptying of the stomach and the absorption of sugars is sometimes effective.

Duodenal ulcer
A raw area in the wall of the *duodenum* (first part of the small intestine), caused by erosion of its inner surface lining. Duodenal ulcers and gastric ulcers (similar raw areas in the lining of the stomach) are also called *peptic ulcers* and have similar causes, symptoms, and treatment.

Duodenitis
Inflammation of the *duodenum* (first part of the small intestine). Duodenitis produces vague gastrointestinal symptoms and no physical signs. The cause is uncertain.

A diagnosis of duodenitis is made by *gastroscopy* (examination of the walls of the duodenum with a flexible viewing instrument passed through the oesophagus, stomach, and pylorus). Gastroscopy shows a diffuse area of inflammation, with redness and swelling of cells in the duodenal lining and often bleeding after contact with the tip of the gastroscope. No direct link has yet been established between gastroscopic findings and the symptoms of duodenitis.

Treatment for duodenitis (which has not been proved to be effective) is similar to that for a duodenal ulcer (see *Peptic ulcer*).

Duodenum

The first part of the small intestine, extending from the pylorus (the muscular valve at the lower end of the stomach) to the ligament of Treitz, which marks the boundary between the duodenum and the jejunum (the second part of the small intestine).

Ducts from the pancreas, liver, and gallbladder feed into the duodenum through a small opening called the ampulla of Vater, which is surrounded by the sphincter of Oddi. Digestive enzymes in the pancreatic secretions and chemicals in the bile are released into the duodenum through this opening.

**LOCATION OF
THE DUODENUM**
The duodenum is about 25 cm long and shaped like a C on its side; it forms a loop around the head of the pancreas.

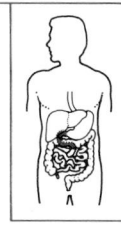

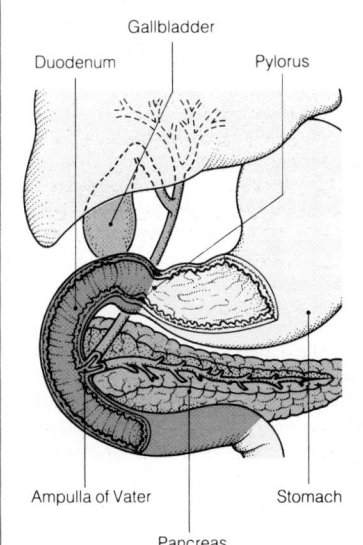

Gallbladder
Duodenum
Pylorus
Ampulla of Vater
Stomach
Pancreas

Dupuytren's contracture

A disorder of the hand in which one or more fingers become fixed in a bent position. In about half the cases, both hands are affected. The disorder is named after the French surgeon who first described it, Baron Guillaume Dupuytren (1777-1835).

The cause is unclear. In most cases there is no apparent cause, although the tendency to develop the disease may in part be inherited. Men over 40 are most often affected.

SYMPTOMS AND SIGNS
The tissues under the skin in the fingers or palm of the hand become thickened and shortened, causing difficulty in straightening the fingers. The disorder often starts as a small, hard nodule on the palm and spreads to form a band or cord of hard tissue under the skin, with puckering of the skin itself. The affected fingers start to bend more and more over a period of months or years. Surgery should be performed when there is any deformity of the fingers. During surgery the bands of thickened tissue are separated from the skin and then cut to free the fingers and allow them to straighten fully. In some patients the disease recurs and further surgery is needed.

Dust diseases

A group of lung disorders caused by the inhalation, usually over several years at work, of dust particles absorbed into the lung tissues. There they may cause *fibrosis* (formation of scar tissue) and progressive lung damage with crippling symptoms.

The main symptoms are a cough and breathing difficulty. It may take at least 10 years of exposure to dusts containing coal, silica, talc, or asbestos before serious lung damage develops (see *Pneumoconiosis*). Hypersensitivity to moulds growing on hay or grain may lead to allergic *alveolitis*.

The incidence and severity of occupational lung diseases have been reduced substantially by preventive measures. Such measures include the use of masks and respirators by workers and the installation of dust extraction machinery. Replacements have been found for especially hazardous substances, such as asbestos.

Workers in relevant industries vary in their susceptibility to dust disease. These people should be under regular medical supervision to ensure that any signs of disease are detected early and serious damage is thus prevented.

Dwarfism

See *Short stature*.

Dydrogesterone

A drug derived from *progesterone hormone* (a natural female sex hormone) which is used to treat a variety

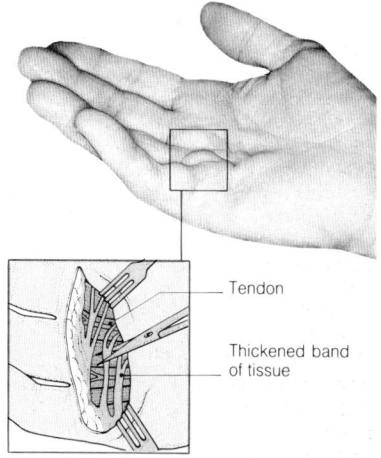

Surgery for Dupuytren's contracture
Bands of tissue under the skin that have become thickened are cut and separated so that the fingers are freed.

of menstrual disorders thought to be caused by a deficiency of this hormone.

Dydrogesterone is prescribed for *premenstrual syndrome* and for absent, irregular, or painful periods (see *Menstruation, disorders of*). It is also given together with an *oestrogen drug* as *hormone replacement therapy* after the menopause. Dydrogesterone is sometimes prescribed for *endometriosis* (a condition in which fragments of tissue that normally line the uterus occur elsewhere in the pelvic cavity). This drug is also given to prevent *miscarriage* in women who have suffered repeated miscarriages.

Dydrogesterone is usually taken on selected days during the menstrual cycle, the exact days depending on the disorder being treated. Possible adverse effects include tenderness of the breasts, swollen ankles, weight gain, and nausea.

Dying, care of the

People who are near death should be given physical and psychological care that will make their final period of life as free from pain, discomfort, and emotional distress as possible.

Today, with good medical care, many deaths, even those from cancer, are pain-free and are associated with little physical discomfort. Emotional distress in the dying can be minimized if understanding and sensitivity are shown by the people who care for them. Carers may include doctors and other medical professionals, counsellors, social workers, clergy, family, and friends. Family and friends should realize that caring for a dying

D

person may cause them great emotional strain. They may also feel guilty because they are unable to do more for the dying person. They, too, may benefit from counselling.

TALKING ABOUT DEATH

Over the last 20 years it has become more common for doctors to tell dying people, particularly cancer patients, the facts relating to their diagnoses. Generally, if a person can discuss the likely outcome of his or her illness and can prepare for death, then dying itself is eased. However, there are people who prefer not to know or who block out the knowledge. The wishes of the patient should be paramount; these wishes may not always be clear and those caring for the patient need considerable perception and understanding. Careful probing may be necessary to ascertain how much a dying person really wants to be told.

Sometimes, even though the dying person has made it clear that he or she would prefer to talk about death, family members feel unable to do so. This may make the patient feel very isolated. Sometimes, a dying person may find it easier to talk to someone who is not a relative. Specially trained people, such as counsellors or members of the clergy, may be able to help promote communication between patient and family.

PHYSICAL CARE

For most dying people, pain is often the most feared problem. Today, however, virtually all pain can be relieved by the use of analgesic drugs (painkillers). Regular, low doses of drugs are given so that pain never builds up and the patient remains alert. Powerful narcotic analgesics, such as morphine and other opiates, are commonly given to relieve severe pain in dying people.

When analgesic drugs are not adequate, other methods may be necessary. These include *nerve blocks* (in which a nerve carrying pain from the body to the brain is interrupted by an injection or surgery), *cordotomy* (severing of nerve fibres in the spinal cord), and *TENS* (transcutaneous electrical nerve stimulation), which is less likely to be effective if narcotic analgesics have been used.

Physical symptoms other than pain may also cause distress. Nausea and vomiting may be a problem when the liver or kidneys have ceased to function adequately. A combination of two or three drugs may occasionally control symptoms. An obstruction in the oesophagus can cause vomiting or dif-

ficulty in swallowing and may need to be relieved by an operation or by *laser treatment* through an *endoscope*. Another common problem in the dying is breathlessness, which may be relieved by morphine.

The patient may develop aches or become stiff from being in bed. Comfort can be improved by keeping the patient as active as possible.

Towards the end, the dying person may become restless and may suffer from breathing difficulty due to *heart failure* or *pneumonia*. These symptoms can be relieved by medication and by placing the patient in a more comfortable position.

PSYCHOLOGICAL CARE

Emotional care is at least as important as the relief of pain. Many people feel anger or depression at the thought of dying; feelings of guilt or regret over the past are also common emotional responses. Ultimately, however, given loving, caring support from family, friends, and others, most terminally ill people come to terms with the thought of death. Sometimes *antidepressant drugs* are prescribed to relieve severe depression.

A great cause of anxiety and worry may be fear of a painful end. Patients should be reassured that adequate pain relief will be maintained at all times and that even when death is very close they need not fear suffering. Most people sink into unconsciousness just before the end and die "in their sleep". Fear of dependency and loss of dignity may also cause worry. The dying person should be allowed to participate as much as possible in family discussions and decisions regarding the future.

Preparing for death may include practical matters, such as writing a will, or less tangible things such as saying "sorry", "thank you", or "goodbye". Confession and reassurance from a priest or spiritual counsellor are also important for some people. Perhaps the most pressing need for the terminally ill person is communication. Relatives, friends, and carers must be willing to share the dying person's concerns.

HOME OR HOSPITAL?

The treatment of most types of cancer requires hospital facilities at some time. However, once an illness has a foreseeable end, many terminally ill people prefer to return home; many families also choose to care for a dying relative at home. Few terminally ill patients require complicated nursing for a prolonged period, and the

sort of loving understanding and emotional care needed may be best provided at home. At home, too, the dying person can maintain some dignity and independence, avoid isolation, and participate in family life. By contrast, a hospital is better equipped to deal with acute illness.

HOSPICES

Hospices are small units, sometimes linked to a general hospital, that have been established specifically to care for the dying and their families. The number of hospices has grown considerably during the last few years. Hospital routine is generally absent; instead, the efforts of the hospice staff, who are specially trained in terminal care, are directed towards the relief of physical and emotional pain. Basic to the hospice philosophy is the idea that dying people and their families need help, care, and understanding. It has been argued that a dying person might find the sight of other people dying depressing, but it has been found that most people who die in a hospice are reassured because death occurs peacefully.

Dys-

A prefix meaning abnormal, difficult, painful, or faulty, as in dysuria (pain on passing urine).

Dysarthria

A *speech disorder* caused by disease or damage to the physical apparatus of speech, or to nerve pathways controlling this apparatus.

Dysarthria differs from *aphasia* (a type of language disorder that affects speech) in that dysarthric patients have nothing wrong with the language centre in the brain. They are able to formulate, select, and write out words and sentences grammatically; it is only vocal expression that causes problems. *Dysphonia* is a speech disability with a more restricted meaning than dysarthria, referring only to defects of sound production caused by some disease or damage to the larynx (voice-box).

CAUSES

Dysarthria is a common feature of many degenerative conditions affecting the nervous system, such as *multiple sclerosis, Parkinson's disease,* and *Huntington's disease.* It also affects some children who have *cerebral palsy.* Dysarthria may result from a *stroke, brain tumour,* or an isolated defect or damage to a particular nerve (such as the hypoglossal nerve that controls movements of the tongue). Structural defects of the mouth, as occur in *cleft lip and palate*, or even ill-fitting false teeth may also affect speech.

TREATMENT
There is no specific treatment for dysarthria. In some cases, drug or surgical treatment of the underlying disease or structural defect may restore the ability to speak clearly. In other instances, patients may benefit from *speech therapy*.

Dyschondroplasia
A rare disorder, also called multiple enchondromatosis, present from birth and characterized by the presence of multiple tumours of cartilaginous tissue within the bones of a limb. Dyschondroplasia is caused by a failure of normal bone development from cartilage. It may affect only one limb. The bones of an affected limb are shortened, resulting in deformity. Rarely, a tumour may become cancerous (see *Chondrosarcoma*).

Dysentery
A severe infection of the intestines, causing diarrhoea (often mixed with blood, pus, and mucus) and abdominal pain. The person may spend hours straining on the toilet, producing little but bloodstained watery mucus.

There are two distinct forms of dysentery. *Shigellosis*, also called bacillary dysentery, is caused by infection with any of a group of bacteria called SHIGELLA. The diarrhoea starts suddenly and is watery; sometimes *toxaemia* (the presence of bacterial toxins in the blood) develops. *Amoebic dysentery* is caused by the protozoan (single-celled) parasite ENTAMOEBA HISTOLYTICA. This form starts more gradually and often persists.

The main risk with dysentery is *dehydration* caused by loss of fluid in the diarrhoea.

Dyskinesia
Abnormal muscular movements caused by a brain disorder. Uncontrollable twitching, jerking, or writhing movements cannot be suppressed and may impair the performance of voluntary movements. The disorder may involve the whole body or may be restricted to a group of muscles.

Different types of dyskinesia include *chorea* (mainly jerking movements), *athetosis* (writhing movements), *choreoathetosis* (a combined form), *tics* (repetitive fidgets), *tremors*, and *myoclonus* (muscle spasms).

Dyskinesia may result from brain damage at birth or may be a side-effect

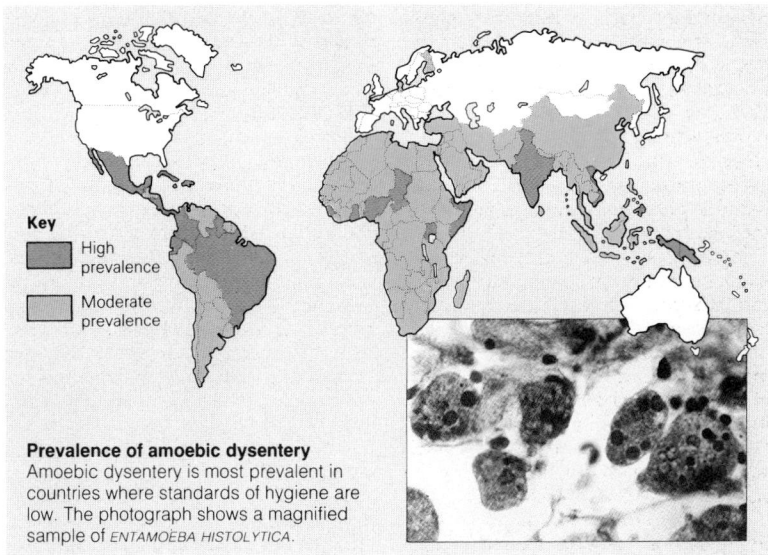

Prevalence of amoebic dysentery
Amoebic dysentery is most prevalent in countries where standards of hygiene are low. The photograph shows a magnified sample of ENTAMOEBA HISTOLYTICA.

Key
High prevalence
Moderate prevalence

of certain drugs, particularly some *antipsychotic drugs* or the antiemetic *metoclopramide*. The affected brain region is a group of linked nerve centres (the *extrapyramidal system*), which includes the *basal ganglia*.

Dyskinesia due to drugs often disappears when drug use is stopped. Otherwise, dyskinesia is difficult to treat. Drugs such as tetrabenazine may help reduce chorea, but often a doctor must prescribe several drugs in turn before one (if any) is effective. (See also *Parkinsonism*.)

Dyslexia
A specific reading disability characterized by difficulty in coping with written symbols. The term is not used to describe other types of reading difficulty, such as problems arising from brain damage or mental handicap, or from speech or visual defects.

Dyslexia does not include reading problems caused by educational or social neglect.

CAUSES AND INCIDENCE
Emotional disturbance, minor visual defects, and failure to "train" the brain have all been suggested as possible causes of dyslexia, but there is now good evidence that a specific, sometimes inherited, neurological disorder underlies true dyslexia. Some 90 per cent of people with dyslexia are male.

SYMPTOMS
The key feature of dyslexia is that in other respects a child with dyslexia has completely normal intelligence. Thus, his or her attainment of reading

skills lags far behind other scholastic abilities and overall IQ. Usually, the child can read numbers or musical notes much more easily than words.

Furthermore, while many young children tend to reverse letters and words (for example, writing or reading p for q, b for d, was for saw, no for on), the majority soon correct such errors. Dyslexic children continue to confuse these symbols. Letters are transposed (as in pest for step) and spelling errors are common. These children may even be unable to read words they can spell correctly. Writing from dictation may be difficult even though they can copy sentences.

TREATMENT
It is important to recognize the problem early to avoid any added frustrations. Specific remedial teaching can help the child develop "tricks" to overcome the deficit, and avoidance of pressure from parents combined with praise for what the child can do is equally important. Given appropriate support and training, sufferers can usually overcome their difficulties, and develop successful careers.

Dysmenorrhoea
Pain or discomfort during or just before a menstrual period. Most teenage girls and young women suffer to some degree from what is called primary dysmenorrhoea. This usually starts two or three years after *menstruation* begins, once ovulation is established. The problem often diminishes after the age of about 25 and is rare following childbirth.

Dysmenorrhoea is known to be associated with the hormonal changes that occur during a period, but the exact mechanism of the link between them remains uncertain. One possibility is that dysmenorrhoea is due to excessive production of, or undue sensitivity to, *prostaglandins,* the hormone-like substances that stimulate muscular spasm of the uterus.

Secondary dysmenorrhoea begins in adult life and is due to an underlying disorder, such as *endometriosis* or *pelvic inflammatory disease.*

Either type of dysmenorrhoea may or may not be accompanied by *premenstrual syndrome* (a bloated feeling, irritability, depression, and other changes that commonly occur in the days preceding menstruation).

SYMPTOMS

Dysmenorrhoea is typically felt as cramp-like pain or discomfort in the lower abdomen, which may come and go in waves. There may also be a dull ache in the lower back and, in some women, nausea and vomiting. In primary dysmenorrhoea the pain starts shortly before a period and usually lasts for less than 12 hours. About 10 per cent of women have symptoms severe enough to interfere with their work or leisure activities. In secondary dysmenorrhoea the pain begins several days before a period and lasts throughout it.

Mild primary dysmenorrhoea is often relieved by *analgesic drugs* (painkillers), such as *aspirin,* or *naproxen* (a prostaglandin inhibitor). Rest in bed with a hot-water bottle is a traditional and sometimes effective remedy. If the condition is severe, symptoms can usually be relieved by suppressing ovulation, with either *oral contraceptives* or other hormonal preparations.

Treatment of secondary dysmenorrhoea depends on the cause.

Dyspareunia

The medical term for painful sexual intercourse. (See *Intercourse, painful.*)

Dyspepsia

The medical term for *indigestion.*

Dysphagia

The medical term for *swallowing difficulty.*

Dysphasia

A term that is sometimes used to describe a disturbance in the ability to select the words with which to speak and write (and/or to comprehend and read). It is caused by dam-age to those regions of the brain concerned with speech and comprehension. (See also *Aphasia.*)

Dysphonia

Defective production of vocal sounds in *speech,* caused by disease or damage to the *larynx* (voice-box) or to the nerve supply to the laryngeal muscles. Dysphonia is distinct from *dysarthria* (in which speech is defective because of damage or disease to other body parts and nerve pathways involved in speech) and from expressive *aphasia* (in which the ability to speak may be profoundly disturbed by damage to the brain's speech centre). (See also *Larynx* disorders box; *Speech disorders.*)

Dysplasia

Any abnormality of growth. The **term** applies to deformities in structures such as the skull (cranial dysplasia) and to abnormalities of single cells (cellular dysplasia). Abnormal cell features include the size, shape, and rate of multiplication of cells.

Dyspnoea

The medical term for shortness of breath. (See *Breathing difficulty.*)

Dysrhythmia, cardiac

A medical term meaning disturbance of heart rhythm, sometimes used as an alternative to arrhythmia. (See *Arrhythmia, cardiac.*)

Dystocia

A term that means difficult or abnormal labour (see *Childbirth*). Dystocia may occur if the baby is very large, or if the mother's pelvis is abnormally shaped or too small for the baby to pass through. Other causes of dystocia include abnormal presentation of the baby (see *Malpresentation*), and ineffective uterine contractions. (See also *Childbirth, complications of.*)

Dystonia

Abnormal muscle rigidity, causing painful spasms, unusually fixed postures, or strange movement patterns. Dystonia may affect a localized area of the body, or may be more generalized.

The most common types of localized dystonia are *torticollis* (painful neck spasm), and *scoliosis* (abnormal sideways curvature of the spine) caused by an injury to the back that produces muscle spasm.

More generalized dystonia occurs as a result of various neurological disorders, including *Parkinson's disease* and *stroke,* and may also be a feature of schizophrenia. Dystonia may be a side-effect of *antipsychotic drugs.*

Dystonia is often difficult to treat but may respond to *anticholinergic*

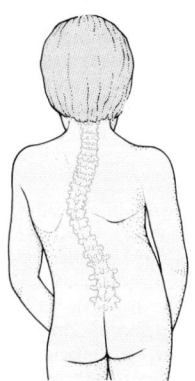

Scoliosis due to dystonia
Injury to the back may result in dystonia and abnormal spasm of the back muscles, which, in turn, may lead to scoliosis (abnormal sideways curvature of the spine).

drugs or *benzodiazepine drugs.* In some cases *biofeedback training* may help. Injections of botulinum toxin, the agent responsible for *botulism,* have proved effective in the treatment of several types of dystonia, including *blepharospasm* (spasmodic contraction of the eyelids) and torticollis. An injection of the toxin into the affected muscles weakens them and will relieve symptoms for as long as several months. Injections can be repeated as necessary.

Dystrophy

Any disorder in which the structure and normal activity of cells within a tissue have been disrupted by inadequate nutrition. The usual cause is poor circulation of blood through the tissue, but dystrophy can also be due to nerve damage or deficiency of a specific enzyme (catalytic protein) in the tissue.

In *muscular dystrophies,* muscle cells fail to develop normally, causing weakness and paralysis. In *leukodystrophies,* there is loss of the sheath surrounding nerves within the brain, causing various disturbances of sensation, movement, and intellect.

Corneal dystrophies are a rare, usually inherited, cause of blindness. In this condition, cells lining the cornea are damaged and the eye's surface becomes opaque.

Dysuria

The medical term for pain, discomfort, or difficulty in passing urine. (See *Urination, painful.*)

E

Ear

The organ of hearing and balance. The ear consists of three parts: the outer ear, the middle ear, and the inner ear. The outer and middle ear are concerned primarily with the collection and transmission of sound. The inner ear is responsible for analysing sound waves; it also contains the mechanism by which the body keeps its balance.

OUTER EAR

The outer ear consists of the pinna (also called the auricle), which is the visible part of the ear, composed of folds of skin and cartilage. The pinna leads into the ear canal (also called the meatus), which is 2.5 cm long in adults and closed at its inner end by the tympanic membrane (eardrum). The part of the canal nearest the outside is made of cartilage. The cartilage is covered with skin that produces wax, which, along with hair, traps dust and small foreign bodies.

The eardrum separates the outer ear from the middle ear. The eardrum is a thin, fibrous, circular membrane covered with a thin layer of skin. It vibrates in response to the changes in air pressure that constitute sound and works in conjunction with the other components of the middle ear.

MIDDLE EAR

The middle ear is a small cavity between the eardrum and the inner ear. It conducts sound to the inner ear by means of a chain of three tiny, linked, movable bones called ossicles. These bones link the eardrum to the oval window in the bony wall that forms the inner side of the middle-ear cavity. The ossicles have names that describe their shapes. The malleus (hammer) is joined to the inside of the eardrum. The incus (anvil) has one broad joint with the malleus (which lies almost parallel to it) and a delicate joint to the third bone, the stapes (stirrup). The base of the stapes fills the oval window, which leads to the inner ear.

The middle ear is cut off from the outside by the eardrum, but it is not completely airtight; a ventilation passage, called the eustachian tube, runs forwards and downwards into the back of the nose. The eustachian tube is normally closed but opens by muscular contraction when we yawn or swallow.

The middle ear acts as a transformer, passing the vibrations of sound from the air outside (which is a thin medium) to the fluid in the inner ear (which is a thicker medium).

INNER EAR

The inner ear is an extremely intricate series of structures contained deep within the bones of the skull. It consists of a maze of winding passages, collectively known as the labyrinth. The front part, the cochlea, is a tube resembling a snail's shell and is concerned with hearing. (For a detailed discussion of how this system works, see *Hearing*.) The rear part (consisting of the saccule, utricle, and three semicircular canals) is concerned with *balance*. The semicircular canals are set at right angles to each other and are connected to a cavity known as the vestibule. The canals contain hair cells bathed in fluid. Some of these cells are sensitive to gravity and acceleration; others respond to the positions and movements of the head (i.e. side to side, up and down, or tilted). The information concerning posture or direction is registered by the relevant cells and conveyed by nerve fibres to the brain. (See also *Ear* disorders box.)

Earache

Pain in the ear, which may originate in the ear itself or may result from a disorder in a nearby structure. Earache is an extremely common symptom, especially in childhood.

CAUSES

The most frequent cause of earache is acute *otitis media* (infection of the middle ear), which occurs most commonly in young children. The pain is

ANATOMY OF THE EAR

The outer ear comprises the pinna and ear canal; the middle ear—the eardrum, malleus, incus, stapes, and eustachian tube; and the inner ear— the vestibule, semicircular canals, and cochlea. Sensory impulses from the inner ear pass to the brain via the vestibulocochlear nerve.

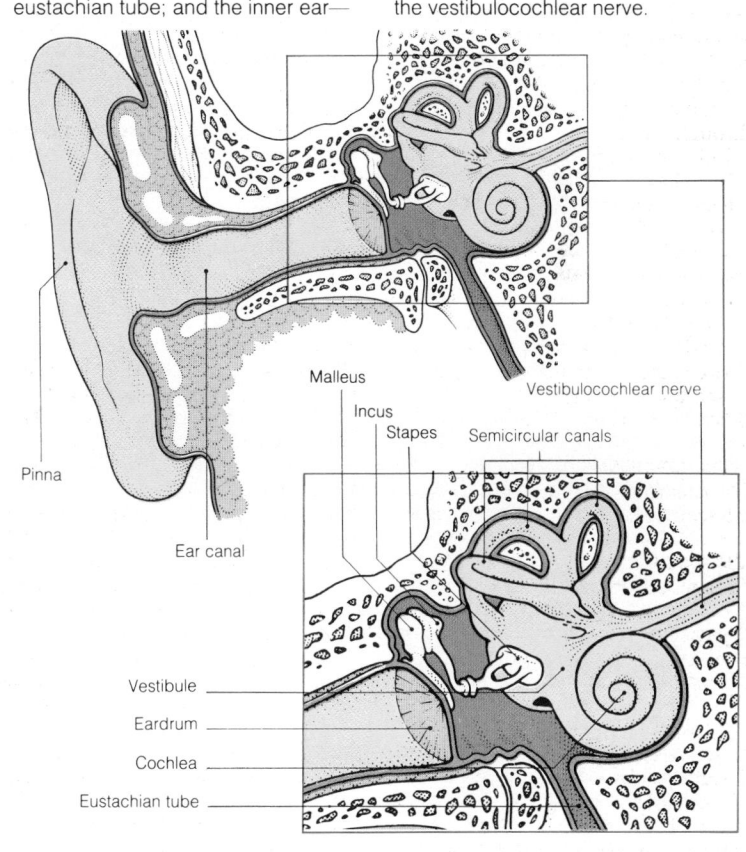

Malleus
Incus
Stapes
Vestibulocochlear nerve
Semicircular canals
Pinna
Ear canal
Vestibule
Eardrum
Cochlea
Eustachian tube

E

DISORDERS OF THE EAR

The ear is susceptible to a large variety of disorders, some of which can lead to *deafness*. *Vertigo* (dizziness associated with a disturbance of balance) may result from some disorders of the inner ear.

CONGENITAL DEFECTS

Very rarely, a baby is born with an absent or extremely narrowed external ear canal, and sometimes the small bones of the middle ear are deformed or absent. Occasionally, the pinna (external ear) is missing or distorted. *Rubella* (German measles) affecting a woman during the first three months of pregnancy can cause severe damage to the baby's hearing apparatus, leading to deafness. Most cases of congenital sensorineural deafness are genetic.

INFECTION

Infection is the most common cause of ear disorders. Infection may occur in the ear canal, leading to *otitis externa*, or may affect the middle ear, causing *otitis media*, which often leads to perforation of the eardrum (see *Eardrum, perforated*). Persistent *glue ear* (build-up of fluid within the middle ear), often due to infection, is the most common cause of hearing difficulties in children.

Middle-ear infection can spread to cause *mastoiditis* (infection of the mastoid process, the bone behind the ear) or *brain abscess*, but these complications have become extremely rare since the introduction of antibiotics.

Virus infection of the inner ear may cause *labyrinthitis* with severe vertigo or sudden hearing loss, or both simultaneously.

INJURY

Cauliflower ear is the result of repeated injury to the pinna. Injury to the external ear canal and perforation of the eardrum can result from poking objects into the ear. A sudden blow, especially a slap, to the ear or a very loud noise may also perforate the eardrum. Prolonged exposure to loud noise or close proximity to a loud explosion can cause *tinnitus* (noises within the ear) and/or deafness. Pressure changes associated with flying or scuba diving can also cause minor damage and pain (see *Barotrauma*).

TUMOURS

Tumours in the ear are rare, but occasionally a *basal cell carcinoma* (rodent ulcer) or a *squamous cell carcinoma* will affect the pinna. The latter may also involve the ear canal. Cancers of the middle and inner ears are extremely rare. *Acoustic neuroma* is a benign (nonmalignant), slow-growing tumour of the acoustic nerve that may press on structures within the ear to cause deafness, tinnitus, and imbalance. *Cholesteatoma*, a growing collection of skin cells and debris, is not a tumour, but may be equally dangerous.

OBSTRUCTION

Ear-canal obstruction is most often caused by dried *earwax*, but may also result from otitis externa. In children, a frequent cause is putting a foreign body into the ear (see *Ear, foreign body in*).

DEGENERATION

Deafness in many elderly people is due to *presbyacusis*, deterioration of the hair cells in the cochlea.

POISONING/DRUGS

The inner ear is especially sensitive to damage by certain classes of drugs. The most important—the aminoglycoside *antibiotics* group—include such drugs as neomycin and gentamicin. These drugs can cause damage to the cochlear hair cells, especially if used in high concentration and particularly in the presence of kidney disease, which can delay the excretion of the drugs from the body.

Other drugs that can damage ear function include quinine and the salicylates (including aspirin) and the *diuretic drugs* frusemide, ethacrynic acid, and bumetanide.

OTHER DISORDERS

In *otosclerosis*, a hereditary condition, the base of one of the small bones in the middle ear becomes fixed, causing deafness. *Menièrè's disease* is an uncommon disorder in which deafness, vertigo, and tinnitus result from the accumulation of fluid within the labyrinth in the inner ear.

INVESTIGATION

The function of hearing is investigated by various tuning-fork and audiometric *hearing tests*, which reveal different types and levels of hearing loss. The external ear canal and the eardrum may be examined with an *otoscope* and mirror; an otoscopic microscope may also be used.

The function of the balancing mechanism of the inner ear is investigated by observing *nystagmus* (jerky eye movements) when the head is placed in different positions or the whole body rotated, and when the ear is syringed with hot or cold water (*caloric tests*). These tests may be refined by *electronystagmography*.

likely to be severe and stabbing; there may also be loss of hearing and a raised temperature. If the eardrum bursts, the discharge of fluid may produce immediate relief from pain.

Another common cause of earache is *otitis externa* (inflammation of the outer ear canal), which is often caused by infection. Infection may affect the whole canal or it may be localized, sometimes taking the form of a boil or abscess. The earache may be accompanied by irritation in the ear canal, and by a discharge, and there may be slight hearing loss.

A much rarer cause of earache is *herpes zoster* infection, which causes blisters in the ear canal. The earache may persist for weeks or months after the infection has cleared up.

Intermittent earache may also occur in people with dental problems, *tonsillitis*, throat cancer (see *Pharynx, cancer of*), pain in the lower jaw or neck muscles, and other disorders affecting areas near the ear. Earache in such cases occurs because the ear and many nearby areas are supplied by the same nerves; the pain is said to be "referred" to the ear.

INVESTIGATION

After inspecting the outer ear, the doctor will examine the ear canal and eardrum with an *otoscope* and, if necessary, a binocular microscope. The mouth, throat, and teeth are also examined. In some cases, X-rays and other tests may need to be carried out (see *Ear, examination of*).

TREATMENT
Analgesic drugs may be given to relieve pain. Other treatment depends on the underlying cause of the earache. *Antibiotic drugs* may be prescribed for an infection. Pus in the outer ear may need to be aspirated (sucked out), usually as an outpatient procedure. Pus in the middle ear may require draining through a hole made in the eardrum, an operation known as *myringotomy*.

Ear, cauliflower

See *Cauliflower ear*.

Ear, discharge from

An emission of fluid from the ear, also known as otorrhoea. The discharge may be watery or thick, clear or coloured, odourless or foul-smelling, intermittent or continuous.

A discharge from the ear may be caused by infection of the outer ear (see *Otitis externa*). It is also commonly caused by perforation of the eardrum (see *Eardrum, perforated*), usually as a result of infection of the middle ear (see *Otitis media*). In very rare cases, following fracture of the skull (see *Skull, fracture of*), *cerebrospinal fluid* or blood may be discharged from the ear.

INVESTIGATION AND TREATMENT
Any discharge from the ear should be reported to a doctor. A swab of the discharge will be taken and sent for laboratory analysis to identify the cause of any infection. *Hearing tests* may be performed.

X-rays of the bones of the skull will be taken if there has been a *head injury* or if a serious type of middle-ear infection is suspected.

Treatment depends on the cause and usually includes *antibiotic drugs*.

Eardrum, perforated

Rupture or erosion of the eardrum, usually as a result of infection. Perforation of the eardrum often causes brief, intense pain. There may be slight bleeding and a discharge from the ear (see *Ear, discharge from*).

Perforation of the eardrum usually leads to some reduction in hearing (although such an effect may be very slight).

CAUSES AND INCIDENCE
Most commonly, the eardrum is perforated as a result of a build-up of pus in the middle ear due to uncontrolled acute *otitis media* (infection of the middle ear).

Perforation of the eardrum may also be associated with *cholesteatoma* (a chronic disease of the middle ear). Another less common cause of perforation is injury, such as may result from the insertion of a sharp object into the ear, a blow to the ear (usually a hard slap), a nearby explosion, *barotrauma* (pressure damage resulting from flying or diving), or a fracture to the base of the skull. Very rarely, perforation of the eardrum is caused by a tumour of the middle ear.

In some cases, a doctor may deliberately puncture the eardrum to drain the middle ear (see *Myringotomy*).

Perforation of the eardrum was much more common before *antibiotic drugs* became widely available.

DIAGNOSIS
Diagnosis is confirmed by examination of the ear (see *Ear, examination of*). *Hearing tests* may be performed to assess any hearing loss.

TREATMENT
Anyone who suspects a perforated eardrum should cover the ear with a clean, dry pad (to prevent infection from entering the middle ear) and seek medical help. *Analgesic drugs* (painkillers) may be taken if required.

The doctor will prescribe *antibiotic drugs* to treat, or sometimes to prevent, infection. Most perforations due to acute infection or injury heal quickly, usually within a month. If the perforation has failed to heal or close sufficiently within six months, a *myringoplasty* (an operation to repair the eardrum) may be performed.

Surgery is always necessary to treat perforation associated with the disorder cholesteatoma.

Ear, examination of

A doctor will examine the ear to investigate the possible causes of the following symptoms: *earache*, discharge from the ear (see *Ear, discharge from*), hearing loss, a feeling of fullness in the ear, disturbance of *balance*, *tinnitus* (noises in the ear), or swollen or tender lymph nodes (see *Glands, swollen*) below or in front of the ear.

The doctor can inspect only the pinna (the visible outer ear), the ear canal, and the eardrum. To investigate the middle and inner ears, more specialized tests are required.

HOW IT IS DONE
The doctor begins by examining the pinna for any evidence of swelling, tenderness, ulceration, or deformity and examines the skin above and behind the ear for signs of previous surgery. To inspect the ear canal and

eardrum, the doctor usually uses an *otoscope* (a viewing instrument for examining the ear). If necessary, a more magnified, three-dimensional image can be obtained by using a binocular microscope.

To obtain images of the middle and inner ears, the doctor may arrange for *X-rays*, *tomography*, *CT scanning*, or *MRI* to be carried out. Hearing and balance may require assessment by means of *hearing tests*, *caloric tests*, and *electronystagmography*.

Ear, foreign body in

The external ear canal is a common location for foreign bodies. Children often insert small objects, such as beads, peas, or stones, into their ears. It is also possible for insects to fly or crawl into the ear.

TREATMENT
SMALL OBJECTS These must always be removed by a doctor. Under no circumstances should removal ever be attempted by poking with cotton buds, hair-grips, or similar objects; these efforts usually drive the object farther into the ear canal.

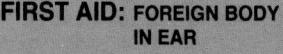

FIRST AID: FOREIGN BODY IN EAR

DO NOT
■ attempt to dislodge the object by probing. Small objects must be removed by a doctor.
■ pour liquid into the ear unless you are certain the object is an insect.

TO REMOVE AN INSECT

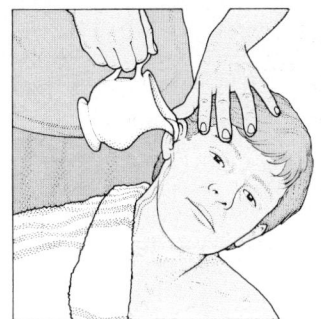

Tilt the victim's head so that the affected ear is facing upwards. Pour lukewarm water into the ear and the insect may float to the surface. If this fails, call your doctor.

E

The physican will remove the object either by *syringing* the ear or by grasping the object with a pair of fine-toothed forceps. A brief general anaesthetic may be required if the object is impacted, as often occurs with organic foreign bodies, such as beans, which swell when moistened by ear secretions.

INSECTS An insect can sometimes be removed from the ear by getting the person to tilt his or her head so that the affected side is uppermost and then pouring olive oil or lukewarm water into the ear. If this is not successful, a doctor will need to syringe the ear after killing the insect with chloroform or drowning it with oil. It is impossible for insects to penetrate to the brain.

Ear, nose, and throat surgery
See *Otorhinolaryngology*.

Ear piercing
Making a hole in the earlobe or, occasionally, another part of the external ear, to accommodate an earring. Ear piercing was once performed with a needle, but the risk of transmitting diseases through the use of unsterile needles caused this method to be replaced by a special ear-piercing gun.

HOW IT IS DONE
A local anaesthetic is not necessary, since the procedure causes only minor discomfort. The earlobe is pierced by a stud, fired into it by the gun, which does not come into contact with the ear. The studs are of gold or gold-plate (cheaper metals can cause contact *dermatitis*), are kept sealed in a sterile pack before use, and are not handled during the procedure.

For six weeks after insertion, the studs must be cleaned regularly with hydrogen peroxide or surgical spirit to prevent infection; the studs are kept in the ears and turned twice daily to prevent the hole from closing.

Ears, pinning back of
See *Otoplasty*.

Earwax
A yellow or brown secretion, also known as cerumen, produced by glands in the outer-ear canal. In most people, wax is produced in only small amounts, comes out on its own, and causes no trouble; in other people, so much wax forms that it regularly obstructs the canal.

Excess earwax may produce a sensation of fullness in the ear and, if the canal is blocked completely, partial deafness. These symptoms are made worse if water enters the ear and makes the wax swell. Prolonged blockage may also inflame the skin of the canal, causing irritation.

TREATMENT
Wax that causes blockage or irritation should be removed by a doctor. A firm plug of wax can be removed using a ring probe, a right-angled hook, or *forceps*. If the wax is too soft for this, it can be softened further with oil and then flushed out with a syringe containing warm water (see *Syringing of ears*). If there is a possibility that the eardrum may be damaged, the doctor will use suction instead of syringing.

A doctor will sometimes suggest that a patient should soften his or her own earwax with warmed olive oil or almond oil or with a commercially available preparation. Cotton buds should never be used as they can push wax deep into the canal, making matters worse.

Ecchymosis
The medical term for a *bruise.*

ECG
The abbreviation for electrocardiogram, a record of the electrical impulses that immediately precede contraction of the heart muscle. The waves produced are known as the P,Q,R,S, and T waves.

An ECG is a useful means of diagnosing disorders of the heart, many of which produce deviations from normal electrical patterns. Among these disorders are *coronary artery disease, coronary thrombosis, pericarditis* (inflammation of the membrane surrounding the heart), *cardiomyopathy* (heart muscle disorders), *myocarditis* (inflammation of the heart muscle), and arrhythmias (see *Arrhythmia, cardiac*).

Echocardiography
A method of obtaining an image of the structure of the heart using *ultrasound* (inaudible, high-frequency sound waves). The sound waves are reflected differently by each part of the heart, resulting in a complex series of echoes which can be detected and displayed visually.

WHY IT IS DONE
Echocardiography is a major diagnostic technique used to detect structural, and some functional, abnormalities of the heart wall, the heart valves, and the heart's large blood vessels. Blood flow across valves is also measured.

The procedure is especially valuable for studying disorders of the heart valves. Abnormal opening and closing of the valves can be detected because they deviate from normal patterns of valve movement. Other diagnostic uses include detection of congenital heart disease (see *Heart disease, congenital*), various abnormalities of the large blood vessels, *cardiomyopathy* (heart muscle disorders), *aneurysms* (ballooning of the heart wall or the walls of blood vessels), *pericarditis* (inflammation of the membrane that surrounds the heart), and the presence of a blood clot within a heart chamber.

HOW IT IS DONE
Echocardiography is harmless and the patient feels nothing; it has the added advantage of producing recordings without having to place an instrument inside the patient's body.

The transducer (the instrument that sends out and receives sound signals) is placed on the chest in a position that allows its sound waves to reach the structures under investigation. The echoes are detected, amplified, and then displayed visually as a series of lines on an oscilloscope screen or a paper tape. This information is interpreted by cardiologists as a picture of the heart and its valves and the way they are working.

Echocardiography has become increasingly more sophisticated in the past 20 years. Multiple moving transducers and computer analysis allow images to be generated that give clear anatomical pictures of the heart and information about the movement and condition of the heart muscle, valves, and pericardium. The investigation may be performed at the bedside and is free of risk to the patient, making it valuable for the very sick.

Doppler echocardiography measures the velocity of blood as it flows through the heart. Images that show both normal and abnormal blood flow may be generated, and enhanced by colour, allowing an assessment to be made of the functional importance of structural abnormalities such as *septal defects* and *valvular heart disease.*

Echolalia
The compulsive repetition of what is spoken by another person. The tone and accent of the speaker are copied as well as the actual words. Echolalia may be a symptom of *schizophrenia* and sometimes occurs in people who suffer from *mental handicap* or from *autism.* Echolalia may be accompanied by echopraxia (imitating the behaviour of another person).

THE ELECTROCARDIOGRAM (ECG)

Electrocardiography causes no discomfort. Electrodes connected to a recording machine are applied to the chest, wrists, and ankles. The machine displays the electrical activity in the heart as a trace on a moving graph or on a screen. Any abnormality is thus revealed to the doctor. To the right are shown normal and abnormal recordings.

An ECG can be taken at home, in the doctor's surgery, or in the hospital; a 24-hour record can be obtained from a tape recorder worn by the patient.

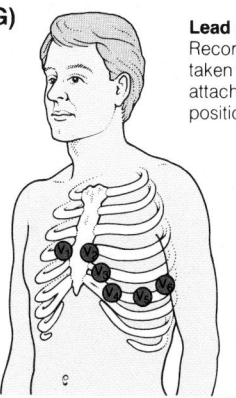

Lead positions
Recordings are taken with a lead attached to these positions.

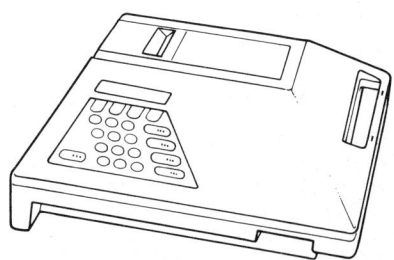

Portable electrocardiograph
A modern, lightweight, portable ECG machine. Leads from the machine are attached to the chest, wrists, and ankles using conducting jelly.

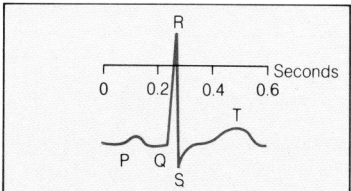

Normal ECG
This tracing shows the electrical activity preceding one normal heartbeat. The vertical axis shows the current flowing towards the recording lead. The rise at P occurs just before the atria (upper heart chambers) begin to contract, the QRS "spike" occurs just before the ventricles (lower chambers) begin to contract, and the rise at T occurs as the electrical potential returns to zero.

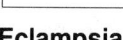

Normal rhythm
The heart chambers are contracting with regularity.

Ventricular fibrillation
Here, the contractions of the lower heart chambers are extremely irregular.

Complete heart block
The upper and lower heart chambers are beating independently.

Atrial fibrillation
Caused by the upper heart chambers beating fast and irregularly.

Eclampsia

A rare, serious condition of late pregnancy, labour, and the period following delivery. Eclampsia is characterized by seizures (convulsions) in the woman, sometimes followed by coma and death; eclampsia also threatens the life of the baby. The disorder occurs as a complication of moderate or severe (but not mild) *pre-eclampsia*, a condition of late pregnancy that is marked by *hypertension* (high blood pressure), *proteinuria* (protein in the urine), and *oedema* (accumulation of fluid in the tissues).

CAUSES

In spite of intensive investigation, the cause of eclampsia and pre-eclampsia remains unknown. Eclampsia is thought to be caused by cerebral oedema (accumulation of fluid in the brain tissue) consequent on pre-eclampsia. Pre-eclampsia was formerly thought to be due to a placental toxin (poison) but is now thought to be due to an abnormality in the *immune response* to the pregnancy.

Eclampsia occurs more commonly in women who have had little or no *antenatal care* because the development of pre-eclampsia in these women may go unrecognized and therefore untreated.

INCIDENCE

About half of all cases develop in late pregnancy, one third during labour, and the rest after delivery.

SYMPTOMS AND SIGNS

In eclampsia the symptoms that characterize severe pre-eclampsia are present. Before the onset of seizures, the woman may suffer from headache, confusion, blurred vision, and abdominal pain. The seizures consist of violent, rhythmic, jerking movements of the limbs caused by involuntary contraction of the muscles; there may also be breathing difficulty caused by constriction of the muscles of the larynx. The seizures may sometimes be followed by coma.

TREATMENT

The seizures are treated by ensuring that the woman can breathe properly

(sometimes by inserting an *endotracheal tube* down her throat) and by giving *anticonvulsant drugs*, which prevent further seizures.

The baby's condition is monitored throughout. Rapid delivery (often by emergency *caesarean section*) is usually performed because the condition is likely to improve once the baby has been born.

OUTLOOK

In the past, many babies failed to survive eclampsia, because of lack of oxygen in the uterus. Nowadays, the outlook for the baby depends partly on the stage of pregnancy at which the condition occurs.

After delivery, the mother's blood pressure usually returns to normal within a week and proteinuria clears within six weeks. In a small number of cases, however, the woman develops serious complications before, during, or after delivery. These may include *heart failure, kidney failure, liver failure, intracerebral haemorrhage, pneumonia*, or *pulmonary oedema*.

E

Econazole

An *antifungal drug*. Econazole is used in cream form to treat fungal skin infections (see *Athlete's foot; Tinea*), and in cream or pessary form to treat vaginal *candidiasis*.

This fast-working drug usually begins to act within two days. Skin irritation is a rare adverse effect.

ECT

The abbreviation for electroconvulsive therapy, which uses electric shocks to induce *seizures* as a treatment for severe *depression*. Anaesthesia and *muscle-relaxant drugs* are used to minimize movements of the body and the effects of ECT are limited primarily to the brain.

WHY IT IS USED

ECT is now used almost exclusively to treat severe depressive illness that has become life-threatening because of accompanying weight loss and neglect. It is used less widely to treat *postnatal depression*, catatonic *schizophrenia*, and some cases of *mania* that have not responded to other treatments. ECT is not used to treat people with severe physical illness or those who have had a recent *myocardial infarction* (heart attack).

HOW IT IS DONE

The patient is given a general anaesthetic and a muscle-relaxant drug before two padded electrodes are applied to the temple, one on each side or both on the same side. A controlled electric pulse is delivered to the electrodes from a small machine until a brain seizure occurs. The seizure is indicated by brief muscular rigidity, followed by twitching of the limbs and eyelids. Afterwards, patients experience only mild discomfort similar to the discomfort felt after a minor dental operation.

Treatment usually consists of six to 12 seizures (two or three per week).

OUTLOOK

If a true brain seizure has been induced at each session, the patient's condition usually begins to improve by the third treatment, often dramatically. Temporary *amnesia* (memory loss) is a possible side-effect. ECT usually relieves depression more rapidly than drug treatment.

Ecstasy

A *designer drug*, related to the amphetamines, that was widely but illegally used in the late 1980s and early 1990s. The drug is sold in tablet form in clubs and discotheques, although its possession is an offence. Taken by mouth,

ecstasy makes people feel lively, alert, sociable, and happy, and apparently gives them energy. Most people seem able to take the drug safely; a few react badly, becoming confused, having a raised temperature, and eventually losing consciousness; convulsions may occur. At least seven young people died in Britain in 1992 after taking ecstasy. Repeated use seems to carry a risk of liver damage.

Ectasia

A medical term meaning widening, usually used to refer to a disorder affecting a duct that carries secretions from a gland or organ. For example, mammary duct ectasia—a rare disorder that affects women mainly around the time of the menopause—is widening of the ducts that carry secretions from the tissues of the breast to the nipple.

-ectomy

A suffix denoting surgical removal. Tonsillectomy is surgical removal of the tonsils.

Ectoparasite

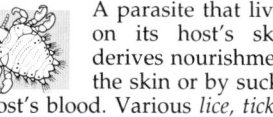 A parasite that lives in or on its host's skin and derives nourishment from the skin or by sucking the host's blood. Various *lice, ticks, mites*, and some types of *fungi* are occasional ectoparasites of humans. By contrast, endoparasites live inside the body.

Ectopic

A medical term used to describe a structure that occurs in an abnormal location or position, or an activity that occurs at an abnormal time.

Ectopic heartbeat

A contraction of the heart muscle that is out of the normal timed sequence. An ectopic heartbeat occurs shortly after a normal beat and is followed by a longer than usual interval.

Ectopic beats can occur in a heart that is otherwise functioning normally and may cause no symptoms. Multiple ectopic beats can sometimes cause *palpitations*.

After a *myocardial infarction* (heart attack), the occurrence of multiple ectopic beats is a sign of damage to the conduction system of the heart muscle. Multiple ectopic beats may lead to ventricular *fibrillation*, a rapid uncoordinated heartbeat that can cause collapse and death.

Multiple ectopic beats that are causing palpitations, or that occur after a

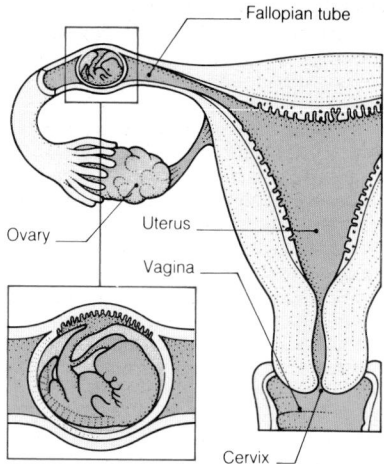

Location of an ectopic pregnancy
The pregnancy usually develops in the fallopian tube; occasionally it develops in the ovary, abdominal cavity, or cervix.

myocardial infarction, are often treated with an *antiarrhythmic drug*. (See also *Arrhythmia, cardiac*.)

Ectopic pregnancy

A pregnancy that develops outside the uterus, most commonly in the *fallopian tube*, but sometimes in the ovary or, rarely, in the abdominal cavity or cervix. As the pregnancy develops, it may damage or rupture surrounding tissue, causing serious bleeding.

About one in every 200 pregnancies is ectopic. Ectopic pregnancy is a life-threatening condition that requires emergency treatment. A very few women still die in the UK each year as a result of ectopic pregnancy.

CAUSES

The fertilized ovum (egg) may become stuck in the fallopian tube if there is a *congenital* abnormality of the tube, or if the tube is damaged in any way. Damage may result from infection (see *Pelvic inflammatory disease*) or from surgery on the fallopian tubes.

A pregnancy that occurs following the failure of some methods of contraception has an increased risk of being ectopic. Ectopic pregnancy has been associated with use of an *IUD* (intrauterine contraceptive device), progesterone-only *oral contraceptives*, hormonal postcoital contraception (see *Contraception, postcoital*), and sterilization operations, especially if the fallopian tubes have been cauterized (see *Sterilization, female*).

SYMPTOMS AND SIGNS

Most ectopic pregnancies are discovered in the first two months, often before the woman realizes she is pregnant. In most cases a menstrual period is missed, but, in about 20 per cent of affected women, menstruation occurs. Symptoms of ectopic pregnancy usually include severe pain in the lower abdomen and vaginal bleeding which may be mistaken for a period. Rupture or internal bleeding cause symptoms of *shock*—pallor, sweating, weakness, and faintness.

DIAGNOSIS AND TREATMENT
Death is unusual unless the condition is not recognized. In most cases a *pregnancy test* and an *ultrasound* scan will lead to the diagnosis being made without delay; it will be confirmed by *laparoscopy*. Surgical treatment is usually possible using *minimally invasive techniques*. The surgeon removes the embryo (which is usually already dead), the placenta, and any damaged tissue at the site of the pregnancy. Any torn blood vessels are repaired and, if the fallopian tube cannot be repaired, it is removed. Many doctors prefer to remove the tube because of the risk of another ectopic pregnancy. If blood loss is severe, *blood transfusions* are needed.

OUTLOOK
It is still possible to have a normal pregnancy even if one fallopian tube has been removed, although the chances of conception are slightly reduced. Women with two damaged tubes may require *in vitro fertilization* to achieve an intrauterine pregnancy.

Ectropion
A turning outwards of the eyelid so that the inner surface is exposed.

INCIDENCE AND CAUSES
Ectropion is most common in elderly people, usually affecting the lower lid and due to weakness of the muscle surrounding the eye.

The condition may also be caused by the contraction of scar tissue in the skin near either lid. Ectropion also often follows *facial palsy,* in which the muscles surrounding the eye (and other facial muscles on that side) are paralysed.

SYMPTOMS AND SIGNS
Even slight ectropion interferes with normal drainage of tears by distorting the opening of the tear duct. Chronic *conjunctivitis* may result, with redness, discomfort, and overflow of tears so that the skin becomes damp and inflamed. Constant wiping tends to pull the lid farther from the eye.

TREATMENT
Surgery to tighten the lid by removing a wedge of tissue is simple and effec-

tive in the early stages of ectropion. Plastic surgery may be needed if the condition is long-standing.

Eczema
An inflammation of the skin, usually causing itching and sometimes accompanied by scaling or blisters. Some forms of eczema are better known as *dermatitis* (such as seborrhoeic dermatitis, contact dermatitis, and photodermatitis). Eczema is sometimes caused by an *allergy,* but often occurs for no known reason.

TYPES
ATOPIC ECZEMA This chronic, superficial inflammation occurs in people who have an inherited tendency towards allergy. They, or members of their family, may also have other allergies, such as *asthma* or allergic *rhinitis* (hay fever). Dietary treatment—excluding certain foods or food additives—is sometimes helpful.

Atopic eczema is common in babies and often appears between the ages of two months and 18 months. An intensely itchy rash occurs, usually on the face, in the inner creases of the elbows, and behind the knees. The skin often scales in these areas, and small red pimples may appear. As the baby scratches, the pimples begin to ooze and join to form large weeping areas. Infection may occur, particularly in the nappy area.

For mild cases, treatment consists of applying *emollients,* such as petroleum jelly, which help keep the skin in the infected area soft. In severe cases, ointments containing *corticosteroid drugs* may be prescribed, and *antibiotic drugs* may be given for infection. *Antihistamine drugs* may be prescribed to reduce itching, particularly if it keeps a baby awake at night. The baby should be prevented from becoming too hot, which aggravates the condition. Only cotton clothing should be in direct contact with the skin.

The condition often clears of its own accord as a child grows older, although it may come and go for several years. Most children outgrow atopic eczema by puberty.

NUMMULAR ECZEMA This type usually occurs in adults. The cause is unknown. Nummular eczema takes the form of circular, itchy, scaling patches anywhere on the skin, similar to *tinea* (ringworm), from which the eczema needs to be distinguished. Corticosteroid drugs may be applied to the affected skin to help reduce inflammation, although the disorder is persistent and often resistant to treatment.

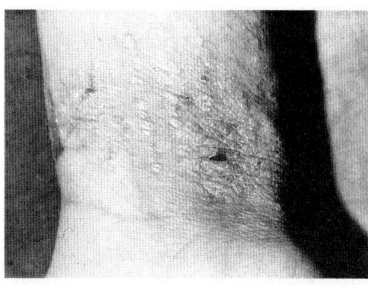

Atopic eczema
An example of atopic eczema on the creases of the inner wrist, showing the characteristic pimples and raw, scaling skin. Because the rash is intensely itchy, scratching is usually inevitable and aggravates the condition.

HAND ECZEMA This type is usually a result of irritation by substances such as detergents and dishwashing liquid, but may occur for no ascertainable reason. Itchy blisters, up to about 2.5 cm across, develop, usually on the palms, and the hand may be covered with scales and cracks. Tests are performed to check for allergy.

Hand eczema usually improves if rubber gloves are worn over white cotton gloves when in contact with any irritants. The hands should be thoroughly patted dry after washing. An unscented hand cream should be applied several times a day. If severe, corticosteroids may be prescribed for the inflammation and antibiotics may be given for infection.

STASIS ECZEMA In people with varicose veins, the skin on the legs may become irritated, inflamed, and discoloured. The most important factor is swelling of the legs, which may be controlled with compression bandages or stockings. Corticosteroid ointments may give temporary relief.

GENERAL TREATMENT
To reduce irritation and the likelihood of scratching, a soothing ointment should be applied to the affected areas, which should then be covered by a dressing to prevent scratching. Absorbent, nonirritating materials such as cotton should be worn next to the skin; irritating fabrics such as wool, silk, and rough synthetics should be avoided.

Edentulous
Without teeth, either because they have not yet grown or because they have fallen out or been removed.

EEG
The abbreviation for electroencephalogram. An EEG records the minute electrical impulses produced by the

activity of the brain. The technique of electroencephalography was first used in medicine in 1928, although it had been known since the 19th century that electrical impulses could be recorded from animal brains.

WHY IT IS DONE

An EEG indicates, by the frequency of the recorded activity, the mental state of the subject—that is, whether he or she is alert, awake, or asleep. Also, by revealing characteristic wave patterns, the EEG can help in diagnosing certain conditions, especially *epilepsy* and certain types of *encephalitis*, *dementia*, and *brain tumour*.

Electroencephalography can also be used to monitor the condition of patients during surgery and to assess the depth of *anaesthesia*. It is also used as a test for *brain death*, but it is not required to make the determination.

Effusion

The escape of fluid through the walls of a blood vessel into a tissue or body cavity, often as a result of a vessel being inflamed or congested. For example, *pleural effusion*, a symptom of *heart failure*, occurs when raised blood pressure in the veins leads to fluid being forced out of the blood and through the walls of capillaries into the pleural cavity around the lungs.

Effusion, joint

The accumulation of fluid in a joint space, causing swelling, limitation of movement, and usually pain and tenderness. A joint is enclosed by a capsule lined with a membrane called the synovium. This membrane normally secretes small amounts of fluid to lubricate the joint, but if it is damaged or inflamed (e.g. by *arthritis*) it produces excessive amounts of fluid.

TREATMENT

Analgesic drugs (painkillers), *nonsteroidal anti-inflammatory drugs*, and injections of *corticosteroid drugs* help relieve pain and inflammation. The swelling can be reduced by rest, firm wrapping with a bandage, ice-packs, and, when possible, keeping the affected joint

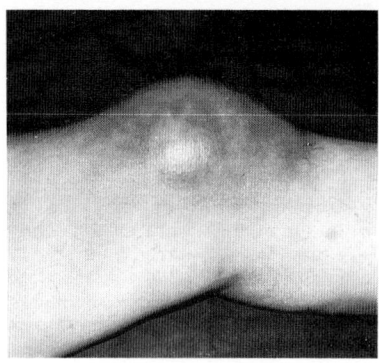

Location of knee joint effusion
Excessive production and accumulation of fluid within a knee joint caused by injury or inflammation.

raised. In some cases, the fluid may need to be aspirated (drawn out) with a hypodermic needle and syringe. *Antibiotic drugs* may also be given if the cause is infective arthritis (also called septic arthritis). *Physiotherapy* may be necessary to restore full movement.

Egg

See *Ovum*.

Ego

The conscious sense of oneself, equivalent to "I". In Freudian *psychoanalytic theory*, this part of the personality maintains a balance between the primitive, unconscious instincts of the *id*, the controls of the *superego* (or conscience), and the demands of the outside world.

Ehlers-Danlos syndrome

An inherited disorder of *collagen*, the most important structural protein in the body. Affected individuals have abnormally stretchy, thin skin that bruises very easily. Wounds are slow to heal and leave paper-thin scars. Sufferers tend to bleed easily from the gums and digestive tract. The joints are exceptionally loose and are prone to recurrent dislocation.

Ehlers-Danlos syndrome is usually (although not always) inherited in an autosomal dominant pattern (see *Genetic disorders*). This means that many affected individuals have an affected parent; each of an affected person's children has a 50 per cent chance of being affected.

There is no known specific treatment for Ehlers-Danlos syndrome, although unnecessary accidental injury, as may occur in contact sports, should be avoided. The outlook for a normal life expectancy is good.

HOW ELECTROENCEPHALOGRAPHY IS DONE

A number of small electrodes are attached to the scalp. Shaving of the scalp is unnecessary. The electrodes are connected to an instrument that measures the brain's impulses in microvolts and amplifies them for recording purposes. The technique is painless, produces no side-effects, and takes about 45 minutes. Recordings are taken with the subject at rest, with eyes open and then shut, during and after *hyperventilation*, and while looking at a flashing light. It is also helpful, especially when epilepsy is suspected, to record activity as the patient goes to sleep.

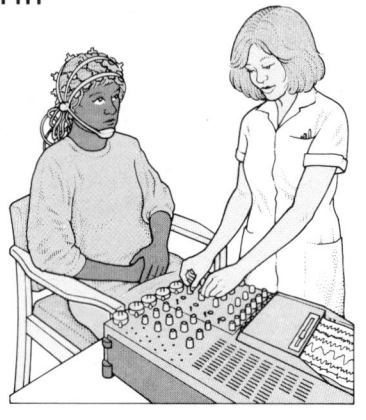

EEG wave patterns

Alpha waves
The prominent pattern of an awake, relaxed adult whose eyes are closed.

Beta waves
The lower, faster oscillation of a person who is concentrating on an external stimulus.

Delta waves
The typical pattern of sleep, but also found in young infants; rarely, they are caused by a brain tumour.

Theta waves
The dominant waves of young children. In adults, they may indicate an abnormality of the brain.

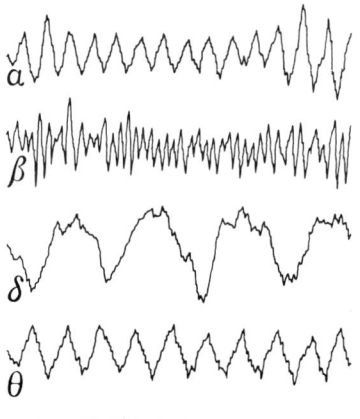

Eisenmenger complex

A condition affecting the heart and lungs in which a heart deformity leads to a build-up of pressure in the right side of the heart (see *Pulmonary hypertension*) that causes the abnormal flow of blood from the right side of the heart to the left side of the heart. Eisenmenger complex most often occurs in people with certain congenital heart defects (see *Heart disease, congenital*), such as uncorrected ventricular *septal defect*.

In people with Eisenmenger complex, deoxygenated blood in the right side of the heart is shunted through the defect into the left side of the heart and recirculated around the body, instead of being sent to the lungs to receive more oxygen. The resultant *hypoxia* (lack of oxygen in the blood) causes *cyanosis* (bluish discoloration of the skin), fainting, and breathing difficulty.

The diagnosis is confirmed by cardiac *catheterization* (the insertion under X-ray control of a thin tube into the heart via a blood vessel) to measure pressure and the composition of *blood gases* within the four heart chambers.

Once Eisenmenger complex has developed, surgical correction of the original heart defect will not help. Drug treatment may help to control symptoms. Most affected people die in their 30s or 40s. A heart-lung transplant may offer new hope to severely disabled patients.

Ejaculation

The emission of *semen* from the penis at *orgasm*. Ejaculation is a reflex action that depends on regular and rhythmic pressure on the penis, usually during intercourse or masturbation. This stimulation acts on spinal nerves and triggers ejaculation.

Shortly before ejaculation the muscles around the epididymides (ducts where sperm are stored), the prostate gland, and the seminal vesicles contract rhythmically, forcing the sperm from the epididymides to move forwards and mix with the secretions from the seminal vesicles and prostate. At ejaculation, this fluid is propelled through the urethra and out of the body.

Because both semen and urine leave the body by the same route, the bladder neck closes during ejaculation. This not only prevents ejaculate from going into the bladder but also stops urine from contaminating the semen. (See also *Reproductive system, male.*)

Ejaculation, disorders of

Conditions in which the normal process or timing of *ejaculation* is disrupted. Disorders of ejaculation are relatively common causes of unhappiness in relationships.

TYPES

PREMATURE EJACULATION In this disorder, ejaculation occurs before or very soon after penetration. Premature ejaculation is the most common sexual problem in men and is especially common in adolescents. Most adult men occasionally experience premature ejaculation, commonly because of overstimulation or anxiety about sexual performance. If premature ejaculation occurs frequently, the cause may be psychological. Sexual counselling and techniques for delaying ejaculation may help to alleviate the problem (see *Sex therapy*).

INHIBITED EJACULATION This is a rare condition in which erection is normal, or even prolonged, but ejaculation is abnormally delayed or does not occur at all. Inhibited ejaculation may be psychological in origin, in which case sexual counselling may help, or it may be a complication of another disorder, such as *diabetes mellitus* or the long-term effects of *alcohol dependence*. Inhibited ejaculation may also occur during treatment with certain drugs, such as some *antihypertensive drugs*.

RETROGRADE EJACULATION In this disorder, the valve at the base of the bladder fails to close during ejaculation. This forces the ejaculate back into the bladder. Retrograde ejaculation may occur as a result of a neurological disease, after surgery on the neck of the bladder, after *prostatectomy* (removal of the prostate gland), or after extensive pelvic surgery. There is no treatment, but intercourse with a full bladder can sometimes lead to normal ejaculation. (See also *Azoospermia*; *Psychosexual dysfunction*; *Sexual problems*.)

Elbow

The joint between the lower end of the *humerus* (upper-arm bone) and the upper ends of the radius and ulna (forearm bones). The elbow joint is stabilized by ligaments at the front, back, and sides. The elbow enables the arm to be bent and straightened, and the forearm to be rotated through almost 180 degrees around its long axis without more than slight movement of the upper arm.

DISORDERS

Disorders include *arthritis* and injuries to the joint and its surrounding muscles, tendons, and ligaments.

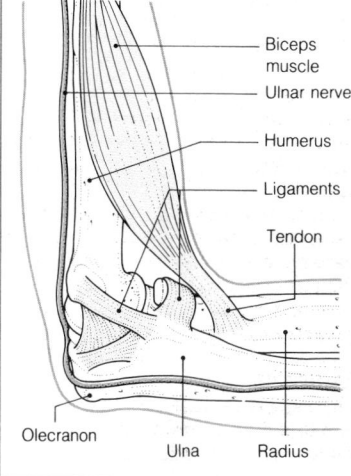

ANATOMY OF THE ELBOW
The elbow is a hinge joint between the lower end of the humerus and the upper ends of the radius and ulna. The biceps muscle bends and rotates the arm at the elbow.

Biceps muscle
Ulnar nerve
Humerus
Ligaments
Tendon
Olecranon
Ulna
Radius

SOFT TISSUE INJURY AND INFLAMMATION Repetitive strain on the tendons of the forearm muscles at the points at which they attach to the elbow (at the bony outgrowths called epicondyles) can lead to an inflammation called *epicondylitis* at these points. The two main types of epicondylitis are *tennis elbow* and *golfer's elbow*. Alternatively, a *sprain* of the joint ligaments can occur, especially in children.

Olecranon *bursitis* occurs over the tip of the elbow in response to local irritation. Repeated overstraightening of the joint can cause damage to the cartilage that lines the joint. Strain on the joint produces an *effusion* (accumulation of fluid within the joint space) or traumatic *synovitis* (inflammation of the membrane that lines the joint capsule).

A sharp blow on the olecranon process (the bony tip of the elbow, also called the "funny bone") may impinge on the *ulnar nerve* as it passes in a groove in this area, causing temporary discomfort—a pins-and-needles sensation and lancing pains that shoot down the forearm into the fourth and fifth fingers.

FRACTURES A fall on to an outstretched hand or on to the tip of the elbow can lead to any of various types of fracture around or at the lower end of the humerus. Children may alternatively sustain an injury to the epiphyses (growing areas) at the ends of the

THE ELDERLY AS A PERCENTAGE OF THE POPULATION (1990)

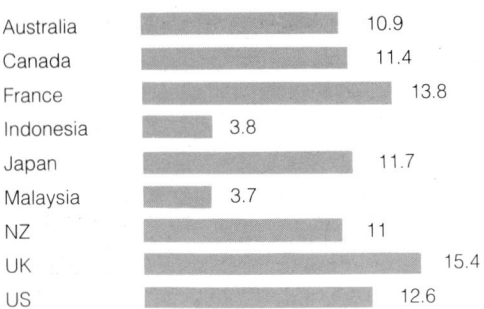

Australia	10.9
Canada	11.4
France	13.8
Indonesia	3.8
Japan	11.7
Malaysia	3.7
NZ	11
UK	15.4
US	12.6

National comparisons
People over 65 now make up more than 10 per cent of the total population in most Western countries. This population pattern results from lower birth rates and increases in life expectancy due to improved medical care.

humerus, radius, or ulna. Dislocation of the elbow can occur at any age as a result of falling on to an outstretched hand; dislocations and fractures of the elbow frequently occur together.

ARTHRITIS *Osteoarthritis,* *rheumatoid arthritis,* and infective arthritis can affect the elbow joint.

Elderly, care of the

As people age they become prone to an increasing number of physical disorders and are more likely to suffer from loneliness and isolation. Efforts to stress personal pride and independence (along with appropriate medical care) can minimize physical and mental deterioration. Sensitive attention to psychological needs can help the elderly enjoy old age and can encourage them to feel that they are still useful members of society.

PHYSICAL CARE

Elderly people often ignore symptoms of illness, either because they do not want to be a nuisance to those caring for them or because they are afraid of being "put away" in a home. Some conditions, such as *hypothyroidism* (underactivity of the thyroid gland) and *anaemia,* which is often due to a poor diet, cause a very gradual deterioration. Such deterioration may incorrectly be assumed to be a natural effect of old age, resulting in failure to diagnose actual medical conditions.

Failing vision and hearing are frequently regarded as inevitable features of old age, but in many cases surgical removal of a *cataract* or provision of a *hearing-aid* can enable the individual to lead a more independent and active life.

To ensure that medical problems are detected early and treated, it is important that carers remain alert to the symptoms and signs of illness. In addition, all people over 65 years of age should have regular check-ups.

PSYCHOLOGICAL CARE

Common causes of *depression* in the elderly are isolation, inactivity, and a feeling of not being wanted. Elderly people can be helped by making them part of family activities. Attending a day-care centre or senior citizen club can provide contact with other people and the opportunity to develop new interests. *Dementia* (loss of normal brain function) becomes more common as a person ages and increases the level of supervision required.

DAY-TO-DAY CARE

Many elderly people prefer to live with their families, ideally in a separate section of the house, where they can have some degree of independence. If this is not possible, they may be able to live near relatives so that help can be provided with daily activities, such as shopping, cooking, and laundry. Assistance with personal care may also be required.

While this type of arrangement may be ideal for the elderly person, the responsibility can be a great strain on other members of the family. Voluntary agencies can sometimes help by providing a daily meal or occasional domestic help.

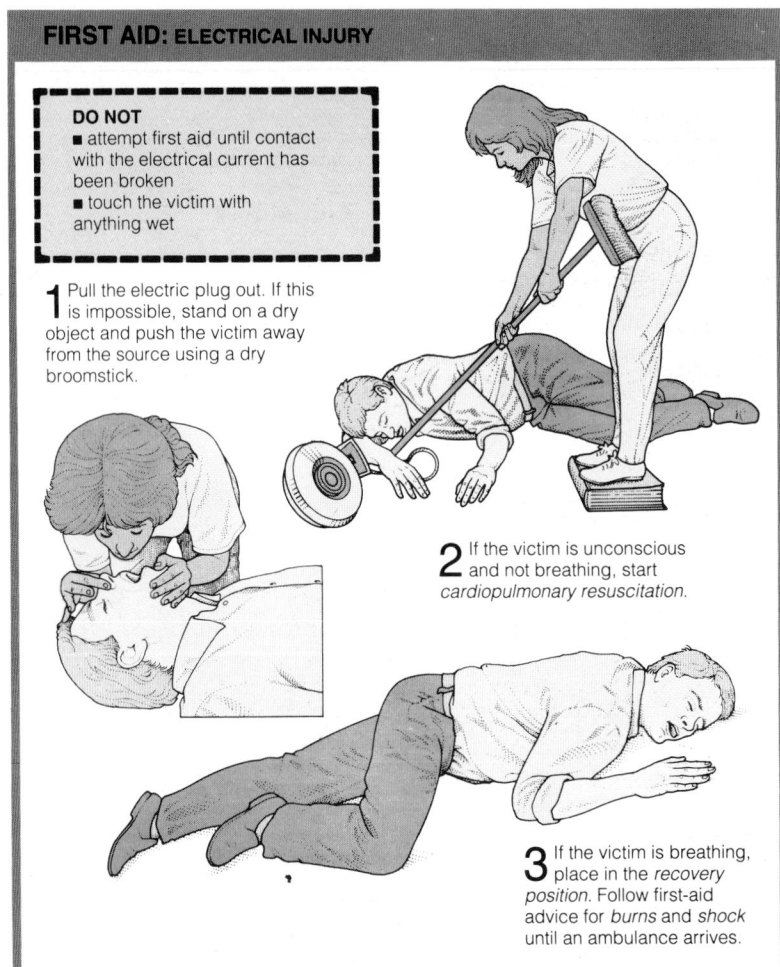

FIRST AID: ELECTRICAL INJURY

DO NOT
■ attempt first aid until contact with the electrical current has been broken
■ touch the victim with anything wet

1 Pull the electric plug out. If this is impossible, stand on a dry object and push the victim away from the source using a dry broomstick.

2 If the victim is unconscious and not breathing, start *cardiopulmonary resuscitation.*

3 If the victim is breathing, place in the *recovery position.* Follow first-aid advice for *burns* and *shock* until an ambulance arrives.

E

The elderly person's home, or that part of the house set aside for his or her use, should be well-heated in winter and cooled in summer to prevent *hypothermia* or *hyperthermia*; a high level of artificial illumination should be provided to make activities such as reading and sewing easier. The risk of falls can be reduced by ensuring that there are no loose rugs or slippery surfaces (see *Falls in the elderly*) and the person living alone can be provided with an alarm that enables him or her to summon help in an emergency.

Sheltered housing is becoming a popular choice for many elderly people. It allows independence while providing discreet supervision and assistance when needed.

Elective
A term used to describe a procedure, usually a surgical operation, that is not essential but can be performed at a chosen time. Because an elective procedure is not an emergency, it is often possible for the patient—in consultation with the doctor—to select the most convenient time for the procedure. Elective surgery includes the correction of nonurgent medical conditions, such as *haemorrhoids* or a *hernia*, as well as some cosmetic procedures, such as *rhinoplasty*.

Electrical injury
Damage to the tissues caused by the passage of an electric current through the body and by its associated heat release.

The internal tissues of the body, being moist and salty, are good conductors of electricity. Dry skin provides a high resistance (several tens of thousands of ohms) to current flow, but moist skin has a low resistance (only a few thousand ohms) and thus allows a substantial current to flow into the body. Serious injury or death from domestic voltage levels is thus more likely in the presence of water. The danger of serious injury is increased if a person is "well-earthed" (i.e. in contact with a good conductor of electricity, such as a bath of water) and decreased if he or she is in a dry environment (especially if he or she is wearing shoes soled with rubber, which is a poor conductor of electricity).

INCIDENCE
Electrical accidents in England and Wales cause just under 100 deaths each year. Many of these deaths occur in the home, as a result of handling a frayed electric flex or using an electri-

cal appliance near water. Some deaths occur among workers in the electrical generating and construction industries as a result of contact with high voltages. Fewer than 10 people die in England and Wales annually as a result of lightning accidents.

Many other people are injured every year, some of them seriously.

PHYSICAL EFFECTS
All except the mildest electric shocks may cause unconsciousness. The extent of tissue damage depends on the size and type of the current flowing through the body. Alternating current (AC) is more dangerous than direct current (DC) because it causes sustained muscle contractions, which, by preventing hand movement, may prevent the victim from releasing his or her grip on the source of the current.

A current as small as one tenth of an amp passing through the heart can bring about a fatal *arrhythmia* (disturbance of the heartbeat). This quantity is about the size of current passing through the filament of a very low-power bulb. The same current passing through the brainstem may cause the heart to stop beating and breathing to cease. Larger currents, generated by high voltages, may also cause charring of tissues, especially at points where the resistance is highest, usually where the current enters and exits from the body.

Electric shock treatment
See *ECT* (electroconvulsive therapy).

Electrocardiography
See *ECG*.

Electrocautery
A technique for destroying tissue by the application of heat produced by an electric current. Electrocautery can be used to remove certain skin blemishes, such as *warts*. (See also *Cauterization; Diathermy; Electrocoagulation*.)

Electrocoagulation
The use of high-frequency electric current to seal blood vessels by heat and thus stop bleeding. Electrocoagulation may be used during all forms of surgery to close freshly cut blood vessels. It is also used to destroy spider naevi and other kinds of abnormal blood vessel formations and to stop nosebleeds. The current is applied through a fine needle or, in surgery, may be delivered through a knife, enabling the surgeon to make bloodless incisions.

Electroconvulsive therapy
See *ECT*.

Electroencephalography
See *EEG*.

Electrolysis
Permanent removal of unwanted hair by means of short-wave electric current, which destroys the hairs' roots.

WHY IT IS DONE
Hair on the face and body can be removed temporarily by shaving or plucking, or by the use of depilatory creams, abrasives, or wax preparations. Electrolysis is the only means of permanent removal.

Before treatment a person should first ensure that the operator is fully trained; incompetent treatment can cause permanent disfigurement.

AREAS THAT CAN BE TREATED
With a few exceptions, electrolysis can be safely used on any part of the body where excessive hair is regarded as unsightly. Its use should be avoided on the lower margins of the eyebrows, where the skin above the eyelids is delicate and easily damaged, and it is questionable whether it should be used on the armpits because of a risk of bacterial infection. Electrolysis has no harmful effect on the breasts (where hair sometimes grows around the areola, the dark area surrounding the nipple) or on the ability of mother or infant to breast-feed.

The legs are not well suited for electrolysis; treatment requires so many sessions that it is too time-consuming and expensive for most people.

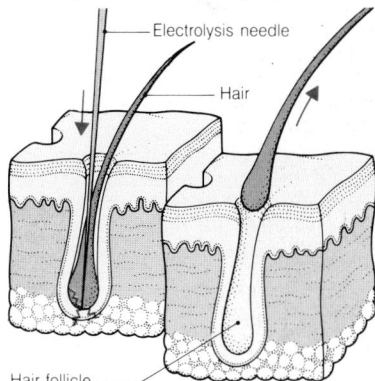

Electrolysis needle

Hair

Hair follicle

How electrolysis is done
To remove each hair, a fine needle is inserted into the follicle and a small electric current is passed through it. The current destroys the root of the hair, which is then pulled out. The procedure may cause some pain, but in skilled hands, it is harmless. If the treatment is successful, there should be no more hair growth from that follicle.

E

Electrolyte

A substance whose molecules dissociate (split) into its constituent *ions* (electrically charged particles) when dissolved or melted. For example, sodium chloride (table salt) dissociates into positive sodium ions and negative chloride ions in water.

Electromyography

See *EMG*.

Electronystagmography

A method of recording the various types of *nystagmus* (abnormal jerky movements of the eye) to investigate their cause. Electrical changes caused by eye movements are picked up by electrodes placed near the eyes and are recorded on a graph for analysis.

Electrophoresis

The movement of electrically charged particles suspended in a *colloid* solution under the influence of an electric current. The direction, distance, and rate of movement vary according to factors such as the size, shape, and electrical charge of the particles.

Electrophoresis can be used to analyse mixtures of substances, particularly to identify different proteins in a mixture. For example, electrophoresis can be used to identify and quantify the various proteins in blood; furthermore, by comparing the results from a particular blood sample with normal values, it is possible to diagnose disorders such as *myeloma*, a tumour of the bone marrow that produces abnormally high levels of a specific *immunoglobulin* in the blood.

Elephantiasis

A disease found in the tropics, characterized by massive swellings of the legs, arms, and scrotum, with thickening and darkening of the overlying skin so that it resembles the skin of an elephant. Most elephantiasis is due to chronic lymphatic obstruction occurring as a feature of *filariasis* (a worm infestation).

ELISA test

A laboratory blood test commonly used in the diagnosis of infectious diseases. ELISA stands for enzyme-linked immunosorbent assay. (See also *Immunoassay*.)

Elixir

A clear, sweetened liquid, often containing alcohol, that forms the basis for many liquid medicines, such as *cough remedies*.

Embolectomy

Surgical removal of an *embolus* (a fragment of material carried in the bloodstream) that has blocked a blood vessel (see *Embolism*).

The embolus may be removed during an operation performed under general anaesthesia. An incision is made in the affected artery and the embolus aspirated (removed through a suction tube).

Alternatively, an embolus may be removed by a procedure known as balloon embolectomy, in which a *balloon catheter* is passed into the affected blood vessel. This procedure may be performed using local anaesthesia.

Embolism

Blockage of an artery by a fragment of material travelling in the bloodstream. The particle causing the blockage is called an embolus and may consist of a blood clot, a bubble of air or other gas, a piece of tissue or tumour, a clump of bacteria, bone marrow, cholesterol, or fat, or any of various other substances.

TYPES

Blood clots are the most common type of embolus and in most cases have broken off from a larger clot that has formed elsewhere in the blood circulation. *Pulmonary embolism* is usually the result of a fragment breaking off from a deep vein *thrombosis* (a blood clot formed in a deep vein, usually in a leg) and being carried via the heart to block an artery supplying the lungs; this is a common cause of sudden, unexpected death. Similar blood clots may form on the lining of the heart after a *myocardial infarction* (heart attack) and then travel to the brain, resulting in a cerebral embolism, which is an important cause of *stroke*.

Air embolism, in which a small artery is blocked by an air bubble, is rare. Fat embolism, in which blood vessels are blocked by fat globules, is a possible complication of a major fracture of the arm or leg. Amniotic fluid embolism, in which some of the fluid that surrounds the baby in the uterus is forced into the mother's circulation, is a rare complication of late pregnancy.

SYMPTOMS

Factors that determine symptoms include the extent of blockage, the size and type of embolus, and the size, nature, and location of the affected blood vessel. In pulmonary embolism the sufferer feels faint and breathless, and has chest pains. If the embolus causes a *stroke*, the symptoms depend on which part of the brain is affected; it may, for example, cause inability to speak, inability to move a part of the body, loss of consciousness, or a disturbance of vision. In the small num-

---

TYPES OF EMBOLISM

Embolisms are named after the part of the circulation affected or the embolus involved (e.g. a fat embolism is caused by fat globules, sometimes released from a bone fracture). When an embolus is released, it is carried through branches of an artery until it becomes lodged. Blood is prevented from reaching parts of the body beyond.

Embolism in the arm
This X-ray of the upper arm was taken after the injection of contrast medium into the blood vessel. It shows, near the top, an embolus obstructing the normal flow of blood through one of the main arteries.

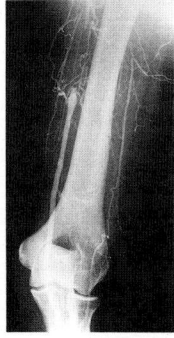

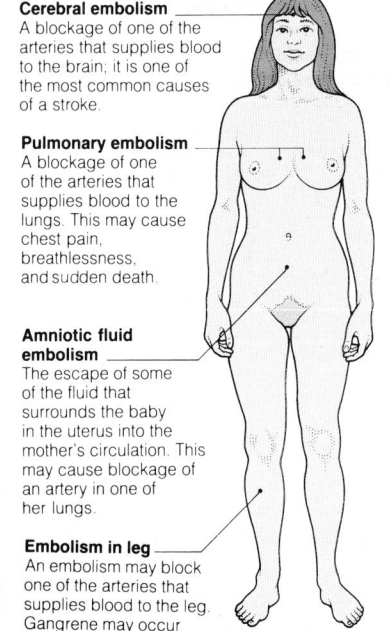

Cerebral embolism
A blockage of one of the arteries that supplies blood to the brain; it is one of the most common causes of a stroke.

Pulmonary embolism
A blockage of one of the arteries that supplies blood to the lungs. This may cause chest pain, breathlessness, and sudden death.

Amniotic fluid embolism
The escape of some of the fluid that surrounds the baby in the uterus into the mother's circulation. This may cause blockage of an artery in one of her lungs.

Embolism in leg
An embolism may block one of the arteries that supplies blood to the leg. Gangrene may occur below the blockage.

ber of serious cases of fat embolism, the patient's heart rate and breathing rate rise dramatically, and there is restlessness and confusion accompanied by drowsiness.

TREATMENT

If a pulmonary or other severe type of embolism causes the person to collapse, emergency life-saving procedures are carried out to maintain breathing and circulation. If the person survives, *embolectomy* (surgery to remove the blockage) may be possible. If surgery is not possible, *thrombolytic drugs* (drugs that dissolve blood clots) and *anticoagulant drugs* (drugs that prevent clot formation) may be administered.

OUTLOOK

In all severe types of embolism, survival depends on the success of resuscitation attempts, the importance of the vessel obstructed, and the speed with which blood flow is re-established. If the source of the embolus is treated, the long-term prospects for the patient are good.

Embolization

Also called therapeutic embolism, the deliberate obstruction of a blood vessel to stop internal bleeding or to cut off blood flow to a tumour.

WHY IT IS DONE

Embolization is increasingly being performed to stop otherwise uncontrollable bleeding, particularly when the patient is too ill to undergo surgery. Among its uses are the control of bleeding from small vessels in the lining of the intestine, often due to a malformation of blood vessels (similar to a birthmark in the skin).

Using the technique to deprive a tumour of its blood supply has several effects. It can relieve the pain caused by the growth; it can cause the tumour to shrivel, making surgical removal easier; or it may stop the tumour from spreading. Embolization may be used to treat tumours that would be difficult to remove surgically, such as tumours in the liver. It is also used to treat certain vascular tumours on the face, such as *haemangiomas*, in preference to surgery that might leave unsightly scars.

HOW IT IS DONE

The procedure is usually carried out by a radiologist with the patient under a general anaesthetic. The first step is to obtain an image of the blood vessel to be blocked and of the vessels leading to it. This image is obtained by means of *angiography*, an X-ray procedure in which a substance that is opaque to X-rays is introduced into the blood vessels through a *catheter* (a flexible tube).

The catheter is then guided, by means of television monitoring, as close as possible to the vessel to be blocked, and the embolus that will block the blood vessel is released. Emboli are made of many materials, such as blood-clotting agents (e.g. fibrin), metal coils, silicone balloons, wool, and medicinal glue.

RISKS

There is always a risk that an embolus may lodge in the wrong blood vessel and cause problems; for example, an embolus that blocks a vessel in the brain may cause a *stroke*. The procedure is still being refined.

Embolus

A fragment of material that travels in the blood circulation and causes obstruction of an artery. An embolus is life-threatening if it blocks the flow of blood through a vital artery (see *Embolism*).

Embrocation

A medication rubbed into unbroken skin to relieve the muscular and joint pain of sprains and strains.

Embryo

The unborn child during the first eight weeks of its development following *conception*; for the rest of the pregnancy it is known as a *fetus*.

Development of the embryo (see illustrated box overleaf) is governed internally by *genes* inherited from the parents, and externally by factors such as the woman's diet and any drugs taken during pregnancy.

THE FIRST TWO WEEKS

The embryo develops from an egg that has been fertilized by a sperm (see *Fertilization*). It starts as a single cell—just large enough to be seen by the naked eye. As the fertilized egg travels along the tube to the uterus, the cell divides in two. These two new cells divide to form four cells. Cell divisions continue, each time doubling the number of cells. The cells form a spherical mass, in the centre of which a hollow depression develops. Within the sphere, the cells then form into two very distinct groups: one makes up the wall lining the sphere; the other expands to form the embryo itself.

On about the sixth day the sphere of cells becomes attached to and then embedded in the lining of the uterus. At the site of attachment the outer layer of cells obtains nourishment from the woman's blood; that part of the outer layer will later develop into the placenta.

Two bubbles form side by side within the cell mass. Between the bubbles a flat disc forms, consisting of layers of cells from which all the baby's tissues and organs will form. The amniotic sac develops around the growing embryo.

THE THIRD WEEK

Early in the third week, the disc of cells becomes pear-shaped. The head of the embryo forms at the rounded end and the lower spine at the pointed end. A group of cells develops along the back of the embryo to form the notochord, a rod of cells that constitutes the basis for the spine. From this time on, the embryo has two recognizable halves that develop more or less symmetrically. The notochord then furrows and the edges grow towards each other before fusing to form the neural tube. Later, the neural tube will develop into the brain and spinal cord.

THE FOURTH WEEK

During the fourth week the embryo becomes recognizable as a mammal. The back grows more rapidly than the front, giving the embryo a C-shape, and a tail becomes visible. Within the embryo, buds of tissue form that will later develop into the lungs, pancreas, liver, and gallbladder.

The neural tube extends towards the head of the embryo, where a broad fold becomes visible that eventually will grow into the brain. The developing ears first appear as pits. Rudimentary eyes develop in the form of stalks. The outer layers begin to form the limb buds and the branchial arches (folds of tissue) that are later to become the jaws and other structures in the neck.

Paired bulges appear on the sides of the neural tube that will become the cartilage, bone, and muscle of the back. On the front of the embryo, just beneath the head, a rudimentary heart develops in the form of a straight tube. As the branchial arches develop, the heart is pushed down into the chest. It is during this period that the embryo is at the greatest risk of birth defects caused by abnormal genetic or external factors (see *Birth defects*).

THE FIFTH WEEK

The external ears become visible, pits mark the position of the developing nose, the upper and lower jaws form, and the limb buds extend, becoming flattened at the end where the hands and feet will develop.

E

THE DEVELOPING EMBRYO

From the time of conception until the eighth week, the developing baby is known as an embryo. At conception, the fertilized egg consists of a single cell, the zygote, which contains genetic material from the sperm and the egg. The zygote divides several times to form a ball of cells, which then implants into the lining of the uterus. At the point of attachment, the outer layer of cells forms the placenta, while a group of cells within one area of the cell ball develops into the embryo. A sac filled with amniotic fluid forms around the embryo to protect it. As the embryo grows, it begins to form features and, by the fifth week, it has developed a recognizable head and limb buds.

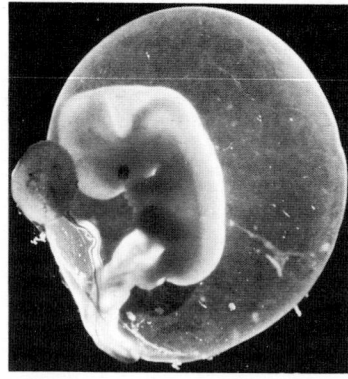

Embryo at about six weeks
The embryo is floating in the amniotic sac. The smaller sac at left (the yolk sac) provides nourishment for the early embryo.

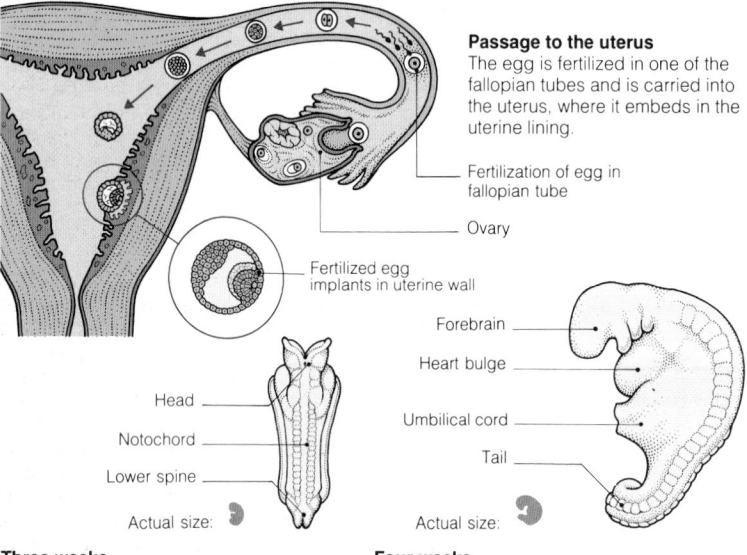

Passage to the uterus
The egg is fertilized in one of the fallopian tubes and is carried into the uterus, where it embeds in the uterine lining.

Fertilization of egg in fallopian tube

Ovary

Fertilized egg implants in uterine wall

Head
Notochord
Lower spine
Actual size:

Forebrain
Heart bulge
Umbilical cord
Tail
Actual size:

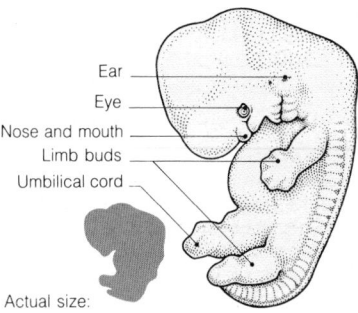

Ear
Eye
Nose and mouth
Limb buds
Umbilical cord
Actual size:

Three weeks
The embryo becomes pear-shaped, with a rounded head, pointed lower spine, and notochord running along its back.

Four weeks
The embryo becomes C-shaped and a tail is visible. The umbilical cord forms and the forebrain enlarges.

Six weeks
Eyes are visible and the mouth, nose, and ears are forming. The limbs grow rapidly from initial tiny buds.

INTERNAL ORGANS AT FIVE WEEKS

All the internal organs (such as the liver, pancreas, stomach, heart, lungs, kidneys, and sex organs) have begun to form by the fifth week. During this critical stage of development, the embryo is highly vulnerable to harmful substances consumed by the mother (such as alcohol and medication), which may cause birth defects.

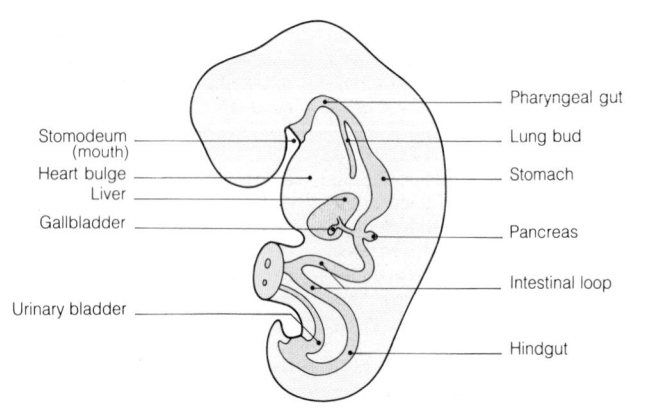

Stomodeum (mouth)
Heart bulge
Liver
Gallbladder
Urinary bladder

Pharyngeal gut
Lung bud
Stomach
Pancreas
Intestinal loop
Hindgut

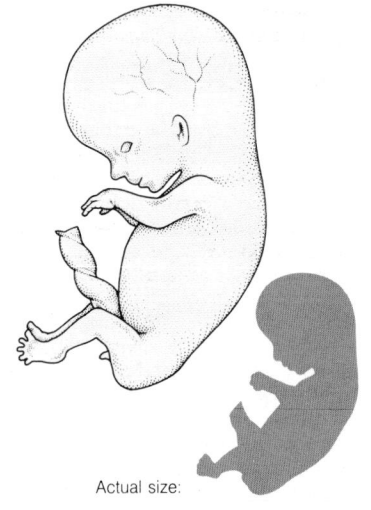

Actual size:

Eight weeks
The face is more "human", the head is more upright, and the tail has gone. Limbs become jointed and digits appear.

The two folds of tissue meet at the front of the embryo and fuse to form the front wall of the chest and abdomen. The umbilical cord develops.

THE SIXTH TO EIGHTH WEEKS
The face becomes recognizably human, the neck forms, the trunk becomes less curved and the head more erect, the tail between the buttocks disappears, the limbs become jointed, and fingers and toes appear.

After eight weeks the embryo is about 2.5 cm long. Most of the internal organs have formed and all the external features are present.

Embryology

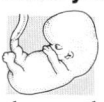 The study of the development and growth of the *embryo* and then the *fetus* from conception through the months of gestation until birth.

Embryology is an essential part of the medical student's training because it leads to a greater understanding of adult anatomy and of the way structural defects in the body may arise. For example, the occurrence of congenital heart defects, such as septal defects ("holes in the heart") and transposition of the main blood vessels, is easier to understand when the stages of fetal heart development are explained.

Embryology was formerly based on the study of animal embryos and dead human embryos at different stages of antenatal development. More recently, details about the nature of physical and chemical processes involved in embryo development have been established by examination of live embryos grown in the laboratory (see *Embryo, research on*).

Embryo, research on

Human *embryos* are grown for a few days (until the first two or three cells divisions have taken place) in specialized laboratories as part of one type of treatment for infertility (see *In vitro fertilization*). Doctors usually fertilize more eggs than they need for this procedure, since they do not know how many will "take" (begin the process of cell division and growth); the surplus embryos at this very early stage may then be frozen for use in later attempts at achieving a pregnancy.

Research on surplus embryos could be directed at improving the results of in vitro fertilization, at finding better methods of contraception, and at detecting genetic disorders at an early stage in pregnancy. However, in several countries, such research has been prohibited, limited to the first 14 days, or is not being carried out

because the doctors concerned have agreed not to do so for ethical reasons.

Emergency

Any condition requiring urgent medical treatment, such as cardiac arrest (heart stoppage), or any procedure that must be performed immediately, such as *cardiopulmonary resuscitation.*

Many emergency cases are dealt with in hospital Accident and Emergency (or Casualty) departments. Doctors and nurses who work in Accident and Emergency departments are specially trained to deal with a wide range of injuries and conditions that require urgent medical attention.

Emesis

The medical term for *vomiting.*

Emetic

A substance that causes vomiting, used to treat some types of poisoning and drug overdose. Emetics work by stimulating the part of the brain that controls vomiting and/or by directly irritating the lining of the stomach.

The most widely used emetic is *ipecacuanha.* Emetics should not be given to a person who is drowsy because he or she may inhale the vomit.

EMG

The abbreviation for electromyogram, a recording of the electrical activity in muscle. Electromyography takes 30 to 60 minutes to perform, depending on the number of muscles to be tested. There are no side-effects.

WHY IT IS DONE
An EMG can reveal the presence of muscle disorders, such as *muscular dystrophy,* or disorders in which the nerve supply to muscle is impaired, such as *neuropathy* or *radiculopathy.* In cases of nerve injury, the actual site of nerve damage can often be located.

HOW IT IS DONE
Electrical activity is measured during muscle contraction and when they are at rest. To detect the electrical impulses, small disc electrodes are attached to the skin surface over the muscle. Alternatively, needle electrodes are inserted into the muscle. The impulses are displayed on an oscilloscope screen and a permanent record can be made on film. Changes in the electrical wave patterns can be used in the diagnosis of certain nerve or muscle disorders.

EMLA

An abbreviation for eutetic mixture of local anaesthetics. This is a cream that is applied to the skin under an

air-excluding dressing (to prevent the cream drying) to produce local *analgesia.* This allows needles to be inserted into blood vessels with less discomfort, particularly in children. It is also used for patients needing repeated cannulation of blood vessels, and in skin grafting.

Emollient

A substance such as olive oil, lanolin, or petroleum jelly that has a soothing, softening effect when applied to the skin, eyes, or mucous membranes (e.g. the lining of the nose and mouth). By forming an oily film, emollients prevent water loss from these surfaces and therefore have a moisturizing effect. Emollients are used in creams, ointments, nasal sprays, and suppositories.

Emotional deprivation

Lack of sufficient loving attention and warm, trusting relationships during a child's early years, leading to difficulty in normal emotional development. Emotional deprivation may result if *bonding* does not occur in the early months of life, if a child is frequently separated from his or her parents for long periods during the first five years, or if parents cannot meet the child's emotional needs.

Emotionally deprived children may be impulsive, crave attention, cannot cope with frustration, and may have impaired intellectual development.

Emotional problems

A common term for a wide range of psychological difficulties. The problems may be due to upbringing, relationships, or psychiatric illness; *anxiety* and *depression* generally predominate.

Empathy

The ability to partake in and understand the thoughts and feelings of another person by comparing them with one's own experiences. In *psychoanalysis* the therapist partly relies on empathy to establish a relationship with a patient.

Emphysema

A disease in which the alveoli (tiny air sacs) in the *lungs* become damaged. The disorder causes shortness of breath and in severe cases can lead to *respiratory failure* or *heart failure.*
CAUSES
In almost all cases, emphysema is caused by cigarette smoking. Atmospheric pollution is sometimes a predisposing factor. In a few cases, a predisposition to emphysema is inher-

E

ited due to a deficiency of a chemical called alpha$_1$-antitrypsin in the lungs; the disease may appear early in life but its development is hastened and intensified by smoking or by exposure to industrial air pollution.

The alveoli, of which there are many millions in each lung, are groups of air sacs at the end of bronchioles (tiny air passages). Through their thin walls, inhaled oxygen is passed into the bloodstream and carbon dioxide is removed from the capillaries to be breathed out. Tobacco smoke and other air pollutants are believed to cause emphysema by provoking the release of chemicals within the alveoli that damage the alveolar walls. Alpha$_1$-antitrypsin is thought to protect against this chemical damage; hence, people with a deficiency of this substance are particularly badly affected. The damage is slight at first, but in heavy smokers it becomes progressively worse; the alveoli burst and blend to form fewer, larger sacs with less surface area, which consequently impairs oxygen and carbon dioxide exchange. Over the years the lungs become less and less elastic, which further reduces their efficiency.

Eventually—sometimes after many years—the level of oxygen in the blood starts to fall, with either of two effects. In some cases *pulmonary hypertension* (raised blood pressure in the pulmonary artery) develops, leading to *cor pulmonale* (enlargement and strain on the right side of the heart) and, subsequently, *oedema* (accumulation of fluid in the tissues), particularly in the lower legs. Other sufferers are able to compensate for oxygen deficiency to some extent by breathing faster. Why individuals react in one way and not the other is not known.

Emphysema is often accompanied by chronic *bronchitis*, also brought on by air pollutants and smoking.

INCIDENCE
No fewer than around 20,000 men and 10,000 women die each year in England and Wales from chronic obstructive lung disease (emphysema and/or chronic bronchitis); only about one quarter of these die from emphysema alone.

SYMPTOMS AND SIGNS
Initially, and for a considerable time in mild cases, there may be no symptoms, but as the disease progresses it results in increasing shortness of breath. At first this may be noticed only when climbing stairs or steep inclines, but gradually it becomes more severe until eventually it occurs after only mild exercise or is present even at rest.

A sign of emphysema is a barrel-shaped chest associated with air being trapped in the outer part of the lungs. There may also be a chronic cough (caused by accompanying bronchitis) and a slight wheeze.

As the disease progresses, sufferers in whom cor pulmonale develops start to turn blue due to oxygen deficiency in the blood and their legs swell because of oedema; these people are known as blue bloaters. Those who breathe rapidly and retain normal colouring are called pink puffers. Many people, however, show signs somewhere between these two extremes. As respiratory and/or heart failure develops, sufferers find it increasingly difficult to breathe.

DIAGNOSIS
The diagnosis is made from the patient's symptoms and signs, from a chest examination, and from various tests. A blood sample from an artery may be analysed to measure the concentration of *blood gases* (oxygen and carbon dioxide). A venous blood sample may be analysed to determine whether the disease is due to alpha$_1$-antitrypsin deficiency. *Chest X-rays* are taken to exclude the possibility of another lung disease being responsible for the symptoms and to determine how great an area of the lungs has been affected. *Pulmonary function tests* are carried out to assess breathing capacity and the efficiency of the alvoli in exchanging gases.

TREATMENT
Because emphysema is incurable—lung tissue that has been damaged cannot be replaced—treatment can only control the disease. The patient must completely stop smoking to prevent further damage. Efficiency of remaining lung tissue may be improved in various ways. *Bronchodilator drugs* are given to widen the bronchioles. Occasionally, *corticosteroid drugs*, taken by inhaler to reduce inflammation in the lungs, are also beneficial. Patients who are shown to have a deficiency of alpha$_1$-antitrypsin may be treated by inhalation of an aerosol containing the enzyme, which has been shown to slow the progression of the disease.

To treat oedema, *diuretic drugs* may be given to reduce the volume of fluid in the body by promoting output through increased urine production.

If the oxygen level of the blood falls considerably, *oxygen therapy* may be needed. Oxygen equipment may be available for use at home.

OUTLOOK
The course of the disease depends on how far it has progressed before the patient gives up smoking. If extensive areas of lung have been damaged or if cor pulmonale has developed, death occurs sooner or later from respiratory and/or heart failure.

Emphysema, surgical
The abnormal presence of air in tissues underlying the skin following injury or surgery. Surgical emphysema most often occurs as a complication of *pneumothorax* (the abnormal presence of air in the pleural cavity between the lung and the chest wall).

Empirical treatment
Treatment given because its effectiveness has been observed in previous, similar cases rather than because there is an understanding of the nature of the disorder and the way the treatment works. In the case of a fever of uncertain origin, for example, a doctor might prescribe antibiotic drugs on the basis of experience with similar cases.

Empyema
An accumulation of pus in a body cavity or in certain organs.

Pleural empyema occurs as a rare complication of a lung infection such as *pneumonia* or *pleurisy*; it may also develop after a severe injury to the chest that penetrates the pleural space. The main symptoms are chest pain, breathlessness, and fever. The diagnosis is confirmed by *chest X-rays* and removal of a sample of pus for laboratory analysis. Treatment is by *aspiration* (removal of the pus by suction) and the injection of *antibiotic drugs*, or by an operation to open the infected cavity and drain the pus.

Empyema of the gallbladder may occur as a complication of *cholecystitis*, when it usually causes abdominal pain, fever, and sometimes jaundice. It is treated by *cholecystectomy* (surgical removal of the gallbladder).

Enalapril
An *ACE inhibitor drug* used in the treatment of *hypertension* (high blood pressure) and *heart failure* (reduced pumping efficiency of the heart). It may be given with a *diuretic drug*. Enalapril was introduced in 1986.

Enamel, dental
The hard outer layer of a tooth that covers and protects the inner structures (see *Teeth*).

Encephalitis

Inflammation of the *brain*, usually caused by a viral infection. In many cases the *meninges* (the membranes that surround the brain) are also affected. An attack may be so mild that it is barely noticeable, but in most cases encephalitis is a serious and potentially life-threatening condition.

CAUSES AND INCIDENCE

The virus most commonly responsible for encephalitis is the *herpes simplex* virus type 1, which also causes cold sores. An increasing number of cases are caused by infection with *HIV* (human immunodeficiency virus), the organism responsible for *AIDS*. Rarely, the condition may be a complication of certain other viral infections, including such diseases as *measles* and *mumps*.

SYMPTOMS AND SIGNS

Encephalitis has variable effects but often starts with headache and fever, and progresses to hallucinations, confusion, paralysis of part or all of the body, and disturbances of behaviour, speech, memory, and eye movement. There is a gradual loss of consciousness and sometimes coma. Epileptic seizures may also occur.

If as well as the brain the meninges are inflamed, the neck usually becomes stiff and the eyes become abnormally sensitive to light.

DIAGNOSIS

Diagnosis is based on symptoms, signs, and the results of *CT scanning* or *MRI* of the brain, an *EEG* (which records the electrical activity of the brain), and a *lumbar puncture* (taking a sample of cerebrospinal fluid from the spinal canal for analysis). Blood tests and, rarely, a brain *biopsy* (removal of a small sample of tissue for analysis) may also be required to confirm the diagnosis.

TREATMENT AND OUTLOOK

The antiviral drug *acyclovir*, administered by *intravenous infusion*, has proved an effective treatment for encephalitis caused by the herpes simplex virus but when the disease results from other viral infections, there is at present no known effective treatment.

Depending on the cause of the encephalitis, some patients fail to recover, some are left with brain damage that results in mental impairment, behavioural disturbances, and persistent *epilepsy*, and others make a complete recovery.

Encephalitis lethargica

An epidemic form of encephalitis (inflammation of the brain). There have been no major outbreaks since the 1920s, although rare sporadic cases still occur. The symptoms are as for encephalitis, with additional lethargy and drowsiness.

About 40 per cent of sufferers died during the major epidemics; many survivors thereafter developed post-encephalitic *parkinsonism*, a movement disorder marked by symptoms such as tremor, rigidity, immobility, and severely disturbed eye movements.

A small number of survivors from the post-World War I epidemics were still alive in the 1970s, when administration of a new antiparkinsonian drug, *levodopa*, brought a remarkable improvement in their conditions. However, after half a century of almost complete immobility, most sufferers were seemingly unable to cope with this "awakening", and lapsed into their former torpid state.

Encephalomyelitis

Inflammation of the *brain* and *spinal cord*, resulting in damage to the *nervous system*. The condition occurs as a complication of about one in 1,000 cases of *measles*, developing a few days after the rash appears. Rarely, it may occur after other viral infections, such as *chickenpox*, *rubella* (German measles), or infectious *mononucleosis* (glandular fever), or it may follow vaccination against *rabies*. *Myalgic encephalomyelitis* is a quite distinct condition, causing fatigue and muscle pains; it usually runs a chronic course for one to two years and sometimes longer.

SYMPTOMS

Symptoms include fever, headache, drowsiness, confusion, epileptic seizures, partial paralysis or loss of sensation, and sometimes coma.

DIAGNOSIS AND TREATMENT

Diagnosis is as for *encephalitis*. Critically ill patients require careful nursing in a hospital. There is no cure for the disease, but *corticosteroid drugs* are given to reduce inflammation and *anticonvulsant drugs* are given to control epileptic seizures.

OUTLOOK

About 10 to 20 per cent of patients die; those who recover may suffer permanent damage to the nervous system, causing mental handicap, *epilepsy*, paralysis, *hypopituitarism* (insufficiency of the pituitary gland), loss of sensation, or incontinence.

Encephalopathy

Any disease or disorder affecting the brain, especially chronic degenerative conditions (see *Brain* disorders box).

Wernicke's encephalopathy is a degenerative condition of the brain caused by a deficiency of thiamine (vitamin B_1); the condition is most common in alcoholics (see *Wernicke-Korsakoff syndrome*).

Hepatic encephalopathy is caused by the effect on the brain of toxic substances which have accumulated in the blood as a result of *liver failure*. Hepatic encephalopathy may cause impaired consciousness, memory loss, personality change, tremors, seizures, stupor, and coma.

Bovine spongiform encephalopathy (BSE) is a new disorder contracted by cows from infected sheep or cattle tissue in their feed. The cause is probably a *slow virus*. BSE causes degeneration of the infected cow's brain and is fatal. Despite public fears, BSE is unlikely to be transmissible to humans.

Encopresis

A type of *soiling* in which children pass normal faeces in unacceptable places after the age at which bowel control is normally achieved (usually when two to three years old).

Endarterectomy

An operation to remove the lining of an artery that is affected by *atherosclerosis* (narrowing by deposits of fatty material). Removing the diseased lining restores normal blood flow to the part of the body supplied by the artery.

WHY IT IS DONE

Endarterectomy is performed to treat *cerebrovascular disease* (in which there is a serious reduction of blood supply to the brain) or to treat *peripheral vascular disease* (in which blood supply to the limbs is impaired).

HOW IT IS DONE

Before surgery, the site of the narrowing is usually first identified by *Doppler ultrasound* and then confirmed by an X-ray procedure called *angiography*, which requires a local anaesthetic. For the operation itself the patient is given a general anaesthetic.

Endarterectomy is a delicate procedure that may take several hours. The operation is performed either endoscopically (see *Endoscopy*) or by open surgery, in which the artery is exposed, clamps are applied, an incision is made, and the diseased lining is removed along with any *thrombus* (blood clot) that has formed. The incision is closed with stitches.

RESULTS

New lining grows in the artery within a few weeks of surgery. The operation

E

E

often brings about a considerable improvement in symptoms (for example, it can greatly reduce pain in the legs in peripheral vascular disease). The long-term effect is more limited, because narrowing of an artery is rarely confined to one site. When narrowing is widespread, *arterial reconstructive surgery* may have to be performed.

Endemic

A medical term applied to a disease or disorder that is constantly present in a particular region or a specific group of people, in contrast to an *epidemic*, which is not generally present but occasionally affects a large number of people. *AIDS*, for example, has become endemic in central Africa and has also spread to many other parts of the world. The lung disease *pneumoconiosis* was formerly endemic in coal miners before government regulations enforced controls over safety levels of coal dust, the causative agent.

Endocarditis

Inflammation of the endocardium (internal lining of the heart), particularly of the heart valves, usually due to infection.

Endocarditis occurs most commonly in people whose endocardium has already been damaged (e.g. by congenital *heart disease* or by *rheumatic fever*), in people whose *immune system* has been suppressed by *anticancer drugs* or by *immunosuppressant drugs*, and in drug abusers who inject drugs intravenously. Endocarditis is also a rare feature of some types of cancer and of some *autoimmune disorders* (e.g. systemic *lupus erythematosus*).

CAUSES AND INCIDENCE

Endocarditis may be caused by bacteria, fungi, or other microorganisms. The microorganisms may be introduced into the bloodstream during cardiac surgery, particularly if artificial materials (e.g. a replacement valve) are inserted. The causative microorganisms may also be introduced during dental treatment (especially tooth extraction) and during surgical and investigative procedures performed on the gastrointestinal and genitourinary systems (e.g. examination of the bladder by *cystoscopy*). The microorganisms that cause endocarditis may also be introduced directly into the bloodstream on dirty needles.

People with an endocardium that is already damaged are particularly vulnerable to endocarditis because clots

that form on the injured surface trap the causative microorganisms, which then multiply rapidly at the site of damage. Intravenous drug abusers are vulnerable to endocarditis, even if their hearts are healthy, because microorganisms from a dirty syringe or from unclean skin at the site of injection are injected and carried to the heart in the bloodstream. People with a suppressed immune system are vulnerable because they have a lowered resistance to infection, and organisms that would normally be harmless can lead to serious infection.

SYMPTOMS

Endocarditis may be subacute or acute. In the subacute form, the disease smoulders undetected, sometimes for many months, during which time it causes serious damage to a heart valve. Symptoms are general and nonspecific; the sufferer may complain of fatigue and weakness, feverishness, night sweats, and vague aches and pains. On examination, the only evident abnormality may be a heart *murmur* that changes from time to time.

Acute endocarditis, which occurs less frequently, comes on suddenly. The patient suffers from severe chills, high fever, shortness of breath, and rapid or irregular heartbeat. The infection progresses quickly and may destroy the heart valves, leading to rapidly progressive heart failure (reduced pumping efficiency).

DIAGNOSIS AND TREATMENT

Any patient suspected of having endocarditis is given a thorough physical examination. Blood samples are taken and sent to the laboratory for analysis. *Cultures* of the blood are examined for bacteria or fungi, and the sensitivity of the organisms to different types of *antibiotic drug* is determined. Tests on the heart may include *ECG*, *echocardiography*, and *angiography*.

Patients are treated with high doses of antibiotic drugs, which are usually given intravenously. Drug treatment, which may last for as long as six weeks, is started in hospital and may be continued at home. *Heart valve surgery* may be needed to replace a valve that has been extensively damaged by infection or to replace an artificial valve. In some cases, heart valve replacement may need to be done as an emergency procedure.

PREVENTION AND OUTLOOK

People at risk of endocarditis because of a heart defect are prescribed antibiotic drugs before undergoing any

procedure that runs a significant risk of introducing bacteria into the bloodstream. People at risk should also be aware of the warning signs of endocarditis and call a doctor should they appear.

Before the introduction of antibiotic drugs, endocarditis was usually fatal. Today, treatment is successful in 65 to 80 per cent of cases.

Endocrine gland

A gland that secretes *hormones* directly into the bloodstream rather than through a duct. Examples of endocrine glands include the *thyroid gland, ovaries*, and *adrenal glands*, which release *thyroxine, oestrogens*, and *hydrocortisone*, respectively. The endocrine glands in the body make up the *endocrine system*. (See also *Exocrine gland*.)

Endocrine system

A collection of glands that produce *hormones* (chemical substances necessary for normal body functioning). The various endocrine glands are shown in the illustrated box.

The hormones produced by the endocrine glands are responsible for numerous body processes, including growth, metabolism, sexual development and function, and response to stress. Any increase or decrease in the production of a specific hormone interferes with the process it controls.

Unlike *exocrine glands*, the secretions of which pass through ducts to local areas, endocrine glands are ductless and release their hormones directly into the bloodstream to be transported to organs and tissues throughout the body.

Endocrinology

The study of the *endocrine system*, including the investigation and treatment of its disorders. A physician who specializes in diseases and disorders of the endocrine glands and the hormones they secrete is called an endocrinologist.

The symptoms and signs of an endocrine disease, such as a *thyroid* disorder or *diabetes mellitus*, may lead a general practitioner to suspect such a disease, but confirmation usually requires referral to an endocrinologist for specialized tests, including measurement of the amounts of various hormones in the blood and urine.

Endodontics

The specialized branch of dentistry concerned with the causes, prevention, diagnosis, and treatment of dis-

ENDOCRINE SYSTEM

The system consists of a collection of hormone-producing glands, many regulated by trophic (stimulating) hormones secreted by the pituitary. The pituitary is itself influenced by hormones secreted by the hypothalamus in the brain. Shown here are the principal glands with a note on the hormones they produce.

Pancreas
This gland secretes insulin and glucagon, which control the body's utilization of glucose.

Adrenal cortex
When stimulated by ACTH, the adrenal cortex produces hydrocortisone, which has widespread effects on metabolism; it also produces androgen hormones and aldosterone, which maintains blood pressure and the body's salt balance.

Ovaries
These produce the hormones oestrogen and progesterone, which influence multiple aspects of female physiology. These processes are controlled by gonadotrophic hormones secreted by the pituitary.

Pituitary gland
The pituitary gland secretes hormones that stimulate the adrenals, thyroid, pigment-producing skin cells, and gonads; it also secretes growth hormone, antidiuretic hormone, prolactin, and oxytocin.

Thyroid gland
This gland produces the hormones thyroxine, triiodothyronine, and calcitonin, which stimulate metabolism, body heat production, and bone growth. Thyroid activity is controlled by TSH, secreted by the pituitary.

Parathyroid glands
These glands secrete parathyroid hormone, which maintains the calcium level in the blood.

Testes
The testes produce testosterone in response to gonadotrophins secreted by the pituitary. A combination of gonadotrophins and testosterone stimulates sperm production and the development of other male characteristics.

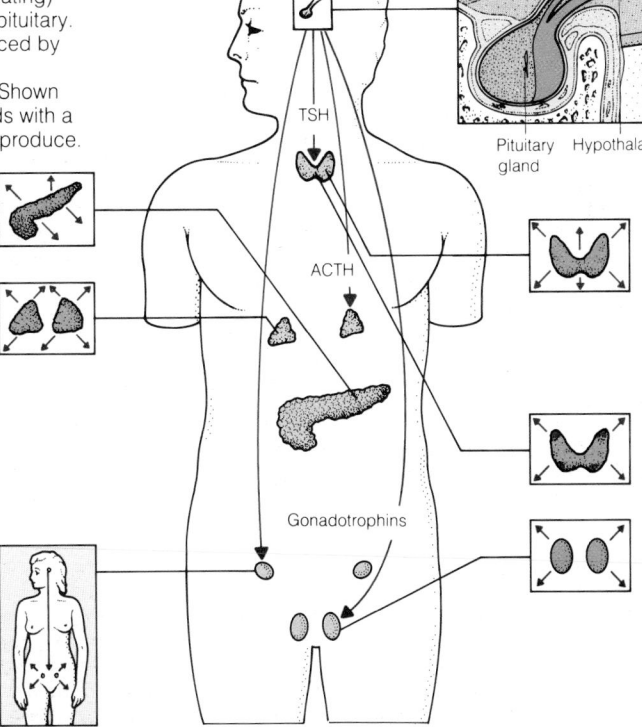

Pituitary gland   Hypothalamus

CONTROL OF HORMONE PRODUCTION

Production of too much or too little hormone by a gland is prevented by feedback mechanisms. Variations in the blood level of the hormones are detected by the part of the brain known as the hypothalamus, which prompts the pituitary to modify its production of trophic (gland-stimulating) hormone accordingly.

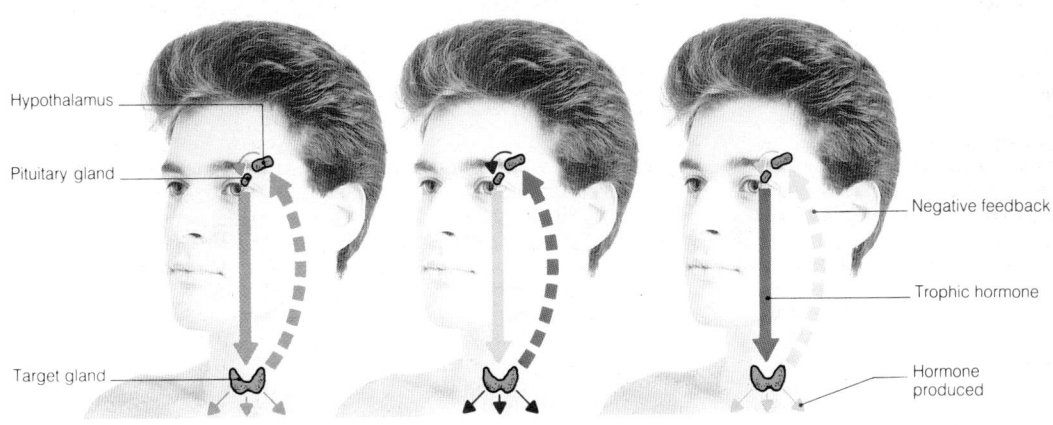

1 The production of hormone by the target gland (in this illustration, the thyroid gland) and of trophic hormone by the pituitary gland is normal.

2 If hormone production by the target gland rises, the feedback effect causes less trophic hormone to be produced, which tends to return the situation to normal.

3 If hormone production by the target gland drops, the feedback lessens and more trophic hormone is produced, which tends to return the situation to normal.

E

ENDOCRINE DISORDERS

In all endocrine disorders, there is either deficient or excess production of a hormone by a gland. Common causes of abnormal hormone production include a tumour or an autoimmune disease affecting a gland, or a disorder of the pituitary or the hypothalamus, which control many other glands. Abnormal hormone production often has a feedback effect on the secretion of trophic (stimulating) hormones by the pituitary and the hypothalamus — as in two of the examples shown. The blood levels of different hormones may need to be measured to pinpoint the cause of a disorder.

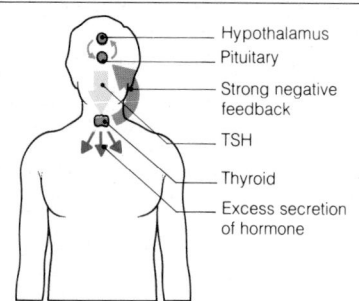

Thyrotoxicosis
This disorder is usually due to an autoimmune disease of the thyroid. Excess hormones cause the symptoms; the output of TSH and its hypothalamic-releasing hormone is reduced, but the thyroid continues to overproduce.

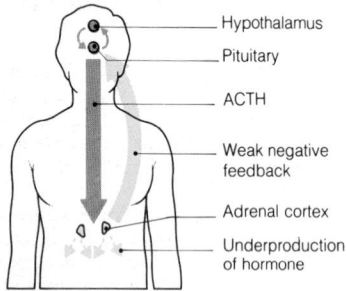

Addison's disease
Symptoms are caused by reduced hormone production by the defective adrenal cortices. Feedback is weak, so the pituitary pours out adrenocorticotrophic hormone (ACTH), but it fails to stimulate the adrenals.

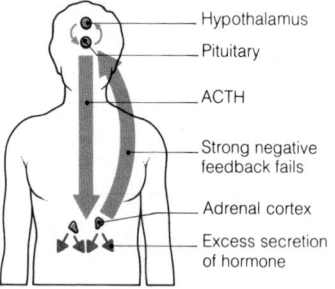

Cushing's disease
This disorder is caused by excess ACTH secretion by a pituitary tumour. This stimulates the adrenal cortices to make excess hydrocortisone, leading to the symptoms of the syndrome. Feedback fails to suppress ACTH secretion.

ease and injury affecting the nerves and pulp in teeth and the periapical tissues in the gum. Common endodontic procedures are *root-canal treatment* and *pulpotomy*.

Endogenous

Arising within the body. For example, an endogenous infection may occur if bacteria from around the anus invade the urinary tract.

Most disorders, however, are *exogenous* (caused by external infections, poisoning, or injury).

Endometrial ablation

A treatment for *menorrhagia* (persistent heavy menstrual blood loss) in which the *endometrium* is removed using an instrument, a hysteroscope, which allows the interior of the uterus to be examined by direct vision. During the operation, most or all of the endometrium is removed; afterwards menstruation either ceases or becomes much less heavy. The procedure has reduced the need for *hysterectomy*.

Endometrial cancer

See *Uterus, cancer of.*

Endometriosis

A condition in which fragments of the *endometrium* (lining of the uterus) are located in other parts of the body, usually in the pelvic cavity.

INCIDENCE AND CAUSE
Endometriosis is most prevalent in women aged 25 to 40 and may cause *infertility*. How endometriosis causes infertility is unknown, but about 10 to 15 per cent of infertility patients have endometriosis and about 30 to 40 per cent of women sufferering from endometriosis are infertile.

The exact cause of endometriosis is uncertain, but in some cases it is thought to occur because fragments of the endometrium shed during *menstruation* do not leave the body with the menstrual flow. Instead, they travel up the fallopian tubes and into the pelvic cavity where they adhere to and grow on any pelvic organ.

These displaced patches of endometrium continue to respond to the menstrual cycle as if they were still inside the uterus, so each month they bleed. This blood cannot escape, however, and causes the formation of slowly growing cysts which may grow as large as a grapefruit. The growth and swelling of the cysts is responsible for much of the pain associated with endometriosis.

SYMPTOMS AND SIGNS
The symptoms of endometriosis vary widely, with abnormal or heavy menstrual bleeding being most common. There may be severe abdominal and/or lower back pain during menstruation, which is often most severe towards the end of a period. Other possible symptoms include dyspareunia (see *Intercourse, painful*) and digestive tract symptoms such as diarrhoea, constipation, or painful defaecation. In rare cases, rectal bleeding occurs at the time of menstruation. In some cases, endometriosis causes no symptoms.

DIAGNOSIS AND TREATMENT
Laparoscopy (examination of the abdominal cavity with a viewing instrument) confirms the diagnosis.

Treatment depends on many factors, including the age and health of the patient, and the severity of the condition. Some cases are mild and require no treatment. In others, endometriosis is suppressed by pregnancy.

Drugs (including *danazol*, *progestogen drugs*, *gonadorelin* analogues, or the combined *oral contraceptive* pill) may be given to prevent menstruation. In severe cases, surgical removal of the cysts may be necessary in addition to drug therapy. A woman who does not want to have children or who is nearing the menopause may consider the possibility of having a *hysterectomy*.

Endometritis

Inflammation of the *endometrium* (uterine lining) due to infection. Endometritis is a feature of *pelvic inflammatory disease* (PID). It may also occur as a complication of abortion or childbirth, after the insertion of an *IUD*, or as the result of a *sexually transmitted disease*.

Symptoms of endometritis include fever, vaginal discharge, and lower abdominal pain. Treatment includes removing any foreign body (such as an IUD or retained placental tissue) and the use of *antibiotic drugs*.

Endometrium

The lining of the inside of the *uterus*. The endometrium contains numerous glands and increases in thickness during the menstrual cycle until ovulation occurs. The surface layers are shed during *menstruation* if conception does not take place.

Endorphins

A group of substances formed within the body that relieve pain. Endorphins have a similar chemical structure to morphine (it is because of this similarity that morphine has an analgesic effect).

In 1973 morphine was found to act at specific sites (called opiate receptors) in the brain, spinal cord, and at other nerve endings. This discovery led to the identification of small protein molecules produced by cells in the body that also act at opiate receptors; these morphine-like proteins were named endorphins (short for endogenous morphines).

Two other small proteins produced within the brain were originally considered to be examples of endorphins, but they have now been reclassified as *enkephalins* because they are released from different nerve endings.

FUNCTIONS

Since their discovery, endorphins have been found at several sites in the body (including the pancreas and testes) as well as in the nervous system. Research is being carried out to determine their full range of functions.

In addition to their analgesic effect, endorphins are thought to be involved in controlling the body's response to stress, regulating contractions of the intestinal wall, and determining mood. They may also regulate the release of hormones from the pituitary gland, notably growth hormone and the *gonadotrophin hormones* (which act on the ovaries or testes).

Addiction and *tolerance* to narcotic analgesics, such as morphine, are thought to be due to suppression of the body's production of endorphins; the withdrawal symptoms that occur when the effects of morphine wear off may be due to a lack of these natural analgesics. Conversely, acupuncture is thought to produce analgesia partly by stimulating the release of endorphins and enkephalins.

Endoscope

A tube-like viewing instrument, with lenses and a light source attached, that is inserted into a body cavity for the purpose of investigating and treating disorders. Some common types of endoscope and their uses are shown in the illustrated box (see overleaf).

Endoscopy

Examination of a body cavity by means of an *endoscope* for purposes of diagnosis or treatment. Many procedures that formerly required major surgery can now be performed much more simply by endoscopy.

Attempts to view the interior of the body through a rigid, lighted, telescope-like tube were made in the early 1900s, but endoscopy really began in the 1930s with the invention of a semi-flexible gastroscope for viewing the stomach. In the 1960s, a second revolution came with the introduction of *fibre-optics* (flexible bundles of glass or plastic fibres along which light is transmitted). This enabled more versatile instruments to be developed and led to the acceptance of endoscopy as a routine part of hospital medicine. A third revolution came in 1986 with the development of small video cameras that could be incorporated into the tip of the endoscope. This permitted the visualization of endoscopic manipulations on a monitor, opening the way to *minimally invasive surgery*, and allowed endoscopic findings to be permanently recorded.

USES

Endoscopy has advanced rapidly, both as a diagnostic aid and as a method of surgery. In diagnosis, virtually any hollow organ or structure can be inspected directly, and endoscopy is often the method of first choice. The operator can inspect and photograph the organ and perform a *biopsy* (removal of a small piece of tissue for microscopic analysis). Endoscopy usually requires only sedation or local anaesthesia, and can therefore be repeated safely at frequent intervals to allow monitoring of a disease's progression and its response to treatment. For example, endoscopy is widely used to follow the effects of treatment on gastric or duodenal ulcers.

SITES OF ENDOMETRIOSIS

Fragments of the *endometrium* may travel from the uterus into the pelvic cavity via the fallopian tubes. They then implant on parts of the pelvic organs (such as the ovaries, vagina, cervix, bladder, and rectum). The patches of endometrium continue to respond to the menstrual cycle and bleed every month, causing the formation of painful cysts, which can be very small or may be as large as a grapefruit.

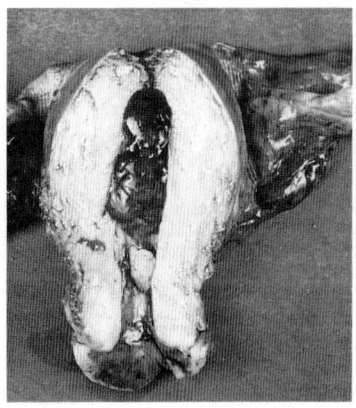

Severe endometriosis
The uterus, fallopian tubes, and ovaries shown above had large cysts around them due to endometriosis. Because the patient was nearing the menopause, the affected organs were surgically removed.

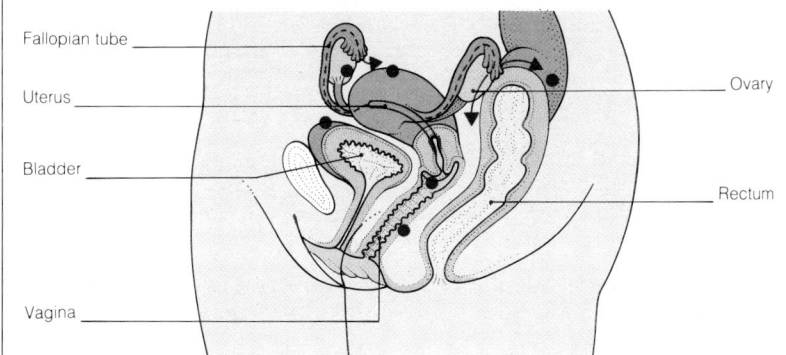

Fallopian tube

Uterus

Bladder

Vagina

Ovary

Rectum

ENDOSCOPES

A typical flexible *fibre-optic* endoscope consists of a bundle of light-transmitting fibres. At one end is the head (featuring a viewing lens and steering device) and a power source. The tip has a light, a lens, and an outlet for air or water. Side channels enable attachments to be passed to the tip. In some endoscopes the tip may contain a camera that transmits a picture electronically to a screen.

A rigid endoscope is a straight, narrow viewing tube with a light source attached.

COMMON TYPES OF ENDOSCOPES

Instruments	Region	Nature
Cystoscope	Bladder	Rigid
Bronchoscope	Bronchi (main airways of the lungs)	Flexible or rigid
Gastroscope	Oesophagus, stomach, and duodenum	Flexible
Colonoscope	Colon (large intestine)	Flexible
Laparoscope	Abdominal cavity	Rigid
Arthroscope	Knee joint	Rigid

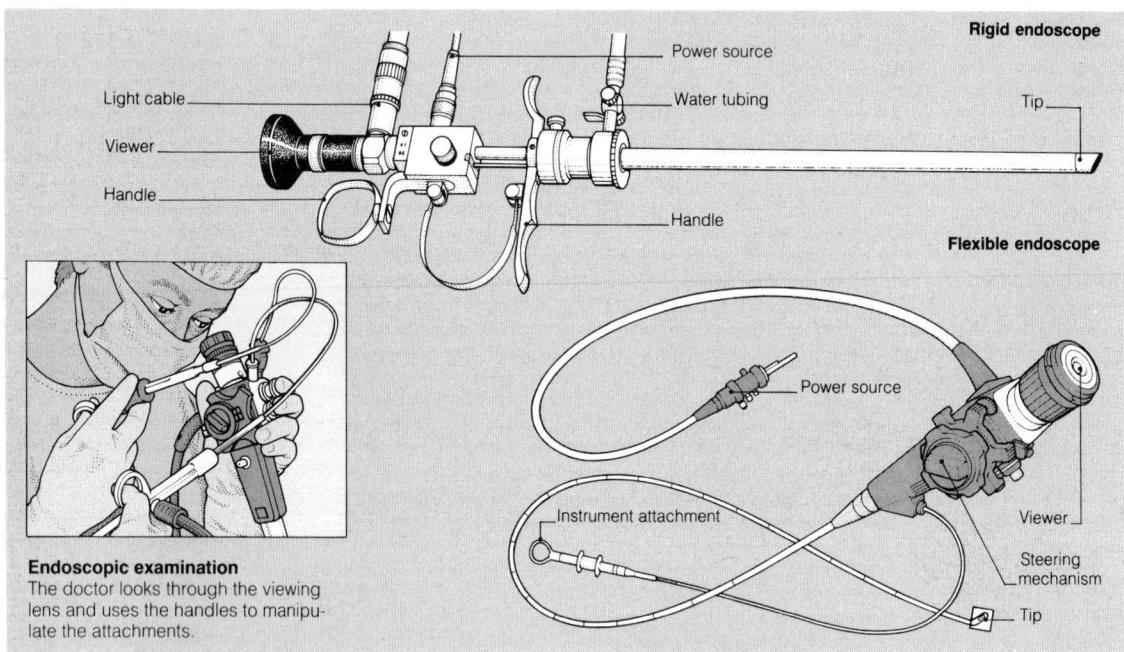

Rigid endoscope

Power source
Light cable
Water tubing
Viewer
Tip
Handle
Handle

Flexible endoscope

Power source
Instrument attachment
Viewer
Steering mechanism
Tip

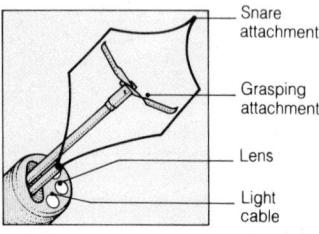

Endoscopic examination
The doctor looks through the viewing lens and uses the handles to manipulate the attachments.

ATTACHMENTS

Various specialized attachments are available for use with the endoscope. They enable the doctor to perform diagnostic and therapeutic procedures such as taking a biopsy specimen (a small piece of tissue for analysis).

Snare attachment
Grasping attachment
Lens
Light cable

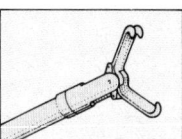

Grasping forceps
Sharp-toothed forceps allow foreign bodies to be grasped firmly and removed.

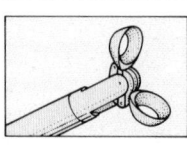

Biopsy forceps
These are used for taking small samples of tissue for microscopic analysis.

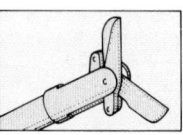

Scissors
Tiny surgical scissors are used for cutting through tissue and removing small growths.

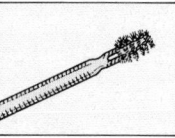

Brushes
Brush attachments are used to obtain cells for cytological examination.

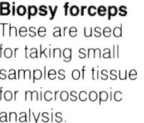

Snare
This thin wire loop, through which an electric current is passed, is used to remove polyps.

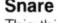

Basket
A wire basket is sometimes used to trap and remove stones from the bile duct.

Many operations are being performed by endoscopy, often transforming a previously major procedure into a minor one. It is valuable in the treatment of acute emergencies such as bleeding from the stomach or the removal of foreign bodies from the lungs or gullet. Operations such as female sterilization, the treatment of torn ligaments or cartilage within the knee joint, and the treatment of infections of the nasal sinuses and polyps, have all become routine endoscopic procedures. (See also *Minimally invasive surgery*.)

Endothelium

The layer of cells that lines the heart, blood vessels, and lymphatic ducts. The cells are squamous (thin and flat), providing a smooth surface that aids the flow of blood and lymph and helps prevent the formation of thrombi (blood clots). (See also *Epithelium*.)

Endotoxin

A poison produced by certain *bacteria* but not released until after the bacteria die; until then the toxin remains in the bacterial cell wall. Released endotoxins cause fever. They also make the walls of capillaries more permeable, causing fluid to leak into the surrounding tissue, sometimes resulting in a serious drop in blood pressure, a condition called endotoxic shock. (See also *Enterotoxin; Exotoxin*.)

Endotracheal tube

A tube passed through the nose or mouth into the trachea (windpipe), usually by an anaesthetist. The endotracheal tube may be provided with an inflatable cuff at its lower end to give an airtight fit which prevents anything other than oxygen or anaesthetic gases entering the lungs. The tube may be made of rubber or various types of plastic.

Endotracheal intubation is performed to ensure that a patient has a clear airway for the delivery of oxygen. It may be necessary if a patient is comatose, is undergoing anaesthesia, or is unable to breathe properly because of a disorder affecting the lungs or airways. An endotracheal tube is used to deliver oxygen to the trachea during artificial *ventilation*.

Enema

A procedure in which fluid is passed into the rectum through a tube inserted into the anus. An enema may be performed as a treatment, to prepare the intestine for surgery, or as an aid to diagnosis.

WHY IT IS DONE

An enema may be given to clear the intestine of faeces either to relieve constipation or in preparation for intestinal surgery. Soap and water were formerly used for this type of enema but today prepacked, small-volume enemas containing medication are used.

Enemas may also be used to administer medicine, such as *corticosteroid drugs* to relieve bleeding and inflammation in *ulcerative colitis* or, less commonly, salt solutions to treat severe *dehydration*.

A barium enema is used as an aid to the diagnosis of disorders of the large intestine (see *Barium X-ray examinations*).

HOW IT IS DONE

No anaesthetic is needed, although the procedure may cause slight discomfort as the fluid stretches the intestine. The patient lies on his or her side with hips raised on a pillow. A catheter (flexible tube) with a soft, well-lubricated tip, is gently inserted into the rectum and the enema fluid, warmed to prevent sudden contraction of the intestine, is slowly introduced through it.

Energy

The capacity to do work or effect a physical change; nutritionists now also refer to the fuel content of a food as its energy content.

There are many different forms of energy—including light, sound, heat, chemical, electrical, and kinetic (the energy possessed by an object by virtue of its motion)—and most of them play a role in the body. For instance, the retina converts light energy to electrical nerve impulses, thereby making vision possible. Muscles use chemical energy—obtained from food—to produce kinetic energy (movement) and heat.

Energy is measured in units called calories and joules. One calorie is defined as the amount of energy needed to raise the temperature of 1 g of water by 1°C; 1 calorie is equivalent to about 4.2 J (therefore, 1 J equals approximately 0.24 calories). Because the calorie and the joule are very small, more practical units in dietetics are the kilocalorie (kcal) which is 1,000 calories, sometimes called simply a Calorie (C), and the kilojoule (1,000 joules, or 1 kj).

TERMINOLOGY

The total chemical energy in a food is gross energy. After an allowance is made for the approximately five per cent that is not digested, the remainder is digestible energy. After allowing for loss in the urine (nitrogen compounds from proteins), the remainder is metabolizable energy (see *Metabolism*). *Carbohydrates* and *proteins* provide 4 kcal per g; *fats* provide 9 kcal per g.

In general, the energy liberated from the breakdown of *nutrients* is stored as chemical energy in the form of *ATP* (adenosine triphosphate) molecules. The energy in these molecules is then available to power processes that consume energy, such as muscle contraction or the building up of complex substances needed for repair and maintenance of body structures.

Energy requirements

The amount of *energy* needed by a person for cell *metabolism*, muscular activity, and growth. This energy is provided by the breakdown of *carbohydrate, fat,* and *protein* in the diet and by stored nutrients in the liver, muscles and adipose tissue.

ENERGY EXPENDITURE

Energy is needed to keep the heart beating and the lungs functioning and to maintain body temperature. The rate at which these processes use energy is known as the basal metabolic rate (BMR). The BMR accounts for three quarters of the total daily expenditure of energy of the average sedentary person. Any form of movement increases energy expenditure above the BMR.

Additional energy is needed during growth to provide for extra body tissue. During pregnancy and lactation the mother's energy requirement increases because she must be able to meet the needs of the baby as well as her own.

When more energy is ingested as food than is spent, the surplus is stored and there is usually a gain in weight. When less is consumed than is spent, there is usually a loss of weight as the body stores are used up. (See also *Nutrition; Obesity*.)

Engagement

The descent of the head of the fetus into the mother's pelvis. In a woman's first pregnancy, engagement usually occurs by the 37th week but, in subsequent pregnancies, it may not occur until labour begins. Rarely, engagement may fail to occur—if, for example, the baby's position in the uterus is abnormal, the baby's head is too big for the mother's pelvis, or if there is *placenta praevia* (abnormal position of the placenta across the opening of the uterus).

E

Engorgement

Overfilling of the breasts with milk. Engorgement is common a few days after childbirth, when the milk supply arrives quickly and forcibly (see *Breast-feeding*). The condition causes the breasts and nipples to become swollen and tender. This makes it not only painful for the mother to feed the baby but can make it very difficult for the baby to suck. Engorgement can make a woman more likely to suffer from *mastitis* (inflammation of the breast). The problem can be relieved by *expressing milk*.

Enkephalins

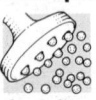

A group of small protein molecules produced in the brain and by nerve endings elsewhere in the body (in the digestive system and adrenal glands, for example). Enkephalins have an analgesic (painkilling) effect and are also thought to produce sedation, to affect mood, and to stimulate motivation.

Enkephalins were initially considered to be *endorphins* (endogenous morphines), but it has since been discovered that they are released by different nerve endings and that they differ slightly chemically.

Enophthalmos

A sinking inwards of the eyeball. Enophthalmos is most commonly caused by fracture of the floor of the orbit (bony cavity making up the eye socket), or alternatively by shrinkage of the eye itself due to the formation of scar tissue following inflammation or injury.

Enteric-coated tablet

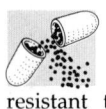

A form of drug preparation consisting of a tablet, the surface of which is covered with a substance that is resistant to the action of stomach juices. Enteric-coated tablets pass undissolved through the stomach into the small intestine, where the covering dissolves and the contents are absorbed.

Such tablets are used either when the drug might harm the stomach lining (as may occur with certain corticosteroid drugs, such as prednisone) or when the stomach juices may destroy the efficacy of the drug, as can happen with sulphasalazine.

The drawback of some enteric-coated tablets is that they may pass through the gastrointestinal tract without dissolving.

Enteric fever

An alternative name for either *typhoid fever* or *paratyphoid fever*.

Enteritis

Inflammation of the small intestine. Enteritis may result from infection, particularly *giardiasis* and *tuberculosis*, or from *Crohn's disease*, which is sometimes called regional enteritis. Enteritis usually causes diarrhoea. (See also *Gastroenteritis; Colitis*.)

Enteritis, regional

Another name for *Crohn's disease*.

Enterobiasis

The medical term for infestation of the intestines by the small roundworm *ENTEROBIUS VERMICULARIS*. (See *Threadworm infestation*.)

Enterostomy

An operation in which a portion of small or large intestine is joined to another part of the gastrointestinal tract or to the abdominal wall. When part of the *colon* (large intestine) is brought through an incision in the abdominal wall to allow the discharge of faeces into a bag attached to the skin, the operation is called a *colostomy*; when the ileum (last section of the small intestine) rather than the colon is used, the procedure is called an *ileostomy*.

Enterotoxin

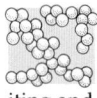

A type of *toxin* (poison released by certain bacteria) that inflames the lining of the intestine, causing vomiting and diarrhoea.

Staphylococcal *food poisoning* is caused by eating food contaminated with an enterotoxin produced by staphylococci bacteria; the toxin is resistant to heat and is therefore not destroyed by cooking. The bacteria themselves do not need to be alive or even present for this type of food poisoning to occur.

The severe intestinal purging that occurs in *cholera* is caused by an enterotoxin that is actually produced in the intestine by the cholera bacteria. (See also *Endotoxin; Exotoxin*.)

Entropion

A turning in of the margins of the *eyelids* so that the lashes rub against the *cornea* and the *conjunctiva*.

CAUSES

Entropion is sometimes congenital (present from birth), especially in fat babies. It is common in the elderly, when weakness of the muscles surrounding the lower part of the eye allows the lower lid plate to turn inwards. Entropion of the upper or lower lid may be caused by scarring on the inner surface of the lid—for example, due to *trachoma*.

SYMPTOMS AND SIGNS

Entropion is often recognized by the sufferer or by his or her family. The lower lid margin is rolled inwards so that the lashes are concealed, which sometimes irritates the conjunctiva. When gentle pressure is applied with the fingertip over the lid, the margin pops out, revealing the lashes again.

COMPLICATIONS

In later life, entropion can cause irritation, conjunctivitis, or corneal ulceration. Untreated, persistent entropion may permanently damage the cornea and cause problems with vision and, in some people, blindness.

TREATMENT

Entropion in babies does not disturb the eye and nearly always disappears spontaneously within a few months. In the elderly or in sufferers from trachoma, surgery to correct the entropion prevents damage to the cornea.

ENT surgery

See *Otorhinolaryngology*.

Enuresis

The medical term for bed-wetting. Enuresis is a common phenomenon; about 10 per cent of children still wet the bed at the age of five years, and many of these continue to do so until the age of eight or nine. A slightly higher number of boys than girls are bed-wetters, and the problem tends to run in families.

CAUSES

In most cases, bed-wetting is due to slow maturation of nervous system functions concerned with control of the bladder. Occasionally it results from psychological stress. In a small number of bed-wetters, there is a specific physical cause—for example, a structural abnormality of the *urinary tract* present from birth, *diabetes mellitus, urinary tract infection,* or a nervous system defect, such as *spina bifida* or spinal cord damage. In each of these cases, the child also has difficulty with daytime bladder control (see *Incontinence, urinary*).

INVESTIGATION

A physical examination, *urinalysis* (urine testing), and other procedures, such as *ultrasound scanning* and *urography* (X-ray imaging of the urinary tract), may be performed. *Cystometry* (a test of bladder function) is also occasionally carried out, usually only on older children who have daytime problems as well.

TREATMENT

In the absence of an ascertainable cause, or until the problem can be more fully investigated, treatment starts with training the child to pass urine regularly during the day. This helps the child to recognize when the bladder is full, even during sleep. Systems such as rewarding the child with a star on a chart for each dry night are often successful.

If such simple measures fail to work, a special night-time alarm system may be recommended by the doctor. The basic system consists of a pad, placed in the child's bed between the lower sheet and the mattress, that is sensitive to humidity changes and triggers a loud alarm when urine is passed. Smaller alarms are now available that do not need pads under the sheet. The alarm awakens the child, who can then use the toilet. Eventually, the child wakes whenever urine is about to be passed. Alarms are said to be successful with over two thirds of bed-wetting children over seven years old.

Other measures include getting the child to go to the toilet each night immediately before bed, and waking him or her to use the toilet two or three hours after going to bed. Some types of *antidepressant drugs* have also been used successfully, but many doctors do not prescribe them because the drugs generally cause side-effects and are dangerous in overdose.

Parents should not punish a child for bed-wetting or focus undue attention on it, as this may only make the child more anxious and the problem worse. The majority of bed-wetting children eventually become dry at night.

Environmental medicine

The study of the effects on health of natural environmental factors, such as climate, altitude, sunlight, and the presence of various minerals. Working environments are studied separately (see *Occupational medicine*).

CLIMATE

There is convincing evidence that particular types of illness respond well to certain climates. For example, sufferers from chest disorders, such as chronic *bronchitis* and *asthma,* usually obtain some relief from their symptoms in a warm, relatively dry climate. In Europe, where most respiratory complaints are more common in winter, sufferers may benefit from spending their winters in a warm environment. Until the development of specific drug treatment in the 1940s, the prime treatment for pulmonary *tuberculosis* was to move the patient to a mountain sanatorium to enjoy the cool, clean, dry air.

ALTITUDE

Although mountainous regions have much less atmospheric pollution, they are not necessarily beneficial to health because the air becomes thinner as altitude increases. People with a chest disease who ascend quickly (over a few days) from sea level to 1,500 m may find that their breathing difficulty worsens. Above about 3,000 m, breathing becomes difficult even for healthy people. Rapid ascent from sea level to 3,600 m higher carries the risk of altitude sickness (see *Mountain sickness*), which can produce symptoms ranging from sleeplessness and nausea to coma or death. Only a small number of communities in the high Andes live permanently above that level but tourists climbing mountains in Africa and the Himalayas may develop altitude sickness.

Sustained living seems to be impossible above 6,000 m because at that level the blood cells increase to compensate for lack of oxygen. This strains the heart and causes a predisposition to thrombosis (abnormal blood clotting).

SUNLIGHT

White people who live in sunny climates may suffer ill effects from repeated exposure to sunlight, including wrinkling of the skin and an increased risk of *cataracts* and of skin cancers, such as *basal cell carcinoma* and malignant *melanoma*, and the precancerous condition solar *keratosis.* These risks have been increased by damage caused by environmental pollutants to the protective layers of ozone in the upper atmosphere.

E

THE GROWING IMPORTANCE OF ENVIRONMENTAL MEDICINE

Large areas of the world are naturally hostile to humans and were, in the past, avoided. Today exploitation of natural resources has lured people into these regions and has highlighted the importance of environmental medicine.

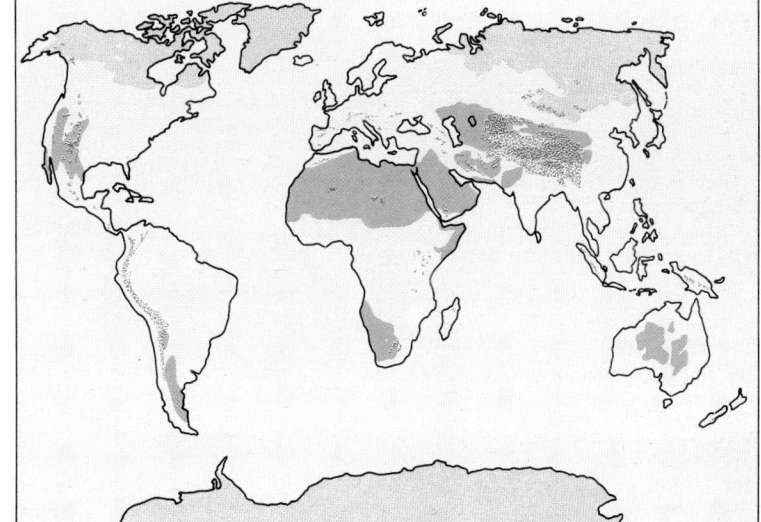

Key

Desert regions

Cold regions with average winter temperature below −23°C

Mountain regions above 3,000 m

E

MINERALS

Variations in the distribution of certain *minerals* in the environment are known to have an effect on health. For example, there is a slightly higher than average incidence of cancers in areas where the radioactive gas *radon* is emitted (from granitic rocks). In contrast, there is a lower than average incidence of *dental caries* in populations in regions where the water has a high *fluoride* content.

Enzyme

A protein that regulates the rate of a chemical reaction in the body. There are thousands of enzymes, each with a different chemical structure. It is this structure that determines the specific reaction regulated by an enzyme. To function properly, many enzymes need an additional component called a coenzyme, which is often derived from a *vitamin* or *mineral*.

Every cell in the body produces various enzymes; different sets of enzymes occur in different tissues, reflecting their specialized functions. For example, the *pancreas* produces the digestive enzymes lipase, protease, and amylase; among the numerous enzymes produced by the *liver* are some that metabolize drugs.

INDUCTION AND INHIBITION

Enzyme activity is influenced by many factors. Liver enzyme activity is increased by certain drugs, such as *barbiturate drugs*, which affect the rate at which other drugs are metabolized by the liver. This effect, known as enzyme induction, is responsible for many important drug interactions (see *Drug*).

Conversely, many drugs inhibit or block enzyme action. Some *antibiotic drugs* destroy bacteria by blocking bacterial enzymes while leaving human ones unaffected. Similarly, some *anticancer drugs* work by blocking enzymes in tumour cells, affecting normal body cells to a lesser degree.

ENZYMES AND DISEASE

Measuring enzyme levels in the blood can be useful for diagnosing disorders of certain organs or tissues. For example, the level of heart enzymes is raised after a *myocardial infarction* (heart attack) because the damaged heart muscle cells release enzymes into the bloodstream; muscle enzyme levels are raised in *muscular dystrophy*; and liver enzymes—measured in *liver function tests*—may be raised as a result of certain liver disorders.

Many inherited metabolic disorders, such as *phenylketonuria*, galac-tosaemia, and *G6PD deficiency*, are caused by defects in, or deficiencies of, specific enzymes.

ENZYMES AND TREATMENT

Enzymes can play a valuable role in treating certain diseases and disorders. Pancreatic enzymes may be given as digestive aids to patients with *malabsorption* related to pancreatic disease; enzymes that loosen sputum (phlegm) in the airways may be given to people with chronic lung disease; enzymes such as *streptokinase* and *tissue-plasminogen activator* are used to treat acute *thrombosis* (especially in the coronary arteries) and arterial *embolism* (especially pulmonary embolism). Papain from the papaw fruit can be used in the dressing of wounds and ulcers because it dissolves dead tissue and coagulated blood and may thus reduce bruising and swelling.

HOW ENZYMES WORK

An enzyme is a protein that acts as a catalyst for a chemical change in the body — that is, it greatly speeds up the rate at which the change occurs. The change may be a small modification to the structure of a substrate (chemical) in a body tissue, the splitting of a substrate, or the joining of two substrates.

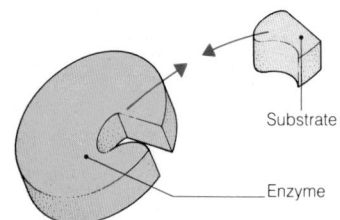

1 The shape of an enzyme determines its activity. It will combine only with a specific substrate that has molecules of a complementary shape.

Substrate
Enzyme

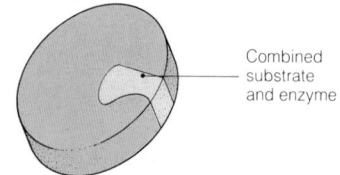

2 When enzyme and substrate combine, their interaction causes a chemical change within the substrate — in this case, splitting it into two products.

Combined substrate and enzyme

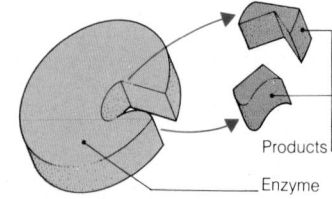

3 After the reaction, the enzyme molecule is unchanged and can move on to combine with another substrate molecule and repeat the process.

Products
Enzyme

Ependymoma

A rare type of *brain tumour* that occurs most often in children. It is a *glioma*, a tumour arising from the glial (supporting) cells within the nervous system. The symptoms, methods of diagnosis, and treatment of ependymomas are the same as for other types of brain tumour.

Ephedrine

A drug that stimulates the release of *noradrenaline* (a type of *neurotransmitter* released from nerve endings).

Ephedrine is prescribed as a *decongestant drug* to treat nasal congestion, and sometimes as a *bronchodilator drug* to treat asthma. Ephedrine eye-drops relieve redness of the eye by narrowing blood vessels that have become widened in response to minor irritation. Occasional uses include the relief of motion sickness and of enuresis (bed-wetting) in children.

Epicanthic fold

A vertical fold of skin extending from the upper eyelid to the side of the nose. Epicanthic folds are a normal feature in Orientals but are rare in other races, except in babies, in whom they usually disappear as the nose develops. Epicanthic folds are a feature of *Down's syndrome*.

The folds can be removed by minor cosmetic surgery.

Epicondylitis

A painful inflammation of an epicondyle, one of the bony prominences of the *elbow* at the lower end of the humerus (upper-arm bone). Various forearm muscles that bend or straighten the wrist or fingers are attached by *tendons* to the epicondyles. Overuse of these muscles can lead to epicondylitis due to repeated tugging of the tendons at their point of attachment to the bone.

Epicondylitis affecting the prominence on the outer side of the elbow, caused by overuse of the muscles that straighten the fingers and wrist, is called *tennis elbow*. When the prominence on the inner side of the elbow is affected, caused by overuse of muscles that bend the fingers and wrist, it is called *golfer's elbow*.

Epidemic

A medical term applied to a disease that for most of the time is rare in a community but that suddenly spreads rapidly to affect a large number of people. Epidemics of new strains of *influenza* are probably the most common, occurring periodically when the influenza virus changes to a form to which the population has no resistance. (See also *Endemic*.)

Epidemiology

The study of disease as it affects groups of people, as opposed to individuals. Originally, as its name suggests, epidemiology dealt mainly with epidemics of infectious diseases (such as cholera, plague, and influenza) and outbreaks of infections (such as gastroenteritis) associated with food poisoning. More recently, it has been applied to widespread noninfectious diseases, such as cancer and heart disease.

Members of a population (or, in comparative studies, populations) under study are carefully counted and defined in terms of each person's race, sex, age, occupation, social class, marital status, and the like. Then the *incidence* of the disorder (the number of new cases per week, month, or year) and its *prevalence* (the number of people with the disorder at any given time) are determined. These observations may be repeated at regular intervals to detect changes occurring over time. The result is an exact statistical record which often yields many valuable findings.

Groups that spend all their lives in one defined area often provide more useful information than very mobile populations whose environments change considerably over the course of their lives. For example, a high incidence of cancer of the oesophagus has been found among the inhabitants of one region of China and in remote parts of Iran. These groups have been studied intensively in a search for the foods or other agents responsible.

COMPARATIVE EPIDEMIOLOGY
Comparative epidemiology is proving to be a most potent weapon in the attempt to understand better cancer, heart disease, and other widespread diseases that afflict people in devel-

oped countries today. Two or more groups are chosen—one having, the other not having, a characteristic that may affect the frequency of a disease. For example, in a study of the link between smoking and lung cancer, one group may consist of smokers and the other of nonsmokers; the proportion with cancer in each group is then calculated. In such cases, the epidemiologist is careful to make the two groups as nearly identical as possible in other respects, carefully matching such factors as age, sex, weight, and socioeconomic status.

Another approach is to compare a group of people having a certain disease, such as hypertension (raised blood pressure), with a control group of people without the condition but similar in other respects; the aim is to isolate identifying factors, such as obesity, which differ between the two groups.

The links discovered by comparative epidemiology—such as the correlation of a high level of fish oils in the diet and low prevalence of heart disease—do not demonstrate cause and effect. For example, epidemiologists have discovered that the prevalence of heart disease is high in countries in which most people have a car. This association obviously does not mean that owning a car causes heart disease, but because such ownership suggests a more sedentary lifestyle, the link reinforces the belief that lack of exercise increases the risk of heart disease.

Epidermolysis bullosa

A group of rare, inherited conditions in which blisters appear on the skin after minor damage. The disorder has a wide range of severity, from a type in which blisters form on the feet in hot weather, to a form in which there is widespread blistering and scarring.
CAUSES
The condition is caused by a genetic defect which may show either an autosomal dominant or an autosomal recessive pattern of inheritance (see *Genetic disorders*). It is diagnosed by means of a skin *biopsy* (removal of a small amount of skin for microscopic analysis).
OUTLOOK
No special treatment for the condition is available, although injury to the skin should be avoided and simple protective measures should be taken to prevent the rubbing of affected areas when blisters appear.

The outlook varies from a gradual improvement in mild cases to progressive serious disease in the most severe cases. Parents of affected children should obtain *genetic counselling* so that the risks of later children being affected can be calculated.

Epididymal cyst

A harmless swelling, usually painless, that may develop in the *epididymis*, located at the upper rear part of the testis. Small cysts are very common in men over the age of 40 and need no treatment. Rarely, they may become tender or may enlarge and become uncomfortable, in which case it may be necessary to have an operation to remove them surgically.

Epididymis

A long, coiled tube connecting the vasa efferentia (small tubes leading from the testis) to the vas deferens (the sperm duct leading to the urethra). Sperm cells produced in the testis pass slowly along the epididymis, maturing there until they are capable of fertilizing an egg. They are then stored in the seminal vesicles until *ejaculation* takes place.

Disorders affecting the epididymis include *epididymo-orchitis* (inflammation of the epididymis and testis) and

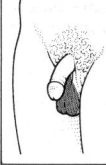

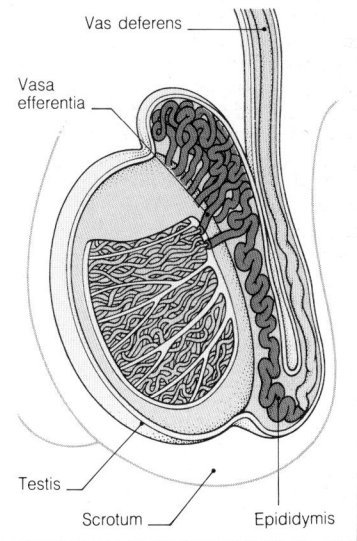

LOCATION OF THE EPIDIDYMIS
The epididymis runs along the back of the testis and links the vasa efferentia to the vas deferens.

Vas deferens

Vasa efferentia

Testis

Scrotum

Epididymis

E

epididymal cysts (fluid-filled swellings in the epididymis). Infection or injury can block the epididymis; if this occurs in both testes, infertility can result.

Epididymitis
See *Epididymo-orchitis.*

Epididymo-orchitis
Acute inflammation of a *testis* and its associated *epididymis* (the coiled tube that carries sperm away from the testis). Epididymo-orchitis is characterized by severe pain and swelling at the back of the testis and is accompanied by swelling and redness of the *scrotum* in severe cases.

The inflammation is caused by infection. Often there is no obvious source of infection, but sometimes the cause is a bacterial *urinary tract infection* that has spread via the vas deferens (sperm duct). In rare cases, epididymo-orchitis results from the spread of *tuberculosis.*

DIAGNOSIS
The symptoms of severe pain and swelling are similar to those of torsion of the testis, in which the testicular cord becomes twisted and blocks its own blood supply (see *Testis, torsion of*). An exploratory operation may be necessary to make a firm diagnosis and to save the testis. In some cases testicular scans may be helpful.

TREATMENT
Treatment is with *antibiotic drugs* and rest. If there is an underlying urinary tract infection, its cause is investigated. The tuberculous form of the disease usually responds to drugs used to treat other forms of tuberculosis. It may take several months for the testis to return to its normal size. (See also *Orchitis.*)

Epidural anaesthesia
A method of pain relief in which a local anaesthetic is injected into the epidural space (the space around the membranes surrounding the spinal cord) in the middle and lower back to numb the nerves that supply the chest and the lower half of the body.

Epidural anaesthesia is used to relieve pain during and after surgery, to relieve pain during *childbirth,* and in some cases to control cancer pain.

The anaesthetic is usually introduced into the epidural space via a catheter (flexible, fine tube), which is left in place to allow further doses of anaesthetic to be given as necessary. Epidural anaesthesia may be combined with a light general anaesthetic.

Epiglottis
The flap of cartilage lying behind the tongue and in front of the entrance to the *larynx* (voice-box). At rest, the epiglottis is upright and allows air to pass through the larynx and into the rest of the respiratory system. During swallowing it folds back to cover the entrance to the larynx, preventing food and drink from being inhaled.

Epiglottitis
A rare but serious and sometimes fatal infection that mainly affects children between the ages of two and six. Caused by the bacterium HAEMOPHILUS INFLUENZAE, it results in sudden inflammation and swelling of the *epiglottis* (the flap of cartilage at the back of the tongue that closes off the *larynx* and *trachea* during swallowing). The swollen epiglottis obstructs breathing. If the condition is not recognized and treated promptly, it can cause death by suffocation.

SYMPTOMS
The illness comes on suddenly within a few hours. The child becomes feverish, develops stridor (noisy breathing), has difficulty swallowing, and drools because he or she cannot swallow saliva. Breathing becomes increasingly difficult and the child prefers to sit upright in an attempt to make breathing easier. Within a few hours of the onset of the illness, the child may develop cyanosis (bluish discoloration of the skin and mucous membranes) and become semiconscious due to lack of oxygen.

DIAGNOSIS
The symptoms and signs of epiglottitis resemble those of *croup;* expert

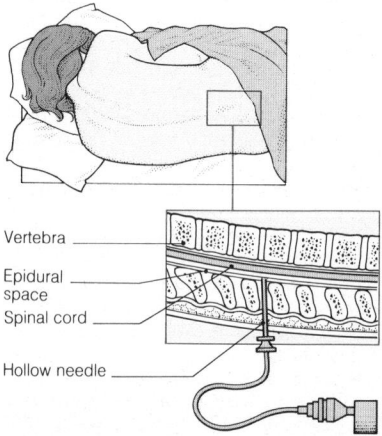

Vertebra
Epidural space
Spinal cord
Hollow needle

Administering an epidural anaesthetic
The anaesthetic is injected into the epidural space (the region surrounding the spinal cord within the spinal canal).

assessment by an experienced paediatrician may be necessary to distinguish between them. For this reason, any child who becomes feverish and develops noisy breathing should be seen by a doctor as soon as possible. If he or she suspects epiglottitis, the child will be admitted to hospital. In hospital, X-rays of the neck are usually taken to help confirm the diagnosis.

TREATMENT
An *endotracheal tube* is usually passed through the nose or mouth and into the trachea in order to maintain breathing; artificial *ventilation* may be needed. Intravenous *antibiotic drugs* (usually *ampicillin* and/or *chloramphenicol*) are used to cure the infection. With prompt treatment the outlook is good; recovery usually takes place within a week.

A vaccine against the HAEMOPHILUS INFLUENZAE bacterium type B is now included in the routine schedule of childhood *immunization*; this should reduce the frequency of the illness.

Epilepsy
A tendency to recurrent seizures or temporary alteration in one or more brain functions.

Seizures are defined as transient neurological abnormalities caused by abnormal electrical activity in the brain. Human activities, thoughts, perceptions, ideas and emotions are normally the result of the regulated and orderly electrical excitation of nerve cells in the brain. During a seizure, a chaotic and unregulated electrical discharge occurs. In some cases, a stimulus such as a flashing light sets off this abnormal sequence, but often seizures appear without any obvious trigger.

Many people with epilepsy lead normal lives and have no symptoms between seizures. Some can tell when an attack is imminent as they experience an aura (a restless, irritable, or uncomfortable feeling) shortly before the attack.

CAUSES
Seizures are a symptom of brain dysfunction and, like symptoms in other parts of the body, can result from a wide variety of disease or injury. Seizures may occur in association with *head injury,* birth trauma, brain infection (such as *meningitis* or *encephalitis*), *brain tumour, stroke,* drug intoxication, drug or alcohol withdrawal, or a *metabolic disorder.* A tendency to seizures may develop for no obvious reason or there may be an inherited predisposition.

FIRST AID: EPILEPTIC SEIZURE

DO NOT
- restrain the victim or place anything in the mouth
- attempt to move the victim unless he or she is in danger of further injury

1 Carefully loosen tight clothing around the neck.

2 When the attack is over, place the victim in the *recovery position* and allow him or her to regain consciousness.

INCIDENCE

About one person in 200 suffers from epilepsy. The disorder usually starts in childhood or adolescence. Many people outgrow epilepsy and do not require medication.

TYPES

Epileptic seizures can be classified into two broad groups—generalized and partial seizures.

The form a seizure takes depends on the part of the brain in which it arises and on how widely and rapidly it fans out from its point of origin.

Generalized seizures, which cause loss of consciousness, affect the whole body and may arise over a wide area of the brain. There are two main types of generalized seizure—grand mal and absence (petit mal) seizures.

Partial seizures are usually caused by damage to a more limited area of the brain. Partial seizures are divided into simple seizures and complex seizures. In either of these types, the electrical disturbance may spread and affect the whole brain, causing a generalized seizure.

GRAND MAL During this type of generalized seizure the person falls down unconscious and the entire body stiffens and then twitches or jerks uncontrollably. There may be an initial cry; breathing is then absent or very irregular during the seizure. Following the seizure, the muscles relax, and bowel and bladder control may be lost. The person may feel confused and disoriented and perhaps have a headache; often he or she will want to sleep. These effects usually clear in several hours. The person usually has no memory of the event. Prolonged seizures, referred to as status epilepticus, can be fatal without emergency treatment.

ABSENCE SEIZURES (PETIT MAL) This type of generalized seizure, in which there is a momentary loss of consciousness without abnormal movements, occurs mainly in children. There is a blank period lasting from a few seconds to up to half a minute or so, during which the sufferer is unaware of anything. To the onlooker, it may appear that the person is simply daydreaming or inattentive, and the attack may even pass unnoticed. Absence seizures may occur hundreds of times daily and can markedly impair school performance.

SIMPLE PARTIAL SEIZURES Consciousness is maintained in this type of partial seizure. An abnormal twitching movement, tingling sensation, or even hallucination of smell, vision, or taste, occurs without warning and lasts several minutes.

Jacksonian epilepsy is a type in which twitching occurs and spreads slowly from one part of the body to another on the same side. Sufferers retain awareness during the event and can recall the details.

COMPLEX PARTIAL SEIZURES In this type of seizure, also known as *temporal lobe epilepsy*, conscious contact with the surroundings is lost. There may be abnormal behaviour that is not easily recognized as being due to epilepsy. The sufferer becomes dazed and may not respond if addressed. Involuntary actions, such as fumbling with buttons or lip smacking, sometimes occur. These actions are called automatisms and (rarely) can take more bizarre forms. The person typically remembers little, if any, of the event.

PREVENTION

Many epileptics experience seizures at times of extreme fatigue or stress. Infectious illnesses, especially if fever is present, also lower the seizure threshold. By avoiding these situations and taking prescribed medication regularly, epileptics can reduce the frequency of seizures. Occasionally, epileptics discover a distracting technique that can abort a seizure once the aura has begun.

DIAGNOSIS

In making the diagnosis, the doctor seeks as much information as possible about the attacks. Since patients frequently do not have recall, information may be obtained from witnesses.

After a complete examination of the nervous system, the doctor usually orders an *EEG* to help with the diagnosis. It is important to realize that the EEG cannot always absolutely confirm or refute the diagnosis of sei-zures, and that the results must be weighed in the light of the person's symptoms and signs.

In some cases, an *ECG* (electrical monitoring of the heartbeat) is performed to exclude cardiac *arrhythmias* as a cause of loss of consciousness in an adult. *CT scanning* or *MRI* of the brain and *blood tests* may also be performed.

TREATMENT

Opinion is divided on whether a single seizure should be treated; doctors agree that people with recurrent seizures should take *anticonvulsant drugs*.

Anticonvulsant drugs are the first line of treatment for epilepsy, and, in almost all cases, they lessen the frequency of seizures. The drugs may have unpleasant side-effects, including drowsiness and impaired concentration. The doctor will attempt to find the one drug that works best, but, with very severe epilepsy, a combination may be needed to control seizures. If no seizures occur for two to three years (depending on their cause), the doctor may suggest reducing or stopping drug treatment.

Rarely, surgery may be considered if it is thought that a single area of brain damage (usually in the temporal lobe) is causing the seizures and if medication is ineffective.

OUTLOOK

If epilepsy develops during childhood and there is a definite family history of the disease, the chances are good that the problem will decrease after adolescence; it may even disappear altogether. However, seizure control is likely to be more difficult in temporal lobe epilepsy or if the disorder has been brought about by severe brain damage.

One third of those in whom epilepsy develops eventually grow out of the condition and experience no further seizures. Another third find that the seizures become less frequent in response to treatment. The conditions of the last third stay the same.

Sufferers from epilepsy are usually able to work, but the disorder may limit their choice of jobs. There are restrictions on obtaining a driving licence. It is advisable, unless the seizures are very well controlled, to avoid high-risk jobs involving heights or dangerous machinery and sports such as skiing.

Many epileptics carry a special card, tag, or bracelet that states they have epilepsy. Epileptics are recommended to advise colleagues on what to do if a seizure occurs.

E

DEALING WITH AN EPILEPTIC SEIZURE

Most major epileptic seizures last only a minute or two and demand little of the bystander. All that is necessary is to let the attack run its course and to ensure that the person is in no physical danger and can breathe while he or she is unconscious.

The person should not be held down, nor should his or her movements be restrained. Any tight clothing around the neck should be loosened and something soft placed beneath the head. The mouth should not be forced open and no object wedged between the teeth. Once the convulsions have ceased, the victim should be put into the *recovery position*.

An ambulance should be called if the seizure continues for more than five minutes, if another seizure immediately follows the first one, or if consciousness is not regained a few minutes after the seizure has ended.

Epiloia

See *Tuberous sclerosis*.

Epinephrine

The American name for *adrenaline*.

Epiphora

See *Watering eye*.

Epiphysis

Either of the two growing ends of the long bones (femur, tibia, fibula, ulna, radius, and humerus) of the limbs. The epiphysis is separated from the diaphysis (shaft of the bone) by a layer of cartilage, called the epiphyseal plate or growth plate.

During childhood and adolescence, bones grow as the result of *ossification*, a process in which cartilage cells multiply and absorb calcium to develop into bone. In this way, the cartilage in the ephiphyseal plate is gradually replaced by new bone.

Epiphysis, slipped

See *Femoral epiphysis, slipped*.

Episcleritis

A localized patch of inflammation affecting the outermost layers of the *sclera* (the white of the eye) immediately under the *conjunctiva* (the transparent membrane covering the sclera).

Episcleritis usually occurs for no known reason and generally affects middle-aged men. It may be a complication of *rheumatoid arthritis*. The purplish patch of inflammation is oval, slightly raised, and less than 1 mm across. It may cause a deep, dull, aching pain that tends to be worse at night. During the day there may be *photophobia* (abnormal sensitivity of the eyes to light).

The condition usually disappears by itself within a week or two but may recur. Symptoms may be relieved by eye-drops or ointment containing a *corticosteroid drug*.

Episiotomy

A surgical procedure in which an incision is made in the *perineum* (the tissue between the vagina and the anus) to facilitate the delivery of a baby. After delivery, the cut tissues are stitched back together.

WHY IT IS DONE

Until recently, many obstetricians advocated its use almost routinely on the grounds that a surgical cut will heal better than a tear, and that women who have had episiotomies will experience less trouble later in life from stretching of the vagina. The majority view nowadays seems to be that episiotomies should be performed only when there are clear reasons for it.

An episiotomy is advisable if the perineum fails to stretch up over the baby's head and/or a large perineal tear looks likely. It prevents a ragged tear that is more painful, more difficult to repair, and more commonly leads to complications. Episiotomy is usually necessary in a *forceps delivery*, because the instruments occupy additional space in the vagina, and in a *breech delivery*, in which there is little opportunity for gradual stretching of the perineal tissues.

An episiotomy is usually performed if the baby is suffering from *fetal distress* (the effects of receiving insufficient oxygen during labour), because episiotomy speeds delivery. An episiotomy is also usually performed to reduce pressure on the baby's head during a premature birth.

In most cases, however, the naturally elastic vagina should not have to be cut to allow a normal delivery. Small tears probably cause less damage and pain than an episiotomy.

HOW IT IS DONE

As the baby's head descends through the maternal pelvis and begins to stretch the perineum, local anaesthetic is injected into the area (unless the woman has already been given an anaesthetic).

Scissors are used to make a cut extending from the back wall of the vagina through the perineal skin and muscles. This cut may be directed to the side of (mediolateral), or in a direct vertical line with, the anus (midline).

HOW IT IS REPAIRED

An episiotomy is usually repaired shortly after delivery of the baby. The woman lies on her back with her feet in stirrups. The perineum is thoroughly cleaned and more local anaesthetic is injected if necessary. The vagina is inspected to assess the size of the incision and to see whether further tears have occurred. The wound is repaired in layers, usually with absorbable sutures.

RECOVERY PERIOD

The woman can walk as soon as she wishes. Occasionally, *ice-packs* and *analgesic drugs* are required. The perineum should be kept clean and care taken to avoid *constipation*. Absorbable sutures dissolve after about 10 days and thus do not require removal. In most cases, healing is straightforward. Discomfort in the region of the scar may be felt for some weeks.

Epispadias

A rare *congenital* abnormality in which the opening of the *urethra* is not in the glans (head) of the *penis*, but on the upper surface of the penis. The penis may also curve upwards.

Surgery is carried out in infancy, using tissue from the foreskin to reconstruct the urethra and create a penis

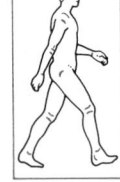

LOCATION OF THE EPIPHYSIS
Each epiphysis is situated at the ends of the long bones of the body and is separated from the shaft of the bone by an epiphyseal plate.

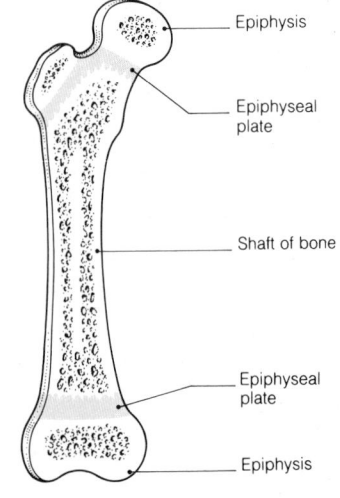

Epiphysis

Epiphyseal plate

Shaft of bone

Epiphyseal plate

Epiphysis

that will allow satisfactory sexual intercourse in adult life. Sometimes more than one operation is needed to correct the condition. (See also *Hypospadias*.)

Epistaxis
The medical term for a *nosebleed*.

Epithelium
The cells, occurring in one or more layers, that cover the entire surface of the body and that line most of the hollow structures within it. (Structures that are not lined with epithelium are the blood vessels, lymph vessels, and the inside of the heart, which are lined with *endothelium*, and the chest and abdominal cavities, which are lined with *mesothelium*.)

Epithelium varies in cell type and thickness according to the function it performs. There are three basic cell shapes: squamous (thin and flat), cuboidal, and columnar. These structures may vary further. In the respiratory tract, for example, epithelial cells bear brush-like filaments called cilia that create a current in the surrounding fluid. This current propels dust particles from inhaled air back up the bronchi and trachea.

Most internal organs lined with epithelium are covered with only one layer of cells, but the skin, which is subjected to more trauma, consists of many layers with a dead outer layer of cells that is constantly being shed.

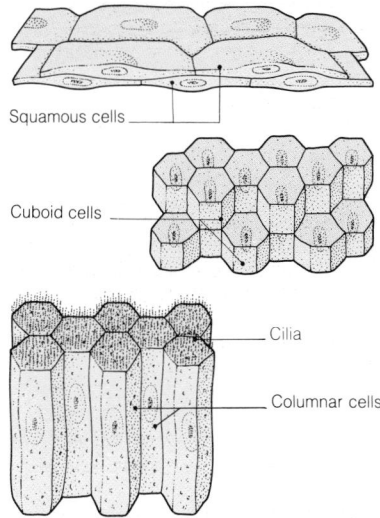

Squamous cells

Cuboid cells

Cilia

Columnar cells

Types of epithelium
The cells of the epithelium vary in shape and size according to function. The three basic types are squamous, cuboidal, and columnar.

Epoetin
A genetically engineered preparation of the human hormone erythropoietin, which is produced in the kidneys and stimulates the bone marrow to manufacture red blood cells. Lack of erythropoietin in *kidney failure* may cause serious *anaemia*, but this responds to treatment with epoetin. The hormone is also used to treat itching associated with *uraemia*, as well as the anaemia that often occurs in chronic disorders such as *rheumatoid arthritis*. It has been used (illegally) by some athletes in an attempt to improve their stamina.

Epstein-Barr virus
A virus that causes infectious *mononucleosis*; the virus is also associated with *Burkitt's lymphoma* and cancer of the *nasopharynx*.

ERCP
The abbreviation for endoscopic retrograde cholangiopancreatography, an X-ray procedure for examining the *biliary system* and the pancreatic duct. ERCP is used mainly when *ultrasound scanning, CT scanning,* or *MRI* fail to provide a sufficiently detailed image.
HOW IT IS DONE
ERCP is usually an outpatient procedure and takes 20 to 40 minutes. No food or drink is taken for eight hours before the examination. A *sedative* drug is usually given and a local anaesthetic applied to the throat.

An *endoscope* (a flexible viewing tube with a lens and light attached) is passed down the oesophagus, through the stomach, and into the *duodenum* (the upper part of the small intestine). The endoscope operator then passes a catheter (fine, flexible tube) through the endoscope into the ampulla of Vater (the opening in the duodenum that leads to the common bile duct and pancreatic duct). He or she then passes a radiopaque contrast medium (one that shows up on X-ray film) through the catheter to fill the pancreatic duct and all the ducts of the biliary system. X-rays are taken that show any abnormalities in the ducts.

If disease is detected, it can sometimes be treated at the same time. For example, stones obstructing the lower end of the common bile duct can be removed by using an attachment on the endoscope to widen the duct. If there is a suspected tumour at the ampulla, the endoscope can be used to perform a *biopsy* (removal of a small sample of tissue for analysis) or brushing of cells for cytological examination (see *Cytology*).

Erection
The hardness, swelling, and elevation of the *penis* that occurs in response to sexual arousal or physical stimulation. Erections are also common during sleep and may occur for no obvious reason in very young boys.

The penis contains three cylinders of erectile tissue with a network of blood vessels controlled by the spinal nerves. During an erection, the penis becomes filled with blood as the vessels dilate (widen) to allow increased blood flow. Muscles around the vessels contract and prevent blood from leaving, so maintaining the erection.

Erection, disorders of
Conditions in which the normal process of erection is disrupted, including total or partial failure to attain or maintain erection (see *Impotence*), persistent erection without sexual desire (see *Priapism*), and bowed erection (see *Chordee*).

Ergocalciferol
An alternative name for vitamin D$_2$ (see *Vitamin* D), also called calciferol.

Ergometer
A machine that measures the amount of physical work done and the body's response to a controlled amount of exercise. An ergometer makes continuous recordings, during and immediately after activity, of heart-rate and rhythm (using an *ECG*), blood pressure, the rate of breathing, and the volume of oxygen taken up from the surrounding air.

Ergometrine
A drug given after *childbirth, miscarriage,* or *abortion* to control loss of blood from the uterus. Ergometrine is usually given in a single injection but tablets may also be needed in some cases. The drug works by causing the muscles of the uterus to contract, which compresses the blood vessels and thus reduces bleeding.

Ergot
A product of CLAVICEPS PURPUREA, a fungus that grows on rye and various other cereals. Ergot contains several *alkaloids* (nitrogen-containing substances) with medicinal and poisonous effects.

The most important drugs produced from ergot are *ergotamine*, used to treat migraine, and *ergometrine*, used to control blood loss from the uterus following childbirth, miscarriage, or abortion.

Before it was known that ergot was a poison, bread made with contaminated rye caused outbreaks of ergot poisoning. The effects included gangrene of the toes and fingers, seizures, mental disorders, and, in some cases, death.

Ergotamine

A drug used in the prevention and treatment of *migraine*. It works by constricting the dilated blood vessels surrounding the brain and is used as an alternative to *analgesic drugs* (painkillers).

Ergotamine is most effective if taken during the early warning stages of a migraine attack. Once the headache and nausea of migraine are present, it is less likely to be effective and may even increase the nausea.

Erosion, dental

Loss of enamel from the surface of a tooth as a result of attack by acids or other chemicals. The first sign of enamel loss is a dull, frosted appearance. As the condition progresses, smooth, shiny, shallow cavities form.

Erosion affecting the outer surfaces of the front teeth is most often caused by excessive consumption of citrus fruits, fruit juices, or carbonated drinks; it also sometimes occurs in people who use acid in industrial processes. Erosion mainly affecting the inner surfaces of the molar teeth may be caused by frequent regurgitation of acidic fluid from the stomach—for example, in people suffering from *acid reflux* or *bulimia*.

Erosion may be combined with, and also accelerate, *abrasion* (mechanical wearing away of teeth) and attrition (wearing down of the chewing surfaces), leading to extensive damage to many teeth. (See also *Caries, dental*.)

Eroticism

The character and emotive nature of sexual excitement. The term derives from the ancient Greek for "desire", personified and deified as Eros. Sexual arousal may be stimulated by thoughts, by the touching of the erogenous zones (especially the mouth, breasts, genitals, and anus), or by a variety of other sensations (such as the look and feel of certain clothes, the scent of a perfume, or the sound of a piece of music).

In *psychoanalytic theory*, eroticism is contrasted with *narcissism* (self love). Eroticism is a mature love that can be fulfilled only when the loved one is also satisfied. Narcissism is typical of immature personalities and is a love that merely wishes to satisfy itself.

Eruption

The process of breaking out or appearing, as of a skin rash or a new tooth.

Eruption of teeth

The process by which developing *teeth* move through the jaw and gum to project into the mouth.

DECIDUOUS DENTITION

Deciduous teeth (also called primary or milk teeth) usually begin to appear when a baby is about six months old. In most cases, the lower front teeth are the first to erupt. Occasionally, a baby is born with one or two teeth already visible. Other babies do not have any teeth visible until they are about nine months old. All 20 deciduous teeth usually erupt by the time the child is three years old. Infants may suffer a mild general upset at the time of eruption (see *Teething*).

PERMANENT DENTITION

Permanent teeth (the secondary teeth) generally begin erupting when a child is six years old. The first permanent molars erupt towards the back of the mouth and appear in addition to, rather than replacing, the deciduous teeth. Children and parents are often unaware that these are permanent teeth.

The eruption of permanent teeth nearer the front of the mouth is preceded by reabsorption of the roots of the deciduous teeth, which become loose and detach. The succeeding permanent tooth emerges a few weeks after its deciduous predecessor is detached and falls out.

TOOTH ERUPTION

The top diagrams show the approximate ages at which particular deciduous teeth usually appear. The ages at which specific types of permanent teeth usually appear are shown in the lower diagrams. Red denotes erupting teeth; grey denotes erupted deciduous teeth; white denotes erupted permanent teeth.

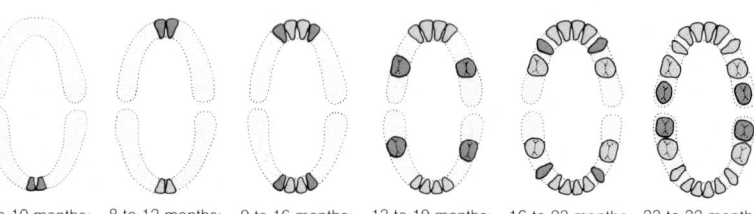

| 6 to 10 months: lower central incisors | 8 to 12 months: upper central incisors | 9 to 16 months: lateral incisors | 13 to 19 months: first molars | 16 to 23 months: canines | 23 to 33 months: second molars |

Deciduous teeth
The full deciduous set (left) consists of eight incisors, four canines, and eight molars. They usually start erupting at six months.

Permanent teeth
The full set of permanent teeth (below) consists of eight incisors, four canines, eight premolars, and 12 molars. They usually start erupting at six years.

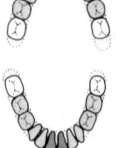 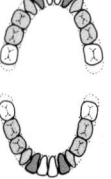 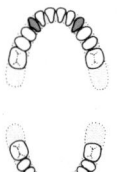 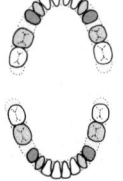 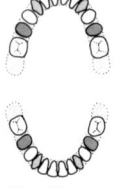 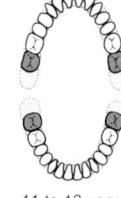 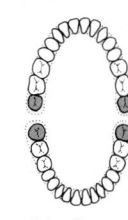

| 6 to 7 years: first molars | 6 to 8 years: central incisors | 7 to 9 years: lateral incisors | 9 to 12 years: canines | 10 to 12 years: first premolars | 10 to 12 years: second premolars | 11 to 13 years: second molars | 17 to 21 years: third molars |

Wisdom teeth (the last molar teeth) usually erupt between the ages of 17 and 21, but in some people never appear. In others, wisdom teeth are impacted (blocked from erupting) because of insufficient space in the jawbone (see *Impaction, dental*).

Erysipelas

An infection, usually of the face, caused by streptococcal bacteria, which are thought to enter the skin through a small wound or sore. Young children and the elderly are most often affected.

The disorder starts abruptly with malaise, fever, headaches, and vomiting. Itchy, red patches appear on the face and spread across the cheeks and the bridge of the nose to form an inflamed area with raised edges. Within this area, pimples develop that first blister, then burst, and then crust over.

Treatment is with *penicillin drugs*, which usually clear the condition within a week. (See also *Cellulitis*.)

Erythema

A term meaning redness of the skin. Disorders of which skin redness is one feature include *erythema multiforme*, *erythema nodosum*, *lupus erythematosus*, *erythema ab igne*, and erythema infectiosum (*fifth disease*).

Erythema can have many causes, including *blushing*, *hot flushes*, *sunburn*, raised temperature, and inflammatory, infective, or allergic skin conditions such as *acne*, *dermatitis*, *eczema*, *erysipelas*, *rosacea*, and *urticaria* (nettle rash).

Erythema ab igne

Red mottled skin that may also be dry and itchy, caused by exposure to strong direct heat. Erythema ab igne is most common on the shins, due to sitting too close to a fire, or on the abdomen, due to hugging a heating pad or a hot-water bottle.

Dryness and itching of the skin can often be relieved by an *emollient* (soothing cream). The redness usually fades in time, although it rarely disappears completely.

Erythema infectiosum

See *Fifth disease*.

Erythema multiforme

An acute inflammation of the skin, and sometimes of the internal mucous membranes (the thin moist tissue that lines bodily cavities), sometimes accompanied by generalized illness. Erythema multiforme means literally "skin redness of many varieties".

CAUSES AND INCIDENCE

The disease can occur as a reaction to certain drugs (including *penicillin drugs*, *sulphonamide drugs*, *salicylate drugs*, and *barbiturate drugs*), or may accompany certain viral infections (such as *herpes simplex* causing cold sores) or bacterial infections (such as *streptococcal infections* causing sore throat). Pregnancy, *vaccination*, and *radiotherapy* are other possible causes. However, half of all cases occur for no apparent reason. The disease is most common in children and young women.

SYMPTOMS

A symmetrical rash of red, often itchy spots, similar to the rash of measles, erupts on the limbs and sometimes on the face and the rest of the body. The spots may blister or may progress to form raised, red, pale-centred wheals—so-called target lesions. Those affected may have fever, sore throat, headache, and/or diarrhoea.

In a severe form of erythema multiforme, called Stevens-Johnson syndrome, the mucous membranes of the mouth, eyes, and genitals become inflamed and ulcerated.

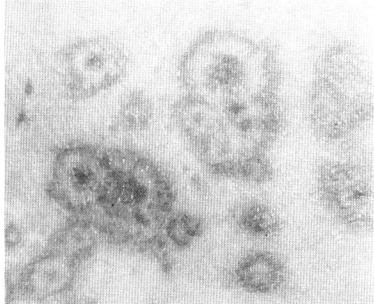

The rash of erythema multiforme
The spots of this rash are usually itchy and have a bull's-eye appearance, with concentric rings of different shades of red around a pale centre.

TREATMENT

If the treatment for some other disorder is believed to be the cause of the erythema, the treatment will be withdrawn. Any causative illness will be treated if possible. In some cases, *corticosteroid drugs* are given to reduce inflammation and irritation. Patients suffering from Stevens-Johnson syndrome are given *analgesic drugs* (painkillers), plenty of fluids (sometimes intravenously), *sedative drugs*, and sometimes corticosteroid drugs.

Erythema multiforme usually clears within five to six weeks, although it may recur. Stevens-Johnson syndrome normally responds to treatment, but in some cases the patient may become seriously ill as a result of shock or of inflammation spreading within the body.

Erythema nodosum

A condition characterized by an eruption of red-purple swellings on the legs in association with another illness. It is most common between the ages of 20 and 50 and affects women more than men.

CAUSES AND INCIDENCE

The most common cause of erythema nodosum is a *streptococcal infection* of the throat, but the condition is also associated with other diseases, most commonly *tuberculosis* and *sarcoidosis*, and may occur as a reaction to certain drugs, including *sulphonamide drugs*, *penicillin drugs*, and *salicylate drugs*. In about one third of cases, no cause can be discovered.

SYMPTOMS

The swellings, which range from 1 to 10 cm in diameter, are shiny and tender and occur on the fronts of the shins, thighs, and, less commonly, the arms. Joint and muscle pains and fever also usually occur.

TREATMENT

Effective treatment of any underlying condition clears the swellings. Bed rest, *analgesic drugs* (painkillers), and, occasionally, *corticosteroid drugs* may be necessary. The condition usually subsides within a month.

Erythrasma

A bacterial skin infection, caused by the organism CORYNEBACTERIUM, which affects the groin, armpits, and skin between the toes. Affected areas are raised above the rest of the skin and are irregularly shaped. On white skin, affected areas look red-brown; on dark skin, they may look either lighter or darker than the normal skin. There are usually no other symptoms. Erythrasma is more common in people with *diabetes mellitus*.

Erythrasma is diagnosed by inspecting the skin under a special light, called Wood's light, which shows up the affected areas as red fluorescent patches. The condition generally clears when treated with *erythromycin*.

Erythrocyte

Another name for a red blood cell (see *Blood cells*).

E

E

Erythroderma

See *Exfoliative dermatitis*.

Erythromycin

ANTIBIOTIC
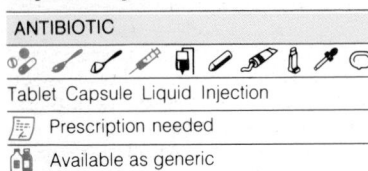
Tablet Capsule Liquid Injection
Prescription needed
Available as generic

An *antibiotic drug* used to treat infections of the skin, chest, throat, and ears. Erythromycin is particularly useful in the treatment of *pertussis* (whooping cough) and *legionnaires' disease*. In children under eight years old, erythromycin is a useful alternative to *tetracycline*, which can cause permanent staining of developing teeth.

Possible adverse effects include nausea, vomiting, abdominal pain, diarrhoea, and an itchy rash.

Eschar

A scab on the surface of the skin formed to cover damage caused by a burn, abrasion, severe scratching, or some skin diseases and infections.

Esmarch's bandage

A broad, rubber bandage wrapped around the elevated limb of a patient to force blood out of the blood vessels towards the heart; this enables surgery to be performed more easily in a blood-free area.

The Esmarch's bandage is wrapped from the toes or fingers upwards, and a pneumatic (inflatable) tourniquet is then applied to the thigh or upper arm to stop blood from returning to the limb. The Esmarch's bandage is removed, leaving the inflated tourniquet in position during surgery.

Esotropia

A term for a convergent *squint*. One eye looks directly at an object while the other eye turns inwards.

ESR

The abbreviation for erythrocyte sedimentation rate, which is the rate at which red blood cells sink towards the bottom of a test tube. Because the ESR is increased in certain disorders, it is a useful aid to diagnosis and can also be used to monitor the effect of treatment.

HOW IT IS DONE
Whole blood collected from the person on whom the test is being performed is mixed with anticoagulant (a chemical that prevents the blood from clotting) in a test tube and left undisturbed at a constant temperature for one hour.

The red blood cells, which can be seen as a dark red clump, settle to the bottom of the tube, leaving the clear, straw-coloured plasma at the top. The ESR is the number of millimetres the red cells fall in one hour.

RESULTS
The ESR is increased if the level of fibrinogen (a type of protein) in the blood is raised. Fibrinogen is raised in response to inflammation, especially when caused by infection or an *autoimmune disease,* such as *temporal arteritis*. The ESR is also increased if levels of *immunoglobulins* (another type of protein) are very high, as occurs in *multiple myeloma*.

ESWL

Extracorporeal shock wave lithotripsy (see *Lithotripsy*).

Ethambutol

A drug used in conjunction with other drugs in the treatment of *tuberculosis*. Ethambutol rarely causes side-effects, although occasionally it may cause inflammation of the optic nerve, resulting in blurred vision.

Ethanol

The chemical name for the *alcohol* in alcoholic drinks; it is also called ethyl alcohol.

Ether

A colourless liquid that produces unconsciousness when inhaled. Ether (full name, diethyl ether) was the first general anaesthetic to be introduced. It was administered on a gauze mask placed over the patient's nose and mouth.

Ethics, medical

A code of behaviour that addresses the relationships between doctor and patient, and among doctors. Medical ethics covers a wide range of behaviour, including involvement with patients and their families, professional competence, public image, and commercial behaviour. Ethical standards in the UK are enforced by the *General Medical Council*.

Doctors must not abuse their relationship of trust with patients. In particular, they must not enter into sexual relationships with patients and must maintain in confidence information learned from patients. They must give clear priority to their patients' interests.

Doctors are expected to develop and maintain their skills and to update their knowledge to the standard of their colleagues. They should not refer patients to unlicensed practitioners of alternative medicine. Fees should conform to recognized schedules; all forms of fee splitting or rebates are unacceptable. In addition, it is against ethical standards for a doctor to be dependent on alcohol or drugs.

The doctor should ensure that the patient not only consents to all procedures, investigations, and treatments, but that this consent is based on an unbiased and full explanation of any risks, drawbacks, and alternatives that might be considered.

Any time a patient is asked to enrol in a research study, the investigator should see that consent is full and free, and that patients do not feel pressured to agree because of a sense of gratitude owed to the doctor for previous treatment. Research on children or on patients who are mentally handicapped should, in general, be considered only when there is a reasonable prospect that the person concerned will benefit from the investigation and that the risks and any discomfort inherent in the research are minimal.

Ethical considerations are also important in the care of the dying, in the termination of pregnancy, in the care of children born with major physical and mental handicaps, and in the care of patients with mental disorders.

Ethinyloestradiol

A synthetic form of the female sex hormone oestradiol. It is most commonly used in *oral contraceptives,* in which it is combined with a *progestogen drug.* Ethinyloestradiol is also prescribed to stimulate sexual development in female *hypogonadism* (underdevelopment of the ovaries) and in the treatment of symptoms caused by the *menopause,* such as hot flushes and sweating (see *Hormone replacement therapy*). Ethinyloestradiol is also used to treat menstrual disorders (see *Menstruation, disorders of*).

Ethosuximide

An *anticonvulsant drug* used to treat petit mal (a type of *epilepsy*). Ethosuximide is often prescribed in preference to other anticonvulsant drugs because, unlike some of them, it rarely causes drowsiness or liver damage. Ethosuximide may, however, cause nausea and vomiting and in rare cases affects the production of blood cells in the bone marrow and causes aplastic anaemia (see *Anaemia, aplastic*).

Ethyl alcohol

Another name for ethanol, the *alcohol* in alcoholic drinks.

Ethyl chloride

A colourless, flammable liquid once used as a general anaesthetic and now occasionally used as an *analgesic drug* (painkiller).

Applied to the skin as a spray, ethyl chloride quickly evaporates and, as a result, makes the skin feel so cold that any pain or irritation is reduced. It may be used to numb an area of skin before a minor surgical procedure, such as lancing a boil, and is sometimes used to alleviate the pain that arises from sprained or strained muscles or ligaments.

Ethyl chloride is also used in the treatment of *larva migrans,* a hookworm infection acquired from cats and dogs.

Etretinate

A drug chemically related to *vitamin A* that is used in the treatment of severe *psoriasis.* Prescribed only under hospital supervision, etretinate is used when other drugs have failed to help. It works by reducing the production of keratin, the protein that forms the hard, outer layers of skin. Because of this action, etretinate is also occasionally used to treat other rare skin disorders that cause excessive skin thickening, such as *ichthyosis.*

Symptoms generally improve within four weeks of treatment and the effects may persist for a number of months after the drug therapy has been discontinued.

POSSIBLE ADVERSE EFFECTS
Etretinate can cause liver damage and a rise in blood fats; regular blood tests of liver function and fat levels are therefore usually carried out during treatment. Etretinate should never be taken during pregnancy because of the risk of damage to the developing fetus, and effective *contraception* must be continued for two years after stopping the drug.

Eucalyptus oil

A substance distilled from the leaves of eucalyptus trees. Eucalyptus oil is colourless, with an aromatic, camphor-like smell and a pungent, refreshing taste. The oil is used as a flavouring agent and—applied externally as a rub, inhaled as a vapour, or incorporated in tablets or pastilles—is also used in many proprietary remedies for coughs and colds. There is little evidence that eucalyptus oil has

any curative properties, although it may relieve symptoms.

Eunuch

A man whose testes have been removed or destroyed so that he is sterile and lacks male hormones. The term was used especially to describe boys who were castrated before puberty to make them suitable for guarding harems.

A male who is castrated before puberty will have characteristic eunuchoid features: broad hips, narrow shoulders, and undeveloped male secondary *sexual characteristics* (i.e. he will have a small penis, a feminine distribution of body hair, and a high-pitched voice).

Euphoria

A state of confident well-being. Euphoria is a normal reaction to personal success. It can also be induced by drugs, including prolonged use of *corticosteroid drugs.*

Feelings of euphoria with no rational cause may be an indication of brain disease or damage caused by *head injury* (particularly damage to the frontal lobes), *dementia, brain tumours,* or *multiple sclerosis.*

Eustachian tube

The passage that connects each middle *ear* to the back of the nose.

STRUCTURE
The tube is about 36 mm long in an adult. From the middle ear it runs forwards, downwards, and inwards; it ends in the space at the back of the nose just above the soft *palate* (part of the roof of the mouth). A smooth, moist, mucous membrane lines the tube.

FUNCTION
The eustachian tube acts as a drainage passage from the middle ear and maintains hearing by opening periodically to regulate air pressure. The lower end of the eustachian tube opens during swallowing and yawning, thus allowing air to flow up to the middle ear and equalizing air pressure on both sides of the eardrum.

If a change in external pressure is large and rapid, pressure may build up on one side of the eardrum, pushing it inwards or outwards; this is uncomfortable and dulls hearing. Most people have experienced this sensation in response to the increase in pressure that occurs when descending in a plane or going into a tunnel in a car or train. Symptoms can usually be relieved by swallowing hard.

DISORDERS
When a head cold blocks the eustachian tube, equalization cannot occur, which may cause severe pain. Because the displaced eardrum cannot vibrate properly, hearing may be temporarily impaired. A person with a blocked eustachian tube who is subjected to rapid changes in pressure may suffer from *barotrauma* (pressure damage to the eardrum or other structures).

Glue ear (accumulation of secretions in the middle ear) or chronic *otitis media* (middle-ear infection) may occur if the eustachian tube becomes blocked, preventing adequate drainage from the middle ear. These conditions, which often cause partial hearing loss, are more common in children because their adenoids are larger and more likely to block the tube if they become infected. Children's eustachian tubes are also

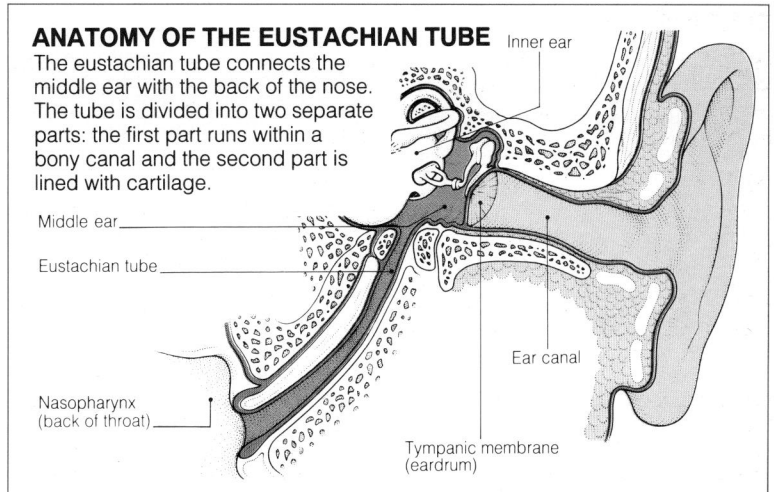

ANATOMY OF THE EUSTACHIAN TUBE

The eustachian tube connects the middle ear with the back of the nose. The tube is divided into two separate parts: the first part runs within a bony canal and the second part is lined with cartilage.

Inner ear

Middle ear

Eustachian tube

Nasopharynx (back of throat)

Ear canal

Tympanic membrane (eardrum)

shorter, making it easier for bacteria to travel from infected areas in the throat to the middle ear.

Euthanasia

The act of killing a person painlessly to relieve his or her suffering. Even when requested by a patient with incurable disease, euthanasia (the literal meaning is "easy death") is against the law in most developed countries.

Euthanasia is distinct from nonintervention, which is the doctor's recognition that, if a patient has an advanced or incurable disease, he or she has a right to refuse medical treatment that would simply prolong the process of dying.

Euthyroid

The term used to describe a person whose *thyroid gland* is functioning normally, or to describe a person who has been successfully treated for *hypothyroidism* (underactivity of the thyroid) or *hyperthyroidism* (overactivity of the thyroid) so that the gland functions normally.

Eversion

A turning outwards. The term is commonly applied to a type of ankle injury or deformity in which the foot is turned outwards.

Evoked responses

The tracing of electrical activity in the brain in response to a specific external stimulus. The responses are much smaller than the impulses recorded by an *EEG* and are a refinement of that technique. Evoked responses were first demonstrated in 1947. Today, with the increased sophistication of computerized electronic technology, evoked responses are a widely used diagnostic tool.

WHY IT IS DONE
The functioning of various sensory systems (e.g. sight, hearing, and touch) can be checked by this technique. The information obtained can be used to reveal abnormalities in the system caused by inflammation, pressure from a tumour, or other disorders, and to confirm the diagnosis of *multiple sclerosis*. The test is extremely sensitive and can often pinpoint the location of a fault.

HOW IT IS DONE
The procedure is painless and usually takes 30 minutes to an hour. A set of small disc electrodes is attached to the scalp in the same way as for an EEG. The electrodes are attached to different parts of the scalp, depending on which sensory system is being tested. The output from the brain is linked to a computer, which produces a print-out after a specific period of stimulation. Analysis is based on the time lapse between stimulus and response; the computer is used to extract this information from the background brain activity that shows up on an EEG.

For testing the visual system, a series of flashes from a stroboscopic light may be used. An example of a more demanding stimulus for the brain, which gives more consistent results, is a board made up of black and white squares constructed so that the colours alternate every second. To test hearing, the ears are subjected to different sounds. To test touch and pain sensations, small electrical stimuli are applied, for example, to a nerve at the wrist.

RESULTS
Testing of evoked responses does not necessarily give an unequivocal diagnosis and is used as a supplement to other tests of the nervous system (e.g. EEG or *EMG*), other investigations, and radiological tests such as *CT scanning* or *MRI*.

Ewing's sarcoma

A rare malignant bone cancer. Ewing's *sarcoma* arises in a large bone, most commonly the femur (thigh bone), tibia (shin), humerus (upperarm bone), or one of the pelvic bones, and spreads to other parts of the body at an early stage.

The condition is most common in children between 10 and 15 years of age; it affects twice as many boys as girls and is only rarely seen in black children.

SYMPTOMS
The affected bone is painful and tender and part of it may swell. The bone may also become weakened and fracture easily. Other symptoms include weight loss, fever, and anaemia.

DIAGNOSIS
The sarcoma is diagnosed by X-rays and a bone *biopsy* (removal of a small piece of bone for analysis). If cancer is found, the complete skeleton is examined by X-rays and *radionuclide scanning*, and the lungs by *CT scanning*, to determine if, and how far, the cancer has spread. Spreading by the time of diagnosis is found in 15 to 20 per cent of cases.

TREATMENT
Treatment is with *radiotherapy* and *anticancer drugs*. Before the introduction of chemotherapy, death usually occurred within two to three years of diagnosis. Today, the chances of survival have improved considerably; 65 per cent of those affected are still alive five years after diagnosis and most of them remain well.

Examination, physical

The part of a medical consultation in which the doctor looks, feels, and listens to various parts of the patient's body in order to assess the patient's condition. The physical examination usually follows history-taking, in which the doctor listens to the patient's complaints and then asks questions. Physical examination and history-taking together may provide the doctor with sufficient information to make a *diagnosis*, or provide clues that will aid the selection of appropriate diagnostic studies.

HOW IT IS DONE
A complete physical examination may be performed if a patient visits a doctor for the first time, if a patient complains of generalized symptoms, or if an examination is required for employment or insurance purposes. A more limited examination will be performed if a patient has a disorder or injury in one part of the body.

The main techniques used by a doctor during a physical examination are inspection, palpation, percussion, and auscultation.

The doctor begins by assessing the patient's general appearance and by looking at any specific problem area, such as a lump, that might be drawn to the doctor's attention.

Most physical examinations include palpation (feeling with the hands), by which the doctor examines relevant parts of the body for signs such as swelling, tenderness, or enlargement of organs.

In some cases, percussion of the chest over the lungs or of other parts of the body may be performed. Percussion is performed by tapping the patient's body with the fingers and listening to the resonance of the sound produced.

Auscultation (listening with a *stethoscope*) may also be needed. This technique is used mainly to listen to sounds made by the heart and lungs, and to listen to the flow of blood through arteries.

The doctor will apply these techniques, sometimes using special equipment, to examine different body systems. For example, he or she may take the pulse or blood pressure, examine the eyes, ears, mouth, throat, and teeth, and assess the strength and coordination of muscles, the mobility of joints, and skin sensation as a reaction to touch and pain.

Excimer laser

An instrument used to reshape the cornea as a treatment for *myopia* (short sight) or long sight. Used since 1983 on tens of thousands of patients, the technique of laser surgery to normalize the sight is claimed to be safe and effective, but its long-term safety has yet to be proved.

Excision

Surgical cutting out of diseased tissue from surrounding healthy tissue, such as the removal of a breast lump or gangrenous skin.

Excoriation

Injury to the surface of the skin or of a *mucous membrane* caused by physical abrasion, such as by scratching. The loss of surface cells causes a raw area to develop.

Excretion

The discharge of waste material from the body. To maintain health, the body must dispose of the by-products of digestion, waste products from the repair of body tissues, and water (to maintain the correct volume of fluid and to remove solid wastes in the form of a solution).

ORGANS OF EXCRETION
The *kidneys* excrete excess nitrogen in the *urine* in the form of urea, along with excess water, salts, some acids, and most drugs.

The *liver* excretes bile, which, as well as containing salts that help emulsify fats in the small intestine, consists of waste products and bile pigments formed from the breakdown of red blood cells. Part of the bile is passed from the body in the *faeces,* which it colours brown.

The large *intestine* excretes undigested food, some salts, and some excess water in the form of faeces.

The *lungs* discharge carbon dioxide and water vapour into the air.

Sweat glands excrete salt and water on to the surface of the skin as a method of regulating the body's temperature.

Exenteration

The surgical removal of all organs and soft tissue in a body cavity in the hope of arresting the growth of a cancer. Exenteration is occasionally performed for cancer in the orbit (the bony structure surrounding the eye) or in the pelvis.

Exercise

The performance of any physical activity that improves health or that is used for recreation or the correction of physical injury or deformity (see *Physiotherapy*). Different types of exercise affect the body in one or more of the following ways: some improve flexibility, some improve muscular strength, some improve physical endurance, and some improve the efficiency of the cardiovascular and respiratory systems. The various effects of different types of exercise are described in the illustrated box (see overleaf).

BENEFITS OF EXERCISE
There is an established association between high levels of aerobic exercise and low incidence of *coronary artery disease.* Regular exercise usually leads to a reduction in blood pressure. It also increases the amount of high-density lipoprotein in the blood, which is thought to help protect against *atherosclerosis* (narrowing of arteries by deposits of fatty material) and *myocardial infarction* (heart attack). Exercise has also been shown to be valuable in relieving the symptoms of *peripheral vascular disease* and of some psychological disorders such as *depression.*

Vigorous work with a muscle or a group of muscles, even if it is of short duration, leads to an increase in the size, strength, and possibly the number of the muscle cells, and an increase in the strength of their ligamentous attachments to bones. Improving the strength of muscles in the back and abdomen can help prevent or ease lower back pain. The increased strength of the muscles and tendons is also a potentially useful insurance against damage due to an unexpected strain.

Vigorous exercise may be a risk for people who are out of condition: an individual who usually never takes exercise, and then attempts a demanding task such as sweeping snow from a driveway, has an increased risk of a myocardial infarction. Professional sportsmen such as footballers have an increased risk of *osteoarthritis* in later life because of repeated minor damage to structures such as the knee and the cervical area of the spine.

Exfoliation

Flaking off, shedding, or peeling from a surface in scales or thin layers, as in *exfoliative dermatitis.*

Exfoliative dermatitis

Inflammation, marked redness, and scaling of the skin over most of the body, also called erythroderma.

Exfoliative dermatitis may be the result of an allergic response to a particular drug or may be caused by the worsening of a skin condition, such as *psoriasis* or *eczema.* Sometimes, exfoliative dermatitis occurs in *lymphoma* and *leukaemia.*

There is a widespread rash with severe flaking of the skin. The loss of surface skin, with exposure of its deeper layers, results in increased loss of water and protein from the body surface. Protein loss may cause *oedema* (accumulation of fluid in tissues) and muscle wasting. Further complications are *heart failure,* due to the pumping of blood through widened blood vessels, and infection.

The treatment and outlook depend on the cause. About 60 per cent of sufferers recover within two to three months; about 30 per cent die as a result of complications; and in the remainder the disease takes a chronic form unresponsive to treatment.

Exhibitionism

The habit of deliberately exposing the genitals to strangers. This form of behaviour is almost always confined to men. The exhibitionist displays his penis to a female passer-by, usually in a secluded spot or from a car or house window with the aim of surprising or frightening the victim.

In 80 per cent of cases, a single court appearance puts an end to the exhibitionist's behaviour. *Psychotherapy* or *behaviour therapy* can sometimes help those who relapse.

Exocrine gland

A gland that secretes substances through a duct on to the inner surface of an organ or on to the outer surface of the body. Examples include the *salivary glands,* which release saliva into the mouth, the *sweat glands,* and the lacrimal glands (see *lacrimal apparatus*), which release tears. The release of exocrine secretions can be triggered by a *hormone* or by a *neurotransmitter.* (See also *Endocrine gland.*)

Exomphalos

A rare birth defect in which a membranous sac containing part of the intestines protrudes through the umbilicus (navel). In mild cases only one or two loops of intestine protrude, but in severe cases most of the abdominal organs are exposed.

THE EFFECTS OF EXERCISE

There are many changes in different body organs during exercise. Muscles require an increase in blood flow because of their greater energy requirements; the heart and lungs work faster and more efficiently. These changes are controlled by the release of the chemicals adrenaline and noradrenaline from the sympathetic nervous system.

The lungs

The rate and depth of breathing increase to ensure sufficient flow of oxygen from the lungs into the blood. This also helps remove additional carbon dioxide produced by muscle cells during exercise.

The joints

Regular exercise helps maintain the mobility of joints. Increased strength in the muscles and tendons around joints makes them more resistant to injury.

The muscles

There is a rise in the chemical activity within muscle cells. The rate of consumption of oxygen and glucose increases.

Flexed muscles

Relaxed muscles

The heart and circulation

The heart beats faster and more powerfully to increase the flow of blood to the working muscles. Blood vessels in the stomach and under the skin are narrowed to compensate for the increased requirements of the muscles.

ECG printouts
Resting heart-rate (above) and during exercise (below)

COMMON TYPES OF EXERCISE

Aerobic 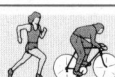	Isometric	Isotonic 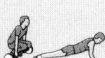	Isokinetic 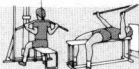
Aerobic exercise is when the body continuously needs to take in additional oxygen to meet the muscles' increased demands. Regular aerobic exercise improves the performance of the cardiovascular and respiratory systems. Jogging, swimming, and cycling are examples of aerobic exercise.	Isometric exercise is exercise without movement, in which one group of muscles exerts pressure against an immovable object or an opposing group of muscles. It is an effective means of increasing muscle strength, but does not exercise the cardiovascular system or help in muscular endurance.	Isotonic exercise is exercise with movement, in which muscle tension is more or less constant and the body works against its own weight or external weights. Isotonic exercise includes weight training and calisthenics (repetitious movements with little or no equipment). It increases muscle strength, size, and endurance.	Isokinetic exercise involves both isotonic and isometric exercise. The muscles move reasonably heavy loads, but are also put through their full range of movement. Isokinetics combines strength training with some aerobic exercise, but requires special equipment.

Also called omphalocele, exomphalos is associated with other birth defects, including intestinal malformations. Many babies with the condition are stillborn or die soon after birth. Exomphalos is treated by surgery. Prior to operation, the covering membranes may be painted with a drying, antiseptic solution to thicken them, making subsequent surgery easier.

Exophthalmos

Protrusion of one or both eyeballs caused by a swelling of the soft tissue in the bony orbit (eye socket). The eyeball is pressed forwards, exposing an abnormally large amount of the front of the eye, forcing the eyelids apart and causing a staring appearance.

CAUSE

The most common cause of exophthalmos is *thyrotoxicosis* (overactivity of the thyroid gland). Other causes include an *eye tumour*, inflammation, or an *aneurysm* (ballooning of an artery) behind the eye; in these cases only one eye is affected.

SYMPTOMS AND SIGNS

Exophthalmos may restrict eye movement and cause *double vision*. In severe cases, the pressure in the orbit may be so high that the blood supply to the optic nerve may be restricted; blindness can result. The lids may be prevented from closing, and vision may become seriously blurred due to drying of the cornea.

TREATMENT AND OUTLOOK

In thyroid exophthalmos, treatment of the thyroid disorder may sometimes relieve the exophthalmos, but often it does not. Early treatment usually returns the vision to normal. Occasionally, surgery to decompress the orbit may be required to relieve pressure on the eyeball and on the optic nerve.

Exostosis

A type of benign *bone tumour* in which there is an outgrowth of bone. Exostosis occurs most commonly at the end of the femur (thigh bone) or tibia (shin).

Exostoses account for 90 per cent of all bone tumours; they affect twice as many men as women. In about 65 per cent of cases the condition is due to hereditary factors; another cause is prolonged pressure on a bone.

SYMPTOMS

In most cases, exostosis produces no symptoms and goes unnoticed. Often it is recognized only after an injury, when it appears as a hard swelling. Occasionally the bony outgrowth presses on a nerve, causing pain or weakness in the affected area (usually when it is beneath a fingernail or toenail).

DIAGNOSIS AND TREATMENT

A preliminary diagnosis based on symptoms and signs can be confirmed by X-ray. Treatment, by surgical removal, is usually performed only if the tumour is causing symptoms or is unsightly.

Exotoxin

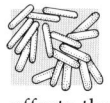 A poison released by some types of bacteria into the bloodstream, from where it causes widespread effects throughout the body. Exotoxins are among the most poisonous substances known. They are produced by certain types of bacteria, such as *tetanus* bacilli (which enter the body through a wound and produce an exotoxin that affects the nervous system to cause muscle spasms and paralysis) and *diphtheria* bacilli (which initially infect the throat, but release an exotoxin that damages the heart and nervous system).

Infections by tetanus, diphtheria, and some other bacteria that release life-threatening exotoxins can be pre-

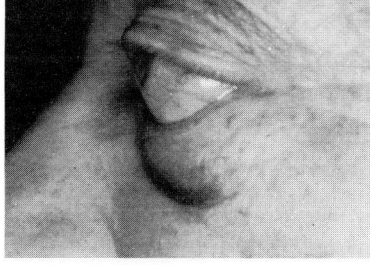

One-sided exophthalmos
The affected eye (shown above) protrudes markedly compared with the normal eye. More commonly, both eyes are affected.

vented by immunization with vaccines consisting of detoxified exotoxins. Treatment of such infections usually includes the administration of *antibiotic drugs* and an *antitoxin* to neutralize the exotoxin. (See also *Endotoxin*; *Enterotoxin*.)

Exotropia

A term for a divergent *squint*. One eye is used for detailed vision and the other is directed outwards.

Expectorants

Cough remedies that encourage the coughing up of sputum (phlegm).

Expectoration

The coughing up and spitting out of sputum (phlegm). (See also *Cough*.)

Exploratory surgery

Any operation to investigate or examine part of the body to discover the extent of known disease or to establish a diagnosis. For example, exploratory *thoracotomy* is performed on the chest and exploratory *laparotomy* on the abdomen.

Exposure

A term used to describe the effects on the body of being subjected to very low temperatures, or to a combination of low temperatures, wetness, and high winds. The primary danger comes from the lowering of body temperature in these conditions (see *Hypothermia*).

The term is also sometimes used to describe subjection to radiation or to a variety of environmental pollutants.

Expressing milk

A technique used by *breast-feeding* women for removing milk from the breasts. Expressing milk may be necessary when the breasts are overfull (see *Engorgement*). A woman may also want to express milk from her breasts so that the milk can be given to the baby in her absence.

Most women find it easier to express milk by hand, but a *breast pump* can be used. Milk should be expressed into a sterilized container and sealed. It will keep for up to 48 hours in a refrigerator. When properly prepared, it can be stored in a freezer for up to six months.

Exstrophy of the bladder

A rare birth defect in which the bladder is turned inside out and is open to the outside of the body through a space in the lower abdominal wall.

EXPRESSING MILK BY HAND
Wash your hands thoroughly before starting, then follow the method below. Repeat the sequence twice on each breast, alternating between breasts. If the breasts are engorged, bathe them in hot water first to help milk flow.

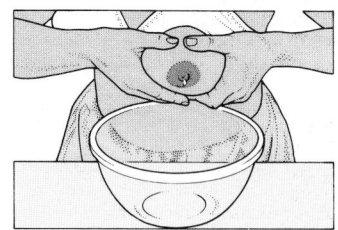

1 Cup the breast in both hands, thumbs on top and fingers underneath. Squeeze the outer part of the breast firmly. Repeat 10 times, moving around the breast.

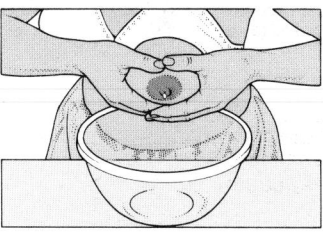

2 Move hands closer to the nipple area and repeat the squeezing movement 10 more times.

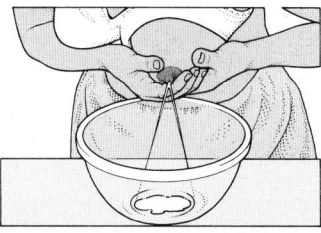

3 Hold the breast in one hand. With the thumb and forefinger of the other hand, squeeze the edge of the areola in and up so that milk squirts out. Move your hand around the areola, squeezing gently and rhythmically for about five minutes.

Usually, there are also other defects, such as *epispadias* (emergence of the urethra through a hole in the shaft of the penis) in males, and failure of the pubic bones to join at the front.

Untreated, an affected child constantly leaks urine. Surgical treatment consists of reconstructing the bladder, if it is big enough, and closing the abdominal wall. If the bladder is very small, it is removed and the urine diverted elsewhere in the abdomen (see *Urinary diversion*).

Extraction, dental

The removal of one or more teeth by a dentist.

WHY IT IS DONE

Extraction may be performed when a tooth is severely decayed, when an abscess has formed, or when a tooth is too badly broken to be repaired by crowning or root canal treatment. Teeth may also be removed if they are causing crowding or malocclusion (incorrect bite), if they are loose because of advanced gum disease, or if they are preventing another tooth from erupting.

HOW IT IS DONE

For most extractions, local anaesthesia is used. General anaesthesia may be used to extract badly impacted wisdom teeth, to extract several teeth at once, or for extremely anxious or mentally handicapped patients or young children.

Most teeth are extracted with dental forceps, which are designed to grasp the root of the tooth. When gentle but firm pressure is applied, the blades cut through the periodontal ligaments (the tough fibrous membranes supporting the tooth in its socket), the socket is gradually expanded, and the tooth is removed. Occasionally the root of the tooth fractures during this procedure, especially if the bone is dense (as in older people) and may need to be removed separately.

If the tooth is especially difficult to remove—for example, if it is impacted, the crown is missing, or the roots are very curved—it may be necessary to cut a small flap into the gum and remove a small amount of nearby bone. The tooth is then extracted and the gum is sutured (stitched).

COMPLICATIONS

Most extractions take place without complications. Occasionally, if a blood clot fails to form in the empty tooth socket, or if the blood clot is dislodged, *dry socket* (infection in the tooth socket) develops. Dislodging a clot can also cause renewed bleeding from the wound; this can be eased by placing a tightly folded handkerchief or a gauze pad on the wound and biting on it gently for about 30 minutes. If bleeding continues, suturing of the tissue around the socket may be necessary.

Extradural haemorrhage

Bleeding into the space between the inner surface of the skull and the external surface of the dura mater, the outer layer of the *meninges* (protective covering of the brain).

CAUSES AND SYMPTOMS

An extradural haemorrhage usually results from a blow to the side of the head that fractures the skull and ruptures an artery running over the surface of the dura mater. The person may momentarily lose consciousness and then apparently recover.

A haematoma (collection of clotted blood) forms and enlarges, increasing pressure within the skull and causing symptoms a few hours or even several days after the injury. The affected person develops a headache that gradually increases in severity; other symptoms include drowsiness, vomiting, seizures, and paralysis on one side of the body. He or she eventually lapses into a coma and, without treatment, may die.

DIAGNOSIS AND TREATMENT

CT scanning confirms the diagnosis. Surgical treatment consists of drilling burr holes in the skull (see *Craniotomy*), draining the blood clot, and clipping the ruptured blood vessel. If the bleeding is diagnosed early (before serious symptoms develop), the outlook is excellent; hence the importance of seeking medical advice and investigation following even a moderate blow to the head (see *Head injury*).

Extrapyramidal system

A network of nerve pathways that links nerve nuclei in the surface of the *cerebrum* (the main mass of the brain), the *basal ganglia* deep within the brain, and parts of the *brainstem*. The system influences and modifies electrical impulses that are sent from the brain to initiate movements in the skeletal muscles.

Damage or degeneration of components in the extrapyramidal system can cause a disturbance in the execution of voluntary (willed) movements and in muscle tone, and can also cause the appearance of involuntary (unwilled) tremors, jerks, or writhing movements. Such disturbances are seen in *Huntington's disease*, *Parkinson's disease*, some types of *cerebral palsy*, and can also occur as a side-effect of taking *phenothiazine drugs*.

Extravert

A person whose interests are constantly directed outwards, to other people and the environment. Extra-verts are active, energetic, sociable, easy to talk to, and have many outside interests and concerns. (See also *Personality*.)

Exudation

The discharge of fluid from blood vessels into a tissue or on to the tissue's surface. An exuded fluid (called an exudate) contains cells and a large amount of protein. Most exudates are produced as a result of *inflammation*. When tissue is inflamed, its small blood vessels become wider and the tiny pores in the vessel walls become enlarged, which allows fluid and cells (mainly white blood cells) to escape.

Eye

The organ of sight. The eye consists of structures that focus an image on to the *retina* at the back of the eye and nerve cells that convert this image into electrical impulses that are carried by the *optic nerve* for interpretation by a specialized region of the brain.

The two eyes work in conjunction under the control of the brain, aligning themselves on an object so that a clear image is formed on each retina. If necessary, the eyes sharpen images by altering focus in an automatic process known as *accommodation*.

The pattern of light falling on the retina stimulates a complex flow of impulses along the optic nerves to the brain. The two optic nerves pass into the skull, meet, partially cross over, and run back, at first on the underside of the brain, and then through its substance to the visual cortex—the area of the back surface of the brain concerned with *vision*.

STRUCTURE

EYEBALL The eyeballs lie in pads of fat within the orbits, bony eye sockets that provide protection from injury. Each eyeball is moved by six delicate muscles, the action of these muscles for both eyes being coordinated by a nerve network in the brainstem.

The eyeball has a tough outer coat, the *sclera* (white of the eye). The front, circular part of the outer coat, the *cornea*, is transparent and protrudes slightly. The cornea serves as the main "lens" of the eye and performs most of the focusing. Behind the cornea is a shallow chamber full of aqueous humour (watery fluid), at the back of which is the *iris* (coloured part) with its *pupil* (central hole) which appears black. Tiny muscles alter the size of the pupil with changes in light intensity to control the amount of light entering the eye.

Immediately behind the iris, and in contact with it, is the crystalline *lens*, suspended by delicate fibres from a circular muscle ring called the ciliary body. Contraction of the ciliary body alters the shape of the lens; this provides the eye with some focusing power additional to that provided by the cornea. Behind the lens is the main cavity of the eyeball, filled with a clear gel (the vitreous humour).

On the inside of the back of the eye is the retina, a complex structure of nerve tissue on which the image formed by the cornea and the crystalline lens falls. The retina requires a constant supply of oxygen and glucose. To meet this need, a thin network of blood vessels, the choroid plexus, lies immediately under it. The *choroid* is continuous at the front with the ciliary body and the iris; these three parts constitute the uveal tract.

CONJUNCTIVA The eyeball is sealed off from the outside by a flexible membrane called the *conjunctiva*, which is firmly secured around the margin of the cornea but lies freely on the sclera over the front third of the globe. It is attached to the skin at the corners of the eye and forms the inner lining of the lids, with a deep cul-de-sac above and below. This arrangement provides a permanent seal while allowing free mobility of the eyeball.

The conjunctiva contains many tiny tear-secreting and mucus-producing glands. They, along with an oily secretion from the meibomian glands in the eyelids, provide the important, three-layer tear film that must constantly cover the cornea and conjunctiva to protect them from damage due to drying out of the cells.

EYELIDS Each lid contains about 30 meibomian glands, with their openings along the lid margin just behind the roots of the lashes. The glands secrete an oil that prevents adhesion of the lid margins during sleep and forms the outer layer of the tear film—a layer that retards evaporation and helps maintain the continuity of the tear film. The blink reflex is protective and helps to spread the tear film evenly over the cornea. This is essential for clear vision. Should the tear film dry out, *corneal abrasion* is more likely.

Just under the skin of the lid is a flat but powerful muscle. Screwing up of the eye in response to danger, contracts this muscle, pushing the globe back into the orbit and covering the eye with a bunched-up mass of tissue.

Eye, artificial

A prosthesis to replace an eye that has been removed. It is worn for cosmetic and psychological reasons.

ANATOMY OF THE EYE

The eye is a complex organ that focuses light-rays to form an image on the retina, which then converts this image into a pattern of nerve impulses that are transmitted to the brain. The cornea and lens focus the light, the pupil controls the amount of light entering the eye, the ciliary body alters the shape of the lens to adjust the focus, and the retina contains millions of nerve cells that respond to light.

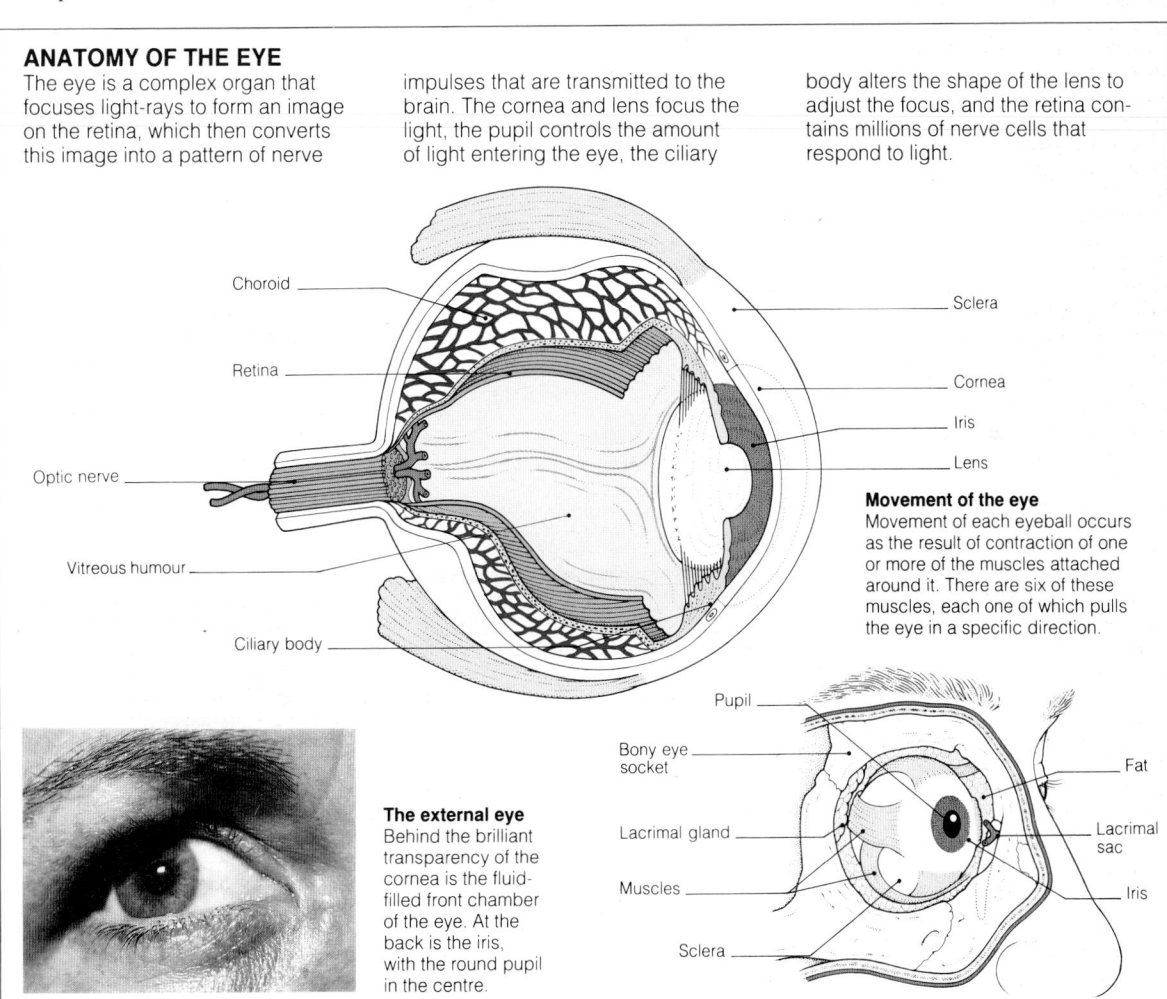

Choroid

Retina

Optic nerve

Vitreous humour

Ciliary body

Sclera

Cornea

Iris

Lens

Movement of the eye
Movement of each eyeball occurs as the result of contraction of one or more of the muscles attached around it. There are six of these muscles, each one of which pulls the eye in a specific direction.

The external eye
Behind the brilliant transparency of the cornea is the fluid-filled front chamber of the eye. At the back is the iris, with the round pupil in the centre.

Pupil

Bony eye socket

Lacrimal gland

Muscles

Sclera

Fat

Lacrimal sac

Iris

E

Often called a "glass eye", the ocular prosthesis is usually a thin, curved, hollow plastic shell. The artificial iris behind the transparent artificial cornea may be produced by hand-painting or using a photograph.

The prosthesis fits neatly behind the eyelids into the cavity from which the natural eye has been removed. Some movement of the artificial eye is achieved by attaching the eye-moving muscles to the remaining conjunctival membrane. In some cases, the eye-moving muscles may be attached to a plastic implant in the eye socket, which allows greater movement of the prosthesis.

Eye-drops

Medication in solution used to treat eye disorders or to aid in diagnosis. Common examples of drugs given in this form are *antibiotic drugs, corticosteroid drugs, antihistamine drugs,* drugs to control *glaucoma* (raised pressure in the eye), and drugs used to dilate (widen) or constrict (narrow) the pupil.

To use eye-drops, first pull the lower lid away from the eye by using a fingertip to draw down the skin below the eye, and then allow drops to fall behind the lid. To reduce the risk of contamination, care should be taken to avoid touching the skin or eye with the dropper.

Eye, examination of

An inspection of the external and internal structure of the eyes either as part of a standard *vision test* or to make a diagnosis when some disorder is suspected.

WHY IT IS DONE

Eye examinations are performed to determine the cause of visual disturbance or other symptoms relating to the eye, and to assess whether or not glasses (or contact lenses) are necessary. Some serious eye disorders, such as *glaucoma,* are symptomless in the early stages and can be detected only by an eye examination.

HOW IT IS DONE

The examination begins with an inspection of the external appearance of the eyes, the lids, and the surrounding skin. A check of eye movements is usually performed. The examiner looks for *squint* and may perform a cover test, which will show if a person has a squint because a squinting eye will move to look directly at a designated object when the other eye is covered. A check of the *visual acuity* (sharpness of vision) in each eye using

a *Snellen chart* (the standard eye testing wall chart) follows. Refraction testing (using lenses of different strengths) may be done to determine what glasses or contact lenses may be needed.

A test of the *visual fields* (extent of the peripheral vision) may also be performed, especially in suspected glaucoma or neurological conditions. *Colour vision* may also be checked because loss of colour perception is an early indication of certain disorders of the retina or optic nerve.

To check for abrasions or ulcers, the conjunctiva and cornea may be stained with *fluorescein* (an orange dye). After staining, conjunctival abrasions appear yellow; corneal abrasions or ulcers show as green areas under white light or fluoresce brilliantly under ultraviolet light.

Applanation *tonometry* (measurement of the pressure within the eye) is an essential test for glaucoma. It is done using a tonometer attached to a slit-lamp microscope.

EQUIPMENT

The *ophthalmoscope* is an instrument used to examine the inside of the eye, especially the retina.

The slit-lamp microscope, with its brilliant illumination and lens magnification, allows meticulous examination of the conjunctiva, cornea, front chamber of the eye, iris, and crystalline lens.

By means of special corneal contact lenses, the magnified view through the slit-lamp microscope may be extended to include the vitreous gel behind the lens and the retina. These contact lenses incorporate mirrors to allow examination of structures at the base of the iris and the front edge of the retina. For a full view of the crystalline lens and the structures behind it, the pupil must be widely dilated with drops, such as tropicamide or cyclopentolate.

Eye, foreign body in

Any material on the surface of the eye or under the eyelid, or an object that penetrates the eyeball. Foreign bodies in the eye are very common; most are easily removed and cause no damage.

CAUSES

Particles of dust are the most common type of foreign body in the eye. Occasionally, a fragment of metal, plastic, or wood may be deflected into the eye—for example, when a person is doing a job in the home or on a car. Rarely, an object travelling at high speed actually penetrates the eyeball—for example, a piece of metal in an industrial accident.

CONDUCTING AN EYE EXAMINATION

During an eye examination, the ophthalmologist checks external appearance, eye movement, visual acuity, visual field, and colour vision. The eyes are checked for the presence of a squint, abrasions, and ulcers. Applanation tonometry and a refraction test are also done.

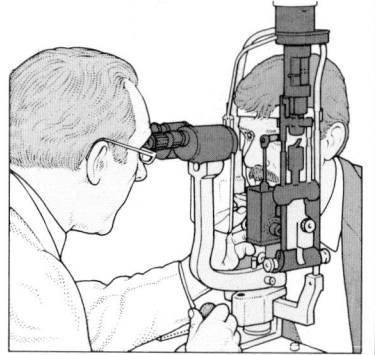

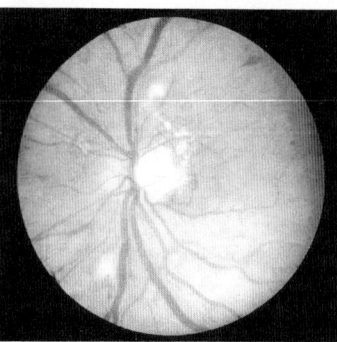

View of retina through ophthalmoscope
The retina (inner back surface of the eye) is examined to assess conditions such as hypertensive *retinopathy,* as seen here.

Z
D A
F X H
P T N D
X A Z F N
H T X U D F
U Z N D F X T
A P H T X Z N U

Applanation tonometry
Measurement of the pressure within the eye is a routine test for glaucoma.

Snellen chart
The chart is used to check visual acuity of each eye; the patient's ability to read letters of different sizes from the same distance is assessed.

SYMPTOMS

A foreign body irritates the eye, causing pain, redness, increased tear production, and usually blepharospasm (uncontrollable closure and squeezing of the eyelid). These symptoms may diminish even if the foreign body remains. Occasionally, there are no symptoms, especially if the eye has been penetrated.

COMPLICATIONS

Some foreign bodies left within the eyeball may change chemically and release damaging ingredients into the substance of the eye, causing blindness. Other foreign bodies may remain whole but may cause infection that leads to blindness. Sympathetic *ophthalmia* is a rare condition that may threaten sight in the uninjured eye.

TREATMENT

Foreign bodies on or in the conjuctiva (the transparent membrane covering the white of the eye and the inside of the eyelids) may be removed at home (see illustrated box).

If a foreign body lies on the cornea (the transparent front part of the eyeball) or may have penetrated the eye, a doctor should be consulted. He or she will examine the eye and eyelids and may insert *fluorescein* (an orange stain) into the eye to show up *corneal abrasions* or sites of penetration. If a penetrating injury is suspected, imaging techniques, such as *ultrasound scanning* or an *X-ray*, may be performed.

A doctor may anaesthetize the surface of the eye with eye-drops containing a local anaesthetic, and then use a sharp spatula to remove a foreign body from the cornea. Metallic objects that have penetrated the eye can sometimes be extracted using a powerful magnet. The eye may be covered with a patch and *antibiotic drugs* in the form of eye-drops or ointment may be prescribed.

Eye injuries

Serious eye injuries may be caused either by penetration of the eye or by a blow to the eye. Often, however, the eye escapes serious injury because it is well-protected by surrounding bone and by the rapid lid-squeeze reflex.

Penetrating injuries are most commonly caused by relatively small objects travelling at high speeds, such as gun pellets, small stones thrown up by rotary lawnmowers, and objects from high-speed machinery used for drilling, sawing, hammering, or grinding. Penetrating injuries can also occur from windscreen glass in car accidents. Foreign bodies within the eye can cause serious problems (see *Eye, foreign body in*).

Blunt trauma to the eyeball, such as a blow from a stick, may cause tearing of the *iris* (coloured part of the eye) or rupture of the *sclera* (white of the eye), with collapse of the eyeball and possible blindness. Lesser injuries may lead to a vitreous haemorrhage (bleeding into the space behind the lens), *hyphaema* (bleeding into the front chamber of the eye), *retinal detachment*, or injury to the trabeculum (the channel through which aqueous humour drains from the eye). Hyphaema affects vision until the blood is reabsorbed. Injury to the trabeculum can lead to *glaucoma*.

Injuries to the centre of the cornea invariably impair vision by causing scarring. Damage to the crystalline lens may cause a *cataract* to form, with resultant loss of vision in that eye. Some injuries also damage the *retina* and the *sclera* at the back of the eye.

Eyelashes, disorders of

The eyelashes are arranged in two rows at the front edge lid and normally curve outwards. Growth in

---

FIRST AID: FOREIGN BODY IN THE EYE

WARNING
Never attempt to remove a particle embedded in the eyeball. Do not remove a foreign body if it is resting on the camera.

LOWER LID

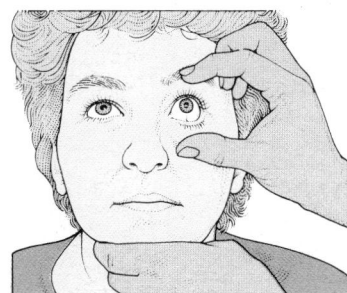

1 Wash your hands. Ask the victim to look up while you separate the lids and examine the eye.

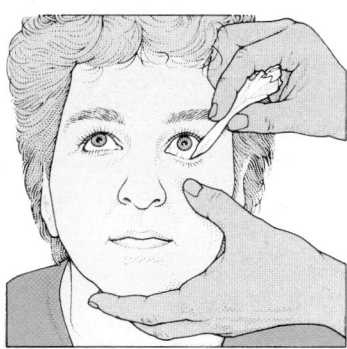

2 First try floating an object out with water; then try lifting it out with the moistened corner of a clean cloth or folded paper.

UPPER LID

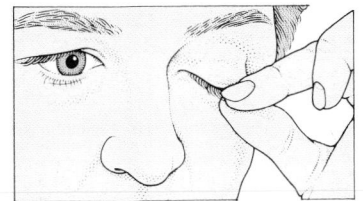

1 Grasp the lashes and carefully draw the upper lid outwards and downwards. If this does not dislodge the object, try floating it off by getting the victim to blink under water.

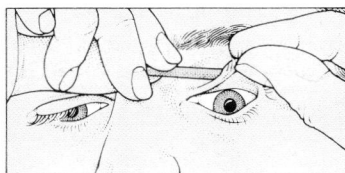

2 If these measures fail, ask the victim to look down while you place a matchstick across the upper lid and fold the lid up over it. Then pick off the object with a clean cloth.

IRRIGATION OF THE EYE

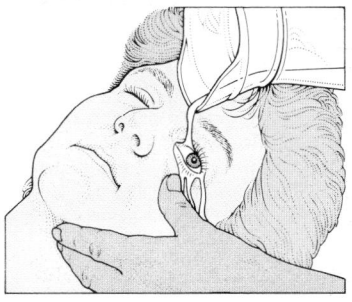

Flush continuously with running water—some corrosives penetrate deeply and take longer to wash out.

DISORDERS OF THE EYE

Many eye disorders are minor, but some lead to serious complications unless treated. (See also *Cornea* disorders box; *Retina* disorders box.)

CONGENITAL DEFECTS

Squint (malalignment of the eyes) is sometimes congenital (present at birth). *Cataracts* (opacity of the lens of the eye) can occur in infants, when the cause may be maternal *rubella* infection early in pregnancy. Very rarely, babies are born with microphthalmos (abnormally small eye) on one or both sides. Vision in a microphthalmic eye is usually very poor. *Nystagmus* (uncontrollable movement in the eyes) is often congenital.

Retinoblastoma is a malignant tumour of the retina that appears in early life and may occur in one or both eyes. Other congenital disorders affecting the eye include *albinism* (absence of pigment) and abnormalities of development of the cornea and retina.

INFECTION

Conjunctivitis, the most common infection, rarely affects vision. In the late stages of neglected conjunctival infection, such as *trachoma* or severe bacterial conjunctivitis, vision can be impaired.

Corneal infections are more serious and can lead to blurred vision or corneal perforation if not treated early. Endophthalmitis (infection within the eye), which may make it necessary to remove the eye surgically, can occur after a penetrating injury, after severe ulceration, (rarely) after major eye surgery, or from infections elsewhere in the body.

IMPAIRED BLOOD SUPPLY

Narrowing, blockage, inflammation, or other abnormalities of the blood vessels of the retina may cause partial or total loss of vision.

TUMOURS

Malignant melanoma of the choroid (the layer of tissue between the retina and the sclera, which is the fibrous outer wall of the eyeball) is the most common primary malignant eye tumour. It can be found without symptoms during routine examinations or can cause a decrease in vision.

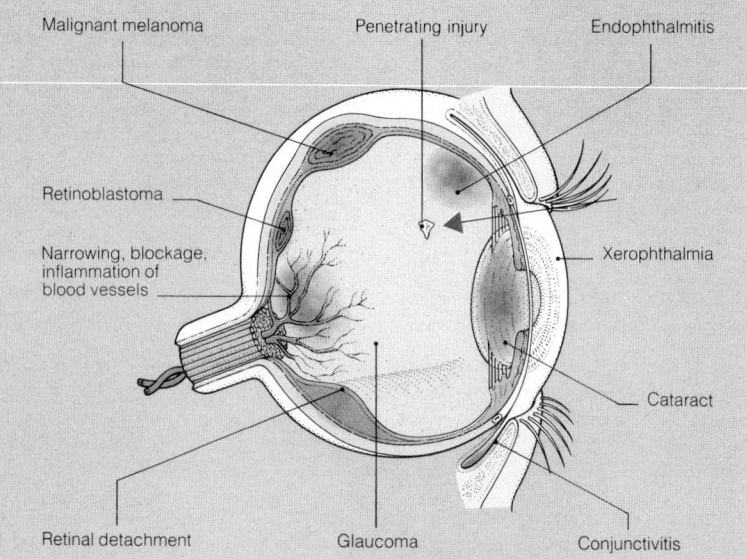

Malignant melanoma — Penetrating injury — Endophthalmitis

Retinoblastoma

Narrowing, blockage, inflammation of blood vessels

Xerophthalmia

Cataract

Retinal detachment — Glaucoma — Conjunctivitis

NUTRITIONAL DISORDERS

Various vitamin deficiencies (particularly vitamin A deficiency) can affect the eye. This may lead to *xerophthalmia* (dryness of the cornea and conjunctiva), night blindness, or, ultimately, *keratomalacia* (corneal softening and destruction).

AUTOIMMUNE DISORDERS

Uveitis (inflammation of the uveal tissues—iris, choroid, and/or ciliary body), when not caused by an infectious agent, may have an autoimmune basis (when the defence mechanisms of the body attack its own tissues). It is common in people with *ankylosing spondylitis* and *sarcoidosis*.

DEGENERATION

Macular degeneration of the retina is common in the elderly. It causes loss of fine, detailed vision, although peripheral vision remains.

Cataract is also common in the elderly; the exact cause is unknown.

OTHER DISORDERS

Glaucoma, a condition in which the pressure in the fluid maintaining the normal shape of the eye is raised, may take various forms. If untreated, glaucoma can lead to permanent loss of vision.

In *retinal detachment*, the retina lifts away from the underlying (choroidal) layer of the eye.

Ametropia is a general term that means the eye has a refractive error (an

error in focusing), such as *myopia* (shortsightedness), *hypermetropia* (longsightedness), or *astigmatism*. None of these is a disease in the ordinary sense of the word; they are caused simply by variations of shape and focusing ability of the eye. *Presbyopia* is the (normal) progressive loss of accommodation (ability to focus at near range) with age. *Amblyopia* (poor vision in one eye without any obvious structural abnormality) is often due to squint.

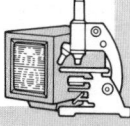

an abnormal direction may be due to injury to the lid or, more commonly, to infection. Occasionally, lashes grow in an abnormal direction for no obvious reason. With age, the lashes become finer and fewer.

Severe *blepharitis* (inflammation of the lid margins) may cause the margins to be so damaged that lash roots are destroyed. *Trachoma*, an infection in which the lid is distorted by scarring, may lead to trichiasis, in which the lashes turn inwards, rub against the cornea, and cause *corneal abrasion*.

Eye, lazy

A popular term for *amblyopia*, in which normal vision has failed to develop in an otherwise healthy eye. The term is also sometimes used to refer to a convergent *squint*.

Eyelid

A fold of tissue at the upper or lower edge of an *orbit* (eye socket). The eyelids provide protection for the eye.

The eyelids are held in position by ligaments attached to the socket's bony edges. They consist of thin plates of fibrous tissue (called the tarsal plates) covered by muscle and a very thin layer of skin. The inner layer is covered by an extension of the *conjunctiva* (the transparent membrane that covers the white of the eye). Along the edge of each eyelid are two rows of eyelashes, which are strong, curved hairs. Immediately behind the eyelashes are the openings of the ducts leading from the meibomian glands, which secrete the oily part of the tear film from within the tarsal plates.

The eyelids act as protective shutters, closing practically instantaneously as a reflex action if anything approaches the eye. The eyelids also act as wipers to smear the tear film across the *cornea* (the transparent front part of the eyeball).

DISORDERS

Disorders include a *chalazion* (a swelling of a meibomian gland), *blepharitis* (inflammation of the edge of the eyelid), and a *stye* (an abscess at the root of one of the eyelashes).

The shape and position of the eyelids are abnormal in a number of disorders, including *entropion* (the eyelid margin turning inwards), *ectropion* (the eyelid margin turning outwards), *ptosis* (a drooping eyelid covering all or part of the eye), and baggy eyelids due to dermatochalasis (excess skin on the lid) or blepharochalasis (excess fat under the skin of the lid).

Myokymia (twitching of the eyelid) is a common phenomenon usually due to fatigue. *Blepharospasm* (tight contraction of the eyelid) is usually caused by a foreign body in the eye.

The skin of the eyelid is a common site for a *basal cell carcinoma*.

Eyelid, drooping

See *Ptosis*.

Eyelid surgery

See *Blepharoplasty*.

Eye, painful red

A very common combination of eye symptoms that may be due to any of several different eye disorders. The presence of pain and redness in one or both eyes requires examination and treatment by a doctor.

Uveitis (inflammation of all or a part of the uvea, such as the iris) is a common cause. The dull, aching pain may be due to swelling within the front of the eye and spasm in muscles around the iris. The redness is caused by widening of blood vessels around the iris.

Another serious cause of pain and redness in one eye is acute closed-angle *glaucoma* (sudden increase in pressure within the eyeball). The pain is severe and may be accompanied by nausea, vomiting, blurred vision, and seeing haloes. There is redness of the white of the eye due to increased blood flow in the surrounding vessels.

Other important causes of painful red eye include *keratitis* (inflammation of the outer protective layer of the eye), usually as a result of a *corneal ulcer*, or a foreign body on the surface of the eye or under one of the eyelids (see *Eye, foreign body in*).

The most common cause of redness and severe irritation (although not strictly pain) affecting the eye is *conjunctivitis*. The redness is due to dilation (widening) of blood vessels in the conjunctiva. The irritation is similar to that caused by grit in the eye. Conjunctivitis can be due to viral or bacterial infections, irritants (such as chemicals), or allergies. Viral conjunctivitis usually eventually affects both eyes and is mildly infectious.

Eye-strain

A term often used to describe aching or discomfort in or around the eye. Eye-strain is not a medical term; the eyes cannot be damaged by being used, by wearing spectacles of the wrong strength, or by not wearing spectacles when they should be worn.

The vague aches that are commonly called eye-strain are usually a form of headache stemming from fatigue, tiredness of muscles around the eye, *sinusitis*, or mild *blepharitis* (inflammation of the eyelid margins) and *conjunctivitis*.

Eye teeth

A common name for canine *teeth*.

Eye tumours

Tumours of the eye are rare. When eye tumours do occur, they are usually malignant and painless.

TYPES AND TREATMENT

RETINOBLASTOMA This is a *congenital* malignant tumour of the retina that occurs in one or both eyes. If the central vision in one eye is affected, the child may have a squint. If the tumour is not discovered in the early stages, it may be seen as a white or yellowish mass in one pupil. Retinoblastoma may sometimes be treated by *radiotherapy*, *laser treatment*, or *cryosurgery* (freezing), but the eye may require removal to prevent spread of the tumour.

MALIGNANT MELANOMA This is a cancer of the choroid layer, under the retina. It usually affects middle-aged and elderly people and is the most common malignant eye tumour. There are no symptoms in the early stages, but the tumour eventually causes detachment of the retina and distortion of vision. Small malignant melanomas can be destroyed by laser treatment, but removal of the eye is often advised to avoid spread of the tumour.

SECONDARY EYE TUMOURS These occur when cancer in another part of the body spreads to the eye. If the secondary tumour grows behind the eyeball, it may cause bulging of the eye. The effect on vision varies, depending on the location and growth rate. Secondary tumours may sometimes be controlled by radiotherapy; the primary tumour will need to be dealt with separately.

BASAL CELL CARCINOMA This is the most common tumour of the eyelid and is believed to be caused by excessive exposure to sunlight. The tumour usually has a small crusty central crater and a hard rolled edge. Although tumours of this type may grow large, they very rarely spread to other parts of the body. In the early stages, a basal cell carcinoma of the eyelid may be treated by surgery, radiotherapy, or cryosurgery. Extensive plastic surgery or removal of the eye may be necessary if the tumour becomes large.

E

F

Face-lift

A cosmetic operation to smooth out wrinkles and lift sagging skin on an aging face to make it look younger. A face-lift is usually performed as an outpatient procedure under a local anaesthetic. The two sides of the face are treated during the same operation.

OUTLOOK

Some bruising of the face is common, but there is usually no pain. The stitches are removed three to five days after the operation. In most cases the scars, which fade within a year, are hidden by natural crease lines or by the hair. The effect of a face-lift usually lasts about five years.

In a few cases, satisfactory healing does not occur because of the accumulation of blood under the skin or because of infection that leads to severe scarring.

Facial nerve

The seventh *cranial nerve*. The facial nerve arises from the pons and medulla oblongata (parts of the *brainstem*) and sends branches to the face, neck, salivary glands, and outer ear.

LOCATION OF THE FACIAL NERVE

Arising from the brainstem, the facial nerve has branches that connect to the outer ear, tongue, salivary glands, and muscles of the neck and face.

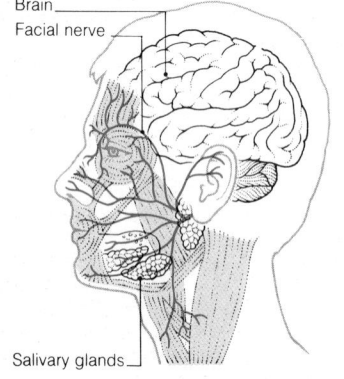

Brain
Facial nerve

Salivary glands

FACE-LIFT

A face-lift is really a skin-lift operation. Its effects are not always permanent. There is some discomfort after a face-lift and the cosmetic effects are not immediately apparent. Care should be taken in choosing a highly reputable surgeon.

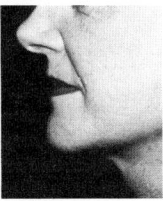

Skin removed

Line of incision

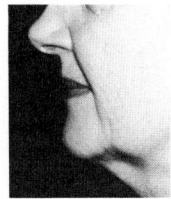

Before and after treatment
The results of most face-lifts are excellent. However, it should be realized that the outcome may not be exactly as expected, and there is always some risk associated with any operation.

How it is done
An incision is made where shown. The skin is undercut as far as the crease running from the nose to the corner of the mouth. It is then pulled upwards and backwards, and its margins are sewn near the hairline.

The facial nerve performs both motor and sensory functions. It controls the muscles of the neck and of facial expression (including muscles in the forehead); it also stimulates secretion by the submandibular and sublingual salivary glands. In addition, the facial nerve conveys taste sensations from the front two thirds of the tongue and carries sensations from the outer ear.

Damage to the facial nerve causes weakness of the facial muscles (see *Facial palsy*) and, in some cases, loss of taste. Such damage is most commonly due to a viral infection. It may also be a feature of a *stroke*; more rarely, damage to the facial nerve may occur as a result of surgery (typically for a tumour) on the parotid gland (one of the salivary glands) or on the ear.

Facial pain

Pain in the face may be due to a variety of causes or may occur for no known reason. In some cases, the cause of pain affects the face directly. In others, a disorder elsewhere in the body results in *referred pain* in the face.

CAUSES

Injury to the face, such as by blows or cuts, is a common cause of facial pain.

Facial pain is also commonly due to infection. *Sinusitis* (inflammation of the air spaces in the facial bones) can cause pain around the eyes and in the cheek bones. The onset of *mumps* can cause pain in the cheeks before any swelling appears in front of and/or below the ears. Pain from a *boil* in the nose or ear may also be felt in the face.

Problems relating to the teeth and jaws are another common cause of facial pain. Pain may be due to dental caries (see *Caries, dental*) or to a tooth abscess (see *Abscess, dental*). In a baby, *teething* can be a painful process. In an adult, facial pain may be due to impacted wisdom teeth (see *Impaction, dental*) or possibly partial dislocation of the jaw (see *Jaw, dislocated*).

Damage to a nerve that supplies the face can result in severe pain. Examples include the knife-like pain that precedes the one-sided rash in *herpes zoster* (shingles), and the intermittent shooting pain of *trigeminal neuralgia* (tic douloureux), which usually affects only one side of the face and is often brought on by touching the face or chewing.

The referral of pain to the face occurs in several disorders. In *angina pectoris* (pain in the chest due to lack of oxygen to the heart), pain may be felt in the jaw. With *migraine* headaches, pain may occur on one side of the face. When facial pain occurs for no reason, it may be a symptom of *depression*.

TREATMENT

Analgesic drugs (painkillers) can provide temporary relief. If facial pain is severe or persistent, however, a doctor or dentist should be consulted.

Facial palsy

Weakness of the facial muscles due to inflammation of or damage to the *facial nerve*. The condition is usually temporary and affects only one side of the face.

CAUSES

Facial palsy is most commonly due to Bell's palsy (named after the Scots surgeon Sir Charles Bell), which occurs for no known reason.

Less commonly, facial palsy is associated with *herpes zoster* (shingles) affecting the ear and facial nerve. Facial palsy may also result from accidental or surgical damage to the facial nerve, or from compression of the nerve by a tumour (e.g. by an *acoustic neuroma* affecting the auditory nerve).

SYMPTOMS

Facial palsy usually comes on suddenly. The eyelid and corner of the mouth droop on one side of the face and there may be pain in the ear on that side. It may be impossible to wrinkle the brow or to close the eye, and smiling is distorted. Depending on which branches of the nerve are affected, taste may be impaired or sounds may seem unnaturally loud.

TREATMENT

Facial palsy often clears up without treatment. Taking *analgesic drugs* may help relieve pain, and exercising the facial muscles may facilitate recovery. In some cases, it may be necessary to tape the eyelid shut at bedtime to avoid *corneal abrasion*.

Bell's palsy is sometimes treated with *corticosteroid drugs* or *ACTH* to reduce inflammation of the facial nerve. Electrostimulation of the nerve is of unproved value. Surgical decompression of the facial nerve is of dubious value in persistent cases of Bell's palsy, but re-routing or grafting of nerve tissue may help people with palsies due to injury or tumour.

Facial spasm

An uncommon disorder in which there is frequent twitching of facial muscles supplied by the *facial nerve*. (This condition is often called a tic, but, in fact, tic is a general term that can refer to spasmodic twitching in any part of the body.) The disorder, which affects mainly middle-aged women, is of unknown cause.

Facies

A medical term for the appearance of the face, as in *adenoid* facies: the dull, open-mouthed expression seen in many children whose nasal passages are blocked due to enlarged adenoids.

Factitious disorders

A group of disorders in which a patient's symptoms mimic those of a true illness but which have in fact been invented by, and are under the control of, the patient. There is no apparent cause other than a wish to receive attention.

The most common type of factitious disorder is *Munchausen's syndrome*, which is characterized by real physical symptoms. In a second form, called *Ganser's syndrome*, there are psychological symptoms.

These disorders differ from *malingering*, in which the person claims to be ill for a particular purpose, such as obtaining time off work or claiming compensation.

Factor VIII

One of the blood proteins (coagulation factors) that takes part in the "coagulation cascade"—an important process in *blood clotting*. Some people with the inherited condition *haemophilia* have a reduced level of factor VIII in their blood and, consequently, have a tendency to abnormal bleeding and to prolonged bleeding when injured.

Freeze-dried concentrates of factor VIII are given to haemophiliacs by regular intravenous injection, which reduces the bleeding tendency and improves the quality of life. Some haemophiliacs administer the treatment themselves at home.

Faecal impaction

A condition in which a large mass of hard *faeces* cannot be evacuated from the rectum. It is usually associated with long-standing *constipation* and dehydrated faeces. Faecal impaction is most common in very young children and in the elderly, especially those who are bedridden.

The main symptoms are an intense desire to pass a bowel movement, pain in the rectum, anus, and centre of the abdomen and, in some cases, watery faeces (which may be mistaken for diarrhoea) that are passed around the impacted mass.

To diagnose the condition, the doctor inserts a gloved finger into the rectum. Treatment is with *enemas* or, if these are ineffective, by manual removal of the faecal mass.

Faecalith

A small, hard, almost stone-like piece of impacted faeces which occasionally forms in a *diverticulum* (a pouch or sac, usually in the large intestine). A faecalith is harmless unless it blocks the entrance to the appendix, causing *appendicitis*, or a diverticulum, causing *diverticulitis*.

Faeces

Waste material from the digestive tract that is expelled through the anus. Solidified in the large intestine, faeces consist of indigestible food residue (roughage, or dietary *fibre*), dead bacteria (which may account for as much as half the weight of the faeces), dead cells shed from the intestinal lining, secretions from the intestine (such as mucus), bile from the liver (which colours the faeces brown), and water.

Examination of the faeces—for colour, odour, consistency, or the presence of blood, pus, fat, parasites, or unusual microorganisms—is important in the diagnosis of digestive tract disorders. (See also *Faeces, abnormal*.)

Faeces, abnormal

Faeces that differ from normal in colour, odour, consistency, or content. The changes may be the result of a harmless condition, but in some cases are due to a disorder of the *digestive system* or to a disorder of a related organ, such as the *liver*.

Diarrhoea (frequent passage of liquid or very loose faeces) may be due simply to anxiety or may be caused by an intestinal infection (see *Gastroenteritis*); by an intestinal disorder such as *ulcerative colitis* or *Crohn's disease*; or by *irritable bowel syndrome*. Loose stools may also indicate *malabsorption*.

Constipation (infrequent passage of very hard faeces) is usually harmless but may be a symptom of a disorder of the large intestine.

Pale faeces may be due to diarrhoea, to a lack of bile in the intestine as a result of *bile duct obstruction*, or to a disease that causes malabsorption (such as *coeliac disease*). In malabsorption, the paleness of the faeces is due to the high fat content. Such faeces may be oily, frothy, foul-smelling, and difficult to flush away.

Dark faeces may simply be the result of unusually large amounts of iron or red wine in the diet. However, if faeces are black, there may be bleeding in the stomach, duodenum, small intestine, or caecum.

Slimy faeces, which contain excessive mucus, may occur for no significant reason, but are sometimes associated with constipation or irritable bowel syndrome. *Enteritis*, *dysentery*, or a tumour (see *Intestine, tumours of*) may also cause slimy faeces, often accompanied by blood.

Blood in the faeces differs in appearance according to the site of bleeding. Blood that originates in the stomach or duodenum is usually passed in the form of black, tarry faeces. Blood due to a disease of the colon, such as ulcerative colitis or a tumour, is red and is usually passed at the same time as the faeces. Blood originating in the rectum or anus, which may be due to tumours or to *haemorrhoids* (piles), is usually bright red; the blood often streaks the faeces but may be visible only on toilet paper or may drip into the toilet bowl.

INVESTIGATION
Severe or persistent abnormality of the faeces should be reported to a doctor. The doctor may ask for a sample of faeces, may perform a *rectal examination*, or may arrange for other tests depending on the suspected diagnosis. (See also *Rectal bleeding*.)

Faeces, blood in the
See *Faeces, abnormal*; *Rectal bleeding*.

Fahrenheit scale
A temperature scale in which the melting point of ice is 32° and the boiling point of water is 212°. On this scale, normal body temperature is 98.6°F (37°C). The scale is named after the German physicist Gabriel Fahrenheit.

To convert Fahrenheit to Celsius, subtract 32 and then multiply by 0.56 (or 5/9). To convert a Celsius temperature to Fahrenheit, multiply by 1.8 (or 9/5) and then add 32. (See also *Celsius scale*.)

Failure to thrive
Failure of expected growth in an infant or toddler, usually assessed by comparing the rate at which a baby gains weight with a standardized growth chart.

Undernourishment may be due to some problem at home, e.g. an unsatisfactory relationship between parent and child. In some cases, the child is actually neglected. Deprived children often have delayed emotional and intellectual development as well as failure to grow.

If a baby fails to gain weight despite receiving an adequate diet and having a stable family background, other conditions may be responsible. Failure to thrive can suggest a serious physical disorder, such as congenital *heart disease*, *kidney failure*, or *malabsorption*.

A baby who fails to thrive is often observed (along with the parent) for a week or two to see how the parent feeds and handles the baby. The baby's diet and weight are carefully monitored. If there are social problems, support for the family can be initiated. (See also *Short stature*.)

Fainting
Temporary loss of consciousness due to insufficient oxygen reaching the brain. The medical term for fainting is syncope.

CAUSES
Fainting often occurs as result of a vasovagal attack, in which overstimulation of the *vagus nerve* causes slowing of the heartbeat and a fall in blood pressure, so reducing the flow of blood to the brain. This type of fainting is usually preceded by sweating, nausea, dizziness, ringing in the ears, dimmed vision, and weakness. Vasovagal attacks are commonly caused by pain, stress, shock, fear, or by being in a stuffy atmosphere that has little oxygen. Other causes include prolonged coughing, straining to defaecate or urinate, or blowing an instrument, particularly the trumpet. Fainting is often attributed to a vasovagal attack in cases where no other cause can be determined.

Fainting may also result from postural *hypotension*, in which pooling of blood in the veins of the legs reduces the amount available for the heart to pump to the brain, with a resultant drop in blood pressure. This may occur when a person stands still for a long time, or suddenly stands up. Postural hypotension is common in the elderly, in sufferers from *diabetes mellitus*, and in people taking *antihypertensive drugs* or *vasodilator drugs*.

In some people, episodes of fainting may be associated with temporary difficulty in speaking or weakness in the limbs; this may indicate a disorder called *vertebrobasilar insufficiency*, in which there is an obstruction to the blood flow in vessels that pass through the neck to the brain. This is one form of *transient ischaemic attack*.

Fainting may be a symptom of *Stokes-Adams syndrome*, in which blood flow to the brain is temporarily inadequate due to cardiac *arrhythmia* (irregularity of the heartbeat), usually associated with a form of *heart block* (interruption of electrical impulses in the heart).

PREVENTION
A person who experiences warning signs of a faint can sometimes avoid fainting by putting his or her head between the knees or, if possible, by lying flat on his or her back with the legs raised.

TREATMENT
Recovery from fainting takes place when normal blood flow to the brain is restored. This usually happens within a couple of minutes because falling to the ground places the head at the same level as the heart. To ensure another attack does not occur, the person should remain lying down for 10 to 15 minutes after regaining consciousness.

If a person fails to regain consciousness within a minute or two of fainting, medical help should be obtained promptly and appropriate first aid

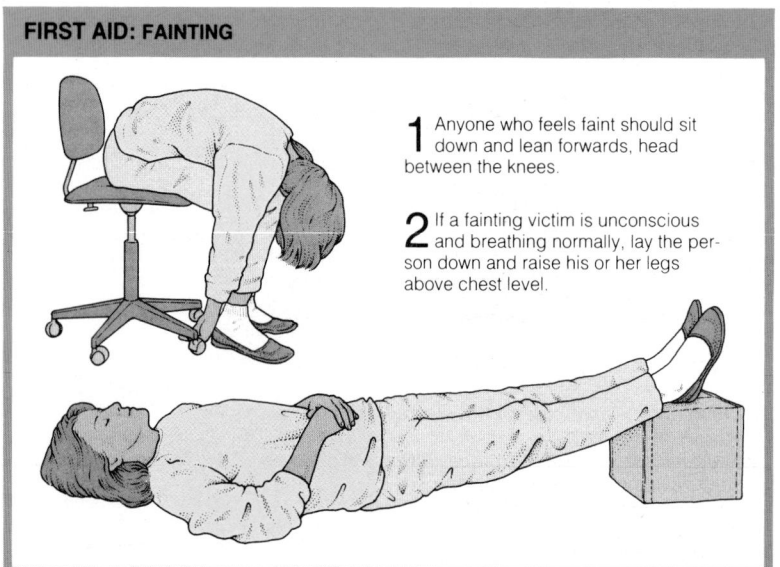

FIRST AID: FAINTING

1 Anyone who feels faint should sit down and lean forwards, head between the knees.

2 If a fainting victim is unconscious and breathing normally, lay the person down and raise his or her legs above chest level.

given (see *Unconsciousness*) until help arrives. Repeated attacks require investigation by a doctor.

Faith-healing

The supposed ability of certain people to cure disease by their possession of a healing force inexplicable to science. The healer usually transmits this supposed force to the sufferer by direct contact, placing his or her hands on the body ("the laying-on of hands"). Often the healer and patient have a deep religious faith and believe the force to be divine. In other cases, no religious faith is involved—only a firm belief in the powers of the healer.

Cures by faith-healing have on occasion been demonstrated to the satisfaction of medical observers. However, people who turn to faith-healing rather than to orthodox medicine may deprive themselves of the possibility of receiving effective treatment for their condition.

Fallen arches

A cause of *flat-feet*, which can develop as a result of weakness of the muscles that support the arches of the foot.

Fallopian tube

The tube that extends from the *uterus* to the *ovary*. The fallopian tube transports eggs and sperm and is where *fertilization* takes place.

STRUCTURE

The funnel-shaped tube is about 7.5 cm long. The narrow end opens into the uterus and the free, expanded end, divided into fimbriae (finger-like projections), lies close to the ovary. Its muscular wall is lined by cells with cilia (hair-like projections).

FUNCTION

The fimbriae sweep up the egg after it is expelled from the ovary. The beating cilia and waves of muscular contractions propel the egg towards the uterus. After intercourse, sperm swim up the fallopian tube from the uterus. The lining of the tube and its secretions sustain the egg and sperm, encouraging fertilization, and nourish the egg until it reaches the uterus.

DISORDERS

Salpingitis is inflammation of the fallopian tube, usually following bacterial infection. It accounts for almost 15 per cent of cases of *infertility*.

Ectopic pregnancy (development of an embryo outside the uterus) most commonly occurs in the fallopian tube. A delay in the passage of the fertilized egg along the tube results in implantation within the tube wall,

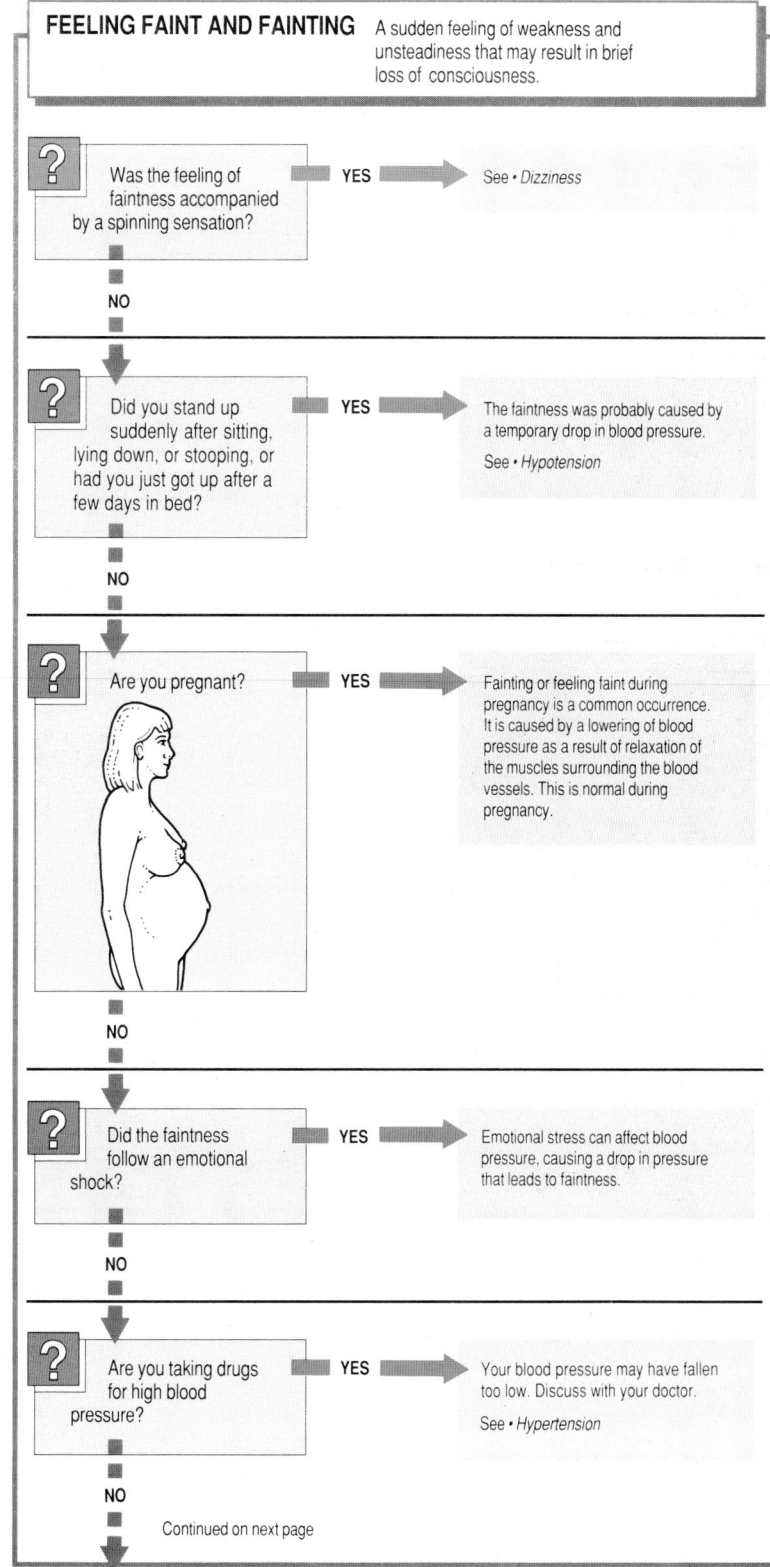

FEELING FAINT AND FAINTING A sudden feeling of weakness and unsteadiness that may result in brief loss of consciousness.

? Was the feeling of faintness accompanied by a spinning sensation?

YES → See • *Dizziness*

NO

? Did you stand up suddenly after sitting, lying down, or stooping, or had you just got up after a few days in bed?

YES → The faintness was probably caused by a temporary drop in blood pressure.
See • *Hypotension*

NO

? Are you pregnant?

YES → Fainting or feeling faint during pregnancy is a common occurrence. It is caused by a lowering of blood pressure as a result of relaxation of the muscles surrounding the blood vessels. This is normal during pregnancy.

NO

? Did the faintness follow an emotional shock?

YES → Emotional stress can affect blood pressure, causing a drop in pressure that leads to faintness.

NO

? Are you taking drugs for high blood pressure?

YES → Your blood pressure may have fallen too low. Discuss with your doctor.
See • *Hypertension*

NO

Continued on next page

F

Are you a diabetic OR has it been an unusually long time since you last ate something?

YES → Low blood sugar is probably causing your faintness. If you are diabetic and have had several such attacks, consult your doctor.

See • *Hypoglycaemia*

NO

Had you spent several hours in strong sunshine or in very hot or stuffy conditions before you felt faint?

YES → You may have heat exhaustion. Lie down and rest in a cool room and drink plenty of fluids.

See • *Heat exhaustion*

NO

Have you noticed one or more of the following symptoms since the attack of faintness?
• numbness and/or tingling in any part of the body
• blurred vision
• confusion
• difficulty speaking
• loss of movement in your arms or legs

YES → Have these symptoms now disappeared?

YES → ☎ **Consult your doctor without delay!**
A temporary decrease in the blood supply to the brain may have caused your symptoms.

See • *Transient ischaemic attack*

NO → ☎ **Consult your doctor without delay!**
A disruption in the blood supply to the brain, caused by a blocked or burst blood vessel, may be the cause of these symptoms.

See • *Stroke*

NO

Are you over 60 years old?

YES → Does turning your head or looking upward suddenly bring on a feeling of faintness?

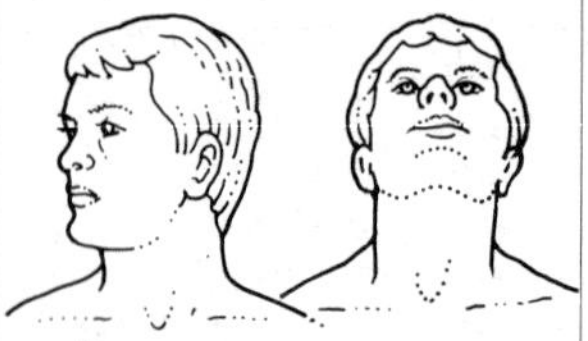

YES → Osteoarthritis of the bones in the neck can cause a feeling of faintness due to pressure on blood vessels passing to the brain. Consult your doctor.

See • *Cervical osteoarthritis*

NO

NO

Continued on next page

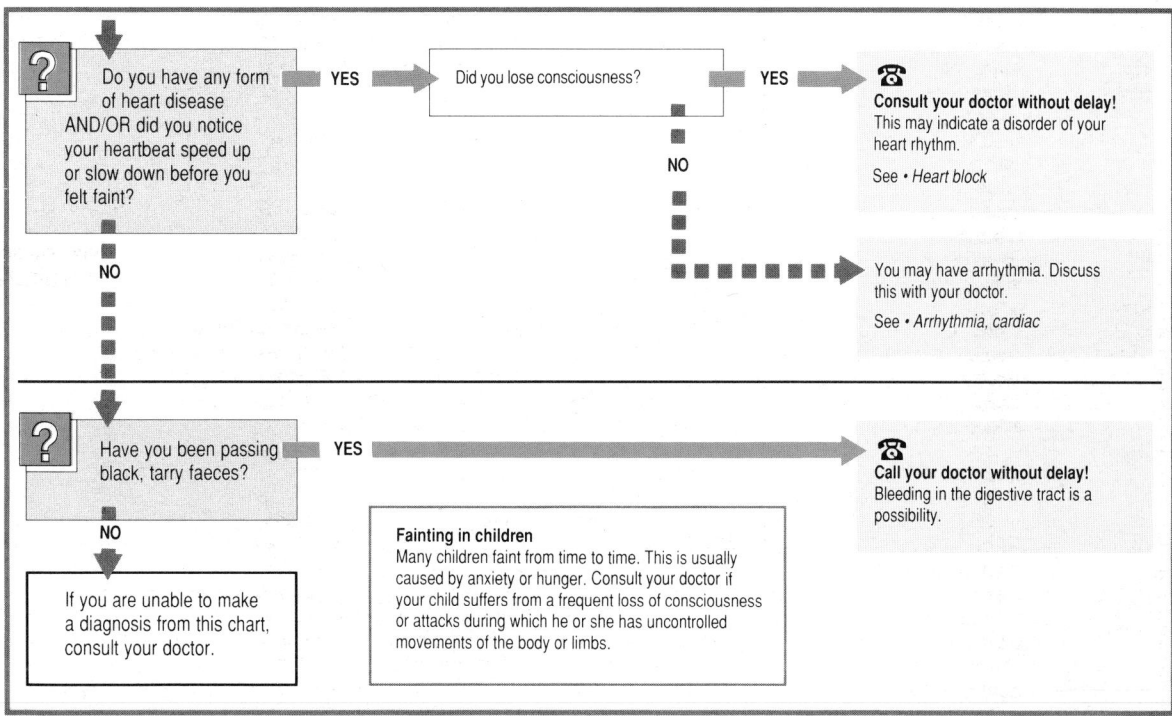

Do you have any form of heart disease AND/OR did you notice your heartbeat speed up or slow down before you felt faint?

YES → **Did you lose consciousness?**

YES → ☎ **Consult your doctor without delay!** This may indicate a disorder of your heart rhythm.

See • *Heart block*

NO → **You may have arrhythmia. Discuss this with your doctor.**

See • *Arrhythmia, cardiac*

NO ↓

Have you been passing black, tarry faeces?

YES → ☎ **Call your doctor without delay!** Bleeding in the digestive tract is a possibility.

NO ↓

If you are unable to make a diagnosis from this chart, consult your doctor.

Fainting in children
Many children faint from time to time. This is usually caused by anxiety or hunger. Consult your doctor if your child suffers from a frequent loss of consciousness or attacks during which he or she has uncontrolled movements of the body or limbs.

---

which is too thin to sustain growth. As the pregnancy progresses, the fallopian tube may rupture and cause internal bleeding.

LOCATION OF THE FALLOPIAN TUBES
Situated in the pelvic cavity, each tube extends from an ovary to the upper part of the uterus.

Uterus
Ovarian ligament
Fallopian tube
Cilia
Fimbriae
Ovary
Broad ligament of uterus

Fallot's tetralogy
See *Tetralogy of Fallot.*

Fallout
See *Radiation hazards.*

Falls in the elderly
The tendency to fall increases steadily with age. Although the majority of falls produce no permanent injury, a significant number of the injuries that do result are ultimately fatal.

CAUSES
Reflex actions in the elderly are much slower than in younger people, and an elderly person who trips or stumbles is often too slow to prevent a fall.

An elderly person may fall either as a result of an accident, commonly caused by a hazard in the home (see illustrated box), or as a result of a medical problem. Medical causes include poor sight, *walking* disorders, cardiac *arrhythmias* (heartbeat irregularities), *hypotension* (reduced blood pressure), *dizziness* for various reasons, *Parkinson's disease*, and the action of various drugs, including *alcohol*, *sleeping drugs*, and *tranquillizer drugs*. Falls sometimes herald the onset of a serious illness, such as *pneumonia*, or *myocardial infarction* (heart attack).

COMPLICATIONS
Broken bones (see *Fracture*) are a common complication of falls in the elderly, especially in women. Not only do women have more falls, they are also more likely to suffer from fractures because their bone strength is reduced as a result of the calcium loss that ordinarily follows the menopause (see *Osteoporosis*).

Falls may sometimes have serious indirect consequences in elderly people. The outlook is particularly grave for those who fall and lie on the floor for more than an hour, particularly if it is cold. This may lead to *hypothermia* (low body temperature) or pneumonia.

A serious fall, or fear of such a fall and the helplessness and dependence it could bring, can have adverse psychological effects on an elderly person, sometimes causing a previously active person to become demoralized and housebound.

ACTION AFTER A FALL
Immediate medical help should be obtained if a person is found unconscious, is in severe pain, is bleeding profusely, is burned, has suspected broken bones, or is showing signs of *shock*. Appropriate first-aid measures should be carried out while awaiting medical help.

PREVENTION
Several simple measures can be taken to guard against falls: ensure that handles in bathrooms and on stairs are

F

PREVENTING FALLS

Half of all falls are accidental, caused by hazards in the home such as poor lighting, worn carpets, rickety handrails, trailing wires, loose rugs and mats, ill-fitting shoes, and inaccessible cupboards. Snow and ice on paths outside are also a major hazard. The illustration shows some of the main hazards in a typical living room, and ways to remedy them.

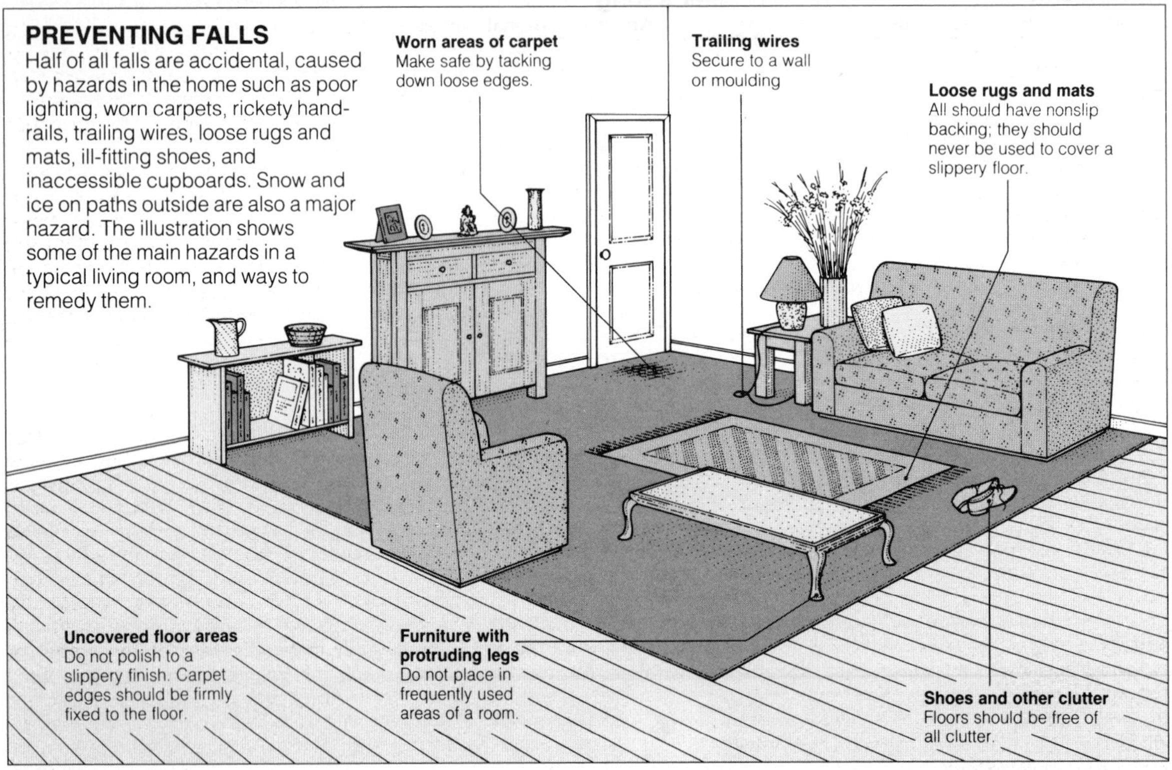

Worn areas of carpet
Make safe by tacking down loose edges.

Trailing wires
Secure to a wall or moulding

Loose rugs and mats
All should have nonslip backing; they should never be used to cover a slippery floor.

Uncovered floor areas
Do not polish to a slippery finish. Carpet edges should be firmly fixed to the floor.

Furniture with protruding legs
Do not place in frequently used areas of a room.

Shoes and other clutter
Floors should be free of all clutter.

secure, good lighting is available, suitable footwear is worn, floor coverings and wiring are safe, and that there is minimal clutter on the floor. Elderly people who live alone can arrange for an alarm system to be installed or for a regular visit by a neighbour. It may also be useful to learn different ways of getting up from the floor.

False teeth
See *Denture*.

Familial
A term applied to a characteristic or disorder that runs in families (that is, it occurs in more members of a particular family than would be expected from the occurrence in the population as a whole). An example of a familial characteristic is male-pattern baldness (see *Alopecia*); an example of a familial disorder is *hyperlipidaemia* (abnormally high levels of fat in the blood).

Familial Mediterranean fever
An inherited condition that affects certain Sephardic Jewish, Armenian, and Arab families. Its cause is unknown. Symptoms usually begin between the ages of five and 15 years. The main symptoms are recurrent episodes of fever, abdominal pain, arthri-

tis, and chest pain. Red skin swellings sometimes occur, and affected people may also suffer psychiatric problems.

Attacks usually last from 24 to 48 hours, but may last longer. Between attacks there are usually no symptoms. There is no specific treatment, but known sufferers are able to reduce the incidence of attacks by taking *colchicine*, a drug usually used to treat gout. Death may eventually occur from *amyloidosis*, which is a complication of the condition.

Family Health Service Authorities
Part of the National Health Service (NHS). Every NHS district has a Family Health Service Authority (FHSA), which is responsible for the administration of the services provided locally by family doctors and by dentists, opticians, and pharmacists.

Complaints may be made to the FHSA about the quality of service provided by family doctors and other health professionals. Conciliation is usually attempted before a formal quasijudicial hearing is arranged.

Family planning
The deliberate limitation or spacing of births. Strategies for family planning

include the different methods of *contraception*, and elective abortion (see *Abortion, induced*).

Decisions concerning family planning are usually made on an individual basis, but some governments have used financial incentives or penalties in an attempt to influence individual decisions. (See also *Birth control*.)

Family therapy
Treatment of the family as a whole rather than treatment of one or more family members on an individual basis. Family therapy is based on the belief that a troubled person should not be seen in isolation from the family unit. The conditions of disturbed children may merely reflect parental conflicts. This approach has become popular in recent years for dealing with the problems of children and adolescents.

Usually the therapist arranges regular meetings with the family in order to find out what feelings lie behind the way parents and children deal with each other. Through discussion and confrontation, these feelings can gradually be changed, leading to greater harmony and understanding.

Famotidine

An *ulcer-healing* drug related to the *antihistamine drugs*. Famatodine reduces the volume of gastric juice and the secretion of acid and pepsin by the stomach. This promotes healing of peptic ulcers and reduces *oesophagitis* (inflammation of the oesophagus).

Famotidine should not be prescibed if there is a possibility of *stomach cancer* or if kidney function is impaired.

Side-effects, which include headaches and dizziness, are uncommon.

Fanconi's anaemia

A rare type of aplastic *anaemia*, characterized by severely reduced production of all types of blood cells by the bone marrow.

Fanconi's syndrome

A rare kidney disorder, occurring mainly in childhood. Various important nutrients and chemicals, such as amino acids, phosphate, calcium, and potassium, are lost in the urine leading to failure to thrive, stunting of growth, and bone disorders such as *rickets*.

Fanconi's syndrome has a wide variety of possible causes, including a number of rare inherited abnormalities of body chemistry; it may also occur as a side-effect of some drugs, such as out-of-date *tetracycline.*

The child may resume normal growth if an underlying chemical abnormality can be corrected. Alternatively, he or she may benefit from a *kidney transplant*. In some cases, neither measure is possible or beneficial and kidney function progressively worsens, leading to death in childhood or early adolescence. The disorder in adults has a much brighter outlook.

Fantasy

The process of imagining events or objects not actually occurring or present. The term also refers to the mental image. Fantasy can give the illusion that wishes have been met. In this sense, it provides satisfaction and can be a means of helping people to cope when reality becomes too unpleasant. Fantasy can also stimulate creative ideas and activities by presenting mental images in new combinations.

Psychoanalysts believe that some fantasies are unconscious and represent certain primitive instincts; these fantasies are always presented to the conscious mind in symbols. For example, the fantasy of returning to the womb might be represented by the image of a cave deep within the earth.

Farmer's lung

 An occupational disease affecting the lungs of farm workers. Farmer's lung is a type of allergic *alveolitis*, in which affected people develop *hypersensitivity* (an excessive allergic reaction) to certain moulds or fungi that grow on hay, grain, or straw. The causative organisms thrive in warm, damp conditions, and outbreaks are most common in areas of high rainfall.

SYMPTOMS

Typical symptoms develop about six hours after exposure to dust containing fungal spores. The symptoms may include shortness of breath and flu-like symptoms of fever, headache, and muscle aches. In single acute attacks, the symptoms persist for about a day. Repeated exposure to the moulds or fungi that provoked the attack may lead to a chronic form of the disease, causing permanent scarring of lung tissues.

DIAGNOSIS AND TREATMENT

The doctor takes a full occupational history and listens through a stethoscope for abnormal sounds in the chest. A *chest X-ray* may show abnormalities; *pulmonary function tests* show that the efficiency of the lungs is reduced. Blood tests for specific *antibodies* indicate exposure to the fungus.

The sufferer should avoid further exposure to mouldy hay or grain; if symptoms persist, *corticosteroid drugs* may be prescribed. Complete recovery can be expected if the disease is diagnosed before permanent lung damage has occurred.

PREVENTION

Farmers can reduce their own and their workers' chances of developing the condition by reducing the water content of hay and grain before storage and by ensuring that storage conditions are cool and dry. Well-ventilated work areas help prevent a build-up of fungal spores in the air; wearing protective masks may help.

Fascia

Fibrous *connective tissue* that surrounds many structures in the body. One layer of the tissue, known as the superficial fascia, envelops the entire body just beneath the skin. Another layer, the deep fascia, encloses muscles, forming a sheath for individual muscles and separating them into groups. The deep fascia also holds in place soft organs, such as the kidneys. Thick fascia in the palm of the hand and sole of the foot have a cushioning, protective function.

Fasciculation

Spontaneous, irregular, and usually continual contractions of a muscle apparently at rest. Unlike the contractions of *fibrillation*, fasciculation is visible under the skin and is described as fine or coarse.

A minor degree of fasciculation is common and is no cause for concern. However, persistent fasciculation with weakness in the affected muscle indicates damage to (or disease of) nerve cells in the spine that control the muscle or nerve fibres that connect the spinal nerves to the muscle; *motor neuron disease* is one such disorder.

Fasciitis

Inflammation of a layer of *fascia* (fibrous connective tissue), causing pain and tenderness. Fasciitis is usually the result of straining or injuring the fascia surrounding a muscle; it most commonly affects the sole of the foot (a condition called plantar fasciitis). Fasciitis may occur in people who suffer from *ankylosing spondylitis* (a rheumatic disorder of the spine) or *Reiter's syndrome* (inflammation of the urethra, conjunctivitis and arthritis).

Treatment consists of resting the affected area and protecting it from pressure (e.g. by wearing cushioned pads in the shoes if the foot is affected). In some cases, injections of *corticosteroid drugs* are given.

Fasciotomy

An operation to relieve pressure on muscles by making an incision in the fascia (fibrous connective tissue) that surrounds them.

WHY IT IS DONE

Fasciotomy is usually performed to treat *compartment syndrome,* a painful condition in which constriction of a group of muscles causes obstruction of blood flow. The condition can result in damage to, or even the death of, affected muscles. Fasciotomy gives the muscles space in which to expand.

The operation is also sometimes performed as a surgical emergency after an injury has caused muscle swelling or bleeding within a muscle compartment.

HOW IT IS DONE

Fasciotomy is performed under a general anaesthetic. An incision is made in the skin over the affected muscle group and then in the underlying fascia to allow the muscles to bulge through. Nonemergency fasciotomy usually requires only a small incision; in an emergency procedure, a much larger incision may be needed.

F

Once the muscles have expanded through the opening, the wound is sewn up. In some cases, the muscles bulge out so much that a *skin graft* is required to repair the incision.

Fasting

Abstaining from all food and drinking only water. In temperate conditions and at moderate levels of physical activity, a person can survive on water alone for more than two months; without food or drink, death usually occurs within about 10 days (survival times are shorter in hot or cold conditions and if activity levels are high).

EFFECTS ON THE BODY

Without food, the energy needed to maintain essential body processes is supplied by substances stored in the body tissues.

About six hours after the last meal, the body starts to use glycogen (a carbohydrate stored in the liver and muscles). This continues for about 24 hours, after which the body adapts to obtaining energy from stored fat and from protein obtained from the breakdown of muscles.

After a few days, most energy is obtained from fat, although some continues to come from muscle breakdown. If fasting continues, the body's *metabolism* slows to conserve energy. As a result of this slowdown, the fat and protein from muscles are consumed more slowly.

In the initial stages of fasting, weight loss is rapid. Later it slows, not only because metabolism slows down, but also because the body starts to conserve its salt supply, which causes water retention. Water that would normally be excreted in the urine is absorbed by the tissues. The accumulated fluid causes oedema (swelling), mainly affecting the legs and abdomen.

In prolonged fasting, the ability to digest food may be impaired or lost entirely because the stomach gradually stops secreting digestive juices. If this occurs, medical supervision may be necessary when eating resumes. Prolonged fasting also halts the production of sex hormones, causing *amenorrhoea* (absence of periods) in women. The body's ability to fight infection deteriorates, and either this or degeneration of the heart muscle may lead to death.

FASTING TO REDUCE WEIGHT

Omitting a main meal each day for a limited period, or occasionally not eating anything for up to 24 hours, may be an effective means of losing weight. However, nobody should go without food for more than 24 hours without consulting a doctor. (See also *Weight reduction*.)

Fatigue

See *Tiredness*.

Fats and oils

Nutrients that provide the body with its most concentrated form of *energy*; 1 g of fat provides 9 kcal (37.8 kJ), whereas 1 g of carbohydrate produces only 4 kcal (16.8 kJ).

Fats, also called lipids, are compounds containing chains of carbon and hydrogen with very little oxygen. Chemically, fats consist mostly of *fatty acids* combined with *glycerol*. They are divided into two main groups, saturated and unsaturated, depending on the proportion of hydrogen atoms. If the fatty acids contain the maximum quantity possible of hydrogen, they are said to be saturated. If there are some sites on the carbon chain unoccupied by hydrogen, they are unsaturated; when many sites are vacant, they are polyunsaturated. Monounsaturated fats are unsaturated fats with one double bond. Animal fats, such as those found in meat and dairy products, are largely saturated, while vegetable fats tend to be unsaturated to varying degrees.

Fats and oils differ in their consistency: fats are usually solid at room temperature but liquefy when heated; oils are usually liquid at ordinary room temperature.

TYPES

Some dietary fats are sources of the fat-soluble vitamins A, D, E, and K and of essential fatty acids. They are mainly triglycerides (combinations of glycerol and three fatty acids) but also comprise other types of fats. Sources in the diet include not only the visible fats (such as butter, margarine, and vegetable oils) but also the so-called invisible fats found in meat, fish, poultry, and dairy products. The oils of certain cold-water ocean fish may protect against *coronary artery disease*.

Structural fats include triglycerides, phospholipids, and sterols. Triglycerides are the main form of fat found in stores of body fat (adipose tissue). These stores act as an energy reserve as well as providing insulation and a protective layer for delicate organs. Phospholipids are structural fats found in cell membranes. Sterols, such as *cholesterol*, are found in animal and plant tissues; they have a variety of functions within the body, often being converted by chemical actions into hormones or vitamins. Phospholipids and sterols are made in the body from the diet and are not themselves essential in the diet.

FAT METABOLISM

Dietary fats are first emulsified by the action of bile salts and then broken down into fatty acids and glycerol by lipase, a pancreatic enzyme. They are absorbed via the lymphatic system before entering the bloodstream.

The lipids are carried in the blood bound to a protein, when they become known as lipoproteins. There are four classes of lipoprotein—chylomicrons, very low-density lipoproteins (VLDLs), high-density lipoproteins (HDLs), and low-density lipoproteins (LDLs). LDLs and VLDLs contain large amounts of cholesterol, which they carry through the bloodstream and deposit in cells. The HDLs pick up cholesterol and carry it back to the liver for processing and excretion. (See also *Nutrition*.)

Fatty acids

Organic acids, containing carbon, hydrogen, and oxygen, that are constituents of *fats and oils*. There are more than 40 different fatty acids found in nature, distinguished by their constituent number of carbon and hydrogen atoms.

Certain fatty acids cannot be synthesized by the body and must be provided by the diet. These fatty acids are linoleic, linolenic, and arachidonic acids, sometimes referred to collectively as the essential fatty acids and at one time called vitamin F. Strictly speaking, only linoleic acid is essential, since the body can make the other two from linoleic acid obtained from food. (See also *Nutrition*.)

Favism

A disorder characterized by an extreme sensitivity to the broad bean *VICIA FABA* (fava). If an affected person eats these beans, a chemical in the bean causes rapid destruction of his or her red blood cells, leading to a severe type of anaemia (see *Anaemia, haemolytic*).

Favism is uncommon except in some areas of the Mediterranean, especially lowland Greece, where up to 10 per cent of the population is affected. Favism is an inherited condition caused by a sex-linked *genetic disorder*. Affected people have a defect in a chemical pathway within their red blood cells that helps to protect the cells from injury. This defect is called *G6PD deficiency* (glucose-6-phosphate dehydrogenase deficiency).

Children in any family with a history of favism should be screened for the condition at an early age. If the disorder is found, they must avoid broad beans and certain drugs (including some *antimalarial drugs* and *antibiotic drugs*) that can have a similar destructive effect on their red blood cells. A list of drugs to avoid can be obtained from a doctor when the disorder is diagnosed. With these precautions, affected people are able to remain in good health.

Febrile

Feverish or related to *fever*, as in febrile *convulsions* which occur mainly in young children who have high temperatures.

Feeding, artificial

Administration of nutrients other than by mouth, usually through a tube inserted into the stomach or small intestine. Occasionally, a tube is inserted directly into the stomach or jejunum (upper part of the small intestine) by surgical means. This is called enteral nutrition. If the gastrointestinal tract is not functioning, food must be introduced into the bloodstream by *intravenous infusion*. This technique is known as total parenteral nutrition.

WHY IT IS DONE

Tube feeding may be necessary for people who have gastrointestinal disorders (such as those resulting in *malabsorption*) or disorders affecting the nervous system or kidneys. Premature babies often require tube feeding if their sucking reflexes are undeveloped, as do burn or fever patients because of their increased nutritional requirements.

Intravenous feeding is usually necessary when large areas of the absorbing surface of the small intestine have been damaged by disease or have been surgically removed.

HOW IT IS DONE

TUBE FEEDING Suitable food mixtures or preparations of predetermined levels of nutrients are administered via a narrow plastic tube. The tube is passed through the patient's nose (guided via the nasopharynx to the oesophagus) and into either the stomach or the duodenum.

If tube feeding is the sole means of nutrition, it must provide all of the essential nutrients (and adequate fluids) to meet the person's daily needs, which can vary markedly.

There are two alternative methods of tube feeding—continuous drip feeding and bolus feeding. Continuous drip feeding is generally preferred because it is tolerated better by patients. Bolus feeding allows rapid administration of a set amount of nutrients at intermittent periods throughout the day. In both methods the rate of flow can be controlled by a pump.

The tube is usually left in place for adults and older children, but for infants and young children it may be removed and later reinserted for each feeding.

INTRAVENOUS FEEDING This method is generally used only when tube feeding is impractical or ineffective; its main drawback is the risk of introducing infection directly into the bloodstream or of blocking a blood vessel. In some cases, there may be problems affecting the liver or gallbladder.

Nutrient preparations are given into an arm vein or directly into a large central vein near the heart via a *catheter* (thin, flexible tube) inserted under local anaesthetic and strict *aseptic technique*. Intravenous feeding is sometimes used to supplement feeding by mouth, but can if necessary provide all the nutrients needed to meet a patient's requirements.

Feeding, infant

A baby grows more rapidly in its first year than at any future time in its life. A good diet is essential for healthy growth and development.

BREAST- OR BOTTLE-FEEDING

NUTRITIONAL REQUIREMENTS During the first four to six months, most babies' nutritional requirements are met by milk alone, whether by *breast-feeding* or *bottle-feeding*. Both human milk and artificial milk (cow's milk modified to resemble human milk) contain carbohydrate, protein, fat, vitamins, and minerals in similar proportions (see *Milk* for components), but human milk is the food of choice because it provides these nutrients in the perfect blend as well as containing *antibodies* and white blood cells that protect the baby against infections.

After the baby is six weeks old, supplementary *vitamin D* should be given to breast-fed babies; multivitamin drops containing vitamins A and C in addition to vitamin D are usually given. Most bottle-fed babies do not need extra vitamins because modified dried cow's milk preparations are supplemented with vitamins. Additional vitamins should, however, be given

to bottle-fed babies who are at risk of *rickets* (e.g. Asian babies in northern climates).

At six months a baby can be safely taken off artificial milk and fed with unchanged cow's milk. Supplementary vitamins should then be given until the baby is established on a mixed diet.

If a baby seems unable to tolerate milk of any kind (see *Food allergy; Food intolerance*), a doctor should be consulted; he or she may recommend a preparation based on soya beans, vegetable oils, glucose, sucrose, corn syrup, modified meat protein, and other substances. Babies should not be fed skimmed milk, or semi-skimmed milk, which has relatively too much protein and minerals and insufficient calories compared with whole milk.

EMOTIONAL REQUIREMENTS For healthy emotional development, a baby requires warmth, security, and contentment; the act of feeding plays an important part in meeting these needs. Breast-feeding is again preferable in this respect because it establishes an intimate bond between mother and child, but bottle-feeding is a perfectly satisfactory alternative if the baby is cuddled and talked to while he or she is fed.

INTRODUCING SOLIDS

Solid foods, initially in the form of purees and cereals, should be introduced into an infant's diet at some time between the ages of three and six months, depending on the baby's birth weight and rate of growth. By six months the baby should be eating some true solids, such as chopped up meat and vegetables. The accompanying chart (overleaf) gives the optimum times for the introduction of solids, but a baby's general contentment also provides some guide. A rapidly growing baby who is unable to drink enough milk to satisfy his or her hunger should be given the more concentrated calories of solid food.

Many parents prefer to give their infants home-prepared purees rather than prepared foods. In this case, there are important things to remember: salt and other additives should not be used, since too much salt and other minerals can dangerously overburden a baby's kidneys. Sugar, too, should be kept to a minimum in the diet; a baby easily learns to have a "sweet tooth", which will lead to future dental decay; for the same reason, babies should not be given bottles of sweetened drinks.

A baby can live healthily on a vegetarian diet (one that contains no meat or fish) provided eggs are included, but a baby fed on a vegan diet (one that also excludes dairy produce and eggs as well as all other animal products) is at risk of severe malnutrition. A vegan diet makes it very hard to obtain enough calories, calcium, essential fatty acids, vitamins (especially the fat-soluble vitamins A, D, E, and K, and vitamin B_{12}), and protein. Overall, it is a very bad diet for infants and growing children whose nutrient requirements are relatively much greater than adults'.

FEEDING PROBLEMS

Any difficulties associated with milk usually appear within the first month.

Some babies have an intolerance to certain foods; reactions can include vomiting, diarrhoea, or allergic rashes. For this reason, solids should be introduced one by one so that any that cause problems can be identified.

Prolonged crying after feeds may mean that the baby needs help bringing up wind, that artificial milk is not being digested properly, or that the baby has colic (see *Colic, infantile*). (See also *Nutritional disorders*.)

Femoral epiphysis, slipped

Displacement of the upper *epiphysis* (growing end) of the *femur* (thigh bone). Such displacement is rare, usually affects those between the ages of 11 and 13, and occurs more often in boys, in obese children with delayed sexual and physical development, and in children who grow rapidly.

While the bone is still growing, the epiphysis is separated from the shaft of the bone by a plate of cartilage. This constitutes a zone of relative weakness in the bone, so that a fall or other injury, even a minor one, can cause the epiphysis to slip out of position.

SYMPTOMS

A limp develops and the child feels pain in the knee rather than in the hip. The leg tends to turn outwards and hip movements are restricted.

TREATMENT

An operation is performed under general anaesthesia to manipulate the displaced parts of bone back into position and fix them together with metal pins. To prevent possible damage to the other thigh, it, too, may be strengthened with pins during the same operation.

OUTLOOK

Surgery usually provides an effective repair and prevents further accidents of the same type. However, after the

injury, the hip tends to be more susceptible than normal to *osteoarthritis*. In rare cases, the hip becomes stiff and painful.

Femoral nerve

One of the main nerves of the leg. The femoral nerve is made up of fibres from nerves in the second, third, and fourth segments of the lumbar spinal cord. The nerves emerge from the lower back region of the spine and run down into the thigh, where they branch to supply the skin and muscles of the front of the thigh. The nerve branches that supply the skin convey sensation; the branches that supply the muscles stimulate contraction of the *quadriceps muscle* of the thigh, causing the knee to straighten.

Damage to the femoral nerve (which impairs the ability of the knee to straighten) is usually caused by a

slipped disc in the lumbar region of the spine (see *Disc prolapse*). Damage may also occur as the result of a backward dislocation of the hip or, rarely, as a result of a *neuropathy*.

Femur

The medical name for the thigh-bone, the longest bone in the body. The lower end hinges with the tibia (shin) to form the knee joint. The upper end is rounded into a ball (head of the femur) that fits into a socket in the pelvis to form the hip joint. The head of the femur is joined to the bone shaft by a narrow piece of bone called the neck of the femur. The neck of the femur is a point of structural weakness and a common fracture site (see *Femur, fracture of*).

The femur can be felt through the skin at two sites. At the lower end, the bone is enlarged to form two lumps

APPROXIMATE AGES FOR INTRODUCING SOLIDS		
4 months	At second breast- or bottle-feed offer one or two teaspoons of	vegetable or fruit puree or cereal.
4½ months	At second breast- or bottle-feed offer two teaspoons of cereal. At third breast- or bottle-feed offer	two teaspoons of vegetable or fruit puree.
5 to 6 months	*Early morning* Breast- or bottle-feed. *Breakfast* Two teaspoons of cereal and mashed hard-boiled egg yolk, followed by breast- or bottle-feed. *Lunch* One teaspoon of meat or fish puree with three teaspoons of	strained vegetables. Offer water or well-diluted fruit juice instead of milk. *Mid-afternoon* Mashed banana or other soft fruit followed by usual milk feed. *Dinner* Breast- or bottle-feed if the baby is still hungry.
6 to 7 months	*Early morning* Breast- or bottle-feed. *Breakfast* Two teaspoons of cereal with well-cooked scrambled egg. Offer cow's milk from a cup. *Lunch* Offer minced or mashed	food instead of pureed. Give meat or fish with some vegetables, then offer yogurt and fruit. Give a drink of water or well-diluted fruit juice. *Late afternoon/dinner* Meat or cheese sandwich. A drink of cow's milk.
7 to 8 months	*Early morning* Offer a drink of water or well-diluted fruit juice instead of milk. *Breakfast* Cereal and hard-boiled egg with wholemeal bread and butter. A drink of cow's milk.	*Lunch* Cheese, fish, or minced meat with mashed vegetables. Pudding or fresh fruit. A drink of water or well-diluted fruit juice. *Late afternoon/dinner* Meat or cheese sandwich. A drink of cow's milk.
9 to 12 months	*Early morning* A drink of water or well-diluted fruit juice. *Breakfast* Cereal, then well-cooked egg or fish with wholemeal toast and butter. A drink of cow's milk.	*Lunch* Chopped meat or fish, or cheese, with vegetables. Pudding or fresh fruit. A drink of water or well-diluted fruit juice. *Late afternoon/dinner* Meat or cheese sandwiches. A drink of cow's milk.

(the condyles) that distribute the weight-bearing load on the knee joint. On the outer side of the upper end of the femur is a protuberance called the greater trochanter.

The shaft of the femur is surrounded by powerful muscles whose principal functions are to move the hip and knee joints. The shaft is also well supplied with blood vessels; because of this, a fracture can result in considerable blood loss.

LOCATION OF THE FEMUR
The femur extends from the hip joint, down the thigh, to the knee joint.

- Greater trochanter
- Neck of femur
- Femur
- Condyles
- Tibia

Femur, fracture of

The symptoms, treatment, and possible complications of a fracture of the femur (thigh-bone) depend on whether the bone has broken across its neck (the short section between the top of the shaft and the hip joint) or across the shaft.

FRACTURE OF NECK OF FEMUR
This type of fracture, often called a broken hip, is very common in elderly people, especially in women suffering from *osteoporosis* (thinning of the bone) and is usually associated with a fall. The incidence of this type of fracture doubles approximately every seven years after the age of 65, so that by the age of 90 one woman in four has suffered this type of fracture.

In a fracture of the neck of the femur, the broken bone ends are often considerably displaced; in such cases there is usually severe pain in the hip and groin (made worse by movement)

and the leg cannot bear any weight. Occasionally, the broken ends of bone become impacted (wedged together). In this case there is less pain and walking is often still possible, which may delay reporting of the injury and detection of the fracture.

DIAGNOSIS AND TREATMENT Diagnosis of a suspected fracture is confirmed by X-ray. If the bone ends are displaced, an operation under general anaesthesia is necessary, either to realign the bone ends (a procedure called reduction) and to fasten them together with metal screws, plates, or nails, or to replace the entire head and neck of the femur with a metal or plastic substitute (see *Hip replacement*). Both procedures produce a stable repair, and hip and knee movement can be resumed immediately.

If the bone ends are impacted, the person is kept in bed for a few weeks to prevent any jarring movement that might dislodge the bones. The fracture heals naturally without surgery, but supervised exercise is necessary to maintain hip and knee mobility. X-rays are taken periodically to determine how well the fracture is healing.

With either type of repair, walking is started with the aid of crutches, progresses to walking with a walking frame, walking with a stick, and, finally, without aid.

COMPLICATIONS These depend on the site of the fracture. A break at the union of the neck and shaft may result in hip deformity (see *Coxa vara*). A fracture across the neck itself may damage the blood supply to the head of the femur, causing the head to crumble (a condition called avascular necrosis). As a result, the bone ends may fail to fuse, or *osteoarthritis* may develop in the joint. In either case, more surgery (usually hip replacement) is required. Osteoarthritis may also develop even if avascular necrosis does not occur.

FRACTURE OF SHAFT OF FEMUR
This type of fracture usually occurs when the femur is subjected to extreme force, such as in a road traffic accident. In most cases, the bone ends are considerably displaced, causing severe pain, tenderness, and swelling.

DIAGNOSIS AND TREATMENT Diagnosis of this injury is confirmed by X-ray. With a fractured femoral shaft there is often substantial blood loss from the bone. In most cases, the fracture is repaired by an operation (under general anaesthesia) in which the two ends of the bone are realigned and

fastened together with a long metal pin. However, sometimes the bone ends can be realigned by manipulation, and surgery is not necessary. After realignment of the bones, the leg is supported with a *splint* and put in *traction* to hold the bone together correctly while it heals.

Following both types of treatment, supervised exercise and massage of the knee, ankle, and foot is started to prevent the joints from becoming stiff. The progress of healing is checked regularly by X-rays; when it is complete, weight bearing and walking is started gradually.

COMPLICATIONS These include failure of the bone ends to unite or successful fusion of the broken ends at the wrong angle, infection of the bone, or damage to a nerve or artery. All of these complications usually require more surgery. A fracture of the lower end of the shaft can result in permanent stiffness of the knee.

Fenbufen

A *nonsteroidal anti-inflammatory drug* (NSAID). Fenbufen is used to relieve pain and stiffness caused, for example, by *rheumatoid arthritis*, *osteoarthritis* and *gout*. Fenbufen is also used to reduce pain and help speed recovery following muscle and ligament sprains.

This drug is said to be less likely to cause bleeding in the stomach than some other NSAIDs but to be more likely to cause a rash.

Fenoprofen

A *nonsteroidal anti-inflammatory drug* (NSAID). Fenoprofen is used to relieve pain and stiffness caused, for example, by *rheumatoid arthritis*, *osteoarthritis*, and *gout*. Fenoprofen is also used in the treatment of muscle and ligament sprains; it reduces pain and helps speed recovery. In common with all NSAIDs, fenoprofen may have side-effects, especially irritation of the stomach.

Ferrous sulphate

Iron sulphate (see *Iron*).

Fertility

The ability to produce children without undue difficulty.

MALE FERTILITY
A man's fertility depends on the production of normal quantities of healthy *sperm* in the testes, and on the ability to achieve *erection* and to ejaculate *semen* into the vagina during *sexual intercourse*.

F

The *testes*—under the influence of *gonadotrophin hormones* from the pituitary gland—produce hundreds of millions of sperm. The large output is necessary for normal fertility because only about one in 80,000 sperm ejaculated into the vagina reaches a fallopian tube (see *Fertilization*).

Normal fertility also requires a large proportion of the sperm to be healthy. After ejaculation, the sperm must be able to pass through the hostile environment of acid secretions in the vagina, to penetrate a barrier of mucus around the cervix, and to swim into the fallopian tubes.

Men become fertile at puberty and usually remain so (although to a lesser degree) well into old age.

FEMALE FERTILITY

The ability of a woman to conceive depends on normal *ovulation* (the monthly production of a healthy *ovum* by one of the *ovaries*) and the ovum's unimpeded passage down a fallopian tube towards the uterus; on thinning of the mucus surrounding the mouth of the cervix to enable sperm to penetrate more easily; and on changes in the lining of the uterus that prepare it for the implantation of a fertilized ovum. These processes are in turn dependent on normal production of gonadotrophins by the pituitary gland, and on production of the sex hormones *oestrogen* and *progesterone* by the ovaries.

Women become fertile at puberty and remain so until the *menopause*, which usually occurs during a woman's 40s or 50s. (See also *Fertility drugs*; *Infertility*.)

Fertility drugs

A diverse group of hormonal or hormone-related drugs used in certain circumstances to treat some cases of female and male *infertility*.

In women, fertility drugs may be prescribed when abnormal hormone production by the pituitary gland or ovaries disrupts *ovulation* or causes mucus around the cervix to become so thick that sperm cannot penetrate it.

In men, fertility drugs are less effective, but may be used when abnormal hormone production by the pituitary gland or the testes interferes with normal sperm production. (See also *Clomiphene*; *Gonadotrophin hormones*; *Infertility*; *Testosterone*.)

Fertilization

The union of a *sperm* and an *ovum* (egg). In natural fertilization (see illustrated box), the sperm and ovum unite

after *sexual intercourse*. Fertilization may also occur as a result of semen being artificially introduced into the cervix (see *Artificial insemination*), or may take place in the laboratory (see *In vitro fertilization*).

Fetal alcohol syndrome

A combination of *congenital* defects resulting from high *alcohol* consumption by the mother during *pregnancy*.

Even small amounts of alcohol may be harmful in pregnancy, because (like *tobacco-smoking*) alcohol seems to affect fetal growth. The risks of *miscarriage* and *birth defects* may also be increased. Fetal alcohol syndrome, however, is a rare condition, which occurs only if there is persistent alcohol consumption during pregnancy. It has been reported in approximately one third of infants born to mothers with chronic *alcohol dependence* who go on drinking throughout pregnancy. It may occur in babies of women who consistently drink the equivalent of as little as 30 millilitres of pure alcohol (the equivalent of two mixed drinks or two to three bottles of beer or glasses of wine) per day. While there is no evidence that an occasional glass of wine or beer is dangerous, the accepted medical advice is that women should abstain completely from alcohol during early pregnancy.

The affected baby has diminished growth, delayed mental development, a small head, a small brain, and small eyes with short eye slits. He or she may have a cleft palate, a small jaw, heart defects, and joint abnormalities. As a newborn, the baby sucks poorly, sleeps badly, and is irritable. In effect, he or she is suffering from alcohol withdrawal.

Almost one fifth of affected babies die during the first few weeks of life; many who survive are physically and mentally handicapped to some degree.

Fetal circulation

Blood circulation in the fetus is different from the normal circulation after birth (see *Circulatory system*). The fetus neither breathes nor eats, so oxygen and nutrients are obtained—via the *placenta* and *umbilical cord*—from the mother's blood. The other fundamental difference in circulation is that blood bypasses the lungs in the fetus.

Oxygen and nutrients enter the fetal blood in the placenta, an organ embedded in the inner lining and wall of the uterus and connected to the fetus by the umbilical cord. The oxygenated blood flows to the fetus

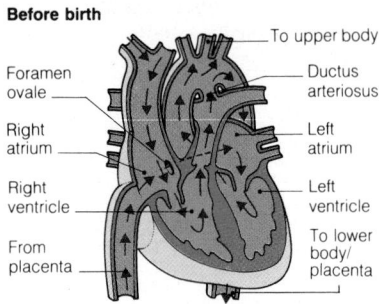

Before birth

Foramen ovale

Right atrium

Right ventricle

From placenta

To upper body

Ductus arteriosus

Left atrium

Left ventricle

To lower body/placenta

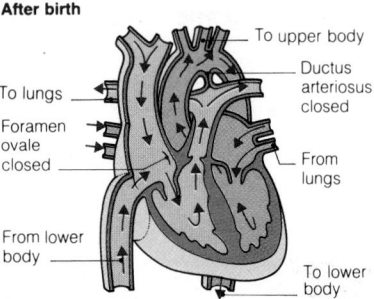

After birth

To lungs

Foramen ovale closed

From lower body

To upper body

Ductus arteriosus closed

From lungs

To lower body

Fetal heart circulation
In the fetus, blood passes from the right atrium of the heart to the left atrium through the foramen ovale. Another channel, the ductus arteriosus, allows blood to pass from the pulmonary artery to the aorta. Both channels close after birth.

along a vein in the umbilical cord, then enters the right atrium (right upper chamber) of the heart, after which, instead of flowing to the lungs, it bypasses them. It does this by flowing into the left atrium through a hole called the foramen ovale.

The blood then passes to the left ventricle (left lower chamber), from where it is pumped to the upper parts of the body to provide the tissues with oxygen. It then returns to the heart, flowing into the right atrium and from there into the right ventricle. (After birth, blood pumped from this ventricle passes via the pulmonary artery to the lungs for reoxygenation and elimination of carbon dioxide and other wastes.) However, in the fetus, the blood is only partly deoxygenated at this stage and has more tissues to supply with oxygen. Bypassing the lungs again, it flows from the pulmonary artery into the aorta; it does this through a channel called the ductus arteriosus which, like the foramen ovale, closes after birth.

The aorta carries the blood to the lower parts of the body, from where, completely deoxygenated, it is carried by two arteries in the umbilical cord to the placenta. There, carbon dioxide

F

THE PROCESS OF FERTILIZATION

Fertilization occurs when the head of a sperm penetrates a mature ovum in a fallopian tube. After penetration, the nuclei (which contain the genetic material) of the sperm and ovum fuse, and the body and tail of the sperm drop off. The newly fertilized ovum, called a zygote, then forms an outer layer that is impenetrable to other sperm. The zygote undergoes repeated cell divisions as it passes down the fallopian tube, so that, by the time it reaches the uterus, it has grown into a solid ball of cells called a morula. It then develops an inner cavity with a small cluster of cells to one side; this is called a blastocyst.

FERTILE PERIOD

Ovulation occurs about halfway through the menstrual cycle (14 to 16 days before the start of a period), after which the released ovum is available for fertilization for about two days. Sperm can also live for approximately two days, so the peak fertile period is about four days.

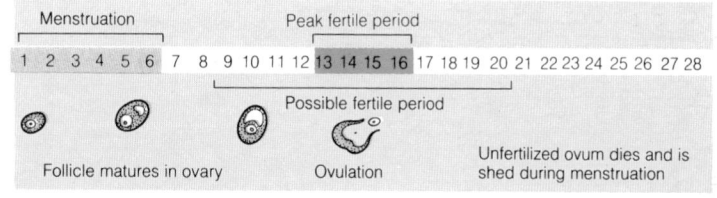

Follicle matures in ovary — Ovulation — Unfertilized ovum dies and is shed during menstruation

Peak and possible fertile periods

Although the peak fertile period is about four days, the possible fertile period may last seven to 12 days, due to variations in how long the ovum and sperm can survive and the timing of ovulation. The illustration shows the peak and maximum possible fertile periods in a 28-day cycle.

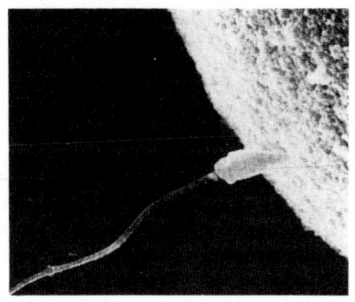

Sperm and ovum
A single sperm penetrates the ovum, thereby fertilizing it. To achieve this, the sperm releases enzymes that dissolve a path through the ovum's outer layers.

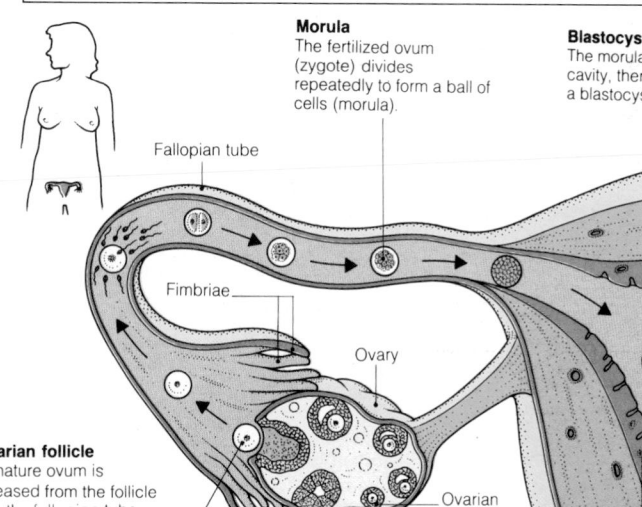

Morula
The fertilized ovum (zygote) divides repeatedly to form a ball of cells (morula).

Blastocyst
The morula develops a cavity, thereby becoming a blastocyst.

Fallopian tube

Fimbriae

Ovary

Ovarian follicle
A mature ovum is released from the follicle into the fallopian tube

Ovarian follicle

Uterus

JOURNEY OF THE SPERM

When semen is ejaculated into the vagina, as many as 500 million sperm are released, most of which are capable of fertilizing an ovum. But, as they travel upwards (propelled by their whip-like tails), more than half are killed by acidic vaginal secretions; many more die during the journey up through the cervix and uterus and into the fallopian tubes. The journey can take from one to five hours, and, in the end, only a few thousand sperm have survived.

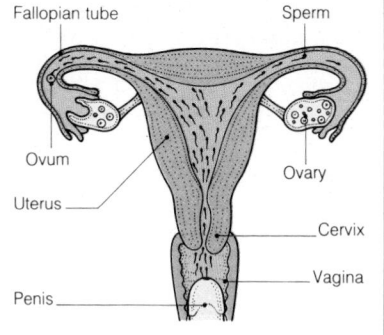

Fallopian tube — Sperm

Ovum

Uterus

Ovary

Cervix

Vagina

Penis

Lifespan of sperm
A sperm can live in a fallopian tube for up to 48 hours, during which time it is capable of fertilizing an ovum.

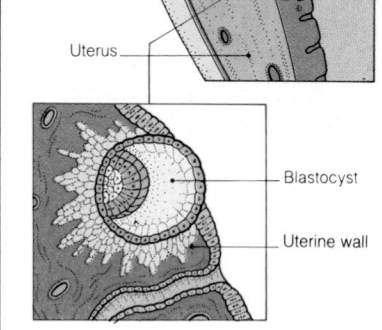

Blastocyst

Uterine wall

Blastocyst
The blastocyst embeds in the uterine wall (implantation), where it develops into an embryo and also forms the placenta.

F

and other waste products diffuse into, and are carried away by, the mother's blood and are excreted by the mother.

In rare cases, the foramen ovale or ductus arteriosus fails to close after birth, causing a congenital heart disorder (see *Heart disease, congenital*).

Fetal distress

Physical stress experienced by a fetus during labour as a result of not receiving enough oxygen. The most stressful period of labour for a baby is during a contraction, when the uterus tightens and thus reduces the baby's supply of oxygen from the placenta. If, in addition, there are problems with the labour, such as the mother's losing blood or having a pelvis too small for the size of the baby's head, the amount of oxygen reaching the baby may be inadequate.

MONITORING
Fetal distress causes the baby's heart-rate to slow, which shows as a dip on a cardiotocograph (see *Fetal heart monitoring*). Alternatively, a distressed baby may show no variability in heart-rate. This is in contrast to a healthy baby, whose heart-rate varies within a normal range of from 120 to 160 beats per minute. The obstetrician and midwife keep a close watch on the heart-rate and, if necessary, may obtain a blood sample from the baby's scalp for analysis. *Acidosis* (high acidity) indicates that the baby is not getting enough oxygen. The amniotic fluid around the baby is examined for signs of *meconium* because passing of these fetal faeces can be an indication of fetal distress.

DELIVERY
Fetal distress sometimes occurs as a temporary episode, but if acidosis is severe, the distressed fetus may need to be delivered promptly—by *caesarean section* if oxygen shortage occurs during the first stage of labour, and by *forceps delivery* or *vacuum extraction* during the second stage. (See also *Childbirth*.)

Fetal heart monitoring

Use of an instrument to record and/or listen to an unborn baby's heartbeat during pregnancy and labour. Some form of monitoring of fetal well-being is performed during labour in all hospitals.

WHY IT IS DONE
In pregnancy, monitoring is carried out at intervals if tests indicate that the placenta is not functioning normally or if the baby's growth has been slow. Uterine contractions or other stimuli,

such as reflex kicking, increase the heart-rate in a healthy fetus; the midwife or obstetrician can detect this using a fetal heart monitor.

During labour, monitoring can detect *fetal distress*, caused by the baby's not receiving enough oxygen. A fetus deprived of oxygen usually has an abnormal heart-rate. Fetal monitoring can detect this abnormality and allows the obstetrician to take appropriate action, which may include emergency delivery procedures.

HOW IT IS DONE
In the simplest form of fetal heart monitoring, the midwife or obstetrician uses a special fetal stethoscope to listen to the baby's heartbeat.

In a more sophisticated version, known as cardiotocography, an electronic fetal heart-rate monitor is used to make a continuous paper or sound recording of the heartbeat together with a recording of uterine contractions. The heartbeat is picked up either externally by an *ultrasound* transmitter strapped to the mother's abdomen or, as an alternative during labour, internally by an electrode attached to the baby's head and linked to the recording device by a wire inserted through the mother's vagina. The fetal heartbeat is amplified and heard as a beeping noise or printed as a paper trace. The mother's uterine contractions are measured and recorded either by an external pressure gauge strapped to the mother's abdomen or by an internal plastic tube that is inserted through the vagina into the amniotic fluid.

ADVANTAGES AND DISADVANTAGES
Electronic fetal monitoring has the advantage of giving the doctor a minute-by-minute assessment of the baby's condition. Many obstetricians are convinced that babies are less likely to become hypoxic (deprived of oxygen) during labour with continuous monitoring and that monitoring therefore results in the bringing to birth of healthier babies.

However, routine electronic fetal monitoring has been controversial for a number of reasons. Critics have claimed that it limits maternal mobility during labour and that it leads to overdiagnosis of fetal distress and therefore to unnecessary caesarean sections. Critics also claim that external monitoring unnecessarily exposes healthy babies to ultrasound and that internal monitoring may increase the risk of infection during labour without resulting in improvement in the outcome of low-risk pregnancies.

Fetishism

Reliance on special objects in order to achieve sexual arousal. Fetishism is thought to be rare and restricted to men; because of the nature of the practice, there are no reliable statistics.

The objects need not have an obvious sexual meaning; they include shoes, gloves, rubber or leather garments, and parts of the body such as the feet or ears. It seems that once a particular fetish has led to successful orgasm, it becomes increasingly difficult to obtain sexual satisfaction without it. Nevertheless, many fetishists are able to have a stable sexual relationship, provided their partners join in the practice.

CAUSES
Fetishism usually has no obvious cause, although it may, rarely, result from certain forms of brain damage. According to psychoanalysts, the origin may be a childhood *fixation* of sexual interest upon some aspect of the mother's body or appearance.

TREATMENT
As long as fetishism does not impair sexual or social life, there is no reason for any form of medical interference. Treatment is needed only if the behaviour is causing distress or if there are persistent criminal acts, such as stealing underwear.

Fetoscopy

A procedure for directly observing a fetus inside the uterus by means of a fetoscope, a type of *endoscope* (viewing instrument). The fetoscope can also be used to take samples of fetal blood and tissue for analysis and to permit treatment of some fetal disorders.

WHY IT IS DONE
Fetoscopy is used to diagnose various *congenital* abnormalities and *genetic disorders* before the baby is born. Because the technique carries some risks, it is performed only if there is a greater-than-normal chance that the baby will have some abnormality (for example, if the mother has already had an abnormal baby or if there is an established family history of genetic disorders).

Fetoscopy allows a close-up look at the developing fetus, particularly the face, limbs, genitals, and spine, and can detect abnormalities, such as spinal column defects, facial defects, and limb defects. By attaching additional instruments, the fetoscope can also be used for the surgical correction of some defects, such as certain urinary system disorders. (See also *Amniocentesis; Chorionic villus sampling*.)

F

DEVELOPMENT OF THE FETUS

By the 32nd week of pregnancy, the internal organs of the fetus are almost fully mature and it is perfectly formed. In most cases, the fetus has turned to lie head-down in the pelvis.

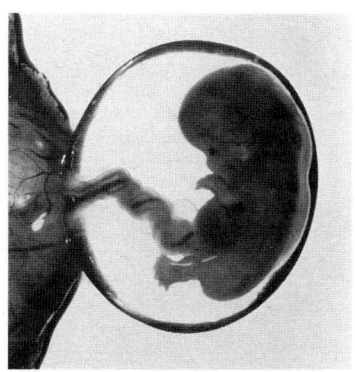

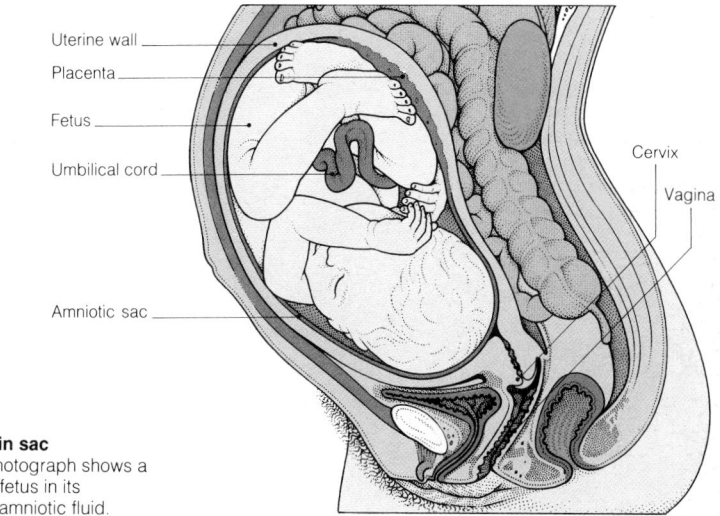

Uterine wall
Placenta
Fetus
Umbilical cord
Amniotic sac
Cervix
Vagina

Fetus in sac
This photograph shows a young fetus in its sac of amniotic fluid.

GROWTH OF THE FETUS FROM 8 TO 40 WEEKS

Between the eighth week and term (40th week), the length of the fetus increases by 20 times; its weight increases by about 1,700 times.

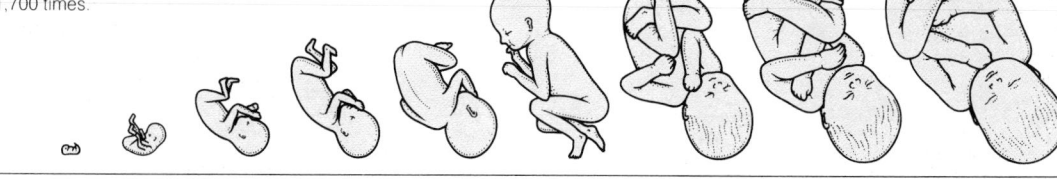

Week	8	12	16	20	24	28	32	36	40
Length	2.5 cm	7.5 cm	16 cm	25 cm	33 cm	37 cm	40.5 cm	46 cm	51 cm
Weight	2 g	18 g	135 g	340 g	570 g	900 g	1.6 kg	2.5 kg	3.4 kg

Fetus

The unborn child from the end of the eighth week after conception until birth. For the first eight weeks, the unborn child is called an *embryo*.

The fetus develops in the mother's *uterus* in a sac filled with *amniotic fluid*, which cushions it against injury. The oxygen and nutrients the fetus needs are supplied through the *placenta*, an organ embedded in the inner wall of the uterus and attached to the fetus by the umbilical cord. (See also illustrated box.)

Fever

Known medically as pyrexia, a fever is defined as a body temperature above 37°C, measured in the mouth, or 37.7 °C, measured in the rectum.

A fever may be accompanied by other symptoms, such as shivering, headache, sweating, thirst, a flushed face, hot skin, and faster than normal breathing. In some cases there may be rigors (attacks of severe shivering followed by drenching sweats and a sudden fall in body temperature). *Confusion* or *delirium* sometimes occurs with fever, especially in the elderly; a very high fever may also cause seizures (see *Convulsions, febrile*) or *coma*, especially in children.

CAUSES
Most fevers are caused by bacterial or viral infections, such as *typhoid fever, tonsillitis, influenza,* or *measles*. In these cases, proteins called pyrogens are released when the white blood cells of the body's defence system fight the microorganisms responsible for the illness. These pyrogens act on the temperature-controlling centre in the brain, causing it to raise body temperature in an attempt to destroy the invading microorganisms.

Fever may also occur in noninfectious conditions, such as *dehydration,* *thyrotoxicosis* (a condition that results from overactivity of the thyroid gland), *myocardial infarction* (heart attack), and *lymphoma* (a tumour of the lymphatic system). The function of fever is not understood in such cases. (See also *Fever* symptom chart.)

TREATMENT
A doctor should be consulted if a fever lasts more than three days or if there are worrying accompanying symptoms, such as severe headache with stiff neck, abdominal pain, or pain when passing urine. Prompt medical advice is also necessary if fever occurs in a baby who is less than six months old, in a child with a history of febrile convulsions, or in an elderly person.

Antipyretic (fever-reducing) drugs, such as *aspirin* (adults only) and *paracetamol,* may be given to treat fevers due to infections; such drugs also help relieve any aches and pains accompanying the fever. Otherwise, treatment

F

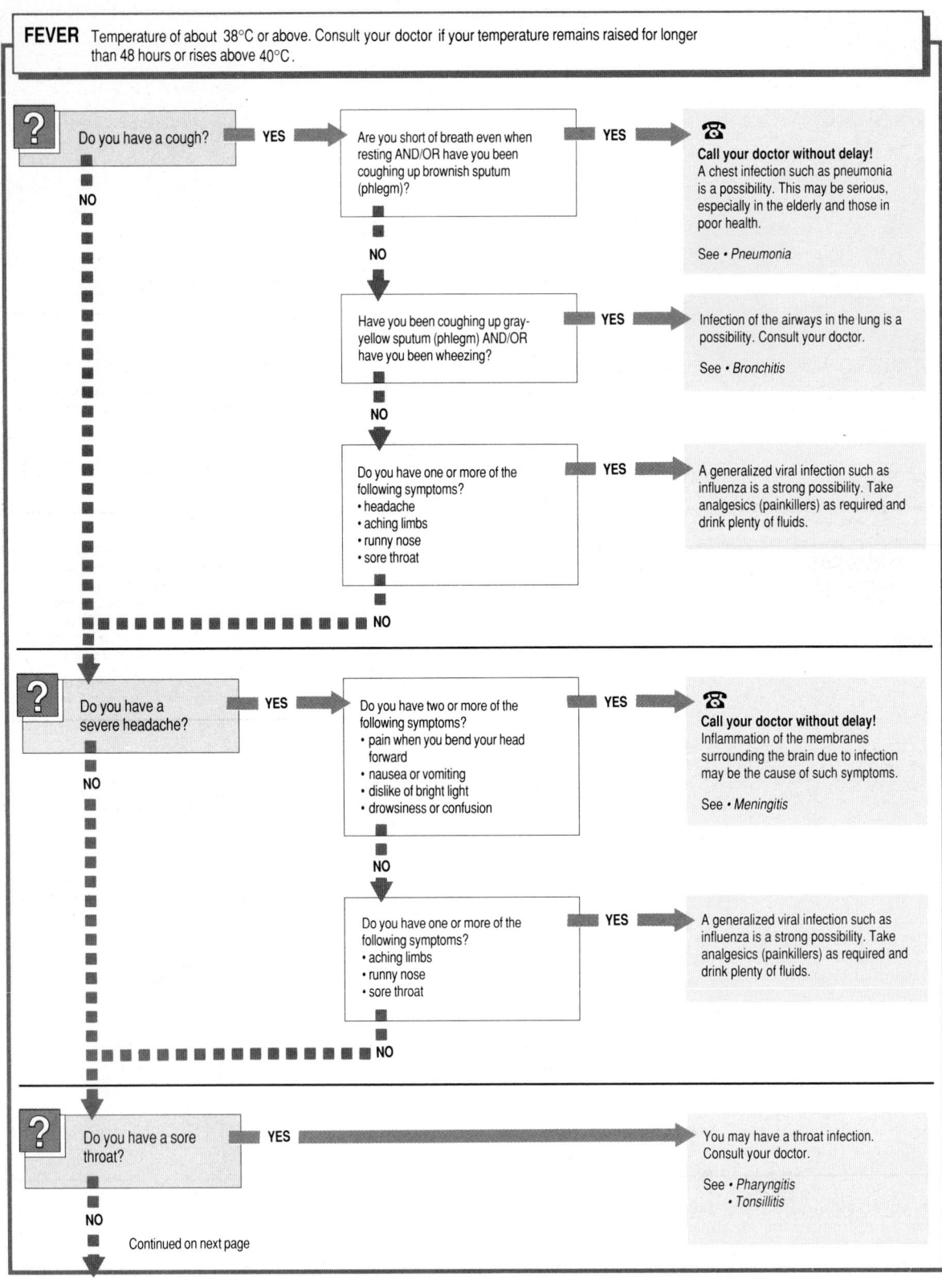

FEVER Temperature of about 38°C or above. Consult your doctor if your temperature remains raised for longer than 48 hours or rises above 40°C.

? Do you have a cough? — **YES** →

Are you short of breath even when resting AND/OR have you been coughing up brownish sputum (phlegm)? — **YES** →

☎
Call your doctor without delay!
A chest infection such as pneumonia is a possibility. This may be serious, especially in the elderly and those in poor health.

See • *Pneumonia*

NO ↓

Have you been coughing up gray-yellow sputum (phlegm) AND/OR have you been wheezing? — **YES** →

Infection of the airways in the lung is a possibility. Consult your doctor.

See • *Bronchitis*

NO ↓

Do you have one or more of the following symptoms?
• headache
• aching limbs
• runny nose
• sore throat
— **YES** →

A generalized viral infection such as influenza is a strong possibility. Take analgesics (painkillers) as required and drink plenty of fluids.

NO

? Do you have a severe headache? — **YES** →

Do you have two or more of the following symptoms?
• pain when you bend your head forward
• nausea or vomiting
• dislike of bright light
• drowsiness or confusion
— **YES** →

☎
Call your doctor without delay!
Inflammation of the membranes surrounding the brain due to infection may be the cause of such symptoms.

See • *Meningitis*

NO ↓

Do you have one or more of the following symptoms?
• aching limbs
• runny nose
• sore throat
— **YES** →

A generalized viral infection such as influenza is a strong possibility. Take analgesics (painkillers) as required and drink plenty of fluids.

NO

? Do you have a sore throat? — **YES** →

You may have a throat infection. Consult your doctor.

See • *Pharyngitis*
    • *Tonsillitis*

NO

Continued on next page

F

? Do you have one or more of the following symptoms?
• pain in the small or side of the back
• abnormally frequent urination
• pain when passing urine
• pink or cloudy urine

YES → ☎ **Consult your doctor without delay!**
An acute infection of the kidney or bladder may be the cause of this.

See • *Cystitis*
• *Glomerulonephritis*
• *Pyelonephritis*

NO

Fever in children
A fever is usually caused by infection from a virus or bacterium. However, a child may also become feverish if allowed to become overheated. Do not give aspirin; use an aspirin substitute. A raised temperature causes a child's forehead to feel hot and causes increased sweating and a general feeling of being ill. Normal temperature may vary from 36 to 37.5°C. Minor fluctuations within this range are no cause for concern if your child seems otherwise well.

If your baby's temperature rises above 39°C, whatever the suspected cause, call your doctor at once. High temperature can lead to seizures in some babies.

? Have you recently returned from a stay in a hot country?

YES → ☎ **Consult your doctor without delay!**
A tropical disease that is rare in this country is a possibility.

See • *Malaria*
• *Typhoid fever*

NO

? Have you spent most of the day in strong sunlight or in very hot conditions?

YES → Exposure to heat may have caused your temperature to rise. In most cases your temperature will return to normal after you have rested for an hour or so in a cool room. Drink plenty of fluids. Call your doctor at once if the fever continues to rise.

NO

? Are you a woman? **YES** → Have you had a baby within the past two weeks? **YES** → ☎ **Call your doctor without delay!**
Puerperal infection, although rare today, is a possible cause of fever after childbirth. It occurs when the uterus and/or vagina become infected after delivery. If, however, you also have pain or redness of the breast, you may have a breast infection.

See • *Breast-feeding*
• *Mastitis*
• *Puerperal sepsis*

NO

NO

Do you have pain in the lower abdomen AND/OR have you had an unusually heavy or unpleasant-smelling vaginal discharge? **YES** → An infection of the uterus and/or fallopian tubes is a possible cause of such symptoms. Consult your doctor.

See • *Salpingitis*

NO

If you are unable to make a diagnosis from this chart, consult your doctor.

is directed towards the underlying cause (for example, giving *antibiotic drugs* for a bacterial infection).

Febrile convulsions can often be prevented by cooling the entire body, either in a lukewarm bath or by sponging with lukewarm water, as soon as the fever starts.

Fibre, dietary

Indigestible plant material in food. Dietary fibre includes certain types of polysaccharides, cellulose, hemicelluloses, gums, and pectins (see *Carbohydrates*) and also lignin.

STRUCTURE

Cellulose, hemicelluloses, and lignin form the main structural components of plant cell walls. Pectins and gums are viscous (sticky) substances in plant sap. Together, these five substances provide the plant with a structure that is stable and partly rigid. Humans do not possess the necessary enzymes to digest these substances, which pass through the digestive system virtually unchanged and cannot be used as a source of energy. Some substances in dietary fibre are fermented by bacteria in the large intestine to produce acids and gas.

FUNCTION

Some components of dietary fibre have the capacity to hold water and thus add bulk to the faeces, which then pass through the intestines more easily, aiding normal bowel function. For this reason, dietary fibre can be effective in treating *constipation* and disorders such as *diverticular disease*. Dietary fibre may also be useful in the treatment of *irritable bowel syndrome*.

The easiest way to increase the amount of fibre in the diet is to increase the intake of unrefined carbohydrate foods such as wholemeal bread, cereals, and grains, root vegetables, and fruits. (See also *Nutrition*.)

Fibre-optics

The transmission of images through bundles of thin, flexible, glass or plastic threads that propagate light by total internal reflection. This means that all the light from a powerful external source travels the full length of the fibre without losing its intensity.

Fibre-optics has led to the development of *endoscopes*, instruments that enable structures deep within the body to be viewed directly. One bundle of fibres carries light to the penetrative end of the instrument and a parallel bundle transmits the image of what is illuminated to the viewer's eye or to a still or video camera. The

GOOD SOURCES OF FIBRE (per 100 g portion)

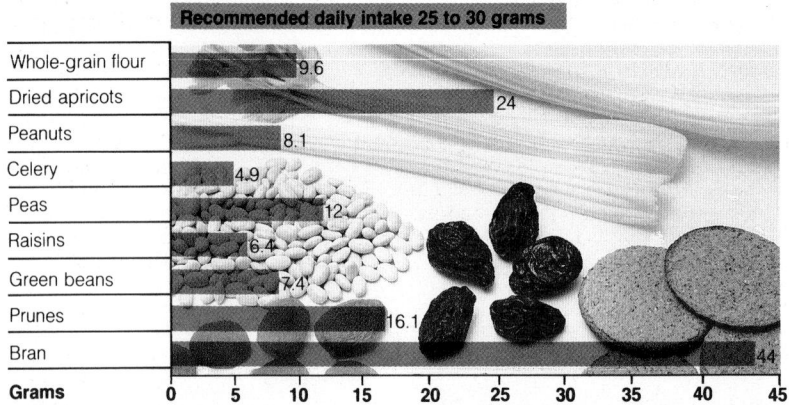

	Recommended daily intake 25 to 30 grams	
Whole-grain flour	9.6	
Dried apricots	24	
Peanuts	8.1	
Celery	4.9	
Peas	12	
Raisins	6.4	
Green beans	7.4	
Prunes	16.1	
Bran	44	

Grams 0 5 10 15 20 25 30 35 40 45

Essential for the efficient working of the digestive system, fibre is usually eaten as fruit or grains. Among the best sources are bran, apricots, prunes, and whole-grain bread. Eating sufficient fibre in food can reduce constipation.

flexibility of the fibres allows them to be passed through the loops of the large intestine or down through the curve of the stomach and into the duodenum without distorting the image. (See also *Endoscopy*.)

Fibrillation

Localized, spontaneous, rapid contractions of individual muscle fibres. Unlike *fasciculation* (a similar muscular "quivering"), fibrillation cannot be seen under the skin. In skeletal muscles, fibrillation is detected by an *EMG* (electromyogram). In heart muscle it is detected by an *ECG* (electrocardiogram).

Fibrillation usually occurs after a nerve supplying a muscle is destroyed, which causes the affected muscle to become weak and waste away. Fibrillation of the heart muscle is caused by disruption of the spread of nerve impulses through the muscle wall of a heart chamber. As a result, the chamber no longer contracts as a single unit; instead, it produces a rapid, irregular rhythm (see *Atrial fibrillation; Ventricular fibrillation*).

Fibrinolysis

The breakdown or dissolution of fibrin, the principal component of any blood clot. Fibrin is a stringy protein that is formed in blood from a precursor substance, fibrinogen, as the end product of coagulation. Along with platelets and red blood cells, fibrin forms the final clot that plugs and seals a damaged blood vessel wall (see *Blood clotting*).

In addition to the coagulation system, blood contains a fibrinolytic system, the end-product of which is an enzyme called plasmin, formed from a precursor called plasminogen. Plasmin acts directly to break up fibrin filaments with the effect thus of dissolving clots.

The fibrinolytic system is activated in parallel with the coagulation system when a blood vessel is damaged. It helps restrain clot formation in blood vessels (thus helping to prevent clots from blocking blood vessels) and eventually dissolves a clot once a broken blood vessel wall has healed. *Thrombosis* (abnormal clot formation) occurs only if there is a disturbance in the balance between mechanisms that promote clot formation, such as sluggish blood flow, and those, such as fibrinolysis, that restrain clot formation or dissolve blood clots.

Fibrinolytic drugs

Drugs used to dissolve blood clots. (See *Thrombolytic drugs*.)

Fibroadenoma

A benign, fibrous tumour found commonly in the breast. Fibroadenomas of the breast are painless, firm, round lumps, usually 1 to 5 cm in diameter, and movable. Fibroadenomas occur most often in women under 30 and are more common in black women. Multiple tumours may develop in one or both breasts.

Removal is performed under either a local or a general anaesthetic. After removal, lumps believed to be fibroadenomas are examined by a pathologist to rule out the small chance of *breast cancer*.

Fibroadenosis

Overgrowth of glandular and fibrous tissue in the breasts, causing pain, tenderness, swelling, and cysts or other lumps in the breast. This common disorder is also known as benign mammary dysplasia, chronic mastitis, fibrocystic disease of the breast, cystic mastitis, or benign breast disease. The development of fibroadenosis may be related to fluctuating levels of female sex hormones; it is most common in women between the ages of 30 and 50.

SYMPTOMS

Fibroadenosis usually causes one or both breasts to become lumpy and tender. There may be either diffuse lumpiness of the breasts or a single breast lump, usually affecting the upper, outer part of the breast. There may also be a feeling of heaviness in an affected breast and occasionally a discharge from the nipple. The symptoms are worse during the second half of the menstrual cycle.

DIAGNOSIS AND TREATMENT

Mammography or a *biopsy* (removal of a sample of tissue for microscopic analysis) may be performed to rule out the possibility of *breast cancer*.

No specific treatment is generally required, but *diuretic drugs* may help relieve symptoms. If symptoms are severe, *progestogen drugs, danazol,* or *bromocriptine* may be prescribed. Any cysts in the breasts may be aspirated (drained using a needle and syringe).

Women with fibroadenosis should examine their breasts carefully each month (see *Breast self-examination*) so that any changes can be reported promptly to a doctor.

Fibrocystic disease

A term that is used to refer either to the inherited disorder *cystic fibrosis,* characterized by the secretion of abnormal mucus by various glands and by recurrent respiratory infection, or to the presence of single or multiple benign tumours or cysts in the breast (see *Fibroadenosis*).

Fibroid

A benign tumour of the *uterus.* Fibroids consist of smooth muscle bundles and *connective tissue* that grow slowly within the uterine wall. As a fibroid enlarges, it may grow within the muscle so that the uterine cavity is distorted, or it may protrude from the uterine wall into the uterine cavity but remain attached by a stalk. Fibroids may be as small as a pea or as large as a grapefruit, and there may be one or more of them.

INCIDENCE AND CAUSE

Fibroids are among the most common tumours, occurring in about 20 per cent of women over 30. They appear most often in women aged 35 to 45 and seldom before the age of 20.

The cause of fibroids is unknown, but it is thought to be related to an abnormal response to *oestrogen hormones. Oral contraceptives* containing oestrogen can cause fibroids to enlarge, as can *pregnancy.* Decreased oestrogen production after the *menopause* usually causes them to shrink.

SYMPTOMS

In many cases there are no symptoms, especially if a fibroid is small. If a fibroid grows and erodes the lining of the uterine cavity, it may cause heavy or prolonged menstrual periods; severe bleeding can lead to iron-deficiency *anaemia.* Large fibroids may exert pressure on the bladder, causing discomfort or frequent passing of urine, or on the bowel, causing backache or constipation. Occasionally, a fibroid attached to the uterine wall becomes twisted and causes a sudden pain in the lower abdomen. Fibroids that distort the uterine cavity may be responsible for recurrent miscarriage or infertility.

DIAGNOSIS

Symptomless fibroids are often discovered during a routine pelvic examination. When fibroids are thought to be the cause of menstrual disturbances or responsible for other symptoms, *ultrasound scanning* can confirm the diagnosis.

TREATMENT

Small, symptomless fibroids usually require no treatment, but regular examinations may be necessary to determine whether they are growing. Surgery is required for fibroids that cause serious symptoms or complications. A *hysterectomy* (removal of the uterus) is sometimes considered if there are large numbers of fibroids. Myomectomy (shelling out the fibroid from its capsule) saves the uterus and is another alternative.

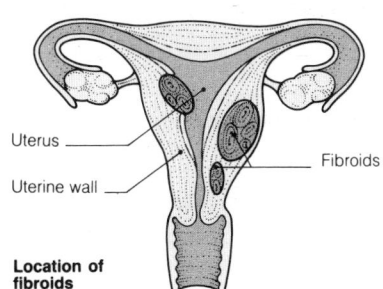

Uterus

Fibroids

Uterine wall

Location of fibroids

Fibroma

A benign tumour of the cells that make up *connective tissue* (material that surrounds body structures and holds them together). For example, a neurofibroma is a tumour of the cells that surround nerve fibres (see *Neurofibromatosis*). An ovarian fibroma is a tumour of the cells that surround the follicles from which ova (eggs) develop. Treatment is not required unless the tumour is causing symptoms.

Fibrosarcoma

A rare, malignant (cancerous) tumour of the cells that make up *connective tissue* (material that surrounds body structures and holds them together). A fibrosarcoma may develop from a *fibroma* (a benign tumour of connective tissue) or it may be malignant from the start.

A fibrosarcoma most often develops in tissues around the muscles in a limb but can also affect a bone or the cells around nerve fibres. The tumour can spread to damage nearby structures.

A fibrosarcoma causes a localized swelling, which may not be noticed at first, depending on its site and how deep it is. Occasionally, widened veins appear on the skin over the growth; the fibrosarcoma may feel warm or may pulsate.

Treatment is by surgical removal or *radiotherapy*; this may be only temporarily successful if cells from the tumour have spread via the bloodstream to start growths elsewhere in the body.

Fibrosis

An overgrowth of scar tissue or *connective tissue* (material that surrounds body structures and holds them together).

Fibrous tissue may be formed as an exaggerated healing response to injury, infection, or inflammation. It can also result from a lack of oxygen in a tissue, usually due to inadequate blood flow through it—for example, in heart muscle damaged by a *myocardial infarction* (heart attack).

In fibrosis, specialized structures (such as kidney cells or muscle cells) are replaced by fibrous tissue, which causes impaired function of the organ concerned. An overgrowth of fibrous tissue can compress hollow structures, as occurs in *retroperitoneal fibrosis,* in which the ureters (tubes draining urine from the kidneys into the bladder) become blocked. Fibrous tissue formed within a muscle after a tear shortens the muscle and disrupts

F

the normal contraction of fibres. This increases the likelihood of further tears unless the muscle is stretched and exercised.

Fibrositis

Pain and stiffness in the muscles. Fibrositis is not a medical term, and some doctors refuse to recognize the condition because investigation usually fails to reveal any detectable reason for the symptoms.

Tension and bad posture may cause the condition, which seems to occur more often in anxious people and in those who spend time sitting in a cramped position. Sometimes, an attack occurs after an infection or new exercise. Fibrositis is most common in middle-aged and elderly people.

SYMPTOMS
Pain and stiffness may be felt in the neck, shoulders, chest, buttocks, knees, and back. There is usually no restriction of movement. Tender areas can sometimes be felt in the affected muscles. In some cases, the attacks (which are generally worse in cold, damp weather) are accompanied by exhaustion and disturbed sleep.

TREATMENT
Analgesic drugs (painkillers), hot baths, massage, and relaxation exercises usually relieve the pain and stiffness. Exercises to improve posture, starting with a gradual programme to tone the muscles, may help prevent attacks. (See also *Back pain*.)

Fibula

The outer and thinner of the two long bones of the lower leg. The fibula is much narrower than the other lower-leg bone, the *tibia* (shin), to which it runs parallel and to which it is attached at both ends by ligaments. The top end of the fibula does not reach the knee, but the lower end extends below the tibia and forms part of the *ankle*.

The main function of the fibula is to provide an attachment for muscles. It provides little supportive strength to the lower leg, which is why pieces of bone can safely be taken from it for grafting elsewhere in the body.

FRACTURE
The fibula is one of the most commonly broken bones. Fracture of the fibula just above the ankle may occur with a severe ankle sprain as a result of a violent twisting movement. *Pott's fracture* is fracture of the fibula just above the ankle combined with dislocation of the ankle and sometimes with fracture of the tibia.

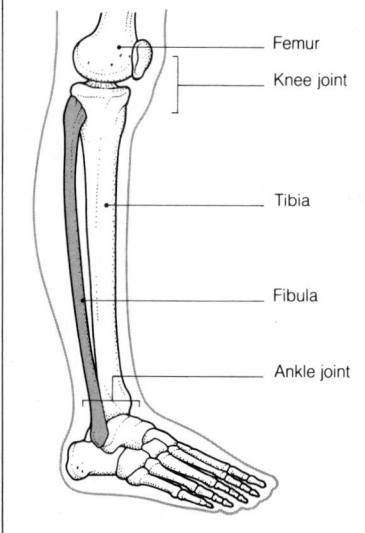

LOCATION OF THE FIBULA
The fibula lies beside the tibia on the outside of each lower leg.

- Femur
- Knee joint
- Tibia
- Fibula
- Ankle joint

A suspected fracture of the fibula is X-rayed to confirm the diagnosis. In some cases the lower leg is immobilized in a plaster *cast* to allow the bone to heal. If the fracture occurs in the middle portion of the fibula, immobilization may not be needed. If the fracture is severe (especially if it is accompanied by dislocation of the ankle), surgery may be necessary to fasten the broken pieces of bone with metal pins.

A fractured fibula may take up to six weeks to heal, depending on its severity and the age of the patient.

Fifth disease

An infectious disease of childhood that causes a widespread rash. It is also known as "slapped cheek" disease or as erythema infectiosum. Fifth disease is the least well-known of the five common childhood infections.

Fifth disease affects children between the ages of two and 14 and usually occurs in small outbreaks in the spring. It is caused by a virus known as parvovirus. The incubation period is four to 14 days.

SYMPTOMS AND TREATMENT
The rash starts on the cheeks as separate, rose-red, raised spots, which subsequently converge. Within a few days the rash spreads in a lacy pattern over limbs but only sparsely on the trunk. It is often accompanied by mild fever. The rash usually clears after about 10 days but may recur over several weeks. Adults, who contract the disease only rarely, may have joint pain and swelling.

The only treatment required is bed rest, plenty of clear fluids, and *paracetamol* to reduce any fever.

Fight-or-flight response

The physical response when the sympathetic division of the *autonomic nervous system* is aroused. The fight-or-flight response is common to all animals, including man, and is a reaction to sensing a threat of any kind. The physiological changes occur in response to fear and also in *anxiety disorders*. *Adrenaline, noradrenaline,* and other hormones are released from the adrenal glands and the nervous system, leading to a raised heart-rate, dilation of the pupils, the hair standing on end, and increased flow of blood to the muscles. All these responses make the body more efficient in either fighting or fleeing the apparent danger.

Filariasis

A group of tropical diseases caused by various parasitic worms or their larvae, which are transmitted to man by insect bites. Adult females, which vary in length from 2 to 50 cm, produce thousands of microfilariae (larvae) which are carried throughout the body in the bloodstream. Blood-sucking insects (primarily certain species of mosquito, fly, and midge) ingest the microfilariae while feeding on blood from infected people and transmit them by biting others.

Filariasis is prevalent in tropical Africa, Indonesia, the South Pacific, coastal Asia, southern Arabia, southern Mexico, and Guatemala.

TYPES AND SYMPTOMS
Some species of worm live in the lymphatic vessels. Swollen lymph nodes and recurring attacks of fever are early symptoms. Inflammation of lymph vessels results in localized *oedema* (an accumulation of fluid in the tissues, causing swelling). Following repeated infections, the affected area—commonly a limb or the scrotum—becomes enormously enlarged and the skin becomes thick, coarse, and fissured, leading to a condition known as *elephantiasis*.

The larvae of another type of worm invade the eye, causing blindness (see *Onchocerciasis*). A third type, which may sometimes be seen and felt moving just beneath the skin, causes *loiasis*, characterized by irritating and sometimes painful areas of oedema called calabar swellings.

DIAGNOSIS AND TREATMENT

The diagnosis of filariasis is confirmed by microscopic examination of blood for the presence of microfilariae.

A three-week course of the *anthelmintic drug* diethylcarbamazine most often cures the infection, but may cause a reaction marked by fever, sickness, and muscle and joint pains.

PREVENTION

Where the resources are available, filariasis can be controlled by the administration of diethylcarbamazine preventively and by the use of insecticides, repellents, nets, and protective clothing to help avoid insect bites. (See also *Roundworms; Insects and disease.*)

Filling, dental

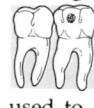

The process of replacing a chipped or decayed area of tooth with an inactive material. The term is also used to describe the restorative (filling) material itself. Amalgam, a hard-wearing mixture of silver, mercury, and other metals, is generally used for back teeth, where the filling will not show. Tooth-coloured plastic material, porcelain, or acrylic is more likely to be used for front teeth. Other substances, such as gold, are also sometimes used.

WHY IT IS DONE

When enamel is damaged, bacteria can invade the dentine beneath and eventually attack the pulp (blood vessels and nerves), causing the tooth to die. Teeth should be repaired as early as possible, ideally when only the enamel is affected. Filling also restores a tooth's original shape, which is important for appearance and also to maintain a correct bite.

HOW IT IS DONE

If the filling required is large or in a sensitive area, the dentist will numb the surrounding gum with a local anaesthetic. Any soft, decayed material is scooped out with sharp instruments. A high-speed drill is used to remove harder material and to shape a hole that will hold the filling securely. While the dentist works, a suction tube placed in the patient's mouth draws away saliva; the cavity is kept as dry as possible with occasional bursts of compressed air.

If the pulp is almost exposed, the bottom of the cavity is lined with a sedative paste to protect the sensitive pulp from pressure and temperature

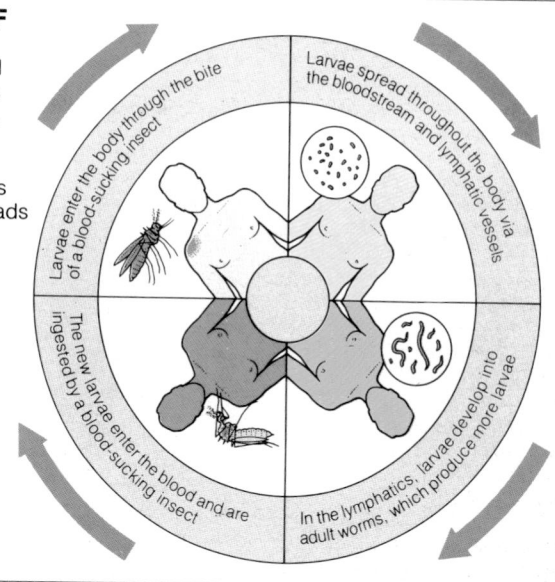

THE CYCLE OF FILARIASIS

Filariasis is caused by parasitic worms and/or their larvae. There are several stages in the development of this infection as it spreads through the body.

Larvae enter the body through the bite of a blood-sucking insect

Larvae spread throughout the body via the bloodstream and lymphatic vessels

The new larvae enter the blood and are ingested by a blood-sucking insect

In the lymphatics, larvae develop into adult worms, which produce more larvae

changes. If one or more of the walls of the tooth is missing through extensive decay, a matrix (steel band) may be placed around the tooth to support the filling. The dentist mixes the amalgam (or other filling material), which at first has a gummy consistency, and packs it into the cavity, smoothing the surface. The filling sets sufficiently to allow the matrix to be removed after a few minutes. The amalgam hardens completely over the next 24 hours.

If a front tooth is chipped, the dentist may use a *bonding* technique in which the tooth's surface is etched with a mild acid solution and plastic or porcelain tooth-coloured material is then attached to the roughened surface, shaped, polished, and finished.

OUTLOOK

Amalgam fillings have a limited life and may need to be replaced after about 10 years. Occasionally, a filling needs to be replaced earlier—for example, if decay has spread under the filling, either because of poor fit or due to recurrent decay. Occasionally, fillings are dislodged or fractured.

Film badge

A device that enables hospital staff members to monitor their exposure to *radiation*. Film badges are worn by those who perform X-ray procedures and radiotherapy. A badge consists of a piece of photographic film in a holder worn on the clothing. The film has a fast (sensitive) emulsion on one side and a slow emulsion on the other. Small doses of radiation blacken only

the fast emulsion; higher doses start to blacken the slow emulsion and make the fast emulsion opaque.

Finasteride

Finasteride is a specific *enzyme* inhibitor that metabolizes testosterone into the more potent androgen, dihydrotestosterone. It is used to treat benign prostatic enlargement (see *Prostate, enlarged*), improving urinary flow. Adverse effects include impotence, and decreased libido and ejaculate volume.

Finger

One of the digits of the *hand*. Each finger has three phalanges (finger bones) and the thumb has two. The phalanges join at hinge joints moved by muscle tendons that flex (bend) or extend (straighten) the finger. The tendons are covered by synovial sheaths that contain fluid, enabling the muscles to work without friction. A small artery, vein, and nerve run down each side of the finger. The entire structure is enclosed in skin with a *nail* at the tip.

DISORDERS

Congenital disorders include *polydactyly* (extra fingers), *syndactyly* (fused fingers), or missing fingers. Sometimes the skin membrane between the fingers is very long and deep, giving an appearance of *webbing*.

Finger injuries are common, particularly *lacerations, fractures,* and tendon ruptures. *Mallet finger* occurs when the extensor tendon along the back of the finger is pulled from its attachment after a blow to the fingertip.

F

STRUCTURE OF A FINGER
The phalanges (bones) are joined at hinge joints and are moved by tendons.

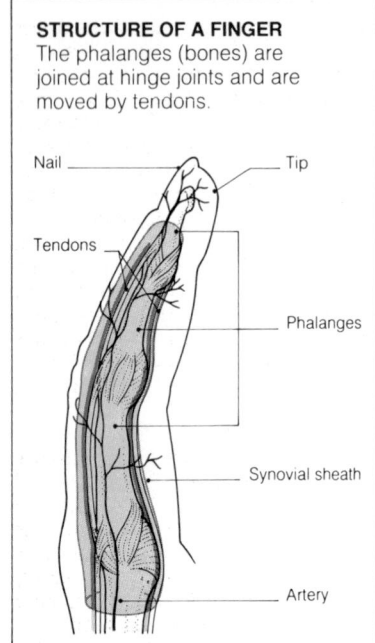

Nail — Tip

Tendons

Phalanges

Synovial sheath

Artery

Inflammation due to *rheumatoid arthritis* or *osteoarthritis* may affect the finger joints, causing stiffness, pain, swelling, and deformity. The flexor tendons, which run along the front of the fingers, may become inflamed and stuck in the tendon sheath, causing *trigger finger*.

Infections may occur in the finger pulp at the tip; *paronychia* (infection of the tissue around the nail) sometimes follows a minor cut.

Altered control of the muscles in the walls of the vessels and impaired blood supply to the hands and fingers may cause *Raynaud's disease*. Dactylitis is a spindle-shaped swelling of the fingers, which occurs in *sickle cell anaemia* and is an uncommon feature of tuberculosis and syphilis.

Clubbing of the fingers may occur as a sign of chronic lung disease, lung cancer, and some forms of congenital heart disease.

Tumours of the finger are rare but may occur in *chondromatosis*, a condition characterized by multiple benign cartilage tumours.

Finger-joint replacement
A surgical procedure in which artificial joints made of metal, plastic, or silicone rubber are used to replace finger joints destroyed by disease.
WHY IT IS DONE
The main use of the operation is to relieve pain and to restore some degree of movement to hands that have been crippled by *rheumatoid arthritis*, which destroys the cartilage, bone, and lining of joints, leaving them weak and unstable.

Less commonly, surgery is performed to relieve pain and to improve mobility in joints in which *osteoarthritis* has destroyed the cartilage and created new bone.
HOW IT IS DONE
The operation is performed under local or general anaesthetic. Several finger joints are usually treated simultaneously.

An incision is made to expose the joint; the ends of the two diseased bones in the joint are cut away, along with diseased cartilage. An artificial joint is then inserted into the bone ends. The tissue covering the joint and the overlying skin are sewn up and the finger is immobilized in a splint until the wound has healed.
RECOVERY PERIOD
The hand is bandaged and raised in a sling to prevent swelling. The stitches are removed after about 10 days, after which the patient is encouraged to move the fingers and return to normal activities. Exercises for the fingers may be required later to maintain finger function.
RESULTS
The procedure is usually successful in relieving pain and enabling the patient to use his or her hands again. However, it can rarely restore normal movement to the hand because joint diseases affect not only bones and cartilage in the joints, but also surrounding tissue that contributes to the flexibility of joints.

Fingerprint
An impression left on a surface by the pattern of fine curved ridges on the skin of the fingertips. The ridges occur in four main patterns—loops, arches, whorls, and compounds (combinations of the other three). It is on these ridges that fingerprint classification is based.

In law, fingerprints are accepted as a means of identification, since no two people—not even identical twins—have the same fingerprints. (See also *Genetic fingerprinting*.)

First aid
The treatment of any injury or sudden illness given before professional medical care can be provided.
MINOR INJURIES
Most first aid consists of treating minor injuries, such as small *wounds*, *sprains*, foreign bodies in the eye (see *Eye, foreign body in*), minor *burns*, and *fractures*. Coping with these injuries requires proficiency in applying *bandages*, *dressings*, and *splints*.
EMERGENCY FIRST AID
The aims of first-aid treatment in an emergency are to preserve life, to prevent the condition from worsening, to protect the individual from further harm, to aid recovery, to provide reassurance to victim and family, and to make the ill or injured person as comfortable as possible.

The role of the person giving first aid is to assess the situation, to give immediate and appropriate treatment, and to arrange for the ill or injured person to be seen by a doctor or taken to hospital without delay. Additionally, the person administering first aid should find out as much as possible about the events surrounding the accident or injury from the victim or from bystanders.

If the victim is unconscious or losing consciousness, the person giving first aid must first ensure that the airway is clear, that breathing is satisfactory (by checking breathing rate), and that the circulation is good (by checking pulse and skin colour). Airway, breathing, and circulation are easily remembered by the letters ABC.

The *recovery position* helps maintain an open airway in an unconscious person who is breathing. *Artificial respiration* is necessary if a patient is not breathing. *Cardiopulmonary resuscitation* is essential if the person is not breathing and has no heartbeat. Any significant *bleeding* must be controlled by the rescuer applying pressure at the appropriate *pressure point*.

No severely injured or ill person should be moved without trained help unless life is in immediate danger. This especially applies to anyone with a suspected *spinal injury*. The person should be covered to keep him or her warm, and any tight or constricting clothing should be loosened.

If many people are injured, the person giving first aid must establish an order of priority for their care. Highest priority is for those who have no pulse, are breathing with difficulty or not at all, are unconscious, or bleeding severely. Such people may die unless immediate treatment is given.

First-aid training is provided by various organizations, which award certificates to all those who have attended courses and thereafter passed an examination. (See also *Childbirth* emergency box; *Choking;*

FIRST AID: FIRST-AID KIT

1	Sticking plasters	**7**	Elastic bandages	**13**	Snub-ended scissors
2	Aspirin or paracetamol	**8**	Adhesive tape	**14**	Antiseptic cream
3	Absorbent sterile gauze bandages	**9**	Torch	**15**	Antiseptic wipes
4	Foil or "space" blanket	**10**	Box of sterile cottonwool	**16**	Hydrogen peroxide (3% solution) or surgical spirit
5	Triangular bandage	**11**	Round-ended tweezers	**17**	Syrup of ipecacuanha
6	Calamine lotion	**12**	Safety pins		

Drowning; Frostbite; Heatstroke; Hypothermia; Poisoning. First-aid treatment for other specific conditions appears under the appropriate heading—for example, *Epilepsy; Nosebleeds.*)

Fistula

An abnormal passage from an internal organ to the body surface or between two organs.

Fistulas may be congenital (present from birth) or may be acquired as a result of tissue damage. Congenital types include *tracheoesophageal fistulas*, branchial fistulas (see *Branchial disorders*), and thyroglossal fistulas (see *Thyroglossal disorders*). Acquired fistulas may result from injury, infection, or cancer. Some types of *arteriovenous fistula* (between an artery and a vein) are constructed artificially to provide ready access to the blood circulation, which may be necessary in people who are having *dialysis*.

Fistulas of the urinary tract, which open from the urethra or bladder to the perineum (the area between the anus and the genitals) may be a complication of radiotherapy to the pelvis or a complication of damage caused by

a difficult childbirth. Such fistulas may cause urinary *incontinence* or *urinary tract infection.*

Fistulas between the intestine and the skin may occur in *Crohn's disease* and may also occur as complications of abdominal surgery. The intestinal contents may escape through an opening to the skin or through a surgical wound.

Some types of fistula close spontaneously, but most need to be cut out and repaired surgically.

Fit

See *Seizure.*

Fitness

Having the capacity for physical work so that normal daily activities can be performed without exhaustion. Fitness depends on strength (the ability to exert force for pushing, pulling, lifting, and other bodily functions), flexibility (the ability to bend, stretch, and twist through a full range of movements), and endurance (the ability to maintain a certain amount of effort for a certain period of time).

HOW FITNESS IS ACHIEVED

Because cardiovascular fitness is the precondition for all other forms of fitness, aerobic exercise, which increases the efficiency of the body's use of oxygen, is the basis for any fitness programme. Exercises to develop flexibility and strength should be combined with aerobic exercise for a total fitness programme. Although fitness training has cumulative effects that build up over many months (provided that there is a sustained increase in activity levels), the effects are specific to the muscles used and the ways in which they are used. A variety of activities is necessary to achieve a general training effect.

BENEFITS OF FITNESS

A person who is fit has a better chance of avoiding *coronary artery disease* and preventing the effects of age and chronic disease. When the body is fit, the maximum work capacity is increased, endurance is increased, and a particular task utilizes a smaller proportion of the work capacity.

The strength, endurance, and efficiency of the heart is also increased by exercise. A fit heart pumps 25 per cent more blood per minute when at rest and over 50 per cent more blood per minute during physical exertion than an unfit heart. A fit person's heart normally beats 60 to 70 times a minute; an unfit person's heart beats 80 to 100 times per minute. The heart of a fit person is more efficient than that of an unfit person and is therefore less subject to strain. (See also *Aerobics; Exercise.*)

Fitness testing

A series of exercises designed to determine an individual's level of *fitness*, primarily cardiovascular fitness and muscle performance.

WHY IT IS DONE

Fitness testing is usually performed to determine a person's level of fitness before starting an exercise programme. It also determines whether or not a person will be at risk when starting to exercise, particularly following a *myocardial infarction* (heart attack). Fitness testing is also done periodically to assess and monitor progress during an exercise programme.

HOW IT IS DONE

The tests are usually carried out by a doctor in his or her office or in the outpatient department of a hospital. A physical examination is usually performed, including measurements of height, weight, and body fat. Blood

451

and urine tests may be carried out, including an analysis of blood *cholesterol* and high-density and low-density lipoprotein content, since high cholesterol levels are related to *atherosclerosis* (narrowing of arteries by deposits of fatty material).

One test involves measuring the performance of the heart during physical work. The heart's efficiency at pumping blood is measured using the pulse rate (number of heartbeats) per minute. The more efficient the heart, the slower it works during exercise and the quicker it returns to normal afterwards. The pulse is taken at rest, and then the heart performance is measured during exercise at one or more intensities. This exercise may include step climbing, riding a stationary bicycle, or walking or running on a treadmill. After a specific period, the exercise is stopped and the pulse is taken to determine how hard the heart is working at its maximum level. The pulse is usually taken again after a minute to determine how long it takes for the heartbeat to return to normal. The blood pressure response to exercise also gives useful information to the doctor and patient.

Another type of exercise test involves measuring a person's overall performance in a standard exercise. This is most suitable for monitoring progress through an exercise programme and for setting goals. The test may be based either on measuring the distance covered in a fixed time or the time needed to cover a fixed distance. (See also *Aerobics; Exercise.*)

Fixation

A term used by Sigmund Freud to describe the attachment of a person's libido (sexual drive or interest) to real or imagined events during early childhood. Freud suggested that young children go through various stages related to certain parts of the body. These stages were called the oral, anal, and phallic stages because putting things in the mouth, concern about faeces, and playing with the penis or clitoris were prominent behaviours during the different stages. In modern *psychoanalytic theory*, childhood stages are viewed within the context of the child's early relationships, starting with the mother.

EFFECTS
Fixations are unconscious and exist to some extent in all human beings; experiences from childhood are seen as permanently affecting the adult's thoughts and feelings. However,

when the fixations are very powerful, resulting from especially traumatic relationships or series of events or experiences, they lead to the sort of behaviour that would be expected from an immature child. Regression (going back) to one of these early stages is thus regarded by some analysts as the underlying cause of certain emotional disorders.

Flail chest
A type of chest injury, usually resulting from a road traffic accident or from violence. In flail chest, multiple rib fractures, usually at the front and side of the chest, produce an isolated portion of the chest wall. This portion moves in when the victim breathes in and moves out when he or she breathes out; this motion is opposite to the normal direction.

The injury may severely impair the efficiency of breathing and result in collapse due to *respiratory failure* and *shock*. It makes breathing and coughing very painful, which can increase the likelihood of chest infection and collapse of the lung (see *Atelectasis*).

TREATMENT
Emergency treatment consists of turning the person on to the affected side or supporting the flail segment by firm strapping. In the most severe cases, the patient may need immediate admission to an intensive care unit, where artificial *ventilation* can be maintained. This treatment is continued for about 10 days until the ribs are sufficiently healed.

Flat-feet
A condition, usually affecting both feet, in which the arch is absent and the sole rests flat on the ground. The medical term for this condition is the Latin equivalent: pes planus.

CAUSES
Almost everyone is born with flat-feet. The arches form gradually as supportive ligaments and muscles in the soles of the feet develop, and are not usually fully formed until about the age of six.

In some people, however, the ligaments and muscles are weak for unknown reasons and the feet remain flat. Less commonly, the arches do not form because of a hereditary defect in the structure of the small bones of the foot.

Flat-feet can also be acquired in adult life because of fallen arches, sometimes as the result of a rapid increase in weight. Flat-feet may also be caused by a weakening of the mus-

cles and ligaments that support the arch, which sometimes occurs in a neurological or muscular disease such as *poliomyelitis*.

SYMPTOMS AND TREATMENT
Most flat-feet—due to ligaments and muscles that have never developed fully—are usually painless and require no treatment. When the condition is caused by a defect in the foot bones or develops in adult life, the feet may ache when walking or standing. A few affected children require an operation to correct the bones in the feet. In adults, treatment consists of wearing arch supports in the shoes and performing exercises to strengthen the weakened ligaments and muscles.

Flatulence
Abdominal discomfort or fullness, relieved by belching or passage of wind through the anus. Flatulence is a feature of many gastrointestinal conditions, in particular *dyspepsia, irritable bowel syndrome*, and disease of the *gallbladder.*

When a person is in an upright position, most swallowed air passes back up the oesophagus to be expelled through the mouth. When a person is in a prone position, the air may pass through the intestine and anus instead. Gas formed in the intestine is passed only through the anus.

Flatus
Gas passed through the anus, commonly called "wind". Gas is formed in the large intestine as a result of the action of bacteria on carbohydrates and amino acids in digested food; the gas consists of hydrogen, carbon dioxide, and methane. Air may be swallowed while eating and enter the stomach or intestine. Excessive swallowing of air, known as aerophagy, may occur during rapid eating or at times of stress.

Large amounts of gas may cause considerable abdominal discomfort, which may be relieved by the passage of wind through the anus or by defaecation. Normal amounts of gas may cause abdominal discomfort in people whose intestines are abnormally sensitive. (See also *Flatulence.*)

Flatworm
 Any species of worm that has a flattened shape—as opposed to a *roundworm* or nematode, which has a cylindrical shape. Flatworms are also sometimes called platyhelminths.

Two types of flatworm are parasites of humans—cestodes (tapeworms) and trematodes (flukes and schistosomes). (See also *Tapeworms*; *Liver fluke*; *Schistosomiasis*.)

Flea bites
See *Insect bites*.

Flies
See *Insects and disease*.

Floaters
Fragments perceived to be floating in the field of vision. Floaters move rapidly with eye movement but drift slightly when the eyes are still. They do not usually affect vision.

Most floaters are shadows cast on the retina by microscopic structures in the *vitreous humour*, a jelly-like substance that lies behind the lens. In older people, the vitreous humour tends to shrink slightly and detach from the retina, often causing conspicuous floaters, which usually decrease with time.

The sudden appearance of a cloud of dark floaters, especially if accompanied by bright light flashes, suggests *retinal tear* or *retinal detachment*. A large red floater that obscures vision is usually due to a *vitreous haemorrhage*.

Flooding
A technique used in *behaviour therapy* for treating *phobias*.

Floppy infant syndrome
A condition in which a baby's muscles lack normal tension or tone. There are many possible causes and careful medical examination and investigation are required. (See *Hypotonia in infants*.)

Floppy valve syndrome
See *Mitral valve prolapse*.

Floss, dental
Soft nylon or silk thread, waxed or unwaxed, used to remove dental *plaque* and food particles from between the teeth and around the line of the gum.

Flow cytometry
A test that reveals the arrangement and amount of *DNA* (genetic material) within cells as a means of diagnosing malignancy. The pattern of DNA in cancer cells is different from that of normal cells. The test is helpful in distinguishing benign from malignant cells, and also in monitoring the effects of *anticancer drug* treatment. (See also *Cytology*.)

Flu
See *Influenza*.

Flucloxacillin
A *penicillin drug*. Flucloxacillin is usually prescribed to treat *staphylococcal infections*, such as wound and skin infections and certain types of pneumonia.

Fluctuant
A term used medically to describe the movement within a swelling when the swelling is palpated (examined by touch). Such a movement is a sign that the swelling contains liquid (such as pus in an abscess).

Fluke
 A type of flattened worm, also called a trematode, which may infest humans or animals. The two main diseases caused by flukes are *liver fluke* infestation, which occurs worldwide, and *schistosomiasis*, a common and debilitating tropical disease.

Fluorescein
A harmless orange dye used in *ophthalmology* as an aid to the diagnosis of certain types of *eye* disorders.

Fluorescein drops can be applied to the eye to check for the presence of conjunctival abrasions, which show up yellow when stained, or of *corneal abrasions* or *corneal ulcers*, which look green under white light or fluoresce brilliantly under ultraviolet light.

The dye is also used in a technique known as fluorescein angiography, which shows details of the blood circulation in the *retina* and *choroid* (the innermost layers of the eye). For this technique, a sterile solution of fluor-

escein is injected into a vein, and then photographs of the retina, using blue light and a green filter on the camera, are taken while the fluorescein is passing through the blood vessels in the eye.

Fluoridation
The addition of *fluoride* to the water supply as a means of reducing the incidence of dental *caries* (tooth decay). Some areas have naturally high levels of fluoride in the drinking water; in other areas, fluoride may be added to bring the concentration up to a recommended level of 0.7 to 1.2 parts per million. Fluoridation began in the US in the 1940s. In the UK, decisions to add fluoride to drinking water are made by the local authorities; in 1988 the authorities that had opted to add fluoride remained in the minority. Although considerable political controversy has surrounded fluoridation programmes, there is no firm evidence that fluoridation at the recommended level has any harmful effects.

Fluoride
A mineral compound that is useful in helping prevent dental *caries* (tooth decay). Fluoride is thought to work by strengthening the mineral composition of the tooth enamel (see *Teeth*), making it more resistant to acid attacks. Fluoride may also reduce the acid-producing ability of microorganisms in dental *plaque*.

Fluoride that is ingested during the formation of teeth produces a lifelong beneficial effect because it is incorporated into the developing tooth substance. Children who drink fluoridated water from birth have up

---

HOW TO USE DENTAL FLOSS

Floss should be used as an adjunct to toothbrushing to remove plaque and food particles from gaps between teeth and around gums. Care should be taken to avoid damaging the gum margins.

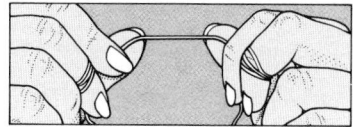

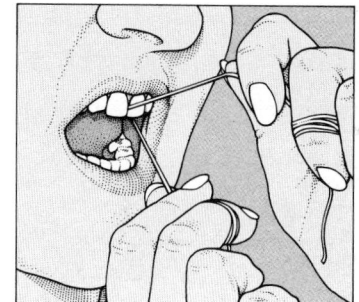

1 Break off a generous length of floss (about 50 cm) and wrap the ends around one finger of each hand. Do not use the same length of floss twice.

2 Holding the floss taut, guide it gently into the gap between the teeth until it reaches the gum line. Then rub the sides of each tooth with the floss using an up-and-down motion.

F

F

to 65 per cent fewer cavities and 90 per cent fewer extractions during childhood than those who have drunk water with less than the recommended fluoride level.

Water supplies may naturally provide sufficient fluoride (the recommended level is 0.7 to 1.2 parts per million) or it may be added (see *Fluoridation*). If the fluoride level is too low, children can be given drops or tablets.

Fluoride is also beneficial to both children and adults when applied directly to the teeth. The dentist may treat children's teeth by painting on a fluoride solution or holding a fitted tray filled with fluoride gel against the teeth for a few minutes. Fluoride mouthwashes and toothpastes are available for use at home.

Ingestion of excess fluoride during tooth formation may lead to *fluorosis*.

Fluorosis

Mottling of the tooth enamel caused by ingestion of excess *fluoride* as the *teeth* are formed. In very severe cases, mottling is so great that the enamel develops unsightly brown stains. Such cases usually occur only where the fluoride level in water is much greater than the recommended level. Fluorosis can occur in other areas if excessive additional fluoride is consumed—for instance, in the form of fluoride tablets.

Mild white mottling of the teeth may occur in a small percentage of children ingesting water at the recommended level, but this form of fluorosis does not usually impair appearance.

Fluorouracil

An anticancer drug used in the treatment of cancers of the breast, bladder, ovaries, and intestine.

Flurazepam

A *benzodiazepine drug* used in the treatment of *insomnia*.

Flush

Reddening of the face and sometimes the neck, caused by dilation of the blood vessels near the skin's surface. Flushing may occur during *fever*. *Hot flushes* are common at the *menopause*.

Foam, contraceptive

See *Spermicide*.

Foetus

An alternative spelling for *fetus*.

Folic acid

A *vitamin* essential for the production of red *blood cells* by the *bone marrow*.

Folic acid is contained in a variety of foods, particularly liver and raw vegetables; adequate amounts are usually included in a normal diet.

During pregnancy, folic acid plays an important part in fetal growth—in the development of the nervous system and in the formation of blood cells. Research studies have shown that the incidence of *neural tube defects* is much reduced if women take folic acid supplements (0.4 mg per day) for a month before conception and during the first 12 weeks of pregnancy. Women at high risk are recommended to take a higher dose of 5 mg per day.

Folic acid deficiency is a cause of megaloblastic *anaemia*, which causes symptoms such as fatigue, depression, and pallor. Deficiency can occur during any serious illness or can result from a poor diet, especially in people who drink large amounts of alcohol.

Folie à deux

A French term used to describe the unusual occurrence of two people's sharing the same psychotic illness (see *Psychosis*). Commonly the two are closely related (e.g. a married couple or a brother and sister) and share one or more paranoid *delusions*. If the sufferers are separated, one of them almost always quickly loses the symptoms, which have been imposed or communicated by the dominant, and genuinely psychotic, partner.

Folk medicine

Any form of medical treatment based on popular tradition, including the charming of warts, the use of copper bracelets to treat rheumatism, and ear-piercing to improve eyesight. These remedies have in common their support by local conviction and lack of a professional practitioner. By contrast, the diagnostic and healing techniques used by a witch doctor are known as traditional medicine; those used by a chiropractor or a homeopathist are known as *alternative medicine*.

Follicle

A small cavity in the body. Examples are *hair* follicles, pits on the surface of the skin from which hair grows, and ovarian follicles, fluid-filled cavities in the female *ovary* in which ova (eggs) develop.

Follicle-stimulating hormone

A *gonadotrophin hormone*, also known as FSH, produced and secreted by the pituitary gland.

Folliculitis

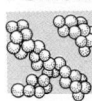

Inflammation of one or more hair follicles as a result of a *staphylococcal infection*. Folliculitis may occur almost anywhere on the skin. It is commonly found on the neck, thighs, buttocks, or armpits, causing a *boil*, or it may affect the bearded area of the face, leading to the development of pustules (see *Sycosis barbae*).

Treatment is with *antibiotic drugs*. The infection often spreads to other members of the family. To prevent this or to control an outbreak that has already occurred, each person should wash frequently and use a separate face-cloth and towel; clothes worn next to the skin should be washed daily in boiling water.

Fomites

Inanimate objects, such as clothing, books, bed linen, or a telephone receiver, which are not harmful in themselves, but which may be capable of harbouring bacteria, viruses, parasites, or other harmful organisms and thus may convey an infection from one person to another.

Fomites mainly transmit respiratory infections, such as influenza. The singular is fomes.

Fontanelle

One of the membrane-covered spaces between the bones of a baby's skull. At birth, the bones of the skull are not yet fully fused and two soft areas between the skull bones can be felt on

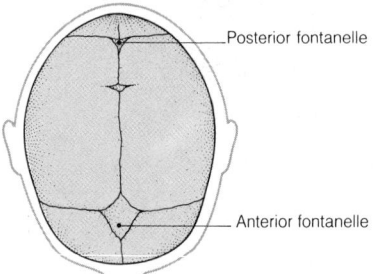

Location of the fontanelles
There are two soft areas on the baby's skull—the anterior fontanelle is diamond-shaped, the posterior fontanelle is triangular.

the scalp. These soft areas are the anterior (front) fontanelle, which is diamond-shaped, about 2.5 cm in diameter, and usually closes up by the age of 18 months, and the posterior (rear) fontanelle, which is triangular, about 6 mm in diameter, and closes up within about two months of birth.

DISORDERS

It is normal for the fontanelles to bulge and become tense when a baby cries. However, persistent tension at other times may indicate an abnormality, particularly *hydrocephalus* (an accumulation of fluid within the baby's skull). A sunken fontanelle may be a sign of *dehydration*. If a fontanelle is abnormally large or takes a long time to close, the cause may be a brain abnormality or a disorder, such as *rickets*, affecting the skull bones. Early closure of the fontanelles results in deformity called *craniosynostosis*.

Occasionally, a third fontanelle is present between the other two; this occurs in *Down's syndrome*. Some babies have extra bones in the anterior fontanelle; this is not abnormal. The extra bones fuse into the skull when the gap closes.

Food additives

Any substance added to food for the purposes of preservation or to improve its acceptability. Contrary to popular belief, not all food additives are artificial; sugar and salt are probably used more commonly than any others. Any additive must be officially approved before being accepted for use in food processing.

TYPES AND USES

Additives fall into four main groups: those that preserve food and affect its "keeping" quality, those that affect texture, those that affect appearance and taste, and miscellaneous additives, such as rising and glazing agents, flour "improvers", and antifoaming agents.

Preservatives, such as sodium nitrate, are added to food to control the growth of bacteria, moulds, and yeasts, especially those that might contaminate the food after it has left the manufacturer. Other additives, such as antioxidants, improve the keeping quality of the food by preventing undesirable changes (such as by stopping rancidity in foods containing fat).

Additives that improve texture include emulsifiers, stabilizers, thickeners, and gelling agents. They alter the "mouth feel" and consistency of food. Lecithin, which occurs naturally in all animal and plant cells, is an emulsifier added to margarine to prevent separation.

Appearance and taste are often improved by the use of colourings, flavourings, sweeteners, and flavour enhancers. Colours and flavours are used mainly to compensate for losses during processing, to strengthen existing colours or flavours, and to ensure standardization in products. *Artificial sweeteners*, such as saccharin and aspartame, are used in place of sugar, especially in products designed for diabetics or slimmers.

RISKS

Food additives are carefully monitored and regulated; there is no evidence that any additives in general use can harm the population as a whole. However, even though an additive may be harmless to most people, it may produce an allergic reaction in others. The best known flavour enhancer, *monosodium glutamate* (MSG), may cause *Chinese restaurant syndrome*. Tartrazine, a widely used yellow food colouring, produces an allergic reaction in a very small number of people.

Additives are sometimes blamed for causing *hyperactivity* in children, but most doctors believe that the majority of hyperactive children are not allergic to food additives.

Food allergy

An inappropriate or exaggerated reaction of the *immune system* to a food. Sensitivity to cow's milk protein is a fairly common food allergy in young children. Other foods most commonly implicated in food allergy include wheat, fish, shellfish, and eggs. Allergy to food is much more common than allergy to food additives.

Food allergy is more common in people who suffer from other forms of *allergy* or *hypersensitivity*, such as *asthma*, allergic *rhinitis* (hay fever), and *eczema*.

Immediate reactions, occurring within an hour or sometimes minutes of eating the trigger food, include lip swelling, tingling in the mouth or throat, vomiting, abdominal distension, abnormally loud bowel sounds, and diarrhoea.

The only effective treatment of food allergy is to avoid the offending food. (See also *Food intolerance*.)

Food-borne infection

Any infectious illness caused by eating food contaminated with viruses, bacteria, worms, or other organisms.

CAUSES

There are two main mechanisms by which food can become infected.

First, many animals that are kept or caught for food may harbour disease organisms in their tissues or internal organs. If meat or milk from such an animal is eaten without being tho-

FOOD ADDITIVES

Antioxidants	Comments	Possible use in
E 300–302	L-ascorbic acid/ascorbates (vitamin C)	Fruit drinks
E 307	Synthetic alpha-tocopherol	Cereal-based baby foods
E 322	Lecithins	Low-fat spreads

Colours		
*E 102	Tartrazine (yellow/orange)	Soft drinks
*E 104	Quinoline yellow (greenish/yellow)	Smoked fish
E 160	Carotenes/Annatto (orange)	Cheese

Emulsifiers and stabilizers		
E 406	Agar (extracted from seaweed)	Ice cream
E 412	Guar gum (extracted from cluster beans)	Packet soups
E 440	Pectin (occurs naturally in fruits and plants)	Jams, preserves

Preservatives		
*E 210–219	Benzoic acid/benzoates	Fruit products
*E 220–227	Sulphur dioxide/sulphites	Meat products
*E 249–252	Nitrites/nitrates	Cooked and cured meats

*Warning – may produce reactions in susceptible people

Most additives approved by the EEC or EU have been given an E number, which must be listed by type and name and/or by number on food labels. Some examples of food additives and foods in which they are used are shown above. Antioxidants improve the keeping qualities of certain foods by preventing undesirable chemical changes. Preservatives also improve keeping quality, but by inhibiting growth of microorganisms. Emulsifiers and stabilizers improve the texture of foods.

roughly cooked or pasteurized, the organisms may cause illness in their human host. In the UK, the only common infection of this type is *food poisoning* from improperly cooked meat, poultry, fish, shellfish, or eggs.

Second, food may be contaminated with disease organisms spread from an infected person or animal—usually by flies moving from faeces to food.

PREVENTION
Food-borne infections can be controlled or prevented by adequate sanitation and sewage treatment; by multiple laws and regulations that govern animal husbandry, the production of food in farms and factories, and its subsequent storage and distribution; and by generally high standards of personal hygiene with regard to handling and eating of food.

In some less affluent parts of the world, many of these controls do not exist and the chances of a food-borne infection are thus much higher. When visiting such countries, it is wise to avoid certain foods, particularly salads, any meat or fish that looks suspect or not thoroughly cooked, shellfish, milk, butter, cream, and ice cream. Raw fruits and vegetables are generally safe once the exterior peel or skin has been removed.

Immunization is available against certain food-borne and water-borne infections, such as *typhoid fever* and *cholera*, but immunization usually provides only partial protection and is no substitute for good food hygiene. (See also *Water-borne infection*.)

Food fad

A like or dislike of a particular food or foods that is carried to extremes. A food fad may lead to an undue reliance on, or avoidance of, a particular foodstuff.

Fads are especially common in toddlers and adolescents and in those under stress. For most people, food fads are not serious since they are either short-lived or restricted to a limited number of foods. However, when food fadism or food aversion has an obsessional quality about it, or is persistent, it may be indicative of a more serious eating disorder. (See also *Anorexia nervosa; Bulimia*.)

Food intolerance

An adverse reaction to a food or food ingredient that occurs each time the substance is eaten, that is not due to a psychological cause or to *food poisoning*, and that does not affect the *immune system*.

CAUSES
Food intolerance is mainly of unknown cause, but is sometimes due to various unknown irritants, *toxins*, or *food additives*. The condition may be associated with an adverse reaction to foods such as green peppers, fried foods, or onions. Food intolerance can be caused by an inborn or acquired biochemical defect, such as *lactase deficiency* (an inability to digest milk sugar).

Food poisoning

A term used for any illness of sudden onset, usually with stomach pain, vomiting, and diarrhoea, suspected of being caused by eating contaminated food. Most cases are the result of contamination of food by bacteria or viruses.

Food poisoning is usually suspected when, for example, several members of a household (or customers at a restaurant) become ill after eating the same food.

TYPES AND CAUSES
Food poisoning can be classified, according to cause, into infective and noninfective types. Some foods can cause poisoning of either type. For example, shellfish such as mussels, clams, and oysters can become contaminated by bacteria or viruses, by toxins acquired from poisonous plankton (tiny marine animals and plants), or by chemical pollutants in the water.

BACTERIAL CAUSES In the UK, food-borne illness is on the increase despite educational programmes and legislation to improve the general standards of food hygiene. Up to 30,000 cases of bacterial food poisoning occur annually. The bacteria commonly responsible belong to the groups called *SALMONELLA* and *CAMPYLOBACTER*, certain strains of which are able to multiply rapidly in the intestines to cause widespread inflammation. Food poisoning due to *LISTERIA* is in addition now being increasingly recognized (see *Listeriosis*).

Some farm animals, especially poultry, commonly harbour bacteria responsible for food poisoning. If frozen poultry is not completely thawed before being cooked, or is not cooked thoroughly, it is liable to cause poisoning. Eggs laid by affected poultry may also contain disease-causing bacteria. Fresh eggs are unlikely to be heavily contaminated, but eggs stored for more than three weeks should be well cooked, especially before being eaten by babies, the sick, or the elderly.

Bacteria may also be transferred to food from the excrement of infected animals or people, either by flies or by the handling of food by an infected person—especially if the hands have not been washed after using the toilet. If contaminated food is left for any time in warm conditions, a large colony of bacteria may develop without obvious food spoilage.

Some types of bacteria cause the formation of toxins which may be difficult to destroy even with thorough cooking. Toxin-forming strains of *STAPHYLOCOCCUS*, for example, may spread to food from a septic abscess on a food-handler's skin. The organism *CLOSTRIDIUM PERFRINGENS* is resistant to heat and may survive in precooked foods, such as stews and pies, which are not correctly stored. *Botulism* is a very uncommon, life-threatening form of food poisoning caused by a bacterial toxin and now mostly associated with defective home preservation of food.

VIRAL CAUSES The viruses that most commonly cause food poisoning are astravirus, rotavirus, and Norwalk virus (a common contaminant of shellfish). These cause food poisoning when raw or partly cooked foodstuffs have been in contact with water contaminated by human excrement.

NONINFECTIVE CAUSES These include poisonous mushrooms and toadstools (see *Mushroom poisoning*), and fresh fruit and vegetables that have been contaminated with high doses of insecticide. Chemical poisoning can also occur if food has been stored in an unsuitable container—for example, if a container that has previously held a poison is used to store food, or if acidic fruit juice is kept in a metal container made partly of zinc.

Various exotic foods (for example, the puffer fish, considered a delicacy in Japan, or cassava, a staple food in many tropical countries) can also cause moderate to lethal poisoning if improperly prepared and cooked.

SYMPTOMS
The onset of symptoms varies according to the cause of poisoning. Symptoms usually develop within 30 minutes in cases of chemical poisoning, between one and 12 hours in cases of bacterial toxins, and between 12 and 48 hours with most bacterial and viral infections. Symptoms vary considerably according to how badly the food was contaminated, but usually include nausea, vomiting, diarrhoea, stomach pain, and, in severe cases, *shock* and collapse.

INFECTED ANIMAL PRODUCTS

Some animals harbour disease organisms (e.g. bacteria, worms, and parasites) in their tissues and these may cause infection if meat or dairy products are consumed raw or improperly cooked. Beef, pork, and fish tapeworm infestations, salmonella poisoning, and (rarely) brucellosis can be transmitted in this way.

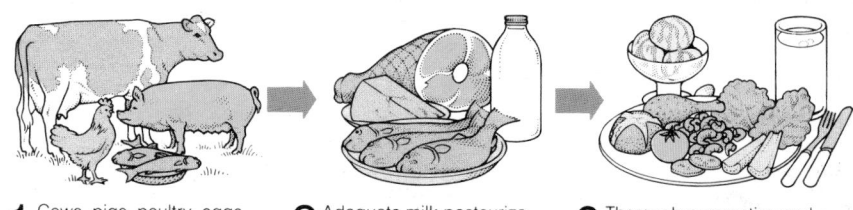

1 Cows, pigs, poultry, eggs, fish, and shellfish are sources of bacterial, viral, or worm infection or infestation.

2 Adequate milk pasteurization and inspection of meat and fish before sale prevents most infections and infestations of this type.

3 Thorough preparation and cooking of meats, fish, shellfish, poultry, and eggs further reduces the risk of infection.

F

FOOD CONTAMINATION

Intestinal infections may be spread from person to person if organisms in faeces contaminate food, directly or indirectly. This can occur if vegetable crops are sprayed with sewage, flies settle on faeces and then on food, or if food is handled by a person who has not washed his or her hands.

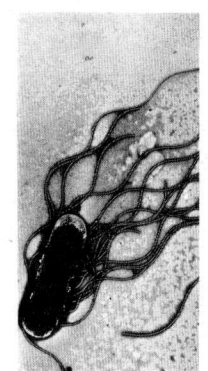

Contaminating organism
The photograph (left), taken through an electron microscope, shows a typical *SALMONELLA* bacterium. The organism uses its many flagellae (whip-like structures) to move. *SALMONELLA* is a common contaminant of poultry, eggs, and egg products and may cause severe food poisoning.

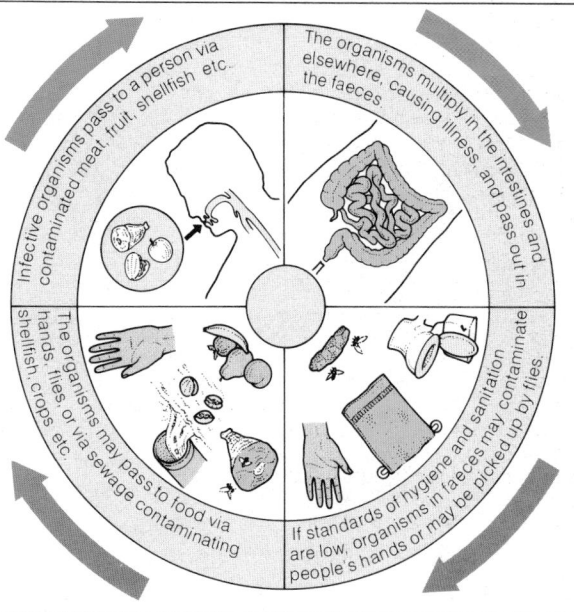

The symptoms of botulism are markedly different, affecting the nervous system and causing difficulty in speaking, visual disturbances, muscle paralysis, and vomiting.

DIAGNOSIS

The diagnosis of bacterial food poisoning can usually be confirmed from a culture of a sample of the person's vomit or faeces. Chemical food poisoning can often be diagnosed from a description of what the person has eaten, and from analysis of a sample of the suspect food, if available.

TREATMENT

Mild cases can be treated at home. The affected person should eat no solid food but should drink plenty of fluids, which should include some salt and sugar to replace what is being lost (see *Rehydration therapy*).

If vomiting and diarrhoea are severe, or if an affected person collapses, medical assistance should be sought. If possible, samples of food left from a recent meal should be kept; they may help pinpoint the cause and possibly prevent a widespread outbreak of poisoning.

Hospital treatment may be necessary in severe cases. If poisoning by a chemical or bacterial toxin is suspected, gastric *lavage* (washing out the stomach) may be carried out. Otherwise, treatment usually concentrates on preventing or treating dehydration; fluids and electrolytes (salts) are given by mouth or intravenously.

Except for botulism and some cases of mushroom poisoning, most food poisoning is not serious. Recovery generally occurs within three days.

PREVENTION

Some simple measures can virtually eliminate the chances of food poisoning. Hands should always be washed before handling food, and fresh vegetables and fruit rinsed in clean water. Cutting boards and implements used on raw meat should also be rinsed before they are used for other food. Frozen poultry should always be completely thawed before cooking and then should be well cooked. Because raw meat and poultry carry disease-causing organisms, it is important to wash the hands immediately after handling these foods and before proceeding with further food preparation. Such organisms are destroyed by proper cooking.

Ask for advice on the preparation of any food that is unfamiliar to you.

Suspect items—such as mussels that do not open when boiled, bulging tin cans, or any food that smells or looks obviously spoiled—should be rejected. People who preserve food at home should take care to sterilize food thoroughly by heating it in a pressure cooker at 120°C for 30 minutes. (See also *Cholera*; *Dysentery*; *Typhoid fever*.)

Foot

The foot has two vital functions—to support the weight of the body in standing or walking and to act as a lever to propel the body forwards.

STRUCTURE

The largest bone of the foot is the *calcaneus* (heel-bone); it is jointed with the talus, the second largest bone. In front of the talus and calcaneus is a series of smaller bones—the navicular, cuboid, and cuneiform. These in turn are jointed with five long bones called the metatarsals. The phalanges are the bones of the toes; the big toe has two phalanges, all the other toes have three.

Tendons passing around the ankle connect the muscles that act on the various bones of the foot and toes. The main blood vessels and nerves pass in front of and behind the inside of the ankle joint to supply the foot. The undersurface of the normal foot forms a natural arch which is supported by ligaments and muscles. Fascia (fibrous tissue) and fat form the sole of the foot, which is covered by a layer of tough skin.

DISORDERS

Injuries to the foot commonly result in *fracture* of the metatarsals and phalanges. The calcaneus may fracture following a fall from a height on to a hard surface.

Deformities of the foot are fairly common and include *talipes* (club-foot), *flat-feet*, and *claw-foot*. Another common deformity is a *bunion*, which is a thickened *bursa* (fluid-filled pad) overlying the joint at the base of the big toe.

A number of disorders can affect the skin of the foot. *Corns* are small areas of thickened skin and are usually caused by tight-fitting shoes. *Plantar warts* (verrucas) are warts that develop on the skin on the sole. *Athlete's foot*, a fungal infection, mainly affects the skin between the toes, causing it to become itchy, sore, and cracked. *Gout*, a fairly common type of arthritis, often affects the joint at the base of the big toe or one of the joints in the foot. Ingrowing of the toenail (see *Toenail, ingrowing*) commonly affects the

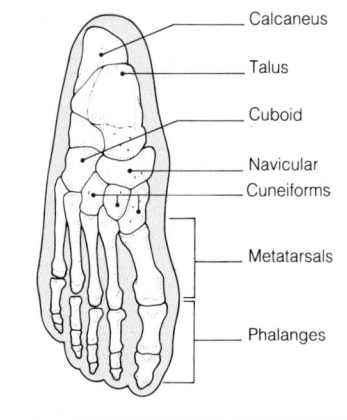

ANATOMY OF THE FOOT
An adult has 26 bones in each foot—one eighth of the total number in the entire skeleton. The calcaneus is attached to the talus above. In front are the navicular, cuboid, and cuneiform bones, which are attached to the metatarsals. Phalanges form the toes.

Calcaneus
Talus
Cuboid
Navicular
Cuneiforms
Metatarsals
Phalanges

nail of the big toe, causing inflammation of the surrounding tissues and *paronychia* (infection of these tissues). *Foot-drop* (inability to raise the foot properly) may be due to damage to the muscles in the leg that perform this movement or to the nerves that supply these muscles.

Foot-drop

A condition in which the foot cannot be raised properly. It hangs limp from the ankle joint, causing it to catch on the ground when walking.

CAUSES

Neuritis (inflammation of a nerve) affecting the nerves that supply muscles that move the foot is a common cause of foot-drop; it may be due to *diabetes mellitus*, *multiple sclerosis*, or to a *neuropathy*. Weakness in the foot muscles can also result from pressure on a nerve root as it leaves the spinal cord, due perhaps to a *disc prolapse* (slipped disc) or, rarely, to a tumour.

TREATMENT

Treatment is of the underlying cause, but in many people the weakness persists. A foot-drop splint (see *Caliper splint*) can be worn to keep the foot fixed in place when walking.

Foramen

A natural hole or passage in a bone or other body structure, usually to allow the passage of nerves or blood vessels.

The foramen magnum is the large opening in the base of the skull through which the spinal cord passes.

Forceps

A tweezer-like instrument used for handling tissues or equipment during surgical procedures. Various types of forceps are designed for specific purposes. For example, forceps used for holding or removing wound dressings have scissor handles to make manipulation easier, and tissue forceps have fine teeth at the tip of each blade so that tissues can be handled delicately during operations. (See also *Forceps delivery*; *Forceps, obstetric*.)

Forceps delivery

The use of forceps (see *Forceps, obstetric*) by an obstetrician to ease out the baby's head during a difficult birth (see *Childbirth*). *Vacuum extraction* may be used as an alternative.

WHY IT IS DONE

Forceps delivery is used if the mother is overtired or unable to push out her baby unaided, or if the baby is showing signs of *fetal distress*. (If fetal or maternal distress occurs before the second stage of labour begins, a *caesarean section* rather than forceps delivery is necessary.)

Forceps are used to control the head in *breech delivery* (in which the baby's buttocks are delivered before the head) to prevent a too-rapid delivery. Forceps are also used if the baby's head is stuck in the middle of the mother's pelvis and needs to be rotated to make delivery possible. This type of delivery, called a mid-forceps delivery, requires extreme skill on the part of the obstetrician; a *caesarean section* is sometimes performed instead.

HOW IT IS DONE

The mother is given an *analgesic drug* (painkiller) and either local or *epidural anaesthesia*. She then lies on her back, with her legs raised in stirrups, and her bladder may be emptied with a *catheter*. The obstetrician then examines the mother. Forceps can be applied only if the cervix (neck of the uterus) is fully dilated and the baby's head is engaged in the pelvis. An *episiotomy* (making of a cut in the perineum) is usually performed before a forceps delivery.

The forceps blades are placed on either side of the baby's head, just in front of the ears. If the baby's chin points downwards, gentle traction is applied to the forceps and the baby is delivered. If the chin is pointing side-

COMMON FOREIGN BODIES IN CHILDREN

Children constantly experiment with objects in the environment. They frequently place small objects into their mouths, noses, or ears. As a result, a swallowed or stuck foreign body is a common occurrence. It is wise to keep all small objects well out of reach of children.

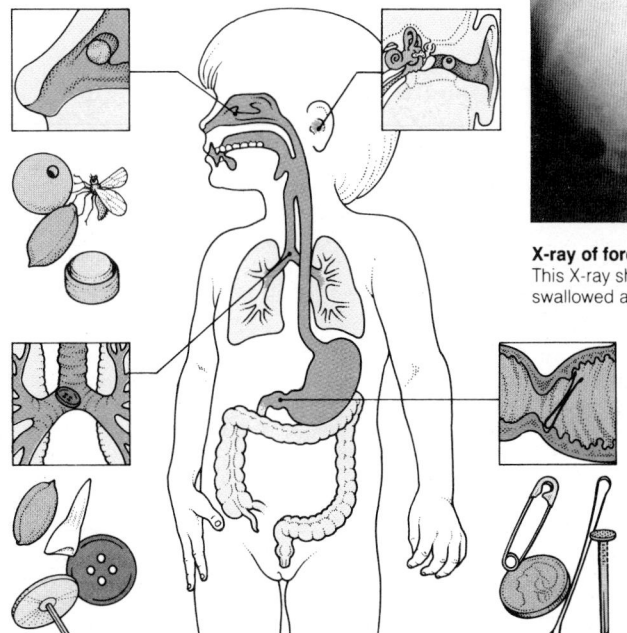

Ear and nose
Attempting to remove a foreign body from the ear can be dangerous because of the risk of pushing the object further in. The doctor uses a syringe, suction, or forceps. A foreign body in the nose may be taken out with forceps by the doctor; an older child may be able to blow it out while the other nostril is blocked.

Lungs
Inhaled objects such as peanuts or teeth may become lodged in the bronchi and cause obstruction of air flow, resulting in pneumonia or lung collapse. Symptoms may include choking, coughing, and breathing difficulty. If the child is choking, call an ambulance or take him or her to hospital immediately.

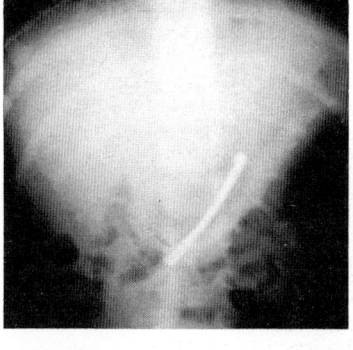

X-ray of foreign body
This X-ray shows that the child has swallowed a closed hair-grip.

Stomach
Foreign bodies commonly found in the stomach include coins, batteries, marbles, and buttons. Most small, smooth objects pass safely out of the body in faeces, but an object that has failed to pass through the body after seven to 10 days, or sharp objects or batteries, usually require removal by endoscopy or surgery.

---

ways or upwards, rotation of the head is usually necessary before traction can be applied; in such cases, rotation forceps are used.

RECOVERY PERIOD
After a forceps delivery, care is similar to that following a spontaneous (unassisted) vaginal delivery. Sometimes there is greater bruising of the perineum, but this usually heals rapidly and can be eased by the application of ice-packs. After a forceps delivery, the baby may have forceps marks on the face but these disappear after a few days. The length of stay in hospital for both mother and child is usually the same as after a spontaneous vaginal delivery.

Forceps, obstetric
Surgical instruments used in *forceps delivery* to deliver the head of a baby in a difficult labour.

Obstetric forceps consist of two blades that cup the baby's head. Each blade is joined to a separate handle and the two handles are fitted together; when assembled, the blades are separated by a fixed distance (see illustrated box).

Foreign body
An object that is present in an organ, opening, or passage of the body but that should not be there. A foreign body may enter the body accidentally (by inhalation or swallowing, for example) or it may be deliberately introduced. Common sites include the airways (see *Choking*), ear (see *Ear, foreign body in*), eye (see *Eye, foreign body in*), rectum, urethra, and vagina.

Splinters or other objects that enter via the skin and become embedded in body tissues are also classed as foreign bodies. (See also illustrated box.)

Forensic medicine
The branch of medicine concerned with the law, especially criminal law. The forensic pathologist is a doctor who specializes in the examination of bodies when circumstances suggest

OBSTETRIC FORCEPS
The two wide, blunt blades are designed to fit around the baby's head. The handles lock together so that the blades are held apart.

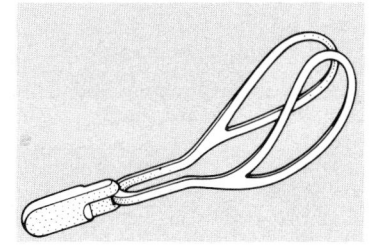

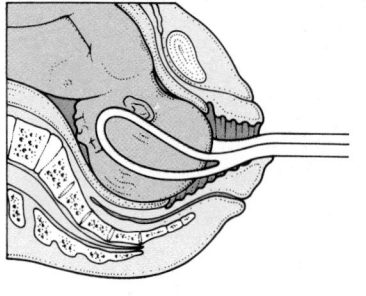

Positioning
The forceps blades lie along the sides of the baby's head just in front of the ears.

death was unnatural (i.e. suicide, homicide, or an accident). The examination usually includes an assessment of the time of death (from data such as the temperature of the corpse and its state of decomposition), deduction of the likely nature of any weapon used (from study of the injuries), and matching of blood, hair, and skin from the victim with those on any weapons, on the clothing of suspects, or on parts of a vehicle.

Forensic pathologists may also be asked to examine victims of alleged sexual assault or child abuse. They also consult in cases of poisoning and possible drug deaths.

Forensic scientists use laboratory methods to study body fluids (such as blood, semen, and saliva) found on or near the victim and compare the fluids with those from suspects. They are also trained in ballistics and the identification of fibres from clothing.

In addition, forensic scientists may advise on *blood groups* and *genetic fingerprinting* in criminal investigations and in cases of disputed paternity.

Foreskin

The popular name for the prepuce, the loose fold of skin that covers the glans of the *penis* when it is flaccid and which retracts during erection.

At birth, the foreskin is attached to the glans and slowly separates over the first three to four years of life. No attempt should be made to retract the foreskin in a young boy. If tightness persists after the age of five, there is no need to consult a doctor unless the child is unable to pass urine normally or suffers from recurrent infection (because the glans can not be cleaned adequately).

In some societies, the foreskin is routinely removed from newborn boys, an operation called *circumcision*, usually for religious or hygienic reasons. Circumcision may be performed at any age as a treatment for disorders of the foreskin.

DISORDERS

In *phimosis*, the foreskin remains persistently tight after the age of five, causing difficulty in passing urine and ballooning of the foreskin. There may be recurrent *balanitis* (infection and inflammation of the glans and foreskin). Erection is often painful, which is why the condition is frequently discovered only at puberty.

In the related disorder *paraphimosis*, the foreskin becomes stuck in the retracted position, causing painful swelling of the glans.

Forgetfulness

Inability to remember. (See *Memory*.)

Formaldehyde

A colourless, pungent, irritant gas. In medicine, a solution of formaldehyde and a small amount of alcohol in water—a preparation known as formalin—is used to preserve tissue specimens or to harden them (a procedure called fixation) before they are stained and examined. Formalin is also used as a *disinfectant* and as a constituent of building glues. In a few people, formaldehyde causes an allergic reaction affecting the skin or lungs.

Formication

An unpleasant sensation, as if ants were crawling over the skin. Formication may occur following abuse of certain drugs, such as alcohol, cocaine, or morphine. Scratching of the skin may cause a rash and occasionally lead to an incorrect diagnosis of a skin disease.

Formula, chemical

A way of expressing the constituents of a chemical in symbols and numbers. Every known chemical substance has a formula. Water, for example, has the formula H_2O, indicating that it is composed of molecules of two hydrogen atoms (H_2) and one oxygen atom (O).

Fracture

A break in a bone, most commonly caused by a fall. A bone is usually broken directly across its width, but can also be fractured lengthwise, obliquely, or spirally.

TYPES OF FRACTURE

Fractures are divided into two main types: closed (or simple) and open (or compound). In a closed fracture the broken bone ends remain beneath the skin and little or no surrounding tissue is damaged; in an open fracture one or both bone ends project through the skin. Fractures may also be classified according to the shape or pattern of the break (see box).

If the two bone ends have moved apart, the fracture is termed displaced; in an undisplaced fracture the ends remain in alignment and there is simply a crack in the bone.

CAUSES AND INCIDENCE

Most fractures are caused by a sudden injury that exerts more force on the bone than it can withstand. The force may be direct, as when a finger is hit by a hammer, or indirect, as when twisting the foot exerts severe stress on the *tibia* (shin).

Some diseases, such as *osteoporosis* and certain forms of cancer, weaken bone so much that it takes only a minor injury—or none at all—for the bone to break. This type of fracture is termed pathological.

Common sites of fracture include the hand, the wrist (see *Colles' fracture*), the *ankle joint*, the *clavicle* (collarbone), and the neck of the femur or hip (see *Femur, fracture of*), usually as a result of a fall.

Elderly people are the most prone to fractures because they fall more and because their bones are fragile.

SYMPTOMS AND SIGNS

There is usually swelling and tenderness at the fracture site, and, in some cases, deformity or projection of bone ends. The pain is often severe and is usually made worse by movement.

FIRST-AID TREATMENT

Anyone suffering a suspected or known fracture should be taken to hospital; if the injured person cannot walk, medical help should be summoned. Do not try to force back a displaced bone yourself.

Treat severe bleeding (see *Bleeding, treatment of*), covering any open wounds with a clean dressing. Move the patient as little as possible. *Splinting* is usually necessary, especially if the injured person needs to be moved or if there is a long delay before help arrives. If an injured arm can be bent comfortably across the chest, splint it first and then apply a *sling*. If *spinal injury* is suspected, do not move the person at all unless his or her life is in immediate danger.

Do not give the injured person any food or liquid in case a general anaesthetic is needed later.

PROFESSIONAL TREATMENT

X-rays are taken to confirm the diagnosis and to provide a clear picture of the type of fracture and the degree of any displacement or malalignment.

Bone begins to heal immediately after it has broken. The first aim of treatment is therefore to ensure that the bone ends abut each other and are in alignment so that the bone will retain its previous shape after the fracture heals. Displaced bone ends are manoeuvred back into position—a procedure known as reduction. The bone may be manipulated through the skin (closed reduction) under a local or general anaesthetic. Alternatively, the bone may be repositioned through an incision under general anaesthesia (open reduction).

FRACTURES: TYPES AND TREATMENT

There are two main types of fractures: simple (closed) and compound (open). Within these two categories are several other types, three of which are illustrated here.

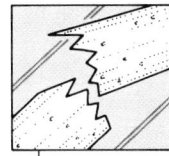

Compound fracture
A sharp piece of bone punctures the skin and is therefore exposed to organisms. There is a high risk of infection.

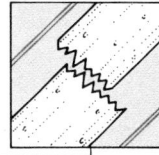

Transverse fracture
This may result from a sharp, direct blow or be a stress fracture caused, for example, by prolonged running.

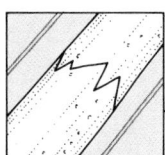

Simple fracture
The broken bone does not break the skin. Because organisms do not come into contact with the fracture, infection is rare.

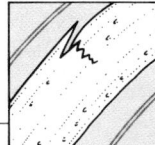

Greenstick fracture
This type usually occurs in children. Sudden force causes only the outer side of the bent bone to break.

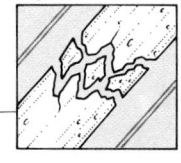

Comminuted fracture
The bone shatters into more than two pieces. This fracture is usually caused by severe force, such as in a car accident.

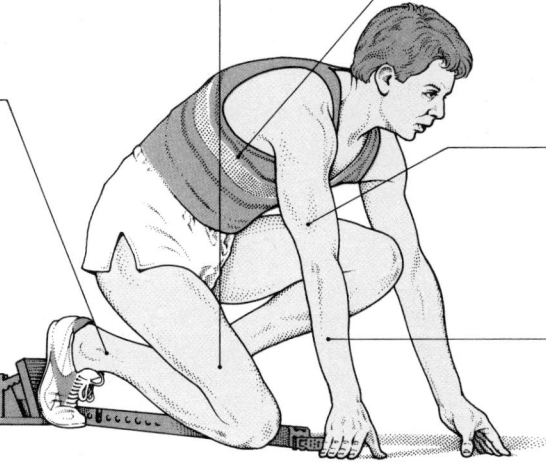

REPAIR OF FRACTURES

There are various ways of repairing fractures depending on the particular bone, the severity of the fracture, and the age of the patient.

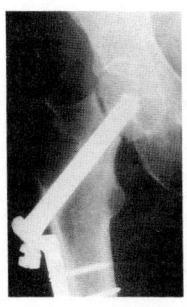

Internal fixation
The photograph (left) shows immobilization of an unstable ankle fracture by the insertion of metal screws across the bone ends.

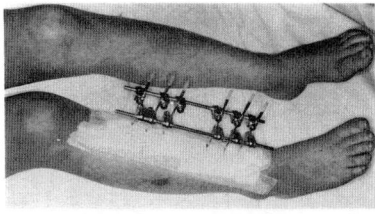

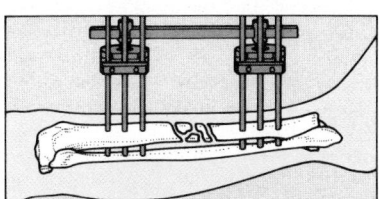

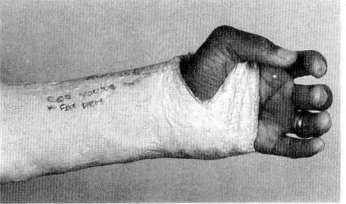

External fixation
Immobilization may be achieved by means of a plaster cast (above) or, in cases such as an unstable fracture of the tibia (left and above left), through the use of metal pins inserted into the bone on either side of the break and locked into position on an external metal frame.

THE BONE HEALING PROCESS

After a fracture, the bone starts to heal immediately. Any displacement of the bone ends must therefore be corrected without delay to minimize deformity.

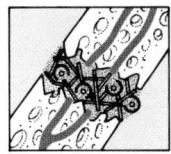

2 Macrophages invade the fracture site to remove wound debris. Fibroblasts then create a mesh to form a base for new tissue.

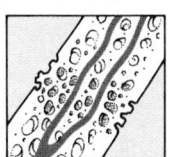

4 Remodelling takes place, with more dense, stronger bone laid down. New blood vessels have formed.

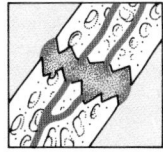

1 A blood clot forms between the bone ends, sealing off the ends of the damaged vessels.

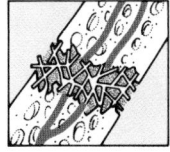

3 New bone (callus) is laid down between the bone ends and over the fracture line.

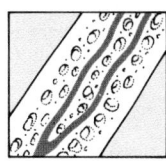

5 Over a period of weeks, the bone returns to its former shape.

F

Once the fracture has been reduced, the bone is immobilized to allow the broken pieces to reunite firmly.

In some cases the ends of the fractured bone may be fixed together by metal pins inserted through the skin and into the bone and kept in position by attachment to an external frame (external fixation); once the fracture has healed, the pins and frame are removed. In other cases an operation is done to open up the injury site and fasten together the bone pieces with metal screws, nails, plates, rods, or wires (internal fixation).

RECOVERY PERIOD

The time taken for fractures to heal varies considerably and depends on many factors. Fractures mend much more easily in children than in adults, and in babies they can heal in as little as two weeks. In an adult a weight-bearing bone, such as the tibia, may take up to six months to knit together completely; bones that do not bear weight, such as the *radius* (one of the lower-arm bones) and clavicle (collarbone), generally take no longer than eight weeks.

COMPLICATIONS

Most fractures heal without problem. Healing is sometimes delayed because the blood supply to the affected bone is inadequate (as a result of damaged vessels) or because the bone ends are not close enough together. If the fracture fails to unite, internal fixation or a *bone graft* may be required.

Occasionally, bone ends reunite at the wrong angle. If this causes deformity, an operation may be necessary to break the bone again, set it correctly, and fix it with nails. *Osteomyelitis* is a possible complication of open fractures and may be difficult to cure.

REHABILITATION

Physiotherapy plays an important part in rehabilitation after a fracture because complete immobility of a bone for a prolonged period can result in loss of muscle bulk, stiffness in nearby joints, and *oedema* (accumulation of fluid), with a risk of permanent disability. The patient is encouraged to begin gradually using the affected part as soon as is safely possible, and is given exercises that will restore flexibility to the joints and strength to the muscles. (See also *Monteggia's fracture; Pelvis; Pott's fracture; Rib, fracture of; Skull, fracture of.*)

Fracture, dental

A break in a *tooth*. Tooth fractures are most commonly caused by falling on to a hard surface or by being hit in the mouth by a hard object, as may occur when playing sports. Front teeth that project more than normal are especially vulnerable to accidental fracture. Fractures may involve the crown or the root of the tooth, or both. In most cases, only the enamel (the hard, brittle covering of the crown) is fractured.

Fractures of the enamel or of the enamel and dentine can usually be repaired by dental *bonding*; in some cases, a replacement crown may be fitted (see *Crown, dental*). If the pulp of a tooth is damaged, *pulpotomy* may be performed. Fractures of the root of a tooth may be treated by splinting (see *Splinting, dental*), by *root-canal treatment*, by the fitting of a replacement crown over the root, or by removing the tooth (see *Extraction, dental*).

Fragile X syndrome

An inherited defect of the X *chromosome* that causes *mental handicap*. Fragile X syndrome is the most common cause of mental handicap after *Down's syndrome*.

The disorder occurs within families according to an X-linked recessive pattern of inheritance (see *Genetic disorders*). Although males are mainly affected, women are able to carry the genetic defect responsible for the disorder and pass it on to some of their sons, who are affected, and some of their daughters, who in turn become carriers of the defect.

Approximately one in 1,500 men is affected by the condition; one in 1,000 women is a carrier. In addition to being mentally handicapped, affected males are generally tall, physically strong, have a prominent nose and jaw, increased ear length, large testes, and are prone to epileptic seizures. About one third of female carriers show some intellectual impairment.

There is no treatment for the condition. If a woman has a history of the syndrome in her family, it is useful to seek *genetic counselling* regarding the risk of a child's being affected.

Freckle

A tiny patch of pigmented skin, often round or oval in shape. Freckles occur on sun-exposed areas of skin and tend to become more numerous as a result of continued exposure. The tendency to freckling is inherited and occurs most in fair and red-haired people.

Freckles are harmless, but people with highly freckled complexions should avoid excess sunlight and should use *sunscreens*.

Free-floating anxiety

Vague apprehension and tension associated with *generalized anxiety disorder*.

Frequency

See *Urination, frequent*.

Freudian slip

A slip of the tongue or a minor error in action that could be what the person really wanted to say or do. The term, also called a parapraxia, is derived from Sigmund Freud's book "The Psychopathology of Everyday Life". As the error tends to be laughed off, Freud saw the process as a compromise between the fulfilment of an unconscious wish and the conscious effort to repress it.

Freudian theory

A discipline developed by Sigmund Freud (1856–1939), a Viennese neurologist. The theory developed out of his treatment of neurotic patients using hypnosis and later the interpretation of dreams. This formed the basis of his technique of *psychoanalysis*. Freud believed that feelings, thoughts, and behaviour were controlled by unconscious wishes and conflicts and that problems occurred when these desires were not fulfilled or the conflicts remained unresolved.

According to Freud, the conflicts originated in childhood and persisted into adulthood. The essence of his theory concerns early psychological development, particularly sexual development. Freud defined a number of stages—oral, anal, and genital (representing the areas of the body on which an infant's attention becomes fixed at different ages)—and three components of personality—the *id*, *ego*, and *superego* (based respectively on pleasure, reality, and moral and social constraints). The classic Freudian model sees all behaviour as having its roots in unconscious instincts, but ultimately being determined by the interplay between the id, ego, and superego. (See also *Psychoanalytic theory; Psychotherapy.*)

Friar's balsam

A name for tincture of benzoin. Friar's balsam is used as an *inhalation* for the relief of nasal congestion, acute rhinitis, sinusitis, and to loosen coughs. It is available over-the-counter.

Friedreich's ataxia

A very rare inherited disease in which degeneration of nerve fibres in the spinal cord causes *ataxia* (loss of coordinated movement and balance). The disease is the result of a genetic defect, usually of the autosomal recessive type (see *Genetic disorders*). It affects about two people per 100,000.

SYMPTOMS

Symptoms first appear in late childhood or adolescence. The main symptoms are unsteadiness when walking, clumsy hand movements, slurred speech, and rapid, involuntary eye movements. In many cases there are also abnormalities of bone structure and alignment.

TREATMENT AND OUTLOOK

There is as yet no cure for the disease. Once symptoms have developed, the disease becomes progressively more severe, and, within 10 years of onset, more than half the sufferers are confined to wheelchairs. If *cardiomyopathy* (heart muscle disease) develops, it may contribute to an early death. People who have blood relatives with Friedreich's ataxia may benefit from *genetic counselling* before deciding whether to have children.

Frigidity

Lack of desire for or inability to become aroused during sexual intercourse (see *Sexual desire, inhibited*). The term has been used almost exclusively with reference to women and is now being discouraged because of its negative connotations—blaming a woman for something that may exist only in the mind of her partner. (See also *Orgasm, lack of*.)

Frostbite

Damage to tissues caused by extremely cold temperatures. Frostbite can affect any part of the body that is not properly covered, but the nose, ears, fingers, and toes are most susceptible. The lower the temperature, the shorter the time required to cause damage; wind and blizzard conditions also harm more quickly.

The first symptoms are a pins-and-needles sensation, followed by complete numbness. The skin appears white, cold, and hard, and then becomes red and swollen. If only the skin and immediately underlying tissues are damaged, recovery may be complete. If blood vessels are affected, *gangrene* (tissue death) can follow. After the tissue has thawed, blisters form and some areas of skin eventually become black, indicating that the tissue is dead. In such cases, the damage is permanent and amputation of the affected part may be necessary.

TREATMENT

Frostbite must be treated promptly but thawing should be undertaken only when there is no risk of further freezing. The person should be sheltered from the cold and the affected parts warmed as quickly as possible by immersing them in water at 40°C. Movement of the affected parts should be avoided; massage is not helpful. (See also first-aid box.)

Frottage

The act of rubbing against another person to achieve sexual arousal. Also called frotteurism, it is usually carried out in a densely packed crowd where a man rubs his (clothed) genitals against a woman's buttocks or thigh. Such men commonly indulge in other sexual *deviations*, may have an abnormal interest in buttocks (see *Fetishism*), and are unable to form successful sexual relationships.

Frozen section

A method of preparing a *biopsy* specimen (tissue removed for microscopic examination) that provides a rapid indication of whether or not the tissue is malignant. Frozen section does not yield sufficient detail for routine use and cannot replace the more lengthy conventional preparation of biopsy specimens. It was formerly used to provide information while a patient was undergoing surgery, but has now been largely superseded by other techniques, such as aspiration biopsy, which can be performed before the operation.

WHY IT IS DONE

Frozen section is primarily used to determine whether *breast lumps* are benign or malignant. It can also be used to check whether thyroid or intestinal tumours are malignant, and to diagnose *lymphomas*.

HOW IT IS DONE

Frozen section is performed during a surgical procedure and provides information that will allow the surgeon to decide whether or not further tissue should be removed before the operation is completed.

The surgeon removes a sample of tissue and sends it to the pathology laboratory for analysis. The sample is quickly frozen in liquid nitrogen, cut into very thin sections, placed on a glass slide, and stained so that the cells can be examined under the

---

FIRST AID: FROSTBITE

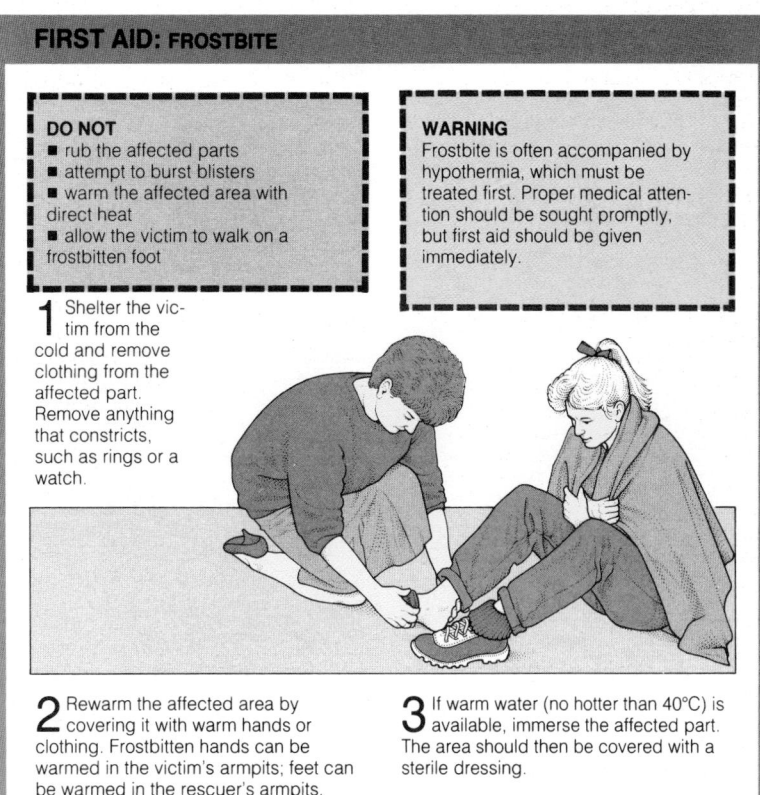

DO NOT
- rub the affected parts
- attempt to burst blisters
- warm the affected area with direct heat
- allow the victim to walk on a frostbitten foot

WARNING
Frostbite is often accompanied by hypothermia, which must be treated first. Proper medical attention should be sought promptly, but first aid should be given immediately.

1 Shelter the victim from the cold and remove clothing from the affected part. Remove anything that constricts, such as rings or a watch.

2 Rewarm the affected area by covering it with warm hands or clothing. Frostbitten hands can be warmed in the victim's armpits; feet can be warmed in the rescuer's armpits.

3 If warm water (no hotter than 40°C) is available, immerse the affected part. The area should then be covered with a sterile dressing.

microscope. The entire process takes about 20 minutes. Information about the sample is then conveyed to the operating theatre and the surgeon decides what action is needed.

Frozen shoulder

Stiffness and pain in the *shoulder*, making normal movement of the joint impossible. In severe cases, the shoulder may be completely rigid and pain may be intense.

Frozen shoulder is caused by inflammation and thickening of the lining of the capsule in which the joint is contained. The problem usually develops for no known reason, but in some cases it follows a minor injury to the shoulder, a *stroke*, chronic *bronchitis*, or *angina pectoris*.

The condition mainly affects middle-aged people, and there is a higher-than-average incidence among people with *diabetes mellitus*.

TREATMENT
Moderate symptoms can be eased by exercise and by taking *analgesic drugs* (painkillers) and *nonsteroidal anti-inflammatory drugs*, and by applying *ice-packs* to the shoulder or using a heat lamp. In severe cases, injections of *corticosteroid drugs* into the joint may be required to relieve pain. Manipulation of the joint under a general anaesthetic can also restore mobility, but carries the risk of initially increasing pain in the joint.

Whatever the severity and treatment, recovery is usually slow.

Frusemide

A *diuretic drug* commonly used to treat *oedema* (fluid retention) and *hypertension* (high blood pressure). When given by injection, frusemide has a rapid effect. It is therefore often used in emergencies to treat *pulmonary oedema* (fluid in the lungs).

Frustration

A deep feeling of discontent and tension because of unresolved problems, unfulfilled needs, or because the path to a goal is blocked. In a person who is mentally healthy, frustration can be dealt with in a socially acceptable way. In less well-adapted people, it may lead to *regression* (childlike behaviour), *aggression*, or *depression*.

FSH

Abbreviation for *follicle-stimulating hormone*, a *gonadotrophin hormone* (one that stimulates the gonads—the ovaries and testes) produced by the anterior part of the pituitary gland.

Fugue

An episode of altered consciousness in which a person apparently purposefully wanders away from home or work and, in some cases, adopts a new identity. When the fugue ends, the affected person has no recollection of what has occurred.

Fugues may last for hours or days. During a short fugue, the sufferer may be confused and agitated. During a longer fugue, behaviour may appear normal but there may be accompanying symptoms, such as hallucinations, feeling unreal, or an unstable mood.

Fugues are uncommon. Causes include *dissociative disorders*, *temporal lobe epilepsy*, *depression*, *head injury*, and *dementia*. (See also *Amnesia*.)

Fulminant

A medical term used to describe a disorder that develops and progresses suddenly and with great severity. The term is usually applied to an infection that has spread rapidly through the bloodstream to affect several organs and cause a high fever.

The term may also be applied to types of arthritis in which many joints are painful and stiff and deformities appear soon after the onset of symptoms, or to a cancer that has spread rapidly to cause dramatic weight loss and debility.

Fumes

See *Pollution*.

Functional disorders

A term for illnesses in which there is no evidence of organic disturbance even though physical performance is impaired.

Fungal infections

Diseases of the skin or other organs caused by the multiplication and spread of *fungi*. Fungal infections, also known as mycoses, range from the mild and unnoticed to the severe and sometimes fatal. (In addition to infections, fungi can also cause allergic disorders, such as *asthma* and allergic *alveolitis*.)

CAUSES
Some fungi are harmlessly present all the time in areas of the body such as the mouth, skin, intestines, and vagina, but are prevented from multiplying through competition from bacteria. Other fungi are dealt with by the body's *immune system* (defences against infection).

Fungal infections are more common and serious in people who are taking long-term *antibiotic drugs* (which destroy the bacterial competition) and in those who are taking *corticosteroid drugs* or taking *immunosuppressant drugs* (used to suppress the immune system). Fungal infections more commonly affect people with an immune deficiency disorder, such as *AIDS*. Such infections are described as *opportunistic infections* because they take advantage of the victim's lowered defences. Some fungal infections are also more common in people with *diabetes mellitus*.

Fungi that cause skin infections thrive in warm, moist conditions, such as may occur between the toes and in the genital area.

TYPES
Fungal infections can be broadly classified into superficial infections (those that affect the skin, hair, nails, genital organs, and the inside of the mouth); subcutaneous infections (those beneath the skin); and "deep" infections (those affecting internal organs, such as the lungs or, more rarely, the liver, bones, lymph nodes, brain, heart, or urinary tract).

SUPERFICIAL INFECTIONS The main superficial fungal infections are *candidiasis* (thrush) and *tinea* (including ringworm and athlete's foot), both of which are very common. Candidiasis is caused by the yeast CANDIDA ALBICANS and usually affects the genitals or inside of the mouth. Tinea affects external areas of the body.

SUBCUTANEOUS INFECTIONS These are rare. The most common is called *sporotrichosis* and may follow contamination of a scratch. Most other conditions of this type occur mainly in tropical countries, the most important being *mycetoma* (sometimes called Madura foot).

DEEP INFECTIONS These are rare or uncommon (although becoming more common), but can be a serious threat to people who have an immune deficiency disorder or who are taking immunosuppressant drugs. Fungal infections of this sort include *aspergillosis*, *histoplasmosis*, *cryptococcosis*, and *blastomycosis*, all caused by different fungi. The fungal spores enter the body by inhalation into the lungs. Candidiasis can also spread from its usual sites to infect the oesophagus, urinary tract, and numerous other internal sites.

Fungi

Simple parasitic life-forms including moulds, mildews, yeasts, mushrooms, and toadstools. There are more

FUNGAL DISEASES

The skin, genitals, and nails are common sites of fungal infection. Examples of types include *tinea* (ringworm) and *candidiasis* (thrush). Fungi also (rarely) infect the lungs and other internal organs to cause a more serious disease. They may also cause allergic lung disease, such as farmers' lung.

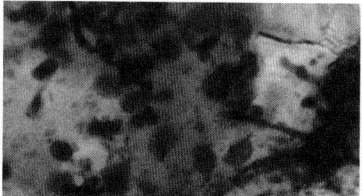

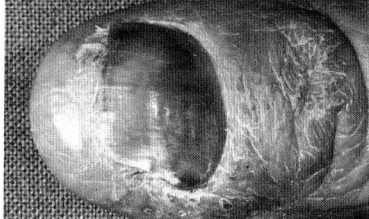

Fungal nail infection
This condition most often affects people whose hands are frequently immersed in water. It is liable to last for years. Antifungal medications benefit some people.

Colony of fungal cells
The microscope photograph (left) shows a colony of yeast cells in a skin fragment.

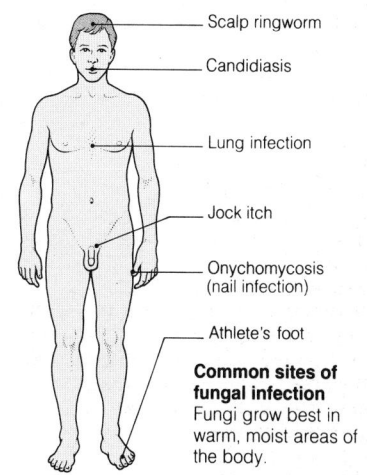

Scalp ringworm
Candidiasis
Lung infection
Jock itch
Onychomycosis (nail infection)
Athlete's foot

Common sites of fungal infection
Fungi grow best in warm, moist areas of the body.

F

FUNGAL GROWTH

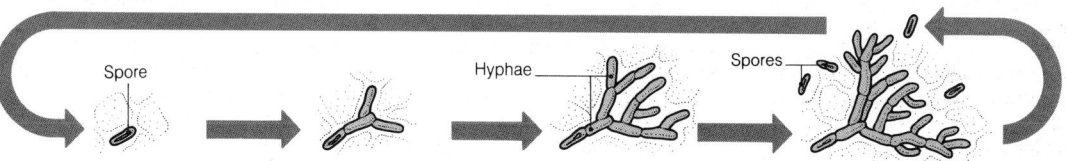

Spore   Hyphae   Spores

1 Many fungal colonies originate from spores that have been carried in the air and have settled at a suitable site for growth.

2 If nutrients are available and other conditions (such as temperature) are favourable, a spore starts to divide.

3 The cells of many fungi divide to form a network consisting of branched chains of tubular filaments called hyphae.

4 Eventually a colony may start forming its own spores. They may be carried to new sites to set up new growths.

than 100,000 different species of fungi worldwide. Of these, most are either harmless or positively beneficial to human health, including various yeasts used in baking and brewing, some moulds that are the source of certain *antibiotic drugs*, and various edible mushrooms and truffles that are considered gastronomic delicacies in many parts of the world. There are, however, also a number of fungi that can cause sometimes fatal disease and illness in humans. The study of fungi and fungal diseases is known as mycology.

Some fungi, notably the yeasts, occur as colonies of individual cells. In others, the cells divide to form chains of tubular filaments called hyphae, which are organized into a complex network called a mycelium. With some soil-living fungi, parts of the mycelium form into large fruiting bodies, seen as mushrooms or toadstools. Many fungi form minute bodies called spores, which are like seeds. These spores can be carried in the air and, if they settle in a suitable location with nutrients available, they

divide to form a new mycelium; the moulds that eventually form on exposed food are a type of mycelium. Fungal spores are ever-present in the air and soil.

FUNGI AND DISEASE
Fungi can cause illness and disease in a variety of ways.

First, the fruiting bodies of some soil-living fungi contain toxins that can produce direct poisoning if eaten (see *Mushroom poisoning*).

Second, certain fungi that infect food crops produce dangerous toxins that can cause a type of food poisoning if contaminated food is eaten. The best known of these are a fungus that infects rye and other cereals and produces a toxin called *ergot*, and another that grows on peanuts and produces the poison *aflatoxin*. Ergot poisoning is rare today, but chronic aflatoxin poisoning from eating mouldy peanuts is a suspected cause of liver cancer in some regions of Africa.

Third, the inhaled spores of some fungi can cause a persistent allergic reaction in the lungs, known as allergic *alveolitis*. Farmers' lung, caused by

spores from mouldy hay, is an example of such a reaction. Fungal spores are also sometimes responsible for other allergic disorders such as *asthma* and allergic *rhinitis* (hay fever).

Fourth, some fungi are able to invade and form colonies within the lungs, in the skin, beneath the skin, or sometimes in various tissues throughout the body, leading to conditions ranging from mild skin irritation to severe, even fatal, widespread infection and illness (see *Fungal infections*).

Fungicidal
A term describing an ability to kill *fungi*. (See *Antifungal drugs*.)

Funny-bone
Popular term for the small area at the back of the *elbow* where the ulnar nerve passes over a prominence of the humerus (upper-arm bone). A blow to the nerve causes acute pain, numbness, and a tingling sensation in the forearm and hand.

Furuncle
Another name for a *boil*.

G

G6PD deficiency

An inherited disorder that affects the chemistry of red blood cells, making them prone to damage by infectious illness or certain drugs or foods.

CAUSES AND INCIDENCE

G6PD deficiency is caused by the production within red blood cells of abnormal molecules of an enzyme (a type of protein) called glucose-6-phosphate dehydrogenase. Because the molecules of this substance are defective, they cannot carry out their normal function, which is to help in a chemical process that protects the cells from damage.

The disorder is the result of an abnormality in the affected person's genetic material and is inherited in an X-linked recessive pattern (see *Genetic disorders*). This means that most of those affected are male, but women may carry the defective gene in a hidden form and pass it on to some of their sons. The disorder is very rare in people of northern European stock but affects as many as 15 per cent of southern Europeans and black males.

The drugs that can precipitate haemolysis (red cell destruction) in affected people are listed in the accompanying table. In one form of G6PD deficiency, known as *favism*, affected people are extremely sensitive to a chemical in broad beans, which they must avoid eating.

SYMPTOMS

A few days after taking a precipitating drug or food, or during the course of an infectious illness, a person with G6PD deficiency develops symptoms of haemolytic *anaemia* (such as jaundice, fatigue, headaches, shortness of breath on exertion, and sometimes darkening of the urine due to the destruction of red blood cells).

DIAGNOSIS AND TREATMENT

The presence of G6PD deficiency can be established by a blood test. The deficiency cannot be treated but any episode of haemolytic anaemia caused by a drug can be halted by stopping use of the drug. Full recovery then takes place within a few days.

Anyone with a history of G6PD deficiency in the family should ask for a screening test before taking any of the incriminated drugs. If the test result is positive, these drugs should be avoided. Anyone known to have the condition should also seek prompt treatment for any infectious illness to prevent a haemolytic crisis.

GABA

Common abbreviation for gamma-aminobutyric acid, a *neurotransmitter* (chemical released from nerve endings that conveys messages within the nervous system). GABA controls the flow of nerve impulses by blocking the release of other neurotransmitters (e.g. *noradrenaline* and *dopamine*) that stimulate nerve activity. The activity of GABA is increased by *benzodiazepine drugs* and by *anticonvulsant drugs*.

It has been suggested that people with *Huntington's disease* (a hereditary disease characterized by mental handicap and involuntary movements) have insufficient GABA-producing nerve cells in the brain centres that coordinate movement.

Gait

The style or manner of *walking*. Some neuromuscular disorders are evaluated on the basis of altered gait.

Galactorrhoea

Spontaneous, persistent production of milk by a woman who is not pregnant or lactating (producing milk after childbirth), or, very rarely, production of milk by a man.

CAUSES

Lactation is initiated by a rise in the level of *prolactin* (a hormone produced by the pituitary gland). Galactorrhoea is caused by an excessive amount of prolactin being secreted as a result of a *pituitary tumour* or as a result of other endocrine diseases, such as *hypothyroidism*. Certain *antipsychotic drugs* (such as chlorpromazine) and some

brain diseases (for example, *meningitis*) may be associated with increased prolactin production. However, in about 50 per cent of cases, no cause can be found.

SYMPTOMS AND SIGNS

The breast secretion is obviously milk-like. If it is of any other colour or bloodstained, another cause (such as a breast tumour) should be suspected. Excessive levels of prolactin may also adversely affect the ovaries, causing *amenorrhoea* (absence of menstrual periods) or *infertility*. If the underlying cause is a pituitary tumour, the symptoms may include headache and visual disturbances.

TREATMENT

Surgery or *radiotherapy* may be required if there is a pituitary tumour, but the symptoms are often controlled and the size of the tumour decreased by treatment with *bromocriptine*.

In addition to treating the underlying cause, hormone or drug therapy may be used to suppress prolactin and thus prevent milk production. Bromocriptine, which suppresses prolactin production, can successfully treat galactorrhoea when the cause is unknown, and may also allow the subsequent return of periods and fertility.

Galactosaemia

An extremely rare inability of the body's biochemical system to change galactose (a sugar derived from the milk sugar lactose) into glucose because of the absence of an enzyme in the liver. Galactosaemia is caused by an autosomal recessive genetic defect (see *Genetic disorders*).

SYMPTOMS

Galactosaemia causes no symptoms at birth, but jaundice, diarrhoea, and vomiting soon develop and the baby fails to gain weight. If untreated, the condition results in liver disease, *cataract* (opacity in the lens of the eye), and *mental handicap*.

DRUGS TO BE AVOIDED BY PEOPLE WITH G6PD DEFICIENCY

Class	Drugs to avoid
Antimalarial drugs	Primaquine, chloroquine, quinine*, dapsone
Antibacterial and antibiotic drugs	Nitrofurantoin, sulphonamides (such as co-trimoxazole and sulphacetamide), chloramphenicol*, nalidixic acid
Analgesics (painkillers)	Aspirin*
Miscellaneous	Vitamin K (water-soluble form), probenecid, quinidine*

*These drugs do not usually cause problems in the type of G6PD deficiency that affects black people.

DIAGNOSIS AND TREATMENT

The diagnosis is confirmed by urine and blood tests. Feeding with a special lactose-free milk leads to dramatic improvement; normal milk must be avoided throughout life.

Gallbladder

A small, pear-shaped sac situated underneath the liver, to which it is attached by fibrous tissue. *Bile* produced by the liver passes to the gallbladder by means of a small tube, the cystic duct. This duct branches off from the bile duct, which carries bile from the liver to the duodenum.

Within the gallbladder, bile is stored and concentrated (by absorption of its water content through the gallbladder walls). When food passes from the stomach to the duodenum, secretin and cholecystokinin (gastrointestinal hormones) cause the gallbladder to contract and expel bile into the duodenum, where the bile emulsifies fats contained in the food. (See also *Biliary system.*)

Gallbladder cancer

A rare cancer of unknown cause, occurring mainly in old age. It usually occurs in gallbladders with *gallstones,* but affects only a minute number of gallstone sufferers. The incidence of this cancer is less than three new cases per 100,000 population per year.

The cancer may cause *jaundice* and tenderness in the upper right abdomen but is sometimes symptomless. It is diagnosed by *ultrasound scanning;* occasionally, the cancer is discovered during surgery on the gallbladder.

Cancer of the gallbladder is treated by removal of as much of the tumour as possible. The cancer has often invaded the liver by the time it is detected, making the outlook poor.

Gallium

A metallic element whose radioactive form is used in *radionuclide scanning* (a technique for obtaining images of internal organs). Gallium is injected into the bloodstream and, about 72 hours later, scanning is performed.

ANATOMY OF THE GALLBLADDER

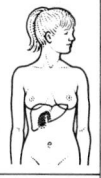

A small, muscular sac that lies under the liver. The gallbladder expels bile via the common bile duct into the duodenum.

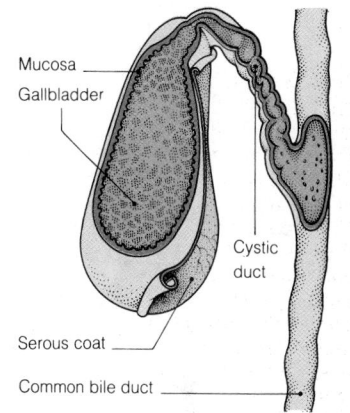

Mucosa
Gallbladder
Cystic duct
Serous coat
Common bile duct

G

DISORDERS OF THE GALLBLADDER

The gallbladder rarely causes problems in childhood or early adulthood but, from middle age onwards, the increasing occurrence of gallstones can sometimes give rise to symptoms.

Because the digestive system can function normally without a gallbladder, its removal has little known long-term effect.

CONGENITAL AND GENETIC DEFECTS

Abnormalities present from birth may include no gallbladder, an oversized gallbladder, or two gallbladders; these defects rarely cause problems.

METABOLIC DISORDERS

The principal gallbladder disorder, with which most other problems are associated, is the formation of *gallstones.* Gallstones are common, but only about 20 per cent of people with gallstones have symptoms or complications. Attempts by the gallbladder to expel the stone or stones can cause severe *biliary colic* (abdominal pain). There are three main types of gallstones: cholesterol gallstones, pigment gallstones, and mixed gallstones. The great majority are cholesterol or mixed gallstones, and women are affected up to four times as often as men, depending on their age and nationality. Every year

thousands of people develop gallstones. Many people carry "silent" gallstones, which produce no symptoms.

INFECTION AND INFLAMMATION

If a gallstone becomes stuck in the outlet from the gallbladder, the trapped bile may irritate and inflame the gallbladder walls and the bile itself may become infected. This is called acute *cholecystitis.* The first symptom may be biliary colic, which is followed by fever and abdominal tenderness.

Repeated attacks of biliary colic and acute cholecystitis can lead to chronic cholecystitis, in which the gallbladder becomes shrunken and thick-walled and ceases to function. Rarely, the gallbladder may become inflamed without the presence of gallstones —a condition that is called acalculous cholecystitis.

Occasionally, cholecystitis proceeds to a condition in which the gallbladder fills with pus, called *empyema* of the gallbladder. This can cause a high fever and severe abdominal pain.

TUMOURS

Gallbladders harbouring *gallbladder cancer* usually contain gallstones. However, this cancer is extremely uncommon compared to the high prevalence of gallstones.

OTHER DISORDERS

In rare cases where a gallbladder is empty when a stone obstructs its outlet, it may fill with mucus secreted by the gallbladder walls, resulting in a distended, mucus-filled gallbladder known as a *mucocele.*

INVESTIGATION

Gallbladder problems are investigated by physical examination and techniques such as *ultrasound scanning, radionuclide scanning,* or *cholecystography* (X-rays of the gallbladder after it has been filled with radiopaque substance). Blood tests may also be carried out.

Gallium tends to accumulate in tumours and pus; its main uses in scanning are to detect malignant diseases, such as *Hodgkin's disease,* and abscesses or areas of *osteomyelitis.*

Gallstones

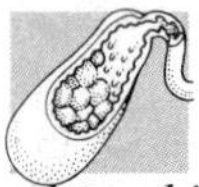

Round or oval, smooth or faceted lumps of solid matter found in the *gallbladder* (the sac under the liver where bile is stored and concentrated). Gallstones are sometimes found in the bile ducts (which connect the gallbladder and liver to the duodenum). In these cases, the symptoms can be severe. There may be one to 10 or more stones, ranging in size from about 1 to 25 mm across. Gallstones composed principally of *cholesterol* are the most common type, but some contain a high content of bile pigments and other substances, such as calcium compounds.

CAUSES AND INCIDENCE

Gallstones develop when an upset occurs in the chemical composition of bile. This most commonly occurs when the liver either puts too much cholesterol into the bile (which occurs in obesity) or fails to put in enough of the detergent substances that normally keep cholesterol in solution.

Excess cholesterol in the bile may lead to the formation of solid cholesterol fragments, which may build up to form stones. In some cases, this process may be triggered by bacteria within the gallbladder. Fasting for long periods may help gallstones to develop by causing bile to stagnate in the gallbladder.

Gallstones are rare in childhood and become progressively more common with age. Up to four times as many women as men are affected, depending on their age and nationality; autopsies show that 20 per cent of all women have gallstones when they die.

Risk groups include overweight people and women who have had many children. Use of oral contraceptives may cause gallstones to form earlier than they would otherwise.

PREVENTION

People should avoid becoming overweight and should limit their consumption of sugar and fat. Some experts believe a high intake of fibre helps prevent gallstones and that drinking one alcoholic drink a day has a protective effect.

SYMPTOMS

Only about 20 per cent of gallstones cause symptoms or complications. Symptoms commonly begin only when a gallstone gets stuck in the duct leading from the gallbladder. This causes *biliary colic* (intense pain in the upper right side of the abdomen or between the shoulderblades) and may make the sufferer feel sick and possibly vomit. Indigestion made worse by fatty foods often seems to be associated with gallstones. Flatulence is common. Other possible complications include *cholecystitis* (inflammation of the gallbladder) and *bile duct obstruction* leading to jaundice.

DIAGNOSIS AND TREATMENT

Ultrasound scanning can detect 95 per cent of gallstones and is therefore the first test to be performed. An older and slightly less sensitive method is X-ray oral *cholecystography,* which utilizes an iodine-containing dye taken by mouth. Blood tests may also be performed. If the doctor suspects that the gallstones may have escaped into the bile ducts, *cholangiography* may be carried out.

Stones that are not causing symptoms are usually left alone, since they are unlikely to cause problems. When symptoms do occur, the choice of treatment depends on factors such as the severity of the symptoms and the patient's age and general health.

The gallbladder and stones may be removed by *cholecystectomy,* which is now usually performed laparoscopically (see *Minimally invasive surgery*); recovery is much quicker than after the conventional, open operation. In some cases, ultrasonic shock waves (see *Lithotripsy*) are used to shatter stones, after which the fragments pass into the bowel and cause no further problems. Treatment with drugs such as *chenodeoxycholic acid* or *ursodeoxycholic acid* can slowly dissolve stones, but may cause side-effects such as diarrhoea; also, stones tend to recur when treatment is stopped.

Gambling, pathological

Chronic inability to resist impulses to gamble, resulting in personal or social problems. Most gamblers can stop at a given point; pathological or "compulsive" gamblers seem unable to control the amount they spend and are unable to stop even when they continue to lose. The urge to gamble is so great that tension can be relieved only by more gambling. Family problems, bankruptcy, and crime may be the consequences.

Gamma-globulin

A substance prepared from human blood that contains *antibodies* against most common infections. (See *Immunoglobulin injections.*)

Ganglion

A group of nerve cells that have a common function; the spinal nerves have ganglia close to their roots, and the *basal ganglia* in the brain are concerned with the control of muscular movements.

The term ganglion is also used to describe a cystic swelling associated with the sheath of a *tendon.* It is a common condition and usually occurs on the wrist, although a finger or foot may sometimes be affected. The cyst, which contains thick fluid derived from the synovial fluid that lubricates tendons and joints, can vary from the size of a small pea to, rarely, the size of a golf ball.

A ganglion may disappear spontaneously; if it does not, treatment is usually necessary only if the cyst is painful or unsightly. The fluid may be sucked out with a needle and syringe, but ganglions treated in this way commonly recur. The best treatment is surgical removal, after which ganglions rarely occur.

Gangrene

Death of tissue, usually as a result of loss of blood supply. Gangrene can affect a small area of skin, but can also affect, for example, a finger or even a substantial portion of a limb.

SYMPTOMS

Pain is felt in the dying tissues, but once they are dead they become numb. The affected skin and underlying tissue turn black. Bacterial infection may develop, causing the gangrene to spread and give off an unpleasant smell. There may be redness, swelling, and oozing pus around the blackened area.

There are two types of gangrene (dry and wet). In dry gangrene there is usually no bacterial infection; the deprived area dies because its blood

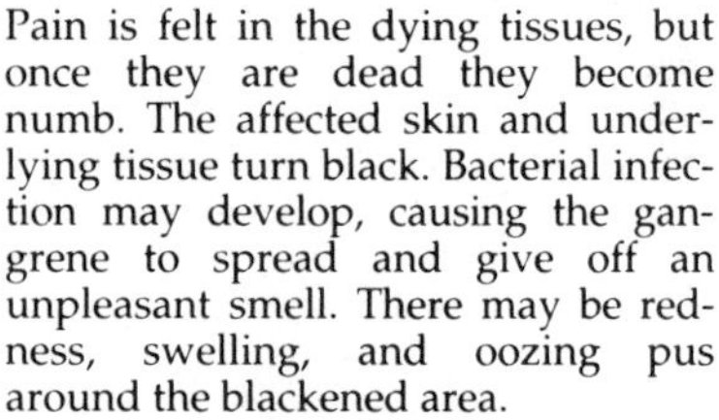

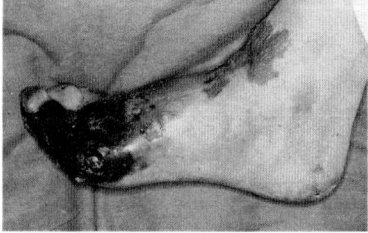

Gangrene of the foot
This photograph shows a foot with an extensive area of dead tissue, with blackening of the overlying skin.

supply is blocked. This type of gangrene does not spread to other tissues. It may be caused by *arteriosclerosis, diabetes mellitus, thrombosis,* an *embolism,* or *frostbite.* Wet gangrene develops when dry gangrene or a wound becomes infected by bacteria. A particularly virulent type—known as gas gangrene—is caused by a dangerous strain of bacteria that destroys muscles and produces a foul-smelling gas. Gas gangrene has caused millions of deaths in war.

TREATMENT
Treatment of dry gangrene consists of improving circulation to the affected body part before it is too late. If the tissue becomes infected, the patient is given *antibiotic drugs* to prevent wet gangrene from setting in.

If wet gangrene is diagnosed, *amputation* of the affected part is unavoidable. Usually, some of the adjacent living tissue must be removed as well.

Ganser's syndrome
A rare, *factitious disorder* in which a person seeks, consciously or unconsciously, to mislead others regarding his or her mental state. Ganser's syndrome occurs most often in prisoners. A characteristic of the disorder is the giving of "approximate answers" (e.g. twice two equals five); the choice of an answer near the correct one suggests that the person knows the real response. The sufferer also displays symptoms that simulate *psychosis,* such as episodes of intense agitation or stupor.

Gardnerella vaginalis
A bacterium commonly found in the vaginal discharge of women with non-specific *vaginitis.*

Gargle
A liquid preparation to wash and freshen the mouth and throat, usually not meant to be swallowed. Gargles may contain mouth fresheners, flavourings, *antiseptics,* or local anaesthetics. Those containing antiseptics and local anaesthetics relieve the irritation associated with sore throats, but do not cure the underlying cause. The home remedy of gargling with salt water is usually equally effective.

Gas-and-air
A mixture of *nitrous oxide* and *oxygen,* used chiefly as an *analgesic drug* (painkiller) during *childbirth.* It is usually available in premixed cylinders and may be self-administered, through a gas mask, as required.

Gastrectomy
Removal of the whole stomach (total gastrectomy) or, more commonly, a part of the stomach (partial gastrectomy). Gastrectomy is a major operation requiring hospitalization and extensive post-operative care.

WHY IT IS DONE
Total gastrectomy is a rare operation used to treat some *stomach cancers.* Partial gastrectomy is fairly common. It is usually performed to deal with *peptic ulcers* (ulcers of the stomach or duodenum), especially ulcers that have failed to heal after changes in diet or drug treatment, ulcers that bleed very badly or perforate (make a hole in) the stomach or duodenal wall. In the treatment of duodenal ulcers, partial gastrectomy may be combined with *vagotomy* (cutting of the nerves to the acid-secreting part of the stomach) to prevent more ulcers. Partial gastrectomy is sometimes performed to treat cancers located near the stomach's outlet.

HOW IT IS DONE
A general anaesthetic is given and the stomach emptied by means of a *nasogastric tube* (a tube passed through the nose down the oesophagus into the stomach). Different gastrectomy procedures are shown in the illustrated box below.

RECOVERY PERIOD
After the operation, the nasogastric tube is left in position to allow digestive secretions to drain. When the volume of these secretions diminishes and normal *peristalsis* (the rhythmic contractions that force food through the digestive system) returns, the patient is given small amounts of water. If these do not cause abdominal

---

TYPES OF GASTRECTOMY

There are several different types of gastrectomy operations. In total gastrectomy, the whole stomach is removed; in partial gastrectomy, between one half and two thirds of the stomach is removed. There are two common types of partial gastrectomy operation—the Billroth I and the Billroth II.

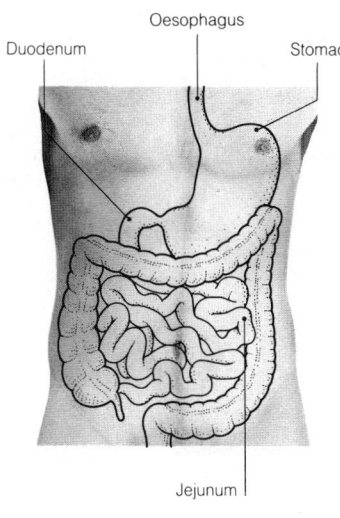

Oesophagus
Duodenum
Stomach
Jejunum

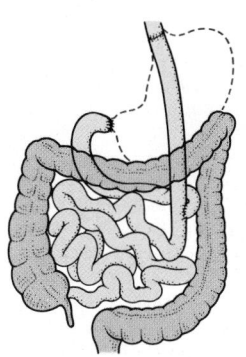

Total gastrectomy
The whole stomach is removed and the oesophagus is joined directly to the jejunum (the middle section of the small intestine).

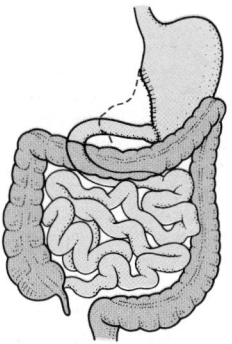

Billroth I gastrectomy
The remaining part of the stomach is joined to the duodenum (the first part of the small intestine).

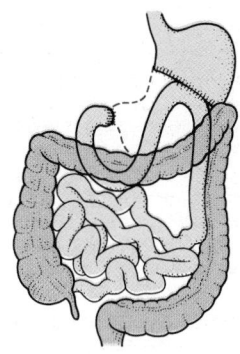

Billroth II gastrectomy
The surgeon performs a *gastroenterostomy* (a procedure in which the stomach is joined to the jejunum) and seals the end of the duodenum to form a blind loop.

pain or nausea, the nasogastric tube is removed. The intake of fluids is gradually increased and, within a few days, a light diet can be started.

COMPLICATIONS

Only about 10 per cent of patients suffer complications requiring further treatment after partial gastrectomy. There is a higher risk of complications after total gastrectomy.

Because removal of the stomach disturbs normal digestion, post-gastrectomy syndromes (side-effects after gastric surgery) develop in some patients. The most troublesome are fullness and discomfort after meals; formation of an ulcer at the new junction between stomach and small intestine; regurgitation of bile, which may lead to *gastritis* (inflammation of the stomach), *oesophagitis* (inflammation of the oesophagus), and vomiting of bile; diarrhoea; and *dumping syndrome* (sweating, nausea, dizziness, and weakness felt soon after eating a meal because food leaves the stomach too quickly). These side-effects usually disappear in time, but diet and drug treatment or another operation may be necessary.

Other complications include *malabsorption* (a reduced ability to absorb food, minerals, and vitamins), which may lead to *anaemia* or *osteoporosis* (thinned bones). After total gastrectomy, patients cannot absorb vitamin B_{12} and are therefore given monthly injections for the rest of their lives.

Gastric erosion

A break in the surface layer (mucosa) of the membrane lining the stomach. If a break extends deeper than this layer, it is called a gastric ulcer (see *Peptic ulcer*). Gastric erosion occurs in some cases of *gastritis* (inflammation of the stomach lining).

CAUSES AND SYMPTOMS

The causes of gastric erosions are not clear, but many cases are the result of the ingestion of *alcohol, iron tablets, aspirin,* or other *nonsteroidal anti-inflammatory drugs* (NSAIDs), such as indomethacin or naproxen. The stress of serious illness, such as *septicaemia* or *kidney failure,* or of *burns* may bring on a gastric erosion.

Often there are no symptoms, although erosions may bleed, resulting in *vomiting blood* or *melaena* (black faeces containing blood). Slight but persistent blood loss may eventually cause *anaemia.*

DIAGNOSIS AND TREATMENT

Gastric erosions are diagnosed by *gastroscopy* (examination of the stom-

ach by means of a flexible viewing instrument), which reveals small bleeding points in the stomach lining.

Gastric erosions usually heal completely in a few days when treated with *antacid drugs* and with *ulcer-healing drugs,* such as cimetidine, ranitidine, or famotidine.

Gastric ulcer

A raw area in the wall of the stomach caused by a breach of its inner surface lining. (See *Peptic ulcer.*)

Gastritis

Inflammation of the mucous membrane that lines the stomach. The illness may be acute, occurring as a sudden attack, or chronic, developing gradually over a long period.

CAUSES

Acute gastritis may be caused by irritation of the stomach lining by a drug, most commonly *aspirin*; by *alcohol*; by infection of the stomach by a bacterium of the HELICOBACTER genus; or by extreme physical stress such as *head injury*, severe *burns*, or the development of *liver failure.*

Chronic gastritis may be caused by prolonged irritation of the stomach by alcohol, *tobacco-smoking,* or *bile*; by an *autoimmune disorder* that damages the stomach lining (see *Anaemia, megaloblastic*); or by degeneration of the stomach lining with age.

SYMPTOMS

Gastritis produces similar symptoms to a gastric ulcer, with which it may be confused. Symptoms include discomfort in the upper abdomen (often aggravated by eating), nausea, and vomiting. In acute gastritis, the faeces may be blackened by blood lost from the stomach; in chronic gastritis, slow blood loss may cause anaemia (see *Anaemia, iron-deficiency*), resulting in symptoms such as pallor, tiredness, and breathlessness.

DIAGNOSIS

The diagnosis is made using *gastroscopy* (direct examination of the stomach lining through a flexible viewing instrument called a gastroscope). A stomach *biopsy* (removal of a sample of tissue for analysis) may be performed at the same time, using an attachment at the end of the gastroscope. Microscopic examination of the sample indicates the type of inflammation. The correlation between the microscopic findings and the symptoms is not always clear.

TREATMENT

A person with gastritis should take *paracetamol* and not *aspirin* for pain

relief, should avoid alcohol, and should not smoke. *Ulcer-healing drugs,* especially *bismuth* preparations, may help heal the inflamed stomach lining.

Gastroenteritis

Inflammation of the stomach and intestines, often causing sudden and sometimes violent upsets. The illness does not usually last for more than two or three days and the sufferer tends to recover without any specific treatment other than replacement of lost fluid and salt. *Dysentery, typhoid fever, cholera, food poisoning,* and *travellers' diarrhoea*—as well as many milder stomach upsets—are all forms of gastroenteritis.

CAUSES AND INCIDENCE

Gastroenteritis is an extremely common cause of mild illness in developed countries and a major cause of death in some developing ones, especially among infants.

The illness may be caused by any of a variety of bacteria, bacterial toxins, viruses, and other small organisms that have contaminated food or water supplies. There are also a number of noninfectious causes of gastroenteritis—for example, *food intolerance,* very spicy foods, certain irritant drugs and poisons, and excessive intake of alcohol. In many people, *antibiotic drugs* cause symptoms similar to those of gastroenteritis because the drugs can upset the balance of bacteria that occur naturally in the intestines.

SYMPTOMS

The onset and severity of symptoms depends on the type and concentrations of the microorganisms, food, or toxic substance causing the illness. Appetite loss, nausea, vomiting, cramps, and diarrhoea are the symptoms; these may come on gradually, but more often appear suddenly. The combination of symptoms may be so mild that they cause little disruption to daily routine, or the attack may be so severe that *dehydration, shock,* and collapse occur. Severe symptoms are most likely in babies and the elderly.

DIAGNOSIS

In mild attacks, no detailed inquiries or investigations are usually made, but in more serious cases the doctor may try to find out if other people have been affected and may ask about food that has been eaten and any recent travel abroad.

TREATMENT AND OUTLOOK

Mild cases are treated at home. The affected person should rest, preferably in bed, and take plenty of fluids in frequent small amounts. If much fluid is being lost by vomiting and diarrhoea, *rehydration therapy* to replace lost fluids is necessary. Ready-prepared salt and glucose rehydration mixtures can be obtained from chemists. If commercial preparations are not available, the patient may be given a solution of one teaspoon of salt and eight teaspoons of sugar in a litre of water. No solid food should be eaten until symptoms subside.

If the illness is severe, hospital treatment may be necessary. Fluids may be given by *intravenous infusion* to replace the vital body salts lost by vomiting and diarrhoea. After the acute phase, water and then other clear fluids are given by mouth; if these fluids do not cause further upset, a bland diet is introduced. Treatment with *antibiotic drugs* is reserved for specific bacterial infections such as typhoid fever.

In most cases the illness subsides gradually without any special measures; recovery is usually complete with no complications.

PREVENTION
Care taken in food preparation and hygiene can substantially reduce the chances of gastroenteritis (see *Food poisoning; Food-borne infection*). Some protection against typhoid fever and cholera can be acquired by vaccination before travelling to countries where these diseases occur. Avoidance of substances known to cause upset will minimize noninfectious attacks.

Those caring for a person with the symptoms of gastroenteritis should be scrupulous about personal hygiene to prevent the illness from spreading.

Gastroenterology

The study of the *digestive system* and the diseases and disorders affecting it. The major organs involved include the mouth, oesophagus, stomach, duodenum, small intestine, colon, and rectum. Diseases of the liver, gallbladder, and pancreas are also included in this specialty.

A specialist in this branch of medicine is called a gastroenterologist. The work of the gastroenterologist has been revolutionized in recent years by the development of fibre-optic *endoscopes*. Much of the gastrointestinal tract can now be visualized directly by these instruments and samples can be taken for laboratory examination.

The gastroenterologist, whenever possible, treats patients by advising on diet and lifestyle and/or by prescribing medication; if necessary, the gastroenterologist refers patients for surgical treatment.

Gastroenterostomy

A surgically created connection between the stomach and the jejunum (the middle two thirds of the small intestine). Gastroenterostomy is occasionally combined with partial *gastrectomy* (removal of the lower part of the stomach).

WHY IT IS DONE
The operation was formerly performed as part of the treatment of a duodenal ulcer (see *Peptic ulcer*) but is now rare. The purpose of gastroenterostomy is to allow food to pass directly from the stomach to the small intestine, thereby avoiding faulty emptying arising as a complication of *vagotomy*, or permitting a bypass around a duodenum that is scarred and obstructed.

Gastrointestinal hormones

A group of hormones released from specialized endocrine cells in the stomach, pancreas, and intestine that controls various functions of the digestive organs. Gastrin, secretin, and cholecystokinin are probably the best documented of these hormones. (See illustrated box.)

Other gastrointestinal hormones released by the intestine include motilin, neurotensin, and enteroglucagon; their precise functions are still being studied.

DISORDERS
Disorders produced by gastrointestinal hormones are relatively rare. The most notable example is a tumour of gastrin-secreting cells in the pancreas or the wall of the intestine, a condition called *Zollinger-Ellison syndrome*.

Gastrointestinal tract

The part of the *digestive system* that consists of the *mouth, oesophagus, stomach,* and *intestine*; it excludes the liver, gallbladder, and pancreas.

Gastroscopy

Examination of the lining of the oesophagus, stomach, and duodenum (the first part of the small intestine) by means of a type of *endoscope* (a long, flexible viewing instrument) called a gastroscope or oesophago-gastroduodenscope, inserted through the mouth.

WHY IT IS DONE
Gastroscopy is used to investigate symptoms, such as severe pain in the upper abdomen or bleeding from the upper gastrointestinal tract, and to look for disorders of the oesophagus, stomach, and duodenum. The procedure may also be used to assess how these disorders are responding to treatment. Gastroscopy is used to identify the source of bleeding and sometimes to treat bleeding sites in

G

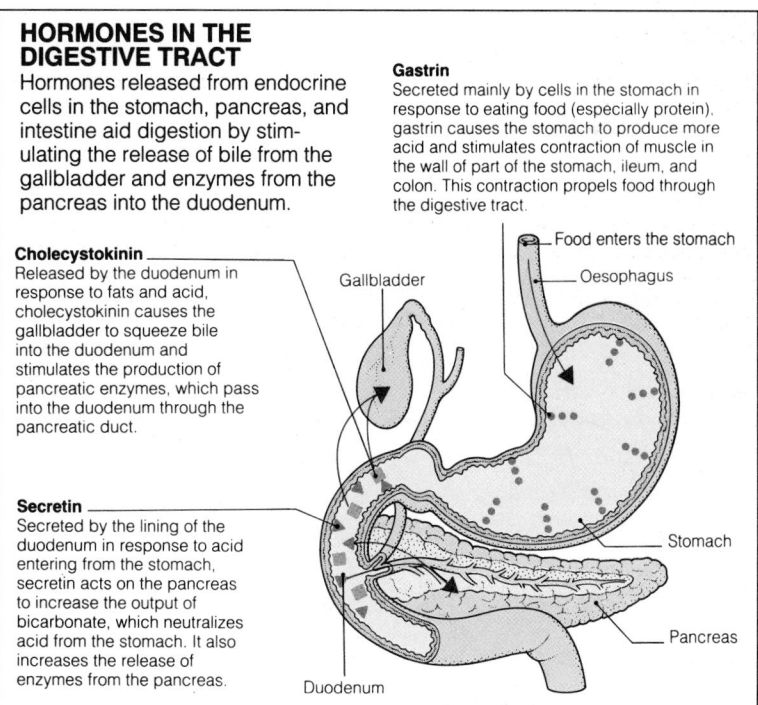

HORMONES IN THE DIGESTIVE TRACT

Hormones released from endocrine cells in the stomach, pancreas, and intestine aid digestion by stimulating the release of bile from the gallbladder and enzymes from the pancreas into the duodenum.

Cholecystokinin
Released by the duodenum in response to fats and acid, cholecystokinin causes the gallbladder to squeeze bile into the duodenum and stimulates the production of pancreatic enzymes, which pass into the duodenum through the pancreatic duct.

Secretin
Secreted by the lining of the duodenum in response to acid entering from the stomach, secretin acts on the pancreas to increase the output of bicarbonate, which neutralizes acid from the stomach. It also increases the release of enzymes from the pancreas.

Gastrin
Secreted mainly by cells in the stomach in response to eating food (especially protein), gastrin causes the stomach to produce more acid and stimulates contraction of muscle in the wall of part of the stomach, ileum, and colon. This contraction propels food through the digestive tract.

Food enters the stomach
Gallbladder
Oesophagus
Stomach
Pancreas
Duodenum

G

the oesophagus, the stomach, and the duodenum.

A video camera is often incorporated into the tip of the endoscope so that the stomach's interior may be viewed on a screen. Various attachments to the instrument enable the doctor to remove *biopsy* samples (small amounts of tissue for microscopic examination).

A gastroscope may be used for procedures such as injecting *oesophageal varices* (abnormally enlarged veins in the oesophagus) or *oesophageal dilatation* (stretching) of an *oesophageal stricture*. A gastroscope is also used to ease the passage of a gastric feeding tube through the skin (see *Gastrostomy*).

HOW IT IS DONE

The procedure is performed when the stomach is empty; patients should therefore fast for at least six hours beforehand. A *sedative drug* is usually given to relax the patient, and a local anaesthetic may be sprayed on to the back of the throat. A general anaesthetic may be used for particularly anxious patients or if elaborate investigations or treatments are required.

Diagnostic examinations usually last for five to 20 minutes. Some discomfort may be felt as the tube passes down the throat, which may be sore afterwards.

Complications from gastroscopy are rare. Most are caused by inhalation of vomit or adverse reactions to sedative drugs.

Gastrostomy

A surgically produced opening in the stomach, usually connecting the stomach to the outside so that a feeding tube can be placed in the stomach or passed into the small intestine.

Gastrostomy may be performed on people starving due to oesophageal cancer (see *Oesophagus, cancer of*) or unable to chew and swallow due to a *stroke* or other neurological disease. (See also *Feeding, artificial*.)

Gaucher's disease

A *genetic disorder* inherited as an autosomal recessive, in which the lack of an enzyme, glucocerebrosidase, leads to accumulation of a fatty substance, glucosylceramide, in the liver, spleen, bone marrow, and sometimes in the brain. Several types of the disease, of variable severity, are all now treatable by regular injections of the missing enzyme. This is, however, very expensive to produce.

Gauze

An absorbent, open-weave fabric, usually made of cotton. For medical purposes it is usually sterilized and sealed in a package.

Gauze is often used as a *dressing* for wounds, absorbing blood and other oozing fluids. It can be applied dry or can be immersed in an *antiseptic* fluid or cream; a bandage or adhesive tape is used to hold it in place. Gauze is usually not used to dress skin ulcers because it tends to stick to moist surfaces, and can dislodge new tissue when it is removed.

Surgeons sometimes insert pieces of gauze into wounds during surgery to soak up blood and keep the operation site clear.

Gavage

The process of feeding liquids through a *nasogastric tube* (one passed into the stomach through the nose). (See *Feeding, artificial*.)

Gavage also refers to hyperalimentation (treating a patient by excessive feeding beyond appetite requirements).

Gay bowel syndrome

A combination of conditions affecting the anus, rectum, and colon that occurs mainly, but not exclusively, in male homosexuals.

The conditions in gay bowel syndrome result from various types of sexual activity, such as penile-anal contact, oral-anal contact, and fisting (insertion of the fist into the rectum).

The syndrome includes noninfectious disorders, such as *haemorrhoids, polyps*, foreign bodies in the rectum, and injury to the anus and rectum. *Proctitis* (inflammation of the rectum) is common and there may also be *anal fistulas*, rectal abscesses, and rectal ulcers. Infections occurring in gay bowel syndrome include anal warts (see *Warts, genital*), *amoebiasis*, viral *hepatitis, gonorrhoea, syphilis, shigellosis*, and *lymphogranuloma venereum*.

Gemfibrozil

A drug that lowers the levels of fats (lipids) to reduce the risk of atherosclerosis, which leads to coronary heart disease and stroke. It is usually given to people with *hyperlipidaemia* only after a low fat diet has failed to reduce blood fat levels significantly. Gemfibrozil may cause nausea and diarrhoea, and should not be taken by persons with kidney or liver disease.

Gender identity

The inner feeling of maleness or femaleness. Gender identity is not necessarily the same as biological sex. It is fixed within the first two to three years of life and is reinforced during puberty; once established, it usually cannot be changed. Gender role is the public declaration of gender identity—that is, the image people present outwardly that confirms their inner feelings about their gender.

Gender identity problems occur when a person has persistent feelings of discomfort about his or her sexual identity. *Transsexualism* is the most common example of this problem.

Gene

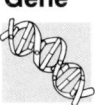

A unit of the material of heredity. In physical terms, a gene consists of a short section of the substance *DNA* (deoxyribonucleic acid) contained within the nucleus of a cell. In functional terms, a particular gene has a specific influence on the workings of a cell; the activities of the same gene in many different cells specify a particular physical or biochemical feature of the whole body (e.g. hair colour or a chemical step in the digestion of food).

Every human cell holds, within its nucleus, more than 50,000 different genes. Through the sum of their effects, genes influence and direct the development and functioning of all organs and systems within the entire body. In short, they provide an instruction manual or programme for growth, survival, reproduction, and possibly also for aging and death.

Each of a person's cells (with the exception of egg and sperm cells) contains an identical set of genes. This is because all the cells are derived, by a process of division, from a single fertilized egg, and with each division the genes are copied to each offspring cell. Within any cell, however, some genes are active and others are idle, according to the specialized nature of the cell (e.g. different sets of genes are active within liver cells and nerve cells).

If the genes from any two people (other than identical twins) are compared, they always show a number of differences. These differences account for all or much of the variation among people in such aspects as gender, height, skin, hair and eye colour, and body shape, and in susceptibility to certain diseases and disorders (see *Inheritance; Genetic disorders*). Genes also influence intelligence, personality, physical and mental talents, and behaviour, although the extent of their contribution here is less clear-cut because environment and learning also play an important role.

GENE STRUCTURE AND FUNCTION

The physical material of inheritance, DNA, is an extremely long, chain-like structure. Together with some protein, it makes up the 23 pairs of *chromosomes* in the nuclei of all cells. A gene corresponds to a small section of DNA within a chromosome.

All genes fulfil their function, or exert an influence in cells or in the body at large, by directing the manufacture of particular proteins. (See illustrated box overleaf.)

Although many proteins have a particular structural or catalytic role in the body, others are synthesized solely for the purpose of influencing the activity of other genes, which they are able to switch "on" or "off". The genes responsible for making these proteins are termed "control" genes. The whole process of development and growth can be thought of as being programmed by the sequential switching "on" or "off" of particular genes; this control programme is exceedingly complex.

The activities of control genes help differentiate, for example, between nerve and liver cells, where quite different sets of genes are active or idle. If the control genes are disrupted, cells may lose their specialist abilities and begin to multiply out of control; this is the probable mechanism by which cancers and other tumours are started (see *Carcinogenesis; Oncogenes*).

MUTANT GENES

Whenever a cell divides, copies of all of its genetic material are made for the two daughter cells by the process of DNA replication (see *Nucleic acids*) and chromosomal division (see *Meiosis; Mitosis*). However, the copying process is not perfect, and very occasionally a fault occurs, leading to a *mutation* (change) in the nucleic acid sequence; this, in turn, alters the structure of the DNA in one of the daughter cells—and thus leads to a change in one of its genes. This mutant gene is then passed on each time the cell subsequently divides. If a gene mutation occurs during the formation of an egg or sperm cell that later takes part in fertilization, the person who develops from the fertilized egg will have the mutant gene present in each of his or her cells.

Carrying a mutant gene can have various effects. In some cases, it affects the structure of the protein whose manufacture is directed by the gene. Depending on the importance of the protein and the change in its structure, this usually has a disadvantageous effect, ranging from mild to lethal. Moreover, the mutant gene may be passed on to some of the person's own children. Diseases or disorders that result from such mutant genes are termed *genetic disorders*. Very rarely, genetic mutations occur that have a positively beneficial effect.

ALLELES, DOMINANCE, AND RECESSIVENESS

The consequences of inheriting a mutant gene are influenced by further factors. For every protein in the body, there are normally two genes capable of directing the manufacture of that protein—one inherited from the mother and one from the father. These may or may not be identical. The two genes are carried at the same location on each of a pair of chromosomes. If one of the genes mutates, leading to production of an altered protein, it can often be "masked" by the presence of a normal gene on the other chromosome of the pair.

In fact, the gene at any particular location on a chromosome can exist in any of various forms, called alleles, consisting usually of a normal form and one or more mutant forms, which cause the production of altered proteins. If the effects of a particular allele mask or override those of the allele at the same location on its partner chromosome, it is said to be dominant. The masked allele is recessive.

Dominant genetic traits, such as brown eyes and blood group A, are those in which the allele producing the trait needs to be present only in a single dose for it to have an outwardly apparent effect. Recessive traits, such as blue eyes and blood group O, are those in which an allele for the trait must usually be present in a double dose for it to have an outward effect.

WHERE DO YOUR GENES COME FROM?

A person's genes are inherited from his or her parents. Half come from the mother and half from the father via the egg and sperm cells. Each parent provides a different selection, or "mix", of his or her genes to each child; this accounts for the marked differences in appearance, health, and personality among most brothers and sisters. Everyone holds a copy of his or her genes within each body cell.

Gene transmission
In this diagram, only eight genes are shown—in reality, each cell in the body contains about 50,000 genes. Half of them come from the mother and half from the father—thus a quarter of the genes originate from each of the four grandparents.

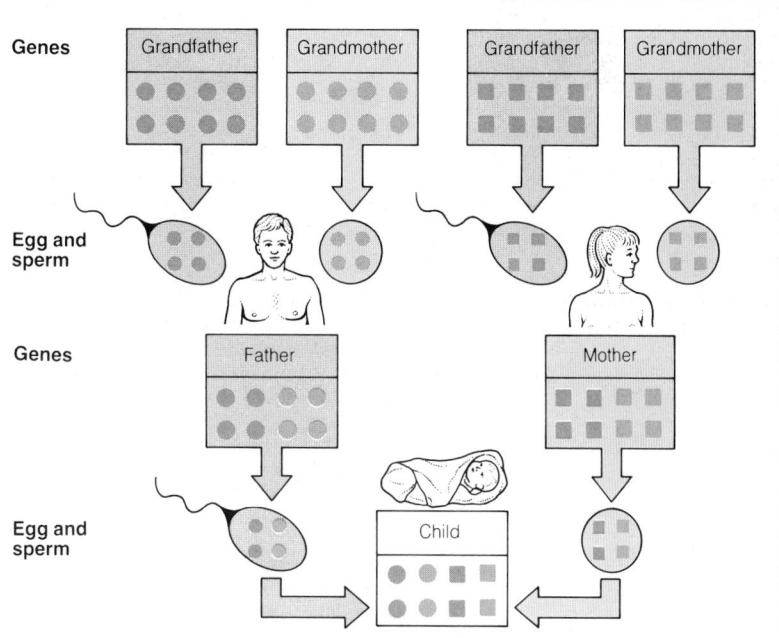

WHAT GENES ARE AND WHAT THEY DO

Genes are units of hereditary material contained in a person's cells. They hold information for all aspects of bodily growth and development, exerting their effects by directing the manufacture of proteins. All of a person's genes come from his or her parents. The physical differences between people, such as in eye, hair, and skin colour, arise from slight differences in gene structure.

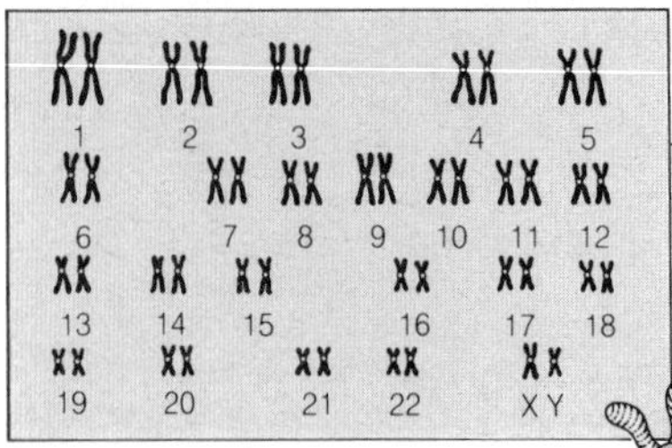

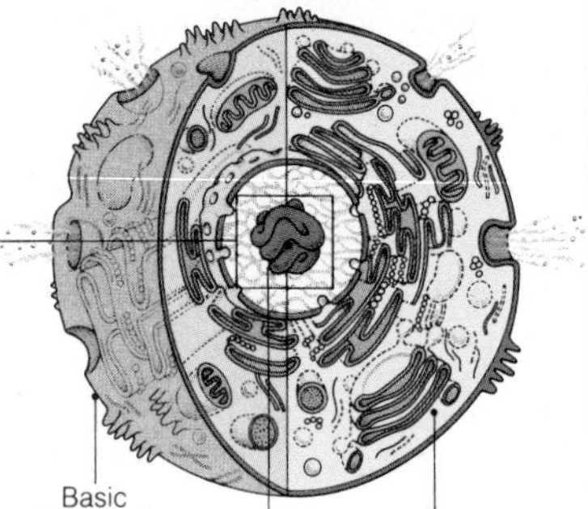

G

DNA PRINTOUT

Through painstaking laboratory research, the exact structure of many genes is now known.

```
TTC-GAG-CAT-CTG-GGG-ATG-
TCA-TGT-CCT-TCA-TCG-TTT-
TGA-TTA-CCG-ACC-CCA-TCG-
TAT-GAC-ACG-CAA-GTT-CCG-
CGG-TCA-CGC-ACG-TCA-TGT-
GGG-GAC-TCG-TAA-TCA-CGT-
CAA-GCG-AGT-TTA-AAT-AGA-
CGA-CGC-AGC-TTT-GAA-TTC-
TAT-AAC-TAC-TAA-CTG-TTA-
TTG-TTA-TGT-GAT-GGG-TTA-
ATG-AGC-GGA-GTG-CAT-TAT-
```

This printout shows a small part of the DNA base sequence in the gene that codes for the protein trypsin, a digestive enzyme.

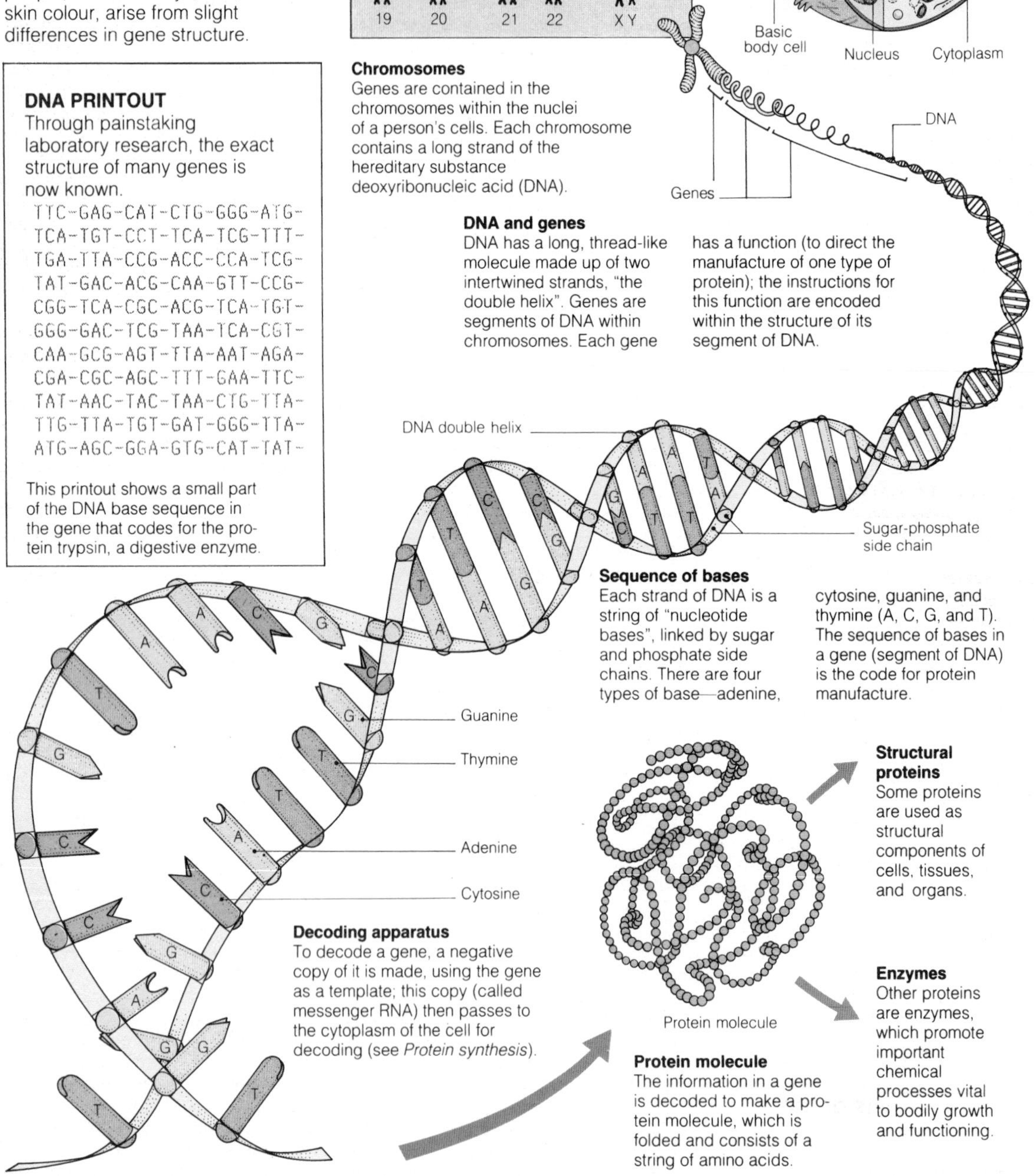

Chromosomes

Genes are contained in the chromosomes within the nuclei of a person's cells. Each chromosome contains a long strand of the hereditary substance deoxyribonucleic acid (DNA).

Basic body cell
Nucleus
Cytoplasm
Genes
DNA

DNA and genes

DNA has a long, thread-like molecule made up of two intertwined strands, "the double helix". Genes are segments of DNA within chromosomes. Each gene has a function (to direct the manufacture of one type of protein); the instructions for this function are encoded within the structure of its segment of DNA.

DNA double helix

Sugar-phosphate side chain

Sequence of bases

Each strand of DNA is a string of "nucleotide bases", linked by sugar and phosphate side chains. There are four types of base—adenine, cytosine, guanine, and thymine (A, C, G, and T). The sequence of bases in a gene (segment of DNA) is the code for protein manufacture.

Guanine
Thymine
Adenine
Cytosine

Decoding apparatus

To decode a gene, a negative copy of it is made, using the gene as a template; this copy (called messenger RNA) then passes to the cytoplasm of the cell for decoding (see *Protein synthesis*).

Protein molecule

Protein molecule

The information in a gene is decoded to make a protein molecule, which is folded and consists of a string of amino acids.

Structural proteins

Some proteins are used as structural components of cells, tissues, and organs.

Enzymes

Other proteins are enzymes, which promote important chemical processes vital to bodily growth and functioning.

The patterns by which various traits and disorders are passed on from parents to children, including the further complication of sex-linked and multifactorial inheritance and disorders, are discussed under *Inheritance* and *Genetic disorders*. Medical advice on genetic matters—for example, to parents on the chances of an intended child being affected by a particular genetic disorder—is the province of *genetic counselling*.

Generalized anxiety disorder

A neurotic illness in which the main symptoms are chronic and persistent apprehension and tension about nothing in particular ("free-floating anxiety"). There may also be physical reactions such as trembling, sweating, lightheadedness, and irritability.

Symptoms may be so severe that they interfere with everyday living and require medical attention. Psychological treatments (such as *psychotherapy*) or drugs may be helpful, although *sedative drugs* and *tranquillizer drugs* are kept to a minimum because dependence can result. (See also *Anxiety; Anxiety disorders*.)

General Medical Council

The statutory body set up in 1858 to enable people to distinguish between phony or quack doctors and those with a sound, supervised, scientific training. The General Medical Council (GMC) maintains the "Medical Register", which includes the names of all doctors who have fulfilled its educational requirements, i.e. been trained by a recognized medical school.

The GMC maintains not only educational standards but also behavioural ones; it is the GMC that forbids doctors to commit adultery with their patients, practise while under the influence of drink or drugs, or fall below acceptable levels of competence. Any member of the public who believes a doctor has broken the rules set out in the GMC's guidelines may make a formal complaint. The GMC has legal powers to investigate such complaints and if a doctor's behaviour is held to have amounted to "professional misconduct" he or she may be suspended or permanently removed from the Register—or, in popular terms, "struck off".

General paralysis of the insane

The late stage of mental and physical deterioration that occurs in untreated or unsuccessfully treated *syphilis*.

General practice

The term used in Britain to describe the medical care provided by most doctors working outside hospitals.

Virtually all general practitioners in Britain work within the National Health Service, although they are independent contractors rather than salaried employees. Most work in partnerships or groups, sharing premises that they either own or rent from the local authority. Many practices nowadays employ quite large numbers of staff, including receptionists and nurses; increasingly often nurses carry out routine treatments, perform screening tests, and give practical advice on health promotion.

General practitioners are paid under the terms of a complex contract, which includes some basic allowances and expenses, together with a fee for each patient registered with the doctor. There are financial incentives for doctors to achieve high rates of immunization and of screening tests such as *cervical smears*.

The essential feature of British general practice is that the patient has a personal doctor and, if neither moves house or dies, the patient may go on seeing the same doctor for many years. The continuity of care this ensures is widely seen as an important advantage of the system.

Generic drug

A medicinal drug marketed under its official medical name (its generic name) rather than under a patented brand name. In the UK, generic names are chosen by the Nomenclature Committee of the British Pharmacopoeia, which includes doctors, pharmacologists, pharmacists, and chemists.

Genetic code

The inherited instructions, contained in chemical form within the nuclei of cells, that specify the activities of cells and thus the development and functioning of the whole body. The term "genetic code" is also used more widely to include the system by which the instructions are copied from a cell to its offspring, the chemical basis by which the instructions are encoded, and the "key" by which the coded instructions are translated.

The basis of the genetic code is contained within molecules of the long, chain-like substance deoxyribonucleic acid (DNA). DNA, along with some protein, makes up the *chromosomes* present in the nuclei of cells. A particular *gene*, or unit of inheritance, corresponds to a section of DNA within a chromosome. Each gene contains the coded instructions for a cell to manufacture a particular protein, which may be an *enzyme* with a vital role in the cell's activities or may have some other function or structural use in the body. Most biochemical activity in the body stems from the manufacture of proteins under the guidance of genetic coding.

Little was known about how bits of DNA could specify the manufacture of proteins until the chemical structure of DNA was worked out in 1953. It was found that DNA consists of two long intertwined strands (the "double helix"), each consisting of a sequence of simple chemicals called nucleotide bases. Four different types of base, labelled A, C, G, and T, occur in DNA. The sequence of these bases along particular sections of one of the strands provides the instructions for protein manufacture.

The bases A, C, G, and T can be thought of as the letters of the code. Their sequence along a section of DNA (for example, CGGATCCTAGTTGATCATGAC) would be completely meaningless without the key to the code, employed by the cell's decoding apparatus. This decoder reads the bases three at a time, and each triplet of bases codes for a particular amino acid, the chemical unit from which proteins are made. For example, the base sequence ACG in a section of DNA codes for the amino acid cysteine and the sequence TGA codes for threonine. As triplets of nucleotide bases are read in turn, the corresponding amino acids are brought together and linked, and, as a complete sequence of bases is read, a chain of amino acids (a polypeptide chain) is formed. This may be a protein molecule itself or may form part of a larger protein structure. Certain base triplets, found at the end of gene sequences, code for termination of *protein synthesis*.

A complication of the system is that the decoding apparatus does not read directly from DNA but from an intermediary substance, messenger *RNA* (ribonucleic acid). The DNA acts as a template for RNA manufacture which in turn provides the coded instructions necessary for protein synthesis.

See *Nucleic acids* for a description of the process by which DNA is copied and passed on from each cell to its offspring (and via egg and sperm cells to a new individual).

Genetic counselling

Guidance given (usually by a doctor with experience in genetics) to a person or persons who are considering having a child but are concerned because there is a blood relative (perhaps a previous child) with an inherited disorder, or because they are at risk for some other reason of bearing a child with such a disorder.

In most cases, genetic counselling entails predicting the chances of recurrence of a condition that has already affected one or more members of a family. Such counselling depends on a correct diagnosis of the disorder. The counsellor can then explain why the disorder occurred and how it is inherited.

Genetic counselling also includes discussing the outlook for an affected child, advising couples about contraception if they decide not to have children or not to have any more children, and discussing the alternative routes to parenthood.

WHO IS COUNSELLED?

Counselling is important for parents of a child with a *genetic disorder*, such as cystic fibrosis or haemophilia, or a *chromosomal abnormality*, such as Down's or Turner's syndrome. Counselling may be useful if a child is born with *birth defects*, such as a cleft lip or congenital heart disease, and may be helpful in many other conditions, such as epilepsy, mental handicap, or abnormal sexual development. Counselling may be useful for prospective parents if there is a history of any of these conditions in a blood relative, or if a woman has had several *miscarriages* or *stillbirths*.

Genetic counselling may also be advisable in cases of first-cousin marriages and advanced maternal age.

HOW IT IS DONE

Genetic counselling may be provided by a clinical geneticist, by a paediatrician, or by the family doctor.

The counsellor makes a pedigree (family tree), which includes details of any diseases in the family, blood relationship between partners, or history of miscarriages. Information from death certificates or postmortem reports of relatives may also be needed.

When a couple have already had an abnormal child, the counsellor will ask if there was any exposure to radiation or drugs during pregnancy, or injury to the child at birth, as these can cause abnormalities in otherwise healthy families. The counsellor examines the affected child and his or her parents and arranges for any necessary tests, such as *chromosome analysis*. Certain conditions, such as Down's syndrome, sometimes result from abnormalities in the parents' chromosomes.

For many genetic disorders, it is now possible to establish with some certainty whether or not the parents of an affected child are "carriers" of a defective gene, which can significantly affect the chances of recurrence. Although the actual genes are not identified, DNA markers (fragments of genetic material known to be close to the defective gene on a chromosome) have been identified, and these can be looked for on the parents' chromosomes by advanced laboratory techniques (see *Genetic probe*), which are becoming more readily available.

Virtually every case investigated by a genetic counsellor is unique. Several factors may influence the chances of a disorder recurring, and, in some cases, complex mathematical calculations must be carried out to estimate the risk for a couple.

WHAT IT CAN OFFER

When a couple have had an abnormal child, an important aspect of counselling is the explanation of how it occurred and how the child will progress, including the chances of the child having children and whether they, too, will be affected.

Otherwise, advice consists mainly of an estimate of the risk of occurrence or recurrence of the disorder in question. The couple's decision to have children or to have more children of their own depends partly on how they view the risk estimate; and also on other factors, such as the severity of the disorder, the burden an affected child would place on the family, and the availability of alternative routes to parenthood.

The decision on the best course of action is left to the parents after they have had detailed discussions with the counsellor and feel satisfied that they understand the condition in question and its implications.

When there is a significant risk of producing an abnormal child, the parents may choose to try for a healthy child (allowing the pregnancy to continue to term only if no abnormality is found during antenatal testing). Techniques for the accurate identification of genetic disorders are now available very early in pregnancy, sometimes using fetal blood cells recovered from the mother's blood, and at no risk to the fetus. In other cases, the diagnosis may be made by *chorionic villus sampling* or *amniocentesis*. In such cases, an induced *abortion* may be chosen if an abnormality is found.

Alternatively, a couple at risk of having children with a particular condition, such as muscular dystrophy, may decide to use *in vitro fertilization* to conceive, and have genetic tests carried out on the embryos. Only those embryos without the genetic abnormality are implanted in the woman's uterus.

If a couple decide against having children, options for parenthood include adoption and *artificial insemination* by donor (the mother's egg is fertilized by donor sperm). The latter is worth considering if both parents are carriers of a rare inherited condition or if the father has a dominant genetic disorder.

Genetic disorders

Any disorder caused, wholly or partly, by a fault or faults in the inherited, genetic material in a person's cells—that is, in the *genes*, which are formed from *DNA* (deoxyribonucleic acid) and make up the *chromosomes* in the cells. A large number of diseases have a genetic cause.

Many genetic disorders are apparent at birth and are thus also *congenital*. However, the terms genetic and congenital are not synonymous; many genetic defects do not become apparent until many years after birth, and many congenital abnormalities are not genetic in origin.

Many people with a genetic disorder have one or more relatives affected by the same disorder—that is, the disorder is also *familial*. However, there are also occasions when a child is born unexpectedly with a genetic disorder (that is, with no previous family history). There are a number of mechanisms by which this can occur.

CAUSES AND TYPES

Abnormal genetic material can lead to disorders or disease because genes control the manufacture in cells of *enzymes* and other proteins that play roles of varying importance in cells and the body as a whole. If the genetic material is defective, abnormal proteins (or abnormal amounts of proteins) may be produced, causing disturbances in body chemistry that lead to disease.

For a person to exhibit a genetic disorder, the abnormality in the genetic material must usually be present in each of his or her cells, which means that it must also have been present in either the egg or the sperm cell (or both) from which the individual was derived. There are two ways in which this can happen. The first is that one or both parents carried a defect in their own genetic material; the second is

UNIFACTORIAL GENETIC DISORDERS

Autosomal dominant
In these disorders, the defective gene must be present in only a single dose to cause outward abnormality. Each child of an affected person usually has a 1 in 2 chance of inheriting the defective gene and of being affected and a 1 in 2 chance of being unaffected.

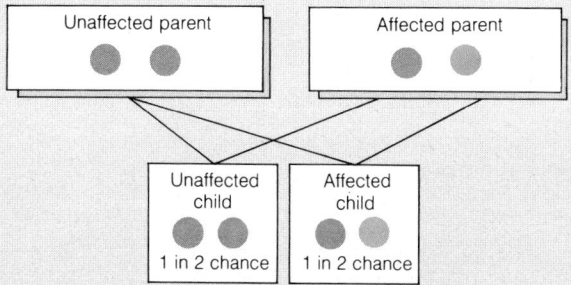

Examples
Achondroplasia
Familial polyposis
Hereditary spherocytosis
Huntington's disease
Marfan's syndrome
Neurofibromatosis
Polycystic kidney (adult type)
Tuberous sclerosis

Key
○ Defective gene
● Normal gene

Autosomal recessive
Here, a defective gene must be inherited in a double dose to cause abnormality. Usually both parents of an affected person are unaffected carriers of the defective gene. Each of their children has a 1 in 4 chance of being affected and a 2 in 4 chance of being a carrier.

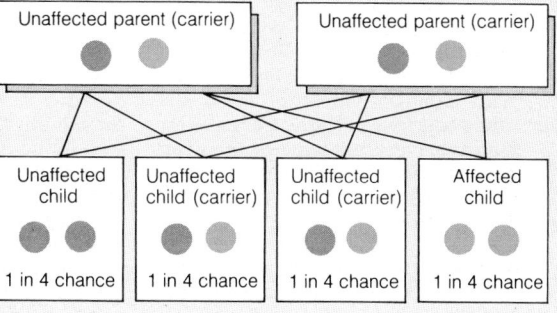

Examples
Albinism (oculocutaneous)
Cystic fibrosis
Friedreich's ataxia
Galactosaemia
Hurler's syndrome
Phenylketonuria
Sickle cell anaemia
Tay-Sachs disease

Key
○ Defective gene
● Normal gene

X-linked recessive
These conditions are caused by defects on the X chromosome usually leading to outward abnormality in males only, where the defect cannot be masked by a second, normal, X chromosome. Women can be carriers of the defect and half their sons may be affected.

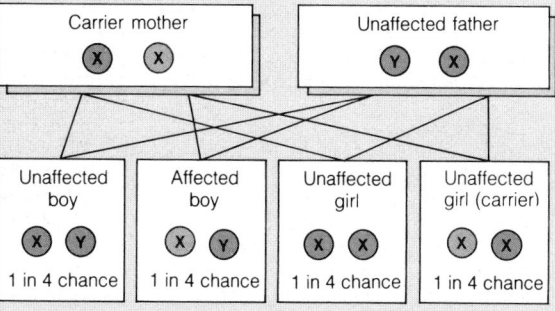

Examples
Christmas disease
Colour blindness (most types)
Fragile X syndrome
G6PD deficiency
Haemophilia
Muscular dystrophy (Duchenne)

Key
(X) Defective X chromosome
(X) Normal X chromosome
(Y) Y chromosome

that a *mutation* (a change in the genetic material) occurred during the formation of the egg or sperm cell. Mutations are one of the mechanisms by which a child affected by a genetic disorder can be born into a family that has never had a known history of genetic disorders. With some of the more common genetic disorders, such as Duchenne *muscular dystrophy*, about one third of cases are due to new mutations.

Genetic disorders fall into three broad classes: *chromosomal abnormalities*, unifactorial defects, and multifactorial defects. In the first, a child is born with an abnormal number of whole chromosomes, or extra or missing bits of chromosomes, in the cells.

Since chromosomes contain many genes, this can lead to multiple disturbances and disorders.

Unifactorial disorders are caused by a single defective gene or pair of genes; these disorders are distributed among the members of an affected family according to relatively simple laws of inheritance. Multifactorial disorders are caused by the additive effects of several genes, along with environmental factors; the pattern of inheritance is less straightforward.

UNIFACTORIAL DISORDERS
These disorders are rare, but there are many of them, and in total they cause a considerable amount of disability.

All unifactorial genetic disorders are the result of defects in a gene, or in

a pair of genes, controlling the production of a particular protein. They can be divided into two groups—called sex-linked and autosomal disorders—according to whether the affected gene or genes are located on the sex chromosomes (nearly always the X chromosome) or on any of the other 22 pairs of chromosomes, which are known as autosomes (see *Chromosomes*).

Autosomal disorders generally affect both sexes equally and are further divided into two groups, called autosomal dominant and autosomal recessive, according to whether the defective gene needs to be present in a single or double dose to cause an outward abnormality.

Sex-linked disorders show a bias in their incidence among the sexes. Most are of one type—X-linked recessive disorders—and primarily affect males. Some examples of the three varieties of unifactorial disorder are shown in the table on the previous page.

AUTOSOMAL DOMINANT DISORDERS With these disorders, a person needs to carry the defective gene in only a single dose for it to have an outwardly apparent effect. Such individuals are termed *heterozygotes* with respect to the gene, which means they carry one normal copy and one defective copy of the gene. Because the defective gene is dominant—that is, it overrides the normal gene—its presence usually leads to an outward abnormality (but not always a severe one).

Some affected people have inherited the defective gene from one of their parents. In other cases, there is no family history of the condition and the defect has usually arisen as a result of a mutation.

If an affected individual has children, each one has a 50 per cent chance of inheriting the defective gene and of being affected. Often these disorders appear in each of several generations, finally disappearing only when the affected individuals in a generation have no affected children or no children at all.

AUTOSOMAL RECESSIVE DISORDERS People who manifest these disorders have always acquired the particular gene defect in a double dose—they are said to be *homozygotes* with respect to the defective gene. In most cases, both parents of an affected person are heterozygotes—they carry the defective gene in a single dose along with a normal gene. But, because the defective gene is recessive and "masked" by the normal gene, the parents display no outward abnormality.

With all autosomal recessive defects, the number of such carriers in the population always outnumbers those actually affected. For example, with *cystic fibrosis* (the most common disorder of this type), one in 22 of the population is a carrier of the defective gene, but only one person in 2,000 is born with the condition. The majority of carriers are unaware of the fact and have no family history of the condition—the defective gene has been passed on to them silently over many generations. When two carriers have children and one is born with an autosomal recessive condition, the manifestation of the defect thus usually comes as a complete surprise.

Because both parents are carriers, any subsequent child will have a one in four chance of also being affected.

X-LINKED RECESSIVE DISORDERS In these conditions, the defective gene is on the X chromosome. Women have two X chromosomes in their cells; men have only one, which they inherit from their mothers and pass on to their daughters.

When a woman inherits the defective gene in a single dose, its effect is masked by the normal gene on her other X chromosome because it is recessive and she displays no outward abnormality. She is a heterozygote carrier of the defective gene. However, when a male inherits the defective gene, there is no normal gene on a second X chromosome to mask it, and he will thus display the abnormality.

The familial pattern of these disorders is as follows. Affected males far outnumber affected females and in all cases have inherited the genetic defect from their mother (who is a carrier). They pass the defective gene to none of their sons but to all of their daughters, who become carriers in turn. Carrier females transmit the defective gene on average to half their sons, who are affected, and to half their daughters, who become carriers in turn. This type of disorder cannot be passed on by an unaffected male. Thus, the pattern is for some of the males in an affected family to have the disorder, while the females in the family are either known or possible carriers.

MULTIFACTORIAL DISORDERS
A large number of disorders fall into this category—including *asthma*, insulin-dependent *diabetes mellitus*, *schizophrenia*, and a number of conditions present at birth, such as *talipes* (clubfoot) and *cleft lip and palate*.

In each case, susceptibility to the disorder is thought to be determined by a number of different genes which, along with environmental influences, have an additive effect. The degree to which susceptibility to each of these various disorders is determined by genes has been estimated and is termed *heritability*.

AFFECTED FAMILIES
The underlying cause of genetic disorders (defects in genes) cannot be treated. However, there are a number of methods by which the chances of a child being born with a genetically based disorder can be reduced.

If a couple are considering having children and if either of them or any of their parents or close blood relatives has a genetically based disorder, they would be wise to obtain *genetic counselling*. This is especially important if the couple have had a child with a genetically based condition.

The options can be assessed once the couple's own genetic make-up has been established, and include testing the embryo in early pregnancy and terminating the pregnancy if the disorder is present. Another option is *in vitro fertilization*, where tests are carried out on embryos before implantation; donor eggs or sperm may be used. Steady progress is also being made in the treatment of genetic disorders by techniques such as enzyme replacement therapy or *bone marrow transplant*.

Genetic engineering
A branch of genetics concerned, in its broadest sense, with the alteration of the inherited, genetic material carried by a living organism, in order to produce some desired change in the characteristics of the organism.

In practice, the main application of genetic engineering so far has been to mass-produce a variety of substances—all proteins of various sorts—that have uses in medical treatment and diagnosis. The function of any *gene* is to control the production of a particular protein in a living cell. If the gene responsible for synthesizing a useful protein can be identified, and if it can be inserted into another cell that can be made to reproduce rapidly, then a colony of cells containing the gene can be grown. The colony will then produce the protein in large amounts.

WHY IT IS DONE
Genetic engineering has been used for producing some human hormones (notably *insulin* and *growth hormone*), proteins such as *factor VIII* (used to treat *haemophilia*), and *tissue plasminogen activator* (used to dissolve blood clots). Substances made in this way are free of any risk of contamination with viruses such as *HIV* or the agent that causes *Creutzfeldt-Jakob disease* and are, therefore, safe to use in treatment.

HOW IT IS DONE
The main technique for the mass-production of useful proteins by genetic engineering is called recombinant *DNA* technology. DNA (deoxyribonucleic acid) is the genetic material in cells that controls the manufacture of different proteins.

The first step is to identify a specific gene within the DNA of a cell that controls the manufacture of a particularly useful protein. This involves a number of highly sophisticated laboratory techniques. The next step is either to extract the gene from the cell or, if the exact chemical structure of the gene can be worked out, to synthesize it.

The final step is to introduce the gene into the DNA of a suitable recipient cell. *Enzymes* can be used to split the recipient cell's DNA at a certain site and so produce a gap into which the gene can be spliced (hence the term recombinant DNA).

The types of cells or organisms suitable for such genetic alteration are those that can subsequently be made to reproduce rapidly and indefinitely. The most popular organisms to date have been the common intestinal bacterium *ESCHERICHIA COLI* and various yeasts, but cells of other organisms, including human cancer cells, have also been used with success.

OUTLOOK

In view of the ease with which some of the bacteria and other organisms used for genetic engineering can reproduce, and the possibility of accidentally creating and liberating highly dangerous microorganisms, doubts have frequently been expressed about the dangers of "tampering with nature" in this way. These dangers are real but are well recognized by researchers in the field, who have produced stringent codes of practice and regulations to ensure safety.

In the future, it may be possible to extend genetic engineering to the manipulation of human genetic material to treat *genetic disorders*.

Genetic fingerprinting

A technique, also known as DNA fingerprinting, which is able to reveal relationships between individuals. Genetic fingerprinting, which was first used in 1984, can be used to prove paternity (see *Paternity testing*) or to identify a criminal suspect by comparing DNA samples.

DNA is the genetic material contained in all living cells and can be extracted from blood, semen, and other body tissues. A pattern of chemical signals within the DNA molecule is unique to each person (except for identical twins) and this unique pattern can be used to provide the genetic "fingerprint".

HOW IT IS DONE

A sample, usually a blood sample, is taken from the suspected person and DNA is extracted from it. The DNA is cut into fragments by an *enzyme* and the fragments are separated into bands in an agar gel by a process

called electrophoresis. The band pattern is transferred to a nylon membrane, after which a radioactive DNA "probe" is added; the probe binds to specific sequences of DNA on the membrane. X-ray film is placed next to the membrane to detect the radioactive pattern. The film is developed and the unique pattern of bands, known as the genetic fingerprint, becomes visible.

USES

The genetic fingerprint in one sample can be compared with the genetic fingerprint in samples taken from another individual or in forensic samples. In this way, genetic fingerprinting can be used to resolve cases of disputed paternity or maternity, showing with certainty whether an individual is or is not the parent of a particular child. Such information may be needed, for example, to resolve civil paternity disputes or to provide further evidence in immigration disputes.

Genetic fingerprinting has important applications in forensic science. Forensic samples may be analysed to identify or eliminate suspects. For example, a blood sample at the scene of a crime or a semen sample in a rape case can be analysed and its genetic fingerprint compared with that of a suspect's sample.

Genetic probe

A specific fragment of *DNA* (deoxyribonucleic acid) used in laboratory tests to determine whether particular gene defects or genetic "markers" are present in a person's or a fetus's genetic material (i.e. the DNA contained in the *chromosomes* of all cells).

Genetic probes have their main use in antenatal diagnosis of *genetic disorders*, and in investigating whether individuals with a family history of a genetic disorder carry the defective gene themselves. This is appropriate for dominant genes that cause disease in adult life, and for recessive genes that do not cause disease in healthy gene carriers but may be passed on by them to their children who would develop the disease.

Some genetic probes detect the abnormal gene directly, and this type of probe can be used to diagnose genetic disorders. However, many defective genes cannot be identified directly, and gene probes have to be used to demonstrate genetic markers, which are themselves harmless, but may be inherited along with a particular defective gene. The inheritance

of the defective gene can be predicted by tracking the genetic markers through an individual family.

One of the main laboratory techniques using genetic probes involves isolating DNA from the chromosomes of cells from the person or fetus being tested. This DNA is split up using *enzymes* in a test tube, and the fragments are fixed on to a filter. A radioactively labelled sequence of DNA (the probe) is added, and this will bind to the gene or marker sequence in the DNA of the individual being tested. This binding can then be visualized as a variety of patterns on an X-ray film.

Genetics

The study of *inheritance*—that is, how the characteristics of living organisms are passed from one generation to another, the chemical basis by which such characteristics are determined, and the causes of the similarities and differences among individuals of one species or between different species. More particularly, genetics includes the study of *DNA* (deoxyribonucleic acid), the substance in cells that determines the characteristics of an organism, and of genes, which are units of inheritance corresponding to specific bits of DNA.

Particular branches of human genetics include population genetics, which studies the relative frequency of various genes in different human races; molecular genetics, which is concerned with the structure, function, and copying of DNA from one cell to another, and also how *mutations* (changes) occur in DNA; and medical or clinical genetics, which is concerned with the study and prevention of *genetic disorders*.

Genital herpes

See *Herpes, genital*.

Genitalia

The reproductive organs, especially the external (visible) ones. The male genitalia include the *penis, testes* (within the *scrotum*), *prostate gland, seminal vesicles,* and associated ducts, such as the *epididymis* and *vas deferens*. The female genitalia include the *ovaries, fallopian tubes, uterus, vagina, clitoris, vulva,* and *Bartholin's glands*.

Genitalia, ambiguous

A group of conditions, also known as intersex, in which the external sex organs are not clearly male or female,

G

G

or in which the external sex organs resemble those of people with the opposite chromosomal sex.

A person with ambiguous genitalia may have true *hermaphroditism*, in which they possess both testicular and ovarian tissue, or *pseudohermaphroditism*, in which they possess only testicular or ovarian tissue. These disorders of sexual differentiation may result from an abnormality of the sex chromosomes, an abnormality of the testes or ovaries, or a hormonal disorder (see *Sex determination*).

Genital ulceration

An eroded area of skin on the *genitalia*. In men, the ulcer may be on the skin of the penis or scrotum; in women, it may be on the vulva or within the vagina.

CAUSES

The most common cause of genital ulceration is a *sexually transmitted disease*. The early stages of *syphilis* are characterized by a hard chancre, a painless ulcer at the site where the bacteria penetrated the skin. The HERPES SIMPLEX virus may cause painful, fluid-filled blisters to develop on the genitalia; infection of the blisters by bacteria can cause ulceration (see *Herpes, genital*). *Chancroid* is a common tropical bacterial infection that causes painful genital ulcers. *Granuloma inguinale*, also common in the tropics, is a bacterial infection that causes painless genital ulcers. *Lymphogranuloma venereum* is a viral infection resulting in blisters that occasionally ulcerate.

Genital ulceration may also develop as a result of injury or damage, which may occur during sexual intercourse.

Behçet's syndrome is a rare condition that causes tender, recurrent ulcers in the mouth and on the genitals. Cancer of the penis or vulva may cause a painless ulcer with raised edges that turn outwards.

Genital ulceration may also sometimes be a side-effect of drugs.

Genital warts

See *Warts, genital*.

Genito-urinary medicine

The branch of medicine concerned with *sexually transmitted diseases* and their effects on the *reproductive system*, *urinary tract*, and other parts of the body. There is some overlap between this specialty and *urology* (which deals with reproductive system disorders in men) and *gynaecology* (which is concerned with reproductive system disorders in women).

Genome, human

The detailed map of the position and function of every one of the 100,000 *genes* on the 23 pairs of human *chromosomes*, together with the differences (alleles) in individual genes that are responsible for human variations, such as hair colour, and for *genetic disorders*. Several thousand genes, most of which were those altered in common genetic disorders, had been identified by the late 1980s, when a decision was made to decipher the complete human genome. The project should be completed by the year 2000.

Gentamicin

An *antibiotic drug* given by injection to treat serious infections, or in the form of drops or ointment to treat eye or ear infections.

Gentamicin cannot be given by mouth because it is inactivated by the digestive process. It is given by injection, often in combination with other antibiotic drugs, to treat serious infections, such as *meningitis, septicaemia* (blood poisoning), and *endocarditis* (inflammation of the heart lining). Because gentamicin can damage the kidneys or inner ear, blood tests may be performed during treatment to determine gentamicin levels in the blood and so allow careful monitoring of the dose.

Gentian violet

A purple dye used mainly by microbiologists to make bacteria visible under the microscope. Gentian violet also has antiseptic properties and was formerly used to treat burns, boils, carbuncles, fungal infections, and mouth ulcers.

Genu valgum

The medical term for *knock-knee*.

Genu varum

The medical term for *bowleg*.

Geriatric medicine

The medical specialty that is concerned with care of the elderly. Many diseases and disorders affecting the elderly may occur in patients of all ages, but older people tend to respond differently to sickness and treatment. For example, *aging* is associated with a progressive decline in the functioning of the major organs—the heart, lungs, kidneys, liver, and brain. Consequently, an infection in one of these organs or elsewhere in the body that would cause only minor illness in a young adult might be life-threatening in an older person. Any illness in an elderly person may cause a temporary but marked slowing of thought processes, and may lead to *confusion* and other features that may be mistaken for *dementia*. This is due to the added stress that is placed on the brain during the illness. Furthermore, many drugs are eliminated from the body by the liver or the kidneys and, if these organs are affected by aging, dosages of drugs may require modification in order to avoid dangerous side-effects.

A geriatrician is a doctor who has had special training in care of the elderly sick. He or she takes particular care not to give excessive doses of drugs and also tries to avoid moving patients away from familiar surroundings unless hospital admission is essential. The geriatrician is also involved in preparing patients to cope with everyday tasks as well as possible after they leave hospital, and will make contact with social services and voluntary agencies. (See also *Rehabilitation*.)

Germ

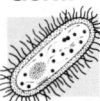

The popular term for any microorganism that causes disease. Examples include *viruses* and *bacteria*. In medicine, the word germ is used to describe simple, undifferentiated cells that are capable of developing into specialized tissues, such as the cells of the early embryo.

German measles

Another name for *rubella*.

Germ cell tumour

A growth comprised of immature sperm cells in the male testis or of immature ova (eggs) in the female ovary. A seminoma is one type of germ cell tumour (see *Testis, cancer of*).

Gerontology

The study of *aging* in all its aspects (developmental, biological, medical, sociological, and psychological). The specialty that treats the medical problems of the elderly is called *geriatric medicine* or geriatrics.

Gestalt theory

A school of psychology based on the idea that a sense of wholeness is more important than the individual bits and pieces of perception and behaviour. It was founded in Germany early this century by a group that adopted the name gestalt, meaning "form", "pattern", or "configuration". In a broad sense, gestalt refers to any idea based on the notion that the whole is more than the sum of its parts.

In studying emotional states and social issues, Gestalt theory emphasizes viewing things as a whole rather than breaking them down into collections of stimuli and responses. Gestalt therapy became popular as a means of coping with personal problems and is still practised today by some therapists; this type of therapy aims to increase self-awareness by looking at all aspects of an individual within his or her environment.

Gestation
The period from *conception* to birth, during which the developing infant is carried in the uterus.

Gestation normally lasts around 270 days, about nine months. Because of the difficulty in determining the precise date of conception, doctors time pregnancies from the first day of the last normal menstrual period, giving a gestation period of 284 days. (See also *Childbirth; Embryo; Fetus; Pregnancy*.)

Giardiasis
An infection of the small intestine, caused by the protozoan (single-celled) parasite *GIARDIA LAMBLIA*. Giardiasis is most common in tropical areas and in people who have visited the tropics. Recently it has become more common in developed countries, mainly affecting homosexual men, people living in institutions, and preschool children in nurseries. Giardiasis is spread by contaminated food or water or by direct contact with an infected person.

SYMPTOMS
About two thirds of those infected have no symptoms. When symptoms do occur they begin one to three days after the parasite has entered the body. The person has violent attacks of diarrhoea accompanied by flatus (wind); the faeces are foul-smelling, may be greasy, and tend to float in the toilet bowl. Abdominal discomfort, cramps, and swelling, loss of appetite, and nausea may also occur. In some cases, the infection becomes chronic.

DIAGNOSIS AND TREATMENT
The infection is diagnosed from microscopic examination of a sample of faeces for the presence of the parasites. If there is any doubt, a *jejunal*

biopsy (removal of a small sample of tissue for microscopic analysis) may be carried out.

Acute giardiasis usually clears up without treatment. However, drug treatment with *metronidazole* quickly relieves symptoms and prevents the spread of infection.

PREVENTION
Infection can be prevented by thorough hand washing before handling food and by avoiding food or water that could possibly be contaminated.

Giddiness
See *Dizziness*.

Gigantism
Excessive growth (especially height) resulting from overproduction, during childhood or adolescence, of growth hormone by a tumour of the *pituitary gland*. Untreated, the tumour may eventually destroy the pituitary gland and cause death during early adult life. If the tumour develops after growth has stopped, the result is *acromegaly* rather than gigantism.

Oversecretion of growth hormone from early life can result in an individual attaining an immense height. The tallest documented giant in medical history, Robert Wadlow, reached a height of 2.72 m before he died, aged 22. Such instances are rare, however. By far the most common reason for a child being tall is that his or her parents are tall. Other rare causes of excessive height in childhood are *Marfan's syndrome* and *thyrotoxicosis*.

DIAGNOSIS AND TREATMENT
The diagnosis of gigantism is made when *brain imaging* and blood tests confirm the presence of a pituitary tumour and excessive amounts of growth hormone. The condition may be treated with *bromocriptine*, a drug that blocks the release of growth hormone, or by surgery or *radiotherapy* to remove or destroy the tumour.

Gilbert's disease
An inherited disorder that affects the way in which *bilirubin* is processed by the *liver*.

Gilbert's disease is common, affecting about two per cent of the population. Usually there are no symptoms, but mild jaundice, sometimes with malaise, anorexia, and abdominal pain, may be brought on by an illness. Sufferers are otherwise healthy. No treatment is necessary.

Gilles de la Tourette's syndrome
A rare disorder of movement, named after the French neurologist who first described it in 1885, now commonly termed Tourette syndrome. It starts in childhood with repetitive grimaces and tics, usually of the head and neck, sometimes of the arms, legs, and trunk. Involuntary barks, grunts, or other noises may appear as the disease progresses. In about half the cases, the sufferer has episodes of coprolalia (using foul language).

The syndrome is more common in males, and is probably underdiag-

G

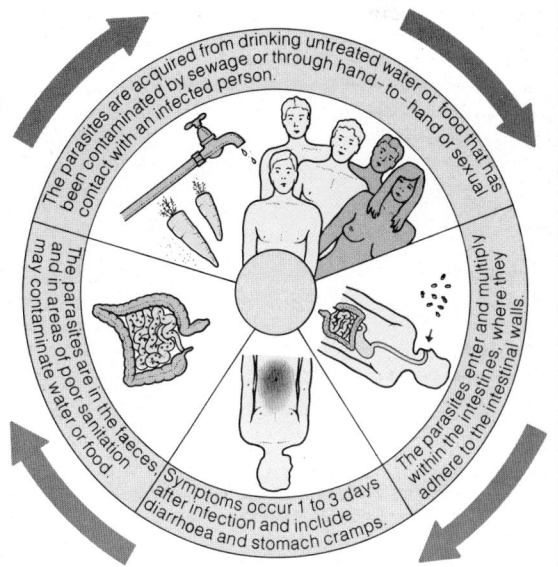

HOW GIARDIASIS IS SPREAD
Giardiasis is spread by contaminated water or food, or by personal contact. This parasitic infection is most common in the tropics, but recently it has become a more frequent occurrence in developed countries, especially among groups of preschool children.

nosed because of its strange symptoms. It is usually of lifelong duration but *antipsychotic drugs*, such as *haloperidol*, can provide effective relief in some cases.

Gingiva

The Latin name for the *gums* surrounding the base of the teeth.

Gingivectomy

Surgical removal of part of the gum margin. Gingivectomy may be used to treat severe cases of gingival *hyperplasia* (thickening of the gums), a condition usually caused by the anticonvulsant drug *phenytoin*. Gingivectomy is also used to remove pockets of infected gum formed during the advanced stages of *periodontitis* (gum disease).

Gingivectomy is performed by a dentist using local anaesthetic. After surgery, the newly exposed area around the base of the teeth may initially be sensitive; the exposure also makes the teeth appear to be longer. There are no complications as long as scrupulous *oral hygiene* is maintained after surgery.

Gingivitis

Inflammation of the gingiva (gums), often due to infection. Gingivitis is a reversible stage of gum disease.

CAUSES

Gingivitis is usually caused by the build-up of dental *plaque* (a sticky deposit of bacteria, mucus, food particles, and other irritants) around the base of the teeth. It is thought that toxins produced by bacteria within the plaque irritate the gums, causing the gums to become infected, tender, and swollen. Gingivitis can result from injury to the gums, usually from rough toothbrushing or flossing.

INCIDENCE

Mild gingivitis is very common in young adults. Pregnant women and people with *diabetes mellitus* are susceptible because of changes in their hormone levels.

SYMPTOMS

Healthy gums are pink or brown and firm; in people with gingivitis, they become red-purple, soft, shiny, and swollen. The gums bleed easily, especially during toothbrushing, and are often tender.

PREVENTION AND TREATMENT

Good *oral hygiene* is the main means of preventing and treating gingivitis. Teeth should be thoroughly brushed with a *fluoride* toothpaste at least once a day and preferably after all meals;

dental floss should be used at least once a day. A dentist should be consulted at least once a year so that dental plaque and *calculus* (mineralized plaque) can be removed (see *Scaling, dental*). The dentist may recommend a mouthwash for use at home.

COMPLICATIONS

Untreated gingivitis may damage gum tissue around the base of the teeth, leading to the formation of pockets in which plaque and calculus can collect. Bacteria within the plaque may cause inflammation to spread, eventually leading to chronic *periodontitis*, an advanced stage of gum disease in which the supporting tissues of the teeth and the surrounding bone become eroded, loosening the teeth.

Acute ulcerative gingivitis may develop due to invasion of tissue by *anaerobic* bacteria in people with chronic gingivitis, especially those with lowered resistance to infection (see *Gingivitis, acute ulcerative*).

Gingivitis, acute ulcerative

Painful bacterial infection and ulceration of the gums, also known as acute necrotizing ulcerative gingivitis, trench mouth, Vincent's stomatitis, or Vincent's disease.

CAUSES AND INCIDENCE

The condition is caused by abnormal growth of microorganisms which usually exist harmlessly in small numbers in gum crevices. Predisposing factors include poor *oral hygiene*, smoking, throat infections, and emotional stress. In many cases acute ulcerative gingivitis is preceded by *gingivitis* or by *periodontitis*. The condition is relatively rare, primarily affecting young adults aged 15 to 35.

SYMPTOMS

The symptoms appear over the course of a day or two. The gums become sore and inflamed and bleed at the slightest pressure. Crater-like ulcers, which bleed spontaneously, develop on the gum tips between teeth, and there is a foul taste in the mouth, bad breath, and sometimes swollen lymph nodes. As the disease advances, ulcers spread along the gum margins and into deeper tissues. Occasionally, the infection spreads to the lips and the lining of the cheeks, resulting in destruction of tissues (see *Noma*).

TREATMENT

The dentist usually prescribes a mouthwash containing hydrogen peroxide to relieve pain and inflammation. After a few days, when the gums are less tender, scaling (see *Scaling, dental*) is performed to remove

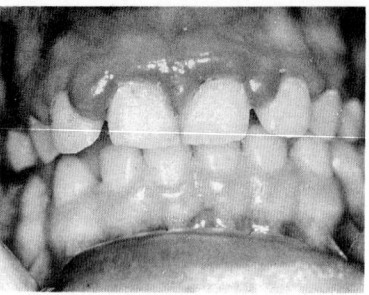

Example of gingivitis
The gums around the bases of the upper teeth are puffy, shiny, and tender. They overhang the teeth margins. Affected gums often bleed when brushed.

dental *plaque* and *calculus* from the teeth. In severe cases, the antibacterial drug *metronidazole* may be prescribed to control infection.

Regular follow-up visits to the dentist may be necessary. Counselling may focus on maintaining oral hygiene, giving up smoking, or learning to cope with stress.

Gland

A group of specialized cells that manufacture and release chemical substances, such as *hormones* and *enzymes*, for use in the body.

There are two main types of glands: endocrine and exocrine. *Endocrine glands* do not have ducts and thus release their secretions directly into the bloodstream; examples include the pituitary, thyroid, and adrenal glands. *Exocrine glands* have ducts and release their secretions either on to the surface of the skin or into a hollow structure such as the mouth or digestive tract; examples include the sebaceous glands, which secrete sebum on to the skin, and the salivary glands. The pancreas releases endocrine secretions (insulin) and exocrine secretions (cholecystokinin).

Lymph nodes (collections of cells in the *lymphatic system*) are sometimes referred to as glands. Strictly speaking, this is an incorrect usage of gland because lymph nodes do not secrete chemical substances. However, they do release white blood cells, which play an important role in fighting infections and in allergic reactions.

Glanders

An infection of horses caused by the bacterium *PSEUDOMONAS MALLEI*, which is only very rarely transmitted to humans.

Initial symptoms include mild fever, headache, general aches and pains, and possibly some generalized swelling of the lymph nodes. Ulcers or abscesses may develop where bacteria entered through the skin; if entry of bacteria was through the lungs, *pneumonia* may develop. In severe cases, *septicaemia* (blood poisoning) may then follow. Treatment is with *antibiotic drugs*.

Glands, swollen

Enlargement of the *lymph nodes* (glands) as a result of inflammation and/or proliferation of white blood cells within them. The medical term for this is lymphadenopathy.

CAUSES

Swollen glands are a very common symptom and are usually caused by a minor infection. Children are especially prone to swollen glands as a result of infections, partly because the lymphatic system plays a more important part in combating infections in childhood than in adult life. Swollen glands may also be caused by an allergic reaction (see *Allergy*).

Rarer causes of swollen glands include *Hodgkin's disease* and other forms of *lymphoma* (lymph gland tumour), *leukaemia* (cancer of the white blood cells), or a *metastasis* (secondary cancer that has spread from elsewhere in the body).

When the underlying cause affects a limited area, swollen glands also tend to be localized; for example, a throat

Common sites of swollen glands
The three most common sites where swollen glands can be felt are in the neck, armpit, and groin.

infection may result in swelling only of the lymph glands in the neck.

Swollen glands near the surface of the skin—in the groin or neck, for example—are usually felt as tender, slightly warm lumps. However, swelling of deeper glands, such as those in the lungs or abdomen, is almost invariably unnoticeable.

INVESTIGATION AND TREATMENT

In many cases, the cause of swollen glands is obvious from the presence of a localized infection or something such as a bee sting that has caused an allergic reaction. In other cases, the accompanying symptoms usually indicate the cause; for example, swollen glands with a sore throat, fever, and tiredness suggest infectious *mononucleosis* (glandular fever) or, rarely, HIV infection (see *AIDS-related complex*).

If swollen glands persist or there is no obvious cause, tests may be necessary. These may include a blood count, chest X-rays to look for swollen glands in the lungs, or a *biopsy* (removal of tissue for microscopic analysis) of an affected lymph node.

Treatment depends on the underlying cause. *Antibiotic drugs* may be given for an infection, *antihistamine drugs* for an allergy, and *radiotherapy* and/or *anticancer drugs* for a tumour.

Glandular fever

See *Mononucleosis, infectious*.

Glasses

Simple optical devices used to correct focusing errors in the eyes so that clear vision is achieved. The lenses are made of glass or plastic and the shape and thickness are chosen during an eye test (see *Vision tests; Myopia*).

TYPES OF LENSES

Lenses may be convex (outwardly curved), concave (inwardly curved), or cylindrical (see illustrated box overleaf). Most are single-vision lenses, but bifocal or trifocal lenses, with smaller areas differing in power from the main lens, are common. Varifocal lenses, with power increasing gradually from the centre to one edge, are becoming popular. Lenses may have a permanent tint or may incorporate chemicals that produce darkening on exposure to light.

Glass eye

See *Eye, artificial*.

Glaucoma

A condition in which the pressure of the fluid in the *eye* is so high that it causes damage. A minimal pressure is

required to maintain the shape of the eyeball, but excessive pressure may result in the compression and obstruction of the small blood vessels that nourish the fibres of the *optic nerve*. The result is nerve fibre destruction and gradual loss of vision.

TYPES AND CAUSES

The most common form is chronic simple (open-angle) glaucoma, which rarely occurs before the age of 40 and often causes no symptoms until blindness is advanced. It is due to a gradual blockage of the outflow of aqueous humour (fluid in the front compartment of the eye) over a period of years, causing a slow rise in pressure. This type tends to run in families.

In acute (closed-angle) glaucoma, there is a sudden obstruction to the outflow of aqueous humour from the eye and the pressure rises suddenly. Subacute glaucoma causes similar but transient bouts of acute glaucoma.

Congenital glaucoma is due to a structural abnormality in the drainage angles of the eyes.

Glaucoma can also be caused by injury to the eye, or by a serious eye disease such as *uveitis, lens dislocation,* or adhesions (abnormal bands of tissue) between the iris and the cornea.

INCIDENCE

Glaucoma is one of the most common major eye disorders in people over 60; it is responsible for about 15 per cent of blindness in adults in the UK. Nearly two per cent of people over the age of 40 have chronic simple glaucoma. The incidence rises with age and about 10 per cent of people over 70 have abnormally raised pressure within the eye, often causing little or no damage.

SYMPTOMS AND SIGNS

Chronic simple glaucoma often causes no symptoms because the gradual loss of peripheral vision is not apparent to the affected person. Only late in the disease, when there is severe, irreversible damage, may the person be aware of some visual loss.

The symptoms of acute glaucoma include a dull, severe, aching pain in and above the eye, some fogginess of vision, and (in subacute bouts) the perception of haloes (rainbow rings around lights) at night. Nausea and vomiting may occur and the eye may become red and have a partly dilated pupil and a hazy cornea.

DIAGNOSIS

Chronic simple glaucoma often causes no symptoms and is usually detected only by routine eye examinations. Applanation *tonometry* (measuring the

WHY GLASSES ARE USED

For *hypermetropia* (longsightedness), convex (or plus) lenses are needed. Sufferers of *presbyopia* also need plus (magnifying) lenses. *Myopia* (shortsightedness) requires concave (or minus) lenses.

LONGSIGHTEDNESS

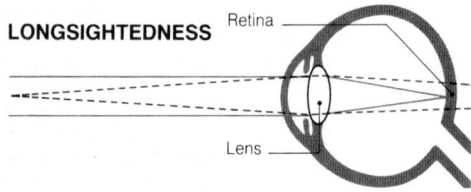

Before correction
Longsightedness occurs when focusing power is inadequate. Light from a distant object is focused on the retina, but light from a close object is focused behind it.

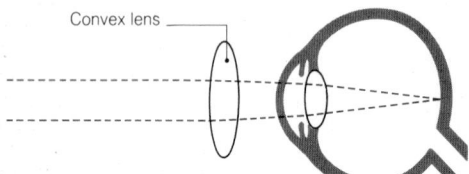

After correction
Convex magnifying (or plus) lenses cause the light from the close object to focus on the retina.

SHORTSIGHTEDNESS

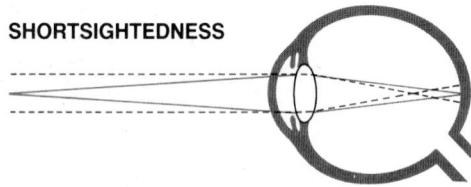

Before correction
Distant objects are blurred, because the focusing power of the eye is too great. Light from the distant object is focused in front of the retina.

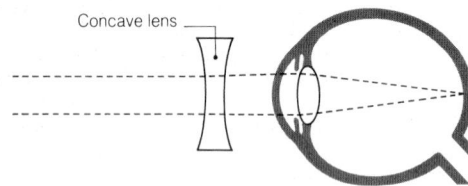

After correction
Concave weakening (or minus) lenses are used to cause the light from the distant object to focus on the retina.

ASTIGMATISM

The surrounding surfaces of the cornea are steeper in one direction than in the other. The correcting lenses are designed with additional curvature in one meridian. The lenses are then set accurately in the frame of the glasses so that the steepest curves correspond to the flattest meridian of the cornea. Both concave lenses for myopia and convex lenses for hypermetropia and presbyopia can be designed in this way to correct astigmatism.

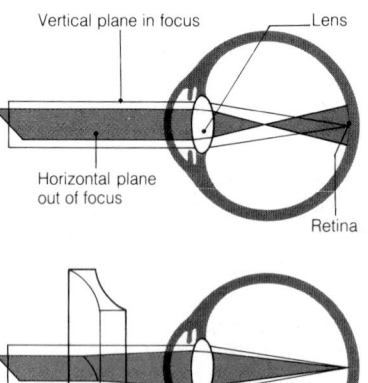

pressure in the eye) is an essential check for glaucoma, especially if there is a family history of the disorder. Use of an *ophthalmoscope* to examine the back of the eye may show an abnormal optic nerve. Visual field testing and gonioscopy (examination of the drainage angle) can also be important.

TREATMENT
Chronic simple glaucoma can usually be controlled with eye-drops (e.g. *timolol* twice daily), which reduce the pressure in the eye. Repeated tonometry and visual field testing may be carried out to ensure that the glaucoma is being controlled; if necessary, other eye-drops will be given. If drops fail to control the pressure, tablets or long-acting capsules may also be prescribed. The medicines for treatment of chronic simple glaucoma usually need to be continued for life since, if they are stopped, the pressure generally rises. If medicines fail to reduce the pressure in chronic simple glaucoma, and if there is a continuing loss of visual field or vision, surgery may be necessary to open up the blocked drainage channel or to create an artificial channel for the aqueous humour.

Acute glaucoma is a medical emergency calling for urgent treatment. Various treatments (eye-drops, pills, liquids, intravenous fluids) are given to try to reduce the very high pressure in the eye. Usually, after the pressure is controlled, surgery is necessary for the treatment of acute glaucoma to try to prevent a further attack. This is usually a peripheral *iridectomy*, fashioning a small opening at the periphery of the iris so that aqueous humour can drain more easily. The iridectomy is often curative but, if the drainage angle was damaged by the attack, drug treatment may be needed to control the pressure after surgery. Other types of surgery, as for chronic simple glaucoma, may be necessary.

OUTLOOK
The pressure rise of glaucoma can normally be prevented by treatment, but early diagnosis and treatment are needed in order to prevent any impairment of vision.

Glibenclamide

An oral *hypoglycaemic drug* used to treat non-insulin-dependent *diabetes mellitus*. Glibenclamide stimulates the pancreas to produce *insulin*, which promotes the uptake of glucose (sugar) into muscle and fat tissue, thereby lowering the level of glucose in the blood.

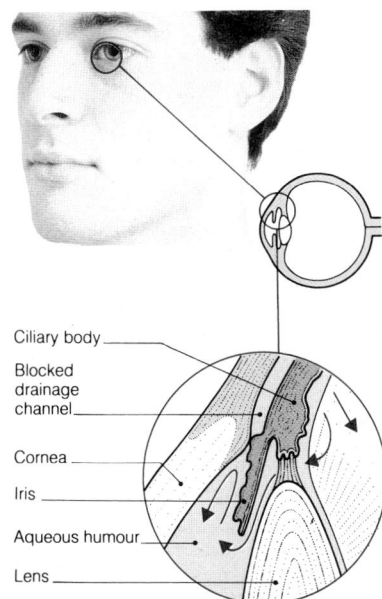

Acute closed-angle glaucoma
This type of glaucoma is caused by an unduly narrow angle between the iris and the back of the peripheral cornea. Dilation of the pupil may therefore lead to a sudden complete blockage of the outflow, causing a rapid increase in pressure in the eyeball.

Ciliary body
Blocked drainage channel
Cornea
Iris
Aqueous humour
Lens

Glioblastoma multiforme

A fast-growing and highly malignant type of *brain tumour*. Glioblastoma multiforme is a type of *glioma*, a tumour arising from glial (supporting) cells within the brain. Most glioblastomas develop within the cerebrum (the main mass of the brain).

There are about 400 to 500 new cases of glioblastoma multiforme each year in the UK. The cause is unknown.

Symptoms, diagnosis, and treatment are as for other types of brain tumour. Despite treatment, the outlook is poor, with few patients surviving more than two years.

Glioma

A type of *brain tumour* arising from the supporting glial cells within the brain.

Gliomas make up about 60 per cent of all primary brain tumours (originating from the brain rather than spread from elsewhere). There are about 1,800 new cases each year in the UK.

Types of glioma include *astrocytoma*, *glioblastoma multiforme* (a highly malignant variety of astrocytoma), *ependymoma* and *medulloblastoma* (more common in children), and *oligodendroglioma*. Symptoms, diagnosis, and treatment are as for other types of brain tumour.

Globulin

Any of a group of proteins characterized by being insoluble in water but soluble in dilute salt solutions; *antibodies* (also known as *immunoglobulins*) are an example.

TYPES
Globulins in plasma can be divided into three main groups, known as alpha-, beta-, and gamma-globulins.

Alpha-globulins include alpha$_1$-antitrypsin and haptoglobin. The former is an *enzyme* produced by the lungs and liver; deficiency is associated with *hepatitis* in children and *emphysema* (a lung disorder) in young adults. Haptoglobin is found in the blood plasma, where it binds together *haemoglobin* (the oxygen-carrying protein in red blood cells) and prevents it from being excreted in the urine by the kidneys. Various other alpha-globulins are produced as a result of inflammation, tissue damage, *autoimmune disorders* (in which the immune system attacks the body's own tissues), or certain cancers.

Beta-globulins consist mainly of low-density lipoproteins (LDLs), substances involved in the transport of fats in the blood circulation, and transferrin, which carries iron in the blood. The amount of beta-globulins is increased in certain types of *hyperlipidaemia* (a condition in which abnormally high levels of fats are present in the blood).

All of the gamma-globulins are antibodies, which are proteins produced by the immune system in response to infection, as part of an allergic reaction, and after an organ transplant. Gamma-globulins may also be produced in any disorder that causes persistent inflammation of an organ, such as *rheumatoid arthritis* or *cirrhosis* of the liver. Certain conditions, such as *multiple myeloma*, result in the production of large amounts of a specific gamma-globulin.

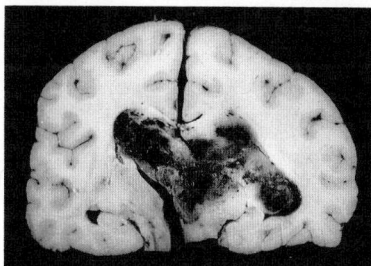

Cross-section of a brain
This photograph (taken from an autopsy specimen) shows a large area of brain infiltrated by a glioma (dark colour).

Globus hystericus

A condition, also called globus pharyngis, in which there is an uncomfortable feeling of a "lump in the throat". This lump is felt to interfere with swallowing and breathing, sometimes so much so that the sufferer is convinced that he or she cannot breathe. Respiration comes in sighs or gasps, anxiety increases, and *hyperventilation* (rapid breathing) and symptoms of a *panic attack* often ensue. Some patients insist that their Adam's apple has become larger or displaced in some way.

In most cases there is no physical basis for these attacks, which occur most commonly in people who are feeling anxious or depressed. The condition is not life-threatening. Breathing in and out of a small paper bag fitted tightly around the nose and mouth will alleviate the symptoms brought on by hyperventilation.

Unless a physical cause is found, treatment is by reassurance, breath-control training, and, in some instances, psychological treatments (e.g. *psychotherapy*). Use of *antianxiety drugs* or *antidepressant drugs* to treat the condition is rarely helpful.

Glomerulonephritis

Inflammation of the glomeruli (filtering units of the *kidney*). Both kidneys are affected, although not all the glomeruli are affected simultaneously. Damage to the glomeruli hampers the removal of waste products, salt, and water from the bloodstream, which may cause serious complications.

CAUSES AND INCIDENCE
The incidence of glomerulonephritis differs markedly around the world, mainly because some common tropical diseases (such as *malaria* and *schistosomiasis*) are important causes. Although these diseases are rarely responsible for glomerulonephritis in developed countries, glomerulonephritis is still the most common cause of chronic *kidney failure* in the US and Europe.

Some types of the disease are caused by the patient's *immune system* making *antibodies* to eliminate microorganisms—usually bacteria responsible for an infection, such as a *streptococcal infection* of the throat. These antibodies combine with bacterial *antigens* to form particles called immune complexes, which circulate in the bloodstream and become trapped in the glomeruli; this triggers an inflammatory process that may damage the glomeruli and

G

G

prevent them from working normally. Glomerulonephritis also occurs in some *autoimmune disorders*, such as systemic *lupus erythematosus* (a chronic disease of connective tissues).

SYMPTOMS

Mild forms of glomerulonephritis may produce no symptoms and the disease may be discovered only when a urine sample is tested for some other reason. In some cases, glomerulonephritis comes to light only when kidney failure has reached an advanced stage and causes symptoms due to the accumulation of waste products and fluid that are usually eliminated in the urine.

Some sufferers experience a dull ache over the kidneys. The urine may become bloodstained because damaged glomeruli can allow red blood cells into the urine. Proteinuria (loss of protein into the urine) may cause *oedema* (accumulation of fluid in body tissues), causing swelling of parts of the body (see illustrated box). Such swelling may cause mild puffiness around the eyes. The combination of proteinuria, low albumin (protein) in the blood, and oedema, is called *nephrotic syndrome*. *Hypertension* (high blood pressure) may develop and is a possibly serious complication of glomerulonephritis.

In some cases, glomerulonephritis is severe and sudden, so that kidney failure develops over a few days; sufferers often notice that they are passing very small quantities of urine.

DIAGNOSIS

There are many types of glomerulonephritis and the same cause may produce different types in different individuals. Diagnosis involves *urinalysis* (microscopic and chemical analysis of urine) and *kidney biopsy* (removal of a small amount of kidney tissue for microscopic analysis). *Kidney-function tests* may also be performed to measure how well the kidneys are removing waste products and how much protein is being lost in the urine.

TREATMENT

Treatment usually involves admission to hospital and depends on the type and severity of the disease.

Children with nephrotic syndrome usually respond to treatment with *corticosteroid drugs*, such as prednisolone. Glomerulonephritis following a streptococcal infection usually clears up after the infection is successfully treated with *antibiotic drugs*.

In general, adults respond less well to treatment but eventual kidney failure may sometimes be prevented

or delayed. Drugs may be prescribed to control hypertension and a special diet may be given to reduce the kidneys' load. A few patients with severe glomerulonephritis respond to treatment with *immunosuppressant drugs* (which dampen the body's natural defence system) or *plasmapheresis* (which rids the bloodstream of immune complexes and substances that damage the glomeruli).

Glomerulosclerosis

Scarring that occurs as a result of damage within the glomeruli (filtering units of the *kidney*).

Mild glomerulosclerosis occurs normally with age; a 10 per cent decrease in kidney function is common each decade after the age of 30. However, even a 75 per cent reduction is compatible with a normal life.

Glomerulosclerosis may occur in some severe types of *glomerulonephritis* that are difficult to treat and in which damage progresses to destroy the kidneys. Typically, sufferers develop severe *proteinuria* (the presence of protein in the urine) and severe *oedema* (accumulation of fluid in body tissues), resulting in swelling of parts of the body.

Glomerulosclerosis is also found in some people with *diabetes mellitus*. It is seen in reflux nephropathy (kidney damage associated with backflow of infected urine from the bladder) and in some people with *hypertension* (high blood pressure). Intravenous drug abuse may cause glomerulosclerosis. The condition has also been found in some people with *AIDS*.

Glomus tumour

A small, painful, bluish swelling in the skin, usually on a finger or toe near or under the nail, which is tender to touch and more painful if the limb is hot or cold. Glomus tumours result from an overgrowth of glomus bodies, structures with numerous nerve endings that normally control blood flow and temperature in the skin. The tumours are surgically removed.

Glossectomy

Removal of all or part of the *tongue*. Glossectomy may be performed to treat *tongue cancer* although this condition is more commonly treated by *radiotherapy*. If a large part of the tongue is removed, speech is impaired and eating is difficult. A liquid diet is then necessary.

THE EFFECTS OF GLOMERULONEPHRITIS

The glomeruli are damaged as a result of inflammation. Red blood cells and protein leak into the urine.

Protein loss from the circulation causes fluid to accumulate in body tissues, causing oedema.

Kidney

Kidney tubule

Damaged glomerulus
Red blood cells
Protein
Urine travels toward the bladder

Cross-section of a damaged glomerulus
Damage to the glomerulus causes red blood cells and protein to pass into the urine, which may be bloodstained.

Normal tissue
Water
Blood
Protein

Swollen tissue
Water
Blood
Protein

Healthy tissue
Through osmotic pressure, protein molecules in the blood draw back water lost to surrounding tissues.

Oedema
If protein is lost into the urine, there is a fall in osmotic pressure and more water escapes into surrounding tissues, causing swelling.

Glossitis

Inflammation of the *tongue*. The tongue feels sore and swollen and looks red and smooth; adjacent parts of the mouth may also be inflamed.

Glossitis occurs in various forms of *anaemia* and in *vitamin B* deficiency. Other causes include infection of the mouth (especially by *herpes simplex*), irritation by dentures, and excessive use of alcohol, tobacco, or spices. A congenital form of glossitis affects the middle portion of the back of the tongue.

Treatment is for the underlying cause. Self-help measures include maintaining good *oral hygiene*, by not smoking, and by avoiding acidic or spicy foods that aggravate the soreness. Regular rinsing of the mouth with a salt solution may help.

Glossolalia

Speaking in an imaginary language that has no actual meaning or syntax. Some Christians regard glossolalia as a sign of possession by the Holy Spirit; scientists tend to view it as a form of *hypnosis* or *hysteria*. (See also *Neologism*.)

Glossopharyngeal nerve

The ninth *cranial nerve*. This nerve performs both sensory and motor functions. It conveys sensations, especially taste, from the back of the tongue, regulates secretion of saliva by the parotid gland, and controls movement of the throat muscles.

Glottis

The part of the *larynx* (voice-box) that consists of the vocal cords and the slit-like opening between them.

Glucagon

A hormone produced by the *pancreas* that opposes the action of *insulin*. Glucagon stimulates the breakdown of glycogen (a carbohydrate stored in the liver and muscles) into glucose (sugar). The glucose is then released into the bloodstream, where it is available as a source of energy for cells anywhere in the body. Glucagon thus regulates the level of glucose in the blood; when the level falls, glucagon is released from the pancreas.

USE AS A DRUG

Glucagon is extracted from the pancreas of pigs or cows for use as a drug. It is given by subcutaneous (under the skin) injection in the emergency treatment of people with *diabetes mellitus* who are unconscious as a result of hypoglycaemia (low blood sugar).

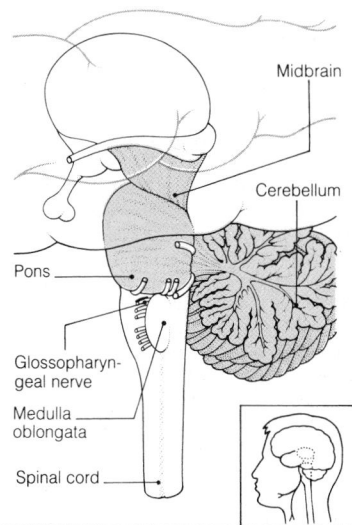

LOCATION OF THE GLOSSOPHARYNGEAL NERVE
The nerve arises from the medulla oblongata and branches to the tongue, parotid gland, and pharynx.

Midbrain

Cerebellum

Pons

Glossopharyngeal nerve

Medulla oblongata

Spinal cord

Glucagon produces recovery within 15 to 20 minutes; the patient is then given glucose by mouth to prevent a relapse. Nausea and vomiting are occasional adverse effects.

Glucocorticoids

Hormones produced by the cortex (outer layer) of the *adrenal glands* that affect carbohydrate metabolism by increasing the blood sugar level and the amount of glycogen in the liver. The principal glucocorticoid is *hydrocortisone* (also called cortisol), which also has a *mineralocorticoid* (affecting the body's sodium and potassium balance) effect.

Glucose

A simple sugar (monosaccharide) produced by the digestion of starch and sucrose; also called dextrose. Glucose is a fruit sugar, present in fruits and fruit juices together with fructose. It is the chief source of energy for the body and is carried to all tissues in the blood. The term blood sugar refers to glucose in the bloodstream.

BLOOD SUGAR LEVELS

Despite wide variation in carbohydrate intake (and, therefore, large fluctuations in the amount of glucose in the body), the blood sugar level is normally kept within narrow limits. This is achieved by the actions of several hormones, notably *insulin, glucagon, adrenaline, corticosteroid hormones*, and *growth hormone*. If the blood sugar level is abnormally high (known as *hyperglycaemia*), it may cause *glycosuria* (glucose in the urine). An abnormally low blood sugar level is called *hypoglycaemia*.

Insulin, released by the pancreas in response to increased blood sugar levels, lowers the level by stimulating the uptake of glucose by cells. Inside the cells, glucose may be "burned" to produce energy, converted to *glycogen* for storage (mainly in the liver and muscles), or used in the production of triglycerides (fats).

Glucagon is released by the pancreas when the blood sugar level is low. It stimulates the breakdown of stored glycogen to glucose, which is then released into the bloodstream.

Adrenaline and corticosteroid hormones released by the adrenal glands in response to stress have the same basic effect as glucagon—that is, they stimulate the release of glucose to increase the blood sugar level.

Glue ear

Accumulation of fluid in the middle-ear cavity, causing impaired hearing. Persistent glue ear is most common in children. It is often accompanied by enlarged *adenoids* and frequently occurs with viral upper respiratory tract infections, such as the common *cold*. Usually both ears are affected. The condition is also known as otitis media with effusion, persistent middle-ear effusion, and secretory otitis media.

CAUSES

The mucus-secreting lining of the middle-ear cavity sometimes becomes overactive, producing large amounts of sticky fluid. If there is blockage of the *eustachian tube*, which links the middle ear to the back of the nose, the fluid cannot drain away. The fluid subsequently accumulates and interferes with the movement of the delicate bones in the middle ear.

SIGNS

The first, and often the only, sign is some degree of *deafness*. The child may be unaware of this and, unless his or her unresponsiveness is noticed by parents or teachers, the condition may pass undetected.

DIAGNOSIS

Glue ear is sometimes first detected through *hearing tests*, which should be carried out routinely on all children. Once any hearing loss is detected or suspected in a child, a doctor uses an

G

G

otoscope (viewing instrument) to examine each eardrum for the characteristic changes in appearance and colour that occur in glue ear.

TREATMENT
In mild cases the patient is given nose drops containing *decongestant drugs* to unblock the affected eustachian tube, so that the fluid can drain through it.

When the condition is severe, a *myringotomy* (a surgical opening in the eardrum) and insertion of *grommets* (small tubes) may be needed. Removal of the adenoids may also be required (see *Adenoidectomy*).

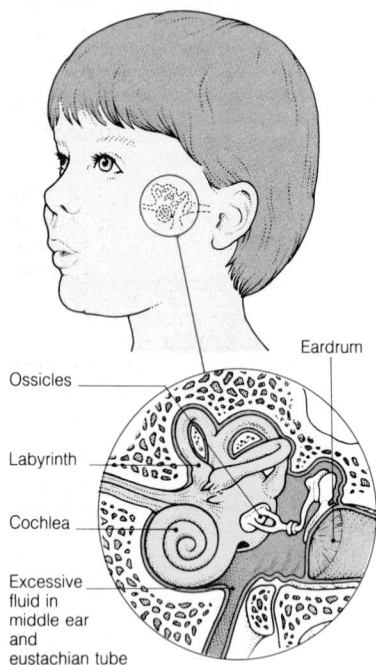

Ossicles

Eardrum

Labyrinth

Cochlea

Excessive fluid in middle ear and eustachian tube

Effects of glue ear
In this condition, sticky fluid in the middle ear prevents free movement of the eardrum and ossicles, causing deafness.

Glue-sniffing
See *Solvent abuse*.

Gluten

A combination of gliadins and glutenins (types of proteins) formed when certain cereal flours (most notably wheat flour) are mixed with water. Sensitivity to part of the gliadin in gluten causes *coeliac disease*.

Gluten enteropathy
See *Coeliac disease*.

Gluten intolerance
See *Coeliac disease*.

Gluteus maximus
The large, powerful muscle in each of the buttocks which helps give them their rounded shape. The gluteus maximus is responsible for moving the thigh sideways and backwards.

Glycerol
A colourless syrupy liquid which has a sweet taste. Glycerol, also known as glycerine, is used in several drug preparations and in the food processing industry.

Glycerol is prepared commercially from *fats* and *oils*; it is an essential constituent of triglycerides (simple fats). The triglyceride molecule consists of one molecule of glycerol combined with three molecules of fatty acids.

In the form of rectal *suppositories*, glycerol relieves *constipation* by softening hard faeces. Glycerol is used in moisturizing creams to help prevent dryness and cracking of the skin (for example, it is used to protect the nipples during breast-feeding). Glycerol is also used in ear-drops to help soften earwax prior to syringing of the ears, and in *cough remedies* to help soothe a dry, irritating cough.

Glyceryl trinitrate
A *vasodilator drug* used to treat and prevent symptoms of *angina pectoris* (chest pain due to inadequate blood supply to the heart).

Glyceryl trinitrate may cause a headache, flushing, and dizziness. Adverse effects are usually relieved by a reduction in the dose; this can be achieved by putting a tablet under the tongue and then spitting it out when sufficient of the preparation has dissolved to cause the chest pain to cease.

Glycogen
The principal *carbohydrate* storage material in the body. Glycogen is a polysaccharide, consisting of many glucose molecules linked to form long chains, and is found mainly in the liver and in muscles.

Glycogen plays an important role in controlling blood sugar levels. When there is too much sugar (glucose) in the blood, the excess is converted to glycogen. This conversion (controlled by *insulin* and *corticosteroid* hormones) takes place chiefly in the liver and in muscles. When the blood sugar level is low, glycogen is converted back to glucose (a process that is regulated by the hormones *glucagon* and *adrenaline*) and released into the bloodstream.

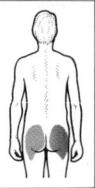
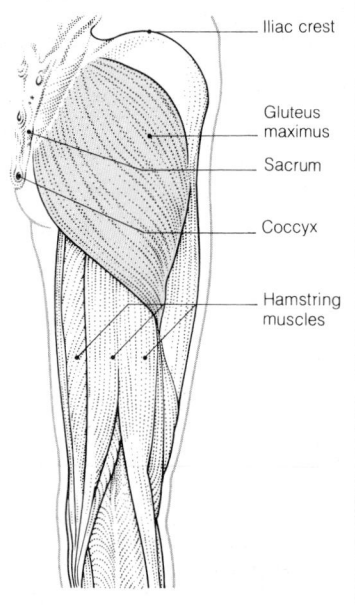

LOCATION OF THE GLUTEUS MAXIMUS
The top is attached to the sacrum, coccyx, and pelvis. The lower part is attached to the femur (thigh-bone).

Iliac crest

Gluteus maximus

Sacrum

Coccyx

Hamstring muscles

Glycosuria
The presence of *glucose* in the urine. Glycosuria results from failure of the *kidneys* to reabsorb glucose back into the bloodstream after the blood has been filtered. Glycosuria by itself does not necessarily indicate that a serious condition is present.

CAUSES
In the normal filtering process in the kidneys, glucose is removed from the bloodstream along with many other normal blood constituents and unwanted waste products. The filtered fluid passes down the many tubules of the kidneys, where wanted substances are reabsorbed and returned to the bloodstream and unwanted substances are excreted as urine. In most healthy people, glucose is one of the substances that is almost completely reabsorbed.

Glycosuria may be caused by failure of the kidneys to reabsorb all the glucose because of *hyperglycaemia* (an abnormally high level of glucose in the blood), as in *diabetes mellitus*.

Alternatively, glycosuria may occur if the kidney tubules have been damaged and are unable to reabsorb even normal amounts of glucose. Damage to the tubules may be a result of rare *metabolic disorders* present from birth or be a consequence of *drug poisoning* or heavy metal poisoning.

Glycosuria also occurs in some healthy people who have kidneys that are unable to reabsorb all the glucose filtered out of the bloodstream. This condition tends to run in families. Glycosuria often occurs during pregnancy as a consequence of hormonal changes; this is usually not serious provided there are no other symptoms and blood glucose is normal.

DIAGNOSIS AND TREATMENT

Glycosuria may be found during a routine examination or if the doctor is performing specific tests because diabetes mellitus is suspected. Urine can be tested for glucose by using a chemically impregnated strip that changes colour when it comes in contact with glucose. Treatment depends on the underlying cause.

Goitre

Enlargement of the *thyroid gland*, visible as a swelling on the neck.

CAUSES

The thyroid gland may enlarge (without any disturbance of its function) at puberty, during pregnancy, or as a result of taking *oral contraceptives*. In many parts of the world the main cause of a goitre is lack of sufficient *iodine* in the diet. The thyroid requires the iodine to produce the hormone thyroxine; a deficiency causes swelling of the thyroid.

A condition known as toxic goitre develops in *Graves' disease* and in other forms of *hyperthyroidism* (overactivity of the thyroid gland) that lead to *thyrotoxicosis*. Typical features of thyrotoxicosis include warm, dry skin, increased appetite, weight loss, tremor, insomnia, and occasional muscle weakness and agitation.

A goitre is also a feature of different types of *thyroiditis* (inflammation of the thyroid gland), including *Hashimoto's thyroiditis* (an autoimmune disorder) and de Quervain's thyroiditis, both of which damage the gland.

Other causes of goitre include a tumour or nodule in the gland and, in rare cases, *thyroid cancer*. A goitre can also be caused by drugs given to treat overactivity of the thyroid gland.

SYMPTOMS

A goitre can range in size from a barely noticeable lump to an enormous swelling, depending on the cause. Large swellings may press on the oesophagus or trachea, making swallowing or breathing difficult.

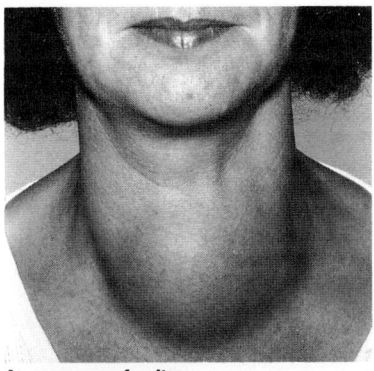

Appearance of goitre
The thyroid may become enlarged for various reasons, including dietary deficiency of iodine, inflammation, or an autoimmune disorder affecting the gland.

DIAGNOSIS AND TREATMENT

Diagnosis is based on the nature of the swelling and any accompanying symptoms. *Thyroid-function tests*, including blood tests and *radionuclide scanning*, may be carried out to determine the activity of the thyroid gland. X-rays may be taken to investigate accompanying symptoms.

A goitre that is not caused by disease may eventually disappear or may be so small that it does not require treatment. However, a large or unsightly goitre, or one that is causing difficulty with swallowing or breathing may require total or partial removal (see *Thyroidectomy*).

If iodine deficiency is identified as the cause, the patient will be advised to eat more fish and iodized salt, which are both rich in iodine. When a goitre is the result of disease, treatment will be for the underlying disorder. If a drug is the cause, the goitre usually disappears once the course of treatment is over.

Gold

An *antirheumatic drug* used to treat *rheumatoid arthritis* and, occasionally, arthritis arising as a complication of *psoriasis*. Gold is usually prescribed in severe cases after a *nonsteroidal anti-inflammatory drug* (NSAID) has proved ineffective.

HOW IT WORKS

Gold has an anti-inflammatory action that relieves joint pain and stiffness and may prevent further damage.

POSSIBLE ADVERSE EFFECTS

A common adverse effect of gold is *dermatitis* (skin inflammation); if itching occurs, the drug is usually withdrawn. Gold may damage the kidneys, liver, and bone marrow. Blood tests

are performed during treatment to check the function of these organs.

Gold may cause loss of appetite, nausea, diarrhoea, abdominal pain, and, occasionally, *anaphylactic shock* (a serious allergic reaction that requires emergency treatment).

Golfer's elbow

A condition caused by inflammation of the epicondyle (bony prominence) on the inner side of the *elbow*, at the site of attachment of some forearm muscles. The inflammation causes pain and tenderness at the inner side of the elbow and sometimes in the forearm.

Golfer's elbow is caused by overuse of these muscles, which act to bend the wrist and fingers. Activities that can cause the condition include gripping and twisting (such as using a screwdriver) or playing golf with a faulty grip or swing.

TREATMENT

Treatment consists of resting the elbow, applying ice-packs, and taking *analgesic drugs* (painkillers) and/or anti-inflammatory tablets. If the pain is severe or persistent, injection of a *corticosteroid drug* may be helpful.

If the pain is caused by a sport, it is wise to stop playing for a week or two and to seek advice about technique.

Gonadorelins

Drugs that are analogues of gonadorelin, the hypothalmic-releasing hormone that stimulates the pituitary gland to secrete the *gonadotrophin hormones*, *luteinizing hormone*, and *follicle-stimulating hormone*. Drugs such as buserelin and goserelin, having a closely similar structure to gonadorelin, suppress the release of the natural hormone, thereby reducing the secretion of the pituitary hormones. These drugs are used to treat *endometriosis* and hormone-dependent cancers including *breast cancer* and *prostate cancer*.

Gonadotrophin hormones

Hormones that stimulate cell activity in the gonads (*ovaries* and *testes*). Gonadotrophins are essential for female and male fertility. The two most important gonadotrophins are follicle-stimulating hormone (FSH) and luteinizing hormone (LH), which are secreted by the *pituitary gland*. Another gonadotrophin, HCG (see *Gonadotrophin, human chorionic*), is produced by the placenta.

GONADOTROPHIN HORMONE THERAPY

Synthetic HCG is used in the treatment of recurrent *miscarriage* and certain types of female and male

G

489

infertility. Menotrophin (a gonadotrophin extracted from the urine of postmenopausal women) contains both FSH and LH and is used in the treatment of female infertility due to a failure to ovulate.

Gonadotrophin, human chorionic

A hormone produced by the *placenta* in early *pregnancy*. Human chorionic gonadotrophin (HCG) stimulates the *ovaries* to produce *oestrogen* and *progesterone*, hormones needed to maintain a healthy pregnancy.

HCG is excreted in the urine; its measurement forms the basis of most pregnancy tests (a high level confirming pregnancy).

HCG THERAPY

HCG extracted from the urine of pregnant women is given by injection to treat certain types of *infertility*. Along with *clomiphene* tablets, which stimulate gonadotrophin release from the pituitary, HCG may induce *ovulation* in women who have not been ovulating. In men, HCG has been used in an attempt to increase sperm production.

HCG is occasionally given to prevent *miscarriage* in women whose production of progesterone is deficient.

HCG is also prescribed for the treatment of cryptorchidism (see *Testis, undescended*) in young boys, although surgical correction is usually required.

Gonads

The sex glands—the *testes* in men and the *ovaries* in women. The testes, situated in the scrotum, produce sperm and secrete the hormone *testosterone*. The ovaries, situated in the abdomen, release usually one ovum (egg) from either the right or the left ovary each month and secrete the hormones *oestrogen* and *progesterone*.

The activities of the gonads—both male and female—are regulated by *gonadotrophin hormones* released by the pituitary gland.

Gonorrhoea

One of the most common *sexually transmitted diseases*, popularly known as "the clap". Gonorrhoea occurs throughout the world.

CAUSES AND INCIDENCE

Gonorrhoea, caused by the bacterium NEISSERIA GONORRHOEAE, is most often transmitted during sexual intercourse, including oral or anal sex. An infected woman may also transmit the disease to her baby during childbirth.

Gonorrhoea is the second most common sexually transmitted disease

in the UK, after *nonspecific urethritis* and it is most prevalent among young adults who have had multiple sexual partners. 50,000 cases are reported from STD clinics in the UK each year.

SYMPTOMS AND SIGNS

Gonorrhoea has a short incubation period of two to 10 days. In men, symptoms usually include a urethral discharge and pain on passing urine. About 60 per cent of infected women have no symptoms; if symptoms are present, they usually consist of a vaginal discharge or a burning sensation when passing urine.

Infection acquired through anal sex causes gonococcal *proctitis* (inflammation of the rectum and anus). It causes pain and anal discharge in only about 10 per cent of infected people. Oral sex with an infected person may lead to gonococcal *pharyngitis*, which may cause sore throat but often causes no symptoms. A baby exposed to infection in the mother's reproductive tract during childbirth may acquire gonococcal *ophthalmia*, a severe inflammation affecting one or both eyes.

COMPLICATIONS

Untreated gonorrhoea may spread to other parts of the body. In men, it may cause *prostatitis* (inflammation of the prostate) or *epididymo-orchitis* (inflammation of the epididymides and testes), affecting fertility. In women, untreated gonorrhoea affects the fallopian tubes, causing *pelvic inflammatory disease* (PID). Damage to the fallopian tubes causes increased susceptibility to further episodes of PID, increases the risk of an *ectopic pregnancy* occurring in a fallopian tube, and may lead to *infertility*.

Gonococcal bacteria may occasionally spread through the bloodstream to cause gonococcal *arthritis*, with pain and swelling of joints around the body. Multiplication of bacteria in the bloodstream causes *septicaemia*, producing generalized symptoms and signs, including fever and malaise. Rarely, gonococcal septicaemia affects the brain or heart and may cause death.

DIAGNOSIS

Many disorders can cause a urethral or vaginal discharge, and laboratory tests are necessary to confirm a diagnosis of gonorrhoea. Tests are carried out on a sample of the discharge or on swabs taken from the urethra, cervix, and sometimes the rectum.

TREATMENT

Gonorrhoea is treated with an antibiotic, usually a *penicillin drug*, such as procaine penicillin or *ampicillin*. If the infection is caused by penicillin-resis-

tant NEISSERIA GONORRHOEAE or if the infected person is allergic to penicillin, other antibiotics, such as cefotaxime, ciprofloxacin or spectinomycin, may be used. After treatment, tests are performed to ensure that the infection has been cured.

OUTLOOK

Treatment for gonorrhoea is effective but does not protect against reinfection. Sexual partners must be told that they might have gonorrhoea even if they have no symptoms; many clinics have counsellors (known as contact tracers or health advisers) who identify and inform all people who might have been infected by the patient.

Goodpasture's syndrome

A rare condition characterized by *glomerulonephritis* (inflammation of the filtering units of the kidney), coughing up blood, and *anaemia*. Goodpasture's syndrome is a serious disease; unless treated early it may lead to life-threatening bleeding into the lungs and progressive *kidney failure*.

Goodpasture's syndrome is an *autoimmune disorder* (one in which the body's *immune system* attacks its own tissues). *Antibodies* are formed that attack the capillaries (tiny blood vessels) in the lungs and kidneys, eventually resulting in inflammation and disruption of the normal functioning of the lungs and kidneys.

The disease usually affects young men, but can develop in women and at any age.

TREATMENT

Sometimes the disease responds to treatment with *immunosuppressant drugs* (drugs that hamper the normal working of the body's immune system) and *plasmapheresis* (a procedure for removing unwanted antibodies from the blood plasma).

People who suffer from severe and repeated attacks require treatment by *dialysis* (a technique for removing waste products from the blood) and, eventually, a *kidney transplant*.

Gout

A metabolic disorder that causes attacks of *arthritis*, usually in a single joint. Gout may be associated with kidney stones (see *Calculus, urinary tract*) which may lead to *kidney failure*.

SYMPTOMS AND SIGNS

An acute attack of gout usually affects a single joint, most commonly the joint at the base of the big toe, but it can affect other joints, including the knee, ankle, wrist, foot, and small joints of the hand.

The affected joint is red, swollen, and extremely tender; the pain reaches a peak level of intensity within 24 to 36 hours. The redness and swelling may spread and be confused with *cellulitis* (inflammation of tissues beneath the skin). The pain is so intense that the sufferer may not be able to stand on an affected foot or even tolerate the pressure of bedclothes on it. Sometimes there is a mild fever.

The first attack usually involves only one joint and lasts a few days. Some people never have another attack, but most have a second attack between six months and two years after the first. After the second attack, more and more joints may be involved, and there may be constant pain due to damage to the joint from chronic inflammation.

TREATMENT

Pain and inflammation in gout can be controlled with large doses of a *nonsteroidal anti-inflammatory drug* (NSAID). *Colchicine* is sometimes prescribed if NSAIDs are not considered suitable. For maximum benefit, treatment should start as soon as an attack begins; patients prone to recurrent attacks should carry their gout medicine with them. As the inflammation subsides, usually within two to three days, the dose is gradually reduced and finally stopped. If an attack of gout is not responding to treatment with an NSAID or colchicine, a *corticosteroid drug* may be injected into the affected joint.

Increased levels of purine (a product of *DNA*) can raise the level of uric acid in the blood. Although a strict low-purine diet is not necessary, people with gout should avoid foods that are high in purine, such as liver and other offal, poultry, and pulses. Heavy consumption of alcohol should also be avoided because it may precipitate an acute attack.

Many people never have more than a few attacks of gout, and further treatment is usually unnecessary. If attacks are recurrent, the frequency can be reduced by lowering the urate levels with drugs that either inhibit the formation of uric acid (such as *allopurinol*) or increase the excretion of uric acid by the kidneys (uricosuric drugs, such as *probenecid* and *sulphinpyrazone*). If the level of uric acid in the blood is very high, drug treatment will need to be continued for life to prevent the possible development of *hypertension* (high blood pressure) or kidney disease.

GOUT

Gout is a common joint disease, affecting 10 times more men than women. In men it occurs at any time after puberty; in women it usually occurs only after the menopause. There is often a family history of the disorder. Hyperuricaemia (excess uric acid in the blood) leads to formation of uric acid crystals in joints; crystals may also be deposited in soft tissues in the ears and around tendons.

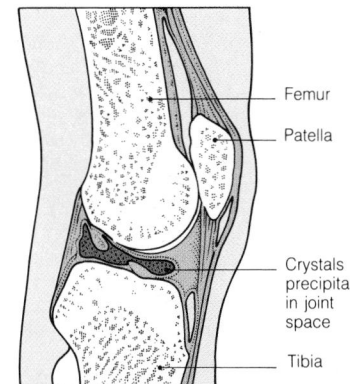

Crystal precipitation
Crystals of uric acid precipitate into the joint space and surrounding tissues of the knee, causing intense inflammation and extreme pain.

Femur
Patella
Crystals precipitate in joint space
Tibia

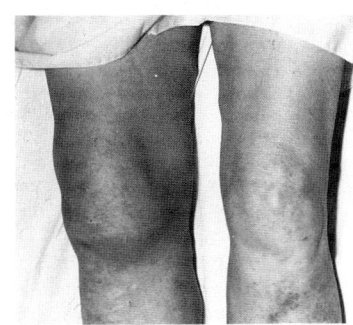

Appearance of gout
Deposition of uric acid crystals in the joint space has caused inflammation and obvious swelling of the affected right knee.

DIAGNOSIS

Gout is considered as a diagnosis whenever an attack of arthritis affects a single joint. A blood test is usually performed; a high level of uric acid suggests gout.

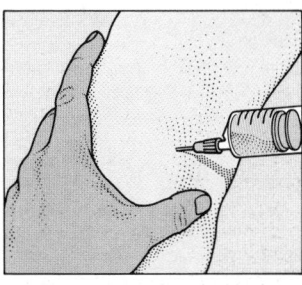

Aspiration
Fluid is aspirated (removed through a needle into a syringe) from the swollen knee joint and examined under a microscope.

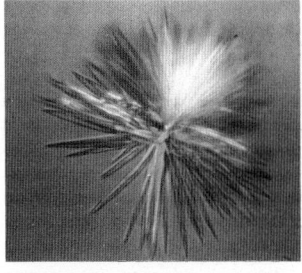

Microscopic evidence
The presence of uric acid crystals confirms the diagnosis.

Grafting

The process of transplanting healthy tissue from one part of the body to another (autografting), from one person to another (allografting or homografting), or from an animal to a person (xenografting).

Grafting is used to repair or replace diseased, damaged, or otherwise defective tissues or organs. Those that are most commonly transplanted (see *Transplant surgery*) include the skin (see *Skin graft*); bone (see *Bone graft*); bone marrow (see *Bone marrow trans-* plant); the cornea of the eye (see *Corneal graft*); the kidney (see *Kidney transplant*); the heart (see *Heart transplant*); the heart and lungs (see *Heart-lung transplant*); the liver (see *Liver transplant*); the heart valves (see *Heart-valve surgery*); and blood vessels and nerves (see *Microsurgery*).

COMPLICATIONS

With autografting, the grafted tissue is usually assimilated at the new site without any trouble and soon grows into the surrounding tissue to provide a good repair.

G

G

Problems occur, however, with allografting and xenografting, both of which are usually carried out to replace rather than repair tissue. Xenografting is not performed clinically except for the use of porcine (pig) heart valves. The major disadvantage of allografting is that the recipient's defence system automatically attempts to reject the foreign cells of the donor's tissue and to destroy them in the same way that it would invading microorganisms. The only exceptions are grafts between identical twins (because their tissue matches exactly) and corneal grafting (because the cornea has no blood supply and therefore no white blood cells and antibodies to act as a defence system).

To overcome rejection, as close a match as possible between the tissues of recipient and donor is sought (see *Tissue-typing*). *Immunosuppressant drugs* are given to suppress the body's defence system—although this can cause other problems, such as decreased kidney function. The immunosuppressant drug *cyclosporin*, introduced in the mid-1980s, has been very effective in the control of rejection and *graft-versus-host disease*.

Graft-versus-host disease

A common complication of a *bone marrow transplant*. Graft-versus-host disease is caused by cells called cytotoxic T-*lymphocytes*, present in the transplanted marrow, attacking the transplant recipient's tissues. Lymphocytes form part of the *immune system* and normally play a beneficial role by attacking cells recognized as foreign. However, in transplant procedures, this activity is harmful.

Graft-versus-host (GVH) disease may occur soon after an organ transplant or may appear some months later. The first sign of the disease is usually a skin rash. This may be followed by diarrhoea, abdominal pain, jaundice, inflammation of the eyes and mouth, and breathlessness. Most patients recover within a year, but some gradually get weaker and thinner and about one third die.

Graft-versus-host disease can be prevented by giving *immunosuppressant drugs*, such as *cyclosporin*, to all transplant recipients. If the disease develops, it is treated with *corticosteroid drugs* and with other immunosuppressant drugs. It may be possible to prevent GVH in bone marrow transplants by removing cytotoxic T-cells from the donor marrow before the transplant is performed.

Gram's stain

An iodine-based stain widely used in bacteriology to help differentiate between various types of bacteria. It is also known as Gram's iodine.

There are several different methods of Gram staining. Basically, however, the specimen is stained with gentian violet, followed by a solution of Gram's stain, and then treated with a decolorizing agent such as acetone. Finally, the specimen is counterstained with a red dye. Bacteria that retain the dark violet stain are known as gram-positive, whereas those that lose the violet stain after decolorization but take up the counterstain (causing them to appear pink) are gram-negative. Examples of gram-positive bacteria include several species of STREPTOCOCCUS, STAPHYLOCOCCUS, and CLOSTRIDIUM; gram-negative bacteria include VIBRIO CHOLERAE (which causes cholera) and various species of SALMONELLA.

Grand mal

A type of epileptic seizure in which the sufferer, sometimes after warning symptoms, cries out, falls to the ground unconscious, and has generalized jerky muscle contractions. The seizure may last for a few minutes. The person usually remains unconscious for a time and may have no recall of the seizure on awakening. (See also *Epilepsy*.)

Granulation tissue

A mass of red, moist, granular tissue that develops on the surface of an ulcer or open wound during the process of healing. The tissue consists mainly of fibroblasts (which make collagen) and numerous small blood vessels. (See also *Healing*; *Wound*.)

Granuloma

An aggregation of cells, of a type associated with chronic inflammation.

CAUSES AND TYPES

Granulomas usually occur as a reaction to the presence of certain infectious agents or to a foreign body, but may occur in conditions of unknown cause.

Certain infections, such as *tuberculosis*, *brucellosis*, *leprosy*, and *syphilis*, although caused by different bacteria, give rise to infective granulomas in many different organs of the body. *Sarcoidosis*, a condition of unknown cause, is also characterized by granulomas in different organs. Granulomas may also occur in parasitic and fungal infections.

A foreign body granuloma can occur as a reaction to inorganic material, such as dust, talcum powder, dirt, or a suture. A pyogenic granuloma is a common benign skin tumour which develops on exposed areas following minor injury and often occurs on the hands of gardeners. The swellings are raised, red, moist, and tender and often disappear gradually without treatment. Pyogenic granulomas can be removed surgically, or by *electrocautery* or *cryosurgery*.

Many other, largely unrelated, conditions are also described as granulomas. For example, a dental granuloma is a swelling arising from poorly fitting false teeth; another type of granuloma is a benign growth on the iris. (See also *Granuloma annulare*; *Granuloma inguinale*; *Granuloma, lethal midline*.)

Granuloma annulare

A harmless skin condition characterized by a circular, raised area of skin, occurring most commonly in children, usually on the knuckles or fingers, and less commonly on the upper part of the feet or on the elbows or ears. The raised area spreads slowly outwards to form a ring, 2.5 to 7.5 cm in diameter, with raised edges and a flattened centre. Rarely, several of these ring-like patches occur over a wider area. The cause is unknown.

The diagnosis of granuloma annulare is often made simply from its appearance but may be confirmed by means of a skin *biopsy* (removal of a small sample of tissue for microscopic investigation). No treatment is necessary. In most cases, the affected skin heals completely over a period of several months or years.

Granuloma inguinale

A *sexually transmitted disease* that causes ulceration of the genitals. The infection is caused by bacteria-like organisms called Donovan's bodies. Granuloma inguinale is common in certain parts of the tropics, although it is very rare in developed countries. There are only about 20 cases a year reported in the UK, mainly in travellers from the tropics.

The first symptoms are painless, raised nodules on the penis or labia or around the anal area. The nodules gradually ulcerate and then form red, raised areas that are usually painless. These areas sometimes contain pus and, if left untreated, may eventually heal with extensive scarring.

Diagnosis is based on finding Donovan's bodies in a *biopsy* sample (tissue removed for microscopic analysis) from a sore. The antibiotic drugs *tetracycline* or *gentamicin* are effective treatments.

Granuloma, lethal midline
A rare disorder of unknown cause in which the nose and other facial structures become inflamed and eventually destroyed by progressive damage to the skin and underlying tissues.

Patients with midline granuloma are usually in their 40s or 50s; women are affected more often than men. The first symptoms are usually caused by ulceration within the nose. Tissue destruction may spread to the facial sinuses, the gums, and the orbits (eye sockets).

The most effective treatment is *radiotherapy*, which usually halts the progression of the disease and may improve symptoms for years.

Graves' disease
A disorder characterized by toxic *goitre* (an overactive and enlarged thyroid gland), excessive production of thyroid hormones leading to *thyrotoxicosis*, and sometimes *exophthalmos* (bulging eyeballs). Graves' disease is an *autoimmune disorder* (a disorder in which the *immune system* attacks the body's own tissues).

Gravida
The medical term for a pregnant woman. The term is often combined with a prefix to indicate the total number of pregnancies (including the present one). For example, a primigravida is a woman who is pregnant for the first time, and a secundigravida is one who is pregnant for the second time; multigravida is a general term for a woman who has been pregnant at least once before.

Gray
An SI (International System of Units) unit of radiation dosage (see *Radiation units* box).

Grey matter
Regions of the central nervous system (*brain* and *spinal cord*) consisting principally of closely packed and interconnected nuclei of nerve cells, rather than their filamentous projections or axons, which make up the white matter.

In the brain, grey matter is primarily found in the outer layers of the *cerebrum* (the main mass of the brain and the region responsible for advanced mental functions) and in some regions deeper within the brain. Grey matter also makes up the inner core of the spinal cord.

Grief
An intensely unhappy and painful emotion, usually caused by loss of a loved one. (See *Bereavement*.)

Grip
The *hand* is particularly well-adapted for gripping, with an opposable thumb (i.e. one that is able to touch each of the fingers), specialized skin on the palm and fingers to provide adhesion, and a complex system of muscles, tendons, joints, and nerves that enables precise movements of the digits.

The hand can perform two basic grips: grasping, which is a strength hold that involves the whole hand, and pinching, which is a precision hold using the thumb and a finger. Both grips are controlled by a combination of long muscles in the forearm and short muscles in the hand itself.

Gripping ability can be reduced by any condition that causes muscular weakness or impairment of sensation in the palms or fingers (e.g. a *stroke* or *nerve injury*) or by disorders that affect the bones or joints of the hand or wrist, such as *arthritis* or a *fracture*, or by traumatic loss of a finger.

Grippe
A term of French origin for any illness resembling *influenza*. The term was once used commonly in English-speaking as well as French-speaking countries.

Griseofulvin
A drug given by mouth to treat *tinea* infections (a group of fungal infections) which have not responded to antifungal creams or lotions. Griseofulvin is particularly useful in the treatment of infections affecting the scalp, beard, palms, soles of the feet, and nails.

Common side-effects are headache, loss of taste, dry mouth, abdominal pain, and *photosensitivity* (increased sensitivity of the skin to sunlight). During long-term treatment, griseofulvin may cause liver or bone marrow damage; blood tests may be carried out to check the function of these organs.

Groin
The hollow between the lower abdomen and top of the thigh. (See also *Groin, lump in the*; *Groin strain*.)

Groin, lump in the
A swelling in the hollow between the lower abdomen and the top of the thigh. The most common cause of a lump in the groin is enlargement of a lymph node as a result of an infection (see *Glands, swollen*). Another common cause is a *hernia*, in which abdominal contents protrude through a weak area in the abdominal wall.

Other possible causes of a lump in the groin include an *abscess* (a pus-filled sac), a *lipoma* (a painless benign tumour of fat cells), or an undescended testis (see *Testis, undescended*). Rarely, a lump in the groin may be due to a *varicose vein* or to an *aneurysm* (balloon-like swelling of an artery).

INVESTIGATION AND TREATMENT
The cause of a lump in the groin can usually be ascertained by physical examination by a doctor. Treatment depends on the cause.

Groin strain
Pain and tenderness in the groin due to overstretching of a muscle, typically while running or participating in sports. The muscles commonly affected are the adductors (on the inside of the thigh), which help to rotate and flex the thigh and pull it inwards, and the rectus femoris (at the front of the thigh), which also flexes the thigh.

Pain and tenderness in the groin that mimics pain due to muscle strain may sometimes be caused by *osteoarthritis* in the hip or lower spine, *osteitis pubis* (inflammation of the pubic bones, situated at the front and base of the spine), or an inguinal *hernia* (a protrusion of abdominal contents through a weak area in the abdominal wall).

INVESTIGATION AND TREATMENT
Groin strain is difficult to treat and recovery may be slow. When the cause is obviously a simple muscle strain, treatment is by *physiotherapy*. However, if another cause is suspected, or if what was thought to be a muscle strain does not respond to physiotherapy, tests such as *X-rays* may be required. An X-ray may show that a muscle has pulled a small piece of bone away from the pelvis; surgery to wire the bone back into position may then be necessary.

Grommet tube
A small tube that may be inserted through the eardrum during a *myringotomy* (a procedure in which an incision is made in the eardrum) in order to treat *glue ear* in children.

The grommet equalizes the pressure on both sides of the eardrum, permitting mucous fluid to drain down the eustachian tube into the back of the throat. Tubes are usually allowed to fall out on their own as the hole in the eardrum closes, which generally occurs between six and 12 months after insertion. Children with grommets need not take any special precautions when swimming, since water rarely enters the ears and seems to do no harm.

Group therapy

Any treatment of emotional or psychological problems in which groups of patients meet regularly with a therapist. Interaction among members of the group is thought to be therapeutic and for certain problems is considered to be more effective than the traditional patient-therapist relationship.

A typical therapy group consists of eight to 10 people. The members meet for an hour or more once or twice a week to discuss their problems with one another, guided by a therapist.

Group therapy may be useful for people with personality problems and for sufferers from *alcohol dependence, drug dependence, anxiety disorders* and eating disorders (such as *anorexia nervosa* and *bulimia*).

Growing pains

Vague aches and pains that occur in the limbs of children. The pains are usually felt at night and most often affect the calves of children aged between six and 12 years old. The cause of growing pains is unknown, although they do not seem to be related to the process of growth itself.

Growing pains are of no medical significance and require no treatment, although they may interfere with the child's sleep and may alarm parents. If pain is severe or associated with other symptoms, such as joint swelling or malaise, a doctor should be consulted.

Growth

An abnormal proliferation of cells within a localized area (see *Tumour*); the increase in height and weight as a child develops (see *Growth, childhood*).

Growth, childhood

The period of most rapid growth occurs before birth, during embryonic and fetal development. After birth, although growth is still very rapid in the first few years of life, especially in the first year, the rate of growth steadily decreases. At the onset of *puberty* there is another major period of growth and development which continues until full adult height is reached, usually at about 16 or 17 in girls and 19 to 21 in boys. In general, increase in weight follows the same pattern as increase in height.

Significant variations occur within the typical overall growth pattern. For example, baby boys grow faster than girls until the age of about seven months, after which girls grow faster. Girls continue to grow more rapidly until about four years of age, when the growth rate becomes the same, and remains so until puberty. Overall, girls tend to be shorter than boys at all ages until puberty, when they become taller for a few years because they enter the pubertal growth spurt earlier. But because puberty is later in boys, their final height is greater.

Growth is not simply a process of becoming taller and heavier. The body shape also changes because different areas grow at different rates. At birth, the head is already about three quarters of its adult size; the head grows to almost full size during the first year. Thereafter, it becomes proportionately smaller because the body grows at a much faster rate. The limbs grow faster than the trunk during early childhood but more slowly during puberty.

Different tissues also grow at different rates. For example, lymphatic tissue grows rapidly until just before adolescence, when it begins to shrink. The brain also grows quickly during the early years, but reaches about nine tenths of its adult weight by the age of five, after which its growth rate decreases markedly.

FACTORS THAT INFLUENCE GROWTH

Growth can be influenced by heredity and by environmental factors, such as nutrition, general health, and emotional welfare. Hormones also play an important role, particularly *growth hormone, thyroid hormones*, and, at puberty, the *sex hormones*.

A child with taller-than-average parents also tends to grow to above-average height because of the effects of heredity. However, this may be counteracted by poor health or undernutrition. In infancy, weight is the best indicator of health and nutrition. Thereafter, height is equally important. Regular measurement of height, weight, and, in babies, head circumference, provides an invaluable record of a child's growth rate.

A chronic illness, such as *cystic fibrosis*, will retard growth if it is un-

CHANGES IN BODY PROPORTIONS BETWEEN BIRTH AND ADOLESCENCE

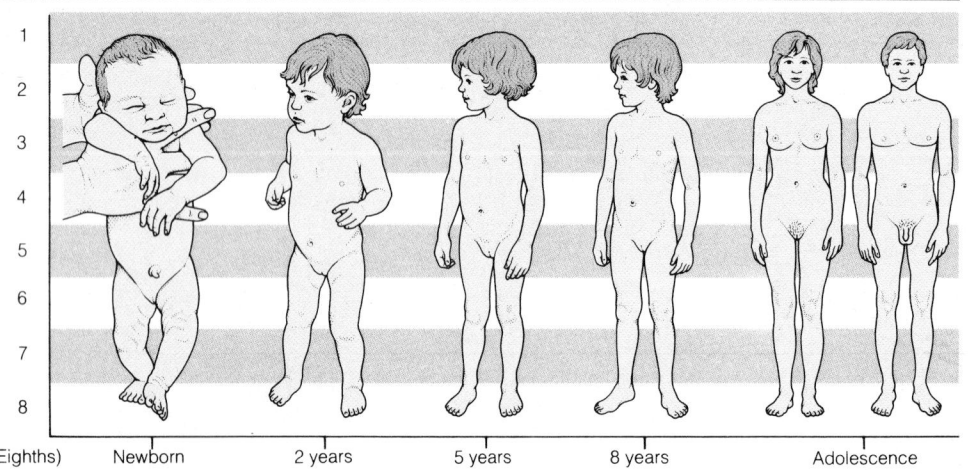

(Eighths)   Newborn   2 years   5 years   8 years   Adolescence

If the body is divided into eight equal parts, it can be seen that proportions change radically in relation to the body's overall length. For example, a newborn baby's legs account for only three eighths of his or her height while an adolescent's legs account for one half. A newborn's head accounts for as much as a quarter of his or her height while an adolescent's head accounts for only one eighth.

GROWTH CHART: BOYS 1 TO 18 YEARS

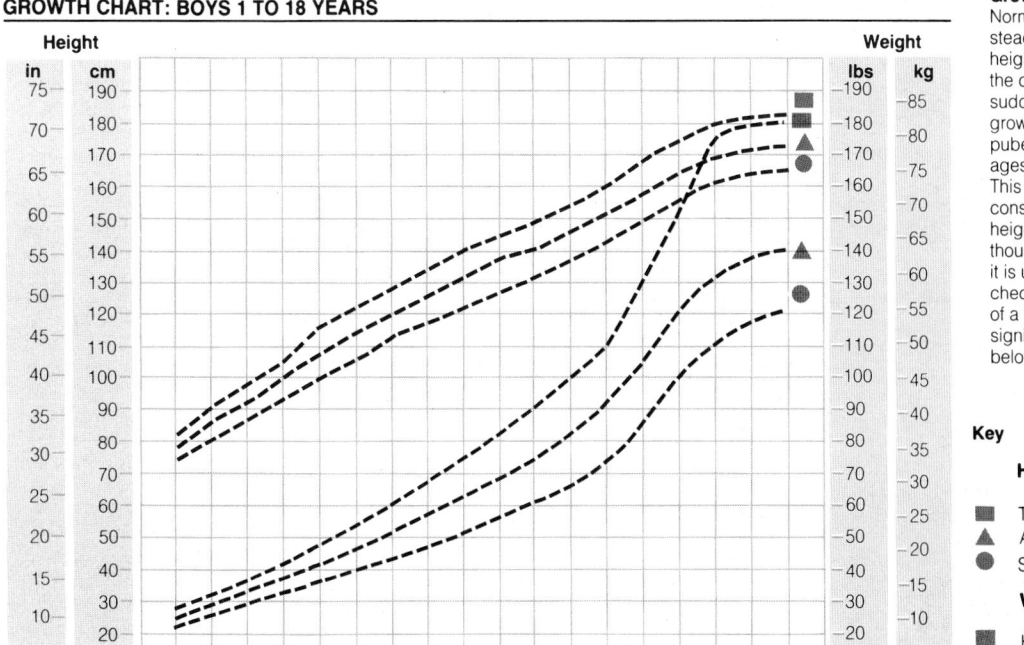

Height
in / cm

Weight
lbs / kg

Age (years)

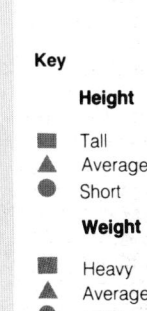

Growth in boys

Normally, there is a steady increase in height and weight until the onset of puberty. A sudden spurt in growth occurs during puberty (between the ages of 13 and 16). This chart was constructed using the height and weight of thousands of children; it is used by doctors to check whether growth of a particular boy is significantly above or below average.

Key

Height

■ Tall
▲ Average
● Short

Weight

▦ Heavy
▲ Average
● Light

GROWTH CHART: GIRLS 1 TO 18 YEARS

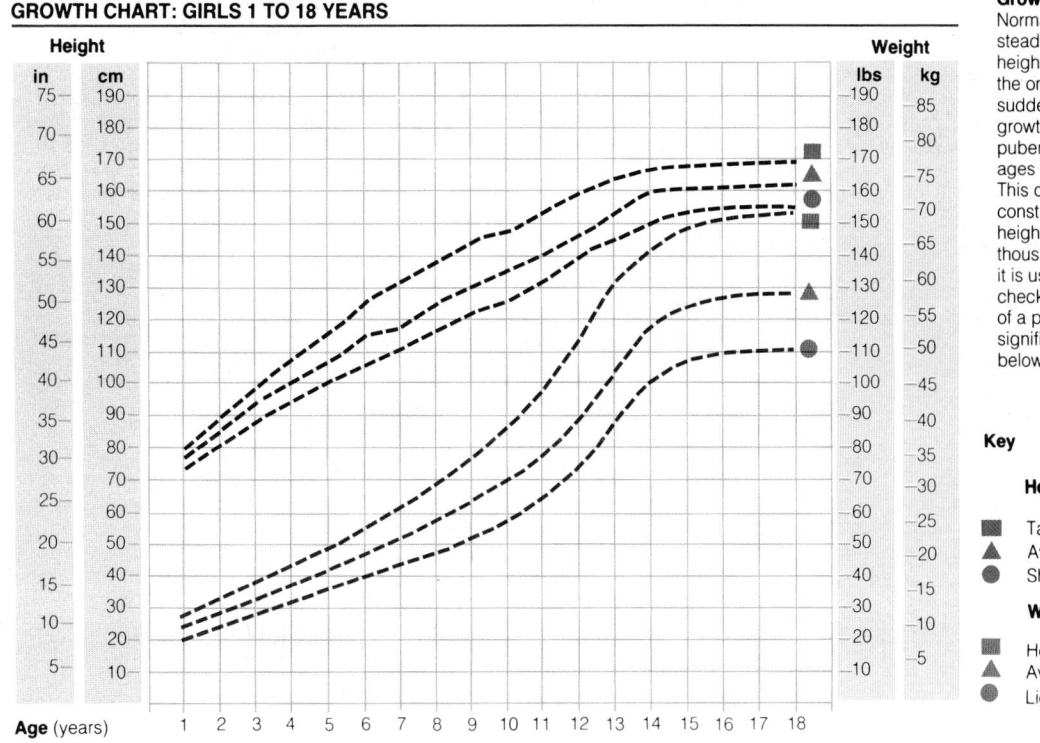

Height
in / cm

Weight
lbs / kg

Age (years)

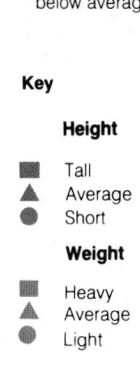

Growth in girls

Normally, there is a steady increase in height and weight until the onset of puberty. A sudden spurt in growth occurs during puberty (between the ages of 11 and 14). This chart was constructed using the height and weight of thousands of children; it is used by doctors to check whether growth of a particular girl is significantly above or below average.

Key

Height

■ Tall
▲ Average
● Short

Weight

▦ Heavy
▲ Average
● Light

detected. Even a minor illness can slow growth, although the growth rate usually catches up when the child recovers. In some cases, slow growth may be the only sign that a child is ill, malnourished, emotionally distressed or deprived. However, there is wide individual variation in the growth rate, and *short stature* does not necessarily indicate poor health. Slow growth in a child requires assessment by a paediatrician.

Abnormally rapid growth is rare. Usually, it is a familial trait but it may occasionally indicate an underlying disorder, such as a pituitary gland tumour causing *gigantism*. (See also *Age; Child development*.)

Growth hormone

A substance produced by the *pituitary gland* that stimulates normal body growth and development by altering chemical activity in cells. Growth hormone stimulates the production of protein in muscle cells and the release of energy from the breakdown of fats. Oversecretion of growth hormone may result in *gigantism* or *acromegaly*.

GROWTH HORMONE THERAPY

In the past, growth hormone was extracted from human corpses, and very rarely this led to the transmission of the brain disorder, *Creutzfeldt-Jakob disease*. The hormone is now genetically engineered and is completely safe. Growth hormone therapy is used to treat *short stature* when the underlying cause is a pituitary gland disorder. It is also used for children with genetic disorders associated with short stature, such as Turner's syndrome. Treatment is usually started in early childhood. Growth hormone is sometimes given with an anabolic *steroid*, which also promotes tissue growth.

POSSIBLE ADVERSE EFFECTS

There is a slight risk that *diabetes mellitus* may develop during treatment. Some people produce *antibodies* to growth hormone, but this does not seem to reduce its effectiveness.

Guar gum

A gum extracted from the cluster bean (CYAMOPSIS TETRAGONOLABA). Guar gum is not digested in the body and is therefore classed as dietary fibre. It is used as an aid to controlling the blood sugar level in people with *diabetes mellitus*. Guar gum granules are either sprinkled on food or dissolved in water to form a thick gel for drinking.

HOW IT WORKS

Guar gum forms a sticky solution in the stomach and slows the movement of nutrients from there into the small intestine. This action slows the rate at which glucose is absorbed from the small intestine into the bloodstream, thus preventing a sudden rise in the blood sugar level after a meal. There is no evidence that guar gum is effective as a slimming aid.

POSSIBLE ADVERSE EFFECTS

Guar gum has an unpleasant taste and may cause flatulence, nausea, and abdominal discomfort.

Guillain-Barré syndrome

A rare form of damage to the peripheral nerves (see *Peripheral nervous system*) that causes weakness of the limbs. The nerves become inflamed, particularly where their roots leave the spine, impairing both movement and sensation. The disease is also known as acute polyneuritis and ascending paralysis.

CAUSES AND INCIDENCE

The cause of the disease is believed to be an allergic reaction to an infection, usually viral; the nerves are inflamed by *antibodies* produced by the reaction. In most cases the disease develops two or three weeks after the onset of an infection, usually an infection of the upper respiratory tract, such as a sore throat or influenza, or a gastrointestinal upset. In 1976, an epidemic occurred in the US following mass vaccination against swine flu. The incidence is about 900 cases per year in the UK.

SYMPTOMS

Weakness, often accompanied by numbness and tingling, usually starts in the legs and spreads to the arms. The weakness becomes progressively worse and may develop into paralysis. The muscles of the face and those controlling speech, swallowing, and breathing may also be affected, causing difficulty with these activities.

DIAGNOSIS

Diagnosis of Guillain-Barré syndrome is made from the patient's symptoms and signs, from the results of electrical tests to measure how fast nerve impulses are being conducted, and from a *lumbar puncture*, in which a sample of cerebrospinal fluid is taken from the spinal canal for analysis.

TREATMENT AND OUTLOOK

Patients are treated in hospital, where their condition can be closely monitored. *Intubation* (insertion of a breathing tube down the throat) and mechanical *ventilation* may be necessary to aid breathing. *Plasmapheresis* (in which blood plasma is withdrawn from the patient, treated to remove antibodies, and replaced) or treatment with *immunoglobulin* may be employed in severe cases.

Most people recover completely without specific treatment, but some are left with permanent weakness in affected areas and/or suffer from further attacks of the disease.

Guilt

A painful feeling that arises from the awareness of having broken a moral or legal code. Guilt is self-inflicted, unlike shame, which depends on how others view the transgression. Some psychoanalysts see guilt as a result of the prohibitions of the *superego* (conscience) that were instilled by parental authority in early life. Others see guilt as a conditioned response to actions that in the past have led to punishment.

Feeling guilty from time to time is normal. However, feeling very guilty for no reason or experiencing guilt at an imagined crime is one of the main symptoms of psychotic *depression*.

Guinea worm disease

A tropical disease caused by a female parasitic worm more than 1 m long. Infection is the result of drinking water containing the water flea CYCLOPS, which harbours larvae of the worm. The larvae pass through the intestinal wall and mature in body tissues. After about a year, the adult female worm, now pregnant, approaches the surface of the skin, and creates an inflamed blister that bursts, exposing the end of the worm.

The disease occurs in Africa, South America, the Caribbean, the Middle East, and India.

SYMPTOMS AND TREATMENT

Urticaria (nettle rash), nausea, vomiting, and diarrhoea often develop while the blister is forming.

The traditional remedy is to wind the worm gently from the skin on to a small stick. Once the worm is out, the condition usually clears up.

The drugs *thiabendazole* and niridazole are given to reduce inflammation and make extraction of the worm safer, *antibiotic drugs* are given to control secondary infection, and the patient is immunized against *tetanus*. The disease can be controlled if the local population can be instructed in methods for filtering water supplies, and if they can avoid contaminating surface sources such as supplies of fresh rainwater.

Gullet

The common name for the *oesophagus*.

Gum

Also called the gingiva, the soft tissue surrounding the *teeth* that protects underlying structures and helps keep the teeth tightly in position in the *jaw*. The gingival margin, a cuff of gum 2 mm thick, fits tightly around the base of the teeth and is anchored within the bony socket by the periodontal ligaments.

Normal healthy gums are pink or brown and are firm. Careful *oral hygiene,* including daily brushing and flossing, is needed to avoid gum disease, especially on reaching middle age.

DISORDERS

Gingivitis (an early, reversible stage of gum disease, characterized by inflammation of the gums) may occur if dental *plaque,* which contains bacteria, is allowed to collect around the base of the teeth. Bleeding gums are nearly always a symptom of gingivitis; rarely, they are due to *leukaemia* or *scurvy* (vitamin C deficiency). Bruised gums are more likely to be caused by a *bleeding disorder.* Gingival *hyperplasia* (fleshy thickening of the gums) occurs most commonly as a side-effect of treatment with *phenytoin* (an anticonvulsant drug).

Untreated gingivitis may lead to chronic *periodontitis,* the advanced stage of gum disease, in which infected pockets form between the gums and the teeth.

Gumboil

See *Abscess, dental.*

Gumma

A soft tumour that is characteristic of the late stages of untreated *syphilis* but is now extremely rare in the UK.

Gut

A common name for the *intestine.*

Guthrie test

A blood test performed routinely on babies between the eighth and 14th day after birth to check for *phenylketonuria.* This is an inherited disorder in which the *amino acid* phenylalanine accumulates in the blood and tissues, usually leading to severe brain damage unless treated. The Guthrie test measures the amount of phenylalanine in the blood.

HOW IT IS DONE

The baby's heel is pricked with a needle and a few drops of blood are soaked on to a piece of absorbent filter paper. The paper is then placed on a nutrient medium containing bacteria whose growth is activated by phenylalanine. The size of the area of bacterial growth that appears is directly related to the concentration of phenylalanine in the blood.

RESULTS

A concentration of phenylalanine above 20 mg per ml indicates that phenylketonuria may be present; other, more accurate tests are performed to confirm the diagnosis.

The Guthrie test may also be used to screen for other disorders of amino acid metabolism, such as tyrosinaemia, one of several other disorders in which phenylalanine accumulates in the blood.

Gynaecology

The medical specialty concerned with the female *reproductive tract.* Gynaecology is involved with the investigation and treatment of menstrual problems (see *Menstruation, disorders of*), *infertility, sexual problems,* problems relating to the *menopause,* and other problems affecting the female reproductive tract, such as uterine *fibroids, ovarian cysts,* and cervical *polyps.* Gynaecologists also give advice about methods of *contraception.* Treatments include drug therapy and surgical procedures, such as *dilatation and curettage* (D and C) and *hysterectomy* (removal of the uterus).

Gynaecology covers disorders of early pregnancy, such as recurrent *miscarriage,* although the management of pregnancy falls within the specialty of *obstetrics.* In the UK, specialists in gynaecology are also specialists in obstetrics.

Gynaecomastia

Enlargement of one or both breasts in the male, almost always due to an excess of the female sex hormone *oestrogen* in the blood.

CAUSES

Oestrogen, which is responsible for female secondary *sexual characteristics,* is produced in large quantities in women, but is also produced in small amounts in all men (just as all women produce small amounts of male sex hormones). In some males, however, an abnormal amount of oestrogen is produced, usually for reasons that are not fully understood, but sometimes because of disease.

Gynaecomastia is quite common at *puberty,* taking the form of a slight swelling in one or both breasts, often accompanied by some tenderness. A young boy with gynaecomastia is likely to be worried and embarrassed; he should be reassured that his masculinity is not threatened and that the problem will soon pass. Gynaecomastia of this mild, temporary kind can also occur at birth.

If the condition develops later—most commonly when a man is over the age of 50—the enlargement may be greater, especially in an already obese man. Such cases are usually not serious, but investigation is necessary to rule out the possibility of an underlying disease. This disease could be *cirrhosis* of the liver, in which the liver is unable to break down oestrogen; a tumour of the testis (see *Testis, cancer of*), which can raise the level of oestrogen in the blood; or, if only one breast is affected, *breast cancer,* in which case the swelling is caused by the presence of a tumour.

Adult gynaecomastia, which sometimes affects only one breast, can also occur when synthetic hormones and some drugs, such as *digoxin, spironolactone* and *cimetidine,* change the balance of sex hormones in the blood.

DIAGNOSIS

A doctor may arrange for blood tests. If cancer is suspected, a *biopsy* (removal of the entire lump or a piece of tissue for analysis) will be performed; early treatment is essential if the cause is breast cancer.

TREATMENT

The treatment depends on the underlying cause. If a drug is responsible, an alternative drug will be prescribed if possible; otherwise, the gynaecomastia must be weighed against the effects of withdrawing the drug treatment, which may in itself be undesirable.

If there is no underlying disease, the swelling usually subsides without treatment, although it may take a few years. A man who is embarrassed by enlarged breasts may prefer to have cosmetic surgery.

If the swelling is moderate, an operation can be performed that leaves only a small, unnoticeable scar around part of the areola (the dark skin surrounding the nipple). In many cases, this operation can be carried out under a local anaesthetic as an outpatient procedure. *Mammoplasty,* an operation more frequently performed on women, is used when breast enlargement is severe. This operation takes longer, requires a general anaesthetic, and leaves extensive and obvious scarring.

G

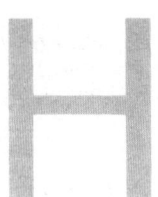

H₂-receptor antagonists

A group of *ulcer-healing drugs* related to the *antihistamine drug* group. The name is an abbreviation for histamine₂-receptor antagonists. These drugs work by blocking the action of the chemical *histamine* at specific *receptors* (sites on a cell's surface), preventing release of acid in the stomach. Acid reduction promotes the healing of *peptic ulcers* and relieves symptoms of *oesophagitis*. (See also *Cimetidine*; *Ranitidine*; *Famotidine*.)

Habituation

The effect of becoming accustomed to an experience. In general, the more a person is exposed to a stimulus, the less he or she is aroused by it. Experiments have shown that frightening pictures make the pulse rate rise less the more they are seen. People can also become habituated to certain drugs, and need increasing amounts to receive the same effect (*tolerance*).

Haem-

A prefix indicating blood, as in *haemoglobin* (an important protein in red blood cells).

Haemangioblastoma

A rare type of *brain tumour* that consists of blood-vessel cells. Haemangioblastomas usually develop as cysts in the *cerebellum*. They are slow-growing and usually benign. Haemangioblastomas most commonly affect children and young adults.

The principal symptoms are headache, vomiting, *ataxia* (incoordination), and *nystagmus* (abnormal jerky movements of the eyes).

A haemangioblastoma can be clearly distinguished from the surrounding brain tissue and can usually be removed surgically. In most cases, surgical removal of the tumour results in a complete cure.

Haemangioma

A birthmark caused by an abnormal distribution of blood vessels. Haemangiomas may be flat or raised.

Port-wine stains are large, flat, purple-red marks, which are permanent and can be unsightly. In rare cases, port-wine stains are associated with abnormalities in the blood vessels of the brain (see *Sturge-Weber syndrome*).

Small, flat marks, often known as stork marks or stork bites, are common in newborn babies, particularly on the back of the neck. Most begin to fade about three weeks after birth.

Raised bright red haemangiomas, often called strawberry marks, usually enlarge rapidly during the first few weeks after birth. After the age of about six months, the redness gradually fades and the lump subsides. Approximately 50 per cent of these marks disappear by the time the child is five years old; 90 per cent disappear by the age of nine.

Some raised haemangiomas are tinged blue by venous blood. These haemangiomas affect deeper tissues than strawberry marks but usually disappear during childhood.

COMPLICATIONS AND TREATMENT
Haemangiomas do not usually require treatment unless they are causing a particular problem. If a haemangioma starts to bleed, medical advice should be sought; meanwhile, the bleeding can be controlled by firm pressure with a clean handkerchief.

A haemangioma that bleeds persistently may require removal, especially if it is on the lip or tongue, where it may easily be bitten, or if it is on the vulva (external female genitalia) or anus, where it is subject to repeated pressure. A haemangioma on the face may need to be removed if it is causing distress.

Removal is carried out by *laser treatment*, *cryosurgery* (destruction of tissue by extreme cold), *radiotherapy*, *embolization*, or *plastic surgery*. If removal is not possible, some haemangiomas can be disguised with cosmetics.

Haemarthrosis

Bleeding into a *joint*, causing the capsule that encloses the joint to swell.
CAUSES
Haemarthrosis is usually the result of severe damage to a joint, such as a torn capsule, torn ligaments, or fracture of a bone forming part of the joint. The most common cause is a sports injury to the knee.

A rarer cause is a *bleeding disorder*, such as *haemophilia* (in which failure of the blood-clotting mechanism causes abnormal bleeding). Any joint may be affected and bleeding into the joint

may occur spontaneously or be caused by even the slightest knock. Overuse of *anticoagulant drugs* can cause haemarthrosis.
SYMPTOMS AND SIGNS
Haemarthrosis causes a joint to swell immediately after injury; swelling that occurs 12 to 24 hours later is probably caused by *synovitis* (inflammation of the lining of the joint). In addition to swelling and pain, haemarthrosis may cause the joint to stiffen into a fixed position as a result of spasm in surrounding muscles.
DIAGNOSIS AND TREATMENT
As a first-aid measure, *ice-packs* may be used to reduce swelling and pain. If swelling occurs after an injury, fluid is withdrawn from the joint through a needle to relieve pain and allow analysis of the fluid to diagnose the condition. *X-rays* may be necessary if a fracture is suspected. Haemophiliacs are given *factor VIII* to promote blood clotting.

To prevent further bleeding, the doctor will bandage the joint and advise resting it in an elevated position; cells in the joint capsule gradually absorb any remaining blood. Surgery, such as repair of a *ligament*, is sometimes necessary.

Repeated haemarthrosis may damage the surfaces of the joint, causing *osteoarthritis*, which is characterized by persistent pain and stiffness.

Haematemesis

The medical term for *vomiting blood*.

Haematology

The study of *blood* and its formation, and the investigation and treatment of disorders affecting the blood and the *bone marrow*.

Microscopic examination and counting of blood and bone marrow cells are essential procedures in diagnosing different types of blood disorders, such as *anaemia* or *leukaemia*. Analysis of blood is used in the diagnosis of a wide range of disorders as well as specific blood disorders.

Haematoma

A localized collection of blood (usually clotted) caused by bleeding from a ruptured blood vessel. A haematoma may occur almost anywhere in the body and, depending on the site and amount of accumulated blood, may vary in seriousness from a minor to a potentially fatal disorder.
TYPES
Less serious types include subungual haematoma (under a fingernail or toe-

nail), haematoma auris (in the tissues of the outer ear, better known as *cauliflower ear*), and perianal haematoma (under the skin around the anus). The accumulated blood presses on the surrounding tissues, which may cause considerable pain. In such cases, a doctor may lance and drain the haematoma to relieve the pressure and thus alleviate the pain. Most haematomas disappear on their own within a few days.

Among the more serious types are those that press on the brain, notably extradural and subdural haematomas (see *Extradural haemorrhage; Subdural haemorrhage*). These types of haematoma are usually due to an injury that ruptures a blood vessel just under the skull and may be fatal unless they are treated promptly.

Haematoma auris

The medical term for *cauliflower ear*.

Haematuria

Red blood cells in the *urine*. Blood in the urine may be readily visible or the presence of small amounts of blood may give the urine a smoky appearance. In some cases the blood is not visible to the naked eye.

CAUSES

Haematuria can be caused by blood entering the urine at any point along the *urinary tract*, from the kidney to the urethral opening. Almost any disorder of the urinary tract can cause haematuria. *Urinary tract infection* is one of the most common causes; *prostatitis* may cause haematuria in men. Cysts, *kidney tumours, bladder tumours*, and stones (see *Calculus, urinary tract*) may cause blood in the sufferer's urine, as can *glomerulonephritis*, in which the glomeruli (the filtering units of the kidney) become inflamed. *Bleeding disorders* may also cause blood to appear in the urine.

INVESTIGATION

If the blood is not visible to the naked eye, it may be discovered during a urine test when the urinary sediment is examined under the microscope. Urine dip-sticks have a small patch that is impregnated with a dye at one end; when dipped in urine containing blood, the patch turns blue.

To determine the cause of blood in the urine, it may be necessary to obtain images of the urinary tract by *ultrasound scanning, CT scanning*, or intravenous *urography*. These tests usually detect conditions such as cysts, stones, and tumours. If bladder disease is thought to be the cause, a *cystoscopy* (direct examination of the bladder through a viewing instrument passed through the urethra) is performed. If a kidney tumour seems likely, *angiography* may be performed to show the blood vessels of the kidney, although this technique has been largely replaced by CT scanning.

Haemochromatosis

An inherited disease (also known as "bronze diabetes") in which too much dietary iron is absorbed. Excess iron gradually accumulates in the liver, pancreas, heart, testes, and, to a lesser extent, in other organs.

CAUSES

The disease occurs almost exclusively in men. Women are very rarely affected because they regularly lose iron in their menstrual blood. Although haemochromatosis is known to be genetic in origin, the exact method of inheritance is unclear. Male relatives of an affected person are more likely than average to develop the disease.

SYMPTOMS AND COMPLICATIONS

Haemochromatosis rarely causes problems until middle age. A loss of sexual drive and a reduction in the size of the testes are often the first signs. Eventually, excess iron causes liver enlargement and *cirrhosis* (chronic liver damage), deficient insulin production by the pancreas leading to *diabetes mellitus*, bronzed skin coloration due to iron pigment deposition under the skin (hence the alternative name), cardiac *arrhythmia* and other heart disorders, and, during the late stages of the disease, *liver failure* and *liver cancer*.

DIAGNOSIS AND TREATMENT

The diagnosis is based on *blood tests*, which reveal a high level of iron in the blood, and a *liver biopsy* (removal of a small sample of tissue for analysis), which shows the abnormal presence of iron.

Haemochromatosis is treated by withdrawal of blood from a vein (*venesection*). Initially, the procedure is performed once or twice a week. After the iron level has returned to normal, venesection is required only three or four times a year.

In young men, treatment can prevent the development of complications; in people who have fully developed haemochromatosis, regular venesection can prolong life. Drug treatment with *chelating agents*, such as desferrioxamine, has been investigated as an alternative to venesection. (See also *Haemosiderosis*.)

Haemodialysis

One of the two means of *dialysis* (removal of waste products from the blood by means of artificial filtration) used to treat *kidney failure*.

Haemoglobin

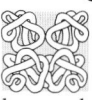 The oxygen-carrying pigment found in red *blood cells*. Haemoglobin binds with oxygen to form oxyhaemoglobin, a compound that gives oxygenated blood its bright red colour. There are 350 million haemoglobin molecules in the average blood cell, and each can carry four molecules of oxygen. Haemoglobin is found in many animals—from insects and worms to birds, fish, and mammals.

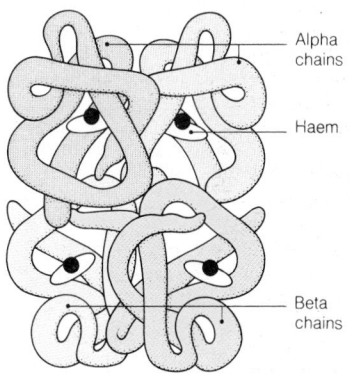

Structure of haemoglobin
Each molecule contains four globin chains—two alpha and two beta. Each chain carries a haem component capable of binding oxygen.

STRUCTURE

Haemoglobin is a large molecule made in the *bone marrow* from two components, haem and globin.

The composition of haemoglobin molecules varies, giving rise to normal and abnormal forms of haemoglobin. Haemoglobin F is the normal form in fetal life. This is replaced during infancy by the normal adult forms, haemoglobin A and A_2.

FUNCTION

The principal function of haemoglobin is to combine with and transport oxygen from the lungs and deliver it to all body tissues, where it is required to provide energy for the chemical reactions of all living cells. Carbon dioxide, which is produced as the waste product of these reactions, is transported to the lungs for excretion during breathing out.

DISORDERS

Some defects in haemoglobin production result from a *genetic disorder*; such defects are subdivided into errors of haem production, known as *porphyrias*, and those of globin production, known as *haemoglobinopathies*. Other defects, such as some types of *anaemia*, have a nongenetic cause.

Haemoglobinopathy

A term used to describe a variety of *genetic disorders* in which there are errors in the production of globin chains (components of *haemoglobin*, the oxygen-carrying substance in the blood).

In some types of haemoglobinopathy, abnormal globin chains are produced, giving rise to abnormal haemoglobin molecules. This is the underlying defect in *sickle cell anaemia*. In other types, normal globin chains are produced, but in abnormal amounts. This is the underlying defect in the *thalassaemias*. Combined forms also occur.

The haemoglobinopathies cause anaemia and chronic sickness in millions of people in Asia, Africa, Mediterranean countries, and the Caribbean, and in many people of these racial origins living in northern Europe and the US.

Haemoglobinuria

The presence in the *urine* of *haemoglobin* (the oxygen-carrying pigment in the blood).

Haemoglobin is mainly contained within red blood cells, although a small amount is free in the blood plasma. Excessive *haemolysis* (breakdown of red cells), which may be caused by heavy exercise, cold weather, falciparum *malaria* (blackwater fever), and haemolytic *anaemia*, increases the concentration of free haemoglobin in the plasma. The excess of free haemoglobin in the plasma is excreted in the urine.

Haemolysis

The destruction of red *blood cells*. Haemolysis is the normal process by which old red blood cells that have lost their elasticity are destroyed, mainly in the *spleen*. This process releases iron for recycling in new red cells. *Bilirubin*, a waste product of haemolysis, is excreted into the *bile* by the liver.

Abnormal haemolysis in which red blood cells are destroyed prematurely may cause anaemia and jaundice (see *Anaemia, haemolytic*).

Haemolytic anaemia

See *Anaemia, haemolytic*.

Haemolytic disease of the newborn

Excessive *haemolysis* (destruction of red blood cells) in the fetus and newborn infant by *antibodies* produced by the mother. Haemolytic disease of the newborn is most often caused by *Rhesus incompatibility*—a blood group incompatibility between mother and baby, named after the Rhesus monkey in which the Rhesus (Rh) factor was first discovered.

A milder form of the disease may result from ABO and other blood group incompatibilities.

CAUSE

Haemolytic disease may occur if the woman's blood is Rh negative, if she is carrying a baby whose blood is Rh positive, and if she has previously had a baby whose blood was Rh positive. A previous miscarriage, induced abortion, or *amniocentesis* in which the fetus's blood was Rh positive can also sensitize the woman. In each of these situations, blood has passed at some stage from the fetus to the woman. This causes the woman to produce Rh antibodies (directed against the Rh-positive blood cells) because her *immune system* recognizes the fetal blood cells as "foreign". In a first pregnancy, Rh antibodies do not form sufficiently to harm the baby. During any subsequent pregnancy, however, Rh antibodies form early on and may cross the placenta and attack the fetal blood cells.

A mismatched *blood transfusion* (giving Rh-positive blood to a woman who is Rh-negative) also sensitizes the woman to produce Rh antibodies.

DIAGNOSIS

All pregnant women have their blood groups tested at the first antenatal check. Rh-negative women are tested for Rh antibodies at this visit and again at 28 and 36 weeks' gestation; they are tested more frequently if there has been a previous pregnancy.

If a pregnant woman shows rising levels of Rh antibodies, amniocentesis is performed at intervals to measure *bilirubin* levels in the *amniotic fluid*. Bilirubin is a breakdown product of red blood cells and the level of bilirubin thus indicates the severity of haemolysis in the fetus.

SYMPTOMS AND SIGNS

In mild cases, the newborn baby becomes slightly jaundiced during the first 24 hours of life (due to excess bilirubin in the blood) and slightly anaemic. In more severe cases, the level of bilirubin in the blood may increase to a dangerous level, causing

a risk of *kernicterus* (a type of brain damage). The most severely affected babies have marked anaemia while still in the uterus, become very swollen (hydrops fetalis), and are often stillborn.

TREATMENT

If the condition is very mild, no treatment is required. In other cases, the aim is to deliver the baby before anaemia becomes severe. This usually means *induction of labour* between 35 and 39 weeks' gestation.

If the baby is severely affected before he or she is mature enough to be delivered safely (after 30 weeks' gestation), fetal blood transfusions may be necessary. Rh-negative blood is injected into the fetal umbilical vein, the fetal heart, or the fetal abdominal cavity. The procedure is monitored by *ultrasound scanning*. Transfusions of blood given in this way may need to be repeated several times until the baby has reached a size when labour may be safely induced.

After the baby is born, frequent blood tests are performed to assess jaundice and anaemia. *Phototherapy* (light treatment that converts bilirubin in the skin into a water-soluble form that is more easily excreted from the body) and plenty of fluids help reduce the jaundice. If the bilirubin level becomes dangerously high, exchange transfusion (by which blood is removed from the baby and replaced by Rh-negative blood) is performed.

PREVENTION AND OUTLOOK

Haemolytic disease of the newborn is far less common since the introduction and use of *anti-D (Rh_o) immunoglobulin* in the early 1970s. This preparation is given by injection to any Rh-negative woman within 72 hours of childbirth, miscarriage, or elective abortion, and destroys Rh-positive blood cells from the fetus before they have had time to sensitize the woman's immune system.

Improved general obstetric and paediatric care has also resulted in a reduction in the severity of the cases that still occur.

Haemolytic-uraemic syndrome

A rare disease in which red *blood cells* are destroyed prematurely and the kidneys are severely damaged, causing *kidney failure*. Haemolytic-uraemic syndrome occurs mainly in infants and young children.

CAUSES

The precise cause of the disorder is unknown. It is thought that the lining of small blood vessels in the kidneys becomes damaged, causing small clots to form. These clots cause *haemolysis* (breakdown of red cells) as blood flows past them, leading to *anaemia*. The resultant damage to the kidneys causes them to fail. Haemolytic-uraemic syndrome often occurs in epidemics and appears to be triggered by a bacterial or viral infection.

SYMPTOMS AND SIGNS
The onset of the disease is sudden, with headache, fatigue, shortness of breath, and sometimes jaundice. Little urine is passed and what is passed may contain blood. Severe *hypertension* (high blood pressure) is common and may cause *seizures.*

DIAGNOSIS AND TREATMENT
Blood and urine tests are performed to determine the degree of kidney damage. *Dialysis* is necessary until the kidneys have recovered. *Antihypertensive drugs* are given to lower blood pressure. Transfusions of red blood cells may be given to control the anaemia. In severe cases, transfusion or exchange of plasma (the fluid in which blood cells are suspended) may be required to prevent continual clotting of blood and excessive breakdown of red cells. Most children make a full recovery.

Haemophilia
An inherited *bleeding disorder* caused by a deficiency of a particular blood protein. Haemophiliacs (who are almost always male) suffer recurrent bleeding, usually into their joints. Bleeding may occur spontaneously or after injury. Before the transmission mechanisms of *HIV* infection were understood, many haemophiliacs became infected with the virus as a direct result of treatment of their condition. Some have developed *AIDS.*

INCIDENCE AND CAUSES
About one male in 10,000 is born with haemophilia. The deficient blood protein, known as *factor VIII*, is one of a series of proteins essential to the process of *blood clotting.*

The lack of factor VIII is due to a defective gene, which shows a sex-linked pattern of inheritance (see *Genetic disorders*). Affected males pass the defective gene on to none of their sons but to all of their daughters, who are carriers of the condition. Some of the sons of carrier females may be affected, and some of the daughters of carriers may themselves be carriers. Many haemophiliacs have an uncle, brother, or grandfather also affected. About one third of cases have no family history of haemophilia.

SYMPTOMS
The severity of the disorder differs markedly among affected individuals. Most bleeding episodes involve bleeding into joints and muscles. The episodes often start when an affected child reaches weight-bearing age as a toddler. Bleeding episodes are painful and, unless treated promptly, can lead to crippling deformities of the knees, ankles, and other joints.

Injury and even minor operations such as tooth extraction may lead to profuse bleeding. Internal bleeding can give rise to symptoms such as *haematuria* (blood in the urine) or extensive bruises.

DIAGNOSIS
Haemophilia is diagnosed by *blood-clotting tests,* which reveal that factor VIII activity is abnormally low. A different type of blood test can be used to determine whether or not a woman is a carrier. *Amniocentesis* or *chorionic villus sampling* can be used to diagnose haemophilia in a fetus.

TREATMENT
Fifty years ago most haemophiliacs did not survive to adulthood; today, bleeding episodes can be controlled by infusions of concentrates of factor VIII. Regular infusions can be given as a preventive treatment. Alternatively, factor VIII may be given as soon as possible after the start of a bleeding episode. Patients can be shown how to administer the treatment themselves. Serious or unusual bleeding episodes may require hospitalization.

Although the use of factor VIII has considerably improved the quality of life for many haemophiliacs, the transmission of infections via factor VIII concentrates caused considerable problems in the 1980s. At that time, factor VIII was produced from large supplies of donor blood (2,000 to 5,000 individual donations) and, despite efforts to screen donors, the supplies were sometimes contaminated with viruses. Haemophiliacs commonly became infected with hepatitis B and C (see *Hepatitis, viral*) and, in the early years of the AIDS *pandemic* (before its cause was identified), many also became infected with HIV; many thousands of haemophiliacs and their sexual partners developed, and died from, AIDS. More recently, effective screening techniques for these viruses, and heat treatment of the factor VIII prepared from blood donations, have combined to reduce these risks to very low levels. A genetically-engineered factor VIII became available in the early 1990s, and as this preparation comes

into general use all risk of virus infection from factor VIII will be eliminated.

OUTLOOK
A child who has haemophilia should avoid activities with a risk of injury, including contact sports, such as football. Activities such as swimming and walking should be encouraged.

Haemophiliacs who test positive for HIV should take the usual precautions against transmitting the virus and are advised not to have children. Haemophiliacs who do not test positive for HIV and the female relatives of haemophiliacs should obtain *genetic counselling* before starting a family.

Haemophilus influenzae
A bacterium responsible for many cases of two serious infectious childhood diseases, *epiglottitis* and *meningitis*. A vaccine for the commonest variety, HAEMOPHILUS INFLUENZAE B, is now available and was included in the routine schedule of childhood immunizations from 1993 onwards.

Haemoptysis
The medical term for *coughing up blood.*

Haemorrhage
The medical term for *bleeding.*

Haemorrhoidectomy
The surgical removal of *haemorrhoids.*

WHY IT IS DONE
This operation may be carried out if simpler methods of treatment, such as banding, fail to resolve the problem. Haemorrhoidectomy tends to be reserved for people who have large, prolapsing, bleeding haemorrhoids.

HOW IT IS DONE
Stages in a haemorrhoidectomy are shown in the illustrated box.

RECOVERY PERIOD
Laxative drugs are given after the operation to soften the stools to make them easier to pass. Nonnarcotic *analgesic drugs* (painkillers) and warm baths ease discomfort. Complete healing occurs after three to six weeks. Avoidance of constipation can frequently prevent recurrences.

COMPLICATIONS
Bleeding is a possible complication. A slight loss of sensation in the anal area may impair the ability to control release of wind.

Haemorrhoids
Swollen veins in the lining of the anus. Haemorrhoids may occur close to the anal opening, in which case they are called external haemorrhoids. They may also occur higher in

H

the anal canal, in which case they are called internal haemorrhoids. In some cases, haemorrhoids protrude outside the anus, in which case they are called prolapsing haemorrhoids.

CAUSES AND INCIDENCE
Haemorrhoids are very common, particularly during pregnancy and immediately after childbirth. Some people have a congenital weakness of the veins in the anus which makes the development of haemorrhoids more likely. Haemorrhoids are caused by increased pressure in the veins of the anus, usually due to straining to pass hard faeces. Such faeces may result from a diet that contains too many highly refined foods and that lacks sufficient fibre.

SYMPTOMS
Rectal bleeding and increasing discomfort, even pain, on defaecation are the most common features. Prolapsed haemorrhoids often produce a mucous discharge and itching around the anal opening. A complication of prolapse is thrombosis and strangulation (in which a clot forms in the vein, the vein does not spring back into position in the anus, and its blood supply is reduced); this can cause extreme pain. Iron-deficiency *anaemia* may result from prolonged bleeding.

DIAGNOSIS
Proctoscopy (inspection of the rectum with a viewing instrument) is usually performed to exclude the possibility of cancer (see *Anus, cancer of*; *Rectum, cancer of*) and other disorders of the anus and rectum.

TREATMENT
Mild cases are controlled by drinking fluids, eating a high-fibre diet, and establishing regular toilet habits. Rectal suppositories and creams containing *corticosteroid drugs* and local anaesthetics help reduce swelling and pain. More troublesome haemorrhoids may be treated by *sclerotherapy* (injection of an irritant liquid) or *cryosurgery* (application of extreme cold), which cause the swollen veins to shrivel, or by banding (see illustrated box). These procedures may be performed on an outpatient basis.

Prolapsing haemorrhoids generally require a *haemorrhoidectomy*.

Haemosiderosis
A general increase in iron stores in the body. Haemosiderosis may occur after repeated blood transfusions or, more rarely, as a result of excessive intake of iron. Haemosiderosis does not usually affect the function of body organs.

REMOVING HAEMORRHOIDS
In the procedures shown below, the patient is usually first given a laxative so that the lower bowel is clear of faeces. Either general or epidural anaesthesia is given before a haemorrhoidectomy is performed.

BANDING HAEMORRHOIDS

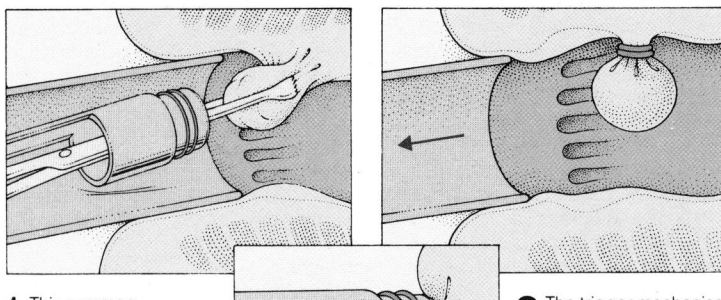

1 This common, simple, and effective procedure is usually painless (causing no more than a mild ache afterwards) and no anaesthesia is required. The patient lies on one side, the proctoscope is positioned, and the haemorrhoid is grasped with the forceps.

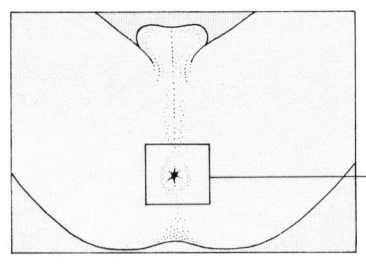

2 Gentle traction is applied to draw the mass into the drum and the banding instrument is pressed into the anal wall.

3 The trigger mechanism of the banding instrument is fired and the bands are squeezed off on to the neck of the haemorrhoid. The proctoscope is withdrawn, leaving the haemorrhoid with its base tightly constricted by the bands. The haemorrhoid then withers and drops off painlessly within a few days.

HAEMORRHOIDECTOMY

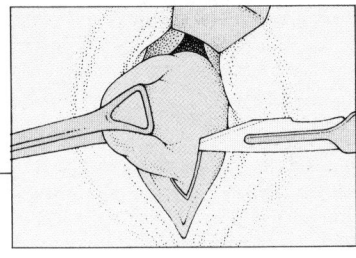

Using general or epidural anaesthesia, the patient is examined with a proctosigmoidoscope to exclude a diagnosis of tumour. The patient is then placed in the *lithotomy position*. The haemorrhoid is clamped, placed under traction, secured with a suture, and then removed with a knife.

Haemospermia
The medical term for blood in the semen (see *Semen, blood in the*).

Haemostasis
The arrest of bleeding. There are three main natural mechanisms by which bleeding is stopped after injury. First, small blood vessels constrict (narrow) when damaged, thus lessening the "gaps" through which blood can flow. Second, blood cells called platelets aggregate (clump) and plug the bleeding points. Third, the blood plasma coagulates, forming filaments of a substance called fibrin. These filaments enmesh blood cells at the bleeding points and contract to form a solid clot that seals the damaged blood vessel (see *Blood clotting*). Defects in any of the three natural mechanisms of haemostasis can cause a *bleeding disorder*. (See also *Bleeding, treatment of*.)

Haemostatic drugs
A group of drugs used to treat *bleeding disorders* and to control bleeding.

Preparations of clotting factors are an important type of haemostatic drug. Clotting factors are present naturally in the body to aid *blood clotting* but are deficient in certain disorders. For example, preparations of factor VIII are used to treat *haemophilia*; factor IX is used to treat *Christmas disease*. The clotting factor is injected after abnormal bleeding to stimulate clotting, or before surgery to reduce the risk of excessive bleeding.

Other commonly prescribed haemostatic drugs include *vitamin K* preparations (used to treat an overdose of certain *anticoagulant drugs*) and aminocaproic acid, which disrupts *fibrinolysis* (the body's mechanism for dissolving blood clots).

Haemostatic preparations of gelatine and cellulose may be applied to the skin or gums to stop bleeding (e.g. after tooth extraction).

Haemothorax

A collection of blood in the pleural cavity (the space between the chest wall and the lung).

Haemothorax is most commonly caused by chest injury, but it may arise spontaneously in people with defects of blood coagulation or, occasionally, as a result of cancer.

Symptoms include pain in the affected side of the chest and the upper abdomen and breathlessness. The pulse-rate may be raised. If extensive, haemothorax may compress the lung and cause partial lung collapse. Blood in the pleural space tends to remain fluid and can be aspirated (withdrawn through a needle).

Hair

A thread-like structure composed of dead cells containing *keratin* (a fibrous protein that is also the main constituent of the nails and outer skin layer). Hair has little practical function in humans.

STRUCTURE

The root of each hair is embedded in a tiny pit in the skin called a hair follicle. Each shaft of hair consists of a spongy semihollow core (the medulla), a surrounding layer of long, thin fibres (the cortex), and, on the outside, several layers of overlapping cells (the cuticle). During the growing phase of a hair the root is firmly enclosed by live tissue called a bulb, which supplies the hair with keratin; the bulb is the pale swelling that sometimes can be seen when a hair is pulled out. The upgrowth of dead cells and keratin from the root forms the hair.

TYPES

There are three types of human hair. From the fourth month of gestation, the fetus is covered with downy hair called lanugo, which is shed during

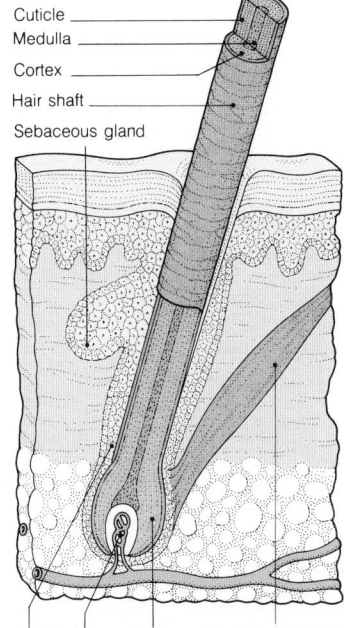

THE STRUCTURE OF A HAIR
The hair shaft contains dead cells and keratin (a type of protein). The root is embedded in the skin.

Cuticle
Medulla
Cortex
Hair shaft
Sebaceous gland

Follicle   Root   Bulb   Erector pili muscle

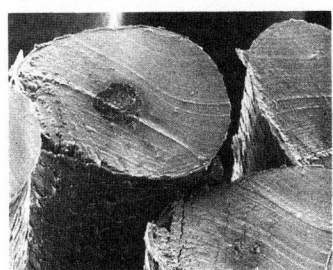

Cross-section through hairs
The central medulla, cortex, and outer cuticle can all be clearly differentiated in this microscope photograph.

the ninth month. After birth and until puberty, vellus hair, which is fine, short, and colourless, covers most of the body. The third type, terminal hair, is thicker, longer, and often pigmented; it grows on the scalp, the eyebrows, and the eyelashes. At puberty, terminal hair replaces vellus in the pubic area and the armpits. In most men and some women the process continues on the face, limbs, and trunk (see *Hirsutism*).

COLOUR AND TEXTURE

Hair colour is determined by the amount of pigment called *melanin* in the hair shaft. Melanin is produced by cells called melanocytes at the base of the hair follicle. Red melanin is responsible for red and auburn hair, black melanin for all other colours. If cells receive no pigment, the cortex of each hair becomes transparent and the resulting hair appears white.

The degree of curliness of a hair depends on the cross-section shape of its follicle.

DISORDERS

Many hair disorders appear to be purely cosmetic, but they can also be a symptom of a more serious underlying disorder.

Brittle hair, which breaks easily and splits at the ends, is usually due to excessive shampooing, combing, or blow-drying. Occasionally, brittle hair can be a sign of severe vitamin or mineral deficiency, or may indicate *hypothyroidism* (underactivity of the thyroid gland). Very dry hair is often the result of excessive use of heated rollers or curling irons, or frequent perming, tinting, or bleaching; it can also be caused by malnutrition.

Ingrown hairs occur primarily in black people or in people with very curly hair. The free-growing end of the hair penetrates the skin near the follicle. Ingrown hairs often cause severe inflammation.

Hairball

A ball of hair in the stomach. Also known as a trichobezoar, it is found in people who nervously pull, suck, or chew their hair. (See *Bezoar*.)

Hairiness, excessive

See *Hirsutism*; *Hypertrichosis*.

Hair removal

Hair is usually removed from different parts of the body for cosmetic reasons. It may also be shaved from around an incision site to allow thorough cleansing before surgical operations.

HOW IT IS DONE

The method used depends on the part of the body involved and the degree of permanency required.

Shaving removes hair at skin level and is suitable for the legs, for armpit and pubic hair, and for the facial beard in men. Shaving is quick and safe, but the hair soon grows back.

Depilatory creams dissolve the hair just below the skin surface, creating a smoother effect than shaving. However, depilatories may cause irritation and should be used with caution on sensitive areas. Waxing is suitable for the legs and face. The wax

H

HAIR GROWTH

Scalp hair grows about a centimetre per month. There are about 300,000 hairs on the scalp, though there is considerable individual variation. The exact number depends on the number of hair follicles, which is established before birth. Each hair goes through alternating periods of growth and rest. On average, a person sheds 100 to 150 scalp hairs a day.

Growth phase Hair shaft

At the start of a growth phase (which, on the scalp, lasts about three years for each hair), the hair root stimulates the growth of a bulb and then a shaft.

Root
Bulb

Rest phase Old hair falls out

During the rest phase (which lasts about three months on the scalp), the bulb retracts from the root and eventually the hair falls out. A new hair begins to grow in the same follicle.

New hair forms

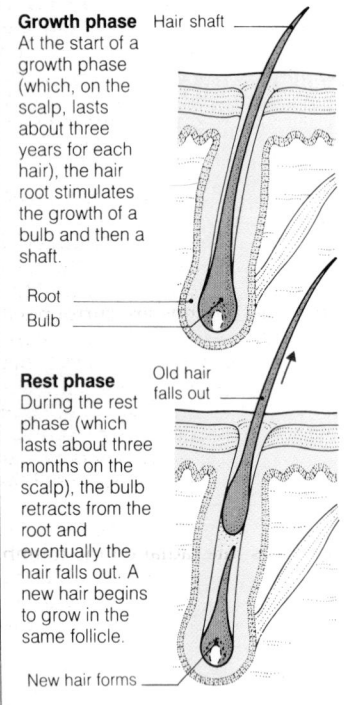

is applied to the area and peeled off, pulling out the hair with it. Plucking with tweezers is suitable for small areas. After each of these methods, hair takes several weeks to regrow.

Permanent removal of hair requires *electrolysis*, in which an electric current is used to destroy the growing part of the hair. Electrolysis is very time-consuming and expensive, and is usually used only for small areas.

Hair transplant

A cosmetic operation in which hairy sections of scalp are removed and transplanted to hairless areas to treat *alopecia* (baldness).

HOW IT IS DONE
One or a combination of the following techniques may be employed.
PUNCH GRAFTING This is the most common method of hair transplantation; it

is performed using a local anaesthetic and is an outpatient procedure. A punch is used to remove small areas of bald scalp, about 6 mm across, which are replaced with areas of hairy scalp. The grafts are taped into position until natural healing takes effect.

STRIP GRAFTING This requires a general anaesthetic and is carried out in hospital. Strips of bald skin are cut from the top of the head, and strips of hairy scalp are stitched in their place.

FLAP GRAFTING This is often used to form a new hairline. It is similar to strip grafting, except that flaps of hairy skin are lifted, swivelled, and stitched to replace areas of bald skin.

MALE PATTERN BALDNESS REDUCTION This relatively new technique consists of cutting out areas of bald skin and then stretching surrounding areas of hair-bearing scalp to replace the bald areas.

RESULTS
The success of hair transplantation varies. The hair in punch grafts often falls out after transplantation, leaving unsightly patches for several months until new hair grows. Also, hair does not always grow properly in the areas from which graft skin is taken. Even successful transplants do not last indefinitely; after a time, the transplanted areas also become bald.

Half-life

The time taken for the activity of a substance to reduce to half its original level. The term is usually used to refer to the time taken for the level of *radiation* emitted by a radioactive substance to decay to half its original level. The concept of half-life is useful in *radiotherapy* for assessing how long material will stay radioactive in the body.

Half-life is used in pharmacology to refer to the length of time taken by the body to eliminate half the quantity of a drug in the bloodstream.

Halitosis

The medical term for bad breath. Halitosis is occasionally a sign of illness, but is usually simply a result of smoking, drinking alcohol, eating garlic or onions, or poor oral and dental hygiene. Neither constipation nor indigestion is a cause.

Persistent bad breath not caused by any of these may be a symptom of mouth infection, *sinusitis*, or certain lung disorders, such as *bronchiectasis*.

Hallucination

A perception that occurs when there is no external stimulus (for example, hearing voices or seeing faces when

there is no one there). Hallucination differs from an *illusion*, in which a real stimulus is present but has been misinterpreted (thinking that the ticking of a clock is a bomb, for example).

TYPES AND CAUSES
Auditory hallucinations (the hearing of voices) are the most common type. They are a major symptom of *schizophrenia*, but may also be caused by *manic-depressive illness* and certain brain disorders. Visual hallucinations (seeing visions) are most often found in states of *delirium* brought on either by a physical illness (such as *pneumonia*) or by alcohol withdrawal (see *Delirium tremens*). *Hallucinogenic drugs*, such as mescaline, are another common cause. Hallucinations of smell are often a sign of *temporal lobe epilepsy*, especially when the epilepsy is caused by a tumour. Hallucinations of touch and taste are uncommon and probably occur mainly in people with schizophrenia. There is evidence that people subjected to *sensory deprivation* or to overwhelming physical stress hallucinate temporarily.

Hallucinogenic drug

A drug that causes a *hallucination*. Hallucinogens include certain drugs of abuse, also called psychedelic drugs, such as *LSD*, *marijuana*, *mescaline*, and *psilocybin*. Alcohol may also have an hallucinogenic effect if taken in large amounts; hallucinations also occur during alcohol withdrawal. Certain prescription drugs, including *anticholinergic drugs*, *levodopa*, and *timolol*, may cause takers to have hallucinations in rare instances.

Hallux

The medical name for the big *toe*.

Hallux rigidus

Loss of movement in the large joint at the base of the big toe due to *osteoarthritis*. The condition often follows an injury. The joint is usually tender and swollen, and pain is worse during walking or running.

Hallux rigidus, which may be mistaken for *gout*, is diagnosed if X-rays reveal degeneration of the joint. Treatment consists of resting the toe and wearing an insert in the shoe to support the front of the foot and to reduce movements of the toe during walking. Surgery is sometimes required.

Hallux valgus

A deformity of the big toe in which the joint at the base projects out from the foot and the top of the toe turns inwards. The condition, which is more common in women, is usually associated with wearing narrow, pointed shoes with high heels, but is sometimes caused by an inherited weakness in the joint. A hallux valgus often leads to the formation of a *bunion* (a firm, fluid-filled, sometimes painful swelling over the joint) or to *osteoarthritis* in the joint.

Treatment is required only if the bunion becomes very large or persistently inflamed or if the osteoarthritis causes pain and limits foot movement. In this case, the toe may be straightened by means of *osteotomy* (surgery to remove part of a bone and realign its ends) or *arthrodesis* (surgery to fuse the bones of a joint).

Haloperidol

An *antipsychotic drug* used in the treatment of mental illnesses such as *schizophrenia* and *mania*.

Haloperidol is also given to control the symptoms of *Gilles de la Tourette's syndrome* (a rare neurological disorder) and may be used, in small doses, to sedate aggressive or hostile people with *dementia*.

POSSIBLE ADVERSE EFFECTS
Adverse effects include drowsiness, lethargy, weight gain, dizziness, and, more seriously, *parkinsonism* (a neurological disorder that causes symptoms such as abnormal involuntary movements and stiffness of the face and limbs).

Halothane

A colourless liquid inhaled as a vapour to induce and help maintain general anaesthesia (see *Anaesthesia, general*). In rare cases it may cause *arrhythmia* (abnormal heart rhythm) or liver damage.

Hamartoma

A benign, tumour-like mass consisting of an overgrowth of tissues that are normally found in the affected part of the body.

Hamartomas are common in the skin (the most common type is a *haemangioma*, an overgrowth of blood vessels in the skin), but also occur in the lungs, heart, or kidneys.

Hammer-toe

A deformity of the *toe* (usually the second toe) in which the main toe joint stays bent. A painful *corn* often develops on this joint because of pressure from the overlying shoe. Hammer-toe is caused by an abnormality of the tendons in the toe.

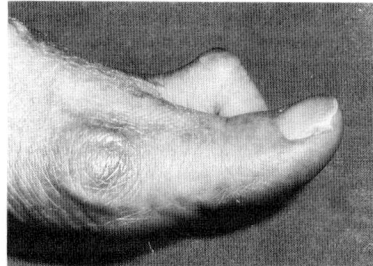

Appearance of hammer-toe
This photograph shows the typical appearance of a hammer-toe, in which one of the joints of the second toe is fixed in a bent position.

A protective felt pad usually eases pressure on the joint and thus relieves pain. If pain persists, the deformity may require surgical correction.

Hamstring muscles

A group of muscles at the back of the thigh. The upper ends of the hamstring muscles are attached by tendons to the pelvis; the lower ends are attached by tendons called hamstrings to the tibia and fibula. The hamstring muscles bend the knee and swing the leg backwards from the thigh.

DISORDERS
Tearing of the hamstring muscles is common in sports, particularly in sprinting. The injury happens suddenly and is very painful. Bruising over the area develops several days later. Repeated strenuous exercise may cause a sprain of the muscles, with pain coming on gradually (see *Overuse injury*). Both types of injury can often be prevented by warming-up exercises.

Sciatica (pain down the back of the leg caused by pressure on the sciatic nerve) may be particularly severe in the hamstring muscles.

Painful spasms of the hamstring muscles can also sometimes occur as a protective response to a knee injury; by restricting movement of the damaged knee joint, the muscle spasms limit further injury.

Hand

The hand, which is the most versatile part of the body, allows humans (and other primates) to hold and manipulate objects. This ability is primarily due to the fact that the fingers and thumb can move independently and can form an effective *grip*.

STRUCTURE
The hand is made up of the wrist, palm, and fingers (see below).

Movements of the hand are achieved mainly by tendons that attach the muscles of the forearm to the bones of the hand. These tendons are surrounded by synovial sheaths containing a lubricating fluid that prevents friction. Other movements are controlled by short muscles in the palm of the hand; some of these muscles make up the prominent areas along the sides of the hand from the bases of the thumb and little fingers to the wrist.

Blood is supplied to the hand by two arteries (the radial on the thumb side of the wrist and the ulnar on the little finger side) and is carried away by veins that are prominent on the back of the hand.

Sensation and movement in the hand are controlled by the radial, ulnar, and median nerves.

THE SKELETAL STRUCTURE OF THE HAND AND WRIST

Four of the eight wrist bones (carpals) articulate with the radius and ulna. The rest are connected to the five bones of the palm (metacarpals), each of which articulates with a phalanx.

Trapezium bone
Trapezoid bone
Capitate bone
Hamate bone
Scaphoid bone
Pisiform bone
Lunate bone
Triquetral bone

Carpals

Radius

Ulna

Phalanges   Metacarpals

H

DISORDERS

Because they are so frequently used, the hands are susceptible to injury, including cuts, burns, bites, fractures, and, occasionally, tendon injuries. *Dermatitis* is also common, since the hands are exposed to a considerable variety of irritating agents.

The hand may be affected by contracture, a deformity caused by shrinkage of tissues in the palm of the hand (see *Dupuytren's contracture*) or damage to muscles in the forearm (see *Volkmann's contracture*). Degeneration of a synovial sheath on the upper side of the wrist may cause a harmless swelling known as a *ganglion*.

Osteoarthritis commonly attacks the joint at the base of the thumb, rendering it painful and immobile. *Rheumatoid arthritis* may cause deformity by attacking the joints at the base of the fingers and rupturing tendons.

Handedness

Preference for using the right or left hand. Some 90 per cent of healthy adults use the right hand for writing; two thirds prefer the right hand for most activities requiring coordination and skill. The rest are either left-handed or ambidextrous (able to use both hands equally well). There is no male-female difference in the proportions preferring each hand.

It is uncertain why all humans are not simply ambidextrous. Up to the age of about 12, it is possible to switch handedness if a person's dominant hemisphere of the brain is damaged.

CAUSES

Inheritance is probably the most important factor in determining handedness. Studies have shown a greater number of nerves going to one side of the brain even in the newborn. A child made to use the right hand despite natural preference, however, may "become" right-handed. In earlier times, left-handed people were considered to be unlucky or evil (the word sinister is derived from the Latin word for left), so children were trained to be right-handed. Even today, so many people are naturally right-handed that the pressure to conform is high, especially in some cultures where the left hand is that used for wiping the anus after defaecation. Some left-handed people may subconsciously resent the change when forced to use the right hand.

Handedness is related to the division of the brain into two hemispheres, each of which controls movement and sensation on the opposite side of the body. In most right-handed people, the speech centre is in the left hemisphere, so that a *stroke* affecting this side of the brain causes *aphasia* (speech impairment) as well as paralysis and weakness of the right arm and leg. In 70 per cent of left-handed people, the speech centre is on the right, and left hemisphere damage does not cause aphasia.

EFFECTS OF HANDEDNESS

It is not clear whether handedness is related to special abilities. Left-handed tennis players or bowlers seem to succeed because their shots or balls come from an unusual angle. Although the left brain is related to verbal ability and logical reasoning, and the right to emotional and spatial awareness, there is no evidence that more artists are left-handed or more philosophers right-handed.

Hand-foot-and-mouth disease

A common infectious disease of toddlers, caused by a virus known as a coxsackievirus. Hand-foot-and-mouth disease often occurs in small epidemics in nursery schools, usually in the summer months.

The illness is usually mild and lasts only a few days. Symptoms include blistering of the palms, soles, and inside of the mouth, reluctance to eat, and a slight fever. There is no treatment other than mild *analgesic drugs* (painkillers) to relieve the discomfort of the blisters. The illness is unrelated to foot-and-mouth disease in cattle.

Handicap

The extent to which a physical or mental *disability* (loss or impairment of a faculty) interferes with normal functioning and causes the person to be disadvantaged.

The management and treatment of a handicap involves assessment of the specific disability, the provision of suitable aids, specific educational help, and, if necessary, longer-term support in an appropriate setting.

Hangnail

A strip of skin torn away from the side or base of a fingernail, exposing a raw, painful area. Hangnails usually occur after frequent immersion in water has dried the skin on the fingers. Biting the nails is another common cause. The raw area may become infected and develop into a *paronychia*.

A hangnail should be trimmed with scissors and covered until it heals. The condition may be prevented by applying a moisturizing cream.

Hangover

The unpleasant effects sometimes experienced on waking after overindulgence in *alcohol*. Characterized by headache, nausea, vertigo, and depression, the severity of a hangover is determined by the amount and type of alcohol consumed. Brandy and red wine have high concentrations of congeners (secondary products of alcohol fermentation), which may produce bad hangovers.

Alcohol increases urine production and some of the symptoms of a hangover are due to mild dehydration; drinking a large quantity of water before going to sleep may help. Recovery from a hangover is usually just a matter of time, but people suffering from *alcohol dependence* may experience more severe and persistent hangovers or they may suffer from withdrawal symptoms. (See also *Alcohol intoxication*.)

Hansen's disease

A chronic bacterial infection, also known as leprosy, that damages nerves, mainly in the limbs and facial area, and may also lead to skin damage. Untreated Hansen's disease can have severe complications, which include blindness and disfigurement. Contrary to popular belief, Hansen's disease is not highly contagious.

CAUSES

Hansen's disease is caused by a bacterium, MYCOBACTERIUM LEPRAE, spread in droplets of nasal mucus. A person is infectious to others only during the first stages of the disease. Only people living in prolonged close contact with an infected person are at risk of infection. This, along with the fact that only three per cent of the population are susceptible to Hansen's disease at all, means that there is no justification for the practice (still prevalent in some countries) of isolating people with the disease.

INCIDENCE

Worldwide, there are about 20 million sufferers from Hansen's disease, mostly in Asia, Central and South America, and Africa. Probably fewer than 20 per cent of these have access to treatment. A small number of cases (fewer than 20) are diagnosed each year in the UK. In all these cases, the infection is contracted while the sufferer is temporarily abroad.

SYMPTOMS AND SIGNS

Hansen's disease has a very long incubation period—about three to five years. Most of the destructive effects on nervous tissue are caused not by bacterial growth but by a reaction of the body's *immune system* to the organisms as they die.

There are two main types of Hansen's disease: the lepromatous type, in which the damage is widespread, progressive, and severe; and the tuberculoid type, which is milder.

Initially, damage is confined to peripheral nerves, which supply the skin and muscles. Skin areas supplied by affected nerves become lighter or darker and sensation and sweating in these areas are reduced.

As the disease progresses, the peripheral nerves swell and become tender. Hands, feet, and facial skin eventually become numb and muscles become paralysed.

Complications include loss of all sensation in the hands and feet, so that accidental burns or injuries are not noticed, leading to extensive scarring or even to loss of fingers or toes. Muscle paralysis can lead to further deformity. Damage to the facial nerve means that the eyelids cannot be closed; the cornea dries and ulcerates, leading to blindness. Alternatively, direct invasion by bacteria may lead to inflammation of the eyeball, again leading to blindness. The disability caused by the combined effects of blindness and loss of touch sensation is extremely severe.

Cartilage and bone in the nose are often eroded, and bones elsewhere in the body may be destroyed.

The testes may atrophy (waste), leading to sterility.

DIAGNOSIS
Early diagnosis of the disease is essential to prevent permanent disfigurement and disability. A provisional diagnosis is made from a physical examination of the patient; the presence of the bacteria is confirmed by a skin *biopsy* (removal of a sample of tissue for analysis).

TREATMENT
Drug treatment may be with a combination of dapsone, rifampicin, and clofazimine, which kills most of the causative bacteria within a few days. Any damage that has already occurred, however, is irreversible. Patients cease to be infectious soon after treatment starts.

Prevention of damage to the feet and other insensitive areas—through the use of proper footwear and health education—is very important. *Plastic surgery* may be helpful for people with facial deformities. Nerve and tendon transplants may improve the function of damaged limbs.

OUTLOOK
With so many sufferers in poor countries, the battle against Hansen's disease has only just begun. Experimental vaccines against Hansen's disease are under trial.

Hardening of the arteries
The popular term for *arteriosclerosis*, the most common form of which is *atherosclerosis*.

Hare lip
A common term for the *birth defect* in which there is a split in the upper lip due to failure of the two sides to fuse during fetal development. Also called cleft lip, it is often associated with a similar failure of the two halves of the palate to join. (See *Cleft lip and palate*.)

Hashimoto's thyroiditis
An *autoimmune disorder* in which the body's immune system develops *antibodies* against its own thyroid gland cells. As a result, the thyroid gland becomes unable to produce enough *thyroid hormones*, a condition called *hypothyroidism*.

The principal symptoms are tiredness, muscle weakness, and weight gain. A goitre (enlargement of the thyroid gland) develops.

The diagnosis is confirmed by blood tests to measure the level of thyroid hormones and to detect the presence of thyroid antibodies. Treatment consists of thyroid hormone replacement therapy, which is continued for life. If a goitre persists despite drug treatment, surgery may be necessary.

Hashish
Another name for *marijuana*.

Hay fever
The popular name for a seasonal form of allergic rhinitis. (See *Rhinitis, allergic*.)

Headache
One of the most common types of pain. A headache is only very occasionally a symptom of a serious underlying disorder.

The pain of a headache does not come from the brain, which contains no sensory nerves, but arises from the *meninges* (the membranes around the brain) and from the scalp and its blood vessels and muscles. The pain is produced by tension in, or stretching of, these structures.

The pain may be felt all over the head or may occur in only one part—for example, in the back of the neck, the forehead, or one side of the head. Sometimes the pain moves to another part of the head during the course of the headache. The pain of headache may be superficial or deep, throbbing or sharp, and there may also be accompanying or preliminary symptoms, such as nausea, vomiting, and visual or sensory disturbances.

TYPES
Many headaches are simply the body's response to some adverse stimulus, such as hunger or a change in the weather. These headaches usually clear up in a few hours and leave no after-effects.

Tension headaches, caused by tightening in the muscles of the face, neck, and scalp as a result of stress or poor posture, are also common. They may last for days or weeks and can cause varying degrees of discomfort.

Some types of headache are especially painful and persistent but nevertheless are not an indication of a progressive underlying disorder. *Migraine* is a severe, incapacitating headache preceded or accompanied by visual and/or stomach disturbances. Cluster headaches cause intense pain behind one eye and may wake the sufferer nightly for periods of weeks or months.

CAUSES
Common causes of headache include *hangover*, irregular meals, prolonged travel, poor posture, a noisy or stuffy work environment, excitement, and excessive sleep. Recent research has shown that certain foods (such as cheese, chocolate, and red wine) trigger migraine attacks in susceptible people. *Food additives* may also cause headache. Other causes include *sinusitis, toothache, head injury*, and *cervical osteoarthritis*. Some headaches are due to overuse of *analgesic drugs* (painkillers) and disappear when the drugs are stopped. Among the rare causes of headache are *brain tumour, hypertension* (high blood pressure), *temporal arteritis* (inflammation of arteries in the face, neck, and scalp), *aneurysm* (ballooning of a blood vessel, in this case in the brain), and increased pressure within the skull.

INVESTIGATION
If headaches are persistent, without obvious cause, and do not respond to self-help treatment, medical advice should be sought. The doctor will ask about the nature and site of the pain and at what intervals the headaches occur. A careful general physical and neurological examination will be performed. *CT scanning* or *MRI* (magnetic

H

HEADACHE Pain in the head that may be anything from mild to severe and incapacitating.

Is your temperature 38°C or above? — **YES** → Many feverish illnesses may cause a headache.
See • *Fever*

NO ↓

Have you injured your head within the past few days? — **YES** → **Are you feeling unusually drowsy AND/OR have you felt nauseated or been vomiting?** — **YES** → ☎ **EMERGENCY! GET MEDICAL HELP NOW!** This suggests the possibility of a brain injury.
See • *Extradural haemorrhage*

NO ↓ (from drowsy question)
A persistent headache is common following a head injury.
See • *Head injury*

NO ↓

Have you felt nauseated or been vomiting? — **YES** → **Do you have severe pain in and around one eye AND is your vision in that eye blurred?** — **YES** → ☎ **Call your doctor without delay!** This suggests the possibility of raised pressure inside the eye.
See • *Glaucoma*

NO ↓

Do you have two or more of the following symptoms?
• pain when you touch your chin to your chest
• dislike of bright light
• drowsiness or confusion
— **YES** → ☎ **EMERGENCY! GET MEDICAL HELP NOW!** These symptoms suggest the possibility of a brain injury or irritation of the meninges.
See • *Subarachnoid haemorrhage*

NO ↓

Have you suddenly begun to have a severe throbbing pain in one or both temples? — **YES** → ☎ **Consult your doctor without delay!** Inflammation of the arteries in the head is a possibility, especially if you are over 50.
See • *Temporal arteritis*

NO ↓

Was the pain one-sided or preceded by disturbed vision? — **YES** → You may have a migraine.
See • *Migraine*

NO

Continued on next page

NO ↓

508

H

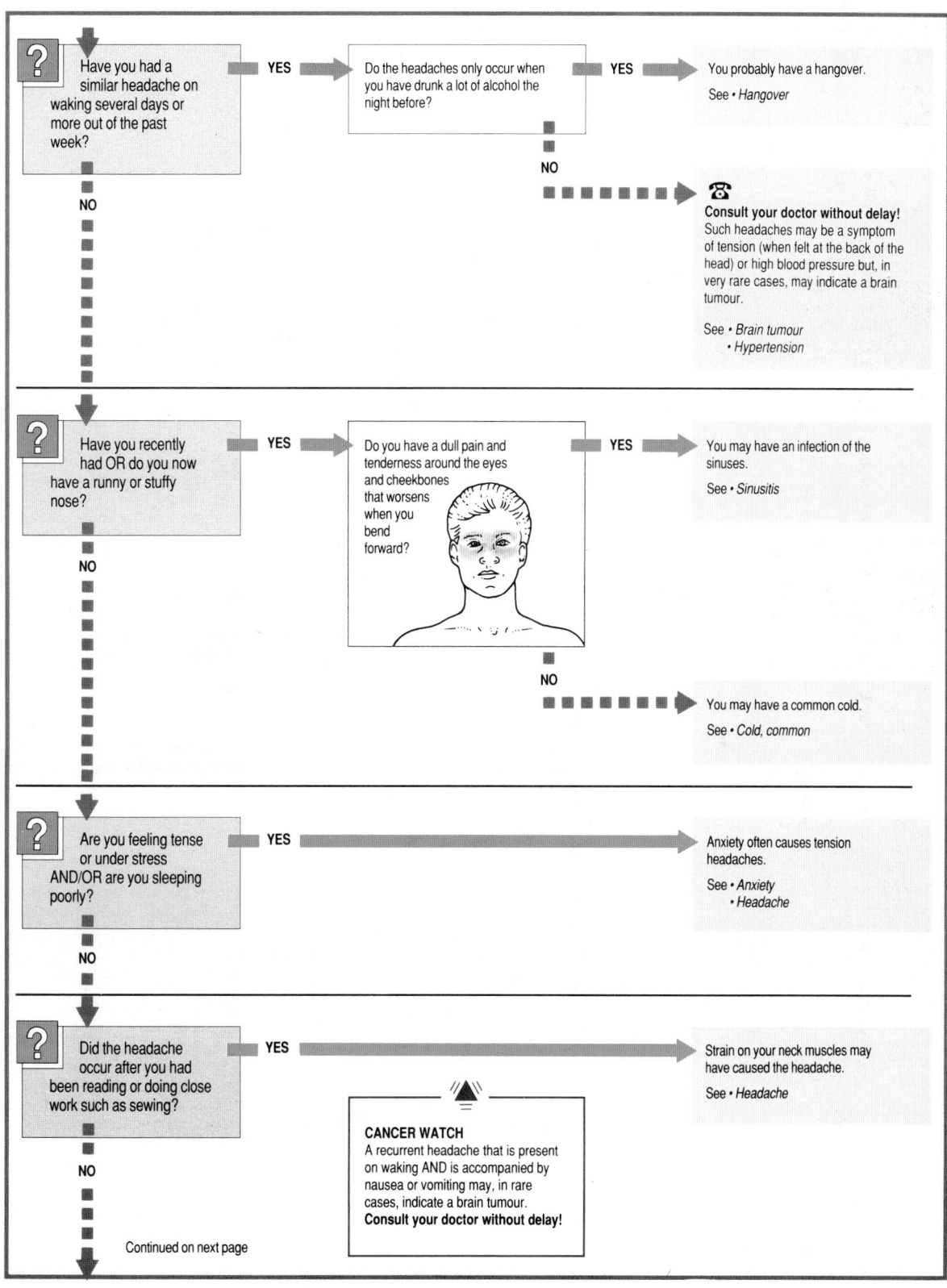

Have you had a similar headache on waking several days or more out of the past week?

YES → **Do the headaches only occur when you have drunk a lot of alcohol the night before?**

YES → You probably have a hangover.

See • *Hangover*

NO ┄┄→ ☎

Consult your doctor without delay!
Such headaches may be a symptom of tension (when felt at the back of the head) or high blood pressure but, in very rare cases, may indicate a brain tumour.

See • *Brain tumour*
   • *Hypertension*

NO

Have you recently had OR do you now have a runny or stuffy nose?

YES → **Do you have a dull pain and tenderness around the eyes and cheekbones that worsens when you bend forward?**

YES → You may have an infection of the sinuses.

See • *Sinusitis*

NO ┄┄→ You may have a common cold.

See • *Cold, common*

NO

Are you feeling tense or under stress AND/OR are you sleeping poorly?

YES → Anxiety often causes tension headaches.

See • *Anxiety*
   • *Headache*

NO

Did the headache occur after you had been reading or doing close work such as sewing?

YES → Strain on your neck muscles may have caused the headache.

See • *Headache*

CANCER WATCH
A recurrent headache that is present on waking AND is accompanied by nausea or vomiting may, in rare cases, indicate a brain tumour.
Consult your doctor without delay!

NO

Continued on next page

H

? Did any of the
following apply in the
12 hours before the
headache started?
• you were exposed to
strong sunlight
• you were in stuffy, smoky,
or noisy surroundings
• you drank more alcohol
than usual
• you missed a meal

YES ➡ Headaches are often brought on by
such circumstances and are usually
no cause for concern.

NO

? Are you currently
taking any medicines
AND/OR are you taking
the birth-control pill?

YES ➡ Certain drugs can cause headaches
as a side effect. Discuss promptly
with your doctor.

NO

If you are unable to make a
diagnosis from this chart and
the headache persists overnight
or if you have other symptoms,
consult your doctor.

resonance imaging) may be carried out if a neurological cause for the headaches is suspected.

TREATMENT

Prevention is more important than treatment; many of the known causes can easily be avoided, particularly if the sufferer knows what triggers the headaches. Once a headache has started (provided it is not a migraine or cluster headache), one or more of the following measures should ease the pain: relaxing in a hot bath; lying down; avoidance of aggravating factors (such as excessive noise or a stuffy room); stretching and massaging the muscles in the shoulders, neck, face, and scalp; taking a mild analgesic drug; and sleeping.

Head-banging

Persistent, rhythmic banging of the head, usually against a wall or hard object. Head-banging occurs in mentally handicapped people, particularly children and adolescents in institutions that provide little or no stimula-

tion. Head-banging is a form of self-stimulation and is also an attention-seeking device. It may lead to serious injury. Protective headgear and *behaviour therapy* may help.

Head-banging also occurs in some normal toddlers, often when they are frustrated or angry, or as a comfort when going to sleep. It may sometimes occur during sleep.

Most children grow out of head-banging. In the majority of cases, the problem is best ignored, but if head-banging is severe or persistent a doctor should be consulted.

Head injury

Injury to the head may occur as a result of traffic accidents, sports injuries, falls, assault, accidents at work and at home, or bullet wounds. Most people have a minor head injury at least once in their lives, but very few of the injuries are severe enough to require treatment. One per cent of all deaths are caused by head injury, half as a result of traffic accidents.

A head injury can damage the scalp, skull, or brain. Minor injuries cause no damage to the underlying brain. Even when there is a *skull fracture*, or the scalp is split, the brain may not be damaged. However, a blow may severely shake the brain, sometimes causing *brain damage*, even when there are no external signs of injury.

A blow often bruises the brain tissue, causing death of some of the brain cells in the injured area. When an object actually penetrates the skull, foreign material and dirt may be implanted into the brain and lead to infection. A blow or a penetrating injury may tear blood vessels and cause *brain haemorrhage* (bleeding in or around the brain). Head injury may cause swelling of the brain; this is particularly evident after bullet wounds because their high velocity causes extensive damage. If the skull is fractured, bone may be driven into the underlying brain.

SYMPTOMS AND SIGNS

If the head injury is mild, there may be no symptoms other than a slight headache. In some cases there is *concussion*, which may cause confusion, dizziness, and blurred vision (sometimes persisting for several days). More severe head injuries, particularly blows to the head, may result in unconsciousness that lasts longer than a few minutes, or *coma*, which may be fatal.

Post-concussive *amnesia* (loss of memory of events that occurred after an accident) may occur, especially if the skull has been fractured. This amnesia usually lasts more than an hour after consciousness is regained. There may also be pretraumatic amnesia (loss of memory of events that occurred before the accident). The more serious the injury to the brain, the longer unconsciousness and amnesia are likely to last.

After a severe brain injury, a person may suffer some muscular weakness or paralysis and loss of sensation.

Symptoms such as persistent vomiting, pupils of unequal size, double vision, or a deteriorating level of consciousness suggest progressive brain damage.

INVESTIGATION

Any person suffering loss of consciousness, however brief, should be seen by a doctor. The person may be hospitalized for observation; *skull X-rays* are performed to identify any fracture. If a brain haemorrhage is suspected, *CT scanning* may be carried out.

TREATMENT

Cuts to the scalp may require stitching. People whose consciousness is deteriorating will be kept under close observation. If a blood clot forms inside the skull, the clot may be life-threatening and will require surgical removal; severe skull fractures may also require surgery.

OUTLOOK

Recovery from minor head injuries may take several days if there are persistent symptoms of concussion. Survival following major head injuries has been improved by advances in nursing and medical care, but permanent physical or mental disability (including changes in personality) may follow if there has been permanent damage to the brain. Epileptic seizures sometimes occur after a severe head injury (especially after a penetrating injury, severe skull fracture, or serious brain haemorrhage). Recovery from a major head injury may be very slow, but victims may continue to show signs of progressive recovery for as long as five years.

Head lag

The backward flopping of the head that occurs when an infant is placed in a sitting position. Head lag is obvious in the newborn because the neck muscles are still weak, but by four months of age the baby can hold his or her head upright in line with the trunk. The disappearance of head lag is a measure of motor development (see *Child development*); good control of the head is essential before a baby can learn to sit.

Heaf test

A type of *tuberculin test*.

Healing

The process by which the body repairs bone, tissue, or organ damage caused by injury, infection, or disease. In popular usage, the term means simply "restoring to health".

THE HEALING PROCESS

The initial stages of healing are the same for all parts of the body. After injury, the blood forms clots in damaged areas of tissue. White blood cells, *enzymes*, *histamine*, other chemicals, and *proteins* from which new cells can be made accumulate at the site of damage. Fibrous tissue is laid down within the blood clot to form a supportive structure. Any dead cells are broken down and absorbed by the white blood cells. Some tissues, such as bone, are then able to regenerate by

proliferation of the cells that remain around the damaged area. In such cases, the original structure and function are fully restored.

Other tissues, such as nerve tissue, may be unable to proliferate. In other cases, there may be an inadequate blood supply or persistent infection that prevents tissue regeneration. In these cases, the fibrous tissue that forms in the blood clot may develop into tough scar tissue, which keeps the tissue structure intact but may impair its function (e.g. the restriction of movement that sometimes happens after a muscle tear).

WOUND HEALING

The body repairs skin wounds by one of two processes: healing by first intention and healing by second intention.

Healing by first intention occurs when the edges of the wound are close together and there has been minimal loss of tissue. If the wound is deep, the edges of the skin may need to be held together with stitches or a butterfly bandage. The blood that seeps from the edges of the wound forms a clot which becomes the base on which scar tissue is laid down. When healing is complete, only a fine scar remains.

Healing by second intention occurs when the edges of the wound are not brought together. In this slower type of healing, pink *granulation tissue* grows from the exposed tissue. This granulation tissue is eventually covered by skin, which grows over the wound from the cut edges. By the time healing is complete, the granulation tissue has developed into tough scar tissue.

Health

At its simplest, health is the absence of physical and mental disease. However, the wider concept promoted by the World Health Organization is that all people should have the opportunity to fulfil their genetic potential. This includes the ability to grow and develop physically and mentally without the impediments of inadequate nutrition or environmental contamination, and to be protected as much as possible against infectious diseases. (See also *Diet and disease*; *Health hazards*.)

Health centre

A building owned by a local authority and leased to one or more groups of doctors as premises for their general practices. The centre may also include

premises for a pharmacist and for other health professionals, such as opticians and chiropodists. A health centre differs from a group practice medical centre, which is collectively owned by the doctors rather than by the local authority.

Health food

The term applied to products that are meant to promote health, including unprocessed and wholefood products, organically grown fruits and vegetables, and dietary supplements. The term is misleading because it suggests that only "health foods" are good for people. In fact, a healthy diet is based on sound *nutrition*.

Health hazards

Environmental factors that are known or suspected to cause disease. Some health hazards are obvious, such as contamination of water supplies or food with sewage or other effluents, and pollution of the air with smoke or poisonous chemicals. Others are less apparent—for example, radioactivity (which is detectable only with special instruments) and sunlight.

TYPES

For people in developing countries, in other words for the majority of the world's population, the main hazards come from lack of access to safe, pure water, from inadequate means of disposal of sewage and domestic refuse, and from insufficient or contaminated food. Foods contaminated with microorganisms, such as bacteria and moulds, present far greater health hazards than those associated with the additives that are used in developed countries to combat such contamination. Nevertheless, food-borne illness in the UK is on the increase despite educational programmes and legislation to improve general standards. (See *Food additives*; *Food-borne infection*; *Food poisoning*.)

There are four other main types of health hazard, all of which are present in both developed and developing countries. First, there are the numerous *infectious diseases* transmitted by contact or by insects or other animals. (See *Bacteria*; *Fungal infections*; *Insects and disease*; *Viruses*; *Zoonoses*.) The second type comprises work-related hazards, such as industrial *accidents*, and a wide variety of occupational disorders, e.g. *asbestosis*, *pneumoconiosis*, *lead poisoning*, cancers associated with exposure to chemicals. (See *Occupational disease and injury*.)

H

H

HEARING

The ears are the organs of hearing. Each ear has three separate regions—the outer ear, middle ear, and inner ear. Sound waves are channelled through the ear canal to the middle ear, from where a complex system of membranes and tiny bones conveys the vibrations to the inner ear. A part of the auditory nerve converts the vibrations to nerve impulses, which are then transmitted to the brain.

To function properly, the eardrum must have equal air pressure on each side so that it can vibrate freely. Pressure is equalized via the eustachian tube, which runs from the back of the throat to the middle ear.

ROUTE TO THE BRAIN

Auditory sensations are picked up by nerve fibres in the cochlea and travel along the auditory nerve to the medulla. From there, they pass via the thalamus to the superior temporal gyrus—the part of the cerebral cortex involved in receiving and perceiving sound.

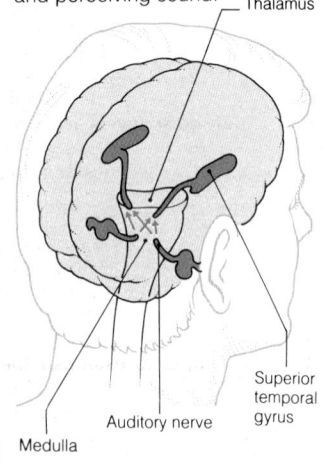

Thalamus

Superior temporal gyrus

Auditory nerve

Medulla

Outer ear
The pinna (the visible part of the ear) channels sound waves into the outer-ear canal (auditory canal) toward the eardrum. Hairs and waxy cerumen line the canal.

Malleus (hammer) and incus (anvil)
The malleus, attached to the eardrum, transmits vibration to the incus.

Stapes (stirrup) and oval window
The incus in turn transmits vibration to the stapes and the oval window membrane.

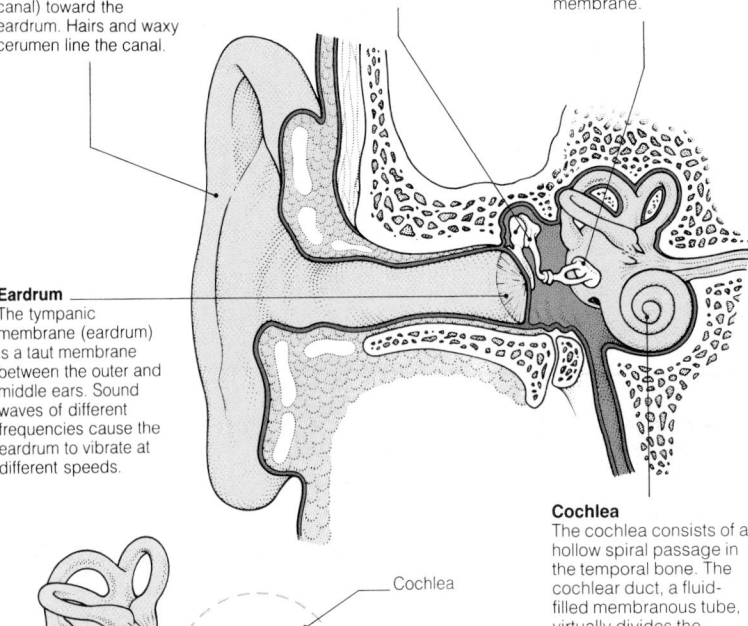

Eardrum
The tympanic membrane (eardrum) is a taut membrane between the outer and middle ears. Sound waves of different frequencies cause the eardrum to vibrate at different speeds.

Cochlea
The cochlea consists of a hollow spiral passage in the temporal bone. The cochlear duct, a fluid-filled membranous tube, virtually divides the cochlea lengthwise; it is full of microscopic hairs that stimulate nerve cells in response to sound vibrations, transmitted through the oval window.

Function of cochlea

Inside the cochlea (shown uncoiled), the first part of the basilar membrane responds most to high-frequency vibrations; the far end registers only lower frequencies.

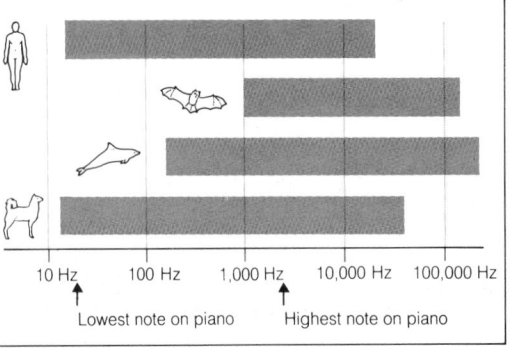

Cochlea

Oval window

Basilar membrane

Nerve fibres

COMPARISON OF FREQUENCY RANGES

Different animals are able to hear different ranges of sound frequencies. The diagram shows the normal ranges of sound, in hertz (cycles per second), that can be heard by a human, a bat, a dolphin, and a dog.

10 Hz   100 Hz   1,000 Hz   10,000 Hz   100,000 Hz

Lowest note on piano   Highest note on piano

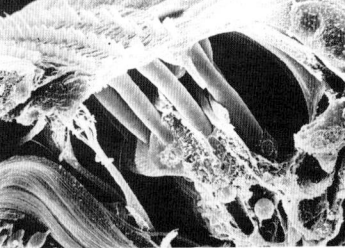

Electron micrograph of inner ear
The section shows four rows of hair cells, which convert sound waves into electrical impulses to be sent to the brain.

The third category of hazards includes those associated with domestic and social life, such as accidents in the home or on the road, and injuries and other hazards, such as drowning, from recreational activities. In many developed countries, domestic and traffic accidents are the most important risks to health in early adult life. *Alcohol* and *tobacco-smoking* are other major hazards to health.

Finally, there are many types of global environmental hazard, including sunlight (see *Sunlight, adverse effects of*), cosmic radiation and background radioactivity (see *Radiation hazards*), and *pollution* of the environment.

Hearing
The sense that enables sound to be perceived. The *ear* (the organ of hearing) transforms the sound waves it receives into nerve impulses that pass to the *brain*.

MECHANISM OF HEARING
Almost all sound is heard by a mechanism known as air conduction (see illustrated box). This process is supplemented by a secondary form of hearing called bone conduction, in which sound waves set up vibrations in the skull bones that pass directly to the inner ear. This form of hearing affects the way a person hears his or her own voice.

HEARING DISORDERS
Problems with hearing (from minor sound distortions to total inability to hear) result when any part of the sound-transmitting and analysing mechanism is damaged (see *Deafness*).

Hearing-aids
Electronic devices that improve hearing in people with certain types of *deafness*. A hearing-aid consists of a tiny microphone (to pick up sounds), an amplifier (to increase their volume), and a tiny speaker (to transmit sounds to the ear).

HOW IT WORKS
A tiny microphone collects sound and transforms it into electric current. The amplifier increases the strength of the current and feeds it along a tube to an earpiece, which fits into the outer-ear canal (or, more rarely, on to the bone behind the ear) and converts the current back to sound (which has now been amplified).

A volume control on the aid, usually operated by turning a tiny wheel, enables the level of incoming sound to be adjusted. The aid is designed at the factory to amplify those pitches for which the user

has the most loss. Further modifications of this sort may be made by the hearing-aid dispenser.

TYPES
The most common types of hearing-aid are inconspicuous. The mechanical parts, along with a battery to power them, are contained in a small plastic case that fits comfortably behind the ear, in the side-piece of a pair of glasses, or entirely within the ear canal. Aids that fit entirely in the ear are most popular today.

More powerful aids that amplify sound to a greater degree are also available but are now rarely used. In these aids, the microphone, amplifier, and battery are contained in a larger case worn on the body; the current is carried to the earpiece by a thin wire.

Some people with conductive deafness, especially if there is inflammation or discharge in the ear canal, may be given a bone-conduction hearing-aid. This type of hearing-aid may be fitted to a glasses frame or hair-band.

Most modern hearing-aids include switches that enable normal reception of sound by the microphone to be replaced by a process known as electromagnetic induction. This process picks up transmitted speech in telephones and in public buildings that have been equipped for the purpose. The greatest advantage of electromagnetic induction is that it obscures amplified background noise.

Other devices available for the hard-of-hearing include amplified telephone receivers, flashing lights

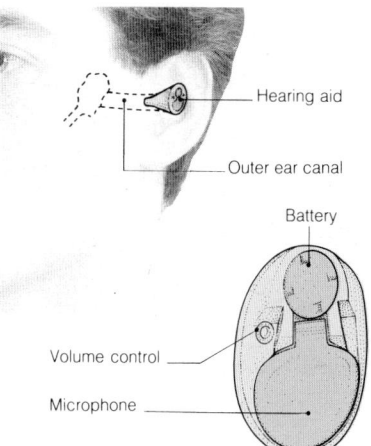

Hearing-aids
Hearing-aids amplify sound waves for people who have impaired hearing. Many hearing-aids include an earpiece, a microphone, an amplifier, a volume control, and a battery.

instead of doorbells and telephone bells, vibrators that respond to sound, headphones for television sets, teletypewriters, and guide dogs for the deaf. (See also *Cochlear implant*.)

Hearing loss
A deterioration in the ability to perceive sound. See *Deafness*.

Hearing tests
Tests performed to determine whether a person's hearing is impaired, the degree of impairment, and what part of the *ear* may be causing the problem. The main types of hearing test are described in the table (overleaf).

WHY THEY ARE DONE
Hearing tests are performed as part of a routine assessment of *child development*. They are sometimes carried out during a general medical examination, and may be performed regularly to check the hearing of people exposed to high noise levels at work.

Hearing tests may be necessary if a person complains of impaired hearing or in cases of suspected hearing loss, such as if a child's speech development is poor or if an elderly person appears to be suffering from *dementia*. A hearing test can also help determine the cause of *tinnitus* and dizziness.

AIMS OF TESTING
The doctor attempts to establish the extent and pattern of any hearing deficit by testing the person's ability to hear sounds at different frequencies and volumes. The lowest level at which a person can hear and repeat words (the speech reception threshold) is tested, as is the ability to hear words clearly (speech discrimination). The doctor also tries to ascertain whether any hearing loss is conductive or sensorineural in type (see *Deafness*). Test results enable the doctor and patient to decide on appropriate treatment, if necessary.

Heart
The muscular pump in the chest which, throughout life, beats continuously and rhythmically to send blood to the lungs and to the rest of the body. During an average lifetime, the heart contracts more than 2,500 million times.

STRUCTURE
Much of the heart consists of a special type of muscle, called myocardium. The myocardium, given sufficient oxygen and nutrients, contracts rhythmically and automatically without any other stimulus.

TYPES OF HEARING TEST

Tests	Function	
Tuning fork tests	These tests are used to determine whether hearing loss is conductive or sensorineural. In the Rinne test, the patient is asked whether the sound is louder with the vibrating tines held near the opening of the ear canal (air conduction) or with the base of the fork held against the mastoid bone (bone conduction). In a normal ear or in one with sensorineural loss,	air conduction is greater than bone conduction. In conductive loss, bone conduction is greater than or equal to air conduction. Weber's test, in which the base of the fork is placed on the forehead, is useful for diagnosing unilateral hearing loss. If hearing loss is conductive, the patient hears the tuning fork better in the ear with the poorer hearing.
Pure-tone audiometry	This is a test in which an audiometer is used to generate sounds of varying frequency and intensity. The audiometer is an electrical instrument that measures a person's ability to hear sounds of different frequencies and intensities. Hearing is first assessed by transmitting the sounds through one earphone while the other ear is prevented from hearing them. The sound frequencies range from 250 to 8,000 hertz (cycles per second); for each	frequency, the sound is decreased in intensity until it can no longer be heard. The person whose hearing is being tested gives a signal at the moment when he or she detects each sound, and the results are recorded on a graph called an audiogram. Bone conduction hearing is then assessed using a rubber rod connected to the audiometer (the rod is placed against the mastoid bone behind the ear and kept in place by a headband).
Auditory evoked response	In this form of testing, the brain's response to sound stimulation by the audiometer is analysed by means of electrodes placed on the scalp. This test attempts to evaluate the presence of hearing in a person who is unable to cooperate with other tests (because of mental	handicap, for example). Auditory evoked response is commonly used to assess hearing in very young babies. The test can also help rule out acoustic neuroma (a benign tumour within the auditory canal).
Impedance audiometry	This test is used to determine the type of middle-ear damage occurring in cases of conductive deafness. A probe is fitted tightly into the entrance to the outer-ear canal, sealing it off from outside air pressure and sound. The probe emits a continuous sound. Air is pumped through the probe at varying pressures and, at the same time, a microphone in the probe registers the differing	reflections of sounds from the eardrum as pressure changes in the ear canal. The reflections are recorded on a graph known as a tympanogram. The pattern of differing reflections reveals the extent of elasticity in the eardrum and middle-ear bones, thus indicating the type of disease that is causing the deafness. This device can also measure the air pressure in an air-filled middle ear.

The interior of the heart consists of four distinct chambers. A thick central muscular wall, called the septum, divides the cavity into right and left halves. Each half of the heart consists of an upper chamber, called an atrium, and a larger lower chamber, called a ventricle.

Various large blood vessels emerge from the top and sides of the heart. These vessels deliver blood to the atria or carry blood pumped out by the ventricles.

The internal surface of the heart is lined with a smooth membrane, called endocardium, and the entire heart is enclosed in a tough, membranous bag that is called the pericardium.

FUNCTION

The two sides of the heart have distinct, though interdependent, functions. The right side receives deoxygenated blood from the entire body via two large veins called the venae cavae. This blood arrives in the right atrium and, after transfer to the right ventricle, is pumped to the lungs via the pulmonary artery to be oxygenated (receive oxygen through the *alveoli*) and to lose carbon dioxide. The left side of the heart receives oxygenated blood from the lungs (via the pulmonary veins, which drain into the left atrium); this blood is first transferred to the left ventricle and then pumped to all tissues in the body. The heart can thus be viewed as a dual pump. Nonreturn (one-way) valves situated at the exits from each heart chamber guarantee that blood can flow through the circuit in only one direction (see *Heart valves*).

THE CARDIAC CYCLE

The pumping action of the heart consists of three phases, which together make up a cycle corresponding to one heartbeat. These phases are called diastole, atrial systole, and ventricular systole (see illustrated box, p 516).

To work efficiently, the different parts of the heart must contract in a precise sequence. This sequence is brought about by electrical impulses that emanate from the sinoatrial node, the heart's own pacemaker situated at the top of the right atrium. The electrical impulses are carried partly by the heart muscle itself and partly by specialized nerve fibres.

To avoid bottlenecks developing in the blood circulation, the volume pumped at each stroke by the two sides of the heart must exactly balance each other. However, resistance to blood flow through the general circulation is much greater than resistance to blood flow through the lungs; this means that the left side of the heart must contract much more forcibly than the right side. As a result of this, the muscular bulk of the left side of the heart is greater than that of the right side.

FACTORS AFFECTING HEART-RATE AND OUTPUT

The rate at which the heart beats, and the amount of blood it puts out with each contraction, can vary considerably according to the demands of the body's muscles for oxygen (and thus for blood). At rest, the heart contracts at 60 to 80 beats per minute and puts out about 80 ml of blood at each stroke, thus pumping about 6 litres per minute. However, during extreme exercise, the rate may increase to 200 contractions per minute and the output may increase to almost 250 ml per beat, thereby increasing the total output to 50 litres per minute.

Such changes in heart-rate and output are brought about in two ways.

THE HEART

The heart is positioned centrally in the chest, with its right margin directly underneath the right side of the sternum (breastbone). The rest of the heart points to the left, with its lowest point (the apex) located underneath the left nipple.

The heart acts as a dual pump. Deoxygenated blood from the body arrives, via the vena cava, in the right atrium (upper heart chamber), is transferred to the right ventricle (lower chamber), and is then pumped via the pulmonary artery to the lungs. There it is reoxygenated and returns, via the pulmonary veins, to the left side of the heart. It enters the left atrium, is transferred to the left ventricle, and is then pumped, via a large vessel (the aorta), to all parts of the body.

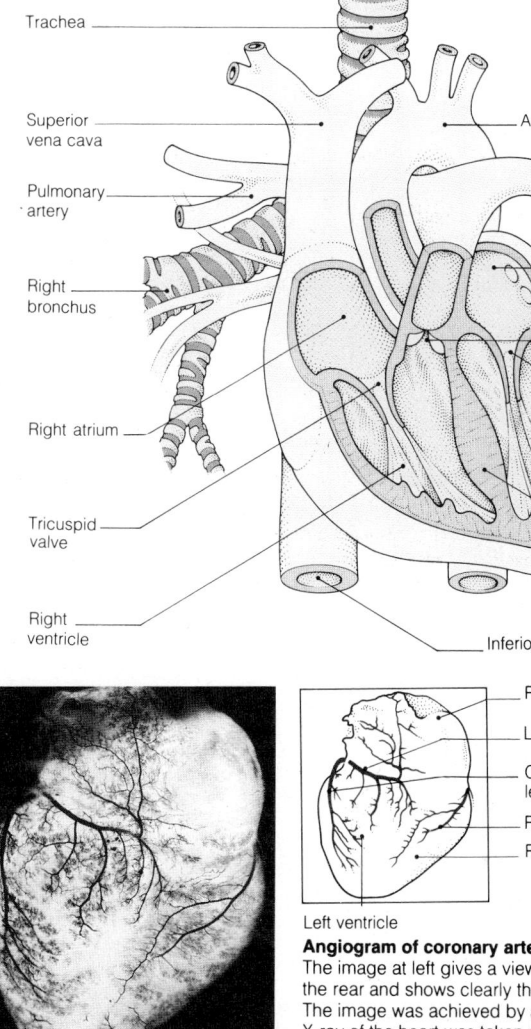

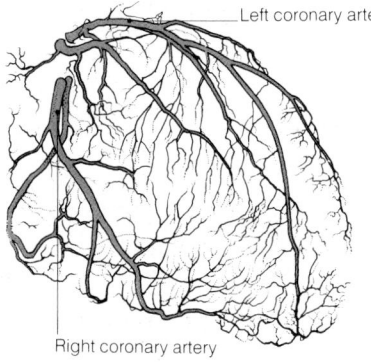

Blood supply

Although the heart muscle is continually pumping blood, it cannot obtain much oxygen from this flow, so it needs its own blood supply. This is furnished by the two coronary arteries, which arise from the aorta. With their branches, these arteries supply the entire heart muscle.

Angiogram of coronary arteries

The image at left gives a view of the heart from the rear and shows clearly the coronary arteries. The image was achieved by angiography—an X-ray of the heart was taken after injecting the coronary arteries with a contrast medium.

First, the heart muscle is able to respond automatically to any increase in the amount of blood returned to it from active muscles by increasing its output. This occurs because the more the ventricles are filled with blood during the filling phase of the heart's cycle, the more forcibly they contract during ventricular systole to expel the blood. Second, the heart-rate is under external control of the *autonomic nervous system* (the part of the nervous system concerned with automatic control of body functions). The parts of the autonomic nervous system concerned with heart action are a nucleus of nerve cells called the cardiac centre in the brainstem, and two sets of nerves (parasympathetic and sympathetic) whose activities, controlled by the cardiac centre, exert opposing effects on the heart.

When a person is at rest, it is the parasympathetic nerves—particularly the *vagus nerve*—that are active. Signals carried along the vagus nerve act on the sinoatrial node to slow the heart-rate from its inherent rate of about 140 impulses per minute to a rate closer to 70 per minute (vagal inhibition). During or in anticipation of muscular activity, the vagal inhibition lessens, the heart-rate speeds up, and may speed up even more when the sympathetic nerves come into action. The nerves release *noradrenaline*, which increases the heart-rate and the force of contraction.

The switch from parasympathetic to sympathetic activity is triggered by any influence on the cardiac centre that signals an extra need for increased blood output from the heart. Such influences may include fear or anger, low blood pressure, or a reduction of oxygen in the blood.

Heart, artificial

An implantable mechanical device that takes over the heart's action in pumping blood to maintain the circu-

H

lation. First used in humans in 1985 after years of research in animals, the presently available artificial heart is now seen as a temporary measure to keep a patient alive from a few days to weeks until a *heart transplant* can be performed.

HOW IT WORKS

The type of artificial heart that has so far been used most frequently, but not exclusively, is the Jarvik 7 model. This is a metal and plastic device installed in the patient's chest in place of the diseased heart. During installation, the device is sewn to parts of the patient's own atria (upper chambers) and to the pulmonary artery and aorta (main blood vessels carrying blood out of the heart).

The device is powered by an external machine connected to the device by air lines passing through the chest wall. Pulses of pressure sent through these lines operate the device's pumping action. The patient's movements are restricted by the need to be continuously connected to the machine.

LIMITATIONS AND RISKS

As a temporary measure, the artificial heart has a place in the treatment of life-threatening heart disease, but medical opinion is, at present, strongly against attempts to employ it on a permanent basis. The complications of its use have included *kidney failure*, infection, internal bleeding, mental confusion, and *stroke*. In 1985, after all four US patients in whom an artificial heart had been installed on a permanent basis had died, the researchers decided to concentrate attention on assist devices, which augment rather than replace the damaged heart.

A device known as the intra-aortic balloon pump has been in use since the middle 1970s; it has been found helpful as an alternative method of maintaining the circulation when the heart is badly diseased. The balloon is inflated automatically between each heartbeat to provide extra force to the circulation. This device has the extra advantage of increasing the pressure in the arteries that supply blood to the heart muscle and of relieving the strain on the heart.

Heart attack

See *Myocardial infarction*.

Heartbeat

A contraction of the *heart* that pumps blood to the lungs and the rest of the body. The heartbeat is readily felt on the left side of the chest, where the apex of the left ventricle (lower heart chamber) lies close beneath the skin. The rate at which contractions occur is called the *heart-rate*. The term *pulse* refers to the character and rate of the heartbeat when felt (at the wrist, for example).

Heart block

A common disorder of the *heartbeat* that may lead to episodes of dizziness, fainting attacks, or *stroke*. Heart block is caused by an interruption to the passage of impulses through the specialized conducting system of the heart. Consequently, although the atria beat normally, the ventricles lag behind or contract less often than the atria. This is a completely different problem from the blockage of vessels, e.g. in *atherosclerosis*.

TYPES

There are several grades of heart block. In the least severe form, the delay between the contractions of the atria and ventricles is just slightly longer than normal (called a prolonged P-R interval from its appearance on an *ECG*). Sometimes the delay lengthens with successive beats, until eventually a ventricular beat is dropped. In more severe cases, only a half, a third, or a quarter of the atrial beats is conducted to the ventricles. In complete heart

---

HEART CYCLE

The pumping action of the heart has three main phases for each heartbeat. Each beat is brought about by electrical waves that emanate from the heart's own pacemaker, the sinoatrial node. The electrocardiogram tracing also shows the phases of the cycle.

Diastole
During this resting phase, the heart fills with blood. Deoxygenated blood flows into the right side of the heart; at the same time, oxygenated blood flows into the left side.

Atrial systole
In this second phase, the two atria (upper chambers of the heart) contract simultaneously, squeezing more blood into the two ventricles, which become fully filled.

Ventricular systole
The ventricles contract to pump deoxygenated blood into the pulmonary artery and oxygenated blood into the aorta. When the heart is emptied, diastole begins again.

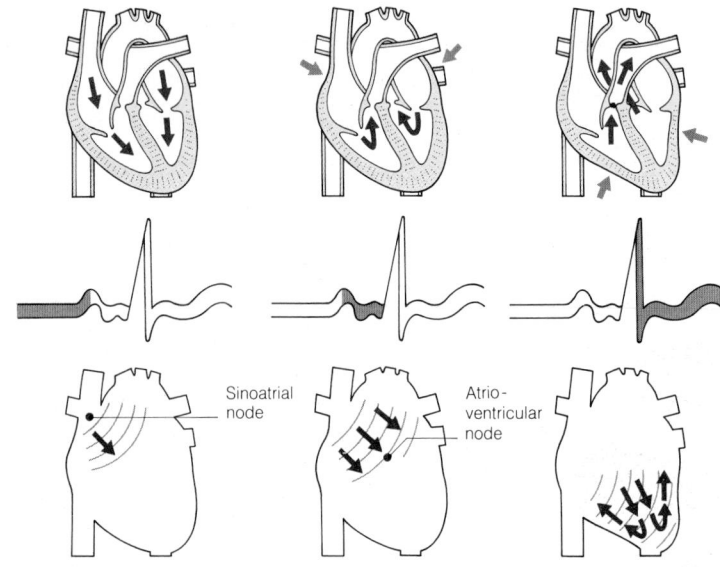

In diastole, the heart muscle is at rest. Towards the end of this phase of the heart cycle, an electrical impulse begins to emanate from the sinoatrial node.

Atrial systole is brought about by the impulse from the sinoatrial node spreading over the atria. The impulse soon reaches another node, the atrioventricular node.

Ventricular systole is brought about by waves of electrical activity carried from the atrioventricular node to all parts of the ventricles by means of special fibres.

DISORDERS OF THE HEART

Heart disorders are by far the most common cause of death in developed countries. They also impair the quality of life of millions of people, restricting activity by causing pain, breathlessness, fatigue, fainting spells, and anxiety. A wide range of conditions can affect the heart by disrupting its pumping action.

GENETIC DISORDERS

In general, inherited or genetic factors do not play a large part in causing heart disorders. However, they do contribute to the *hyperlipidaemias* that predispose a person to *atherosclerosis* and *coronary artery disease*.

CONGENITAL DEFECTS

Structural abnormalities in the heart are among the most common birth defects, but are usually treatable. They result from errors of development in the fetus and include such conditions as *septal defects* ("holes in the heart") and some types of abnormal *heart valves*. (See *Heart disease, congenital*.)

INFECTION

Endocarditis is an infection of the lining of the heart and of the heart valves, usually occurring in people whose hearts have already been damaged by *rheumatic fever* or are abnormal because of some congenital or degenerative disorder. It may also affect drug addicts who inject themselves intravenously with nonsterile needles. The infection may cause damage to and malfunction of any of the heart valves, leading to, for example, *aortic incompetence* (although heart valve disease can also have other causes). Some types of cardiomyopathy are triggered by viral infection; viruses may also cause *myocarditis* (inflammation of the heart).

TUMOURS

Tumours arising from the heart tissues are rare, the most common being the benign *myxoma* (which grows inside one of the chambers of the heart and may interfere with blood flow or valve action). Occasionally a malignant *sarcoma* develops. Secondary tumours, spreading from elsewhere in the body (such as the breast or lung) are more common than primary tumours.

These *metastases* usually grow within the heart muscle or the pericardium (sac that surrounds the heart), but seldom affect the valves. The tumours may produce electrocardiographic (see *ECG*) abnormalities and, if extensive, result in congestive *heart failure*.

MUSCLE DISORDERS

Cardiomyopathy is a general term for disease of the heart muscle itself. One type of cardiomyopathy is inherited; others may be caused by vitamin deficiency or alcohol poisoning, or may be triggered by a viral infection.

Myocarditis is inflammation of the heart muscle. It may be caused by a viral infection or by toxins released during a bacterial infection. Rarely, it results from drugs or radiotherapy.

INJURY

Blunt injury to the heart most often occurs in car accidents through impact with the steering wheel. The heart is compressed between the sternum (breastbone) and the spine and may suffer injury ranging from mild bruising to complete rupture. In immediately fatal car accidents, up to two thirds of the victims have suffered rupture of a heart chamber. Seat-belt use could probably prevent some of these deaths.

Stab wounds to the heart are often fatal within minutes, but, of patients who reach hospital, most survive. Bullet wounds are also very serious; only about 10 per cent of people shot in the heart reach hospital alive.

NUTRITIONAL DISORDERS

The heart muscle is sensitive to severe nutritional deficiency and may become thin and flabby from simple lack of protein and calories. Thiamine (vitamin B_1) deficiency, which is common in chronic alcoholics, causes *beriberi* with congestive heart failure. *Obesity* is another important factor in causing heart disease, probably through its effect on other risk factors such as *hypertension*, *diabetes*, and *cholesterol*.

IMPAIRED BLOOD SUPPLY

The major cause of heart disease in developed countries is impaired blood supply. The coronary arteries (which supply blood to the heart) become narrowed due to *atherosclerosis* and parts of the heart muscle are deprived of oxygen. The result of coronary artery disease may be *angina pectoris* or, eventually, a *myocardial infarction*.

POISONING

The most common toxic substance affecting the heart is alcohol. A large intake for many years may cause a type of cardiomyopathy in which the heart becomes enlarged and heart failure develops. If alcohol intake is stopped, recovery is possible.

DRUGS

Certain drugs may disturb the heartbeat or even cause permanent damage to the heart muscle. These drugs include the anticancer drug doxorubicin, the tricyclic antidepressants, and even many drugs used to treat heart disease.

OTHER DISORDERS

Many common and serious heart disorders may be a complication of some other underlying condition, such as coronary artery disease, cardiomyopathy, or a congenital defect. Such disorders include cardiac *arrhythmia* (a disturbance in the rhythm of the heartbeat), some cases of *heart block* (in which contractions of the upper and lower parts of the heart are not synchronized), and heart failure (inability of the heart to keep up with its workload). Cor pulmonale is a failure of the right side of the heart; it is a consequence of lung diseases (such as *emphysema)*, which increase the resistance to blood flow.

INVESTIGATION

Heart disease and disorders are investigated by such techniques as auscultation (listening to the heart sounds) and *ECG* (electrocardiography); heart *imaging* techniques such as chest X-ray, echocardiography, Doppler colour flow mapping, coronary angiography, *CT scanning*, and *MRI*; cardiac catheterization; blood tests; and, in rare cases, by a *biopsy* of the heart muscle (removal of a small sample of tissue for analysis).

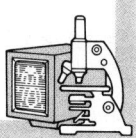

H

TYPES OF CONGENITAL HEART DISEASE

The major malformations are *septal defects*, *coarctation of the aorta*, *transposition of the great vessels*, *patent ductus arteriosus*, *tetralogy of Fallot*, *hypoplastic left heart syndrome*, *pulmonary stenosis*, and *aortic stenosis*. The bars (right) show the incidence of each type of malformation among affected babies.

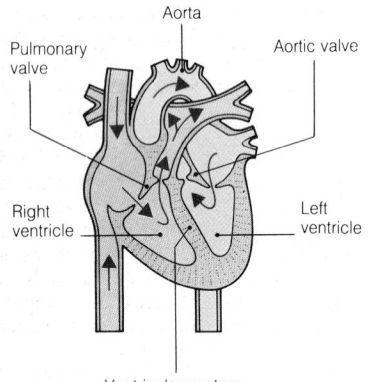

Aorta
Pulmonary valve
Aortic valve
Right ventricle
Left ventricle
Ventricular septum

How blood circulates
Deoxygenated blood (grey) is pumped from the right ventricle into the lungs, where it exchanges carbon dioxide for oxygen. The newly oxygenated blood (pink) enters the left side of the heart and is then pumped out of the left ventricle to all body tissues.

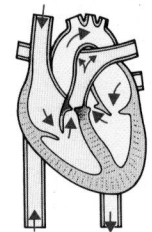

5%

Pulmonary stenosis
This is a narrowing of the pulmonary valve, or (rarely) of the upper right ventricle, which reduces blood flow to the lungs.

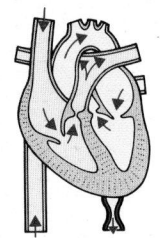

10%

Coarctation of the aorta
In this disorder, localized narrowing of the aorta reduces the supply of blood to the lower part of the body.

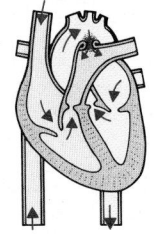

8%

Patent ductus arteriosus
The ductus arteriosus fails to close after birth and blood from the aorta continues to flow through it into the pulmonary artery.

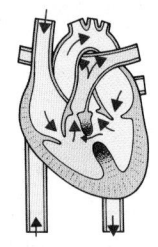

25%

Ventricular septal defect
This is a hole in the ventricular septum, causing blood to flow from the left ventricle to the right and thence to the lungs.

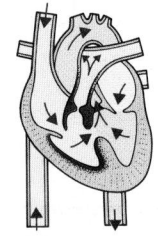

7%

Tetralogy of Fallot
This is a hole in the ventricular septum, pulmonary stenosis, a displaced aorta, and a thickened right ventricle.

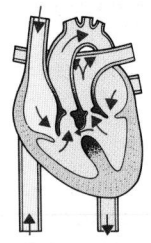

14%

Transposition of the great vessels
Oxygenated blood passes back to the lungs, instead of through the aorta to the body tissues.

---

block, the atria and ventricles beat independently. Thus, while the rate of atrial contraction varies according to the patient's activity, the ventricles contract at a fairly constant rate of about 40 beats per minute.

CAUSES
Heart block may be due to *coronary artery disease*, *myocarditis* (inflammation of heart muscle), an overdose of a *digitalis drug*, *rheumatic fever*, or *syphilitic aortitis*. In about half of all cases of heart block, the patient has no history of heart disease.

SYMPTOMS
A prolonged P-R interval causes no symptoms even though it can be detected on an ECG. Dropped beats may also be symptomless.

In other cases, the rate of the ventricular beat is slower than normal; in complete heart block, the rate does not increase in response to exercise. Sometimes the ventricles are able to compensate by expelling more blood with each contraction. In other cases, the blood output from the ventricles is inadequate, and the patient may become breathless due to *heart failure*, may develop the chest pains of *angina pectoris*, or may faint.

If the ventricular beat becomes very slow, or stops altogether for a few seconds, the patient may black out and have a seizure because insufficient blood reaches the brain. However, the ventricular beat usually restarts within a few seconds. If the delay is prolonged in a person whose brain is affected by atherosclerosis, a stroke may result.

DIAGNOSIS
Heart block may be suspected if a person has a slow, regular heartbeat (below 50 beats per minute) that does not accelerate during exercise. The diagnosis is confirmed by an ECG.

TREATMENT
Some cases of heart block do not require treatment (e.g. if there are no symptoms or if an elderly person has only minor symptoms). Heart block that is causing fainting attacks is usually treated by the fitting of an artificial *pacemaker*, which overrides the natural pacemaker and faulty electrical conducting system in the heart.

Less commonly, heart block may be treated with drugs, such as *isoprenaline*. In most cases, drug treatment is reserved for emergencies or as a temporary measure until an artificial pacemaker can be fitted.

Heartburn

A burning pain in the centre of the chest which may travel from the tip of the sternum (breastbone) to the throat.

Heartburn may be caused by overeating, by eating rich or spicy food, or by drinking alcohol. Recurrent heartburn is a symptom of *oesophagitis* (inflammation of the oesophagus), which is usually caused by *acid reflux* (backflow of stomach acid). Heartburn is often brought on by lying down or by bending forwards.

Occasionally, heartburn may cause chest pain that is mistaken for the pain of heart disease.

Heart disease, congenital

Any heart abnormality that has been present from birth. Congenital heart defects are the most common major malformations compatible with life. Defects may affect the heart chambers, heart valves, or main blood vessels (see illustrated box).

CAUSES AND INCIDENCE

About 800 babies per 100,000 are born with a congenital heart defect. The errors of development leading to defects arise early in the life of the *embryo*. In most cases, there is no known cause. Of known causes, *rubella* (German measles) in the mother is the most common, but can be prevented by vaccination before conception.

Hereditary factors do not seem to be significant. If a couple have an affected child, there is little increased risk of a second child being affected. People born with heart defects have little increased risk of having an affected child. Antenatal diagnosis, using specialized *ultrasound scanning*, is now possible for most defects.

SYMPTOMS AND COMPLICATIONS

The symptoms of congenital heart disease arise from either insufficient or excessive circulation of blood to the lungs or to the body. The defects in heart anatomy can also mean that some deoxygenated blood is pumped to the body instead of to the lungs or some oxygenated blood to the lungs instead of to the body. This is called "shunting". Heart anomalies can result in *cyanosis* (blueness of the skin), breathlessness, or both.

Symptoms may first appear at any time over a wide range of ages, according to the defect. Similarly, recognition of a defect may occur any time from before birth to adulthood.

Apart from cyanosis and breathlessness, an untreated heart defect can cause stunted growth and underdevelopment of the limbs and muscles. Mild respiratory infections may lead to pneumonia. With prolonged cyanosis, *clubbing* (thickening and broadening) of the ends of fingers and toes may develop. If there is insufficient capacity of the heart to increase blood flow during effort, the child may rapidly tire and be unable to take part in physical exercise. In some untreated cases, a serious complication called *Eisenmenger complex* (in which there is increased resistance of the lungs to blood flow) develops.

DIAGNOSIS

Ultrasound scanning of the fetus during pregnancy may be used to examine the heart; many cases of congenital heart disease are first identified at this stage, allowing the timing of treatment to be planned. After birth, any defect suspected on clinical examination will be investigated using procedures such as *chest X-rays*, *ECG*, *echocardiography*, and, less commonly, cardiac *catheterization*.

TREATMENT

Rest, oxygen, and various drugs to assist the circulation and lung function may improve matters for a limited time or sometimes indefinitely. Some conditions, such as small septal defects, may get smaller or disappear on their own. Other defects are likely to worsen, and surgical correction is often a consideration.

Rarely, surgery to correct or relieve a congenital defect may need to be attempted before birth to give the fetus the best chance of survival. More often, surgical correction will be delayed as long as possible to allow the baby to grow. Surgical treatment is now possible for almost all defects; the risk of death from unsuccessful surgery lessens every year. One condition—hypoplastic left heart syndrome (in which the left side of the heart is severely underdeveloped)—can however be treated only by performing a *heart transplant*.

Narrowed heart valves can often be treated by balloon *valvuloplasty*. In this procedure, a special catheter is introduced into the heart to widen the narrowed valve.

In other cases, *open heart surgery*, a heart transplant, or *heart-lung transplant* may be necessary.

OUTLOOK

Following successful heart surgery, recovery to good health with resumption of growth, increased activity, and better appetite follow rapidly, and the child usually has a near-normal life expectancy. Full activities, including sports, are generally possible after three to six months.

Children with heart defects (corrected or uncorrected) are at an increased risk of bacterial *endocarditis*, a potentially dangerous infection of the heart lining and heart valves. To protect against this possibility, children with congenital heart disease are given *antibiotic drugs* before undergoing surgical procedures.

Heart disease, ischaemic

The most common form of heart disease, in which there is a reduced blood supply resulting from narrowing or obstruction of the coronary arteries. (See *Coronary artery disease*.)

Heart failure

Inability of the heart to cope with its workload of pumping blood to the lungs and to the rest of the body. Although heart failure sounds like a life-threatening disorder, the condition is usually treatable and compatible with survival for many years.

TYPES AND CAUSES

Heart failure is usually termed either left-sided or right-sided failure.

LEFT-SIDED FAILURE This may be due to *hypertension* (high blood pressure), *anaemia*, *hyperthyroidism* (overactivity of the thyroid gland), a heart valve defect (such as *aortic stenosis*, *aortic incompetence*, or *mitral incompetence*), or a congenital heart defect (such as *coarctation of the aorta*). In all these conditions, the left side of the heart must work harder to pump the same amount of blood. Sometimes, the extra workload can be compensated for by an increase in the size of the left side of the heart and in the thickness of its muscular walls, or by an increase in heart-rate. Compensation is only temporary, however, and heart failure follows.

Other causes of left-sided heart failure include cardiac *arrhythmias* (irregularities of the heart rhythm), *coronary artery disease*, *myocardial infarction* (heart attack), and *cardiomyopathy* (disease of the heart muscle). In cardiomyopathy, the pumping power of the heart is reduced to a point where it can no longer deal with its normal workload.

Whatever the cause, the left side of the heart fails to empty completely with each contraction or has difficulty accepting blood returning from the lungs. The retained blood creates a back pressure that causes the lungs to become congested with blood. This in turn leads to *pulmonary oedema* (excess fluid in the lungs), of which the main symptom is shortness of breath.

RIGHT-SIDED FAILURE Right-sided failure most often results from *pulmonary hypertension* (raised pressure and resistance to blood flow through the lungs)—itself caused by left-sided failure or by lung disease (such as chronic *bronchitis* or *emphysema*). Right-sided failure can also be due to a valve defect (such as *tricuspid incompetence*) or a congenital heart defect (such as a *septal defect*, *pulmonary stenosis*, or *tetralogy of Fallot*). In all types of right-sided failure, there is a back pressure in the blood circulation from the heart into the venous system, causing swollen neck veins, enlargement of the liver, and *oedema* (accumulation of fluid in the tissues).

H

H

SYMPTOMS

Fatigue is an early symptom of heart failure. Breathing difficulty is the most common symptom of left-sided heart failure and is caused by fluid in the lungs. Breathlessness may first be noticed only during or after exercise, but worsens and is eventually apparent even at rest. The patient may be able to breathe easily only when well propped up in bed. Sometimes he or she may awaken at night with an attack of breathlessness, wheezing, and sweating. Attacks of acute heart failure may subside on their own or may alternatively require urgent, life-saving treatment.

Right-sided heart failure produces less breathlessness and more swelling of the ankles and legs, often with enlargement of the liver and congestion of the intestines, causing discomfort and indigestion.

TREATMENT

Immediate treatment of the heart failure is followed by treatment of its underlying cause.

Immediate treatment consists of bed rest, with the patient sitting up. The patient is given *diuretic drugs*, which increase the output of urine from the kidneys, thus ridding the body of excess fluid and reducing blood volume. *Digitalis drugs*, which slow and strengthen the contractions of the heart, are often given. *Vasodilator drugs*, especially *ACE inhibitor drugs*, reduce the workload on the heart. (Treatment with ACE inhibitors has been shown to prolong life in most cases of heart failure.) *Morphine* is sometimes given as an emergency treatment in acute left-sided failure.

Once the heart failure is treated, attention is directed to treating the underlying cause. If a defective heart valve is responsible, it may be treated by *heart-valve surgery* (although, ideally, defective heart valves should be corrected surgically before severe heart failure develops).

Many other causes of heart failure are also treatable; hypertension and arrhythmias are treated by drug treatment, and congenital septal defects are treated by open heart surgery. However, when the cause is a long-standing cardiomyopathy or chronic lung disease, the outlook is generally not as good.

Heart imaging

Techniques that provide images of the heart and its structure. Imaging is performed to detect structural abnormality, disease, or impaired function.

TYPES

A *chest X-ray* is the simplest and most widely used method of obtaining an image of the heart. An X-ray can show heart size and shape, and whether or not abnormal calcification is present in the valves, major vessels, or the pericardium (membranous bag that surrounds the heart). *Pulmonary oedema* (accumulation of fluid in the lungs) and engorgement (overfilling with blood) of the vessels connecting the heart and lungs are usually detectable on a chest X-ray and may indicate the presence of *heart failure*. Pacemakers and artificial heart valves show up clearly on X-ray and can be checked for position.

Angiography (an imaging technique in which X-rays are taken after the injection of a contrast medium) may be performed to show the heart chambers. Children with complex forms of congenital heart disease, such as *tetralogy of Fallot*, may be investigated by this procedure. Angiography is also performed to evaluate the state of the coronary arteries in patients with *coronary artery disease* and provides information affecting decisions about valve replacement.

Echocardiography (cardiac ultrasound) is most useful as the first step in investigating congenital heart abnormalities or in evaluating valvular or heart wall abnormalities. An ultrasound technique exploiting the *Doppler effect* enables the doctor to measure blood flow across valves.

Radionuclide scanning is a form of imaging that shows only a limited degree of anatomical detail but that provides some information about heart function, such as how well the heart wall moves and how effectively it empties.

The development of more rapid machines for *CT scanning* has made it possible to use this technique to obtain useful information about the heart; earlier scanning machines were too slow to "freeze" a heartbeat.

High-quality images of the heart can also be obtained by *MRI* techniques. These techniques are used, for example, for assessing the results of *coronary artery bypass* surgery. In many cases, MRI techniques may eliminate the need for angiography and for other techniques used to investigate congenital heart disease.

Heart-lung machine

A machine that temporarily takes over the function of the heart and lungs to facilitate certain operations in the chest. Use of the heart-lung machine gives the surgeon more time for operations and prevents the operation site from being obscured by blood.

Operations performed using a heart-lung machine include *open heart surgery*, *heart transplants*, and *heart-lung transplants*.

A heart-lung machine consists principally of a pump (to replace the heart) and an oxygenator (to replace the lungs). The machine is sometimes called a cardiopulmonary bypass or pump oxygenator. Once the machine is connected and working, the patient's heart and lungs are effectively bypassed and the heart can be stopped.

HOW IT WORKS

Blood is taken via cannulas (tubes) inserted into the inferior and superior venae cavae (the main veins draining blood into the heart) and pumped through the oxygenator, which acts as an artificial lung, putting oxygen into the blood and removing carbon dioxide from it. The freshly oxygenated blood is then returned to the arterial circulation via a cannula inserted into the aorta (the main artery carrying blood from the heart) or the femoral artery (a large artery in the leg).

There are two main types of oxygenator. In one type, the blood is passed up a column, through which a gas mixture with a high oxygen content is bubbled. This adds oxygen and removes carbon dioxide. The blood is then treated with a defoaming agent and held in a reservoir until it is returned to the patient. In the second type, called a membrane oxygenator, the blood and gas flow on either side of a thin, semipermeable membrane, through which oxygen passes from gas into blood; carbon dioxide passes in the opposing direction. This method more closely mimics the function of the lungs.

The heart-lung machine also contains a heat exchanger. This may be used to rewarm blood (which loses heat in the machine) before returning it to the patient. In some cases, the heat exchanger is used to cool blood intentionally to cause a drop in the patient's temperature and so give the surgeons more time for the operation (see *Hypothermia, surgical*).

LIMITATIONS

Use of a heart-lung machine tends to damage red blood cells and to cause the blood to clot; these problems are minimized by giving the patient *heparin*, an anticoagulant drug, before the machine is used.

HEART-LUNG TRANSPLANT
In this procedure, both the heart and lungs of a patient are removed and replaced with organs taken from a brain-dead donor. The removed heart can sometimes be given to another patient.

HOW IT IS DONE
Heart and lungs must be removed from both donor and patient; the donor organs are then inserted into the patient.

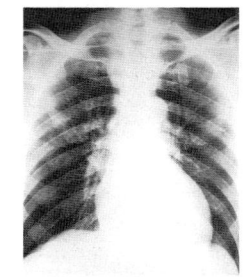

1 The donor heart and lungs must be healthy, and the lungs must match the size of the patient's chest, as measured by chest X-rays.

2 In both donor and patient, the heart and lungs are reached via an incision made in the sternum, and the chest is opened up.

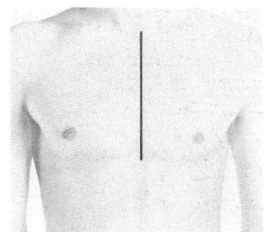

Site of incision

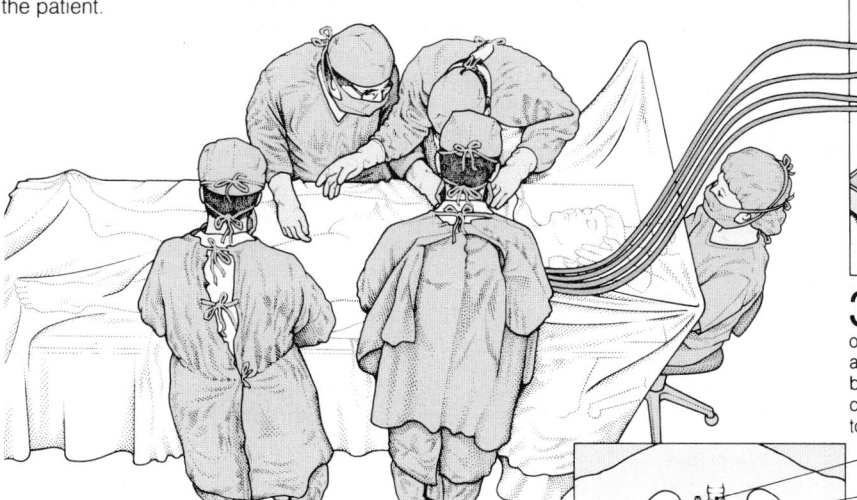

3 The patient is connected to a heart-lung machine. It takes over the function of heart and lungs, oxygenating blood taken from the venae cavae and pumping it back to the body via the aorta.

Trachea

Aorta

Right atrium/Vena cava

4 In both patient and donor, heart and lungs are removed through cuts in the trachea, aorta, and where the heart connects to the venae cavae. The blood vessels linking donor heart and lungs are left intact.

Tracheal reconnection

Aortic reconnection

Right atrium/Vena cava reconnection

5 Insertion of the donor organs into the patient is, in some respects, easier than in the heart transplant, since fewer reconnections have to be made. The main reconnections are between the patient's and donor's tracheas and aortas and between the right atrium of the donor heart and the patient's venae cavae.

WHY IT IS DONE
Subject to availability of a donor, a heart-lung transplant can offer hope to someone who is dying of a terminally chronic lung disease, whether or not he or she is also suffering from heart disease. Diseases treated include *emphysema, cystic fibrosis, sarcoidosis, or interstitial pulmonary fibrosis.* The heart-lung transplant operation has a better success record than that of lung transplant alone.

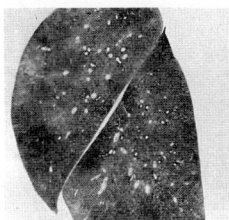 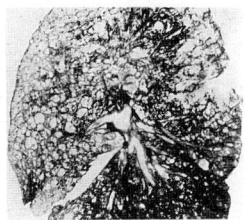

These sections were taken from a healthy lung (left) and an emphysematous lung; transplantation of heart and lungs may give an emphysema patient new hope.

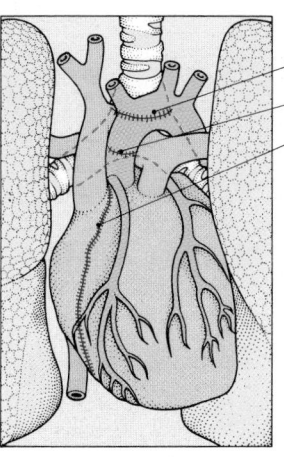

A patient can be kept on a heart-lung machine for only a few hours. Use of the machine reduces the efficiency of the blood supply to the patient's vital organs and thus limits the time available for an operation.

Heart-lung transplant

A procedure in which both the heart and lungs of a patient are removed and replaced with organs from a donor who has been certified brain dead. (See illustrated box for how and why the operation is done).

RISKS AND COMPLICATIONS

The early attempts at heart-lung transplant were unsuccessful. In the early 1980s the risk of donor organ rejection was reduced by the introduction of the drug *cyclosporin*, and by the early 1990s heart-lung transplants had become a standard procedure in specialist centres. Nevertheless, the operation carries substantial risks. Problems may arise from airway obstruction and other lung complications (including *bronchiolitis*) in addition to the risks of organ rejection. Patients face the long-term problems associated with other forms of *transplant surgery*.

Heart-rate

The rate at which the heart beats—that is, contracts to pump blood around the body.

Most people have a heart-rate of between 60 and 100 beats per minute at rest. This rate remains fairly constant throughout life, although it tends to be faster in childhood and to slow slightly with age. Some athletes have a resting rate below 60 beats per minute. Their hearts are very well developed and can pump blood around the body as efficiently at a slow rate as the normal heart can pump it at a faster rate.

Exercise or stress causes an increase in heart-rate. In either case, the increase is due to the release of the hormones *adrenaline* and *noradrenaline* by the adrenal glands and of noradrenaline by the sympathetic nerves around the sinoatrial node, the heart's own pacemaker. A small decrease in heart-rate occurs during total relaxation and sleep.

Many people have a harmless irregularity of heart rhythm in which the rate is more rapid during breathing in than breathing out.

MEASURING HEART-RATE

A doctor uses one of two methods to measure heart-rate and rhythm (the regularity of the beat). One is to feel the pulse (the expansion of an artery in response to contractions of the heart). The other method, which is sometimes more accurate, is to listen with a *stethoscope* placed just below the left nipple (see *Heart sounds*).

A more accurate record of heart-rate and rhythm is provided by an *ECG* (electrocardiogram), which registers the pattern of electrical activity in the heart muscle before each beat.

DISORDERS OF HEART-RATE

A resting heart-rate above 100 beats per minute is termed a *tachycardia* and a rate below 60 beats per minute a *bradycardia*. Tachycardias and bradycardias are considered abnormal when the cause is a condition affecting nerve conduction pathways through the heart or the activity of the sino-atrial node, rather than a response of the heart to exercise or relaxation. (See also *Arrhythmia, cardiac*.)

Heart sounds

The sounds made by the *heart* during each heartbeat. In each heart cycle, there are two main heart sounds, known as the first heart sound and the second heart sound.

The main heart sounds can be heard simply by putting an ear to someone's chest. Using a *stethoscope*, a doctor can hear the heart sounds much more clearly (and may sometimes hear additional sounds or an abnormality of one of the two main sounds). Interpretation of these sounds can be important in the diagnosis of *heart valve* disorders, as well as other heart abnormalities.

The first heart sound is often described as a "lubb". It results from closure of the tricuspid and mitral valves at the exits from the upper chambers of the heart, which occurs when the ventricles (lower chambers) begin contracting to pump blood out of the heart. The second heart sound is a higher-pitched "dupp". This sound, which is caused by closure of the pulmonary and aortic valves at the exits from the ventricles, occurs when the ventricles finish contracting. There is a pause after each lubb-dupp.

In children and young adults, there is often a normal low-pitched third heart sound after the second sound. It is thought to be caused by vibration of the muscle. In people over the age of 40, this sound is abnormal and a sign of heart failure.

Abnormal heart sounds may be a sign of various disorders of the heart. For example, an additional low-pitched sound before the first sound indicates an abnormality of the heart muscle. This sound is often present after a *myocardial infarction* (heart attack). Ejection sounds or "clicks" are high-pitched sounds caused by the abrupt halting of valve opening. These can occur in people with *hypertension* (high blood pressure) or certain heart valve defects. Heart *murmurs* are abnormal sounds caused by turbulent blood flow. They may occur as a result of any of various heart valve defects or types of congenital heart disease.

Heart surgery

Any operation performed on the heart. Heart surgery was a rare and hazardous undertaking until the early 1950s, when an operation called mitral valvotomy became a standard and successful procedure. This operation, performed to correct a narrowed mitral valve, entails passing a finger into the beating heart in order to stretch open the affected valve.

Such "closed" operations on the heart are still occasionally performed, but have largely been superseded in developed countries by *open heart surgery*, in which the heartbeat is deliberately stopped and the heart opened to make repairs. Open heart surgery was made possible by developments such as the controlled cooling of patients for surgery (see *Hypothermia, surgical*) and the introduction in the 1950s of the *heart-lung machine*, which considerably prolonged the time during which the surgeons could work. Open heart surgery allows the treatment of many previously serious or fatal conditions, including most types of heart defect present at birth (see *Heart disease, congenital*) and various disorders of the *heart valves*.

Coronary artery bypass, an operation to treat obstruction of the arteries that supply the heart muscle, was first performed in 1967 and, within five years, was being carried out all over the world. Also in 1967, the first *heart transplant* was performed in South Africa; the results of heart transplant surgery are now much improved largely because of advances in preventing organ rejection.

Another significant development was the introduction in 1979 of balloon *angioplasty* to treat narrowing of the coronary arteries. In some cases, *laser treatment* is used to remove material obstructing an artery.

Angioplasty balloons have also been used to open up narrowed heart valves in cases where the patient is unsuitable for open heart surgery (see *Valvuloplasty*).

Heart transplant

Replacement of a person's damaged or diseased heart by a healthy human heart taken from a donor in whom *brain death* has been certified.

HISTORY

Heart transplantation in animals was first achieved in 1959. The first human heart transplant was performed by Professor Christiaan Barnard in South Africa in 1967. Early results were disappointing, however, and few patients survived more than a month or two. The team led by Professor Norman Shumway at Stanford University, California, began a programme of heart transplants in 1969; by 1984 this team showed that as many as 85 per cent of patients could be expected to survive for at least a year after surgery. The operation is now a standard procedure in many technically advanced countries.

LIMITATIONS

Heart transplantation poses some special problems compared with the more common procedure of kidney transplantation.

First, there can be a problem of timing. Whereas the condition of a patient with kidney failure can be maintained in health by *dialysis* until a donor kidney becomes available, there is no equivalent method for maintaining the condition of someone with a nonfunctioning heart. Hence, a heart transplant is possible only when a suitable donor heart is available at the right time.

Second, heart transplantation has no "fallback" system; if the heart is rejected (attacked by the body's *immune system*), the only hope for the patient is another transplant.

In theory, the mechanical artificial heart (see *Heart, artificial*) is a possible solution to the problems of timing and rejection. In practice, however, no artificial heart has given good enough results to be brought into routine use.

Heart transplant operations are further limited by the fact that they are most likely to succeed if the heart is removed from the donor while it is still beating. One reason for the success of the Stanford heart transplant programme was that California was the first state to allow doctors to certify death while the heart was still beating (provided the brain was irreversibly destroyed by disease or accident). Certification of brain death in a patient connected to an artificial ventilator is now permitted in most developed countries, allowing removal of the heart in optimum condition.

WHY IT IS DONE

Heart transplantation is considered for the treatment of patients with progressive, irremediable heart disease, but who are otherwise in good health. Many such patients have advanced *coronary artery disease*; most of the others have *cardiomyopathy* (disease of the heart muscle).

If the heart disorder is associated with lung disease, a *heart-lung transplant* may be performed.

HOW IT IS DONE

Following its removal from the donor, the heart is chilled in saline to maintain its condition. If necessary, the donor heart can then be transported many miles, often by air, before being implanted into the recipient.

The actual heart transplant operation is no more or less difficult than other major heart surgery. The first step is to connect the patient's major blood vessels to a *heart-lung machine*, which pumps oxygenated blood to the brain and other vital organs while the surgeon operates. Once the blood is bypassed through the heart-lung machine, the surgeon removes the diseased heart, leaving the back walls of the atria (upper heart chambers) in place, and then inserts the donor heart. The major blood vessels are then reconnected, and the new heart can take over from the machine.

OUTLOOK

Once the immediate post-operative period is over, the outlook is good, with more than 80 per cent of patients surviving the first year in some hospitals; there is a death rate of around five per cent per year thereafter. These results are much better than for the surgical treatment of lung or stomach cancer. The main problems are rejection, which can be countered by *immunosuppressant drugs* (such as *cyclosporin*, *prednisone*, and *cyclophosphamide*), and infection, which is always a hazard for people taking immunosuppressant drugs because these drugs weaken the body's defences. (See also *Transplant surgery*.)

Heart valve

A structure at the exit of a *heart* chamber that allows blood to flow out of the chamber, but which prevents backwash. There are four heart valves (one at the exit of each heart chamber). Their correct functioning is vital to the efficiency of the heart as a pump.

The opening and, more particularly, the closing of heart valves during each heart cycle are responsible for *heart sounds*.

DISORDERS

Any of the four heart valves may be affected by stenosis (narrowing), which causes the heart to work harder to force blood through the valve, or by incompetence or insufficiency (leakiness), which makes the valve unable to prevent backwash of blood. These defects cause characteristic *heart murmurs* which can be heard by a doctor.

Valve defects may be present at birth, either alone or with other defects (see *Heart disease, congenital*), or may be acquired later in life. The most common congenital valve defects are *aortic stenosis* and *pulmonary stenosis*.

Acquired heart valve disease is usually the result of degenerative changes or ischaemia (diminished blood supply) affecting part of the heart and leading to aortic stenosis or *mitral incompetence*.

Rheumatic fever was once the main cause of *mitral stenosis*, mitral incompetence, aortic valve defects, and, less commonly, *tricuspid stenosis* and *tricuspid incompetence*. Rheumatic fever is now rare in developed countries but is still prevalent in poorer countries.

Valves may also be destroyed by bacterial *endocarditis*, occurring often in intravenous drug users. Bacterial endocarditis is, however, a possible complication of any valve disorder.

The symptoms and signs of valve disorders vary but disorders commonly lead to *heart failure*, rhythm irregularities (see *Arrhythmias, cardiac*), or symptoms resulting from reduced blood supply to body tissues.

Valve defects may be diagnosed by *physical examination* (including *auscultation* to listen to the heart sounds), chest *X-ray*, *ECG*, *echocardiography*, Doppler echocardiography, and cardiac *catheterization*. Valve defects may be corrected by *heart-valve surgery*.

Heart-valve surgery

An operation to correct a *heart valve* defect or, in many cases, to remove a diseased or damaged valve. A removed valve can be replaced by a mechanical valve (made from metal and plastic), a valve fashioned from human or bovine tissue, a pig valve, or a human valve taken from a corpse.

WHY IT IS DONE

A heart valve may have to be corrected or replaced because it is either stenotic (narrowed) or incompetent (leaky). Surgery is most often performed to treat a disorder of the mitral or aortic valve (which is located on the left side of the heart).

H

In general, heart-valve surgery is considered only when the potential effects of the malfunctioning valve on the heart and on general health are so severe that they will soon be life-threatening. The timing of the operation is crucial and is based on an assessment of the patient's symptoms and the results of tests (such as *ECG*, *chest X-rays*, *echocardiography*, and cardiac *catheterization*).

HOW IT IS DONE

The illustration on this page, right, shows how an aortic valve is replaced.

Valvotomy is an operation in which an instrument or finger is used for the purpose of widening a narrowed valve; *valvuloplasty* is a newer technique, in which a balloon catheter is inserted for the purpose of widening a valve.

RECOVERY AND OUTLOOK

After the operation, the patient is usually kept in an intensive-care unit for 24 hours, followed by a few days in hospital. A longer stay may be necessary if complications develop or if the patient was suffering from severe heart failure before the operation.

Symptoms such as breathlessness may take many weeks to improve and may require continuing medication to maintain the improvement. Some people (those with a mechanical replacement valve and those with heart rhythm abnormalities, for example) require long-term treatment with *anticoagulant drugs* to prevent the formation of blood clots around the new valve, which could become detached and travel to the brain or other organs. All patients need long-term follow-up examinations to ensure that the repaired or replaced valve is working well. In the early 1990s, reports began circulating of the mechanical failure of some versions of a particular design of heart valve, the Bjork Shiley valve. Many patients who had been treated with the potentially defective versions chose to have a replacement fitted to avoid having to live with uncertainty.

Heat cramps

Painful contractions in muscles caused by excessive salt loss due to profuse sweating. Heat cramps are usually brought on by strenuous activity in extreme heat. The condition may occur by itself or as a symptom of *heat exhaustion* or *heatstroke*.

Prevention and treatment consist of taking salt tablets or drinking sufficient quantities of a weak salt solution (a quarter of a level teaspoon of salt to

HEART VALVE REPLACEMENT

Any one of the four heart valves (aortic, pulmonary, mitral, or tricuspid) may require replacing (see diagram below right). Replacement of the aortic heart valve is described in the steps below.

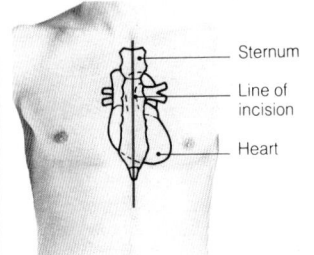

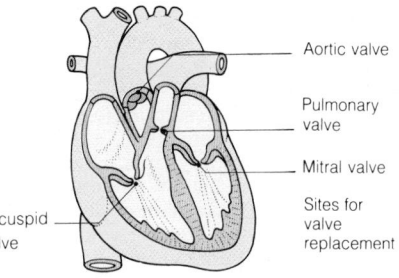

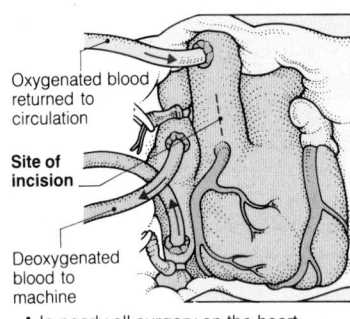

1 In nearly all surgery on the heart valves, the incision into the chest cavity is made through the sternum (breastbone). The patient is put on a *heart-lung machine*, the beating of the heart is stopped, and the heart is opened.

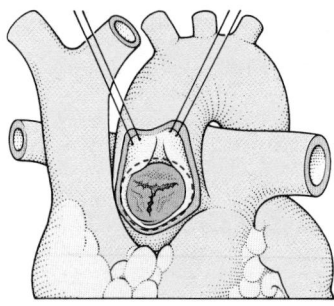

2 The valve is first examined to determine whether it can be repaired or whether it requires replacement. If the latter is necessary (as here), the valve is excised (dotted line indicates where the incision is made).

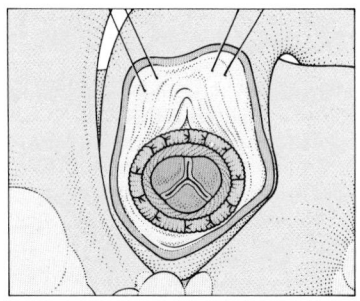

3 A prosthesis is sutured into position and the aorta is closed. The patient is disconnected from the machine and the chest wall is sewn up. The operation takes between two and four hours.

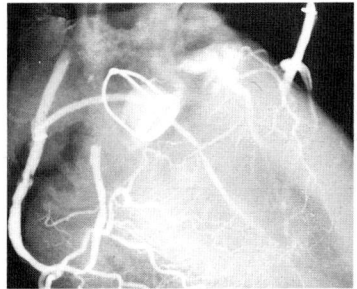

Artificial heart valve in place
This chest X-ray shows the metal components of an artificial heart valve. A ball-and-cage valve has been used to replace the patient's diseased valve.

half a litre of cold water) to keep the urine pale. Too much salt may cause the patient to vomit, thus making the situation worse.

Heat disorders

The body functions most efficiently at a temperature of 37°C; any major deviation disrupts the body processes. Malfunctioning or overloading of the body's mechanisms for keeping its temperature constant may lead to a heat disorder. For example, poor adaptation to heat may lead to *heat cramps*, *heat exhaustion*, or *heatstroke*; excessive environmental heat may result in *prickly heat*. Body functions may also be disrupted by excessive heat production in the body during a high *fever* caused by infection.

TYPES OF REPLACEMENT HEART VALVES

The three main types
There are three main types of replacement valve—biological, mechanical, and homograft. Biological valves are taken from pigs or made from bovine tissue or the patient's own tissue; examples include the Carpentier-Edwards and Ionescu-Shiley valves. Mechanical valves are made from metal, plastic, and carbon fibre. There are two main types—ball-and-cage valves (such as the Starr-Edwards valve) and those with one or more tilting disks (such as the Bjork-Shiley and St. Jude valves). Homografts are human valves that have been removed from people who have died of a disease that does not affect the heart.

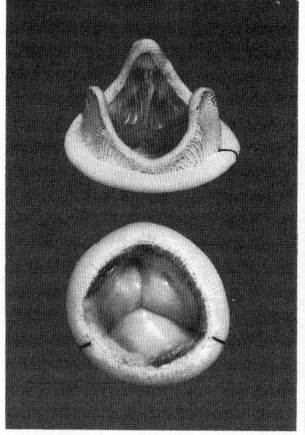
Biological

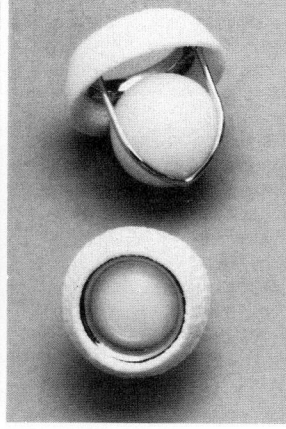
Mechanical

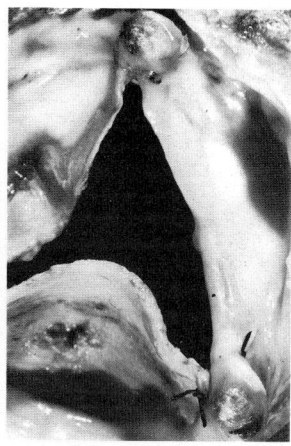
Homograft

H

	Biological	Mechanical	Homograft
Examples	Carpentier-Edwards; Ionescu-Shiley	Starr-Edwards (ball-and-cage); Bjork-Shiley (tilting disk); St. Jude (two tilting disks)	Taken from cadaver
Availability	Readily available	Readily available	Some centres only
Ease of insertion	Routine	Routine	Specialized
Suitable age group	Over 35	All ages	All ages
Duration	About seven years	More than 12 years	More than 12 years
Post-operative drug therapy	Short-term anticoagulants	Lifelong anticoagulants	None necessary
Possible complications	Infection; stroke; damage to blood cells	Infection; stroke; calcification; mechanical failure	Infection; calcification

HEAT REGULATION
The mechanisms by which the body loses unwanted heat to maintain the optimum internal temperature are controlled by the *hypothalamus* (part of the brain). When the hypothalamus is disrupted (e.g. by drugs or a fever) the body may overheat progressively, which may lead to fatal heatstroke if emergency treatment is not given.

When the temperature of the blood rises, the hypothalamus sends nerve impulses to stimulate the sweat glands and dilate (widen) blood vessels in the skin. Sweating itself does not cool the body; the cooling effect is caused by the evaporation of sweat from the skin. Excessive sweating may result in an imbalance of salts and fluids in the body, which may lead to heat cramps or heat exhaustion. Dilation of the blood vessels increases the blood flow near the surface of the skin, thus increasing the amount of heat lost by convection and radiation.

ACCLIMATIZATION
Most heat disorders can be prevented by gradual acclimatization to hot conditions. Full acclimatization takes one to three weeks and involves spending gradually longer periods in the heat, alternating with rest periods in cool conditions. Strenuous exercise should be avoided. Frequent cool baths or showers should be taken and salt tablets (in moderation) or dilute salt solution used (a quarter of a level teaspoon of salt dissolved in half a litre of cold water). It is also helpful to eat a light diet, to avoid alcohol, and to wear loose, lightweight clothes.

Heat exhaustion
Fatigue, sometimes culminating in collapse, caused by overexposure to heat. It is most common in people who are unaccustomed to working in a hot environment, and, unless treated, may develop into *heatstroke*, a potentially life-threatening condition.

CAUSES
There are three main causes of heat exhaustion: insufficient water intake, insufficient salt intake, and a deficiency in the production of sweat, the evaporation of which helps to cool the body.

SYMPTOMS AND SIGNS
Heat exhaustion causes fatigue, faintness, dizziness, nausea, restlessness, headache, and, when salt loss is heavy, *heat cramps* in the legs, arms, back, or abdomen. The skin is usually pale and clammy, breathing is fast and shallow, and the pulse is rapid and weak. There may also be vomiting, and the victim may faint.

PREVENTION AND TREATMENT
Heat exhaustion can usually be prevented by appropriate acclimatization (see *Heat disorders*).

A person who develops heat exhaustion should lie down in a cool place and, if conscious, should take continual sips of a weak salt solution

---

FIRST AID: HEAT EXHAUSTION

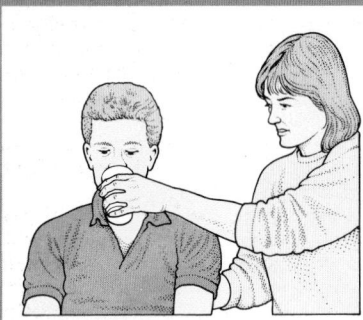

1 Offer plenty of salt solution to drink (about 0.25 teaspoon/0.5 litre) and seek medical help immediately.

2 Lay the victim down in a cool place and raise his or her feet by about 30 cm.

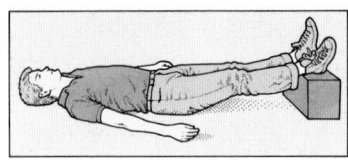

(made up of a quarter of a level teaspoon of salt to half a litre of cold water). If the victim is unconscious, he or she should be placed in the *recovery position* until consciousness returns. Once the patient is conscious, salt solutions can be administered.

With rest and replacement of lost water and salt, a full recovery usually takes place. Victims should, however, consult a doctor because of the risk of heatstroke.

Heatstroke

A life-threatening condition, also called heat hyperpyrexia, in which overexposure to extreme heat and a consequent breakdown of the body's heat-regulating mechanisms cause the body to become dangerously overheated. In some cases, body temperature may reach 41.5°C or more. Without emergency treatment, the victim lapses into coma and death soon follows.

CAUSES
Heatstroke is most commonly brought on by prolonged, unaccustomed exposure to the sun in a hot climate. It is more likely to occur in humid conditions, which reduce the body's ability to cool itself by the evaporation of sweat. Heatstroke can also be caused by working in an extremely hot environment. Susceptibility is greater in people with a disorder of the skin or sweat glands, in people taking *anticholinergic drugs* (which reduce sweating), and in older people in poor health. Overstrenuous activity, unsuitable clothing, overeating, and drinking too much alcohol are sometimes contributory factors.

SYMPTOMS AND SIGNS
Heatstroke is often preceded by *heat exhaustion*, with fatigue, weakness, faintness, and profuse sweating. With the onset of heatstroke itself, sweating diminishes markedly and often stops completely. The skin becomes hot, dry, and flushed, breathing is shallow, and the pulse is rapid and weak. As the condition progresses, body temperature rises dramatically and, without treatment, the victim may quickly lose consciousness and die.

PREVENTION AND TREATMENT
The key to preventing heatstroke is acclimatization (see *Heat disorders*).

If heatstroke develops, emergency medical help should be summoned as soon as possible. Meanwhile, the victim should be wrapped naked in a cold, wet sheet, which should then be kept continuously wet. Alternatively, the victim may be constantly sponged with cold water. Cooling should be increased by fanning. If the victim is unconscious, he or she should be placed in the *recovery position* while being cooled.

Treatment should be continued until the victim's body temperature falls to 38°C or until the body feels cool to the touch. If the victim is conscious, he or she should be given a weak salt solution to sip (a quarter of a level teaspoon of salt dissolved in half a litre of water).

If heatstroke is treated early, the victim usually makes a full recovery. Victims may, however, be at risk of a recurrence.

Heat treatment

The use of heat to treat disease or aid recovery from injury.

Moist heat may be administered by soaking the affected part in a warm bath or by applying a hot *compress* or *poultice*. Dry heat may be applied in the form of a heating pad, a hot-water bottle, or a heat lamp that produces *infra-red* rays.

More precise methods of administering heat to tissues deeper in the body include *ultrasound treatment* and short-wave *diathermy*.

WHY IT IS USED
Heat is used to aid recovery from injury, such as a muscle tear or ligament sprain; by stimulating blood flow, it is thought to help tissues heal more rapidly. In addition, a hot compress is effective in encouraging the formation and the drainage of pus from skin infections.

Heel

The part of the *foot* below the *ankle* and behind the arch. The heel consists of the *calcaneus* (heel bone), an underlying pad of fat, which acts as a protective cushion, and a layer of skin, which is usually thickened as a result of pressure from walking.

FIRST AID: HEATSTROKE

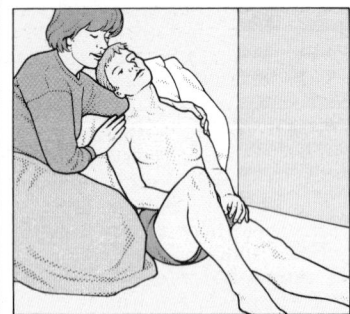

1 Move the victim to a cool, shady place and remove clothing. Place him or her in a half-sitting position and support the head and shoulders (for example, using pillows).

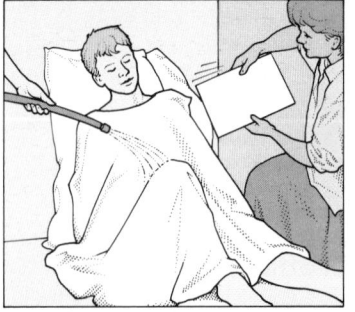

2 Cover the victim with a wet sheet and keep it wet. Fan him or her with a magazine or use an electric fan until the body temperature drops to 38°C. Seek medical help immediately.

Heimlich manoeuvre
A first-aid treatment for *choking*.

Helicobacter pylori
A bacterium found in the stomach of around 40 per cent of Britain's healthy adults and in almost all those who have *peptic ulcers*. The bacterium is thought to damage the mucosal surface of the lining of the stomach and duodenum, thereby allowing gastric acid to cause ulceration. Treatment with antibiotics to eradicate the infection has proved successful in achieving long-term recovery from peptic ulcers.

Heliotherapy
Treatment by exposure to sunlight. Heliotherapy is a form of *phototherapy*.

Helminth infestation
Infection by any species of parasitic worm. (See *Worm infestation*.)

Hemianopia
Loss of one half of the *visual field* in each eye. Hemianopia may be "homonymous" (in which the same side of both eyes is affected by the loss) or "heteronymous" (in which the loss is in opposite sides of the eyes). In either case the visual loss may be temporary or permanent.

Hemianopia is not due to a disorder of the eyes themselves but results from damage to the nerve tracts or brain. Transient homonymous hemianopia in young people is usually caused by *migraine*. In older people it occurs in *transient ischaemic attacks* (symptoms of *stroke* lasting less than 24 hours). Permanent homonymous hemianopia is usually caused by a stroke, but in some cases results from damage to the back of the brain by a tumour, injury, or infection. Hemianopia may also be caused by pressure on the optic nerve from a tumour of the pituitary gland. In this case, the outer half of each eye's visual field is lost.

Hemiballismus
Irregular, uncontrollable, flinging movements of the arm and leg on one side of the body, caused by disease of the *basal ganglia* (part of the brain concerned with coordination). The movements are unpredictable in timing and strength, and may be severe enough to cause injury to the afflicted person or others. (See also *Athetosis*; *Chorea*.)

Hemicolectomy
Surgical removal of half or a major portion of the *colon*. The surgeon may remove either the portion between the beginning of the colon and a point two thirds of the way across the transverse colon, or the portion between this point and the end, either including or excluding the rectum. (See also *Colectomy*.)

Hemiparesis
Muscular weakness or partial paralysis affecting only one side of the body. (See *Hemiplegia*; *Paralysis*.)

Hemiplegia
Paralysis or weakness on one side of the body, caused by damage or disease affecting the motor nerve tracts in the opposite side of the brain. If affected muscles are stiff, the disorder is known as spastic hemiplegia; if the muscles are limp and wasted, the term flaccid hemiplegia is used.
CAUSES
A common cause of hemiplegia is a *stroke*. Other causes include *head injury*, *brain tumour*, *brain haemorrhage*, *encephalitis* (inflammation of the brain), *multiple sclerosis*, complications of *meningitis*, or a *conversion disorder* (a type of psychological disorder).
SYMPTOMS
Paralysis or weakness occurs on only one side of the body. It may affect the arm, leg, part of the trunk, and sometimes the face; one or more sites may be involved at the same time.
TREATMENT AND OUTLOOK
Treatment is directed at the underlying cause and is carried out in conjunction with *physiotherapy* to exercise the affected muscles. The prospects for a person with hemiplegia depend mainly on the cause; in the case of stroke, the outlook depends on age, general health, and the type of stroke. Motivation plays a part, as does the treatment given, but these factors are of less importance than the extent of the brain damage.

Henoch-Schönlein purpura
Inflammation of small blood vessels, causing leakage of blood into the skin, joints, kidneys, and intestine; also called anaphylactoid purpura. The disease is most common among young children, especially boys, and may occur after an infection such as a sore throat. The precise cause of Henoch-Schönlein purpura is not known, but some specialists believe the condition is due to an abnormal allergic reaction to, for example, certain drugs or foods.
SYMPTOMS
The main symptom is a slightly raised, purplish rash on the buttocks and backs of the legs and arms. The joints are swollen and often painful, and colicky abdominal pain may occur. In some cases, intestinal bleeding occurs, resulting in blood in the faeces. The kidneys may become inflamed, resulting in haematuria (blood in the urine) and proteinuria (protein in the urine).
DIAGNOSIS AND TREATMENT
The doctor will arrange for *blood-clotting tests* to rule out the possibility of a *bleeding disorder*.

No specific treatment is usually required except bed rest and mild *analgesic drugs* (painkillers). Most children recover within a month, although complications may arise if inflammation of the kidneys persists. In severe cases, *corticosteroid drugs* may be prescribed.

Heparin
An *anticoagulant drug* used to prevent and treat abnormal *blood clotting*. Heparin is given by injection and is particularly useful as an immediate treatment for deep-vein *thrombosis* or *pulmonary embolism*.
POSSIBLE ADVERSE EFFECTS
Bruising around the injection site is common. Other adverse effects include rash, aching bones, and abnormal bleeding in different parts of the body. Long-term use may cause *osteoporosis* (thinning and weakening of the bones).

Hepatectomy, partial
Surgical removal of part of the *liver*. The liver has remarkable powers of regeneration; up to three quarters of the organ can be removed before it ceases to function.
WHY IT IS DONE
Severe injury to the liver sometimes occurs in road traffic accidents, causing serious bleeding in and death of the damaged area. Surgery is performed to remove the dead tissue.

Benign liver tumours and sometimes *hydatid disease* require partial hepatectomy; rarely, *liver cancer* is also treated in this way.

Hepatectomy, total
Surgical removal of the liver. Hepatectomy is performed as the first stage in a *liver transplant* operation.

Hepatic
Related to the *liver*. For example, the hepatic vein is the vessel that drains blood from the liver.

Hepatitis
Inflammation of the *liver*, with accompanying damage or death of liver cells. Hepatitis is most commonly

caused by viral infection but may also be due to certain drugs, chemicals, or poisons. The condition may be either acute or chronic.

ACUTE HEPATITIS

This form of hepatitis is fairly common with several thousands of cases diagnosed per year in the UK. The most frequent cause is infection with a hepatitis virus, which may be of any of the types A, B, C, D, or E (see *Hepatitis, viral*). Other causes include overdose with drugs, such as *paracetamol*, exposure to certain chemicals, such as dry-cleaning agents, or, rarely, a reaction to certain drugs in normal dosage. Acute hepatitis may also affect heavy drinkers who have progressive liver disease (see *Liver disease, alcoholic*).

SYMPTOMS The most obvious sign of acute hepatitis is *jaundice*. In many cases, jaundice is preceded by a flu-like illness, accompanied by nausea, vomiting, loss of appetite, tenderness in the right upper abdomen, aching muscles, and sometimes joint pain.

In uncommon, severe cases, jaundice may be intense and *liver failure* may develop, with possible effects on other organs (including the brain), resulting in coma and death.

DIAGNOSIS A doctor may strongly suspect acute hepatitis from the symptoms alone, particularly if the patient is in a risk group for exposure to one of the causative viruses, drugs, or chemicals. If drug or chemical poisoning is suspected, blood tests may be performed to identify the cause. *Ultrasound scanning* of the liver may help rule out *bile duct obstruction*, which is another cause of jaundice. *Liver-function tests* can also aid in diagnosis.

TREATMENT In most cases of acute hepatitis, all that can be done is to wait for natural recovery to occur. *Intensive care* may be required if the liver is seriously damaged; rarely, a *liver transplant* is the only hope of saving life. If the disorder is caused by exposure to a chemical or drug, this exposure should be stopped and, in some cases, detoxification using an antidote may be possible. Whatever the cause of the hepatitis, bed rest and a nourishing diet are usually recommended. Recovery usually occurs after a few weeks. Abstinence from alcohol after the illness aids liver regeneration.

CHRONIC HEPATITIS

In some cases, a person fails to recover fully from an episode of acute hepatitis, leading to continued liver cell damage and inflammation. This usually, but not exclusively, occurs with certain types of viral hepatitis.

MAIN TYPES OF VIRAL HEPATITIS

	Viral hepatitis type A (infectious hepatitis)	Viral hepatitis type B (serum hepatitis)
Transmission of infection	Virus is present in faeces of infected people and transmitted to others by faecal contamination of water and food (e.g. through infected people handling food). Faeces are infective from two to three weeks before until eight days after the onset of jaundice. Local epidemics can occur.	These viruses are present in the blood and other body fluids of infected people, many of whom appear to be in normal health. Infection is spread sexually or by sharing hypodermic needles; in the past it was spread by use of contaminated blood and blood products.
Incidence	Worldwide. In the UK, about 2,000 cases are reported annually. In some parts of the world where hygiene is poor, almost everyone has been exposed to this type of hepatitis.	In some parts of Africa and Asia up to 20 per cent of the population are carriers of one or both viruses, often without symptoms. In the UK carrier rates are much lower, but many people were infected in the past by infected transfusions of blood.
Groups at particular risk	Travellers to areas where hygiene standards are poor and prevalence of the virus is high (i.e. parts of Asia, Africa, or South America).	Male homosexuals, people with multiple sexual partners, intravenous drug abusers, health care personnel, or children born to carrier mothers.
Incubation period	Three to six weeks after virus has entered the body.	A few weeks to several months after infection.
Illness	In many cases there is no illness. Otherwise, typical acute hepatitis (flu-like illness with jaundice), usually mild and never progressing to chronic hepatitis.	Typical acute hepatitis, often more severe than with type A virus. Progression to chronic hepatitis and other liver disease may occur. Sometimes, no illness.
Prevention	Recommended for frequent travellers to Africa and Asia. Two doses of vaccine, 2 – 4 weeks apart, then a booster six to 12 months later, gives around ten years' protection.	Screening of blood donors and treatment of donated blood; safe sex and avoidance of blood exchange by drug users. A vaccine is available against hepatitis B for high-risk groups.

Chronic hepatitis may also develop insidiously over a number of years without any acute episodes. Heavy alcohol consumption may be responsible. Other possible causes are an *autoimmune disorder* (in which the body's natural defences attack body tissues), a reaction to a medication, or a metabolic disorder which affects the liver.

Several types of chronic hepatitis are recognized. A type affecting heavy drinkers (see *Liver disease, alcoholic*) and chronic active hepatitis (see *Hepatitis, chronic active*) may both progress to liver *cirrhosis* if untreated. A third type, called chronic persistent hepatitis, is less severe and carries little risk of progression to cirrhosis.

SYMPTOMS The symptoms of chronic hepatitis are usually no worse than a vague feeling of being unwell.

DIAGNOSIS Often the disease remains undetected until the patient has a medical examination and the liver is found to be enlarged, a causative virus or specific *antibody* is found in the blood, or the results of *liver-function tests* are abnormal. A *liver biopsy* (removal of a tissue sample for microscopic analysis) helps the doctor establish the type of chronic hepatitis.

TREATMENT For hepatitis caused by alcohol consumption, total abstinence is the only cure. If strictly observed, this allows complete restoration of liver function. For chronic persistent hepatitis, treatment is not usually needed. For the chronic active form, therapy depends on the precise cause of the disease.

Hepatitis A, B, C, D, and E
See *Hepatitis, viral.*

Hepatitis, chronic active
A type of chronic *hepatitis* in which there is intense and progressive inflammation and destruction of cells surrounding certain structures within the liver. Scar tissue forms and leads to liver *cirrhosis.*

CAUSES
Chronic active hepatitis may be caused in any of four ways—as a result of an *autoimmune disorder* (in which the body's natural defences attack body tissues), a viral infection, a reaction to a drug or chemical, or, rarely, to a *metabolic disorder.*

In the autoimmune type of the disease, antibodies (proteins with a defence role) that inappropriately attack liver cells are formed. This is the most common cause of hepatitis in Northern Europe and one of the most common causes in the US. Women are affected more often than men. Primary biliary cirrhosis may fall into this category.

Viral infection is the most common cause in the UK, most often due to viral hepatitis, caused by either hepatitis B or C viruses (see *Hepatitis, viral*). Men are affected more often than women.

Drugs, including *nitrofurantoin* and *isoniazid,* are a rare cause of chronic active hepatitis. Metabolic disorders that may also cause the disease include *haemochromatosis* and *Wilson's disease.*

SYMPTOMS AND DIAGNOSIS
The disease may cause vague feelings of tiredness, or no symptoms at all. It is diagnosed by *liver biopsy* (removal of a sample of tissue from the liver for microscopic analysis).

TREATMENT
The type of chronic active hepatitis that is caused by an autoimmune disorder is treated with *corticosteroid drugs,* which usually bring some improvement. Viral infections often respond to treatment with *interferon.* In the drug-induced type of the disease, withdrawal of the medication can lead to recovery. For metabolic disturbances, treatment depends on the underlying disorder.

Hepatitis, viral
Any type of *hepatitis* (inflammation of the liver) caused by a viral infection.

TYPES AND CAUSES
Although other viruses may infect the liver as part of a wider infection, certain viruses attack the liver as their primary target. These include five named viruses, hepatitis viruses A, B, C, D, and E, possibly in addition to some others that have not yet been identified. The hepatitis A and E viruses are transmitted mostly by the contamination of drinking water by infected faeces. The E virus is found mostly in developing countries, whereas the A virus is common throughout the world.

Hepatitis B and C viruses are transmitted sexually, and also by blood and blood products. Screening tests for these viruses are now a routine procedure for blood donors; and, as a further precaution, blood products are treated in order to destroy any viruses that could possibly be missed by these tests. As little as ten years ago, most people who needed repeated treatment with blood products—haemophiliacs for example—were infected with one or other of these viruses. Such infections are now very rare but it continues to be possible for the hepatitis B and C viruses to be spread by accidental inoculation of infected blood. The most common causes of accidental inoculation are needle sharing by drug users and the failure of tattooists or acupuncturists to sterilize their needles properly.

Infection with the hepatitis B and C viruses is in many respects more serious than with hepatitis A, since there is a greater risk that the infection will become chronic (see *Hepatitis, chronic active*) and eventually lead to *liver cirrhosis* or *liver cancer.* Carriers of the virus may have few or no symptoms during this time but can infect others.

Screening tests for hepatitis B and C can eliminate virtually any risk of transfusion-associated hepatitis. Hepatitis delta virus can exist only in someone who is already carrying, or has recently been infected with, hepatitis B. It seems to be spread mainly by needle sharing among drug abusers.

SYMPTOMS
Infection with any of the causative viruses may be symptomless or may cause a typical acute *hepatitis* with a flu-like illness followed by jaundice. About 10 per cent of patients infected with hepatitis B, delta, or non-A non-B viruses go on to acquire chronic hepatitis. This rarely, if ever, happens with hepatitis type A.

DIAGNOSIS AND TREATMENT
Diagnosis is usually made by identifying the virus (or antibodies to the virus) in the blood, or in the case of non-A non-B hepatitis, by exclusion of the other types.

There is no specific treatment for any type of viral hepatitis. Bed rest, a nourishing diet, and abstinence from alcohol may speed recovery.

PREVENTION
Vaccine against hepatitis B is available, but is generally recommended only to people who are at high risk of infection, such as health-care workers, children born to carrier mothers, male homosexuals, and drug addicts. Vaccine against hepatitis A is recommended for non-immune, frequent travellers to high-risk areas.

Passive immunization against hepatitis A and hepatitis B by means of *immunoglobulin injections* is also available and can provide some protection. Passive immunization against hepatitis A may be recommended for people travelling for short periods to areas with a high incidence of the disease. The babies of carrier mothers are given hepatitis B immunoglobin after birth to prevent infection while the vaccine (given at the same time) is beginning to build up immunity.

Avoidance of hepatitis A is further helped by observing good hygiene, especially food hygiene, in parts of the world where sanitary standards are low (see *Food-borne infection*). The chances of getting hepatitis B can be reduced by use of a condom during sexual intercourse, by not sharing needles, and by avoiding such activities as tattooing, unless the equipment is sterile.

Hepatoma
A type of *liver cancer.*

Hepatomegaly
Enlargement of the liver, occurring as a result of virtually any type of liver disorder. The enlargement may cause tenderness just beneath the ribs and can be detected by a doctor during the course of a physical examination. (See *Liver* disorders box.)

Herbal medicine
Systems of medical treatment in which various parts of different plants are used in order to treat symptoms and to promote health.

Herbal medicine was the most common medical treatment in most cultures for many centuries.

Heredity

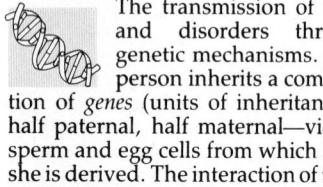

The transmission of traits and disorders through genetic mechanisms. Each person inherits a combination of *genes* (units of inheritance)—half paternal, half maternal—via the sperm and egg cells from which he or she is derived. The interaction of these genes determines the person's inherited characteristics, including, in some cases, disorders or susceptibility to disorders. Half of an individual's genes are passed on, in turn, to each of his or her own children. (See also *Genetic disorders; Inheritance.*)

Heritability

A measure of the extent to which a disease or disorder is the result of inherited factors — as opposed to environmental influences such as diet and climate.

Certain disorders (such as *haemophilia* or *cystic fibrosis*) are known to be caused entirely by hereditary factors. Others (such as occupational disorders) are caused entirely by environmental factors. Between these two extremes are many disorders in which both inheritance and environment probably play a part.

Pinpointing hereditary factors is notoriously difficult. A rough estimate of heritability can be obtained from the known incidence of a disorder in the first-degree relatives (i.e. parents, siblings, and offspring) of affected people and by comparing it with the incidence of the disorder in a population exposed to similar environmental influences. Other estimates of heritability are obtained from studies of identical twins who have been reared apart.

Such studies suggest a relatively high heritability for *schizophrenia, asthma, coronary artery disease,* non-insulin-dependent *diabetes mellitus, ankylosing spondylitis,* and some birth defects, such as *cleft lip and palate, pyloric stenosis,* and *talipes* (club-foot). The heritability for congenital *heart disease* and *peptic ulcer* is low.

Estimates of heritability are useful in *genetic counselling.* (See also *Genetic disorders.*)

Hermaphroditism

A congenital disorder in which both male and female gonads (testes and ovaries) are present and the external genitalia are not clearly male or female. True hermaphroditism is extremely rare and its cause unknown. The majority of affected children are raised as males because the external genitalia usually appear more male than female.

A more common condition is pseudohermaphroditism, in which the gonads of only one sex are present, but the external genitalia may not be clearly male or female. Pseudohermaphroditism is caused by a hormonal imbalance (such as occurs in congenital *adrenal hyperplasia,* for example). Pseudohermaphroditism can usually be treated by appropriate surgery and hormone therapy.

Hernia

The protrusion of an organ or tissue through a weak area in the muscle or other tissue that normally contains it. The term is usually applied to a protrusion of the intestine through a weak area in the abdominal wall.

MAIN TYPES OF ABDOMINAL HERNIA

Inguinal hernia 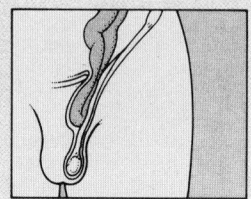	At least 2 per cent of adult males in the UK suffer at some time from this kind of hernia, in which part of the intestine bulges through the inguinal canal (the passage through which the testes descend into the scrotum). The hernia is detected as a bulge in the groin or scrotum; untreated, the hernia may become stuck, so early surgery is generally recommended.
Femoral hernia 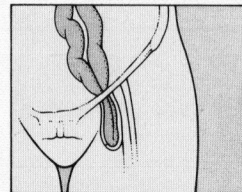	This type of hernia occurs most commonly in obese women; part of the intestine emerges where the femoral vein and artery pass from the abdomen to the thigh. A femoral hernia is noticed as a swelling of the top front of the thigh. Although the hernia itself may be large, its neck is narrow, and the condition can only be corrected by surgery.
Epigastric hernia 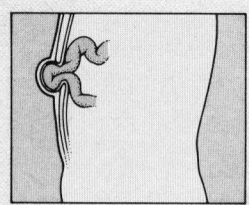	Also called a ventral hernia, an epigastric hernia is caused by a weakness in the muscles of the central upper abdomen; the intestine bulges out at a point between the navel and the breastbone. This form of hernia is three times more common in men than in women and is most likely to occur in people between 20 and 50 years old.
Umbilical hernia 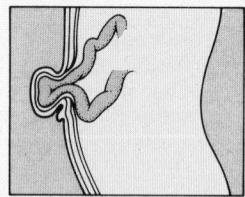	This occurs when part of the intestine protrudes through the abdominal wall at the navel. Babies are the most common sufferers; the hernia can be repaired surgically or it may disappear naturally by about the age of five. A similar problem, a parumbilical hernia, occurs mostly in obese, middle-aged women who have had several children.
Incisional hernia 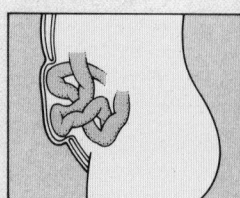	An area of weakness may occasionally develop following a surgical incision in the wall of the abdomen. This area may then develop into an incisional hernia. The defect may become so severe that a large amount of intestine bulges through the abdominal wall; if this happens, a repair using a piece of mesh may be necessary.

The main types of abdominal hernia are shown in the illustrated box. A *hiatus hernia* is a hernia in which the stomach protrudes through the diaphragm into the chest. Very rarely, other organs or tissue (e.g. the brain) may herniate.

CAUSES

Abdominal hernias are usually caused by a *congenital* weakness in the abdominal wall. They sometimes result, especially later in life, from damage caused by lifting heavy objects, substantial weight gain, persistent coughing, or straining to defaecate. Hernias may also develop after surgery.

SYMPTOMS AND COMPLICATIONS

The first symptom of an abdominal hernia is usually a bulge in the abdominal wall. There may also be abdominal discomfort. In some people, the protruding intestine can be pushed back through the abdominal wall. Severe pain occurs when the hernia bulges out and cannot be replaced.

If the blood supply to a twisted, trapped intestine becomes impaired (a condition known as a strangulated hernia), gangrene (tissue death) of the bowel may develop. A strangulated hernia requires urgent treatment.

DIAGNOSIS AND TREATMENT

Hernias are diagnosed by physical examination. If the hernia is causing only slight discomfort and is readily pushed back, a supportive truss may be recommended. Hernias that are painful or impossible to push back are usually treated surgically (see *Hernia repair*).

Hernia repair

Surgical correction of a *hernia*. The procedure is usually performed to treat a hernia of the abdominal wall that is painful or cannot be pushed back. A strangulated hernia requires an emergency operation.

HOW IT IS DONE

Many hernias are repaired on an outpatient basis unless an underlying medical condition necessitates hospitalization. A local, epidural, or general anaesthetic may be used. The surgeon's aim is to push the protruding intestine back into place and then strengthen the weakened muscle wall (see illustrated box). Alternatively, *minimally invasive surgery* is used to repair the hernia laparoscopically, fixing a plastic mesh over the defect from the inside.

RECOVERY AND OUTLOOK

The speed of recovery depends on the surgical technique used, the patient's health, and the type of hernia repaired. Lifting heavy objects should be avoided for three to six months.

The risk of the condition recurring varies with the type of hernia treated. Inguinal and incisional hernias both recur quite commonly; femoral and epigastric hernias only rarely.

Herniated disc

See *Disc prolapse.*

Herniorrhaphy

Surgical correction of a hernia. (See *Hernia repair.*)

Heroin abuse

Nonmedical use of heroin, a *narcotic drug* similar to *morphine*. Heroin is a white or brownish powder that can be smoked, sniffed, or dissolved in water and injected. When used for medical purposes, this drug is generally known as *diamorphine*.

Heroin abuse is a major health problem in many countries. It has many adverse effects on the user and is a sociological and economic problem of immense proportions.

EFFECTS

In addition to having an analgesic (painkilling) effect, heroin produces sensations of warmth, calmness, drowsiness, and a loss of concern for outside events.

Long-term use causes *tolerance* (the need for greater amounts of the drug to have the same effects) and psychological and physical dependence (see *Drug dependence*). Sudden withdrawal of the drug produces symptoms such as shivering, abdominal cramps, diarrhoea, vomiting, sleeplessness, and restlessness. Other common problems of addiction include injection scars, skin abscesses, weight loss, and impotence. Infections, such as with the virus causing hepatitis B and C (see *Hepatitis, viral*) or *AIDS*, are spread by sharing needles. Death commonly occurs from accidental overdose.

Herpangina

A throat infection caused by a type of virus called coxsackie virus. Herpangina most commonly affects young children, but can also occur in adults. The virus is usually transmitted via infected droplets coughed or sneezed into the air. Many people harbour the virus but experience no symptoms.

SYMPTOMS

After an incubation period of two to seven days, there is a sudden onset of fever, loss of appetite, and sore throat. There may also be headache, abdominal discomfort, and vague muscular aches and pains. The throat becomes red and a few small blisters appear,

HERNIA REPAIR

During surgery the hernia is removed or repositioned and the weakened abdominal wall is reinforced with stitching or mesh.

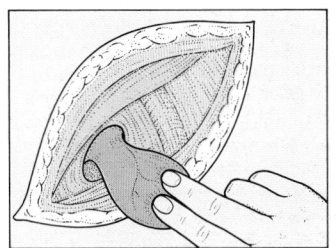

1 The protruding sac of intestine is pushed back into the abdomen or, in some cases (e.g. strangulation), the sac is removed surgically.

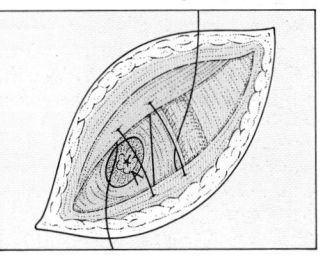

2 The wall of the abdomen may then be repaired by overlapping the edges of the weakened area and securing them with rows of stitching.

LARGE HERNIAS

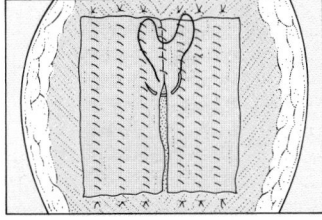

For repair of some large hernias, two mesh leaves are secured by rows of stitching, then joined at the centre.

which enlarge and burst, forming shallow ulcers. The condition usually clears up within a week.

TREATMENT

Usually no treatment is required other than simple *analgesic drugs* (painkillers). There is no specific antiviral therapy available. Antibiotics are generally of no therapeutic value unless a bacterial infection develops as a complication. Recurrent attacks of herpangina may result from infection with different strains of the virus.

H

Herpes

Any of a variety of conditions characterized by an eruption of small, usually painful, blisters on the skin.

When a person is said to be suffering from herpes, the term usually refers to an infection with the *herpes simplex* virus. Forms of the virus are responsible for *cold sores* (painful blisters around the lips) and for the sexually transmitted infection genital herpes, which is characterized by blisters on the sex organs (see *Herpes, genital*). The virus can also cause a number of other conditions affecting the skin, mouth, eyes, brain, or, in rare cases, the whole body.

A closely related virus, the varicella-zoster virus, is responsible for two more conditions in which skin blisters are a feature—*chickenpox* (also known as varicella) and *herpes zoster* (also known as shingles). Like herpes simplex virus, varicella-zoster virus can also affect the eyes or, rarely, may infect the brain or cause a generalized infection throughout the body.

Herpes gestationis and *dermatitis herpetiformis* are among various other conditions in which "herpetiform" (herpes-like) groups of blisters may appear on the skin, but neither is related to herpes simplex or varicella-zoster virus infections.

Herpes, genital

A sexually transmitted disease that produces a painful rash on the genitals. Caused by the *herpes simplex* virus, genital herpes is transmitted by sexual intercourse with an infected person. About 20,000 new cases were reported annually in the UK in the early 1990s.

SYMPTOMS AND SIGNS

After an incubation period of about a week, the virus produces itching, burning, soreness, and small blisters in the genital area. The blisters burst to leave small, painful ulcers, which heal within 10 to 21 days. The lymph nodes in the groin may become enlarged and painful, and the affected person may feel unwell, with headache and fever. Women may find urination very painful if the urine comes into contact with the sores.

TREATMENT

Genital herpes cannot be cured, but the earlier treatment is given, the more likely the treatment will prevent or reduce the severity of an attack. Antiviral drugs, such as *acyclovir,* help make the ulcers less painful and encourage faster healing. Other soothing measures include taking *analgesic drugs* (painkillers) and bathing the area with a salt solution by adding a heaped teaspoon of salt to a pint of water.

Subsequent attacks tend to occur when the patient is anxious or depressed, before menstrual periods, after sexual intercourse, after sunbathing, or when the affected person is run down; these recurrent attacks often clear up quickly with or without treatment. Sexual activity should be avoided until the symptoms have disappeared. If a pregnant woman has an attack of genital herpes when the baby is due, a caesarean section is performed to prevent the baby from being infected during delivery.

OUTLOOK

Once the virus enters the body, it stays there for the rest of the person's life. About 12 to 20 per cent of those affected never have a second attack. Recurrent attacks may be reduced in frequency and severity by treatment with acyclovir. Even without treatment the tendency is for the attacks to become less frequent and less severe.

The herpes virus may have a role in the development of cervical cancer (see *Cervix, cancer of*), women who have had herpes should have a *cervical smear* test every year.

Herpes gestationis

A rare skin disorder of pregnant women, characterized by crops of blisters on the legs and abdomen. The cause is not known and, despite its name, herpes gestationis is not related to any of the disorders caused by the *herpes simplex* viruses.

Severe herpes gestationis is treated with *corticosteroid drugs* in tablet form and may require hospital admission because of the risk of *miscarriage*. The disorder usually clears up completely after the birth of the baby, but tends to recur in subsequent pregnancies.

Herpes simplex

A common and troublesome viral infection, characterized by the appearance of small, fluid-filled blisters. Although most herpes simplex infections are symptomless, mild, or merely irritating, others can be extremely distressing (notably infections affecting the genitals) or, in rare cases, even life-threatening. Herpes simplex infections are *contagious* and usually spread by direct contact with the blisters or the fluid they contain.

TYPES

The virus exists in two forms, known as HSV1 (herpes simplex virus, type 1) and HSV2 (herpes simplex virus, type 2). HSV1 is usually associated with infections of the lips, mouth, and face, whereas HSV2 is often associated with infections of the genitals and infections acquired by babies at birth. However, there is a considerable amount of overlap. Some conditions usually caused by HSV1 are sometimes caused by HSV2 and vice versa.

TYPE 1 VIRUS Most people have been infected with HSV1 by the time they reach adulthood; most of the remainder are infected during adulthood. The initial infection may cause no symptoms or may cause a sometimes severe flu-like illness with mouth ulcers. Thereafter, the virus remains in the nerve cells within the facial area. In many people, the virus is periodically reactivated, causing recurrent *cold sores* that always erupt in the same site (usually around the lips). Cold sores often recur when the temperature at the affected site is raised, such as in a fever or during prolonged exposure to the sun.

Rarely, the virus may infect the fingers, causing an eruption of very painful blisters known as a herpetic *whitlow*. Sometimes the virus may cause an extensive rash of blisters (known as eczema herpeticum) in a person with a pre-existing skin condition such as dermatitis.

If a person with an *immunodeficiency disorder*, such as *AIDS*, or someone who is taking *immunosuppressant drugs* is infected with the virus, it may cause a severe generalized infection that is occasionally fatal.

If the virus gets into an eye, it may cause *conjunctivitis*, which usually lasts only a few days, or, more seriously, a *corneal ulcer*. Very rarely, the type 1 virus may spread to the brain, leading to serious *encephalitis* (inflammation of the brain).

TYPE 2 VIRUS This form of the virus is the usual cause of sexually transmitted genital herpes, in which painful blisters erupt on the sex organs (see *Herpes, genital*). As with cold sores, the blisters recur in some people.

TREATMENT

Treatment of herpes simplex depends on its type, site, and severity. *Antiviral drugs,* such as *acyclovir,* are sometimes helpful, If sores become infected with bacteria, *antibiotic drugs* and bathing in tepid water may be helpful.

Herpes zoster

The medical term for shingles. Herpes zoster is an infection of the nerves that supply certain areas of the skin. This

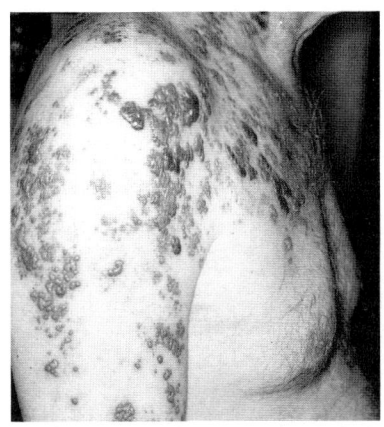

Example of herpes zoster
An extensive rash of crusting blisters over one side of the neck spreads over the shoulder and on to the front of the chest.

disorder causes a painful rash of small, crusting blisters. After the rash heals, pain may persist for months or, rarely, years.

TYPES

Herpes zoster often affects a strip of skin over the ribs on one side. Less commonly, it affects a strip on one side of the neck and arm, or on one side of the lower part of the body. Sometimes, herpes zoster involves one side of the upper half of the face, and the eye may also be affected. Shingles in this area is known as herpes zoster ophthalmicus.

CAUSES

Herpes zoster is caused by the varicella-zoster virus, which also causes *chickenpox*. During an attack of chickenpox, most of the viral organisms are destroyed, but some survive and lie dormant in certain sensory nerves, remaining there for many years. In some people, a decline in the efficiency of the *immune system* (the body's defences against infection) allows the viruses to re-emerge and cause shingles.

The efficiency of the immune system declines with age; this decline is probably accelerated by stress and by the use of *corticosteroid drugs*. Herpes zoster commonly follows a stressful episode.

INCIDENCE

Herpes zoster is a common disease. Every year in the UK, about one person in 350 suffers an attack. The disorder mainly affects people over 50 and the incidence rises with age. Herpes zoster is very common in people whose immune systems have been weakened either by diseases,

such as *lymphoma* or *AIDS*, or by treatment with *immunosuppressant drugs* or *anticancer drugs*.

SYMPTOMS AND SIGNS

The first indication is excessive sensitivity in the area of skin to be affected; this is soon followed by pain, which is sometimes severe and which may, until the rash appears, be mistaken for pleurisy or appendicitis.

After about five days, the rash appears, starting as small, slightly raised, red spots that quickly turn to tense blisters, teeming with viruses. Within three days the blisters have turned yellowish and soon dry, flatten, and crust over. During the next two weeks or so these crusts drop off, often leaving small pitted scars.

The most serious feature of herpes zoster is pain following the attack, a condition known as postherpetic pain. This pain is a consequence of damage to the nerves, causing strong nerve impulses to be constantly produced and passed upwards to the brain. The pain, which affects about one third of sufferers, may be severe and last for months or years. The older the patient and the more pronounced the rash, the more likely it is that the pain will be severe and persistent.

Ophthalmic herpes zoster may be confined to the eyelids and forehead and need not affect the eye itself. But if it does affect the eye, it may cause a *corneal ulcer* or *uveitis*, both of which are potentially serious.

TREATMENT

Provided that treatment is begun soon after the rash appears, *antiviral drugs* (such as *acyclovir*) will reduce the severity of the active stage and minimize nerve damage. If treatment is delayed beyond the early stage of the disease, little can be done to influence the course of the disease or the likelihood of postherpetic pain.

Some relief from pain may be obtained by taking *analgesic drugs*. Many other measures have been advocated for the relief of postherpetic pain, but none has been shown to be consistently effective. Such measures include stimulation of the skin by intermittent rubbing, the passage of alternating electric currents through the skin, local heat, cold spraying, the injection of local anaesthetics, and even surgical cutting of the nerves.

Heterosexuality

Sexual attraction to members of the opposite sex. (See also *Bisexuality*; *Homosexuality, male*; *Lesbianism*.)

Heterozygote

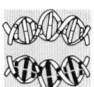

A term used to describe a person whose cells contain two different *genes* controlling a specified inherited trait, in contrast to a *homozygote* who has identical genes controlling that trait. (See also *Inheritance* and *Genetic disorders*.)

Hiatus hernia

A condition in which part of the *stomach* protrudes upwards into the chest through the hiatus (opening) normally only for the oesophagus in the *diaphragm* (the sheet of muscle between the chest and the abdomen).

CAUSES AND INCIDENCE

The underlying cause of hiatus hernia is unknown, but this common condition tends to occur more commonly in obese people (and especially in women in later middle age) and in those who smoke. In some cases, it is present at birth.

SYMPTOMS

Many people have no symptoms, but in some people hiatus hernia affects the efficiency of the muscle at the junction between the *oesophagus* and stomach, permitting *acid reflux* (backflow of acidic juices from the stomach into the oesophagus). This reflux may in turn cause *heartburn*, which is often made worse by bending over or lying down, or *oesophagitis* (inflammation of the oesophagus). The pain of oesophagitis may mimic the pain of *coronary artery disease*.

DIAGNOSIS

Oesophagoscopy (a type of *endoscopy* in which a viewing instrument is passed down the throat into the oeso-

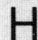 H

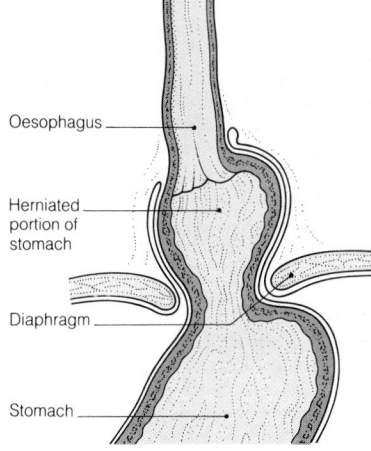

Common type of hiatus hernia
The stomach slides into the chest through the oesophageal hiatus (opening).

Oesophagus

Herniated portion of stomach

Diaphragm

Stomach

phagus) may be performed, and a *biopsy* sample of oesophageal tissue taken for microscopic analysis. A *barium X-ray examination* is usually performed, with the patient tilted head-down; incompetence at the junction between the oesophagus and stomach is indicated if the X-ray shows reflux of the barium into the oesophagus. *Manometry* (the taking of pressure measurements) can confirm the reduced pressure at the junction between the oesophagus and the stomach.

TREATMENT
To alleviate symptoms, the patient should avoid eating large, heavy meals and should never lie down or bend over immediately after a meal. The head end of the bed should be raised to prevent reflux during the night. People who are obese should lose weight and smokers should stop smoking. *Antacid drugs* may be given to reduce stomach acidity and to protect the oesophagus against acid juices.

In severe cases, an operation may be required to return the protruding part of the stomach to the abdomen and to prevent the further reflux of acid stomach contents into the oesophagus.

Hiccup
A sudden, involuntary contraction of the *diaphragm* followed by rapid closure of the *vocal cords* (which causes the characteristic sound). Hiccups, which are also spelled hiccoughs, are extremely common. Most attacks last only a few minutes, consisting of individual hiccups usually with a brief interval between.

CAUSES
In almost all cases, hiccups occur without obvious cause and are not medically significant. Rarely, hiccups may be due to a condition that causes irritation of the diaphragm or of the *phrenic nerves* that supply it. Known causes include *pleurisy, pneumonia,* certain disorders of the stomach or oesophagus, *pancreatitis, alcohol dependence,* and *hepatitis.* Frequent, prolonged attacks of hiccups, which are extremely rare, may lead to severe exhaustion.

TREATMENT
Most minor attacks clear up without treatment. Numerous popular remedies, such as drinking cold water or provoking a sneeze, have been tried with varying success in different people. Drugs, such as *chlorpromazine, haloperidol,* and *diazepam* are sometimes prescribed in severe cases. If

medication fails to cure severe hiccups, surgery on the phrenic nerve to paralyse half of the diaphragm may be performed but this may affect breathing and may not succeed.

Hip
The joint between the *pelvis* and the upper end of the *femur* (thigh bone). The hip is an extremely stable ball-and-socket joint; the smooth, rounded head of the femur fits securely into the acetabulum, a deep, cup-like cavity in the pelvis. Tough ligaments attach the femur to the pelvis, further stabilizing the joint and providing it with the necessary strength to support the weight of the upper body and to take the strain of running, jumping, and other vigorous leg movements. In addition, the ball-and-socket structure of the joint allows the leg a considerable range of movement that is available only because of the unique design of this joint.

DISORDERS
ARTHRITIS *Osteoarthritis* of the hip, one of the most common of all disorders, causes stiffness and pain in the joint, particularly during movement. Occasionally, *ankylosing spondylitis* and rheumatoid arthritis of the hip cause similar problems.

FRACTURE What is commonly called fracture of the hip (most common in elderly people as a result of a fall) is in fact fracture of the head or neck of the femur (see *Femur, fracture of).*

DISLOCATION Congenital dislocation of the hip is remediable (see *Hip, congenital dislocation of).*

Dislocation of the hip by injury is rare and usually results only from extreme force, such as may occur in a road traffic accident.

Dislocation may cut off the blood supply to the head of the femur, causing avascular necrosis (a condition in which the bone dies because of impaired blood supply). It may also injure the sciatic nerve, leading to weakness in the leg.

Hip, congenital dislocation of
A disorder present at birth in which the ball-like head of the femur (thigh bone) fails to fit into the cup-like socket in the pelvis to form a joint but instead lies outside. One or both of the hips may be affected.

CAUSES AND INCIDENCE
The cause of congenital dislocation of the hip is not known, but it is more common in babies born by *breech delivery* and following pregnancies

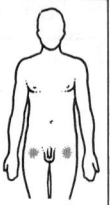

LOCATION OF HIP
The hip is a ball-and-socket joint comprising the dome at the top of the femur (thigh-bone) and the cup-shaped depression in the pelvic bone.

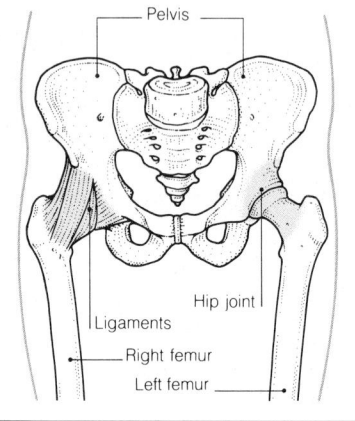

Pelvis

Hip joint

Ligaments

Right femur

Left femur

in which there was *oligohydramnios* (an abnormally small amount of amniotic fluid surrounding the fetus).

About 400 in every 100,000 babies born are affected by instability of the hip joint. In most cases the condition soon corrects itself, but true dislocation does not correct itself. The disorder affects approximately five times as many girls as boys and sometimes runs in families.

DIAGNOSIS
Shortly after birth, and at intervals until walking starts, all babies are given a routine physical examination of the hip to check its stability and range of motion; in many hospitals this is backed up by *ultrasound scanning.* If the condition is not detected in infancy, dislocation may cause a limp when the child is learning to walk.

TREATMENT
If the condition is found in early infancy, light *splints* are applied to the thigh to manoeuvre the ball of the joint into the socket and keep it in position. The splints are worn for two to four months and usually help to correct the problem.

If the condition is not discovered until later in infancy, *traction* is used. The head of the femur is moved into the correct position and kept there by a system of weights and pulleys attached to the leg or by being nursed with the legs raised on a "gallows".

If detection of dislocation is delayed, surgery under a general anaesthetic may be required to correct it. The child must usually stay in hospital for several weeks and wear a plaster *cast* for a few months.

OUTLOOK
Provided the disorder is treated in infancy, the child usually walks normally and there are no after effects. When treatment is delayed, however, there may be lifelong problems with walking. Without treatment, the dislocation often leads to shortening of the leg, limping, and early *osteoarthritis* in the joint.

Hippocratic oath
A set of ethical principles derived from the writings of the ancient Greek physician Hippocrates. The Hippocratic oath is concerned with a doctor's duty to work for the good of his or her patients and to cause no harm, whether by deliberate intent, by prescribing deadly drugs, or by giving advice that might cause death. The oath also covers the principle of confidentiality and condemns abuse of the doctor-patient relationship for sexual purposes.

Hip replacement
A surgical procedure to replace all or part of a diseased hip joint with an artificial substitute.

WHY IT IS DONE
Hip replacement is most often carried out in older people whose joints are stiff and painful as a result of *osteoarthritis*. It may also be needed if *rheumatoid arthritis* has spread to the hip joint, making walking difficult, or if the top end of the femur is badly fractured (see *Femur, fracture of*).

The operation is not usually advised for young patients, since their greater activity puts more strain on the joints and it is not known how long an artificial replacement is likely to last.

HOW IT IS DONE
A procedure for hip replacement is shown in the illustrated box.

RECOVERY PERIOD
The joint remains unstable for a week or two after the operation, and patients must take care not to dislocate the new joint during this time. Patients are advised to sleep on their backs and not to cross their legs, and are taught how to get in and out of the bath without disturbing the joint.

OUTLOOK
Hip replacement is a remarkably successful operation that has transformed the lives of many people who

PERFORMING A HIP REPLACEMENT
In this operation, the surgeon pushes aside or cuts through the surrounding muscles to expose the hip joint. The femur (thigh-bone) is cut and the pelvis is drilled to make room for the two components of the artificial joint. These parts are secured in place, the femur is repaired, and the muscles and tendons are replaced and repaired.

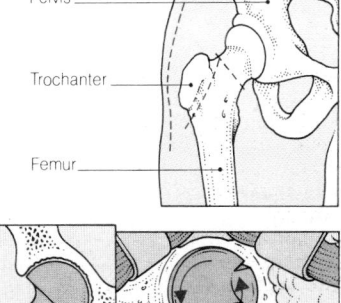
Sites of incision
Pelvis
Trochanter
Femur

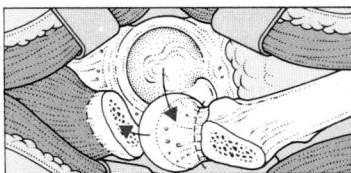

1 The trochanter at the top of the femur is detached, and the hip joint is dislocated to separate the femur and the pelvis. The ball at the top of the femur is then cut away.

2 An instrument known as a reamer is used to make the hollow in the pelvis large enough to make room for the cup-shaped socket formed by the two components of the artificial hip joint.

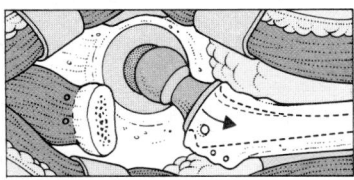

3 A coarse file is used to cut a shaft in the femur, and the ball part of the artificial joint is inserted. The components are fixed in place with a special cement, which binds them to the bone.

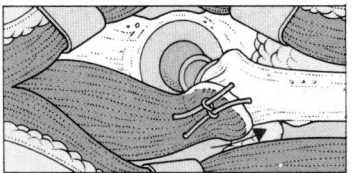

4 The ball is placed in the socket and the trochanter is re-attached to the femur with wires. The muscles and tendons are replaced and repaired, and the incision is then closed.

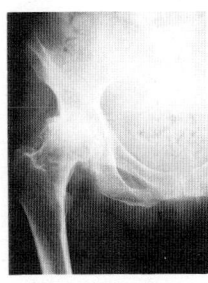
Before
This X-ray shows a hip joint that has been badly damaged by arthritis.

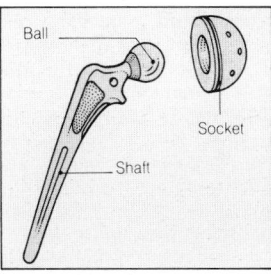
Ball
Socket
Shaft
Components
An artificial hip joint has two parts. The ball and shaft are metal; the socket may be metal or plastic.

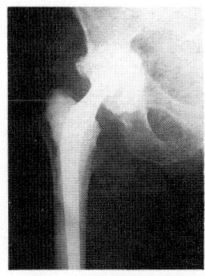
After
This X-ray shows the artificial hip joint in position after surgery.

suffered from severe pain and stiffness. However, with time, a substantial proportion of artificial joints show signs on X-ray of loosening at the cemented union between the bone and the metal. Surgeons and engineers are continuing to develop newer joint designs that do not rely on cement to hold them in place.

Hip, snapping
A fairly common condition in adults in which a characteristic clicking is heard and felt during certain movements of the joint. Snapping hip is generally harmless and does not indicate disease of the hip joint. The noise and sensation are caused by a tendon slipping over the bony prominence on the

outside of the femur when the hip is bent upwards. A snapping hip is different from the clicking that can be heard during examination of the hip of a newborn baby with dislocation of the hip (see *Hip, congenital dislocation of*).

Hirschsprung's disease

A congenital disorder in which a segment of intestine lacks the ganglion cells that control the intestine's rhythmic contractions. The segment without ganglion cells extends up from the lower end of the rectum, usually also involving the last part of the colon. This segment becomes narrowed and blocks the movement of faecal material. As a result, the area of intestine above the narrowed segment becomes widened and convoluted.

Hirschsprung's disease is uncommon and tends to run in families. It occurs about four times more often in boys than in girls.

SYMPTOMS
Symptoms usually appear in infancy or early childhood; they include constipation and bloating. The child usually has a poor appetite and may fail to grow properly.

DIAGNOSIS
A barium enema (see *Barium X-ray examinations*) can show the narrowed segment of the intestine. A *biopsy* (removal of a sample of tissue for microscopic analysis) may be performed during *proctoscopy* (inspection of the rectum with a viewing instrument) or during a surgical procedure. Examination of the biopsy sample will show whether ganglion cells are lacking and thus confirm the diagnosis.

TREATMENT
Treatment involves removing the narrowed intestinal segment and rejoining the normal areas of intestine. Before surgery, a temporary *colostomy* (creation of an artificial outlet for the colon through the abdominal wall) may be necessary if the child is considerably underweight.

Hirsutism
Excessive hairiness, particularly in women. The additional hair is coarse, like a man's, and grows in a male pattern on the face, trunk, and limbs.

CAUSES AND INCIDENCE
Hirsutism occurs in some conditions, such as polycystic ovary syndrome (see *Ovary, polycystic*) and congenital *adrenal hyperplasia*, in which the level of male hormones in the blood is abnormally high. Hirsutism can also be caused by taking anabolic steroids (see *Steroids, anabolic*).

Much more commonly, hirsutism is not a sign of any underlying disorder; it occurs in many normal women, especially after the *menopause*. The condition tends to run in families. Women with dark hair, particularly those of Indian or Hispanic extraction, are particularly likely to be hirsute.

TREATMENT
Hair can be bleached or removed in various ways (see *Hair removal*); the only method of permanent removal is by *electrolysis*. (See also *Hypertrichosis*.)

Histamine
A chemical present in cells (mainly *mast cells*) throughout the body that is released during an allergic reaction (see *Allergy*). Histamine is one of the substances responsible for the swelling and redness that occur in *inflammation*. Histamine also narrows the bronchi (airways) in the lungs, causes itching, and stimulates production of acid by the stomach.

The effects of histamine can be counteracted by *antihistamine drugs*; its action on the acid-forming glands in the stomach is blocked by a group of H_2-*receptor antagonists*.

Histamine$_2$-receptor antagonists
See H_2-*receptor antagonists*.

Histiocytosis X
A rare childhood disease in which there is an overgrowth of a type of tissue cell called a histiocyte. The cause is unknown, but histiocytosis X probably results from a disturbance of the *immune system*.

In the mildest form of the disease, rapid cell growth occurs in one bone only, usually affecting the skull, a clavicle, a rib, or a vertebra, causing swelling and pain. The chances of recovery are good in these cases.

The most severe, and least common, form of the disease affects infants. This form causes a skin rash and enlargement of the liver, spleen, and lymph nodes. The chances of recovery in these cases is poor.

Histocompatibility antigens
A group of proteins that are naturally present within tissues and that have a role in the *immune system* (body's natural defences). The main group of histocompatibility antigens is known as the HLA (human leukocyte antigen) system. A person's tissue type (i.e. the particular set of HLAs in the body tissues) is inherited half from the father and half from the mother. The

main role of HLAs is their defence role against infections and tumours, but they also influence the outcome of organ transplantation (see *Transplant surgery*) and seem to have an effect on individuals' susceptibility to certain diseases.

TYPES AND STRUCTURE
Synthesis of histocompatibility antigens takes place within cells and is under the control of genes. These genes, which are known as the major histocompatibility complex, give rise to several series of antigens, called HLA-A, HLA-B, HLA-C, and HLA-D.

Each histocompatibility antigen is composed of two parts, a constant region (which is the same for all people) and a variable region (which differs among people). The structure of this region is genetically determined (inherited from one of the parents) and can take any of several forms, which have been given numbers. Thus, a particular antigen has a letter (the series it belongs to) and a number corresponding to the form within the series—for example, HLA-A3, HLA-B13, or HLA-C5 types. The number of possible combinations of antigens from the different series is vast, but unrelated people with identical combinations occur at a rate of one in 50,000. By a technique called *tissue typing* every person can be immunologically "fingerprinted".

IMMUNOLOGICAL FUNCTION
Histocompatibility antigens within the series HLA-A, B, and C are present on virtually all living cells in the body. They are essential for the function of certain *lymphocytes* (white blood cells with an immunological function) called killer T cells. The antigens act as a guide for killer T cells to recognize and kill abnormal cells (i.e. virus-infected and tumour cells).

Histocompatibility antigens within the HLA-D series are present on the surfaces of various other cells with a defence role; they influence the interactions of these cells in fighting infection and tumours.

EFFECT IN TRANSPLANTATION
When an organ is transplanted from one person to another, the histocompatibility antigens in the donor organ are generally recognized as foreign and are attacked by the recipient's immune system, leading to rejection. However, if a donor can be found whose HLA types are very similar to those of the recipient (often a blood relative and ideally an identical twin), the chances of rejection occurring are minimized.

DISEASE ASSOCIATION

Certain HLA types occur more frequently in patients with particular diseases than in the rest of the population. For example, *multiple sclerosis* is associated with HLA-A3, *coeliac disease* with HLA-B8, and *ankylosing spondylitis* with HLA-B27.

It is suspected that susceptibility to these diseases is influenced by the HLA types, presumably as a result of their immunological actions. The associations are of interest because they allow identification of individuals at risk and can help in the confirmation of disease.

PATERNITY TESTING

Comparison of HLA types can sometimes show that two people are likely to be related and HLA analysis has therefore sometimes been used in *paternity testing*. This use is now being superseded by modern techniques of *genetic fingerprinting*, which can show relationship with greater certainty.

Histology

The study of tissues, including their cellular structure and function. The main practical use of histology in medicine is in the diagnosis of disease. This often involves obtaining a tissue sample by *biopsy* and examining it under a microscope for abnormalities. The histologist's skill lies in his or her familiarity with the range of normal appearances of tissues and the recognition of the abnormal appearances that occur in different diseases.

Histopathology

The branch of *histology* (the study of tissues) concerned with the effects of disease on the microscopic structure of tissues.

Histoplasmosis

An infection caused by inhaling the spores of HISTOPLASMA CAPSULATUM, a fungus found in soil, particularly in soil contaminated with droppings from birds or bats. Histoplasmosis occurs in parts of the Americas, the Far East, and Africa.

History-taking

The process by which a doctor learns from patients the symptoms of their illnesses and any previous disorders. (See *Diagnosis*.)

HIV

Human immunodeficiency virus. HIV belongs to the class of retroviruses (see *Virus*) and is the cause of *AIDS* and *AIDS-related complex*.

HIV gains access to the body via contaminated blood transfusions, nonsterile needles, or sexual intercourse. A fetus may be infected via the placenta. HIV has an affinity for the *T-lymphocytes*, in which the virus multiplies and, in some cases, destroys function. HIV also attacks the brain and may cause severe damage with *dementia*, although most infected people succumb to AIDS before this.

HIV is an organism of low infectivity; infected people present no threat to the health of their contacts at work or home, except for sexual partners and needle sharers.

The virus that causes AIDS was discovered at the Institut Pasteur in Paris and named the lymphadenopathy associated virus (LAV). In 1984, research workers in the US identified an AIDS virus which they classed as a retrovirus similar to viruses already linked with a rare type of human leukaemia. They named their virus human T cell lymphotropic virus III or HTLV III. The LAV virus and the HTLV virus subsequently proved to be identical and the name now agreed for the organism that causes AIDS is the human immunodeficiency virus or HIV.

More recent research has shown that some AIDS patients in Africa have been infected with a virus that is very similar to HIV. This variant is known as HIV II. A third related virus causes an AIDS-like disease in monkeys. At present, these rarer viruses seem to be found only in Africa.

Hives

An alternative name for *urticaria*.

HLA types

See *Histocompatibility antigens*.

Hoarseness

A rough, husky, or croaking voice, usually caused by interference with the normal working of the vocal cords in the *larynx* (voice box). Most attacks do not last long and clear up of their own accord, but persistent hoarseness requires investigation to exclude the possibility of serious disease.

CAUSES

Hoarseness of limited duration is often due to overuse of the voice (for example, in teachers or singers), which strains small muscles in the larynx. It is also commonly caused by inflammation of the vocal cords as part of acute *laryngitis*, which is usually due to an upper respiratory

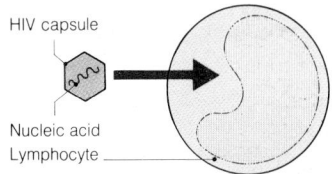

HOW HUMAN IMMUNODEFICIENCY VIRUS (HIV) MULTIPLIES

HIV capsule

Nucleic acid
Lymphocyte

1 HIV, like any virus, consists of some nucleic acid inside a capsule made of protein. The virus invades a lymphocyte (type of white blood cell).

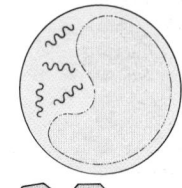

2 The strand of nucleic acid escapes from the capsule and uses the host cell's resources to make copies of itself.

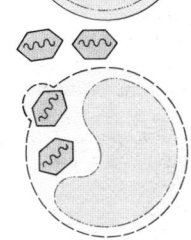

3 Each copy forms a capsule and leaves the host cell, which eventually ceases to function efficiently in fighting disease.

tract infection such as a cold or sore throat. (See overleaf.)

Persistent hoarseness has many possible causes. It may be due to chronic irritation of the larynx (which can be caused by smoking or excessive consumption of alcohol) or to chronic *bronchitis*. Irritation can also be caused by mucus dripping on to the larynx, which may occur in people with nasal *polyps* (harmless growths in the nose), allergic *rhinitis* (hay fever), *sinusitis*, or a deviated *nasal septum* (displacement of the cartilage that separates the two nasal passages).

Polyps on the vocal cords may also cause hoarseness, as may any accidental damage to them during surgery on the thyroid gland. In people with *hypothyroidism* (underactivity of the thyroid gland), hoarseness can result from formation of tissue on the vocal cords.

In young children, hoarseness is a symptom of *croup* (inflammation and narrowing of the airways).

Occasionally, persistent hoarseness in adults has a more serious cause—including cancer of the larynx (see *Larynx, cancer of*). Less commonly, persistent hoarseness is caused by *thyroid cancer* or by *lung cancer*.

HOARSENESS OR LOSS OF VOICE
Any abnormal huskiness in the voice that may be so severe that you can make little or no sound.

Has the hoarseness started within the past three days?

YES → **Do you have or have you just had a cold, cough, or sore throat?**

YES → You probably have inflammation of the vocal cords.
See • *Laryngitis*

NO ↓

Had you been using your voice more than usual just before the hoarseness or loss of voice developed?

YES → Overuse can irritate the vocal cords.
See • *Laryngitis*

NO ↓

Have you recently become tense, nervous, or depressed?

YES → Anxiety can sometimes cause a sudden loss of voice.
See • *Anxiety*

NO

NO ↓

Are you over 40 years old and has your voice deepened?

YES → **Have you noticed two or more of the following symptoms?**
• feeling the cold more than you used to
• dry skin or hair
• weight increase without overeating
• unexplained tiredness

YES → An underactive thyroid gland is a possibility. This is an uncommon problem that is most likely to occur in middle-aged women. Consult your doctor.
See • *Hypothyroidism*

NO

NO ↓

Do you smoke?

YES → Smoking can lead to inflammation of the vocal cords.
See • *Laryngitis*

NO ↓

Have you been drinking alcohol recently?

YES → Drinking alcohol can lead to inflammation of the vocal cords.
See • *Laryngitis*

NO ↓

Self-help
Hoarseness usually clears up after a few days with simple measures such as resting the voice and abstaining from smoking and alcohol.

Continued on next page

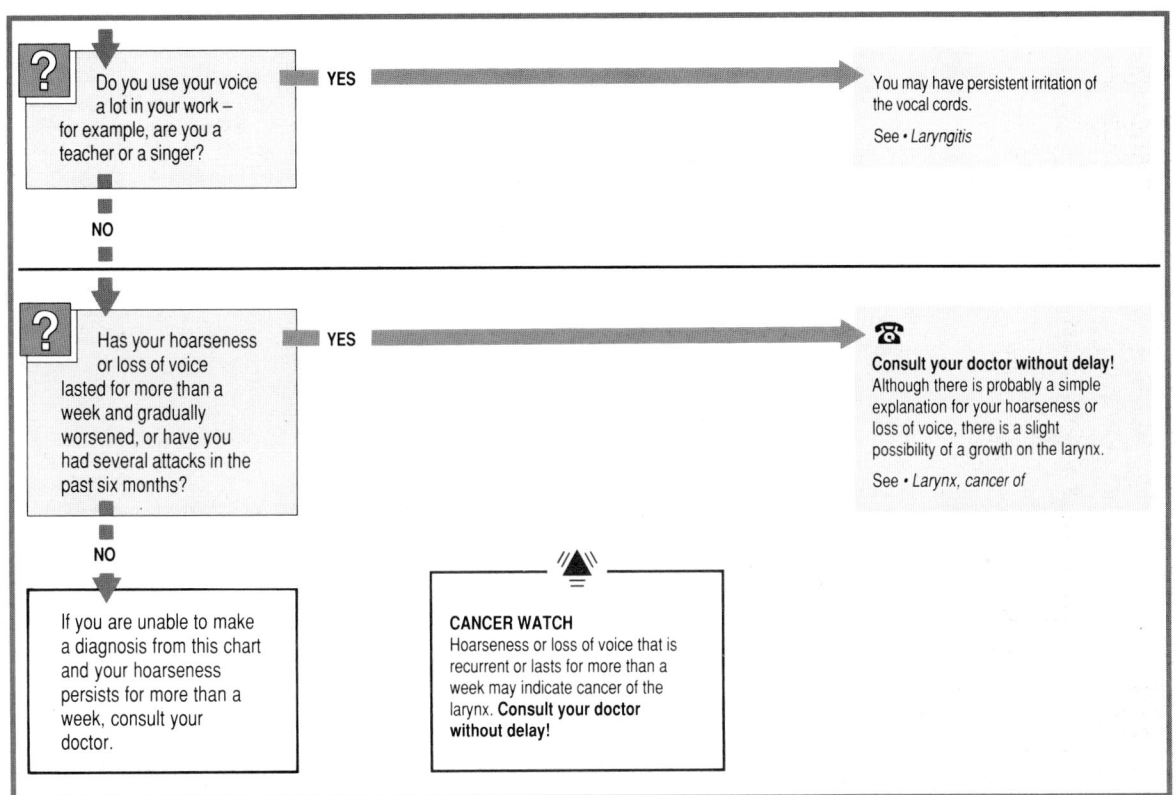

Do you use your voice a lot in your work – for example, are you a teacher or a singer?

YES → You may have persistent irritation of the vocal cords.

See • *Laryngitis*

NO

Has your hoarseness or loss of voice lasted for more than a week and gradually worsened, or have you had several attacks in the past six months?

YES → ☎ **Consult your doctor without delay!** Although there is probably a simple explanation for your hoarseness or loss of voice, there is a slight possibility of a growth on the larynx.

See • *Larynx, cancer of*

NO

If you are unable to make a diagnosis from this chart and your hoarseness persists for more than a week, consult your doctor.

CANCER WATCH
Hoarseness or loss of voice that is recurrent or lasts for more than a week may indicate cancer of the larynx. **Consult your doctor without delay!**

H

SELF-HELP

Anyone suffering from hoarseness believed to be brought on by straining the voice should rest his or her voice until it has returned to normal; otherwise, permanent damage may eventually occur in the vocal cords. Voice training may reduce the likelihood of the hoarseness recurring. Resting the voice, along with not smoking or drinking alcohol, also helps recovery from laryngitis.

INVESTIGATION

It is essential to consult a doctor if hoarseness persists for more than two weeks. In such cases, a *laryngoscopy* (examination of the larynx with a mirror or viewing tube) will be performed to exclude the possibility of cancer (which can be completely cured if diagnosed early).

Hodgkin's disease

Also known as Hodgkin's lymphoma, a malignant disorder in which there is proliferation of cells in the lymphoid tissue (found mainly in the *lymph nodes* and *spleen*) and a resultant enlargement of the lymph nodes. Lymphoid tissue is an important part of the *immune system*. The cause of Hodgkin's disease is unknown.

INCIDENCE

Hodgkin's disease is an uncommon cancer, about 3,000 new cases are diagnosed annually in the UK. This disorder is more common in men than in women, and most commonly develops between the ages of 20 and 30, and between 55 and 70.

SYMPTOMS AND SIGNS

The most common sign is painless enlargement of a group of lymph nodes, typically those in the neck or armpits. Most symptoms are caused by the presence of the enlarged nodes, invasion of other organs by proliferating lymphoid tissue, or impairment of the body's immune system. Thus, there may be a general feeling of illness, with fever, loss of appetite, weight loss, and night sweats. There may also be generalized itching and, rarely, pain after drinking alcohol. Involvement of other organs may cause a diverse range of symptoms (such as breathlessness if the lungs are involved or paralysis if the spine is affected). As the disease progresses, the immune system becomes increasingly impaired and the patient may suffer life-threatening complications from an infection that would normally be trivial.

DIAGNOSIS

Diagnosis of Hodgkin's disease depends on the identification of characteristic cells, called Reed-Sternberg cells, in a *biopsy* specimen (sample of tissue removed for microscopic analysis) from an enlarged lymph node or other affected organ.

Analysis is also made of the relative proportions of other cells in the specimen—including plasma cells, eosinophils, lymphocytes, and granulocytes (all types of white blood cell). This enables the disease to be classified according to its histological type, which is one factor that affects the chances of a cure.

The extent of the disease (known as its *stage*) is also assessed in terms of the number of groups of lymph nodes affected and in terms of any other organs that are involved. This process, called staging, is important for the planning of treatment. Typically, staging includes a *chest X-ray*, *CT scanning* or *MRI* of the abdomen, and a *bone marrow biopsy*.

Other tests may include *laparotomy* (surgical exploration of the abdomen), *liver biopsy, splenectomy,* or *lymphangiography* (X-ray imaging of the lymphatic system) of the abdomen.

TREATMENT AND OUTLOOK

In an early stage, *radiotherapy* is usually curative. If the disease has progressed to involve many organs, however, treatment with *anticancer drugs* is usually recommended and may have to be continued for several months. In some cases, both radiotherapy and drug treatment are used.

The outlook depends on the stage to which the disease has progressed and on the histological type. With current treatment, 75 per cent of patients with newly diagnosed Hodgkin's disease should be cured, and the remainder will have long remissions. (See also *Lymphoma, non-Hodgkin's*.)

Hole in the heart

The common name for a *septal defect*.

Holistic medicine

A form of therapy aimed at treating the whole person—body and mind—not just the part or parts of the body in which symptoms occur. A holistic approach is emphasized by many practitioners of *alternative medicine*, such as homeopathists, acupuncturists, and herbalists.

Holter monitor

A monitoring device that records an electrocardiogram (see *ECG*) continuously for periods of 24 hours or longer. The device is worn by the patient and does not interfere with daily activities. Its use allows the detection and identification of paroxysmal *arrhythmias* (intermittent irregularities in the heartbeat), which cause palpitations or fainting episodes.

Homeopathy

A system of *alternative medicine* that seeks to treat patients by administering small doses of medicines that in a healthy person would bring on symptoms similar to those that the medicine is prescribed to treat.

For example, the homeopathic treatment for diarrhoea would be a very dilute laxative preparation.

Homeostasis

The dynamic processes by which an organism maintains a constant internal environment despite external changes. Homeostasis is a major function of most organs and includes the regulation of blood pressure, body temperature, and blood sugar levels.

Homeostatic mechanisms are vital in the body since tissues and organs can function efficiently only within a narrow range of conditions such as temperature and acidity: homeostasis regulates these by negative feedback. When a certain factor varies from its optimum set point, automatic regulatory mechanisms counterbalance the disturbance and re-establish the internal equilibrium. For example, when the body overheats, sweating is stimulated until the temperature returns to normal. Similarly, when the oxygen level in the blood is low, breathing is stimulated; when blood pressure falls, the heart-rate increases.

Homeostatic mechanisms sometimes malfunction. For example, in malignant *hyperthermia*, the body's thermostat is somehow reset to a higher temperature than normal. In *diabetes mellitus*, blood sugar levels can no longer be regulated because of a malfunction in insulin production.

Homocystinuria

A rare, inherited condition caused by an *enzyme* deficiency. Homocystinuria is a type of inborn error of metabolism (see *Metabolism, inborn errors of*) in which there is an abnormal presence of homocystine (an *amino acid*) in the blood and urine. Affected people are very tall, with long limbs and long, spindly fingers. Some have skeletal deformities, such as spinal curvature, and abnormalities of the eye lens.

Homocystinuria cannot be cured, but some cases may be improved by vitamin B_6 and a special diet.

Homosexuality, female

See *Lesbianism*.

Homosexuality, male

Sexual attraction to other men. Studies of sexuality, such as those of Alfred Kinsey in the 1940s and the Wellcome Trust in 1994, have put the proportion of exclusively homosexual men at between two and five per cent, but many more have had sexual contact with another man at some time.

Homosexuals achieve orgasm in various ways, including oral sex, mutual masturbation, and anal penetration. Each partner may adopt a particular role in the relationship (either active or passive) but more often the roles are interchangeable.

CAUSES

Various behavioural theories have been put forward to explain homosexuality, none having been widely accepted. Research in the early 1990s suggested that a gene on the X chromosome might be an important factor in the cause of homosexuality in at least some men; homosexuality is found in a larger-than-chance number of brothers and male cousins of homosexual men. Its prevalence appears to be much the same in all cultures, with no change over thousands of years, suggesting that homosexuality is a consistent variation in behaviour.

PROBLEMS

Homosexuality is more openly considered nowadays, but some homosexuals feel guilty about their sexual orientation. They may mask their feelings behind apparent heterosexuality or may seek medical help.

Some homosexuals are placed at high risk of *sexually transmitted diseases* by having multiple partners and high rates of sexual activity; it was in homosexual males that the virus responsible for *AIDS* was first identified. (See also *Bisexuality*.)

Homozygote

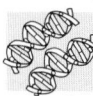

A term used to describe a person whose cells contain two identical *genes* controlling a specified inherited trait, in contrast to a *heterozygote*, whose cells contain two different genes controlling that trait. (See also *Inheritance; Genetic disorders*.)

Hookworm infestation

An infestation of the small intestine by small, round, blood-sucking worms of the species *NECATOR AMERICANUS* or *ANCYLOSTOMA DUODENALE*. The worms are about 12 mm long and have hook-like teeth.

INCIDENCE AND CAUSES

Hookworms infest about 700 million people worldwide, mainly those living in poor countries in the tropics. There is no risk of contracting a hookworm infestation in the UK; visitors to tropical countries may be at risk.

The accompanying illustration shows how hookworms can enter and multiply in the body. In a heavy infestation, there may be several hundred worms in the intestine, consuming up to 50 ml of blood every day.

SYMPTOMS AND COMPLICATIONS

When the larvae penetrate the skin, a red and intensely itchy rash may develop on the feet. This is called ground itch and may last for several days. In light infestations, there may be no further symptoms. In heavier infestations, migration of the larvae through the lungs may produce cough and pneumonia; the presence of adult worms in the intestines may cause vague abdominal discomfort.

By far the most important problem caused by a heavy infestation of hookworms is iron-deficiency *anaemia* due to loss of blood.

DIAGNOSIS AND TREATMENT

Diagnosis is made by microscopic examination of faeces, which can reveal hookworm eggs. *Anthelmintic drugs*, such as *mebendazole*, kill the worms. Treatment also involves improving nutrition with a high-protein diet and correcting anaemia with iron tablets or blood transfusions, if necessary. Elimination of the disease from a community depends on efficient sanitation. (See also *Larva migrans*.)

Hormonal disorders

Conditions that are caused by malfunction of an endocrine gland. See *Endocrine system* and disorders of the *adrenal glands; ovaries; pancreas; parathyroid glands; pituitary gland; testes; thyroid gland.*

Hormonal methods of contraception

See *Contraception, hormonal methods of.*

Hormone

A chemical released into the bloodstream by a particular gland or tissue that has a specific effect on tissues elsewhere in the body.

Many hormones are produced by the glands of the *endocrine system* (the *adrenal glands, ovaries* or *testes, pancreas, parathyroid glands, pituitary gland,* and *thyroid gland*). Hormones are also secreted by other organs, including the kidneys, intestines, brain, and, in women who are pregnant, the *placenta*.

Hormones control numerous body functions, including the *metabolism* (chemical activity) of cells, growth, sexual development, and the body's response to stress or illness. (See the accompanying table on page 543.)

Hormone antagonist

A drug that blocks the action of a *hormone* (chemical messenger released by a gland). *Tamoxifen*, for example, blocks the effects of *oestrogen hormones* and is used in the treatment of some types of breast cancer.

Hormone replacement therapy

The use of a synthetic or natural *hormone* (chemical messenger released by a gland) to treat a hormone deficiency. The term describes the replacement of any deficient hormone, such as giving *thyroid hormones* to treat *hypothyroidism* or *insulin* to treat *diabetes mellitus*. More commonly, hormone replacement therapy refers to the use of *oestrogen hormones* to treat symptoms accompanying the *menopause*.

WHY IT IS DONE

Oestrogen replacement therapy is given to relieve menopausal symptoms such as hot flushes and excessive sweating at night. Oestrogen hormones help prevent atrophic *vaginitis* (thinning and dryness of the vagina), which may make sexual intercourse painful and difficult. Oestrogen hormones also help prevent the development of *osteoporosis* (reduction in bone density) and *atherosclerosis* (narrowing of the arteries by deposits of fatty material).

HOW IT IS DONE

In hormone replacement therapy, oestrogen drugs are usually prescribed in combination with a *progestogen drug* because oestrogen drugs given alone may increase a woman's susceptibility to cancer of the uterus.

The drugs are usually taken orally in a three-stage cycle repeated each month—oestrogen for the first 11 to 14 days, oestrogen and a progestogen for the next seven to 10 days, and no drugs for the last seven days, during which there is often a light menstrual period. Alternatively, oestrogen may be released slowly into the bloodstream from a hormonal *implant* placed under the skin of the abdomen; or from an adhesive patch placed on the skin of the lower trunk. The progestogen is still taken in tablet form.

Therapy is usually given for two to five years, but many women take hormones for much longer to maximize the beneficial effects on their bones and cardiovascular systems. Weight and blood pressure checks, breast and pelvic examinations, and *cervical smear tests*, are carried out regularly to monitor the effects of the therapy. Occasionally, a *biopsy* (removal of a sample of tissue for microscopic analysis) of the lining of the uterus may be carried out to test for cancer.

POSSIBLE ADVERSE EFFECTS

Minor adverse effects include nausea, breast tenderness, fluid retention, and leg cramps. In some women, oestrogen replacement therapy may increase the risk of abnormal blood clotting, and is therefore not usually given to women who smoke heavily or have suffered from *thrombosis, stroke,* liver disease, or severe *hypertension* (raised blood pressure). Women who have had treatment for hormonally-dependent cancers, such as those of the breast or uterus, need careful assessment to balance the benefits and risks of hormone replacement treatment.

HOOKWORM LIFE-CYCLE

Infestation begins with larvae that penetrate the skin or are ingested and enter the bloodstream. They migrate throughout the body, particularly to the small intestine. Adult worms develop and lay eggs, which leave the body in faeces and eventually hatch into larvae.

Head of hookworm
The hookworm uses its sharp, curved, tooth-like structures to cling to the bowel.

The larvae travel to the lungs and are coughed up and swallowed.

In the intestines the larvae develop into adult worms. Eggs produced by the females pass out in the faeces and hatch into larvae in soil.

Larvae burrow through the skin of a person's feet.

Horn, cutaneous

A hard, noncancerous protrusion occasionally found on the skin (usually the face) of elderly people. Horns are slow-growing and vary in colour from yellow to brown to black. They may develop where there was previously a wart on normal skin.

Left untreated, they can grow to a considerable size and may protrude as much as 2 cm. Surgical removal is usually recommended.

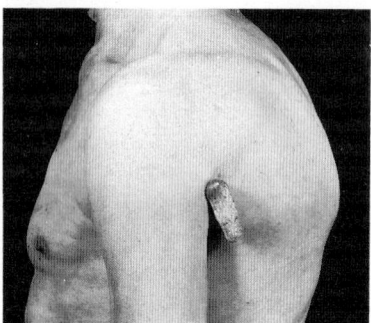

Appearance of cutaneous horn
The horny protuberance that has developed under the arm results from an overgrowth of keratin (a skin protein).

Horner's syndrome

A group of physical signs that affects one side of the face and indicates damage to part of the sympathetic nervous system (see *Autonomic nervous system*). The signs of Horner's syndrome are narrowing of the pupil of the eye, drooping of the lid, and absence of sweating. They are caused by damage to or destruction of sympathetic nerve fibres, usually in the lower part of the neck, and may be the first indication of disease in the area.

Horseshoe kidney

A congenital abnormality in which the two kidneys are fused or joined at the base, forming a horseshoe shape. The condition may be diagnosed antenatally by *ultrasound scanning.*

The joined kidneys usually function normally but may be associated with other congenital kidney abnormalities.

Hospice

A hospital or part of a hospital devoted to the care of patients who are dying (often of cancer). See *Dying, care of the.*

Hospitals, types of

All the really large hospitals in the UK are part of the NHS. However, in the early 1990s many chose to become self-governing trusts, independent of Health Service administration, as part of an NHS reorganization that aimed for increased efficiency by encouraging hospitals to attend to the financial aspects of the care they provided. Many large, old-style hospitals for the mentally ill were closed at this time, with community care becoming the mainstream approach to these patients .

The underlying structure of the NHS remained unchanged, however. Each health district has a general hospital—often a trust—serving a population of 200,000 to 500,000, and providing specialist services in medicine, surgery, obstetrics, gynaecology, and paediatrics. Some more specialist services are concentrated in fewer centres.

Most of the UK's 2,000 private hospitals are, in fact, nursing homes for the elderly infirm. There are around 200 acute hospitals, in which much non-emergency surgery is carried out (around 10 per cent of all such surgery is in the private sector). A few private hospitals provide obstetric care, and around 50 provide inpatient care for the mentally ill or those suffering from *alcohol dependence* or *drug dependence.*

Hot flushes

Reddening of the face, neck, and upper trunk usually caused by decreased *oestrogen hormone* production by the ovaries during or after the *menopause.* Hot flushes may also occur after removal of the ovaries (see *Oophorectomy*). Occasionally, men experience hot flushes after removal of the testes (see *Orchidectomy*), which causes a reduction in testosterone levels.

Hot flushes typically last one to two minutes. They are accompanied by a sensation of heat, are often followed by sweating, and are aggravated by stress. If severe, they can often be alleviated by *hormone replacement therapy.*

Housemaid's knee

Inflammation of the *bursa* (fluid-filled sac) that acts as a cushion over the kneecap. The inflammation is usually caused by prolonged kneeling, but may develop after a blow to the front of the knee. (See also *Bursitis.*)

Human chorionic gonadotrophin

See *Gonadotrophin, human chorionic.*

Humerus

The bone of the upper arm. The smooth, dome-shaped head of the bone lies at an angle to the shaft and fits into a shallow socket in the scapula (shoulder blade) to form the shoulder joint. Below its head, the bone narrows to form a cylindrical shaft. It flattens and widens at its lower end, forming a prominence on each side called an epicondyle. At its base, it articulates with the *ulna* and *radius* (the bones of the lower arm) to form the elbow.

A spiral groove in the shaft of the humerus carries the *radial nerve,* one of the main nerves of the arm.

Humerus, fracture of

Fractures of the *humerus* (the bone of the upper arm) may affect the upper end, the shaft, or the lower end of the bone. The part of the humerus most commonly fractured is the neck of the bone (at the upper end of the humerus, just below the bone's head). This type of fracture most often occurs in elderly people. Fractures of the shaft of the humerus usually affect the middle third of the bone. Such fractures occur in adults of all ages but are uncommon in children. Supracondylar fractures (at the lower end of the bone) occur most commonly in children.

DIAGNOSIS AND TREATMENT
An *X-ray* is performed if any fracture of the humerus is suspected.

A fracture of the neck of the bone usually requires only a *sling* to immobilize the bone; a fracture of the shaft or the lower end of the bone usually needs a plaster *cast.* Most fractures of the humerus heal in six to eight weeks.

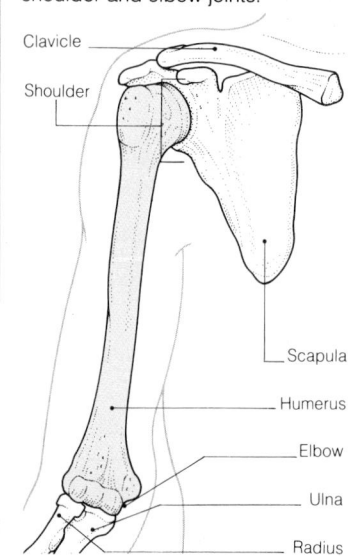

LOCATION OF HUMERUS
The humerus is the bone of the upper arm, located between the shoulder and elbow joints.

Clavicle

Shoulder

Scapula

Humerus

Elbow

Ulna

Radius

H

COMPLICATIONS

Damage to the radial nerve may occur when the shaft of the humerus is fractured. In severe cases, this may result in *wrist-drop*. Fracture of the humerus may be accompanied by damage to the brachial artery. If such damage is undetected, circulation to the arm may be impaired, resulting in *Volkmann's contracture* (a deformity of the forearm and hand due to muscle damage caused by insufficient blood supply). Some supracondylar fractures fail to mend properly—despite all remedial efforts and traction—resulting in deformity of the elbow and an increased risk that *osteoarthritis* will eventually develop.

THE SOURCES AND MAIN EFFECTS OF SELECTED HORMONES

Section of body	Hormone secreted	Effects
Hypothalamus	Releasing hormones	Stimulate hormone secretion by pituitary gland
Pituitary gland	Growth hormone	Stimulates growth and metabolism
	Prolactin	Stimulates milk production after childbirth
	ACTH (adrenocorticotrophic hormone)	Stimulates hormone production by adrenal glands.
	TSH (thyroid-stimulating hormone)	Stimulates hormone production by thyroid gland
	FSH (follicle-stimulating hormone); LH (luteinizing hormone)	Stimulate gonads (ovaries or testes)
	ADH (antidiuretic hormone)	Acts on kidneys to reduce urine production.
	Oxytocin	Stimulates contractions of uterus during labour and ejection of milk during breast-feeding
	MSH (melanocyte-stimulating hormone)	Acts on the skin to promote production of skin pigment (melanin)
Brain	Endorphins; enkephalins	Alleviate pain
Thyroid gland	Thyroid hormone	Increases metabolic rate; affects growth
	Calcitonin	Controls level of calcium in blood
Parathyroid glands	Parathyroid hormone	Controls level of calcium in blood
Thymus	Thymic hormone	Stimulates lymphocyte development
Adrenal glands	Adrenaline; noradrenaline	Prepare body for stress
	Hydrocortisone	Affects metabolism
	Aldosterone	Regulates sodium and potassium excretion by kidneys
	Androgens	Affect growth and sex drive
Kidneys	Renin	Regulates blood pressure
	Erythropoietin	Stimulates erythrocyte production
	Vitamin D	Controls calcium and phosphate metabolism
Pancreas	Insulin; glucagon	Regulate blood sugar level
Placenta	Chorionic gonadotrophin; oestrogens; progesterone	Maintain pregnancy
Gastrointestinal tract	Gastrin; secretin; cholecystokinin	Regulate secretion of some digestive enzymes
Testes	Testosterone	Affects development of male secondary sexual characteristics and genital organs
Ovaries	Oestrogens; progesterone	Affect development of female secondary sexual characteristics and genital organs; control menstrual cycle; maintain pregnancy

The various glands that make up the hormonal system constitute a control and communications network that is complementary to the nervous system. However, instead of using nerve impulses, the glands secrete chemical messengers (hormones) to affect other glands and tissues in various parts of the body. Hormones are carried in the bloodstream to their targets, where they exert their specific effects. This table lists the hormones secreted by different parts of the body and gives a description of their wide-ranging actions.

Humours

Liquid or jelly-like substances in the body. The term usually refers to the aqueous humour (the watery fluid in the front chamber of the *eye*) and the *vitreous humour* (the jelly-like substance in the rear chamber of the eye).

According to early medical theory, four humours—blood, phlegm, black bile, and yellow bile—permeated the entire body, the balance between them determining its state of health.

Hunchback

See *Kyphosis.*

Hunger

A disagreeable feeling caused by the need for food (as opposed to *appetite,* a pleasant sensation felt in anticipation of a meal).

Hunger occurs when the stomach is empty and when the blood sugar level is low. In response to these stimuli, messages from the hypothalamus in the brain cause the muscular wall of the stomach to contract rhythmically, signalling the need for food; if pronounced, these contractions produce hunger pains.

Hunger caused by a low blood sugar level usually results from strenuous exercise. It can also occur in certain diseases, notably in *thyrotoxicosis,* a disorder of the thyroid gland that causes marked speeding-up of body processes, and in insulin-dependent *diabetes mellitus,* in cases where an incorrect balance between insulin and carbohydrate intake causes *hypoglycaemia* (low blood sugar level).

Huntington's disease

An uncommon disease, formerly known as Huntington's chorea, in which degeneration of the *basal ganglia* (paired nerve-cell clusters in the brain) results in *chorea* (rapid, jerky, involuntary movements) and *dementia* (progressive mental impairment). Symptoms do not usually appear until the age of 35 to 50; in rare cases the condition is apparent in childhood.

The disease is due to a defective *gene* on *chromosome* 4, and is inherited as an autosomal dominant disorder. Since the age of onset of symptoms is generally so late, an affected person may have children before realizing that he or she has the disease. Each child has a 50 per cent chance of the condition developing. The disease is present in about 5 to 8 persons per 100,000.

SYMPTOMS

The chorea usually affects the face, arms, and trunk, resulting in random grimaces and twitches and general clumsiness. Dementia takes the form of personality and behaviour changes, irritability, difficulty making decisions, memory loss, and apathy.

When the disease starts in childhood, it may be marked by loss of movement and muscle rigidity.

DIAGNOSIS

Identification of the gene responsible has made accurate diagnosis possible. It has opened up the possibility of telling individual members of families with the disease whether they have inherited the faulty gene (eventually to develop the symptoms and possibly pass on the disease to their children). The ethical implications of offering this knowledge to families are contentious, since many people at risk do not want to know whether they are affected; they may find out, however, through tests performed on other family members (see *Genetic counselling*).

TREATMENT AND OUTLOOK

Sufferers commonly live 15 to 30 years after the onset of symptoms. At present there is no known cure, and treatment is aimed at lessening the chorea with drugs such as tetrabenazine. Identification of the faulty gene and the protein it produces (huntingtin) has encouraged optimism that a treatment will eventually be found.

Hurler's syndrome

A rare, inherited condition caused by an *enzyme* defect. Hurler's syndrome is a type of inborn error of metabolism (see *Metabolism, inborn errors of*) in which there is an abnormal accumulation of substances known as mucopolysaccharides in the tissues.

Affected children may appear normal at birth, but, between six and 12 months of age develop cardiac abnormalities, umbilical hernia, skeletal deformities, and enlargement of the tongue, liver, and spleen. Physical growth is limited and mental development slows, leaving the child mentally handicapped.

The strange physical features of affected children gave the condition its former name of gargoylism.

Hydatid disease

 A rare infestation caused by the larval stage of the small tapeworm ECHINO-COCCUS GRANULOSUS. Larvae most often settle in the liver, lungs, or muscle, causing the development of slowly growing cysts. In rare cases, the brain or other organs are affected.

CAUSE AND INCIDENCE

The illustration on the next page shows how eggs or larvae can enter the body.

Hydatid disease is prevalent only in areas of the world where sheep are managed with the aid of dogs, such as Australia and New Zealand. It is extremely rare in the UK.

SYMPTOMS

Although the infestation is usually acquired in childhood, the cysts grow very slowly, so symptoms, if any, occur mainly in adults. In many cases there are no symptoms.

Cysts in the liver may cause a tender, localized lump or lead to *bile duct obstruction* and jaundice. Cysts in the lungs may press on an airway, causing inflammation; rupture of a lung cyst may cause chest pain, coughing up blood, and wheezing. Cysts in the brain can cause seizures or other symptoms similar to those of a brain tumour. Ruptured cysts may rarely cause *anaphylactic shock* (a severe allergic reaction), which may be fatal.

DIAGNOSIS AND TREATMENT

Hydatid cysts are diagnosed by *CT scanning* or *MRI.* Cysts may be removed surgically. Alternatively, they may be sterilized and then drained. Drug treatments are being investigated.

Hydatidiform mole

An uncommon benign tumour that develops from placental tissue early in a pregnancy in which the embryo has failed to develop normally. A hydatidiform mole, which resembles a bunch of small grapes, is caused by degeneration of the chorionic villi, minute finger-like projections in the placenta. The cause of the degeneration is unknown.

INCIDENCE

A hydatidiform mole is the most common form of trophoblastic tumour. It occurs in about one in 2,000 pregnancies in developed countries; the incidence is much higher in some developing countries. In about three per cent of affected pregnancies the growth develops into a *choriocarcinoma,* a malignant tumour that can invade the walls of the uterus if it is left untreated.

SYMPTOMS, DIAGNOSIS, AND TREATMENT

Vaginal bleeding and excessive morning sickness usually occur.

A hydatidiform tumour shows up on *ultrasound scanning.* Urine and blood tests detect excessive amounts of human chorionic gonadotrophin (see *Gonadotrophin, human chorionic*), which are produced by the tumour.

The tumour can be removed either by suctioning out the contents of the uterus or by a *D and C*. A *hysterectomy* may be considered.

OUTLOOK

There is a small risk that a malignant tumour may develop later; for this reason, tests are performed regularly for several years to determine the levels of human chorionic gonadotrophin in the blood and urine.

A woman should not become pregnant again until her human chorionic gonadotrophin levels have returned to normal for at least a year. There is a one in 75 risk of a recurrence of the condition in a future pregnancy.

Hydralazine

An *antihypertensive drug* which is particularly useful as an emergency treatment for *hypertension*. Hydralazine is also often used when the combination of *diuretic drugs* and *beta-blocker drugs* fails to control high blood pressure.

Hydralazine may cause nausea, vomiting, headache, dizziness, and irregular heartbeat. Less common adverse effects include loss of appetite, rash, and joint pain. When prescribed in high doses over a prolonged period, hydralazine may cause *lupus erythematosus*.

Hydramnios

See *Polyhydramnios*.

Hydrocele

A soft, painless swelling in the *scrotum* caused by the space around a *testis* filling with fluid. A hydrocele is sometimes caused by inflammation, infection, or injury to the testis; occasionally, the cause is a tumour. In most cases, however, there is no apparent cause.

Hydroceles occur very commonly in middle-aged men.

Treatment is rarely necessary. If the swelling is large enough to be uncomfortable or painful, the fluid may be aspirated (drawn off through a hollow needle) under a local anaesthetic. Recurrent swelling may be treated by surgery.

Hydrocephalus

An excessive amount of *cerebrospinal fluid*, usually under increased pressure, within the skull. The term "water on the brain" is a nonmedical phrase which is sometimes used to describe this condition.

Hydrocephalus is often associated with other congenital abnormalities, particularly *spina bifida*.

ORIGINS OF HYDATID DISEASE

The infestation is generally confined to dogs and sheep, but occasionally a child swallows eggs from dog faeces. These hatch into larvae, which migrate through the body, especially to the liver or lungs, to form slow-growing cysts. Symptoms may not appear until years later.

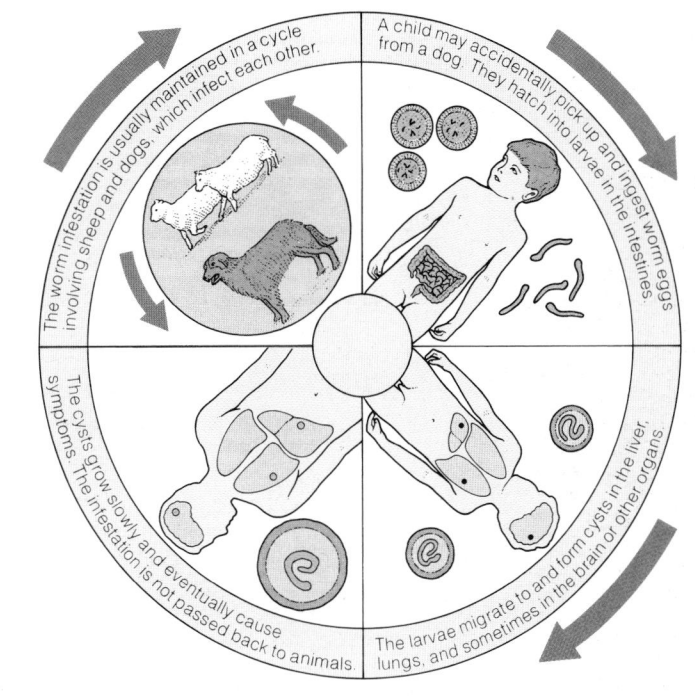

CAUSES

The condition may be *congenital* (present at birth) or may develop as a result of major head injury, brain haemorrhage, infection (*meningitis*, for example), or a tumour.

Hydrocephalus is caused by excessive formation of cerebrospinal fluid, by a block in the circulation of this fluid, or both.

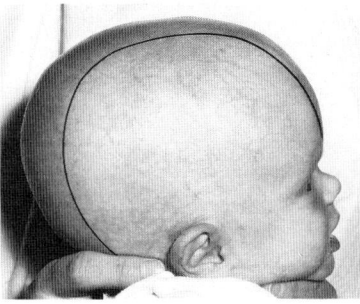

Infant with hydrocephalus
Skull enlargement is due to pressure from excess fluid within the cavities of the brain. To prevent brain damage, the fluid must be drained by means of a tube inserted through a hole made in the skull.

SYMPTOMS

When the condition is congenital, the main feature is an enlarged head that continues to grow at an abnormally fast rate because the bones are not rigid and expand to accommodate the fluid. Other features are rigidity of the legs, *epilepsy*, irritability, lethargy, vomiting, and the absence of normal reflex actions. If the condition is not treated, it progresses to extreme drowsiness, severe brain damage, and seizures, which may lead to the baby's death within a matter of weeks.

When the condition occurs later in childhood or in adulthood, the skull is no longer flexible and symptoms are caused by raised pressure within the skull. Symptoms include headache, vomiting, loss of coordination, and deterioration of mental function.

DIAGNOSIS AND TREATMENT

CT scanning or *MRI* show the location and nature of any obstruction.

In most cases, treatment aims to drain excess fluid away from the brain to another part of the body, such as the peritoneal cavity (lining of the abdomen), where it can be absorbed.

H

Drainage is achieved by means of a valve and *shunt* (tube), which is inserted into the brain through a hole made in the skull. In some cases, the shunt must be left in position for an indefinite period.

In older children and adults, treatment is sometimes only for the underlying cause.

Hydrochloric acid

A strong acid released by the stomach lining. It forms part of the stomach juices and is important in the digestion of proteins. Excessive acid production, which may be stimulated by stress or tobacco smoking, is an important factor in the development of *peptic ulcers*. In *acid reflux* (backflow of stomach acid into the oesophagus), hydrochloric acid may cause *oesophagitis* and heartburn. (See also *Digestive system*.)

Hydrochlorothiazide

A thiazide *diuretic drug* used to reduce *oedema* (fluid retention) in people with *heart failure* (reduced pumping efficiency), *nephrotic syndrome* (a kidney disorder), *cirrhosis* of the liver, and breast tenderness before menstruation. Hydrochlorothiazide is also given to treat *hypertension* (high blood pressure), and is occasionally used to prevent the recurrence of certain types of kidney stones (see *Calculus, urinary tract*).

POSSIBLE ADVERSE EFFECTS

Adverse effects include leg cramps, lethargy, dizziness, rash, and impotence. Hydrochlorothiazide may rarely cause *gout* and may aggravate *diabetes mellitus*.

Hydrocortisone

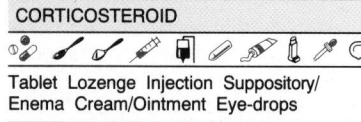

CORTICOSTEROID
Tablet Lozenge Injection Suppository/ Enema Cream/Ointment Eye-drops
Prescription sometimes needed
Available as generic

A *corticosteroid drug* used in creams, sprays, and other *topical* preparations for the treatment of inflammatory or allergic conditions, such as *ulcerative colitis* or *dermatitis*. Hydrocortisone, also called cortisol, is a hormone produced by the *adrenal gland*.

POSSIBLE ADVERSE EFFECTS

Hydrocortisone creams used in excess may cause thinning of the skin. However, if the preparation is dilute, the risk of this is slight.

Hydrogen peroxide

An *antiseptic* solution used to treat infections of the skin or mouth and to bleach hair. Hydrogen peroxide combines with catalase, an enzyme present in the skin and mouth, to release oxygen. This effect kills bacteria and cleanses infected areas. Hydrogen peroxide occasionally causes soreness and irritation.

Hydronephrosis

A condition in which a *kidney* becomes distended (swollen) with urine due to an obstruction in the *urinary tract*. Untreated hydronephrosis can severely damage a kidney and, if both kidneys are affected, it can lead to *kidney failure*.

CAUSES

Many people with hydronephrosis have a *congenital* constriction (narrowing) of the ureter. Obstruction of a ureter may be due to a stone (see *Calculus, urinary tract*), a *kidney tumour*, or, less commonly, a blood clot. In some cases, the kidney becomes distended because of obstruction to the outflow of urine from the bladder due to an enlarged *prostate gland*.

SYMPTOMS AND SIGNS

Acute hydronephrosis, with sudden blockage of the ureter, results in severe pain in the loin. Chronic hydronephrosis, in which the obstruction develops slowly, may cause no symptoms until the ureter has become completely blocked and kidney failure occurs. The kidney may also become infected, resulting in pyonephrosis (pus-filled kidney).

DIAGNOSIS AND TREATMENT

Ultrasound scanning can provide an image of the kidneys and ureter. If the scan reveals an obstruction and if the kidney is still relatively healthy, the blockage is removed or relieved by surgery; the kidney usually resumes normal, or near normal, function. Occasionally, however, a kidney is so badly damaged that it requires removal (see *Nephrectomy*); the remaining kidney, provided it is healthy, will compensate for the loss of the other.

Hydrophobia

A popular term—now almost obsolete—for *rabies*. Meaning "fear of water", hydrophobia refers to the inability to drink that is one of the characteristic symptoms of rabies.

Hydrops

An abnormal accumulation of fluid in body tissues or in a sac (bag-like organ or body structure). Hydrops fetalis,

which may be caused by severe *Rhesus incompatibility*, is marked by generalized *oedema* (fluid collection causing tissue swelling) of the fetus.

Hydrotherapy

The external use of water to treat patients recovering from injury or suffering from lack of mobility. Hydrotherapy includes the use of exercise pools, whirlpool baths, and showers.

People who are unable to bear full weight on a limb (because of arthritis or after a fracture, for example) can often exercise more fully and effectively in a hydrotherapy pool. The buoyant effect of the water allows a greater range of movement and permits fuller use of the limb with little discomfort.

Warm whirlpool baths provide a gentle massage to stimulate areas of the body and relieve stiffness. Cold baths or showers after an injury can reduce blood flow, swelling, and bruising and can help to minimize tissue damage. (See also *Heat treatment; Ice-packs*.)

Hydroxocobalamin

A long-acting synthetic preparation of *vitamin B$_{12}$* given by injection.

Hygiene

The science and practice of preserving health. Today the word is commonly equated with cleanliness, particularly in the sense of personal hygiene. However, in the last century and early years of this century, the term hygiene was widely used as an equivalent to *public health*—the scientific study of environmental influences on health (with particular regard to the provision of pure water supplies, safe sanitation, good housing, and safe conditions in the workplace).

The terms industrial hygiene and occupational hygiene refer to the science of measuring, assessing, and controlling the environment to prevent *occupational disease*.

Hygiene, oral

See *Oral hygiene*.

Hygroma, cystic

A type of *lymphangioma* which may be present around the head and neck, armpits, or groin. Cystic hygromas contain clear fluid. They increase during infancy, usually reaching their maximum size by the age of two, and then gradually disappear. Most are left to disappear naturally, but surgical removal is performed if a cystic hygroma is very unsightly or if it obstructs the airway.

Hymen
The thin fold of membrane surrounding the vaginal opening. The hymen has a central perforation which is usually stretched or torn by the use of tampons or during first sexual intercourse. Once torn, the hymen becomes an irregular ring of tissue around the vaginal opening.

Imperforate hymen is a rare condition in which the hymen has no perforation; at the onset of menstruation, menstrual blood collects in the vagina, causing lower abdominal pain. The condition is easily corrected by a minor operation.

Hyoid
A small, U-shaped bone situated centrally in the upper part of the neck. The hyoid is not joined to any other bone but is suspended by ligaments from the base of the skull. Its function is to provide an anchor point for the muscles of the tongue and for those in the upper part of the front of the neck.

The hyoid is commonly fractured in homicidal strangulation.

LOCATION OF HYOID BONE
The U-shaped hyoid bone provides an anchor for the muscles at the back of the tongue

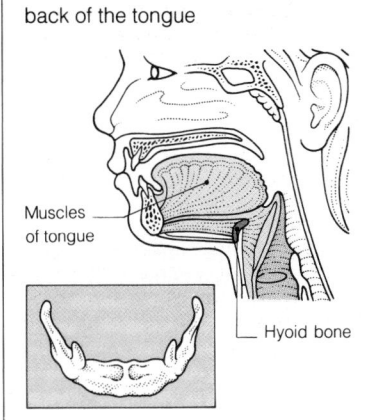

Muscles of tongue

Hyoid bone

Hyoscine
An *anticholinergic drug* prescribed in two distinct forms.

Hyoscine butylbromide is used to relax spasm of the intestinal wall that is the cause of abdominal pain in *irritable bowel syndrome*.

Hyoscine hydrobromide is prescribed to control *motion sickness* and

---

LOCATION OF HYMEN
The membrane that forms the hymen surrounds the opening to the vagina, inside a woman's labia minora.

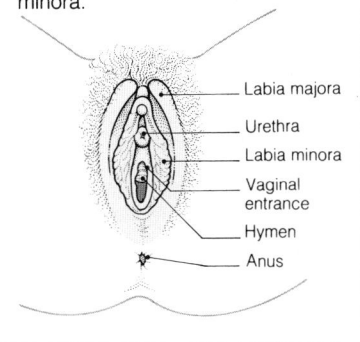

Labia majora
Urethra
Labia minora
Vaginal entrance
Hymen
Anus

---

to reduce nausea in *Ménière's disease*. It is also used in eye-drops to dilate (widen) the pupil before an eye examination or eye surgery. An injection of hyoscine hydrobromide is often given as part of a *premedication* because it dries secretions in the mouth and lungs.

Possible adverse effects of both forms include dry mouth, blurred vision, drowsiness, and constipation.

Hyper-
A prefix meaning above, excessive, or greater than normal, as in *hypertension* (high blood pressure) and *hyperthyroidism* (overactivity of the thyroid gland).

Hyperacidity
A condition in which an excessive amount of acid is produced by the stomach. Hyperacidity is commonly confused with *acid reflux* (which causes a burning sensation in the upper abdomen or lower chest) or *waterbrash* (sudden filling of the person's mouth with a watery fluid). Most people with a duodenal ulcer (see *Peptic ulcer*) produce more acid than normal, and those with *Zollinger-Ellison syndrome* produce vast amounts.

Hyperactivity
A behaviour pattern, also known as attention deficit disorder, in which children have difficulty concentrating and are constantly overactive.

The condition is widely diagnosed in the US but British doctors believe that true hyperactivity is rare.

CAUSES
It has been suggested that some hyperactive children, especially those who are clumsy, may have a subtle

---

form of "minimal" brain damage. However, there is no definite, conclusive evidence. Hyperactive children seem more likely to have fathers who were hyperactive, suggesting that the condition may be partly inherited. Children with *mental handicap, cerebral palsy,* or *temporal lobe epilepsy* may also be hyperactive. Food allergy is widely believed to be a common cause, but research studies suggest that it is involved only rarely.

SYMPTOMS
The main feature of hyperactivity is continual overactivity. Such children are always on the go, full of energy, fidgety, and seem to sleep less than their peers. They also tend to be impulsive and reckless, with no sense of danger, and are usually irritable, emotionally immature, and aggressive. Their attention span is short and, as a result, they do not conform to orderly routine.

Hyperactivity can lead to antisocial acts and to learning difficulty, although IQ is normal. It is not known whether this behaviour is a part of the disorder or simply a result of an affected child's poor attention span and disruptive activity.

DIAGNOSIS
Overactivity in itself does not indicate that a child is hyperactive. A stressful home environment or physical illness may also cause overactivity. It is also true that many of the behavioural problems mentioned are, to some degree, common to all young children. However, when other causes have been eliminated and the behaviour continues past the age of four years, is intense, and is different from that of "normal" children, then it seems reasonable to regard the child as being hyperactive.

TREATMENT
Paradoxically, *stimulant drugs* (such as amphetamines) seem to be the most effective treatment. This suggests that hyperactivity results from "underarousal" of the midbrain, which causes no damping down or control of movements and sensations. Stimulant drugs seem to work by stimulating the midbrain enough to suppress the extra activity. Behaviour therapy and counselling of the child and parents are also useful.

Diets that exclude certain artificial food colourings, additives, or foods benefit very few children.

Hyperactive children should have formal educational and psychological assessment; many need help with reading and spelling.

OUTLOOK

In many cases, hyperactivity disappears completely at puberty. In others, the overactivity subsides and is replaced by sluggishness, depression, and moodiness; these teenagers often fail at school and resort to antisocial behaviour. Sometimes all the symptoms of hyperactivity continue into adult life.

Hyperacusis

An exceptionally developed sense of hearing. Hyperacusis may cause the sensation of pain or discomfort in the ears on exposure to loud noises.

Hyperaldosteronism

A metabolic disorder that is caused by an overproduction of the hormone *aldosterone* by the adrenal glands. See *Aldosteronism*.

Hyperalimentation

Administration of excess amounts of calories, usually intravenously or by stomach tube. (See *Feeding, artificial*.)

Hyperbaric oxygen treatment

A method of increasing the amount of oxygen in the tissues by exposing a person to oxygen at a much higher than normal atmospheric pressure.

WHY IT IS DONE

This technique is occasionally used to treat poisoning from *carbon monoxide*, in which the tissues are starved of oxygen because *haemoglobin* (the oxygen-carrying component of red blood cells) is prevented from taking up oxygen. Hyperbaric oxygen treatment is also used in cases of gas *gangrene*; the bacteria that infect gangrenous tissue cannot survive if they are oxygenated.

HOW IT IS DONE

The patient is placed in a chamber into which oxygen is pumped at up to three times normal atmospheric pressure for no more than three hours. The inhaled oxygen dissolves in the patient's blood.

Hyperbilirubinaemia

A raised blood level of *bilirubin* (a waste product formed from the destruction of red blood cells). Hyperbilirubinaemia may be undetectable except by a blood test, but *jaundice* becomes apparent if the blood bilirubin rises to twice the normal level.

Hypercalcaemia

An abnormally high level of *calcium* in the blood. Minor degrees of hypercalcaemia are quite common in healthy people and probably not significant.

CAUSES

Hypercalcaemia is commonly caused by *hyperparathyroidism* (overproduction of parathyroid hormone, which helps control the blood calcium level).

Cancer may cause hypercalcaemia, either by spreading to bone or by producing abnormal hormones which cause bone to soften, releasing calcium from bone into the blood.

Less commonly, hypercalcaemia is due to excessive intake of *vitamin D*, which helps regulate the absorption of calcium, or to certain inflammatory disorders, such as *sarcoidosis*.

SYMPTOMS

Hypercalcaemia causes nausea, vomiting, lethargy, depression, thirst, and excessive urination. Higher levels of calcium in the blood produce confusion, extreme fatigue, and muscle weakness. If the disorder is untreated and the blood calcium level continues to increase, cardiac arrhythmias (irregularities of the heartbeat), kidney failure, coma, and even death may result. Long-standing hypercalcaemia may cause *nephrocalcinosis* (calcification of the kidney) or kidney stones (see *Calculus, urinary tract*).

DIAGNOSIS AND TREATMENT

The condition is diagnosed by measuring the level of calcium in the blood. If the diagnosis is confirmed, more tests are performed to discover the underlying cause. Any treatment is of the underlying cause.

Hypercapnia

Excessive carbon dioxide in the blood. Carbon dioxide is a waste product of the metabolic processes that produce energy in body cells and is eliminated from the body during *breathing* out. Normally, the amount of carbon dioxide in the blood is maintained within narrow limits. Hypercapnia is caused by failure of mechanisms, such as breathing rate, that normally control blood carbon dioxide levels; it usually leads to respiratory *acidosis*.

Hyperemesis

The medical term for excessive *vomiting*, which may cause dehydration and weight loss. When the condition occurs in pregnancy, it is known as hyperemesis gravidarum.

Hyperglycaemia

An abnormally high level of glucose (sugar) in the blood, occurring in people suffering from untreated or inadequately controlled *diabetes mellitus*. It may also occur in diabetics as a result of an infection, stress, or surgery.

The symptoms of hyperglycaemia are the same as those of diabetes: thirst, the passing of large amounts of urine, *glycosuria* (glucose in the urine), and *ketosis* (an accumulation of ketones in the body). In severe cases, hyperglycaemia may lead to confusion and coma, which require emergency medical treatment with *insulin* and an intravenous infusion of fluids.

Hypergonadism

Overactivity of the gonads (*testes* or *ovaries*) resulting in overproduction of *androgen hormones* or *oestrogen hormones*. Hypergonadism may be caused by disorders of the gonads or by a disorder of the *pituitary gland* that results in overproduction of *gonadotrophin hormone*. During childhood, the condition causes precocious sexual development and excessive growth.

Hyperhidrosis

A term meaning excessive sweating. Hyperhidrosis may be localized, affecting only the armpits, feet, palms, or face. Alternatively, it may be generalized, affecting all areas supplied by *sweat glands*.

CAUSES

Excessive sweating may be caused by hot weather, exercise, or anxiety. In some cases, the condition is due to a disorder, such as an infection, *thyrotoxicosis*, *hypoglycaemia*, or a disorder of the nervous system. More commonly, hyperhydrosis is idiopathic (of unknown cause), usually beginning at puberty and disappearing by the mid-20s or early 30s.

TREATMENT

Sufferers should pay special attention to personal hygiene. Clothing and shoes made of natural materials, such as cotton and leather, tend to be more comfortable than less absorbent materials. Regular use of *antiperspirants* may help. An operation (endoscopic transthoracic sympathectomy) cures excess sweating in the hands, arms, and armpits. The surgeon operates through small incisions in the upper chest, destroying the nerve centres that control sweating in the arms. Patients can leave hospital in less than 48 hours.

Hyperkeratosis

Thickening of the outer layer of the skin due to an increased amount of *keratin* (a tough protein that is the major component of the outer layer of skin). The most common forms of hyperkeratosis are *corns* and *calluses*, caused by prolonged pressure or friction. Hyperkeratosis is a feature of warts on the soles of the feet (see (*Wart, plantar*). It is also a feature of *lichen planus*.

The term hyperkeratosis is sometimes used to describe abnormal thickening of the nails.

Hyperlipidaemias

A group of *metabolic disorders* characterized by high levels of *lipids* (fats) in the blood.

TYPES

Hyperlipidaemias may be classified into six types. These six types are differentiated by the extent to which the blood levels of different forms of lipids are higher than normal (see the table below).

Lipids are carried in the blood in several forms, chiefly *cholesterol*, triglycerides, and lipoproteins. Lipoproteins consist of fat and cholesterol molecules linked to protein molecules. Lipoproteins are classified according to their density, which depends on their relative proportions of cholesterol and protein; the higher the proportion of cholesterol, the lower the density of the lipoprotein. According to this classification, lipo-

proteins are divided into: very low-density lipoproteins (VLDLs), low-density lipoproteins (LDLs), and intermediate-density lipoproteins (IDLs). There are also high-density lipoproteins (HDLs), but these are not involved in the hyperlipidaemias. Chylomicrons (microscopic fat droplets in the blood) are usually also classed as lipoproteins.

CAUSES

Hyperlipidaemias may be inherited or may be a consequence of another disorder, such as *hypothyroidism, alcohol dependence, diabetes mellitus, kidney failure,* and *Cushing's syndrome.* Hyperlipidaemias may also result from treatment with *corticosteroid drugs* or *oestrogen drugs.*

RISKS

Hyperlipidaemias are associated with a number of serious disorders, notably *atherosclerosis* (narrowing of arteries by deposits of fatty material) and *coronary artery disease.* For this reason, if a close relative has, or has had, either of these disorders, particularly if he or she has had a heart attack under the age of 50, other members of the family should be tested.

SYMPTOMS, DIAGNOSIS, AND TREATMENT

The symptoms and treatments for the different types of hyperlipidaemia are shown in the accompanying table. Because many of the types produce similar symptoms, diagnosis usually depends on blood tests to measure the levels of the different lipids.

Treatment depends to some extent on the type of hyperlidaemia, but in all cases is aimed at reducing blood lipid levels and thus lowering the risk of atherosclerosis.

Hypermetropia

Commonly called longsightedness, an error of *refraction* that initially causes difficulty in seeing near objects and then affects distance vision. Hypermetropia tends to run in families.

Hypermetropia is caused by the eye being too short from front to back, so that images are not clearly focused on the retina. Mild or moderate hypermetropia in the young is overcome by *accommodation* (the action of the ciliary muscles to change the shape of the lens), which brings the point of focus forward to produce a clear image.

H

TYPES OF HYPERLIPIDAEMIA

Type	Lipoprotein elevated	Blood cholesterol level	Blood triglyceride level	Symptoms and signs in addition to risk of heart disease	Treatment
I	Chylomicrons	Small elevation	Large elevation	Fatty nodules in skin; abdominal pain; inflammation of pancreas	Diet very low in fats
IIa	Low-density lipoproteins	Small to medium elevation	Normal	Fatty nodules around tendons (especially Achilles tendon and hand tendons) and over joints; white line around rim of cornea	Diet low in saturated fats and cholesterol; cholestyramine, colestipol, or clofibrate may be prescribed.
IIb	Low-density and very low-density lipoproteins	Small to medium elevation	Small elevation	Fatty nodules on eyelids; white line around rim of cornea	Diet low in saturated fats, cholesterol, and carbohydrates; cholestyramine or colestipol may be prescribed.
III	Intermediate-density lipoproteins	Small to medium elevation	Small to medium elevation	Fat deposits in palms and sometimes over joints	Diet low in fats and carbohydrates; clofibrate, nicotinic acid or gemfibrozil may be prescribed.
IV	Very low-density lipoproteins	Normal	Small to medium elevation	Fatty nodules in skin; patient is often obese	Diet low in carbohydrates; weight reduction; clofibrate and sometimes nicotinic acid and gemfibrozil may be prescribed.
V	Chylomicrons and very low-density lipoproteins	Small elevation	Small to medium elevation	Fatty nodules in skin; abdominal pain; inflammation of pancreas; patient may be obese	Diet low in fats and carbohydrates; weight reduction; gemfibrozil and nicotinic acid may be prescribed.

SYMPTOMS AND SIGNS

The error is present from birth, but symptoms generally do not appear until later life. The more severe the hypermetropia, the lower the age at which people experience difficulty viewing close objects, because the power of accommodation declines with age. In time, distant objects also become blurred.

TREATMENT

If necessary, an ophthalmologist may prescribe *glasses* or *contact lenses* with convex lenses which will reinforce focusing power.

Hypernephroma

An alternative and older name for renal cell carcinoma, which is a type of *kidney cancer*.

Hyperparathyroidism

Overactivity of the *parathyroid glands*. These pea-sized glands are embedded in the thyroid gland in the neck and produce parathyroid hormone. This hormone, together with *vitamin D* and *calcitonin* (a hormone produced by the thyroid gland), controls the level of calcium in the body. Overproduction of parathyroid hormone raises the level of calcium in the blood (a condition called *hypercalcaemia*) by removing the calcium from bones. This may lead to bone disorders, for example *osteoporosis*.

In an attempt to normalize the high blood calcium level, the kidneys excrete large amounts of calcium in the urine, which can result in the formation of kidney stones (see *Calculus, urinary tract*).

CAUSES AND INCIDENCE

Hyperparathyroidism is most often caused by a small benign tumour of one or more of the parathyroid glands. In other cases, it occurs when the glands become enlarged for no known reason.

About 40 people per 100,000 suffer from the disorder, which usually develops after the age of 40 and is twice as common in women as in men.

SYMPTOMS

Hyperparathyroidism may cause generalized aches and pains, depression, and abdominal pain. Often, the only symptoms are those caused by kidney stones.

If hypercalcaemia is severe, there may be nausea, vomiting, tiredness, excessive urination, confusion, and muscle weakness.

DIAGNOSIS AND TREATMENT

The condition is diagnosed by X-rays of the hands and skull and by tests to measure the level of calcium, phosphorus, and parathyroid hormone in the blood.

Surgical removal of all abnormal parathyroid tissue usually cures the condition. In some cases, the amount of parathyroid tissue remaining after the operation may be insufficient to meet the body's needs. The affected person may then require treatment for *hypoparathyroidism* (underactivity of the parathyroid glands).

Hyperplasia

Enlargement of an organ or tissue due to an increase in the number of its constituent cells. The new cells are normal, unlike those of a tumour.

HYPERPARATHYROIDISM

In this disorder, the parathyroid glands produce too much parathyroid hormone. Symptoms, signs, and complications of the disorder occur as a result of an increased calcium level in the blood and urine, the loss of calcium from bones, and calcinosis (the formation of calcium deposits in different tissues). Surgical removal of abnormal parathyroid tissue is carried out to prevent complications.

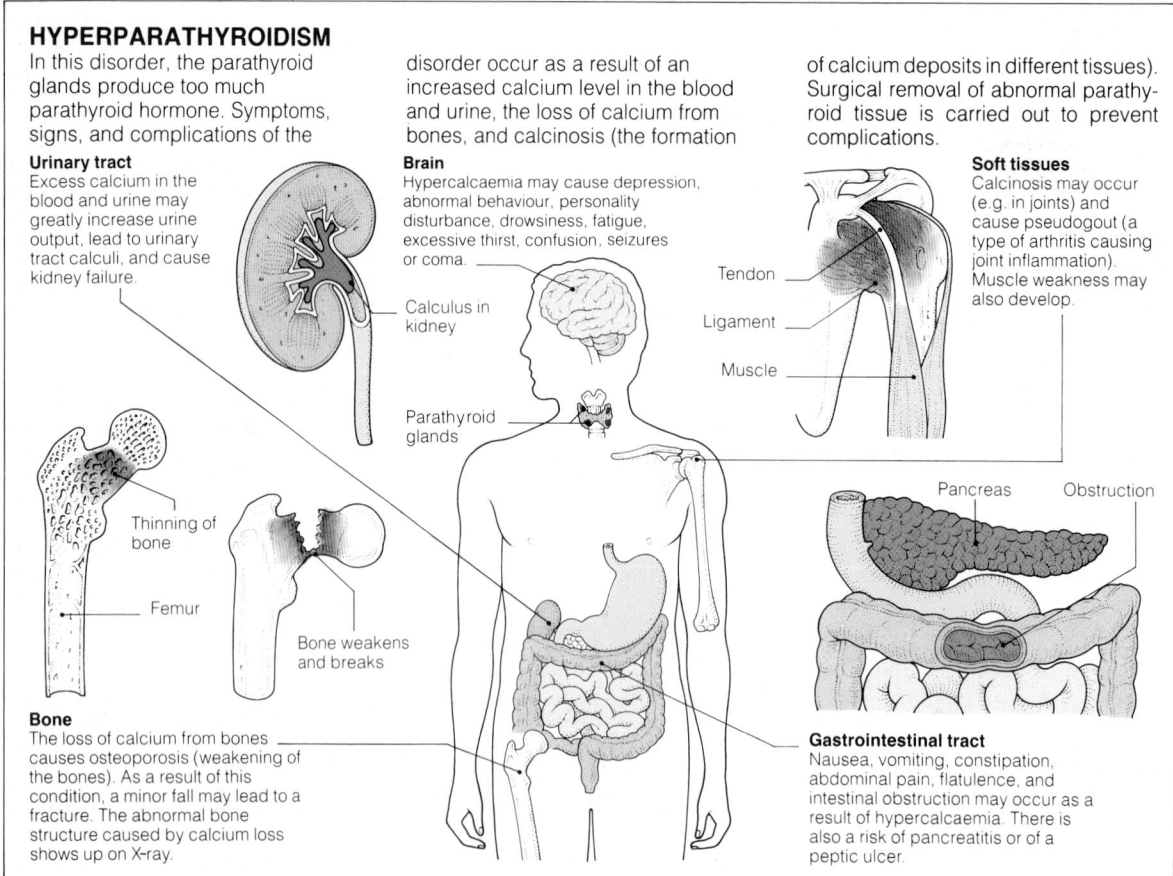

Urinary tract
Excess calcium in the blood and urine may greatly increase urine output, lead to urinary tract calculi, and cause kidney failure.

Brain
Hypercalcaemia may cause depression, abnormal behaviour, personality disturbance, drowsiness, fatigue, excessive thirst, confusion, seizures or coma.

Calculus in kidney

Soft tissues
Calcinosis may occur (e.g. in joints) and cause pseudogout (a type of arthritis causing joint inflammation). Muscle weakness may also develop.

Tendon
Ligament
Muscle

Parathyroid glands

Thinning of bone
Femur

Bone weakens and breaks

Pancreas   Obstruction

Bone
The loss of calcium from bones causes osteoporosis (weakening of the bones). As a result of this condition, a minor fall may lead to a fracture. The abnormal bone structure caused by calcium loss shows up on X-ray.

Gastrointestinal tract
Nausea, vomiting, constipation, abdominal pain, flatulence, and intestinal obstruction may occur as a result of hypercalcaemia. There is also a risk of pancreatitis or of a peptic ulcer.

Hyperplasia is usually the result of hormonal stimulation. It may be a normal occurrence (such as in the enlargement of breast tissue and uterine muscle that occurs during pregnancy) or it may indicate a disorder (such as in hyperplasia of the thyroid or adrenal glands, which may be due to oversecretion of certain pituitary hormones). Hyperplasia of the prostate gland is a common benign condition of men after middle age. (See also *Hypertrophy*.)

Hyperplasia, gingival

Abnormal enlargement of the gums. The condition may be a feature of *gingivitis* (inflammation of the gums), especially when it occurs during pregnancy. Gingival hyperplasia can also develop around the front teeth as a result of persistent breathing through the mouth. The condition can also be caused by *phenytoin*, an anticonvulsant drug used to treat *epilepsy*. Ill-fitting dentures may cause rolls of fibrous gum tissue to form beyond the edges of the dentures.

Enlarged gums should be examined by a dentist; surgical removal of surplus tissue may be necessary.

Hyperpyrexia

A medical term for extremely high body temperature; it is synonymous with hyperthermia. Heat hyperpyrexia is another name for *heatstroke*.

Hypersensitivity

Overreaction of the *immune system* (defence against infection) to an *antigen* (protein recognized as foreign). Hypersensitivity reactions occur only on second or subsequent exposures to particular antigens, after the first exposure has sensitized the immune system. Such reactions have the same mechanisms as those of protective *immunity*. However, while the latter protect against disease, hypersensitivity reactions lead to tissue damage and disease.

Hypersensitivity is closely related to *allergy*, except that only one of the four main types of hypersensitivity reaction (type I) is closely associated with allergic illnesses.

TYPES

The four main types of hypersensitivity reaction are as follows.

TYPE I This type is also called immediate or anaphylactic hypersensitivity. After a first exposure to an antigen (which may be a harmless substance such as grass pollen), *antibodies* (substances that can recognize and bind to the antigen) are formed; these antibodies coat cells called mast cells in various tissues. On second exposure, the antigen and antibodies combine, causing the mast cells to disintegrate and release various chemicals that cause the symptoms of *asthma*, allergic *rhinitis* (hay fever), *urticaria* (nettle rash), *anaphylactic shock* (a severe allergic reaction), or other illnesses of an allergic nature.

TYPE II In this type, antibodies that bind to antigens on cell surfaces are formed, leading to possible destruction of the cells. Type II reactions may be responsible for certain *autoimmune disorders* (in which antibodies attack the body's own tissues) and for some cases of *haemolysis* (red blood cell destruction) triggered by certain drugs.

TYPE III Antibodies combine with antigens to form particles called immune complexes, which can lodge in various tissues and activate further immune system responses, leading to tissue damage. This type of hypersensitivity reaction is responsible for *serum sickness*, for allergic *alveolitis* (a lung disease caused by exposure to the spores of certain fungi), and for the large swellings that sometimes form after booster vaccinations.

TYPE IV This type is also called delayed hypersensitivity. In type IV, sensitized *T-lymphocytes* (a class of white blood cell and an important component of the immune system) bind to antigens and subsequently release chemicals called lymphokines, which promote an inflammatory reaction. Type IV reactions are responsible for contact *dermatitis* and the rash of *measles*; they are important in the body's defence against *tuberculosis* and may also play a part in some "allergic" reactions to drugs.

TREATMENT

Effective treatment of a hypersensitivity reaction depends on its type, cause, and severity. When possible, exposure to the offending antigen should be avoided.

Hypersplenism

Overactivity of the *spleen*, resulting in and associated with blood disease. One of the functions of the spleen is to break down blood cells as they age and wear out. An overactive spleen may begin to destroy cells indiscriminately, causing a deficiency of any of the types of blood cell. In most cases, the spleen will also be enlarged.

Hypersplenism may be primary, occurring for no known reason, but more commonly it is secondary to another disorder in which the spleen has become enlarged, such as *Hodgkin's disease* or *malaria*.

SYMPTOMS AND TREATMENT

A person with hypersplenism is likely to have the symptoms of *anaemia* (due to destruction of red blood cells) or of *thrombocytopenia* (platelet deficiency), and there is sometimes a decrease in resistance to infection due to lack of white cells. There may also be symptoms of an underlying disorder, such as malaria.

Treatment of secondary hypersplenism is aimed at controlling the underlying cause. Primary hypersplenism requires *splenectomy* (removal of the spleen).

Hypertension

Abnormally high *blood pressure* (the pressure of blood in the main arteries). Blood pressure goes up as a normal response to stress and physical activity. However, a person with hypertension has a high blood pressure even at rest. A large number of people have hypertension without even realizing it; because the condition increases the chances of having a *stroke* or of developing heart disease, regular medical checks are advised in order to detect hypertension as early as possible.

Blood pressure is measured by two values, each expressed as millimetres (mm) of mercury (chemical symbol Hg) or mm Hg. The systolic value (the higher value) is the pressure when blood surges into the aorta from the heart; the diastolic value is the pressure when the ventricles (larger heart chambers) relax between beats.

There is no strict dividing line between "normal" and "high" blood pressure, but the World Health Organization defines hypertension as a blood pressure consistently exceeding 160 mm Hg (systolic) and 95 mm Hg (diastolic). A person with a systolic value of 140-160 mm Hg and a diastolic value of 90-95 mm Hg is sometimes referred to as having mild or "borderline" hypertension. However, an elderly person normally has systolic blood pressure readings within or above these values because blood pressure increases with age. Young children usually have blood pressure readings well below these values.

INCIDENCE AND CAUSES

Hypertension is an extremely common condition, affecting 10 to 20 per cent of the UK adult population. The condition is more common in men than in women and its incidence is

H

HYPERTENSION

Hypertension affects 10 to 20 per cent of adults in the UK. It is diagnosed if a person's resting blood pressure is persistently raised. Blood pressure is expressed by two values—the systolic and diastolic pressures—and measured in millimetres of mercury.

Although hypertension rarely causes symptoms, it is a serious condition. Left untreated, it increases the risk of stroke and other disorders. In many cases, there is no obvious cause, but, in some, there is a specific cause, such as a kidney disorder, pregnancy, or use of oral contraceptives. Hypertension is linked to obesity and, in some people, to a high salt intake. Smoking appears to aggravate the effects of hypertension.

H

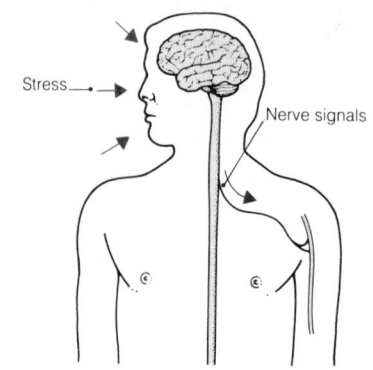

Stress and hypertension
Stress acts on the nervous system, causing blood vessels to constrict and the heart to work harder. Both lead to a temporary rise in blood pressure. Hence, pressure should be measured when a person is relaxed. It is possible (but unproven) that frequent stress may eventually cause hypertension.

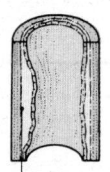

Fatty deposits

Contracted muscle

Atheroma
Hypertension and atherosclerosis, in which arteries are narrowed (left), are closely linked both to each other and to obesity.

Artery wall

Constriction
Factors such as nicotine in tobacco cause artery constriction (left) and a short-term rise in blood pressure that may worsen hypertension.

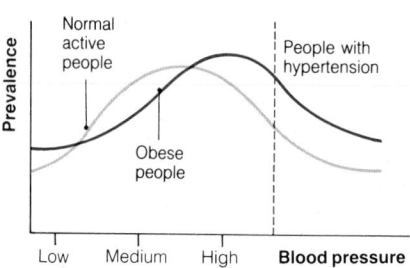

Variation in blood pressure
In any population, blood pressure varies over a wide range in the same way as height. Many people are considered to be hypertensive because they are at the top end of this range (see above). In obese people, the range is similarly wide but shifted towards the top end: hence, more obese people are hypertensive.

COMMON FACTORS AND PREVENTIVE MEASURES

Factors associated with essential hypertension	Age (incidence higher in the elderly)		Family history of the condition		Gender (incidence higher in men than in women)
Factors that may aggravate hypertension	Smoking	Obesity	Excess alcohol intake	Diabetes mellitus	Stress
Self-help and treatment	1. Regular screening of blood pressure is important for early diagnosis and can help to prevent complications 2. Sufferers from essential hypertension should: Reduce weight Not smoke Reduce or stop alcohol intake Reduce salt intake Take regular exercise Learn relaxation. 3. Antihypertensive drugs, prescribed by a doctor, can usually keep high blood pressure under control				

highest in the middle-aged and elderly, although significant numbers of young adults are also hypertensive.

Blood pressure rises as a result of an increase in resistance to the flow of blood in both large and small blood vessels. Resistance increases in the large vessels as they become more rigid with age. Resistance in the smaller vessels depends on the extent to which they are constricted, which is under nerve and chemical control.

About 90 per cent of people with hypertension have no obvious underlying cause for their elevated blood pressure; in such cases it is called essential hypertension. Apart from age and male gender, factors associated with an increased risk of essential hypertension include: tobacco smoking, obesity, excess alcohol intake, a family history of hypertension, a sedentary lifestyle, and a high degree of social and occupational stress. In the other 10 per cent of patients with hypertension, a definite cause is found; it is then called secondary hypertension. Specific causes include various disorders of the *kidneys*, certain disorders of the *adrenal glands*, *pre-eclampsia* (a complication of pregnancy), *coarctation of the aorta* (a type of congenital heart defect), and use of certain drugs. Taking the combined (oestrogen-containing) contraceptive pill appears to increase the risk of hypertension.

SYMPTOMS AND COMPLICATIONS

Hypertension usually causes no symptoms and generally goes undiscovered until detected by a doctor during the course of a routine physical examination. Severe hypertension may sometimes cause headaches, shortness of breath, giddiness and visual disturbances.

Hypertension puts a considerable strain on the heart and blood vessels. Apart from increasing the risk of having a stroke or developing *heart failure* or *coronary artery disease*, high blood pressure may eventually cause kidney damage and *retinopathy* (damage to the retina at the back of the eye). Severe hypertension may cause confusion and seizures.

All these risks increase with the degree of hypertension. For example, for a man in his 40s, each rise of 10 mm Hg in the systolic blood pressure increases the risk of heart disease by about 20 per cent.

DIAGNOSIS

Because of the health risks associated with hypertension, everyone should have their blood pressure checked at least once every five years, and if previous readings have shown borderline or raised blood pressure, more frequently than this. Many family doctors now check the blood pressure of their middle-aged and elderly patients at virtually every consultation.

A diagnosis of hypertension is usually not confirmed until the patient's blood pressure at rest is found to be raised on three separate occasions. However, hypertension is sometimes diagnosed on the first reading if the blood pressure is exceptionally high and accompanied by one of the complications of hypertension, such as retinopathy.

TREATMENT

Occasionally, in the most severe cases of hypertension, immediate admission to hospital for emergency treatment, investigation of the cause, and bed rest, is required.

With mild to moderate hypertension, if no underlying cause (such as a kidney disorder) is found, the first line of attack is alteration of lifestyle. Smokers should stop smoking and drinkers should reduce their consumption of alcohol. Any overweight person with hypertension should make an attempt to reduce weight through restriction of food intake and gradually increased exercise. Regular exercise will help lower the blood pressure in all persons with hypertension as well as protecting against heart disease. The dietary intake of animal fats (contained in milk, cream, cheese, fatty meats and eggs) should be reduced. A restricted intake of salt is also sometimes recommended. All these general health measures may also help to prevent hypertension from developing in the first place.

Some patients find that *biofeedback training* can help to reduce blood pressure. During biofeedback sessions, patients receive continuous monitoring of their blood pressure and gradually learn techniques of relaxation that reduce the pressure.

If self-help measures have no effect, or in the case of more severe hypertension, *antihypertensive drugs* may be prescribed. A large number of different types of antihypertensive drug are available, including diuretics, beta-blockers, vasodilators, ACE inhibitors, and calcium antagonists, which work in different ways on the heart, blood vessels, and nervous system to reduce blood pressure. One or a combination of drugs may be prescribed, leading to satisfactory control of the hypertension in most cases.

Usually, the doctor will wish to monitor the effects of treatment by measurement of blood pressure every two to four weeks, so that adjustment to the drug dosages or regimen can be made if necessary. If any side-effects develop, the doctor should be told, as a more suitable alternative therapy may be available.

In many cases, drug treatment must continue for some years or even for the rest of the patient's life. But this is a small price to pay for the many extra years of life expectancy added through control of hypertension.

Hyperthermia

A medical term for very high body temperature. (See also *Heat stroke*.)

Hyperthermia, malignant

A rapid rise in body temperature to a dangerously high level brought on by general *anaesthesia*. The condition is rare, occurring in only about one in 50,000 operations. In most cases, susceptibility to the condition is inherited; people suffering from certain muscle disorders may also be at risk.

The patient's temperature rises soon after the anaesthetic is given. At the same time, large amounts of *lactic acid* pass from the muscles into the blood, causing *acidosis*. The muscles then stiffen and the patient turns blue; without emergency treatment, seizures and death may follow rapidly.

Malignant hyperthermia may be suspected if the patient does not relax normally during the early, induction stage of anaesthesia, or if he or she shows signs of abnormal muscle contractions after administration of succinylcholine (a chemical used to relax muscles during operations).

TREATMENT

If malignant hyperthermia occurs, the anaesthetic is stopped immediately and the patient is cooled with ice-packs. Pure oxygen and intravenous injections of sodium bicarbonate may be given to counteract acidosis. Injections of dantrolene sodium are given intravenously at five to 10 minute intervals as required.

Hyperthyroidism

Overproduction of *thyroid hormones* by an overactive *thyroid gland*.

CAUSES AND INCIDENCE

The most common form of hyperthyroidism is *Graves' disease*, an *autoimmune disorder* in which the body develops antibodies that stimulate the production of excessive amounts of thyroid hormones. This condition

affects about one per cent of the adult population and is most common in young to middle-aged women. More rarely, hyperthyroidism may be associated with the development of enlarged nodules in the thyroid.

SYMPTOMS AND SIGNS

Symptoms and signs are described in the illustrated box overleaf.

DIAGNOSIS AND TREATMENT

The diagnosis of hyperthyroidism is confirmed by tests to measure the level of thyroid hormones in the blood. The condition may be treated with drugs that inhibit the production of thyroid hormones or by surgical removal of part of the thyroid gland. In older patients, an alternative is a single dose of radioactive iodine, which is taken up by the thyroid and destroys some of its tissue.

Hypertonia

Increased rigidity in a muscle. Hypertonia may be caused by damage to its nerve supply or by cell changes within the muscle itself. Hypertonia causes episodes of continuous muscle spasm (as may occur in the bladder wall, for example, when the outflow of urine is being obstructed by an enlarged prostate gland).

Persistent hypertonia in limb muscles following a *stroke* or major *head injury* causes *spasticity* (increased rigidity). A variable increase in muscle tension associated with abnormal patterns of movement and posture is referred to as *dystonia*.

Hypertrichosis

Growth of excessive hair, often in places that are not normally hairy. Hypertrichosis is often a result of taking certain drugs (including *cyclosporin*, *minoxidil*, and *diazoxide*). The term hypertrichosis is also used to describe hair growth in a coloured, fleshy mole.

Hypertrichosis is not the same as *hirsutism*, which is excessive hairiness, particularly in women, due to abnormal levels of male hormones.

Hypertrophy

Enlargement of an organ or tissue due to an increase in the size, rather than the number, of its constituent cells. For example, skeletal muscles enlarge in response to increased physical demands. (See also *Hyperplasia*.)

Hyperuricaemia

An abnormally high level of *uric acid* in the blood. Hyperuricaemia may lead to the development of *gout* due to the

H

SYMPTOMS AND SIGNS OF HYPERTHYROIDISM

Oversecretion of thyroid hormones produces symptoms associated with overactivity of the body's metabolism. Weight loss, increased appetite, intolerance to heat, and increased sweating are early signs; there may also be tremors and a rapid heart rate. In more severe cases, the thyroid gland is often enlarged and there tends to be physical and mental hyperactivity and wasting of the muscles.

Thyroid gland enlargement
This symptom (known as goitre) may be due to hyperthyroidism. However, it may also be associated with hypothyroidism (underactivity of the thyroid).

Muscle wasting
Severe hyperthyroidism may cause wasting of both skeletal and heart muscle; it may also lead to irregularities of heart rhythm.

Increased appetite
This symptom is a result of the metabolic overactivity that hyperthyroidism causes. Despite increased appetite, there is often weight loss.

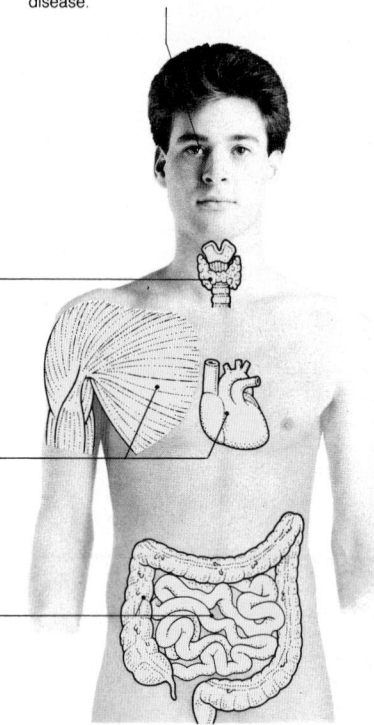

Protruding eyes
This symptom (known as exophthalmos) affects some 30 to 50 percent of people with Graves' disease.

HYPERTHYROID HEART-RATE
The heart-rate may be affected by excessive thyroid hormones, resulting in the heart's beating too rapidly or irregularly.

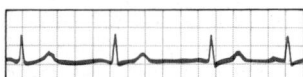

Healthy rhythm
A healthy heart has a regular rhythm and a normal rate of beating.

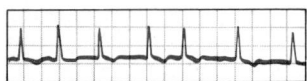

Hyperthyroid rhythm
Hyperthyroidism may cause irregular or too rapid heartbeat.

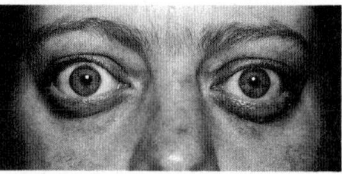

Appearance of exophthalmos
Hyperthyroidism can cause swelling of tissues around the eyes, resulting in a staring appearance.

---

deposition of uric acid crystals in the joints; it may also cause kidney stones (see *Calculus, urinary tract*) and the deposition of crystals elsewhere in the body, especially around joints (see *Tophus*).

CAUSES

Hyperuricaemia may be caused by an inborn error of metabolism (see *Metabolism, inborn error of*), by rapid destruction of cells as part of a disease such as *leukaemia*, or by medication (such as *diuretic drugs*) that reduces the excretion of uric acid by the kidneys. Increased amounts of *purine* (a nitrogen-containing substance) in the diet may raise the level of uric acid in the blood, precipitating gout.

TREATMENT

Drugs, such as *allopurinol* (which reduces uric acid production in cells) and *probenecid* or *sulphinpyrazone* (which increase the excretion of uric acid by the kidneys), may be prescribed for the rest of the patient's life to prevent complications. Foods that are high in purine (such as liver, poultry, and dried peas and beans) should be avoided.

Hyperventilation

Abnormally deep or rapid breathing, usually caused by *anxiety*. Hyperventilation may also occur as a result of uncontrolled *diabetes mellitus*, oxygen deficiency, *kidney failure*, and some lung disorders (such as *pulmonary oedema* and *emphysema*).

Hyperventilation causes an abnormal loss of carbon dioxide from the blood, which can lead to *alkalosis* (increase in blood alkalinity). Symptoms include numbness of the extremities, faintness, *tetany* (painful spasms and twitches of the muscles, especially in the hands and feet), and a sensation of not being able to take a full breath. The effects of alkalosis often add to the already existing feelings of anxiety, and may give rise to "hyperventilation syndrome", in which the sufferer experiences a feeling of impending doom.

Breathing into a plastic or paper bag during an attack may help reduce the loss of carbon dioxide and avoid the risk of alkalosis.

Hyperventilation associated with uncontrolled diabetes or with kidney failure represents the body's efforts to eliminate excess carbon dioxide in dealing with *acidosis*.

Hyphaema

Blood in the front chamber of the *eye*, almost always caused by an injury that ruptures a small blood vessel in the iris or the ciliary body.

Vision is blurred while the blood remains mixed with the aqueous humour, but clears as the red cells sink. In most cases, the blood disappears completely within a few days and vision is fully restored. There is, however, a risk of delayed bleeding three to five days after the injury.

Hypnosis

A trance-like state of altered awareness characterized by extreme suggestibility. Although it was once believed to be a form of sleep, the *EEG* (electrical tracing of brain-wave activity) of a hypnotized person does not show any normal sleep patterns.

HISTORY

A form of hypnotism was first practised by the Austrian physician Franz

Mesmer in the 18th century. Mesmerism (renamed hypnotism after the Greek god of sleep) began to receive attention from many leading members of the medical community in the 19th century. The celebrated Parisian physician Charcot gave public demonstrations, and Freud used hypnosis in his early treatment of hysteria. Hypnotism continues to attract interest, both theoretical and medical, but is used very little in medicine in the UK.

HOW IT IS DONE

For hypnosis to succeed, the subject must first want to be hypnotized. The second requirement is relaxation, so a comfortable chair and a quiet, dimly lit room are usually necessary. The subject is usually asked to fix his or her attention on a particular object while the therapist quietly repeats phrases such as "Be still and listen to my voice" or "Empty your mind of all thoughts". The subject gradually becomes more and more relaxed, eventually losing touch with the environment and hearing only the therapist's voice. At the end of the session, the subject "wakes up" when told to do so.

With training, it is possible for people to practise autohypnosis (self-hypnosis) by repeating certain phrases to themselves or imagining relaxing scenes.

Some people are more easily hypnotized than others, usually those with an intense imaginative life. The ability seems to be related to early childhood experiences and may be partly inherited.

CHARACTERISTICS

Hypnotized subjects wait passively to be told what to do by the therapist and are very suggestible—they touch or hold imaginary objects and act out suggested roles. They do not,

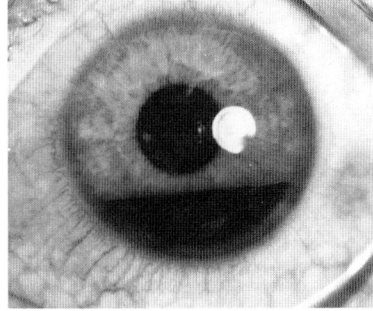

Appearance of hyphaema
Blood that has collected in the front chamber of the eye is clearly visible in front of the iris; hyphaema is usually caused by injury.

however, obey commands to behave in a manner they would normally regard as dangerous or improper.

Attention usually becomes highly selective, so that only one person at a time is heard. Subjects frequently will obey orders to forget everything that has happened during hypnosis, or, alternatively, to remember or repeat behaviour learned while hypnotized (a phenomenon known as posthypnotic suggestion).

THERAPEUTIC USES

Some psychoanalysts use hypnosis as a means of helping patients remember and come to terms with disturbing events or feelings that have been repressed from consciousness. More often, hypnosis is used as a means of helping patients relax. It may be useful in people suffering from *anxiety*, *panic attacks*, or *phobias*, and is sometimes successful in treating addictive habits, such as smoking. Scientific studies are lacking, however, and claims of fantastic cures should be treated with scepticism.

Hypnotic drugs

Drugs that induce sleep. See *Sleeping drugs*.

Hypo-

A prefix meaning under, below, or less than normal, as in hypodermic (under the skin), *hypoglycaemia* (abnormally low blood sugar level), and *hypotension* (lower than normal blood pressure).

Hypoaldosteronism

A rare deficiency of the hormone *aldosterone*, which is produced by the adrenal glands. Hypoaldosteronism may be caused by damage or disease affecting the adrenal glands. The disorder may produce weakness and is treated by the drug fludrocortisone.

Hypocalcaemia

An abnormally low level of *calcium* in the blood. The most common cause is *vitamin D* deficiency, due to a poor diet or, occasionally, to lack of sunshine. Rarer causes include chronic *kidney failure*, which leads to poor absorption of calcium from the diet, and *hypoparathyroidism* (underactivity of the parathyroid glands), resulting in insufficient production of parathyroid hormone, which helps control the level of calcium in the blood.

In mild cases, hypocalcaemia is symptomless. In severe cases, it causes *tetany* (painful spasms and twitches of the muscles, especially in

the hands and feet) due to the effect of low blood calcium on muscle activity. Hypocalcaemia may lead to softening of the bones. In children, such softening takes the form of *rickets*; in adults, it takes the form of *osteomalacia*.

Hypochondriasis

The unrealistic belief or fear that one is suffering from a serious illness, despite medical reassurance.

SYMPTOMS

Hypochondriacs worry constantly about their bodily health and interpret any physical symptom, however trivial, as evidence of a serious disorder. The feared disease may involve many parts of the body or may centre on a particular organ and a single disease, as in *cardiac neurosis* (fear of heart disease). People with hypochondriasis constantly seek medical advice and are likely to undergo numerous tests and treatments.

CAUSES

Hypochondriasis may be a complication of other psychological disorders, including *obsessive-compulsive disorder*, *phobia*, *generalized anxiety disorder*, *schizophrenia*, *depression*, and brain diseases, such as *dementia*.

The cause of hypochondriasis in the absence of an underlying disorder is uncertain. However, it seems to be more common in people who suffered from a true organic illness during childhood or were constantly exposed to sick relatives. The reason for this may be that the hypochondriac becomes programmed to overreact to every bodily feeling. In some cases, however, there there may be an inherited sensitivity to pain. Other factors include social stresses and personality type (typically orderly and obstinate).

TREATMENT

Any underlying mental disorder is treated as required. Hypochondriasis without an underlying cause is more difficult to treat, although an understanding and sympathetic doctor may help relieve distress.

Hypochondrium

The region on each side of the upper abdomen, which is situated below the lower ribs.

Hypoglossal nerve

The 12th *cranial nerve*, which controls movements of the *tongue*. The hypoglossal nerve is rarely damaged. If damage does occur (as a result of a stroke, for example), one side of the tongue becomes paralysed. (See illustrated box overleaf.)

H

H

LOCATION OF HYPOGLOSSAL NERVE

The hypoglossal nerve arises in the medulla oblongata (part of the brainstem), passes through the base of the skull, and runs around the throat to the tongue.

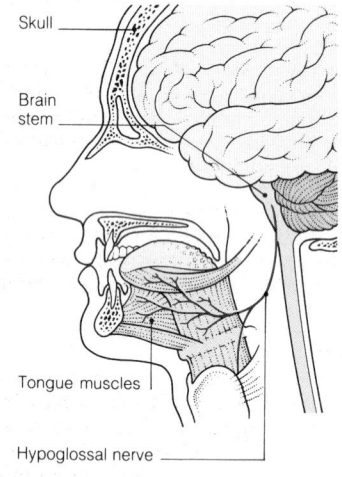

Skull

Brain stem

Tongue muscles

Hypoglossal nerve

Hypoglycaemia

An abnormally low level of glucose (sugar) in the blood. Almost all cases of hypoglycaemia occur in people with insulin-dependent *diabetes mellitus*. In this disease, the pancreas fails to produce enough *insulin* (a hormone that regulates the level of glucose in the blood), resulting in an abnormally high level of glucose. To lower the blood glucose level, diabetics take hypoglycaemic drugs by mouth (see *Hypoglycaemics, oral*) or insulin by injection. Too high a dose of either can reduce the blood glucose to too low a level, thus starving the body cells of energy. Hypoglycaemia can also occur if a person with diabetes misses a meal, fails to eat enough carbohydrates, or takes too much exercise.

Rarely, hypoglycaemia can result from drinking a large amount of alcohol or from an *insulinoma* (an insulin-producing tumour of the pancreas). Some children suffer from hypoglycaemia for no known reason, but in most cases the condition is temporary.

Hypoglycaemia is a serious condition. Failure of the brain to receive sufficient glucose may lead to permanent intellectual impairment.

SYMPTOMS

The principal symptoms include sweating, weakness, hunger, dizziness, trembling, headache, palpitations, confusion, and sometimes double vision. Behaviour is often irrational and aggressive and movements are uncoordinated; this state may be mistaken for drunkenness. The victim may lapse into coma due to extremely low blood sugar.

TREATMENT

Insulin-dependent diabetics should always carry sugar with them (in a convenient form such as sugar lumps or glucose tablets) to take at the first sign of an attack of hypoglycaemia. If it is suspected that an unconscious person has suffered a hypoglycaemic attack, medical help should be summoned immediately. The doctor will give an injection of either glucose solution or the hormone glucagon; the latter counteracts the effects of insulin and raises the blood glucose level by stimulating the conversion of glycogen to glucose.

Hypoglycaemics, oral

COMMON DRUGS

Chlorpropamide Glibenclamide Gliclazide Glipizide Tolazamide Tolbutamide

WARNING

Consult your doctor if you regularly experience symptoms, such as dizziness, nausea, and sweating, that are relieved only by food or a sugary drink. You might be taking too large a dose.

A group of drugs used in the treatment of non-insulin-dependent *diabetes mellitus* when *hyperglycaemia* (raised blood glucose level) cannot be controlled simply by diet.

HOW THEY WORK

Oral hypoglycaemics lower blood glucose levels by increasing the production by the pancreas of *insulin*, a hormone that increases the amount of glucose that is absorbed from the bloodstream into body cells. Insulin rather than oral hypoglycaemics may need to be prescribed temporarily to control the blood glucose level (e.g. during surgery, pregnancy, or a severe illness). Oral hypoglycaemics are of no use in treating insulin-dependent diabetes, in which the pancreas is unable to produce any insulin.

POSSIBLE ADVERSE EFFECTS

Oral hypoglycaemic drugs may cause *hypoglycaemia* (abnormally low blood glucose) if the dosage is too high or if the person has not had enough to eat.

Hypogonadism

Underactivity of the gonads (*testes* or *ovaries*). Hypogonadism may be caused by disorders of the gonads or by a disorder of the *pituitary gland* that results in deficient production of *gonadotrophin hormone*. In men, hypogonadism causes the symptoms and signs of *androgen hormone* deficiency. In women, it causes the symptoms and signs of *oestrogen hormone* deficiency.

Hypohidrosis

Reduced activity of the *sweat glands*. It is a feature of hypohidrotic ectodermal dysplasia, a rare, inherited, incurable condition characterized by reduced production of sweat and usually accompanied by dry, wrinkled skin, sparse, dry hair, small, brittle nails, and conical teeth.

Other causes of hypohidrosis include *exfoliative dermatitis* and some *anticholinergic drugs*.

Hypomania

A mild form of *mania*.

Hypoparathyroidism

Insufficient production of parathyroid hormone by the *parathyroid glands*, which lie behind the *thyroid gland* in the neck. Parathyroid hormone, along with *vitamin D* and *calcitonin* (a hormone produced by the thyroid gland), regulates the level of *calcium* in the body. A deficiency of the hormone results in *hypocalcaemia* (low levels of calcium in the blood).

CAUSES

The most common cause of hypoparathyroidism is accidental removal of the parathyroid glands during surgery on the thyroid gland. The condition may also result from surgery to remove a portion of the parathyroid glands themselves in the treatment of *hyperparathyroidism* (overactivity of the parathyroid glands). Occasionally the parathyroid glands are absent from birth, or they may cease to function for no apparent reason.

SYMPTOMS

The main effect of a low level of calcium in the body is *tetany*, an increased excitability of the nerves that causes uncontrollable, painful, cramp-like spasms of the hands, feet, and sometimes other parts of the body. Very occasionally, general seizures similar to those of an epileptic attack may occur.

DIAGNOSIS AND TREATMENT

The condition is diagnosed by tests to measure the level of calcium and parathyroid hormone in the blood.

If the patient is suffering from an attack of tetany, calcium may be injected slowly into a vein to provide quick relief. To maintain the blood calcium at a normal level, a lifelong course of calcium and vitamin D tablets is necessary (the vitamin D is needed to increase absorption of calcium from the diet). Regular check-ups are necessary to monitor the blood calcium level.

Hypophysectomy

The removal or destruction of the *pituitary gland*.

WHY IT IS DONE

Hypophysectomy is sometimes performed to remove *pituitary tumours*, which can cause various endocrine disorders, such as *acromegaly* and *Cushing's syndrome*.

The operation may also be performed to treat some cancers of the breast, ovary, or prostate gland, the growth of which is stimulated by hormones secreted by the pituitary gland.

HOW IT IS DONE

In some cases, the pituitary gland is removed surgically. The patient is given a general anaesthetic and the gland is removed, usually through the nose. Very large tumours may be removed through an incision into the skull (see *Craniotomy*).

In other cases, the gland may be destroyed by a radioactive implant which can be inserted into the gland by *stereotaxic surgery*.

Hypopituitarism

Underactivity of the *pituitary gland*, resulting in inadequate production of pituitary hormones. Hypopituitarism may lead to deficiency of one or more of the pituitary hormones and thus may produce a variety of effects on the body depending on which hormones are affected.

Possible causes of hypopituitarism are a *pituitary tumour*, an abnormality affecting the *hypothalamus* (part of the brain), or injury to the pituitary gland. Hypopituitarism may also follow surgical treatment or *radiotherapy* of the pituitary gland.

The condition is treated by replacing the deficient hormones.

Hypoplasia

Failure of an organ or a tissue to develop fully and reach its normal adult size.

Hypoplasia, enamel

A defect in tooth enamel. It is usually due to *amelogenesis imperfecta* (a hereditary condition), but may also be caused by vitamin deficiency, injury, or infection of a primary tooth that interferes with maturation of enamel.

Hypoplastic left-heart syndrome

A serious and usually fatal form of congenital *heart disease* that affects about one to two newborn babies in every 10,000 live births. The baby is born with a poorly formed ventricle (pumping chamber) on the left side of the heart and with other heart defects. The aorta (main artery carrying blood from the heart to the body) is malformed and blood can reach it only via a duct (the ductus arteriosus) that links the aorta to the pulmonary artery (blood vessel that transports blood to the lungs).

At birth the baby may seem healthy, but within a day or two the ductus arteriosus closes off and the baby collapses, becoming pale and breathless. There is no effective surgical treatment for the condition and most affected babies die within a week. A few infants have been treated by heart transplantation. The risk of parents having another affected child is small.

Hyposensitization

A preventive treatment of *allergy* to substances such as grass pollens, house-dust mites, and wasp and bee venom. Hyposensitization involves giving gradually increasing doses of an allergen (substance to which the person is allergic). This works by making the *immune system* less sensitive to that substance, probably by causing production of a particular "blocking" *antibody*, which reduces the symptoms of allergy when the substance is encountered.

Before starting treatment, the doctor and patient try to identify trigger factors for allergic symptoms. Skin tests or sometimes blood tests are performed to confirm the specific allergens to which the person has antibodies. Hyposensitization is usually recommended only if the person seems to be selectively sensitive to a specific allergen.

HOW IT IS DONE

A purified extract of a small amount of the allergen is injected into the skin of the arm in a course of injections. The course may need to be repeated annually for a few years.

RISKS

There is a danger of *anaphylactic shock* (a severe allergic reaction) shortly after an injection. Hyposensitization must therefore be performed under close medical supervision.

Hypospadias

A *congenital* defect of the *penis*, occurring in about one in 300 male babies, in which the opening of the *urethra* is situated on the underside of the penis. The urethral opening may be on the glans (head) or the shaft of the penis. In some cases, the penis curves downwards, a condition known as *chordee*, and the foreskin is limited to the front of the penis.

In severe forms of hypospadias the urethral opening lies well back along the penis towards the scrotum. The scrotum may be small, and the testes are undescended (see *Testis, undescended*). In such cases, the true sex of the child may be in doubt.

H

HYPOPLASTIC LEFT-HEART SYNDROME

The heart defects associated with this syndrome are shown (at right) and compared with those of the normal heart (at left). Neither the left ventricle (pumping chamber) nor the aorta is properly formed.

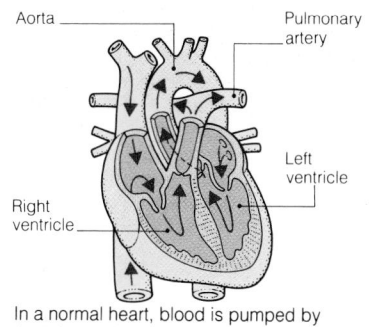

Aorta
Pulmonary artery
Left ventricle
Right ventricle

In a normal heart, blood is pumped by the left ventricle to the body via the aorta. If the left ventricle is poorly formed, blood can reach the body only via the ductus arteriosus, which closes soon after birth.

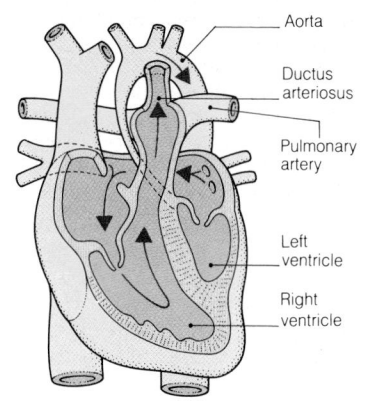

Aorta
Ductus arteriosus
Pulmonary artery
Left ventricle
Right ventricle

TREATMENT

Hypospadias can be corrected by a single operation in which the penis is straightened and a tube of skin (or occasionally bladder lining) is used to create a new urethra that extends to the tip of the penis. The operation is normally performed before the child is two years old; circumcision should not be performed prior to a hypospadias repair because the foreskin may be needed at the operation.

Surgery is usually successful, allowing the child to pass urine normally and, in later years, to have satisfactory sexual intercourse.

Hypotension

The medical term for low *blood pressure*. Some healthy people with a normal heart and blood vessels have blood pressure well below average for their age. Some research studies have suggested that such people have less energy and feel depressed more often than people with normal blood pressures, but most doctors continue to believe that hypotension causes symptoms only when the blood pressure is so low that blood flow to the brain is reduced, causing dizziness and fainting.

In the most common type of hypotension, known as postural hypotension, symptoms occur after abruptly standing or sitting up. Usually, blood pressure increases slightly with these changes in posture; in people with postural hypotension, this normal increase fails to occur. Postural hypotension is sometimes an adverse effect of *antidepressant drugs* or of *antihypertensive drugs* (drugs used to treat high blood pressure). Postural hypotension may also occur in people with *diabetes mellitus,* as a result of nerve damage that disrupts the reflexes controlling blood pressure.

Another type of hypotension develops suddenly as a result of serious burns or injuries that lead to a reduction in blood volume and to *shock.* Acute hypotension may also develop when a disease, such as *myocardial infarction* (heart attack) or *adrenal failure,* leads to shock.

Treatment of hypotension depends on the underlying cause.

Hypothalamus

A region of the *brain,* roughly the size of a cherry, situated behind the eyes and beneath another brain region called the thalamus. The hypothalamus has nerve connections to most other regions of the nervous system.

FUNCTION

The hypothalamus exerts overall control over the sympathetic nervous system (part of the *autonomic nervous system*). In response to sudden alarm or excitement, signals are sent from higher regions of the brain to the hypothalamus, initiating sympathetic nervous system activity. This causes a faster heartbeat, widening of the pupils, an increase in breathing rate and blood flow to muscles (together known as the "fight or flight" response).

Other groups of nerve cells in the hypothalamus are concerned with the control of body temperature, so that, when blood flowing to the brain is hotter or cooler than normal, the hypothalamus switches on temperature-regulating mechanisms (among them sweating or shivering). It receives information from internal sense organs regarding the body's water content and the level of glucose in the blood; if these are too low, the hypothalamus stimulates thirst and appetite for food. The hypothalamus is also involved in regulating sleep, in motivating sexual behaviour, and in determining mood and emotions.

Another role of the hypothalamus is to coordinate the function of the nervous and endocrine (hormonal) systems of the body. The hypothalamus connects with the *pituitary gland* through a short stalk of nerve fibres and controls hormonal secretions from this gland. It does this through direct nerve connections and through specialized nerve cells, which secrete hormones called releasing factors into the blood to travel to the pituitary gland. In this way, the hypothalamus can convert nerve signals into hormonal signals. Thus, the hypothalamus indirectly controls many of the glands of the *endocrine system,* including the pituitary gland, *thyroid gland,* cortex of the *adrenal glands, ovaries,* and *testes.*

DISORDERS

Disorders of the hypothalamus are usually caused by a brain haemorrhage within the hypothalamic region (see *Intracerebral haemorrhage*) or an expanding *pituitary tumour.* Loss of hypothalamic function can have diverse effects, ranging from hormonal disorders to disturbances in temperature regulation, and increased or decreased appetite for food, sex, and sleep.

Hypothermia

A fall in body temperature to below 35°C. Hypothermia causes drowsiness, lowers breathing and heart rates, and may lead to unconscious-

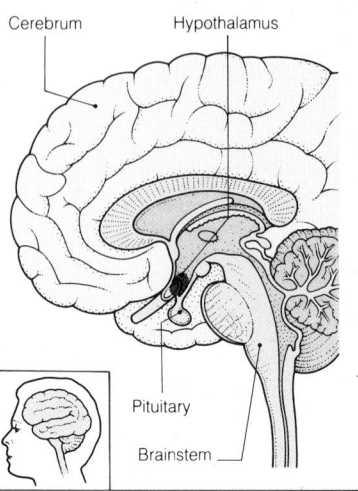

LOCATION OF THE HYPOTHALAMUS
This small area of the forebrain lies under the thalamus and above the pituitary gland.

Cerebrum   Hypothalamus

Pituitary

Brainstem

ness or death. Many victims are elderly people who are unable to keep sufficiently warm in winter.

Hypothermia also includes the deliberate lowering of body temperature during some forms of surgery (see *Hypothermia, surgical*).

CAUSES

Most cases of hypothermia occur in sick elderly people living in poorly heated homes. As the body ages, it gradually loses its sensitivity to cold. An elderly person may not feel cold when the body temperature drops, and as a person gets older, the body becomes increasingly less able to reverse a fall in temperature. The risk of hypothermia is increased if an elderly person has a disorder that reduces the body's heat production (such as *hypothyroidism*), impairs mental function (such as *dementia*), or reduces mobility (such as *arthritis*).

Babies also have an increased risk of suffering from hypothermia, because they lose heat rapidly and cannot easily reverse a fall in temperature.

People of all ages may develop hypothermia as a result of prolonged exposure to extremely cold weather. Hypothermia may develop in only moderately cold conditions if clothing is damp. Victims quite commonly include ill-equipped walkers. Swimming in cold water is another cause of hypothermia. It is now believed that many deaths, which in the past were attributed to drowning, are in fact due to hypothermia. The sea, rivers, and lakes of the UK are for most months of the year cold enough to cause rapid cooling of the body.

Certain drugs may also contribute to the onset of hypothermia. For example, *tranquillizer drugs* (such as chlorpromazine) may lower the level of consciousness and reduce the ability to shiver, which helps protect the body against cold.

SIGNS

A person suffering from hypothermia is usually pale, puffy-faced, and listless, and shows changes in behaviour, such as withdrawal and apathy. The heart-rate is slow and the victim is often drowsy and confused. Areas of the body that are normally warm (e.g. the armpits, the groin) are cold.

In severe hypothermia, breathing becomes slow and shallow, the muscles are often stiff, the victim may become unconscious, and the heart may beat only faintly and irregularly or—especially if the body temperature falls below 32.2°C—it may stop beating altogether.

DIAGNOSIS

The condition is usually obvious from the above signs and the victim's circumstances. To determine how cold the body has become, the rectal temperature is taken with with a special low-reading thermometer. Alternatively, the temperature of the urine may be measured.

TREATMENT

Hypothermia is a medical emergency and anyone who is suspected of suffering from it requires immediate medical attention.

In mild cases, warm drinks and covering the head (from which as much as 20 per cent of the body's heat loss takes place) usually improve the patient's condition.

In more severe cases, treatment varies according to the age of the victim. A young person may be warmed in a hot bath. This method of treatment could, however, prove fatal in an elderly person, whose body might not be able to cope with such rapid warming, which causes a rush of blood to the surface of the body and a consequent reduction in blood supply to the heart and brain.

An elderly victim is usually warmed gradually (at a rate of about 0.6°C per hour) by being covered with layers of heat-reflecting material (space blankets) in a room temperature of 25°C. The patient's rectal temperature is monitored every half hour until temperature, breathing, heart-rate, and level of consciousness improve.

FIRST AID: HYPOTHERMIA

DO NOT
- let the victim walk
- warm the victim by rubbing his or her skin
- give the victim any alcohol
- warm the victim by applying direct heat.

IN BABIES

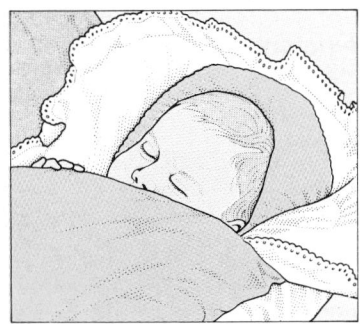

Medical help should be sought immediately. Hypothermia is often difficult to detect. The baby may look pink and healthy, but he or she may be unusually limp and drowsy. Rewarm the baby by keeping him or her well wrapped.

IN ADULTS

1 Seek medical help. If the victim is unconscious and breathing, place in the *recovery position*. If not breathing, begin *artificial respiration*.

2 Move the victim to a warm place. Replace wet clothing with dry, or dry the victim and cover him or her with waterproof material.

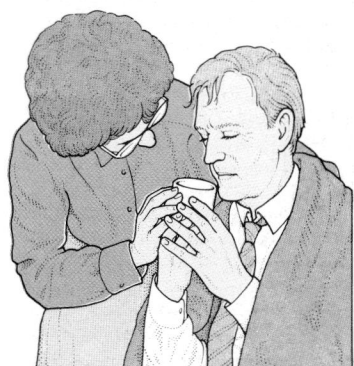

3 If the victim is conscious, give a warm (not hot) drink. Hold the cup or mug if necessary.

4 If the victim is otherwise healthy, place in a warm (not hot) bath.

When hypothermia is severe enough to be life-threatening, victims may be admitted to an intensive care unit for controlled warming. This may be done by withdrawing blood from the patient's circulation, warming it, and returning it to the body. Alternatively, warm fluid may be run into the abdominal cavity.

PREVENTION

An elderly person's living accommodation should be kept at a temperature of at least 18°C. Relatives or neighbours of an elderly person living alone should check that he or she has additional means of keeping warm in winter, including warm blankets and suitable clothing. To reduce heat loss, a warm hat should be worn whenever it is cold.

All elderly people should have a nutritious diet, and should try to eat hot food and to drink warm fluids several times a day.

People walking or climbing in cold weather should carry survival bags, lined with space blankets, into which they can crawl while waiting for help in the event of becoming stranded or an accident occurring.

Hypothermia, surgical

The deliberate reduction of body temperature to prolong the period for which the vital organs can safely be deprived (partly or totally) of their normal blood supply during *open heart surgery*.

Cold reduces the rate of metabolism in cells and tissues and thus increases their tolerance to lack of oxygen.

In the early days of heart surgery, induced hypothermia allowed surgeons to perform quick (eight to 10 minutes) operations on the heart while blood circulation throughout the body was completely stopped.

Today, open heart surgery is usually performed with the general blood circulation maintained by means of a *heart-lung machine*. Nevertheless, mild hypothermia—with the body temperature reduced from 37°C to about 28 to 31°C—is still generally induced as a safety measure. It can allow heart operations to proceed for several hours. A heat exchanger, installed into the machine circuit, can be used to cool the blood before it is returned to the body, thus inducing hypothermia.

During open heart surgery, because the blood supply to the heart is interrupted, the heart muscle itself must also be vigorously cooled. Cooling can be achieved by continuously instilling cold saline at a temperature of about 4°C into the open chest cavity. As a result, damage to the heart muscle from lack of oxygen is minimal, even if an operation lasts several hours.

At the end of the operation, rewarming of the patient is carefully synchronized with restarting the heart and stopping use of the heart-lung machine.

Hypothyroidism

Underproduction of *thyroid hormones* by an underactive *thyroid gland*.

CAUSES AND INCIDENCE

Most cases of hypothyroidism are caused by the body developing *antibodies* against its own thyroid gland (an example of an *autoimmune disorder*) with a resultant reduction in thyroid hormone production. *Hashimoto's thyroiditis* is an example of this phenomenon. More rarely, hypothyroidism may result from surgery to remove part of the thyroid gland or the giving of radioactive iodine as a treatment for *hyperthyroidism* (overactivity of the thyroid).

Hypothyroidism affects about one per cent of the adult population. It is most common in elderly women, although it occurs at all ages and in both sexes.

SYMPTOMS AND SIGNS

Thyroid hormones stimulate energy production, so a deficiency of them causes generalized tiredness and lethargy. There may also be muscle weakness, cramps, a slow heart-rate, dry and flaky skin, hair loss, a deep and husky voice, and weight gain. A syndrome known as *myxoedema*, in which the skin and other body tissues thicken, may develop. In some cases, a *goitre* (enlargement of the thyroid gland) develops, although not all goitres are due to hypothyroidism.

The severity of the symptoms depends on the degree of thyroid deficiency. Mild deficiency may cause no symptoms; severe deficiency may produce all of the above symptoms.

If hypothyroidism occurs in childhood and remains untreated, it may retard growth, delay sexual maturation, and inhibit normal development of the brain.

DIAGNOSIS AND TREATMENT

The disorder is diagnosed by tests to measure the level of thyroid hormones in the blood.

Treatment consists of replacement therapy with the thyroid hormone thyroxine; in most cases, hormone therapy must be continued for life. If this treatment does not cure a goitre, surgery may be required.

Hypotonia

Abnormal muscle slackness. Normally, a muscle that is not being used has a certain inbuilt tension, but in a number of disorders affecting the nervous system (such as *Huntington's disease)* this natural tension or tone is moderately or markedly reduced.

Hypotonia in infants

Excessive limpness in infants. Hypotonia is sometimes known as the floppy infant syndrome.

FEATURES

Hypotonic babies cannot hold their limbs up against gravity and thus tend to lie flat with their arms and legs splayed. Their limbs and joints seem slack when moved by someone else. Floppy babies move around less than normal babies and their mothers may not have felt the baby move much during pregnancy. When held horizontally by the trunk, face downwards, floppy babies hang limply.

CAUSES

Premature infants are naturally more floppy than full-term infants, but normal muscle tension will develop as they mature.

Hypotonia may be caused by a general disorder, such as *hypothyroidism* or *Down's syndrome*. It may also be an early feature of *cerebral palsy* as a result of brain damage, and occurs in disorders of the spinal cord, such as *Werdnig-Hoffman disease,* and in some children with *muscular dystrophy*.

Hypovolaemia

An abnormally low volume of blood in the circulation. Hypovolaemia usually follows severe blood loss, which may occur as a result of injury, internal bleeding, or surgery. It also occurs in other conditions, such as serious burns and severe dehydration.

Hypovolaemia is a dangerous condition because, untreated, it can lead to *shock,* which is potentially fatal.

Hypoxia

An inadequate supply of oxygen to the tissues.

CAUSES

Temporary hypoxia may result from strenuous exercise in which the normal supply of oxygen cannot meet the additional requirements of the tissues.

The condition disappears once exercise has stopped and breathing has reoxygenated the tissues.

More serious causes include impaired breathing (see *Respiratory failure*), usually a result of a lung disorder; *ischaemia* (reduced blood flow to a tissue), which may be due to an artery or heart disorder; and severe *anaemia*, in which the oxygen-carrying capacity of the blood is reduced. Another, rare, cause is *carbon monoxide* poisoning, which prevents the blood from being adequately oxygenated. In severe cases, any of these more serious causes may lead to *anoxia* (complete absence of oxygen in a tissue), which, if prolonged, may cause tissue death.

SYMPTOMS AND SIGNS

Hypoxia in muscles forces the muscle cells to produce energy by *anaerobic* metabolism, which produces lactic acid as a by-product. The build-up of lactic acid causes cramps. Hypoxia in heart muscle may cause the chest pain of *angina pectoris*. Hypoxia of the brain initially causes confusion, dizziness, and incoordination, leading to unconsciousness and death if it persists.

TREATMENT

Severe, potentially life-threatening hypoxia may require treatment by *oxygen therapy* or artificial *ventilation*. Otherwise, the treatment depends on the underlying cause.

Hysterectomy

Removal of the uterus. Hysterectomy is one of the most frequently performed operations in the UK, although many women who would formerly have had a hysterectomy are now being treated by *endometrial ablation*. (See also *Minimally invasive surgery*).

WHY IT IS DONE

Hysterectomy is often performed to treat *fibroids* (benign tumours of the uterus). It is also used to treat cancer of the uterus (see *Uterus, cancer of*) or of the cervix (see *Cervix, cancer of*). Hysterectomy may be performed to relieve *menorrhagia* (heavy menstrual bleeding) or *endometriosis* (a condition in which fragments of the uterine lining occur elsewhere in the pelvis) that have not responded to treatment. Hysterectomy may also be performed to remove a severely prolapsed uterus (see *Uterus, prolapse of*).

TYPES

The most common type of hysterectomy is a total hysterectomy, in which the uterus and cervix are removed. Sometimes, the fallopian tubes and ovaries are removed in addition to the uterus. The operation known as a sub-

H

total hysterectomy, in which the cervix is not removed, is now obsolete. For cervical cancer, a radical hysterectomy (in which the pelvic lymph nodes are also removed) is necessary.

RECOVERY PERIOD

After the operation, a drainage tube may be inserted at the site of the incision. For a few days there may be some vaginal bleeding and discharge and considerable tenderness and pain. The stay in hospital depends on the age and health of the woman and whether there are post-operative problems. Full recovery requires another three to six weeks; sexual intercourse can be resumed about a month after the surgery.

OUTLOOK

After hysterectomy, the woman is unable to bear children; she does not menstruate and needs no contraception. If the ovaries have also been removed from a woman before or around the *menopause, hormone replacement therapy* should be considered.

Many women worry that their sex lives will be affected, but there should be no noticeable change. Early counselling can help dispel fears. Depression is not uncommon if women are inadequately counselled.

Hysteria

A term encompassing a wide range of physical or mental symptoms that are attributed to mental stress.

Derived from the Greek word for uterus, hysteria was once thought to be a physical disorder confined to women. By the 19th century, it was believed to have a psychological origin and was used to describe many seemingly bizarre states (e.g. hallucination, trances, and sleepwalking).

Today, many psychiatrists feel that the term hysteria is no longer helpful in diagnosis. In modern classifications, therefore, the symptoms formerly grouped under this term are now included in the more specific diagnostic categories of *conversion disorder; dissociative disorders; factitious disorders;* and *somatization disorder*.

The term is still sometimes used loosely to describe any difficult or unusual behaviour that does not seem consistent with the symptoms or situation of the patient. Mass hysteria describes the spread of psychologically produced symptoms (such as fainting) from person to person. It usually occurs in schools or institutions of young women in response to group tensions or worries and is often triggered by a charismatic personality.

PERFORMING A HYSTERECTOMY

Hysterectomy may be performed through the abdomen or the vagina. For an abdominal hysterectomy, the incision is made in the lower abdomen (see below). In vaginal hysterectomy, the uterus is removed through an incision at the top of the vagina.

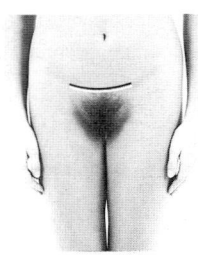

Site of incision for abdominal hysterectomy
The incision is made in the lower abdomen (in this case horizontally) level with the top of the pubic hair.

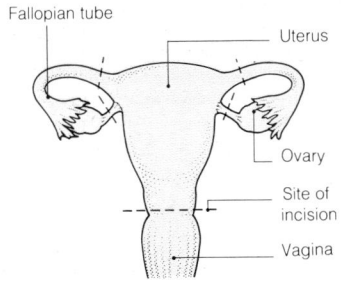

Fallopian tube — Uterus — Ovary — Site of incision — Vagina

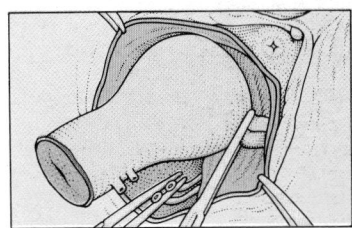

Abdominal hysterectomy
The uterine vessels are clamped. Traction is placed on the top of the uterus and the vessels are tied and then divided. In some cases, the fallopian tubes are cut and the tubes and ovaries left in place.

Vaginal hysterectomy
After a vaginal incision is made, the uterus and cervix are removed (the ovaries cannot be removed in a vaginal hysterectomy). The upper end of the vagina is repaired by stitching.

Hysterosalpingography

An *X-ray* procedure performed to examine the inside of the uterus and fallopian tubes.

WHY IT IS DONE

The examination is performed as part of the investigation of *infertility*. *Laparoscopy* can indicate whether the tubes are blocked, but hysterosalpingography may be needed to determine the site of the blockage, which is most often due to scar tissue caused by a

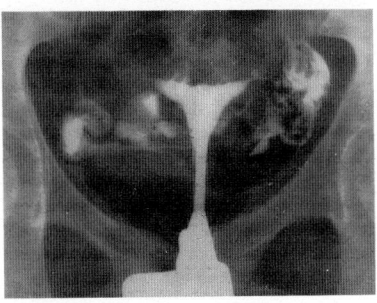

A normal hysterosalpingogram
The X-ray image shows radiopaque substance filling the uterus and passing through the fallopian tubes into the pelvic cavity.

previous infection. Hysterosalpingography also outlines any distortion in the uterus, such as a congenital abnormality or a *fibroid*.

HOW IT IS DONE

The test is an outpatient procedure performed by a radiologist and/or a gynaecologist. It may cause discomfort or a cramp-like pain, so the patient may be mildly sedated.

A plastic or metal *cannula* (tube) is inserted into the cervix (neck of the uterus), a radiopaque contrast medium (one that shows up on X-ray film) is passed through it into the uterus and the fallopian tubes; X-ray pictures are taken to reveal any abnormalities. The procedure takes 10 to 30 minutes.

Hysterotomy

A method of late abortion in which the abdomen and uterus are surgically opened to remove the fetus. Hysterotomy is the most complicated method of abortion and carries the highest risk. It is rarely used today; instead, most late abortions are performed by giving *prostaglandin drugs* to induce labour. (See also *Abortion, induced*.)

Iatrogenic

A term meaning "physician-produced" that can be applied to any medical condition, disease, or other adverse occurrence that results from medical treatment. The development of an iatrogenic condition does not necessarily imply a lack of care or knowledge on the part of the doctor. Many common forms of treatment are seldom, if ever, entirely free of possible unwanted effects. The drowsiness produced by some antihistamine drugs is one example.

Ibuprofen

A *nonsteroidal anti-inflammatory drug* (NSAID) used as a painkiller in the treatment of headache, menstrual pain, and painful injury to soft tissues (such as muscles and ligaments). The anti-inflammatory effect of ibuprofen helps reduce the joint pain and stiffness that occurs in types of arthritis, such as *rheumatoid arthritis* and *osteoarthritis*.

Ibuprofen may cause abdominal pain, diarrhoea, nausea, heartburn, and, rarely, dizziness. It may cause *peptic ulcer*, but is less likely to do so than some other NSAIDs.

Ice-packs

Means of applying ice (in a towel or other material) to the skin to relieve pain, to stem bleeding, or to reduce inflammation. Cold causes the blood vessels to contract, thus reducing the blood flow.

WHY IT IS DONE

Treatment with ice-packs is used to relieve pain in a variety of disorders, including severe *headache*, *haemorrhoids* (piles), and pain in the throat after a *tonsillectomy*. Another common use is after sports injuries to minimize swelling, bruising, and further tissue damage. In the treatment of sports injuries, ice-packs are usually used together with the application of a pressure bandage and the raising of the injured part. Ice-packs may also be used to stop bleeding from small vessels, as in a nosebleed.

HOW IT IS DONE

Ice is wrapped in a wet cloth (to prevent it from burning the skin) and applied to the skin's surface. It is also possible to use special chemical packs that become very cold when they are shaken or struck.

Ichthyosis

A rare, inherited condition in which the skin is dry, thickened, scaly, and darker than normal due to an abnormality in the production of *keratin* (a protein that is the main component of skin). The name ichthyosis is taken from the Greek word "ichthus" (meaning fish); the condition is commonly called fish skin disease.

Ichthyosis usually appears at or shortly after birth and generally improves during childhood. The areas most commonly affected are the thighs, arms, and backs of the hands.

There is no special treatment for ichthyosis, although lubricants and emulsifying ointments help the dryness and bath oils moisten the skin. Washing with soap makes ichthyosis worse and should be avoided. The condition improves in a warm, humid atmosphere.

Icterus

A term for *jaundice*.

Id

One of the three parts of the personality (together with the *ego* and *superego*) described by Sigmund Freud. The id is

Damaged tissue

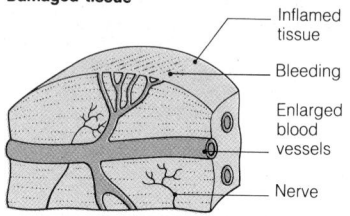

- Inflamed tissue
- Bleeding
- Enlarged blood vessels
- Nerve

Ice-pack application

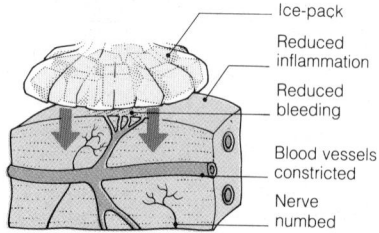

- Ice-pack
- Reduced inflammation
- Reduced bleeding
- Blood vessels constricted
- Nerve numbed

Use of an ice-pack
Applying an ice-pack to an area of damaged tissue helps relieve pain, reduce inflammation and tissue damage, and minimize bleeding and swelling.

the primitive, unconscious store of energy from which come the instincts for food, love, sex, and other basic needs. The id seeks simply to gain pleasure and to avoid pain. (See also *Psychoanalytic theory*.)

Idiocy

An outdated term for the most severe degree of *mental handicap*.

Idiopathic

Of unknown cause. For example, epilepsy for which no specific cause can be found is referred to as idiopathic epilepsy. The word idiopathic comes from Greek "idios" meaning one's own and "pathos" meaning disease.

Idoxuridine

An *antiviral drug* used for the *topical* treatment of *herpes simplex* and *herpes zoster* infections. Idoxuridine may cause irritation of areas to which it is applied. Eye-drops may cause photophobia (abnormal sensitivity to light) and blurred vision.

Ileitis, regional

An old name for *Crohn's disease*.

Ileostomy

An operation in which the *ileum* (lower part of the small intestine) is surgically severed and the end brought through an incision in the abdominal wall and formed into an artificial outlet to allow the discharge of faeces into a lightweight bag attached to the skin. An ileostomy is usually permanent.

WHY IT IS DONE

Permanent ileostomy is usually performed for people with *ulcerative colitis* or *Crohn's disease* whose health, despite drug treatment, continues to deteriorate because of chronic inflammation of the colon. For these people, the only means of restoring health is to perform a *colectomy* (an operation to remove the colon and rectum) followed by an ileostomy.

Temporary ileostomy is sometimes required at the time of partial colectomy (removal of part of the colon) to allow the repair of the colon to heal before waste material passes through it. Temporary ileostomy may also be carried out as an emergency measure in a person who is very ill due to an obstruction high in the large intestine that is preventing the normal passage of faeces. The ileostomy is made above the obstruction and, by allowing waste material to discharge, enables a patient to recover sufficiently to undergo a partial colectomy to remove the obstruction. Temporary ileostomies are closed when the rejoined colon has healed.

HOW IT IS DONE
When the whole of the colon and rectum has been removed, the cut end of the ileum is brought to the surface of the skin through an incision in the abdominal wall.

In the case of a temporary ileostomy, a loop of bowel is brought to the surface and opened so that waste material can pass through. The edges of this opening are then stitched to the skin at the edge of the abdominal incision to create a stoma (an artificial opening). The stoma is usually located on the patient's right side, about 5 cm below the natural waist and away from the hip-bone.

POST-OPERATIVE CARE
For a few days, patients may need to be fed by *intravenous infusion*. After that, the intestine starts to function normally again; semi-liquid waste is discharged through the stoma into a bag that is closely attached to the skin by adhesive seals.

During the convalescent period, patients with permanent ileostomies are given counselling to help them come to terms with an altered body image and the appearance of the stoma. They are also taught the practical aspects of stoma care. There is no muscle control over evacuation of body wastes through the stoma. These wastes are semi-liquid and contain enzymes that can damage the skin around the stoma. For these reasons, it is usually necessary for the bag to be worn at all times. A member of the nursing staff (ideally a stoma-care nurse) teaches the patient how .to empty, change, and dispose of the bag, and how to maintain a good seal between bag and body to protect the skin and prevent leaks.

Full recovery from the operation takes about six weeks, during which time patients should avoid vigorous physical activity.

OUTLOOK
The condition of patients who are given ileostomies after removal of a chronically inflamed colon usually improves dramatically. Because their ability to be active is enhanced, many of these people say they wish they had had the operation years earlier.

Following convalescence, patients should be able to return to their usual employment, lifestyle, and family and social activities. After an ileostomy it is necessary to drink increased

PROCEDURE FOR ILEOSTOMY
Two incisions are made in the abdominal wall (usually on the right side)—a small circular cut for the stoma (most often located about 5 cm below the waist and away from the hip-bone and groin crease) and a vertical cut to give access to the intestine and *mesentery*.

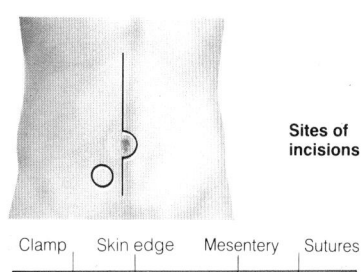

Sites of incisions

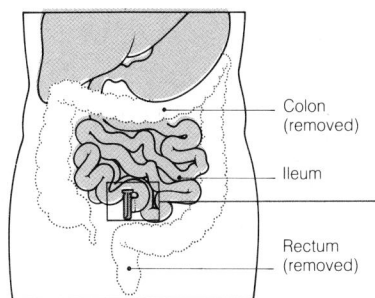

Colon (removed)

Ileum

Rectum (removed)

1 After removal of the colon, the cut end of the ileum is clamped and part of the mesentery is cut to free a short length of ileum for the stoma.

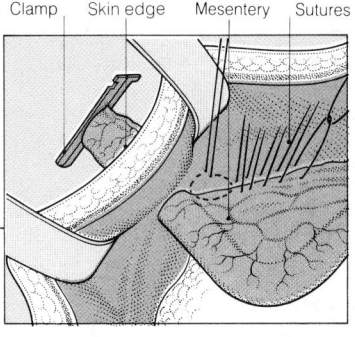

Clamp   Skin edge   Mesentery   Sutures

2 The free end of the ileum is pushed out through the circular incision in the abdomen; the mesentery is then stitched to the inner abdominal wall.

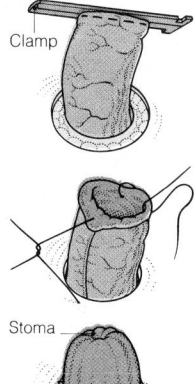

Clamp

Stoma

3 The main vertical incision is closed, and the clamp is removed from the protruding end of the ileum (top). The end of the ileum is then turned back and attached to the abdomen with sutures (middle). When completed, this creates a small protruding stoma (bottom). A temporary ileostomy appliance is usually fitted immediately.

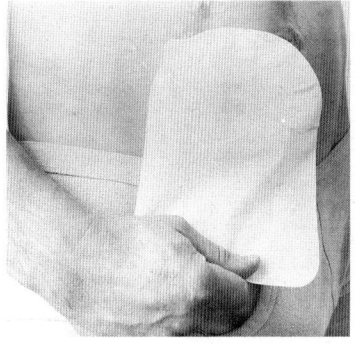

4 After the intestine begins to function normally, an ileostomy bag is fitted around the stoma. The bag is attached closely to the skin by adhesive seals.

amounts of water and to ensure that the intake of salt is adequate, thus compensating for the lack of a colon (the main functions of which are the absorption of water and salt). Apart from this recommendation, it is generally possible to eat a normal diet.

Only an occasional medical check-up is needed to make sure that the stoma is in good condition, although the doctor should always be informed of any change in the function or appearance of the stoma. Occasionally, the channel of the stoma becomes narrowed or prolapses (protrudes too far from the abdomen), requiring surgical correction.

Various attempts have been made to devise ileostomies that require emptying only once or twice a day at fixed times and do not require an external appliance. These devices include internal reservoirs made from loops of small intestine, magnetic closures, and carbon filter systems for gas. However, none is consistently reliable; most patients are still offered a conventional ileostomy.

Ileum
The final, longest, and narrowest section of the small intestine. It is joined at its upper end to the *jejunum* and at its lower end to the large intestine.

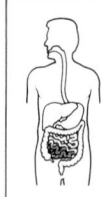

LOCATION OF THE ILEUM

The ileum (the final part of the small intestine) joins the jejunum and caecum (the first part of the large intestine).

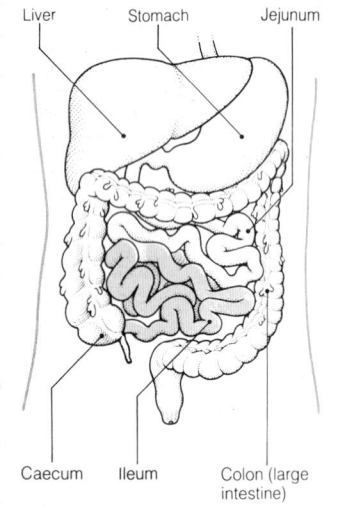

Liver   Stomach   Jejunum

Caecum   Ileum   Colon (large intestine)

The function of the ileum is to absorb nutrients from food that has been digested in the stomach and the first two sections of the small intestine. The millions of *villi* (finger-like projections) that line the ileum considerably increase its surface area and thus its powers of absorption.

DISORDERS

Occasionally, the ileum becomes obstructed—for example, by pushing through a weakness in the abdominal wall (see *Hernia*) or by becoming caught up with scar tissue following abdominal surgery (see *Adhesion*).

Other disorders of the ileum include *Meckel's diverticulum* (a pouch in the ileum wall that may become ulcerated) and diseases in which absorption of nutrients is impaired, such as *Crohn's disease*, *coeliac disease*, tropical *sprue*, and *lymphoma*.

Ileus, paralytic

A failure, usually temporary, of the normal contractility of the muscles of the intestine. As a result, intestinal contents can no longer pass through the body and the intestine becomes obstructed. Paralytic ileus commonly follows abdominal surgery and may also be induced by severe abdominal injury, *peritonitis* (inflammation of the membrane lining the abdomen), internal bleeding, acute *pancreatitis* (inflammation of the pancreas), or interference with the blood or nerve supply to the intestine.

The symptoms of paralytic ileus include a distended (swollen) abdomen, vomiting, and failure to pass faeces. The condition is usually successfully treated by sucking out the intestinal contents through a tube passed through the nose or mouth into the stomach or intestine and by maintaining body fluid levels by *intravenous infusion* (drip).

Illness

Perception by a person that he or she is not well. Illness is a subjective sensation and may have physical or psychological causes. Illness is also sometimes used as a synonym for disease or disorder.

Illusion

A distorted sensation. An illusion is based on misinterpretation of a real stimulus (for example, a pen is seen as a dagger, or the sound of a screeching brake is heard as a scream). An illusion is not the same as an *hallucination* in which a perception occurs without any stimulus.

Usually, illusions are brief and can be understood when explained. They may be due to tiredness or anxiety, to drugs of many sorts, or to certain forms of brain damage. *Delirium tremens* is a classic inducer of illusions.

Imaging techniques

Techniques that produce images of structures within the body that cannot otherwise be seen. Imaging techniques are an invaluable aid in diagnosing abnormalities and disease.

X-RAYS

In 1895 the discovery of *X-rays* revolutionized medical diagnosis by making it possible for the first time to visualize bone, organs, and other internal tissue without opening up the body. The rays are electromagnetic waves of short wavelength. Some are absorbed and others pass through tissues; the shadow that is cast is projected on to a fluorescent screen or a film.

CONTRAST MEDIA X-ray images of bones are distinct, but soft tissues show up less clearly. To overcome this, radiologists from the 1920s onwards began using substances opaque to radiation as part of certain X-ray procedures. When such substances (known as contrast media) are introduced into internal organs, blood vessels, or ducts, they produce (on the X-ray screen or film) an outline of the cavities they fill.

A contrast medium can be introduced into the body in various ways. In *cholecystography* (carried out to examine the gallbladder and common bile duct) and in some *barium X-ray examinations* of the oesophagus, the stomach, and the small bowel, the medium is swallowed in tablet or liquid form. In *bronchography* (used to diagnose various chest disorders) the contrast medium is introduced into the bronchi (airways) connecting the windpipe to the lungs. In *angiography* and *venography*, the contrast medium is injected into an artery or vein, respectively, to provide images of the blood vessels. In intravenous *urography*, the medium injected into a vein in the arm travels to the kidneys and urinary tract. In *ERCP* (by which the pancreatic duct and biliary system are examined), the medium is passed into the ducts by means of a catheter (tube) passed through a channel in an endoscope (a flexible viewing instrument).

SCANNING TECHNIQUES

Since the 1970s, many X-ray imaging techniques have been superseded by newer procedures that are simpler to perform and are safer and more comfortable for the patient. *Ultrasound scanning* consists of passing high-frequency sound waves through the body with a transducer placed against the skin. The waves are reflected to varying degrees by structures of different density, and the pattern of the echoes is electronically recorded on a screen. Ultrasound scanning is the first choice for diagnostic imaging of the gallbladder, female genital tract, and fetus. It also provides remarkably clear pictures of the kidney.

COMPUTERS Many scanning techniques use a computer to provide images. In *CT scanning* (computed tomography scanning), X-rays are passed through the body at different angles. The computer produces cross-sectional images ("slices") of the tissues being examined. In *MRI* (magnetic resonance imaging), the patient is placed in a strong magnetic field and radiofrequency waves are passed through the body. A computer analyses changes in the magnetic alignment of the hydrogen protons of the cells to give an image of the tissues.

CT scanning and MRI are particularly valuable in the diagnosis of brain disorders. So, too, is a more recent technique called *PET scanning* (positron emission tomography scanning),

IMAGING THE BODY

Over the past decade, many new methods of imaging the body have been developed. These new imaging techniques have made it possible to visualize internal structures in a variety of different ways. Today, in addition to conventional X-rays (which show primarily bones), techniques such as CT scanning, radionuclide scanning, ultrasound scanning, MRI, and PET scanning are used to provide detailed diagnostic pictures of soft tissues and organs. The examples given here show some of the different ways in which the kidneys can be imaged.

X-RAYS

Radiopaque contrast media may be utilized to give distinct X-ray images of soft tissues, as in intravenous. urography, which is used to give clear images of the kidneys and urinary tract.

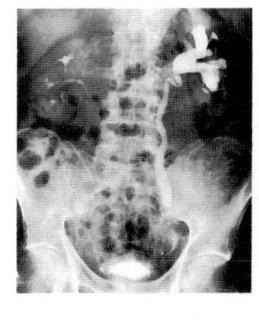
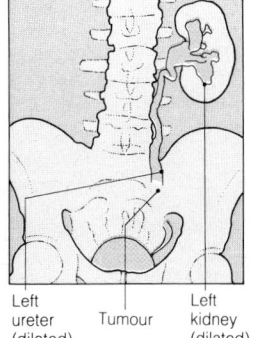

Intravenous urogram
The intravenous urogram (far left) shows the left kidney and ureter, which are visible because they are filled with contrast medium that has been retained due to a tumour obstructing the ureter (see left).

Left ureter (dilated) Tumour Left kidney (dilated)

SCANNING TECHNIQUES

Many new techniques have been developed for imaging the body, particularly the soft tissues. Some of these techniques, such as CT scanning, rely on computers to process the raw imaging data and produce the actual image. Others, such as ultrasound scanning and radionuclide scanning, can produce images without a computer, although one may be used for image enhancement.

Damaged left kidney

Normal right kidney

L   R

Radionuclide scanning
A radioactive substance is introduced into the body, and the radiation emitted is detected by a gamma camera, which converts it into an image. In the scan of the kidneys (left), the left one has taken up little of the radioactive substance (and thus appears faint), which indicates that it is damaged.

Ultrasound scanning

Ultra-high-frequency sound waves reflected from tissues in the body are converted into an image by special electronic equipment. The scan (below left) shows a section through a diseased kidney; the inner tissues (calyx and pelvis) are greatly dilated, and the outer cortex is abnormally thin (see diagram, below right).

CT scanning and MRI

These techniques produce cross-sectional images (slices) of the body. The CT scan (right) shows a greatly dilated right kidney (see diagram, below right).

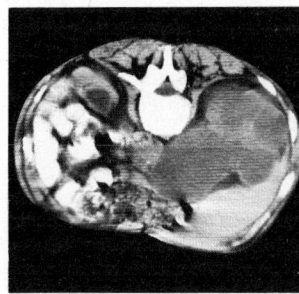

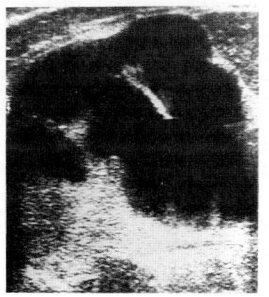

Back   Thin cortex

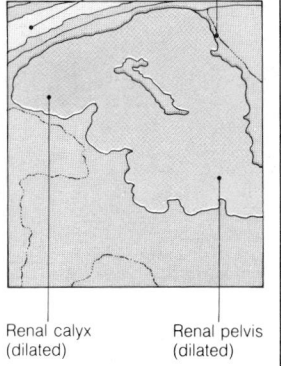

Renal calyx (dilated)   Renal pelvis (dilated)

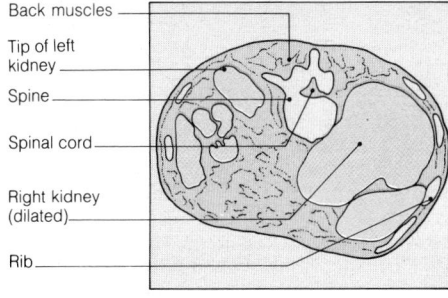

Back muscles

Tip of left kidney

Spine

Spinal cord

Right kidney (dilated)

Rib

in which very short-lived radio-isotopes are introduced into tissues; the paths of gamma rays emitted are analysed by a computer, giving information about brain function and structure.

In *radionuclide scanning*, a gamma camera records, and a computer transforms into images, radiation emitted from tissues into which a radioactive substance has been introduced. The computer may be used to obtain more information from the results.

Imipramine

A tricyclic *antidepressant drug*. Imipramine is most commonly used as a long-term treatment for *depression*, but may take up to six weeks to have a beneficial effect.

Possible adverse effects include excessive sweating, blurred vision, dry mouth, dizziness, constipation, nausea, and, in older men, difficulty passing urine. Overdose, particularly in a child, can be fatal.

Immersion foot

A type of *cold injury* occurring when the feet are wet and cold for a long time. It occurs in people who have been shipwrecked and in soldiers (in whom it is known as trench foot). Initially, the feet turn pale and have no detectable pulse; later, they become red, swollen, and painful, and have a strong pulse.

TREATMENT

If the feet are at the pale stage, they should be gradually and carefully rewarmed; overheating may lead to *gangrene* (tissue death). Conversely, if they are red and swollen, they should be gradually cooled. *Analgesic drugs* (painkillers) may be necessary.

If the condition is ignored and becomes severe, muscle weakness, skin ulcers, or gangrene may develop. Even with mild cases, the feet may be painful and sensitive to cold for several years afterwards.

Immobility

Reduced physical activity and movement. Immobility is particularly harmful in the elderly because it causes muscle wasting and progressive loss of function.

CAUSES

Total immobility is rare; it occurs in coma, which is sometimes the result of *stroke*, *brain tumour*, or major *head injury*. Catatonia is associated with varying degrees of immobility.

Temporary loss of mobility, lasting a few days, occurs during recovery from any serious illness, such as a *myocardial infarction* (heart attack), or from a major surgical procedure.

Fractures in a lower limb may be treated by *traction*, which requires several weeks in bed, or by use of a *cast*, which also hinders mobility.

Loss of mobility may be caused by the symptoms of a specific medical disorder, such as *asthma* or *angina pectoris* (chest pain due to reduced blood supply to the heart muscle). Both these conditions may, in severe cases, be aggravated by exercise. *Arthritis* (inflammation of joints) limits mobility if the hips, knees, ankles, or feet are affected by pain and stiffness. Nervous system disorders that restrict mobility include *hemiplegia* (paralysis on one side of the body), *Parkinson's disease*, and *multiple sclerosis*.

A person may find it difficult to move around because of deteriorating eyesight; alternatively he or she may lack motivation due to *depression* or the effects of alcohol or other drugs (such as *tranquillizer drugs*).

COMPLICATIONS

Total immobility can cause *bedsores*, *pneumonia* due to the build-up of secretions in the lungs, or *contractures* (deformity caused by the shrinkage of tissue).

A common complication of partial immobility is *oedema* (abnormal retention of fluid in body tissues), which causes swelling of the legs because the calf muscles are not pumping the fluid back to the heart via the circulation. Rarely, sluggish blood flow encourages formation of a *thrombus* (abnormal blood clot) in a leg vein.

Obesity is more likely to occur in people who do not exercise. Stiffness tends to develop in any joint that is not being used properly. Muscle wasting and *osteoporosis* (bone thinning) are common problems caused by immobility in the elderly.

TREATMENT

Regular *physiotherapy* and adequate nursing care are important for any person who is totally immobile. Frequent turning and the use of a special mattress and bed reduce the risk of bedsores. Stretching exercises may prevent contractures.

Early mobilization after serious illness or major surgery is usually encouraged to avoid the problems of prolonged bed rest. After a lower limb fracture, walking with the aid of crutches is started as soon as possible.

Aids for the disabled (see *Disability*) can increase mobility in people with leg weakness, stiffness, loss of balance, or poor coordination. If a person is unable to walk despite assistance, exercises may be done in a chair or in bed to keep the muscles and joints in reasonable working order.

Immobilization

An orthopaedic term for techniques used to prevent movement of joints or displacement of fractured bones so that the bones can unite properly. (See *Fracture*.)

Immune response

A defensive reaction of the body to invading microorganisms, cancer cells, transplanted tissue, and other substances or materials that are recognized as antigenic or "foreign" (that is, different from normal body components). The response consists of the production of substances called *antibodies* or *immunoglobulins*, sensitized cells called *lymphocytes*, and other substances and cells that act to destroy the antigenic material. (See also *Immune system*.)

Immune system

A collection of cells and proteins that works to protect the body from potentially harmful, infectious microorganisms (microscopic life-forms), such as bacteria, viruses, and fungi. The immune system also plays a role in the control of *cancer* and is responsible for the phenomena of *allergy*, *hypersensitivity*, and rejection problems after *transplant surgery*.

Some of the main components of the body's immune system are described in the accompanying illustrated boxes.

A newborn child is, to some extent, protected against infection by innate immunity. This consists of physical barriers, such as the skin; substances present in the mouth, urinary tract, or on the eye surface that destroy microorganisms; and *antibodies* or *immunoglobulins* (protective proteins) that have been passed to the child from the mother (including those received in breast milk).

Innate immunity cannot guard against all disease-causing organisms. As the child grows, he or she encounters organisms that overcome the innate defences and thus cause disease. The second line of immune defence, called the adaptive immune system, then comes into play. As the name implies, this system adapts its response specifically to fight each invading organism. In addition, it retains a memory of the invader so

THE INNATE IMMUNE SYSTEM

Each of us has many inborn defences against infection, including external barriers (below), the inflammatory response (right), and phagocyte action (below right). Others include substances called complement (which is activated by and attacks bacteria) and *interferon* (which has antiviral effects).

All these defences are nonspecific and quick-acting. By contrast, the adaptive immune system (see overleaf) mounts specific attacks against particular microbes. These cells are most effective on second exposure to the organisms.

The two parts of the immune system work together; antibodies produced by the adaptive immune system assist phagocyte action.

THE INFLAMMATORY RESPONSE

If microbes break through the body's outermost barriers, inflammation is the second line of defence. Chemicals (such as histamine) are released, prompting the effects shown below, including the attraction of phagocytes to the microbes. The symptoms of inflammation are redness, pain, swelling, and heat.

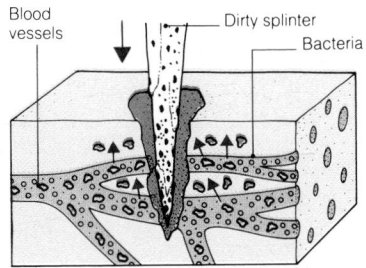

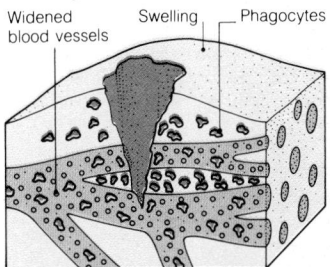

Following tissue injury (here caused by a splinter) and entry of bacteria or other microbes, blood vessels in the area widen and there is increased leakage of fluid from the blood into the tissues. This allows easier access for immune system components that fight the invaders, including phagocytes and soluble factors (such as the group of substances known as complement).

Physical and chemical barriers

These barriers, summarized below, provide the first line of defence against harmful microbes (bacteria, viruses, and fungi).

Eyes
Tears produced by the lacrimal apparatus help wash away microorganisms; tears contain an enzyme (lysozyme) that can destroy bacteria.

Mouth
Lysozyme present in saliva, destroys bacteria.

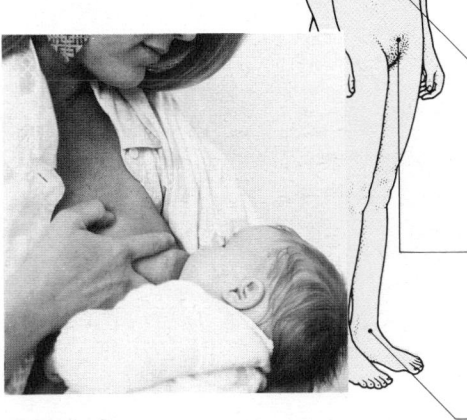

Breast-feeding
Antibodies (proteins with a protective role) formed by the mother against certain microbes are transferred to the baby in breast milk. This action provides some extra immunity until the baby can form his or her own specific antibodies.

Nose
Hairs in the nose help prevent entry of microorganisms on dust particles. This process is assisted by the sneeze reflex.

Respiratory tract
Mucus secreted by cells lining the throat, windpipe, and bronchi traps microbes, which are then swept away by cilia (hairs on cells in the lining) or engulfed by phagocytes (types of white cells). The cough reflex also helps to expel microbes.

Stomach and intestines
Stomach acid destroys the vast majority of microorganisms. The intestines contain harmless bacteria (commensals) that compete with and control the harmful organisms.

Genito-urinary system
The vagina and urethra also contain commensals and are protected by mucus.

Skin
Intact skin provides an effective barrier against most microbes. The sebaceous glands secrete chemicals that are highly toxic to many bacteria.

ACTION OF PHAGOCYTES

These white blood cells are attracted to infection sites, where they engulf and digest microorganisms and debris.

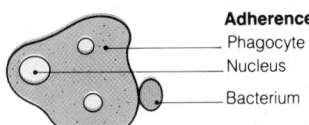

Adherence
- Phagocyte
- Nucleus
- Bacterium

1 The phagocyte contacts and recognizes a microbe as foreign. This process is assisted by chemicals released during inflammation.

Ingestion
- Lysosomes

2 The phagocyte engulfs the microbe in a pouch formed in its membrane. Fluid-filled particles called lysosomes move towards the microbe.

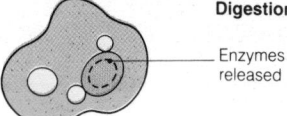

Digestion
- Enzymes released

3 Enzymes within the lysosome are released into the pouch to help digest the microbe. Debris from this process is later ejected.

THE ADAPTIVE IMMUNE SYSTEM

This system is based on cells called lymphocytes. It has two parts. Humoral immunity relies on the production, by B-lymphocytes, of antibodies, which circulate and attack specific microbes. In cellular immunity, cells called T-lymphocytes are activated and attack specific microbes or abnormal cells (such as virally infected or tumour cells).

HUMORAL IMMUNITY

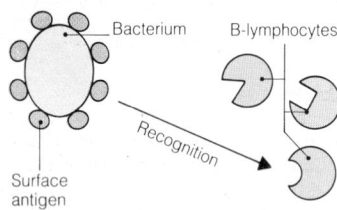

Bacterium • B-lymphocytes • Recognition • Surface antigen

1 A humoral response is started when an antigen (foreign protein)—here on the surface of a bacterium—activates one type of B-lymphocyte.

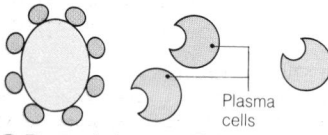

Plasma cells

2 The particular type of B-lymphocyte multiplies, forming cells called plasma cells, which make antibodies designed specifically to attack the bacterium.

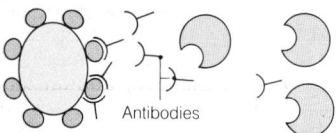

Antibodies

3 After a few days, the antibodies are released and travel to, and attach to, the antigen. This triggers more reactions, which ultimately destroy the bacterium.

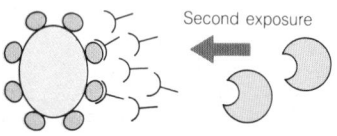

Second exposure

4 Some B-lymphocytes remain in the body as memory cells; if the bacterium enters the body again, they rapidly produce antibodies to halt the infection.

CELLULAR IMMUNITY

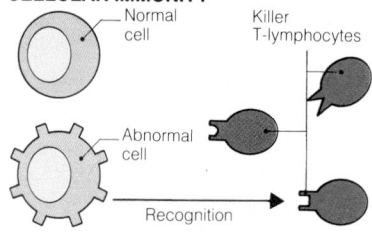

Normal cell • Killer T-lymphocytes • Abnormal cell • Recognition

1 An antigen, here on the surface of an abnormal cell (such as a virus-infected or tumour cell), is identified by, and activates, specific killer (cytotoxic) T-lymphocytes.

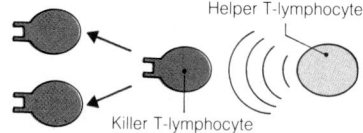

Helper T-lymphocyte • Killer T-lymphocyte

2 With the assistance of helper T cells (another type of T-lymphocyte), the killer T-lymphocytes begin to multiply.

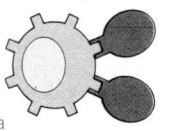

a   b

3 The killer T-lymphocytes travel to, and attach to, the abnormal cells (a), leading to their destruction (b). The T-lymphocytes survive and may go on to kill more targets.

Second exposure

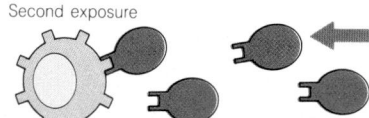

4 Some of the killer T-lymphocytes remain as memory cells, and quickly attack abnormal cells should they reappear (e.g. after reinfection with a virus).

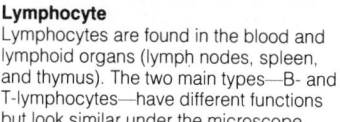

Lymphocyte
Lymphocytes are found in the blood and lymphoid organs (lymph nodes, spleen, and thymus). The two main types—B- and T-lymphocytes—have different functions but look similar under the microscope.

AIDS AND CELLULAR IMMUNITY

HIV—the AIDS virus—disrupts the cellular part of the adaptive immune system.

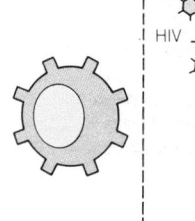
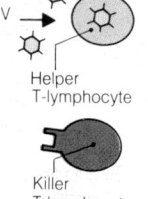

HIV • Helper T-lymphocyte • Killer T-lymphocyte

1 HIV invades and destroys the helper T-lymphocytes, thus preventing the assistance they normally give to killer T-lymphocytes.

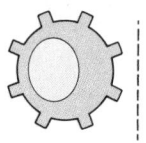
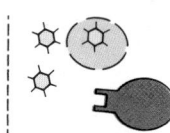

2 As a result, the killer T-lympho-cytes fail to multiply and attack in response to abnormal cells or invading microorganisms.

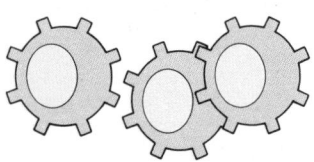

3 Opportunistic viruses and other microbes or tumour cells may thus proliferate unchecked, causing the features of AIDS.

EXAMPLES OF INFECTIOUS ORGANISMS COMBATED

Humoral immunity particularly important against:

Some viruses (e.g. measles)

Many bacteria (e.g. cholera)

Some parasites (e.g. malaria)

Cell-mediated immunity particularly important against:

Many viruses (e.g. herpes simplex)

Some bacteria (e.g. tuberculosis)

Some fungi (e.g. candidiasis)

that defences can be rallied instantly in the future. The person is then said to have acquired immunity to the infection. If the same microorganisms invade again, they are quickly recognized and dealt with (which explains why it is rare for diseases such as measles and diphtheria to affect the same person twice).

The acquisition of immunity in response to an infection can take a few days or weeks to develop; in the interim, a child or adult can become very ill or even die. In the past, many did die. Today, our chance of surviving, recovering from, or totally avoiding infectious diseases is much improved, partly as a result of better general health and nutrition (which bolsters the immune system) and partly through vaccination—artificial *immunization* against specific microorganisms.

INNATE IMMUNITY

The skin provides an impenetrable barrier to the vast majority of infectious agents, most of which can gain entry only via the mucous membranes (i.e. the lining of the mouth, throat, eyes, intestines, vagina, or urinary tract). These areas are protected by the movement of mucus and other fluids (such as tears) and the presence of enzymes (such as lysozyme) that destroy bacteria. If microorganisms penetrate the outer layer of the skin or a mucous membrane, they soon encounter white blood cells called phagocytes (literally, "devouring cells"), which attempt to destroy them, and other types of white cells, such as natural cell-killing (cytotoxic) cells. Microorganisms may also meet naturally produced substances (such as *interferon*) or a group of blood proteins called the complement system, which act to destroy the invading microorganisms.

ADAPTIVE IMMUNITY

The adaptive part of the immune system is extremely complex and only partly understood. Its function is to produce specific defences against a vast range of different invading organisms or tumour cells. Broadly, however, it first must recognize part of an invading organism or tumour cell as an *antigen* (a protein that is foreign or different from any natural body protein).

A response (either humoral or cellular) is then mounted against the antigen. The humoral response consists of the production of soluble proteins, called antibodies or immunoglobulins, manufactured by cells called B-lymphocytes. Cellular responses centre on the activities of cells called T-lymphocytes.

HUMORAL IMMUNITY This type of immunity is particularly important in the defence against bacteria. After a complex recognition process, certain B-lymphocytes are stimulated to multiply. These cells then begin to produce vast numbers of antibodies that are able to bind to the antigens. Once this has occurred, the organisms bearing the antigens are easy prey to phagocytic ("cell-devouring") white cells. Binding of antibody and antigen may also activate the complement system, which increases the efficiency with which phagocytes engulf and destroy the invading organisms.

CELLULAR IMMUNITY This is particularly important in the defence against viruses, some types of parasites that hide within cells, and, possibly, cancer cells. The T-lymphocytes at the centre of cellular immunity are of two types, called helper cells and killer cells. The helper cells play a role in the recognition of antigens. Along with various other functions, they activate the killer cells. Killer lymphocytes lock on to cells that have been invaded by viruses or other parasites which have left recognizable antigens on the cell surfaces. The killer lymphocytes then destroy these parasitized cells. They may act in a similar way against tumour cells and against cells in transplanted tissue.

The memory of the immune system (which provides acquired immunity to certain diseases) relies on the long-term survival of lymphocytes that were activated or sensitized to antigens when these antigens were first encountered.

IMMUNE SYSTEM DISORDERS

The immune system is an essential asset for the protection of the body from infectious agents and probably cancer. In *immunodeficiency disorders*, suppression of the immune system occurs either as a result of an inherited disorder or after infection with certain viruses, including *HIV*, the virus that causes *AIDS*.

In another group of disorders, known as *autoimmune disorders*, the immune system misidentifies the body's own proteins as antigens and mounts an immunological attack against them.

Other disorders occur when the immune system mounts an inappropriate response to what are usually innocuous antigens, such as pollen, causing *hypersensitivity* or *allergy*.

IMMUNOSUPPRESSIVE THERAPY

In certain circumstances, such as after tissue transplants and in people with an autoimmune disorder, it is advantageous to suppress the immune system (especially its adaptive part) through use of *immunosuppressant drugs*. This prevents rejection of the donor organ by lymphocytes and other cells that recognize proteins in the transplanted tissue as antigens.

Immunity

A state of protection against a disease or diseases through the activities of the *immune system*. Innate immunity is present from birth and is the first line of defence against the majority of infectious agents. Acquired immunity is the second line of defence. It develops either through exposure to invading microorganisms (after they have broken through the innate immune defences) or through *immunization.*

Immunization

The process of inducing *immunity* as a preventive measure against certain infectious diseases. The incidence of a number of diseases (e.g. *diphtheria, poliomyelitis*), has declined dramatically since the introduction of effective immunization programmes; one disease (*smallpox*) has been eradicated.

In many countries, including the US (but not the UK), immunization against certain infections is a requirement for entry to school; in the UK the proportion of children immunized rose in the 1980s and early 1990s, partly as a result of incentives being offered to general practitioners to achieve high rates. In most parts of the UK around 90 per cent of schoolchildren are now immunized against the common infections.

IMMUNIZATION AND VACCINATION

Immunization may be active or passive (see diagram). The terms vaccination and active immunization are used interchangeably.

WHO SHOULD BE IMMUNIZED

Some types of immunization, such as immunization against polio, measles, mumps and rubella (see *MMR vaccination*), and against diphtheria, pertussis, and *tetanus* (see *DPT vaccination*), are aimed at the general population, primarily at young children. Others are intended for specific individuals, such as those exposed to dangerous infections during local outbreaks or who are at risk of contracting unusual infections at work (e.g. laboratory technicians or veterinary surgeons).

TYPES OF IMMUNIZATION

There are two main types. In passive immunization, antibodies (protective proteins) are injected and provide immediate, but short-lived protection against specific disease-causing bacteria, viruses, or toxins. Active immunization primes the body to make its own antibodies against such microorganisms and confers longer-lasting immunity.

PASSIVE IMMUNIZATION

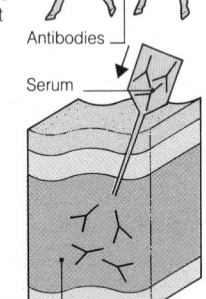

1 Blood is taken from a person or, rarely, an animal previously exposed to a specific microorganism. The blood contains antibodies against that organism.

Antibodies

2 An extract of the blood containing the antibodies (called immune serum or antiserum) is injected into the person to be protected.

Serum

Bloodstream

3 The antibodies help destroy the microorganism if it is present in the blood or enters it over the following few weeks.

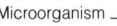

Microorganism

ACTIVE IMMUNIZATION

Vaccine

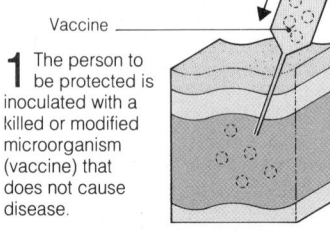

1 The person to be protected is inoculated with a killed or modified microorganism (vaccine) that does not cause disease.

2 The immune system is provoked to make antibodies against the modified microorganism; it also retains a "memory" of the organism.

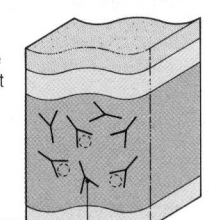

Antibodies

3 If the real microorganism then enters the blood, antibodies are produced in large numbers to halt the infection.

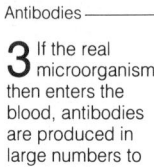

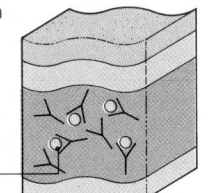

Disease-causing microorganism

tains a large volume of fluid, it may be given in the buttock. Polio vaccine is given orally.

ADVERSE REACTIONS

There are usually no after-effects following immunization. Some vaccines cause pain and swelling at the injection site and may produce a slight fever, a feeling of irritability and malaise, or flu-like symptoms. Young children who develop fever after being immunized should be given *paracetamol*. Some vaccines, such as the measles vaccine, may produce a mild form of the disease.

In very rare cases, severe reactions (such as seizures) occur following immunization. This has led to controversy about the advisability of some types of vaccination, notably against pertussis. However, for most people, the risks of vaccination are much smaller than the risks of damage from the disease.

Although most modern vaccines provide a reliable method of preventing disease, they do not all provide complete protection. *Cholera* and *typhoid fever* vaccinations, in particular, give only partial protection, so other precautions (principally food and water hygiene) must be observed during travel to areas where there is a risk of these diseases.

WHO SHOULD NOT BE IMMUNIZED

Immunization should not be given to any person who suffers from an *immunodeficiency disorder* or widespread cancer. Any person who is taking *corticosteroid drugs* or who has previously had a severe reaction to the same vaccine should not be vaccinated. Some vaccines, (e.g. for typhoid and yellow fever) should not be given to very young children. Vaccination should be delayed if a person has a fever or infection. A number of vaccines should not be given during pregnancy because of the risk to the fetus.

Immunoassay

A group of laboratory techniques that includes ELISA (enzyme-linked immunosorbent assay) and radioimmunoassay. Both are used in the diagnosis of infectious diseases; variants of radioimmunoassay, such as the radioallergosorbent test (RAST) and the radioimmunosorbent test (RIST), are also used in the diagnosis of *allergies* and in the measurement of concentrations of *hormones* in the blood.

ELISA and radioimmunoassay can both determine the presence or absence in a person's blood of a specific protein—such as an *antigen* (a pro-

Immunization before foreign travel may be necessary for entry into certain countries (today, this usually applies only to immunization against *yellow fever*) and to protect the traveller against infection. The traveller should determine a few months before departure which immunizations are necessary or recommended.

The accompanying table gives details of a typical immunization schedule during childhood. (See also *Travel immunization*.)

HOW IMMUNIZATION IS DONE

Most immunizations are given by injection, usually into the tissues under the skin or into the muscle of the upper arm. If the injection con-

TYPICAL CHILDHOOD IMMUNIZATION SCHEDULE

Age	Disease	
2 months	Diphtheria, pertussis (whooping cough),tetanus*, haemophilus influenza b (Hib)	Poliomyelitis†
3 months	Diphtheria, pertussis, tetanus*, haemophilus influenza b	Poliomyelitis†
4 months	Diphtheria, pertussis, tetanus*, haemophilus influenza b	Poliomyelitis†
15 months	Measles, mumps, rubella (German measles)*	Poliomyelitis†
4 to 5 years	Diphtheria, tetanus*	Poliomyelitis†
	*Combined injection	†Oral

tein on the surface of a microorganism or an allergen), a specific *antibody* (a protein formed by the body's *immune system* to protect against a particular type of microorganism or allergen), or other protein, such as a hormone.

The principle underlying these techniques is that, for any specific antibody, there is a specific antigen. If molecules of these two proteins come in close contact, they will bind strongly to each other. Any specific antibody will bind only to its own antigen, and vice versa.

HOW IT IS DONE

First, the surface of a plate or the inside of a test tube is prepared with a covering of the specific protein (antigen or antibody) that will bind to the antibody or antigen whose presence in the blood is to be tested. For example, in the ELISA test for antibody to *HIV* (the virus responsible for *AIDS*), the inside of a test tube is lined with small amounts of antigen from HIV virus.

This surface is then exposed to plasma of the blood; if the antibody (or antigen) under test is present, it will stick strongly to the surface. The surface is then washed and a chemical added that will bind to the bound protein. This chemical is itself linked either to an enzyme called peroxidase (in the ELISA test) or to a radioactive isotope (in radioimmunoassay).

Any excess chemical is washed away, and, if the antibody or antigen was present, either peroxidase or radioactivity is left on the surface. Peroxidase can be detected by adding another chemical that changes colour in its presence; radioactivity can be measured by a gamma counter.

The RIST differs from other types of radioimmunoassay in that the blood serum containing the substance being tested is first mixed with a solution containing the same substance, which has been radioactively labelled. The radioactive and the test versions compete to bind to the test plate. The result is that, after washing, the less radioactivity found on the test plate, the more test substance must have been present in the blood serum.

Immunodeficiency disorders

Disorders in which there is a failure of the *immune system's* defences to fight infection and tumours. Immunodeficiency may be the result of an inherited or a *congenital* defect that interferes with the normal development of the immune system, or may be the result of *acquired* disease that damages the system's function. The result, in either case, is the appearance of persistent or recurrent infection by organisms that would not ordinarily cause disease, poor response to customarily effective treatment, incomplete recovery from illness, and an undue susceptibility to certain forms of *cancer*.

The infections seen in people with immunodeficiency disorders are sometimes called *opportunistic infections* because the microorganisms take advantage of the person's lowered defences. Infections of this type include pneumonia caused by *PNEUMOCYSTIS CARINII*, widespread *herpes simplex* infections, and many *fungal infections*.

INHERITED IMMUNODEFICIENCY

The adaptive part of the immune system (which mounts specific defences against particular microorganisms or tumour cells) has two major prongs. One of these, the humoral system, relies on the production of *antibodies* (or *immunoglobulins*) by B-*lymphocytes*. The other prong is called the cellular system and relies on the activity of T-lymphocytes. Congenital or inherited deficiencies can occur in either of these systems.

Deficiencies of the humoral system include hypogammaglobulinaemia (in which the production of one or more types of immunoglobulin is interfered with) and agammaglobulinaemia (in which there is an almost complete absence of B-lymphocytes and immunoglobulins). The most common type of hypogammaglobulinaemia affects about one person in 600 and usually causes no symptoms or may cause no more than repeated mild attacks of respiratory infection. Agammaglobulinaemia requires regular treatment with *immunoglobulin* if it is not to prove fatal.

Congenital deficiencies of T-lymphocytes may lead to problems such as persistent and widespread *candidiasis* (thrush) affecting the skin, mouth, throat, and vagina.

A combined deficiency of both prongs of the immune system, called severe combined immunodeficiency (SCID), is also known. Affected infants usually die in the first year of life unless treatment can be given by *bone marrow transplant*.

ACQUIRED IMMUNODEFICIENCY

Acquired deficiency of the immune system may result either from disease processes or from damage to the immune system as a result of its suppression by drugs.

Diseases that cause immunodeficiency include infection with *HIV* (human immunodeficiency virus), which leads to *AIDS* (acquired immune deficiency syndrome). Severe malnutrition, especially if there is protein deficiency, and many cancers can also cause immunodeficiency.

Deliberate suppression of the immune system with *immunosuppressant drugs* and *corticosteroid drugs* is usually carried out as part of the treatment of *autoimmune disorders* and after *transplant surgery* to minimize the risk of organ rejection.

IMMUNODEFICIENCY IN THE ELDERLY

A degree of immunodeficiency arises simply as a consequence of age. The *thymus*, which plays an important part in the production of T-lymphocytes, reaches peak size in puberty and steadily shrinks thereafter. This results in a decline in the number and activity of T-lymphocytes with age; there is also a decline in the numbers of B-lymphocytes.

Immunoglobulin

A type of protein found in the blood and in tissue fluids, also known as an *antibody*. Immunoglobulins are produced by cells of the *immune system* called B-lymphocytes. Their function is to bind to substances in the body that are recognized as foreign *antigens* (often proteins on the surface of bacteria and viruses). This binding is a crucial event in the destruction of the microorganisms that bear the antigens.

Immunoglobulins also play a central role in *allergies* and *hypersensitivity* reactions. In this case they bind to antigens that are not necessarily a threat to health, which may provoke an inflammatory reaction.

There are five classes of immunoglobulin; of these, immunoglobulin G (IgG) is the major immunoglobulin in human blood. The IgG molecule consists of two parts, one of which binds to an antigen; the other binds to other cells of the immune system. These other cells are principally white cells called phagocytes, which then engulf the microorganisms bearing the antigen.

The antigen-binding site of the IgG molecule is variable in its structure, the different versions of the molecule being capable of binding to an almost infinite number of antigens.

Immunoglobulins can be extracted from the blood of recovering patients and used for passive *immunization* against certain infectious diseases.

Immunoglobulin injection

Administration of preparations of *immunoglobulins* (*antibodies*) to prevent or sometimes treat infectious diseases. Such preparations are also known as immune globulin or gamma-globulin.

The main use of immunoglobulin injections is in the prevention of viral *hepatitis* (e.g. before travelling to a country where the disease is common). They are also given to prevent *measles* and *rubella* in people who are exposed to these infections and are not already immune to them from previous infection or *immunization*.

Immunoglobulin injections are also given to people with *immunodeficiency disorders* (impaired natural defences).

HOW IT WORKS

Immunoglobulin injections provide immunity to a range of common infectious diseases. They work by passing on antibodies obtained from the blood of large numbers of people who have previously been exposed to these diseases and thus have developed antibodies to them.

POSSIBLE ADVERSE EFFECTS

Immunoglobulin injections may cause rash, fever, and pain and tenderness at the injection site.

Immunology

The discipline concerned with the *immune system*. Immunologists study the functioning of the immune system and investigate and treat disorders of the immune system, including *allergies*, *autoimmune disorders*, and *immunodeficiency disorders* such as *AIDS*.

Specialists in immunology are also concerned with finding ways in which the immune system can be stimulated to provide immunity (principally through the use of *vaccines*).

Immunologists also play an important part in *transplant surgery*, looking pre-operatively for a good immunological match between recipient and donor organ, and suppressing the recipient's immune system after transplantation to minimize the chances of organ rejection.

Immunostimulant drugs

A group of drugs that increase the efficiency of the body's *immune system* (natural defences against infection and abnormal cells). Immunostimulant drugs include *vaccines* (see *Immunization*), and *interferon* and interleukin-2, which are used to treat viral infections and types of cancer.

Immunostimulant *adjuvant drugs* enhance the ability of a vaccine to stimulate the immune system and are

added to the vaccine for this reason. Aluminium phosphate, for example, increases the effectiveness of the *tetanus* vaccine.

Immunosuppressant drugs

COMMON DRUGS
Corticosteroid drugs *Prednisolone   Prednisone*
Cytotoxic drugs *Azathioprine   Chlorambucil Cyclophosphamide   Methotrexate*
Others *Antilymphocyte immunoglobulin Cyclosporin*

A group of drugs that reduce the activity of the body's *immune system* (natural defences). Immunosuppressant drugs are prescribed after *transplant surgery* to prevent the rejection of foreign tissues. They are also given to halt the progress of *autoimmune disorders* (in which the body's immune system attacks its own tissues) when other treatments are ineffective. They are unable, however, to restore tissue that has already been damaged.

HOW THEY WORK

Immunosuppressant drugs work by suppressing the production and activity of *lymphocytes*, a type of white blood cell that plays an important part in fighting infection and in eliminating abnormal cells that may form a malignant tumour.

POSSIBLE ADVERSE EFFECTS

Apart from the individual effects of each type, these drugs increase the risk of infection and of the development of certain cancers.

Immunotherapy

Stimulation of the *immune system* as a treatment for *cancer*. Immunotherapy as a cancer treatment is still largely experimental, but it may prove a useful adjunct to other therapies, such as the use of *anticancer drugs*, in the treatment of *leukaemia*, *lymphoma*, and some other cancers. (The term immunotherapy is also sometimes used to describe *hyposensitization* treatment for *allergy*.)

TYPES

One type of immunotherapy used in the treatment of cancer relies on the use of *immunostimulant drugs*, substances that cause general stimulation of the immune system.

Another technique is to inoculate the patient with tumour cells or cellular extracts, rendered harmless by irradiation, which have been taken from another person suffering from

the same disease. The patient's immune system then produces its own *antibodies*, which attack the tumour cells.

Alternatively, a patient can be given antibodies from another person with the same type of tumour. More recently, monoclonal antibodies (see *Antibody, monoclonal*) directed against tumours have been produced artificially by *genetic engineering*. *Interferon* or chemical poisons can be linked to these antibodies to increase their ability to destroy tumour cells.

LIMITATIONS

One drawback to the administration of some of these anticancer treatments is that they, too, may be recognized as foreign by the person's immune system, causing either allergic reactions (such as serum sickness) or new antibody production, which interferes with anticancer activity.

Impaction, dental

Failure of a tooth to emerge completely from the gum at its normal time of eruption. An impacted tooth remains either fully or partly embedded in bone or soft tissue.

Dental impaction may occur because overcrowding (see *Overcrowding, dental*) leaves little room for the teeth that erupt last (the wisdom teeth and upper canines). Impaction may also occur when a tooth grows in the wrong direction, causing its eruption to be blocked by dense bone.

IMPACTED WISDOM TEETH

These are common, but usually cause no trouble unless they partially penetrate the gum, leaving a flap of tissue over most of the crown. *Plaque*, bacteria, and food debris then collect

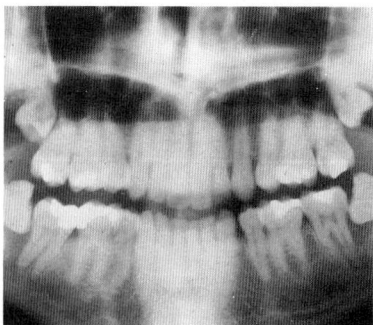

Impacted wisdom teeth
This X-ray shows impacted wisdom teeth lying horizontally in the lower jaw. The impacted teeth are wedged against the adjacent molars and are not able to erupt normally.

between the tooth and the gum, which often becomes inflamed and painful. There may also be swollen *lymph nodes* in the upper neck and difficulty opening the mouth.

Rinsing the area with warm salt water and taking *analgesic drugs* (painkillers) may relieve symptoms but, if infection is present, *antibiotic drugs* are required. A dentist may decide that the tooth requires extraction to prevent more trouble.

IMPACTED UPPER CANINES
These teeth play a much more important part than do wisdom teeth in biting and chewing. If the upper canines are impacted, they are not usually removed, but instead are moved into the correct position by means of an *orthodontic appliance*.

Impetigo
A highly contagious skin infection, common in children, that usually occurs around the nose and mouth.

CAUSES AND INCIDENCE
Impetigo is caused by bacteria entering the skin through a broken area, such as a cut, *cold sore*, or an area affected by *eczema*. The infection occurs more often in warm weather. Impetigo was once extremely com-

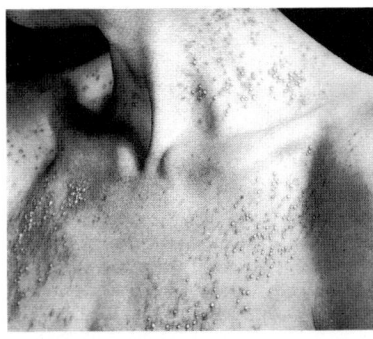

The appearance of impetigo
Fluid-filled blisters appear on the skin (in this case, on the neck and chest). The blisters often burst, releasing fluid that dries to leave pale brown crusts.

mon, but occurs less frequently now because of improved standards of personal hygiene. Small epidemics occasionally occur in schools.

SYMPTOMS AND SIGNS
The skin reddens and small, fluid-filled blisters appear on the surface. The blisters tend to burst, leaving moist, weeping areas underneath; the released fluid dries to leave honey-coloured crusts on the skin. The infected area may spread at the edges

or another patch may develop nearby. In severe cases there may be swelling of the *lymph nodes* in the face or neck; accompanied by fever. Rarely, complications such as *septicaemia* (blood poisoning) or *glomerulonephritis* (a type of kidney inflammation) develop.

TREATMENT
Because impetigo spreads rapidly, it is advisable to consult a doctor. *Antibiotic drugs* in tablet or ointment form usually clear up the problem in about five days. Any loose crusts should be gently washed off with soap and water and the area dabbed dry.

To prevent transmission of the infection, pillowcases, towels, and face-cloths should not be shared and should be boiled after use. Children should not touch affected skin and should stay away from school until the infection clears.

Implant
Any material, natural or artificial, inserted into the body for medical purposes (see illustrated box).

Implantation, egg
Attachment of a fertilized *ovum* (egg) to the wall of the *uterus*. Implantation occurs about six days after *fertil-*

TYPES OF IMPLANTS
Implants may be inserted into various parts of the body. They can be used to replace a diseased structure, to improve appearance, to maintain proper functioning of an internal organ, to treat certain disorders, or to deliver drugs or hormones.

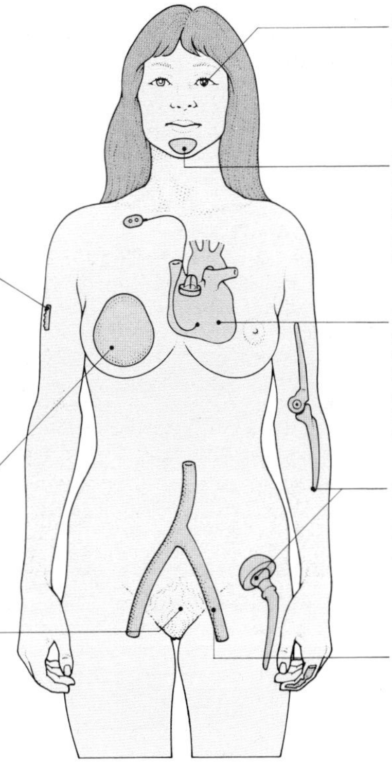

Hormonal
Some hormonal drugs (such as oestradiol and progesterone) can be placed in implants that are inserted under the skin to release the drug slowly over time.

Breast
Silicone implants were widely used to restore breast shape after surgery for cancer, or to increase breast size, but doubts about their long-term safety led to their use declining in the early 1990s.

Therapeutic
Radioactive materials in sealed containers can be inserted into tissue to treat malignant tumours, for example, a cancer of the cervix.

Eye
An implant can be used to replace the lens of the eye after cataract removal, or the entire eyeball if it requires removal because of injury or disease.

Face
Pieces of bone taken from another part of the body, or shaped pieces of silicone, can be implanted on the face to make a receding chin more prominent or to improve the contour at a fracture site.

Heart
Cardiac pacemakers (battery-powered electronic devices connected by wires to the heart muscle) can be implanted in the chest to regulate the heartbeat; diseased heart valves may be replaced with artificial or natural substitutes.

Joints
Diseased joints can be replaced with artificial substitutes to help restore full function. The elbow, the hip, the knee, the finger joints, and the shoulder can all now be treated in this way.

Artery
Diseased sections of artery, such as the lower aorta and upper iliac arteries (shown here), can be replaced or bypassed with artificial tubular materials made from woven or knitted synthetic fibres.

ization, when the blastocyst (early form of embryo) comes into contact with the wall of the uterus. As the cells of the developing *embryo* continue to divide, the outer cell layer penetrates the lining of the uterus to obtain oxygen and nutrients from the mother's blood; later, this layer develops into the *placenta*.

The embryo usually implants in the upper part of the uterus; if it implants low down near the cervix, *placenta praevia* may develop. Rarely, implantation occurs in a fallopian tube, resulting in an *ectopic pregnancy*.

Implants, dental

Posts surgically embedded in the jaw for the attachment of a dental prosthesis (a type of false teeth). Titanium or synthetic materials may be used for the implants.

Implants are useful for people who have lost all their teeth and either are unable to tolerate a traditional *denture* or have lost so much tooth-bearing tissue through injury or disease that a denture would not be stable.

Fitting a dental implant is performed in stages, usually under local anaesthesia. First, holes are drilled in the jaw and posts are inserted into them. Several months later, attachments that protrude above the gum are screwed into the posts. A few weeks later, a prosthesis is fitted.

Impotence

The inability to achieve or maintain an *erection*. Impotence is the most common male sexual disorder, affecting most men at some time in their lives.

CAUSES

In most cases, impotence is caused by psychological factors, which may be temporary (e.g. when caused by fatigue or stress) or long-standing (e.g. when caused by feelings of anxiety and guilt that originated in childhood). Impotence may also be a symptom of severe *depression*.

Approximately 10 per cent of impotence is caused by a physical disorder (e.g. *diabetes mellitus* or a disorder of the *endocrine system*) or by a neurological disorder (e.g damage to the *spinal cord* or an *alcohol-related disorder*). Impotence may be caused by taking various drugs—particularly *antidepressant drugs*, *antipsychotic drugs*, *antihypertensive drugs*, and *diuretic drugs*. Impotence is more common as men get older, possibly because of altered circulation or, very occasionally, lowered levels of the male sex hormone *testosterone*.

DIAGNOSIS AND TREATMENT

Tests may be performed to eliminate the possibility of any physical disorder. A change in medication may sometimes be advised to see whether impotence is affected.

If a physical cause is found, treatment will be given if possible. *Penile implants* help some men whose impotence is caused by disease. Injections of certain *vasodilator drugs*, especially papaverine, may be prescribed in some cases. An attempt will be made to treat depression or *alcohol dependence* if appropriate.

If the cause of impotence is psychological, *counselling* or *sex therapy* (preferably together with the person's partner) may be recommended. Such treatment is successful in more than half the cases of long-term impotence of psychological origin.

Impression, dental

A mould taken of the *teeth*, *gums*, and sometimes the *palate*. A quick-setting material, such as alginate or a rubber compound, is placed in a shaped tray that is eased over the area of which a replica is to be made and left in position until the material has set. After the mould has been removed, plaster of Paris is poured into it to obtain a model of the area. This is then used as a base on which to build a *denture*, *bridge*, or dental *inlay*.

Impressions are also used in *orthodontics* to study the position of the teeth and the structure of the mouth, and to make *orthodontic appliances* to correct irregularities.

Incest

Sexual intercourse between close relatives. Incest is usually considered to include intercourse with a parent, a son or daughter, a brother or sister, an uncle or aunt, a nephew or niece, a grandparent or grandchild.

Incest is illegal or taboo in most societies and against the teaching of many religions. However, the definition of what constitutes incest differs between cultures. This almost univer-

INCIDENCE OF VARIOUS CONDITIONS IN THE UK

Incidence (new cases per 100,000 population per year)	Categorization	Examples
More than 10,000	Extremely common	Common cold
1,000 to 10,000	Very common	Sexually transmitted diseases (all types)
100 to 1,000	Common	Measles Myocardial infarction Stroke
20 to 100	Fairly common	Breast cancer Cancer of colon Gonorrhoea Symptomatic kidney stones Leukaemia Lung cancer
5 to 20	Uncommon	Ovarian cancer Tuberculosis
0.5 to 5	Rare	Anorexia nervosa Hepatitis B Hodgkin's disease Meningococcal meningitis Motor neuron disease Syphilis
0.005 to 0.5	Very rare	Diphtheria Poliomyelitis Acute rheumatic fever Typhoid fever
Less than 0.005	Extremely rare	Botulism Rabies

sal prohibition is probably based on a perceived higher risk of congenital abnormality due to inbreeding.

The actual prevalence of incest is unknown. Research suggests that as many as five to 10 per cent of women have had sexual contact with a father, brother, or other male relative, and that one to two per cent of men have had sexual contact with a male or a female relative.

The existence of *child abuse* involving incest is now well recognized, and support is increasingly available from telephone helplines and from paediatric, psychiatric, and social services. Family counselling may be helpful in some cases; often, however, children are taken into care.

Incidence

One of the two principal measures (the other is *prevalence*) of how common a disease is in a defined population. The incidence of a disease is the number of new cases that occur during a given period (e.g. 17 new cases per 100,000 people per year). Prevalence is the total number of cases of a disease in existence at any one time; it includes both new and old cases. Thus, in 100,000 people, there may be an incidence of, say, 400 cases of a specific type of cancer per year, but a prevalence of 4,000 cases, because the disease lasts an average of 10 years before being cured or causing death.

Incision

A cut made into the tissues of the body by a scalpel (surgical knife). Most incisions are made to gain access to tissue inside the body (usually to repair or remove a diseased organ) or to relieve pressure (e.g. from pus in an abscess).

Standard incision sites for abdominal surgery are shown in the illustrated box.

Incisor

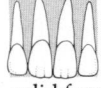 One of the eight front teeth (four in the upper jaw and four in the lower) used for incising (cutting through) solid forms of food. (See *Teeth*.)

Incontinence, faecal

Inability to retain *faeces* in the *rectum*.

CAUSES
A common cause of faecal incontinence, especially in the elderly and in toilet-trained children, is *faecal impaction*, which is often itself caused by long-standing *constipation*. The faeces lodged in the rectum irritate and inflame its lining and, as a result,

faecal fluid and small pieces of faeces are passed involuntarily. Temporary loss of continence may occur at any age in cases of severe *diarrhoea*, when the need to evacuate the bowel becomes too great to withstand.

Less common causes include injury to the anal muscles (as may occur, for example, during childbirth or surgery), *paraplegia* (paralysis of the legs and lower trunk), *mental handicap*, and *dementia*.

TREATMENT
If the underlying cause of faecal impaction is constipation, recurrence may be prevented by a high-fibre diet. Suppositories containing *glycerol* or *laxative drugs* may be recommended. Faecal incontinence in people with dementia or a nerve disorder may be avoided by regular use of enemas or suppositories to empty the rectum.

Incontinence, urinary

Uncontrollable, involuntary passing of *urine*, often due to injury or disease of the *urinary tract*. Urinary incontinence often affects the elderly because the efficiency of the sphincter muscles surrounding the *urethra* declines with age. Women are affected more often than men.

TYPES AND SYMPTOMS
STRESS INCONTINENCE This refers to the involuntary escape of a small amount of urine when a person coughs, laughs, picks up a heavy package, or moves excessively (such as during athletic activity). Stress incontinence is common in women, particularly after childbirth, when the urethral sphincter muscles are stretched.

URGE INCONTINENCE In this type, an urgent desire to pass urine is accompanied by inability to control the bladder as it contracts involuntarily. Urge incontinence may occur when walking or sitting, but is frequently triggered by a sudden change in position. Once urination starts, it continues until the bladder is empty.

TOTAL INCONTINENCE This is a complete lack of bladder control resulting from the total absence of sphincter activity. In rare cases, total incontinence occurs because the urine bypasses the sphincter, as may occur in a person with a vesicovaginal fistula (a hole between the bladder and vagina) or an ectopic ureter (in which the ureter enters the urethra rather than the bladder).

OVERFLOW INCONTINENCE This occurs in chronic *urinary retention*, a condition in which the sufferer is unable to empty the bladder normally, often because of an obstruction such as an enlarged *prostate gland*. The bladder is always full, leading to constant dribbling of the overflow of urine. Relief of the obstruction will restore continence.

ABDOMINAL INCISIONS

Surgery is frequently performed on the abdomen. Standard incision sites provide access to the diseased portion with minimum weakening of the abdominal wall. The most commonly used of these standard incision sites are shown in the diagram below.

Right subcostal
This incision gives access to the gallbladder, bile duct, and upper right part of the colon.

Epigastric
This incision gives access to the stomach and duodenum.

Left paramedian
This incision gives access to many abdominal structures.

Transverse
This incision may be used for upper abdominal surgery on older patients.

McBurney's
This incision is often used for removal of the appendix.

Lower midline
This incision may be used for hysterectomy or caesarean section.

Pfannenstiel
This incision is commonly used for pelvic surgery, particularly prostatectomy, hysterectomy, or caesarean section.

Lower transverse abdominal
This incision provides access to the ureter and to the iliac blood vessels.

Incontinence may be caused by localized disorders of the urinary tract (including infections, bladder stones, or tumours) or by *prolapse* of the uterus or vagina. Incontinence due to lack of control by the brain commonly occurs in the young (see *Enuresis*), the elderly, and those with mental impairment. Damage to the brain or spinal cord by injury or disease also affects bladder control, as does stress, anger, and anxiety. Weak pelvic muscles, a fractured pelvis, or cancer of the prostate can cause incontinence. *Irritable bladder*, in which the bladder muscle contracts intermittently, raises the pressure in the bladder to push some urine out of the urethra; this causes an intense desire to pass urine.

DIAGNOSIS

Urinalysis (examination of the urine) is performed to eliminate the possibility of infection, inflammation, *diabetes mellitus*, or protein loss. *Ultrasound scanning*, intravenous *urography* (X-rays of the kidney and ureters after injection of a radiopaque substance), and X-rays taken while the patient is passing urine (see *cystourethrography*, *micturating*) are used to investigate the possibility of an obstruction. *Cystometry* (measurement of pressure within the bladder) can determine if the bladder is functioning normally or if there is any abnormality of the nerves supplying the bladder. *Cystoscopy* (examination of the urethra and bladder through a viewing instrument) is performed to look for the presence of bladder stones, tumours, or cysts.

TREATMENT

If weak pelvic muscles are causing stress incontinence, *pelvic floor exercises* may help to restore sphincter function. Sometimes, an operation is performed to tighten or lengthen the urethra. In severe cases, an inflatable artificial sphincter may be placed around the urethra; when urination is required, a trigger is pressed to deflate the mechanism in order to allow urine to flow.

Anticholinergic drugs are sometimes used to relax the bladder muscle if irritable bladder is the cause.

If normal bladder function cannot be restored, special incontinence pants (with an internal pad to absorb the urine) can alleviate discomfort. Men can wear a penile sheath leading into a tube connected to a portable urine bag. Some people can avoid incontinence by self-catheterization (see *Catheterization, urinary*) four or five times a day to empty the bladder.

If these measures are unsuccessful and the condition is severe, a *urinary diversion* operation to bypass the bladder may be necessary.

Incoordination

Loss of the ability to produce smooth, harmonious muscular movements, leading to clumsiness and unsteady balance. Incoordination can also mean the failure of a group of organs to work together successfully. (See also *Ataxia*.)

Incubation period

The time during which any *infectious disease* develops, from the point when the infecting organism enters the body until the appearance of symptoms. Different infections have characteristic incubation periods—for example, 14 to 21 days for chickenpox and seven to 14 days for measles. The incubation period for cholera may be as short as several hours.

Incubator

A transparent plastic container in which oxygen, temperature, and humidity levels are controlled to provide premature or sick infants with ideal conditions for survival. An incubator also provides some protection from airborne infection.

Incubators have portholes to allow handling of the baby and smaller holes through which monitoring cables and intravenous and respiratory tubing can pass.

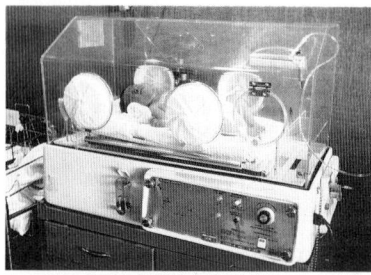

Premature infant in an incubator
Portholes make it possible to handle the infant without disturbing the special conditions provided by the incubator.

Indian medicine

In contrast to Chinese medicine, traditional Indian medicine was based on empirical observation and practice rather than on philosophy. The earliest Indian literature, the Vedas, which date from about 1500 BC, contain detailed descriptions of numerous disorders and their treatments. Ayurvedism, as Vedic medicine is

known, was based largely on herbal treatment, although early Vedic physicians also used simple surgical techniques and invented artificial limbs and eyes.

The Vedic era ended in about 800 BC, but the medical traditions of ayurvedism survived and were further developed (especially the surgical aspect) under the Brahmins, the caste of wise men. As a result, by about 500 AD, Indian medicine had become a scientifically based system with a wide range of surgical techniques (such as operations for cataracts and kidney stones) along with the herbal tradition. The Brahmins, however, cloaked their medical knowledge in theology and superstition and traditional Indian medicine stagnated. Today, most Indian medicine follows Western practices.

Indigestion

A common term covering a variety of symptoms brought on by eating, including *heartburn*, *abdominal pain*, *nausea*, and *flatulence* (excessive wind in the stomach or intestine, causing belching or discomfort). The medical term for indigestion is dyspepsia.

Indigestion refers to discomfort in the upper abdomen, often brought on by eating too much, by eating too quickly, or by eating very rich, spicy, or fatty foods. Nervous indigestion is a common effect of stress. Occasionally, persistent or recurrent indigestion is associated with a *peptic ulcer*, *gallstones*, or *oesophagitis* (inflammation of the oesophagus).

TREATMENT

Self-help treatment includes avoiding foods and situations that bring on symptoms and eating regularly three or four times a day, without rushing. Taking *antacid drugs* or drinking milk may make symptoms subside.

Anyone who takes antacid drugs regularly should see a doctor so that the underlying cause of the problem can be investigated. If abdominal pain persists for more than six hours, or if there are other symptoms, such as prolonged vomiting, vomiting blood (which may appear brown), passing very dark or black faeces, or feeling weak or faint, a doctor should be consulted immediately.

Indomethacin

A *nonsteroidal anti-inflammatory drug* (NSAID) used to relieve pain, stiffness, and inflammation in disorders such as *osteoarthritis*, *rheumatoid arthritis*, *gout*, *ankylosing spondylitis*, and *tendinitis.* Indomethacin is also prescribed to relieve pain caused by injury to soft tissues, such as muscles and ligaments.

Treatment with indomethacin may cause abdominal pain, nausea, heartburn, headache, dizziness, and an increased risk of *peptic ulcer.*

Induction of labour

Use of artificial means to initiate the process of *childbirth.* Labour is induced if the health of the mother or baby would be endangered by allowing the pregnancy to continue. If the pregnancy is not at full term, the risks of induction are weighed against the risks of *prematurity.*

WHY IT IS DONE

The commonest reason for inducing labour is that the pregnancy has continued past the estimated delivery date, which increases the chance of maternal and fetal complications occurring during childbirth. Most obstetricians induce labour if delivery is more than two weeks overdue.

Labour may be induced early if the mother is suffering from *pre-eclampsia,* or if she has chronic *hypertension.* Labour may also be induced if there is Rh incompatibility between the mother and baby (because of the risk of *haemolytic disease of the newborn*) or if there are indications of *intrauterine growth retardation.*

HOW IT IS DONE

The most common technique of inducing labour is to rupture the membrane around the baby to release some of the amniotic fluid. This is sometimes sufficient to start labour. If not, vaginal suppositories containing a *prostaglandin drug* (which stimulates the uterus to contract) may be inserted high in the vagina. Alternatively, an intravenous infusion of *oxytocin* (a hormone that stimulates the uterus to contract) may be used. Careful monitoring of the condition of both mother and baby is important during an induced labour. If attempts to induce labour are unsuccessful, the baby may be delivered by *caesarean section.*

Industrial diseases

See *Occupational disease and injury.*

Infant

A term usually applied to a baby up to the age of 12 months.

Infantile spasms

A rare type of recurrent seizure, also called progressive myoclonic encephalopathy or salaam attacks, that affects babies. Infantile spasms occur most commonly between the ages of four and nine months.

The condition is a form of *epilepsy.* In a seizure, the baby's head suddenly falls forward, the body stiffens, and the limbs bend. Following this, the arms and hands extend and move out. There may be several hundred such spasms per day, each lasting a few seconds and sometimes preceded by a cry. In most cases the seizures are a sign of brain damage and affected babies grow up with severe *mental handicap.*

Infant mortality

The number of infants who die during the first year of life per 1,000 live births. About two thirds of all infant deaths occur during the neonatal period (the first month of life). Most of those who die are very premature (i.e. those born before the 30th week of pregnancy) or have severe *birth defects.*

Infant mortality varies greatly among different countries and among different racial and social groups. A low infant mortality rate reflects good maternal nutrition, good medical and social conditions throughout pregnancy, and good care for the infant after birth. By 1990 the infant mortality rate had fallen to around 8 to 9 per 1,000 live births in Britain—a similar rate to those in Denmark, the Netherlands, and France.

Infarction

Death of an area of tissue caused by *ischaemia* (lack of blood supply). Common examples include *myocardial infarction* (heart attack) and pulmonary infarction, which is lung damage caused by a *pulmonary embolism* (a blood clot that has moved into a vessel in the lung and is obstructing the flow of blood). See also *Necrosis.*

Infection

 The establishment of a colony of disease-causing microorganisms (such as bacteria, viruses, or fungi) in the body. The organisms actively reproduce and cause disease directly by damage to cells or indirectly by toxins they release. Infection normally provokes a response from the *immune system,* which accounts for many of the features of the infection.

Toxic symptoms, such as fever, weakness, and aching joints, are expressions of *infectious disease.* In such cases, the microorganisms are often spread throughout the body (this is called "systemic" infection). Infection may also be localized within a particular tissue or area, often through spread of organisms from parts of the body where they are harmless to parts where they are harmful (e.g. through leakage from the intestines into the abdomen to cause *peritonitis*).

Entry of microorganisms from soil into wounds or during the course of surgical procedures is another common cause of localized infection. In the early days of surgery, infection of internal body cavities was the major (and frequently fatal) risk to the patient. Antiseptic surgical techniques have largely eliminated this problem.

AVOIDANCE

Localized infections (as opposed to infectious diseases) can be avoided by standard hygienic measures, such as keeping the hands clean, not picking at blemishes, washing and covering cuts and grazes, having wounds attended to by a doctor, and seeking regular dental treatment.

SYMPTOMS, DIAGNOSIS, AND TREATMENT

Localized infection is generally followed by *inflammation,* which increases the flow of blood to the infected area, bringing white blood cells and other components of the immune system. Symptoms and signs usually include pain, redness, swelling, formation of a pus-filled abscess at the site of infection, and sometimes a rise in temperature.

Any suspected infection should be brought to the attention of a doctor. Once the nature of the causative microorganism has been discovered, treatment consists of an *antibiotic drug* or other antimicrobial drug.

Infection, congenital

Any infection present at birth that was acquired by the infant either in the uterus or during passage through the birth canal.

INFECTIONS ACQUIRED IN THE UTERUS

Many viruses, bacteria, and other microorganisms can pass from the mother's blood through the placenta and into the circulation of the growing fetus. Particularly serious are organisms responsible for *rubella* (German measles), *syphilis,* and *toxoplasmosis,* and the *cytomegalovirus.* Any of these infections may cause *intrauterine growth retardation.* Further effects depend on the stage of pregnancy at which the infection was acquired. Thus, rubella occurring before 12 weeks may cause *deafness,* congenital *heart disease*, and eye disorders. Some infections in later pregnancy, particularly with a *herpes* virus, may also damage the fetus severely.

A woman who is infected with the HIV virus (responsible for *AIDS*) risks passing the infection on to her baby during pregnancy.

INFECTIONS ACQUIRED DURING BIRTH

These infections are almost always acquired from the mother's vaginal secretions or uterine fluid that has become infected with microorganisms. If the membranes rupture prematurely, the baby is at risk of infection from organisms ascending into the uterus from the birth canal.

Conditions acquired in this way include *conjunctivitis* (sometimes caused by infection with the organisms responsible for *gonorrhoea*), *herpes* infection, a *chlamydial infection*, and infantile *diarrhoea*. *Meningitis, hepatitis B, listeriosis, staphylococcal infections* and *streptococcal infections* may also be acquired in this way. Babies who inhale infected maternal secretions may develop *pneumonia*.

PREVENTION

The risk of a baby's acquiring an infection in the uterus is minimized by immunization against rubella in childhood and by the avoidance, or prompt treatment, of sexually transmitted disease in pregnancy.

If a woman has an active genital herpes infection close to the time of delivery, a *caesarean section* is usually performed, because infection of the newborn baby with herpes simplex virus is particularly serious and commonly fatal.

TREATMENT

If a baby is diagnosed as having an infection at birth, treatment against the infecting agent is started. Any growth retardation that has occurred due to infection in the uterus cannot usually be reversed. Some types of birth defects caused by infection (such as some types of heart defects) are treatable; others (such as congenital deafness) usually are not.

Infectious disease

Any illness caused by a specific microorganism.

INCIDENCE

Infectious diseases are a large and important group of conditions and, until recently, were the major cause of illness and death throughout the world. (In many developing countries, they remain a major cause of death.) Over the last century or so, this situation has changed in the more developed countries as a result of four important advances. First, better methods are employed for controlling the spread of disease organisms—including better sanitation, water purification, housing, pest control, and personal hygiene. Second, many effective *antibiotic drugs* and other antimicrobial drugs have been developed. Third, vaccines and other preparations have been developed to provide immunity to certain infectious diseases (see *Immunization*). Fourth, better general health and nutrition have bolstered immunity and improved survival.

In developed countries, such measures have brought about a dramatic decline in the incidence of some serious diseases (such as *poliomyelitis, diphtheria*, and *tuberculosis*) and the total eradication of *smallpox*. In poorer countries, however, infectious diseases remain a huge problem, for reasons that include lack of resources, ignorance, low standards of public and personal hygiene, the presence of insect transmitters of disease, and, perhaps most importantly, malnutrition. Diseases such as measles may have a mortality of 20 per cent in malnourished children.

CAUSES

Disease-causing organisms fall into a number of well-defined groups. Among the most important are *viruses, bacteria*, and *fungi*, along with three smaller groups, the rickettsiae, chlamydiae, and mycoplasmas. All are relatively simple organisms that can readily multiply in a host's tissues when defences are low. Other groups include the *protozoa* (single-celled animal parasites), *worms*, and *flukes*. These more complex parasites may spend only part of their life-cycle in human tissues; the rest of their life is spent in another animal or in soil. Colonization by worms and flukes (along with external parasites, such as *scabies* and *lice*) may be referred to as an *infestation* rather than an infection. See the accompanying table for examples of transmission mechanisms.

AVOIDANCE

Serious infectious diseases can largely be avoided by measures such as immunization, good hygiene with respect to food and drink and washing the hands after using the toilet, avoiding contact with animal faeces and secretions, and prudence in the choice of sexual partners (or precautions, such as the use of condoms). For travel outside Northern Europe, the US, Canada, Australia, and New Zealand, extra immunizations, and, in some cases, antimalarial tablets and protective measures against insects, may be recommended by your travel agent and confirmed by your doctor.

SYMPTOMS AND DIAGNOSIS

The symptoms of an infectious disease are caused in part by microorgan-

HOW INFECTIOUS DISEASES ARE TRANSMITTED

In developed countries, infectious diseases are usually spread by sexual transmission, airborne transmission, blood-borne transmission, or direct skin contact. In poorer countries, insect-borne, food-borne, and water-borne infection are other important mechanisms of transmission. Certain infections can also pass from a pregnant woman's blood across the placenta into the blood of the fetus.

Cholera bacteria
The comma-shaped bacteria that cause the dangerous infectious disease cholera are spread by contamination of water.

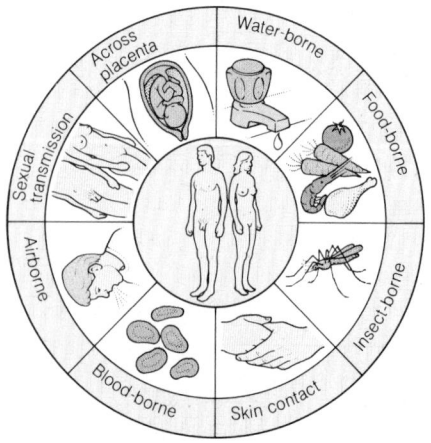

isms damaging cells and tissues, releasing toxins, and drawing on their host's reserves of nutrients; symptoms are also caused by the efforts of the body's defences (including the *immune system*) to destroy the microorganisms. The outcome depends on whether the microorganisms or the defences (sometimes aided by drug therapy) gain the upper hand. The strength of a person's immune system, which reflects his or her general health, strongly influences this outcome.

Fever is a feature in many infectious diseases; symptoms generally are related to the system or organ attacked—for example, cough, diarrhoea, or skin rash.

Apart from diseases in which the symptoms and signs are usually easily

SOME IMPORTANT INFECTIOUS DISEASES

VIRAL INFECTIONS

Infective agent	Transmission	Incubation period	Symptoms	Treatment
AIDS virus infection				
Human immuno-deficiency virus (HIV)	Sexual contact; sharing hypodermic needles; mother to child; infusion of infected blood products	Variable, usually several years	Fever; weight loss; fatigue; diarrhoea; swollen lymph nodes; shortness of breath	Treatment of complicating infections; zidovudine can prolong life expectancy
Chickenpox				
Varicella-zoster virus (herpes zoster virus)	Airborne droplets; direct contact	11 to 21 days	Slight fever; malaise; characteristic rash	Relief of symptoms; acyclovir beneficial in adults
Common cold				
Numerous rhino-viruses; corona-viruses	Airborne droplets; hand-to-hand contact	1 to 3 days	Sneezing; chills; muscle aches; runny nose; cough	Relief of symptoms
Hepatitis, viral				
Hepatitis virus types A, B, C, D, and E	Infected food or water (types A, E); sexual contact; infected blood; sharing needles (types B, C, D)	3 to 6 weeks (types A, E); a few weeks to several months (types B, C, D)	Influenza-like illness; jaundice; many people are asymptomatic	Relief of symptoms; interferon may be beneficial in some cases
Influenza				
Influenza viruses types A, B, or C	Airborne droplets	1 to 3 days	Fever; chills; aches; headache; sore throat; cough; runny nose	Relief of symptoms; fluids
Measles				
Measles virus (a paramyxovirus)	Airborne droplets	7 to 14 days	Fever; cold-like symptoms; characteristic rash; conjunctivitis	Relief of symptoms
Meningitis, viral				
Various viruses	Various methods, including via rodents	Variable	Fever; headache; drowsiness; confusion	Relief of symptoms; acyclovir in some cases
Mononucleosis, infectious				
Epstein-Barr virus	Possibly via saliva	1 to 6 weeks	Swollen glands; fever; sore throat; headache; malaise; lethargy	Relief of symptoms; rest; fluids
Poliomyelitis				
3 polioviruses	From faeces to mouth via hands; airborne droplets	Minor illlness—3 to 5 days. Major illness—7 to 14 days	Minor illness—sore throat; headache; vomiting. Major illness—fever; stiff neck and back; muscle aches; paralysis	Relief of symptoms
Rabies				
Rabies virus (a rhabdovirus)	Bite from infected animal	10 days to 8 months	Fever; general malaise; irrationality; throat spasms; hydrophobia	No effective treatment
Rubella				
Rubella virus	Airborne droplets; mother to child	2 to 3 weeks	Low fever; characteristic rash	Relief of symptoms

CHLAMYDIAL INFECTIONS

Infective agent	Transmission	Incubation period	Symptoms	Treatment
Nonspecific urethritis				
Chlamydia trachomatis	Sexual contact	1 to 4 weeks	Pain on passing urine; watery, mucus discharge	Antibiotics
Psittacosis				
Chlamydia psittaci	Inhalation of dust containing faeces from infected birds	1 to 3 weeks	Flu-like and feverish symptoms; shortness of breath	Antibiotics

RICKETTSIAL INFECTIONS

Infective agent	Transmission	Incubation period	Symptoms	Treatment
Q fever				
Coxiella burnetti	Inhalation of infected dust	7 to 14 days	Sudden onset of fever and sweating; cough; chest pains; headache	Antibiotics
Epidemic typhus				
Rickettsia prowazekii	Bite from infected body louse	About 7 days	Severe headache; high fever; muscle aches; weakness; rash	Antibiotics

BACTERIAL INFECTIONS

Infective agent	Transmission	Incubation period	Symptoms	Treatment
Gonorrhoea				
Neisseria gonorrhoeae	Sexual contact; mother to baby	2 to 6 days	Pain on passing urine; discharge; pain in abdomen	Penicillin; ampicillin; other antibiotics for resistant forms
Meningitis, bacterial				
Neisseria meningitidis (meningococcus); *Streptococcus pneumoniae*; others	Mother to baby via vagina; infection reaching bloodstream from another organ	Less than 3 weeks, could be less than 24 hours	High fever; stiff neck; nausea; confusion	Antibiotic treatment
Pertussis (whooping cough)				
Bordetella pertussis	Airborne droplets	1 to 2 weeks	Runny nose and moderate fever; slight cough leading to characteristic cough spasms	Erythromycin in early stage; small children may require hospital admission.
Pneumonia				
Streptococcus pneumoniae; *Legionella pneumophila*; others	Airborne droplets	1 to 3 weeks	Cough; fever; chest pain; shortness of breath	Antibiotics
Tuberculosis				
Mycobacterium tuberculosis	Airborne transmission; cow's milk	Several weeks to several years	Malaise; weight loss; cough; shortness of breath; chest pain	Various antibiotics; possibly surgery
Typhoid fever				
Salmonella typhi	Food or water contaminated with infected faeces	1 to 2 weeks, sometimes longer	Headache; lethargy, intestinal upsets; very high, prolonged fever	Several effective drugs, but fever takes a long time to control

FUNGAL INFECTIONS

Infective agent	Transmission	Incubation period	Symptoms	Treatment
Tinea				
Epidermophyton spp; *Microsporum* spp; *Trichophyton* spp	Direct contact with infected humans or animals	Variable	Itchy skin patches; patchy hair loss; cracking skin between toes	Antifungal drugs
Meningitis, fungal				
Cryptococcus neoformans	Inhalation of fungus from pigeon droppings	Unknown	Headache; stiff neck; photophobia	Antifungal drugs

PROTOZOAL INFECTIONS

Infective agent	Transmission	Incubation period	Symptoms	Treatment
Amoebiasis				
Entamoeba histolytica	Food or water contaminated by faeces	A few weeks to many years	Severe diarrhoea	Antiprotozoal drugs (e.g. metronidazole)
Giardiasis				
Giardia lamblia	Food or water contaminated by faeces; sexual contact	3 to 40 days	Diarrhoea; abdominal discomfort; bloating	Antiprotozoal drugs (e.g. metronidazole)
Malaria				
Plasmodium falciparum; *Plasmodium vivax*; others	Bite from infected mosquito	10 to 40 days	Chills; high fever; sweating; headache; fatigue	Various drugs (e.g. chloroquine)

recognizable (such as *chickenpox*), diagnosis relies on identifying the causative microorganism. Testing may be by microscopic examination of a specimen of infected tissue or body fluid, by *culture* techniques, or by detecting *antibodies* (proteins manufactured by the body to defend against a particular organism) in the blood (see *Serology*).

A particular problem with infectious diseases is that there is always a time gap (known as the incubation period) between the entry of the microorganisms into the body and the first appearance of symptoms. The incubation period may last from a few hours to several years; during this time, the infected person is likely to pass the microorganism to other people. Furthermore, symptoms may never develop in some infected people, but these people nevertheless continue to carry the disease organisms and unwittingly spread them to others.

As a result, an epidemic can be well established before it is recognized and before control measures are introduced. This can be particularly devastating when the disease is a new one and has a long incubation period and a high mortality (*AIDS* is a classic example).

TREATMENT
The mainstay of treatment is the use of antibiotic and other antimicrobial drugs. Drug treatment must be carefully selected by means of culturing and identifying the causative microorganisms because certain microorganisms are susceptible only to certain drugs. For many viruses, no effective *antiviral drug* is available and treatment relies on supportive measures, such as reducing temperature, maintaining food and fluid intake, etc.

OUTLOOK
Although great strides have been made in the fight against infectious diseases, many problems remain, even in developed countries. The spread of certain diseases (such as sexually transmitted infections) is difficult to control except by modifying human behaviour. For many infections, no effective vaccine has been developed. The majority of viral diseases cannot be effectively combatted with drugs, and some bacteria have developed *resistance* to the drugs available. When a new infectious disease appears, it may be years before an effective vaccine or drug treatment can be devised. In the meantime, large numbers of people may die (once again, AIDS provides the most recent example.)

Infectious mononucleosis
See *Mononucleosis, infectious*.

Inferiority complex
A neurotic state of mind that develops because of repeated hurts or failures in the past. Inferiority complex arises from a conflict between the positive wish to be recognized as someone worthwhile and the haunting fear of frustration and failure. Attempts to compensate for the sense of worthlessness may take the form of aggression and violence, or of overzealous involvement in activities. (See also *Superiority complex*.)

Infertility
The inability to produce offspring. Conception depends on the production of healthy sperm by the man, healthy eggs by the woman, and *sexual intercourse* so that the sperm reach the woman's *fallopian tubes*. There must be no mechanical obstruction to prevent the sperm from reaching the egg, and the sperm must be able to fertilize the egg when they meet (see *Fertilization*). Next, the fertilized egg must be capable of implantation in the uterus (see *Implantation, egg*). Finally, the developing embryo must be healthy and its hormonal environment must be adequate for further

INVESTIGATING INFERTILITY

If no cause for infertility is found after a general check-up and/or a personal interview regarding sexual behaviour, more specialized tests may be performed. Both partners may require testing because infertility can be attributed to one person, to both of them, or to mutual incompatibility.

CAUSES OF INFERTILITY

Conception is a complicated process; the organs involved can be affected in numerous ways, resulting in infertility. Some of the principal underlying causes of infertility—in men and women— are illustrated at right.

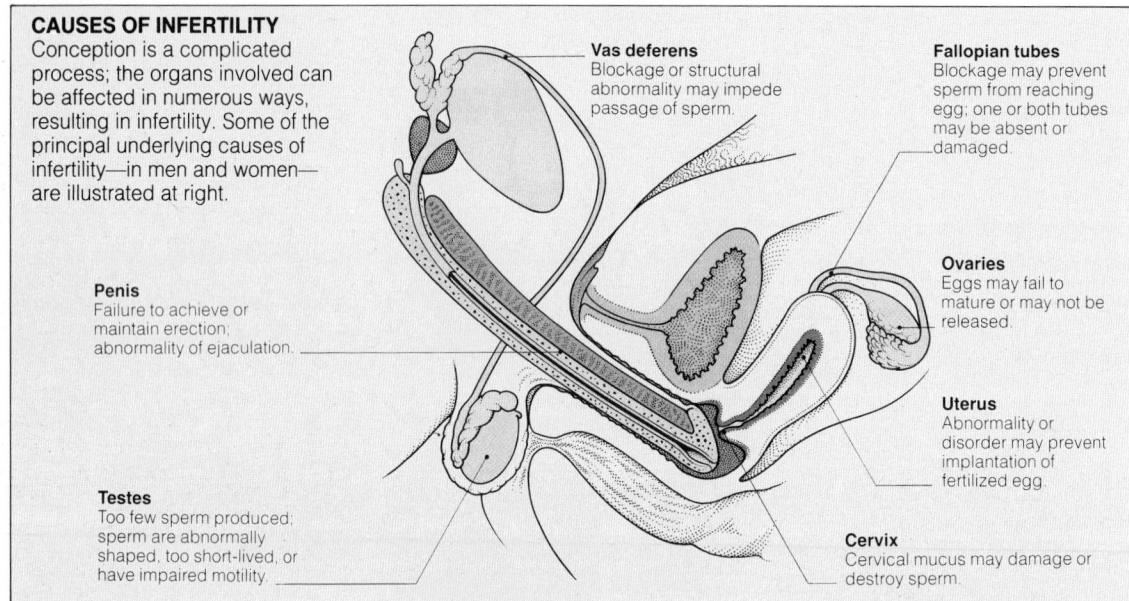

Vas deferens
Blockage or structural abnormality may impede passage of sperm.

Fallopian tubes
Blockage may prevent sperm from reaching egg; one or both tubes may be absent or damaged.

Penis
Failure to achieve or maintain erection; abnormality of ejaculation.

Ovaries
Eggs may fail to mature or may not be released.

Uterus
Abnormality or disorder may prevent implantation of fertilized egg.

Testes
Too few sperm produced; sperm are abnormally shaped, too short-lived, or have impaired motility.

Cervix
Cervical mucus may damage or destroy sperm.

FEMALE INFERTILITY

Investigations to discover the cause of a woman's infertility may include taking a menstrual history, a study of body temperature during the menstrual cycle (below), and/or blood and urine tests to discover whether ovulation is normal, hysterosalpingography (right), or laparoscopy (below right).

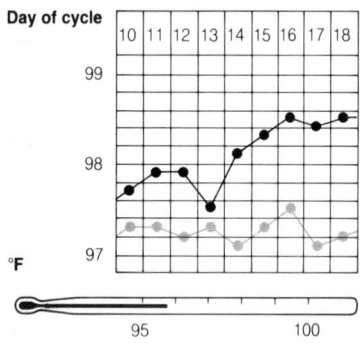

Day of cycle

	10	11	12	13	14	15	16	17	18

99
98
°F 97

95   100

Body temperature and ovulation
Charting a woman's body temperature during her menstrual cycle can indicate abnormalities of ovulation. The chart above shows typical temperature fluctuations during a normal cycle (red line) and those associated with failure to ovulate (grey line).

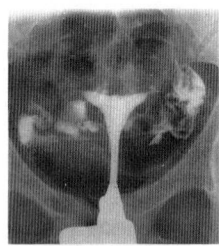

Hysterosalpingography
This X-ray technique is used to visualize the uterus and/or fallopian tubes to determine whether or not there is any abnormality.

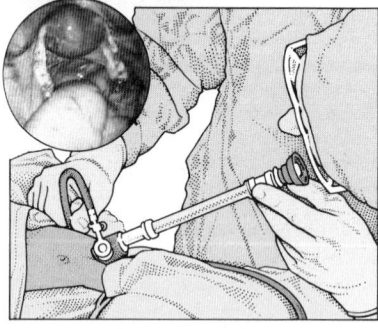

Laparoscopy
In this technique, a laparoscope (a type of viewing tube) is inserted through the abdominal wall to examine the woman's reproductive organs and determine whether an abnormality, such as a cyst or a tumour, is present. The laparoscope view (above) shows a tumour in the left ovary.

MALE INFERTILITY

The first test for investigating male infertility is semen analysis (below). If it reveals a low sperm count, more tests may be needed to investigate the underlying cause.

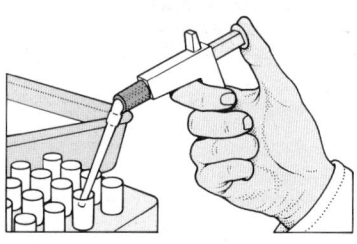

Semen analysis
Semen produced by masturbation is examined as soon as possible for the number, shape, and degree of motility of the sperm. A postcoital semen test may also be performed.

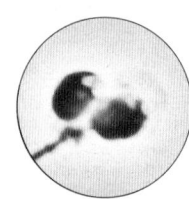

Abnormal sperm
The presence in the semen of large numbers of abnormally shaped sperm, such as the two-headed one (left), may reduce a man's fertility.

development so that the pregnancy can continue to full term. Infertility may result from a disturbance of any of these factors.

INCIDENCE
Infertility is a common problem. As many as one in six couples requires help from a specialist. Infertility increases with age; the older a couple is when trying to conceive, the more difficult it may be.

CAUSES
In rough terms, about 30 per cent of infertility cases are due to factors that affect the man; another 30 per cent are due to factors that affect the woman. In the remaining 40 per cent of cases, infertility is due to both partners.

MALE INFERTILITY The major cause of male infertility is failure to produce enough healthy sperm. *Azoospermia* (in which there is no sperm) and *oligospermia* (in which few sperm are produced) both cause infertility.

In some cases the sperm are malformed or their lifespan after ejaculation is too short for them to travel far enough to reach the egg. Defects in the sperm may be due to a blockage of the spermatic tubes or to damage to the spermatic ducts, usually due to a *sexually transmitted disease*, such as *gonorrhoea*. A *varicocele* (varicose veins in the scrotum) may also be a factor. Abnormal development of the testes due to an endocrine disorder (see *Hypogonadism*) or damage to the testes by *orchitis* (inflammation of the testes) may also cause defective sperm. Toxins, cigarettes, or various drugs can lower the sperm count.

Infertility in men may also be caused by a failure to deliver the sperm into the vagina, as occurs in *impotence* or in disorders affecting ejaculation, such as inhibited ejaculation or retrograde ejaculation (see *Ejaculation, disorders of*).

In rare cases, there may be a chromosomal abnormality (such as *Klinefelter's syndrome*) or a genetic disease (such as *cystic fibrosis*) that causes infertility in men.

FEMALE INFERTILITY Anovulation (failure to ovulate) is the most common cause of female infertility. Failure to ovulate often occurs for no obvious reason. It can be caused by hormonal imbalance, stress, or a disorder of the *ovary*, such as a tumour or cyst.

Blocked fallopian tubes, which frequently occur after *pelvic inflammatory disease*, may prevent the sperm from reaching the egg. The woman may have one tube or no tubes because of a congenital defect or because they were removed surgically (e.g. because

of an *ectopic pregnancy*). Disorders of the uterus (such as *fibroids*) may cause infertility, as can *endometriosis*.

Infertility also occurs if the woman's cervical mucus provides a hostile environment to her partner's sperm by producing antibodies that kill or immobilize them.

Rarely, a chromosomal abnormality (such as *Turner's syndrome*) is the cause of a woman's infertility.

DIAGNOSIS
Tests for infertility are usually carried out if pregnancy has not resulted after a year of regular unprotected intercourse (about 90 per cent of women trying to become pregnant do so within a year).

A physical examination of both the man and the woman will be performed to determine the general state of their health, and to eliminate untreated physical disorders that might be causing the infertility. The partners are interviewed, separately and together, regarding their sexual habits to determine if intercourse is taking place correctly for conception. If the cause of infertility remains undiagnosed after these examinations, additional tests may be performed (see box).

TREATMENT
When no specific cause can be found, improving the general state of health may help. The doctor may suggest changes in diet, (e.g. reducing alcohol intake), and may suggest relaxation techniques and elimination of stress.

Treatment of male infertility is limited. Surgical reversal of vasectomy is possible in some cases. When azoospermia exists, the couple must usually accept their childless state or consider adoption or *artificial insemination* by donor. If the sperm count is low, artificial insemination by the husband may be tried, although its success rate varies. In some cases of male infertility due to a hormonal imbalance, drugs such as clomiphene or *gonadotrophin hormone* therapy may prove useful.

For female infertility, failure to ovulate requires ovarian stimulation with a drug such as clomiphene, with or without a gonadotrophin hormone. Microsurgery can sometimes repair damage to the fallopian tubes if it is not too severe. If surgery on the fallopian tubes is unsuccessful, *in vitro fertilization* is the only way that pregnancy may be possible. Uterine abnormalities or disorders, such as fibroids, may require treatment. If the cervical mucus has proved hostile,

artificial insemination of the husband's semen directly into the cervix can prevent the sperm from coming into contact with the mucus.

In some cases, provided the woman has normal fallopian tubes, treatment may be offered by GIFT (gamete intra-fallopian transfer) or ZIFT (zygote intra-fallopian transfer). In these techniques, the ovaries are stimulated by drugs, and *laparoscopy* is used to recover eggs. In GIFT, the eggs are placed with sperm in the fallopian tubes. In ZIFT, fertilization is observed in the laboratory and an early embryo is put into the tubes.

OUTLOOK
About half the couples professionally treated for infertility achieve a pregnancy. Each couple's chances depend on the cause of the infertility.

Infestation

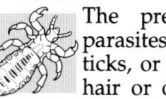 The presence of animal parasites (such as mites, ticks, or lice) in the skin or hair or of worms (such as tapeworms) inside the body.

Infibulation

A form of female circumcision in which the labia majora (the outer lips surrounding the vagina) are removed and the entrance to the vagina narrowed. See *Circumcision, female*.

Infiltrate

Accumulation of substances or cells within a tissue that are either not normally found in it or are usually present only in smaller amounts.

Infiltrate may refer to a drug (such as a local anaesthetic) that has been injected into a tissue or to the build-up of a substance within an organ (such as of fat in the liver caused by excessive alcohol consumption).

Radiologists use the term to refer to the presence of abnormalities, such as the presence of a tumour or signs of pneumonia, on an X-ray.

Inflammation

Redness, swelling, heat, and pain in a tissue due to chemical or physical injury, or to infection.

When body tissues are damaged, specialized *mast cells* release a chemical called *histamine* (other substances are also involved in the inflammatory response, but histamine is believed to be responsible for most of the effects). Histamine increases blood flow to the damaged tissue, which causes the redness and heat. It also makes the blood capillaries more leaky, resulting in fluid oozing out of them and into the tissues, which causes localized swelling. The pain of inflammation is due to stimulation of nerve endings by the inflammatory chemicals.

Inflammation is usually accompanied by an accumulation of white blood cells, which are attracted by the inflammatory chemicals. These white cells help destroy invading microorganisms and are involved in repairing the damaged tissue. Thus, inflammation is an essential part of the body's response to injury and infection.

If inflammation is inappropriate (as in *rheumatoid arthritis* and some other *autoimmune disorders*), it may be suppressed by *corticosteroid drugs* or by *nonsteroidal anti-inflammatory drugs*.

Inflammatory bowel disease
A general term for chronic inflammatory disorders affecting the small and/or large intestine. The cause is unknown. Specific conditions are *Crohn's disease* and *ulcerative colitis*.

Influenza
A viral infection of the respiratory tract (air passages) that causes fever, headache, muscle ache, and weakness. Popularly known as "flu", it is spread by virus-infected droplets coughed or sneezed into the air. Influenza usually occurs in small outbreaks or every few years in epidemics. Outbreaks tend to occur in winter, rapidly spreading, especially in schools and institutions for the elderly.

CAUSES
There are three main types of influenza virus, called A, B, and C. A person who has had an attack caused by the type C virus acquires *antibodies* (proteins made by the *immune system*) that provide immunity against the type C virus for life. Anyone who has been infected with a particular strain of the type A or B viruses acquires immunity to that strain. Both the A- and B-type viruses occasionally alter to produce new strains that may be able to overcome immunity built up in response to a previous attack, thus leading to a new infection.

The type B virus is fairly stable but occasionally alters sufficiently to overcome resistance. A new strain often causes small outbreaks of infection. The type A virus is highly unstable; new strains arise constantly throughout the world. These are the strains that caused the influenza *pandemics* of this century, most notably Spanish flu in 1918, Asian flu in 1957, and Hong Kong flu in 1968.

SYMPTOMS
The classic symptoms of flu (chills, fever, headache, muscular aches, loss of appetite, and fatigue) are brought on by types A and B. Type C causes only a mild illness that is indistinguishable from a common cold. In general, type A is more debilitating than type B.

The general symptoms described, which are more common in adults than in children, are usually followed by a cough (often accompanied by chest pain), a sore throat, and a runny nose. After two days, fever and other symptoms start to subside and, after five days, these symptoms have usually disappeared. Respiratory symptoms persist, however; the sufferer may feel weak and sometimes depressed.

The illness usually clears up completely within seven to 10 days. In rare cases, however, it takes a severe form, causing acute pneumonia that may be fatal within a day or two even in healthy young adults. The Spanish flu epidemic of 1918 killed millions of young adults in all countries of the world.

Type B infections in children sometimes mimic *appendicitis* and have been implicated in *Reye's syndrome*. In babies, the type A virus can cause seizures (see *Convulsions, febrile*).

Secondary bacterial infection is common, particularly in the elderly and in those with lung or heart disease; it may cause fatal *bronchitis, bronchiolitis*, or *pneumonia*.

PREVENTION
Anti-influenza vaccines, containing killed strains of types A and B virus currently in circulation, are available, but have only a 60 to 70 per cent success rate in preventing infection. In addition, any immunity provided is short-lived. Vaccination must be repeated each year just before the start of the influenza season.

It is recommended that older people and anyone suffering from respiratory or circulatory disease be vaccinated, especially if they are living in institutions.

TREATMENT
In all but the mildest cases, a person with influenza should rest in bed in a warm, well-ventilated room. *Analgesic drugs* (painkillers) should be taken to relieve aches and pains and to reduce fever. Warm fluids soothe a sore throat and inhaling steam has a soothing effect on the lungs.

HOW TO USE AN INHALER
With each type, the user puts the nozzle of the inhaler in the mouth, presses the end to release the drug, and simultaneously breathes in through the mouth. If the device is used correctly, the drug is dispersed to the bronchi. A *nebulizer* is a special type of inhaler that delivers the drug as a fine mist through a face-mask.

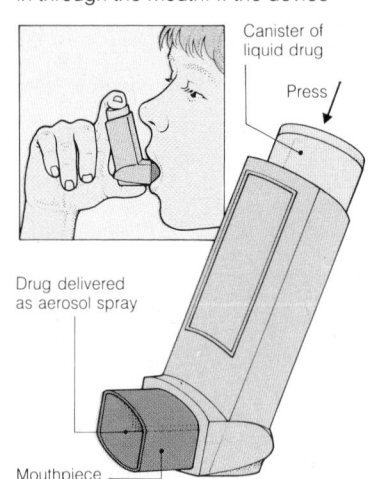

Canister of liquid drug

Press

Drug delivered as aerosol spray

Mouthpiece

Aerosol inhaler
This type of inhaler delivers the drug as an aerosol spray when the user presses the top of the canister.

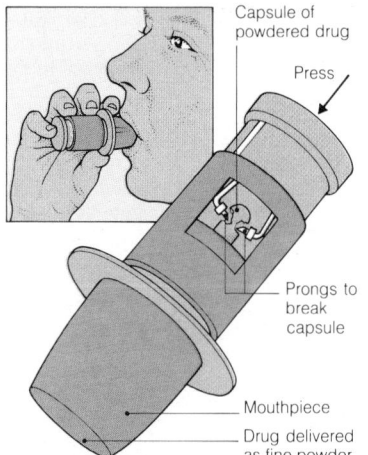

Capsule of powdered drug

Press

Prongs to break capsule

Mouthpiece

Drug delivered as fine powder

Spinhaler
Here, a drug capsule is placed in the end chamber, the top of which is pressed to pierce the capsule and release the drug.

In the case of an elderly person or someone with a lung or heart disease, a doctor should be called as soon as symptoms develop. The antiviral drug amantadine, which can reduce the severity of an attack if given within 24 hours of onset of symptoms, may be given. *Antibiotic drugs* may be used to combat secondary bacterial infection.

Once the fever has abated, the patient can get out of bed, but still needs rest. When he or she has started to regain strength, the return to normal activities should be gradual.

Infra-red

A term denoting the part of the electromagnetic spectrum immediately beyond the red end of the visible light spectrum. Directed onto the skin, infra-red radiation heats the skin and the tissues immediately below it.

The infra-red wave band includes heat waves; an infra-red lamp is one means of giving *heat treatment*.

Infusion, intravenous

See *Intravenous infusion*.

Ingestion

The act of taking any substance (e.g. food, drink, or medications) into the body through the mouth. The term also refers to the process by which certain cells (for example, some white blood cells) surround and then engulf small particles.

Ingrowing toenail

See *Toenail, ingrowing*.

Inguinal

Relating to the groin (the area between the abdomen and thigh), as in inguinal *hernia* (the protrusion of part of the intestine into the muscles of the groin).

Inhalation

The act of taking in breath (see *Breathing*). An inhalation is also a substance, in the form of a gas, vapour, powder, or aerosol, to be breathed in.

Inhaler

A device used for administering a drug in powder or vapour form. Inhalers are used principally in the treatment of various respiratory disorders, including *asthma* and chronic *bronchitis*. Among the medications administered in this way are *bronchodilator drugs* (used to widen the airways) and *corticosteroid drugs* (used to reduce inflammation).

Inheritance

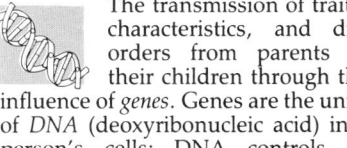 The transmission of traits, characteristics, and disorders from parents to their children through the influence of *genes*. Genes are the units of *DNA* (deoxyribonucleic acid) in a person's cells; DNA controls all growth and functioning of the body. Half of a person's genes come from the mother, half from the father.

Children tend to resemble their parents, particularly in their physical characteristics. However, this resemblance may also apply to mental abilities, mannerisms, personality, and behaviour. In addition, many disorders show a moderate to very notable tendency to "run in families".

Although there is a temptation to ascribe similarities in a family to inheritance, there are equally plausible alternative explanations for many family traits. For example, all the members of a family may be fat not through the influence of genes, but because they all eat the same fattening food and rarely exercise. Children may behave like their mother not because of inheritance, but because they imitate her. Certain abilities and behaviours (e.g. the language a person speaks) are clearly not inherited. Nevertheless, it is accepted that most physical characteristics, many disorders, and some mental abilities and aspects of personality are inherited.

MECHANISMS OF INHERITANCE

Each of a person's cells contains exactly the same genes, which come originally from the egg and sperm cells from which he or she is derived.

The genes in a cell are organized into long strands of DNA called *chromosomes*. The genes controlling most characteristics come in pairs—one gene originating from the father, the other from the mother. Everyone has 22 pairs of chromosomes (called autosomes) bearing these paired genes, in addition to two more chromosomes, the sex chromosomes. Women have two X chromosomes; men have an X chromosome and a Y chromosome.

The inheritance of normal traits and disorders can be divided into those controlled by a single pair of genes on the autosomal chromosomes (unifactorial inheritance); those controlled by genes on the sex chromosomes (sex-linked inheritance); and those controlled by the combination of many genes (multifactorial inheritance).

UNIFACTORIAL INHERITANCE

A large number of variable traits, such as eye colour, blood groups, and the ability to taste certain substances, is thought to be controlled by a single pair of genes. The ways in which these traits are inherited conform to laws first elucidated in the 19th century by the Austrian monk Gregor Mendel. Since then, they have been referred to as the laws of Mendelian inheritance.

Either of the pair of genes controlling a trait may take any of several forms, which are known as alleles. For example, the genes controlling eye colour exist as two main alleles, coding for blue and brown eye colour. Thus, an individual's gene pair for eye colour may be blue/blue (giving blue eyes), brown/brown (giving brown eyes) or brown/blue (also giving brown eyes, because the brown allele is dominant over, i.e. "masks", the blue allele, which is called recessive to the brown allele).

When a couple has a child, only one of the pair of genes controlling a trait is passed to the child from each parent. For example, someone with the brown/blue combination for eye colour has a 50 per cent chance of passing on the blue gene, and a 50 per cent chance of passing on the brown gene, to any child. This factor is combined with the gene coming from the other parent, according to dominant or recessive relationships, to determine the child's eye colour. According to the combination of the parental genes, the numbers of brown- and blue-eyed offspring of a particular couple tend to conform to a certain ratio, in accordance with Mendelian laws (see illustration overleaf).

Similar laws and ratios apply to the inheritance of other traits controlled by single gene pairs, and also to the inheritance of certain *genetic disorders* (e.g. *cystic fibrosis* and *achondroplasia*).

SEX-LINKED INHERITANCE

The most obvious example of sex-linked inheritance is gender itself. Male gender is caused by the existence in males of the genes on the Y chromosome, which is present only in males and is inherited by boys from their fathers. The genes on the Y chromosome almost certainly direct the development of the male primary sex organs (the testes) and all male characteristics derive from the secretion of hormones by these organs.

The X chromosome, on the other hand, is less closely associated with the female sex because it is present in both males (in a single dose) and in females (in a double dose). It seems that female gender is the natural course of development in the absence of the Y chromosome, does not require any extra genes to direct it, and that the X chromosome is concerned with general development.

Any faults in a male's genes on the X chromosome tend to be expressed outwardly, because such a fault cannot (as it can in females) be masked by the presence of a normal gene on a second X chromosome. Faults in the genes of the X chromosome include those responsible for *colour vision deficiency*, *haemophilia*, and other sex-linked inherited disorders, which almost exclusively affect males.

MULTIFACTORIAL INHERITANCE

A number of traits (such as height and build) are believed to be controlled by the combined effects of many genes, along with environmental effects. Using height as an example, a simple model proposes that there are several genes determining a person's stature, some of which are "tall" genes and others "short". A person's height depends on the relative number of tall to short genes.

When two people have children, a child may, in rare cases, inherit all the tall or all the short genes from both parents, and thus be exceptionally tall or short. The laws of chance dictate, however, that, in most cases, a child will inherit a mixture of tall and short genes and thus be in the range of average stature. Nevertheless, the child of tall parents tends to inherit more tall genes than the child of short parents. Dietary and other factors also affect growth so that a person with many short genes may still attain an average stature through good diet.

Multifactorial inheritance, along with the effects of environment, may play a part in causing disorders, such as *diabetes mellitus* and *spina bifida*.

Inhibition

The process of preventing any mental or physical activity. Inhibition in the brain and spinal cord is carried out by special *neurons*, which damp down the action of other nerve cells to keep the brain's activity in balance.

In a psychological sense, certain mental activities can be described as inhibiting other thoughts or reflexes.

In *psychoanalysis*, an inhibition refers to the unconscious restraint of instinctual impulses. Such inhibition may cause symptoms, such as being temporarily unable to write because writing arouses forbidden ideas.

Injection

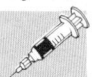 Introduction of a substance into the body from a syringe through a needle. Injections may be intravenous (into a vein), intramuscular (into a muscle), subcutaneous (under the skin), or intra-articular (into a joint).

Injury

Harm to any part of the body. Injury may arise from a wide variety of causes, including physical influences (e.g. force, heat, cold, electricity, vibration, and radiation), chemical causes (e.g. poisons and caustic substances), bites, or oxygen deprivation.

(See *Accidents*; *Bite, animal*; *Bite, human*; *Bleeding*; *Burns*; *Cold injury*; *Dislocation, joint*; *Electrical injury*; *First aid*; *Fractures*; *Head injury*; *Heatstroke*; *Poisoning*; *Radiation sickness*; *Snake bites*; *Soft-tissue injury*; *Spinal injury*; *Sports injuries*; *Sprains*; *Venomous bites and stings*; *Wounds*.)

Ink-blot test

 An outdated psychological test in which the subject was asked to interpret a number of ink blots. The most widely used example was the *Rorschach test*.

Inlay, dental

A filling of porcelain or gold made outside the mouth and used to restore a badly decayed tooth. An inlay may be needed for back teeth or to provide protection for a weakened tooth.

The dentist first makes an angular cavity in the tooth to accept the inlay. A replica of the cavity is then made, generally using a wax *impression*; the inlay is constructed on the replica and cemented in place in the tooth.

Inoculation

The act of introducing a small quantity of a foreign substance into the body, usually by injection, for the purpose of stimulating the *immune system* to produce *antibodies* (protective proteins) against the substance. Inoculation is usually done to protect against future infection by particular bacteria or viruses. (See *Immunization*.)

Inoperable

A term applied to any condition that cannot be alleviated or cured by surgery, such as a very advanced cancer that has spread to many parts of the body or a brain tumour that is not surgically accessible.

Inorganic

A term used to refer to any of the large group of substances that do not contain carbon and to a few simple carbon compounds (e.g. *carbon dioxide* and *carbon monoxide*). Examples of inorganic substances include table salt (sodium chloride) and bicarbonate of soda (sodium bicarbonate).

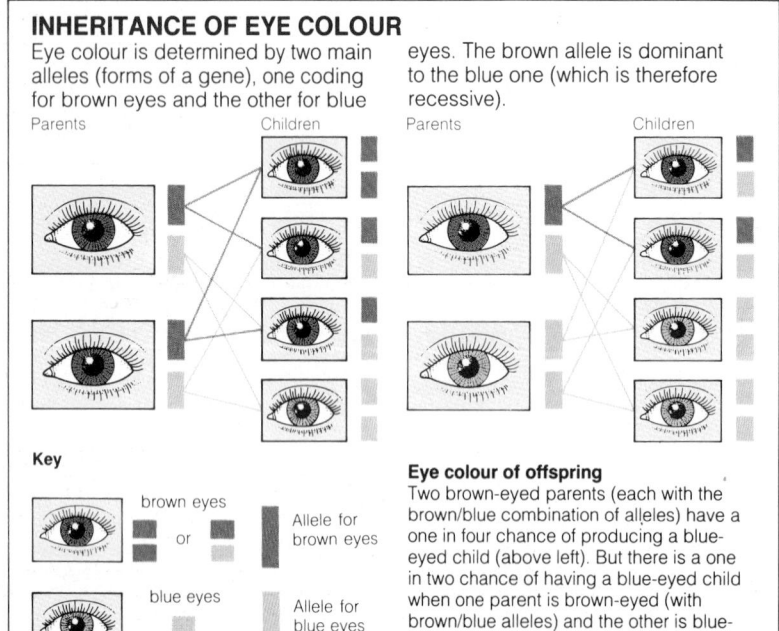

INHERITANCE OF EYE COLOUR

Eye colour is determined by two main alleles (forms of a gene), one coding for brown eyes and the other for blue eyes. The brown allele is dominant to the blue one (which is therefore recessive).

Parents   Children   Parents   Children

Key

brown eyes   or   Allele for brown eyes

blue eyes   Allele for blue eyes

Eye colour of offspring
Two brown-eyed parents (each with the brown/blue combination of alleles) have a one in four chance of producing a blue-eyed child (above left). But there is a one in two chance of having a blue-eyed child when one parent is brown-eyed (with brown/blue alleles) and the other is blue-eyed (above).

Inpatient treatment

Care or therapy received by a patient admitted to a hospital.

Insanity

The common term for serious mental disorder. Today the term insanity has no technical meaning for psychiatrists, but is used in law to indicate a mental state that renders a person not legally responsible for his or her own actions. The "insanity defence" was introduced to ensure that people committing murder as a result of a mental disorder would not be given the death penalty, but would instead receive proper treatment. *Psychosis* now covers serious illnesses formerly denoted by insanity.

Insect bites

Tiny puncture wounds in the skin inflicted by blood-sucking insects, such as mosquitoes, midges, gnats, horseflies, sandflies, fleas, lice, and bedbugs. Small eight-legged creatures called arachnids, which include ticks, spiders, and mites, can cause similar injuries.

Most bites cause only temporary pain (or itching for a day or two) although some people have severe skin reactions. In the tropics and subtropics, insect bites are potentially more serious because certain biting species can transmit disease (see *Insects and disease*).

CAUSES

Insects that bite do so to obtain a blood meal. The mouthparts of biting insects are specially adapted for piercing skin and sucking blood. Insect bites are most common on exposed parts of the head, hands, arms, or legs.

Although mosquitoes (which attack mainly after dark) may be the most troublesome biting insects, many bites blamed on mosquitoes are in fact caused by cat or dog fleas. These fleas inhabit various domestic locations where the pet habitually rests (e.g. carpets, sleeping baskets, or sofas) and, when their normal host is absent, may jump on to humans to feed.

Of the more easily visible insects, horseflies can produce a particularly painful bite, while gnats can be a menace if a swarm is encountered.

SYMPTOMS

All insect bites provoke a reaction in the skin that is primarily an allergic response (see *Allergy*) to substances in the insect's saliva or its faeces, which are often deposited at or near the site of the bite and rubbed in by scratch-ing. Reactions vary from innocuous red pimples to painful swellings (which may weep) or an intensely itching rash. People vary in their reactions to the same biting insect; in some people the reaction may be extremely severe.

AVOIDANCE

Avoiding insect bites can be particularly important for campers and hikers, anyone living in a mosquito-infested area, and travellers or residents in tropical countries.

Bites outdoors can be reduced by wearing trousers, socks, and long-sleeved shirts (especially after dark, when mosquitoes are most active), and by using insect repellents.

Indoors, bites can be reduced by using insect screens over open windows and by spraying bedrooms with aerosols containing pyrethroid insecticides before going to bed. If this fails, it may be necessary to use mosquito nets and slow-burning antimosquito coils that give off pyrethroids.

TREATMENT

Bites or bitten areas should be thoroughly washed with soap and water, and a soothing ointment, such as calamine lotion, should be applied. Scratching should be avoided. If there is a severe reaction, a doctor should be called; a cream containing an *antihistamine drug* may be required.

Severe itching on the scalp or in the pubic hair suggests the possibility of a louse infestation, which is treated with insecticidal lotions (see *Lice*). In the case of flea bites, the entire residence (not just the pet) may require treatment with insecticide to kill the flea population. (See also *Spider bites; Mites and disease; Ticks and disease*.)

Insects and disease

Insects are six-legged animals with a pair of antennae, a firm exterior skeleton, and, in many cases, wings. They include such animals as ants, bees, cockroaches, fleas, flies, lice, and mosquitoes, but not mites, ticks, or spiders, which belong to another animal group, the arachnids. The insects and arachnids both belong to a larger animal group, the arthropods.

DISEASE CAUSED BY INSECTS

There are over one million known species of insects and probably several million that have yet to be identified and named; most are either harmless or positively beneficial to humans. The majority of harmful species cause sickness by attacking crops or stored food, thus contributing to malnutrition and famine.

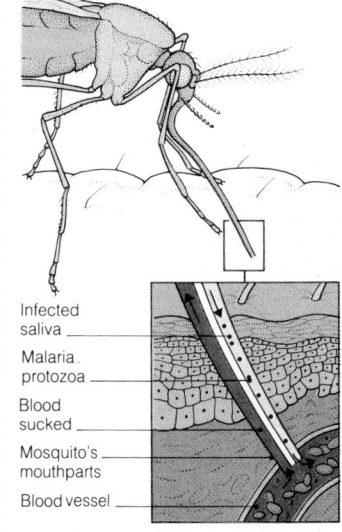

INSECT-BORNE DISEASES

Malaria is by far the most prevalent of the insect-borne diseases, affecting an estimated 200 to 300 million people worldwide.

Infected saliva
Malaria protozoa
Blood sucked
Mosquito's mouthparts
Blood vessel

Transmission of malaria
When an infected *ANOPHELES* mosquito feeds on a person's blood, it injects saliva through its mouthparts; the protozoa that cause malaria enter the blood via the insect's saliva.

Other insects are a more direct cause of illness or disease. Some directly parasitize humans, living under the skin or on the body surface (see *Lice; Chigoe; Myiasis*). Others will sting if provoked, with results that range from moderate discomfort (in most cases) to a severe life-threatening reaction (see *Insect stings*).

The most troublesome insects are flies and various biting insects. Many types of flies settle first on human or animal excrement and then on food to lay eggs or to feed. They can transmit disease organisms from excrement to food via their feet and legs. This is probably important in the spread of intestinal infections such as *typhoid fever* and *shigellosis*.

Insect bites are irritating in themselves, but a much more serious risk is that an insect will spread infectious organisms as a result of its bite. Serious diseases that are spread by biting insects include *malaria* and *filariasis* (transmitted by mosquitoes), *sleeping sickness* (tsetse flies), *leishmaniasis* (sandflies), epidemic *typhus* (lice), and *plague* (rat fleas). Also, various mosquitoes, sandflies, and ticks spread a group of viral illnesses called the arthropod-borne or arboviruses. Such illnesses include *yellow fever*, *dengue*, and some types of viral *encephalitis*.

Organisms picked up when an insect ingests blood from an infected animal or person are able to survive or multiply in the insect. Later, the organisms are either injected into a new human host via the insect's saliva or deposited in the faeces at or near the site of the bite and later rubbed in by the victim.

Most of insect-borne diseases (of which malaria is by far the most important) are confined to the tropics and subtropics.

AVOIDANCE
The avoidance of insect-borne disease is largely a matter of keeping flies off food, discouraging insect bites by the use of suitable clothing and insect repellents, and, in areas of the world where malaria is present, the use of mosquito nets and screens, *pesticides*, and antimalarial tablets.

Insect stings

 A fairly small number of insects (bees, wasps, and hornets) are capable of stinging. Insect venom contains inflammatory substances that cause local pain, redness, and swelling for about 48 hours. Normally, a very large number of stings (hundreds in the case of an adult) must be received for them to be life-threatening. However, about one person in 200 is allergic to insect venom. This means that, after the person's *immune system* has been sensitized by the venom from a sting, one subsequent sting (possibly months or years later) can provoke a severe allergic reaction leading to *anaphylactic shock*. The symptoms may include a severe itchy rash (nettle rash), dizziness, facial and throat swellings, wheezing, vomiting, breathing difficulties, and collapse.

Hyposensitization—a technique for reducing sensitivity to bee or wasp venom (and some other types of allergy)—is recommended for those known to suffer hypersensitivity.

TREATMENT
A bee often leaves its sting sac in the wound. The sac should be gently scraped out with a knife blade or fingernail and not removed by grasping it with fingers or tweezers (which injects more venom). The stung area should be washed with soap and water, a cold compress should be applied, and *analgesic drugs* should be taken to ease the discomfort.

If the symptoms of anaphylactic shock develop, it is essential to seek emergency medical treatment, which initially consists of an injection of *adrenaline*. Any person who is known to be hypersensitive to bee or wasp venom should obtain and carry an emergency kit for the self-injection of adrenaline. In severe cases, the victims of insect stings require *cardiopulmonary resuscitation*.

Any sting in the mouth or throat may be dangerous because swelling may obstruct breathing. Medical assistance should be sought immediately and, if possible, the victim should be given ice cubes to suck. (See also *Scorpion stings*.)

Insecurity
Lack of self-confidence and uncertainty about one's abilities, aims, and relationships with others. Repeated changes of environment (such as frequent moves of home or school) can lead to a sense of insecurity, especially in childhood. A feeling of insecurity may be a feature of *anxiety* and other neurotic mental disorders.

Insight
Being aware of one's own mental state. In a general sense, this means knowing one's own strengths, weaknesses, and abilities.

The term insight also has the specific psychiatric meaning of knowing that one's symptoms are an illness. Loss of insight may be a feature of both psychotic and neurotic disor-

---

FIRST AID: INSECT STINGS AND TICK BITES

INSECT STING

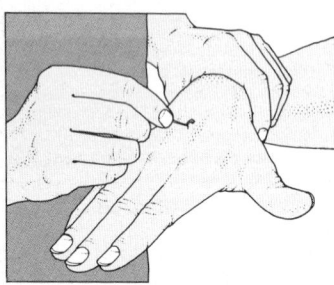

1 Use a needle, knife blade or fingernail to remove the sting and poison sac by scraping them out of the skin. Do not use tweezers because you may squeeze more poison into the wound.

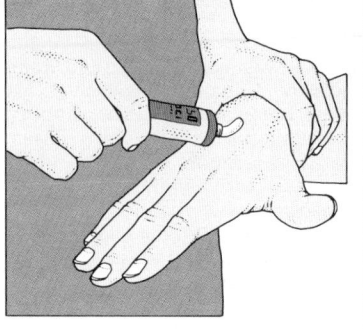

2 Wash the wound with soap and water, and apply a cold compress to reduce swelling. Hydrocortisone cream (if available) applied to the wound will also help to reduce swelling.

TICK BITE

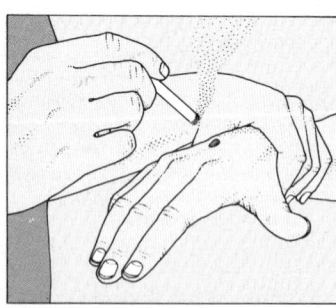

1 If the tick is still clinging to the skin, dislodge it by holding the glowing end of a cigarette or an extinguished match to its body. Do not attempt to pull it off.

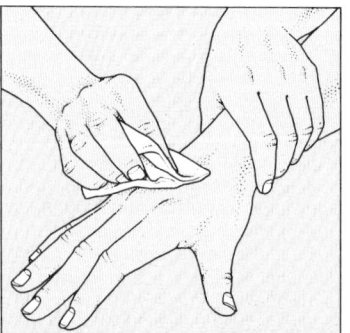

2 Use soap and warm water to wash the area thoroughly. Then rinse and dry the skin gently.

ders. In psychoanalysis, having insight is regarded as an important step towards successful treatment.

In situ

A Latin term meaning "in place". The phrase "carcinoma in situ" is used to describe tissue (particularly of the skin or cervix) that is cancerous only in its surface cells and is completely surrounded by normal cells without any signs of spread to deeper layers.

Insomnia

Trouble in sleeping. People with insomnia may have difficulty in falling asleep or in staying asleep. Most insomnia sufferers also complain of increased daytime fatigue, irritability, and find it difficult to cope. Insomnia is common: as many as one in every three adults may suffer from insomnia at some time in their lives. *Sleeping drugs* are among the most widely used of all medicines.

CAUSES

The most common cause of insomnia is worry about a problem (such as bad news received during the day or a difficult task to cope with the following morning), but other causes are implicated in about half of all cases.

Causes include physical disorders, such as *sleep apnoea, restless legs*, environmental factors (such as noise and light), lifestyle factors (such as too much coffee in the evening, lack of exercise during the day, or keeping erratic hours), or misuse of sleeping drugs (including *benzodiazepine drugs* and *barbiturate drugs*).

Insomnia also can be a symptom of a psychiatric illness. People with *anxiety* and/or *depression* may find it difficult to fall asleep; those suffering from depression typically wake early in the morning. Sleeping much less than usual is common in *mania*, in which the person is so full of drive and energy that he or she does not need much sleep. *Schizophrenia* often causes people to pace about at night, aroused by "voices" or delusions. People with *dementia* or other brain disorders may be afraid in the dark and become restless and noisy, confused by the shadows and sounds of the night.

Withdrawal symptoms from sleeping drugs, *antidepressant drugs*, *antianxiety drugs*, and some illicit drugs (see *Drug abuse*), such as heroin, may cause many weeks of insomnia.

People sometimes mistakenly believe that they are suffering from insomnia because of a misconception about the amount of sleep they need.

In fact, sleep needs vary greatly, with some people requiring less than four hours and others needing more than 10. Some people who think they have insomnia are in fact "out of phase", lying awake for hours after going to bed, but sleeping normally if allowed to sleep late in the morning.

INVESTIGATION AND TREATMENT

An obvious physical or psychological cause for insomnia will be treated. For long-term insomnia with no obvious cause, *EEG* recordings of brain-wave patterns and an assessment of breathing, muscle activity, and other bodily functions during sleep may be useful in discovering the extent and pattern of the problem. Keeping a log of sleep patterns may also be helpful.

Studies have shown that many people with insomnia sleep much more than they think they do. However, they also tend to wake more frequently than normal sleepers. It is the quality, rather than the quantity, of sleep that is the problem in insomnia. People with insomnia should ensure that they are active during the day and should establish a regular routine and time for going to bed each night and waking in the morning. Sleeping drugs should be used only on medical advice.

Instinct

An innate primitive urge. The need for warmth, food, love, and sex, are all forms of instinct, although the instinct for survival is probably the most powerful. An instinct is distinguished from a reflex, which is an involuntary response to a stimulus (such as withdrawing one's hand from a fire).

In animals, instincts often take the form of specific inherited patterns of behaviour. For example, ducks follow their mothers, and beavers build dams—activities that do not appear to have been learned.

Humans have few of these set behaviours, and instincts may be more appropriately regarded as motivators of behaviour. This idea was first developed as a central part of *Freudian theory*. Freud believed that instincts arose from energy aroused in the unconscious. The aim of the instinct was to calm the aroused state by directing the energy onto some outside object (for example, sexual arousal leads to intercourse and orgasm).

Institutionalization

The loss of personal independence that stems from living for long periods in a mental hospital, prison, or other large institution. Apathy, obeying orders unquestioningly, accepting a standard routine, and loss of interests are the main features. Such features are thought to be caused by a lack of rights and personal responsibility, the attitudes of controlling staff, and the effects of drugs.

Care of the long-term sick within the community (as an alternative to hospitalization) is designed to combat the institutionalization process.

Insulin

A *hormone* produced by the *pancreas* in varying amounts depending on the level of glucose (sugar) in the blood. Carbohydrate is absorbed as glucose, increasing the blood glucose level and stimulating the pancreas to produce insulin. Insulin promotes the absorption of glucose into the *liver* and into muscle cells (where it is converted into energy). In the liver, glucose is stored as glycogen, which is reconverted to glucose in response to stress or exercise. Insulin thus prevents a build-up of blood glucose and ensures that various tissues have sufficient amounts of glucose.

Diabetes mellitus occurs when the pancreas produces little or no insulin, causing *hyperglycaemia* (abnormally high blood glucose). An *insulinoma* is a rare benign tumour that causes excessive production of insulin.

INSULIN THERAPY

Insulin supplements have been used in the treatment of diabetes mellitus since 1922. Insulin preparations are produced from pig or ox pancreas or by *genetic engineering* techniques from microorganisms. A variety of short-, intermediate-, or long-acting preparations are available.

Insulin is used in all cases of insulin-dependent diabetes mellitus (total absence of insulin production) and, occasionally, when oral hypoglycaemic drugs (see *Hypoglycaemics, oral*) are unable to control non-insulin-dependent diabetes mellitus (deficient production of insulin), such as during serious illness, major surgery, or pregnancy. Insulin therapy is used to prevent hyperglycaemia and *ketosis* (a build-up of certain acids in the blood), which, in severe cases, may cause coma.

Insulin is given to mimic the body's production of the natural hormone. Insulin injections may be self-administered before meals to act on the increase in blood glucose that occurs after eating. Alternatively, an insulin pump (see *Pump, insulin*) may be used to deliver insulin throughout the day and night; the dose is increased before each meal.

Adjustment of the dose is often needed when there are variations in diet and exercise, and during illness (especially when there has been vomiting). Regular self-monitoring of glucose levels, either by blood or by urine tests, is necessary to ensure adequate control.

POSSIBLE ADVERSE EFFECTS

Insulin injections may cause irritation or dimpling of the skin. Too high a dose will cause *hypoglycaemia* (abnormally low blood glucose) with symptoms (such as dizziness, sweating, irritability, and a feeling of weakness) that are relieved by consuming food or a sugary drink. Severe hypoglycaemia may cause coma, for which emergency treatment with an injection of glucose or *glucagon* (a hormone that opposes the effects of insulin) is necessary.

Allergic reactions to insulin, causing rash or breathing difficulty, are rare. Pig or ox insulin may make the body produce *antibodies* which reduce the effectiveness of the insulin preparation. If this occurs, an alternative preparation should be taken.

Insulinoma

A rare benign tumour of the insulin-producing cells of the *pancreas*. Such a tumour can produce abnormal quantities of *insulin* so that the amount of glucose in the blood (which is reduced by insulin) can fall to dangerously low levels. This is called *hypoglycaemia* and, unless sugar is given immediately, can cause *coma* and death.

Blood insulin levels are normally low during fasting; insulinoma can be diagnosed by finding high levels after a period of fasting. A drug (diazoxide) is administered to prevent hypoglycaemia until surgery can be performed to remove the tumour.

Intelligence

The ability to understand concepts and to reason them out. There is much confusion about the precise definition of intelligence. Many people use the word to mean a special degree of knowledge. The widespread use of *intelligence tests* has led to the idea that intelligence is a single quality.

Many scientists prefer to divide intelligence into various factors. Some see it as having three basic parts—speed of thought, learning, and problem-solving. Others argue that a general factor of intelligence exists, made up of seven special abilities—understanding the meaning of words, fluency with words, working with numbers, visualizing things in space, memory, speed of perception, and reasoning ability. Other researchers go further, dividing intelligence into more than 100 different factors.

Intelligence can also be considered as having three entirely separate forms—abstract intelligence (understanding ideas and symbols); practical intelligence (aptitude in dealing with practical problems, such as repairing machinery); and social intelligence (coping reasonably and wisely with human relationships). Personality plays an important role in this last type of intelligence.

AGE AND INTELLIGENCE

Intelligence, however it is defined, increases up to the age of about six years and then stabilizes. Intelligence quotient (IQ), as measured by intelligence tests, continues to increase to about the age of 26, stays the same until about the age of 40, and then gradually declines (the drop occurring later in a person with an intellectually demanding job).

HEREDITY AND INTELLIGENCE

The role of heredity in intelligence is much argued, but there is no doubt that intelligence is inherited in a manner similar to height. Environment also plays a major part, as does physical health and personality. Intelligent parents tend to have intelligent children, but, even within one family, some children may be brighter than others. Adopted children from deprived social backgrounds, even though they may have IQs closer to their biological than their adopted parents, often score higher than would be expected had they been reared by their biological parents.

Extremes of intelligence occur in *mental handicap* (defined by a low IQ) and in the very gifted (defined by scores over 140).

People with very high IQs are often very successful, but not always. Personality and social adjustment are just as important.

Intelligence tests

Tests designed to provide an estimate of a person's mental abilities.

TYPES

WECHSLER TESTS These are the most widely used of all tests today. There are two basic versions—the Wechsler Adult Intelligence Scale (WAIS) and the Wechsler Intelligence Scale for Children (WISC). Each is divided into verbal and performance sections, which can be used separately or combined to produce an overall score. The verbal sections are concerned with language skills and include measures of vocabulary, general knowledge, verbal reasoning, and verbal memory. The performance sections include

MEASURING INTELLIGENCE

Intelligence is difficult to define precisely and to measure satisfactorily. Nevertheless, various tests have been devised that provide an estimate of a person's mental abilities. Most such tests measure an individual's ability in several areas of mental functioning that are generally thought to be important components or indicators of intelligence—for example, mathematical ability, logical reasoning, vocabulary, comprehension, general knowledge, memory, perceptual ability and pattern recognition, and the ability to understand relationships between concepts or objects. The questions at right are hypothetical examples (at various levels of difficulty) of those that might be asked in a typical intelligence test.

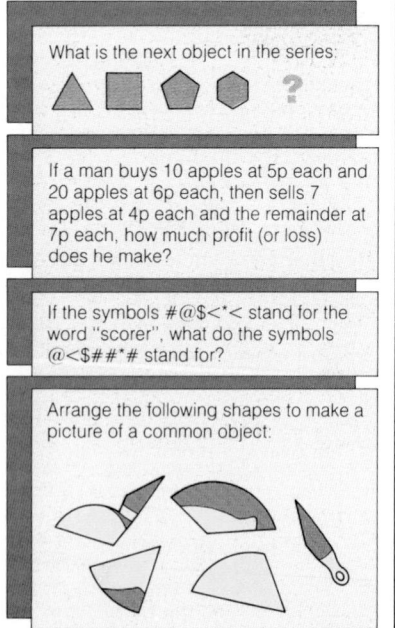

What is the next object in the series:

If a man buys 10 apples at 5p each and 20 apples at 6p each, then sells 7 apples at 4p each and the remainder at 7p each, how much profit (or loss) does he make?

If the symbols #@$<*< stand for the word "scorer", what do the symbols @<$##*# stand for?

Arrange the following shapes to make a picture of a common object:

measures of constructional ability and visual-spatial and perceptual ability (interpretation of shapes).

The performance sections of the test may be used separately for people with language problems. Performance testing can measure basic intellectual ability whereas verbal testing tends to be more culture-bound because it tests skills that reflect social background.

STANFORD-BINET TEST This is a revised version of one of the oldest intelligence tests, devised by the Frenchman Alfred Binet (1857-1911). It is still widely used, mainly as a measure of scholastic ability.

OTHER TESTS Numerous tests that concentrate on testing one particular aspect of intelligence have been devised. The Goodenough-Harris test assesses performance by asking a child to make a picture of a man; the child's score depends on the complexity of the drawing, such as the detail included and the body proportions.

SCORING

In most intelligence tests, scoring is based on the notion of mental age (MA) in relation to actual chronological age (CA), since intelligence normally increases with maturity. The intelligence quotient (IQ) is therefore MA divided by CA, multiplied by 100 to simplify the results. The tests are devised to ensure that three quarters of people have an IQ between 80 and 120. They are also standardized so that the score indicates the same relative ability at different age levels. Regardless of age group, an IQ of 65 indicates that a person is in the bottom one per cent of his or her age group; an IQ of 135 indicates the person is in the top one per cent of his or her age group.

USES

Intelligence tests are useful in predicting whether a person has the ability to cope with certain jobs or to pass certain examinations. They may therefore be used to assess school or job aptitude. However, intelligence tests have been criticized for their alleged bias regarding gender and race. The tests are also used to define the legal notion of *mental retardation* and to assess the effects of *dementia* or other brain disease. In particular, a large difference in verbal and performance scores is helpful in assessing the degree of brain disease. Children with a particular difficulty (such as delayed reading) may be tested to assess the severity and nature of the problem so remedial teaching can be planned.

Intensive care

The constant, close monitoring of seriously ill patients, which enables immediate treatment to be given if the patient's condition deteriorates.

The intensive-care unit of a hospital contains electronic monitoring equipment that allows continuous assessment of vital body functions, such as blood pressure and heart and respiratory rates. The urine output, fluid balance, and blood chemistry of patients in intensive-care units are recorded regularly. Medical and nursing staff are in a high ratio to patients and are specially trained in the techniques of resuscitation.

Intensive care is most often needed for patients who are on artificial *ventilation*, who may be unconscious and not breathing, or suffering from a respiratory illness. Close monitoring in an intensive care unit is also required for people recovering from a *myocardial infarction* (heart attack) or from major surgery, for patients in *shock* who are not responding to emergency treatment, and for those with acute *kidney failure* who require *dialysis*. (See also *Coronary care unit*.)

Inter-

A prefix that means between, as in *intercostal* (between the ribs). (See also *Intra-*.)

Intercostal

The medical term for between the *ribs*, as in the intercostal muscles, thin sheets of muscle between each rib that help expand and contract the chest during breathing.

A TYPICAL INTENSIVE-CARE UNIT

An intensive care unit has a wide variety of sophisticated equipment for constantly monitoring the condition of the seriously ill patient. He or she is likely to be heavily sedated and connected to a ventilator to maintain breathing. Body fluids and blood sugar levels are maintained by intravenous infusion of salts and glucose. Nutrients may also be supplied intravenously. Urine is collected via a catheter. Blood pressure is continuously monitored by an automatic sphygmomanometer. Heart-rate and rhythm are monitored by an ECG machine. Results are often relayed to a central monitoring unit. Monitors are fitted with alarms to alert the staff to any dangerous variation from the normal range. Additionally, other vital functions such as the chemical make-up of the blood are measured frequently.

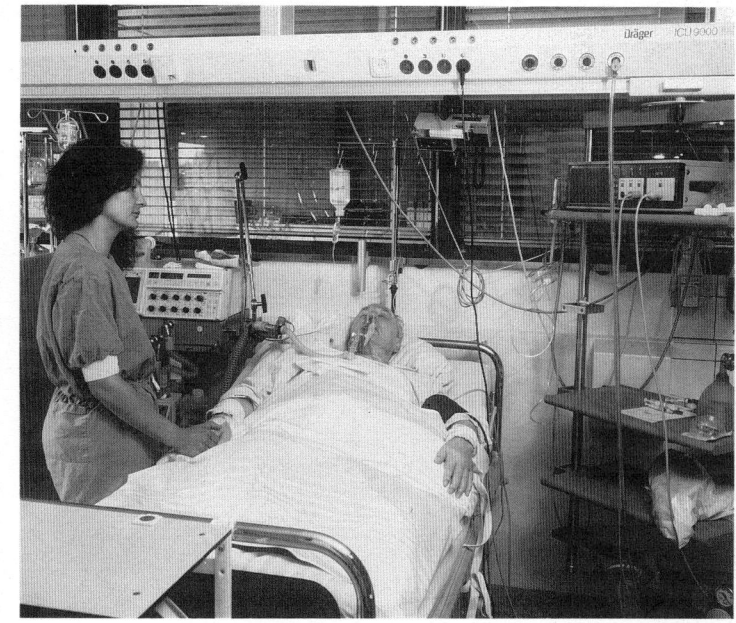

Intercourse, painful

Pain during *sexual intercourse*, known medically as dyspareunia. The problem can affect both men and women, causing pain that may be superficial (around the external genitals) or deep (within the pelvis).

CAUSES

Superficial pain is usually due to a problem that affects the external genitals. *Sexually transmitted diseases* (such as genital *herpes*, *gonorrhoea*, or *chlamydial infections*) cause pain felt on the penis or around the vulval area. *Spermicides* may sometimes cause a burning sensation in both men and women.

In men, superficial pain during sexual intercourse may be caused by anatomical abnormalities, for example *chordee* (bowed erection) or *phimosis* (tight foreskin). *Prostatitis* (inflammation of the prostate gland) may cause a sharp, stabbing pain from the tip of the penis. Prostatitis may also cause a widespread pelvic ache or a burning sensation.

In some women, scarring (after tears from delivery or a poorly healed *episiotomy* repair, for example) may cause painful intercourse. Insufficient vaginal lubrication, especially after the *menopause*, is another cause of painful intercourse in women.

Psychosexual dysfunction may also cause pain during intercourse. For example *vaginismus*, a condition in which the muscles of the vagina go into spasm and thus prevent insertion of the penis, is usually psychological in origin.

In women, deep pain on intercourse is frequently caused by pelvic disorders (such as *fibroids*, *ectopic pregnancy*, or *pelvic inflammatory disease*) or by disorders of the *ovary* (such as *ovarian cysts*).

Endometriosis can cause thickening of tissue within the uterus, resulting in deep pain during intercourse. Varicose veins in the pelvis and

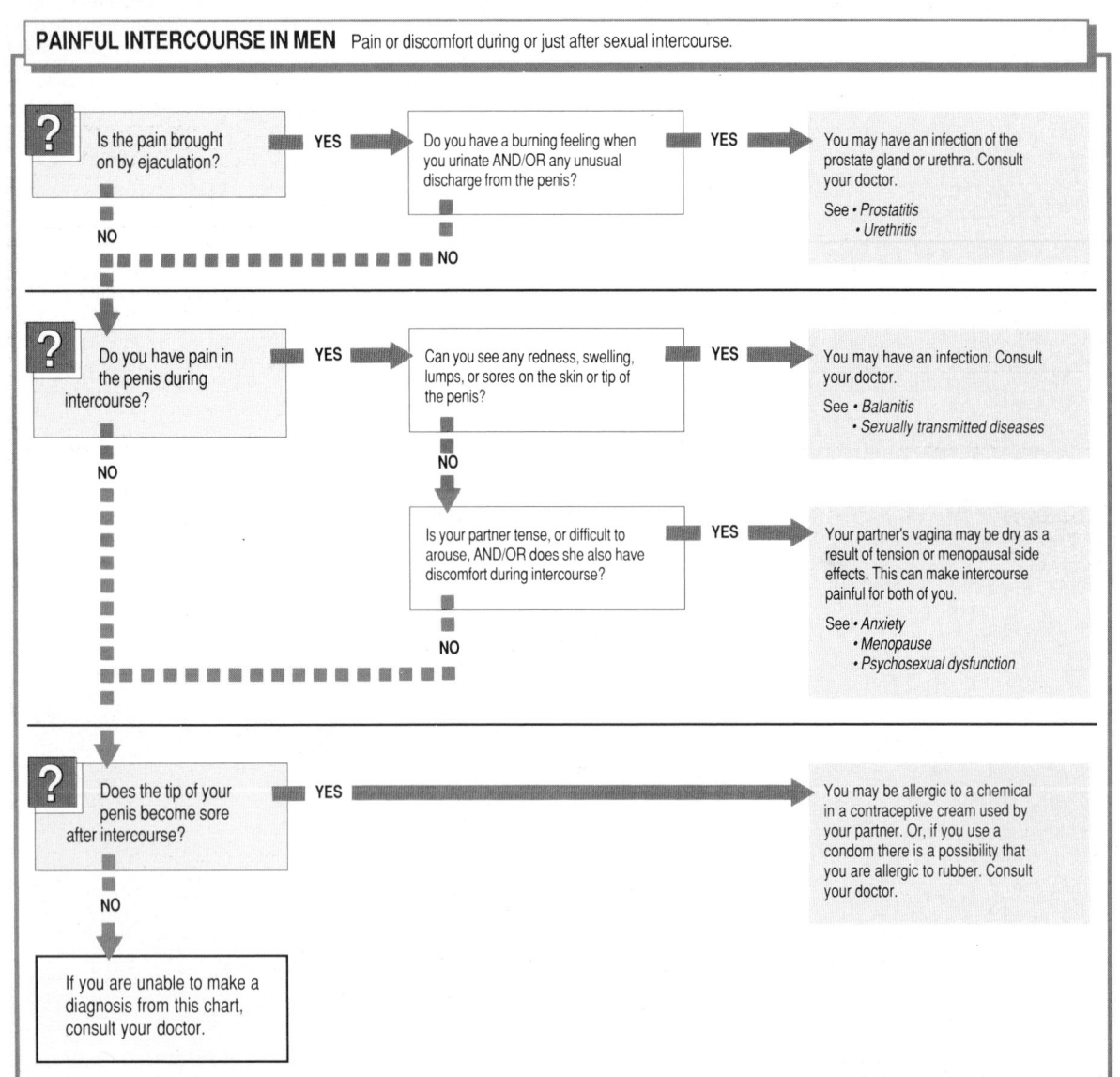

PAINFUL INTERCOURSE IN MEN Pain or discomfort during or just after sexual intercourse.

? Is the pain brought on by ejaculation? — YES — Do you have a burning feeling when you urinate AND/OR any unusual discharge from the penis? — YES — You may have an infection of the prostate gland or urethra. Consult your doctor.

See • *Prostatitis*
    • *Urethritis*

NO / NO

? Do you have pain in the penis during intercourse? — YES — Can you see any redness, swelling, lumps, or sores on the skin or tip of the penis? — YES — You may have an infection. Consult your doctor.

See • *Balanitis*
    • *Sexually transmitted diseases*

NO / NO

Is your partner tense, or difficult to arouse, AND/OR does she also have discomfort during intercourse? — YES — Your partner's vagina may be dry as a result of tension or menopausal side effects. This can make intercourse painful for both of you.

See • *Anxiety*
    • *Menopause*
    • *Psychosexual dysfunction*

NO

? Does the tip of your penis become sore after intercourse? — YES — You may be allergic to a chemical in a contraceptive cream used by your partner. Or, if you use a condom there is a possibility that you are allergic to rubber. Consult your doctor.

NO

If you are unable to make a diagnosis from this chart, consult your doctor.

PAINFUL INTERCOURSE IN WOMEN   Pain or discomfort during or just after sexual intercourse.

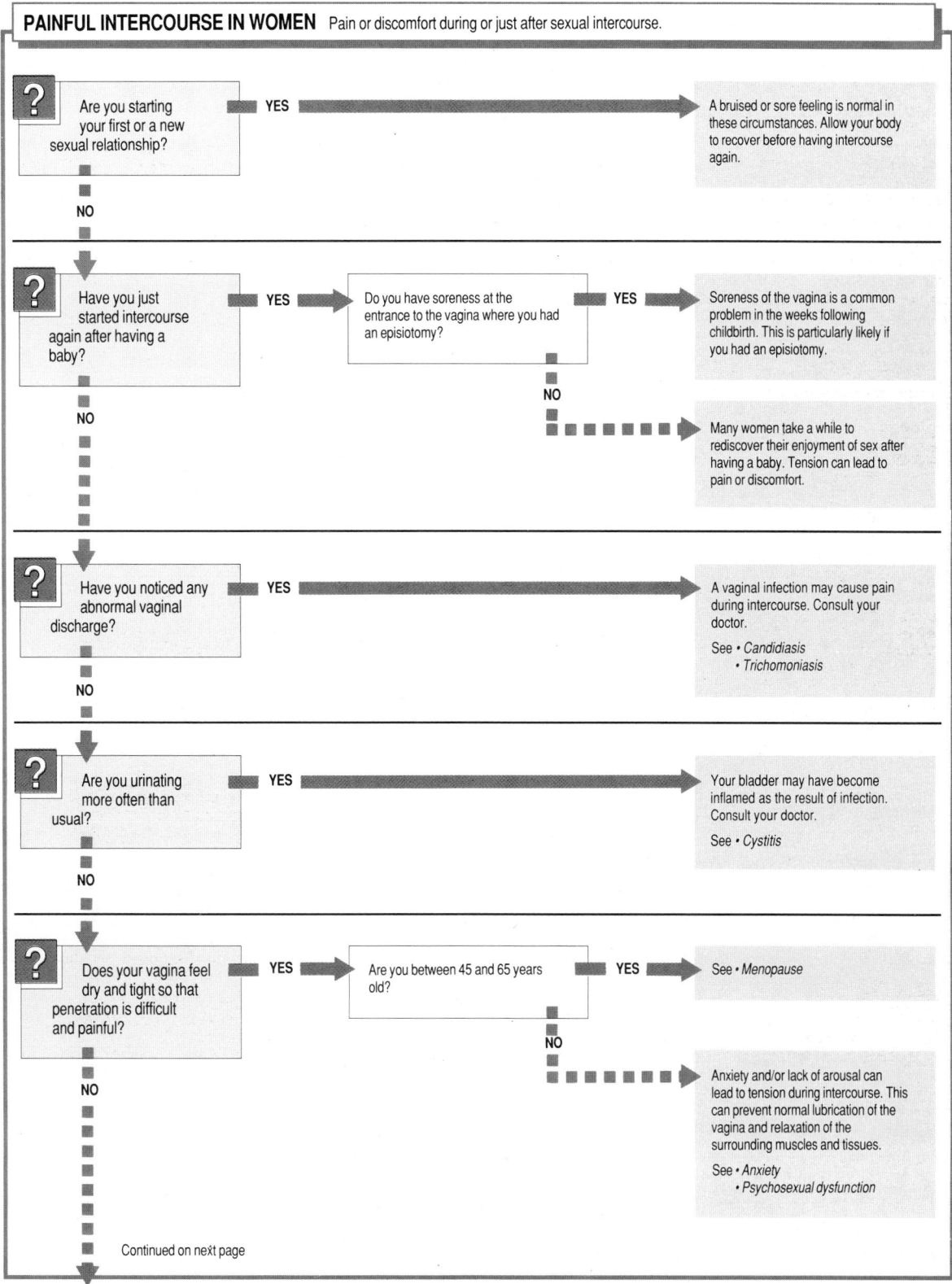

Are you starting your first or a new sexual relationship?

YES → A bruised or sore feeling is normal in these circumstances. Allow your body to recover before having intercourse again.

NO

Have you just started intercourse again after having a baby?

YES → Do you have soreness at the entrance to the vagina where you had an episiotomy?

YES → Soreness of the vagina is a common problem in the weeks following childbirth. This is particularly likely if you had an episiotomy.

NO → Many women take a while to rediscover their enjoyment of sex after having a baby. Tension can lead to pain or discomfort.

NO

Have you noticed any abnormal vaginal discharge?

YES → A vaginal infection may cause pain during intercourse. Consult your doctor.

See • *Candidiasis*
• *Trichomoniasis*

NO

Are you urinating more often than usual?

YES → Your bladder may have become inflamed as the result of infection. Consult your doctor.

See • *Cystitis*

NO

Does your vagina feel dry and tight so that penetration is difficult and painful?

YES → Are you between 45 and 65 years old?

YES → See • *Menopause*

NO → Anxiety and/or lack of arousal can lead to tension during intercourse. This can prevent normal lubrication of the vagina and relaxation of the surrounding muscles and tissues.

See • *Anxiety*
• *Psychosexual dysfunction*

NO

Continued on next page

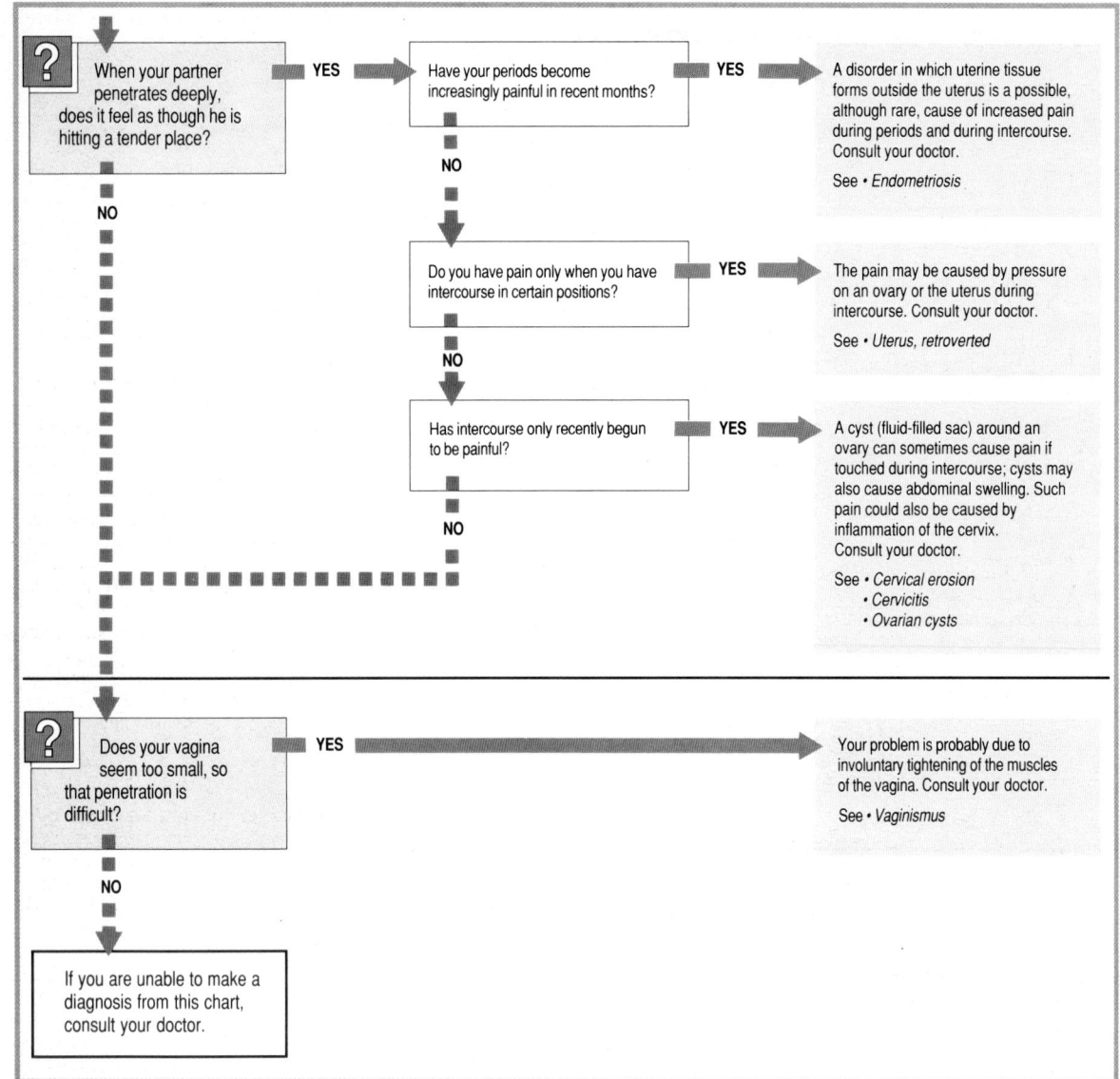

When your partner penetrates deeply, does it feel as though he is hitting a tender place? — **YES** → Have your periods become increasingly painful in recent months? — **YES** → A disorder in which uterine tissue forms outside the uterus is a possible, although rare, cause of increased pain during periods and during intercourse. Consult your doctor.

See • *Endometriosis*

NO ↓

Do you have pain only when you have intercourse in certain positions? — **YES** → The pain may be caused by pressure on an ovary or the uterus during intercourse. Consult your doctor.

See • *Uterus, retroverted*

NO ↓

Has intercourse only recently begun to be painful? — **YES** → A cyst (fluid-filled sac) around an ovary can sometimes cause pain if touched during intercourse; cysts may also cause abdominal swelling. Such pain could also be caused by inflammation of the cervix. Consult your doctor.

See • *Cervical erosion*
• *Cervicitis*
• *Ovarian cysts*

NO

Does your vagina seem too small, so that penetration is difficult? — **YES** → Your problem is probably due to involuntary tightening of the muscles of the vagina. Consult your doctor.

See • *Vaginismus*

NO ↓

If you are unable to make a diagnosis from this chart, consult your doctor.

---

disorders of the *cervix* (such as tumours or infections) can also cause deep pain during intercourse.

Cystitis commonly causes pain during sexual intercourse, especially in women. Other *urinary tract infections* may also cause pain.

TREATMENT

Treatment is directed at the underlying cause of the pain (for example *antibiotic drugs* will combat an infection, while a lubricant will help vaginal dryness). *Analgesic drugs* (painkillers) may also be helpful.

If the discomfort is psychological in origin, special counselling may be required (see *Sex therapy*).

Interferon

The name given to a group of proteins produced naturally by body cells in response to viral infections and other stimuli. Interferon inhibits viral multiplication (see illustration) and increases the activity of natural killer cells—types of *lymphocytes* that form part of the body's *immune system* (natural defences).

USE AS DRUG

Interferons of various types are produced from cultures of human cells, or they may be synthesized in the laboratory from specific *nucleic acids*. They may be given by injection or as a nasal spray.

Interferons are used in the treatment of some types of *leukaemia* and some other cancers including *Kaposi's sarcoma*—a type of skin cancer common in people who have *AIDS*. They are used to treat certain viral infections, including chronic infection with hepatitis viruses B and C (see *Hepatitis, viral*). They are used in combating viral infections in people suffering from *immunodeficiency disorders*. Interferon has also been used in the treatment of *multiple sclerosis*.

Possible adverse reactions to interferons include fever, headaches, lethargy, depression, dizziness, digestive disturbances, and, rarely, hair loss.

HOW INTERFERON FIGHTS VIRAL INFECTIONS

Interferon is part of the body's immune system, providing a defence against many different types of virally infected or tumour cells. It is produced naturally in the body during viral infections, but can also be given as a drug to enhance its natural actions.

VIRAL MULTIPLICATION

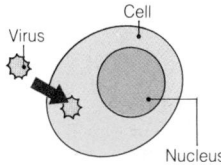

1 A virus can multiply only by first invading one of its host's cells.

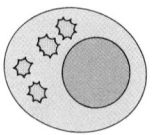

2 The virus takes over the cell's chemical machinery to make copies of itself.

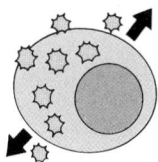

3 The copies of the virus escape to invade more of the host's cells.

HOW INTERFERON WORKS

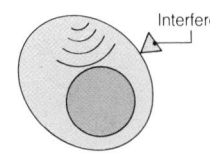

1 Interferon attaches to the membrane of host cells and stimulates them against viral attack.

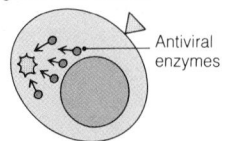

2 If a virus invades a cell primed by interferon, enzymes are produced that impair viral copying.

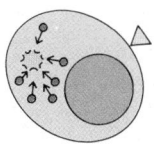

3 Unable to copy itself, the virus is nullified, and the infection is stopped or shortened.

1 Interferon also causes natural killer cells to attack virally infected cells or tumour cells.

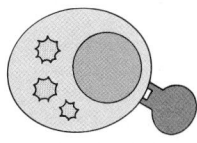

2 A natural killer cell attaches to the abnormal host cell and makes it disintegrate.

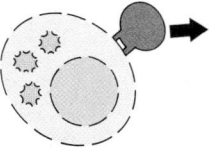

3 The effect of this process is to help limit a viral infection or to slow tumour growth.

Intersex

A group of abnormalities in which the affected person has ambiguous genitalia (abnormal external sex organs that could be of either sex) or external genitalia that have the opposite appearance to the chromosomal sex of the individual. See *Sex determination*.

Interstitial pulmonary fibrosis

Scarring and thickening of the deep lung tissues, leading to shortness of breath. The most important form of interstitial pulmonary fibrosis (IPF) is known as idiopathic IPF, diffuse IPF, or fibrosing alveolitis.

CAUSES

Although the precise cause of idiopathic IPF is unknown, this form of the condition is probably an *autoimmune disorder* (caused by the body's *immune system* attacking its own tissues).

Less common causes of IPF include occupational exposure to mineral dusts and chemical fumes, radiotherapy, reactions to certain drugs, and allergic *alveolitis*.

SYMPTOMS AND DIAGNOSIS

The symptoms of IPF are progressive shortness of breath, cough, chest pain, and clubbing of the fingers, as well as symptoms of any underlying disease. The diagnosis, which is based on symptoms and a physical examination, is confirmed by *chest X-ray* and lung *biopsy* (removal of a sample of tissue for microscopic analysis).

TREATMENT AND OUTLOOK

Treatment of idiopathic IPF often includes *azathioprine* and *corticosteroid drugs*, which suppress the immune system. In other cases, treatment is directed to the underlying cause.

The outlook for recovery is generally poor for occupational dust diseases and for idiopathic IPF, in which the lungs progressively stiffen. Progression of the disease may lead to *heart failure* and *bronchopneumonia*.

When IPF is caused by allergic alveolitis, the condition is more easily treated and the outlook may not be as gloomy.

Interstitial radiotherapy

Treatment of a malignant tumour by inserting radioactive material into the growth or into neighbouring tissue. Using this method, also known as brachytherapy, radiation can be directed to the diseased area more accurately than is possible with radiotherapy using X-rays and there is less risk of radiation damage to healthy tissue.

HOW IT IS DONE

The patient is given a general anaesthetic. Radioactive material (usually artificial radioisotopes) contained in wires or small tubes is then implanted into or near the diseased tissue. If the tumour is in an easily accessible area (such as the mouth), the containers may be pushed in by means of a special needle; for a tumour deep in the body, a surgical procedure is necessary. The material is left in place for variable amounts of time (and sometimes permanently), depending on the radioactive substance and the tumour being treated. (See also *Intracavitary therapy*; *Radiotherapy*.)

Intertrigo

Inflammation of the skin caused by two surfaces rubbing together. Intertrigo is most common in obese people and usually occurs on the inner thighs, in the armpits, on the underside of the breasts, in folds of the abdomen, and between fingers and toes. The affected skin is red and moist. There may be scales or blisters and affected skin may have an odour. The condition is made worse by sweating. Intertrigo is sometimes accompanied by seborrhoeic *dermatitis* or *candidiasis* (thrush).

Treatment consists of weight reduction, keeping affected areas as clean and dry as possible, and, if dermatitis or candidiasis is present, applying a cream containing a *corticosteroid drug* or an *antifungal drug*.

Intestinal imaging

See *Barium X-ray examinations*.

Intestinal lipodystrophy

See *Whipple's disease*.

Intestine

Part of the *digestive system*. The intestine is the major part of the digestive tract and extends from the exit of the stomach to the anus. The intestine

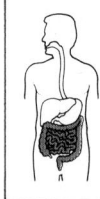

LOCATION OF THE INTESTINE

Situated below the stomach and liver, the intestine occupies much of the central and lower parts of the abdomen.

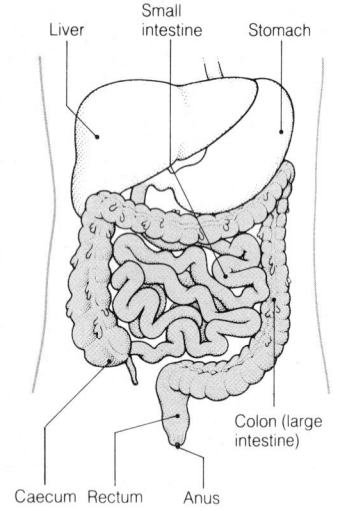

Liver · Small intestine · Stomach

Colon (large intestine)

Caecum · Rectum · Anus

forms a long tube divided into two main sections—the small intestine and the large intestine. The function of the intestine is to break down and absorb food and water into the bloodstream and to carry away the waste products of digestion.

STRUCTURE

The small intestine is about 6.5 m in length and 3.5 cm in diameter. It has three sections—the *duodenum* (a short, curved segment fixed to the back wall of the abdomen) and the *jejunum* and *ileum* (two larger, coiled, and mobile segments). The bile and pancreatic ducts enter the duodenum (see *Biliary system*). The walls of the intestine consist of circular and longitudinal muscles with an internal lining (the mucosa) and an external covering (the serosa). *Peristalsis* (the rhythmic contraction of the muscles) forces partially digested food along the intestine. The mucosa consists of many *villi* (small, finger-like projections) covered with millions of fronds that create a large surface area for the absorption of substances into the blood.

The large intestine, which frames the loops of the small intestine, is about 1.5 m long and 4 to 7 cm in diameter. Unlike the small intestine,

much of it is fixed in position, the muscles run in bands rather than forming a continuous sheet along its length, and there are no internal villi. The main section, the *colon*, is divided into an ascending, a transverse, a descending, and a pelvic portion (the sigmoid colon) that hangs down into the pelvis. The *appendix* hangs from a pouch (the *caecum*) between the small intestine and the colon. The final section before the *anus* is the *rectum*.

FUNCTION

The small intestine is concerned with the digestion of food and the absorption of food into the bloodstream. Some digestion occurs in the stomach, but more digestive enzymes and bile are added to the partly digested food in the duodenum. Glands within the walls of each section of the small intestine produce mucus and more enzymes, all of which help to break down the food into easily absorbable chemical units. The numerous blood vessels in the intestinal walls then carry the digested food to the *liver* for distribution to the rest of the body.

Unabsorbed material leaves the small intestine in the form of liquid and fibre. As this material passes through the large intestine, water, vitamins, and mineral salts are absorbed into the bloodstream, leaving *faeces* made up of undigested food residue, small amounts of fat, secretions from the stomach, liver, pancreas, and intestinal wall, and bacteria. The faeces are compressed and pass into the rectum. Distension of the rectum usually produces the desire to empty the bowel.

Intestine, cancer of

A malignant tumour in the intestine. Both the small and large intestine may develop carcinoid tumours (leading to *carcinoid syndrome*) and *lymphomas*.

Cancer of the small intestine is extremely rare, but cancer of the large intestine is one of the most common of all cancers. In the UK, there are more than 25,000 cases of cancer of the large intestine each year, and this type of cancer accounts for about 20 per cent of all UK cancer deaths. (See *Colon, cancer of; Rectum, cancer of.*)

Intestine, obstruction of

A partial or complete blockage of the small or large intestine. Without treatment, complete obstruction of the intestine is usually fatal.

CAUSES

The most common cause of intestinal obstruction is paralytic ileus (see

Ileus, paralytic), in which the rhythmic muscle contractions of the intestine stop, the intestine dilates, and the intestinal contents are no longer moved along the digestive tract.

Other common causes are a strangulated *hernia*, intestinal *atresia* (a congenital malformation), *stenosis* (narrowing) of the intestine, *adhesions* (bands of scar tissue), *volvulus* (twisting or knotting of the intestine), and *intussusception* (telescoping of a section of intestine).

Intestinal obstruction also occurs in diseases (such as *Crohn's disease, diverticular disease*, and tumours) that affect the intestinal wall. Less commonly, internal blockage of the intestinal canal is caused by impacted food, *faecal impaction, gallstones*, or by some accidentally swallowed object.

SYMPTOMS

The location and degree of obstruction dictate the symptoms.

A blockage in the small intestine usually causes intermittent cramp-like pain in the centre of the abdomen, which tends to be more severe the higher the obstruction. Pain is accompanied by increasingly frequent bouts of vomiting and by failure to pass wind or faeces.

An obstruction in the large intestine, particularly in the colon, causes pain, distention (swelling) of the abdomen, and failure to pass wind or faeces. In some cases, the obstruction is intermittent or partial, allowing faeces to pass and giving temporary abatement of symptoms.

DIAGNOSIS AND TREATMENT

The diagnosis is usually based on the patient's symptoms and on a physical examination. Abdominal *X-rays* will confirm the diagnosis.

The contents of the intestine are removed through a flexible tube passed down the throat. In some cases, surgery may be necessary to correct the obstruction. The actual type of operation depends on the nature and site of the blockage to the flow of intestinal contents.

OUTLOOK

The prospects for a full recovery after surgery are often excellent but they will depend on the cause of the obstruction and on the age and general health of the patient.

Intestine, tumours of

Tumours of the intestine may be cancerous or benign (noncancerous).

Cancerous tumours commonly affect the large intestine (see *Colon, cancer of; Rectum, cancer of*); the small

DISORDERS OF THE INTESTINE

The intestine is subject to various structural abnormalities and to the effects of many infective organisms and parasites; it may also be affected by tumours, impaired blood supply, and other disorders.

CONGENITAL DEFECTS

Babies are sometimes born with an obstruction to the flow of the intestinal contents. This may be due to *atresia* (congenital closure), *stenosis* (narrowing), *volvulus* (twisting of loops of bowel), or blockage by meconium (fetal intestinal contents). Early surgery may be required.

INFECTION AND INFLAMMATION

The general term for inflammation of the stomach and intestines is *gastroenteritis*. This is caused most commonly by viral or bacterial infections, which can range from the trivial to the life-threatening. They encompass many cases of *food poisoning* and travellers' diarrhoea as well as serious diseases such as *typhoid fever* and *cholera*. Protozoal infections (caused by simple, single-celled parasites) include *giardiasis* and *amoebiasis*.

Intestinal worm infestations are exceedingly common worldwide (see *Roundworms; Tapeworms*), although, in the UK, only a few species of worms—including the *threadworm*—are prevalent.

Two important inflammatory conditions of the intestine, not caused by infection, are *ulcerative colitis* (mainly affecting the colon) and *Crohn's disease* (which may affect any part of the digestive tract but usually the small intestine). Sometimes, inflammation is confined to a localized area, such as in *appendicitis* and *diverticular disease*.

TUMOURS

Tumours of the small intestine are rare, but *lymphomas,* carcinoid tumours (producing *carcinoid syndrome*), and benign growths occur. By contrast, tumours of the large intestine are very common (see *Intestine, cancer of*). Certain forms of familial *polyposis* (in which benign polyp-like tumours grow in the colon) may progress to cancer.

IMPAIRED BLOOD SUPPLY

Like other organs, the intestine is dependent on an adequate blood

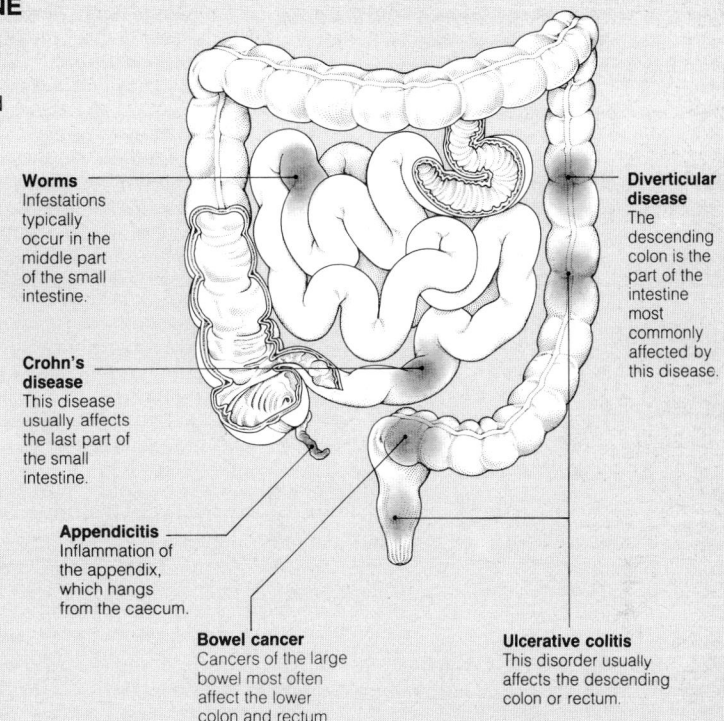

Worms Infestations typically occur in the middle part of the small intestine.

Crohn's disease This disease usually affects the last part of the small intestine.

Appendicitis Inflammation of the appendix, which hangs from the caecum.

Diverticular disease The descending colon is the part of the intestine most commonly affected by this disease.

Bowel cancer Cancers of the large bowel most often affect the lower colon and rectum.

Ulcerative colitis This disorder usually affects the descending colon or rectum.

supply. *Ischaemia* (lack of blood) may result from several causes. Causes include partial or complete obstruction of the arteries in the abdominal wall (from diseases such as *atherosclerosis, thrombosis,* or *embolism*) or from the blood vessels being compressed or trapped, as in *volvulus, intussusception,* or *hernias* (protrusion of intestines through the abdominal wall). Loss of blood supply to a segment of intestine may cause *gangrene* (tissue death) requiring immediate surgery.

OBSTRUCTION

Intestinal obstruction may be caused by pressure from the outside, disease of the intestinal wall (such as cancer, Crohn's disease, or diverticular disease), or internal blockage (such as from *gallstones* or intussusception). One of the most common causes is paralytic *ileus,* in which intestinal contractions cease and the intestinal contents are no longer transported.

OTHER DISORDERS

Peptic ulcer of the duodenum affects about 10 per cent of the population at some time in their lives. Ulceration of the small intestine occurs in typhoid

and Crohns' disease and may cause bleeding into the intestine or even perforation. Ulceration of the large intestine occurs in amoebiasis and in ulcerative colitis.

Diverticula are small pouches protruding from the inside of the bowel. They are usually harmless, but, in diverticular disease, may become inflamed. *Malabsorption* and *coeliac disease* result from changes to the intestinal lining. Finally, *irritable bowel syndrome* is associated with persistent abdominal pain and either constipation or diarrhoea (or both) and is the most common intestinal disorder in Western societies.

INVESTIGATION

Intestinal disorders are investigated by physical examination, and by techniques such as *barium X-ray examination, sigmoidoscopy, colonoscopy,or* occasionally *CT scanning* or *MRI* and by laboratory examination of the faeces or of a *biopsy* specimen taken from the intestinal lining.

intestine is only rarely affected. *Lymphomas* and carcinoid tumours (leading to *carcinoid syndrome*) are cancers that may sometimes occur in the intestine.

Noncancerous tumours of the intestine include *polyps* in the colon, and *adenomas, leiomyomas, lipomas,* and *angiomas* in the small intestine. These noncancerous tumours are usually symptomless and are often discovered incidentally when a *barium X-ray examination* is being performed for some other reason.

Intoxication

A general term for a condition resulting from *poisoning*. Intoxication customarily refers to the effects of excessive drinking (see *Alcohol intoxication*), but also includes *drug poisoning,* poisoning from the accumulation of the by-products of *metabolism* in the body, or the effects of industrial poisons (such as lead intoxication and solvent intoxication).

Intra-

A prefix that means within, as in the term intramuscular (within a muscle). (See also *Inter-*.)

Intracavitary therapy

Treatment of a malignant tumour in a body cavity by placing radioactive material or *anticancer drugs* within the cavity.

Intracavitary *radiotherapy* (also called brachytherapy) is mainly used to treat cancer of the uterus, cervix (neck of the uterus), vagina, or rectum. Radioactive material (usually in the form of artificial radioisotopes embedded in wires or small tubes) is introduced into the cavity and left there for a period of time.

Intracavitary chemotherapy may be used to treat a malignant effusion (a collection of fluid that contains cancerous cells). A needle, sometimes with a catheter (fine tube) attached, is passed through the wall of the abdomen or the chest into the abdominal cavity or pleural cavity (the space around the lungs). The needle is used first to draw off the effusion from the cavity, and then to inject *anticancer drugs* directly into the cavity. (See also *Interstitial radiotherapy*.)

Intracerebral haemorrhage

Bleeding into the brain from a ruptured blood vessel. An intracerebral haemorrhage is one of the three principal main mechanisms by which a *stroke* can occur.

INCIDENCE AND CAUSES

Intracerebral haemorrhage used to be a common cause of stroke, but with improvements in the treatment of *hypertension* (high blood pressure) it now accounts for only one in every 10 strokes. In the UK each year, about one person in 2,500 suffers an intracerebral haemorrhage. Most victims are middle-aged or elderly people with untreated hypertension (high blood pressure) or *atherosclerosis* (narrowing of arteries caused by deposits of fatty material) in the brain. Unlike most cases of *subdural* and *extradural haemorrhage* (bleeding between the surface of the brain and the skull), an intracerebral haemorrhage can occur without any injury or blow to the head.

The ruptured artery is usually in the cerebrum (the main mass of the brain), although sometimes it is in other structures of the brain (such as the cerebellum or the brainstem). The escaped blood seeps outwards, forming a circular or oval mass up to a few centimetres in diameter. As bleeding continues and the volume of escaped blood increases, brain tissue in the blood's path is disrupted and adjacent brain tissues are displaced and compressed.

SYMPTOMS

The symptoms are sudden headache, weakness, and confusion, and often loss of consciousness. Usually the victim falls unconscious to the ground with no warning. Signs resulting from disruption of brain tissue (speech loss, facial paralysis, or one-sided weakness) may develop over periods of minutes or hours.

DIAGNOSIS, TREATMENT, AND OUTLOOK

Diagnosis is by *CT scanning* or *MRI*. Surgical treatment is usually impossible due to the inaccessibility of the rupture, so treatment is aimed at life-support and the reduction of blood pressure.

Large haemorrhages are usually fatal; overall, only about 25 per cent of patients survive. Recurrent bleeding from the same site is uncommon. For the survivor of an intracerebral haemorrhage, rehabilitation and outlook are as for any type of stroke.

Intractable

A term to describe any condition that does not respond to treatment.

Intramuscular

A medical term meaning within a muscle, as in an intramuscular injection, in which a drug is injected deep within a muscle. Such injections are usually given into the upper, outer part of the buttock. The drug is absorbed from the muscle into the bloodstream, which distributes it throughout the body.

Intraocular pressure

The balance between the rate of production and the rate of removal of aqueous humour within the *eye*. It is the intraocular pressure that maintains the shape of the eyeball. Aqueous humour enters the eye from the ciliary body, which constantly produces the fluid, and exits from the drainage angle (a network of tissue between the iris and cornea).

If drainage is impeded, intraocular pressure builds up and leads to *glaucoma*. Intraocular pressure is usually measured by *tonometry* during a routine eye examination. If the ciliary body is damaged (as after prolonged inflammation), less fluid is produced and the eye becomes soft.

Intrauterine contraceptive device

See *IUD*.

Intrauterine growth retardation

Poor fetal growth, usually due to failure of the *placenta* to provide adequate nutrients or sometimes to a fetal defect. Intrauterine growth retardation causes the fetus to be smaller than expected for the length of *gestation*.

CAUSES

Intrauterine growth retardation may be due to a chromosomal defect, such as *Down's syndrome*, which causes the fetus to be "small for dates". A maternal infection, such as *rubella* (German measles), in which the virus passes through the placenta, can also cause poor fetal growth. In most cases, though, the fetus is otherwise normal.

Maternal factors may be responsible for intrauterine growth retardation. For example, *pre-eclampsia, hypertension* (high blood pressure), or chronic *kidney failure* can affect fetal growth, as can the mother's diet. Cigarette smoking is also a major cause, as are malnutrition and alcoholism.

DIAGNOSIS AND TREATMENT

The obstetrician can check whether the uterus is smaller than expected during an antenatal examination; *ultrasound scanning* may be performed to estimate the fetal growth. The mother may be required to rest, and tests of placental function may be needed, including blood tests and electrical *fetal heart monitoring*.

If intrauterine growth retardation is diagnosed, the pregnancy is carefully monitored and the underlying cause of the placental insufficiency treated, if possible. If the baby's growth is slowing, *induction of labour* or a *caesarean section* may be necessary.

OUTLOOK

Because babies suffering intrauterine growth retardation have been chronically undernourished in the uterus, they are usually underweight and may be premature if labour has been induced. Being prone to hypoglycaemia (low blood glucose), *hypothermia*, and infection, they are usually transferred to an *incubator* immediately after birth and provided with special care.

Intravenous

A term meaning within a vein, as in *intravenous infusion* (slow introduction of a substance into a vein) and intravenous *injection* (rapid introduction of a substance into a vein).

Intravenous infusion

The slow introduction of a volume of fluid into the bloodstream. The fluid passes down from a plastic or glass container through tubing into a cannula (thin plastic tube) inserted into a vein, usually in the patient's forearm. The rate at which the fluid drips into the circulation is controlled by an adjustable valve.

An intravenous infusion, commonly known as a drip, is used to give blood (or plasma) to replace that lost in an accident or during an operation (see *Blood transfusion*). An intravenous infusion can also be used to replace or maintain body fluids in patients who are unable to drink or eat. In this case, the fluid is usually a mixture of glucose (sugar) and saline (salt solution). Other uses include the provision of more varied and concentrated nutrients to people unable to digest food normally (see *Feeding, artificial*) and the administration of certain drugs.

Intravenous pyelography

See *Urography*.

Introitus

A general term for the entrance to a body cavity or space, most commonly the vagina.

Introvert

A person more concerned with his or her inner world. Introverts prefer to work alone, are shy, quiet, and withdrawn when under stress. (See also *Extravert; Personality*.)

Intubation

Most commonly, the process of passing an *endotracheal tube* (breathing tube) into the trachea (windpipe). Endotracheal intubation is performed if a patient requires mechanical *ventilation* to deliver oxygen to the lungs—for example, because he or she is in a coma, is anaesthetized, or has severe respiratory disease.

The anaesthetist looks down the patient's throat with a laryngoscope (a viewing instrument) to identify the vocal cords. He or she then passes an endotracheal tube through the patient's mouth and down the throat between the vocal cords into the trachea. Alternatively, the tube may be passed through the nose. The external end of the tube is secured by tape. An inflatable cuff may be used to provide an airtight seal at the bottom of the tube within the trachea.

The term intubation is also used to refer to the placement of a gastric or intestinal tube in the stomach for purposes of suction or the giving of nutrients (see *Feeding, artificial*).

Intussusception

A condition in which part of the intestine telescopes in on itself, forming a tube within a tube (like pulling a shirt sleeve partially inside out), usually resulting in intestinal obstruction (see *Intestine, obstruction of*).

Intussusception most commonly occurs at the junction between the *ileum* (last part of the small intestine) and the *caecum* (the first part of the large intestine).

CAUSES AND INCIDENCE

It is not known exactly why this condition occurs, but in some cases there is a definite association with a recent

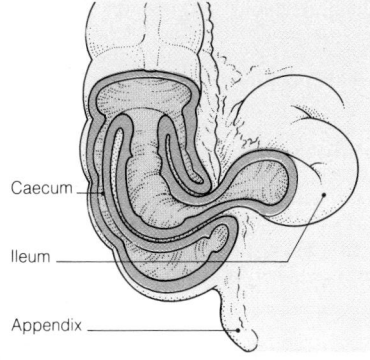

Intussusception
This disorder is characterized by part of the intestine telescoping in on itself. It usually occurs at the junction between the ileum and caecum.

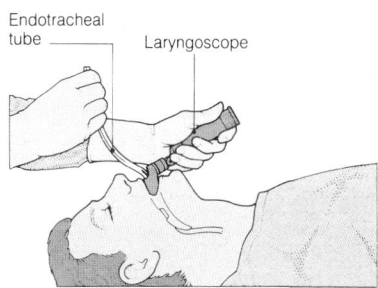

Endotracheal intubation
Guided by an anaesthetist, the endotracheal tube is passed through the patient's mouth and down the throat into the trachea.

infection. In other cases intussusception may start at the site of a *polyp* or *Meckel's diverticulum* (a small, pouch-like projection from the ileum).

Intussusception occurs most commonly in babies after the age of one month. Half of all cases occur in the first year, and three quarters before the age of two. The condition affects approximately two babies per 1,000.

SYMPTOMS

An affected child usually develops severe abdominal colic and screams intermittently. Vomiting is a common feature, and blood and mucus are often found in the faeces. In severe cases of intussusception, the blood supply to the intestine becomes blocked and *gangrene* (tissue death) followed by *peritonitis* (inflammation of the membrane covering the organs in the abdomen) or *perforation* (bursting) may follow.

DIAGNOSIS AND TREATMENT

A barium enema (see *Barium X-ray examinations*) will usually reveal the obstruction. Sometimes the barium enema actually treats the condition; the pressure applied when the enema is introduced can force the prolapsed segment back into position. Otherwise, an operation is carried out. In most cases, the intestine is gently squeezed to push out the inner segment, thus permitting surgery on the cause that led the segment of bowel to telescope.

Invasive

Having the tendency to spread throughout body tissues; the term is usually applied to malignant tumours or to harmful microorganisms. An invasive medical procedure is one in which body tissues are penetrated by an instrument. *Angiography* is an example. (See also *Noninvasive* and *Minimally invasive Surgery*.)

In vitro

The performance of biological processes in the laboratory rather than in the body; in vitro literally means "in glass". Tests successfully carried out in vitro do not always work the same way in the body.

In vitro fertilization

A method of treating *infertility* in which an egg is surgically removed from the ovary and fertilized outside the body. In vitro, which literally means "in glass", refers to the glass Petri dish that is used in the process. The first successful birth as a result of in vitro fertilization (IVF) occurred in England in 1978.

WHY IT IS DONE

In vitro fertilization may be performed when the woman's *fallopian tubes* are permanently blocked or absent. IVF may also be carried out if the man's sperm count is very low or if it is thought that antibodies in the woman's cervical mucus are killing the sperm.

HOW IT IS DONE

Stages in the procedure are shown in the illustrated box.

After IVF, the woman's condition is monitored for a few days to determine if the fertilized eggs have become safely implanted in the uterine wall. Once this occurs, the pregnancy usually continues normally, although the early miscarriage rate is high, and multiple births may occur because more than one of the eggs "takes".

OUTLOOK

It is unlikely that in vitro fertilization will become a widespread treatment of infertility, at least within the near future. Currently, this highly specialized procedure is available only at a small number of centres. It is expensive and the success rate is limited. Recent research has shown that half or more of all eggs have abnormal chromosomes and cannot develop into normal embryos; after fertilization, the eggs begin to divide, but the pregnancy miscarries.

Only about 10 per cent of couples undergoing in vitro fertilization achieve pregnancy on the first attempt, and many attempts may be needed before a successful pregnancy is achieved. Nevertheless, success rates are continuing to improve, and modifications of the technique such as GIFT (see *Infertility*) are simpler and cheaper than the original method.

In vivo

Biological processes occurring within the body. (See also *In vitro*.)

PROCEDURE FOR IN VITRO FERTILIZATION

Fertilization of eggs outside a woman's body can be used to treat some types of infertility. The main stages involved in the procedure of in vitro fertilization are illustrated below.

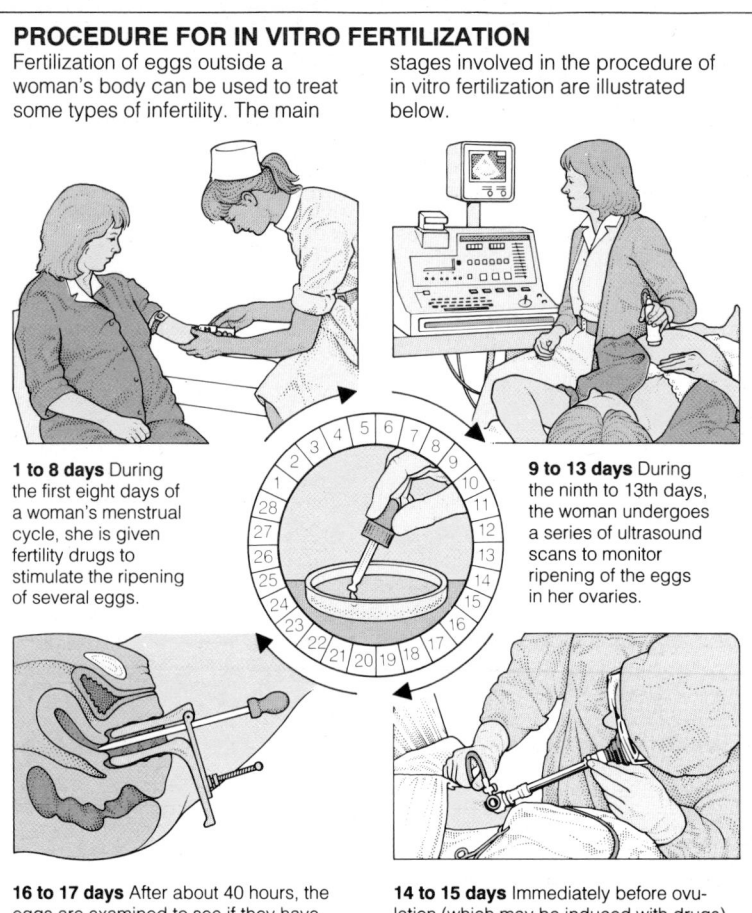

1 to 8 days During the first eight days of a woman's menstrual cycle, she is given fertility drugs to stimulate the ripening of several eggs.

9 to 13 days During the ninth to 13th days, the woman undergoes a series of ultrasound scans to monitor ripening of the eggs in her ovaries.

16 to 17 days After about 40 hours, the eggs are examined to see if they have been fertilized and have started to develop into embryos. If they have, several embryos (usually at the two- or four-cell stage) are placed in the woman's uterus through the vagina.

14 to 15 days Immediately before ovulation (which may be induced with drugs), ripe eggs are removed by laparoscopy or by ultrasound-guided needle aspiration through the vagina or abdomen. The eggs are mixed with the man's sperm in a dish, which is then put in an incubator.

Involuntary movements

Uncontrollable movements of the body, usually affecting the face, head, limbs, and trunk. These movements occur spontaneously and may be slow and writhing (see *Athetosis*); rapid, jerky, and random (see *Chorea*); or predictable, stereotyped, and affecting one part of the body, usually the face (see *Tic*). They may be a feature of a disease (e.g. *Huntington's disease*) or a side-effect of certain drugs used to treat psychiatric conditions.

Iodine

An element essential for the formation of the *thyroid hormones*, triiodothyronine (T_3) and thyroxine (T_4). These hormones control the rate of *metabolism* (internal chemistry) and growth and development. About 100 to 300 micrograms are needed daily. A dietary shortage of iodine may lead to *goitre* (enlargement of the thyroid gland) or to *hypothyroidism* (underactivity of the thyroid gland). Iodine deficiency in the newborn can lead to *cretinism*.

The amount of iodine in food depends on the amount contained in animal feed and the amount in the soil; shortages occur in limestone areas. Shortages can be largely overcome by consuming bread or table salt fortified with iodide or iodate.

MEDICAL USES

Iodine is sometimes given to people who have consumed food or drink contaminated with radioactive iodine. In such cases, absorption by the body of nonradioactive iodine reduces the absorption of the radioactive iodine.

Radioactive iodine is sometimes used to damage, and thus to reduce, the activity of the thyroid gland in cases of *thyrotoxicosis* (a toxic condition resulting from overactivity of the thyroid gland).

Iodine compounds are used as *antiseptics*, in radiopaque contrast media used in some X-ray procedures (see *Imaging techniques*), and in some *cough remedies*.

POSSIBLE ADVERSE EFFECTS

Iodine supplements have possibly caused thyrotoxicosis in some people who have taken them after a long period on a low iodine diet. In rare cases, iodine can cause allergic reactions, e.g. rash, facial swelling, abdominal pain, vomiting, and headache.

Ion

A particle (either an atom or a group of atoms) that carries an electrical charge; positive ions are called cations and negative ions are called anions. Important cations in the body include sodium, potassium, hydrogen, and calcium. Important anions include bicarbonate, chloride, and phosphate.

ROLE IN THE BODY

Many vital body processes depend on the movement of ions across cell membranes. For example, the exchange of sodium for potassium

across the membranes around nerve and muscle cells is the mechanism by which nerve impulses are transmitted and by which muscle contraction occurs. Calcium also plays an important role in muscle contraction as well as being involved in blood clotting and bone growth.

Sodium is the principal cation in extracellular fluid (which surrounds all cells in the body), where it affects the flow of water into and out of cells (see *Osmosis*) and thereby influences the concentration of body fluids.

The levels of sodium, potassium, and calcium are regulated by the kidneys, which control the amount lost from the body in the urine. The level of calcium is also affected by hormonal effects on bones.

The acidity of the blood and other body fluids depends on the level of hydrogen cations, which are produced by various metabolic processes. To prevent these fluids from becoming too acidic, hydrogen cations are neutralized by bicarbonate anions in the extracellular fluid and blood, and by phosphate anions inside cells (see *Acid-base balance*).

ION DISTURBANCES

For the body to function normally, the level of each ion must be maintained within narrow limits; any substantial

deviation can cause symptoms, such as muscle weakness caused by hypokalaemia (too low a level of potassium cations in the blood).

Dehydration caused by insufficient water intake or excessive water loss (from diarrhoea, vomiting, or sweating) increases the concentration of all ions. This may cause thirst, muscle cramps, dizziness, and faintness.

Ionizer

A device that produces *ions* (electrically charged particles). Ionizers that produce negative ions can be used to neutralize positive ions in the atmosphere. Some people believe that use of an ionizer reduces symptoms, such as headaches and fatigue, that may result from a build-up of positive ions generated by electrical machines.

Ipecacuanha

A drug used to induce vomiting in the treatment of *poisoning*. Ipecacuanha (also known as ipecac) is derived from a plant native to South and Central America. Ipecacuanha is not given if poisoning has been caused by corrosive or petroleum-based substances, if the victim is not fully conscious, or if the victim is less than one year old.

IQ

Abbreviation for intelligence quotient, an age-related measure of intelligence (see *Intelligence tests*).

Iridectomy

A procedure performed on the *eye* to remove part of the *iris*. The most common type of iridectomy, known as a "peripheral iridectomy", is usually performed to treat acute *glaucoma*. A small opening is made, surgically or with a laser, near the root (outer edge) of the iris to form a channel through which aqueous humour can drain.

In a complete iridectomy a sector of iris is removed. This type of iridectomy is used, for example, if the iris adheres to the underlying lens.

Iridectomy is sometimes performed to remove tumours and to improve the vision of children who have small central cataracts.

Iridencleisis

A surgical procedure that was used in the 1940s and 1950s to control chronic simple *glaucoma* by creating an artificial channel for the drainage of aqueous humour. Iridencleisis has now largely been replaced by *trabeculectomy*, which is a more reliable surgical procedure.

IMPORTANT IONS AND THEIR ROLES

Cations (positively charged ions)	Major roles in body
Ammonium	Acid-base balance; produced by protein metabolism
Calcium	Nerve conduction; muscle contraction; blood clotting; bone and tooth formation; heart action
Hydrogen	Acid-base balance; component of stomach acid
Magnesium	Nerve conduction; muscle contraction; bone and tooth formation; enzyme activation; protein metabolism
Potassium	Nerve conduction; muscle contraction; water balance; acid-base balance
Sodium	Nerve conduction; muscle contraction; water balance; acid-base balance
Anions (negatively charged ions)	
Bicarbonate	Acid-base balance; neutralizes stomach acid
Chloride	Acid-base balance; water balance; component of stomach acid
Phosphate	Acid-base balance; bone and tooth formation; protein metabolism; energy metabolism; structure of cell membranes

Iridocyclitis

Inflammation of the *iris* and ciliary body. Iridocyclitis is more usually known as "anterior *uveitis*". (See also *Eye* disorders box.)

Iris

The coloured part of the *eye* that lies behind the cornea. The iris is connected at its outer edge to the ciliary body and has a central perforation called the *pupil*, through which light enters the eye and falls on the retina.

The iris is a loose framework of transparent *collagen* (a fibrous protein) and muscle fibres, which constantly contracts and dilates to alter the size of the pupil and to control the amount of light that passes through the pupil and reaches the retina.

LOCATION OF THE IRIS
The iris lies behind the cornea and in front of the lens. The outer edge of the iris is connected to the ciliary body; at the centre is an aperture called the pupil.

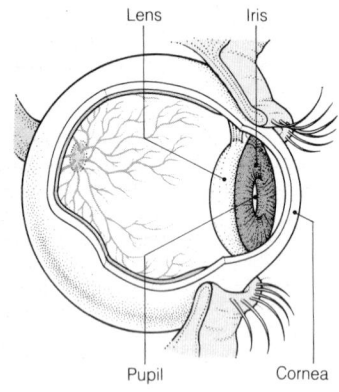

Lens · Iris · Pupil · Cornea

Iritis

An inflammation of the *iris*, now often termed an "anterior *uveitis*".

Iron

A mineral which is essential for the formation of certain *enzymes* (proteins that stimulate chemical reactions), *haemoglobin* (the oxygen-carrying pigment in red blood cells), and *myoglobin* (the oxygen-carrying pigment in muscle cells).

Iron is contained in a variety of foods, such as liver, meat, cereals (especially whole-grain), fish, green leafy vegetables, nuts, and beans. During pregnancy, iron supplements may be necessary for the healthy development of the baby.

Iron deficiency leading to anaemia (see *Anaemia, iron deficiency*) is usually caused by abnormal blood loss, such as from *menorrhagia* (heavy periods) or a *peptic ulcer*, but may also be due to a diet that is low in iron or from which iron is poorly absorbed.

Iron supplements may cause nausea, abdominal pain, constipation, or diarrhoea. They may also colour the faeces black.

Excessive intake of iron over a prolonged period may cause *cirrhosis* of the liver.

Iron-deficiency anaemia

See *Anaemia, iron-deficiency*.

Iron lung

A large machine, properly called a Drinker respirator, formerly used to maintain breathing, especially in people paralysed by *poliomyelitis*. The iron lung has been replaced by less cumbersome and more efficient means of maintaining breathing (see *Ventilation*).

Irradiation

See *Radiation hazards; Radiotherapy*.

Irradiation of food

The treatment of food with ionizing *radiation* to kill bacteria, moulds, insects, and other parasites. Irradiation improves the keeping qualities of food and is a means of controlling some types of *food poisoning*.

Bombarding food with ionizing radiation sterilizes the food by killing microorganisms. However, the process does not destroy bacterial toxins and it may destroy or alter vitamins. It does not render food radioactive. The process is unsuitable for high-fat dairy produce and eggs, in which it causes changes in taste.

Irradiation also inhibits the ripening process and the sprouting of vegetables.

Some countries recommend the irradiation of certain foods, such as poultry, other meats, prawns, some fruits, vegetables, herbs and spices. Categories of prepared foods, such as deep-frozen hospital meals, are irradiated in some countries. Other countries prohibit food irradiation and the importation of irradiated food. There is as yet no way of proving whether food has been irradiated.

The effects of irradiation on food additives and on pesticide residues have not yet been established, nor have the long-term effects of eating irradiated foods.

Irrigation, wound

The cleansing of a deep wound by repeatedly washing it out with a medicated solution or sterile saline.

WHY IT IS DONE
A deep wound is often contaminated with infected foreign material. Unless such a wound is completely cleansed before repair, it may fail to heal, an abscess may form in it, or, in extreme cases, *gangrene* (tissue death) may result. If the wound contains agricultural soil, *tetanus* is a serious risk.

Irritable bladder

Intermittent, uncontrolled contractions of the muscles in the *bladder* wall. Irritable bladder may cause urge incontinence (see *Incontinence, urinary*).

Irritability of the bladder is commonly due to a urinary tract infection

---

IRRIGATION TECHNIQUES
After removal of contaminated tissue, a wound may be cleansed either by forced syringe (or catheter) irrigation or by using an irrigation chamber.

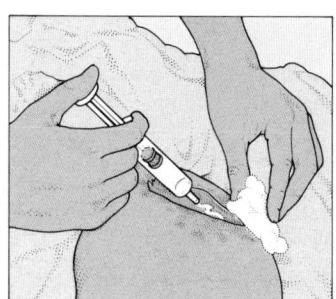

Forced syringe irrigation
A syringe (sometimes with a catheter attached) is used to flush irrigation fluid repeatedly into and out of the wound until the drained fluid is clear.

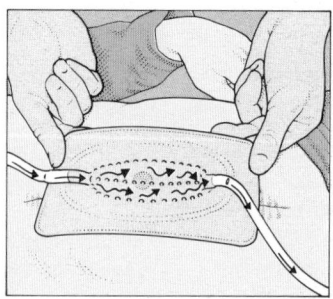

Irrigation chamber
A flexible, plastic irrigation chamber is sealed over the wound; irrigation fluid is then run through the chamber until the drained fluid is clear.

(see *Cystitis*), the presence of a catheter within the bladder, a bladder stone (see *Calculus, urinary tract*), or obstruction to the outflow of urine by an enlarged *prostate gland*. In many cases of irritable bladder, however, no underlying cause for the muscular irritability and spasm is found.

Symptoms may be relieved by *antispasmodic drugs*; other treatment is directed at any underlying cause.

Irritable bowel syndrome

A combination of intermittent abdominal pain and irregular bowel habit (i.e. constipation, diarrhoea, or bouts of each) that occurs in the absence of other diagnosed disease. Other names for the condition are irritable colon syndrome and spastic colon.

Although symptoms subside and even disappear for periods of time, irritable bowel syndrome is usually recurrent throughout life. Although it is not life-threatening and is unlikely to lead to complications, it can cause much distress.

CAUSES AND INCIDENCE

The cause of the condition is not fully understood, but the basic abnormality is a disturbance of involuntary muscle movement in the large intestine. However, there is no abnormality in the intestinal structure and people with irritable bowel syndrome neither lose weight nor become malnourished. Irritable bowel syndrome is the most common disorder of the intestine, affecting 10 to 20 per cent of adults, most of whom do not seek treatment. Nevertheless, the condition accounts for more than half the patients seen by gastroenterologists.

The condition is twice as common in women as in men, usually beginning in early or middle adulthood. Sufferers are often otherwise in good health and have had the condition for some time before seeking medical advice.

A psychological element, particularly anxiety, is believed by some doctors to be the main causative factor; emotional stress tends to exacerbate the condition. However, bowel upset is a normal reaction to stress in many people who do not suffer from the illness.

SYMPTOMS

The symptoms include intermittent cramp-like pain in the abdomen, abdominal distension (swelling), often on the left side, transient relief of pain by bowel movement or passing wind, sense of incomplete evacuation of the bowels, excessive wind, and symptoms aggravated by food. Various other symptoms may also occur (which are not precisely part of the irritable bowel syndrome), such as heartburn, back pain, weakness, faintness, agitation, tendency to tire easily, reduced appetite, and palpitations.

DIAGNOSIS

The initial diagnosis is based on the patient's symptoms and a physical examination. Examination of the faeces, *barium X-ray examination*, and *sigmoidoscopy* (examination of the colon through a viewing instrument passed via the anus) may be performed to exclude conditions, such as cancer (see *Colon, cancer of*; *Rectum, cancer of*) or inflammatory bowel disease (see *Crohn's disease*; *Ulcerative colitis*), that may have similar symptoms.

TREATMENT

A high-fibre diet or bulk-forming agents, such as *bran* or *methylcellulose*, may be recommended for some patients with irritable bowel syndrome. Short courses of *antidiarrhoeal drugs* (such as *loperamide*) may be given for persistent diarrhoea. *Antispasmodic drugs* may be prescribed to relieve muscular spasm. *Hypnosis, psychotherapy*, and *counselling* have proved effective in some cases; most sufferers find treatments that relieve the symptoms but do not cure the disorder.

Ischaemia

Insufficient supply of blood to a specific organ or tissue. Ischaemia is usually caused by disease of the blood vessels, such as *atherosclerosis* (narrowing of arteries by deposits of fatty material), but may also result from injury to a vessel, constriction of a vessel due to spasm of the muscles in the vessel wall, or inadequate blood flow due to inefficient pumping action of the heart.

The symptoms of ischaemia depend on the part of the body affected.

Treatment may include *vasodilator drugs* to widen the blood vessels or, in more severe cases, an *angioplasty* or *bypass operation*.

Isolation

Nursing procedures, also known as barrier nursing, designed to prevent a patient from infecting others or from being infected by them. In either case, the patient is usually isolated in a single room.

TYPES

COMPLETE ISOLATION This is used if a patient has a contagious disease, such as *Lassa fever*, that can be transmitted to others by direct contact and airborne

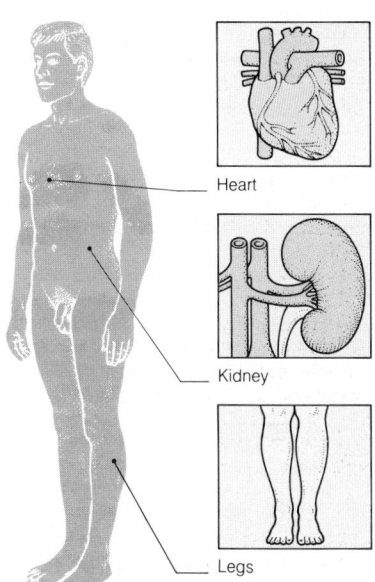

Symptoms of ischaemia
Ischaemia (insufficient blood supply) of the heart causes the chest pain of angina pectoris; ischaemia of blood vessels in the legs may cause a cramp-like pain during exercise. Ischaemia may also affect the kidneys (causing kidney failure) or the brain (resulting in a stroke).

germs. All staff wear masks, gowns, caps, and gloves, which afterwards are incinerated or sterilized. Bed linen, eating utensils, bedpans, and any other items that come into contact with the patient are also sterilized and, even though they wear gloves, staff members must wash their hands thoroughly after each nursing task.

PARTIAL ISOLATION This is carried out if the patient's disease is transmitted in a more limited way—for example, only by respiration (as in *tuberculosis*) or only by contact with infected skin (as in *impetigo*) or faeces (as in *cholera*). In these cases, some of the precautions taken in complete isolation nursing are unnecessary.

REVERSE ISOLATION This technique, also known as reverse barrier nursing, is used to protect a patient whose resistance to infection has been severely lowered. The air supply to the room is filtered. Visiting is drastically limited. All staff and visitors wear caps, gowns, masks, and gloves. Bed linen and all items used by the patient are sterilized. When these measures do not give enough protection (such as after a *bone marrow transplant*), the patient is placed in an isolator (plastic tent) or special cubicle.

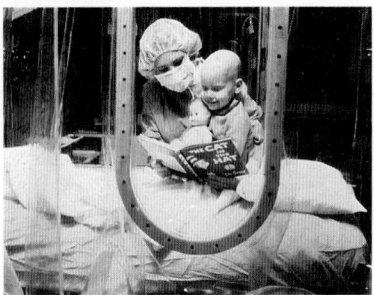

Child being nursed in an isolator
The plastic tent and strict sterilization procedures protect the patient from infection.

Occasionally, long-term reverse isolation is needed for patients with severe combined immunodeficiency (SCID) (see *Immunodeficiency disorders*); these patients are born without normal defences against infection.

Isoniazid

An *antibacterial drug* used to prevent and treat *tuberculosis*. As a preventive measure, isoniazid may be given to close contacts of people suffering from tuberculosis. To treat the disease, isoniazid is given in combination with other antibacterial drugs, usually for at least six months.

Adverse effects, which are rare, include nausea, fatigue, numbness, twitching, and insomnia. Because isoniazid may increase the amount of pyridoxine (vitamin B_6) lost from the body, supplements of this vitamin may be given to avoid the possibility of nerve damage.

Isoprenaline

A drug that is given by injection for the emergency treatment of patients in whom a heart disorder has caused slowing of the heart-rate. Isoprenaline is often given as an interim measure to increase the heart-rate before a *pacemaker* can be implanted.

Isoprenaline also widens the airways in people with asthma, but this drug is now only rarely used to treat asthma because many other *bronchodilator drugs* are less likely to cause adverse effects.

Adverse effects of isoprenaline include dry mouth, dizziness, nervousness, headache, palpitations, and chest pain.

Isosorbide

A long-acting *nitrate drug* that acts as a *vasodilator drug*. Isosorbide is used to reduce the severity and frequency of *angina pectoris* (chest pain due to

impaired blood supply to heart muscle). This drug is also given to treat severe *heart failure* (reduced pumping efficiency).

Adverse effects include headache, hot flushes, and dizziness.

Isotope scanning

See *Radionuclide scanning*.

Isotretinoin

A drug derived from *vitamin A* used in the treatment of severe *acne* when other treatments have proved ineffective. Isotretinoin works by reducing the formation of sebum (natural skin oils) and keratin (a tough protein that is the major component of the outer layer of skin).

POSSIBLE ADVERSE EFFECTS
Isotretinoin may cause itching, dryness and flaking of the skin, and cracking of the lips. Rarely, it may cause liver damage and an increased risk of *coronary artery disease* and *peripheral vascular disease*. Isotretinoin may damage a developing fetus; pregnancy should be avoided during treatment and for at least three months after taking the drug.

Ispaghula

A bulk-forming *laxative drug* commonly used to treat *constipation*, *diverticular disease*, and *irritable bowel syndrome*. Ispaghula is taken by mouth; as it travels through the intestine, it absorbs a large volume of water from surrounding blood vessels, thereby softening and increasing the volume of the faeces.

Ispaghula is also used to reduce the frequency and to increase the firmness of the faeces in people with chronic, watery *diarrhoea* and to control the consistency of bowel movements in patients who have had a *colostomy* or an *ileostomy*.

Possible adverse effects of ispaghula include flatulence, abdominal distension, and discomfort.

Itching

An intense, distracting irritation or tickling sensation in the skin which may be generalized (felt all over the skin's surface) or localized (confined to one area). The reason for the sensation is not fully understood.

Itching is the most prominent symptom of many skin diseases, but does not itself necessarily indicate an underlying skin disorder. People differ in their tolerance to itching, and a person's threshold can be altered by stress, emotions, or other factors.

Itching is worse when the skin is warm and when there are few distractions, making it more noticeable at night.

CAUSES
GENERALIZED ITCHING Excessive bathing, which removes the skin's natural oils and may leave the skin excessively dry and scaly, is a common cause of itching. Some people experience itching after taking certain drugs, such as cocaine, codeine, and some antibiotics. Soap, detergents, and roughly textured clothing (e.g. clothing made from wool) also produce itching in some people.

Many elderly people suffer for no apparent reason from dry, itchy skin, especially on their backs. A similar condition affects some younger people in cold weather. Itching commonly occurs during pregnancy.

Many skin conditions produce an itchy rash—for example, *chickenpox*, *urticaria* (nettle rash), *eczema*, and fungal infections (see *Tinea*). Less common causes include *psoriasis* or *dermatitis herpetiformis*.

Generalized skin itchiness can be a result of *diabetes mellitus*, *kidney failure*, *jaundice*, and thyroid disorders. Disorders of the blood (such as *leukaemia*) and of the lymphatic system (for example, *Hodgkin's disease*) occasionally cause itching.

LOCALIZED ITCHING Pruritus ani (itching around the anal region) occurs in adults, particularly those with such problems as *haemorrhoids*, *anal fissure*, and persistent diarrhoea. Pruritus ani often results from irritation caused by overzealous cleansing after defaecation. *Worm infestation* is the most likely cause of itching in children.

Another form of intense skin irritation confined to one area occurs in pruritus vulvae, which affects the external genitalia in women. The condition may be due to *candidiasis*, hormonal changes (at puberty, pregnancy, and the menopause), or to use of spermicides or vaginal suppositories, ointments, and deodorants.

Lice and *scabies* infestations cause intense itching. *Insect bites*, too, can produce intense skin irritation.

TREATMENT
Specific treatment depends on the underlying cause, if known. Cooling lotions, such as *calamine*, relieve irritation; *emollients* reduce dryness.

Soaps often irritate itchy skin, especially if a rash is visible. Soaps should be used only when necessary; a mild cleansing lotion or water alone is often sufficient to keep most of the skin adequately clean. Itchy skin should be handled very gently. Scratching temporarily relieves itching, but makes the itching worse in the long run. The scratching habit can be suppressed by applying a soothing lotion, ointment, or wet compress to the affected areas when the urge to scratch occurs.

-itis

A suffix meaning "inflammation of". Virtually every organ or tissue in the body can suffer inflammation (the most common form of tissue disorder), so "-itis" is by far the most common word ending in medicine. An example of its use is *bronchitis* (inflammation of the bronchi).

The term -itis is applied strictly to cases of inflammation with redness, pain, heat, and swelling. The term should not be used loosely to imply general disorder, for which the ending "-opathy" is appropriate.

IUCD

An abbreviation for intrauterine contraceptive device (see *IUD*).

IUD

An abbreviation for intrauterine contraceptive device. An IUD, alternatively called an IUCD or coil, is a mechanical device inserted into the uterus for purposes of *contraception*. IUDs are not recommended for some groups of women, but for others they are an efficient and acceptable method of contraception. The failure rate for IUDs is about two to three per cent.

The IUDs licensed for current use in the UK are all plastic devices with either copper or silver incorporated to improve effectiveness. Some women are still using devices made only of plastics. Most IUDs have a plastic string which, following insertion of the device, comes through the cervix into the vagina. The string makes removal easier and indicates the presence of the IUD.

HOW THEY WORK

Although it is not definitely known how IUDs function, it is thought that the main effect is to inhibit the implantation of a fertilized egg in the wall of the uterus (see *Implantation, egg*).

HOW THEY ARE USED

An IUD may be inserted by a general practitioner, family planning doctor, or gynaecologist. The device can be inserted any time during the menstrual cycle, but the preferred time is during or just after menstruation (because it is unlikely that the woman is pregnant and because the cervix is easier to handle). After a full-term pregnancy, a woman should wait for at least six weeks before having an IUD inserted.

An IUD is inserted through the vagina and cervix into the uterine cavity. Most IUDs are loaded in a small plastic tube that is inserted through the cervical canal; the device is gently pushed out by means of a plunger. Once an IUD is in place, it provides immediate protection. The woman should check once or twice a week that the string is present. If it is not, the string has probably curled up into the uterus, but it is possible that the IUD has been expelled.

IUDs containing copper need to be replaced every three to five years.

WHO SHOULD NOT USE IUDS

Women who have never been pregnant are more likely to have complications than women who have had children. Women with no previous pregnancies usually have more pain on insertion, higher expulsion rates, and a heavier menstrual flow. A woman with *fibroids* may be advised not to have an IUD. Any woman with a history of pelvic disease or infection of the fallopian tubes should not use an IUD. Women with many partners (or whose partner has other sexual partners) are at risk of *pelvic inflammatory disease* (PID) and should probably avoid IUDs. Young women have a higher infection rate than older women. Women with heavy or painful periods may find the IUD makes their symptoms worse.

COMPLICATIONS

Immediately after insertion, there may be bleeding, pain, or vaginal discharge. Menstrual periods after insertion may be heavier and more painful than before.

Women who become pregnant despite having an IUD have a higher rate of *ectopic pregnancy*. PID may be severe and lead to permanent infertility. A rare complication of IUD use is a perforated uterus, in which the device works its way through the wall of the uterus into the abdominal cavity.

IVF

See *In vitro fertilization*.

IVP

The abbreviation for intravenous pyelography, also known as intravenous *urography*.

IVU

The abbreviation for intravenous *urography* (an imaging technique).

THE IUD (INTRAUTERINE CONTRACEPTIVE DEVICE)
The IUD, also known as the IUCD, is basically a small plastic contraceptive device inserted into the uterus through the cervix. IUDs are thought to work by preventing the implantation of fertilized eggs in the uterus.

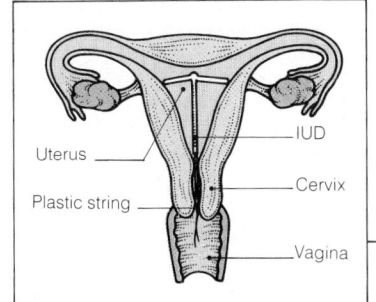

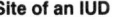

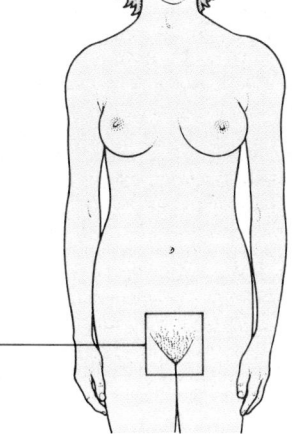

Site of an IUD
An IUD is inserted into the uterus; it has a plastic string that hangs down through the cervix and into the vagina. All types of

IUDs can be inserted—by specially trained personnel—in family planning clinics, hospitals, or general practitioners' surgeries.

Jakob-Creutzfeldt disease
See *Creutzfeldt-Jakob disease.*

Jaundice
Yellowing of the skin and the whites of the eyes caused by an accumulation of the yellow-brown *bile* pigment *bilirubin* in the blood. Jaundice is the chief sign of many disorders of the *liver* and *biliary system.* Many babies develop jaundice soon after birth (see *Jaundice, neonatal*).

TYPES AND CAUSES
Bilirubin is formed from *haemoglobin* (the oxygen-carrying pigment in red blood cells) when old red cells are broken down, mainly by the *spleen.* The pigment is absorbed from the blood by the liver, where it is made soluble in water and is excreted in bile. The process can be upset in any of three ways, causing the main types of jaundice: haemolytic, hepatocellular, and obstructive.

HAEMOLYTIC JAUNDICE In haemolytic jaundice, the amount of bilirubin produced is too great for the liver to process. This is caused by excessive *haemolysis* (breakdown of red cells), which can have many causes (see *Anaemia, haemolytic*). A type of jaundice similar to haemolytic jaundice can develop as a result of a mild liver disorder called *Gilbert's disease.*

HEPATOCELLULAR JAUNDICE In hepatocellular jaundice, bilirubin builds up in the blood because its transfer from liver cells to bile is prevented, usually as the result of acute *hepatitis* (inflammation of the liver) or *liver failure.*

OBSTRUCTIVE JAUNDICE In obstructive jaundice, also known as cholestatic jaundice, bile is prevented from flowing out of the liver because of blockage of the bile ducts (see *Bile duct obstruction*) due to disorders such as *gallstones* or a tumour. Obstructive jaundice can also occur if the bile ducts are not present (as in *biliary atresia*) or have been destroyed within the liver (for example, in primary *biliary cirrhosis*). As a result, *cholestasis* (stagnation of bile in the liver) occurs and bilirubin is forced back into the blood.

SYMPTOMS AND SIGNS
In some cases, such as in acute hepatitis, jaundice is only one of several signs and symptoms. In other cases, such as in Gilbert's disease, it may be the sole sign of a disorder.

Obstructive jaundice is usually accompanied by two other characteristic features: pale faeces and dark urine. The faeces are pale because bilirubin, which normally colours faeces brown, does not reach the intestine; the urine is dark because large amounts of water-soluble bilirubin are filtered into it from the blood. Bilirubin may also be deposited in the skin, causing itching.

In haemolytic jaundice, the colour of both urine and faeces is normal. In hepatocellular jaundice, the faeces are normal but the urine may be dark.

DIAGNOSIS AND TREATMENT
If excessive haemolysis is suspected, *blood tests* are carried out to determine the amount of water-insoluble bilirubin. A *blood smear* indicates whether large numbers of immature red cells are present; if they are, haemolysis is the suspected cause of the jaundice.

To diagnose hepatocellular jaundice, the blood is tested and a *liver biopsy* (removal of a small sample of tissue for analysis) may be performed.

If the doctor suspects obstructive jaundice, *ultrasound scanning, liver function tests,* and *cholangiography* may be carried out to determine if the bile ducts are diseased or blocked.

In all cases, treatment is for the underlying cause.

Jaundice, neonatal
Yellowing of the skin and whites of the eyes in the newborn period, due to the accumulation of *bilirubin* (a yellow-brown *bile* pigment) in the blood. Many babies develop *jaundice* during the first few days after birth; premature babies are especially prone to the condition.

In the newborn period, jaundice is usually due to immaturity of the *liver,* resulting in failure of the liver to excrete bilirubin efficiently. This form of jaundice is usually harmless and disappears towards the end of the first week.

Much less commonly, jaundice in babies is caused by *haemolytic disease of the newborn, G6PD deficiency,* infection, *hepatitis* (inflammation of the liver), *hypothyroidism* (underactivity of the thyroid gland), or *biliary atresia.*

DIAGNOSIS AND TREATMENT
Diagnosis is based on physical examination. In some cases, blood tests, urine tests, *ultrasound scanning,* and other tests may be performed.

Treatment depends on the underlying cause. Jaundiced babies usually require extra fluids and may be treated with *phototherapy.* In severe cases, exchange transfusion (a type of *blood transfusion*) may be necessary. If severe neonatal jaundice is not treated promptly, *kernicterus* (a form of brain damage) may occur.

Jaw
The lowest and only mobile bone of the face, also known as the mandible. The term jaw sometimes includes the bone that extends from the inner rims of the eyes to the mouth, more commonly known as the *maxilla.*

The mandible is U-shaped as seen from above and bears the lower teeth on its upper surface. It is connected to the base of the *skull* at the *temporomandibular joints,* which can be felt in the cheek just in front of the earlobe. Powerful muscles, arising from the temple on either side, attach to the jaw for movements needed in chewing and biting; other muscles allow side-to-side and downward movement.

Jaw, dislocated
Displacement of the lower *jaw* from one or both of the *temporomandibular joints* (the joints between the jaw and the base of the skull). A dislocated jaw is usually caused either by a blow or by yawning.

ANATOMY OF THE JAW
The U-shaped, mobile bone of the face meets the skull in front of the ears at the temporomandibular joint. The jaw bears teeth on its upper surface.

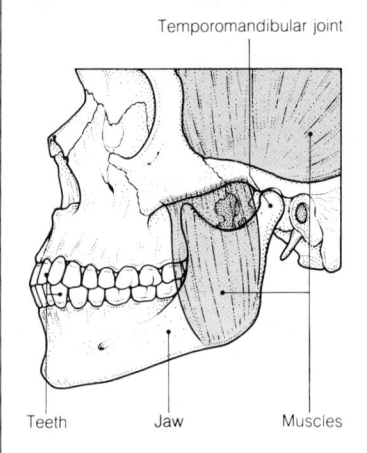

The jaw is the most commonly dislocated joint because it is very unstable. Once dislocation has happened, it tends to recur.

SYMPTOMS
There is pain in front of the ear on the affected side or sides and the jaw projects forwards. The mouth cannot be fully closed and, as a result, the victim drools and has difficulty eating and speaking.

TREATMENT
A second person can easily correct the dislocation. He or she should stand in front of the victim, place a thumb on the lower back teeth at each side, and press down. The lower jaw should then click back into position. To avoid causing injury when the teeth snap shut, the thumbs should be wrapped in cloth.

Recurrent dislocation requires an operation to stabilize the joint, such as strengthening the ligaments with stitches. However, surgery is rarely successful in curing the problem.

Jaw, fractured
Fractures of the *jaw* are most often caused by a direct blow to the face. Because of the shape of the jaw, fracture often occurs not only at the site of the blow, but also on the other side of the jaw.

SYMPTOMS
If the fracture is minor, the only symptoms may be some tenderness, pain on biting, and slight stiffness. In more severe injuries, teeth may be loosened or damaged, movement of the jaw may be severely limited, and there may be loss of feeling in the lower lip.

DIAGNOSIS AND TREATMENT
If a fracture is suspected, *X-rays* of the area are taken. Minor fractures are normally left to heal on their own.

For severe fractures in which the bones have become displaced, surgical treatment is required. The bone fragments are first manipulated back into the correct position. Teeth too badly damaged to be saved may require extraction. The jaw is immobilized to allow healing to occur, usually by wiring the upper and lower teeth together. If the patient has no teeth, special dentures can be constructed to hold the wires.

Some fractures cannot be adequately immobilized by this method. In such cases, an incision is made in the skin to expose the jaw bone, holes are drilled in each bone fragment, and wires are inserted and twisted together. The skin incision is sewn up with the wires in position.

RECOVERY PERIOD
If the teeth have been wired together, the patient is given a liquid diet. The wires are usually removed after about six weeks.

Jealousy, morbid
Preoccupation with the sexual infidelity of one's partner. The sufferer, usually a man, becomes convinced that his partner is having an affair.

Morbid jealousy is usually due to *personality disorder*, *depression*, or *paranoia*, but may also occur in those suffering from *alcohol dependence* or organic *brain syndrome*.

Treatment of the underlying disorder may improve the condition, but the outlook is generally poor. Psychiatrists usually recommend separation of the partners, since morbid jealousy is a significant cause of murder.

Jejunal biopsy
A diagnostic test in which a small piece of tissue is removed from the lining of the *jejunum* (the middle, coiled section of the small intestine) for examination under a microscope.

WHY IT IS DONE
The procedure is especially useful in the diagnosis of *Crohn's disease, coeliac disease, lymphoma,* and all other causes of *malabsorption* because these conditions are associated with recognizable changes in the small intestine.

HOW IT IS DONE
The patient may be sedated slightly before the procedure. A small device (Crosby capsule) is attached to a length of fine tubing; both are lubricated and the patient then swallows the capsule. The tube is guided down the oesophagus through the stomach and duodenum until the capsule reaches the jejunum. An *X-ray* is then performed to ensure that the capsule is in the correct position. A syringe is used to withdraw air from the tube and capsule, thereby causing a minute piece of tissue to be sucked into the capsule, where it is sheared off. The tube and capsule are withdrawn and the tissue taken from the capsule for examination.

Jejunum
The middle, coiled section of the small *intestine*, joining the *duodenum* to the *ileum*. It is wider than the ileum and has a thicker wall, but its function is the same—the digestion of food and the absorption of nutrients from it. Among the few disorders that may affect the jejunum are *coeliac disease, Crohn's disease,* and *lymphoma*.

Jellyfish stings

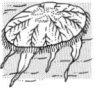

Jellyfish, together with corals, sea anemones, and Portuguese men-of-war, belong to a group of marine animals called coelenterates or cnidarians. These animals have tentacles armed with stinging capsules that discharge when touched. Usually, the result of a sting is no more than an itchy or mildly painful rash, but some jellyfish and Portuguese men-of-war can cause a severe sting. In rare cases, venom entering the bloodstream may cause vomiting, sweating, shock, breathing difficulties, convulsions, and collapse. Dangerous species live mainly in tropical waters.

TREATMENT
If fragments of jellyfish tentacle remain attached to the skin after a sting, vinegar should be applied to inactivate the stinging capsules; tentacle fragments may be removed with adhesive tape. The bare hands should not be used as tentacles may remain capable of causing stings for many hours. *Analgesic drugs* (painkillers) may be taken. A severe reaction requires hospitalization and sometimes *cardiopulmonary resuscitation*. *Antivenoms* for the more dangerous species of jellyfish may be available.

J

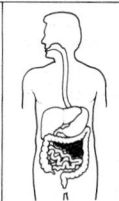

ANATOMY OF THE JEJUNUM
This section of the small intestine joins the duodenum to the ileum. It is wider than the ileum and has a thicker wall.

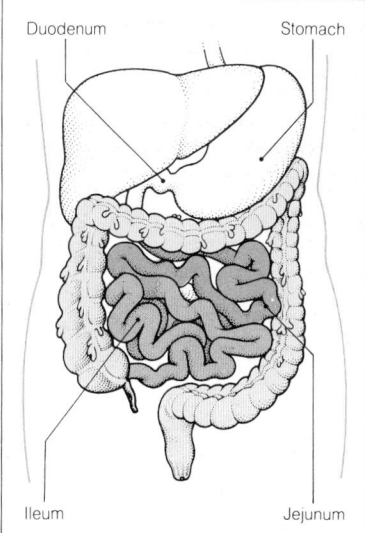

Duodenum

Stomach

Ileum

Jejunum

TYPES OF JOINTS

Some joints are fixed (e.g. the skull) and some allow a little movement (e.g. the vertebrae). Of the mobile joints, the hinge joint is the simplest. Pivot joints allow rotation only, while ellipsoidal joints allow all types of movement except pivotal. Ball-and-socket joints allow the widest range of movement.

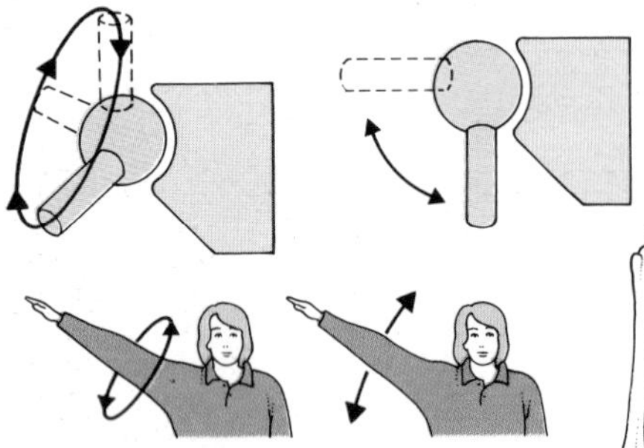

Ball-and-socket joint
A ball-and-socket joint allows the widest range of movement—backwards or forwards, sideways, and rotation. Examples are the hip and shoulder joints.

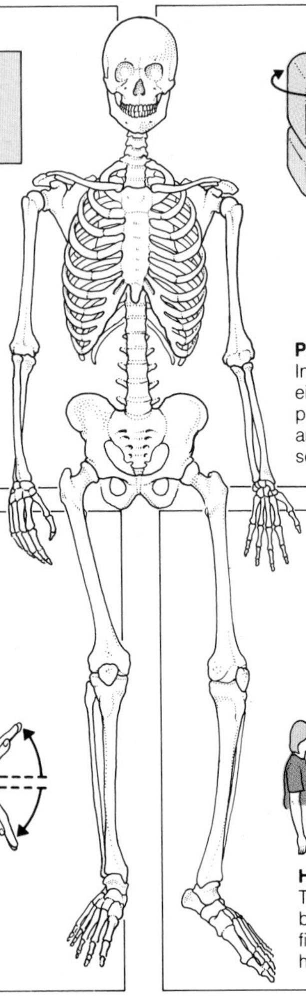

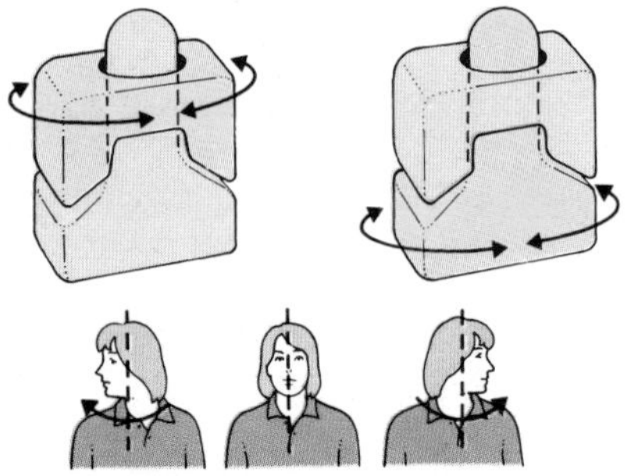

Pivot joint
In a pivot joint, movement is limited to rotation, either by means of a bony projection pivoting within a ring, or a ring pivoting around an axis (e.g. the joint between the first and second vertebrae).

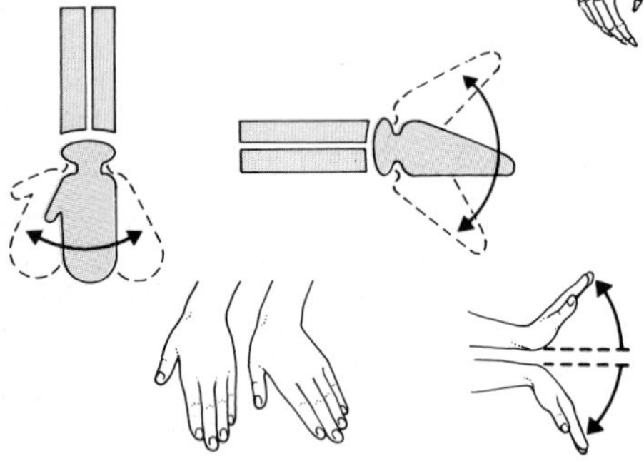

Ellipsoidal joint
In an ellipsoidal joint, an oval-shaped part fits into an elliptic cavity, allowing all types of movement except pivotal (an example is the wrist joint).

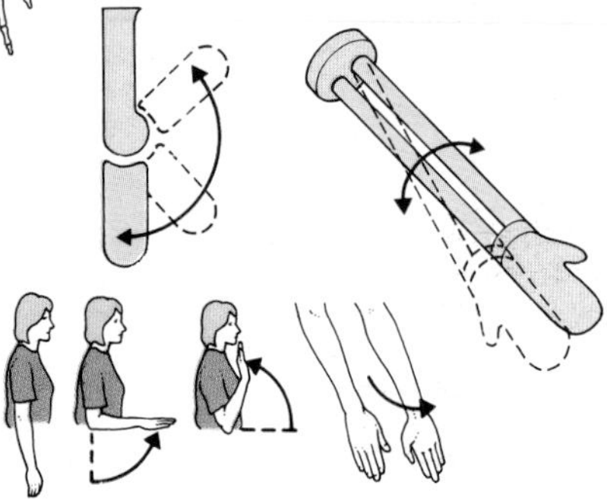

Hinge joint
This is one of the simplest joints; it allows bending and straightening, as in the fingers. The knee and elbow are modified hinge joints that allow some rotation as well.

STRUCTURE OF A FIXED JOINT
Fixed joints are firmly secured by fibrous tissue. The joints between the bones of the skull are an example.

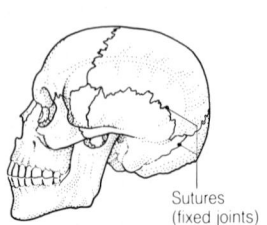

Sutures
(fixed joints)

STRUCTURE OF A MOBILE JOINT
The bone surfaces are coated with very smooth cartilage to reduce friction. The joint is sealed within a tough fibrous capsule lined with synovial membrane, which produces a sticky, lubricating fluid. Each joint is surrounded by strong ligaments that support it and prevent excessive movement. Movement is controlled by muscles that are attached to bone by tendons on either side of the joint. Most mobile joints have at least one bursa (fluid-filled sac) nearby, which cushions a pressure point.

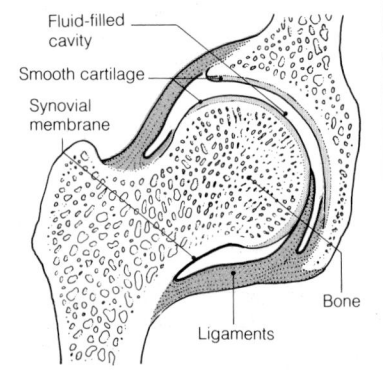

Fluid-filled cavity

Smooth cartilage

Synovial membrane

Bone

Ligaments

Jet-lag

Interruption of the sleep-wake cycle, fatigue, and other symptoms caused by disturbance of normal body rhythms as a result of flying across different time zones.

Symptoms of jet-lag are a desire to sleep during the local day, wakefulness at night, general fatigue, reduced physical and mental activity, and poor memory.

CAUSES

When an air traveller crosses several time zones, his or her "day" (as timed by an external clock) is longer or shorter than 24 hours, depending on the direction of the flight. Many of the traveller's *biorhythms* (natural body rhythms) do not adjust immediately to this shorter or longer day, and this results in jet-lag when the flight is over.

Jet-lag tends to be worse after an eastward flight (which shortens the traveller's day) than after a westward one. It is most likely to affect people over 30 who normally follow an established daily routine.

PREVENTIVE MEASURES

The symptoms of jet-lag can be minimized by drinking plenty of nonalcoholic fluids during the flight and avoiding heavy meals. Also, those flying east should go to bed earlier than usual for a few days before the journey; people flying west should stay up later. It is a good idea, if possible, to arrive in the new time zone in the early evening and to go to bed early.

It may take several days to adjust to a new time zone (about half a day to one day for each time zone that has been crossed). The adjustment can be made easier by breaking up a long journey with a stopover and by resting after the flight.

The pituitary hormone *melatonin* has been shown to play a part in the control of daily rhythms; treatment with this hormone may reduce the severity of jet-lag, but research into this is still at an experimental stage.

Jogger's nipple

Soreness of the nipple caused by the rubbing of clothing against it, usually during sports such as jogging or long-distance running. Jogger's nipple, which affects both men and women, can be prevented by applying petroleum jelly to the nipple before prolonged running. Wearing a clean shirt also helps because sweat can aggravate the condition. Treatment involves covering the nipple with a bandage to reduce rubbing.

Joint

The junction between two or more bones. Most joints are highly mobile, others are fixed or allow only a small amount of movement (see the illustrated box).

DISORDERS

Common joint injuries include *sprains*, damage to the *cartilage*, torn *ligaments*, and tearing of the joint capsule.

Dislocation of a joint is usually caused by injury but is occasionally *congenital*. A less severe injury may cause *subluxation* (partial dislocation). Rarely, the bone ends are fractured, sometimes leading to *haemarthrosis* (bleeding into the joint) or *effusion* (accumulation of fluid in a joint) due to *synovitis* (inflammation of the lining of the joint).

Joints are commonly affected by forms of *arthritis* (inflammation of a joint). *Bursitis* (inflammation of a bursa) may occur as a result of local irritation or strain. Permanent joint deformities may be caused by severe injury or arthritis. Temporary deformities, usually affecting a joint in the legs, may occur during childhood but disappear as growth continues. Surgery may be required to correct certain deformities.

Joint replacement

See *Arthroplasty*.

Joule

The international unit of *energy*, work, and heat. Approximately 4,200 joules (symbol J) or 4.2 kilojoules (kJ) equal one kilocalorie (kcal); 1 kJ equals about 0.24 kcal. (See also *Calorie*.)

Jugular vein

One of three veins on each side of the neck that return deoxygenated blood from the head to the heart. Of the three (internal, external, and anterior) by far the largest is the internal jugular, which arises at the base of the skull, travels down the neck alongside the carotid arteries, and passes behind the clavicle (collarbone), where it joins the subclavian vein (the large vein that drains blood from the arms). The jugular is rarely injured because it lies deep in the structures of the neck.

Jungian theory

Ideas put forward by the Swiss psychiatrist Carl Gustav Jung (1875-1961). Originally an associate of Sigmund Freud, Jung broke away in 1913 to form his own school of analytical psychology, mainly because he did not

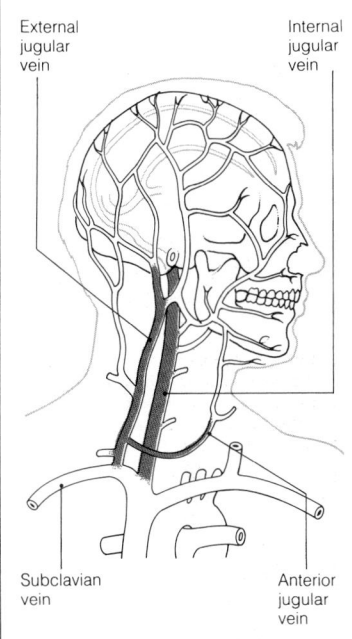

ANATOMY OF THE JUGULAR VEIN
The three veins on each side of the neck that return blood from the head to the heart.

External jugular vein

Internal jugular vein

Subclavian vein

Anterior jugular vein

believe that sexual drive was the only force behind all human activity. Instead, he theorized that certain ideas (called archetypes) inherited from experiences in our distant past were present in each person's unconscious and controlled the way in which each person viewed the world. Jung called these shared ideas the "collective unconscious".

Although Jung believed that each individual also had a "personal unconscious" containing experiences from his or her life, he regarded the collective unconscious as superior. Therapy was therefore aimed at putting people in touch with this source of profound ideas, particularly through the interpretation of dreams.

Jung's therapeutic approach was also based on his theory of personality, which postulated two basic types, the *extravert* and the *introvert*. He believed that one of these types dominates a person's consciousness and that the other must be brought into consciousness and reconciled with its opposite for the person to become a whole individual.

Juvenile arthritis

See *Rheumatoid arthritis, juvenile*.

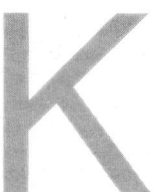

K

Kala-azar

A form of the insect-spread parasitic disease *leishmaniasis*. Kala-azar occurs in many parts of Africa, the Mediterranean area, India, and South America.

Kaolin

An *aluminium* compound used as an ingredient in some *antidiarrhoeal drugs*. Kaolin increases the bulk of the faeces. It is also believed to adsorb *bacteria*, *viruses*, and *toxins* (poisons) from the intestine and transport them through the intestine for excretion in the faeces.

Kaposi's sarcoma

A condition, characterized by malignant skin tumours, which is a prominent feature of *AIDS*. In the past, Kaposi's sarcoma developed slowly and was extremely rare. In patients with AIDS, it is highly aggressive and tumours soon become widespread.

The tumours, consisting of blue-red nodules, usually start on the feet and ankles, spread farther up the legs, and then appear on the hands and arms. In people with AIDS, tumours also commonly affect the gastrointestinal and respiratory tracts, where they may cause severe internal bleeding.

For mild cases of Kaposi's sarcoma, low-dose *radiotherapy* is usually effective. For more severe cases, *anticancer drugs* may be necessary to slow the spread of the tumours.

Kawasaki disease

An acute childhood illness that affects many systems in the body. It is also called mucocutaneous lymph node syndrome. The condition was first observed in Japan in the 1960s. It is becoming increasingly common in western countries. Kawasaki disease usually occurs in the first two years of life. The cause is unknown.

SYMPTOMS

Fever is the first symptom and usually persists for one or two weeks. Other characteristic symptoms are *conjunctivitis*, dryness and cracking of the lips, and swollen *lymph nodes* in the neck. Towards the end of the first week of illness, the palms and soles become red, the hands and feet swell, and a rash similar to that of measles appears over the body. By the end of the second week, the skin at the tips of the fingers and toes peels and the other symptoms subside.

TREATMENT AND OUTLOOK

There is no cure, but *aspirin* may help prevent possible heart complications. Most children make a complete recovery. In about one to two per cent of cases, however, sudden death occurs after the acute phase of the illness, usually due to *coronary artery disease*.

Keloid

A raised, hard, irregularly shaped, itchy scar on the skin. A keloid occurs because of a defective healing process in which an excess of *collagen* (a tough fibrous protein) forms at the site of a healing scar. Keloids occur more commonly in black people than in white people.

Keloids can occur anywhere on the body but are most common over the sternum (breastbone) and over the shoulder. The scars often enlarge after developing and may be unsightly. After several months most keloids flatten and cease to itch.

Injections of *corticosteroid drugs* directly into a keloid may reduce itchiness and cause some shrinkage. Surgical removal is of little use since the new scar that forms is almost always a keloid.

Keratin

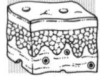 A fibrous protein that is the main constituent of the outermost layer of the *skin*, *nails*, and *hair*. Keratin is a tough substance that is resistant to a wide range of chemical and environmental changes.

Keratitis

Inflammation of the *cornea* (the transparent front part of the eyeball), in contrast to *keratopathy*, noninflammatory disorders of the cornea. Keratitis usually takes the form of a *corneal ulcer*. In interstitial keratitis, which affects about 70 per cent of older children with congenital *syphilis*, the inflammation affects deep corneal tissue.

Symptoms of keratitis include eye pain, excessive watering, blurring of vision, and photophobia (abnormal sensitivity to bright light). If keratitis persists for a long time, blood vessels grow into the cornea.

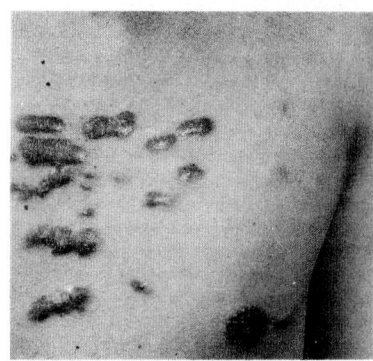

Crop of keloids over the breastbone
These overgrowths of scar tissue usually flatten out and become less noticeable over a period of months or years.

Keratoacanthoma

A harmless skin nodule, which most commonly develops on the face or arm of an elderly person.

A keratoacanthoma initially resembles a small, round wart with a soft centre, and grows rapidly over a period of about eight weeks to reach a maximum size of about 2 cm across. The mature nodule has bulging sides and its centre may have a whitish appearance. Without treatment, the keratoacanthoma slowly disappears after reaching its mature state, but in most cases the patient will prefer to have the nodule removed surgically.

Keratoacanthomas are fairly common. The cause is unknown, but these nodules tend to be more common in people who have had many years of exposure to strong sunlight and in people taking long-term *immunosuppressant drugs*.

Microscopic examination of a small piece of tissue may be necessary to distinguish a keratoacanthoma from a *squamous cell carcinoma* (a form of skin cancer).

Keratoconjunctivitis

Inflammation of the *cornea* associated with *conjunctivitis*. The most common form is epidemic keratoconjunctivitis, caused by a virus that usually causes painful swelling of a small *lymph node* in front of the ear. It is highly infectious and is spread mainly by sharing towels or by unsterile instruments and eye-drops.

The conjunctivitis is often severe, with marked redness, swelling, or destruction of the surface layer of the conjunctiva, leaving a whitish membrane. Seven to 10 days after onset of the disorder, tiny opaque spots resembling snowflakes develop in the cornea. The spots may persist for many months and sometimes interfere with vision.

There is no specific treatment for epidemic keratoconjunctivitis. The corneal opacities can sometimes be minimized by the use of eye-drops containing *corticosteroid drugs*. (See also *Keratoconjunctivitis sicca*.)

Keratoconjunctivitis sicca

A condition of persistent dryness of the *cornea* and *conjunctiva* caused by deficiency in tear production. Commonly referred to as "dry eye", keratoconjunctivitis sicca occurs in *autoimmune disorders* such as *rheumatoid arthritis, Sjögren's syndrome,* and systemic *lupus erythematosus;* all of these conditions can damage the tear-producing glands. Prolonged dryness may cause blurred vision, burning, itching, and grittiness. In severe cases, there may be *corneal ulcers* or scarring of the cornea. The most effective treatment for keratoconjunctivitis sicca is frequent use of artificial tears (see *Tears, artificial*).

Keratoconus

An inherited condition in which abnormal corneal growth causes the central area of the *cornea* to become gradually thinned and conical. The condition affects both eyes.

Keratoconus usually starts around puberty, causing increasing *myopia* (shortsightedness) and a progressive distortion of vision that cannot be fully corrected by glasses. Hard contact lenses improve vision in the early stages but are less effective as the condition progresses.

A *corneal graft* is usually performed when vision has seriously deteriorated and contact lenses are no longer helpful. The results of corneal grafting are generally excellent.

Keratolytic drugs

Drugs that loosen and remove the tough, outer layer of the skin, which is composed mainly of *keratin* (a tough protein). Keratolytic drugs, which include preparations of *urea* and *salicylic acid,* are used in the treatment of skin and scalp disorders, such as *warts,* callosities (see *Callus, skin), acne, dandruff,* and *psoriasis.*

Keratomalacia

A disorder, caused by severe deficiency of *vitamin A,* in which the cornea becomes opaque and ulcerated. Perforation of the cornea is common, often leading to loss of the eye

through infection. Keratomalacia is a common cause of blindness in developing countries. The condition usually occurs only in severely malnourished children and is very rare in developed countries.

Prolonged lack of vitamin A first causes poor vision in dim light, severe dryness of the eyes, and a characteristic foamy patch on the corners of the conjunctiva. There may also be a gritty feeling in the eyelids and abnormal sensitivity to bright light. Treatment with large doses of vitamin A at this stage reverses the effects of the deficiency. Without treatment, the condition leads to irreparable damage and commonly to blindness.

Keratopathy

A general term used to describe a variety of disorders of the *cornea* (the transparent front part of the eyeball).

Actinic keratopathy is damage to the outer layer of the cornea by *ultraviolet light,* either from the sun or from artificial sources, such as sun-lamps or arc-welding torches. The outer layer of the cornea tends to strip off, exposing the nerve endings and causing severe pain. In skiers or mountaineers it is known as snow-blindness.

Exposure keratopathy is damage to the cornea caused by loss of the normal protection afforded by the tear film and the blink reflex. It may occur in a variety of conditions in which the lids inadequately cover the cornea, including severe *exophthalmos, facial palsy,* and *ectropion.*

Keratoplasty

See *Corneal graft.*

Keratosis

A skin growth caused by an overproduction of *keratin* (the tough protein that is the major component of the outer layer of skin). Keratoses occur mainly in the elderly.

TYPES

SEBORRHOEIC KERATOSES Often called seborrhoeic warts, these range from flat, dark brown, rough patches to small, wart-like protrusions and are covered with a greasy, removable crust. Seborrhoeic keratoses occur mainly on the trunk. They are completely harmless but can be unsightly.

SOLAR KERATOSES Small, wart-like, red or flesh-coloured growths that appear on exposed parts of the body as a result of overexposure to the sun over a period of years. Solar keratoses may rarely develop into skin cancer, usually *squamous cell carcinoma.*

TREATMENT

Seborrhoeic keratoses require no treatment unless they are large and unsightly. Solar keratoses must always be removed because of the risk of skin cancer. Removal is usually carried out using *cryosurgery* (the destruction of tissue by extreme cold) or by *curettage.*

Keratosis pilaris

A very common skin condition in which patches of rough skin appear on the upper arms, thighs, and buttocks. The openings of the hair follicles become enlarged by hard plugs of *keratin* (the tough protein that is the major component of the outer layer of skin) and the hairs that grow in them may be distorted.

The condition tends to run in families and occurs most commonly in older children, adolescents, and obese people. It is often worse in winter. Keratosis pilaris is not serious and usually clears up on its own. In severe cases, symptoms can be relieved by rubbing a mixture of salicylic acid and soft paraffin into the affected areas; scrubbing these areas with a loofah may also help.

Keratotomy, radial

A procedure in which radiating incisions are made in the cornea (up to, but not through, its innermost layer) to reduce *myopia* (shortsightedness). It was the first such operation, but other techniques, such as laser reshaping of the cornea, have been developed since. Nevertheless, many thousands of people have had treatment with radial keratomy, mostly with satisfactory results.

Kerion

A red, pustular swelling that develops as a reaction to a fungal infection, usually scalp ringworm (see

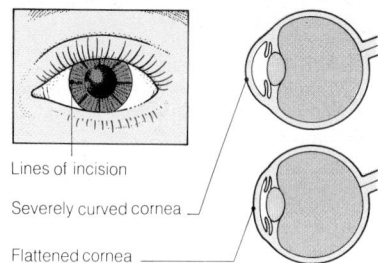

Lines of incision

Severely curved cornea

Flattened cornea

Procedure for keratotomy
Eight or more radial cuts are made in the cornea, avoiding the central zone. During healing, the scars contract, causing the cornea to become flatter and less powerful.

K

Tinea). The inflammation gradually subsides over six to eight weeks but, if severe, may leave a scar and permanent loss of hair from the affected area. Kerion is treated by applying a cream containing an *antifungal drug* to the swelling and by taking the antibiotic drug *griseofulvin*.

Kernicterus

A rare disorder in which newborn, especially premature, infants suffer brain damage as a result of severe jaundice (see *Jaundice, neonatal*). Kernicterus is completely preventable if neonatal jaundice is treated promptly.

In addition to showing signs of jaundice, a baby with kernicterus becomes increasingly listless and may adopt a characteristic posture with the back and neck arched backwards.

Without treatment, affected babies are likely to die at the end of the first week. Less severely affected babies may survive but there will be some degree of permanent brain damage, which may possibly result in a form of *cerebral palsy*.

Ketoconazole

An *antifungal drug* taken by mouth to treat severe *fungal infections* of the lungs, brain, kidney, and lymph glands. Ketoconazole is also applied topically to treat *candidiasis* (thrush) of the skin, mouth, or vagina when other antifungal preparations have proved ineffective.

Ketoconazole tablets may cause nausea (which may be reduced if the drug is taken with food), rash, and, rarely, liver damage.

Ketoprofen

A *nonsteroidal anti-inflammatory drug* (NSAID) prescribed as an *analgesic drug* (painkiller) in the treatment of injury to soft tissues, such as muscles and ligaments. Ketoprofen is also given to reduce joint pain and stiffness in people with types of arthritis, including *rheumatoid arthritis*, *osteoarthritis*, and *ankylosing spondylitis*.

Ketoprofen may cause abdominal pain, nausea, indigestion, and an increased risk of *peptic ulcer*.

Ketosis

A potentially serious condition in which excessive amounts of ketones accumulate in the body. Ketones are substances chemically related to acetone, which is found in solvents such as nail polish remover. Ketosis results whenever glucose is not available to use as a source of energy, which forces the body to use fats instead. This, in turn, leads to fatty acids being released into the blood, where they are converted to ketones.

The underlying causes of ketosis include fasting or starvation, and untreated or inadequately controlled *diabetes mellitus* (in which lack of insulin prevents glucose from being used as fuel). Symptoms and signs include sweet, "fruity"-smelling breath, loss of appetite, nausea, vomiting, and abdominal pain. If the condition is not treated, confusion, unconsciousness, and death may follow.

Ketosis can be diagnosed by a test to detect ketones in the urine. Treatment is the same as for diabetes unless the cause is fasting or starvation, in which case gradual reintroduction of a nutritious diet is usually effective.

Kidney

The organ responsible for filtering the blood and excreting waste products and excess water in the form of *urine*. The kidneys, ureters, bladder, and urethra make up the *urinary tract*.

STRUCTURE

There are two kidneys, each about 10 to 12.5 cm long and about 170 g in weight. They lie in the abdomen below the liver on the right and the spleen on the left. The arteries that supply the kidneys arise directly from the aorta (the main artery of the body leading from the heart). Once within the kidneys, the renal arteries divide into smaller and smaller branches, ending in glomeruli (specialized capillaries that form the filtering units). Each kidney contains about one million glomeruli, which pass the filtered blood through long tubules into the medulla (the central collecting region of the kidney). The glomeruli and tubules make up the nephrons, the functioning units of the kidney. As people age, the number of functioning nephrons is reduced; this process may be speeded up by disease.

FUNCTION

The main functions of the kidney are to regulate blood and *electrolytes* and to eliminate waste products. The most important waste products are those generated by the breakdown of proteins. The kidneys also control the body's *acid-base balance*. When blood and body fluids become too acid or too alkaline, the urine acidity is altered to restore the balance. When excess water is ingested, the kidney excretes it; when water is lost (as a result of diarrhoea or sweating), the kidney conserves it (see *ADH*).

LOCATION OF THE KIDNEYS

The kidneys are situated at the back of the abdominal cavity, just above the waist, on either side of the spinal column. The kidney on the right lies below the liver, while the kidney on the left is situated below the spleen. The arteries that supply the kidneys arise directly from the aorta.

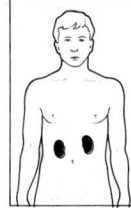

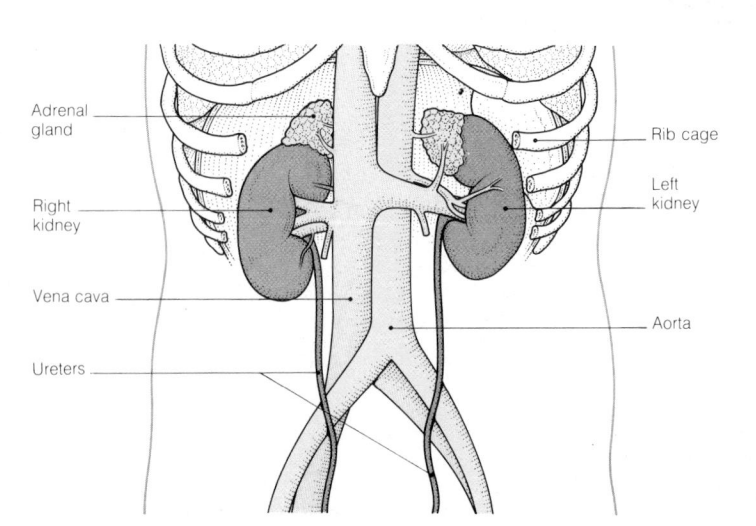

Adrenal gland

Rib cage

Right kidney

Left kidney

Vena cava

Aorta

Ureters

The kidney also produces several hormones, including erythropoietin, which regulates the production and release of red blood cells from the bone marrow. *Vitamin D* is converted into an active hormonal form by the kidney. *Renin*, an enzyme released by the kidney when blood pressure falls, acts on a protein in the blood to produce *angiotensin* (a powerful constrictor of small arteries that helps regulate blood pressure). Angiotensin also controls the release of *aldosterone*, an adrenal hormone that acts on the tubules to promote the reabsorption of sodium and excretion of potassium.

Kidney biopsy

A procedure in which a small portion of *kidney* tissue is removed and examined under a microscope. Kidney *biopsy*, also called renal biopsy, is usually performed as part of the investigation and diagnosis of various kidney disorders, such as *glomerulonephritis*, *proteinuria*, *nephrotic syndrome*, or acute *kidney failure*. It may also be performed to assess the kidneys' response to treatment.

HOW IT IS DONE

There are two basic techniques for performing kidney biopsy: percutaneous (through the skin) and open. The procedure for performing a percutaneous needle biopsy is shown in the illustration.

If a percutaneous needle biopsy is not advisable (e.g. if the patient has a *bleeding disorder* or only one functioning kidney), an open renal biopsy may be performed. With the patient under general anaesthesia, the surgeon makes a small incision in the flank to reveal the kidney and then cuts a small wedge of tissue from the kidney. Biopsy samples of kidney tissue are sent to a pathologist for microscopic examination.

RECOVERY PERIOD

The patient may have slight pain in the back for some hours after the biopsy, and a small amount of blood may be passed in the urine. Provided there are no complications, such as severe bleeding, the patient can return home the following day.

Kidney cancer

A malignant tumour of the *kidney*. Most kidney cancers originate in the kidney itself; in rare instances, cancer may spread to the kidney from another organ.

TYPES

There are three main types of kidney cancer.

RENAL CELL CARCINOMA Also known as hypernephroma or adenocarcinoma, this type of kidney cancer accounts for about 75 per cent of all kidney tumours. It usually occurs after the age of 40 and affects twice as many men as women. The most common symptom is blood in the urine. There may be pain in the loins, a lump in the abdomen, fever, or weight loss. About 25 per cent of patients survive five years or more, the rest dying because the tumour has spread to the lungs, bone, liver, and brain by the time treatment is started.

PERCUTANEOUS KIDNEY BIOPSY

This procedure is performed with a local anaesthetic injected into the skin and tissues over the kidney; it is virtually painless. There is a risk of bleeding from the kidney into the abdominal cavity.

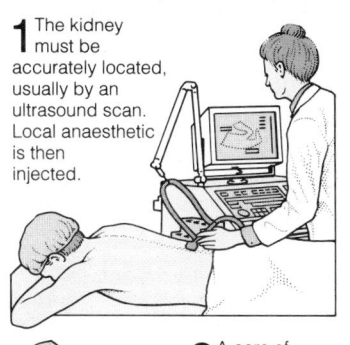

1 The kidney must be accurately located, usually by an ultrasound scan. Local anaesthetic is then injected.

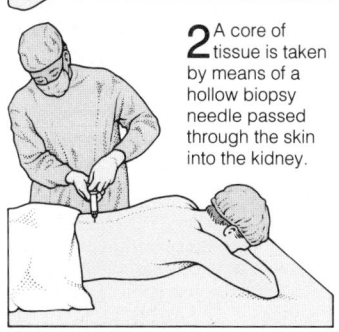

2 A core of tissue is taken by means of a hollow biopsy needle passed through the skin into the kidney.

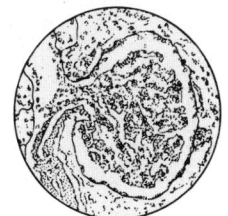

A kidney glomerulus (filtering unit) as seen under a microscope

3 The core of kidney tissue is embedded in wax and cut into thin slices, which are mounted on slides for staining and microscopic examination.

NEPHROBLASTOMA Also called Wilms' tumour, this cancer accounts for approximately 10 per cent of all cancers in children under the age of five; it is rare after that age. Nephroblastoma grows rapidly and is often felt as a lump in the abdomen. This cancer occasionally causes abdominal pain. Nephroblastoma frequently spreads to the lungs, liver, and brain. If treatment is started early, more than 80 per cent of children survive.

TRANSITIONAL CELL CARCINOMA This type of kidney cancer arises from cells lining the renal pelvis. It sometimes develops in tobacco-smokers and in people who have consumed very large quantities of *analgesic drugs* (painkillers) over the course of many years. Blood in the urine is a common symptom; *hydronephrosis* (distension of the kidney with urine) may occur due to blockage of the ureter. Survival rates vary greatly, depending in part on early detection and treatment of the tumour.

DIAGNOSIS AND TREATMENT

Diagnosis is made by *ultrasound*, *CT scanning*, *MRI*, or intravenous *urography*. Treatment consists of *nephrectomy* (removal of the kidney) and sometimes removal of the ureter as well. In the case of a nephroblastoma, nephrectomy is followed by treatment with *anticancer drugs* and, occasionally, by *radiotherapy*.

Kidney cyst

A fluid-filled sac within the *kidney*. Most kidney cysts are noncancerous.

Single kidney cysts probably occur in about half of all people over 50. In some cases, multiple cysts develop in one or both kidneys. Most kidney cysts occur for no known reason and do not usually produce symptoms unless they become large enough to cause pain in the lower back due to pressure.

Kidney cysts also occur in polycystic kidney disease (see *Kidney, polycystic*), a hereditary condition that often leads to *kidney failure* before the age of 50.

DIAGNOSIS AND TREATMENT

Cysts are commonly discovered only when a person is being examined for some other reason. Treatment is not usually necessary. *Aspiration* (withdrawal of fluid by suction) of the cyst may be performed to ensure that there is no malignancy or to relieve severe pain. When the cyst is large, fluid often reaccumulates, requiring surgical removal of the cyst.

K

Kidney failure

The reduction in the ability of the *kidneys* to filter waste products from the blood and excrete them in the *urine,* to control the body's water and salt balance, and to regulate the *blood pressure.* Kidney failure leads to uraemia (a build-up of *urea* and other chemical waste products) and other chemical disturbances in the blood and tissues, leading to symptoms of varying severity.

TYPES AND CAUSES

Kidney failure can be acute (of sudden onset) or chronic (developing more gradually). In acute kidney failure, kidney function usually returns to normal once the underlying cause has been discovered and treated; in chronic failure, function is usually irreversibly lost.

Acute kidney failure most often occurs in people suffering from physiological *shock* as a result of a severe injury or a serious underlying illness. Severe bleeding or burns can reduce blood volume and pressure to the extent that the supply of blood to the kidneys is dramatically reduced. A *myocardial infarction* (heart attack) or acute *pancreatitis* can have a similar effect. The kidneys are particularly susceptible to a reduction in the flow of blood, which can cause damage to the glomeruli (filtering units of the kidneys).

DISORDERS OF THE KIDNEY

The kidneys are susceptible to a wide range of disorders. However, only one normal kidney is needed for good health, so disease is rarely life-threatening unless it affects both kidneys and has reached an advanced stage.

Hypertension (high blood pressure) can be both a cause and effect of kidney damage. Other effects of serious disease or damage include the *nephrotic syndrome* (in which large amounts of protein are lost in the urine and fluid accumulates in body tissues) and acute or chronic *kidney failure.*

CONGENITAL AND GENETIC DISORDERS

Congenital abnormalities of the kidneys are fairly common. In *horseshoe kidney,* the two kidneys are joined at their base. Some people are born with one kidney missing, both kidneys on one side, or a kidney that is partially duplicated and gives rise to two ureters (duplex kidney). These conditions seldom cause problems. In rare cases, a baby is born with kidneys that are so underdeveloped that they are barely functional.

Polycystic disease of the kidneys is a serious inherited disorder in which multiple cysts develop on both kidneys (see *Kidney, polycystic*). In *Fanconi's syndrome* and *renal tubular acidosis* (which are rare), there are subtle abnormalities in the functioning of the kidney tubules, so that certain substances are inappropriately lost in the urine.

IMPAIRED BLOOD SUPPLY

Various diseases may cause damage to, or lead to obstruction of, the small blood vessels within the kidneys, impairing blood flow. *Diabetes mellitus* and *haemolytic-uraemic syndrome* are examples. In physiological *shock,* blood pressure and flow through the kidneys are seriously reduced; this can cause a type of damage known as acute tubular necrosis. The larger blood vessels in the kidney may be affected by *polyarteritis nodosa* and systemic *lupus erythematosus.* In rare cases, there is a defect of the renal artery supplying a kidney, which may lead to hypertension and tissue damage.

AUTOIMMUNE DISORDERS

Glomerulonephritis refers to an important group of autoimmune disorders in which the glomerular filtering units of the kidneys become inflamed. It sometimes develops after infection with streptococcal bacteria.

TUMOURS

Benign *kidney tumours* are rare. They may cause *haematuria* (blood in the urine), although most cause no symptoms. Malignant tumours are also rare. Renal cell carcinoma, the most common type, occurs mostly in adults over 40; nephroblastoma (Wilms' tumour) affects mainly children under four (see *Kidney cancer*).

METABOLIC DISORDERS

Kidney stones are common in middle age. They are usually caused by excessive concentrations of various substances (such as calcium) or lack of inhibitors of crystallization in the urine. In *hyperuricaemia,* there is a tendency for uric acid stones to form (see *Calculus, urinary tract*).

INFECTION

Infection of a kidney is called *pyelonephritis.* An important predisposing factor is obstruction of the flow of urine through the urinary tract, leading to stagnation and subsequent infection spreading up from the bladder. The cause of the obstruction may be a congenital defect of the kidney or ureter, a kidney or ureteral stone, a bladder tumour, or, in a man, enlargement of the prostate gland.

Tuberculosis of the kidney is caused by infection carried by the blood from elsewhere in the body, usually the lungs.

DRUGS

Allergic reactions to certain drugs can cause an acute kidney disease, with most of the damage affecting the kidney tubules. Other drugs may directly damage the kidneys if taken in large amounts for prolonged periods. For example, kidney failure can develop after many years of taking excessive amounts of analgesics. Some potent antibiotics can damage the kidney tubules, producing acute tubular necrosis.

OTHER DISORDERS

Hydronephrosis refers to a kidney swollen with urine as a result of obstruction further down the urinary tract. In the *crush syndrome*, kidney function is disrupted by proteins (released into the blood from severely damaged muscles) that block the filtering mechanisms.

INVESTIGATION

Kidney disorders are investigated by *kidney imaging* techniques such as *ultrasound scanning*, intravenous or retrograde pyelography (see *Urography*), *angiography*, and *CT scanning* or *MRI*, by *kidney biopsy* (removal of a small amount of tissue for analysis); by *blood tests*; and by *kidney function tests*, such as *urinalysis*.

Acute kidney failure may also be caused by obstruction to the urine flow as a result of a stone (see *Calculus, urinary tract, bladder tumour,* or enlarged prostate gland (see *Prostate, enlarged*). Certain rapidly developing types of kidney disease, such as *glomerulonephritis* and *haemolytic-uraemic syndrome,* are other causes of acute kidney failure.

Chronic kidney failure can result from any disease that causes progressive damage to the kidneys, such as *hypertension* (high blood pressure), *diabetes mellitus,* polycystic kidney disease (see *Kidney, polycystic*), or *amyloidosis* (see also *Kidney* disorders box). Longstanding obstruction to the urine flow, due to a stone, tumour, or an enlarged prostate, may also cause chronic kidney failure. Excessive use of *analgesic drugs* (painkillers) over a period of several years is another cause of the condition.

Chronic kidney failure may progress over months or years to an advanced, life-threatening condition called end-stage kidney failure.

SYMPTOMS AND SIGNS
In acute kidney failure, the most noticeable symptom may be a greatly reduced volume of urine. Production of less than 400 ml of urine per day is called *oliguria* and usually means that waste products are not being cleared effectively from the blood. Complete cessation of urine output is called *anuria* and results in a serious build-up of waste products. Some people with kidney failure pass normal amounts of urine despite loss of the filtering and cleansing function of the kidneys; this condition is called nonoliguric acute kidney failure.

Within a short time of the development of acute kidney failure, more symptoms (such as drowsiness, nausea, vomiting, and breathlessness) appear. In many cases, symptoms of the underlying cause of the kidney failure (for example, symptoms of shock such as pale skin and weak pulse) precede those of the kidney failure itself.

Symptoms of chronic failure develop more gradually and may include nausea, loss of appetite, and weakness. Unless the progress of the kidney damage is slowed or arrested, symptoms of end-stage failure may appear (including severe lethargy, weight loss, headache, vomiting, a furred tongue, unpleasant breath, intense, rashless skin itching, and, eventually, collapse, coma, and death).

COMPLICATIONS
Complications of acute kidney failure may include infections such as *pneumonia,* bleeding into the stomach, and deep vein *thrombosis.* In chronic failure, complications due to disturbances in blood chemistry may include high blood pressure (which is both a cause and a result of kidney failure), *anaemia, osteomalacia, hyperparathyroidism* (overactivity of the parathyroid glands), *neuropathy* (nerve disorder), or *myopathy* (muscle disorder).

DIAGNOSIS
A person with suspected kidney failure should undergo *kidney-function tests,* which include measuring the urea and creatinine (two waste products) in the blood; raised levels indicate kidney failure. *Urinalysis* and

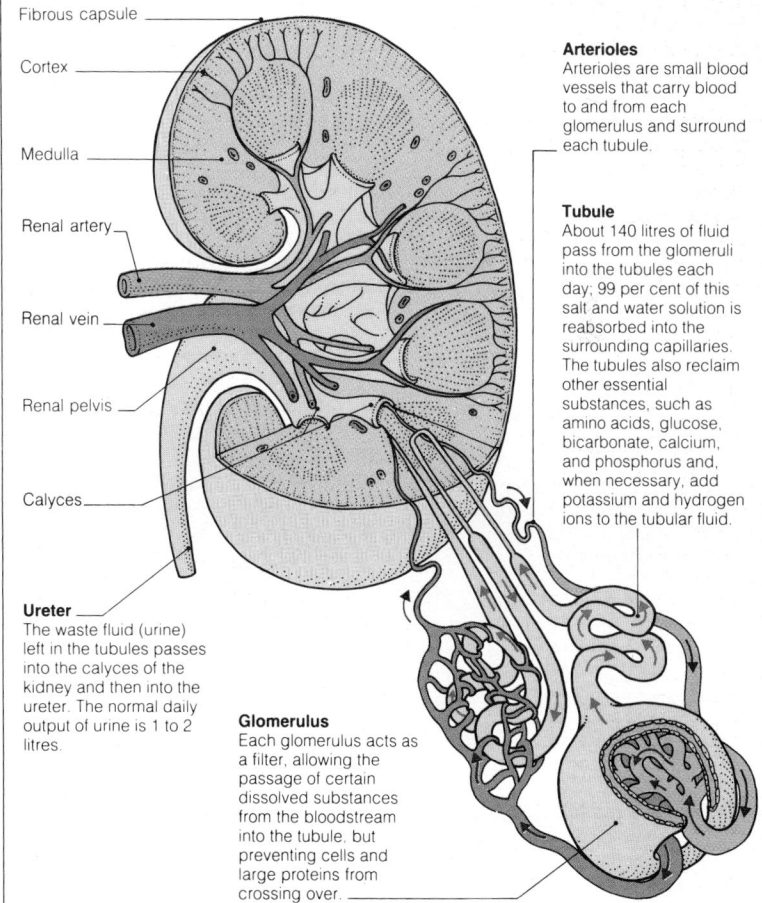

THE FUNCTION OF THE KIDNEY
The kidney is essential to the regulation of the body's fluid balance and acid-base balance. The kidney contains about 1 million nephrons, each of which consists of a glomerulus and a tubule that drain urine into the renal pelvis. Capillaries feed each glomerulus and surround each tubule.

RENAL FUNCTION AND AGE
The efficiency of the kidney diminishes with age as the number of functional nephrons is reduced.

Nephrons per kidney
1,000,000
750,000
500,000
250,000
Age   10 20 30 40 50 60 70 80 90

Fibrous capsule

Cortex

Medulla

Renal artery

Renal vein

Renal pelvis

Calyces

Ureter
The waste fluid (urine) left in the tubules passes into the calyces of the kidney and then into the ureter. The normal daily output of urine is 1 to 2 litres.

Arterioles
Arterioles are small blood vessels that carry blood to and from each glomerulus and surround each tubule.

Tubule
About 140 litres of fluid pass from the glomeruli into the tubules each day; 99 per cent of this salt and water solution is reabsorbed into the surrounding capillaries. The tubules also reclaim other essential substances, such as amino acids, glucose, bicarbonate, calcium, and phosphorus and, when necessary, add potassium and hydrogen ions to the tubular fluid.

Glomerulus
Each glomerulus acts as a filter, allowing the passage of certain dissolved substances from the bloodstream into the tubule, but preventing cells and large proteins from crossing over.

K

blood pressure measurements are also performed. Unless there is an obvious cause of kidney failure (such as severe bleeding), immediate testing is carried out to determine a cause. Techniques include examination of the urine sediment and blood, intravenous *urography*, *kidney biopsy*, *ultrasound scanning*, and *radionuclide scanning*.

TREATMENT

In acute kidney failure, emergency treatment is given for any cause of shock, such as severe bleeding. Blood volume and pressure must be brought back to normal through saline *intravenous infusion* or *blood transfusions*. Surgery may be required for obstruction caused by stones, tumours, or enlargement of the prostate gland. Treatment of other causes may be complex and sometimes controversial, but may include the use of *corticosteroid drugs* and other drugs (as in the treatment of certain forms of glomerulonephritis). *Diuretic drugs* may also be given to improve urine flow and rid the body of excess fluid. In many cases of acute failure, temporary *dialysis* (artificial methods of removing waste products from the blood) may be required until the kidneys recover their function.

Dietary treatment is an important part of the treatment of all types of kidney failure. The diet must be high in carbohydrates and low in protein (the main source of waste products) to reduce the workload on the kidneys; the salt content must also be controlled. Fluid intake is carefully balanced against urine output. If the patient has been taking certain drugs (whose breakdown products are removed from the blood by the kidneys), use of these drugs may be stopped or their dosages reduced.

If hypertension develops, drugs are prescribed to keep the blood pressure under control. In end-stage kidney failure, long-term dialysis or, ideally, a *kidney transplant* is the only satisfactory form of treatment.

OUTLOOK

The outlook varies according to the cause of the failure and the patient's response to treatment. Most people with acute kidney failure eventually make a full recovery, but some require a transplant or lifelong dialysis. In chronic failure, it may be several years before such measures are required. Well over half the people with end-stage kidney failure that is treated by dialysis are able to lead comparatively normal lives for more than five years; a successful kidney transplant improves the outlook.

Kidney-function tests

Tests performed to investigate urinary symptoms and kidney disorders. Kidney-function tests may also be performed as part of a routine investigation before major surgery, or before prescribing drugs that are eliminated by the kidneys. The tests are also performed to determine the function of a transplanted kidney.

TYPES

Urinalysis is a simple kidney-function test. Collected urine is examined under the microscope for blood cells, pus cells, and casts (cells and mucous material that accumulate within the tubules and pass into the urine). Urine may also be cultured to confirm the presence of infection, and may also be tested for substances, such as proteins, that are present only when the kidneys are diseased or damaged.

Kidney function can be assessed by measuring the concentration of substances in the blood (such as *urea* and creatinine) normally eliminated from the body via healthy kidneys. The creatinine clearance test provides an assessment of kidney function by comparing the amount of creatinine in the blood with the amount excreted in the urine over a timed interval, usually 24 hours.

Kidney function may also be assessed by *kidney imaging* techniques, which can help identify whether one or both kidneys are diseased.

Kidney imaging

Techniques for visualizing the kidneys, usually performed for diagnostic purposes.

TYPES

Ultrasound scanning provides remarkably clear pictures of the kidney. It can show an enlarged kidney, indicate the site of any blockage, and show the presence of a cyst or other tumour.

Conventional *X-rays* show the outlines of the kidney and most kidney stones. Intravenous *urography* (in which a radiopaque contrast medium is injected into a vein) gives a good picture of the internal anatomy of the kidney and ureters, as well as the presence of stones. *Angiography* involves injecting a radiopaque substance into the renal arteries or veins to demonstrate the kidneys' blood supply. When a radiopaque substance is injected into the arteries, the technique is known as arteriography. Digital subtraction angiography permits imaging of the renal circulation with less contrast medium and greater safety.

CT scanning and *MRI* provide complete cross-sectional images—generated by advanced computers—of the kidney, and are especially useful for showing abscesses or tumours.

Radionuclide scanning is cheaper than conventional X-rays and exposes the patient to less radiation. The two types usually used for the kidney are the DMSA scan and the DTPA scan. DMSA is a substance given by intravenous injection that binds to the cells of the kidney tubules and gives a single static picture of the kidneys, indicating their relative size, shape, position, and function. DTPA, also given intravenously, is filtered by the glomeruli and passes out in the urine. Pictures are taken at intervals to record its passage through the renal tract. DTPA provides similar information to that provided by the intravenous urogram, although the anatomical details are less clear.

Kidney, polycystic

An inherited disorder in which there are numerous cysts in both *kidneys*. The cysts gradually increase in size until most of the normal kidney tissue is destroyed; cysts may also occur in the liver and, rarely, in other organs. Polycystic kidney disease is distinguished from multiple simple cysts of the kidneys, which occur commonly with age (see *Kidney cyst*).

TYPES

ADULT POLYCYSTIC DISEASE This disorder shows an autosomal dominant pattern of inheritance (see *Genetic disorders*). Symptoms, which may appear at any time (but usually appear in middle age) include abdominal swelling, pain, and *haematuria* (blood in the urine). As the disease progresses, *hypertension* (high blood pressure) and *kidney failure* may result. The kidneys are replaced by very large numbers of small cysts.

JUVENILE POLYCYSTIC DISEASE This rare disorder causes *kidney failure* in infants and young children. It is usually diagnosed at birth because of massive enlargement of the kidneys. Juvenile polycystic disease shows an autosomal recessive pattern of inheritance.

TREATMENT

There is no effective treatment for preserving kidney function in polycystic kidney disease. Symptoms of kidney failure can be treated by *dialysis* (artificial purification of the blood) and *kidney transplant*.

Kidney stone

See *Calculus, urinary tract*.

KIDNEY IMAGING

The various kidney imaging techniques provide invaluable information in the investigation and diagnosis of kidney disorders.

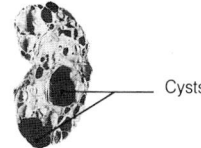

Polycystic kidney
The photograph (left) shows a section through an abnormal kidney from a person with polycystic kidney disease.

Cysts

CT SCANNING AND MRI

These use different scanning methods to produce cross-sectional images displayed as computer-generated pictures. Cystic kidneys are clearly visible on this CT scan.

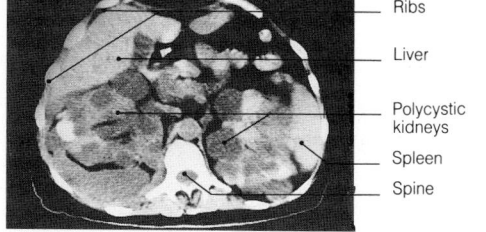

Ribs
Liver
Polycystic kidneys
Spleen
Spine

IVU (INTRAVENOUS UROGRAPHY)

This gives an impression of the anatomy of the kidneys. Here, contrast medium can be seen in the dilated calyces of these abnormal kidneys.

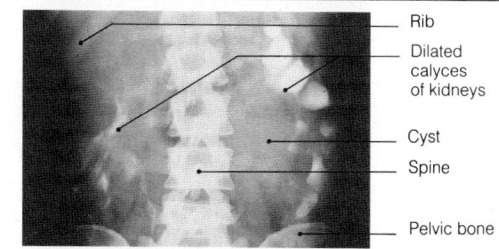

Rib
Dilated calyces of kidneys
Cyst
Spine
Pelvic bone

ULTRASOUND SCANNING

This is a quick technique, which provides clear images of the structure of the kidney. Here, the cysts can be clearly differentiated from the surrounding kidney tissue.

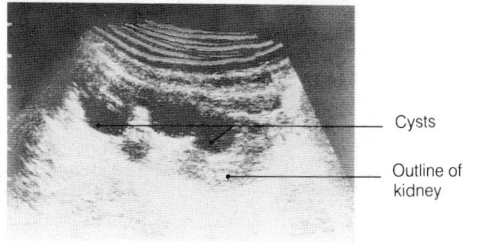

Cysts
Outline of kidney

Kidney transplant

An operation in which the function of a diseased kidney in a person who has chronic *kidney failure* is replaced by a transplanted healthy kidney, either from a living donor or a cadaver. One healthy donor kidney is sufficient to maintain the health of the recipient.

Kidney transplantation is more straightforward than the transplantation of any other major organ and is by far the most commonly performed. Furthermore, the failure of a kidney transplant is much less serious than failure of a heart, liver, or lung transplant because kidney function can be taken over by *dialysis* (artificial purification of the blood).

HOW IT IS DONE
For a description of a kidney transplant operation, see the illustrated box overleaf.

OUTLOOK
Kidney transplants are successful in more than 80 per cent of cases. This figure rises to more than 90 per cent if the donor is a close blood relative. The chief danger is rejection of the donated kidney within the first month or two after transplantation. If the kidney is rejected, the patient returns to dialysis. Further transplants may be attempted if the patient is otherwise in good health. All kidney transplant patients must take *immunosuppressant drugs* for life to prevent rejection.

Kidney tumours

Growths of the kidney. Kidney tumours may be malignant (see *Kidney cancer*) or benign.

Fibromas, lipomas, and *leiomyomas* (which are benign) often cause no symptoms and are sometimes dis-

covered only during kidney surgery performed for another cause. A kidney may be the site of a *haemangioma* (a benign tumour composed of a collection of blood vessels), which may grow very large, and may cause blood to appear in the urine; a kidney haemangioma is sometimes mistaken for cancer.

No treatment is necessary for benign tumours unless they are very large or cause pain or bleeding.

Kilocalorie

The unit of energy equal to 1,000 *calories*, sometimes abbreviated to kcal. In dietetics, a kilocalorie is sometimes called simply a Calorie (or C).

Kilojoule

The unit of energy equal to 1,000 *joules*, abbreviated to kJ. One kcal equals 4.2 kJ.

Kiss of life

A commonly used name for *artificial respiration*.

K

Kleptomania

A recurring inability to resist impulses to steal objects that are not necessarily wanted or needed. The condition is rare, although it is often used by shoplifters and other thieves as an excuse for stealing.

While true kleptomania is rare, shoplifting is sometimes an indication of depressive illness. There is a sense of tension before the theft followed by a feeling of relief while carrying it out. Little thought is given to the consequences, although later the person may suffer from anxiety and depression caused by fear of being caught.

Kleptomania is usually a sign of an immature personality. It may also be caused by *dementia* or result from some forms of brain damage.

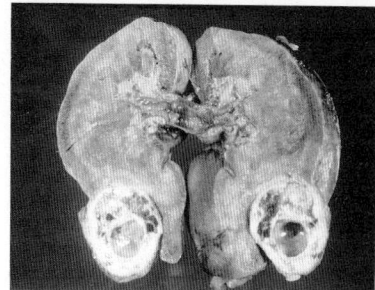

Example of a kidney tumour
A malignant tumour of one kidney (sliced in half). Surgical removal of a malignant kidney tumour is always necessary.

PROCEDURE FOR A KIDNEY TRANSPLANT

The donated kidney comes from a close (living) relative of the patient or from any person who consented to medical use of organs after death (cadaver transplant). The latter are mainly patients who have been declared brain dead. Those dying from head injuries and brain haemorrhage make up the majority of cadaveric donors. To prevent rejection of the kidney by the recipient's *immune system*, the tissue-type and blood group of recipient and donor must be a close match (see *Transplant surgery*).

(see *Transplant surgery*)

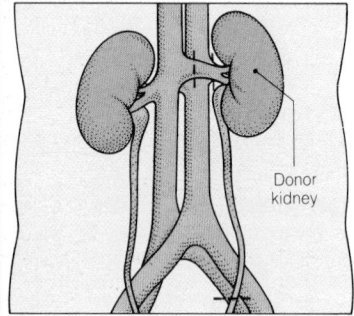

Donor kidney

1 Usually the left kidney is removed from living donors because it has a longer vein than the right and is easier to remove safely. With cadaveric donation both kidneys are used. After removal, the kidneys are flushed with chilled saline solution and an anticoagulant.

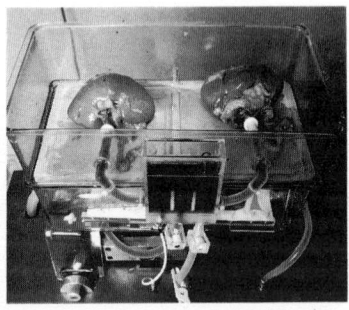

2 Kidneys from a cadaver can be maintained for transplantation by a machine that passes a cooling saline solution through them. The kidneys should be transplanted into the recipients (each kidney usually goes to a separate recipient) as soon as possible, but there is a reasonable success rate if transplantation is delayed for up to 48 hours.

DIALYSIS AND TRANSPLANTATION

A significant proportion of patients with end-stage kidney failure are suitable for a kidney transplant, but many have to remain on dialysis for some time until a suitable donor kidney becomes available. A computer system is used to match donors with the most suitable recipients. The number of available donor kidneys is considerably less than the number of people waiting for a transplant.

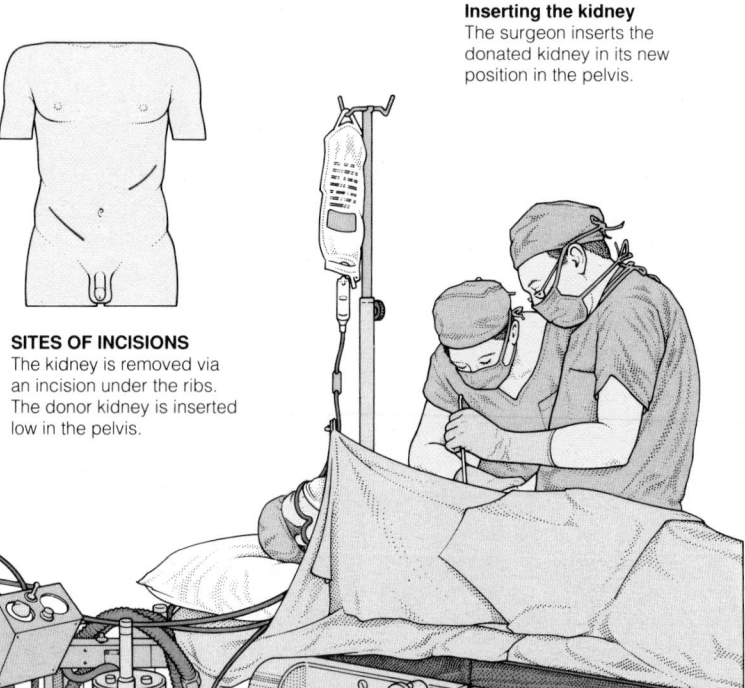

SITES OF INCISIONS
The kidney is removed via an incision under the ribs. The donor kidney is inserted low in the pelvis.

Inserting the kidney
The surgeon inserts the donated kidney in its new position in the pelvis.

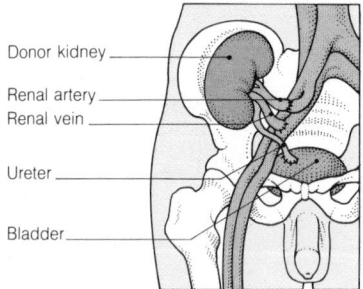

Donor kidney

Renal artery

Renal vein

Ureter

Bladder

3 The donor kidney is usually placed in the pelvis. The renal artery and vein of the donor kidney are joined to a convenient artery (usually a branch of the external iliac artery) and vein of the recipient. The lower end of the donor ureter is connected to the recipient's bladder. The donor kidney usually begins working immediately after transplantation.

THE DONOR (AFTER THE OPERATION)

The health of the donor is not affected by losing one kidney; the remaining kidney enlarges to take over full function. Not unusually afterwards, the donor has a more positive outlook on life.

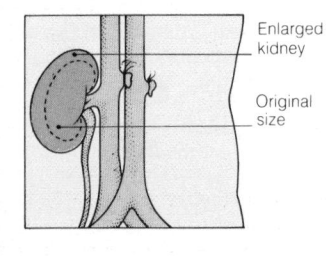

Enlarged kidney

Original size

Klinefelter's syndrome

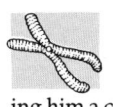

A *chromosomal abnormality* in which a male has one or more extra X *chromosomes* in his cells, giving him a chromosome complement of XXY or, more rarely, XXXY, XXXXY, and so on (instead of XY). Klinefelter's syndrome affects about one in every 500 male infants born. The chances of a baby having the condition increase with the age of the mother.

SYMPTOMS AND SIGNS

The features of Klinefelter's syndrome vary in severity. Often the condition passes unnoticed until puberty, when *gynaecomastia* (breast enlargement) occurs and the testes remain small. Affected males are usually infertile due to *azoospermia* (absence of sperm production). They are usually tall and thin, and the body shape looks female rather than male. The incidence of *mental handicap* is higher in people with Klinefelter's syndrome than in the general population.

DIAGNOSIS AND TREATMENT

Diagnosis is confirmed by *chromosome analysis*. There is no cure for Klinefelter's syndrome. Mastectomy may be performed if gynaecomastia causes psychological distress. Hormonal treatment may be used to induce secondary *sexual characteristics*, such as growth of facial hair. Parents who have had an affected child should receive *genetic counselling*.

Klumpke's paralysis

Paralysis of the lower arm, with wasting of the small muscles in the hand and numbness of the fingers (excluding the thumb) and of the inside of the forearm.

Klumpke's paralysis is caused by injury to the first thoracic nerve (one of the *spinal nerves*) in the brachial plexus (the network of nerves behind the shoulderblade); injury to this nerve is usually the result of dislocation of the shoulder.

Knee

The joint between the *femur* (thighbone) and *tibia* (shin). The *patella* (kneecap) lies across the front of the joint. The knee is a modified hinge *joint*, which is capable of bending, straightening, and slight rotation in the bent position.

STRUCTURE

Two discs of protective cartilage called menisci (see *Meniscus*) cover the surfaces of the femur and tibia. These discs reduce friction between the bones during movement and also increase the stability of the knee. The joint is partly surrounded by a fibrous capsule lined with synovial membrane, which secretes a fluid that allows the cartilage to move freely.

Strong *ligaments* on each side of the joint provide support and limit side-to-side movement. *Cruciate ligaments* within the joint, which cross over each other as they run diagonally between the femur and tibia, provide additional support, prevent overbending and overstraightening of the knee, and limit sliding movement between the bones.

Bursas (fluid-filled sacs) are present above and below the patella and behind the knee. The *quadriceps muscles* (which run along the front of the thigh) straighten the knee; the *hamstring muscles* at the back of the thigh bend the knee.

DISORDERS

Sudden twisting of the knee may cause a ligament sprain or tear a meniscus. If a meniscus is torn and a fragment of the cartilage catches between the surfaces of the joint, the knee may become temporarily locked in one position.

Severe damage to a joint, often as the result of a sports injury, may cause *haemarthrosis* (bleeding into the joint); minor injuries may lead to *synovitis* (inflammation of the joint lining).

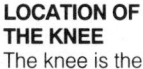
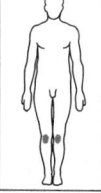

LOCATION OF THE KNEE
The knee is the joint that is situated between the femur and the tibia. The patella lies across the front of the joint.

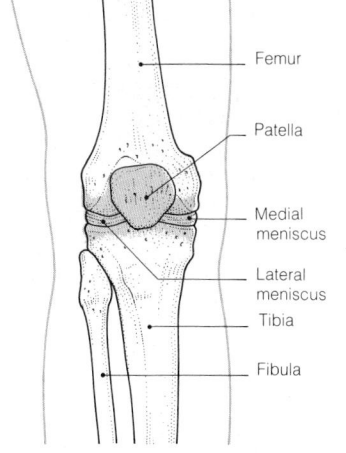

Femur

Patella

Medial meniscus

Lateral meniscus

Tibia

Fibula

Repetitive activity, such as running, may cause inflammation of the tendon below the patella.

Children may suffer from *Osgood-Schlatter disease*, in which the bony tibial tuberosity (the bony prominence below the knee) becomes temporarily inflamed.

Bursitis (inflammation of a bursa) usually occurs in response to local pressure on the front of the knee. Fluid escaping from a bursa behind the knee causes a *Baker's cyst*.

Arthritic conditions most likely to affect the knee are *osteoarthritis, rheumatoid arthritis,* and retropatellar arthritis (inflammation of the undersurface of the patella). A condition similar to retropatellar arthritis, known as *chondromalacia patellae* or anterior knee pain, is common in adolescents.

Fractures of the lower femur, upper tibia, or the patella disrupt normal movement of the knee. A blow to the knee may result in *dislocation* of the patella.

Knock-knee and *bowleg* are common temporary deformities in childhood, which usually disappear as growth continues; in adults, these deformities may be caused by injury or disease.

K

Knee-joint replacement

A surgical procedure to replace a diseased *knee* joint with an artificial substitute. Early replacement knees were simply large hinges. Today, most artificial knees take the form of metal and plastic implants that cover the worn cartilage. The aim of modern knee-joint replacement operations is generally to preserve as much of the original joint as possible.

WHY IT IS DONE

Knee-joint replacement is most often carried out in older people whose knees are severely affected by pain and impaired motion due to *osteoarthritis* or *rheumatoid arthritis*. An artificial knee is not normally recommended for younger patients because it does not restore the full range of movements and is unlikely to withstand vigorous activity.

RECOVERY PERIOD

The plaster *cast* fitted after the operation is usually removed after five days and a programme of exercises is started to strengthen the *quadriceps muscles*. The patient can normally put some weight on the leg after two or three weeks.

OUTLOOK

Improvements that have been made in the design of replacement knee

PROCEDURE FOR A KNEE REPLACEMENT

The surgeon usually makes one long incision, cuts through the joint capsule and synovial membrane, and then pushes aside the patella to reach the joint. Special instruments are used to make precise measurements and to cut away areas of bone so that the artificial knee replacement components will fit and move correctly.

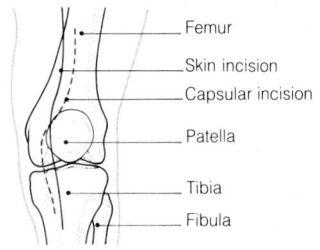

Femur
Skin incision
Capsular incision
Patella
Tibia
Fibula

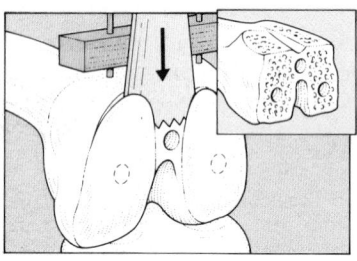

1 The lower end of the femur (thigh-bone) is shaped and holes are drilled into it to accept the femoral component of the prosthesis. Cutting and drilling bones are carried out using special orthopaedic instruments.

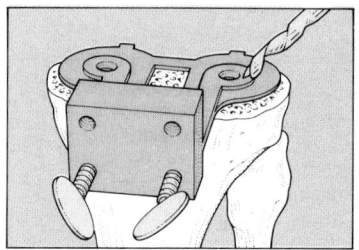

2 The upper end of the tibia (shin-bone) is shaped and holes are drilled into it to accept the tibial component of the prosthesis. The cutting and drilling are again carried out using special orthopaedic instruments.

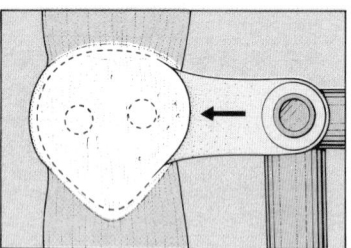

3 The back part of the patella is cut away to leave a flat surface. Small holes are then drilled into this surface to accept the patellar component of the artificial joint.

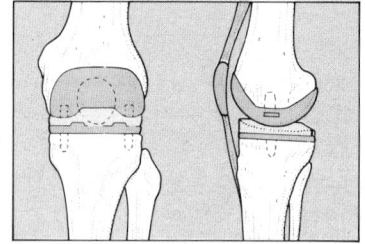

4 Having achieved a satisfactory fit using trial components, the final prosthesis is cemented in place. Excess cement is then removed and a final check is made of the joint movements.

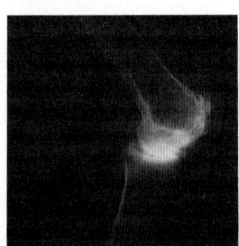

X-ray of arthritic knee
Severe wear and tear of the bone and cartilage can easily be seen on this knee X-ray.

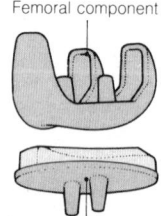

Femoral component

Tibial component

Knee prosthesis
The two main artificial knee components fit over the femur and tibia.

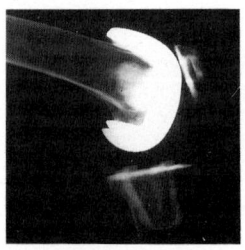

X-ray of artificial knee
This X-ray shows the components of the prosthesis in position after surgery.

joints—and the cements used to fix them—have led to steadily better results. The outcome of a knee-replacement operation is now at least as good as that of a hip replacement: around 90 per cent are functioning well five years after surgery.

Knock-knee

Inward curving of the legs so that the knees touch, causing the feet to be kept farther apart. The condition is known medically as genu valgum.

CAUSES

Knock-knee is a part of normal development in some children and is common between the ages of three and five years. It may also be the result of injury or disease. Among the common causes are diseases that soften the bones (such as *rickets* or *osteomalacia*), *rheumatoid arthritis* or *osteoarthritis* of the knee, or a fracture of the lower *femur* (thigh-bone) or upper *tibia* (shin) that has not healed in a straight, vertical line.

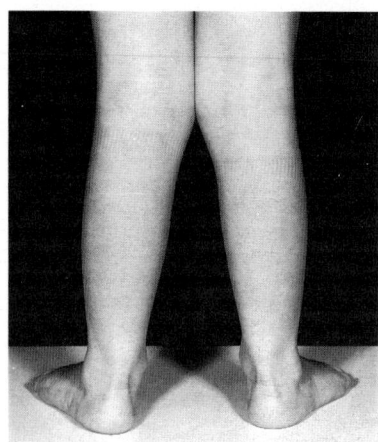

The appearance of knock-knee
This condition is common in toddlers but nearly always disappears by the age of seven.

TREATMENT

In children, knock-knee usually requires no treatment unless it persists after the age of 10, when it may start to strain the joints of the lower leg. Wearing heel wedges in the shoes may help correct the line of the leg, but most people require *osteotomy*, an operation in which the tibia is cut and realigned to straighten the leg.

In adults, treatment consists of osteotomy, or, when the condition has been present for a considerable time, *knee-joint replacement*.

Knuckle

The common name for a *finger* joint.

Koilonychia

A condition in which the *nails* are dry, brittle, and thin, eventually becoming concave (spoon-shaped). Koilonychia may be caused by injury to the nail; koilonychia of the toenails is very common in countries where shoes are not worn. Other causes include iron deficiency *anaemia* and *lichen planus*; rarely, the condition is inherited.

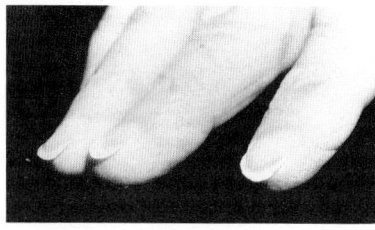

The appearance of koilonychia
In koilonychia, the nails are flattened and look fragile, bending where they protrude past the finger ends.

Koplik's spots

Tiny, grey-white spots within the mouth (on the inner lining of the cheeks) that appear during the incubation period of *measles*. If they are identified, the physician can diagnose measles before the main rash appears.

Korsakoff's psychosis

See *Wernicke-Korsakoff syndrome*.

Kraurosis vulvae

See *Vulvitis*.

Kuru

A progressive and fatal infection of the *brain* that affects some inhabitants of the highlands of New Guinea. Kuru is caused by a virus spread by cannibalism. The condition is now rare.

The disease is caused by a "slow" virus (which causes no signs of disease until many months or years after entry into the body) and the incubation period may be as long as 30 years. Symptoms include progressive difficulty in controlling movements and, eventually, *dementia*.

Kuru has aroused special interest recently because of certain similarities between the causative virus and *HIV* (the virus that causes *AIDS*). It is known that HIV can cause brain changes similar to those in kuru.

Kwashiorkor

A severe type of malnutrition in young children, occurring mainly in poor rural areas in the tropics. Kwashiorkor is chiefly confined to children between one and three years old.

The term kwashiorkor is derived from a Ghanaian word meaning "disease suffered by a child displaced from the breast".

CAUSES

The illness starts when the child is suddenly weaned on to a diet that is low in calories, protein, and certain essential micronutrients such as zinc, selenium, and vitamins A and E. The problem is often exacerbated by a poor appetite due to illness. Measles and other infections common in the tropics precipitate kwashiorkor in undernourished children.

SYMPTOMS AND SIGNS

Children with kwashiorkor have stunted growth, and a puffy appearance due to *oedema* (accumulation of fluid in the tissues). Affected children are apathetic, weak, irritable, and inactive. Their skin sometimes flakes off, leaving a raw, weeping area beneath, and their hair may lose its curliness, become sparse and brittle, and turn from dark to fair.

The liver often enlarges, dehydration may develop (despite the simultaneous presence of oedema), and the child loses resistance against severe infection, which may be fatal. In its severe, advanced stage, the illness is often marked by jaundice, drowsiness, and a fall in body temperature.

TREATMENT

The priorities in severe cases are to keep the child warm, replace lost fluids, and treat any infection. Ini-

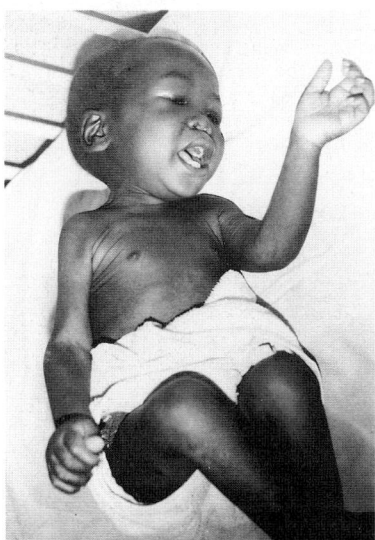

The appearance of kwashiorkor
This small child has a puffy face and legs, is listless, and has sparse hair, all of which are typical features of kwashiorkor.

tially, the child is fed milk (in frequent small amounts) and, if possible, vitamin and mineral tablets. Zinc is given to prevent flaking of the skin. When the oedema has disappeared and the child's appetite has returned, a high-calorie, protein-rich diet is given.

OUTLOOK

Most children treated for kwashiorkor recover, but those less than two years old are likely to suffer permanent stunting of growth. Of the children who are ill enough to be admitted to hospital, about 85 per cent survive. (See also *Marasmus*.)

Kyphoscoliosis

A combination of *kyphosis* (abnormal backward curvature of the spine) and *scoliosis* (curvature of the spine to one side or the other).

Kyphosis

The medical term for excessive backward curvature of the spine. Kyphosis usually affects the spine at the top of the back, resulting in either a hump or a more gradually rounded back. Less commonly, it affects normally forward-curving parts of the spine at the neck and lower back.

K

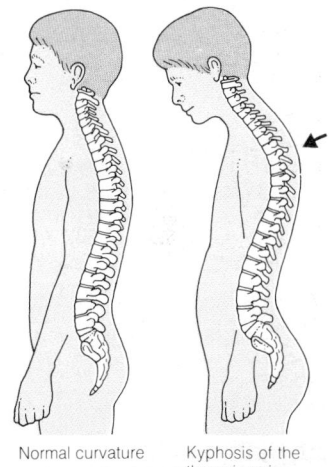

Normal curvature   Kyphosis of the thoracic spine

The appearance of kyphosis
In kyphosis, the thoracic part of the spine is excessively curved, producing a humped (rounded) appearance.

Kyphosis may be caused by any of a variety of spinal disorders, including *osteoporosis* (thinning of bone due to calcium loss), fracture of a vertebra, or a tumour of a vertebra (see *Spine* disorders box). In the past, the main cause of kyphosis was spinal *tuberculosis*. Treatment, which is rarely successful, is of the underlying disorder.

L

Labetalol

A *beta-blocker drug* used to treat *hypertension* (high blood pressure) and *angina pectoris* (chest pain caused by impaired blood supply to the heart).

Possible adverse effects include indigestion, nausea, and, in rare cases, depression and temporary impotence. Labetalol is less likely than some other beta-blocker drugs to cause leg cramps or coldness of the hands and feet.

Labia

The lips of the *vulva* (the female external genitalia) that protect the vaginal and urethral openings. There are two pairs of labia. The outer pair, called the labia majora, are fleshy folds that bear hair and contain sweat glands. The labia majora cover the smaller, hairless inner folds, called the labia minora, which meet to form the hood of the *clitoris*.

Labile

Unstable; likely to undergo change. Vitamins are labile because they are broken down easily by such factors as heat and excess acidity. Blood pressure that has a tendency to fluctuate may be described as labile. In psychiatry, the term is sometimes used to mean emotional instability.

Labour

See *Childbirth*.

Labyrinthitis

Inflammation of the labyrinth (the fluid-filled chambers in the inner *ear* concerned with balance) causing *vertigo*, a sensation that one or one's surroundings are spinning around.

CAUSES

Labyrinthitis is almost always caused by bacterial or viral infection. Viral labyrinthitis may occur during a flu-like illness or during illnesses such as measles or mumps. Bacterial labyrinthitis is commonly caused by inadequately treated *otitis media* (infection of the middle ear), particularly if a *cholesteatoma* (an infected collection of debris in the middle ear) has developed and eroded a pathway into the inner ear. Infection may also reach the inner ear (via the bloodstream) from elsewhere in the body. Less commonly, bacterial labyrinthitis results from a head injury.

SYMPTOMS AND TREATMENT

As well as vertigo, labyrinthitis may cause nausea, vomiting, *nystagmus* (abnormal jerky movements of the eye), *tinnitus* (ringing in the ears), and hearing loss.

Viral labyrinthitis clears up on its own, but symptoms are relieved by *antihistamine drugs* such as meclozine. Bacterial labyrinthitis requires immediate treatment with *antibiotic drugs*; otherwise the infection may lead to permanent *deafness* or spread to cause *meningitis* (inflammation of the membranes covering the brain).

Surgery may be necessary to drain pus from the ear or to remove any cholesteatoma.

Laceration

A torn, irregular wound, as opposed to an *incision*, which is a straight cut. One example of a laceration is the tearing of the perineum (the area between the vagina and anus) that sometimes occurs during childbirth.

Lacrimal apparatus

The system that produces and drains *tears*. The lacrimal apparatus includes the main and accessory lacrimal glands and the nasolacrimal drainage ducts. The main glands secrete tears during crying and when the eye is irritated; the accessory glands maintain the normal tear film.

The main lacrimal glands lie just within the upper and outer margin of

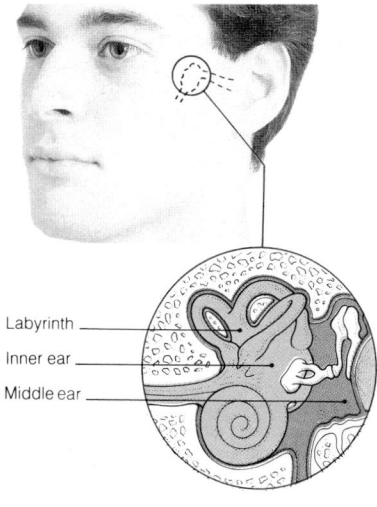

Mechanism of labyrinthitis
In labyrinthitis, inflammation of the fluid-filled chambers (labyrinth) of the inner ear causes disruption of the individual's sense of balance. The inflammation is usually caused by viral or bacterial infection.

the orbit and drain into the *conjunctiva* (the transparent membrane covering the white of the eye and the inside of the eyelids). The accessory glands lie within the conjunctiva, secreting directly on to its surface.

Tears sweep across the front of the eye, and drain through the lacrimal puncta, tiny openings towards the inner end of each eyelid. The puncta are connected by narrow tubes to the lacrimal sacs, which lie in shallow hollows in the lacrimal bones. These bones are situated just within the inner margin of the orbit on either side of the nose. Overlying the lacrimal sacs are flat muscles that compress the sacs during blinking. Leading from the sacs are the nasolacrimal ducts, which run down through the bone to open inside the nose.

The action of blinking sucks away excess fluid by compressing and releasing the lacrimal sacs.

Lactase deficiency

A condition in which lactase, an *enzyme* that is normally present in cells of the small intestine and which breaks down lactose (milk sugar), is missing. Lactase deficiency results in a reduced ability to digest lactose.

TYPES

Lactase deficiency may be present at birth, may develop immediately after weaning, or may not become evident until puberty or later.

LOCATION OF THE LABIA
The labia majora extend forwards from the perineum and fuse at the front at the mons pubis. The labia minora lie within.

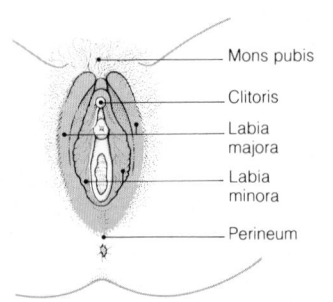

Mons pubis

Clitoris

Labia majora

Labia minora

Perineum

FUNCTIONS OF THE LACRIMAL APPARATUS

Tear production must be sufficient to compensate for evaporation and maintain the tear film. Accessory lacrimal glands in the conjunctiva perform this function. The main lacrimal glands secrete when excess fluid is required. Surplus tears drain into the nose.

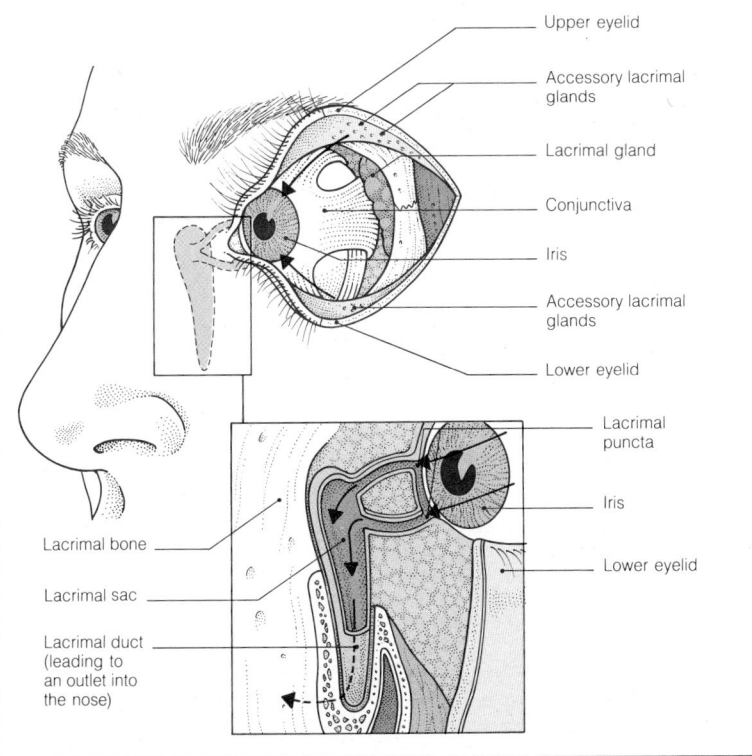

Upper eyelid
Accessory lacrimal glands
Lacrimal gland
Conjunctiva
Iris
Accessory lacrimal glands
Lower eyelid
Lacrimal puncta
Iris
Lower eyelid
Lacrimal bone
Lacrimal sac
Lacrimal duct (leading to an outlet into the nose)

Congenital lactase deficiency is sometimes permanent but is more often temporary. It is caused by delayed enzyme maturation, and occurs especially in premature babies.

Permanent lactase deficiency develops in about 80 to 90 per cent of blacks and Orientals and in about five to 15 per cent of whites. Lactase deficiency may also occur as a complication of intestinal diseases (including *coeliac disease* and *gastroenteritis*); in such cases, the deficiency often disappears as the disease improves.

SYMPTOMS, DIAGNOSIS, AND TREATMENT
Undigested lactose ferments in the intestine and causes severe abdominal cramps, bloating, flatulence, and diarrhoea; weight loss and malnutrition may also occur.

The diagnosis can be confirmed by tests on blood and faeces. Treatment is a lactose-free diet; milk must be avoided but fermented milk products, such as yogurt, can be eaten. Enzyme replacements (which break down lactose either partially or fully) may be used in some cases.

Lactation
The production and secretion of milk after childbirth. (See *Breast-feeding*.)

Lactic acid
A weak acid produced when cells break down glucose by anaerobic metabolism (chemical processes that do not require oxygen) to produce energy. Anaerobic metabolism occurs only when there is too little oxygen for the more usual aerobic metabolism (chemical processes requiring oxygen). For example, lactic acid is produced by muscles during vigorous exercise and is one of the factors that contributes to *cramp*. Lactic acid is also produced in tissues when they receive insufficient oxygen due to impairment of their blood supply in a *myocardial infarction* (heart attack) or *shock*.

Normally, lactic acid is removed from the blood by the *liver*; if lactic acid accumulates, a condition called lactic *acidosis* results.

Lactose
One of the sugars present in milk. Chemically, lactose is a disaccharide *carbohydrate*, a sugar made up of two monosaccharide (simple sugar) units.

Lactose is broken down by lactase (an *enzyme* released by the lining of the small intestine) into the monosaccharides glucose and galactose, which are then absorbed into the bloodstream. People with *lactase deficiency* have a reduced ability to digest lactose.

Lactose intolerance
The inability to digest lactose (milk sugar). Lactose intolerance may be caused by a deficiency of lactase, an enzyme found in the small intestine (see *Lactase deficiency*). Rarely, lactose intolerance occurs in a person who is not deficient in lactase.

Lactulose
A *laxative drug* used to treat *constipation* and *liver failure*. Lactulose causes water to be absorbed into the faeces from the intestinal blood vessels, making the faeces easier to pass. It is useful in the treatment of liver failure because it helps eliminate ammonia from the blood into the faeces.

Lambliasis
Another name for *giardiasis*.

Laminectomy
Surgical removal of part or all of one or more laminae (the bony arches of the *vertebrae*) to expose the *spinal cord*. Laminectomy is performed as the first stage of spinal canal decompression, an operation carried out to relieve pressure on the spinal cord or on a nerve root leading from it (see *Decompression, spinal canal*).

HOW IT IS DONE
An incision is made in the patient's back and the laminae are exposed. Enough of one or more adjacent laminae is then chipped away to give the surgeon access to the cord. Rarely, several complete laminae must be removed. In this case, *spinal fusion* (immobilization of the spine with metal rods or bone grafts) may then be necessary to prevent subsequent instability of the spine.

Lance
To incise (cut) using a *lancet* or a surgical scalpel.

Lancet

A small, pointed, double-edged knife used to open and drain lesions such as boils and abscesses.

Language disorders

Problems affecting the ability to communicate and/or comprehend the spoken and written word. See *Speech; Speech disorders*.

Lanolin

A mixture of a yellow, oily substance obtained from sheep's wool and purified water, used as an *emollient* in the treatment of dry skin. Lanolin is a common ingredient of bath oils and hand creams; it is also used to treat mild *dermatitis*. Occasionally, lanolin may cause an allergic reaction.

Lanugo hair

Fine, soft, downy hair that covers a *fetus*. Lanugo hair first appears in the fourth or fifth month of gestation and usually disappears by the ninth month. It can still be seen in some premature babies.

Lanugo hair sometimes reappears in adults who have cancer, particularly of the breast, bladder, lung, or large intestine. It may also occur in those with *anorexia nervosa* or be a side-effect of certain drugs (especially *cyclosporin*).

Laparoscopy

Examination of the interior of the abdomen using a laparoscope, a type of *endoscope* (viewing instrument). It may be a simple viewing device using a lens and optical fibres, or it may incorporate a small video camera in its tip so that an image may be magnified and viewed on a monitor.

WHY IT IS DONE

Laparoscopy may used in the diagnostic assessment of a patient with acute abdominal pain due, for example, to appendicitis or pancreatitis; surgical procedures such as *appendicectomy* and *cholecystectomy* are now often performed laparoscopically, to avoid the need for large incisions (see *Minimally invasive surgery*). Laparoscopy is widely used in gynaecology for the diagnosis of pelvic pain, and as part of the management of infertility; after stimulation of the ovaries by fertility drugs, several ova may be removed for *in vitro fertilization*. Women are now usually sterilized laparoscopically.

Laparotomy

An operation in which the abdomen is opened to look for the cause of an undiagnosed illness. The term describes any abdominal surgery since, even when the surgeon is operating to treat a known disorder, a thorough examination of the abdomen is carried out.

Laparotomy is now less common than formerly because of the availability of diagnostic procedures such as *CT scanning*, *ultrasound scanning*, and *laparoscopy*.

WHY IT IS DONE

A laparotomy is most often performed nowadays because of problems encountered during laparoscopic surgery. It may be necessary if complications develop that cannot be treated using *minimally invasive surgery*.

HOW IT IS DONE

An incision is made in the abdomen and the abdominal cavity is opened and explored for signs of disease. Any diseased organs are repaired or removed, after which the incision is sewn up.

The recovery period depends upon the nature and extent of the disease discovered and treated.

Larva migrans

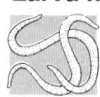

Infections characterized by the presence of the larval (immature) forms of certain worms in the body and by the symptoms caused by movement of the worms.

Visceral larva migrans, better known as *toxocariasis*, is caused by a type of worm that normally parasitizes dogs. Cutaneous larva migrans is caused by larvae of species of hookworm that normally parasitize dogs, cats, or other animals. Also known as creeping eruption, cutaneous larva migrans is contracted by walking barefoot on soil or sand contaminated with animal faeces. The larvae penetrate the skin of the feet and move randomly, leaving intensely itchy red lines which are sometimes accompanied by blistering.

Both types of larva migrans can be treated with *anthelmintic drugs*, such as thiabendazole.

Laryngeal nerve

One of a pair of nerves that carries instructions from the brain to the *larynx* (voice box) and sends sensa-

---

PROCEDURE FOR LAPAROSCOPY

A hollow needle is inserted into the abdomen just below the navel (under anaesthesia), and carbon dioxide gas is pumped through the needle to expand the abdominal cavity. The laparoscope (see below) is then inserted through another incision to view the internal organs. The gas in the abdomen may cause discomfort for a day or two afterwards.

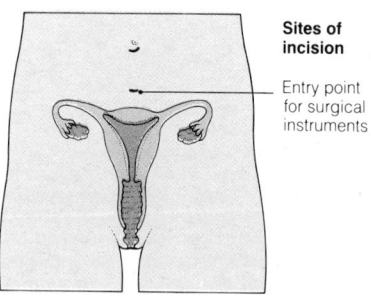

Sites of incision

Entry point for surgical instruments

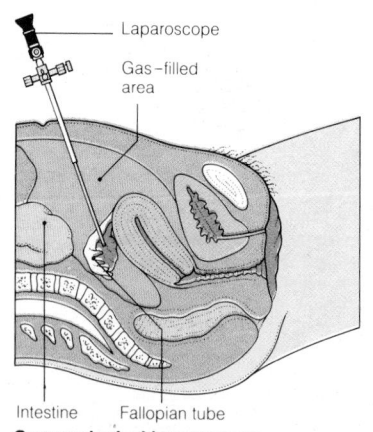

Laparoscope

Gas–filled area

Intestine   Fallopian tube

Gynaecological laparoscopy
Laparoscopy is used in diagnosis and for removing ova for in vitro fertilization. Laparoscopic sterilization is a common sterilization procedure for women.

THE LAPAROSCOPE

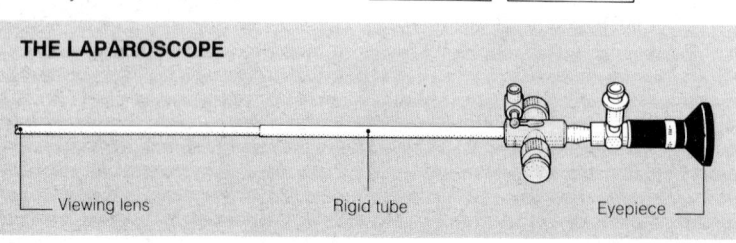

Viewing lens   Rigid tube   Eyepiece

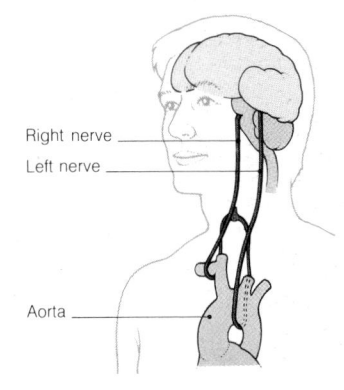

LOCATION OF LARYNGEAL NERVES
Both nerves leave the brain at the base of the skull and pass down the neck. One hooks around an artery behind the right clavicle, the other hooks around the aorta; both return to the larynx.

Right nerve
Left nerve
Aorta

tions from the larynx to the brain. Each nerve leaves the brain through a hole in the base of the skull and passes down the neck. The right laryngeal nerve then hooks around an artery behind the clavicle (collarbone) before returning to the larynx. The left laryngeal nerve travels farther, hooking around the aorta (the major artery leaving the heart) before passing back to the larynx.

Damage to one or both nerves causes *vocal cord* paralysis, resulting in loss of voice and sometimes obstruction to breathing.

Laryngectomy
Surgical removal of all or part of the *larynx* (voice-box) to treat advanced cancer of the larynx (see *Larynx, cancer of*). After the operation, the patient is unable to speak in the usual fashion.

WHY IT IS DONE
If cancer of the larynx is detected early, the prospects of curing it with *radiotherapy* are good. However, large tumours, and those that are not responding to radiotherapy, require surgical removal.

HOW IT IS DONE
With the patient under general anaesthesia, an incision is made in the neck and the larynx is removed. The top of the trachea (windpipe) immediately below the larynx is then sewn to the skin around the surgical wound in the neck to form a permanent opening called a stoma, through which the patient will breathe from then on.

RECOVERY PERIOD
Immediately after the operation, a bell or buzzer and pen and paper are given to the patient so that he or she can communicate. A tube is left in the stoma for a few days so that, as the surrounding tissues heal, they do not close the opening. The air in the patient's room is humidified to reduce the production of mucus in the stoma, and any excess mucus is sucked away.

Initially, all food is passed through a thin tube running from the nose to the stomach. After about 10 days the feeding tube is removed and food (fluid or semi-solid at first) can be taken normally again.

Speed of recovery depends on the patient's age and health and on whether pre-operative radiotherapy has been given.

OUTLOOK
With persistence, the patient can learn from a speech therapist a new way of speaking (called oesophageal speech). Air is swallowed, then expelled in a controlled way; this noise is modulated by the tongue, palate, and lips to form gruff, though distinguishable, words. The technique requires painstaking practice. Alternatively, a silicone tube can be inserted to connect the oesophagus and the trachea; the patient blocks the stoma with a finger, and air is shunted from the lungs into the throat to generate speech; some devices have an automatic valve. Another solution is a vibrating device held in contact with the neck.

Laryngitis
Inflammation of the *larynx* (voice-box) usually caused by infection and resulting in *hoarseness*. Laryngitis may be acute, lasting only a few days, or chronic, persisting over a long period.

CAUSES
Acute laryngitis is usually caused by a viral infection, such as a cold, but it can also be due to an allergy to a drug, pollen, or some other substance.

Chronic laryngitis may be caused by overuse of the voice, by violent coughing, by irritation due to tobacco smoke, alcohol, or fumes, or by damage during surgery.

SYMPTOMS AND SIGNS
Hoarseness is the most common symptom and may progress to loss of voice. There may also be pain or a feeling of discomfort in the throat (especially during swallowing) and a dry, irritating cough. Laryngitis caused by a viral infection is often accompanied by fever and a general feeling of illness.

TREATMENT
A person with laryngitis should rest in bed, avoid tobacco and alcohol, keep the throat lining moist with humidifiers, and take drugs such as *paracetamol* to reduce fever and relieve pain.

If the symptoms do not subside within four or five days, if sputum (phlegm) is coughed up, or if hoarseness persists for several weeks, a doctor should be consulted. *Antibiotic drugs* will be prescribed if there is a bacterial infection. If the doctor suspects a cause other than infection, diagnostic tests may be required, possibly to check for signs of cancer (see *Larynx, cancer of*), which can be cured if treated at an early stage.

Laryngoscopy
Examination of the *larynx* (voice-box) using a mirror held against the back of the palate (indirect laryngoscopy), or a viewing tube called a laryngoscope (direct laryngoscopy). A laryngoscope may be either rigid or flexible.

WHY IT IS DONE
The larynx is inspected when a person complains of persistent hoarseness or has other changes in the voice, when there is persistent stridor (a harsh noise when breathing in), or when someone has difficulty breathing in. Laryngoscopy is also used to examine people who have throat pain or difficulty in swallowing.

INDIRECT LARYNGOSCOPY This technique may be used to detect *laryngitis*, benign or malignant laryngeal tumours, and any reduction of movement in the vocal cords.

DIRECT LARYNGOSCOPY This technique allows the doctor to inspect the larynx in greater detail, and to use an operating microscope. It also allows more elaborate procedures to be performed, such as *biopsy* (removal of a sample of tissue for microscopic analysis), or removal of a foreign body or benign tumour. Direct laryngoscopy is also performed before *intubation*.

HOW IT IS DONE
Indirect and direct laryngoscopy procedures are shown in the illustrated box overleaf.

Laryngotracheobronchitis
Inflammation of the *larynx*, *trachea*, and *bronchi*. Laryngotracheobronchitis is caused by a virus in a quarter to a third of cases; in some other cases, a bacterial infection is involved. Laryngotracheobronchitis can be a mild disorder but can sometimes be life-threatening. It is a common cause of *croup* in young children.

L

L

PROCEDURE FOR LARYNGOSCOPY

There are two techniques. In indirect laryngoscopy, the patient's throat is examined with the use of a mirror. In direct laryngoscopy, the patient's throat is viewed with an instrument called a laryngoscope. If a rigid laryngoscope is used, general anaesthesia is required. Only mild sedation is needed if a flexible laryngoscope is used.

INDIRECT LARYNGOSCOPY

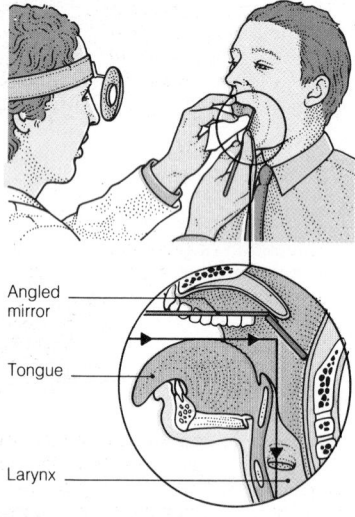

Angled mirror

Tongue

Larynx

The patient sticks out his or her tongue and the doctor rests an angled mirror on the soft palate. A lamp or mirror on the doctor's head illuminates the larynx, which is reflected in the mirror.

DIRECT LARYNGOSCOPY

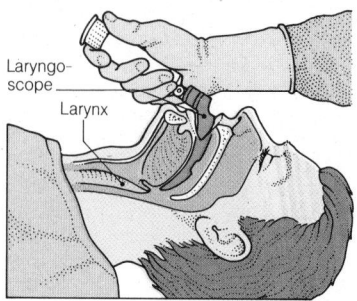

Laryngo-scope

Larynx

A rigid laryngoscope is passed down the throat via the mouth; a flexible laryngoscope is passed via the nostril.

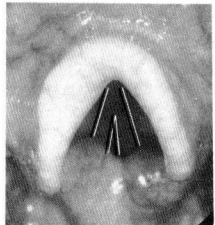

View of larynx
This view was obtained with a laryngoscope. The vocal cords (outlined in red) are at the centre and the epiglottis forms the arc at the top.

LOCATION OF THE LARYNX
The larynx, commonly called the voice-box, is situated deep in the throat between the pharynx and the trachea (windpipe).

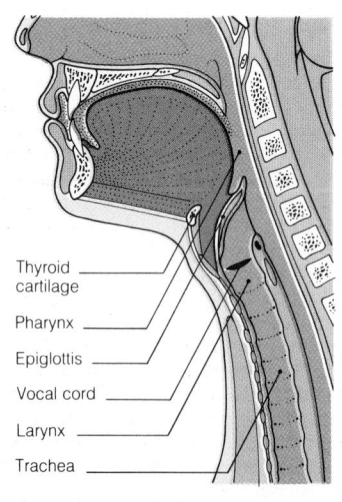

Thyroid cartilage

Pharynx

Epiglottis

Vocal cord

Larynx

Trachea

Larynx
The organ in the throat responsible for voice production and for preventing food from entering the airway during swallowing. Its common name is the voice-box.

STRUCTURE
The larynx, which lies between the *pharynx* (upper part of the airway) and the *trachea* (windpipe), forms part of the tube in the throat that carries air to and from the lungs. It consists of areas of cartilage (tough but flexible tissue), the largest of which is the thyroid cartilage, which projects at the front to form the Adam's apple. Below it, connecting the thyroid cartilage to the trachea, is the cricoid cartilage, which is shaped like a signet ring with the seal at the back. Situated on top of the seal are the two pyramid-shaped arytenoid cartilages. Between them and the interior surface of the Adam's apple stretch two fibrous sheets of tissue, the *vocal cords*, which are responsible for voice production.

Attached to the top of the thyroid cartilage at the entrance to the larynx is the *epiglottis*, a leaf-shaped flap of cartilage that prevents food from entering the larynx during swallowing. The entire larynx is lined with *mucous membrane*.

FUNCTION
The most important function of the larynx is to prevent *choking*. When a person is not eating or drinking, the epiglottis stays upright, keeping the larynx open as part of the airway to the lungs; as soon as swallowing begins, the epiglottis drops like a lid over the larynx, directing food to either side. Closure of the vocal cords also helps protect the airway. The food or drink then passes down the *oesophagus* to the stomach.

The secondary function of the larynx is voice production. Air from the lungs passes through the stretched vocal cords. The resultant vibrations are modified by the tongue, palate, and lips to produce *speech*.

Larynx, cancer of
A malignant tumour of the *larynx* (voice-box), often causing persistent hoarseness. Laryngeal cancer represents about two per cent of all cancers.

CAUSES AND INCIDENCE
The exact causes of laryngeal cancer are not known, but it occurs most commonly in heavy smokers. Laryngeal cancer is also associated with high alcohol consumption.

Laryngeal cancer primarily affects people over 60 and is more common in men than in women.

SYMPTOMS
Hoarseness is the main symptom, particularly when the tumour originates on the vocal cords. A tumour that develops elsewhere in the larynx often passes unnoticed until an advanced stage of the disease, when the tumour causes discomfort in the throat, difficulty in breathing and in swallowing, and the coughing up of blood.

DIAGNOSIS
Laryngoscopy (examination of the larynx with a viewing instrument) reveals any tumour on the larynx. A *biopsy* (removal of a sample of tissue for microscopic analysis) is carried out in hospital under local or general anaesthesia to determine whether the growth is benign or malignant, and also to find out whether or not the lining of the larynx shows any signs of early cancerous change.

TREATMENT
If the tumour is discovered when it is still small, the outcome is usually favourable. A small cancer of the *vocal*

DISORDERS OF THE LARYNX

Disorders affecting the larynx (voice-box) are common. They usually cause *hoarseness* because they interfere with the functioning of the vocal cords. Other symptoms include breathing difficulty, stridor (a harsh noise on breathing in), a painful throat, and coughing. Persistent hoarseness should be reported to a doctor.

CONGENITAL DEFECTS
Rarely, a baby is born with a soft, limp larynx, a condition called laryngomalacia. The main signs are stridor and noisy breathing when feeding. The larynx usually attains a normal firmness by the age of two.

INFLAMMATION
Laryngitis (inflammation of the larynx) is the most common laryngeal disorder in adults; symptoms are hoarseness, fever, and discomfort in the throat. In children, *croup* (inflammation and narrowing of the air passages) is very common up to the age of four. Much rarer is *epiglottitis* (inflammation of the epiglottis, the flap of cartilage that closes the larynx during swallowing). This is a life-threatening disorder in young children.

TUMOURS
Various kinds of benign growth may develop on the vocal cords. The most common is a polyp, a smooth swelling usually caused by smoking, by an infection such as influenza, or by straining the voice. Warts occasionally develop on a child's vocal cords. Both polyps and warts require removal and microscopic analysis to exclude cancer. *Singer's nodes* are small benign growths that can occur on the vocal cords of people who strain their voices. They give the voice a hoarse tone.

Malignant tumours, which cause persistent hoarseness, are usually caused by smoking and/or alcohol use (see *Larynx, cancer of*).

OTHER DISORDERS
A tumour, an infection, or, rarely, throat surgery can damage one or both of the nerves supplying the larynx, causing *vocal cord* paralysis, which results in loss of voice and may interfere with breathing.

INVESTIGATION
Disorders of the larynx are investigated by *laryngoscopy*. Sometimes a *biopsy* sample is taken for pathological analysis; X-rays, especially *tomography*, may provide more information.

---

cords has about a 95 per cent chance of cure. In these cases, *radiotherapy* or *laser treatment* may be used.

For unresponsive and large tumours, partial or total *laryngectomy* (removal of the larynx) is considered unless the patient is frail or elderly. The cure rate varies according to the site and extent of the tumour. Those who have had a laryngectomy must master new techniques for producing speech.

If the tumour has spread throughout the larynx, or to other parts of the throat (or, rarely, other parts of the body), the patient is treated with radiotherapy and *anticancer drugs*. This combination relieves symptoms and often temporarily arrests the progress of the disease.

Laser
A device that produces a concentrated beam of light radiation; laser is an acronym for light amplification by stimulated emission of radiation. A laser beam is parallel, of a single specific wavelength (or sometimes of a narrow band of wavelengths), and coherent (that is, all the crests of the individual waves coincide).

Laser treatment
The use of a *laser* beam in a variety of medical procedures, for example, to cut through tissue, seal small retinal tears, or destroy some tumours.

LOW-INTENSITY TREATMENT
Treatment with low-intensity beams stimulates tissue healing and reduces pain, inflammation, and swelling. It works by improving blood and lymph flow and by reducing the production of *prostaglandins* (hormone-like substances that stimulate inflammation and cause pain). Low-intensity beams are used in the treatment of muscle tears, ligament sprains, and inflamed tendons and joints.

HIGH-INTENSITY TREATMENT
High-intensity treatment destroys cells directly under the beam while leaving adjacent cells undamaged, making it useful in the treatment of some tumours. The beam cuts through tissue and, simultaneously, causes blood clotting, making it a useful surgical tool.

LASERS IN OPHTHALMOLOGY Lasers are used in the treatment of diabetic *retinopathy* (to coagulate, and so prevent bleeding from abnormal blood vessels), to prevent and treat *retinal detachment* (by sealing small tears or areas of degeneration in the retina), to burn a hole in the iris (to reduce excess pressure in the eye in *glaucoma*), and to destroy small tumours of the retina. The laser can also be used to reshape the cornea as a treatment for *myopia* and to restore vision if the lens capsule becomes opaque after *cataract surgery*.

LASERS IN GYNAECOLOGY Laser beams are sometimes used to unblock fallopian tubes by removing scar tissue formed after infection or a *sterilization* procedure. Lasers are also used to destroy abnormal cells in the *cervix*.

OTHER USES Lasers are commonly used to remove small birthmarks and tattoos; they are also effective in removing or improving the appearance of *port-wine stains*. Early malignant tumours of the larynx can be successfully removed without damaging the vocal cords.

Many new applications are currently being investigated. Potential uses include the removal of atherosclerotic *plaque* from inside arteries. It may also be possible to use lasers to disintegrate bladder and kidney stones, and to remove otherwise inaccessible tumours of the brain and spinal cord. (See also illustrated box overleaf.)

Lassa fever

A dangerous infectious disease caused by a virus. Lassa fever, which was first reported in Lassa, Nigeria, in 1969, occurs in occasional outbreaks in West Africa; a small number of cases have been imported into Europe and the US.

In Africa, where the virus is harboured by a type of rat, infection may be acquired by inhaling droplets of an infected rat's urine. Medical and nursing staff are at risk of acquiring the virus from the blood of an infected person or from droplets coughed into the air. However, no one in the UK has ever acquired the disease from an infected person.

L

USE OF A LASER

The concentrated beam of light released by a laser has a variety of medical purposes. When set to low intensity, the laser works to stimulate tissue healing and reduces pain, inflammation, and swelling. At high intensity, the beam destroys cells on which it is focused while leaving adjacent tissue unharmed. It can also cut through tissues without causing bleeding.

Argon laser
Photocoagulation of blood vessels occurs when the blue-green light from this laser is absorbed by haemoglobin.

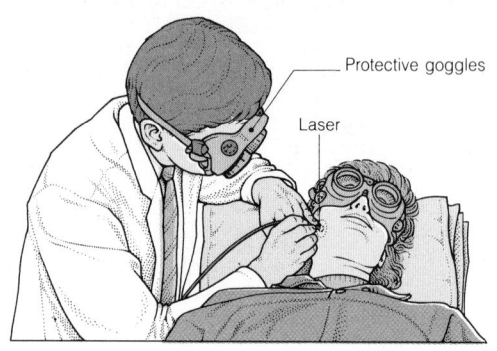

Protective goggles

Laser

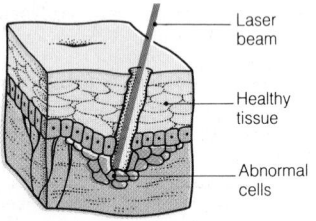

Laser beam

Healthy tissue

Abnormal cells

Focused carbon dioxide laser
This laser is ideal for precision cutting or for destroying abnormal cells because its focused beam leaves surrounding areas of tissue intact.

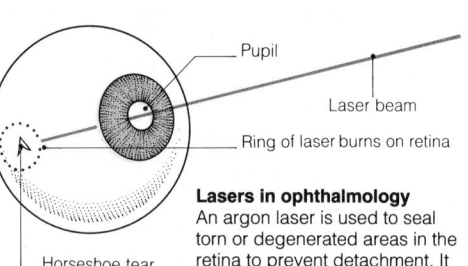

Pupil

Laser beam

Ring of laser burns on retina

Horseshoe tear in retina

Lasers in ophthalmology
An argon laser is used to seal torn or degenerated areas in the retina to prevent detachment. It is also used to treat diabetic retinopathy.

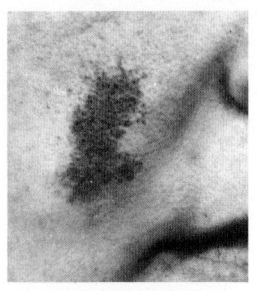

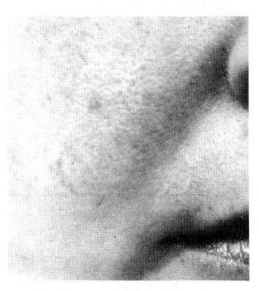

Removing skin blemishes
These photographs, taken before and after laser treatment, show removal of a port-wine stain. In some cases, treatment is less successful, leaving scars.

SYMPTOMS AND TREATMENT

After an incubation period of three to 17 days, the illness starts with fever, headache, muscular aches, and a sore throat. Later, severe diarrhoea and vomiting develop. In extreme cases, the patient's condition deteriorates rapidly in the second week. About one quarter to one third of hospitalized patients die from the illness.

Lassa fever can be diagnosed by a blood test. Infected people must be isolated. Patients are treated by the relief of symptoms and by injections of the *antiviral drug* ribavirin and of serum containing *antibodies* active against the virus.

Lassitude
A term describing a feeling of *tiredness*, weakness, or exhaustion.

Lateral
Relating to, or situated on, one side. Bilateral means on both sides.

Latissimus dorsi
A large, flat, triangular muscle in the back. Its fibres arise from the spines of the lower six thoracic (chest) vertebrae and from the back of the pelvis; they converge on a small tendon that is attached to the humerus (upper-arm bone) just below the shoulder. Contraction of the muscle moves the arm downwards and backwards.

Laudanum
A solution of *opium* once used as a sedative and painkiller and in the treatment of diarrhoea.

Laughing gas
The popular name for *nitrous oxide*, a gas inhaled in combination with oxygen to produce general *anaesthesia*. Laughing gas is so called because of the euphoric effects it produces.

Laurence-Biedl-Moon syndrome
A very rare inherited disorder characterized by increasing *obesity*, *retinitis pigmentosa* that may lead to blindness, *mental handicap*, *polydactyly*, and *hypogonadism*. The condition shows an autosomal recessive pattern of inheritance (see *Genetic disorders*).

Laurence-Biedl-Moon syndrome is probably caused by a disorder of the *hypothalamus* (part of the brain that controls hormone balance). There is no treatment. Parents of an affected child should seek *genetic counselling*.

Lavage, gastric
Washing out the stomach with water, usually to remove poisons.

HOW IT IS DONE

The patient is placed face-down with his or her head below the level of the stomach and turned to one side. A lubricated tube is passed down the oesophagus into the stomach and a funnel is attached to the top. (If the patient is not fully conscious, a tube is also passed down the throat into the trachea to prevent regurgitated water and stomach contents from entering the lungs.) Water is poured into the funnel until the stomach is filled. The top of the tube is then lowered, allowing the fluid in the stomach to drain into a bucket. This process is repeated until the water returns clear. An early sample of fluid from the stomach is kept so that the poison can be analysed. In certain cases, an antidote to the poison (or a neutralizing agent) is added to the water or is passed into the stomach after lavage is finished.

Lavage is not used if a corrosive poison has been swallowed because of the risk that the tube may perforate tissues. Corrosive acids or alkalis may be diluted by giving large amounts of water or milk (see *Poisoning*).

Laxative drugs

WARNING
If constipation lasts for more than a
week, consult your doctor; you may
have a serious underlying disorder.

A group of drugs used to treat *con-stipation*. The use of laxative drugs can often be avoided by eating a diet containing plenty of *fibre*, by drinking plenty of liquids, and by adopting proper toilet habits. Laxative drugs should generally be used only when straining should be avoided (e.g. following childbirth, abdominal surgery, or a *myocardial infarction*). Laxative drugs are sometimes used to clear faeces from the intestine before surgical or investigational procedures.

TYPES
BULK-FORMING LAXATIVES These laxatives increase the volume and softness of faeces by absorbing water in the intestine. Increased bulk stimulates propulsion of faeces through the intestine and makes them easier to pass.

STIMULANT LAXATIVES These drugs stimulate the intestinal wall to contract and as a consequence speed up the elimination of faeces. Because the faeces spend less time in the intestine, less water is reabsorbed into the blood vessels, which helps keep the faeces soft.

LUBRICANT LAXATIVES These substances soften and thus facilitate the passage of faeces. Liquid paraffin is the commonest substance used.

OSMOTIC LAXATIVES These laxatives cause fluid to be retained in the intestine, thus increasing the water content and volume of the faeces.

POSSIBLE ADVERSE EFFECTS
If they are used in excess, laxative drugs may cause diarrhoea. Prolonged treatment may cause dependence on the laxative drug for normal bowel action; laxative use should

therefore be stopped as soon as normal habits are re-established.

Stimulant laxatives and lactulose may cause abdominal cramps and flatulence. Prolonged use of some osmotic laxatives is likely to cause a chemical imbalance in the blood. Lubricant laxatives may coat the intestine, and may also impair vitamin absorption.

Lazy eye
An ambiguous name for the visual defect that commonly results from *squint*. See *Amblyopia.*

Lead poisoning
Damage to the brain, nerves, red blood cells, and digestive system, caused by inhaling lead fumes or swallowing lead salts.

Acute poisoning, which is now relatively rare but sometimes fatal, occurs when a large amount of lead is taken into the body over a short period of time. Chronic poisoning results from small amounts of lead being taken in over a longer period. The body excretes lead very slowly, which therefore accumulates in the body tissues (primarily in the bones). There is some evidence that lead in amounts that are insufficient to cause detectable physical effects may cause mental impairment, particularly in children.

CAUSES AND INCIDENCE
Lead poisoning has occurred in children who have licked or eaten old paint that contains high levels of lead. Adults most at risk include workers in such industries as lead smelting, soldering, demolition, battery manufacture, and pottery glazing. Inhaling the fumes from burning battery casings containing lead may also cause lead poisoning. Eating acidic food or drink that is stored or cooked in lead-glazed or lead-soldered containers has also caused lead poisoning.

The importance of petrol fumes as a cause of lead poisoning is still being debated, but the use of lead-free petrol is reducing the amount of lead in the atmosphere. Few modern paints contain lead.

SYMPTOMS AND SIGNS
Lead poisoning can cause severe, colicky, abdominal pain, diarrhoea, and vomiting. There may also be *anaemia,* loss of appetite, and a blue, black, or grey line along the gum margins. Lead poisoning may also produce weakness or paralysis of the limbs, but such symptoms due to lead poisoning are now almost unknown. Also now very

uncommon is severe lead encephalopathy (disturbance of brain function due to lead poisoning), which may cause headaches, hallucinations, seizures, coma, and even occasionally death.

DIAGNOSIS
Lead poisoning is suspected from the patient's condition and history, and may be confirmed by tests on the blood and urine to measure the levels of lead and other substances produced by the action of lead on the body's cells. Workers exposed to lead should have regular blood tests to detect signs of accumulation of lead in the body before any symptoms develop. In children, *X-rays* may show characteristic areas of thickening in some bones.

TREATMENT
Treatment consists of avoiding further exposure to lead. The doctor may prescribe *chelating agents* to bind to the lead and help the body excrete it at a faster rate. In mild cases, the chelating agent *penicillamine* may be used alone. In more severe cases, penicillamine may be used with other chelating agents, such as edetate calcium di-sodium (calcium EDTA).

Learning
The process by which knowledge or abilities are acquired, or by which behaviour is modified.

Many different theories have been proposed to explain learning. Some, known as behavioural theories, emphasize the role of *conditioning* in learning. Others, known as cognitive theories, are based on the concept that learning occurs through the building of abstract "cognitive" models, using mental capacities such as *intelligence, memory,* insight, and understanding. Social learning theories combine aspects of both behavioural and cognitive learning theories. No one theory can account for the complexities of learning. It is probable that some things are learned by conditioning and others by complex thought processes that take account of many facts.

Learning difficulties
A range of psychological and physical problems that interfere with learning. Learning difficulties may be either general or specific.

Possible causes of a general learning difficulty include borderline or low *intelligence, mental handicap,* and *hyperactivity.*

Examples of specific learning difficulties include *dyslexia* (difficulty in reading), dyscalculia (inability to solve mathematical problems), and dysgraphia (writing disorders). In most cases, the cause of a specific learning disability cannot be ascertained. Some psychologists believe that specific learning difficulties in children of normal intelligence may be caused by forms of *minimal brain dysfunction*, which may be inherited.

Other problems that may cause general or specific learning difficulties include *deafness*, disorders of language or speech (see *Speech disorders*), and disorders of *vision*. Problems with schoolwork caused by emotional or environmental deprivation or by poor teaching are generally not classified as learning difficulties.

ASSESSMENT AND TREATMENT
A child with a suspected learning difficulty will usually be referred for psychological or medical assessment.

Treatment may be medical (such as the correction of a hearing problem), directed at improving language or speech (see *Speech therapy*), or educational (such as extra teaching or placement in a special unit or school).

Leech

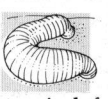

A type of bloodsucking worm with a flattened body and a sucker at each end. Land leeches inhabit tropical forests and can work their way through a person's clothing to attach themselves to the ankles and lower legs. Aquatic leeches live in warm water and attach themselves to swimmers, sometimes penetrating to the bronchi and oesophagus.

Leeches bite painlessly, introducing their saliva into the wound before sucking blood. When they are satiated, they drop off. Leech saliva contains an anticlotting substance, called hirudin, which may cause the wound to bleed for hours after the leech has dropped off. Leeches are thought not to transmit disease.

TREATMENT OF BITES
Attached leeches should be disturbed by applying a lighted match, alcohol, salt, or vinegar. They can then be pulled off gently to prevent the mouthparts from staying attached and becoming infected. A styptic pencil helps stop the bleeding after the leech has been removed. *Endoscopy* (inspection using a viewing instrument) may be necessary to remove leeches from inside the body.

MEDICAL USES
In the past, leeches were attached to the skin to "treat" many illnesses

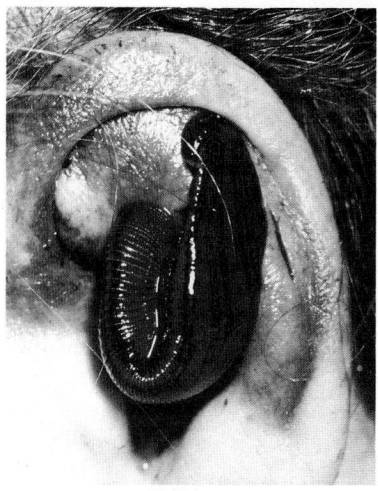

Use of a leech to drain blood
A leech is being used here to drain a haematoma (collection of blood) from a person's outer ear following an injury. Leech bites are painless, but because leech saliva contains an anticlotting agent, the wound may bleed for several hours.

ascribed to excess blood. Today, leeches are sometimes used to drain a *haematoma* (a collection of partially clotted blood) from a wound.

Leg, broken
See *Femur, fracture of; Fibula; Tibia.*

Legionnaires' disease

A form of pneumonia (infection of the lungs) named after an outbreak that caused the death of 29 members of the American Legion who were attending a convention in a Philadelphia hotel in 1976. The bacterium responsible was isolated and named *LEGIONELLA PNEUMOPHILA.* Subsequent tests identified the organism as a common contaminant of water systems which had been responsible for earlier epidemics of pneumonia (the cause of which had not been understood at the time).

CAUSES AND INCIDENCE
The bacterium breeds most readily in warm, moist conditions; in most outbreaks the source of infection has been the water or air-conditioning system in a large public building, including some outbreaks in hospitals. Infection follows the inhalation of droplets of heavily contaminated water (from air-conditioning outlets or showers, for example). Elderly people are particularly at risk.

The disease occurs both in localized outbreaks and as isolated cases.

About 130 to 200 cases occur in England and Wales each year, with about 10 to 40 deaths. More than twice as many men than women are affected, and more than two thirds of the cases occur in people over 50 years of age.

Control of the disease relies on proper disinfection of water systems, together with keeping the water at the correct temperature.

SYMPTOMS AND SIGNS
The first symptoms develop within a week of infection; they include headache, muscular and abdominal pain, diarrhoea, and a dry cough. Over the next few days pneumonia develops, resulting in a high fever, shaking chills, the coughing up of thick sputum (phlegm), drowsiness, and sometimes delirium. Like other types of pneumonia, the illness usually becomes more severe unless treated. This phase lasts about a week, after which either a gradual recovery takes place or progressively serious breathing problems develop.

DIAGNOSIS AND TREATMENT
The patient is admitted to hospital, where analysis of a sample of sputum (cultured on special media) reveals the microorganism responsible for the pneumonia. If the microorganism is *LEGIONELLA PNEUMOPHILA*, the patient is given the antibiotic *erythromycin*, often intravenously, which usually relieves symptoms quickly. Occasionally another antibiotic drug, *rifampicin*, may be required.

OUTLOOK
The outcome of the disease depends on the age and general health of the patient. Younger people generally recover fully, but a substantial proportion of elderly, unfit people die from the illness. Death is usually due to irreversible lung damage.

Leg, shortening of
Shortening of the leg is usually caused by faulty healing of a fractured femur (thigh-bone) or tibia (shin). Other causes are an abnormality present from birth, surgery on the leg, or muscle weakness associated with *poliomyelitis* or some other neurological disorder. Also, a deformity of the hip, knee, or spine may make one leg effectively shorter than the other even if the two are in fact of equal length.

If the difference in leg length exceeds 4 cm, there is usually a noticeable limp; the resultant stress on the lower spine often causes *back pain*. Wearing a shoe with a raised heel can compensate for the shortened leg.

Leg ulcer

An open sore on the leg that fails to heal, usually resulting from poor arterial blood supply to, or venous drainage from, the area. Elderly people are most commonly affected.

TYPES

Venous ulcers (also known as varicose or stasis ulcers) occur mainly on the ankles and lower legs and are caused by valve failure in veins; these ulcers usually appear in conjunction with *varicose veins*.

Bedsores (also called decubitus ulcers) develop on pressure spots on the legs as a result of a combination of poor circulation, pressure, and immobility over a long period.

Leg ulcers may also be due to *peripheral vascular disease*, in which fatty deposits on the inside of arteries or thickening of the arterial walls restrict blood supply to the extremities.

Diabetes mellitus, which increases susceptibility to blood vessel disease and skin infection and impairs sensation, may lead to ulcers.

Ulcers may also develop through neglect of an infected small wound. In the tropics, infection with microorganisms can cause *tropical ulcers*.

PREVENTION AND TREATMENT

Prevention is always easier than cure. In general, anyone susceptible to leg ulcers should attempt to avoid obesity, leg injury, and immobility.

Treatment of leg ulcers, which depends on the cause, should be sought at the earliest sign of trouble. If an ulcer is exuding pus, a wet dressing may be applied under the bandaging. This dressing should be changed only every three to seven days to avoid removing new skin from the area.

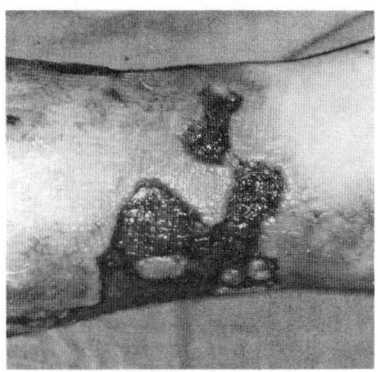

Venous ulcer on leg
This type of ulcer, also known as a stasis ulcer, is caused by impaired drainage of blood from the leg by the veins. It is usually accompanied by oedema (fluid accumulation) in the lower leg.

Leiomyoma

A benign tumour of smooth *muscle* (a type of muscle not under voluntary control). Leiomyomas usually occur in the smooth muscle of the uterus, where they gradually become replaced with fibrous tissue (hence their popular name, *fibroids*). More rarely, leiomyomas develop from smooth muscle in the wall of blood vessels in the skin, where they form tender lumps.

Leiomyomas are usually multiple. Although leiomyomas are not cancerous, they may require surgical removal if they cause symptoms.

Leishmaniasis

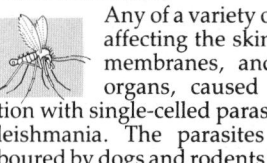 Any of a variety of diseases affecting the skin, mucous membranes, and internal organs, caused by infection with single-celled parasites called leishmania. The parasites are harboured by dogs and rodents in various parts of the world, and are transmitted from infected animals or people to new hosts by the bites of sandflies.

About 12 million people worldwide are thought to be affected. Leishmaniasis is not contracted in the UK, but travellers occasionally contract an infection abroad.

TYPES AND INCIDENCE

The most serious form of leishmaniasis, mainly affecting the internal organs, is called kala-azar or visceral leishmaniasis. It is prevalent in some parts of Asia, Africa, and South America, and also occurs in some Mediterranean countries.

In addition, there are several varieties of cutaneous leishmaniasis (mainly affecting the skin), some of which are prevalent in the Middle East, North Africa, and in the Mediterranean; others occur only in parts of Central and South America.

Travellers can minimize the risk of infection by taking measures to discourage sandfly bites (see *Insect bites*).

SYMPTOMS

Kala-azar causes a persistent fever, enlargement of the spleen, anaemia, and, later, darkening of the skin. The illness may develop any time up to two years after the initial infection, and, unless treated, may be fatal.

The cutaneous forms cause the appearance of a persistent ulcer at the site of the sandfly bite. The ulcer nearly always heals eventually, but can leave an ugly scar. With the South American forms, more extensive tissue damage may occur, often on the face, causing severe disfigurement.

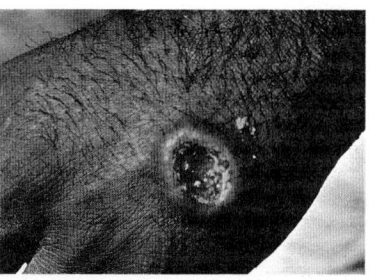

Leishmaniasis ulcer
This skin ulcer, which developed at the site of a sandfly bite, is typical of the lesions found on the skin of people who are suffering from cutaneous leishmaniasis.

DIAGNOSIS AND TREATMENT

Kala-azar is diagnosed by a *bone marrow biopsy* (aspirate) and/or a blood test. The cutaneous forms are diagnosed by identifying parasites in scrapings taken from the edge of affected skin patches. All types of leishmaniasis are treated effectively with drugs, such as sodium stibogluconate, given by intramuscular or intravenous injection.

Lens

The internal optical component of the *eye*, responsible for adjusting focus. Also called the crystalline lens, it is one of two lenses in each eye; the other is the *cornea*, which provides most of the converging power needed to form an image on the *retina*.

L

LOCATION OF THE LENS
This elastic and transparent organ is situated behind the iris and is suspended on delicate fibres from the ciliary body. Its full name—the crystalline lens—differentiates it from the cornea (another lens).

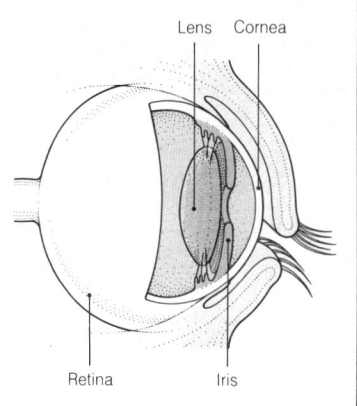

Lens   Cornea

Retina   Iris

The crystalline lens is situated behind the iris and is suspended on delicate fibres from the ciliary body. It is elastic, transparent, and slightly less convex on the front surface than on the back. Changing the curvature of the lens alters the focus so that near or distant objects can be seen sharply (see *Accommodation*).

Opacification of the crystalline lens, from any cause, is called *cataract*. (See also *Lens dislocation*.)

Lens dislocation

Displacement of the eye's crystalline *lens* from its normal position. Lens dislocation is almost always caused by an injury that ruptures some or all of the fibres that connect the lens to the ciliary body. In *Marfan's syndrome*, the fibres are particularly weak and lens dislocation is common.

A dislocated lens may slide sideways, upwards, or downwards, causing severe visual distortion or double vision in the affected eye, or it may slip backwards into the vitreous humour. A lens dislocated forwards through the pupil usually causes a form of *glaucoma* because of closure of the drainage angle of the eye. If the glaucoma is severe, the lens may need to be removed. (See also *Aphakia*.)

Lens implant

A plastic prosthesis used to replace the removed opaque lens in *cataract surgery*. There are many different designs, which may be positioned in front of the iris, clipped to the pupil, or held in place behind the pupil by delicate plastic loops.

A lens implant usually provides excellent distance vision without glasses, but glasses are usually necessary for close vision.

Lentigo

A flat, discoloured area of skin similar to a freckle. Lentigines (the plural of lentigo) are usually light brown and may occur singly or in groups. Unlike freckles they are as common on covered as on exposed parts of the body, and they do not fade in winter. Lentigines are more common in middle-aged and elderly people, especially those who have been exposed to a lot of sun.

Lentigines are harmless and no treatment is necessary. If raised, darker brown areas appear within them, a doctor should be consulted; there is a danger that these areas could develop into malignant melanomas (see *Melanoma, malignant*).

Leprosy

A chronic bacterial infection that causes nerve damage, mainly in the limbs and facial area, and may lead to skin damage. (See *Hansen's disease*.)

Leptospirosis

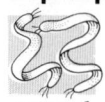 A rare disease caused by a type of spirochaete (spiral-shaped) bacterium harboured by rodents and excreted in their urine. It is also known as Weil's disease. About 20 to 30 cases of leptospirosis are reported in the UK each year.

SYMPTOMS

After an incubation period of one to three weeks, there is an acute illness with fever, chills, an intense throbbing headache, severe muscle aches, eye inflammation, and a skin rash. In most cases, the kidneys are affected, often severely. Liver damage leading to jaundice is also common.

TREATMENT

Antibiotic drugs are effective against the spirochaetes. In about one third of cases improvement is prompt. However, many patients suffer a more persistent illness in which kidney and liver function recover only slowly. In these cases, the nervous system may also be affected, often producing signs of *meningitis* (inflammation of the membranes covering the brain and spinal cord).

Lesbianism

Female homosexuality. According to Alfred Kinsey's studies carried out in the 1940s, about five per cent of women are entirely lesbian in their sexual activity, although some 15 per cent have had, by the age of 45, a homosexual experience. Lesbianism is less common than male homosexuality (see *Homosexuality, male*). Masturbation, oral sex, and mutual rubbing of the clitoris are the usual means of reaching orgasm.

Lesion

An all-encompassing term for any abnormality of structure or function in any part of the body. The term may refer to a wound, infection, tumour, abscess, or chemical abnormality.

Lethargy

A feeling of *tiredness*, drowsiness, or lack of energy.

Leukaemia

Any of several types of cancer in which there exists a disorganized proliferation of white *blood cells* in the bone marrow (the tissue from which all blood cells originate). The production of red blood cells, platelets, and normal white blood cells is impaired as normal cells are crowded out from the marrow by the leukaemic cells (abnormal white cells).

Other organs, such as the liver, spleen, lymph nodes, testes, or brain, may cease to function properly as they become infiltrated by the leukaemic cells. The number of leukaemic cells circulating in the blood may be high.

Leukaemias are classified into acute and chronic types (acute leukaemia generally develops more rapidly than chronic leukaemia). They are also classified according to the type of white cell that is proliferating abnormally. If the abnormal cells are derived from lymphocytes or from lymphoblasts (immature precursors of lymphocytes), the leukaemia is called lymphocytic or lymphoblastic leukaemia. If the abnormal cells are derived from other types of white blood cells or their precursors, the leukaemia is known as myeloid, myeloblastic, or granulocytic leukaemia.

Each year over 5,000 new cases of leukaemia are diagnosed in the UK, and there about 3,500 deaths from this cause. (See also *Leukaemia, acute; Leukaemia, chronic lymphocytic; Leukaemia, chronic myeloid*.)

Leukaemia, acute

A type of *leukaemia* in which the white blood cells produced in excess within the bone marrow are immature cells called blasts. Untreated, acute leukaemia can be fatal within a few weeks to months. Treatment today can often prolong life and may even provide a complete cure.

The abnormal cells may be of two types: lymphoblasts (immature *lymphocytes*) in acute lymphoblastic leukaemia, and myeloblasts (immature forms of other types of white cell) in acute myeloblastic leukaemia. Various subtypes are recognized according to the nature of the abnormal cells.

INCIDENCE AND CAUSES

About 2,500 cases of acute leukaemia are diagnosed annually in the UK. The incidences of the two main types (acute lymphoblastic leukaemia and acute myeloblastic leukaemia) at different ages are shown in the illustrated box (see p.634).

Both types seem to result from a mutation in a single white cell, altering its genetic structure. The cell undergoes an uncontrolled series of

L

divisions until billions of copies of the abnormal cell are present in the bone marrow, blood, and other tissues.

There are a number of possible causes for the original mutation. One type of acute lymphoblastic leukaemia is thought to be caused by a virus similar to the one that causes *AIDS*. Exposure to certain chemicals (such as benzene and some anticancer drugs) and to atomic radiation or radioactive leaks from nuclear reactors can be a cause. Inherited factors may play a part; there is an increased incidence in people with certain genetic disorders (such as *Fanconi's anaemia*) and chromosomal abnormalities (such as *Down's syndrome*). People with certain other blood disorders, such as chronic myeloid leukaemia (see *Leukaemia, chronic myeloid*) and primary *polycythaemia*, are also at increased risk.

SYMPTOMS AND SIGNS
The symptoms and signs of both types of acute leukaemia are caused by overcrowding of the bone marrow by blasts and by infiltration of organs by the abnormal cells. The overcrowding causes the marrow's failure to produce normal blood cells of all types (see illustrated box overleaf).

DIAGNOSIS
The diagnosis of acute leukaemia is based on a *bone marrow biopsy* that confirms an abnormal number of blast cells. The blast cells are sometimes also seen in the blood. When acute lymphoblastic leukaemia is diagnosed, a *lumbar puncture* is usually performed to examine the *cerebrospinal fluid* for the presence of blast cells.

TREATMENT
Treatment includes giving the patient transfusions of blood and platelets, and the use of *anticancer drugs* to kill the leukaemic cells. These drugs tend to make the patient even more susceptible to infection, so powerful *antibiotic drugs* may also be given.

From the beginning of treatment, a catheter (tube) through which all drugs and transfusions are given is commonly inserted into a large vein near the heart. Treatment of leukaemic cells in the cerebrospinal fluid is accomplished by the direct injection of drugs into the fluid and by subsequent *radiotherapy* to the head and spinal cord. Radiotherapy is more commonly given in the treatment of acute lymphoblastic leukaemia than for acute myeloblastic leukaemia.

The course of drug treatment may last for many weeks. When there is no evidence of leukaemic cells in the blood or bone marrow, a state of remission is said to have been achieved. However, without repeated courses of treatment, the leukaemia often relapses (returns). For this reason, the use of drugs is usually continued for many weeks after remission. If the leukaemia relapses after the first remission, a *bone marrow transplant* may be considered. Increasingly, the practice is to offer bone marrow transplantation during the first remission to guard against relapse.

OUTLOOK
The outlook for people with acute lymphoblastic leukaemia is generally better than it is for acute myeloblastic leukaemia, and it is better for children than for adults. Survival rates are shown in the illustrated box overleaf.

Leukaemia, chronic lymphocytic
A type of *leukaemia* caused by proliferation of mature-looking *lymphocytes* (a type of white *blood cell* that plays an important role in the body's *immune system*). Although incurable, the disease is not invariably fatal.

INCIDENCE AND CAUSES
There are about 1,200 new cases of chronic lymphocytic leukaemia diagnosed annually in the UK. Nearly all patients are over 50. The cause of the disorder is unknown.

SYMPTOMS AND SIGNS
Symptoms develop slowly, often over many years. Many cases are discovered by chance when a blood test is performed. In addition to features common to acute forms of leukaemia (see illustrated box overleaf), symptoms and signs may include enlargement of the liver and spleen, persistent raised temperature, and night sweats.

DIAGNOSIS AND TREATMENT
Chronic lymphocytic leukaemia is diagnosed by finding large numbers of lymphocytes, all of the same type, in the blood and on a *bone marrow biopsy*. The severity of the disease is assessed by the degree of liver and spleen enlargement, anaemia, and lack of platelet cells in the blood. In many cases, no treatment is required if the disease is mild. In more severe cases, *anticancer drugs* are given by mouth, sometimes combined with *radiotherapy*. Other measures include transfusions of blood and platelets, *antibiotic drugs* to combat infection, and *immunoglobulin injections* to boost the patient's immune system.

OUTLOOK
The progression of chronic lymphocytic leukaemia is slow. More than half of the patients survive for five years from the time of diagnosis. Eventually, death may result from overwhelming infection but many patients die from causes unrelated to their leukaemia.

Leukaemia, chronic myeloid
A type of *leukaemia*, also known as chronic granulocytic leukaemia, that results from uncontrolled proliferation of the class of white *blood cell* known as granulocytes, neutrophils, or polymorphonuclear leukocytes. Large numbers of these cells, in various stages of maturity, appear in the blood.

INCIDENCE AND CAUSES
There are about 1,000 new cases of chronic myeloid leukaemia diagnosed in the UK each year, mainly among middle-aged to elderly people.

The cause of chronic myeloid leukaemia is not known. However, in most cases, the patient's cells contain a specific *chromosomal abnormality* known as the Philadelphia chromosome. Part of one chromosome is attached to another chromosome.

SYMPTOMS
This type of leukaemia usually has two phases—a chronic phase that may last several years and a more malignant phase, called the blastic or accelerated or acute phase, in which large numbers of immature granulocytes are produced.

During the chronic phase, symptoms develop slowly; they may include tiredness, fever, night sweats, and weight loss. If the number of white cells in the blood rises very high, the blood may become excessively viscous (sticky), impairing the supply of oxygen to various organs. The effects can include visual disturbances and abdominal pain due to death of tissues within the spleen. *Priapism* (persistent, painful erection of the penis) is sometimes a feature.

The symptoms of the second phase are like those of acute forms of leukaemia (see illustrated box overleaf).

DIAGNOSIS AND TREATMENT
The disease is sometimes not apparent until the patient has a blood test for some other reason. The diagnosis is made from the increased numbers of granulocytes in the blood and in the bone marrow (as detected by *bone marrow biopsy*). The presence of the Philadelphia chromosome, found by *chromosome analysis*, may help establish the diagnosis.

Treatment of the chronic phase includes the use of *anticancer drugs*.

L

LEUKAEMIA

In all forms of leukaemia, abnormal white cells proliferate in the bone marrow. There are four main types: acute lymphoblastic leukaemia (ALL), acute myeloblastic leukaemia (AML), chronic lymphocytic leukaemia (CLL), and chronic myeloid leukaemia (CML). Their incidence varies with age (see right). The acute types have a rapid onset. There is a risk of death from overwhelming infection or blood loss, but modern treatment has greatly improved survival rates (below) and may bring a cure.

The chronic forms of leukaemia progress much more gradually but are essentially incurable.

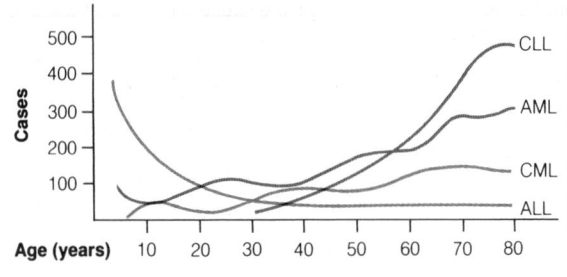

Incidence
The graphs show how the four main types of leukaemia vary in incidence with age. Acute lymphoblastic leukaemia (ALL) is the common type in children, chronic lymphocytic leukaemia (CLL) is the most common over 40

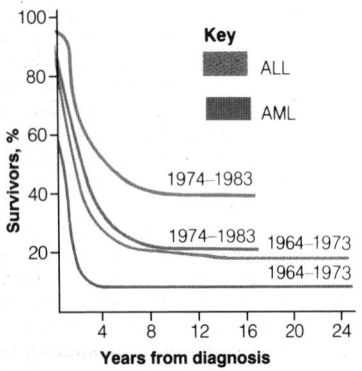

Key
ALL
AML

1974–1983
1974–1983   1964–1973
1964–1973

Survival rates for acute leukaemia
The graphs show survival rates for acute lymphoblastic leukaemia (ALL) and acute myeloblastic leukaemia (AML) for cases diagnosed in the years 1964 to 1973 and 1974 to 1983. The improved survival rates are the result of better treatment.

Symptoms of acute leukaemia
Symptoms are caused partly by the abnormal white cells crowding out the bone marrow (so that it fails to produce sufficient normal blood cells of all types) and partly by the invasion of other body organs by abnormal cells.

Gum bleeding
Gums may bleed as a result of insufficient production of platelet cells by the bone marrow; platelets are needed for the arrest of bleeding.

Bone tenderness
Tenderness of the bones may be felt as the bone marrow becomes packed with immature white cells.

Frequent bruising
Reduced numbers of platelets may lead to bleeding points in the skin and bruising after mild trauma.

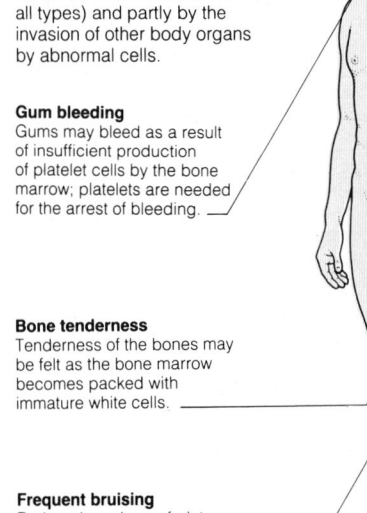

Headache
Headache may be caused by anaemia or by abnormal white cells affecting the nervous system.

Enlarged lymph nodes
The lymph nodes in the neck, armpits, and groin may be swollen with huge numbers of immature white cells. The liver, spleen, and testes may also be swollen.

Anaemia
Anaemia develops if there is insufficient production of red blood cells by the bone marrow. Anaemia causes tiredness, breathlessness on exertion, and pallor.

Infections
White blood cells play a major part in the defence against infection. However, in acute leukaemia, only immature, nonfunctioning white cells are made, so the patient may suffer from repeated chest or throat infections, herpes zoster, or skin and other infections.

HOW LEUKAEMIA ATTACKS THE BODY

Leukaemia is a form of cancer, but with the abnormally growing cells—mutated white blood cells—scattered throughout the body in bone marrow, rather than grouped into a single tumour. The abnormal cells may spill into the blood and may infiltrate and interfere with the function of other organs. But worse, the abnormal cells "take over" the marrow and prevent it from making enough normal blood cells—including normal white cells, red cells, and platelets. This leaves the sufferer highly susceptible to serious infections, anaemia, and bleeding episodes.

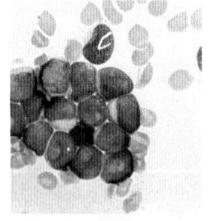

Cell photograph
Shown is blood in acute leukaemia. The large cells are abnormal, immature white cells; the smaller, paler cells are red blood cells.

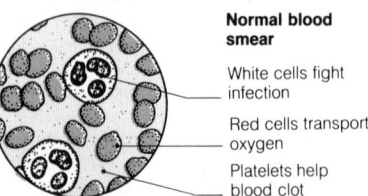

Normal blood smear

White cells fight infection

Red cells transport oxygen

Platelets help blood clot

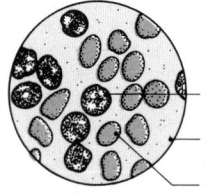

Blood smear in leukaemia

Abnormal white cells—susceptibility to infection

Fewer platelets—bleeding tendency

Fewer red cells – anaemia

Appearance of blood in leukaemia
In leukaemia (above), the blood usually contains many abnormal white cells, and fewer red cells and platelets.

Normal appearance of blood
In a normal blood smear (left), there are large numbers of red cells, many platelets, and a few white cells.

When the disease transforms into the acute phase, treatment is similar to that given for acute leukaemia. If the number of white cells rises very high, the cells may be removed from the patient using a machine known as a cell separator.

Treatment of the acute phase is seldom successful; the patient usually dies of bleeding or infection. *Bone marrow transplants* are now being used in an attempt to cure patients while the condition is still in the chronic phase.

OUTLOOK

The average survival time from first diagnosis is about three years. However, about one fifth of patients survives for 10 years or more. A successful bone marrow transplant may improve the outlook.

Leukocyte

Any type of white *blood cell*.

Leukodystrophies

A rare group of inherited childhood diseases in which the *myelin* sheaths that form a protective covering around many nerves are destroyed.

Diseases within this group include metachromatic leukodystrophy (which causes impaired speech, blindness, paralysis, dementia, and death within a few years), Krabbe's disease (which results in blindness, deafness, seizures, paralysis, and death within one year), and Merzbacher-Pelizaeus disease (which causes progressive incoordination, speech difficulties, paralysis, and mental deterioration from infancy until death, which occurs in early childhood).

Leukoplakia

Raised white patches on the mucous membranes of the mouth or vulva (the area around the vaginal opening). Leukoplakia is due to the thickening of tissue. It is most common in elderly people and is being increasingly found in people with *AIDS*.

CAUSES

Leukoplakia in the mouth, which is most common on the tongue, is usually due to tobacco-smoking (particularly pipe-smoking) or to the rubbing of a rough tooth or denture. It is not known what causes the condition to develop on the vulva.

SYMPTOMS AND TREATMENT

The patches, which develop slowly, cause no discomfort and are usually harmless. Occasionally, they result in a malignant change in the affected tissue. For this reason, leukoplakia should always be reported to a doctor.

Leukoplakia in the mouth may clear up once the cause has been treated. If the condition persists, the patches are removed under a local anaesthetic. Leukoplakia of the vulva is treated in the same way. The removed tissue is examined microscopically for any signs of malignant change. (See also *Mouth cancer*; *Vulva, cancer of.*)

Leukorrhoea

See *Vaginal discharge.*

Levodopa

A drug used in the treatment of *Parkinson's disease*, a neurological disorder caused by deficiency of the neurotransmitter chemical *dopamine* in part of the brain.

HOW IT WORKS

Levodopa is absorbed into the brain and converted into dopamine. Levodopa is usually given in combination with an *enzyme*-inhibitor, such as carbidopa, that reduces the amount of levodopa broken down by the liver before it can reach the brain. This allows a lower dose of levodopa to be given and thereby reduces the risk of adverse effects.

POSSIBLE ADVERSE EFFECTS

Adverse effects include nausea, vomiting, nervousness, and agitation. Prolonged use often impairs the effectiveness of treatment or increases the severity of adverse effects.

Levonorgestrel

A *progestogen drug* used in some *oral contraceptive* preparations.

LH

The abbreviation for luteinizing hormone—a *gonadotrophin hormone* produced by the *pituitary gland*.

LH-RH

The abbreviation for *luteinizing hormone-releasing hormone*. This hormone is released by the *hypothalamus*.

Libido

Sexual desire. Libido is a healthy, normal feeling, especially strong in youth and gradually fading with age. Loss of libido is a common symptom of numerous physical illnesses, and of *depression*, *drug abuse*, and *alcohol abuse*.

The libido theory of the Viennese neurologist and psychoanalyst Sigmund Freud describes sexual development during childhood in terms of oral, anal, and genital stages (representing the areas of the body towards which a child's attention is directed at different ages). Freud believed that

certain neurotic disorders and abnormal sexual behaviours were due to fixation of libido at one of these stages. By contrast, directing the libido (or "love energy") away from oneself and towards other people or objects was seen as a sign of maturity. (See also *Narcissism*; *Sexual desire, inhibited.*)

Lice

Small, wingless insects that feed on human blood. There are three species: PEDICULUS HUMANUS CAPITIS (the head louse), PEDICULUS HUMANUS CORPORIS (the body louse), and PHTHIRUS PUBIS (the crab, or pubic, louse). All lice have flattened bodies and measure up to 3 mm across.

HEAD LICE

These lice live on and suck blood from the scalp. Head lice leave tiny, red spots that itch intensely, leading to scratching, *dermatitis* (skin inflammation), and *impetigo* (a bacterial skin infection). The females lay a daily batch of tiny, pale eggs (nits) that are attached to hairs close to the scalp; the nits hatch in about seven days. The adult lice may live for up to several weeks.

Head lice affect all social classes. Children are most affected, women occasionally, and men rarely. The lice are spread by direct (although not necessarily head-to-head) contact.

Lotions containing malathion, carbaryl, permethrin, and phenothrin kill lice and nits rapidly. The lotion should be washed off 12 hours after application, and a fine-toothed comb used to remove dead lice and nits. Shampoos containing malathion or carbaryl are also effective if used repeatedly over several days. Combs and hairbrushes should be treated with very hot water to kill any attached eggs.

BODY LICE

These lice live and lay eggs on clothing next to the skin. The lice visit the body only to feed. Body lice transmit epidemic *typhus* and *relapsing fever*, diseases that are rare today but which were once common in areas affected by war or natural disaster.

These lice affect only people who rarely change their clothes. Body lice can be killed by placing infested clothes in a hot dryer for five minutes, by washing them in very hot water, or by burning them.

CRAB LICE

These lice live in pubic hair or, more rarely, in armpits, beards, or eyelashes. Crab lice are usually passed from one person to another during sexual contact. (See *Pubic lice.*)

Lichenification

Thickening and hardening of the skin that is caused by repeated scratching. Lichenification is often the result of scratching to relieve the intense itching of disorders such as atopic *eczema* or *lichen simplex*.

Lichen planus

A common skin disease of unknown cause that usually affects middle-aged people. Small, shiny, extremely itchy, pink or purple raised spots appear on the skin of the wrists, forearms, or lower legs. There is often a lacy network of white spots covering the inside lining of the cheeks.

The disease is treated with *corticosteroid drugs*. Creams, sometimes supplemented by injections in severe cases, are used to treat the skin rash. Most cases clear up within 18 months.

Lichen simplex

Patches of thickened, itchy, and sometimes discoloured skin caused by repeated scratching. Typical sites are the neck, wrist, arm near the elbow, and ankles. Lichen simplex is most common in women and is psychological in origin; sufferers often rub the patches (without being aware of doing so) when agitated or under stressful circumstances. A cycle is established in which repeated scratching to relieve itching leads to more skin thickening and itching, which then requires yet more scratching.

Treatment is with oral *antihistamine drugs* and creams containing *corticosteroid drugs* to relieve itching. Sometimes bandaging may be used to protect the skin and so break the cycle. This permits the disorder to subside and the treatment to be effective.

Lid lag

A momentary delay in the normal downward movement of the upper eyelids that occurs when the eye looks down. A characteristic feature of *thyrotoxicosis*, lid lag usually occurs in conjunction with *exophthalmos* (protrusion of the eyeball).

Life expectancy

The number of years a person can expect to live. In most Western countries, life expectancy at birth is about 70 years for men and 75 years for women. This sex difference is thought to be due to the fact that many more men than women smoked in the first half of this century. However, since then, the smoking sex ratio has evened out and there has been an

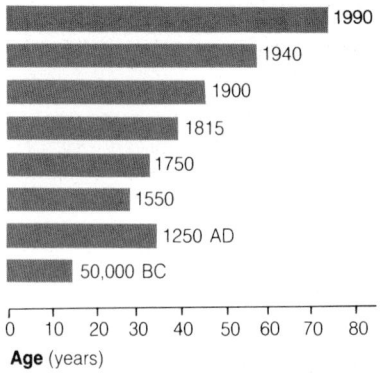

Life expectancy through history
Advances in medicine have dramatically increased life expectancy at birth. Life expectancies in England fluctuated around age 30 to 35 for many centuries, before reaching 40 in the early 19th century and climbing to over 70 in recent decades. Most developed countries follow a similar pattern.

increase in deaths from lung cancer in women. As a result, the sex difference in life expectancy is narrowing.

The expected age of death becomes greater the longer a person lives, so a 70-year-old may have a life expectancy of 15 years; even a 100-year-old can expect to live a year or two.

LIFE EXPECTANCY AND LIFESPAN

Life expectancy should be distinguished from lifespan. Since records began, some old people have lived well beyond 70 years. Gerontologists agree that, in the absence of disease, the average normal lifespan is about 85 years (see *Aging*).

The natural lifespan is determined largely by genetic factors. People whose parents and grandparents lived to be 90 are likely to live to about this age. However, the extent to which individuals fulfil their genetic

potential is affected by environmental factors, such as nutrition and accidents, as well as by disease.

The proportion of the population that attains its natural lifespan depends on the general health of that population, so life expectancy is a good means of comparing the state of health in different countries or in different parts of the same country.

Life expectancy at birth may be as low as 35 years in some developing countries. However, although statistically accurate, this figure is misleading because it reflects the high mortality in infancy. Records show that life expectancy at age 40 is not greatly different around the world.

Life support

The process of keeping a person alive by artificially inflating the lungs (see *Ventilation*) and, if necessary, maintaining the heartbeat with a *pacemaker*.

Ligament

A tough band of white, fibrous, slightly elastic tissue. Ligaments are important components of joints, binding together the bone ends and preventing excessive movement of the joint. Ligaments also support various organs, including the uterus, bladder, liver, and diaphragm, and help maintain the shape of the breasts.

INJURY

Ligaments, especially those in the *ankle joint* and *knee*, are sometimes damaged by injury. Minor sprains are treated with ice, bandaging, and sometimes *physiotherapy*. If the ligament is torn, the joint is either immobilized by a plaster *cast* to allow healing or repaired surgically. Strain of ligaments in the back may cause nonspecific *back pain*, which is usually treated with physiotherapy exercises.

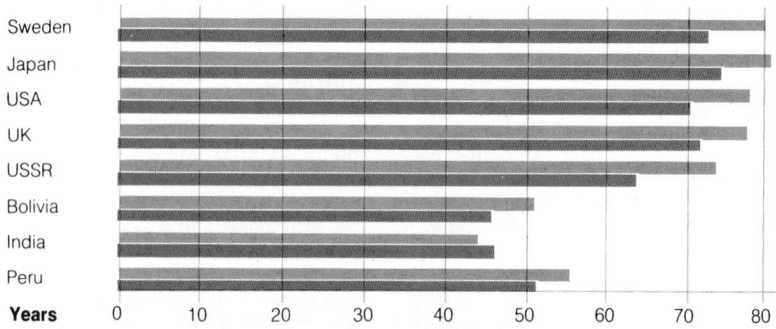

Gender and life expectancy
In rich and poor countries, life expectancy at birth is generally higher for females (grey bars) than males (red). India is an exception.

Nationality and life expectancy
Average life expectancy at birth in most developed countries is now 70 or more; in developing countries it is 40 to 55.

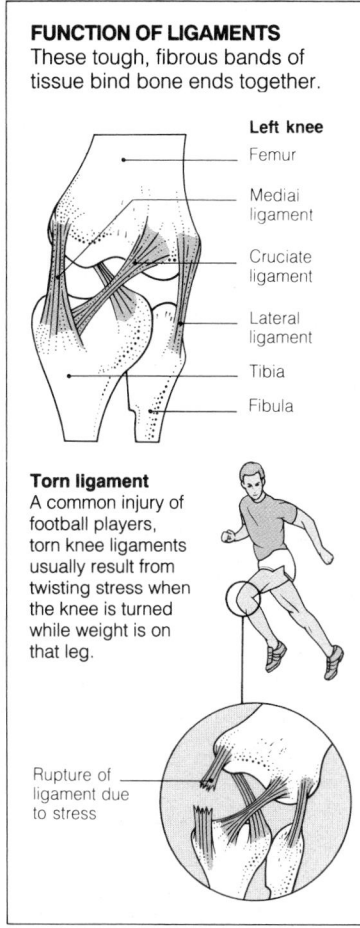

FUNCTION OF LIGAMENTS
These tough, fibrous bands of tissue bind bone ends together.

Left knee

- Femur
- Medial ligament
- Cruciate ligament
- Lateral ligament
- Tibia
- Fibula

Torn ligament
A common injury of football players, torn knee ligaments usually result from twisting stress when the knee is turned while weight is on that leg.

Rupture of ligament due to stress

Ligation
The surgical process of ligating (tying off) a blood vessel to prevent bleeding, or a duct to close it, with a length of thread or other material. The term is used in tubal ligation, a form of sterilization in which the fallopian tubes are tied off (see *Sterilization, female*).

Ligature
A length of thread or other material used for *ligation* (tying off) of a blood vessel or duct.

Lightening
A feeling experienced by many pregnant women when the baby's head descends into the pelvic cavity. Lightening usually occurs in the last three weeks of pregnancy, leaving more space in the upper abdomen and relieving pressure under the ribs.

Light treatment
See *Phototherapy*.

Lignocaine

ANTIARRHYTHMIC LOCAL ANAESTHETIC

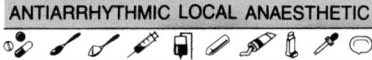

Liquid Injection Intravenous infusion Ointment/Cream/Gel Eye-drops Spray

Prescription generally needed

Available as generic

A local anaesthetic (see *Anaesthesia, local*). Lignocaine is given to numb tissues before minor surgical procedures and as a *nerve block* (to numb the area supplied by a particular nerve). It is also applied topically to relieve discomfort during the insertion of a *catheter* (tube) or an *endoscope* (viewing instrument) or to relieve irritation, for example, from *haemorrhoids*.

Lignocaine is sometimes given by intravenous injection after a *myocardial infarction* (heart attack) to reduce the risk of *ventricular fibrillation* (an irregularity of the heartbeat).

POSSIBLE ADVERSE EFFECTS
High doses given by injection occasionally cause nausea and vomiting.

Limb, artificial
Artificial legs or arms, known medically as limb prostheses. Most artificial limbs are fitted to replace all or part of a limb amputated because of disease or severe injury (see *Amputation*). In some cases, however, they are required as a substitute for limbs missing from birth (see *Limb defects*).

CONSTRUCTION AND MATERIALS
Artificial limbs can be obtained ready-made, but for best results, should be specially made to suit individual needs. A mould taken from the stump of the missing limb is used to make a socket for the top of the prosthesis into which the stump can fit closely and comfortably. The socket, made of wood, leather, or plastic, is attached to the stump by suction or straps.

Each main part of an artificial limb (replacing the natural lower leg, thigh, forearm, or upper arm) is called an extension. The extension consists of an inner strut, which can be made of various materials, covered by foam-rubber that is shaped to match the corresponding part of the natural limb. This unit is enclosed by an outer shell of metal, wood, or leather.

Artificial joints are usually made of plastic and metal and may incorporate sophisticated mechanisms to perform such functions as rotating the wrist, and controlling the length of stride.

Generally, artificial legs are more useful than artificial arms because the straightforward movements of the natural leg are easier to duplicate than the wide-ranging, often intricate, movements of the arm (especially the hand). Even so, the design of artificial hands is now extremely advanced. Electronic circuitry has been developed to pick up muscle and nerve impulses reaching the stump from the spinal cord. The circuitry transforms the impulses into movements of the prosthesis. People with an artificial arm or hand may have several prostheses to perform different functions. (See also illustrated box overleaf.)

Limb defects
Incomplete development of one or more limbs at birth. In some cases, an entire limb is missing. In others, only the hand or foot, or the upper or lower half of a limb, is missing. In a condition called phocomelia, hands, feet, or tiny finger- or toe-buds are attached to limb stumps or grow directly from the trunk. Any combination of limbs may be affected.

Limb defects are rare; the incidence is only about one in every 2,000 live births. The sedative drug *thalidomide* is known to have caused phocomelia in fetuses when taken by pregnant women. Limb defects are sometimes inherited or form part of a syndrome (a group of abnormalities occurring in combination). In many cases, the cause is unknown.

MANAGEMENT
A child with a limb defect usually needs to attend a specialized centre. Paediatricians, occupational therapists, psychologists, social workers, and other experts will treat the condition and advise on the child's development. A prosthetist will fit an artificial limb (see *Limb, artificial*) and teach the child how to use it.

Limbic system
A ring-shaped area in the centre of the brain consisting of a number of connected clusters of nerve cells. The limbic system plays a role in the *autonomic nervous system* (which automatically regulates body functions), in the emotions, and in the sense of smell. The limbic system is extensive, and the different substructures within it have individual names (e.g. the hippocampus, the cingulate gyrus, and the amygdala).

Much of our knowledge of the limbic system comes from study of the behaviour of animals and people known to have damage to or disease in the limbic area of the brain. The

L

L

TYPES OF ARTIFICIAL LIMB

Different types of artificial limbs must restore as much as possible the function of the lost limb, be light enough to be worn comfortably, be easy to put on and take off, and look as normal as possible. Although ready-made prostheses are available and can be quite effective, the best artificial limbs are constructed by specialists and are specially adapted to meet an individual's particular needs.

Initiating movement
The nerve impulses that move the prosthesis originate in the brain and pass via the spinal cord to the stump.

Prosthetic movement
Electronic circuitry in the prosthesis picks up nerve impulses in the stump and causes the prosthesis to move in a near-normal way.

Artificial hands
Many devices are available. The prosthesis on the left is electronically controlled and battery powered; it allows finger and wrist movements. The spade grip on the right is a prosthesis designed to meet a specific need, as are precision tweezers and golf-club grips.

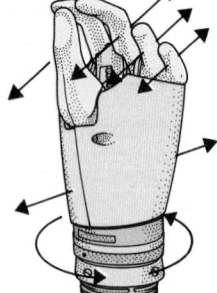

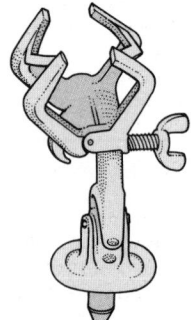

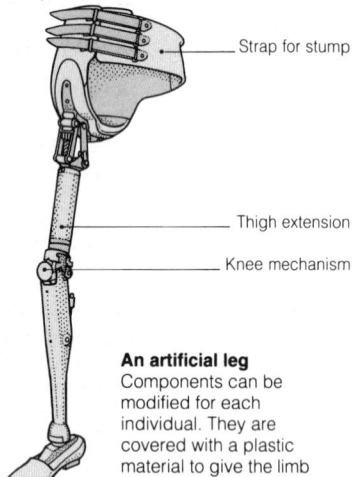

Strap for stump

Thigh extension

Knee mechanism

An artificial leg
Components can be modified for each individual. They are covered with a plastic material to give the limb a natural appearance.

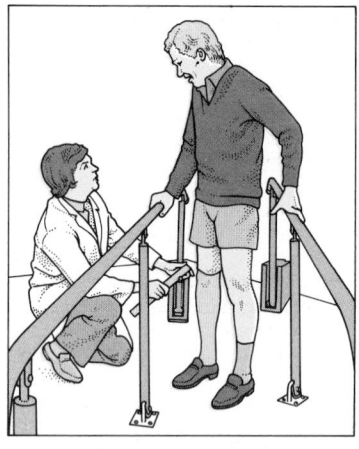

Training with prostheses
Special walking classes enable patients to adjust to their new limbs.

most commonly observed effects are abnormalities of emotional response, such as inappropriate crying or laughing, easily provoked rage, unwarranted fear, anxiety, and depression, and excessive sexual interest.

Limp

An abnormal, uneven pattern of *walking* in which the movements of one leg (or of the pelvis on one side of the body) are different from those of the other. A limp may involve dipping of the pelvis to one side, or failure to straighten the leg fully when the foot is placed on the ground.

Linctus

A bland, glutinous mixture, usually sweetened, given to soothe the irritation caused by an inflamed throat. A simple linctus contains no active drug but linctuses are commonly used as vehicles for various *cough suppressants* (codeine, for example).

Lindane

A drug used in the form of a lotion or cream to treat infestation by *scabies* and some types of *lice*. Lindane, also called gamma benzene hexachloride, is used as a pesticide.

Lindane sometimes irritates the skin and causes itching. In large amounts, it can be toxic, particularly to children. Poisoning can produce vomiting, diarrhoea, convulsions, liver damage, and anaemia.

Linear accelerator

A device for accelerating subatomic particles, such as electrons, to a speed approaching that of light so that they have extremely high energies. A linear accelerator can also be used to generate high-energy X-rays.

In medicine, high-energy electrons or X-rays are used in *radiotherapy* to treat certain cancers. This method causes less damage to the healthy tissue around a tumour than does low-energy radiotherapy.

Liniment

A liquid, rubbed on to the skin to relieve aching muscles and stiff joints. Liniments may contain rubefacients (counter-irritants that increase blood flow beneath the skin), such as wintergreen, turpentine, camphor, or menthol, or certain drugs such as *nonsteroidal anti-inflammatory drugs* (ibuprofen) for example. Liniments should not be taken by mouth or put on broken or inflamed skin.

Lip

One of two fleshy folds around the entrance to the mouth. Externally the lips are covered with skin and internally with mucous membrane, the relative transparency of which allows the red-pink of the underlying capillaries to show through.

The main substructure of the lips is a ring of muscle, whose functions include keeping food in the mouth, helping to produce speech and other sounds (whistling, for example), and kissing. Smaller muscles at the corners of the lips are responsible for facial expression.

DISORDERS

These include chapping (see *Chapped skin*), cheilitis (inflammation, cracking, and dryness), *cold sores* (blisters on the lips due to HERPES SIMPLEX infection), hard chancre (an early sign of *syphilis*), and *lip cancer*.

Lip cancer

A malignant tumour, usually on the lower lip. Lip cancer is largely confined to older people, especially those exposed to a lot of sunlight and those who have smoked cigarettes or a pipe for many years. Lip cancer is the most common form of mouth cancer, but accounts for only about one per cent of all cancers.

SYMPTOMS

A white patch develops on the lip and soon becomes scaly and cracked with a yellow crust. The affected area grows and eventually becomes ulcerated. In some cases, the cancer spreads to the lymph nodes in the jaw and neck.

DIAGNOSIS AND TREATMENT

Any lip sore that persists for longer than a month should be seen by a doctor. Lip cancer (usually a *squamous cell carcinoma*) is diagnosed by *biopsy* (removal of a sample of tissue for microscopic examination).

Treatment is surgical removal, *radiotherapy*, or a combination of both. If the tumour has spread to the lymph nodes in the neck, *neck dissection* and more radiation may be necessary.

Lipectomy, suction

A type of *body contour surgery* in which excess fat is sucked out through a small incision made in the skin.

Lipid disorders

Disorders of metabolism (internal body chemistry) that cause abnormal amounts of *lipids* (fats) in the body. The most common are the *hyperlipidaemia*s, which are characterized by high levels of lipids in the blood. Hyperlipidaemias may be inherited or brought on or aggravated by diet or a disorder. They are potentially serious because they can cause atherosclerosis (narrowing of arteries by deposits of fatty material) and pancreatitis (inflammation of the pancreas). Hyperlipidaemias are usually treated by a diet that is low in cholesterol and saturated fats, and sometimes by lipid-lowering drugs. There are also some very rare lipid disorders due solely to heredity, such as *Tay-Sachs disease*.

Lipid-lowering drugs

COMMON DRUGS

Drugs that act on the liver
Acipimox Bezafibrate Ciprofibrate Fenofibrate Gemfibrozil Nicofuranose Nicotinic acid Pravastatin Probucol Simvastatin

Drugs that act on bile salts
Cholestyramine Colestipol

A group of drugs used to treat *hyperlipidaemia* (abnormally high levels of one or more types of *lipid*, such as *cholesterol*, in the blood). Lipid-lowering drugs are given to reduce the risk of severe *atherosclerosis* (narrowing of the arteries), usually when dietary measures have not worked.

HOW THEY WORK

Some lipid-lowering drugs alter *enzyme* activity in the *liver* to prevent the production of one or more types of lipid from fatty acids. This action reduces the level of lipids in the blood.

Others interfere with the absorption of *bile* salts from the intestine into the blood. Bile salts contain large amounts of cholesterol; a decrease in their concentration in the blood stimulates the liver to convert more cholesterol into bile salts, thus reducing the amount of cholesterol in the blood.

POSSIBLE ADVERSE EFFECTS

Some lipid-lowering drugs that act on the liver cause increased susceptibility to *gallstones*. Those that act on bile salts may cause nausea and diarrhoea.

Lipids

A general term for *fats and oils*. Lipids, or lipins as they are sometimes called, include triglycerides (simple fats), phospholipids (important constituents of cell membranes and nerve tissue), and sterols such as *cholesterol*.

Lipoma

A common *benign* tumour of fatty tissue. Lipomas give rise to slow-growing soft swellings. The tumours may develop anywhere in the body, but most commonly on the thigh, trunk, or shoulder. A person may develop one or many lipomas. The tumours are painless and harmless and do not need treatment, although they may be surgically removed for cosmetic reasons.

Lipoprotein

Particles consisting of a fatty core and a protein outer layer that allow transport of fats into the bloodstream. The protein components are known as apoliproteins. Genetic variations in the structure of apoliproteins and lipoproteins have been shown to play an important part in determining susceptibility to cardiovascular disorders and to *Alzheimer's disease*.

Liposarcoma

A rare cancer of fatty tissue that most commonly develops during late middle age. Liposarcomas usually occur in the abdomen or in the thigh, where they produce firm swellings. The tumours can generally be removed by surgery, but have a tendency to recur.

Lip-reading

A way of understanding words or conversation through the use of visual clues rather than hearing. Lip-reading is invaluable in helping people who are deaf to understand more of what is said to them (see *Deafness*).

HOW IT IS DONE

The basis of lip-reading is that certain speech sounds are produced by characteristic movements, positions, and relationships of the jaw, lips, and tongue. Because there are more than 40 clearly distinct sounds in the English language, facial expression and context are also important.

EFFECTIVENESS

Tests have shown that the proportion of identified words can rise from 20 to 60 per cent after training. Anyone speaking to a deaf person can help improve the effectiveness of lip-reading by speaking slightly more slowly than usual, by not covering the mouth when speaking, and by looking directly at the deaf person.

Liquid paraffin

A lubricant *laxative drug* obtained from petroleum. Liquid paraffin can cause anal irritation, and prolonged use may impair the absorption of vitamins from the intestine into the blood.

Lisp

The most common form of *speech disorder*. A lisp is due to protrusion of the tongue between the teeth so that the "s" sound is replaced by "th". Most children with a lisp have completely normal structures of the mouth and lips. However, sometimes the speech defect is caused by a cleft palate (see *Cleft lip and palate*).

In most children, lisping disappears without treatment. If it persists after the age of about four, *speech therapy* may be considered.

Listeriosis

A bacterial infection common in animals, including cattle, pigs, and poul-

L

try, that may also affect humans. Although the incidence of human listeriosis is low, it appeared to be increasing in the late 1980s. Tighter controls on the storage of cook-chill meals and recommendations that pregnant women should avoid high-risk foods led to a reduced incidence of the disease in the UK in the early 1990s.

Listeriosis is caused by LISTERIA MONOCYTOGENES, a bacterium that is widespread in the environment, especially in soil. Possible sources of human infection include soft cheese, milk, ready-prepared coleslaw and salads, cook-chill foods, and improperly cooked meat. It is normally destroyed at pasteurizing temperatures, but if food is infected and refrigerated, it may continue to multiply. For this reason, chilled food should not be eaten after the "best by" date. Listeriosis can also be spread by direct contact with an infected live animal.

SYMPTOMS

The only symptoms in most affected adults are fever and generalized aches and pains. There may also be sore throat, conjunctivitis, diarrhoea, and abdominal pain. *Pneumonia*, *septicaemia*, and *meningitis* may develop in severe cases. Listeriosis can be life-threatening, particularly in people whose *immune system* is suppressed, in pregnant women, in the elderly, and in the newborn. An unborn child infected through its mother's blood may be stillborn. Listeriosis may be a cause of recurrent miscarrages.

DIAGNOSIS AND TREATMENT

Listeriosis is diagnosed by blood tests and analysis of other body fluids, such as urine. Treatment is with *antibiotic drugs*, such as *ampicillin*. If it is diagnosed and treated at an early stage, the disease can be completely cured. However, severe infection, especially in the newborn, may be fatal.

Lithium

A drug used in the long-term treatment of *mania* and *manic-depressive illness*. Lithium helps prevent mood swings in mania and reduces their frequency and severity in manic-depressive illness.

HOW IT WORKS

Lithium reduces excessive nerve activity in the brain. It is thought to work by altering the chemical balance within certain nerve cells.

POSSIBLE ADVERSE EFFECTS

High levels of lithium in the blood may cause nausea, vomiting, diarrhoea, blurred vision, tremor, drowsiness, rash, and, in rare cases, kidney

damage. Regular blood tests are carried out in order to monitor the level of lithium in the body.

Too much tea and coffee increases the risk of adverse effects. Too much sodium in the diet reduces the effectiveness of treatment.

Lithotomy

Surgical removal of a *calculus* (stone) from the urinary tract, especially from the bladder.

The operation of "cutting for stone" is one of the oldest known surgical procedures. Bladder stones were formerly removed by approaching the organ through incisions between the thighs rather than via the abdomen. The patient would lie back with the knees bent and legs open. Today, this *lithotomy position* is used mainly for gynaecological examinations.

The operations of ureterolithotomy and *pyelolithotomy* (removal of ureteral and kidney stones respectively, by incision) are still occasionally performed. In developed countries, surgical removal of bladder stones is performed only for large stones. Instead, bladder stones are usually crushed and removed by use of a cystoscope (see *Cystoscopy*) or pulverized ultrasonically by *lithotripsy*.

Lithotomy position

Position in which a patient lies on his or her back with the knees bent and wide apart. Once used for *lithotomy* (surgical removal of bladder stones), the position is still used for *pelvic examinations*, childbirth, and many types of pelvic surgery. Stirrups are often used to provide support for the feet and legs.

Lithotripsy

The process of using shock waves or ultrasonic waves to break up *calculi* (stones) for excretion. There are two different procedures—extracorporeal shock-wave lithotripsy (ESWL) and percutaneous lithotripsy.

WHY IT IS DONE

Lithotripsy is used to break up kidney and upper ureteral stones (see *Calculus, urinary tract*) into tiny pieces so that they can be excreted in the urine. The technique is also being used as a treatment for some types of *gallstones*.

ESWL is used to break up smaller stones; percutaneous lithotripsy is used to break up larger stones. Very large stones may be treated with a combination of the two.

HOW IT IS DONE

Both procedures may be performed under general or epidural anaesthetic,

although some machines do not require an anaesthetic at all.

ESWL This technique uses a machine called a *lithotripter* to produce external shock waves to break up stones. X-ray imaging systems are used to show the stone's position and monitor its destruction into a fine sand, which is passed out in the urine or the bile over the following few weeks. ESWL has radically changed the treatment of kidney stones by eliminating the need for surgery in many cases, and is also changing the treatment of gallstones.

PERCUTANEOUS LITHOTRIPSY A nephroscope (a viewing instrument for inspecting the kidney) is inserted into the kidney via a small puncture in the flank. An ultrasonic probe is directed through the nephroscope to break up the stone, and the fragments of stone are then removed through the nephroscope. (See also illustrated box opposite.)

RECOVERY PERIOD

There may be blood in the urine for about 12 hours after treatment. After ESWL there may be some bruising of the skin at the entry and exit points of the shock wave. Most people can return to full activity within a week.

COMPLICATIONS

Ureteral colic (severe spasmodic pain in the side due to obstruction of the ureter by small fragments of stone) may occur after ESWL. Those treated for gallstones may need drug treatment to aid the final elimination of stone residues.

Lithotripter

The machine used in extracorporeal shock-wave *lithotripsy* (ESWL) to disintegrate small *calculi* (stones).

Livedo reticularis

A net-like purple or blue mottling of the skin, usually on the lower legs. It is caused by the enlargement of blood vessels beneath the skin and tends to be worse in cold weather.

Although harmless, the condition is present for life. Livedo reticularis may appear in healthy people, but is more common in those with abnormal sensitivity to cold or in people who have suffered damage to blood vessels just beneath the skin (see *Vasculitis*).

Liver

The largest and one of the most important internal organs, which functions as the body's chemical factory and regulates the levels of most of the main chemicals in blood. The liver is located in the upper right abdominal

LITHOTRIPSY PROCEDURES

Calculi can sometimes be removed without major surgery. Lithotripsy uses ultrasonic or shock waves to break up the calculi. In percutaneous lithotripsy, the calculi are easily removed through a small incision. After extracorporeal shock-wave lithotripsy (ESWL), stone fragments are passed in the urine.

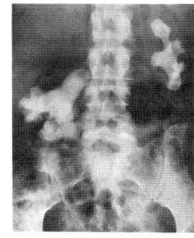

Abdominal calculi
This X-ray shows two staghorn calculi in the kidneys. Before lithotripsy, stones such as these could be removed only by major surgery.

PERCUTANEOUS LITHOTRIPSY

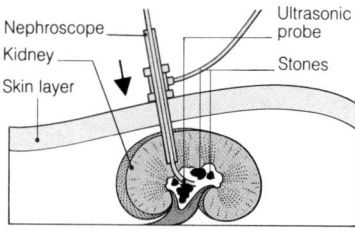

Nephroscope
Kidney
Skin layer
Ultrasonic probe
Stones

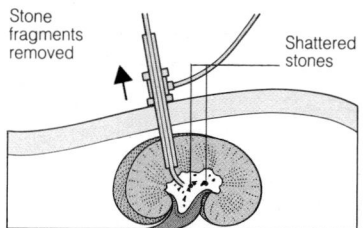

Stone fragments removed
Shattered stones

1 The surgeon first makes a small incision and inserts a nephroscope (a type of viewing tube) into the kidney.

2 A probe is passed through the nephroscope to direct ultrasound waves at the stones, causing them to shatter. Stone fragments are then removed.

EXTRACORPOREAL SHOCK-WAVE LITHOTRIPSY (ESWL)

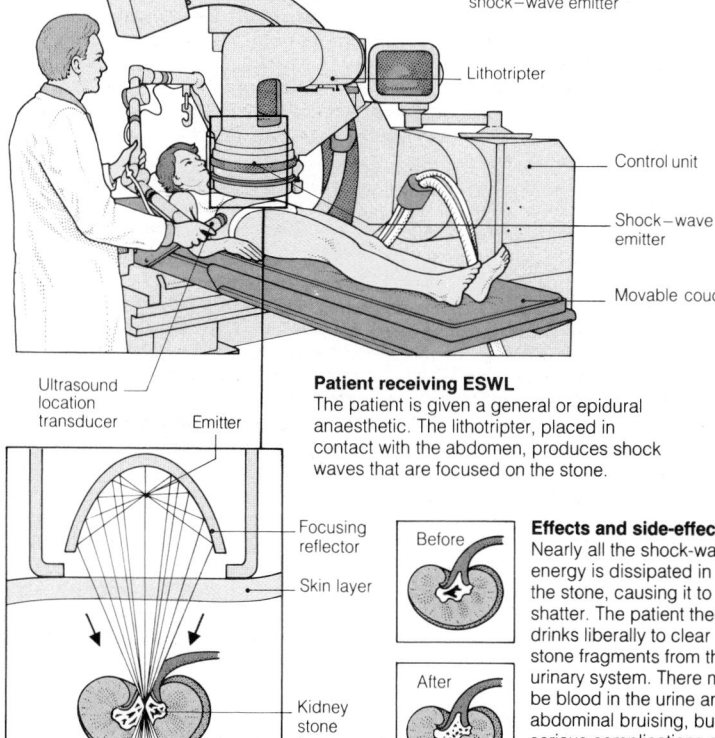

Arm for positioning shock–wave emitter
Lithotripter
Control unit
Shock–wave emitter
Movable couch

Ultrasound location transducer
Emitter
Focusing reflector
Skin layer
Kidney stone fragmented

Patient receiving ESWL
The patient is given a general or epidural anaesthetic. The lithotripter, placed in contact with the abdomen, produces shock waves that are focused on the stone.

Before

After

Effects and side-effects
Nearly all the shock-wave energy is dissipated in the stone, causing it to shatter. The patient then drinks liberally to clear stone fragments from the urinary system. There may be blood in the urine and abdominal bruising, but serious complications are uncommon.

cavity, directly below the diaphragm. In adults, the liver weighs approximately 1 to 1.5 kg.

STRUCTURE

The liver is a roughly cone-shaped, red-brown organ divided into two main lobes. Each lobe consists of many lobules. Surrounding each lobule are branches of the hepatic artery and the portal vein (see illustrated box on p.643). The liver receives oxygenated blood from the hepatic artery and nutrient-rich blood via the portal vein. All the blood from the liver drains into the hepatic veins. The liver cells secrete *bile*, a fluid that leaves the liver through a network of ducts, known as bile ducts. Within the liver, the small bile ducts and branches of the hepatic artery and portal vein form a kind of conduit system called the portal tracts.

FUNCTION

The liver has many functions vital to the body. One is to produce important proteins for blood plasma. These proteins include albumin (which regulates the exchange of water between blood and tissues), complement (a group of proteins that play a part in the *immune system*), coagulation factors (which enable blood to clot when a blood vessel wall is damaged), and globin (a constituent of the oxygen-carrying pigment *haemoglobin*). The liver also produces *cholesterol* and special proteins that help carry fats around the body.

Another function of the liver is to take up glucose that is not required immediately by the body's cells, and store it as glycogen. When the body needs to generate more energy and heat, the liver (under the stimulation of hormones) converts the glycogen back to glucose and releases it into the bloodstream.

The liver also regulates the *blood level* of *amino acids*, chemicals that are the building blocks of proteins. When the blood contains too high a level of amino acids (such as after a meal), the liver converts some of them into glucose, some into proteins, some into other amino acids, and some into *urea*, which is passed to the kidney for excretion in the urine.

Along with the kidneys, the liver acts to clear the blood of drugs and poisonous substances that would otherwise accumulate in the bloodstream. The liver absorbs the substances to be removed from the blood, alters their chemical structure, makes them water soluble, and excretes them in the bile.

L

Bile carries waste products away from the liver and helps in the breakdown and absorption of fats in the small intestine (see *Biliary system*).

Although extremely complex in its functions, the liver is a remarkably resilient organ. Up to three quarters of its cells can be destroyed or surgically removed before it ceases to function.

Liver abscess

A localized collection of pus in the *liver*. The most common causes are a spread of bacteria from intestines inflamed by *diverticulitis* or *appendicitis*, and invasion of the liver by amoebae (single-celled animal parasites) in people infected with *amoebiasis*. In some cases, the source of infection cannot be identified.

An affected person is obviously ill, with a high fever, pain in the upper right abdomen, and (especially if elderly) mental confusion.

DIAGNOSIS AND TREATMENT

Ultrasound scanning usually shows the abscess. The responsible microorganisms can sometimes be identified from a blood sample or from a sample of tissue obtained by aspiration (withdrawal by suction through a needle) of the liver abscess.

A liver abscess can sometimes be treated by aspiration (sucking out the pus), using ultrasound to guide the needle through the abdominal wall. Otherwise, abdominal surgery is necessary to remove the abscess.

Liver biopsy

A diagnostic test in which a small sample of tissue is removed from the *liver*. The procedure is relatively safe, and complications are rare.

WHY IT IS DONE

The main function of the test is to diagnose liver diseases, such as *cirrhosis* and different types of *hepatitis*. A liver biopsy can also help diagnose diseases, such as *lymphomas* and various other types of tumours, which spread throughout the body and affect many organs. Liver biopsy can also provide an important check on the efficacy of treatment of diseases such as chronic active hepatitis.

HOW IT IS DONE

Most liver biopsies are performed under a local anaesthetic. While the patient holds his or her breath, a slim needle is inserted into the liver via a very small incision made over the right lower ribs. The needle is removed together with a small sample

of liver tissue. The structure and cells of the liver tissue are then examined by a pathologist.

A liver biopsy is sometimes performed during the course of another abdominal operation.

Liver cancer

A *malignant* tumour in the *liver*. The tumour may be primary (originating within the liver itself) or secondary (having spread from elsewhere). There are two main types of primary tumour—a hepatoma, which develops in the liver cells, and a *cholangiocarcinoma*, which arises from cells lining the *bile ducts*.

CAUSES AND INCIDENCE

Hepatomas are the most common form of cancer worldwide. They are closely linked to infection with hepatitis B (see *Hepatitis, viral*), which is common throughout Africa, the Middle East, and the Far East. In the UK, hepatitis B is a relatively uncommon infection, so the incidence of hepatomas is quite low: there are about 700 new cases in the UK annually. When a hepatoma does occur, it is usually a complication of *cirrhosis* of the liver.

Secondary liver cancer is relatively common in the UK (about 20 times more common than primary cancer). This type of cancer often originates from cancers in the stomach, pancreas, or large intestine, which may have been small and caused no symptoms (and so remained undiagnosed until they had spread to the liver).

SYMPTOMS AND SIGNS

The most common symptoms of any liver cancer are weight loss, loss of appetite, and lethargy. Many sufferers also have pain in the upper right abdomen. The later stages of the disease are marked by *jaundice* and *ascites* (fluid in the abdomen).

DIAGNOSIS

Liver tumours are usually detected as a result of *ultrasound scanning* that reveals abnormal areas in the liver. The diagnosis is confirmed by *liver biopsy* (removal of a small sample of liver tissue for microscopic analysis).

About 80 per cent of hepatomas raise the production of a substance called *alpha-fetoprotein* by the liver; measurement of the blood level of this protein is used as a screening test in geographical areas where the cancer is common. *Angiography* (X-rays obtained after injecting a radiopaque substance into an artery) is also used to detect hepatomas too small to be seen by other scanning techniques.

LOCATION OF THE LIVER

The liver is a roughly cone-shaped, red-brown organ that occupies the upper right-hand portion of the abdominal cavity. It lies immediately beneath the diaphragm, to which its upper side is attached. Its base is in contact with the stomach, right kidney, and intestines. Tucked within a depression on the underside of the liver is the gallbladder.

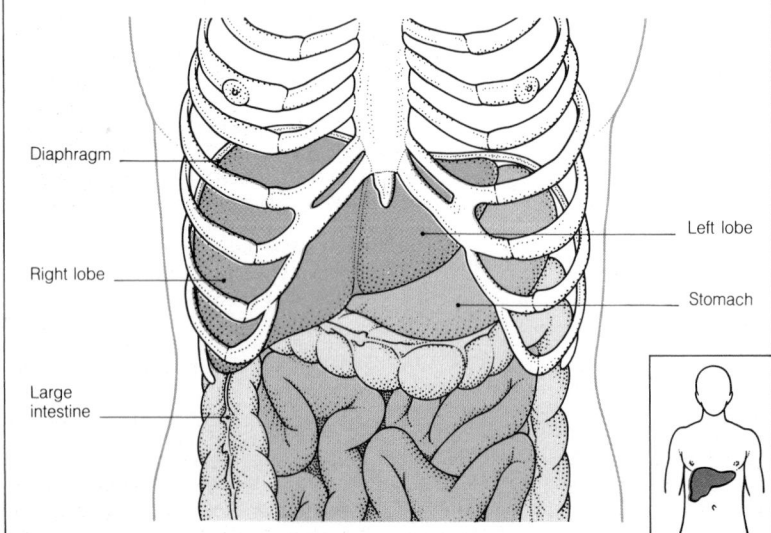

Diaphragm

Right lobe

Large intestine

Left lobe

Stomach

TREATMENT

A hepatoma usually remains confined to the liver for a long time. In cases where cirrhosis is not also present (which is rare in the UK), complete removal of the tumour, leading to cure, is sometimes possible. In other cases, *anticancer drugs* can help the patient survive longer. A *liver transplant* may occasionally be considered.

There is no cure for secondary liver cancer, but anticancer drugs can help slow the progress of the disease. Tying off or blocking the hepatic artery or one of its branches to deprive the tumour of its blood supply has been attempted, as has placing a catheter into the artery to administer anticancer drugs continuously.

Liver, cirrhosis of
See *Cirrhosis*.

Liver disease, alcoholic
Damage to the *liver* caused by persistent heavy *alcohol* consumption, with progression to *cirrhosis* of the liver (severe structural damage and loss of function) and death.

TYPES
Excess fat accumulation in the liver affects almost everyone with a moderate to high alcohol consumption. However, this condition is completely reversible through abstinence and, if reversed, carries a low risk of progression to cirrhosis.

Some persistent drinkers develop acute or chronic *hepatitis*. Individual liver cells are destroyed and there is inflammation and scarring of the liver. In people who continue to drink, there is a high risk (about 90 per cent) of progression to cirrhosis; in most people who stop drinking, the liver returns to normal. Cirrhosis is irreversible, but abstinence often leads to improvement in liver function.

CAUSES AND INCIDENCE
Until the 1960s, alcoholic liver damage was thought to be caused mainly by the malnutrition associated with alcohol dependence rather than by alcohol itself. It is now accepted that alcohol is directly toxic to the liver.

There is a clear relationship between the total amount of alcohol consumed in a population and the incidence of cirrhosis. The prevalence of alcoholic liver disease has been rising rapidly in most developed countries since about 1960, and the increase has been particularly steep in women. In the UK, around 6,000 people die each year as a result of alcoholic cirrhosis of the liver.

A person who consumes a daily average of 200 ml of alcohol (contained, for example, in about three quarters of a bottle of whisky or two and a half bottles of wine) has a 50 per cent chance of developing cirrhosis within 20 years. A much lower daily average intake of 45 ml of alcohol (con-

tained, for example, in four single whiskies or four glasses of wine) in a man, or half that amount in a woman, still carries a substantial risk.

SYMPTOMS AND DIAGNOSIS
The first symptoms or signs of liver damage are the same as those of hepatitis or cirrhosis. *Liver-function*

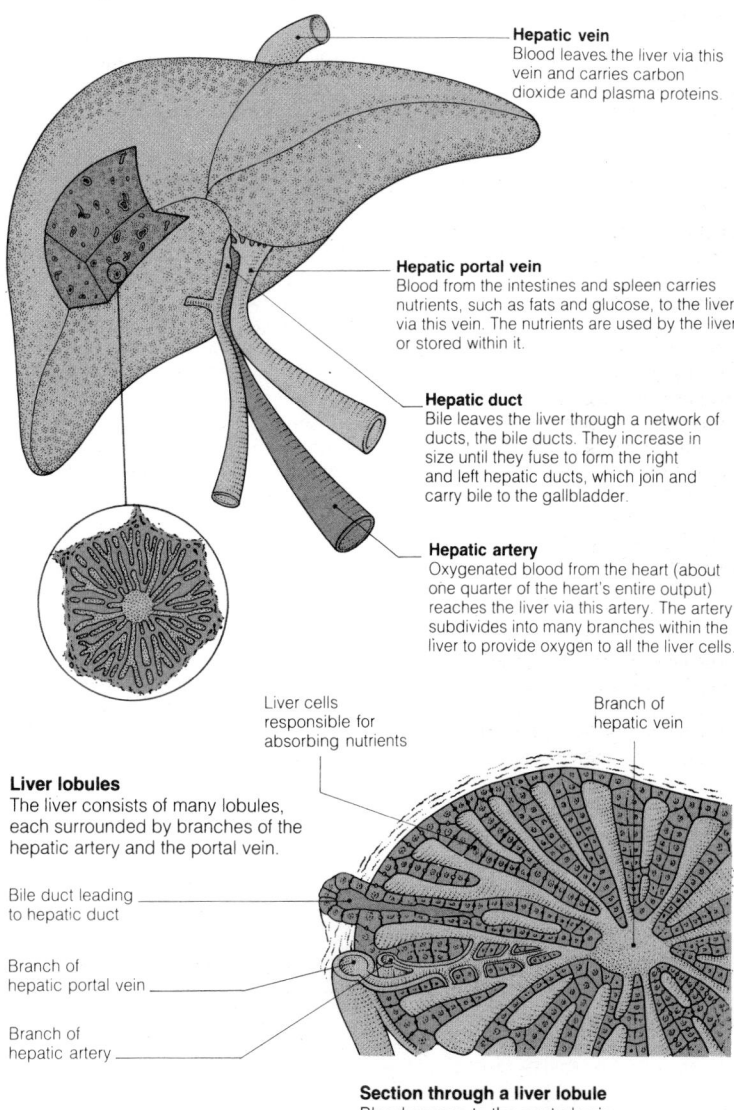

LIVER STRUCTURE AND FUNCTION
The liver is a large organ with numerous functions. It absorbs oxygen and nutrients from the blood, and regulates the blood's glucose and amino-acid levels. It helps break down drugs and various toxins, and manufactures important proteins, such as albumin and blood coagulation factors. The liver also produces bile, which removes waste products and helps process fats in the small intestine.

Hepatic vein
Blood leaves the liver via this vein and carries carbon dioxide and plasma proteins.

Hepatic portal vein
Blood from the intestines and spleen carries nutrients, such as fats and glucose, to the liver via this vein. The nutrients are used by the liver or stored within it.

Hepatic duct
Bile leaves the liver through a network of ducts, the bile ducts. They increase in size until they fuse to form the right and left hepatic ducts, which join and carry bile to the gallbladder.

Hepatic artery
Oxygenated blood from the heart (about one quarter of the heart's entire output) reaches the liver via this artery. The artery subdivides into many branches within the liver to provide oxygen to all the liver cells.

Liver cells responsible for absorbing nutrients

Branch of hepatic vein

Liver lobules
The liver consists of many lobules, each surrounded by branches of the hepatic artery and the portal vein.

Bile duct leading to hepatic duct

Branch of hepatic portal vein

Branch of hepatic artery

Section through a liver lobule
Blood passes to the central vein via pathways between cells.

tests show a characteristic pattern of abnormalities, and *liver biopsy* (removal of a sample of tissue for microscopic analysis) may be recommended to identify the precise type of damage.

TREATMENT AND OUTLOOK

Abstinence from alcohol is the only method of returning the liver to normal or improving its function and prolonging life expectancy. Treatment methods are as for *alcohol dependence.*

Liver failure

A complication of acute *hepatitis* (inflammation of the *liver*) in which there is such a severe impairment of liver function that it affects other organs, particularly the brain. Liver failure may also refer to a critical stage in *cirrhosis* of the liver.

SYMPTOMS

The principal symptoms of acute liver failure are those of the underlying hepatitis; later, symptoms of brain dysfunction develop. Disturbance of brain function probably occurs because the liver fails to break down certain substances (such as ammonia) that build up in the blood and then poison or alter the transmission of nerve messages in the brain. Symptoms may include agitation and restlessness, followed by drowsiness, confusion, and coma—a condition known as hepatic *encephalopathy.*

When liver failure accompanies cirrhosis, other complications, such as *ascites* (fluid in the abdomen) and internal bleeding, may develop in addition to hepatic encephalopathy. The symptoms of brain dysfunction develop more slowly, with recurrent episodes of drowsiness or confusion. These episodes are frequently precipitated by bacterial infections or by changes in drug treatment or diet.

DIAGNOSIS AND TREATMENT

A diagnosis is made from the patient's history, a physical examination, *liver-function tests*, and tests for viruses that can cause acute hepatitis.

Treatment of acute liver failure consists of skilled intensive care. There is no specific cure, although the use of *antibiotic drugs* and *lactulose* can reduce the number of intestinal bacteria, which are one of the main sources of toxic ammonia entering the bloodstream. A *liver transplant* is occasionally possible and suitable for certain patients. Only about a quarter of patients survive acute liver failure.

When brain dysfunction complicates cirrhosis, treatment of precipitating causes (such as infection) often leads to an improvement.

Liver fluke

 Any of various species of flukes (small, flattened, worms) that infest the *bile ducts* within the *liver.*

The only fluke of any importance in the UK is *FASCIOLA HEPATICA*, which causes the disease fascioliasis. The adult flukes normally infest sheep and produce eggs that are passed in the sheep's faeces. The eggs are eaten by snails, from which immature forms of the fluke emerge. They then become encysted (enclosed in a sac) on aquatic vegetation, particularly watercress. The disease is now only very rarely seen in the UK.

Fascioliasis has two stages. During the first stage, young flukes migrate through the liver, causing liver tenderness and enlargement, fever, night sweats, and sometimes a rash. In the second stage, adult worms are present in the bile ducts. This may lead to *cholangitis* (inflammation of the bile ducts) and *bile duct obstruction*, which can cause *jaundice.* In minor infections, there may be no symptoms. The disease is diagnosed from the pre-

sence of fluke eggs in the patient's faeces. Treatment with the *anthelmintic drug* praziquantel may be effective.

Another species of liver fluke, *CLONORCHIS SINENSIS*, is common in the Far East. Infection is typically acquired by eating raw or undercooked freshwater fish. The symptoms and treatment are broadly similar to those for fascioliasis.

Liver-function tests

A series of tests of blood chemistry that can detect changes in the way the *liver* is making new substances, breaking down and/or excreting old ones, and whether liver cells are healthy or being damaged. The tests are widely used to help in the diagnosis of liver disease, and to assess responses to treatment.

Liver-function tests are particularly useful in distinguishing between acute and chronic liver disorders and between *hepatitis* (liver inflammation) and *cholestasis* (obstruction to the flow of bile). The most commonly performed tests are described in the accompanying table.

TABLE OF LIVER-FUNCTION TESTS

Test	Significance
Serum bilirubin	Bilirubin is the yellow breakdown product of red blood cells that is passed to the liver and excreted in bile. It is the substance that gives the yellow colour to the skin in jaundice. A high bilirubin level in the blood may indicate defective processing of bile by the liver or obstruction to bile flow.
Serum albumin	Albumin is one of the main proteins in blood. Made by the liver, one of its actions is to hold fluid inside the blood vessels. A low level is found in many chronic liver disorders and is often associated with ascites and ankle oedema (fluid collection in the abdomen and around the ankles).
Serum alkaline phosphatase	Alkaline phosphatase is an enzyme found in bile. The blood level of this enzyme rises when there is obstruction to the flow of bile (cholestasis).
Serum aminotransferases (transaminases)	The aminotransferases are enzymes released from liver cells into the blood when the liver cells are damaged. The levels will be raised in acute and chronic hepatitis.
Prothrombin time	A normal result in this test of blood clotting depends on the presence in the blood of a protein made by the liver from a fat-soluble vitamin, vitamin K. The test result can be abnormal in two kinds of disorders—when the protein is not made because of liver cell damage, and when there is a blockage to bile flow in the liver, causing a lack of bile in the intestines (which interferes with fat and vitamin K absorption).

DISORDERS OF THE LIVER

By far the most common cause of liver disease in the UK and other developed countries is excessive consumption of alcohol (see *Liver disease, alcoholic*). Alcohol-related disorders, which include alcoholic *hepatitis* and *cirrhosis*, outnumber all other types of liver disorder by at least five to one.

Worldwide, the pattern of liver disease is different. In parts of Africa and Asia, up to 20 per cent of the population are carriers of the hepatitis B virus; (see *Hepatitis, viral*) in these parts of the world, the most important liver disorders are virus-induced cirrhosis and primary *liver cancer*.

Apart from alcohol- and virus-induced liver disease, the liver may be affected by congenital defects, bacterial and parasitic infection, circulatory disturbance, metabolic disorders, poisoning, and autoimmune processes.

Liver failure (complete loss of liver function) may occur as a result of acute hepatitis, poisoning, or cirrhosis. Enlargement of the liver (hepatomegaly) and *jaundice* are two common signs of liver disease.

CONGENITAL DEFECTS

Defects of liver structure at birth principally affect the bile ducts. A choledochal cyst is a malformation of the hepatic duct (formed from the union of all the small bile ducts in the liver) which may obstruct the flow of bile in infants (causing jaundice); it requires removal. In *biliary atresia*, the bile ducts are absent, again causing jaundice.

INFECTION AND INFLAMMATION

Hepatitis is a general term for inflammation in the liver; it may be caused by viruses such as the hepatitis A, B, C, D, and E viruses (see *Hepatitis, viral*). Bacteria may spread up the biliary system towards the liver to cause *cholangitis* or *liver abscess*. Parasitic diseases that may affect the liver include *schistosomiasis, liver fluke*, and *hydatid disease* (caused by various types of worm or fluke) and *amoebiasis* (caused by a single-celled parasite).

POISONING AND DRUGS

Apart from alcohol, many drugs and toxins are broken down by the liver, damaging liver cells in the process. Suicidal overdose with the painkilling drug paracetamol causes severe liver damage, which may not be obvious until up to two days after the overdose. Some medications, even in normal doses, can cause acute or chronic hepatitis by a direct toxic effect or through drug allergy.

Poisoning by certain types of mushrooms can cause acute liver failure (see *Mushroom poisoning*).

AUTOIMMUNE DISORDERS

Liver cells and bile ducts can be targets for autoimmune reactions (in which the body's immune system attacks its own tissues). A gradual destruction of liver cells is the main problem in autoimmune chronic active hepatitis (see *Hepatitis, chronic active*). The slowly progressive bile duct damage that occurs in primary *biliary cirrhosis* and sclerosing cholangitis possibly also has an autoimmune basis.

METABOLIC DISORDERS

The two main metabolic disorders affecting the liver are *haemochromatosis* (in which there is too much iron in the body) and *Wilson's disease* (in which there is too much copper).

TUMOURS

The liver is a common site of malignant tumours that have spread from cancers of the stomach, pancreas, or large intestine. Enlargement of the liver and spleen is a common feature of *leukaemias* and *lymphomas*. Primary tumours of the liver are much less common. (See *Liver cancer*.)

OTHER DISORDERS

In *Budd-Chiari syndrome*, the veins draining the liver become blocked by blood clots, causing painful swelling of the liver and severe *ascites* (collection of fluid in the abdomen). Obstruction of the portal vein is one cause of *portal hypertension* (high blood pressure in the portal vein), which can lead to *oesophageal varices* (swollen veins in the oesophagus) and ascites. Portal hypertension is also one of the usual complications of cirrhosis.

Hepatitis
Inflammation of the liver may be caused by one of the hepatitis viruses, alcohol, or various poisons.

Amoebiasis
Infection by amoebic parasites can cause painful abscesses in the liver.

Liver cancer
Malignant tumours may arise from the liver itself or may spread from cancer elsewhere in the body.

Choledochal cyst
This congenital malformation blocks the flow of bile through the hepatic duct.

L

INVESTIGATION

Disorders of the liver may be investigated by physical examination, *liver biopsy, liver-function tests, ultrasound scanning*, and *CT scanning* and *MRI*.

Liver imaging

A technique that produces images of the *liver, gallbladder, bile ducts,* and blood vessels supplying the liver to detect abnormality or disease.

TYPES

CONVENTIONAL X-RAY TECHNIQUES *Cholecystography* and *cholangiography* are techniques in which a contrast medium (an iodine-containing substance that is opaque to X-rays) is introduced to show up *gallstones,* tumours, and blockages. *ERCP* (endoscopic retrograde cholangiopancreatography) is an alternative method of examining the *biliary system* by means of a contrast medium; it is especially useful in detecting blockage or narrowing of a bile duct or pancreatic duct by a stone or tumour.

Angiography shows up the blood vessels in the liver. It can be used to confirm the diagnosis of a *haemangioma* or to plan the treatment of liver tumours and other disorders.

SCANNING TECHNIQUES *Ultrasound scanning* is the most widely used of all liver imaging techniques. It is simple, safe, noninvasive, and produces excellent images, particularly of gallstones. *CT scanning* and *MRI* provide good images, and are commonly used to add further information to that provided by an ultasound scan.

Radionuclide scanning can indicate the presence of a cyst or a tumour. It is also useful in recording the progress of radioactive isotopes as they are excreted from the liver in bile.

Liver transplant

Replacement of a diseased *liver* with a healthy liver removed from a donor who has been declared brain dead. Liver transplantation is a technically difficult procedure, but it has now become routine in specialist centres around the world and is the only curative treatment for irreversible liver failure. The chances of long-term survival are now close to those of *kidney transplants,* but the main problem remains the shortage of donor organs.

WHY IT IS DONE

Transplantation is worth considering only for people with life-threatening or severely debilitating liver disease. However, if the disease process is too advanced, the person is unlikely to survive the operation. An assessment must be made of the likely length of survival and the quality of life with and without the operation.

In adults, the best results are obtained in the treatment of advanced liver *cirrhosis* in people with long-standing chronic active *hepatitis* or primary *biliary cirrhosis.* In acute *liver failure,* there can be difficulty in obtaining donor organs at an appropriate time, but people with a slightly less acute illness and those with *Budd-Chiari syndrome* have been successfully treated. People with primary *liver cancer* are rarely considered for transplantation because there is a high risk that the tumour will recur.

In children, congenital *biliary atresia* is the most common reason for liver transplantation.

HOW IT IS DONE

The donor organ is obtained from someone who has suffered *brain death* but whose liver is still healthy. The organ can be stored in cold salt solutions for a few hours.

A general anaesthetic is given and the recipient's abdomen is opened. The diseased liver is removed, the donor organ is inserted in its place, and the major blood vessels and common bile duct are reconnected.

RECOVERY PERIOD

The first few days after the operation are spent in an *intensive-care* unit. *Immunosuppressant drugs* (particularly *cyclosporin*) are given to reduce the risk of rejection.

OUTLOOK

In some cases rejection of the donor organ occurs and a second transplant operation provides the only hope. There is now a 60 to 80 per cent chance of surviving one year, and more than half of the people receiving a liver transplant now survive for five years. The quality of life is generally excellent, with most people returning to near normal activity within a few weeks of the operation.

Living will

A written declaration, signed by an adult person of sound mind, that instructs his or her doctors to withhold or withdraw life-sustaining treatment if he or she suffers from an incurable and terminal condition.

In some countries, legislation has been passed giving legal effect to living wills. In the UK, however, no such law has been passed, although campaigners for the legalization of euthanasia have called for its introduction. The existence of a document drawn up by a solicitor would have no legal force, but it might influence a doctor's decision.

Lobe

One of the clearly defined parts into which certain organs, such as the brain, liver, lungs, and thyroid gland, are divided. The term may also be used to describe any projecting, flat, pendulous part of the body, such as the earlobe.

Lobectomy

An operation to cut out a lobe in the brain (see *Lobotomy, prefrontal*), liver (see *Hepatectomy, partial*), lungs (see *Lobectomy, lung*), or thyroid gland (see *Thyroidectomy*).

Lobectomy, lung

An operation to remove one of the lobes of the *lung.* Lobectomy is usually performed to remove a malignant tumour, but may also be used to treat localized *bronchiectasis* that has not responded to medical treatment. In the past, lobectomy was carried out to treat *tuberculosis,* which is today treated by drugs.

After lobectomy, the remaining lobes expand to fill the chest cavity.

HOW IT IS DONE

With the patient under a general anaesthetic, a curved incision is made, starting under the armpit and extending across the back, following the line of the lower edge of the shoulder-blade. The muscles are cut through and the ribs are spread apart (or one is removed) to expose the lung. The blood vessels and bronchus (main airway) leading to the diseased lobe are then tied off and divided, and the lobe is removed. Before the incision is sewn up, a tube is inserted into the pleural space surrounding the lung to drain off fluid. The tube is usually removed after 24 hours.

The operation usually requires a hospital stay of several weeks; full recovery may take several months.

Lobotomy, prefrontal

The cutting of some of the fibres linking the frontal lobes to the rest of the *brain.* Prefrontal lobotomy was extensively used in the 1940s and 1950s to treat serious psychiatric disorders. However, the operation often resulted in harmful personality changes and is now used only as a last resort to treat people with severe, chronic depression. (See also *Psychosurgery.*)

Lochia

The discharge after childbirth of blood and fragments of uterine lining from the site where the placenta was attached. The discharge is bright red for the first three or four days and then becomes paler. The amount of lochia decreases as the placental site heals and usually ceases within six weeks.

Locked knee

A temporary inability to move the *knee* joint. A locked knee may be caused by a torn knee cartilage or by *loose bodies* in the joint.

Lockjaw

A painful spasm of the jaw muscles that makes it difficult or impossible to open the mouth. Lockjaw is the most common symptom of *tetanus*.

Locomotor

Relating to movement of the extremities, as in locomotor *ataxia*, the incoordinated movements and lurching gait that occur in the later stages of untreated syphilis.

Lofepramine

A tricyclic *antidepressant drug* that is used in the long-term treatment of *depression*. Lofepramine is less likely to cause sedation than many other antidepressant drugs.

Loiasis

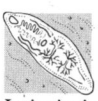
A form of the tropical parasitic disease *filariasis* that is caused by an infestation by the worm LOA LOA. Loiasis is transmitted by the bite of CHRYSOPS flies. The adult worms, which are between 3 and 7 cm long, travel beneath the skin, producing itchy areas of inflammation known as Calabar swellings. The worms may also sometimes be seen moving across the front of the eye. Loiasis is treated with a course of diethylcarbamazine, which destroys the worms.

Loin

The part of the back on each side of the spine between the lowest pair of ribs and the top of the pelvis.

Loose bodies

Fragments of bone, cartilage, or capsule linings that are free to move within a *joint*. Loose bodies may occur whenever there is any damage to a joint, as in *osteoarthritis* (degeneration due to wear and tear), fracture, or *osteochondritis dissecans* (fragmentation of bone and cartilage due to disrupted blood supply).

SYMPTOMS AND SIGNS
Loose bodies are usually troublesome only if they lodge between joint surfaces, where they cause the joint to lock (usually only briefly), resulting in severe pain. The joint usually swells several hours later. Although the swelling subsides, further locking and swelling can recur at any time.

DIAGNOSIS AND TREATMENT
X-rays or *arthroscopy* (inspection of the interior of a joint through a viewing instrument) reveal whether loose bodies are present.

Gentle manipulation may be required to unlock the joint. If locking occurs frequently, the loose bodies may be removed during arthroscopy or by surgery.

Longsightedness

See *Hypermetropia*.

Loperamide

An *antidiarrhoeal drug* used in the treatment of recurrent and sudden bouts of diarrhoea. Loperamide is also given to help regulate bowel action in people who have had an *ileostomy*.

Loperamide occasionally produces a rash. Other rare adverse effects, such as fever, abdominal cramps, and bloating, are often difficult to distinguish from symptoms of the disorder causing the diarrhoea.

Lorazepam

A *benzodiazepine drug* that is used in the treatment of *insomnia* and *anxiety*. If use of lorazepam is suddenly stopped after it has been taken regularly for more than three weeks, there may be withdrawal symptoms (see *Drug dependence*).

Lordosis

Inward curvature of the *spine*, which is normally present to a minor degree in the lower back. Lordosis in the lower back can become exaggerated by poor posture (especially in someone who is overweight and also has weak abdominal muscles) or by *kyphosis* (backward curvature of the spine) above the lower back.

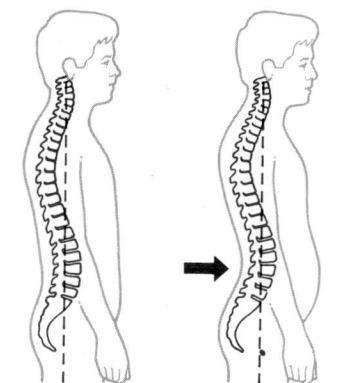

Normal and abnormal lordosis
The normal inward curvature of the spine (left) is exaggerated in abnormal lordosis (right).

Once pronounced lordosis has developed, it is usually a permanent condition and can lead to *disc prolapse* or *osteoarthritis* of the spine.

Loss of normal lordosis in the lower back or neck can occur when the back or neck muscles are in spasm. The condition corrects itself once the cause is successfully treated.

Lotion

A liquid drug preparation applied to the skin. Lotions have a cooling, soothing effect and are useful for covering large areas. Examples of drugs prepared as a lotion include *calamine* and *betamethasone*, which are used to treat skin inflammation.

LSD

A synthetic *hallucinogenic drug* (drug that produces hallucinations) derived from ergot (a type of fungus). LSD is the abbreviation for lysergic acid diethylamide. The drug has no medical role. Its distribution and manufacture is controlled by the Misuse of Drugs Act because of the drug's high potential for abuse.

LSD sometimes produces "bad trips" in which a person experiences panic, fear, and physical symptoms, such as nausea, dizziness, and weakness. In severe cases, sedation in hospital may be necessary for several days. There may also be "flashbacks" to previous trips months or even years afterwards.

Although there is no evidence that LSD causes *psychosis* (mental illness characterized by a loss of contact with reality), it may act as a trigger in a person predisposed to mental illness. There is also evidence that LSD damages chromosomes.

Ludwig's angina

A rare bacterial infection of the floor of the mouth that becomes life-threatening as it spreads to the throat. The affected tissues become inflamed, swell, and harden.

The disorder is usually caused by an infected tooth or gum and is most common in people with poor *oral hygiene*. It generally results in fever, pain, and swelling in the mouth and neck, and difficulty in opening the mouth and swallowing.

If the condition is not treated immediately with *antibiotic drugs*, the swollen tissues of the throat may cause difficulty in breathing. *Tracheostomy* (making a hole in the windpipe and inserting a tube through it) may be necessary to prevent asphyxiation.

Lumbago

A general term for lower *back pain*. Lumbago is a symptom that may be caused by various disorders, but in many cases no definite cause is found.

Lumbago may be caused by an intervertebral *disc prolapse*. It may also arise if a bit of *synovium* (thin membrane lining the capsule surrounding a joint) is caught between the surfaces of a small intervertebral joint, or if there is momentary *subluxation* (incomplete dislocation) of an intervertebral joint with straining of *ligaments*. Lumbago is often caused by a sudden turning or bending movement but may also begin gradually.

Lumbago is often aggravated by movement and relieved by rest. Treatment is usually bed rest, with additional measures as appropriate. (See also *Lumbosacral spasm*.)

Lumbar

Relating to the part of the back between the lowest pair of ribs and the top of the pelvis. The lumbar region of the *spine* consists of the five lumbar vertebrae between the lowest (12th) thoracic vertebra and the sacrum.

Lumbar puncture

A procedure in which a hollow needle is inserted into the lower part of the spinal canal to withdraw *cerebrospinal fluid* (the watery liquid that surrounds the brain and spinal cord) or to inject drugs or other substances. Lumbar puncture is used less often since the development of *CT scanning* and *MRI* (magnetic resonance imaging) as diagnostic tests.

WHY IT IS DONE
The main use of the lumbar puncture is to examine cerebrospinal fluid to diagnose and investigate disorders of the brain and spinal cord (such as *meningitis* and *subarachnoid haemorrhage*). The procedure is also used to inject drugs into the fluid (such as *anticancer drugs* to treat *leukaemia* and malignant diseases of the central nervous system). Another use of lumbar puncture is to inject a contrast medium that will show up on X-ray (see *Myelography*) to produce images of the spinal cord. Lumbar puncture can also be used to inject a local anaesthetic to achieve extensive anaesthesia without loss of consciousness.

HOW IT IS DONE
The patient lies on his or her side, chin on chest and knees drawn up to pull the vertebrae (bones of the spine) apart. The area of skin overlying the lumbar vertebrae at the base of the spine is anaesthetized with a local anaesthetic. A hollow needle is then inserted between two of the vertebrae and into the spinal canal and is used to withdraw cerebrospinal fluid or to inject drugs, an anaesthetic, or a contrast medium.

After the needle is removed, the puncture site is covered with sterile tape. The procedure takes less than 20 minutes. Lumbar puncture usually causes no discomfort although some people may have a headache for a short time afterwards.

Lumbosacral spasm

Prolonged, excessive tightening of the muscles that surround and support the lower part of the *spine*. Lumbosacral spasm is a cause of *back pain* and may occasionally result in temporary *scoliosis* (curvature of the spine to one side). Treatment may include bed rest, *analgesic drugs* (painkillers), and *muscle-relaxant drugs*.

Lumen

The space within a tubular organ. The term is most commonly used to refer to the cavity of the intestine.

Lumpectomy

An operation to treat breast cancer (see *Mastectomy*).

Lunacy

An outdated term for serious mental disorder. It was coined because of the belief that phases of the moon ("luna" in Latin) could bring on mental illnesses, especially illnesses that seemed to come and go. Patients were called lunatics and mental hospitals were known as lunatic asylums.

Lung

The main organ of the *respiratory system*. The two lungs supply the body with the oxygen needed for *aerobic* metabolism and eliminate the waste product carbon dioxide.

LOCATION AND STRUCTURE OF THE LUNGS

The lungs lie in the chest within the rib-cage. Air entering the body via the nose and mouth travels down the trachea to the main bronchi, which divide into smaller bronchi and then into bronchioles. These in turn lead to alveoli, where the oxygen/carbon dioxide exchange takes place. During expiration (breathing out), air leaves the body by the same routes.

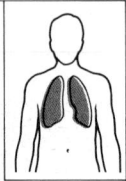

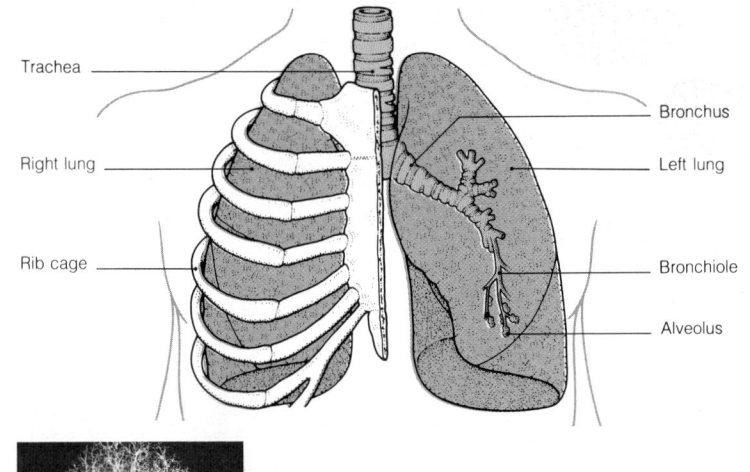

Trachea

Right lung

Rib cage

Bronchus

Left lung

Bronchiole

Alveolus

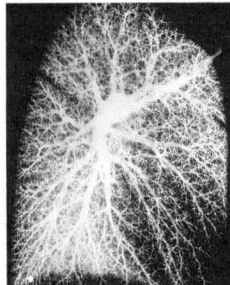

Blood vessels in a lung
The tiniest "twigs" of this extensive blood vessel "tree" form into capillaries that surround the alveoli (air sacs) in the lung. Oxygen and carbon dioxide are exchanged between the alveoli and the capillaries.

STRUCTURE

The *trachea* (windpipe) branches in the chest into two main *bronchi* (air passages), which supply the left and right lungs. The main bronchi divide again into smaller bronchi and then into bronchioles, which lead to air passages that open out into grape-like air sacs called *alveoli*. It is through the thin walls of the alveoli that gases (notably oxygen and carbon dioxide) diffuse into or out of the blood.

Each lung is enclosed in a double membrane called the *pleura*, which allows the lungs to slide freely as they expand and contract during *breathing*. (See also *Respiration*.)

Lung cancer

The most common form of *cancer* in the UK, lung cancer is the leading cause of cancer deaths in men and the second most common cause (after breast cancer) in women. There were about 35,000 deaths from lung cancer in 1993 in England and Wales. The peak age for lung cancer is 65 to 75 years. The disease is uncommon before the age of 40.

CAUSES

Smoking cigarettes is the main cause of lung cancer. The more cigarettes smoked per day and the lower the age at which smoking started, the greater the risk of lung cancer. Smokers of cigars or pipes have a lower risk of developing lung cancer than people who smoke cigarettes, but they still have a significantly higher risk than do nonsmokers (see *Tobacco-smoking*). Passive smoking (the inhalation of tobacco smoke by nonsmokers) has also been shown to increase the risk of developing lung cancer.

Living in an environment with a high level of air pollution or working with substances such as radioactive minerals or asbestos may cause some cases of lung cancer.

TYPES

There are several types of lung cancer, the most common being squamous cell carcinoma, small cell carcinoma (also called oat cell carcinoma), adenocarcinoma, and large cell carcinoma; each has a different growth pattern and response to treatment. The squamous cell, small cell, and large cell types are all strongly associated with tobacco use; the relationship between adenocarcinoma and tobacco use is less clear.

SYMPTOMS AND SIGNS

The first and most common symptom is a cough, occurring in about 80 per cent of people with lung cancer. About half of all people with lung cancer have a chronic cough due to *bronchitis*. Other symptoms include coughing up blood, shortness of breath, chest pain, and wheezing.

Lung cancer can spread locally to affect tissues immediately surrounding the lungs, or can spread to other parts of the body, especially the liver, brain, and bones. Pain may occur in these sites, and weight loss is a common symptom. Local spread may cause the collapse of a lung (see *Atelectasis*) or *pneumonia* (inflammation of the lung) or may affect the pleura (membrane covering the lung), causing *pleural effusion* (excess fluid between the lung and chest wall).

DIAGNOSIS

Lung cancer may be suspected from the patient's symptoms and from a

L

DISORDERS OF THE LUNG

The lungs are continuously exposed to airborne particles, such as bacteria, viruses, and allergens, all of which can cause lung disorders. Most of these disorders do not interfere with oxygen supply; those that do are a major threat to health.

INFECTION

Infective disorders are common, especially *tracheitis* (inflammation of the lining of the windpipe) and *croup* (a virus infection of young children). *Bronchitis* (inflammation of the bronchi), *bronchiectasis* (swelling of the bronchi), and *bronchiolitis* (inflammation of the bronchioles) commonly follow colds or *influenza*. *Pneumonia* (inflammation of the lung) is usually caused by infection by viruses or bacteria. Fungal infections of the lungs, such as *aspergillosis*, *actinomycosis*, *histoplasmosis*, and *candidiasis*, are relatively uncommon.

ALLERGIES

Bronchial *asthma*, in which the muscles of the bronchi contract and obstruct the free passage of air, often occurs in sensitized people exposed to pollens, house mites, fungal spores, animal *dander*, and many other agents. Allergic *alveolitis* (inflammation of the alveoli) may be caused by many organic dusts, such as mouldy hay.

TUMOURS

Lung cancer is one of the most common of all malignant tumours; in most cases it is associated with cigarette smoking. Secondary malignant tumours, which have spread from other parts of the body to the lungs, are common. However, benign tumours affecting the lung are uncommon.

INJURY

Lung injury usually results from penetration of the chest wall. *Pneumothorax* (air in the pleural cavity) and *haemothorax* (blood in the pleural cavity) are usually caused by a penetrating injury; either may cause collapse of the lung. Injury can also occur from the inhalation of poisonous dusts, gases, or toxic substances. *Silicosis* and *asbestosis* are caused by inhalation of silica and asbestos, respectively; they may lead to progressive *fibrosis* of the lung.

IMPAIRED BLOOD AND OXYGEN SUPPLY

The most serious disorder is *pulmonary embolism*, in which a blood clot formed in one of the major veins breaks free and is carried to the lungs. The clot may block the pulmonary arteries and cause death. Heart failure may cause *pulmonary oedema*, in which the lungs become filled with fluid. *Respiratory distress syndrome*, which may affect newborn babies or adults, has many causes. In this condition, leakage of fluid into the alveoli seriously interferes with the oxygen supply. *Emphysema*, in which the walls of the alveoli break down so that the area for oxygen exchange is reduced, is frequently seen in people suffering from chronic bronchitis and asthma.

INVESTIGATION

Lung disorders are investigated by *chest X-ray*, *CT scanning*, *bronchoscopy*, *pulmonary function tests*, *sputum* analysis, *blood tests*, and physical examination. Sometimes a biopsy of lung tissue is taken for analysis.

physical examination. In most cases, however, the cancer is discovered when a *chest X-ray* shows a characteristic shadow on the lung.

To confirm the diagnosis, tissue must be examined microscopically for the presence of cancerous cells (see *Cytology*). The simplest test is to examine samples of sputum (phlegm), because cancer cells may have been shed into the airways and appear in the sputum. A *bronchoscopy* (inspection of the bronchi with a viewing instrument) is usually performed to examine the condition of the lungs. A *biopsy* (removal of a sample of tissue for microscopic analysis) may be performed during bronchoscopy. Alternatively, cells for biopsy may be obtained through a needle inserted into the chest, or the chest may be opened up to allow surgical removal of part of the tumour.

TREATMENT
If lung cancer is diagnosed at an early stage, *pneumonectomy* (removal of the lung) or *lobectomy* (removal of part of the lung) may be performed. Surgery is usually possible only when the cancer is still fairly small and confined to one lung, and when the patient's general condition enables a major operation to be performed. *Anticancer drugs* and *radiotherapy* may be used to contain the spread of the tumour or to destroy cancerous cells, and are the usual treatment for small cell carcinoma.

OUTLOOK
Overall, less than 10 per cent of lung cancer patients survive for five years after the disease is diagnosed. After surgery, the five-year survival rate is between 15 and 30 per cent; there have been cases of long-term survival in patients treated with anticancer drugs for small cell carcinoma.

The highest chance of cure is obtained when the cancer is discovered and treated early. However, if the cancer has spread beyond the chest, a cure is highly unlikely.

Lung, collapse of
See *Atelectasis*; *Pneumothorax*.

Lung disease, chronic obstructive
The combination of chronic *bronchitis* and *emphysema*, in which there is persistent disruption of air flow into or out of the lungs. Patients who have chronic obstructive lung disease are sometimes described as either pink puffers or blue bloaters, depending on their condition.

Pink puffers are able to maintain adequate oxygen in their bloodstream through an increase in their breathing rate, and hence remain "pink" despite serious lung damage. Pink puffers suffer from almost constant shortness of breath.

Blue bloaters are cyanotic (have a bluish discoloration of the skin and mucous membranes), because of a deficiency of oxygen in the bloodstream, and appear bloated, because of obesity and sometimes *oedema* (accumulation of fluid in body tissues), mainly due to *heart failure* resulting from the lung damage.

Lung-function tests
See *Pulmonary function tests*.

Lung imaging
A technique that provides images of the lungs to aid in the diagnosis of abnormalities or disease.

TYPES
CONVENTIONAL X-RAY TECHNIQUES A *chest X-ray* provides an excellent image of the lungs, from which most lung disorders can be detected. *Tomography* produces a sharp image of a cross-section of an organ at a particular depth and is sometimes used to visualize the interior of a lung that is obscured by an overlying diseased area, or to identify a nodule in the lung more clearly.

In pulmonary *angiography*, a contrast medium (a substance opaque to X-rays) is injected into the pulmonary artery to detect *pulmonary embolism* (blockage by a blood clot). *Bronchography* (in which the contrast medium is injected into the bronchi) was once commonly used to examine bronchi damaged by chronic infections; it has now been largely replaced by *bronchoscopy*. Other imaging techniques are also used to visualize the lungs.

SCANNING TECHNIQUES *CT scanning* and *MRI* provide more detailed images of the lungs than is possible with standard X-rays and play an important role in detecting the presence and spread of *lung tumours*. *Ultrasound scanning* is sometimes used to reveal *pleural effusion* (fluid around a lung).

Other less commonly employed imaging techniques involve the use of *radionuclide scanning* to aid in detecting pulmonary embolism. Digital radiography uses a computer to process a standard X-ray film. The computer removes all unwanted elements (such as the bones of the chest) from the image, leaving a clearer view of the structures to be examined.

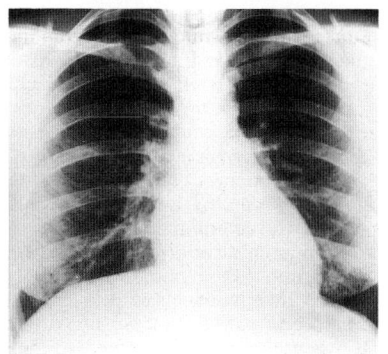
Chest X-ray
This is the most important lung imaging technique. It provides information about the lungs, their blood vessels and main airways.

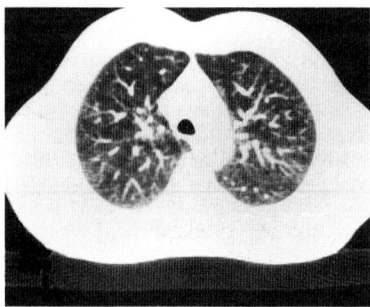
CT scanning
This shows detailed horizontal slices through the lungs. It is useful in showing the extent and spread of lung tumours.

Lung tumours
Growths in the lung, which may be malignant (see *Lung cancer*) or benign. Benign lung tumours are less common than malignant tumours and, unlike malignant tumours, typically affect younger adults and are unrelated to tobacco-smoking.

The most common benign tumour is a bronchial *adenoma*, which arises in the lining of a bronchus. Adenomas often cause bronchial obstruction; coughing up of blood may also occur. Treatment involves surgical removal of the tumour.

Other rare benign tumours include *fibromas* (made up of fibrous tissue) and *lipomas* (made up of fatty tissue). No treatment is necessary unless the tumours are causing problems.

Lupus erythematosus
A chronic disease that causes inflammation of *connective tissue* (material that surrounds body structures and holds them together). The more common type, discoid lupus erythematosus (DLE), affects exposed areas of the

...it occurs ...dwide, although its incidence is higher in certain ethnic groups, such as blacks and Chinese. In high-risk groups the prevalence may be as high as one in 250 women.

SYMPTOMS

The symptoms of both varieties of lupus erythematosus periodically subside and recur with varying degrees of severity.

In DLE the rash starts as one or more red, circular, thickened areas of skin that later scar. They may occur on the face, behind the ears, and on the scalp, sometimes causing permanent hair loss in affected areas.

SLE causes a variety of symptoms common among which is a characteristic red, blotchy, almost butterfly-shaped rash over the cheeks and bridge of the nose. There is no scarring. Most sufferers feel ill, with fatigue, fever, loss of appetite, nausea, joint pain, and weight loss. There may also be *anaemia,* neurological or psychiatric problems, *kidney failure, pleurisy* (inflammation of the lining of the lungs), *arthritis,* and *pericarditis* (inflammation of the membrane surrounding the heart).

DIAGNOSIS

Blood tests and sometimes a skin *biopsy* (removal of a small sample of tissue for microscopic examination) are performed to look for specific *antibodies* that are directed against the body's own tissues.

TREATMENT

Treatment aims to reduce inflammation and to alleviate symptoms; there

...ent of kidney ...r ...ients with drug-induced symptoms usually recover completely after discontinuation of the drug responsible.

Lupus pernio

A variant of the disease *sarcoidosis* in which purple chilblain-like swellings appear on the nose, cheeks, or ears. Lupus pernio more commonly affects women than men.

Lupus vulgaris

A form of *tuberculosis* affecting the skin, especially of the head and neck. Painless, clear, red-brown nodules appear and ulcerate. These eventually heal, leaving deep scars.

Luteinizing hormone

A *gonadotrophin hormone,* also known as LH, produced by the *pituitary gland.*

Luteinizing hormone-releasing hormone

A naturally occurring hormone that is released by the *hypothalamus* in the brain; it is also prepared synthetically as a drug. Natural luteinizing hormone-releasing hormone (LH-RH) stimulates the release of *gonadotrophin hormones* from the *pituitary gland.* Gonadotrophin hormones, in turn, control the production of *oestrogen hormones* and *androgen hormones.*

WHY IT IS USED

Synthetic LH-RH is given to treat abnormally early onset of puberty. It is also currently under investigation as a contraceptive and as a treatment for uterine *fibroids,* prostatic cancer (see *Prostate, cancer of*), and certain types of *breast cancer.*

Synthetic LH-RH reduces the amount of natural gonadotrophins released from the pituitary gland and thus the amount of oestrogen hormones and androgen hormones produced by the ovary and testes. This action reduces the level of cell activity in organs stimulated by these sex hormones, such as the uterus, breast, ovaries, testes, and prostate gland.

POSSIBLE ADVERSE EFFECTS

LH-RH may cause headache, nausea, hot flushes, vaginal dryness, and irregular periods.

Lyme disease

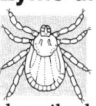 A disease characterized by skin changes, flu-like symptoms, and joint inflammation. It was first described in the community of Old Lyme, Connecticut, in the US in 1975.

CAUSES AND INCIDENCE

Lyme disease is caused by the bacterium BORRELIA BURGDORFERI, which is transmitted by the bite of a tick that usually lives on deer but can infest dogs. The disease is most widely recognized in the US but is also a problem in many parts of Europe, including the heathlands of southern England.

SYMPTOMS AND COMPLICATIONS

At the site of the tick bite, a red dot may appear and gradually expand into a reddened area up to 5 mm across; in some cases, however, the bite passes unnoticed. Symptoms such as fever, headache, lethargy, and muscle pains usually develop, followed by a characteristic joint inflammation, with redness and swelling typically affecting the knees and other large joints.

The symptoms may vary in severity and occur in cycles lasting a week or

corticosteroid drugs are given, ~~and~~ ~~~~ may take longer.

Lymph

A milky body fluid that contains lymphocytes (a type of white blood cell), proteins, and fats. Lymph accumulates outside the blood vessels in the intercellular spaces of body tissues and is collected into the *lymphatic system* to flow back into the bloodstream. Lymph plays an important part in the *immune system* and in absorbing fats from the intestine.

Lymphadenitis

A medical term for inflammation of the lymph nodes, a common cause of lymphadenopathy (swollen glands). See *Glands, swollen.*

Lymphadenopathy

The medical term for swollen lymph nodes (see *Glands, swollen*). A condition called persistent generalized lymphadenopathy, which causes generalized swelling of the lymph nodes, develops in some people infected with HIV (the *AIDS* virus).

Lymphangiography

A diagnostic procedure that enables lymph vessels and lymph nodes (see *Lymphatic system*) to be seen on X-ray film after a contrast medium (a substance opaque to X-rays) has been injected into them.

WHY IT IS DONE

Until recently, lymphangiography was frequently used to determine the extent to which a cancer had spread throughout the body (because lymph nodes trap cancer cells). However, the more straightforward techniques of *CT scanning* and *MRI* also clearly reveal abnormal lymph nodes and

gioma. ~~~~ blisters that may b~~~~ birth but are usually ob~~~~ age of about two years. If the blisters are damaged, they fill with blood, giving a red and white appearance to the lymphangioma. The growth sometimes disappears on its own, but most cases require removal.

accompanied by fever ~~~~ feeling of illness.

Lymphangitis is a clear indication of a serious infection and requires urgent treatment with *antibiotic drugs*. With

---

PROCEDURE FOR LYMPHANGIOGRAPHY

To plan and monitor the progress of treatment for certain types of cancer, such as of the testis or cervix, X-ray pictures of the lymph vessels and nodes can be taken to reveal the spread of the cancer throughout the body. A contrast medium is injected into the foot, from where it travels throughout the lymphatic system. The procedure takes about two and a half hours.

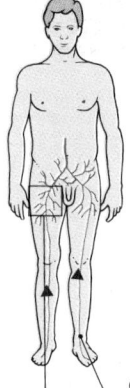

2 After the use of a local anaesthetic, an incision is made over a stained lymphatic vessel in each foot. Contrast medium is injected through a needle into the vessels and passes up the legs, into the groin and abdomen. When the limit of diffusion is reached, the needles are removed and the incisions sewn.

Contrast medium spreading through lymphatic system

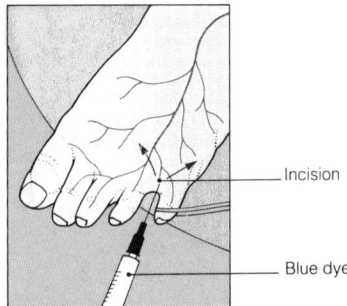

Incision

Blue dye

1 A blue dye is injected through a needle into the web spaces between the toes of each foot, and into the outside of the little toes. The dye spreads rapidly into the tiny lymphatic vessels along the top of the foot, and makes them visible.

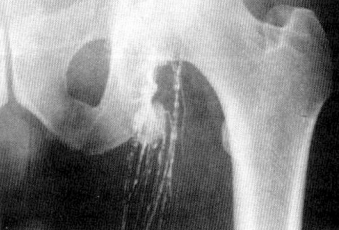

3 The lymph vessels and nodes containing the contrast medium show up clearly on the X-ray pictures. More lymphangiograms are taken after 24 hours.

so. Unless the disease is diagnosed and treated, symptoms may continue for several years, gradually declining in severity. There is usually no permanent damage to joints.

Complications affecting the heart (such as *myocarditis* and *heart block*) or nervous system (such as *meningitis*) occur in some cases.

DIAGNOSIS AND TREATMENT
Anyone in whom the above symptoms develop, particularly after a tick bite, should consult a doctor. The diagnosis of Lyme disease can be confirmed by blood tests.

If diagnosed before joint inflammation occurs, the disease can be quickly cleared up with *antibiotic drugs*. If the disease is more advanced, *nonsteroidal anti-inflammatory drugs* and sometimes *corticosteroid drugs* are given and a cure may take longer.

Lymph
A milky body fluid that contains lymphocytes (a type of white blood cell), proteins, and fats. Lymph accumulates outside the blood vessels in the intercellular spaces of body tissues and is collected into the *lymphatic system* to flow back into the bloodstream. Lymph plays an important part in the *immune system* and in absorbing fats from the intestine.

Lymphadenitis
A medical term for inflammation of the lymph nodes, a common cause of lymphadenopathy (swollen glands). See *Glands, swollen*.

Lymphadenopathy
The medical term for swollen lymph nodes (see *Glands, swollen*). A condition called persistent generalized lymphadenopathy, which causes generalized swelling of the lymph nodes, develops in some people infected with HIV (the *AIDS* virus).

Lymphangiography
A diagnostic procedure that enables lymph vessels and lymph nodes (see *Lymphatic system*) to be seen on X-ray film after a contrast medium (a substance opaque to X-rays) has been injected into them.

WHY IT IS DONE
Until recently, lymphangiography was frequently used to determine the extent to which a cancer had spread throughout the body (because lymph nodes trap cancer cells). However, the more straightforward techniques of *CT scanning* and *MRI* also clearly reveal abnormal lymph nodes and

have largely superseded lymphangiography. Even so, in certain types of cancer (such as cancer of the testis or cervix), the additional information provided by lymphangiography is useful in planning treatment and monitoring its progress.

HOW IT IS DONE
See the illustrated box for stages in the most common type of lymphangiography procedure. Lymphangiography is sometimes performed on the arms to reveal lymph nodes in the upper body.

Lymphangioma
A rare benign tumour of the skin or tongue consisting of a collection of abnormal lymph vessels. It is usually present from birth.

There are two types of lymphangioma. One consists of a group of clear blisters that may be inconspicuous at birth but are usually obvious by the age of about two years. If the blisters are damaged, they fill with blood, giving a red and white appearance to the lymphangioma. The growth sometimes disappears on its own, but most cases require removal.

The other type of lymphangioma, known as a cystic hygroma, is a soft swelling resembling a bunch of small white grapes that grows just beneath the skin (most commonly in the neck). A lymphangioma may become very large and unsightly, and is therefore usually removed when the child is about five years old.

Lymphangitis
Inflammation of the lymphatic vessels as a result of the spread of bacteria (commonly streptococci) from an infected wound. The inflammation is so severe that it causes tender red streaks to appear on the skin overlying the lymphatic vessels. These streaks extend progressively from the site of infection towards the nearest lymph nodes (for example, from an infected finger up the arm towards the lymph nodes in the armpits). The affected nodes become swollen and tender. Lymphangitis is usually accompanied by fever and a general feeling of illness.

Lymphangitis is a clear indication of a serious infection and requires urgent treatment with *antibiotic drugs*. With

---

PROCEDURE FOR LYMPHANGIOGRAPHY
To plan and monitor the progress of treatment for certain types of cancer, such as of the testis or cervix, X-ray pictures of the lymph vessels and nodes can be taken to reveal the spread of the cancer throughout the body. A contrast medium is injected into the foot, from where it travels throughout the lymphatic system. The procedure takes about two and a half hours.

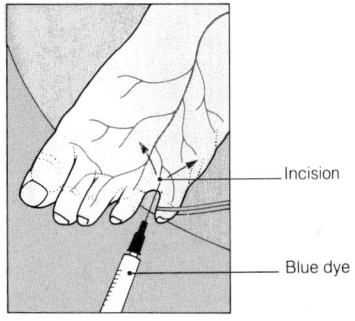

1 A blue dye is injected through a needle into the web spaces between the toes of each foot, and into the outside of the little toes. The dye spreads rapidly into the tiny lymphatic vessels along the top of the foot, and makes them visible.

Incision

Blue dye

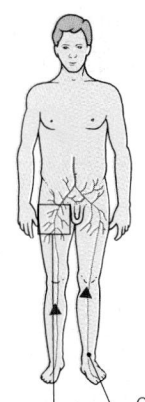

2 After the use of a local anaesthetic, an incision is made over a stained lymphatic vessel in each foot. Contrast medium is injected through a needle into the vessels and passes up the legs, into the groin and abdomen. When the limit of diffusion is reached, the needles are removed and the incisions sewn.

Contrast medium spreading through lymphatic system

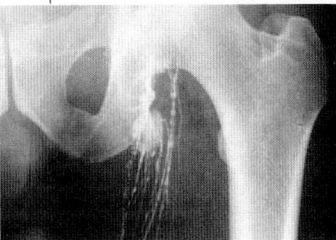

3 The lymph vessels and nodes containing the contrast medium show up clearly on the X-ray pictures. More lymphangiograms are taken after 24 hours.

skin. The more serious and potentially fatal form, systemic lupus erythematosus (SLE), affects many systems of the body (as well as the skin), including the joints and the kidneys.

CAUSES

Lupus erythematosus is an *autoimmune disorder* in which the body's *immune system*, for unknown reasons, attacks the connective tissue as if it were foreign, causing inflammation. It is probable that the disease can be inherited and that hormonal factors play a part. Sometimes the agent that triggers the immune response (for example, a viral infection or sunlight) can be identified. Also, certain drugs can induce some of the symptoms of SLE, particularly in elderly people; the drugs most frequently responsible are hydralazine, procainamide, and isoniazid.

INCIDENCE

Lupus erythematosus affects nine times as many women as men, usually those of childbearing age. It occurs worldwide, although its incidence is higher in certain ethnic groups, such as blacks and Chinese. In high-risk groups the prevalence may be as high as one in 250 women.

SYMPTOMS

The symptoms of both varieties of lupus erythematosus periodically subside and recur with varying degrees of severity.

In DLE the rash starts as one or more red, circular, thickened areas of skin that later scar. They may occur on the face, behind the ears, and on the scalp, sometimes causing permanent hair loss in affected areas.

SLE causes a variety of symptoms common among which is a characteristic red, blotchy, almost butterfly-shaped rash over the cheeks and bridge of the nose. There is no scarring. Most sufferers feel ill, with fatigue, fever, loss of appetite, nausea, joint pain, and weight loss. There may also be *anaemia*, neurological or psychiatric problems, *kidney failure*, *pleurisy* (inflammation of the lining of the lungs), *arthritis*, and *pericarditis* (inflammation of the membrane surrounding the heart).

DIAGNOSIS

Blood tests and sometimes a skin *biopsy* (removal of a small sample of tissue for microscopic examination) are performed to look for specific *antibodies* that are directed against the body's own tissues.

TREATMENT

Treatment aims to reduce inflammation and to alleviate symptoms; there is no cure. *Nonsteroidal anti-inflammatory drugs* may be prescribed to relieve the joint pain, antimalarial drugs for the skin rash, and *corticosteroid drugs* for fever, pleurisy, and neurological symptoms. Cytotoxic *immunosuppressant drugs* are given to patients with kidney damage or severe neurological symptoms. Sufferers whose symptoms are made worse by sunlight should avoid exposure to the sun and should use *sunscreens*.

OUTLOOK

The outlook for patients with SLE has improved dramatically over the past 20 years, although the disease may be life-threatening if the kidneys are affected. With appropriate drug treatment, prolonged survival may be expected for most patients. This improvement may be due to earlier diagnosis, especially of mild cases, and to more effective treatment of kidney problems. Patients with drug-induced symptoms usually recover completely after discontinuation of the drug responsible.

Lupus pernio

A variant of the disease *sarcoidosis* in which purple chilblain-like swellings appear on the nose, cheeks, or ears. Lupus pernio more commonly affects women than men.

Lupus vulgaris

A form of *tuberculosis* affecting the skin, especially of the head and neck. Painless, clear, red-brown nodules appear and ulcerate. These eventually heal, leaving deep scars.

Luteinizing hormone

A *gonadotrophin hormone*, also known as LH, produced by the *pituitary gland*.

Luteinizing hormone-releasing hormone

A naturally occurring hormone that is released by the *hypothalamus* in the brain; it is also prepared synthetically as a drug. Natural luteinizing hormone-releasing hormone (LH-RH) stimulates the release of *gonadotrophin hormones* from the *pituitary gland*. Gonadotrophin hormones, in turn, control the production of *oestrogen hormones* and *androgen hormones*.

WHY IT IS USED

Synthetic LH-RH is given to treat abnormally early onset of puberty. It is also currently under investigation as a contraceptive and as a treatment for uterine *fibroids*, prostatic cancer (see *Prostate, cancer of*), and certain types of *breast cancer*.

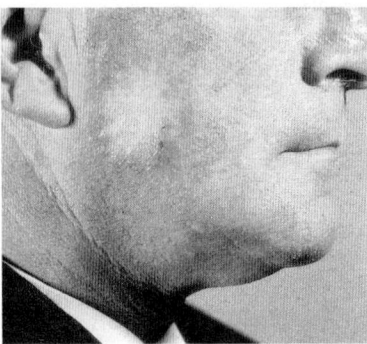

Discoid lupus erythematosus on cheek
The disease causes circular, reddened areas of skin. The patch shown here is healing at its centre to form white scar tissue.

HOW IT WORKS

Synthetic LH-RH reduces the amount of natural gonadotrophins released from the pituitary gland and thus the amount of oestrogen hormones and androgen hormones produced by the ovary and testes. This action reduces the level of cell activity in organs stimulated by these sex hormones, such as the uterus, breast, ovaries, testes, and prostate gland.

POSSIBLE ADVERSE EFFECTS

LH-RH may cause headache, nausea, hot flushes, vaginal dryness, and irregular periods.

Lyme disease

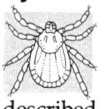

A disease characterized by skin changes, flu-like symptoms, and joint inflammation. It was first described in the community of Old Lyme, Connecticut, in the US in 1975.

CAUSES AND INCIDENCE

Lyme disease is caused by the bacterium BORRELIA BURGDORFERI, which is transmitted by the bite of a tick that usually lives on deer but can infest dogs. The disease is most widely recognized in the US but is also a problem in many parts of Europe, including the heathlands of southern England.

SYMPTOMS AND COMPLICATIONS

At the site of the tick bite, a red dot may appear and gradually expand into a reddened area up to 5 mm across; in some cases, however, the bite passes unnoticed. Symptoms such as fever, headache, lethargy, and muscle pains usually develop, followed by a characteristic joint inflammation, with redness and swelling typically affecting the knees and other large joints.

The symptoms may vary in severity and occur in cycles lasting a week or

L

treatment, the condition usually clears up quickly without complications. (See also *Lymphadenitis*.)

Lymphatic system

A system of vessels (lymphatics) that drains *lymph* from all over the body back into the bloodstream. This system is part of the *immune system*, playing a major part in the body's defences against infection and cancer.

STRUCTURE AND FUNCTION

All body tissues are bathed in a watery fluid derived from the bloodstream. Much of this fluid returns to the bloodstream through the walls of the capillaries, but the remainder (along with cells and small particles such as bacteria) is transported to the heart through the lymphatic system (see illustrated box overleaf).

Situated along the lymphatics are *lymph nodes*, through which the lymph flows. These nodes are, in effect, filters that trap microorganisms and other foreign bodies in the lymph. The nodes contain many lymphocytes (a type of white blood cell), which can neutralize or destroy invading bacteria and viruses. If part of the body is inflamed or otherwise diseased, the nearby lymph nodes become swollen and tender as they limit the spread of the disease (see *Glands, swollen*). If an infection is particularly virulent, the lymphatics may also be inflamed, becoming visible as thin red lines running along a limb (see *Lymphangitis*).

The lymphatic system also plays a part in the absorption of fats from the intestine. While the products of carbohydrate and protein digestion pass directly into the bloodstream, fats pass into the intestinal lymphatics (known as lacteals); the lymph in the lacteals is so rich in fat that it appears milky.

DISORDERS

In some conditions, such as after radical *mastectomy* (which is rarely performed today), the lymphatics to a limb become obstructed, causing lymph to accumulate and the limb to become hard and swollen, a condition known as *lymphoedema*.

Cancer commonly spreads via the lymphatic system. A primary tumour invades the lymphatics and fragments of tumour (metastases) break off and travel to the local group of lymph nodes, where the metastases continue to grow and produce a secondary tumour. This is particularly evident in *breast cancer*, which tends to spread early in the course of the disease to the lymph nodes in the armpit.

Lymph gland

A popular name for a *lymph node*. (See also *Lymphatic system*.)

Lymph node

A small organ lying along the course of a lymphatic vessel; commonly but incorrectly known as a lymph gland.

STRUCTURE AND FUNCTION

Lymph nodes vary considerably in size, from microscopic to about 2.5 cm in diameter. Each node consists of a thin, fibrous outer capsule and an inner mass of lymphoid tissue. Penetrating the capsule are several small lymphatic vessels (which carry lymph into the gland) and a single, larger vessel (which carries it out).

Lymphoid tissue forms *antibodies* and houses *lymphocytes* (a type of white blood cell), both of which play a major role in fighting infection. Lymph nodes also contain macrophages, large cells that engulf bacteria and other foreign particles. The nodes act as a barrier to the spread of infection, destroying or filtering out bacteria before they can pass into the bloodstream. (See also *Glands, swollen*; *Lymphatic system*.)

Lymphocyte

Any of a group of white *blood cells* of crucial importance to the adaptive part of the body's *immune system*. The adaptive portion of the immune system mounts a tailor-made defence when dangerous invading organisms penetrate the body's general defences (such as those provided by other types of white blood cell).

Some lymphocytes retain a memory of invading microorganisms so that the invaders can be dealt with more rapidly when next encountered. It is this memory function that is stimulated by *vaccines*. Lymphocytes protect against the development of tumours and cause rejection of tissue in organ transplants.

TYPES

There are two principal types of lymphocytes. They are called B- and T-lymphocytes.

B-LYMPHOCYTES This type accounts for about 10 per cent of circulating lymphocytes. When an *antigen* (a particular foreign protein, such as a substance on the surface of a bacterium) is encountered by the immune system, certain B-lymphocytes are stimulated to enlarge and undergo cell division, transforming into cells called plasma cells. The plasma cells secrete into the blood vast numbers of tailor-made *immunoglobulins* or *antibodies*

that attach to the antigen on the surface of the microorganism. This starts a process that leads to the destruction of the microorganism. The protective effect of immunoglobulins is called humoral immunity.

T-LYMPHOCYTES This type accounts for more than 80 per cent of circulating lymphocytes. T-lymphocytes are derived from white cells that have at some stage entered the *thymus* gland, where they were "educated" to fulfil a particular function.

There are three main groups of T-lymphocytes: killer (cytotoxic) cells, helper cells, and suppressor cells. The killer T-lymphocytes (like B-lymphocytes) are sensitized and stimulated to multiply by the presence of antigens, in this case by antigens present on abnormal body cells (e.g. cells that have been invaded by viruses, cells in transplanted tissue, and tumour cells). Unlike the B-lymphocytes, the killer cells do not produce antibodies; instead, they travel to and attach to the cells recognized as abnormal. The killer cells then release chemicals known as lymphokines, which help destroy the abnormal cells. This is called cell-mediated immunity.

Helper T-cells enhance the activities of the killer T-cells and B-cells, and also control other aspects of the immune response. In people who are infected with HIV (the *AIDS* virus) these helper T-cells are reduced in number, thus impairing the body's ability to fight certain types of infections and tumours. Suppressor T-cells have the effect of "switching off" the immune response.

MEMORY FUNCTION

Some lymphocytes do not participate directly in immune responses; instead, they serve as a memory bank for the different antigens that have been encountered in the past. These cells may survive for many years.

Lymphoedema

An abnormal accumulation of *lymph* in the tissues, causing swelling of a limb. Lymphoedema occurs if lymphatic vessels are blocked, damaged, or removed, resulting in disruption of the normal drainage of lymph (see *Lymphatic system*).

CAUSES

There are various causes. In the tropical disease *filariasis*, for example, the lymphatic vessels may be blocked by parasitic worms. Blockage may also occur if cancer spreads through the lymphatic system and deposits cancer cells in the lymph vessels.

L

STRUCTURE AND FUNCTION OF THE LYMPHATIC SYSTEM

The lymphatic system is a collection of organs, ducts, and tissues that has the dual role of draining tissue fluid (lymph) back into the bloodstream and of fighting infection. Lymph is drained by a system of channels (the lymphatic vessels). White cells produced by the bone marrow, thymus, and spleen are present in lymph nodes or circulate through the lymphatic system, providing defences against infection.

The lymphatic network

The lymphatic system consists of a network of lymph nodes connected by lymphatic vessels. The nodes generally occur in clusters, mainly around the neck, armpits, and groin.

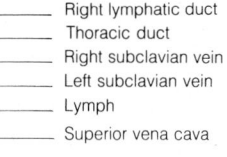

Thoracic duct

Liver

Spleen

Cisterna chyli

Lymph nodes

Lymphatic vessels

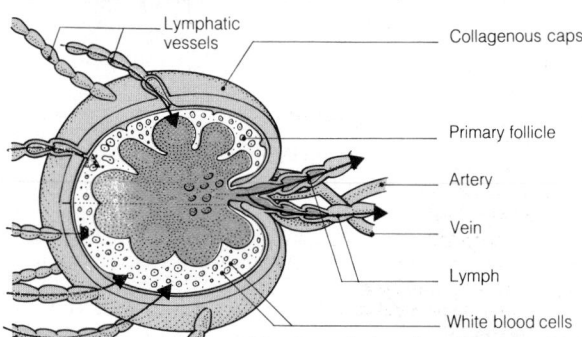

Right lymphatic duct
Thoracic duct
Right subclavian vein
Left subclavian vein
Lymph
Superior vena cava

Lymphatic drainage

Just below the neck, the thoracic duct and the right lymphatic duct drain into the two subclavian veins. These veins unite to form the inferior vena cava, which passes into the heart; in this way, the lymph fluids rejoin the circulation.

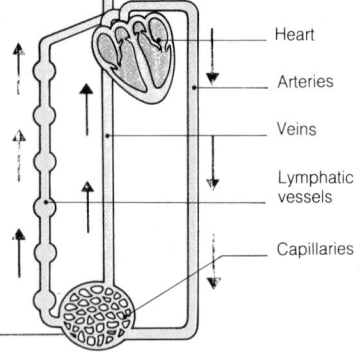

Lymphatic vessels

Collagenous capsule

Primary follicle

Artery

Vein

Lymph

White blood cells

Structure of a lymph node

Any fluid absorbed into the lymphatic system passes across at least one lymph node before it returns to the circulation. The fluid filters through a mesh of tightly packed white blood cells—some of which are grouped into primary follicles consisting of similar cells—which attack and destroy harmful organisms. Every lymph node is supplied by its own tiny artery and vein.

MOVEMENTS OF BODY FLUIDS

Lymph is constantly moving around the body, but the lymphatic system has no central pump equivalent to the heart. Lymph is circulated by the movement of the body's muscles; a system of one-way valves in the lymphatic vessels ensures that it moves in the right direction. Exertion also pushes fluid from body tissues into the bloodstream.

Heart

Arteries

Veins

Lymphatic vessels

Capillaries

Cells   Lymphatic vessel

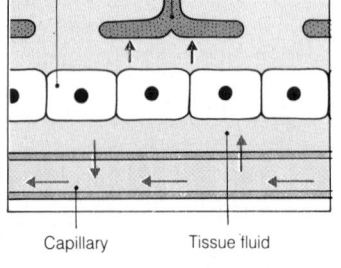

Capillary   Tissue fluid

Fluid exchange

During a 24-hour period, approximately 24 litres of serum-like fluid pass from the bloodstream to the body's tissues. This fluid bathes the cells and provides them with oxygen and nutrients. During the same period of time, approximately 20 litres of fluid pass back from the tissues to the bloodstream, carrying carbon dioxide and other waste products. The remaining 4 litres pass from the tissues to the lymphatic system and return eventually to the circulation from there.

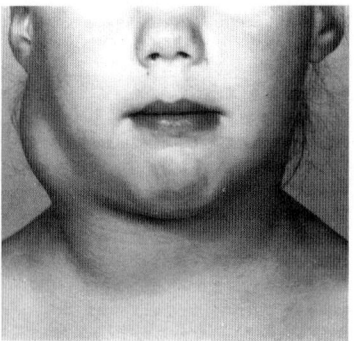

Enlarged lymph nodes

This photograph shows a girl with marked enlargement of the lymph nodes in her neck. In this case, the cause is Hodgkin's disease, a rare cancer that affects the lymph nodes. Enlargement of the nodes may also be due to infection.

Surgical removal of lymph nodes under the arm or in the groin or radiotherapy for a tumour destroys lymph nodes and vessels, sometimes resulting in lymphoedema.

Lymphoedema may also occur for no known cause. It may be present from birth or may develop later in life. Lymphoedema of unknown cause affects twice as many women as men.

SYMPTOMS AND SIGNS

In about 10 per cent of women who have had a radical *mastectomy*, lymphoedema develops in the arm (but not usually in the hand) on the same side as the removed breast. In some such cases, the arm becomes heavy and cumbersome. The incidence of lymphoedema is much lower with newer surgical techniques.

Except after a mastectomy, lymphoedema usually causes swelling of one or both legs. Starting with only a slight, intermittent puffiness around one ankle, the swelling gradually extends up the leg. In about half of all cases, the other leg also becomes affected. The swelling is usually painless, but the leg feels heavy.

In some people the legs enlarge to an unsightly and incapacitating degree, whereas in others the swelling may still be only minimal even 40 or more years after the onset of the lymphoedema.

TREATMENT

There is no known cure for lymphoedema. Treatment consists of taking *diuretic drugs*, massaging the affected limb, wearing an elastic bandage or compression sleeve, and performing exercises with the affected leg or arm elevated. However, these measures usually produce only a slight improvement. In severe cases, when the leg or arm is so large that it causes disability, the swollen tissue and some of the overlying skin may be removed surgically.

Lymphogranuloma venereum

A sexually transmitted disease that is caused by a *chlamydial infection*. The disease is common in tropical countries but rare in the UK (where fewer than 50 cases are diagnosed per year).

The first sign of infection may be a small genital blister that appears between three and 21 days after infection; this blister heals in a few days without leaving a scar. There may also be fever, headache, muscle and joint pains, and a rash.

The lymph glands, particularly in the groin, become painfully enlarged and inflamed. Abscesses may form and ulcers may develop on the skin over the affected glands; the ulcers take several months to heal.

Treatment of lymphogranuloma venereum is with *antibiotic drugs*.

Lymphoma

Any of a group of cancers in which the cells of lymphoid tissue (found mainly in the *lymph nodes* and *spleen*) multiply unchecked.

Lymphomas fall into two categories. If characteristic abnormal cells (Reed-Sternberg cells) are present, the disease is known as Hodgkin's lymphoma. All other types are called non-Hodgkin's lymphoma. (See *Burkitt's lymphoma; Hodgkin's disease; Lymphoma, non-Hodgkin's.*)

Lymphoma, non-Hodgkin's

Any cancer of lymphoid tissue (found mainly in the *lymph nodes* and *spleen*) other than *Hodgkin's disease*.

Non-Hodgkin's lymphomas vary in their malignancy according to the nature and activity of the abnormal cells. Lymphomas are most malignant when the cells are primitive or are poorly differentiated. These cells tend to take over entire lymph nodes quickly. Low-grade (less malignant) lymphomas consist of cells that are better-differentiated.

CAUSES AND INCIDENCE

In most cases of non-Hodgkin's lymphoma, the cause is unknown. Occasionally, the disease is associated with suppression of the *immune system*, particularly after organ transplantation. One type of non-Hodgkin's lymphoma, known as *Burkitt's lymphoma* (common only in the tropics), is thought to be caused by the Epstein-Barr virus; others are suspected to be caused by other viruses.

About 4,000 new cases of non-Hodgkin's lymphoma are diagnosed annually in the UK. Most sufferers are over 50 years old.

SYMPTOMS AND SIGNS

In most patients, there is painless swelling of one or more groups of lymph nodes in the neck or groin. The liver and spleen may enlarge and lymphoid tissue in the abdomen may be affected. Many other organs may become involved, leading to diverse symptoms ranging from headache to skin ulceration.

Unless it is controlled, spread of the disease (often marked by fever) progressively impairs the immune system, leading to death from infections. The patient may also die of an uncontrolled spread of cancer.

DIAGNOSIS

Diagnosis is based on a *biopsy* (removal of a sample for analysis) of lymphoid tissue, usually from a lymph node. The extent of the disease is assessed by a process called staging. A *chest X-ray, CT scanning, MRI, bone marrow biopsy,* and *lymphangiography* (X-rays of the lymph glands) of the abdomen may be required.

TREATMENT AND OUTLOOK

If the lymphoma is confined to a single group of lymph nodes, treatment consists of *radiotherapy*. More usually, the disease is more extensive, and *anticancer drugs* are given. In some cases both forms of treatment are used. When all else fails, a *bone marrow transplant,* along with drugs and/or radiation, may be performed.

About three quarters of patients with a low-grade localized non-Hodgkin's lymphoma survive at least five years. In more severe types of lymphoma that have spread, between 40 and 50 per cent of patients survive for two years or more.

Lymphosarcoma

The former name for a type of what is now called non-Hodgkin's lymphoma (see *Lymphoma, non-Hodgkin's*).

Lypressin

A synthetic preparation of *ADH* (antidiuretic hormone), a hormone that controls the volume of water excreted in the urine. Lypressin is used as a nasal spray to treat *diabetes insipidus* (a deficiency of ADH causing excessive urination and thirst).

Possible adverse effects of lypressin are abdominal cramps, an urge to open the bowels, and nasal congestion which, if severe, may impair the efficiency of treatment.

Lysis

A medical term for breaking down or destruction; the term is usually applied to the destruction of cells by disintegration of their outer membrane. A common example is *haemolysis,* the breakdown of red blood cells. Lysis may be caused by chemical action, such as that of an *enzyme,* or by physical action, such as that of heat or cold. The term lysis is also occasionally used to refer to a sudden recovery from a fever.

Lysozyme

An *enzyme* in tears, saliva, sweat, nasal secretions, breast milk, and many tissues. It destroys bacteria by disrupting their cell walls.

L

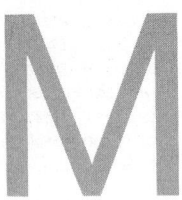

M

Macro-

A prefix meaning large, as in macrophage (a large cell that plays an important part in the body's defence system by engulfing bacteria and other foreign particles) or macroglossia (enlargement of the tongue).

Macrobiotics

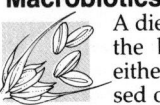
A dietary system based on the belief that foods are either yin or yang (possessed of negative or positive forces, see *Yin and yang*), and that a balance of yin and yang must be maintained for health. Foods are classified as yin or yang according to many factors, including where they are grown, their colour, texture, and taste.

There are several levels of macrobiotic diet; the most extreme consists virtually entirely of whole grains. Eating such a diet may lead to severe malnutrition, *scurvy*, or *anaemia* as a result of the lack of protein, vitamins, and essential minerals.

Macroglossia

Abnormal enlargement of the tongue. Macroglossia is a feature of *Down's syndrome*, of *hypothyroidism* (underactivity of the thyroid gland), and of *acromegaly*. Tumours of the tongue, such as a *haemangioma* or *lymphangioma*, also cause macroglossia, as may *amyloidosis*.

In addition to being unsightly, an abnormally large tongue can cause snoring and is sometimes responsible for *sleep apnoea*. Treatment, if any, depends on the underlying cause.

Macular degeneration

A progressive disorder that affects the central part of the *retina*, causing gradual loss of central vision. Macular degeneration is a painless condition which is common in the elderly. It usually affects both eyes, either simultaneously or one after the other.

The macula is the part of the retina that distinguishes fine detail at the centre of the field of vision. Degeneration begins with partial breakdown

of an insulating layer between the retina and the *choroid* (layer of blood vessels behind the retina). Fluid leakage occurs, and new blood vessels growing from the choroid destroy the retinal nerve tissue and replace it with scar tissue. The effect is a roughly circular area of blindness, increasing in size until it is large enough to obliterate two or three words at normal reading distance. Because of the loss of central vision, the patient has difficulty in seeing people's faces as well as in reading.

With early diagnosis, it is occasionally possible to seal off the leakage by *laser treatment*. In most cases, however, macular degeneration is untreatable but does not lead to complete blindness, because the patient retains vision around the edges of the visual fields.

Macule

A spot that is level with the surface of the skin and discernible only by difference in colour or texture.

Magnesium

An element essential in the diet for the formation of bones and teeth, for muscle contraction, for the transmission of nerve impulses, and for the activation of many *enzymes* (substances that promote biochemical reactions in the body). There is about 35 g of magnesium in an average-sized person, much of it in the bones and teeth.

Sources of magnesium in the diet include cereals (especially wholegrain), nuts, soya beans, milk, fish, and meat.

MAGNESIUM-CONTAINING DRUGS
Magnesium compounds are used in *antacid drugs* and *laxative drugs*: magnesium carbonate and magnesium hydroxide are used in many antacids, magnesium sulphate in laxatives. Magnesium is also a constituent of some mineral supplements.

DEFICIENCY AND EXCESS
Most diets contain sufficient magnesium. Deficiency usually occurs as a result of severe kidney disease, *alcohol dependence*, an intestinal disorder that impairs the absorption of magnesium and calcium, or prolonged treatment with *diuretic drugs* or *digitalis drugs*. Symptoms of deficiency include anxiety, restlessness, tremors, palpitations, and depression. There may also be an increased risk of kidney stones (see *Calculus, urinary tract*) or *coronary artery disease*. Deficiency of the element is treated with magnesium supplements.

Magnesium excess is usually the result of taking too much of a magnesium-containing antacid or laxative, and may cause nausea, vomiting, diarrhoea, dizziness, and muscle weakness. Very large amounts may lead to heart damage or respiratory failure, especially in people with kidney disease. Mild magnesium excess does not usually require treatment. However, anyone who has taken a substantial overdose may require hospitalization so that breathing and heart activity can be monitored (and supported, if necessary) and drugs given to help the body excrete the excess magnesium.

Magnetic resonance imaging
See *MRI*.

Malabsorption

Impaired absorption of dietary nutrients, vitamins, or minerals by the lining of the small intestine.

CAUSES
Malabsorption can be caused by many conditions. In *lactase deficiency*, deficiency of the enzyme lactase in the intestine prevents the breakdown and absorption of lactose (a sugar in milk). In *cystic fibrosis* and chronic *pancreatitis*, damage to the pancreas prevents the production of enzymes required for the digestion and absorption of fats and other nutrients.

In *coeliac disease*, many nutrients cannot be absorbed because of damage to the small intestine by sensitivity to gluten proteins. Uncommon diseases in which the intestinal lining is damaged include *Crohn's disease*, *amyloidosis*, *giardiasis*, *Whipple's disease*, and *lymphoma*.

Removal of portions of the small intestine can cause malabsorption, as can stomach operations that cause food to pass through the digestive tract more quickly than normal.

There are also some disorders that interfere with the passage of bile salts to the small intestine or that interfere with their uptake, thus preventing the breakdown and absorption of fats. These disorders include *bile duct obstruction*, primary *biliary cirrhosis*, and Crohn's disease.

SYMPTOMS AND DIAGNOSIS
Common effects are diarrhoea and weight loss; in severe cases, there may also be malnutrition (see *Nutritional disorders*), *vitamin* deficiency, *mineral* deficiency, or *anaemia*.

The diagnosis may be confirmed by examining faeces for unabsorbed fat, by special tests of carbohydrate absorption (such as the xylose absorption test), and by blood tests to detect anaemia and deficiencies of vitamins, minerals and other nutrients.

To determine the underlying cause of malabsorption, various other tests may be carried out, including *barium X-ray examination* of the small intestine and *jejunal biopsy* (removal of a sample of tissue from the jejunum for microscopic examination).

TREATMENT AND OUTLOOK
Treatment depends on the underlying cause. In most cases, modifications or supplements to the diet return the affected person to health. However, if there is severe, irreversible damage to the lining of the intestine, intravenous infusion of nutrients may be necessary (see *Feeding, artificial*).

Maladjustment
Failure to adapt to a change in one's environment, resulting in an inability to cope with work or social activities. Maladjustment is common and can occur at any age as a reaction to stressful situations (such as starting school, moving house, divorce, physical illness, or retirement). Maladjustment may be expressed by feelings of *depression* or *anxiety*, or by *behavioural problems in children* and adolescents.

Maladjustment is usually temporary, disappearing when the person is removed from the stressful situation or learns to adapt to it.

Malaise
A vague feeling of being unwell. Malaise is a general symptom of little value in diagnosis.

Malalignment
Positioning of *teeth* in the *jaw* so that they do not form a smooth arch shape when viewed from above or below (see *Malocclusion*).

The term malalignment is also used to refer to a *fracture* in which the bone ends are not in a straight line. The ends must then be manipulated back into position so that there is no deformity when the bone heals.

Malar flush
A high colour over the cheekbones, with a bluish tinge caused by reduced oxygen concentration in the blood. Malar flush is considered to be a sign of *mitral stenosis* (narrowing of one of the heart valves), usually following *rheumatic fever*. However, malar flush is not always present in mitral stenosis, and many people with this colouring do not have heart disease.

Malaria

A serious parasitic disease, spread by the bites of *ANO-PHELES* mosquitoes. The disease produces severe fever and, in some cases, complications affecting the kidneys, liver, brain, and blood which can be fatal.

Malaria is prevalent throughout the tropics, affecting up to 300 million people worldwide each year. It is the single most important disease hazard for travellers to warm climates. The World Health Organization has undertaken a massive programme of malaria control, but little progress has been made in the past 20 years. Mosquitoes have developed resistance to insecticides and, in many areas, the malaria parasites have developed resistance to antimalarial drugs.

CAUSES
The parasites responsible for malaria are *protozoa* known as plasmodia. Four species can cause disease in humans: *PLASMODIUM FALCIPARUM*, *PLASMO-DIUM VIVAX*, *PLASMODIUM OVALE*, and *PLASMODIUM MALARIAE*. Each species spends part of its life-cycle in humans and part in *ANOPHELES* mosquitoes (see diagram overleaf).

INCIDENCE
Malaria is a major health problem in much of the tropics (see map overleaf). Children in affected countries suffer repeated infections, and many die. Malaria kills about one million infants and children every year in Africa alone. Most people living in areas where malaria is common acquire some immunity to the disease.

The number of cases diagnosed in England and Wales has risen significantly recently, reaching 2,000 in 1990—with 10 to 12 deaths a year. Most of this rise is attributable to increased travel, especially among immigrants from Asia and Africa returning to their home countries for holidays. Most falciparum malaria infections are contracted in Africa and most of the less dangerous vivax infections occur in visitors and immigrants from the Indian subcontinent.

The chance of contracting malaria within the UK is extremely small. However, cases have occurred among drug users as a result of sharing needles with an infected person, and in people who have received infected blood transfusions.

SYMPTOMS
The period between being bitten by the mosquito and the appearance of symptoms is usually a week or two, but can be as long as a year if the person has been taking antimalarial drugs (which may suppress rather than prevent malaria). Symptoms, which include shaking, chills, and fever, appear only when red blood cells that are infected with parasites rupture to release more parasites into the bloodstream.

The principal symptom of infection is the classic malarial ague (fever). Except in most cases of falciparum malaria, the fever has three stages: a cold stage of uncontrollable shivering (rigors), a hot stage in which the temperature may reach 40.5°C, and finally a sweating stage that drenches the bedding and brings down the temperature. A severe headache, general malaise, and vomiting may accompany the attack. At the end of an attack, the patient is left weak and tired, and sleeps. In many cases, the parasitized red blood cells rupture at the same time in each cycle and the fever develops cyclically, occurring every other day (in vivax and ovale infections) or every third day (in malariae infections).

P. FALCIPARUM infects all ages of red blood cells, whereas the other varieties attack only young or old cells. Falciparum malaria thus affects a greater proportion of the blood cells and is therefore more severe; this form of malaria can be fatal within a few days of the first symptoms. The fever is prolonged and irregular, but symptoms are initially very like those of influenza and the severity of the illness may not be recognized. Red blood cells infected with parasites become sticky and block blood vessels in vital organs, especially the kidneys. The spleen becomes enlarged and the brain may be affected, leading to coma and convulsions. Destruction of blood cells leads to haemolytic anaemia (see *Anaemia, haemolytic*). Kidney failure and jaundice are common complications of falciparum malaria.

Even people who take antimalarial drugs and precautions against bites may contract malaria. Anyone in whom a fever and headache develops after returning from the tropics should see a doctor as soon as possible and mention the trip abroad.

DIAGNOSIS
Malaria is diagnosed by studying blood samples taken at six- to 12-hour intervals; parasites at different stages of development can be clearly seen under a microscope.

TREATMENT
Malaria, especially falciparum malaria, is often a medical emergency that

M

requires admission to hospital. Treatment is with antimalarial drugs. In severe cases, *blood transfusions* may be necessary.

Chloroquine, which eradicates malaria parasites from the blood, is the usual treatment for all types of malaria. However, *quinine* or halofantrine are commonly used to treat chloroquine-resistant falciparum malaria, which is now widespread in many tropical areas. Patients suffering from vivax or ovale malaria must also take *primaquine* to eradicate parasites in the liver. Primaquine may cause haemolytic anaemia in people who have a disorder called *G6PD deficiency.*

PREVENTION

Preventive antimalarial drugs should be taken by all visitors to the tropics, including pregnant women. Drug recommendations are continually updated, and travellers should consult a doctor for up-to-date advice on the choice and dosages of drugs to be taken when visiting different parts of the world.

Chloroquine is often recommended for areas where there is no resistance to this drug; *proguanil* may be preferred for longer-term use because it has fewer side-effects. Drug possibilities for chloroquine-resistant areas include a combination of chloroquine and proguanil, or a more recently developed drug, mefloquine. All antimalarial drugs will need to be taken for some time before visiting a malarious region (usually for one to two weeks), and will also need to be taken for some time afterwards (usually for at least four weeks).

In addition to taking preventive drugs, visitors to the tropics should make every effort to avoid *mosquito bites.* Protective clothing should be worn over the arms and legs in the evening and insect repellents should be used. Other preventive measures against mosquito bites include screens over windows, insecticide sprays, and, if necessary, mosquito nets.

Malformation
A deformity, particularly one resulting from faulty development.

Malignant
A term used to describe a condition that tends to become progressively worse and to result in death. By contrast, a *benign* disorder remains relatively mild and is not usually fatal. The term malignant is primarily used to refer to a cancerous *tumour* that spreads from its original location to establish secondary tumours in other parts of the body, with potentially life-threatening results.

Malignant melanoma
See *Melanoma, malignant.*

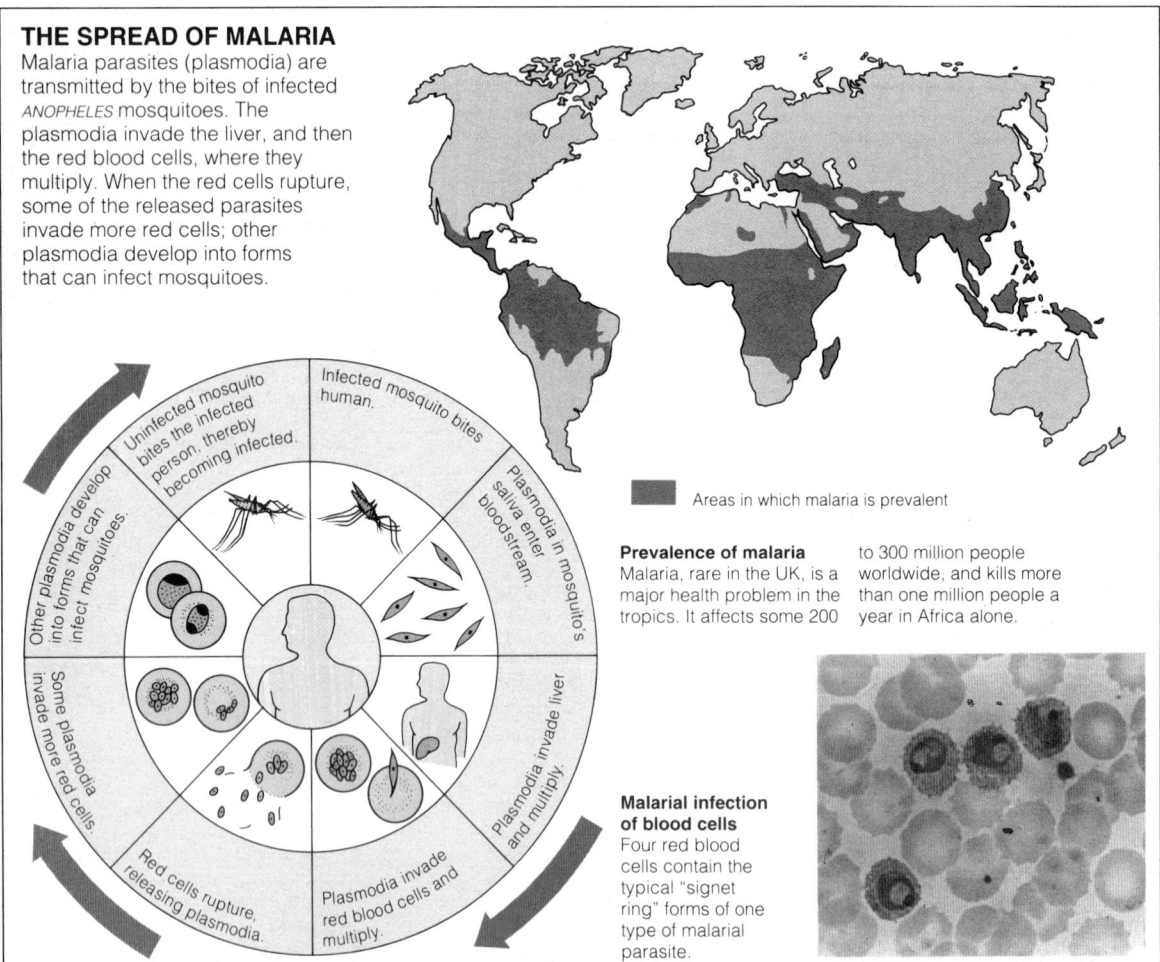

THE SPREAD OF MALARIA
Malaria parasites (plasmodia) are transmitted by the bites of infected *ANOPHELES* mosquitoes. The plasmodia invade the liver, and then the red blood cells, where they multiply. When the red cells rupture, some of the released parasites invade more red cells; other plasmodia develop into forms that can infect mosquitoes.

Areas in which malaria is prevalent

Prevalence of malaria
Malaria, rare in the UK, is a major health problem in the tropics. It affects some 200 to 300 million people worldwide, and kills more than one million people a year in Africa alone.

Malarial infection of blood cells
Four red blood cells contain the typical "signet ring" forms of one type of malarial parasite.

Uninfected mosquito bites the infected person, thereby becoming infected.

Infected mosquito bites human.

Plasmodia in mosquito's saliva enter bloodstream

Plasmodia invade liver and multiply.

Plasmodia invade red blood cells and multiply.

Red cells rupture, releasing plasmodia.

Some plasmodia invade more red cells

Other plasmodia develop into forms that can infect mosquitoes.

Malingering

Deliberate simulation of physical or psychological symptoms for a particular purpose, such as obtaining time off work, avoiding military service, or obtaining compensation. Malingering differs from *factitious disorders*, in which an individual feigns illness for no reason other than a wish to gain the attention associated with illness and being a patient. Malingering is also distinguished from *hypochondriasis*, in which symptoms are not under the individual's voluntary control.

Mallet finger

Injury to the fingertip caused by a heavy blow to the end of the finger that forces the tip from a straight into a bent position. The injury, also called baseball finger, occurs in sports as a result of a ball striking a finger and also in other activities where the fingertip is forcibly bent.

The sudden bending of the extended finger may tear the tendon on the back of the finger, or, if the tendon doesn't "give", may pull off a fragment of bone. In either case, the fingertip is left bent.

Treatment is with an external *splint* or the insertion of a temporary wire through the bones to hold the finger straight. The injury heals over a period of two to three months.

Mallet toe

See *Claw toe*.

Mallory-Weiss syndrome

A condition in which a tear at the lower end of the *oesophagus* causes vomiting of blood. Mallory-Weiss syndrome is particularly common in alcoholics after a bout of excessive drinking accompanied by retching and vomiting. Less commonly, the tear may be produced by violent coughing, a severe asthma attack, or epileptic convulsions. The damage is thought to result from violent contractions of the diaphragm during prolonged retching and vomiting.

DIAGNOSIS AND TREATMENT

Diagnosis is made by passing an *endoscope* (a viewing instrument with a light source and lens attachment) down the oesophagus. The tear generally heals within 10 days and no special treatment is required unless the person has lost a considerable amount of blood, in which case blood transfusions may be necessary.

Malnutrition

See *Nutritional disorders*.

Malocclusion

An abnormal relationship between the upper and lower sets of *teeth* when they are closed. Most people have some teeth that are slightly out of position, but a person is considered to have malocclusion only if the bite (see *Occlusion*) or appearance is

---

CLASSES OF MALOCCLUSION

Unsatisfactory contact between the upper and lower teeth (malocclusion) is of three main classes, shown below.

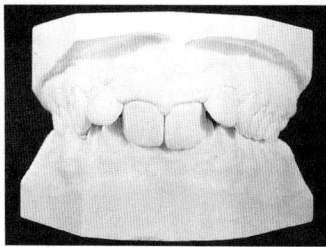

Class 1 malocclusion
In this (the most common) type, the jaw relationship is normal, but, because the teeth are poorly spaced, tilted, or rotated, the upper and lower set do not meet properly.

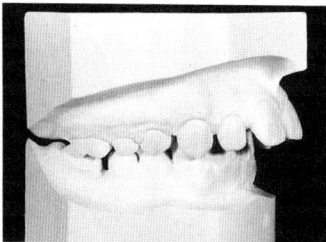

Class 2 malocclusion
In this type—called retrognathism—the lower jaw is too far back; the normal small overbite of the upper incisors is greatly increased, and the molar bite is displaced backwards.

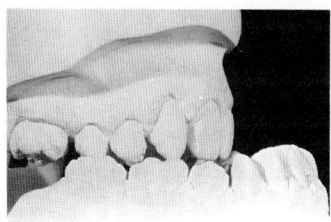

Class 3 malocclusion
In this (the least common) type—called prognathism—the lower jaw is too far forward; the lower incisors meet, or lie in front of, the upper ones, and the molar bite is displaced forwards.

---

adversely affected. There are three basic classes of dental malocclusion (see illustrated box).

CAUSES

Malocclusion usually develops in childhood, when the teeth and jaws are growing. Most cases of malocclusion are inherited; others result from *thumb-sucking* beyond a certain age or from a mismatch between the teeth and jaws (e.g. large teeth in a small mouth, leading to *overcrowding*).

TREATMENT

Treatment, which is usually necessary only if malocclusion is severe, may be carried out to improve appearance, to prevent strain from an abnormal bite (which causes pain, stiffness, and sometimes *arthritis* in the jaw joints), or to make cleaning of the teeth easier and thus help prevent *periodontal disease* and decay (see *Caries, dental*).

It is sometimes possible to correct uneven contacts by smoothing down or building up opposing tooth surfaces. The usual treatment, however, is use of *orthodontic appliances* (braces) to move teeth into the proper position. In cases of dental overcrowding, some teeth may need to be extracted. *Orthognathic surgery* is used to treat severe recession or protrusion of the lower jaw.

Treatment is best carried out in childhood or adolescence, when the teeth and bones of the jaw are still developing. Problems left until adulthood can be treated successfully, but may take longer to correct.

Malpresentation

A condition in which a baby is not in the usual head-first position during *childbirth*. Malpresentation occurs in about five per cent of births.

Types of malpresentation include breech presentation (in which the baby's bottom appears first), face presentation (in which the face rather than the top of the head appears first), and shoulder presentation (which occurs when the baby is lying transversely across the uterus). Breech presentations are the most common form of malpresentation.

A baby lying bottom-first at the onset of labour may be born by *breech delivery* or by *caesarean section*. A baby lying transversely usually requires a caesarean section.

Malta fever

An old name for *brucellosis*.

Mammary gland

See *Breast*.

M

Mammography

An X-ray procedure for examining the *breast*. Mammography is used to investigate *breast lumps* and to screen women for *breast cancer*.

The main value of mammography is that it allows the detection of breast tumours that are too small to be found during a physical examination (see *Breast self-examination*). Successful treatment of breast cancer depends on early detection of malignancy, and research has shown that mammography can significantly increase the early detection rate of breast cancer and can reduce death rates from this cause.

The procedure for mammography is shown in the illustrated box.

Mammoplasty

A cosmetic operation to reduce the size of extremely large or pendulous *breasts,* to enlarge small breasts, or to reconstruct a breast after part or all of it has been removed to treat *breast cancer.* Mammoplasty is performed under general anaesthesia.

BREAST REDUCTION

This procedure reduces the size of the breast and raises it to correct drooping. Incisions are made in the breast and unwanted tissue is removed. Most patients are pleased with the result. The nipple scar and the scar beneath the breast are usually hidden, but the vertical scar is usually evident and may need to be made less obvious by further surgery.

BREAST ENLARGEMENT

The standard surgical method for breast enlargement was, until recently, the insertion of a silicone implant under the skin. However, in the early 1990s, fears about the long-term safety of the implants led to restriction of their use in the US, and surgeons in most other countries have also become more cautious about using them.

Possible complications of the procedure are leakage of silicone from, and hardening of breast tissue around, the implant, and scar formation. Some women who developed autoimmune disorders such as systemic *lupus erythematosus* claimed that

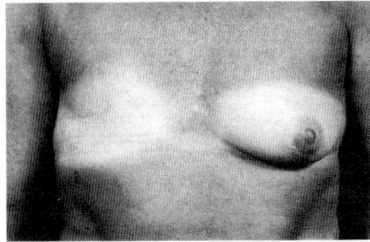

Before

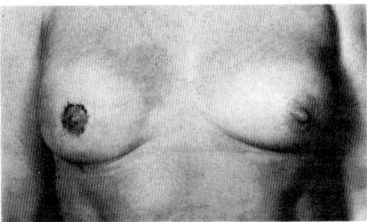

After

Reconstruction of a breast
A breast removed at an earlier mastectomy operation can be reconstructed later using a silicone rubber implant.

their implants were the cause; but this association has not been proved. However, the level of concern was such that, in 1992, the United States Food and Drug Administration restricted the use of implants to women needing breast reconstruction. The main manufacturer of silicone implants, Dow Corning, withdrew from the market that year and set up a compensation fund for women who had suffered side-effects.

BREAST RECONSTRUCTION

The operation is usually carried out at the same time as a *mastectomy.* Surgeons try to remove as little breast tissue as possible, and to restore the normal contours by the insertion of an implant.

Many surgeons continue to believe silicone implants to be satisfactory and safe enough for their use to be continued in these circumstances. Others use a different design of implant filled with materials believed to be safe. On both sides of the Atlantic, trials are in progress to assess the long-term safety of the various choices available for breast reconstruction.

Mandible

The lower *jaw.*

Mania

A mental disorder characterized by episodes of overactivity, elation, or irritability. Mania usually occurs as part of a *manic-depressive illness.*

PROCEDURE FOR MAMMOGRAPHY

Mammography is simple, safe, and causes only slight discomfort. Only low-dose X-rays are used. The breast may be X-rayed from above, the side, or both; sometimes an oblique (angled) view is taken.

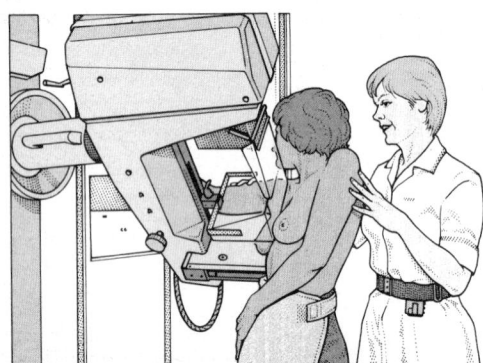

How mammography is done
In the method shown here, the breast is placed on the machine and gently compressed between the X-ray plate below and a plastic cover above. This flattens the breast so that as much tissue as possible can be imaged. Several views may be taken. In another method, the breast hangs freely and is X-rayed from the side.

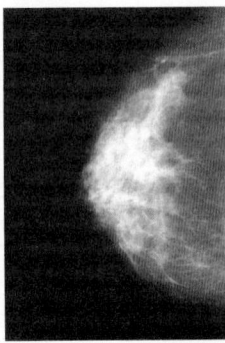 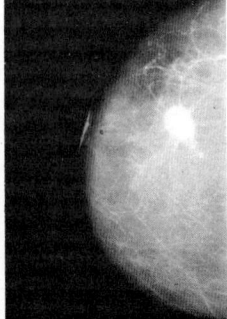

Mammograms
The normal mammogram (far left) shows a side view of a healthy breast, with the milk ducts appearing as denser areas. In the abnormal mammogram (left), an irregular, dense mass in the upper part of the breast indicates a tumour. A biopsy (removal of a tissue sample for analysis) is necessary to determine whether a tumour is cancerous.

PROCEDURE FOR MAMMOPLASTY

One of the most common cosmetic operations, mammoplasty is done to improve the appearance of the breasts by removal of excess fat and skin or by using an implant to increase their size.

BREAST REDUCTION

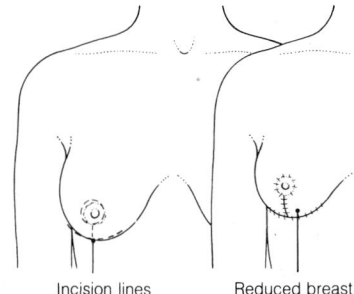

Incision lines   Reduced breast

Incisions are made around the edge of the nipple and in the crease below the breast. These are joined by a third vertical cut. Excess tissue and skin are removed, and the incisions are closed with stitches.

BREAST ENLARGEMENT

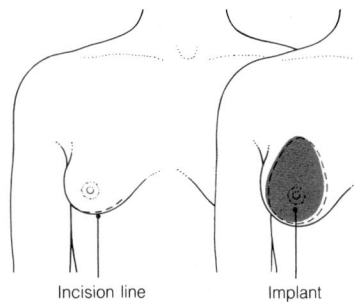

Incision line   Implant

An incision is made in the armpit or along the crease under the breast, and a pocket is created behind the breast to receive the implant. After the implant has been inserted, the incision is stitched.

SYMPTOMS

The primary symptom of mania is an abnormal increase in activity (for example, the sufferer may make elaborate plans for a constant round of social activity). Other symptoms may include: extravagant spending; repeatedly starting new tasks; less need to sleep; increased appetite for food, alcohol, sex, and energetic exercise; outbursts of inappropriate anger, laughter, or sudden socializing; and a grandiose sense of knowing better than others. This may extend to delusions of grandeur (for example, believing oneself to be God). When symptoms are relatively mild, the condition is called hypomania.

Manic attacks usually first appear before the age of 30, and may last for a few days or several months. If attacks begin after the age of 40, they are frequently more prolonged.

TREATMENT

Severe mania often leads to marked social disruption or even violence; hospital admission is usually required. Treatment is generally by means of *antipsychotic drugs*; relapses may be prevented by taking *lithium* or *carbamazepine*.

Manic-depressive illness

A mental disorder in which a disturbance of mood is the major symptom. This disturbance may be unipolar (consisting either of *depression* or *mania*) or bipolar (consisting of a swing between the two states). In a severe form of the illness, sometimes referred to as manic-depressive psychosis, mood swings may be accompanied by grandiose ideas or by extreme negative delusions.

CAUSES

Some disorders affecting the brain, certain drugs, and a clear inherited tendency are all established factors. Research has located at least one of the defective genes responsible on chromosome 11. Mood changes have been linked to changing levels of the chemical *dopamine* in parts of the brain.

PREVALENCE

Depression is very common, affecting about one in 10 men and one in five women at some time in their lives. About a third of these illnesses are severe. By contrast, mania (unipolar or bipolar) is rare, affecting only about eight per 1,000 people, men and women equally.

TREATMENT

Severe manic-depressive illness often requires hospital admission. *Antidepressant drugs* and/or *ECT* (electroconvulsive therapy) are effective in treating depression. *Antipsychotic drugs* such as chlorpromazine and haloperidol are used to control manic symptoms. *Lithium* may be used during remission to prevent a relapse.

Group therapy, family therapy, and individual *psychotherapy* are useful in treating neurotic disorders and in aiding recovery after a severe episode. *Cognitive-behavioural therapy* may also be helpful.

OUTLOOK

Though often crippling in the acute phase, manic-depressive illnesses have a good outlook. Abilities are not affected, and more than 80 per cent of patients recover.

Repeated, severe illnesses, however, or persistent depression, can seriously disrupt life. A significant number of depressed people commit, or attempt to commit, *suicide*, whereas others suffer from social isolation, poverty, and problems caused by *alcohol dependence*. Nevertheless, the widescale use of maintenance treatment with lithium has restored many people with manic-depressive illness to near-normal health.

Manipulation

A therapeutic technique involving the skilful use of the hands to move a part of the body or a specific joint or muscle to treat certain disorders. It is important in *orthopaedics, physiotherapy, osteopathy,* and *chiropractic.*

Doctors and physiotherapists use manipulation to treat deformity and stiffness caused by some disorders of the bones and joints. A general anaesthetic may be necessary in some cases. Manipulation may be used to realign the bones in a displaced *fracture,* to put a joint back into position following a *dislocation,* or to stretch a *contracture* (shortened muscle or tendon). The technique may also be used to increase the range of movement of a stiff joint, usually following injury. Occasionally, manipulation is helpful in the treatment of *frozen shoulder.* Manipulation does not usually relieve stiffness caused by *arthritis* (inflammation of a joint).

Mannitol

An osmotic *diuretic drug* used in the treatment of *oedema* of the brain and *glaucoma,* and to prepare the bowel for *endoscopy.*

Manometry

The measuring of pressure (of either a liquid or gas) by means of an instrument called a manometer.

The simplest type of manometer is a glass U-shaped tube containing mercury, oil, or water. One limb of the tube is connected to the pressure source; the other limb is either open to the atmosphere or closed. Changes in pressure cause the liquid to rise in one limb and to fall in the other. More sophisticated manometers use a

M

coiled spring, diaphragm, or electrical transducer to measure pressure.

Manometry is used to measure *blood pressure* by means of an instrument called a *sphygmomanometer*. Other uses of manometry include measurement of the pressure of *cerebrospinal fluid* in the spinal canal, measurement of pressure at the lower end of the oesophagus in the diagnosis of oesophageal disorders and *hiatus hernia*, and measurement of pressure in the rectum and anus in the investigation of some cases of *constipation* and faecal incontinence (see *Incontinence, faecal*).

Mantoux test

A type of skin test for tuberculosis (see *Tuberculin tests*).

Maprotiline

An *antidepressant drug*. Because maprotiline has a sedative effect, it is useful in *depression* accompanied by anxiety or difficulty sleeping. Maprotiline takes about six weeks to become fully effective. Possible adverse effects include dizziness, drowsiness, palpitations, and rash.

Marasmus

A severe form of protein and calorie malnutrition that usually occurs in famine or semi-starvation conditions. In developing countries, marasmus is widespread in children under three years of age, usually because they have been weaned too early on to an inadequate diet, given inadequate bottle-feeding, or kept too long on unsupplemented breast milk.

Children suffering from marasmus are stunted, emaciated, and usually hungry; they have loose folds of skin on the limbs and buttocks due to loss of muscle and fat. Other signs include sparse, brittle hair, diarrhoea, and dehydration.

DIAGNOSIS AND TREATMENT

Marasmus is diagnosed from a physical examination and the child's dietary history. Treatment consists of keeping the child warm and giving a high-energy, protein-rich diet. Persistent marasmus can cause permanent mental handicap and impaired growth. (See also *Kwashiorkor*.)

Marble bone disease

See *Osteopetrosis*.

March fracture

A break in one of the *metatarsal bones* (long bones in the foot) caused by repeated jarring. Usually affecting the second or third metatarsal, march fracture is caused by running or walking long distances on a hard surface. The name is derived from the high incidence of this fracture in soldiers after long marches.

Pain, tenderness, and swelling occur around the fracture site. *X-rays* may not show the fracture until healing has begun, when callus (new bone) appears as a white shadow. Treatment is rest and, occasionally, immobilization in a plaster *cast*. (See also *Stress fracture*.)

Marfan's syndrome

A rare, inherited disorder of connective tissue (material that surrounds body structures and holds them together) which results in abnormalities of the skeleton, heart, and eyes. The incidence of Marfan's syndrome is about two cases per 100,000 people. The cause is a genetic defect inherited as an autosomal dominant.

SYMPTOMS AND SIGNS

The features of Marfan's syndrome usually appear after the age of 10. Affected people grow very tall and thin, the fingers are long and spidery, the chest and spine are often deformed, and the ligaments, tendons, and joint capsules are weak, leaving the sufferer "double-jointed" and susceptible to joint dislocation. In about 90 per cent of cases, the heart or the aorta (major blood vessel leading from the heart) is abnormal; in more than 60 per cent of sufferers, the lens of the eye is dislocated.

DIAGNOSIS

There are no specific diagnostic tests for Marfan's syndrome. *Echocardiography* may be used to investigate heart abnormalities, and an eye examination may be performed.

TREATMENT AND OUTLOOK

Orthopaedic *corsets* or surgery may be required to correct spinal deformity.

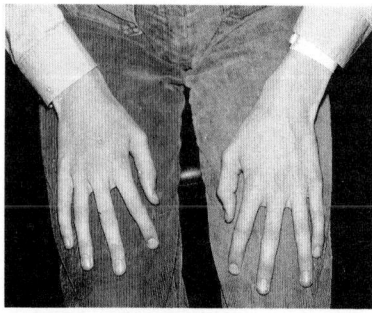

Features of Marfan's syndrome
One of the characteristic features of Marfan's syndrome is long, thin, "spider" fingers (arachnodactyly).

Beta-blocker drugs (propranolol, for example) may help to control heart problems, but heart surgery is necessary in some cases.

Affected people should receive *genetic counselling*; there is a 50 per cent chance that their offspring will inherit the disease. Women with Marfan's syndrome risk heart complications if they become pregnant.

Many sufferers do not live beyond the age of 50, and death is commonly caused by *heart failure* or rupture of an *aortic aneurysm*.

Marijuana

The flowering tops and dried leaves of the Indian hemp plant *CANNABIS SATIVA*. Marijuana contains the active ingredient *THC* (tetrahydrocannabinol), which is found also in cannabis resin (hashish). The chopped leaves are usually smoked as a joint (or reefer) but can be drunk as tea or eaten in food.

EFFECTS

When marijuana is smoked, effects occur within minutes and last for an hour or more. When marijuana is eaten, the effects are not usually felt for half an hour to an hour, and may last for three to five hours.

Physical effects include a dry mouth, mild reddening of the eyes, slight clumsiness, and increased appetite. The main subjective feelings are usually of well-being and calmness, although depression occasionally occurs. Users become dreamy and relaxed, laughing readily and experiencing time as passing very slowly. Sights and sounds become more vivid, imagination increases, and random connections between things seem more relevant.

Large doses may result in panicky states, fear of death, and illusions. Rarely, true psychosis (loss of contact with reality) occurs, producing paranoid delusions, confusion, and other symptoms. These symptoms usually disappear within several days if triggered by the drug, which may merely be acting on an underlying illness. A more permanent state of apathy and loss of concern (known as amotivational syndrome) has been attributed to prolonged, regular use.

There is a possibility that regular users of marijuana may become physically dependent on it. Whether or not the drug causes brain or other physical damage is much debated. Possession and use of marijuana is illegal in the UK.

Marriage guidance

A type of professional therapy for married couples or established partners aimed at resolving problems in relationships. Usually the partners attend sessions together on a regular basis. The counsellor promotes communication and sorts out differences between the partners.

HOW IT IS DONE

Marriage guidance today is largely based on the ideas and methods of *behaviour therapy*. It is assumed that behaviour in a relationship is learned. Another assumption is that both partners are responsible for problems because they have either failed to reinforce desirable behaviour in their partner or have themselves failed to respond with appropriate behaviour.

Therapy starts with an analysis of the good and bad aspects of the relationship. Each of the partners then indicates how he or she would like the other to behave. In some cases, a contract may be drawn up in which each person agrees to do something that the other wants. Alternatively, a system of rewards may be set up in which each partner rewards the other for pleasing or helpful behaviour.

Role play and demonstrations may be used to teach alternative ways of behaving, and training in communication skills given to promote the expression of feelings. If part of the couple's problem is sexual, the counsellor may refer them for *sex therapy*.

Marrow, bone

See *Bone marrow*.

Marsupialization

A surgical procedure used to drain some types of abscess or cyst (e.g. of a *Bartholin's gland* at the entrance to the vagina) and to prevent further abscesses. Marsupialization of a Bartholin's gland abscess involves cutting out part of the abscess wall and a small piece of vaginal tissue, and then forming a pouch by stitching the opened abscess wall to the wall of the vagina.

Marsupialization is also used to treat certain types of cysts affecting the pancreas and liver.

Masculinization

See *Virilization*.

Masochism

A desire to be physically, mentally, or emotionally abused. The term is derived from the name of the 19th-century Austrian novelist Leopold von Sacher-Masoch.

The term masochism is often used specifically to refer to the achievement of sexual excitement exclusively or preferably by means of one's own suffering. Activities include bondage, flagellation, and verbal abuse. The condition is usually chronic, and may even be life-threatening when people increase the severity of their masochistic acts.

Masochists rarely seek professional treatment; when they do, it is usually at the instigation of a spouse who threatens to leave. (See also *Sadism; Sadomasochism*.)

Massage

Rubbing and kneading of areas of the body, usually using the hands. Massage is used to relieve painful muscle spasm, treat muscle injury, reduce oedema (fluid retention in tissue), and, in the treatment of scars, to prevent tethering of skin and underlying tissue. Massage increases blood flow, reduces deep-seated pain by causing counter-irritation of nerve endings in the skin, relaxes muscles, and increases the suppleness of the skin.

Mast cell

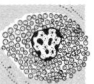 A type of cell, present in most body tissues, that plays an important part in *allergy*. In an allergic response, an allergen stimulates the release of *antibodies*, which attach themselves to mast cells. As a result, the mast cells release substances such as *histamine* (one of the chemicals responsible for producing the symptoms of allergy) into the tissue.

Mastectomy

Surgical removal of all or part of the *breast*. Mastectomy is usually performed to treat *breast cancer* and is often followed by a course of *radiotherapy* or *anticancer drugs*.

The amount of breast and surrounding tissue that is removed depends on the size and location of

M

SELF-MASSAGE

Although massage is most effective when carried out by another person, self-massage can still be useful; for example, it may help to alleviate pain caused by muscular tension.

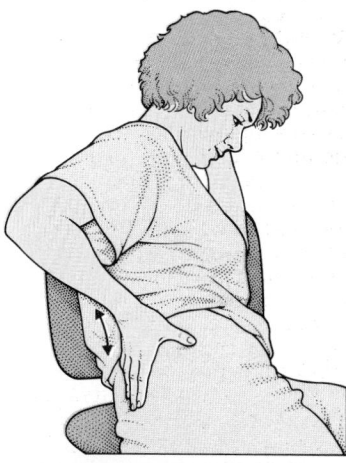

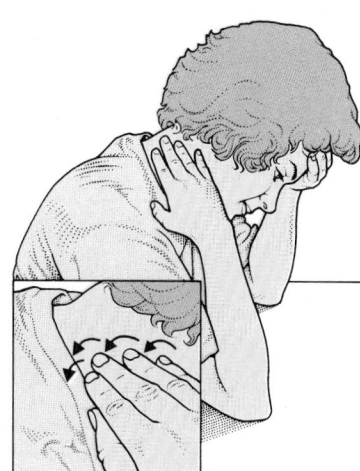

Finger kneading of the neck and foot
For neck massage, the elbows are rested on a firm surface, such as a table, and the head is supported with one hand while the fingertips of the other hand knead the back and side of the neck. After one side of the neck has been massaged, switch hands and massage the other side.

For foot massage, place one thumb over the other and knead the sole from the heel to the ball of the foot.

Kneading the lower back
For self-massage of the lower back, the hands should be placed with the thumbs pointing forwards and the fingertips close together at the back. Firm finger pressure is required to massage this area.

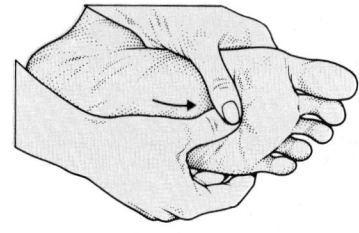

the tumour, on how much the cancer has spread, and on the age and general health of the patient.

TYPES

Until the late 1960s, the standard operation was the radical mastectomy, which involves removal of the affected breast, the chest muscles, underarm lymph nodes, and additional fat and skin from the chest. When some of the chest muscles are left intact, the operation is known as a modified radical mastectomy.

Today, surgeons may recommend lumpectomy (in which only cancerous tissue is removed) or a quadrantectomy (in which one quadrant of the breast is removed). In many cases, however, the treatment is still a mastectomy, which consists of removing the affected breast and sometimes some of the underarm lymph nodes. Sometimes, surgeons leave the overlying skin intact, or leave plenty of surrounding skin to allow the breast to be reconstructed.

HOW IT IS DONE

Each of the operations is performed under a general anaesthetic. For lumpectomy and quadrantectomy, an incision is made over the breast lump, which is cut free and removed together with some of the surrounding breast tissue.

For mastectomy, the incision extends from the armpit to encompass the entire breast. Underlying tissue is then cut free and removed, and a drainage tube is inserted. In all cases, the skin is closed with stitches or clips, which are usually removed after a week. A skin graft is sometimes needed. Some surgeons carry out a subcutaneous mastectomy, in which the skin is left intact and a silicone rubber implant is inserted to preserve the shape of the breast.

RECOVERY PERIOD

Patients may go home one to two days after lumpectomy and quadrantectomy, and can resume most activities within two weeks.

After other operations, the hospital stay is usually several days, and the drainage tube is removed on the second or third day. Analgesic drugs (painkillers) may be necessary for the first week.

OUTLOOK

Healing is usually very good after lumpectomy and quadrantectomy, with no noticeable scarring. Wound infection is uncommon. Skin scars after more radical procedures may be extensive, but usually fade within about a year.

Possible long-term complications, particularly of radical mastectomy, include *lymphoedema* (accumulation of lymphatic fluid in tissues) and stiffness of the arm and shoulder.

If the entire breast has been removed, some form of prosthesis (artificial breast) will be provided. This may be an external prosthesis, or a more permanent internal prosthesis, which may be fitted either immediately or at a later operation (see *Mammoplasty*).

Mastication

The process of chewing food. Mastication consists of two stages. In the first, the canines and incisors (front teeth)

TYPES OF MASTECTOMY

The type of operation depends on many factors, including the site of the tumour and the woman's health.

A small tumour may be treated by lumpectomy; other cases may require more extensive surgery.

LUMPECTOMY

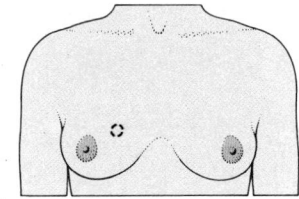

Only the area of cancerous tissue is removed. Lumpectomy is the least invasive procedure and leaves the breast looking normal.

QUADRANTECTOMY

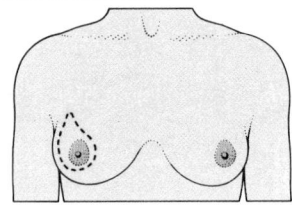

The cancerous tissue plus a wedge of surrounding tissue is removed. The lymph nodes in the armpit may also be removed. The breast is slightly smaller after the operation.

SUBCUTANEOUS MASTECTOMY

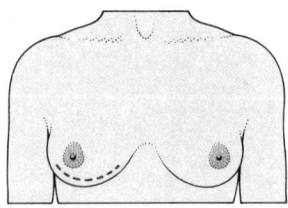

An incision is made under the breast and internal breast tissue is removed, leaving most of the skin intact. The nipple is not involved, but the milk ducts leading to it are cut. In some cases, the appearance of the breast is restored by immediate insertion of some type of implant. More often, however, this is done later.

TOTAL MASTECTOMY

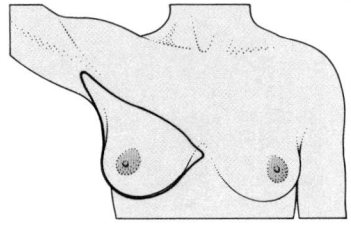

1 A large elliptical incision, encompassing the nipple and sometimes the entire breast, is made. The incision extends into the armpit.

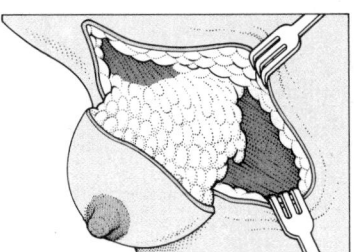

2 All the breast tissue, including the skin and some of the fat, is dissected (cut down) down to the chest muscles. The dissection is continued under the skin into the armpit, to free the upper and outer "tail" of breast tissue with its lymph nodes. All bleeding vessels are tied off before inserting a drainage tube and closing the skin with stitches or clips.

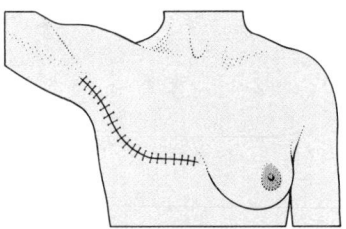

3 The scar after the operation. The woman may wear a prosthesis or may have an implant inserted later.

---

shear the food. In the second, the tongue pushes the food between the upper and lower premolars and molars (back teeth) to be ground by side-to-side and circular movements of the lower jaws. During mastication, saliva is mixed with the food to help break it down for swallowing.

Any food that spills over between the gums and cheeks is scooped up by rhythmic contractions of the cheeks and lips. The muscles of mastication, which attach the lower jaw to the rest of the skull, are controlled by signals from sensory nerves in the mouth to prevent undue stress on tooth-supporting tissues.

Only gross irregularities in the positional relationship of upper to lower teeth (see *Malocclusion*) prevent normal mastication.

Mastitis

Inflammation of *breast* tissue, usually caused by bacterial infection and sometimes by hormonal changes.

CAUSES

Mastitis is usually caused by the entry of bacteria into the breast through the nipple during *breast-feeding*. This type of mastitis is most common during the first month of breast-feeding and is more likely if the nipples are cracked.

Mastitis can also be caused by changes in the levels of sex hormones in the body. This type of mastitis sometimes occurs in the newborn (due to high levels of hormones from the mother's circulation) and at the start of *puberty. Fibroadenosis* (chronic mastitis in which the breasts are tender and lumpy) is also thought to be due to hormonal variations.

SYMPTOMS

Pain, tenderness, and swelling occur in all types of mastitis and may be present in one or both breasts. Bacterial mastitis during breast-feeding causes redness and *engorgement* and may result in a *breast abscess.*

TREATMENT

Mastitis caused by infection is treated with *antibiotic drugs* and *analgesic drugs* (painkillers), and by *expressing milk* to relieve engorgement. Breast-feeding should be continued unless pus begins to drain from the nipple.

Symptoms of mastitis in babies and at puberty usually last for only a few weeks and clear up without specific treatment.

Mastocytosis

An unusual condition, also called urticaria pigmentosa, characterized by numerous itchy, irregular, yellow or orange-brown swellings on the skin. Mastocytosis most commonly occurs on the trunk, and is worse after bathing or scratching.

In some cases, mastocytosis affects many body organs, including the liver, spleen, and intestine. Symptoms, such as diarrhoea, vomiting, and fainting may occur. Very rarely, mastocytosis leads to *anaphylactic shock*, which can be fatal.

Mastocytosis usually begins in the first year of life and disappears by adolescence. Treatment is difficult, although *antihistamine drugs* sometimes help to relieve symptoms.

Mastoid bone

The lower part of the temporal bone of the *skull.* Jutting from the lower part of the mastoid bone is a bony projection called the mastoid process. The mastoid bone is honeycombed with air cells, which are connected to a cavity called the mastoid antrum in the upper part of the mastoid. The mastoid antrum leads into the middle ear. As a result, infections of the middle ear (see *Otitis media*) occasionally spread through the mastoid bone to cause acute *mastoiditis.*

Mastoiditis

Inflammation of the *mastoid bone*, the prominent bone behind the ear.

CAUSE AND INCIDENCE

The disease is caused by the spread of infection from the middle ear (see *Otitis media*) to the mastoid antrum (a cavity in the mastoid bone), and from there to a honeycomb of air cells in the bone.

Mastoiditis has been uncommon since the advent of *antibiotic drugs*, which control middle-ear infection.

SYMPTOMS AND SIGNS

Mastoiditis causes severe pain, swelling, and tenderness behind the ear, as well as pain within the ear. These symptoms are usually accompanied by fever, a creamy discharge from the ear, progressive hearing loss, and some displacement of the outer ear.

COMPLICATIONS

There is always a risk that the infection may spread, causing *meningitis*, a *brain abscess*, or clotting of blood in veins within the brain. The infection may also spread outwards to damage the facial nerve and cause *facial palsy.*

DIAGNOSIS AND TREATMENT

Prompt diagnosis, based on a physical examination, is essential because of the possible complications.

Treatment is with antibiotic drugs, which usually clear up the infection. If

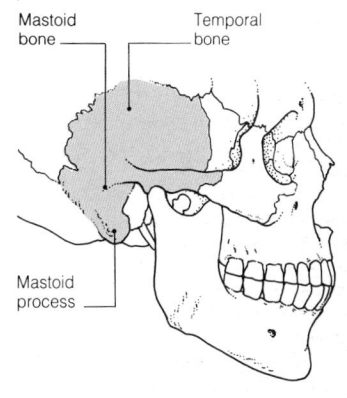

LOCATION OF MASTOID BONE
The mastoid bone is the lower part of the temporal bone. The mastoid process can be felt as a prominence behind the ear.

Mastoid bone

Temporal bone

Mastoid process

the infection persists, an operation known as a mastoidectomy may be necessary. This procedure involves making an incision behind the ear, opening up the mastoid bone, and removing the infected air cells. The wound is then stitched up around a drainage tube, which is removed a day or two later.

Masturbation

Sexual self-stimulation, usually to orgasm. Masturbation is now accepted as a normal behaviour. Over 90 per cent of men and about 65 per cent of women masturbate at some time during their lives. Massaging the penis or clitoris with the hand is the usual method.

There is no evidence that masturbation causes any physical or psychological harm, in spite of the 19th-century belief that it caused insanity, blindness, or other disorders. This notion may have been based on the observation that people who are severely mentally handicapped or suffering from *schizophrenia, dementia*, or other forms of brain damage sometimes masturbate publicly. Such behaviour is a sign not a cause of mental illness.

Maternal mortality

The death of a woman during *pregnancy* or within 42 days of *childbirth, miscarriage*, or induced *abortion*, from any cause related to the pregnancy. The term also describes the number of such deaths per year per 100,000 (or per 1,000 or 10,000) pregnancies.

In previous centuries, women of all social classes commonly died in child-

M

birth; maternal mortality still remains high in developing countries. In developed countries, however, deaths and complications of childbirth have declined dramatically in this century, particularly since about the 1940s. A large proportion of this decline is due to improvements in social conditions (which have resulted in improvements in women's general health); much of the remainder is a result of medical advances in treating the complications of pregnancy and childbirth.

CAUSES

Maternal deaths may occur as a direct result of complications of pregnancy, or as an indirect result of a medical condition that has been aggravated by pregnancy. The principal direct causes include *pulmonary embolism* (blood clots in the lungs), *hypertension* (high blood pressure), *antepartum haemorrhage* or *postpartum haemorrhage*, *ectopic pregnancy* (development of the fetus outside the uterus), *eclampsia* (a condition characterized by seizures during late pregnancy), abortion, miscarriage, or *caesarean section*, and *puerperal sepsis* (infection after childbirth). Important indirect causes are heart disease, *anaemia, hyperthyroidism* (overactivity of the thyroid gland) or *hypothyroidism* (underactivity of the thyroid gland), *diabetes mellitus,* and some cancers.

RELATED FACTORS

Maternal mortality is highest for the first pregnancy, and for the fifth and subsequent pregnancies. It is also greater in women who are younger than 20 or older than 30. Statistically, it is safest for a woman to have her first baby when she is between 20 and 25 years old; it becomes increasingly less safe after the age of 30.

Social factors also play a part; in general maternal mortality is higher among poor, less well-educated women, and among women who do not receive adequate *antenatal care.*

TRENDS

Maternal mortality has decreased considerably since about the 1940s. In the UK, the death rate has fallen from about 60 per 100,000 pregnancies in 1950, to less than 10 per 100,000 in the 1990s. This substantial decline is due largely to social improvements, better obstetric care, the development of *antibiotic drugs* and other drugs to combat infection, and the availability of *blood transfusions.* In addition, because of the ready availability of effective methods of *contraception,* fewer women than formerly have a large number of pregnancies.

Maxilla

One of a pair of bones that forms the upper jaw. At their base the maxillae carry the upper *teeth* and form the roof of the mouth; at the top the maxillae form the floor of the orbits (the eye sockets). Each maxilla contains a large air-filled cavity (called the maxillary sinus) which is connected to the nasal cavity.

DISORDERS

The most common disorder affecting the maxilla is *sinusitis* (inflammation of the mucous membrane that lines the maxillary *sinuses*), usually caused by infection spreading from the nose, less commonly from a tooth. Severe sinusitis occasionally leads to *osteomyelitis* (bone infection).

The maxilla is commonly fractured in road traffic accidents, causing a variety of facial deformities, such as backward displacement of the teeth or caving in of the centre of the face. Immediate surgery to reposition and secure the bones is necessary to prevent permanent disfigurement.

Various kinds of tumours may develop in the maxillary sinus, 80 per cent of which are malignant. Tumours of the maxillary sinus may eventually alter the shape of the jaw, loosen the teeth, block one of the nasolacrimal ducts (causing the eye to water), push the eyeball upwards or outwards, or block the nose and cause a bloody, offensive-smelling discharge. Treatment is by *radiotherapy,* followed by surgical removal of the maxilla.

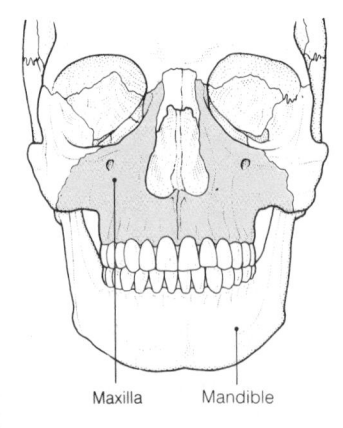

LOCATION OF THE MAXILLA
The maxilla is one of a pair of bones that together form the centre of the face, the upper jaw, and the roof of the mouth.

Maxilla   Mandible

McArdle's disease

A rare *genetic disorder* characterized by muscular stiffness and painful cramps that increase during and after exertion. McArdle's disease is caused by a deficiency of an *enzyme* in muscle cells that stimulates the breakdown of *glycogen* (a complex carbohydrate) to glucose (a type of sugar). This results in a build-up of glycogen in the muscles and prevents the release of glucose (an essential source of energy) during exercise.

Symptoms usually start between the ages of 20 and 30. Myoglobinuria (the presence of muscle cell pigment in the urine) occurs because of the damage to muscle cells; rarely, myoglobinuria is severe enough to cause *kidney failure.* Affected people are usually healthy apart from the need to restrict their exercise.

There is no treatment, although symptoms may be relieved by eating glucose or fructose before exercise.

ME

See *Myalgic encephalomyelitis.*

Measles

A potentially dangerous viral illness that causes a characteristic rash and a fever. Measles affects mainly children but can occur at any age. One attack usually confers lifelong immunity.

CAUSES AND INCIDENCE

The measles virus is highly infective and is spread primarily by airborne droplets of nasal secretions. Infected children can transmit the virus during the eight- to 14-day incubation period to up to one week after the onset of symptoms. Infants under eight months old are rarely affected because they have acquired some immunity from their mothers.

Measles was once very common throughout the world, occurring in epidemics. It is now less common in developed countries due to *immunization.* In the UK, a combined vaccine against measles, mumps, and rubella (see *MMR vaccination*) was included in the standard immunization programme in 1988. Incentives were also introduced to encourage general practitioners to ensure that as many children as possible were immunized; a publicity campaign was aimed at the public to dispel any fears about the safety of vaccines.

In the early 1990s the proportion of children fully immunized rose to 90 per cent or better in most parts of the UK and measles became uncommon. This achievement is important because measles may have rare but serious complications. Measles may also be serious, and sometimes fatal, in children with impaired immunity (such as those being treated for *leukaemia* and those infected with the virus that causes *AIDS*).

In developing countries, measles is still common, accounting for more than one million deaths every year, especially in malnourished children whose defences against infection are seriously impaired.

SYMPTOMS AND SIGNS

The illness starts with a fever, runny nose, sore eyes, and cough, and the sufferer is generally unwell. After three to four days a red rash appears, usually starting on the head and neck and spreading downwards to cover the whole body. The spots sometimes join to produce large red blotchy areas, and the lymph glands may be enlarged. After three days the rash starts to fade and symptoms subside.

The most common complications are ear and chest infections, which usually occur with a return of fever two to three days after the appearance of the rash. Diarrhoea, vomiting, and abdominal pain also occur.

Febrile convulsions are common with measles and are not usually serious (see *Convulsions, febrile*).

A serious complication, occurring in about one in 1,000 cases, is *encephalitis* (inflammation of the brain). Encephalitis causes headache, drowsiness, and vomiting, starting seven to 10 days after the appearance of the rash. Seizures and coma may follow, sometimes leading to *mental handicap* or even death.

Very rarely (in about one in a million cases) a progressive brain disorder, known as subacute sclerosing panencephalitis, develops years after the acute illness.

Measles during pregnancy results in death of the fetus in about one fifth of cases. There is no evidence that measles causes birth defects.

TREATMENT

Plenty of fluids and *paracetamol* should be given to treat the fever. Antibiotic drugs are not required to treat the measles infection itself but may be given to treat bacterial infections that occur as complications.

IMMUNIZATION

Immunization against measles is usually offered at about 15 months of age and produces immunity in about 97 per cent of cases. A booster second shot may be given after school entry. Side-effects of the measles vaccine are generally mild. There may be slight fever, symptoms of a cold, and a rash about one week after vaccination.

The vaccine should not be given to children with any special risk factors (see *Immunization*).

Meatus

A canal or passageway through part of the body. The term usually refers to the external auditory meatus, the canal in the outer *ear* that leads from the outside to the eardrum.

Mebendazole

An *anthelmintic drug* used to treat *worm infestations* of the intestine. Mebendazole is under investigation as a treatment for worms that infest other areas, such as the lungs and liver, as occurs in *hydatid disease*.

Possible adverse effects include abdominal pain and diarrhoea.

Meckel's diverticulum

A common congenital anomaly of the digestive tract in which a small, hollow, wide-mouthed sac protrudes from the *ileum* (the final section of the small intestine). Meckel's diverticulum occurs in two per cent of people.

There are usually no symptoms unless the diverticulum is affected by infection, obstruction, or ulceration. The most common symptom is painless bleeding, which may be sudden and severe, making immediate *blood transfusion* necessary. In some cases, inflammation causes symptoms so similar to those of acute *appendicitis* that the disorder is diagnosed only when abdominal surgery is carried out. A Meckel's diverticulum occasionally causes *intussusception* (telescoping) or *volvulus* (twisting) of the small intestine. Diagnosis may sometimes be made by using technetium *radionuclide scanning*.

Complications are treated by removal of the diverticulum.

Meconium

The thick, sticky, greenish-black faeces passed by infants during the first day or two after birth. Meconium consists of bile, mucus, and shed intestinal cells. After the baby starts feeding, the faeces gradually change in colour and consistency.

Occasionally, the fetus passes meconium into the *amniotic fluid* in the uterus. This is more common in babies who experience *fetal distress* during labour or who are postmature (that is, over 40 weeks' gestation). Meconium in the amniotic fluid may be inhaled

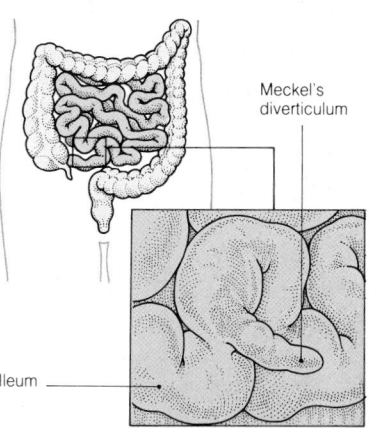

Anatomy of Meckel's diverticulum
In this birth defect, an appendix-like sac protrudes from the ileum (the last section of the small intestine).

when the baby starts to breathe, sometimes blocking the airways and damaging the lungs.

In some babies with *cystic fibrosis*, the meconium is so thick and sticky that it blocks the intestine and causes intestinal obstruction.

Medial

A medical term meaning situated towards the midline of the body. Less commonly, the word medial is used to refer to the middle layer of a body structure, particularly of a blood vessel wall.

Median nerve

One of the main nerves of the arm, which runs down the arm's full length into the hand; it is a branch of the *brachial plexus*.

The median nerve controls the muscles of the forearm and hand, which carry out bending movements of the wrist, fingers, and thumb, and which rotate the forearm palm-inwards. This nerve also conveys sensations from the thumb, index finger, middle finger, part of the ring finger, and the region of the palm at the base of these digits.

DISORDERS

Injury to the shoulder may damage the median nerve at the point where it originates from the brachial plexus. A *Colles' fracture* may damage the median nerve just above the wrist. *Carpal tunnel syndrome* causes pressure that may damage the nerve where it passes through the wrist. The principal symptoms of any damage are numbness and muscle weakness in the areas controlled by the nerve.

M

667

Mediastinoscopy

Investigation of the *mediastinum* (the central compartment of the chest containing the heart, oesophagus, and trachea) by means of an *endoscope* (a viewing tube with a light and lens) inserted into the cavity through an incision in the neck.

Mediastinoscopy is used mainly to perform a *biopsy* (removal of a small sample of tissue for microscopic analysis) of a lymph node to look for disease. Under a general anaesthetic, an incision is made in the base of the neck and an endoscope is passed through it into the mediastinum. A tissue sample is removed by minute blades at the end of the endoscope.

Mediastinum

The space between the lungs, including the structures in that space. The mediastinum extends from the sternum (breastbone) in front to the spine behind, and from the inlet of the thoracic duct (one of the main lymphatic vessels) at the top to the diaphragm at the bottom. The mediastinum contains the *heart*, *trachea* (windpipe), *oesophagus*, *thymus* gland, the major blood vessels entering and leaving the heart, *lymph nodes* and lymphatic vessels, and nerves (including the *vagus nerve* and *phrenic nerve*).

Medical Defence Societies

Nonprofit-making organizations that provide doctors with insurance cover against claims for medical negligence. Medical Defence Societies also advise doctors on all legal aspects of their work, not only claims for negligence, but also disputes about payment and allegations of incompetence or libel. By the late 1980s awards by British courts for damages for medical negligence had increased so much that one Defence Society proposed that doctors should pay much higher premiums. Protests led the government to decide that from 1989 the Crown would accept liability for negligence by hospital doctors employed by the NHS and this ended the crisis.

Medical research organizations

Medical research in the UK is carried out in universities and teaching hospitals, in industry (the pharmaceutical industry in the UK has innovated 10 of the world's top 50 drugs), and in research institutions. It is financed by the Medical Research Council and by medical charities and foundations, such as the Imperial Cancer Research Fund, the British Heart Foundation, the Wellcome Trust, and the Nuffield Laboratories.

Medication

Any substance prescribed to treat disease. (See also *Drug*; *Medicine*.)

Medicine

The study of human diseases; causes, frequency, treatment, and prevention. The term is also applied to any substance prescribed to treat illness.

EARLY HISTORY

In many early cultures, medicine was closely associated with religion; disease was regarded as a punishment from the gods so the victim would turn for help to a priest, who took on the additional function of a medicine man. Medicine probably became separated from religion with the emergence of people skilled in treating injuries such as broken bones and dislocated joints. These healers attracted patients and, in time, apprentices.

By the fifth century BC, the Greek physician Hippocrates had established medicine as a profession with a body of learning and a code of ethics to be passed on to each new generation of physicians (the Hippocratic oath is still used as an ethical guide for the medical profession). The dominant figure after Hippocrates was the second-century, Greek-born Roman physician Galen, who made valuable contributions but whose many false theories about anatomy and physiology were accepted for more than 13 centuries, effectively holding back advances in medical knowledge.

RENAISSANCE DISCOVERIES

With the Renaissance, medicine began to emerge from its long stagnation. In 1543 the Flemish anatomist and physician Andreas Vesalius (1514-1564) produced the first truly accurate anatomical text; in 1628 the English physician William Harvey (1578-1657) first demonstrated the circulation of blood. Also in the 17th century, the Dutch microscopist Antonj van Leeuwenhoek (1632-1723) was first to observe and describe microorganisms and the detailed structure of blood, muscles, and sperm.

MODERN MEDICINE

Despite the medical progress of the Renaissance and notable later achievements, such as the discovery in the late 18th century of the principle of vaccination by the English physician Edward Jenner (1749-1823), it was not until the 19th century that the foundations of modern scientific medicine were laid. This resulted from a realization that medicine needed to become a true science, systematic in its approach and founded on close observation and experimentation. Advances in other disciplines played an important role; the first practical high-powered microscope was developed in the 19th century; the ophthalmoscope (an instrument for examining the eye) was invented in 1851; the first practical thermometer was introduced in the 1860s; and X-rays were discovered in 1895, a discovery that revolutionized diagnosis. These developments, along with the French scientist Louis Pasteur's (1822-1895) work on germ theory, brought about a great advance in the understanding of many diseases.

Curing and controlling disease was not a reality until the 20th century, however, when vaccines were developed against many serious diseases (including typhoid, cholera, and diphtheria); and insecticides and improved sanitation helped control diseases such as malaria, yellow fever, and sleeping sickness.

The early 20th century was also marked by the development of safe anaesthesia, effective surgery, and a steady growth in the number of new drugs. In the late 1930s, the first effective antibacterial drugs (the sulphonamides) were introduced, followed in the 1940s by penicillin, streptomycin, and the tetracyclines; these drugs saved millions of lives.

Among important recent developments are the introduction of diagnostic techniques, such as *MRI*, *CT scanning*, endoscopic examination of the interior of the body (see *endoscopy*), and *ultrasound scanning*. Advances in genetics have opened up the field of genetic counselling for the prevention of inherited disorders, many of which are becoming treatable, due to bioengineering techniques being used to manufacture missing proteins and enzymes.

In the late 1980s, the incorporation of a video camera into the tip of an endoscope made *minimally invasive surgery* possible. For example, the surgeon uses a *laparoscope* to view the interior of the abdomen on a video screen and operates using micro-instruments passed through a small puncture in the abdominal wall. Transplant and implant surgery have become routine.

Today, the boundaries between medicine and other sciences are becoming progressively less distinct;

M

medical research is being increasingly undertaken by scientists who have little or no formal medical training. (See also Landmarks in medicine boxes, this page and overleaf; entries for individual medical, surgical, and scientific specialties.)

Medicine, private

The rich and powerful have always had their personal physicians, but when the *National Health Service* (NHS) was introduced in the UK in 1948 only a tiny fraction of the population chose to continue with a personal contract with their doctors. NHS consultants could choose to work part-time in private practice, and many did; they could admit private patients to beds in "private" wards or blocks in NHS hospitals. However, in the 1950s private practice remained a luxury. In the 1960s, with growing prosperity, many more patients became intolerant of the delays and waiting lists apparently inescapable in the NHS, and private practice grew.

Several organizations, such as the British United Provident Association (BUPA) and Private Patients' Plan, were already offering medical insurance and, as the numbers of their subscribers rose, so did the demand for private treatment—especially *elective* surgery. Private hospitals were built in growing numbers, partly to cater for a demand for British medical expertise from foreigners.

By the late 1980s, around one fifth of all nonemergency surgery was being performed in the private sector. Nevertheless, most people in the UK still use the NHS for their contacts with general practitioners and for the long-term care of the mentally handicapped and mentally ill. In addition, the NHS provides virtually all accident and emergency medical services in the UK.

Medicolegal

Relating to aspects of medicine and law that overlap, particularly to medical matters that come before the courts. Among the matters on which medicolegal experts advise are the laws concerning damages for injuries due to medical negligence or malpractice, medical evidence concerning the extent of injury in a civil action, the use of tests in determining paternity, the mental competence of people who have drawn up wills, and restrictions on the liberty of the mentally ill.

In recent years, new areas of medicolegal study have emerged, notably

LANDMARKS IN MEDICINE: DIAGNOSIS

Date	Development
c.400 BC.	**Disease concept** Introduced by the Greek physician Hippocrates.
1612	**Medical thermometer** Devised by the Italian physician Sanctorius.
c.1660	**Light microscope** Single-lens microscope developed by the Dutch naturalist Antonj van Leeuwenhoek, who discovered microorganisms with it. A practicable compound microscope was not developed until the 19th century.
1810	**Stethoscope** Invented by the French physician René Laennec.
1850–1900	**Germ theory of disease** Proposed by the French scientist Louis Pasteur and developed by the German bacteriologist Robert Koch.
1851	**Ophthalmoscope** Invented by the German scientist Hermann von Helmholtz.
1895	**X-rays** Discovered by the German physicist Wilhelm Roentgen. He also produced the first X-ray picture of the body.
1905	**X-ray contrast medium** First demonstrated (in retrograde pyelography) by Jean Athanase Sicard in Paris.
1906	**Electrocardiograph (ECG)** Invented by the Dutch physiologist Willem Einthoven.
c.1932	**Transmission electron microscope (TEM)** Constructed by the German scientists Max Knoll and Ernst Ruska.
1938	**Cardiac catheterization** First performed by George Peter Robb and Israel Steinberg in New York.
1957	**Fibre-optic endoscopy** Pioneered by the South African-born doctor Basil Hirschowitz at the University of Michigan.
1972	**CT scanner** Invented by the British engineer Godfrey Hounsfield of EMI Laboratories, England, and the South African-born physicist Alan Cormack of Tufts University, Massachusetts.
1975	**Monoclonal antibodies** Large-scale production method developed by the Argentinian-born scientist César Milstein at the Medical Research Council Laboratories, England.
1976	**Chorionic villus sampling** Developed by Chinese gynaecologists as an aid to the early diagnosis of genetic disorders.
1981	**MRI scanner** Developed by scientists at Thorn-EMI Laboratories, England, and Nottingham University.
1985	**PET scanner** Developed by scientists at the University of California.

M

LANDMARKS IN MEDICINE: SURGERY

Date	Development
1545	**Basic surgical principles** Established by the French surgeon Ambroise Paré.
1842	**General anaesthesia** First operation using general anaesthesia performed by the American surgeon Crawford Long, who used ether. In 1845, the American dentist Horace Wells used nitrous oxide (laughing gas) as an anaesthetic. In 1847, the British obstetrician James Simpson introduced chloroform anaesthesia.
1870	**Antiseptic surgery** Pioneered by the British surgeon Joseph Lister, who used a carbolic acid (phenol) spray during surgery to help prevent infection.
1901	**Blood groups** ABO blood groups discovered by the Austrian pathologist Karl Landsteiner, so establishing the basis for safe transfusions.
1951	**Coronary artery bypass graft** First attempted by the Canadian surgeon Arthur Vineberg at the Royal Victoria Hospital, Montreal.
1955	**Kidney transplant** First successful kidney transplant (between identical twins) performed by a team of American surgeons—led by Joseph Murray—of the Harvard Medical School, Massachusetts.
1967	**Heart transplant** First human heart transplant performed by the South African surgeon Christiaan Barnard at the Groote Schuur Hospital, Capetown.
1976	**Coronary angioplasty** Introduced by the Swiss surgeon Andreas Grüntzig at the University Hospital, Zurich.
1987	**Minimally invasive surgery** The first cholecystectomy using laparoscopic techniques under video control was performed by the French doctor, P. Mouret, in Lyon.

LANDMARKS IN MEDICINE: OTHER FORMS OF TREATMENT

Date	Development
c.1270	**Glasses** Thought to have been invented in Italy. Contact lenses were invented in 1887 by the Swiss optician Eugen Frick.
1817	**Dental plate** Introduced by the American dentist Anthony Plantson.
1891	**Baby incubator** Introduced by the French doctor Alexandre Lion.
1901	**Hearing-aid (electric)** Developed by the American inventor Miller Reese Hutchinson. The first truly miniature hearing-aid was introduced in 1952 by the Sonotone Corporation.
1945	**Kidney dialysis machine** Developed by the Dutch surgeon Willem Kolff to treat patients with kidney failure.
1978	**"Test-tube baby"** The first (Louise Brown) was born in England as a result of in vitro fertilization (IVF) techniques developed by the British gynaecologist Patrick Steptoe and the embryologist Robert Edwards.
1979	**Shock-wave lithotripsy** Pioneered by researchers at the University Hospital, Munich.

an individual's right to die (see *Brain death*; *Euthanasia*; *Living will*); the necessity for informed *consent* to any surgical procedure; the legal aspects of *artificial insemination*, *in vitro fertilization*, *sterilization*, and *surrogacy*; and an individual's right to *confidentiality* concerning his or her illness. (For the medical aspects of criminal law, see *Forensic medicine*.)

Meditation
Concentration on an object, a word, or an idea with the intention of inducing an altered state of consciousness. Meditation of different kinds has traditionally been a feature of many religions, particularly Eastern ones.

At its deepest level, meditation can resemble a trance or be an all-engrossing spiritual experience. More commonly, it is a physically calming therapy for body and mind. Some clinical trials have shown that meditation can be a valuable therapy for reducing stress levels and in helping to treat stress-related disorders. The most common form of meditation practised in the west is transcendental meditation (TM), introduced by the Maharishi Mahesh Yogi in the 1960s.

Medroxyprogesterone
A *progesterone* drug used in the treatment of *endometriosis* and certain types of *breast cancer* and uterine cancer (see *Uterus, cancer of*). Medroxyprogesterone is occasionally given to treat menstrual disorders such as mid-cycle bleeding and *amenorrhoea* (absence of menstruation).

Injections of medroxyprogesterone are used as a contraceptive (see *Contraception, hormonal methods of*). Injections are given at three-monthly intervals.

Possible adverse effects include weight gain, swollen ankles, and breast tenderness.

Medulla
The innermost part of an organ or body structure; the adrenal medulla is the central region of an adrenal gland, and the medulla of bone is the bone marrow. The term medulla is also sometimes used to refer to the medulla oblongata (part of the *brainstem* joining the spinal cord).

Medulla oblongata
Also known as the medulla, the medulla oblongata is the lowest part of the *brainstem*; it is situated in the skull between the pons (above) and the spinal cord (below).

Date	Development
1666	**Quinine** The British physician Thomas Sydenham popularized the use of Jesuits' bark (containing quinine) for treating malaria.
1785	**Digitalis** The use of digitalis to treat heart failure described by the British physician William Withering.
1796	**Smallpox vaccination** The first vaccination to be performed, by the British physician Edward Jenner. The first true vaccine (consisting of weakened microorganisms)—against chicken cholera—was developed in 1880 by the French scientist Louis Pasteur.
1805	**Morphine** Extracted from opium and used to relieve pain by the German pharmacist Friedrich Sertürner.
1899	**Aspirin** Developed as a drug by the German scientist Felix Hoffmann.
1911	**Salvarsan** Introduced by the German bacteriologist Paul Ehrlich to treat syphilis.
1928	**Penicillin** Antibacterial action first recognized by the British bacteriologist Alexander Fleming. It was produced as a drug in 1940, by the Australian-born British pathologist Howard Florey and the German-born British biochemist Ernst Chain.
1935	**Sulphonamides** Antibacterial action discovered by the German pharmacologist Gerhard Domagk.
1951	**Oral contraceptive** Developed by the American doctors Gregory Pincus and John Rock, and the Austrian-born American chemist Carl Djerassi.
1959	**Librium (chlordiazepoxide)** The first benzodiazepine minor tranquillizer, introduced by the Swiss pharmaceutical company Hoffmann-LaRoche.
1962	**Nethalide (pronethalol)** The first beta-blocking heart drug, developed by scientists at Imperial Chemical Industries, England.
1984	**Genetically engineered human insulin** Developed by scientists at Genentech, California.
1986	**Zidovudine (originally called AZT)** Introduced for treating AIDS after development by scientists at Burroughs Wellcome Research Laboratories, North Carolina.

Medulloblastoma

A type of malignant *brain tumour* which occurs mainly in children (in whom it is the most common type of brain tumour). The tumour usually arises from the *cerebellum* (a region of the brain concerned with posture, balance and coordination). A medulloblastoma grows rapidly and may spread to other parts of the brain and to the spinal cord.

About 100 cases of medulloblastoma are diagnosed each year in the UK. Typically, a morning headache, repeated vomiting, and a clumsy gait develop, with frequent falls caused by disturbance of the function of the cerebellum. The tumour is diagnosed by *CT scanning* or *MRI* and often responds to *radiotherapy*. This, combined with surgery and the use of *anticancer drugs*, often allows survival for five years or more.

Mefenamic acid

A *nonsteroidal anti-inflammatory drug* (NSAID). Mefenamic acid is used to relieve pain after a minor operation or after injury to soft tissues (such as muscles and ligaments), and to treat joint pain and stiffness caused by types of arthritis, such as *osteoarthritis* and *rheumatoid arthritis*. This drug is also used to relieve *dysmenorrhoea* (painful menstrual periods).

Possible adverse effects of mefenamic acid include abdominal pain, nausea, vomiting, and, after prolonged use, a *peptic ulcer*.

Mega-

A prefix meaning very large, as in *megacolon*, a condition in which the colon (part of the large intestine) is greatly enlarged. The prefix megalo- is synonymous with mega-.

Megacolon

A grossly distended (enlarged) colon (part of the large intestine), usually accompanied by severe, chronic constipation. Megacolon may be present at birth or may develop later in life; it occurs in all age groups.

CAUSES

In children, the main causes of megacolon are *Hirschsprung's disease*, *anal fissures*, and psychological factors that may have developed at the time of toilet-training.

In the elderly, megacolon may be caused by long-term use of powerful *laxative drugs*, particularly those containing senna, rhubarb, or cascara.

People suffering from chronic *depression* or *schizophrenia*, particularly if they live in an institution, often suffer from megacolon. Other, rarer causes include *hypothyroidism*, some neurological disorders (for example, spinal cord injury), and certain drugs (notably the narcotic drugs *morphine* and *codeine*).

SYMPTOMS

The symptoms are severe constipation and abdominal bloating; some sufferers lose their appetite, which may result in weight loss. Occasionally there is diarrhoea, caused by a leakage of semi-liquid faeces around the obstructing hard faeces.

DIAGNOSIS

Megacolon is diagnosed by *proctoscopy* (inspection of the rectum with a viewing instrument), *barium X-ray examination*, and tests of bowel muscle function. If Hirschsprung's disease is suspected, *biopsy* (removal of a small sample of tissue for microscopic examination) of the large intestine may also be performed.

TREATMENT

In severe cases, impacted faeces are removed manually. Often, however, the large intestine can be emptied by saline *enemas*.

M

Megalomania

An exaggerated sense of one's own importance or ability. Megalomania may take the form of a *delusion* of grandeur (such as believing oneself to be Napoleon) or of a desire to organize activities that are expensive, large in scale, and involve many people (for example, leasing an ocean liner for a party). Megalomania is not a formal category of psychiatric illness, although such bizarre ideas and behaviour often occur in *mania*.

-megaly

A suffix meaning enlargement, as in *acromegaly*, a condition in which there is enlargement of the skull, jaw, hands, and feet during adulthood as a result of excessive production of growth hormone by the pituitary gland.

Megestrol

A *progestogen drug* used to treat certain types of *breast cancer* and uterine cancer (see *Uterus, cancer of*). Megestrol is usually prescribed when a tumour cannot be removed by surgery, if a tumour has recurred after surgery, or when other *anticancer drugs* or *radiotherapy* is ineffective.

Possible adverse effects include swollen ankles, loss of appetite, dizziness, headache, rash, and elevation of the blood calcium level.

Meibomian cyst

See *Chalazion*.

Meibomitis

An inflammation of the glands on the eyelid, which causes the normal, oily secretion to thicken. Meibomitis usually affects middle-aged people, often those with *blepharitis* (inflammation of the eyelid), and frequently leads to recurrent meibomian cysts (see *Chalazion*).

Meigs' syndrome

A rare condition in which *ascites* (fluid in the abdominal cavity) and a *pleural effusion* (fluid around one of the lungs) accompany a tumour of the *ovary*. The fluid usually disappears with removal of the tumour.

Meiosis

A special type of cell division that occurs only within the ovaries and testes. The cells that undergo meiotic division are the forerunners of egg and sperm cells.

In meiosis, the *chromosomes* (the inherited genetic material) in the

MECHANISM OF MEIOSIS

In meiosis, a cell in the testis or ovary containing 46 chromosomes divides to form four germ cells (sperm or eggs), each with 23 chromosomes. Germ cells have only half the usual chromosome content because a child can receive only half the genes of each parent.

Key

- ▨ Maternal chromosomes
- ▨ Paternal chromosomes

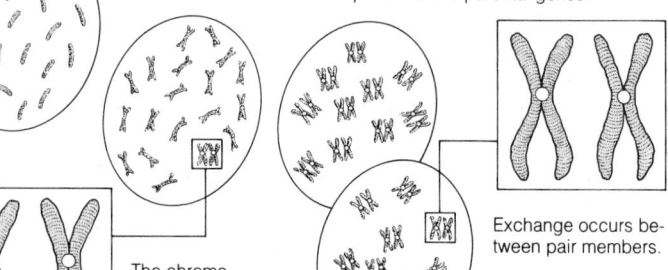

1 The 46 chromosomes in the original cell form 23 pairs (only 10 of the pairs are shown in this sequence). During meiosis, there is exchange of material between pair members, so that each of the germ cells formed receives a unique mix of the parental genes.

Original cell

The chromosomes first double up and then form into pairs.

Exchange occurs between pair members.

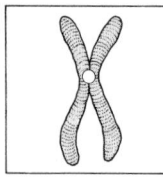

2 After exchange, the cell divides, the two members of each chromosome pair going into separate daughter cells.

First division

Each cell now has one doubled-up chromosome from each of the pairs.

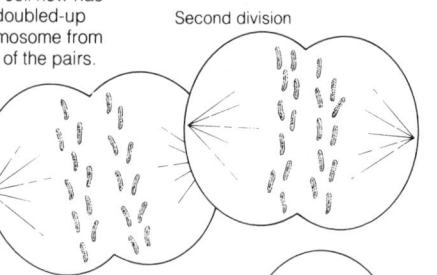

Second division

3 The daughter cells now divide into four germ cells. The doubled-up chromosomes are pulled apart so that each germ cell receives a single (nondoubled-up) chromosome from each of the original pairs.

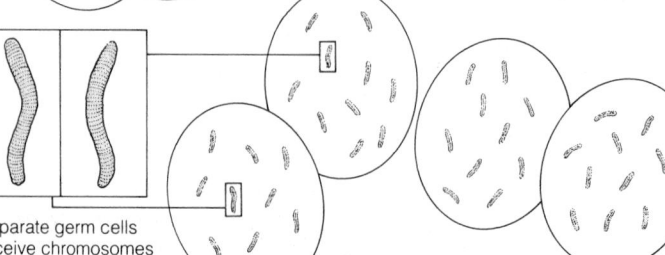

Separate germ cells receive chromosomes containing different genetic mixes.

Germ cells (sperm or eggs)

nucleus of a cell are first duplicated. In the course of two successive cell divisions, the chromosomal material is then divided into four parts, each part going into one of four daughter cells. The four daughter cells each acquire only half of the original cell's chromosomal material, and each daughter cell acquires a different "selection" of this material. Consequently, every egg and sperm formed in the ovary or testis is different in its chromosomal content. As a result of meiosis, parents contribute exactly half of their chromosomal material (genes) to each child, and the selection that each child receives is unique.

Meiosis differs fundamentally from *mitosis*, the more common and simpler method of cell division, in which a cell's chromosomes are exactly duplicated in a single division into two daughter cells.

Melaena

Black, tarry *faeces* caused by bleeding, usually in the upper gastrointestinal tract (oesophagus, stomach, and duodenum). The blood is blackened by the action of secretions during digestion. Melaena is a sign that should never be ignored: it is usually caused by a *peptic ulcer*, but may be an indication of cancer or another disorder of the upper gastrointestinal tract.

Iron, bismuth, or liquorice may also cause blackening of the faeces, which may be mistaken for melaena.

Melancholia

An old term for *depression*, derived from the Greek word for black bile, an excess of which was believed to be the cause of low spirits. The term melancholia is used today to refer to certain symptoms that occur in severe depression. These include loss of pleasure in most activities, lack of reaction to pleasurable stimuli, and inappropriate guilt feelings.

Melanin

The brown or black pigment that gives skin, hair, and the iris of the eyes their colouring. The amount of melanin present in a person depends on race and on exposure to sunlight. The pigment is produced by cells called melanocytes, whose activity is controlled by a hormone secreted by the *pituitary gland* in the brain.

Exposure to sunlight increases the production of melanin, which protects the skin against the harmful effects of ultraviolet rays and causes the skin to darken.

Localized overproduction of melanin in the skin can result in a pigmented spot, most commonly a *freckle* or mole (see *Naevus*).

Melanoma, juvenile

A raised, reddish-brown skin blemish which sometimes appears on the face or legs in early childhood. A juvenile melanoma is a form of *naevus* that grows rapidly up to about 2 cm across. Most juvenile melanomas are harmless. However, if the growth is unsightly, or if the doctor suspects *skin cancer*, the melanoma can be removed surgically.

Melanoma, malignant

The most serious of the three types of skin cancer (the other two being *basal cell carcinoma* and *squamous cell carcinoma*). Malignant melanoma is a tumour of melanocytes, the cells that produce *melanin* (the pigment that colours the skin, hair, and the iris of the eyes).

CAUSES AND INCIDENCE
Malignant melanomas are most common in middle-aged and elderly people with pale skin who have been exposed to strong sunlight for many years. This type of skin cancer is much more common in sunny countries such as Australia and the southern states of the US than in the UK and northern Europe. However, the incidence is rising in the UK and in other countries with similar climates, probably because of the popularity of sunbathing and of holidays in sunny countries. There are now about 2,500 new cases and over 1,000 deaths from this cause in the UK each year.

SYMPTOMS AND SIGNS
The tumour usually develops on exposed skin, but may occur anywhere on the body, including under the nails and in the eye (see *Eye*

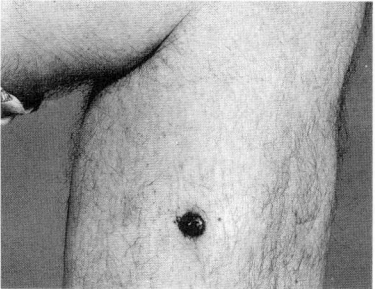

Development of malignant melanoma
Only one mole in a million becomes malignant, but change of shape, darkening, tenderness, pain, itching, or ulceration are warning signs.

tumours). The melanoma usually grows from an existing mole, which may enlarge, become lumpy, bleed, change colour, develop a spreading black edge, turn into a scab, or begin to itch. Occasionally, a malignant melanoma may develop on normal skin.

DIAGNOSIS AND TREATMENT
Because the tumour is highly malignant and often spreads to other parts of the body, early diagnosis is essential. The diagnosis is made by a skin *biopsy* (removal of a small sample of tissue for microscopic analysis).

Treatment consists of surgical removal of the melanoma. To avoid an unsightly scar on exposed areas, a *skin graft* may be carried out at the same time. *Radiotherapy* or *anticancer drugs* may also be necessary.

Melanosis coli

Black or brown discoloration of the lining of the colon, associated with chronic constipation and the prolonged use of certain *laxative drugs*, such as senna, rhubarb, and cascara.

Melanosis coli is most common in the elderly and usually produces no symptoms. The discoloration disappears after the laxatives are stopped. Rarely, the condition is associated with cancer of the colon.

Melasma

See *Chloasma*.

Melatonin

A *hormone* secreted by the *pineal gland* that is thought to play a part in controlling daily body rhythms. Melatonin is currently under investigation for use in preventing *jet-lag*.

Melphalan

An *anticancer drug* used mainly in the treatment of *multiple myeloma* (a cancer of the bone marrow). Melphalan is also prescribed to treat certain types of *breast cancer* and ovarian cancer (see *Ovary, cancer of*).

Possible adverse effects include nausea, vomiting, sore throat, and loss of appetite. Melphalan may also cause aplastic anaemia, abnormal bleeding, and increased susceptibility to infection.

Membrane

A layer of tissue, often very thin, that covers or lines a body surface or forms a barrier. Examples include the *meninges*, which cover the surface of the brain and spinal cord; the *peritoneum*, which lines the abdominal cavity; the tympanic membrane (eardrum),

M

which separates the *ear* canal from the middle ear; and the cell membrane, which forms the boundary of each individual *cell*.

Memory

The ability to remember. Memory is a complex process, usually thought of as having three stages—registration, storage, and recall (see box).

Many factors determine how well something is remembered, including its familiarity and how much attention has been paid to it. Techniques advertised for improving memory are generally based on teaching people methods of improving their coding systems by consciously associating new material with what is already known. For example, a person might be taught to visualize a well-known street and then think of each building as representing a new fact.

MECHANISM OF MEMORY
It is not known where in the *brain* the memory process takes place. There seems to be no set memory area; stimulating the brain with electrodes can evoke different memories from the same site. However, disturbances of the temporal lobe and limbic system

typically cause memory disorders. Stimulation of a particular part of the temporal lobe in patients with *temporal lobe epilepsy* may consistently evoke the same memory.

The mechanisms for storing memory are also unknown. According to one theory, memory may be held in the chemical structure of some substance in brain cells—possibly spare *DNA* that is not being utilized to hold the genetic code. Other theories stress the role of the brain's electrical circuits in memory storage.

A good memory is usually part of a high IQ (see *Intelligence tests*), although some people have extraordinary "photographic" memories that are unrelated to their other intellectual abilities. Even some severely mentally handicapped people have phenomenal memories for specific types of information (the so-called "idiot savant"—learned idiot).

DISORDERS
Disturbances of memory can result from a problem at any of the three stages. Most disturbances are due to failure at the retention or recall stage (see *Amnesia*). In some cases, the problem occurs at the registration stage (e.g. in *mania*, because the person's attention is continually distracted, or in *depression*, because of preoccupation with personal thoughts). Some people with temporal lobe epilepsy have uncontrollable flashbacks of distant past events. The most common disorder of memory is the difficulty in recall that develops with age—so-called benign senile or senescent forgetfulness; this is entirely normal. A more severe loss of memory may be an early symptom of *dementia*.

Memory, loss of
See *Amnesia*.

Menarche
The onset of *menstruation*. Menarche usually occurs around age 13, two or three years after the first physical signs of *puberty* start to appear.

Ménière's disease
A disorder of the inner ear characterized by recurrent *vertigo*, *deafness*, and *tinnitus*. In 80 to 85 per cent of cases, only one ear is affected.

CAUSES AND INCIDENCE
The disease is caused by an increase in the amount of fluid in the membranous labyrinth (the canals in the inner ear that control balance). This increase damages the labyrinth and sometimes the adjacent cochlea (a spiral organ

The cause of Ménière's disease
This condition is caused by excessive fluid in the labyrinth and cochlea, which may become damaged as a result.

that receives sound and transmits it to the brain). The cause of the increase in fluid is not known in most cases. Ménière's disease is uncommon before the age of 50.

SYMPTOMS AND SIGNS
The main symptom is a sudden attack of vertigo, which may be so severe that the person falls to the ground. Vertigo is usually accompanied by nausea, vomiting, nystagmus (abnormal jerky eye movements), and, in the affected ear, deafness, tinnitus, and a feeling of pressure or pain. Attacks, which vary considerably in frequency, may last from a few minutes to several hours; deafness and tinnitus tend to persist between attacks.

DIAGNOSIS AND TREATMENT
Ménière's disease is usually diagnosed from the results of audiometry (see *Hearing tests*), a *caloric test*, and sometimes other tests.

During an attack, the person should rest in bed. An *antiemetic drug* (such as dimenhydrinate or cyclizine) may be given to relieve nausea and tinnitus.

Hearing tends to deteriorate progressively. If deafness becomes total, the other symptoms of the disease usually disappear.

Meninges
The three membranes that cover and protect the *brain* and the *spinal cord*. The outermost layer, the dura mater, is tough and fibrous; it lines the inside of the skull and forms a loose sheath

---

THE STAGES OF MEMORY

Stage 1
In the first stage, known as registration, information is perceived and understood. It is then retained in a short-term memory system that seems to be very limited in the amount of material it can store at one time. Unless refreshed by constant repetition, the contents of short-term memory are lost within minutes, to be replaced by other material.

Stage 2
If information is important enough, it may be transferred into the long-term memory, where the process of storage involves associations with words or meanings, with the visual imagery evoked by it, or with other experiences, such as smell or sound.

Stage 3
The final stage is recall (or retrieval), in which information stored at an unconscious level is brought, at will, into the conscious mind. The reliability of recall depends on how well the material was coded at stage 2.

around the spinal cord. The middle layer, the arachnoid mater, is elastic and web-like; it is separated from the innermost membrane, the pia mater, by the subarachnoid space, which contains *cerebrospinal fluid*. The pia mater is a thin layer that lies directly next to the brain and follows the folds and furrows of its surface.

Inflammation of the meninges, usually from infection, is called *meningitis*. Tumours of the meninges are called *meningiomas*.

Meningioma

A benign *brain tumour* that develops from the meninges (protective coverings of the brain). The tumour arises from cells in the arachnoid (middle layer of the meninges) and usually becomes attached to the dura mater (outer layer).

Meningiomas are rare, with about one new case diagnosed annually per 100,000 population in the UK. They may occur at any age. The tumour expands slowly, sometimes becoming large before it causes symptoms.

SYMPTOMS
These can include headache, vomiting, and impaired mental function from raised pressure within the skull; more specific symptoms include speech loss or visual disturbance due to pressure on the underlying brain tissue. The tumour may invade the overlying bone, causing thickening and bulging of a region of the skull.

DIAGNOSIS AND TREATMENT
Meningiomas can be detected by skull *X-ray*, *CT scanning*, and *MRI*. Because they are usually well demarcated from underlying brain tissue, meningiomas can often be completely removed by surgery. For tumours that cannot be removed surgically, treatment is by *radiotherapy*.

Meningitis

Inflammation of the *meninges* (the membranes that cover the brain and spinal cord) that usually results from infection by any of various microorganisms, usually a virus or a bacterium. Viral meningitis is relatively mild, but bacterial meningitis is life-threatening and requires prompt treatment.

CAUSES
The organisms that cause meningitis usually reach the meninges through the bloodstream from an infection elsewhere in the body. Less common means of transmission are through cavities in the skull from an infected ear or sinuses, or from the air following fracture of the skull.

ANATOMY OF THE MENINGES
The pia mater lies on the brain, separated from the arachnoid mater by the subarachnoid space. The dura mater lines the inside of the skull.

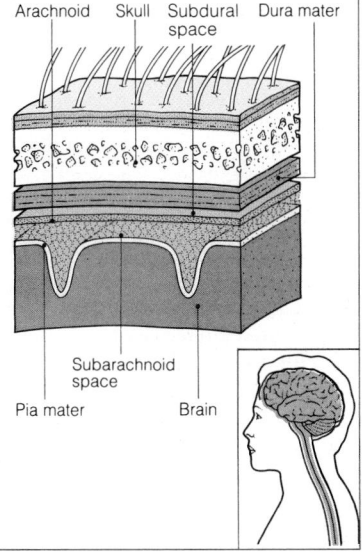

Arachnoid   Skull   Subdural   Dura mater
                    space

Subarachnoid space

Pia mater   Brain

INCIDENCE
Viral meningitis tends to occur in epidemics in the winter months. About 500 cases are notified annually in the UK, but the true incidence is probably much higher than this.

The two most common types of bacterial meningitis are those due to meningococcal infection and *haemophilus influenza*. Both may occur in small epidemics, but more often occur with no apparent explanation. A series of small outbreaks in the west of England in the late 1980s caused widespread concern, but the disease has now become less common again. Vaccination against haemophilus meningitis was introduced into the standard childhood immunization schedule in 1993. Tuberculous meningitis, a less common type of bacterial meningitis, is particularly prevalent among young children in parts of the world where there is a high incidence of *tuberculosis*.

SYMPTOMS
The main symptoms are fever, severe headache, nausea and vomiting, dislike of light, and a stiff neck. In viral meningitis the symptoms are mild and may resemble influenza.

In bacterial meningitis, the main symptoms develop rapidly, sometimes over only a few hours, and are followed by drowsiness and, occasionally, loss of consciousness. In about 50 per cent of cases of meningococcal meningitis there is also a red blotchy skin rash.

In tuberculous meningitis, the sufferer may feel unwell for several weeks before the typical symptoms of meningitis develop.

DIAGNOSIS AND TREATMENT
Meningitis is diagnosed by *lumbar puncture* to remove a small sample of cerebrospinal fluid from the spinal cord for examination.

Viral meningitis requires no treatment. Bacterial meningitis is a medical emergency treated with large doses of intravenous *antibiotic drugs*.

OUTLOOK
Viral meningitis is usually not serious, clears up within a week or two, and leaves no after-effects. Patients with bacterial meningitis who receive prompt treatment usually recover; in a few cases, however, some brain damage occurs.

PREVENTION
Vaccination against the most common type of haemophilus infection has controlled one type of bacterial meningitis, but for most types the most effective protection comes from giving antibiotic drugs to people who have come into contact with sufferers. Vaccination has been unsuccessful in eliminating bacterial meningitis because vaccines exist against only some of the organisms responsible and the protection is of limited duration.

Meningocele

A protrusion of the meninges (protective coverings) of the spinal cord under the skin due to a congenital defect in the spine (see *Spina bifida*). Meningocele is less serious than myelocele, which is protrusion of the spinal cord and of the meninges.

Meningomyelocele

Another name for myelocele (see *Spina bifida*).

Meniscectomy

A surgical procedure in which the whole or part of a *meniscus* (cartilage disc) is removed from a joint, nearly always from the knee.

WHY IT IS DONE
Meniscectomy may be carried out when a meniscus has been damaged (usually due to injury), causing the knee to lock or give way repeatedly. Removing the damaged part of the meniscus cures these symptoms and reduces the likelihood of premature *osteoarthritis* in the joint.

M

M

HOW IT IS DONE

Arthroscopy (in which a viewing instrument is inserted into the joint through a small incision) is performed to confirm that a damaged meniscus is the cause of the symptoms and to locate the area of damage. The damaged portion is removed by means of instruments inserted through the arthroscope. The incision is closed with one stitch and bandaged.

Alternatively, the surgeon may need to open up the knee joint through an incision at the side of the patella (kneecap). After the operation, the wound is stitched and an elastic bandage and a plaster splint are applied over the knee.

RECOVERY PERIOD

After arthroscopic surgery, patients can usually go home later the same day and are able to walk normally within several days.

After an open operation, the patient stays in hospital for a few days. He or she is allowed to put weight on the affected leg after two or three days. The splint is removed after about a week, but normal activities cannot be resumed for four to six weeks.

After either type of meniscectomy, patients should do exercises that strengthen the thigh muscles, which help stabilize the knee.

OUTLOOK

The two types of meniscectomy are about equally effective in relieving symptoms and restoring the knee to normal function, but the scar after an open operation is larger. In either case, there may be an increased risk of osteoarthritis in later life, although the risk is less than if the damaged meniscus had been left in place.

Meniscus

A crescent-shaped disc of cartilaginous tissue found in several joints. The *knee* joint has two menisci; the *wrist* joint and the *temporomandibular joints* of the jaw one each. The main functions of the menisci, which are held in position by ligaments, are to reduce friction during joint movement and to increase joint stability.

Menopause

The cessation of *menstruation;* the term is commonly used to describe the time in a woman's life when physical and psychological changes occur as a result of reduced production of *oestrogen hormones* by the ovaries.

The menopause usually occurs between the ages of 45 and 55. The follicles in the ovaries stop producing ova

(eggs) and less oestrogen is produced. It is this reduced level of oestrogen that causes the problems associated with the menopause. Other hormonal changes include increased amounts of *gonadotrophin hormones* and *androgen hormones* in the blood.

SYMPTOMS AND SIGNS

Hot flushes and night sweats occur in about 70 per cent of all menopausal women. They occur with varying frequency and severity. Women usually have flushes for between two and five years, but sometimes longer. In about 25 per cent of women flushes are so severe that medical help is sought.

Vaginal dryness is the major symptom of 20 per cent of menopausal women. It occurs because the vaginal skin thins and its secretions diminish with the fall in oestrogen levels. The vagina itself shrinks, loses elasticity, and becomes prone to minor infections; sexual intercourse may be more difficult and painful due to dryness (see *Vaginitis*). The neck of the bladder and urethra undergo similar changes, which can result in the "urethral syndrome", in which a need to empty the bladder frequently is felt.

Psychological symptoms—ranging from poor concentration, tearfulness, and loss of interest in sex to a full depressive illness—are often attributed to the menopause; but it is not clear to what extent these are due to the lack of oestrogen or are a reaction to lifestyle changes in middle age.

Changes in *metabolism* (internal body chemistry) also occur during the menopause, but may not cause symptoms until later. The bones become thinner, especially in the first two to five years of the menopause; over a period of 10 to 15 years, *osteoporosis* (a decrease in density and increase in brittleness of the bones) may develop. Other metabolic effects include increased levels of fats in the blood, which may cause an increase in *atherosclerosis* (narrowing of arteries by fatty deposits) and higher incidence of *coronary artery disease* and *stroke.*

TREATMENT

Hormone replacement therapy has proved effective in relieving both the physical and the psychological symptoms of the menopause; it has been shown to prevent the development of osteoporosis and to reduce the risk of heart disease. As the advantages seem to outweigh any drawbacks, many doctors recommend all women to take hormones for a year or two after the menopause. Some recommend longer-term treatment, especially for those with a family history of osteoporosis, and those at risk through having an early menopause or having a slight build.

Menorrhagia

Excessive loss of blood during *menstruation.* The average amount of blood lost during a menstrual period is about 60 ml. A woman with menorrhagia may lose 90 ml or more. Some women often have menorrhagia, but others rarely or never suffer from it.

Menorrhagia may be caused by an imbalance of *oestrogen hormones* and *progesterone hormone,* which control menstruation. This imbalance causes an excessive build-up of endometrium (lining of the uterus).

Any disorder that affects the uterus can cause menorrhagia, including *fibroids, polyps,* the presence of an *IUD,* or a pelvic infection. In some women with menorrhagia no physical cause can be found.

TREATMENT

Treatment depends on the severity of the bleeding, the age of the woman, whether or not she wants children in the future, and on any underlying disorder. Surgical treatment involves a choice of a *D and C* (dilation and curettage), *endometrial resection* (endoscopic removal of the full thickness of the lining of the uterus), or *hysterectomy* (removal of the uterus). Hormones may be prescribed to reduce the amount of bleeding, especially if the

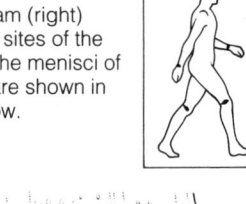

MENISCI
The diagram (right) shows the sites of the menisci. The menisci of the knee are shown in detail below.

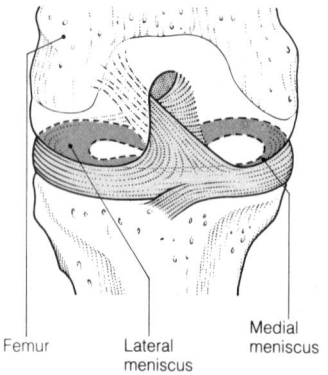

Femur   Lateral meniscus   Medial meniscus

woman is very young. If the condition is severe, a *hysterectomy* (removal of the uterus) may be considered.

A new technique for the treatment of menorrhagia is endometrial ablation, in which an *endoscope* is passed into the uterus and the endometrium is destroyed by *diathermy* or *laser*.

Menotrophin

A *gonadotrophin hormone* given as a drug to stimulate cell activity in the ovaries and testes. Menotrophin is prepared from human menopausal gonadotrophin, which is obtained from urine samples of women who have passed the menopause.

Menotrophin is used together with human chorionic gonadotrophin (see *Gonadotrophin, human chorionic*) in the treatment of certain types of female and male *infertility*. Menotrophin prepares the ovary for ovulation and may help stimulate sperm production.

In women, menotrophin may cause multiple pregnancy, abdominal pain, bloating, and weight gain. In men, it may cause enlargement of the breasts.

Menstrual extraction

A procedure in which the endometrium (the lining of the uterus), which is ordinarily sloughed off during *menstruation*, is removed all at one time. The procedure is also known as menstrual regulation. Menstrual extraction is usually performed to terminate a possible pregnancy.

Menstrual extraction is carried out in the first two weeks after a missed period. It can be performed on an outpatient basis, with or without a local anaesthetic. A plastic tube is inserted into the uterus and the contents, including any embryo if the woman is pregnant, are sucked out.

Menstruation

The periodic shedding of endometrium (lining of the uterus), accompanied by bleeding, that occurs in a woman who is not pregnant. Menstruation identifies the fertile years of a woman's life. Menstrual periods usually begin at puberty (typically between the ages of 11 and 16) and continue until the *menopause* (usually between the ages of 45 and 55).

MECHANISM

Menstruation is the end result of a complicated series of hormonal interactions. At the beginning of the menstrual cycle, *oestrogen hormones* cause the endometrium to thicken to prepare the uterus for the possibility of *fertilization*; this is known as the proliferative or follicular phase.

Ovulation (egg release) usually occurs in the middle of the menstrual cycle and is accompanied by the increased production of *progesterone hormone*. The effect of this hormone is to cause the cells of the endometrium to become swollen and thick with retained fluid. These changes, which occur during the secretory (or luteal) phase of the menstrual cycle, enable a fertilized egg to implant in the endometrium. If pregnancy fails to occur, the production of oestrogens and progesterone from the ovaries diminishes. The fluid-filled endometrium is not required and is shed about 14 days after the start of ovulation. Uterine contractions force the menstrual discharge to be expelled into the vagina.

Blood loss varies from cycle to cycle and from woman to woman, averaging 60 ml. The menstrual cycle, which is counted from the first day of bleeding to the last day before the next menstrual period, lasts between 24 and 35 days in 95 per cent of women, the average being 28 days. The length of bleeding also varies—usually lasting from one to eight days, with the average length being five days.

Menstruation, disorders of

An abnormality in the monthly cycle of menstrual bleeding. Regular *menstruation* depends on the development of a healthy endometrium (lining of the uterus) and the regular cyclical production of *oestrogen hormones* and *progesterone hormone*. This delicate balance is easily upset, making abnormal menstruation one of the most common disorders affecting women. A change in a woman's periods can indicate a problem in the pelvic area, such as *fibroids*, *endometriosis*, or *pelvic inflammatory disease*.

Dysmenorrhoea (painful periods) is the most common disorder. In most women the cause is unknown.

Amenorrhoea (absence of menstruation) is most frequently caused by pregnancy; it may also be caused by a hormonal imbalance, stress, starvation, and *anorexia nervosa*. Polymenorrhoea (too frequent menstruation) occurs when the length of the menstrual cycle is reduced to less than 22 days. It is usually due to a hormone

M

THE MENSTRUAL CYCLE

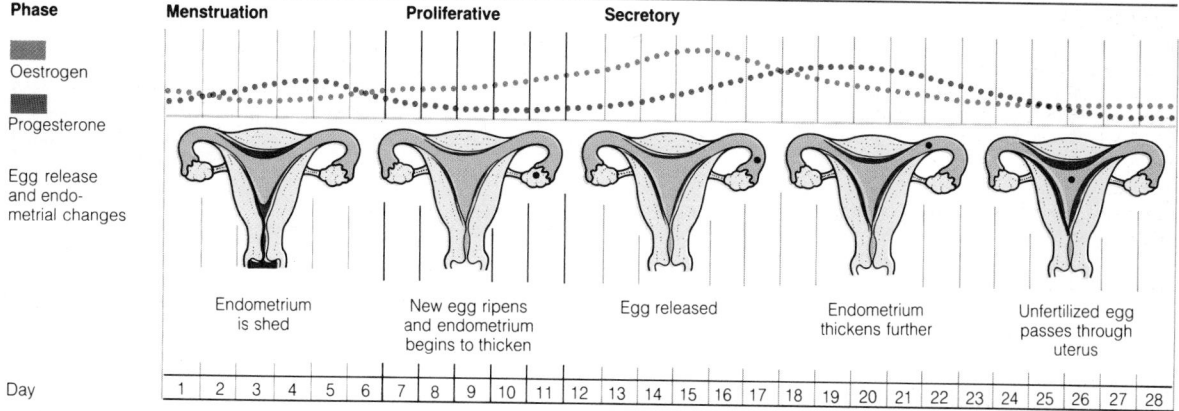

Phase	Menstruation	Proliferative	Secretory

Oestrogen

Progesterone

Egg release and endometrial changes

| Endometrium is shed | New egg ripens and endometrium begins to thicken | Egg released | Endometrium thickens further | Unfertilized egg passes through uterus |

Day | 1 2 3 4 5 6 7 8 9 10 11 12 13 14 15 16 17 18 19 20 21 22 23 24 25 26 27 28

During menstruation, oestrogen and progesterone levels are low, and the unfertilized egg and endometrium are shed. Following menstruation, a pituitary hormone stimulates the ovaries to produce egg follicles. The follicles secrete oestrogen, and one eventually releases an egg. The empty follicle also produces progesterone, which, with oestrogen, prepares the endometrium to receive the egg. If the egg is unfertilized, follicle hormone levels fall and a new menstrual cycle begins.

MENSTRUATION, IRREGULAR

Any variation in the interval between menstrual periods, the duration of bleeding, or the amount of blood lost, or bleeding that occurs in between normal periods, during pregnancy, or after the menopause. An occasional irregular period is generally no cause for concern if it is normal in other respects.

Absent or reduced bleeding

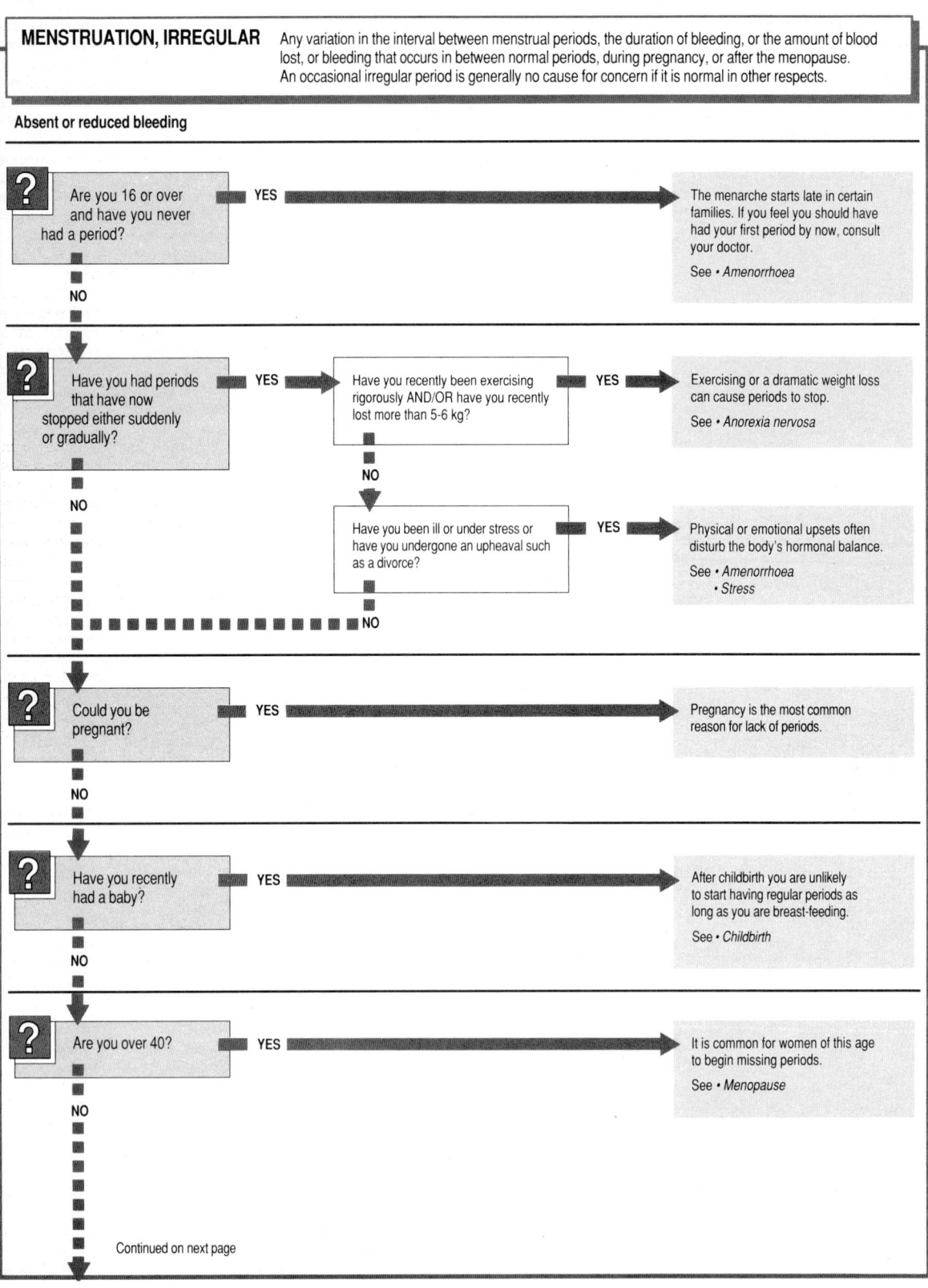

Are you 16 or over and have you never had a period?

YES → The menarche starts late in certain families. If you feel you should have had your first period by now, consult your doctor.

See • *Amenorrhoea*

NO

Have you had periods that have now stopped either suddenly or gradually?

YES → **Have you recently been exercising rigorously AND/OR have you recently lost more than 5-6 kg?**

YES → Exercising or a dramatic weight loss can cause periods to stop.

See • *Anorexia nervosa*

NO

Have you been ill or under stress or have you undergone an upheaval such as a divorce?

YES → Physical or emotional upsets often disturb the body's hormonal balance.

See • *Amenorrhoea*
• *Stress*

NO

NO

Could you be pregnant?

YES → Pregnancy is the most common reason for lack of periods.

NO

Have you recently had a baby?

YES → After childbirth you are unlikely to start having regular periods as long as you are breast-feeding.

See • *Childbirth*

NO

Are you over 40?

YES → It is common for women of this age to begin missing periods.

See • *Menopause*

NO

Continued on next page

M

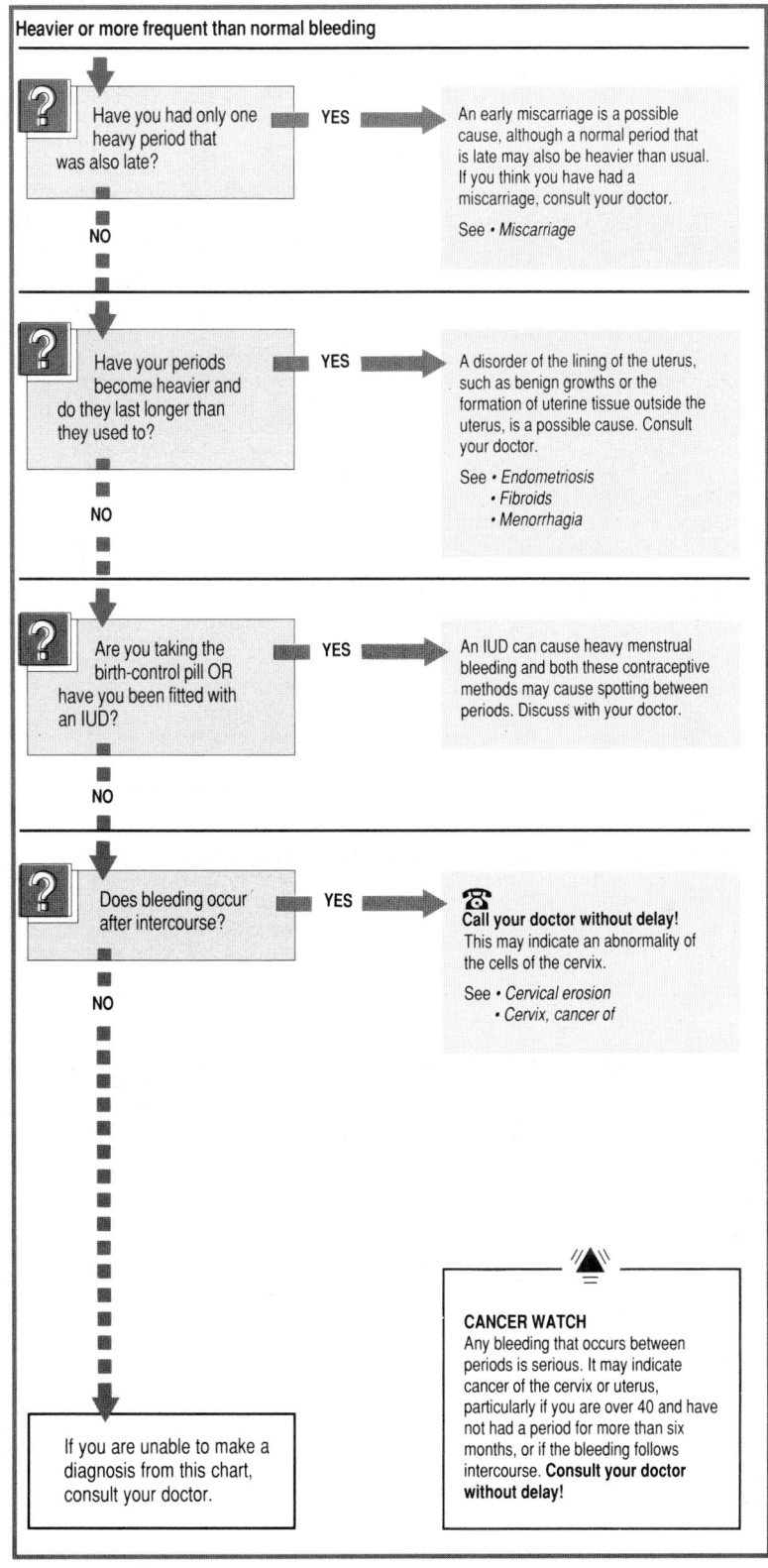

Heavier or more frequent than normal bleeding

Have you had only one heavy period that was also late? — **YES** → An early miscarriage is a possible cause, although a normal period that is late may also be heavier than usual. If you think you have had a miscarriage, consult your doctor.

See • *Miscarriage*

NO

Have your periods become heavier and do they last longer than they used to? — **YES** → A disorder of the lining of the uterus, such as benign growths or the formation of uterine tissue outside the uterus, is a possible cause. Consult your doctor.

See • *Endometriosis*
• *Fibroids*
• *Menorrhagia*

NO

Are you taking the birth-control pill OR have you been fitted with an IUD? — **YES** → An IUD can cause heavy menstrual bleeding and both these contraceptive methods may cause spotting between periods. Discuss with your doctor.

NO

Does bleeding occur after intercourse? — **YES** → ☎ **Call your doctor without delay!** This may indicate an abnormality of the cells of the cervix.

See • *Cervical erosion*
• *Cervix, cancer of*

NO

If you are unable to make a diagnosis from this chart, consult your doctor.

CANCER WATCH
Any bleeding that occurs between periods is serious. It may indicate cancer of the cervix or uterus, particularly if you are over 40 and have not had a period for more than six months, or if the bleeding follows intercourse. **Consult your doctor without delay!**

imbalance. Oligomenorrhoea is the term used if the periods occur infrequently or if the blood loss is scanty.

Menorrhagia (excessive bleeding) may be caused by a hormone imbalance, the presence of an *IUD*, *fibroids*, or *polyps*.

In some women there are extreme variations in the interval between periods, the duration of bleeding, and the amount of blood lost each month (see *Menstruation, irregular*).

Menstruation, irregular
A variation from the normal pattern of *menstruation*. Menstruation is considered to be irregular if there are wide variations in the interval between periods, in the duration of bleeding, or in the amount of blood that is lost.
CAUSES
Disturbance of a woman's menstrual pattern can be caused by stress, travel, or changing the method of contraception. A common cause of irregular menstruation is a disturbance of the balance of *oestrogen hormones* and *progesterone hormone*, which regulate the menstrual cycle. For the first few years after menstruation starts, and for the few years before the *menopause*, the cycles are frequently irregular and ovulation may fail to occur. In some cases, the irregularity is due to unsuspected pregnancy, early miscarriage, or to disorders of the uterus, ovaries, or pelvic cavity. (See also *Vaginal bleeding*.)

Mental handicap
Impaired intellectual function that results in an inability to cope with the normal tasks of life. This term is preferred to the old description of mental retardation.
CLASSIFICATION
To be classified as mentally handicapped, a person usually has an IQ below 70 (see *Intelligence tests*), will have a history of *developmental delay* in childhood, and will have been slow to acquire normal living skills. Within this group (which comprises about two per cent of the population in the UK) there are various degrees of severity of mental handicap, resulting in different levels of disability.
CAUSES
The more severe grades of handicap usually have a specific physical cause; their incidence is the same in all social classes. About a quarter are due to *Down's syndrome*, another quarter to other inherited or congenital conditions (such as *phenylketonuria*), and

M

about one third result from trauma or infection around birth or early childhood. In about 15 per cent of cases the cause is unknown, but the *fragile X syndrome* may account for some.

By contrast, mild mental handicap usually has no specific cause, occurs more commonly in the lower social classes, and seems to run in families. Poverty and malnutrition are probably contributing factors, together with inheritance.

SYMPTOMS
The mildly handicapped usually show no obvious psychological symptoms except slowness in carrying out mental tasks such as arithmetic or problem-solving. Reading is variably impaired.

In more severely handicapped people, speech is limited or absent, and *epilepsy* and other abnormalities of the nervous system are common. Faecal and urinary incontinence and self-injury may also occur.

TREATMENT
There is no specific means of eliminating the intellectual deficit, but special training and behaviour modification can enhance the skills and quality of life of the mentally handicapped. Many mentally handicapped people are cared for in the community rather than in institutions. Family support and counselling can be crucial in preserving a stable home for a handicapped person.

Anticonvulsant drugs may be needed to treat epilepsy, and *antipsychotic drugs* to treat certain types of mental illness.

The incidence of mental handicap should be reduced in future by prevention. Preventive measures include *genetic counselling*, the elimination of infections such as rubella, reducing the intake of alcohol and drugs during pregnancy, and the early identification of fetal abnormalities.

OUTLOOK
There is evidence that mentally handicapped people, even those who are severely impaired, can live rewarding and emotionally stable lives. Handicap is caused not by an absolute limit on achievement, but by delay in acquiring skills; as they grow older, mentally handicapped people often show improvement in personal and social function.

Mental Health Act
The Mental Health Act (1983) details the rights of patients with mental illness and sets out the grounds for detaining mentally ill people against their will. It also outlines forms of legal guardianship and the means

whereby courts can remand to hospital those who have broken the law as a result of mental illness.

Although most people who need psychiatric treatment are voluntarily admitted to hospital, a small proportion (about 10 to 15 per cent) are too disturbed by their symptoms to have insight into their needs. The Act provides a broad definition of "mental disorder" (including "mental illness", "mental impairment", and "psychopathic disorder", but excluding alcohol abuse, drug abuse, and sexual deviancy). When a person is endangering his or her own or other people's health or safety (e.g. threatening harm or suicide, or refusing to eat) because of such a mental disorder, he or she may be compulsorily taken into hospital and given appropriate treatment.

The Act is divided into over 100 sections, defining the rules of such detention. Those most relevant to the process are Sections 2 to 5, which provide the emergency, assessment, and treatment orders. The period of detention permitted under these sections varies in length from 72 hours to six months. In all cases, implementation of a section (sometimes referred to as "sectioning") requires the signature of a doctor and of a relative or an "Approved Social Worker", using a specific Mental Health Act form. Sections lasting for 28 days or up to six months have to be signed by two doctors, one of them a recognized psychiatric specialist. Patients must always be personally interviewed by those signing such sections, and even after admission to hospital they retain the right to appeal to a Mental Health Review Tribunal if they feel they have been unfairly sectioned.

The Mental Health Act commission constantly reviews the welfare of detained patients, many of whom are discharged from sections before formal expiry. The rules concerning hospital orders from courts, and those detained in Special Hospitals for long periods of time, are very detailed. The overall aim of the Act is to ensure the best balance between individual liberty and public or personal safety, while recognizing the "right to treatment" of those unable to judge clearly for themselves.

Mental health legislation has been constantly refined over 200 years in the UK. Regular amendments reflect changes in attitudes to mental illness.

Mental hospital
A hospital specializing in the treatment of psychiatric illness. Formerly

called asylums, many were built in the 19th and early 20th centuries and were of enormous size. They became infamous as institutionalized backwaters filled with chronically ill patients who were commonly neglected and abused. In recent years, many mental hospitals have been closed as part of a trend towards increased care in the community. Still, the debate continues over how much these closures have contributed to the number of homeless people and how best to protect and treat old, long-stay patients (many of whom are homeless) and new, long-stay patients (such as those suffering from *schizophrenia* or advanced *dementia*).

Today, most admissions to mental hospitals are for acute psychiatric illness. People are admitted to remove them from a stressful or harmful home environment, to provide treatment possible only in hospital, or to protect them or others from harm. The majority of these admissions are voluntary, but in some cases detention under the *Mental Health Act* may be necessary.

Mental illness
A general term that describes any form of psychiatric disorder. Mental illness is commonly divided into two broad categories: the more severe *psychoses*, and the less disturbing *neuroses*. Whereas the former are probably caused by complex biochemical brain disease, the latter seem more related to upbringing and personality.

The concept of mental illness is also important, for legal reasons, in determining whether a person can be compulsorily admitted to hospital (see *Mental Health Act*). Mental illness is different from personality disorder or mental handicap but it can also coexist with these other mental disorders.

Mental retardation
See *Mental handicap*.

Menthol
An alcohol prepared from mint oils. Menthol is an ingredient of several over-the-counter inhalation preparations used in the treatment of nasal congestion caused by sinusitis and the common cold.

Meprobamate
An *antianxiety drug* used in the treatment of *anxiety* and *stress*. Meprobamate, which also has a muscle-relaxant effect, is combined with

aspirin to relieve the pain caused by rheumatic disorders (such as *osteoarthritis*) or injury to soft tissues (such as muscles and ligaments).

Because meprobamate has a sedative effect, it may cause drowsiness and dizziness. After long-term use, its sudden discontinuation may cause a severe withdrawal reaction, symptoms of which may include seizures.

Meptazinol

A weak, synthetic narcotic *analgesic drug* used for the short-term relief of moderate to severe pain. Meptazinol is prescribed to relieve pain after surgery, following injury, and during childbirth, and to alleviate the pain caused by kidney stones.

Unlike many other narcotic drugs, meptazinol only rarely causes euphoria and is unlikely to produce dependence. Another advantage over other drugs in this group is that meptazinol is unlikely to cause constipation. Possible adverse effects include nausea, vomiting, and dizziness.

Mercaptopurine

An *anticancer drug* used to treat certain types of *leukaemia* (cancer of white blood cells).

Possible adverse effects of mercaptopurine include nausea, vomiting, mouth ulcers, and appetite loss. Rarely, it may cause liver damage, anaemia, and abnormal bleeding.

Mercury

The only metallic element that is liquid at room temperature. Mercury is used in *thermometers*, *sphygmomanometers* (instruments for measuring blood pressure), and dental *amalgam*. Various compounds of mercury are used in some paints, pesticides, cosmetics, medicines, and in certain industrial processes.

Mercury poisoning

Toxic effects of mercury on the body. Some forms of mercury are absorbed into the body more readily than others and are therefore more dangerous.

If liquid mercury is swallowed, absorption via the intestines is only slight. Swallowing a small amount (e.g. from a broken thermometer) is therefore unlikely to lead to poisoning. However, liquid mercury is highly volatile and gives off a vapour that is readily absorbed into the body via the lungs. Inhalation of mercury vapour—usually as a result of industrial exposure—is the most common cause of poisoning.

Mercury compounds, which are not highly volatile, may cause poisoning by absorption through the skin or intestines.

SYMPTOMS AND SIGNS

Initial symptoms of mercury poisoning depend on the part of the body affected. Mercury compounds that come into contact with the skin may cause severe inflammation. A swallowed mercury compound can cause nausea, vomiting, diarrhoea, and abdominal pain.

After mercury has entered the body, it passes into the bloodstream and later accumulates in various organs, principally the brain and kidneys. Mercury deposits in the brain cause a wide range of symptoms, including tiredness, incoordination, excitability, tremors, numbness in the limbs, and, in severe cases, impairment of vision and very rarely *dementia*. Deposits of mercury in the kidneys may lead to *kidney failure*. Without treatment, severe mercury poisoning may be fatal.

TREATMENT

Mercury poisoning may be treated by giving *chelating agents* (such as penicillamine) to help the body excrete it at a faster rate. In some cases, purification of the blood by haemodialysis (see *Dialysis*) may also be performed, especially if the kidneys have been damaged. Inducing vomiting or pumping out the stomach is helpful only if mercury has been swallowed within the preceding few hours.

Mesalazine

A drug used to treat *ulcerative colitis* in patients who are unable to tolerate *sulphasalazine*. Possible adverse effects include nausea, diarrhoea, abdominal pain, and headache.

Mescaline

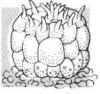 A drug obtained from the Mexican peyote (or peyotl) cactus and classified as a psychedelic or *hallucinogenic drug*. The dried tops of the cactus, known as peyote buttons, have been used for centuries by Mexican and North American Indians in religious ceremonies. In modern times, mescaline has been used to study the mechanism of *psychosis*, because the drug induces temporary psychotic symptoms.

The effects, which generally last for four to eight hours, are similar to those of *LSD* and psilocybin. Effects include illusions, changes in thought and mood, a sense of being in contact with the unknown, intense self-absorption, and an altered sense of time. Although the "trip" is most often pleasant and seemingly insightful, frightening ideas or experiences leading to panic and injury may occur. True psychosis, persisting after the drug has worn off, and addictive craving may occur.

Mesenteric lymphadenitis

An acute abdominal disorder in which *lymph nodes* in the *mesentery* (a membrane that anchors organs to the abdominal wall) become inflamed. Mesenteric lymphadenitis mainly affects children. Its cause is unknown but it may be related to some type of viral infection.

The main symptoms are pain and tenderness in the lower right abdomen, such as occur in appendicitis. There may be mild fever, and sometimes the condition is preceded by a sore throat, chest infection, or swollen lymph nodes in the neck.

The disorder usually clears up rapidly. *Analgesic drugs* (painkillers) may be given to reduce pain and fever. If the sufferer is no better after a few hours or if the symptoms worsen dramatically, a *laparotomy* (surgical opening of the abdominal cavity) may be carried out to rule out the possibility of appendicitis.

Mesentery

A membrane that attaches various organs to the abdominal wall. The term is used particularly to refer to the membranous fold that encloses the small intestine, attaching it to the back of the abdominal wall. The mesentery contains the arteries, veins, nerves, and lymphatic vessels that supply the large and small intestines.

Mesothelioma

A malignant tumour of the *pleura* (the membrane that lines the chest cavity and covers the lungs). There is an increased incidence of mesothelioma in people exposed to asbestos dust (see *Asbestos-induced diseases*).

Mesothelioma may cause no symptoms in some cases, whereas in others it may cause cough, chest pain, and breathing difficulty, especially if a *pleural effusion* (collection of fluid around the lung) develops.

A chest X-ray may show abnormal shadowing; the diagnosis can be confirmed by examination of a sample of fluid from any effusion or by pleural *biopsy* (removal of a sample of tissue for microscopic examination).

M

Surgical removal of a small tumour may result in a complete cure, but the tumour is usually diagnosed only after it has spread over a large area of the pleura. In such cases, there is no effective treatment, although *radiotherapy* may alleviate symptoms.

Mesothelium

A type of *epithelium* (surface cell layer) covering the *peritoneum* (the membrane lining the abdominal wall and covering the abdominal organs), the *pleura* (the membrane lining the chest cavity and covering the lungs), and the *pericardium* (the heart's sac-like covering).

Mestranol

An *oestrogen drug* used in some *oral contraceptives*.

Metabolic disorders

A group of disorders in which some aspect of the body's internal chemistry is disturbed.

Some metabolic disorders result from inherited abnormalities in which a specific *enzyme* (a substance that promotes a metabolic reaction) is absent or deficient or malfunctions in some way (see *Metabolism, inborn errors of*).

Other metabolic disorders result from *endocrine system* disorders in which there is under- or overproduction of a hormone that controls metabolic activity. Examples include *diabetes mellitus*, *Cushing's syndrome*, *insulinoma*, *hypothyroidism* (underactivity of the thyroid gland), and hyperthyroidism (overactivity of the thyroid gland).

Other examples of metabolic disorders are *porphyria*, *hyperlipidaemia*, *hypercalcaemia*, *gout*, and metabolic bone diseases (see *Osteodystrophy*), such as *osteoporosis*, *osteomalacia*, *rickets*, and *Paget's disease*.

Metabolism

A collective term for all the chemical processes that take place in the body. Metabolism is divided into catabolism and anabolism. In a catabolic process, a complex substance is broken down into simpler ones, usually with the release of energy. An example is the "burning" of glucose in body cells to produce energy and the by-products carbon dioxide and water. In an anabolic process, a complex substance is built up from simpler ones, usually with the consumption of energy. The synthesis of complex *proteins* from *amino acids* is an anabolic process.

METABOLIC RATE

The basal metabolic rate (BMR) is the energy required to keep the body functioning at rest (that is, to maintain breathing, heartbeat, body temperature, and other basic body functions). It is measured in joules per square metre of body surface per hour. The metabolic rate increases in response to factors such as exertion, stress, fear, and illness. It is controlled principally by various hormones (such as *adrenaline*, *noradrenaline*, *insulin*, *corticosteroid hormones*, and *thyroid hormones*), which influence the rate at which chemical processes are carried out in body cells. (See also *Metabolic disorders*; *Metabolism, inborn errors of*.)

Metabolism, inborn errors of

Inherited defects of body chemistry. Inborn errors of metabolism are *genetic disorders* in which the disturbance of body chemistry is caused by a single gene defect.

TYPES AND INCIDENCE

There are more than 200 known inborn errors of metabolism, which vary in severity from harmless abnormalities to serious disorders that may cause death in a newborn baby or result in severe physical or mental handicap. Examples include *Tay-Sachs disease*, *phenylketonuria*, *galactosaemia*, the *porphyrias*, *Hurler's syndrome* and various other types of *mucopolysaccharidosis*, Lesch-Nyhan syndrome, homocystinuria, hereditary fructose intolerance, glycogen storage diseases, mucolipidoses, and sphingolipidoses.

Individual disorders are rare. Most affect only one child in every 10,000 to 100,000, but the precise incidence is often unknown because sufferers may have only vague symptoms that are never investigated, or because they die before any characteristic features appear. Collectively, inborn errors of metabolism affect approximately one child in 1,000.

CAUSES

All inborn errors of metabolism are caused by abnormal functioning of a specific *enzyme* (protein that stimulates a chemical reaction) caused by a defect of a single *gene*. Most defects show an autosomal recessive pattern of inheritance (see *Genetic disorders*).

Individual disorders vary in their effects. In some cases the abnormal enzyme is nonfunctional; in others there is some residual activity.

SYMPTOMS AND SIGNS

Symptoms are usually present at or soon after birth, although in some cases they may not appear until later in childhood. Symptoms may include unexplained illness or failure to thrive in a newborn, developmental delay, floppiness, drowsiness, persistent vomiting, or seizures. Signs may include enlarged body organs, bone deformities, anaemia, cataracts, persistent jaundice, unusual body odour, the recurrent development of kidney stones, or a rash brought on by sunlight. An affected child may be intolerant to specific foods.

Miscarriages, stillbirths, or deaths in early infancy suggest the possibility of an error of metabolism.

DIAGNOSIS

Investigations include tests to measure the levels of various substances in the affected child's blood, including *liver-function tests* and *kidney-function tests*. Chemical analysis of a *biopsy* specimen (a small piece of tissue removed from the body) may be performed to check the level and function of a specific enzyme.

Early diagnosis can be important in preventing serious complications. Routine tests are performed on the newborn for some of the more common disorders, such as phenylketonuria. Additional screening may be performed for disorders that are more common in certain countries or racial groups (e.g. Tay-Sachs disease in Ashkenazi Jews).

Certain disorders can now be diagnosed antenatally following *chorionic villus sampling* or *amniocentesis*, allowing for an elective abortion.

TREATMENT

Some inborn errors of metabolism do not require treatment. Some respond to avoidance of a specific environmental factor to which an affected person is abnormally sensitive. For example, avoiding exposure to sunlight may help certain types of porphyria, avoiding food containing phenylalanine is vital in phenylketonuria.

In some cases, the missing enzyme or the protein that it produces can be manufactured using *genetic engineering* techniques. Treatment can then be given to restore the metabolism to normal. Sometimes a vitamin supplement can help compensate for defective enzyme function. If the enzyme concerned is normally made in blood cells then a *bone marrow transplant* may provide a permanent cure. Research is being undertaken into treating inborn errors of metabolism at the gene level, but such treatment is at a very early stage at present.

People with an affected close relative or child may benefit from *genetic counselling* before starting a family or planning another pregnancy.

Metabolite

Any substance that takes part in a metabolic reaction (a biochemical reaction in the body). In the breakdown of glucose to produce energy, the metabolites are glucose, oxygen, carbon dioxide, and water. The term metabolite is sometimes used to refer only to the products of a metabolic reaction. (See also *Metabolism*.)

Metacarpal bone

One of five long, cylindrical bones within the body of the hand. The bones run from the base of each digit to the wrist. On the palm of the hand, the metacarpals are covered by a thick layer of fascia (fibrous connective tissue); on the back of the hand, the metacarpals can be seen and felt through the skin. The heads of the metacarpal bones form the knuckles, standing out prominently when the hand is clenched. Fracture of the metacarpal bones is fairly common, usually as the result of a fall on the hand or a blow to the knuckles.

Metaplasia

A change in tissue resulting from the transformation of one type of cell into another. Usually harmless, but occasionally precancerous, metaplasia can affect the lining of various organs, such as the bronchi (airways) and bladder. Metaplasia of the cervix, which occurs in *cervical erosion*, can be detected by a *cervical smear test*.

Metastasis

A secondary malignant tumour (one that has spread from a primary *cancer* to affect other parts of the body); for example, a metastasis in the liver may arise as a result of the spread of a cancer originating in the colon. The term metastasis also applies to the process by which such spread occurs. The degree of malignancy of a tumour depends largely on its ability to invade surrounding normal tissue and on its ability to send metastases to other parts of the body.

Metastases can spread from one part of the body to another through the lymphatic system, in the bloodstream, or across a body cavity (such as that between the inner and outer layer of the peritoneal membrane in the abdomen).

Metatarsal bone

One of five long, cylindrical bones within the foot. The bones make up the central skeleton of the foot and are held in an arch by surrounding liga-

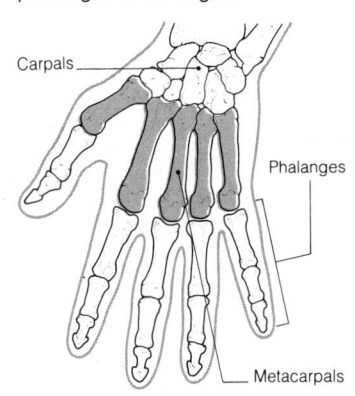

LOCATION OF METACARPAL BONES
The five metacarpals lie between the carpal (wrist) bones and the phalanges of the fingers.

Carpals

Phalanges

Metacarpals

ments. Fracture of the metatarsal bones may be caused by a heavy object falling on the foot, by a twisting injury in which the foot turns over on its outside edge, or by prolonged walking or running on a hard surface (see *March fracture*).

Metatarsalgia

Pain in the foot. Causes include a fracture of one of the *metatarsal bones*, *flatfeet*, or a *neuroma* (benign tumour) of one of the nerves in the foot.

Metatarsophalangeal joint

The joint between each *metatarsal bone* and its adjoining toe bone (see *Phalanges*). The metatarsophalangeal joint at the base of the big toe is commonly affected by *gout* and by *hallux rigidus* (immobility due to *osteoarthritis*). *Hallux valgus* is a deformity of the big toe that may result in a *bunion*.

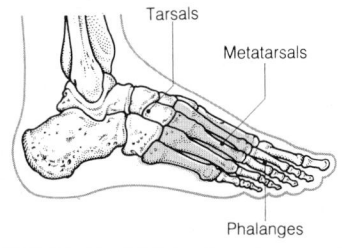

LOCATION OF METATARSAL BONES
The five metatarsals lie between the tarsal bones (which form the ankle and back of the foot) and the phalanges of the toes.

Tarsals

Metatarsals

Phalanges

Metformin

An oral hypoglycaemic drug used in the treatment of non-insulin-dependent *diabetes mellitus*. Metformin lowers the blood sugar level by reducing the production of glucose by cells in the liver and by increasing the sensitivity of cells to *insulin* so that they take up glucose more efficiently from the blood.

Metformin is usually prescribed in addition to another hypoglycaemic drug when that preparation alone has failed to control the diabetes. Possible adverse effects include loss of appetite, a metallic taste in the mouth, nausea, vomiting, and diarrhoea.

Methadone

A synthetic narcotic *analgesic drug* (painkiller) that resembles *morphine*. Methadone causes only mild symptoms when it is withdrawn and is therefore used to relieve withdrawal symptoms in people undergoing a supervised heroin or morphine detoxification programme.

Possible adverse effects include nausea, vomiting, constipation, dizziness, and dryness of the mouth.

Methane

A colourless, odourless, highly flammable gas that occurs naturally in the gas from oil wells and in coal mines, where it is an explosion hazard. "Natural" or "North Sea" gas is composed almost entirely of methane. Methane is also produced by the decomposition of organic matter; it is one of the gases present in intestinal gas (see *Flatus*). By itself methane is not poisonous, in contrast to "coal gas" (which contains carbon monoxide). Cases of gas poisoning are, therefore, much less common than previously. Large quantities of methane may cause death simply by displacing oxygen in the air breathed.

Methanol

A poisonous type of *alcohol* used as a solvent or paint remover, and as an ingredient in some types of antifreeze. Also known as wood alcohol or methyl alcohol, methanol may cause blindness or death if drunk.

POISONING

Methanol is toxic; poisoning usually occurs as a result of drinking it as a substitute for ordinary alcohol (ethanol or ethyl alcohol), although its inebriating effect is weaker.

Symptoms of poisoning, which develop 12 to 24 hours after drinking the methanol, include headache, diz-

M

ziness, nausea, vomiting, and unconsciousness. The symptoms are caused by the breakdown in the liver of methanol into formaldehyde and formic acid. These substances may also damage the retina and the optic nerve, causing blurred vision. If methanol is drunk repeatedly, or if a single large dose is taken, permanent blindness may result.

TREATMENT

If somebody has drunk methanol and is conscious, vomiting should be induced and medical help obtained. Treatment may include pumping out the stomach (see *Lavage, gastric*) and inducing vomiting, although these methods are effective only within about two hours of having drunk the methanol (before it has been absorbed into the bloodstream). In addition, ethanol may be given by injection into the bloodstream because it slows the rate at which the liver breaks down the methanol. An *intravenous infusion* of sodium bicarbonate may be used to neutralize acid products in the blood. Occasionally, purification of the blood by *dialysis* is also necessary.

Methocarbamol

A *muscle-relaxant drug* used to relieve stiffness caused by muscle injury and back pain. Methocarbamol is sometimes given to treat the symptoms of *tetanus* (lockjaw). During prolonged treatment, methocarbamol may cause drowsiness, dizziness, and, in rare cases, liver damage.

Methotrexate

An *anticancer drug* used in the treatment of *lymphoma* (cancer of the lymph nodes) and certain forms of *leukaemia*. Methotrexate is also used to treat some cancers of the uterus, breast, ovary, lung, bladder, and testis. It is sometimes used to treat severe *psoriasis* when other treatments have proved ineffective.

Methotrexate may cause nausea, vomiting, diarrhoea, and mouth ulcers. It may also cause anaemia, increased susceptibility to infection, and abnormal bleeding.

Methyclothiazide

A thiazide *diuretic drug*.

Methyl alcohol

Another name for *methanol*.

Methylcellulose

A bulk-forming *laxative drug* commonly used to treat *constipation*, *diverticular disease*, and *irritable bowel*

syndrome. Methylcellulose is also used to increase the firmness of faeces in chronic watery *diarrhoea* and to regulate their consistency in people who have had a *colostomy* or *ileostomy*.

Methylcellulose preparations are also sometimes used together with appropriate dieting to treat *obesity*. The bulking agent swells to give a feeling of fullness, thus encouraging adherence to a slimming diet.

In eye-drop form, methylcellulose is given to relieve dryness of the eyes caused by exposure to the sun, wind, and other irritants.

POSSIBLE ADVERSE EFFECTS

Methylcellulose may cause bloating, flatulence, and abdominal pain, or even bowel obstruction if sufficient amounts of fluids are not taken.

Methyldopa

An *antihypertensive drug* used in the treatment of *hypertension* (high blood pressure), usually in conjunction with other drugs from this group. Methyldopa is one of the few antihypertensive drugs that is known to be safe to take during pregnancy.

Possible adverse effects of methyldopa include drowsiness, depression, and nasal congestion.

Methylprednisolone

A *corticosteroid drug* used in the treatment of severe *asthma*, skin inflammation, *inflammatory bowel disease*, and types of arthritis, including *rheumatoid arthritis*. Possible adverse effects are typical of drugs belonging to the corticosteroid drug group.

Methysergide

A drug used to prevent *migraine* and cluster *headaches* (recurrent severe headaches). Methysergide is usually given only under hospital supervision when other treatments have been ineffective, and the headaches are seriously disrupting normal life.

Long-term treatment with methysergide may cause abnormal tissue growth in the lungs, around the ureters, or around blood vessels (resulting in chest pain, kidney failure, or leg cramps). Other possible adverse effects include dizziness, drowsiness, nausea, and diarrhoea.

Metoclopramide

An *antiemetic drug* used to prevent and treat nausea and vomiting. Metoclopramide is helpful for the relief of the nausea that sometimes accompanies *migraine* headaches. It is also prescribed to relieve *acid reflux* and to

treat nausea and vomiting caused by *anticancer drugs*, *radiotherapy*, or anaesthetic drugs (see *Anaesthesia, general*).

Metoclopramide is often given with a *premedication* (drug used to relax and sedate a person before an operation) to encourage normal propulsion of food through the stomach, thereby reducing the risk of inhaling vomit when under an anaesthetic.

HOW IT WORKS

Metoclopramide reduces nerve activity in the part of the brain that stimulates vomiting. It also increases the speed with which fluid and food pass from the stomach.

POSSIBLE ADVERSE EFFECTS

Adverse effects of metoclopramide can include dryness of the mouth, sedation, or diarrhoea. Large doses of this drug may cause uncontrollable movements of the face, mouth, and tongue.

Metolazone

A *diuretic drug* used to treat *hypertension* (high blood pressure). Metolazone is also given to reduce *oedema* (fluid retention) in people with *heart failure* (reduced pumping efficiency), kidney disorders, *cirrhosis* of the liver, or *premenstrual syndrome*.

Metolazone is also a useful treatment for certain types of kidney stones (see *Calculus, urinary tract*) because it reduces the amount of calcium excreted in the urine.

Possible adverse effects include weakness, lethargy, and dizziness caused by an increase in the amount of potassium excreted in the urine.

Metoprolol

A cardioselective *beta-blocker drug* used in the treatment of *angina pectoris* (chest pain due to impaired blood supply to heart muscle) and *hypertension* (high blood pressure). Metoprolol is also prescribed to relieve symptoms of *hyperthyroidism* (overactivity of the thyroid gland). It is occasionally given following a *myocardial infarction* (heart attack) to reduce the risk of further damage to the heart.

Possible adverse effects of metoprolol include lethargy, cold hands and feet, nightmares, and rash.

Metronidazole p. 684

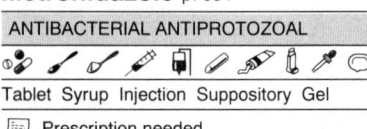

ANTIBACTERIAL ANTIPROTOZOAL				
Tablet	Syrup	Injection	Suppository	Gel

Prescription needed

Available as generic

An *antibiotic drug* that is particularly effective against infections caused by *anaerobic* bacteria (those that do not depend on oxygen), such as a dental *abscess* and *peritonitis*. Metronidazole is also used to treat infections caused by *protozoa*, such as *trichomoniasis*, *amoebiasis*, and *giardiasis*.

Adverse effects include nausea and vomiting, loss of appetite, abdominal pain, and dark-coloured urine. Drinking alcohol during treatment with metronidazole often causes severe unpleasant effects, such as nausea and vomiting, abdominal pain, hot flushes, palpitations, and headache.

Mexiletine

An *antiarrhythmic drug* that is used to treat certain heart-rhythm disorders, usually after a *myocardial infarction* (heart attack). Possible adverse effects include nausea, vomiting, dizziness, and tremor.

Mianserin

An *antidepressant drug* used to treat severe *depression*. This drug also has a sedative effect and is therefore useful in the treatment of depression accompanied by *anxiety* or *insomnia*.

Mianserin usually takes several weeks to become fully effective. Possible adverse effects include a dry mouth, blurred vision, constipation, dizziness, and drowsiness. Prolonged use may, in rare cases, reduce blood cell production in the bone marrow; regular *blood counts* are therefore carried out during treatment.

Miconazole

ANTIFUNGAL			
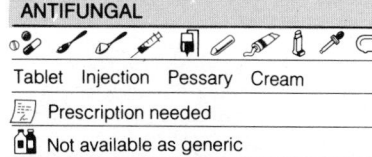
Tablet	Injection	Pessary	Cream
📋 Prescription needed			
💊 Not available as generic			

An *antifungal drug* used to treat *tinea* skin infections, such as ringworm and *athlete's foot*, vaginal *candidiasis* (thrush), and rare fungal infections that affect internal organs.

Miconazole in the form of a cream or vaginal suppository may, in rare cases, cause a burning sensation or a rash. Injections of miconazole may cause nausea, vomiting, and fever.

Micro-

A prefix meaning small, as in microorganisms (minute living organisms, most of which are too small to be seen by the naked eye).

Microangiopathy

Any disease or disorder of the small blood vessels. Microangiopathy may be a feature of various conditions, including *diabetes mellitus*; some kidney diseases, such as *glomerulonephritis* (inflammation of the kidneys' filtering units) or *haemolytic-uraemic syndrome* (premature destruction of red blood cells accompanied by kidney damage); *eclampsia* (a disorder characterized by seizures in late pregnancy); *septicaemia* (blood poisoning); and advanced *cancer*. When microangiopathy accompanies these conditions, the small blood vessels become distorted, resulting in red blood cells becoming damaged or destroyed. This, in turn, leads to a particular type of anaemia that is called microangiopathic haemolytic anaemia (see *Anaemia, haemolytic*).

Another cause of microangiopathy is thrombotic thrombocytopenic *purpura*, a rare, often fatal disease that mainly affects young adults. In this condition, the small blood vessels in many organs throughout the body become blocked and the vessel walls are damaged; haemolytic anaemia, fever, and a patchy, purplish rash known as purpura develop.

Microbe

A popular term for a *microorganism*, especially one that causes disease.

Microbiology

The study of *microorganisms*, particularly those that are pathogenic (disease-causing).

Microbiology began in the 17th century with the discovery by the Dutch microscopist Antonj van Leeuwenhoek (1632-1723) of a wide variety of organisms too small to be seen by the naked eye. However, relatively little progress was made until the 19th century when, largely due to the pioneering work of scientists such as Louis Pasteur (1822-1895) and Robert Koch (1843-1910), it was recognized that microorganisms cause many infectious diseases and are also responsible for processes such as fermentation and decay.

Microbiology continued to progress with the discovery of viruses, the development of *vaccines* and *antibiotic drugs* against many diseases, and studies of the chemical processes that are fundamental to all living cells. Recently, microbiologists have played an important role in the study of genetics by pioneering techniques of *genetic engineering*. In hospitals, microbiologists help identify the infectious organisms responsible for a patient's illness, and also give advice on the sensitivity of these organisms to different drugs.

Microcephaly

An abnormally small head, usually associated with *mental handicap*. Microcephaly may occur if the brain is damaged before birth by, for example, congenital *rubella* (German measles) or if the mother is exposed to X-rays in early pregnancy. Microcephaly may also result from brain damage during birth, or from injury or disease in early infancy.

Microorganism

A tiny, single-celled living organism. Most microorganisms are too small to be seen by the naked eye. In medicine, the most important microorganisms are those that are pathogenic (disease-causing), even though this group constitutes a relatively small minority of the vast number of microorganisms known to exist.

The principal pathogenic microorganisms are *bacteria*, which cause a large number of disorders, including certain types of pneumonia, typhoid, diphtheria, and some types of food poisoning; *viruses* (usually classified as microorganisms although they are not true cells), which cause numerous infections, including AIDS, the common cold, influenza, and measles; *protozoa*, which are the causative agents of various diseases, including malaria, giardiasis, and amoebic dysentery; *fungi*, which cause disorders such as ringworm and thrush; *rickettsiae*, which cause typhus, Rocky Mountain spotted fever, and Q fever; and chlamydiae, which cause various genital, eye, and respiratory infections (see *Chlamydial infections*).

Microscope

An instrument for producing a magnified image of a small object. There are many types of microscopes, ranging from simple, single-lens instruments (magnifying glasses) to compound microscopes and high-powered electron microscopes.

HISTORY

The single-lens microscope may date from as early as the 15th century, but the first truly powerful lenses were probably made by Antonj van Leeuwenhoek (1632-1723). His single-lens microscopes were capable of magnifying up to about 300 times. With

M

them, he discovered microorganisms, thereby founding the science of *microbiology* and providing the basis for the development of the germ theory of disease. Probably the greatest of the early microscopists, however, was the Italian Marcello Malpighi (1628-1694), who is generally regarded as the founder of *histology*.

The compound microscope, which has two lens systems, was developed towards the end of the 16th century. However, the single-lens microscope continued to be widely used until the 19th century, when improvements in optical design and glass technology made the compound microscope a practicable instrument.

Light microscopes continued to be refined, with the development of the phase-contrast microscope, for example. However, the next major advances were instruments that used electrons instead of light—the transmission electron microscope (TEM), invented in the early 1930s, and the scanning electron microscope (SEM), invented in the mid-1960s.

LIGHT MICROSCOPES
Compound microscopes are the most widely used microscopes. They have two lens systems—the objective and the eyepiece—which are mounted at

---

TYPES OF MICROSCOPES

Microscopes are indispensable in medicine. For many purposes, the light microscope, with a magnification of up to 1,500 times, is sufficient. Modern research increasingly requires the much higher magnifications (up to about five million times) of a transmission electron microscope or a scanning electron microscope.

LIGHT MICROSCOPE

Eyepiece
Objective
Specimen
Optical condenser
Focusing knob
Stage
Illuminator

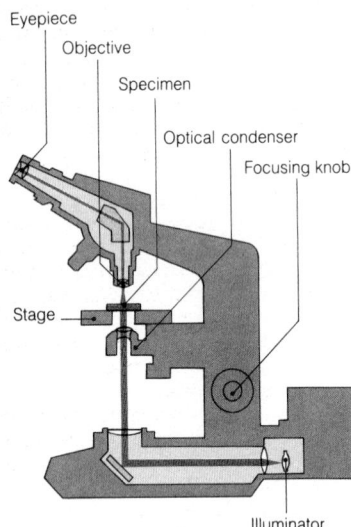

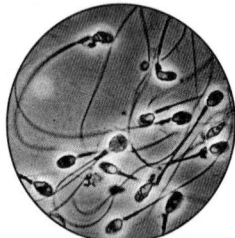

Shown here is a collection of sperm cells.

The compound light microscope
One lens (the objective) forms a magnified image of the specimen; this image is then magnified further by the eyepiece (viewing) lens. The specimen is held on a stage, beneath which is an optical condenser that concentrates light (usually from a built-in illuminator) on to the specimen. Focusing is carried out by altering the distance between the objective and the specimen.

TRANSMISSION ELECTRON MICROSCOPE

Electron gun
Electron beam
Condenser
Specimen
Objective "lens"
Projector "lens"
Viewing binoculars
Fluorescent screen

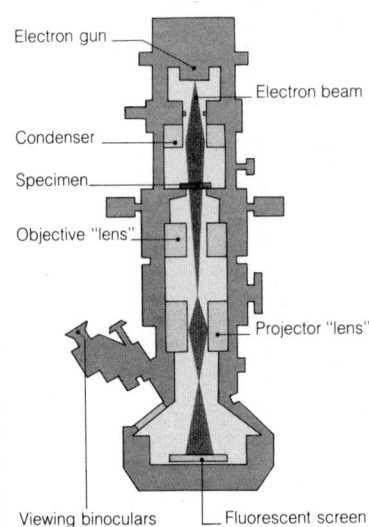

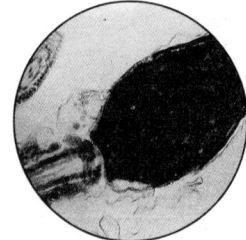

Shown here is the internal structure of a sperm cell.

The transmission electron microscope
An electron beam (generated by a "gun") is concentrated by an electromagnetic condenser, then passes through the specimen. An electromagnetic objective "lens" then produces a magnified "image" of the specimen; this image is further magnified by an electromagnetic projector "lens", which also focuses the image on to a fluorescent screen, where it can be viewed through special binoculars.

SCANNING ELECTRON MICROSCOPE

Electron gun
Electron beam
Condenser
Scanning electromagnets
Fluorescent screen
Detector
Amplifier
Secondary electrons
Specimen

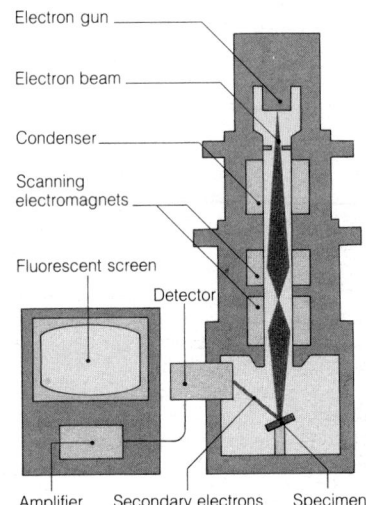

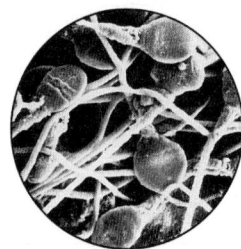

Shown here is the surface structure of sperm cells.

The scanning electron microscope
An electron beam (generated by a "gun") is scanned over the surface of the specimen, causing the emission of a beam of secondary electrons, the intensity of which varies according to the surface features of the specimen. A detector converts the secondary electrons into an electric current, which is then amplified and used to control an electron beam that forms an image on a fluorescent screen.

opposite ends of a tube called the body tube (see illustrated box). There is also a stage to hold the specimen, a light source, and an optical condenser. The maximum practicable magnification of an ordinary light microscope is limited by the wavelength of light to about 1,500 times.

ELECTRON MICROSCOPES
TEMs are similar to light microscopes, except that they use a beam of electrons instead of light, and electromagnetic "lenses" instead of glass ones. Furthermore, because electrons are invisible, the image must be formed on a fluorescent screen or photographic film. Electron microscopes allow much higher magnifications than light microscopes. Modern TEMs can magnify up to about five million times, enabling tiny viruses and large molecules (such as DNA) to be seen.

The SEM works in a different way from the TEM. SEMs have a lower maximum magnification (approximately 100,000 times) than do TEMs. However, unlike TEMs, SEMs produce three-dimensional images. This makes SEMs particularly valuable for studying the surface structures of cells and tissues.

OTHER MICROSCOPES
Phase-contrast and interference microscopes are types of light microscopes with modified illumination and optical systems that make it possible for unstained transparent specimens to be clearly seen. These microscopes are particularly useful for examining living cells and tissues.

Another instrument, the fluorescence microscope, is used to study the chemical composition of cells. In fluorescence microscopy, a specimen that has been selectively stained with fluorescent dyes is illuminated with ultraviolet light, which makes the stained parts glow.

Operating microscopes are low-powered compound microscopes with several modifications. They do not have a stage, and the illumination system is arranged to shine light down on to the living tissues rather than up through the specimen.

USES
The microscope is probably the single most important instrument in biological and medical science. Its applications are vast, ranging from the study of molecular structures to *microsurgery*. Microscopes have enabled scientists to examine both the structure and chemical composition of cells (a study known as *cytology*) and of tissues (histology). Microscopes are also used to investigate diseased tissues (a study known as *histopathology*), thereby playing an important role in diagnosis. And in the operating theatre, microscopes have enabled the development of microsurgery.

Microsurgery
Delicate surgery in which the surgeon views the operation site through a special binocular *microscope* with pedal-operated magnification, focusing, and movements.

Microsurgery technique is used for surgery involving minute, delicate, or not easily accessible tissues. It has strikingly improved the success rate of some operations and made others possible that were previously impracticable. These operations include removing a diseased cataract from the eye and implanting a new lens (see *Cataract surgery*); transplanting a new cornea into the eye (see *Corneal graft*); replacing a diseased stapes (stirrup bone) in the middle ear to treat deafness caused by otosclerosis (see *Stapedectomy*); restoring a severed limb by rejoining disconnected blood vessels and nerves; transplanting toes to replace missing or severed fingers; and unblocking and rejoining obstructed fallopian tubes in the treatment of female *infertility*. (See also illustrated box overleaf.)

Micturition
A term for passing *urine*.

Midbrain
The top part of the *brainstem*, situated above the pons. The midbrain is also called the mesencephalon.

Middle ear
See *Ear*.

Middle-ear effusion, persistent
See *Glue ear*.

Middle-ear infection
See *Otitis media*.

Mid-life crisis
A popular phrase that describes the feelings of distress that affect some people in early middle age (35 to 45 years) after realizing that they are no longer young. The term is used most often to describe men who strive to recapture their sense of youthfulness by having extramarital affairs, suddenly changing jobs, or adopting youthful fashions. Sometimes anxiety or depression, brought on by fears of declining powers and death, can lead to psychiatric illness. Counselling and support are usually effective in helping people to come to terms with the changes of age.

Midwifery
The profession concerned with the assistance of women in *pregnancy* and *childbirth*. A midwife provides care and information throughout pregnancy, supervises labour and delivery, and cares for both mother and baby after the birth.

Registered midwives have met the training standards of the UK Central Council for Midwifery (formerly the Central Midwives Board). Most are registered general nurses who have completed an additional 18-month course in midwifery. Midwives may practise in hospital, health units, or in domiciliary (home delivery) service. They are responsible for normal deliveries, but summon a doctor if an abnormality develops.

Migraine
A severe headache, lasting anything from two hours to two days, accompanied by disturbances of vision and/or nausea and vomiting. A sufferer may experience only a single attack; more commonly, he or she has recurrent attacks at varying intervals.

CAUSES AND INCIDENCE
Migraine occurs in at least 10 per cent of the population and is three times more common in women than in men. It may affect children as young as three years old; 60 per cent of migraine sufferers have their first attack before the age of 20. It is extremely rare for migraine to appear for the first time after the age of 50.

There is no single cause of migraine. It tends to run in families, although the exact mechanism of inheritance is not understood. A number of factors, singly or in combination, may bring on an attack in a susceptible person. These factors may be stress-related (such as anger, worry, excitement, depression, shock, overexertion, changes of routine, and changes of climate), food-related (particularly chocolate, cheese and other dairy products, red wine, fried food, and citrus fruits), or sensory-related (such as bright light or loud noises). Menstruation and the contraceptive pill may also trigger migraine.

TYPES
There are two types of migraine: common and classical. In common migraine, the pain of the headache

M

TECHNIQUES OF MICROSURGERY

Microsurgery started with ophthalmic surgeons, whose demands for more delicate operating instruments led to the adoption of the operating microscope. The results were so favourable that surgeons working in other specialties began to use the technique for intricate operations.

The operating microscope
This surgeon is performing microsurgery with the aid of an operating microscope. The photograph (below) shows a blood vessel as seen through the microscope.

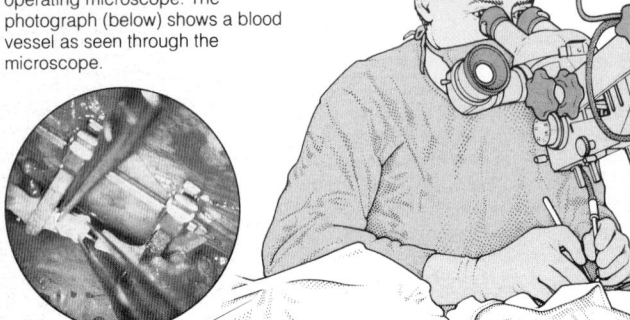

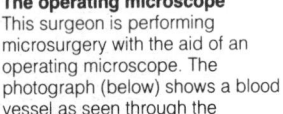

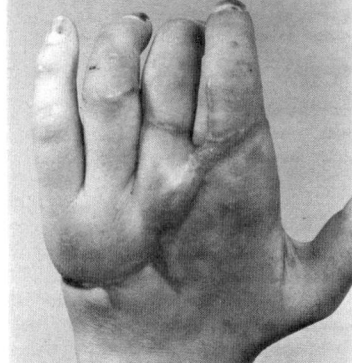

Replantation microsurgery
A major application of microsurgery is the replantation of severed fingers, toes, hands, feet, or even entire limbs. This is successful only if the severed blood vessels and nerves are accurately rejoined so that regeneration occurs.

MAIN AREAS OF OPERATION
Microsurgery is most commonly employed in ophthalmic, vascular, neurological, gynaecological, urological, and otological surgical procedures, in which delicate structures are involved.

Ophthalmology
By using microsurgery, even operations on the delicate retina of the eye are now possible.

Otology
Microsurgery is routinely used for operations on the tiny bones in the middle ear.

Gynaecology
With microsurgery, blockages of the fallopian tubes can often be corrected, restoring fertility.

Urology
A vasectomy (male sterilization) can sometimes be reversed by using microsurgery to rejoin the cut ends of the vas deferens.

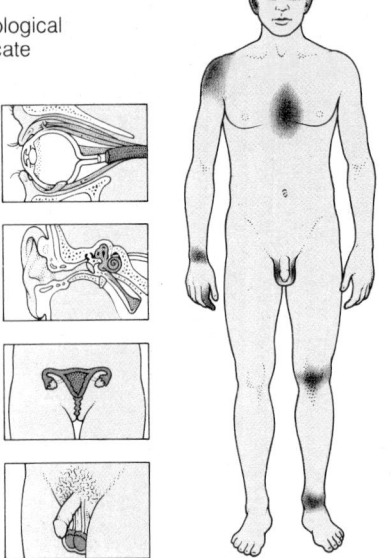

INSTRUMENTS

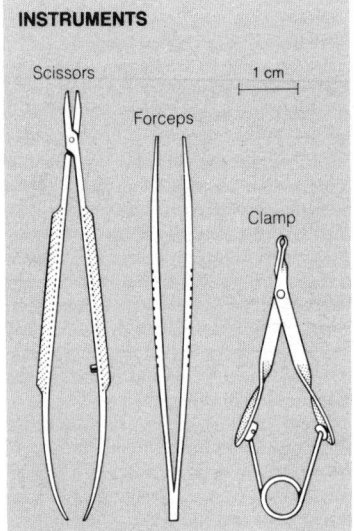

Scissors

1 cm

Forceps

Clamp

Microsurgery is possible only by using extremely delicate operating instruments, such as the fine scissors, forceps, and clamp shown above (their sizes can be judged from the scale bar).

M

develops slowly, sometimes mounting to a throbbing pain that is made worse by the slightest movement or noise. The pain is often, but not always, on only one side of the head and usually occurs with nausea and sometimes vomiting. Many sufferers, particularly children, recover after they have vomited.

Classical migraine is comparatively rare. The headache is preceded by a slowly expanding area of blindness surrounded by a sparkling edge that increases to involve up to one half of the field of vision of each eye. The blindness clears up after about 20 minutes and is often followed by a severe one-sided headache with nausea, vomiting, and sensitivity to light. Other temporary neurological symptoms, such as weakness in one half of the body, may occur.

DIAGNOSIS
Special tests are rarely necessary. The doctor can usually make a diagnosis from the patient's history and a physical examination. If there are accompanying persistent symptoms (such as tingling in a limb) or if the type of headache changes or becomes more severe, a full neurological examination may be carried out to exclude the possibility of a serious condition.

If migraine attacks occur less frequently than once a month, treatment of the acute attack is all that is required. If the attacks are more frequent, preventive treatment may be necessary. The simplest form of prevention is to avoid known trigger factors; keeping a diary can help pinpoint what triggers attacks.

The simplest treatment for a migraine attack is *aspirin* or *paracetamol* plus an *antiemetic drug* (often provided in suppository form). If this combination is not effective, treatment with *sumatriptan* (which acts on the blood vessels in and around the brain) may be prescribed. *Ergotamine* is an alternative treatment. Certain ergotamine preparations may help prevent an attack if taken in the early phases before the headache begins. Most people find that they recover more quickly if they can then sleep in a darkened room.

In cases where migraine attacks occur more frequently than once a month, prophylactic drugs (for example, *beta-blocker drugs* and *calcium channel blockers*) may be prescribed. In virtually all cases, an effective treatment programme can be found; if symptoms persist, however, advice should be obtained from a specialist migraine clinic.

Milia
Tiny, hard, white spots that most often occur in clusters on the upper cheeks and around the eyes of young adults. The cause is usually unknown but they may follow injury or blistering. They are painless and harmless.

Milk
A *nutrient* fluid produced by the mammary gland of mammals. Human milk differs considerably from cow's milk in the proportions of its ingredients. It contains about the same amount of fat, but twice as much lactose (milk sugar) and half as much protein. Virtually all babies can digest milk, but early in childhood some lose the enzyme that breaks lactose down to simpler sugars (see *Lactase deficiency*). Milk allergy occurs in some infants, caused by a *food allergy* or intolerance to the proteins in animal milk. (See also *Breast-feeding*; *Feeding, infant*.)

Milk-alkali syndrome
A rare type of *hypercalcaemia* (abnormally high level of calcium in the blood) accompanied by *alkalosis* (reduced acidity of the blood) and *kidney failure*. Milk-alkali syndrome is caused by excessive, long-term intake of calcium-containing *antacid drugs* and milk. It is most common in people with the symptoms of a *peptic ulcer* and associated kidney disorders.

Symptoms include weakness, muscle pains, irritability, and apathy. Treatment is to reduce the intake of milk and antacids.

Milk of magnesia
A magnesium preparation used as an *antacid drug* and *laxative drug*.

Milk teeth
See *Primary teeth*.

Minamata disease
The name given to a severe form of *mercury poisoning* that occurred in the mid-1950s in people who had eaten fish from Minamata Bay, Japan. The fish contained large amounts of mercury as a result of the water being polluted with industrial mercury waste. By the time the cause of the condition was identified and brought under control, many people had suffered severe nerve damage and some had died.

Mineralization, dental
The deposition of calcium crystals and other mineral salts in developing teeth. (See *Calcification, dental*.)

Mineralocorticoid
The term used to describe a corticosteroid hormone (produced by the cortex of the *adrenal glands*) that controls the amount of salts, including potassium and sodium, excreted in urine. Some corticosteroid hormones (such as *aldosterone*) have only a mineralocorticoid action, whereas others (such as *hydrocortisone*) also have a glucocorticoid effect (that is, they help to regulate the body's use of carbohydrates).

The drug fludrocortisone is used if the adrenal glands produce insufficient amounts of mineralocorticoids.

Minerals
Defined in *nutrition* as chemical elements that must be present in the diet for the maintenance of health. At least 20 minerals are essential. Important among them are potassium, sodium, calcium, magnesium, and phosphorus. Others, such as iron, zinc, and copper, are needed in only tiny amounts (see *Trace elements*). A balanced diet usually contains all the minerals the body requires. (See also tables overleaf showing the main food sources and recommended daily mineral allowances.)

Mineral supplements
Dietary supplements containing one or more *minerals* in tablet or liquid form. Most people obtain adequate amounts of minerals from the diet, and additional amounts are not beneficial. Taken in excess, some mineral supplements may be harmful.

The most commonly used mineral supplement is *iron*, which is used to treat iron-deficiency *anaemia* and is sometimes needed by women who are pregnant or breast-feeding. *Iodine* is sometimes added to salt and bread in areas where there is a risk of iodine deficiency. *Calcium* supplements are sometimes provided during pregnancy and to young children.

Other types of mineral deficiency are rare, with the exception of *magnesium* deficiency, which may result from alcohol dependence, kidney disease, or prolonged treatment with *diuretic drugs* or *digitalis drugs*.

Mineral supplements are sometimes needed by people suffering from an intestinal disorder that impairs the absorption of certain minerals from the diet. (See also individual mineral entries.)

Minilaparotomy
See *Sterilization, female*.

Minimal brain dysfunction
An explanation postulated by some American psychologists for a variety of behavioural and other problems occurring in young children for which a physical cause might be expected but for which none is found.

Minimal brain dysfunction may be a cause of difficulty in concentrating, impulsiveness, *hyperactivity*, and some *learning difficulties*.

Minimally invasive surgery
See p. 48.

Minocycline
A tetracycline *antibiotic drug* used in low doses to treat *acne*. Minocycline can also be used to treat infections of the respiratory or urinary tracts, and to prevent meningococcal *meningitis*.

Minoxidil
A *vasodilator* drug used to treat severe *hypertension* (high blood pressure) when other drugs have been ineffective. Prolonged use can stimulate hair growth, especially on the face. Minoxidil in the form of a lotion is used as a treatment for male-pattern baldness (see *Alopecia*).

M

MINERALS AND MAIN FOOD SOURCES

Mineral	Sources
Calcium	Milk, cheese, butter and margarine, green vegetables, pulses, nuts, soya bean products, hard water
Chromium	Red meat, cheese, butter and margarine, whole-grain cereals and breads, green vegetables
Copper	Red meat, poultry, liver, fish, seafood, whole-grain cereals and breads, green vegetables, pulses, nuts, raisins, mushrooms
Fluorine	Fish, fluoridated water, tea
Iodine	Milk, cheese, butter and margarine, fish, whole-grain cereals and breads, iodized table salt
Iron	Red meat, poultry, liver, eggs, fish, whole-grain cereals and breads
Magnesium	Milk, fish, whole-grain cereals and breads, green vegetables, pulses, nuts, hard water
Phosphorus	Red meat, poultry, liver, milk, cheese, butter and margarine, eggs, fish, whole-grain cereals and breads, green vegetables, root vegetables, pulses, nuts, fruit
Potassium	Whole-grain cereals and breads, green vegetables, pulses, fruit
Selenium	Red meat, liver, milk, fish, seafood, whole-grain cereals and breads
Sodium	Red meat, poultry, liver, milk, cheese, butter and margarine, eggs, fish, whole-grain cereals and breads, green vegetables, root vegetables, pulses, nuts, fruit, table salt, processed foods
Zinc	Red meat, fish, seafood, eggs, milk, whole-grain cereals and breads, pulses

Miosis

Constriction (reduction in size) of the pupil of the *eye*. Miosis may be caused by certain drugs (such as pilocarpine or opium), by a disease affecting the *autonomic nervous system* (such as *Horner's syndrome*), or simply by bright light. A degree of miosis is normal in older people.

Miscarriage

Loss of the fetus before the 28th week of pregnancy or before viability (the ability to survive outside the uterus without artificial support). The medical term for miscarriage is spontaneous abortion.

INCIDENCE

The incidence of miscarriage is difficult to determine, since not all women who miscarry seek medical attention or even realize they are miscarrying. It is estimated that between 10 and 30 per cent of all pregnancies end in miscarriage, with the majority occurring in the first 10 weeks.

CAUSES

A wide range of problems can cause miscarriage. Many miscarriages occur because of abnormalities of the fetus itself, such as *chromosomal abnormalities* or major developmental defects. Severe maternal illness or exposure to toxins may also cause miscarriage. Less common maternal causes include abnormalities such as inadequate progesterone secretion or an *autoimmune disorder*.

After the first three months, miscarriage is less common. Of the three to five per cent of pregnancies that miscarry between 12 and 22 weeks,

RECOMMENDED DAILY ALLOWANCES (RDAs) OF SELECTED MINERALS

	0–6 months	6 months – 1 year	1–3 years	4–6 years	7–10 years	11–14 years	15–18 years	19–22 years	23–50 years	51+ years	Extra needed pregnancy	Extra needed breastfeeding
Calcium (mg)	360	540	800	800	800	1,200	1,200	800	800	800	400	400
Iodine (mcg)	40	50	70	90	120	150	150	150	150	150	25	50
Iron (mg)	10	15	15	10	10	18	18	M 10 F 18	M 10 F 18	10	30–60	A
Magnesium (mg)	50	70	150	200	250	M 350 F 300	M 400 F 300	M 350 F 300	M 350 F 300	M 350 F 300	150	150
Phosphorus (mg)	240	360	800	800	800	1,200	1,200	800	800	800	400	400
Zinc (mg)	3	5	10	10	10	15	15	15	15	15	5	10

Mineral requirements
The table (above) gives the recommended daily allowances (RDAs) of minerals for which amounts have been established; when different, the RDAs for males and females are denoted by M and F.

A Iron requirements while breast-feeding are approximately the same as those for nonpregnant women, but additional iron may be recommended for two to three months after the birth to replenish iron stores depleted by pregnancy.

Units

mg = milligrams (thousandths of a gram)

mcg = micrograms (millionths of a gram)

problems include *genetic disorders, cervical incompetence,* a defect such as a septate (subdivided) uterus, and large uterine *fibroids.* Severe maternal infection or illness can also trigger a late miscarriage.

SYMPTOMS AND SIGNS

The symptoms of miscarriage are cramping and/or bleeding. Light bleeding during the early months of pregnancy occurs in up to half of all pregnancies and is often caused by low placental implantation or *cervical erosion.* Many of these pregnancies continue uneventfully to term.

Heavy bleeding with cramping is generally more serious because it may signal impending miscarriage. Spotting and severe pain can be a symptom of either a threatened miscarriage or an *ectopic pregnancy.* A gush of clear or pinkish fluid may be caused by rupture of the amniotic sac and is a serious sign.

TYPES

Miscarriages are classified medically as different types of abortion.

THREATENED ABORTION The fetus remains alive and has not been expelled from the uterus, despite bleeding from the woman's vagina.

INEVITABLE ABORTION The fetus has died and is being expelled from the uterus. An inevitable abortion may be complete (in which case all the uterine contents are expelled) or incomplete (in which case the fetus and/or placenta are not completely expelled).

MISSED ABORTION The fetus has died but is retained with the placenta in the uterus.

DIAGNOSIS AND TREATMENT

In early pregnancy a woman in whom bleeding and cramping develop is often prescribed bed rest to minimize bleeding. *Ultrasound scanning* may be recommended to determine that the pregnancy is intrauterine (i.e. not ectopic) and that it appears to be progressing normally. A pelvic examination may be performed to find out if the size of the uterus feels appropriate and to see if the cervix is open or closed.

If a miscarriage is incomplete and bleeding is heavy, a *D and C* may be required. If the miscarriage seems complete (i.e. all fetal and placental material has been expelled from the uterus), no further treatment may be needed. Missed abortion requires a D and C or *induction of labour* depending on the duration of the pregnancy. Often, women are given antibiotics and other drugs to minimize bleeding. Rh-negative women are given anti-D(Rh$_0$) immunoglobulin to prevent

Rh complications in any future pregnancies (see *Rhesus incompatibility*).

After the first trimester, any cramping or spotting merits immediate medical attention; at this stage a significant number of possible miscarriages are caused by treatable problems, such as an incompetent cervix, rather than by severe fetal defects.

If there is evidence of an incompetent cervix, the cervix may be stitched shut. Prolonged bed rest may be recommended and uterine relaxants may be administered to women with uterine or cervical abnormalities.

A woman who miscarries three or more times consecutively is called a habitual aborter. Habitual abortion may be caused by genetic, hormonal, or uterine abnormalities, chronic infection, or an autoimmune disease. Evaluation usually includes genetic studies, tests for hormonal problems and infections, and *hysterosalpingography* (X-rays of the uterus and fallopian tubes).

OUTLOOK

The majority of women who miscarry can eventually carry a pregnancy to term. Current diagnostic and treatment measures have made the outlook better than ever before. (See also *Abortion*; *Abortion, elective.*)

Misoprostol

A synthetic *prostaglandin drug* that inhibits gastric secretion. It is used to prevent the development of and to treat *peptic ulcers* associated with *nonsteroidal anti-inflammatory drugs.*

Mites and disease

Mites are small (less than 1.2 mm long), eight-legged animals that resemble tiny spiders. Many species have piercing and blood-sucking mouthparts and may parasitize animals and humans.

Mites can cause problems in a variety of ways. One species, the *scabies* mite, lives solely in human skin, where its burrowing causes an intense itch. Another, the house-dust mite, is common in bedding; inhaling dust containing dead mite parts and faeces can cause *asthma.*

Various other types of mites inhabit grassy areas or affect crops. Chiggers (American harvest mites) can be picked up when walking through thick grass. Their bites can produce an itchy rash. Mites in grain or fruit may cause various types of skin irritation, commonly known as grocers' itch or bakers' itch.

Certain mites transmit diseases, particularly scrub *typhus* and rickett-

sialpox. Both of these diseases are caused by *rickettsiae* (organisms that are intermediate between bacteria and viruses), which normally infect rodents, but which can be transmitted to humans by mites.

The use of insect repellents (such as dimethyl phthalate) is advisable when walking through mite-infested areas.

Mitosis

The way in which most cells divide, so that the *chromosomes* (inherited genetic material) within the nucleus of the original cell are exactly duplicated into two daughter cells.

Each person begins as a single cell (a fertilized egg) and, following successive mitotic divisions of this cell, is born as a multicellular being with trillions of cells, most of which contain exactly the same chromosomal material. Mitotic divisions occur in the body thousands of times every second as dead cells are replaced by new ones formed by the division and multiplication of other cells.

Mitosis can be observed in a cell culture under a microscope. The sequence of events as the original cell divides to form two daughter cells is shown in the illustrated box overleaf.

A minority of cells (in the ovaries and testes) undergoes a fundamentally different type of division that results in the daughter cells receiving only half of the original cell's chromosomal material. This process, called *meiosis*, occurs in the formation of egg and sperm cells.

Mitral incompetence

Failure of the mitral valve of the *heart* to close properly, which allows blood to leak back into the left atrium (upper chamber) when pumped out of the left ventricle (lower chamber). Also known as mitral insufficiency or mitral regurgitation, the disorder may occur in conjunction with *mitral stenosis* (narrowing of the valve).

In mitral incompetence, the left side of the heart must work harder to clear the regurgitated blood. Eventually, left-sided (and later, right-sided) *heart failure* may develop; generally, however, this is not a life-threatening condition. A build-up of blood from the left side of the heart can result in *pulmonary oedema.*

CAUSES AND INCIDENCE

The most common cause (though much less common than it once was) is damage to the valve as a result of *rheumatic fever.* Other causes include *mitral valve prolapse* (floppy valve syn-

M

THE MECHANISM OF MITOSIS

Mitosis is the simplest type of cell division. It provides new body cells to replace those that have died. The new cells each receive an identical copy of the original cell's chromosomes.

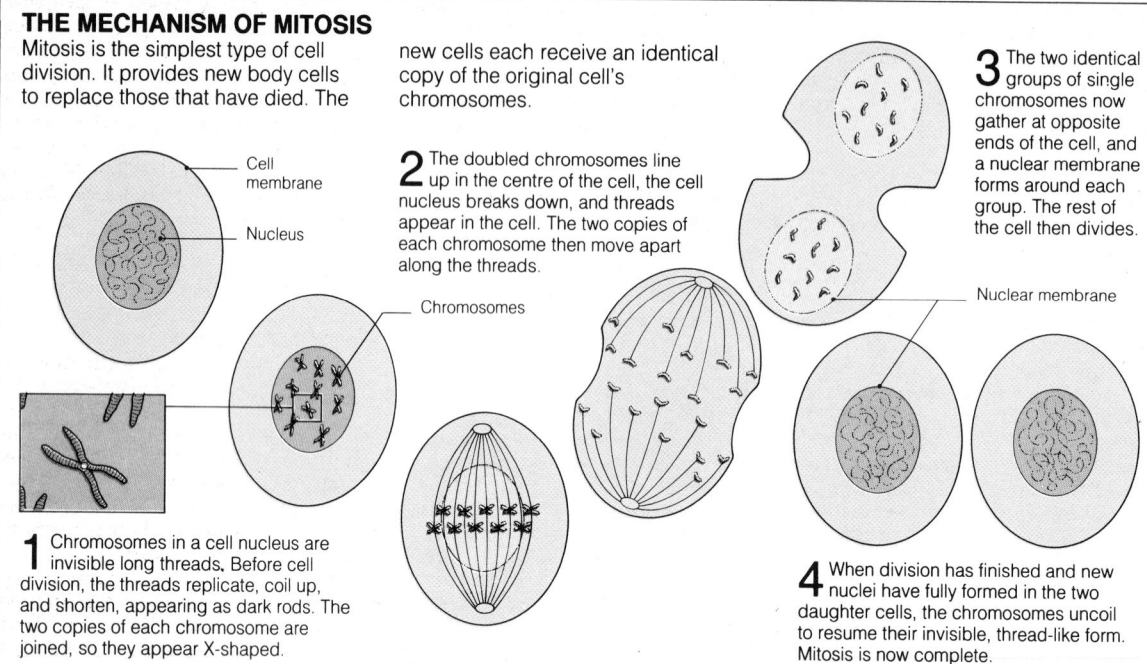

Cell membrane

Nucleus

Chromosomes

1 Chromosomes in a cell nucleus are invisible long threads. Before cell division, the threads replicate, coil up, and shorten, appearing as dark rods. The two copies of each chromosome are joined, so they appear X-shaped.

2 The doubled chromosomes line up in the centre of the cell, the cell nucleus breaks down, and threads appear in the cell. The two copies of each chromosome then move apart along the threads.

3 The two identical groups of single chromosomes now gather at opposite ends of the cell, and a nuclear membrane forms around each group. The rest of the cell then divides.

Nuclear membrane

4 When division has finished and new nuclei have fully formed in the two daughter cells, the chromosomes uncoil to resume their invisible, thread-like form. Mitosis is now complete.

M

drome), damage following a *myocardial infarction* (heart attack), and stretching of the valve due to enlargement of the ventricle in left-sided heart failure. Rarely, the disorder may be present from birth or occurs as part of *Marfan's syndrome*.

SYMPTOMS AND SIGNS

The characteristic symptoms are increasing breathlessness and fatigue, sometimes accompanied by *palpitations*. Later, as right-sided heart failure develops, the ankles swell.

An occasional complication of mitral incompetence is *endocarditis* affecting the valve. Another risk is that a thrombus (blood clot) may form in the left atrium and travel to the brain, resulting in a *stroke*.

DIAGNOSIS

The doctor makes a diagnosis from the patient's history, from a characteristic heart *murmur* heard through a stethoscope, and from the results of chest X-rays, *ECG*, and *echocardiography*. Cardiac *catheterization* is performed in some cases, in particular when surgical correction is being considered.

TREATMENT AND OUTLOOK

If breathlessness is troublesome, a *diuretic drug* may be prescribed to reduce fluid in the lungs and other tissues. *Digitalis drugs* may be given to increase the force of the heart's contraction and to control rhythm disturbances. *Anticoagulant drugs* may be given to prevent the formation of blood clots. Before undergoing dental or other surgery, a person with mitral valve disease should take *antibiotic drugs* to prevent a blood infection that could cause endocarditis.

Heart valve surgery is considered only if severe heart failure develops or if drug treatment fails to prevent the patient's symptoms from becoming severe and disabling.

The outlook for mitral incompetence is good whether it is treated by drugs or by surgery. Breathlessness and fatigue cannot be relieved by treatment once there has been permanent heart damage.

Mitral stenosis

Narrowing of the orifice of the mitral valve in the *heart*. This causes the atrial portion of the left side of the heart to work harder to force blood through the narrowed valve. The consequences are similar to those of *mitral incompetence* (failure of the valve to close properly), which may accompany stenosis.

CAUSES AND INCIDENCE

Mitral stenosis is almost always due to scarring of the valve from an earlier attack of *rheumatic fever*, although in about half the cases there is no medical record of the illness. Mitral stenosis is four times more common in women than in men.

SYMPTOMS AND SIGNS

Symptoms do not usually develop until adulthood, many years after rheumatic fever. The primary symptom is shortness of breath, which at first occurs only on exertion; as the stenosis worsens, breathing difficulty is felt with less exertion and is eventually present when the person is at rest. Other symptoms and signs include *palpitations*, *atrial fibrillation* (rapid uncoordinated, irregular heartbeat), and deeply flushed cheeks. Congestion of the lungs can lead to recurrent chest infections, coughing up of blood, and fatigue.

Possible complications are as for mitral incompetence.

DIAGNOSIS

Mitral stenosis is diagnosed from the patient's history, by a doctor listening to heart sounds through a stethoscope, and by investigations that may include an *ECG*, chest X-rays, echocardiography, and cardiac *catheterization*.

TREATMENT AND OUTLOOK

Drug treatment (with *diuretic drugs* and *digitalis drugs*) is broadly the same as for mitral incompetence, as are the precautions to help prevent infection of the valve (see *Endocarditis*).

If symptoms persist despite drug treatment, balloon *valvuloplasty* may be considered to stretch the defective valve. Alternatively, *heart valve surgery* to repair the valve (a procedure known as mitral valvotomy) or to replace the valve may be performed. The outlook following these treatments is generally good, although they may need to be repeated after several years.

Mitral valve prolapse

A common, slight deformity of the mitral valve, situated in the left side of the *heart*, that can produce a degree of *mitral incompetence* (leakage of the valve). Also known as "floppy valve syndrome", the condition affects up to five per cent of the population and is most common in young to middle-aged women. Mitral valve prolapse causes a characteristic heart *murmur* which may be heard by the doctor through a stethoscope during a routine examination.

The cause of mitral valve prolapse is not known in most cases, although there is some evidence that the condition is inherited. Occasionally, the valve prolapse occurs as a result of *rheumatic fever, coronary artery disease,* or *cardiomyopathy*.

Usually, there are no symptoms and the condition is of no consequence; treatment is not required. Occasionally, however, it may produce chest pain, *arrhythmia* (disturbance of heart rhythm), or leakage of the valve sufficient to cause *heart failure*. These conditions may require treatment with drugs, such as *beta-blocker drugs, diuretic drugs,* or *digitalis drugs,* or, rarely, *heart valve surgery*.

Mittelschmerz

Pain in the lower abdomen that occurs in some women at the time of *ovulation* midway through each menstrual cycle. The pain is usually one-sided and lasts only a few hours; slight spotting (vaginal blood loss) may accompany the pain. Mittelschmerz is usually not severe. However, if it is, *oral contraceptives* may be prescribed to suppress ovulation.

MMR vaccination

Administration of a combined *vaccine* that gives protection against *measles, mumps,* and *rubella* (German measles). The aim of immunization is to eliminate these infections, especially congenital rubella, which can be contracted by an unborn child if the mother is infected during pregnancy. To achieve this aim, at least 90 per cent of children must be vaccinated.

The MMR vaccination was introduced for routine immunization in the UK in October 1988, although it has been in use for some years in other countries, such as the US. The vaccine is now routinely offered to all children in their second year, but can be given at any time after this. Children who have not previously been given the MMR vaccine are offered MMR vaccination at the same time as their pre-school diphtheria, tetanus, and polio boosters. Only a single injection of MMR vaccine is required.

MMR should be given to children who have already been given the measles vaccine on its own, and to children who have had measles, mumps, or rubella unless there is very firm proof that they are already immune. Children who have a personal or close family history of *epilepsy* should also be given the vaccine, but precautions should be taken to ensure the child's temperature is kept down in order to prevent febrile convulsions (see *Convulsions, febrile*) after the vaccination.

Vaccination should be postponed if a child is suffering from an acute feverish illness. Vaccination should not be given to children who have untreated *cancer*, a history of life-threatening allergic reactions, or suppressed immunity (including those who are receiving treatment with *immunosuppressant drugs, radiotherapy* or high-dose *corticosteroid drugs*). Vaccination should not be given within three weeks of another live vaccine, or within three months of an *immunoglobulin injection*. Adult women given the vaccine should avoid pregnancy for at least one month.

POSSIBLE ADVERSE EFFECTS
MMR vaccination is safe and effective. Minor symptoms, such as fever, rash, and malaise, may occur—most commonly, five to 10 days after vaccination. In addition, about one per cent of children develop mild swelling of the *parotid glands* (such as occurs in mumps) three to four weeks after vaccination; this condition is not infectious to others.

Mobilization

The process of making a part of the body capable of movement. Mobilization refers to treatment aimed at increasing mobility in a part of the body that is recovering from injury or affected by disease. Examples include exercises to treat *frozen shoulder* or joint stiffness caused by *arthritis*, and retraining in walking following a *stroke* or *fracture* of the leg.

Surgeons use the term mobilization to refer to the freeing, during an operation, of an organ or structure from surrounding *connective tissue* (material that surrounds body structures and holds them together) and fibrous adhesions (bands of tissue that join normally unconnected parts of the body). For example, in a *cholecystectomy* operation, the gallbladder has to be mobilized from the liver before it can be removed.

Molar

See *Teeth*.

Molar pregnancy

A pregnancy in which a tumour develops from placental tissue and the embryo fails to develop normally. A molar pregnancy may be benign, in which case it is called a *hydatidiform mole*, or malignant, in which case it is called an invasive mole. *Choriocarcinoma* is an invasive mole that tends to spread outside the uterus.

A different type of molar pregnancy occurs after a missed abortion (a type of *miscarriage* in which the dead embryo and placenta are not expelled from the uterus). In this case, the dead tissue is called a carneous mole.

Mole

A type of pigmented *naevus*. See also *Molar pregnancy*.

Molecule

 The smallest complete unit of a substance that can exist independently and still retain the characteristic properties of that substance. Almost all molecules consist of two or more atoms that are linked. A molecule of carbon dioxide comprises one carbon atom linked to two oxygen atoms. Certain unusual molecules, called monatomic molecules, consist of only one atom (e.g. molecules of inert gases such as argon and neon).

Molecules vary enormously in size and complexity. At one extreme are the small, simple ones such as oxygen, which consists of two linked oxygen atoms. At the other extreme are huge, complicated molecules such as *DNA* (deoxyribonucleic acid), which consists of thousands of atoms of carbon, hydrogen, oxygen, nitrogen, and phosphorus linked together to form a double-helix spiral structure.

Molluscum contagiosum

A harmless viral infection characterized by shiny, pearly white papules (tiny lumps) on the skin surface. Each papule is circular, has a tiny central

M

depression, and produces a cheesy fluid when it is squeezed. A crust forms before healing occurs.

The papules appear in groups, or sometimes alone, on the genitals, the inside of the thighs, the face, or elsewhere. Children or, less commonly, adults may be affected. The infection is easily transmitted by direct skin contact or during sexual intercourse. A few thousand cases are reported annually from sexually transmitted disease clinics in the UK.

Molluscum contagiosum usually clears up in a few months, but may require treatment by a doctor.

Mongolian blue spot

A blue-black pigmented spot found singly or in groups on the lower back and buttocks at birth. The spot may be mistaken for a bruise, although it is a type of *naevus*. Mongolian blue spots are common in black or Asian children and are caused by a concentration of melanocytes (pigment-producing cells) deep within the skin. They usually disappear by the time the child is three or four years old.

Mongolism

The outdated name for the disorder now called *Down's syndrome*.

Moniliasis

See *Candidiasis*.

Monitor

To maintain a constant watch on a patient's condition so that any change can be detected early and appropriate treatment given. The term also refers to any device used to carry out monitoring, such as the cardiac monitor used in intensive-care units. A cardiac monitor displays the patient's *ECG* (a record of the heart's electrical activity) on a screen and signals the heart-rate both visually and audibly.

Monoamine oxidase inhibitors

One of the two main types of *antidepressant drug*.

Monoarthritis

Inflammation of a single joint, causing pain and stiffness. Common causes are *osteoarthritis*, *gout*, and infection.

Monoclonal antibody

See *Antibody, monoclonal*.

Mononucleosis, infectious

An acute viral infection characterized by a high temperature, sore throat, and swollen *lymph nodes* (glands), par-

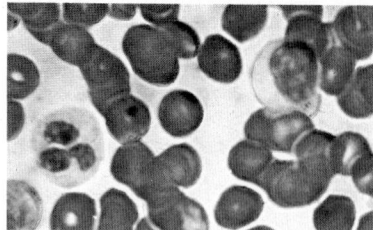

Blood smear in mononucleosis
The large cell with one nucleus, surrounded by many red blood cells, is an atypical lymphocyte (it is bigger than normal). Such cells are a feature of mononucleosis.

ticularly in the neck (hence its common name, glandular fever).

CAUSES AND INCIDENCE

Infectious mononucleosis is caused either by the Epstein-Barr virus or cytomegalovirus, both members of the herpesvirus family. The disease develops only if the virus is encountered for the first time at an age when the response of the body's *immune system* is most vigorous (that is, during adolescence and early adult life). The peak incidence of the illness occurs between ages 15 and 17. Each year, tens of thousands of young people in the UK develop the illness. Kissing is thought to be a common method of transmitting the virus.

Once in the body, the virus multiplies in the *lymphocytes* (white blood cells that form part of the immune system). Lymphocytes are also called mononuclear cells. When infected with the virus, the lymphocytes alter their appearance and are then referred to as "atypical".

SYMPTOMS AND SIGNS

The illness usually starts with a fever and headache, followed by swelling of the lymph nodes in the neck, armpits, and groin and by a severe sore throat due to tonsillitis. The enlarged, inflamed tonsils make swallowing difficult and, in rare cases, may obstruct breathing. Occasionally, mild liver damage may occur, leading to jaundice for a few days. A doctor may feel an enlarged spleen in the upper left part of the abdomen.

DIAGNOSIS

The diagnosis is often obvious from the symptoms and from examination of a *blood smear*, which shows many atypical lymphocytes in the blood. A test for the infection—the heterophil antibodies test—may also be carried out. This test looks for antibodies (proteins produced by the immune system to counter the virus) that possess the unique ability to cause clump-

ing of red cells taken from sheep's blood. More specific tests are also available when the diagnosis is in doubt.

TREATMENT AND OUTLOOK

Almost all patients recover after four to six weeks without drug treatment. If the antibiotic *ampicillin* is given in the mistaken belief that the patient has a bacterial infection, it may produce a rash and worsening of symptoms. Rest is needed for a month or so to allow the body's immune system to destroy the virus. In rare cases, *corticosteroid drugs* are required to reduce severe inflammation, particularly if breathing is obstructed by swollen tonsils. For a period of two or three months after recovery, patients often feel depressed lack energy and feel very sleepy during the day.

Monorchism

The presence of only one testis. Unless a testis has been removed by surgery (see *Orchidectomy*), the most probable cause of monorchism is a *congenital* absence. The term monorchism should not be used to describe a testis that has not descended into the scrotum (see *Testis, undescended*).

Monosodium glutamate

A *food additive* frequently used as a flavour enhancer and seasoning. Monosodium glutamate (MSG) is the sodium salt of an amino acid, derived from protein. Until recently, MSG was suspected to be the cause of *Chinese restaurant syndrome*, in which a sense of pressure in the face, pain in the chest, and a feeling of burning in the head and upper trunk comes on 20 minutes after a meal and lasts for about 45 minutes. Clinical trials have shown that MSG does not produce exactly this symptom pattern, although it may occasionally cause symptoms in sensitive people.

Monteggia's fracture

Fracture of the *ulna* (the bone on the inner side of the forearm) just below the elbow, with dislocation of the *radius* (the bone on the outer side of the forearm) from the *elbow* joint. Monteggia's fracture can be caused by a fall on to the arm or by a blow to the back of the upper arm.

Treatment usually requires an operation through two incisions on either side of the forearm. The fractured bone-ends of the ulna are realigned and fixed with a plate and screws or a long nail to restore the length of the forearm. Then the head of the radius

M

is replaced in the elbow joint. The incisions are sewn up and the limb is immobilized in a plaster *cast* until the fracture has healed, which usually takes about 12 weeks.

Moon face
The rounded facial appearance that is a feature of *Cushing's syndrome*.

Morbid anatomy
Also known as pathological anatomy, the study of the structural changes that occur in body tissues as a result of disease, especially the changes that are visible to the naked eye during a postmortem examination (in contrast to the tissue changes that are visible only through a microscope).

Morbidity
The state or condition of being diseased. In medical statistics, the morbidity ratio is the proportion of diseased people to healthy people in a community.

Morbilli
Another name for *measles*.

Morning-after pill
See *Contraception, postcoital*.

Morning sickness
See *Vomiting in pregnancy*.

Moron
An outdated term, derived from the Greek word for dull, for a person with mild *mental handicap*.

Morphine
The best known narcotic *analgesic drug* (painkiller), derived from the unripe seed pods of the opium poppy.
WHY IT IS USED
Morphine is given to relieve severe pain caused by *myocardial infarction* (heart attack), major surgery, serious injury, and cancer. It is occasionally used as a *premedication* (a drug used to prepare a person for surgery).
HOW IT WORKS
Morphine blocks the transmission of pain signals at specific sites (called opiate receptors) in the brain and spinal cord, thereby preventing the perception of pain. It also induces a sense of well-being or euphoria.
POSSIBLE ADVERSE EFFECTS
Morphine causes drowsiness, dizziness, constipation, nausea, vomiting, and confusion.
ABUSE
The euphoric effects of morphine are addictive and have led to its abuse.

Short-term use is unlikely to cause *drug dependence*. Long-term abuse leads to a craving for the drug and *tolerance* (the need for greater amounts to have the same effect). It also causes physical dependence, with severe flu-like symptoms, such as profuse sweating, shaking, and abdominal cramps, when the drug is suddenly withdrawn (see *Withdrawal syndrome*).

Morphoea
A condition in which one or more hard, flat, round or oval patches develop on the skin. Morphoea is a type of *scleroderma* (a disease in which there is progressive hardening of tissues), but it is confined to the skin.

The skin patches of morphoea are white or reddish, measuring up to several centimetres in diameter. They usually occur on the trunk, neck, hands, or feet. Loss of hair or ulceration at the affected site may also occur. The condition most often affects middle-aged women.

Morphoea is harmless but can be disfiguring. There is no treatment.

Mortality
The death rate, that is, the number of deaths per 100,000 (or, occasionally, per 1,000 or 10,000) of the population per year. The total mortality is made up of the individual mortality from different causes (such as accidents, coronary artery disease, and cancer). The study of differences in these proportions between one country and another, or different periods in the same country, can offer valuable information about the comparative state of health of a population or about disease trends.

Mortality is often calculated for specific groups. For example, *infant mortality* measures the deaths of live-born infants during the first year of life; perinatal mortality measures the deaths (including all stillbirths) during the first week (or sometimes month) of life.

Standardized mortality compares the death rate in an occupational or

M

MAJOR CAUSES OF DEATH IN ENGLAND AND WALES (1992)*

Cause	Male deaths	Female deaths
Circulatory system disorders	122,000	132,000
Coronary heart disease	79,000	67,000
Cerebrovascular disease	25,000	41,000
Other circulatory diseases	18,000	24,000
Cancer	76,000	70,000
Lung	22,000	10,500
Breast	—	14,000
Prostate	8,700	—
Brain	1,700	1,200
Lymphatic	5,000	4,700
Other cancers	38,600	39,600
Accidents	10,723	5,958
Road accidents	2,848	1,210
Falls	1,327	1,941
Fires	272	227
Drowning	193	66
Other accidents	6,083	2,514
Diabetes mellitus	3,500	4,500
Nervous system disorders	4,400	8,600
Infections	1,400	1,300
Respiratory disorders	29,000	30,000
Pneumonia	9,400	17,000
Chronic obstructive airways disease	17,000	11,000
Other respiratory disorders	2,600	2,000
Suicide	3,000	900
Other causes	61,577	41,242
Total	311,600	294,500

*excluding deaths in infants under four weeks old

socioeconomic group with that for the entire population. It is a useful indicator of the relative safety of an occupation, or of whether a specific socioeconomic group is at particular risk. (See also table showing Major causes of death, previous page; *Life expectancy; Maternal mortality*.)

Mosaicism

The presence of two (or more) groups of cells containing different chromosomal material within one person.

Usually, each of a person's body cells contains 46 *chromosomes*. They include the two sex chromosomes (XX in females and XY in males). In a mosaic person, some cells may contain 46 and others 45, 47, or other numbers of chromosomes. The probable cause in most cases is a fault in cell division early in embryonic life. The diagnosis is made by *chromosome analysis* of skin or white blood cells.

Mosaicism can give rise to syndromes associated with *chromosomal abnormalities* (such as *Down's syndrome* and *Turner's syndrome*). A girl with Turner's syndrome mosaicism has some cells with a normal chromosome complement and others missing an X sex chromosome. About three per cent of Down's syndrome children have mosaicism and carry a mixture of normal cells and others containing the extra number 21 chromosome.

Depending on the proportion of abnormal cells and the type of abnormality, people with mosaicism range from looking physically normal to having features typical of a chromosomal abnormality syndrome. People with mosaicism are often less severely affected than those with the abnormality in all their cells.

Mosquito bites

Mosquitoes are flying insects found throughout the world. The females bite humans or animals to obtain the blood needed to produce eggs, which are laid and hatched in stagnating water. Mosquitoes are therefore most prevalent around marshes, ponds, reservoirs, and water tanks, especially after a rainy period. Male mosquitoes do not bite.

Mosquitoes are a nuisance simply because of their bites. However, the main problem with mosquitoes is disease transmission—particularly in the tropics. During a bite, a mosquito may acquire infectious organisms from the blood of an infected person; the organisms multiply within the insect and are transferred to another person during a subsequent bite.

DANGEROUS MOSQUITOES

Mosquito	Appearance	Habits	Diseases transmitted
ANOPHELES species	Head and body in straight line and at an angle to surface	Mainly rural; bite at night	Malaria; filariasis
CULEX species	Body parallel to surface; head bent down; whining flight; brown colour	Urban or rural; bite in evening or at night	Viral encephalitis; filariasis
AEDES species	Body shape as for CULEX, but tropical species are black and white	Urban or rural; bite during day	Dengue; yellow fever; viral encephalitis

The main disease-transmitting mosquitoes belong to three groups: *ANOPHELES, AEDES,* and *CULEX*. They have varying appearances and habits and transmit different diseases (see chart).

TREATMENT
Mosquito bites should be washed with soap and water, and a soothing cream applied. A doctor should be consulted if mosquito bites cause a severe skin reaction.

PREVENTION
Protective measures against mosquitoes (to limit the chances of infection) should be taken in the tropics and subtropics and in any area where the insects are rampant. The most effective measures are the wearing of long sleeves and socks at dusk to reduce the amount of exposed skin, placing mosquito screens over windows, and the use of insect-repellent sprays or slow-burning coils that release a smoke containing insecticide. A mosquito net that surrounds the bed is of value in preventing mosquitoes from biting during sleep.

Attempts to control mosquitoes in the tropics have included direct attack with insecticides, efforts to limit breeding areas, and even the release of vast numbers of sterilized male mosquitoes. However, these efforts have achieved only limited success. (See also *Insect bites; Insects and disease*.)

Motion sickness

A condition produced in some people by road, sea, or air travel. In its mildest form, motion sickness may be only a feeling of slight uneasiness or discomfort, and a headache; in severe cases, there may be distress, excessive sweating and salivation, pallor, nausea, and vomiting.

Motion sickness is caused by the effect of any repetitive pronounced movement on the organ of balance in the inner ear. Other factors also play a part, however. Anxiety based on previous attacks, a stuffy or fume-laden atmosphere, a full stomach, or the sight of food can make the condition worse. So, too, can focusing on nearby objects; sufferers should try to look at a point on the horizon.

PREVENTION
Various *antiemetic drugs* are available to prevent or help control motion sickness. Some, such as *hyoscine*, are available as adhesive patches worn on the skin; others, such as cyclizine, are usually taken orally about an hour before the start of the journey. Some drugs for motion sickness may cause drowsiness and increase the effects of alcohol. Some people obtain relief by wearing an acupressure band on the wrist.

Motor

A term used to describe anything that brings about movement, such as a muscle or a nerve. It is usually applied to nerves (including those in the part of the brain called the cerebral cortex) that stimulate muscles to contract and thereby produce movement.

Motor neuron disease

A group of disorders in which there is degeneration of the *nerves* within the *central nervous system* that control muscular activity. This leads to weakness and wasting of the *muscles*. The cause of motor neuron disease is unknown.

TYPES

AMYOTROPHIC LATERAL SCLEROSIS Also known as ALS or Lou Gehrig's disease, this is the most common type of

M

motor neuron disease. About one or two cases of ALS are diagnosed annually per 100,000 people in the UK. The disease usually affects people over the age of 50 and is more common in men. About five to 10 per cent of cases run in families.

In most cases, the first symptom is weakness in the hands and arms, accompanied by wasting of the muscles. There may also be *fasciculations* (spontaneous, irregular contractions of small areas of muscle), and muscle cramps or stiffness. In some cases, symptoms begin in the legs. Wherever the disease first appears, all four extremities soon become involved. ALS does not affect sensation or bladder function.

Other types of motor neuron disease include progressive muscular atrophy and progressive bulbar palsy, which both start with patterns of muscle weakness that differ from typical ALS but usually develop into ALS.

CHILDHOOD TYPES Two types of motor neuron disease start in childhood or adolescence, and in most cases are inherited.

Werdnig-Hoffman disease, also called infantile progressive spinal muscular atrophy, affects infants at birth or soon afterwards; with rare exceptions, muscle weakness becomes progressively worse, leading to death within several months to several years.

A less severe type is chronic spinal muscular atrophy, which may begin any time during childhood and adolescence. This type causes progressive weakness but may not lead to serious disability.

DIAGNOSIS
The diagnosis of motor neuron disease may be confirmed by various tests, including *EMG* (measurement of electrical activity in muscles), muscle *biopsy* (removal of a sample of tissue for microscopic analysis), blood tests, *myelography* (X-ray examination of the spinal cord after injection of a radiopaque substance), *CT scanning,* or *MRI.*

TREATMENT AND OUTLOOK
Motor neuron disease typically goes on to affect the muscles involved in breathing and swallowing. Involvement of these muscles usually leads to death within two to four years of onset. However, about 20 per cent of sufferers survive for more than five years, and about five per cent for more than 10 years.

Nerve degeneration cannot be slowed down, but *physiotherapy* and use of various aids may help reduce

disability. In the late stages of the disease, the sufferer cannot speak, swallow, or move, but maintains intellect and awareness. Psychological and physical support are needed, and may be provided at home or in a *hospice.*

Mould

 Any of a large group of *fungi* that exist as many-celled, filamentous colonies. Some moulds are the source of antibiotic drugs, such as penicillin. Others can cause disease, such as *aspergillosis.*

Mountain sickness
An illness that can affect mountain climbers, hikers, or skiers who have ascended too rapidly to heights above about 2,400 m or, more commonly, to above 3,000 m.

CAUSES
Mountain sickness is caused by the reduced atmospheric pressure—and thus reduced oxygen—at high altitude, but the exact mechanism by which reduced pressure leads to illness is not fully understood. Broadly, reduced oxygen in the blood, along with other changes in blood chemistry, affects the nervous system, muscles, heart, and lungs.

At higher altitudes the blood flow through the lungs and to the brain is greater than normal; this, combined with an apparent increase in the permeability (leakiness) of blood vessels, can lead to *oedema* (accumulation of fluid) in these organs.

Mountain sickness is more likely the younger the person, the faster the ascent, and the higher the altitude.

PREVENTION
A person ascending to an altitude above 2,400 m should do so gradually, stopping for a day or two's rest after each further ascent of 600 to 900 m. Ascending higher during the rest day is permissible, provided a return to the lower level is made before night.

SYMPTOMS AND SIGNS
In most cases, mountain sickness is mild and short-lived, with symptoms such as headache, nausea, dizziness, and impaired mental processes. No further ascent should be made until the symptoms disappear.

Some cases are more severe. Sufferers develop a condition known as high-altitude pulmonary oedema, in which fluid builds up in the lungs, leading to severe breathlessness, cough, and the production of frothy sputum (phlegm). In some cases, a condition known as cerebral oedema

develops, in which fluid builds up around the brain, causing severe headache, vomiting, unsteadiness, confusion, hallucinations, seizures, and sometimes coma.

FIRST AID AND TREATMENT
In serious cases, the victim must be brought down from the mountain and taken to a hospital as quickly as possible. Any delay can result in brain damage and death. The administration of pure oxygen, if available, can help. In hospital, *diuretic drugs* are often given to help reduce oedema.

The condition of patients with high-altitude pulmonary oedema often improves rapidly after descending a few hundred metres. Patients with cerebral oedema may take days or weeks in hospital to recover.

Mouth
The oral cavity. The mouth is the first part of the *digestive system,* where food is broken down for swallowing (see *Mastication*). It is also used in *breathing,* and converts vibrations produced by the *larynx* (voice-box) into *speech.*

STRUCTURE
The roof of the mouth consists of a hard bony *palate* at the front and a soft fleshy palate behind. Most of the floor of the mouth is formed by the *tongue,* which contains specialized cells, sensitive to taste, known as taste-buds. Surrounding the palate and tongue are the *teeth,* which are set in the shock-absorbent tissue of the *gums.* Enclosing them all are the cheeks and *lips,* which contain a ring of muscle that helps keep food in the mouth. The inside of the mouth is lined with mucous membrane, which is lubricated with saliva produced by three pairs of *salivary glands.*

DISORDERS
The most common deformities of the mouth, other than alignment of the teeth (see *Malocclusion*), are *cleft lip and palate* (a split in the upper lip and a gap in the roof of the mouth). The latter may occur alone or together.

Infections of the mouth are common. Examples include an abscess around the root of a tooth (see *Abscess, dental*) and oral *candidiasis* (thrush), a fungal infection that produces sore, cream-coloured patches on the lining of the mouth. Noninfective conditions that also cause discoloration include *leukoplakia* (in which there are thickened white or grey patches) and *lichen planus* (in which a white network of raised tissue develops).

Extremely common are *mouth ulcers,* painful white or yellow open sores

M

that may develop anywhere on the mucous membrane within the mouth. *Cysts* (swellings filled with fluid or semi-solid material) sometimes occur on the lining of the cheek; *ranula* are cysts on the floor of the mouth.

Any lump, sore, or ulcer in the mouth that persists for more than three or four weeks should be seen by a doctor. In rare cases, the abnormality is an early sign of a malignant growth (see *Mouth cancer*).

Mouth cancer

Malignant tumours affecting the lips, tongue, and oral cavity. *Lip cancer* and *tongue cancer* are the most common types of mouth cancer. Less commonly affected by cancer are the floor of the mouth, the salivary glands, the inside of the cheeks, the gums, and the palate.

CAUSES AND INCIDENCE

The main predisposing causes of mouth cancer are poor *oral hygiene*, drinking alcoholic spirits, and *tobacco-smoking*. The risk to pipe and cigar smokers is as great, or greater, than the risk to cigarette smokers; chewing tobacco and inhaling snuff also predispose to mouth cancer. Irritation from ill-fitting dentures or jagged teeth are other predisposing factors.

Oral cancers represent about five per cent of all malignancies. Men are affected twice as commonly as women, and most cases occur in men over the age of 40.

SYMPTOMS AND SIGNS

Mouth cancer usually starts with a whitish patch, called *leukoplakia*, or a small lump. These may be accompanied by a burning sensation, but are usually painless. As the tumour grows, it may develop into an ulcer or a deep, hard-edged fissure (crack), which may bleed and erode surrounding tissue. In its advanced stages, mouth cancer is usually painful.

DIAGNOSIS

Any lump, discoloured patch, or other tissue change in the mouth that does not clear up within a month should be reported to a doctor. In some cases, a dentist is the first person to detect a cancerous change. The diagnosis is based on a *biopsy* (removal of a small sample of tissue for microscopic analysis).

TREATMENT AND OUTLOOK

Treatment consists of surgical removal of all cancerous tissue, *radiotherapy*, or a combination of both. Extensive surgery may result in facial disfigurement and problems with eating and speaking, which may require

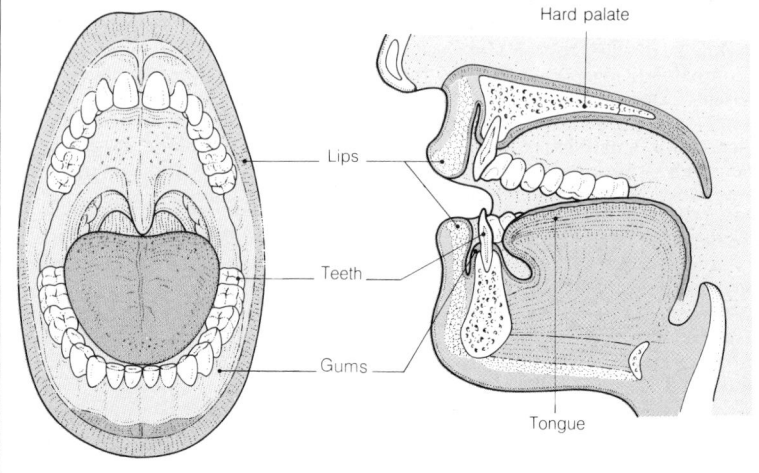

ANATOMY OF THE MOUTH

The mouth has a complicated structure, reflecting its various functions. For example, the tongue, lips, teeth, and palate play an essential role in speech production. Together with the salivary glands, the same mouth parts also play a role in eating and drinking.

Hard palate
Lips
Teeth
Gums
Tongue

reconstructive surgery. Radiotherapy sometimes damages the salivary glands (see *Mouth, dry*).

The rate of spread of oral cancer varies according to the site. When oral cancer in any form is detected and treated early, the outlook is good, resulting in a cure in three quarters of cases. More than half the people with oral cancer survive for more than five years after treatment.

Mouth, dry

The result of inadequate production of saliva. Dry mouth is usually a temporary condition caused by fear, infection of a *salivary gland*, or the action of *anticholinergic drugs*.

Permanent dry mouth is rare. It can occur, for unknown reasons, as part of *Sjögren's syndrome* or it may result from *radiotherapy* given to treat a tumour of the mouth. Permanent dryness of the mouth is in most cases accompanied by difficulty in swallowing and speaking, interference with taste, and tooth decay. Dry mouth may be partly relieved by spraying the inside of the mouth with artificial saliva.

Mouth-to-mouth resuscitation

See *Artificial respiration*.

Mouth ulcer

An open sore caused by a break in the *mucous membrane* that lines the mouth. Mouth ulcers take the form of round or oval, shallow, white, grey, or yellow spots with an inflamed red border. They may occur singly or in clusters anywhere in the mouth.

TYPES

The most common type of mouth ulcer is an aphthous ulcer (see *Ulcer, aphthous*), which may occur on the inside of the cheek or lip or on the tongue. Also common are ulcers caused by the *herpes simplex* virus, which also causes *cold sores*.

Rare types of mouth ulcer include those occurring in *Behçet's syndrome*, *tuberculosis*, *syphilis*, acute ulcerative *gingivitis*, *leukaemia*, *anaemia*, and drug allergy.

A mouth ulcer may be an early stage of *mouth cancer*. Any ulcer that fails to heal within a month, or that recurs, should be seen by a doctor. *Blood tests* and/or a *biopsy* (removal of a small sample of tissue for microscopic analysis) may be required to determine the cause of the ulcer.

Mouthwash

A solution for rinsing the mouth. Various medicinal claims are made for mouthwashes, but many do no more than leave the mouth feeling fresh and, if used vigorously, remove loose food debris from the teeth (an effect that can be achieved with water). If used for a prolonged period, mouthwashes may irritate the mouth.

Some mouthwashes are useful in certain circumstances. When the

M

gums are too tender for proper tooth-brushing, as occurs in some types of *gingivitis* (inflammation of the gums), a mouthwash containing *hydrogen peroxide* can help clean the teeth by its foaming action.

When routine dental hygiene is impossible, as is the case after oral surgery, a mouthwash containing *chlorhexidine*, used as directed by the dental surgeon, is effective against bacteria in dental *plaque* (the sticky coating on the teeth).

Fluoride mouthwashes help prevent dental caries, probably by strengthening tooth enamel, and possibly also by acting directly against plaque.

A mouthwash of warm salt water can help ease painful inflammation caused by tooth disorders, such as impacted wisdom teeth (see *Impaction, dental*) or *dry socket* (infection at the site of a tooth extraction).

Antiseptic mouthwashes intended to combat *halitosis* (bad breath) are usually ineffective because they do not treat the cause of the problem.

Movement

Bodily movements include skeletal movements and movements of soft tissues and body organs. All movement is brought about by the actions of various types of *muscles*.

SKELETAL MOVEMENTS

The simplest skeletal movement consists of a change in the relative position of two *bones*, brought about by shortening of a muscle attached to the two bones and acting across a *joint*. Simultaneously, other muscles and soft tissues, such as skin, *tendons*, and *ligaments*, are stretched.

More complex skeletal movements involve many bones, joints, and muscles, which are arranged to allow an enormous range of possible actions, from turning a screwdriver to turning a somersault. Even in a fairly simple movement, several muscles are active, some contracting to initiate and maintain a movement while others that oppose the movement contract to help prevent sudden, uncontrolled movement.

All voluntary (willed) skeletal movements are initiated in the part of the *cerebrum* (the main mass of the brain) called the motor cortex. Signals are sent down the spinal cord along nerve fibres, and from there along separate nerve fibres to the appropriate muscles. Control relies on information supplied by sensory nerve receptors, in the muscles and elsewhere, that record the position of

MOVEMENT

During life, movement occurs constantly throughout the body. All visible movements are caused by the shortening of muscles, usually for only brief periods at a time. All movement is either voluntary (willed) or involuntary (automatic).

SKELETAL MOVEMENT

This always involves moving bones relative to one another. Many muscles are involved. Some act to brace certain bones so that different bones can be moved by other muscles.

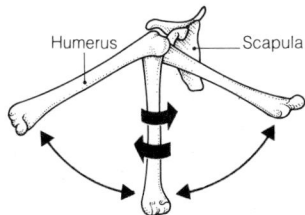

Combined rotation and displacement

Arm movements
A ball-and-socket joint, the shoulder allows movements in all directions.

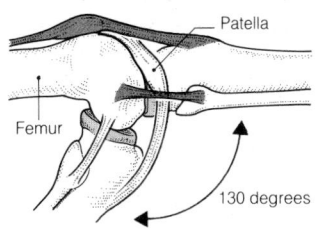

Knee movement
A hinge joint, the knee allows movement (through an arc of about 130 degrees) in only one plane.

EYE MOVEMENT

Six muscles work together on the eyeball to give a range of smooth, precise movements. The eye can move through an arc of about 100 degrees horizontally and about 80 degrees vertically.

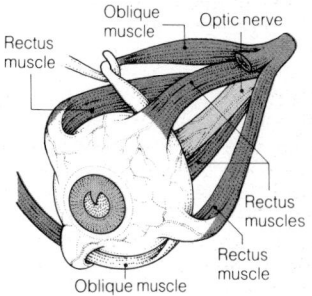

Eye muscles
The four rectus eye muscles run directly from the eyeball; the oblique muscles are attached to and pull on the eyeball at an angle.

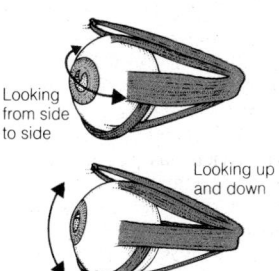

Looking from side to side

Looking up and down

Actions of the eye muscles
Two rectus muscles control side-to-side eye movements. The other muscles control up-and-down and rotational movements.

INVOLUNTARY MOVEMENT

Many movements are not under voluntary control but are regulated by the autonomic nervous system. One example is the beating of the heart, which automatically speeds up in response to increased demands for oxygenated blood by body tissues and slows down again when these demands decrease. Another example is peristalsis (see right).

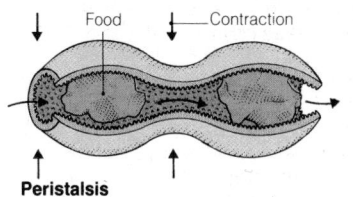

Food — Contraction

Peristalsis
This is an example of movement caused by involuntary muscle action. Waves of contraction pass along muscles in the intestinal wall, forcing the contents forwards and preventing obstruction.

M

the different parts of the body and the amount of contraction in each muscle. This information is integrated in specific areas of the brain (including the cerebellum and basal ganglia) that control coordination, initiation, and cessation of movement. Learning complex sequences (such as piano playing) involves the establishment of unconscious patterns of nerve activity in the cerebellum.

Skeletal movements can also occur as simple *reflexes* in response to certain sensory warning signals. In these instances, the movement is automatic and less controlled, involving far fewer nerve connections.

OTHER MOVEMENTS

Not all body movements involve the skeleton. Movements of the eyes and tongue are brought about by contractions of muscles attached to soft tissues. Again, they may be voluntary movements or reflexes. Movements of the internal organs are involuntary; they include the *heartbeat* and *peristalsis* (rhythmic contractions of the walls of the digestive tract).

DISORDERS

Disorders of the nervous system, muscles, joints, or bones may impair movement. (See *Nerve injury*; *Neuropathy*; *Brain* disorders box; *Spinal cord*; *Muscles* disorders box.)

Moxibustion

A form of treatment, often used in conjunction with *acupuncture*, in which a cone of wormwood leaves (moxa) or certain other plant materials is burned just above the skin to relieve internal pain. The burning material is thought to act as a counter-irritant, relieving deep-seated pain by irritating nerve endings in the skin.

MRI

Magnetic resonance imaging. MRI is a diagnostic technique that provides high-quality cross-sectional or three-dimensional images of organs and structures within the body without using X-rays or other radiation.

HOW IT WORKS

During the imaging, the patient lies inside a massive, hollow, cylindrical magnet. The nuclei (protons) of the body's hydrogen atoms normally point in random directions. In a magnetic field, however, these atoms line up parallel to each other, like rows of tiny magnets. If the hydrogen nuclei are then knocked out of alignment by a strong pulse of radio waves, they produce a detectable radio signal as they fall back into alignment.

MAGNETIC RESONANCE IMAGING (MRI)

A valuable diagnostic technique, MRI has been in use since the early 1980s. The patient lies down surrounded by a massive electromagnet and is exposed to short bursts of powerful magnetic fields and radio-waves. The bursts stimulate protons (hydrogen nuclei) in the patient's tissues to emit radio signals, which are detected and analysed by computer to create an image of a "slice" of the patient's body.

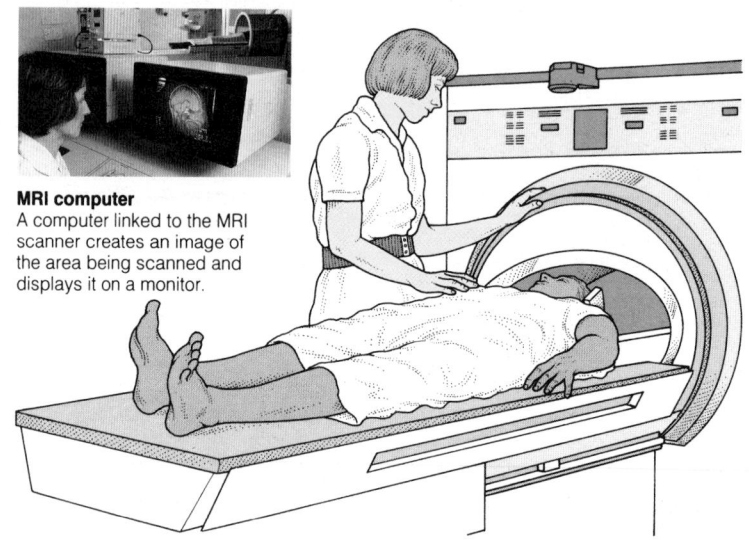

MRI computer
A computer linked to the MRI scanner creates an image of the area being scanned and displays it on a monitor.

THE SCANNING PROCESS

An MRI scanner consists of a powerful electromagnet, a radio-wave emitter, and a radio-wave detector. A plane of the body is selected for imaging and the electromagnet is turned on.

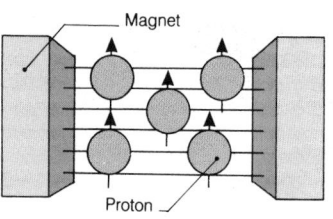

Magnet

Proton

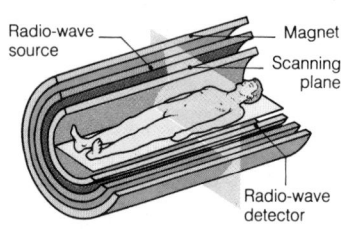

Radio-wave source

Magnet

Scanning plane

Radio-wave detector

1 Normally, the protons (nuclei) of the body's hydrogen atoms point randomly in different directions, but under the influence of the scanner's powerful magnetic field they align themselves in the same direction.

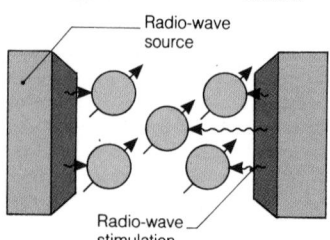

Radio-wave source

Radio-wave stimulation

2 Next, the radio-wave source emits a powerful pulse of radio-waves, the effect of which is to knock the protons out of alignment.

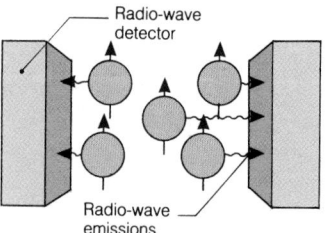

Radio-wave detector

Radio-wave emissions

3 However, milliseconds later, the protons realign themselves, emitting faint radio signals as they do; these signals are picked up by the scanner's radio-wave detector.

Magnetic coils in the machine detect these signals and a computer changes them into a cross-sectional or three-dimensional image based on the strength of signal produced by different types of tissue. Tissues that contain a lot of hydrogen (such as fat) produce a bright image; those that contain little or no hydrogen (such as bone) appear black.

WHY IT IS DONE

Images from MRI are similar in many ways to those produced by *CT scanning*, but MRI usually gives greater contrast between normal and abnormal tissues.

MRI is especially useful in studying the brain and spinal cord. White and grey matter, which are relatively poorly differentiated in CT scans, are distinct and well-defined in MRI scans. MRI provides clear images of tumours of the brain and spinal cord. Also shown clearly by MRI is the internal structure of the eye and ear.

MRI also produces detailed images of the heart and major blood vessels, provides images of blood flow, and is useful for examining joints and soft tissues, particularly in the knee. The role of MRI in imaging the abdominal organs is less established.

HOW IT IS DONE

MRI is usually an outpatient procedure. During the examination the patient must lie still; children may be given a general anaesthetic. A scan usually takes about half an hour.

RISKS

There are no known risks or side-effects to MRI. The technique does not use radiation and can therefore be performed repeatedly with no known adverse effects. However, any person fitted with a pacemaker, hearing aid, or other electrical device should tell his or her doctor before undergoing MRI, since the scanner may interfere with these devices.

OUTLOOK

MRI is not as widely available as CT scanning, but it has become routine in specialist hospitals, especially those for the investigation of nervous diseases. Magnetic resonance spectroscopy, a variation on MRI using other chemical elements, is being developed as a means of investigating the functioning of structures such as muscle and the heart.

MS

The abbreviation for *multiple sclerosis*.

MSG

The abbreviation for the food additive *monosodium glutamate*.

Mucocele

A swollen sac or cavity within the body that is filled with mucus secreted by its inner lining. A mucocele of the appendix is caused by narrowing of the opening of the appendix into the intestine. A mucocele of the gallbladder, sometimes called hydrops of the gallbladder, may be caused by a gallstone obstructing its outlet.

Mucolytic drugs

Drugs that make sputum (phlegm) less sticky and easier to cough up. An example is *acetylcysteine*.

Mucopolysaccharidosis

A group of inherited metabolic disorders (see *Metabolism, inborn errors of*). The best known of these disorders is *Hurler's syndrome;* others include Hunter's, Sanfillippo's, Morquio's, Maroteaux-Lamy, and Scheie's syndromes. The mucopolysaccharidoses are rare, collectively affecting about one child in 10,000.

All mucopolysaccharidoses are *genetic disorders* in which there is an abnormality of a specific *enzyme*. This abnormality affects the way carbohydrates are handled within body cells, leading to an accumulation in the tissues of unwanted substances called mucopolysaccharides.

Depending on the disease, features include abnormalities of the skeleton and/or the central nervous system (brain and spinal cord) with mental handicap and, in some cases, a characteristic facial appearance. There may also be clouding of the cornea, liver enlargement, and joint stiffness.

No specific treatment is available. Some children with Hurler's syndrome have been successfully treated by a *bone marrow transplant,* which provides them with a continuing source of the deficient enzyme.

Some mucopolysaccharidoses usually cause death during childhood or adolescence. Mild varieties may allow a reasonably normal life. Parents with a seriously affected child should receive *genetic counselling* concerning the risk of any future child being affected and information on whether antenatal diagnosis of the disorder is possible.

Mucosa

Another term for *mucous membrane*.

Mucous membrane

The soft, pink, skin-like layer that lines many of the cavities and tubes in the body, including the respiratory tract, digestive tract, the urinary and genital passages, and eyelids. Mucous membranes secrete a mucus-containing fluid which keeps body structures moist and well-lubricated. The fluid is produced and released on to the surface of the mucous membrane by millions of specialized cells, called goblet cells, situated within the membrane.

Mucus

The thick, slimy fluid secreted by *mucous membranes*. Mucus moistens, lubricates, and protects those parts of the body lined by mucous membrane, such as the digestive, respiratory, and genital tracts. Mucus eases swallowing, lubricates food as it passes through the digestive tract, prevents stomach acid from damaging the stomach wall, and prevents *enzymes* from digesting the intestine. In the respiratory tract, mucus moistens inhaled air and traps smoke and other foreign particles in the airways (to keep them out of the lungs). Mucus also facilitates sexual intercourse.

Mucus method of contraception

See *Contraception, natural methods of*.

Multiple myeloma

A malignant condition of middle to old age, also called myelomatosis. Multiple myeloma is characterized by the uncontrolled proliferation and disordered function of cells called plasma cells in the *bone marrow*.

Plasma cells are a type of B-*lymphocyte* (class of white blood cell) responsible for producing *immunoglobulins*, which normally help protect against infection. In multiple myeloma, the proliferating plasma cells produce an excessive amount of a single type of immunoglobulin while production of other types is impaired, making the patient prone to infection.

Multiple myeloma is rare. About 1,500 cases are diagnosed annually in the UK.

SYMPTOMS AND SIGNS

Proliferation of the abnormal plasma cells within bone causes pain and destruction of bone tissue. If the *vertebrae* are affected, they may collapse and compress nerves, causing symptoms such as numbness or paralysis. The level of calcium in the blood may increase markedly as bone is destroyed, as may the level of one or more of the immunoglobulins secreted by the plasma cells. These changes in the blood may damage the kidneys, leading to *kidney failure*.

M

In addition to the increased risk of infection, patients may suffer from *anaemia* and have a tendency to abnormal bleeding if healthy bone marrow is replaced by malignant plasma cells.

DIAGNOSIS, TREATMENT, AND OUTLOOK

The disease is diagnosed by a *bone marrow biopsy* (removal of a sample of tissue for microscopic analysis), which reveals an abnormal appearance; by blood or urine tests, which show an excess of specific immunoglobulins; and by X-rays, which indicate areas of destroyed bone.

Treatment includes the use of *anticancer drugs* to reduce the number of abnormal plasma cells, *radiotherapy* of diseased areas of bone, and various supportive measures, including *blood transfusions* to correct anaemia, *antibiotic drugs* to combat infections, and *analgesic drugs* to relieve pain.

The severity of the illness and the outlook vary, but only about one fifth of patients survive for four years or longer from the time of diagnosis.

Multiple personality

A rare disorder in which a person has two or more distinct personalities, each of which dominates at different times. The personalities are almost always very different from each other and are often total opposites, as in the story of Dr. Jekyll and Mr. Hyde.

Although multiple personality is often called split personality, a phrase also used to describe *schizophrenia*, the two disorders are unrelated. The split in schizophrenia is between thought and feeling.

Multiple pregnancy

See *Pregnancy, multiple.*

Multiple sclerosis

A progressive disease of the central *nervous system* in which scattered patches of *myelin* (the protective covering of nerve fibres) in the brain and spinal cord are destroyed. This causes symptoms ranging from numbness and tingling to *paralysis* and *incontinence*. The disease was formerly called disseminated sclerosis.

The severity of multiple sclerosis (MS) varies markedly among sufferers. It is characterized by a multiple, patchy pattern of disabilities, variable in site and time, with dramatic, unpredictable improvements. A patient may be severely disabled one week and apparently normal the next.

CAUSES

The cause of multiple sclerosis remains unknown. It is thought to be an *autoimmune disorder* in which the body's defence system begins to treat the myelin in the central nervous system as foreign, gradually destroying it, with subsequent scarring and damage to some of the underlying nerve fibres.

There seems to be a genetic factor since relatives of affected people are eight times more likely than others to contract the disease. Environment may also play a part—it is five times more common in temperate zones (such as Europe and the US) than in the tropics. Spending the first 15 years of life in a particular area seems to determine future risk—so that migrants from the UK to South Africa, for example, have a higher rate of the disease than their children born in South Africa. It is thought that a virus picked up by a susceptible person during this early period of life may be responsible for the disease's later development.

INCIDENCE

Multiple sclerosis is the most common acquired (not present at birth) disease of the nervous system in young adults. In the relatively high-risk temperate areas the incidence is approximately one in every 1,000 people. The ratio of women to men sufferers is three to two.

SYMPTOMS AND SIGNS

Multiple sclerosis usually starts in early adult life. It may be active briefly and then resume years later. The symptoms vary according to which parts of the brain and spinal cord are affected. Spinal cord damage can cause tingling, numbness, or a feeling of constriction in any part of the body. The extremities may feel heavy and become weak. *Spasticity* (increased rigidity) and paralysis sometimes develop. The nerve fibres to the bladder may be involved, causing incontinence.

Damage to the white matter in the brain may lead to fatigue, vertigo, clumsiness, muscle weakness, slurred speech, unsteady gait, blurred or double vision, and numbness, weakness, or pain in the face.

Symptoms may occur singly or in combination and may last from several weeks to several months. In some sufferers, relapses may be precipitated by injury, infection, or physical or emotional stress.

The severity of attacks varies considerably from one person to another. In some people, the disease consists of mild relapses and long symptom-free periods throughout life, with very few permanent effects. In others, a series of flare-ups leave some disability, but there is then no further deterioration. Some sufferers become gradually more disabled from the first attack and are bedridden and incontinent in early middle life. A few people suffer gross disability within the first year.

A person paralysed by multiple sclerosis may have additional problems, such as painful muscle spasms, urinary tract infections, constipation, skin ulceration, and changes of mood between euphoria and depression.

DIAGNOSIS

There is no single diagnostic test for multiple sclerosis, but typical appearances on *MRI*, of patchy damage to white matter, strongly suggest that the disease is present. *Evoked response tests* on the eyes, which measure the speed at which impulses travel along the optic nerve, also provide strong evidence.

TREATMENT

The search for a cure is still in progress. Many patients claim to have benefited from modifications to the diet, including the addition of sunflower or evening primrose oils. Treatment with *interferon* has been shown to slow the progress of the disease (which is measured by repeated examinations using MRI). Clinical trials are in progress in several countries to assess the long-term value of interferon treatment, which is expensive. Treatment with *hyperbaric oxygen*, which was acclaimed as effective in the 1970s and 1980s, was eventually shown by clinical trials to be of little value.

Individuals suffering from MS should be encouraged to adopt as positive an outlook as possible, and to lead as active a life as their disabilities allow. *Corticosteroid drugs* may be prescribed to alleviate the symptoms of an acute episode; other drugs may be given to control specific symptoms, such as incontinence and depression. *Physiotherapy* often helps strengthen muscles, and various aids can help patients maintain mobility and independence.

Multivitamins

A group of over-the-counter preparations containing a combination of *vitamins* that are used to supplement the intake of vitamins in the diet. (See *Vitamin supplements.*)

Mumps

An acute viral illness, mainly of childhood. The chief symptom is inflammation and swelling of one or both of the *parotid glands* situated just inside

FEATURES OF MULTIPLE SCLEROSIS

This disease can affect any area of the white matter of the brain and spinal cord. The plaques of demyelination are areas in which the fatty myelin sheaths of the nerve fibres have been destroyed. Affected fibres cannot conduct nerve impulses, so functions such as movement and sensation may be lost. The patchy distribution of plaques causes very varied effects.

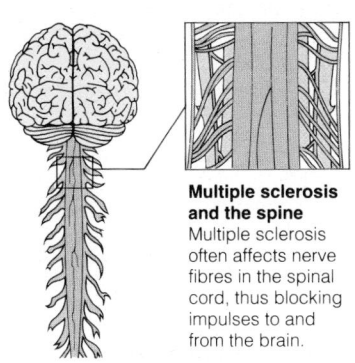

Multiple sclerosis and the spine

Multiple sclerosis often affects nerve fibres in the spinal cord, thus blocking impulses to and from the brain.

Effects of multiple sclerosis

The fibre of the nerve tract is not usually destroyed. But the loss of insulating myelin and its replacement by neuroglia alters normal ion movements, so that the fibre can no longer conduct impulses.

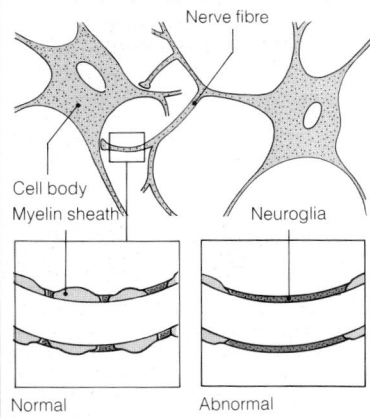

Nerve fibre

Cell body
Myelin sheath

Neuroglia

Normal   Abnormal

RANGE OF OUTLOOKS IN MULTIPLE SCLEROSIS

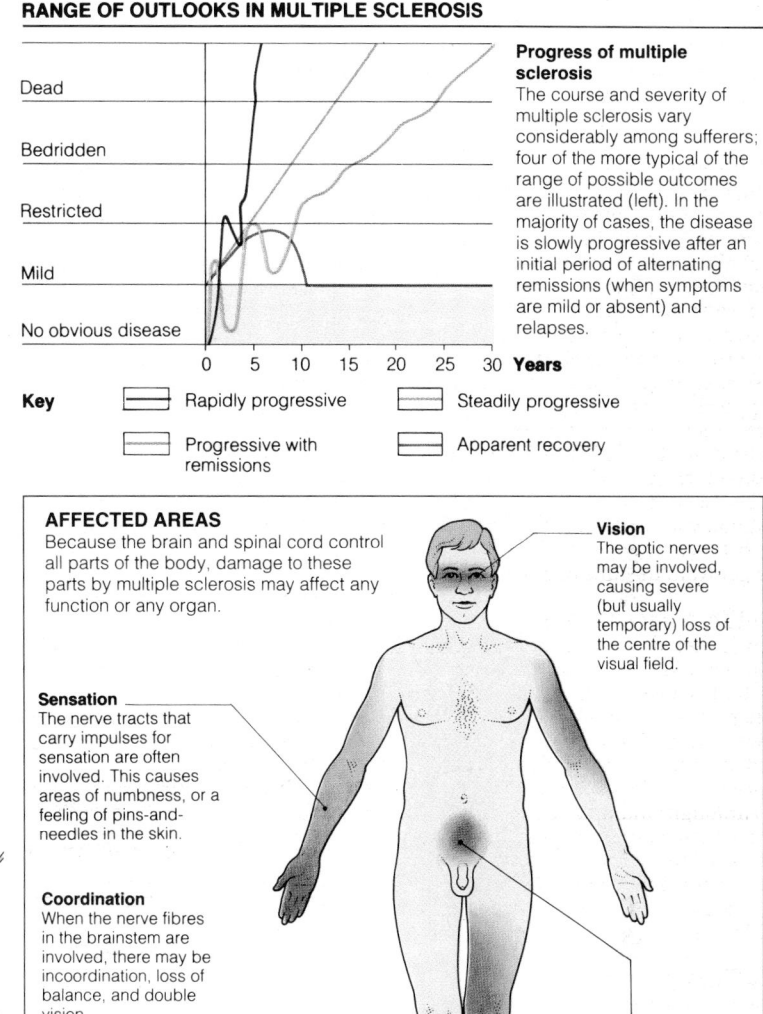

Progress of multiple sclerosis

The course and severity of multiple sclerosis vary considerably among sufferers; four of the more typical of the range of possible outcomes are illustrated (left). In the majority of cases, the disease is slowly progressive after an initial period of alternating remissions (when symptoms are mild or absent) and relapses.

Key

Rapidly progressive

Steadily progressive

Progressive with remissions

Apparent recovery

AFFECTED AREAS

Because the brain and spinal cord control all parts of the body, damage to these parts by multiple sclerosis may affect any function or any organ.

Vision
The optic nerves may be involved, causing severe (but usually temporary) loss of the centre of the visual field.

Sensation
The nerve tracts that carry impulses for sensation are often involved. This causes areas of numbness, or a feeling of pins-and-needles in the skin.

Coordination
When the nerve fibres in the brainstem are involved, there may be incoordination, loss of balance, and double vision.

Movement
Plaques on the long motor nerve tracts in the brain or spinal cord may affect walking, sometimes causing dragging of one leg or a feeling of weakness.

Bladder
In those severely affected by multiple sclerosis, spinal cord damage often leads to incontinence due to loss of sphincter control in the bladder.

M

the angle of the jaw. Serious complications are uncommon. However, in teenage and adult males, mumps can be a highly uncomfortable illness in which one or both *testes* become inflamed and swollen. One attack of mumps confers lifelong immunity to future attacks.

CAUSES AND INCIDENCE
The mumps virus is spread in airborne droplets. There is an incubation period of two to three weeks between infection and the appearance of symptoms. It is possible for an affected person to spread the virus to others for about a week before and up to two weeks after the symptoms appear. The majority of infections are acquired at school or from infected family members.

With the introduction into the UK (in 1988) of *MMR vaccination*, the disease has become much less common. In most parts of the country 90 per cent or more of children have now been vaccinated against the disease, and epidemics no longer occur.

SYMPTOMS AND COMPLICATIONS
Many infected children have no symptoms, or they may feel only slightly unwell and have some discomfort in the region of the parotid glands. In more serious cases,

M

the child first complains of pain in this region and has difficulty in chewing; the glands on one or both sides then become swollen, painful, and tender. Fever, headache, and swallowing difficulty may develop, but the temperature falls after two to three days and the swelling subsides within a week to 10 days. When only one side is affected, the second gland often swells as the swelling of the first gland subsides.

An occasional complication of mumps is *meningitis*, which can cause headache, photophobia (abnormal sensitivity to light), drowsiness, fever, and stiff neck. Mumps meningitis usually clears up without there being any long-term effects. A less common complication of mumps is *pancreatitis*, which causes abdominal pain and vomiting.

In males after puberty, *orchitis* (inflammation of the testis) develops in about a quarter of cases. Only one testis is usually affected, becoming swollen, tender, and painful for two to four days. Subsequently, the affected testis may shrink to smaller than normal size. In rare cases, mumps orchitis affects both testes, very occasionally leading to *infertility*. There is no evidence that mumps contracted during pregnancy has any effect on the fetus.

DIAGNOSIS AND TREATMENT
Mumps is usually diagnosed from the patient's symptoms. The diagnosis may be confirmed by measuring *antibodies* to the mumps virus in the blood or by culturing the virus from samples of saliva or urine.

There is no specific treatment, but an affected child may be given *analgesic drugs* (painkillers) and plenty to drink. In moderate to severe cases, the child may need to stay in bed during the first few days of the illness and should not go to school until symptoms have subsided.

For males with severe orchitis, a doctor may sometimes prescribe a stronger painkiller, and *corticosteroid drugs* to reduce inflammation.

IMMUNIZATION
MMR vaccine includes a safe and effective mumps vaccine in combination with vaccines for measles and rubella. It is given routinely in the UK to children in their second year. MMR vaccine may also be given at any time after this age but should not be given before the age of one. Mumps vaccine should not be given to anyone with risk factors for vaccination (see *Immunization*).

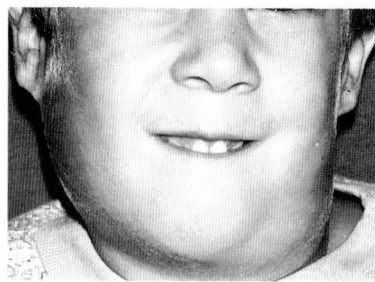

Appearance of mumps
The swelling, especially if present on both sides, may give the affected child a somewhat hamster-like appearance.

Males after puberty who have never had mumps or never been immunized against it should avoid contact with any infected person. If symptoms of mumps do develop, passive immunization with an *immunoglobulin* injection may provide some protection against the development of orchitis.

Munchausen's syndrome

A form of chronic *factitious disorder* in which the sufferer complains of physical symptoms that are pretended or self-induced. Sufferers are not *malingering*, they simply want to play the patient role. Most afflicted people are repeatedly hospitalized for investigations and treatment.

Pain in the abdomen, bleeding, neurological symptoms (such as dizziness and blackouts), skin rashes, and fever are the usual complaints. Sufferers typically invent dramatic, but often plausible, histories and, once in the hospital, behave disruptively. Many show evidence of self-injury or of previous treatment (such as numerous scars or detailed medical knowledge). In Munchausen's syndrome by proxy, parents cause factitious disorders in their children.

It is difficult to determine the causes of Munchausen's syndrome; when challenged, sufferers may deny any allegations of deception or may immediately discharge themselves from hospital. Treatment is aimed at protecting sufferers from unnecessary operations and treatments.

Murmur

A sound caused by turbulent blood flow through the *heart*, as heard by a doctor through a *stethoscope*. Murmurs are a separate phenomenon from other types of normal or abnormal *heart sounds*, which are caused mainly by sudden acceleration or deceleration of blood movement.

Heart murmurs are not necessarily a sign of disease, but an unusual sound is regarded as an indication of possible abnormality in the blood flow. Apart from "innocent" murmurs, the most common cause of extra blood turbulence is a disorder of the heart valves, such as stenosis (narrowing) or incompetence (leakage) with regurgitation. Murmurs can also be caused by some types of congenital heart disease (see *Heart disease, congenital*), such as a *septal defect* (hole in the heart) or *patent ductus arteriosus*, by *pericarditis* (inflammation of the membrane around the heart), or by other, rarer, conditions, such as a *myxoma* in a heart chamber.

By noting the location on the chest wall at which the murmur is best heard and the timing of the murmur in relation to the basic heart sounds, and by considering these factors in conjunction with other signs and symptoms, the doctor can usually arrive at a diagnosis, which may be confirmed by *echocardiography*.

Muscle

A structure composed of bundles of specialized cells capable of contraction and relaxation to create movement, both of the body itself in relation to the environment and of the organs within it. There are three types of muscle: skeletal, smooth, and cardiac.

SKELETAL MUSCLE
The largest part of the musculature consists of skeletal (voluntary) muscles; the body contains more than 600 such muscles.

Skeletal muscles are classified according to the type of action they perform. An extensor opens out a joint, a flexor closes it; an adductor draws a part of the body inwards, an abductor moves it outwards; a levator raises it, a depressor lowers it; and constrictor or sphincter muscles surround and close orifices.

Skeletal muscles are composed of groups of muscle fibres in an orderly arrangement. A small muscle may be made up of only a few bundles of fibres, while the major muscles in the body (such as the gluteus maximus that forms the bulk of the buttock) are made up of hundreds of bundles. A muscle fibre is made up of even smaller longitudinal units, called myofibrils, the basic working units of which are microscopic filaments of actin and myosin (two proteins that control contraction).

Movement of the skeletal muscles is under the voluntary control of the

THE BODY'S MUSCLES

The most prominent muscles in the body are the skeletal muscles, which account for 40 to 45 per cent of body weight. These muscles are called voluntary because they are under conscious control; some important voluntary muscles are indicated on the illustration below.

Many internal organs, such as the heart and intestines, also consist partly or entirely of involuntary muscle, which is not under conscious control.

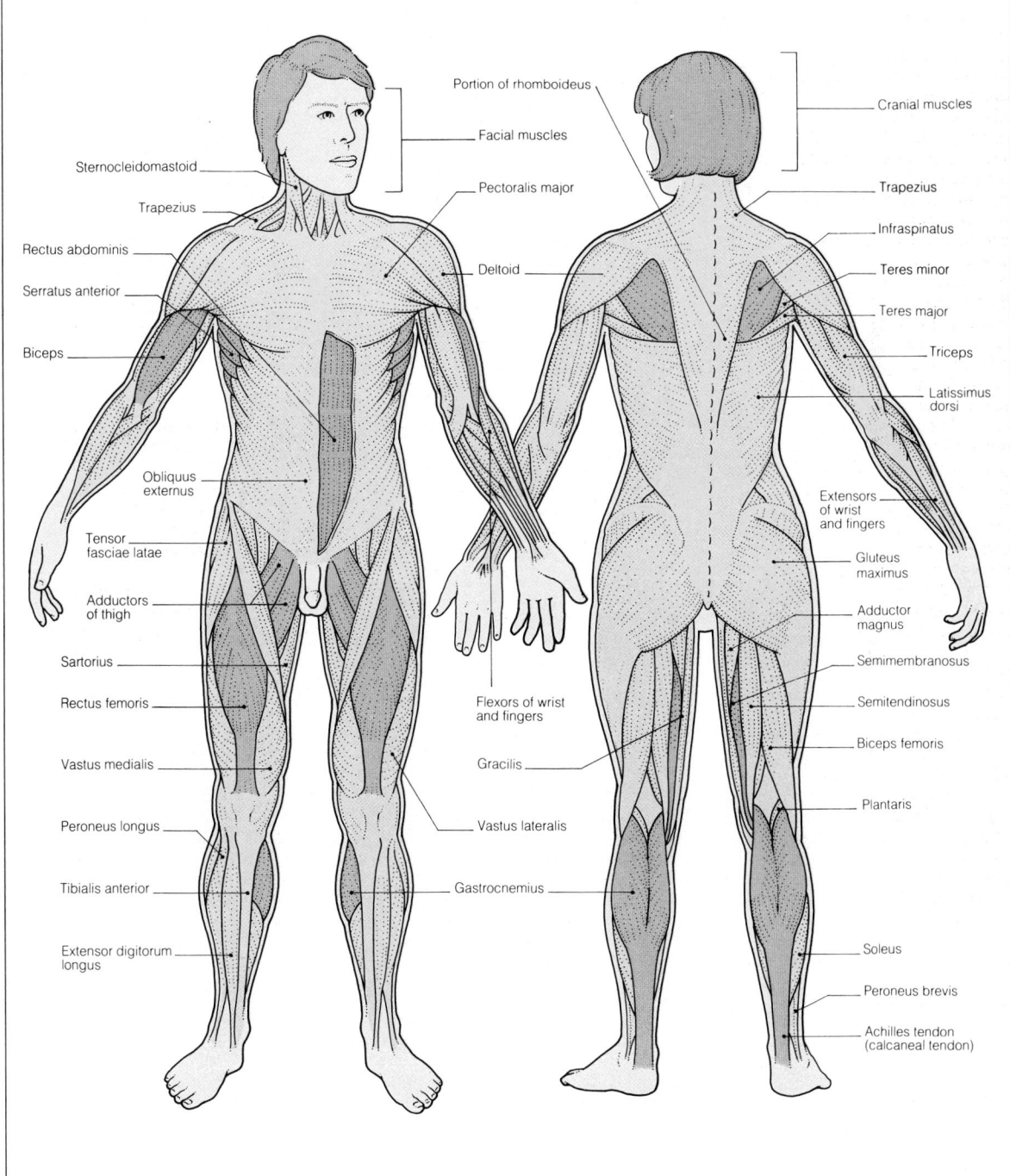

Portion of rhomboideus
Facial muscles
Sternocleidomastoid
Pectoralis major
Trapezius
Rectus abdominis
Deltoid
Serratus anterior
Biceps
Obliquus externus
Tensor fasciae latae
Adductors of thigh
Sartorius
Rectus femoris
Vastus medialis
Peroneus longus
Tibialis anterior
Extensor digitorum longus
Flexors of wrist and fingers
Gracilis
Vastus lateralis
Gastrocnemius

Cranial muscles
Trapezius
Infraspinatus
Teres minor
Teres major
Triceps
Latissimus dorsi
Extensors of wrist and fingers
Gluteus maximus
Adductor magnus
Semimembranosus
Semitendinosus
Biceps femoris
Plantaris
Soleus
Peroneus brevis
Achilles tendon (calcaneal tendon)

M

brain. Each muscle fibre is supplied with a nerve ending that receives impulses from the brain. The nerve impulses stimulate the muscle by releasing *acetylcholine*, a type of *neurotransmitter* (chemical released from nerve endings). This starts a chain of chemical and electrical events, involving sodium, potassium, and calcium ions, which results in the filaments of myosin sliding over the actin filaments in much the same way as an extendable ladder moves when it is being closed. This movement of myosin over actin filaments causes the muscle to contract (shorten).

Each muscle contains a set of specialized nerve fibres that register the force of contraction; another set in the tendon gauge the stretch. The information received by these fibres is transmitted to the brain and is vital in limiting muscle action.

Skeletal muscle is maintained in a state of partial contraction—called muscle tone. *Spasticity* is one form of abnormally increased muscle tone.

Skeletal muscle activity is affected by changes in chemical composition of the fluid surrounding the muscle cells. A fall in potassium ions causes muscle weakness; a decrease of calcium ions causes muscle spasm.

SMOOTH MUSCLE

This type of muscle is concerned with the movements of internal organs, such as *peristalsis* in the intestine and contractions of the uterus during childbirth. Many other parts of the body, such as the bronchi of the lungs, the bladder, and the walls of blood vessels, also contain smooth muscle.

Smooth muscle is composed of long, spindle-shaped cells. In most hollow organs, these cells are arranged in bundles organized in an outer longitudinal layer and an inner circular one. However, the mechanism of contraction relies on the same sliding action of actin and myosin as in skeletal muscle.

The nerve supply to smooth muscle comes from the *autonomic nervous system*, which is not under conscious control. Hence, its alternative name—involuntary muscle. Nerves from the autonomic nervous system penetrate into the muscle, where they divide into many branches. Neurotransmitter release from these nerves initiates the process that leads to contraction.

As well as responding to neurotransmitters, smooth muscle also responds to various *hormones*, to the stretch of individual muscle fibres, and to changes in the chemical composition of the fluid surrounding the fibres (e.g. changes in acidity).

CARDIAC MUSCLE

This type of muscle, also called myocardium, is found only in the *heart*; it has unique properties that enable it to contract rhythmically about 100,000 times a day to propel blood through the circulatory system. The structure of cardiac muscle resembles that of skeletal muscle.

Contraction of cardiac muscle is stimulated by the autonomic nervous system, by hormones, and by the stretching of muscle fibres.

To act as an efficient pump, the muscles of the heart must contract in an orderly, regular manner. Separate muscle fibres are joined end to end by areas of extensive folds that allow contractions to be transmitted rapidly from one fibre to another. The stimulus for cardiac muscle contraction is initiated in an area of the right atrium (called the sinoatrial node), which stimulates a regular rate of contrac-

tion. Specialized conducting cells in cardiac muscle form a network capable of transmitting nerve impulses throughout the cardiac muscle fibres, spreading the contraction through both atria and then both ventricles alternately (see *Heart*).

MUSCLE MOVEMENT

Contraction makes a muscle shorter and draws together the bones to which the muscle is attached.

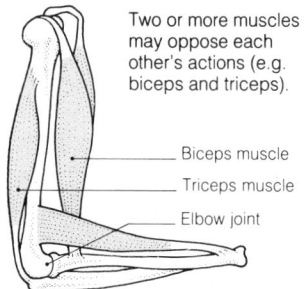

Two or more muscles may oppose each other's actions (e.g. biceps and triceps).

Biceps muscle
Triceps muscle
Elbow joint

Controlled movement at the elbow relies on coordinated relaxation and contraction of the biceps and triceps.

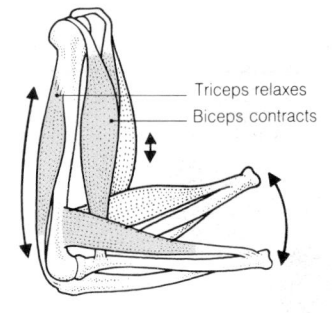

Triceps relaxes
Biceps contracts

MUSCLE TYPES

Skeletal and cardiac muscles appear striped under the microscope, unlike smooth muscles.

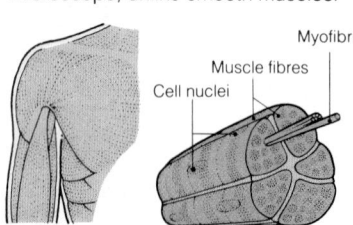

Myofibril
Muscle fibres
Cell nuclei

Skeletal muscle
Skeletal muscle consists of bundles of fibres (muscle cells), each containing contractile elements (myofibrils).

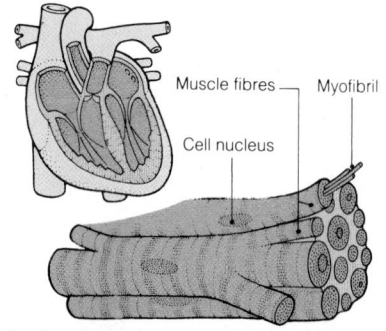

Muscle fibres — Myofibril
Cell nucleus

Cardiac muscle
Cardiac muscle contains short, branching cells that interconnect to help spread the signals that cause contraction.

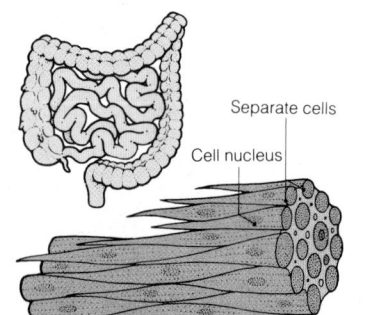

Separate cells
Cell nucleus

Smooth muscle
Smooth muscle consists of more loosely woven, tapering cells. Contraction is slower than in other muscle types.

M

Muscle-relaxant drugs

A group of drugs used to relieve *muscle spasm* and *spasticity*. Muscle-relaxant drugs are often used in combination with an *analgesic drug* (painkiller) to relieve muscle stiffness caused by types of *arthritis*, *back pain*, or a disorder of the *nervous system*, such as a *stroke* or *cerebral palsy*. Muscle-relaxant drugs are occasionally used to relieve muscle rigidity caused by injury.

HOW THEY WORK

Except for *dantrolene*, muscle-relaxant drugs partly block nerve signals from the brain and spinal cord that stimulate muscles to contract.

Dantrolene acts directly on muscles by interfering with the chemical activity in muscle cells that is necessary for muscle contraction.

POSSIBLE ADVERSE EFFECTS

Because muscle-relaxant drugs reduce the strength of muscle contraction, they may cause weakness which is noticed when performing certain activities. Also, some muscle-relaxant drugs cause drowsiness. In rare cases, dantrolene causes liver damage.

Muscle spasm

Sudden involuntary contraction of a muscle. Muscle spasm is a normal reaction to pain and inflammation around a joint. Common causes of muscle spasm include muscle *strain*, other musculoskeletal injuries, pressure on a nerve from a *disc prolapse*, poor posture, and stress.

Treatment is usually directed at the cause of the spasm. In some cases, *muscle-relaxant drugs* may also be needed. (See also *Spasticity*.)

Muscular dystrophy

A group of muscle disorders, due to genetic defects, which lead to slow but progressive degeneration of muscle fibres. Different forms of muscular dystrophy are classified according to the age at which the symptoms

---

DISORDERS OF MUSCLE

The most common muscle disorder is injury, followed by symptoms caused by a lack of blood supply to a muscle (including the heart). In addition, there are a number of other, rarer disorders of muscle.

GENETIC DISORDERS

The *muscular dystrophies* cause progressive weakness and disability. Some types appear at birth, some in infancy, and some develop as late as the fifth or sixth decade.

One type of *cardiomyopathy*, a general term for disease of the heart muscle, is inherited.

INFECTION

The most important infection of muscle is *gangrene*, which may complicate deep wounds (especially those contaminated by soil). *Tetanus* is acquired in a similar way, causing widespread muscle spasm through the release of a powerful toxin.

Viruses (especially influenza B) may also infect muscles (causing *myalgia*, as may the organism causing *toxoplasmosis*. *Trichinosis* is an infestation of muscle with the worm TRICHINELLA SPIRALIS, which is acquired by eating undercooked meat (usually pork).

INJURY

Muscle injuries, such as tears and *strains*, are very common; they cause bleeding into the muscle tissue. Healing leads to formation of a scar in the muscle, which shortens its natural length. Blunt muscle injury may result in *haematoma* formation from bleeding into the muscle. Rarely, bone may form in the blood clot, causing *myositis* ossificans.

TUMOURS

Primary muscle tumours may or may not be cancerous. Noncancerous tumours are called *myomas*, those affecting smooth muscle are *leiomyomas*, and those affecting skeletal muscle are rhabdomyomas. Myomas of the uterus (see *Fibroids*) are among the most common of all tumours. Cancerous tumours are called myosarcomas and are very rare; cancers of the skeletal muscle are known as *rhabdomyosarcomas*.

Secondary tumours, which spread from a primary site of cancer elsewhere in the body, very rarely involve muscle.

HORMONAL AND METABOLIC DISORDERS

Muscle contraction depends on the maintenance of proper levels of sodium, potassium, and calcium in and around muscle cells. Any alteration in the concentration of these substances affects muscle function. For example, a severe drop in the level of potassium (hypokalaemia) causes profound muscle weakness and may stop the heart. A drop in blood calcium (hypocalcaemia) causes increased excitability of muscles and, occasionally, spasms.

Thyroid disease is often associated with muscle disorders, the most common being a swelling of the small muscles that move the eyes, causing a bulging eyeball (see *Exophthalmos*).

Adrenal failure causes general muscle weakness.

IMPAIRED BLOOD SUPPLY

Muscles depend on a good blood supply for normal function. *Cramp* is usually caused by a lack of blood flow, sometimes associated with severe exertion. *Peripheral vascular disease*, which restricts the blood supply,

causes *claudication* (muscle pain on exercise). *Angina pectoris* (chest pain caused by lack of blood supply to heart muscle) occurs in *coronary artery disease*.

The *compartment syndrome* is pain in muscles as a result of pressure that limits their blood supply. It may be brought on by injury or exercise, and occurs most often in athletes with well-developed muscles.

POISONS AND DRUGS

Several toxic substances can damage muscle. They include alcohol, which can cause damage following a prolonged drinking bout. Other substances that may cause muscle damage include aminocaproic acid, chloroquine, clofibrate, emetine, and vincristine.

AUTOIMMUNE DISORDERS

Myasthenia gravis is a disorder of transmission of nerve impulses to muscles; it usually begins by causing drooping of the eyelids and double vision. Other diseases with an autoimmune basis that may affect muscles are *lupus erythematosus*, *rheumatoid arthritis*, *scleroderma*, *sarcoidosis*, and *dermatomyositis*.

INVESTIGATION

Muscle disorders are investigated by *EMG* (electromyography), which measures the response of muscles to electrical impulses, and by muscle *biopsy* (removal of a sample of tissue for analysis).

M

DUCHENNE MUSCULAR DYSTROPHY: A TYPICAL FAMILY TREE

Key

Unaffected male

Affected male

Carrier female

? Possible carrier female

Unaffected female

Affected males always inherit the gene for the disorder from their mothers, who are carriers of the gene, although unaffected themselves. About half the sons of carriers are affected; the other sons are neither affected nor carriers. The

daughters of carriers have a 50 per cent chance of being carriers themselves; complex blood tests provide the only means of knowing whether or not a certain daughter (or granddaughter) is a muscular dystrophy carrier.

appear, the rate at which the disease progresses, and the way in which it is inherited. (See box for main types.)

INCIDENCE
All forms of muscular dystrophy are rare. Duchenne muscular dystrophy is the most common and most severe type, affecting about one in 3,000 boys. It is inherited through a recessive, sex-linked gene (see *Genetic disorders*) so that only males are affected and only females can pass on the disease. Other types of muscular dystrophy include Becker's, limb-girdle, facioscapulohumeral, and myotonic dystrophies. These may affect children and adults and are due to autosomal or to sex-linked defects.

DIAGNOSIS
Identification of the gene for Duchenne muscular dystrophy has made diagnosis possible in most cases even before symptoms develop. Once muscle weakness is apparent other tests become useful, including measurement of muscle *enzymes* and an *EMG* (a test for electrical activity in the muscles).

TREATMENT AND OUTLOOK
There is no effective treatment for muscular dystrophy. An affected child should remain active for as long as possible to keep the healthy muscles in good condition. Sufferers should not be allowed to become overweight. Surgery to the heel tendons may assist walking in some

cases. The long-term outlook depends on the type of muscular dystrophy.

PREVENTION
Families in which a child or adult has developed any form of muscular dystrophy should receive *genetic counselling*. Rapid progress is being made in the understanding of the genetic defects responsible and how the muscles become affected. Reliable tests are now available in most cases to determine whether or not family members are carriers of a defective gene; those found to carry the gene may be offered help if they are planning to have children. *IVF* may be used to ensure that any children born do not have the disease. Antenatal *chorionic villus sampling* and termination of a pregnancy may also be considered.

Musculoskeletal
Relating to muscle and/or bone. The musculoskeletal system is the bony skeleton of the body and the hundreds of muscles attached to it.

Mushroom poisoning
There are many species of poisonous mushrooms and toadstools in the UK, but only some of them cause poisoning. Many of the others have an unpleasant taste and are thus unlikely to be eaten in sufficient amounts to cause problems.

TYPES, SYMPTOMS, AND TREATMENT
Most fatal cases of mushroom poisoning in the UK are caused by *AMANITA PHALLOIDES* (the death cap), which bears a superficial resemblance to the edible field mushroom. There are some clear differences, however. The death cap grows in deciduous woods (mainly beech and oak), has a yellow-olive-coloured cap, and, most importantly, has white gills on the underside of its cap (not pink-brown as on the edible field mushroom).

The death cap and one or two related species, such as *AMANITA VIROSA* (the destroying angel), contain highly poisonous peptides called amanitins, which attack cells in the lining of the small intestine, the liver, and, occasionally, the kidneys. Symptoms such as severe abdominal pain, vomiting, and diarrhoea usually develop eight to 14 hours after eating the mushroom. Later, there may be liver enlargement and jaundice; about 10 to 15 per cent of victims die of *liver failure* (this stage of the poisoning resembles acute viral hepatitis). There is no effective antidote. Treatment consists of supportive measures in hospital. For those who survive the poisoning, recovery is usually fairly rapid after about one week's illness.

Another species, *AMANITA MUSCARIA*, or fly agaric, is very similar in shape to the death cap but has a red cap flecked with white. Symptoms of poisoning, which appear within 20 minutes to two hours, may include drowsiness, visual disturbances, delirium, muscle tremors, and nausea and vomiting. Treatment of this type of mushroom poisoning, and of other types in which symptoms develop rapidly, is by gastric lavage (see *Lavage, gastric*) and the administration of activated charcoal. Full recovery usually occurs within 24 hours.

"Magic" mushrooms are a species containing the hallucinogenic substance *psilocybin*. As well as hallucinations, these mushrooms may cause high fever in children, which requires medical attention. The effects usually subside within four to six hours but occasionally they persist longer.

Mutagen
Any physical or chemical agent that, when applied to a group of living cells, increases the rate of *mutation* in those cells. A mutation is a change in the genetic material within a cell, which may, under certain circumstances, give rise to a cancer or a hereditary disease.

M

TYPES OF MUSCULAR DYSTROPHY

Duchenne muscular dystrophy	In this type, the child is slow in learning to sit up and walk, and does so much later than normal. The condition is rarely diagnosed before the age of three, but progresses rapidly. Affected children tend to walk with a waddle and have difficulty climbing stairs. In getting up from the floor, the child "climbs up his legs", pushing his hands against his ankles, knees, and thighs. Sometimes there	is curvature of the spine. Despite their weakness, the muscles (especially those in the calves) appear bulky; this is because wasted muscle is replaced by fat. By about the age of 12, affected children are no longer able to walk; few survive beyond their teenage years, usually dying from a chest infection or heart failure. Affected boys often have below-average intelligence.
Becker's muscular dystrophy	This type produces the same symptoms as the Duchenne type, but starts later in childhood and progresses much more	slowly. Patients often reach the age of 50. Both types of dystrophy have sex-linked inheritance.
Myotonic dystrophy	This form affects muscles of the hands and feet. Infants are floppy and slow to develop. The main feature is that the muscles contract strongly but do not relax easily. Myotonic dystrophy	is associated with cataracts in middle age, baldness, mental retardation, and endocrine problems. The condition has an autosomal dominant pattern of inheritance.
Limb-girdle muscular dystrophy	This type takes different forms. It starts in late childhood or early adult life, and progression is slow. The muscles of the hips and shoulders are mainly	affected. Other nerve and muscle conditions must be eliminated before this form of dystrophy can be diagnosed confidently.
Facioscapulohumeral muscular dystrophy	This form usually appears first between the ages of 10 and 40; it affects only the muscles of the upper arms, shoulder girdle, and face. It is inherited in an autosomal	dominant pattern. In this form of muscular dystrophy, progression of the weakness is slow, and severe disability is rare.

The main mutagens are ionizing *radiation* and some chemicals. The former includes X-rays, cosmic rays, and various emissions (e.g. alpha and beta particles, and gamma rays) from nuclear explosions, radioactive fallout, and reactor leaks (see *Radiation hazards*). Similar types of radiation are also emitted (at very low intensity) by certain rocks.

Many chemical *carcinogens* are thought to cause cancers by altering the genetic material within cells, thus acting as mutagens. Chief among them are chemicals in tobacco smoke.

Mutation

A change in a cell's *DNA* (the genetic material contained in *chromosomes* which provides the coded instructions for the cell's activities). Many mutations are neutral or harmless; some are harmful, giving rise to *cancers*, *birth defects*, and hereditary diseases. Very rarely, a mutation may be beneficial.

CAUSES

A mutation results from a fault in the replication of a cell's DNA in its daughter cells when the cell divides. A daughter cell inherits some faulty DNA, and the fault is copied each time the cell divides, creating a population of cells containing the altered DNA.

Some mutations occur by chance. A steady but low rate of random mutations is caused by natural background *radiation* from the sky and from radioactivity in rocks. Any physical or chemical agent that makes mutations more probable is known as a *mutagen*.

The most important mutagens are various types of high-energy radiation (see *Radiation hazards*), and certain chemicals, including some *carcinogens* (cancer-inducing agents), such as the chemicals in tobacco smoke.

TYPES

Some mutations, known as point mutations, affect only a small part of a section of DNA (called a *gene*). Point mutations may lead to the production of defective enzymes or other proteins in the affected cells, thus disrupting their activities.

In other mutations, entire chromosomes or bits of chromosomes are deleted, added, or rearranged in affected cells. This type of mutation may produce greater disruptive effects than a point mutation.

EFFECTS

The effects of a harmful mutation depend on whether the affected cell is a "germ" cell in an ovary or testis (capable of giving rise to an egg or sperm) or whether it is a somatic cell (one of the other cells in the body).

A mutated somatic cell can, at worst, multiply to form a group of abnormal cells within a particular body region. Often these cells die out, are destroyed by the body's *immune system*, or have only a minor local effect. Sometimes, however, they may form the basis for a tumour.

A mutation in a germ cell can have a dramatically different effect. It may be passed on, via an egg or sperm, to a child, who then carries the mutation in all of his or her cells. This may lead to an obvious birth defect or to an abnormality in body chemistry. Furthermore, the child may pass on the mutation to some of his or her descendants. *Genetic disorders* (such as *haemophilia* and *achondroplasia*) stem originally from point mutations that have occurred to the germ cell of a parent, grandparent, or more distant ancestor. Some of these mutations occur frequently; about one third of all cases of haemophilia are caused by new mutations. *Chromosomal abnormalities* (such as *Down's syndrome*) generally result from mutations in the formation of a parental egg or sperm.

BENEFICIAL MUTATIONS

Very rarely, a mutation in a germ cell confers a survival advantage in the face of some environmental stress. People who inherit this mutation tend to survive longer than their peers; some of their children in turn inherit the mutation and pass it on to succeeding generations. Such mutations tend to become more common in a population over many generations as long as the original environmental stress persists.

An example is the mutation that causes sickle cell trait. Carrying this mutation protects against malaria, so it enhances a child's survival chances where malaria is prevalent. The mutation is common in Africa itself and also affects many people of African origin. A double dose of the mutation (inheriting it from both parents) can lead to *sickle cell anaemia*.

Mutism

Refusal or inability to speak. Mutism may occur as a symptom of profound congenital *deafness*, severe *manic-depressive illness*, catatonic *schizophrenia*, or a rare form of *conversion disorder*. The term may also be applied to the observance of a vow of silence for religious reasons.

Elective mutism describes a rare childhood disorder usually starting before the age of five. The child understands language and speaks properly, but refuses to speak most of the time, preferring to use nods or gestures. A shy, withdrawn personality and anxiety about social situations are important factors. In some cases, mild mental handicap or language problems may be the cause. This condition rarely lasts more than a few months.

Akinetic mutism describes a state of inert passivity that is caused by certain deep-seated tumours of the brain or by *hydrocephalus*. Though conscious and capable of following movements with their eyes, people with akinetic mutism are incontinent, require feeding, and respond at most with a whispered "yes" or "no".

Treatment of mutism depends on the underlying cause.

Myalgia

The medical term for *muscle* pain. Myalgia is common in viral illnesses (such as influenza) and also occurs in a number of rheumatic disorders, such as *rheumatoid arthritis*, systemic *lupus erythematosus*, and *polymyalgia rheumatica*. Myalgia is the main symptom of *polymyositis* and *dermatomyositis*, disorders that cause inflammation of muscle tissue.

Myalgic encephalomyelitis

A disorder of unknown cause characterized by severe muscle fatigue on exertion, also known as ME, post-viral fatigue syndrome, Iceland disease, epidemic neuromyasthemia, and Royal Free disease.

CAUSES AND INCIDENCE

Much debate surrounds the causes and nature of myalgic encephalomyelitis. In particular, there is dispute as to whether the condition is separate from other chronic fatigue syndromes, including that associated with viral infections such as infectious mononucleosis (see *Mononucleosis, infectious*). Some doctors claim that most sufferers have a psychiatric disorder, most often a form of depression, but this explanation is strongly rejected by many people with the disease, and by some doctors researching it.

Myalgic encephalomyelitis sometimes occurs in epidemics, but isolated cases also occur. Females are affected three times more often than males; the peak incidence is between the ages of 30 and 40. The diagnosis became more frequent in the late 1980s as a result of press publicity.

SYMPTOMS

The disorder commonly follows an upper respiratory tract infection or a gastrointestinal infection, from which the sufferer does not fully recover. Fever and headache are followed by muscle pains, tenderness, weakness, and severe muscle fatigue, particularly on exertion. There may also be general malaise, dizziness, nausea, numbness, and a pins-and-needles sensation. Psychological upset, including depression, loss of concentration and memory, sleep disturbances, and panic states are common. The condition usually disappears in time, but in a few cases symptoms persist over a number of years, sometimes exacerbated by stress.

DIAGNOSIS AND TREATMENT

There is, as yet, no diagnostic test for myalgic encephalomyelitis; the diagnosis is reached by excluding other disorders which could account for the symptoms. A full neurological assessment should be made to exclude some rare conditions, such as *myopathies* and myasthenic syndromes. In myalgic encephalomyelitis physical examination and laboratory tests produce normal results, although a high proportion of patients show evidence of recent or current viral infection.

There is no specific curative treatment. Patients may be advised to rest early in the course of the illness, but to take exercise when they feel well enough. Some sufferers may benefit from *psychotherapy*, and some from avoiding alcohol and caffeine. Many patients try self-treatment by diet, or by using antifungal treatments (in the belief that the disease is linked to *candidiasis*).

Myasthenia gravis

A disorder in which the muscles become weak and tire easily. The eyes, face, throat, and limb muscles are most commonly affected. Typically, the sufferer has drooping eyelids, a blank facial expression, and weak, hesitant speech.

CAUSES AND INCIDENCE

Myasthenia gravis is an *autoimmune disorder* in which, for reasons that are not known, the body's *immune system* attacks and slowly destroys the receptors in muscles responsible for picking up nerve impulses. Affected muscles then fail to respond or respond only weakly to nerve impulses.

Myasthenia gravis is a rare disease; two to five new cases per 100,000 people are diagnosed annually in the UK. It affects more women than men (in a ratio of three to two). Although it can occur at any age, myasthenia gravis usually appears between the ages of 20 and 30 in women, and 50 and 70 in men.

SYMPTOMS AND SIGNS

The disease may develop suddenly or gradually. It is extremely variable in the way it affects different people and in how it affects the same person from day to day. The affected muscles become worse with use but may recover completely with rest. Symptom-free periods typically alternate with relapses of the condition.

The eye muscles are the most commonly affected, and most sufferers have drooping eyelids and double vision. Muscle weakness is also common in the face, throat, larynx (voicebox), and neck. This causes difficulty in speaking: the voice becoming weak, hoarse, nasal, and slurred towards the end of a conversation. Chewing and swallowing become more difficult as a meal progresses, so that the sufferer may choke or regurgitate food through the nose. Sometimes the jaw must be supported to prevent it from hanging.

In some people, the arm and leg muscles are also affected, producing difficulty in combing the hair and in climbing stairs. In severe cases, respiratory muscles may be weakened, causing breathing difficulty. Infection, menstruation, medications, stress, and other factors can worsen the condition.

Abnormalities in the *thymus* gland are present in about three quarters of affected people and, in about 10 to 15 per cent of them, a *thymoma* (tumour of the thymus gland) is found.

DIAGNOSIS

The disease is diagnosed by a physical examination, the patient's history, and various tests. The most commonly used diagnostic test involves the injection of the drug edrophonium into a vein. Within a minute, power is temporarily restored to the weak muscles. *EMG*, which detects muscle weakness by measuring the muscle's electrical activity, and blood tests that reveal the presence of certain *antibodies* may also be performed.

In some patients, mainly those over 40, *CT scanning* or *MRI* may be performed to look for a thymoma.

TREATMENT
In mild cases of myasthenia gravis, regular medication with drugs to facilitate the transmission of nerve impulses to the muscles is often sufficient to restore the patient's condition to near normal.

In severe myasthenia gravis, thymectomy (removal of the thymus gland) often considerably improves, and sometimes cures, the condition. Otherwise, regular exchanges of the patient's antibody-containing plasma for antibody-free plasma may be carried out. High doses of *corticosteroid drugs*, which block the immune process, are sometimes given.

OUTLOOK
In mild cases, the sufferer is able to live a comparatively normal life. In a minority of patients, progression of the disease cannot be halted and paralysis of the throat and respiratory muscles may lead to death.

Mycetoma

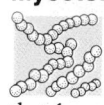 An uncommon tropical infection affecting skin and bone, caused by fungi or by actinomycetes (bacteria that form long chain-like colonies).

The infection is usually confined to one limb and can be highly disfiguring. It produces a hard swelling covered by the openings of multiple drainage channels, through which pus is discharged. The disease organisms form into visible "grains", which are found in the discharge.

Antibiotic drugs are the main treatment if the disease is caused by actinomycetes. Mycetoma caused by fungal infections may be difficult to treat with drugs; surgical removal of diseased tissue may be necessary.

Mycology

The study of *fungi* and *fungal infections.*

Mycoplasma

Any of a group of microorganisms which are the smallest capable of free existence. Mycoplasmas are about the same size as viruses and, like viruses, have no cell wall. However, unlike viruses, mycoplasmas can reproduce outside living cells.

Most types of mycoplasma are harmless to humans, although many cause respiratory diseases in animals such as cattle, sheep, and poultry. One species, MYCOPLASMA PNEUMONIAE, causes a form of *pneumonia* (primary atypical pneumonia) in humans. Pneumonia of this type can be treated effectively with antibiotics, such as *tetracycline drugs*.

Mycosis

Any disease caused by a fungus. (See *Fungi; Fungal infections.*)

Mycosis fungoides

A type of *lymphoma* (cancerous tumour of lymphoid tissue) that primarily affects the skin of the buttocks, back, or shoulders but can also occur in other sites. The cause of this rare disorder is unknown.

In its mildest form, mycosis fungoides produces a red, scaly, rash that does not itch. The rash may spread slowly or remain unaltered for many years. In the more severe forms of the disease, thickened patches of skin and ulcers may develop and *lymph nodes* may enlarge.

DIAGNOSIS AND TREATMENT
A skin *biopsy* (removal of a sample of tissue for examination) is performed to confirm the diagnosis.

Mild cases of the disease are treated with *PUVA* (psoralen drugs plus longwave ultraviolet light treatment) or nitrogen mustard applied to the skin. In more severe cases, *anticancer drugs* may be needed.

Mydriasis

Dilation (widening) of the pupil of the eye. Mydriasis, which occurs naturally in the dark, also occurs if a person is emotionally aroused, after the use of certain eye-drops (such as those containing *atropine*), and after consumption of alcohol.

Adie's syndrome is a benign condition in which one pupil constricts slowly in response to light.

Myectomy

Surgical removal of part or all of a muscle. Myectomy may be performed to alter the power of an eye muscle to correct a *squint*, or to remove a fibroid of the uterus in an operation called a *myomectomy.* Myectomy is also part of the treatment of severely injured and infected muscles.

Myel-

A prefix that denotes a relationship to *bone marrow* (as in *multiple myeloma*, a disorder in which certain bone marrow cells proliferate) or to the *spinal cord* (as in *myelitis*, inflammation of the spinal cord). The prefix myelo- is synonymous with myel-.

Myelin

The fatty material, composed of lipid (fat) and protein, that forms a protective sheath around some types of nerve fibre. Myelin gives the characteristic appearance to the white matter of the brain, which is composed largely of myelinated nerve fibres. In addition to having a protective function, myelin acts as an electrical insulator, thereby increasing the efficiency of nerve impulse conduction.

Abnormal breakdown of myelin is called *demyelination*. It occurs in some diseases of the nervous system, notably *multiple sclerosis*.

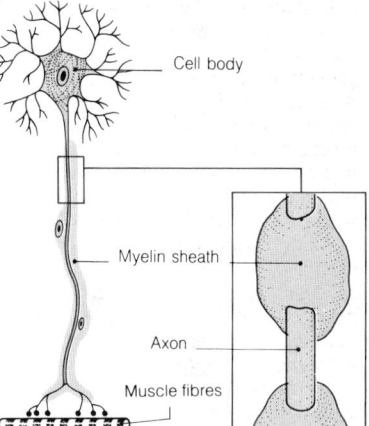

Cell body

Myelin sheath

Axon

Muscle fibres

The myelin nerve sheath
The axon is the conducting fibre of a nerve. To transmit impulses more efficiently, some nerve axons have a myelin sheath.

Myelitis

Inflammation of the spinal cord. Myelitis may be the result of a viral infection—for example, *poliomyelitis* (commonly called polio), *measles*, or *herpes simplex*. The disorder starts suddenly with headache, fever, neck stiffness, and pain in the back and limbs, followed in some cases by muscle pain and weakness, and eventually by paralysis.

Transverse myelitis is a type of myelitis in which there is inflammation of the spinal cord around the middle of the back. The condition may follow a viral illness but often occurs

M

without obvious cause. Common symptoms are back pain and gradual paralysis of the legs. Many people recover, but some are left with *spastic paralysis* of the limbs involved.

Myelocele

A protrusion of the *spinal cord* and its meninges (protective coverings) under the skin due to a congenital defect in the vertebral column (see *Spina bifida*).

Myelography

X-ray examination of the spinal cord, nerves, and other tissues within the spinal canal after injection of a contrast medium (a substance that is opaque to X-rays).

WHY IT IS DONE
In the past, myelography was performed to examine the lower spinal nerves when a *disc prolapse* was suspected; it was also important in diagnosing tumours of the spinal cord, and in locating damaged nerves. Myelography is being replaced today by newer imaging techniques, such as *CT scanning* and *MRI*.

HOW IT IS DONE
The patient lies on the X-ray table. After giving a local anaesthetic, a *lumbar puncture* is performed, using X-ray control to guide a fine needle into the fluid-filled space that surrounds the spinal cord and spinal nerves. A small sample of spinal fluid is withdrawn for testing, and the radiopaque contrast medium is introduced. By tilting the patient head-down, the contrast medium can be moved up the spinal canal. X-ray pictures are then taken of areas where damage is suspected. The entire procedure usually takes 15 to 20 minutes. Afterwards, the patient must lie down for a few hours with the head slightly raised.

Myeloma, multiple

See *Multiple myeloma*.

Myelomatosis

See *Multiple myeloma*.

Myelomeningocele

Another name for myelocele (see *Spina bifida*).

Myelopathy

A term that refers to any disease of the *spinal cord*.

Myelosclerosis

An increase of fibrous tissue within the *bone marrow*, also known as osteosclerosis or myelofibrosis. In myelo-

sclerosis, the ability of the bone marrow to produce blood components is impaired, although this function can be partly taken over by the spleen and liver.

Myelosclerosis may be primary (i.e. occurring without any obvious cause) or secondary (resulting from some other bone marrow disease, such as *polycythaemia* or chronic myeloid *leukaemia*). Primary myelosclerosis most commonly occurs in middle age and has a gradual onset.

The main symptoms of myelosclerosis are those of *anaemia*, caused by impaired red blood cell production by the bone marrow. Enlargement of the spleen, night sweats, itching, loss of appetite, and weight loss are other common symptoms of myelosclerosis. In secondary myelosclerosis, there may be other symptoms connected with the underlying disease.

TREATMENT
Treatment of primary myelosclerosis is aimed at the relief of symptoms, mainly by means of *blood transfusions*. Only 50 per cent of patients survive for more than three years after the onset of the disease. A few patients develop acute leukaemia.

Treatment of secondary myelosclerosis depends on the underlying cause of the condition.

Myiasis

 An infestation of the skin, deeper tissues, or intestines by fly larvae. Myiasis is primarily restricted to tropical regions of the world.

TYPES AND SYMPTOMS
In Africa, the tumbu fly lays eggs on clothing left outside to dry; the larvae that hatch from these eggs penetrate the skin to cause boil-like swellings with a central small hole through which the larva breathes. Various other flies may lay eggs in open wounds, on the skin, or in the ears or nose. Sometimes the larvae penetrate deeply into the tissues, causing considerable destruction. Intestinal infestation can occur after eating contaminated food.

PREVENTION AND TREATMENT
Myiasis can largely be prevented by keeping flies away from food, by covering open wounds, and, in Africa, by thoroughly ironing clothes dried outdoors.

Cutaneous myiasis is treated by placing drops of oil over the swelling caused by the larva. The oil suffocates the larva, which is forced to come to the surface and can then be removed

with a needle. Infestation in deeper tissues may require surgical treatment. Intestinal myiasis can be adequately treated with a laxative.

Myo-

A prefix that denotes a relationship to *muscle* (as in myocarditis, inflammation of the heart muscle).

Myocardial infarction

Sudden death of part of the *heart* muscle, characterized, in most cases, by severe unremitting chest pain. The disorder is popularly known as a heart attack.

Each year in the UK at least 250,000 people have a myocardial infarction, and about 160,000 die from this cause. Myocardial infarction is the single most common cause of death in developed countries.

Men are more likely to suffer a myocardial infarction than women, and smokers are at greater risk than nonsmokers. The children of someone who has died of a myocardial infarction are more likely than average to die from this cause. Other risk factors include increased age, unhealthy diet, obesity, and disorders such as *hypertension* (high blood pressure), *diabetes mellitus*, and *hyperlipidaemias*. Most people who suffer a myocardial infarction have atherosclerosis of the coronary arteries (see illustrated box).

SYMPTOMS AND COMPLICATIONS
The characteristic symptom is sudden pain in the centre of the chest (see illustrated box). The victim may also be short of breath, restless, and apprehensive, have cold clammy skin, feel nauseated or vomit (or both), or lose consciousness.

In mild cases, the pain and other symptoms are slight or do not develop at all (in which case the attack is known as a silent infarct). As a result, the episode usually passes unnoticed and may be discovered only by subsequent tests.

Damage to the heart muscle may be so severe that it leads immediately to *heart failure* (reduced pumping efficiency of the heart). *Arrhythmias* (abnormal heart rhythms) are common. Most people who die of a myocardial infarction do so within the first few hours due to a type of arrhythmia called ventricular fibrillation, which seriously interferes with the heart's pumping action. However, if the person can be brought to a hospital, arrhythmias can be controlled with drugs or electrical *defibrillation*.

M

FEATURES OF MYOCARDIAL INFARCTION

Myocardial infarction, in which an area of heart muscle is deprived of blood supply and suffers tissue death as a result, is a major cause of death in developed countries. Atherosclerosis of the coronary arteries is the cause in most cases of myocardial infarction.

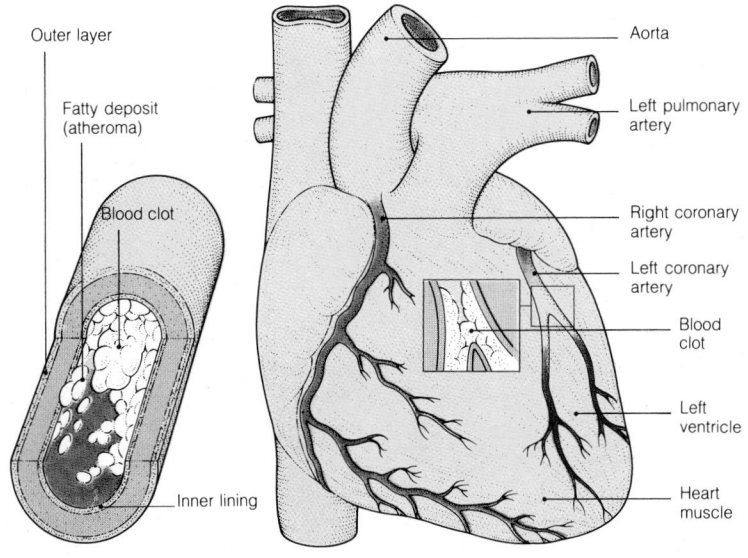

Outer layer

Fatty deposit (atheroma)

Blood clot

Inner lining

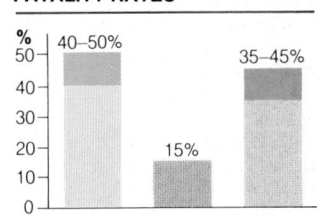

Aorta

Left pulmonary artery

Right coronary artery

Left coronary artery

Blood clot

Left ventricle

Heart muscle

Atherosclerosis

Like all other arteries, the coronary arteries may be affected by atherosclerosis. Patchy plaques of atheroma develop on the inner lining of the arteries, restricting the blood flow and encouraging the formation of blood clots. The clotting results in a sudden stoppage of blood flow to the heart.

OUTLOOK AFTER AN ATTACK

Myocardial infarction is fatal within 20 days in 40 to 50 per cent of cases, and about another 15 per cent die between 20 days and one year of the attack. Further risk persists for years, but a significant number of patients are alive 10 years after an attack.

FATALITY RATES

%
50 40–50%   35–45%
40
30
20   15%
10
0

Key

Patients who die within the first 20 days after the attack

Patients who die between 20 days and one year after the attack

Patients who survive for more than one year after the attack

M

PAIN

Many victims of myocardial infarction have a history of angina pectoris, in which the chest pain is relieved by rest. The pain of infarction usually comes on suddenly, and ranges from a tight ache to intense crushing agony. It lasts for 30 minutes or more, and is not relieved by rest.

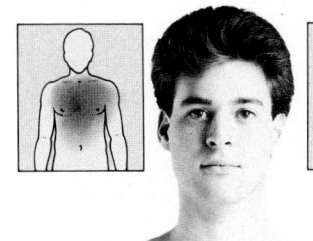
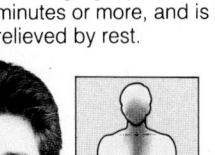
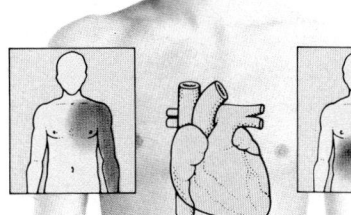

A central chest pressure, ranging from mild to severe, is common to almost every attack of myocardial infarction from coronary obstruction.

In some cases, pain radiates up into the jaw and through to the back. Sometimes, it occurs only in these places.

In many cases, the pain radiates down the left arm; it may cause a sensation of weakness in the arm muscles.

More rarely, angina pectoris may be felt in the upper abdomen. If it occurs only here, it may be mistaken for another disorder.

RISK FACTORS

Uncontrollable factors include a family history of heart disease, old age, and being male.

Habitual cigarette smokers have a substantially increased risk of dying from myocardial infarction.

High blood pressure is a major risk factor, and the risk increases the higher the pressure.

The risk of atherosclerosis and coronary artery disease increases dramatically in those who are more than 30 per cent overweight.

A raised blood cholesterol level (for which there may be a genetic tendency) increases the risk. A high-fat diet is also a factor.

Physical inactivity is also a major risk factor.

M

Possible long-term complications include damage to the mitral valve, leading to *mitral incompetence,* or the development of a weak area in the wall of the heart or in the muscle dividing the two sides of the heart. Complications may require surgery.

DIAGNOSIS

Diagnosis is made from the patient's history and special tests. These include *ECG* and the measurement of *enzymes* released into the blood from damaged heart muscle. Emergency coronary artery *angiography* may be performed if surgery is being considered.

TREATMENT

If a myocardial infarction is suspected, a doctor or ambulance should be called immediately. If the patient is seen within six hours of the onset of symptoms, *thrombolytic drugs* may be given to try and dissolve the blood clot; the sooner this treatment is given, the greater its chances of success. Initial treatment will also include strong *analgesic drugs* (painkillers) and possibly *oxygen therapy. Diuretic drugs* may be given to treat heart failure, which can lead to fluid accumulation in the lungs. *Intravenous infusion* of fluids may be given for shock, and *antiarrhythmic drugs* may be given to control heart rhythm disturbances. *Beta-blocker drugs* are given in some cases to reduce the risk of further muscle damage.

Patients admitted to hospital with an acute myocardial infarction will usually be treated in a *coronary care unit* equipped and staffed to provide 24-hour monitoring of progress. Any cardiac arrhythmias will be recognized and treated immediately. *Angioplasty* (widening of the narrowed coronary arteries) may be performed at an early stage; *coronary artery bypass* grafting may also be considered.

Many patients find the environment of a coronary care unit reassuring. However, some specialists believe they are actually more stressful and recommend that some patients are cared for elsewhere in hospital or at home.

It was once recommended that patients rest in bed for two weeks or more following a myocardial infarction. Today, however, patients are encouraged to be out of bed within four or five days.

OUTLOOK

Once recovery is complete and the patient has left hospital, a full assessment of the heart's condition will be made, usually involving recording an electrocardiogram (see *ECG*) during exercise, and possibly including *radionuclide scanning.* Preventive treatment will be recommended to reduce to a minimum the chances of further attacks. In all cases, patients will be advised to reduce their risk factors (see table on previous page), and to have regular check ups for the rest of their lives. Many go on to lead active lives for at least 10 years after a heart attack.

Myocarditis

Inflammation of the *heart* muscle, usually caused by an infection. Myocarditis is often accompanied by *pericarditis* (inflammation of the outer lining of the heart).

CAUSES

The most common cause of myocarditis is a viral infection, usually due to a coxsackievirus. Mild myocarditis often accompanies viral infections of the lungs. In rare cases, myocarditis is caused by a bacterial infection.

Myocarditis is a characteristic feature of *rheumatic fever.* In rare cases, it is caused by drugs or *radiotherapy.*

In Central and South America, the most common cause of myocarditis is the parasitic infection *Chagas' disease.* Many years after the initial infection, extensive myocarditis leads to progressive heart failure, which is often fatal.

SYMPTOMS AND SIGNS

Myocarditis often causes no symptoms. Rarely, there may be a serious disturbance of the heartbeat, breathlessness, chest pain, and *heart failure* (reduced pumping efficiency of the heart). In severe cases, death may result from *cardiac arrest.*

DIAGNOSIS

Myocarditis may be suspected from the patient's history, which often includes a recent upper respiratory tract infection, and from a physical examination. An *ECG* will show characteristic abnormalities of the heartbeat.

In some cases, a diagnosis is made at a postmortem examination performed after a young person has died unexpectedly during vigorous exercise.

TREATMENT

There is no specific treatment for myocarditis. Bed rest is usually recommended. Exercise should be avoided until an ECG shows a normal pattern. *Corticosteroid drugs* are occasionally prescribed to reduce inflammation.

Myoclonus

Rapid and uncontrollable jerking or spasm of a muscle or muscles, which may occur either at rest or during movement.

Myoclonus may be associated with a disorder affecting the muscles or nervous system. It may occur during an epileptic seizure (see *Epilepsy*) or as a feature of *encephalitis* (inflammation of the brain).

Myoclonus also occurs in healthy people. An example is the twitching of the limbs that often occurs shortly before falling asleep.

Myofacial pain disorder

See *Temporomandibular joint syndrome.*

Myoglobin

The oxygen-carrying pigment in muscles. Myoglobin consists of a combination of iron and protein, and gives muscles their red colour. Like *haemoglobin* (the oxygen-carrying pigment in red blood cells), myoglobin takes up and then stores oxygen, which it releases when the muscle tissues need oxygen to sustain contraction.

The presence of myoglobin in the urine is known as myoglobinuria. Slight myoglobinuria may occur during prolonged, vigorous exercise. Severe myoglobinuria is usually caused by the release of myoglobin from a large area of damaged muscle, such as occurs in *crush syndrome,* and may cause *kidney failure.*

Myoma

A noncancerous tumour of muscle. The most common type of myoma is a *leiomyoma,* which affects the smooth muscle of the intestine, uterus, or stomach.

Myomectomy

Surgical removal of a *myoma* (a noncancerous tumour of muscle). The term is commonly applied to the removal of *fibroids* of the uterus.

Myopathy

A disease of *muscle* that is not caused by disease of the nervous system. Most myopathies are *degenerative disorders; muscular dystrophy* is an example. Others are caused by chemical poisoning, or by a chronic disorder of the *immune system,* or occur as a side-effect of a drug. (See also *Muscle* disorders box.)

Myopia

An error of *refraction* in which near objects can be seen clearly while those in the distance appear blurred. Commonly called shortsightedness, myopia is caused by the *eye* being too long from front to back. As a result, images of distant objects are focused in front of the retina.

Myopia, which tends to be inherited, usually appears around puberty

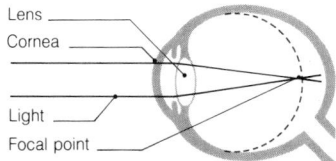

Lens
Cornea
Light
Focal point

Uncorrected myopia
With uncorrected myopia, the images of distant objects are focused in front of the retina and appear blurred.

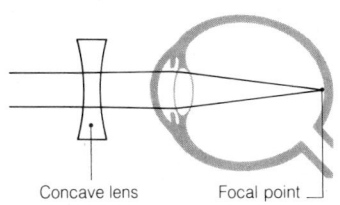

Concave lens   Focal point

Corrected myopia
To see distant objects clearly, the power of the eye must be reduced by a concave (negative) lens.

and increases progressively until the early 20s, when it stabilizes. Myopia that starts in early childhood often progresses into adult life, and may become very severe.

If myopia is detected during a *vision test*, concave *glasses* (or *contact lenses*) may be prescribed to sharpen distant vision. In some cases myopia may be treated surgically by radial keratotomy (see *Keratotomy, radial*) or *laser treatment*.

Myositis
Inflammation of muscle tissue that causes pain, tenderness, and weakness. Types of myositis include *pleurodynia* (a viral infection that affects muscles around the rib-cage), myositis ossificans (in which damaged muscle is replaced by bone), *polymyositis* (inflammation of muscles throughout the body), and *dermatomyositis* (inflammation of muscles plus a rash). Polymyositis and dermatomyositis are *autoimmune disorders*.

Myotomy
A procedure that involves cutting into a muscle. An example is pyloromyotomy—cutting into the muscle surrounding the lower end of the stomach to treat *pyloric stenosis* (narrowing of the stomach's exit).

Myotonia
Inability of a *muscle* to relax after the need for contraction has passed. Myotonia occurs primarily in two forms of myotonic dystrophy: myotonia congenita and dystrophia myotonica. Myotonia congenita starts during infancy and usually improves with age. Dystrophia myotonica is a progressive disorder that starts in early adult life. Drugs, such as procainamide and quinine, may help reduce myotonia.

Myringitis
Inflammation of the eardrum. Myringitis occurs, to some degree, in every case of *otitis media*.

Myringoplasty
Surgical closure of a perforation (hole) in the eardrum (see *Eardrum, perforated*) by means of a tissue graft. Myringoplasty is performed to improve hearing and, sometimes, to stop a recurrent discharge from the ear. The graft is usually taken from the fibrous covering of a muscle in the temple or thigh.

Myringotomy
A surgical opening made through the eardrum to allow drainage of the middle-ear cavity.

WHY IT IS DONE
Myringotomy is usually performed on children to treat persistent *glue ear*, in which a sticky secretion fills the middle-ear cavity. The fluid causes hearing loss, which may become permanent if the condition is not treated before damage occurs.

Before the advent of antibiotics, myringotomy was performed to treat acute *otitis media* (middle-ear infection) by releasing the pus and thereby relieving pressure on the eardrum.

HOW IT IS DONE
With the patient under a general anaesthetic, a small incision is made in the eardrum and most of the fluid is removed by suction. At the same time, a *grommet* (small tube) may be inserted into the eardrum to equalize pressure in the outer and middle ears. In most cases, the patient can leave hospital the following day.

Myxoedema
A condition in which there is thickening and coarsening of the skin and other body tissues (most noticeable in the face, where the lips become swollen and the nose thickened).

Myxoedema often results from *hypothyroidism* (underactivity of the thyroid gland) and in such cases is

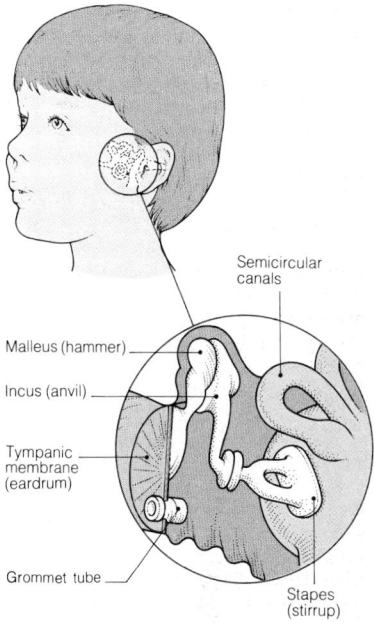

Semicircular canals
Malleus (hammer)
Incus (anvil)
Tympanic membrane (eardrum)
Grommet tube
Stapes (stirrup)

Myringotomy
This operation is performed to treat glue ear. An incision is made in the eardrum, then the thick fluid is sucked out from the middle-ear cavity. A grommet (small tube) may be inserted through the eardrum and into the middle ear to equalize pressure on both sides of the eardrum. Sometimes the adenoids are removed while the patient is having the myringotomy operation.

commonly accompanied by weight gain, hair loss, sensitivity to cold, and mental dullness. The term myxoedema is sometimes used interchangeably with adult hypothyroidism.

Myxoma
A benign, jelly-like tumour composed of soft mucous material and loose fibrous strands. Myxomas usually occur singly, and may sometimes grow very large.

The most common site for a myxoma is under the skin (typically in the limbs or neck). Myxomas may also develop in the abdomen, bladder, or bone. Very rarely, a myxoma may grow inside the heart, where it may lead to the formation of thrombi (blood clots) and to the obstruction of blood flow through the heart. Myxomas can usually be successfully removed by surgery.

Myxomatosis is a highly infectious viral disease of rabbits in which numerous myxomas develop throughout the body; this disease does not affect humans.

M

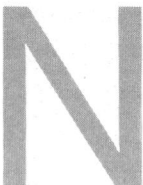

Nadolol

A *beta-blocker drug* used in the treatment of *hypertension* (high blood pressure), *angina pectoris* (chest pain due to impaired blood supply to heart muscle), certain types of *arrhythmia* (irregularity of the heartbeat), and to control symptoms of *hyperthyroidism* (overactivity of the thyroid gland).

Possible adverse effects are typical of other beta-blocker drugs.

Naevus

A skin blemish of various types. Naevi can be flat, slightly raised, or on a stalk, coloured or not coloured, and with or without hair growth. Some naevi are present at birth, others can develop at any age.

TYPES
There are two main groups of naevi: pigmented naevi and vascular naevi.

PIGMENTED NAEVI These are are caused by abnormality or overactivity of melanocytes (skin cells that produce the brown pigment *melanin*).

The most common type of pigmented naevus is a *freckle*, which is a small, flat, light brown to dark brown area which may may occur on any part of the body that is exposed to the sun. A *lentigo* is a light brown spot very similar to a freckle. *Café au lait spots* are another type of light brown pigmented naevus.

Another common type of pigmented naevus is a mole, sometimes called a melanocytic naevus. Moles are brown to dark brown in colour and of different sizes. They are unusual at birth, but commonly develop during childhood and young adulthood. Adults have an average of 15 to 20 moles. In rare cases, moles become cancerous (see *Melanoma, malignant*).

Hairy, pigmented naevi sometimes develop on the shoulders of young men. Another type of pigmented naevus is a halo naevus, in which the skin surrounding the blemish lightens in colour to give a characteristic halo appearance. Juvenile melanomas (see *Melanoma, juvenile*) are red-brown naevi that occur in childhood.

Some naevi have a bluish coloration; these so-called blue naevi are often found on the backs of the hands of young girls. Most black and Asian infants are born with one or more blue-black spots on their lower backs (see *Mongolian blue spot*).

VASCULAR NAEVI These are caused by an abnormal collection of blood vessels. They include port-wine stains and strawberry marks (see *Haemangioma* and *spider naevi*).

TREATMENT
Most naevi are harmless and do not require treatment. However, if a naevus suddenly appears, grows, bleeds, or changes colour, medical advice should be sought without delay to exclude the possibility of *skin cancer*.

Nail

A hard, curved plate on the fingers and toes composed of *keratin* (a tough protein that is also the main constituent of skin and hair). A fingernail takes about six months to grow from base to tip, although there are seasonal growth variations. Toenails take twice as long to grow.

DISORDERS
The nails are susceptible to damage through injury, usually as a result of crushing or pressure on the nail. Sometimes the nails become abnor-

mally thick and curved—a condition called *onychogryphosis* which mainly affects the big toes of elderly people.

Nails may be damaged by bacterial or fungal infections, especially *tinea* and *candidiasis*. In *paronychia* the nail folds are infected. The nails may also be affected by skin disease or by more generalized illnesses.

Examples of the effects of skin disease on the nails include pitting of the nails in *alopecia* areata, pitting and *onycholysis* (separation of the nail from its bed) in *psoriasis*, and scarring and onycholysis in *lichen planus*.

Nail abnormalities may be signs of more generalized disease. Brittle, ridged, concave nails are a sign of iron-deficiency *anaemia*, onycholysis is seen in *thyrotoxicosis*, and fibrous growths on the nails are a sign of *tuberous sclerosis*. Splinter-like black marks develop beneath the nails (denoting bleeding into the nail bed) in *endocarditis* and *bleeding disorders*.

Abnormalities of nail colour may also signify disease. A greenish discoloration may be caused by bacterial infection under the nail; blue nails may be a sign of heart or respiratory disease; and yellow nails that are hard and curved develop in *bronchiectasis* and *lymphoedema*. Nails may also be discoloured by nail polish or nicotine.

DIAGNOSIS AND TREATMENT
Nail disorders are usually diagnosed by inspecting the nails and skin, along with a more extensive physical examination if necessary. Laboratory examination of nail clippings may be performed.

Treatment of nail disorders is difficult. Creams and lotions seldom penetrate sufficiently; oral medication may take months to be effective.

Nail-biting

A common activity that does not indicate any underlying medical condition. Many children bite their nails during their first years at school, but most grow out of it. Nail-biting sometimes continues as a nervous habit in adolescents and adults. Persistent nail-biting may make the nails unsightly and cause pain and sometimes bleeding.

Various preparations with an unpleasant taste can be painted on the nails, but many people become accustomed to the taste.

Nalidixic acid

An *antibiotic drug* used to treat and, occasionally, to prevent *urinary tract infection*. Nalidixic acid is effective

---

ANATOMY OF A NAIL
The nail bed is the area from which the nail grows. At the base of each nail, a half-moon shape, the lunula, is crossed by a flap of skin, the cuticle. The skin that surrounds the nail is the nail fold. The nail is composed of keratin, a tough protein also found in skin and hair.

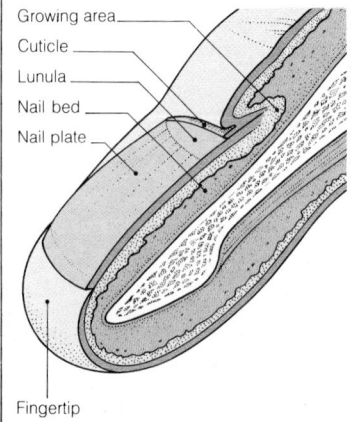

Growing area
Cuticle
Lunula
Nail bed
Nail plate

Fingertip

against some types of bacteria that are resistant to other antibiotics.

Possible adverse effects include nausea, vomiting, increased sensitivity to sunlight, blurred vision, drowsiness, and dizziness.

Naloxone

A drug that blocks the action of *narcotic drugs*. Naloxone reverses breathing difficulty caused by an overdose of a narcotic drug. It is given to people who have been given high doses of a narcotic drug during surgery. Naloxone is also given to newborn babies who have been affected by narcotic drugs given to relieve maternal pain during childbirth.

Possible adverse effects include abdominal cramps, diarrhoea, nausea, vomiting, and tremors.

Nandrolone

An anabolic steroid (see *Steroids, anabolic*). Nandrolone is sometimes used with *growth hormone* in the treatment of *short stature*. It is also used to treat certain types of *anaemia*.

Possible adverse effects include swollen ankles, nausea and vomiting, jaundice, and aggressive behaviour. In men, nandrolone may cause difficulty in passing urine. In women, it may cause irregular menstruation and abnormal hair growth.

Nappy rash

A common condition affecting babies with otherwise healthy skin. Nappy rash results from skin irritation by substances contained in the urine or faeces. Prolonged wetting may also play a part.

Babies vary in their susceptibility to nappy rash. In some babies, it may be the first indication of sensitive skin. Occasionally, skin inflammation is severe. The groin and buttocks may also become infected by bacteria from the baby's faeces or by the fungi that cause *candidiasis* (thrush).

TREATMENT AND OUTLOOK

Prevention is better than cure. The aim is to keep the baby's skin dry for as long as possible. A newborn breast-fed baby passes urine about five to 10 times each day and has a bowel movement after each feeding, so this does present a practical problem. Nappies should be changed frequently and a water-repellent emollient cream applied after each change.

Towelling nappies should be well rinsed and kept soft. Sometimes an ointment containing a mild *corticosteroid drug* may be prescribed to

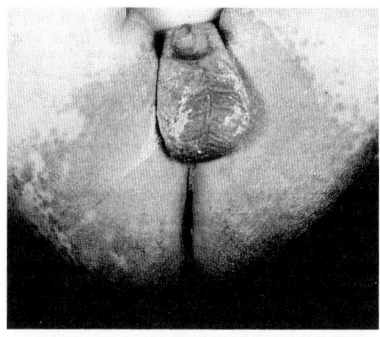

Symptoms of nappy rash
The skin over the buttocks, genitals, and inner thighs becomes red and sore at first, and may progress to blistering.

suppress the inflammation. A corticosteroid is often prescribed in combination with an antifungal drug to kill any candida present.

Naproxen

A *nonsteroidal anti-inflammatory drug* (NSAID). Naproxen is used to relieve joint pain and stiffness in different types of *arthritis*. It is also prescribed to hasten recovery following injury to soft tissues, such as muscles or ligaments.

Possible adverse effects of naproxen include nausea, abdominal pain, and *peptic ulcer*.

Narcissism

Intense self-love. The term is derived from the Greek myth of Narcissus, who so loved to stare at his own reflection in the water that he fell in and drowned. According to *psychoanalytic theory* there is an early stage in child development when the *ego* (self) feels omnipotent. Failure to deal with the frustrations of discovering that this is not so may later result in *neurosis*.

A narcissistic personality disorder is characterized by an exaggerated sense of self-importance, constant need for attention or praise, inability to cope with criticism or defeat, and poor relationships with other people.

Narcolepsy

A *sleep disorder* characterized by chronic, excessive daytime sleepiness with recurrent episodes of sleep occurring several times per day. Attacks may last from a few seconds to more than an hour and may be mildly inconvenient or severely disabling, often interfering with work and daily life. *Cataplexy* (sudden loss of muscle tone without loss of consciousness) occurs in about three quarters of

cases. Other symptoms may include *sleep paralysis* and vivid hallucinations at the onset of sleep or on awakening.

The diagnosis of narcolepsy is made by the examination of an *EEG* (electrical recording of brain activity). In narcolepsy, the REM (rapid eye movement) state, which normally occurs only during *sleep*, intrudes into wakefulness. Narcolepsy is often inherited. Treatment usually involves regular naps, along with *stimulant drugs* to control drowsiness and sleep attacks, and *antidepressant drugs* to suppress cataplexy.

Narcosis

A state of stupor, which is usually caused by a drug (see *Narcotic drugs*) or other chemical. Narcosis resembles sleep, being marked by reduced awareness and by diminished ability to respond to external stimulation. However, unlike someone who is sleeping, a person in narcosis cannot be roused completely.

Narcotic drugs

COMMON DRUGS

Buprenorphine Codeine Diamorphine Dihydrocodeine Morphine Pethidine

A type of *analgesic drug* (painkiller) used to treat moderate and severe pain. Abuse of narcotic drugs for their euphoric effects often causes *tolerance* (the need for greater amounts to have the same effects), and physical and psychological *drug dependence*.

Nasal congestion

Partial blockage of the nasal passage caused by swelling of the *mucus membrane* that lines the *nose*. Swelling of the mucus membrane may be accompanied by the accumulation of thick nasal mucus, which further impedes breathing.

Nasal congestion produces the familiar feelings of a stuffy, "full" nose. There is a frequent desire to blow the nose, but blowing usually has little effect on the congestion.

CAUSES

Nasal congestion is a symptom of the common cold (see *Cold, common*) and of hay fever (see *Rhinitis, allergic*). In these conditions, the swelling is due to inflammation of the membrane that lines the inside of the nose. Inflammation may become persistent in certain disorders, such as chronic *sinusitis* or nasal *polyps*. Nasal congestion may also be caused by certain drugs, such as *reserpine*.

N

TREATMENT

A very simple, effective, and time-honoured method of alleviating nasal congestion is to inhale the steam from a pot of hot water. This loosens the mucus, which enables the sufferer to blow it out through the nose. *Decongestant drugs* in the form of nasal drops and sprays should be used sparingly since prolonged use can make congestion worse. Decongestant tablets and syrups may be recommended for long-term use.

Persistent nasal congestion should be investigated by a doctor.

Nasal discharge

The spontaneous emission of fluid from the *nose*. Nasal discharge is commonly caused by inflammation of the mucous lining and is often accompanied by *nasal congestion*.

In allergic *rhinitis*, the discharge consists of runny, clear mucus. Infection of the nasal passage itself, such as occurs in a cold (see *Cold, common*), or an infection that has spread from the sinuses (see *Sinusitis*) usually causes a thicker discharge of mucus, often mixed with pus. A persistent runny discharge of recent onset may be an early indication of a tumour (see *Nasopharynx, cancer of*).

Bleeding from the nose (see *Nosebleed*) is usually caused by injury or a foreign body in the nose. In rare cases, bleeding from the nose may be a sign of an underlying bleeding disorder or a tumour. A discharge of cerebrospinal fluid from the nose may follow a fracture at the base of the skull (see *Skull, fracture of*).

Nasal obstruction

Blockage of the nasal passage, which interferes with breathing. The blockage may occur on one or both sides of the *nose*.

The most common cause of nasal obstruction is inflammation of the *mucous membrane* that lines the passage (see *Nasal congestion*). Other causes include severe deviation of the *nasal septum*, nasal *polyps*, a *haematoma* (a collection of clotted blood) usually caused by injury, and, rarely, a malignant tumour. In children, enlargement of the *adenoids* is the most common cause of nasal obstruction.

Nasal septum

The central partition inside the *nose* that divides it into two. The nasal septum consists of cartilage at the front and bone at the rear, both of which are covered by *mucous membrane*.

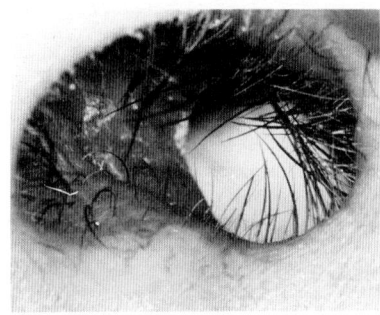

Destroyed nasal septum
This photograph of the left nostril was taken with a light shone into the right nostril. There is a hole in the septum.

DISORDERS

A deviated septum (twisting of the septum to one side) may be present from birth or may be caused by a blow or blows to the nose. The condition is rarely troublesome, but surgery to straighten the septum may be recommended if breathing is obstructed.

Injury may cause a *haematoma* (a collection of clotted blood) to form between the cartilage of the septum and the wall of one nasal cavity. The haematoma may obstruct breathing to varying degrees. Sometimes, a haematoma becomes infected, causing an *abscess*, which may require surgical drainage. Occasionally, an abscess develops on a child's septum without prior injury.

Rarely, a hole may be eroded in the septum by *tuberculosis*, *syphilis*, *Wegener's granulomatosis*, or as a result of sniffing *cocaine*.

Nasogastric tube

A narrow plastic tube that is passed through the nose, down the oesophagus, and into the stomach.

WHY IT IS USED

One of its most common uses is to suck or drain digestive juices from the stomach when the intestine is blocked (as in *pyloric stenosis*) or is not working properly (as may occur after an abdominal operation). A nasogastric tube is also used to give liquid nourishment to very ill patients who cannot eat (see *Feeding, artificial*), to obtain specimens of stomach secretions for examination, and to wash out the stomach after a drug overdose or after swallowing a poison (see *Lavage, gastric*).

HOW IT IS USED

Inserting the tube is a quick, simple procedure that causes little discomfort and does not require an anaesthetic. After it has been lubricated, the tube is passed into one nostril and then, while the patient is swallowing, slid down the throat and into the stomach. To ensure that the tube is in the stomach, a sample of fluid is withdrawn through a syringe and tested on litmus paper for acidity. The stomach contents are then either sucked out through the syringe or a suction device or are allowed to drain freely into a container; fluids for lavage or feeding are introduced through a funnel. If the tube is to be left in place for some time, the protruding end is taped to the face.

Nasopharynx

The passage connecting the nasal cavity behind the *nose* to the top of the throat behind the soft *palate*. Part of the respiratory tract, the nasopharynx forms the upper section of the *pharynx*. During swallowing, the nasopharynx is sealed off (to prevent food from entering it) by the action of the soft palate pressing against the back of the throat.

The nasopharynx contains the lower openings of the *eustachian tubes* (passages connecting the back of the nose to the middle ear) and, in children, the *adenoids*. The adenoids can enlarge to such an extent that the nasopharynx becomes completely blocked, forcing the child to breathe through his or her mouth.

Nasopharynx, cancer of

A malignant tumour that originates in the *nasopharynx* (uppermost part of the throat, behind the nose) and usually spreads to the nasal cavity, nasal sinuses, base of the skull, and lymph nodes in the neck.

Cancer of the nasopharynx is rare in the West but common in the Far East; it is most common between the ages of 40 and 50 and affects twice as many men as women. One cause is believed to be the *Epstein-Barr virus*.

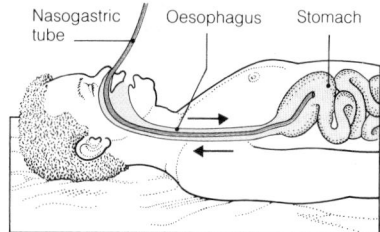

Using a nasogastric tube
The tube is passed via a nostril and the oesophagus into the stomach. Substances may be delivered into the stomach via the tube, or the stomach contents may be removed through it.

N

SYMPTOMS AND SIGNS

Common first signs are recurrent nosebleeds, a persistently runny nose, and voice change. As the tumour spreads, there may also be a bloody nasal discharge, loss of smell, double vision, deafness, paralysis of one side of the face, and severe facial pain.

DIAGNOSIS AND TREATMENT

The diagnosis is made from a *biopsy* (removal of a small sample of tissue for microscopic analysis). *X-rays* may also be taken to determine the extent of the cancer.

Treatment of cancer of the nasopharynx is with *radiotherapy*. The outlook depends on when treatment begins; one third of sufferers survive for more than five years.

National Health Service

The National Health Service (NHS) was introduced in 1948 as the means of providing health care for the whole population.

At that time other European countries had two main types of organized medical systems: the Scandinavian model and the Franco-German model. In the Scandinavian model, the state owned most of the hospitals and the patient received all necessary medical care free at the point of delivery, financed by general taxation. In the Franco-German model, hospitals were mostly owned and run by independent corporations and the fees they charged patients were reimbursed through a system of state-regulated health insurance.

Britain opted for the taxation-based model and took into state ownership virtually all the existing hospitals, including the university teaching hospitals and old-established charitable "voluntary" hospitals, such as Guy's Hospital and St Bartholomew's Hospital, both in London.

The system has changed little despite enormous technological advances in medicine. The NHS is administered by the Department of Health, which oversees the health regions in England, the health region of Wales, and the health boards in Scotland and in Northern Ireland. These regions and boards are responsible for running their hospital and community health-care services.

The first point of contact for a British citizen who wants medical attention is usually a general practitioner or family doctor. These doctors have contracts with the NHS by which they undertake to provide care 24 hours a day, 365 days a year for patients on

their "lists". Some general practitioners still work single-handed but most are now in partnerships and larger group practices. In a typical practice, four or five doctors will have joined together to build or modify premises and to employ receptionists, clerks, nurses, and other members of the practice team. Patients are theoretically free to choose a doctor from those contracted with the local Family Health Service Authority, but many people find that their choice is limited to only a couple of practices close to their homes. General practitioners are reluctant to accept patients who live far away because of practical problems, such as the possible need to visit patients in their own homes. In order to obtain treatment from a general practitioner, a patient must first register with that doctor and be included on his or her list. In partnerships and group practices, a patient will be able to see any of the doctors.

The general practitioner provides diagnoses and treatment for common minor ailments and also assesses more serious disorders. He or she may refer patients for specialist assessment or care at any hospital although, in practice, almost all referrals are to the nearest general hospital. Patients may request specialist referral and the general practitioner will usually agree although he is under no legal obligation to do so.

NHS general hospitals provide a full range of specialist care, including medical specialties, surgery, obstetrics and gynaecology, paediatrics, geriatric care, and psychiatry. A few rare diseases are treated at regional specialist centres and there are also specialist hospitals (usually linked with universities) for complex, rare procedures such as heart transplants. What treatment is needed is decided by the doctors and patients in consultation; when it is provided is a management decision, and a continuing criticism of the NHS is that throughout its history there have been long waiting lists for routine operations, such as the repair of hernias, treatment of varicose veins, and even complex procedures such as heart surgery.

The third area of the NHS is its community services, which include midwifery for women who wish to have their babies born at home, child welfare clinics, ambulance services, the care in the community of the mentally ill, and home helps. The prevention and control of outbreaks of infectious disease, of medically

hazardous pollution, and other aspects of public health also come within the scope of NHS community services through its medical officers for environmental health.

In the early 1990s, several changes were made to the NHS in an attempt to introduce cost-cutting business methods. Hospitals were categorized as providers of health care, while GPs and district health authorities were categorized as purchasers, who were encouraged to shop around among the providers for the best financial, and other, deals possible. Hospitals could opt out of direct control by NHS district authorities and form independent trusts. Some GPs took over the responsibility of managing the available funds for all their patients' treatment, and were able to negotiate terms with their local hospitals. The development of an internal market for health care was expected to improve efficiency, but the changes were introduced during a period of economic recession, and caused considerable controversy. At the time of going to press, the reform process was still under way, strongly supported by some and opposed by others.

Natural childbirth

See *Childbirth, natural.*

Naturopathy

A form of *alternative medicine* based on the principle that disease is due to the accumulation of waste products and toxins (poisons) in the body, and that symptoms reflect the body's attempt to rid itself of these substances. Practitioners of naturopathy believe that health is maintained by avoiding anything artificial or unnatural in the diet or in the environment.

Nausea

The sensation of needing to vomit. Although nausea may occur independently of vomiting, the causes are the same (see *Vomiting*).

Navel

A popular term for the *umbilicus*, the depression in the abdomen that marks the point at which the umbilical cord was attached to the fetus.

Nebulizer

A device used to administer a drug in aerosol form through a face mask or mouthpiece. Nebulizers are used to administer *bronchodilator drugs*, especially in the emergency treatment of an attack of *asthma*. Most patients can

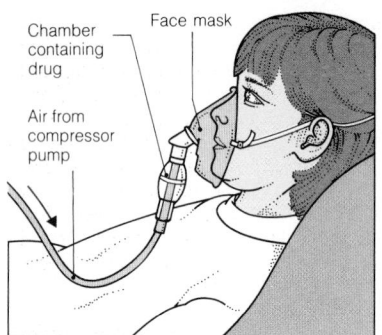

Using a nebulizer
An electric or hand-operated pump sends a stream of air or oxygen across a chamber containing the required drug. This stream of air disperses the drug into a fine mist, which is then conveyed to the face mask and inhaled by the user.

use a nebulizer more easily than a conventional *inhaler* (a pressurized aerosol canister).

Neck

The part of the body that supports the head and serves as a passageway between the head and brain and the body.

The neck contains several vital structures: the *spinal cord* (which carries nerve impulses to and from the brain), the *trachea* (windpipe), the *oesophagus*, and major blood vessels leading to and from the head. Decapitation kills because it cuts through these vital structures. Strangulation kills by compressing major blood vessels and by cutting off the air supply to the lungs.

DISORDERS
INJURY *Torticollis* (wry neck), in which the head is twisted to one side, may result from birth injury to a neck muscle or from skin *contracture* (shrinkage) after burns or other injuries.

Fractures and *dislocations* of any of the vertebrae in the neck can injure the spinal cord, causing paralysis or even death; *whiplash injuries* can also severely damage the spinal cord (see *Spinal injury*).

DEGENERATION The joints between vertebrae may be affected by *cervical osteoarthritis*, causing neck pain, stiffness, and sometimes tingling and weakness in the arm and hand. Similar symptoms may be caused by a *disc prolapse*. In *ankylosing spondylitis*, fusion of the vertebrae may result in permanent neck rigidity.

CONGENITAL DEFECT *Cervical rib* (a small extra rib in the neck) often causes no symptoms until middle age, when it may result in pain, numbness, and a pins-and-needles sensation in the forearm and hand.

OTHER DISORDERS Because structures in the neck are so closely packed, any condition that causes swelling (such as inflammation, allergy, bleeding, or tumours) may, if the swelling is large enough, interfere with breathing or with swallowing.

Enlargement of the lymph nodes usually results from infection, but may be due to other conditions.

Neck pain of unknown origin is very common. As long as neurological symptoms (such as loss of sensation or muscle power) are absent, it is unlikely to be serious. Most sufferers recover within a few weeks.

Neck dissection, radical

A surgical procedure for removing cancerous *lymph nodes* in the neck. The operation is commonly required as part of the treatment of cancer of the tongue, tonsils, or other structures in the mouth and throat.

A flap of skin on the affected side of the neck is raised (under general anaesthetic) to expose the underlying sternomastoid muscle. The muscle is cut through just above the clavicle (collarbone) and lifted up. The entire lymphatic system in the neck (the lymph vessels as well as the lymph nodes) is then removed, together with the internal jugular vein, the lower salivary gland, and other surrounding tissue.

Neck rigidity

Marked stiffness of the neck caused by spasm of the muscles in the neck and spine. Neck rigidity is an important clinical sign of *meningitis* (inflammation of the membranes covering the brain and spinal cord). Severe neck rigidity may cause the head to arch backwards, especially in babies.

Necrolysis, toxic epidermal

A severe, blistering rash in which the surface layers of the skin peel off, exposing large areas of red raw skin over the body.

The effects of toxic epidermal necrolysis are similar to those of a severe third-degree burn, with the same potentially serious risks of widespread infection and loss of body fluid and salts from the exposed body surface.

In newborn babies, the condition is usually caused by staphylococci (a type of bacteria) and is called the scalded skin syndrome. Treatment is with *antibiotic drugs* and sometimes with intravenous fluid replacement.

In adults, the most common cause of toxic epidermal necrolysis is an adverse reaction to a *drug*, particularly a barbiturate, sulphonamide, or penicillin. The condition usually clears up when use of the drug is discontinued. Intravenous fluid replacement is sometimes necessary.

ANATOMY OF THE NECK

The neck contains many important structures, including the larynx, the thyroid and parathyroid glands, many lymph nodes, and the carotid arteries. The upper seven vertebrae of the spine are in the neck; a complex system of muscles is connected to these vertebrae, the clavicles, the upper ribs, and the lower jaw. Contraction of these muscles allows the head to turn and the jaw to open and close.

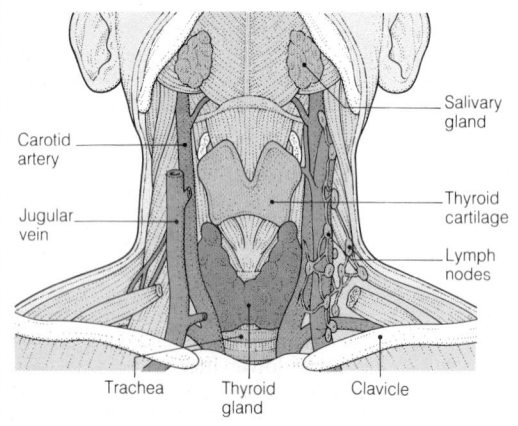

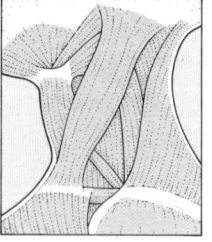

Muscles of the neck
Muscles on the back and side of the neck support and move the head.

Necrophilia

A rare sexual perversion in which orgasm is achieved by means of sexual acts with dead bodies.

Necropsy

A little-used alternative medical term for an *autopsy* (postmortem examination of a body).

Necrosis

The death of tissue cells. Necrosis can occur as a result of *ischaemia* (inadequate blood supply), which may lead to *gangrene*; infection (such as *tuberculosis*); or damage by extreme heat or cold, noxious chemicals (such as acids), or excessive exposure to X-rays or other forms of *radiation*.

The appearance of dead tissue depends on the cause of the necrosis and, usually, on the type of tissue affected. For example, in necrosis due to tuberculosis, the dead tissue is soft, dry, and cheese-like; fatty tissue beneath the skin that has died as a result of damage or infection develops into tough scar tissue that may form a firm nodule.

Nefopam

An *analgesic drug* used to relieve moderate pain caused by injury, surgery, or cancer. Nefopam reduces the perception of pain by the brain but its precise mechanism of action is unclear. Unlike most analgesics that act on the brain, it neither interferes with breathing nor causes euphoria.

Possible adverse effects include nausea, nervousness, dry mouth, and difficulty in sleeping.

Nelson's syndrome

A rare disorder of the *endocrine system* that causes increased skin pigmentation. Nelson's syndrome results from enlargement of the *pituitary gland*, which sometimes follows removal of both *adrenal glands*—an old treatment for *Cushing's disease*.

Nelson's syndrome is treated by *hypophysectomy* (removal or destruction of the pituitary gland).

Nematodes

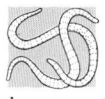 The scientific name for a group of cylindrically shaped worms, some of which can be parasites of humans. (See *Roundworms*.)

Neologism

The act of making up new words that have a special meaning for the inventor. The term also refers to the invented words themselves. Persistent neologism can be a feature of speech in people with *schizophrenia*, in which it occurs with other disordered thoughts.

Neomycin

An *antibiotic drug* used in the treatment of ear, eye, and skin infections, often in combination with other drugs. Neomycin is sometimes given to prevent infection of the intestine prior to surgery. Possible adverse effects include rash and itching.

Neonate

A newly born infant under the age of one month (see *Newborn*).

Neonatology

The branch of *paediatrics* concerned with the care of *newborn* infants and the treatment of their disorders. Problems may be short-term (such as those associated with *prematurity* or with low birthweight) or lifelong (such as *spina bifida*). The neonatologist cares for the baby for the first few weeks of life. After this time, the child's medical care becomes primarily the responsibility of a general paediatrician. In the UK, many neonatologists are also general paediatricians.

Neoplasia

A medical term for *tumour* formation, characterized by a progressive, abnormal multiplication of cells. The term neoplasia does not necessarily imply that the new growth is *malignant*; *benign* tumours also develop as a result of neoplasia.

Neoplasm

A medical term for a *tumour* (any new, abnormal growth). Neoplasms may be *malignant* or *benign*.

Neostigmine

A drug used in the treatment of *myasthenia gravis* (a rare autoimmune disorder that causes muscle weakness). Neostigmine works by increasing the activity of *acetylcholine*, a *neurotransmitter* (chemical released from nerve endings) that stimulates the contraction of muscles.

Possible adverse effects include nausea and vomiting, increased salivation, diarrhoea, abdominal cramps, blurred vision, sweating, muscle cramps, twitching, and rash.

Nephrectomy

Surgical removal of one or both of the *kidneys*.

WHY IT IS DONE

One of the most common reasons for nephrectomy is to remove a malignant tumour (see *Kidney cancer*). A kidney may also be removed if it is not functioning normally due to infection or the presence of stones (see *Calculus, urinary tract*), or is causing severe *hypertension* (high blood pressure). Nephrectomy may also be necessary if a kidney is so badly injured that bleeding cannot be stopped.

HOW IT IS DONE

Nephrectomy is carried out under general anaesthesia. The patient lies on his or her side, bent sharply at the waist over an angled operating table. An incision is made along the lower edge of the ribs, from the spine to the front of the abdomen, in order to expose the kidney. The *ureter* and renal blood vessels are tied off, and the kidney is removed. The incision is stitched up after insertion of a drainage tube, which is left in position for 24 to 48 hours.

OUTLOOK

A person's kidney function becomes virtually normal about six months after removal of a single kidney because the remaining kidney (providing it is healthy) takes over the entire workload. If both kidneys are removed, the patient requires *dialysis* or a *kidney transplant*.

Nephritis

Inflammation of one or both *kidneys*. Nephritis may be caused by infection (see *Pyelonephritis*), by abnormal responses of the *immune system* (see *Glomerulonephritis*), or by metabolic disorders, such as *gout*. (See also *Kidney* disorders box.)

Nephroblastoma

See *Kidney cancer*.

Nephrocalcinosis

The deposition of calcium within the substance of one or both *kidneys*. Nephrocalcinosis is not the same as kidney stones (see *Calculi, urinary tract*), in which calcium particles develop within the drainage channels of the kidney.

Nephrocalcinosis may occur in any condition in which the blood level of calcium is raised—for example, *hyperparathyroidism* (overactivity of the parathyroid gland) and *renal tubular acidosis* (in which the kidney produces urine of lower than normal acidity). Nephrocalcinosis may also develop as a result of taking excessive amounts of certain *antacid drugs* or *vitamin D*.

N

Treatment in nephrocalcinosis is of the underlying cause so that further calcification may be prevented.

Nephrolithotomy

The surgical removal of a *calculus* (stone) from the *kidney* by cutting into the main part of the kidney. Nephrolithotomy may be performed through an abdominal incision, or through a puncture incision made through the skin of the back directly into the kidney (a technique known as percutaneous nephrolithotomy). Instruments are used to grasp and remove the calculus; large calculi may need to be broken up before removal.

Other methods used for removing calculi from the kidneys are *pyelolithotomy* (a surgical procedure in which a calculus is removed through a cut at the renal pelvis) and *lithotripsy* (a nonsurgical procedure in which ultrasonic waves are used to break up calculi for excretion).

Nephrology

The medical specialty concerned with the normal functioning of the *kidneys*, and with the causes, diagnosis, and treatment of kidney disease.

Methods of investigating the kidneys include kidney *biopsy*, *kidney function tests*, and *kidney imaging* techniques (such as intravenous *urography*). Treatment of kidney disorders includes drugs (to control high blood pressure, inflammation, or infection), surgical intervention (for the treatment of stones and tumours), *dialysis* or, in some cases, a *kidney transplant* (for the treatment of advanced kidney disease).

Nephron

The microscopic unit of the *kidney* consisting of a glomerulus (filtering funnel) and a tubule. There are about one million nephrons in each kidney. The nephrons filter waste products from the blood and modify the amount of salts and water excreted in the urine according to the body's needs.

Nephropathy

A term for any disease or damage to the kidneys (see *Kidney* disorders box).

Obstructive nephropathy refers to kidney damage caused by a urinary tract *calculus* (stone), tumour, scar tissue, or pressure from an organ blocking urine flow and creating back pressure within the kidney.

Reflux nephropathy refers to kidney damage caused by backflow of urine from the bladder towards the kidney. It is caused by failure of the valve mechanism at the lower end of the ureter.

Toxic nephropathy refers to damage caused by various poisons or minerals (such as carbon tetrachloride or lead).

Nephrosclerosis

A process in which normal *kidney* structures are replaced with scar tissue. Nephrosclerosis usually represents the final healing stage of any of the various conditions that cause inflammation within the kidney. Examples of such conditions include *diabetes mellitus*, *glomerulonephritis*, and chronic *pyelonephritis*.

Nephrosis

See *Nephrotic syndrome*.

Nephrostomy

The introduction of a small tube into the *kidney* to drain urine to the abdominal surface, thus bypassing the ureter and bladder. Nephrostomy is sometimes performed to aid healing after an operation (typically removal of a *calculus*) on the ureter or kidney-ureter junction.

Nephrotic syndrome

A collection of symptoms and signs that results from damage to the glomeruli (filtering units of the *kidney*), causing severe *proteinuria* (loss of protein from the bloodstream into the urine). Loss of large amounts of protein in the urine lowers the protein content of the blood, resulting in *oedema* (accumulation of fluid in tissues).

CAUSES
Nephrotic syndrome may be caused by *diabetes mellitus*, *glomerulonephritis* (inflammation of the glomeruli), *amyloidosis* (a condition in which amyloid, an abnormal protein, collects in tissues), severe *hypertension* (high blood pressure), reactions to poisons (e.g. lead and carbon tetrachloride), and adverse *drug* reactions.

SYMPTOMS
Oedema causes marked swelling of the legs and face. Fluid may also collect in the chest cavity (producing *pleural effusion*) or within the abdomen (causing *ascites*). Anorexia, lethargy, and diarrhoea may also occur.

TREATMENT
Treatment is of the underlying condition. A low-sodium diet may be recommended, and *diuretic drugs* may be given to reduce oedema. If the concentration of protein in the blood is particularly low, protein may need to be given intravenously.

Nerve

A bundle of nerve fibres which travel to a common location. Nerve fibres, also called axons, are the filamentous projections of many individual *neurons* (nerve cells).

The most obvious nerves in the body are the peripheral nerves, which extend from the *central nervous system* (consisting of the *brain* and *spinal cord*) to other parts of the body.

STRUCTURE
There are 12 pairs of *cranial nerves* (which link directly to the brain) and 31 pairs of *spinal nerves* (which join the spinal cord). All these nerves are peripheral nerves.

In the shoulder and hip regions, the spinal nerves join to form plexuses, from which branch the main nerves to the limbs, such as the median nerve in the arm and the sciatic nerve in the leg. Most nerves divide at numerous points along their length to send branches to all parts of the body, particularly to the sense organs, the skin, skeletal muscles, internal organs, and glands.

FUNCTION
Nerve fibres may have a sensory function, carrying information from a receptor or sense organ at the far end of the nerve towards the central nervous system (CNS), or they may have a motor function, carrying instructions from the CNS to a muscle or to a gland.

Messages are carried by electrical impulses propagated along the fibres. Some nerves carry only sensory or motor fibres, but most carry both.

Nerve functioning is sensitive to cold, pressure, and to a wide variety of injuries (see *Nerve injury*). The peripheral nerves can be damaged by infection, inflammation, poisoning, nutritional deficiencies, and metabolic disorders (see *Neuropathy*).

Nerve block

The injection of a local anaesthetic into or around a nerve to produce anaesthesia (loss of sensation) in a part of the body supplied by that nerve.

WHY IT IS DONE
A nerve block is performed when it is not possible to inject anaesthetic directly into the tissues that are being treated because the area is painfully inflamed or because there is a risk of spreading infection.

Nerve block may also be used to anaesthetize a large area, or an area which is not suitable for injection because it is deep within the body or is covered with bone.

N

HOW IT IS DONE

The local anaesthetic is injected at an accessible area into or around the nerve at a point remote from the area to be treated (for example, the palm of the hand may be anaesthetized by giving injections at sites up the arm, thus blocking the ulnar and the median nerves).

A nerve may be blocked as it leaves the spinal cord. This is done in *epidural anaesthesia*, which is used mainly in childbirth, and in *spinal anaesthesia*, which is used mainly for surgery of the lower abdomen and limbs. A caudal block is a type of nerve block in which an anaesthetic is injected around nerves leaving the lowest part of the spinal cord. It produces anaesthesia in the buttock and genital areas, and is occasionally used in childbirth, especially in a *forceps delivery*.

In a pudendal nerve block, an anaesthetic is injected into nerves passing under the pelvis into the floor of the vagina. This type of nerve block is sometimes used in a forceps delivery. (See also *Anaesthesia, local*.)

Nerve injury

Damage or severance of some or all of the conducting fibres within a *nerve* as a result of trauma. (See *Neuropathy* for nerve damage from causes other than injury.)

Nerves may be damaged in many different injuries, including knife wounds, bullet wounds, penetrating injuries (such as from flying glass, for example), or from accidental contact with powered devices (such as rotary saws and propellers).

PERIPHERAL NERVE INJURY

If injury to a peripheral nerve (i.e. a nerve outside the brain or spinal cord) results in severence of some, but not all, of the individual fibres within the nerve, the cut fibres degenerate on both sides of the injury, leading to loss of power in the muscles and loss of sensation in the skin area supplied by the fibres.

In cases of partial severence in which the ends of the severed fibres are still aligned, new fibres can regenerate along the channels left by the degenerated fibres. These fibres begin to grow within a few days of an injury and continue at a rate of about 2.5 cm per month.

If injury results in total severence of a nerve, the individual fibres try to regenerate but, in the absence of directing channels, simply bunch up to form a lump of tissue; there is no recovery of function.

Regenerating nerve fibres sometimes pass down the wrong channels; as a result, when function is restored, actions may differ from what was intended (for example, an attempt to move the index finger may move the middle finger as well). Movement skills and the interpretation of sensations may need to be relearned.

BRAIN AND SPINAL CORD INJURY

Nerve tracts within the brain and spinal cord are structurally different from the peripheral nerves, and severed fibres in these tracts do not regenerate. For example, it is impossible for vision to be restored if the *optic nerves* are cut.

TREATMENT

Surgery can sometimes repair a severed nerve, but such treatment is possible only for peripheral nerves. Using *microsurgery*, the neurosurgeon ensures that the severed fibres are meticulously brought together and stitched into place with delicate needles and sutures. Careful realignment of the nerve ends gives the fibres the best chance of regenerating along the correct channels. Even with the best surgical repair, recovery is rarely complete.

A programme of *physiotherapy* is needed to keep paralysed muscles healthy and free from *contractures* (abnormal shortening) during the recovery period.

Nerve, trapped

Compression or stretching of a *nerve*, causing numbness, tingling, weakness, and sometimes pain in the area supplied by the nerve.

Common examples of a trapped nerve include *carpal tunnel syndrome*, in which symptoms appear in the thumb, index, and middle fingers as a result of pressure on the median nerve as it passes through the wrist; a *disc prolapse*, in which pressure on the nerve root leading from the spinal cord produces symptoms in the back and legs; and *crutch palsy* (sometimes called Saturday night palsy), in which the radial nerve is pressed against the humerus (upper-arm bone), producing symptoms in the wrist and hand.

A damaged nerve may take some time to heal, causing symptoms to persist. Surgical decompression to relieve pressure on the nerve may be necessary in severe cases.

Nervous breakdown

A popular term used to describe unusual behaviour that is thought to be part of a crisis of severe *anxiety* or tension or part of a psychiatric illness. The term has no technical meaning, but is often applied to people subject to sudden tearfulness, episodes of shouting and screaming, marked social withdrawal, and concern about the possibility of illness.

Nervous energy

A popular term for the increased drive and activity of individuals who are always restless, anxious, and on the go. The term has no technical meaning.

Nervous habit

A nontechnical term for a minor repetitive movement or activity. Sometimes a nervous habit consists of involuntary twitches and facial tics, such as in *Gilles de la Tourette's syndrome* and some forms of *dyskinesia*.

Voluntary nervous habits, such as *thumb-sucking* and nose-picking, are common in young children, but usually disappear naturally with time. Also common is *nail-biting*, which often persists into adult life (20 per cent of adults bite their nails). Such habits are thought to be a means of releasing inner tension.

All nervous habits increase during tension or anxiety, and may be severe in some forms of *depression, anxiety disorder*, or drug withdrawal.

Nervous system

The body's information-gathering, storage, and control system.

STRUCTURE

The nervous system is organized like a computer system that controls a highly complex machine. The central processing unit for the system is the *central nervous system* (CNS), comprising the *brain* and *spinal cord*, which consists of billions of interconnecting *neurons* (nerve cells).

Input of information to the CNS comes from the sense organs. Output (motor) instructions go to the skeletal muscles, muscles controlling speech, internal organs and glands, and the sweat glands in the skin. The cables along which this information is carried are the *nerves* that fan out from the CNS to the entire body. Each nerve is a bundle of the axons (filamentous projections) of many neurons.

In addition to these anatomical divisions of the nervous system, there are various functional divisions. Two of the most important are the *autonomic nervous system*, which is specifically concerned with the automatic (unconscious) regulation of internal body

N

NERVOUS SYSTEM

The nervous system detects and interprets changes in conditions inside and outside the body and responds to them. The central nervous system analyses information and initiates responses; the peripheral nervous system gathers information and carries the response signals. Some responses are involuntary; others are dictated by conscious thought. All nervous system activity consists of signals passed through pathways of inter-connected neurons (nerve cells).

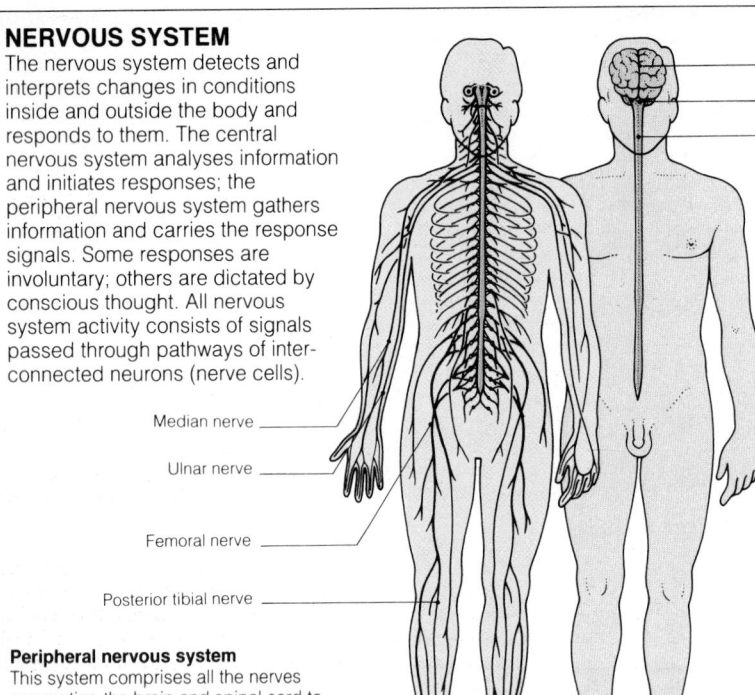

Median nerve

Ulnar nerve

Femoral nerve

Posterior tibial nerve

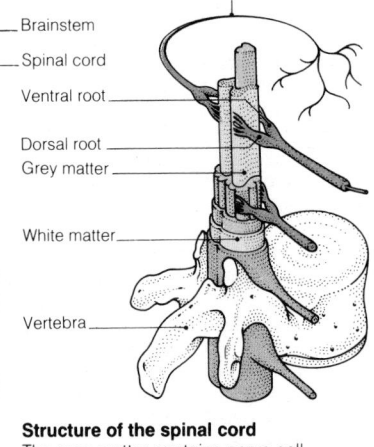

Brain

Brainstem

Spinal cord

Ventral root

Dorsal root

Grey matter

White matter

Vertebra

Spinal nerve

Structure of the spinal cord

The grey matter contains nerve cell bodies; white matter contains their conducting fibres. On joining the cord, spinal nerves split into two. The dorsal root carries sensory fibres; the ventral root carries motor fibres.

Peripheral nervous system

This system comprises all the nerves connecting the brain and spinal cord to the rest of the body. Of these, 31 pairs (the spinal nerves) connect to the spinal cord and 12 pairs (cranial nerves) connect to the brain. The main nerves of the limbs are labelled.

Central nervous system

This system consists of the brain and spinal cord, protected by the skull and spine. The CNS receives input from sense organs and receptors and sends signals to muscles and glands, via the peripheral nervous system.

N

HOW IT WORKS

Some possible events in response to a finger touching a hot object are shown. A receptor sends a message, via a sensory fibre, to the spinal cord. This triggers a signal that travels, via a motor fibre, back to a muscle, which contracts to move the finger. This action is called a reflex arc. Other signals pass to the brain.

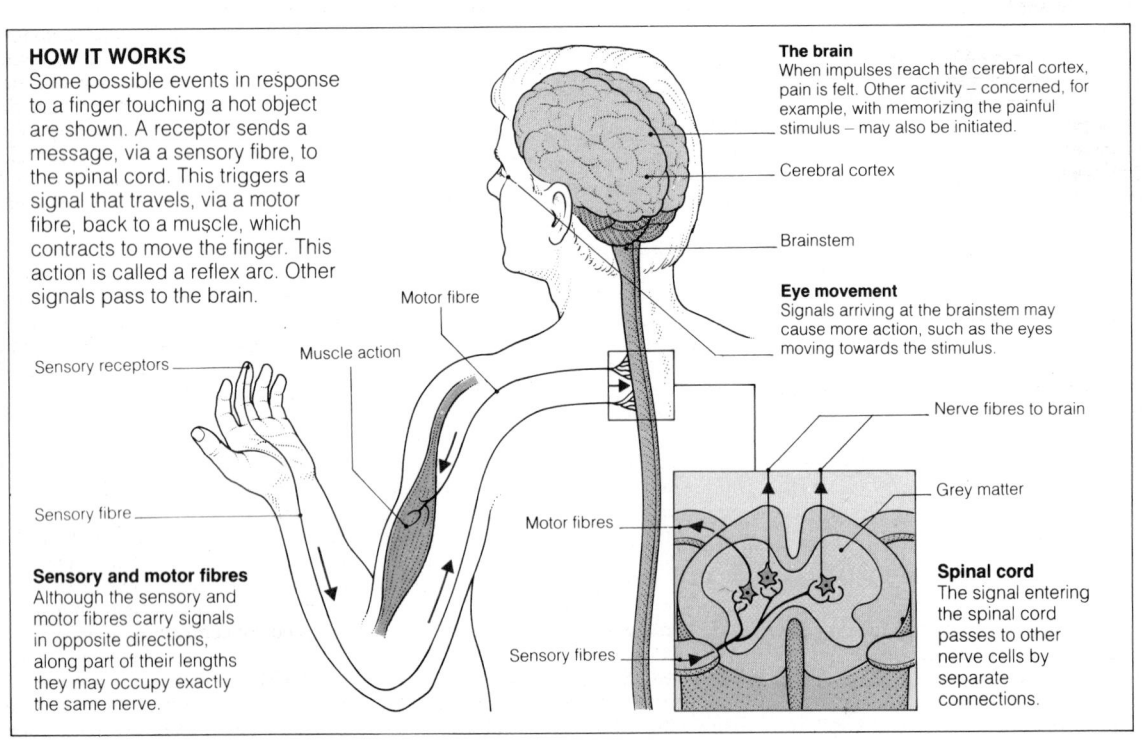

Motor fibre

Muscle action

Sensory receptors

Sensory fibre

Motor fibres

Sensory fibres

The brain

When impulses reach the cerebral cortex, pain is felt. Other activity – concerned, for example, with memorizing the painful stimulus – may also be initiated.

Cerebral cortex

Brainstem

Eye movement

Signals arriving at the brainstem may cause more action, such as the eyes moving towards the stimulus.

Nerve fibres to brain

Grey matter

Sensory and motor fibres

Although the sensory and motor fibres carry signals in opposite directions, along part of their lengths they may occupy exactly the same nerve.

Spinal cord

The signal entering the spinal cord passes to other nerve cells by separate connections.

functioning, and the somatic nervous system, which controls the skeletal muscles responsible for voluntary (willed) movement.

FUNCTION

The overall function of the nervous system is to gather information about the external environment and the body's internal state, to analyse this information, and to initiate appropriate responses aimed at satisfying certain drives. The most powerful drive is for survival. Many survival responses, which range from avoiding physical pain and danger to shivering in response to cold, are initiated unconsciously and automatically by the nervous system.

Other drives are more complex, revolving around a need to experience positive emotions (such as pleasure and excitement) and to avoid negative emotions (such as pain, anxiety, and frustration).

In carrying out its functions, the nervous system has access to many built-in programmes, but it can also improve its performance through *learning*, which relies on *memory*.

The nervous system functions largely through automatic responses to various stimuli (see *Reflex*), although voluntary actions can also be initiated through the activity of higher, conscious areas of the brain. Certain higher functions (such as visual perception, memory storage, thought, and speech production) are extremely complex and not understood in detail. Overall, however, all nervous activity is based on the transmission of impulses through complex networks of neurons.

DISORDERS

Disorders of the nervous system may result from damage to or dysfunction of its component parts (see *Brain* disorders box; *Spinal cord*; *Neuropathy*; *Nerve injury*). Disorders of the nervous system may also be due to impairment of sensory, analytical, or memory functions (see *Vision, disorders of; Deafness; Numbness; Anosmia; Agnosia; Amnesia*), or of motor functions (see *Aphasia; Dysarthria; Ataxia*).

Netilmicin

An *antibiotic drug* usually prescribed only in hospital to treat serious infection, when other antibiotic drugs have been ineffective. In rare cases, netilmicin can damage the inner ear or the kidneys.

Nettle rash

A common name for *urticaria*.

Neuralgia

Pain caused by irritation of, or damage to, a *nerve*. The pain usually occurs in brief bouts, may be very severe, and can often be felt shooting along the affected nerve.

Some types of neuralgia are features of a specific disorder. Sufferers from *migraine* commonly suffer from a form of neuralgia consisting of attacks of intense, radiating pain around the eye. Postherpetic neuralgia is a burning pain that may recur at the site of an attack of *herpes zoster* (shingles) for months or even years after the illness.

Other types of neuralgia result from disturbance of a particular nerve. In glossopharyngeal neuralgia, intense pain is felt at the back of the tongue and in the throat and ear. The structures in this area are served by the glossopharyngeal nerve. The pain may occur spontaneously or may be brought on by talking, eating, or swallowing; its cause is generally unknown. The same is true of *trigeminal neuralgia*, a severe paroxysm of pain affecting one side of the face supplied by the trigeminal nerve.

TREATMENT

Neuralgia is sometimes relieved by *analgesic drugs* (painkillers), such as paracetamol. Glossopharyngeal, trigeminal, and postherpetic neuralgia sometimes respond to *carbamazepine*.

Neural tube defect

A developmental failure affecting the spinal cord or brain in the embryo.

INCIDENCE

Three babies per 2,000 live-born babies in the UK have a neural tube defect. The condition is slightly more common in girls than in boys. Many more fetuses are affected but do not survive to birth. The rate of neural tube defects is higher in the northwest of Britain than in the southeast, and is also higher in the lower social classes.

CAUSES AND OUTLOOK

Early in embryonic development, a ridge of nervous tissue forms along the back of the embryo. As development continues, this material differentiates into the spinal cord and body nerves at the lower end and into the brain at the upper end. At the same time, the bones that make up the spine gradually surround the spinal cord. If any part of this sequence goes awry, many defects can result. The worst is *anencephaly* (total lack of a brain). Much more common is *spina bifida*, in which the vertebrae (spinal bones) do not form a complete ring to protect the spinal cord.

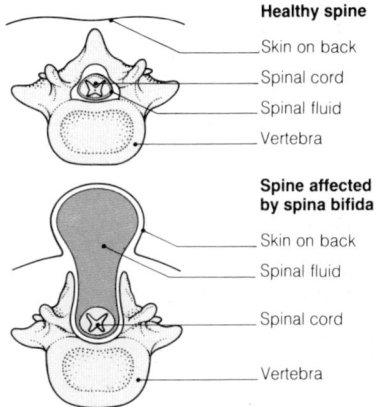

Healthy spine
Skin on back
Spinal cord
Spinal fluid
Vertebra

Spine affected by spina bifida
Skin on back
Spinal fluid
Spinal cord
Vertebra

Neural tube defect
This defect leads to failure of the bony arch to fuse over the back of the spinal cord, thus causing spina bifida.

Genetic factors play a part in neural tube defects, which show multifactorial *inheritance*. Couples who have had an affected child or who have a family history of neural tube defect should seek *genetic counselling*.

Research has shown that the risk of a neural tube defect can be substantially reduced if the mother takes *folic acid* supplements for a month before conception and during the early part of pregnancy.

Ultrasound scanning and *amniocentesis* allow accurate antenatal testing for neural tube defects, and subsequent termination of affected pregnancies. The combination of prevention by folic acid treatment and screening has led to a substantial decline in the numbers of babies born with these defects.

Neurapraxia

A type of *nerve injury* in which the outward structure of a nerve appears intact, but in which some of the conducting fibres have been damaged or have degenerated and thus do not transmit signals to muscles.

Neurasthenia

An outdated term that literally means "nervous exhaustion". It was once used to describe a number of physical and mental symptoms, including loss of energy, insomnia, aches and pains (especially in the chest and abdomen), *depression*, irritability, and reduced concentration.

Neuritis

A term that literally means inflammation of a nerve. True nerve inflammation may be caused by infection (for

N

example by a virus in *herpes zoster* or by a bacterium in *Hansen's disease*). The term neuritis is also often applied to nerve damage or disease from causes other than inflammation. Thus, it has become virtually synonymous with neuropathy, a term for all disorders of the peripheral nerves.

Neuroblastoma

A tumour of the *adrenal glands* or the sympathetic nervous system (part of the *autonomic nervous system*). Most neuroblastomas develop in the adrenal glands or in the sympathetic nerves along the back wall of the abdomen. Less commonly, neuroblastomas develop in the sympathetic nerves of the chest or neck, or, very rarely, in the brain.

Neuroblastomas are the most common extracranial (outside the skull) solid tumour of childhood. About 80 per cent of cases develop during the first 10 years of life, most commonly in the first four years. The incidence is 8.3 cases per one million children.

SYMPTOMS AND SIGNS

The symptoms vary according to the site of the tumour and the extent to which it has spread. Common symptoms include weight loss, general aches and pains, paleness, and irritability. There may also be tumours of the abdomen, neck, eyes, or skin. In some cases, the tumour secretes the hormones *adrenaline* and *noradrenaline*, which may cause diarrhoea, high blood pressure, and flushing of the skin.

DIAGNOSIS

The condition is diagnosed from the symptoms and signs, and from X-rays, blood tests, and urine tests. In some cases, it may be necessary to perform a *biopsy* (removal of a small sample of tissue for microscopic examination) of the bone marrow and any accessible tumours.

TREATMENT AND OUTLOOK

Treatment consists of the surgical removal of the tumour, followed by *radiotherapy* and possibly also by *anticancer drugs*.

The outlook varies greatly because neuroblastomas range from being relatively harmless to highly malignant. Overall, however, about one third of those affected survive for at least five years after treatment.

Neurocutaneous disorders

A group of conditions characterized by abnormalities of the skin as well as abnormalities of the nerves and/or the central nervous system.

The best known of these disorders is *neurofibromatosis*, in which there are brown patches on the skin and numerous fibrous nodules on the skin and nerves. Another example is *tuberous sclerosis*, which is characterized by small skin-coloured swellings over the cheeks and nose, mental deficiency, and epilepsy.

Neurodermatitis

An itchy, eczema-like skin condition caused by repeated scratching. (See also *Lichen simplex*.)

Neuroendocrinology

The study of the interactions between the *nervous system* and the *endocrine system*, which control internal body functions and the way in which the body responds to the external environment.

Neurofibromatosis

An uncommon inherited disorder, also called von Recklinghausen's disease, characterized by numerous neurofibromas (soft, fibrous swellings that grow from nerves) and by *café au lait spots* (pale, coffee-coloured patches) on the skin.

SYMPTOMS AND SIGNS

Neurofibromas may develop anywhere on the skin and sometimes elsewhere in the body. These swellings may be tiny or be as large as several centimetres in diameter. They are sometimes unsightly. Café au lait spots are most common on the skin of the trunk and pelvis.

If neurofibromas occur in the central nervous system, they may cause *epilepsy* and other complications, sometimes affecting vision and hearing. In some cases, neurofibromatosis leads to bone deformities. Rarely, neurofibromas become cancerous.

TREATMENT

Surgical removal of neurofibromas is necessary only if there are complications. Anyone who has this disorder, and parents of an affected child, should seek *genetic counselling* if they are planning a pregnancy.

Neurology

The medical discipline concerned with the study of the *nervous system* and its disorders, particularly with their diagnosis and treatment.

Neurologists are trained to examine the nerves, reflexes, motor and sensory functions, and muscles to determine a disorder's cause and extent. To aid diagnosis, extensive use is made of modern imaging tech-

niques (such as *CT scanning* and *MRI*). In the past, relatively few disorders of the nervous system could be treated effectively. Today, with a better understanding of the biochemical and structural bases of neurological disorders, treatments have been developed for *migraine, Parkinson's disease*, and the control of *pain*. Neurologists have become specialists in the care and support of patients with progressive disorders, such as *multiple sclerosis* and *muscular dystrophy*. (See also *Neuropathology; Neurosurgery*.)

Neuroma

A benign tumour of *nerve* tissue. In most cases, the cause is unknown; rarely, a neuroma develops as a result of damage to a nerve.

A neuroma may affect any nerve in the body. Symptoms vary according to the nerve involved. In most cases, there is intermittent pain in the areas of the body supplied by the affected nerve. The same areas may also become numb and weak if the neuroma develops in a confined space and presses on the nerve.

If symptoms are troublesome, the tumour may be surgically removed. (See also *Acoustic neuroma*.)

Neuron

The term for a nerve cell. The *nervous system* contains billions of neurons, which act in various combinations to do everything from writing a symphony to scratching a fleabite. The neurons are analogous to the wires in a complex electrical machine.

There are three main types of neuron—interneurons, motor neurons, and sensory neurons (see illustrated box opposite).

FUNCTION

The function of a neuron is to "fire" (transmit an electrical impulse along its axon) under certain specific conditions. The electrical impulse causes the release of a chemical called a *neurotransmitter* from the axon terminals. This neurotransmitter may make a muscle cell contract, cause an endocrine gland to release a hormone, or affect an adjacent neuron.

Different stimuli excite different types of neurons to fire. Sensory neurons may be excited by physical stimuli, such as cold, pressure, or light of a certain wavelength. The activity of most neurons is controlled by the effects of neurotransmitters released from adjacent neurons. The ability of a neuron to fire depends on a small difference in electrical potential be-

N

STRUCTURE OF A NEURON

A neuron (nerve cell) consists of a cell body and several branching projections called dendrites. Every neuron has a filamentous projection called an axon (nerve fibre). Axons vary in length from a fraction of a centimetre to about a metre. An axon branches at its end to form terminals, via which signals are transmitted to target cells, such as the dendrites of other neurons, muscle cells, or glands. Bundles of the axons of many neurons are known as nerves or, within the brain or spinal cord, as nerve tracts or pathways.

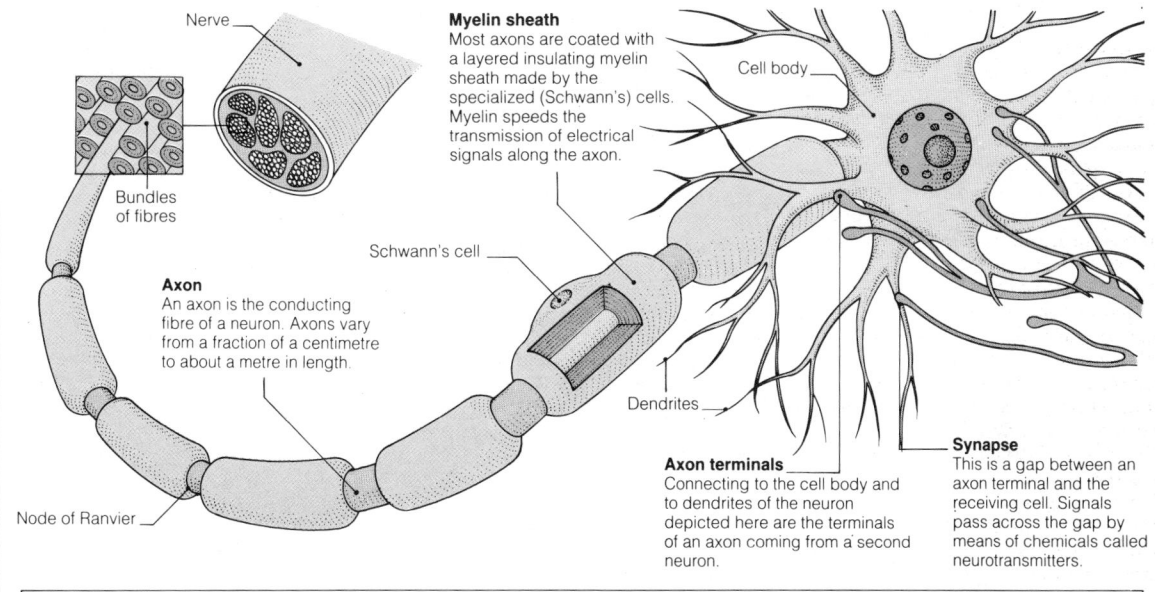

Nerve

Bundles of fibres

Myelin sheath
Most axons are coated with a layered insulating myelin sheath made by the specialized (Schwann's) cells. Myelin speeds the transmission of electrical signals along the axon.

Cell body

Schwann's cell

Axon
An axon is the conducting fibre of a neuron. Axons vary from a fraction of a centimetre to about a metre in length.

Node of Ranvier

Dendrites

Axon terminals
Connecting to the cell body and to dendrites of the neuron depicted here are the terminals of an axon coming from a second neuron.

Synapse
This is a gap between an axon terminal and the receiving cell. Signals pass across the gap by means of chemicals called neurotransmitters.

BASIC TYPES OF NEURON

Sensory neurons carry signals from sense receptors along their axons into the central nervous system (CNS). Motor neurons carry signals from the CNS to muscles or glands; the axon terminals form a motor endplate. Interneurons form all the complex interconnecting electrical circuitry within the CNS itself. For each sensory neuron in the body, there are about 10 motor neurons and 99 interneurons.

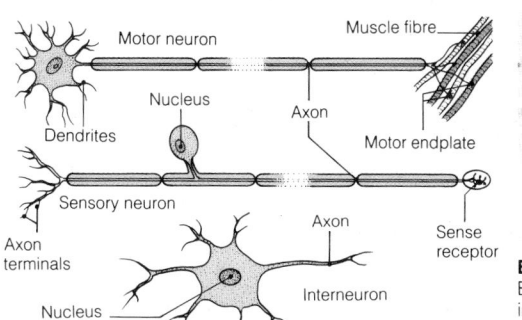

Motor neuron — Muscle fibre
Nucleus — Axon — Motor endplate
Dendrites
Sensory neuron
Axon terminals — Axon — Sense receptor
Nucleus — Interneuron

Brain neurons
Electron micrograph of interneurons in the brain.

N

---

tween the inside and outside of the cell. Under the direct influence of an excitatory neurotransmitter, a sudden change occurs in this potential at one point on the cell's membrane. The change, called an "action potential", then flows along the membrane (and thus along the axon of the cell) at up to 430 kilometres per hour. A neuron may be able to fire in this way several times every second.

Other neurotransmitters stabilize neuronal membranes, preventing an action potential. Thus, the firing pattern of a neuron depends on the balance of excitatory and inhibitory influences acting on it.

LIFESPAN
If the cell body of a neuron is damaged or degenerates, the cell dies and is never replaced. A baby starts life with the maximum number of neurons. The number of neurons decreases continuously thereafter. People seem to be born with an excess number of neurons, so problems arise only when disease, injury, or persistent alcohol abuse affects the *central nervous system*, dramatically increasing the rate of neuron loss.

If a peripheral nerve is damaged, its individual fibres have the ability to regenerate themselves (see *Nerve injury; Neuropathy*).

Neuropathic joint

A joint that has been damaged by a series of injuries, which pass unnoticed because of loss of sensation in the joint due to *neuropathy* (nerve damage caused by disease).

Neuropathic joints develop in a number of conditions, including *diabetes mellitus* and untreated *syphilis*.

When sensation to pain is lost, abnormal stress and strain on a joint do not stimulate the protective reflex spasm of the surrounding muscles; this failure of the protective reflex spasm allows exaggerated movement that can damage the joint. Severe recurrent damage to a joint may lead to *osteoarthritis*, swelling, and deformity. Pain is minimal, however, because of the lack of sensation.

DIAGNOSIS AND TREATMENT
Severe joint degeneration and deformity are visible on *X-rays*. An orthopaedic *brace* or *caliper splint* may be necessary to restrict abnormal joint movement. Occasionally, an *arthrodesis* (a surgical operation to fuse a joint) is performed. The nerve damage is irreversible.

Neuropathology

The branch of *pathology* that is concerned with the causes and effects of disorders of the *nervous system*. (See also *Neurology*).

Neuropathy

Disease, inflammation, or damage to the peripheral *nerves*, which connect the central nervous system (brain and spinal cord), to the sense organs, muscles, glands, and internal organs.

Symptoms caused by neuropathies include numbness, tingling, pain, or muscle weakness, depending on the nerves affected.

TYPES
Most nerve cell axons (the conducting fibres that make up nerves) are insulated by a sheath of a fatty substance called *myelin*, but some are unmyelinated. Most neuropathies arise from damage or irritation either to the axons or to their myelin sheaths. An axon may suffer thinning of, complete loss of, or patchy loss of its myelin sheath. This may cause a slowing of or a complete block to the passage of electrical signals.

Various types of neuropathy are described according to the site and distribution of damage. For example, a distal neuropathy starts with damage at the far end of a nerve (farthest from the brain or spinal cord). A symmetrical neuropathy affects nerves at the same places on each side of the body. Some neuropathies are described according to their underlying cause (for example, diabetic neuropathy and alcoholic neuropathy).

The term neuritis is now used virtually interchangeably with neuropathy. Polyneuropathy (or polyneuritis) literally means damage to several nerves; mononeuropathy (or mononeuritis) indicates damage to a single nerve. *Neuralgia* describes pain caused by irritation or inflammation of a particular nerve.

CAUSES
In some cases of neuropathy there is no obvious or detectable cause.

Among the many specific causes are *diabetes mellitus*, dietary deficiencies (particularly of B vitamins), persistent excessive alcohol consumption, and metabolic upsets such as *uraemia*. Other causes include *Hansen's disease* (leprosy), *lead poisoning*, or poisoning by drugs.

Nerves may become acutely inflamed. This often occurs after a viral infection (e.g. in *Guillain-Barré syndrome*). Neuropathies may result from *autoimmune disorders* such as *rheumatoid arthritis*, systemic *lupus erythematosus*, or *polyarteritis nodosa*. In these disorders, there is often damage to the blood vessels supplying the nerves. Neuropathies may occur secondarily to malignant tumours, such as *lung cancer*, or with *lymphomas* and *leukaemias*. There is also a group of inherited neuropathies, the most common being *peroneal muscular atrophy*.

SYMPTOMS
The symptoms of neuropathy depend on whether it affects mainly sensory nerve fibres or motor nerve fibres.

Damage to sensory nerve fibres may cause numbness and tingling, sensations of cold, or pain, often starting in the hands and feet and spreading towards the centre of the body. Damage to motor fibres may cause muscle weakness and muscle wasting.

Damage to nerves of the *autonomic nervous system* may lead to blurred vision, impaired or absent sweating, episodes of faintness associated with falls in blood pressure, and disturbance of gastric, intestinal, bladder, and sexual functioning, including incontinence and impotence.

Some neuropathies are linked with particular symptoms (e.g. diabetic neuropathy and alcoholic neuropathy may both cause severe pain).

DIAGNOSIS
To determine the extent of damage, studies of nerve conduction are performed, together with *EMG* tests, which record the electrical activity in muscles. To determine the cause of neuropathy, *blood tests*, *X-rays*, nerve or muscle *biopsy* (removal of a small sample of tissue for microscopic analysis), and various other diagnostic tests may be required.

TREATMENT
When possible, treatment is aimed at the underlying cause of the neuropathy. For example, in diabetes mellitus, scrupulous attention to the control of the blood sugar level affords the best chances for recovery. Other people may need to stop drinking alcohol, or, if a nutritional deficiency

has been diagnosed, may be given injections of vitamins such as thiamine (see *Vitamin B complex*).

If treatment is successful and the cell bodies of the damaged nerve cells have not been destroyed, a full recovery from the neuropathy is possible.

Neuropsychiatry

The branch of medicine that deals with the relationship between psychiatric symptoms and neurological disorder. This may include the effects of head injury and alcohol on the brain, or specific disorders such as brain tumours, infections, inherited illnesses, and disorders affecting the brain in childhood and causing mental handicap.

Increasingly, new techniques of *brain imaging* are demonstrating abnormalities of brain structure and function in disorders which produce psychiatric symptoms.

Neurosis

A term commonly used to describe a range of psychiatric disorders in which the sufferer remains in touch with reality.

Neurotic symptoms are distressing to the afflicted person, who is aware of a change from his or her usual psychological state. By contrast, people suffering from psychotic illnesses usually do not recognize that they are ill (see *Psychosis*). Neurotic symptoms generally do not lead to distinctly abnormal behaviour, although they can severely limit work or social activities. They tend to fluctuate in intensity, often in response to social or personal stresses. No physical abnormality has been shown to underlie them.

The major neurotic disorders are mild forms of *depression; anxiety disorders*, including *phobias* and *obsessive-compulsive behaviour; hypochondriasis*; and *dissociative disorders*.

Neurosurgery

The specialty concerned with the surgical treatment of disorders of the *brain, spinal cord*, or other parts of the *nervous system*. Many generalized nervous system disorders do not respond to surgical treatment, but neurosurgery can deal with most conditions in which a localized structural change interferes with nerve function.

Conditions treated by neurosurgery include tumours of the brain, spinal cord, or meninges (membranes that surround the brain and spinal cord), certain abnormalities of the blood vessels that supply the brain, such as an *aneurysm* (balloon-like swelling at a weak point in an artery), bleeding inside the skull (see *Extradural haemorrhage*; *Intracerebral haemorrhage*; and *Subdural haemorrhage*), brain abscess, some birth defects (such as *hydrocephalus* and *spina bifida*), certain types of *epilepsy*, and nerve damage caused by illness or accidents. Neurosurgeons are also concerned with the surgical relief of otherwise untreatable *pain*.

Neurosyphilis

Infection of the brain or spinal cord that occurs in untreated *syphilis* many years after the initial infection.

Damage to the spinal cord due to neurosyphilis may cause tabes dorsalis, characterized by poor coordination of leg movements when walking, urinary incontinence, and intermittent pains in the abdomen and limbs. Damage to the brain may cause *dementia* and muscle weakness, which in rare cases progresses to total paralysis of the limbs (in which case it is called general paralysis of the insane).

Neurotoxin

A chemical that damages nervous tissue. The principal effects of neurotoxic nerve damage are numbness, weakness, or paralysis of the part of the body supplied by the affected nerve.

Neurotoxins are present in the venom of certain snakes (see *Snake bites*), and are released by some types of bacteria (such as those that cause *tetanus* and *diphtheria*). Some chemical poisons, such as arsenic and lead, are also neurotoxic.

Neurotransmitter

A chemical released from nerve endings that transmits impulses from one *neuron* (nerve cell) to another neuron or to a muscle cell. Neurotransmitters are released from nerve endings in response to electrical impulses travelling down neurons. Scores of different chemicals fulfil this function in different parts of the *nervous system* (see illustrated box, above).

Many neurotransmitters, such as *noradrenaline*, act as both neurotransmitters and *hormones*, being released into the bloodstream to act on their target cells at a distance.

TYPES

One of the most important neurotransmitters is *acetylcholine*. This chemical is released by neurons connected to skeletal muscles, causing them to contract, and also by neurons

HOW NEUROTRANSMITTERS WORK

When an electrical impulse travels down a nerve cell axon, it causes the release of a chemical neurotransmitter at the axon terminals. The chemical is not the same in every case; acetylcholine, noradrenaline, dopamine, and serotonin are all important examples.

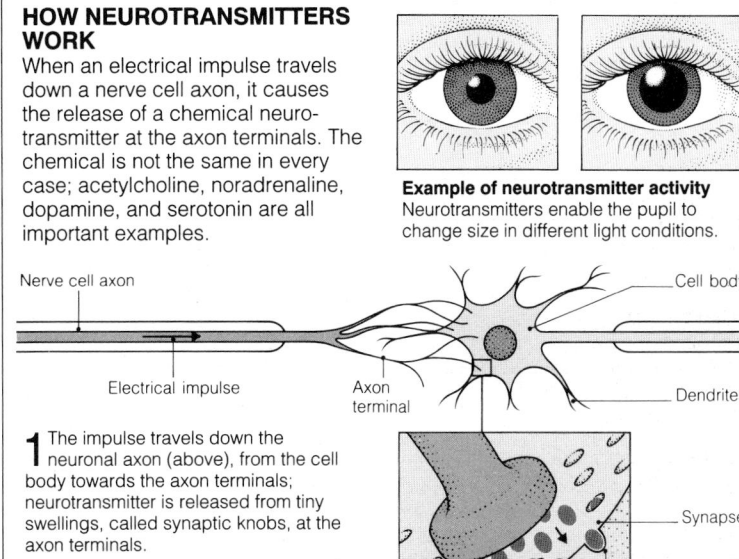

Example of neurotransmitter activity
Neurotransmitters enable the pupil to change size in different light conditions.

Nerve cell axon

Electrical impulse

Axon terminal

Cell body

Dendrites

1 The impulse travels down the neuronal axon (above), from the cell body towards the axon terminals; neurotransmitter is released from tiny swellings, called synaptic knobs, at the axon terminals.

2 The neurotransmitter crosses the gap, or synapse, to the surface membrane of the target cell (right), where it binds to a protein called a receptor.

3 If sufficient target cell receptors are activated by neurotransmitter binding, an impulse is initiated and passes in turn down the target cell's axon (below right).

Synapse

Receptors

Presynaptic membrane (axon terminal)

Postsynaptic membrane (dendrite of target cell)

Neurotransmitter chemical

Electrical impulse to target

that control the sweat glands and the heartbeat. Acetylcholine also transmits messages between neurons in the brain and spinal cord. Interference with the action of acetylcholine on skeletal muscles is the cause of the disease *myasthenia gravis*. It is thought that depletion of the nerve cells that release acetylcholine in the brain may be a factor in *Alzheimer's disease*.

Noradrenaline has an important role in the nervous control of heartbeat, blood flow, and the body's response to stress. This substance is made by the *adrenal glands* as well as being produced by neurons. *Dopamine*, another neurotransmitter, plays an important role in parts of the brain that control movement. Malfunction of the neurons that respond to dopamine is thought to be important in causing *Parkinson's disease*. *Serotonin* is one of the main neurotransmitters in parts of the brain concerned with conscious processes.

In the last 20 years, a new group of neurotransmitters (called neuropeptides) has been discovered. These are small proteins that consist of larger molecules than the previously known neurotransmitters, which consist of very small molecules. The best studied of the neuropeptides are the *endorphins*, used by the brain to control sensitivity to pain.

Newborn

An infant at birth and during the first few weeks of life.

INITIAL EXAMINATION

Immediately after birth, the newborn baby is briefly checked by the nurse, midwife, or doctor in attendance. This examination includes checking the heart-rate with a *stethoscope* and establishment that breathing is normal. The *Apgar score* and other tests are performed to check the baby is in good health. The sex is noted and a check made for any obvious *birth defect*.

NURSING PROCEDURE

The baby is labelled with his or her name and date of birth. A record is also made of the baby's birthweight, length, and head circumference.

At birth, the baby is usually covered with vernix, a white substance that lubricates its passage from the uterus. The vernix is wiped off and the baby is wrapped in a blanket and given to the mother to hold and feed, or is placed in a warm cot. If very small or sick, the baby will be kept in an *incubator* and treated in a neonatal special-care or intensive-care unit.

The frequency of the baby's urine and *meconium* (faeces passed by the newborn) is recorded. During the second week of life, two special blood tests are performed: a blood sample is removed from all babies to check for *phenylketonuria* (see *Guthrie test*) and *hypothyroidism*.

MEDICAL EXAMINATION

Within 24 hours of birth (or sooner if there is any cause for concern), the baby is usually given a complete medical examination by the paediatrician. This examination assesses the baby's general health and identifies any birth defects (such as cleft palate). The skull, eyes, face, abdomen, heart, spine, hips, genitals, and limbs are checked, and the baby's posture, movements, behaviour, cry, reflexes (see *Reflexes, primitive*), and responsiveness are noted.

ABNORMALITIES IN THE NEWBORN

The newborn baby may have a swollen or misshapen head due to pressure during labour. Less commonly, there may be more notable evidence of *birth injury*, such as *cephalhaematoma* (swelling of the scalp caused by bruising around the skull). Most problems caused by the pressure of delivery resolve themselves within a few days.

Jaundice (see *Jaundice, neonatal*) is extremely common in the newborn, especially if the baby is breast-fed. Usually appearing on the second or third day, the jaundice generally disappears over the next few days. In most cases, jaundice in the newborn is harmless. However, the condition may be serious if it appears during the first 24 hours or occurs in a very premature infant.

Some newborn girls have slight vaginal bleeding or discharge, and babies of either sex may have enlargement of the breasts. These harmless conditions are caused by maternal sex hormones that reached the fetus through the placenta. Any extra hormones soon leave the baby's body.

The umbilical cord, which may be painted with antiseptic to prevent infection, usually dries and drops off within a week or so of birth. Infections of the cord stump sometimes occur.

Minor, harmless abnormalities of the newborn include *milia* (tiny, white spots on the face), *haemangioma*, *mongolian blue spot*, and a blotchy, red rash (see *Urticaria, neonatal*) that may occur around the second day. (See also *Prematurity; Postmaturity*.)

Niacin

See *Vitamin B complex*.

Nickel

A metallic element which is present in the body in minute amounts. Its exact role is poorly understood. Nickel is thought to activate certain *enzymes* (substances that promote biochemical reactions). It may also play a part in stabilizing chromosomal material in the nuclei of cells.

Disease due to a deficiency of nickel is unknown. However, exposure to nickel may cause *dermatitis* (inflammation of the skin). *Lung cancer* has been reported in workers in nickel refineries.

Niclosamide

An *anthelmintic drug* used to treat *tapeworm infestation*. Niclosamide causes the tapeworm to loosen its grip on the inner wall of the intestine. The worm is then passed out of the body in the faeces.

Adverse effects include abdominal pain, lightheadedness, and itching.

Nicotinamide

See *Vitamin B complex*.

Nicotine

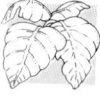 A drug in tobacco which acts as a stimulant and is responsible for dependence on tobacco. Nicotine has no medical use, but certain of its derivatives are used as pesticides.

After inhalation, the nicotine in tobacco smoke passes rapidly into the bloodstream. Nicotine in chewing tobacco is absorbed more slowly through the lining of the mouth. After entering the bloodstream, nicotine acts on the nervous system until the drug is eventually broken down by the liver and excreted in the urine.

EFFECTS

Nicotine acts primarily on the *autonomic nervous system*, which controls involuntary body activities such as the heart-rate. The effects of the drug vary from one person to another, and also depend on dosage and past usage. In someone unused to smoking, even a small amount of nicotine may slow the heart-rate and cause nausea and vomiting. However, in habitual smokers, the drug increases the heart-rate and narrows the blood vessels (the combined effect of which is to raise blood pressure). Nicotine also stimulates the *central nervous system*, thereby reducing fatigue, increasing alertness, and improving concentration.

Regular use of tobacco results in tolerance to nicotine, so that a higher intake is needed for the same effects. This is, however, less noticeable with tobacco than other addictive drugs.

NICOTINE AND DISEASE

Although it is the tar in tobacco smoke that damages lung tissue and causes lung cancer, smoking is also clearly associated with *coronary artery disease*, *peripheral vascular disease*, and other cardiovascular disorders. It is uncertain whether these disorders are caused by the nicotine or by the carbon monoxide content of the smoke.

Excessively large amounts of nicotine can cause poisoning, which may result in vomiting, seizures, and, very occasionally, death.

WITHDRAWAL

Because most smokers are physically dependent on nicotine, stopping smoking commonly causes withdrawal symptoms, such as drowsiness, headaches, fatigue, and difficulty concentrating. To reduce these symptoms in a person who is trying to stop smoking, nicotine may be taken in the form of chewing gum, or absorbed into the bloodstream from impregnated skin patches. (See also *Tobacco-smoking*.)

Nicotinic acid

A form of niacin (see *Vitamin B complex*). Apart from its use as a vitamin supplement, nicotinic acid is also prescribed as a *lipid-lowering drug* and as a *vasodilator drug*. High doses are used to treat certain types of *hyperlipidaemia*. Low doses are used to improve circulation in disorders such as *peripheral vascular disease*.

Adverse effects, which are more common with high doses, include flushing, dizziness, nausea, palpitations, and itching.

Nifedipine

A *calcium channel blocker* used mainly to prevent and treat *angina pectoris*. Nifedipine is also often used to treat *hypertension* (high blood pressure) and disorders affecting the circulation, such as *Raynaud's disease*. Possible adverse effects include *oedema* (accumulation of fluid in tissues), flushing, headache, and dizziness.

Night blindness

The inability to see well in dim light. Many people with night blindness have no discernible eye disease. The condition may be an inherited functional defect of the retina, an early sign of *retinitis pigmentosa*, or a result of vitamin A deficiency.

Nightmare

An unpleasant vivid dream, often accompanied by a sense of suffocation. Nightmares occur during REM (rapid eye movement) *sleep* in the middle and later parts of the night, and are often clearly remembered if the dreamer awakens completely.

Nightmares are very common, especially in children aged between eight and 10, and are particularly likely to occur when the child's breathing is slightly difficult because of a cold or illness, or when there is anxiety over separation from parents or home. In adults, nightmares may be a side-effect of certain drugs, including *beta-blocker drugs* and *benzodiazepine drugs*. Traumatic experiences (such as accidents, torture, or prolonged imprisonment) seem to be particularly associated with disturbing and repeated nightmares. However, there is no specific relationship to psychiatric illness.

Nightmares should not be confused with hypnagogic *hallucinations*, which occur while falling asleep, nor with *night terror*, which occurs in NREM (nonrapid eye movement) sleep and is not remembered the next day.

Night terror

A disorder, occurring mainly in children, consisting of abrupt arousals from sleep in a terrified state. Night terror (also called sleep terror) usually starts between the ages of four and seven, and gradually disappears in early adolescence.

Episodes occur during NREM (nonrapid eye movement) *sleep*, usually half an hour to three and a half hours after falling asleep.

Sufferers wake up screaming in a semiconscious state and remain frightened for some minutes. They do not recognize familiar faces or surroundings, and usually cannot be comforted. Physical signs of agitation, such as sweating or an increased heart-rate, are also common. The sufferer gradually falls back to sleep and has no memory of the event the following day.

Though distressing to parents, night terror in children has no serious significance. In adults, it is likely to be associated with an *anxiety disorder*.

Nipple

The small prominence at the tip of each *breast*. Each of a woman's nipples contains tiny openings through which milk can pass. The nipple and the surrounding areola are darker than the surrounding skin, darkening more and increasing in size during *pregnancy*. Muscle in the nipple allows it to become erect.

DISORDERS

Structural defects of the nipple are rare. One or both nipples may be absent, or there may be additional nipples along a line extending from the armpit to the groin.

An inverted nipple is usually an abnormality of development. It can be corrected by drawing out the nipple between finger and thumb daily for several weeks. Inversion of a previously normal nipple in an adult is much more significant and may be due to *breast cancer*.

Cracked nipples are common during the last months of pregnancy and during the period when a woman is *breast-feeding*. Daily washing, drying, and moisturizing of the nipple

---

LOCATION OF THE NIPPLE

The protrusion at the tip of the breast, surrounded by the areola. Milk ducts emerge at the nipple.

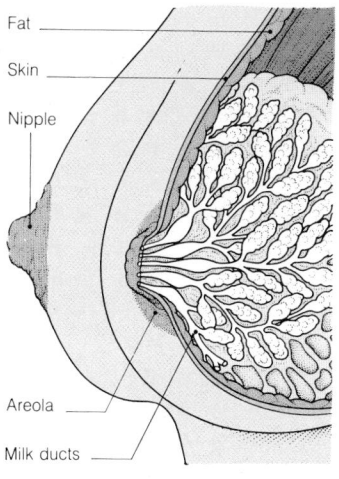

Fat

Skin

Nipple

Areola

Milk ducts

---

can help to prevent cracking. In addition to causing discomfort, cracks may lead to infective *mastitis*.

Papilloma of the nipple is a benign swelling attached to the skin by a stalk. *Paget's disease of the nipple* appears initially as persistent eczema of the nipple. It is caused by a slowly growing cancer arising in a milk duct, and surgical treatment is required.

Discharge from the nipple occurs for a variety of reasons. A clear, straw-coloured discharge may develop in early pregnancy. A milky discharge may occur after the period of breast-feeding is over. *Galactorrhoea* (discharge of milk in someone who is not pregnant or breast-feeding) may be caused by a hormone imbalance; rarely, it may be due to a galactocele (a cyst under the areola). A discharge containing pus indicates a breast *abscess*. A bloodstained discharge may be due to *fibroadenosis* or cancer.

Nitrate drugs

COMMON DRUGS
Glyceryl trinitrate Isosorbide dinitrate

A group of *vasodilator drugs* used in the treatment of *angina pectoris* (chest pain due to impaired blood supply to heart muscle) and severe *heart failure* (reduced pumping efficiency).

Possible adverse effects of nitrate drugs include headache, flushing, and dizziness. *Tolerance* (the need for greater amounts of a drug to have the same effect) may develop when the drug is taken regularly.

Nitrazepam

A *benzodiazepine drug* used in the short-term treatment of *insomnia*. Nitrazepam is long-acting and may cause a hangover effect, with drowsiness and lightheadedness, the following day. Regular use over several weeks can lead to a reduction in its effectiveness as the body adapts.

Nitrazepam can lead to *drug dependence* and to withdrawal symptoms, such as nervousness and restlessness.

Nitrites

Salts of nitrous acid (a nitrogen-containing acid). To preserve meat, sodium nitrite is added in small amounts together with potassium nitrate (saltpetre) and salt to inhibit the growth of potentially harmful bacteria. During the curing process, the nitrate is converted into nitrite which combines with muscle pigment to form the characteristic red colour of

N

cured meats (bacon, salt beef etc.). In large amounts, nitrites can cause dizziness, nausea, and vomiting.

Within the intestine, nitrites are converted to substances called nitrosamines. In laboratory investigations, nitrosamines have been shown to cause cancer in animals. However, there is no conclusive proof that they have the same effect in humans or that eating food containing nitrites is harmful to health.

Nitrofurantoin
An *antibacterial drug* used in the treatment of *urinary tract infection*.

Nitrofurantoin should be taken with food to reduce the risk of irritating the stomach, which can cause abdominal pain and nausea. More serious adverse effects, such as breathing difficulty, numbness, and jaundice, occur rarely.

Nitrogen
A colourless, odourless gas that makes up 78 per cent of the Earth's atmosphere. Atmospheric nitrogen has no biological action, although in scuba diving, bubbles of nitrogen gas may form in body fluids if a diver ascends to the surface too rapidly, causing the "bends" (see *Decompression sickness*).

Although nitrogen gas cannot be utilized by the body, compounds of nitrogen are essential to life. Probably the most important of such compounds are *amino acids*, the building blocks of *proteins*, which represent the fundamental structural substances of all cells and tissues. Because humans cannot make some (so-called essential) amino acids, they must be obtained from the diet in the form of animal and plant proteins. The proteins are then broken down into their constituent amino acids so that they can be absorbed and reconstituted into the specific proteins needed by the body. These processes of protein breakdown and reconstitution produce a variety of nitrogen-containing waste products, primarily *urea*, which is excreted from the body in the urine. (See also *Nitrate drugs; Nitrites*.)

Nitrous oxide
A colourless gas (sometimes called laughing gas) with a sweet smell. Nitrous oxide is used with oxygen to provide *analgesia* (pain relief) and light anaesthesia (see *Anaesthesia, general*) at the site of a serious accident or during dental procedures, childbirth, and minor surgery. For major surgery requiring deeper anaesthesia, a nitrous oxide and oxygen mixture needs to be combined with other drugs.

The advantages of the combination of nitrous oxide and oxygen over other agents are its rapid action and nonflammability. Possible adverse effects include nausea and vomiting during the recovery period.

Nits

The eggs of lice. Both head lice and pubic lice produce eggs, which they glue to the base of the hairs growing from their host's head or pubic area. The nits are tiny, measuring only about 0.5 mm in diameter. They are yellow when newly laid, and white when hatched. Hatching takes place within eight days; the empty eggshells are carried outwards as the hair grows.

Louse infestations are frequently diagnosed from the presence of nits. The distance from the base of hairs to the furthest nits provides a rough approximation of the duration of the infestation. (See *Lice; Pubic lice*.)

Nocardiosis
An infection caused by a fungus-like bacterium. The infection usually starts in the lung and spreads via the bloodstream to the brain and tissues under the skin. The organism that causes nocardiosis is present in the soil in all parts of the world and is acquired by inhalation.

Nocardiosis is rare except in people with *immunodeficiency disorders* or those already suffering from another serious disease.

The infection causes a pneumonia-like illness, with fever and cough. It fails to respond to normal, short-term, antibiotic treatment, and signs of progressive lung damage occur. Brain abscesses may follow. The condition is diagnosed by microscopic examination of sputum (phlegm). Treatment, which may have to be continued for 12 to 18 months, is with *sulphonamide drugs*, sometimes in conjunction with other antibacterial drugs, for example *trimethoprim*.

Nocturia
The disturbance of an individual's sleep at night by the need to pass *urine*. In most people, a moderately full *bladder* does not usually disturb sleep, although light sleepers are more likely than others to wake with the urge to empty their bladders. Drinking alcohol in the evening stimulates urine production and may result in nocturia.

A common cause of nocturia is enlargement of the prostate gland (see *Prostate, enlarged*), which obstructs the normal outflow of urine and causes the bladder to empty incompletely.

Another common cause is *heart failure* (reduced pumping efficiency) leading to the retention of excess fluid in the legs during the day, which is absorbed into the bloodstream when the patient lies down at night and carried to the kidneys to make more urine.

Also common is *cystitis* (inflammation of the bladder), in which irritation of the bladder wall increases its sensitivity so that smaller volumes of urine trigger a desire to pass urine.

Rarer causes of nocturia include *diabetes mellitus*, in which greater volumes of urine are produced both day and night; chronic *kidney failure*, in which the normal ability of the kidney to produce a reduced quantity of more concentrated urine at night is lost; and *diabetes insipidus*, in which the kidneys fail to concentrate the urine owing to lack of a particular pituitary hormone.

Nocturnal emission
Ejaculation that occurs during sleep, commonly called a "wet dream". Nocturnal emission is normal in male adolescents and is a common cause of unnecessary anxiety. Nocturnal emissions may also occur in adult males whose sexual activity is limited.

Node
A small, rounded mass of tissue. The term most commonly refers to a *lymph node*, a normal structure in the lymphatic system. (See also *Nodule*.)

Nodule
A small lump of tissue, usually more than 5 mm in diameter. A nodule may protrude from the skin's surface or it may form deep under the skin. Nodules may be either hard or soft.

Noise
Sound that is disordered and irregular (producing an unpleasant sensation), that is unwanted, or that interferes with the ability to hear.

Hearing may be damaged by exposure to intensely loud noise for a short period (such as an explosion at close range) or by prolonged exposure to lower levels of noise (such as might occur in a machine room or a foundry).

N

COMPARATIVE NOISE LEVELS

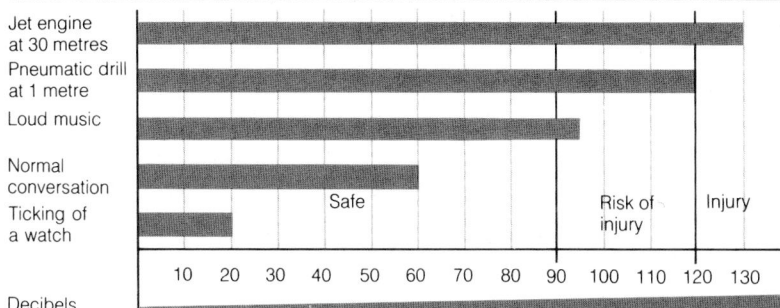

Any noise above 90 decibels may cause damage; the louder the noise, the shorter the time required for damage to occur (see chart).

HOW NOISE DAMAGES HEARING

Exposure to a sudden very loud noise, usually above 130 decibels, can cause immediate and permanent damage. Normally, muscles in the middle *ear* respond to loud noise by altering the stiffness of the ossicles (the chain of bones that pass vibrations to the inner ear), thus reducing their efficiency and damping down the intensity of the noise. But when the noise occurs without warning, these protective reflexes have no time to respond. The full force of the vibrations is carried to the inner ear, causing severe damage to delicate hair cells in the cochlea. Occasionally, loud noises can rupture the *eardrum*.

More commonly, damage from loud noise occurs over a period of time, with gradual destruction of the hair cells of the cochlea and permanent hearing loss.

SYMPTOMS OF NOISE DAMAGE

Sound at 90 decibels or above may cause pain and temporary deafness lasting for minutes or hours. This is a warning that hearing may be damaged unless the source of the noise is removed or unless suitable precautions are taken. Prolonged *tinnitus* (ringing or buzzing in the ears) occurring after a noise has ceased is an indication that some damage has probably occurred.

Prolonged exposure to loud noise leads initially to a loss of ability to hear certain high tones. Later, deafness extends to all high frequencies, and the perception of speech becomes impaired. Eventually, lower tones are also affected.

PREVENTION OF NOISE DAMAGE

Regulations governing maximum noise levels apply to places of work.

People who cannot avoid exposure to loud noise (for example, workers using pneumatic drills) should wear ear protection. People who are persistently exposed to loud noise may have their hearing monitored regularly. Noise from low-flying aircraft may disturb sleep and interfere with social activities such as conversation and listening to music. Regulations exist to control noise levels around airports.

Noma

Also known as cancrum oris, death of tissue in the lips and cheeks caused by bacterial infection. Noma is most often seen in (and largely confined to) young, severely malnourished children in developing countries. It may complicate other diseases, especially *measles*, and sometimes occurs during the last stages of *leukaemia*.

SYMPTOMS

The first symptom is inflammation of the gums and the inner surface of the cheeks. Without treatment, this leads to severe ulceration (with a foul-smelling discharge) and eventual destruction of the bones around the mouth, and loss of teeth. Healing occurs naturally after a time, but scarring may be severe.

TREATMENT

Penicillin drugs and improved nutrition halt the progress of the disease. Plastic surgery may be necessary to reconstruct damaged bones or to improve facial appearance.

Nonaccidental injury

See *Child abuse*.

Noninvasive

A term used to describe any medical procedure that does not involve penetration of the skin or entry into the body through any of the natural openings; examples include *CT scanning* and *echocardiography*. The term non-

invasive is sometimes also applied to benign tumours that do not spread throughout body tissues.

Nonspecific urethritis

Also called nongonococcal urethritis, inflammation of the urethra due to a cause or causes other than *gonorrhoea*. Worldwide, nonspecific urethritis is the most common type of *sexually transmitted disease*. About 150,000 cases are reported from sexually transmitted disease clinics in the UK each year.

CAUSES

The name nonspecific urethritis was given to the disorder at a time when few laboratory tests were available for the detection of microorganisms. Today, almost 50 per cent of cases are known to be caused by CHLAMYDIA TRACHOMATIS (see *Chlamydial infections*); a few are caused by HERPES VIRUS HOMINIS (the virus that causes *herpes simplex*) or TRICHOMONAS VAGINALIS infections (see *Trichomoniasis*). In the remainder of cases, the cause remains unknown.

SYMPTOMS

Nonspecific urethritis has an incubation period of about two to three weeks. In men, the infection usually causes a clear or a purulent urethral discharge often accompanied by pain or discomfort on passing urine. Sometimes these symptoms are very mild or even absent. The equivalent condition in women is called nonspecific genital infection. This does not usually cause symptoms unless there are complications.

DIAGNOSIS AND TREATMENT

Laboratory tests are performed to identify the organism responsible for the infection. Because a woman may have no symptoms, a diagnosis often rests on the fact that she has a male partner with nonspecific urethritis.

Treatment is difficult because in many cases the cause of the infection cannot be determined. The cure rate is approximately 85 per cent. *Antibiotic drugs*, including oxytetracycline and erythromycin, are given. Because relapses are common, however, follow-up visits may be advised for three months after treatment.

COMPLICATIONS

In men, *epididymitis, prostatitis*, and *urethral stricture* (narrowing of the urethra) can occur as complications of nonspecific urethritis.

In women, *salpingitis* (inflammation of the fallopian tubes) and cysts of the *Bartholin's glands* may occur. *Ophthalmia* neonatorum, a type of con-

N

junctivitis, sometimes develops in babies born to women with chlamydial cervicitis.

Reiter's syndrome (in which there is arthritis and conjunctivitis as well as urethritis) occurs as a complication in about five per cent of men who develop nonspecific urethritis.

Nonsteroidal anti-inflammatory drugs

COMMON DRUGS

Diclofenac Diflunisal Fenbufen Fenoprofen Flurbiprofen Ibuprofen Indomethacin Ketoprofen Mefenamic acid Naproxen Piroxicam Tenoxicam

> **WARNING**
> Report abdominal pain, heartburn or indigestion to your doctor.

A group of drugs that produce *analgesia* (pain relief) and reduce inflammation in joints and soft tissues, such as muscles and ligaments. The name nonsteroidal anti-inflammatory drugs is commonly abbreviated to NSAIDs.

WHY THEY ARE USED
NSAIDs are widely used to relieve symptoms caused by types of arthritis, such as *rheumatoid arthritis, osteoarthritis*, and *gout*. They do not cure or halt the progress of disease but improve mobility of the affected joint by relieving pain and stiffness.

NSAIDs are also used in the treatment of back pain, menstrual pain, headaches, pain after minor surgery, and soft tissue injuries.

HOW THEY WORK
NSAIDs reduce pain and inflammation by blocking the production of *prostaglandins* (chemicals that cause inflammation and trigger transmission of pain signals to the brain).

POSSIBLE ADVERSE EFFECTS
NSAIDs sometimes cause adverse effects such as nausea, indigestion, diarrhoea, and *peptic ulcer*.

Noradrenaline

A *hormone* secreted by certain nerve endings (principally those of the *sympathetic nervous system*) and by the medulla (centre) of the *adrenal glands*. Noradrenaline's primary function is to help maintain a constant blood pressure by stimulating certain blood vessels to constrict (narrow) when the blood pressure falls. For this reason, an injection of noradrenaline may sometimes be given in the emergency treatment of *shock* or severe bleeding. (See also *Adrenaline*.)

Norethisterone

A *progestogen drug* used primarily as an ingredient of some *oral contraceptives*. Norethisterone is sometimes prescribed to postpone menstruation.

It is also used to treat *premenstrual syndrome*, menstrual disorders, such as *menorrhagia* (heavy periods), *endometriosis*, and certain types of *breast cancer*. Norethisterone is occasionally given by injection as a long-acting contraceptive.

Possible adverse effects include swollen ankles, weight gain, depression and, rarely, jaundice.

Nortriptyline

An *antidepressant drug* that also has a sedative effect. Nortriptyline is also used in the treatment of nocturnal *enuresis* (bed-wetting) in children over the age of seven years.

Nose

The uppermost part of the respiratory tract and the organ of *smell*.

STRUCTURE
The nose is an air passage connecting the nostrils at its front to the *nasopharynx* (the upper part of the throat) at the rear. The *nasal septum*, which is made of cartilage at the front and bone at the rear, divides the passage into two chambers.

Two small bones, the nasal bones, project from the front of the cranium and form the top of the bridge of the nose; the remainder of the bridge is cartilage. The roof of the nasal passage is formed by bones at the base of the skull, the walls by the maxilla (upper *jaw*), and the floor by the hard *palate*. Projecting from each wall are three conchae (thin, downward-curling plates of bone); the conchae are covered with *mucous membrane*, which considerably increases the surface area of the nasal passage.

The bones surrounding the nose contain air-filled, mucous membrane-lined cavities known as paranasal *sinuses*, which open into the nasal passage. In each wall of the nose is the opening to a nasolacrimal duct, which drains away the tears that bathe the front of the eyeball.

Projecting into the roof of the nasal passage through tiny openings are the hair-like nerve endings of the *olfactory nerves*, which are responsible for the sense of smell.

FUNCTION
One of the main functions of the nose is to filter, warm, and moisten inhaled air before it passes into the rest of the respiratory tract. Just inside the nostrils, small hairs trap large dust particles and even larger foreign bodies and induce sneezing to remove them. Smaller dust particles are filtered from the air by the microscopic hairs of the conchae. All air entering the nose passes over the blood vessels and mucus-secreting cells on the surface

---

ANATOMY OF THE NOSE

The nose is involved in breathing and also in the sense of smell; it is a hollow passage connecting the nostrils and the top of the throat. The upper part of the nose transmits sensations of smell.

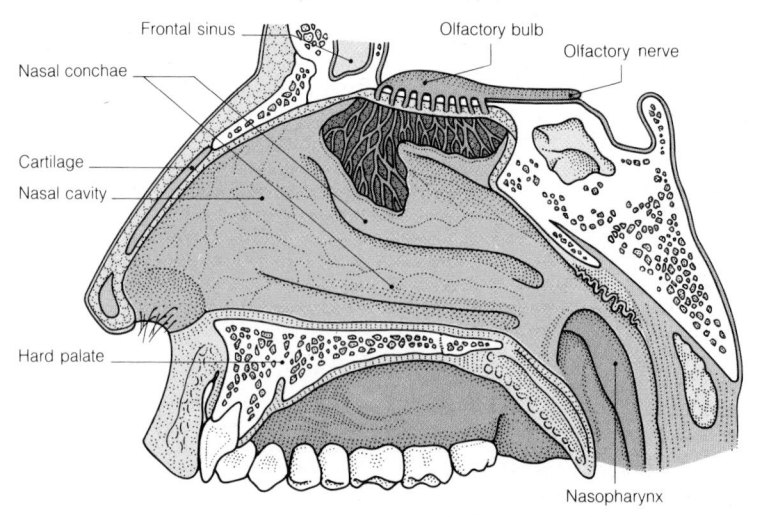

Frontal sinus — Olfactory bulb — Olfactory nerve — Nasal conchae — Cartilage — Nasal cavity — Hard palate — Nasopharynx

DISORDERS OF THE NOSE

The nose is susceptible to a wide range of disorders. Infections and allergic conditions, leading to stuffiness or sneezing and sometimes some loss of smell, are common. Because of its prominent position, the nose is also particularly prone to injury.

CONGENITAL DEFECTS

In choanal atresia, one or both nasal cavities fail to develop fully. If both sides are affected, the baby cannot breathe properly. An abnormality affecting one side may not cause any problems until later in life.

Syphilis that is transmitted to a fetus during pregnancy may lead to a failure of full development of the nasal bones.

INFECTION

The common *cold*, a virus infection, causes inflammation of the lining of the nasal passages and excessive production of mucus, leading to nasal congestion. Small *boils* (infected hair follicles) are common just within the nostril, where they may cause severe pain. Backward spread of infection from the nose occasionally causes *cavernous sinus thrombosis*, a serious condition that, without antibiotics, may be fatal.

TUMOURS

Haemangiomas (benign tumours of blood vessels) commonly affect the nasal cavity in babies. Many disappear spontaneously before puberty.

Basal cell carcinoma and *squamous cell carcinoma* (types of skin cancer) may occur in and around the nostril. The nose may also be invaded by cancers originating in the sinuses.

INJURY

Fracture of the nasal bones (see *Nose, broken*) is a common sports injury that can lead to deformity; it may require corrective surgery. *Nosebleeds* are also common, particularly in children; they may be caused by fragile blood vessels, infection of the lining of the nose, or a blow to the nose.

DRUGS

Repeated sniffing of cocaine interferes with the blood supply to the mucous membrane lining the nose and can cause perforation of the nasal septum. Persistent taking of snuff can irritate or damage the nasal lining.

ALLERGIES

Allergic rhinitis (hay fever) is one of the most common allergies—the most common causative allergens being pollens, animal dander, house mites, and fungal spores. (See *Rhinitis, allergic*.)

OBSTRUCTION

A nasal *polyp* (a projection of swollen mucous membrane) may block a nostril, causing a sensation of congestion.

Young children frequently insert foreign bodies, such as beads, peas, or pebbles, into their nostrils. Objects often become stuck, causing obstruction and a discharge.

INVESTIGATION

To inspect the inside of the nose, the doctor uses a speculum to open up the nostrils. If a fracture is suspected, *X-rays* are taken. For suspected cancer, nasal endoscopy and a *biopsy* are performed.

---

of the conchae. The mucus on the conchae flows inwards, carrying harmful microorganisms and other foreign bodies back towards the nasopharynx so that they can be swallowed and destroyed by the gastric acid in the stomach.

The nose detects smells by means of the olfactory nerve endings, which, when stimulated by inhaled vapours, transmit this information to the olfactory bulb in the brain.

The nose also acts as a resonator, helping to give each voice its individual characteristic tone. (See also *Nose* disorders box.)

Nosebleed

Loss of blood from the mucous membrane that lines the nose, most often from inside one nostril only.

Nosebleeds are most common during childhood, when they are usually insignificant and easily stopped. They occur infrequently in healthy young adults, but become more common and more serious during old age.

CAUSES

The most common causes of a nosebleed are a blow to the nose, fragile blood vessels, or the dislodging of crusts that have formed in the mucous membrane as a result of a common cold or other infection. Rarely, recurrent nosebleeds are a sign of an underlying disorder, such as *hypertension* (high blood pressure), a *bleeding disorder*, or a tumour of the nose or of the paranasal sinuses.

TREATMENT

Most nosebleeds can be controlled by simple first-aid measures (see the illustrated box below).

FIRST AID: NOSEBLEED

WARNING
If a nosebleed starts after a heavy blow to the head, it could indicate a fractured skull. Take the victim to hospital immediately.

1 Sit the victim up, ensuring that he or she leans forward slightly with the mouth held open so that blood or clots do not obstruct the airway.

2 Pinch the lower part of the nostrils for about 15 minutes. The victim should breathe through the mouth.

3 The nostrils should be released slowly and the victim should avoid touching or blowing the nose. If the bleeding has not stopped after 20 minutes, seek medical attention.

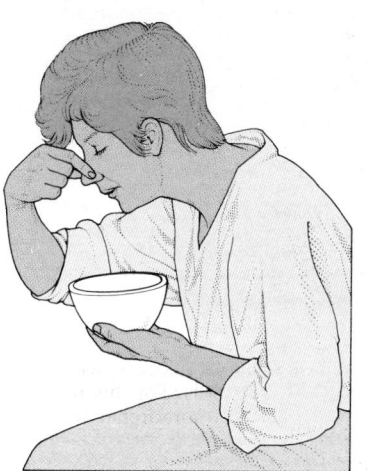

If first-aid treatment fails to stop bleeding within 20 minutes, a doctor should be consulted. He or she may pack the affected nostril firmly with gauze (to apply constant pressure to the wound) or may cauterize the wound. In rare cases, surgery may be needed to stop the bleeding.

Nose, broken

Fracture of the nasal bones or dislocation of the cartilage that forms the bridge of the *nose*. A blow from the side may knock the bones or cartilage out of position or cause displacement of the *nasal septum*. A frontal blow tends to splay the nasal bones outwards, depressing the bridge. Usually, the fracture is accompanied by severe swelling of overlying soft tissue. Such swelling can mask a minor fracture, which may be detected only when *X-rays* are taken.

A fractured nose is painful and remains tender for about three weeks after the injury.

TREATMENT
Resetting is usually carried out either before the swelling has started, or after it has subsided, usually about 10 days after the injury. Occasionally, the displaced bridge can be manipulated into position under a local anaesthetic, but usually a general anaesthetic is needed. A plaster splint is sometimes required during healing.

Nose reshaping
See *Rhinoplasty*.

Notifiable diseases

Medical conditions that must be reported by the doctor responsible for the affected person to the local health authorities.

The notification of certain infectious diseases was gradually introduced in England and Wales around 1900. Notification of certain potentially harmful infectious diseases is important because it enables health officers to take the necessary steps to control the spread of infection (e.g. by isolation or by offering *immunization* to contacts). Notification also allows monitoring of the occurrence of infectious diseases and provides valuable statistics on the *incidence* and *prevalence* of diseases. Such information may be used in formulating health policies such as immunization programmes or improvements in sanitation.

Examples of notifiable infectious diseases are *food poisoning, hepatitis, measles, malaria, tetanus, tuberculosis,* and *pertussis* (whooping cough).

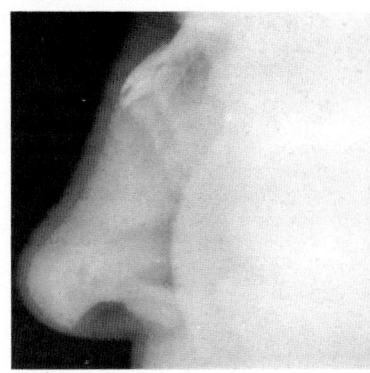

X-ray showing broken nose
The nasal bones under the bridge of the nose and part of the ethmoid bone, which forms the top part of the nasal septum (partition between the two sides of the nose), have been broken.

Some categories of diseases other than infections must also be notified. These include some *birth defects* and certain forms of *handicap*. *Cancers* are registered nationally, and cancer data is now pooled in an international registry. Certain types of *occupational disease* are also notifiable; examples include *lead poisoning, mercury poisoning, cadmium poisoning,* and *anthrax*. (See also *Prescribed diseases*.)

NSAID
The commonly used abbreviation for *nonsteroidal anti-inflammatory drugs*.

NSU
The commonly used abbreviation for *nonspecific urethritis*.

Nuclear energy
The energy released as a result of changes in the nuclei of atoms. It is also known as atomic energy and is principally released in the form of heat, light, and ionizing *radiation*, such as gamma rays.

Nuclear energy is released in certain natural processes, examples of which include the spontaneous decay of naturally occurring radioactive substances (such as uranium ores) and the nuclear reactions that power the sun and other stars. Nuclear energy is also released in man-made devices, for example nuclear reactors and nuclear weapons.

Nuclear magnetic resonance
See *MRI*.

Nuclear medicine
Techniques that use radioactive substances to detect or treat disease. The most important application of nuclear medicine is in diagnosis.

TRENDS IN SELECTED NOTIFIABLE DISEASES

Disease	Cases 1971	1976	1981	1986	1991
Diphtheria	17	2	0	4	2
Dysentery	10,008	5,924	3,352	4,492	9,935
Food poisoning	6,144	8,520	9,397	22,524	52,543
Infective jaundice (hepatitis)	12,621	5,729	9,307	3,498	8,860
Measles	126,041	54,070	48,419	77,181	9,680
Acute meningitis	1,775	1,737	1,309	2,025	2,760
Pertussis (whooping cough)	15,932	3,636	18,336	34,361	5,201
Acute poliomyelitis	6	10	2	3	3
Scarlet fever	12,044	9,337	6,956	6,727	5,665
Tuberculosis	11,128	9,650	7,803	5,795	5,436
Typhoid fever	125	211	183	151	182

This table shows trends in the number of cases of selected notifiable diseases in England over a 20 year period. In general, measles cases had declined by 1991, after a vaccine was introduced in 1968. Pertussis cases had declined again by 1991 after an increase from 1981; this increase was largely due to fewer children being vaccinated in the late 1970s and early 1980s. Note also the large increase in cases of food poisoning.

CASES OF SOME NOTIFIABLE INFECTIOUS DISEASES IN ENGLAND AND WALES (1992)

Disease	Number of cases
Food poisoning	63,347
Dysentery	16,960
Measles	10,628
Infective jaundice (hepatitis)	8,993
Rubella (German measles)	6,212
Tuberculosis	5,798
Scarlet fever	4,645
Acute meningitis	2,571
Pertussis (whooping cough)	2,309
Malaria	1,189
Ophthalmia neonatorum	424
Typhoid fever	201
Paratyphoid fever	81
Acute encephalitis	34
Leptospirosis	28
Cholera	25
Diphtheria	8
Tetanus	6
Typhus	6
Viral haemorrhagic fever	4
Acute poliomyelitis	3
Anthrax	1
Relapsing fever	1
Rabies	0
Lassa fever	0
Marburg disease	0
Plague	0
Yellow fever	0

Radioactive materials, which may be injected or swallowed, are taken up by body tissues or organs in different concentrations, and an instrument called a gamma camera is used to detect and map the distribution of radiation within the body. The technique requires only a small amount of radiation, and produces images that reflect bodily functions—not simply anatomy. (See *Radionuclide scanning*.) In techniques for treatment, higher doses of radiation are used. Diseased tissues are destroyed by exposing them to an external radioactive source or by inserting a radioactive substance

DNA STRUCTURE

A DNA molecule consists of two intertwined strands, the margins of which are chains of sugar and phosphate groups. The chains are linked by pairs of substances called bases, of which there are four types—adenine, guanine, thymine, and cytosine. An adenine on one chain is always paired with thymine on the second: similarly, cytosine is always paired with guanine. The sequence of bases in one chain thus exactly determines the sequence in the other chain.

Nucleotides
Each base, along with the sugar and phosphate groups to which it is attached, forms a unit called a nucleotide.

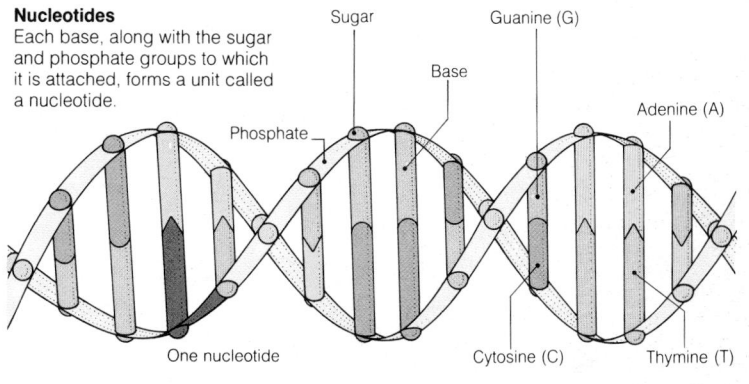

into a body tissue or cavity. (See *Radiotherapy*; *Interstitial radiotherapy*; *Intracavitary therapy*.)

Nucleic acids

Substances found in all living matter that have a fundamental role in the propagation of life. Nucleic acids provide the inherited coded instructions (or "blueprint") for an organism's development; they also provide some of the apparatus by which these instructions are carried out.

There are two types of nucleic acid, called deoxyribonucleic acid (DNA) and ribonucleic acid (RNA). In all plant and animal cells (including humans'), it is the DNA that permanently holds the coded instructions; RNA helps transport, translate, and implement the instructions. The DNA is the main constituent of *chromosomes*, which are carried in the nucleus (central unit) of the cell.

STRUCTURE

DNA and RNA are similar in structure. Both have long, chain-like molecules. The main difference is that DNA usually consists of two intertwined chains, whereas RNA is generally single-stranded.

The basic structure of DNA (see illustrated box) has been likened to a very long rope ladder, the chains of the DNA forming the two sides of the ladder, with interlinking structures between the chains forming the rungs. The ladder is not straight, however, but twisted into a helical (spiral) shape, which gives it great stability. This shape is called a double helix.

If the two DNA chains are separated, it is found that each has a "backbone" (the side of the ladder) consisting of a string of sugar and phosphate chemical groups. Attached to each sugar in this string is a chemical called a base. The base can be any of four types, called adenine, thymine, guanine, and cytosine (or A,T,G, and C), and each forms half of one rung of the DNA ladder. The four bases can occur in any sequence along the chain (a sequence might be, for example, GTCGTATTTAGTCC). The sequence itself, which may be many millions of individual bases long, provides the code for the activities of the cell, just as the sequence of letters on this page provides a message for its readers (see *Genetic code*). Because the two bases that form each rung of the ladder conform to certain pairings (A always pairs with T, and G with C), the sequence of bases on one chain determines the sequence on the second chain. This is of fundamental importance for the copying of DNA molecules when a cell divides.

RNA is like a single strand of DNA, except that the nucleotide base thymine in DNA is replaced by another base, uracil, in RNA, and the sugar and phosphate chain in RNA is chemically slightly different.

FUNCTION

DNA controls a cell's activities by specifying and regulating the synthe-

N

sis of *enzymes* and other proteins in the cell, with different *genes* (sections of DNA) regulating the production of different proteins. For a particular protein to be made, an appropriate section of DNA acts as a template for an RNA chain. This "messenger" RNA then passes out of the nucleus into the cell cytoplasm, where it is decoded to form proteins (see *Genetic code; Protein synthesis*).

When a cell undergoes mitotic division, identical copies of its DNA must go to each of the two daughter cells. The structure of DNA makes this process possible. Starting at one end of the molecule, the two chains separate, or "unzip". As they do so, two more chains are formed (side by side with the original chains) by the linking of free, unlinked, nucleotides that are present in cells. Because only certain base pairings are possible, the new double chains are identical to the original DNA molecule. Thus a dividing cell provides an exact copy of its DNA to its daughter cells. Each of a person's cells carries the same DNA replica that was present in the fertilized ovum, so the DNA message passes from one generation of cells to the next.

Nucleus

The central core, structure, or focal point of an object.

The nucleus of a living *cell* is a roughly spherical unit at the centre of the cell. It contains the *chromosomes* (composed mainly of *nucleic acid*) responsible for directing the cell's activities, and is surrounded by a membrane. This membrane has small pores through which various substances can pass between the nucleus and the cytoplasm (the rest of the cell).

The nucleus of an atom, composed of protons and neutrons, accounts for nearly all the mass of an atom but only a tiny proportion of its volume. *Nuclear energy* is produced through changes in the mass and structure of atomic nuclei.

A nerve nucleus is a group of *neurons* (nerve cells) within the brain and spinal cord that work together to perform a particular function.

Numbness

Loss of sensation in part of the body caused by interference to the passage of impulses along sensory *nerves*.

CAUSES

Numbness can occur naturally and harmlessly (such as when blood supply to a nerve in the leg is cut off temporarily by sitting cross-legged), it can be induced artificially (e.g. by a dentist anaesthetizing a nerve before filling a tooth), or it may be the result of a disorder or damage to the *nervous system* or its blood supply.

Multiple sclerosis can cause loss of sensation in any part of the body through damage to nerve pathways in the central nervous system (CNS). In a *neuropathy*, it is the peripheral nerves (nerves outside the CNS) that are damaged. In a *stroke*, pressure on, or reduced blood supply to, nerve pathways in the brain often causes loss of feeling on one side of the body.

Severe cold, as in *frostbite*, causes numbness by a direct action on the nerves. Numbness may also be a feature of various psychological disorders, such as *anxiety, panic attack*, or a hysterical *conversion disorder*.

DIAGNOSIS AND TREATMENT

Examination by a doctor usually reveals an area of sensory loss or impairment that corresponds to the skin distribution of a single peripheral nerve, several nerves, or a sensory area in the CNS. The distribution of the affected area may suggest the site and mechanism of nerve damage. Treatment, if possible, depends on the underlying cause of the problem.

Nursing

Care of the sick or injured (see *Nursing care*), or an alternative name for *breast-feeding*.

Nursing care

The process of looking after the physical or emotional needs of patients with the aim of restoring, improving, maintaining, or promoting well-being. Nurses assist patients to recover from illness and injury, encourage them to regain their independence, and, in cases of terminal illness, help patients to meet death with as little distress and as much dignity as possible.

Nurses work in hospitals, clinics, health centres, doctors' surgeries, nursing homes, workplaces, schools, and patients' homes. Branches of nursing include general nursing, nursing of the mentally ill or handicapped, nursing of sick children, district nursing, and health visiting. Midwives have special training in antenatal care, childbirth, and postnatal care (see *Midwifery*).

Nursing home

A residential facility for the care of elderly people, or for people with serious illnesses or disabilities.

The rapid increase in the number of elderly people has resulted in an increased need for provision of long-term care. There are currently some 200,000 people aged 65 or over in residential care homes of some kind. Some of these homes are administered by local authorities whereas others are privately run. Registered nursing homes are inspected regularly and must meet certain specified standards of care.

Registered nursing homes differ from private residential homes (where many elderly people may also be cared for) in that they are registered with, and inspected by, local health authorities, and they must provide 24-hour care by qualified nursing staff. Private residential homes, on the other hand, are registered with, and inspected by, the social services. They have no requirement to include qualified nurses on the staff. For this reason, most residential homes are not in a position to provide care for very frail elderly people.

In addition to being well-staffed with registered nurses and support workers, nursing homes must have regular visits from a doctor, provide access to other medical facilities, and also have a pleasant and caring atmosphere.

Most residents in nursing homes suffer from medical conditions related to *aging*, such as *dementia* and *stroke*. Nursing homes usually provide care on a long-term basis, but short-term care is sometimes available for people who are usually nursed at home. (See also *Geriatric medicine*.)

Nutrient

Essential dietary factors, such as carbohydrates, proteins, certain fats, vitamins, and minerals.

Nutrition

The scientific study of food and the processes by which it is digested and assimilated. Until about 30 years ago, nutritionists were mainly concerned with dietary deficiencies and with the minimum amounts of nutrients required for health. In Western societies the focus is now on the dangers of too much fat or sugar in the diet, and the effects of food additives, colourings, and preservatives on health.

A good diet supplies adequate but not excessive quantities of *proteins, carbohydrates, fats, vitamins, minerals*, dietary *fibre*, and water. The basis of a good diet is variety because no one food contains all the nutrients we

NUMBNESS AND TINGLING   Loss of feeling and/or a pins and needles sensation in any part of the body

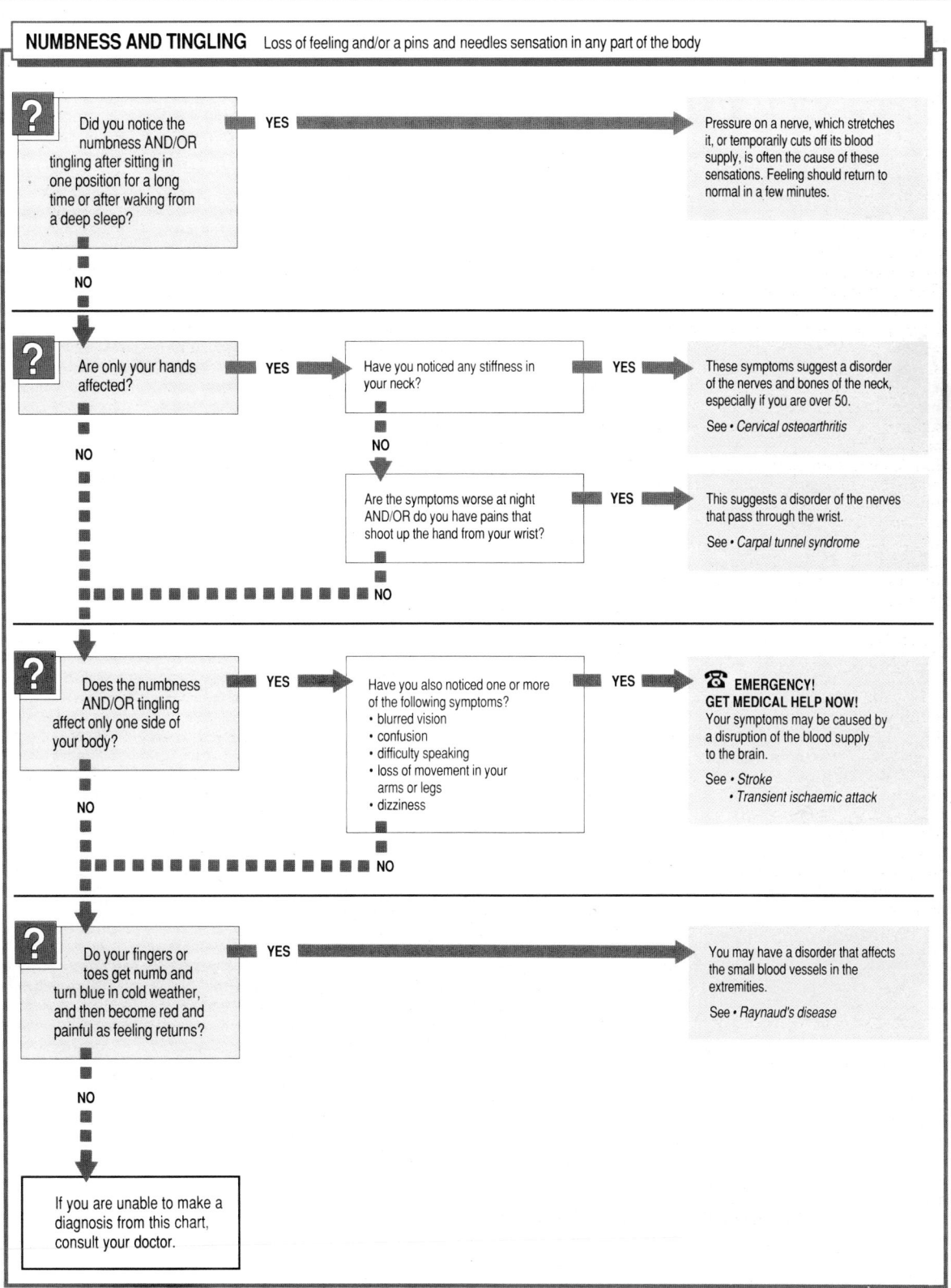

? Did you notice the numbness AND/OR tingling after sitting in one position for a long time or after waking from a deep sleep?

YES → Pressure on a nerve, which stretches it, or temporarily cuts off its blood supply, is often the cause of these sensations. Feeling should return to normal in a few minutes.

NO

? Are only your hands affected?

YES → Have you noticed any stiffness in your neck?

YES → These symptoms suggest a disorder of the nerves and bones of the neck, especially if you are over 50.

See • Cervical osteoarthritis

NO

Are the symptoms worse at night AND/OR do you have pains that shoot up the hand from your wrist?

YES → This suggests a disorder of the nerves that pass through the wrist.

See • Carpal tunnel syndrome

NO

NO

? Does the numbness AND/OR tingling affect only one side of your body?

YES → Have you also noticed one or more of the following symptoms?
• blurred vision
• confusion
• difficulty speaking
• loss of movement in your arms or legs
• dizziness

YES → ☎ EMERGENCY!
GET MEDICAL HELP NOW!
Your symptoms may be caused by a disruption of the blood supply to the brain.

See • Stroke
• Transient ischaemic attack

NO

NO

? Do your fingers or toes get numb and turn blue in cold weather, and then become red and painful as feeling returns?

YES → You may have a disorder that affects the small blood vessels in the extremities.

See • Raynaud's disease

NO

If you are unable to make a diagnosis from this chart, consult your doctor.

N

ESSENTIAL NUTRIENTS

Proteins	The main structural component of tissues and organs. We need proteins for growth and repair of cells. Each protein contains hundreds and sometimes thousands of units called amino acids in specific combinations. In the body there are 20 amino acids; 12 of these are manufactured by the body itself and	the remaining eight are obtained from a balanced diet. A vegetarian diet containing eggs, milk, and cheese provides sufficient amounts of all essential amino acids. A vegan diet, which also excludes dairy products, needs careful planning to prevent protein deficiency (see *Vegetarianism*).
Carbohydrates	The two carbohydrate food groups, sugars and starches, are the main energy sources required for metabolism (chemical processes that take place in cells). Carbohydrates should make up at	least half of the diet. Unrefined (unprocessed) carbohydrates found in cereals and fruit are usually richer in fibre and nutrients than are refined carbohydrates, such as sugar and white flour.
Fats	Fats provide energy for metabolism and are a structural component of cells. Most people in developed countries eat too much fat; fats should constitute no more than 30 per cent of total calorie intake. There are three types of dietary fats: saturated fats (found mostly in meat and dairy products), monosaturated fats (found in olive oil and avocados), and polyunsaturated fats (found in fish and vegetable oils). Saturated fats	tend to increase the amounts of unwanted types of cholesterol in the blood whereas polyunsaturated fats and monosaturated fats have the opposite effect. Studies have indicated that a high level of low-density lipoprotein cholesterol in the blood is associated with coronary artery disease. Our bodies produce enough cholesterol for our needs; any excess is primarily due to eating too much saturated fat.
Fibre	This is the indigestible structural material in plants. Although fibre passes through the intestine unchanged, it is an essential part of a healthy diet. A low-fibre diet may lead to constipation, diverticular disease and other disorders. High-fibre diets (including plenty	of fruit, raw vegetables, grains, and cereals) provide bulk without excess calories. Low-fibre diets tend to be high in refined carbohydrates and fats, and thus are more likely to encourage obesity, heart disease, and other undesirable conditions.
Water	Our bodies are composed of about 60 per cent water. Water constitutes a high proportion of many foods and is essential to maintain metabolism	(chemical processes in cells) and normal bowel function. It also determines the volume of blood in the circulation.
Vitamins	Regulators of metabolism. Vitamins ensure the healthy functioning of the brain, nerves, muscles, skin, and bones. Although vitamins do not supply energy, some enable energy to be released from food. A healthy, balanced diet contains enough vitamins for most people's needs and supplements are not	usually necessary. Indeed, some vitamins (especially A, D, E, and K) are dangerous if taken in excess. The body can store only relatively small amounts of water-soluble vitamins (B and C), but even on a very restricted diet, vitamin deficiency is rare until several months have elapsed.
Minerals	A balanced diet provides enough minerals for most people. Calcium is necessary for the maintenance of healthy teeth and bones. Other minerals, such as zinc and magnesium, are needed in minute amounts to control cell metabolism.	The only mineral commonly required as a supplement is iron, which is used to prevent anaemia in women who have heavy periods. Sodium chloride (table salt) is needed to maintain fluid balance; excess may cause *hypertension*.

need. The daily diet should include foods from each of the four basic food groups: milk and milk products; vegetables and fruits; breads and cereals; meat, eggs, and pulses.

Personal requirements of nutrients and *energy* vary, depending on individual body size, age, sex, and lifestyle. For example, an average woman requires about 2,000 kcal (8,400 kJ) daily compared with about 2,750 kcal (11,550 kJ) for an average man. (See also *Energy requirements*.)

Nutritional disorders

Nutritional disorders may be caused by a deficiency or excess of one or more of the elements of *nutrition*, or by the presence of a *toxin* (poisonous element) in the diet.

NUTRITIONAL DEFICIENCY

A diet that is deficient in *carbohydrate* is almost inevitably also deficient in *protein*, leading to the development of protein-calorie malnutrition. This deficiency is most often seen in Africa and Asia as a result of poverty and famine (see *Kwashiorkor*; *Marasmus*).

Inadequate intake of protein and calories may also occur in people who restrict their diet in an attempt to lose weight (see *Anorexia nervosa*); it can also occur because of mistaken beliefs about diet and health (see *Food fad*) or because of loss of interest in food associated with *alcohol dependence* or *drug dependence*.

Deficiency of specific nutrients is commonly associated with a disorder of the digestive system, such as *coeliac disease*, *Crohn's disease*, or pernicious anaemia (see *Anaemia, megaloblastic*).

NUTRITIONAL EXCESS

Obesity results from taking in more *energy* from the diet than is used up by the body. Nutritional disorders may also result from an excessive intake of *minerals* and *vitamins*. An excessive intake of *fat* is thought to be a contributory factor in *coronary artery disease* and in some forms of *cancer*.

TOXIC EFFECTS

Naturally occurring toxins can interfere with the digestion, absorption, and/or utilization of nutrients, or can cause specific disorders due to their toxic effects (e.g. the *ergot* fungus found on rye can cause ergotism).

Industrial pollutants, pesticides, fertilizers, and other chemicals may also contaminate food.

Nymphomania

A *psychosexual disorder* in which a woman is dominated by an insatiable appetite for sexual activity with nume-

FOOD SOURCES OF ESSENTIAL NUTRIENTS

PROTEIN

Food	Protein content (g of protein per 100 g of food)
Yeast extract	40
Beef, lean, roast	31
Tuna, canned	28
Wheatgerm	27
Cheese, cheddar	26
Chicken, lean, roast	26
Peanuts, shelled, roasted	24
Cod, grilled	17
Cottage cheese, low-fat	13
Brazil nuts, shelled	12
Eggs, boiled	12

FAT

Food	Fat content (g of fat per 100 g of food)
Oils, cooking and salad	100
Butter and margarine	81
Brazil nuts, shelled	67
Peanuts, shelled, roasted	49
Sausage, pork, cooked	42
Beef, lean with fat, roast	40
Low-fat spread	39
Cream, whipping	38
Cheese, cheddar	32
Chocolate, milk	30
Egg yolk	30

CARBOHYDRATE

Food	Carbohydrate content (g of carbohydrate per 100 g of food)
Sugar, white	100
Rice, white, uncooked	87
Cornflakes	84
Pasta, uncooked	84
Honey	81
Flour, white	80
Apricots, dried, stoned	67
Chocolate, milk	57
Beans, haricot, uncooked	45
Bread, wholemeal	37
Prunes	34

FIBRE

Food	Fibre content (g of fibre per 100 g of food)
Bran	44
Apricots, dried, stoned	24
Prunes	14
Peas, boiled	12
Blackcurrants	9
Brazil nuts, shelled	9
Bread, wholemeal	9
Peanuts, shelled, roasted	8
Beans, haricot, uncooked	7
Sweetcorn	6
Celery	5

N

The tables (above) list a selection of foods that are good sources of protein, carbohydrate, fat or fibre, together with the amount of the nutrient concerned in 100 g of each food. The figures given here are averages, because the exact nutrient content of many foods depends on variable factors such as the method of preparation. (See also the articles *Vitamins* and *Minerals*.)

rous different male partners. Nymphomaniacs are often distressed by their own behaviour and their inability to see men as anything other than objects for sexual conquest. Nymphomania is thought to be an expression of some deep psychological disorder.

The equivalent behaviour in men is called satyriasis or Don Juanism. It is said to be caused by intense *narcissism* and by feelings of inferiority.

Nystagmus

A condition in which there is involuntary movement of the eyes; the movement is usually horizontal, but can be vertical or rotatory. In almost all cases, both eyes move together.

CAUSES AND TYPES

In the most common type, called jerky nystagmus, the eyes repeatedly move slowly in one direction and then rapidly in the other, giving a jerking effect. Less commonly, nystagmus is "pendular", with the eyes moving evenly from side to side.

Nystagmus is usually congenital and is not associated with any abnormality of the eyes; the cause is unknown. Because a steady gaze is impossible, there is almost always a moderate to severe defect of visual acuity. Nystagmus also occurs in *albinism* and as a result of any very severe defect of vision present at birth, such as congenital *cataract*.

Persistent nystagmus appearing later in life usually indicates the presence of a disorder of the nervous system (such as *multiple sclerosis*, a *brain tumour*, or an *alcohol-related disorder*) or a disorder of the balancing mechanism in the inner ear. Adult-onset nystagmus is occasionally seen as an occupational disorder in people who work in poor light (coal-miners). Nystagmus may also occur as a normal effect of attempts to follow a sequence of objects rapidly passing the eyes. This phenomenon is known as "optokinetic nystagmus".

Electronystagmography, a method of recording eye movements, may be performed to identify the different types of nystagmus.

Nystatin

ANTIFUNGAL

Tablet Liquid Powder Pessary Cream Ointment

Prescription needed

Not available as generic

An *antifungal drug* used in the treatment of *candidiasis* (thrush). Nystatin may be safely used during pregnancy. High doses of nystatin taken by mouth may cause diarrhoea, nausea, vomiting, and abdominal pain.

Oat cell carcinoma

See *Small cell carcinoma*.

Obesity

A condition in which there is too much body fat. Being obese is not the same as being overweight. A person is usually not considered obese unless he or she weighs 20 per cent or more over the maximum desirable weight for his or her height (see *Weight* tables).

INCIDENCE

It is estimated that about 30 to 35 per cent of the UK population carries too much fat and that about five per cent are obese.

CAUSES

The reasons why some people become obese are unclear. Although obesity occurs when the net energy intake exceeds the net energy expenditure (that is, when more energy is taken in than is being used by the body), overweight people do not always eat more than thin people.

A person's energy requirements are determined partly by his or her basal metabolic rate (the amount of energy needed to maintain vital body functions at rest—see *Metabolism*) and partly by his or her level of physical activity. Obesity may develop in people who have a low basal metabolic rate, or who are less physically active and so need less energy.

It is thought that genetic factors play a part in the development of obesity; children of obese parents are 10 times more likely to be obese than children with parents of normal weight. Some hormonal disorders are accompanied by obesity, but the overwhelming majority of obese people do not suffer from such disorders.

COMPLICATIONS

Obesity increases a person's chance of becoming seriously ill. *Hypertension* (high blood pressure) and *stroke* are twice as likely to occur in obese people than in lean people. *Coronary artery disease* is more common, particularly in obese men under the age of 40. Adult-onset *diabetes mellitus* is five times more common among obese

people, the risk increasing with the degree and duration of obesity. Increasing degrees of extra weight in men are associated with an increased risk of cancer of the colon, rectum, and prostate. With increasing weight, women show a progressive increase in risk of cancer of the breast, uterus, and cervix. *Osteoarthritis* may be aggravated by obesity. Extra weight on the hips, knees, and back places undue strain on these joints. Weight loss does not reverse the disease but does help relieve stress and pain.

TREATMENT

The first line of treatment for obesity is a slimming diet (see *Weight reduction*). An obese person should follow a diet that provides 500 to 1,000 kilocalories less than his or her energy requirements. The body meets this dietary energy deficit by using up some of the excess stored fat. About 0.5 kg of body fat supplies about 3,500 kcal, so a daily deficit of 1,000 kcal would result, on average, in a loss of about 1 kg in a week. Losses of water during the first one to two weeks further increase the loss of weight.

Regular exercise (especially *aerobics*) helps increase weight loss by causing the body to burn extra calories and by increasing the metabolic rate.

Fad diets may cause a dramatic weight loss within a short period of time, but, in almost all cases, the weight is quickly regained when normal eating habits are resumed. The use of drugs as *appetite suppressants* was once popular, but is now rarely recommended by doctors.

Radical procedures are sometimes performed on severely obese people who have failed to lose weight. *Wiring of the jaws* may be carried out to restrict food intake. An operation in which part of the stomach is stapled together may be performed to reduce the size of the stomach and make the person feel full after eating a small amount of food. Intestinal bypass operations, in which a large part of the small intestine is bypassed by cutting the jejunum and joining it to the ileum, are occasionally performed to reduce the length of the digestive tract and allow less food to be absorbed. However, because of the risk of adverse effects, such procedures are attempted only if the person's health is in danger.

OUTLOOK

Some people who have been seriously obese for much of their lives can lose weight without regaining it. As when trying to give up smoking or alcohol, the essential element is motivation.

Obsessive-compulsive disorder

A *neurosis* in which sufferers are constantly troubled by persistent ideas (obsessions) that make them carry out repetitive, ritualized acts (compulsions). Obsessive-compulsive disorder usually starts in adolescence and runs a fluctuating course.

CAUSES AND INCIDENCE

The condition is partly inherited, but environmental factors also play a part. Personality traits of orderliness and cleanliness are said to be related, as is a tendency for other neurotic symptoms. Certain forms of brain damage, especially when due to *encephalitis*, can result in obsessional symptoms.

Obsessive-compulsive disorder is rare, although minor obsessional symptoms probably occur in about one sixth of the population.

SYMPTOMS

People with this disorder usually suffer from both obsessions and compulsions, often accompanied by *depression* and *anxiety*.

Obsessions are recurrent thoughts or feelings that come into the mind seemingly involuntarily. Sufferers regard these thoughts as senseless and sometimes unpleasant, but are unable to ignore or resist them. Thoughts of violence, fears of being infected by germs or dirt, and constant doubts (e.g. whether the front door is shut) are the most common obsessions. One form is obsessional rumination, in which a person broods constantly over a word, phrase, or an unanswerable problem.

Compulsions are repetitive, apparently purposeful acts that are carried out in a ritualized fashion. They are performed for the purpose of warding off fears or relieving anxiety and are thus the physical form of an obsessional state. Sufferers do not usually derive any pleasure from performing the activities, but feel increasingly anxious if they try to resist the compulsion. Handwashing, counting, and checking are the most common compulsions.

Compulsive acts may have to be performed so many times in a particular way that they seriously disrupt work and social life. It may take some sufferers two or three hours just to get up and wash in the morning. In addition, the constant use of soap may irritate the skin.

TREATMENT

In the past, obsessive-compulsive symptoms were treated by *psychoanalysis*. Today, treatment is usually by *behaviour therapy,* sometimes in combination with *antidepressant drugs* (especially *clomipramine*).

OUTLOOK

At least two thirds of all people who have obsessive-compulsive disorder respond well to therapy. Symptoms may recur under stress but can usually be controlled. In severe cases, the affected person may become housebound and severely handicapped by indecision.

Obstetrics

The branch of medicine concerned with *pregnancy* and *antenatal care, childbirth,* and *postnatal care.* Obstetrics also involves the study of the structure and function of the female *reproductive system.* There is thus an overlap with *gynaecology,* and most obstetricians are also gynaecologists.

Obstructive airways disease

See *Lung disease, chronic obstructive.*

Occiput

The lower back part of the head, where it merges with the neck.

Occlusion

Blockage of any passage, canal, opening, or vessel in the body. Occlusion may be the result of disease (in *pulmonary embolism,* for example) or it may be induced for medical reasons (see *Embolism, therapeutic*). The term is also used to refer to the covering of the better-seeing eye during treatment of *amblyopia.*

In dentistry, occlusion is the relationship between the upper and lower teeth when the jaw is shut. In an ideal occlusion: the upper incisors and canines (front teeth) slightly overlap the lower ones; the front two upper incisors are aligned centrally with the front two lower incisors, and the remaining upper teeth are positioned in an alternating pattern relative to the equivalent lower teeth; the outer ridges of the lower premolars and molars (back teeth) fit into the hollows in the corresponding upper teeth.

In practice, very few people have an ideal occlusion, but unless the variation from the ideal is very marked, the arrangement of the teeth usually enables food to be bitten and chewed efficiently. (See also *Malocclusion.*)

Occult

A term meaning hidden or obscure. Occult blood in a sample of faeces is invisible to the naked eye but can be detected by chemical tests.

Occult blood, faecal

The presence in the faeces of blood that cannot be seen by the naked eye but can be detected by chemical tests. It may be a sign of various disorders of the gastrointestinal tract, including *oesophagitis; gastritis* (inflammation of the stomach lining); *stomach cancer;* intestinal cancer (see *Intestine, cancer of*); rectal cancer (see *Rectum, cancer of*); *diverticular disease; polyps* in the colon; *ulcerative colitis;* or the taking of drugs that irritate the stomach or intestine, such as aspirin. Bleeding gums or *haemorrhoids* may also cause occult blood in the faeces, although in most cases of haemorrhoids the blood is visible.

DETECTION

A test on the faeces for occult blood is widely used as a screening test for cancer of the colon. A thin film of faeces is smeared on a chemically coated paper and a drop or two of oxidizing agent is placed on it. If blood is present, the faeces-covered paper turns blue. (See also *Faeces, abnormal; Rectal bleeding.*)

Occupational disease and injury

Illnesses, disorders, or injuries that occur as a result of work practices or of exposure to chemical, physical, or biological factors (such as dusts, poisons, or radiation) in the workplace. The efforts of specialists in this field have made serious occupational diseases much less common than formerly, but new hazards are continually appearing. Overall, occupational diseases still make up an important and fairly common group of conditions (see table overleaf).

TYPES

Some of the main types of occupational diseases are described below.

DUST DISEASES The name *pneumoconiosis* is used to refer to *fibrosis* of the lung that is caused by inhaled inorganic and organic dusts. Pneumoconiosis includes various diseases associated with mining (including coal and quartz mining), china clay processing, metal grinding, and foundry work.

Asbestosis (see *Asbestos-induced diseases*) is a similar hazard in the asbestos, mining, milling, and manufacturing industries, and in the demolition and maintenance of plants and buildings where asbestos has been used. This has been seen particularly in shipbuilding, ship repairing and ship breaking.

Allergic *alveolitis* is a lung condition caused by inhalation of organic dusts (often containing fungal spores). It is often occupationally related (such as *farmers' lung* in agricultural workers).

CHEMICAL POISONING Many industrial chemicals can cause damage to the lungs if inhaled, or to the liver, kidneys, bone marrow, or other organs if they reach the bloodstream via the lungs or skin.

Exposure to the fumes of cadmium (used, for example, in the welding and electroplating industries) may damage the kidneys. Beryllium (used in high-technology industries) can damage the lungs. Lead and its compounds (used in metal processing and other industries) and benzene (used in various industries where solvents are used) can damage the bone marrow, leading to *anaemia* and other blood abnormalities. Carbon tetrachloride and vinyl chloride (used in the manufacture of chemicals and plastics) are causes of liver disease. Many of these compounds can also cause kidney damage.

OCCUPATIONAL SKIN DISEASE Contact *dermatitis* (skin inflammation) can occur as a result of an allergy or of direct irritation by chemicals contacting the skin at work. Many substances may be responsible, from wet cement to chemicals used in the rubber goods industry. Other skin problems may also be occupationally related (for example, severe itching caused by fibreglass, or *squamous cell carcinoma* due to exposure to tar).

RADIATION HAZARDS People with outdoor occupations in sunny climates are at increased risk of skin disease, such as *basal cell carcinoma.*

Workers in the *nuclear energy* industry and in some health-care professions should use precautions to reduce the risk of developing a disease caused by ionizing radiation (see *Radiation hazards*).

INFECTIOUS DISEASES Some rare infectious diseases are more common than average in people with certain occupations. Examples include *brucellosis* and *Q fever* (acquired from livestock) in farmworkers, and *psittacosis* (acquired from birds) in pet-shop owners. *Leptospirosis* is more common than average in sewer workers, miners, ditchdiggers, and fishermen, who acquire the disease from rats, and, increasingly, in farmworkers, who acquire it from cattle. Viral *hepatitis* and *AIDS* are hazards for people who work with blood and blood products.

MISCELLANEOUS Disorders caused by repetitive actions or by overuse of parts of the body range from *writer's cramp* to *carpal tunnel syndrome* and sin-

O

ger's nodes. Raynaud's phenomenon is associated with the handling of vibrating tools. *Deafness* may be caused by exposure to noise, and *cataracts* by exposure to the radiation associated with intense heat.

DIAGNOSIS AND PREVENTION

Sometimes the link between a disease and occupation may be obvious; sometimes it may become apparent only when a patient with mysterious symptoms mentions his or her occupation to the doctor. Part of every medical history is a question regarding the patient's occupation. Even when an occupational disease is suspected, extensive investigation at the workplace may be required to deter-mine the exact cause. In more serious cases, the patient may have to leave his or her occupation. In all cases, measures to prevent a recurrence should be taken. Sufferers may be able to claim benefit under Social Security legislation or may be able to sue an employer for negligence.

Occupational medicine

A branch of medicine concerned with the effects of a person's job on his or her health, and with the effects of health on the capacity to work. Occupational medicine includes the prevention of *occupational disease and injury*, and the promotion of general health in the working population.

Occupational medicine has a long history. As early as the middle ages, it was recognized that miners were at risk of lung diseases caused by dust, and attempts were made to improve their working conditions by increasing ventilation. The scope of occupational medicine widened during the industrial revolution as research revealed the hazards of working with metals, such as lead and mercury, and with various other materials, such as phosphorus.

The occupational physician uses epidemiological techniques (see *Epidemiology*) to analyse patterns of absenteeism, injury, illness, and causes of death in working populations, and

---

SAFETY AT WORK

A major method of preventing occupational disease and injury is the use of suitable protective clothing. This may include an air-filter mask in the presence of dust or fumes; earplugs where there is a noise hazard; eye shields to protect against radiation, chemicals, or metal dust; gloves for handling machinery; protective headgear and reinforced footwear where there is a risk of falling objects.

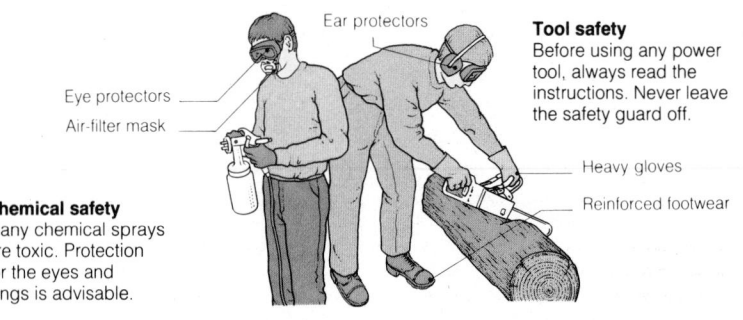

Eye protectors
Air-filter mask

Ear protectors

Tool safety
Before using any power tool, always read the instructions. Never leave the safety guard off.

Heavy gloves
Reinforced footwear

Chemical safety
Many chemical sprays are toxic. Protection for the eyes and lungs is advisable.

OCCUPATIONAL FATAL INJURIES

	Agriculture, forestry, and fishing	Energy and water	Manufacturing industry	Construction industry	Service industry
1981	31	54	123	105	102
1983	29	48	118	118	111
1985	20	46	124	104	99
86/87	27	30	109	99	80
88/89	21	203	94	101	109
90/91	25	27	88	96	110
92/93	18	19	58	63	91

The table above lists the main industries in which occupational fatal injuries to employees (excluding the self-employed) occurred in Britain between 1981 and 1992/93. The Piper Alpha oil-rig disaster was responsible for the high number of fatal injuries in the energy and water industries in 1988/89. Overall, the lowest number of fatal injuries occurred in agriculture, forestry, and fishing.

OCCUPATIONAL DISEASES (1992)

Disease	Employees awarded benefit
Lung diseases (including respiratory cancers)	2,103
Deafness	972
Vibration white finger	2,369
Dermatitis	411
Tenosynovitis and related conditions	649
Nonrespiratory cancers	23
Infectious diseases	12
Other prescribed conditions	91
Total	6,630

The table above shows the numbers of employees (excluding the self-employed) awarded disablement benefit in Britain in 1992 for various occupational diseases. Those suffering from an occupational disease but not awarded benefit are not included.

clinical techniques to investigate and monitor the health of a particular workforce. Health risks can be reduced in two ways: by primary prevention—the reduction of exposure to harmful substances by correct work practices, attention to dust control, use of safe work stations, and the disposal of wastes—and by secondary prevention, which involves regular screening of workers for early evidence of occupational disorders, such as dust diseases or damage to the liver from chemicals.

Today, the occupational physician is also increasingly concerned with psychological stress at work, with the investigation of the hazards (known and unknown) of new technologies, and with promoting healthy personal habits in workers.

Occupational mortality

Death caused by disease contracted at the workplace or by injuries related to a person's work.

The number of deaths from accidents at work in the UK has decreased steadily over the years, reaching about 1,000 deaths annually just before the Health and Safety Executive was set up. The annual death rates (per million at risk) vary with occupations, ranging from five in the manufacture of clothing and footwear to about 1,650 in the offshore oil and gas industries.

In addition, more than 1,000 deaths annually in the UK are attributable to occupational disease—principally to *pneumoconiosis* (dust disease of the lungs) and occupational cancers.

Occupational therapy

Treatment aimed at enabling people disabled by physical illness or a serious accident to relearn muscular control and coordination, to cope with everyday tasks (such as dressing), and, when possible, to resume some form of employment. Treatment, carried out by specially trained therapists, usually starts in hospital and may be continued at an outpatient clinic or in the person's home.

Ocular

Relating to or affecting the *eye* and its structures. The term is also used to refer to the eyepiece of an optical device, such as a microscope.

Oculogyric crisis

A state of fixed gaze, lasting for minutes or hours, in which the eyes are turned in a particular direction (usually upwards). The fixed-eye position is sometimes associated with spasm of the muscles of the tongue, mouth, and neck.

The crisis may occur in people with *parkinsonism* or those who have had *encephalitis*. It may also be induced by drugs (such as *reserpine* or the *phenothiazine* derivatives). An oculogyric crisis is often precipitated by emotional stress.

Oculomotor nerve

The third *cranial nerve*. The oculomotor nerve stimulates only motor functions. This nerve controls all the muscles that move the eye, except for two—the superior oblique muscle (which rotates the eyeball downwards and outwards and is controlled by the *trochlear nerve*) and the lateral rectus muscle (which moves the eye outwards and is controlled by the *abducent nerve*). The oculomotor nerve also supplies the muscle that constricts the pupil, the ciliary muscle (which focuses the eye), and the muscle that raises the upper eyelid.

The oculomotor nerve may be damaged as a result of a fracture of the base of the skull or of a disorder that distorts the brain, such as a tumour. Depending on the severity of damage, the following symptoms may occur: *ptosis* (drooping of the upper eyelid), *squint*, dilation of the pupil, inability to focus the eye, double vision, and slight protrusion of the eyeball.

Oedema

An abnormal accumulation of fluid in the body tissues. Oedema may or may not be visible (as a swelling) and can be either localized (as after an injury) or generalized (as in *heart failure*). Generalized oedema (also called anasarca) was formerly commonly known as dropsy.

WATER BALANCE IN THE BODY

Water accounts for roughly three fifths of body weight and is constantly exchanged between blood and tissues. Water is forced out of the capillaries (tiny blood vessels) and into the tissues by the pressure of blood being pumped around the body. By a reverse process, which depends on the water-drawing power of the proteins in the blood (see *Osmosis*), water is reabsorbed into the capillaries from the tissues. These two mechanisms normally are in balance, keeping the levels of water in the blood and the tissues more or less constant.

Another factor involved in maintaining this balance is the action of the

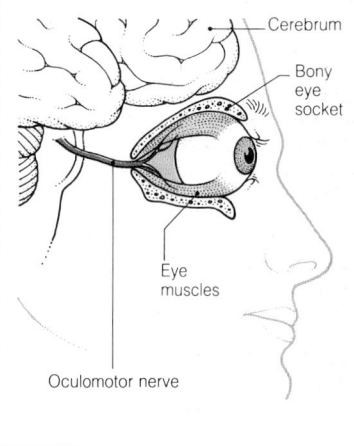

LOCATION OF THE OCULOMOTOR NERVE
The oculomotor nerve originates high in the brainstem and passes forward through a slit in the bony eye socket to reach the muscles that move the eye and eyelids.

Cerebrum

Bony eye socket

Eye muscles

Oculomotor nerve

kidneys, which pass excess salt from the blood into the urine to be excreted from the body.

CAUSES OF OEDEMA

Various disorders can interfere with these processes. Heart failure leads to blood congestion in the veins, creating backward pressure in the capillaries. This backward pressure overcomes osmotic pressure in the capillaries and thus causes more fluid than normal to be forced into the tissues at various places. Backward pressure can also be created by a tumour pressing on veins. The oedema produced is confined to the area drained by the obstructed vein.

In *nephrotic syndrome*, an abnormal loss of protein from the blood, reduces osmotic pressure and prevents enough fluid being drawn from the tissues into the blood. *Kidney failure* prevents salt being excreted from the body, allowing it to accumulate in the tissues and attract water to it.

Other disorders that can cause oedema include *cirrhosis* of the liver, which leads to blood congestion in the veins of the liver, lowers blood protein (and therefore osmotic pressure), and causes salt retention. A deficiency of protein in the diet, as may occur in alcoholics, can also reduce osmotic pressure; oedema in alcoholics may also be due to deficiency of thiamine (vitamin B_1), leading to *beriberi*.

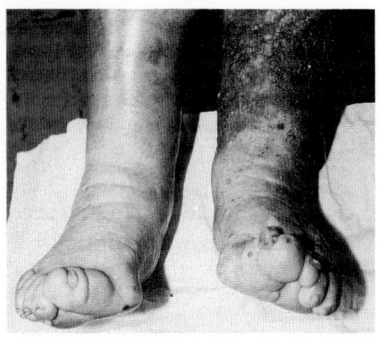

Chronic oedema
An example of chronic oedema, showing the characteristic swelling and stretched, shiny skin. In this patient, the skin of the left leg is also ulcerated.

Injury may cause oedema by damaging capillaries and thus allowing fluid to leak out of them. Blockage of lymphatic vessels may result in *lymphoedema*.

Oedema may also be caused by certain drugs. These include *corticosteroid drugs*, *androgen drugs*, and high-oestrogen *oral contraceptives*, which all act on the kidneys, causing a certain amount of salt retention.

SYMPTOMS AND SIGNS
Until the excess fluid in the body increases by more than about 15 per cent, oedema may show itself only as an increase in weight. After that it is evident as a swelling, often in the lower part of the body (e.g. around the base of the spine and the ankles).

In severe cases, fluid accumulates in one or more of the large body cavities. For example, in *ascites*, fluid collects in the peritoneal cavity of the abdomen, causing abdominal swelling. In *pleural effusion*, fluid fills the pleural cavity of the lungs, resulting in compression of the lungs and in breathing difficulty. In *pulmonary oedema*, the air sacs of the lungs become waterlogged, causing breathing difficulty.

The presence of oedema can be detected by pressing a finger into the swollen area. This action produces an indentation in the skin which slowly flattens out as the fluid seeps back.

TREATMENT
The aim is always to remedy the underlying cause of the oedema. In many cases, however, the underlying cause is not remediable and the only treatment is to make the body excrete the excess fluid by increasing the output of urine by the kidneys. This is done by restricting dietary sodium and by the use of *diuretic drugs*, which may be needed indefinitely.

Oedipus complex
A term used in *psychoanalytic theory* to describe the unconscious sexual attachment of a child for the parent of the opposite sex and the consequent jealousy of, and desire to eliminate, the parent of the same sex. The name is derived from the Greek myth in which, unknowingly, Oedipus kills his father Laius and marries his mother Jocasta.

Sigmund Freud believed that the Oedipus complex (sometimes called the Electra complex in females) was present in all young children and that normal psychological development depended on the child coming to identify with the parent of the same sex and, later, making sexual attachments with members of the opposite sex outside the family.

Oesophageal atresia
A rare *birth defect* caused by a failure of the oesophagus to form correctly during embryonic development. A short section of the *oesophagus* is absent, the part of the oesophagus above the gap terminates in a pouch, and the lower part of the oesophagus, projecting upwards from the stomach, is also blind-ended. In most cases, there is also an abnormal channel, called a *tracheoesophageal fistula*, between one of the sections of oesophagus and the trachea (windpipe). The incidence of oesophageal atresia ranges from one in 1,000 to one in 3,000.

SYMPTOMS AND DIAGNOSIS
The diagnosis may be suspected before birth if the mother has *polyhydramnios* (excess amniotic fluid). The infant cannot swallow saliva or milk, and continuous drooling and regurgitation from the mouth occur. If there is an upper tracheoesophageal fistula, milk may be sucked into the lungs; as a result, attempts at feeding provoke attacks of coughing and cyanosis (a blue-purple skin coloration).

A soft tube inserted into the nose can normally be passed down the oesophagus; in cases of oesophageal atresia, however, this will not be possible. The diagnosis is confirmed by a *chest X-ray* taken after a *radiopaque* tube has been passed as far as possible down the oesophagus.

TREATMENT
Swallowed saliva is sucked out via a tube, and the infant is artificially ventilated. Immediate surgery is necessary. Under a general anaesthetic, the baby's chest is opened, the blind ends of the oesophagus are joined and any tracheoesophageal fistula is closed.

Complications can be prevented by skilled nursing care. Some affected babies do not survive, especially if they are very small or if they also have severe heart disease. If the operation is successful, the baby will develop normally.

Oesophageal dilatation
A procedure to stretch the *oesophagus* after it has become narrowed by disease (see *Oesophageal stricture*), which prevents normal swallowing. The usual cause of the narrowing is swelling and scarring from *oesophagitis* (inflammation of the oesophagus), but the narrowing may also be due to cancer (see *Oesophagus, cancer of*) or *achalasia* (inability of the muscles in the lower oesophagus to relax).

HOW IT IS DONE
The patient must not eat for at least eight hours before the oesophageal dilatation, which is usually carried out under sedation.

First, an *endoscope* (a fine, flexible viewing instrument) is passed through the mouth and down the oesophagus to locate the obstruction. Stretching of the narrowed area is sometimes performed by passing a series of bougies (cylindrical rods with olive-shaped tips) over a guide wire passed down the oesophagus. Increasingly commonly, stretching is now being performed by means of a *balloon catheter* (a fine tube with a balloon at the end), which is passed down the oesophagus. After being inflated, the balloon is kept in position for three minutes and then deflated and withdrawn; the same procedure is repeated later with a larger balloon.

Oesophageal diverticulum
A sac-like outward protrusion of part of the wall of the *oesophagus*.

TYPES
There are two types: a pharyngeal pouch (also called a Zenker's or pulsion diverticulum), and a mid-oesophageal diverticulum (also called a traction diverticulum).

PHARYNGEAL POUCH This type is located at the top of the oesophagus, at its entrance from the pharynx (throat). The pouch usually projects backwards. The cause is a failure of the sphincter (circular muscle) at the entrance to the oesophagus to relax during the act of swallowing, due to muscular incoordination. Instead, the sphincter resists the passage of food. As the powerful throat muscles used for swallowing work against this resistance, part of the lining of the

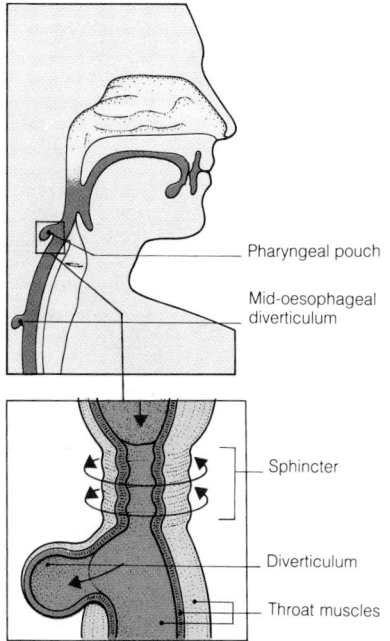

Location of oesophageal diverticulum
The pharyngeal pouch forms at the top of the oesophagus as a reaction to the sphincter's failure to relax during swallowing. The usually symptomless mid-oesophageal diverticulum is a pouch further down the oesophagus.

oesophagus is forced through the oesophageal wall, thus forming the diverticulum.

Once the diverticulum is formed, it gradually enlarges, and food becomes trapped in it, causing irritation, difficulty in swallowing, *halitosis* (bad breath), and regurgitation. The diagnosis is confirmed by a barium swallow (see *Barium X-ray examinations*), and the diverticulum is treated by surgical removal. The sphincter muscle is partly cut at the same time to weaken it and prevent recurrence.

MID-OESOPHAGEAL DIVERTICULUM This disorder consists of a pouch formed further down the oesophagus. It rarely causes symptoms and usually requires no treatment.

Oesophageal spasm
Uncoordinated contractions of the muscles in the *oesophagus*, which fail to propel food effectively down into the stomach. The contractions may be caused by some other oesophageal disorder, such as reflux *oesophagitis*, but in many cases they occur for no apparent reason. Women are affected more often than men. Pain is felt in the chest or upper abdomen and there is difficulty in swallowing. The

symptoms are intermittent and do not worsen.

A barium swallow (see *Barium X-ray examinations*) will show the irregular contractions of the oesophagus and, along with *endoscopy* (passage of a viewing instrument down the oesophagus) and oesophageal *manometry*, can rule out the possibility of a more serious condition, such as a cancer. There is no specific treatment other than for an underlying cause.

Oesophageal stricture
Narrowing of the *oesophagus*, which may cause swallowing difficulty.
CAUSES AND SYMPTOMS
Narrowing may be due to a cancer (see *Oesophagus, cancer of*) or to any of numerous noncancerous causes. These include persistent reflux *oesophagitis*, in which constant irritation from gastric acid causes inflammation and swelling followed by the formation of fibrous scar tissue and narrowing. Prolonged use of a *nasogastric tube* may inflame the oesophagus, leading to a stricture, as may the accidental swallowing of a corrosive liquid.

The symptoms of a stricture are difficulty in swallowing, pain, weight loss, and regurgitation of food.
DIAGNOSIS AND TREATMENT
A barium swallow (see *Barium X-ray examinations*) shows a smooth narrowing of the oesophagus. *Endoscopy* (passage of a viewing instrument down the oesophagus) is used to look at the narrowed area, and a *biopsy* (removal of a sample of tissue for microscopic analysis) is performed to exclude the possibility of cancer.

In most cases, the narrowed area is widened by *oesophageal dilatation*. In rare cases of very severe narrowing over a long segment of the oesophagus (usually due to swallowing corrosives), the affected area may require surgical removal. A loop of colon may be substituted for the removed section, or the ends of the oesophagus may be joined and the stomach brought up into the chest.

Patients who are too old or too frail for surgery may be treated by the insertion of a permanent pliable plastic tube through the narrowed area, or by the creation of a *gastrostomy* (a surgically produced opening in the stomach through which a feeding tube can be placed).

Oesophageal varices
Widened veins in the walls of the lower part of the *oesophagus* and, in some cases, also in the upper part of

the stomach. Oesophageal varices develop as a consequence of *portal hypertension* (increased blood pressure in the portal vein due to liver disease). Blood passing from the intestines to the liver via the portal vein meets increased resistance and is instead diverted through the veins in the walls of the oesophagus and stomach, where the pressure causes the veins to balloon outwards.
SYMPTOMS AND DIAGNOSIS
The affected veins are thin-walled and contain blood at high pressure; they may rupture, causing recurrent episodes of severe haematemesis (vomiting of blood) and melaena (black faeces). Most patients also have other symptoms of chronic liver disease.

Endoscopy (passage of a viewing instrument down the oesophagus) or a barium swallow (see *Barium X-ray examinations*) shows the affected veins bulging from the oesophageal walls.
TREATMENT
Acute bleeding may be controlled by means of a specially designed *balloon catheter*, which is passed into the oesophagus and stomach; the balloon is inflated to press on the bleeding varices. Later, the varices may be treated with intravenous injection of synthetic *ADH* (vasopressin) and/or by injection of a sclerosant—a solution that clots the blood and permanently hardens and seals off the affected veins. Surgery may be performed to lower the pressure in the blood supply to the liver. Recurrent bleeding can sometimes be controlled by other drugs, such as *propranolol*.

Oesophagitis
Inflammation of the *oesophagus*.
TYPES
The two main types are corrosive oesophagitis, caused by swallowing caustic chemicals, and reflux oesophagitis, caused by regurgitation of stomach contents into the oesophagus.

CORROSIVE OESOPHAGITIS The severity of inflammation depends on the caustic chemical swallowed. Chemicals likely to cause very severe corrosive oesophagitis include cleaning or disinfectant solutions. Immediately after swallowing such a chemical, there is severe pain with *shock* and swelling in the throat and mouth. Antidotes are of limited value and gastric lavage (washing out of the stomach) must be avoided as this may only increase the damage. Treatment consists mainly of reducing pain and providing nursing care until the oesophagus heals.

O

REFLUX OESOPHAGITIS This is a very common condition. The main symptom is heartburn (a burning pain in the chest) which worsens on bending over. Symptoms may be worsened by alcohol, smoking, and obesity.

Reflux oesophagitis is caused by poor function of the muscles of the lower oesophagus, which permits reflux (regurgitation) of the stomach's acidic contents into the oesophagus. Poor function of the lower oesophagus may be associated with a *hiatus hernia*, in which the top part of the stomach slides back and forth between the chest and the abdomen.

A less common alkaline form of oesophagitis is caused by the presence of bile in the stomach, which may be a consequence of certain operations, such as partial *gastrectomy*. If the bile flows from the stomach into the oesophagus, it causes inflammation of the oesophagus, which tends to be severe and difficult to treat.

Barrett's oesophagus is a complication of reflux oesophagitis in which tissue normally found in the stomach lining occurs in the oesophagus. This condition may lead to cancer.

DIAGNOSIS
A barium swallow (see *Barium X-ray examinations*) will show reflux of stomach contents, and *endoscopy* of the oesophagus (passage of a viewing instrument down the oesophagus) will show inflammation.

In doubtful cases, special tests may be required. A small tube may be swallowed and a probe positioned in the lower oesophagus to record the acidity over a 24-hour period; alternatively, a dilute acid solution may be introduced into the stomach to see if it reproduces the symptoms.

TREATMENT
The treatment for most cases of persistent oesophagitis is for the sufferer to change his or her diet and lifestyle—to reduce weight, avoid heavy meals, limit alcohol consumption, and stop smoking. *Antacid drugs* may be taken to reduce the acidity of the stomach contents. Elevation of the head of the bed with blocks may be helpful. Sometimes, surgical treatment may be needed for a hiatus hernia.

Severe, chronic oesophagitis of either type can cause an *oesophageal stricture* (narrowing of the oesophagus), which will require prolonged *oesophageal dilatation* and/or extensive surgery.

Oesophagogastroscopy
See *Gastroscopy.*

Oesophagoscopy
Examination of the *oesophagus* by means of an endoscope, a thin, flexible viewing instrument with a light and lenses attached. (See *Gastroscopy.*)

Oesophagus
The muscular tube that carries food from the throat to the stomach.

STRUCTURE
The top end of the oesophagus is the narrowest part of the entire digestive tract (see *Digestive system*) and is encircled by a sphincter (circular muscle) that is normally closed but can open to allow the passage of food. There is a similar sphincter at the point where the oesophagus enters the stomach. The walls of the oesophagus consist of strong muscle fibres arranged in bundles, some circular and others longitudinal. The inner lining of the oesophagus consists of smooth, squamous epithelium (flattened cells).

FUNCTION
The oesophagus acts as a conduit by which liquids and food are conveyed to the stomach and intestines for digestion. Food is propelled downwards towards the stomach by *peristalsis* (powerful waves of contractions passing through the muscles in the oesophageal wall). Gravity plays little part in getting food into the stomach, making it possible to drink whilst upside down. (See also *Swallowing.*)

Oesophagus, cancer of
A malignant tumour of the *oesophagus*, which ultimately causes difficulty in swallowing. Most oesophageal cancers develop in the middle or lower sections of the oesophagus.

CAUSES AND INCIDENCE
The causes of oesophageal cancer are not fully understood, but smoking, a heavy consumption of alcohol, and drinking very hot drinks are thought to be risk factors.

The incidence varies throughout the world. There are about 5,000 cases diagnosed in the UK each year, mainly in people over 50. The cancer is more common in men than in women and more common in black people than in white people. There is a particularly high incidence of oesophageal cancer in parts of the Far East and Iran, where the cancer has been linked to chemicals in certain foods.

SYMPTOMS
Difficulty in swallowing is noticed first with solids and later with fluids (even saliva) and becomes progressively worse. If food cannot pass down the oesophagus it is immediately regurgitated. Rapid weight loss occurs, but no pain develops until the cancer is well advanced. Respiratory infections are common, because regurgitated fluid spills over into the trachea.

DIAGNOSIS
A barium swallow (see *Barium X-ray examinations*) can indicate the site and often the nature of the obstruction of the oesophagus. Definite diagnosis is provided by examination of a *biopsy* sample (a small piece of tissue) obtained through an *endoscope* (viewing instrument) fitted with a tissue-collecting attachment.

TREATMENT AND OUTLOOK
Oesophagectomy (removal of the oesophagus) provides the best hope of cure but is a major undertaking. Incisions are made in the abdomen, chest, and sometimes in the neck. Most of the oesophagus is then removed and the stomach, or sometimes a portion of the colon, is pulled up into the chest and joined to the upper part of the oesophagus.

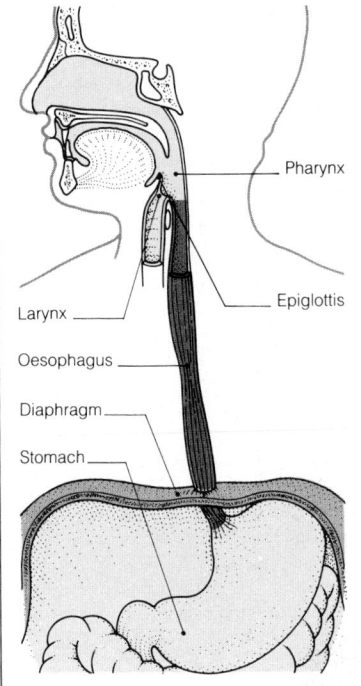

ANATOMY OF THE OESOPHAGUS
A muscular tube that propels food to the stomach from the throat. The upper and lower ends are bounded by sphincters—muscular valves that open to allow food to pass through.

Pharynx

Epiglottis

Larynx

Oesophagus

Diaphragm

Stomach

DISORDERS OF THE OESOPHAGUS

Despite its apparently simple structure, the oesophagus is prone to a number of disorders, most of which lead to difficulty in, or completely prevent, swallowing and/or cause a pain in the chest.

CONGENITAL DEFECTS

Oesophageal atresia is an absence from birth of a section of the oesophagus, with the remaining sections ending in dead ends. It requires urgent surgical correction. Babies are also occasionally born with web-like constrictions of the oesophagus. These are rarely serious enough to require treatment, but may, if necessary, be broken down with a rubber dilator.

INFECTION AND INFLAMMATION

Infections of the oesophagus are uncommon, but may occur in severely immunosuppressed patients whose defences against infection are weakened. The most common infections are *herpes simplex* virus infection or *candidiasis* (thrush) extending downwards from the mouth. Both cause pain on swallowing.

Oesophagitis (inflammation of the oesophagus) is usually due to reflux of the contents of the stomach, causing heartburn (a burning sensation in the chest). A more severe form—corrosive oesophagitis—can occur as a result of swallowing caustic chemicals. Either of these types of oesophagitis may cause an *oesophageal stricture*, with consequent difficulty in swallowing.

INJURY

Apart from the damaging effects of swallowing corrosive chemicals, the most common cause of injury to the oesophagus is severe vomiting and retching, which can occasionally tear the oesophageal lining (and result in bleeding) or in extreme cases lead to rupture. A hard, swallowed *foreign body* can also cause injury and sometimes perforation (formation of a hole) if it penetrates into the oesophageal wall.

TUMOURS

Tumours of the oesophagus are not rare. The initial symptom is usually difficulty in swallowing. About 90 per cent are malignant (see *Oesophagus, cancer of*); the remainder are benign.

OTHER DISORDERS

An *oesophageal diverticulum* is an outwardly protruding sac, usually at the top end of the oesophagus, in which food may collect and cause halitosis (bad breath) and sometimes difficulty in swallowing. *Oesophageal spasm* consists of uncontrollable contractions of the oesophagus, which again may make swallowing difficult. In *achalasia*, the sphincter at the junction between the oesophagus and stomach fails to relax to allow the passage of food, causing pain on swallowing and sometimes regurgitation of food. (See also *Swallowing difficulty*.)

INVESTIGATION

Oesophageal disorders are investigated by barium swallow (see *Barium X-ray examinations*) and by *endoscopy*. Occasionally, a *biopsy* (tissue sample) may be taken for microscopic examination.

For older patients who might not survive this operation, *radiotherapy*, sometimes combined with *anticancer drugs* (particularly cisplatin), can sometimes provide a significant regression of the cancer, relief from symptoms, and even an occasional cure. Some relief from starvation can also be achieved by intubation—the insertion of a rigid tube through the tumour to allow swallowing of liquid or semi-liquid food, or by using a *laser treatment* to burn a passage through an obstructing tumour.

The overall outlook is poor, with only about five per cent of patients surviving for five years; if the cancer is diagnosed early, the outlook is better.

Oestradiol

The most important of the *oestrogen hormones* (female sex hormones), essential for the healthy functioning of the reproductive system and for breast development.

In its synthetic form, oestradiol is prescribed as a tablet to treat symptoms and complications of the *menopause* (see *Hormone replacement therapy*) and to stimulate sexual development in female *hypogonadism* (underdevelopment of the ovaries). It can be taken orally, given by injection, implanted under the skin, or be absorbed through the skin from a transdermal patch.

Oestriol

One of the *oestrogen hormones* (female sex hormones). Oestriol is the predominant oestrogen during pregnancy. Synthetic oestriol is prescribed to treat symptoms and complications of the *menopause* (see *Hormone replacement therapy*) and to stimulate sexual development in female hypogonadism.

Oestrogen drugs

COMMON DRUGS

Dienoestrol Ethinyloestradiol
Oestradiol Oestriol Stilboestrol

WARNING

Tobacco smoking while taking oestrogen drugs significantly increases the risk of abnormal blood clotting, which may cause myocardial infarction, pulmonary embolism, or stroke.

A group of drugs produced synthetically for use in *oral contraceptives* and to supplement or replace the naturally occurring *oestrogen hormones* in the body. Oestrogen drugs are often used in conjunction with *progestogen drugs*.

Oestrogens suppress the production of *gonadotrophin hormones* (hormones that stimulate cell activity in the *ovaries*). High doses of oestrogens may be given as postcoital contraception (see *Contraception, postcoital*) because they prevent conception by blocking the effect of gonadotrophins.

Synthetic oestrogens are used to treat, and in some cases to prevent, symptoms and disorders related to the *menopause*, including atrophic *vaginitis* (dryness of the vagina) and *osteoporosis* (decreased bone density).

Oestrogens may also be used to treat certain forms of infertility, female *hypogonadism* (underdevelopment of the ovaries), menstrual disorders in which there is abnormal bleeding from the uterus, prostatic cancer (see *Prostate, cancer of*), and certain types of *breast cancer*.

POSSIBLE ADVERSE EFFECTS

Oestrogen drugs may cause breast tenderness and enlargement, bloating, weight gain, nausea, reduced sex drive, depression, migraine, and bleeding between periods. Side-effects often subside after two or three months, but, if they persist or are troublesome, a different oestrogen drug may be prescribed. Vaginal creams containing oestrogen should be used sparingly and usually only for a short time to reduce the risk of adverse effects throughout the body.

Oestrogen drugs increase the risk of abnormal blood clotting and are therefore not recommended for people with a personal or family history of *stroke*, *pulmonary embolism*, or deep-vein *thrombosis*, or for people about to undergo surgery. Oestrogen drugs may increase a person's susceptibility to *hypertension* (high blood pressure) and are not usually prescribed if a person has suffered from this disorder in the past. Oestrogens should not be taken during pregnancy as they may adversely affect the fetus.

Oestrogen hormones

A group of *hormones* (chemical messengers released by glands) essential for normal female sexual development and for the healthy functioning of the reproductive system. In women, they are produced mainly in the *ovaries*. Oestrogen hormones are also formed in the *placenta* during pregnancy and, in both men and women, in small amounts in the *adrenal glands*. In men, oestrogens have no known specific function.

Oestrone

One of the *oestrogen hormones*.

Oils

See *Fats and oils*.

Ointment

A greasy, semi-solid skin preparation. Ointments are used to apply drugs to an area of skin or to act as a protective agent. Most ointments contain petrolatum or wax and have an *emollient* (soothing, moisturizing) effect.

Olecranon

The bony projection at the upper end of the *ulna* (the inner bone of the forearm) that forms the point of the *elbow*. The olecranon is commonly known as the "funny bone"; a blow to the nerve that passes across it produces a tingling sensation that passes down the forearm to the fourth and fifth fingertips.

Olfactory nerve

The first *cranial nerve*, which conveys *smell* sensations (as nerve impulses) from the *nose* to the *brain*. Each of the two olfactory nerves detect smells by

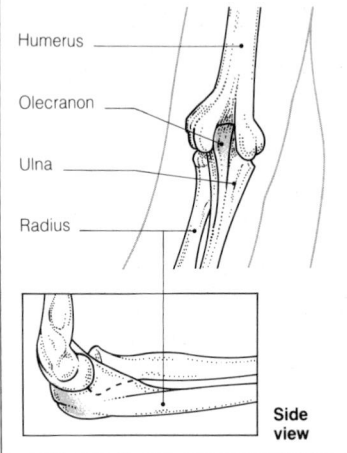

LOCATION OF THE OLECRANON
This is the curved projection at the upper end of the ulna. It acts to prevent elbow overextension.

Humerus

Olecranon

Ulna

Radius

Side view

means of hair-like receptors (nerve endings specialized in detecting stimuli) in the mucous membrane lining the roof of the nasal cavity. Nerve fibres pass from the receptors through tiny holes in the roof of the nasal cavity and come together to form two structures called the olfactory bulbs. From the bulbs, nerve fibres travel to the olfactory centre in the brain.

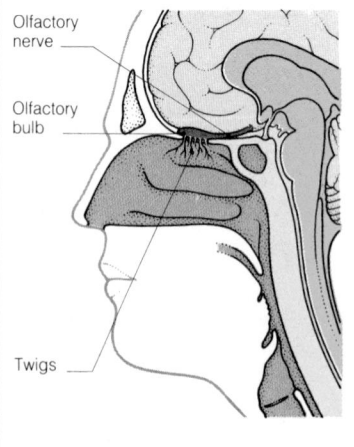

LOCATION OF THE OLFACTORY NERVE
Each olfactory bulb lies on top of a thin bony plate in the roof of the nose and connects to the brain via an olfactory nerve. Nerve twigs pass through the bony plate to enter the nasal lining.

Olfactory nerve

Olfactory bulb

Twigs

Damage to the olfactory nerves, which is usually caused by a head injury, may result in loss or impairment of the sense of smell.

Oligo-

A prefix meaning few, little, or scanty, as in oligospermia (too few sperm in the semen). The prefix olig- is synonymous with oligo-.

Oligodendroglioma

A rare, slow-growing type of primary *brain tumour* that mainly affects young or middle-aged adults. Symptoms, diagnosis, and treatment are as for other types of brain tumour. Surgical removal of the tumour can, in some cases, lead to a complete cure. About one third of patients survive for five years or more.

Oligohydramnios

A rare condition in which there is an abnormally small amount of *amniotic fluid* surrounding the fetus in the uterus during pregnancy.

CAUSES
Amniotic fluid is produced by the *placenta*, swallowed by the fetus, and excreted as fetal urine. Oligohydramnios may occur if the placenta is not functioning properly, as occurs in severe *pre-eclampsia*. Oligohydramnios may also occur if there is an abnormality of the fetal urinary tract.

TREATMENT AND OUTLOOK
In some cases, the underlying disorder can be treated, but sometimes it cannot (particularly if the fetus is abnormal). If oligohydramnios occurs early in pregnancy, it usually results in *miscarriage*. If the condition occurs later in pregnancy, the pressure of the uterus on the fetus may cause a deformity, such as *talipes* (club-foot). If oligohydramnios occurs in an overdue pregnancy, induction of labour or a caesarean section may be performed.

Oligospermia

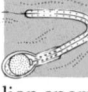

A deficiency in the number of *sperm* per unit volume of seminal fluid; there are normally more than 20 million sperm per millilitre of semen. Oligospermia may be temporary or permanent. It is a major cause of *infertility*, especially when present with certain other disorders of the sperm.

CAUSES
Oligospermia may be caused by a number of different disorders, including *orchitis* (inflammation of a testis), failure of a testis to descend into the scrotum (see *Testis, undescended*), and,

O

infrequently, a *varicocele* (varicose vein of the testis). Stress, cigarette smoking, alcohol abuse, and treatment with some types of drugs may cause temporary oligospermia.

DIAGNOSIS AND TREATMENT

A sperm count is performed as part of *semen analysis*. Treatment is of the underlying cause. *Gonadotrophin hormones* may be prescribed for a short period if the cause of the oligospermia is unknown. (See also *Azoospermia*.)

Oliguria

The production of a smaller-than-normal quantity of *urine* in relation to the volume of fluid taken in. Oliguria may be due simply to excessive sweating without adequate fluid replacement in a hot climate. In other cases, oliguria may be a sign of *kidney failure*.

Olive oil

 An oil obtained from the fruit of the olive tree OLEA EUROPAEA. Warm olive oil may sometimes be used to soften *earwax* before the ears are syringed. Olive oil is also used for its *emollient* (soothing, moisturizing) effect in the treatment of *cradle cap* in babies.

-oma

A suffix that denotes a tumour, as in lipoma, which is a benign tumour of fatty tissue.

Omentum

An apron-like double fold of fatty membrane that hangs down in front of the intestines. In addition to acting as a fat store, the omentum may limit the spread of infection within the abdominal cavity by adhering to the affected area.

Omeprazole

A drug used to treat *peptic ulcer*, reflux *oesophagitis*, and *Zollinger-Ellison syndrome*. Adverse effects include rashes, headache, nausea, diarrhoea, and constipation.

Omphalocele

An alternative name for *exomphalos*.

Onchocerciasis

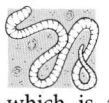 A tropical disease that is caused by infestation with the worm ONCHOCERCA VOLVULUS. The disease, which is a type of *filariasis*, affects more than 20 million people in parts of Africa and Central and South America. Many sufferers are blinded by the disease.

CAUSES AND SYMPTOMS

Onchocerciasis is transmitted from person to person by small, fiercely biting, black simulium flies. These flies breed in, and always remain near, fast-running streams (thus giving the disease its alternative name of "river blindness").

The transmission of the disease and the life-cycle of the worm are shown in the box (below). Blindness can occur as a result of an allergic reaction to dead microfilariae in or near the eyes.

TREATMENT AND PREVENTION

The microfilariae are quickly killed by the drug diethylcarbamazine. This drug must be used with great care, however, because of the severe reactions caused by the dead larvae.

Travellers to areas where the disease is prevalent should take measures to discourage *insect bites*.

Oncogenes

Genes, found in all cells, that are involved in the control of normal cell proliferation. Abnormalities of these genes have been shown to be one of the steps responsible for cells becoming cancerous. Of the full human complement of 50,000 genes, fewer than 100 are probably oncogenes.

Cancerous cells differ from healthy ones in various ways. Their growth is unrestrained, and they infiltrate and destroy normal tissues (see *Cancer*). These differences are induced by *mutations* (alterations) in certain key genes—the oncogenes—which cause them to be "switched on". Switching on of a cell's oncogenes may increase its rate of multiplication, alter its responsiveness to hormonal growth factors, or increase its invasiveness.

Oncogenes may be switched on by the various environmental factors that are known to cause cancer, such as ultraviolet light, radioactivity, tobacco smoke, alcohol, asbestos particles, carcinogenic chemicals, and certain viruses. To transform a cell from normal to malignant seems to require the switching on of between two and four oncogenes. Thus, cancer of the cervix may develop in a woman who smokes and whose cervix has been infected with papillomavirus (a potentially cancer-causing virus), whereas either of these factors by itself might not be sufficient to cause cancer.

Oncology

The study of the causes, development, characteristics, and treatment of *tumours*, particularly *cancers* (malignant tumours). Because there are many different types of tumours, deriving from virtually any tissue in the body, oncology encompasses a range of experimental techniques and investigative approaches. These include surveying the frequency and distribution of tumours, testing new treatments, investigating biochemical processes involved in tumour formation, and studying abnormal genes associated with tumours.

Doctors specializing in the study and treatment of cancer are known as oncologists. They are concerned with

O

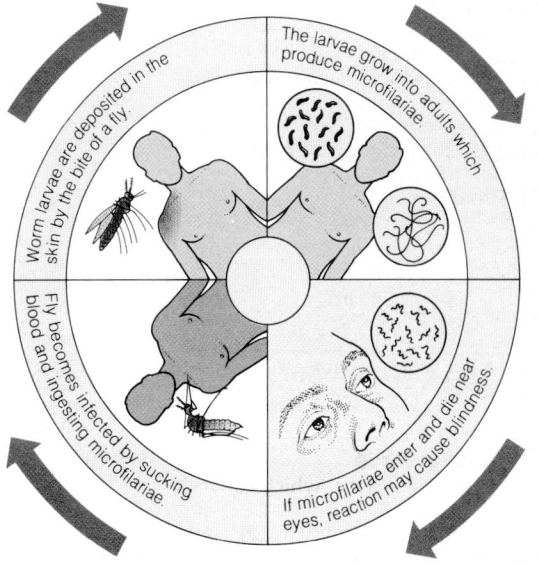

LIFE-CYCLE OF ONCHOCERCIASIS
The infestation is spread by a fly that ingests microfilariae (tiny worms) from an infested person; the worms grow into larvae and are deposited in the skin of a new host when the fly bites.

Worm larvae are deposited in the skin by the bite of a fly.

The larvae grow into adults which produce microfilariae.

If microfilariae enter and die near eyes, reaction may cause blindness.

Fly becomes infected by sucking blood and ingesting microfilariae.

diagnosing the type of cancer and determining its exact location and rate of spread. They will then be responsible for the prescription and monitoring of *radiotherapy* and *anticancer* drug treatment as well as for follow-up care and referral for surgery.

Onychogryphosis

Abnormal thickening, hardening, and curving of the *nails,* which occurs mainly in elderly people. Its cause is unknown, but onychogryphosis is associated with *fungal infection* or with poor circulation.

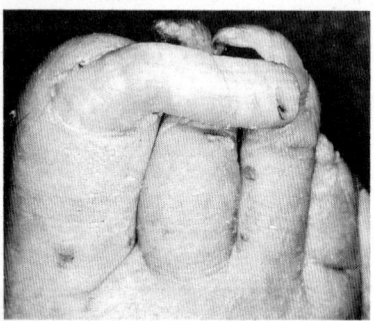

Onychogryphosis
This extraordinary thickening and overgrowth, resembling the claws of the mythological griffin, may affect toenails or fingernails.

Onycholysis

Separation of the *nail* from its bed, beginning at the tip. Onycholysis is a feature of many skin conditions, including *psoriasis, dermatitis,* and some *fungal infections.*

Oophorectomy

Removal of one or both *ovaries.*
WHY IT IS DONE
Oophorectomy is performed to treat *ovarian cysts* or ovarian cancer (see *Ovary, cancer of*). In women under 40, the surgeon attempts to preserve ovarian function by performing only a partial oophorectomy.

Both ovaries may be removed during a *hysterectomy* if disease has spread from the uterus to the ovaries. Removing both ovaries can also reduce the risk of ovarian cancer in women past the menopause. Occasionally, both ovaries may be removed in a patient with *breast cancer,* as the growth of the cancer may be dependent on hormones produced by the ovary.
HOW IT IS DONE
Oophorectomy is performed under general anaesthesia and usually takes less than one hour. The ovaries are removed through an incision in the lower abdominal wall.

RECOVERY PERIOD
There is some pain and tenderness around the operation site. Most activities can be resumed within about a month of surgery, and sexual intercourse after about six weeks.
OUTLOOK
There are usually no adverse effects when one ovary or part of an ovary is removed because *ovulation* and hormone production continue. If both ovaries are removed before the menopause, *hormone replacement therapy* may be necessary.

-opathy

A suffix that denotes a disease or disorder. An example of its use is in the word neuropathy (a disorder of the peripheral nerves). The suffix *-pathy* is synonymous with -opathy.

Open heart surgery

Any operation on the *heart* in which the heartbeat is temporarily stopped and the heart's function is taken over by a mechanical pump.

The early heart surgeons carried out limited operations while the heart continued to beat. In such "closed" operations it was possible, for example, for a surgeon to insert a finger or a specially designed knife into the heart to open the channel of a narrowed valve.

With the development of reliable *heart-lung machines* in the 1950s, much more elaborate heart surgery became possible. Once the pump was connected, the surgeon could open the heart, repair defects, and even reconstruct the main chambers. During the operation, the heart is kept cool through techniques of surgical *hypothermia,* which help to prevent any damage occurring to the heart muscle from lack of oxygen.

The main applications of open heart surgery have been the correction of congenital heart defects (see *Heart disease, congenital*), surgery for heart valve insufficiency or narrowed heart valves (see *Heart valve surgery*), and *coronary artery bypass* surgery.

Operable

A term applied to any condition that is suitable for surgical treatment, such as an accessible benign tumour that requires removal because it is causing symptoms. (See also *Inoperable.*)

Operating theatre

A hospital room in which surgical procedures are performed. The room is designed to reduce the risk of infec-

COMMON SURGICAL OPERATIONS

Operation	Estimated no. performed (England 1990-91)
Removal of uterine contents	182,710
Cystoscopy	113,540
Bone operations	88,765
Tonsils and adenoids	78,430
Inguinal hernia operations	63,540
Hysterectomy	61,050
Myringotomy (eardrum incision)	56,250
Mastectomy	42,610
Arthroplasty (joint replacement)	42,470
Haemorrhoid operations	42,165
Bladder outlet and prostate operations	40,180
Heart surgery	37,780
Gallbladder operations	22,170

tion in open surgical wounds. A ventilation system provides a constant supply of clean, filtered air, the walls and floors are easily washable and are cleaned at least once daily, and there are adjoining rooms with foot- or elbow-operated taps where surgeons, assistants, and nurses use sterile brushes and bactericidal soaps to scrub their hands and forearms before putting on sterile gowns, masks, and gloves. Often built into the walls are light-boxes for viewing images obtained by such techniques as *X-ray, CT scanning,* or *MRI.*
EQUIPMENT
During an operation using general anaesthesia, the anaesthetic machine stands at the head of the operating table (see *Anaesthesia, general*), connected by tubes to oxygen and various anaesthetic gases.

The surgeon's sterile instruments, covered with sterile towels before use, are arranged on stainless steel wheeled tables. There is also a *diathermy* machine, which controls bleeding. If required, other equipment, such as a *heart-lung machine* (which can take over the function of the patient's heart and lungs), is brought into the operating theatre.

OPERATING THEATRE

The operating table can be raised, lowered, and tilted in any direction to allow optimum access to the patient. For some operations, it is best for the surgeon to stand but, during delicate procedures, such as microsurgery, the surgeon usually sits. The operating lamp is designed to give brilliant focal illumination without casting any shadows. The anaesthetic apparatus can maintain breathing in patients who have been given a muscle-relaxant drug.

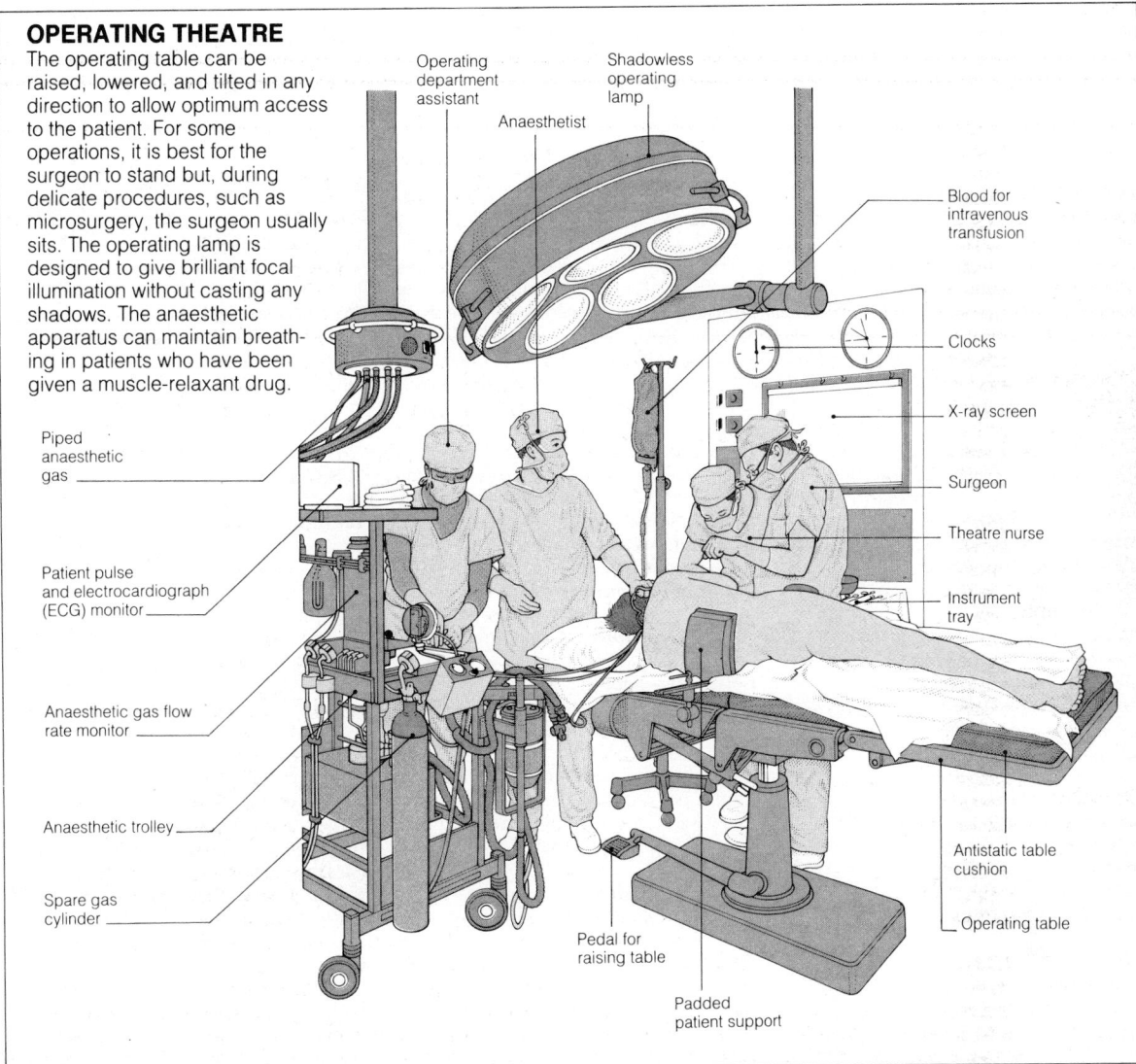

Operating department assistant

Anaesthetist

Shadowless operating lamp

Blood for intravenous transfusion

Clocks

X-ray screen

Surgeon

Theatre nurse

Instrument tray

Piped anaesthetic gas

Patient pulse and electrocardiograph (ECG) monitor

Anaesthetic gas flow rate monitor

Anaesthetic trolley

Spare gas cylinder

Pedal for raising table

Padded patient support

Antistatic table cushion

Operating table

O

Operation

Any surgical procedure, usually carried out with instruments but sometimes using only the hands (as in the manipulation of a simple fracture). Operations range from procedures performed quickly under local anaesthesia (e.g. draining a skin abscess) to surgery lasting several hours performed under general anaesthesia (e.g. a heart or liver transplant).

Ophthalmia

An old term for *Ophthalmitis*.

Ophthalmitis

A term for any inflammatory *eye* disorder. It is also used to describe the following two specific disorders.

Neonatal ophthalmitis (also called ophthalmia neonatorum) is a discharge of pus from the eyes of an infant that starts within 21 days of birth. In many cases the cause is an infection (such as *gonorrhoea* or a *chlamydial infection*) acquired during birth. The condition is treated with *antibiotic drugs*.

Sympathetic ophthalmitis is a rare condition in which a penetrating injury to one eye is followed at least 10 days later by severe *uveitis* (inflammation of the iris and choroid) that threatens blindness in the uninjured eye. The condition can be treated with *corticosteroid drugs*, but in some cases, removal of the injured eye is necessary to save the sight of the other eye.

Ophthalmology

The study of the *eye*, and the diagnosis and treatment of the disorders that affect it. Ophthalmology includes not only the assessment of *vision* and the prescription of *glasses* or *contact lenses* to correct defects, but also the surgery required to treat eye disorders, such as *cataracts*, *glaucoma*, *retinal detachment*, and obstruction of the tear ducts.

Doctors who specialize in care of the eyes are called ophthalmologists. Ophthalmologists frequently work closely with other doctors because many disorders of the retina at the back of the eye are signs of nonoptical disorders, such as *hypertension* (high blood pressure), *atherosclerosis* (narrowing of arteries by fatty deposits), or *diabetes mellitus*. Careful analysis of a person's field of vision (see *Eye, examination of*) can reveal defects that indicate neurological damage, such as that caused by a brain tumour. (See also *Optician; Optometry; Orthoptics*.)

Ophthalmoplegia

Partial or total paralysis of the muscles that move the *eyes*. Ophthalmoplegia may be caused by disease of the muscles themselves (as in *Graves' disease*) or by one of the conditions affecting the brain or the nerves supplying the eye muscles (including *stroke, encephalitis, brain tumour*, and *multiple sclerosis*).

Ophthalmoscope

An instrument used to examine the inside of the *eye*. The ophthalmoscope contains a deflecting prism or a perforated angled mirror, which allows illumination and viewing of the entire area of the retina, the head of the optic nerve, the retinal arteries and veins, and the vitreous humour.

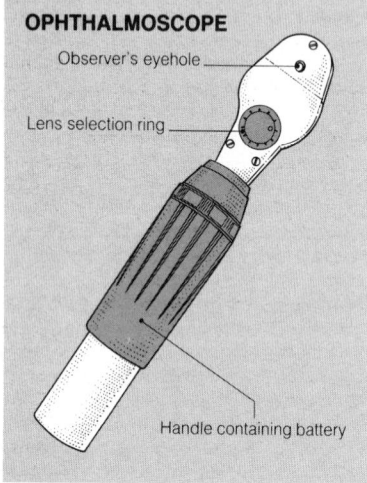

OPHTHALMOSCOPE

Observer's eyehole

Lens selection ring

Handle containing battery

Opiate

Any drug derived from, or chemically similar to, *opium*. The term opiate is also used in the term opiate *receptor* to refer to a specific site on a cell's surface with which opiate drugs combine to initiate their effects.

Opium

A substance obtained from the unripe seed pods of the poppy plant *PAPAVER SOMNIFERUM*. Used as a drug for thousands of years, opium has an analgesic (painkilling) effect and may also cause sleepiness and euphoria.

Opium and its derivatives, which include *codeine* and *morphine*, are among the drugs collectively known as *narcotic drugs*.

Opportunistic infection

Infection caused by organisms that do not usually produce disease in healthy people; or widespread infection by organisms that normally produce only a mild, local infection.

Many of the causative organisms are normally present on or in the human body and cause disease only when the host's *immune system* (natural defences) is impaired. Impairment of the immune system may be due to treatment with anticancer and immunosuppressant drugs, to radiotherapy, or to diseases such as leukaemia. Opportunistic infections also affect premature or malnourished infants and people with *immunodeficiency disorders*.

Opportunistic infections, especially *pneumocystis pneumonia*, are the cause of death in most *AIDS* patients. Many fungal infections, (e.g. *cryptococcosis* and *candidiasis*) and some viral infections (e.g. *cytomegalovirus* and *herpes simplex*) are opportunistic infections.

Opportunistic infections are often unavoidable because the underlying defects in the host's defences cannot easily be rectified. However, treatment with appropriate antimicrobial drugs may be life-saving.

Optic atrophy

A shrinkage or wasting of the *optic nerve* fibres, which results in partial or complete loss of vision. Optic atrophy is caused by disease or injury to the optic nerve and may occur without prior signs of nerve disease, such as inflammation or swelling.

Optic disc oedema

See *Papilloedema*.

Optician

A person who fits and sells *glasses* or *contact lenses*. An optician may be either a dispensing optician (responsible only for fitting and selling glasses or contact lenses) or an ophthalmic optician or optometrist (responsible also for testing for errors of *refraction*).

Ophthalmic opticians are trained to perform eye examinations to test for the degree of *myopia* (shortsightedness), *hypermetropia* (longsightedness), *presbyopia*, or *astigmatism*.

Ophthalmic opticians are not trained to treat disorders of the eye. An optician who suspects that a

patient has an eye disorder will refer him or her to an ophthalmologist. (See also *Ophthalmology; Optometry*.)

Optic nerve

The second *cranial nerve*; the nerve of *vision*. The optic nerve consists of a collection of about one million nerve fibres that transmit impulses from the *retina* (the layer of light receptors at the back of the eye) to the *brain*.

The two optic nerves converge to a junction behind the eyes, where fibres from the inner halves of the retinas cross over. Nerve fibres from the right halves of both retinas pass to the right side of the occipital lobes at the back of the brain, while those from the left halves go to the left side.

Disorders of the optic nerve include *optic neuritis* (inflammation of the optic nerve), and *papilloedema*, which is caused by pressure on the nerve from disease within the orbit (eye socket) or a brain tumour.

Optic neuritis

Inflammation of the *optic nerve*, often causing sudden loss of part of the *visual field*. Optic neuritis is usually accompanied by pain on moving the eyes and tenderness when the eyes are touched. In some cases, however, there may be little or no pain.

The cause of optic neuritis often remains uncertain, but most cases are thought to be due to *demyelination* (destruction of the myelin sheaths) of the optic nerve fibres, which occurs in *multiple sclerosis*. The condition may also result from inflammation or infection of tissues around the optic nerve.

Optic neuritis causes loss of vision, usually in the central part of the visual field. Vision usually improves substantially within six weeks, but each attack causes damage to a proportion of the optic nerve fibres; recurrent attacks usually lead to permanent loss of *visual acuity*.

Treatment with *corticosteroid drugs* may aid the return of vision but seems to have little effect on the long-term outcome of the inflammatory process. (See also *Optic atrophy*.)

Optometry

The practice of assessing *vision* and establishing whether *glasses* or *contact lenses* are needed to correct any visual defect. The eyes are examined by a qualified optometrist who will assess the defect and prescribe and supply appropriate glasses or contact lenses to correct it. Optometrists are not qualified to diagnose or treat actual

O

THE FUNCTION OF THE OPTIC NERVE

Each optic nerve is a bundle of long fibres originating from nerve cells in the retina and passing to the back of the brain. Because of the arrangement of the nerve fibres, disease or injury at any point causes a unique pattern of visual loss. Charting the pattern of visual loss allows accurate location of damage to the nerve.

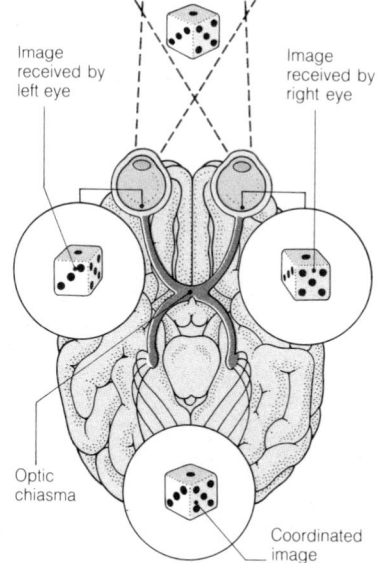

Image received by left eye

Image received by right eye

Optic chiasma

Coordinated image

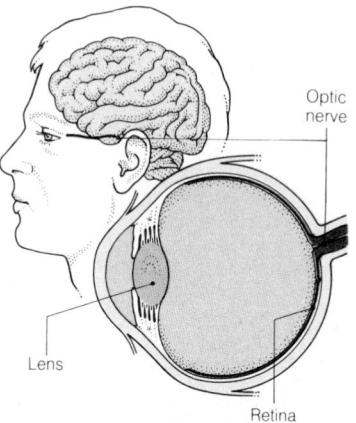

Optic nerve

Lens

Retina

Binocular vision
Because the eyes are a distance apart, they form slightly different images of a nearby object. The fusion of these two images into one provides the illusion of solidity. This is called stereopsis.

disorders of the eye but will refer patients requiring further treatment to an ophthalmologist. (See also *Ophthalmology; Optician.*)

Oral

Concerning the mouth.

Oral contraceptives

COMMON DRUGS

Oestrogens
Ethinyloestradiol Mestranol

Progestogens
Levonorgestrel Norethisterone

WARNING
If you vomit or have diarrhoea while taking an oral contraceptive, follow the advice for missing a pill. If you have missed two consecutive periods, you should have a pregnancy test.

A group of oral drug preparations containing a *progestogen drug*, often combined with an *oestrogen drug*, taken by women to prevent pregnancy. All types of oral contraceptives—combined pills, phased pills, and minipills—are commonly known as "the pill". Combined pills (includ-

ing phased pills) contain an oestrogen and a progestogen. The minipill contains only progestogen.

HOW THEY ARE TAKEN

Combined oral contraceptives need to be taken in a monthly cycle for as long as a woman wishes to avoid pregnancy. The first course of pills is started on the first day of a period or on the fifth day after bleeding starts. Additional contraceptive precautions for the first 14 days are needed if the combined or phased pill is begun on day five, and are usually recommended when starting the minipill.

The way each course of pills is usually taken is described in the illustrated box. Some brands of phased pills contain seven additional inactive pills, which may contain an iron supplement, so that the habit of taking a pill each day is not broken. It is possible to take a combined or a phased pill continuously and thus avoid bleeding, but most doctors do not recommend this. In some women, oral contraceptives may cause menstruation to cease.

MISSING A PILL

For maximum contraceptive effect, each type of pill should be taken at approximately the same time each day. This is particularly important

with the minipill, which should be taken within three hours of the chosen time each day.

A forgotten combined or phased pill should be taken as soon as it is remembered even if this means taking two pills the next day. Pills for the rest of the course should be taken at the correct time. An additional form of contraception should be used for 14 days after missing a pill.

If the minipill is taken more than three hours late, extra precautions should be taken for 14 days.

EFFECTIVENESS

Used correctly, oral contraceptives have a failure rate of less than one pregnancy per 100 woman-years (i.e. the number of pregnancies among 100 women using the method for one year is less than one). Allowing for incorrect use or other factors, the actual failure rates may be as high as between two and three pregnancies per 100 woman-years for the combined or phased pill, and between two and a half and four pregnancies for the minipill.

Certain other drugs (such as *barbiturate drugs, anticonvulsant drugs,* and some *antibiotic drugs*) may impair the effectiveness of oral contraceptives. A woman should always inform her family planning doctor if she is taking other medication.

ADVANTAGES AND DISADVANTAGES

In addition to providing excellent protection against pregnancy, the main advantage of oral contraceptives is that they do not interfere with the spontaneity of sex.

Oestrogen-containing pills protect against cancer of the uterus and ovaries, *ovarian cysts, endometriosis,* and iron-deficiency *anaemia.* They also tend to make periods regular, lighter, and relatively free of menstrual pain.

The main disadvantages of oral contraceptives are that they are medically unsuitable for some women and that they may produce adverse effects.

CONTRAINDICATIONS

Oestrogen-containing pills increase the risk of certain disorders and are not usually prescribed if a woman suffers from *hypertension* (high blood pressure), *hyperlipidaemia* (high levels of fat in the blood), *liver* disease, *migraine, otosclerosis* (an ear disorder), or if she has previously had a *thrombosis* (abnormal blood clot).

The chances of a thrombosis occurring are increased in women who smoke and who are over the age of 35. An oestrogen-containing pill is not usually given during the first few

O

weeks after childbirth or in the four weeks before major surgery because of the increased risk of thrombosis. *Obesity* also makes a woman on the pill more susceptible to thrombosis.

Oral contraceptives are not usually prescribed to a woman who has a personal or family history of heart or circulatory disorders, or who suffers from unexplained vaginal bleeding.

Combined or phased pills may interfere with milk production and should not be taken during breast-feeding. The minipill is usually considered unsuitable for a woman who has had an *ectopic pregnancy*.

POSSIBLE ADVERSE EFFECTS
Oestrogen-containing pills may sometimes cause nausea and vomiting, weight gain, depression, swelling of the breasts, reduced sex drive, increased appetite, cramps in the legs and abdomen, headaches, and dizziness. A more serious adverse effect of these pills is the risk of a thrombosis causing a *stroke* or a *pulmonary embolism*. Oestrogen-containing pills may also aggravate heart disease or cause hypertension, *gallstones*, *jaundice*, and, very rarely, *liver cancer*.

Medical evidence suggests that cancer of the cervix is more common in women taking oestrogen-containing pills, and several studies in the late 1980s pointed to a link between prolonged use of oral contraceptives and the development of breast cancer in women under 35. This may be outweighed by reduced risk of other cancers of the reproductive system.

All forms of oral contraception can cause bleeding between periods, but this is especially true of the minipill. Other possible adverse effects of the minipill are irregular periods, ectopic pregnancy, and ovarian cysts.

There is no evidence that use of an oral contraceptive reduces a woman's fertility permanently (although menstruation may be irregular or absent for some months after stopping the pill). Likewise, there is no evidence that a fetus can be harmed if conceived while the woman is taking the pill or has recently stopped doing so.

Adverse effects usually disappear after a few months of taking the pill. If they persist, it may be necessary to change to a different type of pill or to an alternative method of contraception. Because adverse effects are more likely to occur with high doses of oestrogen, low-oestrogen preparations are prescribed whenever possible. The minipill may be used by women who suffer adverse effects even with low oestrogen doses or who should not take oestrogen drugs for other medical reasons. Women taking oral contraceptives should receive regular check-ups, including blood pressure and weight checks and *cervical smear tests*. (See also *Contraception*.)

Oral hygiene
Measures that keep the *mouth* and *teeth* clean and healthy. Good oral hygiene reduces the incidence of tooth decay (see *Caries, dental*), prevents *gingivitis* and other *gum* disorders, and helps to prevent *halitosis*

HOW ORAL CONTRACEPTIVES WORK
The combined and phased pills increase the levels of oestrogen and progesterone in the body, which interferes with the production by the pituitary gland of two *gonadotrophin hormones* called follicle-stimulating hormone (FSH) and luteinizing hormone (LH). This action in turn prevents ovulation.

The minipill works mainly by making the mucus that lines the inside of the cervix (neck of the uterus) so thick that it is impenetrable to sperm.

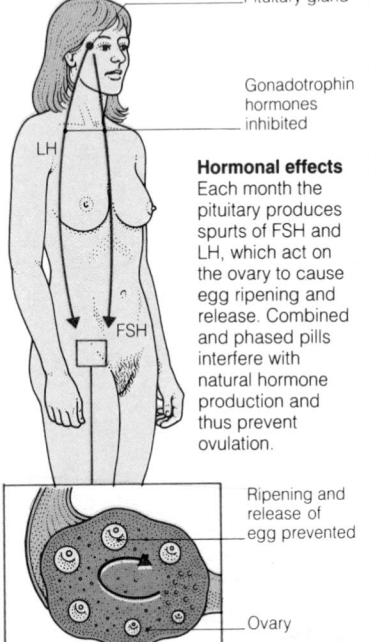

Pituitary gland

Gonadotrophin hormones inhibited

Hormonal effects
Each month the pituitary produces spurts of FSH and LH, which act on the ovary to cause egg ripening and release. Combined and phased pills interfere with natural hormone production and thus prevent ovulation.

Ripening and release of egg prevented

Ovary

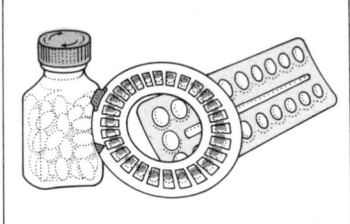

Pill packaging
Most oral contraceptives come in packs that clearly indicate the day on which each pill should be taken.

Effects on eggs
FSH normally brings about egg ripening and LH the egg's release from the ovary; combined and phased pills prevent this.

Combined pill
This pill contains an oestrogen and a progestogen drug in fixed doses. A course usually consists of one pill per day for 21 days, followed by seven pill-free days, during which bleeding may occur. A new course is then started, whether or not bleeding has occurred.

Menstruation

Change   Change

Phased pill—a typical programme
These pills contain both an oestrogen and a progestogen drug, but are divided into two or three groups or phases. The dose of the progestogen drug, and sometimes of oestrogen as well, changes from phase to phase. A course lasts for 21 days followed by seven pill-free days.

Menstruation

Minipill—progestogen only
These pills contain only a progestogen drug in a fixed dose. The pills are taken continuously, one every day with no pill-free days. Bleeding usually occurs during the last few days of each cycle. The minipill has a slightly higher failure rate than the combined and phased pills.

Menstruation

O

(bad breath). Oral hygiene can be broadly divided into personal and professional care.

PERSONAL CARE

The most important aspect of personal oral hygiene is daily removal of dental *plaque* (a sticky, bacteria-containing substance) by thorough *toothbrushing* and use of dental floss (see *Floss, dental*). Use of a *fluoride* mouthwash or of an oral irrigator (a device that produces a forceful jet of water) may also be helpful, but these aids cannot remove plaque or replace brushing and flossing. *Disclosing agents* can help make tooth cleaning more efficient by showing the location of plaque. Dentures must always be kept scrupulously clean by brushing every surface and soaking in a cleansing solution.

PROFESSIONAL CARE

A dentist or a dental hygienist removes stubborn plaque and *calculus* (a hard mineral deposit that forms on the teeth above and below the gums) by *scaling* and polishing. These procedures are usually carried out during a routine check-up; in cases of *periodontal disease*, they may need to be performed more often.

Oral surgery

The branch of surgery concerned with the treatment of deformity, injury, or disease of the teeth, jaws, and other parts of the mouth and face.

All oral surgeons have a degree in general dentistry and further training in oral and maxillofacial (jaw and face) surgery. Many oral surgeons also have medical degrees, although this is not required.

Among the dental procedures carried out by oral surgeons are the extraction of severely impacted wisdom teeth (see *Impaction, dental*) and *alveolectomy* (removal of tooth-bearing bone from the jaw) to improve the fitting of dentures.

More complicated oral surgery includes *orthognathic surgery* to correct deformities of the jaw that result in an abnormal relationship between the upper and lower teeth; repairing a broken jaw; plastic surgery to correct *cleft lip and palate*; and the removal of certain types of benign tumours from tissues within the mouth.

Orbit

The socket in the *skull* that contains the eyeball, protective pads of fat, and various blood vessels, muscles, and nerves. An opening in the back of the orbit allows the *optic nerve* to pass from the eyeball into the *brain*.

LOCATION OF ORBIT

The orbits are the deep cavities in the skull in which the eyeballs and muscles that move the eyes are protectively enclosed.

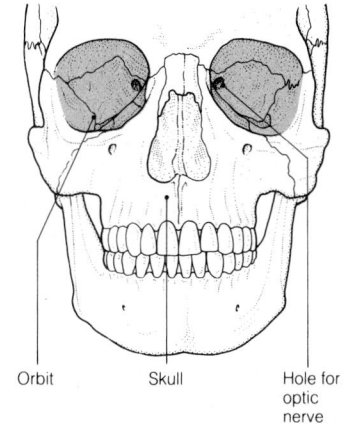

Orbit   Skull   Hole for optic nerve

DISORDERS

INJURY A fracture of the orbit may be caused by a blow of great force, as in a car crash or sports injury. In a fracture of the orbit, the eyeball itself often escapes damage because it is squeezed backwards by protective muscles during reflex blinking. Many such fractures heal without treatment, but some result in facial deformity requiring corrective surgery. Surgery may also be needed to reinforce the floor of the orbit if a fracture causes downward displacement of the eye.

INFECTION Rarely, bacteria infect the fatty tissue lining the orbit, causing orbital *cellulitis*. Usually the infection originates in a nearby sinus, but sometimes it spreads in the blood from a facial infection. The affected eye protrudes and is extremely painful and red. There is also severe swelling of the lids and conjunctiva (the membrane lining the inside of the lids and the white of the eye). Orbital cellulitis is a serious disorder. The pressure on the eye may damage it and there is a slight risk that the infection may spread inwards to cause *meningitis* (inflammation of the membranes covering the brain). Prompt treatment with high doses of *antibiotic drugs* usually clears up the condition.

Orchidectomy

The surgical removal of one or both of the *testes*.

WHY IT IS DONE

Orchidectomy may be performed to treat testicular cancer (see *Testis, can-*

cer of), to treat gangrene due to torsion (see *Testis, torsion of*), or to reduce production of the hormone testosterone as part of the treatment of cancer of the prostate gland (see *Prostate, cancer of*). Because the prostate gland depends on male sex hormones for its normal growth, orchidectomy is often effective in reducing the growth of a prostatic cancer. It is especially effective in controlling the symptoms of secondary tumours in the bones.

HOW IT IS DONE

Under general or spinal anaesthesia, the scrotum is cut open, the blood vessels and nerves leading to the scrotum are cut free, the testis is cut away from surrounding tissue and removed, and the skin is stitched.

After the operation, *analgesic drugs* (painkillers) may be needed and an *ice-pack* may be applied to the scrotum for the first 24 hours to prevent excessive swelling.

OUTLOOK

Complete healing can be expected without complications. Removal of one testis does not affect sex drive, potency, or the ability to have children. The patient is advised to wear an athletic support and to avoid vigorous exercise for a month or so after the operation.

Orchidopexy

An operation in which an undescended testis (see *Testis, undescended*) is brought down into the scrotum. Orchidopexy is usually performed when the boy is between two and five years old to avoid the risk of subsequent infertility or even cancer of the testis (see *Testis, cancer of*).

Under general anaesthesia, an incision is made in the groin and the testis is gently freed and manoeuvred down into the scrotum. The base of the testis is then usually attached to the scrotum with a few stitches to prevent it from retracting. Pain and swelling are relieved with *analgesic drugs* (painkillers). Healing usually takes place without any complications.

Orchitis

Inflammation of a *testis*. Orchitis may be caused by infection with the virus that causes *mumps*.

Orchitis develops in about one quarter of males who contract mumps after puberty. It is characterized by swelling and severe pain in the affected testis and a high fever. In *epididymo-orchitis* (which has different causes), the tube that carries sperm from the testis is also inflamed.

O

Treatment is with *analgesic drugs* (painkillers) and *ice-packs* to reduce swelling and pain; *antibiotic drugs* may be given, but not for mumps orchitis. The condition usually begins to subside after three to seven days. Occasionally, orchitis is followed by shrinking of the testis.

Orf

A skin infection, caused by a pox virus, which is occasionally transmitted to humans from sheep and goats. Orf usually produces a single fluid-filled blister on the arm or the hand. Without treatment, the condition will persist for several weeks. Application of the antiviral drug *idoxuridine* hastens recovery.

Organ

A collection of various *tissues* integrated into a distinct structural unit that performs specific functions. For example, the brain consists of nerve tissue and supporting tissue (called neuroglia) organized to receive, process, and send out information.

Organ donation

The agreement of a person (or his or her relatives) to the surgical removal of one or more organs for use in *transplant surgery*. Most organs used for transplantation are removed immediately after a *donor* has died, but kidneys may also be taken from living donors. Kidney donation by living donors is usually confined to the relatives of transplant patients. Relatives are more likely to have a tissue-type (see *Tissue-typing*) that is compatible with that of the patient. Donation of kidneys by unrelated living donors raises ethical problems, especially when organs are sold.

Before taking a kidney from a living donor, the surgeon will explain carefully the risks of donation, removing the kidney only after the donor has given clear voluntary consent.

The range of organs removed after death is much greater, including the heart, lungs, liver, pancreas, and kidneys. Most organs can be transplanted successfully only if they are removed immediately after death; the best results often require surgical removal of organs before the donor's heart has stopped beating. In practice, this means that most donations of major organs are made from patients who die in an intensive-care unit and are certified as "brain dead" while their heart and lung function is maintained by a machine (see *Death*).

People who want to donate some or all of their organs after death should make their intentions clear to their relatives and sign a donor card. In most Western countries the demand for donated organs is far greater than the supply. Some countries have introduced laws that allow doctors to remove organs after death unless the patient has specifically forbidden it. In practice, doctors are reluctant to carry out such legislation and the supply of donor organs continues to depend on voluntary donations. (See also *Corneal graft; Heart-lung transplant; Heart transplant; Heart valve surgery; Kidney transplant; Liver transplant*.)

Organic

Related to a body *organ*; having organs or an organized structure; or related to *organisms* or to substances from them. In chemistry, the term refers to any of the group of compounds that contain carbon, with the exception of carbon oxides (such as carbon dioxide), carbon sulphides, and metal carbonates (such as calcium carbonate).

The term organic also signifies the presence of disease, in contrast to a *functional disorder* or a *psychosomatic* complaint. (See also *Inorganic*.)

Organic brain syndrome

See *Brain syndrome, organic*.

Organism

A general term for any individual animal or plant. Medically, the most important organisms are humans and disease-causing *microorganisms*, such as *bacteria, fungi, protozoa*, and *viruses*.

Orgasm

Intense sensations resulting from the series of muscular contractions that occur at the peak of sexual excitement. Orgasm is usually followed by physical relaxation and often by drowsiness.

In men, contractions of the muscles of the inner pelvis massage seminal fluid from the prostatic area into the urethra, from which it is forcefully propelled from the urethral orifice (see *Ejaculation*). Following orgasm, the penis becomes soft again and there is a refractory period during which there is no physical response to further sexual stimulation.

Orgasm in women is associated with irregular contractions of the voluntary muscles of the walls of the vagina and, in some women, of the uterus, followed by relief of congestion in the pelvic area. Orgasm usually lasts about three to 10 seconds, but can last up to a minute in some women. It is generally believed that there is no refractory phase in women. Some women experience multiple orgasms if stimulation is continued.

Both men and women may have problems with orgasm (see *Ejaculation, disorders of; Orgasm, lack of*).

Orgasm, lack of

The inability to achieve *orgasm* during sexual activity. Lack of orgasm, also sometimes called anorgasmia, is reported more commonly in women than in men. In either sex, failure to achieve orgasm may result from inhibition of sexual desire (see *Sexual desire, inhibited*), or from an inability to become aroused or to maintain arousal (see *Frigidity; Impotence*). In men, there may be a problem in achieving orgasm despite normal arousal (see *Ejaculation, disorders of*).

In women, lack of orgasm is the most common sexual problem. Between 30 and 50 per cent of women experience difficulty with orgasm at some time in their lives. Some 10 to 15 per cent are unable to achieve orgasm under any circumstances; others experience orgasm only occasionally or under special circumstances.

CAUSES
Lack of orgasm in women during *sexual intercourse* may result from problems with sexual technique, psychological factors, or pain during intercourse (see *Intercourse, painful*).

Problems with sexual technique may be due to inexperience on the part of either the man or the woman, poor sex education, or lack of familiarity with the body's sexual responses. Some women fail to reach orgasm because they do not receive, or do not allow, sufficient foreplay to become properly aroused. In general, women take longer than men to reach orgasm (about 13 minutes for a woman compared to less than three minutes for the average man). In some cases, a woman may experience difficulty in reaching orgasm because of premature ejaculation by her partner. Problems may also arise if a woman has a new partner who is unfamiliar with a woman's sexual responses. Some women are able to achieve orgasm through *masturbation* but not during sexual intercourse.

Psychological factors that may contribute to lack of orgasm in women include anxiety or early sexual trauma. Some women are unable to relax during sex because they are ashamed of their bodies, have sexual inhibitions or deep-seated guilt feelings about sexual pleasure, fear pregnancy, feel uncertain about intimacy, or fear "losing control" during orgasm. Anxiety about sexual performance and psychological pressures to achieve orgasm may have an inhibitory effect, which in time sets up a cycle of failure.

Problems in a long-term relationship may be due to underlying feelings of hostility, boredom, or distrust.

TREATMENT

Women may be helped to achieve orgasm, or to increase its frequency, with *sex therapy* or *marriage guidance*. *Psychotherapy* may help women in whom the problem is related to deep-seated feelings of guilt or insecurity.

Ornithosis

A disease of birds caused by the microorganism CHLAMYDIA PSITTACI. Ornithosis can be transmitted to humans, causing *psittacosis*, a feverish illness accompanied by pneumonia.

Orphan drugs

Drugs that have been developed to treat rare conditions but are not manufactured since the potential sales are small while the cost of performing the necessary safety tests is high. Reluctance to market an orphan drug may increase if the drug is out of patent (i.e. available for other companies to market) or cannot be patented because it is a known substance. In some countries, changes in the law have made it profitable to provide certain orphan drugs.

Orphenadrine

A *muscle-relaxant drug* used to relieve painful muscle spasm caused by injury to soft tissues (such as muscles and ligaments). Orphenadrine is also used to treat *Parkinson's disease*.

Possible adverse effects include dryness of the mouth and blurred vision.

ORT

Oral rehydration therapy is the first-line treatment for diarrhoea and, since its introduction 20 years ago, has transformed the outlook for sufferers of illnesses such as cholera.

A litre of water containing one teaspoonful of salt and eight teaspoonsful of sugar, taken orally, is easily absorbed, replacing lost salts and water. No other treatment is usually needed.

Ortho-

A prefix meaning normal, correct, or straight. It occurs, for example, in the term orthopaedics, which is derived

from the Greek for "straight child" because this branch of surgery was originally concerned with correction of skeletal deformities in children.

Orthodontic appliances

Devices, commonly known as braces, worn to correct *malocclusion* (an abnormal relationship between the upper and lower *teeth*). Braces are most com-

monly fitted during childhood and adolescence when the teeth and jaws are still developing.

WHY THEY ARE USED

Braces are commonly used to correct the position of overcrowded teeth (see *Overcrowding, dental*), which may splay outwards, tilt inwards, or be twisted sideways. Another common use is to correct the position of *buck*

HOW ORTHODONTIC APPLIANCES WORK

The tooth sockets are remarkably responsive to sustained pressure against the teeth. Orthodontic appliances, which may be fixed or removable, provide such pressure. Even gentle pressure applied in a particular direction will move teeth. As they move, bone is remodelled so that the new position is stable.

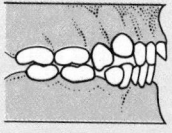

Overcrowding
This is frequently associated with malocclusion (poor alignment between upper and lower teeth). Some teeth have to be extracted to make room for others to be straightened.

FIXED APPLIANCES

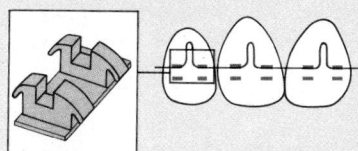

Appearance of brackets and wires
Brackets are fixed appliances cemented to the outer surface of the teeth; they have slots into which arch wires can be fitted.

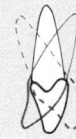

By careful design of the arrangement of wires and springs, force can be exerted in any direction to move a tooth into the desired position.

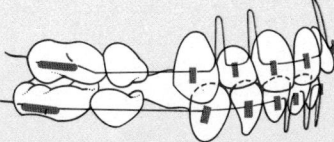

1 Teeth are removed to create space and an appliance made to correct the alignment of the remaining teeth and to close gaps between them.

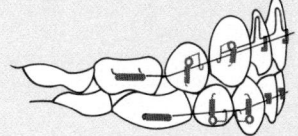

2 Once the teeth in the upper and lower jaws are aligned, the appliance is adjusted to tip or rotate the teeth to give a good appearance and bite.

REMOVABLE APPLIANCES

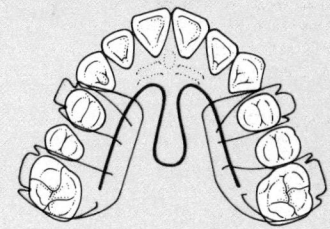

These are easier to keep clean than fixed appliances and are less obtrusive, but they may interfere with speech; their efficiency relies on patients using them as directed. This type exerts pressure to push the teeth at the sides outwards.

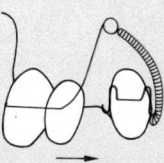

Bow device
This simple wire spring acts by exerting force to straighten the tooth. Many bow devices are more complicated.

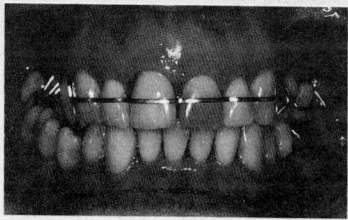

A removable bow
One of the many forms of orthodontic wire appliance, this bow device exerts pressure on the teeth at the sides, which straightens and moves them outwards.

teeth (projecting upper front teeth). Braces can also be used to reposition upper and lower premolars and molars (back teeth) when a faulty relationship between the upper and lower jaws prevents the teeth from meeting properly and interferes with chewing.

TYPES

FIXED APPLIANCES These braces, which cannot be removed by the wearer, exert a continuous pressure and can move teeth in any direction. They are usually fitted to all the upper and/or lower teeth and are used when many teeth need repositioning. The tooth-moving part of a fixed appliance is the arch wire, an adjustable, high-tensile steel wire, threaded through a bracket on each tooth.

To allow extra force to be applied to specific teeth, some brackets may be fitted with small hooks to which headgear (straps that fit around the back and over the top of the head) can be attached when the wearer is in bed.

Fixed appliances are kept in the mouth until the teeth have moved into the correct position, which may take a year or more. Thereafter, a fixed or removable retainer plate may need to be worn for anywhere from six months to five years to hold the teeth in their correct place until tooth and jaw growth stop in late adolescence.

Fixed appliances give more precise control over tooth movement than removable braces, but are more expensive and take longer to fit and adjust. Such appliances also trap dental *plaque* and make cleaning of the teeth more difficult.

Some people can be treated with lingual (also called "invisible") braces, which are fitted to the inner arch (tongue side) of the teeth, and pull rather than push the teeth into place.

REMOVABLE APPLIANCES These braces are used when only one or a few teeth need correcting. They consist of a plastic plate that covers the roof of the mouth (or, much less commonly, the floor of the mouth) with attachments that anchor over the back teeth. Force is applied by means of springs, wire bows, screws, or rubber bands fitted to the plate, sometimes combined with the use of headgear.

Occasionally, a special type of removable appliance is used in younger children before facial growth has stopped. Such braces consist of interconnected upper and lower plates that force the jaw into a position of slight tension against the pull of the surrounding muscles, translating this force to move the teeth.

Potential disadvantages of removable appliances are that their bulk may interfere with speech and that wearers may remove them so often that they become ineffective.

Orthodontics

A branch of *dentistry* concerned with the prevention and treatment of *malocclusion* (an abnormal relationship between the upper and lower *teeth*). In most cases, the orthodontist performs orthodontic procedures on children and adolescents while the teeth are still developing and are relatively manoeuvrable. However, adults may also be able to benefit from orthodontic treatment.

Diagnosis of the exact type of malocclusion involved may require making models of the teeth (see *Impression, dental*) to see clearly how they come together when clenched, taking *X-rays* of the head to relate the position of the teeth to that of the facial bones, and taking X-rays of the jaws to study their structure and relationship.

Orthodontic treatment consists of moving poorly positioned teeth by means of gentle pressure exerted by *orthodontic appliances* (dental braces). In some cases, the orthodontist may first need to extract certain teeth, often the premolars, to provide growing room for the teeth being moved.

Orthognathic surgery

An operation to correct deformity of the jaw and the severe *malocclusion* (an abnormal relationship between the upper and lower teeth) that is invariably associated with it.

HOW IT IS DONE

Orthognathic surgery, which usually requires a stay in hospital, is performed while the patient is under a general anaesthetic.

A jaw that projects too far can be shortened by removing a block of bone from each side and manoeuvring the front of the jaw backwards. A jaw that is too short can be remedied by dividing the bone on each side, sliding the front of the jaw forwards, and inserting bone grafts (taken from elsewhere in the body) into the gaps.

After repositioning, the jaw bones often require splinting (see *Splinting, dental*) until healing occurs.

Orthopaedics

The branch of surgery concerned with disorders of the *bones* and *joints* and their associated *muscles*, *tendons*, and *ligaments*. Orthopaedic surgeons perform many tasks, including setting broken bones and putting on casts; treating joint conditions such as dislocations, slipped discs, arthritis, and back problems; treating bone tumours and birth defects of the skeleton; and surgically repairing or replacing hip, knee, or finger joints.

Orthopnoea

Breathing difficulty brought on by lying flat. Orthopnoea is a symptom of *heart failure* (reduced pumping efficiency) and is caused by *pulmonary oedema* (accumulation of fluid in the lungs). Orthopnoea also occurs with *asthma* and chronic obstructive lung disease (chronic *bronchitis* with or without *emphysema*).

Orthoptics

A technique used to measure and evaluate *squint*, mainly in children. Orthoptics includes assessment of monocular and binocular vision, eye exercises, and measures to combat *amblyopia* (lazy eye).

Os

An anatomical term for a bone, as in os coxae, the hip bone. The term os is also used to refer to an opening in the body, usually the cervical os (entrance to the *uterus*).

Osgood-Schlatter disease

Painful enlargement of the tibial tuberosity, the bony prominence of the *tibia* (shin) just below the knee. Osgood-Schlatter disease occurs most commonly in children (usually boys) aged between 10 and 14. It can be caused by repeated exercise and is a consequence of excessive, repetitive pulling of the *quadriceps muscle* (at the front of the thigh) on the patellar tendon attached to the tibial tuberosity. There is usually pain above and below the knee, which is worse during strenuous activity, and the tibial tuberosity is tender when touched.

The disease usually clears up completely without treatment; if pain is severe, physiotherapy may be recommended, or the knee may be immobilized in a plaster *cast*.

Osmosis

The passage of a solvent (e.g. water) through a semipermeable membrane (one that acts like a sieve) from a less concentrated (weaker) solution to a more concentrated (stronger) one. Osmosis occurs whenever solutions of different strengths are separated by a semipermeable membrane and continues until the solutions are of equal

O

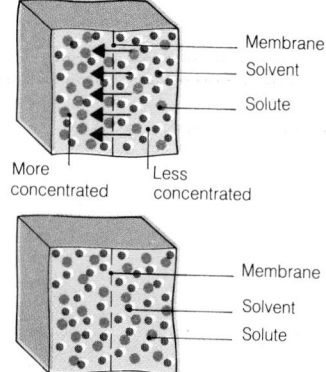

Osmosis

If two solutions, consisting of different concentrations of a solute (e.g. salt) in a solvent (e.g. water), are separated by a semipermeable membrane, solvent moves from the weaker to the stronger solution until the two solutions attain equal concentration.

strength unless the movement of solvent is opposed by applying pressure to the stronger solution. The pressure needed to stop all such movement is called osmotic pressure.

Semipermeable membranes are widespread in the body—they surround all cells. These membranes allow water, salts, simple sugars (such as glucose), and amino acids (but not proteins) to pass through. Consequently, osmosis plays an important part in regulating the distribution of water and other substances.

Ossicle

A small bone, particularly the malleus (hammer), incus (anvil), and stapes (stirrup)—the three tiny bones in the middle *ear* that conduct sound from the eardrum to the inner ear.

Ossification

The process by which *bone* is formed, renewed, and repaired. Ossification begins in the embryo and continues throughout life. There are three main types of ossification: bone growth, during which new bone is formed mainly from *cartilage* at the *epiphyses* (bone ends); bone renewal, which occurs as part of the normal regeneration process; and bone repair, which fuses broken bones after a *fracture*.

Osteitis

Inflammation of bone. The most common cause is infection (see *Osteomyelitis*). Other causes are *Paget's disease* and *hyperparathyroidism* (overactivity of the parathyroid glands).

Osteo-

A prefix that denotes a relationship to bone, as in *osteoporosis*, a condition in which the bones thin and weaken.

Osteoarthritis

A common *joint* disease aggravated by mechanical stress. Osteoarthritis is characterized by degeneration of the cartilage that lines joints or by formation of *osteophytes* (bony outgrowths), which lead to pain, stiffness, and occasionally loss of function of the affected joint.

INCIDENCE

Osteoarthritis occurs in almost all people aged over 60, although not all have symptoms. Various factors lead to the development of osteoarthritis earlier in life, including an injury to a joint or a *congenital* joint deformity. Severe osteoarthritis affects three times as many women as men.

SYMPTOMS

Osteoarthritis causes pain, swelling, creaking, and stiffness of one or more joints. The hips, knees, and spine are most commonly affected. Pain and stiffness may interfere with activities such as walking and dressing, and may disrupt sleep.

Weakness and shrinkage of surrounding muscles may occur if pain prevents the joint from being used regularly. Affected joints become enlarged and distorted by osteophytes, which are responsible for the characteristic gnarled appearance of hands affected by osteoarthritis.

DIAGNOSIS

A diagnosis is generally made from the patient's symptoms, and from a physical examination that reveals joint tenderness, swelling, and pain on movement. An *X-ray* can confirm loss of cartilage and formation of

O

OSTEOARTHRITIS

This differs from rheumatoid arthritis and has a better outlook. It results from excessive wear on joints, sometimes due to obesity or to slight deformity or misalignment of bones in a joint. Inflammation from a disease, such as gout, may also proceed to osteoarthritis. Weight-bearing joints, such as those in the neck, the lower back, and the knees and hips, are the areas most commonly affected by this type of arthritis.

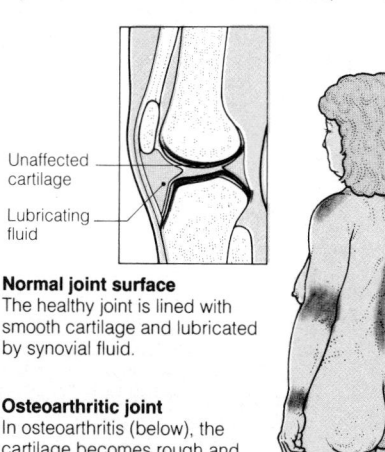

Normal joint surface
The healthy joint is lined with smooth cartilage and lubricated by synovial fluid.

Unaffected cartilage

Lubricating fluid

Osteoarthritic joint
In osteoarthritis (below), the cartilage becomes rough and flaky and small pieces break off to form loose bodies.

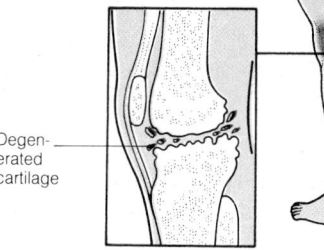

Degenerated cartilage

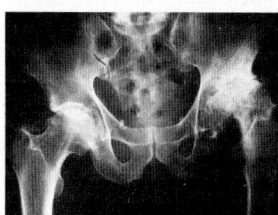

X-ray signs of osteoarthritis
This X-ray shows narrowing of the joint space with osteophyte production and an increase in density of the bone ends.

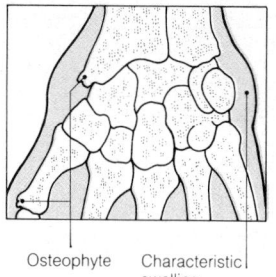

Osteophyte   Characteristic swelling

Osteophytes
These are outgrowths of new bone that tend to occur at the margins of the joint surfaces in osteoarthritis.

osteophytes and can also allow assessment of the extent of the degenerative process.

TREATMENT

There is no cure for osteoarthritis. Symptoms can be relieved by *analgesic drugs* (painkillers) and by *nonsteroidal anti-inflammatory drugs*. An injection of a *corticosteroid drug* can sometimes ease a painful joint. Many sufferers are overweight, and weight loss often gives substantial relief of symptoms. *Physiotherapy*, including exercises and heat treatment, can often relieve symptoms. If the condition is severe, various aids can make coping at home easier (see *Disability*).

Surgical treatment for severe osteoarthritis includes *arthroplasty* (joint-replacement surgery) and *arthrodesis* (immobilization of a joint).

Osteochondritis dissecans

Degeneration of a *bone* just under a joint surface, causing fragments of bone and cartilage to become separated from surrounding bone.

Osteochondritis dissecans commonly affects the knee and usually starts in adolescence. The exact cause is unknown but the disorder is thought to be caused by damage to a small blood vessel beneath the joint surface, which may be initiated by injury. The separated fragment sometimes reattaches but usually forms a *loose body* within the joint. Symptoms include aching discomfort and intermittent swelling of the affected joint. The presence of a loose body may cause locking of a joint.

X-rays show damage to the joint and reveal the presence of any loose bodies. If a fragment has not completely separated, the joint may be immobilized in a plaster *cast* to allow reattachment. Loose bodies of the knee are removed during *arthroscopy*.

The cavity left in the bone by a detached fragment disrupts the smoothness of the joint surface, increasing the likelihood of developing *osteoarthritis* in later life.

Osteochondritis juvenilis

Inflammation of an *epiphysis* (growing area of *bone*) in children and adolescents. The exact cause is unknown, but the condition is thought to be due to disruption of the blood supply to the bone.

There are several distinct types of osteochondritis juvenilis, each involving different bones in the body. *Perthes' disease* affects the epiphysis of the head of the femur (thigh bone).

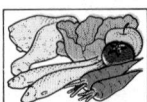
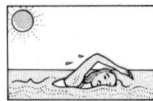
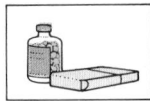

TREATMENT AND SELF-HELP MEASURES IN OSTEOARTHRITIS

The most important self-help measure for sufferers of osteoarthritis is to shed excess weight in order to reduce wear and tear on joints.

In addition, measures to increase muscle power help to stabilize the affected joint, and thereby reduce the symptoms.

Swimming
Regular exercise, to strengthen muscles and maintain joint mobility, can be valuable. Swimming in a heated pool increases muscle power without putting undue strain on joints.

Weight reduction
Eat sensibly, cut sweets and excess carbohydrates out of your diet, or ask your doctor for advice about a reducing diet. Once an ideal weight has been reached, it should be maintained.

Other treatment
Drugs such as aspirin or indomethacin are useful; sometimes corticosteroid injections are advised. There is little evidence that special diets or herbal treatments are effective.

Scheuermann's disease affects epiphyses of several adjoining vertebrae. Other types affect certain bones in the foot and wrist.

SYMPTOMS AND SIGNS

Osteochondritis juvenilis causes localized pain and tenderness and, if the epiphysis forms part of a joint, restricted movement. Inflammation leads to softening of the bone, which may result in deformity because of surrounding pressure. X-rays of the affected area show a patchy appearance and flattening of the bone.

TREATMENT AND OUTLOOK

Immobilization by use of an orthopaedic *brace* or plaster *cast* may be used to relieve pain and reduce the risk of deformity. In some cases of Perthes' disease, an operation is required to relieve the pressure on the diseased bone to prevent more deformity.

The bone usually regenerates within three years and rehardens. In many cases, however, deformity is permanent and increases the likelihood of the development of *osteoarthritis* in later life.

Osteochondroma

A benign *bone* tumour made up of a stalk of bone capped with cartilage. It grows from the side of a bone, usually at the end of a long bone in the region of the knee or shoulder. The osteochondroma develops in late childhood and early adolescence, and stops growing when the skeleton is fully developed.

The tumour, which appears as a hard round swelling near a joint, causes problems only if it interferes with the movement of tendons or the surrounding joint. In such cases, sur-

gical removal may be necessary. Large osteochondromas can interfere with skeletal growth, causing deformity.

Osteochondrosis

See *Osteochondritis juvenilis*.

Osteodystrophy

Any generalized *bone* defect caused by a *metabolic disorder* (an abnormality of the body chemistry). Examples include *rickets*, a childhood condition in which the bones fail to harden properly due to a deficiency of *vitamin D*; *osteomalacia*, the equivalent condition in adults; *osteoporosis* (a decrease in bone density) when it is caused not by aging but by the hormonal disorder *Cushing's syndrome* or by an excessive intake of *corticosteroid drugs*; and bone cysts and reduction of bone mass, which occasionally occur in chronic *kidney failure* or *hyperparathyroidism* (overactivity of the parathyroid glands) due to a disturbance in calcium metabolism in the body.

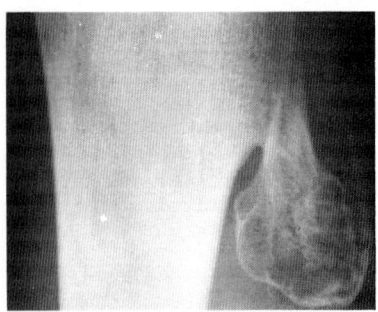

X-ray of osteochondroma
The X-ray shows a typical osteochondroma protruding from the bone. The tumour has a bony stalk and a cap made of cartilage.

An osteodystrophy is usually reversible in adults if the underlying cause can be treated effectively before bone deformity occurs.

Osteogenesis imperfecta

A *congenital* condition characterized by abnormal brittleness of *bones* caused by an inherited defect in the development of the *connective tissue* that forms the basic material of bone. The fragile bones are unusually susceptible to *fractures*.

SYMPTOMS AND SIGNS

Severely affected infants, born with multiple fractures and a soft skull, do not usually survive. Those who are less severely affected suffer from many fractures during infancy and childhood, often caused by only minimal force. A doctor examining such children may sometimes find it difficult to determine whether the cause is osteogenesis imperfecta or *child abuse*. Very mild cases may not be detected until adolescence or later.

A common accompanying sign of the disorder is abnormal thinness of the sclera (whites of the eyes), making them appear blue. In addition, sufferers of osteogenesis imperfecta may be deaf due to *otosclerosis*.

TREATMENT AND OUTLOOK

Fractures are generally treated in the usual way, by immobilization; otherwise, there is no specific treatment for the condition. The fractures usually heal quickly but may cause severe shortening and deformity of the limbs, resulting in stunted, abnormal growth. Skull fractures may cause brain damage or death.

Parents who have a child with osteogenesis imperfecta should seek *genetic counselling* in order to estimate the risk of recurrence in any future pregnancies. Severe osteogenesis imperfecta can be diagnosed prenatally by *ultrasound scanning*.

Osteogenic sarcoma

See *Osteosarcoma*.

Osteoid osteoma

A *bone* disorder in which an abnormal area of bone causes deep pain. An osteoid osteoma measures only about 0.5 cm in diameter, and most commonly affects a long bone of the arm or leg. The diagnosis can be made from an *X-ray*.

Pain, which is typically worse at night, can usually be relieved by *aspirin*. The condition is cured by removing the affected area of bone. (See also *Osteoma*.)

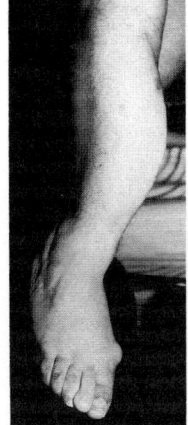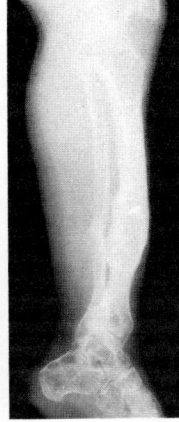

Osteogenesis imperfecta
Affected children may suffer recurrent fractures of the limbs that lead to deformity and shortening, and to abnormal growth. At right is an X-ray of the leg of a sufferer.

Osteoma

A benign tumour of *bone*. An osteoma is hard, usually small, and may occur on any bone. The tumour is usually harmless, but surgical removal may be necessary if an osteoma causes symptoms by pressing on surrounding structures.

Osteomalacia

Softening, weakening, and demineralization of the *bones* in adults due to *vitamin D* deficiency (in children, the condition is called *rickets*).

The development of healthy bone requires an adequate intake of calcium and phosphorus from the diet, but these minerals cannot be absorbed by the body without a sufficient amount of vitamin D. This vitamin is obtained from certain foods and from the action of sunlight on the skin; a deficiency results in softening and weakening of the bones, which then become vulnerable to distortion and *fractures*.

CAUSES

Osteomalacia is usually caused by any of the following, alone or in combination: an insufficient amount of vitamin D in the diet (due to a lack of butter, fortified margarine, fish, eggs, or fish-liver oils), insufficient exposure to sunlight, or inadequate absorption of vitamin D from the intestine (see *Malabsorption*), which may be caused by a disorder such as *coeliac disease* or by intestinal surgery. Rare causes include *kidney failure*, *acidosis* (increased acidity of body fluids), and certain inherited *metabolic disorders*.

Osteomalacia is rare in developed countries. Most commonly affected are people with an inadequate diet, the housebound elderly, and dark-skinned immigrants living in countries that have much less sunlight than their countries of origin.

SYMPTOMS AND SIGNS

Osteomalacia causes pain in the bones (particularly those in the neck, legs, hips, and ribs), muscle weakness, and, if the blood level of calcium is very low, *tetany* (muscle spasms) in the hands, feet, and throat. If the bones become greatly weakened, they may break after a minor injury.

DIAGNOSIS AND TREATMENT

Osteomalacia is diagnosed from the symptoms and signs, along with blood tests, urine tests, and bone *X-rays*. In some cases, a bone *biopsy* (removal of a small sample of bone for microscopic analysis) is performed.

Treatment consists of a diet that is rich in vitamin D and regular supplements of the vitamin. Supplements are usually taken as tablets; if tablets cannot be absorbed by the intestine, injections may be necessary. In some cases of osteomalacia due to malabsorption, calcium supplements may also be taken.

Osteomyelitis

Infection of *bone* and *bone marrow*, usually by bacteria. Osteomyelitis can affect any bone in the body, is more common in children, and most often affects the long bones of the arms and legs and the vertebrae. In adults, the disorder usually affects the pelvis and the vertebrae. In developed countries, adequate nutrition and a generally high resistance to infection have made osteomyelitis, which may be acute or chronic, much rarer than it once was.

ACUTE OSTEOMYELITIS

The infecting microorganism (usually the bacterium STAPHYLOCOCCUS AUREUS) is carried to the bone in the bloodstream, having entered the bloodstream via a skin wound or as a result of infection elsewhere in the body (usually in the nose or throat). The infected bone and bone marrow become inflamed and pus forms, causing fever, severe pain and tenderness in the infected bone, and inflammation and swelling of the skin over the affected area.

The diagnosis may be confirmed by blood *cultures*, bone scanning (see *bone imaging*), and bone X-rays. Treatment is with high doses of *antibiotic drugs* over several weeks or months. With prompt antibiotic treatment, acute

O

osteomyelitis usually clears up completely. If the condition fails to respond to antibiotic treatment, an operation is performed to expose the bone, to clean out the areas of infected and dead bone, and to drain the pus.

CHRONIC OSTEOMYELITIS

This form may develop when an attack of acute osteomyelitis is neglected or fails to respond to treatment. It may also occur after a compound *fracture* or, occasionally, as a result of the spread of *tuberculosis* from another part of the body.

Chronic osteomyelitis causes constant pain in the affected bone. Complications of the disease include persistent deformity and, in children, arrest of growth in the affected bone. In the later stages of the disease (which may have been recurring for many years), *amyloidosis* (harmful deposits of a starchy substance in vital organs) may develop.

Chronic osteomyelitis requires surgical removal of all affected bone, sometimes followed by a *bone graft* to replace the removed bone; antibiotic drugs are also prescribed. If the cause is tuberculosis, antituberculous drugs are prescribed for at least one year after surgery.

Osteopathy

A system of diagnosis and treatment that recognizes the role of the musculoskeletal system (bones, muscles, tendons, tissues, nerves, and spinal column) in the healthy functioning of the human body.

Osteopathy was founded in the US in 1874 by Andrew Taylor Still, MD. It is based on the concept that the human body is a unified organism, in which the musculoskeletal system plays a central role in the patient's well-being. Osteopaths emphasize that all body systems operate in unison, and that disturbances in one system can alter the functions of other systems in the body.

The osteopath uses various manual techniques, as well as traditional diagnostic and therapeutic procedures, to diagnose and treat dysfunction. Manual techniques include manipulation and the application of rhythmic stretching and pressure to restore movement to the joints.

To become a Member of the Register of Osteopaths (MRO) requires completion of a four-year course of study. Properly qualified osteopaths are included on the General Council and Register of Osteopaths (GCRO).

Osteopetrosis

A very rare inherited disorder in which *bones* harden and become more dense. The growth of healthy bone is a balance between the activity of two types of bone cells: bone-forming osteoblasts and bone-reabsorbing osteoclasts. In osteopetrosis, there is a deficiency of osteoclasts, which results in the disruption of normal bone structure.

The mildest form of osteopetrosis may not cause any symptoms. More severe forms can result in greater susceptibility to fractures, stunted growth, deformity, and *anaemia*. Pressure on nerves may cause blindness, deafness, and facial paralysis.

Bone marrow transplants have been attempted on an investigational basis. The transplant supplies the recipient with cells from which healthy osteoclasts might develop.

Osteophyte

A localized outgrowth of *bone* that forms at the boundary of a joint. Osteophytes are a characteristic feature of *osteoarthritis* and are, in part, responsible for the deformity and the restricted movement of affected joints.

Osteoporosis

Loss of protein matrix tissue from *bone*, causing it to become brittle and easily fractured.

Osteoporosis needs to be distinguished from *osteomalacia*, which is demineralization of bone due to vitamin D deficiency. The two conditions may be present at the same time, causing severe bone weakness.

Osteoporosis is a natural part of aging. By the age of 70, the density of the skeleton has diminished by about one third. However, for hormonal reasons, significant osteoporosis is much more common in women than in men. Also, for reasons that are unknown, the disorder is more common in white people than it is in black people.

CAUSES

Bone naturally becomes thinner as a person ages, but women are especially vulnerable to osteoporosis after the *menopause* because their ovaries no longer produce *oestrogen hormones*, which help maintain bone mass.

Other causes of osteoporosis include removal of the ovaries; a diet deficient in calcium, which is essential for bone health; certain hormonal disorders (such as *Cushing's syndrome*) or prolonged treatment with *corticoste-*

roid drugs; and prolonged immobility. Osteoporosis is more common in heavy smokers and drinkers and, for unknown reasons, is associated with chronic *bronchitis* and *emphysema*.

SYMPTOMS AND SIGNS

In many cases, osteoporosis produces no obvious symptoms; the first sign is often a fracture following a fall that would not result in a fracture in a young adult. Typical sites for such fractures are just above the wrist and the top of the femur (thigh bone). Another type of fracture that occurs in osteoporosis is a spontaneous fracture of one or several vertebrae, which causes the bones to crumble, leading to a progressive loss of height or to pain due to compression of a spinal nerve.

DIAGNOSIS

The condition is diagnosed from the symptoms, from bone *X-rays*, and from measurement of bone density by photon absorption (see *Densitometry*).

PREVENTION AND TREATMENT

Bone tissue that has already been lost cannot be easily replaced, but more bone loss can be minimized by preventive measures.

Hormone replacement therapy to compensate for reduced oestrogen production after the menopause has been shown to prevent osteoporosis in women, but the treatment would need to be continued for many years for long-lasting benefits to be obtained. Treatment with biphosphonate drugs will increase bone density, but its long-term effects are still being assessed. Regular, sustained exercise helps to build the bones and maintain their strength.

Both men and women should ensure that their *calcium* intake is adequate. The richest dietary sources of calcium are milk and milk products, green leafy vegetables, citrus fruits, sardines, and shellfish. Calcium tablets may be needed. It is best not to smoke, and to drink alcohol in moderation only.

Osteosarcoma

A malignant tumour of *bone* that spreads rapidly to the lungs and, less commonly, to other areas. Osteosarcoma occurs mainly in adolescents and the elderly. In young people, osteosarcoma develops for no known reason; in elderly people, it is a late, rare complication of *Paget's disease*.

SYMPTOMS

The most common site of the tumour in young people is in a long bone of the leg or arm, or around the knee,

OSTEOPOROSIS

In osteoporosis, the density of bones decreases, and their brittleness increases, although there is no change in size or composition. Women past the menopause are the most commonly affected because their ovaries no longer produce oestrogen, which helps to maintain bone mass. The risk of the condition is greater in a woman who undergoes the menopause early, or whose mother had osteoporosis.

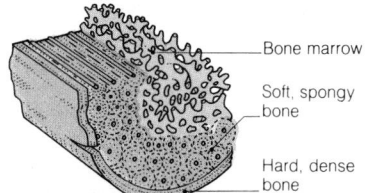

Normal bone cross-section
Bone consists of fibres of collagen (a protein), which give elasticity, and calcium, which gives hardness.

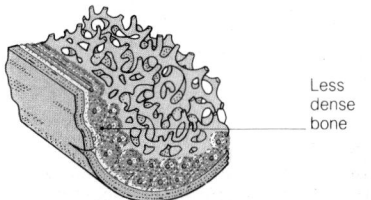

Osteoporotic bone
Thinning is mainly due to loss of collagen, which takes calcium with it. Both hard and spongy bone tissue are affected.

Bone loss with age
The graph on the right shows how the percentage of bone lost increases in both sexes from age 30 onwards, with the losses particularly marked in women after the menopause. By age 75, about half of all women have sustained at least one fracture due to osteoporosis, a much higher proportion than in men.

Spine affected by osteoporosis
The X-ray shows generalized thinning of the vertebrae, giving a characteristic "codfish" appearance to the spine.

hip, or shoulder. The first symptom is usually a painful visible swelling of the affected bone (if it is near the surface) or a deep-seated pain (if the affected bone cannot be felt through the skin).

As a complication of Paget's disease, an osteosarcoma may develop in several bones; its pain may be indistinguishable from that caused by the original disease.

DIAGNOSIS AND TREATMENT
Diagnosis is usually based on *X-rays* of the bone. Other *bone imaging* techniques (e.g. *MRI*) may also be used.

Osteosarcoma is sometimes treated by *radiotherapy*, but it is usually necessary to remove the affected bone surgically. In most cases, this means *amputation* of a limb; in some cases, a prosthesis (see *Limb, artificial*) can be fitted immediately after the amputation. Instead of amputation, it is sometimes possible to remove affected bone and replace it by a *bone graft* or by an artificial bone.

Treatment with *anticancer drugs* is usually given for several months after surgery to destroy any cancer cells that may have spread to other parts of the body. With this additional treatment, the outlook is good; about half of all patients whose disease is discovered early are cured.

Osteosclerosis

Increased *bone* density, usually detected on an *X-ray* as an area of extreme whiteness.

Localized osteosclerosis may be caused by a severe injury that compresses the bone; by *osteoarthritis*, in which bone around affected joints thickens; by chronic *osteomyelitis*, in which healthy bone next to the infected area thickens and becomes more dense; or by an *osteoma* (benign bone tumour), which consists of a hard, dense, usually harmless outgrowth of normal bone tissue.

Osteosclerosis occurs throughout the body in *osteopetrosis*, an inherited bone disorder.

Osteotomy

An operation in which a *bone* is cut to change its alignment or to shorten or lengthen it.

WHY IT IS DONE
Osteotomy is sometimes performed on a *hallux valgus* (a deformity of the big toe) that has caused a *bunion*. Another use is to straighten a long bone that has healed crookedly after a *fracture* or to shorten the uninjured leg after a fractured leg has shortened during healing (see *Leg, shortening of*). Osteotomy can also be used to correct the deformity caused by congenital dislocation of the hip (see *Hip, congenital dislocation of*) when this condition has not been detected and treated early enough to avoid surgery. Osteotomy is also sometimes used to correct *coxa vara* (a hip deformity).

HOW IT IS DONE
Under general anaesthesia, bones are straightened by cutting through them and repositioning the ends; sometimes a wedge of bone is inserted or removed to achieve the correct alignment. Bones can be lengthened by making an oblique cut and displacing the two parts slightly before rejoining them. Bones can be shortened by cut-

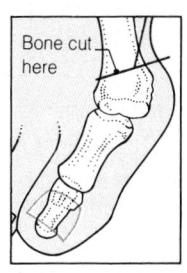
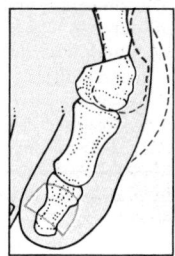

Example of an osteotomy
This procedure is performed to correct a hallux valgus (outward protrusion of the joint at the base of the toe), usually because it has caused a bunion. Part of the top of the first metatarsal bone is removed.

O

ting out a section of bone and rejoining the two parts. After the operation, corrected bones are held in position by a metal plate or nail or by a plaster *cast* or *splint*.

Ostomy

The term used to describe a surgical opening or junction of two hollow organs (e.g. *colostomy* and *ileostomy*).

Otalgia

The medical term for *earache*.

Otitis externa

An *ear* infection causing inflammation of the outer-ear canal, also known as swimmer's ear.

CAUSES

Generalized infection, affecting the whole canal and sometimes also the pinna (external ear), may be caused by fungi, which produce a persistent inflammation known as otomycosis, or by bacteria. Bacterial infection may also cause a localized infection in the form of a *boil*. Sometimes the ear becomes inflamed as part of a generalized skin disorder, such as atopic *eczema* or seborrhoeic *dermatitis*.

Malignant otitis externa is an uncommon and occasionally fatal form of the disorder caused by the bacterium *PSEUDOMONAS AERUGINOSA*. This form usually affects elderly diabetics, whose resistance to infection is reduced, and spreads rapidly into surrounding bones and soft tissue.

SYMPTOMS AND SIGNS

Otitis externa usually causes redness and swelling of the skin of the ear canal, a discharge from the ear, and sometimes an area of eczema around the opening of the ear. The ear may itch only in the early stages, but can become painful. Occasionally, pus blocks the ear, causing deafness.

DIAGNOSIS AND TREATMENT

The doctor examines the ear with an *otoscope* (a viewing instrument) and may take a sample of any pus for laboratory analysis.

Often the only treatment required is a thorough cleaning and drying of the ear by the doctor, sometimes using suction apparatus. In some cases, local application of preparations containing *antibiotic drugs, antifungal drugs*, or *corticosteroid drugs* is needed. Oral antibiotic drugs may be prescribed for the treatment of severe bacterial infections. A person with otitis externa should avoid getting the ear canal wet until the infection has cleared up.

Otitis media

Inflammation of the middle *ear* (the cavity between the eardrum and the inner ear).

CAUSES

The inflammation occurs as the result of a viral or bacterial upper respiratory tract infection extending up the eustachian tube, the passage that connects the back of the nose to the middle ear. The tube may become blocked by the inflammation or sometimes by enlarged *adenoids*, which are often associated with infections of the nose and throat. As a result, fluid produced by the inflammation—along with pus in bacterial infections—is not drained off through the tube but accumulates in the middle ear.

The chronic phase of otitis media (otitis media with effusion) follows an upper respiratory infection that has produced acute otitis media.

INCIDENCE

Children are particularly susceptible to otitis media, partly because of the shortness of their eustachian tubes. About one in six children suffers from the acute form in the first year of life and about one in 10 in each of the next six years. Some children have recur-

rent attacks. Chronic otitis media is much less common because, in most cases, attacks of acute middle-ear infection clear up with treatment.

SYMPTOMS AND SIGNS

Acute otitis media is marked by sudden, severe earache, a feeling of fullness in the ear, deafness, tinnitus (ringing or buzzing in the ear), and fever. Sometimes the eardrum bursts, relieving the pain and resulting in a discharge of pus. In this case, healing usually occurs in a few days.

In chronic otitis media, pus constantly exudes from a perforation in the eardrum and there is some degree of deafness. Complications of the condition include *otitis externa* (inflammation of the outer ear); damage to the bones in the middle ear, causing more deafness (sometimes total) in the affected ear; or a *cholesteatoma* (a matted ball of sometimes infected skin debris). In rare cases, infection spreads inwards from an infected ear, causing *mastoiditis* or a *brain abscess*.

Inadequately treated otitis media may sometimes lead to a continual production of sticky fluid in the middle ear, a condition that is known as *glue ear*.

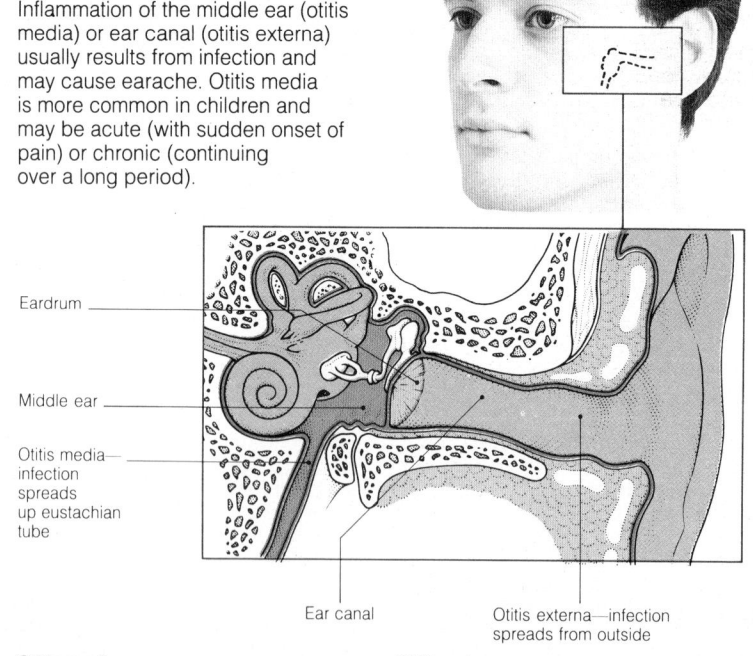

EAR INFECTIONS

Inflammation of the middle ear (otitis media) or ear canal (otitis externa) usually results from infection and may cause earache. Otitis media is more common in children and may be acute (with sudden onset of pain) or chronic (continuing over a long period).

Eardrum

Middle ear

Otitis media—infection spreads up eustachian tube

Ear canal

Otitis externa—infection spreads from outside

Otitis media
This usually occurs through spread of infection from the back of the nose to the middle ear via the eustachian tube.

Otitis externa
The ear canal is susceptible to infection if it is moist (after swimming) or damaged by attempts to remove earwax.

DIAGNOSIS

The diagnosis is usually made from examining the ears with an *otoscope* (a viewing instrument). A swab may be taken of any discharge so that the organism responsible for the infection can be cultured and identified.

TREATMENT

Acute otitis media usually responds to treatment with *antibiotic drugs* and *analgesic drugs* (painkillers).

Chronic otitis media may be treated by *myringotomy* (surgical creation of an opening in the eardrum) and by sucking out pus and infected debris from the ear as necessary. Antibiotic ear-drops may also be needed. A cholesteatoma should always be removed surgically.

Oto-

A prefix that denotes a relationship to the ear, as for example, in *otorrhoea* (a discharge from the ear) and *otosclerosis* (hardening of the ear).

Otoplasty

Cosmetic or reconstructive surgery on the outer *ear*. Otoplasty is usually performed to flatten protruding ears. It may also be done to construct or repair a missing or badly damaged ear.

PROTRUDING EARS

Otoplasty may be performed under general or local anaesthesia. A strip of skin is removed from behind the ear. The underlying cartilage is then remodelled and the two edges of the wound are stitched together, pulling the ear closer to the head. After the operation, a dressing is kept on the ear until the wound has healed, usually 10 to 14 days later, when the stitches are removed. The scar is hidden in the crease between the ear and scalp.

LACK OF AN OUTER EAR

Some children are born with part or all of the outer ear missing, and may also lack an external ear passage; in some cases there is also underdevelopment of the same side of the face.

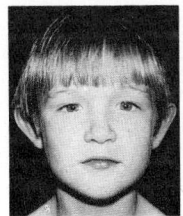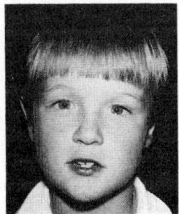

Otoplasty for protruding ears
A strip of skin is removed from behind each ear. The underlying cartilage is remodelled and the edges of the wound are stitched together.

Treatment involves transferring a piece of rib cartilage, which is sculpted to resemble the normal ear, to a pocket of skin where the ear is to be placed. The procedure usually involves three operations. Hearing in the reconstructed ear may be abnormal but if the child has a normal range of hearing in the other ear, no attempt need be made to improve hearing in the reconstructed ear.

Otorhinolaryngology

The surgical specialty concerned with diseases of the *ear*, *nose*, and *throat*. It is commonly known as ENT surgery.

ENT specialists commonly treat *sinus* problems, *otitis media* (middle-ear infection), *glue ear*, *tonsillitis*, and minor hearing loss. Other disorders treated include *otosclerosis*, *Ménière's disease*, airway problems in children, uncontrollable nosebleeds, and cancer of the larynx and sinuses.

Otorrhoea

The medical name for a discharge from the ear (see *Ear, discharge from*).

Otosclerosis

A disorder of the middle *ear* that causes progressive *deafness*. Otosclerosis often runs in families.

CAUSES AND INCIDENCE

Otosclerosis occurs when, for unknown reasons, an overgrowth of bone immobilizes the stapes (the innermost bone of the middle ear). This prevents sound vibrations from being passed to the inner ear, resulting in conductive deafness. In most cases of otosclerosis, both ears are ultimately affected.

About one person in 200 is affected by the disease, which usually starts in early adulthood. It is more common in women than in men and often develops during pregnancy.

SYMPTOMS AND SIGNS

Sound is heard as muffled but is more distinguishable when there is background noise. Affected people tend to talk quietly. Hearing loss progresses slowly over a period of 10 to 15 years and is often accompanied by *tinnitus* (noises in the ear) and rarely by *vertigo* (a spinning sensation). Some sensorineural deafness (caused by damage spreading to the inner ear) may eventually occur, making high tones difficult to hear and causing the sufferer to speak loudly.

DIAGNOSIS AND TREATMENT

The diagnosis is based on abnormal results of *hearing tests*. A *hearing-aid* can markedly improve hearing, but

the condition can be cured only by *stapedectomy* (an operation in which the stapes is replaced by an artificial substitute).

Otoscope

An instrument for examining the *ear*. An otoscope includes magnifying lenses, a light, and a speculum (a funnel-shaped tip that is inserted into the ear canal). The instrument allows easy inspection of the outer-ear canal and the eardrum. With an otoscope it is also possible to detect certain diseases of the middle ear through the semi-transparent eardrum.

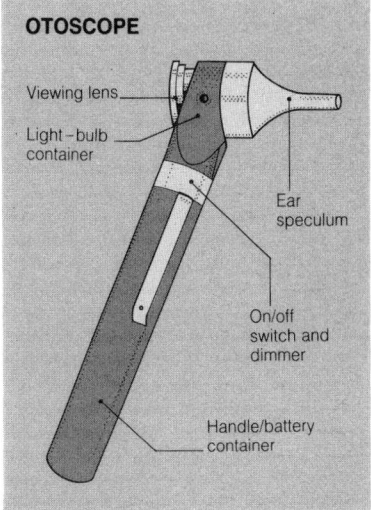

OTOSCOPE

Viewing lens

Light–bulb container

Ear speculum

On/off switch and dimmer

Handle/battery container

Ototoxicity

Toxic damage to the inner *ear*. High doses of certain drugs (especially aminoglycoside *antibiotic drugs*) can damage the cochlea and the semicircular canals in the inner ear, impairing hearing and balance.

Outpatient treatment

Medical care given to a person on a day basis in a hospital or clinic.

Ovarian cyst

An abnormal, fluid-filled swelling in an *ovary*. Ovarian cysts are common and, in about 95 per cent of cases, benign (noncancerous). Many ovarian cysts disappear without treatment.

TYPES

The most common type of ovarian cyst is a follicular cyst, in which the egg-producing follicle of the ovary enlarges and fills with fluid. Cysts may also occur in the corpus luteum, a yellow mass of tissue that forms from the follicle after *ovulation*.

Other types of ovarian cysts include *dermoid cysts* and malignant cysts (see *Ovary, cancer of*).

SYMPTOMS AND SIGNS
Ovarian cysts often cause no symptoms, but some cause abdominal discomfort, pain during intercourse, or menstrual irregularities including *amenorrhoea* (lack of menstruation), *menorrhagia* (heavy periods), or *dysmenorrhoea* (painful periods). Severe abdominal pain, nausea, and fever, which necessitate surgery, may develop if twisting or rupture of an ovarian cyst occurs.

DIAGNOSIS AND TREATMENT
A cyst may be discovered during a routine *pelvic examination*. *Ultrasound scanning* or a *laparoscopy* (an examination of the abdominal cavity through a viewing instrument) may be necessary to confirm the diagnosis as well as to determine the size and position of the cyst.

Simple cysts (which are thin-walled and filled with fluid) often go away on their own. Complex cysts (such as dermoid cysts) do not, and commonly require surgical removal. In many cases, it is only the cyst that needs to be removed, but if a cyst is large it is sometimes necessary for the surgeon to remove the entire ovary (see *Oophorectomy*).

Ovary
One of a pair of almond-shaped glands situated on either side of the *uterus* immediately below the opening of the *fallopian tube*. Each ovary is about 3 cm long and 2 cm wide and contains numerous cavities called follicles in which egg cells (see *Ovum*) develop. In addition to producing ova, the ovaries also produce the female sex hormones *oestrogen* and *progesterone*.

DISORDERS
Absence or failure of normal development of the ovaries is a rare disorder, and one that is usually caused by a chromosomal abnormality (see *Turner's syndrome*).

Oophoritis (inflammation of the ovary) may be caused by the *mumps* virus or by other infections; for example *gonorrhoea* or *pelvic inflammatory disease*.

Ovarian cysts may develop at any age; about 95 per cent of them are benign. Polycystic ovary syndrome (see *Ovary, polycystic*), in which multiple ovarian cysts form, is a disorder thought to be due to the body's inappropriate hormonal stimulation of the ovaries. The cysts may produce small

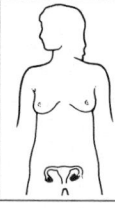

ANATOMY OF THE OVARY
Each ovary consists of glandular cells and egg-producing follicles. After ovulation, each follicle forms a corpus luteum.

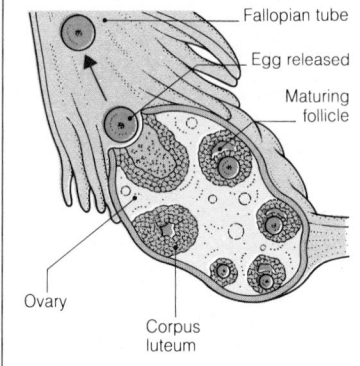

Fallopian tube

Egg released

Maturing follicle

Ovary

Corpus luteum

amounts of male sex hormones, leading to *amenorrhoea* (absence of menstruation), *infertility*, and *hirsutism*.

Cancer of the ovary (see *Ovary, cancer of*) occurs mainly in women over 50 and usually causes few symptoms (if any) in the early stages, although it can cause symptoms similar to those of an ovarian cyst.

Ovarian failure, in which the ovaries cease to function, causes premature *menopause* in about five per cent of all women.

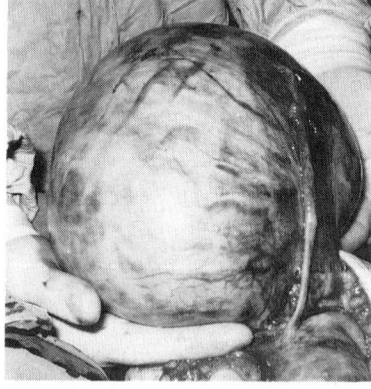

Removal of an ovarian cyst
This photograph shows a surgeon removing a very large ovarian cyst. Most ovarian cysts are much smaller than this.

Ovary, cancer of
A malignant growth of the *ovary*. Cancer of the ovary can occur at any age but is most common after the age of

50. There are about 5,000 cases of this cancer diagnosed in the UK each year. It is three times more common in women who have never had children and less common in women who have taken *oral contraceptives*. The most important risk factor is a family history; the gene responsible is thought to be on *chromosome 17*. Women with relatives who have had the disease should obtain expert advice from a geneticist and may be advised to undergo frequent screening.

The growth may be primary (arising in the ovary) or may be a secondary growth that has spread from another part of the body, often the breast.

SYMPTOMS AND SIGNS
In most cases, ovarian cancer causes no symptoms until it is widespread. The first symptom is usually vague abdominal discomfort and swelling. There may be digestive disturbances, such as nausea and vomiting, abnormal vaginal bleeding, and ascites (excess fluid in the abdominal cavity). A physical examination may reveal a swelling in the pelvis.

DIAGNOSIS AND TREATMENT
Screening for ovarian cancer using *ultrasound scanning* is currently being evaluated in research studies. If the condition is suspected, a *laparoscopy* will usually be performed to confirm the diagnosis and assess how far the tumour has spread.

Treatment is by surgical removal of the growth or as much of the malignant tissue as possible. This usually involves *salpingo-oophorectomy* (removal of the ovaries and fallopian tubes) and *hysterectomy* (removal of the uterus). Surgery is usually followed by *radiotherapy* and *anticancer drugs*.

OUTLOOK
If the growth is confined to the ovaries, 60 to 70 per cent of patients survive for at least five years; if the growth is more widespread, only about 10 to 20 per cent survive for five years. New drug combinations may improve this survival rate, however.

Ovary, polycystic
A condition, also called Stein-Leventhal syndrome, characterized by oligomenorrhoea (scanty menstruation) or *amenorrhoea* (absence of menstruation), *infertility*, *hirsutism* (excessive hairiness), and *obesity*. Often, there are multiple *ovarian cysts*. The condition may sometimes occur in the absence of hirsutism or obesity.

In most women with polycystic ovaries, menarche (the onset of menstruation) occurs at the normal age.

After a year or two of regular menstruation, the periods become highly irregular, and then cease. Hirsutism, which often becomes evident around menarche, occurs in about 50 per cent of cases, as does obesity.

CAUSE
The condition is due to an imbalance between luteinizing hormone (LH) and follicle-stimulating hormone (FSH), which are two *gonadotrophin hormones* produced by the *pituitary gland*; there is excessive stimulation of the ovaries by LH and a relative deficiency of FSH. This results in lack of *ovulation* and in increased production of *testosterone* by the ovaries.

DIAGNOSIS
Tests to determine the level of hormones in the blood are needed to confirm the diagnosis. *Ultrasound scanning* of the ovaries and/or *laparoscopy* (examination of the abdominal cavity with a viewing instrument) may be helpful.

TREATMENT
The condition may be treated with *clomiphene* (an anti-oestrogen drug), *progestogen drugs*, *LH-RH* (luteinizing hormone-releasing hormone), or *oral contraceptives*. In rare cases, surgical removal of a wedge of ovarian tissue is performed. The method of treatment used depends on the severity of the symptoms and on whether the woman wishes to become pregnant.

Women with polycystic ovaries often have a high level of oestrogen in the body, which increases the risk of endometrial cancer (see *Uterus, cancer of*). Treatment with progesterone may be recommended to restore hormonal balance and decrease the risk of this cancer.

Overbite
Overlapping of the lower front *teeth* by the upper front teeth. A slight degree of overbite is normal because the upper jaw is larger than the lower one. In *malocclusion*, overbite may be greater than normal or may be reversed (with the lower teeth projecting in front of the upper ones).

Overbreathing
A common name for *hyperventilation*.

Overcrowding, dental
Excessive crowding of the *teeth* so that they are unable to assume their normal positions in the jaw.

CAUSES
Dental overcrowding is commonly inherited, and may occur either because the teeth are relatively too

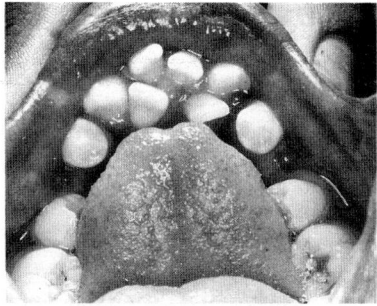

Severe case of overcrowding
The front teeth are crowded together because the two molars, just behind them, have grown too far forward.

large for the jaw or because the jaw is too small to accommodate the teeth.

Overcrowding may also be caused, or be aggravated by, premature loss of primary molar (back) teeth. Premature loss of these teeth can cause the permanent teeth growing beneath them to move out of position and leave insufficient space for the developing permanent teeth further forwards in the mouth.

PROBLEMS
Overcrowding of the teeth may lead to *malocclusion* (an incorrect relationship between the upper and lower teeth). Overcrowding may also prevent certain teeth from erupting through the gum (see *Impaction, dental*). The risk of dental decay (see *Caries, dental*) is increased when the teeth are overcrowded because cleaning of the teeth is more difficult than normal. Difficulty in cleaning the teeth, together with greater stress on tissues supporting the teeth, also increases the risk of *periodontal disease*.

TREATMENT
A dentist or orthodontist decides whether one or more teeth should be extracted to allow room for others to grow. In many cases, the remaining teeth must be fitted with an *orthodontic appliance* to move them into their correct positions.

Overuse injury
A term for any injury that has been caused by repetitive movement of part of the body. An alternative term is *repetitive strain injury*.

A common example of an overuse injury is *epicondylitis*, painful inflammation of one of the epicondyles (bony prominences) at the elbow, caused by the pull of the attached forearm muscles during gardening, painting, or playing certain sports (see *Golfers' elbow; Tennis elbow*).

Overuse injuries of the finger and wrist joints may affect assembly-line workers and typists. Musicians are also prone to a variety of problems; the thumb may be affected in players of woodwind instruments and the neck may be affected in violinists.

Symptoms, which usually disappear with rest, include pain and stiffness in the affected joints and muscles. A recurrence of the injury can sometimes be avoided by a change in the technique used during the causative activity.

Overweight
See *Obesity*.

Ovulation
The development and release of an *ovum* (egg) from a follicle within the *ovary*. Ovulation occurs midway through the menstrual cycle and is regulated by hormones. During the first half of the cycle, follicle-stimulating hormone (FSH) causes several ova to mature in the ovary. At mid-cycle, luteinizing hormone (LH) causes one ripe ovum to be released. The follicle then forms a small mass of yellow tissue called the corpus luteum, which secretes the hormone *progesterone* during the second half of the cycle.

After its release, the ovum travels along the *fallopian tube* and, if *fertilization* does not occur, is shed during *menstruation*. Regular menstruation usually means that ovulation is occurring, except around *puberty* and when nearing the *menopause*.

Some forms of contraception (see *Contraception, natural methods of*) are based on predicting when ovulation occurs each month and avoiding sexual intercourse at this time. Signs of ovulation include a rise in body temperature and changes in the amount and consistency of cervical mucus; there may also be mild abdominal pain (see *Mittelschmerz*).

If a woman does not ovulate, she cannot conceive. Investigation of female *infertility* includes tests to determine whether ovulation occurs.

Ovum
 The egg cell (female cell of reproduction). Each ovum measures about 0.1 mm in diameter. There are about one million immature ova present in each *ovary* at birth; only about 200 per ovary ever mature to be released at *ovulation* during a woman's fertile years. If *fertilization* occurs, the ovum develops into an *embryo*.

O

Oxazepam

A *benzodiazepine drug* used as a short-term treatment for *anxiety*. Like other benzodiazepines, oxazepam may cause dependence if taken regularly for more than two weeks (see *Drug dependence*).

Oxprenolol

A *beta-blocker drug* used in the treatment of *angina pectoris* (chest pain due to inadequate blood supply to the heart muscle), *hypertension* (high blood pressure) and cardiac *arrhythmias* (irregularity of the heartbeat). Oxprenolol may also be prescribed to relieve palpitations and tremor caused by *anxiety* and to control symptoms of *hyperthyroidism* (overactivity of the thyroid gland).

Possible adverse effects are typical of drugs in the beta-blocker group.

Oxygen

A colourless, odourless gas that makes up 21 per cent of the Earth's atmosphere. Oxygen is essential for almost all forms of life, including humans, because it is necessary for the metabolic "burning" of foods to produce energy—a process known as *aerobic* metabolism.

To reach the body cells, where aerobic metabolism takes place, oxygen in the air is absorbed through the lungs and into the blood, where it binds to the *haemoglobin* in red blood cells. In this form, the oxygen is distributed throughout the body, being released from the haemoglobin and taken up by cells in areas where the oxygen level is low.

Oxygen is used therapeutically to treat conditions such as severe *bronchitis* or *hypoxia* (inadequate oxygen in the body tissues). In some cases, high pressure oxygen (see *Hyperbaric oxygen treatment*) is used to treat the bends (*decompression sickness*) or poisoning from *carbon monoxide*. (See also *Ozone*.)

Oxygen tent

A plastic sheet that is placed over a hospital bed to enable a patient to receive *oxygen therapy*. Small oxygen tents, sometimes called croupettes, are occasionally used for infants and toddlers who require humidified (moistened) oxygen but who will not tolerate wearing a face mask. Oxygen is passed into the tent after being humidified by bubbling it through water. Children may find oxygen tents uncomfortably cold or may be frightened by being in an enclosed space.

Oxygen is sometimes administered to infants via a perspex box placed over the head.

Oxygen therapy

Supplying a person with oxygen-enriched air to relieve severe *hypoxia* (inadequate oxygen in body tissues).

In hospitals, oxygen is usually piped to a terminal at the patient's bedside and is administered as necessary through a face-mask or through nasal cannulas (tubes inserted into the nostrils). The concentration of oxygen is varied according to the patient's needs.

People at home can be supplied with oxygen in cylinders for use during acute attacks of hypoxia, as occur in severe *asthma* for example. People with persistent hypoxia due to severe chronic *bronchitis* or *emphysema* may benefit from long-term oxygen therapy. These patients may be supplied with a machine called an oxygen concentrator, which separates oxygen from the air and remixes it in a higher-than-normal concentration. Oxygen-rich air is then piped to different rooms for prolonged inhalation.

People receiving oxygen therapy should not smoke, since smoking not only presents a fire risk but also reduces the oxygen-carrying capacity of the blood and aggravates the underlying condition for which the oxygen is being given. (See also *Hyperbaric oxygen treatment*.)

Oxymetazoline

A *decongestant drug* which is used in the treatment of allergic *rhinitis* (hay fever), *sinusitis*, and the common *cold*. Oxymetazoline has a longer-lasting effect than many other decongestant drugs.

Oxymetazoline may irritate the nose. Prolonged use causes rebound congestion (increased congestion after the drug is withdrawn).

Oxytetracycline

A tetracycline *antibiotic drug*. Oxytetracycline is used to treat *chlamydial infections*, such as *nonspecific urethritis*, *psittacosis*, and *trachoma*. It is prescribed for a variety of other infections, including *bronchitis*, pneumonia caused by *mycoplasma*, *syphilis*, and *cholera*. Oxytetracycline may also be used to treat severe *acne*.

POSSIBLE ADVERSE EFFECTS
Nausea, vomiting, diarrhoea, skin rash, or increased sensitivity of the skin to sunlight are possible adverse effects. Oxytetracycline may discolour developing teeth and is therefore not prescribed for children under 12 or for pregnant women.

Oxytocin

A *hormone* produced by the *pituitary gland*. Oxytocin causes uterine *contractions* during labour and stimulates the flow of milk in women who are *breast-feeding*.

USE AS A DRUG
Synthetic oxytocin can be used to induce childbirth (see *Induction of labour*). It is sometimes used to help expel the placenta (afterbirth) after delivery or to empty the uterus after an incomplete *miscarriage* or a fetal death. Oxytocin is sometimes given as a nasal spray to stimulate milk flow.

POSSIBLE ADVERSE EFFECTS
Contractions may be stronger and more painful than usual, increasing the need for stronger *analgesic drugs* (painkillers). Rare adverse effects, particularly with excessive or prolonged use, include nausea, vomiting, palpitations, seizures, and coma.

Oxyuriasis

An alternative name for enterobiasis or *threadworm infestation*, which is the most common worm infestation in the UK.

Ozena

A severe and rare form of *rhinitis* (inflammation of the mucous membrane in the nose) in which the membrane atrophies (wastes away) and a thick nasal discharge dries to form crusts. Ozena often causes severe *halitosis* (bad breath).

Ozone

A rare form of oxygen, ozone is a poisonous, faintly blue gas that is produced by the action of electrical discharges (such as lightning) on oxygen molecules.

Ozone occurs naturally in the upper atmosphere (about 15 to 30 kilometres above the Earth's surface), where it screens the Earth from most of the sun's harmful ultraviolet radiation. Evidence suggests that the ozone layer is being depleted by various environmental chemicals, notably the chlorofluorocarbons (CFCs) in aerosols. The result of this depletion is that stronger and more potent forms of ultraviolet radiation are now reaching the Earth's surface. Increased ultraviolet levels could lead to an increase in the incidence of skin cancer and cataracts.

O

P

Pacemaker

A device that supplies electrical impulses to the *heart* to maintain the *heartbeat* at a regular rate. A pacemaker consists of a small electronic device and power source connected to the heart via an electrical wire.

In a healthy heart, the heartbeat is maintained by a nucleus of specialized heart tissue called the sinoatrial node, which sends out regular electrical impulses that pass through the heart muscle and trigger heart contractions. An artificial pacemaker is implanted when a person's sinoatrial node is not functioning properly, or when there is some impairment to the passage of the normal electrical impulses (see *Heart block; Sick sinus syndrome*).

The two basic types of pacemaker—fixed rate and demand—are described in the illustrated box. More advanced types can increase the heart-rate during exercise. Devices that can convert an abnormal rhythm back to normal are now also available.

IMPLANTATION

Implantation is carried out under a local anaesthetic. Patients can expect complete healing without complications and should return to normal work and activity as soon as possible. Vigorous exercise should be avoided for two weeks after the operation.

Modern microelectronic circuits require little power, and the lithium batteries used in pacemakers have a long life. Unless the demand on the battery is excessive, a pacemaker will usually operate quite satisfactorily for several years. Battery replacement requires only a minor operation.

PRECAUTIONS

Modern pacemakers are relatively insensitive to interference but may be affected by powerful electromagnetic pulses. Anyone fitted with a pacemaker should avoid powerful radio or radar transmitters and should not pass through security screens at air-

ports. Precautions may also be required if *diathermy* machines are to be used during physiotherapy or surgery. *TENS* is an unsuitable method of pain relief for people with a pacemaker.

Paediatrics

The branch of medicine concerned with the growth and development of children, and with the diagnosis, treatment, and prevention of childhood diseases.

Paediatrics as a specialty is subdivided into neonatology (the care of newborn infants), community paediatrics (preventive medicine and developmental paediatrics), the care of disabled and handicapped children, and other subspecialities, such as paediatric cardiology, neurology, or gastroenterology. The specialty of paediatric surgery is concerned with the diagnosis and treatment of small children with congenital and acquired disorders that may require surgery.

Paedophilia

A sexual perversion in which illegal sexual activity with a prepubertal child is the preferred recurrent means

---

PACEMAKERS

A pacemaker may be external (worn on a belt) or internal (implanted in the chest), like those shown below.

External pacing is used only as a temporary measure. There are two main methods of implantation.

Transvenous implantation

An insulated wire is inserted into a major vein in the neck and guided down into the heart until the electrode at its far end is positioned within the part of the heart muscle to be stimulated. The free end is connected to the pacemaker, which is fitted into a pocket created under the skin of the abdomen or below the collarbone.

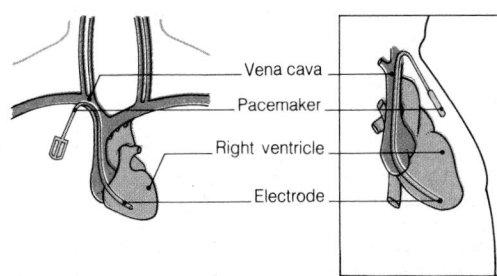

Vena cava

Pacemaker

Right ventricle

Electrode

Side view
The pacemaker is usually well hidden by overlying tissue

Epicardial implantation

The electrode is attached to the outer surface of the part of the heart muscle to be stimulated and the pacemaker is fitted into a pocket constructed underneath the skin of the abdomen.

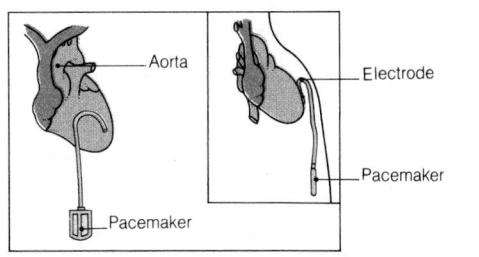

Aorta

Electrode

Pacemaker

Pacemaker

TYPES OF PACEMAKERS

Two main types are shown. In some cases, an external programmer can adjust the rate.

FIXED RATE

Impulse

No response to heartbeat

Fixed-rate pacemaker
This type discharges impulses at a steady rate, irrespective of the heart's activity.

DEMAND

Impulse when beat is missed

Pacemaker suppressed by heartbeat

Demand pacemaker
This type discharges impulses only when the heart-rate slows or a beat is missed. A normal heart-rate and beat suppresses the pacemaker.

of reaching orgasm. Paedophiles are almost exclusively male and may be heterosexual, bisexual, or homosexual. They are rarely diagnosed as suffering from psychosis, but often show personality problems and little concern for the effect of their behaviour on the child.

Paedophiles commonly fantasize about sex with a child. Fondling of children is more common than intercourse. Actual research is rudimentary. However, the incidence of child prostitution and of child sexual abuse within families seems much higher than was previously thought. Nearly 10 per cent of women in some studies have reported some form of sexual interference in childhood or early adolescence. (See also *Child Abuse; Incest*.)

Paget's disease

A common disorder of middle-aged and elderly people in which the normal process of *bone* formation is disrupted, causing the affected bones to weaken, thicken, and become deformed. Also known as osteitis deformans, Paget's disease usually involves only limited areas of the skeleton. The bones usually affected are the pelvis, skull, clavicle (collarbone), vertebrae, and long bones of the leg.

CAUSE AND INCIDENCE

The normal maintenance of healthy bones by the body involves a balance between the actions of cells that break down bone tissue and those that rebuild it. In Paget's disease, this balance is disturbed. The disease varies in frequency from one part of the country to another, suggesting an infective cause, which is thought to be viral. Overall, Paget's disease affects about three per cent of the population over the age of 40, the incidence increasing with age. The disorder has a tendency to run in families and affects more men than women.

SYMPTOMS AND SIGNS

Paget's disease often causes no symptoms and is usually discovered from an *X-ray* taken for some other reason. The most common symptoms are bone pain and deformity, especially bowing of the legs. Affected bones are prone to fracture.

Changes in the skull may lead to leontiasis (distortion of the facial bones that produces a rather lion-like appearance) and to inner-ear damage, sometimes resulting in deafness, tinnitus (ringing in the ear), vertigo, or headaches. Enlarged vertebrae may press on the spinal cord, causing pain and sometimes paralysis of the legs. If the pelvis is affected, severe arthritis of the hips can result. Occasionally, *bone cancer* may develop, and, in rare cases, when many bones are involved, increased blood flow through the affected bones may cause *heart failure*.

DIAGNOSIS

X-rays reveal areas of porous, thickened bone. *Blood tests* that show an elevated level of the *enzyme* alkaline phosphatase (which is associated with bone cell formation) give an indication of the extent and activity of the disease.

TREATMENT AND OUTLOOK

Most people with the disorder do not require treatment, and many others simply need to take *analgesic drugs* (painkillers). In severe cases, the hormone *calcitonin* may be prescribed. It relieves pain, reduces alkaline phosphatase levels, and promotes normal bone formation. Biphosphonate drugs slow the metabolic activity within the bone, reducing both the rates of formation and reabsorption. Surgery may be required to correct deformities or to treat arthritis.

Paget's disease of the nipple

A rare type of *breast cancer* in which the tumour starts in the milk ducts of the nipple. Paget's disease of the nipple looks similar to *eczema* and causes itching and a burning sensation. A sore that will not heal may develop on the nipple. In most cases, only one nipple is affected. Without treatment, the tumour may gradually spread further into the breast.

Anyone who develops eczema of the nipple should consult a doctor, who may arrange for a *biopsy* (removal of a sample of tissue for microscopic examination) to be taken.

Pain

A localized sensation that can range from mild discomfort to an unbearable and excruciating experience. Pain is the result of stimulation of special sensory nerve endings usually following injury or caused by disease.

THE MECHANISM OF PAIN

The basic mechanism of pain is shown in the illustrated box. The skin contains many specialized nerve endings (nociceptors). Stimulation of these receptors leads to transmission of pain messages to the brain. Nociceptors have different sensitivities, some responding only to severe stimulation, such as cutting, pricking, or heating the skin to a high temperature; others respond to warning stimuli, such as firm pressure, stretching, or temperatures not high enough to burn. Pain receptors are present in structures other than the skin, including blood vessels and tendons. Most internal organs have few, if any, nociceptors. The large intestine, for example, can be cut without causing any pain. It does, however, have nociceptors that respond to stretching, which, in severe cases, may cause pain.

PSYCHOLOGICAL ASPECTS OF PAIN

Pain is usually associated with distress and anxiety, and sometimes with fear. People vary tremendously in their pain thresholds (the level at which the pain is felt and the person feels compelled to act). The cause and circumstances of the pain may also affect the way it is perceived by the sufferer. The pain of cancer, because of fear of the disease, may seem much greater and cause more suffering than similar pain resulting from persistent indigestion. Unexplained pain is often worse because of the anxiety it can cause; once a diagnosis is made and reassurance given, the pain may be perceived as less severe.

The experience of pain may be reduced by arousal (e.g. an injury sustained during competitive sport or on the battlefield may go unnoticed in the heat of the moment); strong emotion can also block pain. Some people believe that mental preparation for pain (e.g. in childbirth or in experiments to test pain) can greatly reduce the response.

A person's response to pain is greatly modified by past experience; the outcome of previous episodes of pain may affect the way the individual copes with subsequent pain. Factors such as insomnia, anxiety, and depression, which often accompany incapacitating illness, lower tolerance to pain. Many hospitals now have specialist pain clinics, in which people with severe pain that has proved difficult to control may be assessed and treated. Such patients include those with advanced *cancer* and poorly understood conditions such as *facial pain* and various types of *neuralgia*. Treatment may involve the use of drugs, electrical stimulation (*TENS*), surgery, and sometimes alternative therapies such as *acupuncture* or *hypnosis*. (See also *Pain relief*.)

TYPES OF PAIN

Many adjectives are used to describe different types of pain, such as throbbing, penetrating, gnawing, aching, burning, and gripping. The extent to which a patient is accurately able to

P

describe his or her pain to the doctor is highly variable, even though this can be a vital clue to the diagnosis.

Attempts have been made to categorize pain according to intensity, ranging from a minor cut or sore throat at the lower end of the scale to childbirth or renal colic at the upper.

If the pain comes from an internal organ it is often difficult for the sufferer to pinpoint its origin with any precision. For example, in the early stages of appendicitis, pain may be felt in the region above the navel. In the later stages, when infection has caused inflammation of the perito-

neum (lining of the abdominal cavity), the pain becomes localized above the right groin.

Pain may be felt at a point some distance from the disorder; this phenomenon is known as *referred pain* (see illustrated box). Following amputation of a limb, pain may seem to come

PAIN

Pain mechanisms exist to provide a useful warning of possible injury or to caution against repeating an action that has led to injury. Certain

diseases, such as arthritis and extensive cancer, may set off these same mechanisms, causing chronic pain that has no apparent function.

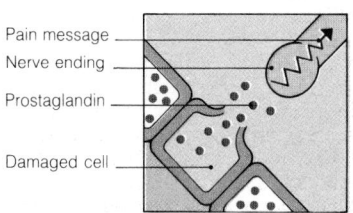

Initiation of pain signals
The signals are set off by stimulation of special nerve endings—by pressure, heat, or release of chemicals, including prostaglandins, by damaged cells.

Reflex action
The nerve pathways that warn of noxious stimuli (through the sensation of pain) may also initiate automatic, reflex actions that help prevent harm.

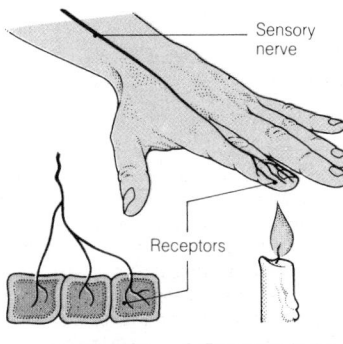

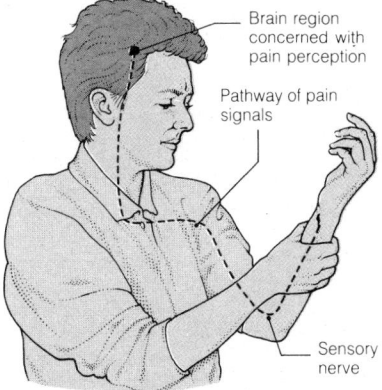

Perception of pain
When an injury occurs, signals pass along nerve pathways concerned with pain, first to the spinal cord and then to the thalamus in the brain; there the pain is perceived.

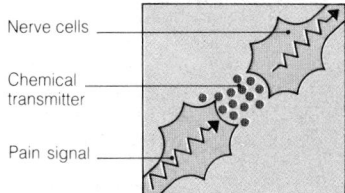

Signal transmission to brain
Within the brain and spinal cord, pain signals pass between nerve cells by means of chemicals that cross the gaps between the cells.

1 Receptors in the fingertip detect heat. Signals are sent along a sensory nerve to the spinal cord.

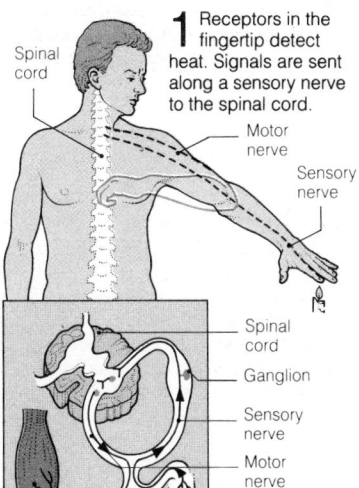

2 The signals arriving in the spinal cord pass instantaneously to a motor nerve that connects to a muscle in the arm. The signals received via the motor nerve cause the muscle in the arm to contract, moving the arm away from the source of danger (the flame).

REFERRED PAIN
A referred pain is one felt in a site other than an injured or diseased part. Sensory nerves from certain body areas converge before they enter the brain, causing confusion about the source of pain signals.

Tooth to ear region
A toothache may be felt in the ear, because the same sensory nerve supplies both parts.

Diaphragm to right shoulder
Inflammation of the diaphragm, often due to pneumonia, may be felt as a pain in the right shoulder.

Heart to left arm
Angina, a pain caused by reduced blood supply to the heart muscle, is often felt in the left shoulder or arm.

Knee to hip
Disorders affecting the knee, such as arthritis, may be felt as pain in the hip.

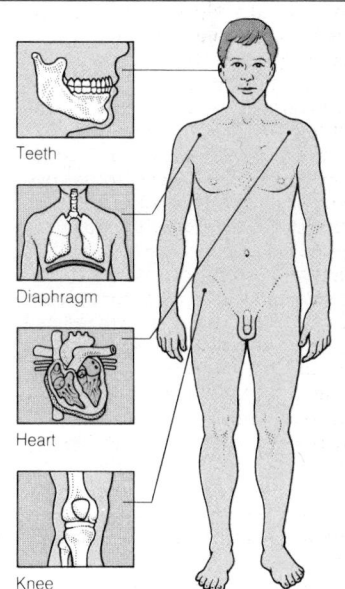

P

from the amputated limb (see *Phantom limb*); in some cases, the person can localize the pain site, such as in a toe despite having had the leg amputated. (See also *Endorphins; Enkephalins*.)

Painful arc syndrome

A condition in which pain occurs when the arm is raised from the side of the body between 45 degrees and 160 degrees.

Painful arc syndrome is usually caused by inflammation of a tendon or a *bursa* around the shoulder joint. The pain is caused by the inflamed tendon or bursa being squeezed between the upper parts of the *scapula* (shoulder-blade) and the *humerus* (upper-arm bone). Treatment includes *physiotherapy* and the injection of *corticosteroid drugs* into the tender area.

Painkillers

See *Analgesic drugs.*

Pain relief

The treatment of *pain*, usually with *analgesic drugs*. Methods of treatment depend on the severity, duration, location, and cause of the pain.

DRUG TREATMENT

Mild analgesic drugs, available over-the-counter, are usually effective in the treatment of mild or moderate pain, such as may be caused by *headache, toothache,* or *dysmenorrhoea* (menstrual pain). *Paracetamol, aspirin* and *codeine* are the most widely used drugs in this group. Pain accompanied by inflammation, as may be caused, for example, by *arthritis* or *sports injuries,* is often alleviated by the administering of a *nonsteroidal anti-inflammatory drug* (NSAID).

Severe pain, such as may be caused by serious injury or kidney stones (see *Calculus, urinary tract*), may require treatment with *narcotic drugs,* such as *morphine* or *pethidine.* Narcotic analgesics are also used to prevent pain after surgery. Long-term use of narcotic analgesics may be necessary to prevent or relieve pain in *cancer.* Narcotic analgesics or local anaesthetic agents may be used to relieve pain during *childbirth.*

NONDRUG TREATMENT

Massage, ice packs, or *poultices* may be used for the relief of localized pain caused by muscle spasm, inflammation, or injury.

Chronic or recurrent pain that has not responded to drug treatment may be relieved by *TENS, acupuncture* or *hypnosis.* TENS is also sometimes used to relieve pain during childbirth.

Surgical procedures are sometimes performed to relieve pain when other treatments have failed. Surgery may involve destruction of nerves that transmit pain (as is done in a *cordotomy*). Alternatively, nerve fibres in the thalamus (the part of the brain that responds to pain) may be cut to prevent perception of pain.

Palate

The roof of the mouth, which separates the mouth from the nasal cavity above. Covered with *mucous membrane,* it consists, in the front, of the hard palate, whose substructure is a plate of bone forming part of the *maxilla* (upper jaw). At the rear is the soft palate, a flap of muscle and fibrous tissue that projects into the *pharynx* (throat). During swallowing, the soft palate presses against the rear wall of the pharynx, preventing food from ascending into the nose.

About one in 500 babies is born with a gap along the midline of the palate (see *Cleft lip and palate*).

Palliative treatment

Therapy that relieves the symptoms of a disorder but does not cure it. For example, treatment for the symptoms of advanced cancer may be palliative rather than curative.

Pallor

Abnormal paleness of the skin and mucous membranes, particularly discernible in the face. Pallor has many possible causes and is only sometimes a symptom of disease.

In some people, pallor is due to a deficiency of the skin pigment *melanin.* Melanin deficiency may occur in people, such as nightworkers or miners, who spend very little time in daylight. It is also a feature of the inherited condition *albinism.*

Pallor may also be caused by constriction (narrowing) of small blood vessels in the skin, which may occur in response to shock, severe pain, injury, heavy blood loss, fainting, or extreme cold. Cutting off the blood flow to the skin ensures that the brain and other vital organs are adequately supplied and that body heat is at least temporarily conserved.

In *anaemia,* pallor results from lack of the blood pigment *haemoglobin* in blood vessels in the skin.

Certain kidney disorders, such as *pyelonephritis* and *kidney failure,* produce a sallow pallor, as does *hypothyroidism.* Rare conditions that give rise to pallor include *lead poisoning.*

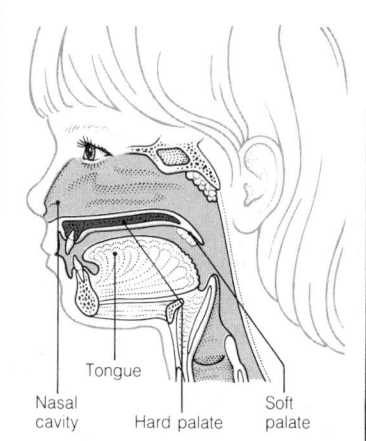

LOCATION OF THE PALATE
The palate forms the floor of the nasal cavity and roof of the mouth, providing a surface against which the tongue can push during chewing and swallowing.

Tongue

Nasal cavity

Hard palate

Soft palate

Palpation

A technique, used in *physical examination,* in which certain parts of the body are felt with the hands. By palpation, the doctor is able to assess the condition of the skin and of the underlying organs.

Palpitation

Awareness of the *heartbeat* or a sensation of having a rapid and unusually forceful heartbeat.

CAUSES

Palpitations are usually felt after strenuous exercise, in tense situations, or after a severe scare, when the heart is beating harder and/or faster than normal. When palpitations are experienced at rest or in a calm mood, they are usually due to *ectopic heartbeats* (premature beats followed by an unusually prolonged pause) and are felt as a fluttering or thumping in the chest, sometimes with a brief but alarming sense that the heart has stopped beating. Ectopic heartbeats do not usually indicate heart disease; they are often caused by drinking alcohol, a high intake of caffeine, or heavy smoking.

Palpitations may be caused by cardiac *arrhythmias* (irregularities of the heartbeat). An example of an arrhythmia is atrial *tachycardia,* a condition in which the heart suddenly starts to beat very rapidly; the affected person may feel faint and breathless. The pulse may be as high as 200 beats per

P

minute but remains regular. In *atrial fibrillation,* the atria (upper chambers of the heart) beat in a disorganized manner and the impulses passed to the ventricles (lower, pumping chambers) are very irregular. *Hyperthyroidism* (overactivity of the thyroid gland) may cause palpitations by speeding up the heartbeat.

DIAGNOSIS AND TREATMENT
If palpitations last for several hours or recur over several days, or if they cause chest pain, breathlessness, or dizziness, a doctor should be consulted as soon as possible, as there may be a serious underlying disorder. Recurrent palpitations may be investigated by means of a 24-hour *ECG* and by *thyroid-function tests.* Treatment depends on the underlying cause.

Palsy
A term applied to certain forms of *paralysis.* Examples are *cerebral palsy, facial palsy,* and Erb's palsy (paralysis of the upper arm and shoulder on one side of the body).

Panacea
A remedy for all diseases; a cure-all. No such remedy is known, despite claims to the contrary made by numerous quacks through the ages.

Pancreas
An elongated, tapered *gland* that lies across the back of the abdomen, behind the stomach. The broadest part of the pancreas (called the head) is situated on the right-hand side, in the loop of the duodenum. The main part of the gland (called the body) tapers from the head, extending towards the left and slightly upwards; the narrower end (called the tail) terminates near the spleen.

STRUCTURE
Most of the pancreas consists of exocrine tissue, embedded in which are "nests" of endocrine cells (the islets of Langerhans). The exocrine cells secrete digestive *enzymes* into a network of ducts that meet to form the main pancreatic duct. This duct joins the common bile duct (which carries bile from the gallbladder) to form a small chamber, called the ampulla of Vater, which opens into the duodenum. The islets of Langerhans are surrounded by many blood vessels into which they secrete *hormones.*

FUNCTION
The pancreas has two functions: digestive and hormonal. The exocrine tissue secretes various digestive enzymes that break down carbo-

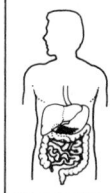

LOCATION OF THE PANCREAS
This organ lies under the stomach, except for its head, which lies within the curve of the duodenum.

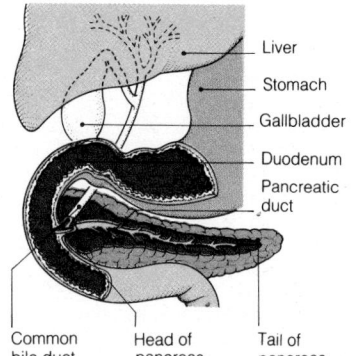

Liver
Stomach
Gallbladder
Duodenum
Pancreatic duct
Common bile duct
Head of pancreas
Tail of pancreas

hydrates, fats, proteins, and nucleic acids (see *Digestive system*). Most of these enzymes are inactive until activated in the duodenum by other enzymes. Also secreted is sodium bicarbonate, which neutralizes stomach acid entering the duodenum. The endocrine cells in the islets of Langerhans secrete the hormones *insulin* and *glucagon,* which regulate the level of glucose in the blood. (See also *Pancreas* disorders box.)

Pancreas, cancer of
A malignant tumour of the exocrine tissue of the *pancreas* (the main tissue in the gland). The cause of the condition is unknown, although it has been linked to heavy smoking and to certain dietary factors, such as a high intake of fats or alcohol.

The incidence of pancreatic cancer has increased threefold during the past 50 years, and there are now about 7,000 cases diagnosed in the UK per year, mostly in people over 50.

SYMPTOMS
The most common symptom is pain in the upper abdomen, often spreading to the back. Other common symptoms are loss of appetite, weight loss, and jaundice. There may also be indigestion, nausea, vomiting, diarrhoea, and tiredness. In most cases, the symptoms do not appear until the cancer is well advanced, often not until it has spread to other parts of the body (typically to the liver or lungs).

DIAGNOSIS
Diagnosis of pancreatic cancer usually requires *ultrasound scanning, CT scanning,* or *MRI* of the upper abdomen, or endoscopic examination of the ducts of the pancreas (see *ERCP*). In some cases, the condition is detected during exploratory surgery on the abdomen (see *Laparotomy, exploratory*).

TREATMENT AND OUTLOOK
If the condition is detected in its early stages, surgical removal of the malignant tissue (see *Pancreatectomy*) along with *radiotherapy* and *anticancer drugs* may result in a cure. However, in most cases the cancer is not diagnosed until it is well advanced, and little can be done apart from relieving the pain with *analgesic drugs* (painkillers), alleviating any other symptoms, and bypassing the growth if it is causing obstruction of the bile duct or bowel. In such cases, the outlook is poor; death occurs in about 90 per cent of the cases within a year of diagnosis.

Pancreatectomy
Removal of all or part of the *pancreas.* Pancreatectomy may be performed to treat *pancreatitis* (inflammation of the pancreas), localized cancer of the pancreas (see *Pancreas, cancer of*), or cancer of the ampulla of Vater (the small chamber formed by the union of the common bile duct and pancreatic duct which opens into the duodenum). Rarely, it is done to treat some endocrine tumours, such as *insulinomas* (insulin-producing tumours).

The amount of the gland that is removed depends on the disorder involved and/or on how much of the pancreas is affected. Obstruction of the pancreatic duct may require removal of only the tail of the gland (the narrower end, nearest the spleen) and the linking of the duct with a small piece of small intestine. Disease of the head of the pancreas (the broader end, situated in the loop of the duodenum) may necessitate removal of both the pancreatic head and the duodenal loop (an operation known as Whipple's operation).

COMPLICATIONS
Pancreatectomy may lead to *diabetes mellitus,* which requires insulin therapy, and *malabsorption,* which requires oral supplements of *pancreatin* (a preparation of digestive enzymes produced by the pancreas).

Pancreatin
An oral preparation of digestive *enzymes* obtained from the pancreas of pigs. Pancreatin is used to supple-

P

DISORDERS OF THE PANCREAS

Serious disruption of pancreatic function occurs only when the secretory tissue of the gland has been damaged or destroyed in advanced disease. The most common pancreatic disorder is *diabetes mellitus*, in which the insulin-producing cells in the gland are destroyed.

CONGENITAL AND GENETIC DISORDERS
About 85 per cent of people with the genetic disorder *cystic fibrosis* produce totally inadequate quantities of pancreatic digestive enzymes, which results in *malabsorption* of fats and proteins. This, in turn, may produce steatorrhoea (excess fat in the faeces) and muscle wasting.

Genetic factors are thought to play some part in diabetes mellitus, although they are not the primary cause of the disease.

Chronic *pancreatitis* (inflammation of the pancreas) may, in rare cases, be hereditary; chronic pancreatitis often causes diabetes.

INFECTION
Acute pancreatitis may result from certain viral infections, especially with the *mumps* or *hepatitis* viruses. Other viruses, such as coxsackieviruses and echoviruses, may also cause pancreatitis. In some cases, coxsackievirus infection may contribute to the development of diabetes.

TUMOUR
Pancreatic cancer is one of the more common cancers (see *Pancreas, cancer of*). It is difficult to diagnose and, in most cases, has spread extensively by the time it is detected.

TRAUMA
Injury to the pancreas—as a result of a blow to the abdomen, for example—may cause acute pancreatitis. The mechanism by which this happens is not fully established, but it is believed that pancreatic enzymes (most of which are inactive until they reach the intestine) are released within the gland and then activated, with the result that they digest the pancreas.

POISONS AND DRUGS
Excessive alcohol intake is a common cause of pancreatitis. It can also be caused by various drugs, such as sulphonamides, oestrogens (including oestrogen-containing contraceptive pills), and thiazide *diuretic drugs*; *corticosteroid drugs* may also cause pancreatitis.

AUTOIMMUNE DISORDERS
The cause of the damage to the pancreas in diabetes mellitus remains controversial. However, there is increasing evidence that, possibly in response to a viral infection, the body's immune system produces *antibodies* (proteins with a role in the defence against infection) that inappropriately attack and destroy the pancreatic cells.

OTHER DISORDERS
Other than alcohol overuse, the condition most commonly associated with pancreatitis is *gallstones*. These occasionally block the exit of the pancreatic duct into the duodenum, which leads to inflammation of the pancreas.

INVESTIGATION
Diagnosis of pancreatic disorders may involve *ultrasound scanning, CT scanning,* or *MRI* of the abdomen, tests to measure levels of pancreatic enzymes in the blood or duodenum, and endoscopic examination of the gland (see *ERCP*).

ment deficiency of these enzymes and thus prevent *malabsorption* of fats, carbohydrates, and proteins. Pancreatin may be required following *pancreatectomy* or by people suffering from pancreatic disorders, such as chronic *pancreatitis*, cancer of the pancreas (see *Pancreas, cancer of*), and *cystic fibrosis*.

Pancreatitis
Inflammation of the *pancreas*, which may be acute or chronic. Acute pancreatitis is less damaging, although attacks may recur. Chronic pancreatitis causes permanent damage to the pancreas due to the formation of fibrous scar tissue.

CAUSES
The main causes of acute pancreatitis are alcohol abuse and *gallstones*. Less commonly, pancreatitis results from a viral infection (such as *mumps* or *hepatitis*), injury (such as may be caused by a strong blow to the abdomen), surgery on the biliary tract, or certain drugs (such as *diuretic drugs* and *sulphonamide drugs*).

Chronic pancreatitis is most commonly caused by alcohol abuse. In rare cases, chronic pancreatitis occurs in people with *hyperlipidaemias* (a group of disorders characterized by high levels of fat in the blood) or *haemochromatosis* (a disorder in which there is an excess of iron in the body). Chronic pancreatitis may also rarely be inherited or result from a severe attack of acute pancreatitis.

SYMPTOMS AND DIAGNOSIS
Acute pancreatitis produces a sudden attack of severe upper abdominal pain, often accompanied by nausea and vomiting. In many cases, the pain spreads to the back. The pain of acute pancreatitis is usually made worse by movement, and may be relieved by adopting a sitting position. An attack usually lasts for about 48 hours and is accompanied by the release of digestive enzymes from the pancreas directly into the blood; measurement of these enzymes is an important diagnostic test. *CT scanning* and *MRI* are very accurate methods of diagnosing acute pancreatitis, provided they are carried out within 72 hours of the onset of symptoms.

Chronic pancreatitis usually produces the same symptoms as acute pancreatitis, although the pain may last from a few hours to several days, and attacks become more frequent as the condition progresses. However, in some cases there may be no pain and the principal signs may be *malabsorption* (due to a deficiency of pancreatic enzymes) or *diabetes mellitus* (due to insufficient *insulin* production by the pancreas). Measuring pancreatic enzyme levels in the blood is of little value in the diagnosis of chronic pancreatitis, although measurement of the output of such enzymes into the duodenum (by means of a fine tube passed through the stomach) may be useful. Abdominal X-rays or scans are the usual diagnostic methods, along with endoscopic examination of the pancreatic ducts (see *ERCP*) to determine the extent of tissue damage.

COMPLICATIONS

If acute pancreatitis causes severe damage to the gland, *hypotension* (low blood pressure), *heart failure, kidney failure, respiratory failure,* and *ascites* (accumulation of fluid in the abdomen) may occur. In some cases, cysts or abscesses may develop in the damaged gland.

Chronic pancreatitis may also lead to the development of ascites and cysts. Other possible complications include obstruction of the common bile duct (see *Bile duct obstruction*), permanent diabetes mellitus, and blood clots in the splenic vein, which drains the spleen and pancreatic veins.

TREATMENT

In acute pancreatitis, fluids and salts are given by *intravenous infusion,* and narcotic *analgesic drugs* are given to relieve pain. In severe cases, peritoneal lavage (washing out the abdominal cavity with sterile fluid) may relieve symptoms. A recurrence of the condition can sometimes be prevented by treating an underlying cause. Occasionally, surgery is needed to remove the pancreas (see *Pancreatectomy*) or to remove any gallstones.

Chronic pancreatitis is treated by providing pain relief, by controlling diabetes mellitus with insulin, and by giving *pancreatin* (a preparation of pancreatic enzymes). In some cases, pancreatectomy may be necessary to relieve pain.

Pancreatography

Imaging of the pancreas or its ducts. The methods used include *CT scanning, MRI, ultrasound scanning,* or the taking of *X-rays* after the injection of a radiopaque contrast medium into the pancreatic ducts either during exploratory surgery or through the use of an endoscope (see *ERCP*).

Pandemic

A medical term applied to a disease that occurs over a large geographical area (sometimes worldwide) and affects a high proportion of the population; a widespread *epidemic.*

Panic attack

A brief period of acute *anxiety*, often dominated by an intense fear of dying or losing one's reason. Panic attacks occur unpredictably at first, but tend to become associated with certain places, such as a crowded supermarket or a cramped lift.

The symptoms begin suddenly and usually include a sense of breathing difficulty, chest pains, palpitations, feeling light-headed and dizzy, sweating, trembling, and faintness. *Hyperventilation* (fast, shallow breathing) often accompanies and worsens the symptoms, leading to *pins-and-needles,* and to feelings of *depersonalization* and *derealization.*

Although unpleasant and frightening, panic attacks last for only a few minutes, cause no physical harm, and are rarely associated with serious physical illness. The symptoms of hyperventilation may be relieved by covering the mouth and nose with a small paper bag and breathing into the bag for a few minutes.

In general, panic attacks are a symptom of an *anxiety disorder, agoraphobia,* or other *phobias* (if they lead to avoidance of certain situations). Less often they are part of a *somatization disorder* or *schizophrenia.* The cause of panic attacks is unknown but increasingly they are treated by *behaviour therapy,* particularly if they are associated with specific phobias. Relaxation exercises may be of some help.

Papain

A naturally occurring mixture of *enzymes,* including one, chymopapain, found in pawpaws. Papain breaks down proteins and has been used to remove clotted blood and dead tissue from wounds and ulcers. Chymopapain is used in *chemonucleolysis* (injection of the enzyme into a prolapsed intervertebral disc).

Papilla

Any small, nipple-shaped projection from the surface of a tissue, such as the mammary papilla (the nipple of the breast) and the lingual papillae (the numerous projections on the surface of the tongue, some of which contain taste buds).

Papilloedema

Swelling of the head of the *optic nerve,* also known as optic disc oedema, which is visible when the eye is examined with an *ophthalmoscope.* Papilloedema usually indicates a dangerous rise in the pressure of *cerebrospinal fluid* in the skull, sometimes caused by a *brain tumour.* Swelling of the head of the optic nerve may also arise from conditions affecting the nerve itself, including damage due to the restriction of blood supply. It may be followed by *optic atrophy.*

Papilloma

A usually nonmalignant tumour, often resembling a wart, that arises

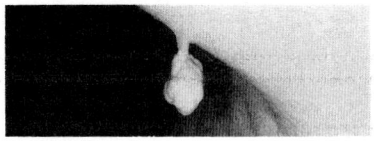

Skin papilloma
This harmless type of growth is common in elderly people. It can easily be snipped off at skin level and the base cauterized by your doctor.

from the *epithelium* (the cell layer that forms the skin and mucous membranes, and that lines most of the hollow organs of the body). Although papillomas may develop from epithelial tissue anywhere in the body, they most commonly affect the skin, tongue, larynx (voice-box), urinary tract, and digestive tract.

Pap smear

See *Cervical smear test.*

Papule

A small, solid, slightly raised area of skin. Papules are usually less than 0.5 cm in diameter and may be raised or flat, have a smooth or warty texture, and be either pigmented or the colour of the surrounding skin. Many skin conditions, including *acne* and *lichen planus*, start with papules.

Par-/para-

Prefixes with several meanings: beside or beyond, as in the parathyroid glands (which are situated behind the thyroid at its sides); closely related to or closely resembling, as in paratyphoid fever (a disease that is similar to typhoid); faulty or abnormal, as in paraesthesia (abnormal sensation); or associated with an accessory capacity, as in paramedical workers (personnel who supplement the work of doctors).

Para-aminobenzoic acid

The active ingredient of many *sunscreen* preparations, also known by its abbreviation PABA.

Paracentesis

A procedure in which a body cavity is punctured with a needle from the outside. Paracentesis is performed to remove fluid for analysis, to relieve pressure due to excess fluid, or to instil drugs. The procedure is quick and relatively painless, and is usually carried out under local anaesthesia.

Paracentesis is most often performed on the abdomen, to aid the diagnosis of conditions causing *ascites*, in which fluid collects in the abdominal cavity. The procedure is also commonly performed on the thorax, and sometimes on other sites, including the pericardium and the scrotum.

Paracetamol

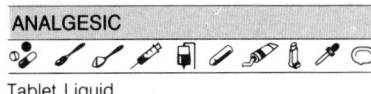

ANALGESIC

Tablet Liquid

 Available over-the-counter

Available as generic

An *analgesic drug* (painkiller). Paracetamol is used to treat mild pain (for example, from headache or toothache) and to reduce fever. It has been widely used since 1955.

Unlike *aspirin*, paracetamol does not cause stomach irritation or bleeding and so is particularly useful as a painkiller for people who suffer from *peptic ulcer* or who cannot tolerate aspirin. Paracetamol may be used with safety to treat children, for whom it is available as a syrup. Paracetamol does not have an anti-inflammatory effect, however, and so is less effective than aspirin as a treatment for injury to soft tissues such as muscles and ligaments.

POSSIBLE ADVERSE EFFECTS
Taken in normal doses, paracetamol may rarely cause nausea or rash. An overdose of paracetamol may cause permanent damage to the liver and can be fatal.

Paraesthesia

Altered sensation in the skin without a stimulus (see *Pins-and-needles*).

Paraffinoma

A tumour-like swelling under the skin caused by prolonged exposure to paraffin. Paraffinomas may occur in the lungs due to inhalation of paraffin, usually in someone who uses liquid paraffin as a laxative. Paraffinomas were an uncommon side-effect of augmentation *mammoplasty* (enlargement of the breast) before silicone replaced paraffin wax in this operation.

Paraldehyde

An unpleasant-smelling sedative drug used to stop prolonged epileptic seizures and occasionally to treat alcohol withdrawal. Paraldehyde can be administered as an enema or by injection. A glass syringe must be used to inject it, because paraldehyde dissolves plastic.

Paralysis

Complete or partial loss of controlled movement caused by the inability to contract one or more *muscles*. Weakness, rather than complete loss of movement, is often referred to as *paresis*. Paralysis may be temporary or permanent, and can affect anything from a small facial muscle to many of the major muscles in the body. Loss of feeling in the affected parts may accompany inability to move them.

TYPES
Paralysis of one half of the body is called *hemiplegia*; paralysis of all four limbs and the trunk is called *quadriplegia*. *Paraplegia* is paralysis of both legs and sometimes part of the trunk. *Palsy* is an outdated term for paralysis; it is still used in the names of certain disorders (such as *cerebral palsy*).

Paralysis may be flaccid, which gives the limbs a floppy disposition, or spastic, in which case the affected parts of the body are rigid.

CAUSES
Muscles that control movement of the body are stimulated to contract by impulses originating in the motor cortex of the *brain*. These impulses travel via the spinal cord and peripheral nerves to reach the muscles. Paralysis may be caused by any form of injury or disorder anywhere along this nerve pathway, or by a muscle disorder.

BRAIN DISORDERS A very common cause of paralysis is a *stroke*, in which damage to part of the brain is caused by bleeding from or blood clotting in a blood vessel that supplies that area of the brain. Because motor nerve fibres cross in the brainstem, paralysis occurs on the side opposite to the site of the brain damage.

Hemiplegia can be caused by any brain disorder in which the portion of the brain that controls movement is damaged—for example, by a *brain tumour*, *brain abscess*, *brain haemorrhage*, *cerebral palsy*, or *encephalitis* (brain infection).

Some forms of paralysis are caused by damage to those parts of the nervous system concerned with the fine control of movement (such as the *cerebellum* and *basal ganglia*). *Parkinson's disease* is caused by lack of dopamine in the basal ganglia.

SPINAL CORD DISORDERS Paralysis can be caused by damage to the spinal cord within a spine fractured in a road traffic accident. Pressure on the spinal cord may cause paralysis in *disc prolapse* or *cervical osteoarthritis*. Muscles supplied by nerves below the damaged area are affected.

Diseases affecting the spinal cord (such as *multiple sclerosis*, *poliomyelitis*, *myelitis*, *Friedreich's ataxia*, *meningitis*, and deficiency of *vitamin* B_{12}) may also cause paralysis.

PERIPHERAL NERVE DISORDERS A group of disorders, known as *neuropathies*, affect the peripheral nerves and cause varying degrees of paralysis. Neuropathies may be caused by a variety of conditions, including *diabetes mellitus*, vitamin deficiency, liver disease, cancer, and the toxic effects of some drugs or metals (such as lead). A neuropathy may also sometimes occur as an inherited disorder.

A type of neuropathy that often causes paralysis of the shoulder, arm, or hand results from injury to the *brachial plexus* (a nerve network that serves the arm and hand).

MUSCLE DISORDERS *Muscular dystrophy* causes progressive muscular weakness and may lead to paralysis. Temporary paralysis sometimes occurs in *myasthenia gravis*.

TREATMENT
The underlying cause is treated if possible. *Physiotherapy* is used to prevent joints from becoming locked into useless positions, which is important in both temporary and permanent paralysis. When the paralysis is temporary (such as in a mild stroke), physiotherapy is used to retrain and strengthen the muscles and joints so that some degree of mobility is possible after recovery.

For paralysed people confined to bed or a wheelchair, nursing care is essential to avoid complications of prolonged *immobility*—such as bedsores, deep vein thrombosis, urinary tract infections, constipation, and limb deformities. (See also *Disability*.)

Paralysis, periodic

A rare, inherited condition that affects young people. Periodic paralysis is characterized by episodes of weakness and paralysis of limb muscles, which occur every six weeks or so and may last from a few minutes to two days. Episodes often begin during the night and wake the sufferer.

The exact cause of periodic paralysis is unknown, although in many cases there is a drop in the level of potassium (which is essential for normal muscle function) in the blood. A meal that is rich in carbohydrates often triggers an attack.

The frequency of attacks can be lessened by reducing the intake of carbohydrates and by taking *acetazolamide* or potassium-sparing *diuretic*

P

drugs. An episode can sometimes be curtailed by taking potassium or by exercising gently at the first sign of muscle weakness. The condition often disappears without treatment by the age of 30.

Paramedic

A term for any health-care worker other than a doctor, nurse, or dentist. Examples of paramedics include physiotherapists, radiographers, and laboratory technicians.

Paranoia

A condition whose central feature is the *delusion* (a false idea not amenable to reasoned argument) that people or events are in some way specially connected to oneself. The term is also used popularly to describe feelings of persecution.

A person suffering from paranoia gradually builds up an elaborate set of beliefs based on the interpretation of chance remarks or events. Typical themes include persecution, jealousy (see *Jealousy, morbid*), love, and grandeur (belief in one's own superior position and powers).

TYPES AND CAUSES
Chronic paranoia may result from brain damage, alcohol abuse, amphetamine abuse, *schizophrenia*, or *manic-depressive illness*. The condition is especially likely to develop in people with paranoid *personality disorder*— suspicious, oversensitive people who seem emotionally cold.

Acute paranoia, lasting for less than six months, may occur in people who have experienced radical changes in their environment, such as immigrants, refugees, or people leaving home for the first time.

In shared paranoia (see *Folie a deux*), delusion develops as a result of a close relationship with someone who already has a delusion.

SYMPTOMS
The feelings and activities of a person with paranoia often seem relatively normal in that they are appropriate to his or her beliefs. There are usually no other symptoms of mental illness apart from occasional *hallucinations*. In time, however, anger, suspicion, and social isolation may mark an increasing change towards difficult and eccentric behaviour. Paranoid individuals rarely see themselves as ill and usually receive treatment only at the instigation of relatives or friends.

TREATMENT AND OUTCOME
When acute illness is treated early with *antipsychotic drugs*, the outlook

is good. In long-standing paranoia, delusions are usually firmly entrenched, although antipsychotic drugs may make them less prominent.

Paraparesis

Partial *paralysis* or weakness of both legs and sometimes part of the trunk. The cause is disease in or injury to the nervous system.

Paraphilia

See *Deviation, sexual*.

Paraphimosis

Constriction of the *penis* behind the glans (head) by an extremely tight foreskin that has been retracted (pulled back), causing swelling and pain. Paraphimosis often occurs as a complication of *phimosis* (an abnormally tight foreskin).

In many cases, the foreskin can be returned manually to its normal position. The swelling in the glans may be reduced by first applying an ice-pack and then squeezing the glans. If manual return proves impossible, an injection or an operation to cut the foreskin may be necessary. *Circumcision* (surgical removal of the foreskin) is usual to prevent recurrence.

Paraplegia

Weakness or *paralysis* of both legs and sometimes of part of the trunk, often accompanied by loss of sensation and by loss of urinary control.

Paraplegia is a result of nerve damage in the *brain* or *spinal cord*. It is usually caused by a motor vehicle accident, sports accident, fall, or gunshot wounds. Twice as many men as women are victims, and the incidence is highest between the ages of 19 and 35 years.

Parapsychology

The branch of *psychology* dealing with experiences and events that cannot be accounted for by scientific understanding. Such paranormal phenomena include telepathy (the communication of thoughts from one person's mind to another), telekinesis (the movement of objects simply by thinking), clairvoyance (the ability to "see" events at a distance without using one's eyes), and precognition (being able to see into the future). These are all forms of extrasensory perception (ESP).

The basis of many paranormal experiences can probably be explained by mental disturbances. Thought broadcasting (in which individuals

have the impression that their thoughts can be heard by others) is a common symptom of *schizophrenia*. Other apparently paranormal experiences are a result of coincidence or self-deception, while some, such as psychic surgery (removal of objects from the body apparently without an incision) are no more than sleight-of-hand trickery.

Paraquat

A poisonous defoliant weedkiller. The forms of paraquat that are generally available to the public are almost harmless, but concentrated solutions used for agricultural purposes can cause potentially fatal poisoning if swallowed, inhaled, or absorbed through the skin.

The main symptom of paraquat poisoning is difficulty in breathing. In severe cases, there may be respiratory failure, acute or progressive lung damage, and kidney failure, which may be fatal.

Marijuana is sometimes contaminated with paraquat. Smoking contaminated supplies can cause any or all of the following: stinging eyes, a burning sensation in the mouth and throat, vomiting, and mouth ulcers.

TREATMENT
If paraquat poisoning is known or suspected, medical help should be obtained immediately. First-aid treatment consists of getting the victim to eat charcoal or fuller's earth (a clay-containing earthy substance), which inactivate paraquat. Medical treatment may include haemodialysis (removal of toxic substances from the blood, see *Dialysis*) and other emergency measures to remove the chemical from the body.

If paraquat has been splashed into the eyes or on to the skin, it should be washed away with plenty of water.

Parasite

Any organism living in or on any other living creature and deriving advantage from doing so, while causing disadvantage to the host. The parasite satisfies its nutritional requirements from the host's blood or tissues or from the host's diet, which allows the parasite to reproduce.

Parasites may remain permanently with their host or may spend only part of their life-cycles in association. Some parasites cause few symptoms, others cause disease and even the eventual death of the host.

Animal parasites of humans include various *protozoa* (single-celled animals), *worms, flukes, leeches, lice, ticks,* and *mites. Viruses* and disease-causing *fungi* and *bacteria* are also essentially parasites. Some types of bacteria actually benefit their hosts (e.g. by helping to control the populations of more harmful organisms) and so are not strictly parasites.

Parasitology

The scientific study of organisms that treat others as their living environment (see *Parasite*), especially the study of their life-cycles and reproductive behaviour, the ways in which they cause disease, and their susceptibility to drug treatment and other methods of halting their multiplication. Although viruses and many types of bacteria and fungi are parasites, their study is conducted under the general title of *microbiology*.

Medical parasitology is concerned primarily with animal parasites of humans, especially the protozoa, worms, flukes, and arthropod parasites (insects and related animals) such as lice and the scabies mite.

Parasuicide

See *Suicide, attempted.*

Parasympathetic nervous system

One of the two divisions of the *autonomic nervous system.* In conjunction with the other division (the sympathetic nervous system), the parasympathetic system controls the involuntary activities of the organs, glands, blood vessels, and other tissues in the body.

Parathion

An agricultural organophosphate insecticide which is highly poisonous to both humans and animals. Poisoning may occur by absorption through the skin (as in agricultural work), by inhalation, or by swallowing.

Symptoms of poisoning include nausea, vomiting, abdominal cramps, involuntary defaecation and urination, excessive salivation and sweating, blurred vision, headache, confusion, and muscle twitching. If poisoning is severe, there may also be difficulty breathing, palpitations, seizures, and unconsciousness. Without treatment, parathion poisoning may be fatal.

TREATMENT
If parathion has been swallowed, treatment consists of inducing vomiting or of washing out the stomach (see *Lavage, gastric*). If poisoning occurred by skin absorption, the victim's clothing is removed and contaminated areas of skin are thoroughly washed.

To counteract the effects of the poison, injections of *atropine* and pralidoxime may be given. It may also be necessary to support the victim's breathing with *oxygen therapy* and/or artificial *ventilation.* With rapid treatment, people may survive doses of parathion much greater than the usual fatal dose, but correct initial diagnosis is essential.

Parathyroidectomy

The surgical removal of abnormal tissue from the *parathyroid glands.* Parathyroidectomy may be performed to treat *hyperparathyroidism* (excess secretion of parathyroid hormone) when it is caused by an *adenoma* (a small, benign tumour) of a parathyroid gland or, less commonly, by a general overgrowth of the glands or by parathyroid cancer.

In the case of an adenoma, usually only one of the glands is involved and needs to be removed. If all the glands are enlarged and overactive, all but one or part of one gland may need to be removed. Removal of all parathyroid tissue leads to *hypoparathyroidism,* causing a dangerously low level of calcium in the blood which may result in *tetany* (painful, cramp-like spasms).

The operation is performed under general anaesthesia. An incision is made in the neck, just beneath the Adam's apple. A section of tissue that is suspected of being abnormal is taken and examined to decide how much parathyroid tissue should be removed. This is then cut out, and the incision sewn up.

The average hospital stay for parathyroidectomy is less than a week. Patients can expect complete healing without complications, although some people need treatment for hypoparathyroidism.

PARASITES

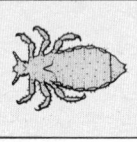 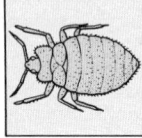 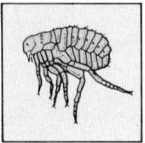 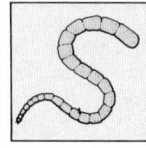 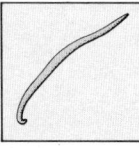

| Head louse | Bedbug | Cat flea | Tapeworm | Hookworm |

ECTOPARASITES (present in skin or on body surface)

Common examples	Activities	How acquired
Head lice Ticks Bedbugs Cat fleas Dog fleas Aquatic leeches	Suck host's blood.	Through contact with other people (lice, scabies mites, warts), animals (ringworm fungi, ticks), vegetation (ticks, mites), or water (aquatic leeches). Bedbugs live in bedroom walls or mattresses and visit humans at night. Cat and dog fleas may visit humans when the pet is absent.
Scabies mites	Burrow in skin.	
Ringworm fungi	Multiply in skin.	
Wart viruses		

ENDOPARASITES (live within body)

Tapeworms Flukes Roundworms Threadworms Hookworms	Adults live in human gut, blood vessels, bile ducts, or elsewhere and produce eggs that are passed out of the body.	By eating infected meat, swallowing eggs on food, contaminating fingers with faecal material, or contact with infected water.
Various disease-causing protozoa, fungi, bacteria, and viruses	Organisms multiply locally or spread throughout the body, causing disease.	By inhalation, water- or food-borne transmission, sexual transmission, or blood-borne infection, among other mechanisms.

Parathyroid glands

Two pairs of oval, pea-sized glands, that lie behind the lobes of the *thyroid gland* in the neck. Some people have only a single parathyroid gland or have extra glands in the neck or chest.

FUNCTION

The glands produce parathyroid hormone, which helps control the level of calcium in the blood. This requires constant regulation, since even small variations from normal can impair muscle and nerve function.

If the level of calcium in the blood drops, the parathyroid glands respond by increasing their output of parathyroid hormone. This causes the bones to release more calcium into the blood, the intestines to absorb more from food, and the kidneys to conserve calcium. These actions quickly restore the blood calcium level. If the blood level of calcium rises, the glands reduce their output of hormone, reversing the above processes.

In rare cases, the parathyroid glands may become overactive (see *Hyperparathyroidism*), causing erosion of the bones and *calculi* (stones) in the urinary tract; or they may become underactive (see *Hypoparathyroidism*), resulting in tetany (painful spasms) or seizures.

Parathyroid tumour

A growth within a *parathyroid gland*. Parathyroid tumours may cause excess secretion of parathyroid hormone into the bloodstream, thereby leading to increased levels of calcium in the blood and to symptoms of *hyperparathyroidism*.

Most parathyroid tumours are benign *adenomas*. Cancers of the parathyroid are very rare and are not highly malignant, although occasionally they may spread to other organs in the body.

TREATMENT AND OUTLOOK

An adenoma that is causing hyperparathyroidism will be surgically removed (see *Parathyroidectomy*). In most cases, surgery gives a complete cure. Occasionally, however, a tumour may recur or the patient may need treatment for *hypoparathyroidism*.

In people who have parathyroid cancer, surgery allows long-term survival without recurrence, provided the entire tumour can be completely removed before it has spread.

Paratyphoid fever

An illness identical in most respects to *typhoid fever*, except that it is caused by a slightly different bacterium, *SALMO-*

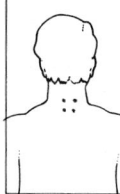

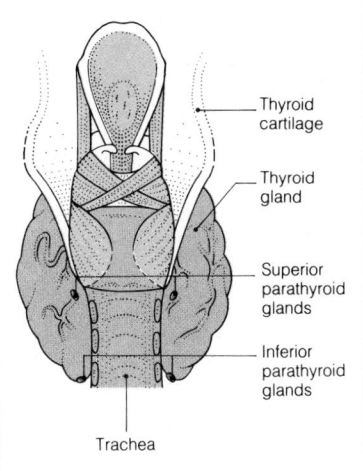

Thyroid cartilage

Thyroid gland

Superior parathyroid glands

Inferior parathyroid glands

Trachea

NELLA PARATYPHI, and is usually less severe. The causative organism is spread in a way similar to the typhoid bacterium, but long-term carriers of infection are less common.

Parenchyma

The functional tissue of an organ, as distinct from accessory structures such as the *stroma* (framework) and the capsule (fibrous outer layer) that hold the organ together.

Parenteral

A term applied to the administration of drugs or other substances by any route other than via the gastrointestinal tract. Examples of parenteral routes of administration include injection into a blood vessel or muscle or insertion of a pessary into the vagina.

Parenteral nutrition

An alternative name for intravenous feeding. (See *Feeding, artificial*.)

Paresis

Partial *paralysis* or weakness of one or several muscles.

Parietal

A medical term that refers to the wall of a part of the body. Examples are the parietal peritoneum (the membrane

that lines the walls of the abdomen and pelvis and the underside of the diaphragm); the parietal bones (the two joined bones that form much of the top, sides, and upper back part of the skull); and the parietal lobes of the brain (the parts of the cerebral hemispheres that are covered by the parietal bones).

Parkinsonism

Any neurological disorder characterized by a mask-like face, rigidity, and slowness of movements. The most common type, which is of unknown cause, is *Parkinson's disease*.

Known causes of parkinsonism include *antipsychotic drugs*, the rare *encephalitis lethargica* infection, *carbon monoxide* poisoning, *cerebrovascular disease*, and the use of certain *designer drugs* of abuse.

Parkinson's disease

A neurological disorder that causes muscle tremor, stiffness, and weakness. The characteristic signs of Parkinson's disease are trembling, a rigid posture, slow movements, and a shuffling, unbalanced walk.

CAUSES AND INCIDENCE

Parkinson's disease is caused by degeneration of or damage to nerve cells within the *basal ganglia* in the brain. The way this affects muscle tension and movement is shown in the illustrated box overleaf.

About one person in 200 has Parkinson's disease. There are about 15,000 new cases a year in the UK. Parkinson's disease occurs mainly in the elderly, and is more common in men than in women. The incidence of Parkinson's disease is lower among smokers than nonsmokers.

SYMPTOMS AND SIGNS

The disease usually begins as a slight tremor of one hand, arm, or leg. In the early stages, the tremor is worse when the hand or limb is at rest; when it is used, the shaking virtually stops.

Later, the disease affects both sides of the body, and causes stiffness and weakness as well as trembling of the muscles. Symptoms include a stiff, shuffling, unbalanced walk that may break into uncontrollable, tiny, running steps; a constant trembling of the hands, more marked at rest and sometimes accompanied by shaking of the head; a permanent rigid stoop; and an unblinking, fixed expression. Eating, washing, dressing, and other everyday activities become very difficult.

The intellect is unaffected until late in the disease, although speech may

P

become slow and hesitant; hand-writing usually becomes very small. Depression is common.

TREATMENT

Although there is no cure for Parkinson's disease, much can be done for sufferers to improve their morale and mobility through exercise, special aids in the home, and encouragement. Organizations exist to provide help and advice for sufferers and their families. No other treatment is usually needed during the early stages.

Later, treatment is with drugs, which minimize symptoms but cannot halt the degeneration of brain cells. Such treatment is often complex because several different types of drugs may need to be administered in various combinations.

Levodopa, which the body converts into *dopamine*, is usually the most effective drug and is often the first to be tried. Its actions may be prolonged if it is combined with benserazide or carbidopa. Treatment with levodopa is usually successful for several years, but its effects gradually wear off. Drugs that may be used in conjunction with, or as substitutes for, levodopa include *amantadine, bromocriptine,* selegiline, and lysuride.

The second main class of drug used is *anticholinergic* agents. Benzhexol and *orphenadrine* reduce tremor and rigidity but cause side-effects such as blurred vision, dry mouth, and difficulty passing urine. They may prove effective, however, as the first treatment for mild symptoms, or in addition to levodopa.

Surgical operations on the brain to reduce tremor and rigidity are little used nowadays but are sometimes recommended for young, active people in otherwise good health. Research began in the 1980s into transplantation of dopamine-secreting tissues into the brain—either the patient's own adrenal glands or tissue taken from fetuses after abortion. The results have been very variable, and the procedure is still at an experimental stage.

OUTLOOK

Untreated, the disease progresses over 10 to 15 years to severe weakness and incapacity. However, with modern drug treatment, patients can obtain considerable relief from the illness and a much improved quality of life. About one third of sufferers eventually show signs of *dementia*.

Paronychia

An infection of the skin fold at the base or side of the *nail*. Paronychia may be acute or chronic. The acute

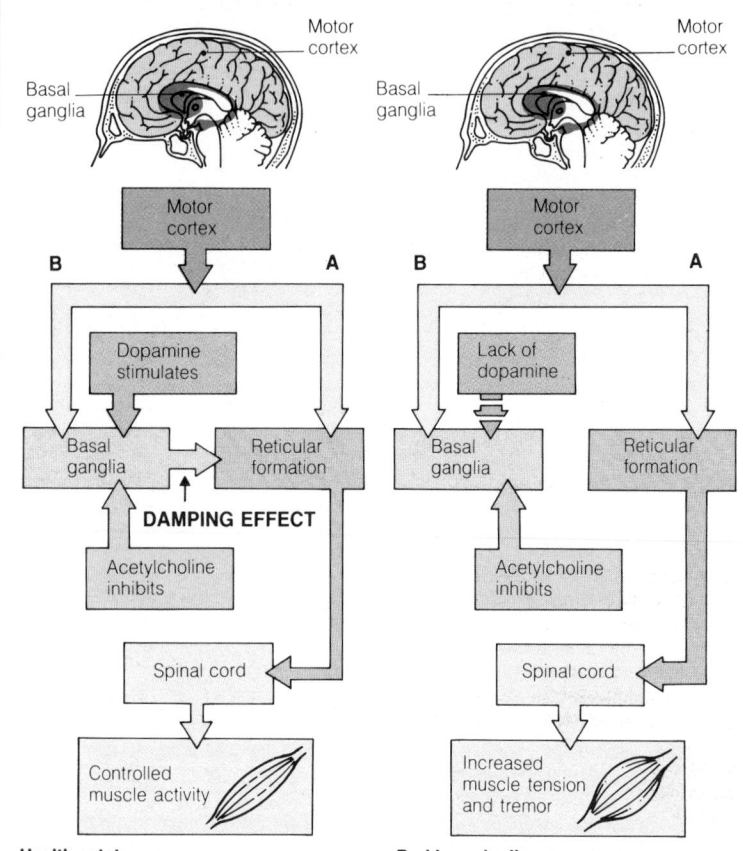

CAUSE OF PARKINSON'S DISEASE

This disorder results from damage, of unknown origin, to the basal ganglia (nerve cell clusters in the brain). The difference between the healthy state and Parkinson's disease is shown below.

Healthy state
During movement, signals pass from the brain's cortex, via the reticular formation and spinal cord (pathway A), to muscles, which contract. Other signals pass, by pathway B, to the basal ganglia; these damp the signals in pathway A, reducing muscle tone so that movement is not jerky. Dopamine, a nerve transmitter made in the basal ganglia, is needed for this damping effect. Another transmitter, acetylcholine, inhibits the damping effect.

Parkinson's disease
In Parkinson's disease, degeneration of parts of the basal ganglia causes a lack of dopamine within this part of the brain. The basal ganglia are thus prevented from modifying the nerve pathways that control muscle contraction. As a result, the muscles are too tense, causing tremor, joint rigidity, and slow movement. Most drug treatments increase the level of dopamine in the brain or oppose the action of acetylcholine.

form is usually caused by bacteria. Chronic paronychia is usually caused by CANDIDA ALBICANS (a yeast).

The condition is most common in women—particularly those who have poor circulation and whose work involves frequent contact with water. Paronychia is also likely to develop in people with skin disease that affects the nail fold.

Treatment is with *antifungal drugs* or *antibiotic drugs*. It is important to keep the hands as dry as possible (by

wearing rubber gloves for wet work and by drying the hands thoroughly each time they are washed). If an abscess forms, surgical drainage may be necessary.

Parotid glands

The largest of the three pairs of *salivary glands* (the other two are the sublingual glands and the submandibular glands). The parotid glands lie, one on each side, above the angle of the jaw, below and in front of the ear. The

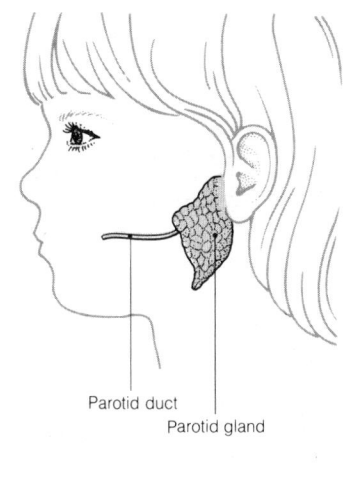

Parotid duct
Parotid gland

parotid glands continuously secrete saliva, which passes along the duct of the gland and into the mouth through an opening in the inner cheek, level with the second upper molar tooth. The output of saliva is increased by the thought, sight, or smell of food.

DISORDERS
Certain conditions, including *dehydration* and *Sjögren's syndrome*, may cause reduced secretion of saliva by the gland, resulting in a dry mouth (see *Mouth, dry*).

Parotitis, inflammation of one or both glands, is usually due to infection with the *mumps* virus but may also be caused by a bacterial infection due to poor oral hygiene, by dehydration, or by severe illness. In some cases, an *abscess* forms in the gland.

Calculi (stones) may block the duct of the parotid gland, causing a painful swelling of the gland. Painless enlargement may be caused by *sarcoidosis*, *tuberculosis*, a *lymphoma*, or a benign tumour. Rarely, carcinoma (a type of malignant *tumour*) of the gland causes a hard, painful growth.

Paroxysm
A sudden attack, worsening, or recurrence of symptoms or of a disease; a *spasm* or *seizure*.

Parturition
The process of giving birth (see *Childbirth*).

Parrot fever
A common name for *psittacosis*.

Pasteurization
The process of heating foods, usually milk and milk products, to destroy pathogenic (disease-causing) micro-organisms and to reduce the number of nonpathogenic organisms, thus protecting against putrefaction and fermentation. The process is named after its inventor, the French scientist Louis Pasteur (1822-1895).

For milk, the conditions are specified by law. Batch pasteurization involves keeping the milk for 30 minutes at a temperature between 62.8°C and 65.6°C. In continuous pasteurization, known as the high-temperature short-time process (HTST), the milk is held for at least 15 seconds at a temperature of at least 71.7°C. Other foods, such as ham, may also be pasteurized to preserve them. In general, pasteurization is preferred to sterilization, which changes the taste and texture of foods.

Patella
The medical name for the kneecap, the triangular bone at the front of the *knee*. The patella is held in position by the lower end of the *quadriceps muscle* (the main muscle at the front of the thigh), and by the patellar tendon, which attaches it to the tibia (shin).

DISORDERS
Dislocation of the patella is usually due to a congenital abnormality, such as underdevelopment of the lower end of the femur (thigh bone) or excessive laxity of ligaments that support the knee. Fracture is usually caused by a direct blow.

Inflammation and roughening of the undersurface of the patella, resulting in knee pain that worsens when bending the knee or climbing stairs, is caused by *chondromalacia patellae* in adolescents and by *arthritis* in adults.

Patent
A term meaning open or unobstructed, as in *patent ductus arteriosus*, a condition in which the ductus arteriosus (a blood vessel that enables blood to bypass the lungs in the fetus) remains open after birth.

The term patent medicine is sometimes used to refer to proprietary drugs protected by a patent.

Patent ductus arteriosus
A *heart* defect in which the ductus arteriosus fails to close at birth. Patent ductus arteriosus accounts for about eight per cent of all heart defects present from birth (see *Heart disease, congenital*), affecting about 60 babies per 100,000.

CAUSES
The ductus arteriosus is a channel between the pulmonary artery and the aorta (two large vessels emerging from the heart). In the fetus, blood pumped by the right side of the heart flows through the ductus arteriosus and bypasses the lungs (see *Fetal circulation*). At or shortly after birth, the ductus usually closes and blood passes to the lungs. In some babies born prematurely or with breathing difficulties, or in babies whose ductus has an abnormal structure, this closure may fail to happen, producing a patent ductus arteriosus. Some of the blood pumped by the left side of the heart and intended for the body is directed via the ductus to the lungs. As a result, the heart must work harder to pump sufficient blood to the body.

SYMPTOMS AND SIGNS
Usually, the defect is not severe enough to cause symptoms. Occasionally, however, when a large amount of blood is misdirected, strain is placed on the heart; as a result, the baby fails to gain weight, becomes short of breath on exertion, and may have frequent chest infections. Eventually, *heart failure* (reduced pumping efficiency) may develop.

DIAGNOSIS AND TREATMENT
The diagnosis is made from hearing a characteristic *murmur* through a stethoscope, from *chest X-rays*, and from an *ECG* and *echocardiography*.

The drug indomethacin often causes the duct to close in premature babies. If this treatment fails, the channel is closed surgically. The operation is straightforward, carries little risk, and enables the child to thrive normally.

Paternity testing
The use of blood tests to help decide whether a particular man is or is not the father of a particular child. Tests are carried out on blood samples taken from the child, from the man who is suspected to be the father, and, sometimes from the child's mother.

WHY IT IS DONE
The investigation may be requested, or ordered by a court, in any of various legal situations in which the paternity of a child is disputed.

HOW IT IS DONE
The blood samples are examined for the presence of various genetically

P

determined substances. These substances may include the proteins found on the surface of red blood cells that determine *blood groups*, other proteins in the blood plasma, *histocompatibility antigens*, and short lengths of *DNA*, the genetic material itself. Comparison of these genetic markers in the different blood samples can provide useful information. For example, if a particular marker is present in the child but not in the mother, it must be determined by a gene present in the real father. If the man who is claimed to be the father does not display this marker in his blood, he can be excluded from paternity.

Techniques have advanced to the stage where it is now possible, through extensive tests, to exclude a wrongly named father in nearly 100 per cent of cases. Until recently it was never possible to prove beyond reasonable doubt that a man was the father of a particular child; the new technique of *genetic fingerprinting* (see illustrated box) has dramatically changed this situation. Using this technique, an investigator may be able to state that the similarities between a man and a child's DNA could have occurred by chance with a probability of just one in 30 thousand million, which would amount to positive proof of paternity.

Patho-
A prefix denoting a relationship to disease, as in pathogen, a disease-causing agent.

Pathogen
Any agent, particularly a *microorganism* (and particularly a parasite bacterium), that causes disease.

Pathogenesis
The processes by which a disease (or disorder) originates and develops. Pathogenesis applies particularly to the cellular and physiological events involved in these processes.

Pathognomonic
A medical term applied to a symptom or sign that is itself characteristic of a specific disease or disorder, and is therefore sufficient to establish a diagnosis. For example, Koplik's spots (small red spots with white centres) on the lining of the mouth are pathognomonic of measles.

Pathological
Relating to disease or to *pathology* (the study of disease).

PATERNITY TESTING USING GENETIC FINGERPRINTING
Genetic fingerprinting is replacing older techniques of paternity testing because it gives a decisive result in more cases.

Blood samples are taken from the mother, child, and suspected father, and some DNA (hereditary material) from each is specially processed.

PATERNITY ESTABLISHED

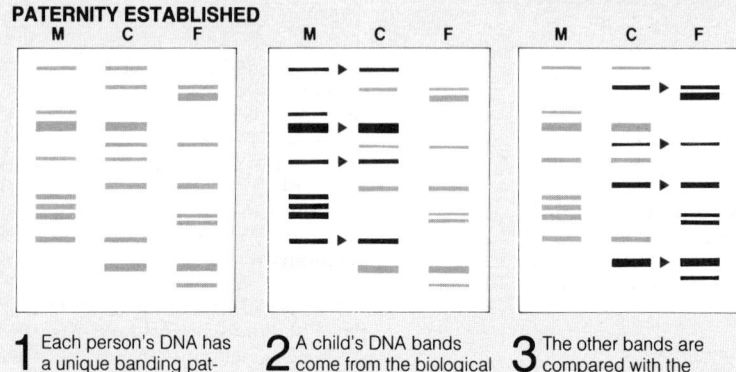

1 Each person's DNA has a unique banding pattern, or "fingerprint", detectable by X-rays after the processing.

2 A child's DNA bands come from the biological parents. First the bands from the mother are identified.

3 The other bands are compared with the suspected father's bands. Here they match, proving paternity.

PATERNITY DISPROVED

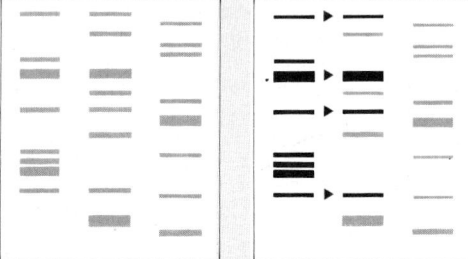

1 The mother's, child's, and suspected father's DNA have different banding patterns.

2 Half the child's DNA bands can be seen to have come from the mother, as before.

3 The other bands are not shared by the suspected father, meaning he is not the biological father.

Key   **M** = Mother   **C** = Child   **F** = Father

Pathology
The study of disease, its causes, mechanisms, and effects on the body. Various factors can cause pathological changes in tissues and cells. These factors include pathogens (disease-causing microorganisms), poisonous chemicals, *radiation*, *inflammation*, degeneration (see *Degenerative disorders*), the accumulation of abnormal substances (see *Infiltrate*), metabolic defects (see *Metabolic disorders; Metabolism, inborn errors of*), *nutritional disorders*, and *carcinogens* (agents that cause *cancer*).

The study of the pathological changes that occur in cells is known as cytopathology (a branch of *cytology*);

histopathology (a branch of *histology*) is concerned with changes in tissues. Both rely on examining cell or tissue samples under the *microscope*.

A doctor who specializes in this subject is called a pathologist. Pathologists conduct the laboratory studies of tissues and cells that help other doctors reach accurate diagnoses, and supervise other laboratory personnel in the testing and microscopic examination of blood and other body fluids.

Pathologists are resposible for conducting autopsies to determine causes of death and to determine what effects a disease or a particular type of treatment has had on the body. It was the growth of postmortem pathology in

P

the 18th and 19th centuries that formed the basis of modern scientific medicine. Study of the body after death enabled a patient's symptoms to be linked with observable changes in the internal organs. It also made it possible for doctors to assess the accuracy of their diagnoses and the effects of their treatment.

Pathology, cellular
Also called cytopathology, the branch of *cytology* concerned with the effects of disease on cells.

Pathology, chemical
Also called clinical biochemistry, the branch of pathology concerned with examining abnormalities in the chemistry of body tissues in disease.

Pathophysiology
The study of the effects of disease on body functions (e.g. how bronchitis impairs lung function).

-pathy
A suffix that denotes a disease or disorder, as in myopathy, any disorder of the muscles.

Peak-flow meter
A piece of equipment that measures the maximum speed at which air can flow out of the lungs. Because narrowed airways slow the rate at which air can be forced from the lungs, a peak-flow meter is useful in assessing the severity of *bronchospasm* (narrowing of the airways in the lungs).

The most common use of a peak-flow meter is to monitor patients with *asthma* and to assess their response to treatment with *bronchodilator drugs*. A peak-flow meter is also useful in confirming whether people with intermittent coughing or breathing difficulty without wheezing have asthma.

People with asthma are encouraged to measure their peak flow every day as a means of monitoring their health, just as diabetics measure their blood sugar level. A diary of readings is kept to record the difference in airflow when symptoms are present and during other times in the day.

The peak flow is measured by taking a deep breath in and then breathing out with maximum effort through the mouthpiece of the meter.

Peau d'orange
A condition in which the skin resembles orange peel. The skin remains a normal colour but develops a dimpled appearance due to retention of fluid in the nearby lymph vessels. Causes of blockage of the lymph vessels include *breast cancer* in the region of the nipple and *elephantiasis*.

Pectoral
A medical term that means relating to the chest, as in the major and minor pectoral muscles.

The pectoralis major is a large, fan-shaped muscle that covers much of the upper part of the front of the chest; it arises from the sternum (breastbone) and cartilages of the second to sixth ribs, and converges on the humerus (upper-arm bone) just below the shoulder. The main function of the pectoralis major is to move the arm across the body.

The pectoralis minor is a smaller, triangular muscle that underlies the pectoralis major; it arises from the third to fifth ribs, and converges on the scapula (shoulderblade), which it moves down and forwards.

Pediculosis
Any type of louse infestation. (See *Lice*; *Pubic lice*.)

Peer review
Processes by which doctors and other scientists review the work, decisions, and writings of their colleagues. Reviewers, who often work anonymously, are commonly known as referees. Manuscripts submitted to scientific journals and requests for research grants are almost always assessed by a process of peer review.

Pellagra
A potentially fatal nutritional disorder caused by niacin deficiency (see *Vitamin B complex*), resulting in dermatitis, diarrhoea, and dementia. Pellagra occurs primarily in poor rural communities in parts of India and southern Africa where people subsist on maize.

CAUSES
Although the niacin content of maize is no lower than that of some other cereals, much of the vitamin occurs in an unabsorbable form unless it is first treated with an alkali such as lime water. (People living in communities in Mexico who prepare the cereal in this way before making tortillas do not suffer from the disease.)

Maize is also low in tryptophan, an amino acid converted into niacin in the body. Disorders such as *carcinoid syndrome* (which increases the breakdown of tryptophan) and *inflammatory bowel disease* (which reduces its absorption from the intestine) may also be a cause.

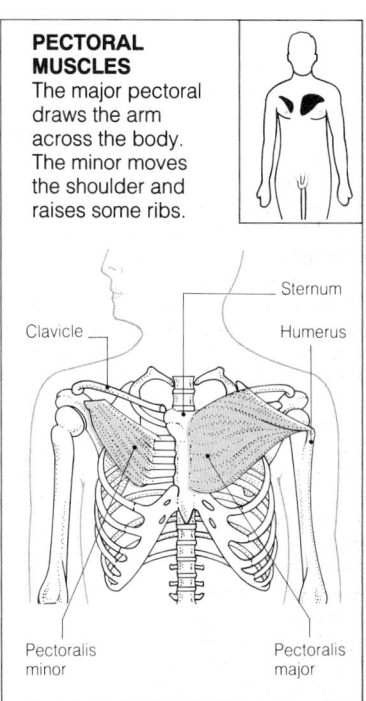

PECTORAL MUSCLES
The major pectoral draws the arm across the body. The minor moves the shoulder and raises some ribs.

Sternum
Clavicle
Humerus
Pectoralis minor
Pectoralis major

SYMPTOMS
The first symptoms are weakness, weight loss, lethargy, depression, irritability, and inflammation and itching where the skin is exposed to sunlight. In acute attacks, weeping (leaking) blisters may develop on the affected skin; the tongue becomes bright red, swollen, and painful.

DIAGNOSIS AND TREATMENT
Pellagra is diagnosed from the patient's condition and dietary history. Daily intake of niacin and a varied diet rich in protein and energy are usually enough to bring about a complete cure.

Pelvic examination
Examination of a woman's external and internal genitalia. A pelvic examination may be performed as part of a general *physical examination*, during contraceptive counselling, or to investigate the cause of symptoms such as abdominal pain, vaginal bleeding or discharge, urinary incontinence, or infertility. During labour, it is performed to help assess the position, descent, and well-being of the baby.

The main aspects of a pelvic examination are shown in the illustrated box on the next page.

Pelvic floor exercises
A programme of exercises to strengthen the muscles and tighten the ligaments at the base of the abdomen.

PROCEDURE FOR PELVIC EXAMINATION

The examination is usually performed with the woman lying on her back with knees bent. If it is carried out because of uterine prolapse or incontinence, she may be asked to lie on her side. The doctor usually begins by inspecting the external genitals for ulceration or swelling and then does an internal examination.

Use of speculum
A speculum is inserted into the vagina to hold apart the vaginal walls; this gives the doctor a clear view of both the vagina and cervix. A *cervical smear* test may also be performed at this time.

Manual examination
The doctor inserts two fingers into the vagina and palpates (feels) the abdomen to evaluate the size and position of the uterus and ovaries, and to detect any abnormal pelvic swelling or tenderness.

These muscles and ligaments, which form the pelvic floor, support the uterus, vagina, bladder, urethra, and rectum. Slackening of the pelvic floor is common during childbirth and is also a part of the aging process.

Performing pelvic floor exercises, especially during pregnancy and following childbirth, tones these structures and may help to prevent prolapse of the uterus (see *Uterus, prolapse of*) and urinary stress incontinence (see *Incontinence, urinary*). Pelvic floor exercises can also sometimes help women who are having difficulty achieving orgasm.

One exercise, carried out during urination, involves stopping and starting the flow of urine several times by contracting and then relaxing the muscles around the vagina, each time for a count of six. Another exercise involves placing two fingers inside the vagina and contracting the muscles around the fingers. The exercises should be done two or three times a day for at least a month.

Pelvic infection

An infection in the female reproductive system. Severe or recurrent pelvic infection is referred to as *pelvic inflammatory disease* (PID). Pelvic infection can result in damage to the fallopian tubes and can cause female *infertility*.

Occasionally, conditions affecting surrounding organs, such as *inflammatory bowel disease*, can damage the female genital tract.

Pelvic inflammatory disease

Infection of the internal female reproductive organs. Pelvic inflammatory disease (PID) is a common cause of pelvic pain in women. The infection may not have any obvious cause, but often occurs after a sexually transmitted disease, such as a *chlamydial infection* or *gonorrhoea*. PID may also occur after miscarriage, abortion, or childbirth. *IUD* users have a higher incidence of PID, as do young, sexually active women.

SYMPTOMS AND SIGNS

Abdominal pain and tenderness, fever, and irregular menstrual periods are common symptoms of PID. The pain often occurs immediately after menstruation and may be worse during intercourse. There may also be malaise, vomiting, or backache.

DIAGNOSIS AND TREATMENT

The doctor may detect tenderness on internal pelvic examination and will take swabs to identify microorganisms that may be causing the condition. A *laparoscopy* (examination of the abdominal cavity using a viewing instrument) may be performed to confirm the diagnosis or to detect any abscess.

Antibiotic drugs are prescribed to clear the infection, and *analgesic drugs* (painkillers) may also be required. If the woman has an IUD, it may need to be removed.

OUTLOOK

Some women have repeated attacks of PID with or without reinfection. PID may cause *infertility* or increase the risk of *ectopic pregnancy*, primarily due to scarring in the fallopian tubes that prevents the egg from travelling down the tube into the uterus.

Pelvic pain

See *Abdominal pain*.

Pelvimetry

Assessment of the shape and dimensions of a woman's pelvis. Pelvimetry is most commonly carried out in about the 37th week of pregnancy to determine whether a woman is likely to have difficulty delivering her baby. Pelvimetry may also be performed after childbirth in women who have required a caesarean section. Such assessment determines whether future deliveries should be vaginal or by caesarean section.

A rough indication of the size of the pelvic outlet can be obtained by manually checking the distance between the ischial tuberosities (the prominent bones in the lower pelvis) during a pelvic examination. More precise measurement is possible using radiological pelvimetry (use of *X-rays* to assess pelvic dimensions).

However, excessive exposure to X-rays in pregnancy may increase the risk of subsequent development of leukaemia or other cancers in unborn children. The procedure is therefore carried out only in certain circumstances, such as a breech presentation, even though the X-ray exposure involved in pelvimetry is minimal.

Pelvis

The ring of bones in the lower trunk, bounded by the coccyx and the hip-bones. The pelvis protects abdominal organs, such as the bladder, rectum, and, in women, the uterus.

STRUCTURE

The pelvis consists of two innominate bones (hip-bones), which are joined by rigid sacroiliac joints to the sacrum (the triangular spinal bone below the lumbar vertebrae) at the back; the hip-bones curve forwards to join at the pubic symphysis at the front. Attached to the pelvis are the muscles of the abdominal wall, the buttocks, the lower back, and the insides and backs of the thighs.

Each innominate bone consists of three fused bones: the ilium, ischium, and pubis. The ilium, the largest and uppermost of these bones, consists of a wide, flattened plate with a long curved ridge (called the iliac crest) along its upper border. The ischium is the bone that bears much of the body weight when sitting. The pubis is the smallest pelvic bone; from the ischium it extends forwards and round to the pubic symphysis, where it is joined to the other pubis bone by tough fibrous tissue. All three bones meet in the acetabulum, the cup-shaped cavity that forms the socket of the hip joint.

The pelvis differs considerably between men and women. In women, the pelvis is generally shallow and broad, and the pubic symphysis joint is less rigid than a man's. These differences facilitate childbirth. In men, the pelvis is usually larger and built more heavily to bear a greater body weight.

DISORDERS

Fractures of the pelvis may be caused by a direct blow, or by a force transmitted through the femur (thighbone). Considerable force is required to cause such a fracture, and it is usually the result of a motor vehicle accident; motorcycle riders are particularly at risk. The fracture itself often heals without problems, but it is frequently accompanied by damage to internal organs within the pelvis, especially the bladder, which may require immediate surgical treatment.

STRUCTURE OF THE PELVIS

The pelvis is a basin-shaped bony structure at the base of the trunk. It consists of the sacrum and coccyx at the back and, at the sides, the two hip-bones, which curve around to meet at the front. The pelvis supports the upper half of the body and protects the lower abdominal organs. The female pelvis is shallower and wider.

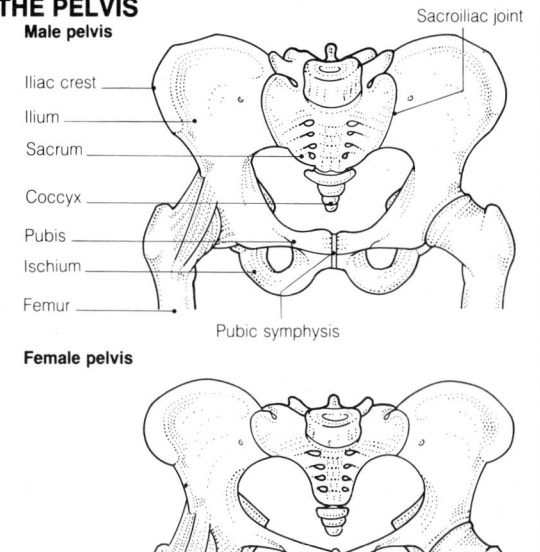

Male pelvis

Iliac crest
Ilium
Sacrum
Coccyx
Pubis
Ischium
Femur

Sacroiliac joint

Pubic symphysis

Female pelvis

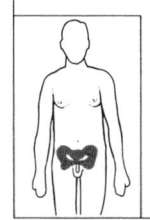

Osteitis pubis (inflammation of the pubic symphysis) is usually caused by repeated stress on the pelvis. It is most common in soccer players as a result of continually kicking a ball. The symptoms include pain in the groin and tenderness over the front of the pelvis. In most cases, the condition clears up with rest.

Pemphigoid

An uncommon, chronic skin disease in which large blisters form on the skin. The blisters in pemphigoid are sometimes intensely itchy, unlike those in *pemphigus*, a similar but more serious disorder. Pemphigoid, which is considered to be an *autoimmune disorder* (one in which the body reacts against its own tissues), primarily affects elderly people.

The diagnosis is confirmed by a skin *biopsy* (removal of a small sample of tissue for microscopic analysis). Treatment is usually a long-term course of *corticosteroid drugs* or, in some cases, *immunosuppressant drugs*.

Pemphigus

An uncommon, serious skin disease in which blisters appear on the skin and on mucous membranes in the mouth and sometimes elsewhere. Pemphigus primarily affects people between the ages of 40 and 60.

SYMPTOMS AND SIGNS

The blisters usually begin in the mouth, and sometimes in the nose, and then appear on the skin. They rupture easily, forming raw, often painful areas that may become infected and that later crust over. Apparently unaffected skin may also blister after gentle pressure. When the blisters occur over a great area of the body, the resultant severe skin loss can lead to secondary bacterial infection and, sometimes, death.

DIAGNOSIS AND TREATMENT

A diagnosis of pemphigus is confirmed by a skin *biopsy* (removal of a small sample of tissue for microscopic analysis).

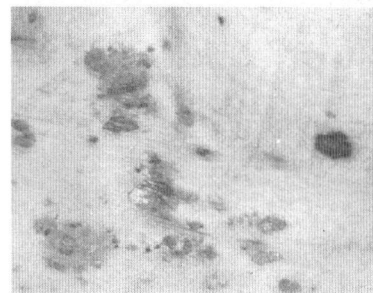

Pemphigus on the back
The typical appearance is of numerous large, raw areas of skin where the fragile blisters have broken down.

P

787

The usual treatment is with *cortico-steroid drugs* given over long periods to keep the disease under control. Other *immunosuppressant drugs* may also help. *Antibiotic drugs* may need to be taken for secondary infections.

Penicillamine

An *antirheumatic drug* sometimes used to treat *rheumatoid arthritis* when symptoms are severe and not relieved by *nonsteroidal anti-inflammatory drugs* (NSAIDs).

Penicillamine is also a *chelating agent* used in the treatment of copper, mercury, lead, or arsenic poisoning. It is used to treat *Wilson's disease* (a rare brain and liver disorder caused by copper deposits in these tissues), primary *biliary cirrhosis* (a liver disorder), and has also been given to people with cystinuria (excessive excretion of cystine in the urine) to prevent stones from forming in the urinary tract.

Penicillamine is not a *penicillin drug*.

POSSIBLE ADVERSE EFFECTS
Penicillamine frequently causes allergic rashes, itching, nausea, vomiting, abdominal pain, and loss of taste. Infrequently, it causes blood disorders or impaired kidney function. Regular blood and urine tests are carried out during treatment.

Penicillin drugs

COMMON DRUGS

Amoxycillin Ampicillin Benzylpenicillin Flucloxacillin Phenoxymethylpenicillin

The first group of *antibiotic drugs* to be discovered. Natural penicillins are derived from the mould PENICILLIUM; other penicillin drugs are synthetic preparations.

Penicillin drugs are used in the treatment of many infections, including *tonsillitis*, *pharyngitis*, *bronchitis*, and *pneumonia*. Penicillins are also given to prevent the recurrence of *rheumatic fever* and to treat bacterial *endocarditis*, *syphilis*, *gonorrhoea*, and acute ulcerative *gingivitis*.

POSSIBLE ADVERSE EFFECTS
The most common adverse effect is an allergic reaction that causes a rash. Any person who has had an allergic reaction to one type of penicillin is not usually prescribed any other type. Another common adverse effect of penicillin drugs is diarrhoea.

Penile implant

A prosthesis inserted into the *penis* to help a man suffering from *impotence* to achieve intercourse. Penile implants

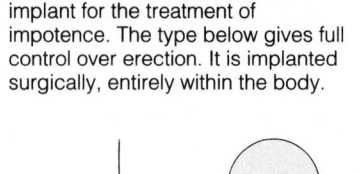

INFLATABLE PENILE IMPLANT

There are various types of penile implant for the treatment of impotence. The type below gives full control over erection. It is implanted surgically, entirely within the body.

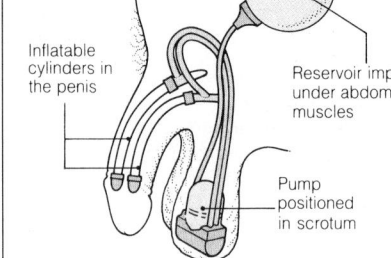

Liquid is pumped from the reservoir

Cylinders fill

Inflatable cylinders in the penis

Reservoir implanted under abdominal muscles

Pump squeezed with fingers

Pump positioned in scrotum

Operation
The device is operated by squeezing the pump in the scrotum. Fluid flows from the reservoir and inflates the cylinders. A small release valve on the pump is pressed to allow the penis to return to a flaccid state.

are usually used only for men who are permanently impotent.

One treatment involves inserting a silicone splint in the tissues of the upper surface of the penis. The penis can be inserted into the vagina, but does not increase in size.

Alternatively, an inflatable prosthesis may be implanted in the penis. This type makes the penis larger and firmer for intercourse and is operated by squeezing a small bulb placed in the scrotum.

Penile warts

See *Warts, genital*.

Penis

The male sex organ through which urine and semen pass. The penis consists mainly of three cylindrical bodies of erectile tissue (spongy tissue full of tiny blood vessels) that run the length of the organ. Two of these bodies, the corpora cavernosa, lie side by side in the upper part of the penis. The third, the corpus spongiosum, lies centrally beneath them, expanding at its end to form the tip of the penis, the glans.

Through the centre of the corpus spongiosum runs the *urethra*, a narrow tube that carries urine and semen out of the body through an opening at the tip of the glans. Surrounding the erectile tissue is a sheath of fibrous connective tissue enclosed by skin. Over the glans, the skin forms a loose fold called the *foreskin*, which is sometimes removed (see *Circumcision*).

DISORDERS
The most common congenital abnormality of the penis is *hypospadias*, in which the urethra opens on the undersurface of the penis anywhere from the base of the glans to the root. In male *pseudohermaphroditism*, which

ANATOMY OF THE PENIS

The corpora cavernosa and spongiosum are the erectile tissues of the penis. A network of nerves controls the blood flow into them.

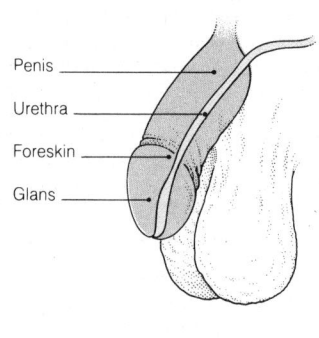

Penis

Urethra

Foreskin

Glans

Cross-section of penis

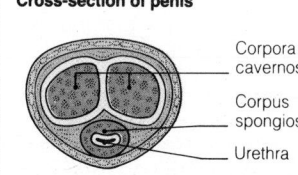

Corpora cavernosa

Corpus spongiosum

Urethra

P

is also a congenital problem, the penis is very small and there is usually also hypospadias.

Balanitis (inflammation of the glans and foreskin) is usually caused by *candidiasis,* although other organisms, including those that cause *gonorrhoea* and *syphilis,* may cause inflammation. Balanitis may lead to *phimosis,* in which the foreskin is abnormally tight, or *paraphimosis,* in which the foreskin retracts at erection but is too tight to move back over the glans.

Penile warts (see *Warts, genital*) are caused by a sexually transmitted virus. Cancer of the penis (see *Penis, cancer of*) is a rare disorder; the incidence is higher in uncircumcised than in circumcised men.

Impotence (failure to attain or maintain an erection) is usually psychological in origin. However, it may be caused by nerve damage associated with *diabetes mellitus, alcohol dependence, atherosclerosis,* or spinal cord injury. Other disorders of the penis include *priapism,* in which an erection is painful and abnormally prolonged, and *Peyronie's disease,* in which the erect penis bends to one side.

Penis, cancer of

A rare form of malignant tumour that is more common in uncircumcised men whose personal hygiene is poor. Viral infection and smoking have both been shown to be additional factors.

The tumour usually starts on the glans (head) of the penis or on the foreskin as a dry, painless, wart-like lump or a painful ulcer, and develops into a cauliflower-like mass. The growth usually spreads slowly, but a highly malignant tumour can spread to the lymphatic glands in the groin within a few months; the glands swell and the skin over them may ulcerate.

Any growth or sore area on the penis that persists for more than two or three weeks should be reported to a doctor. A *biopsy* (removal of a sample of tissue for microscopic analysis) will show whether the condition is due to cancer or to some other cause, such as warts (see *Warts, genital*) or *syphilis.*

Cancer of the penis can generally be treated successfully by *radiotherapy* if it is reported early. Otherwise, surgical removal of part or all of the penis may be necessary.

Pentazocine

A narcotic *analgesic drug* (painkiller) used to relieve moderate or severe pain caused by injury, surgery, cancer, or childbirth.

Possible adverse affects are typical of other narcotic analgesics; they include dizziness, drowsiness, nausea, vomiting, and, rarely, hallucinations. Dependence may develop in people taking high doses for prolonged periods.

Peppermint oil

An oil obtained from the peppermint plant MENTHA PIPERITA. Peppermint oil is prescribed to relieve abdominal colic, particularly in *irritable bowel syndrome.* It may occasionally cause *heartburn.* Peppermint oil is also used as a flavouring in some drug preparations.

Pep pills

A popular name for *stimulant drugs,* particularly *amphetamine drugs.*

Peptic ulcer

A raw area that occurs in the gastrointestinal tract as a result of erosion by acidic gastric juice. Peptic ulcers may occur in the oesophagus, stomach, or duodenum. Rarely, they develop in the jejunum (as occurs in *Zollinger-Ellison syndrome*) or in the ileum (as may occur in *Meckel's diverticulum*). They may be single or multiple, and usually measure about 10 to 25 mm across and about 0.25 mm deep. The typical symptom is a gnawing pain in the abdomen when the stomach is empty.

CAUSES AND INCIDENCE

The lining of the stomach and duodenum is constantly at risk of erosion from the acidic digestive juices. It may be damaged by infection with a bacterium, HELICOBACTER PYLORI, found in the stomachs of around 40 per cent of healthy people but almost 100 per cent of those with peptic ulcers. Infection with helicobacter is much more common in people living in poor socioeconomic conditions. It has been found in 80 per cent of 20-year-olds in countries in Eastern Europe and Asia. In these countries peptic ulcers (and stomach cancers) are also much more common than in Western countries.

Ulcers form in the oesophagus only when acidic juice from the stomach enters it (see *Acid reflux*). Peptic ulcers form in the jejunum when there is a massive outpouring of gastric acid.

Some of the main factors that may be involved in causing peptic ulcer are shown in the illustrated box overleaf. In some people, there is a strong family history of peptic ulceration. Psychological stress may play a part in making an existing ulcer worse.

In the UK, a duodenal ulcer develops in about one in 10 people at some time in their lives; a gastric ulcer

develops in about one in 30. The incidence is about equal in men and women, but more males than females suffer from duodenal ulcers. Middle age is the most likely time for either type of ulcer to develop, although the peak age for the development of duodenal ulcers is somewhat earlier than the peak age for gastric ulcers.

SYMPTOMS

Many people found to have a peptic ulcer suffer no symptoms, but a greater number complain of a burning or gnawing pain in the abdomen, which sometimes wakes them at night. The pain of a duodenal ulcer is often relieved by eating, but usually recurs a few hours later.

Other symptoms accompanying both types of ulcer include loss of appetite (although in some cases a duodenal ulcer increases the appetite), belching, feeling bloated, weight loss, nausea, and vomiting (which usually relieves the pain).

COMPLICATIONS

The most common complication of a peptic ulcer is bleeding from the ulcer. Severe bleeding results in haematemesis (vomiting of blood) and melaena (black faeces), and is a medical emergency. Chronic bleeding may cause iron-deficiency *anaemia.*

Rarely, an ulcer may perforate the wall of the digestive tract and extend to the pancreas, usually causing pain that spreads through to the back. If digestive juices leak through the perforation or if the perforation is on the front wall of the duodenum, the juices may cause *peritonitis* (inflammation of the abdominal lining), producing sudden, severe pain and requiring emergency hospital admission.

Chronic ulcers can cause extensive scarring of the stomach or duodenum, which may narrow the outlet of the stomach into the duodenum (a condition called *pyloric stenosis*) and thus obstruct the passage of food. This may cause vomiting and rapid weight loss.

A small number of gastric ulcers are malignant and should be removed as soon as they are diagnosed.

DIAGNOSIS

The condition can be diagnosed with certainty only after an *endoscopy* (inspection through a viewing instrument) of the stomach and duodenum, which is now standard in most cases. However, a *barium X-ray* may still be preferred in certain circumstances.

TREATMENT

Antacid drugs neutralize excess acidity and assist in the healing of ulcers. Such drugs ultimately relieve pain if

P

SITES AND CAUSES OF PEPTIC ULCER

A peptic ulcer develops in about one in eight people in the UK at some time in their lives. Some of the mechanisms involved in causing ulcers are shown below. Most ulcers respond to self-help measures or to drug treatment, but occasionally surgery is necessary.

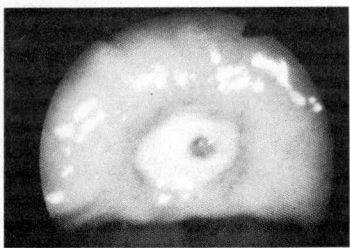

Gastric ulcer
This photograph of an ulcer in the wall of the stomach was taken via a viewing tube passed down the oesophagus.

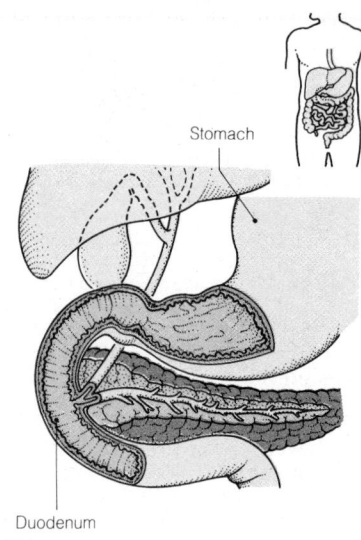

Stomach

Duodenum

Site of ulcers
Peptic ulcers are most common in the first part of the duodenum or lower half of the stomach; oesophageal ulcers also occur.

ULCER CARE

Self-help methods

Avoid smoking, the most important step in self-help.

Avoid drinking alcohol, coffee, and tea.

Avoid using aspirin and nonsteroidal anti-inflammatory drugs.

Eat several small meals a day, at regular intervals, rather than two or three large ones.

Drug treatment

Antacids neutralize acid in the stomach.

H_2 blockers, such as ranitidine, cimetidine, and famotidine, reduce acid secretion by blocking receptors on acid-producing cells.

Antibiotics and bismuth eliminate infection with HELICOBACTER PYLORI, which damages the mucosal lining.

HOW AN ULCER IS FORMED

Acid and pepsin   Mucus

Gastric gland   Epithelial cells

1 Gastric glands in the lining of the stomach secrete acid and the enzyme pepsin, which help break down food. The acid and pepsin would quickly eat away the stomach and duodenum if other cells in the lining did not secrete a protective mucus.

Irritants

Alcohol   Bile   Bacteria   Caffeine   Aspirin

Increased acid secretion

Reduced mucus production

2 Peptic ulcers may be caused by damage to the stomach lining from bacterial infection (from the HELICOBACTER PYLORI bacterium), analgesic drugs, or alcohol combined in some cases with excess acid production. Smoking is another important irritant factor.

Protective wall of epithelial cells broken by acid

Ulcer

3 If damaging influences overcome the protective factors in the stomach or duodenal lining, the mucous layer and mucus-secreting cells are eroded and an ulcer forms. Stress is probably not a prime cause of ulcers but may aggravate an existing ulcer.

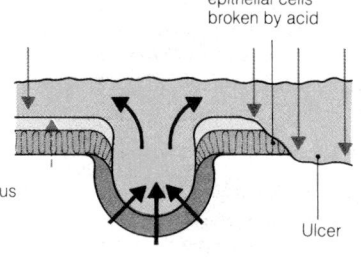

---

taken regularly, and, along with the other self-help measures listed in the illustrated box, may be enough to heal the ulcer. If not, and if symptoms persist, professional treatment will be necessary. This may consist of *antibiotics* and bismuth, to eliminate any infection with HELICOBACTER, or treatment with *ulcer-healing drugs* (such as cimetidine, ranitidine, or famotidine), which reduce acid production.

Either treatment will usually lead to healing of the ulcer and relief of symptoms within six to eight weeks.

If a repeat endoscopy shows that the ulcer has not healed, further treatment may be necessary. Surgery for peptic ulcers is now very rare. If an operation is performed it will usually take the form of a *vagotomy* (cutting of the fibres of the vagus nerve that controls digestive acid production) and pyloroplasty (widening of the outlet of the stomach into the duodenum).

Occasionally, a partial *gastrectomy* (surgical removal of a portion of the stomach) is performed to treat the ulcer and reduce acid production.

Substantial bleeding from an ulcer sometimes requires a *blood transfusion*.

Perforation, peritonitis, or obstruction usually necessitates surgery to correct the problem. In some cases of perforation, however, passing a suction tube into the stomach via the nose to drain off digestive juices may be sufficient treatment. This procedure sometimes allows the perforation to heal of its own accord in the absence of irritation from acidic juices. Peritonitis, however, inevitably requires emergency hospital treatment.

P

Peptide

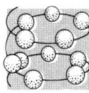

A fragment of protein consisting of two or more *amino acids*. Peptides are formed by the linking of amino acids by chemical bonds (peptide bonds) between the amino and carboxyl groups of adjacent acids. Larger peptides, consisting of many linked amino acids, are known as polypeptides; still longer chains of amino acids, made up of linked polypeptides, are called *proteins*.

Peptides are widely distributed in the body's endocrine and nervous systems. Many *hormones* are peptides, including some *gastrointestinal hormones* and several pituitary hormones, such as *oxytocin*, *ADH* (antidiuretic hormone), and *ACTH* (adrenocorticotrophic hormone). In the nervous system, peptides are found in nerve cells throughout the brain and the spinal cord; examples include *endorphins* and substances involved in the control of the pituitary gland.

Perception

The interpretation of a sensation. People receive information about the environment through the five senses—*taste*, *smell*, *hearing*, *vision*, and *touch*—but the way in which this information is interpreted depends on other factors.

First, the information must be organized into a pattern. In vision, for example, objects must be distinguished from their background and recognized as moving or stationary. Each object then requires identification (e.g. as a chair or a friend), a process that relies on memory. The final interpretation depends on an individual's attitudes, expectations, and mood. Valued objects often appear larger, and hungry people are more likely to notice food sooner than those who have just eaten.

Hallucinations, which are a symptom of *psychosis*, are false perceptions that occur in the absence of sensory stimuli.

Percussion

A diagnostic technique for examining the chest or abdomen by tapping it with the fingers and listening to the resonance of the sound produced. In this way, the condition of internal organs can be deduced. For example, a fluid-filled lung produces a dull note when tapped, and *pneumothorax* (air in the pleural cavity) produces a hollow sound quite distinctive to a doctor. (See also *Examination, physical*.)

Percutaneous

A medical term meaning through the skin. Percutaneous procedures include the injection of drugs into veins, muscles, or other body tissues, and biopsies in which tissue or fluid is removed with a needle.

Perforation

A hole made in an organ or tissue by disease or injury. Among the more common types of perforation due to a disorder are a hole in the wall of the stomach or duodenum (the first part of the small intestine) caused by a *peptic ulcer*, and a rupture of the eardrum, usually caused by middle-ear infection (see *Eardrum, perforated*).

Perforating *wounds* that penetrate through outer layers of tissue to damage an internal organ or cavity usually require exploratory surgery to check for and remove any foreign material.

Peri-

A prefix meaning around, as in pericardium, the membranous sac that surrounds the heart.

Pericarditis

Inflammation of the *pericardium* (the membrane that surrounds the *heart*), leading, in many cases, to chest pain and fever. In addition to inflammation, there may be an effusion (increased amount of fluid) in the pericardial space, which separates the two smooth layers of the pericardium. This excess fluid may compress the heart, restricting its action.

Long-standing inflammation can cause constrictive pericarditis, in which the pericardium becomes scarred, thickens, and contracts, interfering with the heart's action.

CAUSES

Pericarditis has many possible causes. These include certain bacterial, viral, and fungal infections; *myocardial infarction* (heart attack); cancer spreading from a nearby tumour in the lung or breast or by way of the blood from a remote site; and injury to the pericardium from a penetrating wound or after *open heart surgery*. Pericarditis sometimes accompanies *rheumatoid arthritis*, systemic *lupus erythematosus*, and *kidney failure*. It can also occur for no known reason.

SYMPTOMS AND SIGNS

The characteristic symptom of pericarditis is pain behind the sternum (breastbone), sometimes spreading to the neck and shoulders. The pain often becomes more severe if the person takes a deep breath, changes posture, or even swallows; sitting up and leaning forwards sometimes relieves it. Fever is another fairly common symptom.

When pericarditis is due to infection, pus may accumulate in the pericardial space. When, rarely, the cause is a tumour, blood may collect there. If heart action is impeded, heart output and blood pressure fall—a condition known as cardiac tamponade. This results in breathing difficulty and in swollen neck veins. The main symptom of constrictive pericarditis is *oedema* (accumulation of fluid in the tissues) of the legs and abdomen, causing them to swell.

DIAGNOSIS

The condition is diagnosed from information obtained during a physical examination (which includes listening to the heart with a stethoscope), and from the result of an *ECG* and chest *X-rays*. *Echocardiography* may be used to confirm that enlargement of the heart shown on X-rays is due to effusion.

TREATMENT

Treatment is aimed at the underlying cause whenever possible. *Analgesic drugs* (painkillers) or *anti-inflammatory drugs* may be given to relieve pain. If effusion is seriously affecting heart action, the excess fluid is drawn off through a needle inserted through the chest wall into the pericardial space.

Severe constrictive pericarditis may require surgical removal of the thickened pericardium.

Pericardium

The membranous bag that completely envelops the *heart* and the roots of the major blood vessels that emerge from the heart. The pericardium has two layers. The outer layer is tough, inelastic, and fibrous. It is attached to the diaphragm below and to the sternum (breastbone) in front. The inner layer is separated into two sheets. Of these, the inner is firmly attached to the heart and the outer is attached to the fibrous layer. The space between the smooth, inner surfaces of these sheets is called the pericardial space. This contains a small quantity of fluid that lubricates the heart.

Perimetry

A visual field test to determine the extent of peripheral vision. Perimetry, which is not usually done as a routine procedure, may be performed to provide vital information in certain neurological disorders, such as a brain tumour (See *Eye, examination of*.)

P

Perinatal

Relating to the period just before or just after birth. Perinatal is often defined more precisely as the period from the 28th week of pregnancy to the end of the first week after birth. Perinatal mortality is a statistical expression of the number of stillbirths and infant deaths occurring during the first week after birth.

Perinatology

A branch of *obstetrics* and *paediatrics* concerned with the study and care of mother and baby during pregnancy and the early days after birth.

The perinatologist specializes in the management of high-risk pregnancies and births, and in the investigation and treatment of prenatal conditions that might endanger the life or well-being of the fetus, such as *Rhesus incompatibility*, *spina bifida*, or some biochemical disorder. The perinatologist is also skilled in the assessment of placental function and in looking after the health of the expectant mother, who herself may for one reason or another be at risk.

Perineum

The area bounded internally by the pelvic floor (the muscles that form the supportive base of the pelvis) and the surrounding bony structures. The perineum is pierced by the genitourinary and digestive organs. Externally, the perineum is represented by the area between the thighs that lies behind the genital organs and in front of the anus.

Periodic fever

An inherited condition causing recurrent bouts of fever. (See *Familial Mediterranean fever*.)

Period, menstrual

See *Menstruation*.

Periodontal disease

Any disorder of the periodontium (the tissues surrounding and supporting the *teeth*). The most common type of periodontal disease is chronic *gingivitis* (inflammation of the *gums*), which, if untreated, leads to *periodontitis* (inflammation of the periodontal membranes around the base of the teeth and erosion of the bone holding the teeth).

Periodontics

The branch of *dentistry* that is concerned with the study and treatment of diseases that affect the periodontium, (the structures that surround and support the teeth), particularly *gingivitis* (inflammation of the *gums*) and *periodontitis* (inflammation of the periodontium).

A periodontist makes considerable use of *dental X-rays* in diagnosis (to detect loss of bony support in which the teeth are embedded) and is concerned with *preventive dentistry*. Treatment includes dental *scaling*, dental *curettage*, *gingivectomy*, and root planing (removal of *calculus* from the root surface).

Periodontitis

Inflammation of the periodontium (the tissues that support the teeth). There are two types. Periapical periodontitis is a complication of neglected dental *caries* and affects the area around a root tip. Chronic periodontitis is a complication of untreated *gingivitis* (inflammation of the gums). This type affects the whole of the periodontium and is the major cause of tooth loss in adults.

CAUSES
If dental caries is untreated, enamel and the dentine beneath it are eventually destroyed, allowing bacteria to enter the tooth pulp. From there, bacteria spread to the root tip and into the surrounding tissues, sometimes leading to the formation of a dental *abscess*, *granuloma*, or dental *cyst*.

If gingivitis, which is usually the result of poor *oral hygiene*, is neglected, inflamed gum tissue at the base of the teeth becomes damaged and pockets form between the gums and the teeth. Dental *plaque* (a sticky deposit of mucus, food particles, and bacteria) and dental *calculus* (a hard, mineralized coating that forms from plaque and saliva) then collect in these pockets. The bacteria in the plaque and calculus attack the periodontal tissues, causing them to become inflamed and detached from the teeth. The bacteria also eventually erode the bones surrounding the teeth. In time, the teeth become loose in their sockets and fall out.

SYMPTOMS AND SIGNS
In periapical periodontitis, there may be localized toothache, especially when biting. An abscess may cause some bone and ligament destruction, thus causing the tooth to become loose; a large dental cyst may cause visible swelling of the jaw.

In chronic periodontitis, the signs of gingivitis are present (red, soft, shiny, tender gums that bleed easily) along with an unpleasant taste and bad

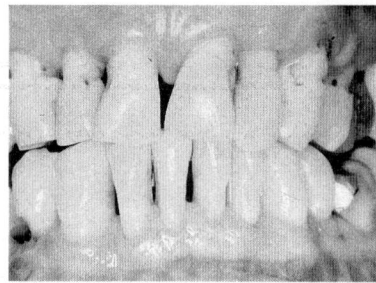

Periodontal disease
The gums are inflamed and have receded. Many of the teeth are eroded at their bases; the tooth sockets may also be decayed.

breath. The deepening pockets in the gums gradually expose the sensitive dentine of the roots of the teeth, causing aching when hot, cold, or sweet foods or liquids are consumed.

Occasionally, there is a discharge of pus from the gums or a gumboil (see *Abscess, dental*); in late stages of chronic periodontitis, there may be bone loss and loosening of teeth.

DIAGNOSIS
In periapical periodontitis, the dentist usually finds a deep cavity beneath a filling, and *dental X-rays* may show bone destruction around the root tip.

The extent of chronic periodontal disease is assessed by measuring the depth of the gum pockets and by taking X-rays to determine the extent of bone loss.

TREATMENT
Periapical periodontitis is treated either by draining pus through the root canal and then cleaning and filling the tooth or, if the tooth cannot be saved, by dental *extraction*. A minor operation may be required to remove dental cysts or large granulomas. Root-canal treatment may also be necessary.

If chronic periodontal disease has not reached an advanced stage, regular, scrupulous cleaning of the teeth can prevent further plaque and calculus formation, and thus halt destruction of the tissues surrounding the teeth. The dentist removes existing plaque and calculus by *scaling* and, in some cases, root planing. In some cases, *gingivectomy* (surgical trimming of the gums) may be required to reduce the size of the gum pockets. Curettage (see *Curettage, dental*) may be carried out to remove the diseased lining from the pocket so that healthy underlying tissue will reattach itself to the tooth. Loose teeth can sometimes be anchored to firmer ones by splinting (see *Splinting, dental*).

P

Period pain

See *Dysmenorrhoea*.

Periosteum

The tissue that coats all the bones in the body except the surfaces inside joints. Periosteum contains small blood vessels that supply nutrients to the underlying bone, and nerves that respond to pain caused by injury or disease. New bone is produced by the periosteum in the initial stages of healing after a *fracture*.

Periostitis

Inflammation of the *periosteum* (connective tissue covering bone). The usual cause is a blow that presses directly on to bone. Rarely, periostitis is caused by infection, such as syphilis. Symptoms include pain, tenderness, and swelling over the affected area of bone.

Peripheral nervous system

All the nerves that fan out from the central nervous system (brain and spinal cord) to the muscles, skin, internal organs, and glands (see *Nerve; Cranial nerves; Spinal nerves*).

Peripheral vascular disease

Narrowing of blood vessels in the legs, and sometimes in the arms, restricting blood flow and causing pain in the affected area. In severe cases, *gangrene* (death of tissue supplied by the vessels) may develop, requiring *amputation* of the limb.

TYPES AND CAUSES
In most cases, peripheral vascular disease is caused by *atherosclerosis*, in which fatty plaques form on the inner walls of arteries. Factors that contribute to the risk of atherosclerosis, such as *hypertension* and inadequately controlled *diabetes mellitus*, are associated with peripheral vascular disease. However, the greatest risk factor is *tobacco-smoking*; more than 90 per cent of patients are, or were, moderate to heavy cigarette smokers.

Diseases affecting the peripheral arteries that are not caused by atherosclerosis include *Buerger's disease*, which mainly affects smokers, and *Raynaud's disease*. Deep vein *thrombosis* and *varicose veins* are diseases of peripheral veins.

SYMPTOMS AND COMPLICATIONS
When narrowing of the arteries develops gradually because of atherosclerosis, the first symptom is usually an aching, tired feeling in the leg muscles when walking. This occurs most often in the calf, but may be felt any-where in the leg. Typically, the pain is relieved by resting the leg for a few minutes, but recurs after roughly the same amount of walking as before. This symptom is called intermittent *claudication*. Prolonged use of the arms may produce a similar symptom.

As the disease worsens, the amount of activity possible before symptoms develop decreases, until eventually pain is present at rest. This pain may be severe and continuous, disturbing sleep. By this stage, the affected leg is dangerously short of blood supply; the foot and lower leg are cold and often numb, the skin is dry and scaly, and *leg ulcers* tend to develop after minor injury. In the final stage there is gangrene, which usually starts in the toes and then spreads up the leg.

Sometimes, sudden arterial blockage occurs. This may be caused by the rapid development of a clot on top of a plaque of atherosclerosis, by a dissecting *aneurysm* (splitting of an arterial wall), or by an *embolism* arising from a clot formed in the heart and carried to obstruct a peripheral artery. Blockage causes sudden severe pain in the affected limb, which becomes cold and either pale or blue. There is no pulse in the limb, and movement and sensation in it are lost.

DIAGNOSIS
The diagnosis is based on blood pressure readings taken at the ankle, calf, upper thigh, and arm, and on blood flow measurements using *Doppler* ultrasound or *plethysmography*.

TREATMENT
Giving up smoking is by far the most important aspect of treatment. Exercise is also extremely important; sufferers should walk for up to an hour each day, stopping whenever claudication occurs and resuming when it stops.

Regular inspection of the feet and scrupulous care of them (ideally by a chiropodist) are essential to prevent infection, which can lead to gangrene. Feet should be washed and stockings changed daily. Shoes should fit well to avoid pressure on the feet, and toenails should be cut straight across.

Surgery on the diseased blood vessels is sometimes required. *Arterial reconstructive surgery* may be performed to bypass affected vessels. *Endarterectomy* may be carried out to remove fatty deposits from blood vessel linings. The newer technique of balloon *angioplasty* is increasingly successfully being used to widen diseased blood vessels in peripheral vascular disease.

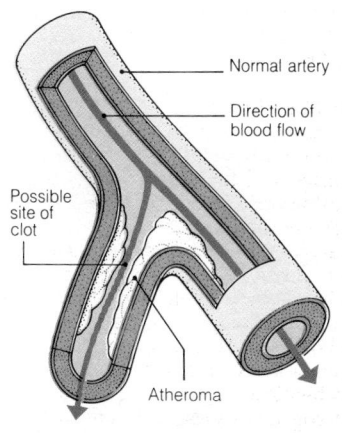

HOW PERIPHERAL VASCULAR DISEASE DEVELOPS
The disease usually starts with the formation of atheromas (fatty plaques) on artery walls. Smokers are among those at highest risk.

Normal artery

Direction of blood flow

Possible site of clot

Atheroma

Clot formation
Clots may form on top of the plaque, restricting blood flow to tissues. This may cause pain and tissue death.

In severe cases in which gangrene has developed, amputation is necessary, usually just below the knee in order to leave a stump suitable for a prosthesis. (See *Limb, artificial*).

Peristalsis

Wave-like movement as a result of rhythmic (but involuntary) contraction and relaxation of the muscles in the walls of the digestive tract and of the *ureters*. Peristalsis is responsible for the movement of food and waste products through the *digestive system* and for transporting urine from the kidneys to the bladder.

Peristalsis in the oesophagus moves food towards the stomach, and is effective even when the body is upside down. In the stomach, peristalsis helps to mix food with gastric juices and moves the partly digested food into the duodenum. In the small intestine, peristalsis changes to a slow back-and-forth churning motion that allows more time for absorption of nutrients.

In the large intestine, peristaltic contractions occur only about once every 30 minutes. Two or three times a day, usually following a meal, a strong, sustained wave of peristalsis passes over the colon. This forces the contents into the rectum and may prompt the urge to defaecate.

HOW PERISTALSIS HAPPENS

The walls of many body passages contain a special type of muscle called smooth muscle. The muscle fibres contract in sequence, sending waves of contraction along the walls of the passage.

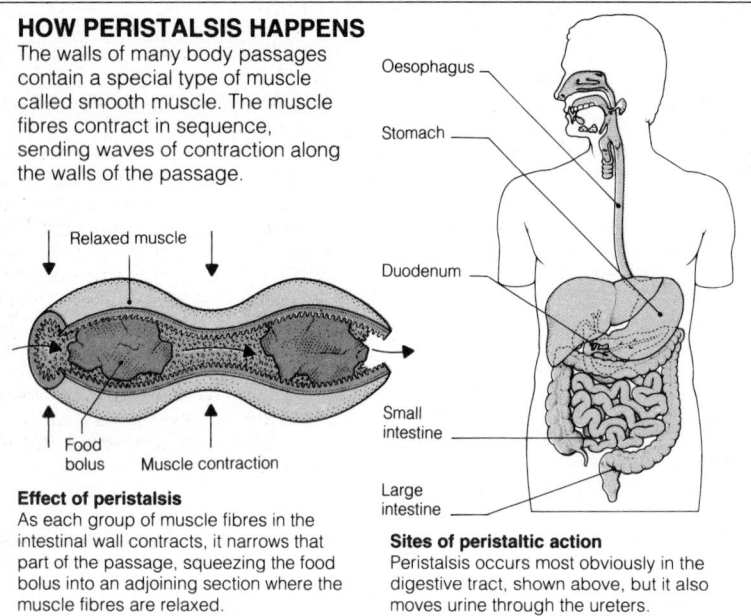

Relaxed muscle

Food bolus   Muscle contraction

Effect of peristalsis
As each group of muscle fibres in the intestinal wall contracts, it narrows that part of the passage, squeezing the food bolus into an adjoining section where the muscle fibres are relaxed.

Oesophagus

Stomach

Duodenum

Small intestine

Large intestine

Sites of peristaltic action
Peristalsis occurs most obviously in the digestive tract, shown above, but it also moves urine through the ureters.

Peritoneal dialysis
See *Dialysis*.

Peritoneum
The two-layered membrane that lines the wall of the abdominal cavity and covers the abdominal organs. The peritoneum contains blood vessels, lymph vessels, and nerves. The large surface area of the peritoneum is equal in size to that of the entire skin.

The most important functions of the peritoneum are to support the abdominal organs, to produce a lubricating fluid that allows the organs to glide smoothly over each other and the abdominal wall, and to protect against infection. The peritoneum also absorbs fluid and acts as a natural filtering system—a function made use of in peritoneal *dialysis*.

The peritoneum may become inflamed as a complication of an abdominal disorder (see *Peritonitis*).

Peritonitis
Inflammation of the *peritoneum* (the membrane that lines the wall of the abdomen and covers the abdominal organs). Peritonitis is a serious, usually *acute*, and painful condition, almost always due to irritation and bacterial infection caused by another abdominal disorder.

CAUSES
The most common cause of peritonitis is *perforation* of the stomach or intestine, which allows bacteria and di-

gestive juices to escape from the digestive tract into the abdominal cavity. Perforation is usually the result of a *peptic ulcer*, *appendicitis*, or *diverticulitis*. Less commonly, intestinal contents may leak into the abdominal cavity after surgery on the intestine. Peritonitis may also be associated with acute *salpingitis*, with *cholecystitis*, or with *septicaemia*.

SYMPTOMS AND SIGNS
Peritonitis is usually marked by severe abdominal pain, which may be either localized (in one place) or generalized (affecting the entire abdomen). In some cases, however, pain may be mild or absent. After a few hours, the muscles in the abdominal wall go into spasm, making the abdomen feel hard, and *peristalsis* (wave-like contractions of the intestinal muscles) stops (see *Ileus, paralytic*). Other symptoms include fever, bloating, nausea, and vomiting. Dehydration and shock may occur.

DIAGNOSIS AND TREATMENT
The condition is diagnosed from a *physical examination* and requires immediate admission to hospital. Prompt surgery may be needed to deal with any underlying cause—for example, removal of a perforated appendix (see *Appendicectomy*) or repair of a perforated peptic ulcer. When the cause of the peritonitis is unknown, a *laparoscopy* or an exploratory *laparotomy* may be performed. *Antibiotic drugs* are often

given, sometimes delaying surgery. Dehydration is treated by an *intravenous infusion* of fluid.

OUTLOOK
In most cases, the patient makes a full recovery following treatment. Occasionally, however, an abscess develops within the abdomen, requiring more surgery. Intestinal obstruction, resulting from the formation of *adhesions* (fibrous bands of scar tissue between loops of the intestine), may occur later.

Peritonsillar abscess
A complication of *tonsillitis*.

Permanent teeth
The second *teeth*, which usually start to replace the primary teeth at about the age of six. There are 32 permanent teeth, 16 in each jaw. Each set of 16 consists of four incisors (biting teeth) at the front, flanked by two canines (eye teeth), and four premolars and six molars (grinding teeth) at the back of the mouth. (See also *Eruption of teeth*.)

Pernicious anaemia
A type of *anaemia* caused by a failure to absorb *vitamin B$_{12}$*, which is essential for normal red blood cell production in the bone marrow. A deficiency leads to the production of abnormal, large, red cells. The vitamin is also essential for normal nerve cell metabolism. (See *Anaemia, megaloblastic*.)

Pernio
An alternative term for *chilblain*.

Peroneal muscular atrophy
A rare, inherited disorder characterized by wasting of the muscles, first in the feet and calves and then in the hands and forearms. The condition, also known as Charcot-Marie-Tooth disease, is a result of degeneration of some of the peripheral nerves. It can affect either sex, but is more common in boys, and usually appears in late childhood or adolescence.

SYMPTOMS AND SIGNS
Wasting of the muscles stops abruptly halfway up the arms and legs, giving them the appearance of inverted bottles; sensation may be lost in the affected areas. Muscle weakness in the legs causes a characteristic high-stepping walk and clawing of the toes.

TREATMENT AND OUTLOOK
No treatment is available but the condition tends to progress so slowly that the sufferer rarely becomes completely incapacitated; sometimes the

P

deterioration stops for no apparent reason. Life expectancy for an affected person is normal.

Perphenazine

A *phenothiazine*-type *antipsychotic drug* used to relieve symptoms in certain psychiatric disorders, such as *schizophrenia* and to sedate agitated or extremely anxious patients. Perphenazine is occasionally used as an *antiemetic drug* to relieve severe nausea and vomiting caused by anaesthesia, *radiotherapy*, chemotherapy, or certain drugs. It has also been prescribed to relieve persistent hiccups.

Possible adverse effects include abnormal movements of the face and limbs, drowsiness, blurred vision, stuffy nose, and headache. Long-term use may cause *parkinsonism*.

Personality

The sum of a person's traits, habits, and experiences. There is much disagreement about precisely what personality is, what defines it, and how it can be assessed. However, the following aspects are usually considered to be important in any definition: temperament, intelligence, and emotion and motivation.

The notion of temperament originates from that of the four ancient humours, which divided people into choleric, melancholic, sanguine, and phlegmatic types. This classification reflects differences in the nature and speed of an individual's responses. For example, some people are easily angered, while others are placid and react slowly. Intelligence defines a person's capabilities in comparison with a theoretical norm, while emotion and motivation describe feelings, attachments to others, moral standards, and aspirations.

The development of personality seems to depend on the interaction of two basic factors: heredity (the qualities a person is born with) and environment (a person's life experiences that affect his or her ways of thinking and behaving).

Personality disorders

A group of conditions characterized by a general failure to learn from experience or to adapt appropriately to changes, resulting in personal distress and impairment of social functioning.

Personality disorders are not forms of illness, but ways of behaving that may become especially obvious during periods of stress. They are usually first recognizable in adolescence and continue throughout life, often leading to *depression* or *anxiety*. Some people realize that they have personality problems; others fail to see their personalities as in any way unusual or difficult, blaming circumstances, bad luck, or other people for their constant failures in life.

TYPES

Specific types of personality disorders are divided into three groups; there is often overlap among types, particularly within each group.

The first group is characterized primarily by eccentric behaviour. Paranoid people show unwarranted suspiciousness and mistrust of others, schizoid people are cold emotionally and have difficulty forming social relationships, and schizotypal personalities show oddities of behaviour similar to those of *schizophrenia*, but less severe.

In the second group, behaviour tends to be dramatic and emotions intensely expressed. Histrionic individuals are very excitable and constantly crave stimulation, narcissists have an exaggerated sense of their own importance (see *Narcissism*), and those with *antisocial personality disorder* consistently fail to conform to the accepted social standards of behaviour. There may be a history of recurrent conflicts with the law.

People in the third group characteristically show anxiety and fear. Included in this group are dependent personalities, who lack self-confidence and cannot function independently (see *Dependence*); compulsive people, who are perfectionists, rigid in their habits, and emotionally cold (see *Obsessive-compulsive disorder*); and passive-aggressive types, who resist demands from others to improve their performances at work and at home.

TREATMENT AND OUTLOOK

The usual forms of treatment are counselling, individual *psychotherapy*, and *behaviour therapy*. Treatment is, however, difficult and patients may not comply. It may prove difficult for people with personality disorders to attain goals, such as avoiding the complications of drug abuse or hospitalization, or maintaining personal relationships and jobs. Drug therapy is used only for treating additional illnesses.

Personality tests

Questionnaires designed to define various *personality* traits or types. Personality tests are used to assist in research, and have been used to assess the suitability of candidates or employees for positions in colleges or industry. The validity and reliability of the tests are uncertain.

The Minnesota Multiphasic Personality Inventory (MMPI) has more than 500 questions, some relating to psychiatric symptoms (such as *depression* or *paranoia*) and others relating to underlying personality traits (such as *intelligence*). Another personality test is said to measure "extraversion-introversion" (how outgoing or reserved a person is) and "neuroticism" (predisposition to developing neurotic illness). Closely related to this test is a third questionnaire, in which a person is rated on pairs of factors, such as tense versus relaxed, or timid versus adventurous.

Perspiration

The production and excretion of sweat from the *sweat glands*. Perspiration is another name for sweat.

Perthes' disease

Inflammation of an epiphysis (growing area) of the head of the *femur*. A type of *osteochondritis juvenilis*, Perthes' disease is thought to be due to disrupted blood supply to the bone.

The condition is most common in children aged from five to 10, especially in boys, and usually affects one hip. Symptoms include pain in the thigh and groin, and a limp on the affected side. Movement of the hip is restricted and painful. X-rays may show flattening, then fragmentation, and, at a later stage, shrinking of the head of the femur.

TREATMENT AND OUTLOOK

Treatment may consist of rest for a few weeks until the pain subsides, followed by splinting of the hip to reduce pressure on the femur, or an operation to change the angle of the head of the femur so that it fits more securely into the pelvis.

Perthes' disease usually clears up by itself within three years, but may leave the hip permanently deformed. Severe deformity may increase the likelihood of *osteoarthritis* later in life.

Pertussis

A distressing infectious disease, also known as whooping cough, which mainly affects infants and young children. The main features of the illness are paroxysms of coughing (during which air is expelled from the chest), often ending in a characteristic "whoop" (during which breath is rapidly drawn in again).

P

CASES OF PERTUSSIS IN ENGLAND AND WALES

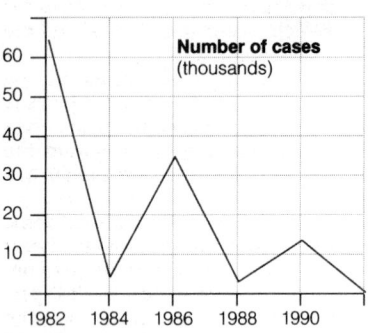

Since the 1980s there has been a general decline in the incidence of pertussis, despite periodic temporary rises.

CAUSES AND INCIDENCE

Pertussis is mainly caused by a bacterium, BORDETELLA PERTUSSIS, that is spread from an infected person to others in coughed-out airborne droplets. The disease leads to inflammation of the entire respiratory tract. The illness occurs worldwide. Infants are susceptible from birth, and the illness is most dangerous in the newborn, especially in premature babies. Adults are occasionally affected. Half of all cases occur before the age of two.

In developed countries, most infants are vaccinated in the first year of life. However, the vaccine is not completely effective in preventing the illness, and not all children are suitable for vaccination. The introduction of vaccination led to a drop in the number of cases in England and Wales from about 100,000 a year to 2,000 in 1972. However, in the early 1970s, many parents in the UK became convinced by press campaigns stating that pertussis vaccine was dangerous and ineffective. The proportion of children vaccinated fell to below 50 per cent and the disease became much more common again, with serious epidemics occurring every four years until the mid 1980s when vaccination rates rose again.

PREVENTION

The belief that pertussis vaccine is ineffective and unacceptably dangerous is now seen to have been mistaken. Because the illness is potentially serious, it is important that as many infants as possible who are suitable for vaccination be vaccinated. The risks of vaccination are far less than the dangers of having pertussis.

The vaccine is usually given in combination with diphtheria and tetanus vaccines (see *DPT vaccination*). In the UK, DPT vaccination is usually given to infants at two, three, and four months of age.

Vaccination against pertussis may cause an infant to become mildly feverish or fretful for a day or two, but this is no cause for concern. Very rarely, in about one in 100,000 cases, an infant may have a severe reaction, with high-pitched screaming or seizures. About one in 300,000 babies may suffer permanent brain damage. To lessen these already very small risks, the vaccine is not given to an infant who has a history of seizures, who has a feverish illness, or who has suffered a previous reaction to the vaccine.

Infants should be kept away from anyone with pertussis.

SYMPTOMS AND COMPLICATIONS

After an incubation period of one to three weeks, the illness starts with a mild cough, sneezing, nasal discharge, fever, and sore eyes; this is the period when the child is most infectious. After a few days, the cough becomes more persistent and severe, especially at night. Whooping occurs in most but not all cases. Sometimes the cough induces vomiting. In infants, there is a risk of temporary *apnoea* (cessation of breathing) after a coughing spasm.

The illness continues for up to 10 weeks and can be exhausting for the whole family, especially if the child's coughing continues at night.

COMPLICATIONS

Coughing may cause nosebleeds and bleeding from blood vessels on the surface of the eyes. Recurrent vomiting may cause *dehydration* and malnourishment. Chest complications include the development of *pneumonia*, *pneumothorax* (a form of collapsed lung), and bronchiectasis (permanent widening of the airways).

DIAGNOSIS AND TREATMENT

Pertussis is usually diagnosed from the symptoms but the causative bacterium can be grown from a swab taken from the back of the nose (per-nasal swab) early in the illness.

Antibiotic drugs are not particularly helpful once the severe coughing stage of the illness has begun. However, if the illness is recognized early, *erythromycin* is often given. This drug reduces the child's infectivity to others and may shorten the length of the illness.

A child with pertussis should be kept warm, given small, frequent meals and plenty to drink, and pro-

tected from stimuli that can cause coughing (such as draughts or smoke). An infant or child who becomes blue or persistently vomits after coughing needs to be admitted to hospital.

Perversion

See *Deviation, sexual*.

Pes cavus

See *Claw-foot*.

Pessary

Any of a variety of devices placed in the vagina. Some types of pessaries are used to correct the position of the uterus (see *Uterus, prolapse of*).

Medications may be given in the form of pessaries, for example to treat vaginal disorders such as *candidiasis* (thrush) or *trichomoniasis*, or to introduce contraceptive *spermicides* into the vagina.

Pesticides

Poisonous chemicals used to eradicate pests of any kind. The most frequently used types are herbicides (weedkillers), insecticides, and fungicides.

Pesticide poisoning, especially in children, may result from swallowing an insecticide or a garden herbicide, such as a chlorate preparation (see *Chlorate poisoning*). Pesticide poisoning also occurs in agricultural workers, often as a result of inhalation or absorption of the chemical through the skin—as in *paraquat* or *parathion* poisoning, for example.

Exposure to pesticides can also occur indirectly, through eating food in which chemicals have accumulated as a result of repeated spraying of crops. Some authorities believe that the result of eating such foods may be insidious long-term damage to health. (See also *DDT*; *Defoliant poisoning*; *Lindane*.)

Petechiae

Red or purple, flat, pinhead spots that occur in the skin or mucous membranes. Petechiae are caused by a localized haemorrhage from small blood vessels. They occur in *purpura* (a group of bleeding disorders) and sometimes in bacterial *endocarditis*.

Pethidine

A synthetic narcotic *analgesic drug* (painkiller) similar to, but less powerful than, *morphine*. Pethidine is given as a *premedication* (a drug used to relax and sedate a person before an operation). It is also used to relieve severe pain after major operations, during childbirth, or, occasionally, in terminal illness.

Since pethidine may cause nausea and vomiting, it is usually given with an *antiemetic drug*.

ABUSE

Pethidine may cause euphoria and is sometimes abused for this effect. Taken regularly, it is likely to cause psychological and physical dependence (see *Drug dependence*).

Petit mal

A type of seizure that occurs in *epilepsy*. Petit mal attacks occur in children and adolescents but rarely persist into adult life. They are characterized by a momentary loss of awareness, occasionally with drooping of the eyelids. Petit mal attacks may occur many times a day, sometimes lasting as long as half a minute each. Treatment is successful with an appropriate *anticonvulsant drug*.

Petroleum jelly

A greasy substance obtained from petroleum, also known as petrolatum or soft paraffin. Petroleum jelly is commonly used as an *ointment* base, as a protective dressing, and as an *emollient* to soothe the skin.

PET scanning

Positron emission tomography, a diagnostic technique based on the detection of positrons (positively charged electrons) emitted by labelled substances introduced into the body. PET scanning produces three-dimensional images that reflect the metabolic and chemical activity of tissues being studied. The images therefore give information about function as well as about structure.

HOW IT WORKS

Substances that take part in biochemical processes in the body are labelled with radioisotopes (radioactive forms of elements, such as carbon 11, nitrogen 13, or oxygen 15). These substances are injected into the bloodstream and are taken up in greater concentrations by areas of tissue that are more metabolically active. In the tissue, the substances emit positrons, which, in turn, release photons. It is the detection of these photons that actually forms the basis of PET scanning.

By surrounding the patient with an array of detectors linked to a computer, the origin of the photons can be computed and a picture built of the distribution of the radioisotope.

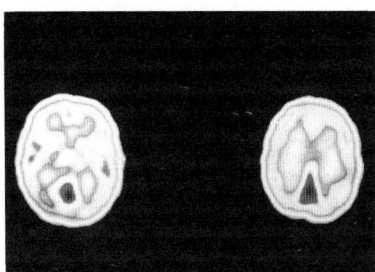

PET scan images of brain sections
Features within the brain appear as light or dark areas according to their uptake of radioactively labelled glucose.

WHY IT IS DONE

PET scanning is particularly valuable for investigating the brain. It is used for detecting tumours (which are more or less metabolically active than surrounding brain tissue), for locating the origin of epileptic activity within the brain, and for examining brain function in various mental illnesses.

OUTLOOK

PET scanning equipment is expensive to buy and operate, and is available in only a few centres. However, because PET scanning can provide valuable information not obtainable by other scanning techniques, most neurological research centres have made arrangements for access to the test for the patients who would most benefit.

Peutz-Jeghers syndrome

An extremely rare, inherited condition in which numerous polyps occur in the gastrointestinal tract and small, flat, brown spots appear on the lips and in the mouth. The syndrome usually produces no symptoms but occasionally the polyps cause abdominal pain, bleed, or lead to *intussusception* (in which the intestine telescopes in on itself and causes obstruction).

Tests may include *barium X-ray examination* and *endoscopy* (inspection through a viewing instrument) of the gastrointestinal tract. Bleeding polyps may be removed.

Peyote

A cactus plant, found in northern Mexico and the southwest of the US, of which the dried blossoms are prepared as a *hallucinogenic* drug. The active ingredient is mescaline, which produces visual hallucinations and altered consciousness lasting for several hours.

Peyronie's disease

A disorder of the *penis* in which there is thickening of part of the sheath of fibrous connective tissue. Peyronie's disease causes the penis to bend at an angle during erection, usually to one side, commonly making intercourse difficult and painful. The disorder most often affects men over 40 and the cause is unknown.

The thickened area can usually be felt as a firm nodule when the penis is flaccid. Eventually, some of the erectile tissue (spongy tissue within the penis responsible for erection) may also thicken.

In some cases, Peyronie's disease improves without treatment. Local injections of *corticosteroid drugs* sometimes improve the condition. If it persists, the thickened area may be removed surgically and replaced with a graft of normal tissue. In some cases, however, this operation creates more scarring and thereby makes the problem worse.

pH

A measure of the acidity or alkalinity of a solution. The pH scale ranges from 0 to 14, 7 denoting neutrality; the smaller the pH value below 7, the more strongly acidic a solution is; the larger the value above 7, the more strongly alkaline it is.

The pH of body fluids must be maintained very near 7.4 (close to neutrality) for the body's metabolic reactions to proceed properly (see *Acid-base balance*). If the pH falls below about 7.3, the condition is called *acidosis*; if it rises above about 7.5, it is called *alkalosis*.

Phaeochromocytoma

A rare tumour of cells secreting the hormones *adrenaline* and *noradrenaline*, which regulate heart-rate and blood pressure. The tumour increases production of these hormones, causing intermittent or sustained *hypertension* (high blood pressure). Phaeochromocytomas may be single or multiple, and usually develop in the medulla (core) of one or both *adrenal glands*. Sometimes they occur in similar tissue in the brain and elsewhere. The tumours may develop at any age but are most common in young to middle-aged adults.

SYMPTOMS AND SIGNS

Most patients have hypertension. At most times, there are usually no other signs or symptoms, but pressure on the area of the tumour, emotional upset, a change in posture, or taking *beta-blocker drugs* can cause a surge of hormones from the tumour. This surge in hormones brings on a sudden rise in blood pressure, rapid pulse,

P

palpitations, headache, nausea, vomiting, clammy skin, and sometimes a feeling of impending death.

DIAGNOSIS AND TREATMENT

Phaeochromocytoma is diagnosed by blood and urine tests to check for excessive adrenaline and noradrenaline and related substances. *CT scanning*, *MRI*, and *radioisotope scanning* may be used to locate tumours.

Treatment consists of surgical removal of the tumours. Before surgery, drugs are usually given to control the patient's blood pressure. The outlook after treatment is very good in almost all cases. In some patients, hypertension recurs and requires treatment with drugs.

Phagocyte

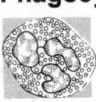 A cell capable of surrounding, engulfing, and digesting microorganisms (such as bacteria and viruses), foreign particles that have entered the body (such as dust inhaled into the lungs), and cellular debris.

Phagocytes form part of the body's *immune system* (natural defences against infection) and are found in the blood, spleen, and lymph nodes, in the alveoli (small air sacs) within the lungs, and elsewhere. Some types of white *blood cells*, especially granulocytes and some monocytes, are "free" phagocytes, able to wander through the tissues and engulf organisms and debris.

Phalanges

The small bones that make up the skeleton of the fingers, thumb, and toes. Each finger has three phalanges, the thumb and big toe have two, and the other toes have three.

Phallus

Any object that may symbolize the male penis.

Phantom limb

The perception that a limb is still present after *amputation*. Impulses from the nerves in the remaining stump are interpreted by the brain as if they were coming from the original limb.

Pharmaceutical

Any medicinal *drug*. The term is also used in relation to the manufacture and sale of drugs.

Pharmacokinetics

The term used to describe how the body deals with a *drug*, including how the drug is absorbed into the blood-stream, distributed to different tissues, broken down, and excreted from the body.

Pharmacology

The branch of science concerned with the discovery and development of drugs; their chemical structure and composition; the ways in which they act in the body; their uses in the prevention or treatment of disease; and with their side-effects and toxicity in long-term treatment.

Pharmacologists continually undertake research to help develop new drugs and find new uses for existing drugs. They are concerned with devising methods of synthesizing naturally occurring drugs, producing and sufficiently testing completely new synthetic drugs, finding new combinations of drugs, and modifying existing drugs to extend or improve their effectiveness.

Most drugs today come in prepackaged forms and dosages, but clinical pharmacologists working in hospitals often develop special preparations to meet special needs, and give advice on dosages, methods of administration, contra-indications and side-effects.

Pharmacopoeia

Any book that lists and describes almost all drugs used in medicine, especially an official national publication, such as the British Pharmacopoeia (BP).

Used as a standard book of reference by doctors and pharmacists, a pharmacopoeia describes sources, preparations, doses, and tests that can be used to identify individual drugs and to determine their purity. Pharmacopoeias may also contain additional information, such as how a drug works, and its possible adverse effects.

Pharmacy

The practice of preparing drugs, making up prescriptions, and dispensing them; the term is additionally used to describe a place where this activity is carried out.

Pharyngeal diverticulum

An alternative term for a pharyngeal pouch. (See *Oesophageal diverticulum*.)

Pharyngeal pouch

An abnormal blind-ending sac that bulges back and down from the top of the oesophagus. (See *Oesophageal diverticulum*.)

Pharyngitis

Inflammation of the *pharynx* (the part of the throat between the tonsils and the larynx), the chief symptom of which is a *sore throat*. Pharyngitis may be acute or chronic.

CAUSES

Pharyngitis is most often caused by a viral infection. Sometimes it is due to a bacterial infection (e.g. a *streptococcal infection*), rarely to *chlamydial infection* or to infection with *mycoplasma*.

Pharyngitis often occurs as part of a cold (see *Cold, common*) or *influenza*, and may also be an early feature of mononucleosis (see *Mononucleosis, infectious*) or *scarlet fever*. *Diphtheria* is a rare, but serious, cause of pharyngitis.

Pharyngitis may also be caused by swallowing substances that scald, corrode, or scratch the lining of the throat. Inflammation of the pharynx can be aggravated by smoking or by excessive consumption of alcohol.

SYMPTOMS AND SIGNS

In addition to a sore throat, there may be discomfort when swallowing, slight fever, earache, and tender, swollen lymph nodes in the neck. In severe acute cases, the fever may be high and the soft palate and throat may swell so much that breathing and swallowing become difficult. One potential complication is oedema (an accumulation of fluid in the tissues) of the larynx (voice-box), which is a life-threatening condition.

TREATMENT

Other than gargling with warm salt water, avoiding lying flat, and taking *analgesic drugs* (painkillers), no treatment is usually required; pharyngitis most often clears up on its own. Antiseptic lozenges and sprays may aggravate the condition and should therefore be avoided.

Particularly severe and/or prolonged sore throats should be reported to a doctor, who may send a throat *swab* sample for analysis and prescribe *antibiotic drugs*. Severe oedema of the larynx may require *intubation* (establishment of an air passage by placing a tube through the larynx into the trachea) or *tracheostomy* (creating an opening in the trachea to insert a breathing tube).

Pharynx

The passage that connects the back of the mouth and the nose to the oesophagus. This muscular tube, lined with *mucous membrane*, forms part of the respiratory and digestive tracts. The uppermost part, the *nasopharynx* (an air passage), connects the nasal

P

cavity to the region behind the soft *palate* of the mouth. The middle section, the oropharynx (a passage for both air and food), runs from the nasopharynx to below the tongue. The lowest portion, the laryngopharynx (a passage for food), lies behind and to each side of the larynx and merges with the oesophagus.

DISORDERS

Acute *pharyngitis* (inflammation of the pharynx), which causes sore throat, is the most common disorder affecting the pharynx. A foreign body, such as a fish-bone, may become lodged in the pharynx, causing pain and *choking*.

A pharyngeal pouch (also called Zenker's diverticulum) is a rare disorder in which a small sac develops in the rear wall of the laryngopharynx (see *Oesophageal diverticulum*).

Malignant tumours of the nasopharynx (see *Nasopharynx, cancer of*), though common in the Far East, are rare in the West, as are cancer of the oropharynx and laryngopharynx (see *Pharynx, cancer of*). The latter two have been linked with smoking and heavy drinking.

Pharynx, cancer of

A malignant tumour of the *pharynx* (the passage that connects the back of the mouth and the nose with the oesophagus). Pharyngeal cancer usually develops in the squamous (flattened, scale-like) cells of the *mucous membrane* which lines the passage. Tumours of the nasopharynx, the uppermost part of the passage, have different causes and symptoms from those occurring elsewhere in the pharynx (see *Nasopharynx, cancer of*).

CAUSES AND INCIDENCE

In the West, almost all pharyngeal cancer is related to smoking (of pipes and cigars as well as cigarettes) and to drinking alcohol. The highest incidence of pharyngeal cancer is in those who both smoke and drink.

The incidence of the disease is about 3,500 cases per year in the UK. The incidence rises with age, and the disorder is more common in men.

SYMPTOMS AND SIGNS

Malignant tumours of the oropharynx (the middle section of the pharynx, running from behind the soft palate to below the tongue) usually cause swallowing difficulty, often with a sore throat and earache. In addition, blood-stained sputum (phlegm) may be coughed up. Sometimes the disease causes no more than the feeling of a lump in the throat or a visible enlarged lymph node in the neck.

LOCATION OF THE PHARYNX
The pharynx, or throat, plays an essential part in breathing and eating and can change shape to help form vowel sounds in speech. It has a mucous membrane lining.

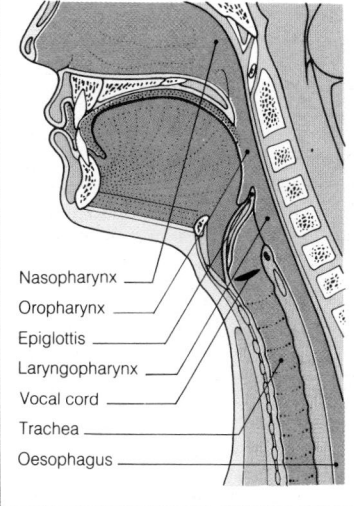

Nasopharynx
Oropharynx
Epiglottis
Laryngopharynx
Vocal cord
Trachea
Oesophagus

Cancer of the laryngopharynx (the lowest part of the pharynx, which lies behind the larynx and merges with the oesophagus) initially causes an uncomfortable sensation of incomplete swallowing. As the tumour spreads, symptoms include a muffled voice, hoarseness, and increased difficulty in swallowing. A sensation of incomplete swallowing may have a different, harmless cause, but this symptom should in all cases be reported to a doctor.

DIAGNOSIS

Diagnosis is made from abnormalities found by *biopsy* (removal of a small sample of tissue for analysis). The biopsy is often performed in conjunction with *laryngoscopy*, *bronchoscopy*, and *oesophagoscopy* (inspection by means of a viewing tube of the larynx, lungs, and oesophagus).

TREATMENT AND OUTLOOK

The growth may be removed surgically or treated with *radiotherapy*. Anticancer drugs may also be given. The outlook varies considerably for each individual patient according to the site and type of tumour, its degree of malignancy, the stage of the disease at the time of treatment, and the age of the patient.

Phencyclidine

A drug of abuse, commonly known as *angel dust*.

Phenelzine

A monoamine oxidase inhibitor *antidepressant drug*. Like other drugs of this type, phenelzine may cause a dangerous increase in blood pressure if taken with certain drugs, foods, or drinks. For this reason, it is usually given only when other antidepressant drugs have proved ineffective.

Phenelzine may cause dizziness and, rarely, jaundice and rash. Headache, unexplained sweating, nausea, and vomiting may indicate a dangerous rise in blood pressure.

Phenobarbitone

A *barbiturate drug* used mainly as an *anticonvulsant drug*. Although phenobarbitone has to some extent been replaced by newer anticonvulsant drugs, it is still often used in combination with *phenytoin* to treat *epilepsy*.

Possible adverse effects from taking phenobarbitone include drowsiness, clumsiness, dizziness, excitement, and confusion.

Phenothiazine drugs

COMMON DRUGS

Chlorpromazine Fluphenazine Perphenazine Thioridazine Trifluoperazine

A group of drugs widely used to treat psychotic illnesses (see *Antipsychotic drugs*) and to relieve severe nausea and vomiting (see *Antiemetic drugs*).

Phenoxymethylpenicillin

A synthetic *penicillin drug*. Phenoxymethylpenicillin is an *antibiotic drug* which is commonly prescribed to treat a variety of bacterial infections, including pharyngitis, tonsillitis, gum infection, and tooth abscess.

Possible adverse effects include rash and nausea. A few people develop a serious allergic reaction in which there is wheezing, breathing difficulty, and swelling around the mouth and eyes.

Phenylbutazone

A *nonsteroidal anti-inflammatory drug* (NSAID) used to relieve the symptoms of *ankylosing spondylitis*. Because of the risk of adverse effects, phenylbutazone is prescribed only under hospital supervision when other similar drugs have proved ineffective. (Phenylbutazone is sometimes given illegally to improve the performance of lame horses.)

POSSIBLE ADVERSE EFFECTS

Phenylbutazone may cause nausea, fluid retention, rash, and *peptic ulcer*.

It may also increase the risk of *blood disorders,* such as agranulocytosis (lack of granulocytes, a type of white blood cell). Regular blood tests are therefore carried out if treatment lasts for longer than one week.

Phenylephrine

A *decongestant drug* commonly used in the treatment of seasonal allergic *rhinitis* (hay fever) and the common *cold.* Phenylephrine has a bronchodilator effect and is included in several preparations used to treat *asthma* and chronic *bronchitis.* In the form of eye-drops, phenylephrine is used to dilate the pupils during examination of or surgery on the eyes.

POSSIBLE ADVERSE EFFECTS
Eye-drops may irritate the eyes. High doses or prolonged use of nasal preparations may cause headache and blurred vision; suddenly to stop taking the drug may lead to worsening of nasal congestion.

Phenylketonuria

An inherited disorder in which the *enzyme* that converts phenylalanine (an amino acid) into tyrosine (another amino acid) is defective. Unless phenylalanine is excluded from the diet, it builds up in the body and causes severe mental handicap.

INCIDENCE AND DIAGNOSIS
About one baby in 16,000 has phenylketonuria (PKU). All newborn babies are routinely given the *Guthrie test* (sometimes called a PKU test), in which a sample of blood is taken from the baby's heel so that the level of phenylalanine can be checked. If the level of phenylalanine is high, more sensitive tests are carried out during the first few weeks of life.

SYMPTOMS AND SIGNS
Affected newborn babies show few signs of abnormality, but unless phenylalanine is avoided they develop neurological disturbances, including *epilepsy,* early in infancy. Affected children have an unpleasant, musty, mousy smell due to the excretion in the sweat and urine of a breakdown product of phenylalanine. Skin, hair, and eye colouring is often lighter than in other members of the family; 90 per cent of affected children have blond hair and blue eyes. Some skeletal changes are associated with phenylketonuria, such as a small head, short stature, and flat feet. About one third to half the patients have eczema.

TREATMENT
The condition is effectively treated by restricting the intake of phenylala-

nine, which is a natural constituent of most protein-containing foods. Babies must be given special milk substitutes. After weaning, they are given a very low-protein, mainly vegetarian, diet. Some doctors believe that a strict low-protein diet should be followed throughout life. Others maintain that a normal diet can be introduced when a child is 10 to 12 years old; the special diet must be reintroduced during pregnancy, to prevent brain damage in the fetus.

Phenylpropanolamine

A *decongestant drug* commonly used in the treatment of seasonal allergic *rhinitis* (hay fever), *sinusitis,* and the common cold.

High doses or prolonged use of phenylpropanolamine may cause anxiety and nausea; suddenly to stop taking the drug may lead to worsening of the congestion.

Phenytoin

An *anticonvulsant drug* commonly used as a long-term treatment for *epilepsy.* Phenytoin is also given to treat *trigeminal neuralgia* and infrequently to control certain types of *arrhythmia* (irregularity of the heartbeat).

Prolonged use of phenytoin may cause slurred speech, dizziness, confusion, and overgrowth of the gums.

Pheromone

An odorous substance, released in minute quantities by an animal, that affects the behaviour or development of other individuals of the same species. Although humans also give off distinctive body odours, it is questionable whether or not these are true pheromones, able to alter the behaviour of other humans.

Phimosis

Tightness of the foreskin, preventing it from being drawn back over the underlying glans (head) of the *penis.*

In uncircumcised males, some degree of phimosis is normal until the age of six months. In some boys it persists for several years, sometimes making it difficult to pass urine and causing the foreskin to balloon out on urination. Phimosis prevents proper cleaning of the glans, leading to *balanitis* (infection of the glans). There may also be an increased risk of cancer (see *Penis, cancer of).* Phimosis makes erection painful and may lead to *paraphimosis* (constriction of the penis behind the glans). Phimosis is treated by *circumcision.*

Phlebitis

Inflammation of a vein, often accompanied by clot formation. The preferred medical name for this condition is *thrombophlebitis.*

Phlebography

The obtaining and interpretation of X-ray images of veins after they have been injected with a radiopaque substance. Phlebography is an alternative name for *venography.*

Phlebotomy

Puncture of a vein for the purpose of removing blood (see *Venepuncture; Venesection.*)

Phlegm

See *Sputum.*

Phobia

A persistent, irrational fear of, and desire to avoid, a particular object or situation. Many people have minor phobias that may cause them some distress but that do not impair their ability to cope with everyday life. It is only when a fear causes significant disturbance and interferes with normal social functioning that it is considered a psychiatric disorder.

TYPES
Simple phobias, also known as specific phobias, are the most common. These may involve fear of particular animals (most often dogs, snakes, spiders, or mice) or of particular situations, such as enclosed spaces (*claustrophobia*), heights, or air travel. Animal phobias usually start in childhood, but other forms may develop at any time. Treatment is not usually required, unless the feared object is so common that it is not easily avoided (e.g. fear of lifts in a person who lives in a large city).

Agoraphobia (fear of open spaces or of entering public places) is a more serious type of phobia, often causing severe impairment and disruption of family life. It is the most common phobia for which treatment is sought. The disorder usually starts in the late teens or early 20s.

Social phobia, which is relatively rare, is fear of being exposed to the scrutiny of others. Examples include fear of eating, speaking, or performing in public, using public toilets, or writing in the presence of others. The disorder usually begins in late childhood or early adolescence.

CAUSES
According to some theories, simple phobias are a form of learned re-

P

sponse (see *Conditioning*). People with such phobias have often been brought up by someone with a similar fear or have had an early frightening experience that has become associated with the feared object or situation. According to other theories, the phobia has a symbolic meaning (e.g. a fear of snakes may result from repressed sexual feelings).

SYMPTOMS
Exposure to the feared object or situation causes intense *anxiety* and sometimes a *panic attack*. Phobic individuals may also suffer from *depression* and generalized anxiety and may indulge in minor obsessional rituals (see *Obsessive-compulsive behaviour*). People with agoraphobia or social phobia may attempt to relieve their anxiety with alcohol, barbiturate drugs, or antianxiety drugs, and may become psychologically dependent on them, thus compounding the problems.

TREATMENT
The most effective treatment is *behaviour therapy*, sometimes combined with *antidepressant drugs*. People with social phobia may benefit from training in social skills.

Phocomelia

A type of *limb defect* in which the feet and/or the hands are joined to the trunk by short, stubby stumps resembling seal fins. The condition is rare and has occurred mostly in children whose mothers took the drug *thalidomide* early in pregnancy.

Phosphates

Salts containing phosphorus and oxygen. Phosphates are an essential part of the diet and are present in many foods, including cereals, dairy products, eggs, and meat.

FUNCTION
About 85 per cent of the body's phosphorus is combined with calcium to form the structure of bone and teeth. The remainder is deposited in small amounts in most of the body's tissues and plays a part in maintaining the acid-alkaline balance of the blood, urine, saliva, and other body fluids. *ATP* (adenosine triphosphate) is a phosphate compound which stores energy for chemical reactions in cells.

DISORDERS
In most people, the kidneys maintain a constant level of phosphates in the body by regulating the amount excreted in the urine. A slight deficiency of phosphates in the diet is compensated for by a reduction in the amount lost in the urine.

Hypophosphataemia (an abnormally low level of phosphates in the blood) may occur in some forms of kidney disease, *hyperparathyroidism*, long-term treatment with *diuretic drugs*, *malabsorption*, or prolonged starvation. It causes bone pain, weakness, seizures, and, in severe cases, coma and death.

DRUG THERAPY
Phosphates may be taken by mouth in the form of drug preparations or milk to treat hypophosphataemia. Phosphates are also used to treat *hypercalcaemia*. Diarrhoea is a possible side-effect of phosphate drugs.

Phosphorus poisoning

There are two forms of phosphorus—yellow and red. Yellow phosphorus is readily absorbed by the body and is highly poisonous. Red phosphorus cannot be absorbed and is nontoxic.

Yellow phosphorus is used in matches, fireworks, some insecticides, and certain rodent poisons. It may cause serious burns if it comes into contact with the skin. Most cases of poisoning occur in industrial workers who accidentally ingest the chemical or inhale its vapour. Acute poisoning, due to absorption of comparatively large amounts of phosphorus over a short period, causes damage to the liver, kidneys, central nervous system, and other organs.

Symptoms of acute phosphorus poisoning include burning abdominal pain, an odour of garlic on the breath, nausea, vomiting, bloody diarrhoea, jaundice, and symptoms of *kidney failure* and *liver failure*. In severe cases, or untreated milder ones, delirium, seizures, unconsciousness, and death may occur within about 48 hours of initial poisoning.

Chronic poisoning, due to taking in small amounts of phosphorus over a relatively long period, may cause gradual destruction of the jawbones (a condition known as phosphonecrosis or phossy jaw), *cirrhosis* of the liver, and kidney damage. This is now very uncommon.

Treatment of acute poisoning consists of washing out the stomach (see *Lavage, gastric*) with copper sulphate, along with injections of calcium and treatment for liver and kidney failure.

Photocoagulation

The destructive heating of tissue by intense light focused to a fine point, as in *laser treatment*. Photocoagulation is used to treat disorders of the retina, especially diabetic retinopathy.

Photophobia

An uncomfortable sensitivity or intolerance to light. Photophobia occurs with some eye disorders, such as *corneal abrasion*, *corneal ulcer*, acute *iritis* (inflammation of the iris), and congenital *glaucoma* (raised pressure in the eyeball). Photophobia is also a feature of *meningitis* (inflammation of the membranes that surround the brain and spinal cord).

Photosensitivity

Abnormal reaction to sunlight. Photosensitivity usually takes the form of a skin rash that occurs as a reaction to the effects of light on the skin. This reaction often occurs because a substance has been ingested, or applied to the skin. Examples of such substances, called photosensitizers, are certain drugs, dyes, chemicals used in perfumes and soaps, and plants such as buttercups, parsnips, and mustard.

Photosensitivity is also a feature of certain disorders that affect internal organs as well as the skin, such as systemic *lupus erythematosus* and *porphyria*. In such disorders, exposure to light may worsen the condition.

TREATMENT
Known photosensitizers should be avoided when possible. If the reaction occurs independently of photosensitizers, a susceptible person should avoid exposure to sunlight, especially between 10 a.m. and 4 p.m. (when the light is at its most intense) and should use *sunscreen* preparations.

Phototherapy

Treatment with light, involving the use of sunlight, nonvisible ultraviolet light, visible blue light, or *lasers*.

Moderate exposure to sunlight is the most basic form of phototherapy. This is helpful in treating about 75 per cent of people with *psoriasis*

A newer form of phototherapy, *PUVA*, combines the use of long-wave ultraviolet light with a *psoralen drug* (e.g. methoxsalen), which sensitizes the skin to light. PUVA is particularly effective in treating psoriasis and is also used in treating some other skin diseases, e.g. *vitiligo* and *mycosis fungoides*. Short-wave ultraviolet light, sometimes combined with application of coal tar, may also be used to treat psoriasis. Several treatments are given; the exposure time is gradually increased according to the reaction of the patient's skin to the therapy.

Visible blue light is used in the treatment of jaundice in the newborn (see *Jaundice, neonatal*), which is caused by

P

accumulation of the bile pigment bili-rubin as a result of an insufficiently developed liver. The light is thought to cause the chemical breakdown of bilirubin, allowing it to be excreted in the urine. With his or her eyes shielded, the infant is completely exposed to the light for 12 hours or more; he or she may need additional fluids to compensate for water loss.

Phototherapy is also used to treat *seasonal affective disorder syndrome*.

Phrenic nerve

Either of the two principal nerves sup-plying the *diaphragm*. Each nerve car-ries motor impulses to, and some of the sensory impulses from, the dia-phragm, and plays an important part in controlling breathing. The phrenic nerves arise from the third, fourth, and fifth cervical nerves in the neck, and pass down through the chest each to one side of the diaphragm. Injury to, or surgical cutting of, one of the nerves results in paralysis of one half of the diaphragm.

The phrenic nerve may be deliber-ately crushed to produce temporary paralysis of the diaphragm after an operation to repair a *hiatus hernia*, or as a rare treatment for intractable *hiccups*. In the past, crushing of the phrenic nerve was performed to treat lung dis-orders such as *tuberculosis*.

Physical examination

See *Examination, physical*.

LOCATION OF PHRENIC NERVES
There are two phrenic nerves, one on each side of the body. Each follows a tortuous course from its origin in the neck, through the chest, to the diaphragm.

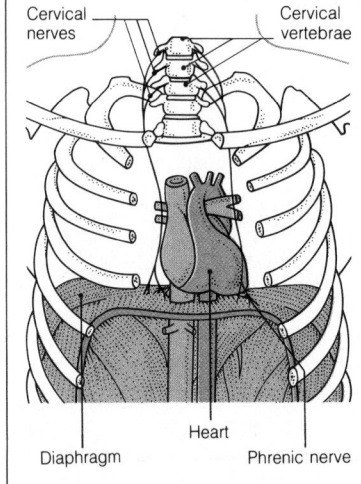

Cervical nerves

Cervical vertebrae

Heart

Diaphragm

Phrenic nerve

Physical medicine and rehabilitation

A branch of medicine concerned with the care of patients who have been disabled as a result either of injuries, or of illness, especially strokes or other neurological disorders.

The doctor responsible for the patient makes a careful assessment before drawing up a rehabilitation programme and enlisting the help of other professionals (for example, phy-siotherapists, nurses, occupational therapists and speech therapists) to help implement it.

Physiology

The study of the functioning of the body, including the physical and chemical processes of its cells, tissues, organs, and systems, and their various interactions. Along with *ana-tomy* (the study of body structure), physiology constitutes the foundation of all medical science.

Strictly, physiology is concerned with normal functioning, but the boundary between normality and abnormality is not always distinct. Thus a specialty has developed called pathophysiology, which is concerned with the functional changes asso-ciated with diseases and disorders. There are also other physiological specialties, such as renal physiology (the study of kidney function), and endocrine physiology (the study of the functions of endocrine glands and their hormone secretions).

Physiotherapy

Treatment of disorders or injuries with physical methods or agents.

Physiotherapy is used to prevent or reduce joint stiffness and to restore

TECHNIQUES OF PHYSIOTHERAPY
Physiotherapy may be given after a stroke, nerve damage, or a fracture, or for muscle pain or arthritis. In addition to the techniques shown, heat and electrical treatments are often used.

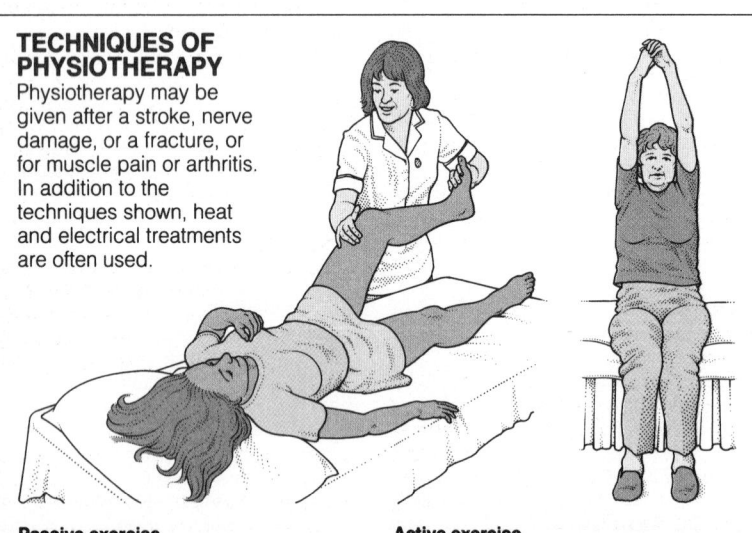

Passive exercise
The therapist moves the affected part. This preserves joint mobility and is valuable after nerve injuries and in the treatment of diseases such as polio.

Active exercise
The patient is taught to contract and relax certain muscle groups or to perform specific movements (e.g. exercising the arm muscles after a stroke).

THERAPEUTIC MASSAGE

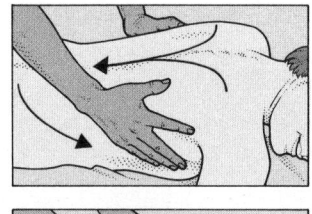

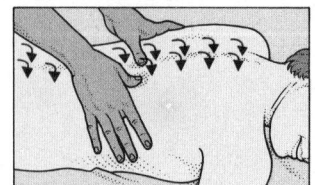

Massage
Massage is given mainly to relieve muscle pain and spasm. Long, sweeping strokes can be alternated with "circling" techniques.

muscle strength in the treatment of arthritis or after a fracture has healed. It is also used to reduce pain, inflammation, and muscle spasm and to retrain joints and muscles after stroke or nerve injury.

Methods of treatment used by physiotherapists include exercises, which may be active or passive (see illustrated box), *massage, heat treatment* (including *ultrasound treatment* and short-wave *diathermy*), cold (see *Ice-packs*), water (see *Hydrotherapy*), and electrical currents (as in *TENS*).

Physiotherapy is also concerned with the maintenance of breathing capacity in people with impaired lung function or the prevention and treatment of pulmonary complications following surgery. Physiotherapists help treat severe respiratory diseases (such as chronic *bronchitis*) and care for the respiratory needs of patients who are on *ventilators* or recovering from major operations. Techniques used include *breathing exercises, percussion, postural drainage*, and the administration of oxygen, drugs, or moisture to the lungs through a *nebulizer*.

Physostigmine

A drug used in the form of eye-drops to treat *glaucoma* (raised pressure in the eyeball).

Pica

A craving to eat substances (such as earth, coal, chalk, or wood) that are not food. Pica sometimes occurs during pregnancy and may be a feature of various nutritional or iron-deficiency disorders. It may also occur in severe psychiatric disorders.

Pickwickian syndrome

An unusual disorder characterized by extreme *obesity*, abnormally shallow breathing, excessive sleepiness, and *sleep apnoea*. It is named after the fat boy Joe in Charles Dickens' "Pickwick Papers". The cause of the disorder is unclear. Symptoms usually improve with weight loss.

PID

See *Pelvic inflammatory disease*.

Pigeon toes

A minor abnormality in which the leg or foot is rotated, forcing the foot and toes to point inwards.

Pigmentation

Coloration of the skin, hair, and iris of the eyes by *melanin* (a brown or black pigment produced by special cells called melanocytes). The greater the amount of melanin present, the darker the coloration. The amount of melanin produced is determined by heredity and by exposure to sunlight. Blood pigments can also colour skin (such as in a bruise).

ABNORMALITIES OF PIGMENTATION

LIGHTENED SKIN Patches of pale skin occur in various skin disorders. In *psoriasis, pityriasis alba*, and *pityriasis versicolor*, skin scales flake off, resulting in loss of melanin. In *vitiligo*, areas of skin stop producing melanin.

The rare, inherited condition *albinism* is caused by generalized melanin deficiency, resulting in pale skin and white hair. In *phenylketonuria*, another genetic condition, sufferers have a reduced melanin level, making them paler-skinned and fairer-haired than other members of the family.

DARKENED SKIN Patches of dark skin mingled with lighter areas may follow an episode of *eczema* or psoriasis, or may occur in pityriasis versicolor. In *chloasma*, hormonal changes cause dark areas to develop on the face; this condition may occur in women who are taking oral contraceptives or during pregnancy or the menopause. Dark facial patches may also be caused by some perfumes and cosmetics, particularly when they contain chemicals that cause *photosensitivity*. Such patches of discoloration usually fade with time.

Permanent areas of pronounced deep pigmentation are usually due to an abnormality of the melanocytes, as is the case with freckles and moles (see *Naevus*). *Acanthosis nigricans*, which may be inherited or acquired, is characterized by dark patches of velvet-like, thickened skin, primarily in body creases.

Darkening of the skin, unrelated to sun exposure, may occur in certain hormonal disorders, such as *Addison's disease* and *Cushing's syndrome*.

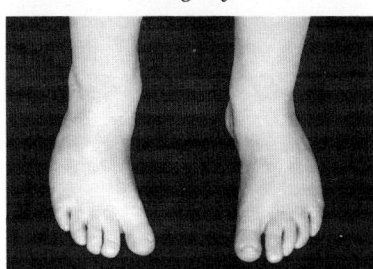

Appearance of pigeon toes
This is a common condition in toddlers. In almost all cases it requires no treatment and corrects itself by about the age of seven.

OTHER SKIN DISCOLORATION Some abnormal skin pigmentation is caused by an excessive blood level of other pigments. An excess of the bile pigment bilirubin in *jaundice* turns the skin yellow, and too much iron in *haemochromatosis* turns the skin bronze. Discoloration may also be caused by an abnormal collection of blood vessels, such as the one that produces a port-wine stain (see *Haemangioma*).

Piles

The common name for *haemorrhoids*.

Pill, contraceptive

See *Oral contraceptives*.

Pilocarpine

A drug obtained from PILOCARPUS plants, used to treat *glaucoma* (raised pressure in the eyeball). Because pilocarpine causes the pupils to constrict, it is also used to reverse dilation (widening) of the pupils (which may be caused by drugs given during surgery or examination of the eyes).

Pilocarpine may initially cause blurred vision, headache, and irritation of the eyes.

Pilonidal sinus

A pit in the skin, often containing hairs, in the upper part of the cleft between the buttocks. Pilonidal sinus is probably caused by hair fragments burrowing inwards. The condition is usually harmless, but the pit can become infected, resulting in recurrent painful abscesses.

Treatment of an infected sinus is by surgical removal of a wide area around the infection; the wound is usually left open to allow slow healing from below. Recurrence of infection is common, and plastic surgery is occasionally required.

Pimozide

An *antipsychotic drug*, which is also used in the treatment of *Gilles de la Tourette's syndrome* (a rare neurological disorder). Pimozide may cause sedation, dry mouth, constipation, and blurred vision.

Pimple

A common name for a small *pustule* or *papule*. Pimples are usually found on the face, neck, or back, particularly in adolescents suffering from *acne*.

Pindolol

A *beta-blocker drug* used in the treatment of *angina pectoris* (chest pain due to inadequate blood supply to heart

P

muscle), *arrhythmias* (irregularities of the heartbeat), and *hypertension* (high blood pressure). In addition, pindolol is currently under investigation for the control of *glaucoma* (raised pressure in the eyeball).

Pindolol is less likely than some beta-blocker drugs to cause *bradycardia* (abnormally slow heartbeat). Otherwise, possible adverse effects are typical of other beta-blocker drugs.

Pineal gland
A tiny, cone-shaped structure within the brain, whose sole function appears to be the secretion of the hormone *melatonin*. The amount of hormone secreted varies over a 24-hour cycle, being greatest at night. Control over this secretion is possibly exerted through nerve pathways from the retina in the eye; a high light level seems to inhibit secretion. The exact function of melatonin is not understood, but it may help to synchronize circadian (24-hour) and other *biorhythms*.

The pineal gland is situated deep within the brain, just below the back part of the corpus callosum (the band of nerve fibres that connects the two halves of the cerebrum). In rare cases, it is the site of a tumour.

Pinguecula
A small, benign, yellowish spot on the *conjunctiva* over the exposed areas of the white of the eye. Pingueculas are sometimes attributed to ultraviolet

radiation in sunlight, and are common in elderly people. In some cases, pingueculas may be removed for cosmetic reasons.

Pink-eye
A common name for *conjunctivitis*.

Pink puffer
A term sometimes used by doctors to describe some patients with chronic lung disease (see *Lung disease, chronic obstructive*).

Pinna
The fleshy part of the outer *ear*, consisting of a flap of cartilage and skin. It is also known as the auricle. The pinna appears to have little practical value; its loss barely affects hearing.

Cosmetic problems affecting the pinna, such as *cauliflower ear*, can usually be corrected by plastic surgery (see *Otoplasty*).

Pins-and-needles
Medically called paraesthesia, a tingling or prickly feeling in an area of skin. It is usually associated with *numbness* (loss of sensation) and occasionally with a burning sensation.

Temporary pins-and-needles is caused by a disturbance in the conduction of impulses through nerves that carry sensation from the skin to the brain (e.g. after sleeping with an arm bent awkwardly under the body). Persistent pins-and-needles may be caused by *neuropathy* (any of a group of nerve disorders).

Pinta
A skin infection occurring in some remote villages in tropical America. The organism responsible, TREPO-NEMA CARATEUM, is closely related to the bacterium that causes *syphilis*. It is uncertain how the disease is transmitted. A large spot, surrounded by smaller ones, appears on the face, neck, buttocks, hands, or feet, and, one to 12 months later, is followed by red skin patches that turn blue, then brown, and finally white. A *penicillin drug* or *tetracycline* clears up the infection, but the skin may be left permanently disfigured.

Pinworm infestation
An alternative name for *threadworm infestation*.

Piperazine
An *anthelmintic drug* used to treat roundworm and *threadworm infestation*. Piperazine paralyses the

worms, which are then expelled with the faeces. The drug is usually taken once a day for seven days to clear threadworms and as a single dose for roundworms. A laxative drug may also be given to speed up the expulsion of the worms.

Possible adverse effects of piperazine include abdominal pain, nausea, vomiting, and diarrhoea.

Piroxicam
A *nonsteroidal anti-inflammatory drug* (NSAID) used to relieve the symptoms of types of arthritis, such as *osteoarthritis, rheumatoid arthritis*, and *gout*. Piroxicam is also used to relieve pain in *bursitis, tendinitis*, and after minor surgery.

Possible adverse effects of piroxicam include nausea, indigestion, abdominal pain, swollen ankles, *peptic ulcer*, and liver problems.

Pituitary gland
Sometimes referred to as the master gland, the pituitary is the most important of the *endocrine glands* (glands that release hormones directly into the bloodstream). The pituitary regulates and controls the activities of other endocrine glands and many body processes (see *Endocrine system*).

STRUCTURE
The pituitary is a pea-sized structure that hangs from the base of the brain, just below the optic nerves, and lies in a cavity in the skull. It is attached by a short stalk of nerve fibres to the

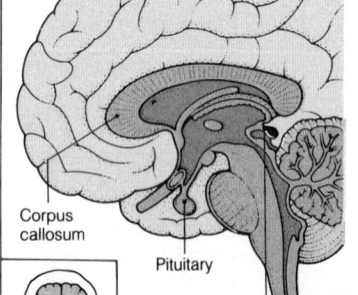

LOCATION OF THE PINEAL GLAND
The pineal gland is situated in the brain, below the rear part of the corpus callosum.

Cerebrum

Corpus callosum

Pituitary

Pineal gland

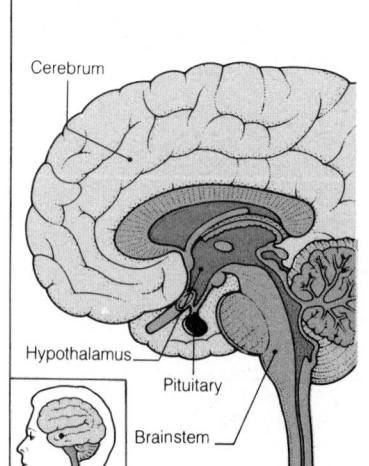

LOCATION OF PITUITARY GLAND
This master gland is itself controlled by the hypothalamus, located immediately above it.

Cerebrum

Hypothalamus

Pituitary

Brainstem

HORMONES SECRETED BY THE PITUITARY GLAND

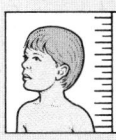

Growth hormone
stimulates cell division and protein synthesis in tissues such as bone and cartilage, leading to growth.

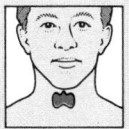

Thyroid-stimulating hormone (TSH)
stimulates the thyroid gland to secrete various hormones vital to body metabolism.

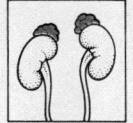

Adrenocorticotrophic hormone (ACTH)
stimulates the adrenal glands to secrete hormones, with multiple effects on metabolism.

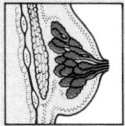
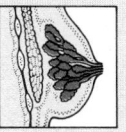

Prolactin
stimulates female breast development, and, in response to sucking of the infant, milk production.

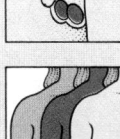

Luteinizing and follicle-stimulating hormones (LH and FSH)
help control the function of male and female sex organs.

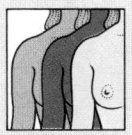

Melanocyte-stimulating hormone (MSH)
controls skin darkening by stimulating pigment cells.

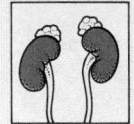

Antidiuretic hormone (ADH)
acts on the kidneys to decrease water loss in the urine and thus reduces urine volume.

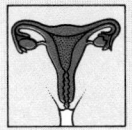

Oxytocin
stimulates contraction of the uterus during childbirth and milk release from the breasts.

hypothalamus, a region of the brain that controls the function of the pituitary by nervous stimulation and by hormone-releasing factors. The pituitary consists of three lobes known from their relative positions as the anterior, intermediate, and posterior.

FUNCTION
The different lobes of the pituitary produce a range of hormones.

The anterior pituitary produces six hormones: *growth hormone*, which stimulates growth; *prolactin*, which stimulates production of milk after giving birth (see *Breast-feeding*); *ACTH* (adrenocorticotrophic hormone), which stimulates hormone production by the adrenal glands; *TSH* (thyroid-stimulating hormone), which stimulates hormone production by the *thyroid gland*; and the *gonadotrophins* FSH (follicle-stimulating hormone) and LH (luteinizing hormone), which stimulate the *gonads*.

The intermediate part of the pituitary secretes one hormone, melanocyte-stimulating hormone (MSH), which controls darkening of the skin.

The posterior pituitary produces two hormones—*ADH* (antidiuretic hormone), which increases reabsorption of water into the blood by the kidneys and therefore decreases urine production; and *oxytocin*, which stimulates contractions of the uterus during labour and the secretion of milk during breast-feeding.

Pituitary tumours
Growths that arise in the *pituitary gland*. Pituitary tumours are rare, comprising about 10 per cent of primary *brain tumours*. Most are benign (noncancerous). However, because the pituitary is situated in a bony hollow at the base of the skull, enlargement of the tumour is upwards, where it tends to press on the *optic nerves*, causing visual field defects.

DISORDERS OF THE PITUITARY GLAND
Any abnormality of the pituitary gland usually means that it produces either too much or too little of one or more hormones, and this causes changes elsewhere in the body. Locally, serious effects may be caused by enlargement of the gland; for example, it may press on the nearby optic nerves and cause visual defects.

CONGENITAL AND GENETIC DISORDERS
Deficiency of *growth hormone* may be a genetic disorder, or it may be due to congenital absence or undergrowth of the pituitary, or to damage to the gland sustained during birth. Whatever the cause, deficiency of growth hormone leads to *short stature*.

Congenital growth hormone deficiency may also be associated with deficiency of other pituitary hormones, notably *ACTH* (adrenocorticotrophic hormone), *gonadotrophin hormones*, and thyroid-stimulating hormone (TSH).

TUMOURS
Pituitary tumours are usually benign but may cause either overproduction of pituitary hormones (hyperpituitarism) or underproduction (hypopituitarism).

INJURY
Birth injury may cause loss of pituitary function, as may head injuries at any age.

IMPAIRED BLOOD SUPPLY
Rarely, the pituitary may suffer deprivation of its blood supply as a result of pressure on its blood vessels from a growing tumour. This may cause a sudden loss of pituitary function, which may be fatal, or a more gradual loss, which produces signs of general underactivity of the gland. A similar deprivation of blood supply may occur as a complication of massive blood loss associated with childbirth (Sheehan's syndrome). This may lead to failure of milk production, and a wide range of secondary effects due to the resultant underactivity of other endocrine glands.

Impaired blood supply may also occur from *vasculitis*, or from pressure on the gland from an *aneurysm* of a nearby artery.

RADIATION
Radiotherapy for a pituitary tumour may cause general underactivity of the gland.

INVESTIGATION
Techniques used to investigate pituitary disorders include analysis of the levels of pituitary hormones in the blood or urine, and of hormones from other endocrine glands under pituitary control; *X-rays*, *CT scanning*, or *MRI* of the pituitary; and *angiography*, to show displacement of blood vessels by a pituitary tumour. A visual field test (see *Vision tests*) may be done.

P

CAUSES AND TYPES

The causes of pituitary tumours are unknown. The most common type is called an endocrine inactive tumour. As it grows, it leads to destruction of some of the hormone-secreting cells in the gland, which causes hypopituitarism (reduced hormone production). This often leads to a failure of sexual function, with cessation of menstrual periods in women and reduced sperm production in men.

Other types of tumours cause the gland to produce too much of a particular hormone. For example, a tumour of the anterior pituitary can cause excess growth hormone production, leading to *gigantism* or *acromegaly*. Too much thyroid-stimulating hormone (TSH) can lead to *hyperthyroidism*. Excess adrenocorticotrophic hormone (ACTH) can cause *Cushing's syndrome*. Finally, an increased production of prolactin can cause *galactorrhoea* (abnormal milk production), absence of menstrual periods, and infertility in women. In men, it can cause impotence, infertility, feminization, and galactorrhoea.

Tumours that affect the posterior pituitary may disrupt production of antidiuretic hormone (ADH) and lead to *diabetes insipidus*.

DIAGNOSIS AND TREATMENT

The diagnosis is made from measurements of the levels of different hormones in the blood and urine, from *CT scanning* or *MRI* of the brain, and usually also from visual field testing (see *Vision tests*).

Treatment may be by surgical excision of the tumour, by *radiotherapy*, by replacement of missing hormones, or by a combination of these techniques. The drug *bromocriptine* is sometimes used to treat pituitary tumours that secrete prolactin or growth hormone because it suppresses production of these hormones.

Pityriasis alba

A common skin condition of children and adolescents in which irregular, fine, scaly, pale patches appear on the face, usually the cheeks. The condition is caused by mild *eczema* and is often more pronounced after exposure to sun because the patches tan poorly. The condition usually clears up with emollients.

Pityriasis rosea

A common mild skin disorder in which flat, scaly-edged, round or oval, dark pink or copper-coloured spots appear over the trunk and upper

arms. The rash may be associated with a viral infection, and is preceded about a week beforehand by a single, larger, round spot (called a herald patch) on the trunk. The condition, which is not contagious, mainly affects children and young adults. Its cause is unknown.

The rash, which lasts for about six to eight weeks, can occasionally cause itching but is otherwise symptomless. Although the rash usually clears up without treatment, a doctor should be consulted to rule out other conditions that cause similar rashes.

Calamine lotion alleviates mild itching; more severe itching can be relieved by *antihistamine drugs*.

Pityriasis versicolor

A common skin condition that produces patches of white, brown, or salmon-coloured finely flaking skin over the trunk and neck. Also known as tinea versicolor, it is caused by colonization of the dead outer layer of skin by a fungus that exists unnoticed on most people's skin. The condition primarily affects young and middle-aged adults and is more common in men. It is not contagious.

The condition is usually noticed because of the contrast in colour between the affected and surrounding skin. Exposure to sunlight can make it more noticeable.

Treatment consists of applying an antifungal cream or lotion at night and washing underclothes and nightclothes thoroughly. It is important to treat the entire trunk, neck, arms, and upper legs each time the preparation is applied. Otherwise, a spot may be missed and the fungus will recur. This treatment usually clears the condition, but the spots may take months to return to normal skin colour.

Pivampicillin

A penicillin-type antibiotic drug. (See *Penicillin drugs*.)

Pivmecillinam

A penicillin-type antibiotic drug used mainly in the treatment of cystitis. (See *Penicillin drugs*.)

Pizotifen

An *antihistamine drug* used to prevent migraine headaches in people who suffer frequent, disabling attacks. The exact mechanism of action is not known but pizotifen is thought to block the effects of the chemicals histamine and serotonin on blood vessels in the brain.

Possible adverse effects include nausea, dizziness, drowsiness, dry mouth, and muscle pains. Pizotifen increases appetite, and prolonged use often causes weight gain.

PKU test

See *Guthrie test*; *Phenylketonuria*.

Placebo

A chemically inert substance given in place of a *drug*. Some doctors may prescribe a placebo if symptoms, such as fatigue, are not caused by an illness that requires drug treatment. The benefit gained from taking a placebo occurs because the person taking it believes it will have a positive effect.

Since the effectiveness of any drug may be due in part to this "placebo effect", which is based on a person's expectations of the drug, many new drugs are tested against a placebo preparation. The placebo is made to look and taste identical to the active preparation; volunteers are not told which preparation they are taking. A comparison of the results enables a more accurate assessment of the drug's efficacy.

Placenta

The organ that develops in the uterus during *pregnancy* and links the blood supplies of the mother and baby.

STRUCTURE

The placenta develops from the chorion (the outermost layer of cells that develops from the fertilized egg). It is firmly attached to the lining of the woman's uterus and is connected to the baby by the umbilical cord. By the end of pregnancy it is about 20 cm wide and 2.5 cm thick. Shortly after the baby is born, the placenta is expelled with other redundant tissues (all together being given the common name, "afterbirth").

FUNCTION

The placenta acts as an organ of respiration and excretion for the fetus. It transfers oxygen from the mother's circulation into the fetus's circulation, and removes waste products from the fetus's blood into the mother's blood for excretion by her lungs and kidneys. The placenta also conveys nutrients from mother to baby.

The placenta produces hormones such as *oestrogen*, *progesterone*, and human chorionic gonadotrophin (HCG; see *Gonadotrophin, human chorionic*). High levels of HCG appear in the woman's urine during early pregnancy and detection of them in the urine forms the basis of *pregnancy*

FUNCTION OF THE PLACENTA

The mother's and baby's blood do not completely mix in the placenta, but are brought sufficiently close so that exchange of nutrients and oxygen (from mother to baby) and waste products (from baby to mother) can occur between the two blood circulations.

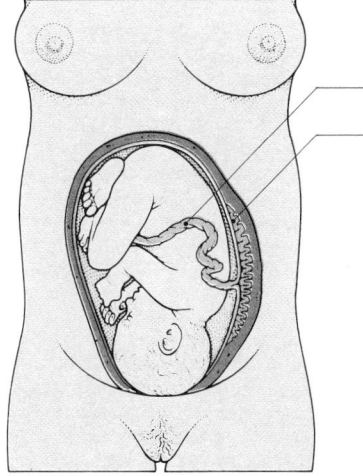

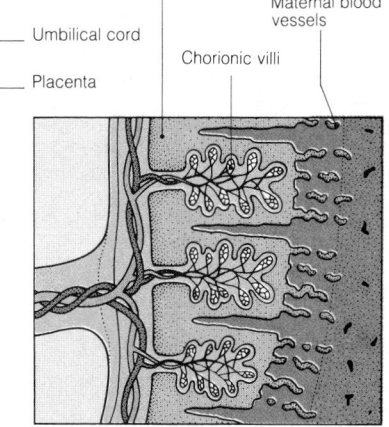

Pool of mother's blood

Maternal blood vessels

Umbilical cord

Chorionic villi

Placenta

How the mother's and baby's blood are brought together
The baby's blood flows via the umbilical cord to the placenta, where it enters numerous tiny blood vessels arranged in "fingers" (chorionic villi). These are surrounded by a pool of maternal blood brought to the placenta by a major artery.

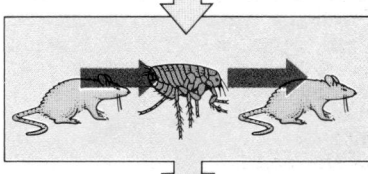

1 The bacterium that causes plague (*Yersinia pestis*) circulates mainly among wild rodents. The bacterium is spread from one rodent to another by rodent fleas.

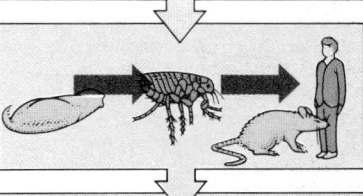

2 Sometimes so many wild rodents die that the fleas transfer to and infest new wild hosts, such as rats, or even humans who enter plague-affected areas.

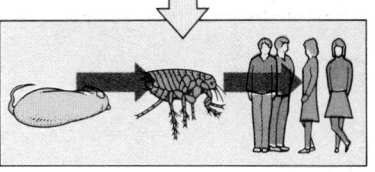

3 The real danger is of plague spreading to, and killing, large numbers of urban rats; rat fleas might then transfer from dead rats to humans en masse, causing an epidemic.

P

---

tests. The hormones enter the mother's blood to help her body adapt to the conditions of pregnancy; they also prepare the breasts for lactation (see *Breast-feeding*).

Placenta praevia
Implantation of the *placenta* in the lower part of the *uterus*, near or over the cervix. Placenta praevia occurs in about one in 200 pregnancies; it is less common in first pregnancies.

The condition varies in severity, depending on how much of the placenta is situated close to the cervix. In some cases, mild placenta praevia is detected during routine *ultrasound scanning* but has no adverse effect on the pregnancy. More severe placenta praevia often causes sudden painless vaginal bleeding in late pregnancy, when placental tissue separates from the uterus.

If the bleeding is slight and the pregnancy still has several weeks to run, bed rest may be all that is necessary. If the bleeding stops, the woman may be allowed to get up but she will probably be advised to remain in hospital until the baby is born because of the risk of sudden severe haemorrhage. The baby is usually delivered by *caesarean section* at the 38th week.

If the bleeding is heavy or if the pregnancy is near term, an immediate delivery is carried out.

Placenta, tumours of
See *Choriocarcinoma*; *Hydatidiform mole*.

Plague
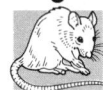 A serious infectious disease that mainly affects rodents but is transmissible to humans by the bites of rodent fleas. Plague has been a scourge to people since early history. One of the largest pandemics (worldwide epidemics) was the "black death" of the 14th century, which killed 25 million people in Europe alone. Today, human plague occurs sporadically in various parts of the world but not in Europe. It can be treated with antibiotic drugs.

CAUSES, TYPES, AND INCIDENCE
The bacterium responsible for the disease, YERSINIA PESTIS, circulates among rodents and their fleas in many parts of the world. The great pandemics of the past were caused by spread of plague from wild rodents to rats in cities and then to humans (via rat fleas) when the rats died. Today, human disease is usually the result of being bitten by fleas from wild rodents. A bite from an infected flea leads to bubonic plague, a form of the disease which is characterized by swollen lymph glands (called "buboes"). Pneumonic plague, which affects the lungs, can occur as a complication of bubonic plague; it is also spread from person to person in infected droplets expelled during coughing.

In recent years, outbreaks of plague have been confined mainly to parts of Africa, South America, and Southeast Asia, but some 10 to 50 cases of human plague occur in the US each year.

PREVENTION
There is a constant risk of plague spreading to urban rat populations, and the main measures to prevent this are rat control and surveillance of the disease in wild rodents. Hikers in

parts of the world where plague is present should not touch rodents or any carcass.

A vaccine against plague is available for people in high-risk occupations.

SYMPTOMS AND SIGNS

Bubonic plague usually starts, two to five days after infection, with fever, shivering, and severe headache. Soon the buboes appear. These are smooth, oval, reddened, intensely painful swellings usually in the groin, less commonly in the armpits, neck, or elsewhere. There may be bleeding into the skin around the buboes, resulting in dark patches. The victim may have seizures and, in about half the cases, will die if not treated. Occasionally, *septicaemia* (blood poisoning) is an early complication and may cause death before buboes appear.

In pneumonic plague, there is severe coughing that produces a bloody, frothy sputum (phlegm) and laboured breathing. Death is almost inevitable unless the disease is diagnosed and treated early.

DIAGNOSIS AND TREATMENT

A sample of fluid taken from a bubo, or of sputum in the case of suspected pneumonic plague, is cultured to confirm the presence of plague bacteria and establish the diagnosis.

Prompt treatment with the antibiotic drugs streptomycin, chloramphenicol, or tetracycline reduces the risk of death to less than five per cent.

All contacts of anyone who has pneumonic plague are watched closely and their temperatures checked regularly for a week. Antibiotic drugs are given as a preventive measure, and at the first suspicion of illness.

Plantar wart

See *Wart, plantar*.

Plants, poisonous

Several species of plants are poisonous to eat or can cause a severe allergic reaction if their leaves brush against the skin.

SKIN CONTACT

Among the plants that can cause skin reactions are nettles, hogweed, poison ivy, and primula. Itching, burning, and blistering may develop at the site of skin contact. In some people, these skin reactions can be extremely severe.

First-aid treatment includes thorough washing of the affected area, sponging with alcohol, and application of calamine lotion. Washing any clothing that may have come in contact with the plant is also advised. In the case of a severe reaction, it is wise to consult a doctor, who may prescribe *corticosteroid drugs* to be taken by mouth or injection.

INTERNAL POISONING

Plants that are poisonous to eat include foxglove, aconite, hemlock, laburnum seeds, and many types of berry, including the berries of deadly nightshade (which are black) and holly (red). Young children are the most commonly affected as a result of eating colourful berries. Symptoms of poisoning vary according to the plant but may include abdominal pain, vomiting, excitement, flushing, breathing difficulties, delirium, and coma. Medical help should be sought at once. The usual treatment is gastric *lavage* and measures to relieve symptoms as they arise.

Fatal poisoning is rare. Children should be taught not to sample berries or any type of wild plant.

Paradoxically, many poisonous plants are also a source of useful drugs. Examples include *atropine* from deadly nightshade and *digitalis drugs* from foxglove. (See also *Mushroom poisoning*.)

Plaque

The term given to an area of *atherosclerosis* (fatty deposits within arteries). The atheromatous plaques give no indication of their presence until they become so large that they reduce blood flow in a vessel or until some disturbance of the surface of the plaque develops, causing *thrombosis* (clotting of blood) at the site. When this occurs in a small or medium-sized vessel, blockage is likely (see *Peripheral vascular disease*). Plaques in the coronary arteries (which supply blood to the heart muscle) are the cause of *coronary artery disease*.

Plaque, dental

A rough sticky coating on the teeth that consists of saliva, bacteria, and food debris. It is the chief cause of tooth decay (see *Caries, dental*) and *gingivitis*; if allowed to accumulate, plaque forms the basis of a hard deposit (see *Calculus, dental*).

Plaque begins to form on teeth within a few hours of cleaning and is responsible for the furry feeling of unbrushed teeth. Salivary mucus, consisting mainly of proteins, forms on the teeth. Bacteria that live in the mouth then multiply within this mucus, gradually building up a layer of plaque. Some of these microorganisms, particularly STREPTOCOCCUS MUTANS, break down the sugar in the remains of carbohydrate food that stick to the mucus, adding to the plaque and also creating an acid that can rapidly erode tooth enamel.

POISONOUS PLANTS

There are numerous different poisonous plants—including some common garden or house plants—in addition to those shown here. Most cases of poisoning occur in young children, who, out of curiosity, eat berries or flowers.

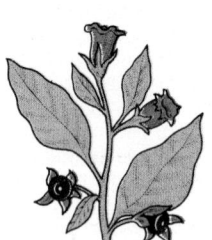

Deadly nightshade
Also known as belladonna, the deadly nightshade is about 1 m high and has shiny black berries. Eating any part of the plant can lead to symptoms such as rash, blurred vision, swallowing difficulty, confusion, and coma.

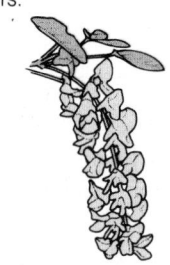

Laburnum
This is a small tree with yellow, pea-shaped flowers. Eating laburnum (especially the seeds) can lead to irritation of the mouth, excessive thirst, vomiting, vertigo, confusion, hallucinations, convulsions, paralysis, and coma.

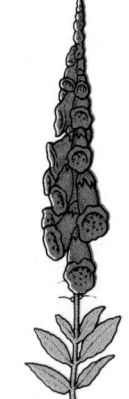

Foxglove
This plant has purplish-pink flowers; it is a source of the heart drug digitalis. Eating the plant irritates the mouth and causes headache, abdominal pain, vomiting, diarrhoea, and disturbance of the heartbeat.

DEVELOPMENT OF PLAQUE

Plaque starts with a deposit of salivary mucus on the teeth. The mucus is colonized by various types of bacteria. Initially, the predominant bacteria are spherical cocci. After a day or two, long filamentous colonies of bacteria spread over the surface of the teeth.

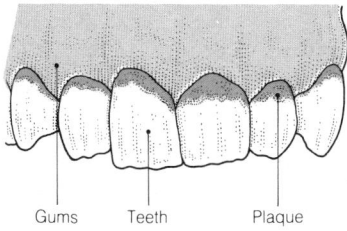

Areas of plaque build-up
Plaque develops predominantly at the margin of teeth and gums. If the gums are inflamed or otherwise unhealthy, the plaque tends to develop more rapidly.

Gums   Teeth   Plaque

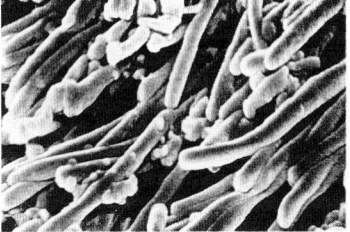

Mature plaque
This picture, taken with a scanning electron microscope, shows a mass of filamentous bacterial colonies in plaque, magnified about 2,000 times.

Plaque should be thoroughly removed at least once a day by *toothbrushing* and use of dental floss (see *Floss, dental*). It can be made more visible by the use of harmless dyes known as *disclosing agents*.

Plasma

The fluid part of *blood* which remains if the blood cells are removed. Plasma is a solution that contains many important nutrients, salts and proteins.

Plasmapheresis

A procedure, also called plasma exchange, for removing or reducing the concentration of unwanted substances in the *blood*. Blood is withdrawn from the patient in the same way as for *blood donation*, and the plasma portion of the blood is removed by special machines called cell separators. The blood cells are then mixed with a plasma substitute and returned to the circulation in the same way as for *blood transfusion*. It usually takes about two hours.

The main use of plasmapheresis is the removal of damaging *antibodies* or antibody-antigen particles (known as immune complexes) from the circulation in some *autoimmune disorders*, such as *myasthenia gravis*, *Goodpasture's syndrome*, and rapidly progressive kidney disease which is sometimes associated with systemic *lupus erythematosus*.

Plasma proteins

All the proteins present in *blood* plasma. Plasma proteins include *albumin*, fibrinogen and other substances important to *blood clotting*, and *immunoglobulins* (proteins with a role in the *immune system*).

Apart from their specific roles, the plasma proteins help maintain blood volume by preventing loss of water from the blood into the tissues. The proteins keep the water in the blood by a phenomenon called osmotic pressure (see *Osmosis*).

Plasminogen activator

See *Tissue plasminogen activator*.

Plaster cast

See *Cast*.

Plaster of Paris

A white powder composed of a calcium compound that reacts chemically with water, giving off heat and producing a paste that can be moulded and shaped before it sets. Plaster of Paris is used for constructing *casts* to immobilize parts of the body and for making dental models (see *Impression, dental*).

Plastic surgery

Any operation carried out to repair or reconstruct skin and underlying tissue that has been damaged or lost by injury or disease, has been malformed since birth, or has changed with aging. Every attempt is made to maintain function of the affected part of the body and to create as natural an appearance as possible.

Operations performed mainly to improve appearance in an otherwise generally healthy person are known as *cosmetic surgery*.

WHY IT IS DONE
Plastic surgery is usually performed to repair damage caused by severe burns or injuries, cancer, certain types of operation, such as *mastectomy* (breast removal), or the effects of aging.

Among the congenital conditions that may require correction by plastic surgery are *cleft lip and palate*, *hypospadias*, and imperforate anus (see *Anus, imperforate*).

HOW IT IS DONE
A variety of techniques is used to provide skin cover for damaged areas, including *skin grafts*, *skin flaps*, *Z-plasty*, and tissue expansion (in which skin is stretched by inserting a silicone balloon beneath the surface which is then gradually increased in size). These techniques may be combined with a *bone graft* or *implants* to provide underlying support.

The scope of plastic surgery has been much broadened over the past 10 years by the use of microsurgical techniques (see *Microsurgery*) to join blood vessels, thus allowing the transfer of blocks of skin and muscle from one part of the body to another.

-plasty

A suffix meaning shaping by surgery; performing *plastic surgery* on. *Rhinoplasty* is plastic surgery on the nose; *mammoplasty* is reshaping or reconstruction of the breast.

Platelet

The smallest type of *blood cell*, also called a thrombocyte. Platelets play a major role in *blood clotting*. A deficiency of platelets (a condition known as *thrombocytopenia*) can cause some types of *bleeding disorders*.

Platyhelminth

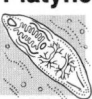 A flat, or ribbon-shaped, parasitic worm. Flukes, *tapeworms*, and schistosomes are types that cause disease in humans. (See *Liver fluke*; *Schistosomiasis*.)

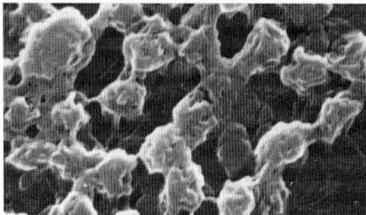

Electron micrograph of platelets
Normal and activated (spiky) platelets can be seen. Activated platelets clump to seal defects in blood vessel walls after injury.

P

Play therapy

A method used in the *psychoanalysis* of young children. Play therapy is based on the principle that all children's play has some symbolic significance.

The child is allowed to choose from the toys, drawing materials, and games in the therapist's room. Watching the child at play helps the therapist diagnose the source of the child's problems; the child can then be helped to "act out" thoughts and feelings that are causing anxiety. An improvement in the child's state may be indicated by changes in play, such as drawing smiling faces.

Plethora

A florid, bright-red, flushed complexion. It may be caused by dilation of blood vessels near the skin surface, or, more rarely, by *polycythaemia* (excessive numbers of red blood cells).

Plethysmography

A method of estimating the blood flow in vessels by measuring changes in the size of a body part. Plethysmography may be used on the penis to establish whether a patient with *impotence* gets an erection during sleep. It is occasionally used in the investigation of deep vein *thrombosis* to detect an obstruction of the blood flow back towards the heart.

Pleura

A thin membrane with two layers, one lining the outside of the *lungs* and the other the inside of the chest cavity. Fluid between the two layers provides lubrication and thus allows smooth, uniform expansion and contraction of the lungs during breathing.

DISORDERS

Pleurisy (inflammation of the pleura) is usually caused by a lung infection, such as *pneumonia* or *tuberculosis*, and may lead to *pleural effusion* (excessive fluid between the layers of the pleura). *Pneumothorax* (air in the pleural cavity) may occur spontaneously or be caused by a penetrating injury.

Pleural effusion

An accumulation of fluid between the layers of the *pleura* (the membrane lining the lungs and chest cavity). Pleural effusion may be caused by *pneumonia, tuberculosis, heart failure, cancer, pulmonary embolism*, or *mesothelioma* (a tumour of the pleura). The effusion may affect one or both sides of the chest.

Pleural effusion causes compression of the underlying lung, leading to breathing difficulty. Diagnosis is confirmed by *chest X-ray*. To determine the cause of the effusion, some of the fluid may be aspirated (removed with a needle and syringe) and examined. A *biopsy* (removal of a tissue sample for microscopic analysis) of the pleura may also be necessary.

Treatment is of the underlying cause. The fluid may need to be drained with a needle or tube to help breathing. In some cases caused by malignancy, *anticancer drugs* are injected into the pleural space to prevent a recurrence.

Pleurisy

Inflammation of the *pleura* (the membrane lining the lungs and chest cavity). Pleurisy is usually caused by a lung infection, such as *pneumonia* or a viral infection of the pleura. Rarer causes include *pulmonary embolism, lung cancer*, and *rheumatoid arthritis*.

Pleurisy causes a sharp chest pain that sometimes travels to the tip of the shoulder on the involved side. The pain, which is worse when breathing in, arises because the two inflamed membranes rub across each other. Treatment is of the underlying cause, along with *analgesic drugs* (painkillers).

Pleurodynia

Pain in the chest usually due to a viral infection. Sometimes called Bornholm disease, pleurodynia is caused by coxsackievirus B and often occurs in epidemics; it usually affects children but can occur at any age.

Symptoms include sudden severe pain in the lower chest or upper abdomen, with fever, sore throat, headache, and malaise. The disease usually settles in three or four days without treatment.

Plexus

A network of interwoven nerves or blood vessels, such as the *brachial plexus* (a network of nerves in the neck and upper arm).

Plication

A surgical procedure in which tucks are taken in the walls of a hollow organ and then stitched to decrease the organ's size. One type of plication is fundoplication, used to treat *hiatus hernia*. In this operation, the fundus (upper part) of the stomach is folded up around the lower end of the oesophagus to create an inkwell-like valve to prevent reflux of gastric acid from the stomach into the oesophagus.

Plummer-Vinson syndrome

Difficulty swallowing caused by the formation of webs of tissue across the upper *oesophagus*, and usually occurring along with severe iron-deficiency *anaemia*. The condition primarily affects middle-aged women.

The diagnosis is made by a barium swallow (see *Barium X-ray examinations*) and by inspection of the oesophagus with an *endoscope* (flexible viewing instrument). Treatment of the anaemia usually relieves symptoms; swallowing is relieved when the web is broken, which often occurs at the time of endoscopy.

Plutonium

A radioactive metallic element which occurs naturally only in infinitesimal amounts in uranium ores; it is produced artificially in breeder reactors by the bombardment of uranium with neutrons. Plutonium is used as a fuel in nuclear reactors and in nuclear weapons, such as the atomic bomb that was dropped on Nagasaki in 1945. The element is highly toxic if it enters the body because of its high rate of *radiation* emission (in the form of alpha particles) and its absorption in bone marrow where it may be retained for many years.

PMS

The abbreviation for *premenstrual syndrome*.

PMT

The abbreviation for premenstrual tension. See *Premenstrual syndrome*.

Pneumaturia

The presence of gas in the *urine*. Pneumaturia usually indicates that a *fistula* (an abnormal connection) has developed between the bladder and the intestine. Such a fistula is an unusual complication of a number of disorders, including *Crohn's disease, cancer*, or *diverticular disease*.

Pneumo-

A prefix meaning related to the lungs, to air, or to the breath. For example, pneumonia is inflammation of the lungs, and pneumothorax is air in the pleural space in the chest.

Pneumoconiosis

Any of a group of lung diseases caused by the inhalation of certain mineral dusts.

Only dust particles smaller than about 0.005 mm in diameter—small enough to reach the smallest air passages and alveoli (air sacs) in the lungs—are likely to cause harm. The dust particles cannot be destroyed within or completely removed from the lungs, so they accumulate and may eventually cause thickening and scarring. The lungs therefore become less efficient in supplying oxygen to the blood.

TYPES, CAUSES, AND INCIDENCE

The main types of pneumoconiosis are coal workers' pneumoconiosis (caused by coal dust), asbestosis (see *asbestos-induced diseases*), and silicosis, caused by dust containing silica (a constituent of sand and many types of rock, and the sole constituent of quartz). Silicosis is a hazard for workers in occupations such as quartz mining, stone cutting, blasting, and tunnel construction.

The risk of developing pneumoconiosis is directly related to the amount of dust inhaled over the years. These diseases primarily affect workers aged over 50, although cases of acute silicosis can occur with 10 months' exposure to a high level of dust.

Other, far less common, types of pneumoconiosis are caused by dusts containing beryllium (used in various high-technology industries), kaolin (from china-clay processing), slate, shale, or haematite (from the mining of iron ore).

The incidence is falling due to better preventive measures (e.g. by enforcing maximum permitted dust levels in industry, by medical surveillance of exposed workers, and by use of protective clothing). In the UK, the numbers of new cases diagnosed annually are approximately 400 with coalworkers' pneumoconiosis, 120 with asbestosis, and fewer than 100 with silicosis. There are about 350 deaths a year from pneumoconiosis, less than one fifth due to asbestosis.

SYMPTOMS AND COMPLICATIONS

Pneumoconiosis is often detected by a *chest X-ray* before it causes any symptoms. If exposure to the dust is stopped at this point, further progression of the disease may be prevented. In other cases, the main symptom initially is shortness of breath, which may gradually get worse.

In severe cases, pneumoconiosis may lead to *cor pulmonale* (right-sided heart failure resulting from lung damage). In a variant of pneumoconiosis, known as progressive massive fibrosis, damage continues relentlessly (mainly affecting the upper parts of the lungs) even though exposure to dust has stopped.

Complications of pneumoconiosis include the development of *emphysema*, and, in people with silicosis, an increased risk of *tuberculosis*. Pneumoconiosis caused by asbestos or haematite is associated with an increased risk of *lung cancer*; smoking increases the risk of cancer.

DIAGNOSIS, TREATMENT, AND OUTLOOK

The diagnosis depends on a history of exposure to dusts, a chest X-ray, medical examination, and *pulmonary function tests*.

There is no treatment for pneumoconiosis apart from treating complications, such as lung infections or cor pulmonale. Further exposure to dust must be avoided.

Anyone in whom pneumoconiosis develops at an early age or in whom progressive massive fibrosis develops at any age is at increased risk of a premature death. Industrial injury benefit can be claimed by anyone in whom pneumoconiosis develops and causes disability.

Pneumocystis pneumonia

 An infection of the lungs that is caused by the microorganism PNEUMOCYSTIS CARINII, a type of protozoan (single-celled) parasite. Pneumocystis pneumonia is an *opportunistic infection* that is dangerous only to people with impaired immunity (resistance) to infection—such as people who are suffering from *AIDS* or *leukaemia*. Pneumocystis pneumonia is a major cause of death in people who have AIDS.

Symptoms include fever, dry cough, and shortness of breath. They may last from a few weeks to a few months. Diagnosis is by examination of the sputum (phlegm) or a lung *biopsy* (removal of a sample of tissue for microscopic analysis). High doses of *antibiotic drugs* may help eradicate the infection, although it may recur.

Pneumonectomy

An operation to remove an entire lung. Pneumonectomy is sometimes performed to treat *lung cancer*. It once was used to treat *tuberculosis*, *bronchiectasis*, and lung infection, but these conditions are usually treated today by drugs or removal of only part of the lung (see *Lobectomy, lung*).

Before a pneumonectomy is performed, *pulmonary function tests* are carried out to make sure that the remaining lung is healthy enough to cope with the increased demands that will be placed on it.

HOW IT IS DONE

Under general anaesthesia, a curved incision is made (starting under the armpit and extending across the back) following the line of the lower edge of the shoulderblade. The muscles are cut through and the ribs spread apart to expose the lung. Sometimes a rib is removed for better exposure. The arteries, veins, and bronchi leading to the lung are tied off and divided, and the lung is removed. A drainage tube is usually inserted into the space between the two layers of *pleura*, and the incision is then stitched.

RECOVERY PERIOD

The drain is usually removed the day after the operation, and the stitches are taken out after about 10 days, when the patient can usually leave hospital. Many patients require artificial *ventilation* for hours to days after the operation. At home, normal activities should be resumed slowly; many people are able to return to work after about two months.

Pneumonia

Inflammation of the *lungs* due to infection. Pneumonia is a common late complication of any serious illness and is the certified cause of about 27,000 deaths in the UK each year. It is more common in males, during infancy and old age, and in those who have reduced immunity to infection (such as alcoholics).

There are two main types: lobar pneumonia and bronchopneumonia. In lobar pneumonia one lobe of one lung is initially affected. In bronchopneumonia, inflammation starts in the bronchi and bronchioles (airways) and then spreads to affect patches of tissue in one or both lungs.

CAUSES

Most cases of pneumonia are caused by viruses or bacteria. Causes of viral pneumonia include adenovirus, respiratory syncytial virus, or a coxsackievirus. The most common bacterial pneumonia is pneumococcal pneumonia caused by STREPTOCOCCUS PNEUMONIAE. Other causes of bacterial pneumonia include HAEMOPHILUS INFLUENZAE, LEGIONELLA PNEUMOPHILIA (see *Legionnaires' disease*), and STAPHYLOCOCCUS AUREUS. Pneumonia may also be caused by a *mycoplasma* (an organism that is intermediate between a bacterium and a virus) or by a *chlamydial infection*; *Q fever* is a type of pneumonia caused by a *rickettsia*.

Rarely, pneumonia may be due to a different type of organism, such as

P

fungi, yeasts, or protozoa. These types usually occur only in people with *immunodeficiency disorders*. For example, *pneumocystis pneumonia*, caused by a protozoon, commonly occurs in people with *AIDS*.

SYMPTOMS AND SIGNS

Symptoms and signs typically include fever, chills, shortness of breath, and a cough that produces yellow-green sputum and occasionally blood. Chest pain that is worse when breathing in may occur because of *pleurisy* (inflammation of the membrane lining the lungs and chest cavity).

Potential complications include *pleural effusion* (fluid around the lung), *empyema* (pus around the lung), and, in rare cases, an *abscess* (collection of pus) in the lung.

DIAGNOSIS

The doctor gives the patient a physical examination, listening to chest sounds through a stethoscope. The diagnosis may be confirmed by a *chest X-ray* and by examination of sputum and of blood for microorganisms.

TREATMENT

Patients with mild pneumonia can usually be treated at home, but hospi-

---

PNEUMONIA

Pneumonia is not a single disease, but the name for several types of lung inflammation caused by infectious organisms. In some cases, accidental inhalation of vomit or a liquid starts the infection. The symptoms, treatment, and outcome vary greatly, depending on the cause and on the general health of the patient.

Lobar pneumonia

In this type, which is rare in most developed countries today, the inflammation is usually confined to just one lobe of one lung—often a lower lobe.

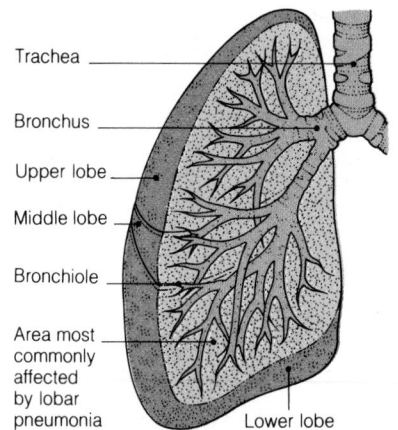

Trachea
Bronchus
Upper lobe
Middle lobe
Bronchiole
Area most commonly affected by lobar pneumonia
Lower lobe

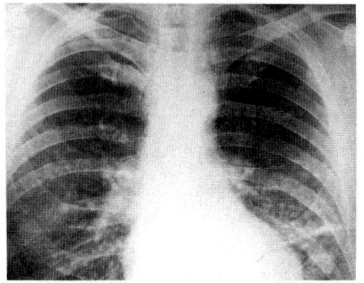

Chest X-ray in bronchopneumonia
The X-ray clearly shows broncho-pneumonia. The blotchy, white areas within the darker areas correspond to patches of inflamed lung.

TYPES, CAUSES, AND TREATMENT OF PNEUMONIA

Types	Causes	Symptoms	Drug treatments	Other treatments
Pneumonias always or usually caused by bacteria				
Lobar pneumonia	*Streptococcus pneumoniae*	Cough, painful breathing, high temperature, rust-coloured sputum	Penicillin	Machine ventilation of the lungs to help breathing may be required in some cases. Physio-therapy to clear sputum out of the lungs may also be needed
Bronchopneumonia	*Haemophilus influenzae* or other organisms	Cough, often a fever, green or yellow sputum	Various antibiotics	
Aspiration pneumonia	Various organisms. Occurs following inhalation of sputum, vomit, liquids, and so on	Fever, cough	Various antibiotics	
Legionnaires' disease	*Legionella pneumophila*	Fever, cough, chest pain, headache, aches and pains	Erythromycin	
Pneumonias not caused by bacteria				
Viral pneumonia	Chickenpox virus, influenza virus, adenovirus and others	Cough, fever, not much sputum	Antibiotics (if lungs become infected by bacteria)	Machine ventilation of the lungs to help breathing may be required in severe cases
Psittacosis	*Chlamydia psittaci*, a bacteria-like organism caught from birds	Cough, raised temperature, not much sputum	Tetracycline or erythromycin	
Q fever	*Coxiella burnetti*, a rickettsia	Cough, raised temperature, not much sputum	Tetracycline or erythromycin	
Mycoplasmal pneumonia	*Mycoplasma pneumoniae*, a bacteria-like organism	Cough, raised temperature, not much sputum	Tetracycline or erythromycin	

P

talization is necessary in severe cases. The drugs prescribed depend on the causative microorganism; they may include *antibiotic drugs* or *antifungal drugs*. *Aspirin* or *paracetamol* may be given to reduce fever. In severe cases, *oxygen therapy* and artificial *ventilation* may be required.

OUTLOOK

Most sufferers recover completely within two weeks. However, some elderly or debilitated people fail to respond to treatment; progressively more lung tissue is affected, and death occurs as a result of *respiratory failure*.

Pneumonitis

A form of inflammation of the *lungs* that may cause coughing, breathing difficulty, and wheezing. Pneumonitis may be due to a wide range of causes, including an allergic reaction caused by inhalation of dust containing animal or plant material (see *Alveolitis*), and exposure to radiation (see *Radiation hazards*). Pneumonitis may also occur as a rare side-effect of some drugs, such as *amiodarone* and *azathioprine*.

Pneumothorax

A condition in which air enters the pleural cavity (the space between the two layers of the *pleura* which cover the *lungs* and the chest wall). The air may enter the pleural cavity from the lungs or from outside the body.

CAUSES

Spontaneous pneumothorax, which usually occurs for no apparent reason, is six times more common in men than in women. Most often, it occurs in thin young adults who have no underlying lung disease; in many cases, it is thought to be due to rupture of a congenital blister at the top of the lung. There is a 30 per cent chance of a recurrence of spontaneous pneumothorax, usually on the same side. Pneumothorax may also be a complication of lung disease (particularly *asthma* or *emphysema*) or it may follow an injury, such as a fractured rib.

A pneumothorax may be caused accidentally when a catheter is inserted into a vein in the neck for intravenous feeding (see *Feeding, artificial*) or to monitor pressure in the heart and circulation.

SYMPTOMS

A pneumothorax may cause chest pain or shortness of breath, the degree of which is proportional to the size of the pneumothorax. Any underlying lung disease will increase breathing difficulty. If there is continual leakage of

air into the pleural space, the pneumothorax may become progressively bigger and produce a tension pneumothorax, which may become life-threatening due to compression of the heart.

DIAGNOSIS AND TREATMENT

A *chest X-ray* confirms the diagnosis. A small pneumothorax in a healthy adult usually disappears within a few days without treatment. A larger one, or a small one in the presence of underlying lung disease, requires treatment. Treatment usually involves removing the air from the pleural cavity through a suction tube inserted through the chest wall for several days. A small pneumothorax can be treated by drawing out the air through a needle and syringe. If the lung fails to expand, or if the pneumothorax recurs, surgery may be required to seal the pleural cavity.

Pocket, gingival

See *Periodontitis*.

Podiatry

A paramedical speciality concerned with the feet (see *Chiropody*).

Podophyllin

A drug used in the treatment of genital warts. It may cause irritation of the treated area and severe toxicity on excessive application.

Poison

A substance that, in relatively small amounts, disrupts the structure and/or function of cells. Although toxin is often used interchangeably with poison, toxin refers strictly and specifically to poisonous proteins produced by pathogenic (disease-causing) bacteria, some animals, and certain plants. (See also *Drug poisoning; Poisoning*.)

Poisoning

Poisons enter the body by various routes. They may be swallowed, inhaled, absorbed through the skin, or injected under the skin (as with an *insect sting* or *snake bite*). Poisons may also originate within the body itself.

For example, bacteria can produce poisonous *endotoxins*, *enterotoxins*, or *exotoxins*. Various disorders, such as *kidney failure*, *liver failure*, and certain *metabolic disorders*, may cause poisonous substances to be produced or to accumulate within the body.

Poisoning may be acute or chronic. In acute poisoning, a large amount of poison enters, or is produced in, the body over a short time (as may occur in *food poisoning*). Chronic poisoning results from the gradual accumulation of a poison that is not eliminated quickly.

P

FIRST AID: POISONING

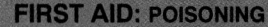

DO NOT
- make the victim vomit if he or she has swallowed corrosives

1 If the victim is conscious, quickly ask what he or she has swallowed.

2 Call an ambulance and say what the victim has taken.

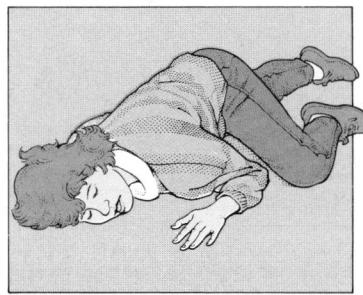

3 If the victim is unconscious but breathing, place him or her in the *recovery position*.

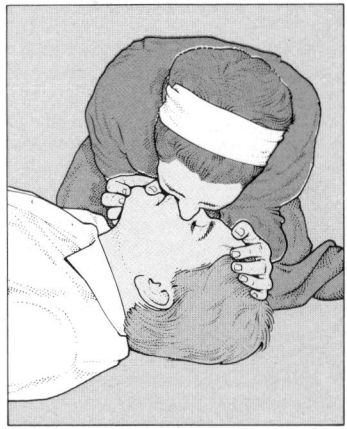

4 If the victim is not breathing, *artificial respiration* is necessary. Use the mouth-to-nose method to avoid contact with the poison.

5 If you are certain the victim has swallowed only tablets or berries, it may help to induce vomiting by placing your fingers at the back of the throat.

P

Inadvertent poisoning is one of the most common types of accident in the home. It occurs principally in young children, although adults sometimes unwittingly poison themselves, often by mistaking the dosage of a prescribed drug (see *Drug poisoning*) or, less commonly, by unthinkingly taking very high doses of certain vitamin or mineral supplements. Exposure to poisonous substances in industry is another important cause of unintentional poisoning in adults. *Drug abuse* is another.

Poisoning may be a deliberate attempt to commit *suicide*. However, many such attempts are unsuccessful or are actually intended to gain sympathy or attention. Taking a drug overdose (often in combination with alcohol, which increases the toxicity of many drugs) is a common method of suicidal poisoning. (See also *Poisoning* first-aid box on previous page; and articles on individual poisons.)

Polio

An abbreviation for *poliomyelitis*.

Poliomyelitis

An infectious disease once known as infantile paralysis but now usually called polio. Poliomyelitis is caused by a virus, which usually provokes no more than a mild illness. However, in more serious cases it attacks the *brain* and *spinal cord*. This may lead to extensive paralysis (including paralysis of the muscles involved in breathing) or may be fatal.

Since the development of effective vaccines in the 1950s, polio has virtually been eliminated from most developed countries, although cases still occur in people who have not been fully vaccinated. Polio also remains a serious risk for unvaccinated people travelling in southern Europe, Africa, or Asia. The WHO is campaigning for polio to be eliminated worldwide by the year 2000.

INCIDENCE OF POLIO

Year	Cases
1985	4
1975	3
1965	91
1955	6,331

Cases: 0   2,000   4,000   6,000   8,000

Since the introduction of routine immunization in 1956, the incidence of polio in the UK has dropped from several thousand cases a year to fewer than 10

There are three closely related polioviruses. Infected people pass large numbers of virus particles in their faeces, from where they may be spread indirectly, or directly via fingers, to food and thus infect others. Airborne transmission also occurs.

In countries where standards of hygiene and sanitation are low, most children become infected early in life, when the infection rarely causes serious illness, and develop immunity. In countries with better standards of hygiene, children do not become immune in this manner; if they are not vaccinated, disastrous epidemics occur. Immunization is thus of vital importance. In the UK, where there has been widespread immunization for over 30 years, the disease is now very rare; a few people each year contract it, often while travelling abroad.

PREVENTION

Vaccination is given during infancy, usually at about two, three, and four months, with a booster dose at about five years (see *Immunization*). The vaccine contains all three types of poliovirus, and immunity develops against each of them. There are two alternative types of vaccine: IPV (inactivated polio vaccine), which contains dead viruses and is given by injection, and OPV (oral poliovirus vaccine), which contains live but harmless strains of virus and is given by mouth. OPV is the vaccine of choice in the UK, except for children who have an *immunodeficiency* disorder, which lowers resistance to infection.

There is an extremely small risk (about one in five million doses) that the live vaccine will cause polio in the vaccinated person or in someone who is a close contact.

SYMPTOMS AND SIGNS

Minor forms of polio are by far the most common. About 85 per cent of children infected with the virus have no symptoms at all. In the rest, after an incubation period of three to five days, there is a short illness with slight fever, sore throat, headache, and vomiting. This lasts for a few days, after which most children recover completely.

In some children, however, after a short period of apparent health there is a major illness with symptoms caused by inflammation of the *meninges* (membranes covering the brain and spinal cord). These symptoms are fever, severe headache, stiffness of the neck and back, and aching in the muscles, sometimes with widespread

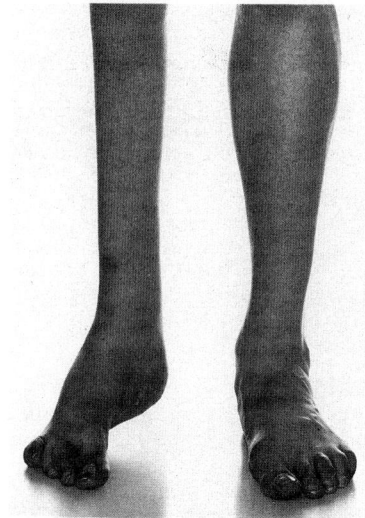

Wasted limb of polio patient
Muscle bulk is severely reduced in the paralysed (right) leg. Muscle function can sometimes be helped by physiotherapy.

twitching. In some cases the condition progresses, often in the course of a few hours, to extensive paralysis of muscles. The legs and lower trunk are the most frequently paralysed. If infection spreads to the brainstem (the lowest part of the brain), the result may be swallowing and breathing problems, or even total loss of these faculties.

DIAGNOSIS

To make a firm diagnosis, the causative virus must be isolated from a sample of cerebrospinal fluid, taken by *lumbar puncture*, or from a throat swab or a sample of faeces. Muscle paralysis combined with an acute feverish illness is so characteristic of severe polio that it usually enables an immediate diagnosis to be made.

TREATMENT

There is no effective drug treatment for polio. Nonparalytic patients do not usually need treatment except for bed rest and *analgesic drugs*. When muscles are paralysed, *physiotherapy* is essential to prevent muscle damage while the virus is active. Later, during convalescence, physiotherapy is needed to help retain muscle function.

When the lower part of the body is paralysed, the bladder does not function properly and may make catheterization (see *Catheterization, urinary*) necessary. Respiratory paralysis requires *tracheostomy* (emergency surgical creation of an opening in the windpipe to insert a breathing tube) and artificial *ventilation*.

OUTLOOK

Recovery from nonparalytic polio is complete. Of those who become paralysed, more than half eventually make a full recovery, more than a quarter suffer only minor permanent muscle weakness, less than a quarter are left with severe disability, and less than one in 10 dies (mainly adults and those in whom the brainstem has been severely affected). Years after extensive paralysis with some recovery, there may be a "postpolio" deterioration with new weakness and pain in some of the recovered muscles.

Pollution

Contamination of the environment by poisons, microorganisms, or radioactive substances.

Serious public concern about pollution developed in the 1950s with the growing realization that *pesticides* were destroying wildlife and disturbing or poisoning the food chain, and that atmospheric nuclear tests were disseminating radioactive fallout over wide areas (see *Radiation*). This concern was strengthened by incidents of industrial pollution, such as the release of mercury waste into Minamata Bay, Japan (see *Minamata disease*); the release into the atmosphere of the poisonous chemical dioxin by a factory explosion in Italy (see *Defoliant poisoning*); damage to seabirds and beaches from oil tanker spillages; and, more recently, from acid rain caused by the burning of coal and oil, and from radioactive fallout from the nuclear reactor explosion at Chernobyl in the former USSR.

A potentially serious pollutant in its long-term effects is *carbon dioxide*, large amounts of which are discharged into the atmosphere by the burning of fossil fuels. The continual increase in the atmospheric carbon dioxide level is producing what is called the "greenhouse effect", which is increasing the average global temperature, and may go on to cause future catastrophic climatic changes.

Another serious pollution effect is the gradual destruction of the *ozone* layer (which blocks harmful ultraviolet radiation from the sun) by various chemicals, notably some CFCs (chlorofluorocarbons). Concern about this effect has led to a reduction in the emission of ozone-depleting chemicals in many developed countries. Other important pollutants include lead (see *Lead poisoning*), cadmium (see *Cadmium poisoning*), and some pesticides, such as *parathion*.

Poly-

A prefix that means many or much, as in polymyositis (inflammation of many muscles) and polyuria (passing of large volumes of urine).

Polyarteritis nodosa

An uncommon disease of medium-sized arteries, also called periarteritis nodosa. Areas of arterial wall become inflamed, weakened, and liable to the formation of *aneurysms* (ballooned-out segments). Many different groups of blood vessels may be involved, including the coronary arteries that supply blood to the heart muscle, or the arteries of the kidneys, intestine, skeletal muscles, and nervous system. The seriousness of the condition depends on which organs are affected and how severely they are affected.

CAUSES AND INCIDENCE

The disease seems to be the result of a disturbance of the *immune system* (body's defences against infection), triggered in some cases by exposure to the *hepatitis B* virus. It may develop at any age but is most common in adults. More men than women are affected.

SYMPTOMS AND COMPLICATIONS

In the early stages the patient has a fever and aching muscles and joints. There is general malaise, loss of appetite and weight, and, if blood vessels supplying nerves are affected, nerve pain. Damage to blood vessels leads to obstruction of the blood supply, causing *hypertension* (raised blood pressure), muscle weakness, ulceration of the skin, and gangrene (tissue death). If the coronary arteries are affected, *myocardial infarction* (heart attack) may occur. Because blood vessels supplying the intestines are frequently affected, a high proportion of patients suffer abdominal pain, nausea and vomiting, and diarrhoea, and pass blood in the faeces.

DIAGNOSIS

Polyarteritis nodosa is diagnosed by finding inflammation in blood vessels in a *biopsy* specimen taken from an affected organ. *Angiography* (X-rays of blood vessels that have been injected with a radiopaque substance) may show areas of narrowing and scarring and/or aneurysms.

TREATMENT AND OUTLOOK

Large doses of *corticosteroid drugs*, sometimes supplemented by *immunosuppressant drugs*, are effective in improving an otherwise unfavourable outlook. Without treatment, few victims of the condition survive for five years; death often occurs from a myocardial infarction, *kidney failure*,

severe bleeding into the intestine, or from complications of hypertension. With modern drug treatment, about 50 per cent of patients survive for five years or more.

Polycystic kidney

See *Kidney, polycystic*.

Polycystic ovary

See *Ovary, polycystic*.

Polycythaemia

A condition characterized by an unusually large number of red cells in the *blood* due to increased production of red cells by the *bone marrow*. This condition usually results from some other disorder or is a natural response to *hypoxia* (reduced oxygen in the blood and tissues). In such cases, it is called secondary polycythaemia. Rarely, it occurs for no apparent reason and is called polycythaemia vera or primary polycythaemia.

SECONDARY POLYCYTHAEMIA

Polycythaemia occurs naturally in people living at (or visiting) high altitudes due to the reduced air pressure and level of oxygen. It can also result from any disorder that impairs the supply of oxygen to the blood (e.g. chronic *bronchitis*). In these cases, the low level of oxygen in the blood stimulates production of the hormone erythropoietin by the kidneys, which in turn stimulates the bone marrow to produce more red cells. The result is an increase in the oxygen-carrying efficiency of the blood, which compensates for the reduced oxygen supply. Descending to sea level, or effective treatment of an underlying disorder, soon returns the person's blood to normal.

Polycythaemia can also be secondary to *liver cancer* or certain kidney disorders that cause excess production of erythropoietin. Treatment of the underlying disorder quickly returns the blood to normal.

POLYCYTHAEMIA VERA

This rare disorder of the bone marrow develops primarily in people over 40. The estimated incidence is about 300 new cases per year in the UK.

The large number of red cells results in an increased volume and thickening of the blood, which may cause headaches, blurred vision, and *hypertension* (high blood pressure). There may also be a flushed skin, dizziness, night sweats, and widespread itching, particularly after a hot bath. Often, the sufferer's spleen is enlarged. There may also be abnormalities in the platelets in the blood, causing a tendency to bleed or to form blood clots. Other complications include *stroke* and, at a late stage, other types of bone marrow disease, such as *myelosclerosis* or acute leukaemia (see *Leukaemia, acute*).

The diagnosis is made from a physical examination and *blood tests* and by ruling out any other causes of polycythaemia. Treatment of polycythaemia vera consists of regular removal of blood through a vein (*venesection*), sometimes in combination with *anticancer drugs* or radioactive phosphorus taken by mouth to control the overproduction of red cells in the marrow.

Treatment enables most patients to survive for 10 to 15 years. Death usually occurs from a stroke or other complication of the disease.

Polydactyly

A *birth defect* in which there is an excessive number of fingers or toes. The extra digits may be fully formed and look like the other fingers or toes or they may be fleshy stumps.

Polydactyly affects about 50 babies in every 100,000. If both parents have polydactyly, there is a one in two chance that each of their children will be affected. Polydactyly often runs in otherwise normal families, but may also occur as part of the *Laurence-Biedl-Moon syndrome* or of other congenital syndromes. If there are no other abnormalities, the condition presents no risk to the child's physical or mental development.

Polydipsia

A medical term for persistent excessive thirst, which occurs, for example, in untreated *diabetes mellitus* and *diabetes insipidus* (see *Thirst, excessive*).

Polyhydramnios

Excess *amniotic fluid* surrounding the fetus during pregnancy. Polyhydramnios occurs in about one in 250 pregnancies.

CAUSES

In many cases, there is no known cause for polyhydramnios. The condition sometimes occurs if the fetus has a malformation (particularly *anencephaly* or *oesophageal atresia*) that makes normal swallowing impossible. Polyhydramnios may also occur if the pregnant woman has *diabetes mellitus*. Polyhydramnios occurs in about 10 per cent of multiple pregnancies.

SYMPTOMS AND SIGNS

In polyhydramnios, an excess of amniotic fluid usually accumulates

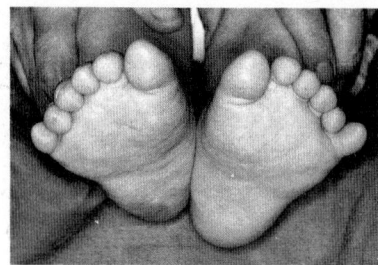

Polydactyly affecting the feet
The extra toes can cause problems with footwear and are usually removed surgically during childhood.

slowly during the second half of the pregnancy, producing symptoms from about week 32. The main symptom is abdominal discomfort. Other possible symptoms are breathlessness and swelling of the legs. The uterus is larger than usual for the duration of the pregnancy.

Less commonly, the fluid accumulates rapidly, causing abdominal pain, breathlessness, nausea, and vomiting. The abdomen becomes tense, the overlying skin is stretched and shiny, and the legs swell. Polyhydramnios may cause premature labour.

DIAGNOSIS

Polyhydramnios is usually evident from the mother's history and a physical examination. *Ultrasound scanning* is needed to detect fetal abnormality or multiple pregnancy.

TREATMENT

Mild cases without fetal abnormality require no treatment other than extra rest. Withdrawal of amniotic fluid via a needle inserted through the abdominal wall can provide temporary relief in severe cases although the procedure may cause premature labour. If the pregnant woman has diabetes mellitus, careful attention must be paid to her diabetic control. If symptoms occur in late pregnancy, *induction of labour* may be performed to deliver the baby early.

Polymyalgia rheumatica

An uncommon disease of elderly people that is marked by pain and stiffness in the muscles of the hips, thighs, shoulders, and neck.

CAUSES AND INCIDENCE

The cause of polymyalgia rheumatica is unknown, but it may be associated with *temporal arteritis*, *rheumatoid arthritis*, systemic *lupus erythematosus*, and, sometimes, cancer.

Polymyalgia rheumatica affects twice as many women as men and is unusual before the age of 50.

SYMPTOMS

The pain and stiffness, which may develop gradually or suddenly, make movement difficult. Morning stiffness is notable and often makes getting out of bed a problem. Weight loss and depression may also occur.

DIAGNOSIS AND TREATMENT

The diagnosis, which is often difficult to confirm, is based on the patient's history, a physical examination, and blood tests (including an *ESR*). If temporal arteritis is suspected, a *biopsy* (removal of a small sample of tissue for analysis) may be performed on an artery at the side of the scalp.

Small doses of *corticosteroid drugs* (higher doses when temporal arteritis is present) usually bring about an improvement in the disorder within a few days. The dosage is gradually reduced and use of the drug may be discontinued within two years.

Polymyositis

A rare disease in which the muscles become inflamed and weak. Polymyositis shares the features of *dermatomyositis* except that there is no rash.

Polymyxins

A group of *antibiotic drugs* derived from the bacterium BACILLUS POLYMYXA. Polymyxins, which include *colistin* and polymyxin B, are commonly given in drop or ointment form to treat eye, ear, and skin infections. They are very infrequently given by injection to treat severe infections because in this form they may cause nerve or kidney damage.

Polyp

A growth that projects, usually on a stalk, from the lining of the nose, the cervix, the intestine, the larynx, or any other *mucous membrane*.

Polyps may need to be removed surgically if they are responsible for symptoms. Some types of polyps are liable to develop into cancer, and are removed whether or not they are causing symptoms.

Polypeptide

A compound that consists of many *amino acids* linked by *peptide* bonds.

Polypharmacy

The practice of prescribing several different drugs to one person at the same time. Drug combinations may be more effective and may reduce the risk of drug resistance. Polypharmacy increases the risk of drug interactions and, thus, the risk of adverse effects.

Polyposis, familial

A rare, inherited disorder, also known as polyposis coli, in which numerous (often a thousand or more) *polyps* are present in the colon and rectum. Without preventive treatment, the development of cancer of the colon (see *Colon, cancer of*) by the age of 40 is almost a certainty.

SYMPTOMS AND DIAGNOSIS

The polyps are not present at birth but usually appear by the age of 10 and may cause bleeding and diarrhoea. However, there are often no symptoms until cancer has developed; it is therefore extremely important that a diagnosis be made as early as possible. The polyps are detected by air contrast *barium X-ray examination* and *colonoscopy* (investigation of the colon with a viewing instrument).

PREVENTION AND TREATMENT

Since there is a 50 per cent chance that the children of an affected parent will inherit the disease, close medical surveillance is necessary from the age of about 10. This screening, by barium examinations and colonoscopy, is performed every two years until the age of about 40, after which time it is unlikely that polyps will appear.

Individual polyps may be cauterized during endoscopic examination. Because there is such a high risk of cancer, more radical treatment may be needed. This often takes the form of total *colectomy* (removal of the entire colon) and the creation of an artificial opening of the ileum (the lower part of the small intestine) through the abdominal wall (see *Ileostomy*). Alternatively, the end of the ileum is joined to the rectum so that a normal passage for bowel movements exists. However, the rectum must be examined regularly to detect polyps, which must be treated immediately before there is a chance for cancerous changes to occur.

Polyuria

See *Urination, excessive*.

Pompholyx

An acute form of *eczema* in which itchy blisters form over the palms and/or soles. The condition, also called dyshydrotic eczema, often develops for no apparent reason but is sometimes due to an allergic response to a substance in contact with the skin. It is associated rarely with *ringworm*.

Treatment is with an astringent, which causes the skin to tighten and dry, or with topical application of a *corticosteroid drug*.

Pons

The middle part of the *brainstem*, situated between the midbrain (above) and the medulla oblongata (below).

Pore

A tiny opening. The term usually describes an opening in the *skin* that releases sweat or sebum (an oily substance secreted by sebaceous glands). Most of the pores from which sebum arises are also *hair* follicles.

Porphyria

Any of a group of uncommon and usually inherited disorders caused by the accumulation in the body of substances called porphyrins. Sufferers often have a rash or skin blistering brought on by sunlight and may have abdominal pain and nervous system disturbances from certain drugs.

CAUSES, TYPES, AND INCIDENCE

Porphyrins are chemicals with a complex structure that are formed in the body during the manufacture of haem—a component of *haemoglobin* (the oxygen-carrying pigment in the blood).

The porphyrias result from blocks in the chemical processes by which haem is formed, resulting in the accumulation of porphyrins. Such blocks are the results of deficiencies of various *enzymes* in the body; these deficiencies are inherited in an autosomal dominant pattern (see *Genetic disorders*). Porphyria due to poisoning is also known.

Six types of porphyria are recognized—acute intermittent porphyria, variegate porphyria, and porphyria cutanea tarda (the more common types); and hereditary coproporphyria, protoporphyria, and congenital erythropoietic porphyria (all very rare). The incidence of each varies throughout the world. The combined prevalence in the UK is unknown, but is probably about one affected person per 10,000 to 50,000 population.

SYMPTOMS AND SIGNS

The different types of porphyria have different features.

ACUTE INTERMITTENT PORPHYRIA This type

usually first appears in early adulthood with attacks of abdominal pain, which may mimic appendicitis. Limb cramps, muscle weakness, and psychiatric disturbances are common. There are no skin symptoms, but the patient's urine turns red when left to stand. A large number of drugs are known to precipitate attacks, including barbiturate drugs, phenytoin, oral contraceptives, and tetracyclines.

VARIEGATE PORPHYRIA This type is similar

in many respects to acute intermittent porphyria, but with blistering of sun-exposed skin. Attacks may be brought on by the same drugs that precipitate acute intermittent porphyria.

PORPHYRIA CUTANEA TARDA This type also

causes blistering of sun-exposed skin, but no abdominal or nervous system disturbance. Wounds are characteristically slow to heal. The urine is sometimes pink or brown. Many cases are precipitated by liver disease, including alcoholic liver disease.

HEREDITARY COPROPORPHYRIA This type of

porphyria is similar to acute intermittent porphyria, with additional skin symptoms in some sufferers.

PROTOPORPHYRIA This type usually

causes mild skin symptoms after exposure to sunlight.

CONGENITAL ERYTHROPOIETIC PORPHYRIA

This type is extremely rare; it is characterized by red discoloration of urine and teeth, excessive hair growth, severe skin blistering and ulceration, and haemolytic *anaemia*. Death may occur in childhood.

DIAGNOSIS AND TREATMENT

The porphyrias are diagnosed by finding abnormal levels of porphyrins in the urine and faeces. More specific tests are available for some types.

Treatment is difficult. Avoiding exposure to sunlight and/or to precipitating drugs is the most important measure. Attacks of acute intermittent porphyria, variegate porphyria, and hereditary coproporphyria can sometimes be helped by administration of glucose or of haematin, which is chemically related to haem. Porphyria cutanea tarda can be helped by the removal of blood through a vein (*venesection*).

Portal hypertension

Increased blood pressure in the portal vein, a large blood vessel that carries blood from the stomach, intestine, and spleen to the liver. The pressure in the veins of the upper stomach and lower oesophagus is raised, causing them to widen (a condition known as *oesophageal varices*) and sometimes to rupture. In addition, fluid is forced from the overloaded portal vein, resulting in *ascites*, an accumulation of fluid in the abdomen.

CAUSES

The most common cause of portal hypertension is the liver disease *cirrhosis*, in which scarring and regenerative tissue in the organ obstruct the portal vein. Another cause is *thrombosis* (abnormal blood clotting) in the

P

vein. This may occur shortly after birth or later in life, when it is usually the result of narrowing of the vein by cirrhosis, compression of the vein by enlarged lymph nodes, or inflammation resulting from an infection. Portal hypertension may also be caused by narrowing of the vein from birth.

Rarely, portal hypertension is due to an abnormal connection between the portal vein and an artery (*arteriovenous fistula*), usually as a result of injury. Portal hypertension can also be caused by increased blood flow from the spleen if disease has caused this organ to enlarge; this is a common cause in the tropics.

SYMPTOMS AND SIGNS

If the veins in the oesophagus and stomach rupture, this causes massive recurrent vomiting of blood and the passing of black faeces. Ascites results in abdominal swelling and discomfort and sometimes difficulty in breathing.

DIAGNOSIS

Portal hypertension is usually diagnosed from the patient's symptoms and signs. The cause can be determined by examining the liver and surrounding blood vessels by means of *ultrasound scanning* and X-ray examination of the blood vessels (see *Angiography*).

TREATMENT AND OUTLOOK

Bleeding from ruptured blood vessels is stopped by sclerotherapy, which comprises the injection of a sclerosant (hardening) solution into or around the veins. This induces inflammation, subsequent scarring, and consequent thickening of the vessels' walls so that the veins are blocked off. Ascites is controlled by restriction of dietary sodium chloride (salt) and by *diuretic drugs*, which increase overall urine production.

In some cases, an operation known as a *shunt* may be carried out to divert blood from the portal vein to some other blood vessel, thus relieving the high pressure.

The outlook depends on how successfully the underlying cause of this condition can be treated.

Port-wine stain

A purple-red birthmark that is level with the skin's surface. A port-wine stain is a permanent and often unsightly type of *haemangioma*. Cosmetic treatment by laser surgery may be possible in some cases.

Positron emission tomography

See *PET scanning*.

PORTAL HYPERTENSION

The most common cause of this condition is liver cirrhosis or some other obstruction to blood flow through the liver. The portal vein becomes congested with blood, and back pressure develops through the system of veins that join the portal vein.

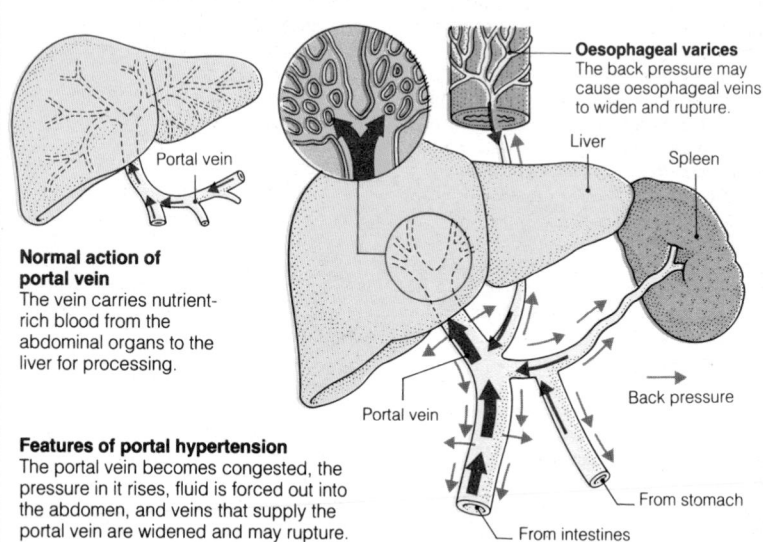

Normal action of portal vein
The vein carries nutrient-rich blood from the abdominal organs to the liver for processing.

Portal vein

Oesophageal varices
The back pressure may cause oesophageal veins to widen and rupture.

Liver

Spleen

Back pressure

Portal vein

From stomach

From intestines

Features of portal hypertension
The portal vein becomes congested, the pressure in it rises, fluid is forced out into the abdomen, and veins that supply the portal vein are widened and may rupture.

Posseting

A term for the regurgitation of small quantities of milk by infants after they have been fed. Posseting is common and harmless.

Postcoital contraception

See *Contraception, postcoital*.

Posterior

Relating to the back of the body. In human anatomy, the term is synonymous with *dorsal*.

Postmaturity

A condition in which a *pregnancy* persists for longer than 42 weeks; the average length of a normal pregnancy is 40 weeks from the first day of the last menstrual period (see *Gestation*). Postmaturity may be due to a family tendency to prolonged pregnancy, or it may be an indication that the head is bigger than the mother's pelvis and that the baby is unable to descend properly (see *Engagement*). Many obstetricians attempt to avoid postmaturity by *induction of labour* as the pregnancy nears 42 weeks' gestation.

COMPLICATIONS

Because the postmature baby is larger than average and the bones of the baby's skull are harder and thus mould less readily, postmaturity is associated with a prolonged labour and an increased likelihood of having a difficult delivery.

The major risk of postmaturity is fetal death and consequent stillbirth; the risk of this occurring doubles by the 43rd week of pregnancy and trebles by the 44th week as compared to the normal 40-week pregnancy. This increase in fetal death rate is in part a consequence of diminished placental efficiency that causes the fetus to be starved of nutrients and oxygen.

Postmature infants tend to have dry skin which cracks and peels and may be more susceptible to infection.

Postmortem examination

Another term for an *autopsy*.

Postmyocardial infarction syndrome

Another name for *Dressler's syndrome*.

Postnasal drip

A watery or sticky discharge from the back of the *nose* into the *nasopharynx* (the uppermost part of the throat, behind the nose). As the fluid trickles down the throat, it may cause a cough, hoarseness, or the sensation that a foreign body is present. Postnasal drip is usually caused by *rhinitis* (inflammation of the mucous membrane in the nose); treatment is of this underlying cause.

Postnatal care

Care of the mother after *childbirth* until about six weeks after delivery.

After delivery the mother's temperature, pulse, and blood pressure are monitored, especially after a *caesarean section* or if there have been any complications, such as *pre-eclampsia* or bleeding.

The length of stay in hospital depends on whether or not there have been any complications. Women used to remain in hospital for up to a week after delivery, but nowadays the length of stay after a straightforward delivery may be only 48 hours or even less. During the hospital stay, a daily check is made for any signs of *puerperal sepsis* (infection of the genital tract after childbirth), including inspection of the *lochia* (vaginal discharge after childbirth). If the woman had an *episiotomy* or tears around the vagina, the wounds are checked daily.

The woman is encouraged to walk as soon as possible after delivery to reduce the risk of *thrombosis* (abnormal blood clotting). If necessary, help is given with feeding techniques (see *Bottle-feeding; Breast-feeding*). There may also be instruction on various abdominal and *pelvic floor exercises*, which can help restore muscle tone.

A final postnatal check-up usually takes place about six weeks after delivery. The obstetrician or GP checks the woman's blood pressure and weight, examines the uterus and bladder to make sure they are in the correct position, and ensures that any wounds are healing properly. Advice on *contraception* may also be given.

Postnatal depression

Depression in a woman after *childbirth*. Postnatal depression is probably caused by a combination of sudden hormonal changes and a variety of psychological and environmental factors. Postnatal depression ranges from an extremely common and short-lived attack of mild depression ("baby blues") to a depressive psychosis in which the woman is very severely depressed and requires admission to hospital to prevent harm to herself or her baby.

MILD DEPRESSION

Probably more than two thirds of mothers have the "blues", which usually start about four to five days after childbirth. The woman feels miserable, discouraged, irritable, sometimes mentally confused, and may cry easily. Apart from hormonal changes, psychological factors may play a role,

including a sense of anticlimax after the birth or an overwhelming sense of responsibility for the baby's care. With reassurance and support from family and friends, the depression usually passes in two or three days.

MORE SEVERE DEPRESSION

In about 10 to 15 per cent of women the depression is more marked and persists for weeks. There may be a constant feeling of tiredness, difficulty in sleeping, loss of appetite, and restlessness. This type of postnatal depression seems more likely to develop if the woman has a strained relationship with her partner, has no support from her family, has financial or other worries, or has a *personality disorder*. At particular risk are women who suffered from depression or anxiety during the pregnancy, first-time mothers, and single parents. In many cases, however, no risk factors are present.

The condition usually clears up of its own accord or responds to treatment with *antidepressant drugs*.

DEPRESSIVE PSYCHOSIS

This severe form of postnatal depression follows about one in 1,000 pregnancies and usually starts two to three weeks after childbirth. Depressive psychosis is marked by severe mental confusion, feelings of worthlessness, threats of suicide or of harm to the baby, and sometimes *delusions*. The woman's moods may change rapidly. Treatment requires admission to hospital, sensitive counselling, and possibly *family therapy*. Antidepressant drugs are often necessary.

Postpartum depression

See *Postnatal depression*.

Postpartum haemorrhage

Excessive blood loss after *childbirth*. Postpartum haemorrhage occurs in about two per cent of all births. It is more common after a long labour, after a multiple birth, or if the woman required general anaesthesia. Before the development of *blood transfusion*, postpartum haemorrhage was a common cause of maternal death.

CAUSES

Most cases of postpartum haemorrhage occur immediately after delivery (primary postpartum haemorrhage) and are due to excessive bleeding from the site where the placenta was attached to the uterus. Such bleeding may be caused by failure of the uterus to contract efficiently after delivery or by the retention of placental tissue within the uterus.

Postpartum haemorrhage immediately after delivery may also be caused by tears anywhere along the birth canal. Tearing is more likely to occur during a *forceps delivery* or a *breech delivery*. In some cases, postpartum haemorrhage occurs because the mother has a *bleeding disorder*.

Occasionally, postpartum haemorrhage occurs with pain and fever between five and 10 days after delivery (secondary postpartum haemorrhage). In these cases, the cause is usually infection of a retained fragment of placenta.

TREATMENT

A blood transfusion may be given to replace lost blood, and emergency treatment may be needed for *shock*. Other treatment depends on the cause of the haemorrhage. Any retained placental tissue may need to be removed under general anaesthetic, an injection of *ergometrine* may be given to stimulate uterine contractions, and any lacerations in the vagina or on the cervix are sutured (stitched). *Antibiotic drugs* are used to treat infection.

Post-traumatic stress disorder

A specific form of *anxiety* that comes on after a stressful or frightening event. Common causes include natural disasters (such as earthquakes), violence, *rape*, torture, and serious physical injury. The condition may also result from military combat, when it is sometimes known as battle fatigue or shell shock.

The symptoms include recurring memories or dreams of the event, a sense of personal isolation, and disturbed sleep and concentration. There may be a deadening of feelings, or irritability and painful feelings of guilt, sometimes building up to form a true depressive illness (see *Depression*). Symptoms may begin immediately after the trauma or may develop many months later. The symptoms are made worse by any reminder of the traumatic experience.

Most people recover given time, emotional support, and counselling. However, prolonged physical deprivation (such as that experienced in a concentration camp) may scar people psychologically for life.

Postural drainage

A technique that enables a person whose lungs are clogged with sputum (phlegm) or other secretions to drain them. The person lies in such a way that the secretions drain by gravity

P

into the trachea (windpipe), from where they are coughed up. Postural drainage is used to treat disorders in which stagnant secretions have become infected (as in chest infections in people suffering from chronic *bronchitis*, *bronchiectasis*, and *cystic fibrosis*).

Postural drainage is sometimes done in association with chest clapping (in which another person gently strikes the chest) intended to loosen sticky secretions.

HOW IT IS DONE

The affected person lies on a bed and each lobe of the lung is drained in turn by the adoption of different postures. The different postures are achieved by lying supine, prone, or on each side; by raising the foot of the bed by varying amounts; and by the use of pillows to elevate different parts of the body. At the same time, the affected person loosens lung secretions by "huffing" (breathing out forcibly) and by raising and lowering the elbows, and sometimes by a helper clapping his or her cupped hand on the affected person's chest wall. A mechanical *vibrator* is sometimes applied to the chest.

Postural hypotension

See *Hypotension*.

Posture

The relative position of different parts of the body at rest or during movement. Good posture consists of efficiently balancing the body weight around the body's centre of gravity in the lower spine and pelvis. It is dependent on the shape of the *spine* and on balanced contraction of *muscles* around the spine and in each limb. Maintaining good posture helps prevent neck pain and *back pain*.

Many people have bad posture as the result of habit, such as sitting slumped in a chair or standing with the shoulders and back hunched. *Obesity* increases the likelihood of bad posture because it increases the strain on muscles. Poor posture may also be caused by neurological disorders (such as *Parkinson's disease*), by muscle disorders (such as *muscular dystrophy*), or by disorders of the joints or bones (such as *ankylosing spondylitis*).

Post-viral fatigue syndrome

See *Myalgic encephalomyelitis*.

Potassium

A mineral which, in combination with *sodium* and *calcium*, maintains normal heart rhythm, regulates the body's water balance, and is responsible for the conduction of nerve impulses and the contraction of muscles.

The body of an average-sized person contains about 140 g of potassium, mainly contained inside the cells. Almost all foods contain potassium, so dietary deficiency is rare. Particularly rich sources include lean meat, whole grains, green leafy vegetables, beans, and many fruits (especially bananas and oranges).

POTASSIUM DEFICIENCY

A low level of potassium in the blood (called hypokalaemia) usually occurs as a result of *gastroenteritis* or some other disorder of the digestive tract that causes loss of gastrointestinal fluids through diarrhoea and/or vomiting. Children are especially vulnerable to this type of potassium loss.

Other potential causes of hypokalaemia include prolonged treatment with *diuretic drugs* or *corticosteroid drugs*; overuse of *laxative drugs*; *diabetes mellitus*; *Cushing's syndrome* (overproduction of corticosteroid hormones by the adrenal cortex); *aldosteronism* (overproduction of the hormone aldosterone by the adrenal cortex); certain kidney diseases; excessive intake of coffee or alcohol; and extremely profuse sweating.

The effects of mild hypokalaemia include fatigue, drowsiness, dizziness, and muscle weakness. In more severe cases, there may be abnormalities of heart rhythm and paralysis of the muscles.

POTASSIUM EXCESS

Much less common than hypokalaemia is an excess of potassium in the blood, a condition called hyperkalaemia. This may be caused by excessive amounts of potassium, usually in the form of supplements to correct hypo-

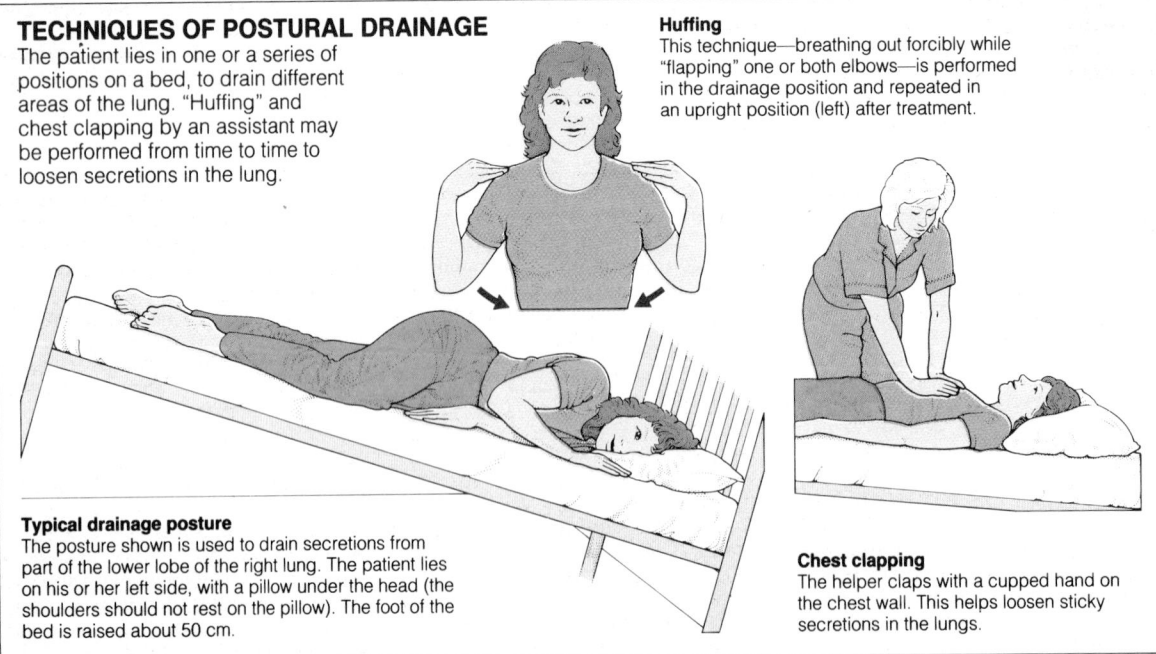

TECHNIQUES OF POSTURAL DRAINAGE

The patient lies in one or a series of positions on a bed, to drain different areas of the lung. "Huffing" and chest clapping by an assistant may be performed from time to time to loosen secretions in the lung.

Huffing
This technique—breathing out forcibly while "flapping" one or both elbows—is performed in the drainage position and repeated in an upright position (left) after treatment.

Typical drainage posture
The posture shown is used to drain secretions from part of the lower lobe of the right lung. The patient lies on his or her left side, with a pillow under the head (the shoulders should not rest on the pillow). The foot of the bed is raised about 50 cm.

Chest clapping
The helper claps with a cupped hand on the chest wall. This helps loosen sticky secretions in the lungs.

P

kalaemia; by severe *kidney failure*; by *Addison's disease*; or by prolonged treatment with potassium-sparing diuretic drugs.

The effects of hyperkalaemia include numbness and tingling, muscle paralysis, heart rhythm disturbances, and, in severe cases, *heart failure*.

Potassium permanganate
A drug that has an *antiseptic* and *astringent* effect, useful in the treatment of *dermatitis* (skin inflammation). Potassium permanganate is sometimes applied on a dressing, may be placed in water as a soak, or may be applied directly to the skin. It can occasionally cause irritation and can stain the skin and clothing.

Potency
The ability of a man to perform *sexual intercourse*; or the strength of a *drug* assessed from its ability to cause certain desired effects.

Pott's fracture
A combined fracture and dislocation of the *ankle* caused by excessive or violent twisting. In a Pott's fracture, the fibula (the outer of the two bones of the lower leg) is broken just above the ankle, and the tibia (shin) also breaks or the ligaments tear, resulting in dislocation.

Treatment consists of manipulating the bones back into position under general anaesthetic, followed by immobilization of the foot, ankle, and lower leg in a *cast* for between eight and 10 weeks. Sometimes metal screws are inserted to hold the bone fragments in place.

Severe fracture-dislocations may result in stiffness of the ankle, and increase the likelihood of *osteoarthritis* developing in later life.

Poultice
A warm pack consisting of a soft, moist substance (such as *kaolin*) spread between layers of soft fabric. Poultices were once widely used for reducing local pain or inflammation, for bringing boils to a head, and for improving local circulation.

Pox
Any of various infectious diseases characterized by blistery skin eruptions (for example chickenpox, cowpox, or smallpox). Pox was formerly a common term for *syphilis* and is still sometimes used as a slang word for this disease.

Praziquantel
An *anthelmintic drug* used to treat *tapeworm infestation*. Adverse effects may include dizziness, drowsiness, and abdominal pain.

Prazosin
A *vasodilator drug* used in the treatment of *hypertension* (high blood pressure). Prazosin is usually given with a *diuretic drug* and sometimes with other antihypertensive drugs.

Prazosin is also used to treat *heart failure* (reduced pumping efficiency) and *Raynaud's phenomenon* (a circulatory disorder).

Prazosin may cause dizziness and fainting by lowering the blood pressure too fast or too much. Other possible adverse effects are nausea, headache, and dry mouth.

Precancerous
A term applied to any condition in which *cancer* has a tendency to develop. There are three types of such conditions. In the first, there are no tumours present but the condition is known to carry an increased risk of cancer. Examples include *ulcerative colitis* (which carries an increased risk of malignant tumours of the colon or rectum) and *Down's syndrome* (which carries an increased risk of *leukaemia*).

In the second type, there are benign tumours that tend to become malignant themselves, such as colonic polyps, or are associated with the development of malignant tumours elsewhere in the body. Examples of this type include *neurofibromatosis* (von Recklinghausen's disease), in which there are large numbers of tumours on the nerves, any of which may become malignant; and *tuberous sclerosis*, in which cancer may develop in the brain, the back of the eye, and various endocrine glands.

The third type comprises disorders that have chronic, sometimes inflammatory or irregular features from the beginning, but which do not always become fully malignant. Disorders within this group include cervical dysplasia (see *Cervix, cancer of*); *leukoplakia* of the mouth (see *Mouth cancer*); and papillomas of the bladder (see *Bladder tumours*).

Predisposing factors
Factors that lead to increased susceptibility to a disease. For example, predisposing factors that make a person more likely to have *coronary artery disease* are a family history of the disease, tobacco-smoking, high blood pres-

sure, high lipid (fat) levels in the blood, being overweight, lack of regular exercise, and mental stress.

Prednisolone

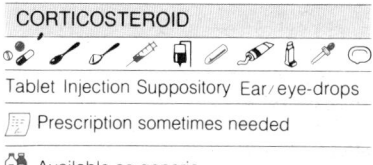

CORTICOSTEROID

Tablet Injection Suppository Ear / eye-drops

Prescription sometimes needed

Available as generic

A *corticosteroid drug* used to reduce inflammation and improve symptoms in a variety of disorders, including *eczema, conjunctivitis, iritis, ulcerative colitis, rheumatoid arthritis,* and *asthma*.

Prednisolone is also used in the treatment of blood disorders, such as *thrombocytopenia* and *leukaemia*.

High doses or prolonged treatment may cause adverse effects typical of corticosteroid drugs, such as facial rounding, *acne, hypertension, osteoporosis, peptic ulcer,* and *diabetes mellitus*.

Prednisone
A *corticosteroid drug* used to reduce inflammation and improve symptoms in a variety of disorders, including *rheumatoid arthritis, ulcerative colitis* and severe *asthma*.

Other disorders that are occasionally treated with prednisone include *Addison's disease* and blood disorders, such as *leukaemia*. Prednisone is also used to prevent organ rejection after *transplant surgery*.

Large doses taken over a prolonged period may cause adverse effects typical of other corticosteroid drugs.

Pre-eclampsia
A serious condition in which *hypertension* (high blood pressure), *oedema* (accumulation of fluid in tissues), and *proteinuria* (protein in the urine) develop in a woman in the second half of pregnancy. Additional symptoms may include headache, nausea and vomiting, abdominal pain, and visual disturbances. The condition is sometimes known as pre-eclamptic toxaemia or PET.

Pre-eclampsia affects about seven per cent of pregnancies. It is more common in first pregnancies and in women aged under 25 or over 35; it is also more common if *diabetes mellitus*, hypertension, or kidney disease is present. Untreated pre-eclampsia may lead to *eclampsia*, which is characterized by seizures; eclampsia may cause maternal or fetal death.

P

TREATMENT

For mild cases of pre-eclampsia, the woman is confined to bed, and *antihypertensive drugs* may be used to reduce blood pressure. If the woman is close to term or if eclampsia is imminent, *induction of labour* or a *caesarean section* may be necessary.

Pregnancy

The period from conception to birth. Pregnancy begins with conception, the *fertilization* of an ovum (egg) by a sperm, and the subsequent implantation of the fertilized egg. The egg develops into the *placenta* and *embryo*, and later into the *fetus*. Most fertilized eggs implant into the uterus. However, very occasionally, an egg implants into an abnormal site, such as a fallopian tube, resulting in an *ectopic pregnancy*, which may develop into an emergency situation. (See illustrated boxes on the stages and features of pregnancy and on the effects of hormones during pregnancy.)

WEIGHT GAIN DURING PREGNANCY

The average increase in pregnancy is 12.7 kg—70 per cent of it occurring during the last 20 weeks. At term, the typical fetus weighs 3.4 kg and the placenta and fluid together weigh another 1.4 kg. The remaining weight is largely due to water retention and increased fat stores. Within six weeks of delivery, most women return to their pre-pregnancy weight.

STAYING WELL

Provided the pregnancy is desired and the woman takes care of herself and has *antenatal care*, there is no reason for her not to feel completely healthy during pregnancy.

A balanced and nutritious diet is important. Appetite will increase, but pregnant women should avoid filling up on high-calorie snacks that are low in nutritional value. It is better to eat frequent, smaller meals. Many doctors prescribe *folic acid* and *iron* supplements during pregnancy.

STAGES AND FEATURES OF PREGNANCY

Pregnancy typically lasts 40 weeks, counted from the first day of the pregnant woman's last menstrual period, and is conventionally divided into three trimesters, each lasting three months. For the first eight weeks following conception, the developing baby is called an embryo; thereafter, it is known as a fetus. It is during the early part of pregnancy (first trimester) that the growing baby is most vulnerable to damage.

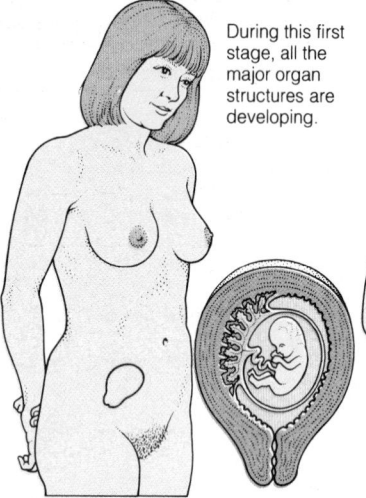

During this first stage, all the major organ structures are developing.

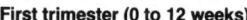

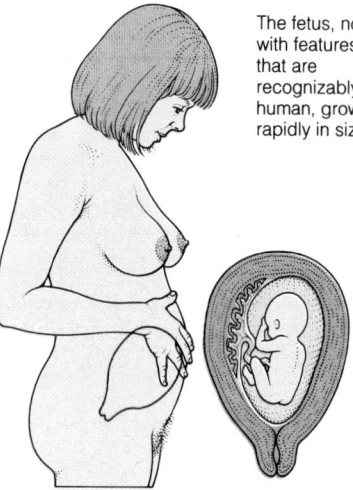

The fetus, now with features that are recognizably human, grows rapidly in size.

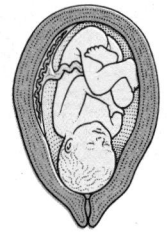

The fetal organs mature in preparation for birth and life outside the uterus.

First trimester (0 to 12 weeks)

The first sign of pregnancy is usually the absence of a menstrual period, though some women have breakthrough bleeding. The breasts start to swell and may become tender as the mammary glands develop to prepare for *breast-feeding*. The nipples start to enlarge and the veins over the surface of the breasts become more prominent. A supportive bra should be worn.

Nausea and vomiting are common, are often worse in the morning, and usually persist for six to eight weeks (see *Vomiting in pregnancy*). Urine is passed more frequently and there is often a creamy white discharge from the vagina. Many women feel unusually tired during the early weeks. Some notice a metallic taste in the mouth or a craving for certain foods. Weight begins to increase.

Second trimester (13 to 28 weeks)

From 16 weeks, the enlarging uterus is easily felt and the woman begins to look noticeably pregnant. The nipples enlarge and darken, and skin pigmentation may deepen. Some women may feel warm and flushed. Appetite tends to increase and weight rises rapidly. Facial features tend to become heavier. By 22 weeks (usually between the 18th and 20th weeks), most pregnant women have felt the baby moving around (sometimes called "quickening").

During the second trimester, nausea and frequency of urination diminish, and the woman may feel generally better and more energetic than during the early weeks. The heart-rate increases, as does the volume of blood pumped by the heart, to allow the fetus to develop properly. These changes put an extra strain on the heart of women who have pre-existing heart disease.

Third trimester (29 to 40 weeks)

In some women, stretch-marks develop on the abdomen, breasts, and thighs. A dark line may appear running from the umbilicus to the pubic hair. *Colostrum* can be expressed from the nipples.

Minor problems are common. Many women become hot and sweat easily, as body temperature rises slightly. More rest may be needed at this stage, though many women find it difficult to find a comfortable position. *Braxton Hicks' contractions* may get stronger.

The baby's head engages (drops down low into the pelvis) around the 36th week in a first pregnancy, but not until a few weeks later in subsequent pregnancies. This "lightening" may relieve pressure on the upper abdomen and on breathing, but increases pressure on the bladder and may result in more vaginal discharge.

Tobacco-smoking and *alcohol* should be avoided throughout pregnancy, and no other drug should be taken except under medical supervision (see *Pregnancy, drugs in*).

Exercise can be continued during pregnancy but strenuous exertion and potentially dangerous sports are generally best avoided.

Sexual intercourse can continue throughout pregnancy (unless there is bleeding or if the waters break). Adopting different positions may make intercourse more comfortable. Libido may decrease during early and late pregnancy, but many women enjoy sex throughout pregnancy.

PROBLEMS DURING PREGNANCY

In addition to the expected features of pregnancy, such as nausea and tiredness, some women experience other minor problems. The symptoms may be troublesome but generally disappear after delivery.

During pregnancy, food passes through the intestine more slowly, which enables more nutrients to be absorbed for the fetus, but which also tends to cause *constipation*. *Haemorrhoids* are fairly common during late pregnancy, as is *heartburn* due to *acid reflux*. The gums may become spongy and bleed easily. *Pica* (a craving to eat substances other than foods, such as clay or coal) is fairly common.

Swollen ankles are common during the second half of pregnancy, especially during the evening. *Varicose veins* may appear in the later months in susceptible women. Leg cramps, backache, and breathlessness are also common during late pregnancy. Pigmentation tends to increase and may cause *chloasma* (commonly called the mask of pregnancy).

Urinary tract infections are more common during pregnancy, and stress incontinence (see *Incontinence, urinary*) may occur, especially during the later weeks. Vaginal *candidiasis* (thrush) is also more common when a woman is pregnant.

Women may find that their moods are more changeable, which may be the result of hormonal effects on the brain. In addition, women often feel more lethargic than usual, and may experience bouts of depression, may be easily annoyed or angered, and may be prone to bouts of crying. On the other hand, some women feel more content during pregnancy.

For complications of pregnancy, see *Antepartum haemorrhage; Diabetic pregnancy; Miscarriage; Polyhydramnios; Pre-eclampsia; Prematurity; Rhesus incompatibility; Vomiting in pregnancy.* (See also *Childbirth; Fetal heart monitoring; Pregnancy, multiple*).

Pregnancy, drugs in

Drugs taken during *pregnancy* may pass from the mother through the placenta to the baby. Although only a few drugs have been proved to cause harm to a developing baby, no drug should be considered completely safe, especially during early pregnancy. For this reason, a pregnant woman should not take any drug (including over-the-counter drugs) without first consulting her doctor.

Drug treatment during pregnancy is usually prescribed only if the poten-

---

EFFECTS OF HORMONES DURING PREGNANCY

A pregnant woman undergoes many changes that enable her to maintain the pregnancy, nourish the baby, and prepare for breast-feeding.

These adaptations are brought about by increased levels of the female sex hormones *oestrogen* and *progesterone*, and by the action of two other

hormones, human chorionic gonadotrophin (HCG) and human placental lactogen (HPL), produced only by the placenta.

EFFECTS OF HORMONES DURING PREGNANCY

Progesterone	Decreases the excitability of smooth muscle, thereby helping to prevent uterine contractions and premature labour. Induces constipation and oesophageal acid reflux as a result of its effects on smooth muscle. Increases body temperature. Affects mood. Increases breathing rate.	**Oestrogens**	Are important for the development of the reproductive system and breasts. Stimulate growth of the uterine muscle to enable the powerful contractions of labour. Increase vaginal secretions. Increase the size of the nipples and help the development of milk glands in the breasts. Increase the production of protein, which is essential for healthy growth of the woman and fetus. Alter collagen and other substances to allow body tissues to soften and stretch in preparation for labour. Relax ligaments and joints. May cause sciatica and backache, and may also contribute to the formation of varicose veins as a result of their effects on body tissue.
Human placental lactogen (HPL)	Increases energy production necessary for fetal development. Causes enlargement of breasts and development of milk glands. Induces temporary diabetes mellitus (gestational diabetes) in susceptible women as a result of its effects on metabolism.		
Human chorionic gonadotrophin (HCG)	Increases energy production necessary for fetal development. Induces gestational diabetes in susceptible women.	**Melanocyte-stimulating hormone (MSH)**	Stimulates pigmentation (in combination with oestrogens), particularly of the nipples. May also produce chloasma (darkening of the facial skin).

tial benefits of treatment outweigh any risk to the baby. Treatment for long-term conditions, such as *epilepsy* or *diabetes mellitus*, is continued during pregnancy but drug therapy may require modification (sometimes even before conception if a woman plans to become pregnant).

Problems in a developing baby may also be caused if a pregnant woman drinks alcohol (see *Alcohol* and pregnancy box), smokes (see *Tobaccosmoking*), or takes drugs of abuse.

POSSIBLE ADVERSE EFFECTS

Drugs taken during the first three months of pregnancy may interfere with the normal formation of the baby's organs, causing *birth defects*.

Drugs taken later in pregnancy may slow the rate at which the baby grows, causing a low birthweight. Or they may damage specific fetal tissue—for example, developing teeth may be damaged by *tetracycline drugs*.

Drugs taken towards the end of pregnancy or during labour and delivery (see *Childbirth* pain relief box) may cause problems for the newborn baby. Narcotic analgesics, for example, may cause breathing difficulty.

Drug abuse during pregnancy can cause serious problems. The babies of women who use *heroin* during pregnancy tend to have a low birthweight and have a higher death rate than normal during the first few weeks after birth. These babies may suffer withdrawal symptoms, such as feeding

and sleeping difficulties, trembling, and seizures. Babies born to women who are intravenous drug abusers have a high risk of being infected with *HIV*, the *AIDS* virus.

Pregnancy, false

An uncommon psychological disorder, medically known as pseudocyesis, in which a woman has the physical signs of pregnancy, including morning sickness, amenorrhoea (lack of periods), breast enlargement, and abdominal swelling. Although the results of *pregnancy tests* prove negative and the fetal heart cannot be heard during examination, the woman remains quite convinced that she is pregnant.

Many women with pseudocyesis are childless or approaching the *menopause* and have an intense desire to have children. Treatment of pseudocyesis may involve *counselling* or *psychotherapy*. (See also *Conversion disorder*.)

Pregnancy, multiple

The presence of more than one fetus in the uterus. Multiple pregnancy can occur if two or more ova (eggs) are released from the ovary and fertilized at the same time. It can also result if a single fertilized ovum divides at an early stage of development. Today, most pregnancies in which there are three or more babies result from the use of *fertility drugs*.

INCIDENCE

Twins occur in about one in 80 pregnancies, triplets in about one in 8,000, and quadruplets in about one in 73,000 pregnancies. Multiple pregnancies are more common in women who are successfully treated with fertility drugs or if a number of already fertilized ova are implanted during *in vitro fertilization*.

DIAGNOSIS AND TREATMENT

During the woman's antenatal examination, the doctor may be able to feel more than one fetus, and may find that the abdomen is larger than expected for the duration of gestation. The doctor may also be able to hear more than one fetal heartbeat when listening through a stethoscope. *Ultrasound scanning* may be used to confirm the diagnosis.

The woman is advised to rest during pregnancy and to increase her protein intake. *Iron* and *folic acid* tablets are usually recommended.

COMPLICATIONS

Hypertension (high blood pressure), *polyhydramnios*, *postpartum haemorrhage*, and *malpresentation* occur more frequently in a multiple pregnancy. *Prematurity* is a common complication, and the weight of each baby is usually less than that of a single baby. Caesarean section is necessary more often than in single pregnancies.

Pregnancy tests

Tests on urine or blood performed to determine whether or not a woman is pregnant; some can be performed at home. Pregnancy tests check for the presence of human chorionic gonadotrophin (see *Gonadotrophin, human chorionic*), produced by the placenta.

HOW IT IS DONE

Urine tests are used most often. Most can detect pregnancy from about two weeks after a missed period, although some of the newer tests can detect pregnancy within a few days of a missed period. The test is usually performed on an early morning midstream urine specimen (because urine is most concentrated at this time). Urine tests are about 97 per cent accurate if the result is positive and about 80 per cent accurate if the result is negative. If the result is negative and there is no menstrual period within about a week, the pregnancy test should be repeated.

Blood tests are normally used only when a very early diagnosis of pregnancy is needed. Blood tests measure the level of human chorionic gonadotrophin in the blood by a laboratory

P

MULTIPLE PREGNANCY

About one pregnancy in 80 is multiple (e.g. twins or triplets). The rate is highest among women in their 30s. Problems arise more often in multiple pregnancies than in single pregnancies. For example, twins are much more likely than single babies to be born prematurely.

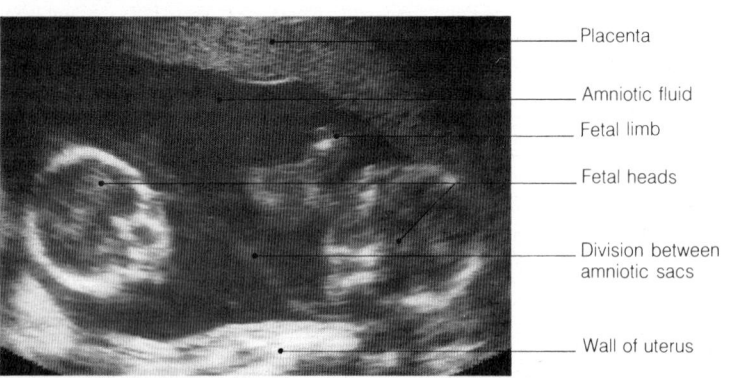

Placenta

Amniotic fluid

Fetal limb

Fetal heads

Division between amniotic sacs

Wall of uterus

Ultrasound scan revealing twins
Ultrasound scanning of the woman's uterus can reveal twins within the first several weeks of pregnancy. Here, two fetal heads, a limb that belongs to the fetus on the right, and the membrane that divides the two amniotic sacs can be seen.

PREGNANCY TEST KIT

Just one of the many types of pregnancy test kit is shown. No kit is 100 per cent accurate. Whether a test indicates pregnancy or gives a negative result despite a missed period, it is wise to consult a doctor for confirmation.

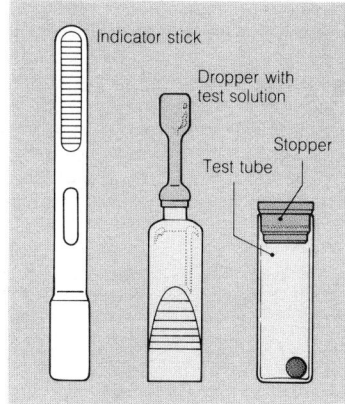

Components of test kit
The kit has three main parts—a dropper tube containing a test solution, a test tube with stopper, and an indicator stick.

Indicator stick
Dropper with test solution
Stopper
Test tube

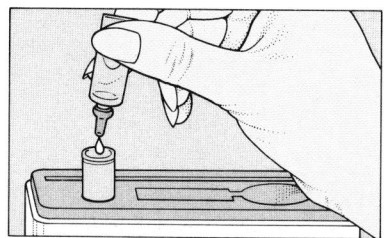

1 The end of the dropper tube is squeezed gently to introduce the test solution into the test tube, which is held upright in a stand provided.

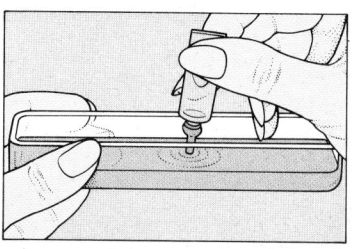

2 The lid of the test kit is used to collect a urine sample early in the morning. Some urine is drawn up into the dropper tube by squeezing and releasing.

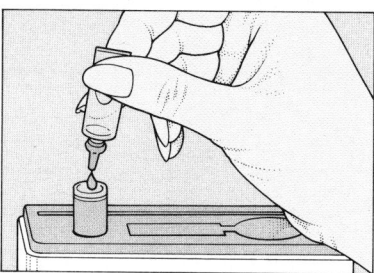

3 Five drops of urine are added to the solution in the test tube. The stopper is put in the test tube, the contents shaken, and the stopper removed.

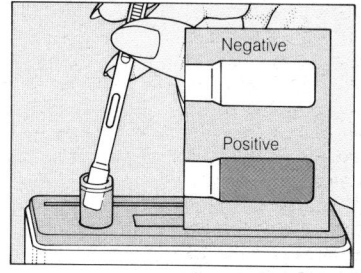

Negative
Positive

4 The indicator stick is placed in the test tube. The result can be read after 30 minutes. If the end of the stick changes colour, it signifies a pregnancy.

technique called *immunoassay*. This produces a result from within nine to 12 days of conception but is more expensive to perform.

Premature ejaculation
See *Ejaculation, disorders of.*

Prematurity
Birth of a baby before 37 weeks' *gestation*. A premature labour carries little risk for the mother, but the premature infant may be less than sufficiently developed to cope with independent life and needs special care.

Prematurity was once a major cause of infant mortality, but improved medical techniques have dramatically increased survival rates for premature babies in developed countries. Approximately five to 10 per cent of babies are born prematurely.

CAUSES
Some 40 per cent of all premature deliveries occur for no known reason. The remainder are due to conditions affecting the mother, the fetus, or the placenta.

Pre-eclampsia is the most common maternal cause of premature labour. Other maternal causes include *hypertension* (high blood pressure), long-standing kidney disease, *diabetes melli-*

tus, and heart disease. Women who have any of these conditions carry an increased tendency to go into labour prematurely, although some mothers tend to deliver prematurely for no apparent reason. However, more commonly, the pregnancy is curtailed early by *caesarean section* or *induction of labour* by the obstetrician to avoid further risk to mother and baby.

Similarly, *antepartum haemorrhage*, which may be caused by separation of the *placenta* from the uterus before the baby is born, may result in premature labour due to the irritant effect of blood within the uterus. Antepartum haemorrhage sometimes makes induction of labour necessary. Other common causes of premature labour are intrauterine infection or premature rupture of membranes.

The most common fetal cause of prematurity is multiple pregnancy (see *Pregnancy, multiple*), a state which accounts for approximately 15 per cent of all premature births. Multiple pregnancy may cause problems in the mother that make caesarean section or induction of labour necessary, or it may cause excessive stretching of the uterus, which stimulates contractions and leads to premature labour. A similar mechanism may occur with *poly-*

hydramnios (excessive amniotic fluid) or if the woman's uterine cavity is smaller than normal.

PREVENTION
If labour begins prematurely, the obstetrician may in some cases attempt to stop labour by administering a drug (such as ritodrine, isoxsuprine, salbutamol, or turbutaline) that has the effect of inhibiting contractions of the uterus.

THE PREMATURE INFANT
The premature infant is not only smaller than a full-term baby but has a characteristic physical appearance—the infant lacks subcutaneous fat, is covered with downy hair called lanugo, and has a very thin, gelatinous skin.

The baby's internal organs are also immature and less than completely developed, making it necessary for the baby to be monitored in a special hospital environment until he or she has developed sufficiently to sustain independent life.

The major complication for a premature infant is *respiratory distress syndrome*, which results from lung immaturity. Other organs, particularly the liver, may also be immature, leading to increased risk of brain haemorrhage, *jaundice*, and *hypo-*

P

glycaemia (low blood sugar). A premature baby has a limited ability to suck and to maintain body temperature. Additionally, the immune system is poorly developed and the baby is more prone to infection.

TREATMENT
Premature infants are usually nursed in a special baby unit that provides intensive care. The baby is placed in an *incubator*, which provides warmth and allows easy observation. Other special care may include artificial *ventilation* to assist breathing, artificial feeding through a stomach tube or into a vein, and treatment with *antibiotic drugs* and *iron* and *vitamin supplements*. The baby is usually kept in hospital until he or she reaches a weight of at least 2.25 kg, is growing satisfactorily, and is capable of feeding well.

OUTLOOK
The survival chances of a premature baby increase with the length of the pregnancy. With modern techniques, some infants now survive even if they are born as early as 23 weeks' gestation and when weighing less than 1 kg, but this remains exceptional. Of babies born at 28 weeks' gestation and given specialist care, approximately 80 per cent survive. Most premature babies catch up with full-term babies before the end of their first year.

Premedication

The term applied to drugs given, often by injection, between one and two hours before an operation to prepare a person for surgery. Premedication usually contains a narcotic *analgesic drug* (painkiller) to help relieve pain and anxiety and to reduce the dose of anaesthetic that will be needed to produce unconsciousness (see *Anaesthesia, general*). An *anticholinergic drug* is often also included because it reduces secretions in the airways and also protects the heart.

Premenstrual syndrome

The combination of various physical and emotional symptoms that occurs in women the week or two before *menstruation*. Premenstrual syndrome (PMS) begins at or after *ovulation* and continues until the onset of menstruation. PMS affects more than 90 per cent of fertile women at some time in their lives and in some women is so severe that work and social relationships are seriously disrupted.

CAUSES
Many theories exist for the cause of PMS. Hormonal changes that occur

PREMATURITY

A premature baby may need to be nursed in an incubator where the temperature and humidity are carefully controlled and the baby can be closely observed. If breathing difficulties develop, they may be treated by artificial ventilation. Very small babies cannot suck so they must be fed intravenously or via a tube passed into the stomach. If jaundice develops, it may be treated by *phototherapy* (light therapy), which breaks up the bilirubin that causes the yellow discoloration of the skin.

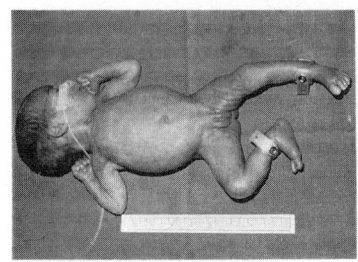

Premature infant
This baby girl was born several weeks prematurely. She is being fed via a flexible tube that passes through the nose and oesophagus into the stomach.

FEATURES AND COMPLICATIONS OF PREMATURITY

Physical features	Complications
Low birthweight (often less than 2.5 kg)	Increased risk of birth injury
Small size	Respiratory distress syndrome
Relatively large head and hands	Recurrent episodes of breathing stoppage
Thin, smooth, shiny skin	Jaundice
Veins visible under the skin	Infection
Little fat under the skin	Poor temperature control
Wizened, wrinkled features	Anaemia
Soft, flexible ear cartilage	Hypoglycaemia (low blood sugar level) and other disturbances of body chemicals
Short toenails (but normal length fingernails)	Rickets
Downy (lanugo) hair	Increased bleeding tendency
Reduced vernix (greasy substance that covers the newborn)	Brain haemorrhage
Protuberant abdomen	Necrotizing enterocolitis (severe intestinal inflammation that may lead to death of intestinal tissue)
Enlarged clitoris (girls)	
Small scrotum (boys)	
Feeble, whining cry	
Irregular breathing	
Poor sucking and swallowing ability	
Tendency to regurgitate	

throughout the menstrual cycle clearly influence PMS, but an imbalance between oestrogen and progesterone levels has not been consistently found. Similarly, deficiencies of *vitamin E*, pyridoxine (see *Vitamin B complex*), *magnesium*, or *prostaglandins* have been suggested but not confirmed.

SYMPTOMS AND SIGNS
The most common emotional symptoms of PMS are irritability, tension, depression, and fatigue. Physical symptoms include breast tenderness, fluid retention, headache, backache, and lower abdominal pain.

TREATMENT
No single method of treatment has proved completely successful. Treatments that may relieve specific symptoms include relaxation techniques to relieve anxiety and tension; *diuretic drugs* to relieve fluid retention; and

dietary changes during the latter half of the menstrual cycle (such as avoidance of salt, caffeine, and chocolate). Taking pyridoxine (vitamin B_6) or evening primrose oil may help some women with breast symptoms, irritability, and depression. *Oral contraceptives* can relieve symptoms by eliminating the normal menstrual cycle. Progesterone supplements are widely used but do not help all women.

Premenstrual tension
See *Premenstrual syndrome*.

Premolar
One of eight permanent grinding *teeth*, two in the upper and two in the lower jaw on each side of the mouth, located between the canines and molars. (See also *Permanent teeth*; *Eruption of teeth*.)

Prepuce
See *Foreskin*.

Presbyacusis
The progressive loss of *hearing* that occurs with age. Presbyacusis is a form of sensorineural *deafness* (degeneration of the hair cells and nerve fibres in the inner ear), which makes sounds less clear and tones, especially higher tones, less audible.

SYMPTOMS AND CAUSES
People with presbyacusis often have difficulty in understanding speech and are usually unable to hear well in the presence of background noise. The severity and progression of the condition vary considerably from person to person (some people who are 80 have far better hearing than others who are only 60).

The natural process of presbyacusis may be exacerbated by exposure to high *noise* levels, by diminished blood supply to the inner ear due to an arterial disease such as *atherosclerosis*, and by toxic damage to the inner ear from certain drugs, such as *aminoglycoside drugs*.

TREATMENT
Hearing-aids can help most people, except for those with a poor ability to discriminate between speech sounds (who therefore have difficulty in understanding what is being said). A person speaking to someone with presbyacusis should remember to speak slowly and clearly. It is also recommended to speak loudly, unless the person with presbyacusis is wearing a hearing-aid.

Presbyopia
The progressive loss of the power of *accommodation* for near vision. The focusing power of the eyes weakens with age until, after about the age of 65, little focusing power remains. Presbyopia is usually noticed around the age of 45 when the eyes cannot accommodate within normal reading distance. Large print can still be seen, but it may be difficult to bring small print into focus unless it is read at arm's length.

Simple reading *glasses* with convex lenses are used to correct presbyopia. Glasses may need to be changed four to five times over the course of about 20 years, until all the focusing is eventually being done by the glasses.

Prescribed diseases
A group of industrial diseases which give sufferers legal entitlement to financial benefit. A claimant has to show that he or she has worked in an occupation that is recognized as increasing the risk of developing a particular disease.

Examples of prescribed diseases include conditions due to physical agents (such as occupational *deafness*), conditions due to biological agents (such as *anthrax*), conditions due to chemical agents (such as *lead poisoning*), and miscellaneous conditions, including *pneumoconiosis* and *byssinosis*. (See also *Notifiable diseases*; *Occupational disease and injury*.)

Prescription
An instruction written by a doctor that directs a pharmacist to dispense a particular drug in a specific dose. A prescription also details how often the drug must be taken, how much is to be dispensed, and any other relevant facts. Drugs that require a prescription (prescription medicines) are available only on the authorization of a doctor because they may be dangerous, habit-forming, or used to treat a disease that needs to be monitored.

All prescriptions must bear the name and address of the patient and the doctor's signature. The pharmacist keeps a record of all prescriptions dispensed.

Preservative
A substance that inhibits the growth of bacteria, yeasts, and moulds and so protects foods from putrefying and fermenting. Examples of preservatives include sulphur dioxide, benzoic acid, salt, sugar, and nitrites. Fat preservatives are termed antioxidants because they inhibit oxidation. (See also *Food additives*.)

Pressure points
Places on the body where arteries lie near the surface and where pressure can be applied to limit severe arterial *bleeding*. Application of pressure at these points will not stop venous bleeding.

Arterial bleeding can be identified because blood from arteries is bright red and is pumped out in regular spurts as the heart beats. To stop

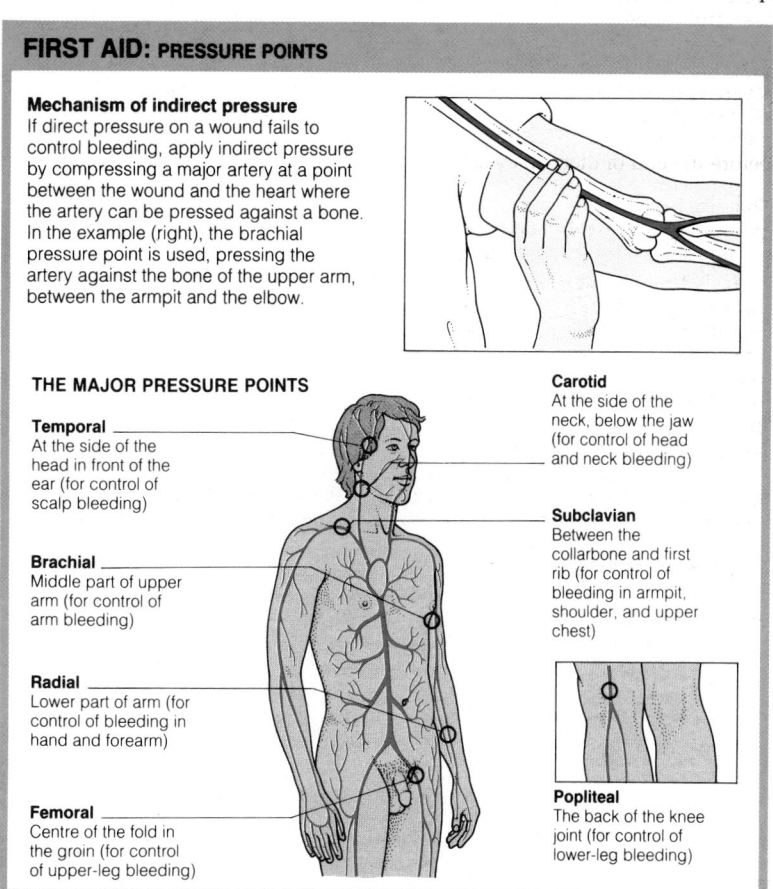

FIRST AID: PRESSURE POINTS

Mechanism of indirect pressure
If direct pressure on a wound fails to control bleeding, apply indirect pressure by compressing a major artery at a point between the wound and the heart where the artery can be pressed against a bone. In the example (right), the brachial pressure point is used, pressing the artery against the bone of the upper arm, between the armpit and the elbow.

THE MAJOR PRESSURE POINTS

Temporal
At the side of the head in front of the ear (for control of scalp bleeding)

Brachial
Middle part of upper arm (for control of arm bleeding)

Radial
Lower part of arm (for control of bleeding in hand and forearm)

Femoral
Centre of the fold in the groin (for control of upper-leg bleeding)

Carotid
At the side of the neck, below the jaw (for control of head and neck bleeding)

Subclavian
Between the collarbone and first rib (for control of bleeding in armpit, shoulder, and upper chest)

Popliteal
The back of the knee joint (for control of lower-leg bleeding)

P

bleeding, pressure is applied by hand to compress the appropriate artery against the underlying bone. (See illustrated box.)

Pressure sores
A common name for *bedsores*.

Prevalence
The total number of cases of a disease in existence at any one time in a defined population. Prevalence is often expressed as the number of cases per 100,000 people. Prevalence is one of the two chief measures of how common a disease is; the other is *incidence*. (See also Prevalence table.)

Preventive dentistry
An aspect of *dentistry* concerned with the prevention of tooth decay and gum disease rather than their treatment. Preventive dentistry consists of encouraging the practice of good *oral hygiene* and a reduced intake of sugary foods, *fluoride* treatment to strengthen tooth enamèl, and *scaling* to remove any accumulated dental *plaque* and *calculus* from the teeth.

Preventive medicine
The branch of medicine that deals with the prevention of disease by public health measures, such as the provision of pure water supplies; by health education to discourage smoking and excess alcohol consumption, to promote exercise, and to advise on a prudent diet; by specific preventive measures, such as immunization against infectious diseases; and by screening programmes to detect diseases such as cancer of the cervix or breast, hypertension (high blood pressure), glaucoma, and tuberculosis, before they cause symptoms.

Most of the increase in the world's population during the 19th century was due to improvements in public health, particularly improvements in the overall standard of nutrition, and the provision of pure water supplies and proper sanitation. Today, these measures remain the priorities of preventive medicine in developing countries, and, along with a programme of immunization in childhood, have been targeted as major objectives by the World Health Organization.

However, in developed countries, the primary objective is to persuade the adult population to adopt a healthier lifestyle. In the UK, many deaths in adults before the age of 65 are preventable, being due to accidents and/or linked to such factors as smoking, an

PREVALENCE OF VARIOUS CHRONIC CONDITIONS IN THE UK

Prevalence (Number of people with the condition per 100,000 population)	Categorization	Examples
More than 25,000	Extremely common	Male pattern baldness Errors of refraction
5,000 to 25,000	Very common	Hypertension (high blood pressure) Osteoarthritis
1,000 to 5,000	Common	Chronic bronchitis Diabetes mellitus (all types) Psoriasis Rheumatoid arthritis
200 to 1,000	Fairly common	Blindness Epilepsy Gout Schizophrenia
50 to 200	Uncommon	Ankylosing spondylitis Down's syndrome Multiple sclerosis Parkinson's disease Ulcerative colitis
5 to 50	Rare	Autism Crohn's disease Cystic fibrosis
Less than 5	Very rare	Albinism Galactosaemia

unhealthy diet, excessive drinking, and insufficient exercise. Adoption of a healthier lifestyle, the wider use of screening for cancers, and measures to reduce accidents could lead to substantial improvements in health.

Priapism
Persistent, painful *erection* of the *penis* without sexual arousal. Priapism is a dangerous condition that requires emergency treatment.

CAUSES

Priapism occurs because blood fails to drain from the spongy tissue of the penis, keeping the penis erect. Possible causes include damage to nerves that control the supply of blood to the penis; a blood disease that causes partial clotting of blood in the penis; and, rarely, blockage of the normal outflow of blood from the penis as a result of an infection (such as *prostatitis* or *urethritis*).

TREATMENT

Urgent treatment is needed because of the risk of permanent damage to the penis. Treatment may involve *spinal anaesthesia* (injection of local anaesthetic into the spinal canal) or withdrawal of blood from the penis through a wide-bore needle.

Prickly heat
An irritating skin rash that is associated with profuse sweating. The medical name for prickly heat, miliaria rubra, literally means "red millet seeds". This term describes the multiple tiny, red, itchy spots that cover the mildly inflamed affected areas of skin. Prickly heat is accompanied by aggravating, prickling sensations. The irritation tends to affect sites on the body where sweat collects, particularly the waist, upper trunk, armpits, and the sides of the elbows.

A milder variety (miliaria crystallina) produces clear, shiny, fluid-filled blisters that tend to dry up quickly without treatment.

CAUSES

The mechanism by which prickly heat is caused is not fully understood, but unevaporated sweat is known to be an important factor. The skin becomes unhealthy and waterlogged. Sweat ducts become blocked with debris and eventually leak sweat into the skin.

TREATMENT AND PREVENTION
Frequent cool showers and sponging of the affected areas relieve the itching; ordinary soap should not be used on affected areas.

Primaquine
A drug used in the treatment of vivax and ovale *malaria*. Primaquine is often given after prophylactic treatment with *chloroquine* has failed to prevent the infection. Primaquine is not effective in preventing a malaria attack but kills the parasites in the liver.

Adverse effects include nausea, vomiting, and abdominal pain. In people with *G6PD deficiency*, primaquine may cause haemolytic *anaemia*.

Primary
A term applied to a disease that has originated within the organ or tissue affected, and is not derived from any other cause or source. Primary liver cancer, for example, is the result of some cancer-producing change in liver cells. Secondary liver cancer results from the spread of cancer cells from another part of the body.

The term primary is also applied to the first of several diseases to affect a tissue or organ in turn. For example, when a viral infection of the lungs is succeeded by a bacterial infection, the viral infection is called primary and the bacterial infection is termed secondary. Primary is also used to mean "of unknown cause".

Primary teeth
The first teeth (also known as deciduous, or milk, teeth), which usually start to appear at the age of six months and are gradually replaced by the permanent teeth from the age of about six years.

There are 20 primary teeth, 10 in each jaw. Each set of 10 consists of four incisors (biting teeth) at the front, flanked by two canines (eye teeth), with four molars (grinding teeth) at the back. (See also *Teeth; Eruption of teeth; Teething.*)

Primidone
An *anticonvulsant drug* used in the treatment of epilepsy and, occasionally, *tremor*. Primidone is usually prescribed with another anticonvulsant. Adverse effects include drowsiness, clumsiness, and dizziness.

Prinzmetal's angina
See *Variant angina.*

Prion
A proteinaceous infectious particle. Prions are small agents that transmit diseases including *Creutzfeldt-Jakob disease* in humans, scrapie in sheep, and bovine spongiform encephalopathy in cattle. Unlike viruses, prions do not contain nucleic acids. They are difficult to destroy, being much more resistant to heat and disinfectants than viruses or bacteria. The prion diseases are all degenerations of the central nervous system and have long incubation periods. As yet, no treatment is available for these diseases.

Probenecid
A drug used in the long-term treatment of *gout* which reduces the level of uric acid in the body by increasing the amount excreted in the urine.

Probenecid also slows the excretion of some *antibiotic drugs* (such as *penicillin* drugs and *cephalosporin drugs*) from the kidneys and is therefore occasionally prescribed with these drugs to boost their levels and thus their effects.

Probenecid may cause nausea and vomiting. It also increases the risk of kidney stones in some people.

Probucol
A *lipid-lowering drug*. Probucol is often prescribed with other lipid-lowering drugs to boost their effect. Treatment is usually monitored by blood tests.

Possible adverse effects include diarrhoea, flatulence, pain in the abdomen, and, rarely, dizziness.

Procainamide
An *antiarrhythmic drug* used in the treatment of certain types of *tachycardia* (abnormally rapid heartbeat): for example, ventricular *arrhythmias* that occur after a *myocardial infarction* (heart attack).

Procainamide may cause nausea, vomiting, loss of appetite, and, rarely, confusion. Prolonged treatment may induce *lupus erythematosus*, causing fever, joint pain, swelling, and rash.

Procaine
A local anaesthetic (see *Anaesthesia, local*) used before surgical or dental treatment and, occasionally, during childbirth. Procaine has largely been replaced by drugs that are quicker to take effect or are longer-acting.

Occasionally, procaine causes an allergic reaction, with a rash or swelling of the face, lips, mouth, or throat. Rare adverse effects of this drug include anxiety, drowsiness, or tinnitus (ringing in the ears).

Procarbazine
An *anticancer drug* particularly useful in the treatment of *lymphomas*. Procarbazine is also used to treat brain tumours and certain cancers of the skin, lungs, and bone marrow.

In addition to the adverse effects typical of anticancer drugs, procarbazine may cause a sudden rise in blood pressure if taken with certain foods or drinks (e.g. cheese and red wine).

Prochlorperazine
A *phenothiazine*-type *antipsychotic drug*. Prochlorperazine is used to relieve the symptoms of certain psychiatric disorders, including *schizophrenia* and mania. In smaller doses, it is also used as an *antiemetic drug* to relieve nausea and vomiting.

Prochlorperazine may cause involuntary movements of the face and limbs, lethargy, dry mouth, blurred vision, and dizziness.

Procidentia
A medical term for severe *prolapse* (displacement of an organ from its normal position in the body), usually of the uterus.

Proctalgia fugax
A severe cramping pain in the *rectum* unconnected with any disease. Proctalgia fugax may be due to muscle spasm, sometimes associated with stress or anxiety. The pain, which may occur at any time, is of short duration and subsides of its own accord.

Proctitis
Inflammation of the *rectum*, causing soreness, bleeding, and sometimes a discharge of mucus and pus. Proctitis commonly occurs with inflammation of the colon as a feature of *ulcerative colitis, Crohn's disease,* or *dysentery.* In cases where inflammation is confined to the rectum, the cause is often unknown. However, especially in male homosexuals, proctitis is sometimes due to *gonorrhoea* or another sexually transmitted disease. Rare causes of proctitis include *tuberculosis, amoebiasis, schistosomiasis,* injury, certain drugs, allergy, or radiation injury.

DIAGNOSIS AND TREATMENT
The diagnosis is made by *proctoscopy* (inspection of the rectum with a viewing instrument). A *biopsy* (removal of a small sample of tissue for laboratory

P

analysis) is sometimes required to determine the exact cause of the rectal inflammation.

Successful treatment of any underlying cause usually clears the problem. *Corticosteroid drugs*, in the form of suppositories or enemas, may relieve symptoms, especially in cases of ulcerative colitis or Crohn's disease.

Proctoscopy

Examination of the *anus* and *rectum* by means of a proctoscope (a rigid viewing instrument) inserted through the anus. A short, flexible sigmoidoscope (see *Sigmoidoscopy*) is sometimes used and is more comfortable for the person being examined.

Procyclidine

An *anticholinergic drug* used in the treatment of *Parkinson's disease*. Procyclidine reduces excessive salivation and muscle rigidity and may improve tremor. Possible adverse effects include dry mouth and blurred vision.

Prodrome

An early warning symptom of illness. For example, a *migraine* headache may be preceded by pins-and-needles in the hands or feet or by an *aura* of visual symptoms. Awareness of a prodrome may enable a migraine headache sufferer to use certain preventive medicines that are far less effective once a headache is established.

Progeria

Premature aging. There are two distinct forms of progeria, both of which are extremely rare.

In Hutchinson-Gilford syndrome, aging starts around the age of four, and by 10 or 12 the affected child has all the external features of old age, including grey hair, baldness, and loss of fat, resulting in thin limbs and sagging skin on the trunk and face. There are also internal degenerative changes, such as widespread *atherosclerosis* (narrowing of the arteries by fatty deposits). Death usually occurs at puberty, most commonly from coronary artery disease.

Werner's syndrome, or adult progeria, starts in adolescence or early adult life and follows the same rapid progression as the juvenile form.

The cause of progeria is unknown, although cells taken from affected people show only a few generations of cell division before they stop reproducing, instead of the 50 or so generations that occur in cells taken from healthy young people.

Progesterone hormone

A female sex hormone essential for the healthy functioning of the female reproductive system. Progesterone is produced in the ovaries during the second half of the menstrual cycle (see *Menstruation*) and by the placenta during *pregnancy*. Small amounts of progesterone are also produced in the adrenal glands and testes.

Following *ovulation*, increased production of progesterone causes the endometrium (lining of the uterus) to thicken in preparation for the implantation of a fertilized egg. If fertilization does not take place, the production of progesterone and also of *oestrogen hormones* falls, resulting in shedding of the uterine lining and the unfertilized egg in the monthly period.

During pregnancy, progesterone is produced by the placenta and causes changes in the mother's body—for example, it contributes to breast changes. Progesterone also passes into the developing baby's circulation, where it is converted in the adrenal glands to *corticosteroid hormones*. At the end of pregnancy, a fall in the level of progesterone helps initiate labour.

Other effects of progesterone produce changes in the cervix and vagina during the menstrual cycle, increased deposition of fat, and increased *sebum* production by glands in the skin.

Progestogen drugs

COMMON DRUGS

Dydrogesterone Ethynodiol diacetate Gestodene Gestronol Hydroxyprogesterone Levonorgestrel Medroxyprogesterone Norethisterone Norgestrel Progesterone

A group of drugs similar to *progesterone hormone*, which includes both natural progesterone and synthetic progesterone derivatives.

WHY THEY ARE USED

Progestogen drugs are used in *oral contraceptives*, either on their own (in the minipill) or with *oestrogen drugs* (in combined and phased pills). Such drugs work by making the cervical mucus impenetrable to sperm, altering the lining of the uterus so that it prevents implantation of fertilized eggs, and reducing *gonadotrophin hormone* production, which may prevent eggs from ripening in either of the ovaries.

Progestogen drugs are also prescribed, sometimes with oestrogen drugs, to treat menstrual problems (see *Menstruation, disorders of*).

In *hormone replacement therapy*, a progestogen drug is used in combination with an oestrogen drug to reduce the risk of cancer of the uterus (see *Uterus, cancer of*), which may occur if oestrogens alone are taken over a long period of time. The progesterone induces the monthly shedding of the uterine lining.

Progestogen drugs are used also to treat *premenstrual syndrome, endometriosis* (a disorder in which fragments of tissue that normally lines the uterus occur elsewhere in the pelvic cavity), and *hypogonadism* (underdevelopment of the ovaries). Progestogen drugs are sometimes effective as *anticancer drugs* in the treatment of certain types of cancers (such as uterine endometrial cancer).

POSSIBLE ADVERSE EFFECTS

Adverse effects include weight gain, *oedema* (accumulation of fluid in tissues), loss of appetite, headache, dizziness, rash, irregular periods, breast tenderness, and, less commonly, *ovarian cysts*.

Prognathism

Abnormal protrusion of the lower jaw or both jaws. If the condition interferes with biting and chewing (see *Malocclusion*) or is disfiguring, *orthognathic surgery* may be performed.

Prognosis

A medical assessment of the probable course and outcome of a disease. It is based on the recorded history of the disease (e.g. 90 per cent of people with small cell carcinoma of the lung die within five years of the condition's developing), the doctor's own experience of treating the disease, and the patient's general condition and age. However, every prognosis is no more than an informed guess, and any patient may prove it wrong.

Progressive

A term used to describe a condition that becomes more severe and/or extensive over time; for example, in progressive muscular atrophy (a type of *motor neuron disease*), weakness and muscle-wasting usually begin in the hands, gradually spread to the arms, shoulders, and legs, and eventually affect the entire body.

Progressive muscular atrophy

A type of *motor neuron disease* in which the muscles of the hands, arms, and legs become weak and wasted and twitch involuntarily. This is a progressively debilitating condition which eventually spreads to other muscles in the body.

P

Proguanil

An antimalarial drug used in the prevention of *malaria* in some parts of the world. Travellers visiting parts where there is a risk of malaria need to start taking proguanil at least 24 hours before leaving home and continue taking it for at least four weeks after returning. In some countries, the malaria parasite has become resistant to proguanil, and another antimalarial drug, such as *chloroquine,* should be taken in combination with proguanil to ensure adequate protection.

Proguanil rarely causes adverse effects. Indigestion, nausea, or vomiting may occur but usually disappears as treatment continues.

Prolactin

A *hormone* produced by the *pituitary gland.* Prolactin, acting with certain other hormones, stimulates the growth and development of the mammary glands (see *Breast*). Secretion of prolactin is increased during *pregnancy,* and helps to initiate and maintain milk production for *breastfeeding.* (See also *Prolactinoma.*)

Prolactinoma

A benign tumour of the *pituitary gland* that causes overproduction of the hormone *prolactin.* In a woman, a prolactinoma may result in *galactorrhoea* (breast secretion at any time other than a few days before childbirth or during breast-feeding), *amenorrhoea* (absence of periods), or *infertility.* In a man, a prolactinoma may cause *impotence* and *gynaecomastia* (breast enlargement). In either sex, it may cause headaches, *diabetes insipidus,* and, if it presses on the optic nerves, gradual loss of the outer field of vision.

The condition is diagnosed from blood tests to measure prolactin levels, and from *CT scanning* or *MRI* of the brain. Treatment may consist of removal of the tumour, *radiotherapy,* or the drug *bromocriptine,* which inhibits prolactin secretion.

Prolapse

Displacement of part or all of an organ or tissue from its normal position. Common structures that prolapse include the uterus (see *Uterus, prolapse of*) and intervertebral discs (see *Disc prolapse*).

Promazine

A *phenothiazine-type antipsychotic drug* used as a sedative drug.

Possible adverse effects of promazine include abnormal movements of the face and limbs, drowsiness, lethargy, dry mouth, constipation, and blurred vision. Long-term treatment may cause *parkinsonism.*

Promethazine

An *antihistamine drug* used to relieve itching in a variety of skin conditions, including *urticaria* (nettle rash) and *eczema.* Promethazine is also used as an antiemetic drug to relieve nausea and vomiting caused by motion sickness and *Ménière's disease.*

Promethazine has a sedative effect and is therefore sometimes used as a premedication (drug used to prepare a person for surgery) and as a short-term sleeping drug for children. Occasionally, promethazine is given to produce sedation during *childbirth.*

Possible adverse effects of promethazine include dry mouth, blurred vision, and drowsiness.

Pronation

The act of turning the body to a prone (facedown) position, or the hand to a palm backwards position. The opposite movements are called *supination.*

Propantheline

An *antispasmodic drug* used in the treatment of *irritable bowel syndrome* and forms of urinary *incontinence.*

Possible adverse effects include dry mouth, blurred vision, and abnormal retention of urine.

Prophylactic

A drug, procedure, or piece of equipment used to prevent disease; the term prophylactic is also sometimes used to refer to a *condom.*

Propranolol

A *beta-blocker drug* used to treat *hypertension* (high blood pressure), *angina pectoris* (chest pain due to inadequate blood supply to the heart muscle), and cardiac *arrhythmias* (irregularities of the heartbeat). It is also used occasionally to reduce the risk of further damage to the heart after *myocardial infarction* (heart attack).

Propranolol is used to relieve symptoms of *hyperthyroidism* (overactivity of the thyroid gland) or of *anxiety,* and to prevent attacks of *migraine.*

Possible adverse effects are typical of other beta-blocker drugs.

Proprietary

A term to describe a drug patented for production by one company. The patent protects the drug's name, ingredients, and process of manufacture.

Proprioception

The body's internal system for collecting information about its position relative to the outside world and the state of contraction of its muscles. This is achieved by means of sensory nerve endings within the muscles, tendons, joints, and sensory hair cells in the balance organ of the inner ear. These structures are called proprioceptors (literally "one's own sensors").

Information from the proprioceptors passes to the spinal cord and brain and is used to make adjustments in the state of contraction of muscles so that posture and balance are maintained. During movement, there is a continuous feedback of information to the brain from the proprioceptors and from the eyes. This helps ensure that actions are smooth and coordinated.

Proptosis

A term for protrusion, particularly of the eyeball (see *Exophthalmos*).

Propylthiouracil

A drug used to treat *hyperthyroidism* (overactivity of the thyroid gland) or to control symptoms of hyperthyroidism in preparation for a *thyroidectomy* (removal of the thyroid gland). Unless an operation is planned, treatment with propylthiouracil is given for at least a year.

Possible adverse effects include itching, headache, rash, and joint pain. Propylthiouracil may reduce the production of white blood cells by the bone marrow and thus increase the risk of infection.

Prostaglandin

One of a group of *fatty acids* that is made naturally in the body and that acts in a similar way to *hormones.* Prostaglandins are divided into broad groups according to their chemical structure. They were first discovered in semen but are now known to occur in many different body tissues, including the uterus, brain, and kidneys. Some prostaglandins are prepared synthetically for use as drugs (see *Prostaglandin drugs*).

EFFECTS

Prostaglandins produce a wide range of effects on the body, including causing pain and inflammation in damaged tissue, protecting the lining of the stomach and duodenum against ulceration, and stimulating contractions in labour (see box overleaf).

Certain drugs counteract the effects of prostaglandins within the body. *Nonsteroidal anti-inflammatory drugs*

P

EFFECTS OF SOME PROSTAGLANDINS

Type	Effect
PGA$_1$	Lowers blood pressure May protect against peptic ulcer
PGD$_2$	Causes inflammation
PGE$_1$	Stimulates contractions of the uterus Lowers blood pressure Reduces stickiness of platelets in blood
PGE$_2$	Causes inflammation Widens airways Increases stickiness of platelets in blood Stimulates contractions of the uterus Protects against peptic ulcer
PGF$_2$	Stimulates contractions of the uterus Narrows airways
PGG$_2$	Causes inflammation
PGI$_2$	Reduces stickiness of platelets in blood

(NSAIDs), *aspirin,* and *corticosteroid drugs* relieve pain and inflammation by reducing prostaglandin production in tissues. Taken long-term, however, NSAIDs and aspirin may increase the risk of a *peptic ulcer,* in part by reducing production of prostaglandins that protect the stomach lining.

Prostaglandin drugs

Synthetically produced *prostaglandins* which have many therapeutic uses.

Dinoprostone and dinoprost are prostaglandins used to stimulate uterine contractions for *induction of labour* at full term, after a fetal death, or to induce a late abortion (see *Abortion, induced*).

Gemeprost is a prostaglandin administered as a vaginal pessary to soften and help dilate the cervix prior to inducing an early abortion.

Alprostadil is an E$_1$ prostaglandin used to treat newborn infants awaiting surgery for certain types of congenital heart disease. It is also being investigated for use in the treatment of *Raynaud's disease.*

Other prostaglandin drugs are under investigation for use in a variety of disorders, including *peptic ulcer.*

Prostate, cancer of

A malignant growth in the outer zone of the *prostate gland.* It is one of the most common cancers in men; over 10,000 cases are diagnosed in the UK each year. Prostate cancer sometimes develops in middle age but most often occurs in the elderly. While its precise cause is unknown, the hormone *testosterone* appears to be involved.

SYMPTOMS AND SIGNS

Symptoms may be caused by enlargement of the prostate (see *Prostate, enlarged*) and include difficulty in starting to pass urine, poor flow of urine, and increased frequency of urination. There may be no urinary symptoms, however, and the first evidence of the disease may be pain in the bones from secondary growths of the cancer. When the tumour causes difficulty in passing urine, the flow of urine may eventually cease completely either because the urethra is totally blocked or because the cancer has spread to the bladder and ureters. In advanced cases, pain may be caused by involvement of nerves in the pelvis or by cancer spreading to bones.

DIAGNOSIS

Screening tests for prostate cancer are still under evaluation. A blood test for a protein, prostate specific antigen, is highly reliable but detects many small cancers that might otherwise have caused no symptoms. Annual rectal examination allows the doctor to assess the size and hardness of the gland. Any doubts will be resolved by *ultrasound scanning* and prostatic *biopsy* (removal of a sample of tissue for microscopic analysis). Blood tests and a bone scan (see *radionuclide scanning*) may be performed to assess whether the cancer has spread.

TREATMENT

If the cancer is small and confined to the prostate gland, and the patient is elderly with a limited life expectancy, no treatment may be recommended; in these circumstances many die from other causes without having any symptoms from the cancer. For younger men in whom a cure is possible, the choice lies between *prostatectomy* (surgical removal of the gland) and *radiotherapy.* If the disease is widespread, it will usually be controllable for several years by reducing the level of testosterone. This may be done by *orchidectomy* (surgical removal of the testes), or by giving *oestrogen drugs,* anti-androgens (drugs that block the action of testosterone), or drugs that block release of the pituitary hormone that regulates the release of testosterone.

Prostatectomy

An operation to remove part or all of the *prostate gland.* Prostatectomy is usually performed when enlargement of the gland is causing obstruction to the flow of urine (see *Prostate, enlarged*). The operation may also be performed to treat cancer of the prostate (see *Prostate, cancer of*) or, occasionally, *prostatitis.*

HOW IT IS DONE

The most common method is transurethral prostatectomy, which is performed during *cystoscopy.* If the prostate gland is very enlarged, retropubic prostatectomy may be performed (see illustrated box).

RECOVERY PERIOD

In rare cases, bleeding after the operation is severe, and *blood transfusions* are required. Blood clots that may form within the bladder can be washed out through the catheter inserted during the operation.

Following removal of the catheter, urination may initially be frequent and sometimes painful; in some cases, there is mild incontinence for a few weeks. Patients are encouraged to drink large amounts of fluid to help to wash out the remaining blood in the urine.

The hospital stay is about four or five days for transurethral prostatectomy and about eight to 10 days for the retropubic operation. After several weeks, patients may resume all activities, including intercourse.

OUTLOOK

Uncommonly, prostatectomy affects potency or sexual sensation. In most cases, the operation causes sterility because semen is expelled backwards into the bladder during orgasm instead of being ejaculated via the penis (a condition known as retrograde ejaculation). Seminal fluid in the bladder is not harmful and is excreted in the urine.

Prostate, enlarged

An increase in the size of the inner zone of the *prostate gland,* also known as benign prostatic hypertrophy. The condition is most common in men over 50. The cause is unknown.

SYMPTOMS AND SIGNS

Symptoms usually develop gradually as the enlarging prostate compresses and distorts the urethra. The flow of urine is obstructed; there is difficulty in starting to pass urine, and the stream of urine is weak.

Initially the bladder muscle becomes overdeveloped to force urine through the obstructed urethra. Event-

P

PROSTATECTOMY—REMOVAL OF THE PROSTATE GLAND

Of the two possible methods of removal shown, the transurethral method is the most commonly used.

It avoids the disadvantages of an abdominal incision and usually permits a shorter stay in hospital.

The retropubic method may be necessary if the prostate is very enlarged or if a cancer is suspected.

TRANSURETHRAL PROSTATECTOMY

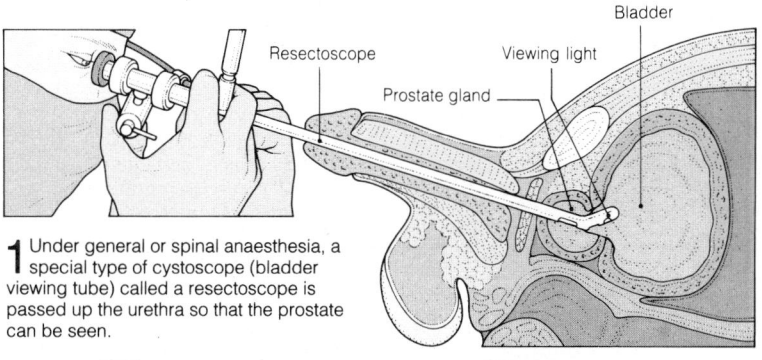

Resectoscope — Viewing light — Bladder — Prostate gland

1 Under general or spinal anaesthesia, a special type of cystoscope (bladder viewing tube) called a resectoscope is passed up the urethra so that the prostate can be seen.

Capsule — Prostate gland — Bladder — Cutting edge

Tissue washed out — Electrode cauterizes bleeding vessels

2 A heated wire loop, or sometimes a cutting edge, is inserted through the resectoscope and used to cut away as much of the prostatic tissue as possible.

3 The pieces of tissue are washed out through the resectoscope and any bleeding vessels are cauterized by means of an electrode passed up the tube.

4 The resectoscope is then withdrawn and a catheter passed via the urethra into the bladder. The catheter is left in place for several days to drain urine from the bladder and allow blood to be washed out.

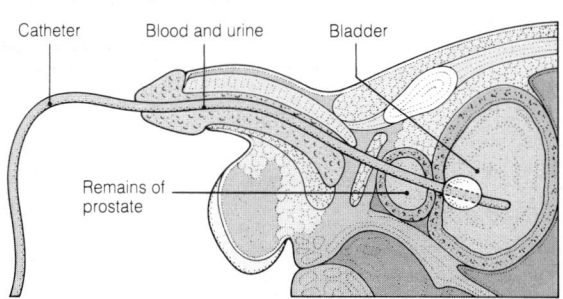

Catheter — Blood and urine — Bladder — Remains of prostate

RETROPUBIC PROSTATECTOMY

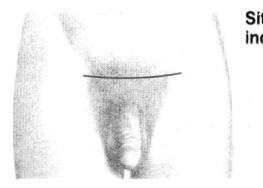

Site of incision

1 Under general anaesthesia, an incision is made in the abdomen to expose the bladder and prostate. The surgeon cuts open the capsule containing the gland.

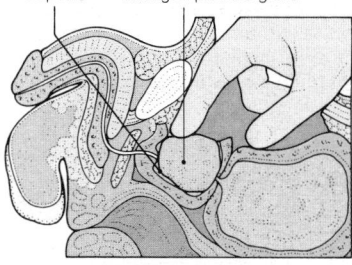

Capsule — Enlarged prostate gland

2 The surgeon then removes the prostatic tissue by hand. Bleeding vessels are cauterized and a catheter is passed up the urethra to drain urine from the bladder.

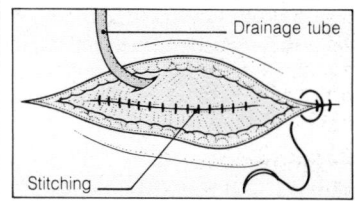

Drainage tube — Stitching

3 A tube is inserted beside the empty capsule to drain fluid and blood; the abdomen is sewn up. The tube and catheter are left in for about a week.

P

---

ually the bladder is unable to expel all the urine (see *Urine retention*) and becomes distended, causing abdominal swelling.

There may be *incontinence* due to overflow of small quantities of urine, and the bladder may become overactive, resulting in frequency of urination (see *Urination, frequent*). This is a sign of bladder muscle failure and usually means surgery is needed.

Severe abdominal pain and the ability to pass only a few drops of urine require immediate treatment.

DIAGNOSIS
Enlargement of the prostate can be detected during a *rectal examination*. The doctor also feels the abdomen for signs of bladder distension.

A sample of urine may be tested for infection and a blood test performed to measure kidney function. *Ultrasound scanning, urography*, and a recording of the strength of urine flow may be performed to give additional information about the severity of the obstruction, and any effects elsewhere in the urinary system, especially the kidneys.

TREATMENT
Mild symptoms of prostatic enlargement do not require treatment; more severe symptoms usually require *prostatectomy* (surgical removal of the prostate gland). Drug treatment with finasteride, which blocks the formation of the active form of *testosterone*, will shrink the gland, but the longterm results of this and other drug treatments have yet to be assessed. Microwave treatment has also been used to shrink the gland, but again long-term results are not yet available.

Prostate gland

A solid, chestnut-shaped organ surrounding the first part of the urethra in the male. The prostate gland is situated immediately under the bladder and in front of the rectum.

The prostate gland produces secretions that form part of the seminal fluid during *ejaculation*. The ejaculatory ducts from the seminal vesicles pass through the prostate gland to enter the urethra.

The prostate gland weighs only a few grams at birth. Enlargement to adult size starts at puberty from the effect of *androgen hormones* and stops at around the age of 20, when it reaches its adult weight of about 20 g. In most men, the prostate begins to enlarge further after the age of 50.

The prostate gland consists of two main zones: an inner zone (which produces secretions responsible for keeping the lining of the urethra moist) and an outer zone (which produces seminal secretions).

DISORDERS

Prostatic problems very rarely occur before the age of 30. *Prostatitis* (inflammation of the prostate) is usually caused by bacterial infection and may be sexually transmitted. It usually affects men in their 30s and 40s, but can occur later in life.

Enlargement of the prostate (see *Prostate, enlarged*) usually affects men over 50 and may interfere with urination by compressing the urethra.

Cancer of the prostate (see *Prostate, cancer of*) is common in old age and may cause symptoms similar to those caused by enlargement of the prostate gland.

Prostatism

Symptoms resulting from enlargement of the prostate gland (see *Prostate, enlarged*).

Prostatitis

Inflammation of the *prostate gland*, usually affecting men between the ages of 30 and 50. Prostatitis is often caused by a bacterial infection that has spread from the urethra. The infection may or may not be sexually transmitted. Presence of a urinary catheter increases the risk of prostatitis.

SYMPTOMS AND SIGNS

Prostatitis causes pain when passing urine and increased frequency of urination; it sometimes causes fever and a discharge from the penis. There may be pain in the lower abdomen, around the rectum, and in the lower back, and blood in the urine.

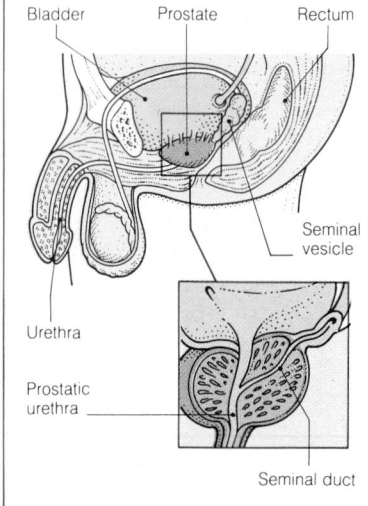
DIAGNOSIS AND TREATMENT

The doctor performs a *rectal examination* by inserting a gloved finger into the rectum; the gland will be tender and enlarged. To investigate the cause of infection, tests are carried out on a urine sample and on urethral secretions obtained after massaging the prostate gland.

Treatment is with *antibiotic drugs*. Despite treatment, the condition may be slow to clear up and tends to recur.

Prosthesis

An artificial replacement for a missing or diseased part of the body. Examples of prostheses used to restore normal function include false legs or arms fitted after amputation (see *Limb, artificial*) or artificial heart valves used to replace valves damaged by disease (see *Heart valve surgery*).

Prostheses are also used for cosmetic reasons. Examples include a breast prosthesis fitted after *mastectomy* (removal of a breast) and glass eyes inserted following removal of diseased eyes (see *Eye, artificial*).

Prosthetics, dental

The branch of *dentistry* concerned with the replacement of missing teeth and their supporting structures. Pros-

---

thetics includes three basic kinds of replacement—partial or complete *dentures* (which are easily removed for cleaning), semipermanent appliances such as overdentures (fittings that are attached over existing teeth), and permanent restorations such as crowns (see *Crown, dental*) and bridges (see *Bridge, dental*).

Proteins

Large molecules that consist of hundreds or thousands of *amino acids* linked (by peptide bonds) to form long chains, which are often folded in various ways. In addition to amino acids, proteins may contain other constituents such as sugars (glycoproteins) and lipids (lipoproteins).

There are two main types of proteins: fibrous and globular. Fibrous proteins are insoluble and form the structural basis of many body tissues, such as hair, skin, muscles, tendons, and cartilage. Globular proteins are soluble and include all *enzymes* (substances that promote biochemical reactions in the body), many *hormones* (such as growth hormone and prolactin) and various proteins in the blood, including *haemoglobin* and *antibodies*. In addition, the *chromosomes* in cell nuclei are formed of proteins linked with *nucleic acids*; proteins linked with lipids constitute a major part of cell membranes (see *Cell*).

PROTEINS AND DIET

Proteins are needed in the diet primarily to supply the body with amino acids. Ingested proteins are broken down in the *digestive system* to amino acids, which are then absorbed and rebuilt into new body proteins (see *Protein synthesis*). Proteins are the only major foodstuff that contains nitrogen. The balance between dietary intake of protein and the excretion of breakdown products from the body (mainly *urea* in the urine) can be followed by measuring the nitrogen intake and the nitrogen output. (See also *Nutrition*.)

Protein synthesis

The formation of *protein* molecules inside cells through the linking of much smaller substances called *amino acids*. Because proteins provide many of the structural components and the *enzymes* that promote biochemical reactions in the body, their manufacture—in the correct numbers and order—is essential to all aspects of development and growth.

Different cells manufacture a different range of proteins. The instructions for their manufacture are held by the hereditary material—the *genes*, which consist of *DNA* (deoxyribonucleic acid)—within the nucleus of the cell. Protein synthesis starts with a gene (a particular length of DNA) acting as a template for the manufacture of a strand of a substance called messenger *RNA*. Like DNA, RNA is a *nucleic acid* and consists of a string of building blocks called nucleotide bases. There are four different types of nucleotide bases; their sequence in the strand of messenger RNA provides the coded instructions (the *genetic code*) for making the particular protein that is required.

The strand of messenger RNA passes out of the cell nucleus, where it is then decoded (see diagram) to form a polypeptide chain (string of amino acids). Several polypeptide chains may be manufactured and combine to form one protein molecule.

The rate of protein synthesis is regulated through adjustments in the amount of the relevant messenger RNA formed within the cell nucleus. Highly complex mechanisms exist for "blocking" or "unblocking" the copying of DNA by messenger RNA; this ensures that the cell makes the right type of proteins, in the right quantities, and at the right time.

Proteinuria

The passage of increased amounts of *protein* in the *urine*. Proteinuria may result from damage to the glomeruli (filtering units in the *kidney*), allowing proteins to leak from the blood into the urine (see *Glomerulonephritis*). Proteinuria may also result from *urinary tract infection* and from damage to the kidney tubules that prevents the normal reabsorption of protein from the urine. Increased protein in the urine may also occur because of a generalized disorder (such as *multiple myeloma*) that causes an increase in the level of protein in the blood.

Proteinuria rarely causes any symptoms, although the urine may appear frothy. The condition is usually discovered during a routine *urine test* or during investigation of an underlying disorder.

Protoplasm

An obsolescent term for the entire contents of a cell, including the cytoplasm and organelles, such as the nucleus. Today, the word protoplasm has largely been replaced by specific terms for the individual cell components (see *Cell*).

STEPS IN PROTEIN SYNTHESIS

Proteins consist of one or more subunits called polypeptides. These are formed, within cells, from building blocks called amino acids, which are provided to each cell as raw materials. The instructions for making polypeptides are encoded in the DNA within the cell nucleus.

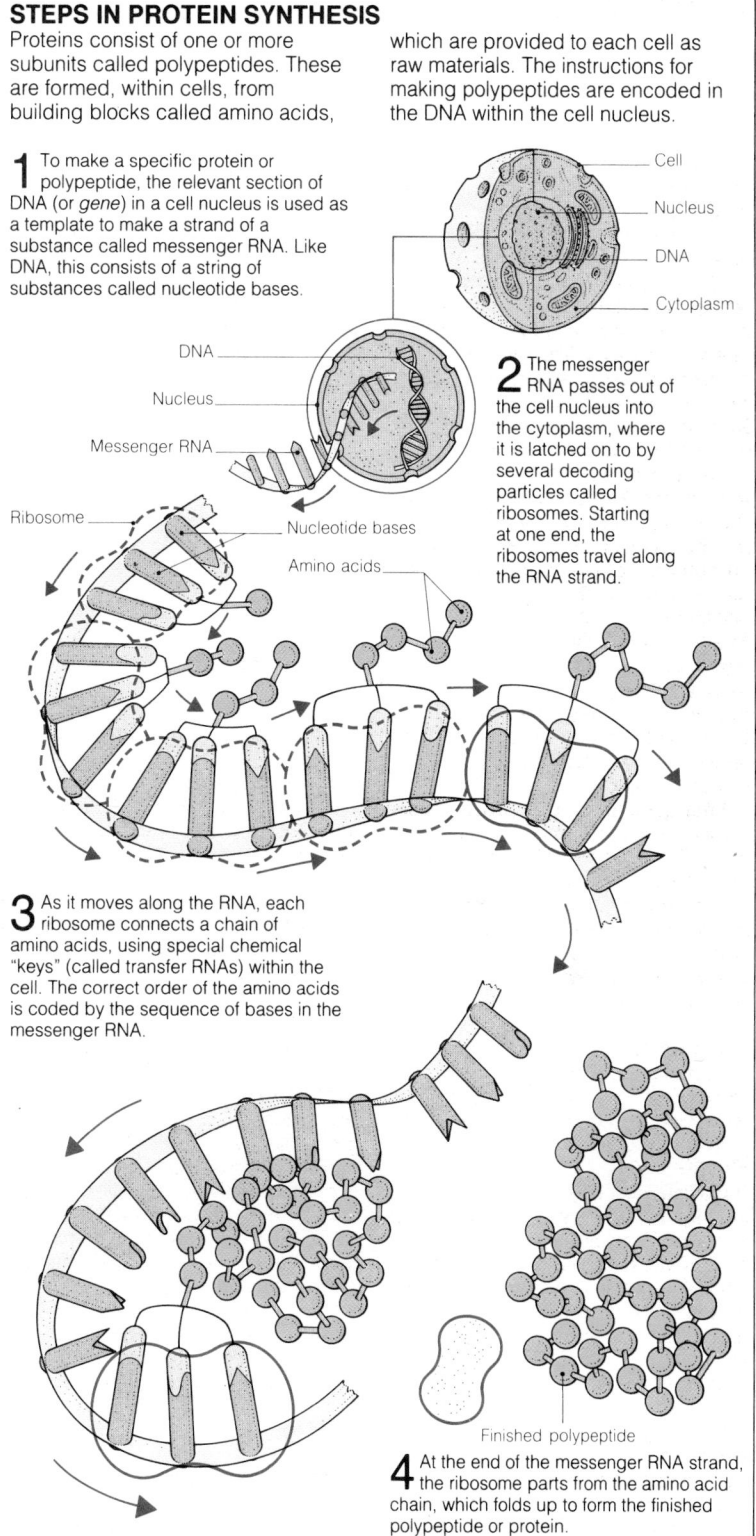

1 To make a specific protein or polypeptide, the relevant section of DNA (or *gene*) in a cell nucleus is used as a template to make a strand of a substance called messenger RNA. Like DNA, this consists of a string of substances called nucleotide bases.

Cell
Nucleus
DNA
Cytoplasm

DNA
Nucleus
Messenger RNA

2 The messenger RNA passes out of the cell nucleus into the cytoplasm, where it is latched on to by several decoding particles called ribosomes. Starting at one end, the ribosomes travel along the RNA strand.

Ribosome
Nucleotide bases
Amino acids

3 As it moves along the RNA, each ribosome connects a chain of amino acids, using special chemical "keys" (called transfer RNAs) within the cell. The correct order of the amino acids is coded by the sequence of bases in the messenger RNA.

Finished polypeptide

4 At the end of the messenger RNA strand, the ribosome parts from the amino acid chain, which folds up to form the finished polypeptide or protein.

P

Protozoa

The simplest, most primitive type of animal; each protozoon consists of a single cell. All types of protozoa are of microscopic size but are bigger than bacteria. The more advanced types are capable of excretion, respiration, and engulfing food particles; they move around through jelly-like movements or the use of whip-like or hair-like attachments called flagella. Some are parasites of larger animals during various stages of their life-cycle.

About 30 different types of protozoa are troublesome parasites of humans. Included among them are the organisms responsible for *amoebiasis* and *giardiasis* (intestinal infections that cause diarrhoea); the sexually transmitted infection *trichomoniasis;* and the insect-borne tropical diseases *malaria, sleeping sickness,* and *leishmaniasis. Toxoplasmosis* (a disease acquired from cats) is also caused by a protozoon.

Protriptyline

An *antidepressant drug.* Protriptyline is especially useful in treating *narcolepsy* or *depression* accompanied by lethargy and tiredness, because it is less likely than other antidepressants to cause drowsiness.

Possible adverse effects include palpitations, anxiety, insomnia, and a rash aggravated by sunlight.

Proximal

A term describing a part of the body that is nearer to a central point of reference, such as the trunk. The hip joint is proximal to the knee; the knuckle is proximal to the fingernail. The opposite of proximal is *distal.*

Prurigo

Thickening and itching of the *skin* due to repeated scratching.

Pruritus

The medical term for *itching.* It is used, for example, in pruritus ani, which is the medical term for itching of the skin around the anus, and pruritus vulvae, which is the term for itching of the external genital area in women.

Pseud-/pseudo-

Prefixes that mean false, as in pseudocyesis (a false pregnancy).

Pseudarthrosis

A term meaning false joint which is used to describe an operation in which the ends of two opposing bones within a joint are removed and a piece of tissue (usually muscle) is fixed between the resulting gap to act as a cushion. This procedure is used to restore mobility and reduce pain when a hip *arthroplasty* (joint-replacement operation) has failed. Pseudarthrosis results in shortening of the affected leg and instability of the joint. A walking aid is usually required.

The term pseudarthrosis also describes a rare condition in children in which congenital abnormality of the bone of the lower half of the tibia (shin) leads to spontaneous fracture without injury. Treatment of this condition consists of inserting a nail through the bone ends and applying a bone graft. If the bone ends fail to unite, amputation of the leg, followed by the fitting of an artificial limb, may be necessary.

Pseudocyesis

See *Pregnancy, false.*

Pseudodementia

A form of severe *depression* in elderly people that mimics *dementia.* Features of both illnesses include intellectual impairment and loss of memory. Nearly one in 10 of those initially thought to be suffering from dementia may turn out to have a depressive illness. Unlike dementia, depression is treatable; many people respond well to *antidepressant drugs.*

Pseudoephedrine

A *decongestant drug* used to relieve *nasal congestion.* Pseudoephedrine is an ingredient in a variety of cough and cold remedies.

High doses of pseudoephedrine may cause anxiety, nausea, dizziness, and, occasionally, hypertension (high blood pressure), headache, and palpitations.

Pseudoepidemic

An outbreak of an illness in a community or in an institution (such as a school) that has no detectable physical cause but is thought to be due to a form of *hysteria.* Typically, the symptoms are vague and mild—headache and a general feeling of sickness—and are induced by group suggestibility combined with anxiety provoked by contact with somebody who already has the symptoms.

Pseudogout

A form of *arthritis* that results from the deposition of calcium pyrophosphate crystals in a joint. The underlying cause of pseudogout is unknown; in rare cases, it is a complication of *diabetes mellitus, hyperparathyroidism,* and *haemochromatosis.*

Symptoms include intermittent attacks of arthritis similar to *gout.* Pseudogout can be distinguished from gout only by examining a sample of the joint fluid under a microscope to identify the crystals, which are different from the urate crystals found in gout. Treatment is with *nonsteroidal anti-inflammatory drugs* (NSAIDs).

Pseudohermaphroditism

A *congenital* abnormality in which the external genitalia resemble those of the opposite sex. Thus, a female pseudohermaphrodite may have an enlarged clitoris resembling a penis and enlarged labia resembling a scrotum. Conversely, a male may have a very small penis and a divided scrotum resembling labia.

In pseudohermaphroditism, an affected person has only ovarian or testicular tissue. This condition thus differs from true *hermaphroditism,* in which an affected person has both. (See also *Sex determination.*)

Psilocybin

An alkaloid present in some types of mushrooms, especially in PSILOCYBE MEXICANA. It is a powerful *hallucinogenic drug* with properties similar to those of *LSD.*

Psittacosis

A rare illness resembling *influenza* that is caused by a microorganism, CHLAMYDIA PSITTACI, and is spread to humans from birds such as parrots, pigeons, or poultry.

The infection is contracted by inhaling dust contaminated by the droppings of infected birds. Most cases occur among poultry farmers, pigeon owners, and people working in pet shops, although anyone who acquires a pet parrot is at slight risk.

SYMPTOMS, DIAGNOSIS, AND TREATMENT
The illness in birds is occasionally serious or even fatal, but often causes no more than lethargy.

Human illness is extremely variable in its features, the most common symptoms being fever, severe headache, and cough, which develop a week or more after exposure to infected birds. Other symptoms include muscle pains, sore throat, nosebleed, lethargy, and depression. In some severe cases, there is also breathing difficulty.

The cause of the condition is often suspected from the patient's occupation; it is diagnosed by finding *antibodies* (proteins with a defence role) specific to the causative organism in the patient's blood.

Treatment with *tetracycline drugs* is usually effective. Without treatment, the illness may continue for several weeks or months before subsiding. Psittacosis may occasionally be fatal if unrecognized and thus not treated.

Psoas muscle

A muscle that bends the hip upwards towards the chest. It is composed of two parts (psoas major and psoas minor) which originate from the lower spine. The lower end of psoas minor is attached to the margin of the pelvis; the lower end of psoas major is joined to the bony prominence just below the neck of the femur (thigh-bone).

A rare disorder of the psoas muscle is an *abscess* (collection of pus), which develops as a complication of *osteomyelitis* (bone infection) of the spine, usually caused by *tuberculosis*.

Psoralen drugs

Drugs containing chemicals called psoralens, which occur in certain plants (such as buttercups) and are present in some perfumes. When absorbed into the skin, psoralens react with *ultraviolet light* to cause darkening or inflammation of the skin. Psoralen drugs may be taken by mouth or applied to the skin.

WHY THEY ARE USED

Psoralen drugs may be used to treat *psoriasis* (a disorder characterized by a scaly rash) and *vitiligo* (a disorder in which patches of skin lose colour).

HOW THEY WORK

Psoralen drugs are used in conjunction with ultraviolet light (a combination that is known as PUVA) as a form of *phototherapy*. This treatment stimulates the production of skin pigment and, in psoriasis, additionally slows the rate at which skin cells grow and multiply.

POSSIBLE ADVERSE EFFECTS

Overexposure to ultraviolet light during psoralen treatment or too high a dose of a psoralen drug may cause redness and blistering of the skin. Psoralens in perfumes may cause a rash when the skin is exposed to ultraviolet light (see *Photosensitivity*). The use of psoralens in suntanning preparations is prohibited in some countries because these chemicals can cause *sunburn*.

LOCATION OF PSOAS MUSCLE

The muscle has two parts—major and minor. The psoas major acts to flex the hip (bend it up towards the trunk) and rotates the thigh inwards. The psoas minor acts to bend the spine down towards the pelvis.

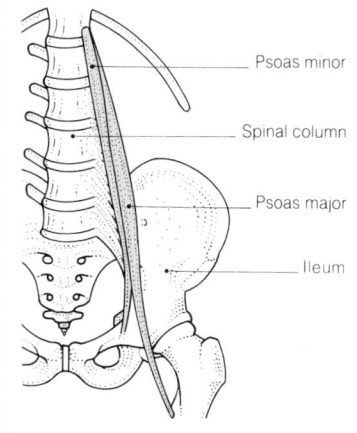

Psoas minor

Spinal column

Psoas major

Ileum

Psoriasis

A common skin disease characterized by thickened patches of inflamed, red skin, often covered by silvery scales. Although psoriasis does not usually cause itching, the affected area may be so extensive that great physical discomfort and social embarrassment may result.

CAUSES AND INCIDENCE

The exact cause of psoriasis is not known but it tends to run in families. Psoriasis occurs in about two per cent of people in the US and Europe and is probably less common in black people and Asians. It affects men and women equally. Psoriasis usually appears between the ages of 10 and 30, but infants occasionally suffer from the condition and it may also sometimes develop in old age.

The underlying abnormality in psoriasis is that new skin cells are produced about 10 times faster than normal. As a result, live cells accumulate and form characteristic thickened patches covered with dead, flaking skin.

Psoriasis tends to recur in attacks of varying severity; attacks may be triggered by a number of factors, such as emotional stress, skin damage, and physical illness.

The skin eruption is sometimes accompanied by a painful swelling and stiffness of the joints, which can be very disabling (see *Arthritis*).

TYPES

The disease has different forms, which may need different treatment.

DISCOID OR "PLAQUE" PSORIASIS In this, the most common form, patches appear on the trunk and limbs, particularly on the elbows and knees, and on the scalp. In addition, the nails may become pitted, thickened, or separated from their beds.

GUTTATE PSORIASIS This form occurs most frequently in children. It consists of numerous small patches that develop rapidly over a wide area of skin, often after a sore throat.

PUSTULAR PSORIASIS This form is characterized by small pustules, which may occur all over the body or be confined to localized areas.

TREATMENT

Mild psoriasis may be helped by moderate exposure to sunlight or an ultraviolet lamp (see *Phototherapy*) and use of an emollient (soothing cream). Moderate attacks are usually treated with an ointment containing *coal tar* or *dithranol*. Other methods of treating psoriasis include *corticosteroid drugs*, *PUVA* (a type of phototherapy), and other drugs, such as *methotrexate*.

Accompanying arthritis is treated with *nonsteroidal anti-inflammatory drugs* (NSAIDs), *antirheumatic drugs*, or methotrexate.

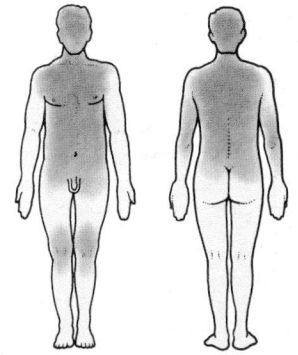

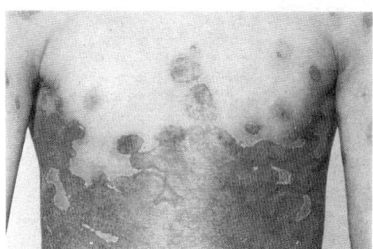

Distribution and appearance of psoriasis
The knees, elbows, scalp, trunk, and back are common sites for psoriasis. The usual appearance is of patches of thickened skin covered by dry, silvery, adherent scales.

P

OUTLOOK

For most people, psoriasis is a long-term condition with no permanent cure, although individual attacks can be completely relieved with appropriate treatment.

Psych-

A prefix meaning mental processes or activities, as in psychology.

Psyche

A term meaning mind (as opposed to body) derived from the ancient Greek for soul or spirit. The most influential description is provided by Freud's *psychoanalytic theory*, which treats the psyche as an organ of the body that is divided into the conscious and unconscious, each with its own functions.

Psychedelic drugs

Drugs, many of which are illicit, that may produce hallucinations, also known as *hallucinogenic drugs*.

Psychiatry

The branch of medicine concerned with the study, prevention, and treatment of mental illness and emotional and behavioural problems. Psychiatry is differentiated from *psychology*, which is principally concerned with the normal mental processes and behaviour of people.

Psychiatry is broad in scope; it approaches the understanding and treatment of mental problems from psychological, social, and physical aspects. Some psychiatrists emphasize that major mental illness is due to genetic and biochemical factors, while psychoanalytically oriented psychiatrists believe that environmental experiences are still the major cause of mental illness. Psychiatrists usually conduct examinations of physical and mental state, and trace the patient's personal and family history to seek the cause of the problem. Laboratory investigations and drug treatments have played an increasingly important role in modern psychiatry.

Within psychiatry there are a number of subspecialties, including child and adolescent psychiatry, community psychiatry (concerned with care of the mentally ill outside psychiatric hospitals), forensic psychiatry (dealing with legal issues, such as rape), neuropsychiatry (relating to brain disorders with mental symptoms), psychiatry of the elderly, and psychiatry of mental handicap (concerned with the psychiatric needs of people with learning disabilities).

Treatment methods in psychiatry may include the use of medication, counselling or *psychotherapy* (individually or in groups), *psychoanalysis*, or *behaviour therapy*.

Psychoanalysis

A treatment for psychiatric disorders based on *psychoanalytic theory*. The system was developed by Sigmund Freud at the beginning of the 20th century as a result of treating, under hypnosis, patients who were supposedly suffering from hysteria. Freud believed that mental disorders were a result of the failure of normal emotional development during childhood. By encouraging the patient to re-enact these years and to verbalize any problems (past or present), Freud believed that important information would emerge from the unconscious mind; the cause of any internal strife would be uncovered and resolved, and the illness would be cured.

Psychoanalysts may have had previous training in various disciplines, including medicine, social work, or psychology, before beginning their training as a psychoanalyst, which usually involves their undergoing analysis themselves.

WHY IT IS DONE

Psychoanalysis can help people with *neurosis* and *personality disorders*. A modified psychoanalytic approach has also been used to treat *psychosis* (when medication is often an important adjunct). Psychoanalysis aims to help the patient understand his or her emotional development and to help the person make appropriate adjustments in particular situations.

HOW IT IS DONE

The treatment involves interviews between a trained analyst and the patient, each lasting perhaps an hour, repeated up to six times a week and continuing for an indefinite period, usually for several years.

Traditionally, the patient lies on a couch with the analyst behind and out of sight. Some therapists prefer to face the patient, who sits in a chair. In dealing with psychotic patients, the structure and reality of face-to-face contact with the psychiatrist is an extremely important element.

The patient is encouraged to talk as freely as possible about his or her life history and any problems that may have occurred in the past or are currently causing concern. This stream of talk is one of free association, with one word or idea leading to another without conscious control so that any

repressed material has the opportunity to surface. The analyst interprets these associations in the light of psychoanalytic theory, paying particular attention to areas of resistance that may contain clues to the person's problem. This leads to different trains of thought, more experiences relived, and sometimes exposure of reasons for symptoms.

Psychoanalysis relies on a number of other key processes. A very close relationship develops with the analyst, who eventually comes to be associated in the patient's mind with important people in his or her history (for example, father, mother, brother, or sister). This experience is called *transference*.

Interpretation of the patient's dreams is another important aspect of the treatment. It is believed that material normally repressed comes to the surface while the patient dreams, usually in the form of symbolic representations (see *Dream analysis*).

The patient is often reluctant to accept the analyst's interpretations and may introduce *defence mechanisms* (such as denial) to cope with the unfolding explanation of his or her behaviour. This reaction is a defence against the anxiety that is stimulated as these repressed conflicts break through into consciousness. Understanding the self-destructive patterns of living is an essential aspect of psychoanalytic treatment.

Psychoanalytic theory

A system of ideas developed by Sigmund Freud early in this century that explains the development of personality and behaviour in terms of unconscious wishes and conflicts.

Psychoanalytic theory has undergone considerable distillation by psychoanalysts over the years. However, its basic concepts and the use of *psychoanalysis* (therapy based on the concepts of psychoanalytic theory) dominated psychiatry until recently.

KEY FEATURES OF FREUDIAN THEORY

Freud placed great emphasis on the importance of sexuality (in its broadest sense) in psychological development. His theory postulates that, during the first 18 months, an infant passes through three phases—oral, anal, and genital—each representing the area of the body to which the child devotes attention at a particular age. After these phases, the child is able to direct attention to people outside himself or herself. Sexual attraction to the parent of the opposite sex develops with consequent desire to eliminate the other parent, who prevents fulfilment of the desire—this is called the *Oedipus complex*.

By the age of five or six, sexual feelings become latent, but re-emerge at *puberty*. At this time, psychological and emotional problems may occur if the individual has not developed normally through the successive stages and has become fixed at a primitive level (see *Fixation*). Problems may also occur if the Oedipus complex has not been successfully dealt with.

Less specifically sexual aspects of psychological development are seen as depending on the interaction among the three parts that make up the personality—the id, ego, and superego. The id is the basic component that guides the individual unconsciously and instinctively towards pleasure; the ego mediates, by conscious reasoning, between internal desires and the reality of the outside world; the superego is also a controlling force but is unconscious, being derived from moral and social standards indoctrinated by parents and other authorities.

It is thought that mental disorders result if conflict between the three aspects of personality cannot be satisfactorily resolved. Freud believed that under normal circumstances tension is dealt with by (among other *defence mechanisms*) repression (in which painful or unacceptable thoughts or memories are kept out of consciousness) and sublimation (in which emotional drives that cannot openly be expressed are channelled into an acceptable activity, such as sport). These normally healthy unconscious processes can become harmful if they occur inappropriately or in excess.

MODERN DEVELOPMENTS
Psychoanalysis has progressed since Freud. In general, modern psychoanalysis is based on the observation that emotional problems for the most part are the result of troubled childhood experiences in the family. The pre-Oedipal problems that are caused by difficulties in the early mother-child relationship are probably even more important than later Oedipal conflicts. Such conflicts may form the basis of later neurotic or psychotic disturbances.

It is necessary for the child to separate from the mother to become an individual and comprehend reality. A healthy mother and father help the child to become an individual. Conflict-ridden parents distort reality and

programme patterns of disturbed self-destructive behaviour. Psychoanalysis in practice attempts to bring to light these unconscious conflicts with the parent (which have led to distortions of reality). The aim is to free the individual from the past and help him or her become a real person in the present. The relationship and interaction between doctor and patient is an essential part of this process.

As the biological basis for psychiatric problems becomes ever more apparent, psychoanalytic theory is decreasing in its influence.

Psychodrama

An adjunct to *psychotherapy* in which the patient acts out certain roles or incidents. These may relate to people closely involved with the patient or may concern situations that he or she finds particularly stressful. The aims of psychodrama are to bring out hidden concerns and to allow a person's disturbing feelings to be expressed. Psychodrama is often carried out with a partner or in a group of patients; music, dance, and mime are also commonly utilized.

Psychogenic

A symptom or disorder that originates from psychological or emotional problems and is not produced or caused by any physical illness.

Psychology

The scientific study of mental processes. Psychology deals with all internal aspects of the mind, such as *memory*, feelings, *thought*, and *perception*, as well as external manifestations, such as *speech* and behaviour. Psychology is also concerned with *intelligence*, *learning*, and *personality* development. Methods employed in psychology include direct experiments, observations, surveys, study of personal histories, and special tests (such as *intelligence tests* and *personality tests*).

Psychologists make an important contribution to the diagnosis and treatment of mental and emotional problems. They play a major part in the use of behaviour therapy, counselling, and in the treatment of behavioural disorders affecting people with a mental handicap. However, because psychologists are not medically qualified, they are not able to prescribe drugs.

Within psychology, a number of different approaches are used. Neuropsychology attempts to relate

human behaviour to brain and body functions. Behavioural psychology studies the ways in which people react to events and learn to adapt accordingly. Cognitive psychology concentrates on thought processes, and is based on the theory that what a person thinks about his or her behaviour is of equal importance to the behaviour itself. Psychoanalytic psychology stresses the role of the unconscious and of childhood experiences (see *Psychoanalytic theory*).

There are many specialized areas within the science. Educational psychologists study learning and intelligence; clinical psychologists are concerned with emotional and behavioural problems; social and industrial psychologists consider the effects of work and the environment on behaviour; and experimental psychologists concentrate on research into new ways of understanding mental events. The emergence of developmental psychology as a specialist area is due to the work of the Swiss psychologist Jean Piaget, who noted that a child's intellectual development passes through certain stages—from simple motor skills to logical and abstract thought.

Psychometry

The measurement of psychological functions. Psychometry includes statistical assessment of intelligence and personality (see *Intelligence tests*; *Personality tests*) as well as numerous methods of testing specific aptitudes, such as memory, logic, concentration, and speed of response. The design of such measurements has become increasingly sophisticated, but the validity of some tests (i.e. whether they measure what they are supposed to measure) is less certain.

Psychoneurosis

A term now used interchangeably with *neurosis*. Neurosis originally referred to any disorder of the nerves; psychoneurosis specifically described nervous disorders associated with psychological symptoms.

Psychopathology

The study of abnormal mental processes. There are presently two main approaches in psychopathology—the descriptive and the psychoanalytic.

Descriptive psychopathology aims to record, as objectively as possible, the symptoms that make up a diagnosis of mental illness. It is particularly concerned with abnormality of *thought*, with mood disturbances, and with the various forms of *hallucination* and *delusion*. The ability to recognize such symptoms when interviewing patients is an important part of the psychiatrist's job.

The psychoanalytic approach is concerned with the unconscious feelings and motives of the individual.

Psychopathy
An outdated term for an *antisocial personality disorder*.

Psychopharmacology
The study of drugs that affect mental states. Since the early 1950s, more effective medications for a range of mental illness have been developed. Particular advances have occurred in the treatment of psychotic illnesses, with the development of *antipsychotic drugs* and *antidepressant drugs*. *Anti-anxiety drugs* have proved to be extremely effective in relieving symptoms in neurotic illness, although the dangers of dependence have been recognized recently.

Psychosexual disorders
A range of conditions related to sexual function. Psychosexual disorders are assumed to stem from psychological problems, although some (e.g. *impotence*) may also be caused by physical injury or illness. Psychosexual disorders include *transsexualism* (a sense that one's anatomical sex is inappropriate), *psychosexual dysfunction* (interference with the normal process of sexual response), and sexual behaviour in which intercourse between consenting adults is not the final aim (see *Deviation, sexual*).

Psychosexual dysfunction
A disorder in which there is interference with the normal process of sexual response in the absence of any known organic cause. Psychosexual dysfunctions are very common in both men and women. They usually start in early adult life, often disappearing spontaneously with experience and increased confidence.

The main dysfunctions affecting men are lack of sexual desire (see *Sexual desire, inhibited*), *impotence*, and premature ejaculation (see *Ejaculation, disorders of*); those affecting women are lack of sexual desire, painful intercourse (see *Intercourse, painful*), *vaginismus*, and lack of orgasm (see *Orgasm, lack of*).

Most psychosexual problems start in early adult life. Some are associated with certain personality traits, including *anxiety* and obsessiveness. Unpleasant early experiences, such as sexual interference in childhood or problems with one's first sexual encounters, are especially likely to inhibit later sexual performance. Unrealistic ideas about normal sexual behaviour or a strict upbringing may also increase the likelihood of sexual problems. Many different kinds of feelings and conflicts (basically nonsexual) can be expressed sexually or can interfere with normal modes of sexual expression.

Psychosexual dysfunctions are common and not usually evidence of serious illness. About 80 per cent of people respond well to *sex therapy*.

Psychosis
A severe mental disorder in which the individual loses contact with reality. Psychosis contrasts with *neurosis*, which describes the milder group of mental illnesses. Neurotic individuals generally know they are ill, but psychotic illness so disturbs the ability to think, perceive, and judge clearly that sufferers often do not realize they are unwell. Psychosis is what people commonly think of as "madness".

TYPES
Three main forms of psychosis are generally recognized: *schizophrenia*, *manic-depressive illness*, and organic brain syndrome (see *Brain syndrome, organic*). However, the symptoms overlap and there is considerable debate about whether each is truly a separate category.

Paranoid illness (see *Paranoia*) is sometimes regarded as a fourth form of psychosis, but many psychiatrists see it as a distinctive disorder.

SYMPTOMS
The main feature of psychotic symptoms is that they may lead the person to view life in a distorted way. Symptoms include *delusions, hallucinations, thought disorders*, loss of *affect* (emotion), *mania*, and *depression*.

CAUSES
It is highly likely that the cause is due to a disorder of brain function.

Research is centred on the role of *neurotransmitters* (chemicals released by nerve endings), such as *dopamine*, and on the importance of the limbic system and frontal lobes of the brain. As yet, no specific physical abnormality that might be isolated by a blood test or X-ray has been clearly related to psychosis. However, a new form of brain imaging, *PET scanning*, may reveal the causes of these disorders.

TREATMENT AND OUTLOOK
Antipsychotic drugs are usually very effective in controlling symptoms. Treatment may need to be long-term, but many sufferers are able to lead normal working lives. In many cases, more extensive rehabilitation is needed, as is continual support for many years.

Psychosomatic
A term used to describe physical disorders that seem to have been caused, or worsened, by psychological factors. Just as a physical reaction (such as crying) may be due to emotion, so it is presumed that worries or unpleasant events can cause physical illness.

For a disorder to be labelled psychosomatic, the psychological factor and physical effect must be closely connected in time and repeatedly related. This is because many chronic illnesses constantly vary in severity, regardless of a person's psychological state, and because there is a tendency to assume that an event was stressful just because a person has become ill.

Common examples of conditions that may fit the psychosomatic label are headache, breathlessness, nausea, *asthma, irritable bowel syndrome, peptic ulcer*, and certain types of *eczema*. (See also *Somatization disorder*.)

Psychosurgery
Any operation on the brain carried out as a treatment for serious mental illness. Psychosurgery is performed only as a last resort to treat severe mental illnesses that have not responded to other forms of treatment.

TYPES
Prefrontal *lobotomy* was once the most widely used form of psychosurgery, but there were often harmful side-effects and this procedure has now been largely replaced by other operations which are safer.

The most commonly performed operations today are forms of *stereotaxic surgery*. In these procedures, a small hole is drilled in the skull above one temple. A diathermy probe is inserted and, under X-ray control, guided to specific areas of the brain, where small cuts are made in nerve fibres. Stereotaxic procedures are most often carried out to relieve severe *depression* or *anxiety* or to treat disabling *obsessive-compulsive disorder*.

Performed less often are the more complex, "open" operations, in which a complete portion of the skull is cut through and lifted up to expose the brain so that specific areas can be removed. Parts of the temporal lobe are cut out to treat *temporal lobe epilepsy*. In rare cases, complete lobes have been removed to treat violent or aggressive behaviour.

OUTLOOK
Psychosurgery has produced good results in some people, enabling those who would otherwise be chronically disabled to lead more useful lives. However, the operations tend to have inconsistent and unpredictable results, and can produce adverse changes in personality and intellect. They remain a controversial form of treatment for psychiatric illness.

Psychotherapy
The treatment of mental and emotional problems by psychological methods. In psychotherapy, the patient talks to a therapist about symptoms and problems and establishes a therapeutic relationship with the therapist.

Any person who uses psychotherapy as a formal method of treatment can be called a psychotherapist. Many psychotherapists have no medical background, but certain personal characteristics are deemed especially important, notably empathy (the ability to understand what a patient is feeling), genuineness (the therapist appears to mean what he or she says), and warmth. The psychotherapist also requires sufficient maturity and experience to be able to cope with the demanding task of dealing with the mental and emotional problems of his or her patients.

WHY IT IS DONE
Psychotherapy is used to help people suffering from *neurosis* or *personality disorders*, as well as individuals with specific personal problems. The aim is to help patients learn about themselves, develop new insights into past and present relationships, and change fixed patterns of behaviour.

HOW IT IS DONE
Treatment varies according to the approach used. *Counselling* is the simplest form of psychotherapy, consisting of advice and psychological support. At the opposite end of the spectrum is *psychoanalysis*, which attempts to explore the deep unconscious feelings and early childhood experiences of the individual (see *Freudian theory*; *Jungian theory*).

Dynamic psychotherapy is based on psychoanalytic principles. The therapist tries to understand and interpret the patient's unconscious messages (without the benefit of formal psychoanalysis) so that the individual can develop a better understanding of his or her underlying feelings and cope with them more effectively.

A course of treatment may be brief, consisting of two or three sessions, or it may extend over many years, depending on the particular problems involved. It may vary in intensity from a simple, supportive approach during a difficult period to an in-depth analysis aimed at reconstructing the personality.

Psychotherapy may involve one person, a couple (see *Marital counselling*), a family (see *Family therapy*), or a group (see *Group therapy*).

Psychotropic drugs
Drugs that have an effect on the mind. Psychotropic drugs thus include *hallucinogenic drugs*, *sedative drugs*, *sleeping drugs*, *tranquillizer drugs*, and *antipsychotic drugs*.

Pterygium
A wing-shaped thickening of the *conjunctiva* (the transparent membrane covering the white of the eye and the inside of the eyelids). Pterygium extends from either side of the eye, across the margin of the cornea towards its centre. The condition is attributed to prolonged exposure to bright sunlight and is common in tropical areas.

If the extension on to the cornea threatens the sufferer's vision, the pterygium should be surgically removed. Occasionally, a prominent pterygium may be removed simply because it causes discomfort. If a pterygium recurs, further treatment may be necessary.

Ptomaine poisoning
An obsolete term for *food poisoning* now known to be caused not by ptomaines—chemical compounds present in decaying foodstuffs—but by bacteria or bacterial poisons.

Ptosis
Drooping of the upper eyelid. The condition may be *congenital* or it may occur later in life, either spontaneously or as a result of injury or disease, such as *myasthenia gravis*. Ptosis is usually due to a weakness of the levator muscle of the upper lid or to interference with the nerve supply to the muscle.

Severe congenital ptosis, in which the drooping lid covers the pupil, should be surgically corrected to avoid

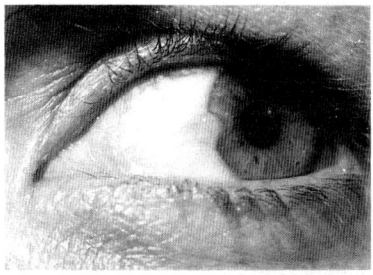

Appearance of pterygium
The conjunctiva has extended beyond the white of the eye to encroach on the cornea (transparent front part of the eye).

the development of *amblyopia* (failure of visual development).

Acquired ptosis without obvious cause may be a sign of a neurological disease, such as a *brain tumour* or a cerebral *aneurysm*, and should be investigated by a doctor.

Ptyalism
See *Salivation, excessive*.

Puberty
The period when secondary sexual characteristics develop and the sexual organs mature, allowing reproduction to become possible. Puberty is the term used for the physical changes that underlie the emotional changes of *adolescence*.

Puberty usually occurs between the ages of 10 and 15 in both sexes; it is initiated by the *pituitary gland* producing hormones (known as *gonadotrophins*) that stimulate the *ovaries* to increase secretion of *oestrogen hormones* and the *testes* to increase secretion of *testosterone*. It is not known what triggers this action by the pituitary gland, but the primary change probably occurs in the part of the brain called the hypothalamus, which controls the pituitary by producing "releasing" and "inhibitory" factors.

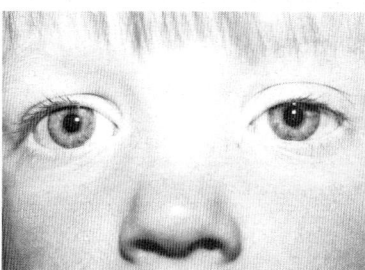

Congenital ptosis in a child
This condition, present from birth, should be corrected surgically to prevent any disturbance of visual development.

Puberty is accompanied by a significant growth spurt and increase in weight. Body weight may double during this period, due primarily to muscle growth in boys and increased fat in girls. The growth spurt occurs later in boys.

PUBERTY IN GIRLS

The first sign of puberty in girls is usually breast budding, which occurs around the age of 11; in about one third of girls, pubic hair appears first. The rate of growth of the two breasts may be unequal but any difference usually disappears by the time full maturity is reached. The first menstrual period usually does not occur for a year or more after the start of puberty, by which time pubic and underarm hair are in the fully developed adult pattern.

Other secondary sexual characteristics, such as the wider pelvis and the female distribution of fat, develop progressively during this period. Puberty is considered to be complete when menstrual periods occur at regular, predictable intervals.

The age at which menstruation starts has decreased during the past century, probably because of a general improvement in nutrition and living standards, but is now stable. Strenuous sports or other hard physical activity (such as ballet) and debilitating disease can also delay the onset of menstrual periods.

PUBERTY IN BOYS

In boys, puberty is heralded by a sudden increase in the rate of growth of the testes and scrotum, followed by the appearance of pubic and facial hair. The penis begins to grow around the age of 13 and reaches its adult size about two years later. However, there is a wide range of variation so that, at the age of 14, some boys may be sexually mature while others still have immature genitals.

The body's increased secretion of testosterone stimulates sperm production and causes the prostate gland and seminal vesicles to mature. It leads to the development of the typical male distribution of hair on the face, chest, and abdomen. The larynx enlarges and the vocal cords become longer and thicker, causing the pitch of the voice to drop.

ABNORMAL PUBERTY

Extremely rarely there are instances in which the normal events of puberty occur at a very young age, sometimes within the first five years of life; the youngest mother on record gave birth to a healthy baby at the age of 5 years 8

CHANGES OF PUBERTY

There is considerable variation in the age of onset of puberty, but girls, on average, undergo puberty earlier than boys. The entire process takes about three to four years to complete. In addition to the sex-specific changes, height and weight both increase rapidly.

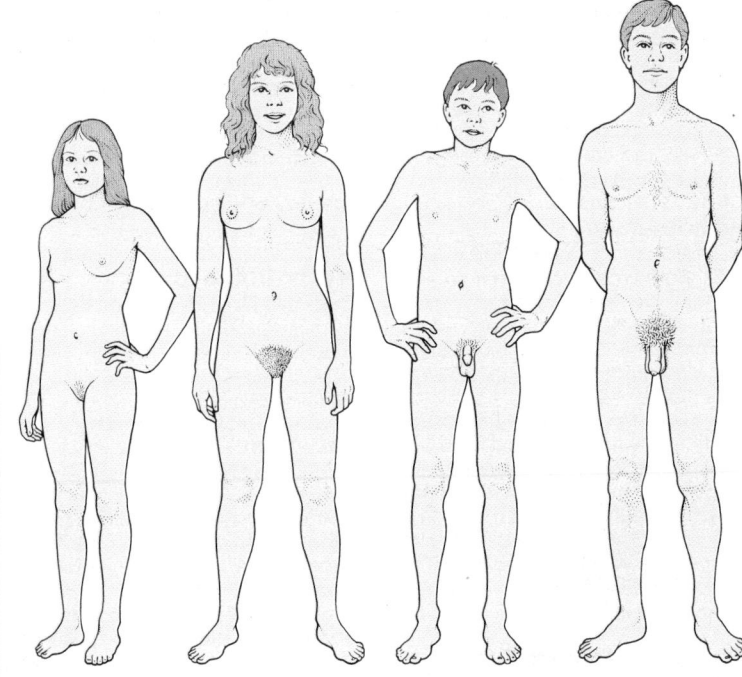

10 to 12 15 to 16   12 to 14 15 to 18

Girls
Puberty most often starts between the ages of 10 and 12 in girls. Major changes include growth of breasts and pubic hair, widening of the hips, enlargement of the uterus, and the onset of menstruation.

Boys
The main changes are enlargement of the sex organs, widening of the shoulders, deepening of the voice, and the growth of facial and pubic hair. The onset is usually between the ages of 12 and 14.

months. Precocious sexual development can occur in either sex. In boys, it may be caused by virilizing hormones from the adrenal gland or by a cyst or tumour in the hypothalamus. In girls, the cause of precocious sexual development is usually not known.

Pubes

The pubic hair or the area of the body covered by this hair.

Pubic lice

 Small, wingless insects that live in the pubic hair and feed on blood. Also called crab lice or crabs (because of their crab-like claws, which they use to grasp hair), they are usually spread by sexual contact. The scientific name for pubic lice is *PHTHIRUS PUBIS*.

Each louse has a flattened body, up to 2 mm across, and can be seen with the naked eye. The females lay minute eggs (called nits) on the hair, where they hatch about eight days later. Pubic lice infestation is not uncommon in the UK; about 10,000 cases are reported from sexually transmitted disease clinics each year.

SYMPTOMS AND SIGNS

Both lice and eggs are visible in the pubic hair. On hairy men the lice may also be found in hair around the anus, on the legs, and on the trunk, and occasionally even in facial hair. The bites sometimes cause itching. Pubic lice can infest children, usually by transmission from parents. In children, lice may attach to the eyelids.

TREATMENT

An insecticide lotion containing lindane (gamma benzene hexachloride) or benzyl benzoate kills the lice and eggs soon after application. An infested person's sexual partner should also be treated; clothes and bedding should be washed in water hotter than 60°C before use.

Public health

A branch of medicine which arose in the 19th century as doctors became aware of the importance of the provision of pure water supplies and safe systems for the disposal of sewage. The medical pioneers in this field instigated the construction of reservoirs and of water and sewage systems. They also turned their attention to working conditions in factories and mines. Measures to control infectious diseases were studied and introduced along with improvements in the care of women during pregnancy and of children in the first few years of life. There were also programmes to improve nutrition and provide immunization against infectious diseases.

Today, the functions of public health are so extensive that they are covered by many different people and agencies, such as Environmental Health Officers, Medical Officers of Environmental Health, the *Public Health Laboratory Service*, and agencies of central government.

Public Health Laboratory Service

An organization comprising 52 laboratories throughout the UK that provide diagnostic testing facilities in cases of suspected infectious disease. The Public Health Laboratory Service is part of the *National Health Service*. The service was set up in World War II to cope with the threat of epidemics associated with bombing, etc. Its current role is the detection and monitoring of infectious diseases (such as measles and typhoid), imported diseases (such as malaria), outbreaks of food poisoning (such as salmonellosis associated with eggs and poultry), and environmental disorders (such as legionnaires' disease).

Pudenda

A term for the external *genitalia*.

Pudendal block

A type of *nerve block* used during childbirth to provide pain relief for a *forceps delivery*. A local anaesthetic (see *Anaesthesia, local*) is injected into either side of the vagina near the pudendal nerve, which passes under the bony prominences on each side of the lower pelvis. The lower part of the vagina becomes insensitive to pain within about five minutes.

Puerperal sepsis

Infection that originates in the genital tract within 10 days after childbirth, miscarriage, or abortion. Puerperal sepsis is rare, occurring in between one and three per cent of pregnancies. Infection usually starts in the vagina and spreads to the uterus.

CAUSES

Infection may be caused by bacteria that normally inhabit the vagina but usually cause harm only if the woman's resistance is low or if placental tissue has been retained in the genital tract. Puerperal sepsis may also be caused by bacteria entering the genital tract from other parts of the body or from outside.

SYMPTOMS AND TREATMENT

The main symptoms are fever, offensive-smelling *lochia* (vaginal discharge after childbirth), headache, chills, and pain in the lower abdomen. If infection spreads to the fallopian tubes (see *Salpingitis*), the tubes may become blocked and cause *infertility*. Further spread of infection may lead to *peritonitis* and *septicaemia*, which may quite rapidly be fatal unless emergency treatment is given.

Treatment includes *antibiotic drugs* and the removal of any remaining placental tissue.

Puerperium

The period of time following *childbirth* during which the woman's uterus and genitals return to their state before the pregnancy.

Pulmonary

Pertaining to the *lungs*. For example, the pulmonary artery is the blood vessel that carries blood from the heart to the lungs.

Pulmonary embolism

Obstruction of the pulmonary artery or one of its branches in the *lung* by an *embolus*, usually a blood clot that originated in a vein in the leg or pelvis as a complication of deep vein thrombosis (see *Thrombosis, deep vein*). If the embolus is large enough to block the main pulmonary artery leading from the heart to the lungs, or if there are many clots, the condition is life-threatening. Pulmonary embolism affects about twice as many women as men; recent surgery, pregnancy, and immobility increase the risk.

SYMPTOMS

Symptoms depend partly on the size of the embolus. A massive embolus that blocks the main pulmonary artery can cause sudden death. Smaller emboli may cause severe shortness of breath, a rapid pulse, dizziness due to low blood pressure, sharp chest pain that is worse when breathing, and coughing up of blood. Small pulmon-

P

PULMONARY EMBOLISM

This condition results when one or more emboli (fragments of material) break off from a blood clot in a vein and are carried, via the heart, to the lungs. The effects depend on the size and numbers of emboli and on the general health of the person's lungs and heart.

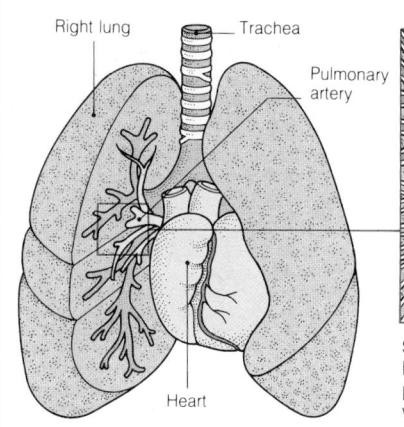

Right lung — Trachea
Pulmonary artery
Heart

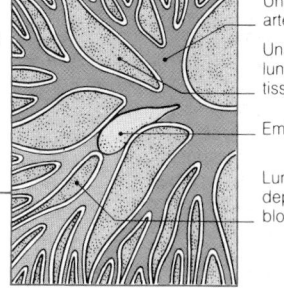

Unaffected artery
Unaffected lung tissue
Embolus
Lung tissue deprived of blood

Site of obstruction
Emboli are carried into the lungs by the pulmonary artery. Most of them lodge within one of the larger or medium-sized arteries and partially deprive a section of lung tissue of blood.

ary emboli may produce no symptoms, but, if they are recurrent, they may eventually lead to *pulmonary hypertension* (increased pressure of blood flow in the lungs).

DIAGNOSIS

Investigation of the lung may include a *chest X-ray, radionuclide scanning*, and pulmonary *angiography*. An *ECG* may show changes in the electrical activity of the heart, and *venography* helps determine the source of the embolus.

TREATMENT

Treatment depends on the size and severity of the embolus. A small embolus gradually dissolves but there is a risk of more emboli developing. *Anticoagulant drugs* (such as heparin and warfarin) are given to reduce the clotting ability of the blood and to reduce the chance of more clots occurring. *Thrombolytic drugs* may hasten the process of clot dissolution. If the embolus is very large, an emergency operation may be necessary in order to remove it.

Pulmonary fibrosis

Scarring and thickening of lung tissue, usually as a result of previous lung inflammation, such as *pneumonia* or *tuberculosis*. Pulmonary fibrosis may occur throughout both lungs (see *Interstitial pulmonary fibrosis*) or may affect only part of one lung.

Shortness of breath is a common symptom. Diagnosis is confirmed by *chest X-ray*. Treatment depends on the underlying cause, but the fibrosis may be irreversible.

Pulmonary function tests

A group of procedures used to evaluate the function of the *lungs* and to confirm the presence of some lung disorders. Pulmonary function tests are also performed before any major operation on the lungs, such as *lobectomy* (removal of a lobe of the lung), to ensure that the person will not be disabled by the reduction in his or her lung capacity.

Spirometry and measurement of lung volume are performed to detect any restriction of normal lung expansion or to detect obstruction of air flow. A *peak-flow meter* is used to assess the degree of *bronchospasm* (narrowing of the airways), while a test of *blood gases* (measurement of the concentration of oxygen and carbon dioxide in the blood) demonstrates the efficiency of the gas exchange in the alveoli in the lungs.

Another test of lung function (diffusing capacity) shows the efficiency

of the lungs in absorbing gas into the bloodstream. This is done by measuring the volume of carbon monoxide breathed out after a low concentration of the gas has been inhaled.

Pulmonary hypertension

A disorder in which the blood pressure in the arteries supplying the lungs is abnormally high. Pulmonary hypertension develops in response to an increased resistance to blood flow through the lungs. To maintain an adequate blood flow, the right side of the heart, which pumps blood to the lungs, must contract more vigorously than was necessary before. This causes an enlargement of the heart's muscle wall. Eventually, right-sided *heart failure* may develop.

CAUSES

Several conditions can lead to increased resistance to blood flow through the lungs. The most important is an inadequate supply of oxygen to the lungs' small air sacs, which may be due, for example, to chronic *bronchitis*. Lack of oxygen causes the small branches of the arteries in the lungs to constrict (narrow) and to thicken their muscular walls, thus causing a permanent increase in resistance. Other causes are *pulmonary embolism* (in which a blood clot blocks off one or several arteries in the lungs), *interstitial pulmonary fibrosis* (thickening and scarring of lung tissue, which can

have many causes) and some types of congenital heart disease (see *Heart disease, congenital*).

Primary pulmonary hypertension is the term used to describe cases in which the cause is not known.

SYMPTOMS AND SIGNS

As long as the enlargement and strengthening of the right side of the heart is sufficient to maintain a normal blood circulation, there is little indication of trouble. But, with the onset of *heart failure* as the right side of the heart fails to meet its workload, symptoms develop. Symptoms include enlargement of veins in the neck, enlargement of the liver, and generalized *oedema* (swelling due to fluid collection in tissues).

TREATMENT

Treatment is directed at the underlying disorder (if known) and to the relief of the effects of right-sided heart failure. *Diuretic drugs* may be valuable in relieving oedema, and sometimes *oxygen therapy* is useful.

Pulmonary incompetence

A defect of the pulmonary valve at the exit of the ventricle (lower, pumping chamber) on the right side of the *heart*. The valve fails to close properly after each contraction of the ventricle, allowing blood pumped out of the chamber to leak back again.

Pulmonary incompetence is a rare type of heart valve defect. When it

---

PULMONARY HYPERTENSION

In this condition, there is increased resistance to blood flow through the lungs (red arrows), usually due to lung disease. The result is a rise in pressure in the pulmonary artery, the right side of the heart (grey lines and arrows), and in the veins that bring blood to the heart.

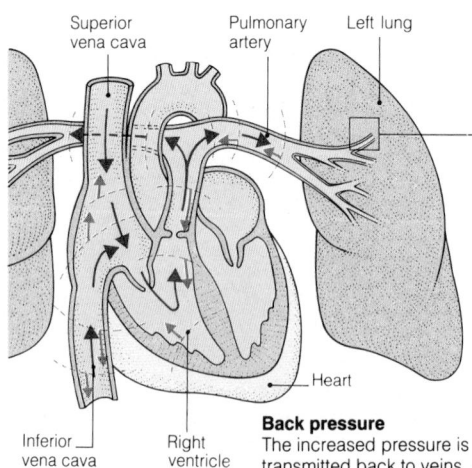

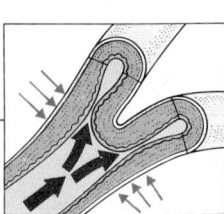

Causes
The most common cause of increased resistance to blood flow through the lungs is constriction of the small arteries in the lungs and thickening of their muscular walls. This thickening usually results from a lung disease such as chronic bronchitis or emphysema.

Back pressure
The increased pressure is transmitted back to veins throughout the body.

does occur, it is usually the result of *rheumatic fever, endocarditis,* or severe *pulmonary hypertension* (raised pressure in the pulmonary artery). Pulmonary incompetence may cause a heart *murmur* that is audible through a stethoscope.

Usually the condition is of little significance. When accompanied by pulmonary hypertension, the eventual result may be right-sided *heart failure*. In such cases, treatment is usually of the pulmonary hypertension rather than an attempt to repair or replace the defective valve.

Pulmonary oedema

Accumulation of fluid in the *lungs*. Pulmonary oedema is usually due to left-sided *heart failure*, which results in a back-pressure of fluid in the lungs. Pulmonary oedema may also be due to chest infection, inhalation of irritant gases (such as sulphur dioxide and chlorine), or to any of the causes of generalized *oedema*.

SYMPTOMS AND SIGNS

The main symptom is breathlessness, which may be very severe. The breathlessness is usually worse when the sufferer lies flat (a symptom known as orthopnoea), and may cause him or her to suddenly waken during the night. There is also a cough that produces frothy sputum, which may be stained pink. Breathing may cause a bubbling sound, or may be wheezy (a condition sometimes called cardiac asthma). Crackling sounds in the patient's chest can be heard through a stethoscope.

DIAGNOSIS AND TREATMENT

Pulmonary oedema is diagnosed by *physical examination*. A *chest X-ray* will clearly indicate the presence of fluid in the lungs.

Treatment with *diuretic drugs* is usually effective. In severe cases, these drugs may need to be given by injection. Other treatment may include the administration of *morphine, oxygen therapy,* and *aminophylline*. In rare cases, artificial *ventilation* may be necessary.

Pulmonary stenosis

A *heart* condition in which the outflow of blood from the ventricle (lower, pumping chamber) on the right side of the heart is obstructed. With pulmonary stenosis, the heart must work much harder than normal to pump blood to the lungs.

The obstruction may be caused by narrowing of the pulmonary valve at the exit of the chamber, by narrowing of the pulmonary artery (large blood vessel beyond the valve) that carries blood to the lungs, or by narrowing of the upper part of the ventricle itself.

CAUSES AND INCIDENCE

Pulmonary stenosis is nearly always congenital (present from birth). About one baby in 8,000 is born with the defect alone or as part of a more complex set of heart defects, called the *tetralogy of Fallot*. Very rarely, pulmonary stenosis develops later in life, usually due to *rheumatic fever*.

SYMPTOMS

In severe cases, a newborn baby's heart begins to enlarge as soon as breathing is established. If the blood supply to the lungs is inadequate, the baby becomes breathless, and damming of blood behind the valve may lead to swelling of the liver and abdomen due to *heart failure*. The baby also may not suck. This is an emergency that can often be helped by surgery.

In less severe cases (which are more common), symptoms may not appear until the child gets older and becomes more active. The main symptom is breathlessness. Marks resembling *chilblains* may appear on the cheeks, hands, and feet as a result of the slower circulation. In mild cases there are no symptoms, and the condition is detected only when a doctor hears a heart *murmur* through a stethoscope.

When pulmonary stenosis exists with other types of heart defect, such as a *septal defect* (hole in the heart), some deoxygenated blood bypasses the lungs and goes back into the general circulation, leading to *cyanosis* (blue-purple skin coloration).

Pulmonary stenosis acquired in later life may lead to the symptoms of heart failure.

DIAGNOSIS

A *chest X-ray* may show enlargement of the heart. *ECG* (measurement of the electrical activity of the heart), *echocardiography*, and Doppler *ultrasound* techniques (imaging of the heart using sound waves) can help diagnose the severity of the narrowing.

TREATMENT

In some cases, a *balloon catheter* is used to relieve the narrowing without the need to open the chest. Alternatively, *heart valve surgery* or other types of *open heart surgery* are often successful.

Pulp, dental

The soft tissue in the middle of each tooth (see *Teeth*). The dental pulp has a rich supply of blood vessels and contains nerves that respond to heat, cold, pressure, and pain.

Pulpectomy

The complete removal of the pulp of a tooth (the soft tissue in the middle of the tooth that contains blood vessels and nerves). Pulpectomy is part of *root-canal treatment*.

Pulpotomy

Removal of the coronal part of the pulp of a tooth (the soft tissue in the middle of the tooth that contains blood vessels and nerves) when it has become inflamed, usually as a result of bacterial infection. The infection is most commonly the result of extensive dental *caries* (tooth decay) or of a dental fracture (see *Fracture, dental*) that exposes the pulp. Successful pulpotomy prevents further degeneration of the pulp.

Under a local anaesthetic, the dentist removes the damaged pulp and covers the wound with a dressing that encourages it to heal. The gap in the overlying dentine and enamel is then sealed (see *Restoration, dental*). If the treatment is unsuccessful, *root-canal treatment* may be required.

Pulse

The rhythmic expansion and contraction of an artery as blood is forced through it, pumped by the *heart*.

The pulse is usually checked during the course of a *physical examination* because it can give clues to the patient's state of health or illness. It is detected by pressing one or more fingers or thumb against the skin over an artery, usually at the wrist, although it can also easily be felt in the neck or the groin. The pulse is sometimes easily visible at the temple or in the neck.

The pulse can be described in terms of its rate (number of expansions per minute), its rhythm, strength, and

P

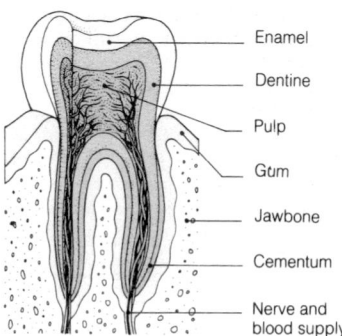

Location of the dental pulp
The pulp forms the soft core at the centre of a tooth. If tooth decay reaches as far as the pulp, the latter degenerates rapidly and must be removed to save the tooth.

Enamel

Dentine

Pulp

Gum

Jawbone

Cementum

Nerve and blood supply

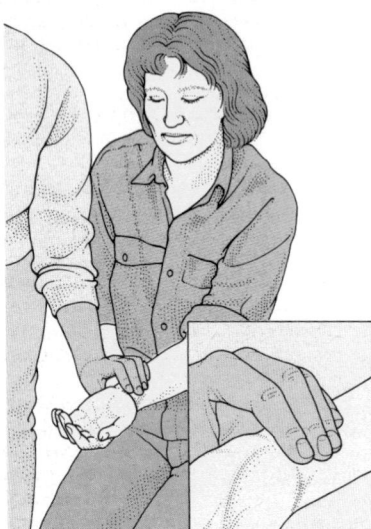

Taking the pulse
Two fingertips are pressed against the wrist just below the base of the thumb to feel the pulse in the radial artery.

whether the blood vessel feels hard or soft. The rate is easily determined by counting the beats in a set period (minimum 15 to 20 seconds) and multiplying to give the beats per minute. The pulse rate usually corresponds to the *heart-rate*, which varies according to the person's state of relaxation or physical activity.

Abnormally high or low rates, or abnormal rhythms, may be a sign of a heart disorder (see *Arrhythmia, cardiac*). When the heart is beating very fast, some of its beats may be too weak to be detectable in the pulse, effectively making the pulse-rate slower than the heart-rate.

If the pulse feels weak, it may be a sign of *heart failure*, *shock*, or an obstruction to the blood circulation. A weak or absent pulse in one or both legs is a sign of *peripheral vascular disease*. The vessel wall should feel soft when the pulse is felt; a wall that feels hard may be a sign of *arteriosclerosis*.

Pump, infusion
A machine for the administration of a continuous, controlled amount of a drug or other fluid through a needle which may be inserted into a vein or under the skin.

An infusion pump consists of a small battery-powered pump that controls the flow of fluid from a syringe into the needle. The pump, which is strapped to the patient, is pre-programmed to deliver the fluid

at a constant rate. If required, it can also be programmed to deliver additional amounts of medication or other fluid at scheduled times.

Infusion pumps are commonly used to administer morphine and other drugs to patients suffering from cancer. They are also used to give insulin to patients who have diabetes mellitus (see *Pump, insulin*).

Pump, insulin
A type of infusion pump (see *Pump, infusion*) used to administer a continuous dose of insulin to some patients with *diabetes mellitus*. The needle is inserted under the skin, usually in the upper arm or abdominal wall. The rate of flow is adjusted so that the level of blood glucose (sugar) is constant.

Punch-drunk
A condition characterized by slurred speech, impaired concentration, and slowed thought processes. It occurs as a result of brain damage caused by several episodes of brief loss of consciousness due to head injury. The name comes from the high incidence of the condition in boxers.

Pupil
The circular opening in the centre of the *iris*. In bright conditions, the pupil constricts (narrows) in order to reduce the amount of light admitted to the *eye*; in dim light, the pupil dilates (widens) to allow more light to reach the retina. Constriction and dilation are controlled by muscles in the iris.

Several drugs affect the size of the pupil. For example, *atropine* eye-drops dilate the pupil and *pilocarpine* eye-drops constrict it.

DISORDERS
The pupil may be congenitally small, irregular in shape, or displaced to one side; there may also be a coloboma (a missing segment or fissure in the iris).

Adie's pupil is a condition in which the affected pupil is larger than the other pupil, with poor constriction in response to light and slow dilation in the dark.

In Argyll Robertson pupil, usually caused by *syphilis*, the pupil is small and irregular, and does not constrict in response to light but does so when an effort at *accommodation* is made.

The pupil is often affected by injury to the iris. This may produce permanent dilation of the pupil or distortion of its shape.

Purgative
A term for a *laxative drug*.

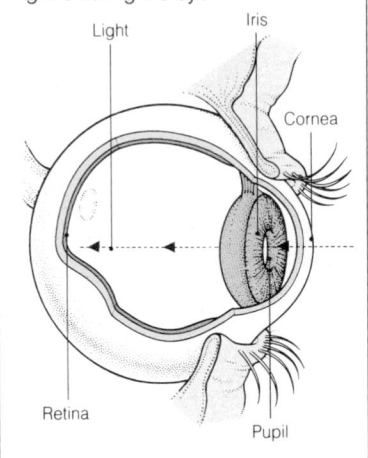

LOCATION OF THE PUPIL
The pupil is the circular opening in the centre of the iris. It can be widened or narrowed by muscles in the iris to adjust the amount of light entering the eye.

Light · Iris · Cornea · Retina · Pupil

Purine
Any of a group of nitrogen-containing compounds synthesized in the body or produced by the digestion of certain proteins. Increased levels of purine can cause *hyperuricaemia* (a raised level of uric acid in the blood), which may lead to *gout*. Foods high in purine include sardines, liver, kidneys, pulses, and poultry. Purine is also present in other substances, including caffeine and theophylline.

Purpura
Any of a group of disorders characterized by purplish or reddish-brown areas or spots of discoloration, visible through the skin, and caused by bleeding within underlying tissues. Purpura also refers to the discoloured areas themselves, which can range from the size of a pinhead to 2.5 cm or so in diameter. The smaller bleeding points are sometimes called *petechiae*; larger, darker areas of discoloration are called ecchymoses or bruises.

TYPES AND CAUSES
There are many different types and causes of purpura.

Common purpura, also often called senile purpura, is the most common of all bleeding disorders, affecting for the most part middle-aged or elderly women. Large discoloured areas appear on the thighs or the back of the hands and forearms. These are caused by thinning of the tissues supporting blood vessels beneath the skin, which as a result rupture easily. Bleeding may also be visible under the membrane that lines the mouth.

Henoch-Schönlein purpura (also called anaphylactoid purpura) is caused by inflammation of blood vessels beneath the skin, sometimes as a result of an allergic reaction. Similar changes may occur in patches within the gastrointestinal tract.

Purpura can also occur as a result of a lack of platelets in the blood—a condition called *thrombocytopenia*. Platelets are the small blood cells that play a crucial role in clotting. A lack of platelets may occur as a result of a disease of the bone marrow (such as *leukaemia* or aplastic *anaemia*), as a side-effect of certain drugs or excessive radiation, or for no apparent reason.

Other types of purpura include that seen in *scurvy* and in forms of the condition caused by damage to blood vessels by certain infections, *autoimmune disorders*, *septicaemia* (blood poisoning), or biochemical disturbances such as uraemia (see *Kidney failure*).

DIAGNOSIS AND TREATMENT

Purpura is investigated by a doctor studying the signs and symptoms and by a full examination and testing of the blood, including *blood-clotting tests*. The state of the blood platelets is of primary interest. It is essential for the doctor to determine exactly the type and cause of the purpura, because treatment depends on the specific type.

Common purpura may be helped by oestrogen *hormone replacement therapy*. Other types may be helped by *corticosteroid drugs* or *immunosuppressant drugs*. In severe cases, *plasmapheresis* (removal of blood, replacement of plasma, and retransfusion) has been effective. Platelet deficiency is treated according to the cause. In some cases, transfusions of platelets must be given. Autoimmune thrombocytopenia (sometimes called

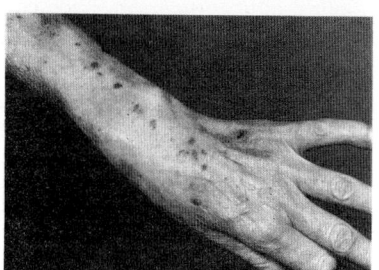

Appearance of senile purpura
This common condition of middle to old age is caused by thinning of the tissues that support blood vessels beneath the skin.

idiopathic thrombocytopenic purpura) is usually treated with corticosteroid drugs or by removal of the *spleen*.

Purulent

A term that means containing, producing, or consisting of *pus*.

Pus

A pale yellow or green, creamy fluid found at the site of bacterial infection. Pus is composed of millions of dead white blood cells, partly digested tissue, dead and living bacteria, as well as minute quantities of other substances. A collection of pus within solid tissue is called an *abscess*.

Among the main pus-forming organisms are streptococci, pneumococci, and *ESCHERICHIA COLI*. Many bacteria produce a distinctive type of pus—for example, *PSEUDOMONAS AERUGINOSA* produces pus with a bluish tinge.

Pustule

A small *skin* blister containing pus. Pustules may occur in a hair follicle or elsewhere in the skin, and may or may not be the result of infection; the pustules in *acne* are noninfective. A *stye* is a pustule at the root of an eyelash.

PUVA

A type of *phototherapy* used to treat certain skin conditions, especially *psoriasis*. PUVA combines the use of a *psoralen drug*, which sensitizes the skin to sunlight, and a controlled dose of long-wavelength *ultraviolet light*. The abbreviation stands for psoralens and ultraviolet A.

Pyelitis

See *Pyelonephritis*.

Pyelography

See *Urography*

Pyelolithotomy

An operation performed to remove a *calculus* (stone) from the kidney. The surgeon approaches the kidney via a longitudinal incision to the right or left of the spine, the junction between the kidney and ureter is cut open, and the calculus is removed with forceps.

Pyelolithotomy is being replaced by *lithotripsy* using ultrasonic waves to break up the stones.

Pyelonephritis

Inflammation of the *kidney*, usually caused by a bacterial infection. Pyelonephritis may be acute, taking the

form of a sudden attack, or chronic, in which repeated or inadequately treated attacks may cause permanent damage to the kidney.

ACUTE PYELONEPHRITIS

Acute pyelonephritis is more common in women and more likely to occur during pregnancy. It usually results when bacteria causing *cystitis* spread up to the kidney.

Symptoms include a high fever, chills, and back pain. Treatment consists of *antibiotic drugs*, which may need to be given by intravenous infusion in severe cases. *Septicaemia* (blood poisoning) is a possible complication.

CHRONIC PYELONEPHRITIS

Chronic pyelonephritis often starts in childhood. It is usually caused by reflux (backflow) of urine from the bladder into one of the ureters, often because the child has a congenital abnormality of the valve where the ureter enters the bladder.

Persistent reflux of urine causes repeated kidney infection, leading, in some children, to inflammation and scarring, which may cause permanent kidney damage. Children in whom recurrent urinary tract infections develop require testing by a doctor. Micturating *cystourethrography* may help identify the presence of reflux so that the underlying abnormality can be corrected surgically.

Possible complications arising from chronic pyelonephritis include *hypertension* (high blood pressure) and *kidney failure*.

Pyloric stenosis

Narrowing of the pylorus (the lower outlet from the stomach) that obstructs the passage of food into the duodenum (the first part of the small intestine). Pyloric stenosis occurs in babies and in adults.

CAUSES AND INCIDENCE

In infants, the condition is caused by a thickening of the pyloric muscle, which occurs, for unknown reasons, soon after birth; about one in every 4,000 babies is affected.

In adults, the narrowing is usually the result of scarring caused by a *peptic ulcer* or of a malignant tumour of the lower stomach (see *Stomach cancer*).

SYMPTOMS AND DIAGNOSIS

Three to four weeks after birth, an affected infant starts projectile vomiting (profuse, forceful vomiting in which the stomach contents may be ejected a distance of several feet) after feeding. Adults with the disorder vomit undigested food several hours after a meal.

PYLORIC STENOSIS IN INFANTS
In infantile pyloric stenosis, the muscle surrounding the outlet from the stomach is abnormally thickened, as shown in the enlarged drawing (below). The condition occurs more often in male than female babies and tends to run in families—infants of a woman who was affected with pyloric stenosis as a baby are liable to develop it.

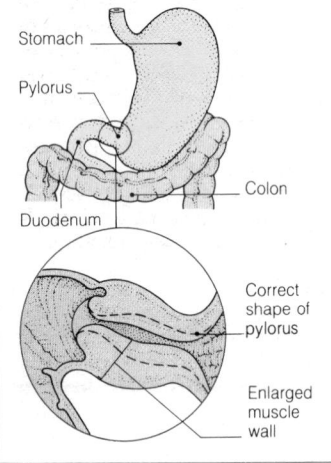

Stomach
Pylorus
Duodenum
Colon
Correct shape of pylorus
Enlarged muscle wall

In an infant, a doctor can feel the thickened muscle through the abdominal wall, but a barium meal (see *Barium X-ray examinations*) may be required to confirm the diagnosis. In adults, pyloric stenosis is diagnosed by a barium meal and *gastroscopy* (examination of the stomach with a flexible viewing instrument).

TREATMENT
Infant pyloric stenosis is sometimes treated with drugs. However, in most cases the only satisfactory treatment is pyloromyotomy: under general anaesthetic, the abdomen is opened and the obstruction relieved simply by making an incision along the length of the thickened muscle.

In adults, surgery is necessary to correct the underlying cause.

Pyloroplasty
An operation in which the pylorus (the outlet from the stomach) is widened to ensure the free passage of food into the intestine. Pyloroplasty may be performed as part of the surgical treatment for a *peptic ulcer*; it prevents tightening of the pyloric muscles following *vagotomy* (cutting of the vagus nerve to reduce stomach acid production).

While the patient is under general anaesthesia, a lengthwise incision is made across the pylorus. The beginning and end of the incision are pushed inwards till they meet, and the opening, which is now at right angles to the original incision, is sewn up. This creates an extra wide passage for the movement of food.

Pyo-
A prefix that denotes a relationship to pus. The prefix py- is also used, as in pyuria, pus in the urine.

Pyoderma gangrenosum
A rare condition characterized by ulcers, usually on the legs, that turn into hard, painful areas surrounded by discoloured skin. Pyoderma gangrenosum occurs as a rare complication in *ulcerative colitis*.

Pyrantel
An *anthelmintic drug* used to treat intestinal *worm infestations*. A single dose of pyrantel is usually sufficient to eradicate the worms. Possible adverse effects include nausea, loss of appetite, and abdominal pain.

Pyrazinamide
A drug sometimes used to treat *tuberculosis*. Possible adverse effects are nausea and an increased risk of gout. There may also be liver damage, resulting in loss of appetite and jaundice.

Pyrexia
A medical term for *fever*.

Pyrexia of uncertain origin
Persistent fever for which no cause is readily apparent despite extensive medical investigations. The cause is usually an illness that is difficult to diagnose or a common disease that presents itself in an unusual way.

Common causes include various viral infections; *tuberculosis*; cancer, particularly *lymphoma* (cancer of the lymphoid tissue); and *collagen diseases*, such as systemic *lupus erythematosus*, *temporal arteritis*, and, in children, Still's disease (see *Rheumatoid arthritis, juvenile*). Another possible cause is a *drug* reaction.

Pyridoxine
Vitamin B_6, one of the B group of vitamins (see *Vitamin B complex*).

Dietary deficiency of this vitamin is very rare but can be induced by various drugs; deficiency causes *neuritis* (nerve inflammation).

Large doses of pyridoxine (50 to 100 mg per day compared with the recommended daily amount of about 2 mg) are sometimes used to treat *premenstrual syndrome* but the results of this treatment are not conclusive.

Pyrimethamine
A drug used to prevent and treat attacks caused by certain strains of *malaria* parasite and also to treat *toxoplasmosis*. Pyrimethamine is usually given in combination with a *sulphonamide drug* or *dapsone*.

Possible adverse effects include loss of appetite, vomiting, and, rarely, rash. Long-term use may reduce blood cell production by the bone marrow, causing *anaemia*, abnormal bleeding, or increased susceptibility to infection.

Pyrogen
A substance that produces *fever*. The term is usually applied to proteins that are released by white blood cells in response to bacterial or viral infections. These proteins act on the temperature-controlling centre within the brain, causing it to raise body temperature. The word pyrogen is also sometimes used to refer to chemicals released by microorganisms—such as bacterial *endotoxins*—which have a similar temperature-raising effect.

Pyromania
A persistent impulse to start fires. The typical person with pyromania becomes fascinated with fires as a child, obtains relief of tension (or even pleasure) from setting fire to something and watching it burn, and has no other motive (such as money) for doing so. The disorder is more often diagnosed in males, and may be associated with a low IQ, alcohol abuse, and sometimes a *psychosexual disorder* (some people seem to be sexually aroused by fires). Pyromania is often difficult to treat; imprisonment is not unusual.

Pyuria
The presence of white blood cells (pus cells) in the *urine*. Pyuria is usually an indication of infection and inflammation in the *kidney* or *urinary tract*.

Microscopic examination and *culture* of the urine are performed to look for a causative microorganism so that appropriate *antibiotic drugs* may be given. In some cases, pyuria occurs when no microorganisms are present and may indicate inflammation of the kidney due to another cause.

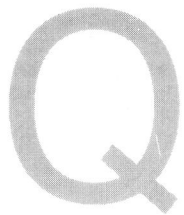

QALY

A quality adjusted life year. QALY is a means of comparing costs and outcomes of treatment for various diseases. Each year of life saved or prolonged is adjusted by a factor, Q, which takes account of how close to normal is the individual's lifestyle before and after treatment. The measure is used by health economists to compare, for example, the relative values of a hip-joint replacement and treating leukaemia (by bone marrow transplantation) or cataract blindness.

Q fever

An uncommon illness with symptoms similar to those of *influenza*. Q fever occurs throughout the world.

CAUSES
The causative organism, COXIELLI BURN-ETTI, is a type of *rickettsia* harboured by farm animals. It occurs in the urine, faeces, milk, flesh, and placentas of infected animals. Q fever may be contracted by inhaling dust contaminated with faeces, urine, or birth products. It may rarely be spread by tick bites.

SYMPTOMS AND SIGNS
About 20 days after infection, the illness begins suddenly with a high fever (that lasts for up to two weeks), severe headache, muscle and chest pain, and cough. A form of pneumonia develops in the second week. Recovery usually follows, but in some cases the disease is prolonged; *hepatitis* develops in one third of these and some suffer *endocarditis*. It is fatal in less than one per cent of cases.

DIAGNOSIS, TREATMENT, AND PREVENTION
Diagnosis of Q fever may be confirmed by a *blood test*. Treatment is with *antibiotic drugs*. An effective vaccine is available for people at risk.

Quackery

A false claim that someone can diagnose and treat disease.

Quadriceps muscle

A muscle with four distinct parts that is located at the front of the thigh, and which straightens the knee.

LOCATION OF THE QUADRICEPS MUSCLE
One upper end attaches to the pelvis; the other two ends attach to the femur. The lower ends merge into a tendon that surrounds the patella and attaches to the tibia.

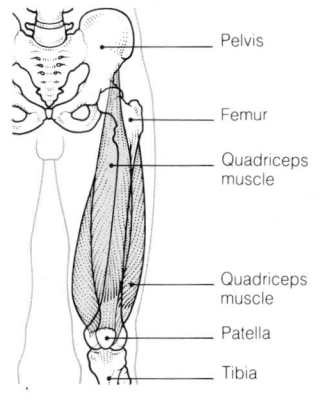

Pelvis
Femur
Quadriceps muscle
Quadriceps muscle
Patella
Tibia

DISORDERS
The most common disorder of the quadriceps is a *haematoma* (a collection of blood) caused by a direct blow. Bruising may follow a few days later. In rare cases, bone forms within the haematoma, restricting movement.

Sudden stretching of the leg may tear the muscle, especially in middle-aged or elderly people. Any knee disorder that brings on pain or swelling, limiting full extension of the leg, causes the quadriceps muscle to begin wasting away within 48 hours, making the knee feel as though it is giving way when weight is placed on the affected leg.

Quadriparesis

Muscle weakness in all four limbs and the trunk. (See also *Quadriplegia*.)

Quadriplegia

Paralysis of all four limbs and the trunk. Quadriplegia may be caused by damage to the *spinal cord* in the neck region. The condition results in loss of feeling and power in the affected parts. (See also *Paraplegia*.)

Quarantine

Isolation of a person recently exposed to a serious infectious disease. The aim is to prevent the spread of a disease by an infected, but symptomless, person.

The term quarantine comes from the Italian word for forty. In the past, ship's crews had to stay at sea for forty days after leaving a port where an epi-

demic illness, such as *cholera, smallpox*, or *plague*, was raging. Later, the forty days was reduced to a period that corresponded more closely to the *incubation period* of the disease involved.

Today, the reduced incidence of most serious infectious diseases and the widespread availability of *immunization* against many of them makes quarantine procedures rarely necessary. In some cases (principally to prevent the spread of *yellow fever*), quarantine has been replaced by compulsory vaccination for travel between certain countries. Contacts of people with highly infectious diseases (such as pneumonic *plague*) may have restrictions placed on their travel in addition to being given preventive immunization. The principal remaining quarantine regulations apply to animals imported into countries, including the UK, that are free from *rabies*.

Quickening

The stage of *pregnancy* when the movements of the fetus are first felt by the pregnant woman. Quickening usually occurs between 16 and 20 weeks of gestation.

Quinine

The oldest drug treatment for *malaria*. Quinine is now used mainly to treat strains of the disease that are resistant to other antimalarial drugs. Large doses are needed and there is a high risk of adverse effects, including headache, nausea, hearing loss, ringing in the ears, and blurred vision.

Quinine is commonly prescribed to help prevent painful leg cramps at night; low doses are used and adverse effects are rare.

Quinolone drugs

COMMON DRUGS

*Acrosoxacin Ciprofloxacin Ofloxacin
Cinoxacin Nalidixic acid Norfloxacin*

A group of *antibiotic drugs*. The first widely used quinolone was *nalidixic acid*, used to treat urinary tract infections. Related compounds have since been produced, which are more active and kill a wider range of bacteria. The quinolone drugs should be used with caution in patients with *epilepsy, liver* and *kidney disorders*, in pregnancy, and during breast-feeding. Common side-effects include nausea, vomiting, abdominal pain, diarrhoea, headache, dizziness, sleep disorders, rash, and blood disorders.

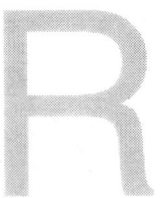

R

Rabies

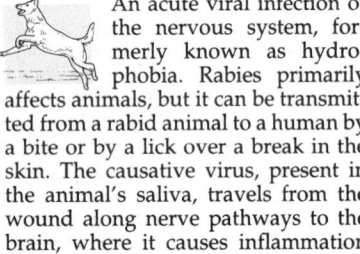

An acute viral infection of the nervous system, formerly known as hydrophobia. Rabies primarily affects animals, but it can be transmitted from a rabid animal to a human by a bite or by a lick over a break in the skin. The causative virus, present in the animal's saliva, travels from the wound along nerve pathways to the brain, where it causes inflammation resulting in delirium, painful muscle spasms in the throat, and other severe symptoms. Once symptoms develop, rabies in humans is usually fatal.

CAUSES AND INCIDENCE

The geographical distribution of rabies, and of some important animal species affected, is shown on the map below. Most human cases result from a bite by a rabid dog. However, the possibility of rabies must be considered whenever any mammal (domestic or wild) bites a human in a country where the virus is present. Rabies may also be acquired from bats; people visiting tropical countries should be cautious when entering caves containing large bat colonies.

Worldwide, there are an estimated 15,000 cases of rabies in humans each year. In the UK, however, cases are extremely rare.

SYMPTOMS AND SIGNS

The incubation period between a bite and the appearance of symptoms is between nine days and many months (the average is four to eight weeks), depending largely on the site of the bite. The first symptoms are slight fever, headache, and loss of appetite, leading to restlessness, hyperactivity, disorientation, and, in some cases, seizures. Often the victim is intensely thirsty, but attempts to drink induce violent, painful spasms in the throat (hence the term hydrophobia). Eye and facial muscles may become paralysed. Coma and death follow three to 20 days after the onset of symptoms.

TREATMENT

Once symptoms have appeared, the features of the disease are treated with sedative drugs and *analgesic drugs* (painkillers). A very small number of people with established rabies are reported to have survived as a result of intensive care aimed at maintaining breathing and the action of the heart. However, the main emphasis must be on preventing the disease.

PREVENTION

Countries free from rabies, such as the UK, impose strict quarantine regulations on the importation of animals.

Any animal bite should be thoroughly cleansed (see *Bites, animal*). If the bite occurs in a country where there is rabies, medical opinion should be sought immediately on whether post-exposure *immunization* is necessary. If so, passive immunization is given with human rabies *immunoglobulin* (ready-made *antibodies* against the rabies virus), and rabies vaccine is given by a course of injections lasting several weeks. Passive immunization is not given to people who have been vaccinated before exposure. Today's vaccines have milder side-effects than those used before 1970.

Every attempt should be made to capture and confine the biting animal. If it appears rabid, it should be killed and its brain examined for microscopic evidence of rabies infection. If no evidence of rabies infection can be found or if a healthy animal remains symptom-free after five days, treatment of the bitten person is stopped.

If immunization is given within two days of the bite, rabies is almost always prevented. The chances of prevention decrease with delay, but immunization can still be effective even weeks or months after a bite.

Rachitic

A term used to describe bony or other abnormalities associated with *rickets* (a bone disease produced by a deficiency of vitamin D). Rachitic is also used to refer to people or populations that are particularly afflicted by rickets.

Rad

A unit of absorbed dose of ionizing radiation (see *Radiation* units box). Rad is an acronym for radiation absorbed dose.

Radial nerve

A branch of the *brachial plexus*. The radial nerve is one of the main nerves of the arm, running down its full length into the hand. The radial nerve controls muscles which straighten the wrist so that the back of the hand is in line with the forearm. The radial nerve

GEOGRAPHICAL DISTRIBUTION OF RABIES

In most rabies-affected areas, the disease circulates mainly among wild animals. Some of the principal animal "reservoirs" of rabies are shown on the right, but other mammals may also be affected—for example, raccoons and bats in North America. Most human cases result from the bite of a rabid dog. The dog may have acquired the virus through contact with a wild animal, but, in some areas, such as the Far East, stray dogs are themselves principal carriers. Vaccinating dogs can largely prevent rabies in humans. A few countries (mainly islands, such as the UK) are rabies-free.

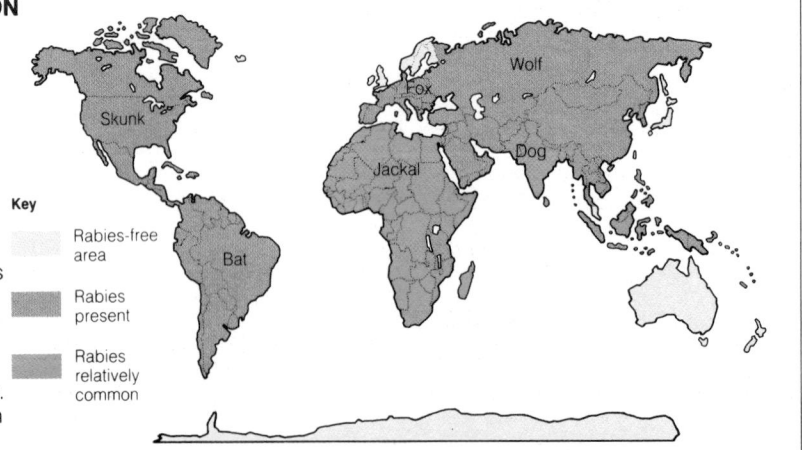

Key

Rabies-free area

Rabies present

Rabies relatively common

also conveys sensation from the back of the forearm; from the thumb, second, and third fingers; and from an area at the base of the thumb.

DISORDERS

The radial nerve winds around the shaft of the humerus (upper-arm bone) and so may be damaged by a fracture of this bone. The nerve may also be damaged by persistent pressure on the armpit (e.g. from a crutch). Such damage may result in *wrist-drop* (inability to straighten the wrist) and numbness in the areas of skin supplied by the radial nerve.

Radiation

The emission of energy in the form of waves or particles. There are two main types of radiation—ionizing and nonionizing. Ionizing radiation is capable of forcibly ejecting one or more of the electrons which orbit the nucleus of an atom, thereby creating an entity called an *ion* that has an electrical charge and is capable of chemical combination with other ions. When ionization occurs in the atoms of molecules that play an important role in the body, it can lead to biological damage.

Nonionizing radiation has a different effect on molecules. It tends to cause excitation of the molecules' constituent atoms (somewhat like shaking them) but it does not impart enough energy to the atoms to displace electrons and form ions.

IONIZING RADIATION

There are three types of ionizing radiation—*X-rays*, gamma rays, and particle radiation.

X-rays are electromagnetic waves (i.e. they are part of the same continuous spectrum—the electromagnetic spectrum—that includes radio waves, *infra-red* radiation, visible light, *ultraviolet light*, and gamma rays) of very short wavelength and very high frequency. They are produced by special electrical machines (X-ray generators). X-rays have no mass and no electrical charge; their penetrating power depends on their energy, which, in turn, depends on the voltage used to generate them. X-rays generated at a few tens of thousands of volts can penetrate only a few millimetres of tissue, whereas those generated at about 100,000 volts are just energetic enough to pass completely through the body and produce X-ray images. X-rays used in *radiotherapy* are generated at several million volts and are sufficiently energetic to destroy deep-seated tumours. They can also destroy other tissues lying in their path.

RADIATION UNITS

Becquerel	The SI unit of radioactivity. One becquerel (symbol Bq) is defined as one disintegration (or other nuclear transformation) per second. Although the number of becquerels is a measure of how strongly	radioactive a particular source is, it takes no account of the different effects of different types of radiation on tissue; for medical purposes, the sievert is generally more useful.
Gray	The SI unit of absorbed dose of ionizing radiation, the gray (symbol Gy) has superseded the rad. One gray is defined as an energy	absorption of 1 joule per kilogram of irradiated material. One gray is equivalent to 100 rads.
Rad	An acronym for radiation absorbed dose, the rad is a unit of absorbed dose of ionizing radiation. One rad is equal to an energy absorption of 100 ergs (an erg is a unit of work or	energy) per gram of irradiated material. The rad has been superseded by the gray (the corresponding SI unit); 1 rad is equivalent to 0.01 grays.
Rem	An acronym for roentgen equivalent man, the rem is the absorbed dose of ionizing radiation that produces the same biological effect as 1 rad of X rays or gamma rays. The rem was introduced as a result of the observation that some types of ionizing radiation, such as neutrons, produce a greater biological effect for an equivalent amount of absorbed energy than X rays or gamma rays. In short, the rem is a measure of the biological effectiveness of irradiation. For X rays and gamma rays, the rem is	equal to the rad. For other types of radiation, the number of rems equals the number of rads multiplied by a special factor (called the quality factor or relative biological effectiveness) that depends on the type of radiation involved. The rem has been superseded by the sievert in the SI system of units; 1 rem is equivalent to 0.01 sieverts.
Sievert	The SI unit of equivalent absorbed dose of ionizing radiation, the sievert (symbol Sv) has superseded the rem. One sievert is the absorbed dose of radiation that	produces the same biological effect as 1 gray of X rays or gamma rays. One sievert is equivalent to 100 rems.

Measurement of radiation levels
In the SI system (the internationally agreed system of units), three main units are used to measure radiation levels—the becquerel, the gray, and the sievert. These three units are defined above, along with two other radiation units (the rad and rem) that have now been largely superseded but are still occasionally used for some purposes.

Gamma rays have almost identical properties to X-rays. The principal difference between the two is that gamma rays are produced by the spontaneous decay of radioactive materials rather than by a machine. They tend to have shorter wavelengths and higher frequencies (and thus greater energies) than X-rays, although there is some overlap between the two.

Particle radiation—unlike X-rays and gamma rays—has mass and may also have electrical charge. It represents parts of atoms, such as electrons (beta particles, which have a negative electrical charge and a very small mass), protons (positively charged particles, each with a mass about 1,800 times that of an electron), or neutrons (particles with the same mass as protons but no electrical charge). It also represents the nuclei of small atoms such as helium (helium nuclei are also known as alpha particles), or even larger atomic nuclei. Particle radiation may be produced during the decay of radioactive atoms or by machines.

SOURCES OF IONIZING RADIATION

Ionizing radiation may originate from natural or man-made sources.

One natural source is cosmic rays, which come from remote parts of the universe as well as from the sun and contribute about 14 per cent of the total radiation exposure in the UK population. These rays consist largely of very high-energy protons, along with a few atomic nuclei (principally helium nuclei). Cosmic rays are highly energetic and not only can irradiate people on the Earth's surface, but also can pass through many metres of soil and rock. The amount of cosmic rays an individual receives depends on the altitude at which he or she lives. A person who is living at an altitude of about 2,000 m, for example, receives more than twice the annual radiation dose of cosmic rays received by a person living at sea level.

Secondary radiation is generated in the upper atmosphere from cosmic rays and consists mainly of gamma rays and high-energy electrons. The annual dose from such secondary radiation varies with latitude, being greatest at the Earth's poles and least at the equator.

The other principal natural source of radiation is radioactivity. Many minerals contain unstable atomic nuclei that spontaneously disintegrate (a process known as radioactive decay), thereby emitting alpha or beta particles and/or gamma rays. The naturally occurring radioactive isotope potassium 40 (isotopes are varieties of an element that are chemically identical but differ in some physical properties) is the principal source of radiation from within the body. Many other natural materials are radioactive and, in some areas, *radon* from soil, rocks, and/or building materials is a major contributor to the annual radiation dose.

Medical X-rays—used to diagnose and/or treat numerous diseases and disorders—are the greatest artificial source of radiation to which the general public is exposed. Radioactive isotopes, also used in diagnosis and treatment, are another medical source of radiation (see *Radionuclide scanning*). Radioisotopes that emit gamma rays are most commonly used (although particle-emitting radioisotopes are also employed); the types selected are usually short-lived to reduce the dose to the patient. In the UK, the average yearly radiation dose from medical sources is about 11 per cent of the total dose of radiation from all sources.

Nuclear reactors are not only potential sources of direct radiation (such as gamma rays and neutrons, which are normally absorbed by thick shielding to prevent them from escaping into the environment), but are also prolific producers of radioactive isotopes. *Uranium* is the most commonly used fuel, often enriched so that it contains more of the fissionable isotope uranium 235 than is present in natural uranium ores. In the reactor it undergoes fission (splitting), thereby producing heat and leaving behind a wide variety of radioactive isotopes. Radioisotopes of iodine, ruthenium, tellurium, and caesium are among those produced in the greatest amounts, although others of greater biological importance, such as *strontium* isotopes, are also produced. In fast-breeder reactors, *plutonium* is used as the main fuel; uranium 238 is the source from which additional plutonium fuel is made.

Nuclear weapons, including atomic bombs of the types used at Hiroshima and at Nagasaki (in which either uranium or plutonium undergoes rapid fission) and hydrogen bombs (which combine nuclear fission and fusion) are intense sources of man-made radiation. However, except for the relatively small battlefield weapons and the "radiation-enhanced" weapon (the so-called neutron bomb), the lethal effects from direct irradiation occur only comparatively near the point of explosion, whereas the lethal effects of blast and heat extend over a considerably larger area.

NONIONIZING RADIATION

The most widespread type of nonionizing radiation is ultraviolet light, a component of sunlight (although much is absorbed by the atmosphere); it is also produced by sun-lamps. This type of radiation can penetrate only superficial layers of body tissue but it causes damage to the RNA (ribonucleic acid) and DNA (deoxyribonucleic acid) molecules in cells, which may lead to skin cancer.

Microwave ovens cook food by means of radio-frequency electromagnetic radiation, which can also heat body tissues and thereby damage them. This type of injury is unlikely to occur because modern appliances are shielded to prevent microwaves from escaping; they also have safety cutoffs to stop radiation emission when the door is opened. Radio and television transmissions are harmless forms of electromagnetic radiation.

The other types of nonionizing radiation to which people are subjected are magnetic fields and *ultrasound*. Weak magnetic fields are generated around all wires carrying electricity, and strong fields are used in medicine for *MRI* (magnetic resonance imaging). The effects of such fields are currently being studied, but there is no evidence that they are harmful. Ultrasound (inaudible high-frequency sound waves) is used in medicine for diagnosis and treatment. Its effects depend on the power used and the duration of exposure. The low power levels and relatively short durations used in medicine are harmless, but exposure to ultrasound at high power levels and/or for a long time may damage tissue. (See also *Radiation hazards; Radiation sickness*.)

Radiation hazards

Hazards from *radiation* may arise from exposure to external sources of radiation (such as *X-rays* or gamma rays) or from the effects of radioactive materials taken into the body. The effects of radiation depend on the dose received, the duration of exposure, and how critical are the organs exposed.

RADIATION DAMAGE

Some forms of radiation damage occur when the total radiation dose exceeds a certain threshold, usually 1 sievert or more (see *Radiation* units box). Examples of such damage include radiation *dermatitis*, *cataracts*, failure of various organs (which may not occur until many years after exposure), or *radiation sickness* (an early reaction to massive irradiation).

In the case of other radiation effects, the severity of damage does not depend upon the specific radiation dose, but the risk that damage will occur increases with increasing doses. *Cancer* is the major example of this type of radiation damage, and is initiated by the mutagenic effect of high-energy radiation. A *mutation* is a change in the genetic material of living cells. Radioactive leaks from nuclear reactors can cause a rise in mutation rates that affects large numbers of people. This may lead to an increase in various cancers, such as forms of *leukaemia*, to *birth defects* in succeeding generations, and to hereditary diseases. Cancer usually develops years after exposure, typically five to 15 years for leukaemia, and 40 years or longer for skin, lung, breast, and other cancers.

The International Commission on Radiological Protection has concluded that the total risk factor for death from radiation-induced cancers is about one in 100 per sievert of radiation absorbed. The risk of genetic damage producing a hereditary disorder within the first two generations fol-

R

lowing irradiation of either parent is also thought to be about one in 100 per sievert, and the additional risk to subsequent generations is thought to be the same.

AVOIDING RADIATION DAMAGE

Radiation damage can be controlled by limiting the exposure of individuals. It is particularly important for people exposed to radiation in the course of their work to have their exposure closely monitored to ensure that it does not exceed what are considered to be safe limits, and that their cumulative radiation exposure is kept below the threshold dose. Younger people and those of reproductive age should have their reproductive organs shielded when having X-rays or *radiotherapy*.

Despite some adverse publicity, there is no evidence of any radiation hazards associated with visual display units (VDUs) or with the *irradiation of food*. VDUs do not emit significant amounts of penetrating radiation, and food which has been irradiated does not itself become radioactive.

Radiation sickness

The term applied to the acute effects of ionizing *radiation* on the whole, or a major part, of the body when the dose is greater than about 1 gray (1 Gy) of X-rays or gamma rays, or 1 sievert (1 Sv) of other types of radiation (see *Radiation* units box).

SYMPTOMS

The effect of exposure to radiation depends critically on the dose and the length of time exposure is maintained. Acute exposures of more than 30 to 100 Gy cause the rapid onset of nausea, vomiting (which may be repeated and severe), anxiety, and disorientation. Within a few hours, the victim usually loses consciousness and dies due to direct damage to the nervous system from the radiation, and to oedema (accumulation of fluid) of the brain; these effects are known as the central nervous system syndrome.

People who have received radiation doses of 10 to 30 Gy also experience an early onset of nausea and vomiting, which tend to start within about two hours of exposure but disappear a few hours later. However, such individuals invariably die within four to 14 days of exposure as a result of radiation damage to the gastrointestinal tract—which causes severe and frequently bloody diarrhoea (known as the gastrointestinal syndrome)—and overwhelming infection due to radiation damage to the *immune system*.

At doses of 1 to 10 Gy, transient nausea and occasional vomiting may occur, but these early symptoms usually disappear rapidly and are often followed by a two- to three-week period of relative well-being. However, by the end of this period, the effects of radiation damage to the bone marrow and immune system begin to appear, with repeated infections (which may be fatal unless treated with antibiotic drugs), and petechiae (pinpoint spots of bleeding under the skin). Some victims may be treated successfully by a *bone marrow transplant* or by isolation in a sterile environment until their own bone marrow recovers.

Radiation damage to other tissues, such as the skin and lining of the respiratory tract, may cause complications, but total-body doses of less than 2 Gy are unlikely to be fatal to an otherwise healthy adult. However, despite the most intensive medical care, few people survive doses of more than 6 Gy.

Radical surgery

Extensive surgery aimed at eliminating a major disease by removing all affected tissue and any surrounding tissue that might be diseased.

In the past, radical surgery was commonly performed in an attempt to cure cancer. Radical *mastectomy* performed to treat *breast cancer*, for example, involved removing the entire affected breast, along with chest muscles, underarm lymph nodes, and other tissue. Such operations are rarely performed today.

Amputation, which is usually performed to prevent the spread of *gangrene* (tissue death), is another form of radical surgery.

Radiculopathy

Damage to the nerve roots that enter or leave the *spinal cord*. Radiculopathy may be caused by *disc prolapse*, spinal *arthritis*, thickening of the meninges (the membranes that cover the brain and spinal cord), and sometimes *diabetes mellitus* or ingestion of heavy metals, such as lead.

Symptoms of radiculopathy are severe pain and, occasionally, loss of feeling in the area supplied by the affected nerves, and weakness, paralysis, and wasting of muscles supplied by the nerves. Treatment is of the underlying cause if possible; otherwise, symptoms may be relieved by *analgesic drugs* (painkillers), *physiotherapy*, or, in some cases, surgery.

Radioactivity

The emission of alpha particles or beta particles and/or gamma rays that occurs when the nuclei of certain unstable substances spontaneously disintegrate. Natural radioactivity is due to the disintegration of naturally occurring radioactive substances, such as uranium ores. However, most elements can be induced to become radioactive by bombarding them with high-energy particles (such as neutrons)—so-called artificial radioactivity. (See also *Radiation*.)

Radiography

The use of *radiation* to obtain images of parts of the body. Radiographers prepare patients for *X-ray* examinations, take and develop X-ray pictures, and assist with other *imaging techniques*.

Radiographers give the patient any special instructions that he or she must follow during the X-ray examination. Once the examination begins, the radiographer is responsible for positioning the patient to provide the best picture of the part under study.

Radiographers also assist radiologists in performing specialized X-ray examinations, such as contrast-medium studies, and carrying out other imaging techniques, such as *radionuclide scanning, ultrasound scanning*, and *MRI*. (See also *Radiology*.)

Radioimmunoassay

A very sensitive laboratory technique that employs radioactive isotopes to measure the concentration of specific proteins in a person's blood.

Proteins that can be detected by radioimmunoassay now include hormones, parts of microorganisms, and antibodies formed against microorganisms or allergy-producing substances. (See *Immunoassay*.)

Radioisotope scanning

See *Radionuclide scanning*.

Radiology

The medical specialty that uses *X-rays, ultrasound, MRI* (magnetic resonance imaging), and *radionuclide scanning* for investigation, diagnosis, and treatment. In general, a radiologist (a doctor who is specially trained and certified in the use of imaging techniques) is seen only on referral from another doctor. Other specialists may also employ radionuclide (radioisotope) scanning for purposes of diagnosis and treatment.

Radiological methods can provide images of almost any organ, system,

R

or part of the body in a *noninvasive* way so that diagnoses can be made and treatment planned or monitored frequently without the patient's needing to undergo exploratory surgery.

Radiological techniques also enable instruments (such as needles and catheters) to be accurately guided into different parts of the body both for diagnosis and, increasingly, for treatment. This subspecialty is known as interventional radiology.

Radiolucent

Almost transparent to *radiation*, especially to X-rays and gamma rays. Objects that are entirely transparent to radiation are termed radiotransparent. Objects that are not transparent to radiation are termed *radiopaque*.

Radionuclide scanning

A diagnostic technique based on the detection of *radiation* emitted by radioactive substances introduced into the body. Different radioactive substances, known as radionuclides, are taken up in greater concentrations by different types of tissue, so that specific organs can be studied. For example, the thyroid gland takes up more radioactive iodine than other parts of the body. The images provided by radionuclide scanning reflect the functioning of an organ better than other techniques, although they provide less anatomical detail.

HOW IT WORKS

A radionuclide substance is swallowed or injected into the bloodstream and accumulates in the target organ. Radiation in the form of gamma rays (similar to X-rays but of shorter wavelength) is emitted from the organ and detected by an instrument known as a gamma camera. The camera contains a scintillation crystal that reacts to gamma rays by emitting minute quantities of light (photons). These are used to produce an image that can be displayed on a screen or in digital (numerical) form.

Using a principle similar to *CT scanning*, cross-sectional images ("slices") can be constructed by a computer from radiation detected by a gamma camera that rotates around the patient. This specialized form of radionuclide scanning is known as SPECT (single photon emission computed tomography).

It is also possible to create moving images with the aid of a computer by recording a series of images immediately following the administration of the radionuclide.

RADIONUCLIDE SCANNING

In this imaging technique, a radionuclide is introduced into the body, where it is taken up in different amounts by different tissues. The radiation emitted by the tissues that take up the radionuclide is then detected by a gamma camera. The radionuclides used may be radioactive varieties of elements that occur naturally in the body (e.g. iodine), or synthetic radioactive elements (e.g. technetium).

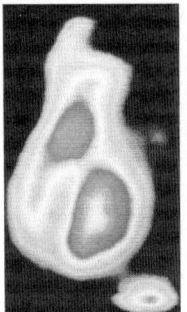

Radionuclide scan of the heart
This image shows radionuclide-labelled red blood cells in the heart. The lower dark area is the left ventricle of the heart.

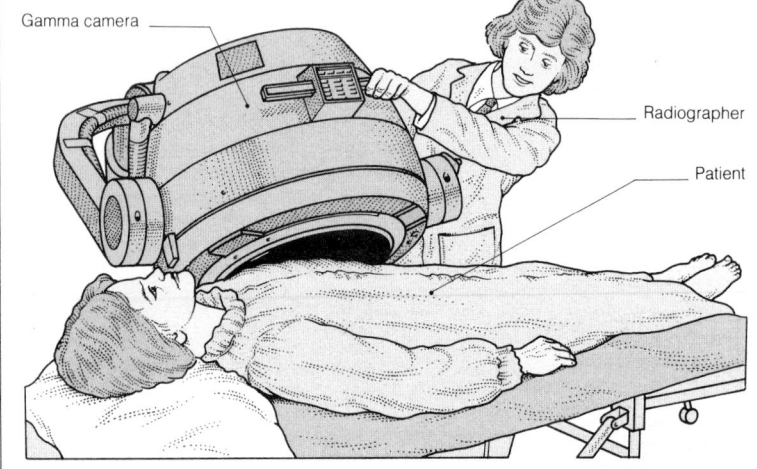

Gamma camera

Radiographer

Patient

WHY IT IS DONE

Radionuclide scanning can detect certain disorders earlier than other imaging techniques because changes in the functioning of an organ often occur before the structure is affected. For example, infection of bone results in increased activity of bone cells, resulting in radionuclide being taken up in greater amounts by diseased bone before structural changes show on conventional X-rays.

The technique is also useful for detecting disorders that affect only function (some thyroid disorders, for example).

Moving images can provide information on functions such as blood flow, the movement of the heart walls, urine flow through the kidneys, and bile flow through the liver.

RISKS

Radionuclide scanning is a safe procedure. It requires only minute doses of radiation and, because the radionuclide is ingested or administered by intravenous injection, it also avoids the risks associated with some X-ray procedures in which a radiopaque

contrast medium is administered by inserting a catheter into the organ (as in cardiac *catheterization* and coronary *angiography*). Moreover, unlike radiopaque contrast media, radionuclides carry virtually no risk to the patient of toxicity or hypersensitivity.

OUTLOOK

Advances in radionuclide scanning depend on the continuing development of radionuclides specific to certain tissues. The fact that monoclonal antibodies (see *Antibody, monoclonal*) can now be produced for use against almost any antigen means that it should be possible to target almost any tissue. Experiments are being carried out using labelled antitumour monoclonal antibodies to assess tumour spread and recurrence.

Radiopaque

Blocking the passage of *radiation*, especially *X-rays* and gamma rays. Many body tissues, with the notable exception of bones, are *radiolucent* (almost transparent to X-rays). For some types of diagnostic X-ray imaging, it is therefore necessary to intro-

R

duce special radiopaque substances into the body to make organs stand out more clearly. In intravenous *urography*, for example, radiopaque iodine compounds are excreted by the kidney into the lower urinary tract to make the structures clearly visible on X-ray photographs.

Radiotherapy

Treatment of *cancer*, and occasionally other diseases, by X-rays or other sources of radioactivity. Sources of this kind produce ionizing *radiation*, which, as it passes through the diseased tissue, destroys or slows down the development of abnormal cells. Provided the correct dosage of radiation is given, normal cells suffer little or no long-term damage. Transient side-effects that develop during treatment are, however, a reflection of acute damage to normal tissue.

WHY IT IS DONE

Radiotherapy has various applications in the treatment of cancer. For example, it may be used on its own in an attempt to destroy all the abnormal cells in various types of cancer, such as cancer of the larynx (see *Larynx, cancer of*), basal cell carcinoma and *squamous cell carcinoma* (two types of skin cancer), cancer of the cervix (see *Cervix, cancer of*), *Hodgkin's disease* (a cancer of lymphoid tissue), and *leukaemia*.

Radiotherapy may also be used in conjuction with other forms of cancer treatment. For example, it is often used after surgical excision of a malignant tumour (such as in the treatment of *breast cancer*) to destroy any remaining tumour cells.

USE OF RADIOTHERAPY

Before treatment, calculations are made of the doses of radiation needed and of the directions from which the rays should be aimed. The areas of the patient's body to be targeted are marked directly on the patient or on a plastic coat that he or she wears. The treatment is usually performed on an outpatient basis, with the patient receiving treatment several times a week.

Radiotherapy machine in use

The patient lies on a table under the machine in a room designed to prevent radiation leakage. A radiographer operates the machine, which sends X-rays, in the predetermined directions and amounts, through the diseased area of the patient's body. The procedure causes no discomfort and usually lasts just a few minutes.

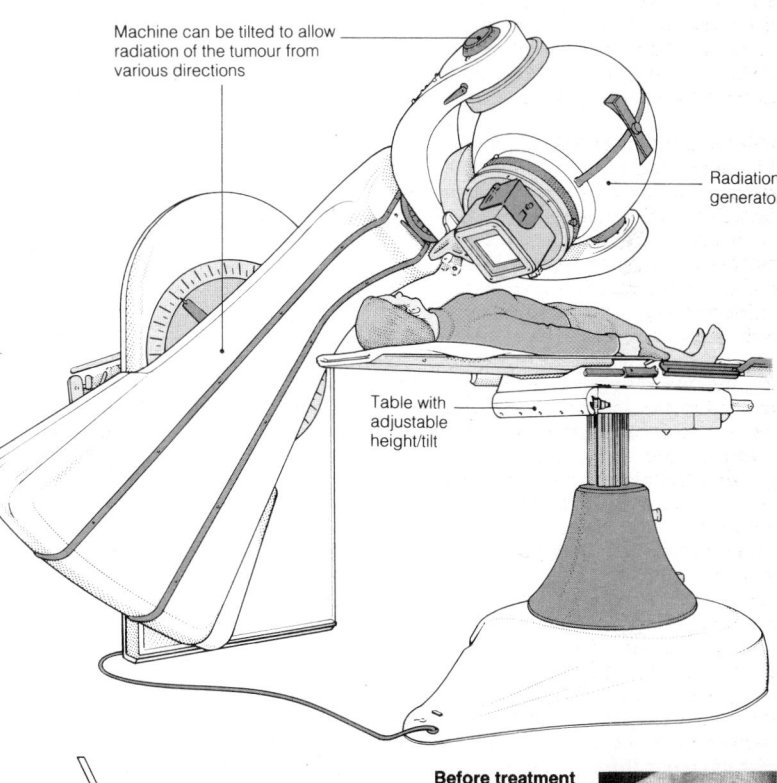

Machine can be tilted to allow radiation of the tumour from various directions

Radiation generator

Table with adjustable height/tilt

EXAMPLES OF RADIOTHERAPY

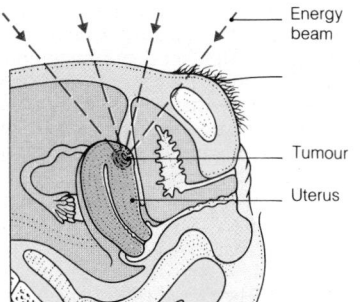

Energy beam

Tumour

Uterus

Rays from different directions

By aiming relatively low-energy rays coming from many directions at a tumour, a large enough dose is achieved in the locality of the tumour to destroy it. Tissues through which the rays pass are unharmed.

Hollow needle

Radioactive pellets

Pituitary gland

Use of radioactive pellets

Another technique is to insert a source of radiation, in the form of tiny radioactive pellets, directly into the tumour via a hollow needle. Pituitary tumours are sometimes treated in this way.

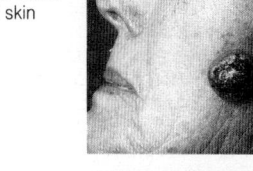

Before treatment
The patient has a malignant skin tumour.

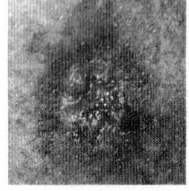

After treatment
The tumour is healing well after radiotherapy.

R

A further use of radiotherapy is to reduce the size of a tumour in order to relieve the symptoms of a cancer that is too far advanced to be curable. Such *palliative* treatment may be directed, for example, at relieving obstruction to swallowing caused by an oesophageal tumour (see *Oesophagus, cancer of*), relieving pain caused by *bone cancer*, and relieving headaches or paralysis caused by a *brain tumour*.

If the benefits of destroying diseased tissue far outweigh the risk of damage to healthy tissue, radiotherapy may be used to treat non-malignant diseases. A common example is use of radioactive iodine to destroy part of an overactive thyroid gland that is producing severe symptoms (see *Thyrotoxicosis*).

HOW IT IS DONE
Some of the main techniques of radiotherapy are shown in the illustrated box on the previous page. Radiation is usually passed through the diseased tissues by means of X-rays (or sometimes electrons) produced by a machine called a linear accelerator. This device has largely supplanted earlier apparatus containing radioactive cobalt, which has the drawback of producing ionizing radiation that is both less intense than the radiation of X-rays and incapable of being shut off.

Some malignant tumours are not treated by radiation from an external source, but by the insertion of radioactive material directly into the growth itself or the surrounding tissue (see *Interstitial radiotherapy*) or alternatively into a body cavity (see *Intracavitary therapy*). Both procedures require an anaesthetic.

Radiation used to treat thyrotoxicosis is given in the form of a liquid containing radioactive iodine. The patient drinks the liquid through a straw, and the radioactive iodine concentrates in the thyroid gland.

COMPLICATIONS
Radiotherapy may produce unpleasant side-effects, including fatigue, nausea and vomiting (for which *antiemetic drugs* may be prescribed), and loss of hair from irradiated areas. Rarely, there may be reddening and blistering of the skin, which can be alleviated by *corticosteroid drugs*.

RESULTS
Radiotherapy cures most cancers of the larynx or skin. The cure rate for other types of cancer varies depending on how early the treatment is begun, but the cure rate can be 80 per cent or higher.

Radium

A rare radioactive metallic element which does not occur naturally in its pure form but is present as various compounds in *uranium* ores, such as pitchblende and carnotite. Radium has four naturally occurring isotopes (varieties of the element that are chemically identical but differ in some physical properties). In order of decreasing abundance they are radium 226, radium 228, radium 224, and radium 223. Artificial radium isotopes have also been produced.

The most important isotope is radium 226, which is produced by the decay of naturally radioactive elements of the uranium series. It is relatively long-lived (with a *half-life* of about 1,600 years), and itself decays to form the gas *radon*, which then decays further to form other, solid, radioactive decay products. During these decay stages, *radiation* is emitted in the form of alpha and beta particles and gamma rays. Radium 226 was formerly used to treat tumours but it has now been superseded by other radioisotopes, such as cobalt 60 and caesium 137.

The use of radium in some luminous paints was discontinued after it was discovered that the radium caused leukaemia and bone tumours in those using the paint.

Radius

The shorter of the two long bones of the forearm; the other is the *ulna*. The radius is the bone on the thumb side of the arm.

LOCATION OF THE RADIUS
The radius is the bone on the outside of the forearm with the palm facing forwards, or on the inside with the palm facing backwards.

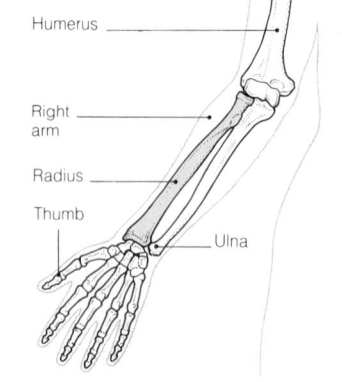

Humerus

Right arm

Radius

Thumb

Ulna

The shaft of the radius has a broad base that articulates with the lower end of the ulna and with the upper bones of the wrist. The disc-shaped head of the radius, which is smaller than the base, articulates with the lower end of the *humerus* (the bone of the upper arm) to form part of the elbow joint.

The radius takes most of the strain when weight is placed on the wrist and is a common site of fractures (see *Radius, fracture of; Colles' fracture*). A fall or blow may sometimes cause dislocation of the radius from the elbow joint along with fracture of the ulna, a condition that is known as *Monteggia's fracture*.

Radius, fracture of

A common type of fracture that may affect the lower end, upper end, or shaft of the *radius* (the shorter of the two long bones in the forearm).

Fracture of the radius just above the wrist is the most common of all fractures in people over 40. It is usually caused by falling on the palm of an outstretched hand, resulting in backward displacement of the wrist and hand (see *Colles' fracture*).

Fracture of the disc-shaped head of the bone just below the elbow joint is one of the most common fractures in young adults. Treatment in such cases consists of removing any blood clot via a syringe and then immobilizing the forearm (bent at a right angle to the upper arm) and the elbow in a plaster *cast* to allow the fracture to heal. If the head of the bone is crushed or splintered, it may need to be removed surgically before the cast is applied. Early movement of the healing arm should be encouraged.

Fracture of the shaft of the radius often results in displacement of the bone ends. An operation is usually required to reposition the bone ends and fix them together with wires or plates and screws. In some cases, however, the bones can be externally manipulated back into position. Once the bones have been repositioned, the limb is immobilized by the use of a plaster cast.

Radon

A colourless, odourless, tasteless, radioactive gaseous element produced by the radioactive decay of *radium*. Radon has three naturally occurring isotopes (varieties of the element that are chemically identical but differ in some physical properties)—radon 219, radon 220, and radon 222.

R

Each of these is short-lived (radon 219 has a *half-life* of about four seconds, radon 220 of about 51 seconds, and radon 222 of about 3.8 days). These isotopes disintegrate—with the emission of *radiation* (in the form of alpha particles)—to form solid radioactive materials known as radon daughters, which themselves emit alpha and beta particles and gamma rays. In addition to radon's naturally occurring radioisotopes, more than a dozen artificial ones have been produced.

The parent sources of radon occur naturally in many materials, such as soil, rocks, and building materials, and the gas is continually released into the atmosphere. As a result, radon makes the largest single contribution (about 32 per cent) to the total radiation exposure of the UK population. This fact has led some researchers to suggest that radon may be a significant causative factor in some cases of cancer (particularly lung cancer). However, this claim has not been demonstrated in the general population. Workers in certain specialized mining industries, such as uranium, fluorspar, and haematite mining (in which radon gas is encountered) have an increased risk of lung cancer.

Ranitidine

An *ulcer-healing drug* belonging to the H_2-receptor antagonist group. It is used to prevent and treat *peptic ulcers* and to treat *oesophagitis*. Possible side-effects include headache, skin rash, nausea, constipation, and lethargy.

Ranula

A cyst in the floor of the mouth which produces a translucent bluish swelling. Ranulas probably arise from damaged *salivary glands*. Treatment is by surgical removal.

Rape

Sexual intercourse with an unwilling partner, which is achieved by the use or the threat of force or violence and against the victim's will, or without the victim's consent. Rape is a criminal offence.

Society, the police, and the courts have in the last decade attempted to do more for rape victims and there is today a greater understanding of the traumatic effects that the crime can have on the victim. Studies have clarified the nature of rape, revealing that, contrary to popular belief, the act most often occurs between people who know each other, is not always accompanied by physical violence, and is not provoked by the victim.

INCIDENCE

Recent years have seen a considerable increase in reported rape cases (see graph). It is difficult to know whether these figures reflect a genuine increase in incidence or a greater willingness on the part of victims to report the crime. Nevertheless, rape is still one of the least reported of all crimes. It is estimated that the majority of rapes are unreported due to the victim's shame, fear of being disbelieved, fear of family rejection, fear of reprisal by the rapist, or fear of the publicity and trauma associated with going through a trial.

MOTIVES

Rape is a violent crime motivated by a need to dominate the victim. The rapist may use forcible sex as one of many forms of abusive, dehumanizing behaviour, being motivated by a profound hostility towards women.

Rape is rarely sexually motivated; it is a crime of dominance, anger and hostility, rather than a crime of passion. There is evidence of a link between alcohol abuse and rape.

About 20 per cent of rapists are reconvicted of sexual offences; up to 80 per cent subsequently commit other crimes and may have a long history of violent crime.

EFFECTS

The rape victim may suffer a variety of physical injuries, usually as a result of beating or choking. Severe injury to the genitals is rare, but there may also be swelling of the labia, bruising of the vaginal walls or cervix, and, occasionally, tearing of the anus or the perineum (the area between the genitals and the anus).

Even in the absence of physical injury, the psychological effects of rape are often severe, including significant *anxiety*, *depression*, or *post-traumatic stress disorder*. Nightmares or daytime flashbacks of the event may also occur.

FORENSIC TESTS

The doctor examining a rape victim performs a physical examination, noting signs of bruising or injury, particularly to the genital area. The examination includes visual inspection of the vaginal canal. A woman is usually present to support the victim.

For laboratory analysis, the doctor collects swabs from any suspected bite marks, from soiled areas of the body, and from the vagina, anus, or throat; fingernail scrapings or clippings; and any torn-out strands of hair from the head or pubic region. Such specimens allow comparisons to be made with samples taken from suspects.

Clothing worn by the victim at the time of the assault is also retained for forensic examination.

TREATMENT

Physical injuries are treated as required. Postcoital contraception (see *Contraception, postcoital*) may be prescribed but, if conception results from the rape, induced *abortion* may be considered. Treatment for *sexually transmitted disease* may be required in some cases.

In the treatment of psychological trauma, rape crisis counselling can be highly beneficial. In some cases, psychiatric support may also be needed. Many victims are now helped by rape support groups organized locally by the social work department of community hospitals.

Rash

A group of spots or an area of red, inflamed skin. A rash is usually temporary and only rarely is a sign of a serious underlying problem. It may be accompanied by itching or fever.

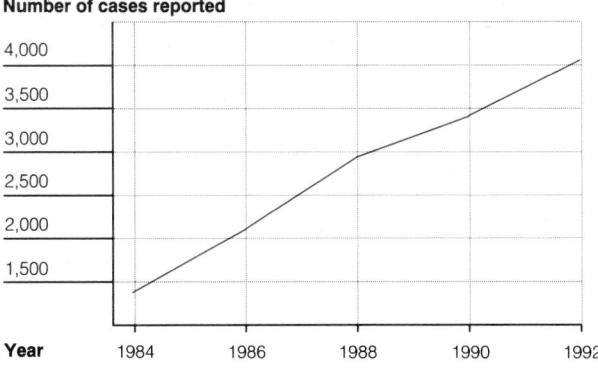

INCIDENCE OF REPORTED RAPE IN ENGLAND AND WALES

Number of cases reported

The graph shows the big increase in rapes reported in England and Wales since 1984. It is difficult to know whether the figures reflect a genuine increase in the incidence of rape or a greater willingness on the part of the victims to report the crime.

RASH WITH FEVER Spots, discoloured areas, or blisters on the skin combined with a temperature of 38°C or above. The most likely cause is one of the childhood infectious diseases.

? Do you have raised, red and itchy spots that turn into blisters?

YES → Chickenpox, a childhood infectious disease caused by the virus that causes herpes zoster, is the likely cause of such symptoms. The rash usually starts on the face and trunk, but may spread to the limbs. Consult your doctor.

See • Chickenpox

NO

? Do you have a rash of dull red spots or blotches?

YES → Do you have two or more of the following symptoms?
• runny nose
• cough
• sore, red eyes

YES → You may have measles, especially if the rash is mainly on your face or trunk and if you did not have the infection as a child. Consult your doctor.

See • Measles

NO

NO

? Do you have a rash of pink spots and is there a tender swelling down the back and sides of your neck?

YES → German measles is possible, especially if you have not already had the disease or been vaccinated against it. Consult your doctor.

See • Rubella

NO

? Do you have a rash of purple spots?

YES → Do you have two or more of the following symptoms?
• vomiting
• headache
• dislike of strong light
• pain when trying to bend your head forward

YES → ☎ **EMERGENCY!**
GET MEDICAL HELP NOW!
Meningitis, inflammation of the membranes surrounding the brain due to viral or bacterial infection, may be the cause of such symptoms.

See • Meningitis

NO

NO → ☎
Call your doctor without delay!
You may have a bleeding disorder caused by infection or by an allergy to a food or drug.

See • Purpura

If you are unable to make a diagnosis from this chart, consult your doctor.

R

RASH WITH ITCHING   Itchy spots or discoloured and/or raised areas of itchy skin.

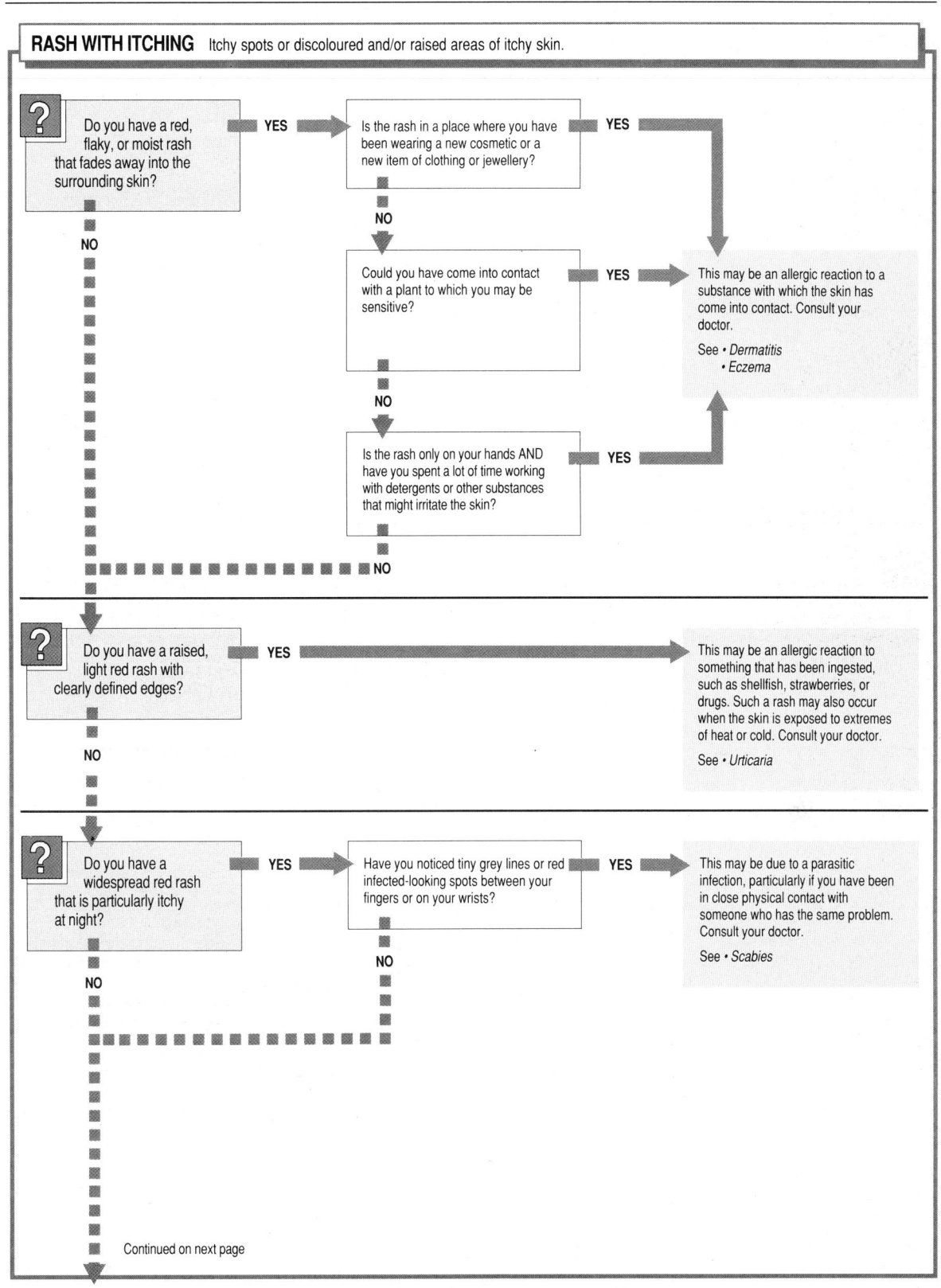

Do you have a red, flaky, or moist rash that fades away into the surrounding skin?

YES → **Is the rash in a place where you have been wearing a new cosmetic or a new item of clothing or jewellery?**

YES →

NO ↓

Could you have come into contact with a plant to which you may be sensitive?

YES →

This may be an allergic reaction to a substance with which the skin has come into contact. Consult your doctor.

See • *Dermatitis*
    • *Eczema*

NO ↓

Is the rash only on your hands AND have you spent a lot of time working with detergents or other substances that might irritate the skin?

YES →

NO

NO ↓

Do you have a raised, light red rash with clearly defined edges?

YES →

This may be an allergic reaction to something that has been ingested, such as shellfish, strawberries, or drugs. Such a rash may also occur when the skin is exposed to extremes of heat or cold. Consult your doctor.

See • *Urticaria*

NO ↓

Do you have a widespread red rash that is particularly itchy at night?

YES → **Have you noticed tiny grey lines or red infected-looking spots between your fingers or on your wrists?**

YES →

This may be due to a parasitic infection, particularly if you have been in close physical contact with someone who has the same problem. Consult your doctor.

See • *Scabies*

NO ↓

NO ↓

Continued on next page

R

R

Do you have one or more red, scaly patches spreading out in a ring?

YES → This could be a fungal infection.
See • *Tinea*

NO

Do you have one or more raised, red spots in a small area?

YES → You may have been bitten by an insect such as a flea or bedbug.
See • *Insect bites*

NO

If you are unable to make a diagnosis from this chart, consult your doctor.

TYPES

A rash may be localized (affecting only a small area of the skin) or generalized (covering the entire body). Doctors also describe rashes according to the type of spots present.

A blistering rash may be either bullous, consisting of large blisters, or vesicular, consisting of small blisters. A pustular rash is made up of pus-filled blisters.

A macular rash consists of spots that are level with the surrounding skin and discernible from it only by a difference in colour or texture.

Nodular and papular rashes are composed of small, raised bumps, which may or may not be the same colour as the surrounding skin.

CAUSES

A rash is the main sign of many childhood infectious diseases (such as *chickenpox* and *scarlet fever*) and of many other infections, ranging from ringworm (see *Tinea*) to *typhus*.

Rashes are a feature of many *skin disorders*, such as *eczema* and *psoriasis*. A rash may also indicate an underlying medical problem. Examples of such rashes include the purple-red spots characteristic of *purpura* (a bleeding disorder); the rash of *scurvy* or *pellagra*, caused by vitamin deficiency; and the rashes appearing in systemic *lupus erythematosus* and other *autoimmune disorders*.

The rashes of *urticaria* (nettle rash) or of contact *dermatitis* may be caused by an allergic reaction to something that has been eaten or with which the skin has come in contact. Drug reactions, particularly to *antibiotic drugs* and *barbiturate drugs*, are also a common cause of rash.

DIAGNOSIS AND TREATMENT

The doctor makes a diagnosis based on the appearance and distribution of the rash, the presence of any accompanying symptoms, and the possibility of allergy (e.g. to drugs).

Any underlying cause is treated if possible. An itching rash may be relieved by a soothing lotion, such as *calamine*, or an *antihistamine drug*.

RAST

An abbreviation for radioallergosorbent test. RAST is a type of radioimmunoassay and is used to detect antibodies to specific allergens. (See *Immunoassay*.)

Rats, diseases from

Rats are shy but potentially aggressive rodents that live close to human habitation; in many cities they outnumber humans. Rats damage and contaminate crops and food stores and can spread disease.

Various microorganisms harboured by rats can cause illness if spread to people. The organisms responsible for *plague* and one type of *typhus* are transmitted to humans by the bites of rat fleas. *Leptospirosis* (Weil's disease) is caused by contact with anything contaminated by rat's urine.

Rat-bite fever is a rare infection, transmitted directly by a rat bite. Either of two types of bacterium may be responsible. Symptoms may include inflammation at the site of the bite and affecting nearby lymph nodes and vessels, bouts of fever, a rash, and, in one type, painful joint inflammation. Antibiotic drugs are effective in treating either type of infection.

Rabies can be transmitted by the bites of infected rats in some parts of the world. *Lassa fever*, another dangerous viral disease, may be contracted from the urine of infected rats in West Africa. Other diseases that can also be transmitted by infected rats in some areas are the viral infection lymphocytic chorio-meningitis, and the bacterial infection *tularaemia*.

Effective control of urban rat populations is important in the prevention of rat-borne epidemic diseases.

Raynaud's disease

A disorder of the blood vessels in which exposure to cold causes the small arteries that supply the fingers and toes to contract suddenly. This action cuts off blood flow to the digits, which become pale. The fingers, usually on both hands, are more often affected than the toes. Young women are the most commonly affected.

When the symptoms develop with no known cause, the disorder is called Raynaud's disease. When symptoms are secondary to some other condition, the disorder is termed *Raynaud's phenomenon*, and there may be more serious long-term consequences.

SYMPTOMS AND SIGNS

On exposure to cold, the digits turn white because of lack of blood. As sluggish blood flow returns, the digits become blue; when they are warmed and normal blood flow is re-established, they turn red. During an attack, there is often a feeling of tingling, numbness, or burning in the affected fingers or toes.

In rare cases, the walls of the arteries gradually thicken, permanently reducing blood flow and eventually leading to painful ulceration or even to *gangrene* (tissue death) at the tips of the affected digits.

DIAGNOSIS AND TREATMENT

The condition is diagnosed from the patient's history. A person with Raynaud's disease should keep the hands and feet as warm as possible. Cigarette smokers should stop smoking because smoking further constricts the arteries. *Vasodilator drugs* may be prescribed to relax the walls of the blood vessels. *Sympathectomy* (an operation in which the nerves that control the diameter of the arteries are cut) has been tried in severe cases.

Raynaud's phenomenon
A circulatory disorder affecting the fingers and toes that shares the mechanism, symptoms, and signs of *Raynaud's disease* but results from a known underlying disorder.

Possible causes of Raynaud's phenomenon include arterial diseases (such as *Buerger's disease, atherosclero-* *sis, embolism,* and *thrombosis*); connective tissue diseases (such as *rheumatoid arthritis, scleroderma,* and systemic *lupus erythematosus*); and various drugs (such as *ergotamine, methysergide,* and *beta-blocker drugs*). Raynaud's phenomenon is a recognized occupational disorder of people who use pneumatic drills, chain saws, or other vibrating machinery; it is sometimes seen in typists, pianists, and others whose fingers suffer repeated trauma.

Treatment is the same as for Raynaud's disease, along with treatment of the underlying disorder.

Reagent
A general term for any chemical substance that takes part in a chemical reaction. The term usually refers to a chemical (or mixture of chemicals) used in chemical analysis or employed to detect a biological substance.

Receding chin
Underdevelopment of the lower *jaw*. The condition can be corrected by facio-maxillary *cosmetic surgery* in one of three ways—lengthening each side of the jaw by inserting a wedge of bone into it, increasing the bulk of the bone at the front of the chin by a bone graft, or implanting a plastic bone substitute at the front of the chin.

Receptor
A general term for any sensory nerve cell—that is, one that converts stimuli into nerve impulses (see illustrated box below).

TYPES OF RECEPTOR
Stimuli are detected by the free endings of sensory nerve cells or by special structures forming the endings of these cells. These respond to specific stimuli (such as light of a certain wavelength) and send a signal indicating the presence of the stimulus to the spinal cord and/or the brain.

Cell surface or chemical receptors (right) are tiny structures on the outer surface of a cell. They allow certain chemicals to bind to the cell and trigger some change within it.

HOW CELL SURFACE OR CHEMICAL RECEPTORS WORK
Most cells have many surface receptors (only one is shown below). Their existence allows the activity of the cell to be influenced from outside.

Skin receptors
The skin contains many types of receptor that respond to stimuli such as pressure, cold, heat, and hair movement, allowing the sensations of touch, temperature, and pain. They include such structures as pacinian corpuscles and Merkel's discs and are all special types of nerve cell ending.

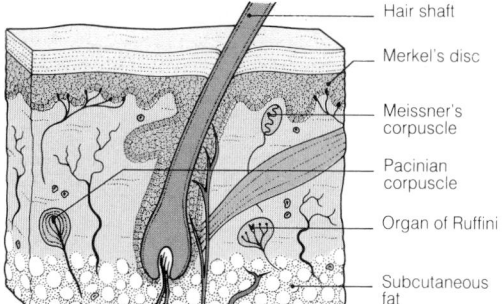

Hair shaft
Merkel's disc
Meissner's corpuscle
Pacinian corpuscle
Organ of Ruffini
Subcutaneous fat

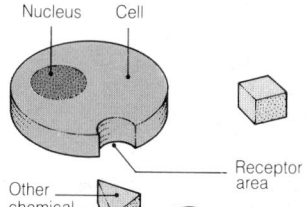

Nucleus   Cell
Other chemical
Receptor area
Hormone molecule

1 A receptor allows only one specific chemical—which may be a hormone or a neurotransmitter substance—to bind to it. The chemical must have a configuration that "fits" the receptor.

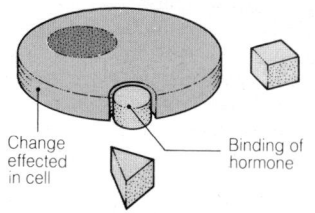

Change effected in cell
Binding of hormone

2 The binding of chemical to receptor alters the outer cell membrane and triggers a change—such as contraction by a muscle cell or increased activity in an enzyme-producing cell.

Receptors in tongue
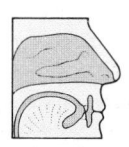
Each taste-bud (below) consists of many receptor cells. Each has surface receptors that respond to chemicals in food.

Receptors in eye
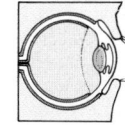
The retina, located at the back of the eye, contains receptor cells, called rods and cones, which are responsive to light.

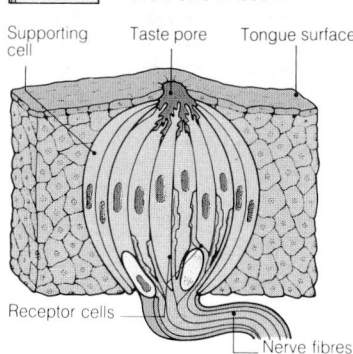

Supporting cell
Taste pore   Tongue surface
Receptor cells
Nerve fibres

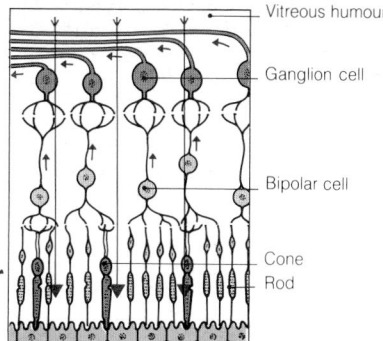

Vitreous humour
Ganglion cell
Bipolar cell
Cone
Rod

R

RECOMBINANT DNA AND GENETICALLY ENGINEERED INSULIN

Genetic engineering can force bacteria to produce human insulin. The insulin gene is obtained (by removing it from human DNA, then purifying it) and spliced into the DNA of a bacterium, causing it to produce human insulin. The bacterium is then cultured for large-scale insulin extraction.

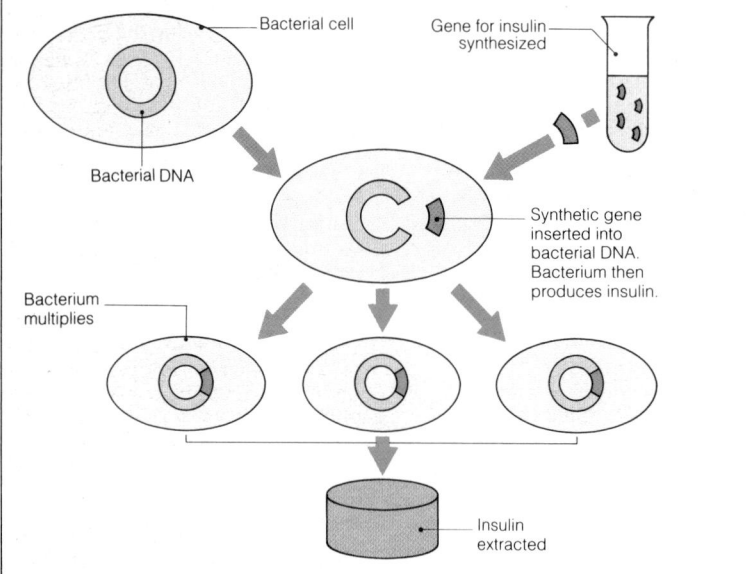

Bacterial cell

Gene for insulin synthesized

Bacterial DNA

Synthetic gene inserted into bacterial DNA. Bacterium then produces insulin.

Bacterium multiplies

Insulin extracted

The term receptor is also used to refer to a specific area on the surface of a cell with a characteristic chemical and physical structure. Many of the natural body chemicals must bind to receptors on cells in order to exert their effects. For example, the hormone adrenaline binds to three different types of receptors (called alpha-, $beta_1$-, and $beta_2$-receptors) which are found on the cells of organs such as the heart and lungs.

Recombinant DNA

A section of *DNA* (genetic material) from one organism that has been artificially spliced into the existing DNA of another organism, often a viral or bacterial cell.

An example of the use of recombinant DNA is the addition of a DNA section containing the genetic code for a hormone such as insulin. If the recipient cell can be encouraged to replicate, large amounts of the hormone can be obtained. (See also *Genetic engineering*.)

Reconstructive surgery

See *Arterial reconstructive surgery*; *Plastic surgery*.

Recovery position

The correct position in which to place a casualty who is breathing while awaiting the arrival of medical help (see accompanying first-aid box).

Rectal bleeding

The passage of blood from the *rectum* or *anus*. Such blood may originate in the rectum or anus, or may come from higher in the gastrointestinal tract. The blood may be mixed with faeces, on the surface of faeces, or passed separately. Blood passed in this way may range in colour from bright red to dark brown or black. The passage of blood may or may not be accompanied by pain. Rectal bleeding requires investigation by a doctor.

CAUSES
The type of bleeding often gives a clue to its origin. *Haemorrhoids* are the most common cause of rectal bleeding in the form of small amounts of bright red blood found on the surface of the faeces or on toilet paper. *Anal fissure, anal fistula, proctitis,* or *rectal prolapse* may also cause this type of bleeding.

Some disorders of the colon, such as *diverticular disease*, may cause dark red faeces. Cancer of the colon (see *Colon,*

cancer of), cancer of the rectum (see *Rectum, cancer of*), or polyps can also cause bleeding. Bloody diarrhoea may be due to *ulcerative colitis, amoebiasis,* or *shigellosis.*

Bleeding high in the digestive tract, usually from a *peptic ulcer,* may cause *melaena* (black, tarry faeces).

DIAGNOSIS
The doctor may be able to make a diagnosis from a *rectal examination. Proctoscopy, sigmoidoscopy, colonoscopy,* and air-contrast *barium X-ray examination* may also be performed.

Rectal examination

Examination of the *anus* and *rectum,* performed to assess symptoms and to check for the presence of tumours of the rectum or *prostate gland.*

A rectal examination is performed as a part of a general *physical examination,* or when a person reports abdominal pain, pelvic pain, or a change in bowel habits. A rectal examination may also be performed if a man complains of urological symptoms and, sometimes (in addition to a pelvic examination), if a woman has gynaecological problems.

The patient usually lies on his or her left side, with the knees bent towards the chest. The doctor inserts a gloved, lubricated finger into the rectum to feel for any tenderness or abnormalities, such as ulcers or growths, and to examine the prostate or cervix, which can be felt through the rectum.

Rectal prolapse

Protrusion outside the *anus* of the lining of the *rectum,* usually brought on by straining to defaecate. The condition causes discomfort, a discharge of mucus, and rectal bleeding.

In infants and young children, prolapse is usually temporary. In elderly people it tends to be permanent because of weakening of the tissues that support the *perineum* (the area between the anus and the external genitals). Rectal prolapse may occur with prolapsing *haemorrhoids.* If the rectal prolapse is large, leakage of faeces may occur.

In younger people, a fibre-rich diet may be all that is necessary to cure the condition. Surgery is sometimes performed, and especially on older people; the operation is not always successful, however.

Rectocele

A bulging inwards and downwards of the back wall of the *vagina* as the *rectum* pushes against weakened tissues

FIRST AID: THE RECOVERY POSITION

DO NOT:
- Leave an unconscious victim by himself or herself.
- Put the victim into the recovery position if you suspect fractures to the neck or spine.

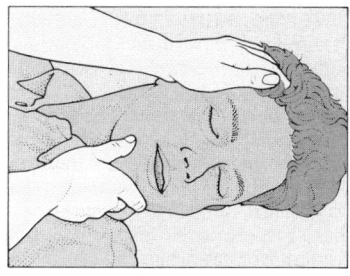

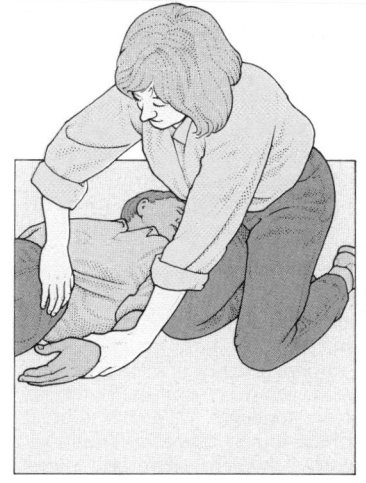

1 Turn the victim's head towards you, tilting it back, to open the airway.

2 Put the arm nearest you by the victim's side and slide it under his or her buttock.

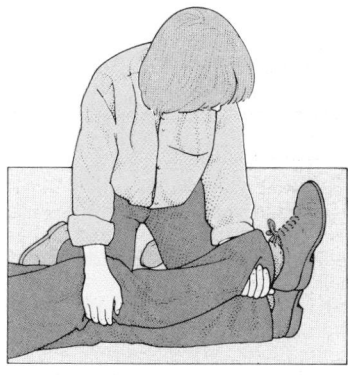

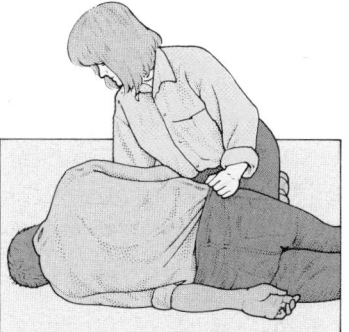

3 Lay the other arm across the chest and cross the leg farthest from you over the near one at the ankle.

4 Grasp clothing at the hip farthest from you with one hand and support the head with the other. Pull the victim towards you to rest against your knees.

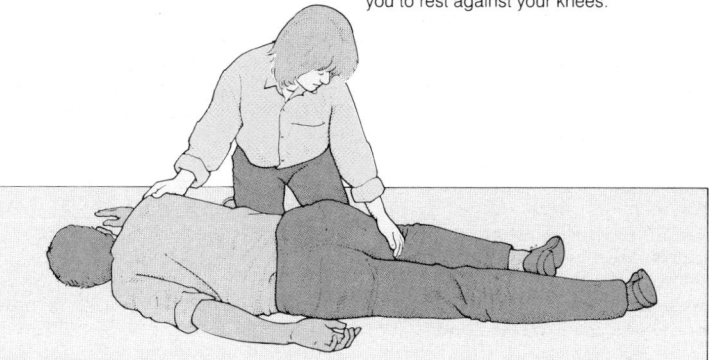

5 Bend the uppermost arm and leg to support the body and stop the victim from rolling on to his or her face. The other arm should now be free. Readjust the head to make sure it is tilted well back and check to see if the airway is clear.

in the vaginal wall. A rectocele is usually associated with a *cystocele* (protrusion of the bladder into the front wall of the vagina) or prolapsed uterus (see *Uterus, prolapse of*).

Depending on its size, a rectocele may cause no symptoms or may lead to constipation by interfering with muscle contraction in the rectum.

Exercises to strengthen the muscles of the pelvic floor may help relieve symptoms (see *Pelvic floor exercises*). If they do not, an operation may be recommended to tighten the tissues at the back of the vagina to improve support for the rectum.

Rectum
A short, muscular tube that forms the lowest part of the large intestine and connects it to the *anus*.

STRUCTURE
Like all of the colon, the very first part of the rectum consists of four layers—the outermost serous layer; the muscular layer; the submucous layer; and the innermost mucous layer, which lubricates the rectum. There is no serous layer in the last 8 to 10 cm of the rectum.

FUNCTION
The rectum collects faeces that have formed in the alimentary tract. Pressure on the wall of the rectum causes nerve impulses to pass to the brain; the urge to defaecate occurs when faeces distend (stretch) the rectum, although defaecation may be voluntarily delayed.

DISORDERS
In rare cases, a baby is born with no rectum or anus (see *Anus, imperforate*).

The rectum may also be affected by various diseases and disorders. These include inflammation (see *Proctitis*), *polyps* (grape-like growths), familial *polyposis* (a condition characterized by numerous polyps that usually become cancerous), and cancer (see *Rectum, cancer of*).

The rectum can become obstructed as a result of narrowing caused by *radiotherapy*, by *granuloma inguinale* (a sexually transmitted disease), or by a pelvic infection. In rare instances, an ulcer develops in the rectum, causing bleeding and discharge. Bleeding and discharge may also result from injury to the rectum caused by anal intercourse or the insertion of foreign objects into the rectum.

Rectal prolapse occurs when the lining of the rectum protrudes outside the anus. In a *rectocele*, the rectum and rear wall of the vagina bulge downwards into the vagina.

R

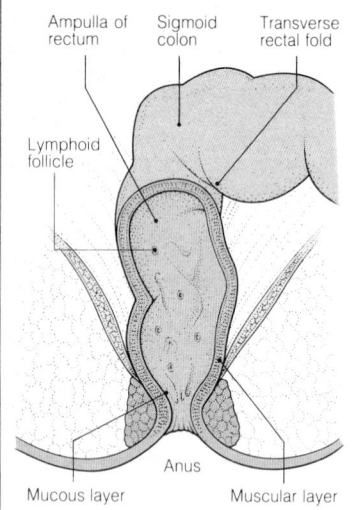

STRUCTURE OF THE RECTUM
The rectum is about 12 cm long; its wall consists mainly of longitudinal and circular muscle. An inner, mucous layer provides lubrication.

Ampulla of rectum

Sigmoid colon

Transverse rectal fold

Lymphoid follicle

Anus

Mucous layer

Muscular layer

Rectal disorders are usually diagnosed by physical examination (see *Rectal examination*) and by examination with a viewing instrument (see *Proctoscopy; Sigmoidoscopy*).

Rectum, cancer of
A malignant tumour in the muscular tube that forms the last part of the large intestine.

CAUSES AND INCIDENCE
The cause of cancer of the *rectum* is unknown, but dietary factors and genetic factors are thought to play a part in its development, as in cancer of the colon (see *Colon, cancer of*). Certain diseases of the colon (e.g. familial *polyposis* and *ulcerative colitis*) increase the risk of colorectal cancer (cancer of the colon and/or rectum).

Colorectal cancer is responsible for about 12 per cent of all cancer deaths in the UK. Rectal cancer accounts for between one quarter and one third of tumours of the large intestine; it is more common in people who are between the ages of 50 and 70.

SYMPTOMS
The earliest symptom may be *rectal bleeding* during defaecation. There may also be a change in bowel habits—diarrhoea or constipation—and a sensation of incomplete emptying of the bowel. Later, pain may

occur. Untreated, the cancer eventually may cause severe bleeding and pain and block the intestine, preventing the passage of faeces. It may also spread to other organs in the pelvis and to other sites, such as the liver.

DIAGNOSIS
A doctor can often detect rectal cancer by a *rectal examination*. The diagnosis is confirmed by *proctoscopy* or *sigmoidoscopy* (examination of the rectum with a rigid or flexible viewing instrument) and *biopsy* (removal of a sample of tissue for microscopic analysis).

TREATMENT
In most cases surgery is performed. If the tumour is in the uppermost part of the rectum, the abdomen is opened, the upper rectum and descending colon are removed, and the two ends are sewn together. To promote healing of the joined bowel, a temporary *colostomy* (which diverts faeces through a surgical opening in the abdomen) may be performed.

If the growth is in the lower rectum, the surgeon performs an operation called an abdomino-perineal resection, in which the abdomen is opened, the colon is cut through above the rectum, an incision is made around the anus, and the entire rectum and anus are removed. The wound is closed and, because there is no longer any outlet for the faeces, a permanent colostomy is created.

Patients who have undergone surgery are examined at regular intervals to ensure that the tumour has not reappeared or spread to other parts of the body.

In elderly or debilitated people unable to undergo major surgery, *diathermy* (the application of high-frequency electric current) may be used to destroy the surface of the tumour and control local symptoms. Other forms of treatment when surgery is not possible are *radiotherapy* and, less often, *anticancer drugs*.

OUTLOOK
The long-term outlook for patients with cancer of the rectum depends on how far the tumour has spread before treatment takes place. About 50 per cent of all people operated on for rectal cancer are alive three years later and almost 40 per cent 10 years later. Survival rates are considerably higher when the disease is treated early.

Red-eye
Another name for *conjunctivitis*.

Reducing
See *Weight reduction*.

Reduction
The process of manipulating a displaced part of the body back to its original position. Reduction may be carried out to realign fractured bone ends (see *Fracture*), to replace a dislocated joint in its socket (see *Dislocation, joint*), or to treat an abdominal *hernia* by pushing the protruding intestine back through the abdominal wall.

Referred pain
Pain felt in a part of the body at some distance from its cause. Referred pain occurs because some apparently remote parts of the body are served by the same nerve or the same nerve root (group of nerves that joins the spinal cord at one point). Nerve impulses that reach the brain from one of these areas may be misinterpreted as coming from another.

Common examples of referred pain are the pain down the inside of the left arm caused by *angina pectoris* or *myocardial infarction*; the pain felt in the tip of the shoulder from irritation of the diaphragm; the pain felt in a testis when the ureter is stretched by a urinary tract *calculus*; and the pain felt in the leg or foot from compression in the spine by a *disc prolapse*.

Reflex
An action that occurs automatically and predictably in response to a particular stimulus, independent of the will of the individual. Both the sensing of the stimulus and initiation of the action are carried out by components of the *nervous system*.

In the simplest reflex, a sensory nerve cell, perhaps at the skin surface, reacts to a stimulus such as heat or pressure. The sensory cell sends a signal along its nerve fibre to the central nervous system (brain and spinal cord). There, the end of the fibre connects to another nerve cell, which becomes stimulated in turn. Activity in this second cell then causes a muscle to contract or a gland to increase its secretory activity. The passage of the nerve signal from original sensation to final action is called a reflex arc.

Sometimes the reflex is more complicated. Sensory signals may be sent from thousands of sensory receptors to groups of nerve cells within the central nervous system. Complex analysis of these signals may be carried out before responses are initiated.

INBORN REFLEXES
Many reflexes are inborn, including those that control basic body func-

R

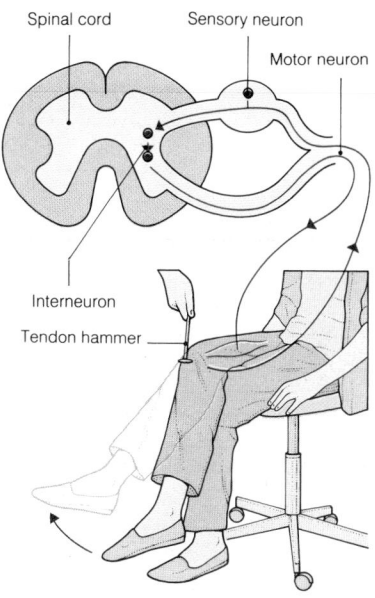

Spinal cord

Sensory neuron

Motor neuron

Interneuron

Tendon hammer

Simple knee-jerk reflex
A tap with a rubber hammer just below the kneecap stretches a tendon of one of the thigh muscles. A signal passes via a sensory neuron (nerve cell) to the spinal cord, activating a motor neuron, which contracts the muscle, jerking the lower leg upwards.

tions. Examples include shivering automatically in response to cold, increased breathing in response to a rise in carbon dioxide in the blood, and contraction of the bladder to expel urine after it has filled beyond a certain point. The part of the nervous system concerned with these processes is called the *autonomic nervous system*. Parts of the *brainstem* and the *hypothalamus* in the forebrain are processing centres for the autonomic nervous system. Some autonomic system reflexes are under partial voluntary (willed) control—emptying of the bladder can be voluntarily delayed for example. Ultimately, however, reflex is stronger than will.

Some inborn reflexes occur only in babies (see *Reflex, primitive*). An example is the grasp reflex when an adult's finger is placed in the palm.

A physical examination usually includes testing several simple, inborn reflexes, such as the knee-jerk, plantar reflex (curling of the toes in response to irritation of the sole of the foot), and constriction of the pupil in response to light. Changes in these reflexes may indicate damage to the nervous system. A full neurological examination also includes the testing of various other reflexes.

The examination of vital reflexes controlled by the brainstem is the basis for diagnosing *brain death*.

CONDITIONED REFLEXES
Reflexes that are acquired as a result of experience rather than being inborn are called conditioned reflexes. They result from the formation of new pathways and connections within the nervous system during life. The process by which these reflexes are acquired is called *conditioning*. One type, operant conditioning, is a particularly important process in *learning*. Once a satisfactory response to a new situation has been discovered (often by a process of trial and error) and repeated several times, it is eventually automatically elicited by that situation or stimulus and thus becomes a sort of reflex. For example, a person walking home from work may follow a familiar route without needing to make any conscious effort to do so.

Reflexology

A form of *alternative medicine* in which the practitioner massages parts of the patient's feet in an attempt to cure disorders affecting other parts of the body.

Reflex, primitive

An automatic movement in response to a stimulus that is present in newborn infants but disappears during the first few months after birth. Primitive reflexes are believed to represent actions that may have been important for survival in earlier stages of human evolution.

Because some of these reflexes can give an indication of the condition of an infant's *nervous system*, they are tested by the paediatrician (a specialist in diseases of children) at the first examinations after birth. Any abnormality of the primitive reflexes may indicate a disorder of the nervous system. Their persistence beyond the expected stage of development may likewise point to a disorder of the developing brain.

The main primitive reflexes are the grasp reflex, the Moro reflex, the tonic neck reflex, the walking or stepping reflex, and the rooting reflex (see illustrated box overleaf).

Reflux

An abnormal backflow of fluid in a body passage due to failure of the passage's exit to close fully. The most common types of reflux are regurgitation of acid fluid from the stomach

into the oesophagus (see *Acid reflux*) and the backflow of urine from the bladder into one or both ureters (vesico-ureteric reflux). Persistent reflux of urine may lead to kidney damage (see *Nephropathy*).

Refraction

The bending of light-rays as they pass from one substance to another. In the *eye*, refraction provides the mechanism by which an image is focused on the retina, thereby permitting *vision*. The term is also used to describe the testing of the eye to determine whether there is any refractive error, such as *myopia, hypermetropia*, or *astigmatism* (see *Vision tests*).

Regenerative cell therapy

A treatment that claims to revitalize the skin. One technique involves the injection of preparations made from a mixture of animals' endocrine glands. Similar claims concerning revitalization have been made for skin creams containing sex hormones or animals' placentas. There is no evidence that any of these treatments works.

Regression

A term used in *psychoanalytic theory* to describe the process of returning to a childhood level of behaviour. Sigmund Freud suggested that human beings progress psychologically through various stages of development from infancy to adulthood. Although disturbed adults may be superficially mature, they may be unconsciously fixated at an earlier level of development. When such people are frustrated or under stress, they undergo regression to immature forms of behaviour, such as thumb-sucking or exposing the genitals. (See also *Fixation*.)

Regurgitation

A backflow of fluid. In medicine, the term is commonly used to describe the return of swallowed food or drink from the stomach into the oesophagus and mouth. The term *acid reflux* is used to describe the backflow of acid juices from the stomach. Regurgitation of milk is very common in babies immediately after feeding, when small amounts of milk are brought up with wind.

The term regurgitation is also used medically to describe the backflow of blood through a *heart valve* that does not close fully because of a disorder, such as *mitral incompetence* or *aortic incompetence*. (See also *Reflux*.)

R

TYPES OF PRIMITIVE REFLEX

Grasping reflex

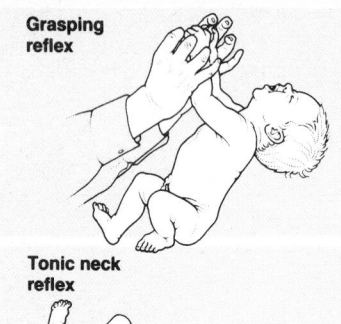

Certain automatic reflexes are present early in life before the baby becomes capable of voluntary movement. These reflexes disappear as the nervous system matures. For about the first four months, any object placed in the infant's palm will be firmly grasped.

Tonic neck reflex

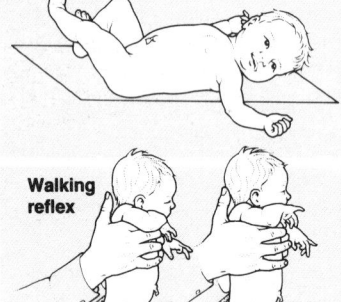

When the young baby turns the head, the arm and leg of that side are stretched out and the arm and leg on the opposite side bend. This reflex normally disappears after the first few months except in premature babies. A strong reflex, persisting for longer than three months, suggests brain damage.

Walking reflex

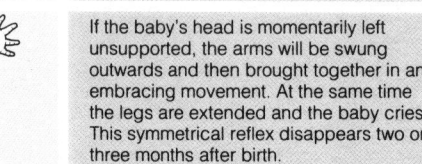

When the baby is held upright with a foot touching the ground, a forward stepping movement is made by each leg as the weight is placed on the other foot. This occurs during the first two months of life and is then lost.

Moro reflex

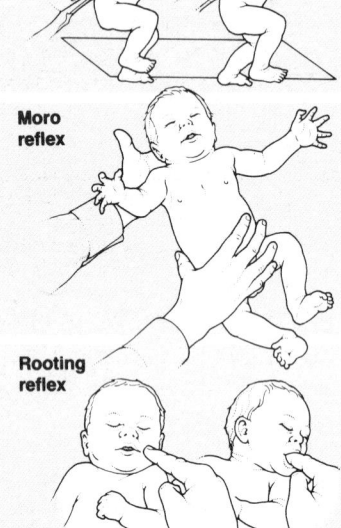

If the baby's head is momentarily left unsupported, the arms will be swung outwards and then brought together in an embracing movement. At the same time the legs are extended and the baby cries. This symmetrical reflex disappears two or three months after birth.

Rooting reflex

This reflex enables the baby to find the nipple. It is evoked by touching the baby's cheek with the fingertip near the corner of the mouth. The head turns so that the finger can enter the mouth. The reflex is best shown if tried near the normal feeding time.

Rehabilitation

Treatment aimed at enabling a person to live an independent life following injury (such as *spinal injury*), illness (such as a *stroke*), *alcohol dependence*, or *drug dependence*. Treatment may include *physiotherapy*, *occupational therapy*, and *psychotherapy*, depending on the problem.

Rehabilitation is often carried out in special centres, some of which are residential. In rehabilitation centres, people from different specialties work together to assess the severity of an individual's *disability* or dependence and develop a tailor-made treatment programme. Industrial rehabilitation centres provide job retraining for people who are unable to return to their previous employment. Drug and alcohol rehabilitation centres help people through the period of withdrawal from the substance they have been addicted to, and also provide psychological support to reduce the risk of relapse.

Rehydration therapy

The treatment of *dehydration* by the administration of fluids and salts by mouth (oral rehydration) or by *intravenous infusion*. The amount of fluid necessary depends both on the person's age and weight, and on the degree of dehydration.

In mild dehydration (which occurs in many young children with *diarrhoea*) rehydration can usually be carried out with solutions given by mouth. Oral rehydration preparations are available commercially in liquid form, or in powder or tablet form to be added to water. The simplest solutions contain only water, sodium chloride, and glucose; others may include potassium and sodium bicarbonate. Any unused solution should be discarded after 24 hours.

If commercial preparations are not available, a home-made oral rehydration solution may be prepared by adding one level teaspoon of salt and eight level teaspoons of sugar to one litre of boiled water (see *ORT*).

In severe dehydration, or if the patient is unable to take fluids by mouth because of nausea or vomiting, an intravenous infusion of saline (sodium chloride) solution, glucose solution, or a combination of both, sometimes supplemented with potassium chloride, may be given in hospital. Additional treatment may be necessary depending on the underlying condition.

Reimplantation, dental

Replacement of a *tooth* in its socket after an accident so that it can become reattached to supporting tissues. Most commonly, it is the front teeth that are involved.

The dentist rinses the tooth in a sterile solution, replaces it in the socket, and maintains it with a splint (see *Splinting, dental*), often for several weeks. Successful reimplantation relies on replacing the tooth soon after the accident (ideally within 30 minutes). The outlook also depends on the age of the patient (the younger the better). Keeping the tooth moist and sterile (e.g. with saliva) also increases the chances of success.

Reiter's syndrome

A condition in which there is a combination of *urethritis*, *arthritis* and *conjunctivitis*. There may also be *uveitis*. Reiter's syndrome is more common in men than in women; it is the most common cause of arthritis in young men.

R

CAUSES AND INCIDENCE

The syndrome usually develops after *nonspecific urethritis*, affecting about two per cent of men with this disorder. It may also occur after an attack of bacillary *dysentery*. Yet although induced by infection, Reiter's syndrome results from an immunological response and usually develops only in people with a genetic predisposition. About 80 per cent of people with the syndrome have the HLA-B27 tissue-type (see *Histocompatibility antigens*).

SYMPTOMS AND SIGNS

Reiter's syndrome usually starts with a urethral discharge followed by conjunctivitis and then arthritis. The arthritis seldom affects more than one or two joints and is often associated with fever and malaise. The affected joints, usually the knee or ankle, are warm, painful, and stiff. Inflammation persists for periods varying from a few days to several months. Tendons and ligaments (especially the Achilles tendon) may become inflamed, as may fibrous tissue in the soles of the feet. Skin rashes are common.

DIAGNOSIS AND TREATMENT

Diagnosis and treatment are based on the symptoms. *Analgesic drugs* and *nonsteroidal anti-inflammatory drugs* relieve pain and inflammation but may have to be taken for a long period. Antibiotic drugs are of no value in treating the arthritis.

OUTLOOK

Relapses occur in about one third of cases, especially after further episodes of nonspecific urethritis.

Rejection

An *immune response* aimed at destroying organisms or substances that the body's adaptive *immune system* recognizes as foreign. Rejection commonly refers to the nonacceptance by the immune system of tissues grafted or of organs transplanted into the body from other sources.

In an attempt to forestall rejection, as close a match as possible is made between the tissues of the donor and the recipient (see *Tissue-typing*). In addition, *immunosuppressant drugs*, such as *azathioprine, corticosteroid drugs*, and *cyclosporin* are given to the recipients of organ transplants to suppress rejection by damping down the activity of the immune system. (See also *Grafting; Transplant surgery*.)

Relapse

The recurrence of a disease after an apparent recovery, or the return of symptoms after a *remission*.

Relapsing fever

An illness caused by infection with spirochaetes (spiral-shaped bacteria) transmitted to humans by ticks or lice and characterized by high fever. Relapsing fever occurs in many parts of the world but not in the UK.

SYMPTOMS AND SIGNS

Relapsing fever starts with a sudden high fever—up to 40°C—accompanied by shivering, headache, muscle pains, nausea, and vomiting. The symptoms persist for three to six days, culminating in a crisis, with a risk of collapse and death. The affected person then apparently recovers but, some seven to 10 days later, suffers another attack. In tick-borne fever, several of these relapses, each progressively milder, are common.

DIAGNOSIS AND TREATMENT

A *blood smear* reveals the presence of the causative spirochaetes. Relapsing fever can be effectively treated with *antibiotic drugs*.

Relaxation techniques

Methods of consciously releasing muscular tension to achieve a state of mental calm. Relaxation techniques can be useful on their own or in conjunction with other forms of therapy.

WHY THEY ARE USED

Relaxation techniques can assist people suffering from *anxiety* symptoms, can help to reduce *hypertension* (high blood pressure), and are a useful means of relieving the stress caused by a busy job or personal problems. They are taught to pregnant women to help them cope with the pain of labour (see *Childbirth, natural*).

TYPES

Active relaxation consists of tensing and then relaxing all the muscles in the body in turn, usually starting with the head and moving down to the feet. Passive relaxation may also be used. This involves clearing the mind of everything else in order to concentrate on a single phrase or sound. Control of the breathing rate (see *Breathing exercises*) is emphasized in both active and passive relaxation techniques. This helps prevent *hyperventilation* (rapid, shallow breathing), which often brings on or worsens anxiety. Taped instructions or *biofeedback training* may help reinforce learning. Once mastered, the techniques can be put into practice in potentially stressful situations.

Traditional methods of concentration, such as *yoga* and *meditation*, employ similar techniques.

Rem

A unit of equivalent absorbed dose of ionizing radiation (see *Radiation* units box). Rem is an acronym for roentgen equivalent man.

Remission

A temporary disappearance or reduction in the severity of the symptoms of a disease, or the period during which this occurs.

Remissions occur in many long-term diseases; the most notable example is *multiple sclerosis*, which typically follows a pattern of alternating remissions and *relapses*. In this disease remissions may initially last for months or even years, but usually become progressively shorter and may eventually become so short as to disappear completely.

Renal

A medical term meaning related to the *kidney*.

Renal biopsy

See *Kidney biopsy*.

Renal cell carcinoma

The most common type of kidney cancer (see *Kidney cancer*).

Renal colic

Spasms of severe pain on one side of the back, usually caused by a kidney stone (see *Calculus, urinary tract*).

The pain of renal colic occurs when kidney stones start to pass down the *ureter*. Stones in the ureter cause a severe pain that extends down to the groin. Sharp intermittent spasms, each usually lasting several minutes, are superimposed on a background of continuous dull pain. There may also be nausea, vomiting, sweating, and blood in the urine.

Renal colic is usually treated with bed rest, plenty of fluids, and injections of an *analgesic drug* (painkiller), such as *pethidine*.

Renal failure

See *Kidney failure*.

Renal transplant

See *Kidney transplant*.

Renal tubular acidosis

A condition in which the kidneys are unable to excrete normal amounts of acid generated by the body's *metabolism* (internal chemistry). In renal tubular acidosis, the blood is more acidic than normal and the urine is less acidic than normal.

R

The cause of renal tubular acidosis is often unknown. Possible causes include kidney damage due to disease, drugs, or a genetic disorder.

Problems that may result from renal tubular acidosis include *osteomalacia* (softening of the bones), kidney stones (see *Calculus, urinary tract*), *nephrocalcinosis* (calcification of the kidney), and hypokalaemia (an abnormally low level of *potassium* in the blood).

Renin

An *enzyme* involved in the regulation of *blood pressure*. When blood pressure falls, the kidneys release renin, which converts an inactive substance called angiotensinogen to the protein *angiotensin* I (also inactive). This protein is then rapidly converted to an active form, angiotensin II, which constricts (narrows) blood vessels and so increases blood pressure. In addition, angiotensin II stimulates the release of the hormone *aldosterone,* which causes the kidneys to retain sodium in the body, thereby helping to increase blood pressure.

Blood pressure can be lowered by drugs that affect the renin-angiotensin system (e.g. *beta-blocker drugs*), which inhibit the production of renin, and *ACE inhibitor drugs* (angiotensin-converting enzyme inhibitor drugs), which interfere with the conversion of angiotensin I to angiotensin II.

Renography

A technique used to measure *kidney* function. Renography is performed quickly and painlessly, and utilizes only a small dose of radiation.

A radioactive substance—either hippuran or pentetic acid—is injected into the bloodstream and passes through the kidney into the urine. Radiation counts are taken continuously during the procedure. The information is recorded graphically as a renogram (a curve of counts per second against time). Both kidneys are examined simultaneously so that a comparison can be made of their function.

Renography is used when obstruction to the passage of urine is suspected. Normally, the radiation count rate increases rapidly for about 30 seconds after injection, rises more slowly for about five minutes, and then decreases as the radioactive substance passes into the bladder. If obstruction is present, the radioactive substance accumulates in the kidney and the count rate continues to rise,

producing a differently shaped renogram. (See also *Kidney imaging.*)

Repetitive strain injury

A type of *overuse injury* affecting keyboard workers and musicians, causing pain and weakness of the wrists and fingers. In the late 1980s and early 1990s, many thousands of people around the world developed symptoms of repetitive strain injury (RSI) and became unable to work. Litigation led to disputes about the proportion of these cases in which there were psychological factors, but the publicity led to improvements in working practices and earlier recognition of the condition. The epidemic showed signs of diminishing by the mid 1990s.

Reproduction, sexual

The process of producing a new generation to continue the existence of a species by the fusion of two cells from different individuals; this is achieved in humans by the fusion of one *sperm* and one *ovum*. This fusion, which is called *fertilization,* is achieved by *sexual intercourse* or *artificial insemination.*

Reproductive system, female

The organs that enable a woman to ovulate (see *Ovulation*), to have *sexual intercourse,* to nourish a fertilized *ovum* until it has developed into a full-grown *fetus,* and to give birth (see *Childbirth*). With the exception of the *vulva* (external genitalia), the female reproductive organs lie within the pelvic cavity.

Ova (eggs) are released at monthly intervals from the *ovaries,* two small egg-shaped glands. The ovaries also secrete female sex hormones (see *Oestrogen hormones*; *Progesterone hormones*), which control the reproductive cycle. Adjacent to each ovary is a *fallopian tube,* which carries ova to the *uterus,* a hollow, pear-shaped organ which is situated between the bladder and the rectum. If, on its journey along the fallopian tube, an ovum is successfully penetrated by a sperm, *fertilization* takes place.

Sperm travel upwards through the *cervix* and uterus on their journey to the fallopian tubes. The cervix projects into the top of the *vagina,* a muscular passage which forms the lower part of the birth canal and receives ejaculated sperm during sexual intercourse. Surrounding and protecting the opening of the vagina are the fleshy folds of the vulva.

The normal functioning of the female reproductive system begins at *puberty* with the onset of *menstruation;* the potential for reproduction ends at the time of the *menopause.*

Reproductive system, male

The organs that enable a man to have *sexual intercourse* and to fertilize ova (eggs) with *sperm.* Sperm and male sex hormones (see *Androgen hormones*) are produced in the *testes,* a pair of ovoid glands suspended in a pouch called the *scrotum.* From each testis, sperm pass into an *epididymis,* a long coiled tube behind the testis, where they

---

FEMALE REPRODUCTIVE SYSTEM

Each month an ovum from one ovary is carried along the fallopian tube. If fertilized, it begins to divide and implants into the lining of the uterus to develop into an embryo. At birth, the baby is forced out via the cervix, the usually narrow passage that forms the neck of the uterus.

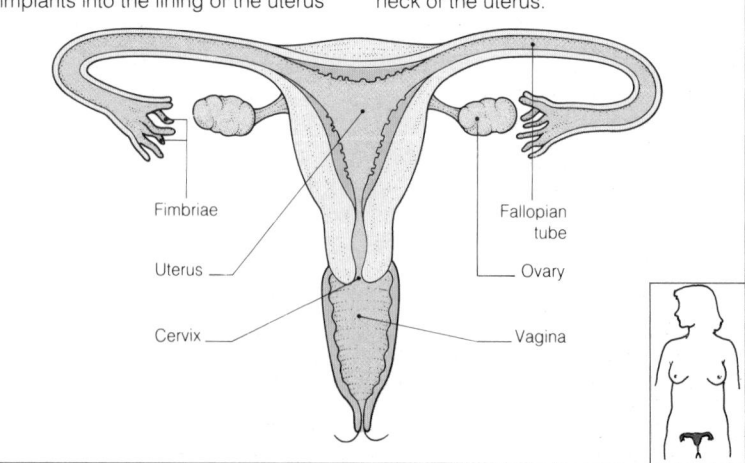

Fimbriae

Uterus

Cervix

Fallopian tube

Ovary

Vagina

R

MALE REPRODUCTIVE SYSTEM

Sperm made in the testis pass via the vas deferens to the seminal vesicle. Secretions from the prostate increase the volume of the semen, which is ejaculated from the penis via the urethra during orgasm.

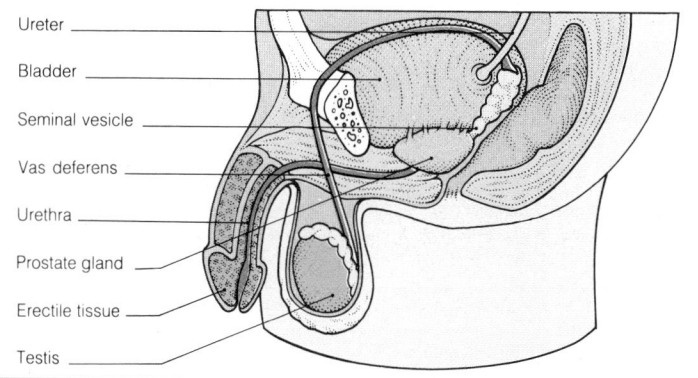

Ureter
Bladder
Seminal vesicle
Vas deferens
Urethra
Prostate gland
Erectile tissue
Testis

slowly mature and are stored. Shortly before *ejaculation,* sperm are propelled from the epididymis into a long duct called the *vas deferens,* which carries the sperm to the seminal vesicles, a pair of sacs that lie behind the bladder. These sacs produce seminal fluid, which is added to the sperm to produce *semen.*

Semen travels from the vesicles along two ducts to the *urethra,* a tube that acts as a passage for urine and for semen. The ducts pass through the *prostate gland,* a chestnut-shaped organ which lies beneath the bladder and surrounds the upper urethra. The prostate produces secretions that are added to the semen.

At *orgasm,* semen is ejaculated from the urethra through the erect *penis,* which during sexual intercourse is placed in the woman's vagina.

Resection

Surgical removal of all or part of a diseased or injured organ or structure. An anterior resection is an operation that removes part of the colon as a treatment for cancer.

Resistance

The ability to oppose. In medical usage, the word resistance has several different meanings.

A resistance to the flow of blood is exerted by the blood vessel walls. This resistance increases as the diameter of blood vessels decreases, whether due to normal physiological processes or to narrowing as a result of disease. An increased resistance leads to a rise in blood pressure.

In *psychoanalysis,* resistance refers to the blocking off from consciousness of repressed material (such as memories or emotions). One task of the psychoanalyst is to help the patient break down this resistance.

Resistance may also refer to an ability to withstand attack from noxious agents (such as poisons, irritants, or microorganisms). A person's resistance to infection is called *immunity.* The degree of immunity varies according to age, nutritional status, general health, the integrity of the person's *immune system,* and previous exposure to infective organisms.

DRUG RESISTANCE

The term drug resistance refers to the ability of some microorganisms to withstand attack from previously effective drugs. Certain bacteria have acquired *genes* (units of hereditary material) that confer protection against specific *antibiotic drugs.* Overuse of these antibiotics encourages the multiplication and spread of the resistant strains, which include some varieties of the organisms responsible for *gonorrhoea, typhoid fever, salmonella* poisoning, *shigellosis* (bacterial dysentery), and other serious infections. Some strains of the parasites that cause *malaria* have become resistant to chloroquine, an important antimalarial drug.

When any dangerous infectious disease can no longer be treated with established remedies, the situation is potentially serious. The development of new drugs has, to date, largely kept pace with the threat. Strategies to prevent the emergence of new resistant strains have included the cyclical use of different antibiotic drugs to treat particular types of infection in hospi-tals. Doctors now try to avoid the indiscriminate prescription of antibiotics, which encourages the emergence of resistance.

Resorption, dental

Loss of substance from *teeth.* Resorption of a tooth may be external (affecting the surface of the root) or internal (affecting the wall of the pulp cavity).

CAUSES AND INCIDENCE

External resorption of tooth roots, which causes the teeth to become loose, is part of the process by which *primary teeth* are shed. It is thought to be activated by pressure from the underlying *permanent teeth* as they erupt (see *Eruption of teeth*).

Some degree of external resorption, affecting the roots, occurs in most adults as part of the aging process. External resorption may also be caused by injury to a tooth, periapical *periodontitis* (inflammation of tissues around the root tip), or pressure from an *orthodontic appliance,* a tumour, or an impacted tooth (see *Impaction, dental*). Completely impacted teeth occasionally undergo resorption of both the crown and the root.

Internal resorption is a rare form of tooth resorption that occurs in about one per cent of adults. The cause is unknown. The condition sometimes spreads outwards from the pulp cavity, producing a pink spot that shows through the crown.

DIAGNOSIS AND TREATMENT

Resorption is usually detected from *dental X-rays.* Treatment of external resorption is of the underlying cause (such as removing an impacted tooth). Internal resorption can usually be successfully halted by *root-canal treatment.*

Respiration

A term for the processes by which oxygen reaches body cells and is utilized by them in *metabolism,* and by which carbon dioxide is eliminated.

The various stages in respiration are described in the illustrated box overleaf. (See also *Respiratory system.*)

Respirator

See *Ventilator.*

Respiratory arrest

Sudden cessation of *breathing.* Respiratory arrest results from any process that severely depresses the function of the respiratory centre in the brain. Causes include prolonged *seizures,* an overdose of *narcotic drugs, cardiac arrest, electrical injury,* serious *head injury, stroke,* or *respiratory failure.*

R

Respiratory arrest leads to *anoxia* (lack of oxygen to tissues) and, if untreated, to cardiac arrest, brain damage, coma, and death. These effects may occur within a few minutes. The victim should be given *artificial respiration* or placed on a *ventilator* without delay. The underlying cause is treated if possible.

Respiratory distress syndrome

A lung disorder that causes difficulty in breathing. Respiratory distress syndrome results in a life-threatening deficiency of oxygen in the blood. The condition affects premature babies (see *Prematurity*) or may occur later in life.

CAUSES AND INCIDENCE

In premature babies, respiratory distress syndrome occurs because the lungs are insufficiently mature to cope with independent breathing. The syndrome occurs because of a deficiency of surfactant, a group of chemicals that normally open or keep open the *alveoli* (tiny air sacs) in the lungs.

In adults, the condition affects people whose lungs have been damaged by disease or injury. The disorder is caused by a stiffening of lung tissue and an increase of fluid in the tissue between the alveoli. The many possible causes include severe *pneumonia*; inhalation of vomit, an irritant gas (such as smoke or chlorine), or a high concentration of oxygen; partial *drowning*; an overdose of a *narcotic drug,* such as heroin or morphine; certain *autoimmune disorders*, and *septicaemia* (blood poisoning).

SYMPTOMS AND SIGNS

The condition starts with an increase in breathing rate. Breathing then becomes laboured and more rapid. Babies with respiratory distress syndrome make grunting noises and draw in the wall of the chest when they breathe. If the condition worsens, progressive deoxygenation of the blood makes the sufferer turn blue. Without treatment, death may eventually result.

DIAGNOSIS AND TREATMENT

Respiratory distress syndrome is confirmed by listening to the lung with a stethoscope, by a *chest X-ray*, and by analysis of *blood gases*. In some cases, other tests may also be needed.

Babies and adults are treated in an *intensive-care* unit. In the early stages, humidified oxygen is given by mask. If respiratory distress increases, an *endotracheal tube* is inserted through the nose or mouth; breathing is then maintained by a *ventilator*. Any underlying cause is treated if possible.

Premature babies who are at risk of respiratory distress syndrome may be given artificial *surfactant* administered directly into the lungs.

OUTLOOK

Respiratory distress is the most common cause of death in premature babies, but with modern intensive care the survival rate for newborn babies with respiratory distress syndrome approaches 90 per cent. For adults with respiratory distress syndrome, the survival rate is between 25 and 50 per cent. Some survivors of respiratory distress syndrome are left with permanent lung damage.

Respiratory failure

A condition in which there is a build-up of carbon dioxide and a fall in the level of oxygen in the blood (see *Hypoxia*). Respiratory failure may be caused by any disorder that disrupts the normal transfer of gases in the blood, including lung disorders (such as *emphysema*, severe *asthma*, or chronic *bronchitis*). Respiratory failure may also be due to damage to the respiratory centre in the brain from an overdose of *narcotic drugs*.

Symptoms include breathlessness, cough, cyanosis (blue discoloration of the skin), an increased respiratory rate, or, less commonly, a reduced respiratory rate.

Respiratory failure usually requires *oxygen therapy*, in which a carefully controlled dose of oxygen is given. In severe cases, the patient must be placed on a *ventilator*. The underlying cause is also treated.

Respiratory function tests

See *Pulmonary function tests*.

Respiratory system

The organs responsible for carrying oxygen from the air to the bloodstream and expelling the waste product carbon dioxide.

Air passes from the *nose* or *mouth*, via various respiratory passages, to millions of balloon-like sacs, the *alveoli,* in the *lungs*. Oxygen in the inhaled air passes through the thin walls of the alveoli into the bloodstream, and carbon dioxide passes from the blood into the alveoli to be breathed out (see *Respiration* box).

Air is inhaled and exhaled by the action of the chest muscles and *diaphragm* (see *Breathing*).

DISORDERS

Disorders of the respiratory system can affect the air passages (causing obstruction of the passage of air into

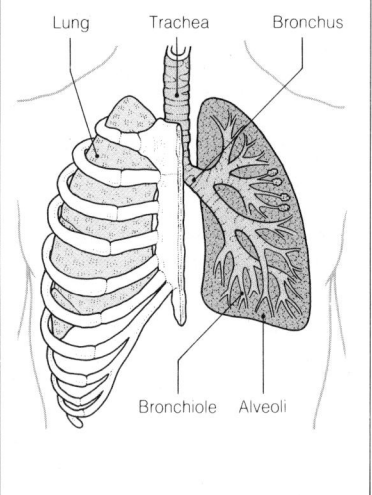

LOCATION OF THE RESPIRATORY SYSTEM
The system includes the upper air passages, lungs, and the muscles that control breathing.

Lung   Trachea   Bronchus

Bronchiole   Alveoli

or out of the lungs) or can affect the lung tissues (resulting in a poor exchange of oxygen and carbon dioxide). The functioning of the respiratory system can also be impaired by disorders, such as *poliomyelitis*, that affect the chest muscles and diaphragm and make inflation of the lungs difficult. (See also *Respiratory tract infection*.)

Respiratory tract infection

Infection of the breathing passages, which extend from the nose to the alveoli. Most of these illnesses, which are classified as upper or lower respiratory tract infections, are caused by viruses or bacteria.

Upper respiratory tract infections affect the nose, throat, sinuses, and larynx. They are among the most common of all illnesses, especially in early childhood. The most familiar upper respiratory tract infections are the common *cold, pharyngitis, tonsillitis, sinusitis, laryngitis*, and *croup*.

Lower respiratory tract infections, which affect the trachea, bronchi, and lungs, include acute *bronchitis*, acute *bronchiolitis*, and *pneumonia*.

Restless legs

A syndrome characterized by unpleasant tickling, burning, prickling, or aching sensations in the muscles of the legs. Symptoms tend to come on at night in bed, although prolonged sit-

R

RESPIRATION

The function of respiration is to provide the energy needed by body cells. Cells obtain this energy mainly by metabolizing glucose with oxygen, and so they require a constant supply of oxygen. In addition, the waste products of the metabolic process—mainly carbon dioxide—must be carried away from the cells.

Respiration includes the breathing of air into the lungs, the transfer of oxygen from the air to the blood, the transport of oxygen in the blood to the body cells, the metabolism of glucose with oxygen in the cells, and the transport of carbon dioxide to the lungs to be breathed out.

During exercise, respiration increases to compensate for higher energy demands by muscle cells.

2 The oxygen-saturated blood passes from the lungs via the pulmonary veins to the left side of the heart.

Carbon dioxide

CO_2

Trachea

Oxygen

O_2

Lung

Aorta

Bronchus

Alveoli

Pulmonary vein

Pulmonary artery

Left side of heart

Right side of heart

Bronchiole

Artery

Vein

Alveolus

Network of capillaries

1 Air, containing oxygen, is breathed into the lungs and enters the alveoli (tiny air sacs). Oxygen diffuses from the air into the blood vessels surrounding the alveoli.

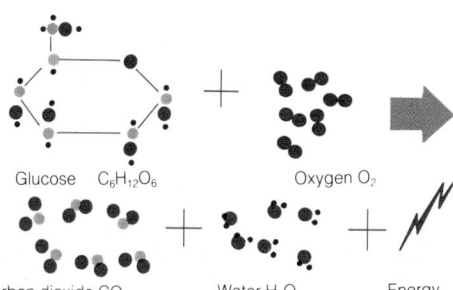

Glucose $C_6H_{12}O_6$

Oxygen O_2

$+$

Carbon dioxide CO_2

Water H_2O

$+$

Energy

6 Carbon dioxide is carried back in the blood to the heart, then to the lungs, where it diffuses into the alveoli and is breathed out of the body.

5 Within body cells, glucose and oxygen take part in a complex series of reactions, which provides energy to power the cells. During this cellular respiration (left), glucose is converted to carbon dioxide and water.

3 From the left side of the heart, the oxygenated blood is pumped via the aorta to the body tissues. The oxygen is carried within the blood by red cells.

O_2

CO_2

Oxygen

Glucose

Blood

Carbon dioxide

Water

Tissues

4 As the blood passes through tissue capillaries, it gives up oxygen (and nutrients such as glucose) to the body tissues and cells and picks up the waste products of cellular respiration—carbon dioxide and water.

BREATHING VOLUMES

One way the body copes with varied demands for oxygen is through changes in breathing volume. The tidal volume—the amount breathed into and out of the lungs at each breath—may vary from 0.5 litre at rest, up to 4.5 litres (near the maximum or vital capacity) during heavy exercise.

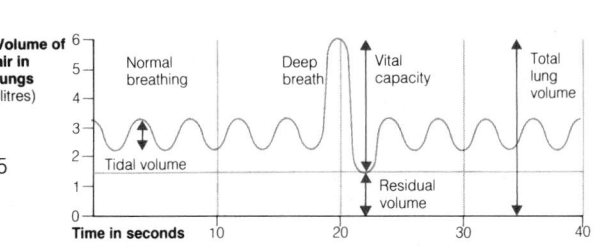

Volume of air in lungs (litres)

Normal breathing

Deep breath

Vital capacity

Total lung volume

Tidal volume

Residual volume

Time in seconds   10   20   30   40

R

ting sometimes triggers the discomfort; relief may be obtained only by movement, such as walking.

Restless legs affects as much as 15 per cent of the population, although many cases are very mild. The condition tends to run in families and is most common in middle-aged women, in people who consume large amounts of caffeine, in smokers, and during pregnancy. It often develops in people with *rheumatoid arthritis*.

The exact cause is unknown; there is no apparent nerve, muscle, or circulatory problem. There is no single cure; some patients benefit from cooling the legs, others from warming them. Treatment with certain drugs, including *levodopa* and *calcium channel blockers* (such as nifedipine) has been found to be effective in some patients.

Restoration, dental

The process of reconstructing part of a tooth that has been damaged by disease or injury. Restoration also refers to the material or substitute part used to rebuild the tooth.

Small areas are usually repaired by first removing the decayed or diseased area and then *filling* the tooth with an inactive material. For more extensive repairs, it may be necessary to fit a dental *inlay* or a *crown*. These are constructed outside the mouth and then cemented into place. For repairing chipped front teeth the dentist may use a *bonding* technique, in which the surface of the tooth is etched with an acid solution and then plastic or porcelain material is attached to the roughened surface.

Restricted growth
See *Short stature*.

Resuscitation
See *Artificial respiration*; *Cardiopulmonary resuscitation*.

Retardation
See *Mental handicap*.

Reticular formation
A network of nerve cells scattered throughout the *brainstem*.

Reticulosarcoma
A term for non-Hodgkin's lymphoma (see *Lymphoma, non-Hodgkin's*).

Retina
The light-sensitive membranous layer that lines the inside of the back of the *eye*, on which images are cast by the *cornea* and *lens*. The retina contains

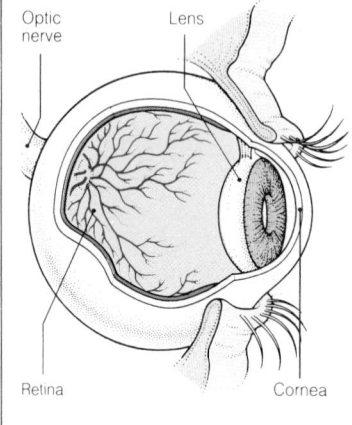

LOCATION OF THE RETINA
The retina is like the light-sensitive film in a camera. It forms a concave membrane over the back inner surface of the eye.

Optic nerve
Lens
Retina
Cornea

specialized nerve cells (the rods and cones) that convert light energy into nerve impulses. The retina also contains a network of connecting and integrating cells, some with very long fibres, that convey these impulses back along the *optic nerve* to the *brain*.

The rods are exceptionally sensitive, responding to very dim light. Cones are less sensitive but are responsible for *colour vision*, producing impulses that vary in strength with the colour of the light striking them.

Near the centre of the retina is the fovea. Here, retinal blood vessels are absent and the light-sensitive cells (almost all cones) are packed so that vision in this area has the highest resolution. (See also *Retina* disorders box.)

Retinal artery occlusion
Blockage of an artery supplying blood to the *retina*, affecting either the main retinal artery or one of its branches. Retinal artery occlusion is most commonly caused by *thrombosis* (abnormal blood clot formation) or *embolism* (a condition in which a clot or fatty deposit is carried by the blood from another area). If the main artery is blocked long enough, the affected eye will become permanently blind. If a small branch is blocked, loss of part of the field of vision will occur.

Retinal detachment
Separation of the *retina* (the light-sensitive inner layer) from the outer layers at the back of the *eye*.

CAUSES
Retinal detachment may follow major injury to the eye, but in most cases the disorder occurs spontaneously. Detachment of the retina is usually preceded by a *retinal tear* (split in the retina), which may be due to natural degeneration or to the pulling away of the retina as a consequence of the contraction of strands in the vitreous humour. As a result of the tear, vitreous fluid collects between the retina and the underlying *choroid* layer, thus separating them.

Detachment is more common in highly myopic (shortsighted) people, who have thinned retinas with areas of degeneration, and in people who have had *cataract surgery*.

SYMPTOMS AND SIGNS
Retinal detachment is painless and the symptoms are exclusively visual. The first indication is the appearance of bright flashes of light, seen at the edge of the field of vision and accompanied by *floaters*. The flashes are caused by strong stimulation of the light-sensitive cells as the tear occurs, and the floaters by the release of blood or pigment into the vitreous humour.

These symptoms do not always occur; the affected person may be unaware of the detachment until a black "drape" obscures vision. This drape descends in a lower detachment, ascends in an upper detachment, enters from the right in a left detachment, and so on.

TREATMENT
Retinal detachment requires prompt medical attention. An ophthalmologist must be consulted before the macula (the site of central vision) becomes detached. Once detachment has occurred, it may not be possible to restore normal central vision.

In the case of an upper detachment (ascending drape), there is a risk that the accumulating fluid will gravitate downwards and strip off the macula; it is therefore safer for the sufferer to lie flat on his or her back. In the case of a lower detachment (descending drape), an upright posture is unlikely to promote any extension of the detachment.

Treatment usually involves surgical repair of the underlying retinal tear. A soft silicone rubber sponge may be sewn in place on the outside of the *sclera* (outer layer of the eye) overlying the detachment. The sponge indents the sclera and leads to absorption of the fluid under the retina, causing the retina to settle back into place. The retina is then fixed in place by cryo-

R

pexy (the application of extreme cold) or *diathermy* (the application of heat), which causes an inflammatory adhesiveness of the underlying tissues. If the macula has not been detached, the results can be excellent.

Retinal haemorrhage

Bleeding into the *retina* (the light-sensitive inner layer at the back of the eye) from one or more blood vessels.

Retinal haemorrhage may be caused by *diabetes mellitus*, which leads to the formation of abnormal, small blood vessels which are fragile and bleed easily. Retinal haemorrhages also occur in *hypertension* (high blood pressure) and *retinal vein occlusion* (blockage of one of the veins that drain blood from the retina).

When the macula (the site of central vision) is involved, vision is severely impaired. Peripheral haemorrhages may pass unnoticed and may be detected only when the eye is examined with an ophthalmoscope.

Retinal tear

The development of a split in the *retina* (the light-sensitive inner layer at the back of the eye), usually caused by degeneration. Retinal tear is more common in people with severe *myopia*

DISORDERS OF THE RETINA

Despite its small size, the retina is subject to a wide variety of disorders, many of which seriously affect the vision or, in some cases, produce blindness.

CONGENITAL AND GENETIC DISORDERS

Colour blindness (see *Colour vision deficiency*), an abnormality of retinal cones (colour receptors in the retina), usually has a genetic basis. Hereditary degenerative disorders of the macula may appear at any age, leading to serious impairment of central vision. Other degenerative disorders of the retina with a genetic basis include *Tay-Sachs disease* and *retinitis pigmentosa*.

Retrolental fibroplasia may result from exposure of a premature baby to excessive oxygen concentration, which causes abnormalities in the retinal vessels.

INFECTION

Toxoplasmosis is an infection of the retina, acquired before birth and recurring later in life, with progressive damage to the retina.

TOXOCARA CANIS is a parasitic worm whose larvae may lodge in the retina and cause severe retinal destruction, producing a white mass resembling a tumour (see *Toxocariasis*). *Onchocerciasis*, an infestation by a tropical worm, may cause severe retinal damage. Bacterial and fungal infections elsewhere in the body can be carried by the blood to the retina. People whose immune systems are impaired are more susceptible to viral infections of the retina.

TUMOURS

Retinoblastoma is a malignant tumour that usually appears in the first three years of life. The affected eye may have visual loss and a visible whiteness in the pupil; *squint* often develops. The tendency to this cancer can be inherited. Secondary malignant tumours, spreading to the eye from primary tumours elsewhere in the body, can occur. A variety of benign tumours occur in the retina. Malignant melanoma can arise from the *choroid* (the layer beneath the retina).

INJURY

The retina may be torn or detached due to severe penetrating or blunt (nonpenetrating) injury (see *Retinal detachment*; *Retinal tear*). Permanent damage may be caused by a retinal burn, sometimes caused by looking directly at an eclipse of the sun.

METABOLIC DISORDERS

Diabetes mellitus may cause *retinopathy*, with fluid leakage and haemorrhage into the retina and with the growth of new, fragile blood vessels on the retinal surface, which bleed readily. Haemorrhage into the vitreous humour may occur from blood vessels, and fibrous tissue can grow forwards on to the humour in cases of "proliferative" retinopathy. This is a major cause of permanent loss of vision.

IMPAIRED BLOOD SUPPLY

Retinal vein occlusion (or *retinal artery occlusion*), a common cause of blindness, results from blockage of the central vein or artery of the retina. Hypertensive retinopathy is damage to the retina caused by high blood pressure, which leads to narrowing and *atherosclerosis* of the retinal arteries, which may both lead to retinal damage.

POISONS

A combination of heavy tobacco-smoking, heavy alcohol intake, and poor nutrition may lead to visual loss. Vitamin deficiency in combination with lead poisoning may cause visual loss. *Methanol* causes widespread and permanent destruction of certain retinal tissues, leading to blindness.

DRUGS

Many drugs can damage the retina, such as *chloroquine*, used in large doses over a long period for the treatment of conditions such as rheumatoid arthritis, and *phenothiazine drugs*, used in the treatment of psychiatric disorders.

OTHER DISORDERS

Age-related *macular degeneration*, causing progressive loss of vision, is common in older people. Retinal detachment often occurs in the absence of injury and may be more common in people with severe *myopia* (shortsightedness).

INVESTIGATION

Retinal disorders are investigated by checking the visual acuity and the visual fields (see *Vision tests*). After dilating the pupils with drops, the retinas are inspected by means of a direct or indirect *ophthalmoscope*. Fluorescein can be injected into a vein, where it is carried by the blood to outline the retinal vessels. Electrophysiological tests can also be carried out to study certain ocular diseases. *Ultrasound* testing can be used to study tumours in or under the retina.

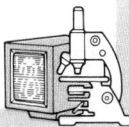

R

(shortsightedness). A retinal tear may also be caused by severe injury to the eye, especially a penetrating injury. *Retinal detachment* usually follows a retinal tear.

If a retinal tear is found before there is any secondary retinal detachment, the hole should be sealed by *laser treatment* or cryopexy (the application of extreme cold).

Retinal vein occlusion

Blockage of a vein carrying blood away from the *retina*, affecting either the main retinal vein or one of its branches. Retinal vein occlusion usually results from *thrombosis* (abnormal blood clot formation) in the affected vein. The condition is more common in people who have *glaucoma* and usually causes disturbance of vision in the affected eye. Retinal vein occlusion may also cause glaucoma and can result in complete blindness.

Retinitis

Inflammation affecting the *retina*. (See also *Retinopathy*.)

Retinitis pigmentosa

A degeneration of the rods and cones of the *retina* (the light-sensitive inner layer) at the back of both eyes. Retinitis pigmentosa usually has a genetic basis, but seldom appears before a person reaches adolescence and may not appear until middle age.

The first symptom of retinitis pigmentosa is usually an awareness that vision in dim light is very poor (night blindness). Testing of the *visual field* shows a ring-shaped area of blindness which, over the course of years, gradually extends to destroy an increasing area of the field. The cones in the macula (the site of central vision) seem more resistant than the peripherally placed rods, so central vision is retained, often for many years. Progression and severity are variable.

An examination of the retinas by ophthalmoscopy shows numerous masses of branching black pigment, distributed in areas corresponding to the extent of visual loss. Affected individuals or the parents of an affected child should seek *genetic counselling*.

Retinoblastoma

A *cancer* of the *retina* (the light-sensitive inner layer at the back of the eye) that affects babies and infants.

An affected eye may be blind, commonly causing a *squint* to develop, which is often the first indication of a retinoblastoma. The tumour may also show itself as a visible whiteness in the pupil. Without early treatment, retinoblastoma can spread from the eye to the orbit (eye socket) and along the *optic nerve* to the brain.

Retinoblastoma occurs in approximately one baby in 20,000. The tendency to develop retinoblastoma has a genetic basis. All the cells of people with this cancer lack part of one of the *chromosomes* in pair number 13. People belonging to families in which there is a tendency to retinoblastoma should seek *genetic counselling*. Newborn infants from affected families should be given regular eye examinations.

The tumour is treated by surgical removal of the affected eye, or by *radiotherapy*. If both eyes are affected, then the eye with the larger tumour may be removed and the other eye given radiotherapy.

Retinoids

See *Vitamin A*.

Retinol

The principal form of *vitamin A* found in the body.

Retinopathy

Disease of the *retina*, usually resulting from either *diabetes mellitus* or alternatively from persistent *hypertension* (high blood pressure).

Diabetic retinopathy is characterized by tiny aneurysms (balloon-like swellings) of the capillaries (tiny blood vessels) in the retina, leakage of fluid from the capillaries, and haemorrhage (bleeding) into the retina. New abnormal blood vessels, which are fragile and bleed readily, grow on the retinal surface. Haemorrhage into the vitreous humour may occur, and fibrous tissue can grow forwards into the vitreous humour. Treatment by *laser surgery* can often halt the progress of the condition.

Hypertensive retinopathy is characterized by narrowing of the retinal arteries. Areas of retina may be destroyed, and haemorrhage and white deposits may occur in the retina. (See also *Retrolental fibroplasia*.)

Retractor

A surgical instrument used to hold an incision open or to hold back surrounding tissue so that the surgeon has free access to the underlying area being operated on. Some retractors are held by the nurse or an assisting doctor; self-retaining retractors have a locking device that keeps them in position without support.

Retrobulbar neuritis

A form of *optic neuritis* in which the inflammation affects the optic nerve behind the eyeball.

Retrolental fibroplasia

Also called retinopathy of *prematurity*, a condition that mainly affects the eyes of premature infants.

Retrolental fibroplasia is usually caused by giving high concentrations of oxygen to premature infants who have a very low birthweight. Excess oxygen causes immature tissues, including those at the margin of the *retina* (the light-sensitive inner layer at the back of the eye), to shut down their blood vessels. When normal oxygen concentrations are resumed, affected retinal tissues sometimes send out strands of new vessels and fibrous scar tissue into the vitreous humour behind the lens. This process may interfere seriously with vision and lead to *retinal detachment*.

Babies with retrolental fibroplasia may be given *laser treatment*.

Retroperitoneal fibrosis

Inflammation and scarring of tissues at the back of the abdominal cavity. Retroperitoneal fibrosis often causes obstruction of the *ureters*, blocking the flow of urine from the kidneys. In severe cases, this obstruction results in *kidney failure*.

Most cases of retroperitoneal fibrosis occur in middle-aged men and are of unknown cause. In some cases, the condition is caused by long-term treatment with *methysergide* (a drug used to treat *migraine*).

Retrosternal pain

Pain in the central region of the chest, in the area of the sternum (breastbone). The most serious cause of retrosternal pain is a *myocardial infarction* (heart attack). More commonly, pain in this region is due to irritation of the *oesophagus* or to *angina pectoris*. (See also *Chest pain*.)

Rett's syndrome

A recently discovered *brain* disorder that only affects girls. This rare condition was first described in the 1960s by an Austrian, Andreas Rett, but became medically recognized only during the 1980s. Rett's syndrome affects about one in every 15,000 female babies born and is thought to be caused by a *genetic disorder*.

The health and development of an affected baby appear normal until symptoms occur, usually when the child is 12 to 18 months old. Skills that had been acquired, such as walking and talking, gradually disappear and the girl becomes progressively handicapped and may show signs of *autism*. Odd, repetitive writhing movements of the hands and limbs are characteristic of the condition, and there are often inappropriate outbursts of crying or laughter.

There is no cure for Rett's syndrome; sufferers need constant care and attention because of the level of handicap. Parents of an affected child should receive *genetic counselling*.

Reye's syndrome

A rare disorder characterized by brain and liver damage following an upper *respiratory tract infection*, *chickenpox*, or *influenza*. Reye's syndrome is almost entirely confined to children under the age of 15.

CAUSES

Evidence suggests that Reye's syndrome is often (but not invariably) related to taking *aspirin* for a viral infection. Doctors now recommend that children should be given *paracetamol* instead of aspirin.

SYMPTOMS AND SIGNS

Reye's syndrome develops as the child is recovering from the infection and starts with uncontrollable vomiting, often with lethargy, memory loss, disorientation, or delirium. Swelling of the brain may cause seizures, deepening coma, disturbances in heart rhythm, and cessation of breathing. Jaundice in Reye's syndrome indicates severe damage to the liver.

TREATMENT

Swelling of the brain is controlled by *corticosteroid drugs* and by intravenous infusions of *mannitol*. *Dialysis* or *blood transfusions* may be carried out to correct the changes in blood chemistry caused by damage to the liver. If breathing stops, the patient is placed on a *ventilator*.

OUTLOOK

With increasing knowledge of the condition, the death rate from Reye's syndrome has dropped dramatically from about 60 per cent to around 10 per cent. The outlook is worse for those who have seizures, lapse into deep coma, and stop breathing. Patients who survive a serious attack may suffer brain damage.

Rhabdomyolysis

Destruction of *muscle* tissue accompanied by the release of *myoglobin* (the oxygen-carrying red muscle pigment) into the blood.

The most common cause of rhabdomyolysis is a severe, crushing muscle injury (see *Crush syndrome*). Other causes include *polymyositis* (a viral infection of muscles) and, rarely, excessive physical exercise.

Rhabdomyolysis usually causes temporary paralysis or weakness of the affected muscle. Except in cases of severe injury, an affected muscle usually regenerates and the condition clears up without treatment.

Rhabdomyosarcoma

A very rare, malignant tumour of *muscle*. Rhabdomyosarcoma may develop during infancy, usually affecting the throat, bladder, prostate gland, or vagina, or it may occur in old age, when it commonly affects a large muscle in the arm or leg. The tumour grows rapidly and spreads to other tissues. Treatment is by surgical removal, combined with *radiotherapy* and *anticancer drugs*.

Rhesus immunoglobulin

See *Anti-D(Rh_o) immunoglobulin*.

Rhesus incompatibility

A mismatch between the blood of a pregnant woman and that of her baby with respect to the Rhesus (Rh) *blood group*. In certain circumstances, this mismatch can lead to *haemolytic disease of the newborn*.

In the past, haemolytic disease of the newborn was a common cause of stillbirth and of hydrops fetalis, a severe and often fatal condition in the newborn resulting from the destruction of fetal blood cells. Haemolytic disease of the newborn due to Rh

sensitization is now becoming rare. This is primarily due to the use of *anti-D(Rh_o) immunoglobulin* to prevent Rh sensitization.

CAUSE

Rh incompatibility results from exposure of a Rh-negative woman to Rh-positive blood. The Rh system (first identified in rhesus monkeys) is based on the presence or absence in the blood of several factors, of which the most important is a substance known as D antigen. The blood of people who are Rh positive contains D antigen whereas the blood of people who are Rh negative does not. Whether an individual has a positive or negative blood type is determined by *genes* (i.e. it is an inherited trait).

Rh incompatibility can arise only when a woman's blood is Rh negative and her baby's blood is Rh positive. This can happen only if the baby's father's blood is also Rh positive. There are usually no problems during a woman's first pregnancy with a baby whose blood is Rh positive. However, as shown in the diagram, the baby may sensitize the woman to Rh-positive blood; if she has a subsequent pregnancy with an Rh-positive baby, there is a risk of haemolytic disease of the newborn. A woman whose blood is Rh negative can also be sensitized if she is mistakenly given a transfusion of Rh-positive blood.

INCIDENCE

Among white people, about one person in six has Rh-negative blood; in about one pregnancy in 11, the mother's blood is Rh negative and the baby's blood is Rh positive. Rh incompatibility is less common in black and

R

HOW Rh INCOMPATIBILITY OCCURS

Without preventive treatment, an Rh-negative woman who is exposed to D antigen (a substance present only in Rh-positive blood) may develop antibodies that will attack the red blood cells of any future Rh-positive babies.

First pregnancy

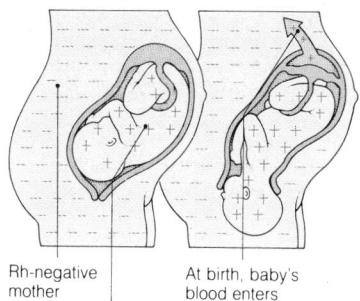

Rh-negative mother

Rh-positive baby

At birth, baby's blood enters mother's circulation

Subsequent pregnancies

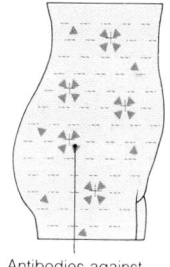

Antibodies against Rh-positive blood formed in mother

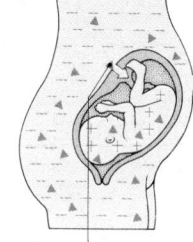

Antibodies cross placenta and destroy red blood cells of subsequent Rh-positive babies

Oriental families than in white families because of a comparative rarity of the Rh-negative blood group in people who are not white.

TREATMENT AND PREVENTION

An injection of anti-D(Rh$_o$) immunoglobulin is given to Rh-negative women soon after the birth of an Rh-positive baby. The injection contains antibodies to Rh factor, which destroy any of the baby's blood cells that may have entered the woman before they have a chance to sensitize her. When given within 72 hours of delivery, the injection prevents Rh sensitization in 99 per cent of cases.

Anti-D(Rh$_o$) immunoglobulin is also given to Rh-negative women after any miscarriage, induced abortion, amniocentesis, or other procedure that might result in exposure of the mother to the fetal blood cells.

If a woman has Rh-negative blood, she is tested for the presence of Rh antibodies at her first antenatal visit and also at subsequent visits. The management of the pregnancy and birth, if antibodies are present and there is a risk to the baby, is as described under *Haemolytic disease of the newborn*.

Rhesus isoimmunization

The development of antibodies formed against Rh-positive blood in a person who has Rh-negative blood. (See *Haemolytic disease of the newborn*; *Rhesus incompatibility*.)

Rheumatic fever

A disease that causes inflammation in various tissues throughout the body. Inflammation of the *joints* is a major feature, but this is less serious in the long term than the risk of permanent heart damage. In some cases, the nervous system is also affected.

Rheumatic fever has now become rare in developed countries, although occasional small outbreaks still occur. It remains an important cause of heart disease in the developing world. Children aged five to 15 years are most commonly affected by rheumatic fever.

CAUSES

Rheumatic fever always follows a throat infection with certain strains of streptococcal bacteria. It is not caused by the presence of the bacteria in the affected tissues but is generally believed to be some form of *autoimmune disorder* (one in which the body's immune system attacks its own tissues) induced by streptococci. The development of rheumatic fever can

usually be prevented by prompt treatment of streptococcal throat infections with *antibiotic drugs*.

SYMPTOMS AND SIGNS

The disease causes fever with pain, inflammation, and swelling of one or more of the larger joints. As one joint improves, symptoms tend to develop in another, although several joints may be affected simultaneously.

If damage to the heart occurs, it develops insidiously; there may be no symptoms until some years later. The heart may be affected in various ways, the most common and most serious being a thickening and scarring of the *heart valves*, leading to narrowing and/or leaking of valves (see *Mitral stenosis*; *Mitral incompetence*). These effects on the heart are permanent and progressive.

Involvement of the nervous system may cause *Sydenham's chorea*, in which there are irregular, uncontrollable, aimless, jerky movements, and usually some emotional upset.

Rheumatic fever may also cause nodules beneath the skin (often over bony prominences) and a rash.

DIAGNOSIS

There are no specific tests for rheumatic fever, but tests may be performed to look for *antibodies* directed against streptococci. The diagnosis may be suspected when arthritis moves from joint to joint, but in other instances the condition may be discovered only after the development of later heart damage, causing *heart failure* or a heart *murmur*.

TREATMENT

As soon as the diagnosis of acute rheumatic fever is made, a *penicillin drug* is used to eradicate streptococci. *Aspirin* or other salicylate drugs are used to control the joint pain and inflammation and to try to minimize heart damage. In some cases, *corticosteroid drugs* may be needed. Sedatives and tranquillizers are helpful in the treatment of Sydenham's chorea.

If heart valve damage occurs, *heart valve surgery* may be needed.

OUTLOOK

The outlook depends on the degree to which the heart has been affected and on whether recurrences can be avoided. The use of penicillin, taken daily for many months or years, may be necessary to prevent further infection with streptococci.

Rheumatism

A popular term for any disorder that causes pain and stiffness in *muscles* and *joints*, including minor aches and

twinges as well as disorders such as *rheumatoid arthritis*, *osteoarthritis*, and *polymyalgia rheumatica*.

Rheumatoid arthritis

A type of *arthritis* (joint inflammation) in which the joints of the fingers, wrists, toes, or other joints in the body become painful, swollen, stiff, and, in severe cases, deformed. The disease usually takes the form of recurrent moderate attacks. The frequency of attacks, the number of affected joints, and the severity of symptoms are variable. Rheumatoid arthritis is medically distinct from *osteoarthritis*.

CAUSES AND INCIDENCE

Rheumatoid arthritis is an *autoimmune disorder* (one in which the *immune system* attacks the body's own tissues). The disease usually starts in early adulthood or middle age but can also develop in children (see *Rheumatoid arthritis, juvenile*) or the elderly.

Rheumatoid arthritis occurs worldwide and affects one to two per cent of the population. It affects two to three times more women than men.

SYMPTOMS AND SIGNS

The onset of the disease is usually gradual, with mild fever and generalized aches and pains preceding specific joint symptoms. In some cases, joint inflammation develops suddenly.

Affected joints become swollen, red, warm, painful, and stiff. Structures around the joint may also become inflamed, resulting in weakness of the ligaments, tendons, and surrounding muscles. The finger joints are the most commonly affected, resulting in a weak grip. *Raynaud's phenomenon* (a condition in which the fingers turn white on exposure to cold) may occur. Swelling of the wrist may cause *carpal tunnel syndrome* (tingling and pain in the fingers caused by pressure on the median nerve). *Tenosynovitis* (inflamed painful tendon sheaths) also sometimes develops in the wrist. Rheumatoid arthritis affecting the feet may cause pain in the toes, arches, and ankles. Other parts of the body sometimes affected by rheumatoid arthritis include the shoulders, knees, and neck joints. Early morning stiffness is common, and sufferers may require help with getting out of bed and dressing.

Soft nodules sometimes develop beneath the skin, especially in areas subjected to physical stress. Some sufferers develop *bursitis*, in which the fluid-filled sac around a joint becomes inflamed. When the knee is affected, a fluid-filled swelling known as a *Baker's*

R

cyst may develop behind it. Many sufferers feel fatigued, partly as a result of the *anaemia* that usually accompanies the disease.

DIAGNOSIS

The diagnosis is based on the patient's condition and medical history, on *X-rays* of affected joints, and on *blood tests* (including a check for specific antibodies known as rheumatoid factor). If rheumatoid factor is absent from a person who otherwise appears to have rheumatoid arthritis, the condition is known as seronegative rheumatoid arthritis.

TREATMENT

Depending on individual requirements, rheumatoid arthritis may be treated by drugs, *physiotherapy, occupational therapy,* or surgery.

Nonsteroidal anti-inflammatory drugs (NSAIDs) may be used to relieve joint pain and stiffness. *Antirheumatic drugs,* such as *gold, penicillamine,* or *sulphasalazine* often slow or arrest the progress of the disease. *Immunosuppressant drugs,* such as *azathioprine* or *corticosteroid drugs,* are given to suppress the body's immune system if antirheumatic drugs fail to control the disorder or if they produce severe side-effects. Corticosteroid drugs may be injected into affected joints to provide local pain relief.

Physiotherapy often plays an important part in the treatment of people with rheumatoid arthritis. Exercising in a warm hydrotherapy pool can lessen muscle spasm and joint stiffness. In some cases, removable splints can be extremely helpful in reducing pain in the hands and wrists. The use of insoles and, if necessary, special surgical shoes can help to relieve pain in the feet.

People disabled by rheumatoid arthritis can also be helped by *occupational therapy.* The occupational therapist can advise sufferers on how to cope with everyday tasks, and can recommend various dressing and household aids (see the illustrated box on physical aids for the disabled that accompanies the *Disability* entry). Severely disabled sufferers may be provided with a *wheelchair.*

In severe cases, surgery may be performed to replace destroyed joints with artificial substitutes (see *Arthroplasty*). Hip and knee replacements are the most common.

As yet there is no evidence that special diets play any significant role in relieving the symptoms of rheumatoid arthritis, but a normal diet supplemented by fish or fish

---

RHEUMATOID ARTHRITIS

One of the most serious forms of joint disease, rheumatoid arthritis may occur as a single episode or a succession of progressively severe attacks. It results from a disturbance in the body's defences against infection, causing these defences to attack various body tissues. In the worst cases, joints are completely destroyed, but modern treatment has reduced the incidence of severe disability.

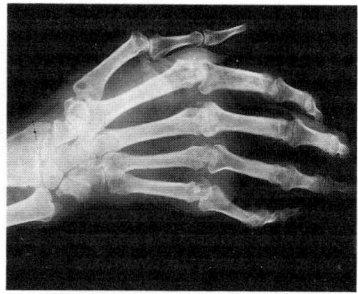

X-ray of the hand in rheumatoid arthritis
Note the destructive changes in the joints and the way the finger bones curve away from the thumb side of the hand.

Affected joints
Rheumatoid arthritis can affect virtually any joint, but especially the fingers, wrists, shoulders, knees, hips, and spinal joints in the neck.

Disease progression
The synovium (membrane lining the capsule of an affected joint) becomes inflamed and thickened (right). Later, inflammation may spread to the cartilage and bone.

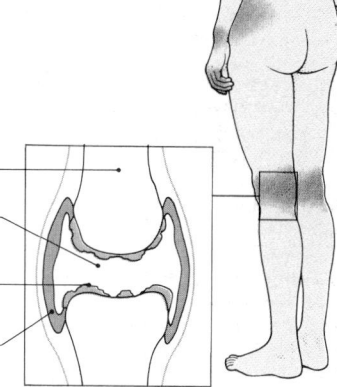

Bone
Inflamed synovium
Cartilage
Capsule

TREATMENT OF RHEUMATOID ARTHRITIS

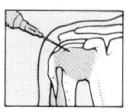

Drug treatment
may include antirheumatic drugs to slow the progress of the disease, nonsteroidal anti-inflammatory drugs to relieve joint pain, and immunosuppressants to dampen the activity of the immune system.

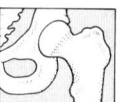

Prostheses
Many joints, such as the hip, can now be replaced with substitutes made from hard-wearing metal and plastic materials. Prostheses may be the only satisfactory solution if a joint becomes seriously damaged.

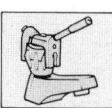

Occupational therapy
can help people who are disabled by rheumatoid arthritis. Sufferers are shown how to cope with everyday tasks, provided with aids for use in the home, and taught principles of joint protection.

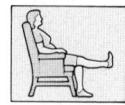

Physiotherapy
aids in the relief of pain and stiffness and helps sufferers to regain use of affected joints and muscles. The doctor or physiotherapist may recommend removable splints to relieve pain in the hands and wrists.

---

oils may be more beneficial than one without. *Acupuncture* may relieve pain, but it has no effect on the course of the disease.

COMPLICATIONS

Severe rheumatoid arthritis may have complications affecting various parts of the body. The covering of the heart may become inflamed, causing *pericarditis.* The small blood vessels may be affected, resulting in poor circulation and the development of ulcers on the hands and feet. Involvement of the lungs may lead to *pleural effusion* or to *pulmonary fibrosis.* The eyes and mouth may become dry (see *Sjögren's syndrome*). The lymph nodes may become enlarged, producing ten-

R

der swellings in the neck, armpit, and groin. The spleen sometimes becomes enlarged, resulting in *hypersplenism* (overactivity of the spleen); the combination of rheumatoid arthritis and hypersplenism is known as Felty's syndrome.

OUTLOOK
Most sufferers must take drugs for the rest of their lives, but effective control of symptoms often allows a near-normal level of activity. Modern methods of treatment have reduced the incidence and severity of deformity and disability.

Rheumatoid arthritis, juvenile

A rare form of *arthritis* (joint inflammation) that affects children. Juvenile arthritis occurs more often in girls than in boys, and most commonly starts between the ages of two and four years or around puberty.

TYPES AND SYMPTOMS
There are three main types of juvenile rheumatoid arthritis.

Still's disease, also called systemic onset juvenile arthritis, starts with an illness in which there is fever, rash, enlarged lymph nodes, abdominal pain, and weight loss. These symptoms last for several weeks, and the joint pain, swelling, and stiffness may not begin for several months.

The other two main types are characterized mainly by joint symptoms. Polyarticular juvenile arthritis causes pain, swelling, and stiffness in many joints. Pauciarticular juvenile arthritis affects four or fewer joints.

DIAGNOSIS
Diagnosis is based on the symptoms and signs and the exclusion of other disorders that can cause joint symptoms in children, such as viral or bacterial infections, rheumatic fever, Crohn's disease, ulcerative colitis, haemophilia, sickle cell anaemia, and leukaemia. Blood tests may help identify the cause of the arthritis. Juvenile rheumatoid arthritis is not diagnosed unless the condition persists for longer than three months.

COMPLICATIONS
Possible complications include short stature, *anaemia*, *pleurisy*, *pericarditis* (inflammation of the outer lining of the heart), and enlargement of the liver and spleen. *Uveitis* (inflammation of the iris and the surrounding muscles in the eye) may develop and, if untreated, may damage vision. Rarely, *amyloidosis* (deposition of a starchy substance in body organs) may occur; if the kidney is involved, *kidney failure* may develop.

TREATMENT
Joint pain and stiffness may be relieved by *aspirin, nonsteroidal anti-inflammatory drugs,* and, in very severe cases, *antirheumatic drugs* (such as gold, penicillamine, chloroquine, or azathioprine) or *corticosteroid drugs*.

Splints may be worn during the day to rest acutely inflamed joints and at night to reduce the risk of deformities. *Physiotherapy* reduces the risk of muscle wasting and contractures (deformities due to shrinkage of tissue). Excessive physical exercise should be avoided and special shoes worn to reduce the risk of foot deformity.

OUTLOOK
In most children the arthritis disappears after several years. However, some are left with joint deformity.

Rheumatoid spondylitis
See *Ankylosing spondylitis.*

Rheumatology
The branch of medicine concerned with the causes, development, diagnosis, and treatment of diseases that affect the *joints, muscles,* and *connective tissue.* Rheumatologists use a variety of investigative techniques, ranging from X-rays of joints to tests of muscle function and blood analysis. Treatment is similarly varied, including drug treatment with anti-inflammatory drugs or analgesic drugs, and physiotherapy.

Rhinitis
Inflammation of the *mucous membrane* that lines the *nose,* usually manifested by some combination of nasal obstruction, nasal discharge, sneezing, and facial pressure or pain.

TYPES
VIRAL RHINITIS This type is a feature of the common cold (see *Cold, common*), and may lead to *sinusitis.*

ALLERGIC RHINITIS Rhinitis due to allergy (see *Rhinitis, allergic*), also known as hay fever, may be seasonal (usually caused by pollens) or occur throughout the year (usually caused by house dust, moulds, or pets). Allergic rhinitis most commonly occurs with vasomotor rhinitis.

VASOMOTOR RHINITIS This may be intermittent or continual. The nose becomes too responsive to stimuli, such as pollutants (e.g. tobacco smoke), changes or extremes in temperature or humidity, some foods, some medicines, or certain emotions. Vasomotor rhinitis is common in pregnancy and in those taking combined *oral contraceptives* or other *oestrogen drugs.*

HYPERTROPHIC RHINITIS This type of rhinitis, characterized by thickening of the nasal mucous membrane and chronic congestion of the nasal veins, can be caused by repeated nasal infections. Hypertrophic rhinitis results in constant stuffiness and sometimes impairment of the sense of smell. In severe cases, treatment may involve surgical removal or shrinkage of part of the swollen tissue.

ATROPHIC RHINITIS This wasting of the mucous membrane can result from aging, from chronic bacterial infections, or from extensive nasal surgery. Other features of atrophic rhinitis include persistent nasal infection, a discharge that dries to a crust, loss of smell, and an unpleasant odour. Treatment is with *antibiotic drugs* and sometimes with *oestrogen drugs.*

Rhinitis, allergic
Inflammation of the *mucous membrane* that lines the *nose* due to *allergy* to pollen, dust, or other airborne substances. Allergic rhinitis, also known as hay fever, causes sneezing, a runny nose, and nasal congestion.

CAUSES
In some people, the inhalation of particles of certain harmless substances provokes an exaggerated response by the *immune system,* which forms *antibodies* against them. These otherwise harmless substances, known as allergens, also trigger the release of *histamine* and other chemicals that cause inflammation and fluid production in the lining of the nose and nasal *sinuses* (air cavities around the nose). The most common of the allergens that cause allergic rhinitis are tree, grass, and weed pollens; moulds; animal skin scales, hair, or feathers; house dust; and house-dust mites.

Pollen-induced allergic rhinitis is seasonal. Tree pollens are most prevalent in spring, grass pollens in summer, and weed pollens in summer and autumn. Sufferers are worst affected on days when the pollen count is high—that is, during hot and windy weather, especially in heavily vegetated, low-lying areas.

People affected by household allergens, such as dust, tend to have less severe symptoms but are affected throughout the year.

INCIDENCE
Allergic rhinitis is a common complaint, affecting as many as five to 10 per cent of the population. It is more common in people who have other allergies, such as *asthma* or *eczema*; like these disorders, it has a tendency to

R

run in families. The condition usually develops before the age of 30 and affects more women than men.

SYMPTOMS AND SIGNS
Exposure to the allergen produces an itching sensation in the nose, palate, throat, and eyes. This is followed by sneezing, stuffiness, a runny nose, and, usually, watering eyes. The eyes may also be affected by *conjunctivitis*, which makes them red and sore.

PREVENTION AND TREATMENT
Skin tests help identify the allergen responsible for the disorder. Once the allergen is known, exposure should be avoided or kept to a minimum, although this is difficult when the cause is pollens.

For mild attacks of allergic rhinitis, occasional use of a *decongestant drug* in the form of a spray or drops may clear up symptoms, but use for more than three or four days can make the condition worse. Many sufferers are helped by taking *antihistamine drugs*, which reduce itching and some degree of nasal congestion and runny nose, but may cause drowsiness. Allergic rhinitis may also be treated with *corticosteroid drugs*, which are available in nasal preparations.

The drug sodium cromoglycate, inhaled regularly throughout the pollen season, may help prevent attacks by blocking the allergic response. Long-term relief of symptoms can sometimes follow desensitization to a particular pollen allergen by a course of injections (see *Hyposensitization*).

Rhinophyma

Bulbous deformity and redness of the *nose* occurring almost exclusively in elderly men. Rhinophyma is a complication of severe *rosacea* (a skin disorder of the nose and cheeks). The tissue of the nose thickens, small blood vessels enlarge, and the sebaceous glands become overactive, making the nose excessively oily.

Rhinophyma can be remedied by an operation. Under a general anaesthetic, the swollen tissue is cut away until the nose is restored to a satisfactory shape. Skin grafting is not necessary because the remaining tissue rapidly regenerates.

Rhinoplasty

An operation that alters the structure of the *nose* to improve its appearance or to correct a deformity caused by injury or disease.

Under either a local or a general anaesthetic, incisions are made within the nose (to avoid visible scars). The

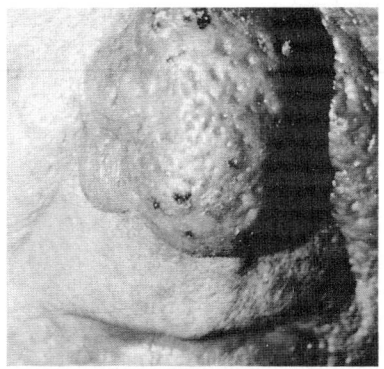

Example of rhinophyma
This disfiguring condition is remedied by paring away the excess tissue. The skin soon regenerates after treatment.

septum (the vertical wall of cartilage and bone that divides the nose) may be altered if breathing passages are blocked. The cartilage and bone of the nasal structure are then reshaped; occasionally, a bone or cartilage graft is used. The nose is finally splinted in position for about 10 days.

Rhinoplasty usually causes considerable bruising and swelling, and the results may not be clearly visible

for weeks or months. Rare complications include recurrent nosebleeds due to persistent crusting at the incision sites and breathing difficulty due to narrowing of the nasal passages.

Rhinorrhoea

The discharge of watery mucus from the nose, usually due to *rhinitis*. Rarely, the discharge consists of cerebrospinal fluid and is due to a head injury. (See *Nasal discharge*.)

Rhythm method

See *Contraception, natural methods of.*

Rib

Any of the flat, curved bones that form a framework for the chest and a protective cage around the heart, lungs, and other underlying organs.

There are 12 pairs of ribs, each joined at the back of the rib-cage to a vertebra in the spine. Their arrangement is shown in the illustrated box. Between the ribs, and attached to them, are thin sheets of muscle that help to expand and relax the chest during breathing. The intercostal spaces between the ribs also contain nerves and blood vessels.

ANATOMY OF THE RIBS

There are seven true ribs attached to the sternum, three false ribs, each attached to a rib above, and two floating ribs on each side. When the ribs are pulled up by the intercostal muscles (between the ribs), they expand the chest, drawing air into the lungs. The front ends of the true ribs are linked to the sternum by cartilages.

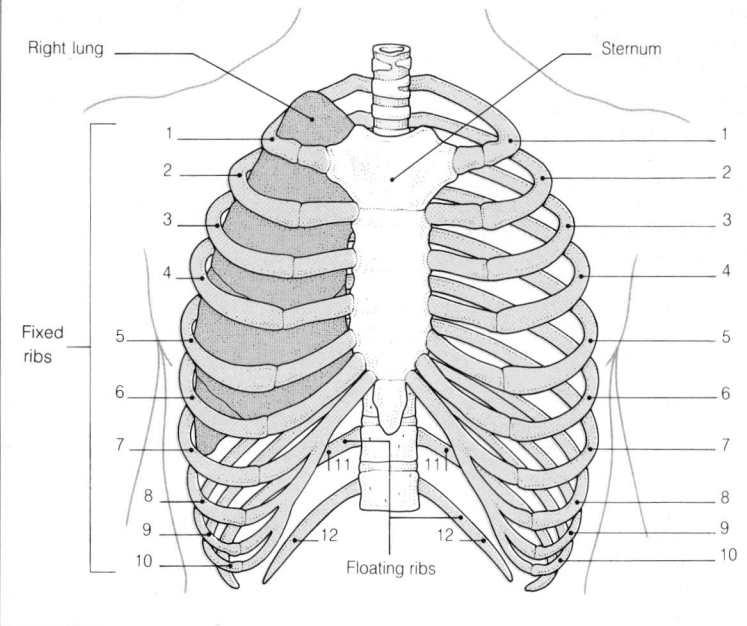

R

879

DISORDERS

The ribs can easily be fractured by a fall or blow (see *Rib, fracture of*).

A rib is one of the more common sites for a benign *bone tumour* or for a *metastasis* (a secondary malignant tumour that has spread from cancer elsewhere in the body).

In rare cases a person is born with one or more extra ribs lying above the uppermost normal rib. Known as *cervical ribs*, the additional ribs may press on nerves supplying the arm or cause other problems.

Ribavirin

A recently introduced *antiviral drug*, also known as tribavirin, that is used in the treatment of infants and children with viral *bronchiolitis* caused by respiratory syncytial virus. Ribavirin is administered by aerosol inhalation or by means of a nebulizer. Adverse effects of the drug are rare.

Clinical trials have shown that ribavirin is also effective against a wide variety of other viral infections, including herpes simplex, hepatitis, and several strains of influenza.

Rib, fracture of

Fracture of a *rib* is usually caused by a fall or blow. It may also be caused by minor stress on the rib-cage, such as that produced by prolonged coughing or even laughing.

The fracture causes severe pain that is made worse by deep breathing, and tenderness and swelling of the overlying tissue. The diagnosis is confirmed by *X-rays*. Pain is relieved by *analgesic drugs* (painkillers) or, occasionally, by an injection of a long-acting, local anaesthetic.

Most rib fractures are undisplaced (i.e. the bone ends remain in alignment) and usually heal easily without specific treatment. Strapping is rarely used to aid healing of broken ribs because it hinders chest expansion and thus increases the risk of *pneumonia*. Instead, the patient is encouraged to take deep breaths while holding the injured side.

A fracture that is displaced or splintered may pierce a lung, thereby causing lung collapse (see *Pneumothorax*). Multiple rib fractures can result in *flail chest* (a type of chest injury in which part of the chest wall moves in the direction opposite to normal during breathing).

Riboflavin

The chemical name of vitamin B_2 (see *Vitamin B complex*).

Rickets

A disease caused by nutritional deficiency that causes deformity of the skeleton during childhood. In rickets, *bones* become deformed because inadequate amounts of *calcium* and *phosphate* are incorporated into them as they grow. A similar deficiency of calcium and phosphate in the bones of adults results in *osteomalacia*.

CAUSES AND INCIDENCE

The most common cause of rickets is deficiency of *vitamin D*, which is vital for the absorption of calcium from the intestines into the blood and for its incorporation into bone. Vitamin D is found in fat-containing animal substances, such as oily fish, butter, egg yolk, liver, and fish-liver oils. There are also small amounts in human and animal milk. Vitamin D is also made in the body through the action of sunlight on the skin.

Rickets occurs primarily in poor countries and in communities where babies (and mothers) receive inadequate vitamin D in the diet and also do not get enough sunlight. Breast milk alone cannot provide all a baby's needs for vitamin D, so a breast-fed baby who gets little sun should be given vitamin D supplements.

Rickets is now rare in developed countries, where vitamin D supplements are often given to infants, where the vitamin is added to margarine, and where most children and babies eat a varied diet and get adequate exposure to the sun. The disorder is seen only in vulnerable groups, such as premature babies, children of Asian parentage living in northern countries including the UK, and some food faddists who avoid foods rich in vitamin D.

Rickets occasionally develops as a complication of a digestive disorder that causes *malabsorption* (failure to absorb nutrients from the intestines). Rickets may also occur in certain rare forms of kidney and liver disease and in children undergoing long-term therapy with types of *anticonvulsant drugs* that interfere with the action of vitamin D.

SYMPTOMS AND SIGNS

The most striking feature of advanced rickets is deformity of the bones, especially of the legs and spine. Typically, there is bowing of the legs and, in infants, flattening of the head as a result of the softness of the skull. Infants with rickets often sleep poorly and show delay in crawling and walking. Other features include *kyphoscoliosis* (spinal curvature), a tendency

to *fractures*, and enlargement of the wrists, ankles, and ends of the ribs. There may also be pelvic pain and muscle weakness.

DIAGNOSIS AND TREATMENT

Rickets is diagnosed from the child's physical appearance and from the results of *X-rays* and *blood tests*.

Rickets due to dietary deficiency is treated with vitamin D supplements, which can restore normal bone growth; in most cases, bone deformities disappear as the child continues to grow. Rickets that occurs as a complication of another disorder, such as malabsorption or kidney disease, is treated according to the cause.

Rickettsia

 A type of parasitic microorganism. Rickettsiae resemble small *bacteria*, but they are able to multiply only by invading the cells of another life form; in this respect they are more like *viruses*.

Rickettsiae are primarily parasites of the arthropods (insects and insect-like animals), such as lice, fleas, ticks, and mites. Such arthropods sometimes transmit rickettsiae to the blood of larger animals (such as rodents, dogs, or humans) in their saliva via bites or in their faeces via a small break in the skin. Human diseases caused by different types of rickettsiae include *Q fever*, *Rocky Mountain spotted fever*, and the various forms of *typhus*.

Rifampicin

An *antibacterial drug* that is used mainly in the treatment of *tuberculosis* and also to treat *leprosy*, *endocarditis*, and *osteomyelitis*. Rifampicin is usually prescribed with other antibacterial drugs because some strains of bacteria quickly develop *resistance* if rifampicin is used alone.

The drug causes harmless, orange-red discoloration of the urine, saliva, and other body secretions. Other possible effects include muscle pain, nausea, vomiting, diarrhoea, jaundice, flu-like symptoms, rash, and itching. This drug interferes with the action of oral contraceptives, so there is a danger of unwanted pregnancy.

Rigidity

Increased tone in one or more *muscles*, which causes them to feel tight; the affected part of the body becomes stiff and inflexible.

Causes of rigidity include injury to a muscle, arthritis affecting a nearby joint, a neurological disorder, such as

Parkinson's disease, or stroke. Rigidity of the abdominal muscles is a sign of *peritonitis*. (See also *Spasticity*.)

Rigor

A violent attack of shivering, often associated with a fever. Rigor may also refer to stiffness or rigidity of body tissues, as in *rigor mortis*.

Rigor mortis

The stiffening of *muscles* that occurs after *death*. Rigor mortis starts some three to four hours after death and is usually complete after about 12 hours; the stiffness then gradually disappears over the next 48 to 60 hours. The greater the amount of physical exertion before death, the sooner rigor mortis begins. Similarly, the sooner rigor mortis begins, the sooner it passes. These facts have important medicolegal implications and, along with other factors, are used to assess the time of death.

Rimiterol

A *bronchodilator drug* used in the treatment of asthma and chronic bronchitis. Possible adverse effects of rimiterol include palpitations, tremor, headache, and hot flushes.

Ringing in the ears

See *Tinnitus*.

Ringworm

A popular name for certain types of fungal skin infections (commonly of the feet, groin, scalp, nails, or trunk). Ringworm is marked by ring-shaped, reddened, scaly, or blistery patches on the skin. (See *Tinea*.)

Ritodrine

A drug used to prevent or delay premature labour (see *Prematurity*) by relaxing the muscles of the uterus. Possible side-effects of ritodrine include tremor, palpitations, nausea, vomiting, chest pain, breathlessness, and hot flushes.

River blindness

See *Onchocerciasis*.

RNA

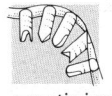

The abbreviation for ribonucleic acid. RNA is one of the two substances that carry the inherited, coded genetic instructions in cells. The other such substance is deoxyribonucleic acid (*DNA*).

In all animal and plant cells, it is DNA that holds a permanent record of

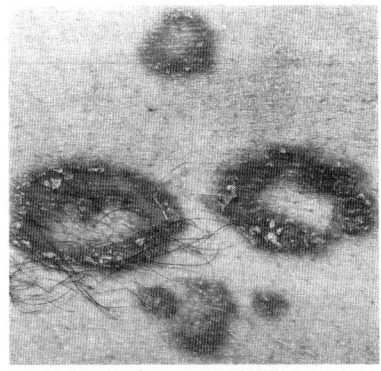

Patch of ringworm
The name arises from the tendency for certain skin fungus infections to spread uniformly outward, leaving normal skin inside the ring.

the instructions; RNA helps decode the instructions. In some viruses, however, the instructions for viral multiplication are held by RNA. (See also *Nucleic acids*; *Protein synthesis*.)

Rocky Mountain spotted fever

A rare, infectious disease causing fever and a rash with spots that spread over the body, darken, enlarge, and bleed. The disease was originally recognized in the Rocky Mountain states of the US but also occurs elsewhere in North and South America. Rocky Mountain spotted fever is caused by a rickettsia (a microorganism similar to a bacterium) and is transmitted from rabbits and other small mammals by tick bites.

The diagnosis can be confirmed by laboratory tests on blood and by tissue samples. Treatment with *chloramphenicol* or *tetracycline* usually cures the disease.

Rodent ulcer

A common name for *basal cell carcinoma*; a type of skin cancer.

Roentgenography

See *X-rays*; *Radiology*.

Role-playing

The acting out of a role (the pattern of behaviour expected of an individual in a given social situation). The conscious adoption of different roles can be a useful technique for learning about oneself, other people, or particular situations.

The phrase "sick role" describes the type of passive behaviour expected and allowed of a patient; people with social or emotional problems may

unconsciously adopt this role as a means of escaping from social obligations and of gaining the sympathy and understanding of others.

Root-canal treatment

A dental procedure performed to save a tooth in which the pulp (the living tissue within a tooth) has died or become untreatably diseased, usually as the result of extensive dental *caries*.

HOW IT IS DONE

X-rays are taken to establish the length of the pulp cavity. Root-canal treatment may be performed after administration of a local anaesthetic. To prevent infection, a *rubber dam* (a small sheet of rubber) is used to isolate the tooth from the saliva.

ROOT-CANAL TREATMENT

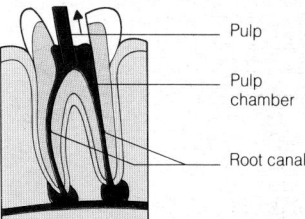

Pulp

Pulp chamber

Root canal

1 A hole is drilled into the crown to remove all material from the pulp chamber. The root canals are then slightly enlarged and shaped with fine-tipped instruments. The procedure is usually monitored by X-rays.

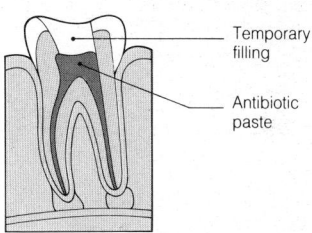

Temporary filling

Antibiotic paste

2 The cavity is washed out, and antibiotic paste and a temporary filling are packed into it. Some days later, the filling is removed and the canals are checked for sterility.

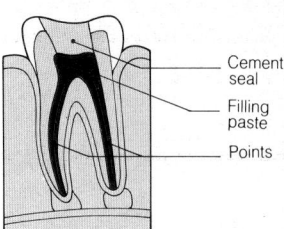

Cement seal

Filling paste

Points

3 When no infection can be detected, the cavity is filled with a sealing paste and/or tapering solid "points" made of gutta-percha resin mixed with zinc and bismuth oxides. The roots are then sealed with cement.

R

The main steps in root-canal treatment are shown in the illustrations, including removal of the pulp, sealing with a temporary filling, checking for infection, and the final filling and sealing of the tooth.

COMPLICATIONS
If the pulp cavity has not been filled completely, bacteria may enter, leading to apical *periodontitis* (inflammation of the tissues around the root tips). It may then be necessary to make an opening in the gum and bone overlying the affected root to allow pus to drain. In some cases, an apicectomy (removal of a small portion of the root tip) and filling of the area with amalgam may necessary.

RESULTS
Teeth whose pulp cavities have been filled may function well for as long as normal teeth. Treated teeth may, however, turn slightly grey; if a tooth is unsightly, its appearance can be restored by bonding (see *Bonding, dental*), by the fitting of an artificial crown (see *Crown, dental*), or by bleaching (see *Bleaching, dental*).

Rorschach test
A psychological test based on the assessment of a person's responses to a standardized set of ink-blot pictures. The test was devised by the Swiss psychiatrist Hermann Rorschach early in the 20th century. It was intended to reveal an individual's attitudes, conflicts, and emotions but is now rarely used. (See also *Personality tests*.)

Rosacea
A chronic *skin* disorder in which the nose and cheeks are abnormally red. The cause of the disorder is usually unknown, but in some cases it results from overuse of *corticosteroid* creams in the treatment of other skin disorders. Rosacea affects about one in 500 people and is most common among middle-aged women.

Rosacea usually begins with temporary flushing, often after drinking a hot beverage or alcohol, eating spicy food, or entering a hot environment. It may then develop into permanent redness of the skin, sometimes accompanied by pustules resembling those of *acne*. In some elderly men, rosacea leads to *rhinophyma* (bulbous swelling of the nose).

TREATMENT
A lengthy course of the antibiotic drug *tetracycline* usually suppresses symptoms but does not cure the disorder. Rosacea tends to recur for five to 10 years and then disappears.

Roseola infantum
A common infectious disease that mainly affects children between the ages of six months and two years. Roseola infantum is probably caused by a virus and is characterized by the abrupt onset of irritability and fever. The temperature may rise as high as 40.5°C. However, on the fourth or fifth day, it drops suddenly back to normal. At about the same time, a rash appears on the trunk, often spreading quickly to the neck, face, and limbs. The rash rarely lasts longer than a day or two. Other symptoms may include a sore throat and enlargement of lymph nodes in the neck.

Occasionally, a child may have a febrile convulsion (see *Convulsion, febrile*) during the course of the fever, but the disease has no serious effects. The only specific treatment is to keep the child cool (by tepid sponging if necessary) and by giving *paracetamol* to reduce the fever.

Rotator cuff
A reinforcing structure around the shoulder joint composed of four muscle tendons that merge with the fibrous capsule enclosing the joint.

The rotator cuff may be torn as the result of a fall. A partial tear may cause *painful arc syndrome* (pain when the arm is lifted in a certain arc away from the body). A complete tear seriously limits the ability to raise the arm and, in cases of severe disability, may require surgical repair.

Roughage
See *Fibre, dietary*.

Roundworms
Also known as nematodes, a class of elongated, cylindrical worms. A dozen or so types are the main parasites of humans (the accompanying table summarizes the main ones). In many cases, the adult worms inhabit the human intestines, usually without causing symptoms unless there is a large number of worms. Sometimes, passage of worm larvae through various parts of the body is the main cause of symptoms. Most types of roundworm infestation are relatively easily treated with *anthelmintic drugs*.

In temperate areas, such as the UK, the only common type of roundworm disease is *threadworm infestation* (which mainly affects children). *Ascariasis*, *whipworm infestation*, *trichinosis*, and *toxocariasis* occasionally occur, although they often cause no symptoms. Some people return from abroad with *hookworm infestation*. In tropical countries, roundworm dis-

DISEASES CAUSED BY ROUNDWORMS (NEMATODES)

Disease	Adult length	Distribution	How acquired
Ascariasis (common roundworm)	15–38 cm	Worldwide	By swallowing worm eggs that have contaminated food or fingers
Enterobiasis (threadworm)	0.2–1.5 cm	Worldwide	By swallowing worm eggs that have contaminated fingers
Trichuriasis (whipworm)	2.5–5 cm	Worldwide	By swallowing worm eggs that have contaminated food or fingers
Ancylostomiasis (hookworm)	1.5 cm	Tropics	By penetration of skin of feet by worm larvae in soil
Strongyloidiasis	0.2 cm	Tropics	By penetration of skin of feet by worm larvae in soil
Toxocariasis	Several cm	Worldwide	By swallowing worm eggs from dirt or dog faeces
Trichinosis (porkworm)	0.1 cm	Worldwide	By eating undercooked pork containing encysted worm larvae
Filariasis	2–50 cm	Tropics	By mosquito and other insect bites

R

eases are much more common; they include those mentioned above and *strongyloidiasis, guinea worm disease,* and different types of filariasis. A diet containing raw fish may lead to infestation with the worms that cause anisakiasis or eustrongyloidiasis.

RSI
The abbreviation for *repetitive strain injury,* a type of *overuse injury.*

Rubber dam
A rubber sheet used to isolate one or more teeth during certain dental procedures. The dam acts as a barrier against saliva and prevents the inhalation of debris or small instruments. To fit a dam, the dentist punches small holes in the sheet for the teeth to protrude, and secures the sheet with clamps and a frame.

Rubefacient
A substance that causes redness of the skin by increasing blood flow to the area. Rubefacients are sometimes included in ointments used to relieve muscular aches and pains. They work by producing counter-irritation (i.e. they cause a less unpleasant sensation that diverts attention from the original pain). Methyl salicylate, menthol, camphor, and turpentine are all examples of rubefacients.

Rubella
A viral infection, also known as German measles (although the similarities with measles are few). Rubella causes a trivial illness in children and a slightly more troublesome one in adults. It is serious only when it affects a woman in the early months of pregnancy, when there is a chance that the virus will infect the fetus and cause any of a range of severe birth defects, known as rubella syndrome.

CAUSES AND INCIDENCE
Apart from mother-to-baby transmission, the rubella virus is spread from person to person in airborne droplets. Symptoms develop after an incubation period of two to three weeks.

Once common worldwide, rubella is now much less prevalent in most developed countries as a result of *immunization* programmes. Until 1988, vaccination against rubella in the UK was targeted at teenage girls and at women planning pregnancies. However, cases of rubella continued to occur in pregnancy (for example, 200 cases in pregnant women during 1986). In October 1988, a combined vaccine against measles, mumps, and

rubella (see *MMR vaccination*) was introduced for infants with the aim of eliminating all these disorders.

SYMPTOMS AND COMPLICATIONS
The infection usually occurs in children aged between six and 12, and is almost invariably mild. A rash appears on the face, spreads to the trunk and limbs, persists for a few days, then disappears. There may be a slight fever and enlargement of lymph nodes at the back of the neck. In some cases, the entire infection passes unnoticed. In adolescents and adults, there may be more marked symptoms, such as headache before the rash appears and a more pronounced fever. The virus may be transmitted to others from a few days before the symptoms appear until one day after they disappear. Polyarthritis (inflammation affecting several joints) is an occasional, short-lived complication, starting after the rash has faded.

CONGENITAL INFECTION
Rubella is a risk to the unborn baby only if the mother is infected during the first four months of pregnancy. The earlier in pregnancy that infection occurs, the more likely the infant is to be affected, and the more serious the abnormalities tend to be. In very early pregnancy, miscarriage may occur.

An affected infant may have one or many defects. The most common abnormalities, in order of frequency, are *deafness,* congenital *heart disease, mental handicap, cataract* and other eye disorders, *purpura, cerebral palsy,* and bone abnormalities. About 20 per cent of affected babies die in early infancy. An affected infant continues to harbour the virus and may infect others via his or her urine, faeces, and saliva for a year or more after birth.

DIAGNOSIS AND TREATMENT
Rubella is easily confused with other viral infections, *scarlet fever,* and *drug* reactions, which may produce similar symptoms. Rubella can be positively diagnosed only by laboratory isolation of the virus from a throat swab or by tests to look for *antibodies* to the virus in the blood. There is no specific treatment for rubella. *Paracetamol* can be given to reduce fever. Treatment of rubella syndrome depends on the particular defects present.

PREVENTION
Rubella vaccine provides effective, long-lasting immunity to the disease; it is now given in the MMR vaccine to all babies at about 15 months of age. Reactions to the vaccine are usually negligible. Rubella infection itself also provides immunity.

Any woman who may become pregnant and is unsure whether or not she has been immunized or has had rubella, should have her immune status checked. If she is not immune, vaccination should be performed.

A nonimmune pregnant woman must avoid contact with anyone who has rubella; if such contact occurs, she should immediately seek a doctor's advice. Passive immunization by *immunoglobulin injection* may help prevent infection of the fetus.

Rubeola
Another name for *measles.*

Running injuries
Disorders resulting from the effects on the body of jogging or running. Such injuries are common but most could be prevented by taking simple precautions. Running injuries most commonly affect the feet and legs.

TYPES
Common types of running injury include *tendinitis* (inflammation of a tendon); *stress fracture* of the tibia (shin), the fibula (the other long bone in the lower leg), or a bone in the foot; and plantar *fasciitis* (inflammation of tissue in the sole of the foot).

Sprinters commonly suffer from tearing of the *hamstring muscles* at the back of the thigh. Long-distance runners are more likely to suffer back pain due to jarring of the spine, tibial *compartment syndrome* (painful cramp in the lower leg caused by muscle compression), or *shin splints* (pain along the inner edge of the tibia).

PREVENTION
Shoes should fit snugly to provide stability but should not cramp the foot; insoles are needed to cushion the jarring force on the legs and spine. Shoes should not be allowed to become worn, because this can cause abnormal positioning of the foot during running, leading to foot strain.

Before running, warming-up exercises should be performed to reduce the risk of injury. Beginners should run short distances at first, and experienced runners should keep their running within sensible bounds. Running should be done in an upright posture, with trunk, neck, and arms relaxed. Long periods of running uphill, downhill, or along the side of a slope should be avoided as they increase stress on the ankle and knee.

Rupture
A common term for a *hernia,* especially an abdominal hernia.

R

S

Sac

A bag-like organ or body structure. For example, the amniotic sac is the thin, membranous, fluid-filled bag that surrounds the fetus.

Saccharin

An *artificial sweetener*.

Sacralgia

Pain in the *sacrum* (the triangular spinal bone below the lumbar *vertebrae*) caused by pressure on a spinal nerve in this area. Sacralgia is usually the result of a *disc prolapse*. In rare cases, it may be due to *bone cancer*. (See also *Back pain*.)

Sacralization

Fusion of the fifth (lowest) lumbar *vertebra* with the upper part of the *sacrum* (the triangular spinal bone below the lumbar vertebrae).

Sacralization may be present at birth, in which case it usually produces no symptoms and is discovered only when an X-ray of the back is taken for some other reason.

A surgical procedure to produce sacralization may be performed to treat a *disc prolapse*, or a condition called *spondylolisthesis*, in which a vertebra is displaced over the one below it. (See also *Spinal fusion*.)

Sacroiliac joint

One of a pair of rigid *joints* between each side of the *sacrum* (the triangular spinal bone below the lumbar *vertebrae*) and each *ilium* (the largest of the bones that form the outer walls of the *pelvis*). The bony surfaces within the joint are lined with cartilage and have a small amount of synovial fluid between them. Strong ligaments between the sacrum and ilium permit only minimal movement at the joint.

The sacroiliac joint may be strained, usually as a result of childbirth or of overstriding when running. Such strains produce pain in the lower back and buttocks. The sacroiliac joint may also become inflamed, a condition called *sacroiliitis*.

Sacroiliitis

Inflammation of a *sacroiliac joint* (one of a pair of joints between each side of the *sacrum* and each *ilium*).

Sacroiliitis can be caused by *ankylosing spondylitis, rheumatoid arthritis, Reiter's syndrome*, or the form of arthritis that occurs with *psoriasis*. In rare cases, sacroiliitis is caused by an infection spread through the bloodstream from elsewhere in the body.

The principal symptom of sacroiliitis is pain in the lower back, buttocks, groin, and back of the thigh. The pain may be accompanied by fever and malaise if the underlying cause is an infection. If the cause is ankylosing spondylitis, pain may be accompanied by stiffness in the back and hips, which is worse after rest and alleviated by exercise.

Sacroiliitis is diagnosed by *X-rays, blood tests*, and, sometimes, scans (see *bone imaging*). If infection is suspected, fluid may be removed from the joint and examined for microorganisms. Treatment is with *nonsteroidal anti-inflammatory drugs* or, if the joint is infected, with *antibiotic drugs*.

Sacrum

The large triangular bone in the lower *spine*. The sacrum's broad upper part articulates with the fifth (lowest) lumbar *vertebra*, and its narrow lower part with the *coccyx*. The sides of the sacrum are connected by the *sacroiliac*

STRUCTURE OF THE SACROILIAC JOINT
The joint forms an interface between the sacrum at the back of the pelvis and the ilium (hip-bone) on each side of the body.

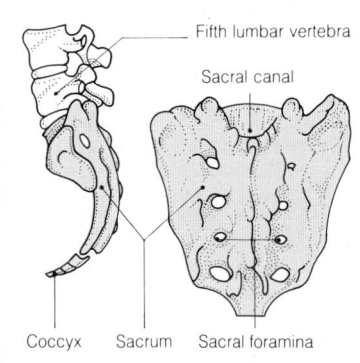

Ilium

Lumbar vertebrae

Sacroiliac ligaments

Sacroiliac joint

Sacrum

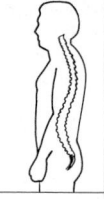

STRUCTURE OF THE SACRUM
The sacrum consists of five vertebrae (spinal bones) that are fused together to form a single solid structure.

Fifth lumbar vertebra

Sacral canal

Coccyx   Sacrum   Sacral foramina

---

joints to each ilium (the largest of the bones that form the *pelvis*). The sacrum thus sits like a wedge in the centre of the back of the pelvis.

DISORDERS
The sacrum is a strong bone and is only rarely fractured. If a fracture does occur, it is usually a result of a fall or of a powerful direct blow to the bone.

Other disorders affecting the sacrum include: *sacralgia* (pain in the sacrum, sometimes due to a *disc prolapse*); *spondylolisthesis*, in which the fifth lumbar vertebra slips over the sacrum; and *sacralization*, in which the sacrum is fused to the fifth lumbar vertebra. (See also *Bone* disorders box; *Spine* disorders box).

Sadism

Pleasure, particularly sexual pleasure, derived from the infliction of suffering or pain on others. Sadism often refers specifically to the attainment of *orgasm* through hurting, humiliating, or torturing someone else. The term is derived from the name of the French writer the Marquis de Sade.

Sadism is more common in men than in women and may be accompanied by *masochism* (a desire to be abused). Sadistic activities include beating, whipping, and tying a victim up, perhaps also with verbal abuse. Rape often has a sadistic basis, but the genuinely sadistic murderer is rare. It is very unusual for sadists to seek help from a psychiatrist. (See also *Sadomasochism*.)

Sadomasochism

Sexual arousal caused by inflicting pain (*sadism*) or by receiving abuse (*masochism*). Sadism and masochism may be combined in an individual, although one trait usually predominates. The sadomasochist is generally male and may practise other sexual *deviations*, such as *fetishism*.

Sadomasochistic literature is a common form of pornography. The practice of sadomasochism may be more widespread than is generally known; biting is a common sex practice. In a broad sense, any relationship in which there is one very dominant and one submissive partner can be said to have sadomasochistic elements.

SADS

The abbreviation for *seasonal affective disorder syndrome*.

Safe period

See *Contraception, natural methods of*.

Safer sex

A term used to describe preventive measures taken to reduce the risk of acquiring a sexually transmitted disease. Safer sex has been publicized recently because of the spread of *HIV* infection, but the same principles apply to reducing the risks of contracting other *sexually transmitted diseases* (STDs), such as *gonorrhoea*, genital herpes (see *Herpes, genital*), and hepatitis B (see *Hepatitis, viral*).

Sexual intercourse is completely safe only if you and your partner are monogamous (have not had sex with anyone else) and neither you nor your partner has an STD. To reduce the risk of acquiring *AIDS*, casual sex and sex with multiple partners should be avoided. People with a higher risk of carrying HIV include: intravenous drug abusers; homosexual and bisexual men; prostitutes; promiscuous men or women; people who received transfusions of blood products before the screening of blood for HIV was introduced (e.g. haemophiliacs); and people from areas where there is a very high incidence of HIV infection (e.g. Central Africa and Haiti).

Known methods of transmitting HIV include vaginal intercourse, anal intercourse, oral sex, sharing sex aids such as vibrators, and any sexual activity that causes bleeding in the vagina or anus. Sex during *menstruation* is particularly dangerous if the woman is a carrier. Any sexual practice that involves contact with urine or faeces also poses a risk.

The virus is thought not to be transmitted during dry kissing, cuddling, caressing, massage, or mutual masturbation (provided the skin is not broken and no semen is ejaculated into or on to the partner's body).

To reduce the risk of acquiring AIDS or any other sexually transmitted disease, a *condom* should be used. If a condom fails to prevent transmission, the cause is most likely to be incorrect use, although condoms do occasionally tear or split, especially during anal intercourse.

Saint Vitus' dance

An outdated term for the disorder now called *Sydenham's chorea*.

Salbutamol

A *bronchodilator drug* used in the treatment of *asthma*, chronic *bronchitis*, and *emphysema*. Because salbutamol also relaxes the muscles in the wall of the uterus, it is also occasionally used in the prevention of premature labour.

Salicylate drugs

A group of drugs with an anti-inflammatory, antipyretic (fever-reducing), and mild analgesic (painkilling) action. *Aspirin* (acetylsalicylic acid), *benorylate*, and *sodium salicylate* are examples of salicylate drugs.

Overdose of drugs in this group causes salicylate poisoning, characterized by hyperventilation (overbreathing), tinnitus (ringing in the ears), deafness, sweating, abnormal bleeding, biochemical disturbances, and, in severe cases, convulsions and coma.

Salicylic acid

A *keratolytic drug* (a drug that loosens and removes the tough outer layer of the skin). Salicylic acid is used to treat skin disorders, including *dermatitis, eczema, psoriasis, dandruff, ichthyosis, acne, warts,* and callosities (see *Callus, skin*). Salicylic acid is also sometimes used to treat *fungal infections*.

Salicyclic acid may cause inflammation and skin *ulcers* if used over a long period or applied to a large area.

Saline

A term meaning salty, or referring to a solution of salt (sodium chloride). Solutions with the same concentration of salt as body fluids are known as normal, or physiological, saline.

HOW TO USE A CONDOM

Using a condom is not a guarantee against transmission of HIV (the AIDS virus) or other sexually transmitted disease, but it does reduce the risks. Whether a condom is used to prevent disease transmission or to prevent conception, it should be used in conjunction with a spermicide preparation.

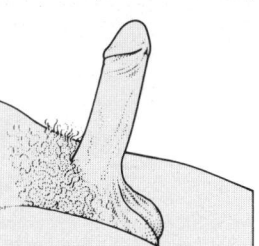 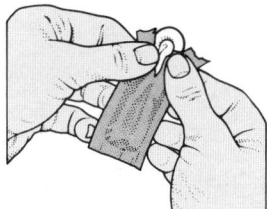 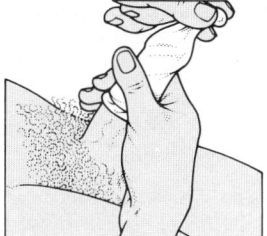 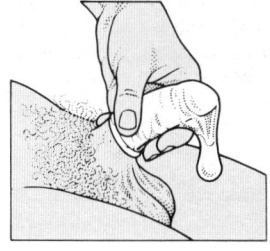

1 The penis should be fully erect before the condom is put on. The condom should be in place before any vaginal or anal penetration by the penis and before oral sex.

2 Use a brand of condom that conforms to British Standards. Do not use one that has no teat, is beyond its "use by" date, or appears to be defective.

3 The teat-end should be squeezed free of air and the condom unrolled fully over the penis. Do not stretch the condom tightly; a tight condom is more likely to burst.

4 The penis should be withdrawn soon after ejaculation. During withdrawal, the base of the condom should be held to prevent spilling the semen.

Normal saline may be given in large amounts by *intravenous infusion* to replace body fluids in cases of dehydration; it is sometimes used in small quantities to dissolve drugs for injection. Normal saline is included in contact lens solutions, which have a close resemblance to natural tears.

Saliva

The watery, slightly alkaline fluid secreted into the mouth by the *salivary glands* and the *mucous membranes* that line the mouth.

Saliva contains the digestive enzyme amylase, which helps break down carbohydrates (see *Digestive system*). Saliva also keeps the mouth moist, lubricates food to aid swallowing, and makes it possible to taste food (taste-buds are stimulated only by dissolved substances).

In addition to amylase, saliva contains minerals (such as sodium, potassium, and calcium), various proteins, mucin (the principal constituent of mucus), urea, white blood cells, and debris from the lining of the mouth.

Salivary glands

Three pairs of glands that secrete *saliva*, via ducts, into the mouth.

The largest pair, the *parotid glands*, lie over the angle of the jaw on each side, just below and in front of the ears; the ducts of these glands run forwards and inwards to open inside the cheeks.

The sublingual glands are situated in the floor of the front of the mouth, where they form a low ridge on each side of the frenulum (the central band of tissue that attaches the underside of the tongue to the floor of the mouth). This ridge has a row of small openings through which saliva is secreted.

The submandibular glands lie towards the back of the mouth close to the sides of the jaw. Their ducts run forwards to open under the tongue on two small swellings, one on each side of the frenulum.

DISORDERS

Among the most common salivary gland disorders is infection of the parotid glands with the *mumps* virus. Another important disorder is the formation of *calculi* (stones) in a duct or within the substance of a gland. A stone in a duct causes a swelling that enlarges during eating because of damming of the flow of saliva; it may also be painful. Surgical removal of a stone in a duct is straightforward, but a stone in a gland itself may necessitate removal of the entire gland.

ANATOMY OF THE SALIVARY GLANDS

Each gland consists of thousands of saliva-secreting sacs. Tiny ducts carry the saliva into the main ducts leading to the mouth.

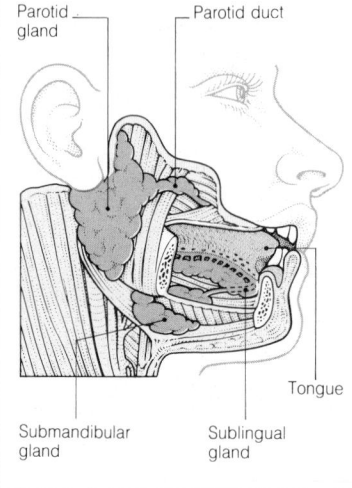

Parotid gland
Parotid duct
Tongue
Submandibular gland
Sublingual gland

Occasionally, the parotid glands are affected by *sarcoidosis*, which may cause considerable swelling. In rare cases, sarcoidosis also affects the facial nerve lying near the gland, which may result in *facial palsy*.

If *oral hygiene* is poor, the salivary glands may become infected by bacteria spreading from the mouth, which can lead to the development of an abscess in the affected glands.

Tumours of the salivary glands are rare, except for a type of parotid tumour which is usually slow-growing, painless, and benign (but which may rarely become malignant).

Insufficient secretion of saliva, causing a dry mouth (see *Mouth, dry*), may result from *dehydration* or *Sjögren's syndrome*. Certain drugs also decrease salivation as a side-effect. (See also *Salivation, excessive*.)

Salivation, excessive

The production of too much *saliva*, sometimes known as ptyalism. Excessive salivation sometimes occurs during pregnancy. It also occurs in a wide variety of disorders.

Excessive salivation commonly occurs in conditions affecting the mouth, including irritation of the inside of the mouth (caused by jagged teeth or ill-fitting *dentures*), dental caries, toothache, gingivitis (inflammation of the gums), *mouth ulcers*, or any

type of painful mouth injury. Digestive tract disorders, such as *oesophagitis* (inflammation of the oesophagus) and *peptic ulcer*, are other possible causes of this symptom.

Excessive salivation may also be caused by a variety of conditions affecting the nervous system, such as *Parkinson's disease, rabies, mercury poisoning*, and overactivity of the parasympathetic division of the *autonomic nervous system* (which controls the salivary glands), usually due to disease or drugs.

In some cases, excessive salivation can be relieved by *anticholinergic drugs*.

Salmonella infections

Infections caused by any of the SALMONELLA group of bacteria. One type of salmonella causes *typhoid fever*; others commonly cause bacterial *food poisoning*. Infants, the elderly, and people who are debilitated are the most likely to be affected.

Reported cases of food poisoning due to salmonella infection increased dramatically in the UK during the 1980s. In many cases, the source of infection was traced to poultry products, particularly hen's eggs and chicken meat. Infection of eggs can originate in the hen's ovaries or may occur as a result of faecal contamination via the egg shell.

SYMPTOMS

Symptoms of salmonella food poisoning usually develop suddenly about 12 to 24 hours after infection. Typical symptoms are malaise, headache, nausea, abdominal pain, diarrhoea, and sometimes shivering and fever. In most cases, symptoms last only two or three days, but may persist longer. *Dehydration* or *septicaemia* (blood poisoning) may occur especially in the very young and old.

DIAGNOSIS AND TREATMENT

Diagnosis is confirmed by isolation of the causative organism in laboratory tests.

Treatment consists mainly of *rehydration therapy* to replace lost fluids. No solid food should be eaten during the first 24 hours of the illness. In severe cases and in babies, fluid replacement by *intravenous infusion* may be necessary. Salmonella food poisoning is treated with *antibiotic drugs* only if the infection has spread into the bloodstream.

PREVENTION

General food hygiene practices should be observed (see *Food poisoning*). People who have had salmonella food poisoning should take particular care with personal hygiene because they may continue to excrete salmonella bacteria in their faeces for as long as six months after infection.

In general, it is advisable to avoid foods that contain raw egg (such as home-made mayonnaise, mousses, and ice cream) that might possibly be contaminated. Salmonella organisms are not killed by light cooking, and eggs should therefore always be well-cooked.

Salpingectomy

Surgical removal of one or both *fallopian tubes*. Salpingectomy may be performed if the tube has become infected (see *Salpingitis*), as a method of contraception (see *Sterilization, female*), or to treat an *ectopic pregnancy*. (See also *Salpingo-oophorectomy*.)

Salpingitis

Inflammation of a *fallopian tube* (the tube from an ovary to the top of the uterus), commonly caused by infection spreading upwards from the vagina, cervix, or uterus. Salpingitis is one feature of *pelvic inflammatory disease*, a general term for inflammation of the internal female pelvic organs.

CAUSES AND INCIDENCE

Salpingitis may be a result of a *chlamydial infection* or a bacterial infection, especially *gonorrhoea*. Although salpingitis usually results from a sexually transmitted disease, it may also follow childbirth, miscarriage, or induced abortion. Other causes include *peritonitis* (inflammation of the abdominal lining), or, rarely, a blood-borne infection, such as *tuberculosis.*

SYMPTOMS AND SIGNS

Symptoms and signs include severe abdominal pain, and fever. The abdomen is very tender and the sufferer is usually most comfortable lying on her back with her legs bent. Vaginal examination is painful.

DIAGNOSIS

The presence of infection may be confirmed by a blood test showing a high number of white blood cells. A culture of a swab sample of the vaginal discharge allows identification of the causative microorganism. *Laparoscopy* (examination of the inside of the abdominal cavity with a viewing instrument) may be performed to confirm the diagnosis and to exclude the possibility of *ectopic pregnancy* or *appendicitis,* which can cause similar symptoms.

COMPLICATIONS

Pus may collect within the fallopian tube itself (a condition known as pyo-

salpinx), sometimes followed by the collection of fluid within the tube (a condition known as hydrosalpinx). A pelvic *abscess* (a collection of pus within the pelvic cavity) sometimes develops.

Occasionally, salpingitis persists despite treatment and causes a variety of symptoms, for example persistent back pain that is worse before menstruation, frequent heavy periods, and pain during intercourse. If the infection damages the inside of the fallopian tubes, ova may be unable to pass the blockage, resulting in *infertility* or an increased risk of an ectopic pregnancy.

TREATMENT

Treatment includes bed rest, fluids, *analgesic drugs* (painkillers), and *antibiotic drugs*. Surgery is performed to drain a pyosalpinx, hydrosalpinx, or pelvic abscess. If infection persists despite treatment with antibiotics, the damaged tubes may be removed, sometimes with the uterus and most of the ovary. (See also *Salpingectomy; Salpingo-oophorectomy*.)

Salpingo-oophorectomy

Removal of one or both *fallopian tubes* and *ovaries*. Salpingo-oophorectomy may be performed to treat persistent *salpingitis* (inflammation of the fallopian tubes) or certain types of benign *ovarian cyst*. It may also be performed together with a *hysterectomy* (removal of the uterus) to treat cancer of the ovary (see *Ovary, cancer of*) or cancer of the uterus (see *Uterus, cancer of*).

Salpingo-oophorectomy is carried out under a general anaesthetic. Removal of the fallopian tube or tubes is a brief, straightforward procedure and the recovery period is short and usually problem-free.

Salt

Any compound of an acid and a base. Popularly, the term usually refers specifically to one such compound: common table salt, known chemically as sodium chloride (see *Sodium*). The term salt may also be applied to any chemical salt or to a mixture of salts used medicinally, such as magnesium sulphate. (See also *Saline*.)

Salve

A term for a healing, soothing, often medicated ointment.

Sandfly bites

Bites of sandflies, which are small delicate, long-legged flies, about 3 mm long, found in most warm parts of the

world. Sandflies can breed in a variety of habitats, including sand, forests, and city rubble.

In some parts of the world, sandflies are harmless, but in other regions sandfly bites can transmit disease to humans. In tropical and subtropical regions sandfly bites may transmit various forms of *leishmaniasis*. In parts of the Mediterranean and Asia, they may transmit the virus responsible for sandfly fever, an influenza-like illness of short duration. In the western Andes, sandfly bites may transmit bartonellosis, causing either joint pain and fever, or a rash, depending on the form of the disease.

Sandflies bite mainly after dusk. In areas where they are numerous, the best protection is to use insect repellents and to wear clothing that covers the arms and legs and is snug at the wrists and ankles (see *Insect bites*).

Sanitary protection

Articles used to protect clothing from bloodstains during *menstruation*. Disposable sanitary napkins or tampons are available in different absorbencies to meet individual needs.

Sarcoidosis

A rare disease of unknown cause in which there is inflammation of tissues throughout the body, especially in the lymph nodes, lungs, skin, eyes, and liver. The disorder occurs mainly in young adults.

SYMPTOMS AND SIGNS

Sarcoidosis may cause a variety of symptoms, including fever, generalized aches, painful joints, arthritis, and painful and bloodshot eyes. Sarcoidosis may also cause enlargement of lymph nodes in the neck and elsewhere, breathlessness, *erythema nodosum* (purplish swellings on the legs), a purplish rash on the face, and areas of numbness. In some cases, there are no symptoms.

Possible complications include *hypercalcaemia* (an abnormally high calcium level in the blood), which may damage the kidneys, and *pulmonary fibrosis* (scarring and thickening of the lung tissues).

DIAGNOSIS AND TREATMENT

A diagnosis may be suggested by a *chest X-ray* that shows enlarged lymph nodes or diffuse shadowing, and by the characteristic rash. A biopsy of the lung, skin, lymph nodes, or liver confirms the diagnosis.

In many cases, no treatment is required. About 90 per cent of patients recover completely within two years,

S

with or without treatment, but the remaining 10 per cent develop a persistent, chronic form of the disease.

Corticosteroid drugs are prescribed to treat persistent fever or persistent erythema nodosum, to prevent blindness in an affected eye, and to reduce the risk of permanent lung damage. *Chloroquine* is sometimes used to treat skin abnormalities.

Sarcoma

A cancer of *connective tissue* (material that surrounds body structures and holds them together).

Types of sarcoma include *osteosarcoma* (arising in bone), *chondrosarcoma* (arising in cartilage), *Kaposi's sarcoma* (which mainly affects the skin and is common in people who have *AIDS*), and *fibrosarcoma*.

Saturated fats

See *Fats and oils*; *Nutrition*.

Scab

A crust that forms on the skin or on a mucous membrane at the site of a healing wound or infected area. A scab is composed of fibrin (a blood protein involved in clotting) and serum (the fluid part of blood) that has leaked from the wound and dried, along with skin scales, pus, and other debris. A similar term is eschar, used in relation to burns.

Scabies

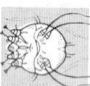 A skin infestation caused by the mite *SARCOPTES SCABIEI*, which burrows into the skin, where it lays eggs. Scabies is highly contagious during close physical contact. The disorder is most common in infants, children, young adults, or in people who are institutionalized.

SYMPTOMS

The mite's burrows can be seen on the skin as tiny, grey, scaly swellings, usually between the fingers, on the wrists and genitals, and in the armpits. Later, reddish lumps may appear on the limbs and trunk. The infestation causes intense itching, particularly at night, and scratching results in the formation of scabs and sores.

TREATMENT

The condition is treated by applying an insecticide lotion, such as *lindane* (also called gamma benzene hexachloride) to all skin below the sufferer's head. The lotion usually kills the mites, but itching may persist for up to two weeks. All sexual contacts and all members of the affected

person's household (even if they show no signs of infestation) should be treated simultaneously.

Scald

A *burn* caused by hot liquid or steam.

Scaling, dental

Removal of dental *calculus* (a hard, chalky deposit) from the teeth, performed to prevent or treat *periodontal disease* (disorders of the gums and other tissues supporting the teeth).

Scaling is carried out with an instrument called a scaler. This may have a sharp, scraping edge or be an ultrasonic model with a tip that vibrates at high speed to chip away the deposit. After scaling, the teeth are usually polished with a mild abrasive paste and motorized buffers.

Scalp

The skin of the head, and its underlying tissue layers, that is normally covered with hair.

Scalp skin differs from other areas of skin in several ways: it is tougher than other skin, and is attached to an underlying sheet of muscle (called the epicranius) that extends from the eyebrows, over the top of the head, to the nape of the neck. This muscle sheet is only loosely attached to the skull, making it comparatively easy for areas of scalp to be torn off (e.g. as a result of catching the hair in machinery). Because the scalp is richly supplied with blood vessels, scalp wounds bleed profusely.

The scalp may be affected by a variety of hair or skin disorders. The most common are *dandruff*; hair loss, particularly in men (see *Alopecia*); *sebaceous cysts*; *psoriasis*; fungal infections, such as ringworm (see *Tinea*); and parasitic infestations, such as *lice*. *Cradle cap*, a harmless form of seborrhoeic *dermatitis* in which greasy, crusty patches appear on the scalp, is common in infants.

Scalpel

A surgical knife for cutting tissue. Scalpels with steel blades are most commonly used, but sharper, diamond or ruby blades are used for some types of surgery, such as for some eye operations.

Scanning techniques

Methods of producing images of body organs by techniques that record, process, and analyse sound waves, radio waves, or X-rays that pass through or are generated by body tissues.

The most widely used scanning technique in medicine is *ultrasound scanning*, in which inaudible, ultra-high-frequency sound waves are passed into the region being examined. These sound waves are reflected more strongly by some structures than others, and the pattern of reflections is detected by one or more transducers and displayed on a screen. Ultrasound was originally developed for the detection of submarines beneath the sea. However, in the past 20 years it has been refined and developed to examine the developing fetus and also the heart, liver, kidney, and other organs.

CT scanning uses X-rays to measure variations in the density of the organ being examined; it compiles an image or picture by computer analysis.

Radionuclide scanning involves the injection into the body of radioactive substances which are taken up in different amounts by different organs. Radioactive iodine, for example, becomes concentrated in the thyroid gland. A radioactivity detector, such as a gamma camera, is positioned near the organ under study, and the pattern of radiation being emitted is recorded and displayed on a screen.

MRI (magnetic resonance imaging) uses a powerful electromagnet to align the nuclei of atoms of hydrogen, phosphorus, or other elements in the body. The nuclei are then knocked out of position by radio waves; in realigning themselves with the magnetic field, the nuclei produce a radio signal that can be detected and transformed into a computer-generated image.

PET scanning (positron emission tomography) is based on the detection of positively-charged particles that are emitted by radioactively labelled substances introduced into the body. A computer is used to build up a three-dimensional image that reflects the chemical activity of the tissue that is being studied.

Scaphoid

One of the *wrist* bones. The scaphoid is the outermost bone on the thumb side of the hand in the proximal row of carpals (the row of wrist bones nearest the elbow).

A fracture of the scaphoid is one of the most common wrist injuries, usually occurring as a result of a fall on an outstretched hand. A characteristic symptom of this injury is tenderness in the space between the two prominent tendons at the base of the thumb on the back of the hand. This symp-

S

tom may be a more positive indication of a scaphoid fracture than an X-ray. Treatment consists of immobilizing the wrist in a *cast.*

An undiagnosed, untreated scaphoid fracture may not heal, which can lead to *osteoarthritis* or, in some cases, to necrosis (death) of part of the bone. These complications may result in persistent pain in the wrist and restriction of its movement.

Scapula
The anatomical name for the shoulderblade. The scapula is a flat, triangular bone situated over the back of the upper ribs. On its rear surface is a prominent spine (which can be felt under the skin) that runs diagonally upwards and outwards to a bony prominence (called the acromion) at the shoulder tip. The acromion articulates with the end of the *clavicle* (collarbone) to form the *acromioclavicular joint.* Just below the acromion is a socket (called the glenoid cavity) into which the head of the humerus (upper-arm bone) fits to form the shoulder joint.

The scapula serves as an attachment for certain muscles and tendons of the arm, neck, chest, and back, and is involved with movements of the arm and shoulder.

Because the scapula is well padded with muscle, great force is required to fracture it. Treatment of a fracture consists of putting the shoulder in a *sling* until the fracture has healed. *Physiotherapy* may be needed to restore movement to the joint.

Scar
Any mark left on damaged tissue after it has healed. Scar tissue forms not only on the skin but on all internal wounds—for example, after a muscle tear or at sites where surgery has been performed.

The body repairs a wound, ulcer, or other lesion by increasing the production of the tough, fibrous protein *collagen* at the site of the damage. This helps form new *connective tissue,* which covers the area of the lesion. If the edges of an incision are brought together when healing takes place, the resultant scar is narrow and pale; if the edges are left apart, the scar is more extensive (see *Healing*).

ABNORMAL SCARS
The term hypertrophic scar is used to describe a large, unsightly scar that sometimes develops at the site of an infected wound. Some people have a family tendency to develop hypertrophic scars for no apparent reason.

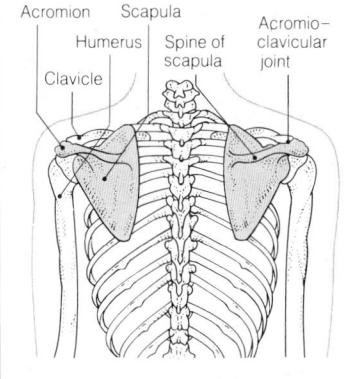

LOCATION OF THE SCAPULAE
The two scapulae are the prominent wing-shaped bones in the upper back. They facilitate many arm and shoulder actions.

Acromion Scapula
Humerus   Spine of   Acromio-
          scapula   clavicular
Clavicle   joint

A *keloid* is a large, irregularly shaped scar that continues to grow in size as the body continues to produce extra collagen after a wound has healed; this type of scar is more common in black people than in white people.

Adhesions are areas of scar tissue that form between unconnected parts of internal organs; they are a potential complication of intestinal surgery.

Scarlatina
Another name for *scarlet fever.*

Scarlet fever
An infectious disease, more common in childhood, that is caused by a strain of streptococcal bacteria. Characterized by a sore throat, fever, and rash, scarlet fever is far less common and far less dangerous than formerly. About 5,000 cases are notified each year in England and Wales.

CAUSES AND SYMPTOMS
The bacteria are spread in droplets coughed or breathed into the air. After an incubation period of usually two to four but sometimes up to seven days, a sore throat, headache, and fever develop. A rash soon appears, caused by a *toxin* released by the bacteria. The rash begins as a mass of tiny red spots on the neck and upper trunk and spreads rapidly. The face is flushed (except for an area around the mouth) and a white coating with red spots may develop on the tongue (called "strawberry tongue"). After a few days this coating comes off to reveal a bright red appearance. Soon afterwards, the fever subsides, the

rash fades, and there is frequently some skin peeling, especially on the hands and feet.

As with other types of sore throat caused by streptococci (see *Strep throat*), there is a risk of *rheumatic fever* or *glomerulonephritis* (inflammation of the filtering units in the kidneys) if the infection is not treated promptly.

DIAGNOSIS AND TREATMENT
The doctor diagnoses scarlet fever from the symptoms and signs and, if necessary, by *culture* of the bacteria from a throat swab.

Treatment is with *antibiotic drugs,* usually penicillin (or erythromycin if the patient is allergic to penicillin). Treatment usually leads to a rapid recovery. During the illness, the patient should rest, drink plenty of fluids, and be given *paracetamol* to relieve discomfort and reduce fever. Some doctors take throat swabs from contacts (such as members of the family) to exclude infection, or may give them a short course of penicillin.

Schistosome
 A type of fluke (flattened worm). Three types of schistosomes are parasites of humans, causing different forms of the tropical disease *schistosomiasis.*

Schistosomiasis
A parasitic disease, also known as bilharzia, that occurs in most tropical countries and afflicts over 200 million people worldwide.

CAUSES AND INCIDENCE
The disease is caused by any of three species of flukes called schistosomes and is acquired from bathing or wading in infested lakes, rivers, and irrigation systems. Forms of schistosome (cercariae) can penetrate the bather's skin and develop within the body into adult flukes (see life-cycle diagram overleaf). Eggs produced by the adult females provoke inflammatory reactions, which in turn may cause symptoms.

The infestation causes bleeding, ulceration, and *fibrosis* (scar tissue formation) in the bladder or intestinal walls; infestation may also cause inflammation and fibrosis in other organs, such as the liver.

SYMPTOMS
Symptoms vary considerably. Some infested people have no symptoms, others become severely ill and suffer serious complications.

The first symptom is usually tingling and an itchy rash where the cercariae have penetrated the skin. Many weeks later, when the adults start producing eggs, an influenza-like illness may develop. Sometimes severe, the illness is marked by high fever, chills, aching, and pains. Subsequent symptoms may include blood in the urine or faeces, abdominal or low back pain, and enlargement of the liver or spleen or both.

Complications of long-term infestation with the schistosome parasite may include liver *cirrhosis*, *bladder tumours*, and *kidney failure*.

DIAGNOSIS AND TREATMENT
The diagnosis is made from a special blood test for *antibodies* to the parasites, and from microscopic examination of a sample of urine or faeces to detect the presence of eggs.

Since the early 1980s, the treatment of schistosomiasis has been revolutionized by use of *praziquantel*, a single dose of which kills the flukes and thus prevents, or limits, damage to internal organs.

PREVENTION
Since no vaccine is available against the disease, visitors to areas where schistosomiasis is present (i.e. much of the tropics) should avoid wading or bathing in any lake, river, or irrigation system.

Control of the disease rests on the provision and use of latrines to avoid contamination of inland water. The Chinese and others have achieved some success through measures directed towards eradicating freshwater snails and through imposing strict sanitary regulations.

Schizoid personality disorder
Inability to relate socially to other people. People with this trait, which is apparent from childhood, are often described as "loners" and have few, if any, friends. They are markedly eccentric, seem to lack warmth or concern for others, and may be vague and apparently detached from normal day-to-day activities.

Schizophrenia develops in about 10 per cent of people who are diagnosed as having a schizoid personality. However, not all people with schizophrenia initially have schizoid personalities. Although the social and employment prospects for schizoid people are severely impaired, some people with schizoid personality disorder do succeed in socially isolated occupations.

Schizophrenia
A general term for a group of psychotic illnesses characterized by disturbances in thinking, emotional reaction, and behaviour. Schizophrenia is sometimes referred to as "split personality" because the sufferer's thoughts and feelings do not relate to each other in a logical fashion. However, the disorder should not be confused with *multiple personality*. Schizophrenia is a disabling illness with a prolonged course that almost always results in chronic ill health and some degree of personality change.

PREVALENCE
Schizophrenia is the most common form of psychotic illness, with a markedly consistent prevalence rate throughout the world of just under one per cent. For reasons that are not understood, schizophrenia is more common in certain geographical areas and in inner-city populations. Onset is usually between the ages of 15 and 30, being, on average, five years later in females than in males; otherwise, the sexes are affected equally.

CAUSES
Inheritance has been shown to play a role in the development of schizophrenia. First-degree relatives (i.e. parents, children, or siblings) of people with schizophrenia have a 10 per cent chance of the illness; more distant relatives have a lower risk. If a person has two parents with schizophrenia or an identical twin with the disorder, he or she has an approximately one in two chance of developing schizophrenia. However, factors other than genetics must also play a part or schizophrenia would inevitably develop in both twins.

Biological studies have shown that certain brain disorders, such as *temporal lobe epilepsy*, *brain tumours*, and *encephalitis*, tend to be related to schizophrenic symptoms. Brain imaging techniques, especially *CT scanning* and *PET scanning*, have revealed abnormalities of structure and function in the brains of people suffering from schizophrenia. It has also been demonstrated that certain drugs, such as *amphetamine drugs*, can cause a schizophrenic illness, and that drugs that block the action of *dopamine* often relieve schizophrenic symptoms.

It seems likely that schizophrenia is possibly worsened by stress in the individual's personal life.

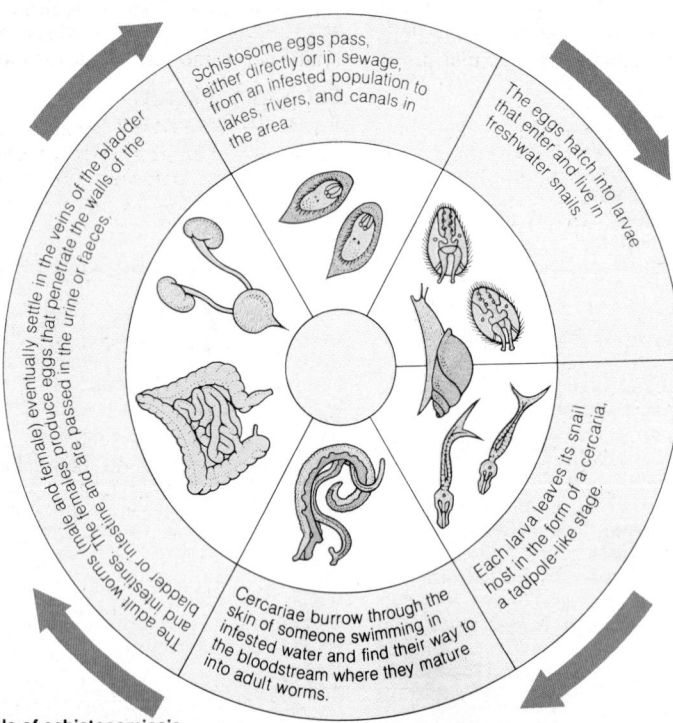

Schistosome eggs pass, either directly or in sewage, from an infested population to lakes, rivers, and canals in the area.

The eggs hatch into larvae that enter and live in freshwater snails.

Each larva leaves its snail host in the form of a cercaria, a tadpole-like stage.

Cercariae burrow through the skin of someone swimming in infested water and find their way to the bloodstream where they mature into adult worms.

The adult worms (male and female) eventually settle in the veins of the bladder and intestines. The females then produce eggs that penetrate the walls of the bladder or intestine and are passed in the urine or faeces.

Cycle of schistosomiasis
The disease affects a large proportion of the population in some parts of the world, such as the Nile valley in Egypt. Many methods have been tried to break the cycle of the disease in affected areas, with varying success. Methods used have included strict sanitary regulations and measures to eradicate freshwater snails.

S

SYMPTOMS

Schizophrenia may begin insidiously, with the individual becoming slowly more withdrawn and introverted, and losing his or her drive and motivation. The change may not be noticed for months or years, until it becomes apparent that the individual is suffering from *delusions* (false ideas that do not respond to reasoned argument) or *hallucinations* (a sensory experience in the absence of an external stimulus). In other cases, the illness comes on more suddenly, usually in response to some external stress.

Delusions may take a variety of forms, ranging from single ideas, such as the belief that one is Jesus Christ or Napoleon, to elaborate delusional systems in which special significance is attached to everyday objects or events. In paranoid schizophrenia, the illness is dominated by delusions of grandeur, persecution, or jealousy.

Hallucinations frequently are experienced as voices that comment on behaviour or thoughts, occasionally in the form of conversations in which the sufferer is referred to as he or she. This type of auditory third person hallucination occurs exclusively in schizophrenia. True visual hallucinations are rare in Western cultures, but distortions of visual perception do occur; faces or objects may look sharper or change shape. Bodily sensations, such as tingling, are common.

Most schizophrenics also suffer from a variety of thought disorders, which impair concentration or clear thinking. Sufferers describe their thoughts as being blocked or inserted into or withdrawn from their minds by some outside force. They may also feel that their thoughts are being broadcast to others.

Disordered thinking is reflected in muddled and disjointed speech. Disturbance of association results in the schizophrenic jumping from one subject to another, seemingly unrelated, one. Inability to think in abstractions often leads to bizarre responses to questions. For example, when a girl was asked why she was turning in a circle, she said she felt she was in a knot and was trying to unravel herself. In some cases, speech disintegrates, becoming a "word salad" of odd phrases, *neologisms* (made-up words), and detached syllables.

In a rare form of schizophrenia, catatonia may occur. Sufferers of catatonic schizophrenia adopt prolonged rigid postures or engage in outbursts of repeated movement.

Symptoms of *manic-depressive illness* may accompany schizophrenia, especially in the early stages. However, as the illness progresses, emotions usually become severely blunted, there is increasing detachment from other people, and there is a loss of interest in hobbies or occupations. Behaviour becomes more eccentric and self-neglect is common.

DIAGNOSIS

For a diagnosis of schizophrenia to be made, the individual must have continuous signs of a profound break with reality and evidence of fragmentation (disorganization) of the personality for at least six months during some time in his or her life. This six-month period must include at least one phase when there are symptoms of hallucinations, delusions, or marked thought disorders.

TREATMENT

The main form of treatment consists of *antipsychotic drugs,* such as *haloperidol,* which reduce the symptoms and make the person more amenable to *psychotherapy.* Some antipsychotic drugs can be given as long-acting *depot injections.* Drug treatment is effective in suppressing the more obvious symptoms of schizophrenia, such as hallucinations, but may result in side-effects, particularly *dyskinesia* (abnormal muscular movements) and tremor.

Schizophrenics may be treated initially in hospital; once the major symptoms are controlled, most sufferers return to the community. Adequate provision of day centres, suitable housing, and vocational opportunities can help to control symptoms, to improve the sufferer's self-reliance, to prevent relapse, and to reduce the stigma attached to mental illness. If the patient is to live at home, the family needs to be provided with support and guidance, since some schizophrenics may be difficult to live with. A certain number relapse, especially if they do not take their medication regularly.

OUTLOOK

Although some 10 per cent of the people who develop schizophrenia remain severely impaired for life, the majority can return to varying degrees of independence. About 30 per cent will return to normal lives and occupations.

The particular form of the illness is important in determining the outlook. Individuals who have schizophrenia combined with manic-depressive symptoms often recover fully, as do many with catatonia. Paranoid schizophrenics, because of the preservation of their personalities, are often able to function well, albeit as somewhat eccentric members of the community. Schizophrenia that comes on slowly, starting around puberty, often causes significant impairment.

Although drugs have improved the outlook for most schizophrenics, inadequate community care frequently results in relapse, neglect, vagrancy, or imprisonment.

Sciatica

Pain that radiates along the *sciatic nerve.* The pain usually affects the buttock and thigh, but sometimes extends down the leg to the foot. In severe cases, the pain may be accompanied by numbness and/or weakness in the affected area.

CAUSES

The most common cause of sciatica is a prolapsed intervertebral disc pressing on a spinal root of the nerve (see *Disc prolapse*). Less commonly, it may be caused by pressure on the nerve from a tumour, abscess, or blood clot, from local muscle spasm, or simply from sitting in an awkward position. Any disorder that involves nerves (such as certain infections, *diabetes mellitus,* or *alcohol dependence*) may affect the sciatic nerve and lead to the development of sciatica.

TREATMENT AND OUTLOOK

Treatment is directed towards the underlying cause, but in many cases the cause is not identified. Thus, treatment consists of measures to relieve the pain, including taking *analgesic drugs* (painkillers) and resting in bed. With such treatment, the pain usually disappears within a few days. In severe cases of sciatica, the pain may persist for several weeks. The condition tends to recur.

S

Sciatic nerve

The main nerve in each leg and the largest nerve in the body. Each sciatic nerve is a branch of the sacral plexus (nerve network) in the pelvis, and is formed from several lumbar and sacral *spinal nerves*. From the sacral plexus, the sciatic nerve passes below the sacroiliac joint (at the back of the pelvis, near the sacrum) and backwards to the buttock, from where it passes behind the hip joint and runs down the back of the thigh. Above the back of the knee, the sciatic nerve divides into two main branches, known as the tibial nerve and the common peroneal nerve.

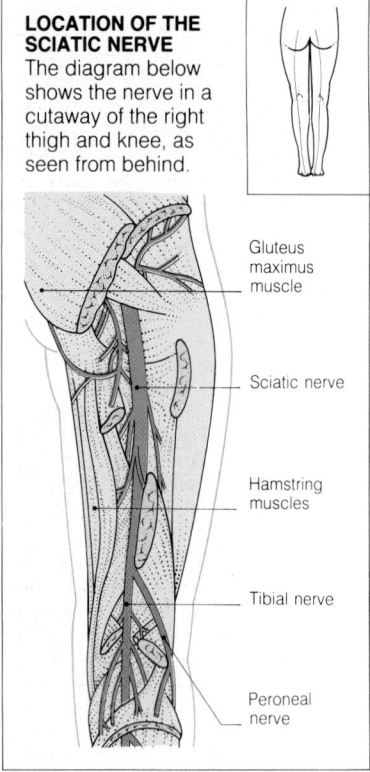

LOCATION OF THE SCIATIC NERVE

The diagram below shows the nerve in a cutaway of the right thigh and knee, as seen from behind.

Gluteus maximus muscle

Sciatic nerve

Hamstring muscles

Tibial nerve

Peroneal nerve

The sciatic nerve supplies the hip joint, many of the thigh muscles, and the skin on the back of the thigh. The tibial and peroneal branches supply the knee and ankle joints, all the muscles of the lower leg and foot, and most of the skin below the knee.

DISORDERS

Probably the most common disorder of the sciatic nerve is *sciatica*, which is often caused by a prolapsed intervertebral disc pressing on a spinal root of the nerve (see *Disc prolapse*). The upper part of the nerve may also be damaged by dislocation of the hip joint, which, in severe cases, may result in paralysis of muscles below the knee and widespread numbness of the skin in that part of the body.

Damage to the peroneal nerve, often due to a fracture of the upper *fibula* (the outer bone of the lower leg), may produce *foot-drop* and numbness of the skin at the side of the lower leg and back of the foot.

The tibial nerve is deeply buried in body tissues and is thus rarely injured. However, this nerve is sometimes damaged by dislocation of the knee, which may cause paralysis of the lower leg and foot, and numbness in the sole of the foot.

Scintigraphy

A less common, alternative name for *radionuclide scanning*.

Scirrhous

A medical term meaning hard and fibrous. The word is usually applied to malignant tumours that have dense, fibrous tissue within them.

Sclera

The white outer coat of the *eye*, visible through the transparent *conjunctiva*. The sclera is composed of dense, fibrous tissue formed from *collagen*, which is strong and protects the inner structures of the eye from injury. The sclera may, however, be penetrated by sharp objects.

Disease of the sclera is uncommon, but *scleritis* (inflammation of the sclera) may occur, usually with a *collagen disease*, such as *rheumatoid arthritis*. The healthy sclera sometimes shows a blue tinge from the underlying *choroid*. If the sclera is exceptionally thin, which occurs in *osteogenesis imperfecta*, this blue appearance is pronounced.

Scleritis

Inflammation of the *sclera* (the white outer coat of the *eye*). Scleritis usually accompanies a *collagen disease*, such as *rheumatoid arthritis*. It also occurs in *herpes zoster* ophthalmicus and in Wegener's granulomatosis. Scleritis may lead to areas of local thinning and possible perforation of the sclera.

Scleritis is usually persistent, but often responds well to eye-drops containing a *corticosteroid drug*. In severe cases, corticosteroids may increase the risk of perforation.

Scleroderma

A rare condition, also known as systemic sclerosis, that can affect many organs and tissues in the body, particularly the skin, arteries, kidneys, lungs, heart, gastrointestinal tract, and joints. Scleroderma is an *autoimmune disorder* (in which the body's immune system attacks its own tissues). Scleroderma is twice as common in women as in men and is most likely to appear between the ages of 40 and 60.

SYMPTOMS AND SIGNS

The number and the severity of symptoms varies dramatically. The most common symptom is *Raynaud's phenomenon* (in which the fingers or toes become white and painful on exposure to cold); this phenomenon may be present for many years without any other symptoms.

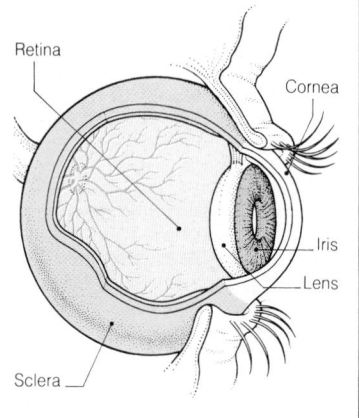

LOCATION OF THE SCLERA

The sclera is about 0.5 mm thick and is continuous with the cornea at the front of the eye. The sclera is extremely tough and protects the inner structures of the eye.

Retina

Cornea

Iris

Lens

Sclera

Also common are changes in the skin, especially of the face and fingers, which becomes shiny, tight, and thickened. There is often puckering around the mouth, giving the sufferer a characteristic mask-like appearance. The pulled skin often leads to difficulty in performing certain manoeuvres, such as bending the fingers or opening the mouth.

In some people, other parts of the body are affected, leading to problems such as difficulty in swallowing, shortness of breath, palpitations, high blood pressure, joint pain, stiffness, and muscle weakness.

There are wide variations from person to person in the degree to which different parts of the body are involved and the rate at which the disease progresses. Progression of scleroderma is often rapid in the first few years and then slows down or even stops. In a small number of people, degeneration is rapid, and leads usually to death from *heart failure, respiratory failure,* or *kidney failure.*

DIAGNOSIS AND TREATMENT

A physical examination is usually sufficient to confirm the diagnosis, but a blood test and a skin *biopsy* (removal of a sample of tissue for microscopic examination) may be performed.

There is no cure for scleroderma, but treatment can relieve symptoms and associated problems. *Vasodilator drugs* and avoiding exposure to cold can relieve Raynaud's phenomenon. *Physiotherapy* may be recommended

S

for joint problems. *Antihypertensive drugs* may be given to treat high blood pressure and *dialysis* may be used to treat kidney failure. *Corticosteroid drugs* are sometimes prescribed if the muscles are involved, but may not be effective.

Scleromalacia
Softening of the *sclera* (the white outer coat of the *eye*). Scleromalacia is commonly a complication of *scleritis* (inflammation of the sclera), especially when scleritis is caused by *rheumatoid arthritis*.

Scleromalacia perforans is a rare, severe form of the condition in which the entire thickness of sclera is involved; the underlying *choroid* layer of the eye bulges through and sometimes perforates the sclera.

Sclerosis
A medical term for hardening of a body tissue. The term is usually used to refer to hardening of blood vessels, as in *arteriosclerosis* (hardening of arteries), or to hardening of nerve tissue due to deposition of abnormal connective tissue, which occurs in the later stages of *multiple sclerosis*.

Sclerotherapy
A method of treating *varicose veins* (swollen, tortuous veins), especially in the legs. *Haemorrhoids* (varicose veins in the anus) and *oesophageal varices* (swollen veins at the bottom of the oesophagus) are also sometimes treated in this way.

In sclerotherapy, the affected vein is injected with a strongly irritant solution (called a sclerosant). This causes inflammation in the lining of the vein, leading to fibrosis (scar tissue formation), and the eventual obliteration of the vein.

Scoliosis
A deformity in which the *spine* is bent to one side. The thoracic (chest) or lumbar (lower back) regions are the most commonly affected.
TYPES AND CAUSES
Scoliosis usually starts in childhood or adolescence and becomes progressively more marked until the age at which growth stops. In many such cases, another part of the spine curves towards the opposite side of the body to compensate for the scoliotic curvature, and resulting in the spine becoming S-shaped. The cause of juvenile scoliosis is unknown; if the condition is not corrected, it may lead to severe deformity.

More rarely, scoliosis develops as a result of a congenital abnormality of the vertebrae (the spinal bones), *poliomyelitis* that has weakened the spinal muscles on one side of the body, or tilting of the pelvis due to one leg being shorter than the other. Occasionally, a spinal injury (such as a *disc prolapse* or ligament sprain) causes temporary scoliosis. In such cases, the spinal curvature appears suddenly and is accompanied by back pain and *sciatica*.
DIAGNOSIS AND TREATMENT
Scoliosis is diagnosed by a physical examination of the spine, hips, and legs, along with X-rays of the spine.

If the cause of the condition is known, treatment is directed towards that cause (e.g. bed rest for a disc prolapse or wearing an orthopaedic shoe with a raised heel to correct a pelvic tilt due to unequal leg lengths).

Scoliosis of unknown cause may not require treatment if the curvature is slight. However, regular measurement of the spine is necessary to assess the progression of the condition. If the scoliosis seems to be worsening—or if the curvature is already marked—it may be treated by immobilization of the spine in a hinged plaster jacket or adjustable metal brace, followed by surgery and bone grafting to fuse the affected spinal vertebrae in a straight line (see *Spinal fusion*). A steel rod with hooks may be used to keep the spine straight until the bones become fused.

Scorpion stings

Scorpions are eight-legged creatures with flexible tails that end in a poison reservoir and a sharp sting. Many species are not dangerous to humans, but some highly venomous species of scorpion are found in North Africa, South America, the southern US, Mexico, parts of the Caribbean, and India.
SYMPTOMS
The effects of many scorpion stings are little worse than a bee sting, with mild to moderate pain and tingling or burning at the site of the puncture wound. With more dangerous species, there may be sweating, restlessness, diarrhoea, and vomiting (caused by stimulation of the *autonomic nervous system*) in addition to severe pain. The venom may also affect the rhythm and strength of the heart's contractions. Fatalities are uncommon in adults; young children and the elderly are at greater risk.

TREATMENT
Any person stung by a scorpion should seek immediate medical attention. If pain is the only symptom, mild *analgesic drugs* (painkillers) and cold compresses may be all that is needed. In severe cases, local anaesthetics and powerful painkillers may be required, and an *antivenom* to deactivate the venom may be administered by intravenous infusion.

Scotoma
An area of abnormal vision within the *visual field*.

Screening
The testing of apparently healthy people with the aim of detecting disease at an early, treatable stage. The ideal screening test is reliable, with a low rate of false-positive results (in which the results of the test are positive even though the people tested do not in fact have the disease) and a low rate of false-negative results (in which the results of the test are negative even though the people tested have the disease). An ideal test is also inexpensive, simple, and acceptable to people, causing neither discomfort nor danger. For a screening test to be of practical use, people found to have the disease must benefit from early diagnosis. For example, screening for unsuspected diabetes is of no use since there is no evidence that the late complications of the disease are lessened by diagnosis before symptoms develop. (See also *Cancer screening*.)

Scrofula
Tuberculosis of the lymph nodes in the neck, often those just beneath the angle of the jaw. Scrofula was once a common disorder, usually caused by drinking contaminated milk. Abscesses would form in the lymph nodes and, after bursting through the skin, leave scars on the neck.

Today scrofula is rare in developed countries. It occasionally develops in Asian or African immigrants in whom the infection has spread from tuberculosis elsewhere in the body. Antituberculous drugs clear up the condition in most cases.

Scrotum
The pouch that hangs behind the penis and contains the *testes*. The scrotum consists of an outer layer of thin, wrinkled skin over a layer of muscle-containing tissue.

Swelling of the scrotum may be caused by an inguinal *hernia*, a swell-

S

ANATOMY OF THE SCROTUM

The scrotum has oil-secreting glands and thinly scattered hairs on its surface. Internally it is divided by a membrane into two halves, each containing a testis.

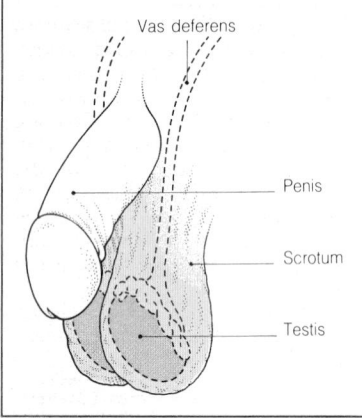

Vas deferens

Penis

Scrotum

Testis

ing of one of the testes, a *hydrocele* (fluid in the sac around one of the testes), or by oedema (accumulation of fluid) in severe *heart failure*.

Scuba-diving medicine

A minor medical specialty concerned with the physiological hazards of underwater diving with self-contained underwater breathing apparatus (SCUBA).

THE MAIN HAZARDS

Most diving hazards stem from the increase in pressure with depth. At a depth of 10 m, the total pressure is twice the surface pressure. At 30 m, it is four times the surface pressure.

MECHANICAL EFFECTS OF PRESSURE CHANGE

During descent, divers must introduce gas into their middle-ear cavities and facial sinuses to prevent damage as the pressure mounts. This mounting pressure is what airline passengers also experience during descent and repressurization (see *Barotrauma*).

Whatever depth they attain, divers must be supplied with breathing mixtures at a pressure equal to the external water pressure. Thus, at 30 m, a diver breathes gas at four times the surface pressure. During ascent, gas in the lungs expands and can rupture the lung tissues if the diver panics and inadvertently holds his or her breath—a serious condition known as pulmonary barotrauma (burst lung). Symptoms of this condition may include coughing up of blood, inability to pass urine, breathing difficulties, and unconsciousness.

TOXIC EFFECTS OF GASES Amateur divers breathe compressed air, which consists mainly of nitrogen and oxygen. These gases are harmless at surface pressures but become toxic at high pressure. Nitrogen impairs the nervous system when air is breathed at depth, causing slowed mental functioning and other symptoms that mimic alcohol intoxication (a condition known as nitrogen narcosis); regulations in the UK allow commercial divers using air to go no deeper than 50 m. Oxygen becomes toxic when air is breathed at increased pressure, when it can cause convulsions or lung damage.

To attain greater depths without risking nitrogen and oxygen poisoning, professional divers use gas mixtures other than air. A typical mixture consists of helium, with only small amounts of oxygen and nitrogen; the helium is relatively nontoxic.

THE BENDS At depth, divers accumulate in their tissues excess quantities of any inert gas they are breathing (nitrogen, if air is being breathed). If pressure is released too quickly (i.e. the diver

ascends too fast) and if a large amount of gas has accumulated because the diver remained at depth for too long, this gas can no longer be held in solution in the tissues and may form bubbles in tissues and in the circulation, causing *decompression sickness*.

OTHER HAZARDS Additional hazards include *hypothermia* (dangerous chilling) due to immersion in cold water, bites or stings from marine animals (see *Bites, animal; Venomous bites and stings*), and risk of *drowning*.

ACCIDENT PREVENTION AND TREATMENT

Any person taking up scuba diving should first receive a medical check-up and undergo thorough training at a recognized diving school.

Pressure-related accidents, such as burst lung and decompression sickness, are treated by recompression of the diver in a special pressure chamber so that any bubbles or pockets of gas in the blood or tissues are reabsorbed. This is followed by slow release of the pressure.

Treatment of other accidents (such as hypothermia and near drowning) is as for nondivers.

RECOMPRESSION CHAMBER FOR DIVING ACCIDENTS

Divers suffering from the bends or other pressure-related accidents are often treated in a recompression chamber. The patient is usually accompanied in the recompression chamber by a doctor.

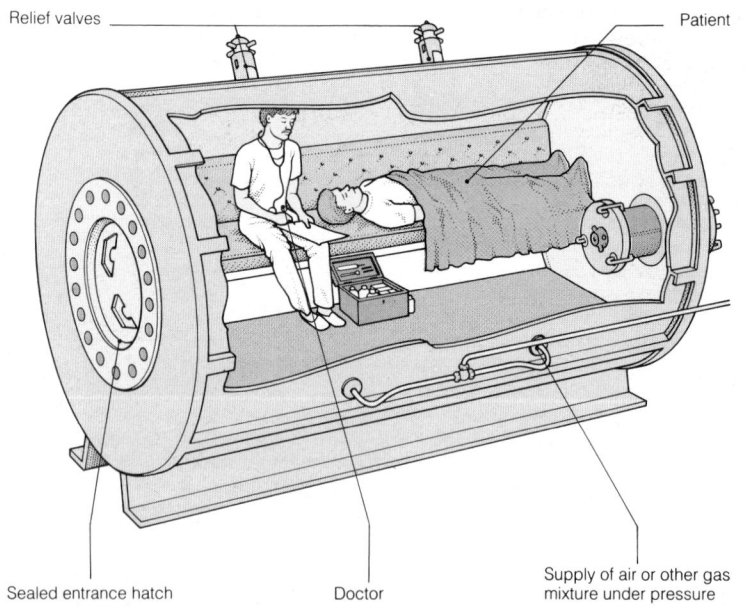

Relief valves

Patient

Sealed entrance hatch

Doctor

Supply of air or other gas mixture under pressure

How it works
A gas mixture (usually air) is pumped into the chamber. As pressure increases, bubbles (pockets of gas) in the diver's tissues are reabsorbed, and symptoms disappear. Once all symptoms have gone, the pressure is slowly released.

S

Scurvy

A disease caused by inadequate intake of *vitamin C*. Scurvy is rare today in developed countries as a result of increased consumption of fresh fruit and vegetables. Body stores of vitamin C give protection against scurvy for about three months.

CAUSES AND SYMPTOMS

Inadequate supplies of vitamin C disturb the body's normal production of *collagen*, which is a protein in *connective tissue* (material that surrounds body structures and holds them together). Collagen continues to be produced in scurvy but is unstable, causing weakness of small blood vessels and poor healing in wounds. Haemorrhages may occur anywhere in the body. They are most obvious in the skin, where they result in widespread bruising. Bleeding from the gums and loosening of the teeth are common; bleeding into muscles and joints also occurs in scurvy, causing pain.

Scurvy is especially serious in children because bleeding into the membranes surrounding the long bones may cause separation of the growing ends of the bones and interference with growth. Major, and sometimes fatal, haemorrhages into and around the brain can occur.

Scurvy is often associated with other vitamin deficiencies, and *anaemia* is common.

PREVENTION AND TREATMENT

A modest intake of fruit (particularly citrus fruit) and vegetables provides the body with sufficient vitamin C to prevent scurvy. Other minor sources are milk, liver, and kidneys.

Scurvy is treated with large doses of vitamin C. Bleeding stops in 24 hours, healing resumes, and muscle and bone pain quickly disappear.

Sealants, dental

Plastic materials applied to the chewing surfaces of the back *teeth* to help prevent decay. The molars and premolars have minute surface grooves in which food debris and bacteria can collect and cause decay (see *Caries, dental*). Sealing the teeth stops harmful material from getting into the grooves. Sealants are of most benefit to children and should be applied as soon as possible after the permanent teeth have erupted.

Teeth to be sealed often require no drilling or anaesthesia. The tooth surface must be acid-etched to roughen it so that the sealant will adhere better (see *Bonding, dental*). The semi-liquid sealant is then applied and is usually hardened by directing a narrow beam of ultraviolet light at the treated tooth for a few seconds.

Some dental sealants are premixed with a chemical activator that causes them to set.

Seasickness

A type of *motion sickness*.

Seasonal affective disorder syndrome

A form of *depression* in which mood changes occur with the seasons. The name seasonal affective disorder syndrome, often abbreviated to SADS, was first used in the 1980s but the disorder is probably as old as man himself. Alternative names are seasonal affective disorder (SAD) and winter depression.

Sufferers from SADS become depressed in the autumn and winter of most years, and then get better in the spring. As many as one person in 20 may be affected to some extent.

Several research studies have shown that people who usually become depressed in the dark cold months of winter may prevent the onset of symptoms by exposing themselves to bright light for two to four hours each morning. The mechanism by which exposure to light has its effects remains unknown.

Sebaceous cyst

A nonspecific term for a large, smooth nodule under the skin (also called a wen if it occurs on the scalp). The most common sites of sebaceous cysts are the scalp, face, ear, and genitals. The cysts contain a smooth, yellow, cheesy material.

Although harmless, sebaceous cysts may grow very large and sometimes become infected by bacteria, in which case they are painful. Large

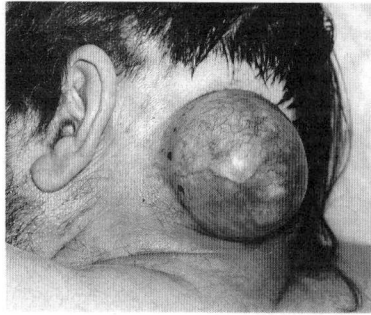

Massive sebaceous cyst
Cysts rarely grow as large as this one, located on the back of the neck. Sebaceous cysts are easily removed surgically.

cysts or cysts that have been infected should be removed under local anaesthetic. The doctor makes a small incision in the skin and removes the cyst. If the entire cyst wall is removed, recurrence is rare.

Sebaceous glands

Minute glands in the *skin* that secrete a lubricating substance called *sebum*. Sebaceous glands either open into hair follicles or discharge directly on to the surface of the skin. They are most numerous on the scalp, face, and anus; they do not occur on the palms of the hands or the soles of the feet. The production of sebum by the sebaceous glands is partly controlled by *androgen hormones* (male sex hormones).

Disorders of the sebaceous glands may lead to *seborrhoea* or *acne* vulgaris.

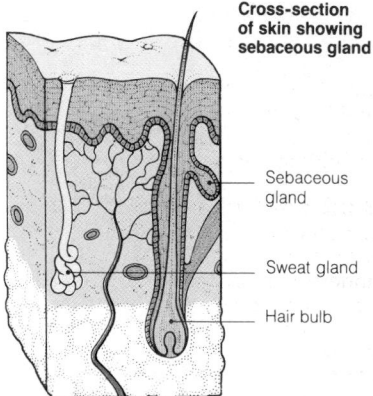

Cross-section of skin showing sebaceous gland

Sebaceous gland

Sweat gland

Hair bulb

Seborrhoea

Excessive secretion of *sebum*, causing increased oiliness of the face and a greasy scalp. The exact cause is uncertain, although *androgen hormones* (male sex hormones) are known to play a part. The condition is most common in adolescent boys.

Seborrhoea usually improves in adulthood without treatment. However, people with seborrhoea are more likely than average to have other skin conditions, particularly seborrhoeic *dermatitis* and *acne* vulgaris.

Seborrhoeic dermatitis

See *Dermatitis*.

Sebum

The oily secretion produced by the *sebaceous glands* of the *skin*. Composed of fats and waxes, sebum lubricates the skin, keeps it supple, and protects it from becoming sodden when immersed in water or cracked when

S

exposed to a dry atmosphere. Sebum also protects the skin from invasion by bacteria and fungi.

Oversecretion of sebum, called *seborrhoea,* causes a greasy skin, and may lead to seborrhoeic *dermatitis* or *acne* vulgaris.

Secondary

A term applied to a disease or disorder that results from or follows another disease (which is called the *primary* disease). For example, secondary *hypertension* (high blood pressure) occurs as a result of some underlying primary disorder, such as a hormonal problem or kidney disease.

Secondary also refers to a *metastasis* (a malignant tumour that has spread from a primary cancer elsewhere in the body).

Secretion

The manufacture and release by a cell, gland, or organ of chemical substances (such as *enzymes* or *hormones*) that are needed for metabolic processes elsewhere in the body. In contrast, *excretion* is the production and release of waste products. The term secretion is also used to refer to the secreted substances themselves.

The secretions of *exocrine glands* (e.g. the salivary glands) are carried away in ducts; the secretions of *endocrine glands* (e.g. the thyroid) are released directly into the bloodstream.

Sectioning

A commonly used term to describe the implementation of a section of the *Mental Health Act.*

Security object

A significant item, such as a special blanket, an old garment, or a favourite soft toy, that provides comfort and reassurance to a young child. In many cases, a child settles down to sleep more easily if his or her security object is near. Some children are unable to sleep without their security objects.

Sometimes referred to as transitional objects, these items represent to the child something part way between a person and a thing. The child may become deeply attached to the object and may become highly distressed if an attempt is made to remove it.

Security objects are often important during the toddler stage and may be used for several years. Most children grow out of the need for such an item by the time they are about seven or eight years old, but close attachments to special toys may persist.

There is no evidence that security objects are in any way harmful. (See also *Thumb-sucking.*)

Sedation

The use of a drug to calm a person. Sedation is used to reduce excessive *anxiety* and occasionally to control dangerously aggressive behaviour. It may also be used as part of *premedication* to produce relaxation before an operation or other uncomfortable procedure. (See also *Sleeping drugs.*)

Sedative drugs

A group of drugs used to produce *sedation* (calmness). Sedative drugs include *sleeping drugs, antianxiety drugs, antipsychotic drugs,* and some *antidepressant drugs.* A sedative drug is often included in a *premedication* (drug given to prepare a person for surgery).

Seizure

A sudden episode of uncontrolled electrical activity in the *brain,* also called a fit. Recurrent seizures are called *epilepsy.* Seizures may be partial or generalized.

In a partial seizure, abnormal electrical activity remains confined to one area of the brain. The affected person may experience tingling or twitching of only a small area of the face, body, or an extremity. Other possible symptoms include *hallucinations,* intense feelings of fear, or *déjà vu.*

In a generalized seizure, abnormal electrical activity spreads throughout the brain. This causes loss of consciousness and features of a grand mal, petit mal, or less common form of generalized seizure.

Seizures may be caused by many different neurological or medical problems, including *head injury, stroke, brain tumour,* infection, metabolic disturbances, withdrawal symptoms in *alcohol dependence,* or an hereditary alcohol intolerance. Whatever the cause, *anticonvulsant drugs* can control or at least reduce the number of seizures.

Selenium

A *trace element* which may help to preserve the elasticity of body tissues. The richest sources are meat, fish, whole grains, and dairy products. The selenium content of vegetables depends on the amount of the mineral in the soil in which they were grown.

DEFICIENCY AND EXCESS
Neither deficiency nor excess of selenium usually has any effect on health.

Excessive intake as a result of taking supplements, occupational exposure,

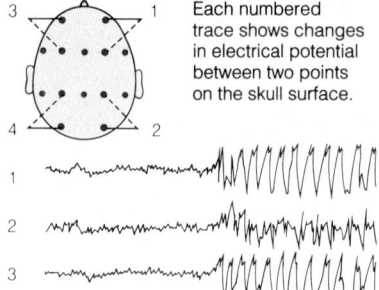

Each numbered trace shows changes in electrical potential between two points on the skull surface.

Normal traces   Abnormal traces during seizure

EEG changes during a seizure
The traces are recordings of electrical activity in a patient's brain, obtained from electrodes placed at various locations on the scalp and linked to an EEG machine. They show the change in activity at the onset of a seizure.

or, rarely, eating vegetables grown in soil with an abnormally high selenium content (as is found in some intensively irrigated areas) may cause a smell of garlic in the breath and urine, and red-orange discoloration or loss of the hair and nails. Some selenium compounds may irritate the skin or, if inhaled, the respiratory tract.

Claims that the selenium content of the diet may influence the risk of developing heart disease have not been substantiated by the results of research studies.

MEDICAL USES
Selenium is a constituent of some *multivitamin* and *mineral* preparations. Selenium sulphide is used in some antidandruff shampoos.

Self-help organizations

Self-help or mutual-aid organizations are usually set up by patients or relatives of those suffering from specific diseases, disabilities, addictions, or emotional problems. The groups may provide individuals with information, emotional support, and, sometimes, financial assistance. Some are also active in raising funds for research, in improving public relations, and in promoting legislation for their cause.

Self-image

An individual's view of his or her own personality and abilities. It is argued that neurotic disorders may stem from incongruity between self-image and how others see one, as, for example, in an *inferiority complex. Psychotherapy* treats neurosis by bringing about a change in the person's perception of

S

the self. Cognitive therapy attempts to improve self-image by changing negative thoughts about oneself.

Self-injury

The act of deliberately injuring oneself. Self-mutilation most often occurs in young adults with *personality disorders,* many of whom are also drug or alcohol abusers, and is three times more common in women.

Self-mutilation usually takes the form of cutting the wrists or burning the forearms with cigarettes. The reasons often given by self-mutilators for their behaviour include aggressive impulses, relief of tension, and sadomasochistic fantasies. Some self-mutilators have had a violent upbringing. People with a *learning difficulty* or a *mental handicap* may use self-mutilation to gain attention or avoid specific situations or demands.

More unusual forms of self-harm, such as gouging out the eyes or mutilating the genitals, are almost always due to *psychosis.* Self-destructive biting is a feature of Lesch-Nyhan syndrome, a rare *metabolic disorder* causing mental handicap.

Semen

Fluid produced by the male on *ejaculation.* Semen is composed of fluid from the seminal vesicles (which produce the greatest part of the semen volume), fluid from the *prostate gland* and Cowper's glands, and *sperm.*

An important constituent of the fluid from the seminal vesicles is fructose (a sugar), which stimulates the sperm to become mobile. The concentration of fructose, the production of sperm, and the volume of the semen is dependent on the presence of the male sex hormone *testosterone.*

Seminal fluid analysis is a procedure performed as part of the investigation of male *infertility.*

Semen, blood in the

A condition in which a small amount of blood is present in the *semen.* Blood in the semen, known medically as haemospermia, is nearly always harmless. The blood, which is usually seen as a darkish stain in the semen at *ejaculation,* usually comes from small blood vessels in the region of the prostate gland or seminal vesicles. In the majority of cases, no cause is found.

Seminal fluid analysis

A method of determining the concentration, shape, and motility (ability to move) of sperm. Seminal fluid analysis is important in the investigation of male *infertility.* It is also performed some weeks after *vasectomy* (male sterilization) to ensure that the semen no longer contains sperm.

The semen specimen is produced by masturbation and should be as fresh as possible for successful analysis in the laboratory. The volume of semen is measured and the specimen examined under the microscope.

Normal semen contains from 20 million to 200 million sperm per millilitre. Seminal fluid analysis may show *oligospermia* (a deficiency in the number of sperm) or *azoospermia* (a complete absence of sperm), altered shape, or diminished motility.

Seminoma

See *Testis, cancer of.*

Senile dementia

See *Dementia.*

Senility

A term meaning old age or, more commonly, the changes in mental ability caused by old age. Many people over 70 suffer from a mild degree of impaired memory and reduced ability to concentrate. This does not mean that the person is developing senile *dementia;* indeed, only five per cent of elderly people become demented.

Senna

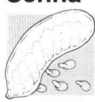

A *laxative drug* obtained from the leaves and pods of the Arabian shrubs CAS-SIA ACUTIFOLIA and CASSIA ANGUSTIFOLIA. Senna stimulates bowel contraction and is used to treat severe *constipation;* it may colour the urine yellow-brown or red.

Sensate-focus technique

A method taught to couples who are experiencing sexual difficulties caused by psychological rather than organic factors. The aim of sensate-focus technique is to make each partner more aware of his or her pleasurable bodily sensations as well as those of the partner, and to reduce anxiety about performance.

The technique is particularly useful in treating loss of sexual desire, failure to become sexually aroused (see *Sexual desire, inhibited*), or inability to achieve orgasm (see *Orgasm, lack of*),

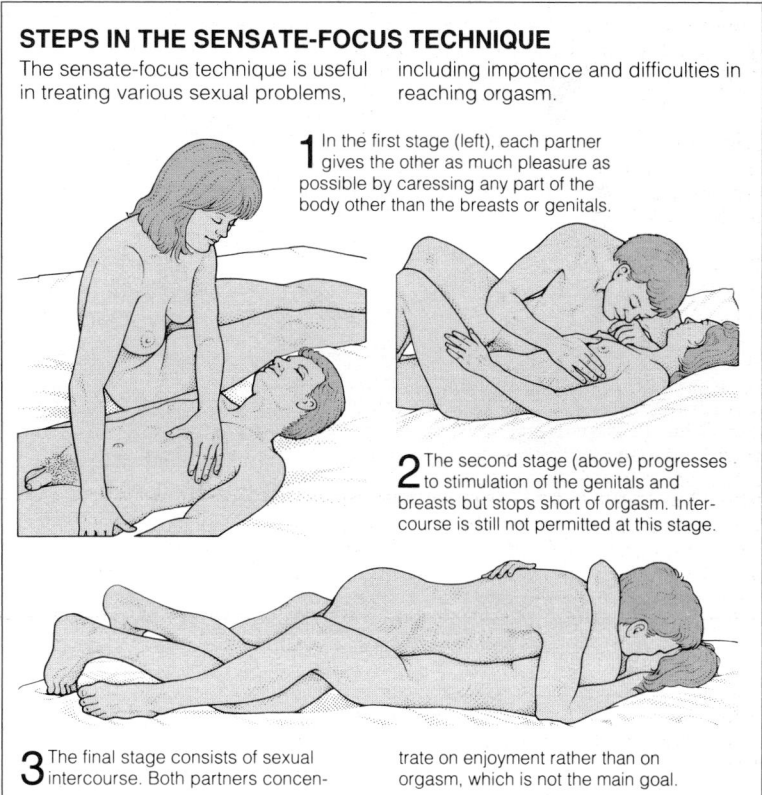

STEPS IN THE SENSATE-FOCUS TECHNIQUE

The sensate-focus technique is useful in treating various sexual problems, including impotence and difficulties in reaching orgasm.

1 In the first stage (left), each partner gives the other as much pleasure as possible by caressing any part of the body other than the breasts or genitals.

2 The second stage (above) progresses to stimulation of the genitals and breasts but stops short of orgasm. Intercourse is still not permitted at this stage.

3 The final stage consists of sexual intercourse. Both partners concentrate on enjoyment rather than on orgasm, which is not the main goal.

S

and in helping men to overcome *impotence* or premature ejaculation (see *Ejaculation, disorders of*).

HOW IT IS DONE

Ideally the technique should be practised in a relaxed romantic setting. It has three stages (see illustrated box). If premature ejaculation is a problem, technique to prevent it can be incorporated (see *Sex therapy*).

EFFECTIVENESS

The sensate-focus technique has an extremely high success rate—between 80 and 98 per cent, depending on the sexual problem.

Sensation

A feeling or impression (such as a sound, odour, touch sensation, or hunger) that has entered consciousness. The senses are the faculties by which information about the external environment and about the body's internal state is collected and brought to the *central nervous system* (the *brain* and *spinal cord*).

SENSORY RECEPTORS

Information is collected by millions of microscopic structures called *receptors*. Receptors are found throughout the body in the skin, muscles, and joints, in the internal organs, in the walls of blood vessels, and in special sense organs, such as the *eye* and inner *ear*. Receptors are attuned to a particular stimulus, such as light of a particular wavelength, chemical molecules of a certain shape, vibration, or temper-

ature. They fire (send an electrical signal) when excited.

Some receptors are the terminals (free nerve endings) of long nerve cell fibres, others are specialized cells that connect to such fibres. When a receptor fires, a signal passes along the appropriate nerve fibre to the spinal cord and/or brain. The principal pathways and destinations of sensory information entering the brain are shown in the diagram. Only a proportion of this information reaches the *sensory cortex* of the brain and is consciously perceived.

THE SPECIAL SENSES

The special senses include *vision, hearing, taste,* and *smell*. The receptor cells for these senses are collected into special organs—the retina in the eyes, the auditory apparatus in the ears, the taste-buds in the *tongue*, and the apparatus for smell in the *nose*. Information from these organs passes directly to the brain via *cranial nerves*. Much of the information passes to the cerebral cortex, although some goes to other areas of the brain (e.g. from the eyes to the *cerebellum*, where it is used to help maintain balance).

INTERNAL AND TOUCH SENSES

These senses include the pain, proprioception (position), pressure, and temperature sensations. Proprioception relies on receptors in the muscles and joints to provide information on the position in space of parts of the body. Pain is one of the most primitive

senses; it warns of noxious stimuli through receptors both at the skin surface and internally.

Many types of receptors are found in the skin. Some are sensitive to pressure, others to the movement of hairs, others to temperature change. Skin receptors are made up of the terminals of nerve fibres, which are wrapped around the roots of hairs, formed into discs, or surrounded by a series of membranes to form onion-like structures (called pacinian corpuscles). Different patterns of stimulation of these receptors give rise to such sensations as pain, tickling, firm or light pressure, heat or cold. Certain skin areas (the lips, palms of the hands, and genitals) have a particularly high concentration of receptors.

Most of the signals from these receptors pass, via the cranial or *spinal nerves* and tracts in the brain or spinal cord, to the *thalamus* and then to two regions of the sensory cortex called the somatosensory cortices. Sensations perceived at certain points within these regions correspond to the parts of the body from which the signals originated. Much larger areas of cortex are devoted to sensations originating from the hands and lips than from less sensitive parts.

Sensation, abnormal

Unpleasant, dulled, or otherwise altered *sensations* without obvious stimulus (e.g. a burning sensation when

PRINCIPAL SENSORY PATHWAYS INTO THE BRAIN

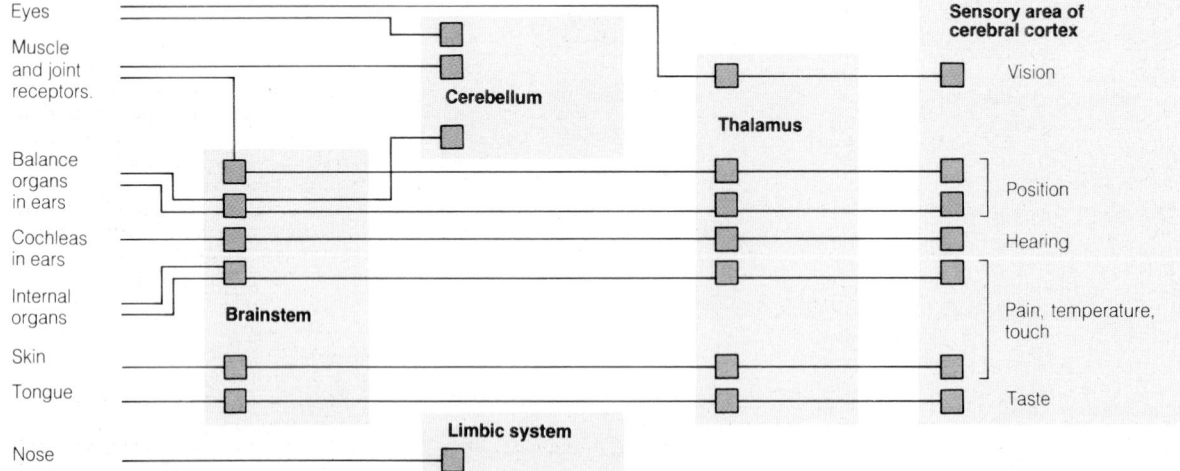

Destinations of sensory information
Some of the information entering the brain passes via the brainstem and/or thalamus to the cerebral cortex (outer surface of the

brain), where sensations are perceived. Other information does not lead to conscious sensation. This includes certain data about body

posture, processed in the cerebellum, and about internal body functioning, processed in the brainstem.

S

there is no source of heat). Abnormal sensations result from damage to, or pressure on, sensory nerve pathways.

TYPES

Numbness and *pins-and-needles* are common abnormal sensations, sometimes combined with *pain* and sometimes occurring with sensations of coldness or burning. *Neuralgia* is characterized by pain with a stabbing, brief, repetitive quality.

More unusual abnormal sensations include a feeling that fluid is trickling down the skin, that part of the body is being constricted by a tight band, or that insects are crawling over the skin (a sensation known as formication).

The special senses can also be impaired or altered by damage to the relevant sensory apparatus or nerve tracts (see *Vision, disorders of; Smell; Deafness; Tinnitus*).

CAUSES

Neuropathy (damage to peripheral nerves) from thiamine deficiency in alcoholics, from *diabetes mellitus*, or from heavy metal (such as lead) poisoning is a common cause of abnormal sensation. The sufferer may complain of tingling or a feeling of walking on cottonwool. The peripheral nerves may also be damaged or irritated by infections such as *herpes zoster* (shingles) or by a tumour pressing on a nerve, often causing severe pain. *Spinal injury, head injury, stroke,* and *multiple sclerosis* are other causes of disruption to nerve pathways in the *brain* or *spinal cord.*

Damage to the *thalamus* (a relay station for sensory pathways in the centre of the brain) can produce particularly unpleasant results, such as a spreading sensation resembling an electric shock that occurs after a simple pinprick. Damage to the parietal lobe in the brain can lead to loss of the ability to locate or recognize objects by touch.

DIAGNOSIS AND TREATMENT

Many tests (including tests of sensation, testing of *reflexes, blood tests, urinalysis,* and *CT scanning, MRI,* or *angiography*) may be required in order to discover the cause of abnormal sensation.

Pressure on or damage to nerves can sometimes be relieved by surgery or by dietary or other treatments to remove or treat the underlying cause. In other cases, severe intractable pain or other abnormal sensation can be relieved only by cutting the relevant sensory nerve fibres or by giving injections to block chemically the transmission of signals along them.

NEUROLOGICAL SENSORY TESTING

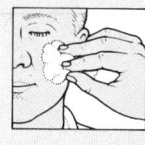

Light touch
With the patient's eyes closed, a piece of cottonwool is brushed lightly across the face.

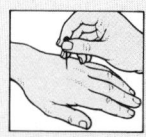

Pinprick
The prick tests pain sensation and may be repeated at different locations on the patient's body.

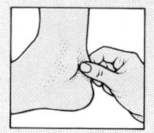

Pain pinch
Pain sense may be further tested by pinching the Achilles tendon at the back of the heel.

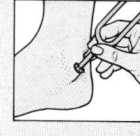

Vibration
A vibrating tuning fork is held against a prominent bone, such as the ankle bone or mastoid bone.

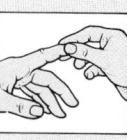

Position sense
The patient, with eyes closed, tells in which direction his or her finger is moved.

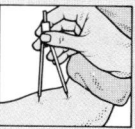

Two-point discrimination
Measures the ability to distinguish two pinpricks from a single prick.

Standard tests
When examining a patient's nervous system, a doctor usually includes several standard tests of touch, position, pain, and vibration senses, such as those above.

Senses
See *Sensation.*

Sensitization
The initial exposure of a person to an allergen or other substance recognized as foreign by the body's *immune system,* which leads to an immune response. On subsequent exposures to the same substance, there is a much stronger and faster immune reaction. This forms the basis of *allergy* and other types of *hypersensitivity* reaction.

Sensory cortex
A region of the outer part of the *cerebrum* (the main mass of the *brain*) in which sensory information comes to consciousness. The sensory cortex contains several layers of linked *neurons* (nerve cells) with complex interconnections.

Pressure, pain, and temperature sensations from the skin, muscles, joints, and internal organs are perceived in regions of the parietal lobe (upper side part of the cerebrum) on both sides of the brain. These regions are called the somatosensory cortices. Taste sensations are also perceived in the parietal lobes. Light, colour, and other visual sensations are perceived in the occipital lobes at the back of the cerebrum; sounds are perceived in the temporal lobes at the sides.

Sensory deprivation
Removing the normal sights, sounds, and physical feelings from a person. Sensory deprivation can produce a variety of mental changes, demonstrated by studies in which volunteers lie immobile in bed (or in a bath of warm water) wearing masks and gloves in a sound-deadened room. After long periods, reported effects generally include feelings of unreality, difficulty in thinking, and *hallucinations; EEG* recordings show a slowing of brain activity.

Prisoners kept in solitary confinement experience similar symptoms, and infants deprived of the companionship and presence of others tend to be disturbed in later life. (See also *Bonding; Emotional deprivation.*)

Separation anxiety
The feelings of distress that a young child experiences when parted from his or her parents or home. Separation anxiety is a normal aspect of infant behaviour which increases in intensity until about two years of age, but is often minimal by the age of three or four. When threatened with separation, the child usually reacts by crying, clinging to the parent, and demanding to be cuddled. Such signs are indicative of *bonding*, which is considered essential to a child's emotional development.

Separation anxiety disorder is a childhood illness in which the reaction to separation is greater than that expected for the child's level of development. The anxiety may manifest itself in the form of headaches, nausea, toothaches, dizziness, or difficulty in sleeping. When separated,

S

the child may worry that he or she will never be reunited with the parents or that they will be killed. Some children refuse to visit friends or to attend school. Separation anxiety disorder may be a feature of *depression*.

Sepsis

Infection of a wound or body tissues with bacteria that leads to the formation of *pus* or to the multiplication of the bacteria in the blood. If the blood becomes infected with bacteria that the *immune system* can prevent from multiplying excessively or can eradicate entirely, the condition is known as *bacteraemia*. However, if bacteria that form toxins are present in the blood in large numbers and are multiplying rapidly, the condition is called *septicaemia* (blood poisoning). (See also *Septic shock*.)

Septal defect

A *heart* abnormality, developed before birth, in which there is a hole in the septum (partition) between the left and right sides of the heart. Commonly known as a hole in the heart, septal defect varies in its effects according to its size and position.

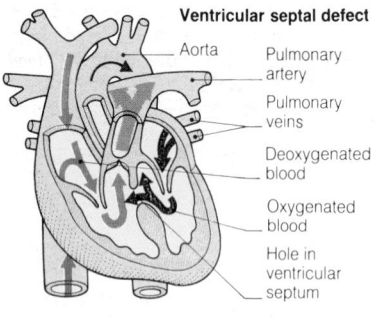

Ventricular septal defect

Aorta

Pulmonary artery

Pulmonary veins

Deoxygenated blood

Oxygenated blood

Hole in ventricular septum

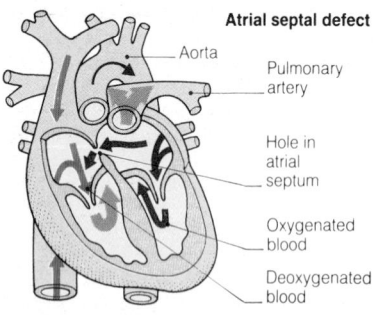

Atrial septal defect

Aorta

Pulmonary artery

Hole in atrial septum

Oxygenated blood

Deoxygenated blood

Two types of septal defect
In both cases, oxygenated blood is forced from the left to the right side of the heart through the hole in the septum. Too much blood passes to the lungs (via the pulmonary artery) and too little to the body tissues (via the aorta).

TYPES
When the hole is in the septum separating the two ventricles (lower chambers of the heart), the abnormality is known as a ventricular septal defect; when it is in the septum between the two atria (upper chambers), it is called an atrial septal defect. In both types, the hole allows some of the freshly oxygenated blood in the left half of the heart (which supplies tissues throughout the body) which is under higher pressure, to flow into the right half, mix with deoxygenated blood, and recirculate through the lungs. If the hole is large, the misdirection of blood results in excessive blood flow through the lungs, with increased pressure in the pulmonary circulation and breathing difficulties.

Some children are born with both atrial and ventricular septal defects; either type may be accompanied by one or more other heart abnormalities and/or other congenital defects.

CAUSES AND INCIDENCE
The precise cause of septal defects is unknown in most cases. (For information on factors influencing the development of congenital heart abnormalities, see *Heart disease, congenital* and *Birth defects*.)

Ventricular septal defects are the most common type of congenital heart abnormality, occurring in about 25 per cent of all cases of congenital heart disease and affecting about 150 babies in every 100,000. Atrial septal defects are less common, affecting about 40 babies per 100,000.

SYMPTOMS AND SIGNS
A small defect of either kind produces little or no effect. With a large ventricular hole, *heart failure* may develop six to eight weeks after birth, causing breathlessness, feeding difficulties, pallor, and sweating. With large atrial defects, however, heart failure may not develop for many years or may not develop at all although there may be some fatigue on exertion.

With both types of defect, *pulmonary hypertension* (high blood pressure in the arteries supplying the lungs) may develop. This is more likely, and occurs at an earlier age, if there is a large ventricular defect.

With a ventricular defect there is also a slight risk of *endocarditis* (inflammation of the lining of the heart); in atrial septal defect, *atrial fibrillation* (rapid, irregular beating of the atria) may occur after the age of 30.

DIAGNOSIS
The diagnosis is based on hearing a heart *murmur* (a type of abnormal

heart sound made by turbulent blood flow) through a stethoscope, followed by a *chest X-ray* and an *ECG*. The diagnosis can be confirmed by Doppler *echocardiography*.

TREATMENT
Atrial septal defects are repaired surgically if they cause symptoms or if examination and tests suggest that complications may develop.

As the child grows, small ventricular holes often become smaller, or even close, on their own. If a large ventricular defect is causing heart failure, it is treated with *diuretic drugs* and with *digitalis drugs*. If the hole does not close spontaneously, it may be repaired by *open heart surgery*, usually before the child reaches school age. The operation has a very high success rate.

OUTLOOK
Modern surgery is so effective in dealing with large septal defects that it enables most affected people to lead normal lives.

Septicaemia

Rapid multiplication of bacteria and the presence of bacterial *toxins* in the blood, a condition commonly known as blood poisoning. As distinct from *bacteraemia* (in which bacteria are present in the blood but do not always multiply), septicaemia is always a serious, and potentially life-threatening, condition.

CAUSES
Septicaemia usually arises through escape of bacteria from a focus of infection somewhere in the body (such as a *urinary tract infection, gastroenteritis, pneumonia, meningitis* or an *abscess*). Septicaemia is more likely in people whose natural resistance to infection has been lowered by an *immunodeficiency disorder* or by *immunosuppressant drugs*, allowing the bacteria to multiply unchecked. Septicaemia is also more likely to develop in drug addicts who use contaminated needles, and in people who have *cancer, diabetes mellitus*, or other debilitating diseases.

SYMPTOMS AND SIGNS
A person with septicaemia develops a high fever, chills, rapid breathing, headache, and, in many cases, clouding of consciousness. Skin rashes or jaundice may occur. In some cases, the hands are unusually warm. In many cases, especially when large amounts of toxins are produced by the circulating bacteria, the sufferer passes into a state of *septic shock*, a life-threatening condition.

S

DIAGNOSIS AND TREATMENT

A diagnosis of septicaemia can be confirmed, and the infective bacteria identified, by growing a *culture* of the organisms from a blood sample.

Treatment is started as soon as septicaemia is suspected. Glucose and/or saline are administered by *intravenous infusion*, and *antibiotic drugs* are given intravenously by infusion or injection. Tests are performed to identify the original site of infection if this is not apparent. Surgery may be necessary in some cases to remove infected material.

Provided the infection is recognized and treated promptly before the development of septic shock, most patients make a full recovery.

Septic shock

A highly dangerous condition in which there is tissue damage and a dramatic drop in blood pressure as a result of *septicaemia* (the multiplication of bacteria and the presence of bacterial *toxins* in the blood).

In many cases, the toxins are the main cause of trouble because they can damage cells and tissues throughout the body, promote clotting of blood in the smallest blood vessels, and seriously interfere with the normal blood circulation. Damage occurs especially to tissues in the kidneys, heart, and lungs. The toxins may cause leakage of fluid from blood vessels and a reduction of the ability of the vessels to constrict, leading to a drop in blood pressure.

CAUSES AND INCIDENCE

Septic shock is most common in people with debilitating disorders, such as *diabetes mellitus*, *cancer*, or liver *cirrhosis*, who also have a focus of infection somewhere in the body (often the intestines or urinary tract) that has led to septicaemia. Progression to septic shock is especially likely in people who have an *immunodeficiency disorder*, in people taking *immunosuppressant drugs*, or in people given prolonged and inappropriate treatment with *antibiotic drugs*. Newborn infants with septicaemia are also particularly susceptible to septic shock.

SYMPTOMS AND SIGNS

The symptoms vary with the extent and site of major tissue damage. Broadly, they are the same as in septicaemia, with additional symptoms including cold hands and feet, often with *cyanosis* (blue-purple coloration) due to slowed blood flow, a weak, rapid pulse, and markedly reduced blood pressure. There may be vomiting and diarrhoea. A poor output of urine may indicate that damage to the kidneys is occurring and that there is a risk of *kidney failure*. *Heart failure* and abnormal bleeding may also develop.

TREATMENT

Septic shock requires immediate treatment, including the use of *antibiotic drugs* and sometimes surgery to remove the focus of infection. Rapid fluid replacement by transfusion and the maintenance of urine flow to prevent the effects of kidney failure are other essential procedures. Measures are also taken to raise the blood pressure and to promote better blood supply to tissues. These measures include *intravenous infusions* and *oxygen therapy*.

Despite treatment, septic shock remains a serious condition; survival rates are no better than 50 per cent.

Septum

A thin dividing wall within or between parts of the body—e.g. the nasal septum is the sheet of cartilage and bone that separates the nostrils.

Sequela

A condition that results from or follows a disease, a disorder, or an injury. The term is usually used in its plural form (sequelae) to refer to the complications of a disease. For example, the sequelae of a common cold may include *bronchitis*, *sinusitis*, and *otitis media* (inflammation of the middle ear).

Sequestration

A portion of diseased or dead tissue separated from, or joined abnormally to, surrounding healthy tissue. The term usually refers to a complication of *osteomyelitis* (bone infection) in which part of a bone dies and becomes separated from healthy bone.

The term sequestration may also refer to a rare congenital abnormality of the lungs in which part of a lobe is not directly connected to a bronchus (airway) but may be connected to surrounding alveoli (air sacs).

Serology

A branch of laboratory medicine concerned with analysis of the contents of blood *serum* (the clear fluid that separates from clotted blood).

Various serological techniques are extremely useful in the diagnosis of infectious diseases. If a person has been exposed to a particular infectious organism, *antibodies* (proteins with a role in immunity) directed specifically against the organism appear in that person's serum some days after exposure. The presence or absence of particular antibodies in the blood can be detected by various laboratory techniques, including *immunoassay* techniques, such as the *ELISA test* and *radioimmunoassay*. The absence of specific antibodies may enable a doctor to exclude a particular infection as the cause of an illness; a rising level of antibodies may give good evidence that a particular infection is present.

Serological techniques are also used to identify the *antigens* (foreign proteins) of infectious organisms by studying the reaction between the antigens (obtained by *culture* of a specimen taken from a patient) and serum samples known to contain certain antibodies. A series of tests may be carried out in which the unknown antigen is added to test tubes containing various *antiserum* preparations which contain specific antibodies; a positive reaction is sometimes revealed by a colour change.

In addition to devising and carrying out diagnostic tests, serologists may be involved in developing antisera for passive *immunization*.

Serologists may also test blood samples for various genetically determined protein markers, including substances that determine *blood groups*. Such tests can help resolve paternity suits (see *Paternity testing*) or cases in which blood left at the scene of a crime can be compared with blood taken from suspects.

Serotonin

A substance found in many tissues, particularly blood platelets, the lining of the digestive tract, and the brain. Serotonin has a variety of effects in the body. It is released from platelets at the site of bleeding, where it constricts small blood vessels, thus reducing blood loss. In the digestive tract, it inhibits gastric secretion and stimulates smooth (involuntary) muscles in the intestinal wall. In the brain, it acts as a *neurotransmitter* (a chemical involved in the transmission of nerve impulses between nerve cells). Serotonin is thought to be involved in controlling states of consciousness and mood; its action in the brain is disrupted by certain hallucinogenic drugs, notably *LSD*.

Serum

The clear fluid that separates from *blood* when it clots. Serum does not contain blood cells or fibrinogen (the

S

protein in blood that helps form clots). It does contain salts, glucose, and other proteins, including various *antibodies* formed by the body's *immune system* to protect against infection.

Serum prepared from the blood of a person (or animal) who has been infected with a microorganism usually contains antibodies that can protect against that organism if the serum is injected into someone else. This is called an *antiserum,* and its use forms the basis of passive *immunization.*

Serum sickness

A short-lived illness that may develop about 10 days after injection with an *antiserum* of animal origin. Virtually all animal sera have been replaced by ones of human origin, which carry no risk; but animal sera are still used to treat *rabies* and *tetanus* in some countries. Serum sickness is a type of *hypersensitivity* reaction similar to an allergic reaction; comparable reactions can occur after taking certain drugs.

CAUSES
Antisera are preparations obtained from human or animal blood that contains specific *antibodies* (substances with a role in immunity). Antisera are sometimes given to protect against dangerous infections. When an antiserum is prepared from animal blood, a protein in the serum may be misidentified by the *immune system* as a potentially harmful *antigen* (foreign protein). In serum sickness, the immune system produces antibodies that combine with the antigen to form particles called immune complexes. These are deposited in various tissues, stimulate more immune reactions, and lead to inflammation and symptoms.

Certain drugs can cause a similar response, although the drug molecules probably combine with a protein in the blood or tissues before they are misidentified as antigens. *Penicillin drugs* are the most important drugs capable of causing serum sickness.

Serum sickness is different from *anaphylactic shock,* another type of hypersensitivity reaction that can also develop in response to antisera, drugs, and other substances. Anaphylactic shock is a more severe, immediate reaction.

SYMPTOMS AND TREATMENT
Symptoms appear a week or two after exposure to the antiserum or drug. There may be an itchy rash, joint pain, fever, and enlarged lymph nodes. In severe cases, a state similar to *shock,* with low blood pressure, develops. Symptoms usually clear up within a few days, provided, in the case of a drug, that its use is stopped.

Soothing lotions can help relieve itching. The doctor may prescribe a *nonsteroidal anti-inflammatory drug* to relieve joint pain and an *antihistamine drug* to shorten the duration of the reaction. In severe cases, a *corticosteroid drug* may be prescribed.

People who have had serum sickness or anaphylactic shock should note the injection or drug to which they are sensitive. A note should also be included in their medical records to warn against future use of the drug.

Sex

Another term for gender and a commonly used term for *sexual intercourse.*

Sex change

Radical surgical procedures, usually combined with sex hormone therapy, that alter a person's anatomical gender. Sex-change operations are performed either on transsexuals (see *Transsexualism*) or on people whose external sex organs are neither completely male nor female (see *Genitalia, ambiguous*).

WHY IT IS DONE
Sex-change operations on transsexuals are performed to give the person a physical appearance that he or she believes coincides with his or her psychological *gender identity.*

Sex-change operations on people with ambiguous genitalia are performed to modify or improve the anatomical appearance and thus provide a more defined sexual identity.

HOW IT IS DONE
TRANSSEXUALS Sex change involves a series of major operations on the genito-urinary tract which are carried out after hormone therapy and extensive counselling.

The male-to-female sex change is the more common procedure. Prosthetic breasts may be implanted to augment breast growth that has been induced by hormone therapy. An operation removes the erectile tissue of the penis and repositions the urethra. The skin of the penis is used to make the lining for a vagina, which is created in the *perineum.* The testes are removed and the skin of the scrotum is used to make the labia.

In the female-to-male sex change, mastectomy is performed to remove the breasts. Afterwards, removal of the uterus and ovaries is carried out. This may be followed by constructing a penis. The female-to-male operation has less satisfactory results than the male-to-female operation.

AMBIGUOUS GENITALIA Operations are usually carried out in infancy. Babies with ambiguous genitalia are assigned a sex as soon as possible after birth, given appropriate surgical and hormonal treatment, and reared as a member of the assigned sex.

Operations on adults who have ambiguous genitalia are uncommon today. In general, they are similar to those performed on transsexuals, with variations depending on the specific anatomical problems.

OUTLOOK
The degree to which transsexuals adjust to their new gender varies. Some make a complete adjustment but others are left with serious psychological problems. Hormone therapy may need to be continued for life to maintain secondary sexual characteristics such as body shape and hair distribution. Female transsexuals can have intercourse but cannot conceive. Males cannot impregnate or ejaculate; they achieve an erection only with mechanical aids (e.g. *penile implants*).

Sex chromosomes

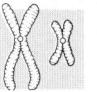 A pair of *chromosomes* that determines an individual's sex. All the cells in a person's body (except for egg or sperm cells) contain a pair of sex chromosomes together with 22 other pairs of chromosomes known as autosomes. In women, the sex chromosomes are of similar appearance and are called X chromosomes. In men, one sex chromosome is an X and the other, a smaller one, a Y. Thus, the normal sex chromosome complement for women is XX, and for men, XY.

FUNCTION
Like all chromosomes, the X and Y chromosomes exert their effects in the body through the activities of their constituent *genes*. These genes contain the coded instructions for chemical processes within cells and for aspects of growth and development within the body as a whole.

The X and Y chromosomes differ in one fundamental way. Genes on the Y chromosome are concerned solely with *sex determination.* Their presence ensures a male, their absence a female. The X chromosome, occurring in both sexes, contains many genes vital to general development and functioning. Absence of the X chromosome is incompatible with life.

The presence of a single X chromosome and 22 pairs of autosomes in the nuclei of ordinary body cells appears to provide the blueprint for general

S

body functioning and development, which seems to have an underlying female pattern. This can be seen in people with *Turner's syndrome*, who have only one sex chromosome, an X. Although full female sexual characteristics never develop, these people are unmistakably female in appearance and identity. Full female sexual characteristics develop only in the presence of a second X chromosome. Addition of a Y chromosome converts the female to the male pattern.

Sex determination

The factors that determine biological sex. The underlying determinants are the *sex chromosomes* in a person's cells—two X chromosomes in females, and one X and one Y chromosome in males. During early life in the embryo, these chromosomes cause the development of different gonads (primary sex organs)—the testes in males and the ovaries in females. In males, the testes then produce hormones that cause the development of a male reproductive tract, including a penis. In females, absence of these male hormones leads to a different pattern of development, with the formation of fallopian tubes, uterus, and vagina. At *puberty*, another surge of hormones from the gonads leads to the development of secondary *sexual characteristics*, such as facial hair in males and breasts in females.

Defects can arise in this process, leading, in some cases, to ambiguous sex. Some people acquire an abnormal complement of sex chromosomes (see *Chromosomal abnormalities*) and all the characteristics of one sex do not develop. In some female fetuses, a metabolic defect causes production of large amounts of male hormones (see *Adrenal hyperplasia, congenital*), causing masculinization of the female genitals (such as enlargement of the clitoris to form an appendage resembling a penis). Conversely, in some male fetuses, male hormones are not produced or they are produced but fail to cause masculinization; the child's genitals are feminized to some degree (the extreme case of this is called *testicular feminization syndrome*). Finally, there are very rare cases of true *hermaphroditism*, in which a child is born with both testicular and ovarian tissue and may have both a vagina and a penis. These ambiguities are different from *transsexualism*, in which a person's biological sex is not in doubt, although it conflicts with his or her psychological disposition.

When an infant is born with ambiguous genitalia, the cause of the ambiguity is investigated and the child is assigned the sex believed to offer the best chance for a healthy life. The decision depends on the possibilities for establishing one sex or another through hormonal and/or surgical treatment. In most cases, a satisfactory male or female appearance and sexual capacity can be achieved. The ability to have children can also be achieved in some cases.

Sex hormones

Hormones that control the development of primary and secondary sexual characteristics and regulate various sex-related functions in the body, such as the menstrual cycle and the production of eggs or sperm. There are three main types of sex hormones—*androgen hormones* (male sex hormones), *oestrogen hormones* (female sex hormones), and *progesterone hormone* (which has the specialized function of preparing for and maintaining *pregnancy*).

Sex-linked inheritance

The process by which a trait or a disorder determined by the *sex chromosomes* in a person's cells, or by the *genes* carried on those chromosomes, is passed to the next generation.

Most people carry two sex chromosomes in their cells. Disorders caused by an abnormal number of sex chromosomes include *Turner's syndrome* (which affects females only and is caused by a missing X chromosome) and *Klinefelter's syndrome* (which affects males only and is caused by one or more extra X chromosomes).

Most other sex-linked traits or disorders are caused by recessive genes on the X chromosome (see *Genetic disorders*). In females, recessive genes for traits or disorders carried on the X chromosome are usually masked by a normal gene on the other X chromosome; males have only a single X chromosome, so no such masking takes place. As a result, X-linked traits or disorders affect many more males than females. Examples of such conditions include *haemophilia*, Duchenne *muscular dystrophy*, and *colour vision deficiency*.

Sex therapy

Counselling for and treatment of *psychosexual dysfunction* (sexual difficulties not due to a physical cause). Sex therapy is usually undertaken in conjunction with *marriage guidance*.

It is estimated that at least 50 per cent of couples experience some form of sexual problem at some stage in their relationships; in most cases, the problem is psychological in origin. Sex therapy can help by changing the general attitude of one or both partners towards sex, by increasing each person's understanding of his or her sexual needs and those of the partner, and by teaching techniques to deal with specific problems. Both partners usually attend the therapy sessions, but individual sex therapy or group therapy may also be useful.

TECHNIQUES

In the *sensate-focus technique*, the couple explores pleasurable, relaxed, sensual rather than sexual, bodily sensations. The goal of this technique is to reduce anxiety about sexual performance and to increase individual awareness of how to give and receive pleasure for at least 15 minutes.

The most common sexual problem in men is premature ejaculation (see *Ejaculation, disorders of*). Two preventive techniques are taught. One is the squeeze technique (see illustration). The other technique requires both partners to stop thrusting a moment before ejaculation is imminent. In either case, once the man has achieved control over the ejaculatory reflex, sexual activity is resumed. The techniques can be repeated as many times as required. They can easily be learned and are highly successful.

A woman who rarely or never experiences orgasm (see *Orgasm, lack of*)

S

THE SQUEEZE TECHNIQUE
This technique is used for treating and preventing premature ejaculation in men.

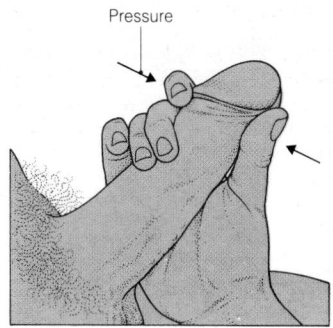

Pressure

Method
Either partner squeezes the penis when the man is about to ejaculate, pressing just beneath the glans (head of the penis) using the thumb and two fingers.

or who has *vaginismus* (spasm of the vaginal muscles, preventing intercourse) may be treated individually, with her partner, or at group therapy sessions. The woman is encouraged to come to terms with her sexuality. She is taught to perform exercises for relaxing and tightening the pelvic muscles (see *Pelvic floor exercises*) and to stimulate the clitoris to achieve orgasm through masturbation.

RESULTS

Sex therapy has proved successful for many sexual problems, with particularly effective results in treating vaginismus, premature ejaculation, lack of orgasm, impotence, and failure to consummate marriage.

Sexual abuse

The subjection of a person to sexual activity that has caused or is likely to cause physical or psychological harm. The victims of sexual abuse are most commonly children or women. The perpetrator is usually an adult male and the activity may be heterosexual or homosexual. Many episodes are unreported or are unrecognized. The causes are badly understood but may be indicative of sexual deviation or of sexual problems in the man.

Forms of sexual abuse range from abnormally affectionate relationships within a family (see *Incest*) to extremely violent sexual assaults, and include the sexual exploitation of children and adolescents who live in or are exposed to an unacceptable sexual environment. When physical sexual abuse of a child is suspected, the child should be interviewed and examined by a trained doctor who is experienced in sexual abuse cases. (See also *Child abuse*; *Rape*.)

Sexual characteristics, secondary

Physical features appearing at *puberty* that indicate the onset of adult reproductive life.

In girls, the earliest secondary sexual characteristic is enlargement of the nipples and breasts. Shortly afterwards, pubic and underarm hair appears, while body fat increases around the hips, stomach, and tops of the thighs to produce the female body shape.

In boys, enlargement of the testes is the first change, followed by thinning of the skin of the scrotum and enlargement of the penis. Pubic, facial, axillary, and other body hair appears, the voice deepens, and muscle bulk and bone size increase.

Sexual desire, inhibited

Lack of sexual desire or of the ability to become physically aroused during sexual activity (see *Sexual intercourse*). Either form of the condition may be physical or psychological.

CAUSES

LACK OF DESIRE A high proportion of women and some men experience loss of sexual desire at some point in their lives. Common physical causes include fatigue, ill health, and vaginal tenderness after childbirth. Certain drugs can also reduce sexual desire, including sleeping pills, antidepressants, antihypertensives, oral contraceptives, and alcohol. Psychological factors include *depression*, anxiety, severe stress, an unsatisfactory relationship with the sexual partner, grief at the death of a sexual partner, an unwanted pregnancy, an abortion, or a traumatic sexual experience such as *rape* or *incest*.

LACK OF PHYSICAL AROUSAL It is rare for a woman or a man to be incapable of physical sexual arousal. The most common reason for failure is poor or insensitive sexual technique on the part of the partner, although hostility, anxiety, guilt about the sex act, or fear of sexual inadequacy may contribute to the problem. In some cases, an individual may simply be unable to respond to a particular partner but be capable of responding to another, making the sexual problem selective rather than general.

TREATMENT

Problems that have a psychological basis or that are caused by the partner's sexual technique can often be successfully treated by *sex therapy* or *marriage guidance*. Sexual problems with a physical or chemical cause often improve once the underlying condition is resolved.

Sexual deviation

See *Deviation, sexual*.

Sexual dysfunction

See *Psychosexual dysfunction*.

Sexual intercourse

A term sometimes used to describe a variety of sexual activities, but more commonly used to refer specifically to the act during which a man inserts his penis into a woman's vagina.

Sexual intercourse provides pleasurable sensations that may result in *orgasm* for one or both partners. The *ejaculation* of *semen* into the woman's reproductive tract is the usual means by which *fertilization* is achieved.

Couples bring many variations to the sexual act in terms of emotions, positions, and techniques used. However, for most couples, kissing, tenderness, and foreplay precede penetration. During sexual intercourse, a series of physiological responses occurs.

PHASES OF INTERCOURSE

Physiologically, intercourse can be divided into four phases—arousal, a plateau phase, orgasm, and resolution (see illustrated box opposite).

DISORDERS

Problems with intercourse may have physical or psychological origins. (See *Intercourse, painful*; *Psychosexual dysfunction*; *Sexual problems*.)

Sexuality

A general term for the capacity, behaviour patterns, impulses, emotions, and sensations connected with reproduction and the use of the sex organs. In biology, sex refers specifically to the anatomical differences between male and female.

Heterosexuality is sexuality directed towards the anatomically opposite sex; in *homosexuality* the attraction is towards the same sex. The term *bisexuality* refers to people who experience sexual attraction to members of either sex. (See also *Gender identity*.)

Sexually transmitted diseases

Infections transmitted primarily, but not exclusively, by sexual intercourse.

HISTORY AND INCIDENCE

Also known as venereal diseases, sexually transmitted diseases (STDs) are acquired more often by people who have many sex partners. Some of the major STDs are also transmitted by blood and thus occur in drug addicts who share needles.

Until about 25 years ago, STDs were thought to be limited to *syphilis*, *gonorrhoea*, *chancroid*, and *lymphogranuloma venereum*. Today, however, these four diseases account for only about 10 per cent of all STDs seen in STD clinics. Other conditions also reported by STD clinics now include *chlamydial infections*, *trichomoniasis*, genital herpes (see *Herpes, genital*), *molluscum contagiosum*, *scabies*, *pubic lice*, genital warts (see *Warts, genital*), HIV infection and *AIDS*. Some other diseases, including viral *hepatitis* and *candidiasis* can also be transmitted by sexual intercourse but are not always STDs.

During World War II, STDs became more prevalent and then declined when the introduction of penicillin provided a cure for syphilis and

S

SEXUAL INTERCOURSE

The term sexual intercourse usually refers to the act during which the male's penis is inserted into the female's vagina. However, some people use the term more broadly to refer to a much wider range of sexual activity. Physiologically, intercourse falls into four main stages—arousal (which generally includes a period of foreplay), a plateau (during which penetration usually occurs), orgasm, and resolution. The duration of each stage of intercourse varies.

Arousal in men
Sexual thoughts, the sight and feel of his partner's body, and foreplay may sexually arouse a man. Blood enters the penis so that it becomes firm and erect.

Plateau phase in men
Vaginal penetration usually takes place during this phase and thrusting movements begin. The penis reaches maximum size and the testes elevate.

Orgasm in men
Muscular contractions in the ducts connecting the testes, prostate, and penis force semen out of the penis, accompanied by intensely pleasurable sensations.

Resolution in men
The penis returns to half its fully erect size and the testes descend.

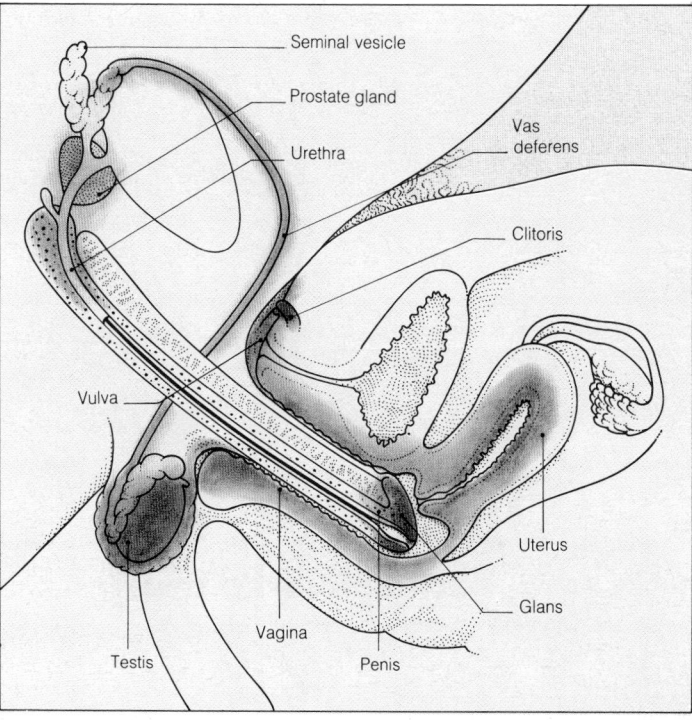

Seminal vesicle
Prostate gland
Urethra
Vas deferens
Clitoris
Vulva
Testis
Vagina
Penis
Uterus
Glans

Arousal in women
Similar factors lead to arousal in women as in men, though foreplay may be more important. The clitoris lengthens, the vagina enlarges, and its walls secrete a lubricating fluid.

Plateau phase in women
Muscular contractions in the walls of the vagina help grip the penis. The uterus rises, and the clitoris may pull back beneath its hood of skin.

Orgasm in women
The walls of the outer part of the vagina contract rhythmically and strongly several times and an intense sensual feeling spreads from the clitoris and throughout the body.

Resolution in women
The clitoris subsides and, more gradually, the vagina relaxes and the uterus falls.

BREATHING RATE
Breaths per minute

50
40
30
20
10

A   P   O   R

HEART-RATE
Beats per minute

250
200
150
100
50

A   P   O   R

BLOOD PRESSURE
Millimetres of mercury (mm Hg)

300
250
200
150
100

A   P   O   R

Key ••• Men ••• Women **A** = arousal **P** = plateau **O** = orgasm **R** = resolution

Breathing rate
Both men and women breathe faster and louder as sexual excitement builds. The rate rises gradually, peaking at about twice the normal rate at orgasm.

Heart-rate
Intercourse provides vigorous exercise for the heart. The heart-rate increases rapidly during arousal, peaks as high as 200 beats per minute at orgasm, then drops.

Blood pressure
Systolic blood pressure rises in a similar pattern to the heart-rate, peaking at orgasm. The rise may be more marked in men than in women.

S

INCIDENCE OF GONORRHOEA IN ENGLAND

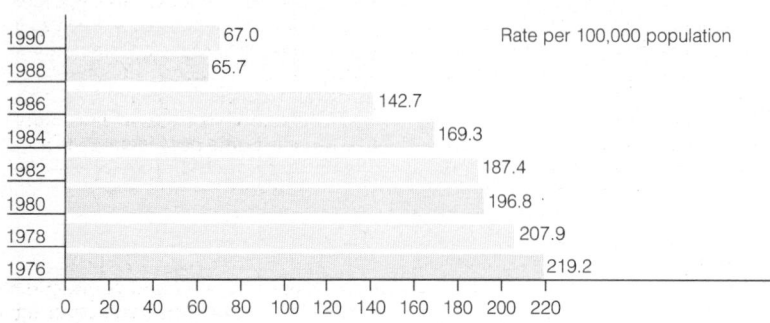

Year	Rate per 100,000 population
1990	67.0
1988	65.7
1986	142.7
1984	169.3
1982	187.4
1980	196.8
1978	207.9
1976	219.2

Gonorrhoea
After a steady decline since the late 1970s, the incidence of gonorrhoea rose slightly in 1990, and it remains one of the more common sexually transmitted diseases.

INCIDENCE OF SYPHILIS IN ENGLAND

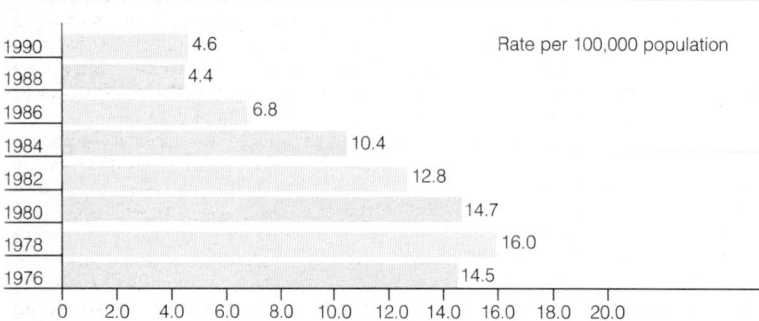

Year	Rate per 100,000 population
1990	4.6
1988	4.4
1986	6.8
1984	10.4
1982	12.8
1980	14.7
1978	16.0
1976	14.5

Syphilis
As with gonorrhoea, the incidence of syphilis generally declined from the late 1970s until 1990, when a slight increase in incidence was recorded.

CUMULATIVE TOTALS OF AIDS CASES REPORTED IN THE UK

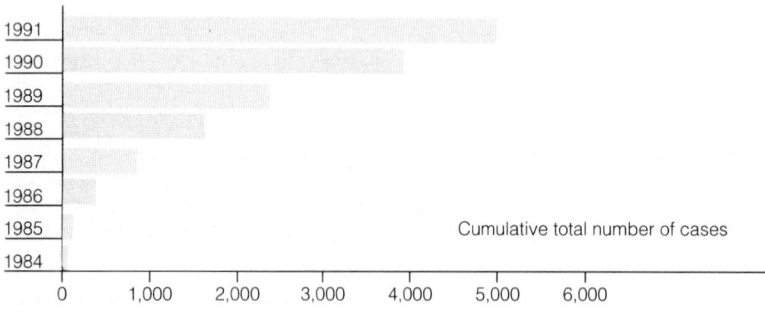

Cumulative total number of cases

Years: 1991, 1990, 1989, 1988, 1987, 1986, 1985, 1984

Axis: 0, 1,000, 2,000, 3,000, 4,000, 5,000, 6,000

AIDS
The graph shows the cumulative total number of AIDS cases reported in the UK up to 1991. In addition, at least 25 times as many people are estimated to be infected with the AIDS virus (i.e. are HIV-positive) than have full-blown AIDS. In the early years of the epidemic, most deaths were in homosexual or bisexual men. More recently, many deaths have been in intravenous drug abusers and, increasingly, in heterosexual women.

gonorrhoea. In the 1960s and 1970s, however, STDs increased again with the introduction of oral contraception. The pill led not only to women having more sex partners, but also to fewer couples using barrier contraceptives, such as condoms, which provide some protection against infection.

In the 1970s, it was recognized that so-called *nonspecific urethritis* was usually due to chlamydia. By the early 1980s a diagnosis of nonspecific urethritis and nonspecific genital infection was being made in about 25 per cent of patients visiting STD clinics; in nearly 50 per cent of these, careful laboratory testing gave evidence of chlamydial infection.

Throughout the 1970s and the early 1980s, most patients with an STD could expect a rapid cure with an antibiotic drug. In the late 1970s, however, it became apparent that certain STDs (notably herpes and hepatitis B) could not be cured by drugs and that herpes could become chronic and hepatitis could be fatal. With the recognition of AIDS in 1982, STDs became a threat to life. Promiscuous sex is now a high-risk activity.

DIAGNOSIS AND TREATMENT
Diagnosis and treatment are given at special STD clinics or from specialists in genito-urinary medicine. The doctor determines which STDs are present (there may be more than one) and then assesses the sensitivity of the infection to various antibiotics. Once drugs have relieved the symptoms, tests are performed to ensure that the patient is no longer infectious.

PREVENTION AND OUTLOOK
To prevent transmitting infection, all recent sexual partners should be traced, examined, and, when necessary, treated. The confidential tracing and treatment of contacts is an essential part of the management of STDs (see *Contact tracing*).

The incidence of most STDs (excluding AIDS) fell in the mid-1980s. But a rise in penicillin-resistant gonorrhoea in some countries in 1988 suggests that the pattern could change again, particularly if people fail to practice *safer sex* techniques.

Sexual problems
Any of a wide variety of difficulties associated with sexual performance or behaviour. A sexual problem may be perceived by both partners in a relationship, by one partner who is affected by a disorder that lies primarily with the other, or by a person worried about his or her own sexual identity or behaviour. Many people consult general practitioners, psychiatrists, or marriage guidance counsellors about sexual problems.

CAUSES
Many problems affecting a person's sexual performance or behaviour are partly or wholly psychological in origin (see *Psychosexual dysfunction; Deviation, sexual; Transvestism*).

S

Sometimes, sexual problems are due to organic disease, such as a disorder affecting blood flow or a hormonal problem. Disorders of the sexual organs may cause pain during intercourse (see *Intercourse, painful*). Sexual performance can be affected by certain drugs, such as *alcohol, antihypertensive drugs,* and *oral contraceptives.*

People with disabilities may have particular sexual problems, which often go unrecognized. Normal sexual desire may be present but gratification may be difficult to achieve because of mobility problems or because the disabled person may be avoided sexually by other people.

The mentally handicapped may not show normal personal control over their sexual behaviour, often because of poor education and social skills.

TREATMENT
Many sexual problems disappear when the underlying cause is treated. In other cases, people may benefit from sex education and counselling.

Sézary syndrome

A rare condition in which there is an abnormal overgrowth of *lymphocytes* (a type of white blood cell) in the skin, liver, spleen, and lymph nodes. Sézary syndrome mainly affects middle-aged and elderly people.

The first symptom is the appearance of red, scaly patches on the skin that spread to form a severe, itchy and flaking rash. There may also be an accumulation of fluid beneath the skin, baldness, and distorted nail growth. Sézary syndrome is sometimes associated with *leukaemia*.

Treatment includes *anticancer drugs* and *radiotherapy*.

Shellfish poisoning

See *Food poisoning.*

Shell shock

See *Post-traumatic stress disorder.*

Shigellosis

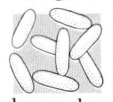 An acute infection of the intestine by bacteria belonging to the genus *SHI-GELLA*. Also known as bacillary dysentery, shigellosis causes diarrhoea and abdominal pain.

CAUSES AND INCIDENCE
The source of infection is the faeces of infected people. The causative bacteria may be spread by an infected person failing to wash the hands after defaecation and then handling food, or by flies in areas of poor sanitation. Endemic in some coun-

tries, shigellosis occurs in isolated outbreaks in the UK, where a few thousand cases are reported annually. It is particularly prevalent in children who attend nurseries, in institutions for the elderly, and in mental hospitals.

SYMPTOMS AND SIGNS
The disease usually starts suddenly, with watery diarrhoea, abdominal pain, nausea, vomiting, generalized aches, and fever. After a few days, the need to defaecate becomes frequent and urgent, and small, watery faeces containing pus and blood are passed. Persistent diarrhoea may cause *dehydration*, especially in babies and older people. Occasionally, *toxaemia* (the presence of bacterial poisons in the blood) develops, resulting in a high fever and sometimes delirium.

The illness usually subsides after a week or so, but in severe cases may last several weeks. Death is rare, usually occurring only in dehydrated babies and older people.

DIAGNOSIS AND TREATMENT
The diagnosis is confirmed by growing a *culture* of the causative bacteria from a sample of faeces.

Hospital treatment may be necessary in severe cases; people with mild infections should stay at home, where precautions should be taken to prevent the spread of infection. Dehydration is treated by *rehydration therapy*. *Antibiotic drugs* may be prescribed.

Shingles

See *Herpes zoster.*

Shin splints

A condition characterized by pain in the front and sides of the lower leg that develops or worsens during exercise. There may also be tenderness over the shin and oedema (accumulation of fluid in tissues) of the surrounding area. Shin splints are a common problem in runners.

CAUSES
Shin splints may be caused by various disorders, including *compartment syndrome* (build-up of pressure in a muscle that may sometimes result from exercise), *tendinitis* (inflammation of a tendon), *myositis* (inflammation of a muscle), a muscle tear, or *periostitis* (inflammation of the outer layer of a bone).

DIAGNOSIS AND TREATMENT
Diagnosis is based on the symptoms, along with an *X-ray* or a radionuclide bone scan (see *Bone imaging*) to exclude the possibility of a *stress fracture* of the tibia (shin-bone), which produces similar symptoms.

In most cases, shin splints clear up after a week or two of rest. However, if the pain is severe or recurrent, other treatment may be necessary, such as a course of *nonsteroidal anti-inflammatory drugs* or *corticosteroid drugs*; infrequently, a surgical operation is performed to alleviate excessive pressure in a muscle. Some people benefit from *physiotherapy* including exercises to stretch and strengthen the legs.

Shivering

Involuntary trembling of the entire body caused by the rapid contraction and relaxation of muscles. Shivering is the body's normal automatic response to cold; it also occurs in association with fever.

When the body becomes cold, temperature-sensitive nerve cells in the *hypothalamus* (part of the brain) act as a thermostat, initiating the shivering reflex. This causes muscles to contract, generating heat. Shivering caused by cold usually disappears as soon as the body is warmed.

Shivering during fever is caused by the release of certain substances by the white blood cells. These substances effectively "reset" the thermostat at a higher point, causing the body to shiver when it needs to lose, rather than retain, heat. The trigger for this release is usually an infection, but fever also occurs in some metabolic, autoimmune, and malignant diseases, and as a side-effect of certain drugs.

Shock

A dangerous reduction of blood flow throughout the body tissues which, if untreated, may lead to collapse, coma, and death. Shock in this sense is physiological shock—different from the mental distress that may follow a physically or emotionally traumatic experience (see *Post-traumatic stress disorder*). Reduced blood pressure is, in most cases, a major factor in causing physiological shock and is one of its main features.

CAUSES
Shock is a common accompaniment to severe injury or illness. It may develop in any situation in which blood volume is reduced (through blood or fluid loss), in which blood vessels are abnormally widened, in which the heart's action is weak, in which blood flow is obstructed, or through a combination of these factors.

Causes include severe *bleeding* or *burns*, persistent *vomiting* or *diarrhoea*, *myocardial infarction* (heart attack), *pul-*

S

907

monary embolism (blockage of blood flow to the lungs), *peritonitis* (inflammation of the abdominal cavity), *spinal injury*, and some types of *poisoning*. *Septic shock* results from bacteria multiplying in the blood and releasing toxins. *Anaphylactic shock* is a type of severe *hypersensitivity* or allergic reaction to an injected substance, such as insect venom or a drug. Shock is made worse by pain and anxiety.

SYMPTOMS

Symptoms of all types of shock include rapid, shallow breathing; cold, clammy skin; rapid, weak pulse; dizziness; weakness; and fainting.

TREATMENT

First aid for shock after an injury includes measures to arrest bleeding (see *Bleeding, treatment of*), maintenance of an open airway, keeping the victim flat, reducing heat loss with blankets, and reassurance. A doctor or ambulance should be called immediately, and no food or drink should be given. Emergency treatment in hospital involves an *intravenous infusion* of fluid or a blood transfusion, *oxygen therapy*, and, if necessary, *morphine* or similar powerful painkillers. Further treatment depends on the underlying cause. (See also *Shock, electric*; *Toxic shock syndrome*.)

Shock, electric

The sensation caused by an electric current passing through the body, and its effects. A mild shock may produce a sense of having been slightly shaken. A current of sufficient size and duration can cause loss of consciousness, cardiac arrest (cessation of the heartbeat), respiratory arrest, burns, and tissue damage. (See also *Electrical injury*.)

Shock therapy

The use of electricity or other agents to produce a sudden and severe disturbance in the nervous system as a means of treating mental illness, particularly severe *depression*. The mechanism of action is unknown.

Only *ECT* (electroconvulsive therapy) is regularly used today. Insulin coma therapy (in which coma was induced by repeated injections of insulin) was a form of shock therapy used in the 1940s and 1950s; it was abandoned because of the risk of permanent, severe brain damage. Another earlier method, involving the use of drugs to stimulate the nervous system, was abandoned because patients often suffered fractures and other injuries due to violent seizures.

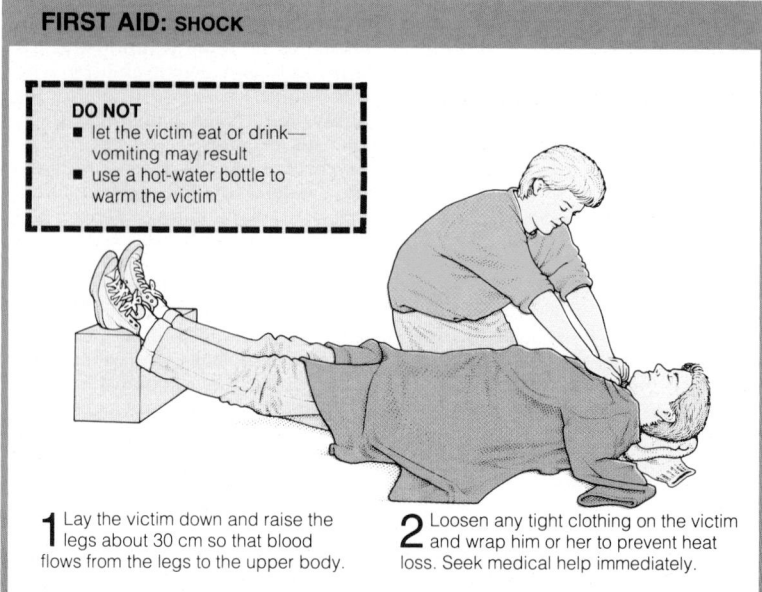

FIRST AID: SHOCK

DO NOT
- let the victim eat or drink— vomiting may result
- use a hot-water bottle to warm the victim

1 Lay the victim down and raise the legs about 30 cm so that blood flows from the legs to the upper body.

2 Loosen any tight clothing on the victim and wrap him or her to prevent heat loss. Seek medical help immediately.

Shortsightedness

See *Myopia*.

Short sight, operations for

See *Keratotomy, radial* and *Laser treatment*.

Short stature

A height significantly below the normal range for a person's age. Short stature is also called dwarfism or, sometimes, restricted growth.

Poor linear growth may be apparent from birth, may become evident in childhood, or may begin at *puberty* if sex hormone production is defective.

CAUSES

There are many causes of short stature, although sometimes no cause is found. Short stature in children is often due to hereditary factors or to slow bone growth. In most cases, growth eventually speeds up, resulting in normal height.

Less commonly, short stature is due to a specific disorder. It may be caused by bone disease, as in untreated *rickets* or *achondroplasia* (a hereditary disorder in which the ends of the limb bones do not grow fully, resulting in disproportionately short limbs).

Certain disorders of the *endocrine system* will cause delayed growth. Examples are deficiency of *growth hormone*, and *hypothyroidism* (thyroid hormone deficiency), which also affects brain development. In these conditions, the ends of the long bones and the small bones of the hands and feet

develop slowly, resulting in delayed bone age (see *Age*).

Emotional deprivation, common in abused or neglected children, chronic malnutrition (undernourishment) and untreated infections, such as *tuberculosis*, may also result in poor growth. Children with such conditions show a *failure to thrive* and are also underweight. *Malabsorption* (impaired absorption of important nutrients, such as protein, trace elements, and vitamins, from the intestine) can also limit growth. Causes include untreated *cystic fibrosis* and *coeliac disease*.

Certain chromosomal disorders are responsible for short stature. In *Down's syndrome*, there is some stunting and in *Turner's syndrome*, the pubertal growth spurt is absent.

Other causes of restricted growth in children include the prolonged use of drugs, particularly *corticosteroid drugs* and *anticancer drugs*. Severe respiratory disease and congenital heart disease, where the supply of oxygen to growing tissues is insufficient, also cause short stature unless they are treated.

INVESTIGATION

The doctor takes into account the parents' height and looks for signs of any possible underlying disease.

Most importantly, the child's growth rate is determined by means of regular measurements of height plotted on a chart. If the growth rate is normal, it indicates that the child's short stature is probably due to heredity or to temporary slow skeletal de-

S

velopment. Slow growth rate suggests that short stature has an abnormal cause. A sudden drop in growth rate can indicate the onset of disease, such as an endocrine disorder affecting the thyroid gland.

Other tests may include *X-rays* to determine bone age and *blood tests* to measure hormone levels.

TREATMENT

Any underlying disorder is treated as appropriate; for example, thyroxine is given if hypothyroidism is diagnosed. Growth hormone is given not only for growth hormone deficiency but may also be used to treat short stature due to disorders such as Turner's syndrome. Growth hormone is sometimes given in combination with the anabolic steroid oxandrolone. (See also *Growth, childhood*.)

Shoulder

The area of the body where the arm attaches to the trunk. The rounded bony surface at the front of the shoulder is the upper part of the *humerus* (upper-arm bone); the bony surfaces that form the top and back of the shoulder are parts of the *scapula* (shoulderblade). The *clavicle* (collarbone) articulates with the acromion (the bony prominence at the outer top part of the scapula) at the *acromioclavicular joint* and extends across the top of the chest to the *sternum* (breastbone), to which it is attached at the sternoclavicular joint.

STRUCTURE OF THE SHOULDER
Three bones meet at the shoulder—the scapula (shoulderblade), clavicle (collarbone), and humerus (upper-arm bone). The shoulder is an example of a ball-and-socket joint.

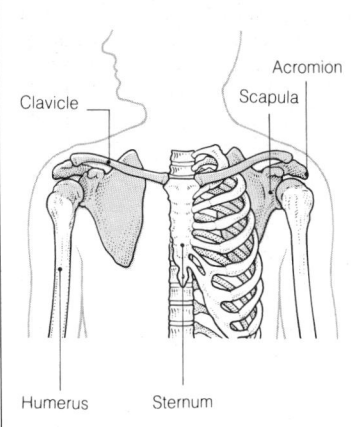

Clavicle

Acromion

Scapula

Humerus   Sternum

Just below the acromion, on the outer wall of the scapula, is a socket (called the glenoid cavity) into which the head of the humerus fits to form the shoulder joint. A *bursa* (fluid-filled sac) under the acromion reduces friction at the joint. The shoulder joint is a ball-and-socket joint with a wide range of movement produced by part of the *biceps muscle*, several small muscles that make up the *rotator cuff*, various muscles in the chest wall, and the *deltoid* muscle (the muscle at the top of the upper arm and shoulder).

DISORDERS

Shoulder injuries are relatively common, including dislocation of the shoulder joint (see *Shoulder, dislocation of*) or of the acromioclavicular joint, and *fractures* of the clavicle or of the upper part of the humerus. Fractures of the scapula are less common.

The shoulder joint may be affected by any joint disorder, including *arthritis* and *bursitis* (inflammation of a bursa). In severe cases, a joint disorder may lead to *frozen shoulder* (a condition in which movements at the joint are extremely restricted). Movement of the shoulder may also be painful and/or restricted as a result of *tendinitis* (inflammation of a tendon) affecting the tendons of the shoulder muscles. Inflammation of a tendon or a bursa around a shoulder joint can cause *painful arc syndrome*, in which pain occurs whilst raising the arm to the side of the body. (See also *Bone disorders box*; *Joints*.)

Shoulderblade

The common name for the *scapula*.

Shoulder, dislocation of

Displacement of the head of the humerus (upper-arm bone) out of the shoulder joint. The most common type of dislocation is a forward and downward displacement, caused by a fall on to an outstretched hand or on to the shoulder itself. A backward dislocation may occur as a result of a powerful direct blow to the front of the shoulder or as a result of violent twisting of the upper arm, such as that caused by an electric shock or a seizure. Either type of dislocation may be accompanied by a fracture, usually of the humerus (see *Humerus, fracture of*).

SYMPTOMS AND DIAGNOSIS

The main symptom is pain in the shoulder and upper arm that is made worse by movement. A forward dislocation often produces obvious deformity of the shoulder; a backward dislocation usually does not.

DISLOCATION OF SHOULDER
In this injury, the rounded head of the humerus (upper-arm bone) has been forced out of its socket just beneath the acromion (tip of the shoulderblade).

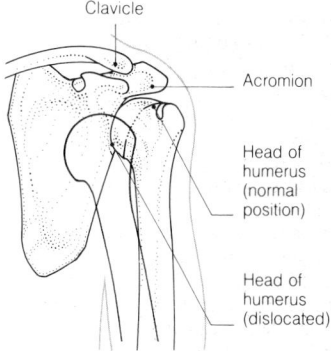

Clavicle

Acromion

Head of humerus (normal position)

Head of humerus (dislocated)

Forward dislocation of left shoulder
A forward and downward dislocation, as shown above, is the most common type.

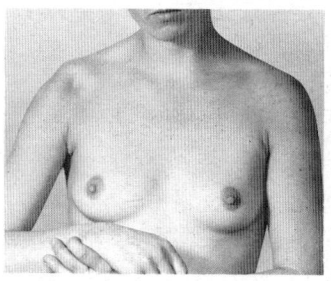

Backward dislocation
A pit can be seen in this woman's right shoulder where the head of the humerus is normally situated.

A dislocation is diagnosed by *X-rays*, which also reveal whether there is an accompanying fracture.

TREATMENT

Treatment is by reduction (manoeuvring the head of the humerus back into the joint socket), which is usually performed under anaesthesia. After reduction, X-rays are taken to ensure the head of the humerus has been correctly repositioned; the shoulder is then immobilized in a sling for about three weeks. When the humerus has been fractured, treatment is usually the same, although the arm may require a longer period of immobilization.

COMPLICATIONS

A dislocation may damage nerves, causing weakness and numbness in the shoulder. Such nerve damage is usually temporary, with full recovery occurring within two to three months.

S

Occasionally, a dislocation damages one of the arteries in the upper arm, causing pain and discoloration of the arm and the hand. In severe cases, *arterial reconstructive surgery* may be necessary.

A violent dislocation may damage the muscles that support the shoulder, making the joint susceptible to recurrent dislocation after only minor injuries. Such cases can often be successfully treated by surgery to tighten one of the supporting muscles.

Shoulder-hand syndrome

Pain and stiffness affecting one shoulder and the hand on the same side of the body; the affected hand may also become hot, sweaty, and swollen. The condition is also known as reflex sympathetic dystrophy. Because of the pain and stiffness, the arm cannot be used properly and the arm muscles may wither as a result of lack of use (see *Sudeck's atrophy*).

The precise cause of shoulder-hand syndrome is unknown, but the condition may occur as a complication of *myocardial infarction* (heart attack), *stroke*, *herpes zoster* (shingles), or a burn or other injury to the shoulder.

In most cases, recovery occurs within about two years. This period may be shortened by *physiotherapy* and treatment with *corticosteroid drugs*. In rare cases, a cervical *sympathectomy* (severing of nerves of the sympathetic nervous system on one side of the neck) is performed.

Shunt

An abnormal or surgically created passage between two normally unconnected parts. The term shunt is usually used to refer to a passage created to relieve abnormal fluid pressure around the brain in *hydrocephalus* or to relieve pressure in the portal veins in *portal hypertension.*

An *arteriovenous fistula* is a shunt between an artery and a vein, which may be created artifically to provide easy access to the bloodstream in people undergoing *dialysis*.

SHUNT FOR HYDROCEPHALUS

The shunt for hydrocephalus consists of two catheters and a valve to prevent backflow. The first catheter is inserted through the skull to drain fluid from the ventricles of the brain. The second is passed into another body cavity, usually the abdominal cavity or the right atrium of the heart, where the excess fluid is absorbed.

This procedure will need to be repeated several times during the first

10 years to replace the catheter as the child grows. In some cases, the shunt may become blocked or infected.

SHUNT FOR PORTAL HYPERTENSION

Various surgical procedures may be used to reduce pressure in the portal system (the veins that carry blood from the digestive organs and spleen to the liver) and thus reduce the risk of bleeding from *oesophageal varices.* Shunts are made by creating a direct link between the portal system and the vena cava. Shunt operations prevent bleeding but do not improve liver function and, in fact, may worsen it. The operation itself carries a fairly high mortality that is related to the severity of the disease. Although bleeding is controlled, it is questionable whether survival is prolonged.

Shy-Drager syndrome

A rare degenerative condition that causes progressive damage to the *autonomic nervous system.* The cause of Shy-Drager syndrome is unknown. The condition begins gradually, affecting people between the ages of 60 and 70, and occurs more commonly in men than in women.

The main symptoms are postural *hypotension* (dizziness and fainting when getting up or after standing still for a long time), urinary incontinence, reduced ability to sweat, impotence, and *parkinsonism* (muscle tremor, rigidity, and slow movements). The condition worsens over several years, leading to disability and sometimes to premature death.

Although there is no cure and no means of slowing the inevitable degeneration, many of the symptoms, particularly the parkinsonism and low blood pressure, can be relieved by drug treatment.

SIADH

An abbreviation for syndrome of inappropriate antidiuretic hormone (secretion). SIADH is a condition in which there is excessive production of *ADH* (antidiuretic hormone), resulting in retention of water and a low level of sodium in the body.

CAUSES

SIADH may be associated with various underlying disorders. These include: cancers, such as small cell carcinoma of the lung (see *Lung cancer*), cancer of the pancreas (see *Pancreas, cancer of*), or *Hodgkin's disease*; certain lung diseases, such as *pneumonia* or chronic obstructive lung disease (see *Lung disease, chronic obstructive*); or brain disorders, such as *encephalitis*, a

brain haemorrhage, or brain damage that results in the pituitary gland's overproducing ADH. Certain drugs, such as chlorpropamide or *oxytocin*, may increase ADH production and lead to SIADH.

SYMPTOMS AND DIAGNOSIS

The symptoms of SIADH include weakness, tiredness, and confusion. The condition is diagnosed from the symptoms and from the results of tests that measure the level of ADH in the blood and compare the concentrations of sodium in the blood and in the urine.

TREATMENT

Treatment includes restriction of water intake, *diuretic drugs* to increase water loss, and saline infusions to increase the concentration of sodium in the body. However, these measures treat only the symptoms; the underlying cause must be treated successfully to bring about a cure.

Siamese twins

Two babies that are born physically joined, also known as conjoined *twins*. The name Siamese twins comes from the first recorded pair, Chang and Eng, who were born in Thailand (formerly Siam) in 1811 and lived for 63 years joined at the hip. Siamese twins are essentially identical twins that fail to separate completely during development from a single fertilized egg. The cause is unknown.

Siamese twins range from two well-developed individuals, connected only by skin and superficial tissue, to a person with only one extra body part (such as an extra leg) as evidence of the second twin. Between these extremes are Siamese twins with two heads and two trunks joined at the waist but with only two legs. In some cases one of the twins is very small and poorly developed. The twins' internal organs and brains may be separate, or some or all of these organs may be shared.

TREATMENT

If the twins survive birth, and if each one is sufficiently developed to function independently, complete separation by surgery may be possible.

Sibling rivalry

A term that describes the intense competition that sometimes occurs between siblings (brothers and/or sisters). It may occur, for example, after the birth of a new baby, when an older sibling constantly seeks to command the parents' attention. Feelings of rivalry may persist through life.

S

Sick building syndrome

A collection of symptoms sometimes reported by people who work in modern office buildings; the symptoms include loss of energy, headaches, and dry, itching eyes, nose, and throat.

The cause of the syndrome is unknown, although it has been attributed to air conditioning, passive exposure to tobacco smoke, loss of natural ventilation and light, and psychological factors, especially frustration at being unable to control physical conditions (e.g. temperature and ventilation) in the working environment. Less convincingly, it has been attributed to fluorescent lighting.

Treatment using environmental agents, such as ionizers, has been unsuccessful. Modification of the working environment may be the best solution.

Sickle cell anaemia

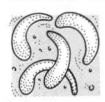 An inherited blood disease that occurs primarily in black people and, less commonly, in people of Mediterranean origin. In sickle cell anaemia, the red cells are abnormal, resulting in a chronic, very severe form of *anaemia* (reduced oxygen-carrying capacity of the blood).

CAUSE

The red cells of affected people contain an abnormal type of *haemoglobin* (oxygen-carrying pigment) called haemoglobin S. In the blood capillaries, where there is less oxygen in the blood, the deficiency of oxygen causes haemoglobin S to crystallize, distorting the red cells into a sickle shape. This makes the cells fragile and easily destroyed, leading to haemolytic anaemia. The abnormal cells are also unable to pass easily through tiny blood vessels, and this difficulty causes intermittent blockage of the blood supply to various organs, causing sickle cell crises.

Sickle cell anaemia occurs in people who have inherited haemoglobin S from both their parents. If haemoglobin S is inherited from one parent, the person has sickle cell trait and is usually free of symptoms. If two such carriers have a child, there is a one in four chance that the child will have sickle cell anaemia, a two in four chance that the child will have sickle cell trait, and a one in four chance that the child will have neither.

INCIDENCE

In the UK, about one in 100 black people of West African origin and one in 200 of West Indian origin suffer from sickle cell anaemia. About one in 10 black people has sickle cell trait.

SYMPTOMS AND SIGNS

The symptoms of sickle cell anaemia usually first appear after the age of six months. Chronic haemolytic anaemia causes fatigue, headaches, shortness of breath on exertion, pallor, and *jaundice*.

Sickle cell crises are sometimes brought on by an infection, cold weather, or dehydration (caused, for example, by prolonged vomiting and diarrhoea), but may also occur for no apparent reason. The crises start suddenly, and attack or damage various parts of the body. The sufferer may experience pains (especially in the bones), blood in the urine (from kidney damage), or damage to the lungs or intestines. The brain may also be affected, leading to *seizures*, a *stroke*, or unconsciousness.

In some children, the *spleen* enlarges and traps red cells at a particularly high rate, causing a severe, life-threatening form of anaemia. From adolescence onwards, the spleen usually shrivels and ceases to function; as a result, affected people are at risk of developing *septicaemia* (blood poisoning) if they are infected by certain types of bacteria, especially pneumococci.

Children with sickle cell anaemia have an increased risk of pneumococcal *pneumonia* and of *gallstones*.

DIAGNOSIS

The diagnosis is made from examination of a specially treated *blood smear* for the presence of sickle-shaped red cells and from *electrophoresis* to check for the presence of haemoglobin S.

TREATMENT

Supportive treatment for sickle cell anaemia includes supplements of *folic acid*, immunization against pneumococcal infections, and *penicillin* to guard against septicaemia.

Life-threatening crises are treated with *intravenous infusions* of fluids for dehydration, *antibiotic drugs* to treat and prevent infections, *oxygen therapy* to increase blood oxygenation, and *analgesic drugs* to relieve severe pain.

If a severe crisis does not respond to the above measures, an exchange *blood transfusion* may be performed to effect a temporary replacement of haemoglobin S. This may be done regularly for people who suffer frequent severe crises. Exchange transfusions may also be carried out during pregnancy, to reduce the risk of a crisis (with possibly fatal consequences for

mother and child), and before surgery, since anaesthesia presents a hazard to people who have sickle cell anaemia (and, to a lesser degree, to those with sickle cell trait).

The only chance of a cure for sickle cell anaemia as yet is a *bone marrow transplant*, a treatment that itself carries a risk to life but offers the prospect of virtually normal health. If the transplant is successful, the red cells produced by the bone marrow will be normal and the anaemia cured. This treatment is available only in specialist centres but has proved successful in around 85 per cent of cases.

OUTLOOK

Until about 30 years ago, sickle cell anaemia usually proved fatal in childhood. Today, although the mortality is still high in those under five years old, improving methods of treatment have enabled more sufferers to survive into adulthood. Some sufferers are now having children.

Black people, and close relatives of anyone with sickle cell anaemia, who do not know whether they carry the sickle cell gene are advised to find out by having a blood test. A couple who both have sickle cell anaemia and/or trait, should obtain *genetic counselling* before starting a family. Tests can be performed in early pregnancy to determine whether a fetus has inherited a double dose of the sickle cell gene and thus will have sickle cell anaemia.

Sick sinus syndrome

Abnormal function of the sinoatrial node (the heart's pacemaker) that leads to episodes of *bradycardia* (slow heart-rate), alternating bradycardia and *tachycardia* (fast heart-rate), or very short episodes of *cardiac arrest* (complete stoppage of the heartbeat). The most common cause is *coronary artery disease*, but the condition can also be caused by a *cardiomyopathy*.

Symptoms include light-headedness, dizziness, fainting, and, occasionally, palpitations.

The diagnosis is confirmed by a 24-hour *ECG* recording. Treatment is usually by *antiarrhythmic drugs* and the fitting of an artificial *pacemaker*.

Side-effect

A reaction or consequence of medication or therapy that is additional to the desired effect. The term usually (although not always) refers to an unwanted or adverse effect. It is not usually applied to the toxic effects produced by a drug overdose, but to a secondary effect of a normal dose.

S

A side-effect may occur if the desired effect of therapy continues beyond the desired limits, such as when bleeding results from treatment with *anticoagulant drugs*. Alternatively, the side-effect may be completely unrelated to the aim of therapy, such as when drowsiness results from *antihistamine drugs* prescribed to alleviate allergic *rhinitis* (hay fever). However, an unwanted side-effect in one circumstance may be a desired effect in another (drowsiness is the desired effect when antihistamines are used as sedatives).

Side-effects that can be expected from the known actions of a particular drug and that can occur in most patients taking that drug are known as type I side-effects. Type II side-effects occur in only a minority of patients and are usually unpredictable —until the doctor discovers the connection between a particular drug and a patient's idiosyncratic response to it. Type II effects may be caused, for example, by a genetic disorder (such as the lack of a specific enzyme that usually inactivates the drug) or by an allergic reaction. Common type II side-effects include a rash, swelling of the face, or jaundice. The occurrence of a type II side-effect usually necessitates withdrawal of the drug. (See also *Drug*.)

Siderosis
Any of a variety of conditions in which there is too much *iron* in the body. Excess iron in the blood or tissues without associated damage is usually called *haemosiderosis*.

SIDS
An abbreviation for *sudden infant death syndrome*.

Sievert
The SI unit of equivalent absorbed dose of ionizing radiation (see *Radiation* units box).

Sight
See *Vision*.

Sight, partial
Loss of vision short of total *blindness*. Partial sight may involve a loss of *visual acuity*, of *visual field*, or of both.

Sigmoid colon
Also known as the pelvic colon, the S-shaped part of the *colon* in the lower abdomen which extends from the brim of the pelvis, usually down to the third segment of the *sacrum* (the triangular bone in the lower spine). The sigmoid colon is connected to the descending colon above and the rectum below.

Sigmoidoscopy
Examination of the *rectum* and the *sigmoid colon* (last parts of the large intestine) with a viewing instrument called a sigmoidoscope or proctosigmoidoscope. Sigmoidoscopy is a form of *endoscopy*.

WHY IT IS DONE
Sigmoidoscopy is performed to investigate symptoms relating to the lower gastrointestinal tract, such as bleeding from the rectum or lower colon, and to look for evidence of disorders, such as polyps (small benign growths), *ulcerative colitis*, or cancer (see *Colon, cancer of*). Attachments on the end of the sigmoidoscope allow a *biopsy* (removal of a small sample of tissue for analysis) to be performed if necessary.

HOW IT IS DONE
Sigmoidoscopy is sometimes performed as a follow-up to a *rectal examination*, in which the doctor examines the rectum with a gloved finger. Sigmoidoscopy may also be preceded by *proctoscopy* (an examination of the anal canal and rectum with a viewing instrument).

The procedure involved, along with a typical view through a sigmoidoscope, is shown in the illustrated box.

Sign
An objective indication of a disease or disorder (e.g. *jaundice*) that is observed or detected by a doctor, as opposed to a *symptom* (e.g. pain), which is noticed by the patient.

Silicone
Any of a specific group of silicon compounds. Silicones are defined as polymeric (long-chain), organic

---

PROCEDURE FOR SIGMOIDOSCOPY

This is an outpatient procedure taking less than half an hour and needing no anaesthetic. Either a rigid or a flexible endoscope (viewing tube) may be used. An *enema* may be given beforehand. The patient lies on the left side with knees drawn up. The entry of the lubricated instrument causes little discomfort.

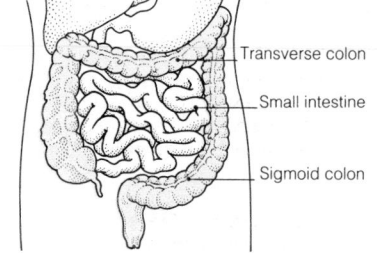

Transverse colon

Small intestine

Sigmoid colon

View through sigmoidoscope

Wall of colon

Flexible sigmoidoscope

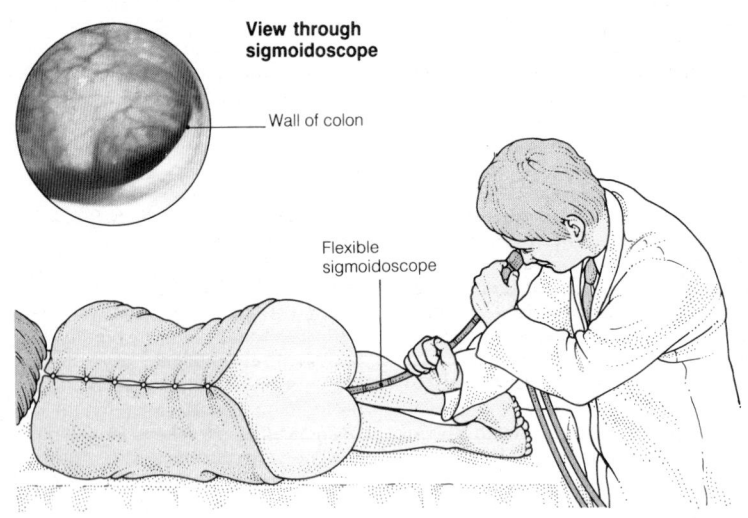

Value of sigmoidoscopy
If the bowel is properly cleared of faeces beforehand and distended by air pumped in through the instrument, a good view of the lining of the rectum and lower colon may be obtained. This area is often affected by benign growths, ulcers, or cancer. Direct observation of disorders allows early diagnosis and treatment.

(carbon-containing) compounds of silicon and oxygen. They exist and are used medically in the form of oils, greases, plastics, or rubbers.

Synthetic silicones are widely used as implants in *cosmetic surgery* because they are resistant to body fluids, permeable to oxygen, and are not rejected by the body. Silicone oil in a silicone rubber bag is used in breast reconstruction or breast enlargement (see *Mammoplasty*).

Silicosis

A lung disease caused by the inhalation of dusts containing silica—a common mineral found in sand, quartz, and various types of rock. (See *Pneumoconiosis*.)

Silver sulphadiazine

An *antibacterial drug* applied as a cream to prevent infection after skin grafts or in burns, leg ulcers, and pressure sores. Side-effects may include permanent grey skin discoloration and allergic reactions such as rashes or itching.

Simvastatin

A *lipid-lowering drug* that acts on liver enzymes that produce *cholesterol*. It may cause bowel upsets, headaches, and, occasionally, muscle pains.

Sinew

A common nonmedical term for a *tendon*, a tough fibrous cord that joins a muscle to a bone.

Singer's nodes

Small, greyish-white lumps or nodules that develop on the vocal cords as the result of constant voice strain. Singer's nodes occur in singers, teachers, politicians, and other people who use their voices excessively, causing hoarseness or loss of voice.

A *biopsy* (removal of a sample of tissue for microscopic examination) may exclude the possibility of there being a malignant tumour (see *Larynx, cancer of*). In acute cases, treatment consists of resting the voice. In chronic cases, surgical removal of the nodes may be necessary. People who develop singer's nodes may benefit from voice training.

Sinoatrial node

The natural pacemaker of the *heart*. The sinoatrial node consists of a cluster of specialized muscle cells within the wall of the right atrium (upper chamber) of the heart. Without any external influence, these cells emit electrical impulses at a rate of 100 per

LOCATION AND FUNCTION OF THE SINOATRIAL NODE

The sinoatrial (SA) node is a small mass of muscle cells in the right atrium of the heart. It sends out impulses at an inherent rate of 100 impulses per minute. External control by the vagus nerve reduces the rate to about 70 per minute. Other mechanisms also affect the rate.

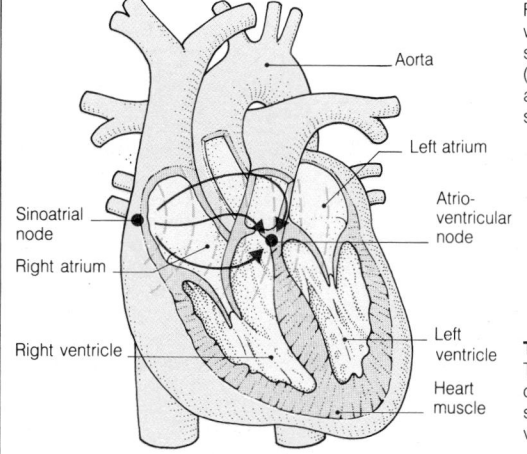

Spread of the impulse
From the SA node, the waves of contraction spread over both atria (pink area) and then to the atrioventricular node serving the ventricles.

Aorta

Left atrium

Atrio-ventricular node

Sinoatrial node

Right atrium

Right ventricle

Left ventricle

Heart muscle

Wave of excitation spreading over atria

Excitation spreading over ventricles

The electrocardiogram
The spread of excitation over the two atria is fairly slow; the spread over the ventricles is rapid.

minute, which initiate the contractions (beats) of the heart. Various hormones and nervous system activities can affect the node, causing it to emit impulses at a different rate, thus slowing down or speeding up the heart. (See also *Heart-rate*.)

Sinus

A cavity within a bone, in particular one of the air-filled spaces, lined with mucous membrane, in the bones surrounding the nose (see *Sinus, facial*, and illustrated box overleaf).

The term sinus also refers to any wide channel that contains blood, such as the venous sinuses in the outermost covering of the brain.

Sinus is also a term for an abnormal, often infected, tract.

Sinus bradycardia

A slow, but regular, heart-rate (less than 60 beats per minute). Sinus bradycardia is caused by reduced electrical activity in the sinoatrial node (the heart's pacemaker). Unlike *heart block*, there is no impairment to the transmission of electrical impulses through the heart. Sinus bradycardia is normal in athletes and in people who exercise regularly; it can be achieved by relaxation techniques.

Sinus bradycardia may also be caused by *hypothyroidism*, by a *myocardial infarction* (heart attack), or by taking certain drugs, such as *beta-blocker* drugs or *digoxin*.

Sinus, facial

Any of the air-filled cavities, lined with mucous membrane, in the bones surrounding the nose. The facial sinuses comprise: the two frontal sinuses in the frontal bone of the forehead just above the eyebrows; the two maxillary sinuses in the cheekbones; the two ethmoidal sinuses, which are honeycomb-like cavities in bones that lie between the nasal cavity and the eye sockets; and the sphenoidal sinuses, which are a collection of air spaces in the large, winged bone behind the nose that forms the central part of the base of the skull. Mucus drains from each sinus along a narrow channel that opens into the nose.

Infection, usually spreading from the nose, may cause *sinusitis* (inflammation of the lining of the sinuses).

Sinusitis

Inflammation of the membrane lining the facial *sinuses* (the air-filled cavities in the bones surrounding the nose) caused by infection. The maxillary sinuses, in the cheekbones, and the ethmoidal sinuses, between the eyes, are the most commonly affected.

CAUSES AND INCIDENCE
Most sinusitis is caused by infection spreading to the sinuses from the nose along the narrow passages that drain mucus from the sinuses into the nose. The disorder is usually the result of a bacterial infection that develops as a complication of a viral infection, such

S

LOCATION AND FUNCTION OF THE SINUSES

The air spaces, or sinuses, in the skull bones lighten the skull and improve the resonance of the voice. The sinuses surround the nose and are lined with mucous membrane. Mucus produced by this membrane drains into the nasal cavity via narrow channels.

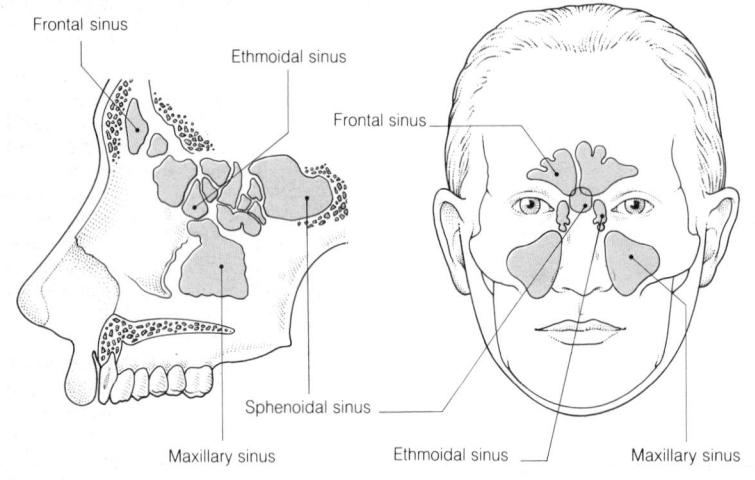

Cross-section through skull

Frontal sinus
Ethmoidal sinus
Frontal sinus
Sphenoidal sinus
Maxillary sinus
Ethmoidal sinus
Maxillary sinus

as the common *cold*. Less commonly, infection may arise from an abscess in an upper tooth (see *Abscess, dental*), from infected water being forced into the sinuses when a person jumps feet first into water without covering the nose, or from a severe facial injury.

Sinusitis is extremely common; many people suffer an attack after every common cold. It seems that once the tendency to sinus infection is established, recurrence is more likely with each cold.

SYMPTOMS AND SIGNS
Sinusitis usually causes a feeling of tension or fullness in the affected area and sometimes a throbbing ache. It may also result in fever, a stuffy nose, and loss of the sense of smell.

A common complication is the formation of pus in the affected sinuses, causing pain and a nasal discharge. Rare complications include orbital cellulitis (see *Orbit*), *osteomyelitis*, and *meningitis*.

DIAGNOSIS AND TREATMENT
X-rays are sometimes taken to determine the location and extent of the disorder; a *culture* may be grown from a lavage (washing) of the maxillary sinus to identify the infective bacteria. *Antibiotic drugs* are given immediately to combat the infection, but the antibiotic chosen may be changed after the result of a culture is known. Use of nose-drops or a spray contain-

ing a *decongestant drug* restores drainage of the sinuses by reducing inflammation of the mucous membranes. Steam inhalations moisten the secretions and are helpful in removing them. If sinusitis persists despite this treatment, surgical drainage of the affected sinuses may be performed.

Sinus tachycardia
A fast, but regular, heart-rate (more than 100 beats per minute). Sinus tachycardia is caused by increased electrical activity in the sinoatrial node (the heart's pacemaker). Such a heartbeat is normal during sudden stressful or anxious moments. It is also normal during exercise and for a short time afterwards. Persistent sinus tachycardia at rest may be caused by fever, *hyperthyroidism*, and other disorders. (See also *Tachycardia*.)

Situs inversus
An unusual condition in which the internal organs are situated in the mirror image of their normal positions. No treatment is required unless there is an associated abnormality of any of the organs, in which case surgery may be necessary. (See also *Dextrocardia*.)

Sjögren's syndrome
A condition in which the eyes and mouth become excessively dry. The nasal cavity, throat and vagina may

also be affected. Sjögren's syndrome tends to occur with certain *autoimmune disorders*, such as *rheumatoid arthritis* or systemic *lupus erythematosus*. The exact cause is unknown. However, because the autoimmune disorder upsets the body's defence system, it begins to destroy the glands that produce lubricating secretions.

Ninety per cent of sufferers are women—mostly middle-aged and often postmenopausal.

The most characteristic and troublesome feature of the condition is *keratoconjunctivitis sicca* (dry eye), which causes itching and burning of the eyes. Artificial tears can be used to moisten the eye. Lack of saliva leads to an increased risk of dental *caries*.

Skeleton
The average human adult skeleton has 213 *bones* (counting each of the nine fused *vertebrae* of the *sacrum* and *coccyx* as individual bones) joined with *ligaments* and *tendons* to form a protective and supportive framework for the attached muscles and underlying soft tissues of the body. In some people, however, there may be a variation in the number of vertebrae or there may be additional small bones (called sesamoids) in tendons around the joints.

STRUCTURE
The skeleton consists of two main parts, known as the axial and appendicular skeletons.

The axial skeleton comprises the *skull*, *spine*, *ribs*, and *sternum* (breastbone). Together, they have a total of 87 bones: 29 in the skull (including the *hyoid* bone and three pairs of auditory *ossicles*); 33 in the spine (seven cervical, 12 thoracic, and five lumbar vertebrae, the five fused vertebrae of the sacrum, and the four fused vertebrae of the coccyx); and 25 in the chest (12 pairs of ribs and the sternum).

The appendicular skeleton consists of the two limb girdles (the *shoulder* and *pelvis*) and their attached limb bones. The appendicular skeleton includes 126 bones, 64 in the shoulders and upper limbs and 62 in the pelvis and lower limbs. There are two bones in each shoulder: the *clavicle* (collarbone) and *scapula* (shoulderblade); three in each arm—the *humerus* (upper-arm bone) and the *radius* and *ulna* (forearm bones); eight *carpals* in each *wrist*; five *metacarpals* in each palm; and 14 *phalanges* in the digits of each hand (two in each thumb and three in each finger).

S

BONES OF THE SKELETON

There are two main parts to the skeleton—the axial and appendicular skeletons (shown below). Some parts, such as the skull and pelvis, consist of several fused or associated bones. The skeleton is not merely an inert framework that supports and protects organs and makes movement possible; the bones are active living structures that constantly produce blood cells and interchange minerals with the blood.

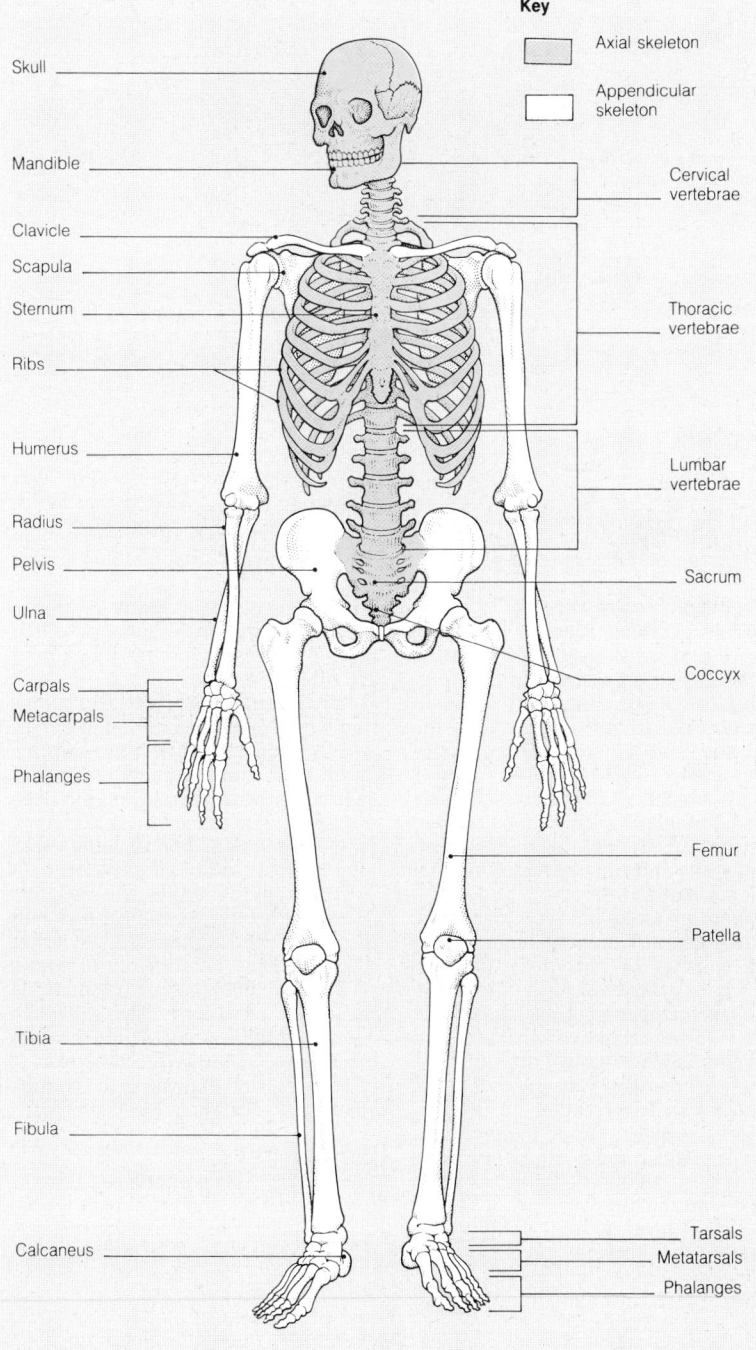

Key

Axial skeleton

Appendicular skeleton

Skull

Mandible

Clavicle

Scapula

Sternum

Ribs

Humerus

Radius

Pelvis

Ulna

Carpals

Metacarpals

Phalanges

Tibia

Fibula

Calcaneus

Cervical vertebrae

Thoracic vertebrae

Lumbar vertebrae

Sacrum

Coccyx

Femur

Patella

Tarsals

Metatarsals

Phalanges

The pelvic girdle consists of two innominate (hip) bones. There are 30 bones in each of the lower limbs: a *femur* (thigh-bone), *patella* (kneecap), and *tibia* and *fibula* (lower-leg bones) in each leg; seven tarsals in the *ankle*, heel (see *Calcaneus*), and back part of the foot; five *metatarsals* in the middle of each foot; and 14 phalanges in the toes (two in each big toe and three in each other toe).

There are only minor differences between the skeletons of men and women. In general, men's bones tend to be slightly larger and heavier than the corresponding bones in women; the female pelvic cavity is wider than that of the male to facilitate childbirth.

The individual bones of the skeleton are connected by three types of *joints*, which differ in the amount of mobility they permit.

FUNCTION

The skeleton plays an indispensable role in movement by providing a strong, stable but mobile framework on which the muscles can act. In effect, it consists of a series of independently movable internal levers on which the muscles can pull to move different parts of the body.

The skeleton also supports and protects body organs, notably the brain and spinal cord, which are encased in the skull and spine, and the heart and lungs, which are protected by the ribs. The ribs also make breathing possible by supporting the chest cavity so that the lungs are not compressed, and by helping in the breathing movements themselves.

The skeleton is not an inert frame, however. It is an active organ that produces blood cells (formed in bone marrow) and acts as a reservoir for minerals such as calcium, which can be drawn on, if required, by other parts of the body.

S

Skin

The outermost covering of body tissue, which protects the internal organs from the environment. The skin is the largest organ in the body. Its cells are continually being replaced as they are lost by wear and tear.

STRUCTURE

The skin consists of a thin outer layer (the epidermis) and a thicker inner layer (the dermis). Beneath the dermis is the subcutaneous tissue, which contains fat. The *hair* and *nails* are extensions of the skin and are composed mainly of *keratin*, which is the main constituent of the outermost part of the epidermis.

EPIDERMIS The epidermis is made up of flat cells that resemble paving stones when viewed under the microscope. Its thickness varies depending on the part of the body, being thickest on the soles and palms and very thin on the eyelids. It is generally thicker in men than in women and normally becomes thinner with age.

The outermost part of the epidermis is composed of dead cells, which form a tough, horny, protective coating. As these dead cells are worn away, they are replaced. The new cells are produced by rapidly dividing living cells in the innermost part of the epidermis. Between the outer and inner parts is a transitional region that consists of both living and dead cells.

Most of the cells in the epidermis are specialized to produce keratin, a hard protein substance that is the main constituent of the tough, outermost part. Some of the cells produce the protective pigment *melanin*, which determines skin colour.

DERMIS The dermis is composed of connective tissue interspersed with various specialized structures, such as hair follicles, *sweat glands*, and *sebaceous glands* (glands that produce an oily substance called *sebum*). The dermis also contains blood vessels, lymph vessels, and nerves.

FUNCTION
The skin's most important function is a protective one. It acts as the main barrier between the environment and the internal organs of the body, shielding them from injury, the harmful rays of sunlight, and invasion from infective agents, such as bacteria.

The skin is a sensory organ containing many cells that are sensitive to touch, temperature, pain, pressure, and itching. It also plays a role in keeping body temperature constant. When the body is hot, the sweat glands cool it by producing perspiration and the blood vessels in the dermis dilate (widen) to dissipate heat; if the body gets cold, the blood vessels in the skin constrict (narrow), which conserves the body's heat.

The epidermis contains a unique fatty substance that makes the skin waterproof—thus making it possible to sit in a bath without soaking up the water like a sponge. The outer epidermis also has an effective water-holding capacity, which contributes to its elasticity and serves to maintain the body balance of fluid and electrolytes. If the water content drops below a certain level, the skin becomes cracked, reducing its efficiency as a barrier.

STRUCTURE OF SKIN

The skin consists essentially of two layers—dermis (true skin), which contains most of the living elements, and epidermis, which is a tough protective covering with an outer layer of dead cells.

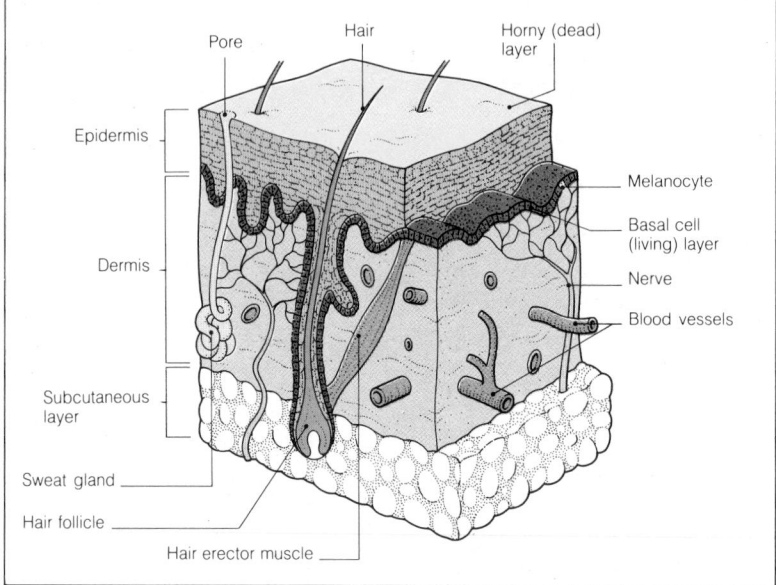

Pore — Hair — Horny (dead) layer

Epidermis

Dermis

Melanocyte

Basal cell (living) layer

Nerve

Blood vessels

Subcutaneous layer

Sweat gland

Hair follicle

Hair erector muscle

Skin allergy

A large number of substances can provoke an allergic reaction through direct contact with the skin of a susceptible person. However, the substance first must have sensitized the person's *immune system* during a previous contact or contacts. If the skin reaction is truly an allergic one, the causative substance produces symptoms only in susceptible people. Many substances that cause skin reactions (fibreglass spicules, for example) are irritant by nature, rather than allergenic, and can affect anyone, not just a sensitive few.

There are two main types of allergic skin reaction. Contact allergic *dermatitis* consists of red, itchy patches, which may blister or form crusts. The patches correspond to the area of contact with the causative substance and develop between a few hours and two days after contact. Substances that can produce such a reaction include adhesives, elastic, nickel in jewellery, some plants, some cosmetics, and chromium salts used in hat and shoe manufacture.

Contact *urticaria* (red, itchy, raised areas on the skin) may develop within a few minutes to half an hour after skin contact with some medications, chemicals, plants, insect saliva (from a bite), and foods such as shellfish.

Urticaria can also be a symptom of an allergic reaction to something eaten, but the majority of cases are probably not allergic in origin. Many drugs can cause skin eruptions, some of which resemble urticaria, but not all of them are allergic in nature.

Atopic *eczema* is an itchy skin condition which is most common in babies and children, particularly those with a family history of allergic-type illnesses such as asthma. Atopic eczema does not seem to be caused by skin contact with an allergen, but in some cases may be the result of a food allergy.

In many skin allergies, the causative substance is obvious and contact with it should be minimized. In other cases, it may be difficult to know which ingredient (e.g. of a cosmetic) is the cause of allergy. The causative agent may be discovered only through exhaustive tests in which the skin is challenged by exposure to various suspected substances (see *Skin tests*).

Skin biopsy

Removal of a portion of diseased skin for laboratory analysis. Skin *biopsy* may be performed when *skin cancer* is suspected or to confirm the diagnosis of certain skin disorders, such as *pemphigus* or *dermatomyositis*.

Under local anaesthesia, the skin is removed with a *scalpel* or a *curette*.

When a highly malignant condition, such as *melanoma*, is suspected, all of the affected area is cut away, together with the skin around and beneath it. Otherwise, only a small portion of skin is removed.

Skin cancer

A malignant tumour in the *skin*. Skin cancer is one of the most common forms of cancer and is becoming more common in Western countries, probably because of the increased exposure of the skin to sunlight that has been fashionable for the past 50 years.

Basal cell carcinoma, squamous cell carcinoma, and malignant *melanoma* are common forms of skin cancer related to long-term exposure to sunlight. *Bowen's disease*, a rare disorder that can become cancerous, may also be related to sunlight exposure. Less common types include *Paget's disease of the nipple* and *mycosis fungoides*; both produce inflammation similar to eczema. *Kaposi's sarcoma* is a type commonly found in *AIDS* patients (although elderly patients may have Kaposi's sarcoma and not have AIDS).

Most skin cancers can be easily cured if treated early, but many people die through delay in seeking treatment. All changed or new skin growths should be seen by a doctor.

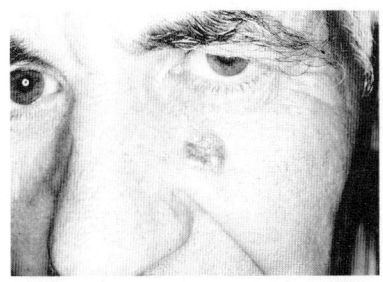

Basal cell carcinoma
This is the most common form of skin cancer. Also called rodent ulcer, it develops most commonly on the face.

Skin flap

A surgical technique in which a section of *skin* and underlying tissue, sometimes including muscle, is moved to cover an area from which skin and deeper tissue have been lost or damaged through injury, disease, or surgery.
WHY IT IS DONE
Unlike a *skin graft*, a skin flap retains its blood supply—either by remaining attached at one end to the donor site or through reattachment of its blood vessels to vessels at the new site. A

TECHNIQUE FOR MOVING A SKIN FLAP

A flap of skin and underlying tissue can be moved to a new site to replace lost tissue; if its blood supply is maintained, the flap will adhere well. Microsurgery to rejoin blood vessels facilitates the technique.

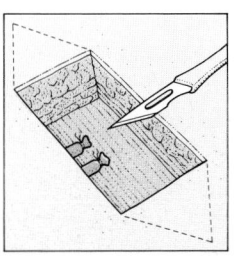

1 The donor area needs a good blood supply if muscle is also to be taken.

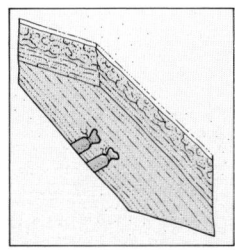

2 The ends of the donor area need to be tapered to allow satisfactory closure.

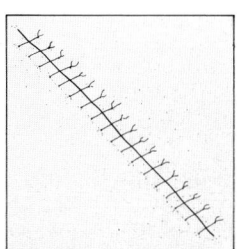

3 The skin may have to be undercut and freed before the wound is closed.

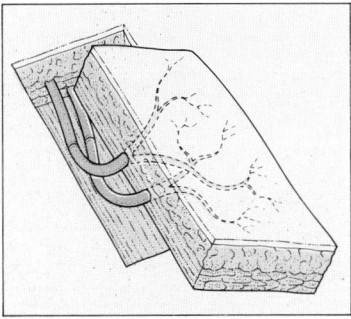

An artery and a vein of suitable size must be available at the recipient site to be joined to blood vessels in the flap.

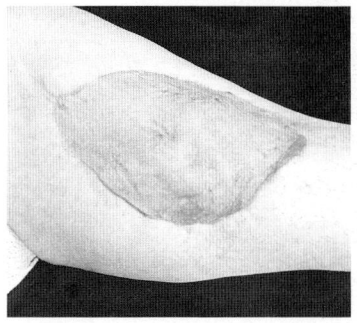

Skin flaps are particularly useful when there has been extensive loss of deep tissue. The results are usually excellent.

---

flap is therefore useful for covering an area, such as exposed bone or tendon, that has lost its blood supply and on which a graft would not "take". Flaps are also used for regions that need thick covering to protect them (e.g. bony prominences like the hip). Since flaps are less likely to contract than skin grafts, they are useful for releasing tension from scarred areas. Flaps may be preferable to grafts because healing and cosmetic results are better.
HOW IT IS DONE
When the area to be covered is relatively small and there is sufficient skin near by, the flap may be left attached at one end and moved by stretching, rotating, or transposing it. Otherwise, the flap is removed from another area of the body and its vessels are attached to new arteries and veins at the site of the graft using microsurgical techniques (see illustrated box). The area left bare by cutting the flap is closed with stitches or, if necessary, by a skin graft. (See also *Microsurgery*.)

Skin graft

A technique used in plastic surgery to repair areas of lost or damaged *skin*. A piece of healthy skin is detached from one part of the body and transferred to the affected area. New cells grow from the graft and cover the damaged area with fresh skin.

Skin taken from an identical twin can be used for a graft, but skin from another person or an animal is soon rejected by the recipient's body (although it may provide useful temporary cover).
WHY IT IS DONE
A skin graft is performed because the area is too large to be repaired by stitching or because natural healing would result in scarring that might be unsightly or restrict movement.
HOW IT IS DONE
Most grafts are performed by removing skin from the donor site and transferring it to the recipient site. There are two basic types of skin graft: split-thickness and full-thickness (see illustrated box overleaf). In some cases,

S

underlying muscle is removed with the full thickness of skin (see *Skin flap*).

RESULTS

All grafts leave scars. Full-thickness grafts yield more natural colour and texture, and contrast less than split-thickness grafts. However, full-thickness grafts are less likely to "take".

Skin patch

See *Transdermal patch*.

Skin peeling, chemical

A cosmetic operation to remove freckles, acne scars, delicate wrinkles, or other surface skin blemishes. A paste containing phenol (carbolic acid) or some other caustic agent is applied to the skin, left for a half hour, and then scraped off. The outer layers of the skin peel away with the paste, thus removing the blemishes.

Because of *photosensitivity*, the raw area must not be exposed to sunlight until new skin layers have fully grown. Permanent discoloration of the skin is common; it may be improved by wearing make-up.

Skin tag

A small, brown or flesh-coloured, protruding flap of skin usually occurring spontaneously, but caused occasionally by unsatisfactory healing of a wound. Anal tags often occur as a complication of *anal fissures* or *haemorrhoids*. Skin tags can usually be removed easily by a doctor.

Skin tests

Procedures for determining the body's reaction to various substances by injecting a small quantity of the substance underneath the skin or by applying it to the skin.

Patch tests are widely used in the diagnosis of contact allergic *dermatitis* (a type of skin allergy). Various suspected substances are applied by means of adhesive patches to the skin. After a specific period of time, the patches are removed and the reactions observed. If one substance has caused reddening or blistering, the person is probably allergic to the substance and should try to avoid it in the future.

Substances injected under the skin may help identify allergens responsible for *asthma*, allergic *rhinitis* (hay fever), or other allergic-type illnesses, even though skin symptoms are not one of the primary features of these conditions. The tests may also be used to test immunity to certain infectious diseases (such as in the *tuberculin test*).

TYPES OF SKIN GRAFT

The two main types of skin graft are split-thickness (in which less than the full thickness of skin is removed from the donor site) and full-thickness. There are advantages to each of these types.

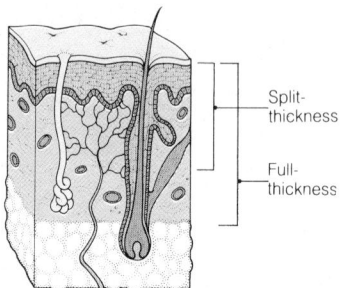

Split-thickness graft
When large areas need to be covered, such as after burns, split-thickness grafts are used and the donor sites are left to regenerate, which they do in a few days. Such sites can be repeatedly harvested.

Full-thickness graft
Full-thickness skin grafts are usually preferred for the face because they more closely match the appearance of normal skin. However, donor sites are limited and must be sutured (stitched).

HOW A FULL-THICKNESS GRAFT IS DONE

Most skin grafts are performed under general anaesthesia. Full-thickness grafts are easily cut with a scalpel. Subcutaneous fat is avoided and any bleeding at the recipient site prevented.

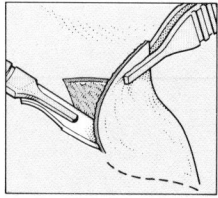

1 Skin for a full-thickness graft is often taken from behind the ear.

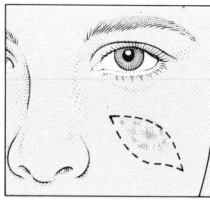

2 The graft must be larger than the area to be covered, to allow for shrinkage.

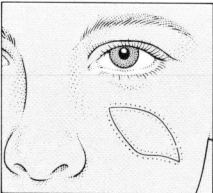

3 Precise fitting and firm pressure are needed to ensure there is a satisfactory "take".

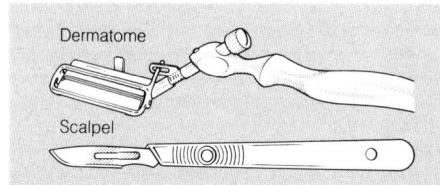

Dermatome

Scalpel

Instruments
Split-skin grafts are cut, usually from the abdomen or thigh, with an instrument called a dermatome. If necessary, the skin can be expanded into a trellis-like mesh on the donor site.

Skin tumours

A growth on or in the *skin* that may be cancerous (see *Skin cancer*) or benign (noncancerous).

Very common types of benign skin tumours include *keratoses* (wart-like growths caused by overproduction of keratin) and squamous *papillomas* (small, raised, sometimes stalked growths). Other benign skin tumours include *sebaceous cysts*, cutaneous horns (hard protrusions from the skin), *keratoacanthomas* (rapidly growing, flesh-coloured nodules), and *haemangiomas* (birthmarks formed by a collection of blood vessels in the skin).

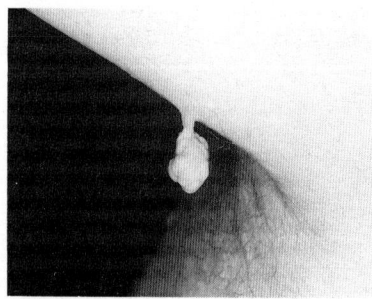

Skin papilloma
This harmless type of tumour is common in elderly people. It can easily be snipped off (and the base cauterized) by a doctor.

S

DISORDERS OF THE SKIN

The skin is the largest and most vulnerable organ of the body. Although skin conditions are seldom life-threatening, many can be severely debilitating and cause psychological problems.

CONGENITAL DISORDERS

A *birthmark* is a type of *naevus* (pigmented skin blemish) present from birth. Naevi include moles, freckles, and *haemangiomas*, such as port-wine stains and strawberry marks.

INFECTION AND INFLAMMATION

Viral infections of the skin include *cold sores*, *warts*, *chickenpox*, *molluscum contagiosum*, and *herpes zoster* (shingles). Bacterial infections include *boils*, *cellulitis*, *erysipelas*, and *impetigo*. Fungal infections, such as *tinea*, cause *athlete's foot* and ringworm.

Inflammation of the skin occurs in *dermatitis* and *eczema*; it may be caused by an allergic reaction to a substance (such as nickel), a detergent, a plant, or a drug. *Psoriasis* is a common and persistent skin disease of unknown cause that consists of large, red patches with silvery, scaly surfaces. *Prickly heat* is an irritating rash that is caused by blockage of the sweat glands.

TUMOURS

Benign (noncancerous) tumours of the skin are extremely common; these include seborrhoeic *keratoses* and most types of naevi. *Bowen's disease* is a skin disorder that may slowly become cancerous. Three common forms of skin cancer are *basal cell carcinoma*, *squamous cell carcinoma*, and malignant melanoma (see *Melanoma, malignant*). Less common skin cancers include *Paget's disease* of

the nipple, *mycosis fungoides*, and *Kaposi's sarcoma*.

INJURY

The skin is vulnerable to many minor injuries, including cuts and bites (see *Bites, animal*; *Insect bites*) as well as more serious *wounds*. *Burns* can be among the most serious of all skin injuries and may cause extensive scarring or death.

HORMONAL DISORDERS

Acne is partly related to the action of androgens (male sex hormones) on the sebaceous glands; it is common among adolescents.

NUTRITIONAL DISORDERS

Deficiency of vitamins A, B, and C can cause *rashes* and other problems.

IMPAIRED BLOOD SUPPLY

Leg ulcers, which are particularly common in the elderly, may be caused by poor blood flow to the skin as a result of *atherosclerosis*, by poor drainage of blood through *varicose veins*, or by the leg swelling associated with heart failure.

DRUGS

Many drugs, including antibiotics, barbiturates, and sulphonamides, may cause a rash. Some cause *urticaria* (hives), others cause *eczema* or a measles-like rash, and some cause *photosensitivity*.

RADIATION

All forms of radiation are potentially damaging to the skin. Overexposure to sunlight (ultraviolet radiation) causes premature aging of the skin and increases the risk of skin cancer (see *Sunlight, adverse effects of*). High doses of other forms of radiation, such as X-rays, may cause severe injury to the skin and may lead to cancer.

AUTOIMMUNE DISORDERS

These disorders include *lupus erythematosus*, a disorder that may affect the skin alone or the skin and other organs; *vitiligo*, characterized by pure white patches and caused by destruction of the skin's pigment cells; *dermatomyositis*, characterized by a specific skin rash and muscle weakness; *morphoea* and *scleroderma*, in which there is progressive hardening of the skin and other tissues; and *pemphigoid* and *pemphigus*, in which large blisters develop on the skin.

OTHER DISORDERS

A *keloid* is an abnormally large and protruding *scar* caused by the continuing production of scar tissue long after healing would usually be complete. *Striae* (stretch-marks) often develop during pregnancy and may also develop as a side-effect of treatment with *corticosteroid drugs*.

Erythema simply means redness and has many possible causes. *Purpura* is a condition in which blood leaks into tissues, giving rise to *petechiae* (tiny pinpoints of blood) or larger bruises.

Xanthelasma are yellowish patches that tend to occur on the eyelids; they are a result of the deposition of cholesterol.

INVESTIGATION
Most skin disorders can be diagnosed from their physical characteristics. A *skin biopsy* (removal of a tissue sample for microscopic analysis) may also be performed, usually to aid in the diagnosis of a skin problem or to exclude skin cancer.

S

Skull

The bony skeleton of the head. The skull encases and protects the brain, houses organs of the special senses, provides points of attachment for muscles, and helps form the first parts of the respiratory and digestive tracts. Many of the bones are hollow, reducing the weight of the skull and adding to the resonance of the voice.

STRUCTURE

The arrangement of the bones in the skull is shown in the illustrated box

overleaf. All the skull bones, except the mandible, are fixed to each other by immovable joints called sutures. The mandible articulates with the temporal bones at the freely movable temporomandibular joints.

Closely associated with, but not strictly part of, the skull are the hyoid (a small bone at the back of the tongue) and the auditory ossicles (the three tiny bones in each middle ear).

The skull's cavities include the cranial cavity (which houses the brain),

the nasal cavity (involved in smell and breathing), and the orbits (which house the eyeballs and their associated muscles). Part of the mouth is also formed by the skull.

Several of the skull bones, notably the maxillas, sphenoid bone, frontal bone, and ethmoid bone, contain *sinuses* (air-filled spaces); these sinuses are called the paranasal sinuses. In addition, there are spaces in the temporal bones that house the structures of the middle and inner ear.

In the cranium, there are many holes for the passage of nerves and blood vessels. Passing through are the *cranial nerves* (which supply most of the sensory structures and muscles of the head and neck) and blood vessels, such as the *carotid arteries* and *jugular veins* (which carry blood to and from the brain). The largest of the holes, called the foramen magnum, is situated in the occipital bone (which forms part of the base and back of the cranium); this hole allows the brainstem to enter the spinal canal, where it continues as the spinal cord.

The skull rests on the first cervical vertebra, called the atlas, which is a ring-shaped bone that articulates with the occipital bone and permits nodding movements of the head. Turning the head is a function of the joint between the atlas and the second cervical vertebra, called the axis. The occipital bone, atlas, and axis are connected by numerous small muscles.

DISORDERS
The skull may be affected by any bone disorder (see *Bone* disorders box) that involves the skeleton, such as *Paget's disease*, but the most common disorder is injury. A blow to the head may cause a fracture (see *Skull, fracture of*), which may result in damage to the brain, and, if a foramen is involved, in damage to a blood vessel or cranial nerve. (See also *Head injury*.)

Skull, fracture of
A break in one or more of the bones of the *skull* caused by injury to the head. A fracture of the skull may be either a closed fracture (also called a simple fracture), in which there is no displacement of the broken pieces, or an open fracture (also called a depressed fracture), in which displacement of the bone fragments occurs.

Because the skull is extremely strong, most skull fractures are closed and cause no complications. However, severe injury to the head may result in an open fracture in which the bone fragments are displaced, usually inwards. In this case, the blood vessels in the *meninges* (the membranes that cover the brain) may be ruptured, resulting in an *extradural haemorrhage* (bleeding into the space between the skull and the outer membrane) or a *subdural haemorrhage* (bleeding into the space between the outer and middle membranes). The resultant blood clot may press on and displace brain tissue. Less commonly, all the meninges may be torn, and the brain itself may be damaged.

SYMPTOMS AND SIGNS
The degree of brain injury does not always correlate with the degree of skull damage. Some injuries cause a skull fracture but little or no brain damage. Other injuries cause severe brain damage even though there is no fracture of the skull.

The symptoms and signs of skull fractures (see *Head injury*) depend mainly on the degree of brain damage sustained. Leakage of cerebrospinal fluid (the liquid that bathes the brain and spinal cord) through the nose or ears indicates rupture of the meninges by a fracture of the base of the skull.

DIAGNOSIS
Any person who has suffered a significant blow to the head—particularly a blow that has caused unconsciousness—should consult a doctor even if there are no symptoms. If the doctor suspects a haemorrhage, *CT scanning* may be performed.

TREATMENT
A person with a closed fracture is hospitalized and observed closely for 12 to 24 hours for signs of complications. If no signs develop, treatment is generally not necessary because the fracture usually heals by itself.

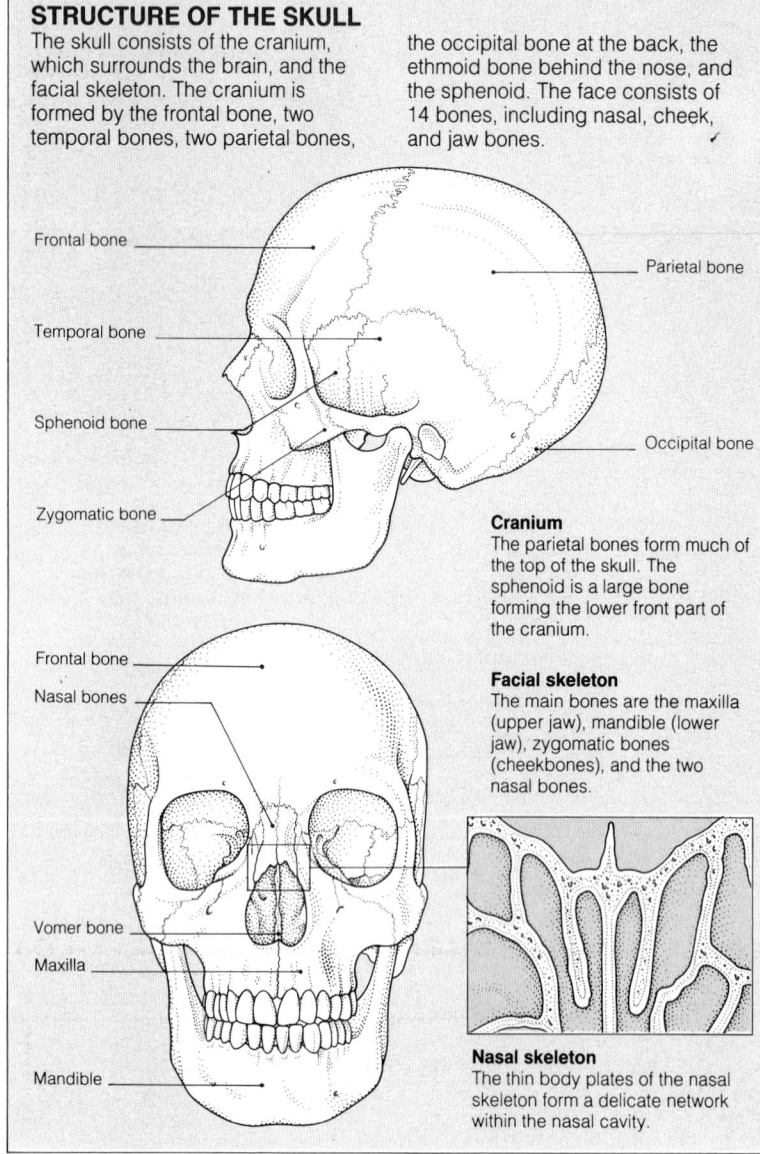

STRUCTURE OF THE SKULL
The skull consists of the cranium, which surrounds the brain, and the facial skeleton. The cranium is formed by the frontal bone, two temporal bones, two parietal bones, the occipital bone at the back, the ethmoid bone behind the nose, and the sphenoid. The face consists of 14 bones, including nasal, cheek, and jaw bones.

Frontal bone
Temporal bone
Sphenoid bone
Zygomatic bone

Parietal bone
Occipital bone

Cranium
The parietal bones form much of the top of the skull. The sphenoid is a large bone forming the lower front part of the cranium.

Facial skeleton
The main bones are the maxilla (upper jaw), mandible (lower jaw), zygomatic bones (cheekbones), and the two nasal bones.

Frontal bone
Nasal bones
Vomer bone
Maxilla
Mandible

Nasal skeleton
The thin body plates of the nasal skeleton form a delicate network within the nasal cavity.

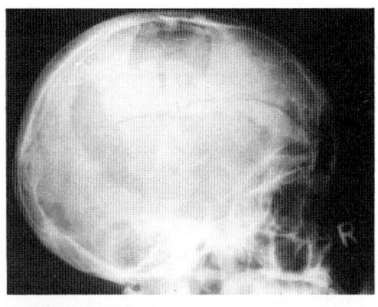

Multiple skull facture
This side-view X-ray shows the cranium smashed into several pieces. Some pieces have been surgically removed.

An open fracture often requires treatment by a neurosurgeon. A haemorrhage may necessitate a *craniotomy* to drain the blood and repair damaged vessels. When deeply depressed fractures have penetrated the meninges and brain tissue, an operation is performed to raise or remove the pieces of fractured bone and repair the damaged tissue. After such an operation, there may be some degree of skull distortion.

Antibiotic drugs are given for all open fractures because of the risk of infection of the meninges (see *Meningitis*) or of the brain itself (see *Encephalitis*).

Skull X-ray

A technique for providing images of the *skull*.

WHY IT IS DONE

X-rays of the skull are usually taken after a *head injury* to look for a fracture (see *Skull, fracture of*) or to locate any foreign bodies in the soft tissues within the skull. A skull X-ray that appears normal does not rule out the possibility of significant brain injury. If such an injury is suspected, or if a skull fracture is found, *CT scanning* of the brain is also performed.

Skull X-rays are useful in the evaluation of a variety of conditions that affect the bones of the skull, such as *pituitary tumours* or metabolic disorders (e.g. *hyperparathyroidism*), and in the evaluation of tumours that have spread to the skull bones.

HOW IT IS DONE

X-rays of the skull are taken from different angles by a radiographer. Depending on the number of views taken, the procedure usually takes about 20 minutes. The X-ray films are interpreted by a radiologist.

SLE

The abbreviation for the disorder systemic *lupus erythematosus*.

Sleep

The natural state of lowered consciousness and reduced *metabolism*. Sleep takes up about one third of an average person's life.

PHYSIOLOGY

EEG recordings of the electrical impulses produced by the brain during sleep show that there are two distinct types of sleep, known as REM (rapid eye movement) and NREM (nonrapid eye movement) sleep. These two types alternate in cycles lasting roughly 90 minutes throughout the sleep period. NREM sleep, which accounts for the major part of sleep, starts with drowsiness; brain waves become increasingly deeper and slower until brain activity and metabolism fall to their lowest level. Dreams are infrequent.

In REM sleep, the brain suddenly becomes more electrically active (with a wave-pattern resembling that of an awake person) and its temperature and blood flow increase. The eyes move rapidly and *dreaming* occurs. REM sleep, also known as paradoxical sleep, periodically interrupts NREM sleep. The first REM period usually takes place 90 to 100 minutes after the onset of sleep and lasts about five to 10 minutes. REM sleep periods increase in length as sleep continues; the last of a night's four or five REM sleep periods may last about an hour. REM sleep occupies about one half of sleep time in babies and about one fifth of sleep time in adults.

FUNCTIONS OF SLEEP

Sleep is a fundamental human need, as is shown by the detrimental effects of *sleep deprivation*. However, it is not understood exactly in what way sleep is beneficial, or why a few, extremely rare individuals sleep very little yet

---

SLEEP PATTERNS

The brain does not rest when a person is sleeping, but there is some reorganization of activity within it.

EEGs (electroencephalograms) and other recordings reveal cyclical patterns to this activity.

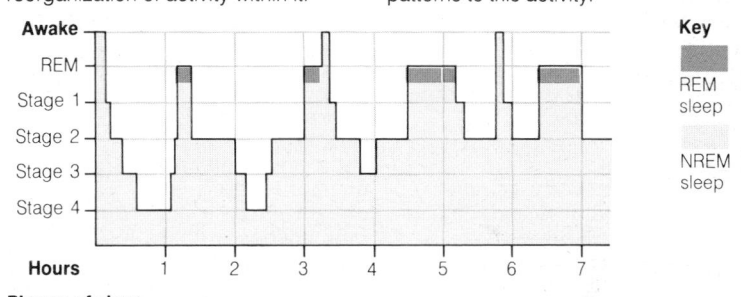

Phases of sleep
There are two types of sleep, REM (rapid eye movement) and NREM (nonrapid eye movement). They can be distinguished by the presence or absence of REMs and by

EEGs or other recordings. The chart shows how a sleeper passes in cycles between the four stages of NREM sleep during the night, with bursts of REM sleep.

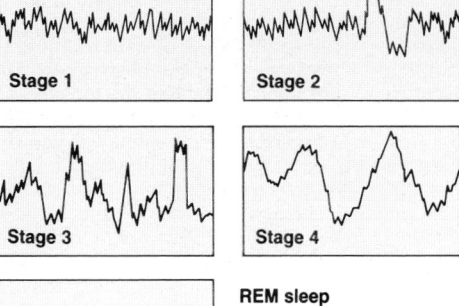

REM sleep
The EEG (left) shows high-frequency, low-voltage waves. People awakened during REM sleep often report dreams.

NREM sleep
This is sometimes called orthodox sleep; in adults it makes up about 80 per cent of the sleeping pattern. It has four stages of progressively greater "depth" of sleep, characterized by EEG waves (left) of increasingly larger voltage (amplitude) and lower frequency (number of waves per second). People awakened during NREM sleep often report they were "thinking" about everyday matters but rarely report dreams.

suffer no ill effects. Apart from the obvious theory that the brain and metabolic processes require periodic rest to function efficiently, it has been suggested that dreaming is necessary to enable the brain to sort out information gathered during waking hours.

SLEEP REQUIREMENTS

The need for sleep decreases with age. A one-year-old baby requires about 14 hours of sleep a day, a child of five about 12 hours, and adults about seven to eight hours. However, these amounts can vary from person to person: some adults need to sleep 10 hours or more a day, while others function efficiently on half that amount or less. As people age, their ability to sustain sleep generally declines. Elderly people tend to sleep less than younger adults at night but doze more during the day.

SLEEP DISORDERS

Sleep disorders are divided into four main categories: difficulty in falling asleep or in remaining asleep (see *Insomnia*); difficulty in staying awake (see *Narcolepsy*; *Sleep apnoea*); disruption in the sleeping/waking cycle as occurs, for example, in shift-workers or people travelling across time zones (see *Jet-lag*); and other problems that interfere with sleep (see *Bed-wetting*; *Night terrors*; *Sleepwalking*).

Sleep apnoea

Episodes of temporary cessation of breathing, lasting 10 seconds or longer, which occur during *sleep*.

People with sleep apnoea may not be aware of having any problem during the night, but they may be excessively sleepy during the day, with poor memory and difficulty in concentrating. This can interfere with work and social activities, and in children, with school performance.

Severe sleep apnoea is a potentially serious condition, because it may result in *hypertension* (high blood pressure), *heart failure* (reduced pumping efficiency), *myocardial infarction* (heart attack), or *stroke*.

TYPES AND INCIDENCE

Sleep apnoea may be classified as obstructive, central, or mixed.

OBSTRUCTIVE SLEEP APNOEA This is the most common type and may affect anyone, but more often middle-aged men. As many as one in 100 men between the ages of 30 and 50 may have the condition. The typical sufferer is overweight and a heavy snorer. People with obstructive sleep apnoea who are very obese and excessively sleepy are said to have *Pickwickian*

syndrome. Obstructive sleep apnoea has been linked with some instances of *sudden infant death syndrome*.

The most common cause of obstructive sleep apnoea is over-relaxation of the muscles of the soft *palate* in the *pharynx* (throat). The muscles sag and obstruct the passage of air during sleep. Obstruction to the passage of air may also be caused by enlarged *tonsils* or *adenoids*, or by an abnormally large tongue or small jaw.

In all cases, the obstruction to air movement usually causes loud snoring. If a complete obstruction occurs, breathing stops. Failure to breathe triggers the brain to restart breathing, and as breathing recommences, a gasp is produced and the person may waken briefly.

CENTRAL SLEEP APNOEA In this form, breathing stops because the diaphragm and chest muscles temporarily cease to work, probably as a result of a disturbance in the brain's control of breathing. Causes include paralysis of the *diaphragm* muscles, and disorders of the *brainstem*. Snoring is not a predominant feature.

MIXED SLEEP APNOEA This is a combined form of sleep apnoea. Usually, there is a short period of central sleep apnoea, followed by a longer period of obstructive sleep apnoea.

TREATMENT

People who are overweight should attempt to lose weight. Alcohol and sleeping drugs should be avoided, as both interfere with the mechanism of breathing and may aggravate sleep apnoea. Tricyclic *antidepressant drugs* may help in milder cases. Some patients with severe sleep apnoea benefit from treatment with continuous positive airway pressure (CPAP). In CPAP, air from a compressor is forced into the airway via a mask worn over the nose. Night-time artificial *ventilation* may be needed.

In some cases, surgical treatment is necessary to relieve obstruction. *Tonsillectomy* (removal of the tonsils), *adenoidectomy* (removal of the adenoids), or *tracheostomy* (creation of an opening into the windpipe, allowing air to flow directly to the lungs) may be performed, depending on the cause of the problem. An operation called uvulo-palato-pharyngoplasty (UPPP) to shorten the soft palate may be recommended in extreme cases.

Sleep deprivation

An insufficient amount of *sleep*. Studies of sleep-deprived volunteers have shown that irritability and a short-

ened attention span may occur after a night in which there was less than three hours' sleep.

After longer periods without sleep, individuals become increasingly unable to concentrate and their performance of tasks deteriorates as they continually slip into short periods of "microsleep". People with epilepsy are more prone to *seizures* after sleep deprivation. Three days or more without sleep may lead to visual and auditory *hallucinations* and, in some cases, to *paranoia*.

Sleep deprivation has been employed as a form of torture, in order to extract confessions, and as a brainwashing technique.

Sleeping drugs

COMMON DRUGS

Benzodiazepines
Flurazepam Nitrazepam Temazepam Triazolam

Others
Chloral hydrate
Chlormethiazole
Promethazine
Zopiclone

A group of drugs used in the treatment of *insomnia*. Sleeping drugs include *benzodiazepine drugs*, *antihistamine drugs*, *antidepressant drugs*, and *chloral hydrate*.

WHY THEY ARE USED

Sleeping drugs may be given to reestablish the habit of sleeping, usually after self-help measures (such as a warm bath or drinking hot milk at bedtime) have not worked. These drugs promote sleep by reducing nerve cell activity within the brain.

HOW THEY ARE USED

Sleeping drugs should always be taken in the smallest effective dose for the shortest period of time. In general, sleeping drugs should be taken for no longer than three weeks and, preferably, not every night.

POSSIBLE ADVERSE EFFECTS

Sleeping drugs may cause drowsiness, unsteadiness, and impaired concentration on waking. These effects can be a particular hazard to the elderly, who are more prone to falls, and can affect a person's ability to drive or to operate machinery.

Long-term use of sleeping drugs may induce *tolerance* (needing a higher dose to have the same effect) and *dependence* (which produces withdrawal symptoms when the person stops taking the drug).

S

Sleeping sickness

A serious infectious disease of tropical Africa caused by the protozoan (single-celled) parasite TRYPANOSOMA BRUCEI. The disease is also known as African trypanosomiasis.

There are two forms. One, occurring in West and Central Africa, is spread primarily from person to person. The other occurs in East Africa and mainly affects wild animals, but is occasionally transmitted to humans. Both forms are spread by the bites of tsetse flies, which transmit the protozoa to people and animals. Within humans, the parasites multiply and spread to the bloodstream, lymph nodes, heart, and brain.

SYMPTOMS AND SIGNS

With both forms of sleeping sickness, a painful nodule develops at the site of the tsetse fly bite.

In the West African form, the disease then takes a slow course, with bouts of fever and lymph node enlargement. After months or years, spread to the brain occurs, causing headaches, confusion, and, eventually, severe lassitude. The victim may become completely inactive, have drooping eyelids, and a vacant expression. Without treatment, coma and death follow.

The East African form runs a faster course. A severe fever develops within a few weeks of infection, and effects on the heart may be fatal before the disease has spread to the brain.

DIAGNOSIS AND TREATMENT

Microscopic examination of the blood, lymph fluid withdrawn from a lymph node, or cerebrospinal fluid obtained by a *lumbar puncture* reveals the presence of the parasites.

Drugs are effective against the parasites but may cause severe side-effects. In most cases, a complete cure can be achieved, although there may be residual brain damage if the infection has already spread to the brain.

PREVENTION

Sleeping sickness is controlled by eradication measures directed against the tsetse fly. Nevertheless, tens of thousands of Africans—and some visitors to safari parks—still contract the disease each year.

To avoid sleeping sickness, visitors to rural parts of Africa should take measures to protect themselves against tsetse fly bites (see *Insect bites*).

Sleep paralysis

The sensation of being unable to move at the moment of going to sleep or when waking up. The experience may

CYCLE OF SLEEPING SICKNESS

The life-cycle of the trypanosomes that cause sleeping sickness is shown. They multiply in a person's blood and lymph vessels and may spread to the brain or heart with serious effects.

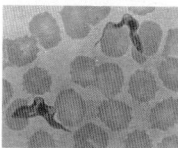

Trypanosomes
The parasites are shown here in blood.

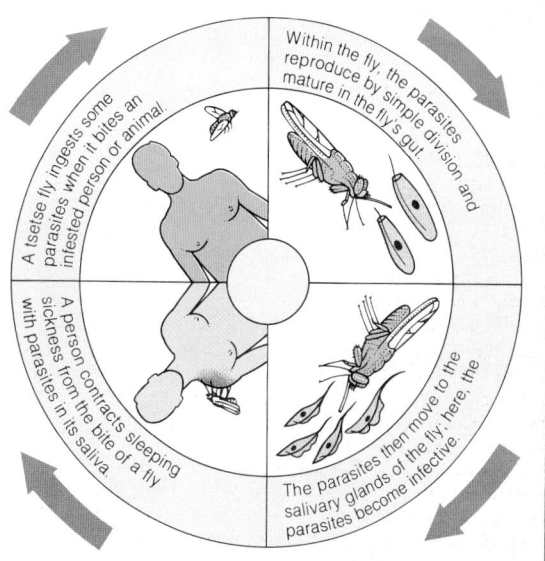

A tsetse fly ingests some parasites when it bites an infested person or animal.

Within the fly, the parasites reproduce by simple division and mature in the fly's gut.

A person contracts sleeping sickness from the bite of a fly with parasites in its saliva.

The parasites then move to the salivary glands of the fly; here, the parasites become infective.

be accompanied by *hallucinations*, which often are frightening. Sleep paralysis most often occurs in people with *narcolepsy*, but occasionally affects otherwise healthy people. Although alarming, the sensation rarely lasts for more than a few seconds. (See also *Cataplexy*.)

Sleep terror

See *Night terror*.

Sleepwalking

Walking while asleep, also known as somnambulism. Sleepwalking occurs during NREM (nonrapid eye movement) *sleep*, or during arousal from this type of sleep, and does not represent the acting out of dreams. Some people show a regular tendency to sleepwalk.

Usually a sleepwalker calmly gets out of bed, wanders around aimlessly for a few minutes, and then goes back to bed. Sometimes sleepwalking arises from a *night terror*, in which case the sleepwalker's behaviour is more frantic and may involve shrieking or thrashing. He or she sometimes talks (usually simple words or phrases) during the sleepwalk, urinates in an inappropriate place, or gets into the wrong bed. Waking the sleepwalker is difficult and unnecessary; steer him or her gently back to bed. Take precautions, such as blocking off the stairs, to avoid injury.

Sleepwalking in children is seldom associated with psychological problems, although it may be aggravated

by anxiety, and tends to disappear naturally with age. Sleepwalking in adults may be related to anxiety, or may be associated with use of sleeping pills, especially in the elderly.

Slimming

See *Weight reduction*.

Sling

A device used to immobilize, support, or elevate an arm. A sling is usually made from a triangular *bandage*, although an emergency sling can be created from a belt, tie, or scarf.

An arm sling may be used as a first-aid measure to support the arm following a fracture, sprain, or other injury (see illustrated box overleaf). A sling may also be used after an operation on the hand or arm, or if the arm is infected.

An elevation sling is a type of sling that is used to hold the hand in a well-raised position to control bleeding or to prevent movement of the arm and shoulder if the clavicle (collarbone) is broken or the shoulder dislocated. This type of sling is applied in a similar fashion to an arm sling, except that the victim's arm is placed across the chest with the fingers nearly touching the opposite shoulder.

Slipped disc

See *Disc prolapse*.

Slipped femoral epiphysis

See *Femoral epiphysis, slipped*.

S

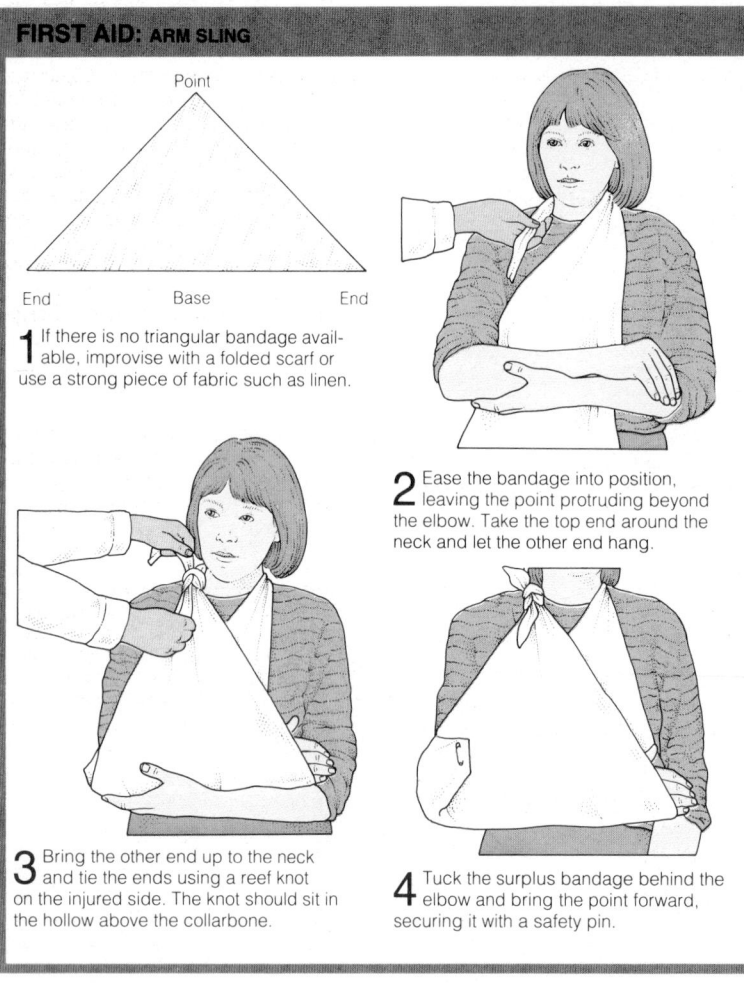

FIRST AID: ARM SLING

Point

End   Base   End

1 If there is no triangular bandage available, improvise with a folded scarf or use a strong piece of fabric such as linen.

2 Ease the bandage into position, leaving the point protruding beyond the elbow. Take the top end around the neck and let the other end hang.

3 Bring the other end up to the neck and tie the ends using a reef knot on the injured side. The knot should sit in the hollow above the collarbone.

4 Tuck the surplus bandage behind the elbow and bring the point forward, securing it with a safety pin.

Slit-lamp
An illuminated microscope that is used to examine the internal structures of the front part of the eye. The use of special lenses allows the slit-lamp to be used to examine the retina. (See also *Eye, examination of.*)

Slough
Dead tissue that has been shed from its original site. Examples of sloughing include the loss of dead skin cells from the skin's surface and the shedding of the lining of the uterus during menstruation. Sloughing also occurs as part of the healing process.

Slow virus diseases
A group of diseases of the central nervous system (brain and spinal cord) that occur many months or even years after infection with a virus. The diseases take a slow course in which there is gradual widespread destruction of nerve tissue. This causes progressive loss of brain function and, at present, a fatal outcome.

Slow virus diseases in humans include *Creutzfeldt-Jakob syndrome*, *kuru*, possibly a form of *Alzheimer's disease*, subacute sclerosing panencephalitis (a complication of *measles*), and possibly the brain disease that occurs in some people infected with *HIV*.

Slow virus diseases in animals include scrapie, which has been known in sheep for many years, and bovine spongiform encephalopathy (BSE) in cows, which is a new disease transmitted in feedstuffs containing contaminated sheep and cattle nervous tissue. These diseases are unlikely to be transmitted to humans.

Small cell carcinoma
The most dangerous and rapidly spreading form of *lung cancer*. Also called oat cell carcinoma, this type of
tumour accounts for about 25 per cent of lung cancers. Most small cell carcinomas reach an inoperable stage by the time a diagnosis is made. The extension of a life by surgery is achieved in about 10 per cent of cases, but, even in these people, the outlook is poor. Spread to other parts of the body is almost inevitable.

Treatment is usually with *anticancer drugs* with or without *radiotherapy*. *Bone marrow transplants* are also currently being tried.

Smallpox
A highly infectious viral disease, common in the 19th century and before, with the distinction of having been totally eradicated by a successful worldwide vaccination campaign. The World Health Organization declared smallpox extinct in 1980.

Smallpox was transmitted from person to person; it was characterized by an illness resembling influenza and a rash that spread over the body and eventually developed into pus-filled blisters. The blisters became crusted and would sometimes leave deeply pitted scars. Complications included blindness, pneumonia, and kidney damage. There was no effective treatment for the disease, which killed up to 40 per cent of its victims.

Eradication was achieved through the cooperative international use of a highly effective vaccine. Eradication was possible because smallpox affected only humans, cases of infection were easily recognized, and victims of the disease were infectious to others only for a short time. These characteristics are shared by some other diseases (e.g. measles, another possible candidate for eradication).

Smallpox vaccination certificates are no longer required for travel abroad, and most countries have discontinued vaccination because there is no longer any risk of the disease and because there is a risk of encephalitis from the vaccine. The virus responsible for smallpox is still maintained at a few research laboratories.

Smear
A specimen for microscopic examination prepared by spreading a thin film of cells on to a glass slide. A common use is in the *cervical smear test*.

Smegma
An accumulation of sebaceous gland secretions beneath the foreskin in an uncircumcised male, usually as a result of poor hygiene.

S

Fungal or bacterial infection of smegma may cause *balanitis* (inflammation of the glans). In a child with *phimosis* (tight foreskin), smegma occasionally hardens into a small stone, known as a smegma pearl. The higher incidence of cancer of the penis in uncircumcised men who smoke may be due to the build-up of cancer-inducing substances in the smegma.

An uncircumcised man should wash his penis daily with the foreskin retracted to prevent an accumulation of smegma.

Smell

One of the five senses. The mechanisms by which smell is perceived are shown in the illustrated box.

DISORDERS

Disturbance of the sense of smell may consist of anosmia (loss of smell, which may be complete or partial, temporary or permanent) or dysosmia (abnormal smell perception). The senses of smell and *taste* are closely connected, so disturbances of smell usually result in disturbances of taste.

Temporary partial anosmia frequently results from inflammation of the nasal mucous membrane, as in the common *cold*, *influenza*, and several forms of *rhinitis*, notably allergic rhinitis (hay fever). Cigarette smoking may also cause anosmia. In hypertrophic rhinitis, the mucous membrane thickens, burying and sometimes distorting the olfactory nerve endings, which may cause permanent anosmia unless the condition is treated. In atrophic rhinitis, the nerve endings waste away, causing some degree of permanent anosmia; there is also a foul-smelling discharge that may overpower other odours.

THE SENSE OF SMELL

The smell receptors are specialized nerve cell endings situated in a small patch of mucous membrane lining the roof of the nose. The axons (fibres) of these sensory cells pass up through tiny perforations in the overlying bone to enter the two elongated olfactory bulbs lying on top of the bone. These bulbs are swellings at the ends of the olfactory nerves; the nerves contain millions of nerve fibres and enter the brain on its lower surface. The olfactory nerves carry sensory information to smell centres situated within the brain.

Smell centres
The centres in the brain concerned with smell include parts of the limbic system and frontal lobes.

Olfactory bulbs
Here, the receptor cell fibres are linked to the nerves that run into the brain.

Nasal cavity
In the nose, hair-like projections from the smell receptor cells lie in the mucous membrane layer.

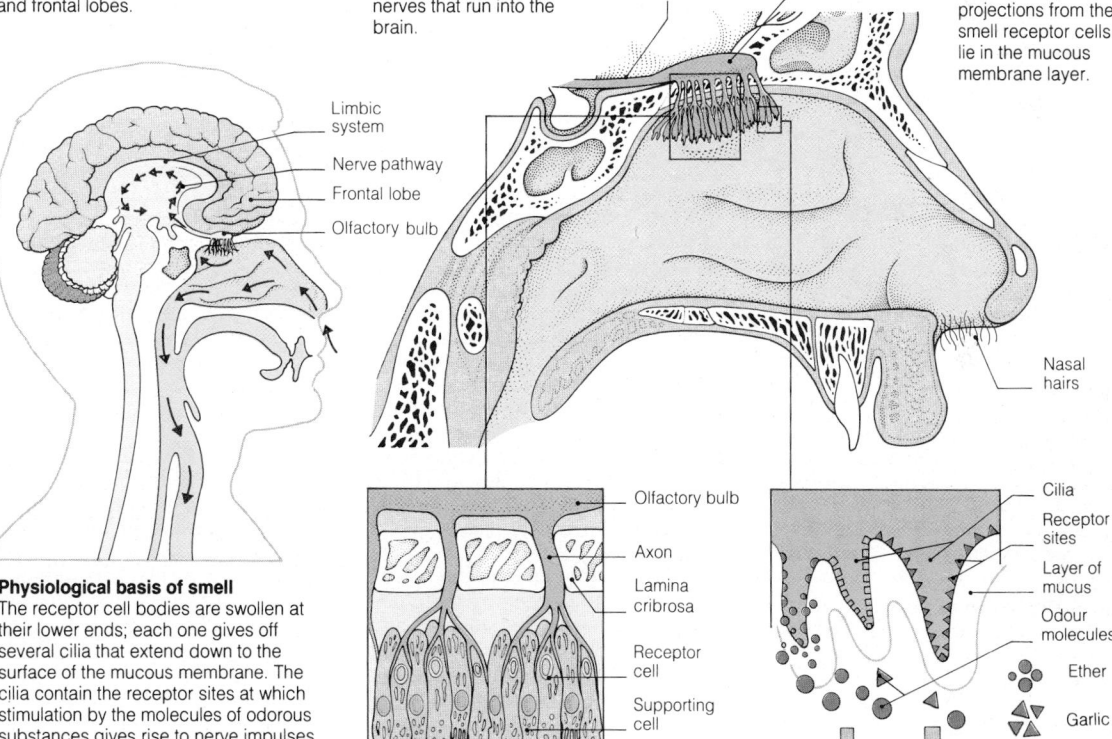

Physiological basis of smell
The receptor cell bodies are swollen at their lower ends; each one gives off several cilia that extend down to the surface of the mucous membrane. The cilia contain the receptor sites at which stimulation by the molecules of odorous substances gives rise to nerve impulses passing up to the brain. We know that we are able to distinguish several thousand different odours, but the exact basis of this high degree of specificity is uncertain. No microscopic difference can be detected among different receptors.

Probable mechanism
The smell process is probably based on a physical "fit" between the odour molecules and the receptor sites. For example, the receptors on some cells may fit only with ether molecules, others with molecules of bleach. The molecules must dissolve in the mucus before they can stimulate the receptors. The sensitivity of the system is remarkable; as few as four molecules can give a recognizable smell.

S

The olfactory nerves can be torn in a head injury. If both nerves are torn, complete permanent anosmia results; during recovery from less severe damage, dysosmia, in the form of illusory bad smells, may occur.

Rarely, anosmia is caused by a *meningioma* (tumour of the meninges, the membranes that surround the brain) or a tumour behind the nose (see *Nasopharynx, cancer of*).

Dysosmia, in the form of illusory, unpleasant odours, may occur as a feature of various psychological disorders, such as *depression* or *schizophrenia*. It may also occur in some forms of *epilepsy* and during "drying out" periods in severe *alcohol dependence*. A person with dysosmia may believe the source of the smell is his or her own body and, despite reassurance to the contrary, may wash excessively and tend to avoid others. (See also *Sensation*.)

Smelling salts
A preparation of *ammonia* that causes a person to withdraw from the pungent substance. Smelling salts were in the past commonly used to prevent fainting or to revive a person who had fainted.

Smoking
See *Tobacco-smoking*.

Snails and disease
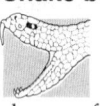
Snails act as host to various types of parasitic flukes (flattened, worm-like animals), which, at different stages in their own life-cycles, infest people. These flukes include *liver flukes* and the parasites responsible for *schistosomiasis* and various other tropical diseases. Control of snail populations can be an important factor in combating these diseases. Edible snails should be cooked thoroughly before being eaten.

Snake bites
Every year, hundreds of thousands of people all over the world are bitten by snakes. However, the chance of death or a serious injury occurring as a result of a bite is relatively small. Most bites are by non-poisonous species, and even the poisonous species only sometimes inject venom when they bite. Furthermore, modern medical treatment is usually effective even in serious cases, provided the victim is transported to hospital quickly. It takes hours or

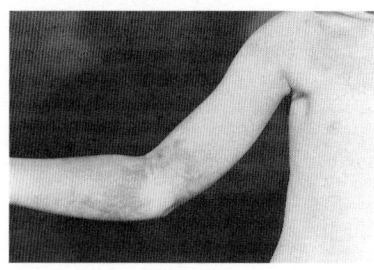

Adder bite on the arm
Following an adder bite, this boy's arm has become bruised and swollen, and the lymph nodes in his armpit have become enlarged.

days, not minutes or seconds, for even the most powerful snake venom to kill a human being.

VENOMOUS SPECIES
Venomous snakes are found mainly in the tropics; the only poisonous snake native to the UK is the adder, a member of the Viperidae (viper family). In the UK, adders bite over 100 people each year, but have caused only about a dozen deaths in the past century.

Around the world, many venomous bites are caused by types of Viperidae. This group of snakes includes lance-headed vipers, water moccasins (cottonmouths), and American rattlesnakes. The saw-scaled or carpet viper, which is native to parts of Africa, the Middle East, and the Indian subcontinent, probably kills more people than any other species of snake.

Other venomous bites are caused by types of Elapidae. This group includes coral snakes, cobras, kraits, and mambas. Cobras alone kill about 10,000 people each year in India.

Venomous bites are also caused by snakes belonging to the Atractaspididae (burrowing asps) and the Hydrophiidae (sea snakes) families, and by a minority (approximately 40 out of 3,000) of types of Colubridae.

EFFECTS OF A BITE
The effects of a venomous bite vary considerably and depend on the type of snake, its size, the amount of venom injected, and the age and health of the victim.

Viperidae make two distinct puncture wounds in the skin. There is an immediate burning pain at the site of the wound, and swelling of the bitten area. Over the next 20 minutes the pain increases in severity and the victim becomes dizzy, nauseated, pale, and sweaty. Blood pressure falls and there is an increase in heart-rate. Thirst, headache, and a pins-and-needles sensation are other common

symptoms. The venom may prevent the blood from clotting, thereby causing bleeding from the fang wounds and bruises beneath the skin. There may also be bleeding from the urinary tract or from the mouth, rectum, or vagina. Internal bleeding further lowers the blood pressure. There is also widespread tissue destruction around the wound.

Elapidae typically make two small puncture wounds with their fangs; they may also chew the skin, producing several wounds. The bite may or may not be painful or become swollen, depending on the species. The venom primarily affects the nervous system. Serious symptoms develop from 10 minutes to eight hours after the bite and may include drooping eyelids, slurred speech, and double vision. The victim becomes drowsy or delirious and may have convulsions. Eventually, if treatment is not given, respiratory paralysis causes death.

TREATMENT
Snake bite victims should receive medical help as quickly as possible. *Antibiotic drugs* and injections of *tetanus* antitoxin are given for all bites, whether venomous or not, to prevent bacterial infection or tetanus.

For a venomous bite, the victim is given an injection of *antivenom* (a serum containing antibodies against the poison). In the most severe cases, kidney *dialysis* to treat *kidney failure*, or artificial *ventilation* to overcome respiratory paralysis may be required. With prompt treatment, most victims of snake bite recover completely.

Sneezing
The involuntary, convulsive expulsion of air through the nose and mouth as a result of irritation of the upper respiratory tract. The irritation may be caused by inflammation of the tract, which occurs in the common *cold*, *influenza*, and allergic *rhinitis* (hay fever); by the presence of mucus; or by inhaling an irritant substance, such as dust or pepper.

Snellen chart
A standard method of measuring *visual acuity* used during *vision tests*. The Snellen chart bears several rows of letters of standard sizes, which are progressively smaller from top to bottom. The chart is set at a distance of 6 metres from the patient. One of the patient's eyes is covered and he or she is then asked to read as far down the chart as possible. The procedure is repeated with the other eye.

S

Normal vision (6/6 vision) requires that all the letters in a line near the bottom of the chart be read correctly. If the person being tested can read only the letters twice as large as those on the 6/6 line (which a normal eye would be able to read at 12 metres), the acuity is said to be 6/12.

Snoring

Noisy breathing through the open mouth during sleep, produced by vibrations of the soft palate. Snoring is usually caused by some condition that hinders breathing through the nose, such as a common *cold*, allergic *rhinitis*, or enlarged *adenoids*. Snoring is more common when a person is sleeping on his or her back because in this position the lower jaw tends to drop open. In some cases, snoring alternates with *sleep apnoea* (temporary cessation of breathing).

Snoring can sometimes be prevented by sewing an object into the nightclothes near the small of the back, thus making it uncomfortable to sleep on the back. Removal of enlarged adenoids will usually cure the condition in children.

Snow-blindness

A commonly used name for actinic *keratopathy*.

Snuff

A preparation of powdered *tobacco* (often with other substances) for inhalation into the nose. Snuff is addictive because it contains *nicotine*, irritating to the nasal lining, which may become abnormally thin and inflamed, and carcinogenic, causing an increased risk of cancer of the nose and throat.

Snuffles

A general term for nasal obstruction, especially in infants suffering from an upper *respiratory tract infection*.

Social skills training

An aspect of behaviour modification by which individuals are encouraged to improve their ability to communicate with others.

Social skills training is an important part of *rehabilitation* for people who have chronic psychiatric and psychological disorders, including *schizophrenia* and *alcohol dependence*, and for people with *mental handicap*.

Role-playing is a commonly used technique in social skills training. During role-play, the person being helped and his or her trainer simulate various social situations, particularly those in which the person feels inadequate or lacks self-assertion. The person is shown how to respond in particular situations, is given a chance to practise, and is told how he or she is performing, sometimes with the aid of a video-recording. Early stages of training may be followed by practice in groups and by trial outings—for example, to a café or shop.

Social skills training is undertaken by psychologists or by other professionals, such as teachers or psychiatric nurses, under their guidance.

Sociopathy

An outdated term for *antisocial personality disorder*.

Sodium

A *mineral* that helps regulate the body's water balance, helps maintain normal heart rhythm, and is involved in the conduction of nerve impulses and the contraction of muscles.

The body of an average-sized person contains about 55 g of sodium. The level of sodium in the blood is controlled by the kidneys, which eliminate any excess of the mineral via the urine.

Almost all foods contain sodium naturally or as an ingredient added during processing or cooking. The principal forms of sodium in food are sodium chloride (table salt) and sodium bicarbonate (baking soda). Apart from table salt, the main dietary sources of sodium are processed foods, cheese, breads and cereals, and smoked, pickled, or cured meats and fish. Pickles and snack foods contain large amounts; sodium is also present in water treated with water softeners.

DEFICIENCY AND EXCESS

Because most foods contain sodium, deficiency is very rare. In fact, most Western diets contain too much sodium. Whereas many nutritionists suggest a daily intake of only 1 to 3 g, the average consumption is 3 to 7 g per day. There is no official recommended daily allowance.

Sodium deficiency is usually the result of excessive loss of the mineral through persistent diarrhoea or vomiting, through profuse sweating, or through prolonged or excessive treatment with *diuretic drugs*. In rare cases, deficiency is due to *cystic fibrosis*, underactivity of the *adrenal glands*, or certain kidney disorders.

Symptoms of deficiency include tiredness, weakness, muscle cramps, and dizziness. In severe cases, there may be a drop in blood pressure, leading to confusion, fainting, and palpitations. Treatment consists of taking sodium supplements. In very hot conditions, sodium supplements may help prevent *heat disorders* by compensating for sodium lost through heavy sweating.

Excessive sodium intake is thought to be a contributory factor in the high incidence of *hypertension* (high blood pressure) in Western countries. In people whose blood pressure is already raised, excessive sodium may increase the risk of heart disease, stroke, and kidney damage. Another adverse effect is fluid retention, which, in severe cases, may cause dizziness and swelling of the legs.

Sodium aurothiomalate

A preparation of *gold*, which is given by injection.

Sodium bicarbonate

An over-the-counter *antacid drug* used to relieve *indigestion*, *heartburn*, and pain caused by a *peptic ulcer*.

Sodium bicarbonate often causes belching and abdominal discomfort. Long-term use may cause swollen ankles, muscle cramps, tiredness, weakness, nausea, and vomiting. Sodium bicarbonate should not be taken by people with *heart failure* or a history of kidney disease.

Sodium cromoglycate

A drug used to treat some types of *asthma*, allergic *rhinitis* (hay fever), allergic *conjunctivitis*, and *food allergy*.

WHY IT IS USED

Sodium cromoglycate is commonly given by *inhaler* to prevent attacks of mild to moderate asthma in children. It is also prescribed for allergic asthma in adults and for asthma induced by exercise or cold air. Sodium cromoglycate has a slow onset of action, taking up to four weeks of regular treatment to produce its antiasthmatic effect. Use of this drug sometimes permits a reduction in the dosage of other drugs taken to relieve attacks. Sodium cromoglycate is not an effective treatment for an acute asthmatic attack.

Taken in the form of a nasal spray, sodium cromoglycate is useful in treating allergic rhinitis. In the form of eye-drops, it treats allergic conjunctivitis, and in the form of capsules it can help in some types of food allergy.

HOW IT WORKS

Sodium cromoglycate works by blocking the release of *histamine* (a chemical released into the body when an allergic reaction occurs).

S

POSSIBLE ADVERSE EFFECTS
Side-effects are generally mild and rarely require treatment to be stopped. Coughing and wheezing on inhalation may be prevented by first using a sympathomimetic *bronchodilator drug*. Throat irritation can be avoided by rinsing the mouth with water after inhalation.

Sodium valproate

An *anticonvulsant drug* used to treat *epilepsy*. Although sodium valproate has less of a sedative effect than many other anticonvulsant drugs, it occasionally causes drowsiness. Other possible side-effects include abdominal discomfort, temporary hair loss, weight gain, and rash. Since prolonged treatment may in rare cases cause liver damage, regular blood tests are usually performed to monitor liver function.

Soft-tissue injury

Damage to one or more of the tissues that surround bones and joints (for example to a *ligament, tendon,* or *muscle*). Soft-tissue injuries include ligament *sprain, tendinitis* (inflammation of a tendon), and muscle *strain.* (See also *Sports injuries.*)

Soiling

Inappropriate passage of *faeces* after the age at which bowel control is achieved (usually at about three or four years of age). The term is usually applied to the accidental passage of soft, unformed faeces into the clothing. More than half of the children with this problem also wet the bed (see *Enuresis*).

Causes of soiling include slowness in developing bowel control, long-standing *constipation* (in which faecal liquid leaks around hard faeces blocking the large intestine), poor *toilet-training,* and psychological stress (caused, for example, by starting school). Soiling is usually distressing to the child, who may hide the messy clothes.

Soiling due to constipation usually responds to treatment. If there is no physical cause, the problem may pass after a discussion involving the child, the parents, and the doctor. If the problem persists, however, *psychotherapy* may be used.

Encopresis is a form of soiling in which children deliberately pass faeces in inappropriate places, such as in their clothing or behind furniture. Such children have no specific physical problem, but often refuse to use a potty or toilet. Encopresis usually improves with time and is rare after the age of 10.

Solar plexus

The largest network of autonomic nerves in the body (see *Autonomic nervous system*). Also known as the coeliac plexus, the solar plexus is situated behind the stomach, where it surrounds the coeliac artery and lies between the adrenal glands. The solar plexus incorporates branches of the *vagus nerve,* the most important component of the parasympathetic nervous system, and the splanchnic nerves. The solar plexus sends out branches to the stomach, intestines, and most other abdominal organs.

Solvent abuse

The practice of inhaling the intoxicating fumes given off by certain volatile liquids. Glue sniffing is the most common form of solvent abuse, but many other substances are used, especially those containing toluene or acetone. The usual method of inhalation is from a plastic bag containing the solvent, but sometimes aerosols are sprayed into the nose or mouth.

INCIDENCE
Solvent abuse is common among boys in poor urban areas. It is usually a group activity that is indulged in for no more than a few months. Solitary abuse over a longer period is frequently associated with delinquency and a disturbed family background. Around 150 deaths from solvent abuse occur each year in Britain.

EFFECTS
Inhalation of solvent fumes produces an effect similar to that of becoming drunk or getting high on drugs, sometimes including hallucinations. Solvent abuse can cause headache, vomiting, stupor, confusion, and coma. Death may occur owing to a direct toxic effect on the heart, a fall, choking on vomit, or asphyxiation by a clinging plastic bag.

Long-term harmful effects include erosion of the membrane lining the nose and throat, and damage to the kidneys, liver, and nervous system. Long-term exposure to benzene (in petrol, cleaning fluids, plastic cements and lacquers, and paint remover) may cause lead poisoning.

DIAGNOSIS AND TREATMENT
The signs of solvent abuse include intoxicated behaviour, a flushed face, ulcers around the mouth, a smell of solvent, and personality changes, such as moodiness and nervousness.

Solvent abusers should be warned of the serious risks to health. Professional counselling may be needed. Acute symptoms resulting from solvent abuse, such as vomiting or coma, require urgent medical attention.

Somatic

A term that means related to the body (soma), as opposed to the mind (psyche), or related to body cells, as opposed to germ cells (eggs and sperm). The term somatic also refers to the body wall, in contrast to visceral (referring to the internal organs).

Somatization disorder

A condition in which a person complains over a period of several years of various physical problems for which no physical cause can be found. The disorder, previously classified as *hysteria,* usually begins before the age of 30 and leads to numerous tests by many doctors. Unnecessary surgery and other treatments often result.

This disorder may be slightly more prevalent in women, many of whom have a family history of *antisocial personality disorder* in male relatives. Symptoms most commonly complained of are neurological (such as double vision, seizures, weakness), gynaecological (painful menstruation, pain on intercourse), and gastrointestinal (abdominal pain, nausea). Associated features may include *anxiety* and *depression,* threats of *suicide,* and various forms of substance abuse.

Physical symptoms in this disorder are caused by underlying emotional conflicts, anxiety, and depression that the affected person is unable to confront and unconsciously displaces on to the body. It is thought that the sufferer finds it easier to view the problem as physical than rather face the emotional conflicts from which he or she is trying to escape. (See also *Conversion disorder; Hypochondriasis.*)

Somatotype

The physical build of an individual. Various attempts have been made to classify people according to body type and to identify corresponding personality traits.

In the 1920s, the German psychiatrist Ernst Kretschmer divided people into three types, each of which he thought was more prone to certain types of mental illness—asthenic (thin) types seemed more likely to have a schizoid personality or schizophrenia; pyknic (stocky) types were more prone to manic-depressive ill-

S

ness; athletic (muscular) types were not associated with any single disorder, but there was more delinquency within this group.

An American psychologist, W. H. Sheldon, working in the 1940s, believed that people did not fit into rigid categories of body type. Instead he identified three structural tendencies (each associated with certain personality traits), which everyone had in different proportions. These were endomorphic—a heavy physique, with poorly developed bones and muscles, associated with a sociable, loving personality; mesomorphic—strong, well-developed bones and muscles, paired with a physical, adventurous personality; and ectomorphic—a tall, thin physique, with light bones and muscles, linked with a restrained, self-conscious personality.

Somatropin

A bio-synthetic *growth hormone*. Somatropin is given to children to treat *short stature* caused by a deficiency of growth hormone.

Somnambulism

See *Sleepwalking*.

Sore

A term used to describe an ulcer, septic wound, or any disrupted area of the skin or mucous membranes.

The word sore is also used adjectivally to describe an area that is tender or painful.

Sore throat

A rough or raw feeling in the back of the throat that causes discomfort, especially when swallowing.

Sore throat is an extremely common symptom, which is usually caused by *pharyngitis*, and occasionally by *tonsillitis*. It may also be the first symptom of the common *cold, influenza, laryngitis,* infectious *mononucleosis,* and many childhood viral illnesses, including *chickenpox, measles,* and *mumps.*

Strep throat, a type of sore throat caused by infection with beta-haemolytic streptococcal bacteria, requires medical attention. Left untreated, strep throat may result in acute *glomerulonephritis* or *rheumatic fever.*

A sore throat can sometimes be relieved by gargling with salt water. Adults may benefit from taking aspirin. If a sore throat persists for more than 48 hours or if a *rash* develops, a doctor should be consulted. Sore throats due to bacterial infection are treated with *antibiotic drugs.*

BODY TYPES AND PERSONALITY

The idea that the features of the psyche (mind) are related to those of the soma (body) is not always borne out in practice. Even so, attempts have been made to relate the two (see below).

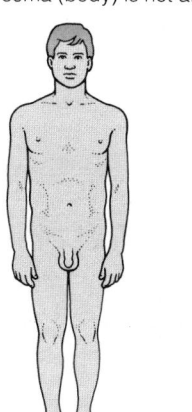 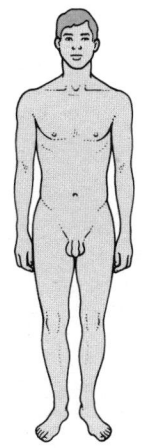 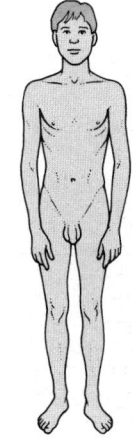

Endomorph
Tends to be sociable, easy-going, pleasure-loving, relaxed, and convivial.

Mesomorph
Is often physically active, strong, athletic, ready for action, and aggressive.

Ectomorph
Is more sensitive, self-conscious, restrained, introspective, and quiet.

Space medicine

A medical specialty concerned with the physiological and pathological effects of space-flight. Space medicine is often linked with the specialty of *aviation medicine.*

During lift-off, there is a large upward acceleration that makes the astronaut feel many times heavier. There is also a tendency for blood to pool downwards. To prevent loss of consciousness as a result of blood draining from the brain, astronauts must lie in a reclining seat and wear a special suit that exerts pressure on certain parts of the body (such as the limbs) and helps maintain blood flow to the head.

Once in stable orbit, the astronaut feels weightless. One effect of weightlessness is on the body's balance mechanisms. Initially, the brain may be unable to make sense of the lack of signals from the balance organ in the inner ear; one manifestation of this is *motion sickness.* Changes also occur in the cardiovascular system (heart and blood vessels) because, in the absence of weight, body fluids are redistributed towards the head. Other effects may include loss of bone and muscle tissue. Such effects could ultimately limit space travel, unless a means can be found to recreate "weight" within spacecraft.

Spasm

An involuntary, often powerful, contraction of a *muscle.* A spasm may affect one or more muscles and may occur once or more; pain is not necessarily an accompanying feature.

Examples of muscle spasms include *hiccups* (in which the diaphragm goes into spasm), muscle cramps (which often affect the muscles in the calves), and *tics* (which frequently affect the facial muscles).

Less commonly, a spasm may be the result of an abnormality in the central nervous system (brain and spinal cord) or a symptom of a muscle disorder. Spasms caused by disease of the nervous system include *myoclonus* and *chorea.* Conditions characterized by spasm include *trigeminal neuralgia* (which affects the muscles of the face and head), *tetany* (spasm caused by a drop of the calcium level in the blood), and *tetanus* (an infectious disease). Rare causes of widespread spasm are *rabies, strychnine poisoning,* and the bite of the black widow spider (see *Spider bites*).

Other types of muscle spasm include *bronchospasm* (contraction of muscles in the small airways of the lungs), which occurs in asthma, and vasospasm (tightening of the muscles in the walls of blood vessels), which occurs in Raynaud's disease.

S

Spasticity

Increased rigidity in a group of *muscles*, causing stiffness and restriction of movement. Spasticity can occur with or without *paralysis* or muscle weakness. In *cerebral palsy*, there is spasticity with paralysis. In *Parkinson's disease* and *multiple sclerosis*, spasticity may occur without paralysis. In *tetanus*, there is spasticity initially of the muscles in the face and neck (lockjaw) and then of other body muscles.

Spastic paralysis

Inability to move a part of the body, accompanied by rigidity of the muscles. Causes of spastic paralysis include *stroke*, *cerebral palsy*, and *multiple sclerosis*. (See also *Paralysis*.)

Specific gravity

Also called relative density, the ratio of the *density* of a substance to that of water. Materials with a relative density of less than 1 are less dense ("lighter") than water; those with a relative density of more than 1 are denser ("heavier") than water. The specific gravity of urine shows if it has a large amount of material dissolved in it (near 1.030) or if it is almost water (near 1.010).

Specimen

A sample of tissue, body fluids (such as blood), waste products (such as urine), or an infective organism taken for the purpose of examination, identification, analysis, and/or diagnosis. The term specimen is also applied to a sample of a tissue or an organism specially prepared for examination under a *microscope*. (See also *Blood tests*; *Urinalysis*.)

SPECT

The abbreviation for single photon emission computed tomography, a type of *radionuclide scanning*.

Spectacles

See *Glasses*.

Speculum

A device for holding open a body orifice (opening) to enable a doctor to perform an examination. A speculum may be made of plastic or metal.

TYPES

There are many types of speculum designed for use on different parts of the body. The speculum used to examine the eardrum is funnel-shaped, with a narrow end inserted into the ear canal and a wide end attached to an *otoscope*. A nasal speculum is used to examine the inside of the nose. The speculum used to hold open the walls of the vagina during a pelvic examination may be shaped either like a duck's bill, with wide, smooth, curved edges and a self-retaining lock to hold it in position, or like a shoehorn bent at both ends at an angle of 90 degrees.

Speech

A system of sounds by which humans communicate.

LANGUAGE AND SPEECH

The terms "speech" and "language" are often used interchangeably, but have different meanings. Language is the representation of objects and ideas by strings of symbols, which form words. These symbols may be speech sounds, written characters, or hand signals. There are two main facets of language ability—understanding the meaning of words (comprehension) and generating words, in grammatical order, to express something meaningful (expression).

Speech is just one method by which language can be communicated to others. Writing and hand signals are others. Each method relies on sequences of muscle movements. Speech involves the muscles used in breathing, the larynx (voice-box), tongue, palate, lips, jaw, and face.

LANGUAGE CENTRES

Language comprehension and expression take place in two areas of the cerebral cortex (the outer layer of the main mass of the brain) known as Wernicke's area and Broca's area. Both are in the dominant cerebral hemisphere (the left hemisphere in most people). In Wernicke's area, incoming messages (heard or read) are scanned and compared with information held in the memory to extract meaning. In Broca's area, words and sentences are composed from vocabulary and from grammatical rules stored in the memory.

SPEECH PRODUCTION

The movement sequences for speech sounds originate from two regions of the cerebral cortex on each side of the brain. These regions are linked to the centre for language expression (Broca's area). The signals for movement pass down nerve pathways to the muscles controlling the larynx, tongue, and other parts involved in speech. The cerebellum (a region at the back of the brain) plays a part in coordinating these movements.

Air from the lungs is vibrated by opening and closing the vocal cords in the larynx. This produces a noise, which is amplified in the hollow cavities of the throat, nose, and sinuses. The sound of vibrated or nonvibrated air is modified by movements of the tongue, mouth, jaw, and lips to produce speech sounds. Vibrated air blown through top teeth resting on lower lips gives "v" or, if the air is not vibrated, "f". Consonants are produced mainly by contact between the tongue, roof of the mouth, teeth, and lips; vowels are produced by changing the shape of the mouth cavity.

LANGUAGE AND SPEECH DEVELOPMENT

Normal development of language and speech in a child depends on maturation of the nervous system and muscles, on the child's exploration of his or her environment, and on interaction with adults. Through play, the child acquires many concepts about different aspects of the world. From adults, the child acquires the verbal labels for objects and concepts that are needed for language development. Normal hearing is, therefore, essential. Language and speech are learned through listening to the speech of others and through monitoring one's own speech.

Stages in the development of language and speech in a child, with the significance of each, are shown in the accompanying table.

Speech disorders

Defects or disturbances can arise in various parts of the nervous system, muscles, and other apparatus involved in *speech*, leading to an inability to communicate effectively. Some of these disorders are, strictly, disturbances of language rather than of speech, since they result from an impaired ability to understand or to form words in the language centres of the brain, rather than from any fault of the apparatus of speech production. Most people with speech disorders can be helped by *speech therapy*.

DISORDERS OF LANGUAGE

Damage to the language centres of the brain (usually as a result of a *stroke*, *head injury*, or *brain tumour*) leads to disorders known as *aphasia* and *dysphasia*. Both children and adults can be affected. The ability to speak and write and/or to comprehend written or spoken words is impaired, depending on the site and extent of the damage.

Delayed development of language in a child is characterized by slowness to understand speech and/or slow growth in vocabulary and sentence

S

structure. Delayed development has many causes, including hearing loss (see *Deafness*), lack of stimulation, or emotional disturbance (see *Developmental delay*). There are, however, considerable variations in speech development in children.

DISORDERS OF ARTICULATION

Articulation is the ability to produce speech sounds; a defect of articulation is sometimes referred to as *dysarthria*. Damage to nerves passing from the brain to muscles in the larynx (voice-box), mouth, or lips can cause speech to be slurred, indistinct, slow, or nasal. The sources of such damage are similar to those that cause aphasia (including stroke, head injury, tumours, *multiple sclerosis, Parkinson's disease*) but the affected regions of the brain are different. Damage to the cerebellum, for example, produces a characteristic form of slurred speech. Structural abnormalities of the mouth, such as cleft palate (see *Cleft lip and palate*) and *malalignment* of the teeth, can also cause poor articulation.

Delayed development of articulation, characterized by an inability to make sounds at appropriate ages, may cause incomprehensible speech. Possible causes are hearing problems or slow maturation of the nervous system. Lisping and lalling (the mispronunciation of "r" as "l") result from poor tongue and lip control.

DISORDERS OF VOICE PRODUCTION

These disorders include hoarseness, harshness, inappropriate pitch or loudness of the voice, and abnormal nasal resonance. In many cases, the cause is a disorder affecting closure of the vocal cords (see *Larynx* disorders box). A voice that is pitched too high or low or that is too loud or soft may be caused by a hormonal or psychiatric disturbance or by severe hearing loss.

Abnormal nasal resonance is caused by too much air (hypernasality) or too little air (hyponasality) flowing through the nose during speech. Hypernasality may result from damage to the nerves supplying the palate (roof of the mouth) or be a result of cleft palate, and causes a deterioration in the intelligibility of speech. Hyponasality is caused by blockage to the nasal airways by congestion or excess mucus and has the sound of someone speaking with a cold.

DISORDERS OF FLUENCY

Nonfluent speech is marked by repetitions of single sounds or whole words and by interruptions in speech; the underlying cause is not understood (see *Stuttering*).

LANGUAGE AND SPEECH DEVELOPMENT IN CHILDHOOD

3 months	Period of babbling begins. The child produces strings of sounds for pleasure. Babbling is important in building sequences of muscle movements	that will be used later to produce meaningful speech sounds.
9 months	The child echoes the speech of others, but words are not yet used with meaning. By listening to and copying adults, the child learns that clusters of	sounds refer to specific objects, people, or situations.
12 to 18 months	The child begins to utter simple words with meaning, often accompanied by gestures. Examples include "bye-bye", "dog", "hot", and "daddy".	Single words are used, with vocabulary gradually increasing from two or three words initially.
18 to 24 months	The child begins to combine concepts to form two-word sentences (e.g. "Hello John" or "That hot!"). By the age of two	years, the child may be using 100 or more different words.
2 to 3 years	The child's sentences become longer (e.g. "I like cake" or "Peter hit Mary"). He or she also begins to incorporate adjectives and adverbs into sentences (e.g. "That's daddy's old coat" or "I want lunch now").	By the age of three years, the average sentence length is four words. Most sounds have developed, with the possible exceptions of "th", "r", "j", "ch", and "sh".
3 years and older	More elaborate sentences with several nouns, verbs in past and future tenses, and linked phrases begin to be used (e.g. "We went to Amy's and we had milk and biscuits" or "I think mummy went downstairs").	However, mistakes are often made (e.g. "What did you played?"), reflecting the child's linguistic immaturity. Language skills continue to develop throughout childhood.

Speech therapy

A form of treatment that attempts to help people with any of a variety of communication problems.

WHY IT IS DONE

Any person with a disturbance of language or a disorder of articulation, voice production, or fluency of speech (see *Speech disorders*) may be helped by speech therapy. Such problems may occur as part of a broader problem, such as a physical *handicap, learning difficulty*, or *hearing loss*. Speech therapists work with all age groups.

HOW IT IS DONE

The therapist—a person trained in the causes, assessment, and treatment of speech and language problems— usually begins by finding out the case history from the client or from a relative or friend, asking how and when the difficulties developed. Relevant medical details are also sought from the client's doctor if necessary.

The client may be asked to provide a sample of speech (which may be recorded) or of writing for detailed analysis. An examination of the physical structures of speech and a *hearing test* may be performed. The therapist may also assess language comprehension by observing the client's reaction to written or spoken requests.

After making an assessment, the therapist decides on the form of treatment, which usually has two parts. First, a programme of exercises is started to improve a specific aspect of language ability or speech performance (e.g. a technique to improve speech fluency). Second, the therapist works with the people most involved with the client (family, teachers, or friends), explaining to them the nature of the difficulties and how they can help. The aim is to create a climate that will provide maximum opportunities for effective communication.

S

Sperm

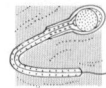

The sex cell of the male, also known as spermatozoon (singular) or spermatozoa (plural), responsible for *fertilization* of the ovum of the female. Sperm are microscopically tiny, measuring 0.05 mm in length.

Sperm are produced within the seminiferous tubules of the *testes* by a process known as spermatogenesis. The production and development of sperm is dependent on the presence of the male sex hormone *testosterone* and of *gonadotrophin hormones* produced by the *pituitary gland*. Sperm production commences at *puberty*.

The original cell from which a sperm develops contains 46 chromosomes, including the XY pair of male sex *chromosomes*. By a process of *cell division* known as *meiosis*, the number of chromosomes in the sperm is halved to 23, including either the X or the Y from the original pair of sex chromosomes. This X or Y is responsible for determining the sex of an embryo that develops after fertilization of the ovum by the sperm (see *Sex determination*).

The final stage of spermatogenesis takes place in the *epididymis*, where each sperm grows a tail that will propel it through the woman's reproductive tract after *ejaculation* during *sexual intercourse*.

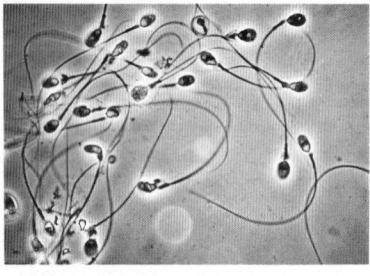

Human sperm magnified 350 times
Each sperm consists of a head that contains the hereditary material and a long, whip-like tail that propels it along.

Spermatocele

A harmless cyst (fluid-filled swelling) of the *epididymis* (the tube that transmits sperm from the testis) containing fluid and sperm.

If a spermatocele grows to a large size or if it becomes uncomfortable, it is usually removed surgically. The operation is straightforward, but may result in an interruption of the passage of sperm through the epididymis, which may render the testis on the affected side infertile.

Spermatozoa

See *Sperm*.

Spermicides

Contraceptive preparations that kill *sperm*. Spermicides are available in the form of creams, gels, foams, and pessaries. They are usually recommended for use with a barrier device, such as a condom or diaphragm, to increase the contraceptive effect (see *Contraception, barrier methods*).

Some spermicides, such as nonoxinol, may offer partial protection against the organisms that cause various *sexually transmitted diseases*, including *gonorrhoea* and *AIDS*.

An uncommon possible adverse effect of spermicides is irritation of the genitals of either partner.

Sphenoid bone

The bat-shaped bone in the centre of the base of the cranium (the part of the *skull* that encases the brain). The central body of the bone contains the sphenoidal sinus (air space) and, in the upper surface, a depression in which the *pituitary gland* is situated. The wings support part of the temporal lobe of the brain (see *Cerebrum*) and form part of the back and side walls of the orbits (eye sockets). Openings in the wings enable the optic and other cranial nerves to pass through.

Spherocytosis, hereditary

An inherited disorder so named because of the large number of unusually small, round, red blood cells (spherocytes) in the circulation. These cells have an abnormal membrane (outer envelope), which makes them fragile and causes them to have a much reduced lifespan because they are readily trapped, broken up, and consumed when blood passes through the *spleen*. At times, the rate of *haemolysis* (red cell destruction) exceeds the rate at which new cells can be made in the bone marrow, leading to *anaemia* (reduced level of the oxygen-carrying pigment *haemoglobin* in the blood due to lack of red cells).

INCIDENCE
Hereditary spherocytosis is the most common form of inherited haemolytic anaemia (see *Anaemia, haemolytic*) in people of northern European extraction. About one person in 4,500 in the UK has the condition. The disorder is inherited in an autosomal dominant pattern (see *Genetic disorders*). Each of an affected person's children has a 50 per cent chance of inheriting the defective gene responsible.

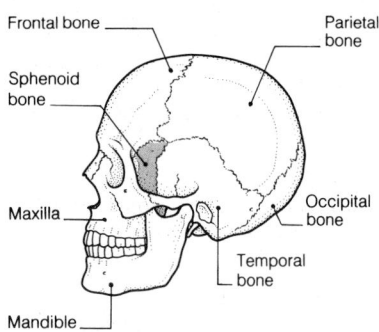

Location of the sphenoid bone
The sphenoid bone is a bat-shaped bone that lies in front of the temporal bones at the base of the skull.

SYMPTOMS
Symptoms of anaemia, (e.g. tiredness, shortness of breath on exertion, and pallor) may develop. Other symptoms include *jaundice*, caused by the high rate of red blood cell destruction, and enlargement of the spleen. Occasionally, there are crises (usually triggered by infection) in which all symptoms worsen. *Gallstones*, caused by the high rate of red blood cell destruction, are a frequent complication.

DIAGNOSIS AND TREATMENT
The diagnosis is made from the presence of spherocytes in the blood of someone with anaemia and from tests to ascertain the structure of the red cell membrane.

The treatment is *splenectomy* (removal of the spleen). The red cells remain abnormally shaped, but the rate at which they are destroyed drops markedly, leading to a striking, and usually permanent, improvement in health. After removal of the spleen, susceptibility to certain bacterial infections increases, necessitating vaccination against pneumococcal infection as well as prompt treatment of infections with *antibiotic drugs*.

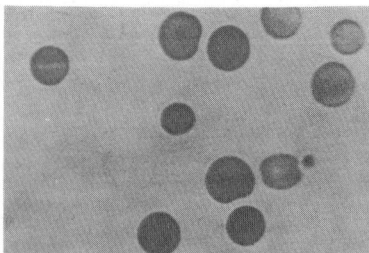

Spherocytes in blood
A person with hereditary spherocytosis has a large number of these unusually small, round, fragile, red cells in the blood.

S

Sphincter

A ring of muscle around a natural opening or passage that acts like a valve, regulating inflow or outflow. An example is the pyloric sphincter at the outlet of the stomach into the duodenum, which controls the stomach's outflow. Another example is the anal sphincter at the rectal outlet, which is partly under voluntary control and permits a voluntary decision on when to empty the bowel.

Sphincter, artificial

A surgically created valve or other device used to treat or prevent urinary or faecal *incontinence*.

An artificial urinary sphincter consists of an inflatable cuff that is inserted around the base of the bladder or upper part of the urethra. When inflated, the cuff prevents urine from leaking from the bladder. The patient deflates the cuff by using a pump, which is usually situated in the scrotum in males or adjacent to the labia in females.

An artificial sphincter to prevent faecal incontinence may be created after removal of the colon and rectum as an alternative to a conventional *ileostomy*. Creation of such a "continent ileostomy" involves using a loop of ileum to create a pouch in which bowel contents collect. Evacuation of faeces is controlled by an artificial sphincter, surgically fashioned from a section of ileum.

A similar continent ileostomy may be provided for a person whose bladder has been removed because of cancer. In such cases, the ureters are joined to a segment of ileum that is formed into a pouch. This procedure is still considered experimental, as are other methods of continent *urinary diversion*.

Sphincterotomy

A surgical procedure that involves cutting the muscle that closes a body opening or that constricts the opening between body passages. In rare cases, sphincterotomy is performed on the anal sphincter to treat an *anal fissure*. It may also be performed on the ampulla of Vater (the opening of the common bile duct into the duodenum) to release an impacted *gallstone*.

Sphygmomanometer

An instrument for measuring blood pressure. A sphygmomanometer consists of a cuff with an inflatable bladder, which is wrapped around a person's upper arm, a rubber bulb to inflate the bladder, and a device that indicates the pressure of blood. This pressure device may consist of a calibrated glass column filled with mercury, a spring gauge and dial, or, in more modern instruments, a digital display. (For an explanation of how a sphygmomanometer is used, see *Blood pressure*.)

Spider bites

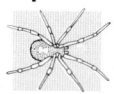 Nearly all spiders produce venom, which they inject, via a pair of fangs, to paralyse and kill their prey. However, only a few species are harmful to humans and none of these is native to the UK.

The hairy tarantula of southern Europe is relatively harmless, although its bite is painful. Spiders whose bites occasionally cause deaths in humans include the black widow spider and the brown recluse spider in North America, the banana spider in South America, and the redback spider and "funnel web" spider in Australia. *Antivenoms* are available for these and many other dangerous spider bites.

Spider naevus

A discoloured patch of skin in the form of a red, raised, pinhead-sized dot from which small blood vessels radiate. A spider naevus is the outward manifestation of a dilated arteriole (small artery) and its connecting capillaries.

Small numbers of spider naevi are common in children and pregnant women. However, in larger quantities, spider naevi may be a sign of an underlying liver disease. (See also *Telangiectasia*.)

Spina bifida

A *congenital* defect in which part of one or more *vertebrae* fails to develop completely, leaving a portion of the *spinal cord* exposed. Spina bifida can occur anywhere on the spine but is most common in the lower back. The severity of the condition depends on how much nerve tissue is exposed.

CAUSES AND INCIDENCE

The cause of spina bifida remains unknown, although vitamin deficiency seems to be one of the main factors involved.

In the UK, the number of babies born with the disorder has been declining recently as screening and prevention programmes have come into general use, but the incidence is still about 30 babies per 100,000 born.

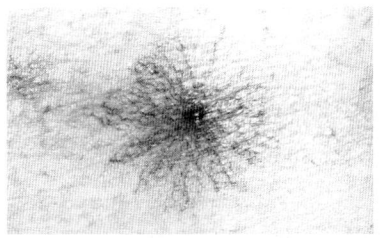

Typical spider naevus
The naevus consists of a tiny, red, raised dot from which widened blood capillaries radiate outwards in all directions.

TYPES

There are four known distinct forms of spina bifida.

SPINA BIFIDA OCCULTA This is the most common and the least serious form. There is little external evidence of the defect apart from a dimple or a tuft of hair over the area of the underlying abnormality. Spina bifida occulta often goes completely unnoticed in otherwise healthy children, although occasionally there are accompanying abnormalities of the lower part of the spinal cord. Symptoms, which include leg weakness, cold and blue feet, and urinary incontinence, may be present from birth or may develop later in life.

MYELOCELE Also known as meningomyelocele, this is the most severe form of spina bifida. The nature of the defect is shown in the box overleaf.

A child with myelocele is usually severely handicapped. The legs are partly or completely paralysed, with loss of sensation in all areas below the level of the defect; hip dislocation and other leg deformities are common. *Hydrocephalus* (excess cerebrospinal fluid within the skull) is common and without treatment may result in brain damage. Associated abnormalities include *cerebral palsy*, *epilepsy*, *mental handicap*, and visual problems. Paralysis of the bladder leads to urinary incontinence or urinary retention, repeated urinary tract infections, and eventual kidney damage. The anus may be paralysed, causing chronic constipation and leakage of faeces.

MENINGOCELE This form is less severe than myelocele. The nature of the defect is shown in the box overleaf.

ENCEPHALOCELE This is a rare disorder, related to spina bifida, in which brain tissue protrudes through the skull. There is usually severe brain damage.

DIAGNOSIS

Closure of the vertebral canal usually occurs within four weeks of concep-

S

tion, meaning that meningomyelocele can often be diagnosed at an early stage in the pregnancy by *ultrasound scanning*. High levels of *alpha-fetoprotein* in the amniotic fluid or maternal blood may indicate spina bifida.

After birth, spina bifida is easy to recognize if there is a protruding sac. Spina bifida occulta can be diagnosed only by an *X-ray* of the spine.

TREATMENT
In cases that are not severe, surgery may be performed to close the defect and thus prevent further damage to the spinal cord. Ideally, the operation should be performed in the first few days of life. If the abnormality is serious, surgery may allow the child to survive, but possibly with severe mental or physical handicap.

If hydrocephalus develops, a *shunt* (tube and valve mechanism) is inserted into the brain to relieve the build-up of fluid.

Urinary retention or urinary incontinence may be relieved by use of a catheter (see *Catheterization, urinary*), which is inserted into the bladder and changed every four to six weeks. Older children may be taught self-catheterization. *Laxative drugs* may be needed.

Physiotherapy encourages mobility and independence; for the more severely affected, wheelchairs and other walking aids may be required. Depending on the degree of disability, special schooling and training for employment may be needed.

PREVENTION
Parents who have had one child with spina bifida should undergo *genetic counselling* if they are considering another pregnancy. During subsequent pregnancies the levels of *alpha-fetoprotein* in the blood and amniotic fluid are measured. Research studies have shown convincingly that the risk of spina bifida is substantially reduced if the mother takes *folic acid* supplements daily for a month before conception, and during the first 12 weeks of pregnancy. Higher doses are recommended for women who have had an affected baby in an earlier pregnancy.

Spinal anaesthesia
Injection of an anaesthetic into the cerebrospinal fluid in the spinal canal in order to block *pain* sensations before they reach the *central nervous system* (brain and spinal cord). It is mainly used during surgery on the lower abdomen and legs.

The procedure is performed by inserting a delicate needle between two vertebrae in the lower part of the

---

TYPES OF SPINA BIFIDA

There are different forms of spina bifida. In one type (spina bifida occulta), the only defect is a failure of the fusion of the bony arches behind the spinal cord. When the bone defect is more extensive, there may be a meningocele, with protrusion of the meninges (the membranes surrounding the cord) or, more seriously, a myelocele, with malformation of the spinal cord itself.

MENINGOCELE

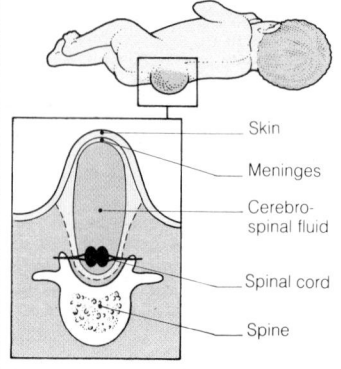

MYELOCELE

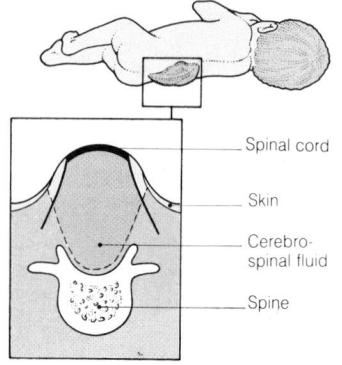

Meningocele
In this type, the nerve tissue of the spinal cord is usually intact; there is skin over the bulging sac and therefore there may be no functional problems. However, repairs are necessary early in life.

Myelocele
In this type, the baby is born with a raw swelling over the spine. It consists of malformed spinal cord, which may or may not be contained in a membranous sac. The child is likely to be very handicapped.

---

spine (see *Lumbar puncture*) and introducing anaesthetic into the cerebrospinal fluid surrounding the spinal cord and its terminal nerve roots. Because the nerves emerging from the spinal cord are bathed in cerebrospinal fluid, they absorb the anaesthetic. The position of the injection and the subsequent controlled spread of the local anaesthetic solution determine the area that is anaesthetized.

After spinal anaesthesia, a headache develops in between one and five per cent of patients. (See also *Epidural anaesthesia*.)

Spinal cord
A cylinder of *nerve* tissue, about 45 cm long and about a finger's width, that runs down the central canal in the *spine*. The spinal cord is a downward extension of the *brain* and, together, they can be considered parts of a single unit—the *central nervous system* (CNS).

STRUCTURE
At the core of the spinal cord is a region with a butterfly-shaped cross section, called the grey matter. This contains the cell bodies of neurons (nerve cells) along with glial (supporting) cells. Some of the nerve cells are motor neurons, whose axons (long,

projecting fibres) pass out of the spinal cord in bundles within the *spinal nerves* and extend to glands or muscles in the trunk and limbs. Others are interneurons (nerve cells contained entirely within the central nervous system), which act to convey messages between other neurons. Also entering the grey matter are the axons of sensory neurons, which have their cell bodies outside the spinal cord. These axons connect with the motor neurons or interneurons.

Surrounding the grey matter are areas of white matter, which consist of bundles of nerve cell axons running lengthwise through the cord.

Sprouting from the spinal cord on each side at regular intervals are two nerve bundles—the spinal nerve roots, containing the fibres of motor and sensory nerve cells. These combine to form the spinal nerves, which emerge from the spine and are the communication cables between the spinal cord and all regions of the trunk and limbs.

The whole of the spinal cord is bathed in *cerebrospinal fluid* and surrounded by a protective sheath, a continuation of the *meninges* that protect the brain.

S

FUNCTION

The nerve tracts that make up the white matter of the spinal cord act mainly as highways for sensory information passing upwards towards the brain (ascending tracts) or motor signals passing downwards (descending tracts). However, the cord is also capable of handling some of the sensory information itself, and of providing appropriate motor responses without recourse to the brain. Many *reflex* actions (such as the knee-jerk reflex) are controlled in this way by the spinal cord.

DISORDERS

The spinal cord may be injured as a result of trauma to the spine (see *Spinal injury*). Severing of an ascending or descending tract interrupts communication between the brain and parts of the body served from parts of the cord below the injury. This can lead to a variety of patterns of *paralysis* and/or loss of sensation, which are usually permanent because nerve cells and fibres within the cord do not regenerate. However, reflexes controlled by the spinal cord are usually maintained.

Pressure on the cord (e.g. by a blood clot, an abscess, or a tumour) can similarly affect movement and sensation. However, the effects of pressure can often be relieved by surgery.

Infections of the spinal cord (including *poliomyelitis*) are relatively rare but can cause serious damage. In *multiple sclerosis*, a degenerative disease, there is patchy loss of the insulating sheaths around nerve fibres.

Spinal fusion

A major surgical procedure to join two or more adjacent *vertebrae*, the bones that make up the *spine*.

WHY IT IS DONE

Spinal fusion is performed if abnormal movement between adjacent vertebrae (as revealed by *X-rays*) causes severe back pain or may damage the spinal cord. Such abnormal movement may be due to various spinal disorders, including *spondylolisthesis*, dislocated facet joints (the movable joints that connect vertebrae), *scoliosis*, *osteomyelitis*, a tumour or injury destroying one or more vertebrae, or *osteoarthritis* causing degeneration of spinal joints.

HOW IT IS DONE

Under general anaesthesia, the affected vertebrae are exposed. *Arthrodesis* (joint fusion) is then carried out, sometimes together with a *bone graft*, using bone chips

---

LOCATION OF THE SPINAL CORD

The cord runs about 45 cm downwards from the brain through a canal in the spine, tapering towards its lower end.

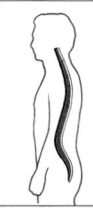

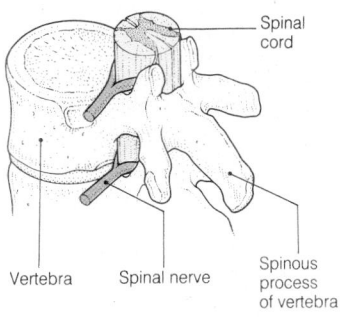

Vertebra   Spinal nerve

Spinal cord

Spinous process of vertebra

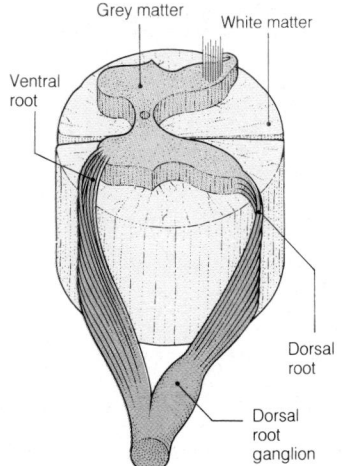

Grey matter   White matter

Ventral root

Dorsal root

Dorsal root ganglion

Structure
The grey matter contains nerve cell bodies, the white matter consists of tracts of nerve fibres. Spinal nerves join the cord at regular intervals.

---

taken from the pelvis. While healing is in progress, the vertebrae are temporarily held together with a plate or screws.

The recovery period includes bed rest for up to six weeks. When mobility is resumed, the patient may initially need to wear a plaster *corset*. Full fusion of the vertebrae takes up to six months.

Results are usually good, but fusing of the vertebrae may place greater strain on the rest of the spine and cause the patient more back pain. The potential gain must be weighed against the risks.

Spinal injury

Damage to the *spine* and sometimes to the *spinal cord*. Injury to the spinal cord may cause loss of sensation, and muscle weakness or *paralysis*.

CAUSES

Spinal injury is usually caused by one of three types of severe force: longitudinal compression, hinging, and shearing. Longitudinal compression, usually due to a fall from a height, crushes the *vertebrae* (spinal bones) lengthwise against each other. Hinging, which can occur in a whiplash injury suffered in a road traffic accident, subjects the spinal column to sudden, extreme bending movements. Shearing, which may occur when a person is knocked over by a motor vehicle, combines both hinging and rotational (twisting) forces.

Any of these forces can dislocate the vertebrae, fracture them, or rupture the *ligaments* that bind them together. In severe dislocations and fractures, the vertebrae, accumulated fluid, or a blood clot may press on the spinal cord, or the cord may be torn or even severed. In all of these cases the function of the spinal cord is impaired or destroyed. An unstable injury is one in which there is a possibility that vertebrae will shift and cause damage, possibly severing the spinal cord. Other injuries are called stable.

SYMPTOMS AND SIGNS

Damage to the vertebrae and ligaments usually causes severe pain and swelling of the affected area. Damage to the spinal cord results in loss of sensation and/or motor function below the site of injury. Injuries below the neck may cause *paraplegia* (weakness or paralysis of the legs and sometimes part of the trunk). Damage to the spinal cord in the neck may result in *quadriplegia* (weakness or paralysis of all four limbs and the trunk) or may be fatal. Weakness or paralysis is often accompanied by loss of bladder or bowel control, resulting in urinary or faecal incontinence or retention.

Pressure on the spinal cord may cause abnormalities of movement, such as muscle weakness or paralysis. It may also cause abnormalities of sensation, such as pain, tingling, or burning sensations.

DIAGNOSIS AND TREATMENT

After an accident in which a spinal injury may have occurred, the victim should be moved only by someone trained in all aspects of first aid. *X-rays* of the spine are carried out to determine whether the spine has been injured and the extent of any damage.

S

In a stable injury, the patient must rest in bed until comfortable movement is possible; he or she may then need to wear an orthopaedic *collar* or *corset* for support or to relieve pain in the injured area.

The priority in an unstable injury is to stabilize the affected bones. If they are dislocated, the surgeon usually manipulates them back into position under general anaesthesia. Some unstable fractures are treated by skeletal *traction* to align the bone ends and hold them in position until healing occurs (which may take up to three months). Other unstable fractures require an operation to fasten the bone ends together permanently with a metal plate or wires.

Research studies have shown that treatment with the drug *methylprednisolone* within a few hours of the injury improves the amount of recovery from spinal cord damage. Surgery may be needed to remove any source of pressure on the cord, but has little part otherwise in the management of neurological problems, since damaged nerve tracts cannot be surgically repaired. Treatment is directed towards preventing the development of problems secondary to the main symptoms. *Physiotherapy* is carried out to stop joints from locking and muscles from contracting as the result of paralysis. Retention of urine or faeces may require *catheterization* or *enemas*.

OUTLOOK
Provided that the spinal cord has not been damaged, recovery is usually complete, although there may be some remaining back pain and stiffness. Even when there is damage, some improvement may occur for up to 12 months. In such cases, the patient's recovery can be aided by a programme of *rehabilitation*. This may include forms of physiotherapy and *occupational therapy*, which can help morale and independence.

Spinal nerves
A set of 31 pairs of *nerves* that connect to the *spinal cord*.
STRUCTURE
The spinal nerves emerge in two rows from either side of the spinal cord and leave the *spine* through gaps between adjacent *vertebrae* (spinal bones). Because the spinal cord runs only two thirds of the way down the spinal canal, the lowest nine pairs of nerves must travel some distance down the canal before finally leaving the spine. These lowest nerves form a "spray" known as the cauda equina.

The distribution and branching of the spinal nerves ensures that all parts of the trunk, arms, and legs are supplied with a network of sensory and motor nerve twigs.
FUNCTION
Like all other nerves, spinal nerves consist of bundles of the axons (long fibres) of individual neurons (nerve cells). Some of these fibres carry information from sensory *receptors* in the skin, muscles, and elsewhere in the body towards the spinal cord; other motor fibres carry signals from the spinal cord to muscles and glands. Just before it connects to the spinal cord, each spinal nerve splits into two bundles, one of which carries only sensory fibres while the other carries only motor fibres. These bundles are sometimes called spinal nerve roots.
DISORDERS
Damage to the shock-absorbing disc of cartilage between two vertebrae sometimes leads to pressure on a spinal nerve root, causing pain (see *Disc prolapse*). Injury to a spinal nerve may lead to loss of sensation and move-

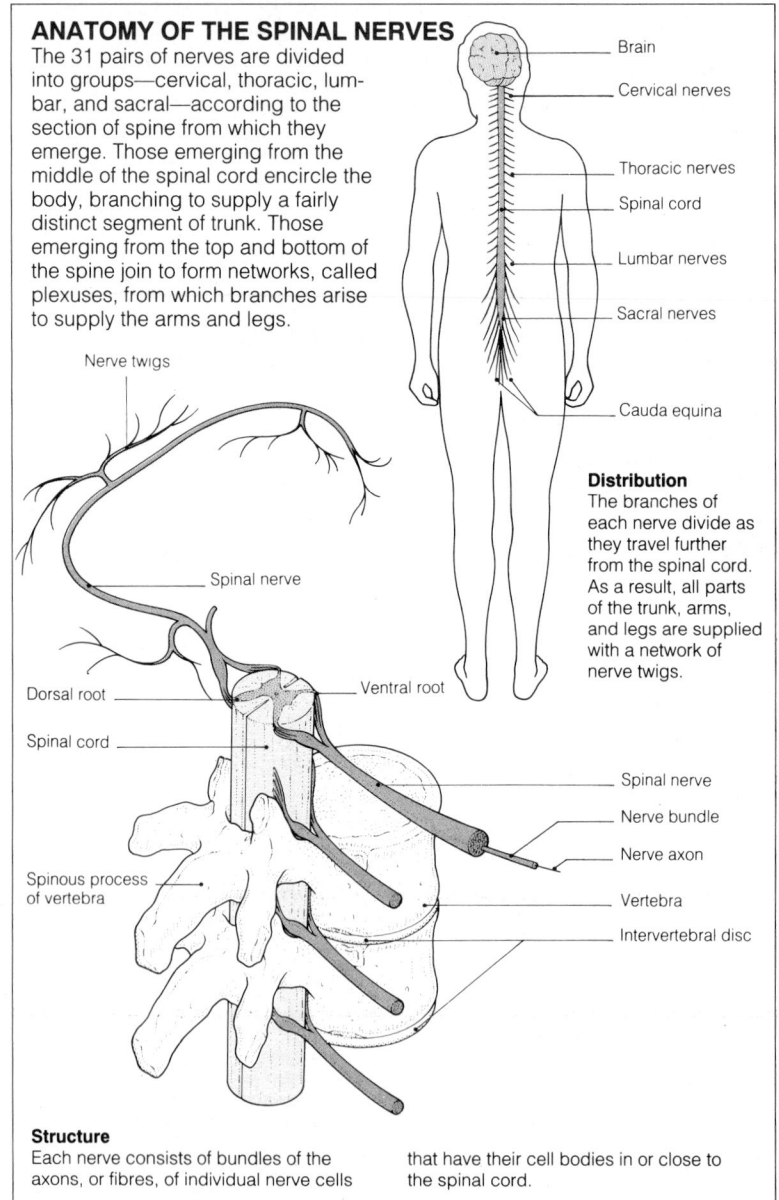

ANATOMY OF THE SPINAL NERVES
The 31 pairs of nerves are divided into groups—cervical, thoracic, lumbar, and sacral—according to the section of spine from which they emerge. Those emerging from the middle of the spinal cord encircle the body, branching to supply a fairly distinct segment of trunk. Those emerging from the top and bottom of the spine join to form networks, called plexuses, from which branches arise to supply the arms and legs.

Brain
Cervical nerves
Thoracic nerves
Spinal cord
Lumbar nerves
Sacral nerves
Cauda equina

Nerve twigs

Spinal nerve

Dorsal root
Spinal cord

Spinous process of vertebra

Ventral root

Spinal nerve
Nerve bundle
Nerve axon
Vertebra
Intervertebral disc

Distribution
The branches of each nerve divide as they travel further from the spinal cord. As a result, all parts of the trunk, arms, and legs are supplied with a network of nerve twigs.

Structure
Each nerve consists of bundles of the axons, or fibres, of individual nerve cells that have their cell bodies in or close to the spinal cord.

S

ment in a part of the body. Damage or degeneration from such causes or from infection, *diabetes mellitus, vitamin deficiency,* or poisoning can lead to neurological symptoms such as pain, numbness, or twitching (see *Nerve injury; Neuropathy*).

Spinal tap

See *Lumbar puncture.*

Spine

The column of bones and cartilage that extends from the base of the skull to the pelvis, enclosing and protecting the *spinal cord* and supporting the trunk and head.

STRUCTURE AND FUNCTION

The spine is made up of 33 roughly cylindrical bones called *vertebrae.* Each pair of adjacent vertebrae is connected by a joint, called a facet joint, which both stabilizes the vertebral column and allows movement in it. Between

each pair of vertebrae lies a disc-shaped pad of tough fibrous cartilage with a jelly-like core (nucleus pulposus) called an intervertebral disc (see *Disc, intervertebral*). These discs cushion the vertebrae during movements such as running or jumping.

In a normal spine the cervical section curves forwards, the thoracic section backwards, the lumbar section forwards (particularly in women), and the pelvic section backwards.

The whole of the spine encloses the spinal cord, a column of nerve tracts running from the brain. Peripheral nerves (see *Peripheral nervous system*) branch off from the spinal cord to every part of the body, their roots passing between the vertebrae.

The vertebrae are bound together by two long, thick ligaments running the length of the spine, and by smaller ligaments between each of the vertebrae.

Several groups of *muscles* are attached to the vertebrae. These muscles control movements of the spine and also help to support it. (See also *Disorders of the spine* box, overleaf.)

Spirochaete

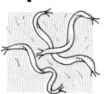

A spiral-shaped bacterium. Spirochaetes cause *syphilis, pinta* and *yaws* (which are both related to syphilis), *leptospirosis, relapsing fever,* and *Lyme disease.*

Spirometry

A *pulmonary function test* used to help diagnose or assess a *lung* disorder or to monitor treatment.

The procedure is shown in the illustrated box. The spirometer records the total volume of air breathed out, known as the forced vital capacity (FVC). It also records the volume of air breathed out in 1 second, known as the forced expiratory volume in 1 second (FEV_1).

In obstructive lung disease (such as *asthma, emphysema,* and chronic bronchitis), the FEV_1/FVC ratio is reduced because the airways are narrowed, thus slowing expiration. In a restrictive lung disease (such as *interstitial pulmonary fibrosis*), the FVC and FEV_1 are reduced almost equally with little

---

STRUCTURE OF THE SPINE

The spine is made up of a column of 33 roughly cylindrical bones called vertebrae. Running through the centre of this bony structure is the spinal cord.

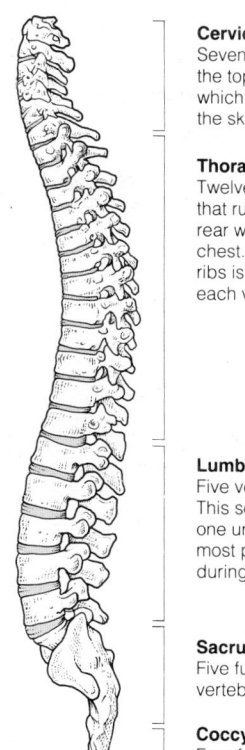

Cervical spine
Seven vertebrae, the topmost of which supports the skull.

Thoracic spine
Twelve vertebrae that run down the rear wall of the chest. A pair of ribs is attached to each vertebra.

Lumbar spine
Five vertebrae. This section is the one under the most pressure during lifting.

Sacrum
Five fused vertebrae.

Coccyx
Four fused vertebrae.

SPIROMETRY

This technique is used to assess certain lung conditions and the patient's response to treatment. It records the rate at which a patient exhales air from the lungs and the total volume exhaled.

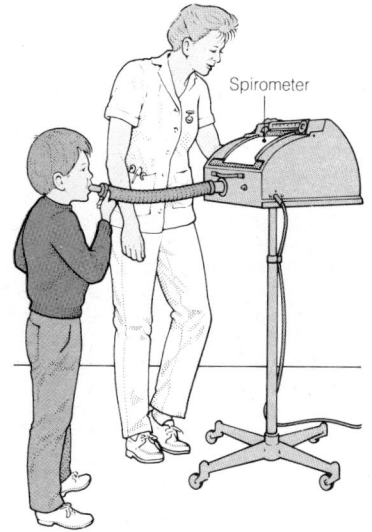

Spirometer

How it is done
The patient exhales forcibly through a mouthpiece into the spirometer. This causes the spirometer to produce a graph like those shown at right.

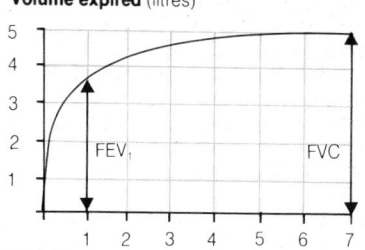

Volume expired (litres)

Time (seconds)

Normal
FEV_1 (forced expiratory volume in the first second) is the volume of air exhaled in the first second and is normally 70 to 80 per cent of FVC (forced vital capacity), the total volume exhaled.

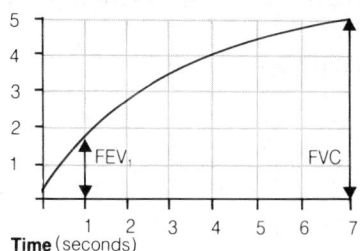

Volume expired (litres)

Time (seconds)

Asthma
A patient with asthma cannot exhale air as fast as normal, due to narrowing of the airways, so FEV_1 is reduced in comparison with FVC.

S

DISORDERS OF THE SPINE

Many disorders of the spine, despite their different causes, result in just one symptom—*back pain*.

CONGENITAL DISORDERS

Some children are born with a gap in the vertebrae that leaves part of the spinal cord exposed. This condition (*spina bifida*) may result in leg paralysis and incontinence.

INFECTION

Osteomyelitis (infection of bone and bone marrow) may in rare cases affect a vertebra, destroying both bone and disc. The most common cause is the spread of an infection, such as *tuberculosis*, from elsewhere in the body.

INFLAMMATION

In *ankylosing spondylitis*, and in some cases of *rheumatoid arthritis*, the joints in the spine become inflamed and later fuse, causing permanent stiffness. *Osteochondritis juvenilis* (inflammation of the growing area of bone in children and adolescents) can affect the vertebrae, when the disease may cause deformity of the spine.

INJURIES

Lifting heavy objects, twisting suddenly, or adopting bad posture can cause any of the following spinal injuries—a sprained ligament, torn muscle, *spondylolisthesis* (dislocated vertebrae), dislocated facet joint, or *disc prolapse* (rupture of the tough outer layer of the disc).

A direct blow, a fall from a height, or sudden twisting can result in fracture of one or more vertebrae. Overexercising the spine can have the same effect (see *Stress fracture*).

TUMOURS

Tumours of the spine are usually malignant; in most cases, they have spread from cancer elsewhere in the body (see *Bone cancer*).

DEGENERATION

Osteoarthritis (degeneration of joint cartilage due to wear and tear) affects the joints in the spines of virtually everyone over 60, particularly people who do heavy manual work or people whose spines have already been affected by disease or injury.

Osteoporosis (thinning and softening of bone), which is most common in older women, can weaken the vertebrae. Under the weight of the trunk, the vertebrae may then fracture.

OTHER DISORDERS

In some people the spine becomes abnormally curved. The excessive curvature may be inwards in the lower back (see *Lordosis*), outwards in the upper back (see *Kyphosis*), or to one side (see *Scoliosis*). Causes include infection, osteoporosis, congenital spine disorder, and muscle disorders.

INVESTIGATION

Spinal disorders are investigated by *X-rays*, *CT scanning*, and *myelography*. Other *bone imaging* techniques, including *MRI*, may sometimes be performed, as may other tests.

---

change in the ratio. This is because lung expansion is limited but the airways are not narrowed.

Spironolactone

A potassium-sparing *diuretic drug*. Combined with thiazide or loop diuretics, it is given to treat *hypertension* (high blood pressure) and *oedema* (accumulation of fluid in tissues).

Spironolactone may cause numbness, weakness, nausea, and vomiting. Less common adverse effects include diarrhoea, lethargy, impotence, rash, and irregular menstruation in women. High doses of spironolactone may cause abnormal breast enlargement in men.

Spleen

An organ that removes and destroys worn-out red blood cells and helps fight infection. Weighing about 200 g, the spleen is a fist-sized, spongy, dark purple organ lying in the upper left abdomen behind the lower ribs.

STRUCTURE

The spleen is covered with a capsule from which many fibrous bands run inwards to give the organ a sponge-like structure. The spaces between the bands are filled with red blood cells, and with *lymphocytes* and *phagocytes* (cells that ingest other cells or foreign particles) which form part of the *lymphatic system*. Blood is supplied to the spleen by a large artery that branches extensively within the organ.

FUNCTION

One of the two main functions of the spleen is to control the quality of circulating red blood cells. It accomplishes this by removing and breaking down all worn-out red cells approximately 120 days after they have been produced in the *bone marrow* and by destroying other red cells that are misshapen or defective. The spleen's other role is to help fight infection by producing some of the *antibodies*, phagocytes, and lymphocytes that destroy invading microorganisms.

In the fetus, the spleen produces red blood cells. After birth, this function is taken over by the bone marrow. However, in certain diseases that affect red cell production in the bone marrow (such as *thalassaemia*), the spleen may resume production.

Despite its functions, the spleen is not an essential organ. If it is removed, its activities are largely taken over by other parts of the lymphatic system, although the individual is more susceptible to infection.

DISORDERS

The spleen enlarges in many diseases. These include: infections, such as malaria, infectious *mononucleosis* (glandular fever), *schistosomiasis*, *tuberculosis*, and *typhoid fever*; blood disorders, such as *leukaemia*, thalassaemia, *sickle cell anaemia* and other diseases that cause haemolytic *anaemia*; and tumours of the spleen, such as *lymphomas* (tumours of lymphoid tissue which may develop in the spleen).

Enlargement of the spleen, which can often be felt as a swelling in the upper left abdomen, is sometimes accompanied by *hypersplenism* (overactivity of the spleen, which reduces the numbers of blood cells).

The spleen is sometimes ruptured by a severe blow to the abdomen, usually in a car crash or by a fall from a height. A rupture is much more likely if the spleen is enlarged or if overlying ribs are fractured. Rupture can cause severe bleeding, which may be fatal. For this reason, the injury requires an emergency operation to remove the spleen (see *Splenectomy*).

S

Splenectomy

Surgical removal of the *spleen.*

WHY IT IS DONE

Splenectomy is usually performed after the spleen has been seriously injured, causing severe haemorrhage. The organ is removed because it is difficult to repair and because, in an adult, its absence has virtually no known ill effects. Its function is largely taken over by other parts of the *lymphatic system* and by the *liver.*

In some cases, the spleen is removed to treat *hypersplenism* and certain types of anaemia, such as hereditary *spherocytosis.* Splenectomy may also be performed during *laparotomy* (surgical exploration of the abdomen) as part of a process, known as staging, by which the extent of *Hodgkin's disease* is assessed.

HOW IT IS DONE

Under general anaesthesia, a vertical or horizontal incision is made in the upper left abdomen, exposing the spleen. After attachments to other tissues have been cut and blood vessels leading into and out of the spleen have been clamped and severed, the organ is removed. The operation takes about an hour.

RECOVERY PERIOD AND OUTLOOK

Patients usually leave hospital six to 10 days after the operation. Complications, such as infection of the operation site, are rare.

In an adult, absence of the spleen slightly increases the risk of contracting infections; children become markedly more susceptible, particularly to pneumococcal *pneumonia.* A child who has undergone a splenectomy should be immunized with pneumococcal vaccine and given long-term *antibiotic drugs.* Healthy fragments of a removed spleen are occasionally reimplanted in a child immediately after splenectomy; in some cases, these fragments regenerate to form an efficient new spleen.

Splint

A device used to immobilize part of the body. Splints may be made of acrylic, polyethylene foam, plaster of Paris, or aluminium. Ambulances may carry inflatable splints. In an emergency, a splint can be constructed from a piece of wood or a rolled-up newspaper secured to the injured part. (See also *Splinting.*)

Splinting

The application of a *splint.* Splinting is used as a first-aid measure (see illustrated box) to prevent movement of a

---

FIRST AID: SPLINTS

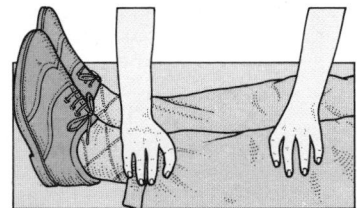

1 If help is coming, do not move the victim but support the limb by placing one hand above the fracture and the other below it.

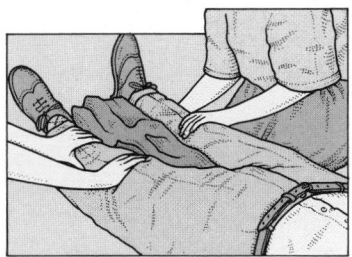

2 If the ambulance is delayed, immobilize the injured leg by using the uninjured leg as a splint. Place padding between the legs, especially between bony prominences (e.g. knees and ankles) and to fill hollows. Gently bring the uninjured leg alongside the injured one. Another person should continue to support the injured limb until immobilization is complete. If it is essential to move the victim, a long, padded splint should also be placed along the outside of the injured leg.

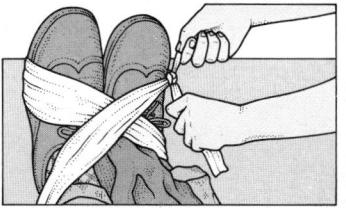

3 Tie the victim's ankles and feet together with a figure-of-eight bandage (which should pass around the splint, if one is being used). Secure the bandage on the uninjured side. If the fracture is near the ankle, it may be necessary to modify the figure-of-eight bandage to avoid bandaging over the fracture site.

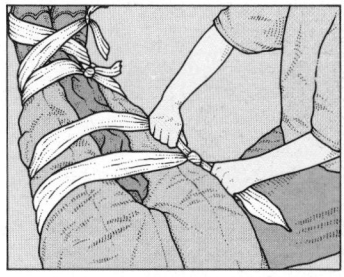

4 Tie other bandages around the knees, and above and below the fracture site. Do not bandage over the fracture site itself, and do not bandage below the fracture if it is near the ankle. If a splint is being used, also bandage around the upper thighs. Tie all knots on the uninjured side.

---

fractured limb or to immobilize a suspected fracture of the spine; this is especially important when the victim is being moved.

Splinting is sometimes required for leg fractures that are being treated by *traction.* Other uses include treatment of finger injuries, such as fracture or *mallet finger,* and of rheumatic disorders affecting the fingers, such as *tenosynovitis* (inflammation of tendon linings) and *rheumatoid arthritis.*

Splinting, dental

The mechanical joining of several teeth to hold them firmly in place while an injury heals or while *periodontal disease* is treated.

Splints may be used to secure teeth that have been fractured (see *Fracture, dental*) or loosened (see *Subluxated tooth*). They may also be used after a tooth has been reimplanted (see *Reimplantation, dental*). Occasionally, teeth

loosened by periodontal disease may be splinted to adjacent, firmer teeth. Splints may also be required after *orthognathic surgery.*

Splints are fashioned directly in the mouth with materials such as wire, quick-setting plastic, and plastic crowns that can be bonded together. (See also *Wiring of the jaws.*)

Split personality

A term used to describe *multiple personality,* in which an individual has two or more personalities, each of which dominates at different times. It is also, incorrectly, used to describe *schizophrenia,* in which the sufferer's feelings and thoughts are not logically related to each other.

Spondylitis

Inflammation of the joints between the vertebrae in the *spine.* Spondylitis is usually caused by *osteoarthritis, rheu-*

S

matoid arthritis, or *ankylosing spondylitis*. In rare cases, it is due to a bacterial infection that has spread from elsewhere in the body.

Spondylolisthesis

The slipping forwards (or occasionally backwards) of a *vertebra* (spinal bone) over the one below it. A forward slippage of the fifth (lowest) lumbar vertebra over the top of the *sacrum* is the most common form of the condition, but it may also occur between the fourth and fifth lumbar vertebrae or between two cervical (neck) vertebrae.

CAUSES AND SYMPTOMS
Lumbar spondylolisthesis, which involves two lumbar vertebrae or the fifth lumbar vertebra and the sacrum, is usually due to *spondylolysis* (in which the bony arch of a lumbar vertebra is abnormally soft and thus liable to slip under stress) or to *osteoarthritis* of the spine (in which the joints between the vertebrae become worn and unstable).

The principal symptoms of lumbar spondylolisthesis include pain in the back that is worse when standing, and *sciatica*.

Cervical spondylolisthesis may be caused by a neck injury, congenital abnormality of the cervical spine, or *rheumatoid arthritis* (in which the supporting ligaments of the cervical spine are weakened or the joints between the vertebrae become worn). The main symptoms are pain and stiffness in the neck and, in severe cases, pain, numbness, or weakness in the sufferer's hands and arms.

DIAGNOSIS AND TREATMENT
Spondylolisthesis is diagnosed by *X-rays* of the spine. Treatment may include *traction*, immobilization of the affected area in a plaster *corset* or orthopaedic *collar*, and *physiotherapy*. In severe and rare cases in which there is nerve compression damage or severe back pain, an operation to fuse the affected vertebrae may be necessary (see *Spinal fusion*).

Spondylolysis

A disorder of the *spine* in which the arch of the fifth (or, rarely, the fourth) lumbar vertebra consists of relatively soft fibrous tissue instead of normal bone. As a result, the arch is weaker than normal and is more likely to be deformed or damaged under stress, which may produce *spondylolisthesis* (forward slippage of a vertebra over the one below it). Otherwise, spondylolysis is usually symptomless.

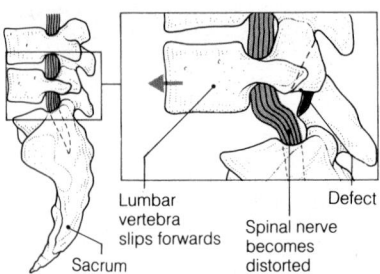

| Lumbar vertebra slips forwards | Defect |
| Sacrum | Spinal nerve becomes distorted |

Normal spine | **Spondylolisthesis**

Lumbar spondylolisthesis
If the lowest lumbar vertebra slips forwards over the sacrum, it may distort or press on a spinal nerve, causing symptoms such as backache or sciatica.

Sponge, contraceptive

A disposable, circular piece of foam impregnated with *spermicide* that is inserted into the vagina as a method of birth control. (See *Contraception, barrier methods*.)

Sporotrichosis

A chronic infection caused by the fungus *SPOROTHRIX SCHENCKII*, which grows on moss and other plants. The infection is most often contracted through a skin wound; gardeners and florists are particularly vulnerable. An ulcer develops at the site of the wound and is followed by the formation of nodules (which can be seen as a chain of protuberances beneath the skin) in lymph channels around the site. Potassium iodide solution taken by mouth usually clears up the infection.

Rarely, in people whose resistance to disease has been lowered, sporotrichosis spreads to the lungs, joints, and various other parts of the body. This condition may require prolonged treatment with the *antifungal drug* amphotericin.

Sports, drugs and

The use of drugs to improve athletic performance has been universally condemned by authorities because it endangers the health of athletes and gives drug users an unfair advantage. Random urine tests to detect abuse are performed in most sports during competition and at other times.

Certain drugs may be taken legitimately by athletes for medical disorders, such as asthma or epilepsy. Care should be taken, however, when using a drug for the treatment of diarrhoea, nasal congestion, or cough because some common medications contain prohibited substances.

TYPES OF DRUGS ABUSED
Four main types of drugs are abused by athletes to enhance physical or mental condition.

STIMULANTS Drugs of this group are taken to prevent fatigue and to increase self-confidence. However, they also impair judgment and may cause excessive aggression, which increases the risk of injury to the user or an opponent.

Stimulants, such as *amphetamine drugs*, carry the risk of causing cardiac *arrhythmias* (irregularities of the heartbeat); prolonged use may cause *heart failure* (reduced pumping efficiency) and increase the risk of a *brain haemorrhage*. Some cold and cough remedies contain low doses of prohibited stimulant drugs and should be avoided before competition.

Caffeine contained in coffee, tea, and cola drinks, and available in tablets, is another popular stimulant. Most authorities only prohibit the use of caffeine in high doses.

HORMONES Two types of hormone drugs may be abused—anabolic steroids (see *Steroids, anabolic*) and *growth hormone*.

Anabolic steroids are substances similar to the male sex hormone testosterone. These drugs are used because they speed the recovery of muscles after strenuous exercise. This permits a more demanding training schedule and causes an increase in muscle bulk and strength. Anabolic steroids are used primarily by weightlifters, by athletes in field events, and by body-builders.

Risks of abusing anabolic steroids include liver damage, liver tumours, and adrenal gland damage. In men they may cause infertility and impotence; in women they may cause *virilization*. If taken during childhood, anabolic steroids may cause *short stature* by affecting the growing areas of bones.

Growth hormone is abused to stimulate growth of muscle; it is likely to cause *acromegaly* (excessive bone growth leading to deformity of the face, hands, and feet) and may cause *diabetes mellitus*.

PAINKILLERS Only narcotic *analgesic drugs* are prohibited but the use of any painkiller (even a weak analgesic such as paracetamol) may aggravate an injury or lead to permanent damage by allowing the individual to participate with his or her pain masked.

BETA-BLOCKER DRUGS *Beta-blocker drugs* are taken to reduce tremor in sports in which a steady hand is vital. Many

S

authorities now prohibit these drugs in the absence of a specific medical disorder that requires them.

Sports injuries

Any injury that arises during participation in sports. Most sports injuries are not actually specific to sports; they can also occur as a result of other activities.

The wide range of sports injuries includes *fractures*, *head injury* (including *concussion*), muscle *strain* or *compartment syndrome*, ligament *sprain*, *tendinitis* (inflammation of a tendon) or tendon rupture, joint *dislocation* or joint *subluxation* (partial dislocation), and injuries to a specific organ, such as an *eye injury*.

Some injuries have a name that includes a sports prefix, but most such injuries can also be caused in ways unrelated to sport. For example, *tennis elbow* (painful inflammation around the outside of the elbow) is a type of *overuse injury* that may occur from playing tennis, but more often results from an activity such as sawing.

TREATMENT

Treatment of a sports injury depends on the body part involved and the severity of the damage. Recovery is not complete until the damaged area is free of pain during exercise. Exercises under the guidance of a sports doctor or physiotherapist may be required to ensure full recovery of movement, balance, and coordination of the injured part and to restore general fitness to reduce the likelihood of further injury. (See also *Sports medicine*.)

Sports medicine

The branch of medicine concerned with assessment and improvement of *fitness* and the treatment and prevention of medical disorders related to sports. Doctors specializing in sports medicine give advice about exercises that improve endurance, strength, and flexibility; perform fitness tests; offer nutritional advice to improve performance; regulate the abuse of drugs by athletes (see *Sports, drugs and*); and provide on-site medical care at sporting events.

Preventive work in sports medicine includes advising the individual on footwear, clothing, and protective equipment to reduce the likelihood of injury, and on fluid requirements to prevent *dehydration*. In addition, the sports doctor advises professional athletes on immunization requirements before competition abroad, and

on coping with *jet-lag* and changes in altitude and climate. In conjunction with a physiotherapist (see *Physiotherapy*), a sports physician diagnoses and treats *sports injuries*.

Spot

A general term for a small lump, mark, or inflamed area on the skin. Many different skin conditions produce particular types of spots, such as *blackheads*, *blisters*, *cysts*, *macules*, *nodules*, *papules*, *pustules*, and *scabs*. Spots may or may not be caused by infection. A collection of spots is known as a *rash*.

Sprain

Tearing or stretching of the *ligaments* that hold together the bone ends in a *joint*, caused by a sudden pull. The fibrous capsule that encloses the joint may also be damaged. The most commonly sprained joint is the *ankle*, which is usually sprained as a result of "going over" on the outside of the foot so that the complete weight of the body is placed on the ankle.

A sprain causes painful swelling of the joint, which cannot be moved without increasing the pain. There may also be spasm (involuntary contraction) of surrounding muscles.

TREATMENT

An *X-ray* of the joint is usually performed to exclude the possibility of a *fracture*. Treatment consists of applying an *ice-pack* to reduce swelling, wrapping the joint with a compression bandage, resting it in a raised position until the pain and swelling begin to subside, and taking *analgesic drugs* (painkillers) to relieve pain. Once the joint is no longer painful, it should be gently exercised.

If ligaments are badly torn, *nonsteroidal anti-inflammatory drugs* may be prescribed to speed healing. In extremely severe cases, surgical repair may be necessary. (For first aid, see the illustrated box overleaf.)

Sprue

A disorder of the intestines that causes failure to absorb nutrients from food. There are two forms of sprue. One occurs mainly in tropical regions (see *Sprue, tropical*); the other, *coeliac disease*, occurs more widely and is due to sensitivity to *gluten*.

Sprue, tropical

A disease characterized by chronic *malabsorption* (impaired absorption of nutrients from the diet by the small intestine) and consequent *malnutrition*

and a type of anaemia caused by deficiency of folic acid and vitamin B_{12} (see *Anaemia, megaloblastic*).

As in *coeliac disease*, villi (frond-like projections) on the lining of the intestine become flattened, decreasing their surface area and so reducing the absorption of nutrients.

CAUSE AND INCIDENCE

The cause of tropical sprue is unknown, but it may result from an infection of the intestine. The disease occurs in tropical regions, predominantly in India, the Far East, and the Caribbean.

SYMPTOMS

Symptoms include loss of appetite, weight loss, an inflamed mouth, sore tongue, and fatty diarrhoea.

DIAGNOSIS AND TREATMENT

The diagnosis is confirmed by a *jejunal biopsy* (removal of a small sample of tissue from the upper small intestine for analysis). The disease responds well to treatment with *antibiotic drugs* and dietary supplements of folic acid, vitamin B_{12}, and, if necessary, other types of vitamins and minerals.

Sputum

Mucous material produced by the cells lining the respiratory tract. Also known as phlegm, sputum is released from glands in the walls of the bronchi (main airways in the lungs).

Sputum production may be increased by infection (see *Respiratory tract infection*), by an allergic reaction (see *Asthma*), or by inhalation of irritants, such as tobacco-smoke (see *Cough, smokers'*). Sputum in the bronchi triggers a reflex *cough*.

The character of sputum varies. A bacterial infection usually causes yellow or green sputum, an allergic reaction usually produces colourless sputum, and *pulmonary oedema* (fluid retention in the lungs) may result in frothy, pink sputum. *Haemoptysis* (blood in the sputum) may be caused by infection or *lung cancer*.

Laboratory tests on sputum include microscopic examination and analysis of a sputum *culture* to identify any bacteria that might be present.

Squamous cell carcinoma

One of the three most common types of skin cancer; the others are *basal cell carcinoma* and malignant *melanoma*.

CAUSES AND INCIDENCE

Squamous cell carcinoma arises from flattened, scale-like cells in the skin, usually in areas that have been exposed to strong sunlight for many years, where solar *keratoses* may have

S

FIRST AID: SPRAINS

WARNING
A severe sprain may be indistinguishable from a broken bone. If
in doubt, treat as a *fracture*.

1 The victim may not be able to move the affected joint or stand up if the knee or ankle is injured. Help the victim into a comfortable position and raise the injured part of the body.

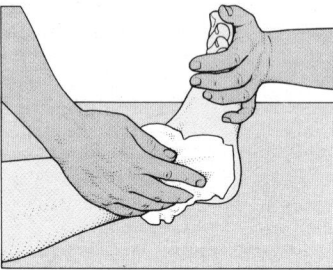

2 If the sprain is recent, apply a cold compress to the affected area and leave for about 30 minutes. This will reduce blood flow and swelling.

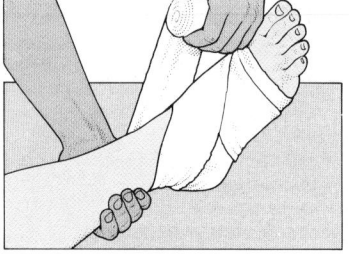

3 Cover the area with a layer of cotton-wool and secure with a bandage. Make two turns around the foot, bring it across the top, and around the ankle.

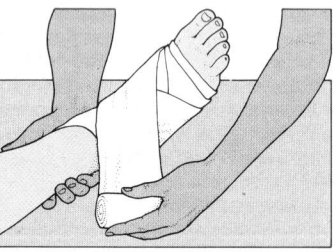

4 Continue figure-of-eight turns, with each turn of the bandage overlapping the previous turn by three quarters of its width.

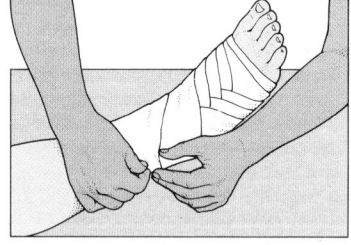

5 Bandage until the foot (not toes), ankle, and lower leg are covered. Secure the loose end. Seek medical aid—an X-ray may be necessary.

developed. This cancer is most common in pale-skinned, fair-haired people over the age of 60. The incidence is also higher than average in people whose work has exposed them to certain substances, such as arsenic, tar, coal, paraffin, or heavy oils.

SYMPTOMS AND SIGNS
The tumour starts as a small, firm, painless lump or patch (usually on the lip, ear, or back of the hand) and slowly enlarges, often resembling a wart or ulcer. Without treatment, the tumour may spread to other parts

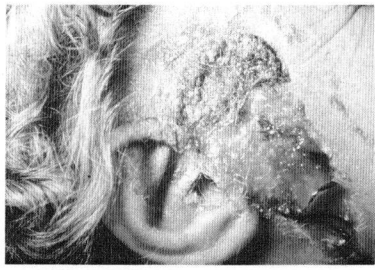

A squamous cell carcinoma
This tumour has spread slowly to cover much of the area in front of the patient's ear. It can be treated by radiotherapy.

of the body and prove fatal. All suspicious skin areas should be reported to a doctor.

DIAGNOSIS AND TREATMENT
The diagnosis is based on a skin *biopsy* (removal of a small sample of tissue for analysis). The tumour is either removed surgically or destroyed by *radiotherapy* or *cryosurgery* (application of extreme cold). Treatment with *anti-cancer drugs* may also be necessary.

Any person who has had a squamous cell carcinoma should limit his or her exposure to sunlight. A follow-up examination is required to check for recurrence.

Squint

A condition in which there is abnormal deviation of one eye in relation to the other. Squint, also known as strabismus, may be convergent, in which one eye is directed too far inwards, or divergent, in which one eye is directed outwards. Less commonly, one eye is directed upwards or downwards relative to the other eye (vertical strabismus).

CAUSES
Many young babies have a squint because the normal mechanism for aligning the two eyes has not yet developed. A squint that starts later in childhood usually results from a breakdown in the development of the mechanism for aligning the eyes; a common contributory factor in such cases is *hypermetropia* (longsightedness), which leads to excessive *accommodation* (adjustment of focus) and causes one eye to turn inwards.

In children who are acquiring the capacity to see simultaneously with two eyes, squint causes double vision because the image in the squinting eye falls on the wrong part of the retina. To avoid such double vision, the brain suppresses the image from the deviating eye, eventually leading to *amblyopia* (reduced sharpness of vision).

In adults, squint may occur as a result of various disorders of the brain, of the nerves controlling the eye muscles, or of the eye muscles themselves. Squint in adults causes double vision, and may be a symptom of *stroke, diabetes mellitus, multiple sclerosis,* tumour, or *hyperthyroidism.*

TREATMENT

Treatment in children up to the age of about six or seven years old may include covering the normal eye with a patch to force the child to use the weak eye. Such patching is designed to encourage normal vision to develop in the affected eye, by enabling the establishment of normal connections between the eye and the brain. Deviation of the squinting eye may be controlled by glasses and/or surgery.

Squint acquired later in life always requires medical investigation of the underlying cause. Persistent double vision due to squint requires special prismatic glasses or surgery.

Even if vision cannot be improved, surgery to improve appearance may be performed at any age.

Stable

Unmoving, fixed, resistant to change, or in a state of equilibrium. A patient's condition is described as stable when it is neither deteriorating nor improving; a stable personality is one that is not susceptible to abnormal behavioural excesses or mental illness. In chemistry, a stable substance is one that is resistant to changes in its chemical composition or physical state, or is not radioactive.

Stage

A term used in medicine to refer to a phase in the course of a disease, particularly in the progression of *cancer.*

In assessing most types of cancer, a method known as staging is used to determine how far the cancer has progressed. The cancer is described in terms of how large the main tumour is, the degree to which it has invaded surrounding tissue, and the extent to which it has spread to lymph glands or other areas of the body. In *Hodgkin's disease,* staging also takes into account whether the lymph nodes on both sides of the diaphragm are affected, and whether the spleen is involved.

Staging not only helps to assess outlook (in general, the more advanced the stage, the worse the outlook) but also the most appropriate treatment. For example, a cancer at a particular stage may respond better to *radiotherapy* than to surgery.

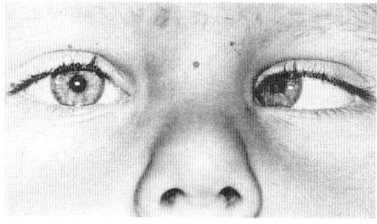

Convergent squint
This child has a convergent squint of the left eye—i.e. the left eye is directed too far inwards (towards the nose).

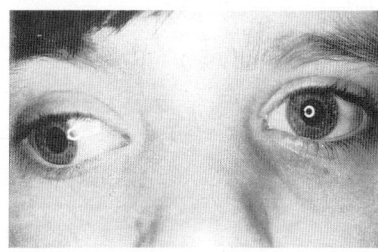

Divergent squint
This child has a divergent squint of the right eye—i.e. the right eye is directed too far outwards (away from the nose).

Staining

The process of dyeing specimens of cells, tissues, or microorganisms so that they are clearly visible or easily identifiable under a *microscope.* Staining is also sometimes carried out to detect or identify certain chemical substances in cells.

Before a specimen can be examined under a microscope, it must be preserved and then sliced or smeared extremely thinly. After these procedures, most specimens are almost transparent, so staining is necessary to make them easily visible.

One of the most commonly used staining techniques is the Papanicolaou stain test, which is used in *cytology* to allow the detection of cancerous and precancerous changes in cells.

Many different stains can be used to identify particular structures or products within cells. A very commonly used stain is haematoxylin and eosin, which is a double stain that colours nuclei blue and cytoplasm pink. Other stains may be used to identify a particular microorganism in tissues or to clarify a diagnosis. A more recent development is the use of special fluorescent dyes that stain specific chemical constituents of cells or tissues; when illuminated with ultraviolet light, the stained constituents glow.

Another commonly used technique, known as immunoperoxidase

staining, involves washing cells with a preparation containing specific types of *antibodies.* These antibodies become attached to specific cell components and chemicals. Tagging of the antibodies with a dye that can be seen under the microscope as red-brown enables the observer to identify certain components or chemicals if they are present within the cells.

Another example of a useful staining technique is *Gram's stain,* which is widely used to identify and differentiate between groups of bacteria.

Stammering

See *Stuttering.*

Stanford-Binet test

A type of *intelligence test.*

Stanozolol

A steroid drug (see *Steroids, anabolic*).

Stapedectomy

An operation on the *ear* to remove the *stapes* (the innermost of the three sound-conducting bones in the middle ear) and replace it with an artificial substitute. Stapedectomy is performed to treat *deafness* caused by *otosclerosis,* a disorder in which the base of the stapes becomes fixed by an overgrowth of spongy bone and can no longer move freely to transmit sound to the inner ear.

HOW IT IS DONE

The operation is performed under local or general anaesthesia. An incision is made so that the eardrum can be folded forwards to allow access to the middle ear. All or most of the stapes is then removed. One end of a plastic or metal prosthesis is inserted into the entrance to the inner ear, and the other end of the prosthesis is attached to the incus (the middle of the three sound-conducting bones in the middle ear). The eardrum is then sewn back in position.

OUTLOOK

Stapedectomy improves hearing considerably in more than 90 per cent of cases. However, in about one per cent of patients, hearing deteriorates or is lost altogether. Because of this risk, a stapedectomy is usually carried out on only one ear at a time.

Stapes

The innermost of the three auditory ossicles (the tiny, sound-conducting bones in the middle *ear*). The stapes, the Latin for stirrup (because of its shape), is the smallest bone in the body. Its head articulates with the

S

incus (the middle auditory ossicle) and its base fits into the oval window in the wall of the inner ear.

In *otosclerosis*, the stapes becomes fixed by an overgrowth of bone and can no longer transmit sound to the inner ear. Hearing loss due to otosclerosis can be cured by an operation known as *stapedectomy*.

Staphylococcal infections

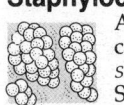 A group of infections caused by *bacteria* of the STAPHYLOCOCCUS genus. Staphylococci, which grow in grape-like clusters, are a common cause of skin infections but can also cause serious internal disorders.

Staphylococcal bacteria are present harmlessly on the skin of most people. If the bacteria become trapped within the skin by a blocked sweat or sebaceous gland, they may cause superficial skin infections, such as *pustules*, *boils*, *abscesses*, *styes*, or *carbuncles*. Infection of deeper tissues may result if the skin is broken (see *Wound infection*). In newborn babies, toxins released by bacteria on the skin can cause a severe, blistering rash called the scalded skin syndrome (see *Necrolysis, toxic epidermal*).

Staphylococcal bacteria are also harmlessly present in the membranes that line the nose and throat. When mucus is not cleared from the lungs, such as after a viral infection, organisms may accumulate in the lungs and cause *pneumonia*.

In menstruating women (particularly those using highly absorbent tampons), toxin-producing staphylococci may colonize the mucous membranes lining the vagina, causing *toxic shock syndrome*. A different type of staphylococcus can cause *urinary tract infection*.

Sometimes staphylococci enter the bloodstream as a result of spread from a skin infection or as a result of introduction from a needle, leading to *septic shock*, infectious *arthritis*, *osteomyelitis*, or bacterial *endocarditis*.

Staphylococcal *food poisoning* is caused by ingestion of toxins produced by the bacteria. A common source of contamination is a pustule on the skin of a food handler.

Starch

See *Carbohydrates*.

Starvation

A condition caused by lack of food over a long period, resulting in weight loss, changes in *metabolism* (body chemistry), and extreme hunger. (See also *Anorexia nervosa; Fasting; Nutritional disorders*.)

Stasis

A slowing down or cessation of flow. For example, in venous stasis there is a reduction or stoppage of blood flow through one or more veins.

Statistics, medical

A science concerned with the collection and analysis of numerical data relating to medicine.

Information on the *incidence* and *prevalence* of various disorders and diseases, both in the general population and among certain groups of the population, is an important aspect of medical statistics. This science also covers such diverse topics as waiting times in outpatient clinics, infection rates after surgery, the frequency of side-effects from drugs, and the evaluation of different types of treatment.

All medical research institutions today employ statisticians to advise on the design and interpretation of medical trials, and on the interpretation of data obtained from such trials. For example, when two treatments are to be compared—or when treatment is to be compared with not giving treatment—the statistician advises on such matters as the number of patients required in the trial to establish a valid conclusion, and on other matters, such as methodology, including how to allocate patients to various treatment groups, how frequently to take measurements of the outcomes of the treatments, and how to analyse the mathematical results. (See also *Statistics, vital*.)

Statistics, vital

Assessment of the health of a country's population, which relies on the collection of data on birth and death rates and on the causes of death (see *Mortality*). In most Western countries today, all deaths are certified (usually by a medical practitioner) and recorded in a national register. They are then classified by cause and analysed according to factors such as age, sex, occupation, social class, and ethnic group.

Comparison of the vital statistics of different countries (or regions within a country) gives a measure of the relative health of their populations as a whole. A detailed comparison may also show variations between social classes or ethnic groups. (See also *Life expectancy; Statistics, medical*.)

Status asthmaticus

A severe and prolonged attack of *asthma*. Status asthmaticus is a serious and potentially life-threatening condition that requires urgent treatment.

Status epilepticus

Prolonged or repeated epileptic seizures without any recovery of consciousness between attacks. Status epilepticus is a medical emergency that may be fatal if not treated promptly. It is more likely to occur if *anticonvulsant drugs* are taken erratically or if they are withdrawn suddenly. (See *Epilepsy*.)

STDs

See *Sexually transmitted diseases*.

Steatorrhoea

The presence of excessive fat in the faeces. Steatorrhoea causes diarrhoea characterized by offensive-smelling, bulky, loose, greasy, pale-coloured faeces, which tend to float in the toilet and are difficult to flush away. Steatorrhoea is a symptom of diseases that interfere with the breakdown and absorption of fat in the diet (notably *pancreatitis* and *coeliac disease*) and of the removal of large segments of small intestine. Steatorrhoea is also a side-effect of some *lipid-lowering drugs*.

Stein-Leventhal syndrome

See *Ovary, polycystic*.

Stenosis

Narrowing of a duct, canal, passage, or tubular organ, such as a blood vessel or the intestine. *Aortic stenosis* is narrowing of the aortic valve opening from the left ventricle (lower chamber of the heart); *pyloric stenosis* is narrowing of the pylorus (the lower outlet from the stomach).

Stereotaxic surgery

Brain operations carried out by inserting delicate instruments through a surgically created hole in the skull and guiding them, with the aid of *X-rays* or *CT scanning*, to a specific area.

WHY IT IS DONE

Stereotaxic procedures are used in the treatment of *pituitary tumours*, in which the gland is cut out or a radioactive implant is inserted into the gland to destroy it.

Other uses include a brain *biopsy* (removal of a small sample of tissue for analysis), insertion of permanent stimulating wires to control otherwise intractable pain, and destruction of areas of the brain to treat disabling

S

neurological disorders, such as severe *depression* (see *Psychosurgery*) or, in rare cases, *temporal lobe epilepsy*. Stereotaxic surgery is also occasionally used to treat people with *Parkinson's disease* in whom severe tremor has not responded to drugs.

HOW IT IS DONE

Under a general or local anaesthetic, an adjustable metal frame is attached to the skull with screws. The area to be treated is located by X-rays or CT scanning and the best position for inserting the instrument is calculated mathematically. The skull is then entered by means of a *burr hole* or *craniotomy*, and the angle of the frame is adjusted to hold and guide a hollow tube into the brain at the correct angle. The required instrument (a needle for biopsies, a scalpel or diathermy probe for cutting or destroying areas) is inserted through the tube and the operation performed; X-rays or scans are taken during the procedure.

Sterility

The state either of being germ-free, or of permanent *infertility*.

Sterilization

A term that refers to the complete destruction or removal of living organisms or to any procedure that renders a person unable to reproduce (see *Sterilization, female; Vasectomy*).

The elimination of microorganisms is vitally important in preventing the spread of infection. It may be achieved by various physical or chemical means, such as by boiling, steaming, or autoclaving (steaming under high pressure); by irradiation with ultraviolet light, X-rays, or gamma rays; or by applying *antiseptics* or *disinfectants*. Liquids can also be sterilized by passing them through extremely fine filters that trap microorganisms as tiny as viruses. Sometimes, more than one method is used (e.g. bed linen may be disinfected and then autoclaved).

Sterilization, female

A usually permanent method of *contraception* in which the fallopian tubes are sealed or cut to prevent a male's sperm from reaching the ova.

Sterilization is a common method of contraception; about 90,000 female sterilizations are carried out each year in England and Wales, most of them in NHS hospitals.

WHY IT IS DONE

Women who have completed their families or who plan not to have children may choose to be sterilized to avoid the inconvenience or side-effects of other methods of contraception. Sterilization may also be chosen by a woman in whom a pregnancy would be a serious threat to health, or in whom there is an unacceptably high risk of children being affected by a serious hereditary disease.

HOW IT IS DONE

The illustrated box shows common procedures for female sterilization, performed using *laparoscopy*.

Alternatively, the surgeon may work directly through a small incision just below the navel. Known as a minilaparotomy, this procedure is carried out in the first few weeks after a woman has given birth. In other cases, the fallopian tubes may be cut and tied off via an incision in the vagina. Alternatively, a hysteroscope (a type of *endoscope*) may be passed through the vagina and into the uterus; the exits of the fallopian tubes into the uterus are then plugged from the inside.

Surgical removal of the uterus (see *Hysterectomy*) or of the fallopian tubes and/or ovaries (see *Salpingectomy; Salpingo-oophorectomy; Oophorectomy*) to treat specific disorders also results in sterilization. These operations are performed through a larger abdominal incision and today are considered too drastic to be performed only for sterilization.

Female sterilization techniques may be performed on an outpatient basis but often the woman is admitted to hospital the day before laparoscopy and discharged the day after the operation.

OUTLOOK

Female sterilization has a very low failure rate (around 0.05 pregnancies per 100 women years of use). If pregnancy does occur after a sterilization operation, there is a greatly increased risk of an *ectopic pregnancy*.

In some cases, microsurgical techniques may succeed in restoring fertility in a woman who has been

---

FEMALE STERILIZATION

Laparoscopic sterilization (below) is the most common method. Both fallopian tubes must be cut, sealed, or otherwise obstructed so that eggs and sperm cannot meet for fertilization to occur.

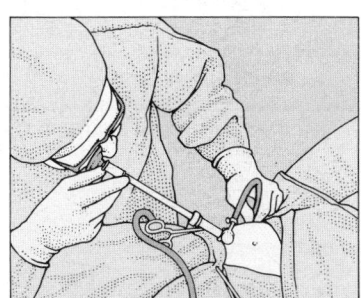

Laparoscopic sterilization
An endoscope (viewing tube) and an operating instrument are passed through separate small incisions in the abdomen.

Instruments
The trocar is a sharp-pointed inner stylus surrounded by a close-fitting tube, the cannula. The instrument can be passed through the abdominal wall. After insertion, the trocar is removed, leaving the hollow cannula in place. Other instruments are passed through the hollow cannula.

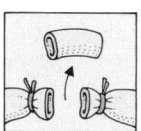

Cutting
A small loop of the fallopian tube may be drawn up, secured by a tight ligature, and then cut off.

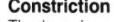

Constriction
The loop is constricted by a tight band. Reversal is possible with this sterilization technique.

Clipping
A plastic or metal clip may be applied to obstruct egg passage. In theory, this method is also reversible.

Cautery
Electrocoagulation (diathermy) can be used to burn through, and thus seal, the fallopian tube.

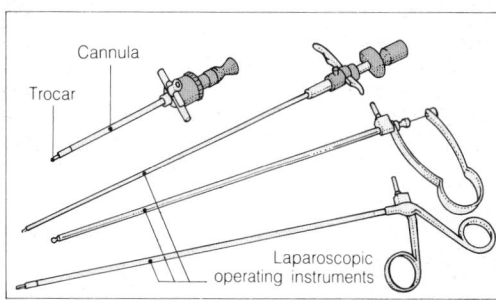

Cannula
Trocar
Laparoscopic operating instruments

S

sterilized; 70 to 75 per cent of women who undergo such surgery later achieve pregnancy.

Sterilization, male
See *Vasectomy*.

Sternum
The anatomical name for the breast-bone, the long, narrow, flat plate of bone that forms the central part of the front of the chest. The sternum consists of three main parts: an upper, triangular portion, called the manubrium; a long, narrow middle part, the body; and, at the lower end, a small, slightly flexible, leaf-shaped projection, the xiphoid process. The upper part of the manubrium articulates with the inner ends of the two *clavicles* (collarbones); attached to the sides of the manubrium and body are the seven pairs of costal cartilages that join the sternum to the *ribs*. Between the manubrium and body is a type of joint known as a *symphysis,* which allows slight movement between these two parts of the sternum when the ribs rise and fall during breathing.

The sternum is very strong and requires great force to fracture it. The

LOCATION OF THE STERNUM
The sternum, or breastbone, is joined to the ribs and clavicles by flexible couplings that allow the chest to move while breathing in and out.

Clavicle

Manubrium

Ribs

Body

Xiphoid process

principal danger of such an injury is not the fracture itself, but the possibility that the broken bone may be driven inwards and damage the heart (which lies behind the sternum).

Steroid drugs
A group of drugs that includes the *corticosteroid drugs,* which resemble hormones produced by the cortex *adrenal glands,* and the anabolic steroid drugs (see *Steroids, anabolic*), which have an effect similar to that of the male sex hormones.

Steroids, anabolic

COMMON DRUGS
Nandrolone Stanozolol

Drugs that have an anabolic (protein-building) effect similar to *testosterone* and other male sex hormones.
WHY THEY ARE USED
Anabolic steroids, by mimicking the anabolic effects of testosterone, build tissue, promote muscle recovery following injury, and help strengthen bones. They are given to treat some types of *anaemia* and, occasionally, to treat postmenopausal women who have *osteoporosis*.
ABUSE
Anabolic steroids have been widely abused by athletes who wish to improve their strength and stamina. This practice has serious risks to health (see *Sports, drugs and*).
POSSIBLE ADVERSE EFFECTS
Adverse effects include acne, *oedema,* damage to the liver, damage to the adrenal glands, infertility, impotence in men, and *virilization* in women.

Stethoscope
An instrument for listening to sounds in the body, particularly those made by the heart or lungs.

The standard stethoscope consists of a Y-shaped flexible plastic tube with an earpiece at the end of each arm of the Y, and a sound-detecting device at the base. One side of this device consists of a thin plastic diaphragm; the other side has a concave bell with a hole in its centre. A doctor presses the diaphragm against a patient's chest or back to hear high-pitched sounds. The concave bell side is placed gently against the skin to allow the doctor to hear low-pitched sounds.

Stevens-Johnson syndrome
A rare skin condition characterized by severe blisters and bleeding in the mucous membranes of the lips, eyes, mouth, nasal passage, and genitals. Stevens-Johnson syndrome is a life-threatening form of *erythema multiforme,* and is believed in many cases to be caused by a *drug* reaction.

Sticky eye
A common description of one of the symptoms of *conjunctivitis* (inflammation of the conjunctival membrane) in which the eyelids tend to become stuck together with discharge.

Stiff neck
A very common symptom, usually due to spasm (involuntary contraction) in muscles at the side or the back of the neck.

In most cases, stiff neck occurs suddenly and for no apparent reason; the symptom is often first noticed upon waking. Stiff neck commonly occurs as a result of a minor neck injury—such as a ligament sprain or *subluxation* (partial dislocation) of a joint between neck vertebrae—that has passed unnoticed but has caused irritation of a nerve; this, in turn, leads to spasm of the neck muscles.

A stiff neck may also result from muscle spasm due to a *disc prolapse* or to a *whiplash injury.*

A relatively rare, but potentially serious, cause of a stiff neck is *meningitis* (infection of the membranes that surround the brain and spinal cord). In such cases, the stiffness is usually accompanied by headache, vomiting, fever, photophobia (abnormal sensitivity to light), and intense pain when bending the neck.
TREATMENT
Mild stiffness of the neck may be relieved by gentle massage, warming, and use of a *liniment.* Severe or persistent stiffness, or stiffness accompanied by symptoms suggestive of meningitis, requires medical attention. (See also *Torticollis.*)

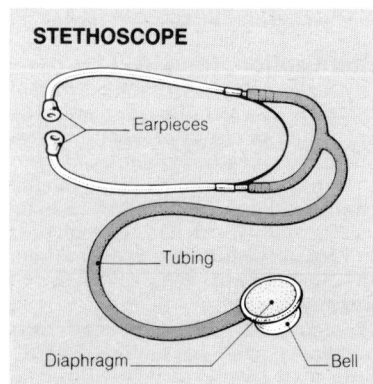

STETHOSCOPE

Earpieces

Tubing

Diaphragm

Bell

S

Stiffness

A term used to refer to difficulty in moving a joint, to restriction of movement in a joint, or to difficulty in stretching a muscle.

Causes of joint stiffness include *arthritis* (inflammation of joint surfaces) and *bursitis* (inflammation of the joint lining). *Rheumatoid arthritis* characteristically causes severe joint stiffness for the first few hours after waking. Causes of muscle stiffness include *cramp* and *spasticity* (increased muscle rigidity).

Stilboestrol

OESTROGEN

°⚬💊 ✏ ✏ 🖊 📱 ⬭ 🖊 🧴 💧 ⬭

Tablet Pessary

📋 Prescription needed

💊 Available as generic

A drug that mimics the natural *oestrogen hormone* oestradiol. Stilboestrol was formerly used as a treatment for threatened miscarriage, but this use has been abandoned as a result of evidence that vaginal cancer may develop many years later in daughters of women who took this drug.

Stilboestrol is still occasionally used to treat cancer of the prostate gland (see *Prostate, cancer of*), but it is now rarely used to treat *breast cancer*. It has been replaced by other *oestrogen drugs* for the treatment of symptoms of the menopause.

Side-effects are as for other oestrogen drugs, particularly nausea, fluid retention, breast enlargement, and increased risk of abnormal blood clotting. Stilboestrol must not be taken during pregnancy.

Stillbirth

Delivery of a dead fetus after the 28th week of *pregnancy*. Stillbirth is also called late fetal death. Stillbirths must be reported and the cause of death recorded on the death certificate.

INCIDENCE

The incidence of stillbirth has decreased dramatically in developed countries over the last 40 or 50 years. In the UK the incidence fell from about 19 stillbirths per 1,000 total births (i.e. live births plus stillbirths) in 1950 to about 5 stillbirths per 1,000 total births in the early 1990s.

As a general rule, stillbirths are more common in poor communities, among older women, and among women who do not receive good *antenatal* care and obstetric care.

CAUSES

The precise cause of stillbirth is unknown in at least one third of cases. Severely malformed babies, particularly those with *anencephaly, spina bifida,* or *hydrocephalus,* account for at least one fifth of stillbirths.

A maternal disorder, such as *antepartum haemorrhage, hypertension* (high blood pressure), or any other condition affecting the function of the *placenta,* may result in stillbirth, often because the fetus is deprived of oxygen. Another cause of stillbirth is severe *Rhesus incompatibility.*

Some infectious diseases (including *measles, chickenpox, influenza, toxoplasmosis, rubella, cytomegalovirus, herpes simplex, syphilis,* and *malaria*) may harm the fetus if contracted during pregnancy. In general, the more severe the infection, the greater the risk of stillbirth. A pregnant woman who is exposed to an infectious disease to which she is not immune should consult her doctor.

PSYCHOLOGICAL EFFECTS

The loss of a baby is deeply distressing. The bereaved parents usually experience a sense of loss that is just as intense as if any other loved person had died, and often they experience feelings of depression, guilt, anger, and inadequacy. Emotional support from friends, relatives, and self-help groups is useful, as is professional counselling.

Still's disease

See *Rheumatoid arthritis, juvenile.*

Stimulant drugs

COMMON DRUGS

Central nervous system stimulants
Caffeine Dexamphetamine Pemoline

Respiratory stimulants
Doxapram

Drugs that increase nerve activity in the *brain* by initiating the release of *noradrenaline,* a type of *neurotransmitter* (chemical released from nerve endings).

TYPES

There are two main groups of stimulant drugs: central nervous system stimulants (including *amphetamine drugs*), which reduce drowsiness and increase alertness by their action on the reticular activating system in the *brainstem*; and respiratory stimulants (see *Analeptic drugs*), which act on the respiratory centre (the area that controls breathing) in the brainstem.

WHY THEY ARE USED

Nerve stimulants are given to treat *narcolepsy* (excessive sleepiness). Paradoxically, they have also been found useful in the treatment of *hyperactivity* in children. Nerve stimulants also suppress the appetite but their use in the treatment of *obesity* is now rarely recommended because of their adverse effects.

Despite the risk of adverse effects, nerve stimulants are sometimes abused because they help prevent fatigue, increase alertness, and may improve self-confidence. Their use by athletes is widely condemned by doctors and prohibited by sports organizations (see *Sports, drugs and*).

POSSIBLE ADVERSE EFFECTS

Effects include shaking, sweating, palpitations, nervousness, sleeping problems, hallucinations, paranoid delusions, and seizures. Long-term use may lead to *tolerance* (the need for greater amounts to have the same effects) and *drug dependence* (withdrawal symptoms on stopping).

Stimulus

Anything that directly results in a change in the activities of the body as a whole or of any individual part (i.e. any agent or event that evokes a response). For example, the sight and smell of food stimulate salivation. Certain nerve cells (known collectively as *receptors*) are specialized to respond to specific stimuli. The rods and cones in the retina of the eye which respond to light are an example of such nerve cell specialization.

Stings

Stinging animals include scorpions and some insects (such as bees and wasps), jellyfish and related marine animals (such as anemones and corals), and some fish (such as stingrays). There are marked differences among these groups in the way the sting is delivered and its effects. (See *Insect stings; Scorpion stings; Jellyfish stings; Venomous bites and stings*.)

Nettles and some other plants carry tiny stinging hairs that hold an irritant liquid. These hairs penetrate and break off in the skin, causing release of the liquid, which has an immediate irritant effect that rarely lasts more than an hour or two. Washing the affected area and applying *calamine* lotion can provide relief. Contact with some other poisonous plants (see *Plants, poisonous*) may result in a more severe allergic reaction, sometimes requiring medical attention.

S

Stitch

A temporary, sudden, sharp pain in the abdomen or side that occurs during severe or unaccustomed exercise, usually running. The cause of a stitch is unknown.

Stitch is also the common name for a suture used to close a wound (see *Suturing*).

Stokes-Adams syndrome

Recurrent episodes of temporary loss of consciousness caused by insufficient blood flow from the heart to the brain. This deficient blood supply is due to irregularity of the heartbeat (see *Arrhythmia, cardiac*), which markedly reduces the pumping efficiency of the heart, or to complete *heart block* (abnormally slow conduction of electrical impulses through the heart muscle), resulting in temporary cessation of the heartbeat.

SYMPTOMS AND TREATMENT

In a typical attack, the sufferer faints suddenly and turns blue if the period of unconsciousness is prolonged. The breathing rate increases and a very slow pulse can be felt. Occasionally, lack of oxygen supply to the brain may cause a *seizure* (convulsion).

In most cases, the heart soon starts beating again, the skin flushes, and consciousness is regained. If this fails to happen, *cardiopulmonary resuscitation* should be carried out promptly to prevent brain damage.

Most people with Stokes-Adams syndrome are fitted with a *pacemaker* to maintain normal heartbeat and prevent future attacks.

Stoma

A term meaning mouth or orifice. A surgically created stoma in the abdomen acts as an artificial anus. A temporary stoma may be used to divert faeces from a healing wound in the intestine. A permanent stoma is created if part of the intestine has been removed. (See also *Colostomy*; *Ileostomy*.)

Stomach

A hollow, bag-like organ of the *digestive system* which is connected to the oesophagus and the duodenum (the first part of the small intestine). The stomach lies in the left side of the abdomen under the diaphragm.

STRUCTURE

The stomach is flexible, allowing it to expand when food is eaten; in an adult, the average capacity is about 1.5 litres. The stomach wall consists of layers of longitudinal and circular

muscle, lined by special glandular cells that secrete gastric juice, and supplied by blood vessels and nerves. A strong muscle at the lower end of the stomach forms a ring called the pyloric sphincter that can close the outlet leading to the duodenum.

FUNCTION

Although the main function of the stomach is to continue the breakdown of food that is started in the mouth and completed in the small intestine, it also acts as a storage organ. If storage were not possible, food would have to be eaten every 20 minutes or so rather than only two or three times a day.

The sight and smell of food and the arrival of food in the stomach stimulate gastric secretion. The gastric juice secreted from the stomach lining contains pepsin (an enzyme that breaks down protein), hydrochloric acid (which kills bacteria taken in with the food and which creates the most suitable environment for the pepsin to work in), and intrinsic factor (which is essential for the absorption of vitamin B_{12} in the small intestine). The stomach lining also contains glands that secrete mucus, which helps provide a barrier to prevent the stomach from digesting itself.

The layers of muscle produce rhythmic contractions about every 20 seconds that churn the food and gastric juice; the combined effect of this movement and the action of the digestive juice convert the semi-solid food into a creamy fluid. This process takes varying lengths of time, depending on the nature of the food. Generally, however, the richer the meal, the longer it takes to be emptied from the stomach. The partly digested food is squirted into the duodenum at regular intervals by the contractions of the stomach and by relaxation of the pyloric sphincter.

Stomach-ache

A common name for discomfort in the upper abdomen. (See *Indigestion*.)

Stomach cancer

A malignant tumour that arises from the lining of the *stomach*, also called gastric cancer.

CAUSES AND INCIDENCE

The cause of stomach cancer remains uncertain but evidence suggests that an environmental factor, probably diet, plays a part. Recent speculation has centred on an association between stomach cancer and eating quantities of salted, pickled, or smoked foods. Certain other factors, such as per-

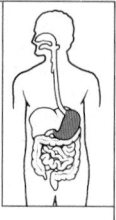

LOCATION OF THE STOMACH
Food enters the stomach from the oesophagus and exits into the duodenum. The stomach lining secretes gastric juice and protective mucus.

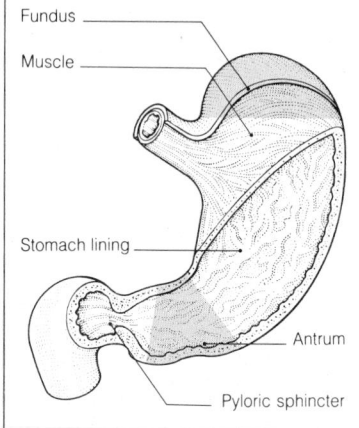

Fundus

Muscle

Stomach lining

Antrum

Pyloric sphincter

Parts of the stomach
The fundus and antrum are two of the main parts of the stomach; the lower oesophageal segment and pyloric sphincters control entry and exit of food.

nicious *anaemia*, partial *gastrectomy*, and belonging to blood group A, seem to increase the risk of developing this cancer.

Stomach cancer rarely affects people under the age of 40 and is more common in men than in women. There is marked geographic variation—with a very high rate of 80 to 90 cases per 100,000 people in Japan compared with 15 to 20 cases per 100,000 people annually in England and Wales, where it causes around 8,000 deaths a year. There has been a dramatic decrease in the worldwide incidence of stomach cancer over the past 50 years.

SYMPTOMS AND SIGNS

The symptoms of stomach cancer (if any) are often indistinguishable from those of *peptic ulcer*. In the advanced stages, there is usually loss of appetite, the sensation that the stomach is filling up quickly, nausea and vomiting, and weight loss.

DIAGNOSIS AND TREATMENT

Diagnosis is usually made by *gastroscopy* (examination of the stomach using a flexible viewing instrument) or by a *barium X-ray examination*. A *biopsy* (removal of a sample

S

DISORDERS OF THE STOMACH

Disorders of the stomach have a variety of causes. Because the stomach is a reservoir, disorders of the emptying of stomach contents occur. Other problems relate to the stomach's role in the preparation of ingested food for digestion.

INFECTION

The large amount of hydrochloric acid secreted by the stomach protects the stomach from some infections by destroying many of the bacteria, viruses, and fungi that are taken in with food and drink. When the protective power is insufficient, a variety of gastrointestinal infections may occur.

TUMOURS

Stomach cancer causes about 13,000 deaths annually in the UK. Early symptoms are often mistaken for *indigestion*, and diagnosis is often delayed until it is too late for a cure. Any change in the customary functioning of the digestive system is important, especially after the age of 50. A persistent feeling of fullness, or pain before or after meals, should never be ignored. Unexplained loss of appetite or frequent nausea should always be reported to a doctor. A tumour in the upper part of the stomach, near the opening of the oesophagus, can cause obstruction and difficulty in swallowing. Sometimes a stomach tumour remains "silent" and the first signs are due to the appearance of secondary growths elsewhere in the body.

Benign (noncancerous) *polyps* can also develop in the stomach.

ULCERATION

The acid and other digestive juices secreted by the stomach sometimes attack the stomach lining. The healthy stomach is prevented from digesting itself mainly by the protective layer of mucus secreted by the lining and by the speed with which damaged surface cells are replaced by the deeper layers. Many influences can upset this delicate balance. One of the most important is excessive acid secretion. The resulting *peptic ulcers* are probably the most common serious stomach disorder. Peptic ulcers are sometimes caused by stress, or by severe injury, such as major burns, accidents, and after surgery and severe infections; often they occur for no apparent reason. The stomach lining can be damaged by large amounts of aspirin or alcohol, sometimes causing *gastritis* (inflammation of the stomach lining). This may eventually lead to ulceration of the stomach lining.

AUTOIMMUNE DISORDERS

Pernicious anaemia is caused by the failure of the stomach lining to produce intrinsic factor, a substance whose role is to facilitate the absorption of vitamin B_{12} (itself necessary for red blood cell formation). Failure to produce the intrinsic factor occurs if there is atrophy of the stomach lining, which also causes failure of acid production. Tests that determine a person's ability to absorb vitamin B_{12} are important in the investigation of this condition. Pernicious anaemia is usually due to an *autoimmune disorder*.

OTHER DISORDERS

Enlargement of the stomach may be caused when scarring from a chronic peptic ulcer occurs at the stomach outlet. It may also be a complication of *pyloric stenosis*, a rare but serious condition in which there is narrowing of the stomach outlet. Rarely, the stomach may become twisted and obstructed, a condition called *volvulus*.

INVESTIGATION

Stomach disorders are investigated primarily by *barium X-ray examinations* and/or *gastroscopy*. Occasionally, a *biopsy* (removal of a tissue sample for microscopic analysis) is performed.

---

of tissue for microscopic examination) of the stomach lining may also be performed using a gastroscope.

The only effective treatment is total *gastrectomy*. However, only about 20 per cent of patients are able to undergo such surgery; in the remainder, the tumour has spread too widely at the time of diagnosis. In inoperable, advanced cases, *radiotherapy* and *anticancer drugs* may be used.

OUTLOOK

If the cancer is detected at a very early stage (before it has spread beyond the stomach lining), a high cure rate is possible. In Japan, where mass screening by gastroscopy is performed, 85 per cent of people are still alive five years after treatment by surgery. In advanced disease, however, the outlook is not good, with less than 10 per cent of patients surviving for longer than five years.

Stomach imaging
See *Barium X-ray examinations*.

Stomach pump
See *Lavage, gastric*.

Stomach ulcer
A raw area in the stomach lining, also called a gastric ulcer. It is a type of *peptic ulcer*.

Stomatitis
Any form of inflammation or ulceration of the mouth. Examples include *mouth ulcers* and *cold sores*.

Stones
Small, hard collections of solid material within the body. Also called calculi, they are formed from substances that are present to excess in fluids such as urine or bile. (See *Calculus, urinary tract*; *Gallstones*.)

Stool
Another word for *faeces*.

Stork mark
A small, flat, harmless, pinkish-red skin blemish found in 30 to 50 per cent of newborn babies. Such marks, which are also called salmon patches, are a type of *haemangioma* usually found around the eyes and at the nape of the neck. Stork marks around the eyes usually disappear within the first year; those at the base of the neck may persist indefinitely.

Strabismus
See *Squint*.

Strain
Tearing or stretching of *muscle* fibres as a result of suddenly pulling them too far. There is bleeding into the damaged area of muscle, causing

S

pain, swelling, and muscle spasm; a bruise usually appears a few days after the injury. Muscle strain of the back is a common cause of nonspecific *back pain*. Strains are most common in athletes.

Treatment may include applying an *ice-pack* to reduce swelling, use of *strapping* or a compression *bandage*, and resting an affected part (in a raised position if appropriate) for 48 hours. *Analgesic drugs* (painkillers) may also be taken to relieve pain. After the rest period, *physiotherapy* including stretching exercises should be started to prevent possible shortening of the muscle due to the formation of scar tissue. In some cases, *nonsteroidal anti-inflammatory drugs* may be prescribed to speed healing.

The risk of muscle strain can be reduced by performing warming-up exercises before any sports activity.

Strangulation

The constriction, usually by twisting or compression, of a tube or passage in the body, blocking blood flow and interfering with the function of the affected organ. Strangulation may occur with a *hernia* or after twisting of the testis (see *Testis, torsion of*).

Strangulation is usually caused by herniation of part of the intestine, either inside the abdomen or externally as in an inguinal hernia, or by *volvulus* (twisting of a piece of intestine). The resulting intestinal obstruction requires an emergency operation (see *Intestine, obstruction of*).

Strangulation of the neck with the hands or with a ligature, such as a cord or scarf, may be deliberate or accidental. The main lethal effect arises from compression of the *jugular veins* in the neck. This prevents blood from flowing out of the brain and head, where it stagnates and its oxygen content is quickly used up. In addition, compression of the *trachea* (windpipe) restricts breathing and impairs oxygenation of the blood. The victim's face becomes congested with blood, turning purple-blue in colour. He or she loses consciousness and, some minutes later, brain damage and death occur from lack of oxygen.

Any constricting ligature must be removed as quickly as possible and medical help summoned. If the victim is not breathing, *artificial respiration* should be performed until an ambulance or doctor arrives.

To prevent accidental strangulation, a child's environment should be kept free of potential ligatures—

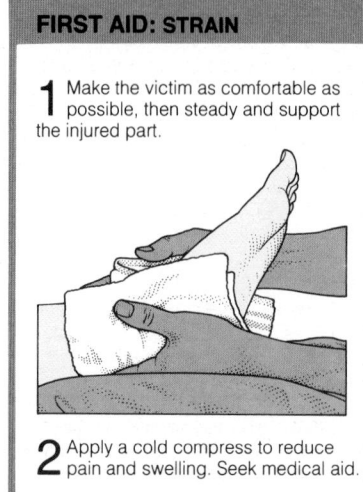

FIRST AID: STRAIN

1 Make the victim as comfortable as possible, then steady and support the injured part.

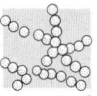

2 Apply a cold compress to reduce pain and swelling. Seek medical aid.

such as cords on toys or clothing, or dangerous restraining apparatus. Children should be discouraged from playing with lassos.

Strangury

A symptom characterized by a painful and frequent desire to empty the bladder, although only a few drops of urine can be passed. Causes of strangury include *prostatitis* (inflammation of the prostate gland), *cystitis*, bladder cancer (see *Bladder tumours*), and bladder stones (see *Calculus, urinary tract*).

Strapping

The application of adhesive tape to part of the body to exert pressure and hold a structure in place.

Strapping is used to reduce pain and swelling caused by soft tissue injuries, such as *sprains* and *strains*. It may also be applied to joints to prevent injury due to excessive movement, or to strengthen a joint that has been injured in order to help prevent recurrence of the injury.

Strawberry naevus

A bright red, raised spot which appears in early infancy. A strawberry naevus is a type of *haemangioma*.

Strep throat

A *streptococcal infection* of the *throat*. Strep throat is most common in children and is spread by droplets (containing the bacteria) coughed or breathed into the air.

In some people, the bacteria cause few or no symptoms, but a proportion suffer a sore throat, fever, general malaise, and enlarged lymph nodes in

the neck. In some cases, toxins released by the bacteria lead to a rash, a condition known as *scarlet fever*.

The diagnosis is usually made by identifying the bacteria in a *culture* grown from a throat swab. The infection is treated with a *penicillin drug* or with another antibiotic drug if the person is allergic to penicillin.

An untreated strep throat infection may lead to the serious complications of *glomerulonephritis* (inflammation in the kidneys) and *rheumatic fever*.

Streptococcal infections

Types of infection caused by *bacteria* of the streptococcus group. Streptococci are spherical bacteria that grow in lines, like beads on a string; they are among the most common disease-causing bacteria in humans.

Certain types of streptococci are present harmlessly in most people's mouths and throats. If the bacteria gain access to the bloodstream (sometimes after dental treatment), they are usually destroyed. However, in some people with heart valve defects there is a risk that bacteria will settle in the heart to cause bacterial *endocarditis*. Another type of streptococcus is normally present harmlessly in the intestines but can spread to cause a *urinary tract infection*.

Other types of streptococci, known as haemolytic streptococci, cause *tonsillitis*, *strep throat*, *otitis media* (middleear infection), *pneumonia*, *erysipelas*, or wound infections. Some haemolytic streptococcal infections may result in *scarlet fever*, and may also give rise to the serious complications of *rheumatic fever* and *glomerulonephritis*. These complications are prevented through prompt treatment with *antibiotic drugs* (usually penicillin).

People in whom rheumatic fever has developed are advised to take an antibiotic drug before, during, and after dental treatment and certain diagnostic and surgical procedures.

Streptokinase

A *thrombolytic drug* used to dissolve blood clots during a *myocardial infarction* (heart attack) or *pulmonary embolism*. Streptokinase is most effective in dissolving newly formed clots. Given by injection in the early stages of a myocardial infarction, streptokinase may limit the amount of damage that is caused to the heart muscle.

Treatment with streptokinase is strictly supervised because of the risk of allergic reaction or excessive bleed-

S

ing. Adverse effects include rash, fever, wheezing, and cardiac *arrhythmias* (irregularities of the heartbeat).

Streptomycin

An *antibiotic drug* used to treat any of a number of uncommon infections, including *tularaemia*, *plague*, *brucellosis*, and *glanders*. Streptomycin is sometimes given in conjunction with a *penicillin drug* to treat *endocarditis* (inflammation of the lining of the heart and heart valves).

Once used to treat a wide range of other infections, streptomycin has now been largely superseded by newer, more effective drugs with less serious side-effects. Discovered in the 1940s, streptomycin was the first effective drug treatment for *tuberculosis*; it is still sometimes used to treat resistant strains of bacteria causing this disease.

POSSIBLE ADVERSE EFFECTS
Most seriously, streptomycin may damage nerves in the inner ear, disturbing balance and causing dizziness, ringing in the ears, and deafness. Other possible adverse effects include numbness of the face, tingling in the hands, headache, malaise, nausea, and vomiting.

Stress

Any interference that disturbs a person's healthy mental and physical well-being. A person may experience stress in response to a wide range of physical and emotional stimuli, including physical violence, internal conflicts, and significant life events (e.g. the death of a loved one, the birth of a baby, or divorce). Some people are more susceptible than others to stress-related medical problems.

EFFECTS
When faced with a stressful situation, the body responds by increasing production of certain hormones, such as *cortisol* and *adrenaline*. These hormones lead to changes in heart-rate, blood pressure, metabolism, and physical activity designed to improve overall performance. However, at a certain level, they disrupt an individual's ability to cope. Less than 20 per cent of people are effective in the face of crises such as fires or floods.

Continued exposure to stress often leads to mental and physical symptoms, such as *anxiety* and *depression*, *indigestion*, palpitations, and muscular aches and pains. *Post-traumatic stress disorder* is a direct response to a specific stressful event. (See also *Relaxation techniques*.)

Stress fracture

A *fracture* that occurs as a result of repetitive jarring of a bone. Common sites include the metatarsal bones in the foot (see *March fracture*), the tibia or fibula (lower-leg bones), the neck of the femur (thigh-bone), and the lumbar region of the spine. Stress fractures are most common among runners, particularly those who run on hard surfaces with inadequate footwear (see *Sports injuries*).

SYMPTOMS AND DIAGNOSIS
The main symptoms include pain and tenderness at the fracture site. Diagnosis is by *X-rays*, although some stress fractures do not show up on X-ray until they have started to heal. Occasionally, a radionuclide bone scan (see *Bone imaging*) may be performed to confirm the diagnosis.

TREATMENT
Treatment consists of resting the affected area for four to six weeks. In some cases, it is also necessary to immobilize the fracture in a plaster *cast*. After recovery, modification of exercise routines and the use of suitably cushioned footwear may help to prevent a recurrence.

Stress ulcer

An acute *peptic ulcer* that sometimes develops after shock, serious burns, severe injuries, or during a major illness. Stress ulcers are usually multiple and are most common in the stomach; they differ from chronic peptic ulcers in that the raw area does not spread deep into the stomach lining.

The exact cause of stress ulcers is unknown. Treatment is primarily preventive; patients in intensive-care units are commonly given *antacid drugs* and/or *H_2-receptor antagonists*.

Stretcher

A frame covered with fabric that is used in first aid for carrying the sick, injured, or deceased. Many stretchers are available, including the standard stretcher, which consists of canvas stretched between two long poles on each side, and the trolley bed, a more sophisticated, adjustable stretcher on wheels carried in ambulances.

Stretchers can be improvised by passing two poles through holes made in the corners of canvas bags, or by rolling up poles in parallel sides of a strong rug or blanket. An overcoat may also be used. Ideally, stretchers should be fairly rigid. The ends of a loaded stretcher should be lifted simultaneously. (See also illustrated box overleaf.)

Stretch-mark

The common name for *stria*.

Stria

Commonly called a stretch-mark, a line on the *skin* caused by thinning and loss of elasticity in the dermis

---

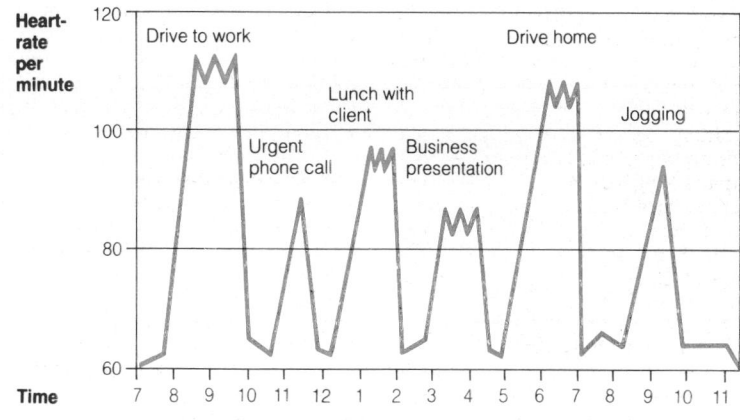

STRESS AND HEART-RATE

The graph shows how a person's heart-rate varies over a typical day. Exercise and stress both activate the body's "fight-or-flight" system and increase heart-rate, but repeated alerting of the system without accompanying physical activity is probably harmful.

Stress levels through the day
Although the home and workplace both present stress, for many city workers the most stressful parts of the day are those spent commuting.

USING A STRETCHER

Stretchers are used to carry injured or seriously ill people to avoid the risk of further injury. Any type of stretcher should be fairly rigid and should always be tested for strength before use.

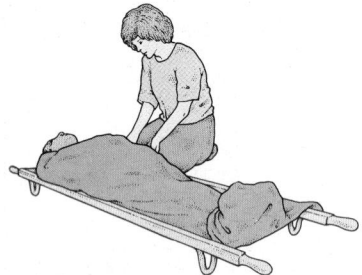

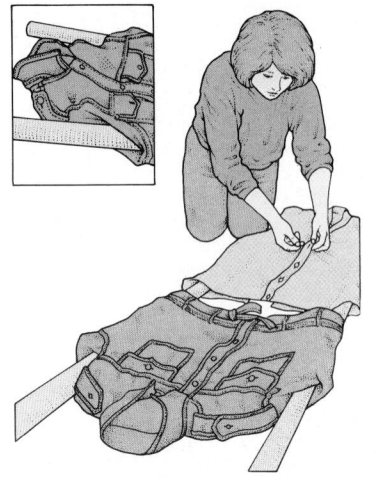

Keeping the victim warm
Place a blanket diagonally on the stretcher. Lift the victim carefully on to the blanket and tuck in the corners.

Improvising a stretcher
Turn the sleeves of two coats inside out. Pass two strong poles through the sleeves and button the coats (see inset).

(lower layer of the skin). Striae first appear as red, raised lines. Later they become purple, eventually flattening and fading to form shiny streaks, usually between 6 and 12 mm wide.

Striae often develop on the hips and thighs during the adolescent growth spurt, especially in athletic girls. They are a common feature of pregnancy, developing in about 75 per cent of pregnant women, and tend to occur on the breasts, the thighs, and the lower abdomen. Purple striae characteristically develop in people with *Cushing's syndrome*.

Striae are possibly caused by an excess of *corticosteroid hormones*. These hormones are known to suppress fibre formation in the skin and to cause *collagen* in the skin to waste away. There is no effective means of prevention or treatment.

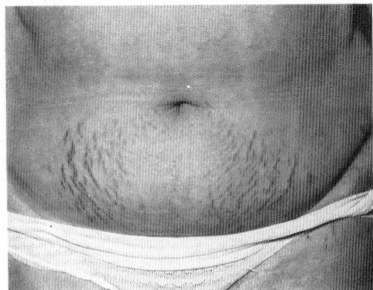

Appearance of striae
Commonly known as stretch-marks, striae often develop on the abdomen, thighs, and breasts of pregnant women.

Stricture

Narrowing of a duct, canal, or other passage in the body. A stricture may result from infection and inflammation; damage to and subsequent formation of scar tissue in or around a passage; development of a tumour; spasm of muscles in a passage wall; or excessive growth of tissue around a passage, which occurs in *prostatism* when the enlarged prostate gland constricts the urethra (the passage between the bladder and outside). In some cases, a stricture is *congenital*.

Stridor

An abnormal breathing sound caused by narrowing or obstruction of the *larynx* or *trachea*.

Stridor is most common in young children. It usually occurs in *croup*, which is caused by a viral infection of the upper airways. A less common, but more serious, cause is the bacterial infection *epiglottitis*. Other causes of stridor include an inhaled *foreign body*, *hypocalcaemia* (a low level of calcium in the blood), and certain disorders of the *larynx*, such as tumours, vocal cord paralysis, and laryngomalacia (softening of the cartilage of the larynx).

Stroke

Damage to part of the *brain* caused by interruption to its blood supply or by leakage of blood through the walls of blood vessels. Sensation, movement, or function controlled by the damaged

area is impaired. Strokes can be fatal and are a leading cause of death in developed countries.

CAUSES

The main types and causes of stroke are shown in the illustrated box.

Certain factors increase the risk of having a stroke. The two most important are *hypertension* (high blood pressure), which weakens the walls of arteries, and *atherosclerosis* (narrowing of arteries by fatty deposits).

Other factors that increase the risk of a stroke include *atrial fibrillation* (a type of heartbeat irregularity), a damaged *heart valve*, and a recent *myocardial infarction* (heart attack). All of these conditions can cause blood clots in the heart which may break off and migrate to the brain. *Polycythaemia* (a raised level of red cells in the blood), *hyperlipidaemia* (a high level of fatty substances in the blood), *diabetes mellitus*, and smoking also increase the risk of stroke by increasing the risk of hypertension and/or atherosclerosis. *Oral contraceptives* increase the risk of stroke in women under 50.

INCIDENCE

In the UK, the overall incidence of stroke is about 200 people per 100,000 population annually. The incidence rises steeply with age and is higher in men than in women.

SYMPTOMS AND SIGNS

Damage to a specific area of the brain impairs bodily sensation, movement, or function controlled by that part of the brain. Some of the possible symptoms and signs are shown in the illustrated box. A stroke that affects the dominant cerebral hemisphere in the brain (usually the left hemisphere) may cause disturbance of language and speech (see *Aphasia*).

Movement on one side of the body is controlled by the cerebral hemisphere on the opposite side. Thus, damage to areas controlling movement in the right cerebral hemisphere results in weakness or paralysis on the left side of the body. Such one-sided weakness or paralysis, known as *hemiplegia*, is one of the most common effects of a serious stroke.

When symptoms last for less than 24 hours and are followed by full recovery, the episode is known as a *transient ischaemic attack* (TIA). Such an attack, which usually lasts for only a few minutes, is a warning signal that a sufficient supply of blood is not reaching part of the brain.

About a third of major strokes are fatal, a third result in some disability, and a third have no lasting ill effects.

S

TYPES AND CAUSES OF STROKE

Stroke may be caused by any of three mechanisms (below). Thrombosis and embolism both lead to cessation of the blood supply to part of the brain and thus to infarction (tissue death). Rupture of a blood vessel in or near the brain may cause an intracerebral haemorrhage or a subarachnoid haemorrhage. Any part of the brain may be affected by a stroke; accordingly, the symptoms vary considerably.

CEREBRAL THROMBOSIS

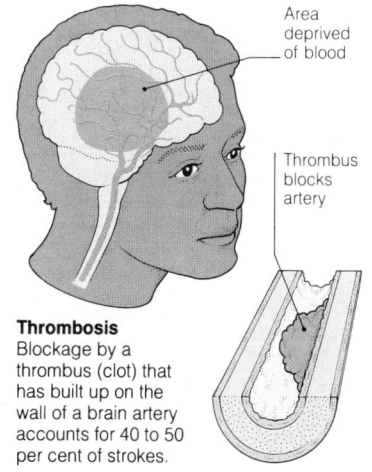

Area deprived of blood

Thrombus blocks artery

Thrombosis
Blockage by a thrombus (clot) that has built up on the wall of a brain artery accounts for 40 to 50 per cent of strokes.

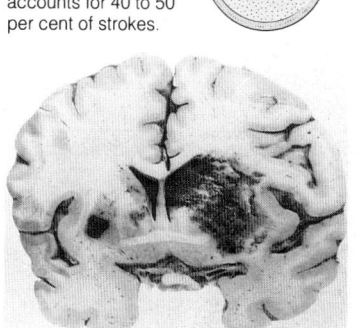

CEREBRAL EMBOLISM

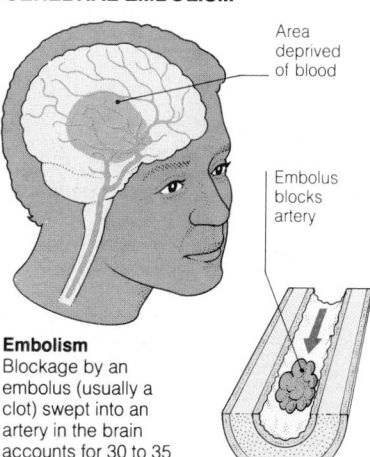

Area deprived of blood

Embolus blocks artery

Embolism
Blockage by an embolus (usually a clot) swept into an artery in the brain accounts for 30 to 35 per cent of strokes.

Tissue death within the brain
The photograph (left) shows a vertical slice through the brain of someone who died of a stroke. A large region of tissue death (dark area), caused by bleeding and oxygen deprivation, can be seen on one side.

HAEMORRHAGE

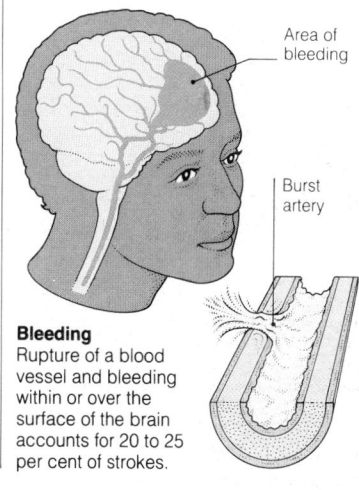

Area of bleeding

Burst artery

Bleeding
Rupture of a blood vessel and bleeding within or over the surface of the brain accounts for 20 to 25 per cent of strokes.

Estimated incidence per 1,000 population

30 —
20 —
10 —

Age   30   40   50   60   70   80   90

Incidence with age
Strokes are rare to uncommon under the age of 60, but thereafter the chances of one occurring increase rapidly.

SYMPTOMS

The symptoms of a stroke usually develop abruptly over minutes or hours, but occasionally over several days. Depending on the site, cause, and extent of damage, any or all of the symptoms shown on the right may be present, in any degree of severity. The more serious cases lead to rapid loss of consciousness, coma, and death or to severe physical or mental handicap, but some strokes cause barely noticeable symptoms.

Hemiplegia
Weakness or paralysis on one side of the body is one of the more common effects of a serious stroke.

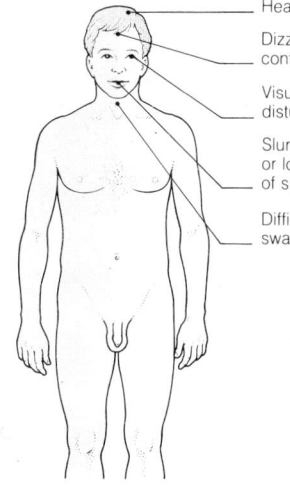

Headache

Dizziness and confusion

Visual disturbance

Slurred speech or loss of speech

Difficulty swallowing

RISK FACTORS

Age

High blood pressure

Atherosclerosis (narrowing of arteries by fatty deposits)

Heart disease

Diabetes mellitus

Smoking

Polycythaemia

Hyperlipidaemia

Use of oestrogens

S

COMPLICATIONS

Possible complications of a major stroke include *pneumonia*, and the formation of blood clots in the veins of the leg (see *Thrombosis, deep vein*), which may travel to the artery supplying the lung to cause a potentially fatal *pulmonary embolism*.

DIAGNOSIS

If someone is thought to have had a stroke, a doctor should be summoned immediately. The doctor will assess whether hospital treatment is advisable or whether the patient is best kept at home.

CT scanning of the brain may sometimes be performed to determine whether the symptoms are caused by a stroke or by some other disorder, such as a *brain tumour, brain abscess, subdural haemorrhage* (bleeding into the space between the outermost and middle membranes covering the brain), or *encephalitis* (inflammation of the brain). A *lumbar puncture* may occasionally be necessary to exclude the possibility of *meningitis* (inflammation of the membranes covering the brain and spinal cord).

To further examine the cause and extent of brain damage, investigations may include an *ECG, chest X-rays, blood tests, angiography,* and, in specialist centres, *MRI*.

TREATMENT

In hospital, patients who are unconscious or semiconscious require a clear airway (breathing passages), feeding by means of *intravenous infusion* or a *nasogastric tube*, and regular changing of position to avoid bedsores or pneumonia. When a stroke has been caused by an embolism, *anticoagulant drugs* or, occasionally, *thrombolytic drugs* may be prescribed. In most cases, *aspirin* is prescribed to reduce the risk of recurrence.

Every effort is made to restore any lost movement or sensation by *physiotherapy* and to remedy any speech disturbance by *speech therapy*.

OUTLOOK

About half of all patients recover more or less completely from their first stroke. Most people paralysed by a stroke learn to walk again. Survivors left with some disability may require *occupational therapy* and aids in the home (see *Disability*). About five per cent of patients require long-term institutional care.

Stroma

The tissue that forms the framework of an organ, as distinct from the functional tissue (called the *parenchyma*)

and the fibrous outer layer that holds the organ together. For example, the stroma of the ovaries is the supporting tissue in which the ovarian follicles (the parenchyma) are embedded. The ovarian stroma consists of fibrous tissue, smooth muscle cells, spindle-shaped cells, and a rich supply of blood vessels.

Strongyloidiasis

An infestation of the intestines by a tiny parasitic worm, STRONGYLOIDES STERCORALIS. The disease is widespread in the tropics, especially the Far East. In the UK, it is occasionally found in refugees and in ex-servicemen who served in the Far East during World War II, but is otherwise rare.

Strongyloidiasis is contracted in affected areas by walking barefoot on soil contaminated with faeces. Worm larvae penetrate the skin of the feet and then migrate, via the lungs and throat, to the small intestine. There they develop into adults, which burrow into the intestinal wall to produce larvae. Most larvae are passed in the faeces, but some enter the skin around the anus to begin a new cycle. Thus, an infestation may persist in one person for more than forty years.

SYMPTOMS

The larvae cause itching and raised red weals where they pass through the skin. In the lungs they may cause *asthma* or *pneumonia*. Intestinal infestation may produce no symptoms but in cases of heavy infestation there may be discomfort, a swollen abdomen, and diarrhoea. Occasionally, an infected person whose *immune system* is depressed dies of complications, such as *septicaemia* or *meningitis*, many years after contracting the infection. Pneumonia may occur more readily in a person whose immune system has been compromised.

TREATMENT

The disease is diagnosed from microscopic examination of a sample of faeces. Strongyloidiasis is treated with an *anthelmintic drug*, usually *thiabendazole*, which eradicates the worms.

Strontium

A metallic element which does not occur naturally in its pure form but is present in various compounds in certain minerals (notably strontianite and celestite), seawater, and marine plants. Strontium is also found in food and, although it is not essential to the body, it is metabolized in a manner similar to calcium and incorporated into bone.

In addition to strontium compounds, there are several radioisotopes (radioactive varieties) of the element, of which strontium 90 is medically the most important. This does not occur naturally, but is produced in relatively large amounts during nuclear fission reactions and is also present in the fallout from some nuclear bomb explosions. Strontium 90 emits *radiation* (in the form of beta particles) for a comparatively long time (the *half-life* of this radioisotope is about 28 years), and accumulates in bone, where the radiation may cause *leukaemia* and/or *bone tumours*.

Other radioisotopes of strontium have also been used in medicine to diagnose and treat bone tumours.

Strychnine poisoning

Strychnine is an extremely poisonous chemical found in the seeds of STRYCHNOS species, a group of tropical trees and shrubs. Although once used as a tonic and general stimulant, strychnine is now no longer used in medicine. Its principal use today is as an ingredient in some rodent poisons; most cases of strychnine poisoning occur in children who accidentally eat such poisons. However, the extremely bitter taste of strychnine and its lack of easy availability makes this form of poisoning rare.

SYMPTOMS AND TREATMENT

The symptoms of poisoning begin soon after strychnine has been ingested. Initial symptoms include restlessness, stiffness of the face and neck, *photosensitivity* (increased sensitivity to light), and increased sensitivity of hearing, taste, and smell. These symptoms are followed by alternating episodes of seizures (fits) and floppiness. Eventually, death may occur from *respiratory arrest*.

The main objectives of treatment are to prevent seizures and to maintain breathing. The victim is given intravenous injections of a *tranquillizer drug* or a *barbiturate drug*, with a *muscle-relaxant drug* if necessary, which counteract the effects of strychnine and help prevent seizures. Breathing may be maintained by a *ventilator*. With prompt treatment, recovery usually occurs in about 24 hours.

Stuffy nose

See *Nasal congestion*.

Stump

The end portion of a limb that remains after *amputation*.

S

Stupor

A state of almost complete *unconsciousness* from which a person can be aroused only briefly and only by vigorous external stimulation. (See also *Coma*.)

Sturge-Weber syndrome

A rare, congenital condition that affects the skin and the brain. Characteristically, a large purple *haemangioma* (a birthmark caused by abnormal distribution of blood vessels) extends over one side of the face, including the eye. A similar malformation of blood vessels in the brain may cause some weakness on the opposite side of the body, progressive *mental handicap*, and *epilepsy*. *Glaucoma* (increased pressure within the eyeball) may develop in the affected eye, leading to partial or complete loss of vision.

The birthmark can be disguised with masking creams; seizures can usually be controlled with *anticonvulsant drugs*. In severe cases, surgery on the affected part of the brain may need to be performed.

Stuttering

A speech disorder in which there is repeated hesitation and delay in uttering words, unusual prolongation of sounds, and repetition of word elements. Stuttering, also known as stammering, usually starts in childhood, beginning before the age of eight in 90 per cent of sufferers.

INCIDENCE
Stuttering occurs in about one per cent of adults. Temporary stuttering is fairly common in children aged two to four. About half the children whose stutter persists until the age of five will continue to stutter in adult life. Stuttering is more common in males, twins, and left-handed people.

SYMPTOMS
The words and sounds that cause problems vary from person to person. The severity of stuttering may be related to circumstances. Some people find that stuttering is worse when they are anxious (such as during public speaking or when using the telephone), while others experience more difficulty when relaxed. Problems rarely occur during singing or reading in unison (possibly because less communication is involved). Some people who stutter also have *tics* and *tremors*.

CAUSES
The cause of stuttering is uncertain, although it has a tendency to run in families. Some researchers believe

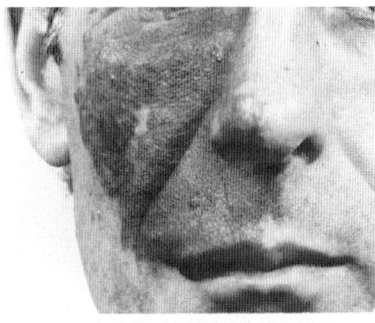

Appearance of Sturge-Weber syndrome
The characteristic flat, purple birthmark extends over the upper part of one side of this man's face.

that stuttering is due to a subtle form of brain damage; others, however, regard stuttering as being primarily a psychological problem.

TREATMENT
Stuttering can often be improved by *speech therapy*. This may include teaching the affected person to give equal weight to each syllable, and use of electronic aids to mask the speaker's voice or to relay speech back to the speaker via headphones.

Stye

Also called a hordeolum, a stye is a small, pus-filled *abscess* near the eyelashes caused by infection.

If a stye is painful, applying warm compresses may help the pus to discharge. Use of an eye ointment containing an *antibiotic drug* can help to prevent a recurrence.

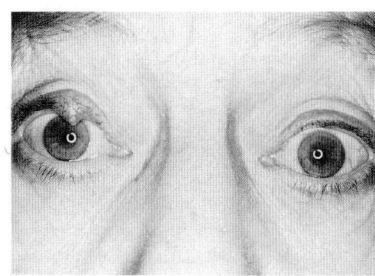

Stye on the upper eyelid
A stye most often forms near the inner corner of an eye but may develop at the base of any of the eyelashes.

Subacute

A medical term applied to a disease that runs a course in time between *acute* and *chronic*. In subacute *endocarditis*, for example, the disease may go undetected for many months during which time it causes severe damage to a heart valve.

Subarachnoid haemorrhage

A type of *brain haemorrhage* in which blood from a ruptured blood vessel spreads over the surface of the brain.

CAUSES AND INCIDENCE
The most common cause of subarachnoid haemorrhage is a burst *aneurysm* (balloon-like swelling of an artery), which commonly occurs on the circular arrangement of blood vessels at the base of the brain. Less commonly, it is due to a ruptured *angioma* (abnormal proliferation of blood vessels within the brain). Bleeding takes place in the space between the arachnoid and the pia mater (the middle and the innermost of the three *meninges* that cover the brain). This space also contains *cerebrospinal fluid*, which becomes mixed with blood.

Subarachnoid haemorrhage usually occurs spontaneously, without any head injury, although it may follow unaccustomed physical exercise. Each year, about five to 10 people per 100,000 suffer a subarachnoid haemorrhage. This form of brain haemorrhage is less common than *intracerebral haemorrhage* (a form of stroke), in which bleeding occurs within the brain itself. Subarachnoid haemorrhage is particularly common in people aged between 35 and 60.

SYMPTOMS
An attack may cause immediate loss of consciousness or a sudden violent headache, often followed by loss of consciousness. If the person remains conscious, other symptoms such as *photophobia* (abnormal sensitivity to light), nausea, vomiting, drowsiness, and stiffness of the neck may develop. Unconscious patients may recover, but attacks during the ensuing days or weeks are common and often fatal.

DIAGNOSIS
The diagnosis is usually made by *CT scanning*. If this is not possible, diagnosis will be confirmed by finding blood in the cerebrospinal fluid after carrying out a *lumbar puncture* investigation. The site of the burst blood vessel is subsequently investigated by *angiography* (X-rays taken after the injection of a radiopaque substance into the bloodstream).

TREATMENT
Treatment consists of general life-support procedures, bed rest, and measures aimed at reducing the risk of recurrence—principally, control of high blood pressure. In many cases, a burst aneurysm is surgically accessible and may be treated by an operation. Aneurysms can be surgically removed, blocked off,

S

or obliterated. Surgery is usually delayed for several weeks after the acute attack.

About one third of patients make a full recovery; another one sixth recover but have some residual disability, such as paralysis, mental deterioration, or epilepsy. The remaining patients (about half) die as a result of the initial or a recurrent attack.

Subclavian steal syndrome

Recurrent attacks of blurred or double vision, loss of coordination, or dizziness caused by reduced blood flow to the base of the brain when one arm (usually the left) is moved. The underlying cause is narrowing of the major arteries that carry blood to the arms (usually due to *atherosclerosis*). The left subclavian artery is particularly affected. Blood supply to the affected arm is reduced but is sufficient provided the arm is kept at rest. When the arm is moved, its muscles require an increased amount of blood, which is diverted from the base of the brain.

A doctor confirms the diagnosis by finding a weak pulse and low blood pressure in the affected arm. *Angiography* (X-rays taken after the injection of a radiopaque substance into the bloodstream) establishes the site of the narrowed artery. Treatment is by *arterial reconstructive surgery*.

Subclinical

A medical term applied to a disorder that produces no symptoms or signs because it is so mild or because it is in the early stages of development. Although a subclinical disorder does not produce symptoms or signs, it may cause damage to organs.

Subconjunctival haemorrhage

Bleeding under the *conjunctiva* (transparent membrane covering the white of the eye). The small blood vessels of the conjunctiva are fragile, poorly supported, and frequently leak. Subconjunctival haemorrhage may occur spontaneously or after coughing or vomiting, which increases pressure in the veins. It is usually harmless and only rarely signals a serious disorder.

Subconjunctival blood disappears without treatment, usually within 10 to 14 days. Recurrences sometimes occur as a result of local weakness in a conjunctival blood vessel.

Subconscious

A term describing mental events (such as thoughts, ideas, or feelings) that one is temporarily unaware of but that can be recalled under the right circumstances. In *psychoanalytic theory*, the subconscious refers to that part of the mind through which information passes on its way from the *unconscious* to the conscious mind.

Subcutaneous

A medical term meaning beneath the skin, as in a subcutaneous injection, one in which a drug is injected into the tissue under the skin.

Subdural haemorrhage

Bleeding into the space between the dura mater, the tough outer layer of the *meninges* (coverings of the brain) and the arachnoid (middle meningeal layer). The trapped blood slowly forms a large haematoma (enlarging blood clot) within the skull. The most common cause is torn veins on the inside of the dura mater following a blow to the head. Subdural haemorrhage most often affects elderly or alcoholic people who have fallen.

SYMPTOMS

The bleeding occurs slowly; it may be weeks or months before the haematoma enlarges sufficiently to cause symptoms by raising pressure within the skull and displacing and pressing on brain tissue. The symptoms, which tend to fluctuate, consist of headache, episodes of confusion and drowsiness, and the development of one-sided weakness or paralysis.

Any person in whom such symptoms develop should consult a doctor immediately. Because the symptoms are similar to those of a *stroke*, it is important that mention be made of any *head injury* that occurred within the previous few months.

DIAGNOSIS AND TREATMENT

The diagnosis is confirmed, and the location of the haematoma investigated, by means of *angiography* (X-rays taken after the injection of a radiopaque substance into the bloodstream) and *CT scanning*.

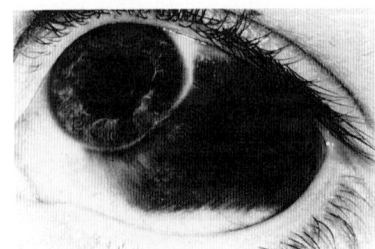

Subconjunctival haemorrhage
The bleeding causes a bright red area to appear in the white of the eye. This may look alarming but is usually harmless.

Surgical treatment is by drilling burr holes into the skull (see *Craniotomy*), drainage of the blood clot, and repair of damaged blood vessels, which usually allows a full recovery if carried out soon enough. (See also *Extradural haemorrhage*.)

Sublimation

The unconscious process by which primitive, unacceptable impulses are redirected into socially acceptable forms of behaviour. Aggression, for example, may be channelled into sports. *Psychoanalytic theory* regards sublimation as a healthy process.

Subluxated tooth

A tooth displaced in its socket as the result of an accident. The upper front teeth are the most vulnerable. The tooth may be depressed deep into the gum, tilted backwards or forwards, and loosened. A dentist can usually manipulate a subluxated tooth back into position, after which it is usually immobilized with a splint (see *Splinting, dental*). If the tooth's blood vessels are torn and the pulp dies, the tooth requires *root-canal treatment*.

Subluxation

Incomplete *dislocation* of a *joint*—that is, displacement of the bony surfaces in a joint so that they no longer face each other exactly but remain in partial contact. In a dislocation, the joint surfaces are displaced so that there is total loss of contact between them. In general, a subluxation causes less damage to the joint and surrounding tissues than does a dislocation.

Normal
The diagram on the left shows the normal position of the bony surfaces in a simple joint, such as the joint in the middle of a finger.

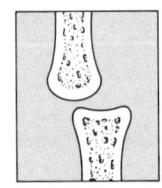

Subluxation
In a subluxation, the surfaces of the bones are slightly displaced from their normal positions relative to each other but are still in contact.

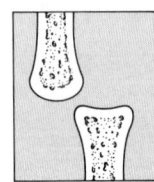

Dislocation
Here, there is almost complete loss of contact between the bone surfaces and, in most cases, considerable damage to surrounding tissues.

S

Submucous resection

An operation to correct a deviated *nasal septum* (the central partition inside the nose) when this is causing breathing difficulty. Under a local or a general anaesthetic, an incision is made in the mucous membrane covering the septum, and displaced cartilage and bone are then cut away. The membrane is closed with absorbable stitches, which do not require removal.

Subphrenic abscess

An *abscess* under the diaphragm.

Substrate

A substance on which an *enzyme* acts. For example, the digestive enzyme amylase acts on the substrate starch (a polysaccharide) and breaks it down into smaller saccharide (sugar) units.

Sucking chest wound

An open wound in the chest wall through which air passes, causing the lung on that side to collapse (see *Lung, collapse of*). The mediastinum (central partition of the chest) may also shift to the other side, causing partial collapse of the other lung.

A sucking chest wound causes severe breathlessness and a life-threatening lack of oxygen. Emergency first-aid treatment is vital. Cover the wound with your hand (or first cover it with a piece of airtight material, such as a plastic bag). It is essential that the wound is kept tightly sealed until medical attention is obtained.

Sucralfate

An *ulcer-healing drug* used to treat *peptic ulcer*. Sucralfate forms a protective barrier over the ulcerated stomach or duodenal lining and thus protects it from further attack by the digestive juices and allows an ulcer to heal.

Antacid drugs should not be taken within an hour of taking sucralfate as they may reduce its effectiveness.

Possible adverse effects include constipation and abdominal pain. Sucralfate may interfere with the absorption of certain drugs, such as *tetracycline drugs* and *digoxin*. In addition, prolonged treatment with sucralfate may impair the absorption of certain vitamins, making supplements necessary.

Suction

The removal of unwanted fluid or semi-fluid material from the body with a syringe and hollow needle or with an intestinal tube and a mechanical pump. Among the many uses of suction are: the clearing of secretions from the throats of newborn babies; clearing the throats of patients who have undergone an operation under general anaesthesia; and the draining of blood and other fluids from the abdominal cavity during or after surgery.

Suction lipectomy

A cosmetic procedure used in *body contour surgery*.

Sudden death

See *Death, sudden*.

Sudden infant death syndrome

The sudden, unexpected death of an infant, which often cannot be explained even after an autopsy. Such deaths, also known as cot deaths, typically occur in apparently healthy babies who seem well when put to bed but are later found dead.

CAUSES AND INCIDENCE

In developed countries, sudden infant death syndrome (SIDS) is the most common form of death between the ages of one month and one year; three quarters of these occur in babies under six months old. SIDS is slightly more common among boys, among second children, and in winter. More deaths seem to occur between midnight and 9 a.m. and at weekends.

Much of the research has been focused on possible risk factors. These include: sleeping face down; *prematurity* and low birth weight; bottle-feeding; cold weather; young, single mothers; smoking, drug addiction, or anaemia in the mother; poor socio-economic background; the death of a sibling as a result of SIDS; and so-called "near miss" infants who have been found near death and have been resuscitated just in time.

Most experts believe there is no single cause of SIDS. It seems probable that some babies die of a sudden overwhelming respiratory infection and others of undetected inborn errors of metabolism (see *Metabolism, inborn errors of*). Most deaths are thought to be caused by some abnormality in the breathing and heart-rate. Abnormal breathing rhythms may be due to a fault in the brainstem, the lungs may have abnormally sensitive airway reflexes, or there may be an abnormality of surfactant (a substance that prevents the air sacs of the lungs from collapsing).

Even though most deaths seem to occur without warning, it is becoming clear that some babies may have been suffering from minor symptoms (such as a cold with a stuffy nose) for several days before death or have shown an inexplicable weight loss.

PREVENTION

Deaths from SIDS have been cut by around one third in the UK and other countries where campaigns have been introduced to persuade mothers to breast-feed, to avoid smoking, and to lay their babies to sleep on their backs. Good obstetric and *antenatal care*, avoiding unnecessary drugs during pregnancy, and close observation of the baby for several days after a minor illness may also be helpful.

Parents of a child who has died from SIDS and parents of "near miss" infants may be reassured by the use of an alarm that sounds if the baby stops breathing. However, there is no evidence that the use of alarms lowers the risk of death, and the number of false alarms that occurs may increase rather than allay the parental anxiety.

EFFECTS

The death of an infant from SIDS is a highly distressing experience.

Grief may manifest itself in a variety of ways, ranging from withdrawal and anger to physical symptoms. There may be feelings of intense guilt, and family relationships may be badly strained by misplaced blame and by severe and persistent grief. Parents may lose confidence in their ability to care properly for any other children. The family should be prepared for a visit from the police and the need for a postmortem examination of the baby. Siblings are also likely to be affected by the death; their grief may be expressed through nightmares, bed-wetting, misbehaviour, or regression to outgrown habits. Some siblings fear they will die in the same way.

Professionals, such as a general practitioner, a paediatrician, a social worker, and a priest, can provide support. Talking to other parents who have been through the same experience can provide great comfort.

Sudeck's atrophy

Swelling and loss of use of a hand or foot after a *fracture* or other injury.

Pain, swelling, and stiffness (especially in the joints) develop in the affected hand or foot about two months after the original injury, usually after the plaster cast has been removed. The nails may stop growing normally and hair on the affected limb may fall out. Despite physiotherapy and attempts to start using the hand or foot again, the symptoms persist.

S

The condition is diagnosed by *X-rays*, which usually show thinning of the bones (see *Osteoporosis*).

Treatment includes elevation of the affected hand or foot, gentle exercise, and *heat treatment*. Complete recovery is usual within about four months. However, if pain persists, a *nerve block* may be tried and, if the block is temporarily successful in relieving pain, *sympathectomy* (an operation to destroy sympathetic nerve pathways) may be attempted. (See also *Shoulder-hand syndrome*.)

Suffocation

A condition in which there is a lack of oxygen due to an obstruction to the passage of air into the lungs. Suffocation may be caused by blockage of the nose and mouth, by blockage of the pharynx or larynx, or by blockage of the trachea. (See also *Asphyxia*; *Choking*; *Strangulation*.)

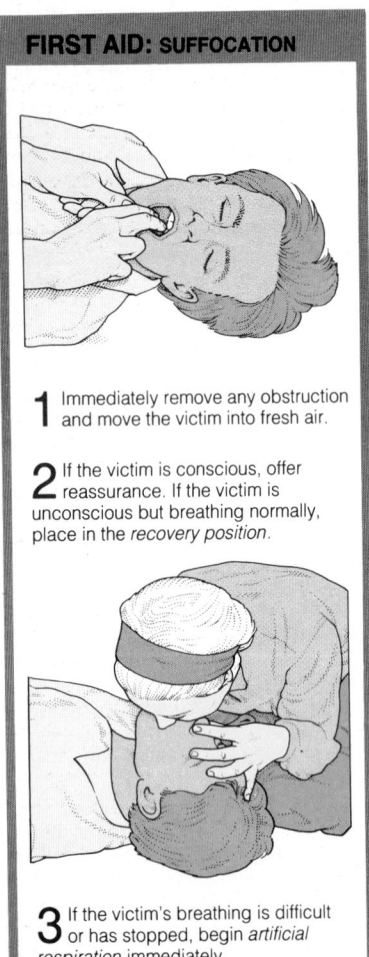

FIRST AID: SUFFOCATION

1 Immediately remove any obstruction and move the victim into fresh air.

2 If the victim is conscious, offer reassurance. If the victim is unconscious but breathing normally, place in the *recovery position*.

3 If the victim's breathing is difficult or has stopped, begin *artificial respiration* immediately.

Sugar

See *Carbohydrates*.

Suicide

The act of intentionally killing oneself. In the UK, suicide accounts for over 4,000 deaths each year.

CAUSES

More than 90 per cent of suicides occur as the result of a psychiatric illness. Suicide victims include about 15 per cent of people suffering from severe *depression*, about 10 per cent of those with *schizophrenia* (particularly young males in the early stages of the illness), about seven per cent of those suffering from *alcohol dependence*, about five per cent of those with an *antisocial personality disorder*, and a small percentage of people suffering from some form of *neurosis*.

Suicide results from a person's reaction to a perceivedly overwhelming problem, such as social isolation, recent death of a loved one (especially a spouse), a broken home in childhood, serious physical illness, growing old, unemployment, financial problems, and drug abuse.

INCIDENCE

The incidence of suicide shows wide variation from one country to another (see table). Published figures may not reflect the true number of suicides in some countries, especially where there are poor systems of reporting deaths or where suicide is considered to be sinful or shameful.

Suicide is most common among the elderly, but recent years have seen a marked increase in the suicide rate among young people. More men than women commit suicide, although women attempt the act more often (see *Suicide, attempted*). Marital status is also a factor. Suicide is most common in divorced people, less so in the single and widowed, and least common in those who are married. For unknown reasons, suicide is more common in spring and summer.

METHODS

The most common method of committing suicide is poisoning, usually by taking an overdose of analgesic drugs (painkillers) or sleeping tablets or by inhaling car exhaust fumes. Violent methods of committing suicide, such as shooting, are far more common in men than in women.

PREVENTION

One myth about suicide is that only people who are not serious about suicide talk about it beforehand. In fact, many people who commit suicide threaten repeatedly to take their own

lives; relatives and friends should always take such threats seriously. Suicidal people usually feel desperately lonely, and the opportunity to talk to a sympathetic, understanding listener is sometimes enough to prevent the despairing act. It was for this reason that suicide prevention centres (notably the Samaritans) were established to provide a 24-hour telephone counselling service for suicidal people.

Following a suicide threat, family or friends should remove any obvious means of committing the act and should watch the person closely. The person's general practitioner or psychiatrist should be consulted immediately so that appropriate treatment may be given. Hospitalization (or frequent sessions with a psychiatrist) may be necessary to provide enough support to help a suicidal person through a crisis period.

Suicide, attempted

Any deliberate act of self-harm that is or is believed to be life-threatening but that in effect proves nonfatal. Most attempted suicides, also known as parasuicides, are carried out in a setting that makes rescue possible. They must therefore be viewed as cries for help by people in extreme distress.

CAUSES AND INCIDENCE

People who attempt suicide constitute a sociologically different group from those who actually kill themselves (see *Suicide*), although there is some overlap between the two. Parasuicide is three times more common in women than in men and is most common in the 15 to 30 age group and in single and divorced people. The rate is highest among people with personality disorders, those who live in deprived urban areas, and those who have problems with alcohol or drugs. Common precipitating factors include an argument with a relative or sexual partner, the recent death of a loved one, financial worries, or severe loss of any kind that results in depression.

Suicide attempts far outnumber actual suicides and, since the 1950s, have become one of the primary reasons for hospital admission. The most common method used is to take an overdose of drugs, most often analgesic drugs (painkillers) or sleeping tablets, often with alcohol.

TREATMENT AND PREVENTION

If someone is discovered to have taken a drug overdose, emergency help should be summoned; if the person is unconscious or not breathing, first-aid

S

SUICIDE RATES (per 100,000 population, age standardized to world population)

Country	Year	Rate
Finland	1991	27.3
Switzerland	1991	24.0
Belgium	1987	16.3
Austria	1991	16.3
Denmark	1991	16.1
France	1990	15.6
Sweden	1989	14.4
Luxembourg	1991	14.2
Czechoslovakia	1990	13.9
Norway	1990	13.6
New Zealand	1989	12.6
Poland	1991	12.6
Germany	1990	11.8
Australia	1988	11.7
Japan	1991	11.5
Canada	1990	11.0
Bulgaria	1991	10.9
USA	1989	10.7
Netherlands	1990	10.2
Portugal	1991	7.4
UK	1991	6.9
Italy	1989	5.1
Greece	1990	2.6

measures should be carried out (see *Drug poisoning*). In other cases, appropriate measures depend on the victim's condition.

All suicide attempts should be treated seriously. Twenty to 30 per cent of people who attempt suicide repeat their attempt within a year, and 10 per cent eventually kill themselves, especially socially isolated men with a physical or mental illness.

The basis of treatment is to provide support, to treat any underlying depression, and to help the person to resolve the difficulties which precipitated the suicide attempt. In some cases, referral for psychiatric help may be necessary but in many cases, the general practitioner can provide the appropriate medical help.

Sulindac

A *nonsteroidal anti-inflammatory drug* (NSAID) used to relieve joint pain and stiffness caused by various types of *arthritis*. Adverse effects are typical of other NSAIDs, including indigestion, *peptic ulcer*, rash and itching, and, rarely, wheezing and breathlessness.

Sulphasalazine

A drug used to relieve inflammation in the intestinal disorders *ulcerative colitis* and *Crohn's disease*. It is also used in cases of resistant *rheumatoid arthritis*.

The drug may cause nausea, vomiting, headache, abdominal pain, loss of appetite, and, occasionally, fever and rash as an allergic reaction. Prolonged treatment may cause *folic acid* deficiency, resulting in *anaemia*.

Sulphinpyrazone

A drug used to treat *gout* (a type of arthritis associated with an excessive level of uric acid in the blood). Sulphinpyrazone does not relieve the symptoms of gout but does reduce the frequency of attacks.

Sulphinpyrazone is also given to reduce *hyperuricaemia* (raised levels of uric acid in the blood) caused by certain drugs, such as thiazide *diuretic drugs* and some *anticancer drugs*. Sulphinpyrazone reduces the amount of uric acid in the blood by increasing the amount excreted in the urine.

POSSIBLE ADVERSE EFFECTS
Adverse effects of the drug include nausea, vomiting, headache, flushing, cloudy or bloodstained urine, rash, itching, wheezing, and breathlessness.

Sulphonamide drugs

COMMON DRUGS

Sulphadiazine Sulphadimidine Sulphamethoxazole

A group of *antibacterial drugs*. Before the large-scale production of *penicillin drugs*, sulphonamide drugs were widely used to treat infectious diseases. Today, they are used mainly to treat urinary tract infections.

The combination drug *co-trimoxazole*, which contains the sulphonamide drug sulphamethoxazole and *trimethoprim*, is used to treat various infections, including *bronchitis*, certain types of *pneumonia*, skin infections, and infections of the middle ear.

Sulphur

A mineral that plays several important roles in the body. Sulphur is a constituent of vitamin B_1 (see *Vitamin B complex*) and several essential *amino acids*. It is needed for the manufacture of *collagen* (which helps to form bones, tendons, and connective tissue) and is a constituent of *keratin* (the chief component of the hair, skin, and nails).

MEDICAL USES
Sulphur is used in some ointments, creams, and skin preparations in the treatment of various skin disorders, including acne, dandruff, psoriasis, scabies, nappy rash, and certain fungal infections.

Sulpiride

An *antipsychotic drug* used in the treatment of *schizophrenia* and *Gilles de la Tourette's syndrome*.

Sumatriptan

A drug that relieves acute attacks of *migraine*. It acts on the same receptors in the brain as 5 hydroxytryptamine, a neurotransmitter and vasoconstrictor, and gives dramatic relief within a few minutes of injection. Sumatriptan may also be taken by mouth. It should not be taken within 24 hours of treatment with the standard migraine drug *ergotamine*, nor should ergotamine be given within six hours of sumatriptan.

Sumatriptan may cause chest pain and tightness, and should not be taken by people with coronary artery disease or other causes of angina. Other side-effects include flushing, dizziness, and feelings of weakness.

Sunburn

Inflammation of the *skin* caused by overexposure to the sun. The *ultraviolet light* in sunlight may destroy cells in the outer layer of the skin and damage tiny blood vessels beneath.

Sunburn is most common in fair-skinned people, whose skin produces only small amounts of the protective pigment *melanin*, and in people who attempt to acquire a tan too quickly in strong sunlight. The affected skin turns red and tender and may become blistered. Several days later the dead skin cells are shed by peeling. In severe cases, sunburn may be accompanied by symptoms of *sunstroke*—such as vomiting, fever, and collapse.

Repeated overexposure to sunlight can cause various adverse effects (see *Sunlight, adverse effects of*).

PREVENTION
Exposure to strong sunlight should be limited to no more than 15 minutes on the first day, particularly in the fair-skinned, and should be increased very gradually. This applies even in hazy conditions. Until a tan is acquired, the skin should be covered or protected with a high protection factor *sunscreen*.

TREATMENT
Calamine lotion or a sunburn cream should be applied to soothe the burned skin, which should be protected from further exposure to the sun until healing takes place. *Analgesic drugs* (painkillers) may be needed to relieve tenderness. A person with severe sunburn should consult a doctor, who may prescribe a cream containing a corticosteroid drug to relieve the symptoms.

Sunlight, adverse effects of

Problems resulting from overexposure to the sun's rays. Some exposure to *ultraviolet light* from the sun is necessary for the body to produce

S

vitamin D. Overexposure can have various harmful effects, particularly in fair-skinned people, who produce only small amounts of the protective skin pigment *melanin*.

Short-term overexposure causes *sunburn* and, in intense heat, can result in *heat exhaustion* or *heatstroke*. Repeated overexposure over a long period can cause premature aging of the skin and wart-like growths called solar *keratoses*. It also increases the risk of *skin cancer*. Exposure should be limited, and the body protected by clothing or *sunscreens*.

Photosensitivity (abnormal sensitivity to sunlight) resulting in a skin rash may occur naturally or may be triggered by taking certain drugs. It may also occur in people suffering from systemic *lupus erythematosus* or *porphyria*.

Exposure to sunlight can also affect the eyes, causing irritation of the conjunctiva. More intense exposure may cause actinic *keratopathy* (damage to the cornea), also called snow-blindness. Symptoms include pain, watering and redness of the eyes, and photophobia; these usually clear up in a few days. Prolonged exposure to bright sunlight may cause *pterygium* (conjunctival thickening). Good sunglasses should be worn to avoid overexposing the eyes to sunlight.

Sunscreens

```
WARNING
Some suntanning preparations do not
contain a sunscreen and therefore
provide no protection against
sunburn.
```

Preparations that help protect the skin from the harmful effects of sunlight (see *Sunlight, adverse effects of*). Sunscreens should be used to help prevent sunburn and not as a substitute for avoiding exposure. Most sunscreens work by absorbing ultraviolet rays, but some (such as titanium dioxide) reflect the sun's rays.

Sunscreen products may be labelled with a sun protection factor (SPF), the highest factor affording the greatest protection. Choice of product should depend on skin type (see box). A sunscreen with a lower SPF may be used once the skin is tanned. During prolonged sunbathing, sunscreens should be reapplied at regular intervals and also after swimming.

Some people are sensitive to the chemicals in sunscreens and develop a rash, most commonly with preparations containing PABA (para-amino-benzoic acid).

Sunstroke

The most common type of *heatstroke*. Sunstroke is usually brought on by overexposure to direct sun in a person who is unaccustomed to a hot climate. It is due to breakdown of the body's heat regulating mechanisms.

Suntan

Darkening of the *skin* after exposure to sunlight. Specialized cells in the outer layer of the skin respond to the *ultraviolet light* in sunlight by producing more of the protective pigment *melanin*. In dark-skinned people, this protective pigment is present in greater amounts. People who spend a lot of time in the sun are likely to experience premature aging and wrinkling of the skin and run a greatly increased risk of *skin cancer*. (See also *Sunlight, adverse effects of*; *Sunburn*.)

Superego

The part of the personality, as described in *psychoanalytic theory*, that is responsible for maintaining an individual's standards of behaviour. Popularly termed the "conscience", the superego arises as a result of a child's incorporating the ideals and moral views of those in authority (usually parents). The superego can create feelings of guilt and anxiety by criticizing the *ego* (the conscious "I") when the ego gives way to the impulses of the *id* (the pleasure seeking part of the personality).

In psychoanalytic theory, an excessively strong superego is said to be the cause of severe, puritanical personality types and of *obsessive-compulsive behaviour*. By contrast, failure to develop an appropriate superego leads to impulsive and immoral behaviour. A harsh, self-punishing superego is said to result from childhood experience with a harsh parent.

Superficial

Situated near the surface, as in the superficial blood vessels (the capillaries that lie near the surface of the skin and play a part in regulating body temperature and in blushing).

Superinfection

A second *infection* that occurs during the course of an existing infection. The term usually refers to an infection by a microorganism that is resistant to drugs being used against the original infection. The second microorganism may be a resistant strain of the first infection, a different pathogen (disease-causing microorganism), or a member of the body's normal flora (microorganisms that are normally present in the body without producing ill effects) that has proliferated excessively because other microorganisms that normally keep it in check have been killed by drug therapy. For example, *tetracycline* therapy may result in superinfection of the mouth, vagina, and/or anus with the fungus that causes *candidiasis* (thrush).

Superiority complex

An individual's exaggerated and unrealistic belief that he or she is better than other people. *Adlerian theory* suggests that a superiority complex develops in some people in response to the natural feelings of inferiority that everyone is born with. In more modern psychoanalytical theories, a superiority complex is considered to be a compensation for unconscious feelings of inadequacy or low self-esteem.

Supernumerary

A term meaning more than the normal number. For example, supernumerary nipples are additional nipples that develop along a line that extends from the armpit to the groin; these extra nipples are not usually associated with underlying glandular tissue. (See also *Supernumerary teeth*.)

RECOMMENDED MAXIMUM EXPOSURE TIMES USING SUNSCREENS

Protection factor	4	8	15
Skin type	Maximum exposure time		
Fair	10 minutes	40 to 80 minutes	1.5 to 2 hours
Medium	50 to 80 minutes	2 to 2.5 hours	5 to 5.5 hours
Dark	1.5 to 2 hours	3.5 to 4 hours	all day
Black	4 hours	all day	all day

S

Supernumerary teeth

One or more *teeth* in excess of the usual number (20 primary and 32 permanent). An extra tooth may be a duplicate of an existing tooth or it may have an abnormal shape and position (usually appearing as a small conical protrusion from the gum above the existing teeth in the upper front jaw).

Supernumerary teeth may interfere with the proper *eruption of teeth* and are therefore usually extracted.

Supination

The act of turning the body to a supine position (lying on the back with the face upward) or of turning the hand to a palm forward position. Movement in the opposite direction to supination is called *pronation.*

Suppository

A solid, cone- or bullet-shaped object containing a drug and an inert substance, usually derived from cocoa butter or another vegetable oil. The suppository is placed in the rectum and melts at body temperature, releasing the active ingredient.

Suppositories are used to treat rectal disorders, such as *haemorrhoids* or *proctitis.* They may also be used to soften faeces and stimulate defaecation. In addition, suppositories may be used to administer drugs into the general circulation via blood vessels in the rectum if vomiting is likely to prevent absorption after oral administration or if the drug would cause irritation of the stomach.

Drugs given by suppository include local anaesthetics, corticosteroids, antiemetics, antibiotics, nonsteroidal anti-inflammatory drugs, and antifungal drugs.

Suppuration

The formation or exudation of *pus.* Suppuration at the site of bacterial infection may result in the accumula-

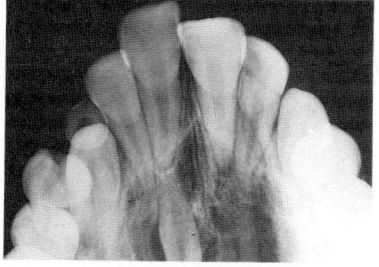

Supernumerary (extra) tooth
This X-ray of the upper jaw shows a supernumerary incisor tooth on the roof of the mouth behind the normal incisors.

tion of pus, forming an *abscess* in solid tissue or a *boil* or *pustule* on the skin. Open sores often suppurate, especially if they are slow to heal, because the exposed underlying tissue tends to become repeatedly infected.

Suprarenal glands

Another name for the *adrenal glands.*

Supraspinatus syndrome

See *Painful arc syndrome.*

Supraventricular tachycardia

An abnormally fast but regular heart-rate that occurs in episodes lasting for several hours or days. In most cases, the heart-rate in supraventricular tachycardia is between 140 and 180 beats per minute, but in rare cases it may be as fast as 300 beats per minute.

Supraventricular tachycardia occurs when abnormal electrical impulses that arise in the atria (upper chambers) of the heart take control of the heartbeat from the *sinoatrial node* (the heart's own natural pacemaker). Symptoms may include palpitations, breathlessness, chest pain, or fainting (see *Stokes-Adams syndrome*).

Diagnosis is made by an *ECG* (electrocardiogram). An attack can sometimes be terminated by *Valsalva's manoeuvre* or by drinking cold water. Recurrent attacks are treated with *antiarrhythmic drugs.* Rarely, the condition may require application of an electric shock to the heart (see *Defibrillation*).

Surfactant

A substance, such as a soap, detergent, or emulsifier, that reduces surface tension; a wetting agent. Pulmonary surfactant is a substance secreted by the alveoli (air sacs) in the lungs, preventing them from collapsing during exhalation. Artificial pulmonary surfactant is often given to very premature babies (see *Respiratory distress syndrome*).

Surfer's nodules

Multiple *exostoses* (bony outgrowths) occurring on bones in the foot and on the tibial tubercle (the bony prominence below the knee at the top of the shin). Surfer's nodules are caused by the repeated banging of the surfboard against the knees and tops of the feet as the surfer kneels to paddle the board. They can be avoided by paddling in a lying position.

Surgery

The treatment of disease, injury, or other disorders by direct physical intervention, usually with instru-

ments. The term is also used to denote those aspects of medical practice that deal with the study, diagnosis, and management of all disorders or injuries treated by operative surgery (as distinct from those treated by drugs, diet, or modification of lifestyle).

Operative surgery involves incision (cutting) into the skin or some other organ, inspection of tissues or organs, removal of diseased tissues or organs, relief of obstruction, replacement of structures in their normal position, redirection of body channels, transplantation of tissues or complete organs, and implantation of mechanical or electronic devices.

Surgery may be minor or major. Minor operations are usually, but not always, performed under local anaesthesia. Major operations are usually performed under general anaesthesia, although local anaesthesia is sometimes used.

Some surgeons, known as general surgeons, perform a variety of operations on almost all parts of the body. Other surgeons specialize in particular branches of surgery, such as orthopaedic surgery, neurosurgery, obstetrics and gynaecology, ophthalmology, gastrointestinal surgery, and plastic surgery. In recent years there has been an increasing trend towards further subspecialization; some surgeons now confine their practices to such narrow limits as surgery of the hand, the cornea, or the skin.

Surgical spirit

A liquid preparation, consisting mainly of ethyl alcohol, that has a soothing and hardening effect when applied to the skin. It is widely used before injections as an *antiseptic* and may also be used to prevent bedsores and to protect the soles of the feet before a long walk or run.

Surrogacy

The agreement by a woman to become pregnant and give birth to a child with the understanding that she will surrender the child after birth to the contractual parents. Surrogacy became publicized with the advent of *in vitro fertilization,* in which the egg and sperm are brought together in the laboratory. The fertilized egg can be transferred to the uterus of any woman who is at the appropriate stage of the menstrual cycle.

Another means of accomplishing surrogacy is through the *artificial insemination* of the surrogate mother with the contracting father's sperm.

S

The ethical and legal aspects of surrogacy have yet to be resolved. In a number of countries a woman who wishes to act as a surrogate for her infertile sister can be helped to do so. Surrogacy for financial reward has been forbidden by law in some countries, including the UK.

Susceptibility

A total or partial vulnerability to an infection, disease, or disorder. In *AIDS*, the *immune system* is impaired and the sufferer is susceptible to a wide range of infections and diseases.

Suture

A type of *joint*, found only between the bones of the *skull*, in which the adjacent bones are mobile during birth but then become so closely and firmly joined by a thin layer of fibrous connective tissue that movement between them is impossible.

The term suture is also used to refer to a surgical stitch (see *Suturing*).

Suturing

The closing of a surgical incision or a wound by sutures (stitches) to promote healing.

MATERIALS USED

Various sterile materials can be used as sutures. These include: catgut (obtained from sheep intestines); linen, silk, or synthetic thread; and stainless steel wire. Suture materials vary considerably in the length of time they retain their strength, the reaction they provoke in tissues, and the likelihood of their allowing minute pockets of infection to form. Certain materials, such as catgut, are absorbable (i.e. they eventually dissolve in the body). The choice of which material to use for an operation is made by the surgeon. The thickness of sutures varies from almost 1 mm, used for the repair of major injuries, to a barely visible 0.01 mm, used for delicate eye and blood vessel surgery.

Most surgical needles are curved and have a point with a cutting edge. The needle is held in a tweezer-like instrument; larger needles may be held with the fingers.

HOW IT IS DONE

The method of suturing a typical incision, and some alternative methods of skin closure, are shown in the illustrated box. Deep incisions or wounds may need to be sutured at several levels to achieve full closure throughout the depth of tissue, thus preventing accumulation of blood in pockets below the surface.

METHODS OF SUTURING

Suturing is carried out under a general or local anaesthetic. The type of stitch used depends on the nature of the wound or incision (two types are shown below). In all cases the surgeon sews the wound edges together to produce minimal distortion of tissue.

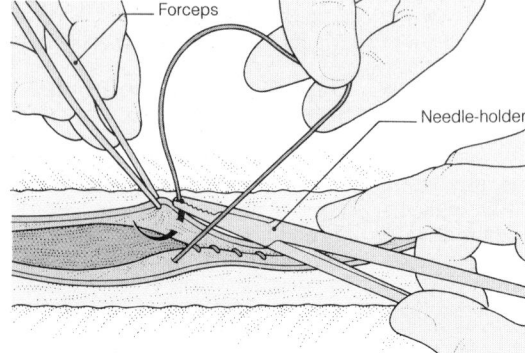
Forceps · Needle-holder

Technique
The surgeon grasps the edge of the wound with forceps held in one hand and, with the other hand, inserts the needle through the skin. In this illustration, the surgeon is shown using a needle-holder, which gives greater control for very fine stitches. In other cases, the needle may be held in the hand.

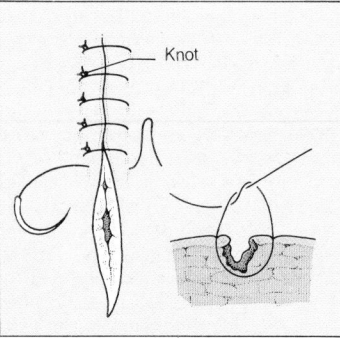
Knot

Standard interrupted sutures
The needle is passed into one skin edge, through the full depth of the wound, and out of the other skin edge. Each stitch is then knotted at the side.

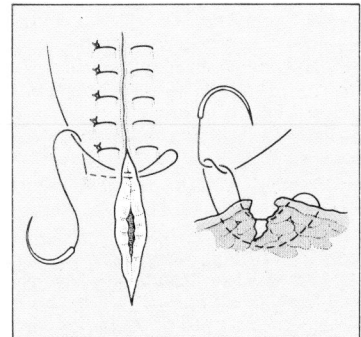

Mattress sutures
For deeper wounds, the needle is passed through the wound twice: first shallowly, close to the skin edges, and then more deeply, farther from the edges.

OTHER METHODS OF CLOSURE

Alternatives to suturing include removable staples and clips 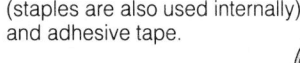 (staples are also used internally) and adhesive tape.

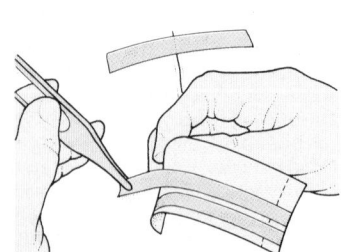

Adhesive tape
When the wound is shallow, tape may be applied directly. For deeper wounds, absorbable stitches are first inserted just below the skin.

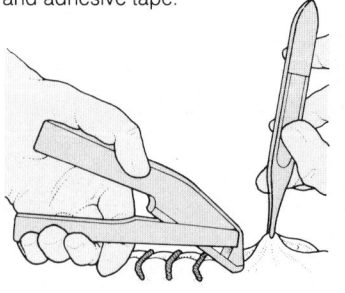

Inserting staples
The wound edges are held up with forceps and equally spaced staples are inserted using an automatic stapling device.

Internal sutures, made of absorbable material, are left in place permanently. Skin sutures are removed by a painless procedure about one to two weeks after insertion.

Swab

A wad of absorbent material used in surgery or to obtain a sample of bacteria from an infected patient.

A surgical swab is commonly a folded piece of cotton gauze held in the hand or in a clamp. It is used to apply cleansing and antiseptic solutions to the skin before an incision is made and to soak up blood and other fluids during an operation. The swab often contains material opaque to X-rays to enable it to be detected if it is accidentally left in the body, an occurrence that is usually prevented by a "swab count" made before the operation begins and again before the patient is stitched up.

A microbiological swab consists of a twist of cottonwool at the end of a thin stick, supplied in a sterile container. The swab is applied to an infected area of the body to absorb pus or mucus, from which a *culture* can be grown to identify infective microorganisms, such as bacteria.

Swallowing

The process by which food or liquid is conveyed from the mouth to the stomach via the oesophagus. The first stage is voluntary (under conscious control), but is so familiar that little thought is given to it. Once food has been well chewed and mixed with saliva (which greatly facilitates swallowing), the tongue pushes it to the back of the mouth and the voluntary muscles in the palate push the food into the pharynx (throat).

The rest of the swallowing process is involuntary (automatic), brought about by a series of *reflexes*; once started, it is rapid, powerful, and difficult to stop. Entry of food into the pharynx causes the epiglottis (a flap of cartilage) to close over the larynx (voice-box) leading to the trachea (windpipe). A sphincter (circular muscle) at the top of the oesophagus relaxes, and the muscles of the pharynx seize the food and squeeze it in the form of a bolus (rounded lump) into the oesophagus. Powerful waves of contraction then pass down the oesophagus, propelling the food towards the stomach. Finally, the muscle at the entry to the stomach (the cardiac sphincter) relaxes and allows the bolus to pass.

Swallowing difficulty

A fairly common symptom with a wide variety of causes, known medically as dysphagia.

CAUSES

Temporary swallowing difficulty may be caused by a foreign object (such as a fish-bone) lodging at the back of the throat or in the oesophagus. Most foreign objects are able to pass on to the stomach, but a scratch in the lining of the throat or oesophagus may cause discomfort. Swallowing difficulty may also result from insufficient production of saliva (see *Mouth, dry*).

Disorders of the oesophagus that may disrupt normal swallowing include *oesophageal spasm* (uncoordinated contractions of the oesophagus), *oesophageal stricture* (narrowing) caused by scarring or a tumour (see *Oesophagus, cancer of*), *oesophagitis* (inflammation), *achalasia* (abnormal contraction of the muscles at the lower end of the oesophagus), or an *oesophageal diverticulum* (an outward protrusion of part of the oesophagus).

Oesophageal atresia (closure or failure of the oesophagus to open) can cause feeding problems in the newborn.

Difficulty in swallowing may also be caused by a nervous system disorder (e.g. *myasthenia gravis*, or *stroke*). It may also have a psychological cause, as in *globus hystericus*.

Pressure on the outside of the oesophagus may obstruct the passage of food. Rarely, pressure is exerted by a *goitre*, an aortic *aneurysm*, or cancer of the bronchus (see *Lung cancer*).

DIAGNOSIS AND TREATMENT

Any person who experiences persistent swallowing difficulty should be examined without delay. Investigations may include *oesophagoscopy* (examination of the oesophagus with a viewing instrument) or barium swallow (see *Barium X-ray examinations*). Treatment depends on the cause.

Swamp fever

Another name for *leptospirosis*, an infectious disease caused by contact with water contaminated by rat's urine. The term has also been applied to *malaria* (swamps being a favourite breeding ground for mosquitoes).

Sweat glands

Minute structures deep within the *skin* that produce sweat. Each gland is made up of a coiled tube, in which the sweat is secreted, and a narrow passageway, which carries the sweat to the skin surface. The average person has about three million sweat glands.

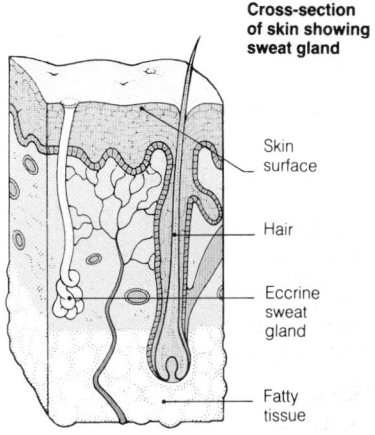

Cross-section of skin showing sweat gland

Skin surface

Hair

Eccrine sweat gland

Fatty tissue

TYPES

There are two types of sweat glands: eccrine and apocrine. Eccrine glands are the most common, especially on the palms and soles; these glands open directly to the skin surface. Apocrine glands, which develop at puberty, occur only in hairy areas, particularly the armpits, pubic region, and around the anus. These glands produce cellular material as well as sweat, and open into a hair follicle before reaching the skin surface.

FUNCTION

Eccrine sweat is composed mainly of water (99 per cent) and minute quantities of dissolved substances, including sodium chloride (salt).

The activity of the sweat glands is controlled by the *autonomic nervous system*. Usually the glands are stimulated to produce sweat to keep the body cool, in which case sweating is heaviest on the forehead, upper lip, neck, and chest. Sweating can also be caused by anxiety or fear, in which case sweat appears mainly on the palms and soles and in the armpits. Sweating also occurs with fevers.

Sweat is odourless until bacteria act upon it, producing *body odour*.

DISORDERS

The most common problem affecting the sweat glands is *prickly heat*, an intensely irritating skin rash caused by blockage of the glands with debris and sweat. Less common disorders include *hyperhidrosis* (excessive sweating), *hypohidrosis* (reduced sweating), and abnormal or excessive skin odour.

Sweating

The process by which the body cools itself. Sweating also occurs as a response to psychological stress or fear. (See *Sweat glands*; *Heat disorders*.)

S

Sweeteners, artificial
See *Artificial sweeteners*.

Swimmer's ear
A common name for *otitis externa*.

Sycosis barbae
Inflammation of the beard area, also called barbers' itch. The condition is caused by infection of the hair follicles, usually with *STAPHYLOCOCCUS AUREUS* bacteria contracted from infected razors and towels. Pus-filled blisters or boils develop around the follicles, sometimes resulting in severe scarring unless they are treated. Treatment is usually with *antibiotic drugs*; growing a beard may help to prevent a recurrence.

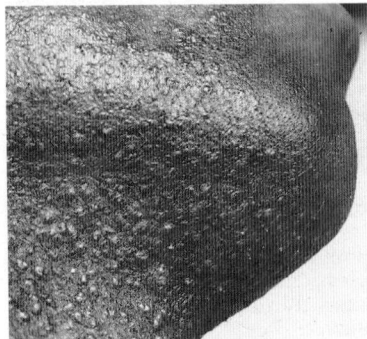

The characteristics of sycosis barbae
Sycosis barbae is caused by folliculitis (infection and inflammation of hair follicles) in the beard area. It tends to affect men with greasy skin, and may be persistent.

Sydenham's chorea
A childhood disorder of the *central nervous system*, formerly called Saint Vitus' dance. The condition is characterized by involuntary (uncontrolled), irregular, jerky movements and usually follows an attack of *rheumatic fever*. Sydenham's chorea is hardly ever seen in the UK today but remains common in developing countries.

Restlessness and irritability usually precede the chorea, which affects the head, face, limbs, and fingers. The involuntary "fidgets" are random and unrepetitive. Voluntary (willed) movements are clumsy and the limbs are often floppy. Early signs are slurred speech and deteriorating handwriting.

Treatment is bed rest and *antibiotic drugs*. Sedation is sometimes necessary if the fidgeting is extreme. The condition usually clears up after two to three months and has no long-term adverse effects. Thereafter, the per-

son may be given antibiotics before surgical or dental treatment to prevent possible heart complications.

Sympathectomy
An operation in which the ganglia (nerve terminals) of sympathetic nerves are destroyed to interrupt the nerve pathway and thus improve blood supply to a limb or relieve chronic pain.

WHY IT IS DONE
The sympathetic nerves form part of the *autonomic nervous system* and control involuntary (automatic) activities in the body, including the widening and narrowing of blood vessels. In *peripheral vascular disease* (a disorder in which the blood vessels in the legs and sometimes in the arms become narrowed), stimulation from the sympathetic nerves produces spasms in the blood vessels that worsen the narrowing. Sympathectomy prevents these spasms from occurring and thus may improve blood supply to the affected area.

The sympathetic nerves also play an important part in producing the sensation of *pain*. In some cases of *causalgia* (a persistent severe pain usually caused by nerve injury), sympathectomy offers the only prospect of relieving the pain.

HOW IT IS DONE
The surgeon may first perform a trial procedure, injecting local anaesthetic into the nerves supplying the affected area. If this provides considerable temporary relief of symptoms, a sympathectomy is usually performed.

Destruction of the nerve ganglia, which lie near the spinal cord, can be accomplished by injecting a sclerosing solution, which causes inflammation and subsequent degeneration of the nerves. Symptoms in the upper part of the body are controlled by an injection into the cervicodorsal sympathetic nerves at the base of the neck. To treat disorders of the lower part of the body, sclerosing solution is injected into the lumbar sympathetic nerves in the middle of the back.

Alternatively, nerve ganglia may be destroyed surgically while the patient is under general anaesthesia. In a cervicodorsal sympathectomy, destruction of the ganglia is achieved through an incision made in the armpit; in a lumbar sympathectomy, the incision runs horizontally from the spine in the lower back almost to the navel.

RESULTS
In general, results depend on the disease for which the procedure is being

performed. A sympathectomy performed to widen blood vessels has variable results. In controlling severe pain, however, the operation usually proves successful. Lumbar sympathectomy in men occasionally results in inability to ejaculate.

Sympathetic nervous system
One of the two divisions of the *autonomic nervous system*. In conjunction with the other division (the parasympathetic nervous system), this system controls many of the involuntary (automatic) activities of the glands, organs, and other parts of the body.

Symphysis
An anatomical term for a type of *joint* in which two bones are firmly joined by tough, fibrous cartilage. Such joints occur between the bodies of the *vertebrae* (the bodies are the parts of the vertebrae that are separated by the intervertebral discs); between the two pubic bones at the front of the *pelvis*; and between the manubrium (upper part) and body (middle part) of the *sternum* (breastbone).

Symptom
An indication of a disease or disorder (such as pain) that is noticed by the sufferer. By contrast, the indications that a doctor notes are called signs. The overall clinical picture, including both symptoms and signs, helps a doctor to identify a particular disease.

Symptoms that prompt a person to obtain medical advice are known as presenting symptoms; such symptoms are not necessarily those that are the first to appear.

The distinction between symptoms and signs is not always clear. For example, fever is experienced by the patient and observed by the doctor. Similarly, in *appendicitis*, pain is a key symptom; tenderness, which is pain felt only when pressure is applied, is a sign generally elicited by the doctor, but which may also be elicited by the patient pressing on his or her own abdomen.

In some conditions, accurate recollection and precise description of symptoms are extremely important for an accurate diagnosis. For example, because physical signs are often absent in *angina pectoris*, diagnosis of this condition may depend almost entirely on the patient's description of the chest pain.

Symptothermal method
See *Contraception, natural methods of*.

Synapse

A junctional connection between two *neurons* (nerve cells) across which a signal can pass. A single neuron may form thousands of these connections with adjacent nerve cells.

A typical neuron has one long fibre (axon) that projects from its cell body, and this splits into several smaller branches and twigs, each ending in a terminal that forms a synapse, usually close to the cell body of an adjacent neuron. At a synapse, the two neurons do not come directly into contact; their surface membranes are separated by a gap known as the synaptic cleft. When an electrical signal passes along a neuronal axon and reaches a synapse, it cannot bridge the cleft directly; instead, it causes the release of a chemical, called a *neurotransmitter*. The neurotransmitter travels across the synaptic cleft and is received at the surface membrane of the next neuron, where it changes the electrical potential of the membrane.

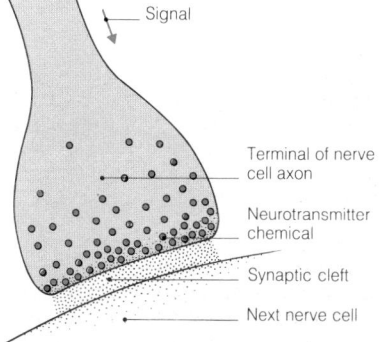

Structure of a synapse
When a signal arrives at the terminal of a nerve cell axon, it causes release of a neurotransmitter, which crosses the synaptic cleft and affects the next cell.

The axonal membrane from which the neurotransmitter is released is called the presynaptic membrane; the neuronal membrane at which it is received is called the postsynaptic membrane. Signals can be transmitted across a synapse in one direction only—from presynaptic to postsynaptic membrane.

A synapse may be excitatory or inhibitory. When a neurotransmitter passes across an excitatory synapse, the effect is to excite the postsynaptic membrane, making it more likely that the receptor neuron will "fire" and propagate an electrical impulse in turn. Inhibitory synapses decrease the excitation of the next neuron.

Most drugs that affect the *nervous system* work as a result of their effects on synapses. Such drugs may affect the release of neurotransmitters (e.g. *reserpine* and *amphetamine drugs*), or they may modify the effects of neurotransmitters on postsynaptic membranes (the mode of action of *atropine* and *beta-blocker drugs*).

Syncope

The medical term for *fainting*.

Syndactyly

A congenital (present at birth) defect in which two or more fingers or toes are joined. The toes of one or both feet are more frequently affected than the fingers.

Syndactyly is often inherited and is more common in males than females. The condition is caused by incomplete development of the digits at the embryo stage, or by constriction of the digits by tissue within the uterus later in fetal development.

In mild cases of syndactyly, the affected fingers or toes are joined only by a web of skin. In more serious cases, the bones of adjacent digits are fused, as is the overlying skin, and there may be only one nail.

Treatment is usually by one or more operations during early childhood to separate the affected digits.

Syndrome

A group of symptoms and/or signs that, occurring together, constitutes a particular disorder. For example, *irritable bowel syndrome* is characterized by a combination of any or all of the following: intermittent pain in the lower abdomen (usually relieved by passing faeces or wind), abdominal swelling, irregular bowel movements (often with a sense of incomplete evacuation of the bowel afterwards), mucus in the faeces, excessive wind, and worsening of symptoms after eating.

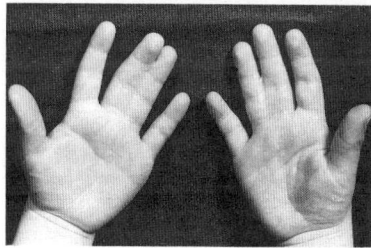

Syndactyly
In this case, the middle and ring fingers of both hands are partly joined. Sometimes, syndactyly occurs in association with other birth defects.

Synovectomy

Surgical removal of the *synovium* (thin membrane lining a joint capsule) to treat recurrent or persistent *synovitis* (inflammation of the synovium), usually in sufferers from severe *rheumatoid arthritis*. The operation is usually performed only if the condition is severely disabling and has not responded to injections of *corticosteroid drugs* or to the taking of *nonsteroidal anti-inflammatory drugs* or *antirheumatic drugs*.

The joint may be opened and the synovium cut away under general anaesthesia, or the operation may be performed by means of *arthroscopy*. After the operation, the joint is kept mobile to inhibit scarring. Synovectomy is a temporary expedient that usually improves symptoms for no more than about two years; further surgery may then be required.

Synovitis

Inflammation of the *synovium* (thin membrane lining a joint capsule). The condition may be acute (of sudden onset and short duration), in which case it is usually caused by an attack of arthritis, injury, overuse of the joint, or infection; or chronic (recurrent or persistent), as in a disorder such as *rheumatoid arthritis*.

The inflammation causes the synovium to secrete an abnormal amount of lubricating fluid, which makes the joint swollen, painful, and often warm and red. To determine the cause of the condition, joint aspiration (removal of fluid from a joint) or a *biopsy* (removal of a sample of the synovium) may be required.

TREATMENT
Symptoms are relieved by rest, supporting the joint with a *splint* or *cast*, *analgesic drugs* (painkillers), *nonsteroidal anti-inflammatory drugs*, and, occasionally, an injection of a *corticosteroid drug*. Any causative infection is treated with *antibiotic drugs*. Chronic synovitis that does not respond to drug treatment or injection may be treated by *synovectomy* (surgical removal of the synovium).

Synovium

A thin membrane that lines the fibrous capsule surrounding a movable *joint*. The synovium also forms a sheath for certain tendons of the hands and feet, lining the fibrous or bony tunnels through which they glide. The membrane secretes synovial fluid, a clear, sticky liquid resembling egg white that lubricates the

S

LOCATION OF SYNOVIUM
Every movable joint is enclosed within a fibrous capsule. The inner lining of the capsule is known as the synovium.

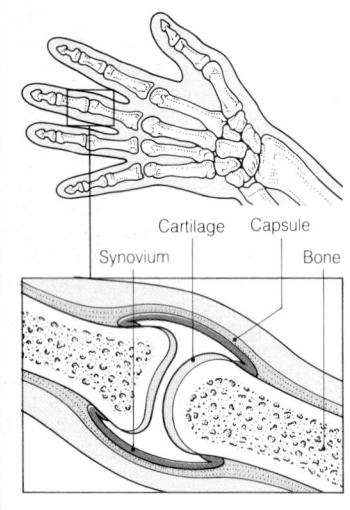

Cartilage   Capsule

Synovium   Bone

Function
The membrane secretes a thick fluid (synovial fluid) that lubricates the joint; the fluid may accumulate and cause pain if the joint is injured.

joint or the tendon. The synovium can become inflamed; in a joint lining this is known as *synovitis*, in a tendon sheath it is known as *tenosynovitis*.

Syphilis
A *sexually transmitted disease* or *congenital* (present from birth) infection of worldwide distribution, first recorded as a major epidemic in Europe in the last decade of the 15th century following the return of Columbus from America. Today, infection is transmitted almost exclusively by sexual contact. Congenital syphilis was once very common but is now very rare. The incidence of syphilis has fallen dramatically since the introduction of penicillin. About 3,500 new cases are reported from sexually transmitted disease clinics in the UK each year.

CAUSES
Syphilis is caused by *TREPONEMA PALLIDUM*, a spirochaete (spiral-shaped bacterium) that penetrates broken skin or *mucous membranes* in the genitalia, rectum, or mouth during sexual intercourse. Infection may also be acquired by kissing or by other intimate bodily contact with an infected person. The risk of infection during a

single contact with an infected person is about 30 per cent. After gaining access, the organism passes quickly by way of the bloodstream and lymphatic system to all parts of the body; within hours, the organism has spread beyond any hope of local treatment.

INCIDENCE
The incidence of syphilis in the UK has remained fairly constant at about 2,000 to 5,000 new cases reported per year since the 1960s. The incidence rose during the 1970s but fell back in the 1980s. The infection is most common in homosexual men.

SYMPTOMS AND SIGNS
Untreated syphilis usually passes through the following stages.

PRIMARY The first symptom is a primary sore (chancre) that usually appears three to four weeks after contact. The chancre is a painless ulcer measuring less than 1 cm in diameter. It has a hard, wet base that is covered with serum teeming with spirochaetes. The ulcer usually develops on the genitals but other possible sites include the anus, rectum, lips, throat, and, very rarely, the fingers. Often, the chancre is inconspicuous and may be missed. The lymph nodes connected with the area containing the chancre become painlessly enlarged and rubbery but are not tender. The chancre heals in four to eight weeks.

SECONDARY Six to 12 weeks after infection, the secondary stage begins. The most obvious feature is a skin rash, which may be transient, recurrent, or may last for months. In white people, the rash is conspicuous, with crops of pinkish or pale red, round spots; in black people, the rash is pigmented and appears darker than the normal skin colour. The rash may be associated with extensive lymph node enlargement. Other possible symptoms include headache, aches and pains in the bones, loss of appetite, fever, and fatigue. The hair may fall out in clumps. Thickened, grey or pink patches called condylomata lata may develop on moist areas of skin and are highly infectious. Meningitis may also develop.

LATENT During this stage, which may last for a few years or may even continue indefinitely, the infected person appears to be normal. However, a few untreated cases proceed, eventually, to tertiary syphilis.

TERTIARY This stage usually starts within 10 years of infection, but may appear as early as three years or as late as 25 years afterwards. The effects are

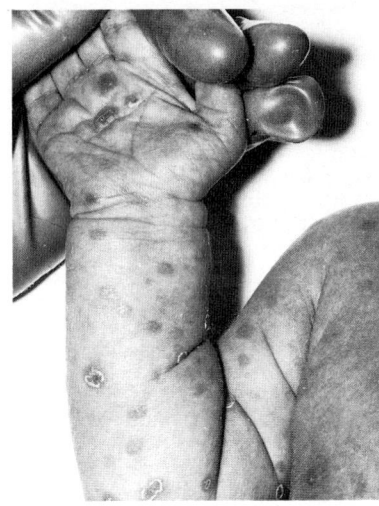

Congenital syphilis
This baby's mother had syphilis during pregnancy. Signs of infection developed in the baby early in life, including a rash, persistent snuffles, bone abnormalities, jaundice, and enlargement of the liver and spleen. Further abnormalities may become apparent years later, such as keratitis (inflammation of the cornea), arthritis, a characteristic facial appearance (with a flat face and saddle-shaped nose), peg-shaped teeth, and mental handicap. Congenital syphilis is rare today: about 65 cases are reported annually in England. Prevention depends mainly on antenatal blood tests.

varied. Tissue destruction, by a process called gumma formation, may involve the bones, palate, nasal septum, tongue, skin, or almost any organ of the body. Among the more serious effects are cardiovascular syphilis, which affects the aorta (the main artery of the body) and leads to aneurysm formation and heart valve disease; neurosyphilis, with progressive brain damage and general paralysis (formerly called general paralysis of the insane); and tabes dorsalis, which affects part of the spinal cord.

DIAGNOSIS
Primary syphilis can be readily diagnosed by finding active spirochaetes during microscopic examination of a smear taken from the chancre serum. Confirmation is given by blood tests, such as the Venereal Disease Research Laboratory (VDRL) test or the fluorescent treponemal antibody absorption test. Secondary, latent, and tertiary syphilis give strongly positive results with these and similar tests. In cases of neurosyphilis, it may be necessary to perform these tests on a sample of cerebrospinal fluid.

S

TREATMENT

All forms of the disease are treated by a course of a *penicillin drug*. Although penicillin is, in general, very safe, the treatment of syphilis is not without danger. More than half of those treated suffer a severe reaction within six to 12 hours, caused by the body's response to the sudden killing of large numbers of spirochaetes. Organ damage already caused by the disease cannot be reversed.

PREVENTION

Promiscuous heterosexual or homosexual intercourse inevitably involves a risk of infection with syphilis. Infection can be avoided by maintaining monogamous relationships. Condoms offer some measure of protection but do not offer absolute protection (see *Safer sex*). People with syphilis are infectious in the primary and secondary stages but not in the latent and tertiary stages.

Syphilis, nonvenereal

A disease caused by the same organism that causes sexually transmitted *syphilis* but that is spread by different means, such as through broken skin and by sharing drinking vessels. Nonvenereal syphilis occurs mainly in the Middle East and Africa. Treatment is with a *penicillin drug*.

Syringe

An instrument for injecting fluid into, or withdrawing fluid from, a body cavity, blood vessel, or tissue. Most syringes consist of a barrel with a plunger at one end and, at the other, a nozzle to which a hollow needle can be attached. The barrel is calibrated to enable the correct dosage of medication to be given. Most modern syringes are disposable plastic instruments that are pre-sterilized and packed in sealed bags.

A hypodermic syringe is, strictly, one used for giving injections just beneath the skin. However, identical instruments are used for intramuscular (into a muscle) and intravenous (into a vein) injections. Thus, the term hypodermic syringe (or sometimes simply syringe) is used for all types.

Syringing of ears

A procedure for removing excessive *earwax* or, less commonly, a foreign body from the outer ear canal (see *Ear, foreign body in*).

The doctor first examines the ear to see if there is a condition (such as a perforated eardrum) that indicates syringing should not be performed. If

there is no such indication, any hard wax may first require softening by putting drops of oil in the ear. The earwax is then washed out using the procedure shown in the illustrated box. Afterwards, the canal is dried, sometimes using alcohol drops. As an alternative to flushing out, wax and other debris may be removed by suction or by small instruments.

Ear syringing may be uncomfortable. Sudden pain or dizziness may indicate a perforation of the eardrum and the need to stop the procedure.

Syringomyelia

A very rare, usually congenital (present from birth), condition in which a cavity forms in the *brainstem* (the low-

EAR SYRINGING

This procedure should be carried out by a doctor or nurse; amateur attempts can damage the eardrum.

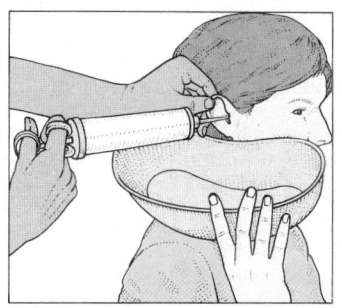

1 The nozzle of a large syringe is placed just inside the ear canal, which is straightened out by pulling the external ear upwards and backwards.

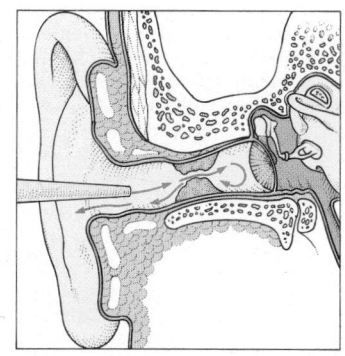

2 A jet of warm water or sodium bicarbonate solution is directed along the upper wall of the patient's ear canal in order to dislodge earwax or a foreign body.

est section of the brain) or at neck level in the *spinal cord*. The cavity gradually expands, filling with cerebrospinal fluid, eventually causing damage to nerve fibres.

The first symptoms usually appear in early adulthood. Affected persons are unable to feel pain or temperature changes in the neck, shoulders, arms, and hands, causing them to suffer injuries without realizing it. The muscles in the same region gradually become weak and wasted, and there is some loss of the sense of touch.

In advanced syringomyelia, there is spasticity (abnormal stiffness and rigidity) in the legs, nasal speech, and sometimes difficulty in swallowing. Many severely affected people are confined to wheelchairs.

No drug treatment is available. In some cases, surgical treatment to relieve pressure in the affected region (see *Decompression, spinal canal*) may arrest what is otherwise an inevitably progressive disease.

System

A group of interconnected or interdependent organs that perform a common function. For example, the parts of the *digestive system* (mouth, salivary glands, oesophagus, stomach, intestines, gallbladder, pancreas, and liver) act together to ingest, break down and absorb food, and to excrete faeces. The term system may also be applied to a method of classification, as in the ABO system for classifying *blood groups*.

Systemic

A term applied to something that affects the whole body rather than a specific part of it. For example, fever is a systemic symptom, whereas swelling is a localized symptom. The term systemic is also applied to the part of the blood circulation that supplies all parts of the body except the lungs.

Systemic lupus erythematosus

See *Lupus erythematosus*.

Systole

A period of muscular contraction of a chamber of the *heart* that alternates with a resting period, called *diastole*. With each *heartbeat*, the atria (upper chambers) contract first, squeezing blood into the ventricles (lower chambers); this is known as atrial systole. The ventricles then contract, pumping blood out of the heart into the arteries; this is known as ventricular systole.

S

T

Tabes dorsalis
A complication of *syphilis*, once common but now rare, that affects the spinal cord, causing abnormalities of sensation, sharp pains, incoordination, and incontinence. Symptoms appear many years after infection.

Tachycardia
A heart-rate of over 100 beats per minute in an adult. Most people have a rate of between 60 and 100 beats per minute, with an average of 72 to 78 beats. Tachycardia occurs in healthy people during exercise, when the heart is stimulated to work faster and thus increase blood flow to muscles. Tachycardia at rest may be caused by *fever, anxiety, hyperthyroidism, coronary artery disease* or any other cause of heart disease or heart failure, a high intake of *caffeine*, or treatment with an *anticholinergic drug* or some *decongestant drugs*. Types of tachycardia include *atrial fibrillation, sinus tachycardia, supraventricular tachycardia,* and *ventricular tachycardia.*

Symptoms of tachycardia may include *palpitations, breathlessness,* and lightheadedness, depending on how fast the heart is beating and on how effectively it is pumping blood.

Tachypnoea
An abnormally fast rate of *breathing*. Tachypnoea may be caused by exercise, anxiety, a lung disorder (such as emphysema), or a cardiac disorder (such as heart failure).

Tacrine
See *Tetrahydroaminoacridine.*

T'ai chi
A Chinese exercise system based on a series of more than 100 postures between which many slow, continuous, deliberate movements occur. T'ai chi is characterized by outer movement and inner stillness; its purpose is to exercise the muscles and achieve integration of mind and body. Devotees believe that continuous flow of movement is important in performing the exercises because it prevents "blockage" of the internal flow of chi—the essential life energy.

Talipes
A *birth defect* in which the foot is twisted out of shape or position. There are many different forms of talipes, all commonly called club-foot. Most cases are thought to be caused by pressure on the baby's feet from the mother's uterus in late pregnancy, but a genetic factor is also present (relatives of affected people have a higher incidence of talipes).

The most common form of talipes is an equinovarus deformity, in which the heel is turned inwards and the rest of the foot bent downwards and inwards. Also, the tibia (shin-bone) may be twisted inwards and there may be underdevelopment of the lower-leg muscles above the affected foot. Talipes equinovarus is twice as common in boys as in girls. In about 50 per cent of cases it affects both feet.

TREATMENT
Talipes equinovarus is treated by repeated manipulation of the foot and ankle, which should begin soon after birth. In some cases, a plaster *cast,* metal *splint,* or adhesive *strapping* may be needed to hold the foot in the corrected position. If these measures are ineffective, an operation to cut the tight ligaments and tendons is performed and the foot is immobilized in a plaster cast for at least three months. If treatment is not carried out before the age of two, the foot cannot be restored to normal, but function can be improved by lengthening a tendon or transferring a tendon from one bone to another (see *Tendon transfer*).

Other types of talipes can usually be corrected by repeated stretching of the foot into a normal position. Occasionally, immobilization of the foot in a plaster cast is required.

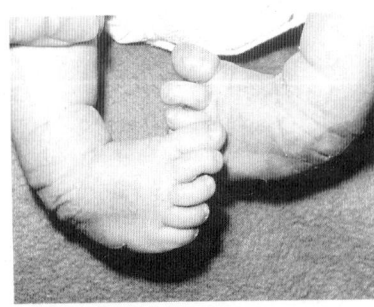

TALIPES EQUINOVARUS
This birth defect affects about one baby in 900. Treatment is by gentle manipulation, repeated several times a day.

Tamoxifen
An *anticancer drug* used in the treatment of certain types of *breast cancer.* Tamoxifen is also sometimes effective in the treatment of other cancers, such as prostate cancer (see *Prostate, cancer of*).

In women of childbearing age, tamoxifen stimulates *ovulation* (egg release) and is therefore occasionally used as a treatment for certain types of *infertility.*

Tamoxifen works by blocking *oestrogen hormone* receptors. It has fewer adverse effects than most anticancer drugs, but may cause hot flushes, nausea, vomiting, swollen ankles, and irregular vaginal bleeding.

Tampon
A plug of absorbent material, such as cottonwool, that is inserted into a wound or body opening to soak up blood or other secretions. The term is most commonly used to refer to a sanitary tampon inserted into the vagina to absorb menstrual blood.

Tamponade
Compression of the *heart.* Tamponade may occur in *pericarditis* (inflammation of the outer lining of the heart) due to the collection of fluid under the lining. Tamponade may also result from the collection of blood and blood clots around the heart after heart surgery or a penetrating chest injury.

Symptoms include breathlessness and, sometimes, collapse because the heart is unable to pump blood efficiently to the lungs and brain. The diagnosis is usually made by *echocardiography.*

Treatment involves immediate removal of any fluid that is pressing on the heart via a hollow needle guided through the chest wall. If blood clots are present, a *thoracotomy* is usually performed to open the chest wall and remove them.

Tan
See *Suntan.*

Tannin
Also known as tannic acid, an organic chemical that occurs in many plants, particularly in tea, oak apples, and the bark of oak, sumac, and mangrove trees.

Tannin has been used in medicine to stop bleeding, to control diarrhoea, and as an antidote to plant poisons. It is no longer used therapeutically because more effective agents are available and because it can cause liver damage. Although tea contains significant amounts of tannin, drinking moderate amounts is unlikely to lead to liver damage. However, it may cause constipation.

Tantrum

An outburst of bad temper, common in toddlers, usually indicating frustration and anger. Tantrums occur in many children between the ages of 15 months and four years, but are especially likely in two-year-olds.

During a tantrum, the child may scream, cry, yell, kick, bang the feet and fists, roll on the floor, go red in the face, spit, and bite. Some toddlers hold their breath during tantrums, sometimes turning blue and, in rare cases, momentarily losing consciousness (see *Breath-holding attacks*).

CAUSES

Tantrums occur at the age when a child starts to gain independence and becomes frustrated by restraints imposed by others, but is not yet able to express these feelings verbally. The outbursts are more likely when the child is tired, and are often brought on by a disagreement between child and parents. Tantrums may start with the birth of another baby, when the older child may believe that the baby is getting all the parents' attention.

Most children have occasional tantrums; frequent outbursts may indicate a *behavioural problem*, which may be due to emotional strain or a communication problem.

TREATMENT

Tantrums should be ignored as much as possible. An angry response will tend to make the child even more excited. Firm and consistent treatment is essential. A child's attention can often be diverted to a game or project. Most children grow out of tantrums when they develop the ability to describe their feelings.

If parents are unable to cope with tantrums, or if a child does not seem to be growing out of them, *child guidance* may be necessary.

Tapeworm infestation

Tapeworms, also called cestodes, are ribbon-shaped parasitic worms that live in human or animal intestines. They are typically acquired by eating undercooked meat or fish. Each adult tapeworm bears suckers or hooks on its head, by which it attaches itself to the intestinal wall. The rest of the worm consists of a chain of flat segments.

CAUSES, TYPES, AND INCIDENCE

Tapeworms in humans have lifecycles that usually also involve another animal host. A typical lifecycle is shown in the illustrated box.

Three large types of tapeworm, acquired by eating undercooked, infected beef, pork, and fish, all have life-cycles of this type. The adults may grow to 6 to 9 m long. All these tapeworms occur worldwide, but, in developed countries, infestations are largely prevented by measures such as adequate meat inspection and sanitary disposal of sewage. In the UK, tapeworm infections usually occur only in people infected abroad.

The much smaller dwarf tapeworm, which is only 2.5 cm long, has a different life-cycle. An infested person may directly cause an infestation of someone else through accidental transfer of worm eggs from faeces to fingers to mouth. The dwarf tapeworm is found worldwide, but especially in the tropics; it primarily affects children.

Humans may act as intermediate hosts to the larvae of a tapeworm for which dogs are the main host. The larvae grow and develop into cysts in the liver and lungs, a condition called *hydatid disease*.

SYMPTOMS

Despite their size, beef, pork, and fish tapeworms rarely cause symptoms, except mild abdominal discomfort or diarrhoea. However, segments of the worm may detach and emerge through the anus or may appear in the faeces. In rare cases, fish tapeworms cause *anaemia*. Dwarf tapeworms can cause diarrhoea and abdominal discomfort.

DIAGNOSIS AND TREATMENT

Tapeworm infestation is diagnosed from the presence of worm segments and/or eggs in the faeces.

Infestations are treated by *anthelmintic* drugs, such as *niclosamide* and *praziquantel*, which effectively kill the tapeworms.

Treatment of pork tapeworms must be carried out carefully because there is a risk that worm eggs will be released and find their way back into the stomach. The patient may then accidentally become the host to the worm larvae, which burrow into the tissues and form cysts. This leads to a condition called cysticercosis, the symptoms of which may include muscle pains and convulsions.

Tarsalgia

Pain in the rear part of the foot, usually associated with *flat-feet*.

Tarsorrhaphy

An operation in which the upper and lower eyelids are sewn together.

WHY IT IS DONE

Tarsorrhaphy may be performed as part of the treatment of *corneal ulcer*. The eyelids act as a bandage to promote healing of the cornea. Tarsorrhaphy is commonly used to protect the corneas in people who cannot close their eyelids because of nerve or muscular disorders or scarring. Tar-

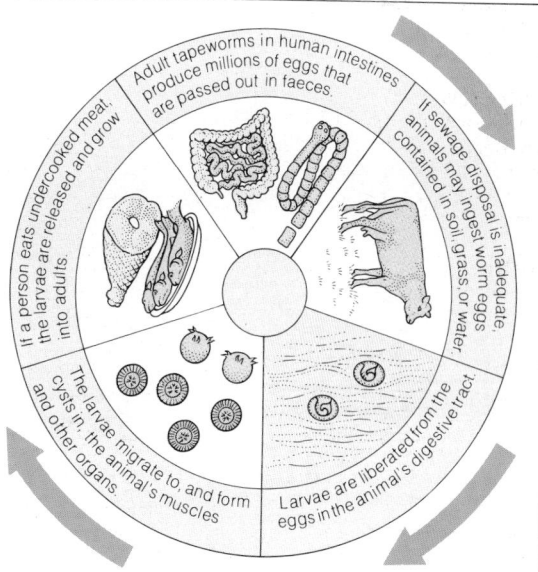

LIFE-CYCLE OF TAPEWORM
Many tapeworms have life-cycles in which the adult and larval worms infest different hosts. In the cycle on the right, the adult worms infest humans and the larvae infest cattle (called the intermediate hosts). Pigs and fish may also act as intermediate hosts to human tapeworms, and humans may act as intermediate hosts to dog and pig tapeworms.

Adult tapeworms in human intestines produce millions of eggs that are passed out in faeces.

If sewage disposal is inadequate, animals may ingest worm eggs contained in soil, grass, or water.

Larvae are liberated from the eggs in the animal's digestive tract.

The larvae migrate to, and form cysts in, the animal's muscles and other organs.

If a person eats undercooked meat, the larvae are released and grow into adults.

T

T

sorrhaphy is also occasionally performed to protect the cornea in people with *exophthalmos*.

HOW IT IS DONE

A strip of tissue is removed from the upper and lower lid edges. The raw surfaces of the lids are then stitched together. By about two or three weeks after the operation, the eyelids have grown together and the stitches can be removed. After having allowed time for the original trouble to clear up, the eyelids are then cut apart and allowed to open.

Tartar

See *Calculus, dental.*

Taste

One of the five special senses. By itself, taste is a relatively crude sense, able to distinguish only between sweet, salty, sour, and bitter. In practice, however, many different flavours can be distinguished because of the combination of the sense of taste and the much more discriminating sense of *smell*. This combination explains why loss of the sense of smell (caused by a common cold, for example) also apparently causes loss of taste (see *Taste, loss of*). The full sensory appreciation of food also involves other factors, such as the appearance of food, which helps stimulate sali-

vation, and the consistency and temperature of the food. The structures on the tongue and the mechanisms involved in taste are shown in the illustrated box.

Taste, loss of

Loss of the sense of *taste*, usually occurring as a result of loss of the sense of *smell*, which contributes greatly to taste.

Loss of taste with loss also of smell is most often caused by inflammation of the nasal passages due, for example, to a common *cold*.

Loss of taste without loss of smell is relatively rare. A possible cause is any

---

THE SENSE OF TASTE

Tastes are detected by special structures called taste-buds, of which everyone has some 10,000, mainly on the tongue, with a few at the back of the throat and on the palate. These taste-buds surround pores within papillae (protuberances) on the tongue surface and elsewhere. Four types of taste-buds exist—sensitive to sweet, salty, sour, or bitter chemicals. All tastes are formed from a mixture of these four elements.

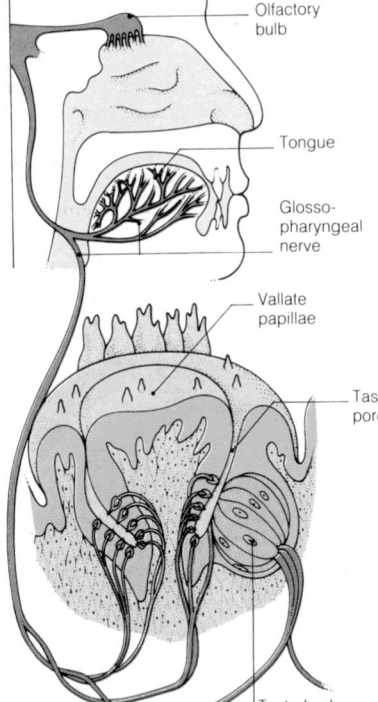

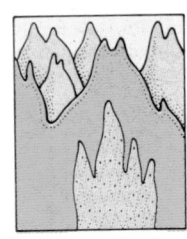

Fungiform papillae
These mushroom-shaped papillae occur in small numbers at random over the tongue surface, mainly in the middle.

Filiform papillae
These smaller peak-shaped protuberances occur in large numbers over all except the back of the tongue's upper surface, and on the palate.

How a substance is tasted
Chemicals in food or drink dissolve in saliva and enter pores in the papillae on the tongue. Around these pores are groups of taste receptor cells—the taste-buds. The chemicals stimulate hairs projecting from the receptor cells, causing signals to be sent from the cells along nerves to taste centres in the brain.

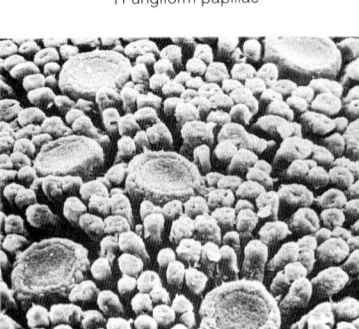

Magnified photograph of tongue surface
This photograph shows large (fungiform) and small (filiform) papillae. Taste-buds are arranged around pores in the surface of the papillae.

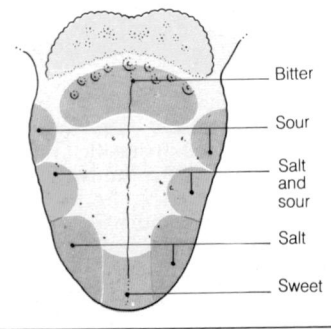

Taste centres on the tongue
Taste-buds sensitive to sweet, salty, sour, or bitter chemicals tend to be grouped into particular areas on the surface of the tongue.

condition that results in a dry mouth (see *Mouth, dry*), because taste-buds can detect the substances responsible for flavours only when those substances are dissolved in saliva.

Complete or partial loss of taste most commonly results from the natural degeneration of the taste-buds with age. It may also result from damage to the taste-buds themselves as a result of *stomatitis* (inflammation of the mouth), *mouth cancer*, *radiotherapy* to the mouth region (which also eliminates salivation by damaging the salivary glands), or the side-effects of certain drugs.

In some cases, loss of taste is caused by damage to the cranial nerves that convey taste sensations to the brain. Nerve damage may occur as a result of a head injury, a tumour of the brain or of the cranial nerves associated with taste, or surgery on the head or neck. In these cases, loss of taste is usually accompanied by facial paralysis.

Disturbances of taste occur in some psychiatric disorders, usually taking the form of taste hallucinations rather than true loss of taste.

Tattooing

The introduction of permanent colours under the surface of the skin, usually to create a picture. Practised for thousands of years, tattooing was originally used as a means of identification. Today it is almost always carried out for decorative purposes.

Tattooing, even by professionals, is potentially dangerous. If the tattooist does not follow strict sterile procedures, the viruses that cause *hepatitis* and *AIDS* may be transmitted through the needles used by the tattooist to introduce the dyes.

Removal of a tattoo is usually difficult and unsatisfactory: a scar almost always results. Small tattoos are best treated by complete removal of the coloured area of skin and the stitching together of the edges of the wound. Larger tattooed areas can sometimes be removed by *dermabrasion* or by *laser treatment*.

Tay-Sachs disease

A serious inherited metabolic disorder that results in early death. Tay-Sachs disease is a type of inborn error of metabolism (see *Metabolism, inborn errors of*). It was formerly known as amaurotic familial idiocy.

CAUSES AND INCIDENCE
Tay-Sachs disease is caused by a deficiency of hexosaminidase A, a certain *enzyme* (a protein essential for regulating chemical reactions in the body). Deficiency results in a build-up of a harmful substance in the brain.

The disease is most common among Ashkenazi Jews. The incidence in this group is around one in 2,500 births, which is 100 times higher than in any other ethnic group. The gene for Tay-Sachs disease is recessive (see *Genetic disorders*) and an Ashkenazi Jew has a one in 25 chance of carrying it. If two carriers marry, there is a one in four chance that they will have an affected child.

SYMPTOMS AND SIGNS
Signs of the illness, which usually appear after the first six months of life, are blindness, dementia, seizures, and paralysis. An exaggerated startle response to sound is an early sign. The disease progresses until the affected child dies, usually before reaching four years of age.

DIAGNOSIS
The diagnosis is based on the clinical history and physical examination; it is confirmed by enzyme analysis of a sample of white blood cells or a sample of skin tissue.

TREATMENT AND PREVENTION
There is no effective treatment for Tay-Sachs disease. Blood-testing programmes for detecting carriers of the gene have been introduced in some countries, including the UK. Carriers and those with an affected child or relative should receive *genetic counselling* before starting a family or planning another pregnancy. If antenatal testing shows that a fetus is affected, the parents may choose to have an abortion and try again for a healthy child.

TB

An abbreviation for *tuberculosis*.

T-cell

One of the two main classes of *lymphocytes* (a type of white blood cell). T-cells play an important role in the body's *immune system*.

Tears

The salty, watery secretion produced by the lacrimal glands, part of the *lacrimal apparatus* of the *eye*. The tear film over the *cornea* and the *conjunctiva* consists of three layers: an inner, mucous layer secreted by glands in the conjunctiva; an intermediate layer of salt water; and an outer, oily layer secreted by the meibomian glands.

The principal function of tears is to keep the cornea and conjunctiva constantly moist. Moisture is essential to maintain transparency of the cornea and to prevent ulceration. By lubricating the surface of the eye, tears aid movement of the eyelid in blinking. Tears also wash away small foreign bodies and contain a natural antiseptic called lysozyme. Another function is their role in expressing emotion.

A deficiency in tear production causes *keratoconjunctivitis sicca* (dry eye). Excessive tear production may cause *watering eye*.

Tears, artificial

Preparations used to supplement inadequate production of tears in *keratoconjunctivitis sicca* and other conditions causing dryness of the eyes. To be effective, artificial tears must be applied at frequent intervals. Artificial tears may also be used to relieve discomfort caused by irritants.

Many preparations contain a preservative that can irritate the eyes. Contaminated preparations may cause serious eye infections.

Technetium

A radioactive metallic element. Technetium does not occur naturally either in its pure form or in compounds, but is produced during nuclear fission reactions. It was the first element to be made artificially (in 1937). Several isotopes (varieties of the element that are chemically identical but differ in some physical properties) have been synthesized, of which the most important medically is a form known as technetium 99m. This radioisotope, incorporated in various chemical substances, is used in *radionuclide scanning* of many of the body's organs, including the brain, heart, lungs, liver, kidneys, and bones.

Teeth

Hard bone-like projections set in the *jaws* and surrounded by the *gums*. The teeth are used for *mastication* (chewing), help people to speak clearly, and also give shape to the face.

Humans have two sets of teeth: the *primary teeth* (of which there are 20) and the *permanent teeth* (of which there are 32). The primary teeth usually erupt between the ages of six months and three years and start to be replaced by the permanent teeth at about the age of six (see *Eruption of teeth*). The arrangement of the teeth is shown in the illustrated box overleaf.

In some people, the teeth fail to grow in the correct relationship to each other, resulting in *malocclusion* (incorrect bite).

T

STRUCTURE AND ARRANGEMENT OF TEETH

At the heart of each tooth is the living pulp, which contains blood vessels and nerves. A hard substance called dentine surrounds the pulp. The part of the tooth above the gum, the crown, is covered by enamel. The roots of the tooth, which fit into sockets in the jawbone, are covered by a sensitive, bone-like material, the cementum. The periodontal ligament connects the cementum to the gums and to the jaw. It acts as a shock absorber and prevents jarring of the teeth and skull when food is being chewed.

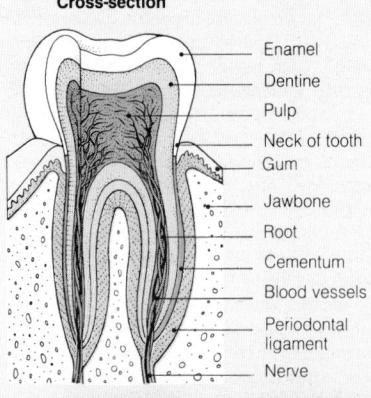

Cross-section

- Enamel
- Dentine
- Pulp
- Neck of tooth
- Gum
- Jawbone
- Root
- Cementum
- Blood vessels
- Periodontal ligament
- Nerve

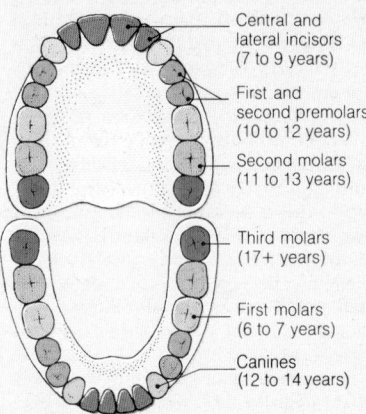

- Central and lateral incisors (7 to 9 years)
- First and second premolars (10 to 12 years)
- Second molars (11 to 13 years)
- Third molars (17+ years)
- First molars (6 to 7 years)
- Canines (12 to 14 years)

The permanent teeth

The illustration above shows the arrangement in the jaw of the permanent teeth—eight incisors, four canines, eight premolars, and 12 molars. The ages when these teeth erupt are indicated.

X-ray of teeth

The panoramic X-ray on the left shows all the teeth of the upper and lower jaw (there are no wisdom teeth) and their surrounding structures. The tooth roots, buried in the jawbones, can be clearly seen; several teeth have been filled.

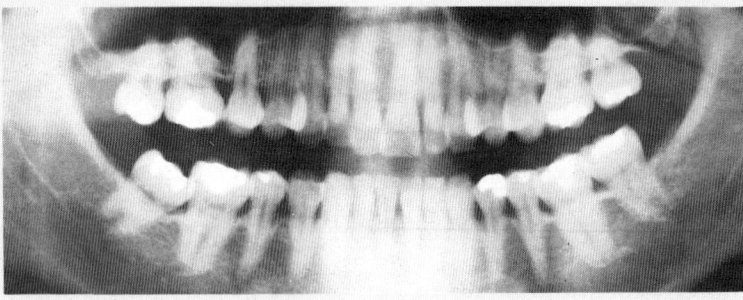

Molars | Premolars | Canines | Incisors | Canines | Premolars | Molars
Third | Second | First

Molars

The molars are large, strong teeth, efficient at grinding food. The third molars, or wisdom teeth, are the last to erupt; in some people, the wisdom teeth never appear.

Premolars

Also known as bicuspids, because of their two distinct edges, the premolars are concerned with grinding food. There are no premolars among the primary (milk) teeth.

Incisors

These teeth have a chisel-shaped, sharp cutting edge that is ideal for biting. The upper incisors overlap the lower incisors slightly when the jaws are closed.

Canines

The canines are sharp, pointed teeth, ideal for tearing food. They are larger and stronger than the incisors, with very long roots. The upper canines are often known as eye teeth.

Although the enamel that covers the crown of each tooth is the hardest substance in the body, it can be eroded when bacteria in the mouth break down carbohydrates in food (see *Caries, dental*). To help prevent decay, good *oral hygiene* is essential, consisting of daily *toothbrushing* and flossing (see *Floss, dental*).

Teeth, care of
See *Oral hygiene*.

Teething
The period when a baby cuts his or her first set of teeth. The primary teeth usually erupt between the ages of about six months and three years (see *Eruption of teeth*).

T

SYMPTOMS AND SIGNS

While teeth are erupting, a baby may be irritable, fretful, clinging, have difficulty in sleeping, and may cry more than usual. Extra saliva may be produced, resulting in dribbling, and the baby tends to chew on anything that he or she can hold.

Before a tooth comes through, the overlying gum may become red and swollen and the erupting tooth can be felt through the gum as a hard lump. When molars (back teeth) erupt, the cheek may feel warm and red on the affected side.

Teething should never be considered the cause of a very high temperature, vomiting, diarrhoea, prolonged loss of appetite, earache, convulsions, cough, or nappy rash. These are symptoms of a disorder and a doctor should be consulted.

TREATMENT

The baby should be given something firm to chew on, such as a piece of apple, or the swollen gum should be rubbed with a finger to ease the irritation. Painkilling dental creams or gels are available for rubbing on the gums.

Telangiectasia

An increase in the size of small blood vessels beneath the surface of an area of skin. Telangiectasia causes redness and an appearance sometimes called "broken veins". The condition is most common on the nose and cheeks. A localized form is the *spider naevus*.

Telangiectasia commonly results from heavy alcohol consumption over many years, or from the loss of supporting tissues in the skin due to overexposure to sunlight. Often, however, there is no obvious cause.

Less commonly, a connective tissue disease, such as systemic *lupus erythematosus* or *dermatomyositis*, is the cause. Telangiectasia may also be a feature of the facial redness of *rosacea*.

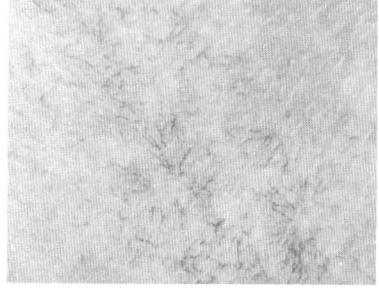

Appearance of telangiectasia
Although sometimes referred to as "broken veins", the blood vessels are in fact simply larger than usual.

Hereditary haemorrhagic telangiectasia is a rare disorder of the blood vessels in which frequent bleeding occurs from small, rounded patches of widened blood vessels around the mouth and nose or elsewhere in the skin or gastrointestinal tract. Frequent bleeding in hereditary haemorrhagic telangiectasia generally results in iron-deficiency *anaemia*.

Telangiectasia is not usually a cause for concern. The only means of removal is electrodesiccation (electrical destruction of the upper layers of the skin) administered by a dermatologist. The procedure is successful only in some cases however.

Temazepam

A *benzodiazepine drug* used in the short-term treatment of *insomnia*.

Temperature

For the body to function optimally, its temperature must be maintained within narrow limits. The generally accepted figure for the average normal body temperature (measured in the mouth) is 37°C. However, in practice, body temperature varies not only among individuals, but also in the same person, being affected by factors such as exercise, sleep, eating and drinking, time of day (lowest at about 3 a.m. and highest at about 6 p.m.), and, in women, the stage of the menstrual cycle (lowest at menstruation and highest at ovulation). In most people, body temperature varies between 36.5°C and 37.2°C. The temperature is higher in the rectum (by about 0.3 to 0.4°C), and lower in the armpit (by about 0.2 to 0.3°C).

TEMPERATURE REGULATION

Body temperature is maintained within optimal limits by the *hypothalamus*, an area of the brain that acts like a thermostat, constantly monitoring blood temperature and automatically activating mechanisms to compensate for changes.

When body temperature falls, the hypothalamus sends nerve impulses to stimulate *shivering*, which generates heat by muscle activity, and to constrict blood vessels in the skin, which reduces heat loss. Conversely, when body temperature rises, the hypothalamus stimulates *sweating* and dilates (widens) blood vessels in the skin to increase heat loss.

A variety of factors—such as infections, certain disorders (notably those of the *thyroid gland*), unusual symptoms of a tumour, and overexposure to cold or extreme heat—may disrupt

the body's heat-regulating system, resulting in *fever, heatstroke*, or, conversely, in *hypothermia*.

Temperature method

See *Contraception, natural methods of*.

Temporal arteritis

An uncommon disease of elderly people in which the walls of the arteries in the scalp that pass over the temples become inflamed. Other arteries in the head and neck may also be affected, as may the aorta (the large artery that carries oxygenated blood from the heart) and its main branches. The inflamed blood vessels become

---

TEMPORAL ARTERITIS

In this disorder, the temporal artery and other arteries in the head are inflamed. Early reporting of symptoms is vital, since, in untreated cases, there is a risk of sudden blindness.

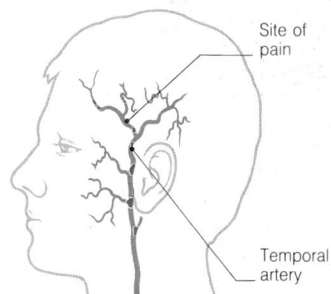

Site of pain

Temporal artery

Telltale symptoms
If the temporal artery is inflamed, it is usually prominent and there is a persistent severe headache and scalp tenderness in the area shown.

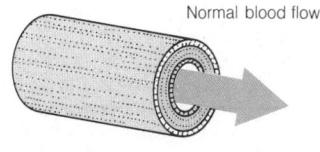

Normal blood flow

Normal artery
A normal artery has a smooth lining, and blood flow is sufficient to meet the needs of the tissues it supplies.

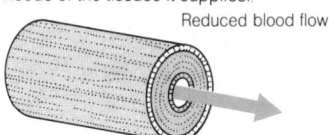

Reduced blood flow

Inflamed artery
In arteritis, the walls of the artery become disrupted and thickened, and blood flow is markedly reduced.

T

narrowed, and blood flow through them is reduced. The disease is also known as giant cell arteritis.

CAUSES AND INCIDENCE

The cause of temporal arteritis is unknown, but it is often associated with *polymyalgia rheumatica* (pain and stiffness in the muscles of the hips, thighs, shoulders, and neck).

In the UK, about 600 cases of temporal arteritis are diagnosed each year. Nearly all sufferers are over 50 years old, and the disease affects more women than men.

SYMPTOMS AND SIGNS

The most common symptom is a headache, usually severe, on one or both sides of the head. The temporal artery (located at the side of the head above the earlobe) may be prominent and the scalp may be tender. In nearly 50 per cent of sufferers, the ophthalmic arteries supplying the eyes may become affected, causing partial loss of vision or even sudden blindness. Other symptoms and signs include low fever, poor appetite, pain on chewing, and lethargy.

Involvement of the aorta or its main branches results in circulatory disorders, such as intermittent *claudication* (pain in the legs on walking) or *Raynaud's phenomenon* (pallor in the fingers on exposure to cold).

DIAGNOSIS AND TREATMENT

Early reporting of symptoms to a doctor is essential because of the risk of blindness. The diagnosis is made by a *biopsy* (removal of a small sample of tissue for analysis) of the temporal artery and by *blood tests* to detect the presence of a raised *ESR* (erythrocyte sedimentation rate).

The disease responds rapidly to a *corticosteroid drug*, which is initially given in high doses to prevent blindness. Most people need to take the drug, at a reduced dosage, for one or two years. If the disease fails to respond to corticosteroid treatment, or if such treatment causes serious side-effects, *immunosuppressant drugs* (such as azathioprine) may be given.

OUTLOOK

With treatment, the disease usually clears up within two years. Most people are not left with any lasting disability. However, if one or both eyes become blind before treatment has become effective, the blindness may be permanent.

Temporal lobe epilepsy

A form of *epilepsy* in which abnormal electrical discharges in the *brain* are confined to one temporal lobe (a local-

---

LOCATION OF THE TEMPORAL LOBE

The temporal lobe forms much of the lower side of each half of the cerebrum (main mass of the brain).

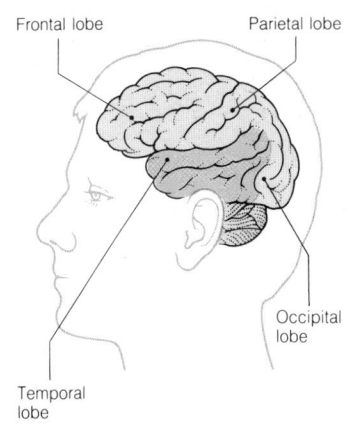

Frontal lobe
Parietal lobe
Occipital lobe
Temporal lobe

---

ized region on the side of the brain). The seizures in temporal lobe epilepsy therefore differ from the generalized disturbances that occur in a grand mal seizure or petit mal (absence seizure).

CAUSE

In most cases there is an area of damage within one of the temporal lobes, which acts as a focus for the abnormal development of electrical discharges in attacks. Damage may be caused by a *birth injury, head injury, brain tumour, brain abscess,* or *stroke*. The temporal lobes are concerned with such functions as smell, taste, hearing, visual associations, and some aspects of memory. Abnormal electrical activity in a lobe may thus cause peculiarities in any of these functions.

SYMPTOMS AND SIGNS

People affected by temporal lobe epilepsy suffer dream-like states that range from partial loss of awareness to total disregard. The person may have unpleasant hallucinations of smell or taste. Also common during attacks is the perception of an illusory scene or the phenomenon of *déjà vu*. There may also be facial grimacing, rotation of the head and eyes, and, often, sucking and chewing movements.

The affected person may perform tasks during the attack but have no memory of them afterwards. An attack may last for minutes or hours before full consciousness returns.

In some cases, a temporal lobe seizure progresses after several seconds or a few minutes to a generalized grand mal seizure.

DIAGNOSIS AND TREATMENT

The principles of investigation and drug treatment for temporal lobe epilepsy are the same as for other types of epilepsy. Surgery to remove the part of the lobe containing the irritating focus for the attacks has been used with success in some cases of temporal lobe epilepsy. However, because of the possible effects on other important functions of the brain, such operations are performed only in severe cases that have not responded to drug treatment.

Temporomandibular joint

A *joint* connecting the mandible (lower *jaw* bone) to the temporal bone of the *skull* (see illustrated box).

Temporomandibular joint syndrome

Pain and other symptoms affecting the head, jaw, and face that are believed to result when the *temporomandibular joints* and the muscles and ligaments that control and support them do not work together correctly. This disorder is often known more simply as TMJ syndrome.

CAUSES

A common cause is spasm of the chewing muscles, often as result of clenching or grinding the teeth due to emotional tension. An incorrect bite, which places additional stress on the muscles, may be a contributing factor.

LOCATION OF THE TEMPOROMANDIBULAR JOINT

The head of the mandible (jawbone) fits into a hollow on the underside of the temporal bone of the skull at the joint.

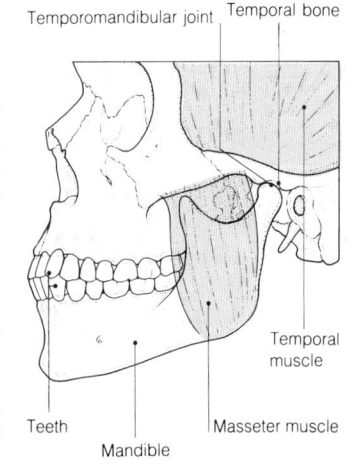

Temporomandibular joint
Temporal bone
Temporal muscle
Masseter muscle
Mandible
Teeth

T

Temporomandibular joint problems may also be caused by displacement of the joint as a result of jaw, head, or neck injuries. In rare cases, *osteoarthritis* is a cause.

SYMPTOMS

Headaches, tenderness of the jaw muscles, and dull, aching facial pain with severe exacerbation in or around the ear are common symptoms of temporomandibular joint syndrome. Difficulty in opening the mouth, "locking" of the jaws, clicking noises as the mouth is opened or closed, or pain caused by opening the mouth wide or by chewing, if persistent, all together or individually, require careful medical diagnosis.

TREATMENT

In most cases, treatment is aimed at eliminating muscle spasm and relieving pain. This may be done by applying moist heat to the face, taking *muscle-relaxant drugs*, massaging the muscles, eating soft foods, or using a device that fits over the teeth at night to prevent clenching or grinding. *Counselling*, *biofeedback training*, and *relaxation exercises* may also help.

The bite may need to be adjusted by the use of a brace or other *orthodontic appliance*, or by occlusal adjustment (grinding down of specific teeth). In very severe cases, surgery on one or both jaw joints may be required.

Tenderness

Pain or abnormal sensitivity in a part of the body when it is pressed or touched. Tenderness experienced during palpation (medical examination by touch) is usually a sign of *inflammation*. For example, *appendicitis* (inflammation of the appendix) causes tenderness of the abdomen; *arthritis* (joint inflammation) causes tenderness around the affected joint. Tenderness is usually associated with swelling, redness, and warmth of the affected part.

Tendinitis

Inflammation of a *tendon*, usually caused by injury. Symptoms include pain, tenderness, and, occasionally, restricted movement of the muscle attached to the affected tendon. A common example is *painful arc syndrome*, which causes pain in the shoulder when the arm is raised between certain angles.

Treatment of tendinitis may include *nonsteroidal anti-inflammatory drugs* (NSAIDs), *ultrasound treatment*, or an injection of a *corticosteroid drug* around the tendon.

Tendolysis

An operation performed to free a *tendon* from *adhesions* (fibrous bands) that surround it and limit its free movement. Such adhesions are usually caused by *tenosynovitis* (inflammation of the inner lining of a tendon sheath).

Tendolysis consists of making a skin incision over the tendon and then splitting open its fibrous sheath. The adhesions are cut away from the tendon surface and the incisions in the sheath and the skin are stitched. Despite surgery, symptoms of tenosynovitis sometimes recur because adhesions form again.

Tendon

A fibrous cord that joins muscle to bone or muscle to muscle. Tendons are strong, flexible, but inelastic. Most are cylindrical; some, such as those attached to the flat muscles of the abdominal wall, consist of sheets of fibres known as aponeuroses.

Tendons are made up principally of bundles of collagen (a white, fibrous protein) and contain some blood vessels. The larger tendons (but not the aponeuroses) also have a nerve supply. Squeezing the tendon hard causes pain; stretching it triggers a *reflex* contraction of the adjoining muscle (e.g. the quadriceps jerk).

FINGER TENDONS

Finger bending and extension are controlled by tendons on either side of the finger; the tendons originate from forearm muscles.

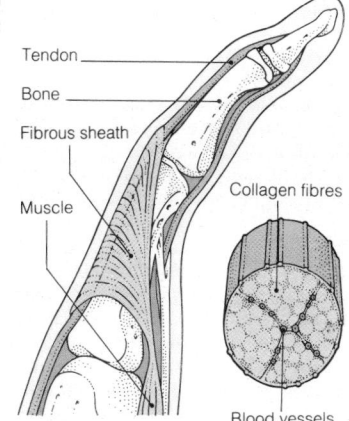

Tendon

Bone

Fibrous sheath

Muscle

Collagen fibres

Blood vessels

Internal structure
A cross-section of a tendon (above right) shows that it consists of numerous parallel bundles of collagen fibres together with some blood vessels.

The tendons in the hands, wrists, and feet are enclosed in synovial sheaths (fibrous capsules) and bathed in a lubricating fluid secreted by the lining of the sheath. These tendons require this additional protection because they do not move in a straight line and, without the fluid, might be subjected to excessive friction.

DISORDERS

Rupture of the *Achilles tendon* can occur during sprinting and jumping when sudden contraction of the calf muscles causes stretching of the tendon. Rupture of a tendon on the back of a finger, resulting in deformity of the fingertip, may be caused by a direct blow to the end of the finger (see *Mallet finger*). In many cases, however, because tendons are so strong, severe stress results in the pulling off of a piece of bone where the tendon is attached, rather than in tearing of the tendon itself.

The long tendon of the biceps muscle in the upper arm may become weakened as a result of repeated rubbing against the humerus (upper-arm bone) and may rupture under even moderate stress. Rupture of tendons in the hands can occur as a complication of *rheumatoid arthritis*.

Tendons in the hand are commonly severed by a deep cut; *tendon repair* using a tendon graft may be required.

Tendinitis, inflammation of a tendon, may follow an injury. *Tenosynovitis*, inflammation of the inner lining of a tendon sheath, usually affects tendons in the hands and wrists and results from overuse. If the outer wall of a tendon sheath is inflamed, the gliding movement of the tendon through the sheath may be restricted, a condition called *tenovaginitis*.

Tendon release
See *Tendolysis*.

Tendon repair

An operation to join the cut or torn ends of a *tendon* or to replace a damaged tendon.

If the cut or torn ends can easily be brought together, they are stitched together with sutures. If the ends are widely separated or contained within a sheath, it may be necessary to insert a tendon graft. Tendons for grafting are taken from elsewhere in the body, usually the foot.

Tendon transfer

An operation to reposition a *tendon* so that it causes a muscle to perform a different function. Tendon transfer

T

may be used to restore function impaired by a deformity, such as *talipes* (club-foot), or by permanent muscle injury or paralysis.

To perform the transfer, the tendon is cut away from its original point of attachment and reattached elsewhere. Tendon transfer causes the muscle to which the tendon is attached to lie in a different position and thus to produce a different body movement when the muscle contracts.

Tenesmus

A feeling of incomplete emptying of the bowel in which the urge to pass faeces is accompanied by ineffective straining. Tenesmus may be a symptom of a disorder of the *rectum*, such as polyps or cancer, or of severe inflammation caused by *ulcerative colitis* or *dysentery*.

Tennis elbow

A condition characterized by pain and tenderness on the outside of the *elbow* and in the back of the forearm. Its medical name is epicondylitis.

Tennis elbow is caused by inflammation of the *tendon* that attaches the extensor muscles (in this case the muscles that straighten the fingers and wrist) to the *humerus*. The condition results from overuse of these muscles, causing constant tugging of the tendon at its point of attachment to the humerus.

Tennis elbow may be caused by playing tennis (or other racquet sports) with a faulty grip, but more commonly it is due to other activities, such as gardening. It is made worse by lifting heavy objects.

TREATMENT
Treatment consists of resting the arm, applying *ice-packs*, and taking *analgesic drugs* (painkillers) and/or *nonsteroidal anti-inflammatory drugs* (NSAIDs).

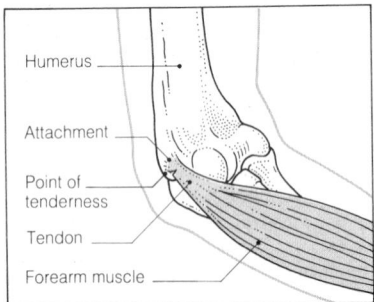

Site of tennis elbow
Pulling of the forearm muscles where they attach to the humerus causes tenderness on the outer side of the elbow.

Ultrasound treatment may help reduce the inflammation. If the pain is severe or persistent, injection of a *corticosteroid drug* may be required. Surgery to release the tendon is occasionally required (see *Tendolysis*).

If the pain has occurred after playing a racquet sport, it is wise to take a break from the sport for a week or two and to consult a professional about playing technique and equipment.

Tenosynovitis

Inflammation of the thin inner lining of the sheath that surrounds a *tendon*. Tenosynovitis is usually caused by excessive friction due to overuse; it is often brought on by working in an awkward position to do a job that involves repetitive movements. A rare cause is bacterial infection. Tendons in the hand and wrist are most commonly affected.

Symptoms include pain, tenderness, and swelling over the tendon. There is also occasionally *crepitus* (a grating noise or sensation) when the tendon is moved. Persistent or recurrent tenosynovitis may lead to restricted movement as a result of the formation of *adhesions* (fibrous bands) between the tendon and its sheath.

TREATMENT
If infection is the cause, *antibiotic drugs* are prescribed. Otherwise, treatment usually consists of *nonsteroidal anti-inflammatory drugs* (NSAIDs) or an injection of a *corticosteroid drug* around the tendon. The hand and wrist may need to be immobilized in a *splint* for a few weeks. If the condition does not improve, surgery may be required to release adhesions (see *Tendolysis*).

Tenovaginitis

Inflammation or thickening of the fibrous wall of the sheath that surrounds a *tendon*. The cause is unknown. Tenovaginitis affecting the sheath of one of the tendons that bends a finger results in *trigger finger*.

TENS

The abbreviation for transcutaneous electrical nerve stimulation. TENS is a method of pain relief achieved by the application of minute electrical impulses to nerve endings that lie beneath the skin. The procedure seems to work by blocking pain messages to the brain by providing an alternative stimulus. TENS is carried out to relieve severe or persistent pain that has not been satisfactorily controlled by *analgesic drugs*. TENS is sometimes used during childbirth.

HOW IT IS DONE
A TENS unit provides electrical impulses to electrodes that are placed on the skin or sometimes surgically implanted. Adjustments of the unit can be made by the patient to achieve best relief.

RISKS
TENS must not be used by anyone with a cardiac *pacemaker*; the electrical impulses from the transmitter may interfere with the pacemaker's action.

OUTLOOK
TENS is beneficial in about 60 per cent of the patients who use it. Pain relief in some people lasts only during stimulation; in others, pain relief persists after treatment.

Tension

A feeling of mental and physical strain associated with *anxiety*. Sufferers feel unpleasantly keyed up, cannot relax, and may have feelings of bottled-up anger. Muscle tension accompanies the mental symptoms and may result in headaches and muscular stiffness and pain, particularly in the back and shoulders. Persistent tension is related to *generalized anxiety disorder*. (See also *Stress*.)

Teratogen

An agent that causes physical abnormalities in a developing *embryo* or *fetus*. Examples of teratogens include the *rubella* virus and the drug *thalidomide*. For a drug to be categorized as teratogenic, there must be evidence that taking the drug during pregnancy causes an increased incidence of *congenital* abnormalities that cannot be explained by other factors. Many chemicals that are known to be teratogenic in some species (such as rats) have not been proved to be teratogenic in humans. Drug-regulatory organizations usually refuse to license drugs for use during pregnancy if they have been found to be teratogenic for any species.

Teratoma

A primary *tumour* consisting of cells that bear no resemblance to those normally found in that part of the body. For example, teratomas that develop in the ovary—one of the most common sites for this type of tumour—often form cysts (called *dermoid cysts*) that may contain skin, hair, teeth, or bone. Other sites in which teratomas may occur include the testes, the pineal gland in the brain, and the mediastinum (the space between the lungs).

T

Terbutaline

A *bronchodilator drug* used in the treatment of *asthma*, chronic *bronchitis*, and *emphysema*. Terbutaline also relaxes the muscles of the uterus, making it useful for the prevention of premature labour (see *Prematurity*).

Possible adverse effects are tremor, nervousness, restlessness, nausea, and, in rare cases, palpitations.

Terfenadine

An *antihistamine drug* used to treat allergic *rhinitis* (hay fever) and allergic skin conditions, such as *urticaria* (nettle rash). Terfenadine has less sedative effect than some other antihistamines and is therefore useful for people who need to avoid drowsiness. Possible adverse effects include nausea, headache, loss of appetite, and rash.

Terminal care

See *Dying, care of the*.

Termination of pregnancy

See *Abortion, induced*.

Testicle

See *Testis*.

Testicular feminization syndrome

A rare inherited condition in which, despite having the external appearance of a female, the affected individual is genetically a male with internal testes. Testicular feminization syndrome is a form of *intersex* and is the most common form of male *pseudohermaphroditism*. It is sometimes alternatively known as androgen resistance syndrome.

CAUSE
Testicular feminization syndrome is caused by a defective response of the body's tissues to *testosterone* (male sex hormone), even though a normal male level of the hormone is produced. The genes that cause testicular feminization syndrome are transmitted on the X chromosome (see *Genetic disorders*). Females can therefore carry the causative genes and transmit them to their sons.

SYMPTOMS AND SIGNS
Affected individuals appear to be girls throughout childhood. Most develop normal female secondary *sexual characteristics* at *puberty*, but menstruation does not occur because there is no uterus and the vagina is short and blind-ending. People with testicular feminization syndrome tend to be tall and are of normal intelligence.

DIAGNOSIS
The condition may be diagnosed before puberty if a girl is found to have an inguinal *hernia* or a swelling in the labia that turns out to be a testis. Otherwise, the diagnosis is usually made at puberty during investigations to find the cause of *amenorrhoea* (failure to menstruate).

The diagnosis is made by *chromosome analysis*, which shows the normal male chromosomal status, and by blood tests, which indicate male levels of testosterone.

TREATMENT AND OUTLOOK
Treatment involves surgical removal of the testes at puberty (because of an increased risk of testicular cancer) and hormonal therapy with *oestrogen drugs*. An affected individual can never be fertile, but can lead an otherwise normal life as a woman.

Testis

One of two male sex organs, also called testicles, that produce *sperm* and the male sex hormone *testosterone*.

The testes are formed within the abdomen near the kidneys early in the development of the male fetus. In response to hormones produced by the mother and to hormones produced in the testes themselves, the testes gradually descend through the inguinal canal in the groin. At birth, they have usually reached the surface of the body, where they hang suspended in a pouch of skin called the *scrotum*.

STRUCTURE
Within each testis are the seminiferous tubules, delicate coiled tubes that produce sperm. The seminiferous tubules lead via the vasa efferentia (small ducts) to the *epididymis*, a structure lying behind the testis in which the newly formed sperm mature. Interstitial cells between the seminiferous tubules produce the male sex hormone testosterone, which passes into small blood vessels in the testis and then into the circulation.

Each testis is protected by a tough, fibrous capsule, the tunica albuginea, and is attached by the spermatic cord, composed of the *vas deferens* (the tube that transports sperm from the epididymis to the urethra) and a number of blood vessels and nerves.

DISORDERS
A direct blow sometimes tears the wall of the testis, resulting in severe pain and bleeding into the scrotal tissue. An operation may be required to drain the blood and repair the testis.

Occasionally, a testis fails to develop completely, does not descend

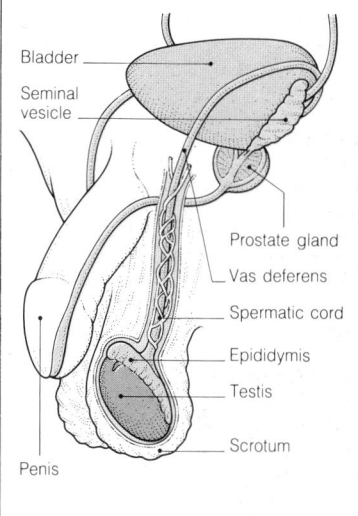

LOCATION OF THE TESTIS
Each testis is suspended in the scrotum by a spermatic cord, which contains the vas deferens, and the arteries, veins and nerves that supply the testis.

Bladder
Seminal vesicle
Prostate gland
Vas deferens
Spermatic cord
Epididymis
Testis
Scrotum
Penis

fully into the scrotum (see *Testis, undescended*), or descends into an abnormal position (see *Testis, ectopic*).

Inflammation of the testis, known as *orchitis*, usually results from infection with the mumps virus. Inflammation of the testis and the epididymis occurs in *epididymo-orchitis*, which is usually caused by a bacterial infection.

Painless swelling of the tissues surrounding the testis usually results from a *hydrocele* (collection of fluid in the scrotum). Other causes of testicular swelling include a *varicocele* (swollen veins within the scrotum), an *epididymal cyst* (fluid-filled swelling of the epididymis), and a *spermatocele* (a sperm-filled swelling of the epididymis).

Torsion of the testis, in which the spermatic cord becomes twisted, cutting off the blood supply to the testis, is most common at the time of *puberty* (see *Testis, torsion of*).

In rare cases, the testis is affected by cancer (see *Testis, cancer of*).

Various conditions affecting the testis may cause a reduction or absence of sperm production; if both testes are affected, *infertility* may result.

Testis, cancer of

A malignant tumour of the *testis*. Cancer of the testis is rare. It occurs most commonly in young to middle-aged

T

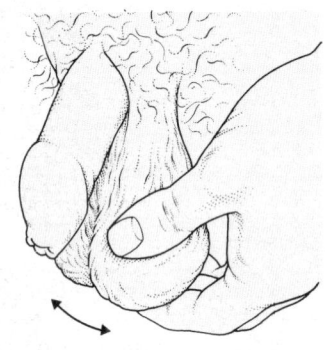
men, and is very rare before *puberty* or in old age. The risk of testicular cancer is higher in men who have a history of undescended testis (see *Testis, undescended*).

TYPES
The most common types of testicular cancer are seminomas and *teratomas*. Seminomas are made up of a single type of cell (probably developing from the cells that produce sperm). Teratomas consist of several different types of cell. Other cancers affecting the testis are extremely rare and develop from testicular tissue or from lymphatic tissue within the testis (see *Lymphoma*).

SYMPTOMS AND SIGNS
Testicular cancer most commonly appears as a firm, painless swelling of one testis. Men are recommended to examine their testes regularly to check for lumps (see illustrated box). In some cases, there may be pain and inflammation.

DIAGNOSIS
The doctor first examines the testis and may perform tests to exclude other causes of testicular swelling (see *Testis, swollen*).

The diagnosis of testicular cancer can be confirmed only by *orchidectomy*

(surgical removal of the testis) and microscopic examination of the testicular tissue. This confirms the presence of cancer and also shows the type of cancer that is present. Other tests, including *CT scanning, MRI, ultrasound scanning,* and *blood tests,* are performed to look for any signs that indicate that the cancer has spread to other parts of the body.

TREATMENT
Orchidectomy may be sufficient to cure testicular cancer in its early stages. However, in patients in whom there is a high risk of spread, preventive treatment, consisting of *anticancer drugs* or *radiotherapy* to lymph nodes in the abdomen, may be carried out even if there are no signs that the disease has spread. Cancer that has spread beyond the testis is usually treated with both orchidectomy and anticancer drugs. Surgery to remove cancerous tissue from the abdomen is occasionally needed.

OUTLOOK
The outlook, which varies according to the type of cancer and how advanced it was when first discovered, is generally good. The cure rate for early testicular cancer is 95 to 100 per cent; the cure rate for advanced disease is 80 to 90 per cent. Provided the other testis is healthy, treatment with radiotherapy and/or anticancer drugs generally does not cause infertility in the remaining testis.

Testis, ectopic
A *testis* that is absent from the *scrotum* because it has descended into an abnormal position, usually in the groin or at the base of the penis. An ectopic testis is most often discovered soon after birth during a routine physical examination. Treatment involves an *orchidopexy,* a surgical operation to place the testis in the scrotum. (See also *Testis, undescended.*)

Testis, pain in the
Even mild injury to the *testis* may result in pain. Usually, no damage is caused, but a direct blow such as a kick may tear the wall of the testis. In this case, the pain is particularly severe, and an operation may be required to drain any accumulated blood and repair the testis.

Severe pain and swelling are a feature of *orchitis* (inflammation of the testis), *epididymo-orchitis* (inflammation of the testis and epididymis), and torsion of the testis (see *Testis, torsion of*). Cancer of the testis (see *Testis, cancer of*) does not usually cause pain.

Pain that seems to come from the testis is occasionally caused by a small kidney stone lodged in the ureter (see *Calculus, urinary tract*).

A doctor can sometimes find no cause for testicular pain; in most of such cases the problem disappears without treatment.

Testis, retractile
A *testis* that is drawn up high into the groin by a pronounced muscle reflex in response to cold or touch. Retractile testis is normal in young children but usually disappears by *puberty*. Failure to feel the testis in the scrotum sometimes causes the condition to be confused with undescended testis (see *Testis, undescended*).

Testis, swollen
Swelling of the *testis* or its surrounding tissues in the *scrotum*, which may or may not be accompanied by pain. Most scrotal swellings are harmless and the testis itself is usually not affected. However, swelling of a testis should always be reported to a doctor to rule out the possibility of a serious underlying disorder.

PAINLESS SWELLING
There are several types of harmless, painless swelling, the most common of which is a *hydrocele* (a collection of fluid in the scrotum). Other usually painless swellings include an *epididymal cyst* (fluid-filled swelling of the epididymis), a *spermatocele* (sperm-filled swelling of the epididymis), a *varicocele* (varicose veins in the scrotum), and a haematocele (a swelling that contains blood and that results from injury).

Cancer of the testis (see *Testis, cancer of*) may also cause a painless swelling in the scrotum, which requires prompt treatment.

PAINFUL SWELLING
Painful swelling of the scrotum may be caused by a sudden event, such as twisting of the spermatic cord (see *Testis, torsion of*) or a direct blow. When associated with fever, the swelling is usually due to infection of the testis (see *Orchitis*) or of the testis and epididymis (see *Epididymo-orchitis*). In very rare cases, a painful swelling is due to cancer of the testis.

Testis, torsion of
Twisting of the spermatic cord, causing acute, severe pain and swelling of the *testis*. Unless the condition is treated within a few hours, the testis is damaged permanently and sperm production ceases.

TORSION OF THE TESTIS
If a testis rotates, veins in the spermatic cord become obstructed and there is severe swelling and pain. Torsion of the testis most commonly occurs around puberty.

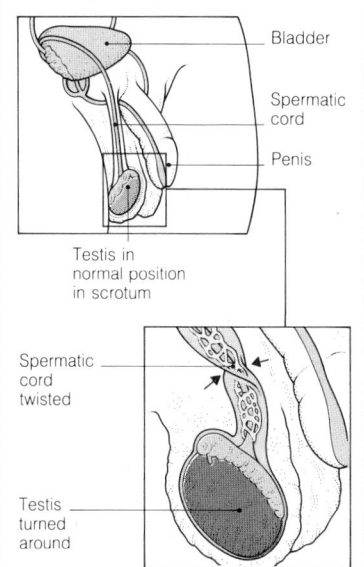

Bladder

Spermatic cord

Penis

Testis in normal position in scrotum

Spermatic cord twisted

Testis turned around

Treatment
Spontaneous untwisting sometimes occurs but unrelieved torsion is dangerous. Torsion must be treated urgently by surgery.

Torsion of the testis is most common around *puberty*, but may also occur in infants or in young adults. The condition is more likely to occur if the testis is unusually mobile within its covering in the *scrotum*.

SYMPTOMS AND SIGNS
Pain develops rapidly and is occasionally accompanied by abdominal pain and nausea. The testis becomes swollen and very tender, and the scrotal skin becomes discoloured.

DIAGNOSIS AND TREATMENT
A diagnosis is made from a physical examination.

Treatment is by surgery. An incision is made in the skin of the scrotum and, if the diagnosis is confirmed, the testis can be immediately untwisted. If blood flow resumes, the testis is anchored in the scrotum with small stitches to prevent a recurrence of the problem. If irreversible damage exists, *orchidectomy* (removal of the testis) is performed. In all cases, the other testis is also anchored to the scrotum to prevent torsion on that side.

OUTLOOK
Recovery from the operation is rapid. If treatment was prompt, the testis recovers completely. Even if one testis is removed, the other is usually capable of maintaining fertility.

Testis, undescended
A *testis* that has failed to complete its normal passage from within the abdomen to the *scrotum*. Not all testes that are absent from the scrotum are undescended (see *Testis, ectopic*; *Testis, retractile*). Undescended testis is found in about one per cent of full-term and in up to 10 per cent of premature male babies. Usually, only one testis fails to descend. In many cases, an undescended testis descends of its own accord within several months of birth; an undescended testis rarely, if ever, descends of its own accord after this time.

CAUSES AND SYMPTOMS
The final descent of the testis through the inguinal canal to the scrotum is controlled by hormones from the mother and from the testis itself. If these stimuli do not have an effect, the spermatic cord (which carries the vas deferens and the blood vessels to the testis) fails to lengthen sufficiently to allow full descent. Alternatively, a normal testis may be prevented from reaching the scrotum by the presence of fibres that interrupt its route and cause it to remain in the groin.

An undescended testis does not develop normally and is not capable of normal sperm production. If both testes are undescended, *infertility* results. A testis that fails to descend normally is at increased risk of testicular cancer (see *Testis, cancer of*).

DIAGNOSIS AND TREATMENT
The diagnosis is made during examination of the newborn or later in infancy. It is rare for the condition to remain unnoticed into adult life.

Treatment is by *orchidopexy*, an operation in which the undescended testis is lowered into the scrotum. Surgery within the first few years of life gives the testis the best chance of developing normally. If the undescended testis is very poorly developed and the other testis is normal, the undescended testis is removed.

Test meal
A procedure used to measure the output of acid by the *stomach*. The name test "meal" derives from the fact that gruel used to be given to stimulate the stomach to secrete fluid. Today, an injection of *histamine* or more commonly of pentagastrin (a synthetic preparation of the hormone gastrin) is given instead.

In some instances, an *insulin* test (in which an injection of insulin is given) is performed to confirm the completeness of a *vagotomy* (an operation in which the vagus nerve is cut).

HOW IT IS DONE
A *nasogastric tube* is passed via the nose into the stomach after an overnight fast, and an initial sample of gastric fluid is sucked up through the tube. The injection is then given and further samples of stomach fluid are taken at intervals for a period of up to two hours. The samples are analysed for the amount of hydrochloric acid they contain.

RESULTS
High levels of acid are found in people with a duodenal ulcer (see *Peptic ulcer*) or *Zollinger-Ellison syndrome*. Absence of acid is characteristic of pernicious anaemia (see *Anaemia, megaloblastic*).

An insulin test done following a complete vagotomy will not result in the normal secretion of gastric acid that would occur if the vagus nerve were intact.

Testosterone
The most important of the *androgen hormones* (male sex hormones). Testosterone stimulates bone and muscle growth and sexual development. It is produced by the *testes* and in very small amounts by the *ovaries*.

DRUG THERAPY
Synthetic or animal testosterone is used to stimulate *puberty* or to treat *infertility* in males suffering from deficiency caused by disorders of the testes or *pituitary gland*. Testosterone was formerly used in the treatment of *breast cancer* but is now rarely used for this purpose.

Excess testosterone given to stimulate puberty may interfere with normal growth or cause over-rapid sexual development. In males, testosterone may cause *priapism* (painful, persistent erection). In females, high doses of testosterone may cause deepening of the voice, excessive hair growth, or hair loss. Treatment with some orally-administered forms of testosterone may cause liver damage.

Tests, medical
Medical tests may be performed to investigate the cause of a person's symptoms and thus establish a *diagnosis*, to monitor the course of a disease, or to assess a patient's response to treatment. Tests are also sometimes

performed on apparently healthy people to find disease at an early stage; this is known as *screening*.

To be of value, a medical test must be reasonably accurate in identifying or excluding the presence of a particular disease. The degree of accuracy is based on three factors: sensitivity, specificity, and predictive value.

Sensitivity is the ability of a test to show a positive (abnormal) value when the disease being tested for is actually present. A test that always detects a specific disease is said to have 100 per cent sensitivity. One that shows positive results in only 80 people out of a hundred who have the disease is said to have 80 per cent sensitivity; the 20 per cent of the cases missed on the test reflect the false-negative test results.

Specificity is the extent to which a test shows false-positive results in healthy people. For example, a test that shows false results in 20 per cent of the people tested is said to have 80 per cent specificity.

Sensitivity and specificity may vary with the controls used in different laboratories and with the criteria for normal values.

The third measure of a test's accuracy is its predictive value. This is determined by a mathematical formula that includes the number of times the test is accurate (the true-negative test results plus the true-positive test results) and the total number of tests performed. The predictive value thus determines the probability that a patient who has a positive test result actually has the disease or, conversely, that a patient who has a negative test result does not have the disease. The predictive value is dependent on the *prevalence* of the disease in the group being tested; when a disease is rare, a positive result is much more likely to be significant.

There is tremendous variation in accuracy among tests. For example, the faecal occult blood test (see *Occult blood, faecal*) used to detect cancer of the stomach or intestine is very sensitive; a person whose test results are negative (normal) is unlikely to have the disease. However, the test is not highly specific and many people whose test results are positive (abnormal) do not have the disease. More tests are required to confirm the diagnosis before any remedial treatment is performed.

An *ECG* to diagnose acute *myocardial infarction* (heart attack) is reasonably specific. A person whose test results are positive is almost definitely affected and is admitted to an intensive-care unit for treatment. However, the test is not sensitive; about half the people with severe chest pain who have negative test results may also need treatment.

The best tests have both high specificity and high sensitivity, and therefore high predictive value. Today's tests for *syphilis*, for example, have almost 100 per cent predictive value; they almost always show a positive result in someone who has the disease and a negative result in someone who does not have the disease.

Tetanus

A serious, sometimes fatal, disease of the *central nervous system* (brain and spinal cord) caused by infection of a wound with spores of the bacterium *CLOSTRIDIUM TETANI*.

TYPES OF MEDICAL TESTS

Brain and nervous system	EEG
	Evoked responses
	Hearing tests
	Vision tests
	Lumbar puncture
	Intelligence tests
		Myelography
		Brain imaging
		  CT scanning
		  MRI
		  PET scanning

Skin, bones, and muscles	EMG Biopsy	Bone imaging X-rays
Endocrine system and metabolism	Thyroid-function tests Thyroid scanning	Blood tests Urinalysis
Blood and immune system	Blood tests Lymphangiography	Skin tests Bone marrow biopsy

Heart and circulation	Heart imaging
	  Chest X-ray
	  Angiography
	  Echocardiography
	  Venography
		ECG
		Catheterization, cardiac
		Cardiac stress test

Lungs	Pulmonary function tests
	  Blood gases
	  Peak-flow meter
	  Spirometry
		Chest X-ray
		Bronchoscopy

Biliary system	Liver-function tests
	Liver imaging
	  Ultrasound scanning
	  Cholangiography
		Cholecystography
		ERCP
		Liver biopsy

Gastrointestinal tract	Endoscopy
	  Colonoscopy
	  Gastroscopy
		Barium X-ray examinations
		Jejunal biopsy
		Occult blood, faecal

Urinary tract	Kidney imaging Urography Ultrasound scanning	Urinalysis Kidney-function tests Cystoscopy
Reproductive system	Pregnancy tests Hysterosalpingography Mammography Ultrasound scanning Laparoscopy	Amniocentesis Cervical smear test Chorionic villus sampling Chromosome analysis Seminal fluid analysis

The table above lists some commonly performed medical tests, classified according to the body system they are used to study. Each test listed in the table has its own entry. Only some of the most important imaging techniques for each body organ have been included; a complete list appears in the appropriate imaging article.

T

CAUSES AND INCIDENCE

The spores live mainly in soil and manure, but are also found in the human intestine and elsewhere. If spores that have entered the body through a wound infect tissues that are poorly supplied with oxygenated blood, they multiply and produce a *toxin* that acts on the nerves controlling muscle activity.

About half a million cases of tetanus occur worldwide each year; in the UK, fewer than 20 cases are reported annually. All occur in nonimmunized people, mostly in those aged over 50. In developing countries, tetanus often causes death in newborn infants as a result of contamination of the umbilical stump by spores.

PREVENTION

DPT vaccination (combined immunization against diphtheria, pertussis, and tetanus) is given routinely in the UK during childhood. Thereafter, tetanus immunization booster shots are recommended every 10 years. Any wound, particularly a deep or dirty one, should be cleaned and treated with an *antiseptic*.

SYMPTOMS AND SIGNS

The most common symptom is *trismus* (stiffness of the jaw, commonly known as lockjaw), which makes it difficult to open the mouth. Other symptoms include stiffness of abdominal and back muscles, and contraction of facial muscles, producing a fixed, mirthless smile. There may also be a fast pulse, slight fever, and profuse sweating. Eventually, painful muscle spasms develop. If these affect the larynx or chest wall, *asphyxia* may result. The spasms usually subside after 10 to 14 days.

DIAGNOSIS AND TREATMENT

The diagnosis is made from the patient's symptoms and signs, and a course of tetanus *antitoxin* injections is started. Severe cases may require a *tracheostomy* (insertion of a breathing tube into the windpipe) and maintenance of respiration using a *ventilator*. Given prompt treatment, most people recover completely.

Tetany

Spasms and twitching of the *muscles*, most commonly those in the hands and feet, although the face, larynx (voice-box), or spinal muscles may also be affected. Initially, the spasms are painless; if the condition persists, they tend to become increasingly painful. In some cases, muscle damage eventually results if the underlying cause is not treated. Tetany is a symptom of a biochemical disturbance in the body, and should not be confused with *tetanus*, an infection.

The most common cause of tetany is *hypocalcaemia* (a low level of calcium in the blood), which may be due to a diet lacking in vitamin D. Other causes include hypokalaemia (a low blood level of *potassium*), which is commonly a result of prolonged diarrhoea or vomiting; *hyperventilation* (abnormally deep or rapid breathing), which is most often a result of anxiety; or, more rarely, *hypoparathyroidism* (underactivity of the parathyroid glands).

Tetracycline drugs

COMMON DRUGS

Minocycline Oxytetracycline Tetracycline

A group of *antibiotic drugs* commonly used in the treatment of *acne*, *bronchitis*, *syphilis*, *gonorrhoea*, *nonspecific urethritis*, and certain types of *pneumonia*. Tetracyclines are also prescribed for some other infections, such as *cholera*, *brucellosis*, and *Rocky Mountain spotted fever*.

Possible adverse effects include nausea, vomiting, diarrhoea, and, less commonly, rash and itching. Tetracyclines may discolour developing teeth and are therefore not usually prescribed for children under the age of 12 or for pregnant women. Tetracyclines may worsen kidney function in people suffering from a kidney disorder.

Tetrahydroaminoacridine

A drug, also known as tacrine, that is used to treat *Alzheimer's disease*. The level of the brain chemical *acetylcholine* is low in people with this disease, and treatment with tetrahydroaminoacridine increases acetylcholine production. The drug does not, however, affect the underlying brain degeneration.

Clinical trials with tetrahydroaminoacridine have shown that when it is given in high doses it improves some symptoms, such as memory loss, but it may cause impaired liver function and many patients cannot tolerate its continued use. The long-term results of treatment with tetrahydroaminoacridine are still uncertain.

Tetralogy of Fallot

A form of congenital *heart disease* in which there are four coexisting heart anomalies: displacement of the aorta, narrowing of the pulmonary valve, a hole in the ventricular septum, and thickening of the wall of the right ventricle (see diagram). As a result of these defects, blood pumped to the body from the heart is insufficiently oxygenated, which typically leads to *cyanosis* (bluish-purple coloration) and breathlessness. Tetralogy of Fallot occurs in about 1 in 1,000 babies.

SYMPTOMS AND SIGNS

Affected infants appear normal at birth, although disturbance of blood flow in the heart can be detected as *murmurs* by a doctor using a stethoscope. Severely affected babies may become cyanosed and breathless early in life. Less severely affected children may show a gradual increase in the degree of cyanosis and breathlessness. In such children, spells of cyanosis may be brought on by feeding, exertion, or infections. Other symptoms include failure to gain weight and poor development.

In older children who remain untreated, *clubbing* of the fingers and toes is usually evident. Another fea-

NORMAL HEART

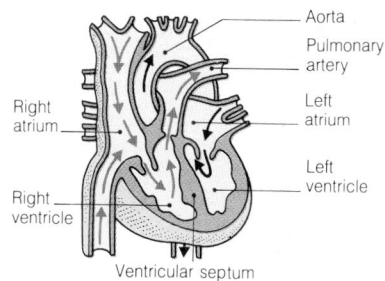

- Aorta
- Pulmonary artery
- Left atrium
- Left ventricle
- Right atrium
- Right ventricle
- Ventricular septum

TETRALOGY OF FALLOT

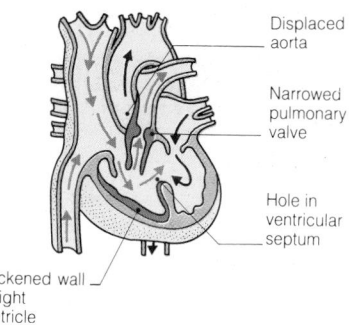

- Displaced aorta
- Narrowed pulmonary valve
- Hole in ventricular septum
- Thickened wall of right ventricle

Defects in tetralogy of Fallot
The four defects are shown above. Insufficient blood passes to the pulmonary artery and lungs to be oxygenated, and the large volume of blood pumped to the body via the aorta is therefore lacking in oxygen.

T

ture in older children is the adoption, after exertion, of a squatting position, knees up to the chest, to help them recover from breathlessness.

DIAGNOSIS

The condition is suspected from the child's symptoms and from a physical examination. A chest *X-ray* shows a characteristic shape of the heart. An *ECG*, echocardiogram (see *Echocardiography*), and in some cases cardiac *catheterization* are performed in order to determine the severity of the abnormality.

TREATMENT AND OUTLOOK

Surgery is necessary for permanent correction of the disorder. The optimal time for surgical repair is before the child starts school. A temporary procedure is usually performed first. A duct is created between the aorta and pulmonary artery so that some of the blood pumped into the aorta is diverted to the lungs. Subsequently, corrective *open heart surgery* is performed. The narrowed pulmonary artery is widened and the hole in the heart is closed. If this corrective operation is successful, no further surgery should be necessary.

Tetraplegia

An alternative name for *quadriplegia* (*paralysis* in all four limbs).

Thalamus

A structure within the *brain* consisting of an egg-shaped mass of nerve tissue, about the size of a walnut. The two thalami sit at the top of the *brainstem* and are connected by many tracts to all parts of the brain.

FUNCTION

The thalamus is an important relay centre for sensory information flowing into the brain. Different clusters of nerve cells within the thalamus receive information from the sense organs, such as the eyes and ears, and, via the spinal cord, from touch and pressure receptors in the skin. Some basic sensations, such as *pain*, may actually reach consciousness within the thalamus. Other types of sensory information are processed and relayed to parts of the cerebral cortex (outer layer of the brain), where the sensations are perceived.

The thalamus seems to act as a filter, selecting only information of particular importance from the mass of sensory signals entering the brain. This is important for the ability to concentrate on a particular task. Certain centres within the thalamus may also play a part in long-term memory.

LOCATION OF THE THALAMUS

The two thalami are situated deep within the brain, just above the brainstem.

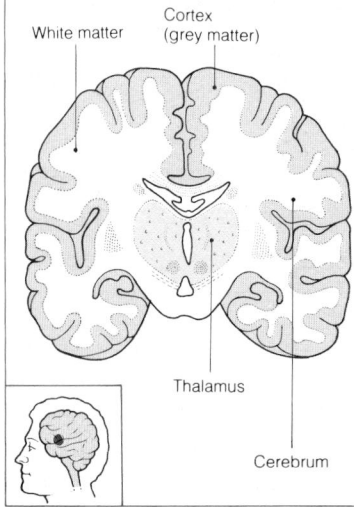

White matter

Cortex (grey matter)

Thalamus

Cerebrum

DISORDERS

Damage to the thalamus due to a *stroke* or *brain tumour* usually causes loss of sensation, but in some cases causes heightened sensitivity to pain, temperature, and other sensory stimuli.

Thalassaemia

A group of inherited *blood* disorders in which there is a fault in the production of *haemoglobin*, the oxygen-carrying substance that is synthesized in the *bone marrow* for incorporation into red blood cells. Many of the red cells produced are fragile and rapidly haemolysed (broken up), leading to anaemia (see *Anaemia, haemolytic*).

Thalassaemia is prevalent in the Mediterranean region, the Middle East, and Southeast Asia, and in families originating from these areas.

CAUSES, TYPES, AND INCIDENCE

The haemoglobin of healthy people contains two pairs of globins (protein chains), known as alpha chains and beta chains. In thalassaemia, synthesis of either the alpha or the beta chains is reduced, causing an imbalance between the alpha and beta chains in much of the haemoglobin that is produced.

Abnormal haemoglobin production in thalassaemia is caused by inheritance of a defective *gene*. Most commonly, it is the production of beta chains that is disturbed, leading to beta-thalassaemia. This condition is inherited in an autosomal recessive

pattern (see *Genetic disorders*). If a person inherits one defective gene for the disease, he or she is said to have beta-thalassaemia minor or thalassaemia trait, which is never severe. If two defective genes are inherited—one from each parent—the result is a much more severe condition called beta-thalassaemia major, or Cooley's anaemia. If two people with the minor trait have offspring, each child has a one in four chance of suffering from beta-thalassaemia major.

Alpha-thalassaemia is much less common than the beta type. If there is a severely reduced production of alpha chains, the lack of normal haemoglobin is incompatible with life and an affected infant dies within a few hours of birth. Lesser degrees of alpha-thalassaemia also occur.

SYMPTOMS

Beta-thalassaemia major produces the symptoms of haemolytic anaemia, including fatigue and shortness of breath with *jaundice* and enlargement of the *spleen* due to the rapid break-up of red blood cells. These symptoms first appear three to six months after birth. In untreated cases, to compensate for the reduced lifespan of red cells, the bone marrow expands greatly and may cause bones to grow abnormally. This leads to a characteristic enlargement of the skull in untreated patients. Normal body growth is arrested and, without treatment, death occurs during early childhood.

In the forms of alpha-thalassaemia compatible with life, there are also symptoms of anaemia but these are generally less severe.

DIAGNOSIS AND TREATMENT

The diagnosis of beta-thalassaemia major is made from microscopic examination of the blood, which shows many small, pale red blood cells, and from other blood tests that show reduced levels of adult haemoglobin in the blood.

Treatment is with blood transfusions, which should allow an affected child to grow normally. In addition, the spleen may be removed when the child is older (see *Splenectomy*). However, as each blood transfusion is administered, some iron is absorbed and eventually the internal organs become overloaded with iron, a condition known as *haemosiderosis*. This can lead to liver *cirrhosis*, to gland disorders such as *diabetes mellitus*, and to *heart failure*, which is a frequent cause of death in young adults with the disease. Compounds called *chelating agents* can help to reduce the iron overload. A *bone marrow transplant* offers a cure for the disease, but the procedure carries its own mortality risk.

OUTLOOK

Parents or other close relatives of a child with thalassaemia, and any person known to have beta-thalassaemia minor (thalassaemia trait), may derive benefit from *genetic counselling*. Beta-thalassaemia major can now be diagnosed by *antenatal screening* techniques; parents may choose to have the pregnancy terminated if a fetus is severely affected.

Thalidomide

A *sleeping drug* that was withdrawn in the UK in 1961 after it was found to cause limb deformities in many of the babies born to women given this drug during pregnancy. Thalidomide is currently under investigation for use in treating certain forms of *Hansen's disease* (leprosy).

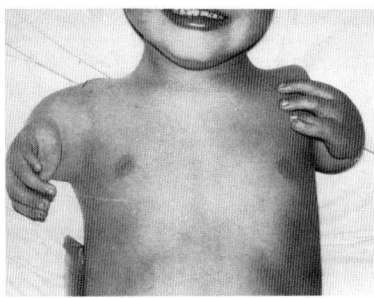

Thalidomide child
Phocomelia (stunted limbs) was a common result of the action of thalidomide on the fetus at an early stage of development.

Thallium

A rare metallic element that does not occur naturally in its pure form but is present (in minute amounts) as various compounds in certain ores of zinc and lead. Accidental poisoning may occur from swallowing rat poison and is characterized by loss of hair, disorders of the nerves in the limbs, and disturbance of the stomach and intestines.

Thallium 201 (an artificial radioactive isotope of the element) is sometimes used in *radionuclide scanning* of the heart. In this role, it reveals areas of heart muscle that have a poor blood supply or that have been damaged by a *myocardial infarction* (heart attack).

THC

The abbreviation for tetrahydrocannabinol (dronabinol), the active ingredient in *marijuana*. This drug is used to treat nausea and vomiting in cancer patients undergoing radiotherapy or anticancer drug treatment.

Theophylline

A *bronchodilator drug* used primarily in the treatment of *asthma* and to prevent attacks of *apnoea* (cessation of breathing) in premature infants. Theophylline may also be used to treat *heart failure* because it stimulates the heartrate and increases excretion of urine.

Possible adverse effects include dizziness, nausea, vomiting, diarrhoea, palpitations, and seizures.

Therapeutic

A term meaning related to treatment. The therapeutic dose of a drug is the amount required to have the most beneficial effect.

Therapeutic community

A method of treating antisocial behaviour that entails patients living together as a group in a nonhospital environment usually under the supervision of medical and nursing staff. Therapeutic communities are used for treating people suffering from *drug dependence, alcohol dependence*, and certain *personality disorders*.

Staff and patients share all decisions at regular group meetings, and unacceptable behaviour and its effects are confronted and discussed openly. All aspects of day-to-day activity thus provide a focus for learning appropriate social and interpersonal skills. (See also *Social skills training*.)

Therapy

The treatment of any disease or abnormal physical or mental condition. Examples of therapy include *radiotherapy* for cancer and *psychotherapy* for certain psychiatric disorders.

Thermography

A technique in which temperature patterns on the surface of the skin are recorded in the form of an image.

WHY IT IS DONE

Thermography provides clues to the presence of diseases and abnormalities that alter the temperature of the skin, such as circulatory problems, inflammation, and tumours. However, because so many conditions affect skin temperature, further examination and tests are necessary to confirm the underlying cause.

HOW IT IS DONE

Two techniques are used in thermography to detect skin temperature. In one, a special camera or scanner picks

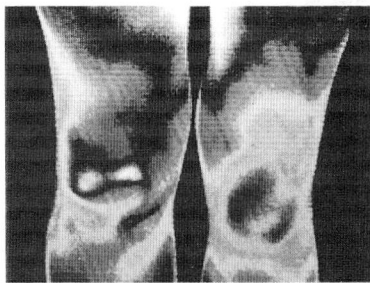

Thermographic image of the knees
Areas with different surface temperatures show up as different shades in thermographic images. Excess heat indicates either inflammation or rich blood flow.

up infra-red radiation naturally emitted from the skin. In the other, sheets of special temperature-sensitive liquid crystals are applied to the skin and change colour in response to changes in temperature.

RESULTS

Thermography is a safe technique. Results have not proved sufficiently reliable for thermography to fulfil hopes that it might prove useful as an early screening test for breast cancer.

Thermometer

An instrument used to measure *temperature*. A traditional clinical thermometer consists of a glass capillary tube (a tube with a very fine bore) that is sealed at one end and has a mercury-filled bulb at the other. Different styles of thermometer may be used to measure the temperature in the mouth, armpit, and rectum.

Clinical thermometers may be calibrated in *Celsius* (centigrade), *Fahrenheit*, or sometimes both. The wall of the thermometer is thickened on one side to form a cylindrical lens that makes the mercury easier to see.

When the bulb of the thermometer is placed in the mouth, armpit, or rectum, the mercury expands up the capillary tube. The thermometer is removed and the body temperature—indicated by the level of the mercury—is then read against a scale on the glass. There is a small kink in the capillary tube just above the bulb to prevent the mercury from moving down the tube when the thermometer is removed. Before the thermometer can be used again, the mercury must be shaken back down into the bulb.

A modern version of the traditional clinical thermometer uses an electronic probe connected to a digital readout display, and these devices give an almost instantaneous reading.

T

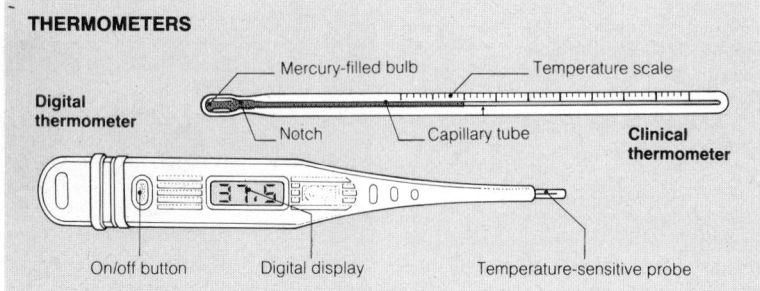

THERMOMETERS

Digital thermometer

Mercury-filled bulb

Temperature scale

Notch

Capillary tube

Clinical thermometer

On/off button

Digital display

Temperature-sensitive probe

In recent years, there has been a trend towards using disposable skin thermometers that employ heat-sensitive chemicals that change colour at specific temperatures. Disposable skin thermometers are generally less accurate than the mercury or digital types because they are more likely to be affected by external factors, such as the temperature of the environment.

Thiabendazole

An *anthelmintic drug* used to treat *worm infestations*, including *strongyloidiasis*, *trichinosis*, and *toxocariasis*.

Thiabendazole may cause dizziness, loss of appetite, nausea, vomiting, headache, drowsiness, and diarrhoea. Rarely, an allergic reaction to the drug occurs, leading to fever, rash, facial swelling, and, in severe cases, causing collapse.

Thiamine

See *Vitamin B complex*.

Thiopentone

A *barbiturate drug* that is widely used as a general anaesthetic (see *Anaesthesia, general*). Thiopentone is given by intravenous injection and quickly produces unconsciousness. The effects of thiopentone are, however, relatively short-lived, and a different anaesthetic agent is therefore used to maintain anaesthesia.

Thioridazine

An *antipsychotic drug* used to treat *schizophrenia* and *mania*. Its tranquillizing effect reduces the abnormal experiences of patients who suffer from these conditions, and helps relieve their *anxiety* and *depression*.

Thioridazine may cause *dyskinesia* (abnormal movements) but is less likely to do so than some other antipsychotic drugs. Drowsiness, dry mouth, muscle stiffness, and dizziness may occur. High doses of thioridazine taken over long periods may damage the retina.

Thirst

The desire to drink. Thirst is one means by which the amount of water in the body is controlled (the other is the volume of urine excreted).

Thirst is stimulated by an increase in the concentration of salt, sugar, or certain other substances in the blood. Concentration of these substances in the serum (the liquid portion of blood) rises if fluid intake falls or if dietary intake of the substances (most commonly salt) increases. As the concentrated blood passes through the *hypothalamus* in the brain, special nerve receptors are stimulated, inducing the sensation of thirst.

Thirst is also stimulated if the volume of blood decreases as a result of sweating, vomiting, diarrhoea, severe bleeding, or extensive burns. Thirst may also be caused by a dry mouth, even when a person is adequately hydrated; in such cases, thirst can usually be relieved merely by moistening the mouth.

Damage to the hypothalamus (as a result of a head injury, for example) may cause loss of the desire to drink and consequent *dehydration*.

Thirst, excessive

A strong and persistent need to drink, most commonly due to *dehydration*. Excessive thirst is a symptom of untreated *diabetes mellitus* and *diabetes insipidus*. Other causes of excessive thirst include *kidney failure*, treatment with certain drugs (such as *phenothiazine drugs*), and severe blood loss. Abnormal thirst may also be psychological in origin, a condition known as psychogenic polydipsia.

Thoracic outlet syndrome

A condition in which pressure on the *brachial plexus* (the nerve roots that pass into either arm from the neck) causes pain in the arms and shoulders, a pins-and-needles sensation in the fingers, and weakness of grip and other hand movements.

Severe symptoms are usually caused by a *cervical rib*, which is an extra rib above the first rib that is linked to the first rib by a fibrous band of tissue which presses on the brachial plexus. Thoracic outlet syndrome may also result from pressure on the brachial plexus due to drooping shoulders, an enlarged scalenus muscle in the neck, or a tumour. The condition is made worse by lifting and carrying heavy loads or by an increase in body weight.

Treatment usually involves exercises to improve posture. *Nonsteroidal anti-inflammatory drugs* and *muscle-relaxant drugs* are sometimes helpful. Severe cases may be treated by surgical removal of the first rib.

Thoracic surgery

A surgical specialty concerned with operations on organs within the chest cavity, excluding the heart. Thoracic surgery is concerned particularly with disorders of the *lungs, oesophagus,* and trachea (windpipe).

Thoracotomy

An operation in which the chest is opened to provide access to organs in the chest cavity.

WHY IT IS DONE

A thoracotomy is usually performed to allow a surgeon to operate on a diseased *heart, lung,* or other organ in the chest cavity, such as the *oesophagus*. It may also be carried out as an emergency procedure following a severe chest injury.

HOW IT IS DONE

There are two types of thoracotomy: lateral and anterior. Both are performed under general anaesthesia.

A lateral thoracotomy provides access to the lungs, major blood vessels, and oesophagus. A curved incision is made from between the shoulderblades, around the side of the trunk beneath the armpit, to just below the nipple. The necessary operation is then performed. Afterwards, a drainage tube is inserted into the pleural cavity (the space between the membrane covering the lung and the membrane lining the chest wall) to allow fluid to drain and to prevent the lung from collapsing. The incision is then closed with stitches.

An anterior thoracotomy provides access to the heart and coronary arteries. A vertical incision is made from between the clavicles (collarbones) at the base of the neck to the lower end of the sternum (breastbone). The sternum is divided with a saw and prised

T

apart. The heart is then exposed and the necessary surgery performed. Following insertion of a drainage tube into the pleural cavity, the sternum is closed with strong stitches (sometimes wire) and the overlying skin is sewn up.

RECOVERY PERIOD

Despite drainage, secretions in the air passages often cause breathing problems after surgery. To clear the passages, the patient is encouraged to breathe deeply and cough and is given *physiotherapy*. The drainage tube is usually removed within 48 hours after surgery.

Thorax

The medical name for the chest. The thorax extends from the base of the neck to the *diaphragm muscle* and is supported and protected by the *ribs, sternum* (breastbone), and *vertebrae* (spinal bones). The main structures in the thorax are the *heart, lungs, oesophagus,* and large blood vessels such as the *aorta* and pulmonary arteries.

Thought

A mental activity that enables humans to reason, form judgments, and solve problems. The essential features of thought are the substitution of symbols (in the form of words, numbers, or images) for objects, the formation of these symbols into ideas, and the arrangement of ideas into a certain order in the mind. A person's thoughts are represented to others by speech, writing, and behaviour.

Aspects of thought that can be examined or tested include speed and efficiency, content of ideas, and the logical relationship between ideas. (See also *Thought disorders*.)

Thought disorders

Abnormalities in the structure or content of *thought* as reflected in a person's speech, writing, or behaviour.

In the thought disorder characteristic of *schizophrenia*, sometimes referred to as formal thought disorder, associations lose their logical connection. The individual may jump from one subject to another that is apparently unrelated, or may make indirect associations or "clang" associations (the relating of words that sound the same rather than connect logically).

Other thought disorders that occur in schizophrenia include the invention of new words (see *Neologisms*), thought blocking (sudden interruption in the train of thought), experiencing thoughts as being inserted into or withdrawn from the mind by some outside force, and auditory *hallucinations*, in which a voice is heard dictating or repeating the subject's thoughts.

An inability to think clearly and coherently occurs in all types of *confusion*, including *dementia* and delirium. Rapidly jumping from one idea to another ("flight of ideas") as a result of a loosening of associations is characteristic of *hypomania* and *mania*. In *depression*, the opposite occurs: thinking becomes slow, there is a lack of ideas and associations, and a tendency to dwell in great detail on trivial subjects. Recurrent ideas that seem to come into a person's mind involuntarily are characteristic of *obsessive-compulsive behaviour*.

Delusions (false beliefs that do not respond to reasoned argument), which occur in schizophrenia and other psychotic illnesses, may be an expression of distorted thinking.

Threadworm infestation

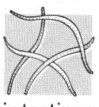 A common infestation with a small parasitic worm, *ENTEROBIUS VERMICULARIS*, that lives in the intestines. This species is also sometimes called pinworm.

CAUSES, INCIDENCE, AND SYMPTOMS

Threadworms primarily affect children and are the most common worm parasite of children in temperate areas. Possibly one fifth of all children in the UK are affected at any time.

The female adult threadworms are white and about 10 mm long. They lay eggs in the skin around the anus, and their movements cause tickling or itching in the anal region, often at night, which may cause the child to scratch. Eggs are transferred directly via the fingers to the mouth to cause reinfestation, or are carried on toys or blankets to other children. Swallowed eggs hatch in the intestine and the worms reach maturity after a period of two to six weeks.

DIAGNOSIS AND TREATMENT

Adult worms can sometimes be seen in the faeces or on the buttocks.

ANATOMY OF THE THORAX

The heart, lungs and large blood vessels (such as the aorta) occupy almost all of the thoracic cavity; part of the oesophagus and trachea are also in the thorax. The thoracic contents are protected and supported by the ribs, sternum (breastbone), and vertebrae.

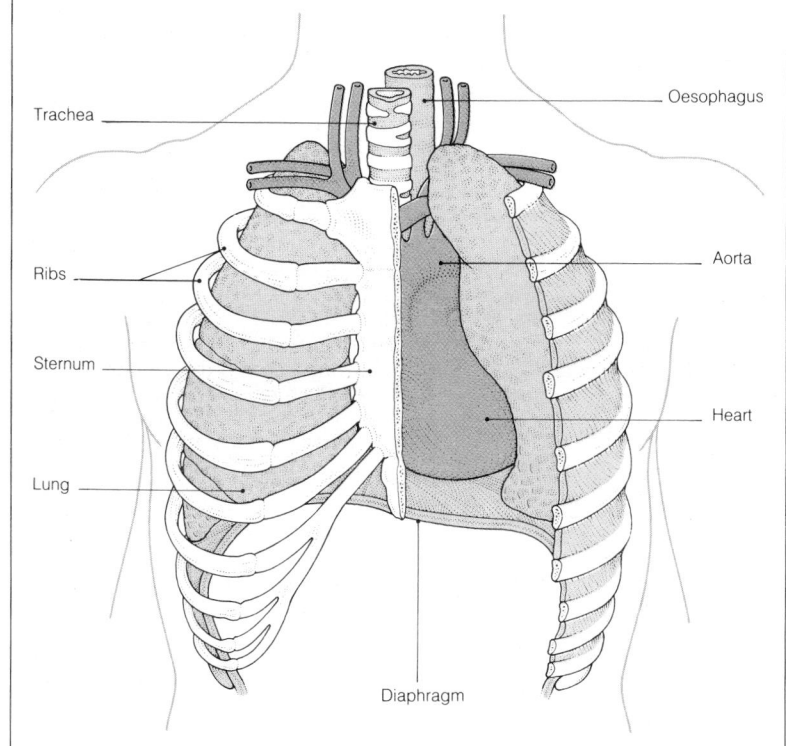

Trachea

Ribs

Sternum

Lung

Diaphragm

Oesophagus

Aorta

Heart

T

CYCLE OF THREADWORM INFESTATION

The adult worms live in the large intestine, from where the females migrate to lay eggs around the anal region. Eggs may be transferred to the mouth (via fingers, sheets, or toys), are swallowed, and hatch to start a new infestation. Occasionally, in a girl, an adult worm migrates into the vagina or bladder, leading to a discharge or to cystitis.

Eggs are swallowed and move through the intestines, where they hatch into larvae.

Larvae develop into adults in the intestine, from where female worms migrate.

Female worms lay eggs around the anus at night, causing itching and scratching in the area.

Worm eggs are accidentally transferred from child's anus to mouth via fingers.

Threadworm eggs for microscopic examination can be obtained by applying a piece of sticky paper to the anal area.

Ointments may be used to relieve anal itching. A doctor may prescribe an *anthelmintic drug*, which, in combination with good hygiene, usually clears up the problem. Treatment of all members of the family is advisable.

Preventive and self-help measures include the wearing of pyjamas to discourage scratching, keeping the fingernails short, and washing the hands scrupulously before all meals. Sheets and nightwear should be changed frequently, washed at high temperature, and ironed.

Thrill

A vibrating sensation felt when the flat of the hand is held against the front of the chest. A thrill is caused by abnormal blood flow in the *heart* due to a diseased heart valve or to some form of congenital *heart disease*. A thrill is always accompanied by an audible heart *murmur*.

Throat

A popular term for the *pharynx*, the passage running down from the back of the mouth and nose to the upper part of the *oesophagus* and the opening into the *larynx* (voice-box). The term throat is also used to refer to the front of the neck. (See also *Sore throat*.)

Throat cancer

See *Pharynx, cancer of*.

Thrombectomy

The removal of a *thrombus* (blood clot) that is partly or completely blocking a blood vessel.

Thrombectomy may be performed as an emergency procedure if a thrombus is blocking a major artery (such as one supplying blood to the brain, lungs, or intestines). It may also be performed as a precautionary measure if there is a risk of an *embolus* (fragment) breaking off from a thrombus and being carried into the bloodstream to block an artery.

Before surgery, the site of the thrombus is established by *angiography* and the patient is given *anticoagulant drugs* (drugs that prevent the blood from clotting). With the patient under general anaesthesia, incisions are made to uncover the affected blood vessel. The blood vessel is then opened and the thrombus aspirated (sucked out). The incision is closed with delicate stitches.

Thromboangiitis obliterans

Another name for *Buerger's disease*.

Thrombocytopenia

A reduction in the number of *platelet* cells in the blood. Because platelets play a vital role in the arrest of bleeding (by plugging any small breaks that develop in the walls of blood vessels), thrombocytopenia causes a tendency to bleed, especially from the smaller blood vessels. The result may be thrombocytopenic purpura (abnormal bleeding into the skin).

CAUSES AND SYMPTOMS

Thrombocytopenia may be caused by a reduced rate of production of platelets by the *bone marrow* or by a fast rate of destruction of the platelets.

In a form of thrombocytopenia known as idiopathic thrombocytopenic purpura (ITP), the underlying cause is not apparent. However, this type of thrombocytopenia commonly follows a viral infection and may be an *autoimmune disorder* in which the infection triggers destruction of the platelets by the immune system. ITP occurs mainly in children and young adults. The symptoms may include purple bruises or bleeding points in the skin, nosebleeds, *haematuria* (blood in the urine), bleeding in the mouth, and *menorrhagia* (heavy menstrual bleeding). There is a small risk of *brain haemorrhage*, the warning signs for which are headache and dizziness.

Thrombocytopenia can be a feature of *leukaemia*, *lymphoma*, other malignant diseases, megaloblastic *anaemia*, systemic *lupus erythematosus*, or *hypersplenism* (overactivity of the spleen). Another possible cause is the rare disorder thrombotic thrombocytopenic purpura (TTP), which also causes damage to the kidneys and the brain and spinal cord. Thrombocytopenia may also occur after exposure to X-rays or radiation, in severe fevers, and as a reaction to certain drugs.

DIAGNOSIS

Thrombocytopenia is diagnosed from the patient's symptoms and from the presence of low numbers of platelets when a *blood count* is performed. A diagnosis of ITP is made by excluding other possible causes.

TREATMENT AND OUTLOOK

Any underlying disease will be treated if possible, and any causative drug withdrawn.

Children with ITP may not require treatment, but most adults are given *corticosteroid drugs*. In most cases, ITP lasts a few days to a few weeks before clearing up, although sometimes, particularly in adults, the bleeding tendency may recur from time to time. If ITP persists for many weeks or becomes recurrent, *splenectomy* (removal of the spleen) may be performed, giving a lasting cure in about three quarters of cases.

Thromboembolism

The blockage of a blood vessel by a fragment that has broken off from a thrombus (blood clot) and been carried elsewhere in the circulation. (See also *Thrombosis*; *Embolism*.)

T

Thrombolytic drugs

COMMON DRUGS

Alteplase Anistreplase Streptokinase

A group of drugs, also sometimes known as fibrinolytic drugs, used to dissolve blood clots occurring in *thrombosis, embolism,* and *myocardial infarction* (heart attack).

Thrombolytic drugs work by increasing the blood level of plasmin (an enzyme that dissolves fibrin, the main constituent of blood clots).

Treatment with thrombolytic drugs is carefully monitored because of the risk of abnormal bleeding. An allergic reaction, causing rash and breathing difficulty, may also occur.

Thrombophlebitis

Inflammation of part of a vein, usually near the surface of the body, along with clot formation in the affected segment. The condition can occur after minor injury to a vein (such as after an injection or intravenous infusion) and is particularly common in intravenous drug abusers. Thrombophlebitis can develop as a complication of *varicose veins* and also in blood vessel disorders such as *Buerger's disease.*

There is obvious swelling and redness along the affected segment of vein, which is extremely tender when touched. Fever and malaise often occur. Serious complications are uncommon, although sometimes far more dangerous clot formation develops in deeper veins (see *Thrombosis, deep vein*).

Treatment includes use of a crepe bandage to give gentle support, *nonsteroidal anti-inflammatory drugs,* and, if infection of the vein is suspected, *antibiotic drugs.*

Thrombosis

The formation of a thrombus (blood clot) within an intact blood vessel. Clotting is a normal response that prevents bleeding when a blood vessel wall is injured. Thrombus formation is abnormal if it occurs when a vessel wall has not been cut or punctured.

A thrombus within an artery may eventually grow to block the artery, preventing blood and oxygen from reaching the organ or tissue supplied by the artery. Thrombi of this type are an important cause of death and disability in developed countries. A thrombus that forms within one of the arteries supplying the heart muscle, a condition known as coronary thrombosis, is the usual cause of *myocardial*

infarction (heart attack). A thrombus within one of the arteries supplying the brain, a condition known as cerebral thrombosis, is a common cause of *stroke.*

Thrombi may also block arteries supplying blood to the legs, kidneys, retinas, intestines, and other organs, sometimes causing severe damage and symptoms such as pain and loss of function. Another danger is that an embolus (fragment of thrombus) may break off and be carried in the bloodstream to block an important blood vessel perhaps at some distance from its site of origin.

Thrombi sometimes form in veins—either in inflamed veins near the surface, a condition known as *thrombophlebitis,* or in deeper veins (see *Thrombosis, deep vein*). In deep vein thrombosis, the risk of large emboli breaking off and being carried to the heart and lungs is particularly serious, the result potentially fatal.

CAUSES

In the blood there is a fine balance between the mechanisms that encourage and discourage clotting, so there is neither a tendency to bleed nor to form clots (see *Blood clotting*). Thrombosis can occur if there is an upset in favour of clotting.

In arteries, the clotting process may be encouraged by a build-up of atheroma (fatty deposits) on blood vessel walls. Any of the factors that encourage *atherosclerosis*—such as smoking, obesity, *diabetes mellitus,* or *hypertension* (high blood pressure)—is similarly associated with an increased tendency to form clots. Clot formation may also be encouraged by damage to blood vessel walls from inflammation, which occurs in *arteritis* and phlebitis. Abnormal clotting may also be due to spread of infection in the blood, either to local blood vessels or throughout the circulation in *septicaemia* (spread and multiplication of bacteria through the blood).

A clotting tendency may result from an increase in the level of coagulation factors in the blood, which may occur in pregnancy or when using *oral contraceptives.* A clotting tendency may also result from a liver disease that leads to deficient production of antithrombin, an anticlotting factor. Any circumstance that causes a slowing down of blood flow to a particular area (such as inactivity during a long air flight, or general anaesthesia induced for a surgical operation) may also result in a clotting tendency.

SYMPTOMS AND DIAGNOSIS

An arterial thrombus may cause no symptoms until it impairs the flow of blood through a blood vessel. At this point it may cause reduced function of the organ or tissue supplied by the blood vessel and, in some cases, severe pain. Venous thrombosis may also cause pain and swelling.

When thrombosis is a suspected cause of symptoms, it is investigated by *angiography* or by *venography* (X-rays of blood vessels taken after the injection of a radiopaque substance).

TREATMENT

Treatment may include the use of *anticoagulant drugs,* which discourage clotting, or *thrombolytic drugs,* which help break down clots that have already formed. *Nonsteroidal anti-inflammatory drugs* are often given to relieve the inflammation of thrombophlebitis. Other treatment, such as *antibiotic drugs* if infection is the cause of thrombosis, may be necessary. In cases where a clot is life-threatening, surgical removal may be required (see *Thrombectomy*).

Thrombosis, deep vein

The formation of a thrombus (blood clot) within deep-lying veins, usually in the legs.

CAUSES AND INCIDENCE

Deep vein thrombosis is generally caused by a combination of sluggish blood flow through one part of the body and some condition that increases the natural tendency of the blood to clot.

Sluggish blood flow occurs when a person lies or sits still for long periods. An increase in the level of coagulation factors in the blood, which occurs after an operation or injury, during pregnancy, and in women taking *oral contraceptives,* causes an increased tendency for the blood to clot.

An increased tendency to form clots can also occur as a result of *polycythaemia* (increased numbers of red cells in the blood), severe infection, liver disease, and certain types of cancer. Deep vein thrombosis is common in people with *heart failure* and in those who have had a *stroke* or who are immobilized for long periods. Other causes include injury to the veins or the spread of *thrombophlebitis* (inflammation and clot formation in superficial veins) to deeper veins. Age and obesity both predispose to thrombosis.

SYMPTOMS AND COMPLICATIONS

If a deep vein thrombosis occurs somewhere other than in a leg, there are often no symptoms. Clots in the leg veins may cause symptoms such as pain, tenderness, swelling, discoloration, and ulceration of the skin, depending on the site and extent of the clots (see illustrated box).

Deep vein thrombosis is not always of serious significance. However, if clots are extensive, part of a clot may break free and be carried up to the heart and from there to the lungs, where it may block an artery. This is called a *pulmonary embolism* and is always a serious condition.

DIAGNOSIS

The presence and extent of deep vein thrombosis is diagnosed by *venography* (introduction of a radiopaque substance into the veins followed by X-rays) and by a type of *radionuclide scanning* called the radioactive fibrinogen test. Doppler *ultrasound scanning* may also be used to detect thrombi.

TREATMENT

Treatment depends on the site and extent of the blood clots. If they are small, confined to the calf, and the patient is mobile, treatment may be unnecessary, as the clots often break up spontaneously. In some cases, *anticoagulant drugs* may be given to prevent extension of the clots. In other cases, *thrombolytic drugs*, which actively dissolve the clots, may be given. If there is a high risk of a clot breaking off and causing a pulmonary embolism, *thrombectomy* may be performed to remove the clot surgically.

PREVENTION

The incidence of deep vein thrombosis has been reduced by encouraging people to get up as soon as possible after an operation or childbirth. If a person is immobilized for a long period, he or she should wiggle the toes and flex the ankles and knees to keep the blood moving. Blood flow in the legs of an immobilized person may also be stimulated by the pumping up and down of inflatable bags around the legs.

When an operation is performed on someone thought to be particularly susceptible to deep vein thrombosis, anticoagulant drugs may be given.

Thrombus

A blood clot that has formed inside an intact blood vessel—as distinct from one that has formed to seal the wall of a blood vessel after injury.

A thrombus is life-threatening if it grows to obstruct the blood supply to an organ such as the heart or brain. Even a thrombus in a less vital blood vessel can be dangerous because it may produce *gangrene* in part of an organ or extremity served by the blood vessel, or lead to *embolism*, in

---

DEEP VEIN THROMBOSIS

Thrombi, or clots, tend to form when blood flow is sluggish and in circumstances (such as pregnancy) in which there is a rise in the level of coagulation factors in the blood. Once a clot has formed, it may provide a site for further clotting, so that a long, snaky clot may grow along the length of a vein. Thrombi form most commonly in the leg veins and may interfere with the drainage of blood from a leg (below right), causing signs and symptoms of varying severity.

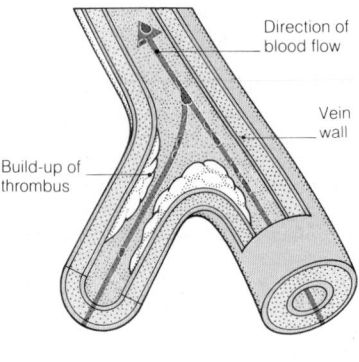

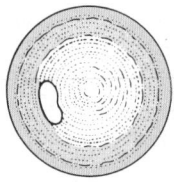 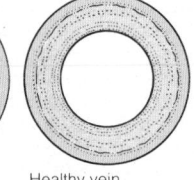

Partly blocked vein   Healthy vein

Normal and obstructed vein
Thrombi tend to form at points where a vein lining is damaged and may then grow to obstruct blood flow. The main danger is that a piece of clot will detach and be carried to the heart and lungs to cause a potentially fatal obstruction.

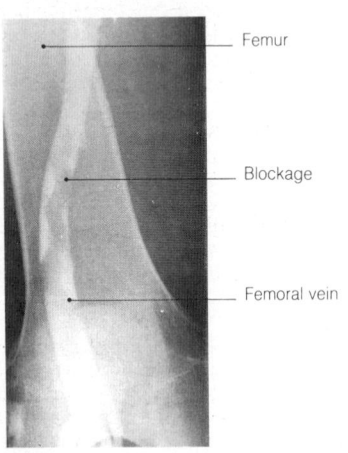

Example of deep vein thrombosis
This venogram shows a thrombus blocking the femoral vein just above the knee.

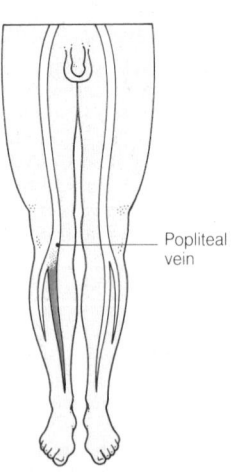

Calf vein thrombosis
When clots are localized in the calf and popliteal veins, there is usually some pain in the calf but there may be little swelling.

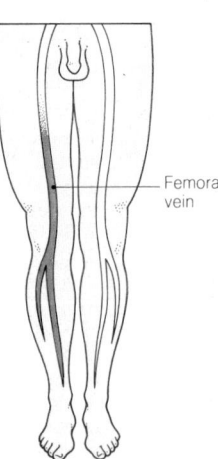

Femoral vein thrombosis
If clots are present in the femoral vein as well as calf veins, there is usually pain and swelling up to the region above the knee.

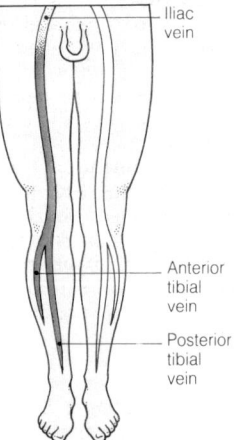

Iliac vein thrombosis
Clots in the iliac vein may affect drainage of blood from the whole leg, causing severe pain and swelling in the leg.

T

which a fragment of the thrombus breaks off and is carried to obstruct the blood circulation elsewhere. (See also *Blood clotting*; *Thrombosis*.)

Thrush
A common name for the fungal infection *candidiasis*.

Thumb-sucking
A common habit in young children. For the young child, thumb-sucking provides comfort (especially before falling asleep), oral gratification, amusement if the child is bored, and reassurance, especially in periods of stress, such as the birth of a new baby in the family.

Thumb-sucking tends to decrease after the age of about three. Only a few children do not grow out of the habit by six or seven. In general, it is best for parents to ignore a child's thumb-sucking; constant reprimands may make the habit worse.

COMPLICATIONS
In most cases, there is no evidence that thumb-sucking is harmful. However, *malocclusion* (incorrect bite) of the second teeth may develop if the habit continues after about the age of seven. The effect on the teeth is usually only temporary; their position improves considerably or even returns completely to normal after thumb-sucking stops. In severe cases, treatment with an *orthodontic appliance* may be recommended.

Thymoma
A tumour of the *thymus* gland. Thymomas are rare and are classified according to the type of thymus tissue from which they arise. An epithelial thymoma, arising from *epithelium*, is a slow-growing tumour that rarely spreads to other parts of the body. A lymphoid thymoma arises from lymphoid tissue, eventually resulting in generalized non-Hodgkin's *lymphoma*. A granulomatous thymoma consists of a mixture of epithelial and lymphoid tissue, and closely resembles *Hodgkin's disease*. The other main type of thymoma is a thymic *teratoma* (a tumour consisting of tissue that is not normally found in the thymus), which is usually benign in women but malignant in men.

Thymomas may affect function of the *immune system*, causing increased susceptibility to infection. They are commonly associated with *myasthenia gravis* (an autoimmune disease), which can sometimes be cured by removal of the thymoma.

Thymoxamine
A *vasodilator drug* occasionally used in the treatment of *Raynaud's disease*. Possible adverse effects of thymoxamine include nausea, diarrhoea, hot flushes, headache, and dizziness.

Thymus
A gland that forms part of the *immune system*. The thymus is situated in the upper part of the chest, behind the sternum (breastbone), and consists of two lobes that join in front of the trachea (windpipe). Each lobe is made up of lymphoid tissue consisting of tightly packed *lymphocytes*, *epithelium*, and fat.

The thymus plays a part in the body's immune response from about the 12th week of gestation until puberty. The gland gradually enlarges until puberty, when it begins to shrink. Lymphoid and epithelial tissues are gradually replaced by fat, although some glandular tissue remains until after middle age.

The function of the thymus is to condition lymphocytes to become *T-cells* and thus take part in the body's defence against viruses and other infections.

DISORDERS
Abnormal enlargement of the thymus may occur in several conditions, including *myasthenia gravis*, *acromegaly*, *thyrotoxicosis*, and *Addison's disease*. Myasthenia gravis is also sometimes associated with *thymomas*

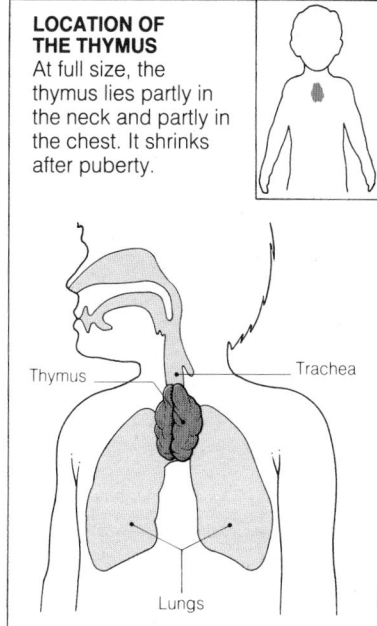

LOCATION OF THE THYMUS
At full size, the thymus lies partly in the neck and partly in the chest. It shrinks after puberty.

Thymus — Trachea

Lungs

(tumours of the thymus). In children, *immunodeficiency disorders* may arise as a result of abnormal development of the thymus.

Thyroglossal disorders
Congenital defects arising from failure of the thyroglossal duct to disappear during embryonic development. In the *embryo*, this duct runs from the base of the tongue to the thyroid gland in the neck. Abnormal development may cause the duct to persist in its entirety or partly as a cyst.

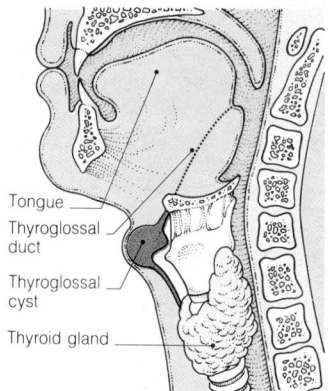

Tongue
Thyroglossal duct
Thyroglossal cyst
Thyroid gland

Thyroglossal duct and cyst
The thyroglossal duct, lying between the tongue and the thyroid, sometimes persists after fetal life, and a cyst may form.

A thyroglossal cyst almost always becomes infected and swollen, a condition that may be mistaken for an abscess. Infection may lead to formation of a thyroglossal fistula (abnormal passage between the cyst and the surface of the neck).

Because of the danger of repeated infection, a thyroglossal cyst or fistula should be completely removed surgically, along with any remaining parts of the thyroglossal duct.

Thyroid cancer
Cancer of the *thyroid gland* is relatively rare, accounting for only about one per cent of all cases of cancer. In most cases, the cause of the condition is unknown, although it is one of the cancers associated with exposure to radioactive fallout. Thyroid cancer has one of the highest cure rates of all types of cancer.

SYMPTOMS AND SIGNS
A thyroid cancer is usually first noticed as a single, firm nodule in the neck. The tumour may grow slowly or rapidly, depending partly on the particular type of cancer and partly on the age of the patient (growth tends to be

T

slower in younger people). Thyroid cancers are painless in many cases; symptoms arise when tumours press on other structures in the neck. Such symptoms may include severe hoarseness or loss of voice, caused by pressure on the nerves to the larynx (voice-box), or difficulty in swallowing, caused by pressure on the pharynx (throat). Spread of the cancer to the lymph nodes, which often occurs at an early stage, causes enlargement of the nodes. Advanced cancers are usually hard and irregularly shaped and are often firmly attached to adjacent structures in the neck.

DIAGNOSIS
A doctor's initial physical examination cannot differentiate between a cancerous and a noncancerous nodule. For this reason, single thyroid nodules are always imaged (see *Thyroid scanning*). In some cases, tissue is removed for microscopic analysis either by a needle *biopsy* or surgically. If there are several nodules, they are likely to be benign rather than cancerous.

TREATMENT
Treatment is usually by total *thyroidectomy* (surgical removal of the entire gland); occasionally, it is also necessary to remove surrounding tissues. The loss of thyroid tissue results in a lack of natural *thyroid hormones*, and patients usually need to take thyroxine for the rest of their lives. Such supplements may also help to control *metastases* (secondary growths).

In virtually all cases, treatment with radioactive *iodine* is used after surgery. Because it is selectively taken up and concentrated in the thyroid, radioactive iodine has the advantage of destroying any residual cancer while leaving normal body tissue undamaged. This treatment may be repeated at one- to five-year intervals if any residual tissue is detected.

OUTLOOK
If thyroid cancer is diagnosed and treated at an early stage (even if local spread has occurred), the outlook is generally good.

Thyroidectomy
Surgical removal of all or part of the *thyroid gland*.

WHY IT IS DONE
Thyroidectomy is performed to treat *thyroid cancer*, some cases of *hyperthyroidism* that cannot be controlled by drugs, *goitre* (enlargement of the thyroid gland) that is causing breathing or swallowing difficulties or unsightly swelling, or a benign tumour of the thyroid gland.

SUBTOTAL THYROIDECTOMY
This operation entails removal of only part of the thyroid. The parathyroids (at the rear of the gland) are left intact.

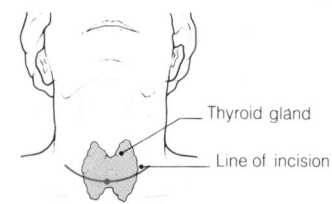

Thyroid gland

Line of incision

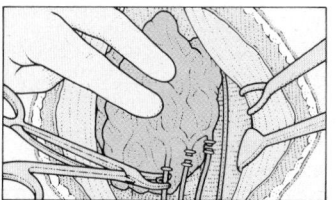

1 After administration of a general anaesthetic, an incision is made in the neck. Layers of skin and muscle are then drawn aside to expose the thyroid gland underneath.

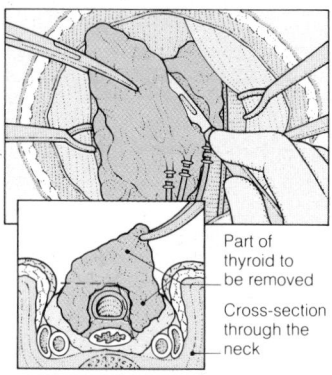

Part of thyroid to be removed

Cross-section through the neck

2 Once the front of the gland has been detached from its blood supply, much of it is cut away (with care taken not to damage nearby nerves), and bleeding vessels are sealed.

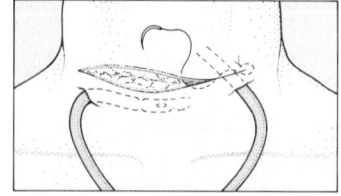

3 Tubes are sometimes placed in the site of the removed gland to drain blood that accumulates. The muscle and skin layers are replaced and the incision closed with sutures or clips.

HOW IT IS DONE
With the patient under general anaesthesia, an incision is made in the neck and all or part of the thyroid gland is removed. A common form of operation to remove part of the thyroid (subtotal thyroidectomy) is shown in the illustrated box.

RECOVERY PERIOD
The wound usually heals quickly. The stitches and drainage tube can usually be removed within a few days of the operation, after which the patient leaves hospital.

Removal of all—or a large part—of the thyroid gland necessitates lifelong hormone replacement therapy with *thyroid hormones*.

COMPLICATIONS
There is a very small risk of damage to structures close to the thyroid gland. Injury to the nerve supplying the vocal cords can lead to hoarseness; damage to the *parathyroid glands* can result in a low calcium level in the blood and *tetany* (painful muscle spasms in the hands, feet, and face). After the operation, careful monitoring is required to ensure that hormone levels are in the normal range.

Thyroid-function tests
A group of procedures used to evaluate the function of the *thyroid gland* and to detect or confirm any disorder of the gland.

Thyroid function can be measured by carrying out *blood tests* to determine the level of thyroxine (T_4) and triiodothyronine (T_3) in the blood. A sample of blood is taken from the patient's vein and the serum (liquid part of the blood) is tested.

The main function of the thyroid gland is to convert tyrosine (an amino acid) and *iodine* into T_4 and T_3. One way of measuring thyroid function is therefore to measure the rate at which iodine is accumulated by the gland. This can be done by introducing into the body a radioactive isotope of iodine (or *technetium*, which behaves in a similar way to iodine) and then measuring the level of radioactivity in the gland (see *Thyroid scanning*).

The thyroid secretes T_4 and T_3 into the bloodstream under the direct control of thyroid-stimulating hormone (TSH) from the *pituitary gland*. Measurement of the amount of TSH in the blood provides a sensitive means of diagnosing thyroid malfunction. Various indices created by ratios of T_3 and T_4 enable the specialist to give a more accurate diagnosis of the patient's condition.

T

Thyroid gland

One of the main *endocrine glands*, which helps regulate the body's energy level. The thyroid gland is situated in the front of the neck, just below the larynx (voice-box). It consists of two lobes, one on each side of the trachea (windpipe), joined by a narrower portion of tissue called the isthmus.

STRUCTURE

Thyroid tissue is composed of two types of secretory cells: follicular cells and parafollicular cells (or C cells). Follicular cells, which make up most of the gland, are arranged in the form of hollow, spherical follicles. These cells secrete the iodine-containing hormones thyroxine (T_4) and triiodothyronine (T_3). The space inside the follicles is filled with a yellow, semifluid, colloid material that is essential for the production of T_4 and T_3.

Parafollicular cells occur singly or in small groups in the spaces between the follicles. These cells secrete the hormone *calcitonin*. Also between the follicles are numerous blood capillaries, small lymphatic vessels, and connective tissue.

FUNCTION

T_4 and T_3 play an important role in controlling body *metabolism*. Calcitonin acts in conjunction with parathyroid hormone to regulate calcium balance in the body. (See also *Thyroid gland* disorders box; *Thyroid hormones*.)

LOCATION OF THE THYROID GLAND

This major gland lies at the base of the neck just in front of the trachea (windpipe).

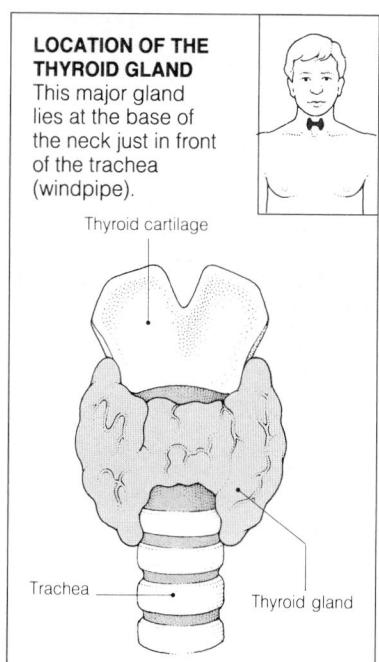

Thyroid cartilage

Trachea

Thyroid gland

Thyroid hormones

The hormones thyroxine (T_4), triiodothyronine (T_3), and *calcitonin*, produced by the *thyroid gland*.

FUNCTION

T_4 (the hormone produced in greatest amounts by the thyroid gland) and T_3 regulate *metabolism* (the chemical activity in cells that releases energy from nutrients or uses energy to create other substances, such as proteins). In children, these hormones are also essential for normal physical growth and mental development.

Calcitonin acts in conjunction with parathyroid hormone (secreted by the *parathyroid glands*) to regulate the level of calcium in the body.

REGULATION

T_4 AND T_3 The secretion of T_4 and T_3 by the thyroid is controlled by a hormonal feedback system involving the *pituitary gland* and *hypothalamus*.

CALCITONIN The secretion of calcitonin by the thyroid is regulated directly by the level of calcium in the blood. Raised blood calcium stimulates calcitonin secretion, stimulating deposition of calcium in bone and thereby reducing the calcium level; decreased blood calcium inhibits calcitonin output to help increase the calcium level. This feedback regulation occurs independently of the pituitary gland or hypothalamus.

DEFICIENCY AND EXCESS

Insufficient thyroid hormone production is known as *hypothyroidism*. The symptoms include tiredness, dry skin, hair loss, weight gain, constipation, and sensitivity to cold. In childhood, deficiency of thyroid hormone may cause *cretinism* (a condition characterized by severe growth retardation, coarseness of the facial features and mental impairment).

CONTROL OF THYROID HORMONE PRODUCTION

(Raised blood levels of thyroid hormones)

Bloodstream
If blood levels of the thyroid hormones T_3 and T_4 rise, they decrease the sensitivity of the pituitary to thyrotrophin-releasing hormone (TRH), secreted by the hypothalamus.

Hypothalamus
Secretes TRH.

Pituitary gland
The pituitary becomes less sensitive to TRH, so it secretes less thyroid-stimulating hormone (TSH).

Thyroid gland
In response to lowered TSH stimulation, the thyroid reduces its production of the hormones T_3 and T_4.

Bloodstream
The blood levels of T_3 and T_4 thus gradually fall back to normal.

(Reduced blood levels of thyroid hormones)

Bloodstream
If blood levels of the thyroid hormones T_3 and T_4 fall, the hypothalamus is stimulated to produce more TRH.

Hypothalamus
Increases secretion of TRH.

Pituitary gland
In response to stimulation by TRH, the pituitary increases production of TSH.

Thyroid gland
In response to increased TSH stimulation, the thyroid increases its production of T_3 and T_4.

Bloodstream
The blood levels of T_3 and T_4 thus gradually rise back to normal.

Why control is necessary

The blood levels of the hormones T_3 (triiodothyronine) and T_4 (thyroxine) produced by the thyroid must be kept within narrow limits, otherwise hyperthyroidism or hypothyroidism may result. The control systems above exist to achieve this balance but certain disorders may interfere with the system.

T

DISORDERS OF THE THYROID GLAND

The function of the thyroid gland is controlled by both the pituitary gland and the hypothalamus, so thyroid disorders may be due not only to defects in the gland itself, but also to disruption of the hypothalamic-pituitary hormonal control system. Thyroid disorders may cause symptoms due to overproduction of thyroid hormones (*hyperthyroidism*), underproduction of these hormones (*hypothyroidism*), or enlargement or distortion of the gland. *Myxoedema*, *Graves' disease*, and *Hashimoto's thyroiditis* are the common disorders of thyroid function. *Goitre* (enlargement of the thyroid gland) may sometimes occur without any accompanying abnormality of thyroid function.

CONGENITAL DEFECTS

In rare cases, the thyroid gland is missing completely at birth, producing severe *cretinism*. However, congenital thyroid deficiency more often takes the form of underdevelopment or maldevelopment, in which there is sufficient hormone-producing thyroid tissue to avoid cretinism but insufficient tissue to produce normal amounts of hormones. If untreated, this may lead to juvenile myxoedema.

Sometimes the thyroid develops in an abnormal position in the neck; in rare cases, this causes difficulty in swallowing or breathing.

GENETIC DISORDERS

A genetic disorder may impair the thyroid's ability to secrete hormones. The low blood level of thyroid hormones results in greatly increased secretion by the pituitary gland of thyroid-stimulating hormone (TSH), which, in turn, causes the thyroid to enlarge. This is one way in which a goitre may develop.

INFECTION

Thyroid infection is uncommon, but sometimes occurs as a complication of infection elsewhere in the body. The resulting *thyroiditis* may require treatment with antibiotics. If an abscess forms, a minor operation may be necessary to open and drain it. Viral infection of the thyroid can cause temporary hyperthyroidism as well as an extremely painful gland.

Tumours
Most lumps in the thyroid are benign, and some thyroid cancers are not highly malignant. A stone-hard, rapidly-growing lump is an indication of thyroid cancer.

Autoimmune diseases
These are common causes of thyroid disorders. In Hashimoto's thyroiditis, much of the thyroid's glandular tissue is replaced by masses of lymphocytes.

Goitre
Enlargement of the thyroid (goitre) may result from hormonal imbalances at puberty or during pregnancy. Goitre may also be due to autoimmune disease, or, rarely, to iodine deficiency.

TUMOURS

Thyroid tumours may be benign or malignant. Thyroid *adenomas* are benign tumours that may secrete thyroid hormone, sometimes in sufficient amounts to cause hyperthyroidism. *Thyroid cancers* vary greatly in their malignancy and rate of growth. They are relatively rare but may be suspected if a single firm or hard lump can be felt in the gland. One particular type of thyroid tumour secretes the hormone calcitonin.

AUTOIMMUNE DISORDERS

Graves' disease is a form of thyroid overactivity whose chief feature is hyperthyroidism. The disease is thought to be due to the body producing an "autoantibody" that stimulates the thyroid to secrete excessive amounts of hormones. Autoantibodies are also believed to be associated with certain other thyroid disorders, notably Hashimoto's thyroiditis, in which the antibodies damage glandular cells.

MYXOEDEMA

Deficiency of thyroid hormone (hypothyroidism) may be associated with Hashimoto's thyroiditis or atrophy of the thyroid, or may be a consequence of treatment for hyperthyroidism. The result is myxoedema, a condition in which the skin becomes dry and thickened, and facial features become coarse. Constipation, cold intolerance, and fatigue are other common symptoms. In many cases, the cause of myxoedema is not known.

HORMONAL DISORDERS

Hormonal changes during puberty or pregnancy are a relatively common cause of a minor degree of goitre, which usually subsides when hormone levels return to normal. Hyperthyroidism due to excessive production of TSH by the pituitary gland is rare but can occur as a result of a pituitary tumour.

NUTRITIONAL DISORDERS

Because iodine is necessary for the production of thyroid hormone, deficiency of this mineral may lead to goitre. Severe iodine deficiency in children may cause myxoedema. These problems can be avoided by using table salt that contains iodine.

RADIATION

Irradiation of the head or neck increases the likelihood of thyroid tumours, although it may be 25 years or more until such tumours develop.

INVESTIGATION

Suspected disturbances of thyroid function are investigated initially by taking a medical history and performing a physical examination. Blood samples may also be taken for *thyroid-function tests*, in which the levels of thyroid or pituitary hormones are measured, and the gland itself may be imaged by various *thyroid scanning* techniques. In some cases, such as a suspected thyroid tumour, a fine-needle *biopsy* may be carried out to obtain a sample of thyroid tissue for examination under the microscope.

T

Overproduction of thyroid hormones is known as *hyperthyroidism*. Symptoms of hyperthyroidism include fatigue, anxiety, palpitations, sweating, weight loss, diarrhoea, and intolerance of heat.

DRUG THERAPY

The most commonly used thyroid hormone drugs are the synthetic thyroid hormone preparations levothyroxine and liothyronine. These drugs are used to treat hypothyroidism, to prevent hypothyroidism, to reduce thyroid enlargement in certain types of *goitre*, and to treat *thyroid cancer*.

Because a sudden increase in the body's thyroid hormone level may strain the heart, levothyroxine and liothyronine are usually prescribed in low doses that are gradually increased. Since too high a dose may cause symptoms of hyperthyroidism, regular visits to the doctor are essential; when necessary, blood tests are carried out to monitor the level of thyroid hormones.

Calcitonin is used to treat *Paget's disease*, *osteoporosis*, and *hypercalcaemia*.

Thyroiditis

The medical term for inflammation of the *thyroid gland*. Thyroiditis can be caused by a variety of factors, and occurs in several different forms.

The most common form is *Hashimoto's thyroiditis*, an autoimmune disorder causing *hypothyroidism* (underactivity of the thyroid gland).

Subacute thyroiditis, also known as de Quervain's thyroiditis, is a less common form in which the thyroid becomes tender and painful. Pain, which may be referred (see *Referred pain*) to the jaw, ears, or back of the head, may be accompanied by fever, weight loss, and a general feeling of illness. The precise cause of subacute thyroiditis is unknown. The condition may persist for several months, but in most cases eventually subsides on its own. In severe cases, treatment with *corticosteroid drugs* may be given to reduce the inflammation.

Thyroiditis due to infection is rare; when it does occur, it is usually as a result of an infection that has spread from elsewhere in the body. In some cases, an abscess forms in the gland, which may require surgical drainage.

Rarer still is a condition known as Riedel's thyroiditis or Riedel's struma, in which deposits of dense, fibrous tissue form in the gland and surrounding tissues, resulting in a hardening of the entire area.

Thyroid scanning

Techniques used to provide information about the location, anatomy, and function of the *thyroid gland*. The technique of *radionuclide scanning* is commonly used to investigate disorders of the gland, but *ultrasound scanning* can be useful in some cases.

HOW IT IS DONE

For radionuclide scanning, an injection or an oral preparation containing a radioisotope (radioactive substance) is given, followed after an interval by the recording of images on a gamma camera. The radioisotope preparation usually contains a tiny dose of specially prepared *technetium* or *iodine*, both of which are taken up avidly by thyroid tissue, but hardly at all by other body tissues.

For ultrasound scanning, a transducer producing high-frequency sound waves that penetrate tissue is moved back and forth across the skin over the thyroid gland. Echoes of the sound waves are transformed electronically into an image.

WHY IT IS DONE

Radionuclide scanning reveals the position of any functioning thyroid tissue and is therefore useful in showing whether the gland is abnormally located or absent. The scan also shows the amount of radioisotope taken up by the gland, thus indicating *hyperthyroidism* (overactivity of the thyroid gland) or *hypothyroidism* (underactivity of the thyroid gland).

A radionuclide scan may suggest whether a thyroid nodule or tumour is cancerous or noncancerous and can show whether it is active or inactive. This technique can also detect malignant thyroid tissue that has spread to other parts of the body, therefore playing an important part in planning and in evaluating the treatment of *thyroid cancer*.

Ultrasound scanning is of more limited use because it can show only the structure of thyroid tissue. This technique can be useful in showing whether a *goitre* is solid, cystic (fluid-filled), or a mixture of the two.

Thyrotoxicosis

A term for any toxic condition that results from *hyperthyroidism* (overactivity of the thyroid gland). The term thyrotoxicosis is often used as a synonym for *Graves' disease*.

Thyroxine

The most important *thyroid hormone* produced by the *thyroid gland*. It is represented by the symbol T_4.

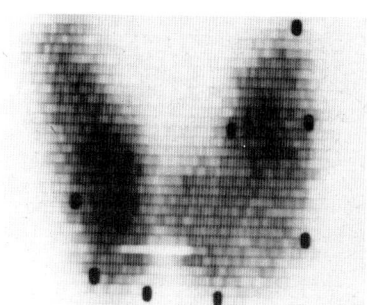

Radionuclide thyroid scanning
In this scan the diffuse darker areas indicate regions of overactive thyroid tissue (the small black ovals are markers).

Tibia

The inner and thicker of the two long bones in the lower leg, also called the shin. The tibia is the supporting bone of the lower leg. It runs parallel to the narrower lower leg bone, the *fibula*, to which it is attached by *ligaments*.

The front surface of the tibia lies just beneath the skin and is easily felt. The upper end articulates with the *femur* (thigh-bone) to form the *knee* joint and the lower end forms part of the *ankle* joint. On the inside of the ankle, the tibia is widened and protrudes to form a large bony prominence called the medial malleolus.

FRACTURE

The tibia is one of the most commonly fractured bones. It may break across

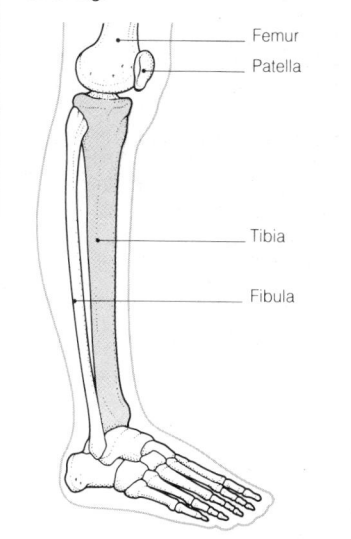

LOCATION OF THE TIBIA
Also called the shin, the tibia can easily be felt beneath the skin of the lower leg.

Femur
Patella
Tibia
Fibula

T

the shaft as a result of a direct blow to the front of the leg, or at the upper end from a blow to the outside of the leg below the knee. Fracture of the lower end of the tibia may accompany dislocation of the ankle and fracture of the fibula in a *Pott's fracture*, caused by violent twisting of the ankle. Prolonged running or walking on hard ground may cause a *stress fracture* of the tibia.

Some fractures of the shaft heal satisfactorily if the leg is immobilized in a plaster *cast*, usually for about six to eight weeks. If the bone ends are displaced or unstable, an operation may be needed to fasten them together with a nail or screw.

Tic

A repeated, uncontrolled, purposeless contraction of a *muscle* or group of muscles, most commonly in the face, shoulders, or arms. Typical tics include pointless blinking, mouth twitching, and shrugging.

Tics are often a sign of a usually minor psychological disturbance. Most develop in childhood, occurring in as many as a quarter of children and affecting three times more boys than girls. Tics are made worse by stress or by drawing attention to them, but often disappear when the child is deeply absorbed or asleep.

Tics usually stop within a year of onset but in some cases persist into adult life. Most can be controlled for short periods of time by will. However, such control is of questionable value because tics appear to release emotional tension.

In rare cases, tics become so severe that they require treatment with *benzodiazepine drugs* or *antipsychotic drugs*. Examples include involuntary contractions of the diaphragm (the muscle that separates the chest from the abdomen), resulting in grunting noises, and *Gilles de la Tourette's syndrome*, a disorder that is characterized by widespread tics and involuntary noises and words.

Tic douloureux

Another name for *trigeminal neuralgia*.

Ticks and disease

Ticks are small, eight-legged animals that feed on blood and sometimes transmit diseases to humans via their bites. Ticks are about 3 mm long before feeding; when bloated with blood, they become much larger. A person may pick up ticks when in various rural habitats, such as long grass, scrub, woodland, or caves. The ticks attach themselves by their mouthparts to the skin of animal or human hosts.

Ticks can spread infectious organisms from animals to humans via their bites. In the UK, the only disease known to be transmitted by ticks is *Lyme disease*. Other diseases transmitted by ticks in various parts of the world include *relapsing fever*, *Rocky Mountain spotted fever*, *Q fever*, *tularaemia*, and certain types of viral *encephalitis*. The prolonged bite of certain female ticks can cause a condition called tick paralysis, in which a toxin in the tick saliva affects the nerves that control movement. In extreme cases, this can lead to paralysis of the respiratory muscles and can be fatal.

Tietze's syndrome

Chest pain localized to an area on the front of the chest wall, usually made worse by movement of the arms or trunk or by pressure from the fingers. Tietze's syndrome is caused by inflammation of one or several *rib* cartilages. Symptoms may persist for several months.

Treatment is with *analgesic drugs* (painkillers) and *nonsteroidal anti-inflammatory drugs*.

Timolol

A *beta-blocker drug* used in tablet form to treat *hypertension* (high blood pressure) and *angina pectoris* (chest pain due to inadequate blood supply to the heart muscle). Timolol is also given after a *myocardial infarction* (heart attack) to prevent further damage to the heart muscle. In eye-drop form, timolol is used to treat *glaucoma*.

Possible adverse effects are typical of other beta-blocker drugs. Eyedrops may cause irritation, blurred vision, and headache.

Tinea

Any of a group of common *fungal infections* of the skin, hair, or nails. Most infections are caused by a group of fungi called the dermatophytes and are often called ringworm.

Tineal infections may be acquired from another person, from an animal, from soil, from the floors of showers, or from household objects, such as chairs or carpets.

The word tinea is sometimes followed by the Latin term for the affected part of the body. For example, tinea pedis affects the feet and tinea cruris affects the groin.

TYPES AND SYMPTOMS

The appearance and symptoms of tinea vary according to the site. The most common type is tinea pedis, also called *athlete's foot*, which causes cracking and itching between the toes.

Tinea corporis (ringworm of the body) is characterized by itchy patches on the body that are usually circular with a prominent edge. Tinea cruris (also commonly called jock itch) produces a reddened, itchy area spreading from the genitals outwards over the inside of the thigh. This form of tinea is more common in males.

Tinea capitis (ringworm of the scalp) causes one or several round, itchy, patches of hair loss on the scalp; it occurs mainly in children and is more common in large cities and overcrowded conditions. Ringworm of the nails, also called tinea unguium or onychomycosis, is often accompanied by scaling of the soles or palms. The nails become thick and turn white or yellow.

DIAGNOSIS AND TREATMENT

Most types of tinea are diagnosed by a doctor from their appearances. However, the diagnosis should be confirmed, and the type of fungus identified, by culturing the organisms in a laboratory. Some scalp infections exhibit fluorescence under a filtered *ultraviolet light* (Wood's light), but most do not.

For most types of tinea, treatment is with *antifungal drugs* in the form of skin creams, lotions, or ointments. However, for widespread infections or those affecting the hair or nails, an antifungal drug in tablet form (usually griseofulvin) may be necessary.

Treatment may be continued for some time after symptoms have subsided to eradicate the fungi and prevent recurrence. For mild infections on the skin surface, there may need to be four to six weeks of treatment; for toenail infections, treatment may be necessary for up to one or two years.

Tingling

See *Pins-and-needles*.

Tinnitus

A ringing, buzzing, whistling, hissing, or other noise heard in the *ear* or ears in the absence of a noise in the environment.

CAUSES

In tinnitus, the *acoustic nerve* transmits impulses to the *brain* not as the result of vibrations produced by external sound waves but, for reasons not fully understood, as the result of stimuli

T

that originate inside the head or within the ear itself. The condition is almost always associated with hearing loss, particularly with deafness due to *presbyacusis* and continuous exposure to loud noise.

Tinnitus can occur as a symptom of many ear disorders, including *labyrinthitis*, *Ménière's disease*, *otitis media*, *otosclerosis*, *ototoxicity*, and blockage of the outer ear canal with *earwax*. In rare cases, tinnitus is a symptom of an *aneurysm* or a tumour pressing on a blood vessel in the head. Tinnitus may also be caused by certain drugs, such as *aspirin* or *quinine*, or may follow a *head injury*.

SYMPTOMS
The noise in the ear may sometimes change in nature or intensity. In most cases it is present continuously but the sufferer's awareness of it is usually intermittent. Tolerance of tinnitus varies considerably from one person to another and is largely determined by the sufferer's personality. Many people learn to accept the condition without distress, but some find it almost intolerable.

TREATMENT
Any underlying disorder is treated if possible. Many sufferers make use of a radio, television, cassette player, or headphones to block out the noise in their ears. Some find a tinnitus masker—headphones that play white noise (a random mixture of sounds of a wide range of frequencies)—particularly effective.

Tiredness

A common complaint that is usually the result of overwork or lack of sleep. In some people, persistent tiredness is caused by *depression* or *anxiety*. Tiredness may be due to a more serious condition, such as *anaemia* or *cancer*, but in such cases there are usually also other symptoms.

Tissue

A collection of *cells* specialized to perform a particular function. Examples of tissues include muscle tissue, which consists of cells that are specialized to contract; epithelial tissue, which forms the *skin* and *mucous membranes* that line the respiratory and other internal tracts; nerve tissue, comprising cells specialized to conduct electrochemical nerve impulses; and *connective tissue*, which includes *adipose tissue* (fat), and the various fibrous and elastic tissues (such as tendons and cartilage) that hold the body together.

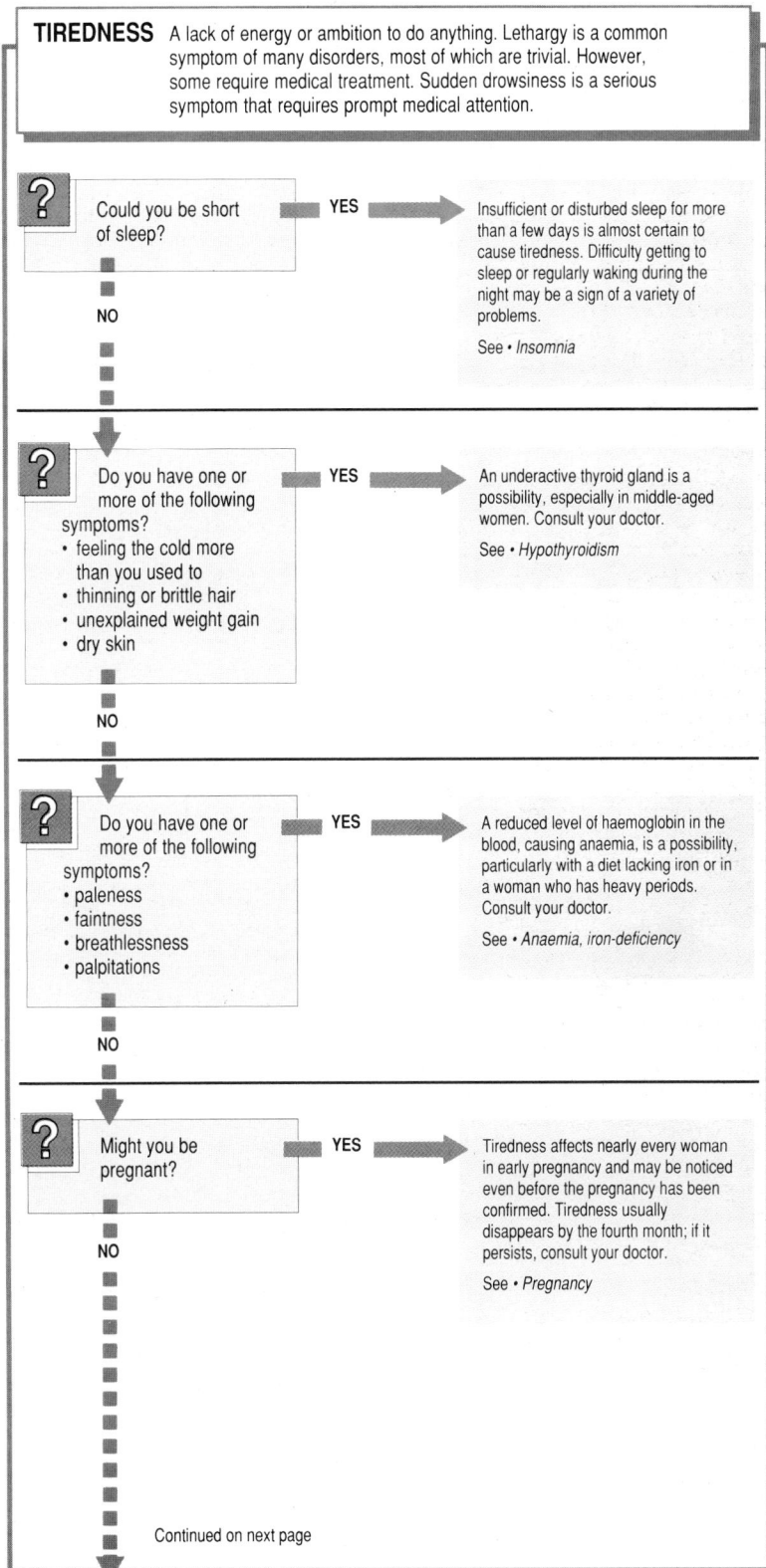

TIREDNESS A lack of energy or ambition to do anything. Lethargy is a common symptom of many disorders, most of which are trivial. However, some require medical treatment. Sudden drowsiness is a serious symptom that requires prompt medical attention.

? Could you be short of sleep? — **YES** → Insufficient or disturbed sleep for more than a few days is almost certain to cause tiredness. Difficulty getting to sleep or regularly waking during the night may be a sign of a variety of problems.

See • *Insomnia*

NO

? Do you have one or more of the following symptoms?
• feeling the cold more than you used to
• thinning or brittle hair
• unexplained weight gain
• dry skin
— **YES** → An underactive thyroid gland is a possibility, especially in middle-aged women. Consult your doctor.

See • *Hypothyroidism*

NO

? Do you have one or more of the following symptoms?
• paleness
• faintness
• breathlessness
• palpitations
— **YES** → A reduced level of haemoglobin in the blood, causing anaemia, is a possibility, particularly with a diet lacking iron or in a woman who has heavy periods. Consult your doctor.

See • *Anaemia, iron-deficiency*

NO

? Might you be pregnant? — **YES** → Tiredness affects nearly every woman in early pregnancy and may be noticed even before the pregnancy has been confirmed. Tiredness usually disappears by the fourth month; if it persists, consult your doctor.

See • *Pregnancy*

NO

Continued on next page

T

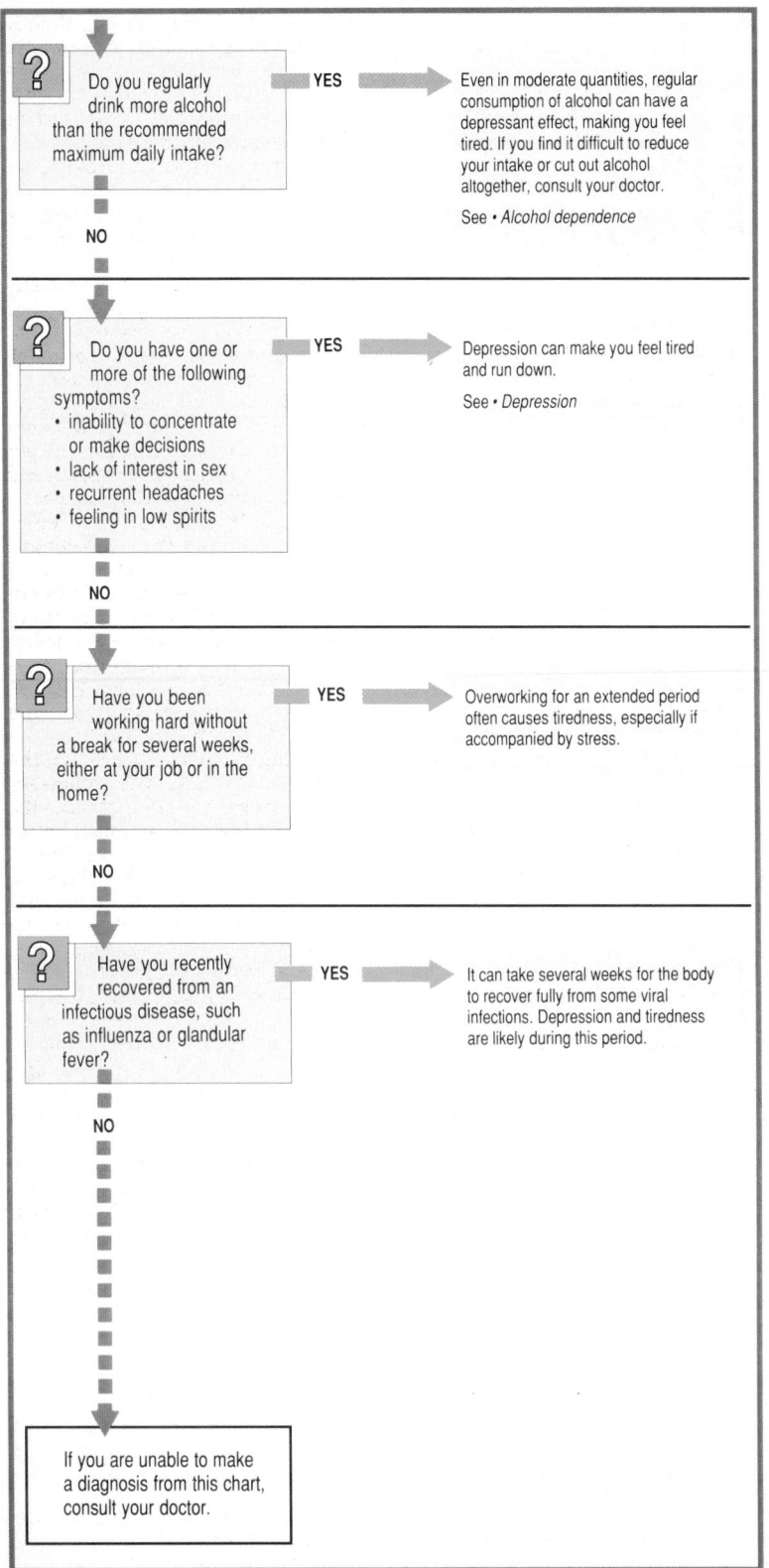

Do you regularly drink more alcohol than the recommended maximum daily intake?

YES → Even in moderate quantities, regular consumption of alcohol can have a depressant effect, making you feel tired. If you find it difficult to reduce your intake or cut out alcohol altogether, consult your doctor.

See • *Alcohol dependence*

NO

Do you have one or more of the following symptoms?
- inability to concentrate or make decisions
- lack of interest in sex
- recurrent headaches
- feeling in low spirits

YES → Depression can make you feel tired and run down.

See • *Depression*

NO

Have you been working hard without a break for several weeks, either at your job or in the home?

YES → Overworking for an extended period often causes tiredness, especially if accompanied by stress.

NO

Have you recently recovered from an infectious disease, such as influenza or glandular fever?

YES → It can take several weeks for the body to recover fully from some viral infections. Depression and tiredness are likely during this period.

NO

If you are unable to make a diagnosis from this chart, consult your doctor.

Tissue fluid

The watery liquid present in the tiny gaps between body cells, also known as interstitial fluid. Tissue fluid is one component of extracellular fluid (any body fluid outside the cells, including blood and lymph).

To reach cells, oxygen and nutrients must pass from the blood vessels and into the tissue fluid. Similarly, there is a reverse movement of carbon dioxide and other waste products from the cells into the tissue fluid, and then into the bloodstream.

In addition to nutrients and wastes, tissue fluid also contains *ions*. This fluid contains a much higher level of sodium ions, and a much lower level of potassium ions, than intracellular fluid. It is this difference in ion levels that helps control the movement of water into and out of cells by *osmosis*; ion levels also play a role in the transmission of electrical impulses through nerves and muscles.

Tissue fluid is formed by the filtration of liquid out through the walls of the first part of blood capillaries (that is, the part nearest an arteriole), where it is forced out by the high blood pressure. In the last part of capillaries (nearest to a venule), blood pressure is much lower, and tissue fluid passes back into the capillaries; some tissue fluid is also drained away into the lymphatic vessels. Thus, there is a continual flow that keeps the amount of tissue fluid constant. Various disorders—such as *hypertension* (high blood pressure)—may disrupt the balance between formation and drainage of tissue fluid, leading to the accumulation of excess fluid in the tissues, a condition called *oedema*.

Tissue-plasminogen activator

A substance produced by body tissues that prevents abnormal *blood clotting*. Also called TPA, it is produced in small amounts by the inner lining of blood vessels.

DRUG THERAPY

TPA can be prepared artificially by *genetic engineering* techniques for use as a *thrombolytic drug* (a drug that dissolves blood clots), when it is known as alteplase. It is used in the treatment of *myocardial infarction* (heart attack), severe *angina pectoris* (chest pain caused by inadequate blood supply to the heart muscle), and arterial *embolism* (blockage of an artery), including *pulmonary embolism*.

HOW IT WORKS

Given by *intravenous infusion*, TPA dissolves blood clots by converting plas-

T

minogen (a chemical in the blood) to the enzyme plasmin. Plasmin in turn breaks down fibrin, the main constituent of blood clots.

POSSIBLE ADVERSE EFFECTS

Bleeding or the formation of a *haematoma* (collection of blood) may occur at the site of injection. TPA may also cause bleeding elsewhere but this can usually be controlled because TPA has a short-lived action. An allergic reaction to TPA may sometimes occur, although this is less likely than with other thrombolytic drugs. (See also *Fibrinolysis*.)

Tissue-typing

The classification of certain characteristics of the tissues of prospective organ donors and recipients.

WHY IT IS DONE

Tissue-typing is necessary to help match recipient and donor tissues for *transplant surgery*, thus minimizing the risk of rejection of a donor organ by the recipient's *immune system*.

The main features by which a person's immune system distinguishes his or her own tissues from those of other people are called *histocompatibility antigens*. Most important of these are the human leukocyte antigens (HLAs), which are present on the surface of human cells. A person's set of HLAs is inherited and unique to that person (except for identical twins, who have the same set). Hence, perfect tissue matching is achieved only between identical twins. Nevertheless, close relatives often have closely matching HLA types.

HOW IT IS DONE

A person's tissue-type, or HLA "fingerprint", is established by tests in the laboratory on cells from a sample of the person's blood. There are many different possible HLAs and the presence or absence of each must be tested individually. In one of the simpler methods, an *antiserum* containing *antibodies* (substances that react with a particular antigen—in this case, a particular HLA) is added to the test specimen. If the antigen is present, it is detected by an observable colour or other change.

For organ transplantation, once a recipient has been tissue-typed, a selection is made of a donor whose HLA grouping best matches that of the recipient. This helps reduce the chances of *rejection*. It is easiest to find such donors among close relatives.

Titanium dental implants

See *Implants, dental*.

TMJ syndrome

See *Temporomandibular joint syndrome*.

Toadstool poisoning

See *Mushroom poisoning*.

Tobacco

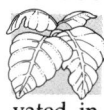 The dried leaf of the plant *NICOTIANA TABACUM*. Indigenous to America, the tobacco plant is now cultivated in many parts of the world. Tobacco is used for *tobacco-smoking*, tobacco-chewing, or as *snuff* by billions of people all over the world.

Tobacco contains a variable percentage of *nicotine*, which is a toxic chemical, and several carcinogenic (cancer-inducing) substances. There is a direct proportion between the amount of tobacco used, the period over which it is used, and the likelihood of cancer. Increased exposure to heavy concentrates of carcinogens in tobacco has been shown to result in an increased risk of tumour development in exposed tissues.

Tobacco smokers have an increased risk of *lung cancer, bladder cancer, kidney cancer*, and pancreatic cancer (see *Pancreas, cancer of*). All tobacco users have an increased risk of cancers of the oral cavity (see *Mouth cancer*), pharynx (see *Pharynx, cancer of*), larynx (see *Larynx, cancer of*) and oesophagus (see *Oesophagus, cancer of*). The majority of people with head and neck cancers have a history of heavy alcohol and tobacco use.

Tobacco-smoking

Despite its practice in Western countries for more than 400 years—and for much longer in some other parts of the world—tobacco-smoking has only relatively recently been accepted as a major health hazard. Much of what is known today about the harmful effects of *tobacco* concerns cigarette-smoking; this is because cigarette smokers have been studied in much greater depth than have either pipe or cigar smokers.

HARMFUL EFFECTS

Lung cancer is probably the best known harmful effect of smoking. More than 30 studies in 10 countries have demonstrated a direct link between smoking and lung cancer. In England and Wales, lung cancer accounts each year for over 100 deaths per 100,000 males; in females the rate is about 40 per 100,000, although this figure is rising. In Scotland, the rates for both sexes are rather higher. Because pipe and cigar smokers tend not to inhale

tobacco smoke, they have a slightly lower risk of lung cancer, although the risk is still significantly greater than for nonsmokers. The risk of developing lung cancer begins to diminish as soon as smoking is stopped.

All forms of tobacco-smoking increase the risk of certain other forms of cancer, including *mouth cancer, lip cancer*, and cancer of the throat (see *Pharynx, cancer of*).

Tobacco-smoking is also directly associated with chronic *bronchitis, emphysema*, and combinations of the two. These diseases, features of which include increasing breathlessness and sometimes the coughing up of sputum, account for about 80 deaths per 100,000 in males and about 30 per 100,000 in females in England and Wales; rates in Scotland are lower.

Another significant harmful effect of smoking is *coronary artery disease*, which is the most common cause of death in middle-aged men in Western countries. The risk of coronary artery disease in a young man who smokes 20 cigarettes a day is about three times that of a nonsmoker, and the risk increases proportionally with the number of cigarettes smoked.

In addition to its effects on the coronary arteries, smoking damages arteries that supply other parts of the body. Smoking may seriously affect the arteries of the legs, leading to *peripheral vascular disease*, which, in severe cases, may necessitate amputation. Also affected by smoking are the arteries of the brain; damage there may result in a *stroke*.

Smoking is extremely harmful during pregnancy. The babies of women who smoke are smaller and less likely to survive than those of nonsmoking mothers. Even after birth, there are hazards for the children of parents who smoke. Such children are more likely to suffer from *asthma* or other respiratory diseases and are more likely to become smokers themselves.

There is also evidence that anybody in the vicinity of a smoker is at increased risk of tobacco-related disorders. Such "passive smokers" also suffer considerable immediate discomfort in the form of coughing, wheezing, and watering eyes.

HOW SMOKING CAUSES HARM

Tobacco contains a variety of different noxious substances, but the dangers of three of them are particularly important.

Nicotine is the substance that causes addiction to tobacco. It acts as a tranquillizer, but also stimulates the re-

T

TOBACCO-SMOKING

About 100,000 deaths per year in the UK are attributed to smoking. The main harmful effects of smoking are respiratory diseases (lung cancer, bronchitis, and emphysema) and cardiovascular diseases (coronary artery disease and peripheral vascular disease).

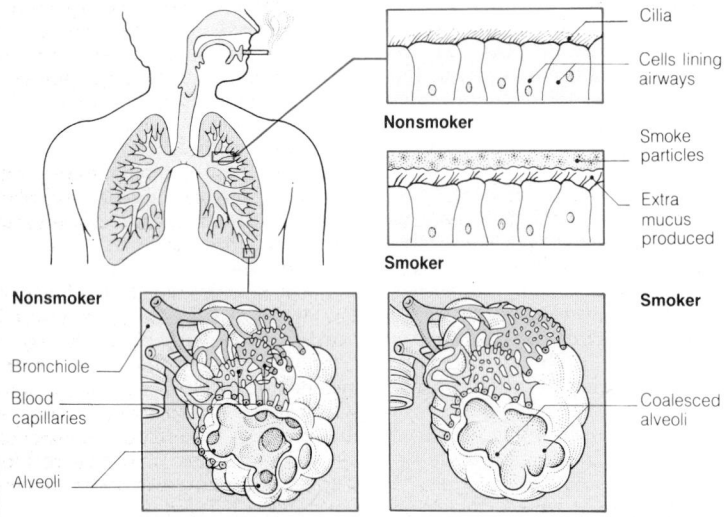

Nonsmoker

Smoker

Cilia
Cells lining airways

Smoke particles
Extra mucus produced

Nonsmoker

Bronchiole
Blood capillaries
Alveoli

Smoker

Coalesced alveoli

How smoking damages the lungs
Smoke particles irritate the lungs' airways, causing excess mucus production (top right). The smoke particles also indirectly destroy the walls of the lungs' alveoli, which coalesce (above right). Both factors reduce lung efficiency. In addition, tar in tobacco smoke has a direct cancer-causing action.

SMOKERS AS A PERCENTAGE OF THE ADULT POPULATION OF THE UK

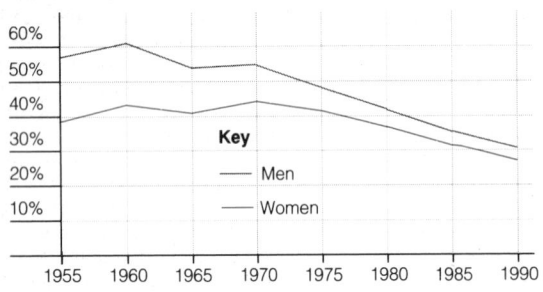

Key
— Men
— Women

Smoking trends
Overall, the proportion of adults (aged over 16) who smoke has decreased since the 1960s. However, this downward trend started later in women than it did in men.

SMOKING-RELATED DEATHS IN THE UK (1990)

Cause	Men	Women	Total
Heart disease	22,382	17,708	40,090
Lung cancer	26,542	11,774	38,316
Chronic bronchitis and emphysema	17,476	8,238	25,714
Total smoking-related deaths	66,400	37,720	104,120

Major health hazards of smoking
The table above gives the estimated numbers of smoking-related deaths by cause and sex in the UK in 1990. Apart from the major killer diseases listed in the table, smoking also causes deaths due to cancers of the mouth, pharynx, larynx, oesophagus, bladder, and pancreas.

lease of *adrenaline* into the smoker's bloodstream, which may explain why some smokers are found to have raised blood pressure.

Tar in tobacco produces chronic irritation of the respiratory system and is thought to be a major cause of lung cancer.

Carbon monoxide passes from the lungs into the bloodstream, where, in competition with oxygen, it easily combines with *haemoglobin* and thus interferes with oxygenation of tissues. In the long term, persistently high levels of carbon monoxide in the blood—which occur in smokers—lead to hardening of the arteries, which in turn greatly increases the risk of *coronary thrombosis*.

STOPPING SMOKING

The most important prerequisite for successfully stopping smoking is an absolute commitment to giving up the habit. The slightest doubt over genuinely wanting to stop is likely to sabotage your efforts. For this reason, simply cutting down the number of cigarettes smoked rarely works; you must decide whether you will continue to smoke or whether you will become a complete nonsmoker.

If you decide to stop smoking, you may find it useful to join a group, to undergo *acupuncture* or *hypnosis*, or to chew nicotine-containing gum. Chewing gum or sucking sweets may help people who miss the oral sensation of smoking.

Many people worry that they will gain weight as a result of stopping smoking. There is a risk that this will occur, because smoking tends to increase the metabolic rate (the rate at which the body "burns" food) and because many people eat more after they stop smoking. However, most doctors agree that being moderately overweight is far less hazardous to health than smoking.

Tobramycin

An *antibiotic drug* used to treat *peritonitis*, *meningitis*, and severe infections of the lungs, skin, bones, and joints. Tobramycin is given by injection, usually in combination with a *penicillin drug*. Eye-drops containing tobramycin are sometimes used to treat *conjunctivitis* and *blepharitis* (inflammation of the eyelids).

High doses of tobramycin given by injection may cause kidney damage, deafness due to inner-ear damage, nausea, vomiting, and headache. Any preparation that contains tobramycin may cause rash and itching.

Tocainide

An *antiarrhythmic drug* that is used to prevent and treat certain irregularities in the pattern of the heartbeat (see *Arrhythmia, cardiac*).

There is a high risk of adverse effects, including nausea, dizziness, tremor, loss of appetite, diarrhoea, confusion, and hallucinations. Prolonged treatment may cause blood disorders such as *thrombocytopenia*.

Tocography

An obstetric procedure for recording muscular contractions of the uterus during *childbirth*. The procedure known as cardiotocography combines tocography with *fetal heart monitoring*.

Tocopherol

A constituent of *vitamin E*. Four tocopherols (alpha, beta, gamma, and delta) and several tocopherol derivatives together make up the substance known as vitamin E. Tocopherols are fat-soluble and occur in many foods. Dietary deficiency of tocopherols is extremely rare.

Todd's paralysis

Weakness in part of the body following some types of epileptic seizure (see *Epilepsy*). The weakness may last for minutes, hours, or occasionally days, but there is no lasting effect. The affected part of the body is usually a part that twitched during the seizure. Todd's paralysis is thought to be caused by damage to, or a tumour in, the motor cortex (the part of the *brain* that controls movement).

Toe

One of the digits of the foot. Each toe has three phalanges (bones), except for the hallux (big toe), which has two. The phalanges join at hinge joints, which are moved by muscle tendons that flex (bend) or extend (straighten) the toe. A small artery, vein, and nerve run down each side of the toe. The entire structure is enclosed in skin with a nail at the top.

The main function of the toes is to maintain balance during walking. People without hands often learn to use their toes to perform tasks usually performed with the fingers.

DISORDERS

Congenital disorders include *polydactyly* (extra toes), missing toes, *syndactyly* (fused toes), or *webbing* (skin flaps between the toes).

Injuries to the toes are fairly common, particularly bruises or fractures. Inflammation of one or several toe

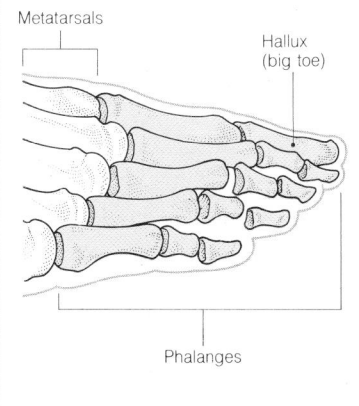

ANATOMY OF THE TOES
Each hallux, or big toe, has two bones called phalanges, which are connected by hinge joints. All the other toes have three phalanges.

Metatarsals

Hallux (big toe)

Phalanges

joints, causing stiffness, pain, swelling, and deformity, may be caused by *osteoarthritis, rheumatoid arthritis* or *gout*.

Infections may occur under the nail as a complication of an ingrowing toenail (see *Toenail, ingrowing*).

Impaired blood supply, usually due to *peripheral vascular disease* (narrowing of arteries in the legs), causes pain and blueness of the toes and can eventually lead to *gangrene*. Numbness and a pins-and-needles sensation in the toes may be caused by damage to peripheral nerves, which is common in *diabetes mellitus*.

A common deformity of the big toe is *hallux valgus*, in which the joint at the base projects outwards while the top of the toe turns inwards. Hallux valgus often results in a *bunion* (a firm, fluid-filled swelling over the joint). Abnormality of a tendon in one of the toes may cause the main joint to remain bent (see *Hammer toe*).

Toenail, ingrowing

A painful condition of a toe (usually the big toe) in which one or both edges of the *nail* press into the adjacent skin, leading to infection and inflammation. The condition usually results from cutting the nail incorrectly, from wearing tight-fitting shoes, and from poor personal hygiene.

TREATMENT AND PREVENTION

Temporary relief from pain can be obtained by bathing the foot once or twice daily in a strong, warm, salt solution; after bathing, the nail should

be covered with a dry gauze dressing. *Antibiotic drugs* may be given to control infection. In some cases, the edge of the affected nail is removed under local anaesthesia.

Unless preventive measures are taken, the problem is likely to recur. The nail should be cut straight across to avoid exposing tender skin that easily becomes infected if a splinter of nail from the cut edge grows into it.

Toilet-training

The process of teaching a young child to acquire complete bowel and bladder control and to make appropriate use of toilet facilities.

WHEN TO START

There is no reason to start toilet-training until the child's nervous system is sufficiently mature. Up to the age of about 18 months, emptying of the bladder and bowel is a totally automatic reaction. The child is not yet able to connect the actions of defaecation and urination with their results, and does not have the ability to control these actions at will.

At around 18 months, a child is able to indicate that he or she has passed urine or a bowel movement, but is not yet aware when he or she is about to do so. At this stage, the child is not quite ready to use the potty, but should become familiar with it, be told what it is for, and practise sitting on it. At around 24 months, the child becomes aware when he or she is about to pass urine or a bowel movement, and says so. At this stage, the child is ready to start using the potty.

USING THE POTTY AND TOILET

Toilet-training should be approached in a relaxed, unhurried manner. The child may rebel if the potty is introduced too early or if he or she is forced to sit on it. Boys initially urinate sitting on the potty but soon learn to urinate standing up.

T

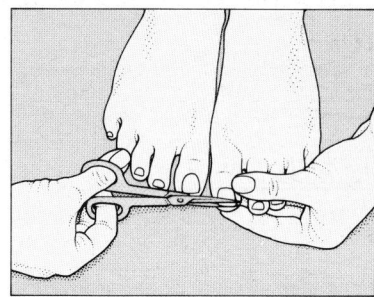

Preventing ingrowing toenails
Cutting the toenails straight across does not damage the skin at the corners of the nails and helps to prevent ingrowing of the nails.

When the child has gained proficiency in using the potty, he or she should be introduced to the toilet. A useful intermediate step is to place the potty near the toilet. The child continues to use the potty for a while, but is taught to use toilet paper and to flush the toilet. When reasonable control has been achieved, the child can be taken out of nappies during the day. Nappies should be worn at night until the child is usually dry on waking.

Children differ in the age at which they become toilet-trained and more so in the age at which they are dry both during the day and at night. A child is unlikely to be completely toilet-trained or to be able to empty the bladder on demand before his or her third birthday. Toilet accidents, particularly wetting, are common up to the age of five because a young child can delay urination for only a few minutes after the initial urge to urinate. Some toilet-trained children may revert to soiling or wetting when anxious or under stress. (See also *Encopresis; Enuresis; Soiling.*)

Tolbutamide

An oral hypoglycaemic drug (see *Hypoglycaemics, oral*).

Tolerance

The need to take increasingly higher doses of a *drug* to attain the same physical or mental effect. Tolerance develops after taking a drug over a period of time and usually results either from the liver becoming more efficient at breaking down the drug or from the body tissues becoming less sensitive to it.

The most familiar example of tolerance occurs in heavy drinkers who become so tolerant of *alcohol* that they are capable of drinking amounts that would render occasional drinkers unconscious. (See also *Alcohol dependence; Drug dependence.*)

Tolmetin

A *nonsteroidal anti-inflammatory drug* (NSAID) used to relieve pain, stiffness, and inflammation in *osteoarthritis, rheumatoid arthritis,* and *ankylosing spondylitis.* Tolmetin is also given to treat pain caused by minor injuries.

Tolnaftate

An *antifungal drug* used to treat and sometimes to prevent the recurrence of types of *tinea,* including *athlete's foot.* Tolnaftate, which is available over-the-counter as a cream, may in rare cases cause skin irritation or rash.

Tomography

An *imaging technique* that produces a cross-sectional image ("slice") of an organ or part of the body.

In *X-ray* tomography, the X-ray machine and film are positioned so that tissue is in focus at one depth only. All background and foreground structures appear blurred. By taking a series of tomograms it is possible to build an outline image of a part of the body which, on an ordinary X-ray film, would be hidden by other structures. For example, tomography is often used to obtain a clear outline of the kidneys during intravenous *urography,* when the kidneys would otherwise be obscured by gas or faecal matter in the intestines.

Most tomography today is performed using computed techniques (see *CT scanning* and *MRI*), which produce extremely accurate and highly detailed images.

-tomy

A suffix denoting the operation of cutting or making an incision, as in thoracotomy, a surgical operation in which the thorax (chest) is opened.

Tone, muscle

The natural tension in the fibres of a *muscle.* At rest, all muscle fibres are maintained in a state of partial contraction by nerve impulses from the spinal cord. This resting muscle tone helps control posture, keeps the eyes open, and allows muscles to contract more efficiently.

Abnormally high muscle tone causes *spasticity,* rigidity, and an increased resistance to movement. Abnormally low muscle tone causes floppiness of the body part (see *Hypotonia; Hypotonia in infants*).

Tongue

A muscular, flexible organ that occupies the floor of the *mouth.*

STRUCTURE AND FUNCTION

The tongue is composed of a mass of muscles covered by *mucous membrane.* These muscles are attached to the mandible (lower jaw) and to the hyoid bone above the larynx. Minute nodules called papillae project from the upper surface of the tongue, giving it a rough texture. Situated between the papillae at the sides and base of the tongue are minute sensory organs called taste-buds, which are responsible for the sense of *taste.*

As well as being the organ of taste, the tongue is essential for *mastication* (chewing), *swallowing,* and *speech.*

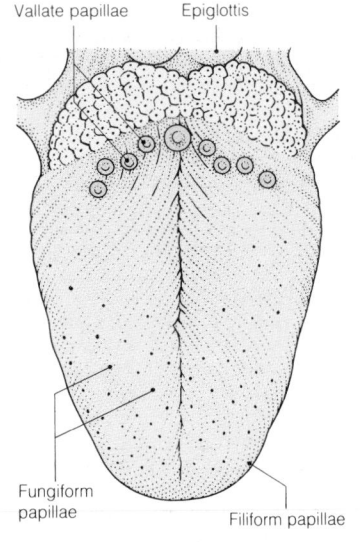

ANATOMY OF THE TONGUE
The tongue consists mainly of muscle; on its surface, it has various types of papillae that contain the taste-buds.

Vallate papillae   Epiglottis

Fungiform papillae

Filiform papillae

DISORDERS

A large tongue is a feature of *Down's syndrome, cretinism,* and *acromegaly.* Temporary enlargement of the tongue as a result of swelling and inflammation occurs in *glossitis.*

Fissures on the tongue are common and usually cause no trouble, but in some cases they are so deep that food particles collect in them, causing discomfort. Unnatural smoothness of the tongue, accompanied by redness and soreness, is a feature of pernicious anaemia (See *Anaemia, megaloblastic*), iron-deficiency anaemia (see *Anaemia, iron-deficiency*), *syphilis,* and *glossitis.*

In rare cases, the papillae on the tongue become elongated and turn black or brown, a condition known as black tongue. This disorder, of which the cause is unknown, is harmless but persistent. The unsightly discoloration can be removed by cleaning the tongue twice a day with a soft toothbrush dipped in an antiseptic mouthwash.

The tongue can be a site for *mouth ulcers* and *leukoplakia* (thickened white or grey patches), a condition that occasionally becomes cancerous (see *Tongue cancer*). Any ulcer or lump on the tongue that does not disappear within about three weeks should be reported to a doctor because of the risk of cancer.

T

Tongue cancer

The most serious type of *mouth cancer* because of its rapid spread. Tongue cancer is one of the two most common types of mouth cancer (the other being *lip cancer*).

Cancer of the tongue mainly affects people over 40. This form of cancer is usually associated with tobacco-smoking and heavy consumption of alcohol, particularly strong spirits; poor oral hygiene is commonly also a contributing factor.

SYMPTOMS AND SIGNS

The edge of the tongue is most commonly affected. The first sign may be a small ulcer with a raised margin, a white patch of thickened tissue known as *leukoplakia,* a deep fissure with hard edges, or a raised, hardened mass. Pain is rare until the cancer is advanced, when there is also excessive salivation, stiffness of the tongue, difficulty in swallowing, and, in some cases, offensive breath.

The tumour may become very large, obstructing the throat and occasionally causing asphyxia. Tongue cancer spreads rapidly to any or all of the following: the gums, the lower jaw, and the lymph nodes in the floor of the mouth and the neck.

DIAGNOSIS AND TREATMENT

Any physical change in the tongue that does not clear up within about three weeks should be reported to a doctor. Cancer is diagnosed by means of a tongue *biopsy* (the removal of a small sample of tissue for microscopic examination).

Small tumours, especially those at the tip of the tongue, are usually removed surgically. Larger tumours or tumours that have spread often require *radiotherapy*. If a tumour is very large and has spread to affect the lymph nodes, the surgeon may remove the whole tongue, the lymph

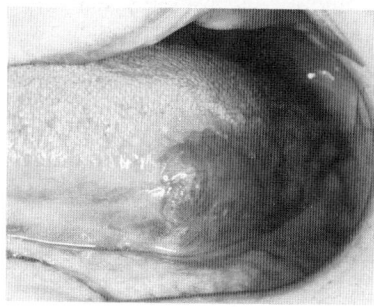

Appearance of tongue cancer
The cancer often starts at the edge of the tongue. It may appear (as here) as a raised mass, as a fissure, or as an ulcer.

nodes, and sometimes the lower jaw, although *anticancer drugs* and occasional radiotherapy in combination may reduce the need for such drastic surgery.

OUTLOOK

Unless the cancer is detected very early, its spread makes the outlook poor. In about half of all sufferers, the lymph nodes are involved by the time of diagnosis. About half of affected women but only a quarter of men survive for five years or more.

Tongue depressor

A flat wooden or metal instrument for holding down the tongue against the floor of the mouth to allow examination of the back of the throat.

Tongue-tie

A minor defect of the *mouth,* also called ankyloglossia, in which the frenulum (the band of tissue attaching the underside of the *tongue* to the floor of the mouth) is too short and extends forwards to the tip of the tongue. There are usually no symptoms other than limited movement of the tongue. In rare cases, the condition causes a speech defect, in which case a minor operation is required to divide the frenulum.

Tonic

One of a diverse group of remedies intended to relieve symptoms such as malaise, lethargy, and loss of appetite. Most tonics contain herbal extracts, vitamins, and minerals. Medical evidence suggests that tonics mainly have a *placebo* effect.

The term tonic is also used adjectivally to relate to muscle tone (see *Tone, muscle*), as in the tonic neck reflex, one of the primitive *reflexes* occurring in newborn babies.

Tonometry

The procedure for measuring the pressure of the fluid within the *eye*. A rise in intraocular pressure is one of the signs of *glaucoma*. Tonometry is usually performed by an ophthalmologist during an eye examination (see *Eye, examination of*).

HOW IT IS DONE

The standard method of measuring pressure in the eye is called applanation tonometry. The ophthalmologist applies a drop of quick-acting anaesthetic and a trace of *fluorescein* to each cornea; he or she then measures the pressure within the eye by means of a tonometer (measuring device) mounted on a *slit-lamp* (light source

with a magnifying viewer). The head of the tonometer is illuminated and touched gently against the anaesthetized cornea. A visible circle of fluorescein-stained tear film is formed, which the ophthalmologist views through the slit-lamp microscope. The force with which the tonometer head is pressed against the cornea is gradually increased until the area of the circle reaches a fixed standard. The force needed to achieve this degree of corneal flattening is a measure of the pressure within the eye.

Tonsil

A pair of oval tissue masses at the back of the throat. The tonsils are made up of lymphoid tissue and form part of the *lymphatic system*, which is an important part of the body's defence against infection. Along with the *adenoids* at the base of the tongue, the tonsils protect against upper *respiratory tract infections*. The tonsils gradually enlarge from birth, reach their maximum size at about seven years of age, and then shrink substantially.

Tonsillitis is a common childhood infection. Rarely, quinsy (an abscess around the tonsil) may develop.

Tonsillectomy

Surgical removal of the *tonsils*.

WHY IT IS DONE

Tonsillectomy was once a common childhood operation; it is now per-

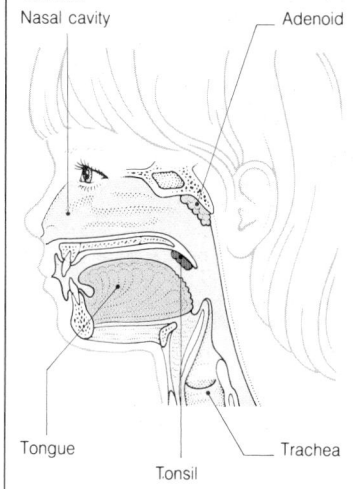

LOCATION OF THE TONSILS
The tonsils can be easily seen on either side of the back of the throat. They reach maximum size at about the age of seven years and then shrink.

Nasal cavity

Adenoid

Tongue

Trachea

Tonsil

T

T

formed only if a child suffers frequent recurrent attacks of severe *tonsillitis*. Less common problems that may necessitate the operation are quinsy (an abscess around the tonsil) or a single tonsil growing larger or becoming deeply ulcerated and therefore coming under suspicion of being malignant. In rare cases, removal of the tonsils may be advised for adolescents or young adults suffering from recurrent bouts of tonsillitis.

HOW IT IS DONE
The operative technique is shown in the illustrated box.

RECOVERY PERIOD
In the first 24 hours after the operation there may be bleeding from the throat; the patient must lie on his or her side to avoid choking and to allow bleeding to be detected. Post-operative pain in the throat and sometimes the ears is common and may require an *analgesic drug* (painkiller). Fluids and soft, easily swallowed foods such as ice cream are usually given for a day or two until the patient can eat normally.

Sore throat, particularly at mealtimes, may persist for up to two weeks after the operation. Full recovery usually takes place within three weeks. In some people, bleeding occurs a week or so after the operation, requiring medical attention and possible readmission to hospital.

PROCEDURE FOR TONSILLECTOMY
Tonsillectomy is most commonly carried out around the age of six or seven. The adenoids may be removed at the same time.

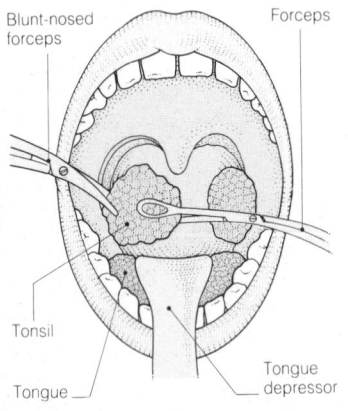

Blunt-nosed forceps

Forceps

Tonsil

Tongue

Tongue depressor

Standard technique
With the patient under a general anaesthetic, the tongue is depressed and the tonsils prised from the back of the throat and then cut away.

Tonsillitis
Inflammation of the *tonsils* due to infection. Tonsillitis mainly occurs in childhood, most children suffering at least one attack.

CAUSES AND INCIDENCE
The function of the tonsils is to help protect against upper *respiratory tract infection*. Sometimes, however, the tonsils themselves become repeatedly infected by the microorganisms they fight. Tonsillitis is most common in children under the age of nine; it also occurs infrequently in adolescents and young adults.

SYMPTOMS AND SIGNS
The main symptoms are a sore throat and difficulty in swallowing (very young children may refuse to eat). The throat is visibly inflamed. Other common symptoms are fever, headache, earache, enlarged and tender lymph nodes in the neck, and unpleasant-smelling breath. Occasionally, the illness causes temporary deafness or quinsy (an abscess around the tonsil). If symptoms persist for more than 24 hours or if pus can be seen on the tonsils, a doctor should be consulted.

TREATMENT
Tonsillitis is treated with bed rest, plenty of fluids, and an *analgesic drug* (painkiller), such as *paracetamol*. In some cases, *antibiotic drugs* may also be prescribed.

Tooth abscess
See *Abscess, dental*.

Toothache
Pain coming from one or more *teeth* and sometimes also from the *gums*, felt as a dull throb or a sharp twinge.

CAUSES
Early dental *caries* (decay) may cause mild toothache when eating sweet or very hot or cold food. More advanced decay or, less commonly, a fracture in a tooth (see *Fracture, dental*) or a deep, unlined filling (see *Filling, dental*) may result in inflammation of the pulp. This usually causes sharp, stabbing pain, which is often worse when the sufferer is lying down.

If the inflammation spreads, periapical *periodontitis* (inflammation of supporting tissues around the root tip) may develop, causing localized pain that is brought on mainly by biting and chewing. A dental abscess (see *Abscess, dental*) may also occur. In this case, pain is severe and often continuous, the gum surrounding the affected tooth is tender and swollen, and there may be swelling of the face and neck accompanied by fever.

Chronic periodontitis, which affects all the supporting tissues around the tooth and which causes the gums to recede, results in aching around exposed tooth roots when hot, cold, or sweet food is eaten. Gums around the affected teeth are tender and swollen.

A filling that is not quite level or a blow to a tooth may also result in inflammation of supporting tissues, causing pain when biting.

Sometimes toothache is not caused by a disorder of the teeth or gums. For example, in *sinusitis* (inflammation of the mucous membrane lining the facial air cavities) pain may be referred to the upper molar and premolar teeth (see *Referred pain*).

TREATMENT
Analgesic drugs (painkillers) may provide temporary relief until a visit to the dentist can be arranged. An emergency appointment should be made if the symptoms suggest there is an abscess. The treatment carried out by the dentist depends on the underlying cause of the toothache.

Toothbrushing
Cleaning of the *teeth* with a brush to remove plaque and food particles from tooth surfaces, and to stimulate the *gums*.

Toothbrushing should be carried out at least once a day using a fluoride *dentifrice* (usually toothpaste); children should brush their teeth after every meal and at bedtime. For complete *oral hygiene*, flossing (see *Floss, dental*) should be performed daily.

A safe and effective toothbrush for general use has an easily gripped handle and soft, round-ended or polished bristles. The size and shape of the head of the brush must allow every tooth to be reached; children need a smaller toothbrush than adults. Toothbrushes should be rinsed after each use and replaced as soon as the bristles become frayed or bent. Interspace brushes, which have small, round heads, are useful for cleaning around *bridges* and fixed *orthodontic appliances*. Electric toothbrushes are also available and may make brushing easier for some people.

Tooth decay
See *Caries, dental*.

Tooth extraction
See *Extraction, dental*.

Toothpaste
See *Dentifrice*.

BASIC TOOTHBRUSHING

Efficient toothbrushing is essential for the preservation of the teeth and the health of the gums. The enemy is plaque, a mixture of food debris, dried saliva, and bacteria, which develops at the gum margins and leads to caries (tooth decay) and gum disease.

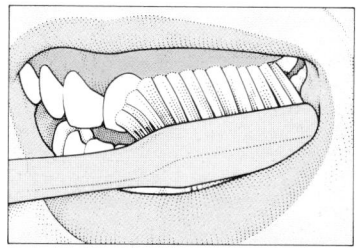

1 With the bristle tips set at 45 degrees to the plane of the teeth, scrub gently along the gum line using short strokes. The bristle tips should do the work.

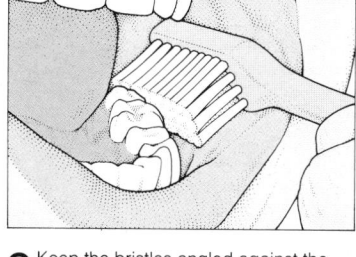

2 Keep the bristles angled against the line of the gums and work over the outer and inner surfaces of the upper and lower teeth. Keep the strokes short.

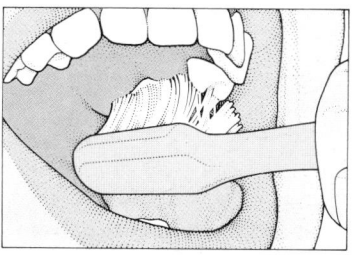

3 Don't forget to scrub over the chewing surfaces of all four sets of premolar and molar teeth. Move slowly over the surfaces, cleaning each tooth in turn.

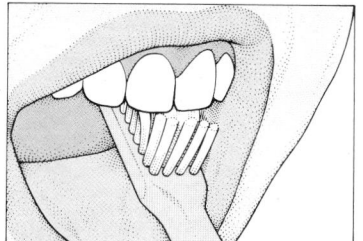

4 Remember to brush the inside surfaces of the front teeth. Hold the brush almost vertical and scrub with an up-and-down movement.

Tophus

A collection of *uric acid* crystals deposited in the tissues, especially around joints (such as the elbow) but occasionally in other places (such as the ear). A tophus is a sign of *hyperuricaemia*, which accompanies *gout*. Tophi may occasionally ulcerate and discharge chalky white material.

Topical

A term describing a *drug* that is applied to the surface of the body, as opposed to being swallowed or injected. Topical refers not only to drugs applied to the skin, but also to those administered into the ear canal, onto the surface of the eye, or as suppositories into the vagina or rectum.

Torsion

A term that means twisting. Almost any structure that is relatively free to move in the body may become twisted, such as the intestine (see *Volvulus*), the spermatic cord from the testis (see *Testis, torsion of*), or a *cyst* on a stalk. One of the principal dangers of torsion is obstruction of the blood supply to the affected part; if this occurs, pain is usually the first symptom. If the torsion is not corrected, tissue death may develop.

Torticollis

Twisting of the neck, causing the head to be rotated and tilted into an abnormal position, in which it remains. Also known as wry neck, torticollis is often accompanied by pain and stiffness in the neck.

CAUSES

The condition usually results from a minor neck injury that causes irritation of cervical nerves and consequent spasm of neck muscles. Torticollis may also result from muscle spasm caused by sleeping in an awkward position or by anxiety. Injury to a neck muscle at birth can also cause torticollis, as can a burn or other injury that has resulted in heavy scarring and contracture (shrinkage) of the skin.

TREATMENT

Treatment for torticollis due to muscle spasm may include wearing an orthopaedic collar (see *Collar, orthopaedic*), *heat treatment*, *ultrasound treatment*, or *physiotherapy*. Injections of the toxin that causes *botulism* will relieve the spasm for several months; this is the preferred treatment in severe cases. When the cause is an injury arising from birth, the muscle is gently stretched several times each day; occasionally, an operation is required to cut the lower end of the muscle.

Touch

The sense by which certain characteristics of objects, such as their size, shape, temperature, and surface texture, can be ascertained through physical contact.

Many types of touch *receptors* are present in the skin. In hairy skin areas, some of the receptors consist of webs of sensory nerve cell endings wrapped around the hair bulbs. These are triggered if the hairs are moved. Other receptors are more common in nonhairy areas of the body, such as the lips and fingertips; these receptors consist of nerve cell endings that may be free or surrounded by bulb-like structures.

Signals from touch receptors pass, via sensory nerves, to the spinal cord, from there to the thalamus in the brain, and on to the *sensory cortex*, where touch sensations are perceived and interpreted.

According to the number and distribution of receptors, the various parts of the body differ in their sensitivity to painful stimuli and in touch discrimination (the ability to distinguish between a single pinprick and two pinpricks placed slightly apart). For example, the cornea is several hundred times more sensitive to painful stimuli than are the soles of the feet. The fingertips are excellent at touch discrimination but relatively insensitive to painful stimuli.

T

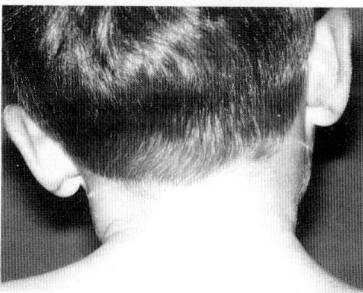

Child with torticollis
The muscles on one side of the neck have gone into spasm, pulling the head over to that side and causing pain.

THE SENSE OF TOUCH

The skin contains many thousands of specialized cells that respond to external stimuli, such as touch, heat, cold, and pressure. These cells (receptors) are divided into two types. One type of receptor consists only of a thin nerve fibre, which may wrap around an individual hair and respond to its movement. The other type has a specialized structure, known as an end organ, surrounding the nerve ending. Some skin receptors consist of several layers of cells attached to one nerve fibre. Others contain several nerve fibres arranged in a loop or coil. Probably several varieties of receptors play a part in each touch modality.

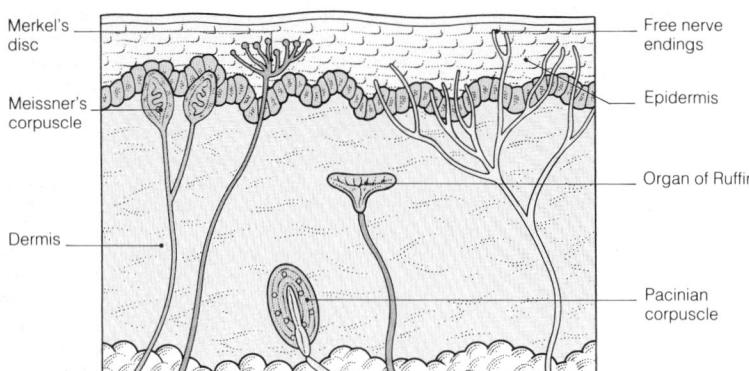

Merkel's disc

Meissner's corpuscle

Dermis

Free nerve endings

Epidermis

Organ of Ruffini

Pacinian corpuscle

Skin receptors
These receptors vary from free nerve endings to corpuscular or bulb-like structures. Individual receptors do not seem to be associated exclusively with any one touch sensation (e.g. cold or pain).

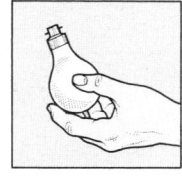

Delicate touch
The ability to detect light contact between an object and the skin. Areas with more receptors are more sensitive.

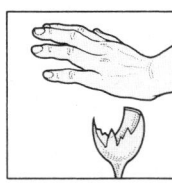

Pain
Pain warns the brain about possible injury from an external stimulus and can trigger a reflex withdrawal.

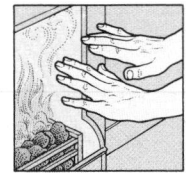

Heat
Some free nerve endings respond specifically to heat. The skin of the wrist is good for testing temperature.

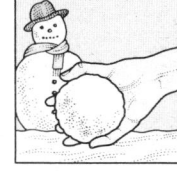

Cold
Cold on the skin is detected by specialized end organs. Extreme cold also stimulates pain receptors.

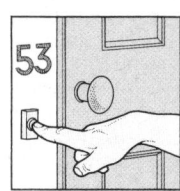

Pressure
A change in pressure on the skin is detected by specialized end organs called pacinian corpuscles.

TOUCH PERCEPTION

General sensations from various parts of the body are perceived at specific points within the brain's cerebral cortex. Highly sensitive body parts, such as the lips and hands, are represented by correspondingly large regions within the cortex.

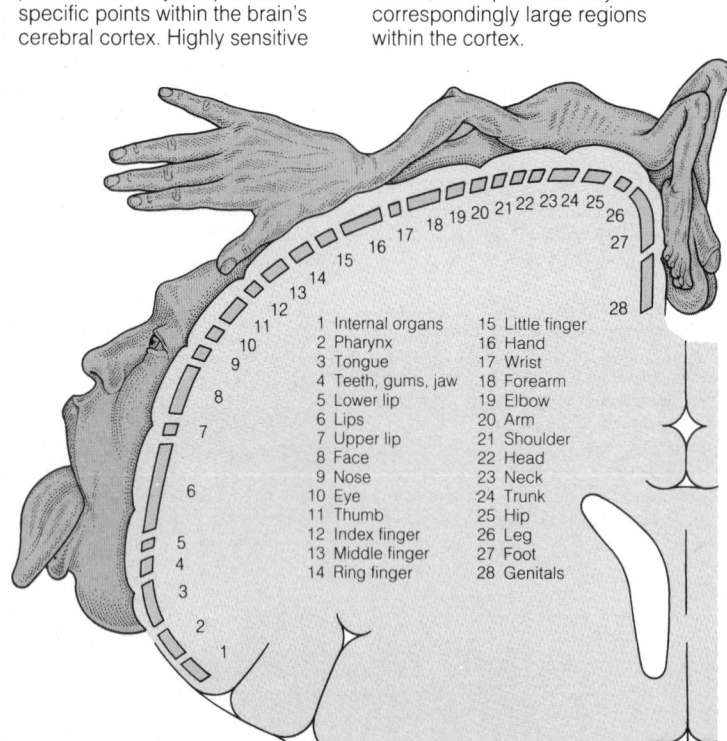

1 Internal organs
2 Pharynx
3 Tongue
4 Teeth, gums, jaw
5 Lower lip
6 Lips
7 Upper lip
8 Face
9 Nose
10 Eye
11 Thumb
12 Index finger
13 Middle finger
14 Ring finger
15 Little finger
16 Hand
17 Wrist
18 Forearm
19 Elbow
20 Arm
21 Shoulder
22 Head
23 Neck
24 Trunk
25 Hip
26 Leg
27 Foot
28 Genitals

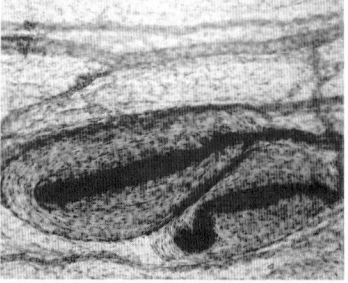

Pacinian corpuscle
These receptors are 1 mm to 4 mm long and occur in hairless areas of skin, especially the fingers.

Touch sense becomes much more developed in people deprived of other senses, particularly blind people; it is this capacity for touch development that is used by systems such as *braille*. (See also *Sensation*.)

Tourette's syndrome
See *Gilles de la Tourette's syndrome*.

Tourniquet
A device placed around a limb to compress blood vessels. A tourniquet may be used to help locate a vein for an intravenous injection or for the withdrawal of blood. By preventing blood from flowing back to the heart, a tourniquet causes veins in the limb below it to swell and become prominent.

An inflatable tourniquet, called an *Esmarch's bandage*, is used to control blood flow in some limb operations. An inflatable tourniquet also forms part of a *sphygmomanometer*, an instrument for measuring *blood pressure*.

Tourniquets have caused more problems than they have solved. In the past, they were used as a first-aid measure to stop severe bleeding. This use is now discouraged because leaving a tourniquet in place for too long can cause *gangrene* (tissue death). First-aid courses now teach the control of bleeding by pressure over the bleeding site (see *Pressure points*), which is usually effective and safer.

Toxaemia
The presence in the bloodstream of *toxins* (poisons) produced by *bacteria*. Toxaemia may be a feature of *septicaemia* (the spread and multiplication of bacteria within the bloodstream from a localized site of infection), but it can also occur without any evidence of bacteria in the blood. Toxaemia with or without septicaemia is sometimes called blood poisoning.

Toxaemia may cause symptoms such as a fever and headache and other symptoms specific to the particular toxin (e.g. muscle spasms caused by the toxin released by *tetanus* bacteria). Toxaemia can lead to the very dangerous condition of *septic shock*, in which there is widespread tissue damage and a drop in blood pressure.

Treatment of toxaemia is as for septicaemia and septic shock—*antibiotic drugs*, removal of a localized site of infection if one can be found, and measures to treat shock, including *intravenous infusions*. For some types of toxaemia, an *antitoxin* may be given. (See also *Toxaemia of pregnancy*; *Toxic shock syndrome*.)

Toxaemia of pregnancy
A disorder of pregnant women characterized by raised blood pressure, tissue swelling, and leakage of protein from the kidneys into the urine (see *Pre-eclampsia*). If severe, toxaemia of pregnancy may progress to seizures and coma (see *Eclampsia*). Toxaemia of pregnancy has some features common to other forms of *toxaemia*, but no toxin has ever been identified.

Toxicity
The property of being poisonous. The term is also used to refer to the severity of adverse effects or illness produced by a *toxin* (a poisonous protein produced by certain bacteria, animals, or plants), by a *poison*, or by a drug overdose (see *Drug poisoning*).

Toxicology
The study of *poisons*, including their chemical composition, preparation, identification, effects on the body, and, where appropriate, their antidotes. (See also *Poisoning*.)

Toxic shock syndrome
An uncommon severe illness caused by a *toxin* produced by the bacterium *STAPHYLOCOCCUS AUREUS*. Toxic shock syndrome was first recognized in the late 1970s and many cases were diagnosed in young women in the early 1980s, particularly in the US. About 70 per cent of cases occur in women who are using vaginal tampons at the time of onset.
CAUSE
Overgrowth of *STAPHYLOCOCCUS AUREUS* bacteria in the vagina and increased production of the toxin they produce have been associated with prolonged use of certain brands of tampons. These brands of highly absorbent tampons have now been taken off the market.

Of the cases that do not occur in association with menstruation, some have been linked to use of a contraceptive cap, diaphragm, or sponge. Other cases arise from skin wounds or infections caused by *STAPHYLOCOCCUS AUREUS* elsewhere in the body.
SYMPTOMS
The onset of toxic shock syndrome is sudden, with high fever, vomiting, diarrhoea, headache, muscular aches and pains, dizziness, and disorientation. A skin rash resembling sunburn develops on the palms and soles, and peels within one or two weeks. The blood pressure may fall dangerously low, and *shock* may develop. Other serious complications include *kidney*

failure and *liver failure*. The mortality is about three per cent, usually due to a prolonged fall in blood pressure or to lung complications.
TREATMENT
Treatment is with *antibiotic drugs*. *Intravenous infusion* may be necessary to treat shock, and more treatment may be needed for complications.

Recurrence is common; women who have had toxic shock syndrome are advised not to use tampons, caps, diaphragms, or sponges.

Toxin
A poisonous protein produced by pathogenic (disease-causing) bacteria, such as *CLOSTRIDIUM TETANI*, which causes *tetanus*; various animals, notably venomous snakes (see *Snake bites*); or certain plants, such as the death cap mushroom *AMANITA PHALLOIDES* (see *Mushroom poisoning*).

Bacterial toxins are sometimes subdivided into three categories: *endotoxins*, which are released only from the inside of dead bacteria; *exotoxins*, which are released from the surface of live bacteria; and *enterotoxins*, which inflame the intestine. (See also *Poison*; *Poisoning*; *Toxaemia*.)

Toxocariasis
 An infestation of humans, usually children, with the larvae of *TOXOCARA CANIS*, a small, thread-like worm that lives in the intestines of dogs. The disease is also sometimes known as visceral larva migrans.
CAUSES AND INCIDENCE
The causes and course of an infestation are shown in the illustrated box on the next page.
PREVENTION
Dogs that live with children should be dewormed regularly: monthly until the dog is six months old, and then annually.
SYMPTOMS AND SIGNS
Usually, infestation in humans causes only mild fever and malaise, which soon clears up. However, following some cases of heavy infestation, *pneumonia* and *seizures* may develop. Another possible complication is loss of vision, which may occur if a larva enters the eye and dies there.
DIAGNOSIS AND TREATMENT
Toxocariasis is diagnosed from sputum (phlegm) analysis, and by a *liver biopsy* (removal of a small sample of the organ for analysis).

Severe cases of toxocariasis require treatment in hospital, where the patient may be given *thiabendazole* (an

T

ORIGINS OF TOXOCARIASIS

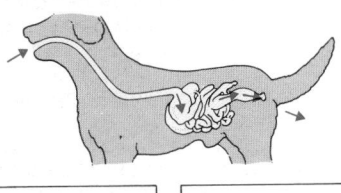

1 A dog (often a puppy) harbouring the small roundworm *TOXOCARA CANIS* in its digestive tract passes large numbers of worm eggs in its faeces, which may contaminate soil.

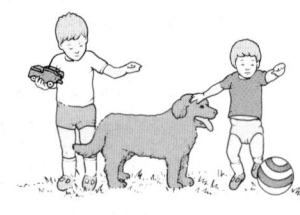

2 Children who play with an infested dog, or with soil contaminated with dog faeces, and who then put their fingers in their mouths, may swallow some of the worm eggs.

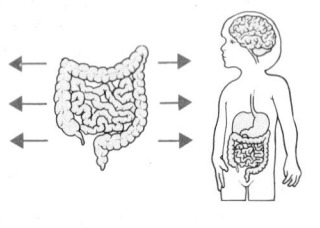

3 The swallowed eggs hatch in the intestines to liberate larvae, which migrate through the tissues to organs such as the liver, lungs, brain, and eyes. They provoke allergic reactions such as asthma and may also have more serious effects, such as loss of vision.

anthelmintic drug) to control the infestation, and an *anticonvulsant drug* to control seizures.

Toxoid

An inactivated bacterial *toxin* (poisonous protein). Inactivation, usually by heat or chemicals, removes the toxicity of the toxin but preserves its property of stimulating antibody production by the *immune system*. Certain toxoids are used to immunize against specific diseases, *diphtheria* or *tetanus* for example.

Toxoplasmosis

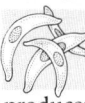

An infection of mammals, birds, and reptiles that is also common in humans. Toxoplasmosis usually produces no ill effects except when it is transmitted by a pregnant woman to her unborn child or in people who have an *immunodeficiency disorder*, such as *AIDS*.

CAUSES AND INCIDENCE
The infection is caused by the protozoan (single-celled microorganism) *TOXOPLASMA GONDII*. Humans are most commonly infected by eating undercooked meat from infected animals. An estimated 25 per cent of pork and 10 per cent of lamb eaten by humans contains toxoplasma organisms. The protozoa also multiply in the intestines of cats, and about one per cent of cats excrete cysts containing toxoplasma eggs in their faeces. Infection in humans can occur through failure to wash the hands after handling the cat or its faeces.

Toxoplasmosis contracted by a woman during pregnancy is transmitted to the child in about one third of cases, often with severe effects.

Infection is extremely common worldwide. However, no more than about 700 to 800 infections annually in the UK lead to recognized illness or effects on the fetus.

SYMPTOMS AND SIGNS
In most cases, the body's *immune system* provides adequate protection against the protozoa, so that the infection produces no symptoms. In some people with a normal immune system, however, the infection causes a feverish illness resembling infectious *mononucleosis*. It may also cause retinitis (inflammation of the retina) and *choroiditis* (inflammation of the blood vessels behind the retina).

Infection of an unborn child during early pregnancy may result in miscarriage or stillbirth. Infants may have enlargement of the liver and spleen, *hydrocephalus*, blindness, mental handicap, and may die during infancy. Infection in late pregnancy usually has no ill effects.

Toxoplasmosis may also take a severe course in people with an immunodeficiency disorder, causing lung and heart damage and severe *encephalitis* (brain inflammation).

DIAGNOSIS AND TREATMENT
The diagnosis is made from *blood tests*. Treatment is necessary only in pregnant women, in children born with severe symptoms, in people with an immune system deficiency, and in

cases of retinitis or choroiditis. Treatment is usually with the antimalarial drug *pyrimethamine* combined with a *sulphonamide drug*.

TPA

The abbreviation for *tissue-plasminogen activator*.

Trabeculectomy

A surgical procedure performed to reduce pressure in the *eye*. Trabeculectomy is used to control *glaucoma* when medication cannot keep the intraocular pressure within safe limits or when, despite medical treatment, loss of *visual field* due to damage to the *optic nerve* is progressing.

Trabeculectomy creates an alternative outlet from the eye for aqueous humour (fluid in the front chamber of the eye) so that a better balance is achieved between the rate of secretion of aqueous humour and its rate of outflow. In this way, the pressure can be kept within normal limits and further damage to the optic nerve fibres is reduced.

HOW IT IS DONE
The *conjunctiva* (mucous membrane covering the front of the eyeball) above the upper edge of the *cornea* is opened and a half-thickness flap of *sclera* (white of the eye) is cut and folded forwards. A small rectangle is removed from the inner layer at the scleral-corneal junction, so that a connection is made into the front chamber of the eye. The outer flap is replaced and secured with delicate stitches and the conjunctiva closed over it.

Trace elements

A group of *minerals* that are required in the diet only in minute amounts to maintain health. The principal trace elements include *chromium, copper, selenium*, and *zinc*. Although only tiny amounts are needed, they are vital to numerous chemical processes in the body. (See also *Nutrition*.)

Tracer

A radioactive substance introduced in to the body so that its distribution, processing, and elimination from the body can be monitored (by using a radiation detector). For example, radioactive iodine may be used as a tracer to study the functioning of the thyroid gland.

Trachea

The anatomical name for the windpipe. The trachea begins immediately below the *larynx* (voice-box) and runs

LOCATION OF THE TRACHEA

The trachea extends down from the larynx for about 10 cm to the point where it divides into the two bronchi.

Nasal cavity

Tongue

Larynx

Trachea

Rings of cartilage

Bronchi

down the centre of the front of the neck to end behind the upper part of the sternum (breastbone), where it divides to form the two main *bronchi*.

The trachea consists of fibrous and elastic tissue and smooth muscle. It also contains about 20 rings of cartilage, which help keep the trachea open even during extremes of neck movement. The lining of the trachea includes cells that secrete mucus (called goblet cells) and other cells that bear minute, hair-like cilia. The mucus helps trap tiny particles in inhaled air; the beating of the cilia moves the mucus upwards and out of the respiratory tract, thereby helping to keep the *lungs* and airways free.

DISORDERS

One of the most common disorders is *tracheitis* (inflammation of the lining of the trachea), which is usually caused by an infection (often by a virus) and is frequently associated with *bronchitis* or *laryngitis*. The principal symptoms are difficult, painful breathing and a harsh cough.

Obstruction of the trachea by an inhaled foreign object is rare because the narrowest part of the upper respiratory tract is the larynx, and any objects that pass through it usually continue through the trachea into a bronchus. However, the trachea may become obstructed by a tumour or narrowed as a result of scarring caused by the prolonged presence of a *tracheostomy* tube inserted to create an artificial airway through the front of the neck. Tracheal obstruction results in breathlessness and produces a loud, harsh, vibrating sound during breathing.

Rarely, a congenital malformation occurs in which a channel forms between the trachea and the oesophagus, situated immediately behind it (a condition called a *tracheoesophageal fistula*).

The trachea is sometimes injured by a direct blow or by strangulation. The seriousness of such an injury depends on the extent to which the airway is obstructed. In extreme cases, the trachea may collapse completely, which may be rapidly fatal unless an emergency tracheostomy is performed to re-establish an airway.

Tracheitis

Inflammation of the *trachea* (the windpipe). Tracheitis is usually caused by a viral infection and aggravated by inhaled fumes, especially tobacco smoke. It often occurs with *laryngitis* and *bronchitis*, a condition known as laryngotracheobronchitis, which is the most common cause of *croup* in young children.

Typical symptoms of tracheitis include a dry cough and hoarseness. In most cases, the condition is of short duration and requires no treatment.

Tracheoesophageal fistula

A rare *birth defect* in which an abnormal passage connects the *trachea* (windpipe) with the *oesophagus*. About three babies per 10,000 are born with a tracheoesophageal fistula. In the most common form, the lower end of the oesophagus connects with the trachea, and the upper end of the oesophagus is underdeveloped, forming a blind-ending pouch.

SYMPTOMS AND SIGNS

The affected baby cannot swallow saliva and as a result drools constantly. During feeding, food is regurgitated and enters the lungs, causing the baby to choke, cough, and sometimes turn blue because of lack of oxygen. The abdomen becomes swollen because inhaled air passes into the stomach through the fistula. The acidic fluid in the stomach passes up into the lungs through the fistula, leading to *pneumonia* and *atelectasis* (lung collapse).

DIAGNOSIS AND TREATMENT

In most cases the condition is discovered soon after birth. Milder forms of tracheoesophageal fistula may not be detected until childhood or even adult life, usually after recurrent attacks of pneumonia. The diagnosis may be confirmed by *chest X-ray* and other radiological studies.

Treatment consists of an operation to close the fistula and to connect the trachea and oesophagus correctly. Before the 1940s, the condition was untreatable; today the survival rate is about 90 per cent.

Tracheostomy

An operation in which an opening is made in the *trachea* (windpipe) and a tube is inserted to maintain an effective airway.

WHY IT IS DONE

Tracheostomy may be performed to treat an emergency or as a planned procedure. Today, acute airway problems are usually handled by an *endotracheal tube* passed via the mouth or nose. A tracheostomy is preferable, however, for the emergency treatment of airway problems (such as a tumour or a foreign body) involving the larynx.

A planned tracheostomy is most commonly performed on a person who has lost the ability to breathe naturally and is undergoing long-term *ventilation* (the pumping of air into the lungs by a machine) or who has lost the ability to keep saliva and other secretions out of the trachea because of coma or a specific airway or swallowing problem. In such cases, tracheostomy is performed after passing an endotracheal tube through the

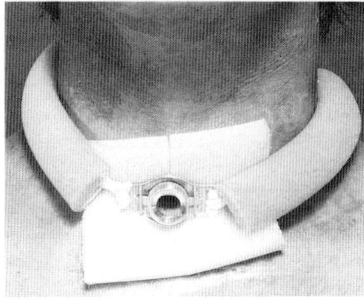

Tracheostomy tube
The tube readily becomes blocked by secretions; it has a metal inner lining that can be removed for cleaning.

T

nose or mouth and into the trachea. Permanent tracheostomy is necessary after *laryngectomy* (surgical removal of the larynx).

HOW IT IS DONE

The operation is carried out under local or general anaesthetic.

An incision is made in the skin overlying the trachea, between the Adam's apple and the clavicles (collarbones). The neck muscles are pulled apart, and the thyroid gland, which surrounds the trachea, is usually severed. A small vertical incision (called a "window") is made in the trachea so that a metal or plastic tube can be inserted. If the patient cannot breathe unaided, the tube is connected to a *ventilator*.

If a laryngectomy is being performed, the cut edges of the trachea are brought forwards and stitched to the edges of the skin wound before the tube is inserted.

RECOVERY PERIOD

For patients who are able to breathe unaided, the air in the room is humidified to reduce the drying of mucus in the airway. Air from a ventilator is humidified before it passes into the tube. Any excessive mucus that accumulates in the airway is sucked away through a catheter inserted into the tube.

While the tube is in place, the patient is usually unable to speak and is therefore provided with a bell or buzzer and with pen and paper for communication. After laryngectomy, the tube is removed after several days, and a permanent opening remains. In other cases, the tube is removed when the patient has recovered from the condition that necessitated the operation, and the opening soon closes and heals.

Tracheotomy

Cutting of the trachea (windpipe). (See also *Tracheostomy*.)

Trachoma

A persistent infectious disease of the *conjunctiva* and *cornea*. Trachoma is caused by an organism, CHLAMYDIA TRACHOMATIS, that is spread by direct contact and possibly by flies (see *Chlamydial infections*). Untreated trachoma leads to complications that may cause blindness. Trachoma is uncommon where standards of personal hygiene are high.

SYMPTOMS AND SIGNS

Infection by CHLAMYDIA TRACHOMATIS causes acute *conjunctivitis*, with pain, *photophobia*, and watering of the

eyes. The eyes become red and inflamed, and the conjunctiva that lines the lids becomes thickened and roughened with scar tissue and studded with small lumps called follicles. Damage to the mucus-secreting cells of the conjunctiva and to the lacrimal (tear-producing) glands may lead to *keratoconjunctivitis sicca* (inflammation and dry eye).

An abnormal growth of blood vessels can extend down from the conjunctiva into the upper part of the cornea, leading to opacity (loss of transparency) and loss of vision. More severe damage to the cornea occurs later when fibrous scarring of the inside of the upper lid causes it to be rolled inwards so that the lashes rub against the cornea, causing ulceration and encouraging secondary bacterial infection. Secondary infection may lead to extensive ulceration, scarring, and even *perforation*, with spread of infection into the eye and permanent loss of vision.

TREATMENT

Antibiotic drugs may be applied to the eye or taken by mouth in an attempt to eradicate the causative organism. No further treatment may be necessary in the early stages of the disease. In established trachoma, however, after scarring has occurred, surgery to correct lid deformities or corneal grafting to restore transparency and vision may be needed.

Tract

A group of organs that form a common pathway to perform a particular function. For example, the urinary tract comprises the kidneys, ureters, bladder, and urethra, which together form a series of connected structures for the removal of waste products from the body.

The term tract also refers to a bundle of nerve fibres that have a common function, as in the pyramidal tract, a bundle of nerve fibres in the spinal cord that carry nerve impulses from the brain to the muscles.

Traction

A procedure in which part of the body is placed under tension to correct the alignment of two adjoining structures or to hold them in position.

WHY IT IS DONE

The most common use of traction is in the treatment of a *fracture* in which muscles around the bone ends are pulling the bones out of alignment. Fractures of the shaft of the *femur* (thigh-bone) are most likely to be treated in this way. Traction is also used to align and immobilize unstable fractures of the cervical spine (neck) when any movement of the vertebrae might damage the spinal cord (see *Spinal injury*).

HOW IT IS DONE

To apply traction to a lower limb fracture, the person lies on a bed with the

---

TRACTION FOR FEMORAL FRACTURE

Because of the power of the thigh muscles and their tendency to go into spasm, fractures of the femur (thigh-bone) tend to override.

Without traction to prevent this, the bone would heal with overlapping ends and the leg would be permanently shortened.

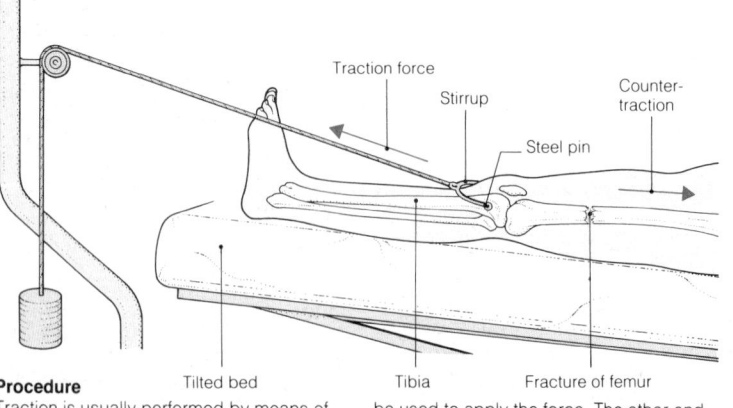

Traction force

Counter-traction

Stirrup

Steel pin

Procedure

Tilted bed

Tibia

Fracture of femur

Traction is usually performed by means of a narrow steel pin through the upper end of the tibia (shin), to which a steel stirrup is attached so that a cord and weight can

be used to apply the force. The other end of the femur must be immobilized (or countertraction applied) to keep the fractured bone ends aligned.

injured limb supported by attachments from an overhead frame. The upper end of the fractured bone is held immobilized while the lower end is pulled in a straight line away from it by a system of weights and pulleys. The traction grip is obtained by a pin inserted through the tibia (shin) or through a plaster cast applied to the limb. For spinal fractures, the patient lies flat on a firm surface and weights are attached to tongs inserted into holes drilled on either side of the skull. Both limb and spinal fractures are maintained in continuous traction until healing has occurred.

Training

A programme of *exercises* undertaken to prepare for a particular sport. Training may be concentrated on improving particular skills or on improving physical *fitness*.

Fitness training should include both *aerobic* and anaerobic exercises, which together build up strength, flexibility, and endurance (the capacity to exercise for long periods).

Interval training is a type of fitness programme in which a particular exercise, such as running a set distance at a timed pace, is repeated several times with a rest period between. Circuit training consists of performing a set number of different exercises, such as push-ups, sit-ups, and step-ups, one after the other.

The selection of an appropriate training programme requires specialized assessment and advice. Self-imposed training schedules may be damaging to health; for example, bone and muscle disorders may develop in runners if their training is unsupervised.

Trait

Any characteristic or condition that is inherited (determined by a *gene* or genes). Blue or brown eye colour, dark or light skin, body proportions, and nose shape are all examples of genetic traits.

The majority of common traits (such as eye colour) have no obvious effect on health. Others may have marginally advantageous effects in particular environments (such as dark skin in a sunny climate) or mildly disabling effects (such as *colour vision deficiency*). Severely handicapping traits, such as *cystic fibrosis* or *osteogenesis imperfecta*, are individually rare, but the fact that there are many different types means that they are collectively quite common (see *Genetic disorders*).

The term trait is also sometimes used in a more restricted sense to describe a mild form of a recessive genetic disorder. For example, a person who inherits the sickle cell gene in a single dose is said to have sickle cell trait. A double dose of the same gene causes the much more serious *sickle cell anaemia*.

Trance

A sleep-like state in which consciousness is reduced, voluntary actions are lessened or absent, and bodily functions are diminished. A trance usually results from separation of a group of mental processes from the rest of the mind rather than from any physical brain disturbance.

Trances are claimed to be induced by *hypnosis* and have been reported as part of a group experience, particularly in a religious context. Trances are sometimes a feature of *catalepsy, automatism*, and petit-mal *epilepsy*.

Tranquillizer drugs

Drugs with a sedative effect, subdivided into major tranquillizers (see *Antipsychotic drugs*) and minor tranquillizers (see *Antianxiety drugs*).

Transcutaneous electrical nerve stimulation

A method of pain relief achieved by the application of minute electrical impulses to nerve endings under the skin. (See *TENS*.)

Transdermal patch

A type of dressing that releases a drug when in contact with the skin.

Transference

The unconscious displacement of emotions from people who were important during one's childhood, such as parents, to other people when one is an adult. Transference is important in *psychoanalysis*.

Transfusion

See *Blood transfusion*.

Transfusion, autologous

See *Blood transfusion, autologous*.

Transient ischaemic attack

A brief interruption of the blood supply to part of the *brain* that results in temporary impairment of vision, speech, sensation, or movement. Typically, the episode lasts for several minutes or, at the most, for a few hours. Any attack with effects that last for more than 24 hours is called

a *stroke*. Transient ischaemic attacks (TIAs) can be the prelude to a full-scale stroke.

CAUSES
Some TIAs occur when an artery supplying the brain becomes temporarily blocked by a flake of clotted blood carried from elsewhere in the bloodstream (see *Embolism*). Other attacks are caused by narrowing of an artery due to *atherosclerosis*.

SYMPTOMS AND SIGNS
Symptoms occur suddenly, and vary widely, according to the site and duration of the interruption to the flow of blood to the brain. Common symptoms include weakness or numbness in an arm or leg, *aphasia* (disturbance of language functions), dizziness, or partial blindness. An attack is always followed by full recovery.

DIAGNOSIS
Diagnostic testing may include *CT scanning* to rule out the possibility of a brain tumour or a subdural *haematoma* (a swelling containing blood), which sometimes produce TIA-like symptoms. Blood tests to look for blood-clotting abnormalities may also be done. Other tests, including *ultrasound scanning*, digital subtraction *angiography*, or conventional angiography, may be used to look at the vessels for evidence of atherosclerosis. In some cases, the heart is studied as a possible source of blood clots.

TREATMENT
Treatment is aimed at preventing a major stroke, which occurs within five years in from one quarter to one third of the patients with TIA. Possible treatments include *endarterectomy*, *anticoagulant drugs*, or *aspirin* (which reduces the stickiness of platelets in the blood). Aspirin has consistently been proved effective in clinical trials.

Transillumination

A procedure sometimes carried out during physical examination of a lump or swelling. Light from a small torch is shone against one side of the lump; if light can be seen on the other side, the doctor knows that the lump contains clear fluid because fat or other tissue would block the light. For example, a *hydrocele* (a fluid-containing swelling in the scrotum) allows light to pass, whereas a *varicocele* (a mass of enlarged veins) in the scrotum does not.

Translocation

A rearrangement of the *chromosomes* inside a person's cells. Translocation is a type of *mutation* (change in the

T

EFFECT OF CHROMOSOMAL TRANSLOCATION

A translocation is a rearrangement of the chromosomes in body cells. A person carrying a translocation may show no abnormality but there is a risk of his or her child having a chromosomal abnormality.

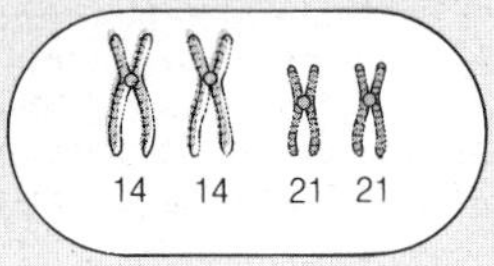

Normal cell
A body cell normally contains 22 paired chromosomes (called autosomes) plus two sex chromosomes (XX in women and XY in men). Just two pairs of autosomes—numbers 21 and 14—are shown here.

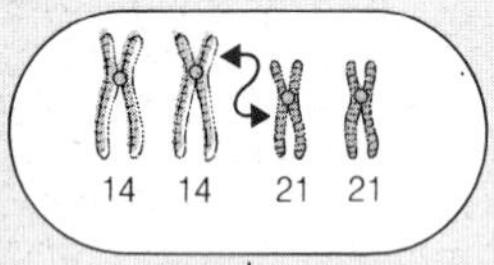

Example of translocation
In a typical translocation, a large part of one chromosome is joined to a large part of another. Here, most of chromosome number 21 and chromosome number 14 join together.

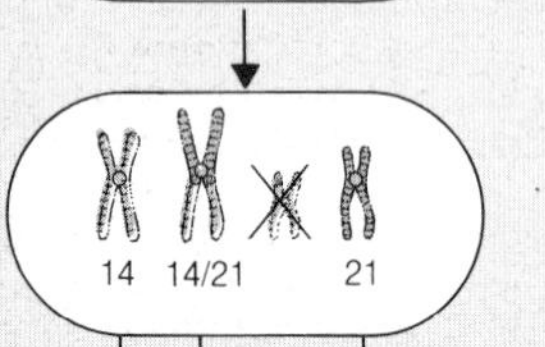

Balanced translocation (parent)
The remaining bits of chromosomes 21 and 14 disappear. If, as here, the translocation is balanced—that is, the total amount of chromosomal material is normal or near normal—no outward abnormality is seen.

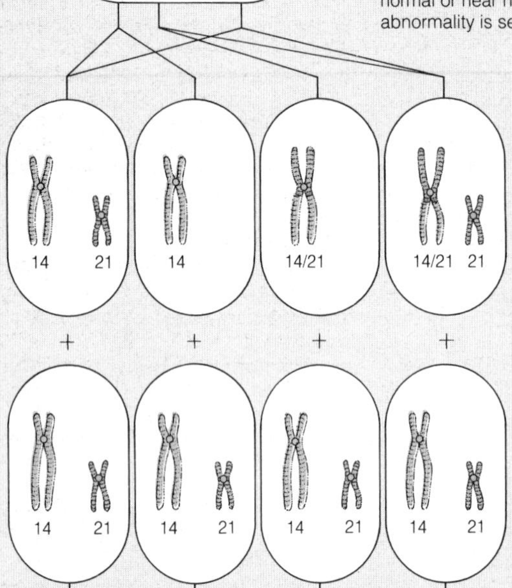

Eggs or sperm produced
A parent with the above translocation makes four types of egg or sperm. They are (from left)—normal, missing a chromosome 21, carrying joined chromosomes 14 and 21, and the same with an extra chromosome 21.

Normal egg or sperm
An egg or sperm from the parent with the translocation combines with one from the other parent, which has one number 21 and one number 14 chromosome. Any of the four outcomes below may result.

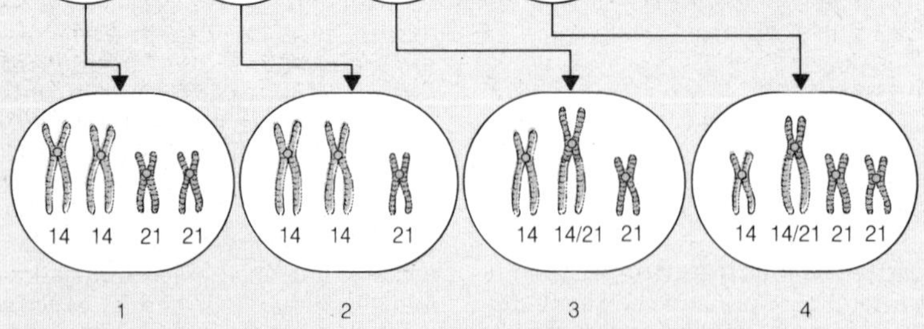

Child
The child may have (1) normal chromosomes, (2) a missing chromosome 21 (incompatible with life), (3) a balanced translocation (like the parent), and (4) effectively, an extra chromosome 21, leading to Down's syndrome. In the last case, the parents may benefit from genetic counselling.

genetic material). Sections of chromosomes may be exchanged, or the main parts of two chromosomes may be joined. A translocation may be inherited or be acquired as the result of a new mutation.

Often, because there has been no net loss or gain of chromosomal material within the person's cells, a translocation has no outward effect, and causes no abnormality. However, the translocation can mean that some of the person's egg or sperm cells carry too much or too little chromosomal material, which leads to a risk of a *chromosomal abnormality*, such as Down's syndrome, in the person's children (see illustrated box).

When a chromosomal abnormality occurs, the child's and the parents' chromosomes are checked to discover whether a translocation is the cause (see *Chromosome analysis*). *Genetic counselling* can help determine the risk of another child's being affected and can provide advice about antenatal diagnosis.

Transmissible

A term meaning capable of being passed from one person to another, or from one organism to another of the same or a different species. The term may be applied to an *infectious disease* or to an inherited *genetic disorder*.

Transplant surgery

The replacement of a diseased organ or tissue with a healthy, living substitute. The organ is usually taken from a person who has just died. Some transplanted kidneys (less than 10 per cent in the UK) are taken from living relatives of the patient (see *Organ donation*).

Around the world about 150,000 major organs have been transplanted, mostly in the past 10 to 15 years. About 80 per cent of patients are alive and well one year after the transplantation of a major organ, such as the heart or liver, and most survive at least five years.

The earliest successful transplant operation was *corneal grafting*, carried out early this century. The cornea is not affected by the *rejection* process (the automatic attempt by the body's *immune system* to reject foreign cells and destroy them) because it has no blood supply, and therefore no white blood cells and antibodies to bring about rejection.

Kidney transplantation was shown to be technically possible in the 1950s, but early transplant operations ended

TRANSPLANTS PERFORMED IN THE UK IN 1993

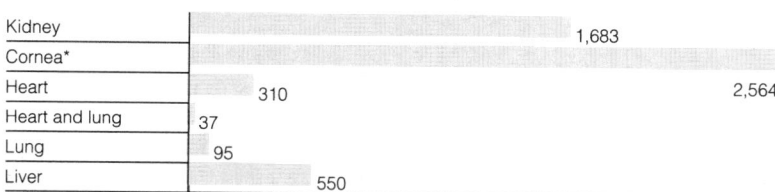

Kidney	2,564
Cornea*	1,683
Heart	310
Heart and lung	37
Lung	95
Liver	550

*This figure is an estimate because not all corneal transplants are registered

Factors affecting transplant numbers

The table above shows the provisional numbers of cadaveric transplants performed within the NHS in 1993. (A cadaveric transplant is one in which the organ for transplantation is taken from a person who has just died.) The number of specific transplant operations performed depends partly on demand (i.e. on how many people would benefit from receiving a transplant) and partly on the availability of donor organs. Strict selection of potential organ recipients is usually necessary because of shortages of suitable donor organs and because only relatively few specialist centres have the facilities and expertise required for carrying out transplant operations.

in failure because of rejection. In the 1960s, however, *corticosteroid drugs* and cytotoxic agents (see *Anticancer drugs*) were found to suppress the rejection response, making transplantation practicable. The discovery in the 1970s and introduction in the early 1980s of *cyclosporin*, a more effective *immunosuppressant drug*, substantially improved success rates.

A second important factor in improving the results of transplant surgery has been the steady improvement in techniques for matching donors and recipients. Organ transplantation proceeds most smoothly when the donor and recipient share most of the same tissue-types (see *Histocompatibility antigens; Tissue-typing*). Matching of tissue-types has become less important, however, since the introduction of cyclosporin.

A third factor that has contributed to higher success rates is the development of techniques for organ preservation. After removal from the donor, the organ is washed with an oxygenated fluid and cooled; this reduces the risk of damage due to lack of blood. Nevertheless, it is still important to keep to a minimum the time the organ is deprived of a normal blood supply. In most cases of heart or liver transplantation, the organs are removed from the donor while the heart is still functioning, but after *brain death* has been certified.

Every patient who undergoes an organ transplant operation must take immunosuppressant drugs indefinitely; this damping down of the body's natural defences exposes him or her to a greater risk of infection, especially with fungi (see *Fungal infections*) and protozoal *parasites*. Patients undergoing long-term immunosuppressant treatment are also at increased risk of certain types of cancer, especially *lymphomas*. (See also *Heart transplant; Heart-lung transplant; Liver transplant; Kidney transplant*.)

Transposition of the great vessels

A form of congenital *heart disease* in which the two major vessels that carry blood away from the heart—the aorta and the pulmonary artery—are in each other's normal position. This means that, unless the baby also has a septal defect (hole in the heart) through which blood can flow, insufficient oxygenated blood is supplied to the body's tissues. Transposition of the great vessels occurs in about 40 babies per 100,000 born.

SYMPTOMS

Cyanosis (blueness of the skin) usually develops and the baby becomes increasingly short of breath; the baby also feeds poorly. Symptoms vary in severity according to the amount of oxygenated blood passing through the septal opening.

DIAGNOSIS AND TREATMENT

A firm diagnosis can be made only after a *chest X-ray, ECG, echocardiography*, and cardiac *catheterization* (in which a catheter is introduced into the heart via a blood vessel).

The cardiac catheter may be used to make a hole in the septum. Alternatively, emergency surgery may be performed to create or enlarge an existing septal hole. These techniques allow enough oxygenated blood to reach the body tissues and keep the child alive. Later, reconstructive *open heart surgery* is performed to create a nearly normal circulation.

Transsexualism

A rare disorder in which a person feels persistently uncomfortable about his or her anatomical sex, and wishes to live as a member of the opposite sex. Usually developing in early adulthood, transsexualism is much more common in men than in women. The condition may be associated with a disturbed child-parent relationship and may follow a period of cross-dressing (see *Transvestism*).

Features associated with transsexualism include *personality disorder, alcohol dependence, drug dependence, anxiety, depression*, and work problems. In many transsexuals, sexual drive is quite low. Some transsexuals are actively homosexual.

Transsexualism should be distinguished from the delusion (false belief not responding to reasoned argument) of belonging to the other sex, which sometimes occurs in *schizophrenia*, and from physical *intersex* (in which there are congenital abnormalities of the sexual structures).

Transsexuals commonly seek hormonal or surgical treatment to bring about a physical *sex change*. A careful psychiatric evaluation and physical examination are necessary before such treatment is undertaken.

Transvestism

A persistent desire by a man to dress in women's clothing, also called cross-dressing. Transvestism commonly starts in childhood with secret masturbation while dressed in the underwear of a female relative. Transvestism should be differentiated from female impersonation, which does not involve the component of sexual arousal.

Transvestism ranges from the occasional wearing of female underclothes to constant, public dressing in women's clothes and extensive involvement in transvestite subculture. For some individuals, cross-dressing serves to relieve anxiety; for others it provides sexual excitement. Occasionally, transvestism develops into *transsexualism*.

Transvestites rarely seek medical or psychiatric treatment. Most transvestites are heterosexual and have a sexual relationship with a female partner who knows and can accept the cross-dressing as a special need. A crisis may occur, however, if transvestism is accidentally revealed to a partner or family member. Psychiatric intervention in such cases consists of helping the partner and family to understand

T

that transvestites are not dangerous and that their behaviour does not break the law.

Tranylcypromine
A monoamine-oxidase inhibitor *antidepressant drug* used mainly in patients with severe depression.

Trapezius muscle
A large, diamond-shaped *muscle* that extends from the back of the skull to the lower part of the thoracic spine (the part of the spine in the chest) and, at its broadest point, across the width of the shoulders.

At the shoulders, the trapezius is attached to the top and back of the scapula (shoulderblade) and to the outermost part of the clavicle (collarbone). Along its midline, the trapezius is also attached by ligaments to the vertebrae (spinal bones).

The trapezius muscle helps support the neck and spine. It is also involved in movements of the arm. When an arm is raised, the trapezius on that side contracts, thereby causing the scapula to rotate.

Trapped nerve
See *Nerve, trapped.*

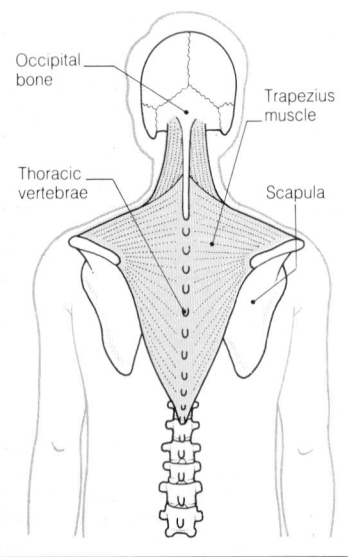

LOCATION OF THE TRAPEZIUS MUSCLE
The trapezius is a large, diamond-shaped muscle in the upper part of the back. It helps to support the neck and head, and is also involved in raising the arms.

Occipital bone

Trapezius muscle

Thoracic vertebrae

Scapula

Trauma
A physical injury or a severe emotional shock. The psychological condition that can result from physical or emotional trauma is known as *post-traumatic stress disorder.*

Trauma surgery
See *Traumatology.*

Traumatology
Emergency treatment of patients suffering from acute trauma (physical injury), commonly as a result of road traffic accidents, industrial accidents, domestic accidents, shootings, or stabbings.

In cases of life-threatening trauma, the priorities are to prevent *asphyxia* by maintaining a clear airway, to arrest *bleeding*, to treat *shock*, and to deal with major chest wounds affecting the heart or lungs. If there are abdominal injuries, an exploratory operation called a *laparotomy* or, in the case of head injuries, a *craniotomy,* may be required. Multiple injuries require coordinated treatment by different specialists.

Once the patient's condition is stable, other injuries, such as fractures and superficial cuts, are treated. (See also *Accidental death.*)

Travel immunization
Any person planning to travel outside Europe, the US, Canada, Australia, and New Zealand may need immunizations before departure. Few immunizations are now compulsory for international travel. Nevertheless, some immunizations are advisable for the traveller's own protection.

Travel agents and tour operators often include information about which immunizations may be required. Also, there is a useful leaflet on this subject obtainable from local DH offices. Travellers are recommended to consult a doctor about individual requirements. If necessary, the doctor can check the latest immunization recommendations for particular destinations.

The doctor needs information on the countries to be visited, the duration and nature of the visit, particularly whether the traveller will be going into remote areas or remaining in major cities, and the individual's previous immunization history. Most UK citizens will have received childhood immunization against certain diseases, such as diphtheria, pertussis (whooping cough), tetanus, and polio (see *Immunization*). However, for

some people who intend to travel to certain specific destinations, booster doses are advisable.

With knowledge of the individual's medical history, the doctor can decide if there are grounds for not administering a particular vaccine. Children under one year old are not usually given certain travel vaccines, notably those against yellow fever, cholera, and typhoid. In general, infants should receive their routine childhood immunizations before travelling abroad.

Having established the individual's needs, the doctor will work out an appropriate schedule of injections. Some vaccines must be given in two or three doses several weeks apart, so it is wise to consult your doctor at least two to three months before departure. People who travel a lot may find it convenient to ensure that their immunizations are kept regularly up to date.

No vaccine is available against *malaria*, a potentially fatal infection, but drugs taken by mouth will give highly effective protection.

Traveller's diarrhoea
An affliction of people visiting foreign countries. Episodes of diarrhoea range in severity from inconvenient to debilitating. Known by a variety of colourful names, such as Spanish tummy, Montezuma's revenge, Delhi belly, and the Tokyo trots, all are forms of *gastroenteritis.*

Travel sickness
See *Motion sickness.*

Trazodone
An *antidepressant drug.* Trazodone has a strong sedative effect and is particularly useful in the treatment of *depression* that is accompanied by *anxiety* or *insomnia.* Possible adverse effects include drowsiness, constipation, dry mouth, dizziness, and, rarely, *priapism* (painful, persistent erection).

Treatment
Any measure taken to prevent or cure a disease or disorder or to relieve symptoms. Examples include *drug* treatment, *radiotherapy, surgery,* bed rest and *physiotherapy.*

Trematode
The scientific name for any *fluke* or *schistosome* (flattened worm that may parasitize humans).

Trembling
See *Tremor.*

GUIDELINES FOR TRAVEL IMMUNIZATION

Immunization	Reason for immunization	Effectiveness
Yellow fever	Compulsory for entry to some countries and advisable for visits to others within yellow fever zones in Africa and South America. May also be needed when travelling from yellow fever zones to some Asian countries.	Almost 100 per cent protection for at least 10 years. Certificate provided.
Cholera	Occasionally compulsory for entry to some countries in Asia and Africa. Also advisable when travelling to many other Asian and African countries.	Gives moderate protection for six months. Other precautions against cholera needed in epidemic areas.
Typhoid fever	Recommended when travelling anywhere outside Europe, the US, Canada, Australia, and New Zealand for anyone who has not received immunization or a booster within the past three years.	Gives moderate protection for about three years, after which a booster is needed.
Tetanus	Advisable for anyone who has not received childhood immunization or a booster within the past 10 years.	Highly effective, with booster needed every 10 years.
Polio- myelitis	Advisable for anyone who has not received childhood immunization or a booster within the past 10 years.	Highly effective, with booster needed every 10 years.
Hepatitis A	Recommended for protection against viral hepatitis type A when travelling to any country where hygiene and sanitary standards are low.	Highly effective.
Measles	Advisable for anyone who has not received childhood immunization and who has not had measles.	Highly effective; gives lifelong protection.
Diphtheria	Advisable for anyone who has not received childhood immunization and who is shown by a test to be nonimmune.	Highly effective.
Hepatitis B Rabies Meningitis	Recommended only for people who are at special risk because of their occupation or the nature of their visit abroad.	All highly effective.
Smallpox	No longer necessary as the disease has been eradicated.	

Tremor

An involuntary, rhythmic, oscillating movement in the *muscles* of part of the body, most commonly the hands, feet, jaw, tongue, or head. Tremor is caused by rapidly alternating contraction and relaxation of the muscles.

Occasional temporary tremors are experienced by almost everyone, usually at times of heightened emotion, and are due to increased production of the hormone *adrenaline*.

A slight persistent tremor unrelated to any disease is common in elderly people. Another type of persistent tremor not associated with disease is known as essential tremor. This is a fine-to-moderate tremor (six to 10 movements per second) that runs in families and may be temporarily relieved by a small amount of alcohol or by taking *beta-blocker drugs*. Both these types of tremor increase when the affected part of the body is moved.

Some types of persistent tremor indicate an underlying disorder. Coarse tremor (four to five muscle movements per second) present at rest but reduced during movement is often a sign of *Parkinson's disease*. An intention tremor (tremor that is worse on movement of the affected part) may be a sign of *cerebellar ataxia*. Other disorders marked by tremor include *multiple sclerosis, Wilson's disease, mercury poisoning, thyrotoxicosis,* and hepatic *encephalopathy*.

Tremor may also be caused by drugs, among them *amphetamine drugs, antidepressant drugs, antipsychotic drugs, lithium,* and *caffeine*. Withdrawal from some drugs, including *alcohol*, may also result in tremor. The so-called morning shakes may be an indication of *alcohol dependence*.

Trench fever

An infectious disease that was common among troops in the trenches of World War I and World War II, but is now rare or unknown in most parts of the world. Like epidemic *typhus*, which it resembles, the disease is caused by *rickettsiae* (microorganisms similar to bacteria) spread by body *lice*. The symptoms include headache and muscle pains as well as fever, which may occur in bouts. Trench fever is treated with *antibiotic drugs*.

Trench foot

See *Immersion foot*.

Trench mouth

See *Gingivitis, acute ulcerative*.

Trephine

A hollow, cylindrical instrument with a saw-toothed edge used for cutting a circular hole, usually in bone. Trephines are most often used to bore holes in the skull to form a removable flap before operations on the brain.

Perforation of the skull to relieve excess pressure is a recent innovation and is part of conventional surgery. Ancient peoples used trephines on the skull (as evidenced by the skulls found by paleontologists) but the reason they did so is unknown; most likely it was done by witch doctors to encourage the release of evil spirits.

Tretinoin

A drug chemically related to *vitamin A*, which is applied to the skin to treat *acne* and certain skin disorders characterized by scaling and thickening, such as *ichthyosis*. Tretinoin is also being evaluated as a treatment for the

T

wrinkling of the skin with age, especially in people who have been exposed to strong sunlight.

Tretinoin may aggravate acne in the first few weeks of treatment but usually improves the condition within three to four months. In some people, tretinoin causes skin irritation and peeling. Excessive exposure to sunlight while using tretinoin may aggravate any irritation and lead to *sunburn*. In rare cases, tretinoin may bleach or darken the skin.

Trial, clinical

A test on human volunteers of the effectiveness and safety of a drug, or a systematic comparison of alternative forms of medical or surgical treatment for a particular disorder. Clinical trials are also used to test the usefulness of new medical or surgical appliances, dressings, or equipment.

In the development of new drugs, clinical trials follow *animal experimentation* that mainly evaluates toxic effects; clinical trials are usually undertaken at a late stage before the manufacturer proceeds to commercial production. The purpose of clinical trials is to demonstrate that the new drug is effective, safe, and superior to, or at least as good as, existing drugs. Such trials are also useful in revealing effects that may not have been suspected from results of the animal tests.

Careful precautions are necessary to ensure that the results of clinical trials are not misleading. Trials that fail to eliminate the effects of personal bias or the *placebo* effect may be of little value. For these reasons, most clinical trials are carried out in the form of randomized, *controlled trials*. Sometimes trials of this kind give conflicting results, in which case a meta-analysis of all the trials may be done, distilling a verdict from the whole body of research on the topic.

Triamcinolone

A *corticosteroid drug* used to treat inflammation of the mouth, gums, skin, and joints. Triamcinolone is also used to treat *asthma* and certain blood disorders, such as *thrombocytopenia* and *leukaemia*.

Triamterene

A potassium-sparing *diuretic drug*. Triamterene is used with thiazide or loop diuretics to treat *hypertension* (high blood pressure) and *oedema* (accumulation of fluid in tissues). Possible adverse effects include nausea, vomiting, weakness, and rash.

Tribavirin

An *antiviral drug* also known as ribavirin. It is given by inhalation to infants, especially when they have other serious diseases, for the treatment of severe *respiratory tract infections*. It is also effective in treating *lassa fever*.

Triceps muscle

The name (meaning "three heads") of the *muscle* at the back of the upper arm. At the upper end of the triceps, one of the three heads is attached to the outer edge of the scapula (shoulderblade); the other two heads are attached to either side of the upper part of the humerus (upper-arm bone). The lower part of the triceps is attached by a large *tendon* to the olecranon process of the ulna (the bony prominence at the back of the elbow). Contraction of the muscle straightens the arm. (See also *Biceps muscle*.)

Trichiasis

An alteration in the direction of growth of the eyelashes in which the lashes grow inwards towards the eyeball. The abnormally directed lashes can rub against the eye, causing severe discomfort and sometimes damage to the *cornea*. Trichiasis can result from the inflammation and scarring that occurs in *trachoma*. Severe scar-

---

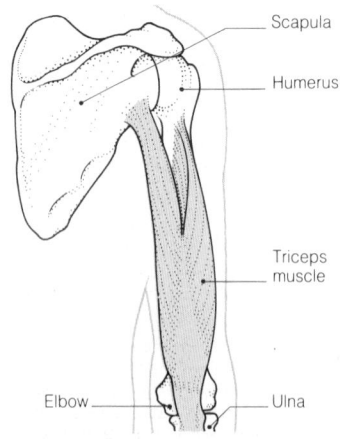

LOCATION OF THE TRICEPS MUSCLE
This muscle at the back of the upper arm functions to straighten the elbow joint, thus opposing the action of the biceps at the front of the upper arm.

Scapula

Humerus

Triceps muscle

Elbow

Ulna

---

ring may lead to *entropion* (turning in of the lid margin).

Temporary treatment involves removal of the offending lashes, but the lashes regrow and may again cause pain and damage. Permanent treatment may be by *electrolysis* to destroy the growth follicles of the eyelashes involved, or by minor surgical adjustment of the lid margin.

Trichinosis

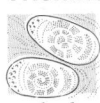 An infestation with the larvae of a tiny worm, TRICHINELLA SPIRALIS, usually acquired by eating undercooked pork, ham, or sausages.

CAUSES AND INCIDENCE
Larvae are present as cysts in the muscles of infested animals, such as pigs, dogs, and rats. Worldwide, infestation of humans is largely confined to pork-eating populations. It is rare in the UK.

If a person eats the raw or undercooked meat of an infested animal, the larvae are released from the cysts and develop into adults in the person's intestines. The adult worms discharge fresh larvae, which travel around the body in the bloodstream to various tissues and organs, including the heart and brain, and to the muscles, where they form cysts.

The principal preventive measure is thorough cooking of all pork products. Freezing to a temperature below −18°C for 24 hours also kills the larvae.

SYMPTOMS AND COMPLICATIONS
Slight infestation usually causes no symptoms; heavy infestation may cause diarrhoea and vomiting within a day or two, followed, a week or so later, by more symptoms as new larvae circulate through the body. Symptoms may include fever, swelling around the eyelids, and severe muscle pains, which may last for several weeks. In most people, the symptoms subside and gradually disappear. Very rarely, an infected person becomes seriously ill and may die.

DIAGNOSIS AND TREATMENT
Trichinosis may be suspected by a doctor from the symptoms. The diagnosis is confirmed by *blood tests*, which detect antibodies to the larvae, or by a muscle *biopsy* (removal of a sample of tissue for microscopic analysis), which shows the larvae themselves.

The disease is treated with an *anthelmintic drug* (usually *thiabendazole*) that kills adult worms in the intestines and attacks larvae in the tissues. *Corticosteroid drugs* are given to reduce inflammation. This generally leads to recovery within a few days to weeks.

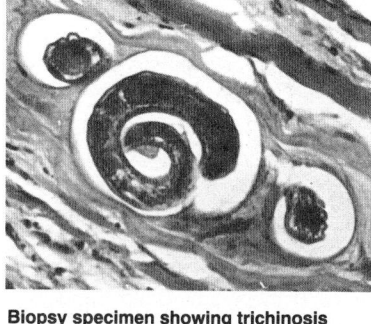

Biopsy specimen showing trichinosis
This photomicrograph of a section of a patient's muscle shows a cyst formed by a TRICHINELLA SPIRALIS larva.

Trichomoniasis

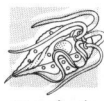

An infection caused by the protozoan (single-celled microorganism) *TRICHO-MONAS VAGINALIS*. Trichomoniasis is a common cause of *vaginitis* in women. In most cases, the infection is sexually transmitted, but it is occasionally contracted indirectly, such as from an infected towel. Trichomoniasis is less commonly reported in men, in whom the infection affects the urethra but usually does not cause symptoms. Occasionally, trichomoniasis is transmitted by a woman to her baby during the process of childbirth.

Trichomoniasis, which itself is not a serious condition, may occur in conjunction with other sexually transmitted diseases. About 20,000 cases of trichomoniasis are reported annually from sexually transmitted disease clinics in the UK.

SYMPTOMS AND SIGNS
In women, the causative organism may inhabit the vagina for years without causing symptoms. If symptoms do occur, they include painful inflammation of the vagina and vulva, and a profuse, yellow, frothy, offensive discharge. Sexual intercourse may be painful. Men usually have no symptoms but some suffer from urethral discomfort and signs of *nonspecific urethritis*.

DIAGNOSIS AND TREATMENT
The diagnosis is made from a laboratory examination of a sample of the vaginal discharge or of swabs taken from the urethra. Diagnosis is usually difficult in men.

Treatment is with *metronidazole*, which usually clears up the condition. An infected person's sexual partner or partners should be traced, examined, and treated at the same time to prevent reinfection.

Trichotillomania

The habit of constantly pulling out one's own hair. Trichotillomania can be associated with severe *mental handicap* or with a psychotic illness, such as *schizophrenia*. It may also occur in psychologically disturbed children as an outward expression of anxiety and frustration.

The sufferer typically pulls, twists, and breaks off chunks of hair from the scalp, leaving bald patches; occasionally, pubic hair is pulled out. Children sometimes eat the removed hair, which may form a hairball in the stomach, known medically as a trichobezoar (see *Bezoar*).

Treatment depends on the cause and may consist of *psychotherapy* or *antipsychotic drugs*.

Tricuspid incompetence

Failure of the tricuspid valve of the *heart* to close properly, allowing blood to leak back into the right atrium (upper chamber) during contractions of the right ventricle (lower chamber). This lowers the pumping efficiency of the heart. The condition is also known as tricuspid insufficiency.

CAUSES AND INCIDENCE
Tricuspid incompetence is usually due to an increased workload on the right side of the heart as a result of *pulmonary hypertension* (high pressure in the blood supply to the lungs). This causes the right ventricle to distend and leads to widening of the opening in which the tricuspid valve is situated.

In rare cases, tricuspid incompetence occurs in people who have had *rheumatic fever*. It may also result from bacterial infection of the heart in intravenous drug abusers. In both these

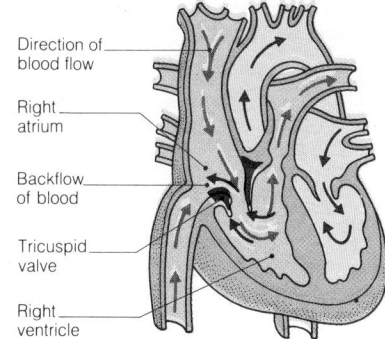

Defect in tricuspid incompetence
The tricuspid valve lies between the atrium and ventricle in the right side of the heart. Incompetence means that when the right ventricle contracts, some blood escapes back into the right atrium.

Labels on figure: Direction of blood flow · Right atrium · Backflow of blood · Tricuspid valve · Right ventricle

groups of people, tricuspid incompetence may be accompanied by other heart valve disorders.

SYMPTOMS
The tricuspid incompetence causes symptoms of right-sided *heart failure*, notably *oedema* (fluid collection and swelling) affecting the ankles and abdomen. The liver is congested with blood and is swollen and tender. Veins in the neck are distended.

DIAGNOSIS AND TREATMENT
The condition is diagnosed from the patient's symptoms, from a characteristic *murmur* heard through a stethoscope, and by tests that may include an *ECG, chest X-rays, echocardiography,* and cardiac *catheterization*.

Treatment for heart failure, with *diuretic drugs* and *ACE inhibitor drugs*, often clears up the symptoms. If symptoms persist, *heart valve surgery* may be performed to repair or replace the malfunctioning valve.

Tricuspid stenosis

Narrowing of the opening of the tricuspid valve in the *heart* between the right atrium (upper chamber) and right ventricle (lower chamber). Tricuspid stenosis is an uncommon type of heart valve disorder. When it does occur, it is usually in a person who has previously had *rheumatic fever*. Tricuspid stenosis may also occur in intravenous drug abusers as a result of bacterial infection of the heart.

Tricuspid stenosis is usually accompanied by other types of heart valve disorder, such as *mitral stenosis*.

The right atrium must work harder to pump blood through the narrowed valve, causing it to enlarge. The symptoms are very similar to those of *tricuspid incompetence*; the condition is diagnosed by the same procedures.

Drug treatment is given with *diuretic drugs* to reduce *oedema* (accumulation of fluid in tissues) and sometimes a *digitalis drug* to increase the force of the heart's contractions. If symptoms persist, *heart valve surgery* may be carried out to repair or replace the defective valve.

Trifluoperazine

An *antipsychotic drug* used principally in the treatment of *schizophrenia*.

Trigeminal nerve

The fifth *cranial nerve*. The trigeminal nerves, one of each side, arise from the pons (part of the *brainstem*). Each nerve divides into three main branches, which then subdivide into a complete network of nerves.

T

LOCATION OF THE TRIGEMINAL NERVE

The trigeminal nerve splits into three main branches. The ophthalmic nerve supplies most of the scalp, the upper eyelid, tear gland, and cornea; the maxillary nerve supplies the upper jaw; and the mandibular nerve supplies the tongue, lower jaw, and jaw muscles.

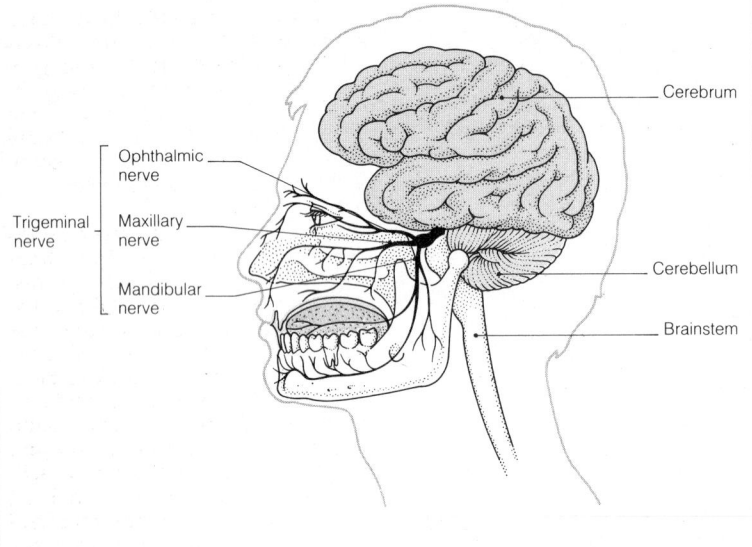

Trigeminal nerve
- Ophthalmic nerve
- Maxillary nerve
- Mandibular nerve

Cerebrum

Cerebellum

Brainstem

The trigeminal nerves and their branches supply sensation to the face, scalp, nose, teeth, lining of the mouth, upper eyelid, sinuses, and front two thirds of the tongue. They also stimulate contraction of the jaw muscles responsible for chewing, and control the production of saliva by the salivary glands and of tears by the lacrimal glands.

Damage to, or disease in, one area supplied by a branch of the trigeminal nerve may cause *referred pain* in another area supplied by a different branch of the nerve. For example, sinusitis (infection of the sinuses) may cause toothache.

Trigeminal neuralgia

A disorder of the trigeminal nerve (fifth *cranial nerve*) in which episodes of severe, stabbing pain affect the cheek, lips, gums, or chin on one side of the face. The pain is very brief (lasting only a few seconds to minutes) but is often so intense that the sufferer is unable to do anything for the duration of the attack. The pain often causes wincing and for this reason is commonly called tic douloureux (literally, "painful twitch").

Trigeminal neuralgia is unusual under the age of 50. When the condition occurs in younger people, it may be associated with *multiple sclerosis*.

Attacks occur in bouts that may last for weeks at a time. Pain-free intervals between attacks tend to become shorter with time.

The cause of trigeminal neuralgia is uncertain. The pain nearly always starts from one trigger point on the face and can be brought on by touching the face, washing, shaving, eating, drinking, or even talking.

Treatment is difficult. *Carbamazepine* suppresses the pain in most sufferers, but a few people develop resistance to the drug or are unable to tolerate a high enough dosage to relieve the pain. If drug treatment fails, several surgical options are available.

Trigger finger

Locking of one or several fingers in a bent position. Forcible straightening of an affected finger usually causes an audible click.

Trigger finger is caused by inflammation of the fibrous sheath that encloses the *tendon* of the affected finger and is accompanied by localized swelling of the tendon. When the finger is bent, the enlarged tendon is forced out of the narrowed mouth of the sheath and is then unable to re-enter it. There is usually tenderness at the base of the affected finger. In addition, a small swelling may be felt over the tendon.

Treatment of trigger finger involves either the injection of a *corticosteroid drug* into the sheath to reduce inflammation, or a surgical procedure to widen the opening of the sheath.

Trimeprazine

An *antihistamine drug* used mainly to relieve itching in allergic conditions, such as *urticaria* (nettle rash) and atopic *eczema*. Because trimeprazine has a sedative effect, it is useful in the relief of itching that interferes with sleep. Trimeprazine is also used as a *premedication* to sedate children before surgery.

The adverse effects of trimeprazine are typical of other antihistamines, although trimeprazine is more likely to cause drowsiness.

Trimethoprim

An *antibacterial drug* prescribed for a wide variety of infections. Trimethoprim is used on its own to treat *urinary tract infection*, *prostatitis*, and *bronchitis*. The drug *co-trimoxazole* is a combination of trimethoprim and another antibacterial drug, *sulphamethoxazole*.

Possible adverse effects of trimethoprim include rash, itching, nausea, vomiting, diarrhoea, and sore tongue.

Trimipramine

A tricyclic *antidepressant drug*. Trimipramine has a strong sedative effect and is used to treat *depression* accompanied by *anxiety* or *insomnia*.

Possible adverse effects include dry mouth, blurred vision, dizziness, constipation, and nausea.

Triple vaccine

See *DPT vaccination*.

Triprolidine

An *antihistamine drug* used to treat allergies, such as allergic *rhinitis* (hay fever) and *urticaria* (nettle rash). Tri-

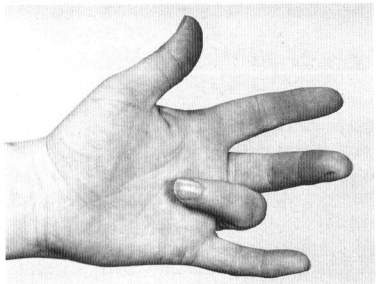

Appearance of trigger finger
The disorder is caused by inflammation of the sheath of one of the tendons involved in controlling the finger's movements.

prolidine is also a common ingredient of *cough remedies* and *cold remedies*. It is occasionally given to treat or prevent allergic reactions to *blood transfusions* or certain foods.

Possible adverse effects include dry mouth, dizziness, difficulty in passing urine, and, in children, *hyperactivity*.

Trismus

Involuntary contraction of the *jaw* muscles, resulting in the mouth's becoming tightly closed, a condition commonly known as lockjaw.

Trismus may occur as a symptom of *tetanus, tonsillitis, mumps,* acute ulcerative *gingivitis,* an abscess around a back tooth (see *Abscess, dental*), nasopharyngeal cancer (see *Nasopharynx, cancer of*), or *Parkinson's disease.* Occasionally, trismus is psychological in origin; for example, it sometimes occurs in *anorexia nervosa.*

Treatment of trismus is of the underlying cause.

Trisomy

The presence, within a person's cells, of an extra chromosome so that there are three *chromosomes* of a particular number, instead of the usual two. The result can range from the death and miscarriage of an affected embryo to a range of physical abnormalities in a live-born child.

CAUSES AND INCIDENCE
A trisomy may result from a fault by which an extra chromosome gets into an egg or sperm cell during the cell's formation. If an affected egg or sperm takes part in fertilization, the resulting embryo also has an extra chromosome, causing trisomy. Most types of trisomy are more common with advanced maternal age.

By far the most common trisomy in live-born infants is trisomy 21, also called *Down's syndrome* (formerly called mongolism), in which there are three number 21 chromosomes. Much less common are trisomy 18 (Edwards' syndrome) and trisomy 13 (Patau's syndrome). Trisomy 8 and trisomy 22 are extremely rare. Partial trisomies, in which only part of a chromosome is in triplicate, have also been found.

SYMPTOMS
All full trisomies cause multiple abnormalities, such as skeletal and heart defects, facial anomalies, and mental deficiency. Babies with full trisomies other than Down's syndrome usually die early in infancy. The effect of a partial trisomy is variable, depending on how much extra chromosomal material is present.

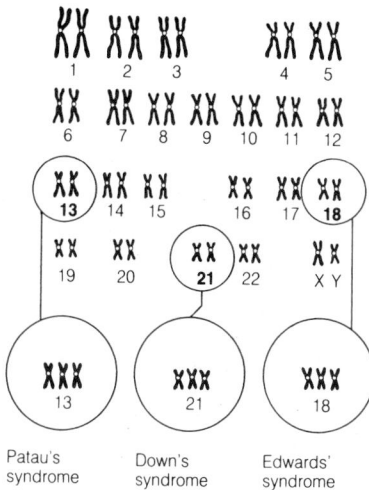

Patau's syndrome   Down's syndrome   Edwards' syndrome

Types of trisomy
In all trisomies a child has three, instead of the usual two, chromosomes of a particular number. Down's syndrome is by far the most common trisomy.

DIAGNOSIS AND TREATMENT
Trisomies are diagnosed by *chromosome analysis* of cells. There is no specific treatment for these disorders. Parents of an affected baby should obtain *genetic counselling* to assess the risk of a future child being affected. Antenatal diagnosis, particularly by means of *amniocentesis* and chromosome analysis of the cells obtained, can be performed if a pregnancy is considered to be at risk.

Trisomy 21 syndrome

A set of abnormalities caused when a child has three, instead of the usual two, number 21 chromosomes in each of his or her cells. It is better known as *Down's syndrome.*

Trochlear nerve

The fourth *cranial nerve.* The trochlear nerves, one on each side, arise from the midbrain (part of the *brainstem*) and pass through the skull to enter the eye sockets through gaps in the skull bones. Each trochlear nerves supplies only one eye muscle: the superior oblique muscle. Contraction of this muscle rotates the eye downwards and outwards.

Damage to the trochlear nerve (as a result of a skull fracture, for example) may lead to *double vision.*

Trophoblastic tumour

A growth arising from the tissues that develop into the placenta. The most common type of trophoblastic tumour

is a benign growth called a *hydatidiform mole.* A malignant trophoblastic tumour that spreads outside the uterus is called a *choriocarcinoma.*

Tropical diseases

Many diseases are virtually confined to tropical areas. In most cases, this is not due primarily to tropical geographical factors (such as temperature, humidity, or disease-carrying insects), but to the fact that large populations in many tropical countries live in poverty and squalor.

DISEASES OF POVERTY
Malnutrition is one of the major causes of illness in the tropics. Apart from causing nutritional deficiency disorders, a poor diet weakens the body's ability to fight infectious diseases such as *measles* and *diphtheria.* Overcrowded living conditions are a cause of such diseases as *tuberculosis.*

Low standards of public health administration, food inspection and handling, and a lack of sanitary facilities, which encourage water and soil contamination with human excrement, are the cause of a vast number of diseases, including *typhoid fever, shigellosis, cholera, amoebiasis,* and *tapeworm infestation.* Most of these

LOCATION OF THE TROCHLEAR NERVE
This nerve emerges from the brain and supplies a muscle that rotates the eye down and outwards.

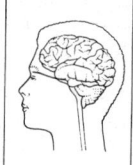

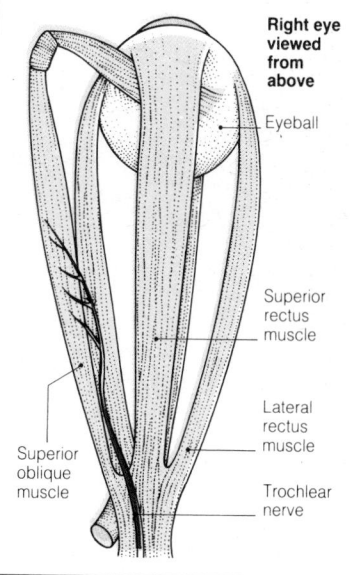

Right eye viewed from above

Eyeball

Superior rectus muscle

Lateral rectus muscle

Trochlear nerve

Superior oblique muscle

T

diseases were common in temperate zones before improvements in public health and sanitation. Only some diseases, such as *hookworm infestation* and *schistosomiasis*, appear to be related to temperature or soil conditions found only in the tropics in addition to the lack of community sanitation and walking barefoot.

DISEASES SPREAD BY INSECTS

Some tropical diseases depend on the coincidence of a parasite and a specific insect *vector* (agent responsible for spread) such as a mosquito. These diseases include *malaria, yellow fever, sleeping sickness,* and *leishmaniasis.* It is worth noting, however, that at least some of the relevant insect vectors can survive in temperate zones; malaria was once common in parts of southern England.

LIGHT AND HEAT

Certain conditions arise as a result of exposure to tropical sunlight. The most common is skin damage from *ultraviolet light,* leading to wrinkling, loss of elasticity, and an increased tendency to *skin cancer,* especially in white people with fair colouring. Ultraviolet light also damages the outer tissues of the eye (the conjunctiva and the cornea) and may lead to the development of *pinguecula* and *pterygium.* Undue exertion in the tropics, with inadequate water intake and salt replacement, may lead to *heat exhaustion*; prolonged exposure to high temperatures may lead to *heatstroke.*

Tropical ulcer

An area of persistent skin and tissue loss caused by infection, a condition that occurs mainly in tropical regions. The ulcers are most common in people who are malnourished.

The classic form of tropical ulcer results from contamination of a cut or abrasion (usually on a foot or leg) by a mixture of various types of bacteria. Infections spread beneath the skin, and the affected tissue dies and is shed, leaving the ulcer in place.

Treatment consists of thorough cleaning of the ulcer, which is then dressed; the patient also needs *antibiotic drugs* and a nourishing, protein-rich diet. With this treatment, the ulcer usually heals, although it may leave some scarring and deformity.

Similar types of ulcer can occur as a result of more specific infections, such as *diphtheria* of the skin, cutaneous *leishmaniasis,* and *yaws.* Treatment is as described above, except that drug therapy may vary according to the causative organisms.

To avoid tropical ulcers, it is particularly important to wash any cuts, sores, or abrasions thoroughly and cover them with a sterile dressing.

Tropicamide

A drug used to dilate the *pupil* before an eye examination and, occasionally, before eye surgery. Rare adverse effects include blurred vision, increased sensitivity to light, stinging, dry mouth, flushing, and *glaucoma* (increased pressure in the eye).

Trunk

The central part of the body, comprising the thorax (chest) and abdomen, to which the head and limbs are attached. The term trunk also refers to any large blood vessel or nerve from which smaller vessels or nerves branch off.

Truss

An elastic, canvas, or padded metal appliance used to hold an abdominal *hernia* (protrusion of part of the intestine through a weakened area in the abdominal wall) in place. The hernia is pushed back through the abdominal wall before the truss is put on, usually while the person lies down. A truss may be used to treat a hernia that is causing discomfort or is unsightly in people who are waiting for an operation to repair the hernia or who are unfit for surgery.

Trypanosomiasis

A tropical disease caused by protozoan (single-celled) parasites known as trypanosomes. In Africa, trypanosomes spread by tsetse flies are the cause of *sleeping sickness.* In South America, other trypanosomes, spread by beetle-like insects, are the cause of *Chagas' disease.*

Tsetse fly bites

 Tsetse flies are found in Africa, where they spread the parasitic disease *sleeping sickness.* They are brown, about the size of houseflies, and have a projecting proboscis (feeding apparatus). The bites of tsetse flies can be painful. Measures to minimize the risk of bites include use of insecticide sprays and protective clothing impregnated with insect repellent.

T-tube cholangiography

An *imaging technique,* also called operative or post-operative choledochography, performed to check that there are no residual *gallstones* in the common bile duct after *cholecystectomy* (surgical removal of the *gallbladder*).

The T-shaped rubber tube used in this type of cholangiography is inserted when the gallbladder is removed. The short arms of the T are inserted into the common bile duct, and the main body of the tube is brought out through a small incision in the abdomen.

T-tube cholangiography is carried out eight to 10 days after surgery on the gallbladder. Contrast medium is injected into the T-tube and *X-rays* are taken. If no residual gallstones are found, the T-tube is removed. Otherwise, the tube is left until a decision is made concerning treatment to remove the gallstones.

Tubal ligation

See *Sterilization, female.*

Tubal pregnancy

See *Ectopic pregnancy.*

Tubercle

Any of several small, nodular masses apparent in tissues that have been infected by the bacterium that causes *tuberculosis.* Such tubercules are grey and semi-transparent.

The term tubercle (or tuberculum or tuberosity) also refers to any small, rounded protrusion on the surface of a bone. For example, the tibial tubercle is a bump at the top of the *tibia* (main bone of the lower leg), immediately below the knee.

Tuberculin tests

Skin tests used to determine whether or not a person has been previously infected with *tuberculosis.* Tuberculin tests are performed in the diagnosis of suspected tuberculosis and are also carried out before *BCG vaccination.*

HOW THEY ARE DONE

The skin of the forearm is first cleaned with alcohol. A small dose of tuberculin (a purified protein extracted from the bacteria that cause tuberculosis) is then introduced into the skin by one of various techniques. In the Mantoux test, tuberculin is injected into the skin with a needle. In the Heaf test, a drop of tuberculin is put on the forearm and a spring-loaded device with a circle of sharp prongs is used to force the tuberculin through multiple tiny punctures in the skin. The tests are nearly painless.

RESULTS

The forearm is examined after a few days and the skin reaction at the test site noted. If there is no change in the

T

skin, the reaction is said to be negative. This indicates that the person has never been exposed to and has no immunity against tuberculosis. If the test area of skin becomes red, hard, and raised, the reaction is positive. A positive reaction indicates previous exposure to tuberculosis, either through BCG vaccination or through actual infection.

Tuberculosis

An infectious disease, commonly called TB, caused in humans by the bacterium MYCOBACTERIUM TUBERCULOSIS. Tuberculosis was once common worldwide and was a major killer in childhood and early adult life. In Europe in the mid-19th century, it was responsible for about a quarter of all deaths. Its incidence fell until the 1980s, but people infected with HIV are highly susceptible to tuberculosis and the disease is becoming more common again in communities with high rates of HIV infection. In parts of Africa, as many as half of all new cases of tuberculosis are in people who are HIV positive.

CAUSES
Infection is passed from person to person in airborne droplets (which are produced by coughing or sneezing). The bacteria breathed into the *lungs* then multiply to form an infected "focus". In a high proportion of cases, the body's *immune system* then halts the infection and healing occurs, leaving a scar.

In about five per cent of cases, however, the primary infection does not resolve. Spread occurs via the vessels of the *lymphatic system* to the lymph nodes. Sometimes at this stage bacteria enter the bloodstream and spread to other parts of the body; this is called miliary tuberculosis and may occasionally be fatal. In some people, the bacteria go into a dormant state in the lungs and other organs, only to become reactivated many years later. Progressive damage may then occur, such as the formation of cavities in the lungs.

In some cases, the primary infection is not in the lungs but in the lymph nodes (particularly of the neck), intestines, bones, kidneys, or other organs.

INCIDENCE
Worldwide, there are 30 million people with active tuberculosis; about three million die from the disease annually. Tuberculosis is most prevalent where resistance has been lowered by disease or malnutrition.

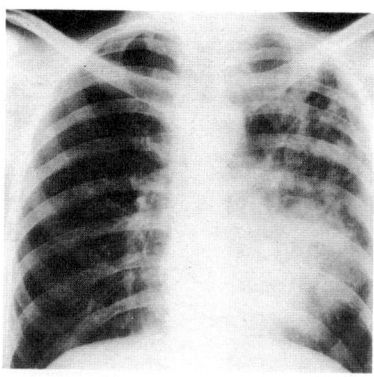

Chest X-ray showing tuberculosis
The right lung appears normal, but the left lung shows dense opacities (white areas) adjoining the heart shadow.

The incidence of tuberculosis in England and Wales was about 6,000 new cases annually in the late 1980s. The disease is more common in deprived city areas, in the elderly, in close contacts of a person suffering from tuberculosis, and in people suffering from *immunodeficiency disorders*, *diabetes mellitus*, or *alcohol dependence*. Tuberculosis is about 25 times more common in immigrants from the Indian subcontinent, who produce more than one third of all new cases in England and Wales.

PREVENTION
In the UK, an important preventive measure against tuberculosis is the use of *BCG vaccination* in high-risk groups and in children at about the age of 13. Another preventive measure is *contact tracing* so that relatives and close friends of a tuberculosis victim can be examined, X-rayed, and given a *tuberculin test*. Contact tracing thus makes it possible to detect tuberculosis at an early stage and reduce the risk of spreading the infection to other people.

SYMPTOMS AND COMPLICATIONS
Because tuberculosis usually affects the lungs, the main symptoms include coughing (sometimes bringing up blood), chest pain, shortness of breath, fever and sweating (especially at night), poor appetite, and weight loss. The main complications of tuberculosis of the lungs are *pleural effusion* (collection of fluid between the lung and the chest wall), *pneumothorax* (air between the lung and the chest wall), and, in some cases, progression of the disease to death.

DIAGNOSIS
The diagnosis is made from the patient's symptoms and signs, and

from a *chest X-ray* and tests on the sputum (phlegm) and skin. The chest X-ray is almost always abnormal. The upper parts of the lung are most commonly affected and may show cavities. Old healed areas of tuberculosis often remain as persistent shadows.

The sputum is examined for tuberculosis organisms. Attempts are also made to grow the bacteria from the sputum or other body fluids, although this procedure can take as long as six weeks. A tuberculin test may be carried out. A positive test result indicates that the person has either been immunized against tuberculosis or has been infected. Occasionally, *bronchoscopy* or the removal and examination of a piece of tissue (e.g. from a lymph node) may be necessary to make a firm diagnosis.

TREATMENT AND OUTLOOK
Modern drugs are very effective against tuberculosis, but in many parts of the world the bacteria are becoming resistant to some of these drugs and treatment needs to be monitored carefully. Ideally, at least three drugs should be given at the same time to reduce the risk of resistance. In the UK, a common treatment is three or four drugs daily for two months, followed by two drugs (usually *isoniazid* and *rifampicin*) for a further four to seven months. An adverse drug reaction (usually a rash or fever) develops in about five per cent of patients, who then require a modification of treatment. Blood tests are often performed to ensure that the drugs are not causing toxic effects on the liver.

Provided the full course of treatment is taken, the majority of patients are fully restored to health and suffer no recurrences.

Tuberosity

A prominent area on a *bone* to which *tendons* are attached. For example, the gluteal tuberosity is a ridge on the upper back part of the shaft of the femur (thigh-bone) to which tendons of part of the gluteus maximus muscle are attached. Other bones with tuberosities include the ischium (one of the three fused bones that form the pelvis), the humerus (upper-arm bone), and the radius and the ulna (lower-arm bones).

Tuberous sclerosis

An inherited disorder affecting the skin and *nervous system*. The most typical skin feature of tuberous sclerosis is adenoma sebaceum (an acne-like condition of the face) but a variety of

T

other skin conditions may also occur. Affected people characteristically suffer from *epilepsy* and *mental handicap*, although intelligence may be normal in mild cases. Other associated problems include the development of noncancerous tumours, especially of the brain, kidney, retina, and heart.

There is no cure for tuberous sclerosis. Treatment, including *anticonvulsant drugs* and the removal of tumours, is aimed at relieving troublesome symptoms. Seriously affected people may not live beyond the age of 30. *Genetic counselling* is recommended for affected families who are considering having children. In some cases, the gene for tuberous sclerosis can be detected in the fetus at an early stage in the pregnancy, allowing for the possible termination of pregnancy.

Tuboplasty

An operation in which a damaged fallopian tube is repaired to treat *infertility*. Tuboplasty is performed if a tube has become scarred and blocked, usually following *salpingitis* (infection of the fallopian tubes) or *pelvic inflammatory disease*. The procedure is sometimes performed using *microsurgery* techniques.

The fertility rate following tuboplasty varies from less than five to about 50 per cent, depending on the severity of the problem and on whether there are other reasons for the infertility. *Ectopic pregnancy* is more common in women who have had diseased tubes or tuboplasty than in those with healthy fallopian tubes.

Tularaemia

An infectious disease of wild animals, such as rabbits and squirrels, that is occasionally transmitted to humans. Tularaemia does not occur in the UK, but some cases are reported in other parts of Europe and in the US.

CAUSES AND INCIDENCE

Humans may be infected through direct contact with an infected animal or its carcass, in which cases the causative bacteria enter the body via a cut or abrasion in the skin. Tularaemia can also be acquired through a bite from an infected tick, flea, fly, or louse or, in rare cases, by eating infected meat.

Tularaemia is diagnosed by a blood test that detects *antibodies* formed against the bacteria. Treatment is with *antibiotic drugs*. Without treatment, tularaemia is fatal in about five per cent of cases; with treatment, the fatality rate is less than one per cent.

Tumbu fly bites

A cause of *myiasis* (skin infestation with fly larvae) in Africa.

Tumour

By strict definition, any swelling. In its more usual meaning, tumour is synonymous with neoplasm and refers to an abnormal mass of tissue that forms when cells in a specific area reproduce at an increased rate. Tumours may be *malignant* (cancerous) or *benign* (noncancerous).

Malignant tumours invade surrounding tissues and may also spread via the bloodstream or lymphatic system to form a secondary growth (called a *metastasis*) elsewhere in the body. *Cancer* is the general term used to refer to all types of malignant tumours. A malignant tumour that arises from epithelial tissues (such as skin) is termed a *carcinoma*; one that arises from connective tissue (such as muscle, bone, or fibrous tissue) is called a *sarcoma*.

Benign tumours usually grow slowly and do not metastasize, although they may sometimes be multiple. They tend to remain confined within a fibrous capsule, making surgical removal relatively straightforward. However, benign tumours may grow large enough to cause damage by pressing on nearby structures, which can be particularly dangerous in confined spaces, such as when they form inside the skull.

At the microscopic level, one essential difference between benign and malignant tumours is that benign tumours retain many of the features of the tissue from which they arise. In contrast, malignant tumours tend to comprise small, rapidly growing cells that form masses of tissue with fewer recognizable features of the tissue from which they originate.

Tumour-specific antigen

A substance secreted by a specific type of *tumour* (or class of tumours) that is detectable in the blood. Tumour-specific antigens, also known as tumour-associated antigens, do not provide conclusive results when screening for malignant tumours because most of the substances can also be produced in nonmalignant conditions. Repeated measurements of the levels of tumour-specific antigens are, however, helpful in monitoring a patient's response to therapy.

Examples of tumour-specific antigens include carcinoembryonic antigen and *alpha-fetoprotein*, which are both produced by immature fetal tissue and known as onco-fetal antigens. Carcinoembryonic antigen is produced in abnormal amounts by about half of all tumours of the colon, stomach, breast, lungs, and pancreas. Alpha-fetoprotein levels in blood serum are raised in 70 per cent of cases of hepatoma (a primary *liver cancer*) and in most cases of *teratoma* of the testis (see *Testis, cancer of*).

Tunnel vision

Constriction of the *visual field* so that only objects straight ahead can be clearly seen.

CAUSES

The most common cause of tunnel vision is chronic simple *glaucoma*, in which raised pressure within the eye results in the destruction of *optic nerve* fibres. As a result of this destruction, peripheral vision is gradually lost until the visual field is reduced to only a few degrees across.

Tunnel vision may also be caused by a tumour or other brain disorder that interferes with the fibres that connect the *optic nerve* to the brain. *Pituitary tumours*, for example, can press on the point where the optic nerves come together, causing loss of the right half of the right eye's visual field and the left half of the left eye's visual field. *Retinitis pigmentosa* (retinal degeneration) may cause the loss of peripheral vision and lead to the development of tunnel vision.

Turner's syndrome

A disorder caused by a *chromosomal abnormality*.

INCIDENCE AND CAUSES

Approximately one in 3,000 live-born girls is born with Turner's syndrome. The chromosomal abnormality may arise in one of three ways. Most affected females have only 45 chromosomes compared with the normal complement of 46, the missing chromosome being one of the X chromosomes. Sometimes, however, both X chromosomes are present but one is defective. Occasionally, the condition arises as a type of *mosaicism*, in which some cells are missing one X chromosome, some have extra chromosomes, and others have their normal number of chromosomes.

SIGNS

The main features of the syndrome are shortness of stature, webbing of the skin of the neck, absence or very retarded development of secondary sexual characteristics (see *Sexual characteristics, secondary*), amenorrhoea (absence of menstruation), *coarctation of the aorta*, abnormalities of the eyes and bones, and a degree of *mental handicap*. Without treatment, the average adult height is 1.35 metres.

TREATMENT

Coarctation of the aorta is treated by surgery at an early age. Menstruation may be induced by *oestrogen drugs* but sufferers continue to be infertile. To increase the girl's final height, growth hormone may be given.

Twins

Two offspring resulting from one pregnancy. Twins may develop from a single ovum (egg) or from two ova.

Monozygotic or monovular (identical) twins develop when a single, fertilized ovum divides completely and equally at an early stage of development; if this division is incomplete it results in *Siamese twins* (also known as conjoined twins). Monozygotic twins share the same placenta. Although one is often much bigger than the other at birth, they are always of the same sex and look remarkably alike.

Twins from two ova are called dizygotic or binovular twins. The ova from which they develop may be released by the same or different ovaries; fertilization of the two ova occurs simultaneously. Each dizygotic twin has its own placenta. The twins may be of the same or of different sexes, and may look quite different.

Twins occur in about one in 80 pregnancies. Dizygotic twins are more likely to occur in older women, in women who have had many previous pregnancies, and in women who have a history of twins in the family; they are also more common in Africa and Asia. These factors do not have any bearing on the incidence of monozygotic twins.

Twins face greater difficulties from the start. Deaths are more frequent before, during, or just after birth. When rearing twins, especially monozygotic twins, it is important to emphasize that they are two individuals not half of a pair. (See also *Pregnancy, multiple.*)

Twins, conjoined

Another name for *Siamese twins*.

Twitch

See *Fasciculation*; *Tic*.

Tylectomy

A term sometimes used for lumpectomy (removal of a lump), especially in *breast cancer*. (See *Mastectomy*.)

TWO TYPES OF TWINS

During each menstrual cycle, either one ovum or a small number of ova may be released. If one ovum is fertilized and the two cells formed from its first division develop independently, the result is identical twins. If two ova are fertilized and mature normally, nonidentical twins result.

IDENTICAL TWINS

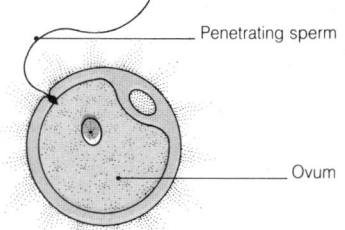

Identical twins come from a single fertilized ovum. When the ovum splits, the two cells formed develop independently.

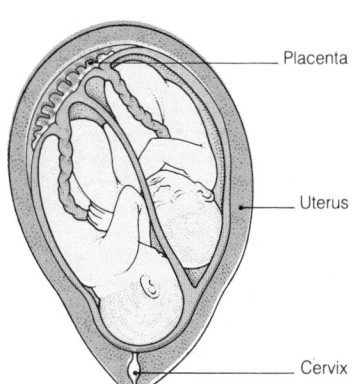

The result is a pair of genetically identical twins sharing the same placenta. They are monozygotic, or monovular, twins.

NONIDENTICAL TWINS

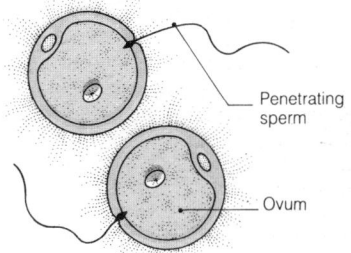

Nonidentical twins come from two separate ova that have been fertilized by two separate sperm.

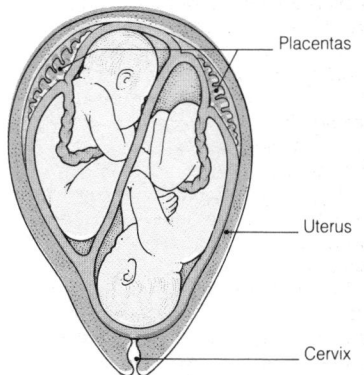

The resulting individuals are genetically distinct and have separate placentas. They are dizygotic, or binovular, twins.

Tympanometry

A type of *hearing test*.

Tympanoplasty

An operation on the ear to treat conductive *deafness* by repairing a hole in the eardrum (see *Myringoplasty*) or by repositioning or reconstructing diseased ossicles.

WHY IT IS DONE

In a healthy ear, sound waves are conducted from the eardrum to the oval window of the inner ear by a chain of three bones called ossicles. Chronic *otitis media* (middle-ear infection) can fuse these bones in position or erode them, interfering with sound conduction. In such cases, tympanoplasty offers the only chance of restoring some of the lost hearing.

HOW IT IS DONE

Under general anaesthesia, an incision is made to provide access to the middle ear. Viewing the ear through an operating microscope, the surgeon then repositions or repairs the chain of ossicles. This may involve reshaping and transposing one of the bones, replacing an ossicle with a plastic substitute, grafting an ossicle taken from a donor, or fashioning an ossicle from cartilage. The bones are then reset in position and the eardrum repaired.

RESULTS

Tympanoplasty results in a considerable improvement in hearing in the majority of patients, but a successful outcome of the operation cannot be guaranteed in some instances. (See also *Stapedectomy*.)

T

Tympanum
Part of the *ear*, comprising the middle-ear cavity (tympanic cavity) and eardrum (tympanic membrane).

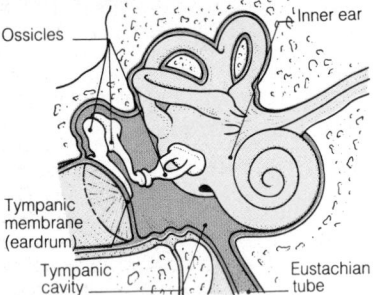

Anatomy of the tympanum
The tympanic cavity contains three movable bones (malleus, incus, and stapes), which transmit sound from the tympanic membrane (eardrum) to the inner ear.

Typhoid fever
An infectious disease contracted by eating food or drinking water contaminated with the bacterium *SAL-MONELLA TYPHI*. An almost identical disease, *paratyphoid fever*, is caused by related bacteria.

CAUSES AND INCIDENCE
The infection is contracted from the faeces of a person who has the disease or who is a symptomless carrier of the causative bacteria. In areas of poor sanitation, typhoid is commonly spread by the contamination of drinking water with sewage, or by flies carrying the bacteria from infected faeces to food. Elsewhere, infection is usually due to the handling of food by typhoid carriers. Shellfish that have been contaminated by sewage are an occasional source of typhoid.

During the development of the disease, the bacteria pass from the intestines into the blood, and then to the spleen and liver, where they multiply. The organisms are excreted from the liver, accumulate in the gallbladder, and are released in enormous numbers into the intestine. Carriers, after recovering from typhoid fever, may continue to harbour typhoid bacteria in the gallbladder and shed them in the faeces for many years.

Typhoid is uncommon in developed countries but epidemics occur regularly in developing countries. There are usually fewer than 200 cases a year in England and Wales, most of which are acquired abroad.

PREVENTION
Typhoid is a *notifiable disease*, and people with the disease should be medically isolated.

Immunization against typhoid is generally advisable before travelling anywhere outside northern Europe, North America, Australia, and New Zealand. The vaccine is given in two doses, followed every three years by a booster dose. Typhoid immunization often causes swelling and pain at the site of injection, lasting for one to two days.

The vaccine does not provide complete protection; travellers at risk should drink only boiled water or bottled drinks and take care over what they eat (see *Food-borne infection*).

SYMPTOMS AND SIGNS
Typhoid has an incubation period of seven to 14 days. The course of the infection varies from a mild upset to a major life-threatening illness. The first symptom is usually severe headache, followed by fever, loss of appetite, malaise, abdominal tenderness, constipation, and often delirium. Constipation soon gives way to diarrhoea. During the second week of the illness, small, raised pink spots can be seen on the chest and abdomen for several days, and there is enlargement of the liver and spleen.

The illness usually clears up within four weeks. However, if treatment is delayed, severe, and sometimes fatal, complications may develop. Possible gastrointestinal complications include intestinal bleeding, and *perforation* of the intestine leading to *peritonitis*. Among other possible complications are *urinary tract infection* and *kidney failure*.

DIAGNOSIS AND TREATMENT
The diagnosis is confirmed by obtaining a *culture* of typhoid bacteria from a sample of blood, faeces, or urine, or by a *blood test* that reveals the presence of *antibodies* against typhoid bacteria.

Either *chloramphenicol* or *amoxycillin* usually brings the disease under control within a few days and prevents complications; severely ill patients may require supplementary treatment with *corticosteroid drugs*. An operation may be needed if widespread peritonitis or severe bleeding develops.

Given early diagnosis and proper treatment, the outlook is usually excellent, although relapses are common within a few weeks of treatment.

Typhus
 Any of a group of infectious diseases, with similar symptoms, caused by *rickettsiae* (microorganisms similar to bacteria) and spread by insects or similar animals.

TYPES
Of the various types of typhus, epidemic typhus is historically the most important. This disease formerly occurred in epidemics that killed hundreds of thousands of people in times of war, famine, or other natural disasters. Today, epidemic typhus is rare except in some highland areas of tropical Africa and South America. Epidemic typhus is spread between humans by body lice, which ingest the causative organism, *RICKETTSIA PRO-WAZEKI*, from the blood of infected people, and deposit infected faeces on to the skin of other people. The rickettsiae are introduced into the bloodstream by scratching.

Endemic typhus, also called murine typhus, is a disease of rats that is occasionally spread to humans by fleas; sporadic cases occur in North and Central America. Scrub typhus is spread by mites and occurs in India and Southeast Asia.

PREVENTION
Epidemic typhus can be prevented through control of human louse infestation with insecticides. A vaccine also exists against the disease. Preventive measures are especially important in crowded conditions following natural disasters.

Other types of typhus can be prevented by taking measures, such as the use of protective clothing, to discourage bites by fleas, mites, or ticks.

SYMPTOMS AND SIGNS
In epidemic typhus, severe headache, back and limb pain, coughing, and constipation develop suddenly and are followed by high fever, confusion, a rash similar to that of measles, prostration, a weak heartbeat, and, in many cases, delirium. Without treatment, death may occur from *septicaemia, heart failure, kidney failure*, or *pneumonia*.

Other types of typhus have similar symptoms and signs, and similar complications.

DIAGNOSIS AND TREATMENT
Particular types of typhus fever are diagnosed by tests that can detect blood products formed in reaction to the rickettsial organisms. Typhus fevers are treated with *antibiotic drugs*. Other measures may be required to relieve severe symptoms and to treat complications. Convalescence is often slow, particularly in the elderly.

Typing
A general term for procedures by which blood or tissues are classified. (See *Blood groups*; *Tissue-typing*.)

T

U

Ulcer

An open sore on the *skin* or on a *mucous membrane* that results from the destruction of surface tissue. Ulcers may be shallow, or deep and crater-shaped, and are usually inflamed and painful.

Skin ulcers most commonly occur on the leg (see *Leg ulcer*), usually as the result of inadequate blood supply to, or drainage from, the limb. Among the rarer forms of skin ulcers are *basal cell carcinomas*, which are a form of skin cancer.

Ulcers on mucous membranes most commonly develop within the digestive tract, occurring in the mouth (see *Mouth ulcer*), the stomach or the duodenum (see *Peptic ulcer*), or in any part of the small or large intestines (see *Ulcerative colitis*).

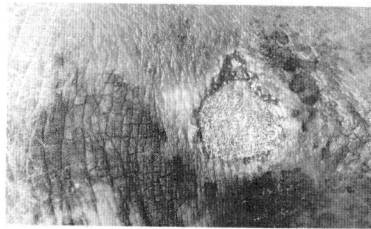

Ulcer on the forehead
An ulcer on this area of the skin is often due to a basal cell carcinoma—a type of skin cancer that is easily treated.

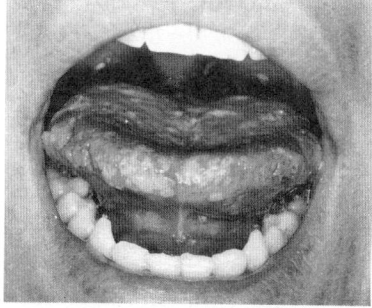

Ulcers in the mouth
Aphthous ulcers are common, painful, and typically last for one to two weeks. Most heal well, without leaving scars.

The skin or mucous membranes of the genitalia may also be affected by ulcers (see *Genital ulceration*). Most genital ulcers are caused by sexually transmitted disease. Examples of this type of ulcer are hard chancres, which develop during the first stage of *syphilis,* and soft chancres (see *Chancroid*).

Ulcers may also develop on the cornea, the transparent covering at the front of the eyeball (see *Corneal ulcer*).

Ulcer, aphthous

A small, painful *ulcer* that occurs alone or in a group on the inside of the cheek or lip or underneath the tongue.

INCIDENCE

Minor aphthous ulcers affect about 20 per cent of the population at any given time. They are most common between the ages of 10 and 40 and affect women more than men. The most severely affected people have continuously recurring ulcers; others have just one or two ulcers per year.

SYMPTOMS

Each ulcer is usually small and oval with a grey centre and a surrounding red, inflamed halo. The ulcer usually lasts for one to two weeks.

CAUSES

The ulcer may be a hypersensitive reaction to haemolytic streptococcus bacteria, which have often been isolated from aphthous ulcers. Other factors commonly associated with the occurrence of these ulcers are minor injuries (such as at an injection site or from a toothbrush), acute stress, and allergies (such as allergic *rhinitis*). In women, ulcers are most common during the premenstrual period. Ulcers may also be more likely to occur if other members of the family suffer from recurrent ulceration.

TREATMENT

Analgesic mouth gels or mouth-washes may ease the pain of an aphthous ulcer. Some ointments form a waterproof covering that protects the ulcer while it heals. Ulcers will heal by themselves if left alone, but a doctor may prescribe an ointment containing a *corticosteroid drug* or a mouthwash containing a *tetracycline drug* to speed up the healing process.

Ulceration

The formation or presence of one or more *ulcers*.

Ulcerative colitis

Chronic inflammation and ulceration of the lining of the *colon* and *rectum*. The disease sometimes begins by affecting only the rectum.

CAUSES AND INCIDENCE

The cause of ulcerative colitis is unknown. In the UK, the disease affects between 40 and 50 people per 100,000. It is most common in young and middle-aged adults.

SYMPTOMS AND SIGNS

The main symptom is bloody diarrhoea; the faeces may also contain pus and mucus. In severe cases, diarrhoea and bleeding are extensive and there may be abdominal pain and tenderness, fever, and general malaise. The incidence of attacks varies considerably. Most commonly, attacks occur at intervals of a few months; however, in some cases, symptoms are either continuous or occur infrequently.

One of the main dangers of severe ulcerative colitis is *anaemia*, caused by blood loss. Other complications include a toxic form of *megacolon* (an abnormally enlarged colon), which may become life-threatening; rashes; mouth ulcers; *arthritis*; and *conjunctivitis* or *uveitis*. In addition, people whose entire colon has been inflamed for more than 10 years are at increased risk of developing cancer of the colon (see *Colon, cancer of*).

DIAGNOSIS

The diagnosis is based on examination of the rectum and lower colon (see *Sigmoidoscopy*) or of the entire colon (see *Colonoscopy*) with a viewing instrument, or by a barium enema (see *Barium X-ray examinations*). During sigmoidoscopy or colonoscopy, a biopsy (removal of a small sample of tissue for microscopic analysis) may be performed. Samples of faeces may also be taken for analysis to exclude the possibility of infection (by bacteria or parasites) as a cause of the symptoms. *Blood tests* may be required.

People who have had ulcerative colitis for many years require periodic colonoscopy and biopsy to check for the development of cancer.

TREATMENT

In most cases, medical treatment effectively controls the disease. Treatment usually consists of *corticosteroid drugs* (to control symptoms by reducing inflammation) and *sulphasalazine* and its derivatives (to maintain long-term freedom from symptoms). The newer derivatives of sulphasalazine, such as *mesalazine* and olsalazine, have fewer side-effects and are generally preferred.

Colectomy (surgical removal of the colon) may be required if inflammation is extensive, severe, and uncontrollable; colectomy is required for most patients with toxic megacolon.

U

This operation usually produces a dramatic improvement in the patient's health, although he or she is usually left with an *ileostomy* (an opening in the surface of the abdomen through which the faeces are passed).

Ulcer-healing drugs

COMMON DRUGS

H₂-receptor antagonists
Cimetidine Famotidine Nizatidine Ranitidine

Others
Antacids Bismuth subnitrate Carbenoxolone Misoprostol Omeprazole Pirenzepine Sucralfate

A group of drugs that are used to treat and prevent stomach and duodenal ulcers (see *Peptic ulcer*).

HOW THEY WORK
Ulcer-healing drugs work in several distinct ways.

H₂-receptor antagonists work by blocking the effects of histamine, an action that reduces acid secretion in the stomach and thus promotes the healing of ulcers. *Antacid drugs* taken regularly may be effective in healing duodenal ulcers, because they neutralize the excess acid. *Omeprazol* and misoprostol directly reduce acid secretion.

Other ulcer-healing drugs, such as *sucralfate*, are believed to form a protective barrier over the ulcer, thereby giving the underlying tissues time to heal. Eradication of HELICOBACTER PYLORI infection by treatment with a combination of *bismuth* and *antibiotic drugs* usually results in healing with a low risk of relapse, and is the preferred treatment for recurrent ulceration.

The choice of ulcer-healing drugs depends on the length of time symptoms have been present and the appearances of the ulcer at endoscopy. In many cases of recent onset, a course of acid-blocking drugs or antacids will give rapid relief. Recurrent ulcers usually require antibiotic treatment.

POSSIBLE ADVERSE EFFECTS
Adverse effects may include confusion, headaches, and dizziness. These drugs may mask the symptoms of *stomach cancers*, and are therefore not usually prescribed for periods longer than two months unless the possibility of cancer has been ruled out.

Ulna

The longer of the two bones of the forearm; the other is the radius. With the palm forwards, the ulna is the inner bone (i.e. nearer the trunk) running down the forearm on the side of the little finger.

The upper end of the ulna articulates with the radius and extends into a rounded projection (which is called the *olecranon* process) that fits around the lower end of the humerus (upper-arm bone) to form part of the *elbow* joint. The lower end of the ulna is rounded and articulates with the carpals (*wrist* bones) and lower part of the radius.

Ulna, fracture of

Fractures of the *ulna* typically occur across the shaft or at the *olecranon* process (the rounded projection at the tip of the elbow).

A shaft fracture is usually caused by a blow to the forearm or a fall on to the hand. Sometimes the radius is fractured at the same time (see *Radius, fracture of*). An operation is usually needed to reposition the broken bone ends and fix them together, using either a plate and screws or a long nail down the centre of the bone. The arm is then immobilized in a plaster *cast*, with the elbow at a right angle, until the fracture heals.

A fracture of the olecranon process is usually caused by a fall on to the elbow. If the bone ends are not displaced, the arm is immobilized in a plaster cast that holds the elbow at a right angle; if they are displaced, they are fitted together during a surgical operation and fixed with a metal screw; if the bone is broken into several pieces, the smallest fragments are removed and the *triceps* muscle is reattached to the broken end of the ulna.

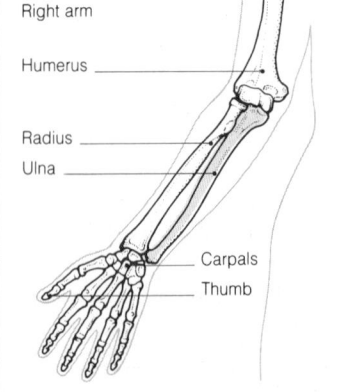

LOCATION OF THE ULNA
The ulna hinges at the elbow on the inner side of the lower end of the humerus (upper-arm bone). It is less mobile than the radius.

Right arm

Humerus

Radius

Ulna

Carpals

Thumb

Ulnar nerve

One of the principal *nerves* of the arm, running down its full length into the hand. A branch of the *brachial plexus*, the ulnar nerve controls muscles that move the thumb and fingers. It also conveys sensation from the fifth and part of the fourth fingers, and from the palm at the base of these digits.

DISORDERS
A blow to the *olecranon* process (the rounded projection at the tip of the elbow), over which the ulnar nerve passes, causes a pins-and-needles sensation and pain in the forearm and in the fourth and fifth fingers.

Persistent numbness and muscle weakness in areas controlled by the nerve may be caused by pressure from an abnormal bony outgrowth from the *humerus* (upper-arm bone). This may be due to *osteoarthritis* or to a fracture of the humerus. If an operation is not performed to relieve the pressure, the hand muscles controlled by the nerve may become permanently damaged, resulting in a *claw-hand*.

Ultrasound

Sound with a frequency greater than the human ear's upper limit of perception—that is, higher than 20,000 hertz (cycles per second). Ultrasound used in medicine for diagnosis or treatment is typically in the range of one million to 15 million hertz (see *Ultrasound scanning; Ultrasound treatment*).

Ultrasound scanning

A diagnostic technique in which very high frequency sound waves (inaudible to the human ear) are passed into the body, and the reflected echoes are detected and analysed to build a picture of the internal organs or of a fetus in the uterus. The procedure is painless and considered safe.

Also called sonography, ultrasound scanning was originally a spin-off from naval sonar (used to detect submarines in World War II) and was first used medically in the 1950s, when it produced still images; most modern scanners produce moving pictures, which are easier to interpret.

HOW IT WORKS
The illustrated box explains how ultrasound scanners work and are operated.

WHY IT IS DONE
Ultrasound waves pass readily through soft tissues and fluids, making this procedure particularly useful for examining fluid-filled organs (such as the uterus in pregnancy, and the gallbladder) and soft organs (such as the liver). Ultrasound

U

waves cannot, however, pass through bone or gas. They are thus of limited use for examining regions that are surrounded by bone (such as the adult brain) or that contain gas (such as the lungs or intestines).

OBSTETRIC USES One of the most common uses of ultrasound is to view the uterus and fetus in pregnancy.

Ultrasound scanning is often performed about 16 to 18 weeks into the pregnancy, but may be performed at any stage. If the date of conception is known, the scan shows whether the fetus is of the expected size; conversely, fetal size can help establish the accurate date of conception and therefore predict the expected date of delivery. The scan also reveals whether there is a multiple pregnancy (see *Pregnancy, multiple*). It is also possible to identify certain gross abnormalities, such as *anencephaly* or *spina bifida*. Congenital *heart disease* can sometimes be detected, enabling the baby to be delivered in a hospital that specializes in correcting such defects soon after birth. The scan also shows the position of the placenta. If the placenta is in a position that could obstruct normal childbirth (a condition known as *placenta praevia*), delivery by *caesarean section* may be necessary.

Scans earlier in pregnancy may be performed if the doctor suspects an *ectopic pregnancy* (presence of an embryo outside the uterus), *hydatidiform mole* (abnormal tumour in the uterus), impending *miscarriage*, or early death of the fetus.

Ultrasound is also vital for the procedure of *amniocentesis* (removal of amniotic fluid via a needle for analysis) and is used during *chorionic villus sampling* (removal of tissue from the placenta for analysis). A scan shows the position of the fetus and placenta before either of these procedures and also helps in guiding the needle into the uterus.

Later in pregnancy, a scan may be carried out if the growth rate of the fetus seems slow, if fetal movements cease or are excessive, or if the mother experiences vaginal bleeding. For high-risk or overdue pregnancies, a scan may be carried out before delivery to check on fetal size, development, and position in the uterus, the amount of amniotic fluid, and to recheck the position of the placenta.

NONOBSTETRIC USES In the newborn child, ultrasound can be used to scan the brain, via a gap (the anterior fontanelle) in the skull, to investigate *hydrocephalus* or to diagnose a *brain tumour* or brain haemorrhage.

Echocardiography is a type of ultrasound technique used to look at the heart. This technique is particularly useful for investigating congenital heart disease and disorders of the heart valves.

The liver can be clearly viewed by ultrasound, which can be used to diagnose liver disorders such as *cirrhosis*, cysts, abscesses, or tumours. Ultrasound shows the presence of

HOW ULTRASOUND SCANNING WORKS

Ultrasound waves are emitted by a device called a transducer, which is placed on the skin over the part of the body to be viewed. The transducer contains a crystal that converts an electric current into sound waves. The waves used have frequencies in the range of 1 to 15 million hertz. At these high frequencies, the waves can be focused into a fine parallel beam, which passes through a "slice" of the body if the transducer crystal is made to oscillate back and forth. Some of the waves are reflected at tissue boundaries, so a series of echoes is returned. The transducer also acts as a receiver, converting these echoes into electrical signals, which are processed and displayed on a screen to give a two-dimensional image of the scanned body slice. By moving the transducer, different slices through the body can be seen.

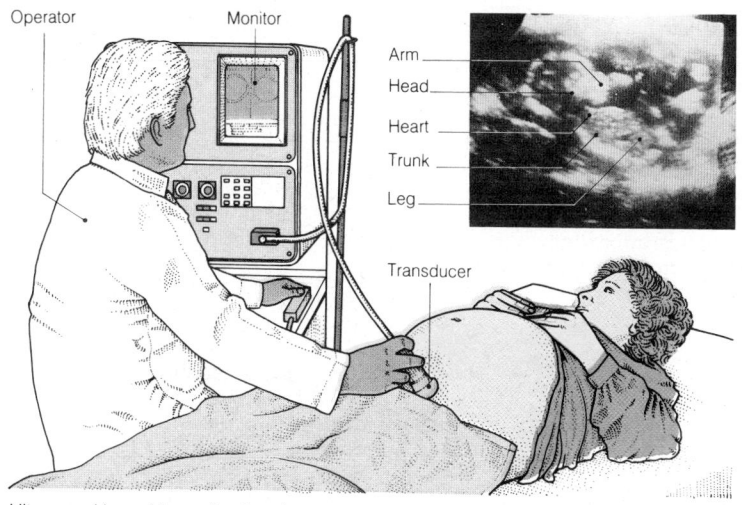

Operator — Monitor — Arm — Head — Heart — Trunk — Leg — Transducer

Ultrasound has wide applications in medicine and is especially useful in obstetrics. It offers no known risk to the baby. By moving the transducer across the outer wall of the abdomen, views of the growing fetus are obtained from various angles, so it is possible to screen for abnormalities.

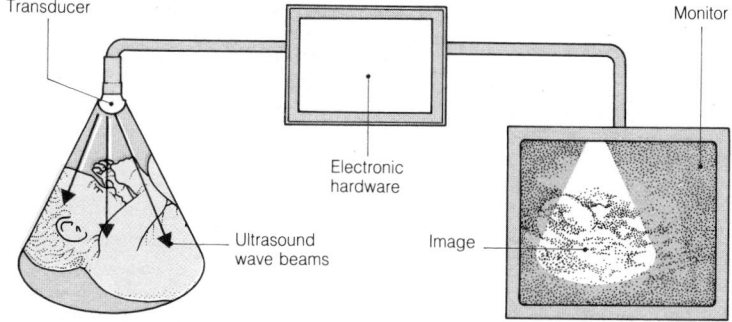

Transducer — Monitor — Electronic hardware — Ultrasound wave beams — Image

Parts of an ultrasound scanner
The transducer emits a beam of high frequency waves, which are passed through a slice of the body; the echoes are picked up by the transducer and converted by the electronic hardware into an image displayed on the monitor.

U

gallstones in the gallbladder or bile ducts. In a patient with *jaundice*, a scan can help establish whether the jaundice is due to obstruction of the bile ducts or to liver disease. The pancreas can be scanned for cysts, tumours, or *pancreatitis*, and the kidneys for congenital defects, cysts, tumours, and *hydronephrosis* (swelling due to obstruction to the outflow of urine). Other organs that may be scanned by ultrasound for diagnostic purposes (primarily to look for cysts, solid tumours, or foreign bodies) include the thyroid gland, breasts, bladder, testes, ovaries, spleen, and eyes.

Ultrasound scanning is also used during needle *biopsy* (insertion of a very thin hollow needle into an organ to remove cells, tissue, or fluid for examination) to help guide the needle accurately to a specific spot.

ELECTROMAGNETIC SPECTRUM

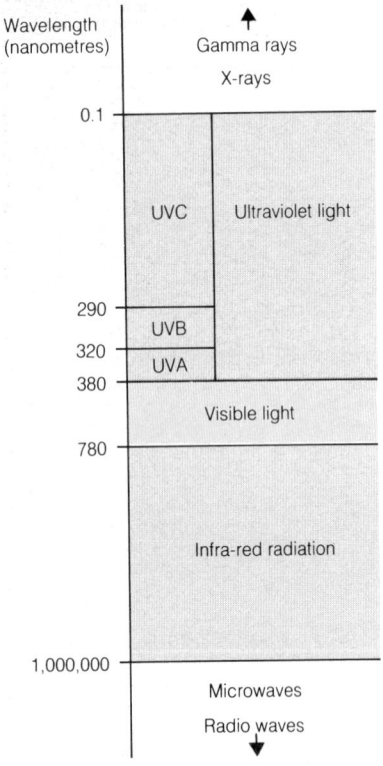

Ultraviolet light in the spectrum
Different types of electromagnetic radiation are defined according to their wavelengths. The diagram shows the different types—which together make up the electromagnetic spectrum—and their wavelength limits in nanometres (one nanometre equals one thousand-millionth of a metre). Ultraviolet light is the part of the electromagnetic spectrum between visible light and X-rays.

Doppler ultrasound is a modified form of ultrasound that exploits the *Doppler effect* (the change in pitch that occurs when a sound source is moving relative to the detector) to investigate moving objects. One important use of Doppler ultrasound is to examine the fetal heartbeat. Doppler ultrasound is also used in the technique, sometimes called angiodynography, by which information can be obtained about the rate of blood flow through blood vessels. This procedure enables the doctor to detect narrowing of vessels or turbulence in the flow of blood.

HOW IT IS DONE
For a scan in early pregnancy, the woman is usually asked not to pass urine for a few hours beforehand; a full bladder helps improve the view of the uterus by displacing nearby loops of intestine. For a liver or gallbladder scan, the patient is usually asked to fast for several hours beforehand.

Clothing over the region to be scanned is removed, and oil or jelly is smeared over the skin to achieve good contact when the transducer is passed back and forth over the skin. During the scan, which takes about 15 minutes (or sometimes less), the patient can usually lie back and watch the images appearing on the screen.

The ultrasonic waves produce no detectable sensation. When a scan is performed in conjunction with a technique involving insertion of a needle, a local anaesthetic is used and there is usually little or no discomfort.

Ultrasound treatment
The use of high-frequency sound waves to treat *soft-tissue injuries* (such as injuries to ligaments, muscles, and tendons). The treatment reduces inflammation and speeds up healing. It is thought to work by improving blood flow in tissues under the skin.

During treatment, there may be a feeling of warmth and a slight tingling sensation. Occasionally, severe pain occurs if the sound waves are pointed at a bone surface just under the skin.

Ultraviolet light
Invisible light from the part of the electromagnetic spectrum immediately beyond the violet end of the visible light spectrum (i.e. between visible light and *X-rays*). Long wavelength ultraviolet light (i.e. that nearest visible light) is often termed UVA; intermediate wavelength ultraviolet light is designated UVB; and short wavelength ultraviolet light (i.e. that nearest X-rays) is called UVC.

Ultraviolet light occurs naturally in sunlight, but much of it—including all UVC and much UVB (both of which are potentially harmful)—is absorbed by the *ozone* layer of the atmosphere. The ultraviolet light that reaches the earth's surface, mainly UVA with some UVB, is responsible for the tanning and burning effects of sunlight and for the production of *vitamin D* in the skin. However, it is the ultraviolet component of sunlight that can have harmful effects (see *Sunlight, adverse effects of*), such as *skin cancer*, especially in fair-skinned people.

Suntan lamps, which produce ultraviolet light artificially, are designed to emit only UVA rays. In practice, however, they also give off a small amount of UVB light and may pose a significant health risk. Ultraviolet light is also produced by certain other types of equipment, such as welding torches, carbon arcs, and lasers. Special precautions, such as the use of goggles, should always be taken when using such equipment.

MEDICAL USES
Ultraviolet light is sometimes used in *phototherapy* to treat certain skin conditions, such as *psoriasis and vitiligo*, and also jaundice of the newborn (see *Jaundice, neonatal*).

A mercury-vapour lamp (Wood's light) can also be used to produce ultraviolet light artificially. This light is used to diagnose certain skin conditions, such as *tinea*, because it causes the infected area to fluoresce.

Umbilical cord
The rope-like structure connecting the fetus to the *placenta* that supplies oxygen and nutrients from the mother's

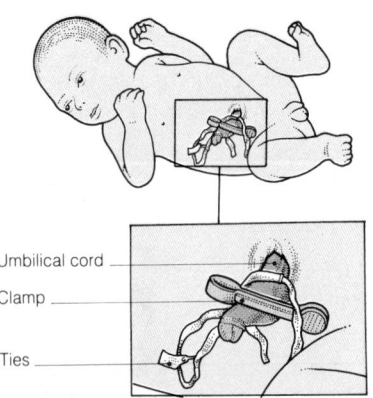

Umbilical cord
Clamp
Ties

Umbilical cord after birth
The cord ceases to function after birth and is clamped and cut; the baby now obtains oxygen through his or her own lungs.

circulation. The umbilical cord is usually 40 to 60 cm long and consists of a jelly-like substance in which two arteries and a vein are embedded.

Several minutes after delivery, the umbilical cord is clamped and then cut about 2.5 cm from the baby's abdominal wall. The stump falls off within a couple of weeks, leaving a scar called the *umbilicus* (navel).

DISORDERS

In rare cases, the umbilical cord protrudes down through the mother's cervix during labour. This is dangerous because the baby's oxygen supply can be cut off. Prompt delivery, by *caesarean section* or a *forceps delivery*, is necessary. Sometimes the cord pulls tightly around the baby's neck during delivery, but can usually be freed by slipping it over the baby's head.

Rarely, there is only one artery in the umbilical cord. This condition may be associated with birth defects.

The newborn baby's umbilical stump sometimes becomes infected and may ooze pus. This condition, called omphalitis, generally begins during the first week of life. Treatment involves gently wiping the umbilicus with sterile cottonwool and water. Treatment with *antibiotic drugs* may also be necessary.

Quite commonly, a fleshy protuberance called a *granuloma* grows on the umbilical stump, sometimes as a result of chronic infection. Umbilical granulomas may be destroyed by local application of silver nitrate. Umbilical polyps (also called umbilical adenomas) are shiny, bright red, raspberry-like growths which may also appear in the newborn period. Such polyps may require surgical removal.

Umbilicus

The scar on the abdomen that marks the site of attachment of the *umbilical cord* to the fetus. The umbilicus is commonly called the navel.

DISORDERS

An umbilical *hernia* is a soft swelling at the umbilicus caused by protrusion of the abdominal contents through a weak area of the abdominal wall.

Umbilical hernias are quite common in newborn infants, occurring twice as commonly in boys as in girls. When the baby cries, the swelling increases in size and may cause discomfort. Umbilical hernias usually disappear without treatment by the time a child is about two years old. If an umbilical hernia has not disappeared spontaneously by the age of about four, surgery may be necessary.

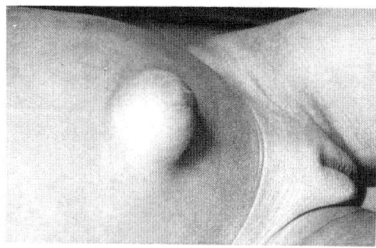

Umbilical hernia
This condition, present from birth, is due to a localized weakness in the abdominal wall. It usually disappears without treatment.

Occasionally, umbilical hernias develop in adults, especially in women following childbirth. Surgery may be necessary if such hernias are large, persistent, or disfiguring.

In rare cases, a discharge from the umbilicus develops due either to an infection or to an abnormal connection between the umbilicus and the urinary, biliary, or intestinal tract. Possible causes of the abnormal connection, which can be corrected surgically, include a birth defect, cancer, or tuberculosis.

Occasionally, benign or malignant tumours develop in the umbilicus. Such tumours may be secondary to cancers in the breast, colon, ovary, or stomach.

In rare cases, women develop *endometriosis* in the umbilicus, causing it to bleed periodically. Surgery may be necessary in such cases.

Unconscious

A specific part of the mind in which ideas, memories, perceptions, or feelings that a person is not currently aware of are stored and actively processed. The contents of the unconscious mind are not easily retrievable,

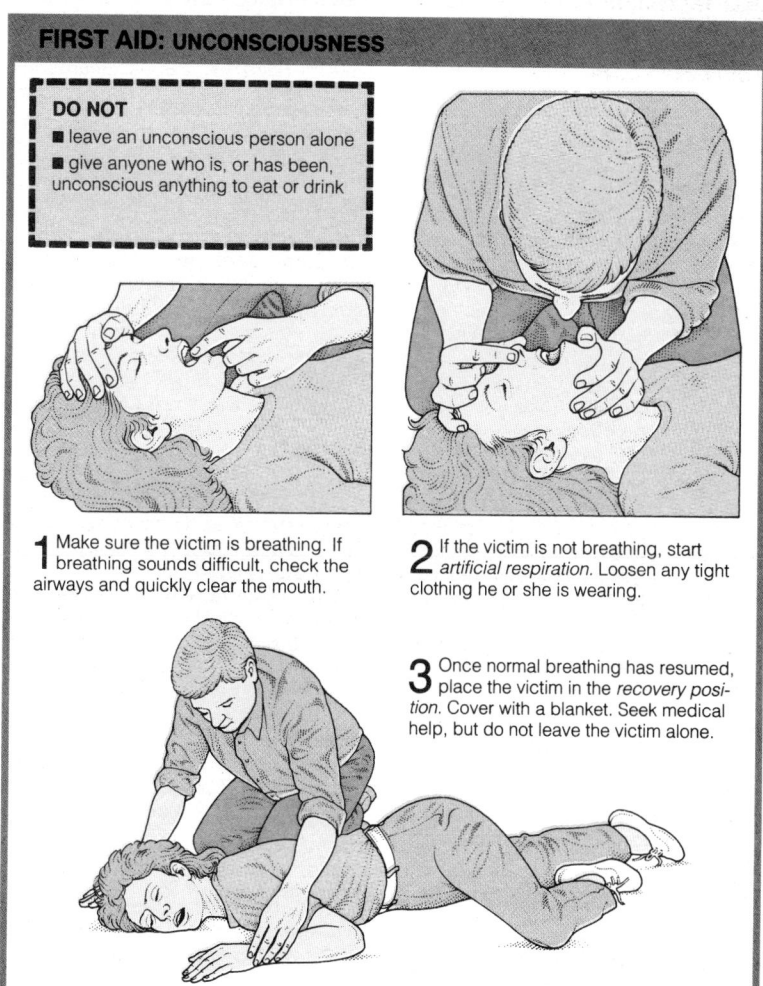

FIRST AID: UNCONSCIOUSNESS

DO NOT
- leave an unconscious person alone
- give anyone who is, or has been, unconscious anything to eat or drink

1 Make sure the victim is breathing. If breathing sounds difficult, check the airways and quickly clear the mouth.

2 If the victim is not breathing, start *artificial respiration*. Loosen any tight clothing he or she is wearing.

3 Once normal breathing has resumed, place the victim in the *recovery position*. Cover with a blanket. Seek medical help, but do not leave the victim alone.

U

in contrast to those of the *subconscious*. *Freudian theory* stresses the importance of the unconscious in determining behaviour and causing neurotic symptoms. *Jungian theory* describes a collective unconscious, inherited by every person and derived from experiences in our distant past.

Unconsciousness

Abnormal loss of awareness of the self and of one's surroundings, resulting from a reduced level of activity in the reticular formation of the *brainstem*. *Sleep* is a normal state of altered consciousness from which a person can be roused easily; an unconscious person can be roused only with difficulty or not at all. Unconsciousness may be brief and light, as in *fainting*, or deeper and more prolonged (see *Coma*). The term *concussion* refers to a brief transient state of unconsciousness following a head injury.

Underbite

See *Prognathism*.

Unsaturated fats

See *Fats and oils*.

Uraemia

The presence of excess *urea* and other chemical waste products in the *blood*. Uraemia results from *kidney failure*.

Uranium

A radioactive metallic element which does not occur naturally in its pure form but is widely distributed in various compounds in ores such as pitchblende, carnotite, and uraninite.

Natural radioactive decay of uranium yields a series of radioactive products, including *radium* and *radon*, and progresses ultimately to lead. During the various decay stages, *radiation* is emitted as alpha and beta particles and gamma rays. In addition to its *radiation hazards*, uranium is chemically poisonous, causing damage to the urinary system.

Urea

A waste product of the breakdown of proteins and the main nitrogenous (nitrogen-containing) constituent of *urine*. Proteins in food are digested in the intestine to form *amino acids*, which are absorbed into the bloodstream and transported to the *liver*. In the liver, amino acids in excess of the body's requirements are converted into urea, which is transported by the bloodstream to the *kidneys* and excreted in the urine.

The kidneys are usually highly efficient at eliminating urea from the body. A high-protein diet increases the amount of urea produced. Healthy kidneys are able to cope with increased urea production, but *kidney failure* impairs the kidneys' ability to eliminate urea and leads to *uraemia* (abnormally high blood levels of urea). For this reason, measurement of urea levels in the blood is one of the routine *kidney-function tests*.

Urea is also formed in the body from the breakdown of cell proteins. If there is a large increase in urea from this source (due, for example, to severe tissue damage resulting from injury or surgery), the kidneys are sometimes unable to cope and uraemia results.

Certain conditions (such as liver damage) may lead to a decrease in the blood level of urea. Blood levels of urea also fall during pregnancy, when the blood is more dilute than usual.

MEDICAL USES
Urea is used in various creams and ointments to moisturize and soften the skin in the treatment of disorders such as *psoriasis*, atopic *dermatitis*, *ichthyosis*, and other conditions in which the skin is dry and scaly. Occasionally, urea is used as an osmotic *diuretic drug*, primarily to reduce pressure in the skull due to cerebral *oedema* or to reduce pressure in the eye caused by *glaucoma*.

Ureter

One of the two tubes that carry *urine* from the *kidneys* to the *bladder*. Each ureter is about 25 to 30 cm long. The walls of the ureters have three layers: a fibrous outer layer; a muscular middle layer; and an inner watertight layer (known as transitional epithelium). Each ureter is supplied by blood vessels and nerves.

Urine flows down the ureters partly due to gravity but mainly as a result of the pumping action known as peristalsis in which wave-like contractions pass several times a minute through the muscular ureter walls. Each ureter enters the bladder via a tunnel in the bladder wall, which is angled to prevent reflux (backflow) of urine into the ureter when the bladder muscle contracts.

DISORDERS
Some people are born with double ureters, on one or both sides of the body, usually in association with partial duplication of the kidney on an affected side. Double ureters may be completely distinct along their entire

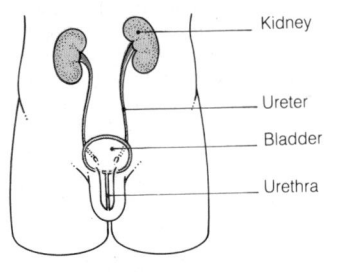

ANATOMY OF THE URETER
The ureters are tubes that carry urine from the kidneys to the bladder. They enter the back of the bladder at an angle.

- Kidney
- Ureter
- Bladder
- Urethra

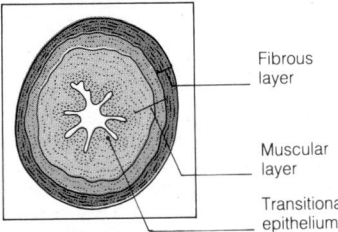

- Fibrous layer
- Muscular layer
- Transitional epithelium

Cross-section
Each ureter has three layers: a fibrous outer layer, a muscular middle layer, and an inner transitional epithelium.

length or may join to form a Y shape. In many cases, ureteric duplication causes no problems, but there may be a tendency for urine to reflux up one of the tubes if the duplicated ureters enter the bladder separately. There may also be problems, such as *incontinence* or infection, if a ureter enters the urethra or the vagina instead of the bladder. Corrective surgery can be performed if necessary.

Spasms of the ureter may result if a stone (see *Calculus, urinary tract*) passes down or becomes stuck in a ureter. This extremely painful condition is commonly known as *renal colic*.

Ureteritis is an inflammatory condition of the ureter, which may be caused by blockage of the ureter by a stone, or by the spread of infection from the bladder.

Ureteric colic

See *Renal colic*.

Ureterolithotomy

The surgical removal of a stone (see *Calculus, urinary tract*) that is stuck in a *ureter* (tube that carries urine from a kidney to the bladder). In some cases, calculi are removed by means of *cystoscopy* or *lithotripsy* rather than by ureterolithotomy.

U

HOW IT IS DONE

Ureterolithotomy is preceded by intravenous *urography* to locate the calculus. With the patient under general anaesthesia, the surgeon makes an abdominal incision and feels the ureter to locate the calculus. The ureter is then opened with a longitudinal cut, the calculus is removed with forceps, and a check is made for more calculi. The ureter and abdomen are then sewn up, leaving a tube inserted into the abdomen to drain any urine that leaks from the ureter. This tube is removed four or five days later and the patient can then leave hospital.

Urethra

The tube by which *urine* is excreted from the *bladder*. In females, the urethra is short and opens to the outside just in front of the vagina between the labia minora. In males, the urethra is much longer. It is surrounded by the prostate gland at its upper end and then forms a channel through the length of the penis. The location and relative length of the male and female urethras are shown in the illustrated box.

DISORDERS

Although urethral infections, scarring, and congenital abnormalities occur in both sexes, these disorders are much more common and serious in males than in females.

In male infants, a urethral valve is sometimes present. This is a flap that arises from the lining of the urethra and impedes the flow of urine. The resulting bottleneck causes back pressure on the *kidneys* as urine overfills the bladder, ureters, and collecting ducts of the kidneys. Permanent and severe damage to the kidneys can occur if the urethral valve is not removed surgically.

Urethritis (inflammation of the urethra) may be due to infection, irritation, or minor injury. Inflammation may be followed by scarring and formation of a *urethral stricture* (a narrowed section of the urethra).

The male urethra is easily damaged in accidents involving pelvic injury and may require surgical repair. Injury to, or surgery on, the urethra may lead to urethral stricture.

Urethral dilatation

A procedure in which a *urethral stricture* (narrowed urethra) in a male is widened by means of a slim, round-tipped instrument inserted through the opening of the urethra at the tip of the penis. Urethral dilatation is performed under either local or general anaesthesia. The procedure may need to be repeated.

Urethral discharge

A fluid that flows from the *urethra* in some cases of *urethritis* caused by infection. In *gonorrhoea*, the discharge is yellow and purulent (pus-containing); in other types of infection the discharged fluid is clear.

Urethral stricture

An uncommon condition in which the male *urethra* becomes narrowed and sometimes shortened along part of its length as a result of shrinkage of scar tissue within its walls.

CAUSES AND SYMPTOMS

Scar tissue may form after injury to the urethra or after persistent *urethritis* (inflammation of the urethra). In the past, urethritis was most commonly due to *gonorrhoea*, but modern antibiotic treatment has made strictures from this cause uncommon.

A urethral stricture may make it difficult or painful to pass urine or to ejaculate, and may cause some deformation of the penis when erect.

In some cases, a urethral stricture may lead to kidney damage due to back pressure from the build-up of urine. A urethral stricture may also encourage the development of *urinary tract infection*.

TREATMENT

A urethral stricture is usually treated by *urethral dilatation* (widening of the urethra by inserting a slim, round-tipped instrument through the urethral opening at the tip of the penis). If dilatation fails, an instrument called a urethrotome may be inserted to cut through the scar tissue. In some cases, a urethral stricture may be completely removed and the urethra reconstructed by plastic surgery.

Urethral syndrome, acute

A set of symptoms of uncertain cause experienced by some women and, very rarely, by some men. The symptoms consist of pain and discomfort in the lower abdomen, a frequent urge to pass *urine*, and, in women, pain around the vulval region. Middle-aged women are the most commonly affected by this syndrome.

In most cases, the doctor cannot discover any causative infection, and the patient's *kidney* function and *urinary tract* anatomy are normal. Emotional and psychological factors may contribute. In women who have gone through the menopause, the symptoms may be due to inflammation of the vulva associated with thinning of tissues (see *Vulvitis*).

Treatment may be difficult. Cases due to vulvitis may be relieved by use of *oestrogen drugs* or *corticosteroid drugs* in cream form. Antiseptic creams and strong soaps should be avoided because they may cause irritation or an allergic reaction that worsens the symptoms. Scrupulous personal hygiene and a high fluid intake are usually recommended.

Urethritis

Inflammation of the *urethra*, usually due to an infection but sometimes having other causes.

LOCATION OF THE URETHRA

The urethra is the tube through which urine is passed from the bladder. There is no voluntary muscle in the urethra. The flow of urine is controlled by muscles in the wall and outlet of the bladder.

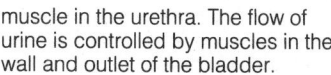
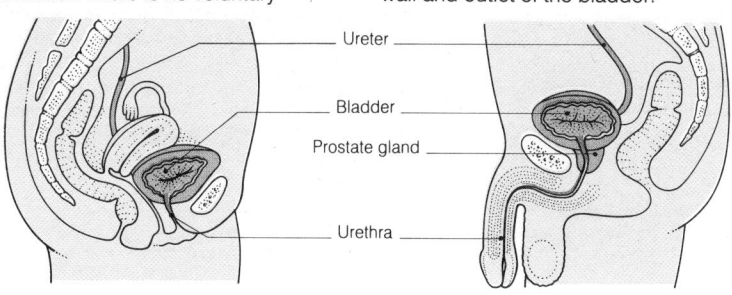

Ureter
Bladder
Prostate gland
Urethra

Urethra in a woman
The female urethra is short—about 4cm long—and runs down to open to the exterior just in front of the vagina.

Urethra in a man
The male urethra is about 18–20cm long. It passes through the prostate gland and along the full length of the penis.

U

CAUSES

Urethritis may be caused by various infectious organisms, including the bacterium that causes *gonorrhoea*. *Nonspecific urethritis* may be caused by any of a large number of different types of microorganisms, including bacteria, yeasts, and *chlamydial infection*. Bacteria from the skin or rectum sometimes spread to infect the urethra.

Urethritis may also be caused by damage from an accident or from a surgically introduced catheter or cystoscope (viewing instrument for examining the bladder). Other possible causes include exposure to irritant chemicals, such as antiseptics and some spermicidal preparations.

SYMPTOMS AND COMPLICATIONS

Urethritis causes a burning sensation and pain when passing urine. The pain can be severe and is sometimes likened to passing small fragments of broken glass. The urine may be blood-stained and, particularly when gonorrhoea is the cause, there is often a yellow, pus-filled, discharge.

Urethritis may be followed by scarring and the formation of a *urethral stricture* (narrowing of a section of the urethra), which can make the passing of urine difficult.

TREATMENT

Infections are treated with an appropriate *antibiotic drug*. Antibiotic treatment may also be needed if bacterial infection follows urethritis due to a noninfective cause. Urethral strictures are usually treated by the technique of *urethral dilatation*.

Urethrocele

An anatomical abnormality caused by a weakness in the tissues in the front wall of the *vagina*. This weakness allows the overlying *urethra* to bulge backwards and downwards into the vagina. A urethrocele may be congenital (present from birth), may develop after *childbirth*, or may be associated with *obesity*.

A urethrocele may cause difficulty in emptying the bladder and pain during sexual intercourse (see *Intercourse, painful*). It also increases susceptibility to *urinary tract infection*.

The usual treatment for a urethrocele is a surgical operation to tighten the tissues at the front of the vagina, thus giving the urethra better support (see *Vaginal repair*).

-uria

A suffix relating to *urine*, as in *protein-uria*, the term for presence of protein in the urine.

Uric acid

A waste product of the breakdown of *nucleic acids* in body cells. A small amount of uric acid is also produced by the digestion of foods rich in nucleic acids, such as liver, kidneys, and other offal.

Most uric acid produced in the body passes, via the bloodstream, to the *kidneys*, which remove the acid from the blood and excrete it in the urine. However, some uric acid passes into the intestine, where it is broken down by bacteria into chemicals which are excreted in the faeces.

The kidneys of a healthy person maintain blood levels of uric acid within acceptable limits. When uric acid excretion is disrupted, it may result in *hyperuricaemia* (abnormally high levels of uric acid in the blood), which, in turn, may lead to *gout* or kidney stones (see *Calculi, urinary tract*). Causes of hyperuricaemia include kidney disease, *leukaemia*, haemolytic *anaemia*, genetic disorders in which an enzyme involved in uric acid excretion is lacking, and certain drugs, including some *diuretic drugs* and *anticancer drugs*.

Urinal

A container for *urine*, useful for bedridden men (women use a *bedpan*). Also known as a urinal is an appliance for men suffering from urinary *incontinence*, which consists of a thick rubber tube connected by a plastic tube to a drainage bag strapped on the leg.

Urinalysis

A battery of tests on a patient's *urine*, including measurements of the urine's physical characteristics (such as colour, concentration, and cloudiness), microscopic examination, and chemical testing. Urinalysis can be used to check kidney function and to detect and diagnose *urinary tract* and other disorders.

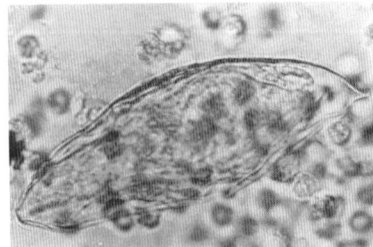

Schistosome egg in urine
The tropical disease schistosomiasis may be diagnosed by the finding of schistosome (worm) eggs on urinalysis.

TYPES OF TESTS

MICROSCOPIC EXAMINATION Microscopy of urine may reveal *haematuria* (red blood cells in the urine), indicating damage to the glomeruli (filtering units of the kidneys) or some other disorder of the kidneys or urinary tract. Fragments of protein and kidney cells, called casts, in the urine may indicate various types of kidney disease. *Urinary tract infection* results in the presence of pus or bacteria in the urine. Crystals in the urine indicate the possibility of an inborn error of metabolism (see *Metabolism, inborn errors of*) or susceptibility to stones (see *Calculi, urinary tract*). The parasitic disease *schistosomiasis* may be diagnosed from the presence of worm eggs in the urine.

CULTURE If a single drop of fresh urine is spread thinly on the surface of a nutrient gel and incubated, any bacteria present will multiply and produce colonies. The appearance of these colonies under microscopic examination allows the microbiologist to identify the organism causing a urinary tract infection.

CHEMICAL TESTS A range of simple stick or strip tests is available to show the presence of various substances in the urine, and to measure properties of the urine, such as its acidity and concentration (ratio of dissolved substances to water). These tests rely on a simple colour change when the stick or strip is dipped into the urine. Substances tested for include glucose (a high level usually means that the patient has *diabetes mellitus*), blood, protein, and bile. Detection of human chorionic gonadotrophin in the urine is the basis of many *pregnancy tests*. Urine tests are also useful in determining whether a person has been taking a particular drug. (See also *Kidney-function tests*.)

Urinary diversion

Any surgical procedure performed to allow passage of urine when the normal outlet channel of the *urinary tract*, via the bladder and urethra, is obstructed or cannot be used, or when the bladder has been surgically removed.

TEMPORARY DIVERSION
Temporary urinary diversion is sometimes required when passage of urine is blocked by enlargement of the *prostate gland* or by *urethral stricture*. In such cases, a small opening is made through the abdominal wall just above the pubic bone, and a tube is passed directly into the bladder (see *Catheterization, urinary*). Temporary

U

URINARY DIVERSION USING ILEAL CONDUIT

This is a standard operation performed when the bladder has been removed or is seriously malfunctioning and beyond hope of repair. A midline incision in the abdomen is used; before making it, the surgeon creates an opening through the abdominal wall in a good position for later attachment of the collecting bag.

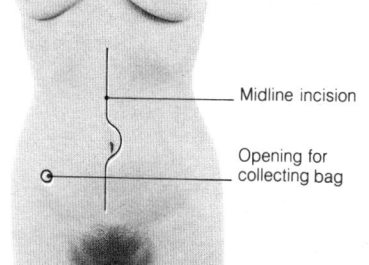

Midline incision

Opening for collecting bag

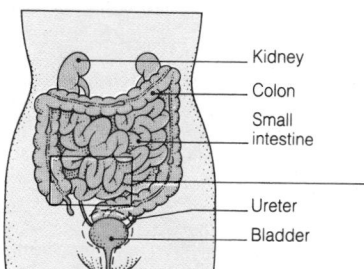

Kidney
Colon
Small intestine
Ureter
Bladder

1 A short length is cut out of the ileum (the lower part of the small intestine), retaining the mesentery (supporting folds of tissue) and the essential blood vessels that supply the freed section.

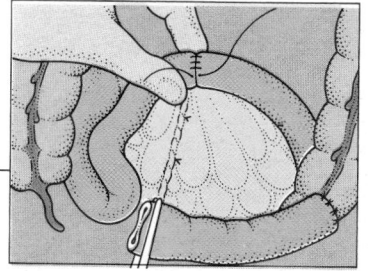

2 The cut ends of the intestine are stitched together to re-establish continuity. One end of the freed length of intestine is closed and the other end is temporarily clamped.

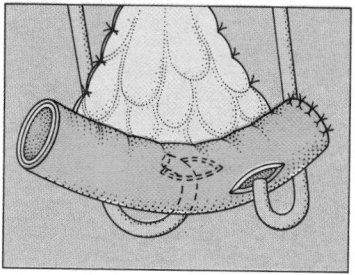

3 The ureters are now implanted into the isolated length of ileum. The open end of this segment is brought through the abdominal wall and stitched in place.

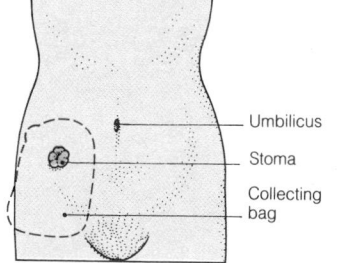

Umbilicus
Stoma
Collecting bag

4 A collecting bag for receiving the patient's urine is fixed with adhesive around the new stoma (opening) in the wall of the abdomen.

diversion is also required after some operations on the urinary tract; a small tube is introduced into the kidney and brought to the abdominal surface, bypassing the ureters and allowing healing to take place.

PERMANENT DIVERSION

Permanent urinary diversion is needed when the bladder has been removed, usually to treat advanced bladder cancer, or when neurological control of the bladder is severely disturbed, such as after severe spinal injury. Permanent diversion may also be required if there is an irreparable *fistula* (abnormal opening) between a female patient's bladder or urethra and the vagina.

Permanent diversion is usually achieved by creating what is known as an ileal conduit (see illustrated box). A section of the ileum is removed to create a substitute bladder, into one end of which the surgeon implants the ureters. The other end of the substitute bladder is then brought out through an incision in the abdominal wall, as in an *ileostomy*. The patient wears a bag attached to the skin to collect urine.

In recent years, the use of so-called continent urinary diversions has been investigated. These permit the patient to control the drainage of urine by periodically emptying an internal ileal conduit pouch with a catheter, there-

by permitting a degree of continence. Initial results have been encouraging, although this treatment is still considered experimental.

Urinary retention

Inability to empty the *bladder* or difficulty in doing so. Urinary retention may be complete, in which case urine cannot voluntarily be passed at all (although some may leak out), or incomplete, in which case some urine may be passed but the bladder fails to empty completely.

CAUSES

Retention may be due to an obstruction to the flow of urine. This problem predominantly affects males. Causes include *phimosis* (tight foreskin), *urethral stricture*, a stone in the bladder (see *Calculus, urinary tract*), *prostatitis* (inflammation of the prostate), enlargement of the prostate (see *Prostate, enlarged*), or a tumour of the prostate (see *Prostate, cancer of*). In women, urinary retention may result from pressure on the urethra from uterine *fibroids* or from a fetus in the uterus. In either sex it may be due to a *bladder tumour*.

Alternatively, retention may be due to defective functioning of the nerve pathways concerned with the sensing of bladder enlargement and with the triggering of bladder emptying. This may be induced by a general or spinal anaesthetic, by drugs that act on the bladder, or by surgery. Defective nerve functioning may also be due to injury to the nerve pathways or to disease of the spinal cord.

SYMPTOMS AND COMPLICATIONS

Except when nerve pathways are defective, complete urinary retention causes discomfort and pain in the lower abdomen, which may be severe. The filled bladder can be felt on examination as a swelling above the pubic bone. Chronic or partial retention, by contrast, may not cause any serious symptoms and the sufferer may be unaware of it.

There is a risk that retention will lead to kidney damage from back pressure up the urinary tract. Incomplete emptying often leads to a *urinary tract infection*.

TREATMENT

Urinary retention is treated by inserting a drainage tube into the bladder, usually via the urethra (see *Catheterization, urinary*). The cause of the retention is then investigated if it is not already known. When obstruction is the cause, it can usually be treated; if nerve damage is the cause, the pros-

U

pects are less hopeful; permanent or intermittent catheterization is sometimes necessary in such cases.

Urinary system

See *Urinary tract.*

Urinary tract

The part of the body concerned with the formation and excretion of *urine.* The urinary tract consists of the *kidneys* (with their blood and nerve supplies), renal pelvises (funnel-shaped ducts that channel urine from the kidneys), *ureters, bladder,* and *urethra.*

The kidneys make urine by filtering blood. The urine collects in the renal pelvises and then passes down the ureters into the bladder by the actions of gravity and peristalsis (wave-like contractions of the walls of the ureters). Urine is then stored in the bladder until a sufficient amount is present to stimulate micturition (passage of urine). When the bladder contracts, the urine is expelled from the body through the urethra.

Urinary tract infection

An infection anywhere in the *urinary tract. Urethritis* (inflammation of the urethra) may be caused by mechanisms other than infection, but *cystitis* (inflammation of the bladder) and *pyelonephritis* (inflammation of the kidneys) are nearly always caused by a bacterial infection.

Urethral infections are more common in men than women. However, infections further up the urinary tract are more common in women because of the shorter female urethra.

CAUSES

Urethritis is often due to a *sexually transmitted disease,* such as *gonorrhoea* or *nonspecific urethritis.* Other urinary tract infections are usually caused by organisms that have spread from the rectum, via the urethra, to the bladder or kidneys. Infections can also be carried to the urinary tract in the blood.

In men, there is often an identifiable predisposing factor, usually some condition that impairs the drainage of urine, such as an enlarged prostate gland (see *Prostate, enlarged*) or a *urethral stricture.* In women, urinary tract infections often occur without any identifiable underlying cause. Such infections are, however, more common during pregnancy.

In both sexes, urinary tract infection may be caused by a stone (see *Calculus, urinary tract*), a *bladder tumour,* or a congenital abnormality of the urinary tract, such as a double kidney on one side. Defective bladder emptying as a result of *spina bifida* or of damage to the spinal cord in a *spinal injury* leads almost inevitably to urinary tract infection.

The risks of a urinary tract infection can be reduced by careful personal hygiene, by drinking plenty of fluids, and by regular emptying of the bladder.

SYMPTOMS

Urethritis causes a burning sensation when passing urine. Cystitis causes a frequent urge to pass urine, lower abdominal pain, *haematuria* (blood in the urine), and, in many cases, general malaise with a mild fever. Pyelonephritis causes pain in the loins and high fever.

COMPLICATIONS

Urethritis can lead to scarring of the urethra and formation of a *urethral stricture.* Cystitis does not usually produce complications unless infection spreads up to the kidneys. Without proper treatment, pyelonephritis can lead to permanent kidney damage, *septicaemia* (spread of infective organisms to the blood), and *septic shock.* If a calculus in a kidney is the underlying cause of infection, it may grow rapidly during the course of the infection.

DIAGNOSIS

Infection is diagnosed by examination of a *culture* of a few drops of urine. The urine specimen is taken midstream to avoid contamination of the specimen by organisms that normally live in the last part of the urethra.

Further investigation is usually needed for men who have any urinary tract infection or for women suffering from recurrent cystitis or pyelonephritis. Such investigation is performed by *urography* (an X-ray procedure for examining the urinary tract after injection of a radiopaque contrast medium) or by *ultrasound scanning.*

TREATMENT

Most urinary tract infections are treated with *antibiotic drugs*; the specific drug used depends on the type of infection.

Urination, excessive

The production of more than about 2.5 litres of *urine* per day. Excessive urination is known medically as polyuria.

CAUSES

Excessive urination is sometimes due to psychiatric problems, which may cause a person to drink compulsively. The high intake of fluid leads inevitably to a high urine output.

Various diseases may cause abnormal amounts of certain substances to be excreted in the urine; these substances draw water with them, increasing the urine volume. The most important disease in this group is *diabetes mellitus,* in which excess glucose in the blood spills into the urine. Certain kidney diseases, known as salt-losing states, lead to excessive salt loss in the urine, with an accompanying increase in volume.

In the disorder known as central *diabetes insipidus,* excessive urination results from reduced production of ADH (antidiuretic hormone) by the pituitary gland. This leads to a marked increase in urine volume because ADH normally acts on the kidneys to concentrate the urine. In nephrogenic diabetes insipidus, which may result from various kidney disorders, normal amounts of ADH are produced but the kidneys fail to respond to it.

DIAGNOSIS

Any person who passes large quantities of urine should consult a doctor.

In a compulsive drinker, urine volume soon drops if water intake is restricted, but no such drop occurs in a patient with diabetes insipidus. Central diabetes insipidus improves after administration of synthetic ADH, but nephrogenic diabetes insipidus does not.

In patients with diabetes mellitus, the glucose level in the blood and urine is high; in salt-losing patients, an excessive amount of sodium is detectable in the urine.

TREATMENT

Treatment of excessive urination depends on the underlying cause. (See also *Urination, frequent.*)

Urination, frequent

The passing of urine more frequently than usual, also called simply "frequency". Most people pass urine an average of four to six times daily and only occasionally need to urinate at night. A marked increase in this rate constitutes frequency.

In some cases, frequency is the inevitable result of excessive production of urine (see *Urination, excessive*). In other cases, the total volume of urine produced is not high or may even be lower than usual.

Frequency is commonly due to *cystitis* (inflammation of the bladder) caused by infection. Reducing fluid intake in such cases has the effect of making the urine more concentrated (and thus more irritant), which increases urinary frequency. Sufferers from cystitis should drink more than usual, not less.

U

THE URINARY TRACT

Also known as the urinary system, the urinary tract consists of the kidneys, in which urine is formed to carry away waste materials from the blood; the ureters, which transport the urine from the kidneys; the bladder, where the urine is stored until it can be conveniently disposed of; and the urethra, through which the bladder is emptied to the outside. The kidneys require a large blood supply and are connected close to the body's main artery, the aorta. More than a litre of blood passes through the kidneys every minute.

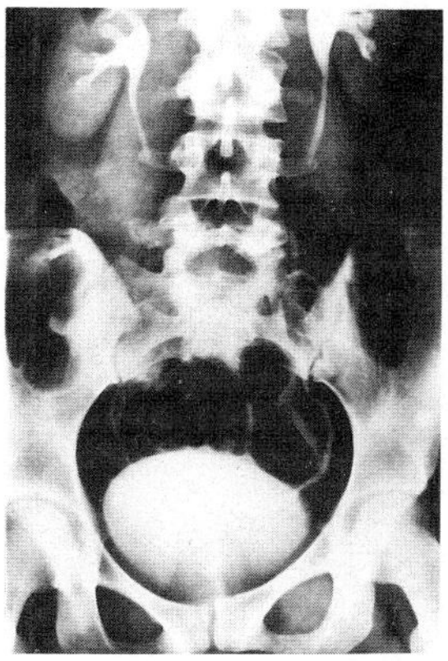

X-ray showing urinary tract

The X-ray on the left, taken using the technique of intravenous urography, shows (as lighter areas) the calyces and pelvis of each kidney, the ureters and bladder, as well as the bones of the lower spine and pelvic girdle.

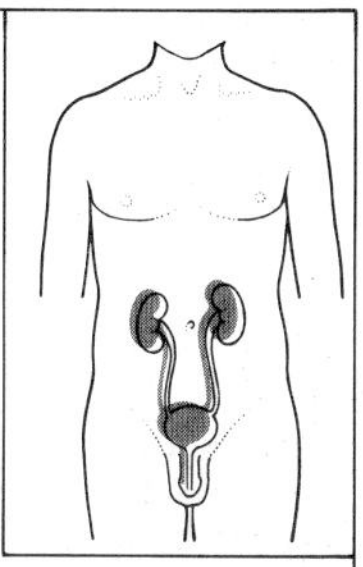

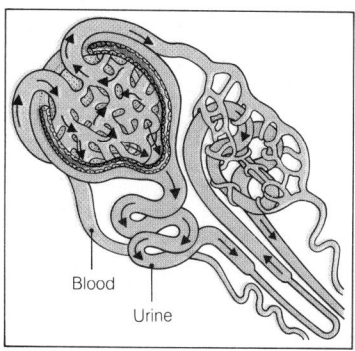

The filtering units
Each kidney has about one million of these units, which form dilute urine by filtering the blood.

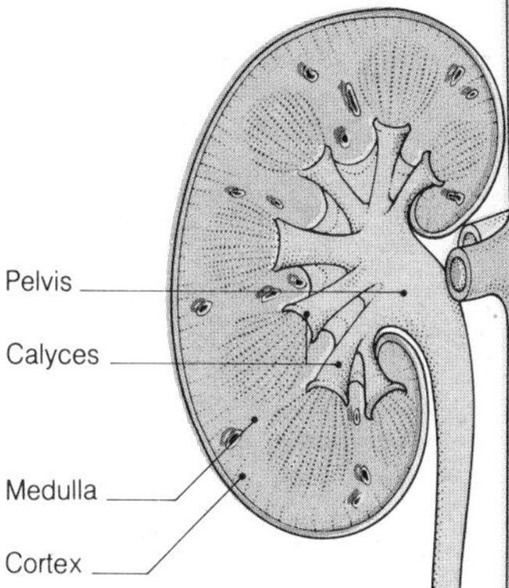

Blood

Urine

COMPOSITION OF URINE

Urine consists almost entirely of water, with only small amounts of urea (the main waste product), other waste products (e.g. creatinine and uric acid), and sodium chloride (salt).

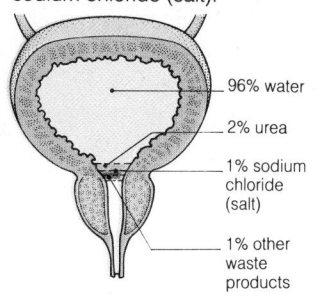

- 96% water
- 2% urea
- 1% sodium chloride (salt)
- 1% other waste products

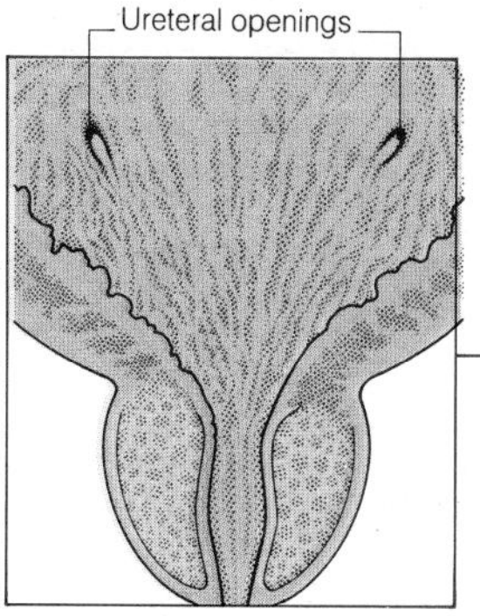

Interior of bladder
The two ureteral openings and the urethral orifice form a triangle at the base of the bladder. In males, the urethra runs through the body of the prostate gland situated below the bladder.

Pelvis

Calyces

Medulla

Cortex

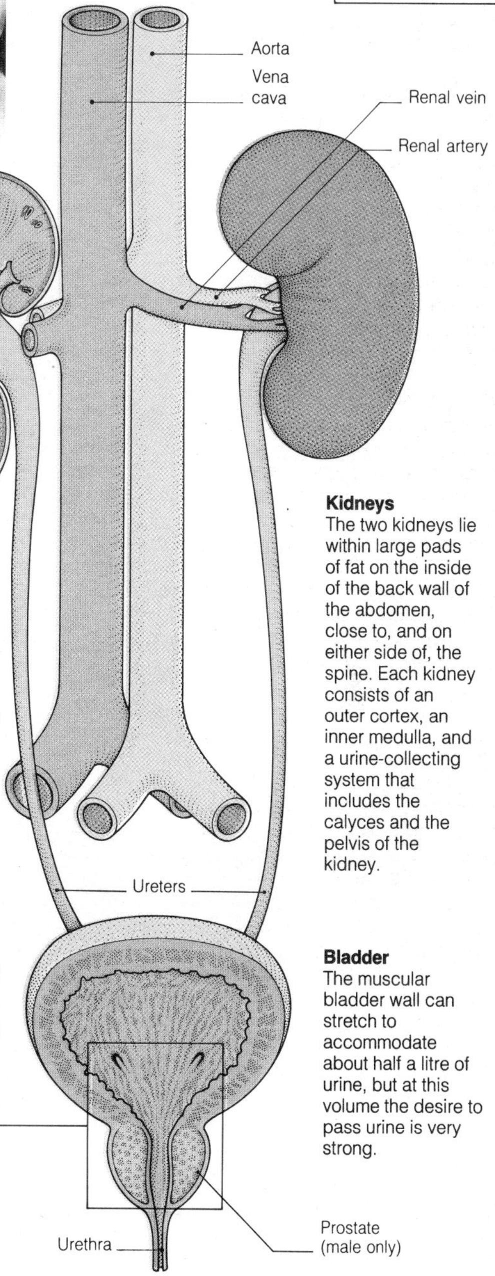

Collecting system

From the tubules that lead from the filtering units, much of the water and some other substances are reabsorbed into the blood. The remaining, more concentrated, urine runs into collecting ducts and then into the pyramid-shaped calyces of the kidney and the kidney pelvis. From there, the urine passes into the ureter.

Ureteral openings

Aorta

Vena cava

Renal vein

Renal artery

Kidneys

The two kidneys lie within large pads of fat on the inside of the back wall of the abdomen, close to, and on either side of, the spine. Each kidney consists of an outer cortex, an inner medulla, and a urine-collecting system that includes the calyces and the pelvis of the kidney.

Ureters

Bladder

The muscular bladder wall can stretch to accommodate about half a litre of urine, but at this volume the desire to pass urine is very strong.

Prostate (male only)

Urethra

U

Anxiety is a common cause of increased frequency. Other causes include stones in the bladder (see *Calculi, urinary tract*), an enlarged prostate gland (see *Prostate, enlarged*) in men, and, in rare cases, a *bladder tumour*. Some people who are suffering from *kidney failure* also notice that they pass urine more frequently, particularly during the night.

Treatment of urinary frequency is always of the underlying cause once it has been diagnosed.

Urination, painful

Pain or discomfort when passing urine, also known medically as *dysuria*. The pain is often described as having a burning or scalding quality. Sometimes it is preceded by difficulty in starting the flow. Pain after the flow has ceased, with a strong desire to continue, is called *strangury*.

The most common cause of dysuria is *cystitis* (inflammation of the bladder), especially in women. Dysuria may also be caused by a *bladder tumour* or stone (see *Calculus, urinary tract*), especially if blood clots or small stones or crystals are passed in the urine. Strangury is usually due to spasm of an inflamed bladder wall, but may also be caused by bladder stones.

Other possible causes of dysuria include *urethritis* (inflammation of the urethra), often due to *gonorrhoea*; in men, *prostatitis* (inflammation of the prostate gland) or *balanitis* (inflammation of the glans of the penis); and in women, vaginal *candidiasis* (thrush) or an allergy to vaginal deodorants.

Mild discomfort when passing urine may be caused by highly concentrated urine, which may result from fever or excessive sweating.

Dysuria may be investigated by physical examination, *urinalysis, urography*, or *cystoscopy*. (See also *Urethral syndrome, acute*.)

Urine

The pale yellow fluid produced by the *kidneys* and excreted from the body via the *ureters, bladder*, and *urethra*. Waste products and excess water or chemical substances are eliminated from the body in the urine.

URINE PRODUCTION

Urine is produced by the filtration of blood through the kidneys. The filtering units of the kidneys remove about 110 litres of watery fluid from the blood every day. Nearly all of this fluid is then reabsorbed into the blood; the remainder is passed from the body as urine.

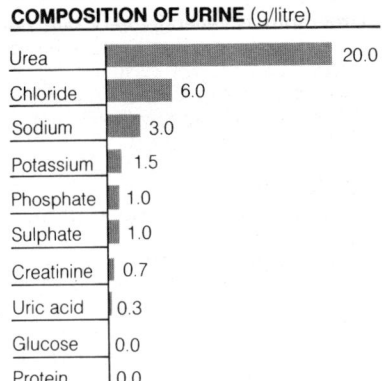

COMPOSITION OF URINE (g/litre)

Urea	20.0
Chloride	6.0
Sodium	3.0
Potassium	1.5
Phosphate	1.0
Sulphate	1.0
Creatinine	0.7
Uric acid	0.3
Glucose	0.0
Protein	0.0

Composition of urine
The chart shows the normal average contents of urine, other than water. The main waste products excreted are urea, creatinine, and uric acid. Variable amounts of sodium, chloride, hydrogen, and other ions are excreted to adjust the body's water, salt and acid-base balance.

A healthy adult may produce between about 0.5 and 2 litres of urine per day. The minimum volume of urine needed to remove all waste products is about 0.5 litre; any volume produced above this level consists of excess water. A high fluid intake increases the amount of urine produced; a high fluid loss from sweating, vomiting, or diarrhoea leads to reduced production.

COMPOSITION

The average composition of urine excreted by a healthy person is shown in the diagram.

The volume, acidity, and salt concentration of the urine are carefully regulated by hormones such as *ADH* (antidiuretic hormone), *atrial natriuretic peptide*, and *aldosterone*. These hormones act on the kidneys to ensure that the body's water, salt, and *acid-base balance* (acidity or alkalinity of the blood and tissue fluids) is kept within narrow limits.

Measurements of the composition of urine are useful in the diagnosis of a wide variety of conditions, from kidney disease and diabetes to pregnancy (see *Urinalysis*).

Urine is normally sterile when passed and has only a faint odour. The unpleasant smell of stale urine is due to the action of bacteria, which causes the release of ammonia.

Urine, abnormal

Urine may be produced in abnormal amounts or may have an abnormal appearance or composition.

ABNORMAL VOLUME

Production by an adult of more than about 2.5 litres of urine per day is unusual unless he or she is drinking excessively or has a disease (see *Urination, excessive*).

Abnormally low urine production (*oliguria*) of less than about 0.4 litre per day may occur in severe *dehydration* and in cases of acute *kidney failure*. It also occurs when the kidneys are not receiving their normal blood supply due, for example, to *heart failure, shock*, or advanced liver disease.

No production of urine by the kidneys (*anuria*) may occur in extreme cases of kidney damage. However, lack of the passage of urine from the bladder is more commonly caused by obstruction in the lower part of the urinary tract as a result of a *bladder tumour*, stone (see *Calculus, urinary tract*), or an enlarged prostate gland (see *Prostate, enlarged*).

ABNORMAL APPEARANCE

Cloudy urine may be due to a *urinary tract infection*, in which case it may have an offensive smell. Urinary tract calculi can also produce cloudy urine, which is not necessarily infected. Cloudy urine may be caused by the presence of certain salts, such as phosphates. In rare instances, *lymph* enters the urine and gives it a milky appearance.

Slight *haematuria* (blood in the urine) produces a smoky appearance. Larger amounts of blood produce easily recognizable red urine, which may contain clots. Red urine is not always due to blood, however. Some dyes used in confectionery may be excreted in the urine, and a wide variety of drugs can discolour it (for example, rifampicin turns urine orange). People who eat beetroot may pass red urine. In some patients with *porphyria*, the urine turns red if it is left to stand; in some patients with *jaundice*, the urine is orange or brown. Frothy urine, particularly if the froth persists after shaking, may contain an excess of protein.

ABNORMAL COMPOSITION

In *diabetes mellitus*, the excess glucose present in the blood spills into the urine, causing *glycosuria*. In *glomerulonephritis* (inflammation of the filtering units of the kidneys) and in *nephrotic syndrome*, there may be excess protein present in the urine (*proteinuria*). In *kidney failure*, the total amount of waste products in the urine (such as urea) is reduced.

Other kidney disorders, such as *Fanconi's syndrome* and *renal tubular*

U

acidosis, may make the urine too acid or too alkaline, or may cause it to contain excess amino acids, phosphates, salt, or water.

Urine tests

See *Urinalysis.*

Urography

A procedure for obtaining *X-ray* pictures of the *urinary tract* (kidneys, ureters, and bladder), also known as pyelography. The technique involves the introduction into the bloodstream of a radiopaque medium that shows up on X-rays when it is excreted by the kidneys, ureters, and bladder.

WHY IT IS DONE

Urography is performed, for example, to investigate recurrent *urinary tract infections, haematuria* (blood in the urine), and suspected stones (see *Calculi, urinary tract*).

Urography is also performed to discover whether kidney disease is the cause of *hypertension* (high blood pressure) in a young person.

HOW IT IS DONE

INTRAVENOUS UROGRAPHY (IVU) The patient is told not to drink for four hours before the IVU, and is given a laxative to empty the bowel.

With the patient lying down, X-rays of the abdomen are taken. An *iodine*-based contrast medium is then injected into the bloodstream via a vein in the arm, from where it travels to the kidneys and urinary tract. Further X-rays are taken immediately after the injection, and then five, 10, and 30 minutes later. Between the five- and 10-minute X-rays, pressure may be applied to the abdomen to improve the definition of the central cavities of the kidneys. After the bladder has filled with contrast medium, the patient is asked to urinate while another X-ray is taken.

RETROGRADE PYELOGRAPHY Under anaesthesia, a cystoscope (a type of viewing instrument) is passed into the bladder (see *Cystoscopy*). A fine tube is then threaded through the cystoscope and up the ureter to the kidney. A small quantity of contrast medium is injected and X-rays are taken.

RESULTS

The X-rays obtained by IVU allow the radiologist to see the size, shape, and position of the kidneys, the course of the ureters, the size and position of the bladder, and whether there are any obvious obstructions in the ureters. The X-ray taken after urination shows whether or not the bladder has emptied completely.

COMPLICATIONS

Urography is generally very safe, but must not be used in people who are sensitive to iodine. With retrograde pyelography, there is a risk of aggravating any infection that may be present in the urinary tract.

Urokinase

A *thrombolytic drug* prepared from human urine or from a *culture* of human kidney tissue. Urokinase is given to dissolve blood clots in people who have had a recent *myocardial infarction* (heart attack) or *pulmonary embolism*. Given by injection in the early stages of a myocardial infarction, urokinase may limit the extent of damage that is caused to the heart muscle.

Treatment with urokinase is strictly supervised due to a risk of excessive bleeding. Urokinase sometimes produces a mild allergic reaction that causes rash or fever.

Urology

A branch of medicine concerned with the structure, functioning, and disorders of the *urinary tract* in males and females, and of the *reproductive system* in males.

Problems that are investigated and treated by urologists include congenital abnormalities of the urinary tract, *incontinence, urinary retention, urinary tract infection, bladder tumours,* and stones (see *Calculi, urinary tract*). Many urological problems are treated by surgery.

Investigative techniques commonly used in urology include *urography, cystoscopy, ultrasound scanning, cystometry,* and *urinalysis.*

Urticaria

A *skin* condition, also known as nettle rash or hives, characterized by the development of itchy weals (raised white or yellow lumps surrounded by an area of red inflammation). Weals vary considerably in size, and large ones may merge to form irregular, raised patches. The rash is most common on the limbs and trunk but may appear anywhere on the body.

Urticaria usually lasts for no more than a few hours, but some people develop a persistent or recurrent form of the disorder. Urticaria sometimes occurs with *angioedema* (an allergic condition in which swelling occurs in various parts of the body). *Dermographism* is a less common form of urticaria in which weals form after the skin is stroked.

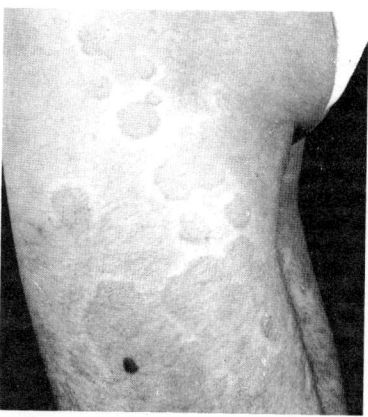

Appearance of urticaria
This skin condition is characterized by itchy weals with a white or yellow centre and an outer area of inflammation.

CAUSES

The cause of urticaria is often not known. Of known mechanisms, the most common is an allergic reaction (see *Allergy*) in which the chemical *histamine* is released from skin cells, causing fluid to leak from tiny blood vessels into the skin tissues. Urticaria often results from an allergic reaction to a particular kind of food (such as milk, eggs, shellfish, strawberries, or nuts), *food additive* (such as tartrazine, a food colorant), or *drug* (such as penicillin or aspirin).

Urticaria may also be caused by exposure to heat, cold, or sunlight. Less commonly, urticaria may be associated with another disorder, such as *vasculitis,* systemic *lupus erythematosus,* or *cancer.*

TREATMENT AND PREVENTION

Itching can be relieved by applying *calamine* lotion or by taking *antihistamine drugs.* More severe cases may require *corticosteroid drugs.* Identifying and avoiding known trigger factors can help prevent future allergic reactions. Even if the cause cannot be identified, however, a tendency to urticaria often disappears in time without any treatment.

Urticaria, neonatal

A very common skin condition, also known as erythema neonatorum or toxic erythema, that affects newborn infants. Neonatal urticaria consists of a blotchy rash in which raised white or yellow lumps are surrounded by ill-defined red areas of inflammation. The rash usually appears on the second day after birth, occurring predominantly over the face, chest, arms,

U

and thighs. The cause of neonatal urticaria is unknown. No treatment is necessary and the rash usually clears up within a few days.

Uterine muscle relaxants

Drugs used in selected cases to delay the premature delivery of a *fetus*. Beta-2-adrenoceptor stimulants, such as fenoterol and *salbutamol,* relax the muscle of the *uterus* in the same way as they act in *bronchial asthma.* Their main effect is to permit a delay of up to 48 hours, during which time treatment may be given with *corticosteroid drugs* to improve the chances of survival of the fetus. Treatment with uterine muscle relaxants may sometimes substantially postpone labour in the period between 24 and 33 weeks' gestation.

Uterus

The hollow, muscular organ of the female *reproductive system* in which the fertilized *ovum* (egg) normally becomes embedded and in which the *embryo* and *fetus* develop. It is also commonly known as the womb.

The uterus is situated in the pelvic cavity, behind the bladder and in front of the intestines.

STRUCTURE

The uterus of a nonpregnant woman measures 7.5 to 10 cm in length and weighs about 60 to 90 g. In shape, it resembles an upside-down pear. The lower, narrow part of the uterus opens into the *vagina* at the *cervix* (neck of the uterus); the upper part opens into the *fallopian tubes.*

In most women, the uterus is anteverted (tilts forwards) at an angle of 90 degrees to the vagina. In about 20 per cent of women, the uterus is retroverted (tilts backwards; see *Uterus, retroverted*).

The uterus is lined with *endometrium,* which is a specialized type of tissue that undergoes changes during the menstrual cycle. The endometrium builds up under the influence of hormones from the ovary. When hormonal support is withdrawn at the end of each menstrual cycle, the blood supply to the endometrium is cut off and the layer of tissue is shed (see *Menstruation*).

During *pregnancy,* the uterus expands in size to accommodate the growing baby. Muscle bulk also increases dramatically. At full-term, the uterus weighs about 1 kg, and the powerful uterine muscles expel the baby through the birth canal (see *Childbirth*).

After the *menopause,* the endometrium atrophies (becomes thinner), and the uterine muscle and connective tissue are reduced.

Uterus, cancer of

A malignant growth in the tissues of the *uterus.* Cancer of the uterus affects two main sites—the cervix (see *Cervix, cancer of*) and the *endometrium* (lining of the uterus). In rare cases, the uterine muscle is affected by a type of cancer known as a leiomyosarcoma. The term uterine cancer is more usually taken to refer only to cancer of the endometrium.

INCIDENCE AND CAUSES

In the UK, endometrial cancer is the third most common cancer of the female reproductive tract. There are about 3,500 new cases diagnosed annually, compared with over 4,000 new cases of *ovarian cancer* and over 4,000 of cervical cancer.

Endometrial cancer occurs more commonly in women who have had an excess of *oestrogen hormone* in their systems, particularly if *progesterone hormone* levels are low. Factors that may raise the oestrogen level include obesity, a history of failure to ovulate, or long-term taking of oestrogen hor-

---

ANATOMY OF THE UTERUS

The nonpregnant uterus lies deep in the pelvis immediately behind and above the urinary bladder and in front of the rectum. It is usually tilted forwards at an angle to the vagina, and is curved downwards slightly. When the bladder is full, the uterus is pushed up and back.

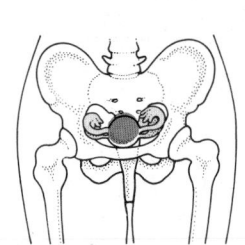
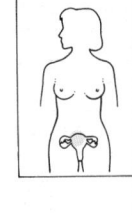

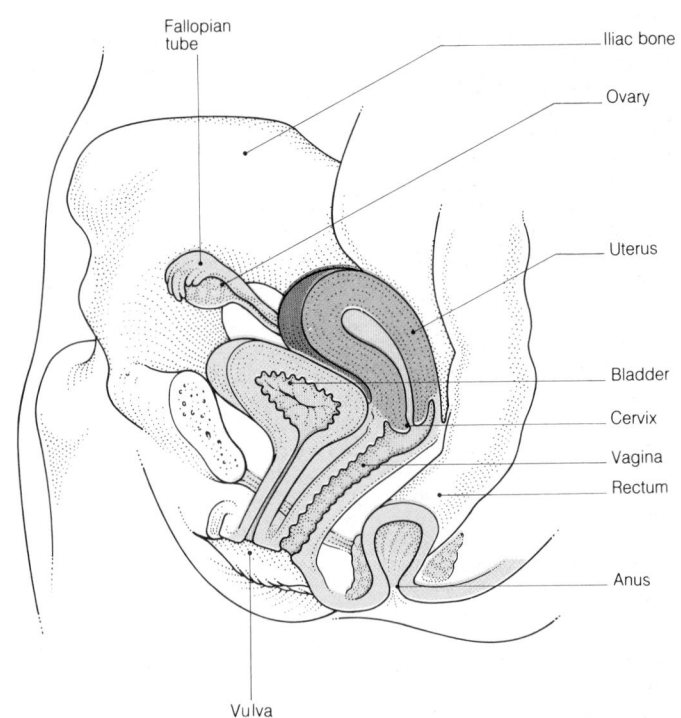

Fallopian tube · Iliac bone · Ovary · Uterus · Bladder · Cervix · Vagina · Rectum · Anus · Vulva

The uterus is a thick-walled organ that consists mainly of muscle. The fallopian tubes enter on both sides of the uterus just below its uppermost point. The small uterine cavity is lined with a mucous membrane called the endometrium, which undergoes changes during the different phases of the menstrual cycle. The cervix is lined with a flatter mucous membrane identical to that of the vagina.

U

DISORDERS OF THE UTERUS

Conditions that affect the uterus include congenital disorders, infection, benign or malignant growths, and hormonal imbalances that may affect menstrual flow.

CONGENITAL DISORDERS

In embryonic life, the uterus develops in two halves, which fuse along the midline. One per cent of women have a congenital malformation of the uterus, usually resulting from a fusion error. Malformation is not usually serious, but may predispose a woman to premature labour, *breech* presentation, or retention of the placenta after childbirth. Less commonly, the uterus may be absent, or there may be separate right and left halves, each with its own cervix and vagina. If a congenital malformation makes it difficult or impossible for a woman to conceive or to carry a pregnancy to term, surgical correction may be necessary.

INFECTION AND INFLAMMATION

Endometritis (infection and inflammation of the lining of the uterus) may originate in the uterus or be caused by infection spreading from elsewhere in the reproductive tract, such as the cervix or fallopian tubes. Endometritis may also develop if placental fragments are retained after childbirth or a *miscarriage*.

TUMOURS

Benign tumours of the uterus include *polyps* and *fibroids*. Malignant tumours include cancer of the endometrium (see *Uterus, cancer of*).

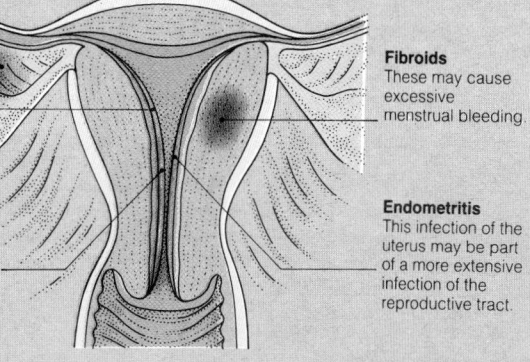

Endometriosis The lining of the uterus may grow in abnormal places.

Polyps These may arise from the cervix or endometrium. If polyps bleed, they require investigation.

Cancer of the endometrium This is a relatively common cancer in women; it causes abnormal bleeding.

Fibroids These may cause excessive menstrual bleeding.

Endometritis This infection of the uterus may be part of a more extensive infection of the reproductive tract.

Tumours may also affect placental tissue. Such tumours include *hydatidiform mole*, which is usually benign, and *choriocarcinoma*, which is malignant.

HORMONAL DISORDERS

Excessive production of *prostaglandins* by the uterus may lead to *dysmenorrhoea* (painful periods) or *menorrhagia* (heavy periods).

Hormonal disorders affecting the *ovary* or other organs may disrupt the normal build-up of endometrium during the menstrual cycle, causing menstrual disorders (see *Menstruation, disorders of*), especially *amenorrhoea* (absence of periods) or irregular, heavy bleeding.

INJURY

Injury to the uterus is rare, except following surgery, particularly an *abortion*. In rare cases, the uterus may be perforated by an *IUD*.

OTHER DISORDERS

The uterus may move from its normal position (see *Uterus, prolapse of*).

Adenomyosis (invasion of the uterine muscle by endometrium) may lead to dysmenorrhoea, menorrhagia, and pain during intercourse.

Endometriosis (the presence of endometrium outside the uterus) may be symptomless or may be associated with dysmenorrhoea, menorrhagia, painful intercourse, and *infertility*.

INVESTIGATION

A physical examination may be followed by *blood tests*, a *biopsy* (removal of a sample of tissue for microscopic analysis), imaging of the uterus by *hysterosalpingography* or *ultrasound scanning*, or *laparoscopy* (examination of the abdominal cavity through a viewing tube).

---

mones if these are not balanced by taking *progestogen drugs*.

Unlike cervical cancer, which is rare among women who have not had sexual intercourse, endometrial cancer may occur in virgins; it is more common in women who have had few or no children. Use of *oral contraceptives* lowers the risk of endometrial cancer.

SYMPTOMS AND SIGNS

The first symptom of endometrial cancer in a woman after the menopause is usually a bloodstained vaginal discharge. In a younger woman, the first symptom may be *menorrhagia* (heavy periods), bleeding between periods, or bleeding after sexual intercourse. A variety of other conditions can also cause such bleeding.

DIAGNOSIS

Diagnosis must be made from a sample of uterine lining obtained either by *biopsy* or by *D and C* (dilatation and curettage). A *cervical smear test* is not an effective screening test for cancer of the uterus.

TREATMENT

Very early endometrial cancer is usually treated by simple *hysterectomy* and removal of the fallopian tubes and ovaries. Some surgeons recommend removal also of lymph nodes in the pelvis and abdomen. If the cancer has spread, *radiotherapy* may be recommended. Treatment with *anticancer drugs* may also be used.

With early treatment, the five-year survival rate is over 80 per cent.

Uterus, prolapse of

A condition in which the *uterus* descends from its normal position down into the *vagina*. The degree of prolapse varies from first degree prolapse, in which there is only slight displacement of the uterus, to third degree prolapse, in which the uterus can be seen outside the vulva. Third degree prolapse is also known as procidentia.

Related conditions include *cystocele* (in which the bladder bulges into the front wall of the vagina); *urethrocele* (in which the urethra bulges into the front wall of the vagina; and *rectocele* (in which the rectal wall bulges into the back wall of the vagina). A general term for these conditions is pelvic relaxation. Prolapse of the uterus

U

PROLAPSE OF THE UTERUS

This condition is caused by weakening and slackness of the various ligaments, muscles and connective tissues that help to keep the uterus in position in the pelvis. Prolapse of the uterus, which is more common in women who have had children, may occur in conjunction with a rectocele or cystocele. There are three degrees of uterine prolapse, as shown below.

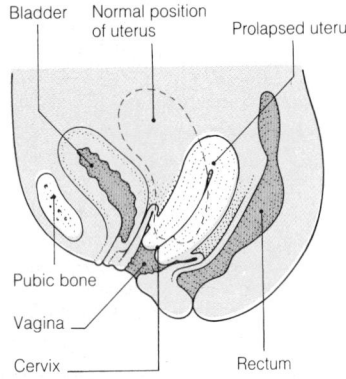

First degree prolapse
In this, the least severe degree of prolapse, strain causes the cervix (neck) of the uterus to move farther down in the vagina; however, it remains well within the vagina.

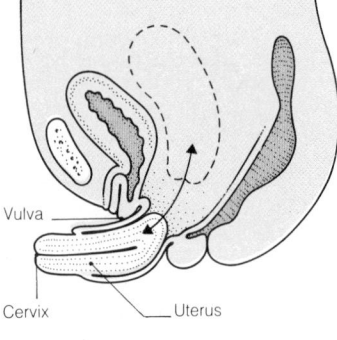

Third degree prolapse
The whole uterus projects outside the vulva. The surface of the cervix and the everted vaginal wall eventually dry out and are replaced by thick white tissue.

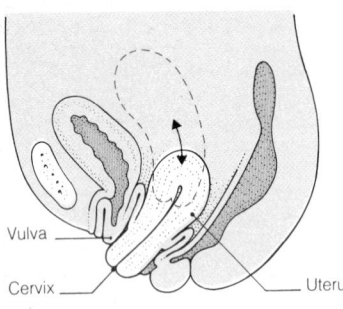

Second degree prolapse
The cervix protrudes beyond the vulva during straining, but retracts on relaxation. The vagina is partly everted (turned inside out).

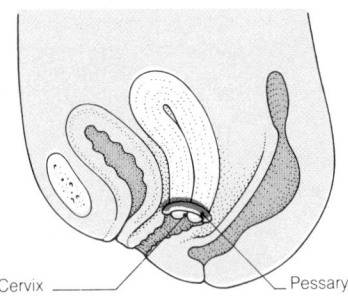

Treatment of prolapse
The uterus may be held in position by a plastic pessary inserted into the vagina; alternatively, a hysterectomy or vaginal repair may be performed.

wards. In severe cases, the uterus is visible from the outside. Other symptoms, such as leakage of urine or difficulty in passing urine or faeces, may result from an accompanying cystocele, urethrocele, or rectocele.

DIAGNOSIS
Prolapse of the uterus is diagnosed by physical examination. In some cases, it is discovered during a routine *pelvic examination*. Investigation of the urinary system may be necessary if the bladder is also prolapsed.

PREVENTION AND TREATMENT
Pelvic floor exercises strengthen the muscles of the vagina and thus reduce the risk of a prolapse, especially following childbirth.

If prolapse is severe, a vaginal *hysterectomy* (removal of the uterus through the vagina), along with tightening of the support ligaments and, in some cases, *vaginal repair* may be recommended. For women who do not want surgery, or who are not fit enough to undergo general anaesthesia, a plastic ring-shaped *pessary* may be inserted into the vagina to hold the uterus in position. Such pessaries need to be replaced under medical supervision at regular intervals.

Uterus, retroverted

A condition in which the *uterus* inclines backwards rather than forwards. A retroverted uterus was formerly believed to be the cause of various gynaecological symptoms. It is now generally considered to be a harmless variation of the normal.

CAUSES AND INCIDENCE
About 20 per cent of women have a uterus that is retroverted. Retroversion occurs in some women because the uterus has stayed in the retroverted position usual in infancy rather than becoming anteverted (tilting forwards) as it matures. In others, the position of the uterus changes after childbirth—either becoming retroverted when it was previously anteverted, or vice versa. Less commonly, retroversion of the uterus is caused by a disease, such as a tumour, scarring as a result of *endometriosis*, or *pelvic inflammatory disease*.

SYMPTOMS
Retroversion usually causes no symptoms, but an underlying disease may produce symptoms such as *dysmenorrhoea* (painful periods), painful intercourse, and *infertility*.

DIAGNOSIS AND TREATMENT
A retroverted uterus is diagnosed by physical examination of the pelvis (see *Pelvic examination*).

always occurs with some degree of vaginal relaxation, but vaginal relaxation may occur without any prolapse of the uterus.

CAUSES AND INCIDENCE
Normally, the uterus is kept in position by supporting *ligaments*. Stretching of these ligaments (for example, during childbirth) is the most common cause of uterine prolapse. Retroversion of the uterus (see *Uterus, retroverted*) makes such a prolapse more likely.

Prolapse occurs most commonly in middle-aged women who have had children, although it can occur in childless women. The condition was more common in the past when women had more pregnancies and were in poorer general health. Prolapse is aggravated by obesity.

SYMPTOMS
There are often no symptoms, but sometimes there is a dragging feeling in the pelvis or a sensation that something is being displaced down-

U

RETROVERTED UTERUS

In about 80 per cent of women, the uterus is anteverted (tilted forwards). In addition, the body of the organ is anteflexed (bent forwards). In simple retroversion, the organ is tilted back, but not bent back. A retroverted uterus may also be retroflexed (bent back). Retroversion may or may not cause symptoms.

ANTEFLEXION

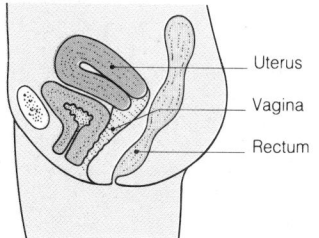

- Uterus
- Vagina
- Rectum

RETROVERSION

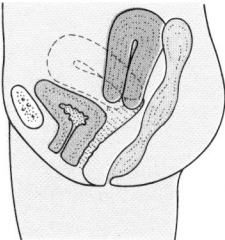

RETROFLEXION

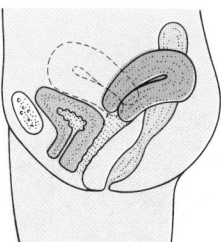

Anteflexion
The illustration shows the usual position of the uterus, lying bent and tilted forwards, at right angles to the vagina.

Retroversion
A retroverted uterus that can easily be anteverted by manipulation seldom causes any symptoms.

Retroflexion
If the retroversion and retroflexion are the result of disease, there are usually symptoms. Intercourse may be painful.

Treatment is unnecessary if there are no symptoms. In the rare cases in which a retroverted uterus does cause symptoms, the gynaecologist may manipulate the uterus into a forward position and then insert a plastic vaginal pessary to hold the uterus in place. If this procedure relieves the symptoms, surgery may be performed to change the position of the uterus permanently.

If an underlying gynaecological disease is suspected of being the cause of the retroversion, *laparoscopy* (examination of the abdominal cavity through a viewing instrument) may be suggested.

LOCATION OF THE UVEA

The uvea consists of the iris, ciliary body, and choroid.

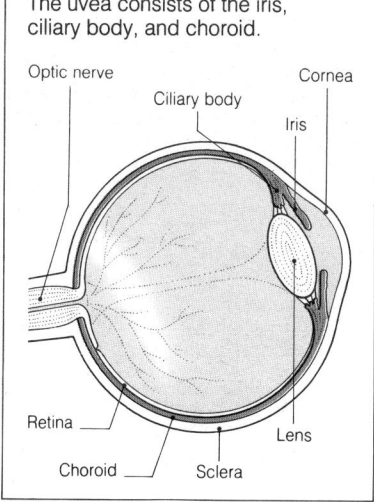

- Optic nerve
- Cornea
- Ciliary body
- Iris
- Retina
- Lens
- Choroid
- Sclera

Uvea

Part of the *eye*, comprising the *iris* (the pigmented area around the pupil), the ciliary body and its muscle that focuses the lens, and the *choroid* (the blood-vessel-containing layer just under the retina).

The uvea contains many blood vessels. In the iris, these supply the active muscles that control the dilation (widening) and constriction (narrowing) of the pupil. The blood vessels in the choroid supply oxygen and nutrients to the retina.

Pigment cells give the eye its colour and improve optical efficiency. In the uvea, pigment cells are concentrated in the back layer of the iris and scattered throughout the choroid. (See also *Uveitis*.)

Uveitis

Inflammation of the *uvea*, which may seriously affect vision. Uveitis may affect any part of the uvea, including the iris (when it is called iritis), the ciliary body (when it is known as cyclitis), or the choroid (when it is called choroiditis).

CAUSES

Uveitis is most commonly caused by an *autoimmune disorder*. Infections that sometimes cause uveitis include *tuberculosis* and *syphilis*.

TREATMENT

Treatment involves monitoring the inflammation with a *slit-lamp*. *Corticosteroid drugs*, usually in the form of eye-drops, are given to relieve inflammation. Eye-drops containing a substance related to *atropine* are given to block nerve impulses to the muscles of the iris and ciliary body. Other drugs may be given to treat uveitis that is due to infection.

Uvula

The small, conical, fleshy protuberance that hangs from the middle of the lower edge of the soft palate. The uvula is composed of muscle and connective tissue, with a covering of mucous membrane. Some people are born with a bifid (forked) uvula. This is of little significance, but may be associated with cleft palate (see *Cleft lip and palate*).

LOCATION OF THE UVULA

This conical fold of loose, wet tissue hangs down from the middle of the soft palate.

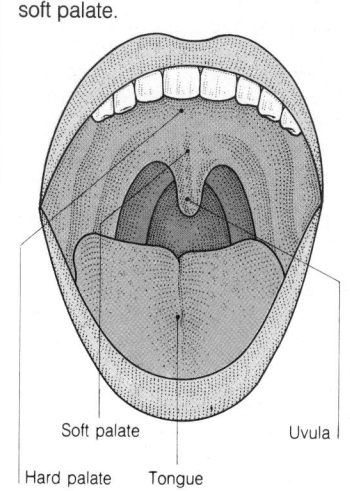

- Soft palate
- Uvula
- Hard palate
- Tongue

U

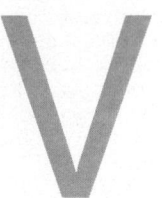

Vaccination

One of the main types of *immunization* (a procedure to stimulate or bolster the body's *immune system*). Vaccination is another term for active immunization, in which killed or weakened microorganisms are introduced into the body, usually by injection. These microorganisms sensitize the immune system so that if disease-causing organisms of the same type later enter the body, they are quickly destroyed through the action of *antibodies* or by other immune mechanisms.

Vaccination does not encompass the other main type of immunization procedure—passive immunization—in which ready-made antibodies are given by injection to provide short-term immunity.

Vaccine

A preparation given to induce *immunity* against an infectious disease. A vaccine works by sensitizing the body's *immune system* to a particular disease-causing bacterium, bacterial toxin, or virus. If the particular infectious agent invades the body at a later time, the sensitized immune system quickly produces *antibodies*, which help destroy either the agent itself or the toxin it produces.

Most vaccines are preparations containing the organisms (or parts of the organisms) against which protection is sought. So that these organisms themselves do not cause disease, they are killed or weakened. The term "live attenuated organisms" describes strains of organisms that have been rendered harmless. Attenuation is achieved either by artificially altering their genes or by successively infecting laboratory animals, thus producing small changes in the organisms which considerably reduce the ability of the organisms to cause disease without reducing their ability to induce immunity. Other vaccines contain chemically modified bacterial *toxins*. Again, modification removes the dangerous qualities of the toxin without affecting the immune features.

Vaccines are now available to protect against a wide variety of infectious diseases. Examples of live attenuated vaccines are those given to protect against *measles*, *mumps*, and *rubella* (see *MMR vaccination*), *yellow fever*, and *poliomyelitis*. *Diphtheria* and *tetanus* vaccines contain inactivated bacterial toxins. *Cholera*, *typhoid fever*, *pertussis*, *rabies*, and *influenza* vaccines contain killed organisms. *Hepatitis B* vaccine is now produced by *genetic engineering*.

Vaccines are usually given by injection into the upper arm. Oral polio vaccine is given on a sugar lump or by drops on the tongue. Some vaccines require several doses, spaced some weeks apart; others require only one dose. The effectiveness of vaccines varies from near total protection in most cases, to only partial or weak protection (for example, against typhoid fever or cholera). The duration of effectiveness also varies from a few months to lifelong. (See also *Immunization*.)

Vacuum extraction

An obstetric procedure to facilitate delivery of a baby. Vacuum extraction was introduced in the 1950s as an alternative to *forceps delivery*. It may be used if the second stage of labour (see *Childbirth*) is prolonged, if the mother becomes exhausted, or if the baby shows signs of *fetal distress*. Vacuum suction techniques are also used to perform early abortions (see *Abortion, induced*).

HOW IT IS DONE

Vacuum extraction is performed using an instrument called a ventouse, or vacuum extractor, consisting of a suc-

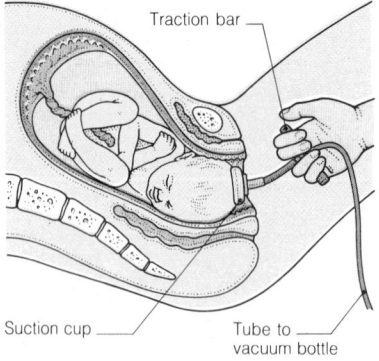

Traction bar

Suction cup

Tube to vacuum bottle

Technique of vacuum extraction
Once the suction cup is attached to the baby's head, the obstetrician pulls on the traction bar during each contraction, and the baby is drawn out through the vagina.

tion cup connected to a vacuum bottle. The cup is placed on the baby's head in the birth canal and the vacuum machine is turned on; this sucks the baby's scalp firmly into the cup. The obstetrician draws the baby out of the mother's vagina by gently pulling on the cup with each uterine contraction.

Delivery by vacuum extraction is generally slower than with forceps, but there is less risk of damage to the mother's genital tract. The baby is born with a swelling on the scalp, but this disappears after a few days, usually without treatment.

Vagina

The muscular passage, forming part of the female *reproductive system*, that connects the *cervix* (neck of the uterus) with the external genitalia.

STRUCTURE

The vagina is 7 to 10 cm in length, the back wall being slightly longer than the front. The vagina is H-shaped in cross-section. The muscular walls have a ridged inner surface and are richly supplied with blood vessels. The walls are usually in contact with each other, except during sexual arousal and intercourse when they become engorged with blood.

FUNCTION

The vagina has three functions. It is a receptacle for the penis during *sexual intercourse*, bringing sperm closer to an ovum for fertilization; it provides an outlet for blood shed at *menstruation*; and, during *childbirth*, it stretches considerably to allow the baby to pass through.

DISORDERS

Vaginal discharge is a common symptom, which may indicate a disorder in the vagina or cervix.

Congenital abnormalities include vaginal atresia (partial or complete absence of the vagina) and blocking of the external opening of the vagina by an imperforate *hymen*.

Infections (see *Vaginitis*) and prolapse of the vagina (see *Cystocele*; *Urethrocele*; *Rectocele*) are the most common disorders. Cancer of the vagina occurs very rarely.

In *vaginismus*, sexual intercourse and pelvic examination are rendered impossible by abnormal (and painful) spasm of the muscles around the vaginal entrance.

Vaginal bleeding

Bleeding, via the *vagina*, that may come from the *uterus*, the *cervix*, or from the vagina itself.

STRUCTURE OF THE VAGINA

The vagina has muscular walls, which are highly elastic to allow intercourse and childbirth; it has a ribbed inner lining that secretes a lubricating fluid during sexual arousal and intercourse.

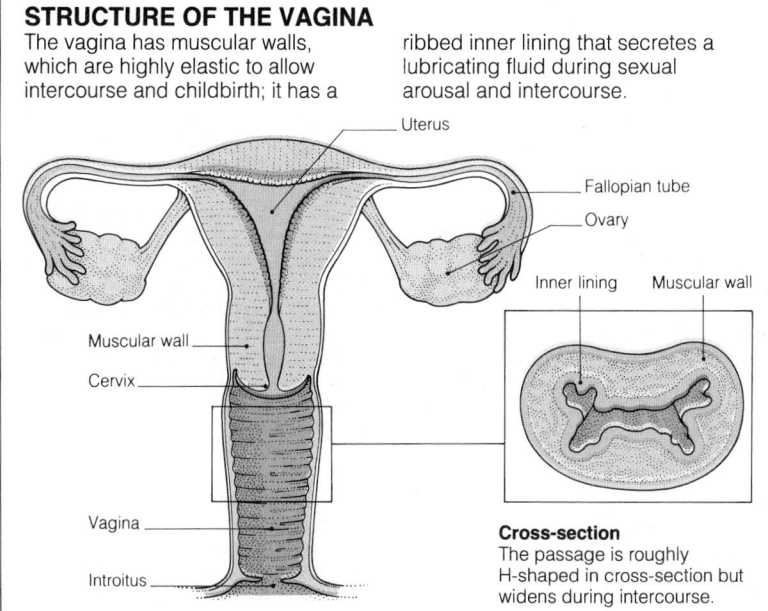

Cross-section
The passage is roughly H-shaped in cross-section but widens during intercourse.

The most common source of bleeding is the uterus and the most likely reason for it is *menstruation*. From puberty to the menopause, menstrual bleeding usually occurs at regular intervals. However, problems may occur with either the character or the timing of the bleeding (see *Menstruation, disorders of*).

Nonmenstrual bleeding from the uterus may be due to a variety of causes. Hormonal drugs, such as *oral contraceptives*, can cause spotting (see *Breakthrough bleeding*). Other possible causes include *endometritis* (infection of the uterine lining), endometrial cancer (see *Uterus, cancer of*), and *fibroids*. Bleeding from the uterus may also occur during pregnancy. In the early months, bleeding may be a sign of threatened *miscarriage*. Later in pregnancy, it may indicate serious problems with the placenta, such as *placenta praevia* or placental abruption (see *Antepartum haemorrhage*).

Bleeding from the cervix may be due to *cervical erosion*, in which case it may occur after sexual intercourse. *Cervicitis* (infection of the cervix) and *polyps* may also cause bleeding. More seriously, bleeding from the cervix may be a sign of cervical cancer (see *Cervix, cancer of*).

Vaginal bleeding originating from the walls of the vagina is less common than bleeding from the uterus or the cervix. The most likely cause is injury during intercourse, especially after the menopause, when the walls of the vagina become thinner and more fragile. In extreme cases, the vaginal wall in women after the menopause may be so fragile that bleeding occurs without any apparent precipitating cause. Occasionally, severe *vaginitis* causes vaginal bleeding. In rare cases, vaginal bleeding is caused by cancer of the vagina.

Any bleeding not caused by menstruation should be investigated by a doctor. Infections can be treated with *antibiotic drugs*. Breakthrough bleeding can be prevented by the adjustment of hormone dosages. Fragile vaginal walls can be helped by use of a cream containing *oestrogen drugs*. Growths, such as polyps, fibroids, or cancer of the uterus or cervix, may require surgical treatment.

Vaginal discharge
The normal or abnormal emission of secretions from the *vagina*.

Some mucous secretion from the walls of the vagina and from the cervix is normal in the reproductive years. The amount and nature of the discharge varies considerably from woman to woman and at different times in the menstrual cycle (see *Menstruation*). *Oral contraceptives* can increase or decrease the discharge, and secretions are usually greater during pregnancy. Sexual stimulation, with or without intercourse, also produces increased vaginal discharge.

Discharge may be abnormal if it is excessive, offensive-smelling, yellow or green, or if it causes itching. Abnormal vaginal discharge often occurs in *vaginitis*, and may be caused by various microorganisms. Infection with the fungus CANDIDA ALBICANS causes a thick, white discharge (see *Candidiasis*). Infection with the protozoan parasite TRICHOMONAS VAGINALIS causes a profuse green-yellow discharge (see *Trichomoniasis*). A forgotten tampon or a retained pessary may cause a profuse and highly offensive discharge. Very rarely, a vaginal discharge may occur in childhood; this is usually the result of infection or a foreign body. Abnormal vaginal discharge is often accompanied by vaginal and vulval itching.

Treatment depends on the cause. Infections are treated with an *antibiotic drug* or *antifungal drug*. Foreign bodies are removed.

Vaginal itching
Irritation in the *vagina*, which commonly occurs with *vulval itching*.

In many cases, vaginal itching is a symptom of *vaginitis*, which may result from infection or from an allergic reaction to chemicals in deodorants, spermicides, creams, and douches. Vaginal itching is very common after the *menopause*, when it is caused by low oestrogen levels.

Depending on the cause, treatment for vaginal itching may be with *antibiotic drugs* or hormones, sometimes taken orally and sometimes applied in the form of a cream.

Vaginal repair
An operation, also known as colporrhaphy, to correct prolapse (displacement) of the vaginal wall.

TYPES
There are two different types of vaginal repair operations: anterior colporrhaphy and posterior colpoperineorrhaphy. Either type may be accompanied by a vaginal *hysterectomy* if the uterus is also prolapsed (see *Uterus, prolapse of*).

ANTERIOR COLPORRHAPHY This operation is performed for prolapse affecting the front wall of the vagina.

The repair is performed through the vagina. A triangle of vaginal skin is removed, with its base towards the uterus. Supporting stitches are inserted through the skin at one side of the triangle, across the gap, and through the skin at the other side. The tissues are then drawn together, narrowing the vagina.

V

POSTERIOR COLPOPERINEORRHAPHY This procedure is performed for prolapse of the back wall of the vagina.

The repair is performed through the vagina. Triangles of skin are removed from the vagina and from the perineum (the area between the genitals and the anus), with the bases of the triangles at the vaginal opening. The perineal muscles are stitched tightly together and the skin on each side of the triangles is brought together and stitched, thereby narrowing the vagina.

Vaginismus

Painful, involuntary spasm of the muscles that surround the entrance to the *vagina*, interfering with *sexual intercourse*. When penetration is attempted, the woman's pelvic floor muscles tighten and virtually close the vaginal entrance, making penetration very painful; her legs may straighten and come together. This spasm also usually occurs when a doctor attempts a vaginal examination, which may therefore have to be carried out under anaesthesia.

CAUSES
Vaginismus usually occurs in women who fear that penetration will be painful. Often they have been previously unable to insert a tampon or a finger into the vagina. A traumatic experience with painful penetration, such as *rape* or a history of sexual abuse as a child (see *Child abuse*), may predispose a woman to vaginismus. Chronic *vaginitis* may result in painful intercourse and lead to vaginismus. Sufferers may also be particularly sensitive to the stretching sensation that occurs during penetration, which may trigger a spasm when intercourse is first attempted. A vicious circle of anxiety and spasm is then established.

In some women, a contributing factor may be underlying guilt or fear associated with the sexual act due to a restrictive upbringing or an inadequate sex education.

DIAGNOSIS
The doctor first examines the woman to ensure that she does not have any anatomical abnormalities of the *vagina* that might be causing pain, leading to spasm. Common causes of vaginal pain are infections such as *candidiasis* and, in older women, atrophy (thinning of the vaginal lining) due to low hormone levels.

TREATMENT
Any medical problem that is contributing to vaginismus is given appropriate treatment.

Vaginismus is commonly treated by use of a series of graded dilators, which the woman introduces into her vagina. Starting with the smallest size, she practises inserting and removing the instrument, also learning to relax and tighten her vaginal muscles with the dilator in place. Over the course of several treatment sessions, the size of the dilator is gradually increased until the woman is comfortable with the largest size (about the size of the average erect penis). Sexual intercourse can then be attempted.

Results of treatment are usually excellent, with the woman experiencing no discomfort during penetration. (See also *Intercourse, painful; Psychosexual dysfunction*.)

Vaginitis

Inflammation of the *vagina*. Vaginitis may be caused by infection, allergic reaction, hormone deficiency associated with aging, or the presence of a foreign body, such as a forgotten tampon in the vagina.

Vaginal infection is commonly caused by the fungus CANDIDA ALBICANS (see *Candidiasis*) or the protozoan parasite TRICHOMONAS VAGINALIS (see *Trichomoniasis*), both of which cause irritation and *vaginal discharge*. Another common form of vaginitis, known as nonspecific vaginitis, is caused by bacteria that normally inhabit the vagina. In nonspecific vaginitis, these bacteria multiply for unknown reasons (possibly through stress or a change of sexual partner) and cause an offensive, fishy-smelling vaginal discharge.

Vaginitis may also be caused by a reaction to the spermicidal creams often used with barrier contraceptives, to chemicals in vaginal douches, or to the ingredients of soaps, bath oils, or bath salts.

After the *menopause*, the lining of the vagina becomes thin and dry and prone to inflammation. Such inflammation, known as atrophic vaginitis, is due to a reduction in the production of *oestrogen hormones*.

TREATMENT
Infections are treated with *antibiotic drugs* or *antifungal drugs* as appropriate. In cases of allergy, irritant agents should be avoided. Any foreign body should be removed and any secondary infection treated with antibiotic drugs. Atrophic vaginitis is treated with *oestrogen drugs* in cream or tablet form. (See also *Vulvitis; Vulvovaginitis*.)

Vagotomy

An operation in which the *vagus nerve*, which controls production of digestive acid by the stomach wall, is cut to treat some cases of *peptic ulcer*.

HOW IT IS DONE
The operation is performed under general anaesthesia. An incision is made in the upper abdomen to expose the two branches of the vagus nerve, which lie in front of and behind the lower oesophagus. In many cases, all the nerve fibres of the vagus nerve are then cut (a procedure known as a truncal vagotomy). Less commonly, only some of the nerve fibres are cut (procedures known as selective vagotomy and highly selective vagotomy).

A *pyloroplasty* (surgical widening of the lower outlet of the stomach) or a *gastrojejunostomy* (surgical creation of a connection between the stomach and jejunum) is usually performed with either a truncal or a selective vagotomy (but not with a highly selective vagotomy). These accompanying procedures are needed to allow free emptying of the stomach because a truncal or a selective vagotomy interferes with the normal emptying of the stomach.

RECOVERY PERIOD
After the operation the patient is given fluids by *intravenous infusion*

TECHNIQUE OF VAGOTOMY
One branch of the vagus nerve acts to increase the secretion of acid and pepsin into the stomach. Vagotomy reduces this secretion and helps to heal peptic ulcers.

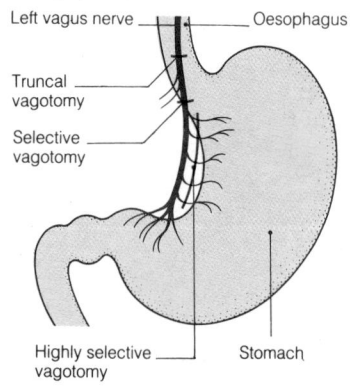

Left vagus nerve — Oesophagus
Truncal vagotomy
Selective vagotomy
Highly selective vagotomy — Stomach

Types
In a truncal vagotomy all the fibres of the vagus nerve are cut. In selective and highly selective vagotomies, only nerve fibres that supply the stomach are cut.

V

until the gastrointestinal tract can accept swallowed fluids (usually after two or three days).

OUTLOOK

The operation cures peptic ulcers in about 90 per cent of cases, but occasionally there are troublesome side effects, including diarrhoea and *dumping syndrome* (premature passing of food from the stomach into the intestine, causing a feeling of weakness and bloating after meals).

Vagus nerve

The 10th *cranial nerve* and the principal component of the parasympathetic division of the *autonomic nervous system*. The vagus nerve is the longest of the cranial nerves, and it branches most extensively. It emerges from the medulla oblongata (part of the *brainstem*), passes through the neck and chest to the abdomen, and has branches to most of the major organs in the body, including the larynx (voice-box), pharynx (throat), trachea (windpipe), lungs, heart, and much of the digestive system.

COURSE OF THE VAGUS NERVE

There are two vagus nerves, right and left. The right vagus nerve supplies the rear portion of the stomach; the left vagus nerve supplies the front portion of the stomach.

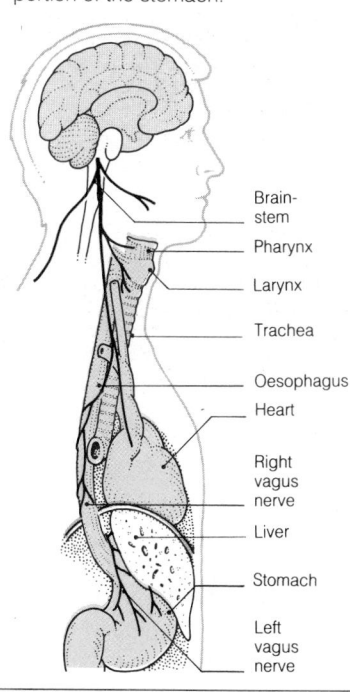

Brain-stem

Pharynx

Larynx

Trachea

Oesophagus

Heart

Right vagus nerve

Liver

Stomach

Left vagus nerve

The vagus nerve acts on target organs by releasing *acetylcholine*, causing narrowing of the bronchi and slowing of the heart-rate. Acetylcholine also stimulates the production of stomach acid and pancreatic juice; stimulates the activity of the gallbladder; and increases *peristalsis* (the rhythmic, muscular contractions that move food through the digestive tract).

Branches of the vagus nerve supply the muscles of the larynx and trachea and are thus involved in the actions of swallowing, coughing, sneezing, and speech quality.

DISORDERS

Overactivity of the vagus nerve increases the production of stomach acid, which is a factor in the development of a *peptic ulcer*. Some cases of peptic ulcer may be successfully treated by a *vagotomy* (an operation to cut part of the vagus nerve).

The vagus nerve may be damaged by an infection (such as *meningitis*), tumour, or stroke. In most such cases, the *glossopharyngeal nerve* (the ninth cranial nerve) and the *accessory nerve* (the 11th cranial nerve) are also affected. The possible effects of such damage include impairment or complete loss of the gag reflex, difficulty in swallowing, and hoarseness. In severe cases, death may result.

Valgus

The medical term for outward displacement of a part of the body.

Valproic acid

See *Sodium valproate*.

Valsalva's manoeuvre

A forcible attempt to breathe out when the airway is closed. Valsalva's manoeuvre may be performed without conscious effort or it may be carried out as a deliberate action.

The manoeuvre occurs naturally when an attempt is made to breathe out while holding the *vocal cords* tightly together. This happens when lifting a heavy object, straining on the toilet, and at the beginning of a sneeze.

When it is performed deliberately by pinching the nose and holding the mouth closed, Valsalva's manoeuvre is useful in preventing pressure damage to the eardrums because it forces air through the ducts leading to the middle-ear cavities (see *Barotrauma*).

Valve

A structure that allows fluid or semifluid material to flow in one direction through a tube or passageway but

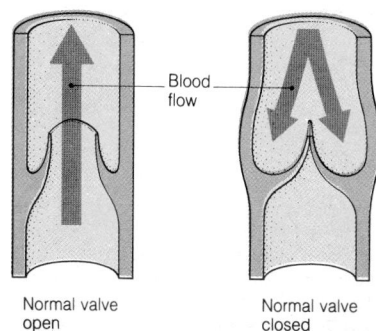

Normal valve open

Normal valve closed

Blood flow

Valves in the circulatory system
The valves are flaps that open to allow blood to flow in one direction but close to prevent blood flow in the opposite direction.

closes to prevent reflux in the opposite direction. The most important valves in the body are at the exits from the *heart* chambers and in the *veins*. By ensuring that blood flows in one direction only, these valves are vital to the *circulatory system*; without them, the circulation of blood could not occur.

There are also small valves in the vessels of the *lymphatic system*. The muscular rings at the junction of the stomach and duodenum and between the small and large intestines are also sometimes called valves. In fact, these structures are flow-regulating devices and do not prevent backflow.

Defects of the *heart valves* include stenosis (narrowing) and/or incompetence (inability to prevent backflow). Either defect can lead to *heart failure*. Incompetence of the valves in the veins—most commonly in the legs—causes *varicose veins*.

Valve replacement

A surgical operation to replace a defective or diseased heart valve. (See *Heart valve surgery*.)

Valvotomy

An operation performed to correct a stenosed (narrowed) *heart valve*. Cuts are made, or pressure applied, to separate the flaps of the valve where they have joined and thus to reduce the degree of narrowing.

In the past, valvotomy operations were usually performed, with the heart still beating, by means of a dilating instrument or even a finger introduced into the heart via an incision. Today, valvotomy is usually performed with the heart opened up (see *Heart valve surgery*). Balloon *valvuloplasty* is a newer technique for treating a narrowed valve without the need to open the chest.

V

Valvular heart disease

A defect of one or more of the valves in the heart. (See *Heart valve*.)

Valvuloplasty

A reconstructive or repair operation on a defective heart valve (see *Heart valve surgery*).

Valvuloplasty can be performed as an open-heart operation (in which the patient is connected to a *heart-lung machine* and the heart opened up). However, the newer technique of balloon valvuloplasty makes it possible to treat a stenosed (narrowed) valve without opening the chest. A *balloon catheter* is passed through the skin into a blood vessel and from there to the heart. Inflation of the balloon via the catheter may then help separate the flaps of a narrowed valve.

Vaporizer

A device for converting a drug or water into an aerosol (fine spray) so that medication can be taken by inhalation or so that inhaled air can be moistened. A common example of a vaporizer is an *inhaler*, used to administer *bronchodilator drugs* and *corticosteroid drugs* in the treatment of asthma and other respiratory disorders. Vaporizers are also used to moisten air breathed by children with croup.

Variant angina

A form of *angina* that causes chest pain at rest, often during sleep. The pain may be associated with breathlessness and palpitations. The cause is thought to be narrowing of the coronary arteries by muscular spasm in their walls. Treatment with *calcium channel blockers* or *nitrates* is usually effective.

Varicella

Another name for *chickenpox*.

Varices

Enlarged, tortuous, or twisted sections of vessels, usually veins. Varices is the plural of varix. A vein affected by varices is called a *varicose vein*. Although varicose veins can occur anywhere in the body, they most commonly occur in the legs. *Oesophageal varices* are enlarged veins in the lower end of the oesophagus.

Varicocele

Varicose veins surrounding the *testis*. Varicocele is a very common condition that affects about 10 to 15 per cent of men. It almost exclusively affects the left testis and is usually harmless, although there may be aching discomfort in the *scrotum* or an abnormally low sperm count.

Diagnosis is confirmed by examination of the scrotum while the patient is standing. The aching may be relieved by wearing an athletic support or tight underpants. Surgery to divide and tie off the swollen veins is sometimes performed if the sperm count is low.

Varicose veins

Enlarged, tortuous, or twisted superficial *veins* (veins just beneath the skin). Varicose veins in the legs are the best-known type. Examples of varicosities in other parts of the body include *haemorrhoids* (in the anus), *oesophageal varices* (in the oesophagus), and *varicoceles* (in the scrotum).

CAUSES
There are two main systems of veins in the legs—the deep veins, which lie among the muscles and carry about 90 per cent of the blood, and the superficial veins, which are often visible just under the skin and are less well supported by other surrounding tissues.

After oxygenating the tissues of the legs, the circulating blood is collected by the leg veins and pumped upwards by contractions of the leg muscles. The blood then passes, via connecting veins, to veins in the abdomen, which return it to the heart.

Valves in the veins prevent blood from draining back down the leg under the force of gravity. However, these valves must support a high column of blood and, in many people, they become defective, causing pooling of blood in the superficial veins, which become swollen and distorted. Factors that may contribute to the development of varicose veins include *obesity*, hormonal changes and pressure on the pelvic veins during *pregnancy*, hormonal changes at the *menopause*, and standing for long periods of time.

Thrombophlebitis (inflammation and clotting of blood in veins) or deep vein *thrombosis* (clotting of blood in the deeper veins) may sometimes be associated with varicosities.

INCIDENCE
Varicose veins are extremely common, affecting about 15 per cent of adults. Women are affected more often than men. The disorder tends to run in families.

SYMPTOMS AND SIGNS
The most common sites for varicose veins are the backs of the calves and the insides of the legs. The veins are blue, visibly enlarged, prominent, and tortuous.

Some people have no symptoms, but others experience a severe ache in the affected area (made worse by prolonged standing), swelling of the feet and ankles, and persistent itching of the skin. These symptoms become progressively worse during the day and can be relieved only by sitting with the legs raised. In women, symptoms are often most troublesome just before menstruation, potentially exacerbating premenstrual syndrome.

In severe cases, tissues in the leg become starved of oxygen and nourishment. This causes the skin to become thin, hard, dry, scaly, and discoloured, and may lead to the formation of *leg ulcers*.

Injury to a large varicose vein may cause severe bleeding. (Such bleeding can be stopped by keeping the affected leg raised and by applying moderate pressure; a doctor should then be consulted.)

DIAGNOSIS AND TREATMENT
Varicose veins in the legs are diagnosed from a physical examination performed while the patient remains standing.

For many people, the only treatment needed is the wearing of elastic support stockings, regular walking, as little standing still as possible, and sitting with the feet up.

In more severe cases, *sclerotherapy* may be carried out. The vein is first emptied of blood, then an irritant solution is injected into the varicose veins. After injection, firm pressure is applied to press the walls of the veins together. Compression is maintained by tight bandaging. The consequent scarring and blockage of the injected veins cause the venous blood to be diverted into other, healthy veins.

If varicose veins are very painful, ulcerated, or prone to bleed, they may require removal by an operation known as stripping (see illustrated box). The operation usually takes about half an hour. The patient must keep the leg bandaged for several weeks afterwards.

Both sclerotherapy and surgery are usually successful, but varicose veins may later develop elsewhere.

Variola

Another name for *smallpox*. The term variolation was once used to describe smallpox vaccination.

Varus

The medical term for an inward displacement of part of the body.

VARICOSE VEINS

When valves in the veins work correctly, the weight of the blood column is well distributed. When valves fail, some veins become engorged with blood and swell.

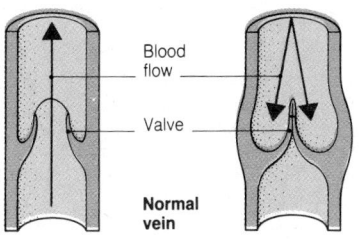

Blood flow

Valve

Normal vein

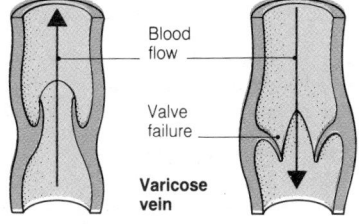

Blood flow

Valve failure

Varicose vein

How varicosities are caused
In a normal vein, valves stop blood from draining down due to gravity. If valves fail, blood is able to pool downwards.

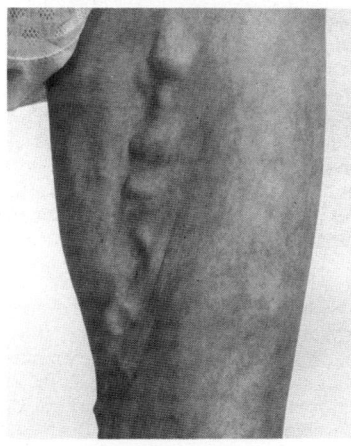

Appearance of varicose vein
This varicosity of the saphenous vein on the inside of the thigh shows the typical tortuous, swollen appearance.

STRIPPING A VEIN

Vein stripping is performed only in severe cases when the valves in the main surface veins are shown to be malfunctioning (and there are symptoms) or the skin is ulcerated. Visible varicosities usually occur in the branches of the vein and these may have to be treated separately.

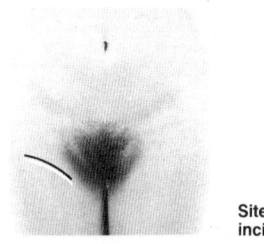

Site of incision

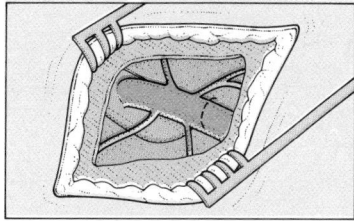

1 Here the greater saphenous vein and its four main upper branches are exposed by an incision in the groin.

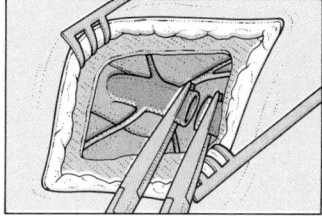

2 The vein is clamped and cut and both free ends tied off. The four branches are also securely tied off and cut. If branches remain, the operation may fail.

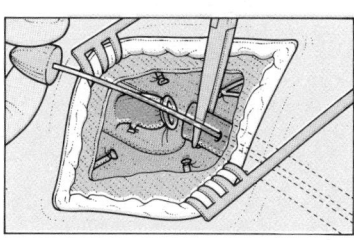

3 A small hole is made in the top of the vein and a flexible wire is passed down the vein to the calf or ankle and brought out through a small incision.

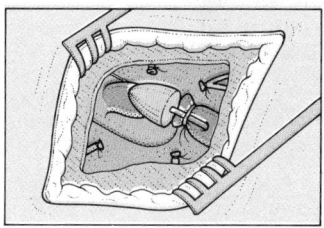

4 The upper end of the wire has a specially shaped metal head; the vein is tied firmly to the wire just below the head.

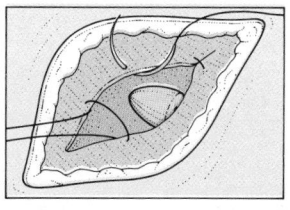

5 The upper incision is closed and the vein is then removed by pulling the wire out through the lower incision. The

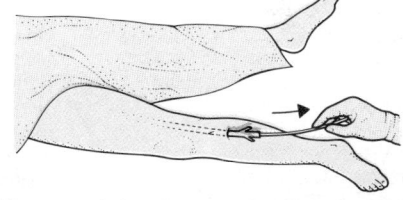

vein bunches up on the stripper and its branches tear off as it does so. Bleeding is not usually severe.

Vascular

Relating to the blood vessels (see *Circulatory system*).

Vasculitis

Inflammation of blood vessels. Vasculitis usually leads to damage to the lining of vessels, with narrowing or blockage, so that the blood flow is restricted or stopped. As a result, the tissues supplied by the affected vessels are also damaged or destroyed by *ischaemia* (lack of blood supply and, therefore, oxygen).

Vasculitis is thought to be caused in most cases by minute bodies in the circulating blood. These tiny bodies, known as immune complexes, consist of *antigens* (foreign materials, such as components of microorganisms) bound to *antibodies* that have been formed in response to the antigens. Normally, the immune complexes are destroyed by *phagocytes* (types of white blood cell), but sometimes they adhere to and settle in the walls of the blood vessels, where they cause severe inflammation.

In at least some cases, the antigens are known to be *viruses*.

Vasculitis is the basic disease process in a number of conditions, including *polyarteritis nodosa*, *erythema nodosum*, *Henoch-Schönlein purpura*, *serum sickness*, *temporal arteritis*, and *Buerger's disease*.

Vas deferens

A narrow tube on each side of the body that carries and stores *sperm* released from one *testis* and *epididymis*. The plural form of the term is vasa deferentia.

Each vas deferens is about 60 cm long and passes into the *prostate gland* at the base of the bladder to connect to a tube from the seminal vesicles to form the ejaculatory duct. Sperm and seminal fluid are passed through this duct into the urethra during *ejaculation*.

A *vasectomy* (male sterilization) involves blocking each vas deferens to prevent the passage of sperm.

Vasectomy

The operation of male sterilization. Vasectomy is a minor surgical procedure that consists of cutting the *vas deferens* (the duct that carries sperm from one testis to the seminal vesicle) on each side of the body. After the operation, the man continues to ejaculate as normal, but the *semen* no longer carries *sperm*, which are reabsorbed within the testes.

WHY IT IS DONE
Male sterilization provides a method of *contraception* that is safe and close to

---

LOCATION OF THE VAS DEFERENS
The vas deferens passes from the epididymis, up and around the bladder, before entering the prostate, where it connects to a tube from the seminal vesicle to form the ejaculatory duct.

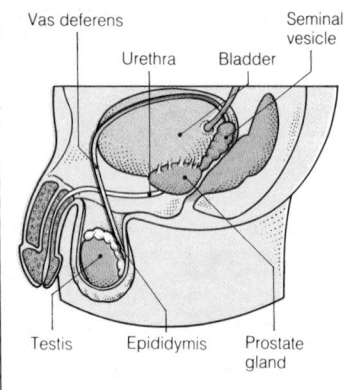

Vas deferens · Seminal vesicle · Urethra · Bladder · Testis · Epididymis · Prostate gland

---

HOW VASECTOMY IS PERFORMED
This operation blocks the passage of sperm from the testes but does not prevent the prostate and other glands from secreting the fluids that form most of the semen. Hence it has little effect on the volume of the ejaculate and no effect on orgasm.

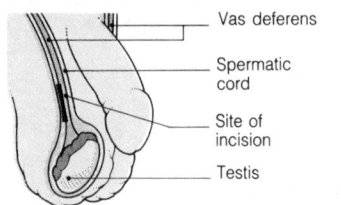

Vas deferens · Spermatic cord · Site of incision · Testis

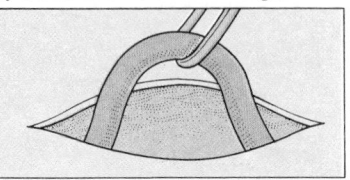

1 Incisions are made on both sides near the root of the penis; the vas deferens is cut free of the spermatic cord. Blood vessels are avoided.

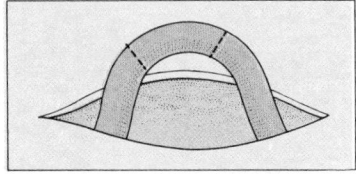

2 A loop of the vas deferens is freed and brought out through the incision. There are now several possibilities; usually, a length of the vas is cut out.

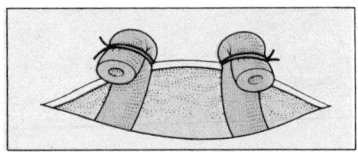

3 To prevent the cut ends from rejoining, they are often bent back and tightly closed with ligatures. They are then pushed back into the spermatic cord.

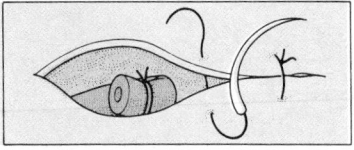

4 The skin incision is now closed with three or four sutures. When the local anaesthetic wears off, there is usually a mild, dull, aching pain for a few days.

---

100 per cent effective; the risk of problems or complications is lower than for female sterilization. However, vasectomy is often irreversible, and the decision to have it performed should be carefully considered by the man and his partner.

HOW IT IS DONE
The operation is performed on an outpatient basis under a local anaesthetic. The basic steps are shown in the illustrated box. The procedure takes 15 to 20 minutes.

RECOVERY PERIOD
The patient should rest for 24 hours. There may be slight bruising of the *scrotum* and/or bleeding from the external wound for a few days. To relieve any pain, *paracetamol* should be taken rather than *aspirin*, which can prolong bleeding.

Most men return to work within a few days, and sexual relations can be resumed as soon as the man is able, often within a week to 10 days. For two weeks, tight-fitting underpants or a jockstrap should be worn to support the scrotum.

After a vasectomy, a man remains fertile until the sperm already present in the vas deferens are ejaculated or

die. Only after two consecutive specimens of semen are analysed (about three months after the operation) and found to be sperm-free is a man considered sterile. Until that time, either he or his partner needs to use some other form of contraception.

OUTLOOK
In one in approximately 2,000 cases, sperm reappear (often long after the patient has been pronounced sterile) because the severed parts of a vas deferens reunite. If this occurs, the man can safely undergo another vasectomy operation.

Although most men who have a vasectomy experience no sexual problems as a result, the operation very rarely causes psychological problems that affect sexual performance. If *counselling* or *psychotherapy* fails to clear up these problems (or if a man strongly regrets that he has been sterilized) it may be possible to have the operation reversed. About 50 per cent of all reversal operations are successful.

Vasoconstriction

Narrowing of blood vessels, causing reduced blood flow to a part of the body. Vasoconstriction under the skin

V

occurs in response to cold and reduces heat loss from the body. It also occurs due to a fall in blood pressure in physiological *shock*. Vasoconstriction is also caused by *decongestant drugs*, which relieve *nasal congestion* by reducing blood flow to the lining of the nose.

Vasodilation

Widening of blood vessels, causing increased blood flow to a part of the body. Vasodilation under the skin occurs in response to hot weather and increases heat loss from the body. It also occurs as a response to *vasodilator drugs* and *alcohol*.

Vasodilator drugs

A group of drugs that widen blood vessels. Vasodilator drugs include *ACE inhibitor drugs, calcium channel blockers, nitrate drugs,* and *sympatholytic drugs*.

WHY THEY ARE USED

Vasodilator drugs are used to treat disorders in which abnormal narrowing of blood vessels reduces blood flow through tissues, impairing the supply of oxygen. Such disorders include *angina pectoris* (chest pain caused by inadequate blood supply to heart muscle) and *peripheral vascular disease* (poor blood flow in limbs).

Vasodilator drugs are also used to treat *hypertension* (high blood pressure) and *heart failure* (reduced pumping efficiency). Drugs of the vasodilator group are also occasionally prescribed in the treatment of senile *dementia*, although they rarely improve symptoms.

HOW THEY WORK

Vasodilator drugs widen blood vessels by relaxing surrounding muscles within the walls of the vessels; calcium channel blockers and nitrate drugs have a direct action on these muscles; sympatholytic drugs block the nerve signals that stimulate muscular contraction; and ACE inhibitors interfere with enzyme activity in the blood—an action that reduces the production of angiotensin II (a chemical that narrows blood vessels).

POSSIBLE ADVERSE EFFECTS

All vasodilator drugs may cause flushing, headaches, dizziness, fainting, and swollen ankles.

Vasopressin

An alternative name for *ADH* (antidiuretic hormone).

Vasovagal attack

Temporary loss of consciousness due to sudden slowing of the heartbeat, usually brought on by severe pain, stress, shock, or fear. A vasovagal attack, which is a common cause of *fainting* in healthy people, is a result of overstimulation of the *vagus nerve*, which helps to control breathing and blood circulation.

VD

The abbreviation for venereal disease, another general term for *sexually transmitted disease*.

Vector

An animal that transmits a particular *infectious disease*. A vector picks up disease organisms from a source of infection (such as an infected person's or animal's blood or faeces), carries them within or on its body, and later deposits them where they infect a new host, directly or indirectly.

Mosquitoes, fleas, lice, ticks, and flies are the most important vectors of disease to humans. When an organism develops or completes part of its life-cycle inside a vector, this vector is called a biological vector. For example, mosquitoes are biological vectors for malarial parasites, which develop and multiply inside the insect and are injected into the blood of a new host by the mosquito's bite.

When a vector is not essential to the life-cycle of a disease organism, it is called a mechanical vector. For example, flies may act as mechanical vectors of *shigellosis* (bacterial dysentery) by carrying the bacteria on their legs from infected faeces to food.

Vegetarianism

Eating a diet that excludes meat and fish, and sometimes all other animal products. Human beings do not need to eat meat or animal products to maintain health as long as the nutrients supplied by plant foods provide a balanced diet (see *Nutrition*).

TYPES

There are three main types of vegetarian diet. In a lacto-ovovegetarian diet all types of fish and meat are excluded, but milk, milk products and eggs are allowed. A lactovegetarian diet is basically the same, except that eggs are also excluded. A vegan diet excludes all foods of animal origin, including milk and milk products.

V

TYPES OF VASODILATOR DRUGS

The different types of vasodilator drugs work in various ways to prevent or reduce the contraction of muscle cells in blood vessel walls, thus helping to widen the blood vessels.

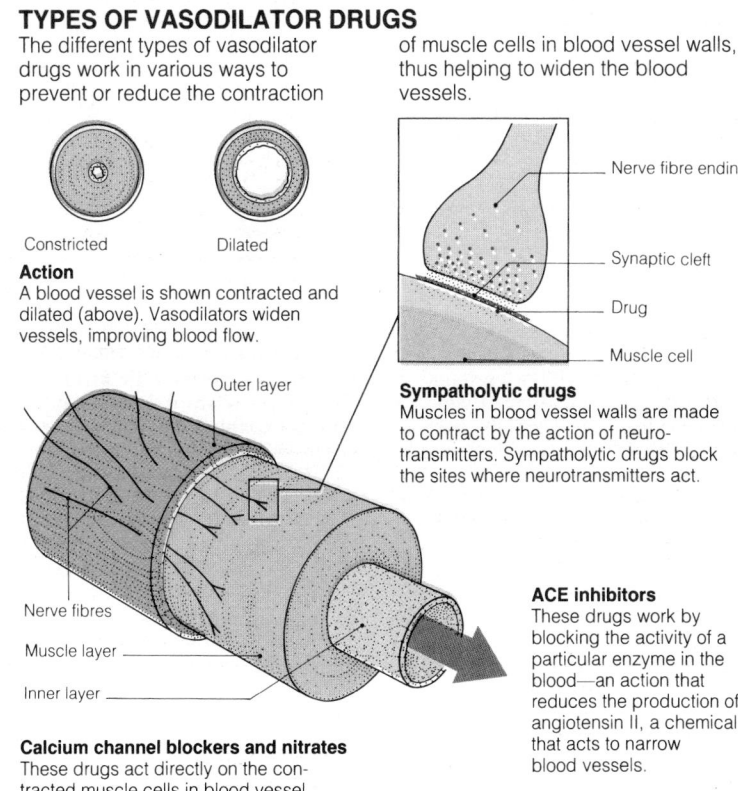

Constricted   Dilated

Action

A blood vessel is shown contracted and dilated (above). Vasodilators widen vessels, improving blood flow.

Outer layer

Nerve fibres

Muscle layer

Inner layer

Calcium channel blockers and nitrates

These drugs act directly on the contracted muscle cells in blood vessel walls, causing them to relax.

Nerve fibre ending

Synaptic cleft

Drug

Muscle cell

Sympatholytic drugs

Muscles in blood vessel walls are made to contract by the action of neurotransmitters. Sympatholytic drugs block the sites where neurotransmitters act.

ACE inhibitors

These drugs work by blocking the activity of a particular enzyme in the blood—an action that reduces the production of angiotensin II, a chemical that acts to narrow blood vessels.

DIETARY RISKS

Although animal products are not essential to the human diet, any restriction on food choice calls for special care. Problems have arisen on vegan diets from a deficiency of *vitamin B₁₂*, giving rise to megaloblastic anaemia (see *Anaemia, megaloblastic*) because this vitamin is found virtually only in animal foods. Nowadays, vitamin B₁₂ can be obtained from preparations made from extracts of certain types of yeast or from fermentation liquors.

Vegans, unlike lactovegetarians, cannot benefit from calcium-rich milk and milk products and must rely on less rich sources of calcium, such as grains, nuts, legumes, seeds, and dark-green leafy vegetables.

Although the iron in plant foods is poorly absorbed compared with that from meat, vegetarians and vegans do not appear to suffer from *iron* deficiency, possibly because their diets are rich in *vitamin C*, which assists the absorption of iron.

A properly planned vegetarian diet contains sufficient protein.

BENEFITS

Vegetarian diets are relatively rich in fibre (see *Fibre, dietary*), which may help protect against *diverticular disease* and cancer of the intestine (see *Colon, cancer of; Rectum, cancer of*). Vegetarian diets are also unusually low in *fats*, especially saturated fats which are considered to be a contributory factor in *coronary artery disease* and possibly in some forms of cancer. Vegetarian diets are also likely to contain less *sodium* and more *potassium* than that of a meat-eater, and there is evidence that vegetarians have lower blood pressures than people who eat meat.

Vegetative state

A term sometimes used to describe a type of indefinite deep *coma*. Although the eyes may be open and occasional random movements of the head and limbs may occur, there are no other signs of consciousness and no responsiveness to stimuli. Only basic functions, such as breathing and heartbeat, are maintained.

Vein

A vessel that returns blood towards the *heart* from the various organs and tissues of the body.

The majority of veins carry deoxygenated (blue) blood. This blood collects in small vessels called venules in the tissues. The venules join to form veins, which deliver the blood to the two largest veins in the body, the venae cavae. The venae cavae then carry the deoxygenated blood to the right side of the heart to be pumped to the lungs.

The main exceptions to this design are the pulmonary veins in the chest, which carry oxygenated blood from the lungs to the left side of the heart. Another special vein is the portal vein, which carries nutrient-rich blood from the intestines to the liver.

The walls of veins, like those of arteries, consist of a smooth inner lining, a muscular middle layer, and a fibrous outer covering. However, blood pressure in veins is much lower than blood pressure in arteries. Correspondingly, the walls of veins are thinner, less elastic, less muscular, and weaker. Veins collapse when empty, whereas arteries do not.

The inner linings of many veins contain folds, which act as valves, ensuring that blood can flow only towards the heart. The blood is helped on its way through the veins by pressure on the vessel walls from the contraction of surrounding muscles. (See also *Circulatory system*.)

Veins, disorders of

The most common disorder affecting a *vein* is a *varicose vein*, in which the vein becomes enlarged, tortuous, or twisted. Varicose veins occur most commonly in the legs, where they are caused by failure of the valves farther up the vein. *Oesophageal varices* are varicose veins in the lower part of the oesophagus. These commonly result from back pressure through the circulation from *cirrhosis* of the liver. *Haemorrhoids* are varicose veins in the anus.

Inflammation of a vein is called phlebitis. This condition is almost always associated with a tendency to blood clotting in the affected vein, in which case it is called *thrombophlebitis*. Clot formation in the small veins near the surface is not significant, although clots may cause swelling and tenderness. However, clots that form in deeper, larger veins (see *Thrombosis, deep vein*) may become widespread, increasing the risk that part of a clot will break off and block an important artery elsewhere in the body.

The blood pressure in veins is much lower than the blood pressure in arteries, causing an injured vein to bleed much more slowly than an artery of the same size. Bleeding from injured veins can usually be stopped by applying gentle pressure to the vein. It is also possible to stop bleeding from

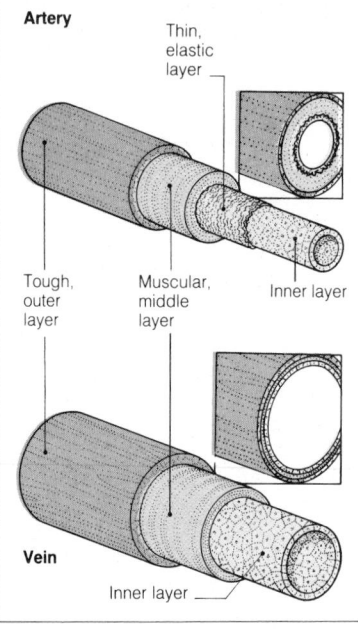

STRUCTURE OF A VEIN AND AN ARTERY

Like arteries, the walls of veins have a smooth inner layer, a muscular middle layer, and a fibrous outer layer. However, the walls are thinner and less muscular than those of arteries.

Artery

Thin, elastic layer

Tough, outer layer

Muscular, middle layer

Inner layer

Vein

Inner layer

veins (but not from arteries) by raising an injured part of the body above the level of the heart.

Vena cava

Either of two very large *veins* into which all the circulating venous (deoxygenated) blood drains. The two venae cavae (the superior vena cava and the inferior vena cava) deliver venous blood to the right atrium (one of the upper chambers of the *heart*) for pumping to the lungs. Each vena cava measures nearly 2.5 cm in diameter.

The superior vena cava starts at the top of the chest, behind the lower edge of the right first rib and close to the sternum (breastbone). It travels some 7.5 cm downwards, passing through the pericardium (outer lining of the heart) before connecting to the right atrium. The superior vena cava is formed from the right and left brachiocephalic veins, which themselves are formed from union of the subclavian veins (draining blood from the arms), the jugular veins (draining blood from the head), and several minor veins. The superior vena cava also receives blood from the azygos vein, which

V

drains much of the chest. The superior vena cava thus collects blood from the whole of a person's upper trunk, head, neck, and arms.

The inferior vena cava starts in the lower abdomen, in front of the fifth lumbar vertebra, and travels some 25 cm upwards in front of the spine, behind the liver, and through the diaphragm before joining to the right atrium. It is formed from the union of the two common iliac veins, which receive blood from the legs and pelvic organs. The inferior vena cava also receives blood from the hepatic vein, which drains the liver, and the renal veins, which drain the kidneys.

Venepuncture

A common procedure in which a *vein* is pierced with a needle to withdraw blood or to inject fluid. It is usually performed on a vein in the forearm.

HOW IT IS DONE

A *tourniquet* is applied to the upper arm, causing the veins to swell. A suitable vein, usually a large one that can be easily felt through the skin, is selected. The overlying skin is cleaned with alcohol, and a sterile needle is inserted into the vein. For taking blood or injecting medication, the needle has a syringe attached. For *intravenous infusion*, a cannula (narrow tube) is inserted into the vein via the needle; the needle is then withdrawn, and tubing for the fluid to flow through is attached to the cannula.

After the required amount of fluid has been injected or withdrawn, the needle or cannula is removed. The area is then covered with a piece of cottonwool and firm pressure applied for a minute or two until any bleeding has stopped.

Venepuncture is not usually painful but may cause some discomfort. Slight bruising may appear at the venepuncture site but usually fades in a few days.

Venereal diseases

See *Sexually transmitted diseases*.

Venereology

The medical discipline concerned with the study and treatment of *sexually transmitted diseases*.

Venesection

The process of withdrawing blood from a *vein*, also called phlebotomy, for *blood donation* or for therapeutic bloodletting. Regular bloodletting is used in the treatment of *polycythaemia* (a disorder in which the blood is too thick); in *haemochromatosis* (a disorder of body iron chemistry) to reduce the amount of iron in the body; and very occasionally in some types of *heart failure* to reduce the blood volume and ease the heart's workload.

Venography

A diagnostic procedure, also known as phlebography, that enables *veins* to be seen on an *X-ray* film after they have been injected with a substance opaque to X-rays.

WHY IT IS DONE

Venography is used to detect anatomical abnormalities or diseases of the veins themselves—such as narrowing or blockage from *thrombosis* (abnormal clot formation) or a tumour—as well as disease or injury in organs that are supplied by the veins. The procedure is also used to evaluate the extent of disease before planning treatment.

The veins most frequently studied are those in the leg, usually because of suspected deep vein thrombosis (see *Thrombosis, deep vein*). Other commonly studied veins include the axillary veins in the arm, the superior and inferior venae cavae (the main veins leading to the heart), and the renal veins (leading from the kidney).

HOW IT IS DONE

Contrast medium is injected either through a needle directly into the veins to be examined or, if the veins are not readily accessible, through a catheter that has been guided, under X-ray control, along the venous system to the required vein. A sequence of X-ray pictures is taken so that blood flow along the veins can be studied. Leg venography takes about 20 minutes to perform; other types may take longer.

The newer technique of digital subtraction *angiography* adds to the information obtained through use of computer analysis to process images and remove unwanted shadowing.

LOCATION OF THE VENAE CAVAE

All the circulating blood, after being pumped to the body, returns to the heart via the venae cavae. The superior vena cava collects blood from the whole of the upper trunk, head, neck, and arms. The inferior vena cava drains blood from all parts of the body below the chest.

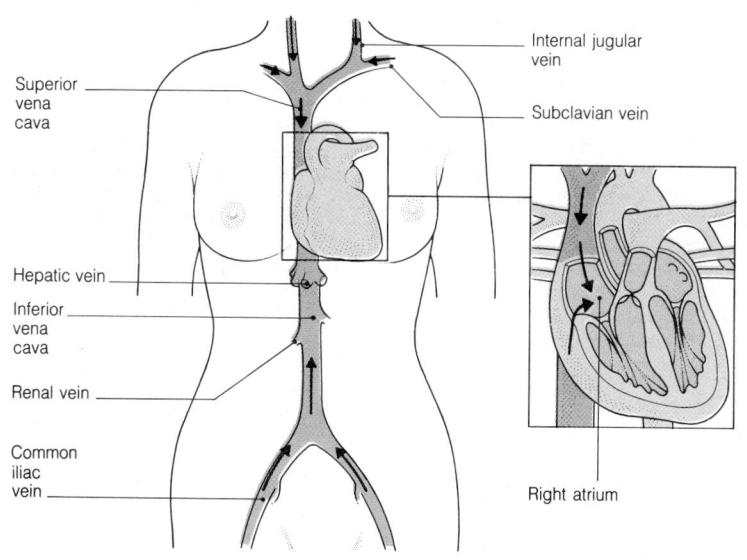

Superior vena cava

Hepatic vein

Inferior vena cava

Renal vein

Common iliac vein

Internal jugular vein

Subclavian vein

Right atrium

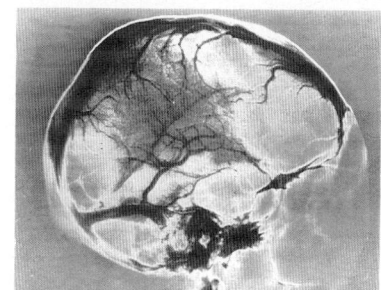

Venogram showing veins within the skull
This X-ray image of a skull shows both the veins and the venous sinuses (dark areas), which are wide blood drainage channels.

Venomous bites and stings

The injection of venom (poison) by certain animals via their mouthparts (bites) or some other injecting apparatus (stings). Often, these venoms are carried for purely defensive purposes to discourage predators. Sometimes they are used to kill or immobilize prey. It is rare for a venomous animal to attack a person unless cornered, provoked, stepped on, or otherwise disturbed.

Specific *antivenoms* are available to treat many, though not all, animal venoms. In cases of serious poisoning, administration of antivenom can sometimes be life-saving.

TYPES OF VENOMOUS ANIMAL

For the better known types of venomous bites and stings, see *Insect stings*; *Jellyfish stings*; *Scorpion stings*; *Snake bites*; *Spider bites*. Other venomous animals include certain species of centipedes, millipedes, and fish.

CENTIPEDES AND MILLIPEDES Centipede bites can cause severe pain and local swelling but are not a danger to life. Certain millipedes secrete, and sometimes squirt out, an irritating liquid that may be dangerous if it enters the eyes. First aid is by thorough irrigation with water.

FISH STINGS Venomous fish inflict stings by means of certain fins or specialized spines on their bodies. Examples of venomous fish include weeverfish, scorpion fish, lionfish, and stonefish. Of these, only weeverfish are found off the coast of the UK; most of the venomous species of fish live in tropical waters, where they are a danger to swimmers, waders, snorkellers, and scuba divers.

Ventilation

The use of a machine called a *ventilator* to take over *breathing*, and thus maintain life, in a person who lacks or who has lost the ability to breathe in the natural way.

WHY IT IS DONE

Arrested or severe impairment of breathing may be caused by damage to the respiratory centre in the *brainstem* due to *head injury*, brain disease, or an overdose of *narcotic drugs*. Breathing difficulties may also be due to damage to or malfunctioning of the breathing mechanism as a result of chest injury, respiratory disease, a nerve or muscle disorder, or major chest or abdominal surgery. Occasionally, difficulties arise as a result of problems during general *anaesthesia*. Severely premature babies with *respiratory distress syndrome* may also need ventilation for a period until their lungs develop sufficiently to cope with breathing unaided.

HOW IT IS DONE

Artificial ventilation is usually carried out in an *intensive-care* unit or *operating theatre*. The patient is connected to the ventilator by means of an *endotracheal tube* passed through the nose or mouth into the trachea (windpipe); if prolonged ventilation is likely to be required, a tube is inserted into an opening made in the trachea, an operation called a *tracheostomy*. Conscious patients, and those nearing the end of anaesthesia, are usually given muscle-relaxant and sedative drugs to prevent them from resisting the insertion and irritant presence of the tube.

During ventilation, the patient's *blood gases* (the amount of oxygen and other gases in the patient's blood) are checked by analysing blood samples; *X-rays* are taken to assess the state of the lungs; and the pulse, blood pressure, heart rhythm, and temperature are monitored.

The patient is unable to eat or drink when connected to the ventilator. Fluids are therefore given by *intravenous infusion*. Drugs may need to be given in the same way.

The patient's inability to cough may cause secretions to accumulate in the lungs. These are removed by suction apparatus, and intensive *physiotherapy* is given to prevent the secretions from building up again.

When the patient begins to recover, he or she is disconnected from the ventilator and allowed to breathe naturally for increasingly longer and more frequent periods. After the blood gases have returned to a normal level during spontaneous breathing, the patient is taken off the ventilator permanently.

Ventilator

A device, also known as a respirator or a life-support machine, used for the artificial *ventilation* of a patient who lacks or who has lost the ability to breathe naturally.

A ventilator is an electrical pump connected to an air supply that works like bellows. The pump can be adjusted to vary the proportion of oxygen in the pumped air and to regulate the amount of air delivered according to the needs of the patient. The air is pumped through a humidifier, which adds sterile water vapour to prevent the lungs from drying out;

TECHNIQUE OF ARTIFICIAL VENTILATION

Machine-assisted breathing may be needed when a person has lost the ability to breathe naturally—often following a severe head injury, narcotic drug overdose, or in various other medical emergencies. It may also be needed when a muscle relaxant has been given during an operation as part of a general anaesthetic.

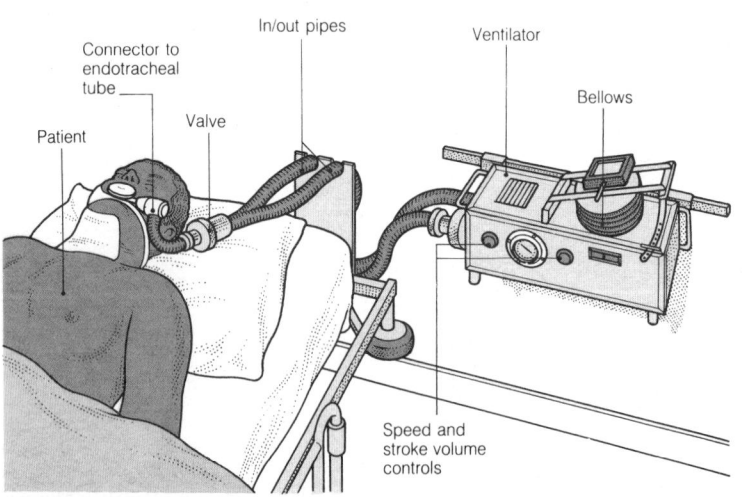

Connector to endotracheal tube

In/out pipes

Ventilator

Patient

Valve

Bellows

Speed and stroke volume controls

Procedure
The air is delivered to the patient's lungs via a tube inserted into the windpipe. After each inflation, the air is expelled by the natural elasticity of the lungs. Fluids and drugs must be given to the patient by intravenous infusion.

V

the air is directed through a tube passed down the patient's trachea (windpipe) to inflate the lungs. The air is then expelled by the natural elasticity of the lungs and rib-cage. A valve on the ventilator prevents the expelled air from re-entering the lungs.

Ventilatory failure

A life-threatening condition in which the amount of carbon dioxide in the blood rises and the amount of oxygen falls due to disruption of the normal exchange of gases between the air in the lungs and the blood. Ventilatory failure may be due to lung damage, which reduces the area through which gas exchange can occur. Treatment may be given in the form of drugs to stimulate respiration or by artificial *ventilation*. (See also *Respiratory failure*.)

Ventouse

See *Vacuum extraction*.

Ventral

Relating to the front of the body, or describing the lowermost part of a body structure when a person is lying face-down. In human anatomy, ventral means the same as anterior. The opposite of ventral is *dorsal* (or posterior).

Ventricle

A cavity or chamber. Both the *heart* and *brain* have anatomical parts known as ventricles.

The brain has four ventricles: one in each of the two cerebral hemispheres (which make up the cerebrum, or main mass of the brain); a third at the centre of the brain, above the brainstem; and a fourth situated between the brainstem and the cerebellum. These cavities are filled with cerebrospinal fluid and are linked by ducts so that the fluid can circulate through them. The cavities are lined in part with tuft-like clusters of blood vessels called the choroid plexus, derived from vessels in the *meninges*, which secrete the *cerebrospinal fluid*.

The heart has two ventricles. These are the lower, pumping chambers of the heart, which receive blood from the atria (upper heart chambers) and pump it to the lungs and to the rest of the body.

Ventricular ectopic beat

A type of cardiac *arrhythmia* (abnormal heart rhythm) in which abnormal heartbeats are initiated from electrical impulses in the *ventricles* (lower chambers of the *heart*). In the normal heart, beats are initiated from electrical impulses in the sinoatrial node in the right atrium (upper heart chamber).

CAUSES

Many people, especially older people, have occasional ventricular ectopic beats that do not signify any disorder. Ventricular ectopic beats may be also caused by *myocardial infarction* (heart

attack), *heart failure,* disturbances of body chemistry, or *digitalis drugs.*

SYMPTOMS

Ventricular ectopic beats often cause no symptoms. Sometimes, a ventricular ectopic beat causes the sensation that the heart has stopped for a second and then restarts with a thump.

DIAGNOSIS AND TREATMENT

Ventricular ectopic beats may be detected on an *ECG* (measurement of electrical activity of the heart) as a broad, bizarre-looking wave (see illustrated box overleaf).

If a person has frequent ventricular ectopic beats that cause symptoms, or has beats that arise from more than one site in the ventricles, treatment with an *antiarrhythmic drug* may be required.

Ventricular fibrillation

A life-threatening cardiac *arrhythmia* (abnormal heart rhythm) in which the *heart* has rapid, uncoordinated, and ineffective contractions. Ventricular fibrillation is caused by abnormal *heartbeats* initiated by electrical activity in the ventricles (lower heart chambers). It is a common complication of *myocardial infarction* (heart attack) and may also be caused by electrocution or drowning. The heart ceases to pump blood effectively and the condition is fatal unless the normal heart rhythm is quickly restored.

The diagnosis of ventricular fibrillation is confirmed by *ECG* (measurement of electrical activity of the heart) which shows broad, irregular waves (see illustrated box overleaf).

Treatment is with *defibrillation* (administration of an electric shock to the heart) and *antiarrhythmic drugs*. *Cardiopulmonary resuscitation* may be an interim life-saving measure.

Ventricular tachycardia

A serious cardiac *arrhythmia* (abnormal heart rhythm) in which each heartbeat is initiated from electrical activity in the ventricles (lower heart chambers) rather than the sinoatrial node in the right atrium (upper heart chamber). The result is an abnormally fast heart-rate of between 140 and 220 beats per minute.

Ventricular tachycardia is caused by serious heart disease, such as *myocardial infarction* (heart attack) or *cardiomyopathy*. It may last for a few seconds or for several days. Diagnosis is confirmed by *ECG* (recording of the electrical activity of the heart), which shows broad, regular abnormal waves (see illustrated box overleaf).

LOCATION OF THE VENTRICLES

The location of the ventricles in the brain (seen from above) and in the heart are shown below. Of the heart ventricles, the right ventricle pumps blood to the lungs, the left pumps blood to the rest of the body.

VENTRICLES IN THE BRAIN

Together, these four irregularly shaped cavities contain about 25 ml of cerebrospinal fluid.

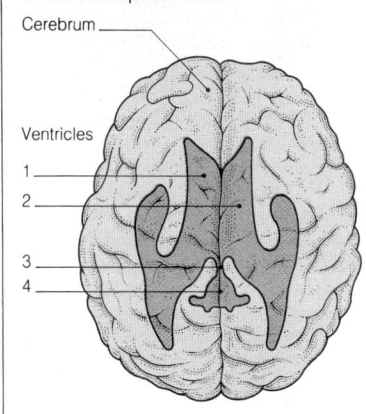

Cerebrum

Ventricles

1
2

3
4

VENTRICLES IN THE HEART

The ventricles of the heart are the large, lower chambers, separated by a muscular wall, the septum.

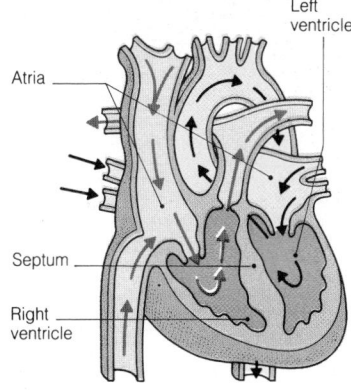

Left ventricle

Atria

Septum

Right ventricle

V

TYPES OF VENTRICULAR ARRHYTHMIA

The ventricles (lower chambers) of the heart usually beat regularly in response to excitatory waves spread from the upper chambers. If rhythm disturbances (which may be associated with heart disease) occur, they are visible on an electrocardiograph (ECG) recording.

Normal heartbeat

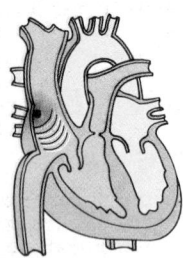

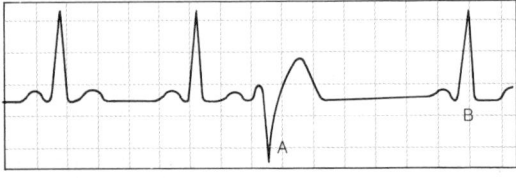

Normal heartbeat

This is the normal ECG appearance of the heartbeat. The regular spikes coincide with beats of the ventricles (lower heart chambers). The small rises before each spike coincide with contractions of the atria (upper chambers).

Ventricular ectopic beat

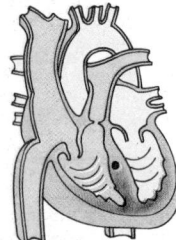

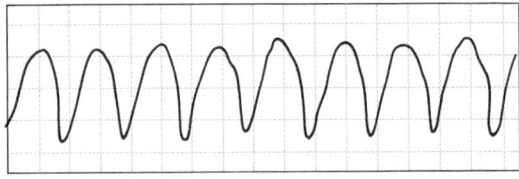

Ventricular ectopic beat

Here there is an abnormal beat, which has a broad, bizarre-looking waveform on the ECG; it occurs just before the expected normal beat. To the patient, the heart may seem to stop at time A and restart with a thump at time B.

Ventricular tachycardia

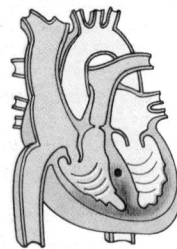

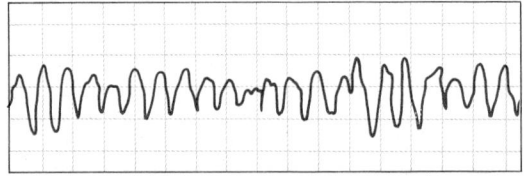

Ventricular tachycardia

Here there is a rapid succession of abnormal beats, caused by an abnormal focus of electrical activity in a ventricle. It usually indicates serious underlying heart disease. The rate of beating may be very high—up to 220 beats per minute.

Ventricular fibrillation

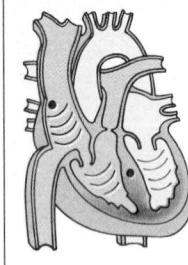

Ventricular fibrillation

This pattern is seen only when the heart is in a state of virtual arrest, usually after a heart attack, with the ventricles twitching in a rapid and totally irregular manner. Unless a normal rhythm can be restored, the condition is rapidly fatal.

Emergency treatment is with *defibrillation* (administration of an electric shock to the heart) or by injection of an *antiarrhythmic drug*, such as *lignocaine*. Use of the drug is usually continued by mouth for several months.

Verapamil

A drug that acts as a *calcium channel blocker* used in the treatment of *hypertension* (high blood pressure), *angina pectoris*, and certain types of *arrhythmia* (abnormal heart rhythm).

Possible adverse effects include headache, facial flushing, dizziness, ankle swelling, and constipation.

Vernix

The white, greasy, cheese-like substance that covers the skin of a newborn baby. Vernix consists of fatty secretions and dead cells. It is thought to protect the baby's skin and insulate against heat loss before birth. Vernix lubricates the passage of the baby through the birth canal.

Verruca

The Latin name for a *wart*. The term is commonly applied to warts on the soles of the feet, known medically as plantar warts.

Version

A change in the direction in which a *fetus* lies so that a *malpresentation*, most often a breech (bottom-down) presentation, becomes the normal cephalic (head-down) presentation. Version is also the term for the obstetric procedure used to change the presentation of a fetus.

Many breech babies undergo version spontaneously, especially before the 34th week of pregnancy. If this does not occur, the obstetrician may be able to manipulate the fetus into the cephalic position by a procedure called external version. With one hand on the mother's abdomen over the baby's head and the other over the baby's buttocks, the obstetrician very gently attempts to rotate the baby, bringing its head down into the mother's pelvis. External version is performed between the 34th and 37th week of pregnancy and can be done with or without general anaesthesia. Drugs may be used to relax the uterus.

External version carries small risks of inducing premature labour (see *Prematurity*), rupture of the membranes, *antepartum haemorrhage*, or knotting of the umbilical cord. The risks of external version must be weighed against those of vaginal breech delivery and of *caesarean section*.

In internal version, the obstetrician turns the fetus by reaching inside the uterus. Internal version is rarely done except in the case of a second twin who is not in the normal position after delivery of the first twin.

Vertebra

Any of the 33 approximately cylindrical bones that form the *spine*. There are seven vertebrae in the cervical spine in the neck; 12 vertebrae in the thoracic

V

spine in the chest; five vertebrae in the lumbar spine in the lower back; five fused vertebrae in the *sacrum*; and four fused vertebrae in the *coccyx* (see illustrated box). Between each pair of separate vertebrae is an intervertebral disc (see *Disc, intervertebral*).

Vertebrobasilar insufficiency

Intermittent episodes of dizziness, double vision, weakness, and difficulty in speaking caused by reduced blood flow to parts of the *brain*.

The obstruction to blood flow is usually caused by *atherosclerosis* (narrowing of arteries by fatty deposits) of the basilar and vertebral arteries and other arteries in the base of the brain. Vertebrobasilar insufficiency sometimes precedes a *stroke*.

Vertigo

An illusion that one or one's surroundings are spinning, either horizontally or vertically. Vertigo is a common complaint, but only rarely is it a sign of an underlying disorder. The term is sometimes used erroneously to describe the sensation of *dizziness* or faintness.

CAUSES

Vertigo results from a disturbance of the semicircular canals in the inner *ear* or the nerve tracts leading from them. It can occur in healthy people when sailing, on amusement park rides, or even when watching a film. Astronauts in zero gravity experience vertigo when moving their heads.

Severe vertigo, usually accompanied by other symptoms, may indicate a number of diseases. *Labyrinthitis* (inflammation of the semicircular canals) causes sudden vertigo accompanied by vomiting and unsteadiness. Labyrinthitis often occurs in conjunction with an infection, such as *influenza* or *otitis media* (infection of the middle ear), and usually clears up as the infection subsides. *Ménière's disease* is a more serious condition characterized by attacks of vertigo that are sometimes severe enough to cause the sufferer to fall to the ground. The attacks of vertigo may be accompanied by severe vomiting, *tinnitus* (noises in the ears), *nystagmus* (jerky eye movements), and unsteadiness.

Elderly people with *atherosclerosis* often suffer from vertigo as a result of suddenly moving the head. Vertigo is less commonly caused by a tumour of the *brainstem* or by *multiple sclerosis*. Vertigo may also be psychological in origin, in which case it is usually associated with *agoraphobia* (fear of open spaces).

INVESTIGATION

If disease is the suspected cause of vertigo, the doctor performs an examination of the ears, eyes, and nervous system, sometimes including *CT scanning* of the brain.

TREATMENT

Vertigo that comes on suddenly is usually assumed to be due to labyrinthitis and is treated with bed rest and with *antihistamine drugs* or *anticholinergic drugs*. If vertigo persists for more than a few days, the sufferer should walk as much as possible to

---

LOCATION AND STRUCTURE OF THE VERTEBRAE

The 33 vertebrae are arranged as shown. Apart from the top two, they all have a similar structure. The topmost cervical vertebra (the atlas) has no body. The second (the axis) forms a pivot on which the atlas can rotate, allowing the head to be turned in all directions.

The spine

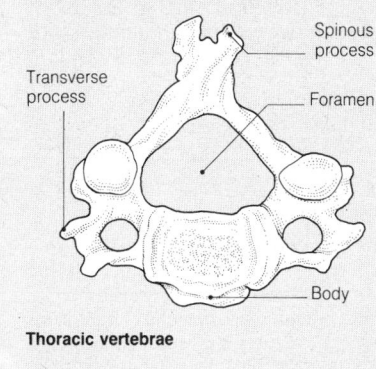

Cervical vertebrae (7)

Thoracic vertebrae (12)

Lumbar vertebrae (5)

Sacral vertebrae (5)

Coccygeal vertebrae (4)

Cervical vertebrae

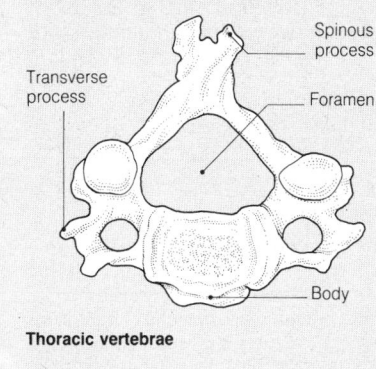

Transverse process

Spinous process

Foramen

Body

Thoracic vertebrae

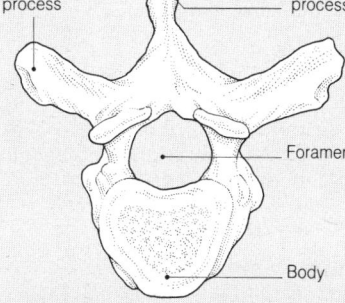

Transverse process

Spinous process

Foramen

Body

Lumbar vertebrae

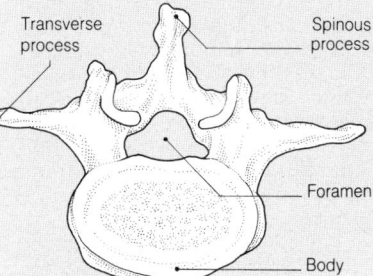

Transverse process

Spinous process

Foramen

Body

Arrangement
The vertebrae fall into five groups—cervical, thoracic, lumbar, sacral, and coccygeal. The top 24 are separated by discs of cartilage.

Structure
Three typical vertebrae are shown above. The foramen in each is the channel through which the spinal cord runs. The processes serve as muscle attachments.

V

allow the body to develop compensatory measures. In some cases, antihistamine drugs may be prescribed to prevent recurrent attacks.

Vesicle

A small skin blister, usually filled with clear fluid, that forms at the site of skin damage. The term vesicle is also used to refer to any small sac-like structure in the body (e.g. the seminal vesicles, which store seminal fluid).

Vestibulitis

Inflammation of the nasal vestibule (the part of the nasal cavity just inside the nostril), usually as a result of bacterial infection.

Vestibulocochlear nerve

The eighth *cranial nerve* concerned with *balance* and *hearing*. Each vestibulocochlear nerve (one on each side) carries sensory impulses from the inner *ear* to the brain, which it enters between the pons and the medulla oblongata (parts of the *brainstem*). The vestibulocochlear nerve consists of two parts—the vestibular nerve and the cochlear nerve (the latter is also sometimes known as the acoustic nerve or auditory nerve).

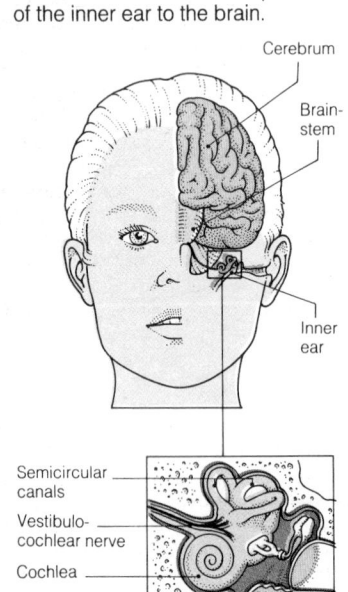

LOCATION OF THE VESTIBULOCOCHLEAR NERVE
This nerve conducts sensory impulses concerned with hearing and balance from different parts of the inner ear to the brain.

Cerebrum
Brainstem
Inner ear
Semicircular canals
Vestibulocochlear nerve
Cochlea

The vestibular nerve carries sensory impulses from the semicircular canals in the inner ear to the *cerebellum* in the brain, which, in conjunction with information from the eyes and joints, controls balance. The cochlear nerve carries sensory impulses from the cochlea (the snail-shaped part of the inner ear responsible for detecting sound) to the hearing centre in the brain, where the impulses are interpreted as sounds.

DISORDERS
A tumour of the cells that surround the vestibulocochlear nerve (see *Acoustic neuroma*) may cause loss of balance, *tinnitus* (ringing or other noises in the ear), and *deafness*. Deafness may also result from damage to the vestibulocochlear nerve, which is sometimes due to an infection, such as *meningitis* or *encephalitis*, or to an adverse reaction to a drug, such as *streptomycin*.

Viability

The capability of independent survival and development. A normal human fetus is widely accepted to be viable from 28 weeks' gestation onwards. However, fetuses born as early as the 23rd to 24th week now commonly survive after care in a neonatal intensive-care unit.

Vibrator

A mechanical device applied to the body to tone or relax muscles and to massage the skin. Vibrators may also be used as an aid to sexual stimulation (possibly during *sex therapy*) or as an alternative to sexual intercourse for inducing orgasm.

Villus

A minute finger-like projection from a membranous surface, particularly one of the countless millions of them that occur on the mucous lining of the small *intestine*. Although villi are present in all three sections of the small intestine, they are largest and most numerous in the duodenum and jejunum (the first and second parts), where most of the absorption of digested food occurs.

STRUCTURE
Each intestinal villus contains a small lymph vessel and a network of capillaries (tiny blood vessels). The outer surface of each villus is covered with hundreds of hair-like structures (called microvilli) which increase the surface area of the small intestine to an area approximately equal to that of a tennis court.

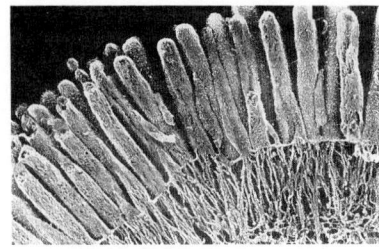

Microvilli in the intestine
This scanning electron micrograph shows numerous microvilli projecting from a single cell in the lining of the small intestine.

FUNCTION
The function of the intestinal villi is to provide a large surface area for the absorption of food molecules into the blood and lymphatic systems. Food particles that are broken down into small molecules by digestive enzymes reach the bloodstream via the capillaries of the villi.

Vincent's disease

A severe form of gingivitis in which bacterial infection causes painful ulceration of the gums (see *Gingivitis, acute ulcerative*). This condition is also sometimes called acute necrotizing ulcerative gingivitis, trench mouth, or Vincent's stomatitis.

Viraemia

The presence of *virus* particles in the blood. Viraemia can occur at certain stages in a variety of viral infections.

Some viruses, such as those responsible for viral *hepatitis*, *yellow fever*, and *poliomyelitis*, may simply be transported in the bloodstream. Symptoms arise when virus particles enter and start multiplying in target tissues rather than from the viraemia.

Other viruses, such as the *rubella* virus and *HIV* (the virus that causes *AIDS*), exist within lymphocytes (types of white blood cell), which they use as a place to multiply as well as a means of spreading.

If viraemia is a feature of a viral infection, there is a risk that the infection may be transmissible in blood or blood products, or by insects that feed on blood.

Virginity

The physical state of not having experienced *sexual intercourse*.

Virilism

Masculine characteristics that affect the physical appearance of a woman. Virilism is caused by excessive levels

V

of *androgen hormones*. Androgens are male sex hormones which, in women, are normally secreted in small amounts by the adrenal glands and ovaries. Raised levels of these hormones induce various changes in women, including *hirsutism* (excessive hair growth); a male-pattern hairline with balding at the temples; disruption or cessation of menstruation; enlargement of the clitoris; loss of normal fat deposits around the hips; development of the arm and shoulder muscles; and deepening of the voice as a result of enlargement of the larynx. (See also *Virilization*.)

Virility

A term used to describe the quality of maleness, especially in sexual characteristics and performance.

Virilization

The process by which *virilism* occurs in women as a result of overproduction of *androgen hormones* (male sex hormones) by the adrenal glands and/or ovaries. This process, in turn, may be caused by various underlying conditions, such as certain *adrenal tumours*, polycystic ovary (see *Ovary, polycystic*) and some other *ovarian cysts*, or congenital *adrenal hyperplasia* (a rare genetic disorder).

Virion

A single, complete, virus particle. (See *Viruses*.)

Virology

The study of *viruses* and the *epidemiology* and treatment of diseases caused by viruses. In a more restricted sense, virology also means the isolation and identification of viruses to diagnose specific viral infections. To achieve this, a tissue or fluid sample must be obtained for analysis. Depending on the suspected virus, the type of sample studied may be a specimen of faeces, sputum, blister fluid, blood, urine, cerebrospinal fluid, or even a brain biopsy specimen.

Unlike bacteria, viruses cannot be grown in a culture medium; they can multiply only within living cells. For this reason viruses must be grown in cultures of cells, which can be any of many types of animal or human cell that can easily be made to multiply in test tubes. The cell culture is exposed to the specimen or fluid sample that contains the virus, and the cells are then observed for distinctive changes that occur when they are infected with certain viruses.

Alternatively, virus particles or components of viruses can sometimes be detected directly in specimens by the use of *staining* techniques or an electron microscope. Sometimes, the virus particles must first be made to clump together by adding an *antiserum* (*antibodies* obtained from the blood of someone who has had the viral infection, and which will bind to the virus particles). *Immunoassay* techniques, in which "labelled" antibodies are added to the specimens and detected if they have bound to virus cell components, are another possible means of detecting infection.

Another method of diagnosing viral infections is to look for antibodies produced by the *immune system* to combat the viruses. A rapidly rising level of antibodies to a particular virus can provide good evidence of infection. Antibodies can be detected by immunoassay and by other laboratory techniques (see *Serology*).

Virulence

The ability of a microorganism to cause disease. Virulence can be assessed by measuring what proportion of the population exposed to the microorganism develops symptoms of disease, how rapidly the infection spreads through body tissues, or by the mortality from the infection.

Viruses

The smallest known types of infectious agent. Viruses are about one half to one hundredth the size of the smallest *bacteria*, from which they differ in having a much simpler structure and method of multiplication. Viral infections range from the trivial, such as *warts*, the common cold (see *Cold, common*), and other minor respiratory tract infections, to extremely serious diseases, such as *rabies* and *Lassa fever*. Viral infection also leads to the development of *AIDS*, and probably to various *cancers*.

NATURE OF VIRUSES

It is debatable whether viruses are truly living organisms or just collections of large molecules capable of self-replication under very specific favourable conditions. Their sole activity is to invade the cells of other organisms, which they then take over to make copies of themselves. Outside living cells, viruses are wholly inert. They are incapable of activities typical of life, such as metabolism (internal processing of nutrients).

The number of different kinds of virus probably exceeds the number of

types of all other organisms. Viruses parasitize all recognized life-forms. Not all viruses cause disease, but many do.

STRUCTURE AND REPLICATION OF VIRUSES

A single virus particle (virion) consists simply of an inner core of *nucleic acid* surrounded by one or two protective shells (capsids) made of protein. These capsids are built from a number of identical protein subunits arranged in a highly symmetrical form, usually either as a 20-faced solid (an icosahedron) or as a spiral tube. Surrounding the outer capsid may be another layer called the viral envelope, which also consists mainly of protein. The viral envelope is often lost when the virus invades a cell.

The nucleic acid at the core is called the genome and consists of a string of *genes* that contain coded instructions for making copies of the virus. Depending on the type of virus, the nucleic acid may be either *DNA*, in which there are two complementary, intertwined strands of nucleic acid (the double helix), or *RNA*, consisting of a single strand.

The basic process by which a virus replicates is shown in the illustrated box overleaf. Different viruses employ different strategies, some highly complex, to make copies of themselves once they have invaded a host cell. During replication of the viral nucleic acid, the viral genes may first have to code the manufacture of special *enzymes* called polymerases or transcriptases to assist in replication; alternatively, the virus may borrow these enzymes from the host cell. Sometimes the viral genome must invade the nucleus of the host cell and incorporate itself into the cell's *chromosomes* (genetic material) before it is able to replicate.

Sometimes, if the viral genome invades the nucleus of the host cell, it may not replicate immediately but may "hide" there, perhaps becoming reactivated months or years later. The viral genome may also interact with the cell's chromosomes—a process that may convert the host cell into a tumour cell.

TYPES

Viruses that cause human disease are grouped into more than 20 large families; the most important are shown in the table overleaf.

In recent years, special attention has been paid to the family of retroviruses, which include *HIV* (human immunodeficiency virus), the agent responsible for AIDS. HIV is an RNA

V

VIRUSES AND DISEASE

All viruses have the same basic structure (right), but they come in various shapes and sizes. Examples from the main families are shown below (some in cross-section). All are tiny—from about 15 to 300 nanometres in diameter (one nanometre equals one thousand-millionth of a metre); most are so small that they can be seen only with an electron microscope. All types of viruses can multiply only within cells of their host (far right).

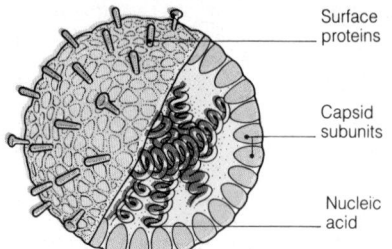

Surface proteins

Capsid subunits

Nucleic acid

Structure of a typical virus particle
Nucleic acid in the centre is surrounded by one or more capsids made of protein subunits.

VIRAL REPLICATION

The sequence below shows how a virus multiplies. The signs and symptoms of viral infection are caused by the virus interfering with or destroying the host's cells.

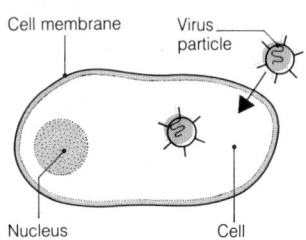

Cell membrane   Virus particle

Nucleus   Cell

1 The virus particle first attaches itself to and then injects itself into the host cell.

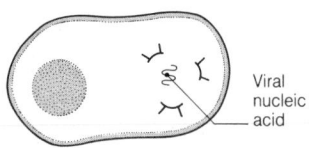

Viral nucleic acid

2 The viral capsid breaks down and the viral nucleic acid (DNA or RNA) contained inside is released.

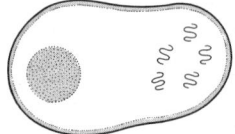

3 The viral nucleic acid replicates itself; the new copies are made from raw materials in the host cell.

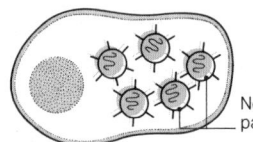

New particles

4 Each of the new copies of the viral nucleic acid now directs the manufacture of a capsid for itself.

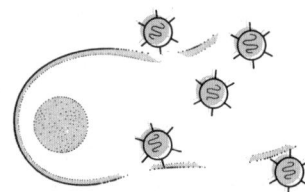

5 The newly formed virus particles are released in large numbers, and the host cell may be destroyed.

TYPES OF VIRUS

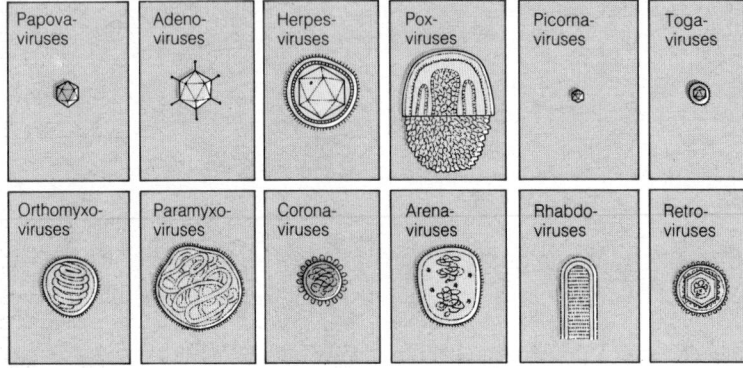

Family	Examples of conditions or diseases
Papovaviruses	Warts
Adenoviruses	Respiratory and eye infections
Herpesviruses	Cold sores, genital herpes, chickenpox, herpes zoster (shingles), glandular fever, congenital abnormalities (cytomegalovirus)
Poxviruses	Cowpox, smallpox (eradicated), molluscum contagiosum
Picornaviruses	Poliomyelitis, viral hepatitis type A, respiratory infections, myocarditis
Togaviruses	Yellow fever, dengue, encephalitis
Orthomyxoviruses	Influenza
Paramyxoviruses	Mumps, measles
Coronaviruses	Common cold
Arenaviruses	Lassa fever
Rhabdoviruses	Rabies
Retroviruses	AIDS, degenerative brain diseases, and (possibly) various kinds of cancer

V

virus and, after invading a cell, first manufactures an enzyme called reverse transcriptase, which it needs to make copies of itself. Research into this enzyme may reveal a means of attacking HIV.

HOW VIRUSES CAUSE DISEASE

Viruses gain access to the body by all possible entry routes. They are inhaled in droplets; swallowed in food and fluids; passed through the punctured skin in the saliva of feeding insects or rabid dogs or on infected needles; viruses are accepted directly by the mucous membranes of the genital tract during sexual intercourse and by the conjunctiva of the eye after accidental contamination.

Many viruses begin to invade cells and multiply near their site of entry. Some enter the lymphatic vessels and may spread to the lymph nodes, where many are engulfed by white blood cells. Some, such as HIV, invade and then multiply within *lymphocytes* (a type of white cell). Many pass from the lymphatics to the blood and within a few minutes are spread to every part of the body. They may then invade and start multiplying within specific target organs such as the skin, brain, liver, or lungs. Other viruses travel along nerve fibres to their target organs.

Viruses cause disease in a variety of ways. First, they may destroy or severely disrupt the activities of the cells they invade, possibly causing serious disease if vital organs are affected. Second, the response of the body's *immune system* to viral infection may lead to symptoms, such as fever and fatigue, or to a disease process. In particular, antibodies produced by the immune system may attach to viral particles and circulate as immune complexes in the bloodstream. The antibodies may then be deposited in various parts of the body and cause inflammation and severe tissue damage. Third, by interacting with the chromosomes of their host cells, viruses may cause cancer. Fourth, a virus may cause disease by weakening the cell-mediated arm of the immune system (i.e. the activity of T-lymphocytes). This is how HIV works, invading and disrupting one type of T-lymphocyte so that the body's normal defences against a wide range of infections are lost.

VIRUSES AND CANCER

The chromosomes in all normal body cells contain 50 or more genes (known as *oncogenes*) that are necessary for the growth or *differentiation* of the cells.

Certain retroviruses contain almost identical oncogenes. In the process of replication, these viruses may modify the chromosomes of the host cell. A small mutation in these can "switch on" the oncogenes inappropriately, thus prompting the cell to begin unrestrained division, leading to the formation of tumours.

To date, this process has been found to cause many cancers in animals but only one type of cancer in humans. The virus responsible is similar to the AIDS virus and can cause *leukaemia* in the person it infects. However, other viruses are known to be at least potentially cancer-producing in humans, and this is a major area of research.

RESISTANCE TO VIRUSES

The immune system deals fairly rapidly with most viruses. Each mechanism of the immune system may be involved in resisting a viral attack—including white cells (macrophages) that engulf the viral particles, and lymphocytes that produce antibodies against the virus or attack virally infected cells. This leads to recovery from most viral infections within a few days to weeks. Furthermore, the immune system is often sufficiently sensitized by the infection to make a second illness from the same virus rare (as is the case with *measles*).

With some viruses, however, the speed of the attack is such that serious damage or even death may occur before the immune system can adequately respond (as is the case with rabies and some cases of *poliomyelitis*). In other cases, a virus is able to dodge or hide from the immune system, so that the infection becomes chronic or recurrent. This is common with many *herpes* virus infections (such as genital herpes and shingles) and with viral hepatitis B (see *Hepatitis, viral*). Finally, the AIDS virus, by weakening the immune system, leaves the body open to many *opportunistic infections*.

FIGHTING VIRAL DISEASE

Viruses are more difficult than bacteria to combat with drugs because it is difficult to design drugs that will kill viruses without also killing the cells they parasitize. Nevertheless, there has been progress in the development of antiviral agents, especially against the herpes group of viruses (see *Antiviral drugs*). Such drugs may work by helping to prevent viruses from entering cells or by interfering with their replication in cells.

Interferon refers to a group of natural substances, produced by virus-infected cells, that protect uninfected cells. Some interferons can now be produced artificially (by means of *genetic engineering*) and have been tried in the treatment of various viral infections, including the common cold and viral hepatitis B.

Otherwise, treatment of viral infections depends largely on alleviating the patient's symptoms and trusting the body's immune defences to bring about a cure.

A much more fruitful area in the fight against viruses is *immunization*. One viral disease, *smallpox*, has already been eradicated worldwide through a coordinated vaccination programme. Highly effective vaccines are also now available to prevent many others, including poliomyelitis, measles, *mumps, rubella,* hepatitis types A and B, *yellow fever,* and rabies.

Viscera

A collective term used to describe the internal organs.

Viscosity

The resistance to flow of a liquid or gas; the "stickiness" of a fluid. The viscosity of the blood affects its ability to flow through small blood vessels. An increase in the viscosity of the blood—caused by an increase in the proportion of red blood cells—increases the risk of *thrombosis* (abnormal clot formation).

Vision

The faculty of sight. Vision involves two main components—the *eye* and the *brain*.

When light-rays reach the eye, most of the focusing is done by the cornea. However, the eye also has an automatic fine-focusing facility, known as *accommodation*, that operates by altering the curvature of the crystalline *lens*. Together, these two systems provide sufficient optical power to form an image on the *retina*. The light-sensitive rods and cones in the retina convert the elements of this image into nerve impulses that, after preliminary processing in the retina, pass into the visual cortex of the brain via the *optic nerves*. The rods, which are proportionally more concentrated at the periphery of the retina, are highly sensitive to light but not to colour. The colour-sensitive cones are concentrated more at the centre of the retina (see *Colour vision*).

Accurate alignment of the two eyes is achieved by coordination of the motor nerve impulses to the six tiny

V

THE SENSE OF VISION

Vision starts in the retina, the membrane at the back of the eye that contains the light-sensitive rod and cone cells. Much of the rest of the eye is concerned with focusing light, in the right quantities, on to the retina. Huge amounts of data are sent from the retina via the optic nerves to the brain for analysis.

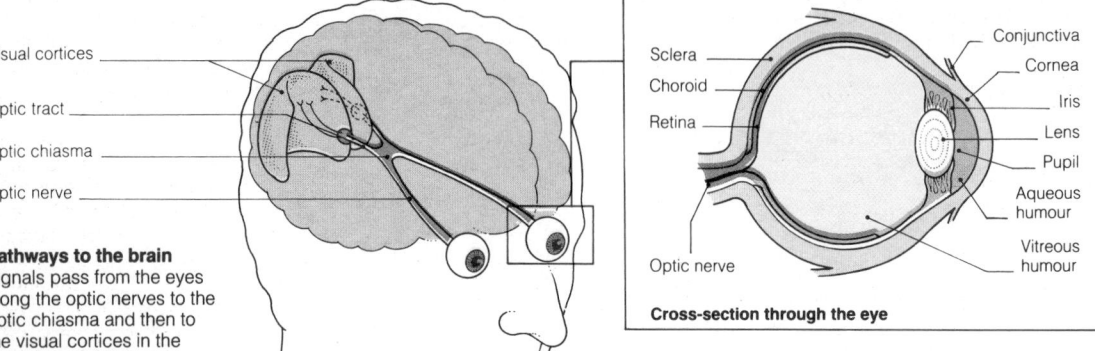

Visual cortices

Optic tract

Optic chiasma

Optic nerve

Sclera
Choroid
Retina

Conjunctiva
Cornea
Iris
Lens
Pupil
Aqueous humour
Vitreous humour

Optic nerve

Cross-section through the eye

Pathways to the brain

Signals pass from the eyes along the optic nerves to the optic chiasma and then to the visual cortices in the brain. There is some crossover of nerve fibres at the optic chiasma, so both sides of the brain receive signals from both eyes.

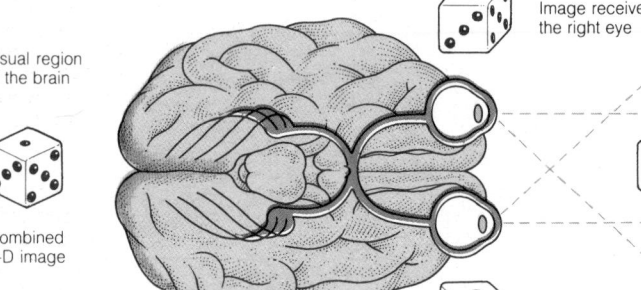

Image received by the right eye

Visual region of the brain

Combined 3-D image

Image received by the left eye

Stereoscopic vision

The two eyes receive slightly different views of all but the most distant objects; information from the two images is compared and processed in the brain to give a single 3-D interpretaton of the object.

IMAGE RECEPTION

The light-rays from an object stimulate a group of receptors in the retina within an area that has the same shape as the object but is upside down. The brain automatically interprets the image the right way up.

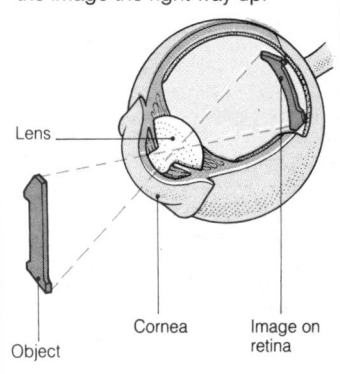

Lens

Object

Cornea

Image on retina

EYEBALL MOVEMENTS

To maintain the image of any moving object on the centre of the retina, precise eyeball movements, achieved by the six muscles shown below, are necessary. The muscles act to swivel the eyeball in the directions indicated (the right eye is shown). The muscles always act in groups.

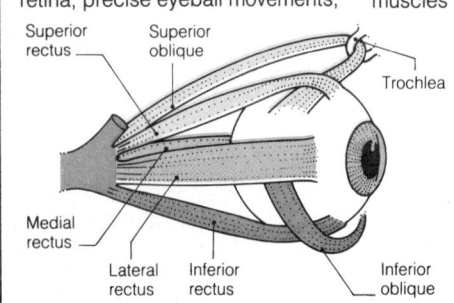

Superior rectus
Superior oblique
Trochlea

Medial rectus

Lateral rectus
Inferior rectus
Inferior oblique

Inferior oblique
Upwards, outwards, and anticlockwise rotation

Lateral rectus
Outwards

Superior oblique
Downwards, outwards, and clockwise rotation

Superior rectus
Upwards, inwards, and clockwise rotation

Medial rectus
Inwards

Inferior rectus
Downwards, inwards, and anticlockwise rotation

V

muscles that move each eye. This coordination is achieved in the brain, which correlates information from several sources, taking into account the brain's perception of the images, the position of the head, the position of the eyes relative to the head, and the position of the two eyes relative to each other.

Accurate alignment of the two eyes allows the brain to fuse the images from each eye, but because each eye has a slightly different view of a given object, the brain obtains information that is interpreted as solidity or depth. This stereoscopic vision is important in judging distance.

Vision, disorders of

The most common visual disorders are due to simple errors of *refraction*, such as *myopia*, *hypermetropia*, and *astigmatism*. The blurring of vision from refractive errors can almost always be corrected by *glasses*. Defects of vision that cannot be eliminated in this way may have any of a wide variety of causes, including loss of binocular fusion (which can cause *double vision* or *amblyopia*), disorders of the *eye* or *optic nerve*, disorders of the nerve pathways that connect the optic nerves to the *brain*, and disorders of the brain itself.

VISUAL DEFECT FROM EYE AND OPTIC NERVE DISORDERS

Eye or optic nerve disease often affects vision in only one eye or in the two eyes to different degrees. Any interference with the transparency of the eye affects vision. Loss of transparency may result from corneal opacities (clouding of the cornea) following infection, ulceration, or injury; from *cataract* (opacification of the crystalline lens); or from *vitreous haemorrhage* (bleeding into the gel of the eye behind the lens).

Defects near the centre of the retina cause loss of the corresponding parts of the *visual field* of the affected eye. This is especially serious if the central part of the retina, where sharp *visual acuity* exists, is involved (see *Macular degeneration*). Peripheral retinal damage, which occurs in the early stages of chronic simple *glaucoma* or *retinitis pigmentosa*, may not cause noticeable visual disturbance if sharp central vision is unaffected.

Floaters (freely moving shadows perceived in the field of vision) are usually of no significance, but necessitate an eye examination. Floaters may signify a *retinal tear* or haemorrhage, or they may herald a *retinal detachment*, especially if accompanied by bright flashing lights at the periphery of the field of vision.

A defect in the optic nerve in front of the optic nerve crossing causes visual disturbance in one eye only, which often takes the form of a central *scotoma* (a blind spot in the centre of the field of vision). This condition can be due to *optic neuritis*.

VISUAL DEFECT FROM NERVE PATHWAY DISORDERS

Disorders of one of the nerve pathways behind the optic nerve crossing always affect both eyes. This is because half of the fibres from each optic nerve—those from the inner half of each retina—cross over before they reach the back of the brain. Each pathway thus has contributions from both eyes, and any interruption thus causes loss of part of the visual field of each eye.

VISUAL DEFECT FROM BRAIN DISORDERS

Severe damage to one side of the visual area of the brain, such as from loss of blood supply in *stroke*, causes loss of the inner half of the field of vision of the eye on the same side and of the outer half of the field of the other eye. This condition, in which half of the field of vision is lost, is known as *hemianopia*.

Visual disturbance may also arise from involvement of the areas of the brain concerned with the psychological and associational aspects of vision. Disorders of these functions may cause visual *agnosia* (failure to recognize objects), visual *perseveration* (in which a scene continues to be perceived after the direction of gaze has shifted), or visual hallucinations.

Vision, loss of

An inability to see, which may develop slowly or suddenly, and may be temporary or permanent, depending on the cause. Vision loss may affect one or both eyes. It can cause complete blindness, or may affect only peripheral (side) vision or only central vision. A person suffering from loss of central vision is usually aware of the fact, since it prevents reading and discernment of fine detail. However, loss of peripheral vision may pass unnoticed by the sufferer until it is well advanced and causes clumsiness.

SLOW VISION LOSS

A progressive loss of visual clarity is common with advancing age as a result of loss of transparency of the crystalline lenses of the eyes (see *Cataract*). Other common causes of gradual loss of vision are *macular degeneration* and chronic simple *glaucoma*, and complications of *diabetes mellitus*. Gradual visual loss may also be due to progressive opacity of the cornea from *keratopathy* (disease of the cornea) of any kind, or to progressive distortion from *keratoconus* (a conical deformity of the cornea). *Retinitis pigmentosa* causes a variable degree of visual loss in both eyes.

SUDDEN VISION LOSS

Sudden loss of vision may be caused by optical, vascular, or neurological disorders. *Hyphaema* (bleeding into the aqueous humour) usually results from injury; the blood can block the normal passage of the light to the retina. Severe *uveitis* (inflammation of the uvea) may cause serious reduction in vision. *Vitreous haemorrhage* (bleeding into the gel of the eye) and retinal disorders, such as *retinal haemorrhage*, may also reduce vision suddenly.

Optic neuritis (inflammation of the optic nerve) can severely reduce vision in one eye. Any damage to the nerve connections between the eyes and the brain, or to the visual area of the brain itself, can cause loss of peripheral vision. Damage may sometimes be a result of *embolism*, *ischaemia*, tumour, inflammation, or injury.

Vision tests

The part of an eye examination that determines if there is any reduction in the ability to see. Most vision tests are tests of *visual acuity* (sharpness of central vision). Tests of *visual field* (the total area of vision when looking ahead) may also be performed in order to assess disorders of the eye and the nervous system. Refraction tests are done to discover whether the patient has a refractive error (i.e. an error that can be corrected with glasses), such as *hypermetropia*, *myopia*, or *astigmatism*. Refraction tests also show whether a person has *presbyopia* (a deficiency in the power of accommodation).

VISUAL ACUITY TESTS

Visual acuity is tested, one eye at a time, using a *Snellen chart*. In the test, the patient attempts to read letters of standard sizes from a standard distance of six metres.

REFRACTION TESTS

Retinoscopy is one type of refraction test. In this technique, a narrow beam of light is projected into the eye, from a distance of about 65 cm, by an instrument that allows the tester to observe the light reflected back through the pupil from the retina. Small movements of the light are made in various

V

directions. The appropriate correction can be determined from the power and type of lenses needed to neutralize the movement of the light.

Refinement of the degree of refractive correction needed can be achieved by determining the person's subjective response to changes in his or her vision brought about by the use in continuous succession of slightly different lenses.

ACCOMMODATION TESTS

The power of accommodation (ability to focus on near objects) may be measured by correcting any refractive error with *glasses*, and then determining the nearest distance at which very small print can be read.

VISUAL FIELD TESTS

Visual field tests can indicate disorders of the peripheral parts of the retinas, of the optic nerves, or of the optical pathways that convey nerve impulses from the eyes to the back of the brain. Most visual field tests involve the use of large black screens or white hollow bowls. The patient's head is secured, one eye is covered, and the other is directed to a point at the centre of the inside of the bowl. Small spots of light are projected on to the inner surface of the bowl; the spots appear for brief periods in various places or are moved inwards from the periphery. The person being tested responds when he or she sees the spot. (See also *Eye, examination of.*)

TYPES OF VISION TESTS

These tests are performed to measure a number of variables—the acuity of a patient's distance vision and the power of the lenses he or she may need (visual acuity and refraction tests), the extent of peripheral vision (visual field tests), and the ability to focus on near objects (accommodation tests).

VISUAL ACUITY TESTS

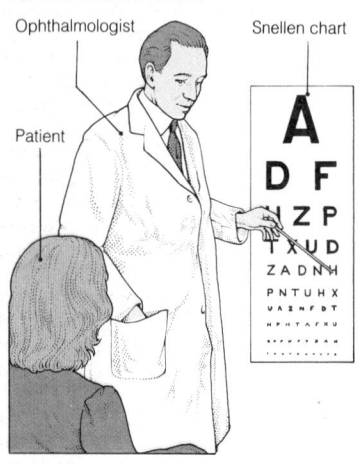

These tests use the familiar Snellen chart. Visual acuity is measured according to how far down the chart the patient can read accurately.

REFRACTION TESTS

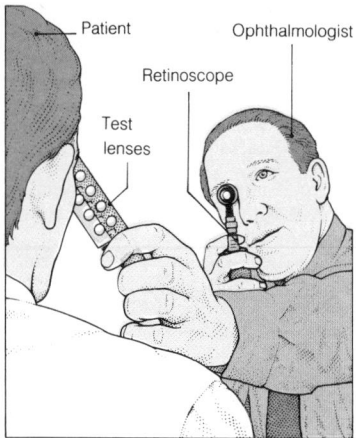

The effect of lenses on movements of light reflected from the eye (as the light source is moved) is observed to help calculate the corrective glasses needed.

ACCOMMODATION TESTS

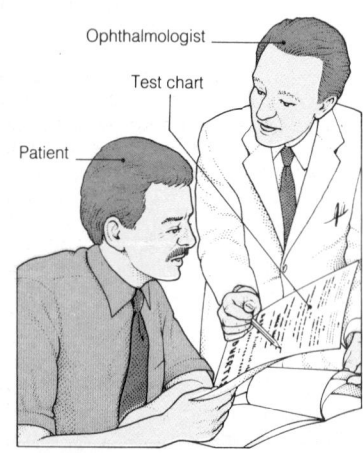

After any distance-focusing ability has been corrected with glasses the ability to read small print close-up is measured to test accommodation.

VISUAL FIELD TESTS

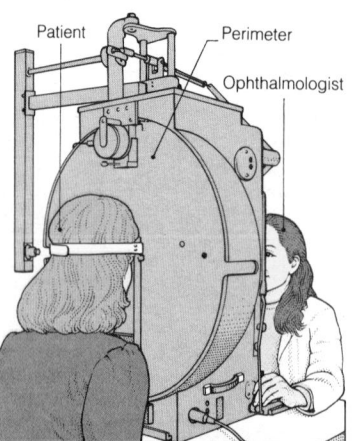

One eye is fixed straight ahead, the other covered, and lights are shone on to a white bowl or screen in front of the patient to find the field of vision of each eye.

Visual acuity

Sharpness of *vision*. Visual acuity is concerned with sharpness (discrimination) of central vision, not with the extent or clarity of the peripheral vision (see *Visual field*). A person's visual acuity is measured during a *vision test*.

Refractive errors (errors that can be corrected with glasses), such as *myopia, hypermetropia,* and *astigmatism,* are the most common cause of poor visual acuity. Poor visual acuity for near objects occurs in *presbyopia.*

Visual field

The total area in which visual perception is possible while looking straight ahead. The visual fields normally extend outwards over an angle of about 90 degrees on either side of the midline of the face, but are more restricted above and below, especially if the eyes are deep-set or the eyebrows are prominent. The visual fields of the two eyes overlap to a large extent so that a defect in the field of one eye may be concealed if both eyes are open (see illustrated box).

The level of *visual acuity* (sharpness of vision) in the visual field is much lower in areas remote from the point at which one is looking directly. For instance, it is impossible to read fine print as little as 5 degrees to one side of the fixation point. This is especially apparent to people with *macular degeneration,* who have no central vision and must therefore use other parts of the visual field.

Partial loss of visual field is less obvious than loss of central vision;

V

THE VISUAL FIELDS

The field of vision of each eye (with the head and eyes immobile) extends through an angle of about 130 degrees and is divided into an area that overlaps with the visual field of the other eye (binocular vision) and an area that can be seen only by one eye.

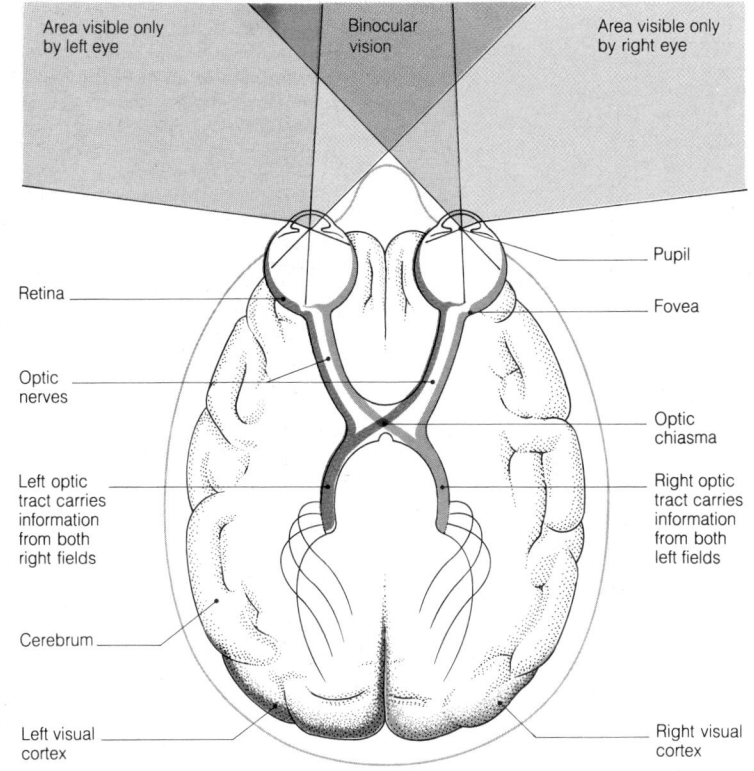

Area visible only by left eye

Binocular vision

Area visible only by right eye

Retina

Optic nerves

Left optic tract carries information from both right fields

Cerebrum

Left visual cortex

Pupil

Fovea

Optic chiasma

Right optic tract carries information from both left fields

Right visual cortex

Route of visual signals
Note that all light from the fields left of centre of both eyes (grey) falls on the right sides of the two retinas; and information about these fields goes to the right visual cortex. Information about the right fields of vision (pink) goes to the left cortex. Data about the area of binocular vision go to both cortices.

even people with extensive visual field loss, such as from *glaucoma* or *stroke*, may be unaware of it if they still have sharp central visual acuity. (See also *Vision, disorders of; Vision tests*.)

Vital sign

An indication that a person is still alive. Vital signs include chest movements caused by breathing, the presence of a pulse (which indicates that the heart is beating), and the constriction of the pupil of the eye when it is exposed to a bright light. A doctor certifies *death* on the basis of the absence of all these signs. Additional tests, such as measurement of brain activity, may also be required in certain circumstances, notably if the patient is on a life-support system.

Vitamin

Any of a group of complex organic substances that are essential in small amounts for the normal functioning of the body. With few exceptions (niacin and vitamin D), the body cannot manufacture these substances itself, making it necessary to obtain them from the diet. There are 13 vitamins—A, C, D, E, K, B_{12}, and the seven vitamins discussed under the heading of *vitamin B complex* (thiamine or B_1, riboflavin or B_2, niacin, pyridoxine or B_6, pantothenic acid, folic acid, and biotin or vitamin H). Each vitamin is present in many different foods. Vitamin D is also produced in the skin when it is exposed to sunlight, and niacin is made by the body from tryptophan (an *amino acid*).

A varied diet that includes different types of foods is likely to contain adequate amounts of all the vitamins, and supplements are not usually necessary. However, a doctor may recommend *vitamin supplements* in certain circumstances, such as for young children, some women who are pregnant or breast-feeding, and for people taking certain *lipid-lowering drugs*, which reduce intestinal absorption of vitamins, or other drugs that interfere with vitamin function.

TYPES
Vitamins can be categorized as fat-soluble or water-soluble vitamins.

FAT-SOLUBLE VITAMINS The fat-soluble vitamins (A, D, E, and K) are absorbed with fats from the intestine into the bloodstream and then stored in fatty tissue (mainly in the liver). They are not normally excreted in the urine.

Body reserves of some of these vitamins may last for several years and a daily intake is therefore not usually essential; in fact, an excessive intake of a fat-soluble vitamin from pharmaceutical preparations may be harmful, especially vitamin D.

Deficiency of a fat-soluble vitamin is usually due to a disorder in which intestinal absorption of fats is impaired (see *Malabsorption*) or to a prolonged poor or restricted diet.

WATER-SOLUBLE VITAMINS The water-soluble vitamins are C, B_{12}, and the members of the B complex. The body can store only a limited amount of these and they are rapidly excreted in the urine if taken in greater amounts than the body requires. A regular intake is therefore essential to prevent a deficiency. Vitamin B_{12} is an exception because it is stored in the liver and these stores last for several years.

Deficiencies of water-soluble vitamins are thus more likely to occur than fat-soluble vitamin deficiencies. Foods that contain water-soluble vitamins should be eaten daily; moreover, prolonged cooking, storage, and processing tend to damage these vitamins, so fresh or lightly cooked foods are the best sources. Frozen fruits and vegetables can also be a good source of water-soluble vitamins. Taking very large amounts of water-soluble vitamins does not usually cause toxic effects although adverse reactions to very large doses of vitamin C and pyridoxine have been reported.

FUNCTION
The role of all the vitamins in the body is not fully understood. Most vitamins have been found to have several important actions on one or more

V

body systems or functions, and many are involved in the activities of *enzymes* (substances that promote chemical reactions in the body). See also articles on individual vitamins.

Vitamin A

A fat-soluble *vitamin* essential for normal growth, for the formation of bones and teeth, for cell structure, for night vision, and for protecting the linings of the respiratory, digestive, and urinary tracts against infection.

Vitamin A is absorbed by the body in the form of retinol. This is found in animal foods, such as liver, fish-liver oils, egg yolk, and dairy produce, and is also added to margarines. *Carotene*, which is converted into retinol in the body, also provides a good source of vitamin A. Carotene is present in green vegetables, tomatoes, and various fruits, such as oranges, plums, and peaches. It is especially abundant in carrots.

DEFICIENCY

Vitamin A deficiency is rare in developed countries. In most cases it is due to failure of the intestine to absorb sufficient quantities of the vitamin as a result of *malabsorption*, which may be due to damage, *cystic fibrosis*, or obstruction of the bile duct. Vitamin A deficiency may also occur as an adverse effect of long-term treatment with certain *lipid-lowering drugs*. Deficiency is common in some developing countries due to a combination of low dietary levels of retinol and low dietary levels of fat, which is essential for the absorption of both retinol and carotene.

The first symptom of deficiency is night blindness (inability to see in dim light), followed by dryness and inflammation of the eyes, *keratomalacia* (damage to the cornea), and eventually blindness. Deficiency also causes reduced resistance to infection, dry rough skin, and, in children, stunted growth.

Worldwide, there are half a million new cases of *xerophthalmia* (dry eye caused by vitamin A deficiency) each year; half of these result in blindness.

EXCESS

Prolonged, excessive intake of vitamin A can result in a condition called hypervitaminosis A. This condition most commonly occurs as a result of taking large quantities of self-prescribed vitamin supplements. (To avoid the risk of overdose, manufacturers of the vitamin limit the potency of their preparations.)

Symptoms of hypervitaminosis A include headache, nausea, loss of appetite, peeling of the skin, hair loss, and, in women, irregular menstruation. In extreme cases, the liver and spleen become enlarged. Excessive intake during pregnancy may cause birth defects. In infants, the condition may cause skull deformities, which disappear if the diet is corrected.

Excessive intake of carrots can give rise to a harmless orange coloration of the skin; this is known as carotenaemia and vanishes when the diet is corrected.

MEDICAL USES

Several compounds, known as retinoids, which are chemically related to retinol have recently been under investigation for inhibiting the growth of certain types of tumours; the results so far are conflicting.

RECOMMENDED DAILY ALLOWANCES (RDAs) OF SELECTED VITAMINS

	Birth-6 months	6 months -1 year	1-3 years	4-6 years	7-10 years	11-14 years	15-18 years	19-22 years	23-50 years	51+ years	Extra needed pregnancy	Extra needed breast-feeding
Folic acid (mcg)	30	45	100	200	300	400	400	400	400	400	400	100
Niacin (mg)	6.0	8.0	9.0	11	16	M 18 F 15	M 18 F 14	M 19 F 14	M 18 F 13	M 16 F 13	2.0	5.0
Pyridoxine (mg)	0.3	0.6	0.9	1.3	1.6	1.8	2.0	M 2.2 F 2.0	M 2.2 F 2.0	M 2.2 F 2.0	0.6	0.5
Riboflavin (mg)	0.4	0.6	0.8	1.0	1.4	M 1.6 F 1.3	M 1.7 F 1.3	M 1.7 F 1.3	M 1.6 F 1.2	M 1.4 F 1.2	0.3	0.5
Thiamine (mg)	0.3	0.5	0.7	0.9	1.2	M 1.4 F 1.1	M 1.4 F 1.1	M 1.5 F 1.1	M 1.4 F 1.0	M 1.2 F 1.0	0.4	0.5
Vitamin A (mcg) 1	420	400	400	500	700	M 1,000 F 800	M 1,000 F 800	M 1,000 F 800	M 1,000 F 800	M 1,000 F 800	200	400
Vitamin B$_{12}$ (mcg)	0.5	1.5	2.0	2.5	3.0	3.0	3.0	3.0	3.0	3.0	1.0	1.0
Vitamin C (mg)	35	35	45	45	45	50	60	60	60	60	20	40
Vitamin D (mcg) 2	10	10	10	10	10	10	10	7.5	5.0	5.0	5.0	5.0
Vitamin E (mg) 3	3.0	4.0	5.0	6.0	7.0	8.0	M 10 F 8.0	M 10 F 8.0	M 10 F 8.0	M 10 F 8.0	2.0	3.0

1 RDA expressed in mcg of retinol (a form of vitamin A). 1 mcg of retinol (a unit called a retinol equivalent, or RE) equals 6 mcg of beta-carotene (another form of vitamin A).

2 RDA expressed in mcg of cholecalciferol (one of the forms of vitamin D). 10 mcg of cholecalciferol equals 400 international units (IU) of vitamin D.

3 RDA expressed in mg of alpha-tocopherol (one of the forms of vitamin E). 1 mg of alpha-tocopherol equals 1 alpha-tocopherol equivalent (1 alpha-TE).

Units
mg = milligrams (thousandths of a gram)

mcg = micrograms (millionths of a gram)

Vitamin requirements
The table (above) gives the recommended daily allowances (RDAs) of vitamins for which amounts have been established; when different, the RDAs for males and females are denoted by M and F.

V

The drug *tretinoin* (a derivative of vitamin A) is effective in the treatment of severe *acne*.

Vitamin B

See *Vitamin B₁₂*; *Vitamin B complex*.

Vitamin B₁₂

Also known as cyanocobalamin, vitamin B₁₂ plays a vital role in the activities of several *enzymes* (substances that promote chemical reactions in the body). Vitamin B₁₂ is important in the production of the genetic material of cells (and thus in growth and development), in the production of red blood cells in bone marrow, in the utilization of folic acid (a constituent of the *vitamin B complex*) and carbohydrates in the diet, and in the functioning of the nervous system.

Foods rich in vitamin B₁₂ include liver, kidney, chicken, beef, pork, fish, eggs, and dairy products.

DEFICIENCY AND EXCESS

A balanced diet contains sufficient amounts of vitamin B₁₂ for the body's needs. Deficiency of vitamin B₁₂ is almost always due to an inability of the intestine to absorb the vitamin, most commonly as a result of pernicious anaemia (see *Anaemia, megaloblastic*). Less commonly, deficiency of vitamin B₁₂ may be an effect of *gastrectomy* (removal of all or part of the stomach), result from *malabsorption* due to an intestinal disorder, or be a consequence of following a vegan diet (one that excludes all kinds of animal products).

The principal effects of vitamin B₁₂ deficiency are megaloblastic anaemia, a sore mouth and tongue, and symptoms caused by damage to the spinal cord, such as numbness and tingling in the limbs. There may also be depression and loss of memory.

No harmful effects are known to occur as a result of a high intake of vitamin B₁₂.

Vitamin B complex

A group of *vitamins* that consists of thiamine (vitamin B₁), riboflavin (vitamin B₂), niacin, pantothenic acid, pyridoxine (vitamin B₆), biotin (vitamin H), and folic acid. *Vitamin B₁₂* is discussed separately.

THIAMINE

This vitamin plays a vital role in the activities of various *enzymes* (substances that promote chemical reactions in the body) involved in the utilization of *carbohydrates* and consequently in the functioning of the nerves, muscles, and heart.

Particularly good sources of thiamine include wheat-germ, bran, whole-grain or enriched cereals, wholemeal breads, brown rice, pasta, liver, kidney, pork, fish, beans, nuts, and eggs.

Those susceptible to deficiency include elderly people on a poor diet relatively rich in sugar and white flour products, those suffering from *hyperthyroidism* (overactivity of the thyroid gland), those with disorders of *malabsorption*, and those with severe *alcohol dependence*. Deficiency may also occur as a result of severe illness, major surgery, or serious injury.

Mild thiamine deficiency may cause tiredness, irritability, loss of appetite,

VITAMINS AND MAIN FOOD SOURCES

Fat-soluble	Good sources
Vitamin A	Liver; fish-liver oils; egg yolk; milk and dairy products; margarine; various fruits and vegetables (such as oranges and carrots)
Vitamin D	Cod-liver oil, oily fish (such as sardines, herring, salmon, and tuna); liver; egg yolk; margarine
Vitamin E	Vegetable oils (such as corn, soya bean, olive, and sunflower oils); nuts; meat; green, leafy vegetables; cereals; wheat-germ; egg yolk
Vitamin K	Green, leafy vegetables (especially cabbage, broccoli, and turnip greens); vegetable oils; egg yolk; cheese; pork; liver
Water-soluble	
Thiamine (vitamin B₁)	Wheat-germ; bran; whole-grain or enriched cereals; wholemeal bread; brown rice; pasta; liver; kidney; pork; fish; beans; nuts; eggs
Riboflavin (vitamin B₂)	Brewer's yeast; liver; kidney; milk; cheese; eggs; whole grains; enriched cereals; wheat-germ
Niacin	Liver; lean meat; poultry; fish; nuts; dried beans; enriched cereals; bread; wheat-germ; potatoes
Pantothenic acid	Liver; heart; kidney; fish; egg yolk; wheat-germ; most vegetables; most cereals
Pyridoxine (vitamin B₆)	Liver; chicken; pork; fish; whole grains; wheat-germ; bananas; potatoes; dried beans
Biotin (vitamin H)	Liver; peanuts; dried beans; egg yolk; mushrooms; bananas; grapefruit; watermelons
Folic acid	Green, leafy vegetables; mushrooms; liver; nuts; dried beans; peas; egg yolk; wholemeal bread
Vitamin B₁₂ (cyanocobalamin)	Liver; kidney; chicken; beef; pork; fish; eggs; milk; cheese; enriched cereals
Vitamin C	Citrus fruits; tomatoes; green, leafy vegetables; potatoes; green peppers; strawberries; blackcurrants

Vitamin needs

A varied diet usually provides all vitamin needs. For vegans (who eat no animal products), vitamins B₁₂ and D may be lacking; these vitamins can be obtained from supplements or, in the case of vitamin D, through adequate exposure to sunlight.

V

and sleep disturbances. Severe deficiency may cause abdominal pain, constipation, depression, memory impairment, and *beriberi* (which may be fatal); in sufferers of chronic alcohol dependence, it may cause *Wernicke-Korsakoff syndrome*.

Excessive intake of thiamine is not known to cause harmful effects.

RIBOFLAVIN

Riboflavin is essential for the activities of various enzymes involved in the breakdown and utilization of carbohydrates, fats, and proteins, the production of energy in cells, the utilization of other B vitamins, and the production of hormones by the adrenal glands.

Particularly good sources of riboflavin are liver and milk, also eggs, whole grains, and brewer's yeast.

People susceptible to deficiency include those taking phenothiazine *antipsychotic drugs*, tricyclic *antidepressant drugs*, or oestrogen-containing *oral contraceptives*, those with malabsorption disorders, or those with severe alcohol dependence. Riboflavin deficiency may also occur as a result of serious illness, major surgery, or severe injury.

Prolonged deficiency of riboflavin may cause chapped lips, soreness of the tongue and corners of the mouth, and certain eye disorders, such as *amblyopia* (poor visual acuity) and *photophobia* (abnormal sensitivity to bright light).

Excessive intake of riboflavin is not known to cause harmful effects.

NIACIN

This consists of nicotinic acid and nicotinamide, and does not have a designated vitamin number. Niacin plays an essential role in the activities of various enzymes involved in the metabolism of carbohydrates and fats, the functioning of the nervous and digestive systems, the manufacture of sex hormones, and the maintenance of healthy skin.

The principal dietary sources of niacin include liver, lean meat, poultry, fish, nuts, and dried beans. Niacin is present in cereals in a chemically-bound form that is not absorbed by the body; part is liberated and becomes available when the cereal is baked. Niacin can be made in the body from tryptophan (an *amino acid* present in proteins).

Most cases of deficiency are due to malabsorption disorders or to severe alcohol dependence. Prolonged niacin deficiency causes *pellagra*, the principal symptoms of which include

soreness and cracking of the skin, inflammation of the mouth and tongue, and mental disturbances; pellagra can be fatal.

Excessive intake of niacin is not known to cause harmful effects.

PANTOTHENIC ACID

Pantothenic acid is essential for the activities of various enzymes involved in the metabolism of carbohydrates and fats, the manufacture of corticosteroids and sex hormones, the utilization of other vitamins, the functioning of the nervous system and adrenal glands, and normal growth and development.

Pantothenic acid is present in almost all vegetables, cereals, and animal foods. Particularly rich sources of this vitamin include liver, heart, kidney, fish, egg yolk, and wheat-germ.

A dietary shortage is almost never seen; deficiency usually occurs as a result of malabsorption disorders or severe alcohol dependence. Deficiency may also sometimes occur as a result of severe illness, major surgery, or serious injury. The principal effects of deficiency include fatigue, headache, nausea, abdominal pain, numbness and tingling, muscle cramps, and susceptibility to respiratory infections. In severe cases, a *peptic ulcer* may develop.

Excessive intake of pantothenic acid is not known to have harmful effects.

PYRIDOXINE

This vitamin plays a vital role in the activities of various enzymes and hormones involved in the breakdown and utilization of carbohydrates, fats, and proteins, in the manufacture of red blood cells and antibodies, in the functioning of the digestive and nervous systems, and in the maintenance of healthy skin.

Good dietary sources of pyridoxine include liver, chicken, pork, fish, whole grains, wheat-germ, bananas, potatoes, and dried beans. Pyridoxine is also manufactured in small amounts by intestinal bacteria. Groups susceptible to deficiency include elderly people on a poor diet, people with a malabsorption disorder, people with severe alcohol dependence, and people who are being treated with certain drugs (including *penicillamine* and *isoniazid*).

Deficiency of pyridoxine may cause weakness, irritability, depression, skin disorders, inflammation of the mouth and tongue, cracked lips, anaemia, and, in infants, seizures.

Excessive intake—100 times or more above the normal daily intake—

has been reported to cause *neuritis*. Doses of 50 to 100 mg per day are said to be helpful in relieving symptoms of premenstrual syndrome but the results are not clear.

BIOTIN

Biotin is essential for the activities of various enzymes involved in the breakdown of fatty acids and carbohydrates and for the excretion of the waste products of protein breakdown.

Biotin is present in many foods. Particularly rich sources of this vitamin include liver, peanuts, dried beans, egg yolk, mushrooms, bananas, grapefruit, and watermelon. Biotin is also manufactured by bacteria present in the intestines.

Deficiency may occur during prolonged treatment with *antibiotic drugs* or *sulphonamide drugs*. It may also result from long-term high consumption of raw egg whites, which contain a substance that interferes with the intestinal absorption of biotin. Otherwise, no dietary shortage has been observed. The principal symptoms of biotin deficiency include weakness, tiredness, poor appetite, hair loss, depression, inflammation of the tongue, and eczema.

Excessive intake of biotin is not known to cause harmful effects.

FOLIC ACID

This vitamin plays a vital role in the activities of various enzymes involved in the manufacture of *nucleic acids* (the genetic material of cells) and therefore in growth and reproduction, in the production of red blood cells, and in the healthy functioning of the nervous system.

The principal dietary sources of folic acid include green leafy vegetables, mushrooms, liver, nuts, dried beans, peas, egg yolk, and wholemeal bread.

A varied diet that includes fresh vegetables and fruit generally provides enough folic acid for the body's needs. Mild deficiency is relatively common, but can usually be corrected by increasing the daily consumption of foods containing folic acid. More severe deficiency may occur during pregnancy or breast-feeding, in premature or low-birthweight infants, in people undergoing *dialysis*, in people with certain blood disorders, *psoriasis*, malabsorption disorders, or severe alcohol dependence, and in people taking certain drugs, including *anticonvulsant drugs*, antimalarial drugs, oestrogen-containing oral contraceptive drugs, and some *analgesic drugs* (painkillers), *corticosteroid drugs*, and sulphonamide drugs.

V

The principal effects of folic acid deficiency include anaemia, sores around the mouth, a sore tongue, and, in children, poor growth.

Folic acid supplements taken just before conception, and for the first 12 weeks of pregnancy, have been shown to reduce the risk of the fetus having a *neural tube defect*.

Vitamin C

Also known by its chemical name, ascorbic acid, a vitamin that plays an essential role in the activities of various *enzymes* (substances that promote chemical reactions in the body). Vitamin C is important for the growth and maintenance of healthy bones, teeth, gums, ligaments, and blood vessels; in the production of certain *neurotransmitters* (chemicals responsible for the transmission of nerve impulses between nerve cells) and of adrenal gland hormones; in the response of the *immune system* to infection; in wound healing; and in the absorption of *iron*.

The principal dietary sources of vitamin C are fruits and vegetables. Citrus fruits, tomatoes, green leafy vegetables, potatoes, green peppers, strawberries, and blackcurrants are particularly rich sources. Considerable amounts of vitamin C are lost during the processing, cooking, or keeping warm of foods.

DEFICIENCY

Dietary deficiency of vitamin C is rare. Slight deficiency may occur as a result of a serious injury or burn, major surgery, use of *oral contraceptives*, fever, or continual inhalation of carbon monoxide (a constituent of tobacco-smoke and traffic fumes). More pronounced deficiency is usually caused by a very restricted diet.

Mild deficiency may cause weakness, general aches and pains, swollen gums, and *nosebleeds*. Severe deficiency leads to *scurvy* and *anaemia*.

EXCESS

Large doses of vitamin C are taken by some people in the belief that they prevent the common cold, but there is no convincing evidence to support this belief. Excessive intake of vitamin C is not usually harmful unless the daily dose is more than about 1 g, when it may cause nausea, stomach cramps, diarrhoea, and, occasionally, kidney stones.

Vitamin D

The collective term for a group of related substances—including ergocalciferol (vitamin D_2), and cholecalciferol (vitamin D_3)—that play several vital roles in the body. Vitamin D helps regulate the balance of *calcium* and *phosphate*, aids the absorption of calcium from the intestine, and is essential for strong bones and teeth.

Good sources of vitamin D include oily fish (such as sardines, herring, salmon, and tuna), liver, and egg yolk; vitamin D is also added to margarines. In the body, vitamin D is formed by the action of ultraviolet rays in sunlight on a specific chemical in the skin.

DEFICIENCY

Deficiency may occur in people on a poor diet; in premature infants; in those deprived of sunlight, such as night-workers; and in dark-skinned people, particularly those living in foggy urban areas, who do not absorb enough ultraviolet rays.

Deficiency also occurs in certain disorders, most commonly those in which intestinal absorption of the vitamin is impaired (see *Malabsorption*). Other causes include liver disorders, kidney disorders, and some genetic defects. Prolonged use of certain drugs, such as *phenytoin* (an anticonvulsant drug), may also result in vitamin D deficiency.

Deficiency in young children causes *rickets* (a condition in which there is poor bone formation). Long-term deficiency in adults leads to *osteomalacia* (the adult equivalent of rickets, in which the bones lose calcium and become very fragile).

EXCESS

Excessive intake of vitamin D disrupts the balance of calcium and phosphate in the body and leads to *hypercalcaemia* (an abnormally high level of calcium in the blood). Symptoms of an excessive vitamin D intake include weakness, abnormal thirst, increased urination, gastrointestinal disturbances, and depression. An excess of vitamin D may also lead to abnormal calcium deposits in the soft tissues, kidneys, and blood vessel walls. In children, vitamin D excess may cause growth retardation.

Vitamin E

The collective term for a group of substances—of which alpha-tocopherol is the most important—that play several vital roles in the body, principally concerned with protecting fats from oxidation.

Vitamin E is essential for normal cell structure, for maintaining the activities of certain *enzymes* (substances that promote chemical reactions in the body), and for the formation of red blood cells. This vitamin also protects the lungs and other tissues from damage by pollutants, helps prevent red blood cells from being destroyed by poisons in the blood, and is believed to slow aging of cells.

The principal dietary sources of vitamin E are vegetable oils, nuts, meat, green leafy vegetables, cereals, wheat-germ, and egg yolk.

DEFICIENCY

Dietary shortages rarely occur; deficiency usually occurs only through impaired intestinal absorption (see *Malabsorption*), in certain liver disorders, and in premature infants.

Vitamin E deficiency leads to the destruction of red blood cells, which eventually results in *anaemia*. In infants, deficiency causes irritability and oedema (accumulation of fluid in body tissues).

EXCESS

Prolonged, excessive intake of vitamin E may cause abdominal pain, nausea and vomiting, and diarrhoea. It may also reduce intestinal absorption of vitamins A, D, and K, which, in severe cases, may produce symptoms of deficiency of these vitamins.

Vitamin K

A *vitamin* that is essential for the formation in the liver of substances that promote blood clotting.

The principal dietary sources of vitamin K are green leafy vegetables (especially cabbage, broccoli, and turnip greens), vegetable oils, egg yolk, cheese, pork, and liver. Vitamin K is also manufactured by bacteria that live in the intestine.

DEFICIENCY AND EXCESS

Dietary deficiency rarely occurs. Deficiency may develop in people suffering from *malabsorption* disorders in which intestinal absorption is impaired, from certain liver disorders, and from chronic diarrhoea. Deficiency may also develop as a result of prolonged treatment with *antibiotic drugs* (which destroy intestinal bacteria). Newborn infants lack the intestinal bacteria that produce vitamin K and are therefore routinely given supplements to prevent deficiency.

Deficiency of vitamin K reduces the ability of the blood to clot. This may cause nosebleeds, seeping of blood from wounds, and bleeding from the gums, intestine, and urinary tract. In rare, very severe cases, brain haemorrhage may result.

Excessive intake of vitamin K is not known to cause harmful effects.

V

Vitamin supplements

A group of dietary preparations containing one or more *vitamins*.

Most people do not usually need vitamin supplements (see *Nutrition*). Eating a variety of foods provides adequate amounts of all vitamins. Excessive amounts of some vitamins (especially A and D) may sometimes be harmful.

MEDICAL USES

Vitamin supplements are used to treat diagnosed vitamin deficiency, to prevent vitamin deficiency in susceptible people, and to treat certain medical disorders.

In developed countries, deficiency most commonly occurs in people on a poor diet, such as those with severe *alcohol dependence* or *drug dependence*, those on a low income, and elderly people who are not eating properly. A vegan diet (one that excludes all animal products) may sometimes result in vitamin deficiency. Deficiency may also result from *malabsorption*, *liver disorders*, and *kidney disorders*.

Vitamin supplements are also used to prevent deficiency during periods of increased requirements, such as pregnancy, breast-feeding, and infancy. They are also given to people who are taking certain drugs that may impair the absorption of vitamins, to those suffering from serious illness or injury, or to people who have had major surgery. People who are being fed intravenously or via a tube (see *Feeding, artificial*) are also likely to need vitamin supplements.

Certain vitamins are used to treat some conditions that are not specific deficiency disorders. Vitamin D, for example, is used in the treatment of *osteoporosis* and vitamin A derivatives are prescribed for severe *acne*.

There is no clear medical evidence to support the claims that vitamin C helps to prevent or cure the common cold, that vitamin B$_6$ helps relieve premenstrual syndrome, or that vitamin E improves well-being.

Vitiligo

A common disorder of *skin* pigmentation in which patches of skin lose their colour. Depigmented white patches are particularly obvious in dark-skinned people, occurring most commonly on the face, hands, armpits, and groin. Affected skin is particularly sensitive to sunlight.

Vitiligo is thought to be an *autoimmune disorder* that causes an absence of melanocytes, the specialized cells responsible for secreting the skin

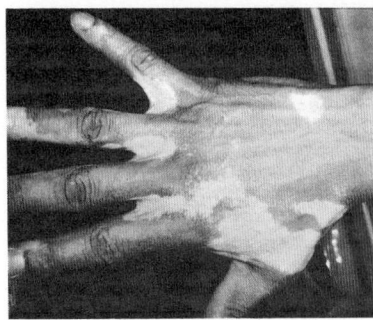

Vitiligo affecting the right hand
Loss of pigment is the only skin change that occurs. The usual remedy is to mask the white patches with cosmetics.

pigment *melanin*. The condition may occur at any age but usually develops in early adulthood. It affects about one in 200 people. Spontaneous repigmentation occurs in about 30 per cent of cases.

TREATMENT

Make-up may be used to disguise areas of vitiligo; in mild cases, no further treatment may be necessary. *Phototherapy* using *PUVA* induces significant repigmentation in more than 50 per cent of cases, but many treatments are required. Creams containing *corticosteroid drugs* may also help. If areas of vitiligo are extensive, chemicals may be used to remove pigment from remaining areas of normal skin.

Vitreous haemorrhage

Bleeding into the *vitreous humour*, the gel-like substance that fills the main cavity of the *eye* between the crystalline lens and the retina. A common cause of vitreous haemorrhage is diabetic *retinopathy*, in which new, fragile blood capillaries that bleed readily form on the retina.

Any bleeding into the vitreous humour is likely to affect vision; a major haemorrhage into the centre of the gel causes very poor vision for as long as the blood remains. Blood released into the periphery of the vitreous humour may be reabsorbed and the transparency of the gel restored, but a large haemorrhage may persist for months or never clear.

Vitreous humour

The transparent, gel-like body that fills the large rear compartment of the *eye* between the crystalline lens and the retina. The vitreous humour consists almost entirely of water. Under certain conditions, it can exert sufficient pull on the retina to cause *retinal tears* and *retinal detachment*.

Vivisection

The performance of a surgical operation on a live animal, particularly for research purposes. (See also *Animal experimentation*.)

Vocal cords

Two fibrous sheets of tissue in the *larynx* (voice-box) that are responsible for voice production. The cords are attached at the front to the inner surface of the thyroid cartilage (Adam's apple) and at the rear to the arytenoid cartilages.

The so-called true vocal cords are the cords that vibrate and make sound; the false vocal cords are merely folds in the larynx, just above the true vocal cords, that have nothing to do with sound production.

Most of the time the vocal cords lie apart, forming a V-shaped opening called the glottis through which air is breathed. Vocal sounds are produced when the cords tighten, close, and vibrate as air expelled from the lungs passes between them. Alterations in the tension of the cords produce sounds of different pitch, which are modified by the tongue, palate, and lips to produce *speech*. (See also *Larynx, disorders of*.)

Voice-box

See *Larynx*.

Voice, loss of

Inability to speak normally due to a disorder affecting the *vocal cords* or, rarely, to a psychological problem. Loss of voice may be partial or total, temporary or permanent.

Partial loss of voice, also known as dysphonia, is fairly common and may be caused by any condition that interferes with the normal working of the vocal cords.

Temporary loss of voice commonly results from straining of the muscles of the *larynx* (which control the vocal cords) through overuse of the voice. Temporary dysphonia also often results from inflammation of the vocal cords in *laryngitis*.

Persistent or recurrent dysphonia may be due to *polyps* (benign growths) on the vocal cords, thickening of the vocal cords as a result of *hypothyroidism*, or, less commonly, to interference with the nerve supply to the muscles of the larynx as a result of cancer of the larynx (see *Larynx, cancer of*), thyroid gland (see *Thyroid cancer*), or oesophagus (see *Oesophagus, cancer of*). In rare cases, the vocal cords themselves or the nerves supplying them

V

LOCATION OF THE VOCAL CORDS

The vocal cords are located at the top of the larynx (voice-box). Their top edges stretch between the thyroid cartilage at the front and the arytenoid cartilages at the back. If brought close together, the cords vibrate and emit sounds as air passes between them.

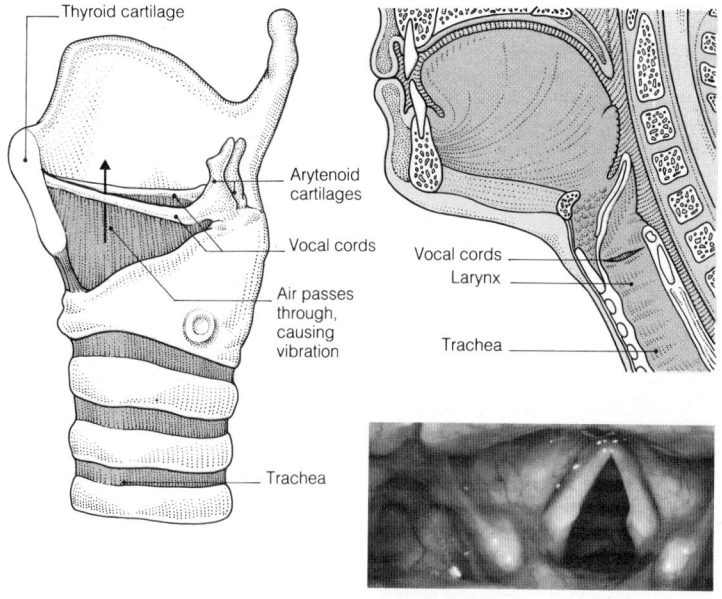

Thyroid cartilage

Arytenoid cartilages

Vocal cords

Air passes through, causing vibration

Trachea

Vocal cords
Larynx
Trachea

Action
For voice production, the cords are brought close together by muscles that act on the arytenoid cartilages.

View of vocal cords
This photograph shows the two vocal cords in their position at rest: spaced apart to form a V-shaped opening.

may be accidentally damaged during a surgical operation performed to treat thyroid cancer, resulting in permanent dysphonia.

Total loss of the voice, known as *aphonia*, is rare and is usually of psychological origin. (See also *Hoarseness*; *Larynx, disorders of*.)

Volkmann's contracture

A disorder in which the wrist and fingers become permanently fixed in a bent position. Volkmann's contracture occurs as a result of ischaemia (inadequate blood supply) in the forearm muscles that control the wrist and fingers.

CAUSES

Ischaemia in the forearm muscles may be caused by damage to the brachial artery as a result of a displaced fracture of the humerus (see *Humerus, fracture of*) or of dislocation of the *elbow*. Ischaemia may also follow any forearm injury that leads to *oedema* (retention of fluid within tissues), with consequent swelling of tissues and compression of blood vessels.

SYMPTOMS

Initially, the fingers become cold, numb, and white or blue. Finger movements are weak and painful, and no pulse can be felt at the wrist. Unless treatment is started within a few hours, the characteristic wrist and finger deformity develops.

TREATMENT

Any displaced bones are first manipulated back into position under general anaesthetic. If blood flow to the affected hand fails to improve, an operation is performed in which the tissues in the forearm are cut open to relieve pressure on the underlying muscles. Blockage of the artery may be relieved by injecting a *vasodilator drug* or by cutting open the artery and removing part of the lining. Occasionally, a section of damaged artery is cut out and replaced by a graft taken from a vein.

If there is permanent deformity, *physiotherapy* may restore function to an acceptable level. In severe cases, surgery may be required to shorten the bones in the forearm, to cut away

damaged muscle, and to transplant healthy muscle from another part of the forearm. This procedure is sometimes accompanied by *arthrodesis* (fusion) of the wrist joint.

Volvulus

Twisting of a loop of *intestine* or, in rare cases, of the *stomach*. Volvulus is a serious condition that causes obstruction of the passage of intestinal contents (see *Intestine, obstruction of*) and a risk of *strangulation*. If strangulation occurs, blockage of the blood flow to the affected area leads to potentially fatal *gangrene*.

The symptoms of volvulus are severe *colic* followed by vomiting.

Volvulus may be present from birth or may be a result of *adhesions* (bands of scar tissue). It is more common in Africa and Asia than in Europe or North America, possibly because of an association between volvulus and a very high-fibre diet.

Volvulus requires emergency treatment. In most cases, surgery is necessary to treat the condition.

Vomiting

Involuntary forcible expulsion of stomach contents through the mouth. Vomiting is usually preceded by nausea, pallor, sweating, excessive salivation, and slowing of the heart-rate.

MECHANISM

Vomiting occurs when the vomiting centre in the *brainstem* is activated. Activation of the vomiting centre may occur as the result of information passing directly to it from the frontal lobes of the brain, the digestive tract, or the balancing mechanism in the inner ear when these mechanisms are either damaged or disturbed. The centre may also be activated by the chemoreceptor trigger zone, also in the brainstem, which is itself stimulated by the presence in the blood of poisons or certain other substances.

Once activated, the vomiting centre sends messages to the diaphragm (the sheet of muscle separating the chest from the abdomen), which presses sharply downwards on the stomach, and to the wall of the abdomen, which presses inwards. Simultaneously, the pyloric sphincter between the base of the stomach and the intestine closes and the region between the top of the stomach and the oesophagus relaxes. As a result, the stomach contents are expelled upwards through the oesophagus. As this happens, the larynx (voice-box) is tightly closed by the epiglottis (the flap of cartilage at

V

its entrance) to prevent vomit from entering the trachea (windpipe) and causing choking.

CAUSES

Vomiting commonly happens after overindulgence in food or alcohol. It is also a common adverse effect of many drugs and often follows general anaesthesia (see *Anaesthesia, general*).

Vomiting may also result from disorders of the stomach or intestine that result in inflammation, irritation, or distension (swelling) of either organ. Such disorders include *peptic ulcer*, acute *appendicitis*, *gastroenteritis*, and *food poisoning*. Less commonly, vomiting is a symptom of intestinal obstruction due to *pyloric stenosis*, *intussusception*, or a tumour of the digestive tract.

Vomiting may also be caused by inflammation of organs associated with the digestive tract, such as the liver (see *Hepatitis*), the pancreas (see *Pancreatitis*), and the gallbladder (see *Cholecystitis*).

Another possible cause of vomiting is raised pressure within the skull, which may be due to *encephalitis*, *hydrocephalus*, a *brain tumour*, or a *head injury*. When the rise is rapid, it causes sudden, extremely forceful vomiting, often without any prior nausea. Vomiting is a common feature of *migraine*.

Vomiting is also a common feature of disorders affecting the balancing mechanism within the inner ear, such as *Ménière's disease* and acute *labyrinthitis*, or of disturbance of the mechanism by unusual movement, such as that experienced on a boat (see *Motion sickness*).

Disorders of the *endocrine system*, such as *Addison's disease*, may cause vomiting, as do disturbances of hormone production in early pregnancy (see *Vomiting in pregnancy*).

Vomiting is sometimes a symptom of a metabolic disorder, such as ketoacidosis (excessive production of ketones and acids), which may be due to poorly controlled *diabetes mellitus*.

Internal bleeding from the oesophagus, stomach, or duodenum, or swallowing blood from a nosebleed, can also result in *vomiting blood*.

Vomiting sometimes occurs as a reaction of disgust to a situation or food. It may also be a symptom of a psychological or emotional problem or be part of the psychiatric disorders *anorexia nervosa* or *bulimia*.

INVESTIGATION AND TREATMENT

Persistent vomiting requires investigation by a doctor. Treatment depends on the underlying cause. Do not eat or drink or take any unnecessary medication during the active phase of vomiting. *Antiemetic drugs* may be prescribed.

Vomiting blood

Known medically as haematemesis, vomiting blood is a symptom of bleeding from within the digestive tract. It usually occurs as a result of a serious disorder of the oesophagus, stomach, or duodenum.

Vomiting blood may be caused by a tear at the lower end of the oesophagus (see *Mallory-Weiss syndrome*), bleeding from *oesophageal varices* (widened veins in the oesophagus and upper stomach), severe erosive *gastritis* (inflammation of the stomach lining), *peptic ulcer*, or, in rare cases, *stomach cancer*. Blood can also be vomited if it is swallowed during a nosebleed.

Vomited blood may be dark red, brown, black, or resemble coffee grounds (as a result of the action of stomach acid). Depending on the extent of internal bleeding and the quantity of stomach contents, the blood may either streak the vomit or constitute a major part of it. Vomiting blood is often accompanied by *melaena* (the passing of black, tarry faeces).

The underlying cause of vomiting blood is investigated by *endoscopy* (inspection through a viewing instrument) of the oesophagus and stomach, or by *barium X-ray examinations*. If blood loss is severe, *blood transfusion* and possibly surgery to stop the bleeding may be needed.

Vomiting in pregnancy

Nausea and vomiting in early *pregnancy* are extremely common. These symptoms are experienced by about half of all pregnant women.

The vomiting usually starts before the sixth week of pregnancy and continues until about the 12th week; in some cases it occurs throughout pregnancy. The probable cause is activation of the vomiting centre in the brain due to changed hormone levels during pregnancy.

Vomiting occurs most commonly in the morning, often after waking (hence its common name, morning sickness), but can occur at any time. It is sometimes precipitated by emotional stress, travelling, or food. Sufferers may find it helpful to eat small, regular meals.

In rare cases, the vomiting becomes severe and prolonged, a condition known as hyperemesis gravidarum. This can cause dehydration, nutritional deficiency, alteration in blood acidity, liver damage, and weight loss. Immediate hospital admission is required to replace lost fluids and chemicals by *intravenous infusion*, to rule out the possibility of any serious underlying disorder, and to control the vomiting (although *antiemetic drugs* are avoided if possible).

Von Recklinghausen's disease

Another name for *neurofibromatosis*.

Von Willebrand's disease

An inherited lifelong *bleeding disorder* with similarities to *haemophilia*.

CAUSES AND INCIDENCE

Von Willebrand's disease is caused by a defective *gene* and is usually inherited in an autosomal dominant pattern (see *Genetic disorders*). A person needs to inherit only one copy of the defective gene to suffer from the disease. As many as one person in 1,000 is believed to have the gene but its effects are variable. Unlike haemophilia, the disease affects equal numbers of males and females.

The gene defect leads to a reduced concentration in the blood of a substance called von Willebrand factor. This factor plays a dual role in the arrest of bleeding. It helps platelets in the blood to plug injured blood vessel walls, and it forms part of *factor VIII* (a substance that is vital to blood coagulation). In the absence of von Willebrand factor, neither blood coagulation nor platelet plug formation can proceed normally, so there is a tendency to bleed.

SYMPTOMS

The symptoms may include excessive bleeding from the gums and from cuts and nosebleeds. Women may suffer from *menorrhagia* (excessive menstrual bleeding). In some cases, symptoms are minimal. In the most severe forms, deep bleeding into joints and muscles may be a problem.

DIAGNOSIS

The disease is diagnosed by *blood-clotting tests*, which show a long bleeding time, and by measurements that reveal reduced levels of von Willebrand factor in the blood.

TREATMENT

Bleeding episodes can be prevented or controlled by the giving of desmopressin (a substance resembling *ADH*), which raises the body's natural production of von Willebrand factor. Another possible treatment is the administration of cryoprecipitate (a

V

VOMITING Forceful expulsion of stomach contents that usually has a simple explanation, such as irritation of the stomach by infection or overindulgence in food or alcohol. However, it may be a sign of a more serious disorder, particularly if there are accompanying symptoms. Vomiting may or may not be preceded by nausea.

Have you had severe abdominal pain that has not been relieved by the vomiting? — **YES**

☎ **EMERGENCY!**
GET MEDICAL HELP NOW!
A serious abdominal condition, such as appendicitis or a perforated duodenal ulcer, may cause such symptoms.

See • *Appendicitis*

NO

Have you vomited red blood, or black or dark brown matter that resembles coffee grounds? — **YES**

Treatment for vomiting
If you have been vomiting, provided you suspect no serious cause, try the following self-help measures:
• Eat no solid food until your nausea and vomiting subside.
• Drink plenty of clear (nonalcoholic) fluids in small sips even if you cannot keep anything down for long.
• Do not smoke.
• Do not take aspirin.

If you vomit repeatedly for more than 24 hours, or if more symptoms develop, consult your doctor.

☎ **EMERGENCY!**
GET MEDICAL HELP NOW!
This could be caused by bleeding somewhere in the digestive tract.

NO

Do you have diarrhoea AND/OR is your temperature 38°C or above? — **YES**

This may be caused by an infection of the digestive tract. If symptoms persist, consult your doctor.

See • *Gastroenteritis*

NO

In the past few hours, have you done any of the following? — **YES**
• overeaten
• eaten large amounts of rich, creamy, or spicy food
• consumed a large amount of alcohol

Inflammation of the stomach lining often occurs as the result of overindulgence. Consult your doctor if you have recurrent attacks.

See • *Gastroenteritis*

NO

Have you eaten anything that may have gone bad or to which you may be allergic? — **YES**

Poisoning by food contaminated by bacteria or by poisonous chemicals or by food to which you are allergic may be responsible for the vomiting.

See • *Food poisoning*

NO

Continued on next page

V

Do you have a headache?

YES → Have you had a head injury within the past 24 hours?

    YES → ☎ **EMERGENCY!**
GET MEDICAL HELP NOW!
You may have a brain injury.

    NO ↓

Do you have one or more of the following symptoms?
- pain when you bend your head forward
- dislike of bright light
- drowsiness or confusion

    YES → ☎ **EMERGENCY!**
GET MEDICAL HELP NOW!
These symptoms suggest the possibility of a serious brain disorder.

See • *Meningitis*
      • *Subarachnoid haemorrhage*

NO

NO

Was your headache preceded by visual distortion, weakness of an extremity, and/or nausea AND is the headache one-sided (sometimes with blurred vision and nasal stuffiness)?

YES → The symptoms are probably due to a migraine attack. Consult your doctor.

See • *Migraine*

NO

Do you have severe pain in or around one eye AND is your vision blurred?

YES → ☎
Consult your doctor without delay!
These symptoms suggest the possibility of acute glaucoma, in which excess fluid causes increased pressure in the eye; this is particularly likely if you are over 40.

See • *Glaucoma*

NO

Before you vomited, did everything around you seem to spin?

YES → Disorders of the inner ear cause vomiting and dizzy spells. Consult your doctor.

See • *Labyrinthitis*
      • *Ménière's disease*

NO

> **Vomiting and the Pill**
> If you are taking the birth-control pill and suffer from an attack of vomiting, your protection against conception may be reduced. Continue to take your pills as usual, but use an extra form of contraception until you start a new packet of pills.

Continued on next page

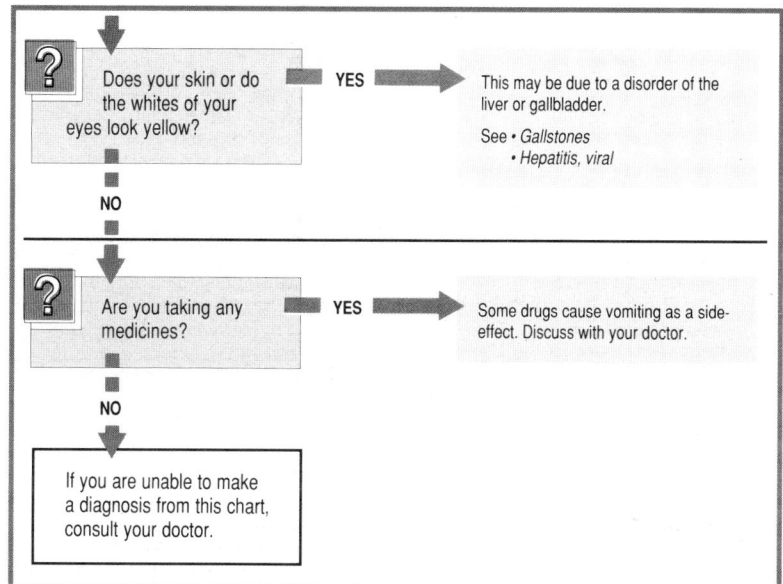

Does your skin or do the whites of your eyes look yellow?

YES → This may be due to a disorder of the liver or gallbladder.
See • *Gallstones*
• *Hepatitis, viral*

NO

Are you taking any medicines?

YES → Some drugs cause vomiting as a side-effect. Discuss with your doctor.

NO

If you are unable to make a diagnosis from this chart, consult your doctor.

preparation obtained from normal blood plasma), which is a rich source of von Willebrand factor.

Voyeurism

The repeated observation of unsuspecting people who are naked, in the act of undressing, or engaging in sexual activity. Commonly called Peeping Toms, voyeurs become sexually aroused through the act of looking and have no wish to engage in sexual activity themselves. Orgasm is achieved (usually by masturbation) while watching or remembering the witnessed events. In its severe form, voyeurism is the only way in which orgasm is achieved.

Vulva

The external, visible part of the female genitalia. The vulva comprises the *clitoris* and two pairs of skin folds called *labia*.

The most common symptom of a disorder affecting the vulva is *vulval itching*, known medically as pruritus vulvae. Itching of the vulva often occurs with vaginal itching.

Various generalized skin disorders, such as *dermatitis*, may affect the vulva. Specific vulval conditions include genital warts (see *Warts, genital*), *vulvitis, vulvovaginitis*, and cancer (see *Vulva, cancer of*).

Vulva, cancer of

A rare disorder that most commonly affects postmenopausal women. Cancer of the vulva may be preceded by

vulval itching, but in many cases the first symptom is a lump or painful ulcer on the vulva.

A diagnosis of vulval cancer is made by *biopsy* (removal of a small sample of tissue for laboratory analysis). Treatment is by surgical removal of the affected area. The outlook depends on how soon the cancer is diagnosed and treated.

Vulval itching

A term for irritation of the *vulva* (the female external genitalia), also known as pruritus vulvae.

Most commonly, vulval itching is due to an allergic reaction to chemicals in deodorants, spermicides, creams, and douches. Itching is also very common after the *menopause*, when it is due to low levels of *oestrogen hormone*. Vulval itching may also be caused by a vaginal discharge due to an infection of the vagina (see *Vaginitis*). A group of vulval skin changes, collectively called vulval dystrophies (see *Vulvitis*), can cause itching of the vulva.

Treatment of vulval itching may be in the form of *antibiotic drugs* or hormones, sometimes taken orally and sometimes applied in cream form.

Vulvitis

Inflammation of the *vulva*, which may have a variety of different causes.

Infections that may cause vulvitis include *candidiasis*, genital herpes (see *Herpes, genital*), and warts (see *Warts, genital*). Infestations with *pubic lice* or *scabies* are other possible causes.

Vulvitis may also occur as a result of changes in the vulval skin. These changes tend to affect women after the menopause, although there is no apparent cause. They may take the form of red or white patches and/or thickened or thinned areas that may be inflamed. Formerly called a variety of names, such as kraurosis vulvae and lichen sclerosus et atrophicus, these conditions are now generally known as vulval dystrophy.

Other possible causes of vulvitis are allergic reactions to soap, cream, or detergent, excessive vaginal discharge, or urinary *incontinence*.

TREATMENT
Treatment depends on the cause. A combination of drugs applied to the vulva along with good hygiene is the usual remedy. In some cases of vulval dystrophy, a *biopsy* (removal of a small sample of tissue for laboratory analysis) may be carried out to exclude the slight possibility of cancer. (See also *Vulvovaginitis; Vaginitis*.)

Vulvovaginitis

Inflammation of the *vulva* and *vagina*. Vulvovaginitis is usually due to the infections *candidiasis* or *trichomoniasis*, which cause a profuse vaginal discharge that also affects the vulva. In children, nonspecific infection may occur. (See also *Vaginitis; Vulvitis*.)

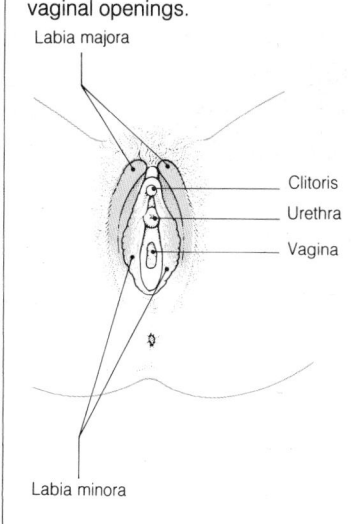

ANATOMY OF THE VULVA
The outer skin folds (labia majora) are usually in contact. If parted, they reveal the clitoris and inner folds (labia minora), which enclose the urethral and vaginal openings.

Labia majora

Clitoris

Urethra

Vagina

Labia minora

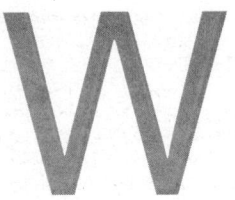

W

Walking

Movement of the body in one direction by lifting the feet alternately and bringing one foot into contact with the ground before the other starts to leave it. The manner of walking, known as gait, is determined by body shape, size, and posture, and often reflects the individual's personality. A normal pattern of walking is shown in the illustrated box.

Walking is controlled by nerve signals from the motor cortex (part of the *cerebrum* of the brain) and by signals from the *basal ganglia* and the *cerebellum*, located at the back of the brain. The signals are sent via the spinal cord to nerve cells and from there are carried by nerve fibres to the muscles. In response to changes in position, the cerebellum also receives information from the muscles, joints, eyes, and the balance organ in the inner ear. This information is used to adjust new signals sent to the muscles by the brain to ensure balance and coordinated movement.

Some of the nerves that control walking are located in a very primitive part of the brain. This may account for the walking reflex that occurs in newborn babies in which the legs move automatically in a walking motion when the child is held upright and the sole presses on a surface (see *Reflex, primitive*). The age at which children walk varies enormously.

DISORDERS

Abnormal gait may be caused by muscle weakness, by abnormalities of the skeleton, or by joint stiffness, causing immobility in the lower limbs or spine. Abnormal gait may also be the result of neurological disorders that affect the central control of locomotion and the balance and input of information to the nervous system from muscles and joints.

Different disorders affect walking in a variety of ways; the doctor can often gain clues to the underlying cause of a disorder by observing the way in which a person walks.

MUSCULAR CAUSES Any condition that causes wasting or loss of any of the muscles connected to the legs or feet may cause abnormal walking. In *muscular dystrophy*, the legs are held wide apart and the person waddles because of weakness of the buttock muscles. In *poliomyelitis* or after severe muscle injury, weakness of individual groups of muscles may cause limping because of unbalanced muscle action.

SKELETAL CAUSES Congenital deformities of the foot, such as *talipes* (clubfoot), may prevent normal walking. In talipes equinovarus, for example, the heel cannot be brought to the ground and a characteristic limping gait results. Congenital dislocation of the hip (see *Hip, congenital dislocation of*) that has not been detected in infancy may be noticed only when the child starts to walk—the foot on the affected side is placed flat on the ground while the opposite knee is flexed. *Scoliosis* (deformity of the spine) can also result in abnormal gait.

During a stage in their growth, children often develop *knock-knee* or *bowleg*. These conditions may produce a strange walk, but both usually disappear within several years.

Synovitis of the hip is a common cause of limping in children, most often in boys between the ages of two and 12 years. The limp, which is accompanied by pain of varying severity, starts suddenly and lasts for only a few days or weeks. Another common cause of limping in boys, usually between the ages of five and

---

THE MECHANICS OF WALKING

Many different muscles take part in the walking process. They contract in a complex, rhythmic sequence in response to programmes of signals sent from the motor cortex in the brain. Feedback of information from the muscles and joints to the brain helps to ensure that the gait is smooth, steady, and coordinated.

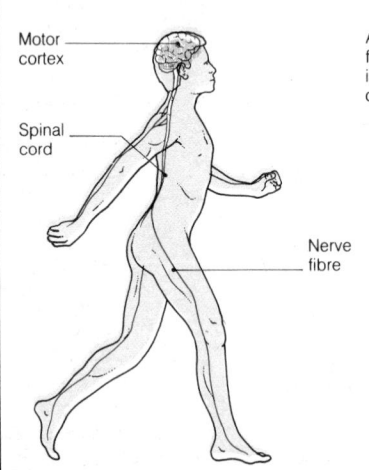

Route of the signals
The signals for walking originate in the motor cortex and are carried via the spinal cord and nerve fibres to muscles.

Motor cortex
Spinal cord
Nerve fibre

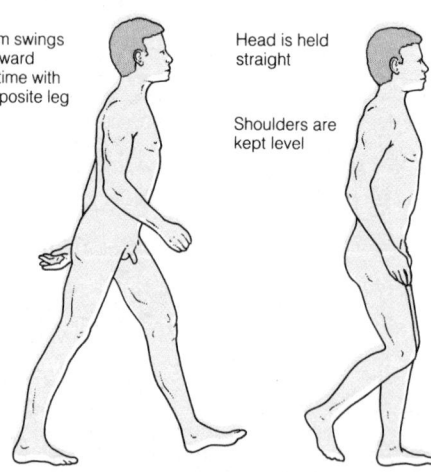
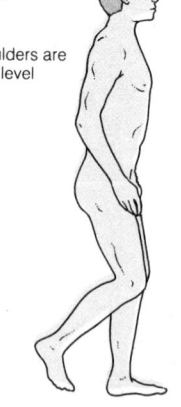

Arm swings forward in time with opposite leg
Head is held straight
Shoulders are kept level

1 As the left foot touches the ground, the right arm swings forward and the right foot shifts on to tiptoe.

2 Once the left foot is fully planted on the ground and supporting the body, the right foot is raised.

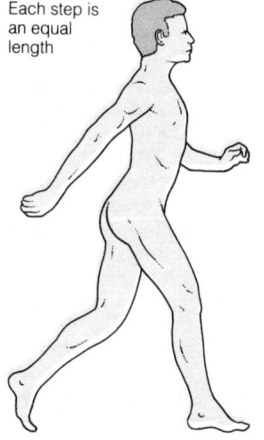

Each step is an equal length

3 A sequence of muscle contractions advances the right leg, and the left arm swings forward.

10, is *Perthes' disease*. The limp may or may not be painful. Young adolescents may develop a painful limp as a result of a slipped epiphysis (see *Femoral epiphysis, slipped*).

Other causes of limp include a painful *bone tumour* and *arthritis*.

Bone shortening may follow fracture or disease of one of the long bones of the leg (the *tibia*, *fibula*, or *femur*). This condition always causes an abnormal gait, usually with a dip of the body to the shortened side.

NEUROLOGICAL CAUSES Among the most common of the neurological causes is *stroke*, which commonly results in *hemiplegia* (paralysis or weakness of one side of the body). Because the affected leg is held stiffly extended, it must be swung outwards and forwards in walking. When both legs are affected by weakness (a condition known as paraparesis), they are held extended and pressed together at the thighs so that only short steps are possible and the toes scrape along the ground. In some people with paraparesis, the legs cross with each step, which produces a characteristic scissor movement.

In *parkinsonism* there is difficulty in starting to walk; the body is bent forwards at the waist and hips, with bending at the knees and ankles. The steps are short and shuffling with the feet barely clearing the ground. As progress continues, the steps become more and more rapid, and the person may eventually fall unless assisted.

Other disorders, including severe peripheral *neuritis*, *multiple sclerosis*, tertiary *syphilis*, and various forms of *myelitis*, may damage the sensory nerves or the spinal cord. The damage causes loss of information to the brain about the position of the joints, resulting in a characteristic gait. The body is bent forwards and the eyes are fixed on the ground, the legs are held wide apart, and the feet are carried much higher than normal and thrown forwards with sudden movements. People affected in this way are critically dependent on vision for walking; the gait becomes even worse if vision is defective.

Disease of the cerebellum or of the balancing mechanisms in the inner ears, such as *Ménière's disease*, may cause severe loss of balance and instability so that the affected person walks cautiously, with the legs apart, sometimes lurching to one side as though intoxicated (see *Ataxia*). In *chorea*, the gait may be bizarre and dance-like, with sudden thrusting

WALKING AIDS

Various types of walking aids are available for different forms and degrees of disability. The choice depends on such factors as whether the person is usually healthy or chronically disabled and whether the disability affects one or both of the person's legs.

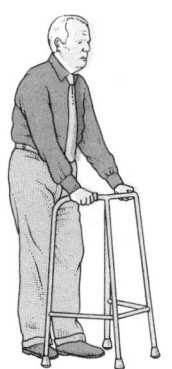
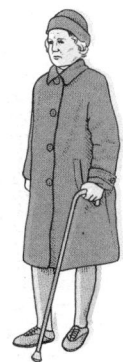
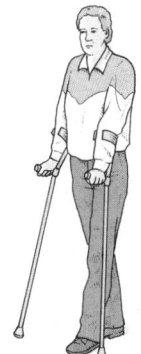
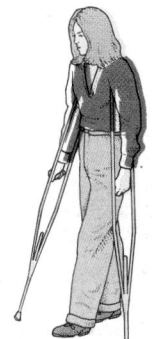

Walking frame   Walking stick   Elbow crutches   Full-length crutches

Walking frame and walking stick
Frames are useful for people affected by weakness on both sides, sticks for those who have one-sided weakness or pain.

Elbow and full-length crutches
Elbow crutches are often useful for people recovering from strokes, full-length crutches for those with leg injuries.

HOW TO USE CRUTCHES
Crutches are suitable only for people who are able to support their weight on at least one leg.

There are various ways of using crutches, as shown in the illustrations below.

FOUR-POINT WALKING

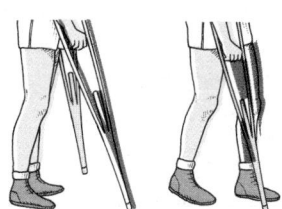

The feet and crutch tips are well separated, and one point is moved at a time. There are two possible sequences—right crutch, left foot, left crutch, right foot (above) or right then left crutch, right then left foot.

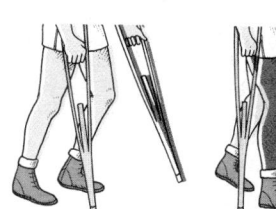

THREE-POINT WALKING

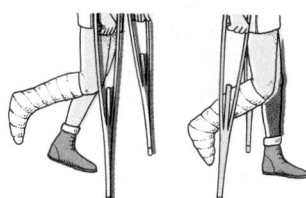

The crutches are advanced together while the person balances on one or both feet; the weight is then borne by the crutches while the feet are moved.

TWO-POINT WALKING

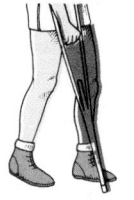
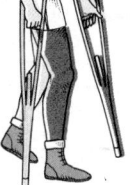

In two-point walking with crutches, the person moves the left foot and right crutch forward together, followed by the right foot and left crutch.

W

movements of the hips and twisting of the trunk and limbs. The steps are irregular and of varying length.

Walking aids

Equipment for increasing the mobility of people who have a disorder that affects *walking*. Support from a walking aid may be required by people with *arthritis* or other diseases affecting mobility, by those recovering from an injury (such as a *fracture* or *sprain*), or by those who are waiting to be fitted with a prosthesis (artificial limb) after an amputation.

WALKING FRAMES

Walking frames provide a very stable form of support and may be useful for people with severe balancing problems or for those who are affected by weakness, pain, or stiffness on both sides. However, walking frames tend to get in the way of the feet, allowing only slow progress.

Walking frames are usually made of a light, strong alloy and have four rubber-tipped legs in order to prevent sliding. They can be supplied with wheels on the front legs to make manoeuvring easier.

CRUTCHES

Crutches provide greater mobility than a walking frame, but they are suitable only for people who are able to support their own weight. Crutches are often used by people who need to avoid placing weight on an injured leg or foot while healing takes place. Body weight should be taken by the hands through the cross-bar of each crutch.

Full-length crutches are usually used by otherwise healthy people who have suffered a bone fracture or a severe strain or sprain of a joint, ligament, or tendon of a lower extremity. Body weight should not be taken through the armpits with full-length crutches, because this can cause radial nerve palsy.

Elbow crutches are sometimes useful because they allow gradual progression from a high degree of support to almost natural walking. People with arthritis in their upper limbs should not use elbow crutches because the additional strain on the joints may make the arthritis worse.

Crutches are usually made of a light alloy and are rubber-tipped. There are various ways of using crutches (see illustrated box on previous page).

WALKING STICKS

Walking sticks are most commonly used by people who have weakness, pain, or stiffness on one side. They are usually made of wood and have various types of handles to suit different grips. Lightweight aluminium sticks, whose length can easily be adjusted, are also available. A walking stick should have a rubber tip (or ferrule) to prevent slipping. For extra stability, walking sticks with three or four small feet on the end of the shaft can be used; such sticks are called tripods or quadropods.

A walking stick of the correct length should always be used, permitting an upright posture with the elbow slightly bent. It is generally best to walk with the stick on the strong side so that the stick is forward when the foot on the weak side comes forward. However, if one side is very weak, the stick may be held on the weak side, close to the leg, and moved with it, acting as a type of splint.

ELECTROMUSCULAR STIMULATION

Computer-controlled electromuscular stimulation of the leg muscles to facilitate walking in quadriplegics and paraplegics is being investigated.

Walking, delayed

Most children walk by around 15 months of age. Delayed walking may be suspected if the child is unable to walk unassisted by 18 months. (See *Developmental delay*.)

Warfarin

> **WARNING**
> Always check with your doctor before taking any other drug with warfarin since many drugs interfere with its anticlotting action.

An *anticoagulant drug* used to treat and prevent abnormal *blood clotting*. Warfarin is used to treat *thrombosis*, to prevent *stroke* and to treat *transient ischaemic attack*. It is also prescribed to prevent blood clotting after heart valve replacement (see *Heart valve surgery*), in some *heart valve disorders*, or in persistent *atrial fibrillation*.

Warfarin works by inhibiting the formation of *vitamin K*-dependent clotting factors in the liver. Because warfarin is fully effective only after several days, a faster-acting anticoagulant, such as *heparin*, is usually also prescribed during the first few days.

POSSIBLE ADVERSE EFFECTS

Warfarin may cause abnormal bleeding in different parts of the body; regular blood-clotting (prothrombin time) tests are therefore carried out to allow careful regulation of dosage. Warfarin may also cause nausea, loss of appetite, abdominal pain, and rash.

Wart

A very common, contagious, harmless growth on skin or mucous membranes. Warts affect only the topmost layer of skin. They do not have roots, seeds, or branches. The black dots that are sometimes evident are capillaries that have become clotted due to the rapid skin growth caused by the wart virus.

TYPES

Warts are caused by the human papillomavirus, HPV, of which at least 30 different types are known. These cause diferent types of warts at various sites, such as the hands or genitals; HPV 16, for example, causes changes in the uterine cervix.

COMMON WARTS These are firm, sharply defined, round or irregular, flesh-coloured to brown growths, up to about 6 mm in diameter. They often have a rough surface.

Common warts usually appear on sites subject to injury (such as the hands, face, knees, and scalp), particularly in young children.

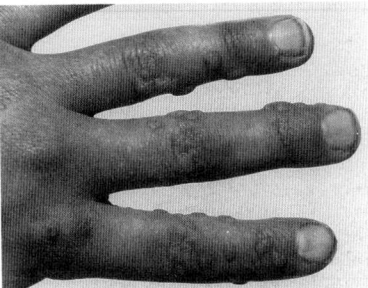

Common warts on hand
Warts often grow in crops. In time, they disappear spontaneously but they can be removed by freezing.

FLAT WARTS Flat-topped, flesh-coloured lumps that occur mainly on the wrists, the backs of the hands, and the face. These warts may itch.

DIGITATE WARTS Growths, sometimes dark in colour, that have finger-like projections.

FILIFORM WARTS Long, slender growths that may occur on the eyelids, armpits, or neck.

PLANTAR WARTS These are flat warts on the sole of the foot (see *Wart, plantar*). They are flattened simply as a result of the pressure placed on them; otherwise, they are just like other warts.

GENITAL WARTS These extensive, pink, cauliflower-like areas may occur on the genitals of men or women (see *Warts, genital*). Genital warts should be treated promptly. There is some evidence that warts infecting a

W

woman's cervix may predispose her to cervical cancer. It is important that both sexual partners be checked and rechecked since the infection can pass back and forth between them. Condoms can sometimes prevent transmission of the causative virus. Warts in the genital region of young children may be a sign of sexual abuse.

TREATMENT

About 50 per cent of warts disappear in six to 12 months without any treatment; warts other than genital and painful plantar warts are often left to disappear naturally.

Common, flat, and plantar warts can be treated in various ways. They can sometimes be destroyed by the application of a wart-removing liquid or special plaster. Several treatments may be needed and sometimes a wart returns. Warts are also commonly treated by *cryosurgery*, in which liquid nitrogen is used to freeze the wart solid. As it thaws, a blister forms, lifting the wart off. Alternatively, *electrocautery*, *curettage*, or *laser treatment* may be used.

Wart, plantar

A hard, horny, rough-surfaced area on the sole of the foot caused by a virus called a papillomavirus. Plantar warts, also commonly known as verrucas, may occur singly or in mosaic-like clusters.

Infection is usually acquired from contaminated floors in swimming pools and communal showers. Because of pressure from the weight of the body, the wart is flattened and forced into the skin of the sole, sometimes causing discomfort or pain when walking.

TREATMENT

Many plantar warts disappear without treatment, but some persist for

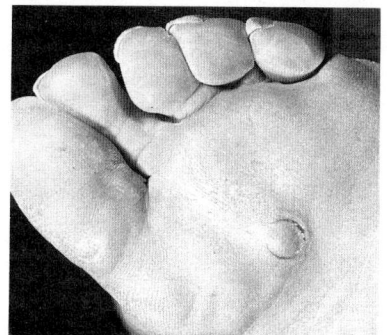

Typical plantar wart
This type of wart may need treatment—a doctor may pare it down with a scalpel and apply a corrosive paint.

years or may recur. To relieve discomfort, a foam pad may be worn in the shoe. Plantar warts can be removed by *cryosurgery*, *electrocautery*, *curettage*, *laser treatment*, or by applying salicylic acid plasters.

Warts, genital

Soft warts that grow in and around the entrance of the vagina and the anus and on the penis. Genital warts are transmitted by sexual contact and are caused by a papillomavirus. There may be an interval of up to 18 months between infection and the appearance of the warts.

Over 40,000 cases of genital warts are reported annually from sexually transmitted disease clinics in the UK.

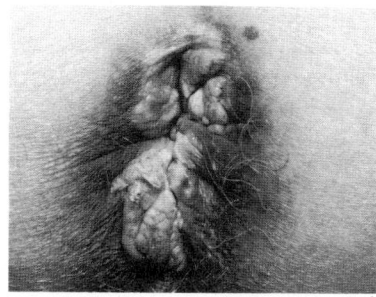

Genital warts around the anus
These growths are painless but need treatment—usually by the application of podophyllin or by surgical removal.

Genital warts have been linked with cases of cervical cancer (see *Cervix, cancer of*). A woman who has had genital warts—or whose partner has had genital warts—should have annual *cervical smear tests*.

Genital warts may be removed by surgery or by the application of *podophyllin*. However, there is a tendency for the warts to recur.

Wasp stings

See *Insect stings*.

Water

Although only a simple chemical (molecularly, two atoms of hydrogen bonded to one of oxygen—H_2O), water is essential to all forms of life. Some simple life-forms, such as certain microorganisms, can survive in a state of suspended animation for years or decades without water. However, even they require water to carry out functions such as growth and reproduction.

Water is the most common chemical in the human body (and also one of the most abundant substances on

Earth). Water accounts for about 99 per cent of all the molecules in the body, but for a comparatively smaller percentage of the total body weight (about 60 per cent in an average man). Thus, a man weighing 70 kg contains about 42 litres of water, of which about 28 litres are within the body cells themselves and 14 litres are extracellular. Of the extracellular water, about 3 to 4 litres are in the blood plasma, lymph, and cerebrospinal fluid; the remaining 10 to 11 litres are in *tissue fluid*.

ROLE IN THE BODY

Water is essential to life because it provides the medium in which all metabolic reactions take place (see *Metabolism*). It also provides the medium for the transportation of chemical substances, such as *ions*, in the body. The blood plasma carries water to all body tissues; it also carries excess water from tissues for elimination from the body by the *liver*, *kidneys*, *lungs*, and *skin*. The interchange of water between the blood and tissue cells occurs via the tissue fluid, which bathes all the individual cells. The passage of water in the tissue fluid into and out of cells takes place by a process called *osmosis*.

WATER BALANCE IN THE BODY

Intake (litres)

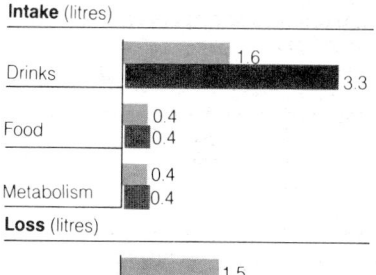

Drinks	1.6	3.3
Food	0.4 / 0.4	
Metabolism	0.4 / 0.4	

Loss (litres)

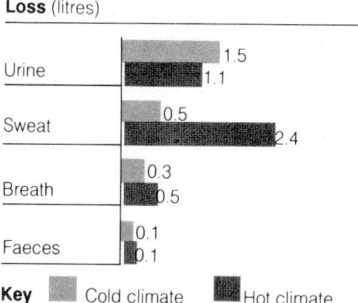

Urine	1.5 / 1.1	
Sweat	0.5	2.4
Breath	0.3 / 0.5	
Faeces	0.1 / 0.1	

Key ▨ Cold climate ■ Hot climate

W

Water intake and loss
The charts show average intake of water from various sources and losses in urine, sweat, and so on. In cool climates, people tend to drink more than the amount required to satisfy thirst; the excess water is lost in urine. In hot climates, large amounts of water are lost in sweat, and an increase in fluid intake is essential to avoid dehydration.

WATER BALANCE

Water is taken into the body not only by drinking, but also in food. A small amount of water is actually formed within the body by the metabolism of food.

Water is lost from the body in the *urine* and *faeces*, as water vapour breathed out, and by *sweating*. The amount passed out of the body in the urine depends largely on the amount of fluid drunk; the amount lost as sweat depends on physical activity and the external temperature.

The amount of water in the body must remain within relatively narrow limits for the proper functioning of metabolic processes; this balance is achieved by the activities of the kidneys, which control the balance between fluid intake and output by regulating the amount of water excreted from the body in the urine. The minimum daily urinary output necessary to remove waste products is about 0.5 litres, although most healthy adults usually produce about 1.5 litres of urine a day. The amount produced in excess of the minimum is controlled mainly by *ADH* (antidiuretic hormone), which is produced by the posterior portion of the pituitary gland and acts on the kidneys to reduce water excretion.

The body's water balance is also regulated in another way. If there is an excessive amount of any substance (such as sugar or salt) dissolved in the blood that must be excreted by the kidneys, extra water is needed to accomplish this function. This may lead to *dehydration* despite increased production of ADH, but is usually compensated for by increased water intake as a response to thirst.

In some disorders, such as *kidney failure* or *heart failure,* insufficient water is excreted in the urine, resulting in *oedema* (abnormal accumulation of water in body tissues).

Water-borne infection

Any disease caused by infective or parasitic organisms transmitted via water. Infections can be contracted if infected water is drunk, if it contaminates food, or if individuals swim or wade in it.

DRINKING WATER

Worldwide, contamination of drinking water is an important mode of transmission for various diseases, including hepatitis A (see *Hepatitis, viral*), many viral and bacterial causes of *diarrhoea, typhoid fever, cholera, amoebiasis,* and some types of *worm infestation.*

Contamination results from the discharge of human or animal excretory products containing infective organisms into rivers, lakes, reservoirs, or wells used as a source of water supply. The discharge may be direct or in the form of untreated sewage. It can also occur through leakage between sewage and water supply systems. This could happen, for example, in a city affected by a major earthquake.

In developed countries, such as the UK, the risks of water-borne infection are minimized through measures such as adequate sanitary facilities, sewage treatment and disposal, and the sterilization and testing of water before it is supplied to homes. Tap water is usually safe to drink therefore (unless there is a specific warning not to drink it).

In developing countries, sanitary facilities, sewage disposal, and water treatment may be inadequate. As a consequence, members of the population are more likely to carry the types of disease organisms spread by water. It is therefore best not to drink tap water in such countries and always to regard with suspicion any water taken directly from rivers, lakes, and wells.

AVOIDANCE OF INFECTION The accompanying table summarizes safe and suspect sources of drinking water in developed and developing countries. If safe tap water is unavailable, bottled or canned water or drinks of well-known brand names are usually safe; do not put ice made from suspect water into drinks. Rainwater is usually free of infective organisms provided it is not allowed to stand for a long period before drinking.

Water that may be infected should be sterilized before drinking. The most reliable method is to boil it for five minutes. Boiling kills any infective organisms present. If boiling is impractical, the alternative is to filter the water and then to sterilize it chemically. Filtering is necessary to remove suspended particles, which can harbour disease organisms and interfere with sterilization. Various types of filters are available; some remove bacteria and other infective organisms as well as inanimate particles. The manufacturer's instructions should be followed carefully. For chemical sterilization, purifying tablets that contain chlorine or iodine are used. Water should be left for 20 to 30 minutes after treatment before being used.

Vegetables or other foods that have been washed in suspect water should not be eaten unless they have been thoroughly cooked or peeled. (See also *Food-borne infection.*)

IMMERSION IN WATER

Swimming in polluted water is liable to cause an ear infection (see *Otitis externa*). The risk can be minimized by shaking the head from side to side after swimming to clear water out of the outer ear canals.

Most swimmers inadvertently swallow some water. If the water is contaminated, there is a risk of contracting any of the diseases transmitted in polluted drinking water. It is therefore advisable to avoid swimming in rivers that may be polluted with sewage (for example, downstream of towns) or in the sea near large coastal resorts.

A form of *leptospirosis* is caused by contact with water contaminated by rat's urine; sewage workers, canal workers, and more recently, trout farmers are most at risk.

In tropical countries, swimming or wading in rivers, lakes, and ponds is very inadvisable due to the risk

SAFETY OF WATER AND OTHER DRINKS FOR CONSUMPTION

	Developed countries	Developing countries
Usually safe	Tap water from public supply; rainwater; canned or bottled drinks; springwater	Canned or bottled drinks of well-known brands; rainwater
Suspect	Water direct from rivers, streams, lakes, ponds, canals, and wells	Tap water (cities); springwater
Very suspect	Obviously polluted water (i.e. cloudy in appearance or with an unpleasant smell)	Tap water (rural areas); water direct from rivers, streams, lakes, ponds, and canals

Safe and suspect water
Water from any source that falls into the suspect or very suspect categories should be sterilized. Techniques include boiling, filtering, and chemical treatment.

W

of contracting *schistosomiasis* (also known as bilharzia), a serious disease caused by a fluke that can burrow through the swimmer's skin. Swimmer's itch is caused by a similar type of fluke, which burrows into the skin and causes an itchy rash.

OTHER MECHANISMS OF WATER-BORNE INFECTION
Fish (particularly shellfish) that live in polluted water may collect infective organisms in their bodies. Such fish must be expertly cleaned and prepared and then promptly and thoroughly cooked to avoid possible hepatitis, cholera-like illnesses, *food poisoning*, or a *tapeworm infestation*.

Legionnaires' disease is a type of pneumonia caused by a bacterium that can contaminate the water systems of large buildings. It is not apparently contracted from actually drinking contaminated water; the route of infection seems to occur via inhalation of water from showers or from the water used in some air-conditioning systems.

Waterbrash
Sudden filling of the mouth with tasteless saliva. It is not to be confused with *acid reflux* (the regurgitation of gastric juices), which has an unpleasant, sour taste. Waterbrash is usually accompanied by other symptoms, such as abdominal pain before a meal. It usually indicates a disorder of the upper gastrointestinal tract.

Waterhouse-Friderichsen syndrome
A serious, but very rare, condition that is caused by infection of the bloodstream by bacteria of the meningococcus group. The main feature is bleeding into the adrenal glands, which leads to acute *adrenal failure* and to *shock*. Waterhouse-Friderichsen syndrome is often associated with *meningitis*.

Watering eye
An increase in the volume of the tear film, usually producing epiphora (overflow of *tears*). Watering may be caused by excess tear production due to emotion or to conjunctival or corneal irritation. It may also be caused by an obstruction to the channel that drains tears from the eye. (See also *Lacrimal apparatus*.)

Water intoxication
A condition caused by excessive water retention in the *brain*. The principal symptoms are headaches, dizziness,

nausea, confusion, and, in severe cases, seizures and unconsciousness.

Various disorders can disrupt the body's water balance, leading to accumulation of water in body tissues, including the brain. Such disorders include *kidney failure*, liver *cirrhosis*, severe *heart failure*, diseases of the *adrenal glands*, and certain lung or ovarian tumours that produce a substance with a similar action to *ADH* (antidiuretic hormone).

There is also a risk of water intoxication for about 48 hours after surgery, because the stress of an operation leads to increased ADH production. Water intoxication may also occur during induction of labour with *oxytocin*, which has an action similar to that of ADH.

Water on the brain
A nonmedical term for *hydrocephalus*.

Water on the knee
A popular term for accumulation of fluid within or around the knee joint. The most common cause is *bursitis* (inflammation of a bursa, one of the fluid-filled sacs that cover and cushion pressure points in the body). Another possible cause is fluid within the knee joint (see *Effusion, joint*).

Water retention
The accumulation of fluid in body tissues (see *Oedema*).

Water tablets
See *Diuretic drugs*.

Wax bath
A type of *heat treatment* in which hot, liquid wax is applied to part of the body to relieve pain and stiffness in inflamed or injured joints. Wax baths are most commonly used to treat sufferers from *rheumatoid arthritis*.

A wax bath is given by dipping the body part into wax kept at a temperature of 50 to 55°C. The limb is held in the wax for a few seconds and then withdrawn; the wax solidifies, forming a thin layer. The procedure may be repeated until the wax coating is about 10 mm thick. The treated area is wrapped in a plastic sheet and blanket to retain the heat. After 20 minutes, the wax is peeled off and exercises are performed to encourage movement in the treated joints.

Weakness
A term used to describe a general lack of vigour or strength, which is a common symptom of a wide range of con-

ditions, including *anaemia, emotional problems,* and various disorders affecting the heart, nervous system, bones, joints, and muscles. When associated with emotional disorders (such as depression), weakness may represent a lack of desire or ambition rather than a lack of muscle strength.

More specifically, the term weakness is used to describe loss of power in certain muscle groups, which may or may not be accompanied by muscle wasting and loss of sensation. (See also *Paralysis*.)

Weaning
The gradual substitution of solid foods for milk or milk formula in an infant's diet (see *Feeding, infant*).

Webbing
A flap of skin, as between adjacent fingers or toes. Webbing is a common congenital abnormality that often runs in families and which may affect two or more digits. Although mild webbing is completely harmless, surgical correction may be performed for cosmetic reasons. In severe cases of webbing, adjacent digits may be completely fused (see *Syndactyly*). Webbing of the neck may be a feature of *Turner's syndrome*.

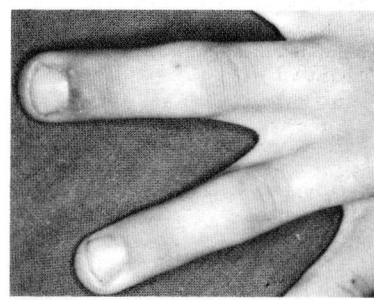

Webbing of the fingers
This curious feature is often an inherited trait, appearing in each of several generations of a family. Most cases are completely harmless and do not require treatment.

Wegener's granulomatosis
A rare disorder in which *granulomas* (nodular collections of abnormal cells) associated with areas of chronic tissue inflammation due to *vasculitis* (inflammation of the blood vessels) develop in the nasal passages, lungs, and kidneys.

CAUSES AND SYMPTOMS
The cause of the condition is unknown, but it is thought to be an *autoimmune disorder* (a disorder in which the body's natural defences attack its own tissues).

W

The principal symptoms include a bloody discharge from the nose, coughing (sometimes with the production of bloodstained sputum), breathing difficulty, chest pain, and blood in the urine. There may also be loss of appetite, weight loss, weakness, fatigue, and joint pains.

DIAGNOSIS AND TREATMENT

A diagnosis usually requires the microscopic examination of a *biopsy* sample of abnormal tissue, which may be taken from inside the nose, from a lung, or from a kidney.

Treatment is with a combination of *immunosuppressant drugs*, such as *cyclophosphamide* or *azathioprine*, and *corticosteroid drugs* to alleviate the symptoms and, in some cases, to help bring about a *remission* in the disease process.

OUTLOOK

With prompt treatment, most people recover completely within about a year, although *kidney failure* develops in some sufferers.

Without treatment, various complications may occur, including perforation of the nasal septum, causing deformity of the nose; inflammation of the eyes; a rash, nodules, or ulcers on the skin; and damage to the heart muscle, which may be fatal.

Weight

The heaviness of a person or object. In children, weight is a routine index of *growth*. At all ages, divergence from the normal weight for height may have medical implications. Measurement of an individual's weight is part of a routine physical examination. Many people routinely measure their own weight at home on bathroom scales. Ideally, a person should be weighed before breakfast, either naked or wearing light clothing.

Weight can be compared to charts standardized for an individual's height, age, and sex. If weight is below 80 per cent of the standard weight for height, the individual's *nutrition* is probably inadequate as a result of poor diet or disease.

In healthy adults, weight remains more or less stable because energy intake from the diet matches energy expenditure used to fuel all body activities (see *Metabolism*). *Weight loss* or weight gain occurs if the net balance is disturbed.

Obesity can be most easily assessed in terms of weight for height. A person is considered to be obese if his or her weight is 20 per cent more than that given in a standard weight-for-

WEIGHT TABLE: MEN

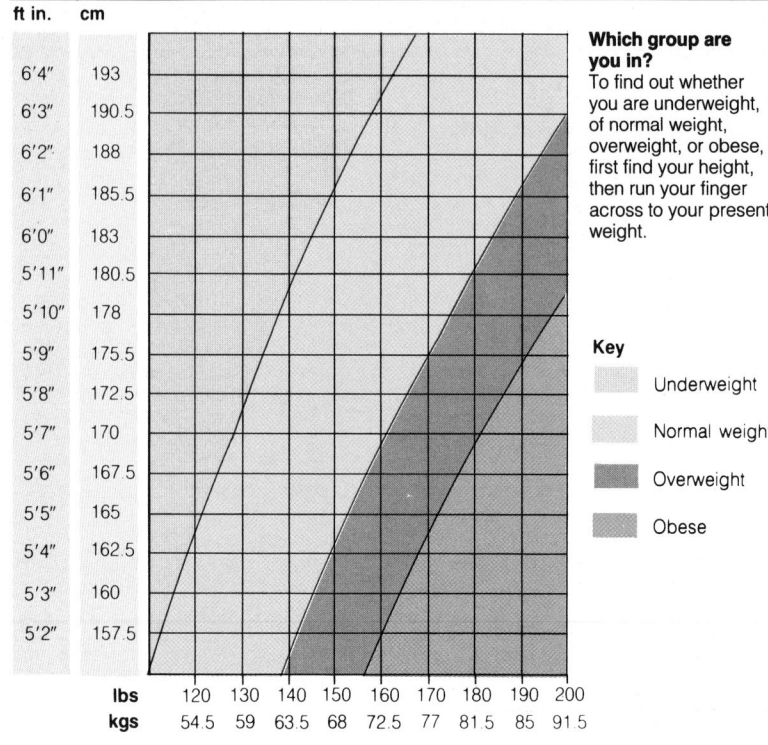

Which group are you in?
To find out whether you are underweight, of normal weight, overweight, or obese, first find your height, then run your finger across to your present weight.

Key
Underweight
Normal weight
Overweight
Obese

WEIGHT TABLE: WOMEN

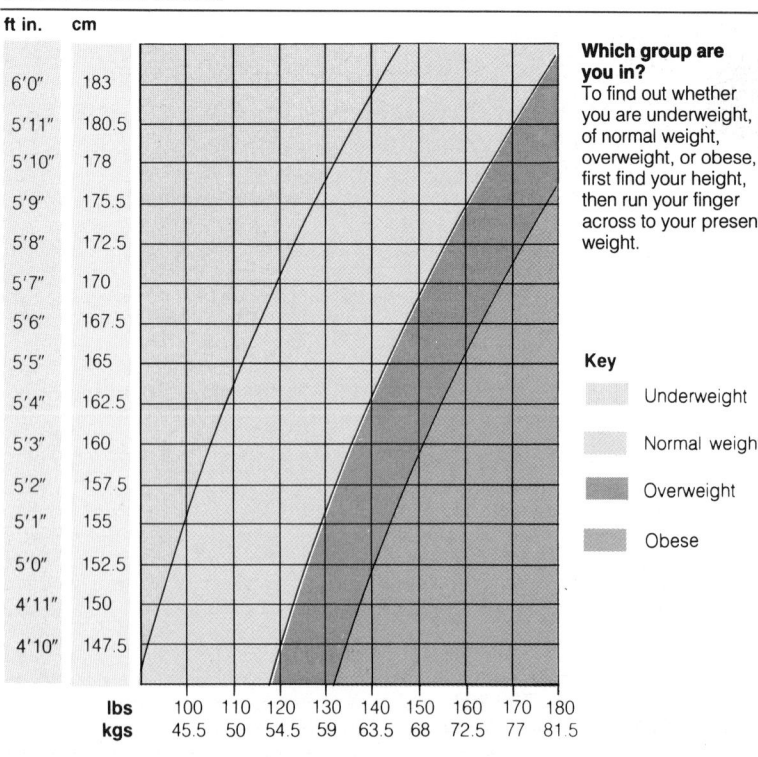

Which group are you in?
To find out whether you are underweight, of normal weight, overweight, or obese, first find your height, then run your finger across to your present weight.

Key
Underweight
Normal weight
Overweight
Obese

WEIGHT LOSS

Minor fluctuations in weight as a result of temporary changes in the level of exercise taken or the amount of food eaten are normal. More drastic, unintentional weight loss, especially when combined with other symptoms such as loss of appetite, usually requires medical attention.

Is your appetite as good as ever? — **YES** →

Have you noticed two or more of the following symptoms?
- excessive sweating
- weakness or trembling
- unexplained tiredness
- bulging eyes

— **YES** →

An overactive thyroid gland is a possibility, especially if you are a woman. Consult your doctor.

See • *Graves' disease*
    • *Hyperthyroidism*

NO ↓

Have you noticed one or more of the following symptoms?
- unusually frequent or abundant urination
- increased thirst
- unexpected tiredness
- genital itching

— **YES** →

This may be due to diabetes mellitus, a hormonal disorder in which insufficient insulin is produced by the pancreas.

See • *Diabetes mellitus*

NO →

If you feel well, there is probably no serious cause for your weight loss. However, if your weight continues to drop, discuss this with your doctor to exclude the slight possibility of a serious underlying disorder.

NO ↓

CANCER WATCH
There is a possibility of cancer if weight loss and loss of appetite are combined with abdominal pain OR a change in bowel habits. **Consult your doctor without delay!**

Have you noticed one or more of the following symptoms?
- recurrent diarrhoea
- recurrent constipation
- recurrent abdominal pain
- blood in the faeces
- recurrent nausea or vomiting

— **YES** →

Consult your doctor without delay!
A disorder of the digestive tract may be responsible.

See • *Crohn's disease*
    • *Intestine, cancer of*
    • *Irritable bowel syndrome*
    • *Malabsorption*
    • *Peptic ulcer*
    • *Stomach cancer*

Signs of weight loss
If you lose weight without deliberately attempting to slim down, you should always take the matter seriously, especially if other symptoms suggest the possibility of illness. If you do not weigh yourself regularly, the following signs may indicate that you have lost weight:
- people remark on your changed appearance
- your cheeks become sunken
- your trousers or skirts become loose around the waist
- your collars fit more loosely
- you need a smaller bra

Continued on next page

W

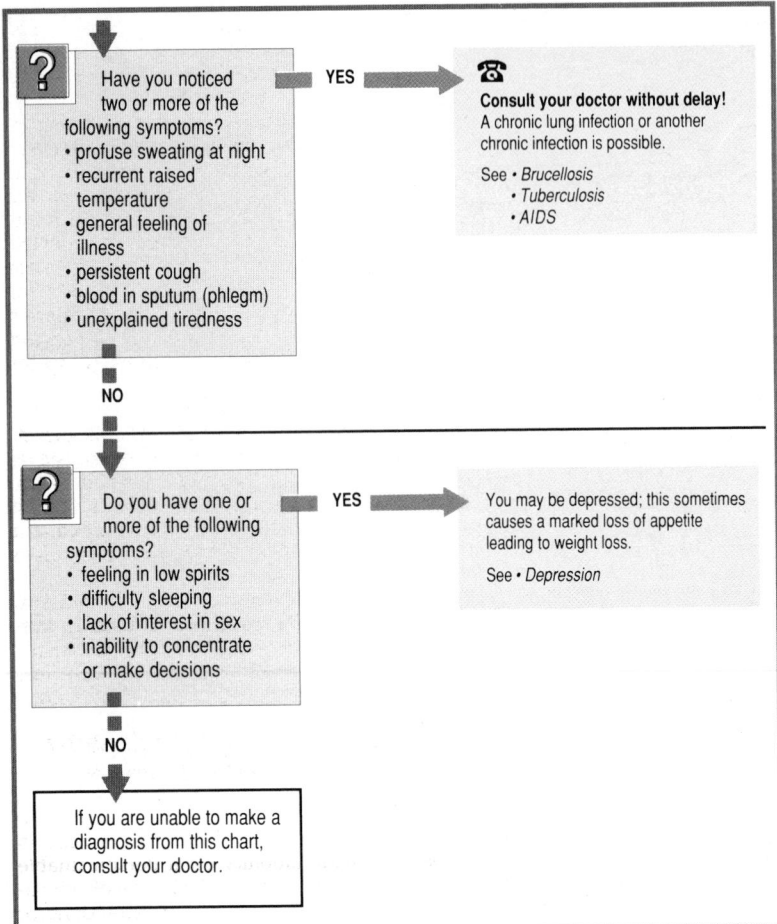

Have you noticed two or more of the following symptoms?
- profuse sweating at night
- recurrent raised temperature
- general feeling of illness
- persistent cough
- blood in sputum (phlegm)
- unexplained tiredness

YES

☎ **Consult your doctor without delay!**
A chronic lung infection or another chronic infection is possible.

See • *Brucellosis*
• *Tuberculosis*
• *AIDS*

NO

Do you have one or more of the following symptoms?
- feeling in low spirits
- difficulty sleeping
- lack of interest in sex
- inability to concentrate or make decisions

YES

You may be depressed; this sometimes causes a marked loss of appetite leading to weight loss.

See • *Depression*

NO

If you are unable to make a diagnosis from this chart, consult your doctor.

---

height table. An alternative method of assessment is to use the body mass index, also called Quetelet's index, which is obtained by dividing weight in kilograms by the square of height in metres; a body mass index above 27 (i.e. above the 85th percentile) constitutes obesity.

Weight loss
Loss of body weight occurs any time there is a decrease in the net balance of energy intake compared with energy expenditure. This decrease may be due to deliberate *weight reduction*, to a change in diet, or to a change in activity level. Weight loss may also occur as a symptom of a wide range of disorders.

CAUSES
Many diseases disrupt the appetite and may lead to weight loss by reducing the intake of energy. *Depression* reduces the motivation to eat, *peptic ulcer* causes pain and may lead to food avoidance, and some kidney disor-ders cause loss of appetite due to the effect of *uraemia* (raised levels of urea in the blood). In *anorexia nervosa* and *bulimia*, complex psychological factors affect the individual's eating pattern.

Energy intake may also be affected by digestive disorders. Persistent *vomiting* due to *gastroenteritis*, for example, leads to weight loss. Cancer of the oesophagus (see *Oesophagus, cancer of*) or *stomach cancer* causes loss of weight, as does the *malabsorption* of nutrients that occurs in certain dis-orders of the intestine or pancreas.

Disorders that increase the rate of metabolic activity in cells cause weight loss by increasing the expenditure of energy. These disorders include any type of *cancer*, chronic infection such as *tuberculosis*, and *hyperthyroidism* (overactivity of the thyroid gland). Untreated *diabetes mellitus* also causes weight loss, initially due to a greater fluid loss from the increase in urine output and as a result of loss of energy from glycosuria (glucose in the urine);

eventually, a wasting of tissue mass causes weight loss as fat stores are broken down.

Unexplained weight loss may be a sign of disease and should always be investigated by a doctor. A working diagnosis may be established by means of a careful patient history and a physical examination. Symptoms and signs usually suggest a specific cause, which permits the doctor to select appropriate tests.

Weight reduction
The process of losing excess body fat. A person who is severely overweight (see *Obesity*) is more at risk of suffering from various illnesses, such as *diabetes mellitus*, *hypertension* (high blood pres-sure), and heart disease.

HOW IT IS DONE
The most efficient way to lose weight is to eat less. To lose weight, people should eat 500 to 1,000 kcal (2,100 kJ to 4,200 kJ) a day less than their energy requirements. This should result in a weight loss of between 0.5 and 1 kg per week until a desirable weight is achieved. The rate of weight loss may be faster during the first one to two weeks of a weight reduction diet because of the loss of water that occurs during this period.

Exercise forms an important part of a reducing regime, burning excess energy and improving muscle tone. Some people believe *aerobics* speed up the metabolism after exercising, but this is probably true only for regular and strenuous exercise like that undertaken by an athlete in training.

FAD DIETS
Many people who are trying to lose weight want to do so quickly; they may follow fad diets that provide severely restricted energy intakes. Although there may be a rapid weight loss in the beginning, most of these diets do not work in the long term and the lost weight usually returns.

A number of liquid diets providing about 330 kcal (1,400 kJ) per day have been developed. Some doctors are concerned about the effects of these liquid diets. Any diet that provides less than 1,000 kcal (4,200 kJ) per day should be undertaken only under medical supervision.

Weil's disease
Another name for *leptospirosis*.

Welder's eye
Acute *conjunctivitis* and *keratopathy* (corneal damage) caused by the intense *ultraviolet light* radiation

W

RECOMMENDATIONS FOR WEIGHT REDUCTION

Cut down drastically on all visible fats, such as butter, margarine, cream, and cooking oils, as well as the invisible	fats present in pastries, biscuits, and cakes. Choose low-fat milk, cheeses, and yogurts.
Choose lean cuts of meat and avoid processed meat such as salami. Grill or	roast meat without adding fat instead of frying.
Eat more boiled legumes (e.g. lentils and beans), which provide protein but	contain very little fat.
Avoid refined carbohydrates such as sugar (sucrose) as well as refined	grain products such as white flour and white rice.
Increase your consumption of unrefined carbohydrates. Eat wholemeal bread,	whole-grain rice and cereals, fresh fruit, and plenty of vegetables.
Reduce your intake of alcoholic	drinks, which are high in calories.

Dietary recommendations for weight loss
Careful choice of the right types of food—and, in particular, the avoidance of items with a high calorie content per unit of weight (mainly fats)—makes it easier to achieve a low-calorie diet without necessarily having to reduce the bulk of the food you eat.

that is emitted by the electric welding arc. Welder's eye results from failure to wear adequate eye protection while welding.

Wen
A name for a *sebaceous cyst*.

Werdnig-Hoffmann disease
A very rare inherited disorder of the *nervous system* that affects infants. Also known as infantile spinal muscular atrophy, Werdnig-Hoffmann disease is a type of *motor neuron disease*. Werdnig-Hoffmann disease affects the nerve cells in the spinal cord that control muscle movement. Its underlying cause is unknown.

Marked floppiness and paralysis occur during the first few months. Affected babies move less than normal babies and sometimes the mother recalls being aware of reduced fetal movements before the baby was born. Severely affected infants tend to lie still in a frog-like position with the knees bent up and turned out. The muscles of the face are unaffected, with the result that the child has an alert expression that is in sharp contrast to his or her physical helplessness. The baby becomes increasingly floppy and deformed over the following few months. The muscles that control breathing and feeding are also affected, and this usually causes death before the child is three years old.

There is no cure for Werdnig-Hoffmann disease. Treatment aims to keep the affected infant as comfortable as possible.

Wernicke-Korsakoff syndrome
An uncommon *brain* disorder almost always due to the malnutrition that occurs in chronic *alcohol dependence*. Occasionally, Wernicke-Korsakoff syndrome is caused by malnutrition occurring in other conditions, such as *cancer*.

CAUSES
Wernicke-Korsakoff syndrome is caused by deficiency of thiamine (vitamin B$_1$, see *Vitamin B complex*), which affects the brain and nervous system. The thiamine deficiency is probably caused by the combined effects of poor eating habits and an inherited defect in thiamine metabolism.

SYMPTOMS
The disease consists of two stages—Wernicke's encephalopathy and Korsakoff's psychosis—each characterized by particular symptoms.

Wernicke's encephalopathy usually develops suddenly and produces *nystagmus* (abnormal jerky eye movements) and other abnormal eye movements, *ataxia* (difficulty in coordinating body movements, especially walking), slowness, and confusion. Sufferers also usually have signs of *neuropathy*, such as loss of sensation, a pins-and-needles sensa-

tion, or impaired reflexes. The level of consciousness progressively falls and may lead to coma and death unless treated.

Korsakoff's psychosis may follow Wernicke's encephalopathy if treatment is not begun soon enough. Symptoms consist of severe *amnesia* (memory loss), apathy, and disorientation. Recent memory is affected more than distant memory, sufferers often not being able to remember what they did even a few minutes previously. Confabulation (invention of stories) may occur to make up for gaps in memory.

TREATMENT AND OUTLOOK
Wernicke's encephalopathy is a medical emergency. If the diagnosis is even suspected, high doses of intravenous thiamine are given to the patient immediately. This treatment reverses most of the symptoms, often within a few hours.

In the absence of prompt treatment, Korsakoff's psychosis is usually irreversible, leaving the sufferer permanently handicapped by memory loss and in need of continual supervision.

Wernicke's encephalopathy
See *Wernicke-Korsakoff syndrome*.

Wheelchair
A chair mounted on wheels used to provide mobility for a person unable to walk. The simplest type of wheelchair is pushed by an attendant or hand-propelled by the disabled person. Manual wheelchairs have small wheels with casters at the front and large, narrow wheels at the back; these wheelchairs are designed so that the hand-rims can be easily gripped by a disabled person.

Powered wheelchairs are battery-operated and controlled electronically by finger pressure or, if necessary, by chin pressure or breath control. The battery provides power for six to eight hours and is recharged overnight by connection to an electrical outlet. Wheels are usually small with wide, low-pressure tyres. Several different types of powered chair are available. Those suitable for outdoor use are capable of negotiating raised obstructions but are usually too wide and long for convenient use indoors; conversely, indoor models are lighter and more compact but they cannot mount pavements.

Wheelchairs may be made of lightweight metal (such as titanium or an alloy) and are often foldable for easy storage in the boot of a car.

W

Wheeze

A high-pitched, whistling sound produced in the chest during breathing; it is caused by narrowing of the airways. A wheeze may be loud enough to be heard by those in the room with the sufferer or just audible with a stethoscope. Wheeze is a feature of *asthma* and also occurs in *bronchitis*, *bronchiolitis*, and *pulmonary oedema* (accumulation of fluid in the lungs). Inhalation of a foreign body, such as a peanut, into the airways may also cause a wheeze. (See also *Breathing difficulty*.)

Whiplash injury

An injury to the soft tissues, *ligaments*, and spinal joints of the neck caused by the neck's being bent forcibly and violently forwards and then backwards or vice versa. Whiplash injury most commonly results from sudden acceleration or deceleration, as in a car collision. However, some degree of whiplash to the neck occurs in all forms of head injury.

Damage to the spine usually involves minor *sprain* of a neck ligament, or *subluxation* (partial dislocation) of a cervical joint. Occasionally, a ligament may rupture or there may be a fracture of a cervical vertebra (see *Spinal injury*). Characteristically, pain and stiffness in the neck are much worse 24 hours after the injury.

Treatment may include immobilization in an orthopaedic *collar*, *analgesic drugs* (painkillers), *muscle-relaxant drugs*, and *physiotherapy*. Recovery is usually complete but it can take several weeks before full pain-free neck movement is possible.

Whipple's disease

A rare disorder that may affect many organs. Also called intestinal lipodystrophy, Whipple's disease causes a variety of symptoms and signs, including malabsorption (impaired absorption of nutrients by the small intestine), diarrhoea, abdominal pain, progressive weight loss, joint pains, swollen lymph nodes, abnormal skin pigmentation, anaemia, and fever. The condition most commonly occurs in middle-aged men.

The precise cause of Whipple's disease remains unknown but it is probably due to an unidentified bacterial infection. Diagnosis is by *jejunal biopsy* (removal of a small sample of tissue from the jejunum for microscopic analysis). Affected tissues are found to contain macrophages (a type of scavenging cell) containing rod-shaped bacteria. Treatment is with *antibiotic drugs* for at least one year. Attempts to correct nutritional deficiencies that have arisen from malabsorption are made with dietary supplements.

Whipple's operation

A type of *pancreatectomy* in which the head of the pancreas and the loop of the duodenum are surgically removed. It is named after the US surgeon Allen Whipple (1881-1963).

Whipworm infestation

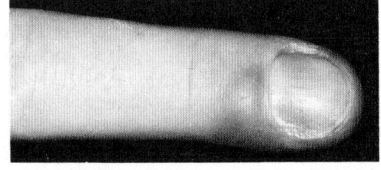 The whipworm is a small, cylindrical whip-like worm, between 2.5 and 5 cm long, that can live in the human large intestine.

The life-cycle of the whipworm is shown in the illustrated box. A light infestation causes no symptoms. A heavy infestation can cause abdominal pain, diarrhoea, and, sometimes, *anaemia*, because the worms consume a small amount of the host's blood every day. The condition is diagnosed by finding whipworm eggs during an examination of faeces.

Treatment is with *anthelmintic drugs*, such as *mebendazole*, which usually bring about a satisfactory cure; heavy infestations may require more than one course of treatment.

Whitehead

A very common type of skin blemish (see *Milia*).

Whitlow

An abscess on the fingertip or, rarely, on the toe. The most common type is an acute *paronychia*. A whitlow causes the finger to swell and become extremely painful and sensitive to pressure and touch. It may be caused by the virus that causes *herpes simplex* or by a bacterium, which usually enters the body through a cut.

A whitlow caused by bacterial infection may be treated with *antibiotic drugs* or, if the infection is severe, by incision and drainage in a minor surgical procedure under local anaesthesia. A whitlow caused by the virus that causes herpes simplex is treated by the application of an *antiviral drug*; such whitlows should not be incised and drained because of the high risk of spreading the infection.

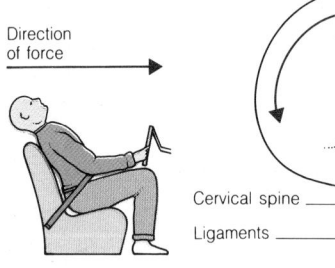

Herpetic whitlow
This extremely painful finger infection, caused by the herpes simplex virus, may be helped by applying an antiviral ointment.

CAUSE OF WHIPLASH INJURY

This injury to the neck section of the spine may occur when a car is subjected to a sudden violent force and the occupant's body is restrained in the seat but his or her head is not restrained.

Sudden acceleration
Here, there is a sudden force from behind (usually due to another vehicle's striking the rear of the car). As the body accelerates forwards, the head jerks violently backwards relative to the body, stretching and bending the neck; the head then rebounds forwards.

Sudden deceleration
Here, there is a sudden violent force from the front towards the back of the vehicle, due, for example, to a collision with a tree. The seat belt restrains the body, but the head continues to move forwards, stretching the neck; the head then rebounds backwards.

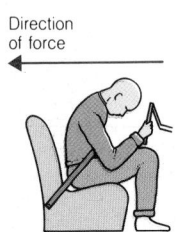

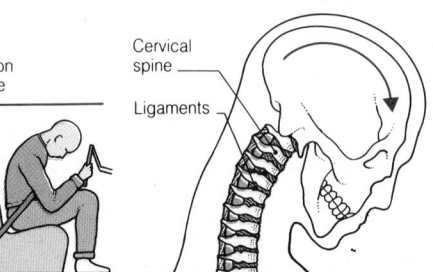

Direction of force

Cervical spine

Ligaments

Direction of force

Cervical spine

Ligaments

W

LIFE-CYCLE OF WHIPWORM

Whipworm infestation (known medically as trichuriasis) occurs worldwide and is particularly common in the tropics. In the UK, whipworm infestation mainly affects immigrants and residents of mental institutions; up to 1,000 cases are identified annually. Adult whipworms are 2.5 to 5 cm long. They may live in a person's intestine for up to 20 years. Most infestations do not cause symptoms.

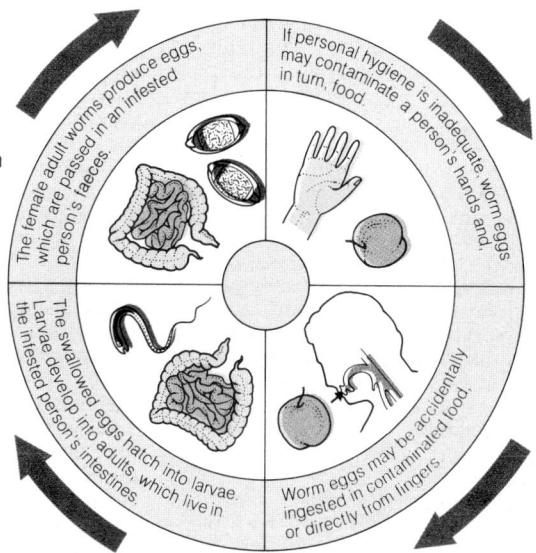

The female adult worms produce eggs, which are passed in an infested person's faeces.

If personal hygiene is inadequate, worm eggs may contaminate a person's hands and, in turn, food.

The swallowed eggs hatch into larvae. Larvae develop into adults, which live in the infested person's intestines.

Worm eggs may be accidentally ingested in contaminated food, or directly from fingers.

A very rare complication of an untreated whitlow is *osteomyelitis*, a serious bacterial infection of the bone and bone marrow.

Whooping cough
See *Pertussis*.

Wife beating
Repeated deliberate physical injury inflicted by a husband on his wife. The term wife beating is also sometimes applied loosely to violence between non-married partners.

PREVALENCE
About one third of all reported assaults are by males on their female partners, and about one third of women filing for divorce describe physical abuse. There is little doubt that many cases of wife beating go unreported. In about 20 per cent of reported cases the abuse continues for more than 10 years.

CAUSES
Husbands who abuse their wives have usually learned domestic violence from their parents' behaviour, have an immature personality and low self-esteem, and acquire aggressive attitudes from their peer groups. Aggravating factors include *alcohol dependence*, *drug abuse*, *stress*, and obsession with the partner's sexual fidelity (see *Jealousy, morbid*).

Abused women in many cases stay with their partners for a combination of reasons, the most common of which are feelings of personal inadequacy, a sense of guilt leading to the belief that the violence is justified, fear of the social stigma involved in telling others about the abuse, underlying love for the partner, financial dependence, unwillingness to break up the family, social isolation, and *depression* which produces apathy.

MANAGEMENT OF THE PROBLEM
Shelters have been opened in some areas to provide a temporary refuge for abused women and their children. In addition, a system that provided abused women with adequate financial support would make it less difficult for them to leave their partners. *Marriage guidance* also has a role, provided the couple wishes to address the problem openly.

Will, living
See *Living will*.

Wilms' tumour
A type of *kidney cancer*, also called nephroblastoma, that occurs mainly in children.

Wilson's disease
A rare, inherited disorder in which copper accumulates in the liver and is slowly released into other parts of the body. Eventually, Wilson's disease causes severe damage to both the liver and the brain.

SYMPTOMS AND SIGNS
Symptoms, which vary in severity from person to person, usually first appear in adolescence but sometimes occur as early as five or as late as 50. The toxic effects of copper on the liver can cause various disorders, progressing from *hepatitis* to *cirrhosis*. Accumulation of copper in the brain causes progressive problems ranging from mild intellectual impairment to crippling rigidity, tremor, and dementia.

DIAGNOSIS AND TREATMENT
The diagnosis is based on analysis of blood and urine and a liver *biopsy* (removal of a small sample of tissue for microscopic analysis) to discover the amount of copper in the body.

Wilson's disease requires lifelong treatment with *penicillamine*, a drug that binds with copper and thus enables it to be excreted. If started soon after the onset of symptoms, penicillamine can sometimes improve liver and brain function. If the disease is discovered before toxic effects produce symptoms, the drug may be able to prevent them from developing.

Wind
A common name for gas in the gastrointestinal tract, which may be expelled through the mouth (see *Belching*) or passed through the anus (see *Flatus*).

Babies often swallow air during feeding which, unless they are "winded", can accumulate in the stomach and cause discomfort. A baby's wind can be brought up by gently patting or rubbing the baby's back.

Windpipe
A common name for the *trachea*.

Wiring of the jaws
Immobilization of the jaws by means of metal wires to allow a fracture of the jaw to heal or as part of a treatment for *obesity*. In the most commonly used method, thin, hairpin-shaped wires with a central eyelet (closed loop) are wound around pairs of adjacent teeth; about six wires are fixed to teeth in the

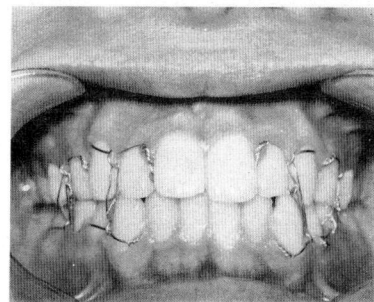

Wired jaws
A total of eight pairs of teeth have been wired together to immobilize the jaw while a fracture heals.

W

upper and lower jawbones. Wires are then threaded through opposing pairs of upper and lower eyelets and twisted together to hold the jaws in a rigid position.

When a fracture is being treated, the jaws are kept wired in a fixed position for about six weeks. For promoting weight loss, the jaws are wired for as long as a year. In both cases, the person is unable to chew and can take only a liquid or semi-liquid diet. For weight loss purposes, the diet is calorie controlled and the patient is kept under medical supervision. This form of diet treatment, though effective while the jaws are wired, usually fails when the overweight person resumes his or her previous eating habits.

Wisdom tooth

One of the four rearmost *teeth*, also known as third molars. In most people, the wisdom teeth erupt between the ages of 17 and 21. However, in some people, one or more fails to develop or to erupt. In many cases, wisdom teeth are unable to emerge fully from the gum as a result of overcrowding (see *Impaction, dental*).

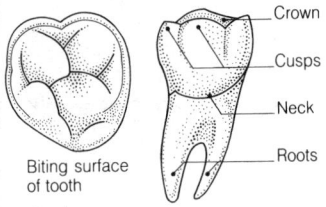

Crown

Cusps

Neck

Roots

Biting surface of tooth

Structure of wisdom tooth
Like other molars, each wisdom tooth has strong roots and a bulky crown with many cusps and an extensive grinding surface.

Witches' milk

A thin, white discharge from the nipple of a newborn infant. Witches' milk occurs quite commonly and is usually accompanied by enlargement of one or both of the baby's breasts. The discharge is caused by maternal hormones that entered the fetus's circulation through the placenta. Witches' milk is harmless and usually disappears spontaneously within a few weeks.

Withdrawal

The process of retreating from society and from relationships with others. Withdrawal is usually indicated by aloofness, lack of interest in social activities, preoccupation with one's own concerns, and difficulty in communicating with others.

Withdrawal is also a term applied to the psychological and physical symptoms that develop on discontinuing a substance on which a person is dependent (see *Withdrawal syndrome*).

Withdrawal bleeding

Vaginal blood loss that occurs when the body's level of *oestrogen hormones*, *progesterone hormone*, or *progestogen drugs* drops suddenly.

Menstruation is a form of withdrawal bleeding because it is preceded in the menstrual cycle by falling levels of both oestrogen and progesterone. The withdrawal bleeding that occurs at the end of each month's supply of combined *oral contraceptive* pills mimics menstruation, but is usually shorter and lighter. Discontinuation of an oestrogen-only or progestogen-only preparation also produces bleeding, which may differ from normal menstruation in amount and duration.

Withdrawal method

See *Coitus interruptus*.

Withdrawal syndrome

A group of unpleasant mental and physical symptoms that are experienced when a person stops using a drug on which he or she is dependent (see *Drug dependence*).

In general, any drug that causes euphoria or that relieves pain or anxiety can cause dependence and withdrawal symptoms of varying degrees. Withdrawal syndromes most commonly result from *alcohol dependence*, *tobacco-smoking*, *narcotic drug* dependence, or regular use of *tranquillizer drugs*. Other drugs that may lead to withdrawal symptoms include *amphetamine drugs*, *cocaine*, *marijuana*, and *caffeine*.

TYPES

ALCOHOL Withdrawal symptoms start six to eight hours after the last drink and may last four to seven days. Common symptoms include trembling of the hands and tongue, sweating, nausea, anxiety, and sometimes cramps and vomiting. More severe symptoms include seizures (see *Delirium tremens*), confusion, and hallucinations. Withdrawal symptoms may be frightening and frequently result in a resumption of drinking. Many alcohol-dependent people need a drink in the morning to ward off the minor withdrawal syndrome that is experienced on waking.

NARCOTIC DRUGS *Heroin* or *morphine* withdrawal syndrome starts eight to 12 hours after the last dose and may

last for seven to 10 days. At first, a craving for the drug is the most prominent feature, accompanied by restlessness, sweating, running eyes and nose, and yawning. As the syndrome progresses, a variety of other symptoms appear, including diarrhoea, vomiting, abdominal cramps, dilated pupils, loss of appetite, gooseflesh (the origin of the term "cold turkey"), irritability, tremor, weakness, and depression.

Other narcotic drugs, such as *codeine* and some prescription *analgesic drugs*, cause withdrawal symptoms similar to those produced by heroin or morphine. Lower doses may produce withdrawal symptoms that are less intense and that develop more slowly.

TRANQUILLIZERS Withdrawal syndrome from *barbiturate drugs* and *meprobamate* begins from 12 to 24 hours after the last dose and has many similarities to alcohol withdrawal. The first symptoms are usually tremor, anxiety, restlessness, and weakness, sometimes followed by delirium, hallucinations, and, in some cases, seizures. A period of prolonged sleep occurs just before the symptoms clear up, which is between three and eight days after onset, depending on the drug.

Withdrawal from *benzodiazepine drugs* may begin much more slowly (up to 14 days after the last dose) and can in some cases be life-threatening.

TOBACCO-SMOKING Withdrawal symptoms from *nicotine* (the substance in tobacco responsible for dependence) develops gradually over 24 to 48 hours. In addition to a desperate desire to smoke, the most common symptoms are irritability, difficulty in concentrating, frustration, headaches, and restless anxiety.

OTHER DRUGS Discontinuation of an amphetamine drug or cocaine results in lethargy, extreme tiredness, and dizziness. Cocaine withdrawal may also lead to severe depression, and sometimes to other physical symptoms, such as tremor and sweating.

Chronic marijuana users have reported various withdrawal symptoms, including tremor, sweating, nausea, vomiting, diarrhoea, irritability, and sleep disturbances.

Symptoms of caffeine withdrawal, consisting of tiredness, headaches, and irritability, may occur in people accustomed to drinking large quantities of tea, coffee, or caffeine-containing soft drinks. The onset of these symptoms usually occurs several hours after the last drink of caffeine-containing liquid.

W

FIRST AID: WOUNDS

> **DO NOT**
> ■ attempt to remove the
>   object from the wound.

FOREIGN BODY

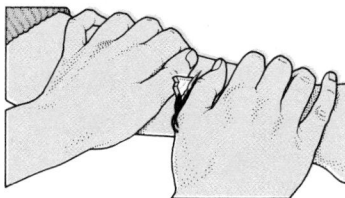

1 Apply direct pressure above and
below the object. Lay the victim down
and raise and support the limb.

2 Lightly drape a piece of gauze over
object and wound and place a ring pad
over it. Or use cottonwool to build up a pad
around the wound. It should be high enough
to prevent pressure on the object.

Ring pad

1 Place a narrow bandage across one
hand. Wind one end once or twice
around your fingers to make a loop.

2 Bring the other end through the loop,
wind it repeatedly around the loop,
pulling it tight each time.

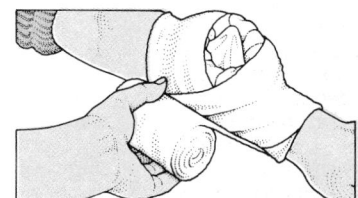

3 Secure with a roller bandage. Make
two straight turns, overlapping the
pad, on either side. Then continue with
diagonal turns until the pad is held firmly.
Take the victim to hospital.

DEEPER WOUNDS

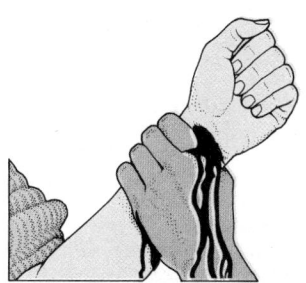

1 Examine the wound for foreign
bodies; if there is none, apply direct
pressure to control bleeding by pressing
on the wound with the fingers or palm.
Lay the victim down and raise the injured
part higher than the chest and heart.

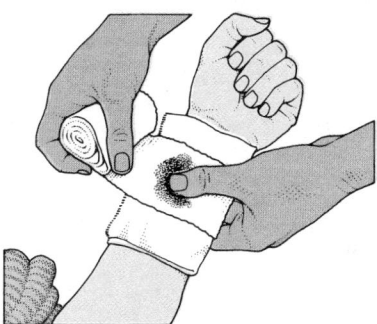

2 Put a sterile, unmedicated dressing over
the wound so that it extends well beyond
the edges of the wound. Secure the dressing
firmly with a bandage.

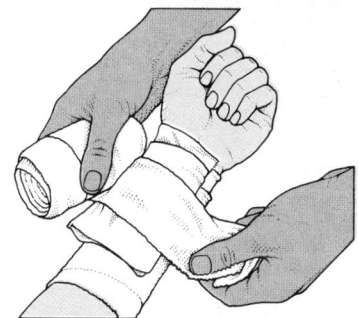

3 If the blood seeps through, do not
remove the bandage, but put more
dressing and another bandage on top.
Watch for *shock* and seek medical help.

CUTS AND SCRAPES

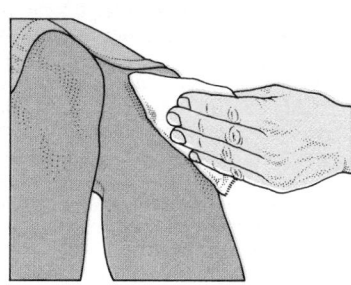

1 Rinse the wound under cold, running
water. Then, using cottonwool, gauze
or antiseptic wipes, clean around the
wound. Work outwards, using a clean pad
for each stroke.

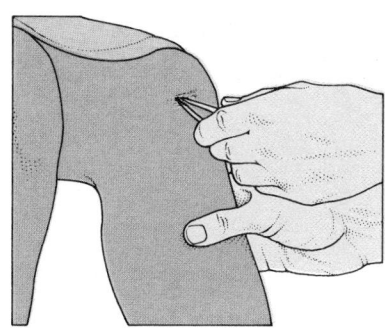

2 Remove any loose foreign bodies, such
as metal, glass, or gravel, with the gauze
or cottonwool, or with tweezers.

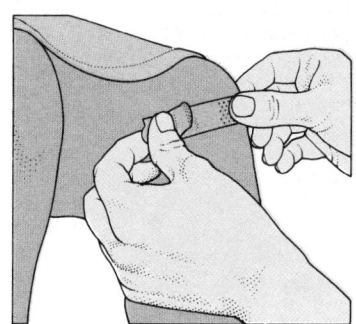

3 Dry the surrounding area and dress
the wound. If it is small, use an adhesive dressing. Otherwise, make a dressing
with a piece of gauze and cottonwool.
Secure with a bandage.

TREATMENT
Severe withdrawal syndromes require medical treatment. Symptoms may be suppressed by giving the patient small quantities of the drug he or she had been taking. More commonly, however, a substitute drug is given, such as *methadone* for narcotic drugs or *diazepam* for alcohol. The dose of the drug is then gradually reduced. This substitution process requires careful adjustment and can be safely managed only in a medical setting.

Wobble board
A balancing board used during *physiotherapy* to improve muscle strength and coordination in the feet, ankles, and legs. A wobble board is sometimes used after an ankle sprain to reduce the risk of a recurrence.

A wobble board consists of a smooth flat surface with a rocker attached to its underside. The rocker may be cylindrical, so that the board will only rock in one plane, or it may be spherical, allowing movement in all directions.

Womb
See *Uterus*.

Word blindness
See *Alexia*; *Dyslexia*.

World Health Organization
The World Health Organization (WHO) was established in 1948 as an agency of the United Nations with responsibilities for international health matters and public health. Its headquarters are in Geneva, Switzerland; there are also regional offices for Europe, Africa, North America, South America, Southeast Asia, the Eastern Mediterranean, and the Western Pacific (including Australia).

The WHO has campaigned effectively against certain infectious diseases, notably smallpox (which was declared to have been eradicated throughout the world in 1980), tuberculosis, and malaria. Its other functions include sponsoring medical research programmes, organizing a network of collaborating national laboratories, and providing expert advice to its 160 member states on matters such as health service organizations, family health, the use of medicinal drugs, the abuse of drugs, and mental health. The organization's current strategy is described in its campaign "Health for all by the year 2000". The plan gives specific targets for basic public health measures, such as the provision of piped water supplies and other basic sanitation, the universal provision of immunization of children against infectious diseases, and reductions in the use of tobacco and alcohol.

Worm infestation
Several types of worm, or their larvae, can exist as parasites of humans. These worms range in size from the microscopic to many metres in length and may live in the intestines, blood, lymphatic system, bile ducts, or organs such as the liver. Worms are more common than is realized; in many cases, they cause few or no symptoms, and a person may have an infestation for many years without realizing it. Other worms can cause chronic, sometimes severe and debilitating, illness.

There are two main classes of worm—the *roundworms*, which have long, cylindrical bodies, and the platyhelminths, which have flattened bodies. The platyhelminths are further subdivided into the cestodes (tapeworms) and trematodes (flukes).

Worm diseases found in developed countries include *threadworm infestation*, *ascariasis*, *whipworm infestation*, and *toxocariasis* (all caused by different types of roundworm); infestation with *liver flukes*; and some types of *tapeworm infestation*. However, apart from threadworm infestation, these are all very uncommon in the UK. Important types of worm diseases occurring in tropical regions include *hookworm infestation, filariasis*, and *guinea worm disease* (all caused by roundworms); and *schistosomiasis* (caused by a type of fluke).

Worms may be acquired by eating undercooked, infected meat, by contact with soil or water containing worm larvae, or by accidental ingestion of worm eggs (via the fingers or food) from soil contaminated by infected faeces.

The diagnosis of a worm infestation may be alarming but most types can be easily eradicated with *anthelmintic drugs* (see box below).

Wound
Any damage to the skin and/or underlying tissues caused by an accident, act of violence, or surgery. Wounds in which the skin or mucous membrane is broken are called open; those in which they remain intact are termed closed.

TYPES
Wounds can be divided into the following five broad categories: an incised wound; an abrasion (or graze); a *laceration*; a penetrating wound; and a contusion (see illustrated box on the facing page).

Many penetrating wounds and some contusions are deceptive in appearance, showing little external sign of damage but involving serious internal injury. Low-velocity gunshot injuries cause tissue damage all along the path of the projectile. High-velocity gunshot injuries may also damage distant structures as a result

---

DRUGS USED TO TREAT WORM INFESTATIONS

Infestation	Drug
Threadworm	Mebendazole, piperazine, pyrantel
Common roundworm (ascariasis)	Mebendazole, piperazine, pyrantel
Whipworm	Mebendazole
Hookworm	Bephenium, mebendazole, pyrantel
Strongyloidiasis	Mebendazole, thiabendazole
Toxocariasis	Diethylcarbamazine, thiabendazole
Tapeworm	Niclosamide, praziquantel
Filariasis	Diethylcarbamazine
Schistosomiasis	Praziquantel

Anthelmintic drugs
Drugs such as those listed above are the main treatment for worm infestations. Usually just one or two doses are required but sometimes longer treatment is needed. Laxatives may also be given to aid expulsion of worms living in the intestines.

W

TYPES OF WOUNDS

Wounds can be divided into the following categories: incised wounds, in which the skin is cleanly cut (e.g. surgical incisions); abrasions (or grazes), in which surface tissue is scraped away; lacerations, in which the skin is torn (e.g. animal *bites*); contusions, in which the underlying tissues are damaged by a blunt instrument; and penetrating wounds (e.g. stab or gunshot wounds).

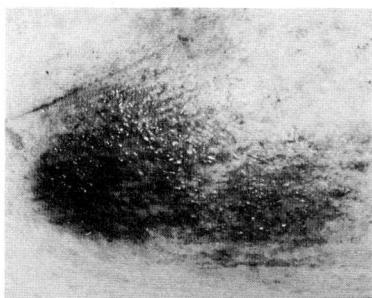

Abrasion on the arm
Abrasions usually result from sliding falls and may contain dirt. They should be carefully cleaned and dressed.

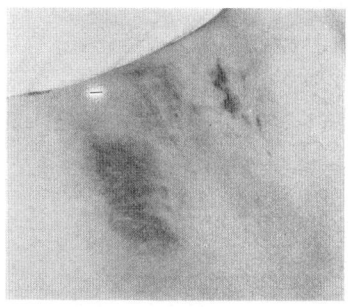

Contusion from a seat belt
Although the skin remains intact in this type of wound, there may be damage to the underlying tissues.

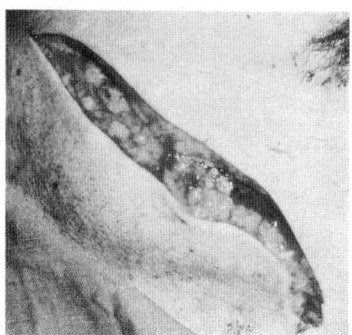

Knife wound down the side of the face
This is a deep incised wound, cleanly cut, and likely to heal with minimal scarring once its edges have been stitched.

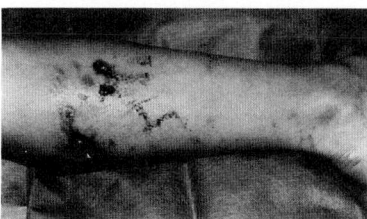

Dog-bite lacerations on the arm
Such wounds are usually cleaned and then left open to heal. Antibiotic and antitetanus treatment may be given.

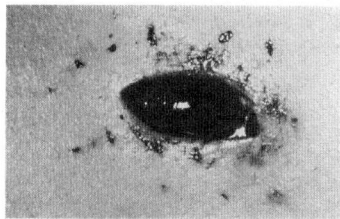

Penetrating stab wound to the chest
A penetrating wound such as this may appear small, but the knife may have punctured organs deep in the body.

of shock waves travelling through body tissues. In stab wounds, vital organs may be perforated and major blood vessels may be severed. In contusions, the liver, spleen, or kidney may be ruptured and cause severe internal bleeding.

TREATMENT

Many minor wounds can be treated by first-aid measures (see *Bleeding, treatment of; Dressings*; and Wounds first-aid box).

More extensive or deeper wounds require professional treatment, which varies according to the type of wound. If the wound contains any foreign material or dead tissue, this is removed; the wound is then cleansed with an antiseptic solution to decrease the risk of *wound infection*.

New, clean, incised wounds may be closed by *suturing* (stitching), and usually heal with minimal scarring. Lacerations may need to have the jagged skin edges cut away before they are stitched. Small incised wounds can be closed by taping the edges together; this is a very useful method of closure, especially in children. Contaminated wounds are usually left open in order to prevent abscess formation.

Deep wounds in which there is extensive tissue damage and/or a high risk of infection are usually filled with layers of sterile gauze and covered with a bandage for four or five days. If, after this time, there is no sign of infection and the skin edges can be brought together without tension, the wound may be stitched. Otherwise, the wound may be left open and allowed to heal on its own.

Penetrating wounds or contusions may require an exploratory operation on the abdominal cavity (see *Laparotomy*) or the chest cavity (see *Thoracotomy*). Damage to blood vessels, nerves, or bones often necessitates repair by specialized surgical techniques, such as *microsurgery*. If there has been extensive loss of skin, *skin grafting* may be required. (See also *Healing*.)

Wound infection

Any type of *wound* is susceptible to the entry of bacteria; the resultant infection can delay healing, result in disability, or cause death. Infection of a wound is indicated by redness, swelling, warmth, pain, and sometimes the presence of pus and the formation of an *abscess*. Wound infection may

sometimes result in complications due to local spread of infection to adjacent organs or tissue, or to distant spread of infection via the blood.

SURGICAL WOUNDS

About five to 10 per cent of surgical wounds become infected. Primary infection—occurring during the operation itself or while dressing the wound afterwards—is a common occurrence despite routine *aseptic technique* (the creation of a germ-free environment). *Antibiotic drugs* are therefore administered as a preventive measure for 24 hours after surgery. Infection is more likely to develop in obese patients or those with reduced natural defences against infection, such as the elderly and those suffering from cancer.

For surgery in which there is a higher-than-average risk of infection (such as an intestinal operation) or in which infection would have particularly serious consequences (such as a joint-replacement operation), the patient is given antibiotic drugs as a preventive measure.

NONSURGICAL WOUNDS

Of nonsurgical wounds, those most likely to become infected are wounds sustained in an agricultural accident

W

STRUCTURE OF THE WRIST

The wrist is a complex joint that allows the hand to be bent forward and backward relative to the arm (through an angle of almost 180 degrees) and also moved side to side (through about 70 degrees).

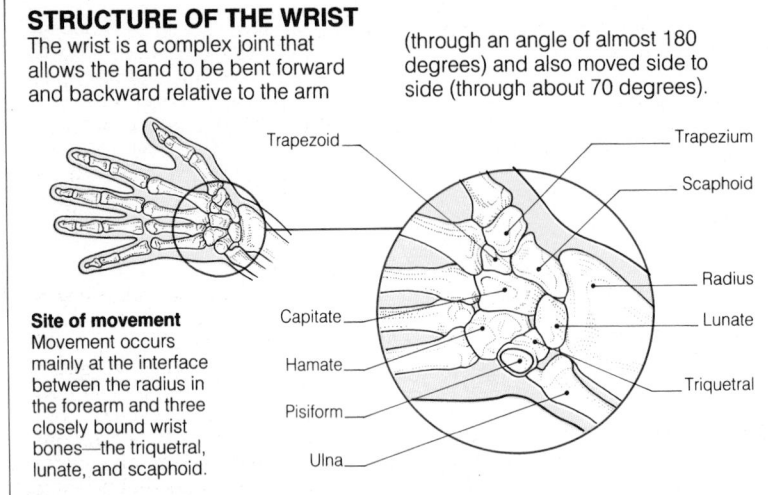

Site of movement
Movement occurs mainly at the interface between the radius in the forearm and three closely bound wrist bones—the triquetral, lunate, and scaphoid.

Labels: Trapezoid, Trapezium, Scaphoid, Capitate, Radius, Hamate, Lunate, Pisiform, Triquetral, Ulna

---

or by soldiers in battle. There is a risk of infection by the soil-borne bacterium CLOSTRIDIUM TETANI, which causes the serious, sometimes fatal, infection *tetanus*, or of infection by related bacteria, such as CLOSTRIDIUM PERFRINGENS, which cause gas *gangrene*.

In dealing with any serious nonsurgical wound, the doctor attempts to prevent infection by removing any foreign material or dead tissue from the wound, thoroughly cleaning it with an antiseptic solution, and giving antibiotic drugs. In addition, if there is a risk that the wound might be contaminated with soil, an anti-tetanus injection is given unless the patient has received one within the previous five years.

TREATMENT
Once infection is discovered, a sample of blood or pus is taken and the patient is given an antibiotic drug. When a *culture* of the causative bacteria has been grown, treatment may need to be changed to a more appropriate antibiotic. Any abscess should be drained surgically.

Wrinkle

A furrow in the *skin*. Wrinkling is a natural feature of aging caused by a loss of skin elasticity. Wrinkles are most obvious on the face and other exposed parts of the body but occur all over the skin. Premature deep wrinkling is usually caused by overexposure to the ultraviolet rays in sunlight.

Despite the claims made for various "rejuvenating" skin preparations, no treatment can permanently restore skin elasticity. Nevertheless, treatment with some *vitamin A* derivatives is being evaluated as a means of reducing wrinkling. A *face-lift* smoothes out wrinkles by stretching the skin, but the operation's effects last only about five years.

Wrist

The joint between the *hand* and the arm. The skeleton of the wrist consists of eight bones (known collectively as the carpus) arranged in two rows—the scaphoid, lunate, triquetral, and pisiform bones, which articulate with the radius and ulna (bones of the forearm); and the trapezium, trapezoid, capitate, and hamate, which are connected to the bones of the palm. The bones of the carpus articulate with each other.

Many tendons, which connect the forearm muscles to the fingers and thumb, run across the wrist. The extensor tendons, which straighten the fingers, are on the back of the wrist; the flexor tendons, which bend the fingers, are on the front. These tendons pass under ligaments to prevent them from springing away from the wrist. The gap between the ligaments and tendons at the front of the wrist is known as the carpal tunnel.

Also passing across the wrist are the arteries and nerves supplying the muscles, bones, and skin of the hand and fingers.

DISORDERS
Wrist injuries may lead to serious disability by limiting hand movement. This is especially likely to occur with fractures of the scaphoid bone, which often fail to heal, and with injuries in which the tendons or nerves in the wrist are severed.

A common wrist injury in adults is *Colles' fracture*, in which the lower end of the radius is fractured and the wrist and hand are displaced backwards. In young children, similar displacement results from a fracture through the epiphysis (growing end) of the radius. A *sprain* can affect ligaments at the wrist joint, but most wrist sprains are not severe.

Pressure on the median nerve as it passes through the carpal tunnel causes numbness, tingling, and pain in the thumb, index, and middle fingers (see *Carpal tunnel syndrome*). Damage to the radial nerve, which may be caused by fracture of the humerus (upper-arm bone), results in *wrist-drop* (inability to straighten the wrist).

Other conditions that may affect the wrist include *tenosynovitis* (inflammation of the inner lining of a tendon sheath) and *osteoarthritis* (degenerative joint disease).

Wrist-drop

Inability to straighten the *wrist*, so that the back of the hand cannot be brought into line with the back of the forearm. This causes weakness of grip because the hand muscles can function efficiently only when the wrist is held straight.

Wrist-drop is caused by damage to the *radial nerve*, usually at a point where it passes beneath the armpit or where it winds around the *humerus* (upper-arm bone). The radial nerve may be damaged by prolonged pressure in the armpit (see *Crutch palsy*) or by a fracture of the humerus (see *Humerus, fracture of*).

Treatment involves holding the wrist straight. In some cases, this may be achieved by means of a simple splint. However, if damage to the radial nerve is permanent, the usual treatment is *arthrodesis* (surgical fusion) of the wrist bones in a straight position.

Writer's cramp

An inability to write as a result of spasm of the muscles of the hand (see *Cramp, writer's*).

Wry neck

Abnormal tilting and twisting of the head. Wry neck may be due to various causes, including injury to, or spasm of, the muscles on one side of the neck (see *Torticollis*).

W

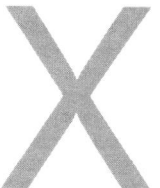

Xanthelasma

Yellowish deposits of fatty substance in the eyelids which are sometimes associated with *hyperlipidaemias* (a group of disorders in which there are raised levels of fats in the blood). Xanthelasmas may be removed by a simple surgical procedure performed under a local anaesthetic. (See also *Xanthomatosis*.)

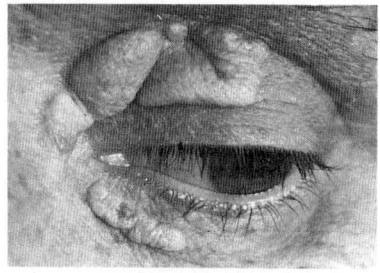

Appearance of xanthelasma
These fatty deposits around the eyes are common in elderly people but are usually of no more than cosmetic importance.

Xanthoma

A yellowish deposit of fatty material in the skin, often on the elbow or buttock. Xanthomas may be associated with *hyperlipidaemias* (a group of disorders in which there are raised levels of fats in the blood). (See *Xanthomatosis*.)

Xanthomatosis

A condition in which deposits of yellowish, fatty material occur in various parts of the body, particularly in the skin, internal organs, corneas, brain, and tendons. The deposits may occur only in the eyelids, a condition known as *xanthelasma*. The most important feature of xanthomatosis is the tendency for fatty material to be deposited in the linings of blood vessels, leading to generalized *atherosclerosis*. Xanthomatosis is often associated with *hyperlipidaemias* (a group of disorders in which there are raised levels of fats in the blood).

Treatment aims to lower the levels of fats in the blood. This is achieved by means of a diet that is low in *cholesterol* and high in polyunsaturated fat, and by treatment with drugs.

X chromosome

A *sex chromosome*. Every normal female body cell has a pair of X chromosomes; every normal male body cell has one X chromosome and one Y chromosome, whereas each sperm carries either an X or a Y chromosome. Abnormal genes on X chromosomes cause *X-linked disorders*.

Xeroderma pigmentosum

A rare, inherited skin disease. The skin is normal at birth, but *photosensitivity* (extreme sensitivity to sunlight) causes it to become dry, wrinkled, freckled, and prematurely aged by about the age of five. Benign skin tumours and *skin cancers* also develop. Xeroderma pigmentosum is often accompanied by eye problems, such as *photophobia* and *conjunctivitis*.

Treatment consists of protecting the skin from sunlight by wearing protective clothing and using *sunscreens*. Skin cancers are usually treated surgically or with *anticancer drugs*.

Xerophthalmia

An *eye* disorder in which *vitamin A* deficiency causes the conjunctiva and cornea to become abnormally dry. Without treatment, xerophthalmia may progress to *keratomalacia*, a condition in which there is severe damage to the cornea.

Xerostomia

Abnormal dryness of the mouth (see *Mouth, dry*).

Xipamide

A thiazide *diuretic drug* used to treat oedema (accumulation of fluid in tissues) and high blood pressure.

Possible adverse effects of xipamide include dizziness and mild gastrointestinal disturbances.

Xiphisternum

An alternative name for the xiphoid process, the small, leaf-shaped projection that forms the lowest of the three parts of the *sternum* (breastbone).

X-linked disorders

Sex-linked *genetic disorders* in which the abnormal gene or genes—the causative factors—are located on the X chromosome, and in which almost all those affected are males; *colour vision deficiency* and *haemophilia* are examples. (See also *Fragile X syndrome*.)

X-rays

A form of invisible electromagnetic energy of short wavelength that is produced when high-speed electrons strike a heavy metal. X-rays were discovered in 1895 by Wilhelm Conrad Roentgen. From the time of their discovery, X-rays have been used to an increasingly important degree in medicine both for diagnosis and for treatment.

WHY THEY ARE USED
X-rays can be used to produce images of bones, organs, and internal tissues. Low doses of X-rays are passed through the tissues and cast images—essentially shadows—on to film or on to a fluorescent screen. The X-ray image, also known as a radiograph or roentgenogram, shows any structural changes in the area that is being examined.

X-rays have the potential to damage living cells, especially those that are dividing rapidly. Because cancer cells divide rapidly, high doses of radiation are used (along with other forms of radiant energy) for treating cancer (see *Radiotherapy*).

HOW THEY WORK
X-rays are produced artificially by bombarding a heavy metal tungsten target with electrons in a device known as an X-ray tube (or Coolidge tube). The X-rays that are emitted travel in straight lines and radiate outwards in all directions from a point on the target. In an X-ray machine, the X-ray tube is surrounded by lead casing, except for a small aperture through which the X-ray beam emerges.

Each of the body's tissues absorbs X-rays in a predictable way. Bones, which are dense and contain calcium, absorb X-rays well. In contrast soft tissues—skin, fat, blood, and muscle, for example—absorb X-rays to a lesser extent. Thus, when an arm, for instance, is placed in the path of an X-ray beam, the X-rays pass readily through the soft tissues but penetrate the bones much less easily. As a result, the arm casts a shadow on to film or on to a fluorescent screen, with the bone appearing white and the soft tissues dark grey.

THE X-RAY EXAMINATION
When a patient arrives for an X-ray examination, the radiographer explains the procedure. The patient undresses to expose the area to be X-rayed and must remove any objects that might produce an image on the film, such as jewellery, hair-grips, dentures, or a wig.

X

X-RAY EXAMINATION

Probably the best-known of all imaging techniques, X-rays are also one of the most useful, particularly for imaging the skeleton, the chest, and body conduits such as the blood vessels and digestive tract (after a radiopaque material has been introduced into them). Modern X-ray equipment is designed to produce high-quality images at the lowest possible radiation dose to the patient.

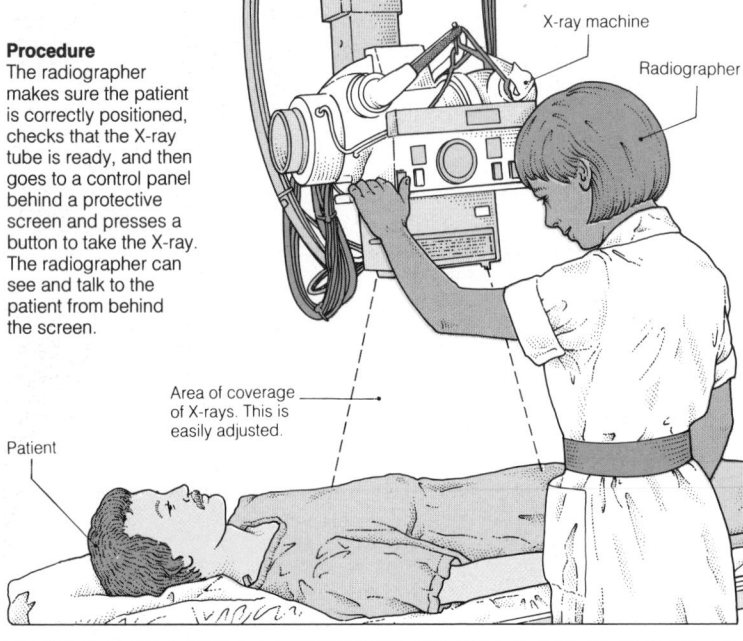

Procedure
The radiographer makes sure the patient is correctly positioned, checks that the X-ray tube is ready, and then goes to a control panel behind a protective screen and presses a button to take the X-ray. The radiographer can see and talk to the patient from behind the screen.

X-ray machine

Radiographer

Area of coverage of X-rays. This is easily adjusted.

Patient

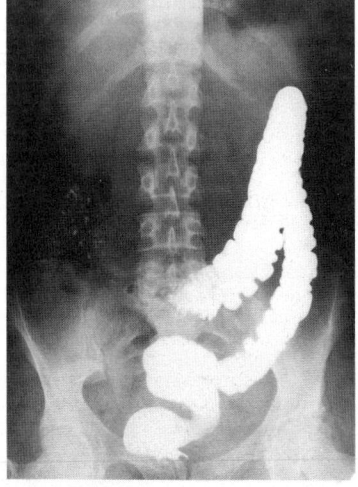

Barium enema
This X-ray shows the lower part of the large intestine outlined by a radiopaque contrast medium containing a barium compound.

The position of the patient when the X-ray is taken is carefully chosen to provide the clearest view of the part under examination, although this position may require modification if the patient is very ill or in severe pain.

The X-ray film is usually contained in a flat cassette; the patient lies, sits, or stands with the region to be examined in contact with the cassette. To avoid getting a blurred image, the patient must keep still while the X-ray is taken. Every effort is made to keep the patient comfortable and relaxed and to use the shortest possible exposure time—usually just a fraction of a second. If necessary, the region under examination can be supported or immobilized.

When the patient is in the correct position, the film is in place, and the X-ray tube is ready, the radiographer leaves the room for a few moments and presses the exposure button on the control panel to take the X-ray.

Once the X-ray film has been developed, it is interpreted by a radiologist. Some disorders, such as fractures, are immediately recognizable; others, such as some tumours, may take more time to assess.

SPECIAL X-RAY TECHNIQUES

Hollow or fluid-filled parts of the body often do not show up well on X-ray film unless they first have a contrast medium (a substance that is opaque to X-rays) introduced into them. Contrast-medium X-ray techniques are used to look at the gallbladder (see *Cholecystography*), the bile ducts (see *Cholangiography*), the urinary tract (see *Urography*), the gastrointestinal tract (see *Barium X-ray examinations*), the blood vessels (see *Angiography*; *Venography*), the spinal cord (see *Myelography*), and the spaces within joints (see *Arthrography*).

X-rays can be used to obtain an image of a "slice" through an organ or part of the body by using a technique known as *tomography*. More detailed and accurate images of a body slice are produced by combining tomography with the capabilities of a computer (see *CT scanning*).

X-RAY SAFETY

Large doses of radiation can be extremely harmful and even small doses carry some risk (see *Radiation hazards*). Modern X-ray film, equipment, and techniques are designed specifically to produce high-quality images with the lowest possible radiation exposure to the patient. The possible hazard of genetic damage can be minimized by using a lead shield to protect the patient's reproductive organs from the X-rays. X-ray examinations are generally avoided if there is any possibility of pregnancy. Radiographers and radiologists wear a *film badge* to monitor their exposure to radiation. (See also *Imaging techniques*; *Radiography*; *Radiology*.)

X-rays, dental

See *Dental X-rays*.

Xylometazoline

A *decongestant drug* used to relieve nasal congestion caused by a common *cold*, *sinusitis*, or hay fever (see *Rhinitis, allergic*). Available in nose-drops or nasal sprays, xylometazoline works by narrowing the small blood vessels in the lining of the nose. It is also used as an ingredient of eye-drops in the treatment of allergic *conjunctivitis*.

Excessive use of xylometazoline may cause headache, palpitations, or drowsiness. Long-term use may cause nasal congestion to become worse when the drug is stopped.

X

USING X-RAYS TO LOOK AT THE BODY

X-rays are perhaps the most widely used method of imaging the body. When passed through body tissues on to photographic film, X-rays cast images of internal structures, allowing alterations in silhouette to be seen. Soft tissues do not show up as well as bone on X-rays, but, by using a contrast medium, they too can be visualized. New computer techniques produce even clearer, more detailed images.

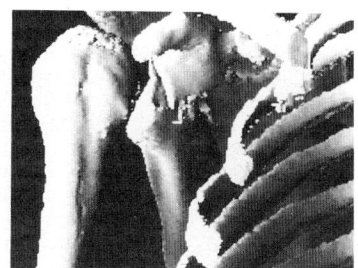

3-D CT scan
A computer can transform X-ray images of body slices into a three-dimensional image of part of the body. This scan shows a badly damaged shoulderblade.

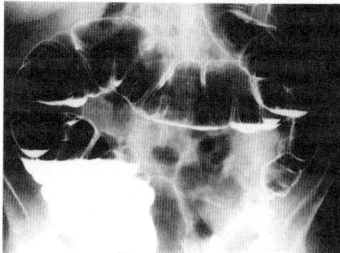

Barium X-ray
Introducing barium, which is opaque to X-rays, into the large intestine allows it to be visualized.

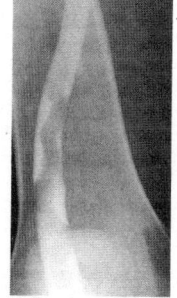

Venography
This technique for examining veins involves injecting them with a contrast medium before they are X-rayed. The femoral vein shown here (in the foreground) is partly blocked by blood clots.

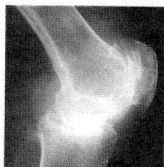 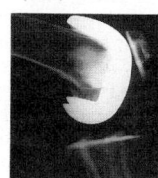

X-rays of knee joint
The X-ray at left shows erosion of bone and cartilage. The parts of an artificial knee are seen in the X-ray at right.

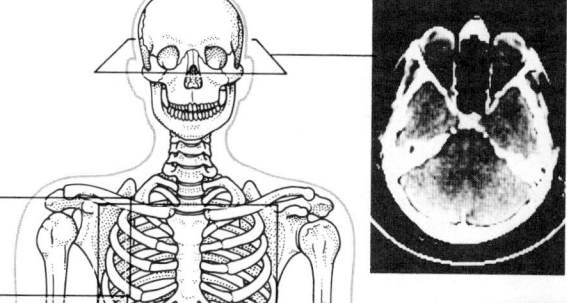

CT scan
Combined use of a computer and X-rays produces cross-sectional images. In this brain scan, the eyes and nose are seen at the top; the central light area represents the brainstem.

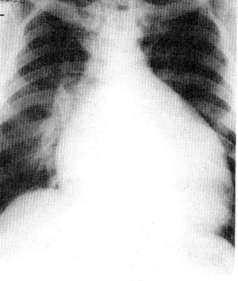

Chest X-ray
This heart appears enlarged due to accumulation of fluid around it.

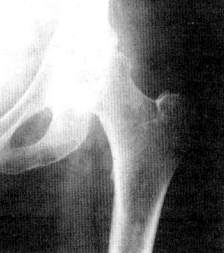

X-ray of hip joint
This X-ray of an osteo-arthritic hip shows almost complete degener-ation of the cartilage.

 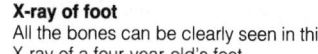

X-ray of foot
All the bones can be clearly seen in this X-ray of a four-year-old's foot.

X

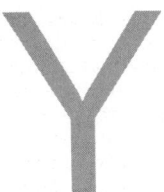

Y

Yawning

An involuntary act, usually associated with drowsiness or boredom, in which the mouth is opened wide and a slow, deep breath taken through it. Yawning is accompanied by a momentary increase in the heart-rate, slight narrowing of some tiny blood vessels, and, in many cases, watering of the eyes (possibly because of pressure on the tear glands as a result of the facial movements).

The purpose of yawning is unknown, but one theory suggests it is triggered by raised levels of carbon dioxide in the blood; thus, its purpose could be to reduce the level of carbon dioxide and to increase the level of oxygen in the blood.

Yaws

A disease found throughout poorer subtropical and tropical areas of the world that is caused by a spirochaete (spiral-shaped bacterium) very similar to that which causes syphilis. Yaws is not, however, a sexually transmitted disease. The infection is almost always acquired in childhood.

Three or four weeks after infection, a single, highly infectious, itchy, raspberry-like growth appears at the site of infection. Scratching spreads the infection and leads to the development of more growths elsewhere on the skin. Without treatment, the

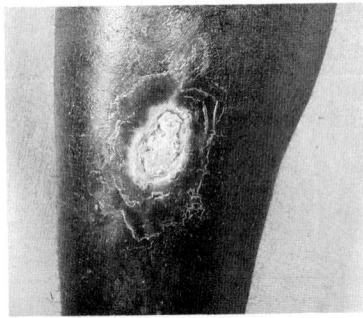

Yaws ulcer on leg
Yaws is an infection that mainly affects the skin and bones. Ulceration and tissue destruction may occur in advanced cases.

growths heal slowly over the course of about six months. Recurrence of the growths is common.

Yaws can be cured by a single large dose of a *penicillin drug*. In about 10 per cent of untreated cases, widespread tissue loss eventually occurs. This may lead to gross destruction of the skin, bones, and joints of the legs, nose, palate, and upper jaw.

Y chromosome

A *sex chromosome* that is present in every normal male body cell, paired with an X chromosome.

Yeasts

Types of *fungi*. Certain yeasts can cause infections of the skin or mucous membranes. The most important disease-causing yeast is CANDIDA ALBI-CANS, which causes *candidiasis*.

Yellow fever

 An infectious disease of short duration and variable severity caused by a virus transmitted by mosquitoes. In severe cases, the skin of the sufferer becomes yellow from *jaundice*—hence the name yellow fever.

CAUSES
Today, yellow fever is contracted only in Central America, parts of South America, and a large area of Africa. In forest areas, various species of mosquitoes may spread the infection from monkeys to humans. In urban areas, it is transmitted between humans by AEDES AEGYPTI mosquitoes.

PREVENTION
Eradication of the causative mosquito from populated areas has greatly reduced the incidence of yellow fever. Vaccination confers long-lasting immunity and should always be obtained before travel to affected areas. A vaccination certificate is required for entry to many countries where the disease is prevalent or when travelling from these areas.

A single injection of the vaccine gives protection for at least 10 years. Children under one year old should not be vaccinated. Reactions to the vaccine are rare and usually trivial.

SYMPTOMS AND SIGNS
Three to six days after infection, there is sudden onset of fever and headache, often with nausea and nosebleeds. Characteristically, despite the high fever, the heart-rate is very slow. In many cases, the patient recovers in about three days.

In more serious cases, the fever is higher and there is severe headache and pain in the neck, back, and legs. Damage may occur rapidly to the liver and kidneys, causing jaundice and *kidney failure*. This may be followed by a stage of severe agitation and delirium, leading to coma and death.

DIAGNOSIS AND TREATMENT
During epidemics, diagnosis is easy. A diagnosis can be confirmed by using blood tests to isolate the causative virus or to find *antibodies* to the virus.

No drug is effective against the yellow fever virus; treatment is directed at maintaining the blood volume. Transfusion of fluids is often necessary. In mild and moderate cases, the outlook is excellent and complications are few. Relapses do not occur and one attack confers lifelong immunity. Overall, however, about 10 per cent of victims die.

Yin and yang

Fundamental concepts in traditional *Chinese medicine* and philosophy. Yang embodies positive, active, "male" qualities and thus complements yin, which embodies negative, passive, "female" qualities. The concepts of yin and yang are also central to the theoretical basis of *macrobiotics*.

Yoga

A system of Hindu philosophy and physical discipline. The main form of yoga practised in the West is hatha-yoga, in which the follower adopts a series of poses, known as asanas, and uses a special breathing technique. This maintains flexibility of the body, teaches physical and mental control, and is a useful *relaxation technique*.

If attempted by people in poor health or practised incorrectly, yoga may pose health hazards, such as back disorders, *hypertension* (high blood pressure), and *glaucoma* (increased pressure in the eye).

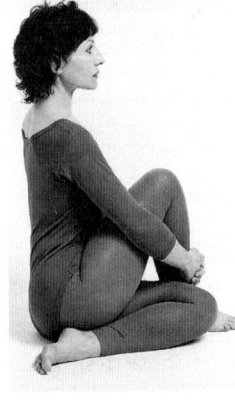

Yoga pose
This photograph shows a stage of the full twist asana, which is excellent for promoting flexibility.

Z

Zidovudine

An *antiviral drug*, formerly known as azidothymidine or AZT. Zidovudine was approved for use in the treatment of *AIDS* in 1987.

WHY IT IS USED

Zidovudine is used to treat serious AIDS-related conditions, such as *pneumocystis pneumonia* and infections of the brain and nervous system caused by *HIV* (the AIDS virus). Zidovudine does not cure these conditions but may prolong remissions or improve symptoms. For example, it may reduce lymph node swelling and promote weight gain. Although zidovudine slows the progress of AIDS, relapse commonly occurs after several months of treatment.

Conflicting results have emerged from research into the use of zidovudine in people infected with HIV but without symptoms. Early trials suggested that the treatment postponed the onset of AIDS-related illnesses, but later studies showed there was little or no effect on overall survival, and the postponement of AIDS had to be balanced against the side-effects of the treatment.

HOW IT WORKS

Zidovudine blocks the action of the *enzyme* that stimulates the AIDS virus to grow and multiply. Clinical trials have shown that the resultant reduction in virus activity leads to an increase in the production and number of T-helper lymphocytes (a type of white blood cell). This in turn improves the *immune system's* efficiency, making the occurrence of *opportunistic infections*, such as candidiasis (thrush), less likely. Zidovudine does not appear to stop the growth of other viruses.

POSSIBLE ADVERSE EFFECTS

By reducing the number of red blood cells produced, zidovudine often causes severe *anaemia*, requiring blood transfusion. For this reason, regular blood tests are performed and the drug is withdrawn if the blood count is dangerously low. Too high a dose of zidovudine may cause restlessness, insomnia, and fever.

Zidovudine also impairs the absorption and thus the effectiveness of *trimethoprim* and sulphamethoxazole, the antibiotic drugs used to treat pneumonia in people who have AIDS.

Zinc

A *trace element* that is essential for normal growth, development of the reproductive organs, normal functioning of the prostate gland, healing of wounds, and the manufacture of proteins and nucleic acids (the genetic material of cells). Zinc also controls the activities of more than 100 enzymes and is involved in the functioning of the hormone insulin.

Small amounts of the element are present in a wide variety of foods; particularly rich sources include lean meat, wholemeal breads, whole grain cereals, dried beans, and seafoods.

DEFICIENCY

Zinc deficiency is rare. Most cases occur in people who are generally malnourished. Deficiency may also be caused by any disorder that causes *malabsorption*, by *acrodermatitis enteropathica* (a disorder of zinc absorption), or by increased zinc requirements due to cell damage (for example, as a

result of a burn or in *sickle cell anaemia*). Symptoms of deficiency include impairment of taste and loss of appetite; in severe cases, there may also be hair loss and inflammation of the skin, mouth, tongue, and eyelids. In children, zinc deficiency impairs physical growth and delays sexual development.

EXCESS

Prolonged, excessive intake of zinc (usually through supplements) may interfere with the intestinal absorption of *iron* and *copper*, leading to a deficiency of these minerals and resultant symptoms of nausea, vomiting, fever, headache, tiredness, and abdominal pain.

MEDICAL USES

Zinc compounds, such as *zinc oxide*, are included in many preparations for treating skin and scalp disorders.

Zinc oxide

An ingredient of many skin preparations that has a mild *astringent* (drying) action and a soothing effect. Zinc oxide is used to treat painful, itchy, or moist skin conditions (such as eczema, bedsores, and nappy rash) and to ease the pain caused by hae-

A SELECTION OF ZOONOSES (DISEASES CAUGHT FROM ANIMALS)

Animal	Disease	Animal	Disease
Bat	Histoplasmosis Rabies	Horse	Glanders
Cat	Toxoplasmosis Cat-scratch fever Fungal infections	Pig	Trichinosis Pork tapeworm Brucellosis
Cow	Brucellosis Beef tapeworm Q fever Cowpox	Rabbit	Tularaemia
Dog	Rabies Toxocariasis Mite infestations Fungal infections	Rat	Leptospirosis Rat-bite fever
Chicken	Salmonella infection Psittacosis	Sheep	Liver fluke Anthrax

Relative importance

With the exception of fungal infections and mites caught from pets, all the diseases listed above are rare or unknown in the UK. Several of the diseases may be caught from animals that are used as food (pigs and cows, for example) but such diseases are prevalent mainly in countries in which food hygiene regulations and/or practices are lax. Rabies, probably the most serious zoonosis, can be caught from various animals in addition to those listed above—foxes, skunks, and mongooses, for example.

Z

morrhoids and insect bites or stings. It also blocks the ultraviolet rays of the sun (see *Sunscreens*).

Zinc oxide is also used to thicken lotions and creams, making them easier to apply.

Zollinger-Ellison syndrome

A rare condition characterized by severe and recurrent *peptic ulcers* in the stomach, duodenum, and upper small intestine. Zollinger-Ellison syndrome is caused by one or several tumours, usually found in the *pancreas*, that secrete the hormone gastrin. This hormone stimulates the stomach and duodenum to produce large quantities of acid, which leads to ulceration. The high levels of acid in the digestive tract also cause diarrhoea and steatorrhoea (abnormally fatty faeces) in almost half the people with Zollinger-Ellison syndrome.

The condition often goes unrecognized until surgery for the peptic ulcers is rapidly followed by a recurrence of the ulceration. Once suspicion is aroused, the doctor performs blood tests; high levels of gastrin are usually sufficient to confirm the diagnosis.

The tumours are most often cancerous, although of a slow-growing type. If possible, the tumour or tumours are removed surgically; otherwise, total *gastrectomy* (surgical removal of the stomach) is necessary.

Zoonosis

Any infectious or parasitic disease of animals that can be transmitted to humans. Many disease organisms can infect only humans or particular animals, but zoonotic organisms are more flexible and can adapt themselves to many different species.

Zoonoses are usually caught from animals closely associated with humans, either as pets (such as dogs, cats, or parrots), food sources (such as pigs or cattle), or scavenging parasites (such as rats). Examples include *toxocariasis* (from dogs), *cat-scratch fever* and some *fungal infections* (from cats), *psittacosis* (from parrots or other birds), *brucellosis* (from cows, goats, or pigs), *trichinosis* (from pigs), and *leptospirosis* (from rats). *Rabies* can infect virtually any mammal, but dog bites are a common cause of human infection worldwide. (See the box on the previous page.)

Other zoonoses are transmitted from animals less obviously associated with humans, usually by insect *vectors*. For example, some cases of

TECHNIQUE OF Z-PLASTY

This relatively simple plastic surgery technique is carried out to revise unsightly scars or to relieve skin tension caused by scar contracture. It can be particularly useful for dealing with facial scars or scars that cross natural skin creases.

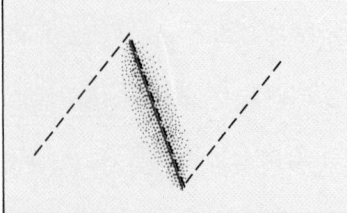

1 Three incisions are made, forming a Z. The central incision is made lengthwise through the scar.

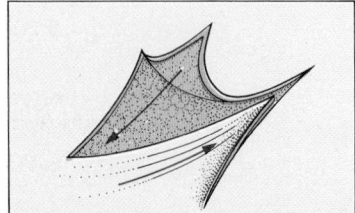

2 Two triangular flaps are developed by cutting skin away from underlying tissue, and the flaps are then transposed.

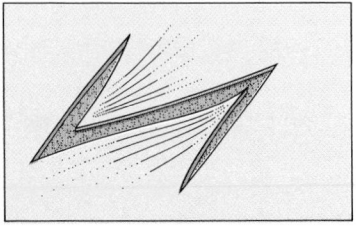

3 This manoeuvre creates a new Z, of which the central arm is at right angles to the original direction of the scar.

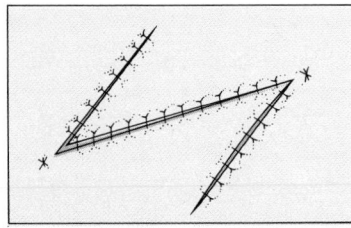

4 The flaps are sutured in place. With careful planning, the suture lines can be hidden in natural skin creases.

yellow fever are transmitted from forest monkeys to humans via the bites of mosquitoes. (See also *Dogs, diseases from; Cats, diseases from; Rats, diseases from; Insects and disease.*)

Z-plasty

A technique that is used in *plastic surgery* to change the direction of a scar so that it can be hidden in natural skin creases or to relieve skin tension caused by *contracture* of a scar. Z-plasty is especially useful for revising unsightly scars on the face and for releasing scarring across joints, such as on the fingers or in the armpits, that may restrict normal movement or cause deformity.

A Z-shaped incision is made with the central arm of the Z along the scar. Two V-shaped flaps are created by cutting the skin away from underlying tissue. The flaps are then transposed and stitched. The procedure has the effect of redistributing tension perpendicular to the original defect.

Zygote

The cell produced when a *sperm* fertilizes an *ovum*. A zygote, measuring about 0.1 mm in diameter in humans, contains all the genetic (hereditary) material for a new individual—half coming from the sperm and half from the ovum.

The zygote travels down one of the woman's *fallopian tubes* towards the uterus, dividing as it does so. After about a week, the mass of cells (now called a blastocyst) implants into the lining of the uterus, and the next stage of embryological growth begins. (See also *Embryo; Fertilization.*)

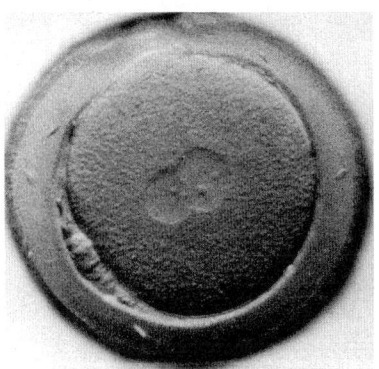

Appearance of a zygote
The photograph shows a human egg just after fertilization by a sperm. The two circular areas at the centre are the nuclei of the sperm and egg merging.

Z

DRUG GLOSSARY
AND INDEX

DRUG GLOSSARY

The drug glossary includes all the most important generic drugs, a broad range of brand-name drugs, and the various vitamins, minerals, and other substances that may be used as drugs. The generic names are the official names for drugs, which are chosen by the Nomenclature Committee of the British Pharmacopoeia Commission. Drug brand names are chosen by individual manufacturers.

If a generic drug has a separate entry within the encyclopedia, the page number of this entry is given directly after the drug's name. If a drug belongs to a group of drugs that has an encyclopedia entry, this information is given in the glossary together with the relevant page number. If a generic drug belongs to a drug group that does not have an encyclopedia entry, the glossary tells you the disorder or disorders for which the drug you are looking up is most commonly used, and gives appropriate page references. In the case of brand-name drugs, glossary entries give the equivalent generic drug names and appropriate page references to entries within the main part of the encyclopedia. If a brand-name drug contains several generic drugs, or if its ingredients do not have separate entries, the glossary will direct you to appropriate drug group or disorder entries.

This selection of drugs is designed to reflect a wide diversity of drugs for the treatment or prevention of disease. Inclusion of any drug does not imply BMA endorsement; similarly, exclusion does not indicate BMA disapproval.

A

Abidec a brand-name multivitamin 702

Acarbose 59, a generic drug used in the treatment of non-insulin-dependent (type 2) diabetes mellitus 348

Accupro a brand name for quinapril, an ACE inhibitor drug 61

Accuretic a brand-name preparation containing a mixture of quinapril, an ACE inhibitor drug 61, and hydrochlorothiazide 546

Acebutolol 60, a generic beta-blocker drug 164

Acemetacin a generic nonsteroidal anti-inflammatory drug 734

Acepril a brand name for captopril 231

Acetazolamide 61, a generic drug for the treatment of glaucoma 483

Acetic acid 61, an ingredient of antiseptics 119

Acetohexamide 61, a generic hypoglycaemic drug 556

Acetomenaphthone a generic drug used in multivitamin preparations 702

Acetoxyl a brand name for benzoyl peroxide 163

Acetylcholine 61, a chemical neurotransmitter 729 also used to induce miosis 690

Acetylcysteine 61, a generic drug used as an antidote for paracetemol 778 overdose. Also used as a mucolytic drug 701

Acezide a brand-name preparation containing captopril 231 and hydrochlorothiazide 546

Achromycin a brand-name tetracycline drug 981, a type of antibiotic drug 114

Acipimox a generic lipid-lowering drug 639

Acitretin a generic drug with similar actions to etretinate 417, used to treat psoriasis 837

Aclacin a brand name for aclarubicin, an anticancer drug 115

Aclarubicin a generic anticancer drug 115

Acnecide a brand-name preparation containing benzoyl peroxide 163

Acnegel a brand name for benzoyl peroxide 163

Acnidazil a brand-name preparation containing benzoyl peroxide 163 and miconazole 683

Acnisal a brand-name preparation containing salicylic acid 885

Acrivastine a generic antihistamine drug 118

Acrosoxacin 64, a generic quinolone drug 849 used to treat gonorrhoea 490

Actal a brand-name antacid preparation 111

ACTH 64, a type of hormone 541

Actifed Compound a brand-name decongestant drug 335

Actilyse a brand-name thrombolytic drug 987

Actinac a brand-name preparation containing chloramphenicol 268 and hydrocortisone 546 used to treat acne 62

Actinomycin D another name for dactinomycin, a generic anticancer drug 115

Actonorm a brand-name antispasmodic drug 120

Actraphane 30/70, Human a brand name for insulin 589

Actrapid, Human a brand name for insulin 589

Actron a brand-name preparation containing aspirin 137 and paracetamol 778

Acupan a brand name for nefopam 721

Acyclovir 66, a generic antiviral drug 120

Adalat a brand name for nifedipine 730

Adalat Retard a brand name for nifedipine 730

Adcortyl a brand name for triamcinolone 1014

Adexolin a brand-name preparation containing vitamins A 1062, C 1065, and D 1065

Adifax a brand name for dexfenfluramine,

an appetite suppressant drug 127

Adizem a brand name for diltiazem 359

Adrenaline 70, a hormone 541 used to treat acute allergic reactions and glaucoma 483

Adriamycin a brand name for doxorubicin 371

AeroBec a brand name for beclomethasone 160

Aerocrom a brand name for sodium cromoglycate 927

Aerolin a brand name for salbutamol 885

Afrazine a brand name for oxymetazoline 770

Agarol a brand-name laxative preparation 629 containing liquid paraffin 639 and phenolphthalein 1119

Akineton a brand name for biperiden, used to treat Parkinson's disease 781

Albendazole a generic drug used to treat hydatid cysts 544

Alclometasone a generic corticosteroid drug 312

Alcobon a brand name for flucytosine, an antifungal drug 117

Alcuronium a generic muscle-relaxant drug 707 used in general anaesthesia 99

Aldactide a brand-name diuretic preparation 364 containing spironolactone 938 and hydroflume-thiazide 1110

Aldactone a brand name for spironolactone 938

Aldesleukin a generic anticancer drug 115

Aldomet a brand name for methyldopa 684

Alexan a brand name for cytarabine, an anticancer drug 115

Alfacalcidol a generic derivative of vitamin D 1065

Alfa D a brand name for alfacalcidol, a derivative of vitamin D 1065

Alfentanil a generic analgesic drug 102 used in general anaesthesia 99

Algicon a brand-name antacid preparation 111

Alginate a generic reflux suppressant added to antacids 111

Alginic acid a generic reflux suppressant added to antacids 111

Algitec a brand-name preparation containing cimetidine 278 and alginic acid 1097

Alimix a brand name for cisapride 281

Alka-Seltzer a brand-name analgesic preparation 102 containing aspirin 137 and sodium bicarbonate 727

Alkeran a brand name for melphalan 673

Allantoin a generic derivative of uric acid 1030, used in skin preparations

Allbee with C a brand-name multivitamin 702

Allegron a brand name for nortriptyline 734

Aller-eze a brand name for clemastine, an antihistamine drug 118

Alloferin a brand name for alcuronium, a muscle-relaxant drug 707 used in general anaesthesia 99

Allopurinol 87, a generic drug used to treat gout 490

Allyloestrenol a generic progestogen drug 830

Almodan a brand name for amoxycillin 94

Alomide brand-name eye-drops containing lodoxamide, used in the treatment of allergic conjunctivitis 296

Alophen a brand-name laxative preparation 629 containing phenolphthalein

Alphaderm a brand name for hydrocortisone 546

Alpha tocopheryl acetate another name for vitamin E 1065

Alphavase a brand name for prazosin 821

Alphodith a brand name for dithranol 364

Alphosyl a brand name for coal tar 283

Alprazolam 88, a generic antianxiety drug 114

Alprostadil a generic prostaglandin drug 832 used to treat congenital heart disease 519

Alrheumat a brand name for ketoprofen 612

Altacite a brand name for hydrotalcite, an antacid preparation containing aluminium 88 and magnesium 656

Alteplase a generic thrombolytic drug 987

Alu-Cap a brand-name antacid drug 111

Aludrox gel a brand name for aluminium hydroxide 89

Aludrox SA a brand-name antacid 111 and antispasmodic preparation 120

Aluhyde a brand-name antispasmodic drug 120

Aluminium acetate a generic astringent 139

Aluminium chloride 89, a generic antiperspirant 118

Aluminium hydroxide 89, a generic antacid drug 111

Alupent a brand name for orciprenaline, a bronchodilator drug 215

Alvedon a brand name for paracetamol 778

Alvercol a brand-name preparation containing alverine, an antispasmodic drug 120, and sterculia, a generic bulk-forming substance used as an anti-diarrhoeal drug 116 and a laxative drug 629

Alverine a generic anti-spasmodic drug 120

Amantadine 90, a generic antiviral drug 120 also used to treat Parkinson's disease 781

Ambaxin a brand name for bacampicillin, a penicillin drug 1098

AmBisome a brand name for amphotericin B 94

Amethocaine a generic local anaesthetic 101

Amfipen a brand name for ampicillin 94

Amikacin a generic antibiotic drug 114

Amikin a brand name for amikacin, an antibiotic drug 114

Amil-Co a brand-name diuretic preparation 364 containing amiloride 92 and hydrochlorothiazide 546

Amilmaxco a brand-name diuretic preparation 364 containing amiloride 92 and hydroclorothiazide 546

Amiloride 92, a generic potassium-sparing diuretic drug 364

Amilospare a brand name for amiloride 92

Aminoglutethimide 92, a hormone antagonist 541 used to treat Cushing's syndrome 325 and breast cancer 205

Aminophylline 92, a generic bronchodilator drug 215

Amiodarone 92, a generic antiarrhythmic drug 114

Amitriptyline 92, a generic antidepressant drug 116

Amix a brand name for amoxycillin 94

Amlodipine 92, a generic calcium channel blocker 224

Ammonium chloride a generic drug used as an expectorant 421 and also to alter the acidity of the urine 1034

Amnivent a brand name for aminophylline 92

Amoram a brand name for amoxycillin 94

Amorolfine a generic antifungal drug 117

Amoxapine 94, a generic antidepressant drug 116

Amoxil a brand name for amoxycillin 94

Amoxycillin 94, a generic penicillin drug 788, a type of antibiotic drug 114

Amoxymed a brand name for amoxycillin 94

Amphotericin B 94, a generic antifungal drug 117

Ampicillin 94, a generic penicillin drug 788, a type of antibiotic drug 114

Ampiclox a brand-name preparation containing ampicillin 94 and cloxacillin 283

Amrit a brand name for amoxycillin 94

Amsacrine a generic anticancer drug 115

Amsidine a brand name for amsacrine, an anticancer drug 115

Amylobarbitone a generic barbiturate 156 sleeping drug 922

Amytal a brand name for amylobarbitone, a barbiturate 156 sleeping drug 922

Anacal a brand-name preparation used to treat anal irritation 121

Anadin a brand-name preparation containing aspirin 137 and quinine 849

Anadin Extra, Anadin Extra Soluble brand-name preparations containing aspirin 137 and paracetamol 778

Anadin Ibuprofen a brand name for ibuprofen 562

Anafranil, Anafranil SR brand names for clomipramine 282

Anapolon 50 a brand name for oxymetholone, an anabolic steroid 946

Andrews Answer a brand name for paracetamol 778

Andrews Antacid a brand-name antacid preparation 111

Androcur a brand name for cyproterone 326

Anectine a brand name for suxamethonium, a muscle-relaxant drug 707 used in general anaesthesia 99

Anestan a brand-name preparation containing ephedrine 408 and theophylline 983

Anethaine a brand name for amethocaine, a local anaesthetic 101

Anexate a brand name for flumazenil, a drug used to reverse the sedative effects of benzodiazepine drugs 163

Angettes-75 a brand-name preparation containing aspirin 137, used to prevent thrombosis 987

Angilol a brand name for propranolol 831

Angiopine a brand name for nifedipine 730

Angiozem a brand name for diltiazem 359

Anhydrol Forte a brand name for aluminium chloride 89

Anistreplase a generic thrombolytic drug 987

Anodesyn a brand-name preparation containing ephedrine 408, lignocaine 637, and allantoin 1097, used to relieve anal itching 121

Anquil a brand name for benperidol, an antipsychotic drug 119

Antabuse a brand name for disulfiram 364

Antazoline a generic drug used to treat allergic conjunctivitis 296

Antepsin a brand name for sucralfate 957

Anthisan a brand-name antihistamine preparation 118

Anthranol a brand name for dithranol 364

Antihaemophilic factor a blood protein used to promote blood clotting 183

Antipressan a brand name for atenolol 140

Anturan a brand name for sulphinpyrazone 958

Anugesic-HC a brand-name preparation used to relieve anal itching 121

Anusol-HC a brand-name preparation used to relieve anal itching 121

APP a brand-name anti-spasmodic preparation 120

Apresoline a brand name for hydralazine 545

Aprinox a brand name for bendrofluazide 163

Aprotinin a generic drug used to promote blood clotting 183

Apsifen a brand name for ibuprofen 562

Apsin VK a brand-name penicillin drug 788, a type of antibiotic drug 114

Apsolol a brand name for propranolol 831

Apsolox a brand name for oxprenolol 770

Aquadrate a brand-name emollient preparation 397

Arachis oil a generic preparation used to treat scaly skin 914

Aramine a brand name for metaraminol, a vaso-constrictor drug 1046 used in the treatment of acute hypotension 558

Arbralene a brand name for metoprolol 684

Aredia a brand name for disodium pamidronate, a generic biphosphonate drug 171 used in the treatment of hyper-calcaemia 548 due to cancer

Arelix a brand name for piretanide, a loop diuretic drug 364 used to treat hypertension 551

Argipressin a synthetic form of vasopressin 1047

Arpicolin a brand name for procyclidine 830

Arpimycin a brand name for erythromycin 416

Arret a brand name for loperamide 647

Artane a brand name for benzhexol, used to treat Parkinson's disease 781

Arthrofen a brand name for ibuprofen 562

Arthrosin a brand name for naproxen 717

Arthrotec a brand name for diclofenac 356

Arthroxen a brand name for naproxen 717

Artracin a brand name for indomethacin 576

Arythmol a brand name for propafenone, an anti-arrhythmic drug 114

Asacol a brand name for mesalazine 681

Ascabiol a brand name for benzyl benzoate, used to treat scabies 888

Ascorbic acid another name for vitamin C 1065

Asendis a brand name for amoxapine 94

Aserbine a brand-name preparation used to treat leg ulcers 631

Asilone a brand-name antacid preparation 111

Askit a brand-name preparation containing aspirin 137

Asparaginase a generic anticancer drug 115

Aspav a brand-name analgesic 102 preparation containing aspirin 137, and papaveretum 1118

Aspirin 137, a generic analgesic drug 102

Aspro a brand name for aspirin 137

Astemizole a generic antihistamine drug 118

AT 10 a brand name for vitamin D 1065

Atarax a brand name for hydroxyzine, an anti-anxiety drug 114 also used to treat pruritus 836

Atenix a brand name for atenolol 140

AtenixCo a brand-name preparation containing atenolol 140 and chlorthalidone, a thiazide diuretic drug 364

Atenolol 140, a generic beta-blocker drug 164

Atensine a brand name for diazepam 356

Ativan a brand name for lorazepam 647

Atracurium a generic muscle-relaxant drug 707 used in general anaesthesia 99

Atromid-S a brand name for clofibrate 282

Atropine 143, a generic anticholinergic drug 115

Atrovent a brand name for ipratropium bromide, a bronchodilator drug 215

Audicort a brand-name preparation containing neomycin 721 and triamcinolone 1014 used to treat ear infections 383

Augmentin a brand-name antibiotic preparation 114 containing co-amoxiclav (a mixture of amoxycillin 94 and clavulanic acid, a drug used to enhance the effect of amoxycillin)

Auranofin 143, a generic antirheumatic drug 119

Aureocort a brand-name preparation containing triamcinolone 1014 and chlortetracycline, a tetracycline drug 981

Aureomycin a brand-name tetracycline drug 981, a type of antibiotic drug 114

Aventyl a brand name for nortriptyline 734

Avloclor a brand name for chloroquine 269

Avomine a brand name for promethazine 831

Axid a brand name for nizatidine, an ulcer-healing drug 1024

Azactam a brand-name antibiotic preparation containing aztreonam 149

Azamune a brand name for azathioprine 149

Azapropazone a generic nonsteroidal anti-inflammatory drug 734

Azatadine a generic antihistamine drug 118

Azathioprine 149, a generic immunosuppressant drug 572

Azelaic acid a generic drug used to treat acne 62

Azelastine a generic antihistamine drug 118 available as nasal spray for allergic rhinitis 878

Azidothymidine the former name for zidovudine 1093

Azithromycin 149, a generic antibiotic drug 114

Azlocillin a generic penicillin drug 788, a type of antibiotic drug 114

AZT an abbreviation of azidothymidine, the former name for zidovudine 1093

Aztreonam 149, a generic antibiotic drug 114

B

Bacampicillin a generic penicillin drug 788, a type of antibiotic drug 114

Bacitracin a generic antibacterial drug 114

Baclofen 150, a generic muscle-relaxant drug 707

Bactrim a brand name for co-trimoxazole 313

Bactroban a brand-name antibacterial 114 nasal preparation containing mupirocin 1115

Bambec a brand name for bambuterol 156

Bambuterol 156, a generic bronchodilator drug 215

Banocide a brand-name anthelmintic drug 113

Baratol a brand-name antihypertensive drug 118

Barquinol HC a brand-name preparation containing hydrocortisone 546

Baxan a brand-name cephalosporin 247, a type of antibiotic drug 114

Baycaron a brand name for mefruside, a thiazide diuretic drug 364

Beclazone a brand name for beclomethasone 160

Becloforte a brand name for beclomethasone 160

Beclomethasone 160, a generic corticosteroid drug 312

Becodisks a brand name for beclomethasone 160

Beconase a brand name for beclomethasone 160

Becotide a brand name for beclomethasone 160

Bedranol SR a brand name for propranolol 831

Belladonna 163, a generic anticholinergic drug 115

Benadon a brand name for pyridoxine 848, part of the vitamin B complex 1063

Bendogen a brand name for bethanidine 166, an antihypertensive drug 118

Bendrofluazide 163, a generic thiazide diuretic drug 364

Benemid a brand name for probenecid 829

Benerva a brand name for thiamine 984, part of the vitamin B complex 1063

Benethamine penicillin a generic penicillin drug 788, a type of antibiotic drug 114

Benoral a brand-name analgesic drug 102

Benorylate 163, a generic analgesic drug 102

Benoxyl a brand name for benzoyl peroxide 163

Benperidol a generic antipsychotic drug 119

Benserazide a generic drug administered with levodopa 635 to treat Parkinson's disease 781

Benylin Expectorant a brand-name cough remedy 314

Benylin Paediatric a brand-name cough remedy 314 for children

Benzagel a brand name for benzoyl peroxide 163

Benzalkonium chloride a generic skin antiseptic 119

Benzhexol a generic drug used to treat Parkinson's disease 781

Benzocaine a generic local anaesthetic 101

Benzoic acid a generic antifungal preparation 117

Benzoin tincture an aromatic resin added to inhalations 585

Benzoyl peroxide 163, a generic skin antiseptic 119 used to treat acne 62

Benzthiazide a generic thiazide diuretic drug 364

Benztropine a generic drug used to treat Parkinson's disease 781

Benzydamine a generic analgesic drug 102

Benzyl benzoate a generic drug used to treat scabies 888

Benzylpenicillin a generic penicillin drug 788, a type of antibiotic drug 114

Berkatens a brand name for verapamil 1053

Berkmycen a brand name for oxytetracycline 770

Berkolol a brand name for propranolol 831

Berkozide a brand name for bendrofluazide 163

Berotec a brand-name bronchodilator preparation 215

Beta-Adalat a brand-name preparation containing atenolol 140 and nifedipine 730

Beta-Cardone a brand-name beta-blocker drug 164

Beta-carotene another name for vitamin A 1062

Betadren a brand name for pindolol 803

Betadur CR a brand name for propranolol 834

Betagan a brand name for levobunolol, a beta-blocker drug 164 used as eye-drops

Betahistine 165, a generic drug used to treat Ménière's disease 674

Betaloc a brand name for metoprolol 684

Betamethasone 165, a generic corticosteroid drug 312

Beta-Prograne a brand name for propranolol 834

Betaxolol a generic beta-blocker drug 164 used to treat glaucoma 483

Bethanechol a generic drug used to treat urinary retention 1031

Bethanidine 166, a generic antihypertensive drug 118

Betim a brand name for timolol 994

Betnelan a brand name for betamethasone 165

Betnesol a brand-name preparation containing betamethasone 165

Betnesol-N a brand-name preparation containing betamethasone 165 and neomycin 721

Betnovate a brand-name preparation containing betamethasone 165

Betnovate-C, Betnovate-N brand-name preparations containing beta-methasone 165

Betoptic a brand-name beta-blocker drug 164 used to treat glaucoma 483

Bezafibrate a generic lipid-lowering drug 639

Bezalip a brand-name lipid-lowering drug 639

Bicillin a brand name for procaine penicillin, a penicillin drug 788

Biltricide a brand name for praziquantel 821

BiNovum a brand-name oral contraceptive 755

Biogastrone a brand name for carbenoxolone 231

Biophylline a brand name for theophylline 983

Bioplex a brand name for carbenoxolone 231

Bioral Gel a brand name for carbenoxolone 231

Biorphen a brand name for orphenadrine 759

Biotin part of the vitamin B complex 1063

Biperiden a generic drug used in the treatment of Parkinson's disease 781

Bisacodyl a generic stimulant laxative drug 629

Bismag a brand-name preparation containing sodium bicarbonate 927

Bismuth 173, an element

BiSoDol a brand-name preparation containing sodium bicarbonate 927

Bisoprolol a generic beta-blocker drug 164

Blemix a brand name for minocycline 689

Bleomycin a generic anticancer drug 115

Blocadren a brand name for timolol 994

Bolvidon a brand name for mianserin 685

Bonefos a brand name for sodium clodronate, a biphosphonate drug 171

Brelomax a brand name for tulobuterol, a bronchodilator drug 215

Bretylate a brand name for bretylium, an anti-arrhythmic drug 114

Bretylium a generic anti-arrhythmic drug 114

Brevibloc a brand name for esmolol, a beta-blocker drug 164

Brevinor a brand-name oral contraceptive 755

Bricanyl a brand name for terbutaline 977

Brietal Sodium a brand name for methohexitone, a drug used for general anaesthesia 99

Britiazim a brand name for diltiazem 359

Britlofex a brand name for lofexidine, used to relieve withdrawal symptoms following the use of narcotic drugs 1084

Brocadopa a brand name for levodopa 635

Broflex a brand name for benzhexol, a drug used to treat Parkinson's disease 781

Brolene a brand-name preparation containing propamidine isethionate, a drug used to treat eye infections 426

Bromazepam a generic antianxiety drug 114

Bromocriptine 213, a generic drug used to treat Parkinson's disease 781

Brompheniramine a generic antihistamine drug 118

Bronchodil a brand-name bronchodilator drug 215

Brufen a brand name for ibuprofen 562

Buccastem a brand name for prochlorperazine 829

Buclizine a generic antiemetic drug 117

Budesonide 217, a generic corticosteroid drug 312

Bufexamac a generic drug used to treat mild skin inflammation 919

Bumetanide 217, a generic loop diuretic drug 364

Bupivacaine a generic local anaesthetic 101

Buprenorphine a generic narcotic drug 717, a type of analgesic drug 102

Burinex a brand-name diuretic drug 364

Burinex-K a brand-name diuretic drug 364 with potassium 820

Buscopan a brand name for hyoscine butylbromide 547

Buserelin a generic gonadorelin drug 489 used in the treatment of endometriosis 402 and cancer of the prostate 832

Buspar a brand-name non-benzodiazepine antianxiety drug 116

Buspirone hydrochloride a generic antianxiety drug 116

Busulphan a generic anticancer drug 115

Butacote a brand name for phenylbutazone 799

Butobarbitone a generic barbiturate drug 156, a type of sleeping drug 922

C

Cafadol a brand-name preparation containing paracetamol 778 and caffeine 221

Cafergot a brand-name preparation containing a mixture of ergotamine 414 and caffeine 221, used to treat migraine 687

Caffeine 221, a generic stimulant drug 947

Calabren a brand name for glibenclamide 484

Caladryl a brand-name preparation containing diphenhydramine 360 and calamine 223

Calamine 223, a generic preparation used to soothe skin irritation 919

Calcichew a brand-name chewable preparation containing calcium 224

Calcichew D3 a brand-name chewable preparation containing calcium 224 and vitamin D 1065

Calcidrink a brand-name preparation containing calcium 224

Calciferol 223, another name for vitamin D 1065

Calcilat a brand name for nifedipine 730

Calcimax a brand-name multivitamin 702

Calciparine a brand-name drug containing heparin 527

Calcipotriol a vitamin D derivative for topical application in psoriasis 837

Calcisorb a brand name for sodium cellulose phosphate, used to treat hypercalcaemia 135

Calcitare a brand name for calcitonin 223

Calcitonin 223, a generic drug used to treat bone disorders 193

Calcitriol a derivative of vitamin D 1065

Calcium 224, an essential mineral

Calcium-500 a brand-name preparation containing calcium 224

Calcium and Ergocalciferol tablets a preparation containing calcium 224 and vitamin D 1065

Calcium carbonate a generic antacid drug 111

Calcium chloride a form of calcium 224

Calcium Folinate tablets a preparation containing folinic acid, used to counteract complications following treatment with methotrexate 684

Calcium gluconate a form of calcium 224

Calcium Lactate tablets a generic calcium 224 supplement

Calcium Leucovorin a preparation containing folinic acid, used to counteract complications following treatment with methotrexate 684

Calcium Resonium a brand name for poly-styrene sulphonate resins, used to remove excess potassium from the blood 820

Calcium-Sandoz a brand-name preparation containing calcium 224

Calgel a brand-name preparation containing lignocaine 637

Calimal a brand name for chlorpheniramine 269

Calmurid HC a brand-name preparation containing hydro-cortisone 546

Calpol a brand name for paracetamol 778

Calsynar a brand name for salcatonin, a synthetic form of calcitonin 223

CAM a brand-name bronchodilator drug 215

Camcolit 250 a brand name for lithium 640

Camphor a generic drug used to relieve skin irritation 919

Canesten a brand name for clotrimazole 283

Canesten HC a brand-name preparation containing clotrimazole 283 and hydrocortisone 546

Cannabis 230, a central nervous system depressant 246

Cantil a brand-name antispasmodic drug 120 containing mepenzolate, used to treat irritable bowel syndrome 603

Capasal a brand-name preparation used to treat dandruff 331

Capastat a brand name for capreomycin, an antibacterial drug 114 used in the treatment of tuberculosis 1019

Capitol a brand-name preparation used to treat dandruff 331

Caplenal a brand name for allopurinol 87

Capoten a brand name for captopril 231

Capozide a brand-name preparation containing captopril 231 and hydrochlorothiazide 546

Capreomycin a generic antibacterial drug 114 used in the treatment of tuberculosis 1019

Caprin a brand name for aspirin 137

Captopril 231, a generic ACE inhibitor drug 61

Carace a brand name for lisinopril, an ACE inhibitor drug 61

Carace Plus a brand-name preparation containing lisinopril, an ACE inhibitor drug 61, and hydrochlorothiazide 546

Carbachol a generic drug used to treat glaucoma 483

Carbamazepine 231, a generic anticonvulsant drug 116

Carbaryl a generic drug used to treat lice 635

Carbellon a brand-name preparation used to treat flatulence 452

Carbenicillin a generic penicillin drug 788, a type of antibiotic drug 114

Carbenoxolone 231, a generic ulcer-healing drug 1024

Carbidopa a generic drug used in combination with levodopa 635 in the treatment of Parkinson's disease 781

Carbimazole 232, a generic drug used to treat thyrotoxicosis 993

Carbocisteine a generic mucolytic drug 701

Carbo-Cort a brand-name preparation containing coal tar 283 and hydrocortisone 546

Carbo-Dome a brand name for coal tar 283

Carbomix a brand name for activated charcoal 256

Carboplatin a generic anticancer drug 115 related to cisplatin 281

Carboprost a generic drug used in the treatment of blood loss after delivery, see Childbirth, complications of 264

Cardene a brand-name calcium channel blocker 224

Cardura a brand name for doxazosin, an antihyper-tensive drug 118

Carisoma a brand name for carisoprodol, a muscle-relaxant drug 707

Carisoprodol a generic muscle-relaxant drug 707

Carmustine a generic anticancer drug 115

Carteolol a generic beta-blocker drug 164 used to treat glaucoma 483

Carylderm a brand-name preparation containing carbaryl, used to treat pediculosis 785

Cascara a generic stimulant laxative drug 629

Castor oil 239, a generic stimulant laxative drug 629

Catapres a brand-name antihypertensive drug 118 containing clonidine 283

Caved-S a brand-name combined ulcer-healing drug 1024

CCNU a brand name for lomustine, an anticancer drug 115

Cedocard a brand name for isosorbide dinitrate, a form of isosorbide 604, a vasodilator drug 1047

Cefaclor a generic cephalosporin 247, a type of antibiotic drug 114

Cefadroxil a generic cephalosporin 247, a type of antibiotic drug 114

Cefixime a generic cephalosporin 247, a type of antibiotic drug 114

Cefizox a brand name for ceftizoxime, a cephalosporin 247, a type of antibiotic drug 114

Cefodizime a generic cephalosporin 247, a type of antibiotic drug 114

Cefotaxime a generic cephalosporin 247, a type of antibiotic drug 114

Cefoxitin a generic cephalosporin 247, a type of antibiotic drug 114

Cefpodoxime a generic cephalosporin 247, a type of antibiotic drug 114

Cefsulodin a generic cephalosporin drug 247

Ceftazidime a generic cephalosporin 247, a type of antibiotic drug 114

Ceftizoxime a generic cephalosporin 247, a type of antibiotic drug 114

Ceftriaxone a generic cephalosporin 247, a type of antibiotic drug 114

Cefuroxime a generic cephalosporin 247, a type of antibiotic drug 114

Celance a brand name for pergolide, used in the treatment of Parkinson's disease 781

Celectol a brand name for celiprolol, a beta-blocker drug 164

Celevac a brand name for methylcellulose 684

Celiprolol a generic beta-blocker drug 164

Centyl K a brand-name preparation containing bendrofluazide 63 and potassium 820

Cephalexin a generic cephalosporin 247, a type of antibiotic drug 114

Cephamandol a generic cephalosporin 247, a type of antibiotic drug 114

Cephazolin a generic cephalosporin drug 247

Cephradine a generic cephalosporin 247, a type of antibiotic drug 114

Ceporex a brand name for cephalexin 246

Cerebrovase a brand name for dipyramidol 360

Cervagem a brand name for gemeprost, a prostaglandin drug 832 used to ripen and soften the cervix before induction of abortion 57

Cesamet a brand name for nabilone, an antiemetic drug 117

Cetirizine a generic antihistamine drug 118

Cetrimide a type of antiseptic 119

Charcoal 256, used in the emergency treatment of some types of poisoning

Chemotrim a brand name for co-trimoxazole 313

Chendol a brand name for chenodeoxycholic acid 256

Chenodeoxycholic acid 256, a naturally occurring chemical used to dissolve gallstones 468

Chenofalk a brand name for chenodeoxycholic acid 256

Chloractil a brand name for chlorpromazine 269

Chloral hydrate 268, a generic sleeping drug 922

Chlorambucil 268, a generic anticancer drug 115

Chloramphenicol 268, a generic antibiotic drug 114

Chlordiazepoxide 268, a generic antianxiety drug 114

Chlorhexidine 268, a type of antiseptic 119

Chlormethiazole a generic sleeping drug 922

Chlormezanone a generic antianxiety drug 114

Chloromycetin a brand name for chloramphenicol 268

Chloroquine 269, a generic drug used to treat malaria 657

Chlorothiazide a generic thiazide diuretic drug 364

Chlorpheniramine 269, a generic antihistamine drug 118

Chlorpromazine 269, a generic antipsychotic drug 119

Chlorpropamide 269, a generic drug used to treat diabetes mellitus 348

Chlortetracycline a generic tetracycline drug 981, a type of antibiotic drug 114

Chlorthalidone a generic diuretic drug 364

Cholecalciferol 270, another name for vitamin D 1065

Choledyl a brand-name preparation containing choline theophyllinate, a bronchodilator drug 215

Cholestyramine 273, a generic lipid-lowering drug 639

Choline salicylate a generic analgesic drug 102 used in some mouth gels

Choline theophyllinate a generic bronchodilator drug 215

Chromium 275, an essential mineral

Chymotrypsin an enzyme used to relieve soft-tissue inflammation 928

Cicatrin a brand-name anti-infective skin preparation 915

Cidomycin a brand name for gentamicin 480

Cilastatin used together with imipenem, an antibiotic drug 114, to delay the metabolism of imipenem by the kidneys

Cilazapril a generic ACE inhibitor drug 61

Cilest a brand-name oral contraceptive 755 containing ethinyl-oestradiol 416 and norgestimate, a progestogen drug 830

Cimetidine 278, a generic ulcer-healing drug 830

Cinazière a brand name for cinnarizine 278

Cinnarizine 278, a generic antihistamine drug 118

Cinobac a brand-name drug used to treat urinary tract infections 1032

Cinoxacin a generic antibacterial drug 114

Ciprofibrate a generic lipid-lowering drug 639

Ciprofloxacin a generic antibacterial drug 114

Ciproxin a brand-name anti-bacterial preparation 114 containing ciprofloxacin

Cisapride 281, a generic drug that stimulates gastric motility

Cisplatin 281, a generic anticancer drug 115

Citanest a brand name for prilocaine, a local anaesthetic 101

Citramag a brand-name preparation containing magnesium citrate, used to empty the bowel before radiological examination and surgery

Citrical a brand-name preparation containing calcium 224

Claforan a brand-name preparation containing cefotaxime, a cephalosporin drug 247

Claradin a brand name for effervescent aspirin 137

Clarithromycin a generic antibiotic drug 114 related to erythromycin 416

Clarityn a brand-name preparation containing loratadine, an anti-histamine drug 118

Clavulanic acid a generic drug used to enhance the effect of some penicillin drugs 788

Clemastine a generic antihistamine drug 118

Climagest a brand-name preparation containing oestradiol 749 and norethisterone 734

Climaval a brand name for oestradiol 749

Clindamycin 282, a generic antibiotic drug 114

Clinicide a brand name for carbaryl, used to treat lice 635

Clinitar a brand name for coal tar 283

Clinoril a brand name for sulindac 959

Clioquinol a generic antibacterial 114 and antifungal drug 117

Clobazam a generic benzodiazepine 163 anti-anxiety drug 114

Clobetasol a generic corticosteroid drug 312

Clobetasone a generic corticosteroid drug 312

Clofazimine a generic drug used to treat leprosy 632

Clofibrate 282, a generic lipid-lowering drug 639

Clomid a brand name for clomiphene 282

Clomiphene 282, a generic drug used to treat female infertility 581

Clomipramine 282, a generic antidepressant drug 116

Clonazepam 282, a generic anticonvulsant drug 116

Clonidine 283, a generic antihypertensive drug 118

Clopamide a generic thiazide diuretic drug 364

Clopixol/Clopixol Acuphase brand names for zuclopenthixol, an antipsychotic drug 119

Clorazepate a generic antianxiety drug 114

Clotrimazole 283, a generic antifungal drug 117

Cloxacillin 283, a generic penicillin drug 788, a type of antibiotic drug 114

Clozapine a generic antipsychotic drug 119

Clozaril a brand name for clozapine, an antipsychotic drug 119

Coal tar 283, an ingredient in preparations used to treat psoriasis 837, eczema 389, and dandruff 331

Co-amilofruse a preparation containing the generic drugs amiloride 92 and frusemide 464

Co-amilozide a preparation containing the generic drugs amiloride 92 and hydrochlorothiazide 546

Co-amoxiclav a preparation containing the generic drugs amoxycillin 94 and clavulanic acid, a drug used to enhance the effect of amoxycillin 94 and some other penicillin drugs 788

Cobadex a brand-name hydrocortisone 546 cream

Cobalin-H a brand name for hydroxocobalamin 546

Co-Betaloc a brand-name preparation containing hydrochlorothiazide 546 and metoprolol 684

Cocaine 284, a generic central nervous system stimulant 947

Co-careldopa a preparation containing the generic drugs carbidopa and levodopa 635

Co-codamol a preparation containing the generic drugs codeine 285 and paracetamol 778

Co-codaprin a preparation containing the generic drugs aspirin 137 and codeine 285

Cocois a brand-name ointment containing coal tar 283, salicylic acid 885, and sulphur 959

Codafen Continus a brand-name preparation containing ibuprofen 562 and codeine 285

Codalax a brand name for co-danthramer, a stimulant laxative drug preparation 629

Codalax Forte a brand name for co-danthramer, a stimulant laxative drug preparation 629

Coda-Med a brand-name preparation containing paracetamol 778 and codeine 285

Codanin a brand-name preparation containing paracetamol 778 and codeine 285

Co-danthramer a stimulant laxative drug preparation 629 containing the generic drugs danthron and poloxamer "188"

Co-danthrusate a stimulant laxative drug preparation 629 containing the generic drugs danthron and docusate

Codeine 285, a generic narcotic drug 717, a type of analgesic drug 102

Co-dergocrine a preparation containing a mixture of certain vasodilator drugs 1047

Codis 500 a brand-name analgesic preparation containing aspirin 137 and codeine 285

Co-dydramol a preparation containing the generic drugs paracetamol 778 and dihydrocodeine, a narcotic analgesic drug 102

Co-fluampicil a preparation containing the generic drugs flucloxacillin 453 and ampicillin 94

Cogentin a brand name for benztropine, a drug used to treat Parkinson's disease 781

Cojene a brand-name analgesic preparation containing aspirin 137 and codeine 285

Colchicine 286, a generic drug used to treat gout 490

Colestid a brand-name lipid-lowering drug 639

Colestipol a generic lipid-lowering drug 639

Colifoam a brand-name preparation containing hydrocortisone 546

Colistin 287, a generic polymyxin 816, a type of antibiotic drug 114

Collodion a substance used in certain skin preparations 915

Colofac a brand name for mebeverine, an antispasmodic drug 120

Colomycin a brand name for colistin 287

Colpermin a brand name for peppermint oil 789, used in the treatment of irritable bowel syndrome and diverticular disease

Colven a brand-name antispasmodic drug 120

Co-magaldrox an antacid preparation containing the generic drugs aluminium hydroxide 89 and magnesium hydroxide 111

Combantrin a brand name for pyrantel 848

Combidol a brand name for chenodeoxycholic acid 256

Comixo a brand name for co-trimoxazole 313

Comox a brand name for co-trimoxazole 313

Complement Continus a brand name for pyridoxine 848

Concavit a brand-name multivitamin preparation 702

Concordin a brand name for protriptyline 836

Condyline a brand name for podophyllotoxin 813

Conjugated oestrogens a combination of female sex hormones 903 used to treat symptoms of the menopause 676

Conotrane a brand-name barrier cream 159

Conova 30 a brand-name oral contraceptive 755

Contac-400 a brand-name preparation containing phenylpropranolamine 800 and chlorpheniramine 269

Convulex a brand name for sodium valproate 928

Copholco a brand-name cough remedy 314, containing pholcodine and menthol 680

Copper 306 an essential element

Co-prenozide a preparation containing the generic drugs oxprenolol 770 and cyclopenthiazide 326

Co-proxamol 306, an analgesic drug preparation 102 containing the generic

drugs dextropropoxyphene 348 and paracetamol 778

Coracten a brand name for nifedipine 730

Cordarone X a brand name for amiodarone 92

Cordilox a brand name for verapamil 1053

Corgard a brand name for nadolol 716

Corgaretic a brand-name preparation containing bendrofluazide 163 and nadolol 716

Corlan a brand name for hydrocortisone 546

Coro-Nitro a brand name for glyceryl trinitrate 488

Corsodyl a brand name for chlorhexidine 268

Cortelan a brand-name corticosteroid drug 312

Corticotrophin 312, another name for ACTH 64

Cortisol 312, another name for hydrocortisone 546

Cortisone 312, a generic corticosteroid drug 312

Cortistab a brand name for cortisone 312

Cortisyl a brand name for cortisone 312

Corwin a brand name for xamoterol, a drug used in the treatment of mild heart failure 519

Cosalgesic a brand-name analgesic preparation containing dextropropoxyphene 348 and paracetamol 778

Cosmegen Lyovac a brand name for dactinomycin, an anticancer drug 115

Cosuric a brand name for allopurinol 87

Co-tenidone a preparation containing the generic drugs atenolol 140 and chlorthalidone, a thiazide diuretic drug 364

Co-trimoxazole 313, an antibacterial drug preparation 114 containing the generic drugs sulphamethoxazole 959 and trimethoprim 1016

Coversyl a brand name for perindopril, an ACE inhibitor drug 61

Covonia a brand-name cough remedy containing dextromethorphan 348, guaiphenesin 314 and menthol 680

Covonia for Children a brand-name cough remedy containing dextromethorphan 348 and menthol 680

Cremaffin a brand-name preparation containing liquid paraffin 639 and magnesium hydroxide 111

Creon a brand name for pancreatin 775

Crisantaspase a generic anticancer drug 115

Cromogen a brand name for sodium cromoglycate 927

Crotamiton a generic drug used to relieve pruritus 836 including pruritus after scabies 888

Crystal violet another name for Gentian violet 480

Crystapen a brand name for benzylpenicillin, a penicillin drug 788

Cullen, Mrs a brand-name analgesic preparation containing aspirin 137

Cupanol a brand name for paracetamol 778

Cuplex a brand-name combined preparation containing salicylic acid 885 used to remove warts 1074

Cuprofen a brand name for ibuprofen 562

Cyanocobalamin another name for vitamin B_{12} 1063

Cyclandelate a generic vasodilator drug 1047

Cyclimorph a brand-name analgesic preparation containing morphine 695, and cyclizine, an antiemetic drug 117

Cyclizine a generic anti-emetic drug 117

Cyclofenil a generic drug used to treat infertility 581

Cyclogest a brand-name progesterone 830 vaginal pessary

Cyclopenthiazide 326, a generic thiazide diuretic drug 364

Cyclopentolate a generic drug used in eye-drops to produce cycloplegia 326

Cyclophosphamide 326, a generic anticancer drug 115

Cyclo-Progynova a brand-name preparation containing oestradiol

749 and norgestrel, a progestogen drug 830

Cycloserine a generic drug used to treat tuberculosis 1019

Cyclosporin 326, a generic immunosuppressant drug 572

Cyklokapron a brand-name drug used to promote blood clotting 183

Cymalon a brand name for sodium citrate, a drug used to relieve discomfort in urinary tract infection 1032

Cymevene a brand name for ganciclovir, an antiviral drug 120

Cyproheptadine a generic antihistamine drug 118 also used as an appetite stimulant drug 127

Cyprostat a brand name for cyproterone acetate 326

Cyproterone acetate 326, a generic synthetic sex hormone 903

Cystemme a brand name for sodium citrate, a drug used to relieve discomfort in urinary tract infection 1032

Cystoleve a brand name for sodium citrate, a drug used to relieve discomfort in urinary tract infection 1032

Cystopurin a brand name for potassium citrate, a drug used to relieve discomfort in urinary tract infection 1032

Cystrin a brand name for oxybutynin, used to treat frequent urination 1032

Cytacon a brand name for vitamin B_{12} 1063

Cytamen a brand name for cyanocobalamin 325

Cytarabine a generic anticancer drug 115

Cytosar a brand name for cytarabine, an anticancer drug 115

Cytotec a brand name for misoprostol 691

D

Dacarbazine a generic anticancer drug 115

Dactinomycin a generic anticancer drug 115

Daktacort a brand-name preparation containing hydrocortisone 546 and miconazole 685

Daktarin a brand name for miconazole 685

Dalacin C a brand name for clindamycin 282

Dalivit a brand-name multivitamin preparation 702

Dalmane a brand name for flurazepam 454

Dalteparin a generic anticoagulant drug 116

Danazol 331, a generic drug used to treat endometriosis 402

Daneral-SA a brand name for pheniramine, an antihistamine drug 118

Danol a brand name for danazol 331

Danol-1/2 a brand name for danazol 331

Danthron a generic stimulant laxative drug 629

Dantrium a brand name for dantrolene 332

Dantrolene 332, a generic muscle-relaxant drug 707

Daonil a brand name for glibenclamide 484

Dapsone 332, a generic drug used to treat leprosy 632

Daranide a brand-name drug used to treat glaucoma 483

Daraprim a brand name for pyrimethamine 848

Davenol a brand-name cough remedy 314 containing carbinoxamine, an antihistamine drug 118, ephedrine 408, and pholcodine 1119

Day Nurse a brand-name cold remedy containing dextromethorphan 348, paracetamol 778, and phenylpropanolamine 800

DDAVP a brand name for desmopressin, a drug used to treat diabetes insipidus 348

Debrisoquine a generic antihypertensive drug 118

Decadron a brand name for dexamethasone 347

Decadron Shock-Pak a brand name for dexamethasone 347

Deca-Durabolin-100 a brand name for nandrolone 717

Decazate a brand name for fluphenazine, an antipsychotic drug 119

Declinax a brand name for debrisoquine, an antihypertensive drug 118

Decortisyl a brand name for prednisone 821

Delax a brand-name laxative preparation 629 containing liquid paraffin 639 and phenolphthalein 1119

Delfen a brand-name spermicide 932

Deltacortril Enteric a brand name for prednisolone 821

Deltastab a brand name for prednisolone 821

Demeclocycline a generic antibiotic drug 114

Demix a brand name for doxycycline 371

Demser a brand name for metirosine used in the treatment of phaeo-chromocytoma 797

De-Nol a brand name for bismuth 173

De-Noltab a brand name for bismuth 173

Depixol a brand-name preparation containing flupenthixol, an anti-psychotic 119 and antidepressant drug 116

Depo-Medrone a brand name for methyl-prednisolone 684

Deponit a brand name for glyceryl trinitrate 488

Depo-Provera a brand name for medroxy-progesterone 670

Depostat a brand-name progestogen drug 830 used to treat breast cancer 205

Dequalinium a generic antifungal drug 117 used to treat mild oral infections 577

Derbac-M a brand name for carbaryl, a drug used to treat lice 635

Dermonistat a brand name for miconazole 685

Dermovate a brand name for clobetasol, a cortico-steroid drug 321

Dermovate-NN a brand-name preparation containing clobetasol, a corticosteroid drug 312, neomycin 721, and nystatin 741

Deseril a brand name for methysergide 684

Desipramine a generic tricyclic antidepressant drug 116

Desmopressin a generic drug used to treat diabetes insipidus 348

Desmospray a brand name for desmopressin, a drug used to treat diabetes insipidus 348

Desogestrel a generic progestogen drug 830

Desonide a generic corticosteroid drug 312

Desoxymethasone a generic corticosteroid drug 312

Deteclo a brand-name tetracycline drug 981, a type of antibiotic drug 114

De Witt's Analgesic a brand name for paracetamol 778

Dexamethasone 347, a generic corticosteroid drug 312

Dexamphetamine 347, a generic central nervous system stimulant drug 947

Dexa-Rhinaspray a brand-name combined preparation used to treat infections of the nose 735

Dexedrine a brand name for dexamphetamine 347

Dexfenfluramine a generic appetite suppressant drug 127

Dextromethorphan 348, a generic cough remedy 314

Dextromoramide 348, a generic narcotic drug 717, a type of analgesic drug 102

Dextropropoxyphene 348, a generic analgesic drug 102

Dextrose 348, a type of sugar

DHC Continus a brand name for dihydrocodeine, a narcotic drug 717

Diabetamide a brand name for glibenclamide 484

Diabinese a brand name for chlorpropamide 269, an oral hypoglycaemic drug 556

Dialar a brand name for diazepam 356

Diamicron a brand name for gliclazide, a hypoglycaemic drug 556

Diamorphine 353, another name for heroin

Diamox a brand name for acetazolamide 61

Dianette a brand-name preparation containing cyproterone acetate 326 and ethinyloestradiol 416

Diaphine a brand name for diamorphine, a narcotic analgesic drug 102

Diarphen a brand-name preparation containing diphenoxylate 360 and atropine 143

Diarrest a brand name for dicyclomine, a generic antispasmodic drug 120 used to treat irritable bowel syndrome 603

Diazemuls a brand name for diazepam 356

Diazepam 356, a generic benzodiazepine 163 antianxiety drug 114

Diazoxide a generic antihypertensive drug 118

Dibenyline a brand name for phenoxybenzamine, an antihypertensive drug 118

Dichlorphenamide a generic drug for the treatment of glaucoma 483

Diclofenac 356, a generic nonsteroidal anti-inflammatory drug 734

Diclomax a brand name for diclofenac 356

Diclozip a brand name for diclofenac 356

Diconal a brand-name analgesic preparation containing dipipanone, a narcotic analgesic drug 102, and cyclizine, an antiemetic drug 117

Dicyclomine a generic antispasmodic drug 120 used to treat irritable bowel syndrome 603

Dicynene a brand name for ethamsylate, a drug used to promote blood clotting 183

Didronel a brand-name preparation containing etidronate, used in the treatment of Paget's disease 772

Dienoestrol a generic oestrogen drug 749 used to treat menopausal vaginitis 1042

Diethylcarbamazine a generic anthelmintic drug 113

Diethylpropion a generic appetite suppressant drug 127

Difflam a brand-name preparation used to relieve soft-tissue inflammation 928

Diflucan a brand name for fluconazole, an antifungal drug 117

Diflucortolone a generic corticosteroid drug 312

Diflunisal 357, a generic nonsteroidal anti-inflammatory drug 734

Digitoxin 359, a generic digitalis drug 359

Digoxin 359, a generic digitalis drug 359

Dihydrocodeine a generic narcotic drug 717, a type of analgesic drug 102

Dihydroergotamine a generic drug used to treat migraine 687

Dihydrotachysterol another name for vitamin D 1065

Dihydroxycholecalciferol another name for vitamin D 1065

Dijex a brand-name antacid preparation 111

Diloxanide furoate a generic drug used to treat amoebiasis 93

Diltiazem 359, a generic calcium channel blocker 224

Dilzem a brand name for diltiazem 359

Dimenhydrinate a generic antihistamine drug 118

Dimercaprol a generic drug used to treat metal poisoning 813

Dimethicone a silicone-based substance used in barrier creams 159 and in antacids 111

Dimethindene a generic antihistamine drug 118

Dimetriose a brand name for gestrinone, a drug used to treat endometriosis 402

Dimotane a brand name for brompheniramine, an antihistamine drug 118

Dimotapp a brand-name nasal decongestant preparation containing brompheniramine, an antihistamine drug 118, phenylephrine 800, and phenylpropranolamine 800

Dimyril a brand-name cough remedy 314

Dindevan a brand name for phenindione, an anticoagulant drug 116

Dinoprost a generic prostaglandin drug 832 used to stimulate uterine contractions in childbirth 261 and induced abortion 57

Dinoprostone a generic prostaglandin drug 832 used to stimulate uterine contractions in childbirth 261 and induced abortion 57

Diocalm Junior a brand-name preparation used in rehydration therapy 866

Dioctyl a brand-name stimulant laxative drug 629

Dioderm a brand name for hydrocortisone 546

Dioralyte a brand-name preparation used in rehydration therapy 866

Diovol a brand-name antacid preparation 111

Dipentum a brand name for olsalazine 751

Diphenhydramine 360, a generic antihistamine drug 118

Diphenoxylate 360, a generic antidiarrhoeal drug 116

Diphenylpyraline a generic antihistamine drug 118

Dipipanone a generic narcotic drug 717, a type of analgesic drug 102

Dipivefrine a generic drug that is converted to adrenaline 70 and has similar actions to that hormone

Diprivan a brand name for propofol, a drug used in general anaesthesia 99

Diprosalic a brand-name combination preparation containing betamethasone 165 and salicylic acid 885

Diprosone a brand name for betamethasone 165

Dipyridamole 360, a generic drug used to treat abnormal blood clotting 183

Dirythmin SA a brand name for disopyramide 364

Disalcid a brand name for salsalate, a nonsteroidal anti-inflammatory drug 734

Disipal a brand name for orphenadrine 759

Disodium etidronate a generic drug used to treat Paget's disease 772

Disodium pamidronate a generic biphosphonate drug 171 used in the treatment of hyper-calcaemia 548 due to cancer

Disopyramide 364, a generic antiarrhythmic drug 114

Disprin a brand name for aspirin 137

Disprol a brand name for paracetamol 778

Distaclor a brand name for cefaclor 244

Distalgesic a brand name for co-proxamol 306

Distamine a brand name for penicillamine 788

Distaquaine V-K a brand-name penicillin drug 788, a type of antibiotic drug 114

Distigmine a generic drug used to treat urinary retention 1031 and myasthenia gravis 710

Disulfiram 364, a generic drug used to treat alcohol dependence 82

Dithranol 364, a generic drug used to treat psoriasis 837

Dithrocream a brand name for dithranol 364

Dithrolan a brand-name preparation containing dithranol 364 and salicylic acid 885

Ditropan a brand name for oxybutynin used to treat frequent urination 1032

Diumide K a brand-name preparation containing frusemide 464 and potassium 820

Diurexan a brand name for xipamide 1089

Dixarit a brand name for clonidine 283

Dobutamine a generic drug used to treat heart failure 519 and shock 907

Docusate a generic laxative drug 629

Do-Do a brand-name preparation containing guaiphenesin, a cough remedy 314

Dolmatil a brand name for sulpiride 959

Dolobid a brand name for diflunisal 357

Doloxene a brand name for dextropropoxyphene 348, a narcotic analgesic drug 102

Doloxene Compound a brand-name analgesic preparation containing dextropropoxyphene 348, aspirin 137, and caffeine 221

Domical a brand name for amitriptyline 92

Domperidone 368, a generic antiemetic drug 117

Dopacard a brand name for dopexamine, a drug used to treat heart failure 519

Dopamet a brand name for methyldopa 684

Dopamine 369, a natural neurotransmitter used to treat heart failure 519 and shock 907

Dopexamine a generic drug used to treat heart failure 519

Dopram a brand name for doxapram, a respiratory stimulant drug 947

Doralese a brand name for indoramin, an anti-hypertensive drug 118

Dormonoct a brand name for loprazolam, a benzodiazepine drug 163

Dothapax a brand name for dothiepin 370

Dothiepin 370, a generic antidepressant drug 116

Dovonex a brand name for calcipotriol, a vitamin D derivative for topical application in psoriasis 837

Doxapram a generic respiratory stimulant drug 947

Doxazosin a generic antihypertensive drug 118

Doxepin a generic tricyclic antidepressant drug 116

Doxorubicin 371, a generic anticancer drug 116

Doxycycline 371, a generic tetracycline drug 981, a type of antibiotic drug 114

Doxylamine a generic antihistamine 118 sleeping drug 922

Doxylar a brand name for doxycycline 371

Dozic a brand name for haloperidol 505

Dramamine a brand name for dimenhydrinate, an antihistamine drug 118

Drapolene a brand name antiseptic 119 skin cream containing benzalkonium chloride 1099

Driclor a brand-name preparation containing aluminium chloride 89

Dristan a brand-name analgesic preparation containing aspirin 137, chlorpheniramine 269, and phenylephrine 800

Drogenil a brand name for flutamide, used in the treatment of cancer of the prostate 832

Droleptan a brand name for droperidol, an antipsychotic 119 and antiemetic drug 117

Droperidol a generic antipsychotic 119 and antiemetic drug 117

Dryptal a brand name for frusemide 464

DTIC-Dome a brand name for dacarbazine, an anticancer drug 115

Dulcolax a brand name for bisacodyl, a stimulant laxative drug 629

Duofilm a brand-name preparation used to treat warts 1074

Duovent a brand-name preparation containing two bronchodilator drugs 215, fenoterol and ipratropium bromide

Duphalac a brand name for lactulose 623

Duphaston a brand name for dydrogesterone 379

Durabolin a brand name for nandrolone 717

Duracreme a brand-name spermicide 932

Duragel a brand-name spermicide 932

Duromine a brand name for phentermine, an appetite suppressant drug 127

Dyazide a brand-name preparation 364 containing hydrochlorothiazide 546 and triamterene 1014

Dydrogesterone 379, a generic progestogen drug 830

Dynese a brand-name antacid preparation 111

Dysman a brand name for mefenamic acid 671

Dyspamet a brand name for cimetidine 278

Dytac a brand name for triamterene 1014

Dytide a brand-name diuretic preparation containing triamterene 1014 and benzthiazide, a thiazide diuretic drug 364

E

Ebufac a brand name for ibuprofen 562

Econacort a brand-name preparation containing hydrocortisone 546 and econazole 388

Econazole 388, a generic antifungal drug 117

Ecostatin a brand name for econazole 388

Ecothiopate a generic drug used to treat glaucoma 483

Eczederm a brand-name emollient preparation 397

Edecrin a brand name for ethacrynic acid, a loop diuretic drug 364

Edrophonium chloride a generic drug used in the diagnosis of myasthenia gravis 710

Efamast a brand name for gamolenic acid, used for symptomatic relief of tenderness of the breast 208

Efcortelan, Efcortesol brand names for hydro-cortisone 546

Effercitrate a brand name for potassium citrate, a drug used to relieve discomfort in urinary tract infection 1032

Efudix a brand name for fluorouracil 454

Elantan LA a brand name for isosorbide mononitrate, a form of isosorbide 604

Elavil a brand name for amitriptyline 92

Eldepryl a brand name for selegiline, a drug used to treat Parkinson's disease 781

Eldisine a brand name for vindesine, an anticancer drug 115

Electrolade a brand-name preparation used in rehydration therapy 866

Elkamol a brand name for paracetamol 778

Elocon a brand name for mometasone, a corticosteroid drug 312

Eltroxin a brand name for thyroxine 993

Eludril a brand-name preparation containing amethocaine, a local anaesthetic 101, and chlorhexidine 268

Emblon a brand name for tamoxifen 968

Emcor a brand name for bisoprolol, a beta-blocker drug 164

Emeside a brand name for ethosuximide 417

Emflex a brand name for acemetacin 61

Eminase a brand name for anistreplase, a thrombolytic drug 987

Emla a brand-name preparation containing lignocaine 637 and prilocaine, a local anaesthetic 101

Enalapril 398, a generic ACE inhibitor drug 61

En-De-Kay a brand name for fluoride 453

Endoxana a brand name for cyclophosphamide 326

Enduron a brand name for methyclothiazide 684

Enflurane a generic drug used in general anaesthesia 99

Enoxaparin a generic anticoagulant drug 116

Enoximone a generic drug used in the treatment of heart failure 519

Entamizole a brand-name drug used to treat amoebiasis 93

EP a brand-name preparation containing paracetamol 778 and codeine 285

Epanutin a brand name for phenytoin 800

Ephedrine 408, a generic decongestant drug 335

Epifoam a brand-name preparation containing hydrocortisone 546

Epifrin a brand name for adrenaline 70

Epilim a brand name for sodium valproate 928

Epirubicin a generic anticancer drug 115

Epoetin 413, a synthetically prepared hormone used in the treatment of anaemia 95

Epogam a brand name for gamolenic acid, a drug

used in the treatment of eczema 389

Epoprostenol a generic anti-coagulant drug 116

Eppy a brand name for adrenaline 70

Eprex a brand name for epoetin 413

Equagesic a brand-name analgesic drug 102 containing aspirin 137

Equanil a brand name for meprobamate 680

Eradacin a brand name for acrosoxacin 64

Ergocalciferol another name for vitamin D 1065

Ergometrine 413, a generic drug used to control uterine bleeding after childbirth 261

Ergotamine 414, a generic drug used to treat migraine 687

Erwinase a brand name for crisantaspase, an anticancer drug 115

Erycen a brand name for erythromycin 416

Erymax a brand name for erythromycin 416

Erythrocin a brand name for erythromycin 416

Erythrolar a brand name for erythromycin 416

Erythromid a brand name for erythromycin 416

Erythromycin 416, a generic antibiotic drug 114

Erythroped a brand name for erythromycin 416

Erythropoietin 413, a hormone used in the treatment of anaemia 95

Eserine another name for physostigmine 803

Esidrex a brand name for hydrochlorothiazide 546

Eskamel a brand-name preparation containing sulphur 959

Eskazole a brand name for albendazole, a drug used to treat hydatid cysts 544

Eskornade a brand-name decongestant preparation 335 containing phenyl-propanolamine 800 and diphenylpyraline, an antihistamine drug 118

Esmolol a generic beta-blocker drug 164

Estracombi a brand-name preparation containing oestradiol 749 and norethisterone 734

Estracyt a brand name for estramustine, an anti-cancer drug 115

Estraderm TTS a brand-name preparation containing oestradiol 749

Estradurin a brand-name preparation containing polyestradiol, a long-acting oestrogen drug 749 used as an anticancer drug 115

Estragest TTS a brand-name preparation containing oestradiol 749 and norethisterone 734

Estramustine a generic anticancer drug 115

Estrapak a brand-name preparation containing oestradiol 749 and norethisterone 734

Ethacrynic acid a generic loop diuretic drug 364

Ethambutol 416, a generic drug used to treat tuberculosis 1019

Ethamsylate a generic drug used to promote blood clotting 183

Ethinyloestradiol 416, a generic oestrogen drug 749

Ethionamide a generic drug used to treat tuberculosis 1019 and leprosy 632

Ethoheptazine a generic narcotic drug 717, a type of analgesic drug 102

Ethosuximide 416, a generic anticonvulsant drug 116

Ethynodiol diacetate a generic progestogen drug 830

Etidronate disodium see disodium etidronate

Etodolac a generic nonsteroidal anti-inflammatory drug 734

Etomidate a generic drug used in general anaesthesia 99

Etoposide a generic anticancer drug 115

Etretinate 417, a generic drug used to treat psoriasis 837

Eudemine a brand name for diazoxide, an anti-hypertensive drug 118

Euglucon a brand-name hypoglycaemic drug 556

Eugynon-30 a brand-name oral contraceptive 755 containing ethinyl-oestradiol 416 and levonorgestrel 635

Eumovate a brand-name corticosteroid preparation 312 containing clobetasone

Eumovate-N a brand-name preparation containing clobetasone 312 and neomycin 721

Eurax a brand-name preparation containing crotamiton, a drug used to relieve pruritus 836 including pruritus after scabies 888

Eurax-Hydrocortisone a brand-name preparation containing hydrocortisone 546 and crotamiton, a drug used to relieve pruritus 836

Evaphol a brand name for pholcodine, a cough remedy 314

Evorel a brand-name preparation containing oestradiol 749

Exelderm a brand name for sulconazole, an antifungal drug 117

Exirel a brand name for pirbuterol, a broncho-dilator drug 215

Ex-lax a brand name for phenolphthalein, a stimulant laxative drug 629

Exocin a brand name for ofloxacin, an antibiotic drug 114

Exolan a brand name for dithranol 364

Expelix a brand name for piperazine 804

Expulin a brand-name cough remedy containing chlorpheniramine 269, menthol 680, pholcodine, 1119, and pseudo-ephedrine 836

Expurhin Paediatric a brand-name preparation containing chlorphen-iramine 269, ephedrine 408, and menthol 680

Eye-Crom brand-name eye-drops containing sodium cromoglycate 927

F

Fabahistin a brand name for mebhydrolin, an antihistamine drug 118

Fabrol a brand name for acetylcysteine 61

Famel a brand name for pholcodine, a cough remedy 314

Fam-lax a brand-name preparation containing phenolphthalein, a laxative drug 629

Famotidine 435, a generic ulcer-healing drug 1024

Fanalgic a brand name for paracetamol 778

Fansidar a brand name for pyrimethamine 848, an antibacterial drug 114

Farlutal a brand name for medroxyprogesterone 670

Fasigyn a brand-name antibacterial drug 114

Faverin a brand name for fluvoxamine, an antidepressant drug 116

Fectrim a brand name for co-trimoxazole 313

Fefol a brand-name preparation containing folic acid 454 and iron 602

Fefol-Vit a brand-name preparation containing iron 602 and vitamin B complex including folic acid 1063

Fefol-Z a brand-name preparation containing iron 602, folic acid 454, and zinc 1093

Felbinac a generic non-steroidal anti-inflammatory drug 734

Feldene a brand name for piroxicam 804

Felodipine a generic calcium channel blocker 224

Femeron a brand name for miconazole 685

Femigraine a brand-name analgesic preparation containing aspirin 137 and cyclizine, an antiemetic drug 117

Feminax a brand-name preparation containing paracetamol 778, codeine 285, and hyoscine 547

Femodene, Femodene ED brand-name oral contraceptives 755 containing ethinyloestradiol 416 and gestodene, a progestogen drug 830

Femulen a brand-name oral contraceptive containing ethynodiol diacetate, a progestogen drug 830

Fenbid a brand name for ibuprofen 562

Fenbufen 439, a generic nonsteroidal anti-inflammatory drug 734

Fenbuzip a brand name for fenbufen 439

Fenfluramine a generic appetite suppressant drug 127

Fennings Children's Cooling Powders a brand name for paracetamol 778

Fenofibrate a generic lipid-lowering drug 639

Fenoprofen 439, a generic nonsteroidal anti-inflammatory drug 734

Fenopron a brand name for fenoprofen 439

Fenostil Retard a brand name for dimethindene, an antihistamine drug 118

Fenoterol a generic bronchodilator drug 215

Fenox a brand name for phenylephrine 800

Fentanyl a generic analgesic drug 102 used in general anaesthesia 99

Fentazin a brand-name antipsychotic drug 119

Feospan a brand name for iron 602

Ferfolic SV a brand-name preparation containing folic acid 454 and iron 602

Fergon a brand-name preparation containing iron 602

Ferrocap a brand name for iron 602

Ferrocap-F 350 a brand-name preparation containing folic acid 454 and iron 602

Ferrocontin Continus a brand name for iron 602

Ferrocontin Folic Continus a brand-name preparation containing iron 602 and folic acid 454

Ferrograd a brand name for iron 602

Ferrograd C a brand-name preparation containing iron 602 and vitamin C 1065

Ferrograd Folic a brand-name preparation containing folic acid 454 and iron 602

Ferromyn a brand name for iron 602

Ferrous fumarate a form of iron 602

Ferrous gluconate a form of iron 602

Ferrous glycine sulphate a form of iron 602

Ferrous succinate a form of iron 602

Ferrous sulphate a form of iron 602

Fersaday a brand name for iron 602

Fersamal a brand name for iron 602

Fertiral a brand name for gonadorelin 489

Fesovit Z a brand-name preparation containing iron 602, zinc 1093, vitamin B complex 1063, and vitamin C 1065

Filair a brand name for beclomethasone 160

Filgrastim a generic drug used to treat deficiency of white blood cells in blood disorders 185

Finasteride 449, a generic drug used in the treatment of benign prostatic enlargement 832

Flagyl a brand name for metronidazole 684

Flamazine a brand-name antibacterial drug 114

Flavoxate a generic anti-spasmodic drug 120 used for symptoms of urinary tract infections 1032

Flaxedil a brand name for gallamine trithiodide, a generic muscle-relaxant drug 707 used in general anaesthesia 99

Flecainide a generic antiarrhythmic drug 114

Flemoxin Solutab a brand name for amoxycillin 94

Fletchers' Enemette a brand-name laxative drug containing docusate 629

Flexin Continus a brand name for indomethacin 576

Flixonase a brand name for fluticasone, a cortico-steroid drug 312

Flixotide a brand name for fluticasone, a cortico-steroid drug 312

Flolan a brand name for epoprostenol, an anticoagulant drug 116

Florinef a brand name for fludrocortisone, a cortico-steroid drug 312

Floxapen a brand name for flucloxacillin 453

Flu-Amp a brand name preparation containing ampicillin 94 and flucloxacillin 453

Fluanxol a brand-name antipsychotic 119 and antidepressant drug 116

Fluclomix a brand name for flucloxacillin 453

Fluclorolone a generic corticosteroid drug 312

Flucloxacillin 453, a generic penicillin drug 788, a type of antibiotic drug 114

Fluconazole a generic antifungal drug 117

Flucytosine a generic antifungal drug 117

Fludrocortisone a generic corticosteroid drug 312

Flumazenil a generic drug used to reverse the sedative effects of benzodiazepine drugs 163

Flumethasone a generic corticosteroid drug 312

Flunisolide a generic corticosteroid drug 312

Flunitrazepam a generic benzodiazepine 163 sleeping drug 922

Fluocinolone a generic corticosteroid drug 312

Fluocortolone a generic corticosteroid drug 312

Fluor-a-day a brand name for fluoride 453

Fluoride 453, a mineral used to help prevent dental caries 236

Fluorigard a brand name for fluoride 453

Fluorometholone a generic corticosteroid drug 312

Fluorouracil 454, a generic anticancer drug 115

Fluothane a brand name for halothane 505

Fluoxetine a generic antidepressant drug 116

Flupenthixol a generic antipsychotic 119 and antidepressant drug 116

Fluphenazine a generic antipsychotic drug 119

Flurandrenolone a generic corticosteroid drug 312

Flurazepam 454, a generic benzodiazepine 163 sleeping drug 922

Flurbiprofen a generic nonsteroidal anti-inflammatory drug 734

Flurex a brand-name preparation containing paracetamol 778 and phenylephrine 800

Flurex Bedtime a brand-name preparation containing diphen-hydramine 360, paracetamol 778, and pseudoephedrine 836

Fluspirilene a generic antipsychotic drug 119

Flutamide a generic drug with actions similar to cyproterone acetate 326 used to treat cancer of the prostate 832

Fluticasone a generic corticosteroid drug 312

Fluvoxamine a generic antidepressant drug 116

FML a brand name for fluorometholone, a corticosteroid drug 312

FML-Neo a brand-name preparation containing fluorometholone, a corticosteroid drug 312, and neomycin 721

Folex-350 a brand-name preparation containing folic acid 454 and iron 602

Folic acid 454, a vitamin 1062

Folicin a brand name for folic acid 454 and iron 602

Folinic acid a generic drug used to counteract complications following treatment with methotrexate 684

Follicle-stimulating hormone 454, a natural hormone 541 used to treat infertility 581

Fomac a brand name for mebeverine, a generic antispasmodic drug 120

Forceval a brand-name preparation containing multivitamins 702 and minerals 689

Formaldehyde 460, a substance used in preparations for removing warts 1074

Formestane a generic anticancer drug 115

Fortagesic a brand-name preparation containing paracetamol 778 and pentazocine 789

Fortral a brand name for pentazocine 789

Fortum a brand name for ceftazidime, a generic cephalosporin drug 247

Foscarnet a generic antiviral drug 120

Foscavir a brand name for foscarnet, an antiviral drug 120

Fosfestrol a generic anticancer drug 115

Fosinopril a generic ACE inhibitor drug 61

Fragmin a brand name for dalteparin, an anticoagulant drug 116

Framycetin a generic aminoglycoside 92, a type of antibiotic drug 114

Framycort a brand-name antibacterial 114 and corticosteroid preparation 312

Framygen a brand-name antibacterial preparation 114

Franol a brand-name preparation containing ephedrine 408 and theophylline 983

Franol Plus a brand-name bronchodilator drug 215

Franolyn Chesty a brand name for dextromethorphan 348

Franolyn Expect a brand-name preparation containing ephedrine 408 and theophylline 983

Frisium a brand-name antianxiety drug 114

Froben a brand name for flurbiprofen, a nonsteroidal anti-inflammatory drug 734

Fru-Co a brand name for co-amilofruse, a mixture of amiloride 92 and frusemide 464

Frumax a brand name for frusemide 464

Frumil a brand-name preparation containing amiloride 92 and frusemide 464

Frusemide 464, a generic loop diuretic drug 364

Frusene a brand-name preparation containing triamterene 1014 and frusemide 464

Frusid a brand name for frusemide 464

FSH 464, the abbreviation for follicle-stimulating hormone 454

Fucibet a brand-name preparation containing betamethasone 165 and fusidic acid, an antibiotic drug 114

Fucidin a brand-name antibiotic drug 114

Fucidin H a brand-name preparation containing hydrocortisone 546 and fusidic acid, an antibiotic drug 114

Fucithalmic a brand name for fusidic acid, an antibiotic drug 114

Fulcin a brand name for griseofulvin 493

Full Marks a brand name for phenothrin, used to treat lice 635

Fungilin a brand name for amphotericin 94

Fungizone a brand name for amphotericin 94

Furadantin a brand name for nitrofurantoin 732

Furamide a brand-name drug used to treat amoebiasis 93

Fusidic acid a generic antibiotic drug 114

Fybogel a brand name for ispaghula 604

Fybogel Mebeverine a brand-name preparation containing mebeverine, a generic antispasmodic drug 120, and ispaghula 604

Fynnon a brand name for aspirin 137

G

Gabapentine a generic anticonvulsant drug 116

Galake a brand name for co-dydramol, a preparation containing the generic drugs paracetamol 778 and dihydrocodeine, a narcotic analgesic drug 102

Galcodine a brand-name cough remedy containing codeine 285

Galenamet a brand name for cimetidine 278

Galenamox a brand name for amoxycillin 94

Galenphol a brand name for pholcodine, a cough remedy 314

Galfer a brand name for iron 602

Galfer FA a brand-name preparation containing iron 602 and folic acid 454

Galfer-Vit a brand-name preparation containing iron 602 and vitamins 1062

Galfloxin a brand name for amoxycillin 94

Gallamine trithiodide a generic muscle-relaxant drug 707 used in general anaesthesia 99

Galpseud a brand name for pseudoephedrine 836

Gamanil a brand name for lofepramine 647

Gamma benzene hexachloride another name for lindane 638

Gamma globulin 468, a preparation of antibodies used in immunization 569

Gamolenic acid a generic drug used for symptomatic relief of breast tenderness 208. Also claimed to improve eczema 389

Ganciclovir a generic antiviral drug 120

Ganda a brand-name eye-drop preparation containing guanethidine, a generic antihypertensive drug 118, and adrenaline 70

Garamycin a brand name for gentamicin 480

Gardenal a brand name for phenobarbitone 799

Gastrils a brand-name antacid preparation 111

Gastrobid Continus a brand name for metoclopramide 684

Gastrocote a brand-name antacid drug 111 containing aluminium hydroxide 89 and sodium bicarbonate 927

Gastroflux a brand name for metoclopramide 684

Gastromax a brand name for metoclopramide 684

Gastron a brand-name antacid drug 111 containing aluminium hydroxide 89 and sodium bicarbonate 927

Gastrozepin a brand name for pirenzepine, an ulcer-healing drug 1024

Gaviscon a brand-name antacid preparation containing alginic acid, a reflux suppressant, magnesium trisilicate, an antacid drug 111, aluminium hydroxide 89, and sodium bicarbonate 927

G-CSF an abbreviation for recombinant human granulocyte-colony stimulating factor, another name for filgrastim 1107

Geangin a brand name for verapamil 1052

Gelcosal a brand-name preparation containing coal tar 283 and salicylic acid 885

Gelcotar a brand name for coal tar 283

Gelusil a brand-name drug used to treat flatulence 452

Gemeprost a generic prostaglandin drug 832 used to ripen and soften the cervix before induction of abortion 57

Gemfibrozil 472, a generic lipid-lowering drug 639

Genisol a brand-name preparation used to treat dandruff 331, eczema 389, and psoriasis 837 affecting the scalp

Genotropin a brand name for somatropin 929, a synthetically prepared growth hormone 496

Gentamicin 480, a generic antibiotic drug 114

Gentian mixture, acid and alkaline generic appetite stimulant drugs 127

Gentian violet 480, a dye used to treat skin infections 919

Genticin a brand name for gentamicin 480

Gentisone a brand-name preparation containing gentamicin 480 and hydrocortisone 546

Gestanin a brand name for allyloestrenol, a progestogen drug 830

Gestodene a generic progestogen drug 830

Gestone a brand name for progesterone 830

Gestrinone a generic drug used to treat endometriosis 402

Gestronol a generic progestogen drug 830

Givitol a brand-name preparation containing iron 602, vitamin B complex 1063, and vitamin C 1065

Glibenclamide 484, a generic hypoglycaemic drug 556

Glibenese a brand name for glipizide, a hypoglycaemic drug 556

Gliclazide a generic hypoglycaemic drug 556

Glipizide a generic hypoglycaemic drug 556

Gliquidone a generic hypoglycaemic drug 556

Glucagon 487, a hormone 541 used to treat hypoglycaemia 556

Glucobay a brand name for acarbose 59

Gluco-lyte a brand-name preparation used in rehydration therapy 866

Glucophage a brand name for metformin 683

Glurenorm a brand name for gliquidone, a hypoglycaemic drug 556

Glutaraldehyde a generic drug used to treat warts 1074

Glutarol a brand name for glutaraldehyde, a drug used to treat warts 1074

Glycerin another name for glycerol 488

Glycerol 488, a generic drug used to relieve constipation

Glyceryl trinitrate 488, a generic vasodilator drug 1047

Glycopyrronium bromide a generic anticholinergic drug 116

Glypressin a brand name for terlipressin, a synthetic preparation of ADH 67

Glytrin a brand name for glyceryl trinitrate 488

Gold 489, a generic drug used to treat rheumatoid arthritis 131

Golden Eye Drops a brand-name preparation containing propamidine isethionate used to treat eye infections 426

Gonadorelin 489, a generic drug that has the action of pituitary gonadotrophins

Gonadotrophin, human chorionic 490, a gonadotrophin hormone 489

Gonadotraphon LH a brand name for human chorionic gonadotrophin 490

Gopten a brand name for trandolapril, an ACE inhibitor drug 61

Goserelin a generic anticancer drug 115

Gramicidin a generic aminoglycoside 92, a type of antibiotic drug 114

Graneodin a brand-name antibiotic preparation 114 containing neomycin 721 and gramicidin 1109

Granisetron a generic antiemetic drug 117

Granocyte a brand name for lenograstim, a granulocyte stimulating factor 492

Gregoderm a brand-name preparation containing hydrocortisone 546, neomycin 721, nystatin 741, and polymyxin 816

Griseofulvin 493, a generic antifungal drug 117

Grisovin a brand name for griseofulvin 493

Growth hormone 496, a hormone 541 used in the treatment of short stature

GTN 300-mcg a brand name for glyceryl trinitrate 488

Guaiphenesin a generic expectorant 421

Guanethidine a generic antihypertensive drug 118

Guanor Expectorant a brand-name cough remedy 314

Guarem a brand name for guar gum 496

Guar gum 496, a plant substance used to treat diabetes mellitus 348 by controlling the level of blood sugar

Guarina a brand name for guar gum 496

Gyno-Daktarin a brand name for miconazole 685

Gynol II a brand-name spermicide 932

Gyno-Pevaryl a brand name for econazole 388

H

Haelan a brand-name preparation containing flurandrenolone, a corticosteroid drug 312

Haelan-C a brand-name preparation containing flurandrenolone, a corticosteroid drug 312, and clioquinol, an antibacterial 114 and antifungal drug 117

Halciderm Topical a brand-name preparation containing halcinonide, a corticosteroid drug 312

Halcinonide a generic corticosteroid drug 312

Haldol a brand name for haloperidol 505

Halfan a brand name for halofantrine, a drug used to treat uncomplicated chloroquine-resistant falciparum malaria 657

Half-Betadur CR a brand name for propranolol 831

Half-Beta-Prograne a brand name for propranolol 831

Half-Inderal LA a brand name for propranolol 831

Halibut liver oil a fish oil containing vitamin A 1062 and vitamin D 1065

Halofantrine a generic drug used to treat uncomplicated chloroquine-resistant falciparum malaria 657

Haloperidol 505, a generic antipsychotic drug 119

Halothane 505, a generic drug used in general anaesthesia 99

Halycitrol a brand-name preparation containing vitamin A 1062 and vitamin D 1065

Hamarin a brand name for allopurinol 87

Harmogen a brand-name oestrogen drug 749

Haymine a brand-name preparation containing chlorpheniramine 269 and ephedrine 408

HCG an abbreviation for human chorionic gonadotrophin 490

Hedex a brand name for paracetamol 778

Hemabate a brand name for carboprost, a drug used to treat blood loss after delivery, see Childbirth, complications of 264

Heminevrin a brand-name sleeping drug 922

Heparin 527, a generic anticoagulant drug 116

Hep-Flush a brand-name preparation containing heparin 527

Hepsal a brand-name preparation containing heparin 527

Heroin another name for diamorphine 353

Herpid a brand name for idoxuridine 562

Hetrazan a brand name for diethylcarbamazine, an anthelmintic drug 113

Hexachlorophane a type of antiseptic 119

Hexamine a generic drug used to treat urinary tract infection 1032

Hexopal a brand name for nicotinic acid 730

Hibiscrub a brand-name preparation containing chlorhexidine 268

Hibisol a brand-name preparation containing chlorhexidine 268

Hibitane a brand name for chlorhexidine 268

Hill's Balsam a brand-name cough remedy 314 containing pholcodine 1119

Hioxyl a brand name for hydrogen peroxide 546

Hiprex a brand name for hexamine, a drug used to treat urinary tract infections 1032

Hirudoid a brand-name preparation used to treat skin inflammation 919

Hismanal a brand name for astemizole, an anti-histamine drug 118

Histalix a brand-name preparation containing diphenhydramine 360 and menthol 680

Homatropine a generic anticholinergic drug 115

Honvan a brand name for fosfestrol, an anticancer drug 115

Hormonin a brand name for oestradiol 749

HRF a brand name for gonadorelin 489, a generic drug that has the action of pituitary gonadotrophins

Human Actraphane 30/70 a brand-name insulin preparation 589

Human Actrapid a brand-name insulin preparation 589

Human chorionic gonadotrophin 490, a hormone used to treat infertility 581

Human Initard 50/50 a brand-name insulin preparation 589

Human Insulatard a brand-name insulin preparation 589

Human Mixtard 30/70 a brand-name insulin preparation 589

Human Monotard a brand-name insulin preparation 589

Human Protaphane a brand-name insulin preparation 589

Human Ultratard a brand-name insulin preparation 589

Human Velosulin a brand-name insulin preparation 589

Humatrope a brand name for somatropin 929, a synthetically prepared growth hormone 496

Humegon a brand-name preparation containing follicle-stimulating hormone 454 and luteinizing hormone 651

Humulin a brand name for insulin 589

Hydergine a brand name for co-dergocrine, a preparation containing a mixture of vasodilator drugs 1047

Hydralazine 545, a generic antihypertensive drug 118

Hydrea a brand name for hydroxyurea, an anticancer drug 115

Hydrenox a brand name for hydroflumethiazide, a thiazide diuretic drug 364

Hydrocal a brand-name preparation containing hydrocortisone 546 and calamine 223

Hydrochlorothiazide 546, a generic thiazide diuretic drug 364

Hydrocortisone 546, a generic corticosteroid drug 312

Hydrocortistab a brand name for hydrocortisone 546

Hydrocortisyl a brand name for hydrocortisone 546

Hydrocortone a brand name for hydrocortisone 546

Hydroflumethiazide a generic thiazide diuretic drug 364

Hydrogen peroxide 546, a type of antiseptic 119

Hydromet a brand-name preparation containing methyldopa 684 and hydrochlorothiazide 546

HydroSaluric a brand name for hydrochloro-thiazide 546

Hydrotalcite a generic antacid drug containing aluminium 88 and magnesium 656

Hydroxocobalamin 546, a synthetic form of vitamin B_{12} 1063

Hydroxychloroquine a generic derivative of chloroquine 269

Hydroxycholecalciferol another name for alfacalcidol, a derivative of vitamin D 1065

Hydroxyethylcellulose a substance used in eye-drops to supplement inadequate production of tears 971

Hydroxyprogesterone a generic progestogen drug 830

Hydroxyurea a generic anticancer drug 115

Hydroxyzine a generic antianxiety drug 114 also used to treat pruritus 836

Hygroton a brand name for chlorthalidone, a thiazide diuretic drug 364

Hygroton-K a brand-name diuretic preparation containing chlorthalidone, a thiazide diuretic drug 364, and potassium 820

Hyoscine 547, a generic anticholinergic drug 115

Hypnomidate a brand name for etomidate, a drug used in general anaesthesia 99

Hypnovel a brand name for midazolam, a benzo-diazepine drug 163

Hypotears a brand-name eye preparation containing polyvinyl alcohol, used to supplement inadequate production of tears 971

Hypovase a brand name for prazosin 821

Hypromellose an ingredient of artificial tear preparations 971

Hypurin a brand name for insulin 589

Hytrin a brand name for terazosin, an antihypertensive drug 118

I

Ibrufhalal a brand name for ibuprofen 562

Ibugel a brand-name topical preparation containing ibuprofen 562

Ibular a brand name for ibuprofen 562

Ibuleve a brand-name topical preparation containing ibuprofen 562

Ibumed a brand name for ibuprofen 562

Ibuprofen 562, a generic nonsteroidal anti-inflammatory drug 734

Ichthammol a generic preparation used to treat eczema 389

Idarubicin a generic anticancer drug 114

Idoxene a brand-name eye ointment containing idoxuridine 562

Idoxuridine 562, a generic antiviral drug 120

Iduridin a brand name for idoxuridine 562

Ifosfamide a generic anticancer drug 115

Ilosone a brand name for erythromycin 416

Ilube a brand-name eye preparation containing acetylcysteine 61 used to supplement inadequate production of tears 971

Imbrilon a brand name for indomethacin 576

Imdur a brand name for isosorbide 604

Imigran a brand name for sumatriptan 959

Imipenem a generic antibiotic drug 114

Imipramine 566, a generic antidepressant drug 116

Immunoglobulin 571, a preparation of antibodies used in immunization 569

Immunoprin a brand name for azathioprine 149

Imodium a brand name for loperamide 647

Imperacin a brand name for oxytetracycline 770

Imtack a brand-name preparation containing isosorbide dinitrate 604

Imunovir a brand-name antiviral drug 120

Imuran a brand-name immunosuppressant drug 572

Indapamide a brand-name thiazide diuretic drug 364

Indaxa a brand name for indapamide, a thiazide diuretic drug 364

Inderal, Inderal LA brand names for propranolol 831

Inderetic a brand-name preparation containing bendrofluazide 163 and propranolol 831

Inderex a brand-name preparation containing bendrofluazide 163 and propranolol 831

Indocid, Indocid R brand names for indomethacin 576

Indolar SR a brand name for indomethacin 576

Indomax a brand name for indomethacin 576

Indomethacin 576, a generic nonsteroidal anti-inflammatory drug 734

Indomod a brand name for indomethacin 576

Indoramin a generic antihypertensive drug 118

Infacol a brand-name preparation containing dimethicone, used in the treatment of infantile colic 287

Initard 50/50 a brand name for insulin 589

Innovace a brand name for enalapril 398

Innozide a brand-name preparation containing enalapril 398 and hydrochlorothiazide 546

Inosine pranobex a generic antiviral drug 120

Inositol part of the vitamin B complex 1063

Inoven a brand name for ibuprofen 562

Insulatard a brand name for insulin 589

Insulin 589, a hormone 541

Intal a brand name for sodium cromoglycate 927

Intal Compound a brand name preparation containing isoprenaline 604 and sodium cromoglycate 927

Interferon 594, a generic antiviral 120 and anticancer drug 115

Intraval Sodium a brand name for thiopentone 984

Intron A a brand name for interferon 594

Intropin a brand name for dopamine 369

Iodine 600, an essential mineral

Ionamin a brand name for phentermine, an appetite suppressant drug 127

Ionil T a brand-name shampoo used to treat dandruff 331

Ipecacuanha 601, a generic drug used to induce vomiting in the treatment of drug overdose 377 and poisoning 813

Ipral a brand name for trimethoprim 1016

Ipratropium bromide a generic bronchodilator preparation 215

Iprindole a generic antidepressant drug116

Iron 602, an essential mineral

Isclofen a brand name for diclofenac 356

Isib a brand name for isosorbide mononitrate 604

Isisfen a brand name for ibuprofen 562

Ismelin a brand name for guanethidine, a generic antihypertensive drug 118

Ismo a brand name for isosorbide 604

Isocarboxazid a generic antidepressant drug 116

Isoconazole a generic antifungal drug 117

Isoflurane a generic drug used in general anaesthesia 99

Isogel a brand name for ispaghula 604

Isoket a brand name for isosorbide dinitrate 604

Isometheptene mucate a generic drug used to treat migraine 687

Isomide a brand name for disopyramide 364

Isoniazid 604, a generic drug used to treat tuberculosis 1019

Isoprenaline 604, a generic bronchodilator drug 215

Isopto Alkaline a brand-name artificial tear preparation 971

Isopto Atropine a brand name for atropine 143

Isopto Carpine a brand name for pilocarpine 803

Isopto Frin a brand-name artificial tear preparation 971 also containing phenylephrine 800

Isopto Plain a brand name artificial tear preparation 971

Isordil a brand name for isosorbide dinitrate 604

Isosorbide 604, a generic vasodilator drug 1047

Isosorbide dinitrate a form of isosorbide 604

Isosorbide mononitrate a form of isosorbide 604

Isotrate a brand name for isosorbide mononitrate 604

Isotretinoin 604, a generic drug derived from vitamin A 1062 used to treat acne 62

Isotrex a brand name for isotretinoin 604

Ispaghula 604, a generic laxative drug 629

Isradipine a generic calcium channel blocker drug 224

Istin a brand name for amlodipine 92, a calcium channel blocker 224

Itraconazole a generic antifungal drug 117

Ivermectin a generic anthelmintic drug 113

J

Jackson's All Four a brand-name cough remedy containing guaiphenesin 314

Jectofer a brand name for iron 602

Jexin a brand name for tubocurarine, a muscle-relaxant drug 707 used in general anaesthesia 99

Joy-rides a brand name for hyoscine 547

Junifen a brand name for ibuprofen 562

Junior Lemsip a brand-name preparation containing paracetamol 778 and phenylephrine 800

Junior Meltus Dry Cough a brand-name cough remedy 314 containing dextromethorphan 348 and pseudoephedrine 836

Junior Meltus Expectorant a brand-name cough remedy 314 containing guaiphenesin 1109

Junior Mu-Cron a brand-name cough preparation containing ipecacuanha 601 and phenyl-propanolamine 800

K

Kabiglobulin a brand name for human immunoglobulin 571

Kabikinase a brand name for streptokinase 950

Kalspare a brand-name preparation containing triamterene 1014 and chlorthalidone, a thiazide diuretic drug 364

Kalten a brand-name preparation containing atenolol 140, amiloride 92, and hydrochloro-thiazide 546

Kanamycin a generic antibiotic drug 114

Kannasyn a brand name for kanamycin, an antibiotic drug 114

Kaodene a brand-name preparation containing codeine 285 and kaolin 610

Kaolin 610, a generic ingredient of some antidiarrhoeal drugs 116

Kaopectate a brand-name antidiarrhoeal drug 116

Kapake a brand-name preparation containing paracetamol 778 and codeine 285

Karvol a brand-name drug used as an inhalant 585

Kay-Cee-L a brand-name potassium supplement 820

Kefadol a brand name for cephamandole, a cephalosporin drug 247

Keflex a brand name for cephalexin 246

Kefzol a brand name for cephazolin, a cephalo-sporin drug 247

Kelfizine W a brand-name sulphonamide drug 959

Kemadrin a brand name for procyclidine 830

Kemicetine a brand name for chloramphenicol 268

Kenalog a brand name for triamcinolone 1114

Kerlone a brand name for betaxolol, a beta-blocker drug 164

Kest a brand-name laxative preparation 629 containing magnesium sulphate 1113 and phenolphthalein 1119

Ketamine a generic sedative drug used in general anaesthesia 99

Ketoconazole 612, a generic antifungal drug 117

Ketoprofen 612, a generic nonsteroidal anti-inflammatory drug 734

Ketorolac a generic nonsteroidal anti-inflammatory drug 734

Ketotifen a generic antihistamine drug 118 used to prevent asthma attacks 138

Ketovail a brand name for ketoprofen 612

Ketovite a brand-name vitamin supplement preparation 1066

Kiditard a brand name for quinidine, a generic antiarrhythmic drug 114

Kinidin Durules a brand name for quinidine, a generic antiarrhythmic drug 114

Klaricid a brand name for clarithromycin, an antibiotic drug 114 related to erythromycin 416

KLN a brand-name preparation containing kaolin 610

Kloref a brand-name potassium supplement 820

Kolanticon a brand name for dicyclomine, an antispasmodic drug 120 used to treat irritable bowel syndrome 603

Konakion a brand name for vitamin K 1065

Kwells a brand name for hyoscine 547

Kytril a brand name for granisetron, an antiemetic drug 117

L

Labetalol 622, a generic beta-blocker drug 164

Labophylline a brand name for theophylline 983

Labrocol a brand-name beta-blocker drug 164

Lacidipine a generic calcium channel blocker 224

Lactic acid a naturally occurring acid used in wart treatments 1075

Lactitol a generic osmotic laxative drug 629

Lactulose 623, a generic laxative drug 629

Ladropen a brand name for flucloxacillin 453

Lamictal a brand name for lamotrigine, an anti-convulsant drug 116 used in the treatment of epilepsy 410

Lamisil a brand name for terbinafine, an antifungal drug 117

Lamotrigine a generic anticonvulsant drug 116 used in the treatment of epilepsy 410

Lamprene a brand name for clofazimine, a drug used to treat leprosy 632

Lanolin 624, a generic preparation used in the treatment of dry skin 915

Lanoxin a brand name for digoxin 359

Lanoxin-PG a brand name for digoxin 359

Lansoprazole a generic drug used in the treatment of peptic ulcer 789 and reflux oesophagitis 747

Lanvis a brand name for thioguanine, an anticancer drug 115

Laractone a brand name for spironolactone 938

Laraflex a brand name for naproxen 717

Larapam a brand name for piroxicam 804

Laratrim a brand name for co-trimoxazole 313

Largactil a brand name for chlorpromazine 269

Lariam a brand name for mefloquine, used to prevent and treat chloroquine-resistant falciparum malaria 657

Larodopa a brand name for levodopa 635

Lasikal a brand-name diuretic preparation containing frusemide 464 and potassium 820

Lasilactone a brand-name preparation containing spironolactone 938 and frusemide 464

Lasipressin a brand-name preparation containing penbutolol, a beta-blocker drug 164, and frusemide 464

Lasix + K a brand-name diuretic preparation containing frusemide 464 and potassium 820

Lasma a brand name for theophylline 983

Lasoride a brand-name diuretic drug 364

Laxoberal a brand-name laxative preparation containing sodium picosulphate 629

Laxose a brand name for lactulose 623

Ledercort a brand name for triamcinolone 1114

Lederfen, Lederfen F brand names for fenbufen 439

Ledermycin a brand-name tetracycline drug 981, a type of antibiotic drug 114

Lederspan a brand name for triamcinolone 1014

Lem-Plus, Lemsip brand-name preparations containing paracetamol 778 and phenylephrine 800

Lenium a brand name for selenium sulphide 896

Lentard MC a brand name for insulin 598

Lentaron a brand name for formestane, an anticancer drug 115

Lentizol a brand name for amitriptyline 92

Leucovorin another name for folinic acid, a drug used to counteract complications following treatment with methotrexate 684

Leukeran a brand name for chlorambucil 268

Leuprorelin a generic drug used in the treatment of cancer of the prostate 832 and endometriosis 402

Levamisole a generic anthelmintic drug 113

Levobunolol a generic beta-blocker drug 164 used as eye-drops

Levodopa 635, a generic drug used to treat Parkinson's disease 781

Levonorgestrel 635, a generic progestogen drug 830

Levophed a brand name for noradrenaline 734

Lexotan a brand name for bromazepam, an antianxiety drug 114

Lexpec a brand name for folic acid 454

Lexpec with Iron a brand-name preparation containing iron 602 and folic acid 454

Lexpec with Iron-M a brand-name preparation containing iron 602 and folic acid 454

Libanil a brand name for glibenclamide 484

Librium a brand name for chlordiazepoxide 268

Librofem a brand name for ibuprofen 562

Lidifen a brand name for ibuprofen 562

Lignocaine 637, a generic local anaesthetic 101

Li-Liquid a brand name for lithium 640

Lindane 638, a generic drug used to treat scabies 888 and lice 635

Lingraine a brand name for ergotamine 150

Lioresal a brand name for baclofen 150

Liothyronine a generic synthetic thyroid hormone 991

Lipantil a brand name for fenofibrate, a lipid-lowering drug 639

Lipostat a brand name for pravastatin, a lipid-lowering drug 639

Liquid paraffin 639, a generic laxative preparation 629

Liquifilm Tears a brand-name eye preparation containing polyvinyl alcohol used to supplement inadequate production of tears 971

Liquorice a naturally occurring substance occasionally used to treat peptic ulcer 789

Lisinopril a generic ACE inhibitor drug 61

Liskonum a brand name for lithium 640

Litarex a brand name for lithium 640

Lithium 640, a generic drug used to treat manic-depressive illness 661

Livial a brand name for tibolone 994

Lobak a brand-name preparation containing paracetamol 778 and chlormezanone, an antianxiety drug 114

Loceryl a brand name for amorolfine 94

Locoid a brand name for hydrocortisone 546

Locorten-Vioform brand-name ear-drops containing clioquinol, an antibacterial 114 and antifungal 117 drug, and flumethasone, a cortico-steroid drug 312

Lodine a brand name for etodolac, a nonsteroidal anti-inflammatory drug 734

Lodoxamide a generic drug used in eye-drops to treat allergic conjunctivitis 296

Loestrin 20, Loestrin 30 brand-name oral contraceptives 735 containing ethinyl-oestradiol 416 and norethisterone 734

Lofepramine 647, a generic antidepressant drug 116

Lofexidine a generic drug used to relieve withdrawal symptons 1084 following the use of narcotic drugs

Logiparin a brand-name anticoagulant drug 116 containing tinzaparin

Logynon, Logynon ED brand-name oral contraceptives 755 containing ethinyloestradiol 416 and levonorgestrel 635

Lomotil a brand-name antidiarrhoeal drug 116 containing diphenoxylate 360 and atropine 143

Lomustine a generic anticancer drug 115

Loniten a brand name for minoxidil 689

Loperamide 647, a generic antidiarrhoeal drug 116

Lopid a brand name for gemfibrozil 472, a lipid-lowering drug 639

Loprazolam a generic benzodiazepine drug 163

Lopresor a brand name for metoprolol 684

Lopresoretic a brand-name preparation containing metoprolol 684 and chlorthalidone, a thiazide diuretic drug 364

Loratadine a generic antihistamine drug 118

Lorazepam 647, a generic benzodiazepine 163 sleeping drug 922

Lormetazepam a generic benzodiazepine drug 163

Loron a brand name for sodium clodronate, a biphosphonate drug 171

Losec a brand name for omeprazole 751, used in the treatment of peptic ulcer 789 and reflux oesophagitis 747

Lotriderm a brand-name preparation containing betamethasone 165 and clotrimazole 283

Loxapac a brand name for loxapine, an anti-psychotic drug 119

Loxapine a generic antipsychotic drug 119

Ludiomil a brand name for maprotiline 662

Lugol's solution a brand-name preparation used to treat hyperthyroidism 553

Lurselle a brand name for probucol 829

Lustral a brand name for sertraline, an anti-depressant drug 116

Lyclear a brand name for permethrin, used to treat lice 635

Lymecycline a brand-name tetracycline drug 981, a type of antibiotic drug 114

Lypressin 655, a generic synthetic preparation of ADH 67

Lysuride a generic drug used in the treatment of Parkinson's disease 781

M

Maalox a brand-name antacid drug 111

Maalox Plus a brand-name antacid drug 111

Maclean a brand-name antacid drug 111

Macrobid a brand name for nitrofurantoin 732

Macrodantin a brand name for nitrofurantoin 732

Madopar a brand-name preparation containing levodopa 635

Magaldrate a generic antacid drug 111

Magnapen a brand name for co-fluampicil, a preparation containing the generic drugs ampicillin 94 and flucloxacillin 453

Magnesium 656, a mineral

Magnesium carbonate a generic antacid drug 111

Magnesium hydroxide a generic antacid drug 111

Magnesium oxide a generic antacid 111 and laxative drug 629

Magnesium sulphate a generic laxative drug 629

Magnesium trisilicate a generic antacid drug 111

Malathion a generic drug used to treat pediculosis 785 and scabies 888

Malix a brand-name hypoglycaemic drug 556

Maloprim a brand name for pyrimethamine 848

Manerix a brand name for moclobemide, an antidepressant drug 116

Manevac a brand-name laxative containing senna 897

Mannitol 661, a generic osmotic diuretic drug 364

Manusept a brand-name antiseptic 119 containing triclosan

Maprotiline 662, a generic antidepressant drug 116

Marcain a brand-name epidural anaesthestic 102

Marevan a brand name for warfarin 1074

Marplan a brand name for isocarboxazid 116

Marvelon a brand-name oral contraceptive 755 containing ethinyl-oestradiol 416 and desogestrel, a progestogen drug 830

Masnoderm a brand name for clotrimazole 283

Maxepa a brand-name drug used to treat hyperlipidaemia 549

Maxidex a brand name for dexamethasone 347

Maxitrol a brand-name preparation containing dexamethasone 347

Maxivent a brand name for salbutamol 885

Maxolon a brand name for metoclopramide 684

Maxtrex a brand name for methotrexate 684

Mebendazole 667, a generic anthelmintic drug 113

Mebeverine a generic antispasmodic drug 120

Mebhydrolin a generic antihistamine drug 118

Mectizan a brand name for ivermectin, an anthelmintic drug 113

Medazepam a generic benzodiazepine 163 antianxiety drug 114

Medicoal a brand name for activated charcoal 256

Medihaler-epi a brand name for adrenaline 70

Medihaler-Ergotamine a brand name for ergotamine 414

Medihaler-Iso a brand name for isoprenaline sulphate 604

Medised a brand-name analgesic drug 102

Medrone a brand name for methylprednisolone 684

Medroxyprogesterone 670, a generic progestogen drug 830

Mefenamic acid 671, a generic nonsteroidal anti-inflammatory drug 734

Mefloquine a generic drug used to prevent and treat chloroquine-resistant falciparum malaria 657

Mefoxin a brand name for cefoxitin, a cephalosporin drug 247

Mefruside a generic thiazide diuretic drug 364

Megace a brand name for megestrol 672

Megestrol 672, a generic progestogen drug 830

Melleril a brand name for thioridazine 984

Melphalan 673, a generic anticancer drug 115

Menadiol another name for vitamin K 1065

Menophase a brand-name preparation containing mestranol 682 and norethisterone 734

Menotrophin 677, a generic gonadotrophin hormone drug 489 containing follicle-stimulating hormone 454 and luteinizing hormone 651

Menthol 680, an extract from mint used in inhalations 585 and in skin preparations 914

Menzol a brand name for norethisterone 734

Mepacrine a generic drug used to treat giardiasis 481

Mepenzolate a generic antispasmodic drug 120

Mepranix a brand name for metoprolol 684

Meprobamate 680, a generic antianxiety drug 114

Meptazinol 681, a generic analgesic drug 102

Meptid a brand name for meptazinol 681

Mequitazine a generic antihistamine drug 118

Merbentyl a brand name for dicyclomine, an antispasmodic drug 120 used to treat irritable bowel syndrome 603

Mercaptopurine 681, a generic anticancer drug 115

Mercilon a brand-name oral contraceptive 755 containing ethinyl-oestradiol 416 and desogestrel, a progestogen drug 830

Mesalazine 681, a generic drug used to treat ulcerative colitis 287

Mesna a generic drug used together with certain anticancer drugs 115

Mesterolone a male sex hormone 903

Mestinon a brand-name drug used to treat myasthenia gravis 710

Mestranol 682, a generic oestrogen drug 749

Metalpha a brand name for methyldopa 684

Metamucil a brand name for ispaghula 604

Metaraminol a generic vasoconstrictor drug 1046 used in the treatment of acute hypotension 558

Meted a brand-name shampoo containing salicylic acid 885 and sulphur 959

Metenix 5 a brand-name thiazide diuretic drug 364

Meterfolic a brand-name preparation containing iron 602 and folic acid 454

Metformin 683, a generic drug used to treat diabetes mellitus 348

Methadone 683, a generic narcotic drug 717, a type of analgesic drug 102

Methenamine another name for hexamine, a generic drug used to treat urinary tract infection 1032

Methionine a generic drug used to treat paracetamol overdose 778

Methixene a generic anticholinergic drug 115

Methocarbamol 684, a generic muscle-relaxant drug 707

Methohexitone a generic sedative drug used in general anaesthesia 99

Methotrexate 684, a generic anticancer drug 115

Methotrimeprazine a generic antipsychotic drug 119

Methoxamine a generic vasoconstrictor drug 1046 used in the treatment of acute hypotension 558

Methoxsalen a generic psoralen drug 837

Methyclothiazide 684, a generic thiazide diuretic drug 364

Methylcellulose 684, a generic bulk-forming laxative drug 629

Methylcysteine a generic mucolytic drug 701

Methyldopa 684, a generic antihypertensive drug 118

Methylphenobarbitone a generic anticonvulsant drug 116

Methylprednisolone 684, a generic corticosteroid drug 312

Methyl salicylate a generic analgesic preparation 102 used to treat muscle and joint pain

Methysergide 684, a generic drug used to prevent migraine 687

Metipranolol a generic beta-blocker drug 164 used to treat glaucoma 483

Metirosine a generic antihypertensive drug 118 used in the treatment of phaeochromocytoma 797

Metoclopramide 684, a generic antiemetic drug 117

Metolazone 684, a generic thiazide diuretic drug 364

Metopirone a brand name for metyrapone, a drug used in the treatment of Cushing's syndrome 325

Metoprolol 684, a generic beta-blocker drug 164

Metosyn a brand-name corticosteroid drug 312

Metramid a brand name for metoclopramide 684

Metriphonate a generic drug used in the treatment of schistosomiasis 889

Metrodin a brand name for urofollitrophin, containing follicle-stimulating hormone 454

Metrogel a brand name for metronidazole 684

Metrolyl a brand name for metronidazole 684

Metronidazole 684, a generic antibiotic drug 114

Metrotop a brand name for metronidazole 684

Metyrapone a generic drug used in the treatment of Cushing's syndrome 325

Mexiletine 685, a generic antiarrhythmic drug 114

Mexitil a brand name for mexiletine 685

Miacalcic a brand name for salcatonin, a synthetic form of calcitonin 223

Mianserin 685, a generic antidepressant drug 116

Micolette Micro-Enema a brand-name preparation containing sodium citrate for use in constipation 297

Miconazole 685, a generic antifungal drug 117

Micralax Micro-enema a brand-name preparation containing sodium citrate for use in constipation 297

Microgynon 30 a brand-name oral contraceptive 755

Micronor a brand-name oral contraceptive 755

Microval a brand-name oral contraceptive 755

Mictral a brand name for nalidixic acid 716

Midamor a brand name for amiloride 92

Midazolam a generic benzodiazepine drug 163 used for premedication 826

Midrid a brand-name drug used to treat migraine 687

Mifegyne a brand name for mifepristone, a drug used to induce abortion 57

Mifepristone a generic drug used to induce abortion 57

Migrafen a brand name for ibuprofen 562

Migraleve a brand-name drug used to treat migraine 687

Migravess a brand-name drug used to treat migraine 687

Migril a brand-name preparation containing ergotamine 414

Mildison a brand name for hydrocortisone 546

Milk of magnesia 689, a brand-name antacid preparation 111

Milpar a brand-name preparation containing liquid paraffin 639 and magnesium hydroxide 111

Milrinone a generic drug used in the treatment of heart failure 519

Minihep a brand name for heparin 527

Min-I-Jet Adrenaline a brand name for adrenaline 70

Min-I-Jet Atropine Sulphate a brand-name preparation containing atropine 143

Min-I-Jet Bretylium Tosylate a brand-name preparation containing bretylium, an antiarrhythmic drug 114

Min-I-Jet Calcium Chloride a brand-name preparation containing calcium 224

Min-I-Jet Frusemide a brand name for frusemide 464

Min-I-Jet Isoprenaline a brand name for isoprenaline 604

Min-I-Jet Morphine Sulphate a brand-name preparation containing morphine 695

Minims Amethocaine brand-name eye-drops containing amethocaine, a local anaesthetic 101

Minims Artificial Tears brand-name eye-drops containing hydroxy-ethylcellulose, used to supplement inadequate production of tears 971

Minims Atropine brand-name eye-drops containing atropine 143

Minims Benoxinate brand-name eye-drops containing oxybuprocaine, a local anaesthetic 101

Minims Chloramphenicol brand-name eye-drops containing chloramphenicol 286

Minims Cyclopentolate brand-name eye-drops containing cyclopentolate, used to produce cycloplegia 326

Minims Gentamicin brand-name eye-drops containing gentamicin 480

Minims Homatropine Hydrobromide brand-name eye-drops containing homatropine, a generic anticholinergic drug 115

Minims Metipranolol brand-name eye-drops containing metipranolol, a beta-blocker drug 164 used to treat glaucoma 483

Minims Neomycin Sulphate brand-name eye-drops containing neomycin 721

Minims Phenylephrine Hydrochloride brand-name eye-drops containing phenylephrine 800

Minims Pilocarpine brand-name eye-drops containing pilocarpine 803

Minims Prednisolone brand-name eye-drops containing prednisolone 821

Minims Tropicamide brand-name eye-drops containing tropicamide 1018

Minitran a brand name for glyceryl trinitrate 488

Minocin a brand name for minocycline 689

Minocycline 689, a generic tetracycline drug 981, a type of antibiotic drug 114

Minodiab a brand-name drug used to treat diabetes mellitus 348

Minoxidil 689, a generic vasodilator drug 1047

Mintec a brand name for peppermint oil 789

Mintezol a brand name for thiabendazole 984

Minulet a brand-name oral contraceptive 755 containing ethinyl-oestradiol 416 and gestodene, a progestogen drug 830

Miradol a brand name for paracetamol 778

Miraxid a brand-name penicillin drug 788, a type of antibiotic drug 114

Misoprostol 691, a generic drug used in the prevention and treatment of peptic ulcers 789 associated with the use of nonsteroidal anti-inflammatory drugs 734

Mithracin a brand name for plicamycin, an anticancer drug 115

Mithramycin another name for plicamycin, a generic anticancer drug 115

Mitobronitol a generic anticancer drug 115

Mitomycin a generic anticancer drug 115

Mitomycin C Kyowa a brand name for mitomycin, an anticancer drug 115

Mitoxana a brand name for ifosfamide, an anticancer drug 115

Mitozantrone a generic anticancer drug 115

Mivacron a brand name for mivacurium, a muscle-relaxant drug 707 used in general anaesthesia 99

Mivacurium a generic muscle-relaxant drug 707 used in general anaesthesia 99

Mixtard 30/70 a brand name for insulin 589

Mobiflex a brand name for tenoxicam 976, a nonsteroidal anti-inflammatory drug 734

Mobilan a brand name for indomethacin 576

Moclobemide a generic antidepressant drug 116

Modalim a brand name for ciprofibrate, a lipid-lowering drug 639

Modecate a brand-name antipsychotic drug 119

Moditen a brand-name antipsychotic drug 119

Modrasone a brand name for aclomethasone 80

Modrenal a brand name for trilostane, a drug used in the treatment of Cushing's syndrome 325

Moducren a brand-name beta-blocker drug 164

Moduret-25 a brand-name preparation containing amiloride 92 and hydrochlorothiazide 546

Moduretic a brand-name preparation containing amiloride 92 and hydrochlorothiazide 546

Mogadon a brand name for nitrazepam 731

Molipaxin a brand name for trazodone 1012

Mometasone a generic corticosteroid drug 312

Monaspor a brand name for cefsulodin, a cephalosporin drug 247

Monit a brand name for isosorbide 604

Mono-Cedocard a brand name for isosorbide 604

Monocor a brand name for bisoprolol, a beta-blocker drug 164

Monoparin a brand name for heparin 527

Monoparin Calcium a brand name for heparin 527

Monosulfiram a generic drug for scabies 888

Monotard, Human a brand name for insulin 589

Monotrim a brand name for trimethoprim 1016

Monovent a brand name for terbutaline 977

Monphytol a brand-name antifungal preparation 117 containing undecenoates 1126

Moorland a brand-name antacid preparation 111

Morphine 695, a generic narcotic drug 717, a type of analgesic drug 102

Motens a brand name for lacidipine, a calcium channel blocker 224

Motilium a brand name for domperidone 368

Motipress a brand-name antidepressant drug 116

Motival a brand-name antidepressant drug 116

Motrin a brand name for ibuprofen 562

Movelat a brand-name preparation used to relieve soft-tissue inflammation 928

MST Continus a brand name for morphine 695

Mucaine a brand-name antacid drug 111

Mucodyne a brand-name mucolytic drug 701

Mucogel a brand-name antacid drug 111

Mu-Cron a brand-name preparation containing paracetamol 778 and phenylpropanolamine 800

Multiparin a brand name for heparin 527

Mupirocin a generic anti-bacterial preparation 114

Mustine a generic drug used to treat Hodgkin's disease 539

Myambutol a brand name for ethambutol 416

Mycardol a brand-name drug used to treat angina 106

Mycifradin a brand name for neomycin 721

Mycota a brand-name antifungal preparation 117 containing undecenoates 1126

Mydriacyl a brand name for tropicamide 1018

Mydrilate a brand name for cyclopentolate, used as eye-drops to produce cycloplegia 326

Myelobromol a brand-name anticancer drug 115

Myleran a brand-name anticancer drug 115

Mynah a brand name for ethambutol 416

Myocrisin a brand-name drug containing gold 489

Myotonine chloride a brand-name drug used to treat urinary retention 1031

Mysoline a brand name for primidone 829

Mysteclin a brand-name preparation containing amphotericin 94 and tetracycline 981

N

Nabilone a generic antiemetic drug 117

Nabumetone a generic nonsteroidal anti-inflammatory drug 734

Nacton a brand name for poldine methylsulphate, an antispasmodic drug 120

Nadolol 716, a generic beta-blocker drug 164

Nafarelin a generic gonadorelin drug used to treat endometriosis 402

Naftidrofuryl a generic vasodilator drug 1047

Nalbuphine a generic analgesic drug 102

Nalcrom a brand name for sodium cromoglycate 927

Nalidixic acid 716, a generic antibiotic drug 114

Nalorex a brand name for naltrexone, a drug that blocks the action of narcotic drugs 717

Naloxone 717, a generic drug that blocks the action of narcotic drugs 717

Naltrexone a generic drug that blocks the action of narcotic drugs 717

Nandrolone 717, a generic anabolic steroid 946

Naphazoline a generic decongestant drug 335

Napratec a brand-name preparation containing naproxen 717 and misoprostol 691

Naprosyn a brand name for naproxen 717

Naproxen 717, a generic nonsteroidal anti-inflammatory drug 734

Narcan a brand name for naloxone 717

Nardil a brand name for phenelzine 799

Narphen a brand name for phenazocine, an analgesic drug 102

Naseptin a brand-name antibacterial 114 nasal preparation containing chlorhexidine

Natrilix a brand name for indapamide, a thiazide diuretic drug 364

Natulan a brand name for procarbazine 829

Navidrex a brand name for cyclopenthiazide 326

Navispare a brand-name preparation containing amiloride 92 and cyclopenthiazide 326

Navoban a brand name for tropisetron, an antiemetic drug 117

Nebcin a brand name for tobramycin 998

Nedocromil a generic drug used to prevent asthma attacks 138

Nefopam 721, a generic analgesic drug 102

Negram a brand name for nalidixic acid 716

Neocon 1/35 a brand-name oral contraceptive 755 containing ethinyl-oestradiol 416 and norethisterone 734

Neo-Cortef a brand-name preparation containing hydrocortisone 546 and neomycin 721

Neo-Cytamen a brand name for hydroxo-cobalamin 546

Neogest a brand-name oral contraceptive 755 containing norgestrel, a progestogen drug 830

Neo-Medrone a brand name for methyl-prednisolone 684

Neo-Mercazole a brand name for carbimazole 232

Neomycin 721, a generic antibiotic drug 114

Neo-NaClex a brand name for bendrofluazide 163

Neo-NaClex-K a brand-name preparation containing bendrofluazide 163 and potassium 820

Neosporin brand-name eye-drops containing neomycin 721, polymyxin B 816, and gramicidin 1109

Neostigmine 721, a generic drug used to treat myasthenia gravis 710

Neotigason a brand name for acitretin 62

Nepenthe a brand name for morphine 695

Nephril a brand name for polythiazide, a thiazide diuretic drug 364

Nericur a brand name for benzoyl peroxide 163

Nerisone a brand name for diflucortolone, a corticosteroid drug 312

Netillin a brand name for netilmicin 725

Netilmicin 725, a generic antibiotic drug 114

Neulactil a brand name for pericyazine, an antipsychotic drug 119

Neupogen a brand name for filgrastim, used to treat deficiency of white blood cells, see Blood disorders 185

Neurontin a brand name for gabapentin, an anticonvulsant drug 116

Niacin 730 part of the vitamin B complex 1063

Nicabate brand-name patches containing nicotine 730

Nicardipine hydrochloride a generic calcium channel blocker 224

Niclosamide 730, a generic anthelmintic drug 113

Nicofuranose a generic drug used to treat hyperlipidaemia 549

Nicorette brand-name chewing gum or patches containing nicotine 730

Nicorette Plus brand-name chewing gum or patches containing nicotine 730

Nicotinamide part of the vitamin B complex 1063

Nicotine 730, a stimulant drug 947 found in tobacco

Nicotinell TTS brand-name patches containing nicotine 730

Nicotinic acid 730, another name for niacin, part of the vitamin B complex

Nicoumalone a generic anticoagulant drug 116

Nifedipine 730, a generic calcium channel blocker 224

Nifensar XL a brand name for nifedipine 730

Niferex a brand name for iron 602

Night Nurse a brand-name preparation containing dextromethorphan 348, paracetamol 778, and promethazine 831

Nikethamide an analeptic drug 102

Nimodipine a generic calcium channel blocker 224

Nimotop a brand name for nimodipine, a calcium channel blocker 224

Nipent a brand name for pentostatin, an anticancer drug 115

Nipride a brand name for sodium nitroprusside, a vasodilator drug 1047

Nitoman a brand name for tetrabenazine, a drug used to treat movement disorders 699-700

Nitrazepam 731, a generic benzodiazepine drug 163

Nitrocine a brand name for glyceryl trinitrate 488

Nitrocontin Continus a brand name for glyceryl trinitrate 488

Nitrofurantoin 732, a generic antibacterial drug 114

Nitrolingual a brand name for glyceryl trinitrate 488

Nitronal a brand name for glyceryl trinitrate 488

Nitroprusside abbreviation for sodium nitroprusside, a generic vasodilator drug 1047

Nivaquine a brand name for chloroquine 269

Nivemycin a brand name for neomycin 721

Nizatidine a generic ulcer-healing drug 1024

Nizoral a brand name for ketoconazole 612

Nobrium a brand name for medazepam, a benzodiazepine drug 163

Noctec a brand name for chloral hydrate 268

NODS Tropicamide a brand-name eye preparation containing tropicamide 1018

Noltam a brand name for tamoxifen 968

Nolvadex a brand name for tamoxifen 968

Nonoxinol 9, 10, 11 generic spermicides 932

Nootropil a brand name for piracetam, a drug used in the treatment of myoclonus 714

Noradrenaline 734, a neurotransmitter used to treat acute hypertension 551 and cardiac arrest 234

Norcuron a brand name for vecuronium, a muscle-relaxant drug 707 used in general anaesthesia 99

Norditropin a brand name for somatropin 929, a synthetically prepared growth hormone 496

Nordox a brand name for doxycycline 371

Norethisterone 734, a generic progestogen drug 830

Norflex a brand name for orphenadrine 759

Norfloxacin a generic antibacterial drug 114

Norgalax Micro-enema a brand-name laxative preparation containing docusate 629

Norgestimate a generic progestogen drug 830

Norgeston a brand-name oral contraceptive 755 containing levonorgestrel 635

Norgestrel a generic progestogen drug 830

Noriday a brand-name oral contraceptive 755 containing norethisterone 734

Norimin a brand-name oral contraceptive 755 containing ethinyl-oestradiol 416 and norethisterone 734

Norinyl-1 a brand-name oral contraceptive 755 containing mestranol 682 and norethisterone 734

Noristerat a brand-name injectable contraceptive 305

Normacol a brand-name laxative drug 629 containing sterculia

Normacol Antispasmodic a brand-name antispasmodic drug 120

Normax a brand-name laxative drug 629 containing danthron

Noroxin brand-name eye-drops containing norfloxacin, an antibacterial drug 114

Nortriptyline 734, a generic antidepressant drug 116

Norval a brand name for mianserin 685

Novantrone a brand name for mitozantrone, an anticancer drug 115

Novaprin a brand name for ibuprofen 562

Novasil Plus a brand-name antacid preparation 111

Nozinan a brand name for methotrimeprazine, an antipsychotic drug 119

Nubain a brand-name analgesic drug 102 containing nalbuphine

Nuelin a brand name for theophylline 983

Nu-K a brand name for potassium 820

Nulacin a brand-name antacid drug 111

Numark Cold Relief a brand name for paracetamol 778

Numark Cold Relief with Decongestant a brand-name preparation containing paracetamol 778 and phenylephrine 800

Nurofen a brand name for ibuprofen 562

Nu-Seals Aspirin a brand name for aspirin 137

Nutraplus a brand-name urea 1028

Nutrizym GR a brand name for pancreatin 775

Nuvelle a brand-name preparation containing oestradiol 749 and levonorgestrel 635

Nycopren a brand name for naproxen 717

Nylax a brand-name laxative preparation 629 containing bisacodyl 1099, phenolphthalein 1119, and senna 897

Nystadermal a brand name for triamcinolone 1014

Nystaform a brand-name preparation containing chlorhexidine 268 and nystatin 741

Nystaform-HC a brand-name preparation containing hydrocortisone 546, chlorhexidine 268, and nystatin 741

Nystan a brand name for nystatin 741

Nystatin 741, a generic antifungal drug 117

Nystatin-Dome a brand name for nystatin 741

Nytol a brand name for diphenhydramine 360

O

Octovit a brand-name preparation containing iron 602, multivitamins 702, and minerals 689

Octreotide a generic synthetically prepared hormone, used to treat acromegaly 64 and carcinoid syndrome 234

Ocusert Pilo a brand name for pilocarpine 803

Odrik a brand name for trandolapril, an ACE inhibitor drug 61

Oestradiol 749, a generic oestrogen drug 749

Oestrifen a brand name for tamoxifen 968

Oestriol 749, a generic oestrogen drug 749

Oestrogen 750, a female sex hormone 903

Ofloxacin a generic antibacterial drug 114

Olbetam a brand name for acipimox, a lipid-lowering drug 639

Olive oil 751, an oil used to treat cradle cap 317 and to remove earwax 386

Olsalazine a generic drug used to treat ulcerative colitis 1023

Omeprazole 751, a generic drug used in the treatment of peptic ulcer 789 and reflux oesophagitis 747

Omnopon-Scopolamine a brand-name perioperative analgesic drug 102

Oncovin a brand name for vincristine, an anticancer drug 115

Ondansetron a generic antiemetic drug 117

One-alpha a brand name for alfacalcidol, a derivative of vitamin D 1065

Opas a brand-name antacid preparation 111

Operidine a brand name for phenoperidine, an analgesic drug 102 used in general anaesthesia 99

Opthaine brand-name eye-drops containing proxymetacaine, a local anaesthetic 101

Opilon a brand name for thymoxamine 989

Opium 754, a naturally occurring narcotic drug 717, a type of analgesic drug 102

Opticrom a brand name for sodium cromoglycate 927

Optimine a brand name for azatadine 149

Orabet a brand name for metformin 683

Oral-B Fluoride a brand name for fluoride 453

Oramorph a brand name for morphine 695

Orap a brand name for pimozide 803

Orbenin a brand name for cloxacillin 283

Orciprenaline a generic bronchodilator drug 215

Orelox a brand name for cefpodoxime, a cephalosporin drug 247

Orimeten a brand name for aminoglutethimide 92

Orlept a brand name for sodium valproate 928

Orovite a brand-name preparation containing vitamin B complex 1063 and vitamin C 1065

Orovite 7 a brand-name multivitamin preparation 702

Orphenadrine 759, a generic muscle-relaxant drug 707

Ortho-Creme a brand-name spermicide 932

Ortho-Dienoestrol a brand name for dienoestrol, a generic oestrogen preparation 749 used to treat menopausal vaginitis 1042

Orthoforms a brand-name spermicide 932

Ortho-Gynest a brand name for oestriol 749

Ortho-Gynol a brand-name spermicide 932

Ortho-Novin 1/50 a brand-name oral contraceptive 755 containing mestranol 682 and norethisterone 734

Orudis a brand name for ketoprofen 612

Oruvail a brand-name topical preparation containing ketoprofen 612

Osmolax a brand name for lactulose 623

Ossopan a brand-name calcium preparation 224

Otomize a brand-name ear preparation containing dexamethasone 347 and neomycin 721

Otosporin a brand-name preparation containing hydrocortisone 546, neomycin 721, and polymyxin B 816

Otrivine a brand name for xylometazoline 1090

Otrivine-Antistin brand-name eye-drops containing antazoline, an antihistamine drug 118, and xylometazoline 1090

Ouabain a generic drug similar to the digitalis drugs 359

Ovestin a brand name for oestriol 749

Ovran a brand-name oral contraceptive 755 containing ethinyl-oestradiol 416 and levonorgestrel 635

Ovran 30 a brand-name oral contraceptive 755 containing ethinyl-oestradiol 416 and levonorgestrel 635

Ovranette a brand-name oral contraceptive 755 containing ethinyl-oestradiol 416 and levonorgestrel

Ovysmen a brand-name oral contraceptive 755 containing ethinyl-oestradiol 416 and norethisterone 734

Oxamniquine a generic drug used in the treatment of schistosomiasis 889

Oxatomide a generic antihistamine drug 118

Oxazepam 770, a generic benzodiazepine drug 163

Oxitropium bromide a generic bronchodilator drug 215

Oxivent a brand name for oxitropium bromide, a bronchodilator drug 215

Oxpentifylline a generic vasodilator drug 1047

Oxprenolol 770, a generic beta-blocker drug 164

Oxybenzone a generic sunscreen preparation 960

Oxybuprocaine a generic local anaesthetic 101

Oxybutynin a generic drug used to treat frequent urination 1032

Oxycodone a generic narcotic drug 717, a type of analgesic drug 102

Oxymetazoline 770, a generic decongestant drug 335

Oxymetholone a generic anabolic steroid 946

Oxymycin a brand name for oxytetracycline 770

Oxypertine a generic antipsychotic drug 119

Oxyphenbutazone a generic nonsteroidal anti-inflammatory drug 734

Oxyphenisatin a generic laxative drug 629

Oxyprenix a brand name for oxprenolol 770

Oxytetracycline 770, a generic tetracycline drug 981, a type of antibiotic drug 114

Oxytetramix a brand name for oxytetracycline 770

Oxytocin 770, a type of hormone 541

P

PABA an abbreviation for para-aminobenzoic acid 777, an ingredient in sunscreens 960

Pabrinex a brand-name injectable preparation containing vitamin B complex 1063 and vitamin C 1065

Pacifene a brand name for ibuprofen 562

Padimate O a generic sunscreen ingredient 960

Paldesic a brand name for paracetamol 788

Palfium a brand name for dextromoramide 348

Paludrine a brand name for proguanil 831

Pamergan P100 a brand name for pethidine 796

Pameton a brand name for paracetamol 778

Pamidronate a generic biphosphonate drug 171 used in the treatment of hypercalcaemia 548 due to cancer

Panadeine a brand-name preparation containing codeine 285 and paracetamol 778

Panadol a brand name for paracetamol 778

Panaleve, Panaleve Junior brand names for paracetamol 778

Pancrease a brand name for pancreatin 775

Pancreatin 775, a preparation of pancreatic hormones 541

Pancrex a brand name for pancreatin 775

Pancuronium a generic muscle-relaxant drug 707 used in general anaesthesia 99

Panerel a brand-name preparation containing paracetamol 778 and codeine 285

Panoxyl a brand-name preparation containing benzoyl peroxide 163

Panthenol a form of pantothenic acid, part of the vitamin B complex 1063

Pantothenic acid part of the vitamin B complex 1063

Panzytrat 25 000 a brand name for pancreatin 775

Papaveretum a generic analgesic drug 102

Papaverine a generic vasodilator drug 1047 used in the treatment of impotence 574

Para-aminobenzoic acid 777, an ingredient in sunscreens 960

Paracetamol 778, a generic analgesic drug 102

Paracets a brand name for paracetamol 778

Paracodol a brand-name preparation containing codeine 285 and paracetamol 778

Parake a brand-name preparation containing codeine 285 and paracetamol 778

Paraldehyde 778, a generic anticonvulsant drug 116

Paramax a brand-name preparation containing metoclopramide 684 and paracetamol 788

Paramin a brand name for paracetamol 778

Paramol a brand-name preparation containing paracetamol 778 and dihydrocodeine, a narcotic analgesic 102

Paraplatin a brand name for carboplatin, a generic anticancer drug 115 that is related to cisplatin 281

Parentrovite a brand-name injectable preparation containing vitamin B complex 1063 and vitamin C 1065

Parlodel a brand name for bromocriptine 213

Parmid a brand name for metoclopramide 684

Parnate a brand name for tranylcypromine 1012

Paroxetine a generic antidepressant drug 116

Parstelin a brand-name preparation containing tranylcypromine 1012 and trifluoperazine 1015

Parvolex a brand name for acetylcysteine 61

Pavacol-D a brand name for pholcodine, a cough remedy 314

Pavulon a brand name for pancuronium, a muscle-relaxant drug 707 used in general anaesthesia 99

Pecram a brand name for aminophylline 92

Pemoline a generic central nervous system stimulant drug 947

Penbritin a brand name for ampicillin 94

Penbutolol a generic beta-blocker drug 164

Pendramine a brand name for penicillamine 788

Penicillamine 788, a generic antirheumatic drug 119 and chelating agent 256

Penicillin G another name for benzylpenicillin, a generic penicillin drug 788, a type of antibiotic drug 114

Penicillin V another name for phenoxymethyl-penicillin 799

PenMix a brand-name insulin 589

Pentacarinat a brand name for pentamidine, a generic drug used to treat trypanosomiasis 1018, leishmaniasis 631, and pneumocystis pneumonia 811

Pentaerythritol tetranitrate a generic nitrate drug 731 used to treat angina pectoris 106

Pentamidine a generic drug used to treat trypanosomiasis 1018, leishmaniasis 631, and pneumocystis pneumonia 811

Pentasa a brand name for mesalazine 681

Pentazocine 789, a generic narcotic drug 717, a type of analgesic drug 102

Pentostam a brand name for sodium stibogluconate, a drug used in the treatment of leishmaniasis 631

Pentostatin a generic anticancer drug 115

Pepcid PM a brand name for famotidine 435

Peppermint oil 789, used as a flavouring in some drug preparations and as an intestinal anti-spasmodic 120

Peptimax a brand name for cimetidine 278

Pepto-Bismol a brand-name indigestion

preparation containing bismuth 173

Percutol a brand name for glyceryl trinitrate 488

Perfan a brand name for enoximone, a drug used in the treatment of heart failure 519

Pergolide a generic drug used in the treatment of Parkinson's disease 781

Pergonal a brand-name preparation containing follicle-stimulating hormone 454 and luteinizing hormone 651

Periactin a brand-name antihistamine drug 118

Pericyazine a generic antipsychotic drug 119

Perinal a brand-name preparation containing hydrocortisone 546 and lignocaine 637

Perindopril a generic ACE inhibitor drug 61

Permethrin a generic drug used to treat lice 635

Perphenazine 795, a generic antipsychotic 119 and antiemetic drug 117

Persantin a brand name for dipyridamole 360

Pertofran a brand name for desipramine, a tricyclic antidepressant drug 116

Pethidine 796, a generic analgesic drug 102

Petrolagar a brand name for liquid paraffin 639

Petroleum jelly 797, a greasy substance used as an emollient 397

Pevaryl a brand-name antifungal preparation containing econazole 388

Pharmorubicin a brand name for epirubicin, an anticancer drug 115

Phasal a brand name for lithium 640

Phenazocine a generic analgesic drug 102

Phenelzine 799, a generic monoamine oxidase inhibitor 694 antidepressant drug 116

Phenergan a brand name for promethazine 831

Phenindamine a generic antihistamine drug 118

Phenindione a generic anticoagulant drug 116

Pheniramine a generic antihistamine drug 118

Phenobarbitone 799, a generic barbiturate drug 156

Phenol a type of antiseptic 119

Phenolphthalein a generic laxative drug 629

Phenoperidine a generic analgesic drug 102 used in general anaesthesia 99

Phenothrin a generic drug used to treat lice 635

Phenoxybenzamine a generic antihypertensive drug 118

Phenoxymethylpenicillin 799, a generic penicillin drug 788, a type of antibiotic drug 114

Phensedyl a brand-name preparation containing codeine 285 and promethazine 831

Phensic a brand name for aspirin 137

Phentermine a generic appetite suppressant drug 127

Phentolamine a generic antihypertensive drug 118

Phenylbutazone 799, a generic nonsteroidal anti-inflammatory drug 734

Phenylephrine 800, a generic decongestant drug 335

Phenylpropanolamine 800, a generic decongestant drug 335

Phenytoin 800, a generic drug used to treat epilepsy 410

Phimetin a brand name for cimetidine 278

pHiso-med a brand name for chlorhexidine 268

Pholcodine a generic cough remedy 314

Pholcomed a brand-name cough remedy 314 containing pholcodine 1119

PhorPain a brand name for ibuprofen 562

Phosphates name for salts containing phosphorus used in the treatment of hypophosphataemia 801

Phosphate-Sandoz a brand-name phosphate preparation used to treat hypo-phosphataemia 801

Phyllocontin Continus a brand name for aminophylline 92

Physeptone a brand name for methadone 683

Physostigmine 803, a generic drug used to treat glaucoma 483

Phytex a brand-name antifungal drug 117

Phytocil a brand-name antifungal drug 117

Phytomenadione another name for vitamin K 1065

Picolax a brand-name laxative drug 629 containing sodium picosulphate

Pilocarpine 803, a generic drug used to treat glaucoma 483

Pimozide 803, a generic antipsychotic drug 119 used to treat Gilles de la Tourette's syndrome 481

Pindolol 803, a generic beta-blocker drug 164

Pipenzolate a generic anticholinergic drug 115

Piperacillin a generic penicillin drug 788, a type of antibiotic drug 114

Piperazine 804, a generic anthelmintic drug 113

Piportil Depot a brand name for pipothiazine, an antipsychotic drug 119

Pipothiazine a generic antipsychotic drug 119

Pipril a brand name for piperacillin, a penicillin drug 788

Piptal a brand name for pipenzolate, an anticholinergic drug 115

Piptalin a brand-name preparation containing pipenzolate, an anticholinergic drug 115, and dimethicone, a substance used in antacids 111

Piracetam a generic drug used in the treatment of myoclonus 714

Pirbuterol a generic bronchodilator drug 215

Pirenzepine a generic ulcer-healing drug 1024

Piretanide a generic loop diuretic drug 364

Piriton a brand name for chlorpheniramine 269

Piroxicam 804, a generic nonsteroidal anti-inflammatory drug 734

Pirozip a brand name for piroxicam 804

Pitressin a brand name for vasopressin 1047

Pivampicillin 806, a generic penicillin drug 788, a type of antibiotic drug 114

Pivmecillinam 806, a generic penicillin drug 788, a type of antibiotic drug 114

Pizotifen 806, a generic antihistamine drug 118

Plaquenil a brand name for hydroxychloroquine, a derivative of chloroquine 269

Platet a brand name for aspirin 137

Plendil a brand name for felodipine, a calcium channel blocker 224

Plesmet a brand-name iron preparation 602

Plicamycin a generic anticancer drug 115

Podophyllin 813, a generic drug used to treat warts 1074

Poldine methylsulphate a generic antispasmodic drug 120

Pollon-eze a brand name for astemizole, an antihistamine drug 118

Poloxamer "188" an ingredient of stimulant laxative drugs 629

Polybactrin a brand-name polymyxin drug 816, a type of antibiotic drug 114

Polyestradiol a long-acting generic oestrogen drug 749 used as an anticancer drug 115

Polyfax a brand-name antibacterial preparation 114 containing polymyxin B sulphate 816 and bacitracin 1098

Polymyxin B sulphate a generic polymyxin drug 816, a type of antibiotic drug 114

Polystyrene sulphonate resins ion-exchange resins that may be used to remove excess potassium 820 from the blood

Polytar a brand-name preparation containing coal tar 283

Polythiazide a generic thiazide diuretic drug 364

Polytrim a brand-name preparation containing polymyxin B sulphate 816 and trimethoprim 1116

Polyvinyl alcohol an ingredient of artificial tear preparations 971

Ponderax a brand-name appetite suppressant 127

Pondocillin a brand name for pivampicillin 806

Ponstan a brand name for mefenamic acid 671

Posalfilin a brand-name preparation containing podophyllum 813 and salicylic acid 885

Potassium 820, an essential mineral

Potassium chloride a generic potassium 820 supplement

Potassium citrate a generic drug used to relieve symptoms of urinary tract infection 1031

Potassium clavulanate a generic drug used to enhance the activity of some penicillin drugs 788

Potassium hydroxyquinolone sulphate an ingredient in some anti-infective topical preparations 1003

Potassium permanganate 821, a substance used as an antiseptic 119 and astringent 139

Povidone-iodine a type of antiseptic 119

Powerin a brand-name analgesic preparation containing aspirin 137 and paracetamol 778

Pranoxen Continus a brand name for naproxen 717

Pravastatin a generic lipid-lowering drug 639

Praxilene a brand name for naftidrofuryl, a vasodilator drug 1047

Praziquantel 821, a generic anthelmintic drug 113

Prazosin 821, a generic vasodilator drug 1047

Precortisyl a brand name for prednisolone 821

Predenema a brand-name prednisolone 821 enema

Predfoam a brand-name prednisolone 821 enema

Pred Forte a brand name for prednisolone 821

Prednesol a brand name for prednisolone 821

Prednisolone 821, a generic corticosteroid drug 312

Prednisone 821, a generic corticosteroid drug 312

Predsol a brand name for prednisolone 821

Predsol-N a brand-name preparation containing prednisolone 821 and neomycin 721

Prefil a brand-name appetite suppressant 127

Pregaday a brand-name preparation containing folic acid 454 and iron 602

Pregnavite Forte F a brand-name multivitamin 702, calcium 224, and iron 602 preparation

Pregnyl a brand name for gonadotrophin, human chorionic 490

Prempak-C a brand-name preparation containing an oestrogen drug 749 and norgestrel, a progestogen drug 830

Prepadine a brand name for dothiepin 370

Prepidil a brand name for dinoprostone, a prostaglandin drug 832

Prepulsid a brand name for cisapride 281

Prescal a brand name for isradipine, a generic calcium channel blocker 224

Prestim a brand-name preparation containing bendrofluazide 163 and timolol 994

Priadel a brand name for lithium 640

Prilocaine a generic local anaesthetic 101

Primacor a brand name for milrinone, a drug used in the treatment of heart failure 519

Primalan a brand name for mequitazine, an antihistamine drug 118

Primaquine 829, a generic drug used to treat malaria 657

Primaxin a brand name for imipenem, an antibiotic drug 114

Primidone 829, a generic anticonvulsant drug 116

Primolut Depot a brand name for hydroxyprogesterone, a progestogen drug 830

Primolut N a brand name for norethisterone 734

Primoteston Depot a brand name for testosterone 979

Primperan a brand name for metoclopramide 684

Prioderm a brand name for malathion, used to treat pediculosis 785 and scabies 888

Pripsen a brand-name preparation containing piperazine 804 and senna 897

Pro-Actidil a brand name for triprolidine 1116

Pro-Banthine a brand name for propantheline 831

Probenecid 829, a generic drug used to treat gout 490

Probucol 829, a generic lipid-lowering drug 639

Procainamide 829, a generic antiarrhythmic drug 114

Procainamide Durules a brand name for procainamide 829

Procaine 829, a generic local anaesthetic 101

Procaine penicillin a generic penicillin drug 788, a type of antibiotic

Procarbazine 829, a generic anticancer drug 115

Prochlorperazine 829, a generic phenothiazine 799 and antipsychotic drug 119

Procol a brand name for phenylpropanolamine 800

Proctofoam HC a brand-name corticosteroid preparation 312

Proctosedyl a brand-name corticosteroid preparation 312 and local anaesthetic 101

Procyclidine 830, a generic anticholinergic drug 115

Profasi a brand name for gonadotrophin, human chorionic 490

Proflex a brand name for ibuprofen 562

Progesic a brand name for fenoprofen 439

Progesterone 830, a female sex hormone 903

Progestogen 830, a form of progesterone 830

Proguanil 831, a generic drug used to prevent malaria 657

Progynova a brand name for oestradiol 749

Proleukin a brand name for aldesleukin, an anticancer drug 115

Proluton Depot a brand name for hydroxyprogesterone, a progestogen drug 830

Promazine 831, a generic phenothiazine drug 799, a type of antipsychotic drug 119

Promethazine 831, a generic antihistamine drug 118

Prominal a brand name for methylphenobarbitone, an anticonvulsant drug 116

Prondol a brand name for iprindole, an antidepressant drug 116

Pronestyl a brand name for procainamide 829

Propaderm a brand name for beclomethasone 160

Propafenone a generic antiarrhythmic drug 114

Propain a brand-name analgesic preparation containing paracetamol 778, codeine 285, and diphenhydramine 360

Propamidine a generic drug specific for the treatment of acanthamoeba keratitis, a rare infection of the eye

Propamidine isethionate a generic preparation used to treat eye infections 426

Propanix a brand name for propranolol 831

Propantheline 831, a generic antispasmodic drug 120

Propine a brand name for dipivefrine, which is converted to adrenaline 70 and has similar actions

Propofol a generic drug used in general anaesthesia 99

Propranolol 831, a generic beta-blocker drug 164

Propylthiouracil 831, a generic drug used to treat hyperthyroidism 553

Prosaid a brand name for naproxen 717

Proscar a brand name for finasteride 449

Prostap SR a brand name for leuprorelin 635, used in the treatment of cancer of the prostate 832 and endometriosis 402

Prostigmin a brand name for neostigmine 721

Prostin E2 a brand name for dinoprostone, a prostaglandin drug 832

Prostin F2 alpha a brand name for dinoprost, a prostaglandin drug 832

Protaphane, Human a brand name for insulin 589

Prothiaden a brand name for dothiepin 370

Protriptyline 836, a generic antidepressant drug 116

Provera a brand name for medroxyprogesterone 670

Pro-Viron a brand name for mesterolone, a male sex hormone 903

Proxymetacaine a generic local anaesthetic 101

Prozac a brand name for fluoxetine, an antidepressant drug 116

Proziere a brand name for prochlorperazine 829

Pseudoephedrine 836, a generic decongestant drug 335

Psoradrate a brand name for dithranol 364

Psoriderm a brand-name preparation containing coal tar 283

PsoriGel a brand-name preparation containing coal tar 283

Psorin a brand-name preparation for psoriasis 837 containing dithranol 364, coal tar 283, and salicylic acid 885

Pulmadil a brand name for rimiterol 881

Pulmicort a brand-name corticosteroid drug 312 containing budesonide

Puri-Nethol a brand name for mercaptopurine 681

Pur-In Mix a brand name for insulin 589

Pyopen a brand name for carbenicillin, a penicillin drug 788

Pyrantel 848, a generic anthelmintic drug 113

Pyrazinamide 848, a generic drug used to treat tuberculosis 1019

Pyridostigmine a generic drug used to treat myasthenia gravis 710

Pyridoxine 848, part of the vitamin B complex 1063

Pyrimethamine 848, a generic drug used to treat malaria 657 and toxoplasmosis 1006

Pyrithione zinc a generic preparation used to treat dandruff 331

Pyrogastrone a brand-name ulcer-healing drug 1024

Q

Quellada a brand name for lindane 638

Questran a brand name for cholestyramine 273

Quinalbarbitone a generic barbiturate 156 sleeping drug 922

Quinapril a generic ACE inhibitor drug 118

Quinidine a generic antiarrhythmic drug 114

Quinine 849, a generic drug used to treat malaria 657

Quinocort a brand-name corticosteroid cream 312

Quinoderm a brand-name preparation containing benzoyl peroxide 163 and potassium hydroxy-quinolone sulphate 1119

Quinoped a brand-name preparation containing benzoyl peroxide 163 and potassium hydroxy-quinolone sulphate 1119 used to treat fungal skin infections

R

Ramipril a generic ACE inhibitor drug 61

Ramysis a brand name for doxycycline 371

Ranitidine 857, a generic ulcer-healing drug 1024

Rap-eze a brand-name antacid preparation 111

Rapifen a brand name for alfentanil, an analgesic drug 102 used in general anaesthesia 99

Rapitard MC a brand name for insulin 589

Rapolyte a brand-name preparation used in rehydration therapy 866

Rastinon a brand name for tolbutamide 1000

Razoxane a generic anticancer drug 115

Razoxin a brand name for razoxane, an anticancer drug 115

R.B.C. a brand-name antihistamine 118 preparation

Recormon a brand name for epoetin 413

Redeptin a brand name for fluspirilene, an antipsychotic drug 119

Redoxon a brand name for vitamin C 1065

Refolinon a brand name for folinic acid, used to counteract complications following treatment with methotrexate 684

Regaine a brand name for minoxidil 689

Regulan a brand name for ispaghula 604

Reguletts a brand name for phenolphthalein, a laxative drug 629

Rehibin a brand name for cyclofenil, used to treat infertility 581

Rehidrat a brand-name preparation used in rehydration therapy 866

Relaxit Micro-enema a brand-name preparation containing sodium citrate for use in constipation 297

Relcofen a brand name for ibuprofen 562

Relefact LH-RH a brand name for gonadorelin 489, a generic drug that has the action of pituitary gonadotrophins

Relifex a brand name for nabumetone, a nonsteroidal anti-inflammatory drug 734

Remedeine a brand-name analgesic preparation 102 containing paracetamol 778 and dihydrocodeine 1104

Remegel a brand-name antacid preparation 111

Remnos a brand name for nitrazepam 731

Remoxipride a generic antipsychotic drug 119

Rennie a brand-name antacid preparation 111

Reproterol a generic bronchodilator drug 215

Resiston One a brand-name preparation containing sodium cromoglycate 927 and xylometazoline 1090

Resolve a brand name for paracetamol 778

Resonium A a brand name for sodium polystyrene sulphonate, used to remove excess potassium 820 from the blood

Resorcinol a generic preparation used to treat acne 62

Respacal a brand name for tulobuterol, a broncho-dilator drug 215

Restandol a brand name for testosterone 979

Retin-A a brand name for tretinoin 1013

Retinol 874, the principal form of vitamin A 1062

Retrovir a brand name for zidovudine 1093

Revanil a brand name for lysuride, used in the treatment of Parkinson's disease 781

Rheumacin LA a brand name for indomethacin 576

Rheumox a brand name for azapropazone, a nonsteroidal anti-inflammatory drug 734

Rhinocort a brand name for budesonide, a corticosteroid drug 312

Rhinolast a brand-name preparation containing azelastin, an antihistamine drug 118 available as a nasal spray for allergic rhinitis 878

Rhumalgan a brand name for diclofenac 356

Ribavirin 880, another name for tribavirin 1014

Riboflavin 880, another name for vitamin B 1063

Ridaura a brand name for auranofin 144

Rifadin a brand name for rifampicin 880

Rifampicin 880, a generic antibacterial drug 114

Rifater a brand-name preparation containing pyrazinamide 848 and rifampicin 880

Rifinah 150 a brand-name preparation containing isoniazid 604 and rifampicin 880

Rifinah 300 a brand-name preparation containing isoniazid 604 and rifampicin 880

Rimacid a brand name for indomethacin 576

Rimacillin a brand name for ampicillin 94

Rimactane a brand name for rifampicin 880

Rimactazid a brand-name preparation containing isoniazid 604 and rifampicin 880

Rimadol a brand name for paracetamol 778

Rimafen a brand name for ibuprofen 562

Rimapam a brand name for diazepam 356

Rimapurinol a brand name for allopurinol 87

Rimifon a brand name for isoniazid 604

Rimiterol 881, a generic bronchodilator drug 215

Rimoxallin a brand name for amoxycillin 94

Rinatec a brand name for ipratropium bromide, a bronchodilator drug 215

Risperdal a brand name for risperidone, an antipsychotic drug 119

Risperidone a generic antipsychotic drug 119

Ritodrine 881, a generic drug used to delay premature labour 825

Rivotril a brand name for clonazepam 283

Roaccutane a brand name for isotretinoin 604

Ro-A-Vit a brand name for vitamin A 1062

Robaxin 750 a brand name for methocarbamol 684

Robaxisal Forte a brand-name preparation containing aspirin 137 and methocarbamol 684

Robinul a brand name for glycopyrronium bromide, an anticholinergic drug 115

Robitussin a brand-name cough remedy 314 containing guaiphenesin 1109

Robitussin Plus a brand-name cough remedy 314 containing guaiphenesin 1109 and pseudo-ephedrine 836

Rocaltrol a brand name for calcitriol, a derivative of vitamin D 1065

Roccal a brand-name antiseptic 119 containing benzalkonium chloride 1099

Rocephin a brand name for ceftriaxone, a cephalosporin drug 247

Roferon-A a brand name for interferon 594

Rogitine a brand name for phentolamine, an antihypertensive drug 118

Rohypnol a brand name for flunitrazepam, a benzodiazepine drug 163

Rommix a brand name for erythromycin 416

Ronicol a brand name for nicotinic acid 730

Rosoxacin another name for acrosoxacin 64, a quinolone drug 849 used to treat gonorrhoea 490

Roter a brand-name antacid preparation 111

Rowachol a brand-name drug used to treat gallstones 468

Roxiam a brand name for remoxipride, an anti-psychotic drug 119

Rusyde a brand name for frusemide 464

Rynacrom a brand name for sodium cromoglycate 927

Rynacrom Compound a brand-name preparation containing sodium cromoglycate 927 and xylometazoline 1090

Rythmodan a brand name for disopyramide 364

S

Sabril a brand name for vigabatrin, an anti-convulsant drug 116 used in the treatment of epilepsy 410

Saizen a brand name for somatropin 929, a synthetically prepared growth hormone 496

Salactol a brand-name wart treatment containing lactic acid 1112 and salicylic acid 885

Salamol a brand name for salbutamol 885

Salatac a brand-name wart treatment containing lactic acid 1112 and salicylic acid 885

Salazopyrin a brand name for sulphasalazine 959

Salbulin a brand name for salbutamol 885

Salbutamol 885, a generic bronchodilator drug 215

Salcatonin the generic name for a synthetic form of calcitonin 223

Salicylic acid 885, a generic keratolytic drug 611

Salmeterol a generic bronchodilator drug 215

Salofalk a brand name for mesalazine 681

Salsalate a generic nonsteroidal anti-inflammatory drug 734

Saluric a brand-name thiazide diuretic drug 364

Salzone a brand name for paracetamol 778

Sandimmun a brand name for cyclosporin 326

Sandocal a brand-name calcium supplement 224

Sandoglobulin a brand name for human immunoglobulin 571

Sando-K a brand-name potassium supplement 820

Sandostatin a brand name for octreotide 1117, a synthetically prepared hormone

Sanomigran a brand name for pizotifen 806

Saventrine a brand name for isoprenaline 604

Schering PC4 a brand-name preparation containing levonorgestrel 635 and ethinyloestradiol 416, used for postcoital contraception 304

Scheriproct a brand-name corticosteroid preparation 312 and local anaesthetic 101

Scoline a brand name for suxamethonium, a muscle-relaxant drug 707 used in general anaesthesia 99

Scopoderm TTS brand-name patches containing hyoscine 547

Scopolamine another name for hyoscine 547

Secadrex a brand-name preparation containing acebutolol 60 and hydrochlorothiazide 546

Seconal Sodium a brand name for quinalbarbitone, a barbiturate drug 156

Sectral a brand name for acebutolol 60

Securon a brand name for verapamil hydrochloride 1053

Securopen a brand name for azlocillin, a penicillin drug 788

Seldane a brand name for terfenadine 977

Selegiline a generic drug used to treat Parkinson's disease 781

Selenium 896, an essential mineral

Selenium sulphide a substance used to treat dandruff 331 and pityriasis versicolor 806

Selsun a brand-name preparation used to treat dandruff 331 and pityriasis versicolor 806

Semi-Daonil a brand name for glibenclamide 484

Semitard MC a brand name for insulin 589

Semprex a brand name for acrivastine, an anti-histamine drug 118

Senna 897, a generic stimulant laxative drug 629

Senokot a brand name for senna 897

Septrin a brand name for co-trimoxazole 313

Serc a brand name for betahistine 165

Serenace a brand name for haloperidol 505

Serevent a brand name for salmeterol, a broncho-dilator drug 215

Serophene a brand name for clomiphene 282

Seroxat a brand name for paroxetine, an anti-depressant drug 116

Sertraline a generic antidepressant drug 116

Setlers a brand-name antacid preparation 111

Sevredol a brand name for morphine 695

Silver sulphadiazine 913, a generic antibacterial drug 114

Simeco a brand-name antacid drug 111

Simplene a brand name for adrenaline 70

Simvastatin 913, a generic lipid-lowering drug 639

Sinemet a brand-name preparation containing levadopa 635 used to treat Parkinson's disease 781

Sinequan a brand name for doxepin, an anti-depressant drug 116

Sinthrome a brand name for nicoumalone, an anticoagulant drug 116

Sinutab a brand-name preparation containing paracetamol 778 and phenylpropanolamine 800

Skinoren a brand-name preparation containing azelaic acid used to treat acne 62

Slo-Indo a brand name for indomethacin 576

Slo-Phyllin a brand name for theophylline 983

Sloprolol a brand name for propranolol 831

Slow-Fe a brand name for ferrous sulphate 439

Slow-Fe Folic a brand-name preparation containing iron 602 and folic acid 454

Slow-K a brand name for potassium 830

Slow-Trasicor a brand name for oxprenolol 770

Sno Phenicol a brand name for chloramphenicol 266

Sno Pilo a brand name for pilocarpine 863

Sno Tears a brand-name artificial tear preparation 971

Soda mint tablets a form of sodium bicarbonate 927

Sodium 927, an essential mineral

Sodium Amytal a brand-name barbiturate drug 156

Sodium aurothiomalate 927, a generic drug used to treat arthritis 131

Sodium bicarbonate 927, a generic antacid drug 111

Sodium cellulose phosphate a generic drug used to treat hypercalcaemia 135

Sodium chloride the chemical name for common table salt, used in rehydration therapy 866

Sodium citrate a generic drug used to relieve discomfort in urinary tract infection 1032, and used rectally in constipation 297

Sodium clodronate a generic biphosphonate drug 171 used in the treatment of hyper-calcaemia 548 due to cancer

Sodium cromoglycate 927, a generic drug used to prevent asthma 138

Sodium fluoride a form of fluoride 453

Sodium fusidate a generic antibiotic drug 114

Sodium ironedetate a generic drug used to treat iron-deficiency anaemia 97

Sodium nitroprusside a generic vasodilator drug 1047

Sodium picosulphate a generic laxative drug 629

Sodium stibogluconate a generic drug used in the treatment of leishmaniasis 631

Sodium valproate 928, a generic drug used to treat epilepsy 410

Sofradex a brand-name preparation containing dexamethasone 347 and two antibiotic drugs 114, framycetin 1108 and gramicidin 1108

Soframycin a brand-name preparation containing the antibiotic drugs 114 framycetin 1108 and gramicidin 1109

Solarcaine a brand-name preparation containing benzocaine, a local anaesthetic 101, and triclosan, a type of antiseptic 119

Solpadeine a brand-name preparation containing paracetamol 778 and codeine 285

Solpadol a brand-name preparation containing paracetamol 778 and codeine 285

Solu-Cortef a brand name for hydrocortisone 546

Solu-Medrone a brand name for methyl-prednisolone 684

Solvazinc a brand-name zinc supplement 1093

Somatropin 929, a generic synthetically prepared growth hormone 496

Sominex a brand name for promethazine 831

Somnite a brand name for nitrazepam 731

Soneryl a brand name for butobarbitone, a barbiturate drug 156

Soni-Slo a brand name for isosorbide dinitrate 604

Sorbichew a brand name for isosorbide dinitrate 604

Sorbid SA a brand name for isosorbide dinitrate 604

Sorbitol an artificial sweetener 135 used mainly in diabetic foods

Sorbitrate a brand name for isosorbide dinitrate 604

Sotacor a brand name for sotalol, a beta-blocker drug 164

Sotalol a generic beta-blocker drug 164

Sotazide a brand-name preparation containing sotalol, a beta-blocker drug 164 and hydro-chlorothiazide 546

Sovol a brand-name antacid preparation 111

Sparine a brand name for promazine 831

Spasmonal a brand name for alverine, an antispasmodic drug 120

SP Cold Relief a brand-name preparation containing paracetamol 778 and phenylephrine 800

Spectinomycin a generic antibiotic drug 114

Spectraban a brand-name sunscreen 960

Spiroctan a brand name for spironolactone 938

Spirolone a brand name for spironolactone 938

Spironolactone 938, a generic diuretic drug 364

Spirospare a brand name for spironolactone 938

Sporanox a brand name for itraconazole, an antifungal drug 117

Sprilon a brand-name preparation used for moist skin disorders 919

SRM-Rhotard a brand name for morphine 695

Stabillin V-K a brand name for phenoxy-methylpenicillin 799

Stafoxil a brand name for flucloxacillin 453

Stanozolol 943, a generic anabolic steroid 946

Staril a brand name for fosinopril, an ACE inhibitor drug 61

Staycept pessaries a brand-name spermicide 932

Stelazine a brand name for trifluoperazine 1015

Stemetil a brand name for prochlorperazine 829

Sterculia a generic bulk-forming substance used as an antidiarrhoeal drug 116 and a laxative drug 629

Sterexidine a brand name for chlorhexidine 268

Steri-Neb Cromogen a brand name for sodium cromoglycate 927

Steri-Neb Salamol a brand name for salbutamol 885

Steripod Chlorhexidine a brand name for chlorhexidine 268

Stesolid a brand name for diazepam 356

Stiedex a brand name for desoxymethasone, a corticosteroid drug 312

Stiedex LPN a brand-name corticosteroid drug 312

Stiemycin a brand name for erythromycin 416

Stilboestrol 947, a generic oestrogen drug 749

Streptase a brand name for streptokinase 950

Streptokinase 950, a generic thrombolytic drug 987

Streptomycin 951, a generic antibiotic drug 114

Stromba a brand name for stanozolol 943

Stugeron a brand name for cinnarizine 278

Sublimaze a brand name for fentanyl, an analgesic drug 102

Sucralfate 957, a generic drug used to treat peptic ulcer 789

Sudafed a brand-name expectorant 421 containing pseudo-ephedrine 836

Sudafed-Co a brand-name preparation containing paracetamol 778 and pseudoephedrine 836

Sudafed Expectorant a brand-name expectorant 421 containing guaiphenesin and pseudoephedrine 836

Sudafed Plus a brand-name preparation containing pseudo-ephedrine 836 and triprolidine 1016

Sudocrem a brand-name preparation used to treat nappy rash 717 and pressure sores 828

Sulconazole a generic antifungal preparation 117

Suleo-C a brand-name preparation containing carbaryl used to treat pediculosis 785

Suleo-M a brand name for malathion, used to treat pediculosis 785

Sulfadoxine a generic drug used to prevent and treat malaria 657

Sulfametopyrazine a generic sulphonamide drug 959

Sulindac 959, a generic nonsteroidal anti-inflammatory drug 734

Sulphadiazine a generic sulphonamide drug 959

Sulphadimidine a generic sulphonamide drug 959

Sulphamethoxazole a generic sulphonamide drug 959

Sulphasalazine 959, a generic anti-inflammatory drug 118

Sulphinpyrazone 959, a generic drug used to treat gout 490

Sulphur 959, a mineral used in some preparations

to treat acne 62 and dandruff 331

Sulpiride 959, a generic antipsychotic drug 119

Sulpitil a brand name for sulpiride 959

Sultrin a brand-name preparation containing sulphonamide drugs 959

Sumatriptan a generic drug 959 used in the treatment of migraine 687

Suprax a brand name for cefixime, a cephalosporin drug 247

Suprecur a brand name for buserelin, a gonadorelin drug 489 used in the treatment of endometriosis 402 and cancer of the prostate 832

Suprefact a brand name for buserelin, a generic gonadorelin drug 489 used in the treatment of endometriosis 402 and cancer of the prostate 832

Surgam a brand-name nonsteroidal anti-inflammatory drug 734

Surmontil a brand name for trimipramine 1116

Suscard, Sustac brand names for glyceryl trinitrate 488

Sustamycin a brand name for tetracycline 981

Sustanon a brand name for testosterone 987

Suxamethonium a generic muscle-relaxant drug 707 used in general anaesthesia 99

Symmetrel a brand name for amantadine 90

Synacthen a brand-name drug used to assess function of the adrenal glands 69

Synalar a brand name for fluocinolone, a corticosteroid drug 312

Synalar C a brand-name preparation containing fluocinolone, a cortico-steroid drug 312, and clioquinol, an antibacterial drug 114

Synalar N a brand-name preparation containing fluocinolone, a cortico-steroid drug 312 and neomycin 721

Synarel a brand name for nafarelin, a gonadorelin drug 489 used to treat endometriosis 402

Syndol a brand-name analgesic preparation containing paracetamol 778, codeine 285, and doxylamine, an antihistamine drug 118

Synflex a brand name for naproxen 717

Synkavit a brand-name vitamin-K preparation 1065

Synphase a brand-name oral contraceptive 755 containing ethinyloestradiol 416 and norethisterone 734

Syntaris a brand name for flunisolide, a corticosteroid drug 312

Syntex Menophase a brand-name preparation containing mestranol 682 and norethisterone 734

Syntocinon a brand name for oxytocin 770

Syntometrine a brand-name preparation containing ergometrine 413 and oxytocin 770

Syntopressin a brand name for lypressin 655

Sytron a brand name for sodium ironedetate, used to treat iron-deficiency anaemia 97

T

Tacrine another name for tetrahydroaminoacridine 981

Tagamet a brand name for cimetidine 278

Tambocor a brand name for flecainide, an antiarrhythmic drug 114

Tamofen, Tamofen 20, Tamofen 40 brand names for tamoxifen 968

Tamoxifen 968, a generic anticancer drug 115

Tampovagan Stilboestrol and Lactic Acid a brand-name preparation containing stilboestrol 947 and lactic acid 1112

Tancolin a brand name for dextromethorphan 348

Tanderil a brand-name eye ointment containing oxyphenbutazone, a nonsteroidal antiinflammatory drug 734

Tarcortin a brand-name preparation containing hydrocortisone 546 and coal tar 783

Targocid a brand name for teicoplanin, an antibiotic drug 114

Tarivid a brand name for ofloxacin, an antibacterial drug 114

Tavegil a brand name for clemastine, an antihistamine drug 118

Tazobactam a generic drug used to enhance the effect of some penicillin drugs 788

Tazocin a brand-name preparation containing piperacillin, a penicillin drug 788, and tazobactam 1124

Teejel a brand-name preparation used to treat oral lesions 632

Tegretol a brand name for carbamazepine 231

Teicoplanin a generic antibiotic drug 114

Temazepam 973, a generic benzodiazepine drug 163

Temgesic a brand name for buprenorphin, an analgesic drug 102

Temocillin a generic penicillin drug 788, a type of antibiotic drug 114

Temopen a brand name for temocillin, a penicillin drug 788

Tenchlor a brand-name preparation containing atenolol 140 and chlorthalidone, a thiazide diuretic drug 364

Tenif a brand-name preparation containing atenolol 140 and nifedipine 730

Tenoret-50 a brand-name preparation containing atenolol 140 and chlorthalidone, a diuretic drug 364

Tenoretic a brand-name preparation containing atenolol 140 and chlorthalidone, a diuretic drug 364

Tenormin a brand name for atenolol 140

Tenoxicam a generic nonsteroidal antiinflammatory drug 734

Tensilon a brand name for edrophonium chloride, a drug used in the diagnosis of myasthenia gravis 710

Tensium a brand name for diazepam 356

Teoptic a brand name for carteolol, a beta-blocker drug 164

Terazosin a generic antihypertensive drug 118

Terbinafine a generic antifungal drug 117

Terbutaline 977, a generic bronchodilator drug 215

Terfenadine 977, a generic antihistamine drug 118

Terfex a brand name for terfenadine 977

Terlipressin a generic synthetic preparation of ADH 67

Terpoin a brand-name cough remedy containing codeine 285

Terra-Cortril a brand-name preparation containing hydrocortisone 546 and oxytetracycline 770

Terra-Cortril Nystatin a brand-name preparation containing hydrocortisone 546, nystatin 741, and oxytetracycline 770

Terramycin a brand name for oxytetracycline 770

Tertroxin a brand name for liothyronine, a synthetic thyroid hormone 991

Testosterone 979, an androgen hormone 104

Tetmosol a brand name for monosulfiram, a drug used for scabies 888

Tetrabenazine a generic drug used to treat movement disorders 699-700

Tetrabid-Organon a brand name for tetracycline 981

Tetrachel a brand name for tetracycline 981

Tetracosactrin a generic drug used to assess function of the adrenal glands 69

Tetracycline 981, a generic antibiotic drug 114

Tetrahydroaminoacridine 981 a generic drug used to treat Alzheimer's disease 90

Tetralysal 300 a brand-name tetracycline 981, a type of antibiotic drug 114

T/Gel a brand-name preparation containing coal tar 283

Thalamonal a brand-name preparation containing fentanyl, an analgesic drug 102, and droperidol, an antiemetic drug 117

THC 983, an abbreviation for the active ingredient in marijuana 662

Theo-Dur a brand name for theophylline 983

Theophylline 983, a generic bronchodilator drug 215

Thephorin a brand name for phenindamine, an antihistamine drug 118

Thiabendazole 984, a generic anthelmintic drug 113

Thiamine part of the vitamin B complex 1063

Thioguanine a generic anticancer drug 115

Thiopentone 984, a generic barbiturate drug 156

Thioridazine 984, a generic antipsychotic drug 119

Thiotepa a generic anticancer drug 115

Thymoxamine 989, a generic drug used to treat peripheral vascular disease 793

Thyroxine 993, a generic drug used to treat hypothyroidism 560

Tiaprofenic acid a generic nonsteroidal antiinflammatory drug 734

Tibolone a generic drug used in the treatment of symptoms of the menopause 676

Ticar a brand name for ticarcillin, a penicillin drug 788

Ticarcillin a generic penicillin drug 788, a type of antibiotic drug 114

Tilade Mint a brand name for nedocromil, used to prevent asthma 138

Tildiem a brand name for diltiazem 359

Timecef a brand name for cefodizime, a cephalosporin drug 247

Timentin a brand-name preparation containing ticarcillin, a penicillin drug 788, and clavulanic acid 1101

Timodine a brand-name preparation containing hydrocortisone 546 and nystatin 741

Timolol 994, a generic beta-blocker drug 164

Timoptol a brand name for timolol 994

Tinaderm-M a brand-name preparation containing nystatin 741 and tolnaftate 1000

Tinidazole a generic antibacterial drug 114

Tinset a brand name for oxatomide, an antihistamine drug 118

Tinzaparin a generic anticoagulant drug 116

Tioconazole a generic antifungal drug 117

Tisept a brand name for chlorhexidine 268

Tixylix Cough and Cold a brand-name cough remedy 314 containing chlorpheniramine 269, pholcodine 1119, and pseudoephedrine 836

Tixylix Daytime a brand-name cough remedy 314 containing pholcodine 1119

Tixylix Original a brand-name cough remedy 314 containing pholcodine 1119 and promethazine 831

Tobralex a brand name for tobramycin 998

Tobramycin 998, a generic antibiotic drug 114

Tocainide 999, a generic antiarrhythmic drug 114

Tocopherol 999, a constituent of vitamin E 1065

Tocopheryl another name for vitamin E 1065

Tofranil a brand name for imipramine 566

Tolanase a brand name for tolazamide, a hypoglycaemic drug 556

Tolazamide a generic hypoglycaemic drug 556

Tolbutamide a generic hypoglycaemic drug 556

Tolectin DS a brand name for tolmetin 1000

Tolerzide a brand-name preparation containing sotalol, a beta-blocker drug 164, and hydrochlorothiazide 546

Tolmetin 1000, a generic nonsteroidal anti-inflammatory drug 734

Tonocard a brand name for tocainide 999

Topal a brand-name antacid drug 111

Topicycline a brand-name tetracycline drug 981, a type of antibiotic drug 114

Topilar a brand name for fluclorolone, a corticosteroid preparation 312

Toptabs a brand name for aspirin 137

Toradol a brand name for ketorolac, a nonsteroidal anti-inflammatory drug 734

Totamol a brand name for atenolol 140

Tracrium a brand name for atracurium, a muscle-relaxant drug 707 used in general anaesthesia 99

Tramadol a generic analgesic drug 102

Tramil a brand name for paracetamol 778

Trancopal a brand name for chlormezanone, an antianxiety drug 114

Trandate a brand name for labetalol 622

Trandolapril a generic ACE inhibitor drug 61

Tranexamic acid a generic drug used to promote blood clotting 183

Transiderm-Nitro a brand name for glyceryl trinitrate 488

Tranxene a brand name for clorazepate, an antianxiety drug 114

Tranylcypromine 1012, a generic monoamine-oxidase inhibitor 694 antidepressant drug 116

Trasicor a brand name for oxprenolol 770

Trasidrex a brand-name preparation containing oxprenolol 770 and cyclopenthiazide 326

Trasylol a brand name for aprotinin, a drug used to promote blood clotting 183

Travasept 100 a brand name for chlorhexidine 268

Travogyn a brand name for isoconazole, an antifungal drug 117

Traxam a brand name for felbinac, a nonsteroidal anti-inflammatory drug 734

Trazodone 1012, a generic antidepressant drug 116

Tremonil a brand name for methixene, an anticholinergic drug 115

Trental a brand name for oxpentifylline, a vasodilator drug 1047

Treosulfan a generic anticancer drug 115

Tretinoin 1013, a generic drug used to treat acne 62

Tri-Adcortyl, Tri-Adcortyl Otic brand-name preparations

containing triamcinolone 1014, gramicidin, an antibiotic drug 114, neomycin 721, and nystatin 741

Triadene a brand-name oral contraceptive 755 containing ethinyloestradiol 416 and gestodene, a progestogen drug 830

TriamaxCo a brand-name preparation containing triamterene 1014 and hydrochlorothiazide 546

Triamcinolone 1014, a generic corticosteroid drug 312

Triamco a brand-name preparation containing triamterene 1014 and hydrochlorothiazide 546

Triamterene 1014, a generic diuretic drug 364

Tribavarin 1014, a generic antiviral drug 120

Tribiotic a brand-name antibacterial preparation 114 containing bacitracin 1114, neomycin 721, and polymyxin B 816

Tri-Cicatrin a brand-name preparation containing bacitracin 1114, hydrocortisone 546, neomycin 721, and nystatin 741

Triclofos a generic sleeping drug 922

Triclosan a type of antiseptic 119

Tridil a brand name for glyceryl trinitrate 488

Trientine a generic chelating agent 256 used to treat Wilson's disease 1083

Trifluoperazine 1015, a generic antipsychotic drug 119

Trifluperidol a generic antipsychotic drug 119

Trilostane a generic drug used in the treatment of Cushing's syndrome 325

Triludan a brand name for terfenadine 977

Trimeprazine 1016, a generic antihistamine drug 118

Trimethoprim 1016, a generic antibacterial drug 114

Tri-Minulet a brand-name oral contraceptive 755 containing ethinyloestradiol 416 and gestodene, a progestogen drug 830

Trimipramine 1016, a generic tricyclic antidepressant drug 114

Trimogal a brand name for trimethoprim 1016

Trimopan a brand name for trimethoprim 1016

Trimovate a brand name for clobetasone, a corticosteroid drug 312

Trinordiol a brand-name oral contraceptive 755 containing ethinyloestradiol 416 and levonorgestrel 635

TriNovum, TriNovum ED brand-name oral contraceptives 755 containing ethinyloestradiol 416 and norethisterone 734

Triogesic a brand-name preparation containing paracetamol 778 and phenylpropanolamine 800

Triominic a brand-name preparation containing pheniramine, an anti-histamine drug 118, and phenylpropanolamine 800

Triperidol a brand name for trifluperidol, an antipsychotic drug 119

Tripotassium dicitratobismuthate a generic ulcer-healing drug 1204

Triprolidine 1016, a generic antihistamine drug 118

Triptafen a brand-name preparation containing amitriptyline 92 and perphenazine 795

Trisequens a brand-name preparation containing oestradiol 749 and norethisterone 734

Tritace a brand name for ramipril, an ACE inhibitor drug 118

Trobicin a brand name for spectinomycin, an antibiotic drug 114

Tropicamide 1018, a generic drug used to dilate the pupil of the eye

Tropisetron a generic antiemetic drug 117

Tropium a brand name for chlordiazepoxide 268

Trosyl a brand name for tioconazole, an antifungal drug 117

Tryptizol a brand name for amitriptyline 92

Tubocurarine a generic muscle-relaxant drug 707 used in general anaesthesia 99

Tuinal a brand-name barbiturate 156 sleeping drug 922

Tulobuterol a generic bronchodilator drug 215

Tylex a brand-name preparation containing codeine 285 and paracetamol 778

Tyrozets a brand-name antiseptic lozenge 119

U

Ubretid a brand name for distigmine, used to treat urinary retention 1031 and myasthenia gravis 710

Ucerax a brand name for hydroxyzine, an antianxiety drug 114 also used to treat pruritus 836

Ukidan a brand name for urokinase 1035

Ultradil Plain a brand-name preparation containing fluocortolone, a corticosteroid drug 312

Ultralanum Plain a brand-name preparation containing fluocortolone, a corticosteroid drug 312

Ultraproct a brand-name preparation containing fluocortolone, a corticosteroid drug 312

Ultratard, Human a brand name for insulin 589

Undecenoic acid, undecenonates generic antifungal preparations 117

Uniflu with Gregovite C a brand-name cough 314 and decongestant preparation 335 containing codeine 285, diphenhydramine 360, paracetamol 778, and phenylephrine 800

Unigest a brand-name antacid drug 111

Unihep a brand name for heparin 527

Uniparin, Uniparin Calcium brand names for heparin 527

Uniphyllin Continus a brand name for theophylline 983

Uniroid-HC a brand-name preparation containing hydrocortisone 546 and cinchocaine, a local anaesthetic 101

Unisept a brand name for chlorhexidine 268

Unisomnia a brand name for nitrazepam 731

Univer a brand name for verapamil 1053

Urea 1028, an ingredient of some preparations for treating dry skin 915

Uriben a brand name for nalidixic acid 716

Urispas a brand name for flavoxate, an anti-spasmodic drug 120 used to treat urinary incontinence 575

Urofollitrophin a generic name for an extract containing follicle-stimulating hormone 454

Urokinase 1035, a generic thrombolytic drug 987

Uromide a brand-name drug used to treat urinary tract infection 1031

Uromitexan a brand name for mesna, used together with certain anticancer drugs 115

Ursodeoxycholic acid a generic drug used to treat gallstones 468

Ursofalk a brand name for ursodeoxycholic acid, a generic drug used to treat gallstones 468

Utinor a brand name for norfloxacin, an antibacterial drug 114

Utovlan a brand name for norethisterone 734

V

Vagifem a brand name for oestradiol 749

Vaginyl a brand name for metronidazole 634

Valenac a brand name for diclofenac 356

Valium a brand name for diazepam 356

Vallergan a brand name for trimeprazine 1016

Valoid a brand name for cyclizine, an antiemetic drug 117

Valproic acid see Sodium valproate 928

Valrox a brand name for naproxen 717

Vancocin a brand name for vancomycin, an antibiotic drug 114

Vancomycin a generic antibiotic drug 114

Vansil a brand name for oxamniquine, used in the treatment of schistosomiasis 889

Variclene a brand-name preparation used to treat leg ulcers 631

Varidase Topical a brand name for streptokinase and streptodornase, used in the treatment of leg ulcers 631

Vasaten a brand name for atenolol 140

Vascace a brand name for cilazapril, an ACE inhibitor drug 61

Vascardin a brand name for isosorbide dinitrate 604

Vaseline Petroleum Jelly an emulsion used to treat dry skin 915

Vasocon A brand-name eye-drops containing antazoline, an anti-histamine drug 118, and naphazoline, used in allergic rhinitis 878

Vasogen a brand-name barrier cream 159

Vasopressin another name for ADH 67, a substance used to treat diabetes insipidus 348

Vasoxine a brand name for methoxamine, a vasoconstrictor drug 1046 used in the treatment of acute hypotension 558

Vecuronium a generic muscle-relaxant drug 707 used in general anaesthesia 99

Veganin a brand-name analgesic preparation containing aspirin 137, paracetamol 778, and codeine 285

Velbe a brand name for vinblastine, an anticancer drug 115

Velosef a brand name for cephradine, a cephalosporin drug 247

Velosulin a brand name for insulin 589

Ventodisks a brand name for salbutamol 885

Ventolin a brand name for salbutamol 885

Vepesid a brand name for etopside, an anticancer drug 115

Veracur a brand-name preparation containing formaldehyde 460

Verapamil 1052, a generic calcium channel blocker 224

Veripaque a brand name for oxyphenisatin, a laxative drug 629

Vermox a brand name for mebendazole 667, an anthelmintic drug 113

Verrugon a brand name for salicylic acid 885

Vertigon a brand name for prochlorperazine 829

Verucasep a brand-name preparation used to treat warts 1074

Vesagex a brand-name antiseptic 119, containing cetrimide

Vibramycin, Vibramycin-D brand names for doxycycline 371

Vicks Cold Cure a brand-name cold remedy 286

Videne a brand-name antiseptic 363 containing povidone-iodine

Vidopen a brand name for ampicillin 94

Vigabatrin a generic anticonvulsant drug 116 used in the treatment of epilepsy 410

Vigranon B a brand name for vitamin B complex 1063

Viloxazine a generic tricyclic antidepressant drug 116

Vinblastine a generic anticancer drug 115

Vincristine a generic anticancer drug 115

Vindesine a generic anticancer drug 115

Vioform-Hydrocortisone a brand-name preparation containing hydro-cortisone 546 and clioquinol

Virazid a brand name for tribavirin 1014, a generic antiviral drug 120

Virormone a brand name for testosterone 979

Virudox a brand name for idoxuridine 562

Visclair a brand name for methylcysteine, a mucolytic drug 701

Viskaldix a brand name preparation containing pindolol 803 and clopamide, a thiazide diuretic drug 364

Visken a brand name for pindolol 803

Vista-Methasone a brand name for betamethasone 165

Vitamin A 1062, essential for growth and fertility

Vitamin B Complex 1063, involved in the function of the nerves, muscles, and heart

Vitamin B$_{12}$ 1063, used in the treatment of pernicious anaemia

Vitamin C 1065, essential for maintenance of healthy bones, teeth, and gums

Vitamin D 1065, essential for strong bones and teeth

Vitmamin E 1065, essential for normal cell structure

Vitamin E Suspension a brand-name preparation containing alpha tocopheryl acetate 1065

Vitamin K 1065, essential for the formation of clotting substances in the blood

Vivalan a brand name for viloxazine, a tricyclic antidepressant drug 116

Volital a brand name for permoline, a central nervous system stimulant drug 947

Volmax a brand name for salbutamol 885

Volraman a brand name for diclofenac 356

Voltarol a brand name for diclofenac 356

W

Warfarin 1074, a generic anticoagulant drug 116

Warticon/Warticon Fem a brand name for podophyllotoxin 813

Waxsol a brand-name drug used to remove earwax 386

Welldorm a brand name for chloral hydrate 268

Wellferon a brand name for interferon 594

X

Xamoterol a generic drug used in the treatment of mild heart failure 519

Xanax a brand name for alprazolam 88

Xanthomax a brand name for allopurinol 87

Xipamide 1089, a generic diuretic drug 364

Xuret a brand name for metolazone 684

Xylocaine a brand name for lignocaine 637

Xylometazoline 1090, a generic decongestant drug 335

Xyloproct a brand-name corticosteroid preparation 312 and local anaesthetic 101

Xylotox a brand name for lignocaine 637

Y

Yomesan a brand name for niclosamide 730

Yutopar a brand name for ritodrine 881

Z

Zaditen a brand name for ketotifen, an antihistamine drug 118 used to prevent asthma attacks 138

Zadstat a brand name for metronidazole 684

Zantac a brand name for ranitidine 857

Zarontin a brand name for ethosuximide 416

Zavedos a brand name for idarubicin, an anticancer drug 115

Zestoretic a brand-name preparation containing lisinopril, an ACE inhibitor drug 61, and hydrochlorothiazide 546

Zestril a brand name for lisinopril, an ACE inhibitor drug 61

Zidovudine 1093, a generic antiviral drug 120

Zimovane a brand name for zopiclone 1094

Zinamide a brand name for pyrazinamide 846

Zinc 1093, an essential mineral

Zincef a brand name for cefuroxime, a cephalosporin drug 247

Zincomed a brand-name zinc supplement 1083

Zinc oxide 1093, a substance used in sunscreens 960 and in some preparations for painful, itchy, or moist skin conditions 915

Zinc sulphate an astringent 139

Zineryt a brand name for erythromycin 416

Zinnat a brand-name cephalosporin drug 247, a type of antibiotic drug 114

Zirtek a brand name for cetirizine, an antihistamine drug 118

Zita a brand name for cimetidine 278

Zithromax a brand name for azithromycin 149, an antibiotic drug 114

Zocor a brand name for simvastatin 913, a lipid-lowering drug 639

Zofran a brand name for ondansetron, an antiemetic drug 117

Zoladex a brand name for goserelin, an anticancer drug 115

Zopiclone a generic sleeping drug 922

Zoton a brand name for lansoprazole, used in the treatment of peptic ulcer 789 and reflux oesophagitis 747

Zovirax a brand name for acyclovir 66

Z Span a brand-name zinc supplement 1093

Zuclopenthixol a generic antipsychotic drug 119

Zumenon a brand name for oestradiol 749

Zydol a brand name for tramadol, an analgesic drug 102

Zyloric a brand name for allopurinol 87

INDEX

This index covers the three major parts of the encyclopedia: **Health and Medicine Today;** the **A to Z of Health and Medicine**; and the **Drug Glossary**.

Index entries begin with either a capital or a lower-case letter. Most index entries with an initial capital correspond to titles of entries in the **A to Z of Health and Medicine** or to sections in **Health and Medicine Today**. Other index entries with an initial capital refer you to a **Drug Glossary** entry. With the exception of a few capitalized abbreviations or eponyms, all other index entries have a lower-case first letter.

Index entries that correspond to the titles of encyclopedia entries usually refer you to the page on which the encyclopedia entry starts. (In the case of encyclopedia entries that are simple cross-references to other encyclopedia entries, the index refers you directly to the cross-referenced entries or to major index entries.) Other index entries and all index subentries refer you to the title of an encyclopedia entry or to an illustration title, accompanied by a page number. This number refers to the page where the index topic appears.

Index entries, subentries, or page numbers in *italic* type refer you to illustrations.

A

Abdomen 50
  fluid in: Ascites 136
  removal of fluid from:
    Paracentesis 777
  surgical opening of:
    Laparotomy, exploratory 624
Abdomen, acute 50
abdominal incisions 575
abdominal organs, reversed:
  and Dextrocardia 347
  medical term: Situs inversus 914
Abdominal pain 50
  diagnosing abdominal pain 55
  symptom charts 51, 53
Abdominal swelling 55
  symptom chart 56
Abdominal X-ray 55
abdominoplasty:
  Body contour surgery 190
Abducent nerve 55
  functions of cranial nerves 318
Abduction 55
  descriptive terms in anatomy 104
Abidec 1096
Ablation 57
Abnormality 57
ABO blood classification:
  Blood groups 186
Abortifacient 57
Abortion 57
  spontaneous: Miscarriage 690
Abortion, induced 57
abrasion:
  type of Wound 1086
Abrasion, dental 58
Abreaction 58
Abscess 58
  and Pus 847
Abscess, dental 59
Absence 59
  feature of Epilepsy 411

absorption of nutrients:
  by Digestive system 357;
    Ileum 563
  the digestive process 358
Acanthosis nigricans 59
  causing Pigmentation 803
Acarbose 59
Accessory nerve 59
  functions of cranial nerves 318
Accidental death 59, *60*
Accident-proneness 60
accidents:
  Accidental death 59, *60*
  Accident-proneness 60
  causing Eye injuries 425
  Falls in the elderly 433
  Health hazards 513
  Safety measures 17
acclimatization:
  and Heat disorders 524
Accommodation 60
  and Eye 422; Vision 1052
  loss of: Presbyopia 827
  testing of: *vision tests 1055*
Accupro 1096
Accuretic 1096
Acebutolol 60
ACE inhibitor drugs 61
  effect on Angiotensin 108;
    Renin 868
  examples of: Captopril 231;
    Enalapril 398
  group of Vasodilator drugs 1047
Acemetacin 1096
Acepril 1096
acetabulum:
  part of Hip 534; Pelvis 787
Acetazolamide 61
Acetic acid 61
Acetohexamide 61
Acetomenaphthone 1096
acetone:
  inhalation of: Solvent abuse 928
  excess: Ketosis 612
Acetoxyl 1096
Acetylcholine 61
  action of: Muscle 706; *how neurotransmitters work 729*
  type of Neurotransmitter 729

Acetylcysteine 61
Acezide 1096
Achalasia 61
  causing Swallowing difficulty 963
Achilles tendon 61
  Tendon 975
Achlorhydria 62
Achondroplasia 62
  and Short stature 908
Achromycin 1096
Acid 62
  causes of tooth decay 238
    Decalcification, dental 334;
    Plaque, dental 808
  excess: Peptic ulcer 789;
    Zollinger-Ellison syndrome 1094
  in eye: *disorders of the cornea 308*
  and pH 797
Acid-base balance 62
  regulation of: Kidney 615
Acidosis 62
  causes of: Hypercapnia 548;
    Lactic acid 623
Acid reflux 62
  causes of: Hiatus hernia 533;
    Pregnancy 823
  causing Heartburn 518
acid regurgitation:
  see index entry Acid reflux
Acipimox 1096
Acitretin 1096
Aclacin 1096
Aclarubicin 1096
Acne 62, *63*
  and Sebaceous glands 895
  symptom of: Pimple 803
  treatment of: Isotretinoin 604;
    Tretinoin 1013; Vitamin supplements 1066
Acnecide 1096
Acnegel 1096
Acnidazil 1096
Acnisal 1096
Acoustic nerve 63
  functions of cranial nerves 318
  part of Vestibulocochlear nerve 1054
  testing of: Hearing tests 513

Acoustic neuroma 63
acquired immune deficiency syndrome (AIDS):
  see index entry AIDS
Acrivastine 1096
Acrocyanosis 64
Acrodermatitis enteropathica 64
Acromegaly 64
  cause of: Pituitary tumours 805
Acromioclavicular joint 64
  part of Shoulder 909
acromion:
  and Acromioclavicular joint 64; Shoulder 909
  part of Scapula 889
Acroparaesthesia 64
Acrosoxacin 64
Actal 1096
ACTH 64
  abnormal production of:
    Addison's disease 66;
    Cushing's syndrome 325;
    disorders of the adrenal glands 71; endocrine disorders 402
  normal production of:
    endocrine system 401;
    hormonal system 543;
    Pituitary gland 804
Actifed Compound 1096
Actilyse 1096
actin:
  constituent of Muscle 706
Actinac 1096
Acting out 65
  to achieve Catharsis 241
  and Play therapy 810;
    Psychodrama 839; Role-playing 881
Actinic 65
actinic keratopathy:
  associated with Sunlight, adverse effects of 960
  a disorder of the cornea 308
  type of Keratopathy 611
ACTINOMYCETES bacteria:
  causing Actinomycosis 65;
    Mycetoma 711
Actinomycin D 1096
Actinomycosis 65
  a disorder of the lung 649

Actonorm 1096
Actraphane 1096
Actrapid 1096
Actron 1096
Acuity, visual:
  see index entry Visual acuity
Acupan 1096
Acupressure 65
Acupuncture 65
  and role of Endorphins 403
Acute 66
acute mountain sickness (AMS):
  Mountain sickness 697
acute ulcerative gingivitis:
  see index entry Gingivitis,
    acute ulcerative
Acyclovir 66
  in treatment of Cold sore 287;
    Herpes, genital 532; Herpes
    zoster 533
Adalat 1096
Adalat Retard 1096
Adam's apple 66
  part of Larynx 626
  and Vocal cords 1066
Adcortyl 1096
Addiction 66
  and Alcohol dependence 82;
    Drug dependence 377
Addison's disease 66
  a *disorder of the adrenal glands*
    71; endocrine disorder 402
Adduction 66
  and *descriptive terms in anatomy*
    104
adenine:
  as constituent of Nucleic acids
    737
  and *what genes are and what*
    they do 474
  structure of DNA 39
Adenitis 66
Adenocarcinoma 67
  type of Lung cancer 649
Adenoidectomy 67
Adenoids 67
  anatomy of: Nasopharynx
    718
  and Otitis media 766; Sleep
    apnoea 922
  removal of: Adenoidectomy
    67
Adenoma 67
adenoma sebaceum:
  and Tuberous sclerosis 1019
Adenomatosis 67
adenosine diphosphate (ADP):
  ADP 69
adenosine triphosphate (ATP):
  see index entry ATP
adenovirus:
  causing Pneumonia 811
  viruses and disease 1056
Adexolin 1096
ADH 67
  deficiency of: Urination,
    excessive 1032
  excess: SIADH 910
  function of: Urine 1034; Water
    1075
  production of: *endocrine system*
    401; hormonal system 543;
    Pituitary gland 804

Adhesion 67
  causing Intestine, obstruction
    of 596
  following Peritonitis 794
  type of Scar 889
adhesive bandages:
  Dressings 373
Adie's pupil:
  Pupil 846
Adie's syndrome:
  and Mydriasis 711
Adifax 1096
Adipose tissue 68
  Tissue 995
Adizem 1096
Adjuvant 68
Adlerian theory 68
Adolescence 68
ADP 69
Adrenal failure 69
Adrenal glands 69
  and Corticosteroid drugs 312
  disorders of: *disorders of the*
    adrenal glands 71; endocrine
    disorders 402
  part of *endocrine system 401;*
    hormonal system 543
Adrenal hyperplasia, congenital
    70
  causing Pseudohermaphro-
    ditism 836
Adrenaline 70
  abnormal secretion of:
    Phaeochromocytoma 797
  photomicrograph of adrenaline 43
  in treatment of Anaphylactic
    shock 103; Insect stings 588
Adrenal tumours 70
Adrenocorticotrophic hormone
    (ACTH):
  see index entry ACTH
Adrenogenital syndrome:
  see index entry Adrenal
    hyperplasia, congenital
Adriamycin 1096
AEDES mosquitoes:
  Mosquito bites 696
  transmission of Yellow fever
    1092
AeroBec 1096
Aerobic 71
  and Oxygen 770
Aerobics 71
  and Exercise 419; Exercise and
    fitness 17; Exercise and
    health 20–21; Fitness 451;
    Training 1009
Aerocrom 1096
Aerodontalgia 72
Aerolin 1096
Aerophagy 72
  causing Belching 163;
    Flatulence 452
aerosols:
  CFCs in : Ozone 770;
    Pollution 815
  inhalation of: Solvent abuse
    928
  medical use of: Inhaler 584;
    Vaporizer 1044
Aetiology 72
Affect 72
  abnormal: Psychosis 840

Affective disorders 72
Affinity 72
Aflatoxin 72
  and Fungi 465; Nutritional
    disorders 740
Afrazine 1096
Afterbirth 72
  medical term: Placenta 806
Afterpains 72
agammaglobulinaemia:
  type of Immunodeficiency
    disorder 571
Agar 73
Agarol 1096
Age 73
  see also index entry Aging
Agenesis 73
Agent 73
Agent Orange 73
Age spots 73
Ageusia 73
  common term: Taste, loss of
    970
Aggregation, platelet 73
Aggression 73
  and Inferiority complex 581
Aging 74
  and Age 73; Cancer 228;
    Osteoporosis 764, 765
  Keeping healthy 16
  Exercise in later life 21
Agitation 75
Agnosia 75
Agoraphobia 75
  and Panic attack 777; Vertigo
    1053
  type of Phobia 800
Agraphia 75
Ague 75
  and Malaria 657
AIDS 48, 76
  associated with Haemophilia
    501
  causes of: *causes and prevention*
    of AIDS 78; HIV 537
  and development of Fungal
    infections 464; Kaposi's
    sarcoma 610; Pneumocystis
    pneumonia 811;
    Toxoplasmosis 1006
  effect on *the adaptive immune*
    system 568
  prevention of: *causes and*
    prevention of AIDS 78; Safer
    sex 885
  transmission of: Blood
    transfusion 189
  treatment of: Zidovudine
    (AZT) 1093
AIDS-related complex 79
  see also index entry AIDS
Air 79
Air conditioning 79
  and Legionnaires' disease 630;
    Sick building syndrome 911
air conduction:
  in Hearing 513
  testing of: *types of hearing test*
    514
Air embolism 79
  type of Embolism 394
air-fluidized therapy units:
  care of burn patients 218

Air pollution:
  Pollution 815
air pressure:
  and Aviation medicine 148;
    Eustachian tube 417
  changes of: Barotrauma 159;
    Mountain sickness 697
Air swallowing:
  see index entry Aerophagy
air travel:
  and Aviation medicine 148
  causing Barotrauma 159
  conditions affecting passenger
    suitability for air travel 148
Airway 79
Airway obstruction 79
Akathisia 80
Akinesia 80
akinetic seizure:
  common term: Drop attack 373
Akineton 1096
Albendazole 1096
Albinism 80
  symptoms of: Nystagmus 741;
    Pallor 774; Pigmentation 803
Albumin 80
  production of: Liver 641
  type of Plasma protein 809
Albuminuria 80
Alclometasone 1096
Alcobon 1096
Alcohol 80
  alcohol and the body 81
  alcohol and pregnancy 82
  consumption 16
    and Heatstroke 526; Noc-
    turia 732; Sleep apnoea 922
  Smoking and drinking 22–23
  see also index entries Alcohol
    dependence; Alcohol
    intoxication; Alcohol-related
    disorders
Alcohol dependence 82
  Alcoholics Anonymous 83
  associated with Child abuse
    260; Suicide 958; Suicide,
    attempted 958
  leading to Delirium tremens
    337; Dementia 338;
    Wernicke-Korsakoff
    syndrome 1081
  see also index entries Alcohol;
    Alcohol intoxication;
    Alcohol-related disorders;
    alcohol withdrawal
Alcoholics Anonymous 83
Alcohol intoxication 83
  alcohol and the body 81
  and Drowning 374; Hangover
    506
  see also index entries Alcohol;
    Alcohol-related disorders
Alcoholism:
  see index entry Alcohol
    dependence
Alcohol-related disorders 84
  and Alcohol consumption 16;
    Smoking and drinking
    22–23
  examples: Cardiomyopathy
    235; Cirrhosis 279; Dementia
    338; Encephalopathy 399;
    Fetal alcohol syndrome 440;

Alcohol-related disorders
(continued)
Gastritis 470; *disorders of the liver 645;* Liver disease, alcoholic 643; Neuropathy 728; Pancreas, cancer of 775; Pancreatitis 776; Wernicke-Korsakoff syndrome 1081
see also index entries: Alcohol dependence; Alcohol intoxication
alcohol withdrawal:
Alcoholics Anonymous 83
causing Delirium tremens 337; Epilepsy 410; Withdrawal syndrome 1084
see also index entry Alcohol dependence
Alcuronium 1096
Aldactide 1096
Aldactone 1097
Aldesleukin 1097
Aldomet 1097
Aldosterone 84
and Angiotensin 108; Renin 868; Urine 1034
effect on Kidney 615
excess: Conn's syndrome 297
Aldosteronism 84
see also index entry Aldosterone
Alexan 1097
Alexander technique 85
Alexia 85
Alfacalcidol 1097
Alfa D 1097
Alfentanil 1097
Algicon 1097
alginate:
use of: Antacid drugs 111; Impression, dental 574
Alginate 1097
Alginic acid 1097
Algitec 1097
Alienation 85
Alignment, dental 85
Alimentary tract 85
see also index entry Digestive system
Alimix 1097
Alkali 85
in eye: *disorders of the cornea 308*
and pH 797
alkaline phosphatase:
abnormal blood levels of: Paget's disease 772
measurement of: *liver-funtion tests 644*
Alkaloids 85
Alkalosis 85
cause of: Hyperventilation 554
and pH 797
Alka-Seltzer 1097
Alkeran 1097
Alkylating agents 85
Allantoin 1097
Allbee with C 1097
Allegron 1097
alleles:
and Gene 473; Inheritance 585
Aller-eze 1097

allergen:
allergy and the body 86
and Sensitization 899
see also index entry Allergy
allergic reaction:
see index entry Allergy
allergic rhinitis:
Rhinitis, allergic 878
Allergy 85
allergy and the body 86
causing Anaphylactic shock 103; Asthma 138; Conjunctivitis 296; Rhinitis, allergic 878; Urticaria 1035
to Cephalosporins 247; Drug 376; Insect bites 587
Food allergy 455
and Hypersensitivity 551; Immune system 566
treatment of: Antihistamine drugs 118; Corticosteroid drugs 312; Hyposensitization 557; Triprolidine 1016
see also index entry allergen
Alloferin 1097
allografting:
Grafting 491
Allopathy 87
Allopurinol 87
in treatment of Arthritis 132
Allyloestrenol 1097
Almodan 1097
Alomide 1097
Alopecia 87
treatment of: Minoxidil 689
Alophen 1097
alpha₁-antitrypsin:
and Emphysema 398
type of Globulin 485
alpha chains:
and Thalassaemia 982
Alphaderm 1097
Alpha-fetoprotein 88
and Amniocentesis 39
in diagnosis of Down's syndrome 371; Liver cancer 642; Spina bifida 934
type of Tumour-specific antigen 1020
alpha particles:
type of Radiation 851
Alpha tocopheryl acetate 1097
Alphavase 1097
Alphodith 1097
Alphosyl 1097
Alprazolam 88
Alprostadil 1097
Alrheumat 1097
ALS (amyotrophic lateral sclerosis):
type of Motor neuron disease 696
Altacite 1097
Alteplase 1097
Alternative medicine 88
and Ethics, medical 416; Folk medicine 454
Altitude sickness:
alternative term: Mountain sickness 697
Alu-Cap 1097
Aludroxgel 1097

Aludrox SA 1097
Aluhyde 1097
Aluminium 88
Aluminium acetate 1097
aluminium chloride 89
aluminium hydroxide 89
Alupent 1097
Alvedon 1097
Alveolectomy:
Alveoloplasty 89
Alveolitis 89
Alveoloplasty 89
Alveolus, dental 89
Alveolus, pulmonary 89
damage to: Emphysema 397
part of Lung 648; Respiratory system 870
Alvercol 1097
Alverine 1097
Alzheimer's disease 90
causing Dementia 338
role of Neurotransmitter 729
treatment of: Tetrahydroaminoacridine 981
Amalgam, dental 90
constituent of: Mercury 681
in treatment of Caries, dental 236
use of: Filling, dental 449
Amantadine 90
in treatment of Influenza 584
Amaurosis fugax 91
Ambaxin 1097
Ambidexterity 91
and Handedness 506
AmBisome 1097
Amblyopia 91
causes of: Ptosis 841; Squint 942; deficiency of Vitamin B complex 1063
a *disorder of the eye 426*
treatment of: Occlusion 743
Ambulance 91
Amelogenesis imperfecta 91
effect on Calcification, dental 223
Amenorrhoea 91
a *disorder of menstruation 678*
Amethocaine 1097
Amfipen 1097
Amikacin 1097
Amikin 1097
Amil-Co 1097
Amilmaxco 1097
Amiloride 92
Amilospare 1097
Amino acids 92
as constituent of Proteins 834
constituent of: Nitrogen 732
metabolism of: Liver 642
as source of Urea 1028
Aminobenzoic acid 1097
Aminoglutethimide 92
Aminoglycoside drugs 92
side-effect of: Ototoxicity 767
types of Antibiotic drugs 114
Aminophylline 92
Aminosalicylic acid 1097
Amiodarone 92
Amitriptyline 92
Amix 1097
Amlodipine 92

Ammonia 92
from breakdown of Urine 1034
Ammonium chloride 1097
Amnesia 92
Amniocentesis 39, 92
and Genetic counselling 476
in diagnosis of Down's syndrome 371; Rhesus incompatibility 875
and Genetic analysis 39
using Ultrasound scanning 1025
Amnion 93
Amnioscopy 93
Amniotic fluid 93
analysis of: Amniocentesis 39, 92
deficiency of: Oligohydramnios 750
Amniotic sac 93
and Embryo 395
Amniotomy 93
Amnivent 1097
amoeba:
causing Colitis 287
see also index entry Amoebiasis
Amoebiasis 93
cause of: Protozoa 836
causing Liver abscess 642; Rectal bleeding 862
prevalence of: *prevalence of amoebic dysentery 381*
treatment of: Amoebicides 94; Metronidazole 684
type of Dysentery 381
Amoebic dysentery:
see index entry Amoebiasis
Amoebicides 94
Amoram 1097
Amorolfine 1097
Amoxapine 94
Amoxil 1097
Amoxycillin 94
Amoxymed 1097
Amphetamine drugs 94
causing Schizophrenia 890
and Withdrawal syndrome 1084
Amphotericin B 94
in treatment of Cryptococcosis 323; Sporotrichosis 940
Ampicillin 94
Ampiclox 1097
amplifier:
in Hearing aids 513
ampulla of Vater:
anatomy of: Biliary system 168; Duodenum 379; Pancreas 775
Amputation 94
leading to Phantom limb 798
in treatment of Osteosarcoma 765; Peripheral vascular disease 793
treatment of: Limb, artificial 637; *types of artificial limb 638;* Prosthesis 834
Amputation, congenital 94
Amputation, traumatic 95
Amrit 1097

AMS (acute mountain sickness):
Mountain sickness 697
Amsacrine 1097
Amsidine 1097
amygdala:
part of Limbic system 637
amylase:
constituent of Saliva 886
function of: *the digestive process 358*
Amylobarbitone 1097
Amyloidosis 95
causing Nephrotic syndrome 722
as complication of Familial Mediterranean fever 434; Rheumatoid arthritis, juvenile 878; Osteomyelitis 763
Amyotrophic lateral sclerosis:
type of Motor neuron disease 696
Amyotrophy 95
Amytal 1097
anabolic effect:
of Androgen hormones 105; Steroids, anabolic 946
Anabolic steroids:
Steroids, anabolic 946
anabolism:
in Biochemistry 169; Metabolism 682
Anacal 1097
Anadin 1097
Anadin Extra, Anadin Extra Soluble 1097
Anadin Ibuprofen 1097
Anaemia 95
types and causes of anaemia 96
causes of: Hookworm infestation 541; Spherocytosis, hereditary 932; deficiency of Vitamin B complex 1063; deficiency of Vitamin C 1065; deficiency of Vitamin E 1065
and Hypersplenism 551; Rheumatoid arthritis 876
symptoms of: Glossitis 487; Pallor 774
Anaemia, aplastic 96
Anaemia, haemolytic 97
types and causes of anaemia 96
see also index entry Haemolytic disease of the newborn
Anaemia, iron-deficiency 97
types and causes of anaemia 96
Anaemia, megaloblastic 98
types and causes of anaemia 96
Anaemia, pernicious 99
anaemia, sickle cell:
Sickle cell anaemia 911
Anaerobic 99
anaerobic exercise:
in Training 1009
Anaesthesia 99
complications of: Sickle cell anaemia 911
see also index entries Epidural anaesthesia; Spinal anaesthesia
Anaesthesia, dental 99

Anaesthesia, general 99
techniques for general anaesthesia 100
development of: *landmarks in medicine: surgery 670*
operating theatre 753
Anaesthesia, local 101
see also index entries EMLA; Epidural anaesthesia; Spinal anaesthesia
Anaesthetics 102
Anafranil, Anafranil SR 1097
Anal dilatation 102
Anal discharge 102
anal disorders:
disorders of the anus 121
examples: Anal fissure 102; Anal fistula 102; Anal stenosis 103; Anus, cancer of 121; Anus, imperforate 121; Crohn's disease 320; Haemorrhoids 501; Threadworm infestation 985
symptoms of: Itching 604; Rectal bleeding 862
Analeptic drugs 102
Anal fissure 102
a disorder of the anus 121
symptom of: Rectal bleeding 862
Anal fistula 102
a disorder of the anus 121
and Rectal bleeding 862
Analgesia 102
see also index entry Analgesic drugs
Analgesic drugs 102
how analgesics work 103
examples: Aspirin 137; Benorylate 163; Codeine 285; Heroin 536; Ibuprofen 562; Methadone 683; Morphine 695; Narcotic drugs 717; Nonsteroidal anti-inflammatory drugs 734; Opium 754; Paracetamol 778; Pentazocine 789; Pethidine 796; Sodium salicylate 928
overuse causing Headache 507
anal itching:
a disorder of the anus 121
Itching 604
anal phase:
and Fixation 452; Psychoanalytic theory 838
anal sphincter:
Sphincter 933
Anal stenosis 103
a disorder of the anus 121
Anal stricture:
see index entry Anal stenosis
anal tags:
type of Skin tag 918
Analysis, chemical 103
Analysis, psychological:
Psychoanalysis 838
Anaphylactic shock 103
and Allergy 85; Hypersensitivity 551
causes of: Hyposensitization 557; Insect stings 588
type of Shock 907

anaphylactoid purpura:
alternative term: Henoch-Schönlein purpura 527
Anapolon 50 1097
anasarca:
alternative term: Oedema 745
Anastomosis 104
Anatomy 104
Anatomy and pathology 28
Ancylostomiasis:
alternative term: Hookworm infestation 540
Andrews Answer 1097
Andrews Antacid 1097
Androcur 1097
Androgen drugs 104
Androgen hormones 105
Anectine 1097
Anencephaly 105
diagnosis of: Ultrasound scanning 1024
and Neural tube defect 725
Anestan 1097
Anethaine 1097
Aneurysm 105
treatment of: Arterial reconstructive surgery 130; Neurosurgery 728
types of aneurysm 106
Anexate 1097
Angel dust 106
Angettes-75 1097
Angiitis:
type of Vasculitis 1045
Angilol 1097
Angina 106
Angina pectoris 106
a disorder of the heart 517; disorder of muscle 707
symptom of: Chest pain 251
treatment of: Beta-blocker drugs 164; Calcium channel blockers 224; Isosorbide 604; Nadolol 716; Nifedipine 730; Nitrate drugs 731; Pindolol 803; Propranolol 831; Vasodilator drugs 1047
Angioedema 107
associated with Urticaria 1035
treatment of: Chlorpheniramine 269
angiogram:
see index entry Angiography
Angiography 107, *108*
in diagnosis of Subarachnoid haemorrhage 955
type of Contrast X-ray 32
type of: Digital subtraction angiography 32
uses of: Neurology 726; Kidney imaging 616
Angioma 108
causing Subarachnoid haemorrhage 955
angioneurotic oedema:
alternative term: Angioedema 107
Angiopine 1098
Angioplasty, balloon 108
procedure for balloon angioplasty 109
use of: Heart surgery 522

Angiotensin 108
and Kidney 615; Renin 868; Vasodilator drugs 1047
angiotensin-converting enzyme (ACE) inhibitors:
ACE inhibitor drugs 61
Angiozem 1098
Anhidrosis 109
Anhydrol Forte 1098
Animal experimentation 109
Animals, diseases from:
Zoonosis 1094
anion:
and Acid 62
type of Ion 601
Anisometropia 110
a disorder of the eye 426
Anistreplase 1098
Ankle joint 110
and Clonus 283
disorders of: Pott's fracture 821; Sprain 941
ankles, swollen:
feature of Pregnancy 823; Oedema 746
ankyloglossia:
alternative term: Tongue-tie 1001
Ankylosing spondylitis 110
treatment of: Indomethacin 576; Ketoprofen 612
and Sacroiliitis 884
a disorder of the spine 938
Ankylosis 110
Anodesyn 1098
Anodontia 110
Anomaly 111
ANOPHELES mosquitoes:
Mosquito bites 696
transmission of Malaria 657
Anorexia 111
alternative term: Appetite, loss of 127
Anorexia nervosa 111
and Bulimia 217
symptoms of: Lanugo hair 624; Weight loss 1080
Anorgasmia 111
common term: Frigidity 463
feature of Psychosexual dysfunction 840
Anosmia 111
absence of Smell 925
anovulation:
causing Infertility 581
Anoxia 111
and Hypoxia 560
Anquil 109
Antabuse 1098
Antacid drugs 111
example: Sodium bicarbonate 927
in treatment of Hiatus hernia 533
Antazoline 1098
Antenatal care 112
Antenatal screening 113
see also index entry Pregnancy
Antenatal screening *112*, 113
types of screening tests 25
antenatal surgery:
in treatment of Heart disease, congenital 517

Antepartum haemorrhage 113
Antepsin 1098
Anterior 113
    alternative term: Ventral 1051
Anthelmintic drugs 113
    examples: Mebendazole 667;
        Niclosamide 730; Piperazine
        804; Praziquantel 821;
        Pyrantel 848; Thiabendazole
        984
    in treatment of Hookworm
        infestation 540; Threadworm
        infestation 985; Whipworm
        infestation 1082
    *drugs used to treat worm
        infestations 1086*
Anthisan 1098
Anthracosis 113
Anthranol 1098
Anthrax 113
Antianxiety drugs 114
    examples: Alprazolam 88;
        Chlordiazepoxide 268;
        Diazepam 356; Lorazepam
        647; Meprobamate 681
    and Psychopharmacology 840
Antiarrhythmic drugs 114
    examples:Amiodarone 92;
        Disopyramide 364;
        Mexiletine 685;
        Procainamide 840;
        Tocainide 999
Antibacterial drugs 114
    examples: Nitrofurantoin, 732;
        Sulphonamide drugs 959;
        Trimethoprim 1016
    see also index entry Antibiotic
        drugs
Antibiotic drugs 114
    examples: Aminoglycoside
        drugs 92; Ampicillin 94;
        Cefaclor 244; Cephalexin
        246; Cephalosporin drugs
        247; Chloramphenicol 265;
        Clindamycin 282; Cloxacillin
        253; Colistin 287; Doxy-
        cycline 371; Erythromycin
        416; Gentamicin 480;
        Metronidazole 684;
        Minocycline 689; Nalidixic
        acid 716; Oxytetracycline
        770; Penicillin drugs 788;
        Polymyxins 816;
        Tetracycline drugs 981;
        Tobramycin 998
    see also index entry
        Antibacterial drugs
Antibody 115
    alternative term:
        Immunoglobulin 571
    as constituent of Serum 901
    in diagnosis of Infectious
        disease 585
    function of: Immune response
        566; Immune system 566; *the
        adaptive immune system 568;
        the innate immune system 567*
    and Immunization 569; How
        immunization works 26;
        Immunodeficiency disorders
        571; Immunotherapy 572;
        Plasmapheresis 809; Vaccine
        1040

    production of: Lymphocyte
        653
    use of: Gamma-globulin 468;
        Immunoassay 570;
        Radioimmunoassay 853;
        Serology 901
Antibody, monoclonal 115
    production of: *landmarks in
        medicine: diagnosis 669*
    use of: Immunotherapy 572
Anticancer drugs 115
    examples: Aminoglutethimide
        92; Chlorambucil 268;
        Cisplatin 281;
        Cyclophosphamide 326;
        Doxorubicin 371;
        Mercaptopurine 681;
        Methotrexate 684;
        Procarbazine 829
    in treatment of Leukaemia 632;
        Lung cancer 649
Anticholinergic drugs 115
    examples: Atropine 143;
        Hyoscine 547
Anticoagulant drugs 116
    examples: Heparin 226;
        Warfarin 1074
    use of: Heart valve surgery
        523; Thrombectomy 986;
        Thrombosis 987
Anticonvulsant drugs 116
    examples: Ethosuximide 417;
        Phenobarbitone 799;
        Phenytoin 800; Primidone
        829; Sodium valproate 928
Antidepressant drugs 116
    examples: Maprotiline 662;
        Nortriptyline 734;
        Phenelzine 799;
        Protriptyline 836;
        Tranylcypromine 1012;
        Trazodone 1012;
        Trimipramine 1016
    and Psychopharmacology 840
Antidiarrhoeal drugs 116
    examples: Kaolin 610;
        Loperamide 647
    see also index entry ORT
Antidiuretic hormone (ADH):
    see index entry ADH
Antidote 117
Anti-D(Rh$_o$) immunoglobulin
    117
    in prevention of Haemolytic
        disease of the newborn 500
    and Rhesus incompatibility
        875
Antiemetic drugs 117
    examples: Metoclopramide
        684; Prochlorperazine 829
Antifreeze poisoning 117
Antifungal drugs 117
    examples: Clotrimazole 283;
        Ketoconazole 612;
        Miconazole 685; Nystatin
        741; Tolnaftate 1000
Antigen 118
    and Immune response 566;
        Immune system 566; *the
        adaptive immune system 568;
        the innate immune system 567*;
        Immunoassay 570;
        Immunoglobulins 571;

    Serology 901; Tissue-typing
        997
Antihaemophilic factor 1098
Antihistamine drugs 118
    examples: Chlorpheniramine
        269; Promethazine 831;
        Terfenadine 977;
        Trimeprazine 1016;
        Triprolidine 1016
    and Histamine 536
    in treatment of Conjunctivitis
        296; Rhinitis, allergic 878
Antihypertensive drugs 118
    examples: Captopril 231;
        Hydralazine 545;
        Methyldopa 684
Anti-inflammatory drugs 118
antimalarial drugs:
    examples: Chloroquine 269;
        Quinine 849
    Malaria 657
    and Travel immunization 1012
anti-oestrogen drug:
    example: Tamoxifen 968
antioxidants:
    types of Food additives 455
Antiperspirant 118
    constituent of: Aluminium 88
Antipressan 1098
Antipsychotic drugs 119
    examples: Chlorpromazine
        269; Haloperidol 505;
        Perphenazine 795;
        Thioridazine 984;
        Trifluoperazine 1015
    and Psychopharmacology 840
Antipyretic drugs 119
Antirheumatic drugs 119
    examples: Chloroquine 269;
        Penicillamine 788
Antiseptics 119
    examples: Hydrogen peroxide
        546; Iodine 600; Potassium
        permanganate 820
    and Sterilization 945
Antiserum 119
antisocial behaviour:
    and Acting out 65
    see also index entry Antisocial
        Personality disorder
Antisocial personality disorder
    119
    and Somatization disorder 928;
        Suicide 958
    type of Personality disorder
        795
Antispasmodic drugs 120
    examples: Atropine 143;
        Propantheline 831
antithrombin:
    and Blood clotting 183
Antitoxin 120
Antitussive drugs 120
    alternative term: Cough
        remedies 316
Antivenom 120
    in treatment of Jellyfish stings
        607; Scorpion stings 893;
        Snakebites 926; Venomous
        bites and stings 1050
Antiviral drugs 120
    examples: Acyclovir 67;
        Amantadine 90; Idoxuridine

    562; Interferon 594;
        Zidovudine 1093
Antral irrigation 120
Anturan 1098
Anugesic-HC 1098
Anuria 120
    feature of Kidney failure 614
    and Urine, abnormal 1034
Anus 121
    and Rectum 863
    see also index entry anal
        disorders
Anus, cancer of 121
Anus, imperforate 121
    and Rectum 863
    treatment of: Plastic surgery
        809
Anusol-HC 1098
Anxiety 121
    causing Chest pain 257;
        Insomnia 589; Irritable bowel
        syndrome 603; Night terror
        731; Panic attack 777; Sleep-
        walking 923; Torticollis 1003
    treatment of: Relaxation
        techniques 867
    see also index entry
        Antianxiety drugs
Anxiety disorders 122
Aorta 122
    abnormalities of: *types of
        congenital heart disease 518;*
        Marfan's syndrome 662
    *location and structure of the aorta
        123*
    part of Circulatory system 279,
        280
Aortic incompetence 122
    and *disorders of the heart 517*
Aortic stenosis 123
Aortitis 124
Aortography 124
Apap 1097
Aperient 124
    type of Laxative drug 629
Apgar score 124
    in assessment of Newborn 729
Aphakia 124
Aphasia 124
    type of Speech disorder 930
Apheresis 125
    and Blood donation 184
Aphonia 125
    common term: Voice, loss of
        1066
Aphrodisiacs 125
aphthous ulcer:
    Ulcer, aphthous 1023
Apicectomy 125
Aplasia 125
Aplastic anaemia:
    Anaemia, aplastic 96
Apnoea 125
Apocrine gland 125
    type of Sweat gland 963
Apolipoprotein 125
    and Alzheimer's disease 90
Aponeurosis 125
    and Tendon 975
Apoplexy 125
    modern term: Stroke 952
Apothecary 126
APP 1098

Appendicectomy 126
Appendicitis 126
  causing Pelvic infection 786;
    Peritonitis 794
  treatment of: Appendicectomy
    126
Appendix 127
  removal of: Appendicectomy
    126
  see also index entry
    Appendicitis
Appetite 127
  and Hypothalamus 558
Appetite, loss of 127
  and Anorexia nervosa 111
Appetite stimulants 127
Appetite suppressants 127
  example: Amphetamine drugs
    94
Apraxia 127
Apresoline 1098
Aprinox 1098
Aprotinin 1098
Apsifen 1098
Apsin VK 1098
Apsolol 1098
Apsolox 1098
aptitude testing:
  part of Psychometry 839
APUD cell tumour 128
Aquadrate 1098
aqueous humour:
  part of Eye 423
arachidonic acid:
  type of Fatty acid 436
Arachis oil 1098
Arachnodactyly 128
  feature of Marfan's syndrome
    662
Arachnoiditis 128
arachnoid mater:
  layer of Meninges 675
  tumour of: Meningioma 675
arachnoid tumour:
  type of Meningioma 675
Aramine 1098
arboviruses:
  and Insects and disease 587
Arbralene 1098
ARC:
  abbreviation for AIDS-related
    complex 79
arcus juvenilis:
  and Arcus senilis 128
Arcus senilis 128
Aredia 1098
Arelix 1098
areola:
  part of Breast 204; Nipple 731
Argipressin 1098
Argyll Robertson pupil:
  Pupil 846
arm:
  bones of: Humerus 542;
    Radius 856; Ulna 1024
  disorders of: Humerus,
    fracture of 542; Radius,
    fracture of 856; Shoulder,
    dislocation of 909; Shoulder-
    hand syndrome 910; Ulna,
    fracture of 1024
  joints of: Elbow 391; Shoulder
    909; Wrist 1088

and *movement* 699
  muscles of: Biceps muscle 166;
    Triceps muscle 1014
Aromatherapy 128
Arousal 128
Arpicolin 1098
Arpimycin 1098
Arret 1098
Arrhenoblastoma 128
Arrhythmia, cardiac 128, *129*
  a *disorder of the heart 517*
Arrowroot 129
Arsenic 129
  causing Squamous cell
    carcinoma 941
Artane 1098
arterial blood sampling:
  type of Blood test 188
arterial lining, removal of:
  medical term: Endarterectomy
    399
Arterial reconstructive surgery
  130
  in treatment of Subclavian
    steal syndrome 956
Arteries, disorders of 130
  leading to Stroke 952;
    Subarachnoid haemorrhage
    955; Thrombosis 987
  see also index entry
    Atherosclerosis
Arteriography 130
  type of Angiography 107
Arteriole 130
  part of Circulatory system 279,
    280
Arteriopathy 130
  common term: Arteries,
    disorders of 130
Arterioplasty 130
  alternative term: Arterial
    reconstructive surgery 130
Arteriosclerosis 130
  see also index entry
    Atherosclerosis
Arteriovenous fistula 130
  type of Fistula 451
Arteritis 131
Artery 131
  part of Circulatory system 279,
    280
  and Pulse 845
  see also index entry Arteries,
    disorders of
Arthralgia 131
Arthritis 131, *132*
  causing Stiffness 947
  as complication of Obesity
    742
  effect on Joints 609
  and Paget's disease 772;
    Reiter's syndrome 866
Arthrodesis 132
  in treatment of Neuropathic
    joint 727
Arthrofen 1098
Arthrography 132
Arthrogryposis:
  Contracture 305
Arthropathy 132
Arthroplasty 132
  and Pseudarthrosis 836
Arthrosin 1098

Arthroscopy 132
  how arthroscopy is done 133
  in diagnosis of Loose bodies
    647; Osteochondritis
    dessicans 762
  use of: Meniscectomy 676
Arthrotec 1098
Arthroxen 1098
artificial body part:
  alternative term: Prosthesis 834
  and Heart valve surgery 523;
    Hip replacement 535;
    Knee-joint replacement 619;
    Limb, artificial 637; *types of
    artificial limb 638*
  see also index entry Implant
Artificial insemination 133
  and Surrogacy 961
Artificial kidney 134
  use of: Dialysis 44, 351;
    procedure for dialysis 352
Artificial respiration 134
Artifical sweeteners 134
artificial tears:
  Tears, artificial 971
Artracin 1098
arytenoid cartilages:
  part of Larynx 626
  and Vocal cords 1066; *location
    of the vocal cords 1067*
Arythmol 1098
Asacol 1098
asbestos:
  as Carcinogen 233
  causing Lung cancer 649;
    Mesothelioma 681
  see also index entry Asbestos
    induced diseases
Asbestos-induced diseases 135
  and *disorders of the lung 649*;
    Pneumoconiosis 810
Asbestosis:
  Asbestos-induced diseases 135
Ascabiol 1098
Ascariasis 135
  life cycle of the ascaris worm 136
  cause of: Roundworms 882
ascending colon:
  part of Intestine 595
Ascites 136
  feature of Liver failure 644;
    Pancreatitis 777; Portal
    hypertension 817
Ascorbic acid 136
  alternative term: Vitamin C
    1065
Asendis 1098
Aseptic technique 136
  in prevention of Wound
    infection 1087
Aserbine 1098
Asilone 1098
Askit 1098
Asparaginase 1098
aspartame:
  an Artificial sweetener 134
Aspav 1098
Asperger's syndrome 137
Aspergillosis 137
  a Fungal infection 464; *disorder
    of the lung 649*
Aspermia:
  Azoospermia 149

Asphyxia 137
Aspiration 137
  for *biopsy procedures 170;* Bone
    marrow biopsy 194
aspiration pneumonia:
  type of *pneumonia 812*
Aspirin 137
  an Analgesic drug 102
  associated with Reye's
    syndrome 875
  causing Gastritis 470; Occult
    blood, faecal 743
  landmarks in medicine: drugs 671
  in treatment of Transient
    ischaemic attack 1009
Aspro 1098
Assay 137
Astemizole 1098
Astereognosis 137
Asthenia 138
  modern term: Weakness 1077
Asthenia, neurocirculatory:
  alternative term: Cardiac
    neurosis 234
Asthma 138
  and Allergy 85; Rhinitis,
    allergic 878
  assessment of: Peak-flow
    meter 785
  Status asthmaticus 939
  treatment of: Aminophylline
    92; Hydrocortisone 446;
    Inhaler 585; Nebulizer 719;
    Prednisolone 821;
    Salbutamol 885; Sodium
    cromoglycate 927
Asthma, cardiac 139
Astigmatism 139
  a *disorder of the eye 426*
  treatment of: Contact lenses
    299; *why glasses are used 484*
Astringent 139
Astrocytoma 139
Asylum 139
  modern term: Mental
    hospital 680
Asymptomatic 139
Asystole 140
  causing Cardiac arrest 234
AT 10 1098
Atarax 1098
Ataxia 140
Atelectasis 140
Atenix 1098
AtenixCo 1098
Atenolol 140
Atensine 1098
Atheroma 140
  and Atherosclerosis 140;
    Plaque 808
  leading to Thrombosis 987
  treatment of: Arterial
    reconstructive surgery 130
Atherosclerosis 140
  and Arteries, disorders of 130;
    disorders of the heart 517;
    hypertension 551; Plaque 808;
    disorders of the retina 872
  *arterial degeneration in
    atherosclerosis 141*
  in Down's syndrome 370
  leading to Ischaemia 603;
    Peripheral vascular disease

Atherosclerosis (continued)
793; Raynaud's
phenomenon 860; Stroke 952
treatment of: Arterial
reconstructive surgery 130;
Endarterectomy 399
Athetosis 141
resulting from Kernicterus
612
Athlete's foot 142
cause of: Tinea 994
treatment of: Miconazole 685
Ativan 1098
atlas bone:
and Skull 919
location and structure of the
vertebrae 1053
atmospheric pressure:
see index entry air pressure
atomic bomb:
and Nuclear energy 736;
Radiation 851
atomic energy:
and Nuclear energy 736;
Radiation 851
atomic radiation:
see index entry Radiation
Atony 142
atopic eczema:
and Skin allergy 916
type of Eczema 389
Atopy 142
ATP 142
and ADP 69; Energy 405
constituent of: Phosphates
801
Atracurium 1098
Atresia 142
causing Intestine, obstruction
of 596
Atrial fibrillation 142
causing Palpitation 774
type of Arrhythmia, cardiac
128
Atrial flutter 142
type of Arrhythmia, cardiac
128
Atrial natriuretic peptide 143
effect on Urine 1034
atrial septal defect:
Septal defect 900
atrioventricular node:
anatomy of Heart 515; Vena
cava 1048
and cardiac arrhythmia 128;
heart cycle 516
Atrium 143
part of Heart 515
Atromid-S 1098
atrophic rhinitis:
type of Rhinitis 878
Atrophy 143
Atropine 143
Atrovent 1098
Attachment 143
Audicort 1098
Audiogram 143
Audiology 143
Audiometry 143
types of hearing test 513
auditory evoked response:
Evoked responses 418
types of hearing test 513

Auditory nerve 143
and functions of cranial nerves
318
part of Vestibulocochlear
nerve 1054
auditory ossicles:
parts of Ear 383
Augmentin 1098
Aura 143
feature of Epilepsy 410
Auranofin 143
Aureocort 1098
Aureomycin 1098
Auricle 143
alternative term: Pinna 804
part of Ear 383
Auriscope 144
Auscultation 144
use of: Examination, physical
418
Autism 144
feature of Rett's syndrome 875
Autoclave 145
use of: Sterilization 945
autograft:
Corneal graft 307
Grafting 491
Autoimmune disorders 145
and Immune system 566
examples: Addison's disease
66; Dermatomyositis 345;
Diabetes mellitus 348;
Graves' disease 493;
Hashimoto's thyroiditis 507;
Hypothyroidism 560; Lupus
erythematosus 650;
Myasthenia gravis 710;
Pernicious anaemia 794;
Polymyalgia rheumatica 816;
Polymyositis 816;
Rheumatoid arthritis 876;
Scleroderma 892; Temporal
arteritis 973; Vitiligo 1066
treatment of: Azathioprine
149; Plasmapheresis 809
Automatism 146
feature of Epilepsy 411
Autonomic nervous system 146
functions of the autonomic
nervous system 147
divisions of: Parasympathetic
nervous system 780;
Sympathetic nervous system
964
part of Nervous system 723
Autopsy 146
autosomes:
and Chromosomal
abnormalities 275; Genetic
disorders 476; Inheritance
585
Autosuggestion 146
avascular necrosis:
complication of Femur,
fracture of 439
Aventyl 1098
Aversion therapy 148
and Behaviour therapy 162
Aviation medicine 148
Avitaminosis 149
Avloclor 1098
Avomine 1098
Avulsed tooth 149

Avulsion 149
Axid 1098
Axilla 149
axillary nerve:
part of Brachial plexus 197
axis bone:
and Skull 920
location and structure of the
vertebrae 1053
Axon 149
part of Neuron 726; structure of
a neuron 727
Ayurvedism:
type of Indian medicine 576
Azactam 1098
Azamune 1098
Azapropazone 1098
Azatadine 1098
Azathioprine 149
in treatment of Rheumatoid
arthritis 877; Wegener's
granulomatosis 1077
Azelaic acid 1098
Azelastine 1098
azidothymidine (AZT):
new name: Zidovudine 1093
Azithromycin 149
Azlocillin 1098
Azoospermia 149
diagnosis of: Seminal fluid
analysis 897
feature of Klinefelter's
syndrome 619
AZT 149
new name: Zidovudine 1093
Aztreonam 149
azygos veins:
anatomy of: Vena cava 1048

B

Babinski's sign 150
baby:
Birthweight 173
Bottle-feeding 196
Breast-feeding 206
Childbirth 261
Child development 264,
266–267
Fetus 443
Infant 577
Neonatal care 44
Newborn 729
Postmaturity 818
Pregnancy 822
Prematurity 825
Twins 1021
Baby blues 150
medical term: Postnatal
depression 819
Bacampicillin 150
type of Penicillin drug 788
bacillary dysentery:
alternative term: Shigellosis
907
Bacilli 150
types of Bacteria 152
Bacitracin 1098
Back 150
reducing strain on the back 153

Spine 937
see also index entries back
disorders; Back pain
backache:
symptom chart 151
see also index entry Back pain
Backbone:
Spine 937
back disorders:
disorders of the spine 938
see also index entry Back pain
Back pain 150, 153
causes of: Disc prolapse 362;
Fibroid 447; Lumbosacral
spasm 648; disorders of the
spine 938; Tension 976
symptom chart 151
Baclofen 150
Bacteraemia 152
and Sepsis 900; Septicaemia
900
Bacteria 152
causing bacterial infections 580;
Food poisoning 456;
Infection 577; Infectious
disease 578; Staphylococcal
infections 944; Streptococcal
infections 950
culturing of: Culture 323;
culturing and testing bacteria
155
examples: Bacilli 150; common
types of bacteria 154;
Salmonella 886; Spirochaete
937
producing Endotoxin 405;
Enterotoxin 406; Exotoxin
421; Toxin 1005
staining of: Gram's stain 492
study of: Bacteriology 154
type of Microorganism 685
bacterial meningitis:
see index entry Meningitis
Bactericidal 154
types of: Antibacterial drugs
114; Antibiotic drugs 114
Bacteriology 154
see also index entry Bacteria
Bacteriostatic 155
types of: Antibacterial drugs
114; Antibiotic drugs 114
Bacteriuria 155
Bactrim 1098
Bactroban 1098
Bad breath:
medical term: Halitosis 504
Bagassosis 155
causing Alveolitis 89
Baker's cyst 155
affecting Knee 619
and Rheumatoid arthritis 876
Balance 155
affected by Acoustic neuroma
63; disorders of the ear 384;
Streptomycin 951; Vertigo
1053
control of: Cerebellum 247; Ear
383; Vestibulocochlear nerve
1054
Balanitis 156
affecting Penis 789
Baldness:
medical term: Alopecia 87

ball-and-socket joint:
  in Hip 534
  types of joints 608
balloon angioplasty:
  Angioplasty, balloon 108
Balloon catheter 156
  in treatment of Pulmonary
    stenosis 845
balloon tuboplasty:
  type of Tuboplasty 1020
balloon valvuloplasty:
  type of Valvuloplasty 1044
Balm 156
Bambec 1098
Bambuterol 156
Bandage 156
  first aid: applying bandages 157
  type of Dressing 373
Banocide 1098
Baratol 1098
barber's itch:
  medical term: Sycosis barbae
    964
Barbiturate drugs 156
  examples: Phenobarbitone 799;
    Thiopentone 984
  and Withdrawal syndrome
    1084
Barium X-ray examinations 157,
  158
  type of Contrast X-ray 34
Barnard, Christiaan:
  landmarks in medicine: surgery
    670
Barotrauma 159
Barquinol HC 1098
Barrett's oesophagus:
  complication of Oesophagitis
    748
barrier contraceptives:
  see index entry Contraception,
    barrier methods of
Barrier cream 159
  in prevention of Chapped skin
    256
Barrier method 159
  see also index entry
    Contraception, barrier
    methods of
Barrier nursing 159
bartholinitis:
  disorder of Bartholin's glands
    159
Bartholin's cyst:
  disorder of Bartholin's glands
    159
Bartholin's glands 159
Basal cell carcinoma 160
  cause of: Occupational disease
    and injury 743
  and Eyelid 428; *disorders of the*
    nose 735
  treatment of: Radiotherapy 855
  type of Skin cancer 917;
    disorder of the skin 919
Basal ganglia 160
  and Huntington's disease 544;
    Parkinson's disease 781
basal metabolic rate (BMR):
  and Energy requirements 405;
    Metabolism 682
base:
  and Acid-base balance 62

alternative term: Alkali 85
  constituent of Nucleic acids
    737
basophil cells:
  and Allergy 85
basophil leukocyte:
  type of Blood cell 182
Battered baby syndrome 160
  Child abuse 260
Baxan 1098
Baycaron 1098
B-cell:
  type of Lymphocyte 653
BCG vaccination 160
  in prevention of Tuberculosis
    1019
Beclazone 1099
Becloforte 1099
Beclomethasone 160
Becodisks 1099
Beconase 1099
Becotide 1099
Becquerel:
  a *radiation unit 851*
Bed bath 160
Bedbug 160
Bedpan 160
Bedranol SR 1099
Bed rest 161
Bedridden 161
Beds, hospital 161
Bedsores 161
  and Nursing care 738
  treatment of: Zinc oxide 1093
  type of: Leg ulcer 631
Bed-wetting 162
  medical term: Enuresis 406
Bee stings:
  Insect stings 588
Behavioural problems in
  children 162
  and Conduct disorders 295;
    Diet and disease 356
  type of: Tantrum 969
Behaviourism 162
behaviour modification:
  by Behaviour therapy 162;
    Conditioning 295; Learning
    629
Behaviour therapy 162
  method of: Conditioning 295
  use of: Marriage guidance 663
Behçet's syndrome 163
Belching 163
  and Indigestion 576
Belladonna 163
Bell's palsy 163
  alternative term: Facial palsy
    429
Benadon 1099
Bendogen 1099
Bendrofluazide 163
Bends 163
  cause of: Nitrogen 732
  medical term: Decompression
    sickness 334
  and Scuba-diving medicine
    894
Benemid 1099
Benerva 1099
Benethamine penicillin 1099
Benign 163
Benoral 1099

Benorylate 163
Benoxyl 1099
Benperidol 1099
Benserazide 1099
Benylin Expectorant 1099
Benylin Paediatric 1099
Benzagel 1099
Benzalkonium chloride 1099
Benzhexol 1099
Benzocaine 1099
Benzodiazepine drugs 163
  causing Withdrawal syndrome
    1084
  examples: Chlordiazepoxide
    268; Diazepam 356;
    Lorazepam 647; Oxazepam
    770
  introduction of: *landmarks in*
    medicine: drugs 671
Benzoic acid 1099
Benzoin tincture 1099
Benzoyl peroxide 163
  in treatment of Acne 63
Benzthiazide 1099
Benztropine 1099
Benzydamine 1099
Benzyl benzoate 1099
Benzylpenicillin 1099
Bereavement 163
Berger's disease:
  form of Glomerulonephritis
    485
Beriberi 164
  cause of: deficiency of Vitamin
    B complex 1063
Berkatens 1099
Berkmycen 1099
Berkolol 1099
Berkozide 1099
Berotec 1099
Berylliosis 164
beryllium:
  causing Berylliosis 164
Beta-Adalat 1099
Beta-blocker drugs 164
  abuse of: Sports, drugs and
    940
  how beta-blockers work 165
  development of: *landmarks in*
    medicine: drugs 671
  examples: Acebutolol 60;
    Atenolol 140; Labetalol 622;
    Metoprolol 684; Nadolol 716;
    Pindolol 803; Propranolol
    831; Timolol 994
  in treatment of Migraine 688
Beta-Cardone 1099
Beta-carotene 1099
Betadren 1099
Betadur CR 1099
Betagan 1099
beta-globulins:
  types of Globulin 485
Betahistine 165
Betaloc 1099
Betamethasone 165
beta particles:
  type of Radiation 855
Beta-Prograne 1099
beta-receptors:
  and *how beta-blockers work 165*
  types of Receptors 861
Betaxolol 1099

Bethanechol 1099
Bethanidine 166
Betim 1099
Betnelan 1099
Betnesol 1099
Betnesol-N 1099
Betnovate 1099
Betnovate-C, Betnovate-N 1099
Betoptic 1099
Bezafibrate 1099
Bezalip 1099
Bezoar 166
Bi- 166
bicarbonate ion:
  type of Ion 601
Bicarbonate of soda:
  Sodium bicarbonate 927
Biceps muscle 166
Bicillin 1099
Bicuspid 166
Bifocal 166
  type of Glasses 483
big toe:
  medical term: Hallux 504
Bilateral 166
Bile 166
  and Biliary system 167; *function*
    of the biliary system 168
  constituent of: Bilirubin 168
  production of: Liver 641
  storage of: Gallbladder 467
Bile duct 166
  part of Biliary system 167
  and *function of the biliary system*
    168; Intestine 595
Bile duct cancer:
  medical term:
    Cholangiocarcinoma 270
Bile duct obstruction 166
  cause of: Gallstones 468
  causing Jaundice 606
Bilharzia 167
  alternative term:
    Schistosomiasis 889
Biliary atresia 167
  a disorder of the liver 645
Biliary cirrhosis 167
  a disorder of the liver 645
Biliary colic 167
  cause of: Gallstones 468
  a disorder of the gallbladder 467
Biliary system 167
  functions of: Bile 166; *function*
    of the biliary system 168
  parts of: Bile duct 166;
    Gallbladder 467; Liver 640
Biliousness 168
Bilirubin 168
  and Anaemia 96
  in Blood 181
  causing Jaundice 606;
    Kernicterus 612
  as constituent of Bile 166
  excess of: Hyperbilirubinaemia
    548
Billings' method 169
Billroth's operation 169
  types of gastrectomy 469
Biltricide 1099
Binet test 169
  type of Intelligence test 590
binge eating:
  feature of Bulimia 217

binocular vision:
mechanism of: *the function of the optic nerve 754; the sense of vision 1058*
BiNovum 1099
Bio- 169
Bioavailability 169
Biochemical analysis 37
Biochemistry 169
Biofeedback training 169
Relaxation techniques 867
Biogastrone 1099
Biomechanical engineering 169
Biophylline 1099
Bioplex 1099
Biopsy 38, 169
biopsy procedures 170
in diagnosis of Breast cancer 206; Cancer 227; Lung cancer 650; Oesophagus, cancer of 748; Pharynx, cancer of 799; Proctitis 829; Rectum, cancer of 864; Sprue, tropical 941; Stomach cancer 948
and Endoscopy 38, 403; *endoscopes 404;* Sigmoidoscopy 912
types of: Bone marrow biopsy 194; *biopsy of the cervix 253;* Cone biopsy 295; Kidney biopsy 613; Liver biopsy 642; Skin biopsy 916
Bioral Gel 1099
Biorhythms 171
and Jet-lag 609
Biorphen 1099
biotin:
constituent of Vitamin B complex 1063
Biperiden 1099
Biphosphonates 171
Bipolar disorder 171
example: Manic-depressive illness 661
birds, diseases from:
examples: Alveolitis 89; Histoplasmosis 537; Psittacosis 836
Birth:
see index entry Childbirth
Birth canal 171
Birth control 171
methods of: Coitus interruptus 286; Contraception 301; Contraception, barrier methods of 302; Contraception, hormonal methods of 304; *methods of contraception 303;* Contraception, natural methods of 304; Contraception, postcoital 304; Family planning 434; Sterilization, female 945; Vasectomy 1046
birth-control pill:
Oral contraceptives 755
Birth defects 172
causes of: Chromosomal abnormalities 275; Genetic disorders 476; Pregnancy, drugs in 823

and Embryo 395; Infant mortality 577; Newborn 729
Birth injury 173
and Newborn 730
Birthmark 173
treatment of: Cryosurgery 322; Laser treatment 47, 627
types of: Haemangioma 498; Naevus 716; Port-wine stain 818
Birthpool 173
birth rates:
Statistics, vital 944
Birthweight 173
and Prematurity 825; Sudden infant death syndrome 957
Bisacodyl 1099
Bisexuality 173
and Sexuality 904
Bismag 1099
Bismuth 173
causing Melaena 673
BiSoDol 1099
Bisoprolol 1099
Bite (dentistry):
abnormality of: Malocclusion 659
affected by Thumb-sucking 989
medical term: Occlusion 743
Bites, animal 173
first aid: insect stings and tick bites 588
types of: Insect bites 587; Snake bites 926; Spider bites 933; Venomous bites and stings 1050
Bites, human 174
Black death 174
modern term: Plague 807
Black eye 174
black faeces:
see index entry Faeces, abnormal
Blackhead 174
feature of Acne 63
Blackout 174
Fainting 430
Black teeth:
Discoloured teeth 362
Blackwater fever 174
Bladder 174
anatomy of the bladder 175
disorders of the bladder 176
and Catheterization, urinary 242
investigation of: Cystometry 329; Cystoscopy 329
part of Urinary tract 1032, *1033*
removal of: Cystectomy 326
stone in: Calculus, urinary tract 224
Bladder cancer:
Bladder tumours 175
bladder control:
in children: Developmental delay 348; Toilet-training 999
defective: Disc prolapse 362; Enuresis 406; Incontinence, urinary 575
Bladder tumours 175
causing Incontinence, urinary 575

blastocyst:
development of: *the process of fertilization 441;* Zygote 1094
blastomycosis:
type of Fungal infection 464
Bleaching, dental 176
bleaching, hair:
Hair 503
Bleeding 177
causing Hypotension 558; Hypovolaemia 560; Kidney failure 614; Shock 907
and Menstruation 677; Nosebleed 735; Placenta praevia 799; Postpartum haemorrhage 819; Uterus, cancer of 1037; Varicose veins 1044
stopping: Bleeding, treatment of 178; Blood clotting 183; *how blood clots 184;* Haemostasis 502; Pressure points 827
see also index entry Bleeding disorders
Bleeding disorders 177
and Blood clotting 183; Platelets 809
diagnosis of: Blood-clotting tests 183
treatment of: Blood products 188; Factor VIII 429; Haemostatic drugs 502
types of: Christmas disease 275; Haemophilia 501; Thrombocytopenia 986; Von Willebrand's disease 1068
Bleeding gums:
Gingivitis 482
bleeding, rectal:
Rectal bleeding 862
bleeding time:
measurement of: Blood-clotting tests 183
Bleeding, treatment of 178
Pressure points 827
in Shock 907
Blemix 1099
Bleomycin 1099
Blepharitis 178
causing Eyelashes, disorders of 425
Blepharoplasty 178, 179
Blepharospasm 179
spasm of Eyelid 428
Blind loop syndrome 179
Blindness 179
causes of: Cataract 240; Cavernous sinus thrombosis 244; Chloroquine 269; Corneal abrasion 307; Filariasis 448; Glaucoma 483; Keratomalacia 611; Onchocerciasis 751; Tay-Sachs disease 971; Trachoma 1008
and *disorders of the cornea 308; disorders of the eye 426; disorders of the retina 873*
partial: Transient ischaemic attack 1009
temporary: Migraine 687

types of: Colour vision deficiency 292; Night blindness 731
Vision, loss of 1059
Blind spot 180
blinking, abnormal:
Tic 994
Blister 180
bloating:
Abdominal swelling 55
and Faeces, abnormal 429; Hirschsprung's disease 536
Blocadren 1099
Blocked nose:
Nasal congestion 717
Nasal obstruction 718
Blocking 181
Blood 181
andBloodclotting184
Circulatory system 279, *280*
constituents of: Blood cells 181; *constituents of blood 182;* Haemoglobin 499; Lymphocyte 653; Plasma 809; Plasma proteins 809; Platelet 809; Serum 901
disorders of: Bleeding disorders 177; *disorders of the blood 185*
blood alcohol levels:
alcohol and the body 81
blood calcium levels:
abnormally high: Hypercalcaemia 548; Hyperparathyroidism 550
abnormally low: Hypoparathyroidism 550
regulation of: Calcitonin 223; Calcium 224; Parathyroid glands 781; Vitamin D 1065
blood cancer:
medical term: Leukaemia 632
Blood cells 181
constituents of blood 182
disorders of the blood 185
and Haemoglobin 499
types of: Lymphocyte 653; Platelet 809
blood cholesterol levels:
see index entry blood lipid levels
blood clot:
causing Embolism 394; Thrombosis 987; Thrombosis, deep vein 987; *deep vein thrombosis 988*
medical term: Thrombus 988
removal of: Embolectomy 394; Thrombectomy 966
type of Embolus 395
see also index entry Blood clotting
Blood clotting 183
how blood clots 184
Blood-clotting tests 184
and Calcium 224; Factor VIII 429; Fibrinolysis 446; Vitamin K 1065
Coagulation, blood 283
disorders of: Bleeding disorders 177; *disorders of the blood 185*

prevention of: Anticoagulant
drugs 116
see also index entry blood clot
Blood-clotting tests 184
in diagnosis of Purpura 846
blood coagulation:
see index entry Blood clotting
blood, coughing up:
see index entry Coughing up
blood
Blood count 184
Blood culture:
Culture 323
Blood donation 184
and AIDS 79; Blood
transfusion 189; Blood
transfusion, autologous 189;
Haemophilia 501; Hepatitis,
viral 529
blood fat levels:
see index entry blood lipid
levels
Blood film 186
blood flow:
in Circulatory system 279, *280*
disorders of: Arteries,
disorders of 130; Ischaemia
603; Veins, disorders of 1048
investigation of:
Plethysmography 810
and Resistance 869
Blood gases 186
blood glucose levels:
and Diabetes mellitus 348;
*living with diabetes mellitus
349;* Glucose 487
effect on: Glucagon 487;
Hypoglycaemics, oral 556;
Insulin 589
high: Hyperglycaemia 548
low: Hunger 544;
Hypoglycaemia 556
Blood groups 186
blood group compatibility 187
in Blood transfusion 189;
Forensic medicine 459;
discovery of: *landmarks in
medicine: surgery 670*
and Paternity testing 783;
Rhesus incompatibility 875
blood in faeces:
see index entries Faeces,
abnormal; Rectal bleeding
blood in urine:
medical term: Haematuria 499
bloodletting:
medical term: Venesection
1049
Blood level 187
blood lipid levels:
and Cholesterol 273; Coronary
artery disease 310; Diet and
disease 356; Fats 18; Fats
and oils 436; Oral
contraceptives 755
high: Hyperlipidaemias 549
reduction of: Lipid-lowering
drugs 639
testing of: Other screening
tests 27
Blood loss:
see index entries Bleeding;
Bleeding, treatment of

Blood poisoning 187
causing Toxaemia 1005
medical term: Septicaemia 900
from Sepsis 900
Blood pressure 187
high: Hypertension 551, 552
low: Hypotension 558; Shock
907
measurement of: *taking the
blood pressure 24;*
Sphygmomanometer 933
regulation of: Angiotensin 108;
Renin 868
and Sodium 927
Blood products 188
and AIDS 77; Hepatitis, viral
529
types of: Factor VIII 429;
Immunoglobulins 571
use of: Haemostatic drugs 502;
Immunization 569
Blood smear:
Blood film 186
blood sugar levels:
see index entry blood glucose
levels
Blood tests 188
for AIDS 77; Blood groups 186
types of: Blood-clotting tests
184; Blood count 184; Blood
film 186; Prostate, cancer of
832
Blood transfusion 189
leading to AIDS 77; Hepatitis,
viral 529
type of: Blood transfusion,
autologous 189
uses of: Bleeding, treatment of
178; Haemolytic disease of
the newborn 500;
Haemophilia 501;
Leukaemia, acute 633;
Leukaemia, chronic 633;
Malaria 658; Shock 907
Blood transfusion, autologous
189
blood urea levels:
measurement of: Kidney
function tests 616
and Urea 1028
Blood vessels 190
and Circulatory system 279,
280
disorders of: Arteries,
disorders of 130; Bleeding
disorders 177; Veins,
disorders of 1048
examples of: Aorta 122; Vena
cava 1048
investigation of: Angiography
101
joining: Anastomosis 104
narrowing of: Vasoconstriction
1046
types of: Arteriole 130; Artery
131; Capillary 231; Vein 1048
widening of: Vasodilation
1047
blood volume:
abnormally low:
Hypovolaemia 560; Shock
907
and Blood 181

blood, vomiting:
see index entry Vomiting
blood
Blue baby 190
cause of: Heart disease,
congenital 519
and Cyanosis 325
Blue bloater 190
and Emphysema 397
blue skin:
medical term: Cyanosis 325
Blurred vision 190
causes of: Multiple sclerosis
702; Neuropathy 728;
Polycythaemia 815; Vision,
disorders of 1059
tests for: Vision tests 1059;
types of vision tests 1060
Blushing 190
B-lymphocyte:
part of Immune system 568
type of Lymphocyte 653
BMR:
see index entry basal
metabolic rate
body chemistry:
medical term: Metabolism 682
study of: Biochemistry 169;
Physiology 802
body "clock":
Biorhythms 171
Body contour surgery 190
body imaging:
see index entry Imaging
techniques
Body odour 190
causes of: Hyperhidrosis 548;
Metabolism, inborn errors of
681
and Sweat glands 963
treatment of: Antiperspirant
118; Deodorant 342
body temperature:
see index entry Temperature
Boil 191
compound: Carbuncle 233
multiple: Folliculitis 454
Bolus 191
and Swallowing 963
bolus feeding:
type of Feeding, artificial 437
Bolvidon 1099
Bonding 191
and Separation anxiety 899
Bonding, dental 191
Bone 192
disorders of the bone 193
growth of: Epiphysis 412;
Vitamin A 1062; Vitamin C
1065; Vitamin D 1065
features of: Foramen 458;
Periosteum 793; Sinus 913;
Tuberosity 1019
formation of: Ossification 761
and Skeleton 914; *bones of the
skeleton 915*
structure of: *the structure of
bone 192;* Calcium 224;
Phosphates 801
type of: Ossicle 761
Bone abscess 192
bone age:
Age 73

bone, broken:
see index entry Fracture
Bone cancer 192
diagnosis of: Bone imaging 194
types of: Chondrosarcoma 273;
Ewing's sarcoma 418;
Fibrosarcoma 447; Multiple
myeloma 701; Osteosarcoma
764
see also index entry Bone
tumour
bone conduction:
and Deafness 332; Hearing
513
bone, cutting of:
Osteotomy 765
Bone cyst 193
bone density:
decrease of: Osteoporosis 764;
increase of: Osteopetrosis 764;
Osteosclerosis 765; Paget's
disease 772
measurement of:
Densitometry 339
Bonefos 1099
bone, fracture of:
see index entry Fracture
Bone graft 193
in treatment of Osteomyelitis
763
type of Plastic surgery 809
Bone imaging 194
methods of: Radionuclide
scanning 854; *a radionuclide
bone scan 35;* X-rays 1089
bone implant:
use of: Plastic surgery 809
bone, infection of:
causing Osteomyelitis 763
diagnosis of: Radionuclide
scanning 854
leading to Sequestration 901
bone, inflammation of:
medical term: Osteitis 761
in Osteochondritis juvenilis
762; Osteomyelitis 763
Bone marrow 194
production of Blood cells 182
Bone marrow biopsy 194
Bone marrow transplant 46, 194
*performing a bone marrow
transplant 195*
complication of: Graft-versus-
host disease 492
in treatment of Anaemia 96;
Anaemia, aplastic 96;
Genetic disorders 478;
Immunodeficiency
disorders 571; Leukaemia,
acute 633; Leukaemia,
chronic myeloid 635;
Lymphoma, non-Hodgkin's
655; Radiation sickness 853;
Sickle cell anaemia 911
type of Transplant surgery 47
bone pain:
feature of Osteoid osteoma
763; Osteomalacia 763;
Osteomyelitis 763; Paget's
disease 772; Sickle cell
anaemia 911
bones, brittle:
see index entry Brittle bones

bone scanning:
see index entry Bone imaging
bones, deformed:
causes of: Fracture 460;
Metabolism, inborn errors of
682; Osteochondritis
juvenilis 762; Osteogenesis
imperfecta 763;
Osteomalacia 763; Paget's
disease 772; Rickets 880
bones, hard:
feature of Osteopetrosis 764
bones, soft:
feature of Osteomalacia 763;
Rickets 880; deficiency of
Vitamin D 1065
bones, weak:
feature of Osteogenesis
imperfecta 763;
Osteomalacia 763;
Osteoporosis 764; Paget's
disease 772; Rickets 880
Bone tumour 196
cause of: Strontium 954
types of: Chondromatosis 273;
Osteochondroma 762;
Osteoma 763
see also index entry Bone
cancer
Booster 196
Travel immunization 1012
Vaccine 1040
Borborygmi 196
Borderline personality disorder
196
Bornholm disease 196
alternative term: Pleurodynia
810
Borofax 1098
Bottle-feeding 196
and Feeding, infant 437
Botulism 196
type of Food poisoning 456
bovine spongiform
encephalopathy (BSE):
Encephalopathy 399
Bowel 197
medical term: Intestine 596
opening into: Colostomy 290;
Ileostomy 562
removal of: Colectomy 287
bowel control:
in children: Developmental ·
delay 346; Toilet-training
999
defective: Disc prolapse 362;
Incontinence, faecal 575
bowel habit, change of:
and Abdominal pain 50
causes of: Diverticular disease
365; Rectum, cancer of 863
investigation of: Barium X-ray
examinations 157
Bowel movements, abnormal:
Faeces, abnormal 429
Bowel sounds:
medical term: Borborygmi 196
Bowen's disease 197
type of Skin cancer 917
Bowleg 197
medical term: Varus 1044
resulting from Rickets 880
and Walking 1072

Brace, dental:
Orthodontic appliances 759
Brace, orthopaedic 197
brachial artery:
damage to: Humerus, fracture
of 543
Brachialgia 197
Brachial plexus 197
branches of: Radial nerve 850;
Ulnar nerve 1024
damage to: Klumpke's
paralysis 619; Thoracic
outlet syndrome 984
brachytherapy:
type of Interstitial
radiotherapy 595
Bradycardia 197
and Heart-rate 522
type of Arrhythmia, cardiac
128
Braille 197, 198
aids for the blind 179
Brain 198
anatomy of: Basal ganglia 160;
Brainstem 202; location of the
brainstem 203; structure of the
brain 199; Cerebellum 247;
Cerebrospinal fluid 248;
Cerebrum 249; Cranial
nerves 318; Hypothalamus
558; Limbic system 637;
Meninges 674; structure of a
neuron 727; Pineal gland 804;
Pituitary gland 804;
Thalamus 982; Ventricle
1051
disorders of the brain 200
part of Central nervous system
246; Nervous system 723,
724
Brain abscess 198
causes of: Mastoiditis 665;
Nocardiosis 732
treatment of: Neurosurgery 726
brain biopsy:
by Stereotaxic surgery 944
Brain damage 201
causes of: DPT vaccination
372; Encephalitis 399; Head
injury 510; Hypoglycaemia
556; Kernicterus 612; Lead
poisoning 629; Meningitis
675; Skull, fracture of 920;
Stroke 952
causing Cerebral palsy 248;
Coma 293; Paralysis 778;
Schizophrenia 890
and Concussion 294; Nerve
damage 723
Brain death 201
and Organ donation 758
brain dysfunction:
in Alzheimer's disease 90;
Dementia 338; Epilepsy 410;
Liver failure 644
and Brain damage 201;
disorders of the brain 200
Minimal brain dysfunction 689
brain, electrical activity in:
and Concussion 294; Sleep 922
investigation of: EEG 389
Brain failure:
Brain syndrome, organic 203

Brain haemorrhage 201
causing Paralysis 778
types of: Extradural
haemorrhage 422;
Intracerebral haemorrhage
598; Subarachnoid
haemorrhage 955; Subdural
haemorrhage 956
Brain imaging 202
methods of: CT scanning 35,
323; MRI 36, 700; PET
scanning 37, 797;
Ultrasound scanning 1025
brain, impaired blood supply to:
and Cerebrovascular disease
249; Stokes-Adams
syndrome 948; Stroke 952;
Transient ischaemic attack
1009
brain, lack of:
medical term: Anencephaly
105
brain, oedema of:
in Mountain sickness 697;
Radiation sickness 853
treatment of: Betamethasone
166; Mannitol 661; Urea 1028
Brainstem 202
location of the brainstem 203
Brain syndrome, organic 203
Brain tumour 204
causing Paralysis 778
diagnosis of: PET scanning 37,
797; Ultrasound scanning
1025
treatment of: Neurosurgery 728
types of: Glioma 485;
Medulloblastoma 671;
Meningioma 675;
Oligodendroglioma 750
Bran 203
source of Fibre, dietary 446
in treatment of Irritable bowel
syndrome 603
Branchial disorders 203
Brash, water:
Waterbrash 1077
Braxton Hicks' contractions 204
stages and features of pregnancy
822
Breakbone fever 204
medical term: Dengue 339
Breakthrough bleeding 204
Breast 204
disorders of the breast 205
Nipple 731
Breast abscess 204
complication of Mastitis 665
Breastbone:
medical term: Sternum 946
Breast cancer 205
detection of: Breast self-
examination 207;
Mammography 660
features of: Paget's disease of
the nipple 772; Peau
d'orange 785
treatment of: Gonadorelins
489; Mastectomy 663;
Megestrol 672; Radiotherapy
855; Tamoxifen 968
see also index entry Breast
reconstruction

breast engorgement:
feature of Breast-feeding 206;
Mastitis 665
Breast enlargement:
medical term: Mammoplasty
660
procedure for mammoplasty 661
see also index entries breast
growth (female); breast
growth (male)
Breast-feeding 206
causing Mastitis 665
Feeding, infant 437
breast growth (female):
and Puberty 841; changes of
puberty 842
breast growth (male):
associated with Cirrhosis 281;
Klinefelter's syndrome 619
causes of: Prolactinoma 831;
Spironolactone 938
medical term: Gynaecomastia
497
breast implant:
use of: Mammoplasty 660;
procedure for mammoplasty
661
breast, inflammation of:
medical term: Mastitis 665
Breast lump 207
cause of: Mastitis 665
detection of: Breast self-
examination 207
see also index entry Breast
cancer
Breast pump 207
breast quadrantectomy:
type of Mastectomy 664
Breast reconstruction:
type of Mammoplasty 660
procedure for mammoplasty 661
Breast reduction:
type of Mammoplasty 660
procedure for mammoplasty 661
breast, removal of:
medical term: Mastectomy 663
Breast, self-examination 207
Breast tenderness 208
a disorder of the breast 205
Breath-holding attacks 208
feature of Tantrum 969
Breathing 208
abnormally deep: Anxiety 121;
Hyperventilation 554
abnormally rapid: Anxiety 121;
Hyperventilation 554; Panic
attack 777; Tachypnoea 968
abnormal rhythms: Apnoea
125; Cheyne-Stokes
respiration 257; Sleep
apnoea 922; Sudden infant
death syndrome 957
noisy: Croup 321; Stridor 952;
Wheeze 1082
see also index entries
Breathing difficulty;
breathing stoppage
Breathing difficulty 209
feature of Alveolitis 89;
Asthma 138; Atelectasis 140;
Bronchitis, acute 213;
Bronchitis, chronic 214;
Choking 269; Diphtheria

362; Emphysema 397; Epiglottitis 410; Guillain-Barre syndrome 496; Heart block 516; Heart disease, congenital 519; *disorders of the heart 517*; Heart failure 519; Histoplasmosis 537; Hyperventilation 554; Larynx, cancer of 626; Lung cancer 649; Mitral incompetence 691; Myasthenia gravis 710; Panic attack 777; Pneumoconiosis 810; Pneumonia 811; Pneumonitis 813; Pneumothorax 813; Pulmonary embolism 843; Pulmonary fibrosis 844; Pulmonary oedema 845; Pulmonary stenosis 845; Respiratory distress syndrome 870; Septal defect 900; Tobacco-smoking 997; Transposition of the great vessels 1011

symptom chart 210

Breathing exercises 209

breathing passages, infection of: Respiratory tract infection 870

breathing stoppage: causes of: Airway obstruction 79; Choking 269 feature of Apnoea 125; Cheyne-Stokes respiration 257; Sleep apnoea 922 and Respiratory arrest 869 treatment of: Artificial respiration 134

Breathlessness 211 see also index entry Breathing difficulty

breech birth: see index entry Breech delivery

Breech delivery 211 causing Birth injury 173 *delivering a breech baby 212* and Malpresentation 659

Brelomax 1099

Bretylate 1099

Bretylium 1099

Brevibloc 1099

Brevinor 1099

Bricanyl 1099

Bridge, dental 212 Prosthetics, dental 834

Brietal Sodium 1099

Bright's disease 212 alternative term: Glomerulonephritis 485

Britiazim 1099

British Dental Association 212

British Medical Association 212

Britlofex 1099

Brittle bones 212 causes of: Osteogenesis imperfecta 763; Osteomalacia 763; Osteoporosis 764 following Menopause 676

brittle nails: and Koilonychia 621

Brocadopa 1099

Broca's area of brain: function of: Speech 930

Broflex 1099

Broken tooth: Fracture, dental 462

Broken veins: Telangiectasia 973

Brolene 1099

Bromazepam 1099

Bromides 212

Bromocriptine 213 in treatment of Acromegaly 64; Pituitary tumours 805

Brompheniramine 1099

Bronchiectasis 213 treatment of: Lobectomy, lung 646

bronchiole: Bronchus 216

Bronchiolitis 213 *a disorder of the lung 649*

Bronchitis 213 *a disorder of the lung 649* treatment of: Oxytetracycline 770

Bronchitis, acute 213

Bronchitis, chronic 214

Bronchoconstrictor 215

Bronchodil 1099

Bronchodilator drugs 215 *how bronchodilators work 214* examples: Albuterol 81; Bambuterol 156; Salbutamol 885; Terbutaline 977; Theophylline 983

Bronchography 215

Bronchopneumonia 215 type of Pneumonia 811, *812*

Bronchoscopy 215 in diagnosis of Lung cancer 650 in treatment of Choking 269

Bronchospasm 216

Bronchus 216 part of Lung 649; *location and structure of lung 648* and Vagus nerve 1043

Bronchus, cancer of: Lung cancer 649

bronze diabetes: medical term: Haemochromatosis 499

Brown fat 216

Brucellosis 216

Brufen 1099

Bruise 216 causes of: Bleeding disorders 177; Purpura 846

Bruits 216 detection of: Auscultation 144

Bruxism 216

BSE: Encephalopathy 399

Bubonic plague 216 type of Plague 807

Buccal 2169

Buccastem 1099

Buck teeth 216 treatment of: Orthodontic appliances 759

Buclizine 1099

Budd-Chiari syndrome 217 *a disorder of the liver 645*

Budesonide 217

Buerger's disease 217 causing Raynaud's phenomenon 861

Bufexamac 1099

Bulimia 217 causing Weight loss 1080

bulking agents: in treatment of Irritable bowel syndrome 603 types of Antidiarrhoeal drugs 116

Bulla 217

Bumetanide 217

Bundle branch block: Heart block 516

Bunion 217 cause of: Hallux valgus 505

Buphthalmos 218

Bupivacaine 1099

Buprenorphine 1099

Burinex 1099

Burinex-K 1099

Burkitt's lymphoma 218 type of Lymphoma, non-Hodgkin's 655

Burns 218 causing Contracture 305; Hypotension 558; Hypovolaemia 560; Kidney failure 614; Shock 907 *first aid: treating burns 219*

Burping: alternative term: Belching 163

Burr hole 220

Bursa 220

Bursitis 220 causing Water on the knee 1077 feature of Rheumatoid arthritis 876 treatment of: Piroxicam 804

Buscopan 1099

Buserelin 1100

Buspar 1100

Buspirone hydrochloride 1100

Busulphan 1100

Butacote 1100

Butobarbitone 1100

butter: Fats and oils 436

buttocks: Gluteus maximus 488

Bypass operations 220 in treatment of Ischaemia 603 types of: Coronary artery bypass 308, 309; Shunt 910

Byssinosis 220

transplant 617; Liver transplant 646; Organ donation 758; Transplant surgery 1010

Cadmium poisoning 221 Occupational disease and injury 743

Caecum 221

Caesarean section 221 *procedure for a caesarean section 222* in treatment of Childbirth, complications of 264; Fetal distress 442; Malpresentation 659

Cafadol 1100

Café au lait spots 221 type of Naevus 716

Cafergot 1100

Caffeine 221 causing Palpitation 774; Tachycardia 968 Withdrawal syndrome 1084

caisson disease: modern term: Decompression sickness 334

Calabar swellings: causes of: Filariasis 449; Loiasis 647

Calabren 1100

Caladryl 1100

Calamine 223

Calcaneus 223 part of Foot 458; Skeleton 915

Calcichew 1100

Calcichew D3 1100

Calcidrink 1100

Calciferol 223 se index entry Vitamin D 1065

Calcification 223

Calcification, dental 223

Calcilat 1100

Calcimax 1100

Calcinosis 223

Calciparine 1100

Calcipotriol 1100

Calcisorb 1100

Calcitare 1100

Calcitonin 223

Calcitriol 1100

Calcium 224 abnormal blood levels of: Parathyroidectomy 780; Vitamin D 1065; Tetany 981 deficiency of: Rickets 880; Osteoporosis 764 deposition of: Nephrocalcinosis 721 in treatment of Hypoparathyroidism 556 type of Ion 601

Calcium-500 1100

Calcium and Ergocalciferol tablets 1100

Calcium carbonate 1100

Calcium channel blockers 224 action of: *types of vasodilator drugs 1047* examples: Diltiazem 359; Nifedipine 730; Verapamil 1052 in treatment of Migraine 687

Calcium chloride 1100

C

Cachexia 221

Cadaver 221 use in transplants: Corneal transplant 307; Heart-lung transplant 521; Heart transplant 523; Kidney

Calcium Folinate tablets 1100
Calcium gluconate 1100
Calcium Lactate tablets 1100
Calcium Leucovorin 1100
Calcium Resonium 1100
Calcium-Sandoz 1100
Calculus 224
  alternative term: Stones 949
Calculus, dental 224
  causing Gingivitis 482;
    Periodontitis 792
  and Dental examination 340
  removal of: Periodontics 792;
    Preventive dentistry 828;
    Scaling, dental 888
  resulting from Plaque, dental
    808
Calculus, urinary tract 224
  treatment of: Lithotripsy 45,
    640; *lithotripsy procedures 641*
  urinary tract calculi 225
Calendar method 226
Calf muscles 226
Calgel 1100
Calimal 1100
Caliper splint 226
Callosity:
  Callus, skin 226
Callus, bony 226
Callus, skin 226
  treatment of: Keratolytic drugs
    611
Calmurid HC 1100
Caloric test 226
Calorie 226
  Kilocalorie 617
  unit of Energy 405
Calorie requirements:
  Energy requirements 405
Calorimetry 227
Calpol 1100
Calsynar 1100
CAM 1100
Camcolit 250 1100
Camphor 1100
campylobacter bacterium:
  causing Colitis 287; Food
    poisoning 456
Cancer 227
  incidence of cancer 228
  causes of: Carcinogen 233;
    Carcinogenesis 234;
    Smoking and drinking
    22–23
  diagnosis of: Biopsy 169;
    Cancer screening 25, 230;
    types of cancer test 230
  examples: Bladder tumours
    175; Bone cancer 192; Brain
    tumour 204; Breast cancer
    205; Cervix, cancer of 253;
    Intestine, cancer of 595;
    Kidney cancer 613; Larynx,
    cancer of 626; Leukaemia
    632; Lip cancer 638; Liver
    cancer 642; Lung cancer 649;
    Mouth cancer 698;
    Nasopharynx, cancer of 718;
    Oesophagus, cancer of 748;
    Ovary, cancer of 768; Penis,
    cancer of 789; Uterus, cancer
    of 1036; Vulva, cancer of
    1071

  and Metastasis 683;
  and Obesity 742
  study of: Oncology 751
  treatment of: *treatment of cancer*
    229; Chemotherapy 256;
    Cytotoxic drugs 330;
    Immunotherapy 572;
    Radiotherapy 45, *855*
  type of Neoplasm 721;
    Tumour 1020
  types of: Carcinoma 234;
    Sarcoma 888
Cancerphobia 229
Cancer screening 25, 230
Cancrum oris 230
  alternative term: Noma 733
Candidiasis 230
  affecting Penis 789
  causing Itching 604; *disorders of*
    the lung 649; Vulvitis 1071
  example of Opportunistic
    infection 754
  as a Sexually transmitted
    disease 904; Superinfection
    960
  treatment of: Clotrimazole 283;
    Ketoconazole 612;
    Miconazole 685; Nystatin
    741
  type of Fungal infection 464
Canesten 1100
Canesten HC 1100
Canine tooth:
  Teeth 971
Cannabis 230
  and Marijuana 662
Cannula 230
  use of: Intravenous infusion
    599; Venepuncture 1049
Cantil 1100
Capasal 1100
Capastat 1100
Cap, contraceptive 231
Capgras' syndrome 231
Capillary 231
  part of Circulatory system 279,
    280
Capitol 1100
Caplenal 1100
Capoten 1100
Capozide 1100
Capping, dental:
  Crown, dental 321
Capreomycin 1100
Caprin 1100
Capsule 231
Capsulitis 231
Captopril 231
Caput 231
Carace 1100
Carace Plus 1100
Carbachol 1100
Carbamazepine 231
  in treatment of Trigeminal
    neuralgia 1016
Carbaryl 1100
Carbellon 1100
Carbenicillin 1100
Carbenoxolone 231
Carbidopa 1100
Carbimazole 232
Carbocisteine 1100
Carbo-Cort 1100

Carbo-Dome 1100
Carbohydrates 19, 232
  in Nutrition 738
carbolic acid:
  use of: Skin peeling, chemical
    918
Carbomix 1100
Carbon 232
Carbon dioxide 233
  carbon dioxide laser: *use of a*
    laser 628
  carbon dioxide "snow": Dry
    ice 378
carbonic acid:
  and Acidosis 62
Carbon monoxide 233
  poisoning, effects of: Brain
    damage 201; Hypoxia 560
  poisoning, treatment of:
    Hyperbaric oxygen
    treatment 548
  and Effects of tobacco 22;
    Tobacco-smoking 997
Carbon tetrachloride 233
Carboplatin 1100
Carboprost 1100
Carbuncle 233
Carcinogen 233
  and Carcinogenesis 234
  see also index entry Cancer
Carcinogenesis 234
  and Carcinogen 233
  see also index entry Cancer
Carcinoid syndrome 234
carcinoid tumours:
  in Intestine, cancer of 596
Carcinoma 234
  type of Tumour 1020
Carcinomatosis 234
Cardene 1100
Cardiac arrest 234
  first aid: cardiopulmonary
    resuscitation 237
  and Myocarditis 714;
    Respiratory arrest 869;
    Shock, electric 907; Sick
    sinus syndrome 911
cardiac catheterization:
  see index entry
    Catheterization, cardiac
cardiac compression:
  in *first aid: cardiopulmonary*
    resuscitation 237
cardiac cycle:
  heart cycle 516
Cardiac massage:
  see index entry
    Cardiopulmonary
    resuscitation
cardiac muscle:
  type of Muscle 706
Cardiac neurosis 234
Cardiac output 235
Cardiac stress test 235
Cardiology 235
Cardiomegaly 235
Cardiomyopathy 235
  cause of Death, sudden 333
cardiopulmonary bypass:
  alternative term: Heart-lung
    machine 520
Cardiopulmonary resuscitation
  236

  and Cardiac arrest 234
  first aid: cardiopulmonary
    resuscitation 237
Cardiotocography:
  Fetal heart monitoring 442
Cardiovascular 236
Cardiovascular disorders 236
Cardiovascular surgery 236
Cardioversion 236
  alternative term: Defibrillation
    335
Carditis 236
Cardura 1100
Caries, dental 236
  associated with Nutritional
    disorders 740
  causes of: *causes of tooth decay*
    238; Plaque, dental 808
  causing Toothache 1002
  and Decalcification, dental 334
Carisoma 1100
Carisoprodol 1100
Carmustine 1100
carotenaemia:
  and Carotene 238; Vitamin A
    1062
Carotene 238
  source of Vitamin A 1062
Carotid artery 238
  location of carotid artery 239
carotid body:
  in Carotid artery 238
carotid sinus:
  in Carotid artery 238
carpals:
  part of *the skeletal structure of*
    the hand and wrist 505;
    Skeleton 915; Wrist 1088
Carpal tunnel syndrome 238
carpus:
  alternative term: Wrist 1088
Carrier 239
Car sickness:
  Motion sickness 696
Carteolol 1100
Cartilage 239
  in Joints 609
  removal of: Meniscectomy
    675
  tumours of: Dyschondroplasia
    381
Carylderm 1100
Cascara 1100
Cast 239
Castor oil 239
Castration 239
  and Eunuch 417
catabolism:
  in Biochemistry 169;
    Metabolism 682
Catalepsy 240
Cataplexy 240
Catapres 1100
Cataract 240
  causes of: Galactosaemia 466;
    Metabolism, inborn errors of
    682; Rubella 883
  a *disorder of the eye 426*
  and Radiation hazards 852
  treatment of: Cataract surgery
    240; *procedure for cataract*
    surgery 241; Microsurgery
    687

Cataract surgery 240
    procedure for cataract surgery 241
    and Retinal detachment 872
Catarrh 241
Catatonia 241
    feature of Schizophrenia 890
Catharsis 241
Cathartic 242
Catheter 242
    type of: Balloon catheter 156
    uses of: Catheterization, cardiac 242; Catheterization, urinary 242
Catheterization, cardiac 242
    development of: *landmarks in medicine: diagnosis 669*
    in diagnosis of *disorders of the heart 517*
    use of: Angiography 108
Catheterization, urinary 242
cation:
    and Acid 62
    type of Ion 601
CAT scanning 243
    alternative term: CT scanning 35, 323
Cat-scratch fever 243
Cats, diseases from 243
Cauda equina 243
    and Spinal nerves 936
Caudal 244
Caudal block 244
    type of Nerve block 722
Cauliflower ear 244
Causalgia 244
    treatment of: Sympathectomy 964
Caustic 244
    and Alkali 85
Cauterization 244
Caved-S 1100
Cavernous sinus thrombosis 244
    a *disorder of the nose 735*
Cavity, dental 244
    see also index entry Caries, dental
CCNU 1100
Cedocard 1100
Cefaclor 244
Cefadroxil 1101
Cefixime 1101
Cefizox 1101
Cefodizime 1101
Cefotaxime 1101
Cefoxitin 1101
Cefpodoxime 1101
Cefsulodin 1101
Ceftazidime 1101
Ceftizoxime 1101
Ceftriaxone 1101
Cefuroxime 1101
Celance 1101
Celectol 1101
Celevac 1101
Celiprolol 1101
Cell 244
    abnormal changes in: Cervical smear test 251; Computer-aided diagnosis 294; Dysplasia 382; Oncogenes 751
    cell types 245

coded instructions in:
    Chromosomes 277; DNA 366; Nucleic acids 737; RNA 881
cultures: Culture 323; Virology 1055
replication of: Cell division 246
study of: Cytology 329; *cytology methods 330;* Staining 943
surface receptors: *types of receptor 861*
transformation of: Metaplasia 683
Cell division 246
    and Chromosomes 277
Cellulitis 246
cellulose:
    in Carbohydrates 232; Fibre, dietary 446
Celsius scale 246
Cementum 246
Centigrade scale 246
    modern term: Celsius scale 246
centipedes:
    causing Venomous bites and stings 1050
Central nervous system 246
    part of Nervous system 723, *724*
central nervous system syndrome:
    and Radiation sickness 853
Centrifuge 246
Centyl K 1101
Cephalexin 246
Cephalhaematoma 246, *247*
    associated with Vacuum extraction 1040
    in Newborn 730
Cephalic 247
cephalic presentation:
    and Version 1052
cephalopelvic disproportion:
    causing Childbirth, complications of 264
Cephalosporin drugs 247
Cephamandol 1101
Cephazolin 1101
Cephradine 1101
Ceporex 1101
Cerebellar ataxia 247
Cerebellum 247
cerebral embolism:
    and stroke: *types and causes of stroke 953*
    type of Embolism 394
Cerebral haemorrhage 248
    and stroke: *types and causes of stroke 953*
cerebral oedema:
    see index entry brain, oedema of
Cerebral palsy 248
    associated with Spina bifida 933
    cause of: Kernicterus 612; Rubella 883
    causing Spasticity 930
Cerebral thrombosis 248
    and stroke: *types and causes of stroke 953*

Cerebrospinal fluid 248
    excess of: Hydrocephalus 545
    sampling of: Lumbar puncture 648
    and Spinal cord 934; Ventricle 1051
Cerebrovascular accident 249
Cerebrovascular disease 249
Cerebrovase 1101
Cerebrum 249
    disorders of: Brain damage 201; *disorders of the brain 200;* Brain syndrome, organic 203; Cerebral palsy 248; Dementia 338; Epilepsy 410
    part of Brain 198; Central nervous system 246; Nervous system 723, *724*
    parts of: Basal ganglia 160; Grey matter 493; Meninges 675; Ventricle 1051
Certification 250
Cerumen 250
    common term: Earwax 386
Cervagem 1101
Cervical 250
Cervical cancer:
    see index entry Cervix, cancer of
Cervical erosion 250
Cervical incompetence 251
    causing Miscarriage 690
cervical intraepithelial neoplasia (CIN) classification:
    in Cervical smear test 252
Cervical mucus method 251
    and Contraception, natural methods of 304
Cervical osteoarthritis 251
    causing Paralysis 778
    and Neck 720
Cervical rib 251
    causing Thoracic outlet syndrome 984
    and Neck 720
Cervical smear test 251
    procedure for a cervical smear 252
    and Colposcopy 292; Cytology 329; Screening for cancer 25
    in diagnosis of Cervix, cancer of 255
cervical spine:
    injury to: Whiplash injury 1082
    part of Spine 937
Cervical spondylosis 252
    alternative term: Cervical osteoarthritis 251
Cervicitis 252
    resulting from Nonspecific urethritis 733
Cervix 253
    disorders of the cervix 254
    investigation: Cervical smear test 251
    part of Reproductive system, female 868
Cervix, cancer of 253
    associated with Herpes, genital 532; Warts, genital 1075
    a *disorder of the cervix 254*
    diagnosis of: Cervical smear test 251; Colposcopy 292;

Cone biopsy 295; Cytology 329
    treatment of: Cryosurgery 322
Cesamet 1101
Cestodes 255
    causing Tapeworm infestation 969
    type of Flatworm 452
Cetirizine 1101
Cetrimide 1101
Chagas' disease 255
    causing Myocarditis 714
    type of Trypanosomiasis 1018
Chain, Ernst:
    landmarks in medicine: drugs 671
Chalazion 255
Chancre, hard 255
    feature of Syphilis 966
Chancroid 255
Chapped skin 256
Character disorders:
    Personality disorders 795
Charcoal 256
Charcot-Marie-Tooth disease 256
    alternative term: Peroneal muscular atrophy 794
Charcot's joint 256
Check-up:
    Examination, physical 418
    You and your doctor 32–33
Cheilitis 256
Chelating agents 256
    in treatment of Haemochromatosis 499; Lead poisoning 629; Mercury poisoning 681; Thalassaemia 982
Chemist 256
chemoreceptor trigger zone:
    in Vomiting 1067
Chemotherapy 256
Chemotrim 1101
Chendol 1101
Chenodeoxycholic acid 256
Chenofalk 1101
Chest 256
    medical term: Thorax 985
    removal of fluid from: Paracentesis 777
    surgical opening of: Thoracotomy 985
    X-ray of: Chest X-ray *34, 257*
Chest pain 256
    central: Myocardial infarction 712; Retrosternal pain 874
    diagnosing chest pain 257
    feature of Tietze's syndrome 994
    and Palpitation 774
    symptom chart 258
Chest X-ray 34, 257
Cheyne-Stokes respiration 257
"chi":
    in Chinese medicine 265
Chickenpox 257
    leading to Herpes zoster 533
Chigoe 260
Chilblain 260
Child abuse 260
    and Paedophilia 771
Childbed fever:
    medical term: Puerperal sepsis 843

Childbirth 261
    anaesthesia in: Epidural
        anaesthesia 410; Nerve block
        722; Pudendal block 843
    stages of birth 262
    complications of: Childbirth,
        complications of 264;
        Puerperal sepsis 843
    first aid: emergency childbirth 263
    and Postnatal depression 819
    preparation for: Antenatal care
        112
Childbirth, complications of 264
Childbirth, natural 264
Child development 264, *266–267*
    assessment of: Developmental
        delay 346
Child guidance 265
Chill 265
    medical term: Rigor 881
Chinese medicine 265
Chinese restaurant syndrome
    265
Chiropody 265
Chiropractic 268
Chlamydial infections 268
    causing Lymphogranuloma
        venereum 655; Nonspecific
        urethritis 733; Pelvic
        inflammatory disease 786;
        Pneumonia 811; Psittacosis
        836; Salpingitis 887;
        Trachoma 1008; Urethritis
        1029
    treatment of: Azithromycin
        149; Oxytetracycline 770
    types of: Infectious disease 578;
        Sexually transmitted disease
        904
Chloasma 268
    and abnormal Pigmentation
        803
    associated with Pregnancy
        822
Chloractil 1101
Chloral hydrate 268
Chlorambucil 268
Chloramphenicol 268
    in treatment of Conjunctivitis
        296
Chlorate poisoning 268
Chlordiazepoxide 268
    introduction of: *landmarks in
        medicine: drugs 671*
Chlorhexidine 268
Chlorine 268
Chlormethiazole 1101
Chlormezanone 1101
Chloroform 268
Chloromycetin 1101
Chloroquine 269
    causing *disorders of the retina
        872*
Chlorothiazide 1101
Chlorpheniramine 269
Chlorpromazine 269
    in treatment of Anorexia
        nervosa 111
Chlorpropamide 269
Chlortetracycline 1101
Chlorthalidone 1101
choanal atresia:
    a *disorder of the nose 735*

Choking 269
    first aid: choking 269, 270
    and Larynx 626
Cholangiocarcinoma 270
    type of Liver cancer 642
Cholangiography 270
cholangiopancreatography:
    type of Pancreatography 777
Cholangitis 270
    and *disorders of the liver 645*
Chole- 270
Cholecalciferol 270
    see index entry Vitamin D
Cholecystectomy 270
    *procedure for cholecystectomy
        271*
Cholecystitis 271
    causing Peritonitis 794
    a *disorder of the gallbladder 467*
Cholecystography 272
    in diagnosis of Gallstones 468
cholecystokinin:
    and function of Gallbladder
        467
    a Gastrointestinal hormone
        471
Choledyl 1101
Cholera 272
    travel protection 29
Cholestasis 272
Cholesteatoma 272
    causing Labyrinthitis 622
    following Otitis media 766
Cholesterol 272
    and Amaurosis fugax 91;
        Gallstones 468;
        Hyperlipidaemias 549
    production of: Liver 641
    high blood levels of:
        Atherosclerosis 140;
        Coronary artery disease 310;
        Fats 18; Xanthomatosis 1089
cholesterol tests:
    Other screening tests 27
Cholestyramine 273
Choline salicylate 1101
Choline theophyllinate 1101
Chondritis 273
Chondro- 273
Chondromalacia patellae 273
    affecting Knee 619; Patella
        783
chondromas:
    affecting Finger 449
    leading to Chondromatosis
        273
Chondromatosis 273
Chondrosarcoma 273
Chordee 273
    associated with Hypospadias
        557
Chorea 273
    causing Spasm 929
    affecting Walking 1072
Choreoathetosis 274
Choriocarcinoma 274
    and *disorders of the uterus 1037*
    resulting from Hydatidiform
        mole 544; Trophoblastic
        tumour 1017
Chorion 274
    and development of Placenta
        806

chorionic gonadotrophin, human:
    Gonadotrophin, human
        chorionic 490
Chorionic villus sampling 39, 274
    and Abortion, induced 57;
        Genetic analysis 39
    development of: *landmarks in
        medicine: diagnosis 669*
    in diagnosis of Down's
        syndrome 371; Muscular
        dystrophy 708
Choroid 275
    part of Eye 423; Uvea 1039
Choroiditis 275
choroid plexus:
    in brain: Ventricle 1051
    part of Eye 423
Christian Science 275
Christmas disease 275
chromatin:
    in Chromosomes 277
Chromium 275
Chromosomal abnormalities 275
    and Abortion, induced 57
    causing Down's syndrome
        370; Genetic disorders 476
    diagnosis of: Amniocentesis
        39; Chorionic villus
        sampling 39; Chromosome
        analysis 276; Genetic
        analysis 39
    types of: Mosaicism 696;
        Trisomy 1017
Chromosome analysis 276
    and Amniocentesis 39;
        Chorionic villus sampling
        39; Genetic analysis 39
Chromosomes 277
    in cell: Nucleus 736
    and Amniocentesis 39;
        Chorionic villus sampling
        39; Chromosome analysis
        276; Gene 472; *what genes are
        and what they do 474*; Genetic
        analysis 39; Genome,
        human 480; Inheritance 585
    replication of: Meiosis 672;
        Mitosis 691; *the mechanism of
        mitosis 692*
    structure of: Nucleic acids 737
    translocation of: *effect of
        chromosomal translocation
        1010*; Translocation 1009
    see also index entry
        Chromosomal abnormalities
Chronic 278
Chronic fatigue syndrome:
    Myalgic encephalomyelitis 710
Chronic obstructive lung
    disease:
    Lung disease, chronic
        obstructive 650
chronological age:
    and Age 73; Intelligence tests
        590
chylomicrons:
    in Hyperlipidaemias 549
Chymotrypsin 1101
Cicatrin 1101
Cidomycin 1101
cigarette-smoking:
    see index entry Tobacco-
        smoking

Cilastatin 1101
Cilazapril 1101
Cilest 1101
cilia:
    on Epithelium 413
    in Trachea 1007
Cimetidine 278
Cinazière 1101
Cinnarizine 278
Cinobac 1101
Cinoxacin 1101
Ciprofibrate 1101
Ciprofloxacin 1101
Ciproxin 1101
Circadian rhythm 278
    and Jet-lag 609; Pineal gland
        804
    type of Biorhythm 171
Circulation, disorders of 279
    Arteries, disorders of 130
    Capillary 231
    disorders of the heart 517
    Veins, disorders of 1048
Circulatory system 279, *280*
    and Blood 181; Respiration 869
    parts of: Aorta 122; Arterioles
        130; Artery 131; Capillary
        231; Heart 513; Valve 1043;
        Vein 1048; Vena cava 1048
    see also index entry
        Circulation, disorders of
Circumcision 279
    in treatment of Balanitis 156;
        Paraphimosis 779; Phimosis
        800
Circumcision, female 279
Cirrhosis 279
    and Alcohol and disease 23
    associated with Liver disease,
        alcoholic 643
    causing Gynaecomastia 497;
        Liver failure 644
    diagnosis of: Liver biopsy 642
    a *disorder of the liver 645*
    treatment of:
        Hydrochlorothiazide 546;
        Metolazone 684
Cisapride 281
Cisplatin 281
Citanest 1101
Citramag 1101
Citrical 1101
Claforan 1101
Clap 281
    medical term: Gonorrhoea 490
Claradin 1101
Clarithromycin 1101
Clarityn 1101
Claudication 281
    intermittent: Peripheral
        vascular disease 793
    a *disorder of muscle 707*
Claustrophobia 281
    type of Phobia 800
Clavicle 281
    part of Skeleton 914, *915*
    and Shoulder 909
Clavulanic acid 1101
Claw-foot 281

Claw-hand 281
  and Ulnar nerve 1024
Claw-toe 282
cleft lip:
  common term: Hare lip 507
  feature of Cleft lip and palate
    282
Cleft lip and palate 282
  treatment of: Plastic surgery
    809
cleft palate:
  associated with Hare lip 507
  cause of: Fetal alcohol
    syndrome 440
  feature of Cleft lip and palate
    282
Clemastine 1101
Clergyman's knee 282
  type of Bursitis 220
Climacteric 282
  alternative term: Menopause
    676
Climagest 1101
Climaval 1101
Clindamycin 282
Clinicide 1101
Clinitar 1101
Clinoril 1101
Clioquinol 1101
Clitoridectomy 282
  Circumcision, female 279
Clitoris 282
  enlargement of:
    Pseudohermaphroditism
      836; Sex determination 903;
      Virilism 1055
Clobazam 1101
Clobetasol 1101
Clobetasone 1101
Clofazimine 1101
Clofibrate 282
Clomid 1101
Clomiphene 282
Clomipramine 282
Clonazepam 282
Clone 282
Clonidine 283
Clonus 283
Clopamide 1101
Clopixol/Clopixol Acuphase
  1101
Clorazepate 1102
clostridial infection:
  causing Colitis 287; Food
    poisoning 456;
    Tetanus 980; Wound
    infection 1088
clot:
  see index entries blood clot;
    Blood clotting
Clotrimazole 283
Clove oil 283
Cloxacillin 283
Clozapine 1102
Clozaril 1102
Clubbing 283
  feature of Heart disease,
    congenital 519
  and Finger 449
Club-foot 283
  medical term: Talipes 968
cluster headache:
  type of Headache 507

CNS:
  see index entry Central
    nervous system
CNS stimulants 283
  group of Stimulant drugs 947
Coagulation, blood 283
  see also index entry Blood
    clotting
coal dust:
  and Occupational disease and
    injury 743
  causing Pneumoconiosis 810
Coal tar 283
Co-amilofruse 1102
Co-amilozide 1102
Co-amoxiclav 1102
Coarctation of the aorta 283
  a type of congenital heart disease
    518
Cobadex 1102
Cobalamin 284
  constituent of Vitamin B$_{12}$
    1063
Cobalin-H 1102
Cobalt 284
  constituent of Vitamin B$_{12}$
    1063
  radioactive: Radiotherapy 855
Co-Betaloc 1102
Cocaine 284
  and Withdrawal syndrome
    1084
Co-careldopa 1102
Cocci 284
  types of Bacteria 155
Coccydynia 284
Coccyx 284
  part of Pelvis 787; structure of
    the spine 937
  and Sacrum 884
Cochlea 284
  function of: Hearing 512
  part of Ear 383
  and Vestibulocochlear nerve
    1054
Cochlear implant 284
Co-codamol 1102
Co-codaprin 1102
Cocois 1102
Codafen Continus 1102
Codalax 1102
Codalax Forte 1102
Coda-Med 1102
Codanin 1102
Co-danthramer 1102
Co-danthrusate 1102
Codeine 285
Co-dergocrine 1102
Codis 500 1102
Cod-liver oil 285
Co-dydramol 1102
Coeliac disease 285
  causing Short stature 908
coffee:
  causing Insomnia 589
  constituent of: Caffeine 221
Co-fluampicil 1102
Cogentin 1102
Cognitive-behavioural therapy
  285
Coil 286
  Contraception 301
  methods of contraception 303

effectiveness (failure rates) of
  contraceptive methods 304
  IUD 605
Coitus 286
  common term: Sexual
    intercourse 904, 905
Coitus interruptus 286
Cojene 1102
Colchicine 286
  in treatment of Gout 491
cold agglutinin disorder:
  a disorder of the blood 185
Cold, common 286
  leading to Sinusitis 913
  treatment of: Cold remedies 286
Cold injury 286
Cold remedies 286
Cold sore 286
  cause of: Herpes simplex 532
Colectomy 287
  in treatment of Intestine,
    cancer of 596; Polyposis,
    familial 817; Ulcerative
    colitis 1023
Colestid 1102
Colestipol 1102
Colic 287
Colic, infantile 287
Colifoam 1102
Colistin 287
Colitis 287
Collagen 288
  constituent of: Sulphur 959
  in formation of Scar 889
  in Tendon 975
Collagen diseases 288
  associated with Scurvy 895
  example: Ehlers-Danlos
    syndrome 390
Collarbone 288
  medical term: Clavicle 281
Collar, orthopaedic 288
collective unconscious:
  in Jungian theory 609;
    Unconscious 1028
College of Health 288
Colles' fracture 288
Collodion 1102
Colloid 288
Colofac 1102
Colomycin 1102
Colon 289
  examination of: Colonoscopy
    290; endoscopy of colon 38;
    Sigmoidoscopy 912
  inflammation of: Ulcerative
    colitis 1023
  opening into: Colostomy 290
  part of Intestine 596
  removal of: Colectomy 287;
    Hemicolectomy 527
Colon, cancer of 289
  Intestine, cancer of 595
Colon, disorders of:
  disorders of the intestine 597
Colon, irritable:
  alternative term: Irritable
    bowel syndrome 603
Colonoscopy 290
  in diagnosis of Abdominal
    pain 55; Peutz-Jeghers
    syndrome 797
  endoscopy of colon 38

Colon, spastic:
  alternative term: Irritable
    bowel syndrome 603
colorectal cancer:
  type of Intestine, cancer of
    595
Colostomy 290
  in treatment of Hirschsprung's
    disease 536; Rectum, cancer
    of 864
Colostrum 291
  production of: Breast 204
Colour blindness:
  Colour vision deficiency 292
Colour vision 291
Colour vision deficiency 292
Colpermin 1102
Colposcopy 292
Colven 1102
Coma 293
  causes of: Hypoglycaemia 556;
    Shock 907
  type of Vegetative state 1048
Co-magaldrox 1102
Combantrin 1102
Combidol 1102
Combination drug 293
Comedo 293
  common term: Blackhead
    174
Comixo 1102
Commensal 293
Commode 293
Communicable disease 293
Comox 1102
Compartment syndrome 293
  causing Shin splints 907
  a disorder of muscle 704
  treatment of: Fasciotomy 435
Compensation neurosis 293
Complement 293
  constituent of Blood 181
complement system:
  part of Immune system 569
Complex 294
complexion, florid:
  medical term: Plethora 810
Compliance 294
Complication 294
Comploment Continus 1102
Compos mentis 294
Compress 294
  and Heat treatment 526
Compression syndrome 294
Compulsive behaviour:
  Obsessive-compulsive
    disorder 742
compulsive personality:
  type of Personality disorder
    795
Computed tomography 294
  alternative term: CT scanning
    35, 323
Computer-aided diagnosis 294
Concavit 1102
Conception 294
  failure of: Infertility 581
Concordin 1102
Concussion 294
conditioned reflex:
  and Conditioning 295
  type of Reflex 864
Conditioning 295

Condom 295
  how to use a condom 885
  Contraception, barrier
    methods of 302
  in prevention of AIDS 77;
    Sexually transmitted
    diseases 904
  and Safer sex 885
Condom, female 295
Conduct disorders 295
conductive deafness:
  and Hearing tests 513
  resulting from Otosclerosis 767
  type of Deafness 331
Condyline 1102
Condyloma acuminatum:
  Warts, genital 1075
Cone biopsy 295
  type of *biopsy of the cervix 253*
Confabulation 295
  feature of Wernicke-Korsakoff
    syndrome 1081
Confidentiality 295
Confusion 296
  causes of: Dementia 338;
    Hypoxia 560; Subdural
    haemorrhage 956
congeners:
  causing Hangover 506
Congenital 296
congenital disorders:
  alternative term: Birth defects
    172
  types of: Heart disease,
    congenital 519
Congestion 296
Congestive heart failure:
  Heart failure 519
Conjugated oestrogens 1102
Conjunctiva 296
  disorders of: Conjunctivitis
    296; Pinguecula 804;
    Xerophthalmia 1089
  part of Eye 423
Conjunctivitis 296
  causing Eye, painful red 427
  a *disorder of the eye 426*
  and Reiter's syndrome 866;
    Rhinitis, allergic 878
Connective tissue 297
Connective tissue diseases:
  alternative term: Collagen
    diseases 288
Conn's syndrome 297
  alternative term:
    Aldosteronism 84
  cause of: Adrenal tumours 70
Conotrane 1102
Conova 30 1102
Consciousness 297
  loss of: Fainting 430;
    Unconsciousness 1028;
    Vasovagal attack 1047
Consent 297
  and Ethics, medical 416
Constipation 297
  causes of: Codeine 285; Fibroid
    447; Megacolon 671
  causing Faecal impaction 429
  and Faeces, abnormal 429;
    Hirschsprung's disease 536;
    Soiling 928
  in Pregnancy 822

symptom chart 298
  treatment of: Enema 405;
    Fibre, dietary 446; Lactulose
    623; Laxative drugs 629;
    Methylcellulose 684
Constriction 299
Contac-400 1102
contact dermatitis:
  Dermatitis 344
  and Skin allergy 916
Contact lenses 299
  *care and insertion of contact
    lenses 300*
  invention of: *landmarks in
    medicine: other forms of
    treatment 670*
Contact tracing 301
  and Gonorrhoea 490; Sexually
    transmitted diseases 906
Contagious 301
continent ileostomy:
  and Sphincter, artificial 933
Contraception 301
  methods of contraception 303
  *effectiveness (failure rates) of
    contraceptive methods 304*
Contraception, barrier methods
    of 302
  methods of contraception 303
  in prevention of AIDS 77;
    Sexually transmitted
    diseases 904
  and Safer sex 885
Contraception, hormonal
    methods of 304
  methods of contraception 303
Contraception, postcoital 304
  Oral contraceptives 755
Contraception, natural methods
    of 304
  methods of contraception 303
Contraception, postcoital 304
Contraception, withdrawal
    method of:
  Coitus interruptus 286
Contraceptive 305
  see also index entry
    Contraception
Contraceptive implant 305
contraceptive pill:
  Oral contraceptives 755
Contraceptives, injectable 305
Contractions, uterine 305
  stimulation of: Prostaglandin
    831
Contracture 305
Contraindication 305
contrast media:
  development of: *landmarks in
    medicine: diagnosis 669*
  uses of: Angiography 107;
    Contrast X-rays 34; Imaging
    techniques 562; X-rays 1089
Contrast X-rays 34
  see also index entry contrast
    media
Controlled trial 305
  type of: Double-blind 370
Contusion 305
  type of Wound 1086
Convalescence 305
Conversion disorder 306
Convulex 1102

Convulsion:
  Seizure 896
Convulsion, febrile 306
Cooley's anaemia 306
  type of Thalassaemia 982
Copholco 1102
Copper 306
Co-prenozide 1102
Co-proxamol 306
Coracten 1102
Cordarone X 1102
Cordilox 1102
Cordotomy 306
Corgard 1102
Corgaretic 1102
Corlan 1102
Cormack, Alan:
  *landmarks in medicine: diagnosis
    669*
Corn 306, *307*
  associated with Hammer-toe
    505; Mallet toe 659
Cornea 307
  and Contact lenses 300
  disorders of: *disorders of the
    cornea 308; disorders of the eye
    426*
  function of: Vision 1057; *the
    sense of vision 1058*
  part of Eye 423
  reshaping of: Excimer laser
    419
  see also index entry Corneal
    graft
Corneal abrasion 307
Corneal graft 307
  by Microsurgery 687
  in treatment of Keratoconus
    611; Trachoma 1008
  type of Transplant surgery 46,
    1010
Corneal transplant:
  see index entry Corneal graft
Corneal ulcer 307
  associated with
    Keratoconjunctivitis sicca
    611; Keratomalacia 611
  causes of: Herpes simplex 532;
    Herpes zoster 533
  causing Eye, painful red 427
Coronary 308
  arteries: Heart 513
Coronary artery bypass 308, *309*
  development of: *landmarks in
    medicine: surgery 670*
  in treatment of Myocardial
    infarction 714
Coronary artery disease 310
  associated with Obesity 742;
    Smoking and drinking
    22–23; Tobacco-smoking 997
  Avoiding heart disease 21
  cause of: Plaque 808
  causing Death, sudden 333;
    Sick sinus syndrome 911
Coronary care unit 311
  and Intensive care 44
Coronary heart disease 311
  and Alcohol 82
  see also index entry Coronary
    artery disease
Coronary thrombosis 311
  Thrombosis 987

coronaviruses:
  causing Cold, common 286
  viruses and diseases 1056
Coroner 311
Coro-Nitro 1102
corpora cavernosa:
  part of Penis 788
Cor pulmonale 311
  cause of: Pneumoconiosis 810
  a disorder of the heart 517
corpus callosum:
  part of Cerebrum 249
Corpuscle 311
corpus luteum:
  anatomy of the ovary 768
corpus spongiosum:
  part of Penis 788
Corset 311
Corsodyl 1102
Cortelan 1102
Cortex 312
  cerebral: part of Cerebrum 249
Corticosteroid drugs 312
  causing Cataract 240; Short
    stature 908
  and Cushing's syndrome 325
  examples: Dexamethasone
    347; Hydrocortisone 546;
    Methylprednisolone 684;
    Prednisone 821;
    Triamcinolone 1014
  in treatment of Crohn's
    disease 320; Hepatitis,
    chronic active 529;
    Rheumatoid arthritis 877;
    Rhinitis, allergic 878;
    Temporal arteritis 973;
    Uveitis 1039
Corticosteroid hormones 312
Corticotrophin 312
  alternative term: ACTH 64
Cortisol 312
  alternative term:
    Hydrocortisone 546
Cortisone 312
Cortistab 1102
Cortisyl 1102
Coryza 312
  Cold, common 286
Cosalgesic 1102
Cosmegen Lyovac 1102
Cosmetic dentistry 313
Cosmetic surgery 313
  for Gynaecomastia 497
  and Plastic surgery 809
  types of: Body contour surgery
    190; Face-lift 428;
    Mammoplasty 660;
    Otoplasty 767
Costalgia 313
Cosuric 1102
Cot death:
  Sudden infant death
    syndrome 957
Co-tenidone 1102
Co-trimoxazole 313
Cough 313
  symptom chart 315
  treatment of: Cough remedies
    314
Coughing up blood 314
  causes of: Bronchitis, chronic
    214; Larynx, cancer of 626;

Lung cancer 649;
  Pneumonia 811;
  Tuberculosis 1019
Cough remedies 314
Cough, smoker's 316
  and Tobacco-smoking 997
Counselling 316
  Psychotherapy 841
Coversyl 1102
Covonia 1102
Covonia for Children 1103
Cowpox 317
Coxa vara 317
  treatment of: Osteotomy 765
coxsackievirus:
  causing Hand-foot-and-
    mouth disease 506;
    Pneumonia 811
Crab lice:
  alternative term: Pubic lice
    842
"crack":
  form of Cocaine 284
Cradle cap 317
Cramp 317
  cause of: Lactic acid 623
Cramp, writer's 317
Cranial nerves 318
  Nerve 722
Craniopharyngioma 318
Craniosynostosis 318
Craniotomy 318
  procedure for craniotomy 319
  in treatment of Skull, fracture
    of 914
Cranium 319
  part of Skull 919
Cream 319
Creatinine clearance:
  type of Kidney-function test
    616
Cremaffin 1103
Creon 1103
crepitations:
  detection of: Auscultation
    144
Crepitus 319
Cretinism 319
  causes of: deficiency of Iodine
    600; disorders of the thyroid
    gland 992
Creutzfeldt-Jakob disease 319
  transmitted by Prions 829
cricoid cartilage:
  part of Larynx 626
Cri du chat syndrome 319
Crisantaspase 1103
Crisis 319
Crisis intervention 320
Critical 320
Crohn's disease 320
  treatment of: Sulphasalazine
    959
Cromogen 1103
Crosby capsule:
  use of: Jejunal biopsy 607
Crossbite 320
Cross-eye 320
  appearance of cross-eye 321
  type of Squint 942
Cross-matching 320
  and Blood groups 186; Blood
    transfusion 189

Crotamiton 1103
Croup 321
  associated with Stridor 952
  cause of: Tracheitis 1007
Crowding, dental:
  Overcrowding, dental 769
Crown, dental 321
Cruciate ligaments 321
  part of Knee 619
Crush syndrome 321
crutches:
  causing Crutch palsy 322
  Walking aids 1073, 1074
Crutch palsy 322
Crying in infants 322
Cryo- 322
cryopexy:
  in treatment of Retinal
    detachment 872
cryoprecipitate:
  in treatment of Von
    Willebrand's disease 1068
Cryopreservation 322
Cryosurgery 322
Cryotherapy 323
Cryptococcosis 323
Cryptorchidism 323
  common term: Testis,
    undescended 979
  treatment of: Gonadotrophin,
    human chorionic 490;
    Orchidopexy 757
Cryptosporidiosis 323
Crystal violet 1103
Crystapen 1103
CT scanning 35, 323
  performing a CT scan 324
  development of: landmarks in
    medicine: diagnosis 669
  and Imaging techniques 564;
    imaging the body 565; X-rays
    1090, 1091
  uses of: Brain imaging 202;
    Heart imaging 520; Lung
    imaging 650
CULEX mosquitoes:
  Mosquito bites 696
Cullen, Mrs 1103
Culture 323
  of bacteria: Bacteriology 154
  of chromosomes:
    Amniocentesis 92; Chorionic
    villus sampling 39, 275;
    Chromosome analysis 276
Cupanol 1103
Cuplex 1103
Cupping 324
Cuprofen 1103
Curave 324
Cure 324
  and Faith healing 431
Curettage 324
  uses of: Abortion, induced 57;
    Curettage, dental 325; D
    and C 331
Curettage, dental 325
Curette 325
Curling's ulcer 325
Cushing's syndrome 325
  causes of: disorders of the
    adrenal glands 71; endocrine
    disorders 402; Pituitary
    tumours 805

  causing Hyperlipidaemias 549;
    Pigmentation 803; Stria 952
Cusp, dental 325
Cutaneous 325
Cutdown 325
cuts:
  first aid: wounds 1085
CVS:
  Chorionic villus sampling 39,
    274
Cyanide 325
Cyanocobalamin 325
  alternative term: Vitamin B_{12}
    1063
Cyanosis 325
  feature of Heart disease,
    congenital 519; Respiratory
    failure 870; Septic shock 901;
    Tetralogy of Fallot 981
Cyclandelate 1103
Cyclimorph 1103
Cyclizine 1103
Cyclofenil 1103
Cyclogest 1103
Cyclopenthiazide 326
Cyclopentolate 1103
Cyclophosphamide 326
  in treatment of Wegener's
    granulomatosis 1077
Cycloplegia 326
cycloplegic drug:
  in treatment of Corneal
    abrasion 307
Cyclo-Progynova 1103
Cycloserine 1103
Cyclosporin 326
  use of: Transplant surgery 46,
    1011
Cyclothymia 326
Cyklokapron 1103
Cymalon 1103
Cymevene 1103
Cyproheptadine 1103
Cyprostat 1103
Cyproterone acetate 326
Cyst 326
Cyst-/cysto 326
Cystectomy 326
  how cystectomy is done 327
Cystemme 1103
cystic duct:
  and Bile duct 166; Gallbladder
    467
Cysticercosis 327
  cause of: Tapeworm
    infestation 969
Cystic fibrosis 327
  causing Short stature 908
  inheritance of: Genetic
    disorders 478; unifactorial
    genetic disorders 477
  and disorders of the pancreas 775
cystic hygroma:
  type of Lymphangioma 652
Cystitis 328
  causing Abdominal pain 50;
    Intercourse, painful 592;
    Nocturia 732; Urination,
    frequent 1032; Urination,
    painful 1034
  leading to Nonspecific
    urethritis 733;
    Pyelonephritis 847

  type of Urinary tract infection
    1032
Cystocele 328
  and Uterus, prolapse of 1037
Cystoleve 1103
Cystometry 329
Cystopurin 1103
cystosarcoma phylloides:
  type of Breast lump 207
Cystoscopy 329
  in diagnosis of Incontinence,
    urinary 575
Cystostomy 329
Cystourethrography,
  micturating 329
Cystrin 1103
Cytacon 1103
Cytamen 1103
Cytarabine 1103
-cyte 329
Cyto- 329
Cytology 329
  cytology methods 330
  use of: types of cancer test 230
Cytomegalovirus 330
Cytopathology 330
cytoplasm:
  part of Cell 245
Cytosar 1103
cytosine:
  as constituent of Nucleic acids
    737
  and what genes are and what
    they do 474
  structure of DNA 39
Cytotec 1103
cytotoxic cells:
  part of Immune system 569
  types of Lymphocyte 653
Cytotoxic drugs 330
  types of Anticancer drugs 115

D

Dacarbazine 1103
Dacryocystitis 331
Dactinomycin 1103
dactylitis:
  swelling of Finger 450
Daktacort 1103
Daktarin 1103
Dalacin C 1103
Dalivit 1103
Dalmane 1103
Dalteparin 1103
Danazol 331
D and C 331
  and Abortion, induced 58
  in diagnosis of Uterus, cancer
    of 1037
  in treatment of Menorrhagia
    676
Dander 331
  allergy and the body 86
  causing Allergy 86; Asthma
    138
Dandruff 331
  associated with Blepharitis 178
  cause of: Dermatitis 344
Daneral-SA 1103

Danol 1103
Danol-1/2 1103
Danthron 1103
Dantrium 1103
Dantrolene 332
Daonil 1103
Dapsone 332
Daranide 1103
Daraprim 1103
Davenol 1103
Daydreaming 332
Day Nurse 1103
Day surgery 332
DDAVP 1103
DDT 332
deadly nightshade:
    source of Belladonna 163
    type of Plant, poisonous 808
Deafness 332
    causes of: Acoustic neuroma
        63; Barotrauma 159; Birth
        defects 172; *some possible
        causes of deafness 333;
        disorders of the ear 384;*
        Earwax 386; Glue ear 487;
        Ménière's disease 674; Noise
        732; Otitis media 766;
        Otosclerosis 767; Ototoxicity
        767; Paget's disease 772;
        Presbyacusis 827; Rubella
        883; Streptomycin 951
    causing Developmental delay
        346
    and Cleft lip and palate 282;
        Labyrinthitis 622; Lip-
        reading 639; Tinnitus 994;
        Vestibulocochlear nerve
        1054
    diagnosis of: Hearing tests
        513; *types of hearing test 514*
    treatment of: Cochlear implant
        284; Hearing aids 513;
        Myringotomy 715;
        Stapedectomy 943;
        Tympanoplasty 1021
Death 333
    and Autopsy 146; Brain death
        201; Coroner 311; Dying,
        care of the 379; Forensic
        medicine 459; Life
        expectancy 636; Mortality
        695; Pathology 784
    causes of: Accidental death 59,
        60; Maternal mortality 665;
        Occupational mortality 745
    see also index entries death
        rates; Death, sudden
death rates:
    and *accidental death 60;* Infant
        mortality 577; Maternal
        mortality 665; Mortality 695;
        Occupational mortality 745;
        Statistics, vital 944
Death, sudden 333
    and Sudden infant death
        syndrome 957; Suicide 958
Debility 334
Debridement 334
Debrisoquine 1103
Decadron 1103
Decadron Shock-Pak 1103
Deca-Durabolin-100 1103
Decalcification, dental 334

decapitation:
    Neck 720
Decay, dental:
    alternative term: Caries, dental
        236
Decazate 1103
Decerebrate 334
Deciduous teeth:
    alternative term: Primary teeth
        829
Declinax 1103
Decompression sickness 334
    cause of: Nitrogen 732
    common term: Bends 163
    and Scuba-diving medicine
        894
Decompression, spinal canal
    334
Decongestant drugs 335
    examples: Ephedrine 408;
        Oxymetazoline 770;
        Phenylpropanolamine 800;
        Pseudoephedrine 836;
        Xylometazoline 1090
    in treatment of Rhinitis,
        allergic 878
Decortisyl 1103
Decubitus ulcer:
    common term: Bedsore 161
deep vein thrombosis:
    see index entry Thrombosis,
        deep vein
Defaecation 335
    and Anus 121; Faeces 429;
        Faeces, abnormal 429;
        Peristalsis 793; Rectum 863
    see also index entries
        Constipation; Diarrhoea
defence mechanisms (against
    disease):
    see index entry Immune
        system
Defence mechanisms
    (psychological) 335
    in Bereavement 164
    and Psychoanalysis 838
Defibrillation 335
Defoliant poisoning 335
    and Pollution 815
Deformity 336
Degeneration 336
Degenerative disorders 336
Deglutition 336
    common term: Swallowing 963
Dehiscence 336
Dehydration 336
    causes of: Cholera 272;
        Delirium tremens 337;
        Diarrhoea 353; Fever 443;
        Gastroenteritis 470;
        Hangover 506; Heat
        disorders 525
    causing Thirst, excessive 984;
        Urine, abnormal 1034
    treatment of: Rehydration
        therapy 866
    and Water 1075
Déjà vu 337
    in Seizure 896; Temporal lobe
        epilepsy 974
Delax 1103
Delfen 1103
Delhi belly 337

Delinquency 337
    Behavioural problems in
        children 162
    Child guidance 265
Delirium 337
    and Confusion 296
    feature of Fever 443; Reye's
        syndrome 875
    see also index entry Delirium
        tremens
Delirium tremens 337
    and Alcohol dependence 83;
        Withdrawal syndrome 1084
Delivery 338
    and *stages of birth 262;*
        Childbirth, complications of
        264; Childbirth, natural 264;
        Malpresentation 659
    methods of: Breech delivery
        211; Caesarean section 221;
        *procedure for caesarean section
        222;* Childbirth 261; *first-aid:
        emergency childbirth 263;*
        Forceps delivery 458;
        Vacuum extraction 1040
Deltacortril Enteric 1103
Deltastab 1103
Deltoid 338
    part of Shoulder 909
Delusion 338
    in Dementia 338; Mania 661;
        Megalomania 672; Paranoia
        779; Psychosis 840;
        Schizophrenia 890
Demeclocycline 1103
Dementia 338
    and *alcohol-related disorders 84;*
        Parkinson's disease 781;
        Pseudodementia 836;
        Wilson's disease 1083
    causes of: Alzheimer's disease
        90; Brain syndrome, organic
        203; Cerebrovascular disease
        249; HIV 537
    causing Delusion 338; Insomnia
        589; Kleptomania 617
Dementia praecox 339
    alternative term:
        Schizophrenia 890
Demix 1103
De Morgan's spots 339
Demser 1103
Demyelination 339
    effect on Myelin 711
    feature of Multiple sclerosis
        702
Dendritic ulcer 339
Dengue 339
De-Nol 1103
De-Noltab 1103
Densitometry 339
Density 339
    relative density: Specific
        gravity 930
dental abscess:
    Abscess, dental 59
dental calculus:
    see index entry Calculus,
        dental
dental caries:
    see index entry Caries, dental
dental crowns:
    Crown, dental 321

dental cyst:
    in Periodontitis 792
Dental emergencies 339
Dental examination 340
Dental extraction:
    Extraction, dental 422
dental floss:
    see index entry Floss, dental
dental implants:
    Implants, dental 574
dental impression:
    see index entry Impression,
        dental
dental plaque:
    see index entry Plaque, dental
Dental X-ray 341
Dentifrice 341
    use of: Toothbrushing 1002
Dentine 341
    decay of: Caries, dental 236;
        *causes of tooth decay 238
        structure and arrangement of
        teeth 972*
Dentistry 341
Dentition 342
    alternative term: Eruption of
        teeth 414
    and Permanent teeth 794;
        Primary teeth 829; Teeth
        971; *structure and arrangement
        of teeth 972*
Denture 342
    and Impression, dental 574;
        Prosthetics, dental 834
Deodorant 342
    causing Itching 604; Vaginal
        itching 1041
    in prevention of Body odour
        191
Deoxyribonucleic acid (DNA):
    see index entries DNA;
        Nucleic acids
Dependence 342
    and Addiction 66
    see also index entries Alcohol
        dependence; Drug
        dependence
dependent personality:
    Personality disorders 795
Depersonalization 342
    and Derealization 344
    feature of Panic attack 777
Depilatory 342
    and Hair removal 503
Depixol 1103
Depo-Medrone 1103
Deponit 1103
Depo-Provera 1103
Depostat 1103
Depot injection 343
Depression 343
    causing Insomnia 589;
        Pseudodementia 836; Sexual
        desire, inhibited 904; Suicide
        958; Suicide, attempted 958;
        Weight loss 1080
    in Influenza 584; Manic-
        depressive illness 661;
        Postnatal depression 819;
        Post-traumatic stress
        disorder 819; Pregnancy 822;
        Premenstrual syndrome 826;
        Psychosis 840

and Personality disorders 795;
  Phobia 800
following Rape 857
treatment of: Antidepressant
  drugs 116; Cognitive-
  behavioural therapy 285;
  ECT 388; Exercise 419;
  Imipramine 566; Maprotiline
  662; Protriptyline 836
Dequalinium 1103
Derangement 344
Derbac-M 1103
Derealization 344
associated with
  Depersonalization 342
feature of Panic attack 777
Dermabrasion 344
in treatment of Tattooing 971
Dermatitis 344
  and *allergy and the body 86;*
  Eczema 389; *disorders of the*
  skin 919
  causes of: Allergy 85; Gold
  489; Nickel 730; Skin allergy
  915
  diagnosis of: Skin tests 918
  treatment of: Corticosteroid
  drugs 312; Hydrocortisone
  546; Lanolin 624; Potassium
  permanganate 821
Dermatitis artefacta 344
Dermatitis herpetiformis 344
  and Coeliac disease 285
Dermatology 344
Dermatome 344
Dermatome, surgical 345
Dermatomyositis 345
  type of Autoimmune disorder
  145; *disorder of muscle 707;*
  Myositis 715; *disorder of the*
  skin 919
Dermatophyte infections 345
  alternative term: Tinea 994
dermis:
  part of Skin 915
Dermographism 345
  form of Urticaria 1035
Dermoid cyst 345
  type of Ovarian cyst 767;
  Teratoma 976
Dermoid tumour:
  Dermoid cyst 345
Dermonistat 1103
Dermovate 1103
Dermovate-NN 1103
descending colon:
  part of Intestine 595
Desensitization 345
  use of: Behaviour therapy
  162
Desensitization, allergy:
  Hyposensitization 557
Deseril 1103
Designer drugs 345
Desipramine 1104
Desmoid tumour 346
Desmopressin 1104
Desmospray 1104
Desogestrel 1104
Desonide 1104
Desoxymethasone 1104
Deteclo 1104
Detergent poisoning 346

Development 346
Developmental delay 346
  and Child development 264,
  266–267; Failure to thrive
  430
  resulting from Metabolism,
  inborn errors of 682
deviated septum:
  Nasal septum 718
Deviation, sexual 347
De Witt's Analgesic 1104
Dexamethasone 347
Dexamphetamine 347
  type of Amphetamine drug
  94
Dexa-Rhinaspray 1104
Dexedrine 1104
Dexfenfluramine 1104
Dextrocardia 347
Dextromethorphan 348
Dextromoramide 348
Dextropropoxyphene 348
Dextrose 348
D factor:
  causing Rhesus
  incompatibility 875
DH 348
DHC Continus 1104
Diabetamide 1104
Diabetes, bronze 348
  alternative term:
  Haemochromatosis 499
Diabetes insipidus 348
  and ADH 67
  cause of: Pituitary tumours 805
  causing Urination, excessive
  1032
Diabetes mellitus 348
  causes of: *disorders of the*
  pancreas 775; Pancreatectomy
  775
  causing Gangrene 469;
  Glycosuria 488; Impotence
  574; Itching 604; Leg ulcer
  631; Neuropathy 728;
  Nocturia 732; Paralysis 778;
  Peripheral vascular disease
  793; *disorders of the retina 873;*
  Retinal haemorrhage 873;
  Squint 943; Thirst, excessive
  984; Urination, excessive
  1032; Weight loss 1080
  living with diabetes mellitus 349
  and Hyperglycaemia 548;
  Hypoglycaemia 556; Ketosis
  612; Obesity 742
  in pregnancy: Diabetic
  pregnancy 350
  treatment of: Chlorpropamide
  269; Glucagon 487; Guar
  gum 496; Hypoglycaemics,
  oral 556; Insulin 589; Pump,
  insulin 846
diabetic neuropathy:
  Neuropathy 728
Diabetic pregnancy 350
diabetic retinopathy:
  causing Vitreous haemorrhage
  1066
  treatment of: Photocoagulation
  801
  type of Retinopathy 874
Diabinese 1104

Diagnosis 350
  diagnosing abdominal pain 55
  diagnosing chest pain 257
  Diagnosing disease 30–31
  steps in diagnosing a condition
  351
  Diagnostic techniques 34–39
  Examination, physical 418
  Imaging techniques 564
  imaging the body 565
  landmarks in medicine: diagnosis
  669
  You and your doctor 32–33
Dialar 1104
Dialysis 44, 351
  development of: *landmarks in*
  medicine: other forms of
  treatment 670
  procedure for dialysis 352
  in treatment of Goodpasture's
  syndrome 490; Kidney
  failure 616; Kidney,
  polycystic 616
Diamicron 1104
Diamorphine 353
  and Heroin abuse 531
Diamox 1104
Dianette 1104
Diaphine 1104
Diaphragm, contraceptive 353
  associated with Toxic shock
  syndrome 1005
  Contraception, barrier
  methods of 302
Diaphragm muscle 353
  and Breathing 208
  nerve supply to: Phrenic nerve
  802
  part of Respiratory system 870
diaphysis:
  and Epiphysis 412
Diarphen 1104
Diarrest 1104
Diarrhoea 353
  causes of: Amoebiasis 93;
  Cholera 272; Colitis 287;
  Crohn's disease 320;
  Diverticular disease 365;
  Dysentery 381; Food allergy
  455; Food poisoning 456;
  Gastroenteritis 470;
  Intestine, cancer of 596;
  Irritable bowel syndrome
  603; Polyposis familial 817;
  Shigellosis 907; Typhoid
  fever 1022; Ulcerative colitis
  1023; deficiency of Vitamin
  A 1062
  causing Dehydration 337;
  Incontinence, faecal 575
  symptom chart 354
  treatment of: Antidiarrhoeal
  drugs 116; Colectomy 287;
  Diphenoxylate 360; Kaolin
  610; Rehydration therapy
  866
Diastole 355
  and Heart 514; *heart cycle 516;*
  Systole 967
diastolic blood pressure:
  abnormally high:
  Hypertension 551
  Blood pressure 187

Diathermy 355
  uses of: Operating theatre 752;
  Physiotherapy 803
Diathesis 356
Diazemuls 1104
Diazepam 356
Diazoxide 1104
Dibenyline 1104
Dichlorphenamide 1104
Diclofenac 356
Diclomax 1104
Diclozip 1104
Diconal 1104
Dicyclomine 1104
Dicynene 1104
Didronel 1104
Dienoestrol 1104
die, right to:
  and Euthanasia 418; Living
  will 646
Diet:
  constituents of: Artificial
  sweeteners 134; Calorie 226;
  Carbohydrates 19, 232;
  Cholesterol 272; Energy
  requirements 405; Fats and
  oils 18, 436; Fibre, dietary
  19, 446; Food additives 455;
  Minerals 19, 689; *minerals*
  and main food sources 690;
  recommended daily allowances
  of selected minerals 690;
  Mineral supplements 689;
  Nutrient 738; *essential*
  nutrients 740; food sources of
  essential nutrients 741;
  Nutrition 738; Proteins 18,
  834; Trace elements 1006;
  Vitamin 19, 1061; *vitamins*
  and their sources in the diet
  1063; recommended daily
  allowances of selected
  vitamins 1062; Vitamin
  supplements 1064; Water
  19, 1075
  good dietary habits 357
  Eating well 18–19
  Keeping healthy 16–17
  and Pregnancy 822
  types of: Macrobiotics 656;
  Vegetarianism 1047
  and weight: Fasting 436;
  Obesity 742; Weight 1078;
  Weight reduction 1080; *rules*
  for weight reduction 1081
  see also index entries Alcohol;
  Diet and disease
Diet and disease 356
  infected animal products 457
  Atherosclerosis 140
  Cholesterol 272
  Coronary artery disease 310
  good dietary habits 357
  Eating well 18–19
  Food allergy 455
  Food-borne infection 455
  Food intolerance 456
  Food poisoning 456
  Keeping healthy 16–17
  Nutritional disorders 740
  Obesity 742
  see also index entries Alcohol-
  related disorders: Diet

Dietetics 357
  and Nutrition 738
Diethylcarbamazine 1104
Diethylpropion 1104
Differentiation 357
Difflam 1104
Diffusion 357
Diflucan 1104
Diflucortolone 1104
Diflunisal 357
digestion:
  see index entry Digestive
  system
Digestive system 357
  disorders of: disorders of the
    anus 121; disorders of the
    gallbladder 467; disorders of
    the intestine 596; disorders of
    the liver 645; disorders of the
    oesophagus 749; disorders of
    the pancreas 776; disorders of
    the stomach 949
  functions of: Bile 166; function
    of the biliary system 168; the
    digestive process 358; Enzyme
    408; liver structure and
    function 643; Peristalsis 793;
    Saliva 886
  parts of: Anus 121; Appendix
    127; Bile duct 166; Biliary
    system 167; Caecum 221;
    Colon 289; Duodenum 379;
    Gallbladder 467; Illeum 563;
    Intestine 596; Jejunum 607;
    Liver 640; Mouth 697;
    Oesophagus 748; Pancreas
    775; Pharynx 798; Rectum
    863; Salivary glands 886;
    Stomach 948
Digitalis drugs 359
  landmarks in medicine: drugs 671
Digital subtraction angiography 34
  type of Angiography 108
Digitoxin 359
Digoxin 359
Dihydrocodeine 1104
Dihydroergotamine 1104
Dihydrotachysterol 1104
Dihydroxycholecalciferol 1104
Dijex 1104
Dilatation 359
Dilatation and curettage:
  see index entry D and C
Dilation 359
Dilator 359
  in treatment of Vaginismus
    1042
Diloxanide furoate 1104
Diltiazem 359
Dilzem 1104
Dimenhydrinate 1104
Dimercaprol 1104
Dimethicone 1104
Dimethindene 1104
Dimetriose 1104
Dimotane 1104
Dimotapp 1104
Dimyril 1104
Dindevan 1104
Dinoprost 1104
Dinoprostone 1104
Diocalm Junior 1104
Dioctyl 1104

Dioderm 1104
Dioralyte 1104
Diovol 1104
Dioxin 360
  as constituent of Agent
    Orange 73
  and Defoliant poisoning 335;
    Pollution 815
Dipentum 1104
Diphenhydramine 360
Diphenoxylate 360
Diphenylpyraline 1104
Diphtheria 362
  causing Pharyngitis 798
  and Pertussis 795; Tropical
    ulcer 1018
  prevention of: DPT
    vaccination 371; How
    immunization works 28;
    Vaccine 1040
Dipipanone 1104
Dipivefrine 1104
Diplopia 360
  common term: Double vision
    370
Diprivan 1104
Diprosalic 1104
Diprosone 1104
Dipsomania 360
Dipyridamole 360
Dirythmin SA 1104
Disability 360
  physical aids for the disabled 361
  Handicap 506
  Rehabilitation 866
  and Sexual problems 907
Disalcid 1104
Discharge 361
Disc, intervertebral 361
  part of spine 937
  see also index entry Disc
    prolapse
Disclosing agents 361
  and Oral hygiene 756
  revealing Plaque, dental 808
discoid lupus erythematosus
  (DLE):
  see index entry Lupus
    erythematosus
Discoloured teeth 362
Disc prolapse 362
  cause of: Lordosis 647
  causing Back pain 150;
    Paralysis 778; Radiculopathy
    853; Sciatica 891
  diagnosis of: Myelography 712
  symptoms and treatment of disc
    prolapse 363
  and Spinal nerves 936;
    disorders of the spine 938
  treatment of: Decompression,
    spinal canal 334
Disc, slipped:
  see index entry Disc prolapse
disease:
  causes of: Autoimmune
    disorders 145; Cancer 227;
    Carcinogen 233; Diet and
    disease 356; endocrine
    disorders 402; Genetic
    disorders 476; Iatrogenic
    562; Infection 577; Infection,
    congenital 577; Infectious

  disease 578; some important
    infectious diseases 579–581;
    Inheritance 585;
    Metabolism, inborn errors of
    682; Nutritional disorders
    740; Occupational disease
    and injury 743; Parasite 779;
    Pathogen 784; Pathogenesis
    784; Radiation hazards 852;
    Radiation sickness 853;
    Vector 1047; Zoonosis 1094
  diagnosis of: steps in diagnosing
    a condition 351; Diagnosis
    350; Diagnosing disease
    30–31; Diagnostic techniques
    34–39; landmarks in medicine:
    diagnosis 669; You and your
    doctor 32–33;
    Pathognomonic 784; Sign
    912; Symptom 964; Tests,
    medical 979
  and Illness 564
  nature of: Contagious 301;
    Incubation period 576;
    Morbidity 695; Primary 829;
    Prognosis 830; Secondary
    896; Syndrome 965;
    Transmissible 1010
  occurrence of: Endemic 400;
    Epidemic 409; Incidence 575;
    incidence of cancer 228;
    incidence of various conditions
    in the UK 574; Notifiable
    diseases 736, 737; Pandemic
    777; Prevalence 828;
    Statistics, medical 944;
    Statistics, vital 944
  prevention of: Immunization
    569; Immunization against
    disease 28–29; landmarks in
    medicine: drugs 671;
    Preventive medicine 828;
    Quarantine 849; Vaccination
    1040; Vaccine 1040
  study of: Aetiology 72;
    Environmental medicine
    407; Epidemiology 409;
    Medicine 668; Occupational
    medicine 744; Oncology 751;
    Pathology 784; Pathology,
    cellular 785;
    Pathophysiology 785
  treatment of: Chemotherapy
    256; Drug 375; landmarks in
    medicine: drugs 671; landmarks
    in medicine: surgery 670;
    landmarks in medicine: other
    forms of treatment 670;
    Radiotherapy 855; Surgery
    961; Therapy 983; Treating
    disease 40–41; Treatment
    1012; Methods of treatment
    42–47
  see also index entries Birth
    defects; Immune system;
    Immunity; Mental illness;
    Screening
disease, germ theory of:
  see index entry germ theory of
    disease
Disinfectants 362
  types of: Antiseptics 119
  use of: Sterilization 945

Disipal 1105
Dislocation, joint 362
  and Elbow 392; Hip 534; Hip,
    congenital dislocation of
    534; Jaw, dislocated 606;
    Joint 609; Shoulder,
    dislocation of 909
  partial: Subluxation 956
Disodium etidronate 1105
Disodium pamidronate 1105
Disopyramide 364
disorder:
  see index entry disease
Disorientation 364
  and Cerebrum 249
  in Reye's syndrome 875;
    Wernicke-Korsakoff
    syndrome 1081
displaced fracture:
  Fracture 460
displaced tooth:
  medical term: Subluxated
    tooth 956
Displacement activity 364
Disprin 1105
Disprol 1105
disseminated intravascular
  coagulation:
  type of Bleeding disorder 177
Dissociative disorders 364
Distaclor 1105
Distalgesic 1105
Distamine 1105
Distaquaine V-K 1105
Distigmine 1105
Disulfiram 364
Dithranol 364
Dithrocream 1105
Dithrolan 1105
Ditropan 1105
Diumide K 1105
Diuretic drugs 364
  how diuretic drugs work 365
  examples: Acetazolamide 61;
    Amiloride 92; Frusemide
    464; Hydrochlorothiazide
    546; Mannitol 661;
    Methyclothiazide 684;
    Metolazone 684;
    Spironolactone 938;
    Triamterene 1014
  in treatment of Heart failure
    520
  and Sodium 927
Diurexan 1105
Diurnal rhythms 365
  alternative term: Circadian
    rhythms 278
  type of Biorhythm 171
Diverticula 365
Diverticular disease 365
  causing Peritonitis 794
Diverticulitis 365
  and Diverticular disease 365
Diverticulosis 366
  and Diverticular disease 365
Diving medicine:
  Scuba-diving medicine 894
Dixarit 1105
Dizziness 366
  causes of: Cervical
    osteoarthritis 251;
    Hypotension 558; Hypoxia

560; Shock 907; Subclavian steal syndrome 956; Transient ischaemic attack 1009; Vertigo 1053
symptom chart 367

Djerassi, Carl:
landmarks in medicine: drugs 671

DLE (discoid lupus erythematosus):
see index entry Lupus erythematosus

DMSA scan:
type of Kidney imaging 616

DNA 366
constituent of Chromosomes 277; Gene 472
and disease: Carcinogenesis 234; Radiation 851
function of: *what genes are and what they do 474;* Genetic code 475; Inheritance 585; Protein synthesis 834; *steps in protein synthesis 835*
and Genetic analysis 39; RNA 881
structure of DNA 39
type of Nucleic acid 737

DNA fingerprinting:
alternative term: Genetic fingerprinting 479
use of: Paternity testing 783; *paternity testing using genetic fingerprinting 784*

Dobutamine 1105
Docusate 1105
Do-Do 1105
Dogs, diseases from 368
and Toxocariasis 1005
Dolmatil 1105
Dolobid 1105
Doloxene 1105
Doloxene Compound 1105
Domagk, Gerhard:
landmarks in medicine: drugs 671

Domical 1105
dominance (genetics):
and Genes 473; Inheritance 585

Domperidone 368
Don Juanism:
and Nymphomania 741
Donor 369
and Artificial insemination 133; Blood donation 184; Organ donation 758; Tissue-typing 997; Transplant surgery 46

Dopacard 1105
Dopamet 1105
Dopamine 369
deficiency of: Parkinson's disease 781
excess of: Manic-depressive illness 661
and Schizophrenia 890
type of Neurotransmitter 729
Dopexamine 1105
Doppler colour flow mapping:
in diagnosis of *disorders of the heart 517*

Doppler effect 369
in diagnosis of Aortic incompetence 122; Peripheral vascular disease 793
and Echocardiography 386; Ultrasound scanning 36, 1024

Dopram 1105
Doralese 1105
Dormonoct 1105
Dorsal 369
Dose 369
Dothapax 1105
Dothiepin 370
Double-blind 370
Double vision 370
causes of: Exophthalmos 420; Head injury 510; Multiple sclerosis 702; Squint 942
from nerve damage: Abducent nerve 55; Oculomotor nerve 741; Trochlear nerve 1017

Douche 370
causing Vaginal itching 1041; Vaginitis 1042
Dovonex 1105
Down's syndrome 370, *371*
causing Hypotonia in infants 560; Short stature 908
resulting from Translocation 1010; Trisomy 1017

Doxapram 1105
Doxazosin 1105
Doxepin 1105
Doxorubicin 371
Doxycycline 371
Doxylamine 1105
Doxylar 1105
Dozic 1105
DPT vaccination 371
Drain, surgical 372
Dramamine 1105
Drapolene 1105
Dream analysis 372
in Psychoanalysis 838
Dreaming 372
and Nightmare 731; Sleep 921
dream, wet:
medical term: Nocturnal emission 732

Dressings 373
in treatment of Burns 219
Dressler's syndrome 373
Dribbling 373
of urine: Incontinence, urinary 575
of saliva: Teething 973

Driclor 1105
drill, dental:
use of: Filling, dental 449
drinking:
see index entries Alcohol; Alcohol dependence; Alcohol intoxication; Alcohol-related disorders; Thirst; Thirst, excessive; Water

Drip:
medical term: Intravenous infusion 599

Dristan 1105
Drogenil 1105
Droleptan 1105

drooling:
see index entry Dribbling
Drop attack 373
Droperidol 1105
Dropsy 374
alternative term: Oedema 745
Drowning 374
types of drowning 375
Drowning, dry 375
drowning, partial:
and Respiratory distress syndrome 870
Drowsiness 375
Drug 375
administration of: Compliance 294; Contraindication 305; Cream 319; Depot injection 343; Dose 369; *methods of administering drugs 376;* Drug treatment 42; Inhaler 585; *how to use an inhaler 584;* Injection 586; Intravenous infusion 599; Nebulizer 719; *using a nebulizer 720;* Ointment 750; Pessary 796; Polypharmacy 816; Pump, infusion 846; Suppository 961; Topical 1003; Transdermal patch 1009
development of: Drug sources 42; Drug treatment 40; Genetically engineered drugs 43; *landmarks in medicine: drugs 671;* Natural drugs 42; Synthetic drugs 43
and Drug abuse 376; Pregnancy, drugs in 822
effects of: Drug poisoning 377; Pharmacokinetics 798; Side-effect 911; Tolerance 1000
sources of: Drug sources 42; Genetically engineered drugs 43; Natural drugs 42; Synthetic drugs 43
study of: Pharmacology 798; Psychopharmacology 840
supply of: Drug treatment 42; Pharmacy 798
types of: Generic drug 475; Pharmaceutical 798; Pharmacopoeia 798; Proprietary 831
see also index entry Drug dependence

Drug abuse 376
Drug addiction 377
see also index entry Drug dependence
Drug dependence 377
and Child abuse 260; Endocarditis 400; Sudden infant death syndrome 957; Tolerance 1000; Withdrawal syndrome 1084
drug interactions:
and Compliance 294; Drug 377; Polypharmacy 816
Drug overdose 377
see also index entry Drug poisoning
Drug poisoning 377
and Suicide 958; Suicide, attempted 958

treatment of: Antidote 117; Lavage, gastric 628
drug tolerance:
Tolerance 1000
Drug treatment 40, 42
see also index entries Drug; Treatment
drug trials:
and Animal experimentation 109; Drug treatment 41
types of: Controlled trial 305; Double-blind 370; Trial, clinical 1014
drug withdrawal:
causing Withdrawal syndrome 1084
and Drug dependence 377
dry drowning:
Drowning, dry 375
Dry eye:
medical term: Keratoconjunctivitis sicca 611
Dry ice 378
Dryptal 1105
Dry socket 378
DSM IV 378
DTIC-Dome 1105
DTPA scan:
type of Kidney imaging 616
Dual personality:
type of Multiple personality 702
Duchenne muscular dystrophy:
type of Muscular dystrophy 707
Duct 378
ductus arteriosus:
part of Fetal circulation 440
Dulcolax 1105
Dumbness:
Mutism 710
Dumping syndrome 378
following Vagotomy 1042
duodenal bypass:
medical term: Gastroenterostomy 471
Duodenal ulcer 378
type of Peptic ulcer 789
Duodenitis 378
Duodenum 379
part of Intestine 595
Duofilm 1105
Duovent 1105
Duphalac 1105
Duphaston 1105
duplex kidney:
a disorder of the kidney 614
Dupuytren's contracture 379
Durabolin 1105
Duracreme 1105
Duragel 1105
Duromine 1105
Dust diseases 379
examples: Asbestos-induced diseases 135; Pneumoconiosis 810
type of Occupational disease and injury 743
Dwarfism:
medical term: Short stature 908
Dyazide 1105
Dydrogesterone 379
Dying, care of the 379

dynamic psychotherapy:
Psychotherapy 841
Dynese 1105
Dys- 380
Dysarthria 380
type of Speech disorder 930
dyscalculia:
type of Learning difficulty 630
Dyschondroplasia 381
Dysentery 381
causing Diarrhoea 353;
Proctitis 829
types of: Amoebiasis 93;
Shigellosis 907
dysgraphia:
type of Learning difficulty 630
Dyskinesia 381
Dyslexia 381
type of Learning difficulty 629
Dysman 1105
Dysmenorrhoea 381
and Menstruation, disorders
of 677; *disorders of the uterus
1037*
dysosmia:
defect of Smell 925
Dyspamet 1105
Dyspareunia 382
common term: Intercourse,
painful 592
Dyspepsia 382
common term: Indigestion 576
Dysphagia 382
common term: Swallowing
difficulty 963
Dysphasia 382
and Aphasia 124
Dysphonia 382
and Voice, loss of 1066
Dysplasia 382
detection of: Cervical smear
test 251
in diagnosis of Cervix, cancer
of 253
Dyspnoea 382
common term: Breathing
difficulty 209
Dysrhythmia, cardiac 382
alternative term: Arrhythmia,
cardiac 128
Dystocia 382
Dystonia 382
Dystrophy 382
type of: Muscular dystrophy
707
Dysuria 382
common term: Urination,
painful 1034
Dytac 1105
Dytide 1105

E

Ear 383
disorders of: Cauliflower ear
244; Deafness 332; Earache
383; *disorders of the ear 384;*
Ear, discharge from 385;
Eardrum, perforated 385;
Ear, foreign body in 385;

Earwax 386; Glue ear 487;
Myringitis 715; Otitis
externa 766; Otitis media
766; Otosclerosis 767
examination of: Otoscope 767
noises in: Tinnitus 994
surgery on: Myringotomy 715;
Otoplasty 767;
Stapedectomy 943
Syringing of ears 967
see also index entries Balance;
Hearing
Earache 383
cause of: Otitis media 766
Ear, cauliflower:
Cauliflower ear 244
Ear, discharge from 385
eardrum:
damage to: Eardrum,
perforated 385; Valsalva's
manoeuvre 1043
inflammation of: Glue ear 487;
Myringitis 715
part of Ear 383
surgery on: Myringotomy 715;
Tympanoplasty 1021
Eardrum, perforated 385
causes of: Otitis media 766;
Syringing of ears 967
treatment of: Myringoplasty
715
Ear, examination of 385
Ear, foreign body in 385
Ear, nose, and throat surgery:
Otorhinolaryngology 767
Ear piercing 386
causing Hepatitis, viral 529
Ears, pinning back of:
Otoplasty 767
ears, ringing in:
causes of: Noise 733;
Streptomycin 951
medical term: Tinnitus 994
and Vertigo 1053
Earwax 386
treatment of: Syringing of ears
967
eating, excessive:
and Obesity 742
Ebufac 1105
Ecchymosis:
common term: Bruise 216
eccrine gland:
type of Sweat gland 963
ECG 386
and Cardiac stress test 235;
Coronary artery disease 310;
Heart-rate 522
Holter monitor 540
the electrocardiogram (ECG) 387
invention of: *landmarks in
medicine: diagnosis 669*
Echocardiography 386
in diagnosis of
Cardiomyopathy 236;
Coronary artery disease
311; *disorders of the heart
517;* Pericarditis 791
type of Ultrasound scanning
37, 1025
Echolalia 386
Eclampsia 387
and Pre-eclampsia 821

Econacort 1105
Econazole 388
Ecostatin 1105
Ecothiopate 1105
Ecstasy 388
a type of Designer drug 345
ECT 388
in treatment of Depression
343; Manic-depressive
illness 661
type of Shock therapy 908
Ectasia 388
ectomorphic body type:
a Somatotype 929
-ectomy 388
Ectoparasite 388
Ectopic 388
Ectopic heartbeat 388
Ectopic pregnancy 388
causing Abdominal pain 50
following Pelvic inflammatory
disease 786
and Oral contraceptives 755
Ectropion 389
Eczederm 1105
Eczema 389
of Nipple 731
a disorder of the skin 919
treatment of: Prednisolone
821; Promethazine 831; Zinc
oxide 1093
type of: Pompholyx 817
eczema herpeticum:
and Herpes simplex 532
Edecrin 1105
Edentulous 389
Edrophonium chloride 1105
Edwards, Robert:
*landmarks in medicine: other
forms of treatment 670*
Edwards' syndrome:
and Trisomy 1017
EEG 389
*EEG changes during a seizure 896
how electroencephalography is
done 390*
and Sleep 921
Efamast 1105
Efcortelan, Efcortesol 1105
Effercitrate 1105
Effusion 390
and Pericarditis 791
Effusion, joint 390
Efudix 1105
Egg:
egg and sperm cells 277
medical term: Ovum 769
Ego 390
and Freudian theory 462;
Psychoanalytic theory 838
Ehlers-Danlos syndrome 390
Ehrlich, Paul:
landmarks in medicine: drugs 671
Einthoven, Willem:
*landmarks in medicine:
diagnosis 669*
Eisenmenger complex 391
type of Heart disease,
congenital 519
ejaculate:
and Artificial insemination 133
Ejaculation 391
and Sexual intercourse 904

during sleep: Nocturnal
emission 732
Ejaculation, disorders of 391
ejaculatory ducts:
and Vas deferens 1046
Elantan LA 1105
Elavil 1105
Elbow 391
Eldepryl 1105
Elderly, care of the 392
Eldisine 1105
Elective 393
Electra complex:
and Oedipus complex 746
Electrical injury 393
first aid: electrical injury 392
causing Cardiac arrest 234;
Respiratory arrest 869
electrical power fields:
cause of Brain tumour 203
Electric shock treatment:
ECT 388
electrocardiogram:
see index entry ECG
Electrocardiography (ECG):
see index entry ECG
Electrocautery 393
Electrocoagulation 393
Electroconvulsive therapy:
see index entry ECT
electrocution:
Electrical injury 393
Electroencephalography (EEG):
see index entry EEG
Electrolade 1105
Electrolysis 393
method of Hair removal 504
Electrolyte 394
electromagnetic radiation:
and Colour vision 291;
Radiation 851
electromagnetic spectrum 1026
electromuscular stimulation:
Walking aids 1073
electromyogram:
EMG 397
Electromyography (EMG):
EMG 397
electron microscope:
Microscope 685
types of microscope 686
Electronystagmography 394
Electrophoresis 394
Elephantiasis 394
cause of Filariasis 448
ELISA test 394
and Serology 901
type of Immunoassay 570
Elixir 394
Elkamol 1105
Elocon 1106
Eltroxin 1106
Eludril 1106
Emblon 1106
Embolectomy 394
Embolism 394
in Peripheral vascular disease
793
see also index entry Embolus
Embolization 395
Embolus 395
removal of: Embolectomy
394

and Thrombosis 987
see also index entry Embolism
Embrocation 395
Embryo 395
abnormalities of: Teratogen 976
the developing embryo 396
stages and features of pregnancy
822
see also index entry Fetus
Embryology 397
Embryo, research on 397
Emcor 1106
Emergency 397
Emeside 1106
Emesis:
see index entry Vomiting
Emetic 397
Emflex 1106
EMG 397
in diagnosis of *disorders of*
muscle 707
Eminase 1106
EMLA 397
Emla 1106
Emollient 397
emotion:
abnormalities of: Personality
disorders 795; Psychosis 840;
Schizophrenia 890
and Limbic system 637;
Personality 795
Emotional deprivation 397
causing Short stature 908
and Child abuse 260
Emotional problems 397
Empathy 397
in Psychotherapy 841
Emphysema 397
causes of: Cadmium poisoning
221; Pneumoconiosis 810;
Pulmonary hypertension
844; Tobacco-smoking 997;
Other risks of smoking 22
a disorder of the lung 649
Emphysema, surgical 398
Empirical treatment 398
Empyema 398
emulsifiers:
types of Food additives 455
Enalapril 398
Enamel, dental 398
erosion of: Caries, dental 236
Encephalins:
Enkephalins 406
Encephalitis 399
causes of: Herpes simplex 532;
Measles 667
causing Paralysis 778
spread by Mosquito bites 696
Encephalitis lethargica 399
encephalocele:
in Spina bifida 933
Encephalomyelitis 399
Encephalopathy 399
Encopresis 399
common term: Soiling 928
Endarterectomy 399
En-De-Kay 1106
Endemic 400
Endocarditis 400
affecting Heart valve 523
cause of: Streptococcal
infections 950

following Mitral incompetence
691; Septal defect 900
a disorder of the heart 517
treatment of: Rifampicin 880
endocardium:
lining of Heart 515
Endocrine gland 400
Gland 482
see also index entry Endocrine
system
Endocrine system 400, *401*
endocrine disorders 402
and Gastrointestinal hormones
471; Hormone 541; *the*
sources and main effects of
selected hormones 543
Endocrinology 400
Endodontics 400
Endogenous 402
Endometrail ablation 402
Endometrial cancer:
Uterus, cancer of 1036
Endometriosis 402
causing Abdominal pain 50;
Intercourse, painful 592
sites of endometriosis 403
treatment of: Danazol 331;
Gonadorelins 489;
Hysterectomy 562;
Norethisterone 734
a disorder of the uterus 1037
Endometritis 402
a disorder of the uterus 1037
Endometrium 403
build-up of: Menorrhagia 676
cancer of: Uterus, cancer of 1036
removal of: Endometrial
ablation 402
endomorphic body type:
a Somatotype 929
endophthalmos:
a disorder of the eye 426
Endorphins 403
and Enkephalins 406
type of Neurotransmitter 729;
Peptide 791
Endoscope 403, *404*
use of: Endoscopic surgery 47
see also index entry
Endoscopy
endoscopic retrograde
cholangiopancreatography:
ERCP 413
Endoscopic surgery 47
in treatment of Hyperhidrosis
548
see also index entry
Endoscopy
Endoscopy 38, 403
development of: *landmarks in*
medicine: diagnosis 669
and *endoscopes 404*; Endoscopic
surgery 47; Fibre-optics 446
types of: Arthroscopy 132;
Bronchoscopy 215;
Colonoscopy 290;
Cystoscopy 329; ERCP 413;
Fetoscopy 38, 442;
Gastroscopy 471;
Laparoscopy 624;
Laryngoscopy 625;
Proctoscopy 830;
Sigmoidoscopy 912

Endothelium 405
Endotoxin 405
causing Poisoning 813
fever-causing: Pyrogen 848
Endotracheal tube 405
in treatment of Respiratory
distress syndrome 870
and Ventilation 1050
Endoxana 1106
endurance:
Fitness 451
Sports medicine 941
Enduron 1106
Enema 405
Energy 405
energy expenditure 21
units of: Calorie 226; Joule 609
Energy requirements 405
Enflurane 1106
Engagement 405
Engorgement 406
Expressing milk 421
Enkephalins 406
Enophthalmos 406
Enoxaparin 1106
Enoximone 1106
Entamizole 1106
enternal nutrition:
common term: Feeding,
artificial 437
Enteric-coated tablet 406
Enteric fever:
alternative terms: Paratyphoid
fever 781: Typhoid fever
1022
Enteritis 406
Enteritis, regional:
alternative term: Crohn's
disease 320
Enterobiasis 406
type of Threadworm
infestation 985
enteroglucagon:
type of Gastrointestinal
hormone 471
Enterostomy 406
Enterotoxin 406
causing Poisoning 813
Entropion 406
and Eyelid 428
ENT surgery:
Otorhinolaryngology 767
Enuresis 406
Environmental medicine 407
Enzyme 408
abnormal functioning of:
Metabolism, inborn errors of
682
structure of: Proteins 834
synthesis of: Nucleic acids 737
enzyme-linked immunosorbent
assay (ELISA):
see index entry ELISA test
enzyme replacement therapy:
in treatment of Genetic
disorders 478
eosinophils:
types of Blood cells 182
EP 1106
Epanutin 1106
Ependymoma 408
Ephedrine 408
Epicanthic fold 408

epicondyle:
part of Elbow 391; Humerus
542
Epicondylitis 408
inflammation of Elbow 391
Epidemic 409
Infectious disease 578
widespread: Pandemic 777
Epidemiology 409
epidermis:
part of Skin 915
structure of skin 916
Epidermolysis bullosa 409
Epididymal cyst 409
alternative term: Spermatocele
932
causing Testis, swollen 978
Epididymis *409*
part of Reproductive system,
male 868; Testis 977
and Sperm 932
Epididymitis:
see index entry Epididymo-
orchitis
Epididymo-orchitis 410
cause of: Nonspecific urethritis
733
and Orchitis 757; inflammation
of Testis 977
Epidural anaesthesia 410
and Spinal anaesthesia 934
type of Nerve block 722
Epifoam 1106
Epifrin 1106
Epiglottis 410
part of Larynx 626
Epiglottitis 410
causing Stridor 952
Epilepsy 410
and brain activity: PET
scanning 797
causes of: Head injury 510;
Spina bifida 933; Sturge-
Weber syndrome 955;
Tuberous sclerosis 1020
first aid: epileptic seizure 411
and Infantile spasms 577;
Seizure 896
treatment of: Carbamazepine
231; Neurosurgery 728;
Phenobarbitone 799;
Phenytoin 800; Primidone
829; Sodium valproate 928
types of: Grand mal 492; Petit
mal 797; Status epilepticus
944
Epilim 1106
Epiloia:
Tuberous sclerosis 1019
Epinephrine:
see index entry Adrenaline
Epiphora:
common term: Watering eye
1077
Epiphysis 412
inflammation of: Perthes'
disease 795
premature ossification of:
Achondroplasia 62
Epiphysis, slipped:
Femoral epiphysis, slipped 438
Epirubicin 1106
Episcleritis 412

Episiotomy 412
Epispadias 412
Epistaxis:
    common term: Nosebleed 735
Epithelium 413
    tumour of: Papilloma 777
Epoetin 413
Epogam 1106
Epoprostenol 1106
Eppy 1106
Eprex 1106
Epstein-Barr virus 413
    as a Carcinogen 233
    causing Burkitt's lymphoma
        218; Mononucleosis,
        infectious 694
    and Lymphoma, non-
        Hodgkin's 655
Equagesic 1106
Equanil 1106
equinovarus deformity:
    type of Talipes 968
Eradacin 1106
ERCP 413
Erection 413
Erection, disorders of 413
    assessment of:
        Plethysmography 810
    examples: Chordee 273;
        Impotence 574; Priapism 828
Ergocalciferol 413
    constituent of Vitamin D 1065
Ergometer 413
Ergometrine 413
Ergot 413
    causing Cataract 240
    production of: Fungi 464
Ergotamine 414
erogenous zones:
    Eroticism 414
Erosion, dental 414
Eroticism 414
Eruption 414
Eruption of teeth 414
Erwinase 1106
Erycen 1106
Erymax 1106
Erysipelas 415
    cause of: Streptococcal
        infection 950
Erythema 415
Erythema ab igne 415
Erythema infectiosum:
    Fifth disease 448
Erythema multiforme 415
    form of: Stevens-Johnson
        syndrome 946
Erythema nodosum 415
Erythrasma 415
Erythrocin 1106
Erythrocyte 415
    see also index entries Blood;
        Blood cells
erythrocyte sedimentation rate
    (ESR):
    ESR 416
Erythroderma:
    alternative term: Exfoliative
        dermatitis 419
Erythrolar 1106
Erythromid 1106
Erythromycin 416
Erythroped 1106

erythropoietin:
    effect of: Bone marrow 194
    excess: Polycythaemia 815
    production of: Genetically
        engineered drugs 43;
        Kidney 613
    in treatment of Anaemia 96
Eschar 1106
Eserine 1106
Esidrex 1106
Eskamel 1106
Eskazole 1106
Eskornade 1106
Esmarch's bandage 416
    type of Tourniquet 1005
Esmolol 1106
Esotropia 416
ESP (extrasensory perception):
    Parapsychology 779
ESR 416
Estracombi 1106
Estracyt 1106
Estraderm TTS 1106
Estradurin 1106
Estragest TTS 1106
Estramustine 1106
Estrapak 1106
ESWL 416
    lithotripsy procedures 641
    in treatment of Calculus,
        urinary tract 225
    type of Lithotripsy 45, 640
Ethacrynic acid 1106
Ethambutol 416
Ethamsylate 1106
Ethanol 416
    see also index entry Alcohol
Ether 416
Ethics, medical 416
Ethinyloestradiol 416
Ethionamide 1106
Ethoheptazine 1106
Ethosuximide 416
Ethyl alcohol 417
    see also index entry Alcohol
Ethyl chloride 417
ethylene glycol:
    causing Antifreeze
        poisoning 117
Ethynodiol diacetate 1106
Etidronate disodium 1106
Etodolac 1106
Etomidate 1106
Etoposide 1106
Etretinate 417
Eucalyptus oil 417
Eudemine 1106
Euglucon 1106
Eugynon 30 1106
Eumovate 1106
Eumovate-N 1106
Eunuch 417
Euphoria 417
    cause of: Cocaine 284
Eurax 1106
Eurax-Hydrocortisone 1106
Eustachian tube 417
    blockage of: Glue ear 487;
        Otitis media 766
    and Ear 383; Nasopharynx 718
Euthanasia 418
    and Consent 297
Euthyroid 418

Evaphol 1106
Eversion 418
Evoked responses 418
Evorel 1106
Ewing's sarcoma 418
Examination, physical 418
    You and your doctor 32–33
Excimer laser 419
Excision 419
Excoriation 419
excrement:
    Faeces 429
    and Food-borne infection 455
Excretion 419
Exelderm 1106
Exenteration 419
Exercise 419
    Aerobics 71
    the effects of exercise 420
    Exercise and health 20–21
    Keeping healthy 16–17
    Physiotherapy 802
    in Pregnancy 822
    and Weight reduction 1080
Exfoliation 419
Exfoliative dermatitis 419
exhaustion, nervous:
    alternative term: Neurasthenia
        725
Exhibitionism 419
Exirel 1106
Ex-lax 1106
Exocin 1106
Exocrine gland 419
    Gland 482
Exolan 1106
Exomphalos 419
Exophthalmos 420
Exostosis 421
Exotoxin 421
    causing Poisoning 813
Exotropia 421
Expectorants 421
    types of Cough remedies 314
Expectoration 421
Expelix 1106
Exploratory surgery 421
Exposure 421
exposure therapy:
    type of Behaviour therapy 162
Expressing milk 421
    Breast-feeding 206
Expulin 1106
Expurhin Paediatric 1106
Exstrophy of the bladder 421
extracorporeal shock-wave
    lithotripsy (ESWL):
    see index entry ESWL
Extraction, dental 422
extradural haematoma:
    cause of: Extradural
        haemorrhage 422
    type of Haematoma 498
Extradural haemorrhage 422
Extrapyramidal system 422
extrasensory perception (ESP):
    Parapsychology 779
extraversion-introversion:
    assessment of: Personality
        tests 795
    and Extravert 422; Introvert 599
Extravert 422
    and Jungian theory 609

Exudation 422
Eye 422
    disorders of: Blindness 179;
        Colour vision deficiency 292;
        disorders of the cornea 308;
        disorders of the eye 426;
        disorders of the retina 873;
        Vision, disorders of 1059;
        Vision, loss of 1059
    anatomy of the eye 423
    function of: Colour vision 291;
        Vision 1057; the sense of
        vision 1058; Visual acuity
        1060; Visual field 1060, 1061
    study of: Ophthalmology 753
    see also index entries Eye,
        examination of; Eyelid; eye
        movements; eye muscles;
        eye socket
Eye, artificial 423
eyeball, protruding:
    medical term: Exophthalmos
        420
eyeball, sunken:
    medical term: Enophthalmos
        406
Eye-Crom 1106
Eye-drops 424
eye, dry:
    medical term:
        Keratoconjunctivitis sicca
        611
Eye, examination of 424
    and Tonometry 1001; Vision
        tests 1059; types of vision tests
        1060
Eye, foreign body in 424
    first aid: foreign body in the eye
        425
Eye injuries 425
Eyelashes, disorders of 425
    Trichiasis 1014
Eye, lazy 427
Eyelid 427
    drooping: Ptosis 841
    glands, inflammation of:
        Meibomitis 672
    sewing together: Tarsorrhaphy
        969
    surgery on: Blepharoplasty 178
    swollen: Conjunctivitis 296
    turning inward: Entropion 406
    turning outward: Ectropion 389
Eyelid, drooping:
    medical term: Ptosis 841
Eyelid surgery:
    Blepharoplasty 178
eye movements:
    abnormal: Kernicterus 612;
        Nystagmus 741; Vertigo 1053
    control of: Abducent nerve 55;
        Oculomotor nerve 745;
        Trochlear nerve 1017
    normal: anatomy of the eye 423;
        movement 699; the sense of
        vision 1058
    painful: Optic neuritis 754
    paralysis of: Ophthalmoplegia
        754
eye muscles:
    control of: Abducent nerve 55;
        Oculomotor nerve 745;
        Trochlear nerve 1017

disorders of: Double vision 370; Myasthenia gravis 710
and Eye 422; *anatomy of the eye 423; movement 699; the sense of vision 1058*
Eye, painful red 427
eye socket:
    alternative term: Orbit 757
    component of: Sphenoid bone 932
Eye-strain 427
Eye teeth 427
    structure and arrangement of teeth 972
eye tests:
    see index entry Eye, examination of
Eye tumours 427

F

Fabahistin 1106
Fabrol 1106
face:
    appearance of: Facies 429
    bones of: *structure of the skull 920*
    hair growth on: Androgen hormones 105
    nerve supply to: Facial nerve 428; Trigeminal nerve 1016
    see also index entries Face-lift; Facial pain; Facial palsy; Facial spasm
face-downward position:
    Pronation 831
Face-lift 428
    removal of Wrinkle 1088
    type of Cosmetic surgery 313
facet joint:
    displacement of: Back pain 150
    in Spine 937
face-upward position:
    Supination 961
Facial nerve 428
Facial pain 428
    causes of: Nasopharynx, cancer of 719; Trigeminal neuralgia 1016
Facial palsy 429
    cause of: tumour of Salivary glands 886
    causing Ectropion 389
Facial spasm 429
    and Tetany 981; Tic 994
Facies 429
Factitious disorders 429
Factor VIII 429
    deficiency of: Haemophilia 501
    in Von Willebrand's disease 1068
factor IX:
    deficiency of: Christmas disease 275
    and Haemostatic drugs 503
Faecal impaction 429
    causing Incontinence, faecal 575
Faecalith 429
Faeces 429
    colour of: Bilirubin 169

formation of: Colon 289; Digestive system 359
leakage of: Crohn's disease 320; Faecal impaction 429; Incontinence, faecal 575
see also index entry Faeces, abnormal
Faeces, abnormal 429
    black: Gastritis 470; Indigestion 576; Iron 602; Melaena 673; Oesophageal varices 747; Peptic ulcer 789; Portal hypertension 818
    blood in: Colitis 287; Colon, cancer of 289; Crohn's disease 320; Rectal bleeding 862; Rectum, cancer of 864; Shigellosis 907; Ulcerative colitis 1023
    foul-smelling: Coeliac disease 285
    greasy: Coeliac disease 285; Steatorrhoea 944
    hard: Faecal impaction 429; Faecalith 429
    liquid: Diarrhoea 353
Faeces, blood in the:
    see index entries Faeces, abnormal; Rectal bleeding
Fahrenheit scale 430
Failure to thrive 430
    and Child abuse 261
Fainting 430
    causes of: Heart block 516; Hypotension 558; Neuropathy 728; Shock 908; Vasovagal attack 1047
    symptom chart 431
    and Unconsciousness 1028
Faith healing 431
Fallen arches 431
Fallopian tube 431
    anatomy of: *location of the fallopian tubes 433*
    damage to: Pelvic infection 786; Salpingitis 887
    and Ectopic pregnancy 388; Infertility 583; Sterilization, female 945
    examination of: Hysterosalpingography 561
    part of Reproductive system, female 868
    removal of: Salpingectomy 887; Salpingo-oophorectomy 887
    repair of: Microsurgery 687; Tuboplasty 1020
Fallot's tetralogy:
    Tetralogy of Fallot 981
Fallout:
    Radiation hazards 852
Falls in the elderly 433
    preventing falls 434
False teeth:
    Denture 342
Famel 1106
Familial 434
Familial Mediterranean fever 434
familial polyposis:
    Polyposis, familial 817
Family Health Service Authorities 434

Family planning 434
Family therapy 434
Fam-lax 1107
Famotidine 435
Fanalgic 1107
Fanconi's anaemia 435
Fanconi's syndrome 435
    causing Urine, abnormal 1034
Fansidar 1107
Fantasy 435
Farlutal 1107
Farmer's lung 435
Fascia 435
Fasciculation 435
    cause of: Motor neuron disease 697
Fasciitis 435
fascioliasis:
    infestation with Liver fluke 644
Fasciotomy 435
Fasigyn 1107
Fasting 436
    causing Gallstones 468; Ketosis 612
fat:
    embolism: Embolism 394
    excess body: Obesity 742
    tumour: Lipoma 639
    see also index entry Fats and oils
Fatigue:
    Tiredness 995
Fats and oils 436
    and Fats 18; Glycerol 488
    Nutrition 738
    excess intake of: Coronary artery disease 310; Diet and disease 356; Pancreas, cancer of 775
fat-soluble vitamins:
    types of Vitamin 1061
Fatty acids 436
fatty liver:
    associated with Liver disease, alcoholic 643
Faverin 1107
Favism 436
    cause of: G6PD deficiency 466
Febrile 437
    convulsion: Fever 437
febrile seizure:
    Convulsion, febrile 306
Fectrim 1107
feeding, artificial 437
    by Nasogastric tube 718
    type of: Intravenous infusion 599
Feeding, infant 437
    Bottle-feeding 196
    Breast-feeding 206
    approximate ages for introducing solids 438
feeding, intravenous:
    following Colostomy 290
    type of Feeding, artificial 437
    using Intravenous infusion 599
feet, care of:
    Chiropody 265
    and Diabetes mellitus 350; Peripheral vascular disease 793; Toenail, ingrowing 999
Fefol 1107

Fefol-Vit 1107
Fefol-Z 1107
Felbinac 1107
Feldene 1107
Felodipine 1107
female gender:
    and Chromosomal abnormalities 276; Inheritance 585; Sex determination 903; Sex hormones 903
Femeron 1107
Femigraine 1107
Feminax 1107
Femodene, Femodene ED 1107
Femoral epiphysis, slipped 438
Femoral nerve 438
Femulen 1107
Femur 438
    location of the femur 439
    part of Skeleton 915
Femur, fracture of 439
    causing Leg, shortening of 630
Fenbid 1107
Fenbufen 439
Fenbuzip 1107
Fenfluramine 1107
Fennings Children's Cooling Powders 1107
Fenofibrate 1107
Fenoprofen 439
Fenopron 1107
Fenostil Retard 1107
Fenoterol 1107
Fenox 1107
Fentanyl 1107
Fentazin 1107
Feospan 1107
Ferfolic SV 1107
Fergon 1107
ferric (iron) oxide:
    ingredient of Calamine 223
Ferrocap 1107
Ferrocap-F 350 1107
Ferrocontin Continus 1107
Ferrocontin Folic Continus 1107
Ferrograd 1107
Ferrograd C 1107
Ferrograd Folic 1107
Ferromyn 1107
Ferrous fumarate 1107
Ferrous gluconate 1107
Ferrous glycine sulphate 1107
Ferrous succinate 1107
Ferrous sulphate 439
Fersaday 1107
Fersamal 1107
Fertiral 1107
fertile period:
    the process of fertilization 441
Fertility 439
    effect on: Gonorrhoea 490; Oral contraceptives 756
Fertility drugs 440
    causing Pregnancy, multiple 824
Fertilization 440
    Conception 294
    the process of fertilization 441
    In vitro fertilization 600
    Pregnancy 822
    Reproduction, sexual 868
Fesovit Z 1107

fetal abnormalities:
diagnosis of: Amniocentesis 39, 92; Antenatal care 112; Chorionic villus sampling 39, 274; Fetoscopy 38, 442; Ultrasound scanning 37, 1025
drug-related: Drug 376; Teratogen 976
types of: Birth defects 172; Heart disease, congenital 519
see also index entries Fetus; fetus, death of
Fetal alcohol syndrome 440
fetal cell culture:
and Amniocentesis 39, 92; Chromosome analysis 276
Fetal circulation 440
Fetal distress 442
Fetal heart monitoring 442
Fetishism 442
Fetoscopy 38, 442
Fetus 443
and drugs: Drug 376; Teratogen 976
examination of: Fetoscopy 38, 442
poor growth of: Fetal alcohol syndrome 440; Intrauterine growth retardation 598
movements of: Quickening 849
sex determination of: Amniocentesis 93; Chorionic villus sampling 274
size determination of: Ultrasound scanning 37, 1025
viability of: Ultrasound scanning 1025
see also index entries fetal abnormalities; fetus, death of
fetus, death of
diagnosis of: Ultrasound scanning 1025
and Abortion, induced 57; Miscarriage 691; Stillbirth 947
FEV:
see index entry forced expiratory volume
Fever 443
cause of: Infectious disease 579; Pyrogen 848
symptom chart 444
fever-producing substance:
medical term: Pyrogen 848
Fibre, dietary 19, 446
Diet and disease 357
and Nutrition 738
in treatment of Constipation 299
Fibre-optics 446
use of: Endoscopy 38, 403
Fibrillation 446
fibrin:
and Blood clotting 183; Coagulation, blood 283; Haemostasis 502
breakdown of: Fibrinolysis 446

fibrinogen:
component of Blood 181
in Fibrinolysis 446
type of Plasma protein 809
Fibrinolysis 446
Fibrinolytic drugs 446
alternative term: Thrombolytic drugs 987
Fibroadenoma 446
type of Breast lump 207
Fibroadenosis 447
causing Breast lump 207
Fibrocystic disease 447
Fibroid 447
causing Intercourse, painful 592
treatment of: Hysterectomy 560
a disorder of the uterus 1037
Fibroma 447
Fibrosarcoma 447
Fibrosis 447
and disorders of the lung 649
Fibrositis 448
Fibula 448
part of Skeleton 915
Fifth disease 448
Fight-or-flight response 448
and Hypothalamus 558
Filair 1107
Filariasis 448
causing Lymphoedema 653
the cycle of filariasis 449
type of: Onchocerciasis 751
and Roundworms 883
Filgrastim 1107
Filling, dental 449
Restoration, dental 872
Film badge 449
Finasteride 449
Finger 449
bent: Dupuytren's contracture 379; Volkmann's contracture 1067
bones of: Phalanges 798
clubbing of: Tetralogy of Fallot 981
cold, white: Raynaud's disease 860; Volkmann's contracture 1067
extra: Polydactyly 816
structure of a finger 450
finger tendons 975
joined: Syndactyly 965
movement of: Ulnar nerve 1024
Finger-joint replacement 450
Fingerprint 450
fingerprint, genetic:
see index entry Genetic fingerprinting
First aid 450
arm sling 924
artificial respiration 134
applying bandages 157
bleeding 178
burns 219
cardiopulmonary resuscitation 237
choking (adult) 269
choking (infant and child) 270
dressings 373
electrical injury 392

emergency childbirth 263
epileptic seizure 411
fainting 430
first-aid kit 451
foreign body in ear 385
foreign body in the eye 425
frostbite 463
heat exhaustion 526
heatstroke 526
hypothermia 559
insect stings and tick bites 588
nosebleed 735
poisoning 813
pressure points 827
recovery position 863
shock 908
splints 939
sprains 942
strain 950
suffocation 958
unconsciousness 1027
wounds 1085
fish skin disease:
medical term: Icthyosis 562
fish stings:
Venomous bites and stings 1050
Fistula 451
in Crohn's disease 320
Fit:
see index entry Seizure
Fitness 451
Exercise and health 20–21
Keeping healthy 16–17
Fitness testing 451
Sports medicine 941
Fixation 452
in Psychoanalytic theory 839
Flagyl 1107
Flail chest 452
cause of: Rib, fracture of 880
Flamazine 1107
flashbacks:
cause of: LSD 647
and Memory 674
Flat-feet 452
Flatulence 452
associated with Indigestion 576
Flatus 452
Flatworm 452
alternative term: Platyhelminth 809
Flavoxate 1107
Flaxedil 1107
Flea bites:
Insect bites 587
Flecainide 1107
Fleming, Alexander:
landmarks in medicine: drugs 671
Flemoxin Solutab 1107
Fletchers' Enemette 1107
Flexin Continus 1107
Flies:
Insects and disease 587
Flixonase 1107
Flixotide 1107
Floaters 453
as symptom of Retinal detachment 872
Flolan 1107
Flooding 453
in Behaviour therapy 162

Floppy infant syndrome 453
medical term: Hypotonia in infants 560
Floppy valve syndrome 453
medical term: Mitral valve prolapse 693
Florey, Howard:
landmarks in medicine: drugs 671
Florinef 1107
Floss, dental 453
and Oral hygiene 757; Toothbrushing 1002
in treatment of Plaque, dental 809
Flow cytometry 453
use of: Cytology 330
Floxapen 1107
Flu:
medical term: Influenza 584
Flu-Amp 1107
Fluanxol 1107
Fluclomix 1107
Fluclorolone 1107
Flucloxacillin 453
Fluconazole 1107
Fluctuant 453
Flucytosine 1107
Fludrocortisone 1107
fluid accumulation:
in abdomen: Ascites 136
associated with Nephrotic syndrome 722
in tissues: Oedema 745
treatment of: Diuretic drugs 364
Fluke 453
causing Infectious disease 578; Worm infestation 1086
type of Parasite 779; Platyhelminth 809; Trematode 1012
Flumazenil 1107
Flumethasone 1107
Flunisolide 1107
Flunitrazepam 1107
Fluocinolone 1107
Fluocortolone 1107
Fluor-a-day 1107
Fluorescein 453
in diagnosis of Corneal ulcer 308; disorders of the retina 873
use of: Eye, examination of 424
Fluoridation 453
see also index entry Fluoride
Fluoride 453
and Calcification, dental 223; Caries, dental 236; Toothbrushing 1002
excess of: Fluorosis 454
recommended levels of: Fluoridation 453
Fluorigard 1107
Fluorometholone 1107
Fluorosis 454
Fluorouracil 454
Fluothane 1107
Fluoxetine 1107
Flupenthixol 1107
Fluphenazine 1107
Flurandrenolone 1107
Flurazepam 454
Flurbiprofen 1107

Flurex 1107
Flurex Bedtime 1107
Flush 454
　Blushing 190
　feature of Mitral stenosis 692;
　　Rosacea 882
Fluspiriline 1108
Flutamide 1108
Fluticasone 1108
Fluvoxamine 1108
fly larvae infestation:
　medical term: Myiasis 712
FML 1108
FML-Neo 1108
Foam, contraceptive:
　Spermicides 932
Foetus:
　see index entry Fetus
Folex 350 1108
Folic acid 454
　in prevention of Neural tube
　　defect 725; Spina bifida 934
　in treatment of Sickle cell
　　anaemia 911; Sprue, tropical
　　941
　part of Vitamin B complex 1064
Folicin 1108
Folie à deux 454
　feature of Paranoia 779
Folinic acid 1108
Folk medicine 454
Follicle 454
Follicle-stimulating hormone 454
　causing Ovulation 769
　and contraception: how oral
　　contraceptives work 756
　production of: Pituitary gland
　　805
Folliculitis 454
Fomac 1108
Fomites 454
Fontanelle 454
Food additives 455
　and Nutrition 738
Food allergy 455
　causing Urticaria 1035
　Diet and disease 357
Food-borne infection 455
　infected animal products 457
　and food hygiene 19
　see also index entry Food
　　poisoning
Food fad 456
Food intolerance 456
food irradiation:
　Irradiation of food 602
　and Radiation hazards 853
Food poisoning 456
　and food hygiene 19; Poisoning
　　813
　types of: Botulism 196;
　　Listeriosis 639; Salmonella
　　infections 886;
　　Staphylococcal infections 944
food preservatives:
　types of Food additives 455
Foot 458
　pain in: Metatarsalgia 683
Foot-drop 458
Foramen 458
　in Skull 920
foramen ovale:
　and Fetal circulation 440

forced expiratory volume (FEV):
　measurement of: Spirometry
　　937
forced vital capacity (FVC):
　measurement of: Spirometry
　　937
Forceps 458
Forceps delivery 458
　assisted by Episiotomy 412
　causing Postpartum
　　haemorrhage 819
　using Forceps, obstetric 459
Forceps, obstetric 459
　use of: Forceps delivery 458
Forceval 1108
Foreign body 459
　in ear: first aid: foreign body in
　　ear 385
　in eye: first aid: foreign body in
　　the eye 425
　in nose: disorders of the nose 735
　in wounds: first aid: wounds
　　1085
Forensic medicine 459
foreplay:
　Sexual intercourse 904, 905
Foreskin 460
　part of Penis 788
　removal of: Circumcision 279
　secretions of: Smegma 924
　tight: Paraphimosis 779;
　　Phimosis 800
Forgetfulness:
　Amnesia 92
　Memory 674
Formaldehyde 460
Formestane 1108
Formication 460
　type of Sensation, abnormal
　　899
Formula, chemical 460
Fortagesic 1108
Fortral 1108
Fortum 1108
Foscarnet 1108
Foscavir 1108
Fosfestrol 1108
Fosinopril 1108
fovea:
　and Colour vision 291
　of Retina 872
foxglove:
　source of Digitalis drugs 359
　type of Plant, poisonous 808
Fracture 460
　causes of: Falls in the elderly
　　433; March fracture 662;
　　Stress fracture 951
　causing Malalignment 657
　fractures: types and treatment 461
　susceptibility to: Osteogenesis
　　imperfecta 763;
　　Osteomalacia 763;
　　Osteoporosis 764
　treatment of: Cast 239;
　　Traction 1008
Fracture, dental 462
Fragile X syndrome 462
Fragmin 1108
Framycetin 1108
Framycort 1108
Framygen 1108
Franol 1108

Franol Plus 1108
Franolyn Chesty 1108
Franolyn Expect 1108
Freckle 462
　and Lentigo 632; Melanin 673
　type of Naevus 716
free association:
　in Psychoanalysis 838
Free-floating anxiety 462
　feature of Generalized anxiety
　　disorder 475
Frequency:
　Urination, frequent 1032
Freudian slip 462
Freudian theory 462
Freud, Sigmund:
　and Freudian slip 462;
　　Freudian theory 462;
　　Psychoanalysis 838;
　　Psychoanalytic theory 838
Friar's balsam 462
Frick, Eugen:
　landmarks in medicine: other
　　forms of treatment 670
Friedreich's ataxia 462
　causing Paralysis 778
Frigidity 463
Frisium 1108
Froben 1108
frontal lobe:
　of Cerebrum 249
Frostbite 463
Frottage 463
Frozen section 463
Frozen shoulder 464
　cause of: Bursitis 220
　and Shoulder 909
Fru-Co 1108
fructose:
　type of Carbohydrate 232
Frumax 1108
Frumil 1108
Frusemide 464
Frusene 1108
Frusid 1108
Frustration 464
FSH 464
　see also index entry Follicle-
　　stimulating hormone
Fucibet 1108
Fucidin 1108
Fucidin H 1108
Fucithalmic 1108
Fugue 464
Fulcin 1108
Fulminant 464
Full Marks 1108
Fumes:
　Pollution 815
Functional disorders 464
Fungal infections 464, 581
　cause of: Fungi 465
　causing fungal diseases 465;
　　Infectious disease 578
　treatment of: Antifungal drugs
　　117
Fungi 464
　types of Microorganism 685
　see also index entry Fungal
　　infections
Fungicidal 465
　Antifungal drugs 117
Fungilin 1108

Fungizone 1108
Funny bone 465
　medical term: Olecranon 750
　part of Elbow 391
Furadantin 1108
Furamide 1108
Furuncle 465
Fusidic acid 1108
FVC:
　see index entry forced vital
　　capacity
Fybogel 1108
Fybogel Mebeverine 1108
Fynnon 1108

G

G6PD deficiency 466
GABA 466
Gabapentine 1108
Gait 466
　abnormal: Ataxia 140
　Walking 1072
galactocele:
　affecting Nipple 731
Galactorrhoea 466
　from Nipple 731
　and Pituitary tumours 806;
　　Prolactinoma 831
Galactosaemia 466
galactose:
　abnormal metabolism of:
　　Galactosaemia 466
　type of Carbohydrate 232
Galake 1108
Galcodine 1108
Galen:
　history of Medicine 668
Galenamet 1108
Galenamox 1108
Galenphol 1108
Galfer 1108
Galfer FA 1108
Galfer-Vit 1108
Galfloxin 1108
Gallamine trithiodide 1108
Gallbladder 467
　function of: Bile 166; function of
　　the biliary system 168
　inflammation of: Cholecystitis
　　271; Vomiting 1068
　part of Biliary system 167
　removal of: Cholecystectomy
　　270; procedure for
　　cholecystectomy 271
　role in Typhoid fever 1022
Gallbladder cancer 467
Gallium 467
Gallstones 468
　diagnosis of: T-tube
　　cholangiography 1018
　a disorder of the gallbladder 467
　in disorders of the pancreas 776;
　　Pancreatitis 776;
　　Spherocytosis, hereditary
　　932
　susceptibility to: Lipid-
　　lowering drugs 639
　treatment of: Cholecystectomy
　　270; Lithotripsy 640

Galpseud 1108
Gamanil 1108
Gambling, pathological 468
gamete intra-fallopian transfer
(GIFT):
in treatment of infertility 583
gamma-aminobutyric acid
(GABA):
GABA 466
Gamma benzene hexachloride
1108
gamma camera:
uses of: Nuclear medicine 737;
Radionuclide scanning 854;
Scanning techniques 888
Gamma globulin 468
type of Globulin 485
use of: Immunoglobulin
injections 572
gamma rays:
type of Radiation 851
Gamolenic acid 1108
Ganciclovir 1108
Ganda 1108
Ganglion (swelling) 468
Gangrene 468
and Buerger's disease 217;
disorders of muscle 707;
Tobacco-smoking 997
causes of: Peripheral vascular
disease 793; Polyarteritis
nodosa 815; Raynaud's
disease 860; Thrombus 988;
Tourniquet 1005
Ganser's syndrome 469
Garamycin 1108
Gardenal 1108
Gardnerella vaginalis 469
Gargle 469
gargoylism:
in Hurler's syndrome 544
Gas-and-air 469
gas gangrene:
form of Gangrene 469
occurring in Wound infection
1088
treatment of: Hyperbaric
oxygen treatment 548
gas, intestinal:
causing Flatulence 452
gas in urine:
medical term: Pneumaturia
810
Gastrectomy 469
gastric cancer:
common term: Stomach cancer
948
Gastric erosion 470
gastric lavage:
Lavage, gastric 628
gastric tube:
use of: Intubation 599
Gastric ulcer 470
a type of Peptic ulcer 789
Gastrils 1108
gastrin:
excess: Zollinger-Ellison
syndrome 1094
a Gastrointestinal hormone
471
Gastritis 470
Gastrobid Continus 1108
Gastrocote 1108

Gastroenteritis 470
Gastroenterology 471
Gastroenterostomy 471
Gastroflux 1108
Gastrointestinal hormones 471
Gastrointestinal tract 471
part of Digestive system 357
Gastromax 1108
Gastron 1108
Gastroscopy 471
in diagnosis of Abdominal
pain 55; Pyloric stenosis 848;
Stomach cancer 948
Gastrostomy 472
Gastrozepin 1108
Gaucher's disease 472
Gauze 472
Gavage 472
Gaviscon 1108
Gay bowel syndrome 472
G-CSF 1108
Geangin 1108
Gelcosal 1108
Gelcotar 1108
Gelusil 1108
Gemeprost 1109
Gemfibrozil 472
gender:
genetic basis of: Inheritance
585; Sex chromosomes 902
and Sex determination 903
Gender identity 472
and Sex change 902
Gene 472
a constituent of Chromosomes
277
constituents of: Nucleic acids
737
gene map of chromosome 11, 39
*what genes are and what they do
474*
*where do your genes come from?
473*
and Genetic code 475;
Genetically-engineered
drugs 43; Genetic
engineering 478; Genetic
probe 479; Genetics 479;
Inheritance 585; Mutation
709; Protein synthesis 835
recessive: Sex-linked
inheritance 903
see also index entries DNA;
Genetic analysis; Genetic
counselling; genetic
damage; Genetic disorders;
Genetic fingerprinting
general anaesthesia:
see index entry Anaesthesia,
general
Generalized anxiety disorder 475
General Medical Council 475
General paralysis of the insane
475
feature of Neurosyphilis 729;
Syphilis 966
General Practice 475
Generic drug 475
Drug 375
Genetically engineered drugs 43
Genetic analysis 39
and Blood groups 187; Genetic
fingerprinting 479

see also index entry
Chromosome analysis
Genetic code 475
determining Protein synthesis
835
Genetic counselling 476
for Cystic fibrosis 328; Genetic
disorders 478; Haemophilia
501; Retinoblastoma 874;
Sickle cell anaemia 911;
Spina bifida 934
genetic damage:
and Mutation 709; Radiation
hazards 852
Genetic disorders 476
detection of: Amniocentesis
39, 92; Chorionic villus
sampling 39, 274; Genetic
analysis 39
examples: Achondroplasia 62;
Alzheimer's disease 90;
Charcot-Marie-Tooth
disease 256; Cystic fibrosis
327; Ehlers-Danlos
syndrome 390; Familial
Mediterranean fever 434;
Friedreich's ataxia 462;
G6PD deficiency 466;
Galactosaemia 466;
Gaucher's disease 472;
Gilbert's disease 481;
Haemophilia 501;
Homocystinuria 540;
Huntington's disease 544;
Hurler's syndrome 544;
Marfan's syndrome 662;
McArdle's disease 666;
Mucopolysaccharidosis 701;
Muscular dystrophy 707;
Neurofibromatosis 726;
Osteogenesis imperfecta
763; Osteopetrosis 764;
Peroneal muscular atrophy
794; Peutz-Jehger's
syndrome 797;
Phenylketonuria 800;
Polyposis, familial 817;
Porphyria 817; Sickle cell
anaemia 911; Spherocytosis,
hereditary 932; Tay-Sachs
disease 971; Thalassaemia
982; Tuberous sclerosis 1019;
Wilson's disease 1083
unifactorial genetic disorders 477
see also index entry Genetic
counselling
Genetic engineering 478
of drugs: Genetically
engineered drugs 43
Genetic fingerprinting 479
use of: Paternity testing 783;
*paternity testing using genetic
fingerprinting 784*
genetic markers:
determination of: Genetic
probe 479
and Genetic analysis 39
in Paternity testing 784
Genetic probe 479
use of: Genetic analysis 39
Genetics 479
and Inheritance 585
Genisol 1109

Genital herpes:
Herpes, genital 532
and Sexually transmitted
diseases 904
Genitalia 479
Genitalia, ambiguous 479
see also index entry Intersex
genital phase:
in Psychoanalytic theory 838
genitals, exposing:
Exhibitionism 419
Genital ulceration 480
Genital warts:
Warts, genital 1075
Genito-urinary medicine 480
and Sexually transmitted
diseases 906
Genome, human 480
Genotropin 1109
Gentamicin 480
Gentian mixture, acid and
alkaline 1109
Gentian violet 480
Genticin 1109
Gentisone 1109
Genu valgum 480
common term: Knock-knee
620
example of Valgus 1043
Genu varum 480
common term: Bowleg 197
example of Varus 1044
Geriatric medicine 480
Germ 480
medical terms: Microorganism
685; Pathogen 784
German measles:
Rubella 883
Germ cell tumour 480
germ theory of disease:
Anatomy and pathology 30;
Medicine 668; *landmarks in
medicine: diagnosis 669*
Gerontology 480
and Aging 74; Geriatric
medicine 480
Gestalt theory 480
Gestanin 1109
Gestation 481
see also index entry Pregnancy
gestational diabetes:
and Diabetic pregnancy 350
Gestodene 1109
Gestone 1109
Gestrinone 1109
Gestronol 1109
giant:
Gigantism 481
giant cell arteritis:
alternative term: Temporal
arteritis 973
Giardiasis 481
cause of: Protozoa 836
treatment of: Metronidazole
685
Giddiness:
Dizziness 366
GIFT:
in treatment of Infertility 583
Gigantism 481
cause of: Pituitary tumours
806
Gilbert's disease 481

Gilles de la Tourette's syndrome 481
treatment of: Haloperidol 505; Pimozide 803
type of Tic 994
Gingiva 482
alternative term: Gum 497
Gingivectomy 482
Gingivitis 482
cause of: Plaque, dental 808
and Oral hygiene 756; Periodontal disease 792
Gingivitis, acute ulcerative 482
and Gingivitis 482; Periodontitis 792
gingivostomatitis:
and Cold sore 286
Givitol 1109
Gland 482
Glanders 482
Glands, swollen 483
Glandular fever:
medical term: Mononucleosis, infectious 694
glans:
part of Penis 788
Glasses 483
why glasses are used 484
invention of: landmarks in medicine: other forms of treatment 670
Glass eye:
Eye, artificial 423
Glaucoma 483
acute closed-angle glaucoma 485
associated with raised Intraocular pressure 598; Lens dislocation 632; Retinal vein occlusion 874; Sturge-Weber syndrome 955
causing Tunnel vision 1020
diagnosis of: Eye, examination of 424; Tonometry 1001
a disorder of the eye 426
treatment of: Acetazolamide 61; Physostigmine 803; Pilocarpine 803; Pindolol 804; Timolol 994; Trabeculectomy 1006; Urea 1028
glial cells:
in Cerebrum 249
tumours of: Glioma 485
Glibenclamide 484
Glibenese 1109
Gliclazide 1109
Glioblastoma multiforme 485
Glioma 485
Glipizide 1109
Gliquidone 1109
globin:
constituent of Haemoglobin 499
production of: Liver 641
Globulin 485
and ESR 416
type of Plasma protein 809
Globus hystericus 485
Glomerulonephritis 485
a disorder of the kidney 614
the effects of glomerulonephritis 486
following Scarlet fever 889

Glomerulosclerosis 486
glomerulus:
inflammation of: Glomerulonephritis 485
part of Nephron 722; Kidney 612
scarring of: Glomerulosclerosis 486
Glomus tumour 486
Glossectomy 486
Glossitis 487
inflammation of Tongue 1000
Glossolalia 487
Glossopharyngeal nerve 487
a Cranial nerve 318
Glottis 487
and Vocal cords 1066
Glucagon 487
antagonist to Insulin 590
effect on Carbohydrates 232; Glucose 487; Glycogen 488
production of: Pancreas 775
in treatment of Hypoglycaemia 556
Glucobay 1109
Glucocorticoids 487
Gluco-lyte 1109
Glucophage 1109
Glucose 487
blood levels: Diabetes mellitus 348; living with diabetes mellitus 349; Glucagon 487; Insulin 589
as energy source: Carbohydrates 232
in urine; living with diabetes mellitus 349; Glycosuria 488
glucose-6-phosphate dehydrogenase deficiency: G6PD deficiency 466
glucose-tolerance test:
in diagnosis of Diabetes mellitus 349
Glue ear 487
causing Deafness 332
effects of glue ear 488
treatment of: Grommet tube 493; Myringotomy 715
Glue sniffing:
Solvent abuse 928
Glurenorm 1109
Glutaraldehyde 1109
Glutarol 1109
Gluten 488
allergy to: Dermatitis herpetiformis 344
causing Coeliac disease 285
Gluten enteropathy:
Coeliac disease 285
Gluten intolerance:
Coeliac disease 285
Gluteus maximus 488
Glycerin 1109
Glycerol 488
Glyceryl trinitrate 488
Glycogen 488
metabolism of: Carbohydrate 232; Glucagon 487; Glucose 487; Insulin 589
production of: Liver 641
glycogen storage diseases:
and Metabolism, inborn errors of 682

Glycopyrronium bromide 1109
Glycosuria 488
Glypressin 1109
Glytrin 1109
Gnat bites:
Insect bites 587
Goitre 489
in Hypothyroidism 560
and deficiency of Iodine 600
causing Swallowing difficulty 963
treatment of: Thyroidectomy 990
Gold 489
preparations of: Auranofin 143; Sodium aurothiomalate 927
in treatment of Rheumatoid arthritis, juvenile 878
use of: Crown, dental 321; Filling, dental 449
Golden Eye Drops 1109
Golfers' elbow 489
type of Overuse injury 769
Gonadorelin 1109
Gonadorelins 489
Gonadotrophin hormones 489
and Oral contraceptives 756
production of: Pituitary gland 805
types of: Follicle-stimulating hormone 454; Gonadotrophin, human chorionic 490; Luteinizing hormone 651; Menotrophin 677
Gonadotrophin, human chorionic 490
Gonadotrophon LH 1109
Gonads 490
Ovary 768
Testis 977
underactivity of: Hypogonadism 556
Gonorrhoea 490
affecting Penis 789
causing Pelvic inflammatory disease 786; Salpingitis 887; Urethral discharge 1029; Urethral stricture 1029; Urethritis 1030
incidence of gonorrhoea in England 906
type of Sexually transmitted disease 904
and Urinary tract infection 1032
Goodenough-Harris test:
type of Intelligence test 591
Goodpasture's syndrome 490
treatment of: Plasmapheresis 809
Gopten 1109
Goserilin 1109
Gout 490, 491
cause of: Uric acid 1030
causing Tophus 1003
treatment of: Colchicine 286; Indomethacin 576; Piroxicam 804; Probenecid 829; Sulphinpyrazone 959
Grafting 491
graft rejection:
and Graft-versus-host disease 492; Rejection 867

following Transplant surgery 1010
Graft-versus-host disease 492
Gramicidin 1109
Gram's stain 492
in microscopy: Staining 943
Grand mal 492
type of Epilepsy 411; Seizure 896
Graneodin 1109
Granisetron 1109
Granocyte 1109
Granulation tissue 492
granulocyte:
type of Phagocyte 798
Granuloma 492
in Periodontitis 792
of Umbilical cord 1027
Granuloma annulare 492
Granuloma inguinale 492
Granuloma, lethal midline 493
grasp reflex:
type of Reflex 865; Reflex, primitive 865, 866
Graves' disease 493
a disorder of the thyroid gland 992
Gravida 493
Gray 493
a radiation unit 851
Gregoderm 1109
Grey matter 493
in Brain 198; Spinal cord 934
Grief 493
cause of: Bereavement 164
causing Sexual desire, inhibited 904
Grip 493
Grippe 493
Griseofulvin 493
Grisovin 1109
Groin 493
Groin, lump in the 493
Groin strain 493
Grommet tube 493
in treatment of Glue ear 487
use of: Myringotomy 715
ground itch:
cause of: Hookworm infestation 540
Group therapy 494
Growing pains 494
Growth 494
Growth, childhood 494
growth charts 495
see also index entries Child development; Puberty; Short stature
Growth hormone 496
abuse of: Sports, drugs and 940
deficiency: Short stature 908
production of: Pituitary gland 805
growth, retarded:
Growth, childhood 494
Short stature 908
Grüntzig, Andreas:
landmarks in medicine: surgery 670
GTN 300-mcg 1109
Guaiphenesin 1109
Guanethidine 1109

guanine:
   as constituent of Nucleic acids
      737
   in genes: *what genes are and
      what they do 474*
   structure of DNA 39
Guanor Expectorant 1109
Guarem 1109
Guar gum 496
Guarina 1109
Guillain-Barré syndrome 496
Guilt 496
   and Dying, care of the 380;
      Post-traumatic stress
      disorder 819; Sudden infant
      death syndrome 957
Guinea worm disease 496
Gullet 497
   medical term: Oesophagus 748
Gum 497
   bleeding: Gingivitis 482;
      Gingivitis, acute ulcerative
      482; Scurvy 895
   enlargement of: Hyperplasia,
      gingival 551
   health of: Vitamin C 1065
   inflammation of: Gingivitis
      482; Gingivitis, acute
      ulcerative 482; Salivation,
      excessive 886
   receding: Dental examination
      341
   removal of: Gingivectomy 482
Gumboil
   cause of: Periodontitis 792
   medical term: Abscess, dental
      59
Gumma 497
   feature of Syphilis 966
Gut 497
   Intestine 595
Guthrie test 497
   for the Newborn 730
Gynaecology 497
Gynaecomastia 497
   cause of: Prolactinoma 831
   in Klinefelter's syndrome 619
Gyno-Daktarin 1109
Gynol II 1109
Gyno-Pevaryl 1109
gyri:
   of Brain 198; Cerebrum 249

H

H₂-receptor antagonists 498
Habituation 498
Habsburg jaw 503
Haelan 1109
Haelan-C 1109
Haem- 498
haem:
   constituent of Haemoglobin
      499
Haemangioblastoma 498
Haemangioma 498
   common term: Stork mark 949
   in Newborn 730; Sturge-Weber
      syndrome 955
   and *disorders of the nose 735*

type of Kidney tumour 617;
   Skin tumour 918
Haemarthrosis 498
   of Knee 619
Haematemesis 498
   cause of: Oesophageal varices
      747
   common term: Vomiting blood
      1068
Haematology 498
Haematoma 498
   of brain: Subdural
      haemorrhage 956
   in muscle: *disorders of muscle
      707*; Quadriceps muscle 849
   of Nasal septum 718
   and Tissue-plasminogen
      activator 997
Haematoma auris 499
   common term: Cauliflower ear
      244
haematoxylin and eosin:
   use of: Staining 943
Haematuria 499
   causes of: Bladder tumours
      175; Cystitis 328; Kidney
      cancer 613; Kidney,
      polycystic 616; Sickle cell
      anaemia 911
   and Urine, abnormal 1034
Haemochromatosis 499
   and *disorders of the liver 645*
   causing Pancreatitis 776;
      Pigmentation 802
   treatment of: Venesection 1049
Haemodialysis 499
   type of Dialysis 44, 351
Haemoglobin 499
   abnormal: Sickle cell anaemia
      911; Thalassaemia 982
   function of: Oxygen 770
   and Iron 602
Haemoglobinopathy 500
haemoglobin S:
   in Sickle cell anaemia 911
Haemoglobinuria 500
Haemolysis 500
   causing Anaemia, haemolytic
      97; Haemoglobinuria 500
   example of Lysis 655
   in Spherocytosis, hereditary
      932
Haemolytic anaemia:
   Anaemia, haemolytic 97
Haemolytic disease of the
   newborn 500
Haemolytic-uraemic syndrome
   500
Haemophilia 501
   and Factor VIII 429
   causing Haemarthrosis 498
   type of Bleeding disorder
      177
haemophilia B:
   alternative term: Christmas
      disease 275
HAEMOPHILUS INFLUENZAE 501
   cause of: Epiglottitis 410;
      Meningitis 675
   prevention: *typical
      immunization schedule 28;
      typical childhood
      immunization schedule 570*

Haemoptysis 501
   common term: Coughing up
      blood 314
Haemorrhage 501
   common term: Bleeding 177
Haemorrhoidectomy 501
   removing haemorrhoids 502
Haemorrhoids 501
   causing Occult blood, faecal
      743; Rectal bleeding 862
   and Pregnancy 823
   removal of:
      Haemorrhoidectomy 501;
      removing haemorrhoids 502
   treatment of: Sclerotherapy
      893; Suppository 961
Haemosiderosis 502
Haemospermia 502
   common term: Semen, blood
      in the 897
Haemostasis 502
Haemostatic drugs 502
Haemothorax 503
   and *disorders of the lung 649*
Hair 503
   colour of: Melanin 673
   constituent of: Keratin 610
   follicle: Acne 62; Pore 817
   growth of: *hair growth 504;*
      Minoxidil 689
Hairball 503
hair cells:
   damage to: Noise 733
   part of Ear 383
Hairiness, excessive:
   associated with Ovary,
      polycystic 768; Virilism 1055
   medical terms: Hirsutism 536;
      Hypertrichosis 553
   see also index entry Hair
      removal
hair loss:
   medical term: Alopecia 87
Hair removal 503
   methods of: Depilatory 342;
      Electrolysis 393
Hair transplant 504
Halciderm Topical 1109
Halcinonide 1109
Haldol 1109
Halfan 1109
Half-Betadur CR 1109
Half-Beta-Prograne 1109
Half-Inderal LA 1109
Half-life 504
Halibut liver oil 1109
Halitosis 504
   cause of: Ozena 770
   treatment of: Mouthwash 699;
      Oral hygiene 756
Hallucination 504
   feature of Confusion 296;
      Paranoia 779; Psychosis 840;
      Schizophrenia 891; Sleep
      deprivation 922; Temporal
      lobe epilepsy 974; Thought
      disorders 985
   following Bereavement 164;
      damage to Cerebrum 250
Hallucinogenic drug 504
   examples: LSD 647; Marijuana
      662; Mescaline 681; Peyote
      797; Psilocybin 836

Hallux 504
   common term: big Toe 999
Hallux rigidus 504
Hallux valgus 504
   affecting Toe 999
   causing Bunion 217
Halofantrine 1109
Haloperidol 505
Halothane 505
Halycitrol 1109
Hamarin 1109
Hamartoma 505
Hammer-toe 505
Hamstring muscles 505
   tearing: Running injuries 883
Hand 505
   protection of: Eczema 389;
      Paronychia 782
   and Shoulder-hand syndrome
      910
   spasms of:
      Hypoparathyroidism 556
   weakness of: Carpal tunnel
      syndrome 238
   see also index entry Finger
Handedness 505
hand-eye coordination:
   in old Age 73; Child
      development 265
   and Developmental delay 346
Hand-foot-and-mouth disease
   506
Handicap 506
   Disability 360
handwashing:
   causing Paronychia 782
   continual: Obsessive-
      compulsive disorder 742
   in prevention of Food
      poisoning 457; Shigellosis
      907
Hangnail 506
Hangover 506
   causes of: Alcohol 80; Sleeping
      drugs 922
   causing Headache 507
Hansen's disease 506
   treatment of: Dapsone 332;
      Rifampicin 880
haptoglobin:
   type of Globulin 485
Hardening of the arteries 507
   medical terms: Arteriosclerosis
      130; Atherosclerosis 140
Hare lip 507
   associated with Cleft lip and
      palate 282
Harmogen 1109
Hashimoto's thyroiditis 507
   a disorder of the thyroid gland 992
   symptom of: Goitre 489
Hashish:
   preparation of Marijuana 662
haversian canals:
   part of Bone 192
Hay fever 507
   alternative term: Rhinitis,
      allergic 878
Haymine 1109
HCG (human chorionic
   gonadotrophin):
   Gonadotrophin, human
      chorionic 490

HDL:
see index entry high-density lipoprotein
head:
abnormally small:
Microcephaly 685
flattening of: Rickets 880
parts of: Brain 198; Ear 383; Eye 422; Jaw 606; Mouth 697; Nose 734; Skull 919
see also index entries Headache; Head-banging; Head injury; Head lag
Headache 507
resulting from Brain haemorrhage 202; Cervical osteoarthritis 251; Hangover 506; Head injury 510; Phaeochromocytoma 798; Polycythaemia 815; Spinal anaesthesia 934; Temporal arteritis 974; Yellow fever 1092
symptom chart 508
see also index entry Migraine
Head-banging 510
Head injury 510
causing Brain haemorrhage 202; Cerebral palsy 248; Respiratory arrest 869
treatment of: Ventilation 1050
Head lag 511
head louse:
Lice 635
Heaf test:
Tuberculin tests 1018
Healing 511
acceleration of: Ultrasound treatment 1026
Health 511
Diet and disease 356
good dietary habits 357
Eating well 18–19
Exercise 419
the effects of exercise 420
Exercise and health 20–21
Fitness 451
Keeping healthy 16–17
Nutrition 738
Preventive medicine 828
see also index entry Health hazards
Health centre 511
Health food 511
Health hazards 511
Alcohol 80
Smoking and drinking 22–23
Tobacco-smoking 997
Hearing 512, 513
and Cerebrum 250; Child development 264; Ear 383; Speech 930; Vestibulocochlear nerve 1054
impaired: Cerebral palsy 248; Developmental delay 346; disorders of the ear 384; Noise 732; Speech therapy 931
see also index entries Deafness; Hearing aids; Hearing tests

Hearing aids 513
development of: landmarks in medicine: other forms of treatment 670
in treatment of Presbyacusis 827
see also index entry Deafness
Hearing loss 513
Hearing tests 513
see also index entries Deafness; Hearing; Hearing aids
Hearing tests 513
types of hearing test 514
Heart 513, 515
abnormal position of: Dextrocardia 347
disorders of the heart 517
heart cycle 516
see also index entries Heartbeat; heart covering; heart muscle; Heart-rate; Heart valve
Heart, artificial 515
Heart attack:
see index entry Myocardial infarction
Heartbeat 516
abnormal: Stroke 952; Supraventricular tachycardia 961; Ventricular ectopic beat 1051
abnormal, treatment of: Calcium channel blockers 224; Phenytoin 800
awareness of: Palpitation 774
cessation of: Cardiac arrest 234
normal: Diastole 355; heart cycle 516; Systole 967
see also index entry Heart-rate
Heart block 516
Heartburn 518
causes of: Hiatus hernia 533; Oesophagitis 747
in Pregnancy 823
heart compression:
medical term: Tamponade 968
heart covering:
inflammation of: Pericarditis 791
medical term: Pericardium 791
heart cycle 516
heart disease:
Avoiding heart disease 21
treatment of: Digitalis drugs 359; Weight reduction 1080
types of: disorders of the heart 517; Heart disease, congenital 519; Heart disease, ischaemic 519
see also index entry Coronary artery disease
Heart disease, congenital 519
cause of: Rubella 883
types of congenital heart disease 518
Heart disease, ischaemic 519
heart, enlargement of:
associated with Pulmonary hypertension 844; Pulmonary stenosis 845
medical term: Cardiomegaly 235

Heart failure 519
causes of: damaged Heart valve 523; Septal defect 900; Sleep apnoea 922; Tricuspid incompetence 1015
causing Nocturia 732
and Pulmonary hypertension 844
treatment of: Amiloride 92; Aminophylline 92; Digitoxin 359; Digoxin 359; Hydrochlorothiazide 546; Isosorbide 604; Metolazone 684; Prazosin 821; Venesection 1049
Heart imaging 520
heart lining, inflammation of:
medical term: Endocarditis 400
Heart-lung machine 520
use of: Open heart surgery 752
Heart-lung transplant 521, 522
in treatment of Cystic fibrosis 328
heart murmur:
causes of: Pulmonary incompetence 845; Septal defect 900
Heart sounds 522
Murmur 704
heart muscle:
death of: Coronary artery disease 310; Myocardial infarction 712
disease of: Cardiomyopathy 235
inflammation of: Myocarditis 714
structure of: Muscle 706
Heart-rate 522
abnormally fast: Arrhythmia, cardiac 128; Sinus tachycardia 914; Tachycardia 968; Ventricular tachycardia 1051
abnormally slow: Arrhythmia, cardiac 128; Bradycardia 197; Sick sinus syndrome 911; Sinus bradycardia 913
changes in: Stress 951
and Heart 514
normal: Fitness 451
slowing of: Vagus nerve 1043
see also index entry Heartbeat
heart rhythm:
abnormal: Arrhythmia, cardiac 128
see also index entries Heartbeat; Heart-rate
Heart sounds 522
see also index entry heart murmur
heart stoppage:
Cardiac arrest 234
Heart surgery 522
types of: Angioplasty, balloon 108; Coronary artery bypass 308, 309; heart valve replacement 524; Heart-valve surgery 523; Open heart surgery 752; Valvotomy 1043
Heart transplant 523
landmarks in medicine: surgery 670

Heart valve 523
Valve 1043
heart valve abnormalities:
and Cardiomegaly 235; Pulmonary incompetence 844
diagnosis of: Echocardiography 386
causes of: Rheumatic fever, 876; Streptococcal infections 950
causing Murmur 704
heart valve, mechanical:
in Heart-valve surgery 523
types of replacement heart valves 525
Heart-valve surgery 523
types of: heart valve replacement 524; Valvotomy 1043
Heat cramps 524
Heat disorders 524
Heat exhaustion 525
first aid: heat exhaustion 526
and Sunlight, adverse effects of 960
Heatstroke 526
Heat treatment 526
Physiotherapy 803
Hedex 1109
Heel 526
Heimlich manoeuvre 527
in treatment of Choking 269
HELICOBACTER PYLORI 527
eradication of: Ulcer-healing drugs 1024
Heliotherapy 527
type of Phototherapy 801
Helmholtz, Hermann von:
landmarks in medicine: diagnosis 669
Helminth infestation 527
Worm infestation 1086
helper cells:
of Immune system 569
types of Lymphocyte 653
Hemabate 1109
Hemianopia 527
Hemiballismus 527
Hemicolectomy 527
Heminevrin 1109
Hemiparesis 527
Hemiplegia 527
form of Paralysis 778
and types and causes of stroke 953
Henoch-Schönlein purpura 527
type of Purpura 847
Heparin 527
and Heart-lung machine 520
Hepatectomy, partial 527
Hepatectomy, total 527
Hepatic 527
hepatic encephalopathy:
in Liver failure 644
type of Encephalopathy 399
Hepatitis 527
diagnosis of: Liver biopsy 642
a disorder of the liver 645
and Pancreatitis 776
in Q fever 849
hepatitis A:
travel protection 27

Hepatitis A, B, C, D and E:
see index entry Hepatitis, viral
hepatitis B
type of Hepatitis, viral 529
and Liver Cancer 642
Hepatitis, chronic active 529
hepatitis immunoglobulin:
in prevention of Hepatitis,
viral 529
hepatitis non-A, non-B:
type of Hepatitis, viral 529
Hepatitis, viral 529
a disorder of the liver 645
main types of viral hepatitis 528
Hepatoma 529
type of Liver cancer 642
Hepatomegaly 529
Hep-Flush 1109
Hepsal 1109
herald patch:
in Pityriasis rosea 806
Herbal medicine 529
Heredity 530
and Inheritance 585
Heritability 530
Hermaphroditism 530
and Sex determination 903
Hernia 530
treatment of: Hernia repair
531; Truss 1018
type of: Hiatus hernia 533
Hernia repair 531
Herniated disc:
Disc prolapse 362
Herniorrhaphy 531
alternative term: Hernia repair
531
Heroin 1109
Heroin abuse 531
detoxification: Methadone 683
Pregnancy, drugs in 824
see also index entries Drug
abuse; Drug dependence
Herpangina 531
Herpes 532
Herpes, genital 532
causing Vulvitis 1071
Herpes gestationis 532
Herpes simplex 532
causing Whitlow 1082
and Infection, congenital 578
as Opportunistic infection
754
treatment of: Acyclovir 66;
Idoxuridine 562
Herpes zoster 532
example of herpes zoster 533
treatment of: Acyclovir 66
herpes zoster ophthalmicus:
and Herpes zoster 533
herpetic whitlow 1082
cause of: Herpes simplex 532
Herpid 1109
Heterosexuality 533
Sexuality 904
Heterozygote 533
Hetrazan 1109
Hexachlorophane 1109
Hexamine 1109
Hexopal 1109
hexosaminidase deficiency:
causing Tay-Sachs disease 971
Hiatus hernia 533

causing Heartburn 518
and Phrenic nerve 802
treatment of: Plication 810
Hibiscrub 1109
Hibisol 1109
Hibitane 1109
Hiccup 534
and Phrenic nerve 802
high blood pressure:
medical term: Hypertension
551
high-density lipoprotein (HDL):
and Cholesterol 273; Fats and
oils 436; Hyperlipidaemias
549
Hill's Balsam 1110
Hioxyl 1110
Hip 534
and Pelvis 787
Hip, congenital dislocation of 534
treatment of: Osteotomy 765
and Walking 1072
hippocampus:
part of Limbic system 637
Hippocrates:
and Diagnosis and prognosis
30; Hippocratic oath 535;
Medicine 668; *landmarks in
medicine: diagnosis 669*
Hippocratic oath 535
in history of Medicine 668
Hip replacement 535
and Surgical implants 46
Hip, snapping 535
Hirschowitz, Basil:
*landmarks in medicine:
diagnosis 669*
Hirschsprung's disease 536
Hirsutism 536
Hirudoid 1110
Hismanal 1110
Histalix 1110
Histamine 536
causing Allergy 87;
Inflammation 583; Rhinitis,
allergic 878; Urticaria 1035
production of: Mast cell 663
histamine-blocking drugs:
types of: Antihistamine drugs
118; H_2-receptor antagonists
498; Ulcer-healing drugs
1024
Histamine$_2$-receptor antagonists:
H_2-receptor antagonists 498
Histiocytosis X 536
Histocompatibility antigens 536
and Paternity testing 784
associated with Behçet's
syndrome 163; Coeliac
disease 285
in Tissue-typing 997
Histology 537
and Staining 943
using Microscope 687
Histopathology 537
and Pathology 784
using Microscope 687
Histoplasmosis 537
a Fungal infection 464
history, medical:
see index entry History-
taking

History-taking 537
and Diagnosis 350; *steps in
diagnosing a condition 351;*
Diagnosis and prognosis 30;
Examination, physical 418;
You and your doctor 32–33
HIV 537
and Tuberculosis 1019
causing AIDS 76; AIDS-related
complex 79; Encephalitis
399; Infection, congenital
578
type of Virus 1055
Hives 537
medical term: Urticaria 1035
HLA-B27 tissue type:
and Reiter's syndrome 867
HLA types:
Histocompatibility antigens
536
Hoarseness 537
causes of: Laryngitis 625;
Larynx, cancer of 626;
Thyroid cancer 990
symptom chart 538
Hodgkin's disease 539
type of Lymphoma 655
Hodgkin's lymphoma:
alternative term: Hodgkin's
disease 539
Hoffmann, Felix:
landmarks in medicine: drugs 671
Hole in the heart 540
medical term: Septal defect 900
Holistic medicine 540
Holter monitor 540
Homatropine 1110
Homeopathy 540
Homeostasis 540
Homocystinuria 540
type of Metabolism, inborn
error of 682
homograft:
example: Corneal graft 307
use of: Grafting 491
Homosexuality, female:
Lesbianism 632
Homosexuality, male 540
Sexuality 904
Homozygote 540
and Genetic disorders 478
Honvan 1110
Hookworm infestation 540
hookworm life-cycle 541
and Roundworms 882
hordeolum:
common term: Stye 955
Hormonal disorders 541
endocrine disorders 402
Hormonal methods of
contraception:
Contraception, hormonal
methods of 304
hormonal system:
disorders of: *endocrine disorders
402;* Hormonal disorders 541
*the sources and main effects of
selected hormones 543*
see also index entries
Endocrine system; Hormone
Hormone 541
constituent of: Peptide 791;
Protein 834

measurement of:
Immunoassay 570;
Radioimmunoassay 853
and pregnancy: *effects of
hormones during pregnancy
823*
production of: Endocrine
system 400, *401; the sources
and main effects of selected
hormones 543*
types of: Gastrointestinal
hormones 471; Growth
hormone 496; *the sources
and main effects of selected
hormones 543*
Hormone antagonist 541
Hormone replacement therapy 541
following Menopause 676
in Osteoporosis 764
using Progestogen drugs 830
Hormonin 1110
Horn, cutaneous 542
Horner's syndrome 542
in Klumpke's paralysis 619
hornet sting:
Insect stings 588
Horseshoe kidney 542
a disorder of the kidney 614
Hospice 542
and Dying, care of the 380
Hospitals, types of 542
Hot flushes 542
and Menopause 676
Hounsfield, Godfrey:
*landmarks in medicine:
diagnosis 669*
Housemaid's knee 542
medical term: Bursitis 220
HPV16 (virus):
associated with Cervix, cancer
of 254
HRF 1110
HSV1 (virus):
type of Herpes simplex 532
HSV2 (virus):
type of Herpes simplex 532
Human Actraphane 30/70 1110
Human Actrapid 1110
Human chorionic gonadotrophin
(HCG):
Gonadotrophin, human
chorionic 490
human immunodeficiency virus
(HIV):
see index entry HIV
Human Initard 50/50 1110
Human Insulatard 1110
human leukocyte antigens
(HLAs):
group of Histocompatibility
antigens 536
in Tissue-typing 997
Human Mixtard 30/70 1110
Human Monotard 1110
Human Protaphane 1110
Human Ultratard 1110
Human Velosulin 1110
Humatrope 1110
Humegon 1110
Humerus 542
part of Skeleton 914
and Shoulder 909
Humerus, fracture of 542

humidifier:
  use of: Croup 321; Ventilator 1050
Humours 544
Humulin 1110
Hunchback:
  medical term: Kyphosis 621
Hunger 544
  and Appetite 127
Hunter's syndrome:
  type of Mucopolysaccharidosis 701
Huntington's disease 544
  and GABA 466
Hurler's syndrome 544
  type of Metabolism, inborn error of 682; Mucopolysaccharidosis 701
Hutchinson-Gilford syndrome:
  form of Progeria 830
Hutchinson, Miller Reese:
  landmarks in medicine: other forms of treatment 670
Hydatid disease 544
  origins of hydatid disease 545
  treatment of: Mebendazole 667
Hydatidiform mole 544
  form of Trophoblastic tumour 1017
  leading to Choriocarcinoma 274
  a disorder of the uterus 1037
Hydergine 1110
Hydralazine 545
Hydramnios:
  Polyhydramnios 816
Hydrea 1110
Hydrenox 1110
Hydrocal 1110
Hydrocele 545
  and Testis 977; Testis, swollen 978
Hydrocephalus 545
  diagnosis of: Ultrasound scanning 1025
  and Spina bifida 933
  treatment of: Neurosurgery 729
Hydrochloric acid 546
  production of: Stomach 948
Hydrochlorothiazide 546
Hydrocortisone 546
Hydrocortistab 1110
Hydrocortisyl 1110
Hydrocortone 1110
Hydroflumethiazide 1110
hydrogen:
  Ion 601
Hydrogen peroxide 546
Hydromet 1110
Hydronephrosis 546
  diagnosis of: Ultrasound scanning 1026
  and Kidney cancer 613
Hydrophobia 546
  alternative term: Rabies 850
Hydrops 546
hydrops fetalis:
  cause of: Haemolytic disease of the newborn 500; Rhesus incompatibility 875
HydroSaluric 1110
Hydrotalcite 1110
Hydrotherapy 546
  in Physiotherapy 803

Hydroxocobalamin 546
Hydroxychloroquine 1110
Hydroxycholecalciferol 1110
Hydroxyethylcellulose 1110
Hydroxyprogesterone 1110
Hydroxyurea 1110
Hydroxyzine 1110
Hygiene 546
  and Infection 577
Hygiene, oral:
  Oral hygiene 756
Hygroma, cystic 546
  type of Lymphangioma 652
Hygroton 1110
Hygroton-K 1110
Hymen 547
  imperforate: Vagina 1040
Hyoid 547
Hyoscine 547
Hyper- 547
Hyperacidity 547
Hyperactivity 547
  and Food additives 455
  treatment of: Stimulant drugs 947
Hyperacusis 548
Hyperaldosteronism 548
  alternative term: Aldosteronism 84
Hyperalimentation 548
Hyperbaric oxygen treatment 548
  Oxygen 770
Hyperbilirubinaemia 548
Hypercalcaemia 548
  abnormally high blood level of Calcium 224
Hypercapnia 548
Hyperemesis 548
  excessive Vomiting 1068
hyperemesis gravidarum:
  common term: Vomiting in pregnancy 1068
Hyperglycaemia 548
  abnormally high blood level of Glucose 487
  symptom of Diabetes mellitus 349
  treatment of: Insulin 589
Hypergonadism 548
Hyperhidrosis 548
hyperkalaemia:
  abnormally high blood level of Potassium 820
Hyperkeratosis 548
Hyperlipidaemias 549
  treatment of: Lipid-lowering drugs 639
Hypermetropia 549
  treatment of: why glasses are used 484
Hypernephroma 550
  type of Kidney cancer 613
Hyperparathyroidism 550
  cause of: Parathyroid tumour 781
Hyperplasia 550
Hyperplasia, gingival 551
Hyperpyrexia 551
Hypersensitivity 551
  to Contact lenses 301
  reactions: Immune system 566
  type of: Serum sickness 902

Hypersplenism 551
Hypertension 551, 552
  cause of: Phaeochromocytoma 797
  and disorders of the kidney 614; Peripheral vascular disease 793; Polycythaemia 815
  treatment of: Amiloride 92; Beta-blocker drugs 165; Diuretic drugs 364; Hydrochlorothiazide 546; Labetolol 622; Methyldopa 684; Minoxidil 689; Nadolol 716; Nephrectomy 721; Nifedipine 730; Pindolol 804; Prazosin 821; Propranolol 831; Relaxation techniques 867
hypertensive retinopathy:
  a disorder of the retina 873
Hyperthermia 553
Hyperthermia, malignant 553
Hyperthyroidism 553
  and Pituitary tumours 806; disorders of the thyroid gland 992
  symptoms and signs of hyperthyroidism 554
  treatment of: Nadolol 716; Propranolol 831; Propylthiouracil 831
Hypertonia 553
Hypertrichosis 553
hypertrophic scar:
  type of Scar 889
Hypertrophy 553
  of heart: Cardiomegaly 235
Hyperuricaemia 553
  abnormally high blood level of Uric acid 1030
Hyperventilation 554
  causing Tetany 981
  in Panic attack 777
  treatment of: Relaxation techniques 867
hypervitaminosis A:
  excess of Vitamin A 1062
Hyphaema 554
  appearance of hyphaema 555
  cause of: Eye injuries 425
  causing Vision, loss of 1059
Hypnomidate 1110
Hypnosis 554
  and Freudian theory 462; Trance 1009
Hypnotic drugs 555
  alternative term: Sleeping drugs 922
Hypnovel 1110
Hypo- 555
Hypoaldosteronism 555
Hypocalcaemia 555
  causing disorders of muscle 707
  abnormally low blood level of Calcium 224
Hypochondriasis 555
Hypochondrium 555
hypodermic syringe:
  Syringe 967
hypogammaglobulinaemia:
  and Immunodeficiency disorders 571

Hypoglossal nerve 555
  functions of cranial nerves 318
  location of hypoglossal nerve 556
Hypoglycaemia 556
  abnormally low blood level of Glucose 487
  cause of: Insulin 590
  feature of Prematurity 825
Hypoglycaemics, oral 556
  example: Glibenclamide 484
Hypogonadism 556
  treatment of: Progestogen drugs 830
Hypohidrosis 556
hypohidrotic ectodermal dysplasia:
  causing Hypohidrosis 556
hypokalaemia:
  abnormally low blood level of Potassium 820
  causing disorders of muscle 707
Hypomania 556
  form of Mania 661
Hypoparathyroidism 556
Hypophysectomy 557
Hypopituitarism 557
  cause of: Pituitary tumour 806
Hypoplasia 557
Hypoplasia, enamel 557
Hypoplastic left-heart syndrome 557
Hyposensitization 557
  in treatment of Allergy 87
Hypospadias 557
  abnormality of Penis 788
  treatment of: Plastic surgery 809
Hypotears 1110
Hypotension 558
Hypothalamus 558
  and Pituitary gland 805; control of Temperature 973; Thirst 984
Hypothermia 558
  first aid: hypothermia 559
Hypothermia, surgical 559
  use of: Open heart surgery 752
Hypothyroidism 560
  causing Myxoedema 715
  and Hyperlipidaemias 549; Iodine 600; Pallor 774; disorders of the thyroid gland 992
  in the Newborn 730
Hypotonia 560
Hypotonia in infants 560
Hypovase 1110
Hypovolaemia 560
Hypoxia 560
Hypromellose 1110
Hypurin 1110
Hysterectomy 560
  performing a hysterectomy 561
  and Oophorectomy 752
  in treatment of Fibroid 447; Hydatidiform mole 545; Menorrhagia 677; Uterus, cancer of 1037
Hysteria 561
hysterical amnesia:
  and Dissociative disorders 364

Hysterosalpingography 561
in diagnosis of *disorders of the uterus 1037*
in *investigating infertility 582*
hysteroscope:
use of: Endometrial ablation 402; Sterilization, female 945
Hysterotomy 561
Hytrin 1110

I

Iatrogenic 562
Ibrufhalal 1110
Ibugel 1110
Ibular 1110
Ibuleve 1110
Ibumed 1110
Ibuprofen 562
type of Nonsteroidal anti-inflammatory drug 734
Ice-packs 562
in treatment of Sprain 941
Ichthammol 1110
Ichthyosis 562
Icterus 562
alternative term: Jaundice 606
Id 562
and Freudian theory 462; Psychoanalytic theory 839
in relation to Ego 390; Superego 960
Idarubicin 1110
identical twins:
type of Twins 1021
identity crisis:
in Adolescence 68
Idiocy 562
modern term: Mental handicap 680
Idiopathic 562
IDL:
see index entry intermediate-density lipoprotein
Idoxene 1110
Idoxuridine 562
Iduridin 1110
Ifosfamide 1110
ileal conduit:
use of: Urinary diversion 1030; *urinary diversion using ileal conduit 1031*
Ileitis, regional 562
modern term: Crohn's disease 320
Ileostomy 562
procedure for ileostomy 563
in treatment of Polyposis, familial 817
Ileum 563
location of the ileum 564
part of Intestine 596
surgical opening into: Ileostomy 562
Ileus, paralytic 564
ilium:
part of Pelvis 787

Illness 564
Illusion 564
Ilosone 1110
Ilube 1110
Imaging techniques 564
Diagnosing disease 30–31
Diagnostic techniques 34–39
imaging the body 565
Scanning techniques 888
Imbrilon 1110
Imdur 1110
Imigran 1110
Imipenem 1110
Imipramine 1110
Immersion foot 566
Immobility 566
causing Constipation 299; Osteoporosis 764
leading to Pulmonary embolism 843; Thrombosis, deep vein 987
Immobilization 566
immune complexes:
causing Glomerulonephritis 485; Hypersensitivity 551; Serum sickness 902; Vasculitis 1045
formation of: Viruses 1057
removal of: Plasmapheresis 809
Immune response 566
and Sensitization 899
Immune system 566
function of Antibody 115; Blood cells 182; Immunoglobulin 571; Interferon 594; Lymphocyte 653; Phagocyte 798; Thymus 989
parts of: *the adaptive immune system 568; the innate immune system 567*
Immunity 569
Immunization 28–29, 569
typical childhood immunization schedule 570
Travel immunization 29, 1012; *guidelines for travel immunization 1013*
types of: *types of immunization 570*; Vaccination 1040
using Immunoglobulin injection 572; Vaccine 1040
Immunoassay 570
and Serology 901
immunocomplexes:
see index entry immune complexes
Immunodeficiency disorders 571
leading to AIDS 76; Nocardiosis 732; Opportunistic infections 754
Immunoglobulin 571
alternative term: Antibody 115
function of: Immune system 566; *the adaptive immune system 568*
production of: Lymphocyte 653
type of Plasma protein 809
Immunoglobulin injection 572
Immunology 572
Immunoprin 1110
Immunostimulant drugs 572

Immunosuppressant drugs 572
example: Cyclosporin 326
leading to Fungal infections 464; Opportunistic infections 754
in treatment of Autoimmune disorders 146; Cardiomyopathy 236
uses of: Bone marrow transplant 194; Heart transplant 523; Transplant surgery 46, 1011
immunosuppression:
and Immune system 566
see also index entry Immunosuppressant drugs
Immunotherapy 572
Imodium 1110
Impaction, dental 572
and Eruption of teeth 415
impedance audiometry:
types of hearing test 514
Imperacin 1110
imperforate anus:
Anus, imperforate 121
imperforate hymen:
Hymen 547
Impetigo 573
Implant 573
Mammoplasty 660; Mastectomy 664; Penile implant 788
Surgical implants 46
see also index entry radioactive implants
Implantation, egg 573
and *the developing embryo 396*; Pregnancy 822
Implants, dental 574
Impotence 574
causes of Cystectomy 327; Heroin abuse 531; Neuropathy 728; Prolactinoma 831; Shy-Drager syndrome 910
causing Infertility 583
and Penis 789
treatment of: Penile implant 788; Sensate focus technique 898; Sex therapy 903
type of Psychosexual dysfunction 840
Impression, dental 574
use of: Denture 342
Imtack 1110
Imunovir 1110
Imuran 1110
Incest 574
causing Sexual desire, inhibited 904
and Child abuse 261
Incidence 575
incidence of various conditions in the UK 574
and Prevalence 828
Incision 575
Incisor 578
structure and arrangement of teeth 972
incompetent cervix:
Cervical incompetence 251
Incontinence, faecal 575
cause of: Faecal impaction 429

treatment of: Sphincter, artificial 933
see also index entry Diarrhoea
Incontinence, urinary 575
causes of: Irritable bladder 602; Multiple sclerosis 702; Neuropathy 728; Prostate enlarged 833; abnormality of Ureter 1028
treatment of: Sphincter, artificial 933
Incoordination 576
feature of Ataxia 140
Incubation period 576
of *some important infectious diseases 579–581*
Incubator 576
introduction of: *landmarks in medicine: other forms of treatment 670*
and Neonatal care 44
for the Newborn 730
in treatment of Prematurity 826
incus:
bone in Ear 383
example of Ossicle 761
Indapamide 1110
Indaxa 1110
Inderal, Inderal LA 1110
Inderetic 1110
Inderex 1110
Indian medicine 576
Indigestion 576
Indocid, Indocid R 1110
Indolar SR 1110
Indomax 1110
Indomethacin 576
Indomod 1111
Indoramin 1111
Induction of labour 577
uses of: Childbirth, complications of 264; Postmaturity 818
Industrial diseases:
Occupational disease and injury 743
Infacol 1111
Infant 577
Newborn 729
Infantile spasms 577
Infant mortality 577
Infarction 577
example: Myocardial infarction 712
Infection 577
types of: Food-borne infection 455; Infection, congenital 577
see also index entry Infectious disease
Infection, congenital 577
Infectious disease 578
causes of: Bacteria 152; Fungi 464; Protozoa 836; Rickettsia 880; Viruses 1055; *viruses and disease 1056*
immunity against: Immunity 569
prevention of: Immunization 569; Quarantine 849; Vaccination 1040; Vaccine 1040

transmission of: Cats, diseases
from 243; Dogs, diseases
from 368; Food-borne
infection 455; *infected animal
products 457*; Insects and
disease 587; Rabies 850;
Rats, diseases from 860;
Transmissible 1010; Vector
1047; Zoonosis 1094
type of Health hazard 511;
Occupational disease and
injury 743
types of: Chlamydial
infections 268; Fungal
infections 464; Infection,
congenital 578; *some
important infectious diseases
579–581*; Notifiable diseases
736; Sexually transmitted
diseases 904; *a selection of
zoonoses (diseases caught from
animals) 1093*
infectious hepatitis:
Hepatitis, viral *528, 529*
Infectious mononucleosis:
Mononucleosis, infectious 694
Inferiority complex 581
Infertility 581
causes of: Fibroid 447;
Gonorrhoea 490; Pelvic
inflammatory disease 786;
Prolactinoma 831; Puerperal
sepsis 843; Testis,
undescended 979
following Abortion, induced
58
investigating infertility 582
treatment of: Artificial
insemination 133;
Clomiphene 282;
Gonadotrophin, human
chorionic 490; In vitro
fertilization 600;
Menotrophin 677;
Tamoxifen 968
Infestation 583
Infibulation 583
Infiltrate 583
Inflammation 583
and *the innate immune system
567*
Inflammatory bowel disease 584
Influenza 584
Infra-red 585
cause of Cataract 240
part of *electromagnetic spectrum
1026*
and Thermography 983
Infusion, intravenous:
Intravenous infusion 599
Ingestion 585
Ingrowing toenail:
Toenail, ingrowing 899
Inguinal 585
inguinal hernia:
*main types of abdominal hernia
530*
Inhalation 585
Breathing 209
of medication: Inhaler 585; *how
to use an inhaler 584*;
Nebulizer 719; *using a
nebulizer 720*; Vaporizer 1044

Inhaler 585
how to use an inhaler 584
in treatment of Asthma *138,
139*
Inheritance 585
inheritance of eye colour 586
and Intelligence 590
see also index entries
Chromosomes; Gene
Inhibition 586
Initard 50/50 1111
Injection 586
Injury 586
Ink-blot test 586
type of: Rorschach test 882
Inlay, dental 586
and Restoration, dental 872
innominate bone:
part of Pelvis 787
Innovace 1111
Innozide 1111
Inoculation 586
Inoperable 586
Inorganic 586
Inosine pranobex 1111
Inositol 1111
Inoven 1111
Inpatient treatment 587
inquest:
and Coroner 311
Insanity 587
former term: Lunacy 648
Insect bites 587
and Insects and disease 587
insecticide:
type of Pesticide 796
Insects and disease 587
and Tropical diseases 1017
Insect stings 588
Insecurity 588
insemination, artificial:
Artificial insemination 133
Insight 588
In situ 589
Insomnia 589
treatment of: Lorazepam 647;
Sleeping drugs 922;
Temazepam 973
Instinct 589
Institutionalization 589
Insulatard 1111
Insulin 589
administration of: Pump,
insulin 846
production of: Genetic
engineering 478; *landmarks
in medicine: drugs 671*;
Pancreas 775; Recombinant
DNA 862
in treatment of Diabetes
mellitus 349; Hypoglycaemia
556
insulin coma therapy:
type of Shock therapy 908
insulin-dependent diabetes:
type of Diabetes mellitus 349
Insulinoma 590
treatment of: Pancreatectomy
775
insulin pump:
Pump, insulin 846
Intal 1111
Intal Compound 1111

Intelligence 590
assessment of: Intelligence
tests 590
and Child development 264;
Personality 795
intelligence quotient:
and Intelligence 590
measurement of: Intelligence
tests 591
Intelligence tests 590
and Intelligence 590;
Psychology 839
type of Psychometry 839
Intensive care 44, 591
and Neonatal care 44
of Newborn 730
Inter- 591
interactions, drug:
Drug 376
Intercostal 591
Intercourse, painful 592
leading to Orgasm, lack of 758
symptom chart (men) 592
symptom chart (women) 593
type of Psychosexual
dysfunction 840
Interferon 594
*how interferon fights viral
infections 595*
production of: Immune system
569; Viruses 1057
in treatment of Cold, common
286; Hepatitis, chronic
active 529; Multiple
sclerosis 702
intermediate-density lipoprotein
(IDL):
and Hyperlipidaemias 549
intermittent claudication:
see index entry Claudication
interneuron:
structure of a neuron 727
in Spinal cord 934
type of Neuron 726
Intersex 595
and Genitalia, ambiguous 479;
Transsexualism 1011
type of: Testicular
feminization syndrome 977
interstitial fluid:
alternative term: Tissue fluid
996
Interstitial pulmonary fibrosis
595
causing Pulmonary
hypertension 844
Interstitial radiotherapy 595
type of Radiotherapy 856
Intertrigo 595
Intestinal imaging:
Barium X-ray examinations
157
Intestinal lipodystrophy:
alternative term: Whipple's
disease 1082
Intestine 595
disorders of: Abdominal pain
50; *disorders of the anus 121*;
Colic, infantile 287;
Flatulence 452; Intestine,
cancer of 596; *disorders of the
intestine 597*; Intestine,
obstruction of 596; Intestine,

tumours of 596; Rectum,
cancer of 864
function of: *the digestive process
358*; Peristalsis 793
imaging of: Barium X-ray
examinations 157
part of Digestive system 357
parts of: Anus 121; Appendix
127; Caecum 221; Colon 289;
Duodenum 379; Ileum 563;
Jejunum 607; Rectum 863
surgical joining of:
Anastomosis 104
Intestine, cancer of 596
type of: Rectum, cancer of
864
Intestine, obstruction of 596
causes of: Intestine, cancer of
596; Intussusception 599;
Rectum, cancer of 864;
Volvulus 1067
causing Abdominal swelling
55; Vomiting 1068
Intestine, tumours of 596
see also index entry Intestine,
cancer of
Intoxication 598
Intra- 598
intra-aortic balloon pump:
type of Heart, artificial 516
Intracavitary therapy 598
type of Radiotherapy 856
Intracerebral haemorrhage 598
Intractable 598
Intramuscular 598
Intraocular pressure 598
Intrauterine contraceptive device:
IUD 605
Intrauterine growth retardation
598
Intraval Sodium 1111
Intravenous 599
drug abuse: Drug dependence
377
see also index entry
Intravenous infusion
Intravenous infusion 599
uses of: Feeding, artificial 437;
Rehydration therapy 866
Intravenous pyelography:
type of Urography 1035
intrinsic factor:
absence of: Anaemia,
megaloblastic 98; *disorders
of the stomach 949*
production of: Stomach 948
Introitus 599
Intron A 1111
Intropin 1111
Introvert 599
and Jungian theory 609
Intubation 599
Intussusception 599
cause of: Peutz-Jeghers
syndrome 797
causing Intestine, obstruction
of 596
Invasive 599
In vitro 600
In vitro fertilization (IVF) 600
development of: *landmarks in
medicine: other forms of
treatment 670*

In vitro fertilization (continued)
and Surrogacy 961
in treatment of Genetic
disorders 478; Infertility
583
In vivo 600
Involuntary movements 600
involuntary muscle:
type of Muscle 706
Iodine 600
deficiency of: Goitre 489
dietary: *minerals and main food
sources 690; recommended
daily allowances (RDAs) of
selected minerals 690*
radioactive: Radiation 852
sensitivity to: Urography
1035
in treatment of Thyroid cancer
990
uses of: Radionuclide scanning
854; Radiotherapy 856;
Thyroid scanning 993
Ion 601
production of: Ionizer 601;
Radiation 851
Ionamin 1111
Ionil T 1111
Ionizer 601
ionizing radiation:
type of Radiation 851
radiation units 851
Ipecacuanha 601
Ipral 1111
Ipratropium bromide 1111
Iprindole 1111
IQ 601
and Intelligence 590
measurement of: Intelligence
tests 591
Iridectomy 601
Iridocyclitis 602
Iris 602
disorders of: *disorders of the eye
426;* Eye injuries 425;
Rheumatoid arthritis,
juvenile 878; Uveitis 1039
part of Eye 423; Uvea 1039
and Pupil 846
.   tearing of: Eye injuries 425
Iritis 602
type of Uveitis 1039
Iron 602
deficiency of: Anaemia,
iron-deficiency 97
dietary: *minerals and main food
sources 690; recommended
daily allowances (RDAs) of
selected minerals 690*
excess of: Blood transfusion
189; Haemochromatosis 499;
Haemosiderosis 502;
Siderosis 912
and Melaena 673
Iron-deficiency anaemia:
Anaemia, iron-deficiency 97
Iron lung 602
Irradiation:
Radiation hazards 852
uses of: Radiotherapy 45, 855;
Sterilization 945
Irradiation of food 602
Irrigation, wound 602

Irritable bladder 602
causing Incontinence, urinary
576
a *disorder of the bladder 176*
Irritable bowel syndrome 603
causing Constipation 299;
Diarrhoea 355
a *disorder of the intestine 597*
treatment of: Fibre, dietary
446; Hyoscine 547;
Methylcellulose 684;
Propantheline 831
Ischaemia 603
and Transient ischaemic attack
1009
ischium:
part of Pelvis 787
Isclofen 1111
Isib 1111
Isisfen 1111
Ismelin 1111
islets of Langerhans:
part of Pancreas 775
Ismo 1111
Isocarboxazid 1111
Isoconazole 1111
Isoflurane 1111
Isogel 1111
Isoket 1111
isokinetic exercise:
Types of exercise 20
Isolation 603
and Quarantine 849
Isometheptene mucate 1111
isometric exercise:
Types of exercise 20
Isomide 1111
Isoniazid 604
causing Hepatitis, chronic
active 529
in treatment of Tuberculosis
1019
Isoprenaline 604
Isopto Alkaline 1111
Isopto Atropine 1111
Isopto Carpine 1111
Isopto Frin 1111
Isopto Plain 1111
Isordil 1111
Isosorbide 604
Isosorbide dinitrate 1111
Isosorbide mononitrate 1111
isotonic exercise:
Types of exercise 20
Isotope scanning:
Radionuclide scanning 854
Isotrate 1111
Isotretinoin 604
Isotrex 1111
Ispaghula 604
Isradipine 1111
Istin 1111
Itching 604
medical term: Pruritus 836
treatment of: Calamine 223;
Trimeprazine 1016
-itis 605
Itraconazole 1111
IUCD:
see index entry IUD
IUD 605
and *effectiveness (failure rates) of
contraceptive methods 304*

use of: Contraception 301;
methods of contraception 303
Ivermectin 1111
IVF:
see index entry In vitro
fertilization
IVP 605
type of Urography 1035
IVU 605
Urography 1035

J

Jackson's All Four 1111
Jakob-Creutzfeldt disease:
Creutzfeldt-Jakob disease 319
Jarvik 7:
type of Heart, artificial 516
Jaundice 606
causes of:
Cholangiocarcinoma 270;
Cholangitis 270;
Cholecystitis 271;
Cholestasis 272; Cirrhosis
281; Leptospirosis 632;
Metabolism, inborn errors of
682; Spherocytosis,
hereditary 932; Yellow fever
1092
causing Urine, abnormal 1034
in infants: Haemolytic disease
of the newborn 500;
Newborn 730; Prematurity
825
and Pigmentation 803
treatment of: Phototherapy
802
Jaundice, neonatal 606
and Haemolytic disease of the
newborn 550; Newborn 730;
Prematurity 825
Jaw 606
deformities of: Prognathism
830; Receding chin 861
deformities, treatment of:
Orthognathic surgery 760
disorders of: Burkitt's
lymphoma 218; Jaw,
dislocated 606; Jaw,
fractured 607;
Temporomandibular joint
syndrome 974
and Malocclusion 659
upper jaw: Maxilla 666
see also index entry jaw
muscles
Jaw, dislocated 606
Jaw, fractured 607
treatment of: Wiring of the
jaws 1083
jaw muscles:
anatomy of: *location of the
temporomandibular joint 974*
involuntary contraction of:
Trismus 1017
Jealousy, morbid 607
Jectofer 1111
Jejunal biopsy 607
in diagnosis of Malabsorption
657

Jejunum 607
part of Intestine 596
Jellyfish stings 607
Jenner, Edward:
history of Medicine 668
landmarks in medicine: drugs 671
Jet-lag 609
Jexin 1111
jigger flea:
Chigoe 260
jock itch:
Tinea 994
Jogger's nipple 609
jogging:
causing Jogger's nipple 609
Joint 609
disorders of: Dislocation, joint
362; Effusion joint 390;
Ehlers-Danlos syndrome
390; Gout 490, 491;
Neuropathic joint 727;
Osteoarthritis 761;
Osteochondritis dissecans
762; Rheumatic fever 876;
Rheumatoid arthritis 876;
Subluxation 956
examination of: Arthroscopy
132
examples: Ankle joint 110;
Elbow 391; Hip 534; Knee
619; Shoulder 909; Suture
962; Wrist 1088
false: Pseudarthrosis 836
in Finger 450; Jaw 606; Skull
919; Spine 937; Toe 999
fusion of: Arthrodesis 132
types of joints 608
and *movement 699*
Joint replacement:
medical term: Arthroplasty 132
types of: Finger-joint
replacement 450; Hip
replacement 535; Knee-joint
replacement 619
Joule 609
Joy-rides 1111
Jugular vein 609
part of *circulatory system 280*
and Vena cava 1048
Jungian theory 609
Junifen 1111
Junior Lemsip 1111
Junior Meltus Dry Cough 1111
Junior Meltus Expectorant 1111
Junior Mu-Cron 1111
Juvenile arthritis:
Rheumatoid arthritis, juvenile
878

K

Kabiglobulin 1111
Kabikinase 1111
Kala-azar 610
type of Leishmaniasis 631
Kalspare 1111
Kalten 1111
Kanamycin 1111
Kannasyn 1111
Kaodene 1111

Kaolin 610
 use of: Poultice 821
Kaopectate 1111
Kapake 1111
Kaposi's sarcoma 610
 feature of AIDS 77
Karvol 1111
Kawasaki disease 610
Kay-Cee-L 1111
Kefadol 1111
Keflex 1111
Kefzol 1111
Kelfizine W 1111
Keloid 610
 type of Scar 889
 a *disorder of the skin 919*
Kemadrin 1111
Kemicetine 1111
Kenalog 1111
Keratin 610
 as constituent of Hair 503; Nail
  716; Skin 915
 constituent of: Sulphur 959
Keratitis 610
 causing Eye, painful red 427
 a *disorder of the cornea 308*
Keratoacanthoma 610
 type of Skin tumour 918
Keratoconjunctivitis 610
Keratoconjunctivitis sicca 611
 a *disorder of the cornea 308*
Keratoconus 611
 a *disorder of the cornea 308*
Keratolytic drugs 611
Keratomalacia 611
 a *disorder of the cornea 308*;
  disorder of the eye 426
Keratopathy 611
 disorders of the cornea 308
Keratoplasty:
 Corneal graft 307
Keratosis 611
 leading to Skin tumours 918
Keratosis pilaris 611
Keratotomy, radial 611
Kerion 611
Kerlone 1111
Kernicterus 612
Kest 1111
Ketamine 1111
ketoacidosis:
 causing Vomiting 1068
 type of Acidosis 62
Ketoconazole 612
ketones:
 excess of: Ketosis 612
Ketoprofen 612
Ketorolac 1111
Ketosis 612
 treatment of: Insulin 589
Ketotifen 1111
Ketovail 1111
Ketovite 1111
keyhole surgery:
 Minimally invasive surgery 48
Kiditard 1111
Kidney 612
 disorders of:
  Glomerulosclerosis 486;
  disorders of the kidney 614;
  Nephrocalcinosis 721;
  Nephrosclerosis 722
 drainage of: Nephrostomy 722

 function of: Acid-base balance
  62; *the function of the kidney
  615*; Urine 1034; Water 1076
 investigation of: Kidney
  biopsy 613; Kidney-function
  tests 616; Kidney imaging
  616, 617
 part of Urinary tract 1032, 1033
 part of: Nephron 722
 removal of: Nephrectomy 721
 study of: Nephrology 722
kidney, artificial:
 Dialysis 44, 351; *procedure for
  dialysis 352*
Kidney biopsy 613
Kidney cancer 613
 type of: Wilms' tumour 1083
Kidney cyst 613
 diagnosis of: Ultrasound
  scanning 1026
Kidney failure 614
 as complication of Rheumatoid
  arthritis, juvenile 878
 symptoms of: Thirst, excessive
  984; Urine, abnormal 1034
 treatment of: Dialysis 44, 351;
  Kidney transplant 617
Kidney-function tests 616
Kidney imaging 616, 617
Kidney, polycystic 616
Kidney stone:
 Calculus, urinary tract 224
Kidney transplant 617
 *landmarks in medicine: surgery
  670*
 *procedure for a kidney transplant
  618*
 in treatment of Kidney failure
  616
 type of Transplant surgery 46,
  1010
Kidney tumours 617
 diagnosis of: Ultrasound
  scanning 1026
killer cell:
 and Histocompatibility
  antigens 536; Interferon 594
 part of Immune system 569;
  *the adaptive immune system
  568*
 type of Lymphocyte 653
Kilocalorie 617
 and Calorie 226; Joule 609
Kilojoule 617
 and Joule 609
Kinidin Durules 1112
kissing:
 and Sexual intercourse 904
 in spread of AIDS 77;
  Mononucleosis, infectious
  694; Syphilis 966
Kiss of life 617
 alternative term: Artificial
  respiration 134
Klaricid 1112
Kleptomania 617
Klinefelter's syndrome 619
KLN 1112
Kloref 1112
Klumpke's paralysis 619
Knee 619
 disorders of: Chondromalacia
  patellae 273; *location of knee*

 joint effusion 390; Knock-
  knee 620; Lyme disease 651
 simple knee-jerk reflex 865
 part of Skeleton 915
 parts of: Cruciate ligaments
  321; Meniscus 676; Patella
  783
 surgery on: Meniscectomy 675
 see also index entry Joint
kneecap:
 medical term: Patella 783
Knee-joint replacement 619
 *procedure for a knee replacement
  620*
Knock-knee 620
 example of Valgus 1043
 and Walking 1072
Knoll, Max:
 *landmarks in medicine: diagnosis
  669*
Knuckle 620
 and Metacarpal bone 683
Koch, Robert:
 and Anatomy and pathology
  30; *landmarks in medicine:
  diagnosis 669*; Microbiology
  685
Koilonychia 621
Kolanticon 1112
Kolff, Willem:
 *landmarks in medicine: other
  forms of treatment 670*
Konakion 1112
Koplik's spots 621
Korsakoff's psychosis:
 Wernicke-Korsakoff syndrome
  1081
Krabbe's disease:
 type of Leukodystrophy 635
Kraurosis vulvae:
 type of Vulvitis 1071
Kretschmer, Ernst
 and Somatotype 928
Kuru 621
 type of Slow virus disease
  924
Kwashiorkor 621
Kwells 1112
Kyphoscoliosis 621
Kyphosis 621
 a disorder of the spine 938
Kytril 1112

L

Labetolol 622
Labia 622
 enlargement of:
  Pseudohermaphroditism 836
Labile 622
Labophylline 1112
Labour:
 see index entry Childbirth
Labrocol 1112
laburnum:
 type of Plant, poisonous 808
labyrinth:
 inflammation of: Labyrinthitis
  622
 part of Ear 383

Labyrinthitis 622
 symptoms of: Vertigo 1053;
  Vomiting 1068
Laceration 622
 type of Wound 1086, *1087*
Lacidipine 1112
Lacrimal apparatus 622
 *functions of the lacrimal
  apparatus 623*
lacrimal glands:
 part of Lacrimal apparatus 622
Lactase deficiency 622
 causing Food intolerance 456;
  Lactose intolerance 623
Lactation 623
 and Breast-feeding 206
 suppression of: Bromocriptine
  213
lacteals:
 part of Lymphatic system 653
Lactic acid 623
 causing Cramp 317
Lactitol 1112
lacto-ovovegetarianism:
 type of Vegetarianism 1047
Lactose 623
Lactose intolerance 623
 and Lactase deficiency 622
 causing Diarrhoea 355
lactovegetarianism:
 type of Vegetarianism 1047
Lactulose 623
Ladropen 1112
Laennec, René:
 *landmarks in medicine: diagnosis
  669*
Lambliasis 623
 alternative term: Giardiasis 481
Lamictal 1112
Laminectomy 623
Lamisil 1112
Lamotrigine 1112
Lamprene 1112
Lance 623
Lancet 624
Landsteiner, Karl:
 *landmarks in medicine: surgery
  670*
language:
 and Speech 930; Speech
  disorders 930; Speech
  therapy 931
Language disorders 624
 and Speech disorders 930;
  Speech therapy 931
Lanolin 624
 in treatment of Chapped skin
  256
Lanoxin 1112
Lanoxin-PG 1112
Lansoprazole 1112
Lanugo hair 624
Lanvis 1112
Laparoscopy 624
 and Appendicectomy 126
 in diagnosis of Abdominal
  pain 55; Ovary, cancer of
  768; Salpingitis 887
 uses of: *investigating infertility
  582*; Sterilization, female 945
Laparotomy 624
 in diagnosis of Abdominal
  pain 55; Peritonitis 794

1165

Laractone 1112
Laraflex 1112
Larapam 1112
Laratrim 1112
Largactil 1112
large cell carcinoma:
    type of Lung cancer 649
large intestine:
    see index entries Colon;
        Intestine
Lariam 1112
Larodopa 1105
Larva migrans 624
    causing Toxocariasis 1005
Laryngeal nerve 624
    location of laryngeal nerves 625
Laryngectomy 625
Laryngitis 625
    causing Hoarseness 537
laryngomalacia:
    causing Stridor 952
    a disorder of the larynx 627
laryngopharynx:
    part of Pharynx 799
Laryngoscopy 625
    in diagnosis of Hoarseness 539
    procedure for laryngoscopy 626
    in treatment of Choking 270
    use of: Intubation 599
Laryngotracheobronchitis 625
    feature of: Tracheitis 1007
Larynx 626
    disorders of the larynx 627
    narrowed: Stridor 952
    oedema of: Pharyngitis 798
    removal of: Laryngectomy 625
Larynx, cancer of 626
    causing Hoarseness 537
Laser 627
    Excimer laser 419
Laser surgery 47
Laser treatment 47, 627
    uses of: Cervicitis 253; Cervix,
        cancer of 255; Heart surgery
        522; Laser surgery 47;
        Retinopathy 874; use of a
        laser 628; Tattooing 971
Lasikal 1112
Lasilactone 1112
Lasipressin 1112
Lasix + K 1112
Lasma 1112
Lasoride 1112
Lassa fever 627
Lassitude 628
    feature of Sleeping sickness
        923
    Tiredness 995
Lateral 628
Latissimus dorsi 628
Laudanum 628
Laughing gas 628
Laurence-Biedl-Moon syndrome
    628
Lavage, gastric 628
Laxative drugs 629
    examples: Ispaghula 604;
        Lactulose 623; Liquid
        paraffin 639; Methylcellulose
        684; Senna 897
Laxoberal 1112
Laxose 1112
Lazy eye 629

LDL:
    see index entry low-density
        lipoprotein
Lead poisoning 629
    causing Neuropathy 728
Learning 629
Learning difficulties 629
Ledercort 1112
Lederfen, Lederfen F 1112
Ledermycin 1112
Lederspan 1112
Leech 630
Leeuwenhoek, Antonj van:
    development of Microscope
        685
    history of Medicine 668
    landmarks in medicine: diagnosis
        669
left-handedness:
    and Stuttering 955
    type of Handedness 506
leg:
    bones of: Femur 438; Fibula
        448; Tibia 993
    disorders of: Bowleg 197;
        Femur, fracture of 439; Leg,
        shortening of 630; Leg ulcer
        631; Paraplegia 779; Restless
        legs 870; Sciatica 891; Shin
        splints 907
    joints of: Ankle joint 110; Hip
        534; Knee 619
    muscles of: Calf muscles 226;
        Quadriceps muscle 849
    see also index entry Foot
leg, artificial:
    type of Limb, artificial 637
Leg, broken:
    Femur, fracture of 439
    Fibula 448
    Tibia 993
Legionnaires' disease 630
Leg, shortening of 630
Leg ulcer 631
    treatment of: Calamine 223
Leiomyoma 631
Leishmaniasis 631
    causes of: Protozoa 836;
        Sandfly bites 887
Lem-Plus, Lemsip 1112
Lenium 1112
Lens 631
    disorders of: Cataract 240;
        Lens dislocation 632
    part of Eye 422
    removal of: Cataract surgery
        240; procedure for cataract
        surgery 241
    see also index entries Contact
        lenses; Glasses
Lens dislocation 632
    causing Double vision 370
    feature of Marfan's syndrome
        662
Lens implant 632
    in Cataract surgery 240;
        procedure for cataract surgery
        241
Lentard MC 1112
Lentaron 1112
Lentigo 632
    type of Naevus 716
Lentizol 1112

Leprosy 632
    see index entry Hansen's
        disease
Leptospirosis 632
    and Rats, diseases from 860;
        Water-borne infection 1076
Lesbianism 632
Lesch-Nyhan syndrome:
    associated with Self-injury 897
Lesion 632
Lethargy 632
    Tiredness 995
Leucovorin 1112
Leukaemia 632, 634
    and Radiation hazards 852;
        Strontium 954
    treatment of: Anticancer drugs
        115; Bone marrow
        transplant 194; performing a
        bone marrow transplant 195;
        Mercaptopurine 681;
        Radiotherapy 855
Leukaemia, acute 632
    leukaemia 634
Leukaemia, chronic lymphocytic
    633
    leukaemia 634
Leukaemia, chronic myeloid 633
    leukaemia 634
Leukeran 1112
Leukocyte 635
    type of Blood cell 182
Leukodystrophies 635
Leukoplakia 635
    associated with Mouth cancer
        698; Tongue cancer 1001
Leukorrhoea:
    Vaginal discharge 1041
Leuprorelin 1112
Levamisole 1112
Levobunolol 1112
Levodopa 635
    in treatment of Parkinson's
        disease 782
    type of Synthetic drug 43
Levonorgestrel 635
Levophed 1112
Lexotan 1112
Lexpec 1112
Lexpec with Iron 1112
Lexpec with Iron-M 1112
LH 635
    see also entry Luteinizing
        hormone
LH-RH 635
    abbreviation for Luteinizing
        hormone-releasing hormone
        651
Libanil 1112
Libido 635
    loss of: Sexual desire,
        inhibited 904
Librium 1112
    introduction of: landmarks in
        medicine: drugs 671
Librofem 1112
Lice 635
    eggs of: Nits 732
    type of: Pubic lice 842
Lichenification 636
Lichen planus 636
lichen sclerosus et atrophicus:
    type of Vulvitis 1071

Lichen simplex 636
Lidifen 1112
Lid lag 636
Life expectancy 636
    and Diabetes mellitus 350
    see also index entry lifespan
lifespan:
    and Aging 74; Life expectancy
        636; Keeping healthy 16
Life support 636
    method of: Ventilation 1050
    using Ventilator 1050
Ligament 636
    function of ligaments 637
Ligation 637
Ligature 637
light:
    effects of: Sunburn 959;
        Sunlight, adverse effects of
        959; Suntan 960
    intolerance to: Photophobia 801
    protection from: Sunscreens
        960
    sensitivity to: Photosensitivity
        801
    treatment with: Phototherapy
        801
    type of: Ultraviolet light 1026
Lightening 637
Light treatment:
    medical term: Phototherapy
        801
Lignocaine 637
    in treatment of Cardiac arrest
        234; Venticular tachycardia
        1051
    type of local anaesthetic 101
Li-Liquid 1112
Limb, artificial 637
    types of artificial limb 638
Limb defects 637
    type of: Phocomelia 801
Limbic system 637
limb prosthesis:
    Limb, artificial 637; types of
        artificial limb 638
Limp 638
    and Walking 1072
Linctus 638
Lindane 638
Linear accelerator 638
    use of: Radiotherapy 856
Lingraine 1112
Liniment 638
linoleic acid:
    type of Fatty acid 436
linolenic acid:
    type of Fatty acid 436
Lion, Alexandre:
    landmarks in medicine: other
        forms of treatment 670
Lioresal 1112
Liothyronine 1112
Lip 638
Lipantil 1112
lipase:
    function of: the digestive process
        358
Lip cancer 639
    cause of: Tobacco-smoking 997
Lipectomy, suction 639
    type of Body contour surgery
        190

Lipid disorders 639
Lipid-lowering drugs 639
    examples: Cholestyramine
        273; Gemfibrizol 472;
        Probucol 829
Lipids 639
    and Cholesterol 272; Fats and
        oils 436
Lipodystrophy, intestinal:
    alternative term: Whipple's
        disease 1082
Lipoma 639
Lipoprotein 639
    and Cholesterol 273; Fats and
        oils 436
    excess of: Hyperlipidaemias
        549
Liposarcoma 639
Lipostat 1112
Lip-reading 639
    and Cochlear implant 285;
        Deafness 333
Liquid paraffin 639
Liquifilm Tears 1112
Liquorice 1112
Lisinopril 1112
Liskonum 1112
Lisp 639
Listeriosis 639
Lister, Joseph:
    landmarks in medicine: surgery
        670
Litarex 1112
Lithium 640
    in treatment of Mania 661;
        Manic-depressive illness 661
Lithotomy 640
    types of: Nephrolithotomy
        722; Pyelolithotomy 847;
        Ureterolithotomy 1028
Lithotomy position 640
Lithotripsy 45, 640
    development of: landmarks in
        medicine: other forms of
        treatment 670
        lithotripsy procedures 641
Lithotripter 640
    use of: Lithotripsy 45, 640;
        lithotripsy procedures 641
Livedo reticularis 640
Liver 640
    disorders of the liver 645
    investigation of: Liver biopsy
        642; Liver-function tests 644;
        Liver imaging 646
    liver structure and function 643
    location of the liver 642
    removal of: Hepatectomy,
        partial 527; Hepatectomy
        total 527
Liver abscess 642
    diagnosis of: Ultrasound
        scanning 1025
    feature of Amoebiasis 94
Liver biopsy 642
liver bypass:
    type of Shunt 910
Liver cancer 642
    associated with Polycythaemia
        815
    a disorder of the liver 645
Liver, cirrhosis of:
    and Alcohol and disease 23

Cirrhosis 279
    a disorder of the liver 645
liver damage:
    and Alcohol and disease 23
    disorders of the liver 645
liver disease:
    and Alcohol and disease 23
    disorders of the liver 645
Liver disease, alcoholic 643
    and Alcohol and disease 23
    a disorder of the liver 645
Liver failure 644
    causes of: Cirrhosis 279;
        Mushroom poisoning 708
    a disorder of the liver 645
    treatment of: Lactulose 623
Liver fluke 644
Liver-function tests 644
Liver imaging 646
Liver transplant 646
    in treatment of Hepatitis 528;
        Liver failure 644
Livial 1112
Living will 646
Lobak 1112
lobar pneumonia:
    type of Pneumonia 811, 812
Lobe 646
Lobectomy 646
Lobectomy, lung 646
    in treatment of Lung cancer 650
Lobotomy, prefrontal 646
local anaesthetics 101
Loceryl 1112
Lochia 646
    foul-smelling: Puerperal sepsis
        843
Locked knee 647
    Knee 619
Lockjaw 647
    medical term: Trismus 1017
    symptom of Tetanus 981
Locoid 1112
Locomotor 647
Locorten-Vioform 1112
Lodine 1112
Lodoxamide 1112
Loestrin 20, Loestrin 30 1112
Lofepramine 647
Lofexidine 1112
Logiparin 1113
Logynon, Logynon ED 1113
Loiasis 647
Loin 647
Lomotil 1113
Lomustine 1113
Long, Crawford:
    landmarks in medicine: surgery
        670
longevity:
    see index entries Life
        expectancy; lifespan
Longsightedness:
    medical term: Hypermetropia
        549
Loniten 1113
Loose bodies 647
    feature of Osteochondritis
        dissecans 762
Loperamide 647
Lopid 1113
Loprazolam 1113
Lopresor 1113

Lopresoretic 1113
Loratidine 1113
Lorazepam 647
Lordosis 647
    a disorder of the spine 938
Lormetazepam 1113
Loron 1113
Losec 1113
Lotion 647
Lotriderm 1113
Lou Gehrig's disease:
    type of Motor neuron disease
        696
louse:
    see index entry Lice
low blood pressure:
    see index entry Blood pressure
low blood sugar:
    see index entry blood glucose
        levels
low blood volume:
    see index entry blood volume
low body temperature:
    medical term: Hypothermia 558
low-density lipoprotein (LDL):
    and Cholesterol 273; Fats and
        oils 436
    constitutent of Globulin 485
    excess of: Hyperlipidaemias
        549
Loxapac 1113
Loxapine 1113
LSD 647
    and Serotonin 901
Ludiomil 1113
Ludwig's angina 647
Lugol's solution 1113
Lumbago 648
Lumbar 648
    part of Spine 937
Lumbar puncture 648
    in diagnosis of Sleeping
        sickness 923; Subarachnoid
        haemorrhage 955
Lumbosacral spasm 648
Lumen 648
Lumpectomy 648
    type of Mastectomy 664
lump in the throat:
    medical term: Globus
        hystericus 485
Lunacy 648
Lung 648
    disorders of: Breathing
        difficulty 209, 210; disorders
        of the lung 649
    function of: Breathing 208;
        Respiration 869, 871
    investigation of: Lung imaging
        650; Pulmonary function
        tests 844
    part of Respiratory system 870
    removal of: Lobectomy, lung
        646; Pneumonectomy 811
Lung cancer 649
    cause of: Smoking and cancer
        22; Tobacco-smoking 997
    and Pneumoconiosis 811
    type of: Small cell carcinoma
        924
Lung, collapse of:
    Atelectasis 140
    Pneumothorax 813

Lung disease, chronic
    obstructive 650
lung fibrosis:
    types of: Interstitial
        pulmonary fibrosis 595;
        Pulmonary fibrosis 844
Lung-function tests:
    Pulmonary function tests 844
Lung imaging 650
lung, removal of:
    in Heart-lung transplant 521,
        522
    medical terms: Lobectomy,
        lung 646; Pneumonectomy
        811
lung transplant:
    and Heart-lung transplant 521,
        522
    in treatment of Cystic fibrosis
        328
Lung tumours 650
    type of: Lung cancer 649
Lupus erythematosus 650
    causing Keratoconjunctivitis
        sicca 611; Raynaud's
        phenomenon 861
    feature of: Photosensitivity 801
    treatment of: Plasmapheresis
        809
    type of Autoimmune disorder
        145
Lupus pernio 651
Lupus vulgaris 651
Lurselle 1113
Lustral 1113
Luteinizing hormone (LH) 651
    effect on Ovulation 769
    and Oral contraceptives 756
    production of: Pituitary gland
        805
    type of Gonadotrophin
        hormone 489
Luteinizing hormone-releasing
    hormone (LH-RH) 651
Lyclear 1113
Lymecycline 1113
Lyme disease 651
Lymph 652
    and Lymphatic system 653;
        structure and function of the
        lymphatic system 654
Lymphadenitis 652
    causing Glands, swollen 483
Lymphadenopathy 652
    common term: Glands,
        swollen 483
Lymphangiography 652
Lymphangioma 652
Lymphangitis 652
Lymphatic system 653
    disorders of: Burkitt's
        lymphoma 218; Glands,
        swollen 483; Hodgkin's
        disease 539; Lymphangitis
        652; Lymphoedema 653;
        Lymphoma 655;
        Lymphoma, non-Hodgkin's
        655; Mononucleosis,
        infectious 694
    investigation of:
        Lymphangiography 652
    structure and function of the
        lymphatic system 654

lymph gland 653
  medical term: Lymph node
    653
Lymph node 653
  enlargement of: Glands,
    swollen 483; Mononucleosis,
    infectious 694
  and Lymphatic system 653;
    structure and function of the
    lymphatic system 654
  tuberculosis of: Scrofula 893
Lymphocyte 653
  part of Immune system 569;
    the adaptive immune system
    568
  production of: Spleen 938
  type of Blood cell 182
Lymphoedema 653
Lymphogranuloma venereum
    655
  type of Sexually transmitted
    disease 904
lymphokines:
  causing Hypersensitivity 551
  production of: Lymphocyte
    653
Lymphoma 655
  types of: Burkitt's lymphoma
    218; Hodgkin's disease 539;
    Lymphoma, non-Hodgkin's
    655
  treatment of: Methotrexate
    684; Procarbazine 829
Lymphoma, non-Hodgkin's 655
Lymphosarcoma 655
  alternative term: Lymphoma,
    non-Hodgkin's 655
Lypressin 655
Lysis 655
Lysozyme 655
Lysuride 1113

M

Maalox 1113
Maalox Plus 1113
Maclean 1113
Macro- 656
Macrobid 1113
Macrobiotics 656
Macrodantin 1113
Macroglossia 656
macrophage:
  definition of: Macro- 656
  function of: Lymph node 653
macula:
  see index entry macula lutea
macula lutea:
  disorders of: Macular
    degeneration 656; Retinal
    detachment 872; Retinal
    haemorrhage 873
  function of: Colour vision
    292
Macular degeneration 656
  a disorder of the eye 426;
    disorder of the retina 873;
    Vision, disorder of 1059
Macule 656
Madopar 1113

Magaldrate 1113
Magnapen 1113
Magnesium 656
  minerals and main food sources
    690; recommended daily
    allowances (RDAs) of selected
    minerals 690
Magnesium carbonate 1113
Magnesium hydroxide 1113
Magnesium oxide 1113
Magnesium sulphate 1113
Magnesium trisilicate 1113
Magnetic resonance imaging
    (MRI):
  see index entry MRI
magnetic resonance
    spectroscopy:
  use of: MRI 36, 701
major histocompatibility
    complex:
  and Histocompatibility
    antigens 536
Malabsorption 656
  causing Rickets 880; Weight
    loss 1080
  feature of *disorders of the*
    pancreas 776; Whipple's
    disease 1082
Maladjustment 1113
Malaise 657
Malalignment 657
  bone: Fracture 460
  teeth: Malocclusion 659
Malar flush 657
Malaria 657
  cause of: Protozoa 836
  prevention and treatment of:
    Chloroquine 269;
    Primaquine 829; Proguanil
    831; Pyrimethamine 848;
    Quinine 849
  transmission of: *insect-borne*
    diseases 587; the spread of
    malaria 658; Mosquito bites
    696
Malathion 1113
male gender:
  and Chromosomal
    abnormalities 276; Genetic
    disorders 478; Inheritance
    585; Sex determination 903;
    Sex hormones 903
male-pattern baldness:
  treatment of: Hair transplant
    504; Minoxidil 689
  type of Alopecia 87
male sterilization:
  Vasectomy 1046
Malformation 658
  congenital: Birth defects 172
Malignant 658
Malignant melanoma:
  Melanoma, malignant 673
Malingering 659
Malix 1113
Mallet finger 659
Mallet toe:
  alternative term: Claw-toe 282
malleus:
  bone in Ear 383
  example of Ossicle 761
Mallory-Weiss syndrome 659
  causing Vomiting blood 1068

Malnutrition:
  causes of: Infectious disease
    578; Macrobiotics 656
  causing Immunodeficiency
    disorders 571
  effect on Growth, childhood
    494
  see also index entry
    Nutritional disorders
Malocclusion 659
  treatment of: Orthodontic
    appliances 759
Maloprim 1113
Malpighi, Marcello:
  and Microscope 686
Malpresentation 659
Malta fever:
  modern term: Brucellosis 216
Mammary gland:
  see index entry Breast
Mammography 659
  in diagnosis of Breast cancer
    205
  and Screening for cancer 25
Mammoplasty 660
  procedure for mammoplasty 661
Mandible:
  common term: Jaw 606
Manerix 1113
Manevac 1113
Mania 660
  treatment of: Antipsychotic
    drugs 119; Lithium 640
  type of Psychosis 840
Manic-depressive illness 661
  treatment of: Antipsychotic
    drugs 119; Lithium 640
  type of Psychosis 840
Manipulation 661
Mannitol 661
Manometry 661
Mantoux test 662
  type of Tuberculin test 1018
manubrium:
  part of Sternum 946
Manusept 1113
MAOIs:
  see index entry Monoamine
    oxidase inhibitors (MAOIs)
Maprotiline 662
Marasmus 662
  and Kwashiorkor 621
Marble bone disease
  alternative term: Osteopetrosis
    764
Marcaine 1113
March fracture 662
Marevan 1113
Marfan's syndrome 662
  leading to Aneurysm 105;
    Lens dislocation 632
Marijuana 662
  causing Withdrawal syndrome
    1084
  constituent of: THC 983
Marplan 1113
Marriage guidance 663
  and Sex therapy 903
Marrow, bone:
  Bone marrow 194
Marsupialization 663
Marvelon 1113
Masnoderm 1113

Masculinization:
  alternative term: Virilization
    1055
  and Sex determination 903
Masochism 663
  and Sadism 884;
    Sadomasochism 885
Massage 663
  and Physiotherapy 803;
    techniques of physiotherapy 802
Mast cell 663
  function of: Histamine 536;
    Hypersensitivity 551;
    Inflammation 583
Mastectomy 663
  as part of Sex change 902
  in treatment of Klinefelter's
    syndrome 619
  types of mastectomy 664
Mastication 664
Mastitis 665
  resulting from cracked Nipple
    731
Mastocytosis 665
Mastoid bone 665
  inflammation of: Mastoiditis
    665
Mastoiditis 665
Masturbation 665
  and Orgasm, lack of 758; Sex
    therapy 904
Maternal mortality 665
  and Childbirth 261
Maxepa 1113
Maxidex 1113
Maxilla 666
  part of Skull 919
Maxitrol 1113
Maxivent 1113
Maxolon 1113
Maxtrex 1113
McArdle's disease 666
ME:
  Myalgic encephalomyelitis 710
Measles 666
  prevention of: Immunization
    569; Immunization against
    disease 28; *typical childhood*
    immunization schedule 570;
    MMR vaccination 693;
    Vaccine 1040
  symptom of: Koplik's spots
    621
Meatus 667
Mebendazole 667
Mebeverine 1113
Mebhydrolin 1113
Meckel's diverticulum 667
Meconium 667
  indicating Fetal distress 442
  passing by Newborn 730
Mectizan 1113
Medazepam 1113
Medial 667
Median nerve 667
  part of Brachial plexus 197
Mediastinoscopy 668
Mediastinum 668
Medical Defence Societies 668
medical ethics:
  and Confidentiality 295;
    Ethics, medical 416;
    Hippocratic oath 535

medical history:
  in Diagnosis 350
  see also index entry History-taking
Medical research organizations 668
Medication 668
  and Drug 375
Medicine 668
  and Forensic medicine 459
  history of: *landmarks in medicine: diagnosis 669; landmarks in medicine: drugs 671; landmarks in medicine: surgery 670; landmarks in medicine: other forms of treatment 670*
Medicine, private 669
Medicoal 1113
Medicolegal 669
Medihaler-Epi 1113
Medihaler-Ergotamine 1113
Medihaler-Iso 1113
Medised 1113
Meditation 670
  and Relaxation techniques 867
Medrone 1113
Medroxyprogesterone 670
Medulla 670
Medulla oblongata 670
  part of Brainstem 202
Medulloblastoma 671
Mefenamic acid 671
Mefloquine 1113
Mefoxin 1113
Mefruside 1113
Mega- 671
Megace 1113
Megacolon 671
megaloblastic anaemia:
  Anaemia, megaloblastic 98
Megalomania 672
-megaly 672
Megestrol 672
Meibomian cyst:
  alternative term: Chalazion 255
meibomian glands:
  part of Eye 423
Meibomitis 672
Meigs' syndrome 672
Meiosis 672
  and Chromosomes 278
Melaena 673
  causes of: Oesophageal varices 747; Peptic ulcer 789
  and Rectal bleeding 862
Melancholia 673
Melanin 673
  and colour of Hair 503; Pigmentation 803; Skin 916
  deficiency of: Albinism 80; Pallor 774; Vitiligo 1066
  in prevention of Sunburn 959
melanocytes:
  producing Melanin 673
melanocyte-stimulating hormone:
  production of: Pituitary gland 805
Melanoma, juvenile 673
  type of Naevus 716
Melanoma, malignant 673
  as complication of Lentigo 632

diagnosis of: Skin biopsy 917
of eye: *disorders of the eye 426;* Eye tumour 427
type of Naevus 716; Skin cancer 917
Melanosis coli 673
Melasma:
  alternative term: Chloasma 268
Melatonin 673
  and Biorhythms 171
  production of: Pineal gland 804
Melleril 1113
Melphalan 673
Membrane 673
  of Cell 245
membranes, rupture of:
  as complication of Version 1052
  premature: Childbirth, complications of 264
  use of: Induction of labour 577
Memory 674
Memory, loss of:
  medical term: Amnesia 92
Menadiol 1113
Menarche 674
Mendelian inheritance:
  Inheritance 585
Ménière's disease 674
  a *disorder of the ear 384*
  effect on Balance 155; Walking 1073
  treatment of: Promethazine 831
Meninges 674
  anatomy of the meninges 675
  of Brain 198; Spinal cord 934
  protrusion of: Meningocele 675
Meningioma 675
Meningitis 675
  cause of: *HAEMOPHILUS INFLUENZAE* 501
  causing Stiff neck 946
  as complication of Mastoiditis 665; Mumps 704
  travel protection 27
Meningocele 675
  type of Spina bifida 933, *934*
meningococcal bacteria:
  causing Meningitis 675; Waterhouse-Friderichsen syndrome 1077
Meningomyelocele:
  alternative term: Myelocele 712
  type of Spina bifida 933, *934*
Meniscectomy 675
Meniscus 676
  part of Knee 619
Menopause 676
  and Osteoporosis 764, *765;* Varicose veins 1044
Menophase 1113
Menorrhagia 676
  symptom of Endometriosis 402
  treatment of: Endometrial ablation 402
Menotrophin 677
  type of Gonadotrophin hormone 490
Menstrual extraction 677

menstrual pain:
  medical term: Dysmenorrhoea 381
menstrual periods:
  see index entry Menstruation
menstrual regulation:
  alternative term: Menstrual extraction 677
Menstruation 677
  cessation of: Amenorrhoea 91; Menopause 676; Virilism 1055
  and Sanitary protection 887
  start of: Menarche 674
  see also index entries Menstruation, disorders of; Menstruation, irregular
Menstruation, disorders of 677
  cause of: Ovary, polycystic 768
  examples: Amenorrhoea 91; Dysmenorrhoea 381; Menorrhagia 676; Menstruation, irregular 679
Menstruation, irregular 679
  symptom chart 678
mental age:
  and Intelligence tests 591
mental disorder:
  and Consent 297; Mental Health Act 680; Mental handicap 679; Mental illness 680; Psychiatric treatment 45
Mental handicap 679
  causes of: Cerebral palsy 248; Chromosomal abnormalities 275; Down's syndrome 370; Fragile X syndrome 462; Klinefelter's syndrome 619; Rubella 883; Spina bifida 933; Sturge-Weber syndrome 955; Toxoplasmosis 1006; Tuberous sclerosis 1020; Turner's syndrome 1021
Mental Health Act 680
Mental hospital 680
Mental illness 680
  and Psychiatric treatment 45
Mental retardation:
  see index entry Mental handicap
Menthol 681
Menzol 1113
Mepacrine 1113
Mepenzolate 1113
Mepranix 1113
Meprobamate 680
  causing Withdrawal syndrome 1084
Meptazinol 681
Meptid 1113
Mequitazine 1113
Merbentyl 1113
Mercaptopurine 681
Mercilon 1113
Mercury 681
Mercury poisoning 681
  causing Minamata disease 689
Merzbacher-Pelizaeus disease:
  type of Leukodystrophy 635
Mesalazine 681

Mescaline 681
  source of: Peyote 797
Mesenteric lymphadenitis 681
Mesentery 681
mesmerism:
  modern term: Hypnosis 555
Mesna 1113
mesomorphic body type:
  a Somatotype 930
Mesothelioma 681
Mesothelium 682
messenger RNA:
  see index entry RNA
Mesterolone 1113
Mestinon 1114
Mestranol 682
Metabolic disorders 682
Metabolism 682
Metabolism, inborn errors of 682
Metabolite 683
Metacarpal bone 683
  part of *the skeletal structure of the hand and wrist 505;* Skeleton 914
Metalpha 1114
metal poisoning:
  treatment of: Chelating agents 256
Metamucil 1114
Metaplasia 683
Metaraminol 1114
Metastasis 683
  and Cancer 227; Carcinomatosis 234; Secondary 896; Tumour 1020
Metatarsal bone 683
  part of Foot 458; Skeleton 915
Metatarsalgia 683
Metatarsophalangeal joint 683
Meted 1114
Metenix 5 1114
Meterfolic 1114
Metformin 683
Methadone 683
  in treatment of Withdrawal syndrome 1086
Methane 683
Methanol 683
Methenamine 1114
Methionine 1114
Methixene 1114
Methocarbamol 684
Methohexitone 1114
Methotrexate 684
Methotrimeprazine 1114
Methoxamine 1114
Methoxsalen 1114
Methyclothiazide 684
Methyl alcohol:
  alternative term: Methanol 683
Methylcellulose 684
Methylcysteine 1114
Methyldopa 684
Methylphenobarbitone 1114
Methylprednisolone 684
  in treatment of Spinal injury 936
Methyl salicylate 1114
Methysergide 684
Metipranolol 1114
Metirosine 1114
Metoclopramide 684
Metolazone 684

Metopirone 1114
Metoprolol 684
Metosyn 1114
Metramid 1114
Metriphonate 1114
Metrodin 1114
Metrogel 1114
Metrolyl 1114
Metronidazole 684
Metrotop 1114
Metyrapone 1114
Mexiletine 685
Mexitil 1114
Miacalcic 1114
Mianserin 685
Micolette Micro-Enema 1114
Miconazole 685
Micralax Micro-Enema 1114
Micro- 685
Microangiopathy 685
Microbe 685
    alternative term:
        Microorganism 685
Microbiology 685
Microcephaly 685
Microgynon 30 1114
Micronor 1114
Microorganism 685
    study of: Microbiology 685
microphthalmos:
    a *disorder of the eye* 426
Microscope 685
    development of: *landmarks in*
        medicine: diagnosis 669
    types of microscopes 686
    use of: *microsurgical operation*
        46; Microsurgery 47, 687
Microsurgery 47, 687
    microsurgical operation 46
    techniques of microsurgery 688
    in treatment of Nerve injury
        723
    uses of: Plastic surgery 809;
        Skin flap 917
Microval 1114
microwave ovens:
    and Radiation 852
Mictral 1114
Micturition:
    alternative term: passing Urine
        1034
Midamor 1114
Midazolam 1114
Midbrain 687
    part of Brainstem 202
Middle ear:
    part of Ear 383
Middle-ear effusion, persistent:
    alternative term: Glue ear 487
    and Otitis media 766
Middle-ear infection:
    alternative term: Otitis media
        766
Mid-life crisis 687
Midrid 1114
Midwifery 687
Mifegyne 1114
Mifepristone 1114
Migrafen 1114
Migraine 687
    and Oral contraceptives 756
    treatment of: Ergotamine 414;
        Methysergide 684;

Propranolol 831;
    Sumatriptan 959
    type of Headache 507
Migraleve 1114
Migravess 1114
Migril 1114
Milia 689
    in Newborn 730
Mildison 1114
Milk 689
    abnormal production of:
        Galactorrhoea 466
    and Bottle-feeding 196; Breast-
        feeding 206; Expressing milk
        421
    secretion of: Breast 204
Milk-alkali syndrome 689
Milk of magnesia 689
Milk teeth:
    alternative term: Primary teeth
        829
millipedes:
    causing Venomous bites and
        stings 1050
Milpar 1114
Milrinone 1114
Milstein, César:
    landmarks in medicine: diagnosis
        669
Minamata disease 689
    cause of: Mercury poisoning
        681
mind:
    alternative term: Psyche 838
Mineralization, dental 689
Mineralocorticoid 689
Minerals 19, 689
    minerals and main food sources
        690
    and Nutrition 738; Trace
        elements 1006
    recommended daily allowances of
        selected minerals 690
Mineral supplements 689
Minihep 1114
Mini-I-Jet Adrenaline 1114
Mini-I-Jet Atropine Sulphate
    1114
Mini-I-Jet Bretylium Tosylate
    1114
Mini-I-Jet Calcium Chloride 1114
Mini-I-Jet Frusemide 1114
Mini-I-Jet Isoprenaline 1114
Mini-I-Jet Morphine Sulphate
    1114
Minilaparotomy:
    method of Sterilization, female
        945
Minimal brain dysfunction 689
Minimally invasive surgery 48
    and Day surgery 332;
        Endoscopy 403;
        Laparoscopy 403
    development of: *landmarks in*
        medicine: surgery 670
    use of: Appendicectomy 162;
        Hernia repair 531
    in treatment of Ectopic
        pregnancy 389; Gallstones
        468
Minims Amethocaine 1114
Minims Artificial Tears 1114
Minims Atropine 1114

Minims Benoxinate 1114
Minims Chloramphenicol 1114
Minims Cyclopentolate 1114
Minims Gentamicin 1114
Minims Homatropine
    Hydrobromide 1114
Minims Metipranolol 1114
Minims Neomycin Sulphate 1114
Minims Phenylephrine
    Hydrochloride 1114
Minims Pilocarpine 1114
Minims Prednisolone 1114
Minims Tropicamide 1115
minipill:
    type of Oral contraceptive
        755
Minitran 1115
Minnesota Multiphasic
    Personality Inventory:
    type of Personality test 795
Minocin 1115
Minocycline 689
Minodiab 1115
Mintec 1115
Mintezol 1115
Minulet 1115
Miosis 690
Miradol 1115
Miraxid 1115
Miscarriage 690
    increased risk of: *alcohol and*
        pregnancy 82; Amniocentesis
        39
Misoprostol 691
Mites and disease 691
Mithracin 1115
Mithramycin 1115
Mitobronitol 1115
Mitomycin 1115
Mitomycin C Kyowa 1115
Mitosis 691
    and Chromosomes 278
    mechanism of mitosis 692
Mitoxana 1115
Mitozantrone 1115
Mitral incompetence 691
    disorder of Heart valves 523
mitral regurgitation:
    alternative term: Mitral
        incompetence 691
Mitral stenosis 692
    associated with Malar flush 657
    disorder of Heart valves 523
mitral valve:
    disorders of: Mitral
        incompetence 691; Mitral
        stenosis 692; Mitral valve
        prolapse 693
    part of Heart 514, *515*
Mitral valve prolapse 693
mitral valvotomy:
    type of Heart-valve surgery
        524
Mittelschmerz 693
Mivacron 1115
Mivacurium 1115
Mixtard 30/70 1115
MMR vaccination 693
Mobiflex 1115
Mobilan 1115
Mobilization 693
Moclobemide 1115

Modalim 1115
Modecate 1115
modelling:
    type of Behaviour therapy 162
Moditen 1115
Modrasone 1115
Modrenal 1115
Moducren 1115
Moduret-25 1115
Moduretic 1115
Mogadon 1115
moisturizer:
    type of Emollient 397
Molar:
    structure and arrangement of
        teeth 972
    third molar: Wisdom tooth
        1084
Molar pregnancy 693
Mole 693
    cancerous: Melanoma,
        malignant 673
    type of Naevus 716
Molecule 693
Molipaxin 1115
Molluscum contagiosum 693
Mometasone 1115
Monaspor 1115
Mongolian blue spot 694
    type of Naevus 716
Mongolism 694
    modern term: Down's
        syndrome 370
Moniliasis:
    alternative term: Candidiasis
        230
Monit 1115
Monitor 694
    use of: Coronary care unit 311;
        Intensive care 591
Monoamine oxidase inhibitors
    (MAOIs) 694
    group of Antidepressant drugs
        116
Monoarthritis 694
Mono-Cedocard 1115
monochromatism:
    type of Colour vision
        deficiency 292
Monoclonal antibody:
    Antibody, monoclonal 115
Monocor 1115
monocytes:
    types of Blood cell 182;
        Phagocyte 798
Mononucleosis, infectious 694
Monoparin 1115
Monoparin Calcium 1115
Monorchism 694
monosaccharide:
    type of Carbohydrate 232
Monosodium glutamate 694
Monosulfiram 1115
Monotard, Human 1115
Monotrim 1115
Monovent 1115
Monphytol 1115
mons pubis:
    location of the labia 622
Monteggia's fracture 694
mood:
    abnormalities of: Affective
        disorders 72; Cyclothymia

326; Delirium 337;
Depression 343; Mania 660;
Manic-depressive illness
661; Postnatal depression
819; Premenstrual syndrome
826; Seasonal affective
disorder syndrome 895
and Euphoria 417
medical term: Affect 72
Moon face 695
feature of Cushing's syndrome
325
Moorland 1115
Morbid anatomy 695
Morbidity 695
Morbilli:
alternative term: Measles 666
Morning-after pill:
method of Contraception,
postcoital 304
Morning sickness:
Vomiting in pregnancy 1068
Moron 695
modern term: Mental
handicap 679
Moro reflex:
example of Reflex, primitive
865, 866
Morphine 695
derivative of: Diamorphine 353
landmarks in medicine: drugs 671
Morphoea 695
Morquio's syndrome:
type of Mucopoly-
saccharidosis 701
Mortality 695
see also index entries Death;
death rates
morula:
in the process of fertilization 441
Mosaicism 696
causing Turner's syndrome
1020
Mosquito bites 696
causing Malaria 657
Insects and disease 587
Motens 1115
motilin:
a Gastrointestinal hormone
471
Motilium 1115
Motion sickness 696
treatment of: Promethazine 831
Motipress 1115
Motival 1115
Motor 696
motor cortex:
function of: Cerebrum 250
and Movement 699
motor fibres:
of Nerve 722; Spinal cord 934;
Spinal nerves 936
Motor neuron disease 696
Motrin 1115
Mould 697
causing Alveolitis 89; Rhinitis,
allergic 878
and Diet and disease 357
group of Fungi 464
Mountain sickness 697
Mouret, Dr P:
Landmarks in medicine:
surgery 670

Mouth 697
anatomy of the mouth 698
and Oral hygiene 756
parts of: Gum 497; Lip 638;
Palate 774; Salivary glands
886; Teeth 971; Tongue 1000
Mouth cancer 698
and alcohol-related disorders 84;
Tobacco-smoking 997
Mouth, dry 698
Mouth-to-mouth resuscitation:
Artificial respiration 134
Mouth ulcer 698
Mouthwash 698
Movelat 1115
Movement 699
abnormal: Dyskinesia 381
causing Motion sickness 696
Moxalactam 1107
Moxibustion 700
MRI 36, 700
development of: landmarks in
medicine: diagnosis 669
type of Imaging technique 564;
Scanning technique 888
MS 701
abbreviation for Multiple
sclerosis 702
MSG 701
abbreviation for Monosodium
glutamate 694
MST Continus 1115
Mucaine 1115
Mucocele 701
Mucodyne 1115
Mucogel 1115
Mucolytic drugs 701
use of: Cough remedies 314
Mucopolysaccharidosis 701
Mucosa
alternative term: Mucous
membrane 701
Mucous membrane 701
mucoviscidosis:
alternative term: Cystic
fibrosis 327
Mu-Cron 1115
Mucus 701
in Mucocele 701
secretion of: Mucous
membrane 701; Stomach
948; Trachea 1007
Mucus method of contraception:
Contraception, natural
methods of 304
methods of contraception 303
Multiparin 1115
Multiple myeloma 701
Multiple personality 702
and Split personality 939
Multiple pregnancy:
Pregnancy, multiple 824
Multiple sclerosis 702
causing Optic neuritis 754;
Paralysis 778; Squint 943
features of: Demyelination
339; features of multiple
sclerosis 703
Multivitamins 702
Mumps 702
appearance of mumps 704
complications of: Orchitis 757;
Pancreatitis 776

effect on Parotid glands 783;
Salivary glands 886
prevention of: Immunization
569; typical childhood
immunization schedule 570;
MMR vaccination 693
Munchausen's syndrome 704
Mupirocin 1115
Murmur 704
Murray, Joseph:
landmarks in medicine: surgery
670
Muscle 704
and Aerobics 71
the body's muscles 705
disorders of: disorders of muscle
707; Muscle spasm 707;
Muscular dystrophy 707;
Myalgia 710; Myasthenia
gravis 710; Myopathy 714;
Myositis 715; Myotonia 715;
Rhabdomyolysis 875; Strain
949
muscle movement 706
muscle types 706
removal of: Myectomy 711
tone of: Tone, muscle 1000
type of Tissue 995
muscle enzymes:
abnormal levels of: Muscular
dystrophy 708; Myocardial
infarction 714
types of Enzyme 408
Muscle-relaxant drugs 707
Muscle spasm 707
causing Torticollis 1003
feature of Tetany 981; Multiple
sclerosis 702; Myoclonus 714
muscle tumour:
disorders of muscle 707
types of: Fibroid 447;
Leiomyoma 631; Myoma
714; Rhabdomyosarcoma
875
muscle wasting:
and Atrophy 143
feature of Motor neuron
disease 696; Neuropathy
728; Peroneal muscular
atrophy 794
of Quadriceps muscle 849
Muscular dystrophy 707
causing Paralysis 778
inheritance of: Duchenne
muscular dystrophy 708;
Genetic disorders 477;
Sex-linked inheritance 903
a disorder of muscle 707
types of muscular dystrophy 709
Musculoskeletal 708
Mushroom poisoning 708
type of Food poisoning 456
Mustine 1115
Mutagen 708
Mutation 709
cause of: Mutagen 708
of Gene 473; Oncogenes 751
Mutism 710
Myalgia 710
Myalgic encephalomyelitis 710
Myambutol 1115
Myasthenia gravis 710
causing Paralysis 778

a disorder of muscle 707
treatment of: Neostigmine 721;
Plasmapheresis 809
Mycardol 1115
Mycetoma 711
Mycifradin 1115
Mycology:
study of Fungal infections 464;
Fungi 464
Mycoplasma 711
causing Pneumonia 811, 812
Mycosis 711
alternative term: Fungal
infections 464
and Fungi 465
Mycosis fungoides 711
Mycota 1115
Mydriacyl 1115
Mydriasis 711
Mydrilate 1115
Myectomy 711
Myel- 711
Myelin 711
breakdown of: Demyelination
339; causing Multiple
sclerosis 702
Myelitis 711
Myelobromol 1115
Myelocele 712
type of Spina bifida 933, 934
myelofibrosis:
alternative term:
Myelosclerosis 712
myelography 712
Myeloma, multiple:
Multiple myeloma 701
Myelomatosis:
alternative term: Multiple
myeloma 701
Myelomeningocele:
Myelocele 712
Myelopathy 712
Myelosclerosis 712
Myiasis 712
Myleran 1115
Mynah 1115
Myo- 712
Myocardial infarction 712
causing Shock 907
and Coronary artery disease
310
a disorder of the heart 517
features of myocardial infarction
713
Myocarditis 714
a disorder of the heart 517
myocardium:
muscle of Heart 513
Myoclonus 714
type of Spasm 929
Myocrisin 1115
Myofacial pain disorder:
alternative term:
Temporomandibular joint
syndrome 974
Myoglobin 714
constituent of: Iron 602
myoglobinuria:
feature of McArdle's disease
666
and Myoglobin 714
Myoma 714
a disorder of muscle 707

Myomectomy 714
  in treatment of Fibroid 447
Myopathy 714
Myopia 714
  associated with Retinal
    detachment 872; Retinal tear
    873
  the cause of myopia 715
  treatment of: Contact lenses
    300; Laser treatment 627;
    why glasses are used 484
myosarcoma:
  a *disorder of muscle 707*
myosin:
  constituent of Muscle 704
Myositis 715
  causing Shin splints 907
  types of: Dermatomyositis 345;
    Polymyositis 816
myositis ossificans:
  a disorder of muscle 707
  type of Myositis 715
Myotomy 715
Myotonia 715
Myotonine chloride 1115
Myringitis 715
Myringoplasty 715
Myringotomy 715
Mysoline 1115
Mysteclin 1115
Myxoedema 715
  causing Dementia 338
  feature of Hypothyroidism 560
  a disorder of the thyroid gland 992
Myxoma 715
  a disorder of the heart 517

N

Nabilone 1115
Nabumetone 1115
Nacton 1115
Nadolol 716
Naevus 716
  and Pigmentation 803
  a *disorder of the skin 919*
Nafarelin 1115
Naftidrofuryl 1115
Nail 716
  constituent of: Keratin 610
  disorders of: *fungal diseases*
    465; Koilonychia 621;
    Onychogryphosis 752;
    Onycholysis 752; Toenail,
    ingrowing 999
Nail-biting 716
  causing Hangnail 506
Nalbuphine 1115
Nalcrom 1115
Nalidixic acid 716
Nalorex 1115
Naloxone 717
Naltrexone 1115
Nandrolone 717
Naphazoline 1115
Nappy rash 717
  treatment of: Zinc oxide 1093
Napratec 1115
Naprosyn 1115
Naproxen 717

Narcan 1115
Narcissism 717
  type of Personality disorder
    795
Narcolepsy 717
  a disorder of Sleep 922
  symptom of: Sleep paralysis
    923
Narcosis 717
Narcotic drugs 717
  abuse of: Drug abuse 377;
    Drug dependence 377;
    Heroin abuse 531;
    Withdrawal syndrome 1084
  examples: Codeine 285;
    Diamorphine 353;
    Methadone 683; Morphine
    695; Opium 754;
    Pentazocine 789
  group of Analgesic drugs 102
  overdose, effects of: Drug
    poisoning 378; Respiratory
    arrest 869; Respiratory
    distress syndrome 870
  overdose, treatment of:
    Naloxone 717; Ventilation
    1050
  use of: Pain relief 774
Nardil 1115
Narphen 1115
Nasal congestion 717
  associated with Nasal
    discharge 718
  feature of Cold, common 286;
    Rhinitis 878; Rhinitis,
    allergic 878
Nasal discharge 718
  associated with Nasal
    congestion 718
  causes of: Cold, common 286;
    Influenza 584;
    Nasopharynx, cancer of 719;
    Rhinitis 878; Rhinitis,
    allergic 878
Nasal obstruction 718
Nasal septum 718
  deviated: Nasal obstruction
    718; Submucous resection
    956
  part of Nose 734
  perforated: a *disorder of the nose*
    735; Wegener's
    granulomatosis 1077
Naseptin 1115
Nasogastric tube 718
nasolacrimal ducts:
  part of Lacrimal apparatus 622
Nasopharynx 718
  part of Pharynx 798
Nasopharynx, cancer of 718
National Health Service 719
  and Family Health Service
    Authorities 434
Natrilix 1116
Natulan 1116
Natural childbirth:
  Childbirth, natural 264
Natural drugs 42
  sources of drugs 43
  see also index entry Drug
Naturopathy 719
Nausea 719
  and Vomiting 1067

Navel 719
  medical term: Umbilicus 1027
Navidrex 1116
Navispare 1116
Navoban 1116
Nebcin 1116
Nebulizer 719
  use of: Asthma 139;
    Bronchodilator drugs 215;
    using a nebulizer 720
Neck 720
  stiffness of: Neck rigidity 720;
    Stiff neck 946; Subarachnoid
    haemorrhage 955
  support of: Collar, orthopaedic
    288
Neck dissection, radical 720
Neck rigidity 720
Necrolysis, toxic epidermal 720
Necrophilia 721
Necropsy 721
  alternative term: Autopsy 146
Necrosis 721
necrotizing ulcerative gingivitis:
  alternative terms: Gingivitis,
    acute ulcerative 482;
    Vincent's disease 1054
  complication of Gingivitis 482
Nedocromil 1116
needle sharing:
  and spread of AIDS 77;
    Hepatitis, viral 529; HIV 537
Nefopam 721
negative feedback:
  in *endocrine system 401*
  and Homeostasis 540
Negram 1116
Nelson's syndrome 721
Nematodes 721
  common term: Roundworms
    882
Neocon 1/35 1116
Neo-Cortef 1116
Neo-Cytamen 1116
Neogest 1116
Neologism 721
Neo-Medrone 1116
Neo-Mercazole 1116
Neomycin 721
Neo-NaClex 1116
Neo-NaClex K 1116
Neonatal care 44
  using Incubator 576
Neonate 721
  see also index entry Newborn
Neonatology 721
Neoplasia 721
  formation of Tumour 1020
Neoplasm 721
  alternative term: Tumour 1020
Neosporin 1116
Neostigmine 721
Neotigason 1116
Nepenthe 1116
Nephrectomy 721
  in treatment of Kidney cancer
    613
Nephril 1116
Nephritis 721
Nephroblastoma:
  type of Kidney cancer 613
Nephrocalcinosis 721
Nephrolithotomy 722

Nephrology 722
Nephron 722
  part of Kidney 612
Nephropathy 722
  disorders of the kidney 614
Nephrosclerosis 722
Nephrosis:
  Nephrotic syndrome 722
Nephrostomy 722
Nephrotic syndrome 722
  a disorder of the kidney 614
  treatment of:
    Hydrochlorothiazide 546
Nericur 1116
Nerisone 1116
Nerve 722
  disorders of: Nerve injury 723;
    Neuralgia 725; Neuritis 725;
    Neuroma 726; Neuropathy
    728; Neurotoxin 729
  surgical destruction of:
    Sympathectomy 964
  types of: Cranial nerves 318;
    Spinal nerves 936
  see also index entries Nervous
    system; Neuron
Nerve block 722
  type of Anaesthesia, local 01
Nerve injury 723
Nerve, trapped 723
  example: Carpal tunnel
    syndrome 238
Nervous breakdown 723
Nervous energy 723
nervous exhaustion:
  alternative term: Neurasthenia
    725
Nervous habit 723
Nervous system 723, *724*
  anatomy of: Autonomic
    nervous system 146, *147;*
    Brain 198; Central nervous
    system 246; Cranial nerves
    318; Peripheral nervous
    system 793; Plexus 810;
    Spinal cord 934; *location of*
    the spinal cord 935; Spinal
    nerves 936
  functions of: Hearing 512, *513;*
    Memory 674; Movement
    699; Pain 772, *773;* Reflex
    864; Sensation 898; Smell
    925; Speech 930; Taste 970;
    Thought 985; Touch 1003;
    the sense of touch 1004; Vision
    1057; *the sense of vision 1058*
  and interaction with
    hormones:
    Neuroendocrinology 726
  see also index entries Nerve;
    Neuron
Nethalide:
  development of: *landmarks in*
    medicine: drugs 671
Netillin 1116
Netilmicin 725
Nettle rash:
  medical term: Urticaria 1035
Neulactil 1116
Neupogen 1116
Neuralgia 725
  treatment of: Carbamazepine
    231

neural tube:
  in Embryo 395
Neural tube defect 725
  prevention of: Folic acid 454
  types of: Anencephaly 105;
    Spina bifida 933
Neurapraxia 725
Neurasthenia 725
Neuritis 725
Neuroblastoma 726
Neurocutaneous disorders 726
Neurodermatitis 726
Neuroendocrinology 726
Neurofibromatosis 726
  type of Neurocutaneous
    disorder 726
neurological sensory testing 899
Neurology 726
Neuroma 726
Neuron 726
  anatomy of: Myelin 711;
    structure of a neuron 727
  transmission of impulses:
    Calcium 224;
    Neurotransmitter 729;
    Potassium 820; Sodium 927;
    Synapse 965
  see also index entries Nerve;
    Nervous system
Neurontin 1116
Neuropathic joint 727
Neuropathology 728
Neuropathy 728
  causing Foot-drop 458;
    Paralysis 778; Pins-and-
    needles 804
neuropeptides:
  examples: Endorphins 403;
    Enkephalins 406
  type of Neurotransmitter
    729
Neuropsychiatry 728
Neurosis 728
  assessment of: Personality
    tests 795
  and Suicide 958
  type of Mental illness 680
Neurosurgery 728
Neurosyphilis 729
  complication of Syphilis 966
neurotensin:
  type of Gastrointestinal
    hormone 471
Neurotoxin 729
Neurotransmitter 729
  examples: Acetylcholine 61;
    Endorphins 403;
    Enkephalins 406; GABA 466;
    Noradrenaline 734;
    Serotonin 901
  and Neuron 726; Synapse 965
neutrons:
  type of Radiation 851
Newborn 729
  assessment of: Apgar score
    124; Common screening
    tests 24; Reflex, primitive
    865; *types of primitive reflex
    866*
  blood test: Guthrie test 497;
    heel-prick blood test 25
  care of: Incubator 576;
    Neonatal care 44

disorders of: Birth defects 172;
    Birth injury 173; Haemolytic
    disease of the newborn 500;
    Jaundice, neonatal 606
  faeces of: Meconium 667
Niacin:
  deficiency of: Pellagra 785
  part of the Vitamin B complex
    1064
Nicabate 1116
Nicardipine hydrochloride 1116
Nickel 730
Niclosamide 730
Nicofuranose 1116
Nicorette 1116
Nicorette Plus 1116
Nicotinamide:
  part of Vitamin B complex 1064
Nicotine 730
  and Effects of tobacco 22;
    Tobacco-smoking 997;
    Withdrawal syndrome 1084
Nicotinell TTS 1116
Nicotinic acid 730
  part of Vitamin B complex
    1064
Nicoumalone 1116
Nifedipine 730
Nifensar XL 1116
Niferex 1116
Night blindness 731
  cause of: deficiency of Vitamin
    A 1062
  a disorder of the eye 426
  feature of Retinitis pigmentosa
    874
Nightmare 731
Night Nurse 1116
Night terror 731
  causing Sleepwalking 923
Nikethamide 1116
Nimodipine 1116
Nimotop 1116
Nipent 1116
Nipple 731
  and Breast-feeding 206
  discharge from: Colostrum
    291; Galactorrhoea 466
  disorders of: Jogger's nipple
    609; Paget's disease of the
    nipple 772
  part of Breast 204
Nipride 1116
Nitoman 1116
Nitrate drugs 731
  example: Glyceryl trinitrate 488
  group of Vasodilator drugs
    1047
Nitrazepam 731
Nitrites 731
Nitrocine 1116
Nitrocontin Continus 1116
Nitrofurantoin 732
  causing Hepatitis, chronic
    active 529
Nitrogen 732
  in Scuba-diving medicine 894
Nitrolingual 1116
Nitronal 1116
Nitroprusside 1116
Nitrous oxide 732
  common term: Laughing gas
    628

Nits 732
  eggs of Lice 635
Nivaquine 1116
Nivemycin 1116
Nizatidine 1116
Nizoral 1116
Nobrium 1116
Nocardiosis 732
nociceptors:
  receptors for Pain 772
Noctec 1116
Nocturia 732
  causes of: Cystitis 328; Heart
    failure 519; Prostate,
    enlarged 832
Nocturnal emission 732
Node 732
  type of: Lymph node 653
NODS Tropicamide 1116
Nodule 732
Noise 732
  causing Deafness 332
  comparative noise levels 733
  and Presbyacusis 827
Noltam 1116
Nolvadex 1116
Noma 733
Nonaccidental injury:
  common term: Child abuse
    260
non-A, non-B hepatitis:
  type of Hepatitis, viral 529
non-Hodgkin's lymphoma:
  Lymphoma, non-Hodgkin's
    655
Noninvasive 733
Nonoxinol 9, 10, 11 1116
nonrapid eye movement
    (NREM) sleep:
  see index entry NREM sleep
Nonspecific urethritis 733
  treatment of: Oxytetracycline
    770
  type of Chlamydial infection
    268; Sexually transmitted
    disease 906; Urethritis 1030
  and Urinary tract infection
    1032
Nonsteroidal anti-inflammatory
    drugs 734
  examples: Diflunisal 357;
    Ibuprofen 562;
    Indomethacin 576;
    Ketoprofen 612; Mefenamic
    acid 671; Naproxen 717;
    Piroxicam 804; Tolmetin
    1000
  in treatment of Inflammation
    584; Rheumatoid arthritis
    877
Nootropil 1116
Noradrenaline 734
  type of Neurotransmitter 729
  see also index entry
    Adrenaline
Norcuron 1116
Norditropin 1116
Nordox 1116
Norethisterone 734
Norflex 1116
Norfloxacin 1116
Norgalax Micro-enema 1116
Norgestimate 1116

Norgeston 1116
Norgestrel 1116
Noriday 1116
Norimin 1116
Norinyl-1 1116
Noristerat 1116
Normacol 1116
Normacol Antispasmodic 1116
Normax 1116
Noroxin 1116
Nortriptyline 734
Norval 1116
Nose 734
  damage to lining of: Cocaine
    284
  disorders of: Nasal congestion
    717; Nasal discharge 718;
    Nasal obstruction 718;
    Nosebleed 735; Nose,
    broken 736; *disorders of the
    nose 735*; Rhinitis 878;
    Rhinophyma 879
  function of: Smell 925
  and Nasopharynx 718
  part of: Nasal septum 718
  reshaping of: Rhinoplasty
    879
Nosebleed 735
  feature of Yellow fever 1092
Nose, broken 736
Nose reshaping:
  medical term: Rhinoplasty
    879
Notifiable diseases 736
  *cases of notifiable infectious
    diseases in England and
    Wales 737*
notochord:
  part of Embryo 395
Novantrone 1116
Novaprin 1116
Novasil Plus 1116
Nozinan 1116
NREM (nonrapid eye
    movement) sleep:
  and Sleepwalking 923
  type of Sleep 921
NSAID:
  see index entry Nonsteroidal
    anti-inflammatory drugs
NSU:
  abbreviation for Nonspecific
    urethritis 733
Nubain 1116
Nuclear energy 736
  and Radiation 851
Nuclear magnetic resonance:
  alternative term: MRI 36, 700
Nuclear medicine 736
Nucleic acids 737
  breakdown of: Uric acid
    1030
  as constituents of
    Chromosomes 277; Genes
    472, *474*
  function of: Protein synthesis
    835
  and Genetic code 475
  manufacture of: Vitamin B
    complex 1063
  in Nucleus 738; Viruses 1055,
    1056
  types of: DNA 366; RNA 881

Nucleus 738
  atomic: Nuclear energy 736;
    Radiation 851
  cellular: Cell 245
  cellular constituents of:
    Chromosomes 277; Nucleic
    acids 737
Nuelin 1116
Nu-K 1117
Nulacin 1117
Numark Cold Relief 1117
Numark Cold Relief with
  Decongestant 1117
Numbness 738
  associated with Pins-and
    needles 804
  symptom chart 739
  symptom of Carpal tunnel
    syndrome 238; Cervical
    osteoarthritis 251; Multiple
    sclerosis 702; Raynaud's
    disease 860; Stroke 952;
    Transient ischaemic attack
    1009
  type of Sensation, abnormal
    899
Nurofen 1117
Nursing:
  Breast-feeding 206
  Nursing care 738
Nursing care 738
Nursing home 738
Nu-Seals Aspirin 1117
Nutraplus 1117
Nutrient 738
  sources of: minerals and main
    food sources 690; food sources
    of essential nutrients 741;
    vitamins and main food sources
    1063
  types of: Carbohydrates 19,
    232; Fats and oils 18, 436;
    Fibre, dietary 19, 446;
    Minerals 19, 689; essential
    nutrients 740; Proteins 18,
    834; Trace elements 1006;
    Vitamin 19, 1061; Water 19,
    1075
  see also index entries
    Nutrition; Nutritional
    disorders
Nutrition 738
  and Calorie 226; Dietetics 357;
    Energy requirements 405;
    Food additives 455
  Eating well 18–19
  Keeping healthy 16–17
  of infants: Feeding, infant 437
  recommended daily allowances
    (RDAs) of selected minerals
    690
  recommended daily allowances of
    selected vitamins 1062
  see also index entries
    Nutrient; Nutritional
    disorders
Nutritional disorders 740
  and Anorexia nervosa 111;
    Diet and disease 356; Food
    additives 455; Food allergy
    455; Food-borne infection
    455; Food fad 456; Food
    intolerance 456; Food

poisoning 456;
    Malabsorption 656
  examples: Alcohol-related
    disorders 84; Amblyopia 91;
    Anaemia 95; Beriberi 164;
    Caries, dental 236;
    Keratomalacia 611;
    Kwashiorkor 621; Marasmus
    662; Night blindness 731;
    Obesity 742; Osteomalacia
    763; Pellagra 785; Rickets
    886; Scurvy 895; deficiency
    or excess of Vitamin A 1062;
    deficiency of Vitamin B$_{12}$
    1063; deficiency or excess of
    Vitamin B complex 1063;
    deficiency or excess of
    Vitamin C 1065; deficiency
    or excess of Vitamin D 1065;
    deficiency or excess of
    Vitamin E 1065; deficiency
    of Vitamin K 1065;
    Wernicke-Korsakoff
    syndrome 1081
  see also index entries
    Nutrient; Nutrition
Nutrizym GR 1117
Nuvellle 1117
Nycopren 1117
Nylax 1117
Nymphomania 740
Nystadermal 1117
Nystaform 1117
Nystaform-HC 1117
Nystagmus 741
  a disorder of the eye 426
  and Vertigo 1053
Nystan 1117
Nystatin 741
Nystatin-Dome 1117
Nytol 1117

O

Oat cell carcinoma:
  alternative term: Small-cell
    carcinoma 924
Obesity 742
  associated with Diabetes
    mellitus 348; Hiatus hernia
    533
  and Diet and disease 356;
    Weight 1078; Weight
    reduction 1080
  feature of Pickwickian
    syndrome 803
Obsessive-compulsive disorder
    742
  and Phobia 801; Superego 960
Obstetrics 743
Obstructive airways disease:
  Lung disease, chronic
    obstructive 650
occipital bone:
  part of Skull 920
occipital lobe:
  part of Cerebrum 249
Occiput 743
Occlusion 743
Occult 743

Occult blood, faecal 743
Occupational disease and injury
    743
  Health hazards 511
  safety at work 744
Occupational medicine 744
Occupational mortality 745
Occupational therapy 745
Octovit 1117
Octreotide 1117
Ocular 745
Oculogyric crisis 745
Oculomotor nerve 745
  functions of cranial nerves 318
Ocusert Pilo 1117
Odrik 1117
Oedema 745
  causes of: Cirrhosis 201; Heart
    failure 519; Kidney failure
    614; Kwashiorkor 621;
    Nephrotic syndrome 722;
    Pre-eclampsia 821
  chronic oedema 746
  treatment of: Diuretic drugs
    364
  type of: Angioedema 107
Oedipus complex 746
  and Psychoanalytic theory
    839
Oesophageal atresia 746
  causing Swallowing difficulty
    963
Oesophageal dilatation 746
Oesophageal diverticulum 746
  location of oesophageal
    diverticulum 747
Oesophageal spasm 747
  causing Swallowing difficulty
    963
Oesophageal stricture 747
oesophageal speech:
  following Laryngectomy 625
Oesophageal stricture 747
oesophageal ulcer:
  type of Peptic ulcer 789
Oesophageal varices 747
  as complication of Cirrhosis
    281; Portal hypertension 817
  treatment of: Sclerotherapy
    893; Shunt 910
Oesophagitis 747
  causing Heartburn 518;
    Salivation, excessive 886;
    Swallowing difficulty 963
  resulting from Hiatus hernia
    533
Oesophagogastroscopy:
  Gastroscopy 471
Oesophagoscopy 748
Oesophagus 748
  bleeding in: Melaena 673
  disorders of the oesophagus 749
  narrowing of: Oesophageal
    stricture 747; Swallowing
    difficulty 963
Oesophagus, cancer of 748
  causing Swallowing difficulty
    963; Weight loss 1080
Oestradiol 749
Oestrifen 1117
Oestriol 749
Oestrogen drugs 749
  examples: Mestranol 682;
    Stilboestrol 947

Oestrogen hormones 750
  and Breast cancer 206;
    Tamoxifen 968
  excess: Gynaecomastia 497;
    Uterus, cancer of 1036
  production of: Placenta 806
  in treatment of Osteoporosis
    764; Prostate, cancer of 832
  uses of: Hormone replacement
    therapy 541; Oral
    contraceptives 755
Oestrone 750
Oflaxacin 1117
Oils:
  and Aromatherapy 128
  Fats and oils 436
  type of: Clove oil 283; Cod
    liver oil 285; Eucalyptus oil
    417; Olive oil 751
Ointment 750
Olbetam 1117
Olecranon 750
  part of Elbow 391; Ulna 1024
olfactory bulb:
  part of Olfactory nerve 750
Olfactory nerve 750
  function of: functions of cranial
    nerves 318; the sense of smell
    925
Oligo- 750
Oligodendroglioma 750
Oligohydramnios 750
Oligospermia 750
Oliguria 751
  and Urine, abnormal 1034
Olive oil 751
Olsalazine 1117
-oma 751
Omentum 751
Omeprazole 751
Omnopon-Scopolamine 1117
omphalitis:
  infection of Umbilical cord
    1027
Omphalocele 751
  alternative term: Exomphalos
    419
Onchocerciasis 751
  and disorders of the retina 873
Oncogenes 751
  in Viruses 1057
Oncology 751
Oncovin 1117
Ondansetron 1117
One-alpha 1117
Onychogryphosis 752
Onycholysis 752
onychomycosis:
  type of Tinea 994
Oophorectomy 752
Opas 1117
-opathy 752
Open heart surgery 752
Operable 752
operant conditioning:
  and Learning 629; Reflex 865
  type of Conditioning 295
Operating theatre 752, 753
Operation 753
  see also index entry Surgery
Operidine 1117
Opthaine 1117
Ophthalmia 753

Ophthalmitis 753
Ophthalmology 753
  and Laser surgery 47
Ophthalmoplegia 754
Ophthalmoscope 754
  invention of: *landmarks in medicine: diagnosis 669*
  use of: Eye, examination of 424
Opiate 754
opiate receptors:
  and Endorphins 403
Opilon 1117
Opium 754
  solution of: Laudanum 628
Opportunistic infection 754
  examples: Fungal infections 464; Pneumocystis pneumonia 811
  feature of Immunodeficiency disorders 571
Optic atrophy 754
Optic disc oedema:
  Papilloedema 777
Optician 754
Optic nerve 754
  disorders of: Blindness 179; Optic atrophy 754; Optic neuritis 754; Papilloedema 777; Retrobulbar neuritis 874; Vision, disorders of 1059
  functions of: *functions of the cranial nerves 318; Eye 422; the function of the optic nerve 755; the sense of vision 1058; the visual fields 1061*
Optic neuritis 754
Opticrom 1117
Optimine 1117
Optometry 754
Orabet 1117
Oral 755
Oral-B Fluoride 1117
Oral contraceptives 755
  adverse effects of: Oedema 746; Thrombosis 987
  Contraception, hormonal methods of 304
  development of: *landmarks in medicine: drugs 671*
  methods of contraception 303
  how oral contraceptives work 756
  in treatment of Premenstrual syndrome 826
Oral hygiene 756
oral phase:
  and Fixation 452
  in Psychoanalytic theory 838
Oral surgery 757
Oramorph 1117
Orap 1117
Orbenin 1117
Orbit 757
  part of Skull 919
orbital cellulitis:
  a disorder of the Orbit 757
Orchidectomy 757
  in treatment of Prostate, cancer of 832; Testis, cancer of 978
Orchidopexy 757
  in treatment of Testis, undescended 979

Orchitis 757
  causing Infertility 583; Oligospermia 750
  feature of Mumps 704
Orciprenaline 1117
Orelox 1117
Orf 758
Organ 758
  displacement of: Prolapse 831
  framework of: Stroma 954
  preservation of:
    Cryopreservation 322
  reversed: Situs inversus 914
Organ donation 758
  and Transplant surgery 46, 1010
organelles:
  parts of Cell 245
Organic 758
Organic brain syndrome:
  Brain syndrome, organic 203
"organic" food:
  Health food 511
Organism 758
  cloning of: Clone 282
organ transplants:
  and Organ donation 758; Transplant surgery 46, 1010
Orgasm 758
  facilitation of: Pelvic floor exercises 786; Vibrator 1054
  and Masturbation 665; Sexual intercourse 904, *905*
  see also index entry Orgasm, lack of
Orgasm, lack of 758
  and Psychosexual dysfunction 840
  treatment of: Sensate focus technique 897; Sex therapy 903
  see also index entry Orgasm
Orimeten 1117
Orlept 1117
Ornithosis 759
Orovite 1117
Orovite 7 1117
Orphan drugs 759
Orphenadrine 759
ORT 759
  in treatment of Gastroenteritis 471
Ortho- 759
Ortho-Creme 1117
Ortho-Dienoestrol 1117
Orthodontic appliances 759
  in treatment of Malocclusion 659
Orthodontics 760
Orthoforms 1117
Orthognathic surgery 760
  in treatment of Malocclusion 659; Prognathism 830
  type of Oral surgery 757
Ortho-Gynest 1117
Ortho-Gynol 1117
Ortho-Novin 1/50 1117
Orthopaedics 760
Orthopnoea 760
Orthoptics 760
Orudis 1117
Oruvail 1117
Os 760

Osgood-Schlatter disease 760
Osmolax 1117
Osmosis 760, *761*
osmotic pressure:
  of Blood 181
  and Plasma proteins 809
Ossicle 761
  bones of Ear 383
  surgery on: Stapedectomy 943; Tympanoplasty 1021
Ossification 761
Ossopan 1117
Osteitis 761
osteitis deformans:
  alternative term: Paget's disease 772
osteitis pubis:
  disorder of Pelvis 787
Osteo- 761
Osteoarthritis 761
  feature of: Loose bodies 647
  following Femur, fracture of 439; Lordosis 647; Meniscectomy 675
  treatment of: Ibuprofen 562; Indomethacin 576; Ketoprofen 612; Piroxicam 804; *treatment and self-help measures in osteoarthritis 762*
  type of Arthritis 131
osteoblasts:
  function of: Bone 192
  and Osteopetrosis 764
Osteochondritis dissecans 762
Osteochondritis juvenilis 762
  and *disorders of the spine 938*
  type of: Perthes' disease 795
Osteochondroma 762
Osteochondrosis:
  Osteochondritis juvenilis 762
osteoclastoma:
  type of Bone tumour 196
osteoclasts:
  function of: Bone 192
  and Osteopetrosis 764
Osteodystrophy 762
Osteogenesis imperfecta 763
Osteogenic sarcoma:
  Osteosarcoma 764
Osteoid osteoma 763
Osteoma 763
Osteomalacia 763
  and deficiency of Vitamin D 1065
Osteomyelitis 763
  a *disorder of the bone 193*
  and *disorders of the spine 938*
Osteopathy 764
Osteopetrosis 764
Osteophyte 764
  feature of Osteoarthritis 761
Osteoporosis 764, *765*
  diagnosis of: Densitometry 339
  and Menopause 676; Parathyroid glands 781; *disorders of the spine 938*
  leading to Femur, fracture of 439
  treatment of: Hormone replacement therapy 541; Oestrogen drugs 749; Vitamin supplements 1066
Osteosarcoma 764

Osteosclerosis 765
  alternative term: Myelosclerosis 712
Osteotomy 765
  in treatment of Knock-knee 620
Ostomy 766
Otalgia 766
  common term: Earache 383
Otitis externa 766
  a *disorder of the ear 384*
Otitis media 766
  complication of: Labyrinthitis 622
  a *disorder of the ear 384*
Oto- 767
Otomize 1117
otomycosis:
  feature of Otitis externa 766
Otoplasty 767
Otorhinolaryngology 767
Otorrhoea 767
  common term: Ear, discharge from 385
Otosclerosis 767
Otoscope 767
Otosporin 1117
Ototoxicity 767
Otrivine 1117
Otrivine-Antistin 1117
Ouabain 1117
Outpatient treatment 767
Ovarian cyst 767
  removal of an ovarian cyst 768
Ovary 768
  part of *endocrine system 401; Reproductive system, female 868*
  function of: *the sources and main effects of selected hormones 543*
  removal of: Hysterectomy 560; Oophorectomy 752; Sterilization, female 945
  see also index entry Ovulation
Ovary, cancer of 768
Ovary, polycystic 768
Overbite 769
Overbreathing 769
  medical term: Hyperventilation 554
Overcrowding, dental 769
  causing Malocclusion 659
Overuse injury 769
Overweight:
  Obesity 742
Ovestin 1117
Ovran 1117
Ovran 30 1117
Ovranette 1117
Ovulation 769
  failure of: Infertility 583; Ovary, polycystic 768
  and *the process of fertilization 441;* Menstruation 677
  painful: Mittelschmerz 693
  suppression of: Contraception 301; Dysmenorrhoea 382
Ovum 769
  and Ovulation 769
Ovysmen 1117
Oxamniquine 1117
Oxatomide 1117
Oxazepam 770

Oxitropium bromide 1117
Oxivent 1117
Oxpentifylline 1117
Oxprenolol 770
Oxybenzone 1117
Oxybuprocaine 1117
Oxybutynin 1117
Oxycodone 1117
Oxygen 770
  and Breathing 208;
    Haemoglobin 499; Lung 648
  form of: Ozone 770
  insufficient: Hypoxia 560;
    Mountain sickness 697;
    Suffocation 958
Oxygen tent 770
Oxygen therapy 770
  in treatment of Respiratory
    failure 870
oxyhaemoglobin:
  in Blood cells 181
  form of Haemoglobin 499
Oxymetazoline 770
Oxymetholone 1117
Oxymycin 1117
Oxypertine 1117
Oxyphenbutazone 1117
Oxyphenisatin 1117
Oxyprenix 1117
Oxytetracycline 770
Oxytetramix 1118
Oxytocin 770
  production of: Pituitary gland
    805
  use of: Induction of labour 577
Oxyuriasis 770
  alternative term: Threadworm
    infestation 985
Ozena 770
Ozone 770
  absorption of Ultraviolet light
    1026
  depletion of: Pollution 815

P

PABA:
  abbreviation for Para-
    aminobenzoic acid 777
Pabrinex 1118
Pacemaker 771
  and Brain imaging 202
  interference with: TENS 976
  in treatment of Heart block
    518; Stokes-Adams
    syndrome 948
Pacifene 1118
pacinian corpuscle:
  function of: Sensation 898
  types of receptor 861
Padimate O 1118
Paediatrics 771
  branch of: Neonatology 721
Paedophilia 771
Paget's disease 772
  and Osteosarcoma 764
  treatment of: Biphosphonates
    171
Paget's disease of the nipple 772
  disorder of the Nipple 731

Pain 772, 773
  and Endorphins 403;
    Enkephalins 406;
    Neurotransmitter 729
  type of Sensation 898
  types of: Abdominal pain 50,
    51; Back pain 150, 151, 153;
    Chest pain 256, 258; Earache
    383; Facial pain 428;
    Headache 507, 508; Referred
    pain 864; Toothache 1002
  see also index entry Pain relief
Painful arc syndrome 774
  and Rotator cuff 882;
    Tendinitis 975
Painkillers:
  medical term: Analgesic drugs
    102
  see also index entry Pain relief
Pain relief 774
  in childbirth; pain relief in
    labour and delivery 261
  drug methods: Anaesthesia,
    local 101; Analgesic drugs
    102; Nonsteroidal anti-
    inflammatory drugs 734
  natural: Endorphins 403;
    Enkephalins 406
  nondrug methods:
    Acupuncture 65; Cordotomy
    306; Sympathectomy 964;
    TENS 976
  and Sports, drugs and 940
Palate 774
Paldesic 1118
Palfium 1118
Palliative treatment 774
Pallor 774
Palpation 774
  use of: Examination, physical
    418
Palpitation 774
  causes of: Anxiety 122;
    Arrhythmia, cardiac 129;
    Cardiomyopathy 236
  and Ectopic heartbeat 388
Palsy 775
  alternative term: Paralysis 778
Paludrine 1118
Pamergan P100 1118
Pameton 1118
Pamidronate 1118
Panacea 775
Panadeine 1118
Panadol 1118
Panaleve, Panaleve Junior 1118
Pancreas 775
  disorders of: Pancreas, cancer
    of 775; disorders of the
    pancreas 776; Pancreatitis 776
  imaging of: Pancreatography
    777
  part of Digestive system 357;
    Endocrine system 400, 401
  and production of Glucagon
    487; Hormone 541; the
    sources and main effects of
    selected hormones 543; Insulin
    589
  removal of: Pancreatectomy
    775
Pancreas, cancer of 775
  a disorder of the pancreas 776

Pancrease 1118
Pancreatectomy 775
  in treatment of Pancreas,
    cancer of 775; Pancreatitis
    777
Pancreatin 775
Pancreatitis 776
  causing Kidney failure 614
  a disorder of the pancreas 776
Pancreatography 777
  methods of: CT scanning 323;
    ERCP 413; Ultrasound
    scanning 1026
Pancrex 1118
Pancuronium 1118
Pandemic 777
  and Epidemic 409
Panerel 1118
Panic attack 777
  feature of Phobia 801
Panoxyl 1118
Panthenol 1118
pantothenic acid:
  part of Vitamin B complex
    1064
Panzytrat 25 000 1118
Papain 777
  type of Enzyme 408
Papanicolaou method:
  see index entry Cervical smear
    test
Papaveretum 1118
Papaverine 1118
Papilla 777
  of Tongue 1000
Papilloedema 777
Papilloma 777
papillomavirus:
  as Carcinogen 233
  causing Cervix, cancer of 254;
    Wart 1074; Wart, plantar
    1075; Warts, genital 1075
Pap smear:
  see index entry Cervical smear
    test
Papule 777
  common term: Pimple 803
  feature of Acne 62
Par-/para- 777
Para-aminobenzoic acid 777
  constituent of Sunscreens 960
Paracentesis 777
paracervical block:
  use of: pain relief in labour and
    delivery 261
Paracetamol 778
Paracets 1118
Paracodol 1118
Paraesthesia 778
  common term: Pins-and-
    needles 804
Paraffinoma 778
Parahypon 1109
Parake 1118
Paraldehyde 778
Paralysis 778
  alternative term: Palsy 775
  types of: Hemiplegia 527;
    Paraplegia 779; Quadriplegia
    849
Paralysis, periodic 778
paralytic ileus:
  Ileus, paralytic 564

Paramax 1118
Paramedic 779
Paramin 1118
Paramol 1118
Paranoia 779
  cause of: Sleep deprivation
    922
  feature of: Personality disorder
    795; Psychosis 840
  symptom of: Delusion 338
Paraparesis 779
  type of Paralysis 778
  and Walking 1073
Paraphilia:
  common term: Deviation,
    sexual 347
Paraphimosis 779
  as complication of Phimosis
    800
  a disorder of the Penis 789
  treatment of: Circumcision 279
Paraplatin 1118
Paraplegia 779
  cause of: Spinal injury 935
  type of Paralysis 778
parapraxia:
  common term: Freudian slip
    462
Parapsychology 779
Paraquat 779
  type of Pesticide 796
Parasite 779, 780
Parasitology 780
Parasuicide:
  Suicide, attempted 958
Parasympathetic nervous system
    780
  functions of the autonomic
    nervous system 147
  part of Autonomic nervous
    system 146
  part of: Vagus nerve 1043
Parathion 780
Parathyroidectomy 780
Parathyroid glands 781
  disorders of:
    Hyperparathyroidism 550;
    Hypoparathyroidism 556;
    Parathyroid tumour 781
  part of Endocrine system 400,
    401
  and production of Hormones
    541; the sources and main
    effects of selected hormones 543
  removal of: Parathyroidectomy
    780
Parathyroid tumour 781
Paratyphoid fever 781
  type of Typhoid fever 1022
Paré, Ambroise:
  landmarks in medicine: surgery
    670
Parenchyma 781
  and Stroma 954
Parenteral 781
Parenteral nutrition:
  type of Feeding, artificial 437
Parentrovite 1118
Paresis 781
  type of Paralysis 778
Parietal 781
parietal lobe:
  part of Cerebrum 249

Parkinsonism 781
  cause of: Designer drugs 345
  feature of Shy-Drager
    syndrome 910
  see also index entry
    Parkinson's disease
Parkinson's disease 781
  a *disorder of the brain 200*
  causes of: Neurotransmitter
    729; *cause of Parkinson's dis-*
    ease 782
  features of: Paralysis 778;
    Rigidity 881; Tremor 1013
  treatment of: Amantadine 90;
    Anticholinergic drugs 116;
    Bromocriptine 213; Lev-
    odopa 635
  type of Degenerative disorder
    336
Parlodel 1118
Parmid 1118
Parnate 1118
Paronychia 782
Parotid glands 782
  disorder of: Mumps 702
  location of the parotid glands 783
  types of Salivary glands 886
parotitis:
  a disorder of Parotid glands
    783
Paroxetine 1118
Paroxysm 783
  alternative terms: Seizure 896;
    Spasm 929
Parrot fever 783
  medical term: Psittacosis 836
Parstelin 1118
Parturition 783
  common term: Childbirth 261
Parvolex 1118
passage, blocked:
  medical term: Occlusion 743
passage, narrowed:
  medical term: Stenosis 944
Passive smoking 22:
  causing Lung cancer 649
  and Tobacco-smoking 997
Pasteurization 783
Pasteur, Louis:
  germ theory of disease:
    Anatomy and pathology 30;
    Bacteria 153; Bacteriology
    154; Medicine 668; *landmarks*
    in medicine: diagnosis 669
    landmarks in medicine: drugs 671
  and Pasteurization 783
Patau's syndrome:
  type of Trisomy 1017
patch tests:
  and *allergy and the body 86*
  in diagnosis of Dermatitis 344
  types of Skin tests 918
Patella 783
  disorder of: Chondromalacia
    patellae 273
  part of Knee 619
Patent 783
Patent ductus arteriosus 783
  complication of: Endocarditis
    400
  leading to Heart failure 519
  type of Heart disease,
    congenital *518, 519*

Paternity testing 783
  and Blood groups 187;
    Histocompatibility antigens
    537; Serology 901
  paternity testing using genetic
    fingerprinting 784
Patho- 784
Pathogen 784
  causing Infection 577;
    Infectious disease 578
  examples of: Bacteria 152;
    Fungi 464; Protozoa 836;
    Viruses 1055
  type of Microorganism 685
Pathogenesis 784
Pathognomonic 784
Pathological 784
pathological anatomy:
  alternative term: Morbid
    anatomy 695
Pathology 784
  Anatomy and pathology 30
Pathology, cellular 785
  type of Cytology 329
Pathology, chemical 785
Pathophysiology 785
  type of Physiology 802
-pathy 785
Pavacol-D 1118
Pavulon 1118
Peak-flow meter 785
  in assessment of Asthma 139;
    Bronchospasm 216
  use of: Pulmonary function
    tests 844
Peau d'orange 785
  as symptom of Breast cancer
    205; Elephantiasis 394
Pecram 1118
Pectoral 785
pectoral muscles 785
Pediculosis 785
  infestation with Lice 635;
    Pubic lice 842
peer groups:
  in Adolescence 68
  and Behavioural problems in
    children 162
Peer review 785
Pellagra 785
  cause of: deficiency of Vitamin
    B complex 1064
pelvic colon:
  alternative term: Sigmoid
    colon 912
Pelvic examination 785
  in investigation of *disorders of*
    the cervix 254; Pelvic
    inflammatory disease 786
  procedure for pelvic examination
    786
Pelvic floor exercises 785
  in prevention of Uterus,
    prolapse of 1038
  in treatment of Incontinence,
    urinary 576
Pelvic infection 786
  see also index entry Pelvic
    inflammatory disease
Pelvic inflammatory disease 786
  causes of: Chlamydial
    infections 268; Gonorrhoea
    490; IUD 605

  causing Abdominal pain 54;
    Ectopic pregnancy 388;
    Infertility 583; Intercourse,
    painful 592
Pelvic pain:
  type of Abdominal pain 50
Pelvimetry 786
Pelvis 787
  assessment of: Pelvimetry 786
  and Childbirth, complications
    of 264
  components of: Coccyx 284;
    Sacrum 884
  part of Abdomen 50; Skeleton
    914; *bones of the skeleton 915*
Pemoline 1118
Pemphigoid 787
  a *disorder of the skin 919*
Pemphigus 787
  a *disorder of the skin 919*
Penbritin 1118
Penbutolol 1118
Pendramine 1118
Penicillamine 788
Penicillin drugs 788
  effect on Bacteria 154
  group of Antibiotic drugs 114
  landmarks in medicine: drugs 671
  in treatment of Infectious
    disease 581
Penicillin G 1118
Penicillin V 1118
Penile implant 788
  and Sex change 902
  in treatment of Impotence 574
Penile warts:
  type of Warts, genital 1075
Penis 788
  and Circumcision 279;
    Intercourse, painful 592
  functions of: Ejaculation 391;
    Erection 413; Sexual
    intercourse 904, *905*
  part of Reproductive system,
    male 868, *869*
  parts of: Foreskin 460; Urethra
    1029
Penis, cancer of 789
  associated with Smegma 925
Penmix 1118
Pentacarinat 1118
Pentaerythritol tetranitrate 1118
Pentamidine 1118
Pentasa 1118
Pentazocine 789
Pentostam 1118
Pentostatin 1118
Pepcid PM 1118
Peppermint oil 789
Pep pills 789
pepsin:
  in Stomach 948
Peptic ulcer 789
  and *HELICOBACTER PYLORI* 527
  causing Peritonitis 794; Pyloric
    stenosis 847
  sites and causes of peptic ulcer
    790
  perforated: Abdomen, acute
    50
  recurrent: Zollinger-Ellison
    syndrome 1094
  a *disorder of the stomach 949*

  treatment of: Antacid drugs
    111; Gastrectomy 469;
    Ulcer-healing drugs 1024;
    Vagotomy 1042
Peptide 791
  as constituent of Proteins 834
  constituent of: Amino acids
    92
Peptimax 1118
Pepto-Bismol 1118
Perception 791
  false: Hallucination 504
Percussion 791
  use of: Examination, physical
    418
Percutaneous 791
percutaneous kidney biopsy 613
Percutol 1118
Perfan 1118
Perforation 791
Pergolide 1118
Pergonal 1118
Peri- 791
Periactin 1118
Pericarditis 791
  associated with Dialysis 353;
    Lupus erythematosus 651;
    Rheumatoid arthritis 877
Pericardium 791
  part of Heart 514
Pericyazine 1118
Perimetry 791
Perinal 1118
Perinatal 792
Perinatology 792
Perindopril 1118
Perineum 792
  incision in: Episiotomy 412
Periodic fever 792
  alternative term: Familial
    Mediterranean fever 434
Period, menstrual:
  Menstruation 677
  see also index entries
    Menstruation, disorders of;
    Menstruation, irregular
Periodontal disease 792
Periodontics 792
Periodontitis 792
  causing Toothache 1002
  as complication of Gingivitis
    482
  treatment of: Curettage, dental
    325
periodontium:
  inflammation of: Periodontitis
    792
Period pain:
  medical term: Dysmenorrhoea
    381
Periosteum 793
  inflammation of: Periostitis
    793
  part of Bone 192
Periostitis 793
  causing Shin splints 907
Peripheral nervous system 793
  components of: Cranial
    nerves 318; Spinal nerves
    936
  disorders of: Neuropathy 728
  and Nerve 722
  part of *nervous system 724*

Peripheral vascular disease 793
  causing Leg ulcer 631
  and Tobacco-smoking 997
  treatment of: Angioplasty,
    balloon 108; Vasodilator
    drugs 1047
Peristalsis 793
  in Digestive system 357;
    Intestine 596; Oesophagus
    748; Ureter 1028
  and Muscle 706
  how peristalsis happens 794
  stimulation of: Vagus nerve
    1043
Peritoneal dialysis:
  type of Dialysis 44, 351
Peritoneum 794
  inflammation of: Peritonitis
    794
  part of Abdomen 50
Peritonitis 794
  causing Ileus, paralytic 564;
    Shock 908
  as complication of
    Appendicitis 127; Dialysis
    353; Peptic ulcer 789;
    Puerperal sepsis 843;
    Typhoid fever 1022
Peritonsillar abscess 794
  a complication of Tonsillitis
    1002
Permanent teeth 794
  and Eruption of teeth 414;
    *structure and arrangement of
    teeth 972*
Permethrin 1118
Pernicious anaemia 794
  cause of: deficiency of
    Vitamin B$_{12}$ 1063
  causing Dementia 338
  feature of: Achlorhydria 62
  a disorder of the stomach 949
  type of Anaemia,
    megaloblastic 98;
    Autoimmune disorder
    146
Pernio 794
  common term: Chilblain 260
Peroneal muscular atrophy 794
  type of Neuropathy 728
Perphenazine 795
Persantin 1118
persecution:
  and Delusion 338; Paranoia
    779
Personality 795
  assessment of: Personality
    tests 795
  changes in: Dementia 338;
    Personality disorders 795
  and Intelligence 590
  theories of: Freudian theory
    462; Jungian theory 609;
    Psychoanalytic theory 838
Personality disorders 795
  and Suicide 958; Suicide,
    attempted 958
  treatment of: Psychoanalysis
    838; Psychotherapy 841
Personality tests 795
Perspiration 795
  production of: Sweat glands
    963

Perthes' disease 795
  type of Osteochondritis
    juvenilis 762
  and Walking 1073
Pertofran 1118
Pertussis 795
  *cases of pertussis in England and
    Wales 796*
  prevention of: DPT
    vaccination 371;
    Immunization 569;
    Immunization against
    disease 28–29; *typical
    childhood immunization
    schedule 570*
Perversion:
  alternative term: Deviation,
    sexual 347
Pes cavus:
  common term: Claw-foot 281
pes planus:
  common term: Flat-feet 452
Pessary 796
  causing Vaginal discharge
    1041
  uses of: Abortion, induced 58;
    Uterus, prolapse of 1037
Pesticides 796
  causing Pollution 815
Petechiae 796
  feature of Purpura 846;
    Radiation sickness 853
Pethidine 796
Petit mal 797
  type of Epilepsy 411
Petrolagar 1118
Petroleum jelly 797
PET scanning 37, 797
  development of: *landmarks in
    medicine: diagnosis 669*
  type of Imaging technique 564
  use of: Brain imaging 202
Peutz-Jeghers syndrome 797
Pevaryl 1118
Peyote 797
  source of Mescaline 681
Peyronie's disease 797
pH 797
  see also index entry Acid-base
    balance
Phaeochromocytoma 797
Phagocyte 798
  and Immunoglobulin 571
  part of Immune system 569;
    the innate immune system 567
  in Spleen 938
  type of Blood cell 182
Phalanges 798
  part of Finger 449; *structure of a
    finger 450*; Foot 458; *the
    skeletal structure of the hand
    and wrist 505*; Skeleton 914;
    bones of the skeleton 915; Toe
    999
Phallus 798
  see also index entry Penis
Phantom limb 798
  following Amputation 94
Pharmaceutical 798
  see also index entry Drug
Pharmacokinetics 798
Pharmacology 798
Pharmacopoeia 798

Pharmacy 798
Pharmorubicin 1118
Pharyngeal diverticulum 798
  type of Oesophageal
    diverticulum 746
Pharyngeal pouch 798
  type of Oesophageal
    diverticulum 746
Pharyngitis 798
  a disorder of the Pharynx 799
  symptom of: Sore throat 929
Pharynx 798
  common term: Throat 986
  disorders of: Pharyngitis 798;
    Pharynx, cancer of 799
  part of: Nasopharynx 718
  location of the pharynx 799
Pharynx, cancer of 799
Phasal 1118
Phenazocine 1118
Phencyclidine 799
  common term: Angel dust 106
Phenelzine 799
Phenergan 1118
Phenindamine 1118
Phenindione 1118
Pheniramine 1118
Phenobarbitone 799
Phenol 1119
Phenolphthalein 1119
Phenoperidine 1119
Phenothiazine drugs 799
  causing *disorders of the retina 873*
  examples: Perphenazine 795;
    Prochlorperazine 829;
    Promazine 831
Phenothrin 1119
Phenoxybenzamine 1119
Phenoxymethylpenicillin 799
Phensedyl 1119
Phensic 1119
Phentermine 1119
Phentolamine 11119
phenylalanine:
  causing Phenylketonuria 800
  detection of: Guthrie test 497
Phenylbutazone 799
Phenylephrine 800
Phenylketonuria 800
  causing Mental handicap 680
  diagnosis of: Guthrie test 497
  and Pigmentation 803
  type of Metabolism, inborn
    error of 682
Phenylpropanolamine 800
Phenytoin 800
Pheromone 800
Phimetin 1119
Phimosis 800
  causing Urinary retention 1031
  complication of: Paraphimosis
    779
  a disorder of the Penis 789
pHiso-med 1119
Phlebitis 800
  alternative term:
    Thrombophlebitis 987
Phlebography 800
  alternative term: Venography
    1049
Phlebotomy 800
  alternative term: Venesection
    1049

Phlegm:
  historical usage: Humours 544
  medical term: Sputum 941
Phobia 800
  causing Panic attack 777
  treatment of: Behaviour
    therapy 162
Phocomelia 800
  type of Limb defect 637
Pholcodine 1119
Pholcomed 1119
PhorPain 1119
Phosphates 801
  type of Ion 601
Phosphate-Sandoz 1119
phospholipids:
  types of Fats and oils 436;
    Lipids 639
Phosphorus poisoning 801
Photocoagulation 801
Photophobia 801
  feature of Conjunctivitis 297;
    Corneal abrasion 307;
    Keratitis 610
Photosensitivity 801
  causes of: Chlorpromazine 269;
    Skin peeling, chemical 918
  and Pigmentation 803;
    Sunlight, adverse effects of
    960
  a disorder of the skin 919
Phototherapy 801
  in treatment of Psoriasis 837;
    Vitiligo 1066
  type of: PUVA 847
Phrenic nerve 802
Phyllocontin Continus 1119
Physeptone 1119
Physical examination:
  see index entry Examination,
    physical
Physical medicine and
    rehabilitation 802
Physiology 802
Physiotherapy 802
physique:
  medical term: Somatotype 928
Physostigmine 803
Phytex 1119
Phytocil 1119
Phytomenadione 1119
Piaget, Jean:
  and developmental
    Psychology 839
Pica 803
  feature of Pregnancy 823
Pickwickian syndrome 803
Picolax 1119
PID:
  abbreviation for Pelvic
    inflammatory disease 786
Pigeon toes 803
Pigmentation 803
Piles 803
  medical term: Haemorrhoids
    501
Pill, contraceptive:
  see index entry Oral
    contraceptives
Pilocarpine 803
Pilonidal sinus 803
Pimozide 803
Pimple 803

Pincus, Gregory:
  landmarks in medicine: drugs
  671
Pindolol 803
Pineal gland 804
Pinguecula 804
Pink-eye 804
  medical term: Conjunctivitis
  296
Pink puffer 804
  and Emphysema 398; Lung
  disease, chronic obstructive
  650
Pinna 804
  part of Ear 383
Pins-and-needles 804
  type of Sensation, abnormal
  899
Pinta 804
Pinworm infestation 804
  alternative term: Threadworm
  infestation 985
Pipenzolate 1119
Piperacillin 1119
Piperazine 804
Piportil Depot 1119
Pipothiazine 1119
Pipril 1119
Piptal 1119
Piptalin 1119
Piracetam 1119
Pirbuterol 1119
Pirenzepine 1119
Piretanide 1119
Piriton 1119
Piroxicam 804
Pirozip 1119
pitchblende:
  source of Radium 856;
  Uranium 1028
Pitressin 1119
Pituitary gland 804
  disorders of: *disorders of the*
  pituitary gland 805; Pituitary
  tumours 805
  function of: *the sources and*
  main effects of selected
  hormones 543; hormones
  secreted by the pituitary gland
  805
  and Hypothalamus 558
  part of Brain 198; *endocrine*
  system 401
  removal of: Hypophysectomy
  557
Pituitary tumours 805
  causing Galactorrhoea 466;
  Tunnel vision 1020
  diagnosis of: Skull X-ray 921
  treatment of:
  Hypophysectomy 557
  type of Brain tumour 203
  type of: Prolactinoma 831
Pityriasis alba 806
  and Pigmentation 803
Pityriasis rosea 806
Pityriasis versicolor 806
Pivampicillin 806
Pivmecillinam 806
Pizotifen 806
PKU test:
  alternative term: Guthrie test
  497

Placebo 806
  and Drug 376; Trial, clinical
  1014
Placenta 806
  and *stages of birth 262;*
  Childbirth 264; Chorionic
  villus sampling 39, 274;
  Intrauterine growth
  retardation 598
  development of: Embryo 395;
  the developing embryo 396; the
  process of fertilization 441;
  Implantation, egg 574;
  Pregnancy 822
  functions of: Fetal circulation
  440; *the sources and main*
  effects of selected hormones 543;
  function of the placenta 807;
  effects of hormones during
  pregnancy 823
  position of: Ultrasound
  scanning 1025
Placenta praevia 807
Placenta, tumours of:
  Choriocarcinoma 274;
  Hydatidiform mole 544
Plague 807
  transmission of: Rats, diseases
  from 860
Plantar wart:
  Wart, plantar 1075
Plantson, Anthony:
  landmarks in medicine: other
  forms of treatment 670
Plants, poisonous 808
Plaque 808
  and Atherosclerosis 140;
  arterial degeneration in
  atherosclerosis 141
Plaque, dental 808
  causing Calculus, dental 224;
  Caries, dental 236; Gingivitis
  482; Periodontitis 792
  detection of: Dental
  examination 340; Disclosing
  agents 361
  development of plaque 809
  removal of: Floss, dental 453;
  Oral hygiene 757;
  Toothbrushing 1002
Plaquenil 1119
Plasma 809
  constituents of: Plasma
  proteins 809
  exchange of: Plasmapheresis
  809
  part of Blood 181; *constituent of*
  blood 182
  use of: Bleeding, treatment of
  178
Plasmapheresis 809
  in treatment of Purpura 847
Plasma proteins 809
Plasminogen activator:
  alternative term: Tissue-
  plasminogen activator 996
Plaster cast:
  Cast 239
Plaster of Paris 809
  use of: Cast 239; *fractures: types*
  and treatment 461
Plastic surgery 809
  -plasty 809

Platelet 809
  as *constituent of blood 182*
  deficiency of: Bleeding
  disorders 177; Purpura 847;
  Thrombocytopenia 986
  function of: Blood clotting 183;
  Haemostasis 502
  type of Blood cell 183
Platet 1119
Platyhelminth 809
  causing Tapeworm infestation
  969; Worm infestation 1086
  common term: Flatworm 452
Play therapy 810
Plendil 1119
Plesmet 1119
Plethora 810
Plethysmography 810
  in diagnosis of Peripheral
  vascular disease 793
Pleura 810
  and Lung 649
Pleural effusion 810
  as complication of Pneumonia
  812; Tuberculosis 1019
  feature of Lung cancer 649
Pleurisy 810
  associated with Pneumonia
  812
Pleurodynia 810
  type of Myositis 715
Plexus 810
  examples: Brachial plexus 197;
  Solar plexus 928
Plicamycin 1119
Plication 810
Plummer-Vinson syndrome 810
Plutonium 810
  source of Radiation 852
PMS:
  Premenstrual syndrome 826
PMT:
  Premenstrual syndrome 826
Pneumaturia 810
Pneumo- 810
Pneumoconiosis 810
  causing Occupational
  mortality 745
  and *safety at work 744*
  type of Dust disease 379;
  Occupational disease and
  injury 743
Pneumocystis pneumonia 811
  feature of AIDS 77;
  Immunodeficiency disorders
  571
  type of Opportunistic infection
  754
Pneumonectomy 811
  in treatment of Lung cancer
  650
Pneumonia 811, *812*
  causing Pleurisy 810
  as complication of Pertussis
  796
  a *disorder of the lung 649*
  types of: Legionnaires' disease
  630; Pneumocystis
  pneumonia 811·
Pneumonitis 813
Pneumothorax 813
  as complication of Pertussis
  796; Tuberculosis 1019

a *disorder of the lung 649*
  and Pleura 810
Pocket, gingival:
  cause of: Periodontitis 792
Podiatry 813
Podophyllin 813
  in treatment of Warts, genital
  1075
Poison 813
Poisoning 813
  as method of Suicide 958
  treatment of: Antidote 117;
  Antivenom 120; Charcoal
  256; Chelating agents 256;
  Lavage, gastric 628
poison ivy:
  type of Plant, poisonous 808
Poldine methylsulphate 1119
Polio:
  Poliomyelitis 814
Poliomyelitis 814
  causing Leg, shortening of
  630; Paralysis 778
  effect on Walking 1073
  prevention of: Immunization
  569; *typical*
  childhood immunization
  schedule 570; travel protection
  29; Vaccine 1040
  type of Myelitis 711
pollen:
  and Allergy 85; *allergy and the*
  body 86; Rhinitis, allergic 878
Pollon-eze 1119
Pollution 815
Poloxamer "188" 1119
Poly- 815
Polyarteritis nodosa 815
  type of Arteritis 131
polyarthritis:
  complication of Rubella 883
Polybactrin 1119
Polycystic kidney:
  Kidney, polycystic 616
Polycystic ovary:
  Ovary, polycystic 768
Polycythaemia 815
  a *disorder of the blood 185*
  causing Plethora 810
  treatment of: Venesection 1049
Polydactyly 816
Polydipsia 816
  common term: Thirst,
  excessive 984
Polyestradiol 1119
Polyfax 1119
Polyhydramnios 816
polymorphonuclear leukocyte:
  type of Blood cell 182
Polymyalgia rheumatica 816
  associated with Temporal
  arteritis 974
Polymyositis 816
  causing Rhabdomyolysis 875
  type of Myositis 715
Polymyxin B sulphate 1119
Polymyxins 816
polyneuritis:
  type of Neuropathy 728
polyneuropathy:
  type of Neuropathy 728
Polyp 816

Polypeptide 816
  constituent of: Amino acids 92
  type of Peptide 791
Polypharmacy 816
polyploidy:
  type of Chromosomal
    abnormality 275
polyposis coli:
  alternative term: Polyposis,
    familial 817
Polyposis, familial 817
  complication of: Colon, cancer
    of 289
  treatment of: Colectomy 287
polysaccharide:
  type of Carbohydrate 232
Polystyrene sulphonate resins
  1119
Polytar 1119
Polythiazide 1119
Polytrim 1119
polyunsaturated fats:
  in treatment of Xanthomatosis
    1089
  types of Fats and oils 436
Polyuria:
  common term: Urination,
    excessive 1032
Polyvinyl alcohol 1119
Pompholyx 817
Ponderax 1119
Pondocillin 1119
Pons 817
  part of Brainstem 202
Ponstan 1119
population growth:
  and Birth control 171
Pore 817
Porphyria 817
  features of: Photosensitivity
    801; Urine, abnormal 1034
portal circulation:
  and Liver 641
  part of Circulatory system 279
Portal hypertension 817, *818*
  cause of: Cirrhosis 279
  leading to Oesophageal
    varices 747
  a disorder of the liver 645
Port-wine stain 818
  type of Haemangioma 498;
    Naevus 716
Posalfilin 1119
Positron emission tomography
  (PET):
  see index entry PET scanning
Possetting 818
Postcoital contraception:
  Contraception, postcoital 304
Posterior 818
  alternative term: Dorsal 369
postinfarction syndrome:
  alternative term: Dressler's
    syndrome 373
Postmaturity 818
Postmortem examination 818
  alternative term: Autopsy 146
Postmyocardial infarction
  syndrome 818
  alternative term: Dressler's
    syndrome 373
Postnasal drip 818
Postnatal care 819

Postnatal depression 819
Postpartum depression:
  Postnatal depression 819
Postpartum haemorrhage 819
  causing Maternal mortality 666
Post-traumatic stress disorder
  819
Postural drainage 819
  *techniques of postural drainage
    820*
  in treatment of Bronchiectasis
    213
Postural hypotension:
  type of Hypotension 558
Posture 820
Post-viral fatigue syndrome:
  Myalgic encephalomyelitis 710
Potassium 820
  deficiency of: *disorders of muscle
    707;* Paralysis, periodic 778;
    Tetany 981
  sources of: *minerals and main
    food sources 690*
  type of Ion 601; Mineral 689
Potassium chloride 1119
Potassium citrate 1119
Potassium clavulanate 1119
Potassium hydroxyquinolone
  sulphate 1119
Potassium permanganate 821
Potency 821
  of Drug 375
Pott's fracture 821
  affecting Ankle joint 110;
    Fibula 448; Tibia 994
Poultice 821
Povidone-iodine 1119
Powerin 1119
Pox 821
  alternative term: Syphilis 966
Pranoxen Continus 1119
Pravastatin 1119
Praxilene 1119
Praziquantel 821
Prazosin 821
Precancerous 821
  and Cervix, cancer of 253
Precortisyl 1119
Predenema 1119
Predfoam 1119
Pred Forte 1119
Predisposing factors 821
Prednesol 1119
Prednisolone 821
Prednisone 821
Predsol 1119
Predsol-N 1119
Pre-eclampsia 821
  alternative term: Toxaemia of
    pregnancy 1005
  leading to Eclampsia 387
  type of Toxaemia 1005
Prefil 1119
Pregaday 1119
Pregnancy 822
  and Antenatal care 112;
    Braxton Hicks' contractions
    204; Cervical incompetence
    251; Genetic counselling 476;
    Pregnancy, false 824;
    Pregnancy, multiple 824;
    Stria 951, 952; Twins 1021;
    Vomiting in pregnancy 1068

  causing Abdominal swelling
    55; Amenorrhoea 91;
    Menstruation, irregular 679
  complications of: Antepartum
    haemorrhage 113; Diabetic
    pregnancy 350; Ectopic
    pregnancy 388;
    Haemorrhoids 502;
    Miscarriage 690; Placenta
    praevia 807;
    Polyhydramnios 816;
    Postmaturity 818; Pre-
    eclampsia 821; Prematurity
    825; Pulmonary embolism
    843; Pyelonephritis 847;
    Rhesus incompatibility 875;
    Varicose veins 1044
  confirmation of: Pregnancy
    tests 824
  risks during: *alcohol and
    pregnancy 82;* Pregnancy,
    drugs in 823; Smoking and
    drinking 22–23; Tobacco-
    smoking 997
  stages of: Embryo 395; *the
    developing embryo 396;*
    Fertilization 440; *the process
    of fertilization 441;* Fetus 443;
    *effects of hormones during
    pregnancy 823; stages and
    features of pregnancy 822*
  tests during: Amniocentesis
    39, 92; Antenatal care 112;
    Chorionic villus sampling
    39, 274; Fetal heart
    monitoring 442; Fetoscopy
    38, 442; Ultrasound
    scanning 37, 1024; *how
    ultrasound scanning works
    1025*
  termination of: Abortion,
    induced 57
  see also index entry Childbirth
Pregnancy, drugs in 823
  and *alcohol and pregnancy 82;*
    Teratogen 976; Tobacco-
    smoking 997
Pregnancy, false 824
Pregnancy, multiple 824
  diagnosis of: Ultrasound
    scanning 37, 1025
  leading to Prematurity 825
  and Twins 1021
Pregnancy tests 824
  pregnancy test kit 825
Pregnavite Forte F 1120
Pregnyl 1120
Premature ejaculation:
  Ejaculation, disorders of 391
Prematurity 825, *826*
  feature of Pregnancy, multiple
    824
  and Respiratory distress
    syndrome 870
  treatment of: Incubator 576;
    Neonatal care 44;
    Ventilation 1050
Premedication 826
  and Sedation 896
Premenstrual syndrome 826
  treatment of: Metolazone 684;
    Progesterone drugs 830;
    Vitamin supplements 1066

Premenstrual tension:
  Premenstrual syndrome 826
Premolar 826
  and Eruption of teeth 414;
    Permanent teeth 794;
    *structure and arrangement of
    teeth 972*
Prempak-C 1120
Prepadine 1120
Prepidil 1120
Prepuce:
  common term: Foreskin 460
Prepulcid 1120
Presbyacusis 827
  associated with Tinnitus 995
  a disorder of the ear 384
  type of Deafness 332
Presbyopia 827
  a disorder of the eye 426
Prescal 1120
Prescribed diseases 827
  and Notifiable diseases 736;
    Occupational disease and
    injury 743
Prescription 827
Preservative 827
  type of Food additive 455
pressure measurement:
  scientific term: Manometry 661
Pressure points 827
Pressure sores 828
  alternative term: Bedsores 161
Prestim 1120
Prevalence 828
  and Incidence 575
Preventive dentistry 828
  and Oral hygiene 756
Preventive medicine 828
Priadel 1120
Priapism 828
  cause of: Testosterone 979
  feature of Leukaemia, chronic
    myeloid 633
  a disorder of the Penis 789
Prickly heat 828
  causes of: *disorders of the skin
    919;* Sweat glands 963
Prilocaine 1120
Primacor 1120
Primalan 1120
Primaquine 829
Primary 829
  and Secondary 896
Primary teeth 829
  and Eruption of teeth 414;
    Teeth 971; Teething 972
Primaxin 1120
Primidone 829
primigravida:
  Gravida 493
Primolut Depot 1120
Primolut N 1120
Primoteston Depot 1120
Primperan 1120
Prinzmetal's angina:
  see index entry Variant angina
Prioderm 1120
Prion 829
  causing Creutzfeldt Jakob
    disease 319
Pripsen 1120
Pro-Actidil 1120
Pro-Banthine 1120

Probenecid 829
Probucol 829
Procainamide 829
Procainamide Durules 1120
Procaine 829
Procaine penicillin 1120
Procarbazine 829
Prochlorperazine 829
Procidentia 829
  and Uterus, prolapse of 1037
Procol 1120
Proctalgia fugax 829
Proctitis 829
  associated with Gay bowel
    syndrome 472
  causing Rectal bleeding 862
  treatment of: Suppository 961
Proctofoam HC 1120
Proctoscopy 830
  in diagnosis of Haemorrhoids
    502; Proctitis 829
  and Sigmoidoscopy 912
Proctosedyl 1120
Procyclidine 830
Prodrome 830
Profasi 1120
Proflex 1120
Progeria 830
Progesic 1120
Progesterone hormone 830
  function of: the sources and
    main effects of selected
    hormones 543; effects of
    hormones during pregnancy
    823
  production of: Ovary 768;
    Placenta 806
  type of Sex hormone 903
Progestogen drugs 830
  constituent of Oral
    contraceptives 755
  examples: Megestrol 672;
    Norethisterone 734
  use of: Hormone replacement
    therapy 541
Prognathism 830
  classes of malocclusion 659
Prognosis 830
  Diagnosis and prognosis 30
Progressive 830
Progressive muscular atrophy
  830
  type of Motor neuron disease
    697
Proguanil 831
Progynova 1120
Prolactin 831
  excess of: Prolactinoma 831
  production of: Pituitary gland
    805
Prolactinoma 831
Prolapse 831
  types of: Disc prolapse 362;
    Rectal prolapse 862; Uterus,
    prolapse of 1037
Proleukin 1120
Proluton Depot 1120
Promazine 831
Promethazine 831
Prominal 1120
Pronation 831
Prondol 1120
Pronestyl 1120

pronethalol:
  development of: landmarks in
    medicine: drugs 671
Propaderm 1120
Propafenone 1120
Propain 1120
Propamidine 1120
Propamidine isethionate 1120
Propanix 1120
Propantheline 831
Prophylactic 831
Propine 1120
Propofol 1120
Propranolol 831
  production of: sources of drugs
    43
Proprietary 831
  and Generic drug 475
Proprioception 831
  and Balance 155; Sensation 898
Proptosis 831
  alternative term:
    Exophthalmos 420
Propylthiouracil 831
Prosaid 1120
Proscar 1120
Prostaglandin 831
  effects of some prostaglandins 832
  excess production of: disorders
    of the uterus 1037
Prostaglandin drugs 832
  uses of: Abortifacient 57;
    Abortion, induced 57;
    Induction of labour 577
Prostap SR 1120
Prostate, cancer of 832
  treatment of: Gonadorelins
    489; Hypophysectomy 557;
    Orchidectomy 757;
    Prostatectomy 832, 833;
    Stilboestrol 947
Prostatectomy 832, 833
  in treatment of Prostate,
    cancer of 832; Prostate,
    enlarged 832
Prostate, enlarged 832
  causing Hydronephrosis 546;
    Incontinence, urinary 575;
    Irritable bladder 603; Kidney
    failure 615; Nocturia 732;
    Urinary retention 1031;
    Urinary tract infection 1032
  treatment of: Prostatectomy
    832, 833
Prostate gland 834
  inflammation of: Prostatitis
    834
  part of Reproductive system,
    male 869
prostate specific antigen:
  in diagnosis of Prostate, cancer
    of 832
Prostatism 834
  and Prostate, enlarged 832
Prostatitis 834
  causing Haematuria 499
  as complication of Nonspecific
    urethritis 733
  treatment of: Trimethoprim
    1016
Prosthesis 834
  see also index entries Implant;
    Implants, dental

Prosthetics, dental 834
Prostigmin 1120
Prostin E2 1120
Prostin F2 alpha 1120
protanopia:
  type of Colour vision
    deficiency 292
Protaphane 1120
Proteins 18, 834
  abnormal: Genetic disorders
    476
  analysis of: Electrophoresis
    394
  constituents of: Amino acids
    92; Peptide 791
  dietary: Nutrition 738;
    Vegetarianism 1048
  dietary deficiency of:
    Kwashiorkor 621; Marasmus
    662; Nutritional disorders
    740
  types of: Albumin 80;
    Antibody 115; Enzyme 408;
    Globulin 485;
    Immunoglobulin 571;
    Plasma proteins 809
  in urine: Albuminuria 80;
    Proteinuria 835
  see also index entry Protein
    synthesis
Protein synthesis 834
  and Genetic code 475; what
    genes are and what they do
    474; steps in protein synthesis
    835
Proteinuria 835
  cause of: Nephrotic syndrome
    722
  in pregnancy: Pre-eclampsia
    821
  type of: Albuminuria 80
Prothiaden 1120
protons:
  and Radiation 851
Protoplasm 835
Protozoa 836
  causing Infectious disease 578;
    protozoal infections 581
  types of Microorganism 685
Protriptyline 836
Provera 1120
Pro-Viron 1120
Proximal 836
Proxymetacaine 1120
Prozac 1120
Proziere 1120
Prurigo 836
Pruritus 836
  common term: Itching 604
pruritus ani:
  a disorder of the anus 121
  type of Itching 604
pruritus vulvae:
  common term: Vulval itching
    1071
  type of Itching 604
Pseud-/pseudo 836
Pseudarthrosis 836
pseudoacanthosis nigricans:
  Acanthosis nigricans 59
Pseudocyesis:
  common term: Pregnancy,
    false 824

Pseudodementia 836
Pseudoephedrine 836
Pseudoepidemic 836
Pseudogout 836
Pseudohermaphroditism 836
  and Hermaphroditism 530
  type of: Testicular
    feminization syndrome 977
Psilocybin 836
  type of Hallucinogenic drug
    504
Psittacosis 836
  treatment of: Oxytetracycline
    770
  type of Ornithosis 759
Psoas muscle 837
Psoradrate 1120
Psoralen drugs 837
  use of: Phototherapy 801;
    PUVA 847
Psoriasis 837
  effect on Pigmentation 803
  a disorder of the skin 919
  treatment of: Dithranol 364;
    Methotrexate 684;
    Phototherapy 801; PUVA
    847
Psoriderm 1120
PsoriGel 1120
Psorin 1120
Psych- 838
Psyche 838
Psychedelic drugs 838
  alternative term:
    Hallucinogenic drugs 504
Psychiatric treatment 45
  types of: Behaviour therapy
    162; Psychoanalysis 838;
    Psychotherapy 841
Psychiatry 838
Psychoanalysis 838
  basis of: Freudian theory 462;
    Psychoanalytic theory 838
  and Dream analysis 372;
    Resistance 869; Transference
    1009
  in treatment of Depression
    343; Obsessive-compulsive
    disorder 742; Personality
    disorders 795
  type of Psychiatric treatment
    45; Psychotherapy 841
Psychoanalytic theory 838
  associated with Freudian
    theory 462
  basis of Psychoanalysis 838
  and Oedipus complex 746
Psychodrama 839
Psychogenic 839
Psychology 839
Psychometry 839
  types of: Intelligence tests 590;
    Personality tests 795
Psychoneurosis 839
  alternative term: Neurosis 728
Psychopathology 839
Psychopathy 840
  modern term: Antisocial
    personality disorder 119
Psychopharmacology 840
Psychosexual disorders 840
  see also index entry Sexual
    problems

Psychosexual dysfunction 840
  see also index entry Sexual
    problems
Psychosis 840
  causes of: Designer drugs 345;
    LSD 647; Postnatal
    depression 819
  common terms: Insanity 587;
    Mental illness 680
  treatment of: Antipsychotic
    drugs 119; Psychoanalysis
    838
Psychosomatic 840
Psychosurgery 840
Psychotherapy 841
  in treatment of Depression
    343; Personality disorders
    795; Schizophrenia 891
  type of Psychiatric treatment
    45
Psychotropic drugs 841
Pterygium 841
Ptomaine poisoning 841
  alternative term: Food
    poisoning 456
Ptosis 841
Ptyalism:
  Salivation, excessive 886
Puberty 841
  and Adolescence 68; Growth,
    childhood 494; Menstruation
    677; changes of puberty 842;
    Sexual characteristics,
    secondary 904
Pubes 842
Pubic lice 842
pubis:
  part of Pelvis 787
Public health 843
  and Preventive medicine 828
Public Health Laboratory Service
    843
Pudenda:
  alternative term: Genitalia
    479
Pudendal block 843
  type of Nerve block 723
Puerperal sepsis 843
  and Postnatal care 819
Puerperium 843
Pulmadil 1120
Pulmicort 1120
Pulmonary 843
pulmonary circulation:
  part of Circulatory system 279,
    280
Pulmonary embolism 843
  causing Pulmonary
    hypertension 844; Shock
    907
  complication of Thrombosis,
    deep vein 988
  a disorder of the lung 649
  type of Embolism 394
Pulmonary fibrosis 844
  type of: Interstitial pulmonary
    fibrosis 595
Pulmonary function tests 844
  type of: Spirometry 937
  using Peak-flow meter 785

Pulmonary hypertension 844
  causing Heart failure 519;
    Pulmonary incompetence
    845
  complication of Bronchitis,
    chronic 214; Emphysema
    398; Septal defect 900
Pulmonary incompetence 844
Pulmonary oedema 845
  cause of: Heart failure 519
  type of Oedema 746
Pulmonary stenosis 845
  causing Heart failure 519
  a type of congenital heart disease
    518
Pulp, dental 845
Pulpectomy 845
  in Root-canal treatment 881
Pulpotomy 845
Pulse 845
  abnormal: Arrhythmia,
    cardiac 128; Palpitation
    774
  as measure of Heart-rate
    522
  taking the pulse 846
  weak: Shock 908
Pump, infusion 846
Pump, insulin 846
pump oxygenator:
  alternative term: Heart-lung
    machine 520
punch biopsy:
  a biopsy of the cervix 253
  following Cervical smear test
    252
Punch-drunk 846
  following Concussion 294
punch grafting:
  type of Hair transplant 504
Pupil 846
  constriction of: Miosis 690
  dilation of: Mydriasis 711
  part of Eye 422; Iris 602
Purgative:
  type of Laxative drug 629
Purine 846
Puri-Nethol 1120
Pur-In Mix 1120
Purkinje's cells:
  in Cerebellum 247
Purpura 846
  appearance of senile purpura
    847
  cause of: Thrombocytopenia
    986
  causing Petechiae 796
  feature of Bleeding disorders
    177
  type of: Henoch-Schönlein
    purpura 527
Purulent 847
Pus 847
  collection of: Abscess 58; Boil
    191; Pustule 847
  formation of: Sepsis 900;
    Suppuration 961
  symptom of Infection 577
Pustule 847
  alternative term: Pimple 803

PUVA 847
  in treatment of Mycosis
    fungoides 711; Psoriasis 837;
    Vitiligo 1066
  type of Phototherapy 801
Pyelitis:
  alternative term:
    Pyelonephritis 847
Pyelography:
  see index entry Urography
Pyelolithotomy 847
Pyelonephritis 847
  a disorder of the kidney 614
pyknic body type:
  and Somatotype 928
pyloric sphincter:
  disorder of: Pyloric stenosis
    847
  part of Stomach 948
  type of Sphincter 933
Pyloric stenosis 847
  complication of Peptic ulcer
    789
  pyloric stenosis in infants 848
  a disorder of the stomach 949
Pyloroplasty 848
  and Vagotomy 1042
Pyo- 848
Pyoderma gangrenosum 848
Pyopen 1120
Pyrantel 848
  in treatment of Ascariasis 136
Pyrazinamide 848
Pyrexia:
  common term: Fever 443
Pyrexia of uncertain origin 848
Pyridostigmine 1120
Pyridoxine 848
  part of Vitamin B complex
    1064
Pyrimethamine 848
Pyrithione zinc 1120
Pyrogastrone 1120
Pyrogen 848
  causing Fever 443
Pyromania 848
Pyuria 848

Q

QALY 849
Q fever 849
  cause of: Rickettsia 880
  type of Pneumonia 811
Quackery 849
quadrantectomy:
  type of Mastectomy 664
Quadriceps muscle 849
  and Patella 783
Quadriparesis 849
Quadriplegia 849
  cause of: Spinal injury 935
  type of Paralysis 778
Quarantine 849
Quellada 1120
Questran 1120
Quickening 849

Quinalbarbitone 1120
Quinapril 1121
Quinidine 1121
Quinine 849
  landmarks in medicine: drugs 671
  in treatment of Cramp 317
Quinocort 1121
Quinoderm 1121
Quinolone drugs 849
  examples of: Acrosoxacin 54;
    Nalidixic acid 716
Quinoped 1121

R

Rabies 850
  transmission of: Cats, diseases
    from 243; Dogs, diseases
    from 368
  travel protection 29
Rachitic 850
  see also index entry Rickets
Rad 850
  radiation Dose 369
  a radiation unit 851
radial artery:
  blood supply to Hand 505
Radial nerve 850
  branch of Brachial plexus 197
  and Humerus 542
Radiation 851
  adverse effects of: Cancer 227;
    Carcinogen 233; Cataract
    240; Leukaemia, acute 633;
    Lung cancer 649;
    Occupational disease and
    injury 743; Radiation
    hazards 852; Radiation
    sickness 853; Sunlight,
    adverse effects of 959
  and Environmental medicine
    407; Half-life 504; Infra-red
    585; Nuclear energy 736;
    radiation units 851;
    Radiolucent 854;
    Radiopaque 854; Ultraviolet
    light 1026
  uses of: CT scanning 35, 323;
    performing a CT scan 324;
    Dental X-ray 341; Imaging
    techniques 564; imaging the
    body 565; Interstitial
    radiotherapy 595;
    Intracavitary therapy 598;
    Irradiation of food 602;
    Nuclear medicine 736; PET
    scanning 37, 797;
    Radioimmunoassay 853;
    Radiology 853;
    Radionuclide scanning 35,
    854; Radiotherapy 45, 855;
    Scanning techniques 888;
    X-rays 34, 1089; X-ray
    examination 1090; using
    X-rays to look at the body 1091
  see also index entry
    Radioactivity

Radiation hazards 852
    and Occupational disease and
        injury 743
    see also index entries
        Radiation; Radioactivity
Radiation sickness 853
radiation units 851
radical mastectomy:
    causing Lymphoedema 655
    type of Mastectomy 664;
        Radical surgery 853
Radical surgery 853
Radiculopathy 853
radioactive implants:
    uses of: Interstitial
        radiotherapy 595;
        Intracavitary therapy 598;
        Radiotherapy 45, 856
Radioactivity 853
    and Half-life 504
    sources of: Plutonium 810;
        Radium 856; Radon 856;
        Strontium 954; Technetium
        971; Uranium 1028
    see also index entry Radiation
radioallergosorbent test (RAST):
    see index entry RAST
Radiography 853
Radioimmunoassay 853
    type of Immunoassay 570
Radioisotope scanning:
    Radionuclide scanning 854
Radiology 853
Radiolucent 854
Radionuclide scanning 35, 854
    type of Imaging technique 566;
        Scanning technique 888
    uses of: *imaging the body 565;*
        Liver imaging 646; Thyroid
        scanning 993
    using Technetium 971
Radiopaque 854
Radiotherapy 45, 855
    causing Lymphoedema 655
    in treatment of Leukaemia,
        acute 633; Leukaemia,
        chronic lymphocytic 633;
        Lung cancer 650;
        Retinoblastoma 874
Radium 856
    see also index entry Radiation
Radius 856
    broken: Radius, fracture of
        856
    and Humerus 542; Ulna 1024;
        Wrist 1088
    part of Skeleton 914; *bones of
        the skeleton 915*
Radius, fracture of 856
Radon 856
    see also index entry Radiation
Ramipril 1121
Ramysis 1121
Ranitidine 857
Ranula 857
Rape 857
    causing Sexual desire,
        inhibited 904; Vaginismus
        1042
Rap-eze 1121

rapid breathing, abnormal:
    medical term:
        Hyperventilation 554
rapid eye movement (REM)
    sleep:
        see index entry REM sleep
Rapifen 1121
Rapitard MC 1121
Rapolyte 1121
Rash 857
    symptom charts 858, 859
RAST 860
    type of Immunoassay 570
Rastinon 1121
Rats, diseases from 860
    examples: Lassa fever 627;
        Leptospirosis 632; Plague
        807
Raynaud's disease 860
    treatment of: Nifedipine 731
    type of Peripheral vascular
        disease 793
Raynaud's phenomenon 861
    feature of Rheumatoid
        arthritis 876; Scleroderma
        892
    treatment of: Prazosin 821
Razoxane 1121
Razoxin 1121
R.B.C. 1121
RBC (red blood corpuscle):
    see index entry Blood cells
reading difficulty:
    a Learning difficulty 629
    medical term: Dyslexia 381
Reagent 861
recall:
    stage of Memory 674
Receding chin 861
    treatment of: Cosmetic
        surgery 313
Receptor 861
    and Stimulus 947
recessiveness (genetics):
    and Gene 473; Inheritance
        585
Recombinant DNA 862
    and Genetic engineering
        478
Reconstructive surgery:
    Arterial reconstructive
        surgery 130
    Plastic surgery 809
Recormon 1121
Recovery position 862
    *first aid: the recovery position
        863*
Rectal bleeding 862
    and Faeces, abnormal 430;
        Occult blood, faecal 743
rectal cancer:
    see index entry Rectum,
        cancer of
Rectal examination 862
    in diagnosis of Haemorrhoids
        502; Rectal bleeding 862;
        Rectum, cancer of 864
    techniques of: Proctoscopy
        830; Sigmoidoscopy 912
Rectal prolapse 862

Rectocele 862
    and Uterus, prolapse of 1037
Rectum 863
    disorders of: Proctitis 829;
        Rectal bleeding 862; Rectal
        prolapse 862; Rectum,
        cancer of 864; Ulcerative
        colitis 1023
    part of Intestine 596
    structure of the rectum 864
    see also index entry Rectal
        examination
Rectum, cancer of 864
    diagnosis of: Rectal
        examination 862
    symptoms of: Occult blood,
        faecal 743; Rectal bleeding
        862
red blood corpuscles (RBCs):
    see index entry Blood cells
Redeptin 1121
Red-eye 864
    alternative term:
        Conjunctivitis 296
Redoxon 1121
Reducing:
    Weight reduction 1080
Reduction 864
    in treatment of Fracture 460
Referred pain 864
    Pain 773
Reflex 864
    and *pain 773*
    simple knee-jerk reflex 865
Reflexology 865
Reflex, primitive 865
    types of primitive reflex 866
Reflux 865
    associated with
        Glomerulosclerosis 486
    causing Oesophagitis 747
    type of Nephropathy 722
    type of: Acid reflux 62
Refolinon 1121
Refraction 865
    testing of: Eye, examination of
        424; Vision tests 1059; *1060*
Regaine 1121
Regenerative cell therapy 865
Regression 865
    cause of: Frustration 464
    and Fixation 452
Regulan 1121
Reguletts 1121
Regurgitation 865
    see also index entry Reflux
Rehabilitation 866
Rehibin 1121
Rehidrat 1121
Rehydration therapy 866
Reimplantation, dental 866
Reiter's syndrome 866
    complication of Nonspecific
        urethritis 734
Rejection 867
    complication of Grafting 492;
        Transplant surgery 46, 1010
    and Tissue-typing 997
    prevention of: Azathioprine
        149; Corticosteroid drugs

312; Cyclosporin 326;
        Immunosuppressant drugs
        572
Relapse 867
Relapsing fever 867
Relaxation techniques 867
    examples: Meditation 670;
        Yoga 1092
Relaxit Micro-enema 1121
Relcofen 1121
releasing factors:
    example: Luteinizing
        hormone-releasing hormone
        651
    production of: Hypothalamus
        558
Relefact LH-RH 1121
Relifex 1121
Rem 867
    a radiation unit 851
Remedeine 1121
Remegel 1121
Remission 867
Remnos 1121
REM (rapid eye movement)
    sleep:
        and Dreaming 372
        type of Sleep 921
Remoxipride 1121
Renal 867
Renal biopsy:
    Kidney biopsy 613
Renal cell carcinoma 867
    type of Kidney cancer 613
Renal colic 867
    cause of: Calculus, urinary
        tract 225
    complication of Lithotripsy
        640
Renal failure:
    Kidney failure 614
Renal transplant:
    Kidney transplant 617
Renal tubular acidosis 867
Renin 868
    and Angiotensin 108
    production of: Kidney 613
Rennie 1121
Renography 868
Repetitive strain injury 868
    a type of Overuse injury 769
replantation microsurgery:
    techniques of microsurgery 688
repression:
    as Defence mechanism 335
    in Psychoanalytic theory 839
    and Resistance 869
Reproduction, sexual 868
Reproductive system, female 868
Reproductive system, male 868
    male reproductive system 869
Reproterol 1121
Resection 869
Resistance 869
Resiston One 1121
Resolve 1121
Resonium A 1121
Resorcinol 1121
Resorption, dental 869
Respacal 1121

Respiration 869, *871*
  and Breathing 208; Respiratory
    system 870
Respirator:
  Ventilator 1050
Respiratory arrest 869
  first aid: artificial respiration 134
Respiratory distress syndrome 870
  complication of Prematurity 825
  a disorder of the lung 649
  treatment of: Ventilation 1050
Respiratory failure 870
  causes of: Asthma 138;
    Emphysema 397; Flail chest
    452
  causing Hypoxia 560
  treatment of: Ventilator 1050
Respiratory function tests:
  Pulmonary function tests 844
Respiratory system 870
  function of: Breathing 208;
    Respiration 869, *871*
  parts of: Alveolus, pulmonary
    89; Bronchus 216;
    Diaphragm muscle 353;
    Epiglottis 410; Larynx 626;
    Lung 648; Mouth 697;
    anatomy of the mouth 698;
    Nasopharynx 718; Nose 734;
    Pharynx 798; *location of the
    pharynx 799;* Rib 879;
    Trachea 1006; *location of the
    trachea 1007*
Respiratory tract infection 870
Restandol 1121
Restless legs 870
  causing Insomnia 589
Restoration, dental 872
Restricted growth:
  Short stature 908
Resuscitation:
  Artificial respiration 134
  Cardiopulmonary resuscitation
    236; *first aid: cardiopulmonary
    resuscitation 237*
Retardation:
  Mental handicap 679
Reticular formation 872
  and Arousal 128;
    Consciousness 297;
    Unconsciousness 1028
  location of: Brainstem 202
reticulocyte:
  type of Blood cell 181
Reticulosarcoma 872
  modern term: Lymphoma,
    non-Hodgkin's 655
Retin-A 1121
Retina 872
  disorders of: *disorders of the eye
    426; disorders of the retina 873*
  function of: Vision 1057; *the
    sense of vision 1058*
  part of Eye 422; *anatomy of the
    eye 423*
Retinal artery occlusion 872
Retinal detachment 872
  causing Floaters 453
  following Retinal tear 874
Retinal haemorrhage 873

Retinal tear 873
Retinal vein occlusion 874
Retinitis 874
Retinitis pigmentosa 874
  causing Night blindness 731;
    Tunnel vision 1020
Retinoblastoma 874
  type of Eye tumour 427
Retinoids:
  Vitamin A 1062
Retinol 874
  form of Vitamin A 1062
Retinopathy 874
retinopathy of prematurity:
  alternative term: Retrolental
    fibroplasia 874
retinoscopy:
  type of Vision test 1059
Retractor 874
Retrobulbar neuritis 874
retrograde ejaculation:
  causing Infertility 853
  Ejaculation, disorders of 391
retrograde pyelography:
  type of Urography 1035
Retrolental fibroplasia 874
Retroperitoneal fibrosis 874
Retrosternal pain 874
retroverted uterus:
  Uterus, retroverted 1038
Retrovir 1121
retroviruses:
  example: HIV 537
  types of Viruses 1055
  viruses and disease 1056
Rett's syndrome 874
Reye's syndrome 875
  and Aspirin 137; Influenza 584
Rhabdomyolysis 875
rhabdomyomas:
  disorders of muscle 707
Rhabdomyosarcoma 875
  a disorder of muscle 707
Rhesus immunoglobulin:
  Anti-D(Rh$_o$) immunoglobulin
    117
Rhesus incompatibility 875
  causing Haemolytic disease of
    the newborn 500
  treatment of: Anti-D(Rh$_o$)
    immunoglobulin 117
Rhesus isoimmunization 876
Rhesus (Rh) factors:
  classification of Blood groups
    186
  and Anti-D(Rh$_o$)
    immunoglobulin 117;
    Haemolytic disease of the
    newborn 500; Rhesus
    incompatibility 875
Rheumacin LA 1121
Rheumatic fever 876
  affecting Heart valve 523
  following Scarlet fever 889
  and *disorders of the heart 517*
Rheumatism 876
  types of: Osteoarthritis 761;
    Polymyalgia rheumatica 816;
    Rheumatoid arthritis 876

Rheumatoid arthritis 876, *877*
  associated with Raynaud's
    phenomenon 861; Restless
    legs 872
  treatment of: Azathioprine
    149; Gold 489; Ibuprofen
    562; Indomethacin; 576;
    Ketoprofen 612;
    Penicillamine 788; Piroxicam
    804; Prednisolone 821;
    Prednisone 821;
Rheumatoid arthritis, juvenile 878
Rheumatoid spondylitis:
  Ankylosing spondylitis 110
Rheumatology 878
Rheumox 1121
Rhinitis 878
Rhinitis, allergic 878
Rhinocort 1121
Rhinolast 1121
Rhinophyma 879
  feature of Rosacea 882
Rhinoplasty 879
Rhinorrhoea 879
Rhumalgan 1121
Rhythm method:
  Contraception, natural
    methods of 304
Rib 879
  anatomy of: Skeleton 914; *bones
    of the skeleton 915;* Thorax 985
  disorders of: Flail chest 452;
    Rib, fracture of 880; Tietze's
    syndrome 994
Ribavirin 880
Rib, fracture of 880
Riboflavin 880
  part of Vitamin B complex 1064
ribonucleic acid (RNA):
  see index entry RNA
Rickets 880
  cause of: deficiency of
    Vitamin D 1065
  and Osteomalacia 763
Rickettsia 880
  causing Q fever 849; Rocky
    Mountain Spotted Fever
    881; Typhus 1022
  and Infectious disease 578
Ridaura 1121
Riedel's thyroiditis:
  type of Thyroiditis 993
Rifadin 1121
Rifampicin 880
Rifater 1121
Rifinah 150 1121
Rifinah 300 1121
Rigidity 880
Rigor 881
  symptom of Fever 443
Rigor mortis 881
Rimacid 1121
Rimacillin 1121
Rimactane 1121
Rimactazid 1121
Rimadol 1121
Rimafen 1121
Rimapam 1121
Rimapurinol 1121
Rimifon 1121

Rimiterol 881
Rimoxallin 1121
Rinatec 1121
Ringing in the ears:
  medical term: Tinnitus 994
Ringworm 881
  medical term: Tinea 994
Risperdal 1121
Risperidone 1121
Ritodrine 881
River blindness:
  medical term: Onchocerciasis
    751
Rivotril 1121
RNA 881
  function of: *what genes are and
    what they do 474;* Protein
    synthesis 835
  type of Nucleic acid 737
Roaccutane 1121
Ro-A-Vit 1121
Robaxin 750 1121
Robaxisal Forte 1121
Robb, George Peter:
  *landmarks in medicine: diagnosis
    669*
Robinul 1121
Robitussin 1121
Robitussin Plus 1121
Rocaltrol 1121
Roccal 1121
Rocephin 1121
Rock, John:
  *landmarks in medicine: drugs
    671*
Rocky Mountain Spotted Fever 881
  cause of: Rickettsia 880
Rodent ulcer 881
  alternative term: Basal cell
    carcinoma 160
Roentgenography:
  Radiology 853
  X-rays 1089
Roentgen, Wilhelm Conrad:
  discoverer of X-rays 34, 1089
  *landmarks in medicine: diagnosis
    669*
Roferon-A 1121
Rogitine 1121
Rohypnol 1121
role models:
  in Adolescence 68
Role-playing 881
Rommix 1121
Ronicol 1121
Root-canal treatment 881
rooting reflex:
  example of Reflex, primitive
    865
  types of primitive reflex 866
Rorschach test 882
Rosacea 882
  causing Rhinophyma 879
Roseola infantum 882
Rosoxacin 1121
Rotator cuff 882
  part of Shoulder 909
Roter 1121
Roughage:
  Fibre, dietary 446

Roundworms 882
　transmission of: Cats, diseases
　　from 243
　and Worm infestation 1086
Rowachol 1121
Roxiam 1121
RSI 883
　type of Overuse injury 769
Rubber dam 883
Rubella 883
　and Abortion, induced 57
　causing Birth defects 172;
　　disorders of the ear 384; Heart
　　disease, congenital 519;
　　Infection, congenital 577
　prevention of: MMR
　　vaccination 693; *typical*
　　childhood immunization
　　schedule 570
Rubeola 883
　alternative term: Measles 666
Running injuries 883
Rupture 883
　Hernia 530
Ruska, Ernst:
　landmarks in medicine: diagnosis
　　669
Rusyde 1122
Rynacrom 1122
Rynacrom Compound 1122
Rythmodan 1122

S

Sabril 1122
Sac 884
Saccharin 884
　type of Artificial sweetener 134
Sacralgia 884
Sacralization 884
sacral nerves:
　anatomy of the spinal nerves 936
Sacroiliac joint 884
　inflammation of: Sacroiliitis 884
　part of Pelvis 787
Sacroiliitis 884
Sacrum 884
　and Coccyx 284
　pain in: Sacralgia 884
　part of Pelvis 787; Skeleton
　　914; *bones of the skeleton 915;*
　　structure of the spine 937
Sadism 884
　feature of Sadomasochism 885
Sadomasochism 885
SADS 885
　Seasonal affective disorder
　　syndrome 895
Safe period:
　Contraception, natural
　　methods of 304
Safer sex 885
　and prevention of AIDS 77
safety at work 744
Saint Vitus' dance 885
　modern name: Sydenham's
　　chorea 964

Saizen 1122
Salactol 1122
Salamol 1122
Salatac 1122
Salazopyrin 1122
Salbulin 1122
Salbutamol 885
Salcatonin 1122
Salicylate drugs 885
Salicylic acid 885
Saline 885
Saliva 886
　excessive: Salivation, excessive
　　886
　insufficient: Mouth, dry 698
　production of: Salivary glands
　　886
Salivary glands 886
　types of: Parotid glands 782
salivary stones:
　a disorder of the Salivary
　　glands 886
Salivation, excessive 886
Salmeterol 1122
Salmonella infections 886
　causing Food poisoning 456;
　　Paratyphoid fever 781;
　　Typhoid fever 1022
salmon patch:
　alternative term: Stork mark 949
Salofalk 1122
Salpingectomy 887
Salpingitis 887
　associated with Peritonitis 794
　as complication of Non-
　　specific urethritis 733
Salpingo-oophorectomy 887
Salsalate 1122
Salt 887
　solution of: Saline 885
　see also index entry salt
　　(sodium chloride)
salt (sodium chloride):
　compound of Sodium 927
　excess of: Diet and disease
　　357; Hypertension 553
　loss of: Dehydration 337;
　　Diarrhoea 355; Heat cramps
　　524; Heat disorders 525;
　　Heat exhaustion 525;
　　Urination, excessive 1032
　retention of: Oedema 745
　uses of: Rehydration therapy
　　866; Saline 885
Saluric 1122
Salvarsan:
　development of: *landmarks in*
　　medicine: drugs 671
Salve 887
Salzone 1122
Sanctorius:
　landmarks in medicine: diagnosis
　　669
Sandfly bites 887
　and Insects and disease 588
Sandimmun 1122
Sandocal 1122
Sandoglobulin 1122
Sando-K 1122
Sandostatin 1122

Sanitary protection 887
Sanomigran 1122
Sarcoidosis 887
　variant of: Lupus pernio
　　651
Sarcoma 888
　type of Tumour 1020
Saturated fats:
　and Diet and disease 356;
　　Nutrition 738
　types of Fats 18; Fats and oils
　　436
satyriasis:
　and Nymphomania 741
Saventrine 1122
Scab 888
Scabies 888
Scald 888
　first aid: treating burns 219
　type of Burn 218
scalded skin syndrome:
　cause of: Staphylococcal
　　infections 944
　type of Necrolysis, toxic
　　epidermal 720
Scaling, dental 888
　in treatment of Gingivitis 482;
　　Gingivitis, acute ulcerative
　　482; Periodontitis 792
　use of: Oral hygiene 757;
　　Periodontics 792; Preventive
　　dentistry 828
Scalp 888
　dermatitis of: Cradle cap 317;
　　Dandruff 331
　ringworm of: Tinea 994
　swelling of: Cephalhaematoma
　　246; Sebaceous cyst 895;
　　Vacuum extraction 1040
Scalpel 888
scanning electron microscope
　(SEM):
　type of Microscope 686, 687
Scanning techniques 888
　types of Diagnostic techniques,
　　34–39; Imaging technique
　　564
　types of: CT scanning 323;
　　performing a CT scan 324;
　　MRI 700; PET scanning 797;
　　Radionuclide scanning 854;
　　Ultrasound scanning 1024;
　　how ultrasound scanning works
　　1025
　uses of: Diagnosing disease
　　30–31; *imaging the body 565*
Scaphoid 888
　part of Wrist 1088
Scapula 889
　and Acromioclavicular joint 64
　part of Shoulder 909; Skeleton
　　914; *bones of the skeleton 915*
Scar 889
　abnormal types of: Adhesion
　　67; Desmoid tumour 346;
　　Fibrosis 447; Keloid 610
　formation of: Healing 511
Scarlatina 889
　alternative term: Scarlet fever
　　889

Scarlet fever 889
　associated with Strep throat 950
　cause of: Streptococcal
　　infections 950
Schering PC4 1122
Scheriproct 1122
Schilling test:
　in diagnosis of Anaemia,
　　megaloblastic 99
Schistosome 889
　causing Schistosomiasis 889
　type of Flatworm 453;
　　Platyhelminth 809
Schistosomiasis 889
　cycle of schistosomiasis 890
　type of Water-borne infection
　　1077
Schizoid personality disorder 890
　and Somatotype 928
Schizophrenia 890
　type of Psychosis 840
Sciatica 891
　and *symptoms and treatment of*
　　disc prolapse 363;
　　Spondylolisthesis 940
Sciatic nerve 891
　disorder of: Sciatica 891
　location of the sciatic nerve 892
Scintigraphy 892
　alternative term: Radionuclide
　　scanning 854
Scirrhous 892
Sclera 892
　damage to: Eye injuries 425
　disorders of: Osteogenesis
　　imperfecta 763; Scleritis 892;
　　Scleromalacia 893
　part of Eye 422
Scleritis 892
Scleroderma 892
　symptom of: Raynaud's
　　phenomenon 861
Scleromalacia 893
sclerosing cholangitis:
　type of Cholangitis 270
Sclerosis 893
Sclerotherapy 893
　in treatment of Portal
　　hypertension 818; Varicose
　　veins 1044
Scoline 1122
Scoliosis 893
　affecting Walking 1072
　a disorder of the spine 938
Scopoderm TTS 1122
Scopolamine 1122
Scorpion stings 893
Scotoma 893
　type of Vision, disorder of
　　1059
scratching:
　cause of: Itching 605
　causing Lichenification 636;
　　Lichen simplex 636
Screening 24–27, 893
　types of: Antenatal screening
　　113; *antenatal screening*
　　procedures 112; Cancer
　　screening 230;
　　Mammography 660

Screening (continued)
    uses of: Antenatal care 112;
        Preventive medicine 828
Scrofula 893
Scrotum 893
    anatomy of the scrotum 894
    disorders of: Hydrocele 545;
        Pseudohermaphroditism
        836; Varicocele 1044
    part of Reproductive system,
        male 868, 869
    and Testis 977
Scuba-diving medicine 894
    and Air embolism 79;
        Barotrauma 159;
        Decompression sickness 334
Scurvy 895
    and Bleeding disorders 177
    cause of: deficiency of
        Vitamin C 1065
    symptom of: bleeding Gums
        497
Sealants, dental 895
    use of: Bonding, dental 191
Seasickness 895
    type of Motion sickness 696
Seasonal affective disorder
    syndrome 895
Sebaceous cyst 895
Sebaceous glands 895
    disorders of: Acne 62;
        Blackhead 174; Dermatitis
        344; Seborrhoea 895
    part of Skin 916
    producing Sebum 895
Seborrhoea 895
Seborrhoeic dermatitis:
    type of Dermatitis 344
seborrhoeic wart:
    alternative term: seborrhoeic
        Keratosis 611
Sebum 895
    overproduction of: Seborrhoea
        895
    production of: Sebaceous
        glands 895
Secadrex 1122
Seconal Sodium 1122
Secondary 896
    tumour: Metastasis 683
secondary sexual characteristics:
    Sexual characteristics,
        secondary 904
second teeth:
    Permanent teeth 794
secretin:
    effect on Gallbladder 467
    type of Gastrointestinal
        hormone 471
Secretion 896
secretory otitis media:
    alternative term: Glue ear 487
Sectioning 896
    and Mental Health Act 680
Sectral 1122
Security object 896
    and Attachment 143
Securon 1122
Securopen 1122
Sedation 896

Sedative drugs 896
Seizure 896
    causing Respiratory arrest 869
    feature of Epilepsy 410;
        Withdrawal syndrome
        1084
    types of: Convulsion, febrile
        306; Grand mal 492; Petit
        mal 797
Seldane 1122
Selegiline 1122
Selenium 896
    deficiency of: Kwashiorkor
        621
    type of Trace element 1006
Selenium sulphide 1122
self:
    psychoanalytic term: Ego 390
self-esteem:
    exaggerated: Superiority
        complex 960
    low: Inferiority complex 581
self-governing trust hospitals:
    Hospitals, types of 542
Self-help organizations 896
self-hypnosis:
    method of Hypnosis 555
Self-image 896
Self-injury 897
self-love:
    Narcissism 717
Selsun 1122
SEM (scanning electron
    microscope):
    type of Microscope *686, 687*
Semen 897
    and Ejaculation 391
    production of: Reproductive
        system, male 869
Semen, blood in the 897
semicircular canals:
    function of: Balance 155
    part of Ear 383
Semi-Daonil 1122
seminal fluid:
    constituent of Semen 897
    production of: Reproductive
        system, male 869
Seminal fluid analysis 897
    in diagnosis of Azoospermia
        149; Oligospermia 751
    use of: *investigating infertility
        582*
seminal vesicles:
    part of Reproductive system,
        male 869
seminiferous tubules:
    part of Testis 977
Seminoma:
    type of Testis, cancer of 978
Semitard MC 1122
Semprex 1122
Senile dementia:
    and Alzheimer's disease 90
    Dementia 338
senile purpura:
    type of Purpura 846
Senility 897
Senna 897
Senokot 1122

Sensate-focus technique 897
    type of Sex therapy 903
Sensation 898
    and Perception 791
    see also index entries Hearing;
        Smell; Taste; Touch; Vision
Sensation, abnormal 898
sensation, distorted:
    Illusion 564
sensation, loss of:
    alternative term: Numbness
        738
    induction of: Anaesthesia 99;
        Anaesthesia, dental 99;
        Anaesthesia, general 99;
        Anaesthesia, local 101;
        Nerve block 722
    type of Sensation, abnormal 899
Senses:
    and Sensation 898
    see also index entries Hearing;
        Smell; Taste; Touch; Vision
Sensitization 899
sensorineural deafness:
    assessment of: Hearing tests
        513
    type of Deafness 332
    type of: Presbyacusis 827
Sensory cortex 899
    and Sensation 898
Sensory deprivation 899
    causing Hallucination 504
sensory fibres:
    of Nerve 722; *nervous system
        724;* Spinal cord 934; Spinal
        nerves 936
sensory receptors:
    function of: Sensation 898
    part of *nervous system 724*
    types of receptor 861
sensory testing:
    neurological sensory testing 899
Separation anxiety 899
    causing Nightmare 731
Sepsis 900
Septal defect 900
    type of Heart disease,
        congenital 519
Septicaemia 900
    causing Septic shock 901
    and Puerperal sepsis 843;
        Sepsis 900; Toxaemia 1005
Septic shock 901
    causes of: Septicaemia 900;
        Toxaemia 1005
Septrin 1122
Septum 901
    of nose: Nasal septum 718
    part of Heart 514
Sequela 901
Sequestration 901
Serc 1122
Serenace 1122
Serevent 1122
Serology 901
Serophene 1122
Serotonin 901
    excess of: Carcinoid syndrome
        234
    type of Neurotransmitter 729

Seroxat 1122
Sertraline 1122
Sertürner, Friedrich:
    landmarks in medicine: drugs 671
Serum 901
serum hepatitis:
    Hepatitis, viral *528,* 529
Serum sickness 902
    cause of: Hypersensitivity 551
Setlers 1122
Sevredol 1122
Sex 902
    see also index entries female
        gender; male gender; Sexual
        intercourse
Sex change 902
    in treatment of Transsexualism
        1011
Sex chromosomes 902
    abnormal number of:
        Chromosomal abnormalities
        276
    and Inheritance 585; Sex
        determination 903
    types of Chromosome 277
Sex determination 903
    see also index entry Sex
        chromosomes
Sex hormones 903
Sex-linked inheritance 903
    and Genetic disorders 477;
        Inheritance 585; X-linked
        disorders 1089
Sex therapy 903
    in treatment of Psychosexual
        dysfunction 840
    type of: Sensate-focus
        technique 897
Sexual abuse 904
    types of: Child abuse 260;
        Rape 857
Sexual characteristics, secondary
    904
    development of: Puberty 841;
        changes of puberty 842; Sex
        determination 903
sexual desire, exaggerated:
    medical term: Nymphomania
        740
Sexual desire, inhibited 904
    treatment of: Sensate-focus
        technique 897; Sex therapy
        903
    type of Psychosexual
        dysfunction 840
Sexual deviation:
    Deviation, sexual 347
Sexual dysfunction:
    Psychosexual dysfunction
        840
Sexual intercourse 904, *905*
    and Child abuse 261;
        Deviation, sexual 347; Incest
        574; Rape 857; Sexually
        transmitted diseases 904
    after Hysterectomy 561
    painful: Intercourse, painful
        592; *painful intercourse in men
        592; painful intercourse in
        women 593*

during Pregnancy 823
see also index entry Sexual problems
Sexuality 904
in Psychoanalytic theory 838
and Transsexualism 1011
types of: Bisexuality 173; Heterosexuality 533; Homosexuality, male 540; Lesbianism 632
Sexually transmitted diseases 904
and Contact tracing 301; Rape 857
examples: AIDS 76; *cumulative totals of AIDS cases reported in the UK 906*; Chancroid 255; Chlamydial infections 268; Gonorrhoea 490; *incidence of gonorrhoea in England 906*; Herpes, genital 532; Lymphogranuloma venereum 655; Nonspecific urethritis 733; Pubic lice 842; Syphilis 966; *incidence of syphilis in England 906*; Trichomoniasis 1015; Warts, genital 1075
Sexual problems 906
examples: Ejaculation, disorders of 391; Impotence 574; Infertility 581; *investigating infertility 582*; Intercourse, painful 592; *painful intercourse in men 592*; *painful intercourse in women 593*; Orgasm, lack of 758; Psychosexual dysfunction 840; Sexual desire, inhibited 904; Transsexualism 1011; Vaginismus 1042
treatment of: Penile implant 788; Sensate-focus technique 897; Sex therapy 903
Sézary syndrome 907
shaking:
medical term: Tremor 1013
sheath:
alternative term: Condom 295
Shellfish poisoning:
Food poisoning 456
Shell shock:
Post-traumatic stress disorder 819
Shigellosis 907
and Dysentery 381
shin bone:
medical term: Tibia 993
Shingles:
Herpes zoster 532
Shin splints 907
type of Running injury 883
Shivering 907
and Temperature 973
Shock 907
first aid: shock 908
types of: Anaphylactic shock 103; Electrical injury 393; Septic shock 901; Shock, electric 908; Toxic shock syndrome 1005

Shock, electric 908
first aid: electrical injury 392
type of Electrical injury 393
use of: ECT 388
Shock therapy 908
type of: ECT 388
shock-wave treatment:
medical term: Lithotripsy 45, 640
Shortsightedness:
medical term: Myopia 714
Short sight, operations for:
see index entries: Keratotomy, radial and Laser treatment
Short stature 908
and Growth, childhood 496
treatment of: Growth hormone 496; Nandrolone 717
Shoulder 909
disorders of: Frozen shoulder 464; Painful arc syndrome 774; Shoulder, dislocation of 909; Shoulder-hand syndrome 910
muscles of: Deltoid 338; Rotator cuff 882
a *type of joint 608*
Shoulderblade 909
medical term: Scapula 889
Shoulder, dislocation of 909
and Klumpke's paralysis 619
Shoulder-hand syndrome 910
Shunt 910
and *procedure for dialysis 352*
in treatment of Hydrocephalus 546; Portal hypertension 818; Spina bifida 934
Shy-Drager syndrome 910
SIADH 910
Siamese twins 910
type of Twins 1021
Sibling rivalry 910
Sicard, Jean Athanase:
landmarks in medicine: diagnosis 669
Sick building syndrome 911
Sickle cell anaemia 911
a *disorder of the blood 185*
type of Anaemia, haemolytic 97
Sick sinus syndrome 911
type of Arrhythmia, cardiac 129
Side-effect 911
of Drugs 376
Siderosis 912
SIDS 912
abbreviation for Sudden infant death syndrome 957
Sievert 912
a *radiation unit 851*
Sight:
see index entry Vision
Sigmoid colon 912
examination of: Sigmoidoscopy 912
part of Colon 289; Intestine 596
Sigmoidoscopy 912
in diagnosis of Colitis 288; Colon, cancer of 289; Ulcerative colitis 1023

Sign 912
and Symptom 964; Syndrome 965; Vital sign 1061
Silicone 912
implant: *types of implants 573*
Silicosis 913
a *disorder of the lung 649*
type of Pneumoconiosis 811
Silver sulphadiazine 913
Simeco 1122
Simplene 1122
Simpson, James:
landmarks in medicine: surgery 670
Simvastatin 913
Sinemet 1122
Sinequan 1122
Sinew 913
medical term: Tendon 975
Singer's nodes 913
a *disorder of the larynx 627*
single photon emission computerized tomography (SPECT):
type of Radionuclide scanning 854
Sinoatrial node 913
abnormal functioning of: *cardiac arrhythmia 129*; Sick sinus syndrome 911; Sinus bradycardia 913; Sinus tachycardia 914; Supraventricular tachycardia 961
and Pacemaker 771
part of Heart 514
Sinthrome 1122
Sinus 913
see also index entry Sinus, facial
Sinus bradycardia 913
type of Arrhythmia, cardiac 129
Sinus, facial 913
effect of pressure on: Aviation medicine 148; Barotrauma 159
inflammation of: Sinusitis 913
location and function of the sinuses 914
Sinusitis 913
cause of: Cold, common 286
treatment of: Decongestant drugs 335; Oxymetazoline 770; Phenylpropanolamine 800
Sinus tachycardia 914
type of Arrhythmia, cardiac 129
Sinutab 1122
Situs inversus 914
Sjögren's syndrome 914
causing Keratoconjunctivitis sicca 611; Mouth, dry 698
skeletal muscle:
type of Muscle 704; *the body's muscles 705*
Skeleton 914
bones of the skeleton 915
Skin 915
aging of: Age spots 73; Aging 74; Wrinkle 1088

colour of: Melanin 673; Pigmentation 803
disorders of the skin 919
function of: Sensation 898; Touch 1003; *sense of touch 1004*
structure of: Sebaceous glands 895; *structure of skin 916*; Sweat glands 963
study of: Dermatology 344
Skin allergy 916
Skin biopsy 916
type of Biopsy 170
Skin cancer 917
cause of: Sunlight, adverse effects of 960
treatment of: Cryosurgery 322; Radiotherapy 855
Skin flap 917
use of: Plastic surgery 809
Skin graft 917
types of skin graft 918
use of: Plastic surgery 809
Skinoren 1122
Skin patch:
Transdermal patch 1009
Skin peeling, chemical 918
Skin tag 918
Skin tests 918
in diagnosis of Allergy 86; Rhinitis, allergic 879
type of: Tuberculin tests 1018
Skin tumours 918
disorders of the skin 919
type of: Skin cancer 917
treatment of: Radiotherapy 855
Skull 919
operations on: Burr hole 220; Craniotomy 318; Trephine 1013
part of Skeleton 914; *bones of the skeleton 915*
parts of: Fontanelle 454; Jaw 606; *types of joints 608*; Maxilla 666; Sinus, facial 913; *structure of the skull 920*; Sphenoid bone 932; Suture 962
Skull, fracture of 920
diagnosis of: Skull X-ray 921
type of Head injury 510
Skull X-ray 921
"slapped cheek" disease:
medical term: Fifth disease 448
SLE (systemic lupus erythematosus) 921
see also index entry Lupus erythematosus
Sleep 921
disorders of: Insomnia 589; Jet-lag 609; Narcolepsy 717; Nightmare 731; Night terror 731; Sleep apnoea 922; Sleep paralysis 923; Sleepwalking 923
and Dreaming 372; Snoring 927
ejaculation during: Nocturnal emission 732

Sleep apnoea 922
  causing Insomnia 589
  feature of: Snoring 927
Sleep deprivation 922
Sleeping drugs 922
  types of: Barbiturate drugs
    156; Benzodiazepine drugs
    163; Sedative drugs 896
sleeping sickness (form of
  encephalitis):
  medical term: Encephalitis
    lethargica 399
Sleeping sickness (tropical
  disease) 923
  transmission of: Tsetse fly
    bites 1018
  type of Trypanosomiasis
    1018
Sleep paralysis 923
  feature of Narcolepsy 717
Sleep terror:
  Night terror 731
Sleepwalking 923
"slimmer's disease":
  medical term: Anorexia
    nervosa 111
Slimming:
  Weight reduction 1080
Sling 923
  first aid: arm sling 924
Slipped disc:
  Disc prolapse 362
Slipped femoral epiphysis:
  Femoral epiphysis, slipped
    438
Slit lamp 924
  use of: Eye, examination of
    424
Slo-Indo 1122
Slo-Phyllin 1122
Sloprolol 1122
Slough 924
Slow-Fe 1122
Slow-Fe Folic 1122
Slow-K 1122
Slow-Trasicor 1122
Slow virus diseases 924
  types of: Creutzfeldt-Jakob
    disease 319; Kuru 621
Small cell carcinoma 924
  type of Lung cancer 649
small intestine:
  parts of: Duodenum 379;
    Ileum 563; location of the
    ileum 564; Jejunum 607
  surgical opening into:
    Ileostomy 562; procedure for
    ileostomy 563
  see also index entry Intestine
Smallpox 924
  vaccination against:
    Immunization against
    disease 28; landmarks in
    medicine: drugs 671
Smear 924
  types of: Blood film 186;
    Cervical smear test 251;
    procedure for a cervical smear
    252
Smegma 924

Smell 925
  function of Cerebrum 250;
    Nose 734; Olfactory nerve
    750
  and Taste 970
Smelling salts 926
Smoking:
  of Marijuana 662
  see also index entry Tobacco-
    smoking
smooth muscle:
  type of Muscle 706; the body's
    muscles 705
Snails and disease 926
Snake bites 926
Sneezing 926
Snellen chart 926
  use of: Eye, examination of
    424
Sno Phenicol 1122
Sno Pilo 1122
Snoring 927
  associated with Sleep apnoea
    922
Sno Tears 1122
Snow blindness 927
  type of Keratopathy 611
Snuff 927
  causing Mouth cancer 698
Snuffles 927
Social skills training 927
Sociopathy 927
  modern term: Antisocial
    personality disorder 119
Soda mint tablets 1122
Sodium 927
  type of Ion 601
  see also index entry Salt
Sodium Amytal 1122
Sodium aurothiomalate 927
Sodium bicarbonate 927
Sodium cellulose phosphate 1122
sodium chloride:
  see index entry salt (sodium
    chloride)
Sodium citrate 1122
Sodium clodronate 1122
Sodium cromoglycate 927
  in treatment of Asthma 139;
    Rhinitis, allergic 879
Sodium fluoride 1122
Sodium fusidate 1122
Sodium ironedetate 1122
Sodium nitroprusside 1122
Sodium picosulphate 1122
Sodium stibogluconate 1122
Sodium valproate 928
Sofradex 1122
Soframycin 1122
soft chancre:
  alternative term: Chancroid
    255
  type of Ulcer 1023
soft palate:
  part of Palate 774
  and Uvula 1039
Soft-tissue injury 928
Soiling 928
  type of: Encopresis 399
Solarcaine 1123

solar keratosis:
  type of Keratosis 611
Solar plexus 928
Solpadeine 1123
Solpadol 1123
Solu-Cortef 1123
Solu-Medrone 1123
Solvazinc 1123
Solvent abuse 928
Somatic 928
Somatization disorder 928
Somatotype 928
  body types and personality 929
Somatropin 929
Sominex 1123
Somnambulism:
  Sleepwalking 923
Somnite 1123
Soneryl 1123
Soni-Slo 1123
sonography:
  alternative term: Ultrasound
    scanning 1024
Sorbichew 1123
Sorbid SA 1123
sorbitol:
  type of Artificial sweetener 135
Sorbitrate 1123
Sore 929
Sore throat 929
  causes of: Pharyngitis 798;
    Tonsillitis 1002
Sotacor 1123
Sotalol 1123
Sotazide 1123
Sovol 1123
Space medicine 929
Sparine 1123
Spasm 929
Spasmonal 1123
spastic colon:
  alternative term: Irritable
    bowel syndrome 603
Spasticity 930
  and Muscle 706
Spastic paralysis 930
  feature of Cerebral palsy 248
  type of Paralysis 778
SP Cold Relief 1123
Specific gravity 930
  and Density 339
Specimen 930
  and Biopsy 169; Staining 943
SPECT 930
  type of Radionuclide scanning
    854
  use of: Brain imaging 202
Spectacles:
  Glasses 483
Spectinomycin 1123
Spectraban 1123
Speculum 930
  use of: procedure for a cervical
    smear 252; procedure for pelvic
    examination 786
Speech 930
  delay in: Developmental delay
    347
  language and speech development
    in childhood 931

Speech disorders 930
  types of: Aphasia 124;
    Dysarthria 380; Dysphasia
    382; Dysphonia 382;
    Stuttering 955
speech, oesophageal:
  following Laryngectomy 625
Speech therapy 931
  following Laryngectomy 625;
    Stroke 954
  in treatment of Stuttering 955
Sperm 932
  abnormal production of:
    Azoospermia 149; Infertility
    583; investigating infertility
    582; Oligospermia 750
  investigation of: Seminal fluid
    analysis 897
  production of: Reproductive
    system, male 868, 869; Testis
    977
  role of: Fertility 439;
    Fertilization 440; the process
    of fertilization 441
Spermatocele 932
Spermatozoa:
  see index entry Sperm
sperm duct:
  medical term: Vas deferens
    1046
Spermicides 932
  use of: Contraception, barrier
    methods of 302; Sponge,
    contraceptive 940
Sphenoid bone 932
  part of Skull 919; structure of
    the skull 920
Spherocytosis, hereditary 932
  a unifactorial genetic disorder 477
Sphincter 933
  of Anus 121; Oesophagus 748;
    Stomach 948
  type of Muscle 704
Sphincter, artificial 933
Sphincterotomy 933
Sphygmomanometer 933
  in measurement of Blood
    pressure 187; taking the blood
    pressure 24
Spider bites 933
Spider naevus 933
  type of Telangiectasia 973
Spina bifida 933
  types of spina bifida 934
Spinal anaesthesia 934
spinal canal decompression:
  Decompression, spinal canal
    334
Spinal cord 934
  part of Nervous system 723, 724
  location of the spinal cord 935
  and Spinal nerves 936
  X-ray of: Myelography 712
Spinal fusion 935
Spinal injury 935
  type of: Whiplash injury 1082
Spinal nerves 936
  part of nervous system 724
Spinal tap:
  Lumbar puncture 648

Spine 937
  anatomy of: Coccyx 284; Disc,
    intervertebral 361; Sacrum
    884; Vertebra 1052; *location
    and structure of the vertebrae
    1053*
  disorders of the spine 938
Spirochaete 937
  type of Bacteria 153
Spiroctan 1123
Spirolone 1123
Spirometry 937
  type of Pulmonary function
    test 844
Spironolactone 938
Spirospare 1123
Spleen 938
  overactivity of: Hypersplenism
    551
  removal of: Splenectomy 939
Splenectomy 939
Splint 939
  uses of: Splinting 939;
    Splinting, dental 939
Splinting 939
Splinting, dental 939
Split personality 939
  medical term: Multiple
    personality 702
Spondylitis 939
Spondylolisthesis 940
  a *disorder of the spine 938*
  treatment of: Spinal fusion 935
Spondylolysis 940
  causing Spondylolisthesis 940
spondylosis:
  Cervical spondylosis 252
Sponge, contraceptive 940
  causing Toxic shock syndrome
    1005
  type of Contraception, barrier
    method 302
spontaneous abortion:
  common term: Miscarriage
    690
Sporanox 1123
Sporotrichosis 940
  type of Fungal infection 464
Sports, drugs and 940
Sports injuries 941
Sports medicine 941
Spot 941
  and Rash 857
"spotting":
  alternative term: Breakthrough
    bleeding 204
Sprain 941
  first aid: sprains 942
Sprilon 1123
Sprue 941
  type of: Sprue, tropical 941
Sprue, tropical 941
Sputum 941
Squamous cell carcinoma 941
  type of Lung cancer 649; Skin
    cancer 917
squamous cells:
  of Endothelium 405;
    Epithelium 413
squeeze technique 903

Squint 942
  cause of: Retinoblastoma 874
SRM-Rhotard 1123
Stabillin V-K 1123
Stable 943
Stafoxil 1123
Stage 943
  in diagnosis of Hodgkin's
    disease 539; Lymphoma,
    non-Hodgkin's 655
Staining 943
  using Gram's stain 492
staining, tooth:
  Discoloured teeth 362
Stammering:
  Stuttering 955
Stanford-Binet test 943
  type of Intelligence test 591
Stanozolol 943
Stapedectomy 943
  in treatment of Otosclerosis
    767
Stapes 943
  part of Ear 383
  removal of: Stapedectomy 943
Staphylococcal infections 944
Starch:
  type of Carbohydrate 19, 232
Staril 1123
Starvation 944
  causing Ketosis 612
  Diet and disease 356
Stasis 944
Statistics, medical 944
Statistics, vital 944
Status asthmaticus 944
Status epilepticus 944
  type of Epilepsy 411
Staycept pessaries 1123
STDs:
  abbreviation for Sexually
    transmitted diseases 904
Steatorrhoea 944
Steinberg, Israel:
  *landmarks in medicine: diagnosis
    669*
Stein-Leventhal syndrome:
  Ovary, polycystic 768
Stelazine 1123
Stemetil 1123
Stenosis 944
stepping reflex:
  type of Reflex, primitive 865;
    types of primitive reflex 866
Steptoe, Patrick:
  *landmarks in medicine: other
    forms of treatment 670*
Sterculia 1123
stereoscopic vision:
  and Vision 1059; *the sense of
    vision 1058*
Stereotaxic surgery 944
  use of: Psychosurgery 840
Sterexidine 1123
Sterility 945
  and Infertility 581
Sterilization 945
Sterilization, female 945
Sterilization, male:
  Vasectomy 1046

Steri-Neb Cromogen 1123
Steri-Neb Salamol 1123
Steripod Chlorhexidine 1123
Sternum 946
Steroid drugs 946
Steroids, anabolic 946
  abuse of: Sports, drugs and
    940
Stesolid 1123
Stethoscope 946
  development of: *landmarks in
    medicine: diagnosis 669*
  use of: Auscultation 144; *taking
    the blood pressure 24;*
    Examination, physical 33,
    419
Stevens-Johnson syndrome 946
  type of Erythema multiforme
    415
Sticky eye 946
Stiedex 1123
Stiedex LPN 1123
Stiemycin 1123
Stiff neck 946
  feature of Meningitis 675
  types of: Neck rigidity 720;
    Torticollis 1003
Stiffness 946
  after death: Rigor mortis 881
  of joints: Arthritis 131;
    Rheumatoid arthritis 876
  of muscles: Rigidity 880;
    Spasticity 930
  see also index entry Stiff neck
Stilboestrol 947
Stillbirth 947
  as complication of
    Postmaturity 818
Still's disease:
  Rheumatoid arthritis, juvenile
    878
Stimulant drugs 947
  abuse of: Sports, drugs and
    940
  example: Caffeine 221
  types of: Amphetamine drugs
    94
Stimulus 947
Stings 947
  types of: Insect stings 588;
    Jellyfish stings 607;
    Scorpion stings 893;
    Venomous bites and stings
    1050
Stitch 948
stitch (surgical):
  Suturing 962
Stokes-Adams syndrome 948
Stoma 948
  in Colostomy 290; Ileostomy
    563; Laryngectomy 625
Stomach 948
  disorders of the stomach 949
  function of: *the digestive process
    358*
  hormones of: Gastrointestinal
    hormones 471
  investigations of: Barium X-ray
    examinations 157;
    Gastroscopy 471

  part of Digestive system 357
  removal of: Gastrectomy 469
  surgical opening into:
    Gastrostomy 472
Stomach-ache 948
  Abdominal pain 50, *51;
    recurrent abdominal pain 53;*
    Indigestion 576
Stomach cancer 948
  a *disorder of the stomach 949*
Stomach imaging:
  Barium X-ray examinations
    157
Stomach pump:
  Lavage, gastric 628
Stomach ulcer 949
  type of Peptic ulcer 789; *sites
    and causes of peptic ulcer
    790*
Stomatitis 949
Stones 949
  types of: Calculus, urinary
    tract 224; Gallstones 468
Stool 949
  alternative term: Faeces 429
Stork mark 949
  type of Haemangioma 498
Strabismus:
  Squint 942
Strain 949
  first aid: strain 950
Strangulation 950
Strangury 950
  feature of Urination, painful
    1034
Strapping 950
Strawberry naevus 950
  type of Haemangioma 498
Streptase 1123
Strep throat 950
  cause of: Streptococcal
    infections 950
Streptococcal infections 950
Streptokinase 950
Streptomycin 951
  causing Deafness 332
Stress 951
  associated with *hypertension
    552*
  treatment of: Meditation 670;
    Meprobamate 680;
    Relaxation techniques 867;
    Stress control 17
Stress fracture 951
  type of Running injury 883
stress incontinence:
  Incontinence, urinary 575
Stress ulcer 951
Stretcher 951
  using a stretcher 952
Stretch-mark 951
  medical term: Stria 951
Stria 951
  appearance of striae 952
Stricture 952
Stridor 952
  feature of Croup 321;
    Epiglottitis 410
  investigation of: Laryngoscopy
    625

Stroke 952
  and Alcohol 82
  types and causes of stroke 953
Stroma 954
Stromba 1123
Strongyloidiasis 954
  cause of: Roundworms 883;
    *diseases caused by roundworms
    (nematodes) 882*
Strontium 954
  source of Radiation 852
Strychnine poisoning 954
Stuffy nose:
  Nasal congestion 717
Stugeron 1123
Stump 954
  and Amputation 94; Limb,
    artificial 637; *types of artificial
    limb 638*
Stupor 955
  type of: Narcosis 717
Sturge-Weber syndrome 955
Stuttering 955
St. Vitus' dance:
  modern term: Sydenham's
    chorea 964
Stye 955
Subacute 955
Subarachnoid haemorrhage 955
Subclavian steal syndrome 956
Subclinical 956
Subconjunctival haemorrhage 956
Subconscious 956
  and Consciousness 297;
    Unconscious 1028
Subcutaneous 956
subdural haematoma:
  type of Haematoma 499
Subdural haemorrhage 956
Sublimation 956
  and Psychoanalytic theory 839
Sublimaze 1123
sublingual glands:
  Salivary glands 886
Subluxated tooth 956
Subluxation 956
submandibular glands:
  Salivary glands 886
Submucous resection 957
Subphrenic abscess 957
  type of Abscess 58
substance abuse:
  types of: Drug abuse 376;
    Drug dependence 377;
    Heroin abuse 531; Solvent
    abuse 928
Substrate 957
Sucking chest wound 957
Sucralfate 957
Suction 957
  use of: Ventilation 1050
Suction lipectomy 957
  use of: Body contour surgery
    190
Sudafed 1123
Sudafed-Co 1123
Sudafed Expectorant 1123
Sudafed Plus 1123
Sudden death:
  Death, sudden 333

Sudden infant death
  syndrome 957
Sudden infant death syndrome
  (SIDS) 957
  cause of: Sleep apnoea 922
Sudeck's atrophy 957
Sudocrem 1123
Suffocation 958
Sugar:
  type of Carbohydrate 19, 232
Suicide 958
  suicide rates 959
Suicide, attempted 958
sulci:
  of Brain 198; Cerebrum 249
Sulconazole 1123
Suleo-C 1123
Suleo-M 1123
Sulfadoxine 1123
Sulfametopyrazine 1123
Sulindac 959
Sulphadiazine 1123
Sulphadimidine 1123
Sulphamethoxazole 1123
Sulphasalazine 959
Sulphinpyrazone 959
Sulphonamide drugs 959
  group of Antibacterial drugs
    114
  landmarks in medicine: drugs 671
Sulphur 959
Sulpiride 959
Sulpitil 1123
Sultrin 1123
Sumatriptan 959
Sunburn 959
sunlight:
  abnormal reaction to:
    Photosensitivity 801
  component of: Ultraviolet light
    1026
  effects of: Sunburn 959;
    Sunlight, adverse effects of
    959; Suntan 960
  protection from: Sunscreens
    960
  treatment with: Phototherapy
    801
  and Vitamin D 1065
Sunlight, adverse effects of 959
Sunscreens 960
Sunstroke 960
  type of Heatstroke 526
Suntan 960
Superego 960
  and Freudian theory 462;
    Psychoanalytic theory 839
Superficial 960
Superinfection 960
Superiority complex 960
Supernumerary 960
  teeth: Supernumerary teeth 961
Supernumerary teeth 961
Supination 961
  and Pronation 831
Suppository 961
  use of: Haemorrhoids 502
Suppuration 961
Suprarenal glands 961
  Adrenal glands 69

Supraspinatus syndrome:
  Painful arc syndrome 774
Supraventricular tachycardia 961
  type of Arrhythmia, cardiac
    129
Suprax 1123
Suprecur 1123
Suprefact 1123
Surfactant 961
  abnormality of: Sudden infant
    death syndrome 957
  deficiency of: Respiratory
    distress syndrome 870
Surfer's nodules 961
Surgam 1123
Surgery 961
  and Operating theatre 752;
    Operation 753; Surgical
    implants 46; Surgical
    treatment 46
  history of: *landmarks in
    medicine: surgery 670;*
    Surgical treatment 41
  pain relief during:
    Anaesthesia, dental 99;
    Anaesthesia, general 99;
    *techniques for general
    anaesthesia 100;* Anaesthesia,
    local 101
  types of: Cosmetic surgery
    313; Cryosurgery 322;
    Endoscopic surgery 47;
    Laser surgery 47;
    Microsurgery 47, 687;
    Neurosurgery 728; Plastic
    surgery 809; Transplant
    surgery 46, 1010
Surgical spirit 961
Surmontil 1123
Surrogacy 961
Suscard, Sustac 1123
Susceptibility 962
  and Histocompatibility
    antigens 536
  increase of: Immunodeficiency
    disorders 571
Sustamycin 1123
Sustanon 1123
Suture 962
  of Skull 919
  types of joints 608
  see also index entry Suturing
Suturing 962
Suxamethonium 1123
Swab 963
Swallowing 963
  and Digestive system 359; *the
    digestive process 358*
Swallowing difficulty 963
  causes of: Guillain-Barré
    syndrome 496; Larynx,
    cancer of 626; Myasthenia
    gravis 710; Oesophageal
    atresia 746; Oesophageal
    spasm 747; Oesophageal
    stricture 747; Oesophagus,
    cancer of 748; Pharynx,
    cancer of 799; Plummer-
    Vinson syndrome 810;
    Tonsillitis 1002

investigation of: Barium X-ray
    examinations 157;
    Laryngoscopy 625
  and Accessory nerve 59;
    Vagus nerve 1043
Swamp fever 963
Sweat glands 963
  disorders of: Hyperhidrosis
    548; Hypohidrosis 556
  part of Skin 916
  see also index entry Sweating
Sweating 963
  and Body odour 190; Heat
    disorders 525; Oliguria 751;
    Shy-Drager syndrome 910;
    Water 1076
  feature of Menopause 676;
    Tuberculosis 1019
  see also index entry Sweat
    glands
Sweeteners, artificial:
  Artificial sweeteners 134
Swimmer's ear 964
  medical term: Otitis externa
    766
Sycosis barbae 964
  type of Folliculitis 454
Sydenham's chorea 964
  cause of: Rheumatic fever 876
Sydenham, Thomas:
  landmarks in medicine: drugs 671
sylvian fissure:
  part of Cerebrum 249
Symmetrel 1123
Sympathectomy 964
  in treatment of Hyperhidrosis
    548; Raynaud's disease 861
Sympathetic nervous system 964
  and Hypothalamus 558
  part of Autonomic nervous
    system 146; *functions of the
    autonomic nervous system
    147*
sympatholytic drugs:
  types of Vasodilator drugs
    1047
Symphysis 964
Symptom 964
  and Sign 912; Syndrome 965
Symptothermal method:
  Contraception, natural
    methods of 304
Synacthen 1123
Synalar 1123
Synalar C 1123
Synalar N 1123
Synapse 965
  structure of a neuron 727
  and Neurotransmitter 729
Synarel 1123
Syndol 1124
Syndrome 965
  and Symptom 964
syndrome of inappropriate
  antidiuretic hormone
  secretion:
    SIADH 910

Synflex 1124
Synkavit 1124
Synovectomy 965
synovial sheaths:
    of Hand 505; Tendon 975
Synovitis 965
Synovium 965
    inflammation of: Synovitis 965
    location of synovium 966
    part of Joint 609; *types of joints 608*
    removal of: Synovectomy 965
Synphase 1124
Syntaris 1124
Syntex Menophase 1124
Synthetic drugs 43
    see also index entry Drug
Syntocinon 1124
Syntometrine 1124
Syntopressin 1124
Syphilis 966
    complication of: Neurosyphilis 729
    a Sexually transmitted disease 904
    incidence of syphilis in England 906
    treatment of: *landmarks in medicine: drugs 671*
Syphilis, nonvenereal 967
Syringe 967
Syringing of ears 967
Syringomyelia 967
System 967
Systemic 967
Systemic lupus erythematosus (SLE):
    type of Lupus erythematosus 651
systemic sclerosis:
    alternative term: Scleroderma 892
Systole 967
    and Diastole 355; Heart 514
systolic blood pressure:
    abnormally high: Hypertension 551
    and Blood pressure 187
Sytron 1124

T

T_3:
    type of Thyroid hormone 991
T_4:
    abbreviation for Thyroxine 993
    type of Thyroid hormone 991
Tabes dorsalis 968
    as complication of Neurosyphilis 729; Syphilis 966
Tachycardia 968
    symptom of Coronary artery disease 310
    type of Arrhythmia, cardiac 129

Tachypnoea 968
Tacrine:
    Tetrahydroaminoacridine 981
Tagamet 1124
T'ai chi 968
Talipes 968
    effect on Walking 1072
Tambocor 1124
Tamofen, Tamofen 20, Tamofen 40 1124
Tamoxifen 968
Tampon 968
    causing Toxic shock syndrome 1005; Vaginal discharge 1041; Vaginitis 1042 and tearing of Hymen 547
    type of Sanitary protection 887
Tamponade 968
    cause of: Pericarditis 791
Tampovagan Stilboestrol and Lactic Acid 1124
Tan:
    Suntan 960
Tancolin 1124
Tanderil 1124
Tannin 968
Tantrum 969
    type of Behavioural problem in children 162
Tapeworm infestation 969
    treatment of: Niclosamide 730; Praziquantel 821
    type of Worm infestation 1086
tar:
    as Carcinogen 233
    causing Occupational disease and injury 743; Squamous cell carcinoma 942
    and Effects of tobacco 22; Tobacco-smoking 998
Tarcortin 1124
Targocid 1124
Tarivid 1124
Tarsalgia 969
Tarsorrhaphy 969
    in treatment of Corneal ulcer 308
Tartar:
    alternative term: Calculus, dental 224
tartrazine:
    type of Food additive 455
Taste 970
    associated with Smell 925
    and Facial nerve 428; Glossopharyngeal nerve 487; Tongue 1000
taste-buds:
    part of Tongue 1000
    and *the sense of taste 970*
Taste, loss of 970
Tattooing 971
Tavegil 1124
Tay-Sachs disease 971
    a disorder of the brain 200
Tazobactam 1124

Tazocin 1124
TB:
    abbreviation for Tuberculosis 1019
T-cell 971
    type of Blood cell 182; Lymphocyte 653
Tears 971
    deficiency of: Keratoconjunctivitis sicca 611
    excess of: Watering eye 1077
    production of: Eye 423; Lacrimal apparatus 622; *functions of the lacrimal apparatus 623*
Tears, artificial 971
    in treatment of Keratoconjunctivitis sicca 611
Technetium 971
    use of: Radionuclide scanning 35
Teejel 1124
Teeth 971
    disorders of: Abrasion, dental 58; Calculus, dental 224; Caries, dental 236; Dental emergencies 339; Discoloured teeth 362; Erosion, dental 414; Fluorosis 454; Fracture, dental 462; Impaction, dental 572; Malocclusion 659; Overbite 769; Overcrowding, dental 769; Plaque, dental 808; Subluxated tooth 956; Toothache 1002; *causes of tooth decay 238*
    eruption of: Eruption of teeth 414; Teething 972
    examination of: Dental examination 340; Dental X-ray 341
    extraction of: Extraction, dental 422
    false: Bridge, dental 212; Denture 342; Implants, dental 574; Prosthetics, dental 834
    repairs to: Bonding, dental 191; Crown, dental 321; Filling, dental 449; Inlay, dental 586; Pulpectomy 845; Reimplantation, dental 866; Restoration, dental 872; Root-canal treatment 881; Splinting, dental 939
    straightening of: Orthodontic appliances 759
    structure and arrangement of teeth 972
    types of: Permanent teeth 794; Primary teeth 829
Teeth, care of:
    Oral hygiene 756
teeth, grinding of:
    medical term: Bruxism 216

Teething 972
    and Eruption of teeth 414
Tegretol 1124
Teicoplanin 1124
Telangiectasia 973
    type of: Spider naevus 933
Temazepam 973
Temgesic 1124
Temocillin 1124
Temopen 1124
Temperature 973
    and Heat disorders 524
    high: Convulsion, febrile 306; Fever 443, *444*; Heatstroke 526; Hyperthermia 553; Hyperthermia, malignant 553
    low: Hypothermia 558
    measurement of: Thermometer 983
    during Ovulation 769
    regulation of: Hypothalamus 558; Shivering 907
Temperature method:
    Contraception, natural methods of 304
Temporal arteritis 973
    associated with Polymyalgia rheumatica 816
temporal lobe:
    location of the temporal lobe 974
    part of Cerebrum 249
Temporal lobe epilepsy 974
    treatment of: Psychosurgery 841
    type of Epilepsy 411
Temporomandibular joint 974
    and Jaw 606; Skull 919
Temporomandibular joint syndrome 974
Tenchlor 1124
Tenderness 975
Tendinitis 975
Tendolysis 975
    in treatment of Tenosynovitis 976
Tendon 975
    disorders of: Running injuries 883; Shin splints 907; Sports injuries 941; Tendinitis 975; Tenosynovitis 976; Tenovaginitis 976; Trigger finger 1016
    surgery on: Tendolysis 975; Tendon repair 975; Tendon transfer 975
    type of: Achilles tendon 61
Tendon release:
    medical term: Tendolysis 975
Tendon repair 975
Tendon transfer 975
    in treatment of Talipes 968
Tenesmus 976
Tenif 1124
Tennis elbow 976
Tenoret-50 1124
Tenoretic 1124
Tenormin 1124
Tenoxicam 1124
Tenosynovitis 976

Tenovaginitis 976
TENS 976
  use of: Dying, care of the 380;
    Pain relief 774
Tension 976
  causing Fibrositis 448;
    Headache 507, 508
  feature of Anxiety 122;
    Premenstrual syndrome 826
  see also index entry Stress
Tensilon 1124
Tensium 1124
Teoptic 1124
Teratogen 976
  causing Birth defects 172
Teratoma 976
  and Testis, cancer of 978
Terazosin 1124
Terbinafine 1124
Terbutaline 977
  and Bambuterol 156
Terfenadine 977
Terfex 1124
Terlipressin 1124
Terminal care:
  Dying, care of the 379
Termination of pregnancy:
  Abortion, induced 57
Terpoin 1124
Terra-Cortril 1124
Terra-Cortril Nystatin 1124
Terramycin 1124
Tertroxin 1124
Testicle:
  see index entry Testis
Testicular feminization
  syndrome 977
  and Sex determination 903
Testis 977
  disorders of: Epididymal cyst
    409; Epididymo-orchitis 410;
    Hydrocele 545; Monorchism
    694; Orchitis 757; Testis,
    cancer of 977; Testis, ectopic
    978; Testis, pain in the 978;
    Testis, swollen 978; Testis,
    torsion of 978; Testis,
    undescended 979; Varicocele
    1044
  examination of: self-
    examination of the testis 978
  part of endocrine system 401;
    Reproductive system, male
    868, 869
  producing Sperm 932;
    Testosterone 979
  removal of: Castration 239;
    Orchidectomy 757
Testis, cancer of 977
  detection of: self-examination of
    the testis 978
  treatment of: Orchidectomy
    757
Testis, ectopic 978
  treatment of: Orchidopexy 757
Testis, pain in the 978
Testis, retractile 978
Testis, swollen 978
  causes of: Epididymal cyst 409;
    Hydrocele 545; Mumps 703;

Orchitis 757; Spermatocele
  932; Varicocele 1044
Testis, torsion of 978
Testis, undescended 979
  causing Oligospermia 750
  treatment of: Orchidopexy
    757
Test meal 979
Testosterone 979
  an Androgen hormone 105
Tests, medical 979, 980
  and antenatal screening
    procedures 112; Cancer
    screening 230; Diagnosing
    disease 30–31; Diagnosis
    350; Diagnostic techniques
    34–39; Screening 24–27, 893
"test-tube baby":
  and In vitro fertilization 600
  landmarks in medicine: other
    forms of treatment 670
Tetanus 980
  prevention of: DPT
    vaccination 371; travel
    protection 29
  symptom of: Trismus 1017
Tetany 981
  causes of: Hyperventilation
    554; Hypoparathyroidism
    556; Osteomalacia 763
  causing Spasm 929
Tetmosol 1124
Tetrabenazine 1124
Tetrabid-Organon 1124
Tetrachel 1124
Tetracosactrin 1124
Tetracycline drugs 981
  adverse effects of: Discoloured
    teeth 362; Fanconi's
    syndrome 435
Tetrahydroaminoacridine 981
tetrahydrocannabinol:
  abbreviation for: THC 983
Tetralogy of Fallot 981
  causing Heart failure 519
  a congenital heart disease 518
Tetralysal 300 1124
Tetraplegia 982
  alternative term: Quadriplegia
    849
T/Gel 1124
Thalamonal 1124
Thalamus 982
  function of: Sensation 898
  part of Brain 198
Thalassaemia 982
  a disorder of the blood 185
  type of Haemoglobinopathy
    500
Thalidomide 983
  causing Phocomelia 801
  type of Teratogen 976
Thallium 983
THC 983
  constituent of Marijuana 662
Theo-Dur 1124
Theophylline 983
Thephorin 1124
Therapeutic 983
Therapeutic community 983

Therapy 983
Thermography 983
Thermometer 983, 984
  development of: landmarks in
    medicine: diagnosis 669
Thiabendazole 984
  in treatment of Toxocariasis
    1005; Trichinosis 1014
Thiamine:
  Vitamin B complex 1063
Thioguanine 1124
Thiopentone 984
Thioridazine 984
Thiotepa 1124
Thirst 984
Thirst, excessive 984
  medical term: Polydipsia
    816
  symptom of Diabetes
    insipidus 348; Diabetes
    mellitus 348
Thoracic outlet syndrome 984
Thoracic surgery 984
Thoracotomy 984
Thorax 985
  surgical opening of:
    Thoracotomy 984
Thought 985
Thought disorders 985
  feature of Psychosis 840;
    Schizophrenia 890
Threadworm infestation 985
  cycle of threadworm infestation
    986
Thrill 986
Throat 986
  see also index entry Pharynx
Throat cancer:
  Pharynx, cancer of 799
throat, lump in the:
  medical term: Globus
    hystericus 485
Thrombectomy 986
Thromboangiitis obliterans 986
  alternative term: Buerger's
    disease 217
thrombocyte:
  alternative term: Platelet
    809
  constituents of blood 182
  type of Blood cell 183
Thrombocytopenia 986
  causing Purpura 847
  type of Bleeding disorder
    177
Thromboembolism 986
Thrombolytic drugs 987
  examples: Streptokinase 950;
    Tissue-plasminogen
    activator 996; Urokinase
    1035
  in treatment of Myocardial
    infarction 714; Thrombosis
    987
Thrombophlebitis 987
  alternative term: Phlebitis 800
  and Thrombosis 987
  a Vein, disorder of 1048
Thrombosis 987
  and Arteries, disorders of 130

causes of: Oral contraceptives
  756; Plaque 808; Raynaud's
  phenomenon 861
treatment of: Anticoagulant
  drugs 116; Thrombolytic
  drugs 987
see also index entries
  Thrombophlebitis;
  Thrombosis, deep vein
Thrombosis, deep vein 987, 988
  as complication of Stroke 954
  complication of: Embolism
    394; Pulmonary embolism
    843
  type of Peripheral vascular
    disease 793
  Veins, disorders of 1048
Thrombus 988
  surgical removal of:
    Thrombectomy 986
Thrush 989
  medical term: Candidiasis 230
thumb:
  a Finger 449
  function of: Grip 493
  part of Hand 505
  weakness of: Carpal tunnel
    syndrome 238
Thumb-sucking 989
  in adults: Regression 865
thymectomy:
  in treatment of Myasthenia
    gravis 711
thymine:
  and what genes are and what
    they do 474
  in structure of DNA 39; Nucleic
    acids 737
Thymoma 989
  associated with Myasthenia
    gravis 710
Thymoxamine 989
Thymus 989
  and Lymphocyte 653
  part of the adaptive immune
    system 568
  tumour of: Thymoma 989
Thyroglossal disorders 989
Thyroid cancer 989
  a disorder of the thyroid gland
    992
  treatment of: Thyroidectomy
    990
Thyroidectomy 990
  in treatment of Thyroid cancer
    990
Thyroid-function tests 990
Thyroid gland 991
  disorders of the thyroid gland
    992
  and the sources and main effects
    of selected hormones 543
  part of endocrine system 401
  producing Calcitonin 233;
    Thyroid hormones 991
  removal of: Thyroidectomy
    990
Thyroid hormones 991
  examples: Calcitonin 223;
    Thyroxine 993

and *the sources and main effects of selected hormones 543;* Iodine 600; *disorders of the thyroid gland 992*
Thyroiditis 993
a *disorder of the thyroid gland 992*
type of: Hashimoto's thyroiditis 507
Thyroid scanning 993
thyroid-stimulating hormone:
measurement of: Thyroid-function tests 990
production of: Pituitary gland 805
Thyrotoxicosis 993
treatment of: Iodine 601
type of *endocrine disorder 402*
Thyroxine 993
type of Thyroid hormone 991
Tiaprofenic acid 1124
Tibia 993
part of Skeleton 915
Tibolone 1124
Tic 994
symptom of Gilles de la Tourette's syndrome 481
Ticar 1124
Ticarcillin 1124
Tic douloureux 994
alternative term: Trigeminal neuralgia 1016
tick bites:
first aid: insect stings and tick bites 588
Ticks and disease 994
and Lyme disease 651
Tietze's syndrome 994
Tigason 1113
Tilade Mint 1124
Tildiem 1124
Timecef 1124
Timentin 1124
Timodine 1124
Timolol 994
Timoptol 1124
Tinaderm-M 1124
Tinea 994
causing Athlete's foot 142
common term: Ringworm 881
a *disorder of the skin 919*
treatment of: Antifungal drugs 117
type of Dermatophyte infection 345; Fungal infection 464
Tingling:
alternative term: Pins-and-needles 804
symptom chart 739
Tinidazole 1125
Tinnitus 994
a *disorder of the ear 384*
symptom of Labyrinthitis 622; Ménière's disease 674; Otitis media 766; Otosclerosis 767
Tinset 1125
Tinzaparin 1125
Tioconazole 1125
Tiredness 995

Tisept 1125
Tissue 995
cultivation of: Culture 323
hardening of: Sclerosis 893
storage of: Cryopreservation 322
tissue death:
and Ablation 57; Amputation 94
types of: Gangrene 468; Infarction 577; Necrosis 721
Tissue fluid 996
constituent of: Water 1075
Tissue-plasminogen activator 996
Tissue-typing 997
and Histocompatibility antigens 536
in Organ donation 758; Transplant surgery 1011
Titanium dental implants:
Implants, dental 574
Tixylix Cough and Cold 1125
Tixylix Daytime 1125
Tixylix Original 1125
T-lymphocytes:
causing Graft-versus-host disease 492
infected by HIV 537
part of Immune system 569
type of Blood cell 182; Lymphocyte 653
TMJ syndrome:
Temporomandibular joint syndrome 974
Toadstool poisoning:
Mushroom poisoning 708
Tobacco 997
form of: Snuff 927
Tobacco-smoking 16, 997, *998*
and Birthweight 173; Life expectancy 636; Pregnancy 823; Smell 925
causing Bronchitis, chronic 214; Coronary artery disease 310; Emphysema 397; Gingivitis, acute ulcerative 482; Halitosis 504; Leukoplakia 635; Lip cancer 639; Lung cancer 649; Mouth cancer 698; Myocardial infarction 712; Palpitation 774; Pancreas, cancer of 775; Penis, cancer of 789; Peripheral vascular disease 793; Pharynx, cancer of 799; Stroke 952; Tongue cancer 1001
constituent of: Nicotine 730
Smoking and drinking, 22–23
Tobralex 1125
Tobramycin 998
Tocainide 999
Tocography 999
Tocopherol 999
constituent of Vitamin E 1065
Tocopheryl 1125
Todd's paralysis 999

Toe 999
anatomy of: Foot 458; Phalanges 798
Toenail, ingrowing 999
Tofranil 1125
Toilet-training 999
and Developmental delay 347; Encopresis 399; Enuresis 406; Soiling 928
Tolanase 1125
Tolazamide 1125
Tolbutamide 1000
Tolectin DS 1125
Tolerance 1000
Tolerzide 1125
Tolmetin 1000
Tomography 1000
type of Imaging technique 564; Scanning technique 888; X-ray 1090
type of: CT scanning 323
uses of: *performing a CT scan 324; imaging the body 565; using X-rays to look at the body 1091*
-tomy 1000
Tone, muscle 1000
Tongue 1000
disorders of: Glossitis 487; Leukoplakia 635; Macroglossia 656; Tongue cancer 1001
functions of: Mastication 665; Speech 930; Swallowing 963; *the sense of taste 970*
part of Mouth 697
removal of: Glossectomy 486
Tongue cancer 1001
Tongue depressor 1001
Tongue-tie 1001
Tonic 1001
tonic neck reflex:
a Reflex, primitive 865, *866*
Tonocard 1125
Tonometry 1001
in diagnosis of Glaucoma 483
in measurement of Intraocular pressure 598
use of: Eye, examination of 424
Tonsil 1001
disorders of: Peritonsillar abscess 794; Tonsillitis 1002
removal of: Tonsillectomy 1001; *1002*
Tonsillectomy 1001, *1002*
in treatment of Tonsillitis 1002
Tonsillitis 1002
tooth:
see index entry Teeth
Tooth abscess:
Abscess, dental 59
Toothache 1002
cause of: Caries, dental 236
Toothbrushing 1002, *1003*
part of Oral hygiene 757
and removal of Plaque, dental 809
Tooth decay:
medical term: Caries, dental 236

Tooth extraction:
Extraction, dental 422
Toothpaste:
type of Dentifrice 341
Topal 1125
Tophus 1003
Topical 1003
Topicycline 1125
Topilar 1125
Toptabs 1125
Toradol 1125
Torsion 1003
Torticollis 1003
Totamol 1125
Touch 1003, *1004*
and Sensation 898
Tourette's syndrome:
alternative term: Gilles de la Tourette's syndrome 481
Tourniquet 1005
type of: Esmarch's bandage 416
use of: Venepuncture 1049
Toxaemia 1005
leading to Septic shock 901
Toxaemia of pregnancy 1005
alternative term: Pre-eclampsia 821
Toxicity 1005
Toxicology 1005
Toxic shock syndrome 1005
cause of: Staphylococcal infection 944
Toxin 1005
in blood: Toxaemia 1005
causing Poisoning 813; Septic shock 901
type of Poison 813
Toxocariasis 1005
cause of: Roundworms 882; *origins of toxocariasis 1006*
type of Larva migrans 624
Toxoid 1006
use of: Vaccine 1040
Toxoplasmosis 1006
causing Birth defect 172; Blindness 180
and *disorders of the retina 873*
TPA:
abbreviation for Tissue-plasminogen activator 996
Trabeculectomy 1006
Trace elements 1006
types of Minerals 689
Tracer 1006
Trachea 1006, *1007*
disorders of: Tracheitis 1007; Tracheoesophageal fistula 1007
part of Respiratory system 870
surgical opening into: Tracheostomy 1007
Tracheitis 1007
a *disorder of the lung 649*
Tracheoesophageal fistula 1007
associated with Oesophageal atresia 746

Tracheostomy 1007
  in treatment of Choking 270;
    Ludwig's angina 647;
    Pharyngitis 798; Tetanus 981
    and Ventilation 1050
Tracheotomy 1008
Trachoma 1008
  a disorder of the eye 426
  treatment of: Oxytetracycline
    770
Tracrium 1125
Tract 1008
Traction 1008
Training 1009
  and Fitness 451
Trait 1009
  and Gene 473
Tramadol 1125
Tramil 1125
Trance 1009
Trancopal 1125
Trandate 1125
Trandolapril 1125
Tranexamic acid 1125
Tranquillizer drugs 1009
  types of: Antianxiety drugs
    114; Antipsychotic drugs
    119
  and Drug dependence 377;
    Withdrawal syndrome 1084
Transcutaneous electrical nerve
    stimulation 1009
  see also index entry TENS
Transdermal patch 1009
Transderm-Nitro 1125
Transference 1009
  in Psychoanalysis 838
Transfusion:
  Blood transfusion 189
Transfusion, autologous:
  Blood transfusion, autologous
    189
Transiderm-Nitro 1125
Transient ischaemic attack 1009
  and Fainting 430; Stroke 952
Transillumination 1009
Translocation 1009
  causing Trisomy 1017
  and Chromosomal
    abnormalities 276
  *effect of chromosomal
    translocation 1010*
Transmissible 1010
Transplant surgery 46, 1010
  and Cyclosporin 326; Grafting
    491; Immunosuppressant
    drugs 572; Organ donation
    758; Tissue-typing 997
  development of: *landmarks in
    medicine: surgery 670*
  risks of: Graft-versus-host
    disease 492; Immuno-
    deficiency disorders 571
  *transplants performed in the UK
    in 1988 1011*
  types of: Bone marrow
    transplant 194, *195*; Corneal
    graft 307; Heart-lung
    transplant *521, 522*; Heart
    transplant 523; Kidney

transplant *617, 618*; Liver
    transplant 646
Transposition of the great
    vessels 1011
  *types of congenital heart disease
    518*
Transsexualism 1011
  a Psychosexual disorder 840
  and Sex change 902
Transvestism 1011
Tranxene 1125
Tranylcypromine 1012
Trapezius muscle 1012
Trapped nerve:
  Nerve, trapped 723
Trasicor 1125
Trasidrex 1125
Trasylol 1125
Trauma 1012
  leading to Post-traumatic
    stress disorder 819
Trauma surgery:
  Traumatology 1012
Traumatology 1012
Travasept 100 1125
Travel immunization 29, 1012,
    1013
Traveller's diarrhoea 1012
  type of Gastroenteritis 470
Travel sickness:
  Motion sickness 696
Travogyn 1125
Traxam 1125
Trazodone 1012
Treatment 1012
  *landmarks in medicine: drugs
    671; landmarks in medicine:
    surgery 670; landmarks in
    medicine: other forms of
    treatment 670*
  Methods of treatment 42–47
  Treating disease 40–41
Trematode 1012
Trembling:
  alternative term: Tremor 1013
Tremonil 1125
Tremor 1013
  and Extrapyramidal system
    422
Trench fever 1013
Trench foot:
  alternative term: Immersion
    foot 566
Trench mouth:
  alternative term: Gingivitis,
    acute ulcerative 482
Trental 1125
Treosulfan 1125
Trephine 1013
Tretinoin 1013
Tri-Adcortyl, Tri-Adcortyl
    Otic 1125
Triadene 1125
Trial, clinical 1014
  and Animal experimentation
    109
  type of: Controlled trial 305
    using Double-blind 370
TriamaxCo 1125
Triamcinolone 1014

Triamco 1125
Triamterene 1014
Tribavirin 1014
  also known as Ribavirin 880
Tribiotic 1125
Triceps muscle 1014
Trichiasis 1014
Trichinosis 1014
  *biopsy specimen showing
    trichinosis 1015*
  a disorder of muscle 707
trichobezoar:
  cause of: Trichotillomania 1015
  common term: Hairball 503
  type of Bezoar 166
Trichomoniasis 1015
  causing Nonspecific urethritis
    733; Vaginal discharge 1041;
    Vaginitis 1042
  treatment of: Metronidazole
    685; Pessary 796
  type of Sexually transmitted
    disease 904
Trichotillomania 1015
Tri-Cicatrin 1125
Triclofos 1125
Triclosan 1125
Tricuspid incompetence 1015
  causing Heart failure 519
  disorder of a Heart valve 523
Tricuspid stenosis 1015
  disorder of a Heart valve 523
Tridil 1125
Trientine 1125
Trifluoperazine 1015
Trifluperidol 1125
Trigeminal nerve 1015, *1016*
  functions of cranial nerves 318
  disorder of: Trigeminal
    neuralgia 1016
Trigeminal neuralgia 1016
  type of Neuralgia 725
Trigger finger 1016
  cause of: Tenovaginitis 976
triglycerides:
  formation of: Glycerol 488
  in Hyperlipidaemias 549
  types of Fats and oils 436;
    Lipids 639
triiodothyronine:
  type of Thyroid hormone 991
Trilostane 1125
Triludan 1125
Trimeprazine 1016
Trimethoprim 1016
Tri-Minulet 1125
Trimipramine 1016
Trimogal 1125
Trimopan 1125
Trimovate 1125
Trinordiol 1125
TriNovum, Tri-Novum ED 1125
Triogesic 1125
Triominic 1125
Triperidol 1125
Triple vaccine:
  DPT vaccination 371
Tripotassium dicitratobismuthate
    1125
Triprolidine 1016

Triptafen 1125
Trisequens 1125
Trismus 1017
  feature of Tetanus 981
Trisomy 1017
  type of Chromosomal
    abnormality 275
Trisomy 21 syndrome 1017
  alternative term: Down's
    syndrome 370
Tritace 1125
Trobicin 1125
Trochlear nerve 1017
  functions of cranial nerves 318
Trophoblastic tumour 1017
  type of: Hydatidiform mole
    544
Tropical diseases 1017
Tropical ulcer 1018
Tropicamide 1018
Tropisetron 1125
Tropium 1125
Trosyl 1125
Trunk 1018
Truss 1018
  in treatment of Hernia 531
trust hospitals:
  Hospitals, types of 542
Trypanosomiasis 1018
  types of: Chagas' disease 255;
    Sleeping sickness 923
Tryptizol 1125
Tsetse fly bites 1018
  and transmission of Sleeping
    sickness 923
TSH:
  see index entry thyroid-
    stimulating hormone
T-tube cholangiography 1018
Tubal ligation:
  method of Sterilization, female
    945
Tubal pregnancy:
  alternative term: Ectopic
    pregnancy 388
Tubercle 1018
Tuberculin tests 1018
Tuberculosis 1019
  as complication of
    Pneumoconiosis 811
  diagnosis of: Tuberculin tests
    1018
  prevention of: BCG
    vaccination 160; *travel
    protection 29*
  treatment of: Ethambutol 416;
    Isoniazid 604; Pyrazinamide
    848; Rifampicin 880
  type of bacterial infection 580
  type of: Lupus vulgaris 651
tuberculous meningitis:
  see index entry Meningitis
Tuberosity 1019
Tuberous sclerosis 1019
  type of Neurocutaneous
    disorder 726
Tubocurarine 1125
Tuboplasty 1020
Tuinal 1126
Tularaemia 1020

Tulobuterol 1126
Tumbu fly bites 1020
Tumour 1020
　　alternative term: Neoplasm
　　　721
　　see also index entry Cancer
Tumour-specific antigen 1020
Tunnel vision 1020
Turner's syndrome 1020
　　features of: Amenorrhoea 91;
　　　Short stature 908
　　and Sex chromosomes 903
　　type of Chromosomal
　　　abnormality 276
Twins 1021
　　and Pregnancy, multiple
　　　824
Twins, conjoined 1021
　　alternative term: Siamese
　　　twins 910
Twitch:
　　feature of: Dyskinesia 381
　　types of: Fasciculation 435;
　　　Tic 994
Tylectomy 1021
Tylex 1126
Tympanometry 1021
Tympanoplasty 1021
　　in treatment of Deafness 333
Tympanum 1022
　　part of Ear 983
Typhoid fever 1022
　　prevention of: Immunization
　　　570; Travel immunization
　　　1012, 1013; *travel protection
　　　29*; Vaccine 1040
　　type of *bacterial infection 580*;
　　　Water-borne infection
　　　1076
Typhus 1022
　　cause of: Rickettsia 880
　　transmission of: Rats,
　　　diseases from 860
Typing 1022
　　and Blood groups 186;
　　　Tissue-typing 997
Tyrozets 1126

U

Ubretid 1126
Ucerax 1126
Ukidan 1126
Ulcer 1023
　　examples: Corneal ulcer 307;
　　　Genital ulceration 480; Leg
　　　ulcer 631; Mouth ulcer 698;
　　　Peptic ulcer 789, 790; Ulcer,
　　　aphthous 1023
　　feature of Basal cell carcinoma
　　　160; Noma 733; Pyoderma
　　　gangrenosum 848;
　　　Ulcerative colitis 1023
　　treatment of: Ulcer-healing
　　　drugs 1024
Ulcer, aphthous 1023
Ulceration 1023

Ulcerative colitis 1023
　　features of: Proctitis 829;
　　　Pyoderma gangrenosum
　　　848; Rectal bleeding 862
　　treatment of: Hydrocortisone
　　　546; Prednisolone 821;
　　　Prednisone 821;
　　　Sulphasalazine 959
ulcerative gingivitis:
　　Gingivitis, acute ulcerative 482
Ulcer-healing drugs 1024
　　examples: Antacid drugs 111;
　　　Cimetidine 278; Famotidine
　　　435; Ranitidine 857;
　　　Sucralfate 957
Ulna 1024
　　part of the Skeleton 914, *915*
　　part of: Olecranon 750
Ulna, fracture of 1024
　　and Monteggia's fracture 694
Ulnar nerve 1024
　　and Elbow 391; Funny-bone 465
　　part of Brachial plexus 197
Ultradil Plain 1126
Ultralanum Plain 1126
Ultraproct 1126
Ultrasound 1024
　　type of Radiation 852
　　use of: Lithotripsy 45, 640;
　　　Radiology 853
　　see also index entries
　　　Ultrasound scanning;
　　　Ultrasound treatment
Ultrasound scanning 36, 1024
　　type of Imaging technique 564;
　　　Scanning technique 888
　　*how ultrasound scanning works
　　　1025*
　　use of: Antenatal care 112; *fetal
　　　ultrasound 37; imaging the
　　　body 565*; Radiology 853
Ultrasound treatment 1026
　　use of: Physiotherapy 803
Ultratard, Human 1126
Ultraviolet light 1026
　　causing Sunburn 959
　　and Sunlight, adverse effects
　　　of 959
　　type of Radiation 851
Umbilical cord 1026
　　development of: Embryo 395
　　and Newborn 730
umbilical hernia:
　　disorder of Umbilicus 1027
　　types of abdominal hernia 530
Umbilicus 1027
Unconscious 1027
　　and Subconscious 956
Unconsciousness 1028
　　brief: Concussion 294; Fainting
　　　430
　　first aid: unconsciousness 1027
　　prolonged: Coma 293
Undecenoic acid, undecenoates
　　1126
Underbite:
　　medical term: Prognathism 830
undescended testis:
　　Testis, undescended 979
Uniflu with Gregovite C 1126

Unigest 1126
Unihep 1126
Uniparin, Uniparin Calcium
　　1126
Uniphyllin Continus 1126
Uniroid-HC 1126
Unisept 1126
Unisomnia 1126
Univer 1126
Unsaturated fats:
　　types of Fats 18; Fats and oils
　　　436
uracil:
　　in Nucleic acids 737
Uraemia 1028
　　feature of Kidney failure 615
Uranium 1028
　　source of Radiation 852
Urea 1028
　　constituent of Blood 181;
　　　composition of urine 1034
　　constituent of: Nitrogen 732
　　production of: Liver 641
Ureter 1028
　　obstruction of: Calculus,
　　　urinary tract 224;
　　　Retroperitoneal fibrosis 874
　　part of Urinary tract 1032,
　　　1033
Ureteric colic:
　　Renal colic 867
Ureterolithotomy 1028
Urethra 1029
　　disorders of: Hypospadias 557;
　　　Nonspecific urethritis 733;
　　　Urethral discharge 1029;
　　　Urethral stricture 1029;
　　　Urethritis 1029; Urinary tract
　　　infection 1032
　　part of Penis 788; Urinary tract
　　　1032, *1033*
Urethral dilatation 1029
　　in treatment of Urethral
　　　stricture 1029
Urethral discharge 1029
　　causes of: Gonorrhoea 490;
　　　Nonspecific urethritis 733
Urethral stricture 1029
　　causing Cystitis 328; Urinary
　　　tract infection 1032; Urinary
　　　retention 1031
　　complication of Nonspecific
　　　urethritis 733; Urethritis 1030
　　treatment of: Urethral
　　　dilatation 1029
Urethral syndrome, acute 1029
Urethritis 1029
　　causing Urethral stricture 1029
　　type of Urinary tract infection
　　　1032
　　type of: Nonspecific urethritis
　　　733
Urethrocele 1030
　　and Uterus, prolapse of 1037
urge incontinence:
　　Incontinence, urinary 575
-uria 1030
Uriben 1126
Uric acid 1030
　　and Hyperuricaemia 553;

uricosuric drugs:
　　in treatment of Gout 491
Urinal 1030
Urinalysis 1030
　　urine test 33
　　use of: Kidney-function tests
　　　616
Urinary diversion 1030, *1031*
　　in treatment of Incontinence,
　　　urinary 576
urinary frequency:
　　Urination, frequent 1032
urinary incontinence:
　　Incontinence, urinary 575
Urinary retention 1031
Urinary system:
　　see index entry Urinary tract
Urinary tract 1032, *1033*
　　anatomy of: Bladder 174, *175*;
　　　Kidney 612; Ureter 1028;
　　　Urethra 1029
　　disorders of: *disorders of the
　　　bladder 176*; Calculus,
　　　urinary tract 224, *225*;
　　　Hypospadias 557;
　　　Incontinence, urinary 575;
　　　disorders of the kidney 614;
　　　Nonspecific urethritis 733;
　　　Urethral discharge 1029;
　　　Urethral stricture 1029;
　　　Urethritis 1029; Urinary tract
　　　infection 1032; Urination,
　　　painful 1034
　　function of: *the function of the
　　　kidney 615*; Urine 1034
　　imaging of: Contrast X-rays 34;
　　　Urography 1035
　　study of: Urology 1035
Urinary tract infection 1032
　　causing Irritable bladder 602
　　during Pregnancy 823
　　treatment of: Nalidixic acid
　　　716; Nitrofurantoin 732;
　　　Sulphonamide drugs 959
Urination, excessive 1032
　　at night: Nocturia 732
Urination, frequent 1032
Urination, painful 1034
　　causes of: Cystitis 328;
　　　Gonorrhoea 490; Herpes,
　　　genital 532; Urethritis 1030
Urine 1034
　　constituents of: Urea 1028;
　　　Uric acid 1030; Water 1076
　　production and excretion of:
　　　Urinary tract 1032, *1033*
　　testing of: Urinalysis 1030;
　　　urine test 33
　　see also index entry Urine,
　　　abnormal
Urine, abnormal 1034
　　examples: Anuria 120;
　　　Glycosuria 488;
　　　Haematuria 499; Oliguria
　　　751; Pneumaturia 810
　　and Urination, excessive
　　　1032
Urine tests:
　　Urinalysis 1030; *urine test 33*
Urispas 1126

Urofollitrophin 1126
Urography 1035
  in investigation of Calculus,
    urinary tract 225; *disorders of
    the kidney 614;* Urinary tract
    infection 1032
  type of Contrast X-ray 34;
    Imaging technique 564;
    imaging the body 565; Kidney
    imaging 616, *617*
Urokinase 1035
Urology 1035
Uromide 1126
Uromitexan 1126
Ursodeoxycholic acid 1126
Ursofalk 1126
Urticaria 1035
  treatment of:
    Chlorpheniramine 269;
    Promethazine 831
  type of Skin allergy 916
Urticaria, neonatal 1035
  and Newborn 730
urticaria pigmentosa:
  alternative term: Mastocytosis
    665
Uterine muscle relaxants 1036
Uterus 1036
  and Childbirth 261; *stages of
    birth 262;* Pregnancy 822
  disorders of: *disorders of the
    cervix 254; disorders of the
    uterus 1037*
  part of Reproductive system,
    female 868
  part of: Cervix 253
  removal of: Hysterectomy
    560
Uterus, cancer of 1036
  type of: Cervix, cancer of 253
Uterus, prolapse of 1037, *1038*
  prevention of: Pelvic floor
    exercises 785
  treatment of: Hysterectomy
    560; Pessary 796; Vaginal
    repair 1041
Uterus, retroverted 1038, *1039*
Utinor 1126
Utovlan 1126
Uvea 1039
  inflammation of: Uveitis 1039
Uveitis 1039
  cause of: Herpes zoster 533
  causing Eye, painful red 427
  a disorder of the eye 426
UV light:
  Ultraviolet light 1026
Uvula 1039

V

Vaccination 1040
  and Cowpox 317; Vaccine 1040
  development of: *landmarks in
    medicine: drugs 671*
  in prevention of Infectious
    disease 578
  see also index entry
    Immunization
Vaccine 1040
  as method of Contraception 302
  see also index entries
    Immunization; Vaccination
Vacuum extraction 1040
vacuum suction curettage:
  use of: Abortion, induced 57
Vagifem 1126
Vagina 1040, *1041*
  disorders of: Candidiasis 230;
    Chlamydial infections 268;
    Rectocele 862;
    Trichomoniasis 1015;
    Urethrocele 1030;
    Vaginismus 1042; Vaginitis
    1042
  dryness of: Menopause 676;
    Sjögren's syndrome 914
  function of: Childbirth 261;
    *stages of birth 262; the process
    of fertilization 441;* Sexual
    intercourse 904, *905*
  and *painful intercourse in
    women 593*
  part of Reproductive system,
    female 868
Vaginal bleeding 1040
  causes of: Antepartum
    haemorrhage 113;
    Postpartum haemorrhage
    819; Menstruation 677
vaginal deodorants:
  causing Urination, painful
    1034; Vaginal itching 1041
Vaginal discharge 1041
  causes of: Candidiasis 230;
    Cervical erosion 250;
    Gonorrhoea 490; Pelvic
    inflammatory disease 786;
    Trichomoniasis 1015;
    Uterus, cancer of 1037;
    Vaginitis 1042
  and *stages and features of
    pregnancy 822*
Vaginal itching 1041
Vaginal repair 1041
  in treatment of Uterus,
    prolapse of 1038
Vaginismus 1042
  causing Intercourse, painful
    592
  disorder of the Vagina 1040
  treatment of: Sex therapy 904
Vaginitis 1042
Vaginyl 1126
Vagotomy 1042
  in treatment of Peptic ulcer
    790
Vagus nerve 1043
  functions of cranial nerves 318
  effect on Heart 515
  overstimulation of: Vasovagal
    attack 1047
  surgical cutting of: Vagotomy
    1042
Valenac 1126
Valgus 1043
Valium 1126

Vallergan 1126
Valoid 1126
Valproic acid:
  Sodium valproate 928
Valrox 1126
Valsalva's manoeuvre 1043
  in treatment of Barotrauma
    159; Supraventricular
    tachycardia 961
Valve 1043
  in Veins 1048
  type of: Heart valve 523
  see also index entries Heart;
    heart valve abnormalities;
    Heart-valve surgery
Valve replacement 1043
  see also index entry Heart-
    valve surgery
Valvotomy 1043
Valvular heart disease 1044
  disorder of the Heart valve 523
  see also index entry heart
    valve abnormalities
Valvuloplasty 1044
  type of Heart-valve surgery
    524
Vancocin 1126
Vancomycin 1126
Vansil 1126
Vaporizer 1044
Variant angina 1044
Varicella 1044
  common term: Chickenpox
    257
Varices 1044
  type of: Oesophageal varices
    747
Variclene 1126
Varicocele 1044
  causing Infertility 583;
    Oligospermia 751
  disorder of Testis 977
varicose ulcers:
  type of Leg ulcer 631
Varicose veins 1044, *1045*
  causing Eczema 389
  during Pregnancy 823
  treatment of: Sclerotherapy
    893
Varidase Topical 1126
Variola 1044
  alternative term: Smallpox 924
Varus 1044
vasa efferentia:
  anatomy of: Epididymis 409;
    Testis 977
Vasaten 1126
Vascace 1126
Vascardin 1126
Vascular 1045
Vasculitis 1045
Vas deferens 1046
  anatomy of: Epididymis 409;
    Reproductive system, male
    869; Testis 977
  surgical cutting of: Vasectomy
    1046
Vasectomy 1046
  a method of contraception 303
Vaseline Petroleum Jelly 1126

Vasocon A 1126
Vasoconstriction 1046
Vasodilation 1047
Vasodilator drugs 1047
  examples: Glyceryl trinitrate
    488; Isosorbide 604;
    Minoxidil 689
  in treatment of Ischaemia
    603
Vasogen 1126
vasomotor rhinitis:
  type of Rhinitis 878
Vasopressin 1047
  alternative term: ADH 67
Vasovagal attack 1047
Vasoxine 1126
VD 1047
  alternative term: Sexually
    transmitted disease 904
Vector 1047
  and Zoonosis 1094; *a selection
    of zoonoses 1093*
Vecuronium 1126
vegan diet:
  and Feeding, infant 438;
    Vitamin B_{12} 1063
  type of Vegetarianism 1047
Veganin 1126
Vegetarianism 1047
  and Feeding, infant 438
Vegetative state 1048
Vein 1048
  anatomy of: Valve 1043
  part of Circulatory system
    279, *280*
  X-rays of: Venography 1049
  see also index entry Veins,
    disorders of
Veins, disorders of 1048
  examples: Haemorrhoids 501;
    Oesophageal varices 747;
    Phlebitis 800; Retinal vein
    occlusion 878;
    Thrombophlebitis 987;
    Thrombosis, deep vein 987,
    988; Varicose veins 1044,
    1045
Velbe 1126
Velosef 1126
Velosulin 1126
Vena cava 1048, *1049*
  part of Circulatory system
    279, *280*
Venepuncture 1049
Venereal diseases:
  alternative term: Sexually
    transmitted diseases 904
Venereology 1049
Venesection 1049
  in treatment of Polycythaemia
    816
Venography 1049
  in diagnosis of Thrombosis,
    deep vein 988
Venomous bites and stings
    1050
Ventilation 1050
  and Tracheostomy 1007
  see also index entry
    Ventilator

Ventilator 1050
  in treatment of Respiratory
    distress syndrome 870;
    Respiratory failure 870
  use of: Ventilation 1050
Ventodisks 1126
Ventolin 1126
Ventilatory failure 1051
Ventouse:
  Vacuum extraction 1040
Ventral 1051
Ventricle 1051
  of Cerebrum 249; Heart 514, *515*
Ventricular ectopic beat 1051
  *type of ventricular arrhythmia
    1052*
Ventricular fibrillation 1051
  *type of ventricular arrhythmia
    1052*
ventricular septal defect:
  type of *congenital heart disease
    518*; Septal defect 900
Ventricular tachycardia 1051
  *type of ventricular arrhythmia
    1052*
venule:
  part of Circulatory system 279,
    280
  and Vein 1048
Vepesid 1126
Veracur 1126
Verapamil 1052
Veripaque 1126
Vermox 1126
Vernix 1052
Verruca 1052
  common term: Wart, plantar
    1075
Verrugon 1126
Version 1052
Vertebra 1052, *1053*
  anatomy of: Coccyx 284; Disc,
    intervertebral 361; Sacrum
    884; Skeleton 914, *915*; Spine
    937;
  disorders of: *disorders of the
    spine 938*; Spinal injury 935;
    Spondylolisthesis 940;
    Spondylolysis 940
  fusion of: Sacralization 884;
    Spinal fusion 935
Vertebrobasilar insufficiency 1053
Vertigo 1053
  causes of: *disorders of the ear
    384*; Labyrinthitis 622;
    Ménière's disease 674;
  and Dizziness 366, *367*
Vertigon 1126
Verucasep 1126
very low-density lipoprotein
  (VLDL):
  and Cholesterol 273; Fats and
    oils 436; Hyperlipidaemias
    549
Vesagex 1126
Vesalius, Andreas:
  in history of Anatomy 104;
    Medicine 668
Vesicle 1054
  type of Blister 180

vestibule:
  part of Ear 383
Vestibulitis 1054
Vestibulocochlear nerve 1054
  and *functions of cranial nerves
    318; anatomy of the ear 383*
Viability 1054
Vibramycin, Vibramycin D
  1126
Vibrator 1054
Vicks Cold Cure 1126
Videne 1126
video camera:
  use in Endoscopy 403;
    Laparoscopy 624
Vidopen 1126
Vigabatrin 1126
Vigranon B 1126
Villus 1054
  part of Intestine 596
Viloxazine 1126
Vinblastine 1126
Vincent's disease 1054
  alternative term: Gingivitis,
    acute ulcerative 482
Vincent's stomatitis:
  alternative term: Gingivitis,
    acute ulcerative 482
Vincristine 1126
Vindesine 1126
Vineberg, Arthur:
  *landmarks in medicine: surgery
    670*
Vioform-Hydrocortisone 1126
Viraemia 1054
viral hepatitis:
  Hepatitis, viral 529
viral meningitis:
  see index entry Meningitis
Virazid 1126
Virginity 1054
Virilism 1054
  cause of: Virilization 1055
Virility 1055
Virilization 1055
Virion 1055
  Viruses 1055
Virology 1055
Virormone 1126
Virudox 1126
Virulence 1055
Viruses 1055
  causing disease: Infectious
    disease 578; *viral infections
    579; viruses and disease
    1056*
  study of: Virology 1055
Viscera 1057
visceral larva migrans:
  alternative term: Toxocariasis
    1005
  type of Larva migrans 624
Visclair 1126
Viscosity 1057
Vision 1057, *1058*
  aspects of: Accommodation
    60; Blind spot 180; Colour
    vision 291; Visual acuity
    1060; Visual field 1060,
    1061

and Child development 264,
    266–267
  function of Cornea 307; Eye
    422; *anatomy of the eye 423*;
    Optic nerve 754; Retina
    872
  study of: Ophthalmology
    753
  testing of: Eye, examination
    of 424; Vision tests 1059,
    1060
  see also index entry Vision,
    disorders of
Vision, disorders of 1059
  causes of: *disorders of the
    cornea 308; disorders of the
    eye 426; disorders of the
    retina 873*
  and Developmental delay
    346; Vision, loss of 1059
  examples: Amblyopia 91;
    Anisometropia 110;
    Astigmatism 139; Colour
    vision deficiency 292;
    Double vision 370;
    Floaters 453; Hemianopia
    527; Hypermetropia 549;
    Myopia 714; Night
    blindness 731; Presbyopia
    827; Squint 942; Tunnel
    vision 1020
  treatment of: Contact lenses
    299; Glasses 483, *484*;
    Keratotomy, radial 611
  see also index entries
    Blindness; Vision tests;
    Visual field
Vision, loss of 1059
  see also index entry
    Blindness
Vision tests 1059, *1060*
  and Ophthalmology 753;
    Optometry 754
  types of: Evoked responses
    418; Eye, examination of
    424; Snellen chart 926
Viskaldix 1126
Visken 1126
Vista-Methasone 1126
Visual acuity 1060
  testing of: Eye, examination
    of 424; Snellen chart 926;
    Vision tests 1059, *1060*
  and Visual field 1060, *1061*
  see also index entries Vision;
    Vision, disorders of
Visual field 1060, *1061*
  defects of: Hemianopia 527;
    Macular degeneration 656;
    Optic neuritis 754; Pituitary
    tumours 805; Retinal
    detachment 872; Retinitis
    pigmentosa 874
  testing of: Eye, examination of
    424; Vision tests 1059, *1060*
Vital sign 1061
Vitamin 19, 1061
  and Nutrition 738
  *recommended daily allowances
    of selected vitamins 1062*

*vitamins and main food sources
    1063*
Vitamin A 1062
  and Carotene 238
  source of: Cod-liver oil 285
  see also index entry Vitamin
Vitamin B:
  Vitamin B$_{12}$ 1063
  Vitamin B complex 1063
vitamin B$_1$:
  part of Vitamin B complex
    1063
  see also index entry Vitamin
vitamin B$_2$:
  part of Vitamin B complex
    1063
  see also index entry Vitamin
vitamin B$_6$:
  part of Vitamin B complex
    1063
  see also index entry Vitamin
Vitamin B$_{12}$ 1063
  synthetic form of:
    Hydroxocobalamin 546
  see also index entry Vitamin
Vitamin B complex 1063
  see also index entry Vitamin
Vitamin C 1065
  see also index entry Vitamin
Vitamin D 1065
  source of: Cod-liver oil 285
  see also index entry Vitamin
Vitamin E 1065
  see also index entry Vitamin
Vitamin E Suspension 1127
Vitamin K 1065
  as Haemostatic drug 503
  see also index entry Vitamin
Vitamin supplements 1066
  see also index entry Vitamin
Vitiligo 1066
  disorder of Pigmentation
    803
Vitreous haemorrhage 1066
  cause of: Eye injuries 425
Vitreous humour 1066
  part of Eye 423
Vivalan 1127
Vivisection 1066
  Animal experimentation 109
VLDL:
  see index entry very low-
    density lipoprotein
Vocal cords 1066, *1067*
  disorders of: Hoarseness 537,
    538; Larynx, cancer of 626;
    disorders of the larynx 627;
    Singer's nodes 913; Stridor
    952; Voice, loss of 1066
  part of Larynx 626
Voice-box:
  medical term: Larynx 626
Voice, loss of 1066
  alternative terms: Aphonia
    125; Dysphonia 382
  symptom chart 538
Volital 1127
Volkmann's contracture 1067
Volmax 1127
Volraman 1127

Voltarol 1127
Volvulus 1067
    causing Abdominal pain 54;
        Intestine, obstruction of 596
Vomiting 1067
    excessive: Hyperemesis 548
    induction of: Ipecacuanha 601
    projectile: Pyloric stenosis 847
    symptom chart 1069
    treatment of: Antiemetic
        drugs 117; Perphenazine
        795; Prochlorperazine 829;
        Promethazine 831
    Vomiting in pregnancy 1068
Vomiting blood 1068
    and Abdominal pain 54
    causes of: Cirrhosis 281;
        Mallory-Weiss syndrome
        659; Oesophageal varices
        747; Peptic ulcer 789; Portal
        hypertension 818
Vomiting in pregnancy 1068
vomit, inhalation of:
    causing Choking 270;
        pneumonia 812; Respiratory
        distress syndrome 870
Von Recklinghausen's disease
    1068
    alternative term:
        Neurofibromatosis 726
Von Willebrand's disease 1068
    type of Bleeding disorder 177
Voyeurism 1071
Vulva 1071
    and Bartholin's glands 159
    disorders of: Leukoplakia 635;
        Vulva, cancer of 1071; Vulval
        itching 1071; Vulvitis 1071;
        Vulvovaginitis 1071
    part of Reproductive system,
        female 868
    parts of: Clitoris 282; Labia 622
Vulva, cancer of 1071
vulval dystrophy:
    causing Vaginal itching 1041;
        Vulval itching 1071; Vulvitis
        1071
Vulval itching 1071
Vulvitis 1071
    causing Urethral syndrome,
        acute 1029
Vulvovaginitis 1071

W

WAIS (Wechsler Adult
    Intelligence Scale):
    type of Intelligence test 590
Walking 1072
    in Child development 265
Walking aids *1073*, 1074
Walking, delayed 1074
    type of Developmental delay
        346
Warfarin 1074
Wart 1074
    types of: Verruca 1052; Wart,

plantar 1075; Warts, genital
    1075
Wart, plantar 1075
Warticon/Warticon Fem 1127
Warts, genital 1075
    treatment of: Podophyllin
        813
    type of Sexually transmitted
        disease 904; Wart 1074
Wasp stings:
    type of Insect sting 588
Water 19, 1075
    excessive loss of:
        Dehydration 336;
        Diarrhoea 353; Heat
        disorders 525; Heat
        exhaustion 525
    intake of: Nutrition 738;
        Thirst 984; Thirst,
        excessive 984
    and Ion 601; Osmosis 761
    loss of: Sweat glands 963;
        Urine 1034
    regulation of: ADH 67; Kidney
        612; *the function of the kidney
        615*
    retention of: Oedema 745;
        Water intoxication 1077
    therapeutic use of:
        Hydrotherapy 546
    see also index entry Water-
        borne infection
Water-borne infection 1076
    causing Diarrhoea 353
    and Infectious disease 578;
        Preventive medicine 828
Waterbrash 1077
Waterhouse-Friderichsen
    syndrome 1077
Watering eye 1077
    cause of: Ectropion 389
Water intoxication 1077
Water on the brain:
    medical term: Hydrocephalus
        545
Water on the knee 1077
Water retention 1077
    medical term: Oedema 745
"waters, breaking of the":
    in Childbirth 261
Water tablets:
    medical term: Diuretic drugs
        364
Wax bath 1077
wax, ear:
    Earwax 386
waxing:
    method of Hair removal 503
Waxsol 1127
Weakness 1077
weals:
    feature of Urticaria 1035
Weaning 1077
    and Feeding, infant 437
Webbing 1077
    of neck: Turner's syndrome
        1020
Wechsler tests:
    types of Intelligence tests 590
Wegener's granulomatosis 1077

Weight 1078
    and Obesity 742; Weight
        control 17; Weight loss 1079,
        1080; Weight reduction 1080;
        *recommendations for weight
        reduction 1081*
weightlessness:
    effects of: Space medicine 929
Weight loss 1080
    symptom chart 1079
Weight reduction 1080
    *recommendations for weight
        reduction 1081*
Weil's disease:
    alternative term: Leptospirosis
        632
Welder's eye 1080
Welldorm 1127
Wellferon 1127
Wells, Horace:
    *landmarks in medicine: surgery
        670*
Wen 1081
    alternative name: Sebaceous
        cyst 895
Werdnig-Hoffmann disease 1081
    a Motor neuron disease 697
Werner's syndrome:
    type of Progeria 830
Wernicke-Korsakoff syndrome
    1081
    an *alcohol-related disorder 84*
    and deficiency of Vitamin B
        complex 1064
Wernicke's encephalopathy:
    stage of Wernicke-Korsakoff
        syndrome 1081
"wet dream":
    medical term: Nocturnal
        emission 732
Wheelchair 1081
Wheeze 1082
    associated with Breathing
        difficulty 209
    feature of Asthma 138;
        Bronchitis, acute 213;
Whiplash injury 1082
    injury to Neck 720
    type of Spinal injury 935
Whipple's disease 1082
    symptom of: Malabsorption
        656
Whipple's operation 1082
    type of Pancreatectomy 775
Whipworm infestation 1082
    life-cycle of whipworm 1083
Whitehead 1082
    medical term: Milia 689
white matter:
    of Brain 198; *structure of brain
        199*
    constituent of: Myelin 711
    and Grey matter 493
Whitlow 1082
Whooping cough:
    medical term: Pertussis 795
Wife beating 1083
    and Marriage guidance 663
Will, living:
    Living will 646

Wilms' tumour 1083
    type of Kidney cancer 613
Wilson's disease 1083
    a disorder of the liver 645
Wind 1083
    and Belching 163; Flatus 452
Windpipe 1078
    medical term: Trachea 1006
Wiring of the jaws 1083
    in treatment of Jaw,
        fractured 607; Obesity
        742
WISC (Wechsler Intelligence
    Scale for Children):
    type of Intelligence test 590
Wisdom tooth 1084
    and Eruption of teeth 415
    impacted: Impaction, dental
        572
    *structure and arrangement of
        teeth 972*
Witches' milk 1084
Withdrawal 1084
Withdrawal bleeding 1084
Withdrawal method:
    alternative term: Coitus
        interruptus 286
Withdrawal syndrome 1084
    and Drug dependence 377
Withering, William:
    *landmarks in medicine: drugs
        671*
Wobble board 1086
Womb:
    alternative term: Uterus 1036
wood alcohol:
    chemical term: Methanol 683
    type of Alcohol 80
Word blindness:
    alternative terms; Alexia 85;
        Dyslexia 381
World Health Organization 1086
    and Preventive medicine 828
world population 171
Worm infestation 1086
    and Cats, diseases from 243;
        Dogs, diseases from 368
    treatment of: Anthelmintic
        drugs 113
Wound 1086
    first aid: wounds 1085
    and Healing 511
    types of wounds 1087
Wound infection 1087
    and Sepsis 900
Wrinkle 1088
    treatment of: Face-lift 428
Wrist 1088
    anatomy of: *skeletal structure of
        the hand and wrist 505*
    movements of: *types of joints
        608*
    part of Skeleton 914
Wrist-drop 1088
    cause of: damage to Radial
        nerve 851
    disorder of the Wrist 1088
Writer's cramp 1088
Wry neck:
    medical term: Torticollis 1003

X

Xamoterol 1127
Xanax 1127
Xanthelasma 1089
Xanthoma 1089
Xanthomatosis 1089
Xanthomax 1127
X chromosome 1089
  and Chromosomal
    abnormalities 276;
    Inheritance 585; Sex
    determination 903; Sex-
    linked inheritance 903;
    Sperm 932
  type of Chromosome 278; Sex
    chromosome 902
  see also index entry X-linked
    disorders
Xeroderma pigmentosum 1089
Xerophthalmia 1089
  a *disorder of the eye 426*
Xerostomia 1089
  common term: Mouth, dry 698
Xipamide 1089
Xiphisternum 1089
  part of Sternum 946
xiphoid process:
  alternative term: Xiphisternum
    1089
  part of Sternum 946
X-linked disorders 1089
  examples: Fragile X syndrome
    462; Klinefelter's syndrome
    619; Turner's syndrome 1020
  and Sex-linked inheritance 903
  types of Genetic disorders 477
X-rays 34, 1089
  cause of Cataract 240
  discovery of: *landmarks in
    medicine: diagnosis 669*
  and Film badge 449; Radiation
    hazards 852
  type of Radiation 851
  uses of: Angiography 107;
    Arthrography 132; Barium
    X-ray examinations 157;
    Bone imaging 194; Brain
    imaging 202; Chest X-ray 34,
    257; Cholangiography 270;
    Cholecystography 272; CT
    scanning 35, 323; *performing
    a CT scan 324;* Dental X-rays
    341; Digital subtraction
    angiography 34; ERCP 413;
    Heart imaging 520; Imaging
    techniques 564; *imaging the
    body 565;* Kidney imaging
    616; Liver imaging 646;
    Lung imaging 650;
    Mammography 660;
    Myelography 712;
    Radiography 853; Radiology
    853; Radiotherapy 45, 855;
    Tomography 1000;
    Urography 1035;
    Venography 1049; *X-ray
    examination 1090; using
    X-rays to look at the body 1091*
X-rays, dental:
  Dental X-ray 341
Xuret 1127
Xylocaine 1127
Xylometazoline 1090
Xyloproct 1127
Xylotox 1127

Y

Yawning 1092
Yaws 1092
Y chromosome 1092
  and Chromosomal
    abnormalities 276;
    Inheritance 585; Sex
    determination 903; Sperm
    932
  type of Chromosome 278; Sex
    chromosome 902

Yeasts 1092
  causing Candidiasis 230;
    Fungal infections 464
  types of Fungi 464
Yellow fever 1092
  prevention of: Travel
    immunization 1012;
    *guidelines for travel
    immunization 1013; travel
    protection 29*
  type of Tropical disease
    1018
yellow skin:
  causes of: Carotene 238;
    Jaundice 606; Yellow fever
    1092
Yin and Yang 1092
  in Chinese medicine 265;
    Macrobiotics 656
Yoga 1092
  and Relaxation techniques
    867
Yomesan 1127
Yutopar 1127

Z

Zaditen 1127
Zadstat 1127
Zantac 1127
Zarontin 1127
Zavedos 1127
Zenker's diverticulum:
  disorder of the Pharynx 799
  type of Oesophageal
    diverticulum 746
Zestoretic 1127
Zestril 1127
Zidovudine 1093
  introduction of: *landmarks in
    medicine: drugs 671*
  in treatment of AIDS 79
ZIFT:
  in treatment of Infertility 583

Zimovane 1127
Zinamide 1127
Zinc 1093
  deficiency of: Acrodermatitis
    enteropathica 64
  *recommended daily allowances of
    selected minerals 690*
  sources of: *minerals and main
    food sources 690*
  type of Mineral 689; *essential
    nutrients 740;* Trace element
    1006
Zincef 1127
Zincomed 1127
Zinc oxide 1093
  as constituent of Calamine
    223
Zinc sulphate 1127
Zineryt 1127
Zinnat 1127
Zirtek 1127
Zita 1127
Zithromax 1127
Zocor 1127
Zofran 1127
Zoladex 1127
Zollinger-Ellison syndrome 1094
  feature of: Peptic ulcer 789
Zoonosis 1094
  a selection of zoonoses 1093
Zopiclone 1127
Zoton 1127
Zovirax 1127
Z-plasty 1094
  use of: Plastic surgery 809
Z Span 1127
Zuclopenthixol 1127
Zumenon 1127
Zydol 1127
Zygote 1094
  in *the process of fertilization
    441*
zygote intra-fallopian transfer
    (ZIFT):
  in treatment of Infertility
    583
Zyloric 1127

American Society of Plastic and Reconstructive Surgeons, Inc. *179, 428, 767*; AMI Portland Hospital (Ultrasound Dept.) *824*; Argentum *461, 943, 956, 983, 1075, 1087*

Mr. John Browett *535, 620, 1091*; BUPA Fitness Centre *420*; BUPA Medical Centre *204, 660*

Cemax Inc. *1091*; Dr. M. Curling *252*

Dr. Richard Dawood *158, 192, 1090, 1091*; Professor P. Dieppe and Gower Medical Publishing *491*; Dorling Kindersley (DK)/Paul Fletcher *1092*; DK/Stephan Oliver *21, 38* DK/Susanna Price *24, 32, 33, 40*; DK/Clive Streeter *17, 18, 19*; Dr. R. Doshi, Brook Green Hospital *201, 485*; Dr. Andrew Duncombe, St. Thomas's Hospital Medical School *185, 634*

Edwards Laboratories, Orange County, California *525*

Dr. T. Fowler *90, 199*

Gibbs Dental Division *361, 809*; Glaxo *389, 879*; Mr Brian Glenville *309*

Health Education Authority *22*

The Image Bank *42*; Institute of Orthopaedics, London *74, 736, 761, 762, 765, 877, 1091*

Mr. P.H. Jacobsen, Dental School, Cardiff *212*; Dr. J. R. Jenner *363*; Mr. R.P. Juniper *1083*

KeyMed Ltd *38, 215, 329, 582, 790, 912*

Sue Lloyd *482, 792*; London School of Hygiene and Tropical Medicine *631, 658, 923*

Dr. Francis Matthey *98, 182, 932*; Nancy Durrell McKenna *191, 196, 206, 222, 262, 567*; Penny Miller/ Down's Syndrome Association *371*; Lorraine Miller, Hammersmith Hospital *192*

National Medical Slide Bank *195, 253, 443, 465, 489, 505, 515, 521, 555, 626, 628, 630, 631, 648, 650, 654, 688, 694, 704, 718, 768, 787, 826, 847, 881, 909, 926, 933, 943, 953, 955, 965, 983, 1001, 1003, 1027, 1035, 1045, 1082, 1087*

Vincent Oliver *161*

Philips Medical Systems *36*

Queen Elizabeth Military Hospital, Woolwich (Histopathology Dept., John Boyd Laboratories) *245, 381*; Queen Square Imaging Centre/BUPA *700*

Dr. I.R. Reynolds, Eastman Dental Hospital *659, 759, 769*

Saga Holidays Ltd *17*; Science Photo Library (SPL) *25, 34, 36, 461, 561, 582, 1019*; SPL/Michael Abbey *23*; SPL/ Argentum *1089*; SPL/Dr. Tony Brain *503, 686*; SPL/Dr. Goran Bredberg *512* SPL/CEA-Orsay/CNRI *37, 797*; SPL/CNRI *35, 37, 46, 135, 809, 1049*; SPL/Dr. R. Damadian *36*; SPL/ Division of Computer Research and Technology, National Institutes of Health *39*; SPL/Martin Dohrn *45*; SPL/Don Fawcett *568*; SPL/Fawcett/ Hirokawa/Heuser *1054*; SPL/Prof. C. Ferlaud/CNRI *1067*; SPL/Malcolm Fielding, The BOC Group PLC *44*; SPL/Simon Fraser *48*; SPL/Grave *1004*; SPL/Jan Hinsch *276, 277*; SPL/Manfred Kage *38, 184*; SPL/David Leah *576*; SPL/Francis Leroy *441*; SPL/R. Litchfield *86*; SPL/London School of Hygiene and Tropical Medicine *578*; SPL/Andrew McClenaghan *42*; SPL/Astrid and Hans-Frieder Michler *23, 727*; SPL/Ohio-Nuclear Corporation *35*; SPL/Omikron *970*; SPL/David Parker *26 43, 300*; SPL/Petit Format/CSI *1094*; SPL/Nestlé *396*; SPL/Philippe Plailly *854*; SPL/ John Radcliffe Hospital *1023*; SPL/J.C. Revy *27*; SPL/ David Scharf *686*; SPL/Science Source *604*; SPL/Dr. Karol Sikora *229, 942*; SPL/Dr. Howard Smedley *855*; SPL/St. Bartholomew's Hospital *390*; SPL/St. Mary's Hospital *247*; SPL/Sinclair Stammers *27*; SPL/Dr. Rob Stepney *46*; SPL/James Stevenson *22, 46, 491, 688, 968*; SPL/Alexander Tsiaras *37, 47, 133*; SPL/USDA *457*; SPL/US National Cancer Institute *78*; SPL/John Walsh *587, 686, 932*; SPL/Don Wong *424*; SPL/J.F. Wilson *1066*; Prof. Crispian Scully, Dental School, University of Bristol *238, 341, 972*; Squibb Surgicare Ltd. *290, 563*; St Bartholomew's Hospital *161, 168, 217, 244, 245, 271, 317, 394, 403, 573, 591, 610, 620, 673, 812, 814, 921, 966, 1016, 1025, 1074, 1075, 1091*; St. John's Institute of Dermatology *63, 80, 86, 173, 344, 717, 964*; St. Mary's Hospital Medical School (Audio

Visual Services) *141, 236, 345, 366, 521, 542, 621, 651, 652, 837, 895, 917, 952, 973, 988, 993, 1007, 1091, 1092*; Tony Stone/Chris Harvey *16*; Tony Stone/David Joel *41*; Ron Sutherland *25*; Dr. Paul Sweny *175, 225, 324, 352, 565, 617, 641, 1033*

University of Washington School of Medicine/The Lancet *82*; John Watney *80, 280*; C. James Webb *541, 1015, 1030*; Dr. David Wheeler *352*; Dr. A.R. Williams, Charing Cross and Westminster Medical School *543*; Dr. I. Williams *64, 108, 132, 142, 218, 220, 288, 379, 415, 427, 459, 461, 468, 533, 621, 746, 752, 762, 777, 816, 841, 843, 917, 918, 955, 1023, 1077*; Women's Health Concern *660*

Col. Robert M. Youngson *128, 241, 255, 321, 389, 662, 841*

RESEARCH ACKNOWLEDGMENTS

Dorling Kindersley would like to thank the following organizations, departments, and companies for their help:
Alcoholics Anonymous; ASH; British Association of Electrolysists; British Dental Association; British Nutrition Foundation; BUPA; Department of Health; Institute of Chiropodists; IPPF; Office of Population Censuses and Surveys; Olympus Optical Co.; Royal National Institute for the Blind; SSI Medical Services Ltd., Thorn EMI; United Kingdom Transplant Support Service Authority; Women against Rape